4TH EDITION

SHERRIS MEDICAL MICROBIOLOGY

AN INTRODUCTION TO INFECTIOUS DISEASES

EDITORS

KENNETH J. RYAN, MD
Dean, Academic Affairs
Professor of Pathology
Professor of Microbiology and Immunology
College of Medicine
University of Arizona
Tucson, Arizona

C. GEORGE RAY, MD
Clinical Professor of Pathology
College of Medicine
University of Arizona
Tucson, Arizona

CONSULTING EDITOR

JOHN C. SHERRIS, MD, FRCPATH
Professor Emeritus
Department of Microbiology
School of Medicine
University of Washington
Seattle, Washington

AUTHORS

JAMES J. CHAMPOUX, PHD
Professor and Interim Chair
Department of Microbiology
School of Medicine
University of Washington
Seattle, Washington

W. LAWRENCE DREW, MD, PHD
Professor of Laboratory Medicine
Professor of Medicine
School of Medicine
University of California, San Francisco
Mount Zion Medical Center
San Francisco, California

FREDERICK C. NEIDHARDT, PHD
Frederick G. Novy Distinguished University Professor of
Microbiology and Immunology, Emeritus
University of Michigan
Medical School
Ann Arbor, Michigan

JAMES J. PLORDE, MD
Professor Emeritus
Department of Medicine and
Department of Laboratory Medicine
School of Medicine
University of Washington
Seattle, Washington

CONTRIBUTORS

JOHN J. MARCHALONIS, PHD
Professor and Head
Department of Microbiology and
Immunology
College of Medicine
University of Arizona
Tucson, Arizona

STANLEY FALKOW, PHD
Professor of Microbiology and Immunology
Professor of Medicine
School of Medicine
Stanford University
Stanford, California

MURRAY R. ROBINOVITCH, DDS, PHD
Professor and Chairman
Department of Oral Biology
School of Dentistry
University of Washington
Seattle, Washington

4TH EDITION

SHERRIS MEDICAL MICROBIOLOGY

AN INTRODUCTION TO INFECTIOUS DISEASES

KENNETH J. RYAN, MD
C. GEORGE RAY, MD
EDITORS

McGRAW-HILL
MEDICAL PUBLISHING DIVISION

New York Chicago San Francisco Lisbon London Madrid Mexico City Milan
New Delhi San Juan Seoul Singapore Sydney Toronto

Sherris MEDICAL MICROBIOLOGY, Fourth Edition

234567890 DOW DOW 0987654

ISBN 0-8385-8529-9

NOTICE

Medicine is an ever-changing science. As new research and clinical experience broaden our knowledge, changes in treatment and drug therapy are required. The authors and the publisher of this work have checked with sources believed to be reliable in their efforts to provide information that is complete and generally in accord with the standards accepted at the time of publication. However, in view of the possibility of human error or changes in medical sciences, neither the authors nor the publisher nor any other party who has been involved in the preparation or publication of this work warrants that the information contained herein is in every respect accurate or complete, and they disclaim all responsibility for any errors or omissions or for the results obtained from use of the information contained in this work. Readers are encouraged to confirm the information contained herein with other sources. For example and in particular, readers are advised to check the product information sheet included in the package of each drug they plan to administer to be certain that the information contained in this work is accurate and that changes have not been made in the recommended dose or in the contraindications for administration. This recommendation is of particular importance in connection with new or infrequently used drugs.

This book was set in Times Roman by Progressive Information Technologies. The editors were Janet Foltin and Karen Davis. The production supervisor was Richard Ruzycka. The text designer was Marsha Cohen. The cover designer was Aimée Nordin. The art coordinator was Becky Hainz-Baxter. The index was prepared by Editorial Services. RR Donnelley, Willard, was printer and binder.

This book is printed on acid-free paper.

Library of Congress Cataloging-in-Publication Data

Sherris medical microbiology : an introduction to infectious diseases/Kenneth J. Ryan, C. George Ray, editors.—4th ed.

p. ; cm

Includes bibliographical references and index.

ISBN 0-8385-8529-9 (alk. paper)

1. Medical microbiology. 2. Communicable diseases. I. Title: Medical microbiology. II. Ryan, Kenneth J. (Kenneth James), 1940- III. Ray, C. George, 1934- IV. Sherris, John C. [DNLM: 1. Communicable Diseases. 2. Microbiology. WC 100 S553 2003]

QR46.M473 2003

616′.01—dc21

2003054180

ISBN 0-07-121245-0 (International Edition)

Dedication

To Fritz[a]

[a] Fritz D. Schoenknecht, MD, American microbiologist (1931–1996). Your wit, intellect, music, and twinkle-eyed warnings remain a cherished part of our lives.

CONTENTS

PREFACE

With this fourth edition, *Sherris Medical Microbiology,* which began almost two decades ago as *Medical Microbiology* (1984), retains the same team as the third edition with some redistribution in assignments. The most significant of these is the decision of George Ray to join Ken Ryan as editor. John Sherris continues to act as an advisor to all of us.

The goal of *Sherris Medical Microbiology* remains unchanged from that of the first edition. This book is intended to be the primary text for students of medicine and medical science who are encountering microbiology and infectious diseases for the first time. The organization is the same as the third edition with basic topics followed by chapters on the major bacterial, viral, fungal, and parasitic pathogens. We have tried to strengthen the pathogen presentation style introduced in the third edition. For each virus, bacterium, fungus, or parasite, the most important features of the organism (structure, metabolism, genetics), the disease (epidemiology, pathogenesis, immunity), and the clinical aspects (manifestations, diagnosis, treatment, prevention) are placed in distinct sections and in the same order. The opening to each of these sections is now marked by an icon for the organism 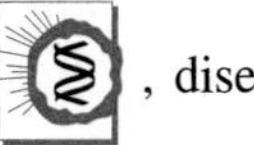, disease, or clinical aspects 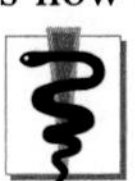. At the juncture between the organism and disease sections, a new feature, the Clinical Capsule, has been introduced. This brief snapshot of the disease is intended to orient the first-time reader before they dive into discussions of pathogenic mechanisms. Fourteen brief chapters at the end summarize the relevant clinical, diagnostic, and therapeutic information into the most common clinical infectious syndromes without the addition of new material. It is hoped that these chapters will be of particular value when the student prepares for case discussions or sees patients.

In *Sherris Medical Microbiology,* the emphasis is on the text narrative, which is designed to be read comprehensively, not as a reference work. In this regard all the pathogenic microorganisms we feel are important are included at a level of detail relevant for medical students. Any added detail in tables and figures is for example or explanation and not intended to be learned. Marginal notations throughout the text have been revised to capsulize major points as an aid for the student during review. A student scanning the red marginal notes will encounter all the major points in a chapter. If a note looks unfamiliar, the relevant text is immediately adjacent.

An overview chapter on the immune response to infection is included for continuity, but it is assumed this subject will be covered by one of the many excellent immunology texts available. The chapter on dental microbiology has been updated to serve the needs of dental students.

Much new material has been included, but in order to keep the student from being overwhelmed, older or less important information has been deleted to keep the size of this book approximately the same as the previous edition. As a rule of thumb, material on classic microbial structures, toxins, and the like has been trimmed unless its role in disease will be explained in the following sections. At the same time, we have tried not to eliminate detail to the point of becoming synoptic and uninteresting. For example, adequate explanation of the pathogenesis of an infectious disease may require discussion of the roles played by multiple proteins, genes, and regulators. Where these features form a coherent picture we have tried to tell the complete story, particularly if it is instructive as a general principle. When details such as the names of proteins and genes have been placed in parentheses, it is a sign the authors feel they need not be memorized.

A saving grace is that our topic is important, dynamic, and fascinating. Who could have predicted that AIDS, which occupied less than a page in the first edition, would in the 1990s become the leading cause of death in young American men and, with this edition, enter a period of drug suppression and hope? Gastritis and ulcers attributed to stress in the past are now being cured by antimicrobial therapy directed against *Helicobacter pylori,* but this bacterium has now been officially declared a carcinogen due to additional links with gastric cancer. Just as we were about to hit the presses, an apparently new infectious disease emerged from the Far East in the form of the severe acute respiratory syndrome (SARS). Never a dull moment! These and many other infectious agents and diseases old and new are described and explained in these pages. The student is invited to read them and begin a lifetime of learning in microbiology, infectious diseases, and medicine.

Kenneth J. Ryan
C. George Ray
Editors

ACKNOWLEDGMENTS

The authors wish to thank Drs. Steve Moseley and Irene Weitzman for selected chapter review and helpful suggestions. Administrative support and manuscript review were provided by Diane Ray, Hildi Williams, Carol Wertman, and Alexa Suslow. We also wish to acknowledge the professionalism of Janet Foltin, Karen Davis, and the McGraw-Hill staff, who took on this complicated new project and completed it with remarkable speed and flexibility.

New illustrations for this edition were prepared under the direction of Becky Hainz-Baxter and Alexander Teshin Associates, whose skill and ability to respond creatively to the diverse needs of this text are gratefully acknowledged. Illustrations prepared by Sam Eng for the mycology and parasitology sections in the first edition have been carried over to this edition, as have many of the illustrations prepared for the second edition by Marilyn Pollack-Senura, and for the third edition by Cindy Tinnes.

Finally, we wish to acknowledge our students, past and present, who provide the stimulation for continuation of this work, and our families who provide the encouragement and support that make it possible.

4TH EDITION

SHERRIS MEDICAL MICROBIOLOGY

AN INTRODUCTION TO INFECTIOUS DISEASES

CHAPTER 1

Overview

KENNETH J. RYAN

> Humanity has but three great enemies: fever, famine and war; of these by far the greatest, by far the most terrible, is fever.
>
> SIR WILLIAM OSLER, 1896*

When Sir William Osler, the great physician/humanist wrote these words, fever (infection) was indeed the scourge of the world. Tuberculosis and other forms of pulmonary infection were the leading causes of premature death among the well to do and the less fortunate. The terror was due to the fact that although some of the causes of infection were being discovered, little could be done to prevent or alter the course of disease. In the 20th century, advances in public sanitation and the development of vaccines and antimicrobials changed this fact (Fig 1-1), but only for the nations that could afford the improvements. As the 21st century begins, the world is divided into countries in which heart attacks, cancer, and stroke have surpassed infection as a cause of death and those in which infection is still the leading cause of death.

A new uneasiness that is part evolutionary, part discovery, and part diabolic has taken hold. Infectious agents once conquered have demonstrated resistance to established therapy, such as multiresistant *Mycobacterium tuberculosis,* and new diseases, such as acquired immunodeficiency syndrome (AIDS), have emerged. The spectrum of infection has widened, with discoveries that organisms once thought to be harmless can cause disease under certain circumstances. Who could have guessed that *Helicobacter pylori,* not even mentioned in the first edition of this book, would be the major cause of gastric and duodenal ulcers and an officially declared carcinogen? Finally, bioterrorist forces have unearthed two previously controlled infectious diseases, anthrax and smallpox, and threatened their distribution as agents of biological warfare. For students of medicine, understanding the fundamental basis of infectious diseases has more relevance than ever.

BACKGROUND

The science of medical microbiology dates back to the pioneering studies of Pasteur and Koch, who isolated specific agents and proved that they could cause disease by introducing the experimental method. The methods they developed lead to the first golden age of microbiology (1875–1910), when many bacterial diseases and the organisms responsible for them were defined. These efforts, combined with work begun by Semmelweis and Lister, which showed how these diseases spread, led to the great advances in public health that initiated the decline in disease and death. In the first half of the 20th century, scientists studied the structure, physiology, and genetics of microbes in detail and began to

*Osler W. *JAMA* 1896;26:999.

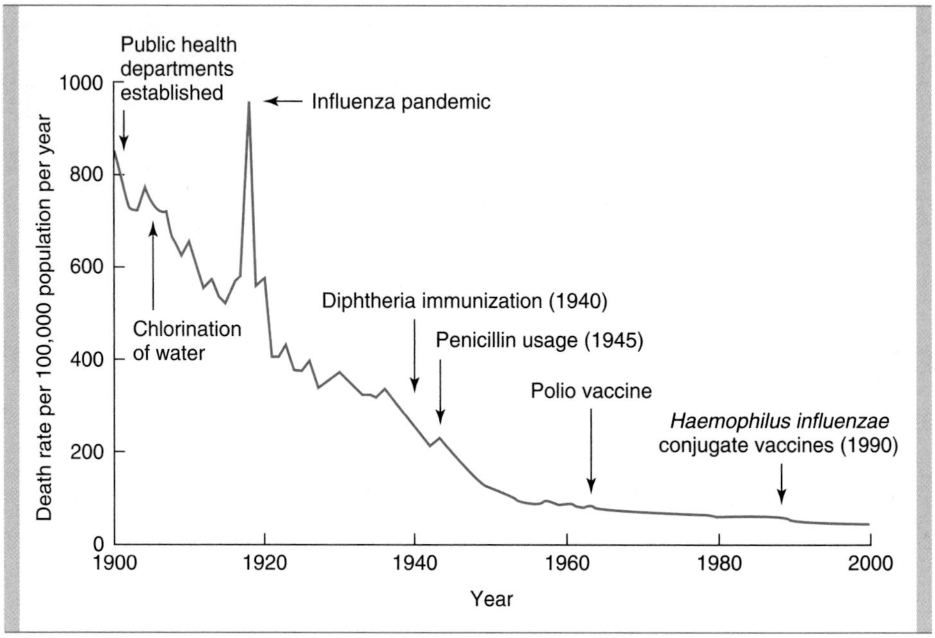

FIGURE 1–1
Death rates for infectious disease in the United States in the 20th century. Note the steady decline in death rates related to the introduction of public health, immunization, and antimicrobial interventions.

answer questions relating to the links between specific microbial properties and disease. By the end of the 20th century, the sciences of molecular biology, genetics, genomics, and proteomics extended these insights to the molecular level. Genetic advances have reached the point where it is possible to know not only the genes involved but understand how they are regulated. The discoveries of penicillin by Fleming in 1929 and of sulfonamides by Domagk in 1935 opened the way to great developments in chemotherapy. These gradually extended from bacterial diseases to fungal, parasitic, and finally viral infections. Almost as quickly, virtually all categories of infectious agents developed resistance to all categories of antimicrobics to counter these chemotherapeutic agents.

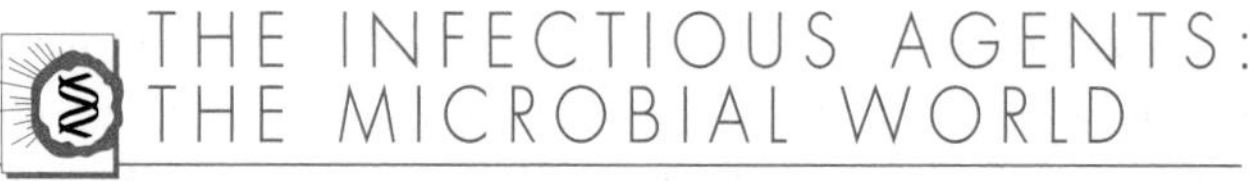

THE INFECTIOUS AGENTS: THE MICROBIAL WORLD

Microbes are small

Microbiology is a science defined by smallness. Its creation was made possible by the invention of the microscope (Gr. *micro,* small + *skop,* to look, see), which allowed visualization of structures too small to see with the naked eye. This definition of microbiology as the study of microscopic living forms still holds if one can accept that some organisms can live only in other cells (eg, all viruses, some bacteria) and others have macroscopic forms (eg, fungal molds, parasitic worms).

Most play benign roles in the environment

Microorganisms are responsible for much of the breakdown and natural recycling of organic material in the environment. Some synthesize nitrogen-containing compounds that contribute to the nutrition of living things that lack this ability; others (oceanic algae) contribute to the atmosphere by producing oxygen through photosynthesis. Because microorganisms have an astounding range of metabolic and energy-yielding abilities, some can exist under conditions that are lethal to other life forms. For example, some bacteria can oxidize inorganic compounds such as sulfur and ammonium ions to generate energy, and some can survive and multiply in hot springs at temperatures above 75°C.

Products of microbes contribute to the atmosphere

Some microbial species have adapted to a symbiotic relationship with higher forms of life. For example, bacteria that can fix atmospheric nitrogen colonize root systems of legumes and of a few trees such as alders and provide the plants with their nitrogen requirements. When these plants die or are plowed under, the fertility of the soil is enhanced by nitrogenous compounds originally derived from the metabolism of the bacteria.

TABLE 1–1

Distinctive Features of Prokaryotic and Eukaryotic Cells

Cell Component	Prokaryotes	Eukaryotes
Nucleus	No membrane, single circular chromosome	Membrane bounded, a number of individual chromosomes
Extrachromosomal DNA	Often present in form of plasmid(s)	In organelles
Organelles in cytoplasm	None	Mitochondria (and chloroplasts in photosynthetic organisms)
Cytoplasmic membrane	Contains enzymes of respiration; active secretion of enzymes; site of phospholipid and DNA synthesis	Semipermeable layer not possessing functions of prokaryotic membrane
Cell wall	Rigid layer of peptidoglycan (absent in *Mycoplasma*)	No peptidoglycan (in some cases cellulose present)
Sterols	Absent (except in *Mycoplasma*)	Usually present
Ribosomes	70 S in cytoplasm	80 S in cytoplasmic reticulum

Ruminants can use grasses as their prime source of nutrition, because the abundant flora of anaerobic bacteria in the rumen break down cellulose and other plant compounds to usable carbohydrates and amino acids and synthesize essential nutrients including some amino acids and vitamins. These few examples illustrate the protean nature of microbial life and their essential place in our ecosystem.

The major classes of microorganisms in terms of ascending size and complexity are viruses, bacteria, fungi, and parasites. Parasites exist as single or multicellular structures with the same eukaryotic cell plan of our own cells. Fungi are also eukaryotic but have a rigid external wall that makes them seem more like plants than animals. Bacteria also have a cell wall, but their cell plan is prokaryotic (Table 1–1) and lacks the organelles of eukaryotic cells. Viruses have a genome and some structural elements but must take over the machinery of another living cell (eukaryotic or prokaryotic) in order to replicate.

Increasing complexity: viruses → bacteria → fungi → parasites

Viruses

Viruses are strict intracellular parasites of other living cells, not only of mammalian and plant cells, but also of simple unicellular organisms, including bacteria (the bacteriophages). Viruses are simple forms of replicating, biologically active particles that carry genetic information in either DNA or RNA molecules, but never both. Most mature viruses have a protein coat over their nucleic acid and sometimes a lipid surface membrane derived from the cell they infect. Because viruses lack the protein-synthesizing enzymes and structural apparatus necessary for their own replication, they bear essentially no resemblance to a true eukaryotic or prokaryotic cell.

Viruses contain little more than DNA or RNA

Viruses replicate by using their own genes to direct the metabolic activities of the cell they infect to bring about the synthesis and reassembly of their component parts. A cell infected with a single viral particle may thus yield many thousands of viral particles, which can be assembled almost simultaneously under the direction of the viral nucleic acid. With many viruses, cell death and infection of other cells by the newly formed viruses result. Sometimes, viral reproduction and cell reproduction proceed

Replication is by control of the host cell metabolic machinery

Some integrate into the genome

simultaneously without cell death, although cell physiology may be affected. The close association of the virus with the cell sometimes results in the integration of viral nucleic acid into the functional nucleic acid of the cell, producing a latent infection that can be transmitted intact to the progeny of the cell.

Bacteria

Smallest living cells

Prokaryotic cell plan lacks nucleus and organelles

Bacteria are the smallest (0.1 to 10 μm) living cells. They have a cytoplasmic membrane surrounded by a cell wall; a unique interwoven polymer called peptidoglycan makes the wall rigid. The simple prokaryotic cell plan includes no mitochondria, lysosomes, endoplasmic reticulum, or other organelles. In fact, most bacteria are about the size of mitochondria. Their cytoplasm contains only ribosomes and a single, double-stranded DNA chromosome. Bacteria have no nucleus, but all the chemical elements of nucleic acid and protein synthesis are present. Although their nutritional requirements vary greatly, most bacteria are free-living, if given an appropriate energy source. Tiny metabolic factories, they divide by binary fission and can be grown in artificial culture, often in less than a day. The Archaebacteria differ radically from other bacteria in structure and metabolic processes; they live in environments humans consider hostile (eg, hot springs, high salt areas) but are not associated with disease.

Fungi

Yeasts and molds are surrounded by cell wall

Fungi exist in either yeast or mold forms. The smallest of yeasts are similar in size to bacteria, but most are larger (2 to 12 μm) and multiply by budding. Molds form tubular extensions called hyphae, which when linked together in a branched network form the fuzzy structure seen on neglected bread. Fungi are eukaryotic, and both yeasts and molds have a rigid external cell wall composed of their own unique polymers, called glucan, mannan, and chitin. Their genome may exist in a diploid or haploid state and replicate by meiosis or simple mitosis. Most fungi are free-living and widely distributed in nature. Generally, fungi grow more slowly than bacteria, although their growth rates sometimes overlap.

Parasites

Range from tiny amoebas to meter-long worms

Parasites are the most diverse of all microorganisms. They range from unicellular amoebas of 10 to 12 μm to multicellular tapeworms 1 meter in length. The individual cell plan is eukaryotic, but the organisms such as worms are highly differentiated and have their own organ systems. Most of the worms have a microscopic egg or larval stage, and part of their life cycle may involve multiple vertebrate and invertebrate hosts. Most parasites are free-living but some depend on combinations of animal, arthropod, or crustacean hosts for their survival.

INFECTIOUS DISEASE

Pathogens are rare

Virulence varies greatly

Of the thousands of species of viruses, bacteria, fungi, and parasites, only a tiny portion are involved in disease of any kind. These are called pathogens. There are plant pathogens, animal pathogens, fish pathogens, as well as the subject of this book, human pathogens. Among pathogens, there are degrees of potency called virulence, which sometimes makes the dividing line between benign and virulent microorganisms difficult to draw. Many bacteria and some fungi are part of a normal flora that colonizes the skin and mucosal surfaces of the body, where most of the time they appear to do no harm. In extreme circumstances, a few of these organisms are associated with mild disease, making them low-virulence pathogens at best. Other pathogens are virtually always associated with disease of varying severity. *Yersinia pestis,* the cause of plague, causes fulminant disease and death in 50 to 75% of individuals who come in contact with it. It is highly virulent. Understanding the basis of these differences in virulence is a fundamental goal of this book. The better students of medicine understand how a pathogen causes disease, the better they will be prepared to intervene and help their patients.

For any pathogen the basic aspects of how it interacts with the host to produce disease can be expressed in terms of its epidemiology, pathogenesis, and immunity. Usually our knowledge of one or more of these topics is incomplete. It is the task of the physician to relate these topics to the clinical aspects of disease and be prepared for new developments which clarify, or in some cases, alter them. We do not know everything, and not all of what we believe we know is correct.

EPIDEMIOLOGY

Epidemiology is the "who, what, when, and where" of infectious diseases. The power of the science of epidemiology was first demonstrated by Semmelweis, who by careful data analysis alone determined how streptococcal puerperal fever was transmitted. He even devised a means to prevent it decades before the organism itself was discovered (see Chapter 72). Since then each organism has built its own profile of vital statistics. Some agents are transmitted by the air, others by food, others by insects, and some spread by the person-to-person route. Some agents occur worldwide, and others only in certain geographic locations or ecologic circumstances. Knowing how an organism gains access to its victim and spreads are crucial to understanding the disease. It is also essential to discovering the emergence of "new" diseases, whether they are truly new (AIDS) or just undiscovered (Legionnaires' disease). Solving mysterious outbreaks or recognizing new epidemiologic patterns have usually pointed the way to the isolation of new agents.

Each agent has its own mode of spread

Epidemic spread and disease are facilitated by malnutrition, poor socioeconomic conditions, natural disasters, and hygienic inadequacy. In previous centuries, epidemics, sometimes caused by the introduction of new organisms of unusual virulence, often resulted in high morbidity and mortality. The possibility of recurrence of old pandemic infections remains, and, in the case of AIDS, we are currently witnessing a new and extended pandemic infection. Modern times and technology have introduced new wrinkles to epidemiologic spread. Intercontinental air travel has allowed diseases to leap continents even when they have very short incubation periods (cholera). The efficiency of the food industry has sometimes backfired when the distributed products are contaminated with infectious agents. The well-publicized outbreaks of hamburger-associated *Escherichia coli* O157:H7 infection are an example. The nature of massive meatpacking facilities allowed organisms from infected cattle on isolated farms to be mixed with other meat and distributed rapidly and widely. By the time outbreaks are recognized, cases of disease are widespread, and tons of meat must be recalled. In simpler times, local outbreaks from the same source would have been detected and contained more quickly.

Poor socioeconomic conditions foster infection

Modern society may facilitate spread

Of course, the most ominous and uncertain epidemiologic threat of these times is not amplification of natural transmission but the specter of unnatural, deliberate spread. Anthrax is a disease uncommonly transmitted by direct contact of animals or animal products with humans. Under natural conditions, it produces a nasty but usually not life-threatening ulcer. The inhalation of human-produced aerosols of anthrax spores could produce a lethal pneumonia on a massive scale. Smallpox is the only disease officially eradicated from the world. It took place so long ago that most of the population has never been exposed or immunized and are thus vulnerable to its reintroduction. We do not know if infectious bioterrorism will work on the scale contemplated by its perpetrators, but in the case of anthrax we do know that sophisticated systems have been designed to attempt it. We hope that we will never learn whether bioterrorism will work on a large scale.

Anthrax and smallpox are new bioterrorism threats

PATHOGENESIS

Once a potential pathogen reaches its host, features of the organism determine whether or not disease ensues. The primary reason pathogens are so few in relation to the microbial world is that being a successful pathogen is very complicated. Multiple features, called virulence factors, are required to persist, cause disease, and escape to repeat the cycle.

Pathogenicity is multifactorial

The variations are many, but the mechanisms used by many pathogens are now being dissected at the molecular level.

The first step for any pathogen is to attach and persist at whatever site it gains access. This usually involves specialized surface molecules or structures that correspond to receptors on human cells. Because human cells were not designed to receive the microorganisms, they are usually exploiting some molecule important for essential functions of the cell. For some toxin-producing pathogens, this attachment is all they need to produce disease. For most pathogens, it just allows them to persist long enough to proceed to the next stage, invasion into or beyond the mucosal cells. For viruses, invasion of cells is essential, because they cannot replicate on their own. Invading pathogens must also be able to adapt to a new milieu. For example, the nutrients and ionic environment of the cell surface differs from that inside the cell or in the submucosa.

Pathogens have molecules that bind to host cells

Invasion requires adaptation to new environments

Persistence and even invasion do not necessarily translate immediately to disease. The invading organisms must disrupt function in some way. For some, the inflammatory response they stimulate is enough. For example, a lung alveolus filled with neutrophils responding to the presence of *Streptococcus pneumoniae* loses its ability to exchange gases. The longer a pathogen can survive in the face of the host response, the greater the compromise in host function. Most pathogens do more than this. Destruction of host cells through the production of digestive enzymes, toxins, or intracellular multiplication is among the more common mechanisms. Other pathogens operate by altering the function of a cell without injury. Cholera is caused by a bacterial toxin, which causes intestinal cells to hypersecrete water and electrolytes leading to diarrhea. Some viruses cause the insertion of molecules in the host cell membrane, which cause other host cells to attack it. The variations are diverse and fascinating.

Inflammation alone can result in injury

Cells may be destroyed or their function altered

IMMUNITY

Although the science of immunology is beyond the scope of this book, understanding the immune response to infection (see Chapter 8) is an important part of appreciating pathogenic mechanisms. In fact, one of the most important virulence attributes any pathogen can have is an ability to evade the immune response. Some pathogens attack the immune effector cells, and others undergo changes that confound the immune response. The old observation that there seems to be no immunity to gonorrhea turns out to be an example of the latter mechanism. *Neisseria gonorrhoeae,* the causative agent of gonorrhea, undergoes antigenic variation of important surface structures so rapidly that antibodies directed against the bacteria become irrelevant.

Evading the immune response is a major feature of virulence

For each pathogen, the primary interest is whether there is natural immunity and, if so, whether it is based on humoral (antibody) or cell-mediated immunity (CMI). Humoral and CMI responses are broadly stimulated with most infections, but the specific response to a particular molecular structure is usually dominant in mediating immunity to reinfection. For example, the repeated nature of strep throat (group A streptococcus) in childhood is not due to antigenic variation as described above for gonorrhea. The antigen against which protective antibodies are directed (M protein) is stable but naturally exists in over 80 types. Each requires its own specific antibody. Knowing the molecule against which the protective immune response is directed is particularly important for devising preventive vaccines.

Antibody or cell-mediated mechanisms may be protective

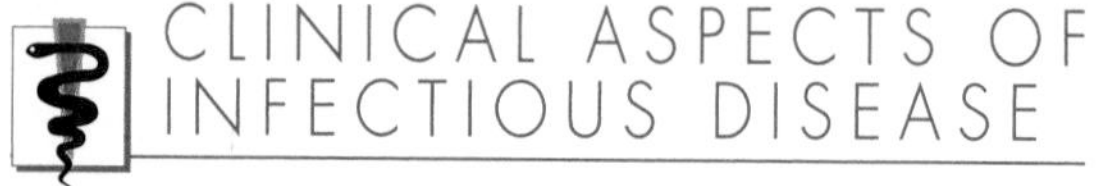

MANIFESTATIONS

Fever, pain, and swelling are the universal signs of infection. Beyond this, the particular organs involved and the speed of the process dominate the signs and symptoms of disease. Cough, diarrhea, and mental confusion represent disruption of three different body

Body system(s) involved dictate clinical findings

systems. On the basis of clinical experience, physicians have become familiar with the range of behavior of the major pathogens. However, signs and symptoms overlap considerably. Skilled physicians use this knowledge to begin a deductive process leading to a list of suspected pathogens and a strategy to make a specific diagnosis and provide patient care. Through the probability assessment, an understanding of how the diseases work is a distinct advantage in making the correct decisions.

DIAGNOSIS

A major difference between infectious and other diseases is that the probabilities described above can be specifically resolved, often overnight. Most microorganisms can be isolated from the patient, grown in artificial culture, and identified. Others can be seen microscopically or detected by measuring the host specific immune response. Preferred modalities for diagnosis of each agent have been developed and are available in clinic, hospital, and public health laboratories all over the world. Empiric diagnosis made on the basis of clinical findings can be confirmed and the treatment plan modified accordingly. The new molecular methods, which detect molecular structures or genes of the agent, are not yet practical for most infectious diseases.

Disease-causing microbes can be grown and identified

TREATMENT

Over the past 60 years, therapeutic tools of remarkable potency and specificity have become available for the treatment of bacterial infections. These include all the antibiotics and an array of synthetic chemicals that kill or inhibit the infecting organism but have minimal or acceptable toxicity for the host. Antibacterial agents exploit the structural and metabolic differences between bacterial and eukaryotic cells to provide the selectivity necessary for good antimicrobial therapy. Penicillin, for example, interferes with the synthesis of the bacterial cell wall, a structure that has no analog in human cells. There are fewer antifungal and antiprotozoal agents because the eukaryotic cells of the host and those of the parasite have close metabolic and structural similarities. Nevertheless, hosts and parasites do have some significant differences, and effective therapeutic agents have been discovered or developed to exploit them.

Antibiotics are directed at structures of bacteria not present in host

Specific therapeutic attack on viral disease has posed more complex problems, because of the intimate involvement of viral replication with the metabolic and replicative activities of the cell. Thus, most substances that inhibit viral replication have unacceptable toxicity to host cells. However, recent advances in molecular virology have identified specific viral targets that can be attacked. Scientists have developed some successful antiviral agents, including agents that interfere with the liberation of viral nucleic acid from its protective protein coat or with the processes of viral nucleic acid synthesis and replication. The successful development of new agents for human immunodeficiency virus has involved targeting enzymes coded by the virus genome.

Antivirals target unique virus-coded enzymes

The success of the "antibiotic era" has been clouded by the development of resistance by the organisms. The mechanisms involved are varied but most often involve a mutational alteration in the enzyme, ribosome site, or other target against which the antimicrobial is directed. In some instances, the organisms acquire new enzymes or block entry of the antimicrobic to the cell. Many bacteria produce enzymes which directly inactivate antibiotics. To make the situation worse, the genes involved are readily spread by promiscuous genetic mechanisms. New agents that are initially effective against resistant strains have been developed, but resistance by new mechanisms usually follows. The battle is by no means lost but has become a never-ending policing action.

Resistance complicates therapy

Mechanisms include mutation and inactivation

PREVENTION

The ultimate outcome with any disease is its prevention. In the case of infectious diseases, this has involved public health measures and immunization. The public health measures depend on knowledge of transmission mechanisms and interfering with them. Water disinfection, food preparation, insect control, handwashing, and a myriad of other

Public health and immunization are primary preventive measures

measures prevent humans from coming in contact with infections agents. Immunization relies on knowledge of immune mechanisms and designing vaccines that stimulate protective immunity.

Attenuated strains stimulate immunity

Live vaccines can cause disease

Immunization follows two major strategies, live and inactivated vaccines. The former uses live but attenuated organisms that have been modified so they do not produce disease but still stimulate a protective immune response. Such vaccines have been effective but carry the risk that the vaccine strain itself may cause disease. This event has been observed with the live oral polio vaccine. Although this rarely occurs, it has caused a shift back to the original Salk inactivated vaccine. This issue has reemerged with a debate over strategies for the use of smallpox immunization to protect against bioterrorism. This vaccine uses vaccinia virus, a cousin of smallpox, and its potential to produce disease on its own has been recognized since its original use by Jenner in 1798. Serious disease would be expected primarily in immunocompromised individuals, who represent a significantly larger part of the population (eg, from cancer chemotherapy, AIDS) than when smallpox immunization was stopped in the 1970s. Could immunization cause more disease than it prevents? The question is difficult to answer.

Purified components are safe vaccines

The safest immunization strategy is the use of organisms that have been killed or, better yet, killed and purified to contain only the immunizing component. This approach requires much better knowledge of pathogenesis and immune mechanisms. Vaccines for meningitis use only the polysaccharide capsule of the bacterium, and vaccines for diphtheria and tetanus use only a formalin-inactivated protein toxin. Pertussis (whooping cough) immunization has undergone a transition in this regard. The original killed whole-cell vaccine was effective but caused a significant frequency of side effects. A purified vaccine containing pertussis toxin and a few surface components has reduced side effects while retaining efficacy.

Vaccines can be genetically engineered

The newest approaches for vaccines require neither live organisms nor killed, purified ones. As the entire genomes of more and more pathogens are being reported, an entirely genetic strategy is emerging. Armed with knowledge of molecular pathogenesis and immunity and the tools of genomics and proteomics, scientists can now synthesize an immunogenic protein without ever growing the organism itself. Such an idea would have astonished even the great microbiologists of the past two centuries.

SUMMARY

Infectious diseases remain as important and fascinating as ever. Where else do we find the emergence of new diseases, together with improved understanding of the old ones? At a time when the revolution in molecular biology and genetics has brought us to the threshold of new and novel means of infection control, the perpetrators of bioterrorism threaten us with diseases we have already conquered. Meeting this challenge requires a secure knowledge of the pathogenic organisms and how they produce disease, as well as an understanding of the clinical aspects of those diseases. In the collective judgment of the authors, this book presents the principles and facts required for students of medicine to understand the most important infectious diseases.

PART I

The Bacterial Cell

CHAPTER 2

Bacterial Structures

CHAPTER 3

Bacterial Processes

CHAPTER 4

Bacterial Genetics

CHAPTER 2

Bacterial Structures

FREDERICK C. NEIDHARDT

This chapter examines the special structural, architectural and chemical features of the prokaryotic (bacterial) cell that contribute to the ubiquity of this large group of organisms and their ability to cause disease in humans. Discussion focuses particularly on the characteristics that distinguish bacteria from the more familiar cells of eukaryotes, which therefore offer the opportunity for medical interventions.

GENERAL MORPHOLOGY, BODY PLAN, AND COMPOSITION

The bacterial cell that is seen today is closer in form to the primordial cells of our planet than is any animal or plant cell. This similarity is misleading, however, because bacteria are the product of close to 3 billion years of natural selection and have emerged as immensely diverse and successful organisms that colonize almost all parts of the world and its other inhabitants. Because bacteria have remained microscopic, it can be concluded that very small size per se is not a disadvantage in nature but rather provides unique opportunities for survival and reproduction. Thus, the first major principle to help us understand bacteria is their small size.

Bacteria are highly successful colonizers

Bacteria are by far the smallest living cells, and some are considered to have the minimum possible size for an independently reproducing organism. Individuals of different bacterial species that colonize or infect humans range from 0.1 to 10 μm (1 $\mu m = 10^{-6}$ m) in their largest dimension. Most spherical bacteria have diameters of 0.5 to 2 μm, and rod-shaped cells are generally 0.2 to 2 μm wide and 1 to 10 μm long. At the lower end of the scale, some bacteria (rickettsias, chlamydia, and mycoplasmas) overlap with the largest viruses (the poxviruses), and at the upper end, some rod-shaped bacteria have a length equal to the diameter of some eukaryotic cells (Fig 2–1). As a shorthand approximation, bacteria are sole possessors of the 1-μm size.

Most bacteria are in the range of 1–10 μm

A wealth of structural detail cannot be discerned in bacteria even with the best of light microscopes because of their small size and because they are nearly colorless and transparent and have a refractive index similar to that of the surrounding liquid. However, shape can easily be discerned with appropriate microscopic techniques, and distinctive shapes are characteristic of broad groupings of bacteria (Fig 2–2). The major forms that can be recognized are spheres, rods, bent or curved rods, and spirals. Spherical or oval bacteria are called **cocci** (singular: **coccus**). Rods are called **bacilli** (singular: **bacillus**). Very short rods that can sometimes almost be mistaken for cocci are called **coccobacilli.** Some rod-shaped bacteria have tapered ends and are therefore termed **fusiform,** whereas others are characteristically club-shaped and may be curved or bent. Spiral-shaped bacteria are called **spirilla** if the cells are rigid and **spirochetes** if they are more flexible and undulating.

Bacteria exhibit a variety of shapes and cell arrangements

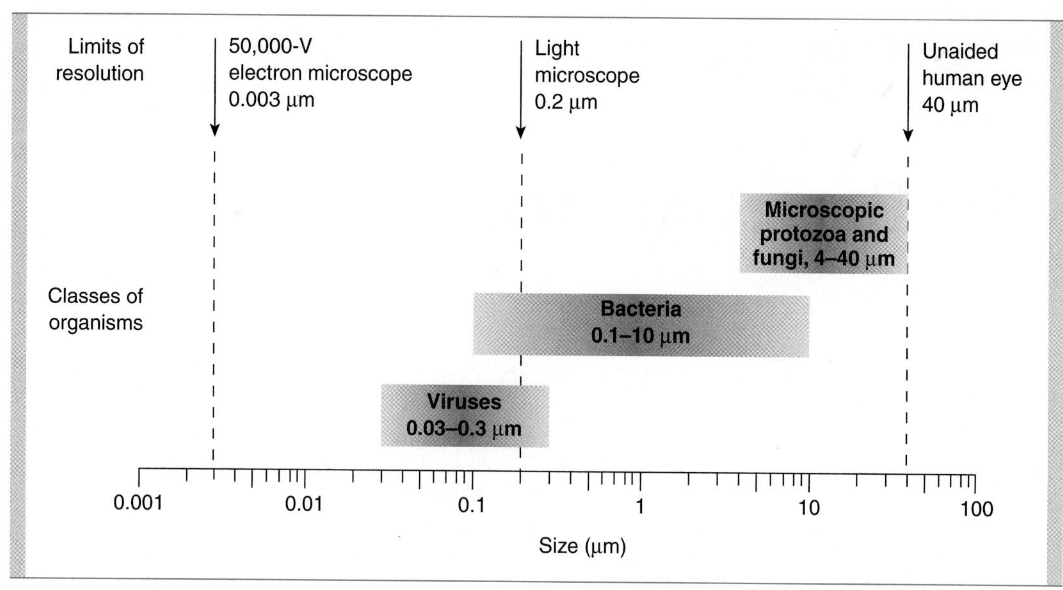

FIGURE 2–1
Relative sizes of microorganisms.

In addition to shape, distinctive arrangements of groups of cells can readily be observed for some bacterial genera (Fig 2–3). The reason one can speak of arrangements of unicellular organisms is that there is a tendency, varying with different genera, for newly divided cells to stick together. The nature of the aggregates formed depends on the degree of stickiness (which can vary with growth conditions) and on the plane of successive cell divisions. Among the cocci, pairs (**diplococci**), chains (**streptococci**), and irregular clusters (**staphylococci**) are found. A few genera of bacteria were named for their distinctive shape or cell arrangement. There are many thousands of species of bacteria, however, so it should be clear that the shape and arrangement of cells cannot be taken far in identifying the particular organism in a given sample or culture. A further caution for medical microbiologists is the tendency of some bacteria to take on altered shapes and arrangements when in contact with various antimicrobics.

Some antimicrobics affect cell morphology

Whatever the overall shape of the cell, the 1-μm size could not accommodate the familiar eukaryotic cell plan. There is insufficient room for mitochondria, nucleus, Golgi apparatus, lysosomes, endoplasmic reticulum, and the like in a cell that is itself only as large as an average mitochondrion. The design of the bacterial cell must thus differ fundamentally from that of other cells. This is precisely the case, and the unique design is designated **prokaryotic.**

Prokaryotic cell design is unique

A generalized bacterial cell is shown in Figure 2–4. The major structures of the cell belong either to the multilayered **envelope** and its **appendages** or to the interior core consisting of the **nucleoid** (or nuclear body) and the **cytosol** (called thus rather than cytoplasm because there is no nucleus; the cytosol is not separated from the genetic material). In contrast to the alien nature of this body plan, the general chemical nature of the bacterial cell is more familiar to a eukaryotic cell biologist. Greater than 90% of its dry mass consists of five macromolecular-like substances similar to those found in eukaryotes: proteins (about 55% of the dry mass); RNA, consisting of the familiar messenger (mRNA), transfer (tRNA), and

Major structures form the envelope, appendages, cytosol, and nucleoid

Chemical nature is similar to eukaryotic cells but with some unique components

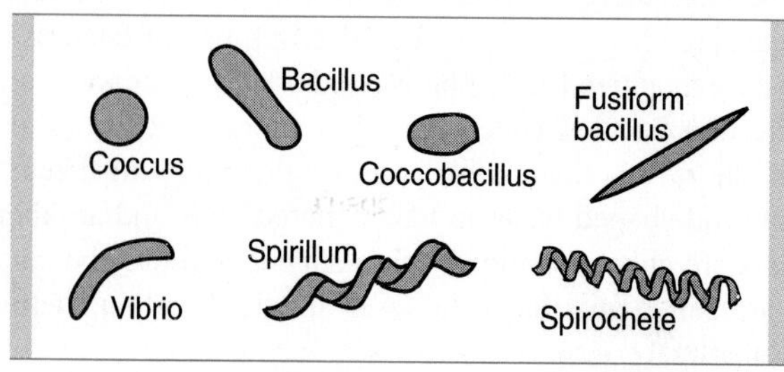

FIGURE 2–2
Shapes of some different bacteria.

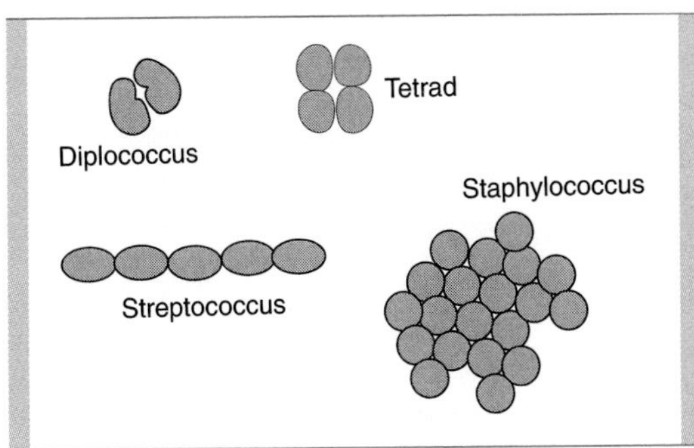

FIGURE 2–3
Arrangement of spherical bacterial cells.

ribosomal (rRNA) types (about 20%); DNA (about 3%); carbohydrate (about 5%); and phospholipid (about 6%). In addition, there are a few macromolecules unique to prokaryotes; a peptidoglycan called **murein** is found in all walled bacteria, and a few other unique molecules (lipopolysaccharide and teichoic acids) are found in specific groups of bacteria.

As we shall see, small size and extraordinarily simple design help explain the success of bacteria in nature. Small size facilitates rapid exchange of nutrients and metabolic byproducts with the environment, whereas simplicity of design facilitates macromolecular synthesis, assembly of cell structures, and formation of new cells by division. Both smallness and simplicity contribute to a distinctive functional property of bacteria—their ability to grow at least an order of magnitude faster than eukaryotic cells. However, at the molecular level, bacteria are far from simple, and it is necessary to learn something of their complexity at this level to understand the ability of some of them to colonize humans or to cause disease.

Small size and simple design facilitate rapid growth

ENVELOPE AND APPENDAGES

As a first approximation, bacteria can be said to have a plain interior and a fancy exterior. The cell core, consisting solely of nucleoid and cytosol, is incredibly simple and almost structureless compared with the interior of a eukaryotic cell. It fits the notion that simplicity facilitates rapid growth. The envelope, on the other hand, is an exceedingly baroque part of the cell, consisting of structures of great complexity that vary in detail among the different major groups of bacteria. This can be readily understood by appreciating three important

Complex structure of cell envelope fits its multiple functions

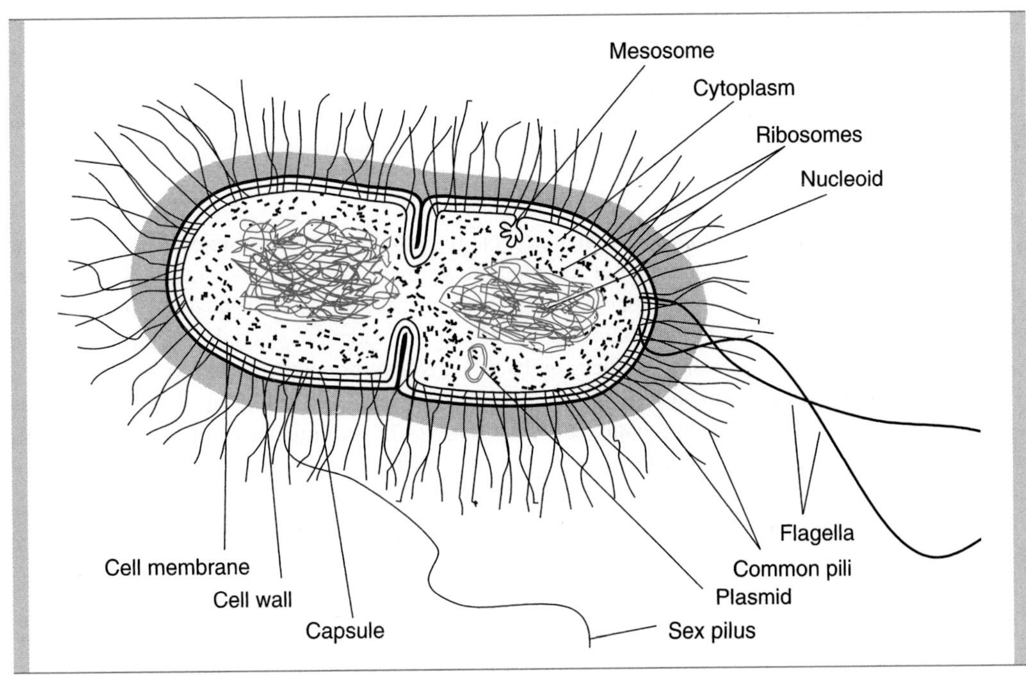

FIGURE 2–4
Schematic of structures of a dividing bacterium.

TABLE 2–1

Components of Bacterial Cells

Structure	Composition	Distribution[a]		
		Gram-Negative Cell	Gram-Positive Cell	Mollicutes (Mycoplasmas)
Envelope				
Capsule (slime layer)	Polysaccharide or polypeptide	+ or −	+ or −	−
Wall		+	+	−
Outer membrane	Proteins, phospholipids, and lipopolysaccharide	+	−	−
Peptidoglycan layer	Murein (+ teichoate in Gram-positive cells)	+	+	−
Periplasm	Proteins and oligosaccharides in solution	+	−	−
Cell membrane	Proteins, phospholipids	+	+	+
Appendages				
Pili (fimbriae)	Protein (pilin)	+ or −	+ or −	−
Flagella	Proteins (flagellin plus others)	+ or −	+ or −	−
Core				
Cytosol	Polyribosomes, proteins, carbohydrates (glycogen)	+	+	+
Nucleoid	DNA with associated RNA and proteins	+	+	+
Plasmids	DNA	+ or −	+ or −	+ or −
Endospore				
All cell components plus dipicolinate and special envelope components		−	+ or −	−

[a] "+" indicates the structure is invariably present, "−" indicates it is invariably absent, and "+ or −" indicates that the structure is present is some species or strains and absent in others.

principles of bacterial functional anatomy: (1) the envelope is responsible for many cellular processes that are the province of the internal organelles of eukaryotic cells, (2) the envelope is the primary site of functions that protect the bacterial cell against chemical and biological threats in its environment, and (3) the envelope and certain appendages make possible the colonization of surfaces by bacteria. Not surprisingly, therefore, more than one fifth of the specific proteins of well-studied bacteria are located in the envelope. Differences in envelope structure and composition (Table 2–1) are the basis of the assignment, described next, of all eubacterial species to one of three major groups: (1) Gram-negative bacteria; (2) Gram-positive bacteria; and (3) wall-less bacteria, including the mollicutes (mycoplasmas) and chlamydia. Figure 2–5 shows schematically these major differences.

Capsule

Hydrophilic capsule gives colonies a smooth appearance, unlike nonmucoid rough variants

Many bacterial cells surround themselves with one or another kind of hydrophilic gel. This layer is often quite thick; commonly it is thicker than the diameter of the cell. Because it is transparent and not readily stained, this layer is usually not appreciated unless made visible by its ability to exclude particulate material, such as India ink. If the

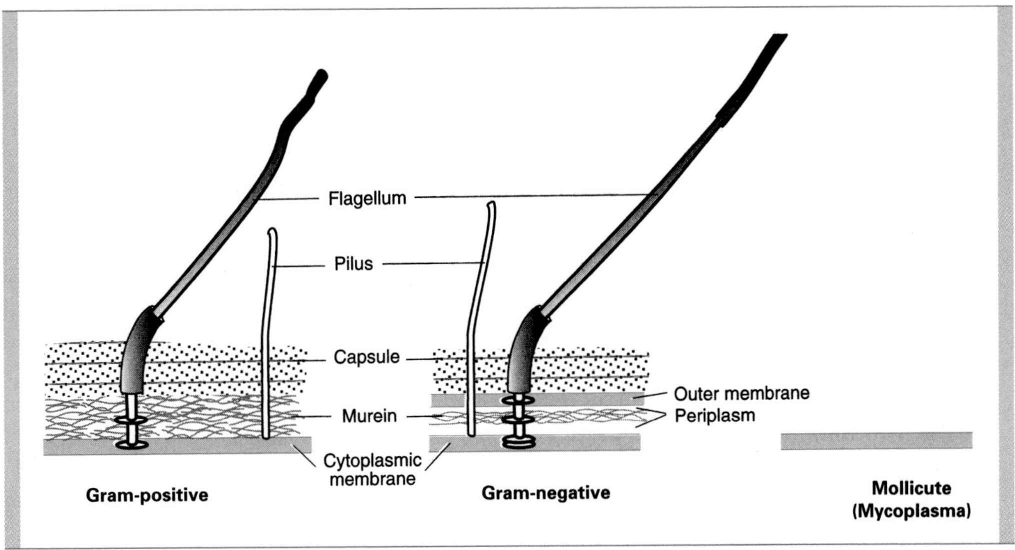

FIGURE 2–5
Schematic representation comparing the envelopes of Gram-positive bacteria, Gram-negative bacteria, and mollicutes.

material forms a reasonably discrete layer, it is called a **capsule;** if it is amorphous in appearance, it is referred to as a **slime layer.** Almost all bacterial species can make such material to some degree. Most capsules or slime layers are polysaccharides made of single or multiple types of sugar residues; some are simple (though unusual) polypeptides, such as the polymer of D-glutamic acid, which forms the capsule of *Bacillus anthracis,* the causative agent of anthrax (see Chapter 18); a few are proteins. When cultured on solid media (see Chapter 15), encapsulated bacteria give rise to smooth, often mucus-like colonies, but unencapsulated variants are common, particularly with long-term laboratory cultivation. Their colonies are nonmucoid and described as "rough."

Capsules can protect bacteria. Within animal and human hosts capsules impede ingestion by leukocytes. *Streptococcus pneumoniae,* the causative agent of pneumococcal pneumonia, in large measure owes its virulence to the ability of its copious polysaccharide capsule to interfere with opsonophagocytosis (see Chapter 17). The pneumococcal polysaccharide, as is the case with most capsular material, is antigenic (see Chapter 8), and when specific antibody attaches to it, phagocytosis can occur. A mouse–pneumococcus experimental model is instructive. Unencapsulated pneumococci are tolerated by mice; however, a single encapsulated cell injected intraperitoneally will kill a mouse unless the mouse has been immunized with capsular material of the specific antigenic type of the infecting pneumococcus, in which case it is protected. More than 80 capsular serotypes of this organism are known, reflecting a diverse genetic capacity of the species to produce capsular polysaccharides of differing chemical structure.

Antiphagocytic effect of some capsules is major virulence determinant

Protection against phagocytosis is only part of the much broader function of bacterial capsules in nature, which is to aid colonization, primarily by assisting the cell to attach to surfaces. For example, the ability of *Streptococcus mutans* and *Streptococcus salivarius* cells to adhere to the surface of teeth is in large measure a function of the polysaccharide capsules of these oral bacteria (see Chapter 62).

Some capsules promote adherence and colonization

Capsules do not contribute to growth and multiplication and are not essential for cell survival in artificial culture. Capsule synthesis is greatly dependent on growth conditions. For example, the capsule made by the caries-producing *S. mutans* consists of a dextran–carbohydrate polymer made only in the presence of sucrose.

Capsule synthesis depends on growth conditions

Cell Wall

Internal to the capsule (if one exists) but still outside the cell proper, a rigid **cell wall** surrounds all eubacterial cells except wall-less bacteria such as the mollicutes (mycoplasmas) and *Chlamydia*. The structure and function of the bacterial wall is so distinctive as to constitute a hallmark of the prokaryotes; nothing like it is found elsewhere. Unlike the capsule, which is dispensable for survival outside the body of the host, the wall has vital functions in all environments. It protects the cell from mechanical disruption and from bursting caused by the turgor pressure resulting from the hypertonicity of the cell interior relative to the environment. The wall provides a barrier against certain toxic chemical and biological agents. In some bacterial species, such as *Streptococcus* (see Chapter 17), it provides a protection from phagocytosis and helps in the binding to eukaryotic cell hosts. Its form is responsible for the shape of the cell.

Unique wall structure prevents osmotic lysis, determines shape, protects against toxins and phagocytosis, and helps in colonization

Bacterial evolution has led to two major solutions to the challenge of constructing a wall that can protect a minute, fragile cell from chemical and physical assault while still permitting the rapid exchange of nutrients and metabolic byproducts required by rapid growth. Long before these solutions were understood in ultrastructural terms, it was recognized that bacteria could be divided into two groups depending on their reaction to a particular staining procedure devised a century ago by the Danish microbiologist Hans Christian Gram. This procedure, the Gram stain, is described in detail in Chapter 15. It depends on the differential ability of ethanol or ethanol–acetone mixtures to extract iodine–crystal violet complexes from bacterial cells. These complexes are readily extracted from one group of bacteria, termed **Gram-negative,** which can be subsequently stained red with an appropriate counterstain. They are retained by the other, termed **Gram-positive,** which are thus stained violet by the retained crystal violet. The positive or negative Gram stain response of a cell reflects which of the two types of wall it possesses.

Gram stain distinguishes two major envelope structures

Virtually all of the eubacteria with walls can be assigned a Gram response. However, the few exceptions include some medically important organisms. For example, the mycobacteria (eg, *Mycobacterium tuberculosis,* the causative agent of tuberculosis) are Gram positive on the basis of their wall structure but fail to stain because of interference by special lipids present in their walls. Most spirochetes, including *Treponema pallidum* (the causative agent of syphilis), although Gram negative by structure, are too thin to be resolved in the light microscope when stained by simple stains.

A few pathogens are not usefully distinguished by Gram stain

Bacteria without walls, whether natural forms (the mollicutes or mycoplasmas) or artificial products of procedures that remove the wall, exhibit a Gram-negative staining response. Furthermore, some bacteria that are Gram positive on the basis of wall structure and staining response may lose this property and appear Gram negative if they have been held under nongrowing conditions. These examples emphasize that being Gram positive is a distinct property that can be temporarily lost because it depends on the integrity of the cell wall; on the other hand, a Gram-negative bacterial cell does not have a staining property to lose.

Cells can lose Gram-positive trait

Gram-Positive Cell Wall

The Gram-positive cell wall contains two major components, peptidoglycan and teichoic acids, plus additional carbohydrates and proteins, depending on the species. A generalized scheme illustrating the arrangement of these components is shown in Figure 2–6.

Major components of Gram-positive walls are peptidoglycan and teichoic acid

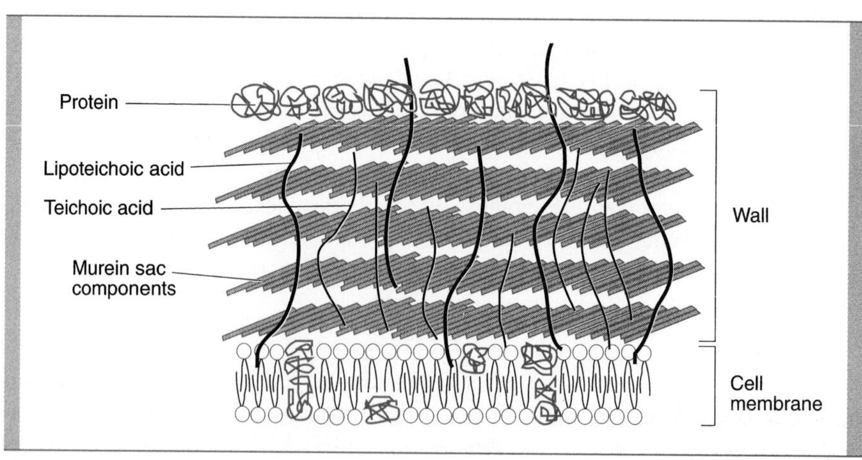

FIGURE 2–6
Schematic representation of the wall of Gram-positive bacteria.

The chief component is **murein,** a peptidoglycan, which is found nowhere except in prokaryotes. Murein consists of a linear glycan chain of two alternating sugars, *N*-acetylglucosamine (NAG) and *N*-acetylmuramic acid (NAM), in 1:4 linkages (Fig 2–7). Each muramic acid residue bears a tetrapeptide of alternating L- and D-amino acids. Adjacent glycan chains are cross-linked into sheets by peptide bonds between the third amino acid of one tetrapeptide and the terminal D-alanine of another. The same cross-links between other tetrapeptides connect the sheets to form a three-dimensional, rigid matrix. The cross-links involve perhaps one third of the tetrapeptides and may be direct or may include a peptide bridge, as, for example, a pentaglycine bridge in *Staphylococcus aureus*. The cross-linking extends around the cell, producing a scaffold-like giant molecule, termed the **murein sac,** or **sacculus.** Murein is much the same in all bacteria, except that there is diversity in the nature and frequency of the cross-linking bridge and in the nature of the amino acids at positions 2 and 3 of the tetrapeptide.

Murein comprises linear glycan chains of alternating NAG and NAM cross-linked in three dimensions by peptide chains

Scaffold-like murein sac surrounds cell

The murein sac derives its great mechanical strength from the fact that it is a single, covalently bonded structure; other features contributing strength are the β-1,4 bonds of the polysaccharide backbone, the alternation of D- and L-amino acids in the tetrapeptide, and extensive internal hydrogen bonding. Biological stability is contributed by components of murein that are not widely distributed in the biological world or in fact are unique to murein. These include muramic acid, D-amino acids, and diaminopimelic acid (an amino acid found in the tetrapeptide of some species). Most enzymes found in mammalian hosts and other biological systems do not degrade peptidoglycan; one important exception is lysozyme, the hydrolase present in tears and other secretions, which cleaves the β-1,4 glycosidic bond between muramic acid and glucosamine residues (see Fig 2–7). On the other hand, bacteria themselves are rich in hydrolases that degrade peptidoglycan, because the murein sac must be constantly expanded by insertion of new chains as the cell grows and forms a cross-wall preparatory to cell division. As we shall learn, disruption of the fine control that bacteria exert over the activity of these potentially

Rare or unique components of murein provide resistance to most mammalian enzymes

Bacterial enzymes insert new murein chains during growth and provide targets for antimicrobics

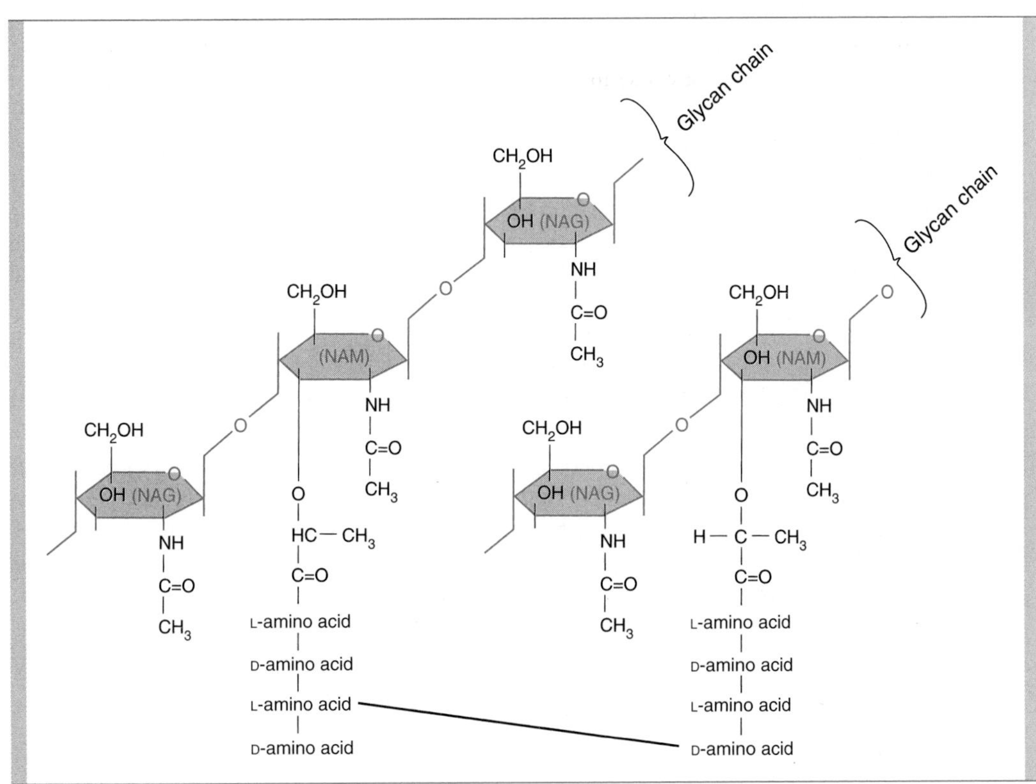

FIGURE 2–7
Schematic representation of the peptidoglycan murein. NAG, *N*-acetylglucosamine; NAM, *N*-acetylmuramic acid.

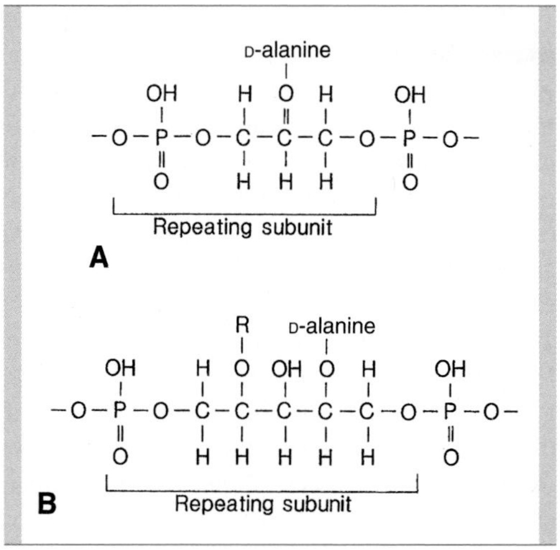

FIGURE 2–8
Schematic reproduction of teichoic acids. **A**. Glycerol teichoic acid. **B**. A ribitol teichoic acid in which R may be glucose or succinate in different species.

lethal enzymes is the means by which a large number of antibiotics and other chemotherapeutic compounds work (see Chapter 13).

Loss of cell wall leads to lysis in hypotonic media or production of protoplasts in isotonic media

The role of the murein component of the cell wall in conferring osmotic resistance and shape on the cell is easily demonstrated by removing or destroying it. Treatment of a Gram-positive cell with penicillin (which blocks formation of the tetrapeptide cross-links and activates the cell's own murein hydrolases) or with lysozyme (which directly hydrolyzes the glycan chains) destroys the murein sac, and the wall is lost. Prompt lysis of the cell ensues. If the cell is protected from lysis by suspension in a medium approximately isotonic with the cell interior, such as 20% sucrose, the cell becomes round and forms a sphere called a **protoplast.** Some protoplasts can grow, and their formation from classic bacteria within patients treated with penicillin-type antibiotics (L-forms) has been postulated to account for some persistent infections. Superficially, protoplasts resemble the mollicutes (mycoplasmas) that are naturally wall-less bacteria.

Teichoic and lipoteichoic acids promote adhesion and anchor wall to membrane

Different teichoic acids occur in different Gram-positive genera

A second component of the Gram-positive cell wall is a **teichoic** acid. These compounds are polymers of either glycerol phosphate or ribitol phosphate, with various sugars, amino sugars, and amino acids as substituents (Fig 2–8). The lengths of the chain and the nature and location of the substituents vary from species to species and sometimes between strains within a species. Up to 50% of the wall may be teichoic acid, some of which is covalently linked to occasional NAM residues of the murein. Of the teichoic acids made of polyglycerol phosphate, much is linked not to the wall but to a glycolipid in the underlying cell membrane. This type of teichoic acid is called **lipoteichoic acid** and seems to play a role in anchoring the wall to the cell membrane and as an epithelial cell adhesin. Teichoic acids are found only in Gram-positive cells and constitute major antigenic determinants of their cell surface individuality. For example, *S. aureus* polysaccharide A is a teichoic acid and *Enterococcus faecalis* group D carbohydrate is a lipoteichoic acid.

Other cell wall components offer protection and promote colonization

Beside the major wall components—murein and teichoic acids—Gram-positive walls usually have lesser amounts of other molecules. Some are polysaccharides, such as the group-specific antigens of streptococci; others are proteins, such as the M protein of group A streptococci. The detailed arrangement of the various antigens in some of the more complex Gram-positive walls is still being worked out, but minor components are thought to protect the peptidoglycan layer from the action of such agents as lysozyme. Some protein components, called **adhesins,** of the cell wall promote colonization by sticking the bacteria to the surfaces of host cells (see Chapter 10).

Gram-Negative Cell Wall

Thin murein sac is imbedded in periplasmic murein gel

The second kind of cell wall found in bacteria, the Gram-negative cell wall, is depicted in Figure 2–9. Except for the presence of murein, there is little chemical resemblance to cell walls of Gram-positive bacteria, and the architecture is fundamentally different. In

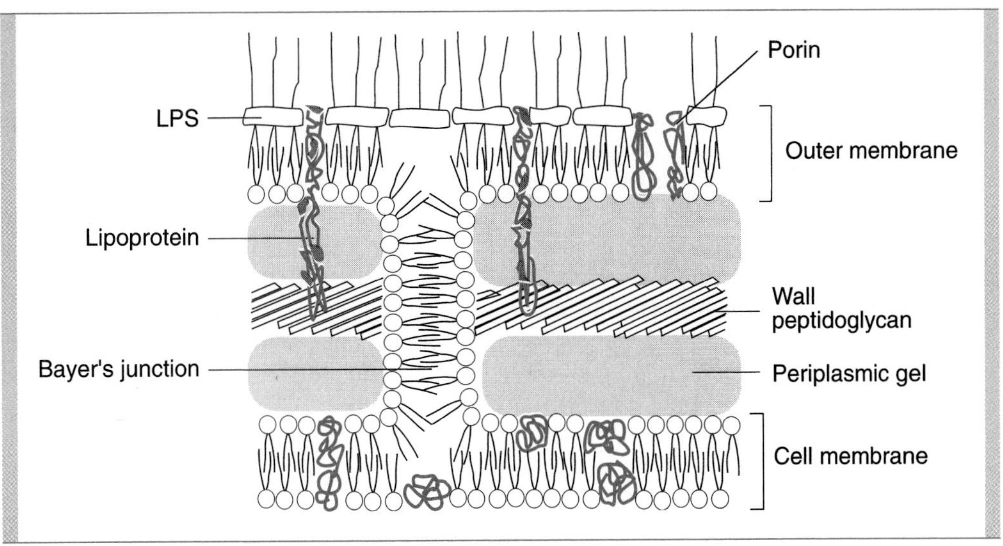

FIGURE 2–9
Schematic representation of wall of Gram-negative bacteria. LPS, lipopolysaccharide with endotoxic properties.

Gram-negative cells, the amount of murein has been greatly reduced, with some of it forming a single-layered sheet around the cell and the rest forming a gel-like substance, the **periplasmic gel,** with little cross-linking. External to this **periplasm** is an elaborate outer membrane.

Historically, the cell wall was regarded as the structure external to the cell membrane (excluding the capsule), and for Gram-positive bacteria this conception is certainly appropriate. Examination of Figures 2–5 and 2–9 shows the dilemma in applying the same term to the Gram-negative envelope. There is some reason to apply the same definition used for the Gram-positive situation, in which case the cell wall of Gram-negative bacteria consists of periplasm with its murein sac plus the outer membrane. This convention is used in Table 2–1 and in the text of this chapter. An alternative convention is to consider that the cell wall of Gram-negative bacteria is simply the structure chemically most like the Gram-positive wall, namely, the thin murein sac, with perhaps its attendant periplasmic gel. The student will quickly realize the underlying truth that **cell wall** is not a very satisfying term. Some microbiologists use cell envelope and envelope layers and avoid using the term cell wall altogether for Gram-negative bacteria.

Gram-negative wall is murein sac plus outer membrane

Earlier electron micrographs had suggested that the small amount of murein in Gram-negative cells, such as *Escherichia coli,* formed a single sheet around the cell, and that this murein sac was floating in a space, the periplasmic space, containing a fairly concentrated solution of proteins and oligosaccharides. Recent evidence modifies this picture and indicates that the "space" is a gel formed by murein peptidoglycan chains with little or no cross-linking.

Whatever its precise nature, the periplasm contains a murein sac, with a unit peptidoglycan structure quite similar to that in Gram-positive cells. Despite its reduced extent in the Gram-negative wall, the murein sac still is responsible for the shape of the cell and is vital for its integrity. As in the case of Gram-positive cells, removing or damaging the peptidoglycan layer leads to cell lysis. If the cells are protected from osmotic lysis during lysozyme or penicillin treatment, they assume a spherical shape. Because such spheres cannot be totally stripped of wall material, they are called **spheroplasts,** in contrast to the protoplasts formed from Gram-positive cells. Spheroplasts of some species can multiply.

Murein sac is responsible for shape and integrity; removal results in spheroplasts

The proteins in solution in the periplasm consist of enzymes with hydrolytic functions (such as alkaline phosphatase), sometimes antibiotic-inactivating enzymes, and various binding proteins with roles in chemotaxis and in the active transport of solutes into the cell (see Chapter 3). Oligosaccharides secreted into the periplasm in response to external conditions serve to create an osmotic pressure buffer for the cell.

Periplasmic proteins have transport, chemotactic, and hydrolytic roles

Gram-negative outer membrane is phospholipoprotein bilayer, of which the outer leaflet is LPS endotoxin

The periplasm is an intermembrane structure, lying between the cell membrane (discussed later) and a special membrane unique to Gram-negative cells, the **outer membrane.** This has an overall structure similar to most biological membranes with two opposing phospholipid–protein leaflets. However, in terms of its composition, the outer membrane is unique in all biology. Its inner leaflet consists of ordinary phospholipids, but these are replaced in the outer leaflet by a special molecule called **lipopolysaccharide** (LPS), which is extremely toxic to humans and other animals, and is called an **endotoxin.** Even in minute amounts, such as the amount released to the circulation during the course of a Gram-negative infection, this substance can produce a fever and shock syndrome called **Gram-negative shock,** or **endotoxic shock.**

Lipid A is toxic moiety of LPS; polysaccharides are antigenic determinants

LPS consists of a toxic **lipid A** (a phospholipid containing glucosamine rather than glycerol), a **core polysaccharide** (containing some unusual carbohydrate residues and fairly constant in structure among related species of bacteria), and **O antigen polysaccharide side chains** (Fig 2–10). The last component constitutes the major surface antigen of Gram-negative cells (which, it is recalled, lack teichoic acids).

Impermeability of outer membrane is overcome by active transport and porins

The presence of LPS in the outer leaflet of the outer membrane results in the covering of Gram-negative cells by a wall that should block the passage of virtually every organic molecule into the cell. Hydrophobic molecules (such as some antibiotics) would be blocked by the hydrophilic layer of O antigen; hydrophilic solutes, including most nutrients, such as sugars and amino acids, would face the barrier created by the

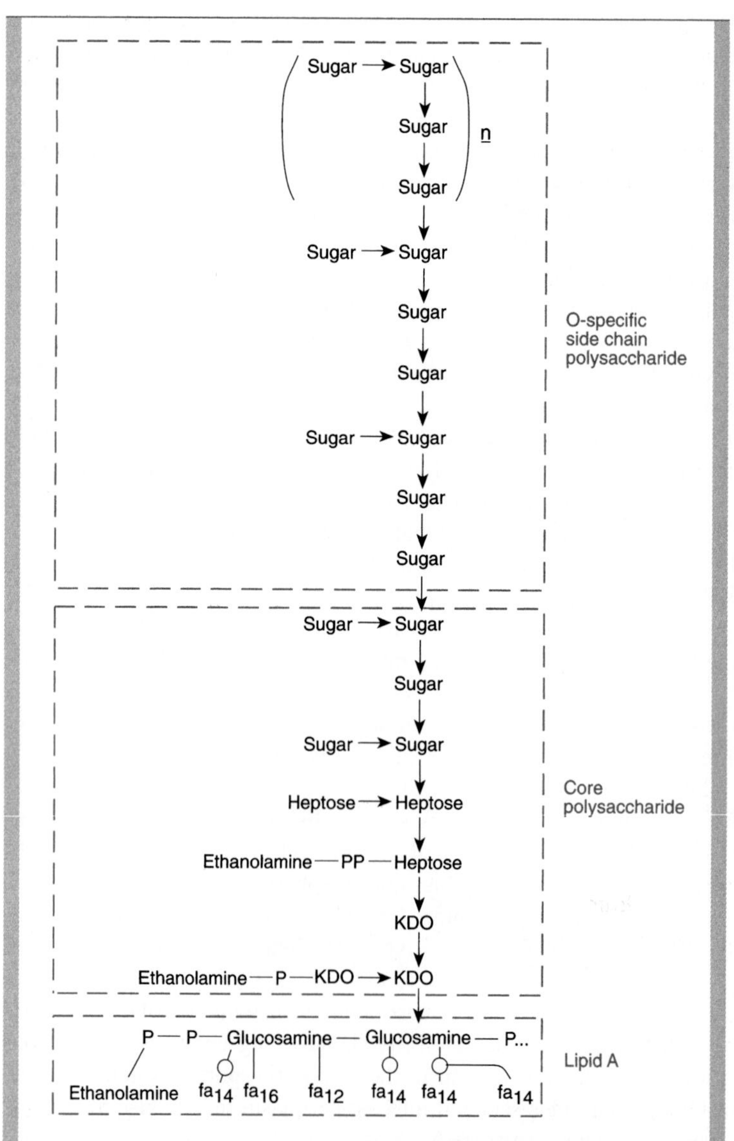

FIGURE 2–10
Schematic representation of lipopolysaccharide. The O-specific side chain is highly variable among species and subspecies and is a major determinant of antigenetic specificity. fa, fatty acid; KDO, ketodeoxyoctanate.

lipid portion of the outer membrane. Clearly this is a trade-off that cannot be made; the Gram-negative cell, for whatever benefit is afforded by possessing a wall with an outer membrane, must make provision for the rapid entry of nutrients. Active transport (described in Chapter 3) is part of the solution, and a particular structural feature of the outer membrane contributes another part. Special proteins, called **porins** or **matrix proteins,** form pores through the outer membrane that make it possible for hydrophilic solute molecules of molecular weight less than about 800 to diffuse through it and into the periplasm.

The outer membrane does not contain the variety of proteins present in the cell membrane, but those that are present are quite abundant. In addition to the porins, there is a protein called **Braun's lipoprotein** or **murein lipoprotein,** which is probably the most abundant outer membrane protein in Gram-negative cells, such as *E. coli.* This protein is covalently attached at its amino end to a lipid embedded in the outer membrane. About one third of these lipoprotein molecules are covalently attached at their carboxyl end to the third amino acid in the murein tetrapeptide. It is believed that this forms the major attachment of the murein layer to the outer membrane of the wall in *E. coli* (see Fig 2–9).

Murein lipoprotein is abundant component that attaches murein sac to outer membrane

The innermost leaflet may well be contiguous in places with the outermost leaflet of the cell membrane (see Fig 2–9), because, at least under the electron microscope, preparations of the outer membrane and the cell membrane can be seen to adhere to each other at **zones of adhesion** (also called **Bayer's junctions**). Other zones of adhesion girding the whole circumference of *E. coli* and related species have been postulated. Because these annular rings tend to form about the cell division septum, they have been called **periseptal annuli.** Their existence is still being examined.

Outer and inner membranes may be adherent in places

In evolving a cell wall containing an outer membrane, Gram-negative bacteria have succeeded in (1) creating the periplasm, which holds digestive and protective enzymes and proteins important in transport and chemotaxis; (2) presenting an outer surface with strong negative charge, which is important in evading phagocytosis and the action of complement; and (3) providing a permeability barrier against such dangerous molecules as host lysozyme, β-lysin, bile salts, digestive enzymes, and many antibiotics.

Outer membrane has many functions

Cell Membrane

Generally the cell membrane of bacteria is similar to the familiar bileaflet membrane, containing phospholipids and proteins, that is found throughout the living world. However, there are important differences. The bacterial cell membrane is exceptionally rich in proteins (up to 70% of its weight) and does not (except in the case of mycoplasmas) contain sterols. The bacterial chromosome is attached to the cell membrane, which plays a role in segregation of daughter chromosomes at cell division, analogous to the role of the mitotic apparatus of eukaryotes. The membrane is the site of synthesis of DNA, cell wall polymers, and membrane lipids. It contains the entire electron transport system of the cell (and, hence, is functionally analogous to the mitochondria of eukaryotes). It contains receptor proteins that function in chemotaxis. Like cell membranes of eukaryotes, it is a permeability barrier and contains proteins involved in selective and active transport of solutes. It is also involved in secretion to the exterior of proteins (exoproteins), including exotoxins and hydrolytic enzymes involved in the pathogenesis of disease. The bacterial cell membrane is therefore the functional equivalent of most of the organelles of the eukaryotic cell and is vital to the growth and maintenance of the cell.

Basic structure of cell membrane is phospholipid–protein bilayer, usually lacking sterols

Membrane has roles in synthetic, homeostatic, secretory, and electron transport processes, and in cell division

Cell membrane is functional equivalent of many eukaryotic organelles

The cell membranes of Gram-positive and Gram-negative cells are similar in composition, structure, and function except for the modification, already described, in Gram-negative cells that places the outer membrane of the wall and the cell membrane in intimate contact (Bayer's junctions).

Flagella

Flagella are molecular organelles of motility found in many species of bacteria, both Gram positive and Gram negative. They may be distributed around the cell (an arrangement called

Flagella are rotating helical protein structures responsible for locomotion

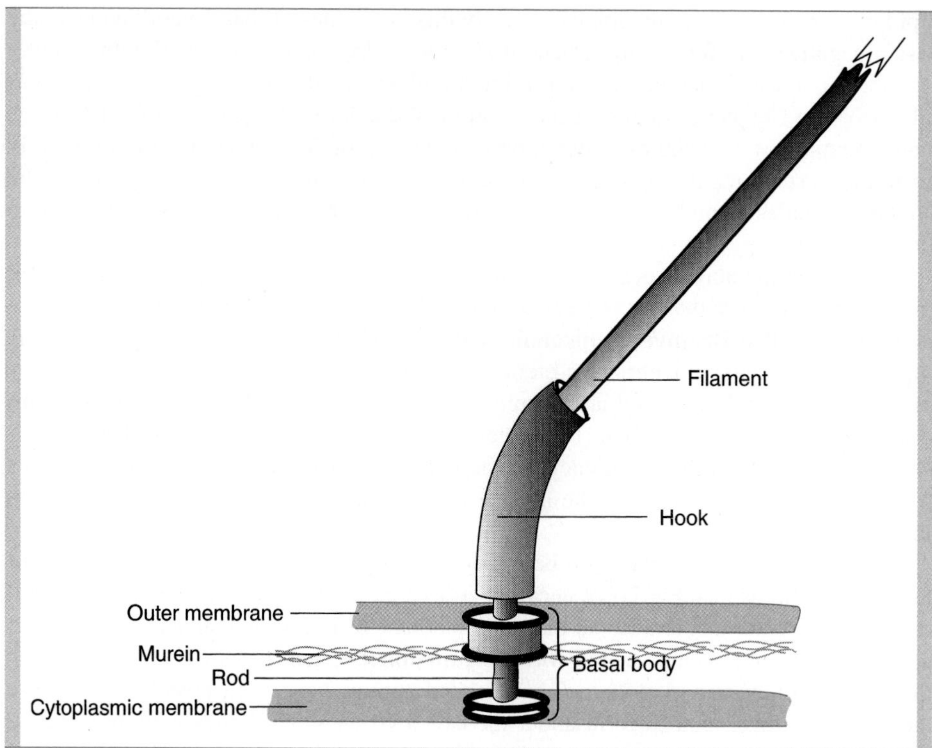

FIGURE 2–11
Schematic representation of the flagellar apparatus. (*After DePamphilis ML, Adler J. Fine structure and isolation of hook-basal body complex of flagella from* Escherichia coli *and* Bacillus subtilis. J Bacteriol *1971;105:384–359.*)

peritrichous from the Greek **trichos** for "hair"), at one pole (**polar** or **monotrichous**), or at both ends of the cell (**lophotrichous**). In all cases, they are individually helical in shape and propel the cell by rotating at the point of insertion in the cell envelope. The presence or absence of flagella and their position are important taxonomic characteristics.

Flagella have bushing rings in cell envelope

Flagellar filament is composed of the protein flagellin

The flagellar apparatus is complex, but consists entirely of proteins, encoded in genes called *fla* (for flagella). They are attached to the cell by a **basal body** consisting of several proteins organized as rings on a central rod (see Fig 2–5). In Gram-negative cells, there are four rings: an outer pair that serve as bushings through the outer membrane and an inner pair located in the peptidoglycan gel and the cell membrane. In Gram-positive cells, only the inner pair is present. The **hook** consists of other proteins organized as a bent structure that may function as a universal joint. Finally, the long **filament** consists of polymerized molecules of a single protein species called **flagellin** (Fig 2–11). Flagellin varies in amino acid sequence from strain to strain. This makes flagella useful surface antigens for strain differentiation, particularly among the Enterobacteriaceae.

Motility and chemotaxis, both important properties contributing to colonization, are discussed in Chapter 3.

Pili

Pili are proteinaceous hair-like projections

Common pili have adherence roles

Male Gram-negative cells of some species have single tubular sex pili

Pili are molecular hair-like projections found on the surface of cells of many Gram-positive and Gram-negative species. They are composed of molecules of a protein called **pilin** arranged to form a tube with a minute, hollow core. There are two general classes, common pili and sex pili (Fig 2–12). **Common pili** cover the surface of the cell. They are, in many cases, **adhesins,** which are responsible for the ability of bacteria to colonize surfaces and cells. To cite only one example, the pili of *Neisseria gonorrhoeae* are necessary for the attachment to the urethral epithelial cells prior to penetration; without pili, the bacterium cannot cause gonorrhea. Thus, common pili are often important virulence factors. In fact, there are at least five different types of common pili (see Chapter 10). Some bacteriologists use the name **fimbriae** to refer to common pili. The sex pilus is diagnostic of a male bacterium and is involved in exchange of genetic material between some Gram-negative bacteria. There is only one per cell. The function of the sex pilus is discussed in Chapter 4.

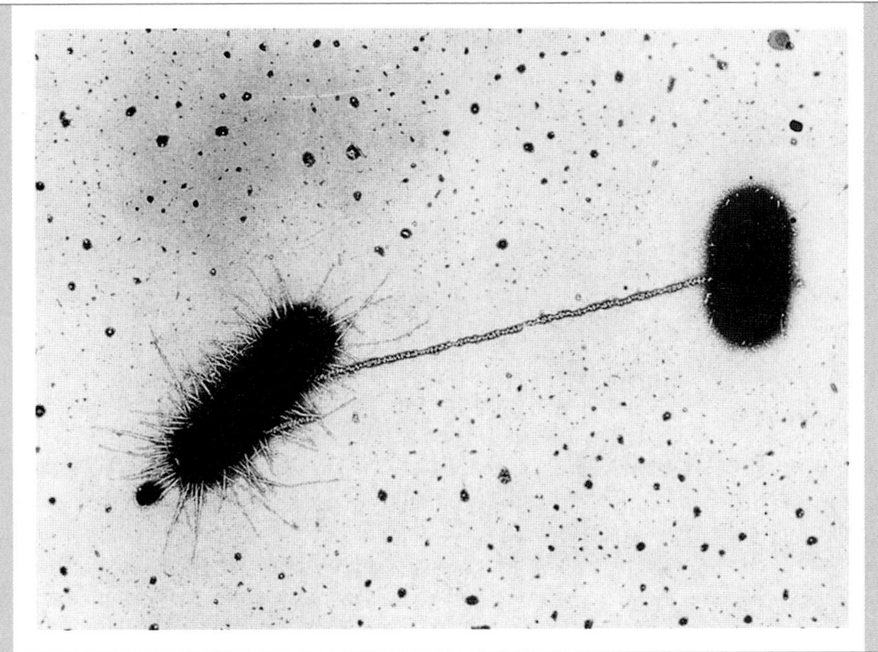

FIGURE 2–12
On the left-hand side is a "male" *Escherichia coli* cell exhibiting many common (somatic) pili and a sex pilus by which it has attached itself to a "female" cell that lacks the plasmid encoding the sex pilus. As discussed in Chapter 4, the sex pilus facilitates exchange of genetic material between the male and female *E. coli*. In this preparation, the sex pilus has been labeled with a bacterial virus that attaches to it specifically. (*Courtesy of Charles C. Brinton and Judith Carnahan.*)

CORE

In contrast to the structural richness of the layers and appendages of the cell envelope, the interior seems relatively simple in transmission electron micrographs of thin sections of bacteria (Fig 2–13). There are two clearly visible regions, one granular (the cytosol) and one fibrous (the nucleoid). In addition, many bacteria possess plasmids that are usually circular, double-stranded DNA bodies in the cytosol separate from the larger nucleoid; plasmids are too small to be visible in thin sections of bacteria.

Cytosol

The dense **cytosol** is bounded by the cell membrane. It appears granular because it is densely packed with ribosomes, which are much more abundant than in the cytoplasm of eukaryotic cells. This is a reflection of the higher growth rate of bacteria. Each ribosome is a ribonucleoprotein particle consisting of three species of rRNA (5 S, 16 S, and 23 S) and about 56 proteins. The overall subunit structure (one 50 S plus one 30 S particle) of the 70 S bacterial ribosome resembles that of eukaryotic ribosomes (which are 80 S, composed of one 60 S and one 40 S particle), but is smaller and differs sufficiently in function that a very large number of antimicrobics have the prokaryotic ribosome as their target.

Cytosol contains 70 S ribosomes and most of cell's metabolic enzymes

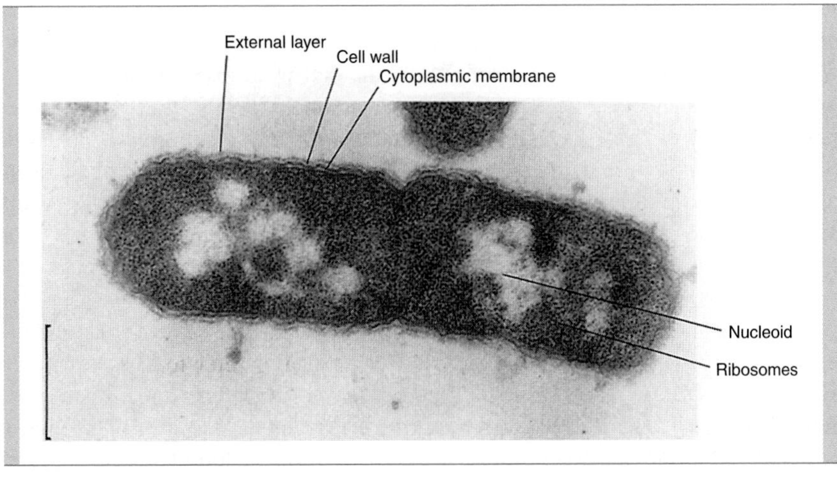

FIGURE 2–13
Electron micrograph of a Gram-negative bacterium. (*Courtesy of the late Dr. E. S. Boatman.*)

The number of ribosomes varies directly with the growth rate of the cell (see Chapter 3). At all but the slowest growth rates about 70% of the ribosomes at any one time exist as polysomes and are engaged in translating mRNA. Except for the functions associated with the cell membrane, all of the metabolic reactions of the cell take place in the cytosol. Accordingly, it is found to be the major location of a great fraction of the 2000 to 3000 different enzymes of the cell. The cytosol of some bacterial species also contains nutritional storage granules called **reserve granules.** The most prevalent kinds consist of glycogen or polymetaphosphate. Their presence and abundance depend on the nutritional state of the cell.

Nucleoid

Nucleoid consists of a large tightly packed circular chromosome of supercoiled double-stranded DNA

Bacteria have no nuclear membrane

Nucleoid may be attached to cell membrane and central structures

The bacterial genome resides on a single chromosome (there are rare exceptions) and typically consists of about 4000 genes encoded in one, large, circular molecule of double-stranded DNA containing about 5 million nucleotide base pairs. This molecule is more than 1 mm long, and it therefore exceeds the length of the cell by some 1000 times. Needless to say, tight packing is necessary, and it is this packing that displaces all ribosomes and other cytosol components from the regions that appear clear or fibrous in electron micrographs of thin sections of bacterial cells (see Fig 2–13). Each region thus contains a chromosome, coated usually by polyamines and some specialized DNA-binding proteins but not with the structural organization of a eukaryotic chromosome. Because it is not surrounded by a membrane, it is not correctly called a nucleus but rather a **nucleoid** or **nuclear body.** The manner in which the DNA molecule is packed to form a nucleoid is not yet totally known. The double-helical DNA chain is twisted into supercoils, and it is suspected that the DNA is attached to the cell membrane. Evidence indicates that the entire chromosome is attached to some central structure, perhaps RNA, at a large number of points (12 to 80), creating folds of DNA, each of which is independently coiled into a tight bundle. Gentle methods of lysing cells permit nucleoids to be isolated as compact particles from which DNA loops can be sprung out.

Cell may contain 2–4 nucleoids depending on growth rate

Each nuclear body corresponds to a DNA molecule. The number of nuclear bodies varies as a function of growth rate; resting cells have only one, rapidly growing cells may have as many as four. As is described in Chapter 4, bacteria are genetically **haploid** for two reasons: (1) because all the chromosomes are identical and are segregated at random into daughter cells, and (2) because when rapidly growing cells slow down and form resting cells, the latter have returned to a single chromosome state.

The absence of a nuclear membrane confers on the prokaryotic cell a great advantage for rapid growth in changing environments. As described in Chapter 3, ribosomes can be translating mRNA molecules even as the latter are being made; no transport of mRNA from where it is made to where it functions is needed.

Plasmids

Plasmids are small, usually circular, double-stranded DNA molecules

Plasmids may encode protective enzymes, virulence determinants, and self-transmissibility

Many bacteria contain small, usually circular, covalently closed, double-stranded DNA molecules separate from the chromosome. More than one type of plasmid or several copies of a single plasmid may be present in the cell. Many plasmids carry genes coding for the production of enzymes that protect the cell from toxic substances. For example, antibiotic resistance is often plasmid determined. Many attributes of virulence, such as production of some pili and of some exotoxins, are also determined by plasmid genes. Some plasmids code for production of a sex pilus by which they promote cell conjugation and thereby accomplish their own intercellular transmission. They are thus "infectious," are nonhomologous to the bacterial chromosome, and provide a rapid method for acquisition of valuable genetic traits. This topic is considered in more detail in Chapter 4.

SPORES

Endospores are hardy, quiescent forms of some Gram-positive bacteria, including important pathogens

Endospores are small, dehydrated, metabolically quiescent forms that are produced by some bacteria in response to nutrient limitation or a related sign that tough times are coming. Very few species produce spores (the term is loosely used as equivalent to endospores), but they are particularly prevalent in the environment. Some spore-forming bacteria are of great importance in medicine, causing such diseases as anthrax, gas gangrene, tetanus, and botulism. All spore formers are Gram-positive rods. Some grow only in the absence of oxygen (eg, *Clostridium tetani*), some only in its presence (eg, *Bacillus subtilis*).

Spore-forming allows survival under adverse conditions

The bacterial endospore is not a reproductive structure. One cell forms one spore under adverse conditions (the process is called **sporulation**). The spore may persist for a long time (centuries) and then, on appropriate stimulation, give rise to a single bacterial cell (**germination**). Spores, therefore, are survival rather than reproductive devices.

Endospore is not a reproductive structure

Spores of some species can withstand extremes of pH and temperature, including boiling water, for surprising periods of time. The thermal resistance is brought about by the low water content and the presence of a large amount of a substance found only in spores, **calcium dipicolinate.** Resistance to chemicals and, to some extent, radiation is aided by extremely tough, special coats surrounding the spore. These include a **spore membrane** (equivalent to the former cell membrane); a thick **cortex** composed of a special form of peptidoglycan; a **coat** consisting of a cysteine-rich, keratin-like, insoluble structural protein; and, finally, an external lipoprotein and carbohydrate layer called an **exosporium.**

Resistance of spore is due to dehydrated state, calcium dipicolinate, and specialized coats

Germination reproduces cell identical to that which sporulated

Sporulation is under active investigation. The molecular process by which a cell produces a highly differentiated product that is incapable of immediate growth but able to sustain growth after prolonged periods (centuries, in some cases) of nongrowth under extreme conditions of heat, desiccation, and starvation is of great interest. In general, the process involves the initial walling off of a nucleoid and its surrounding cytosol by invagination of the cell membrane, with later additions of special spore layers. Germination begins with activation by heat, acid, and reducing conditions. Initiation of germination eventually leads to outgrowth of a new vegetative cell of the same genotype as the cell that produced the spore.

ADDITIONAL READING

Neidhardt FC, Ingraham JL, Schaechter M. *Physiology of the Bacterial Cell: A Molecular Approach.* Sunderland, MA: Sinauer Associates; 1990. A very readable description of the composition, organization, and structure of the bacterial cell is presented in Chapters 1 and 2. A good list of references for further reading is included.

CHAPTER 3

Bacterial Processes

FREDERICK C. NEIDHARDT

This chapter examines how the structural and chemical components of bacteria function in the growth and survival of these cells and in their colonization of the human host.

CELL GROWTH

Growth of bacteria is accomplished by an orderly progress of metabolic processes followed by cell division by binary fission. Therefore, growth requires three complex processes: **metabolism,** which produces cell material from the nutrient substances present in the environment; **regulation,** which coordinates the progress of the hundreds of independent biochemical processes of metabolism to result in an orderly and efficient synthesis of cell components and structures in the right proportions; and **cell division,** which results in the formation of two independent living units from one.

Bacterial growth requires metabolism, regulation, and division by binary fission

Bacterial Metabolism

We do not review in depth the many aspects of (mostly mammalian) metabolism customarily learned in biochemistry courses. Many of the principles, and even some of the details of metabolism, are universal. Indeed, the principle known as the **unity of biochemistry** is underscored by the fact that much of what we know of metabolic pathways is derived from work with *Escherichia coli.* We focus, rather, on the unique aspects of bacterial metabolism that are important in medicine.

The broad differences between bacteria and human eukaryotic cells can be summarized as follows:

1. The metabolism of most bacteria is geared to rapid growth and proceeds 10 to 100 times faster than in cells of our bodies.
2. Bacteria are much more versatile than human cells in their ability to use various compounds as energy sources and in their ability to use oxidants other than molecular oxygen in their metabolism of foodstuffs.
3. Bacteria are much more diverse than human cells in their nutritional requirements, because they are more diverse with respect to the completeness of their biosynthetic pathways.
4. The simpler prokaryotic body plan makes it possible for bacteria to synthesize macromolecules by far more streamlined means than our cells employ.
5. Some biosynthetic processes, such as those producing murein, lipopolysaccharide (LPS), and teichoic acid, are unique to bacteria.

Metabolism of prokaryotic cells is more active, versatile, and diverse than that of human cells

Each of these differences contributes to the special nature of the human–microbe encounter, and each provides a potential means for designing therapeutic agents to modify the outcome of this interaction.

Metabolic reactions accomplish four functions for growth: fueling, biosynthesis, polymerization, and assembly

Bacterial metabolism is highly complex. The bacterial cell synthesizes itself and generates energy for active transport, motility (in some species), and other activities by as many as 2000 chemical reactions. These reactions can be helpfully classified according to their function in the metabolic processes of **fueling, biosynthesis, polymerization,** and **assembly.**

Fueling Reactions

Fueling reactions begin with the entry of substrates

Fueling reactions provide the cell with energy and with the 12 precursor metabolites used in biosynthetic reactions (Fig 3–1).

Nutrients enter despite envelopes that serve as permeability barriers

The first step is the capture of nutrients from the environment. Both Gram-positive and Gram-negative cells have surrounded themselves with envelopes designed in part to exclude potentially harmful substances and, therefore, have had to evolve a number of ways to ensure rapid transport of selected solute molecules through the envelope. Methods used by Gram-negative cells are summarized in Figure 3–2.

Facilitated diffusion involves shuttling by carrier protein

Almost no important nutrients enter the cell by **simple diffusion,** because the cell membrane is too effective a barrier to most molecules (the exceptions are carbon dioxide, oxygen, and water). Some transport occurs by **facilitated diffusion** in which a protein carrier in the cell membrane, specific for a given compound, participates in the shuttling of molecules of that substance from one side of the membrane to the other. Glycerol enters *E. coli* cells in this manner, and in bacteria that grow in the absence of oxygen (anaerobic bacteria, see below) it is reasonably common for some nutrients to enter the cell and for fermentation byproducts to leave the cell by facilitated diffusion. Because no energy is involved, this process can work only with, never against, a concentration gradient of the given solute.

Active transport can move nutrients against concentration gradient

Shock-sensitive transport involves periplasmic binding proteins and ATP-derived energy

Active transport, like facilitated diffusion, involves specific protein molecules as carriers of particular solutes, but the process is energy linked and can therefore establish a concentration gradient (active transport can pump "uphill"). Active transport is the most common mechanism in aerobic bacteria. Gram-negative bacteria have two kinds of active transport systems. In one, called **shock-sensitive** because the working components can be released from the cell by osmotic shock treatments, solute molecules cross the outer membrane either by diffusion through the pores of the outer membrane (as in the case of galactose) or by a special protein carrier (as in the case of maltose). In the periplasm, the solute molecules bind to specific **binding proteins,** which interact with carrier proteins in

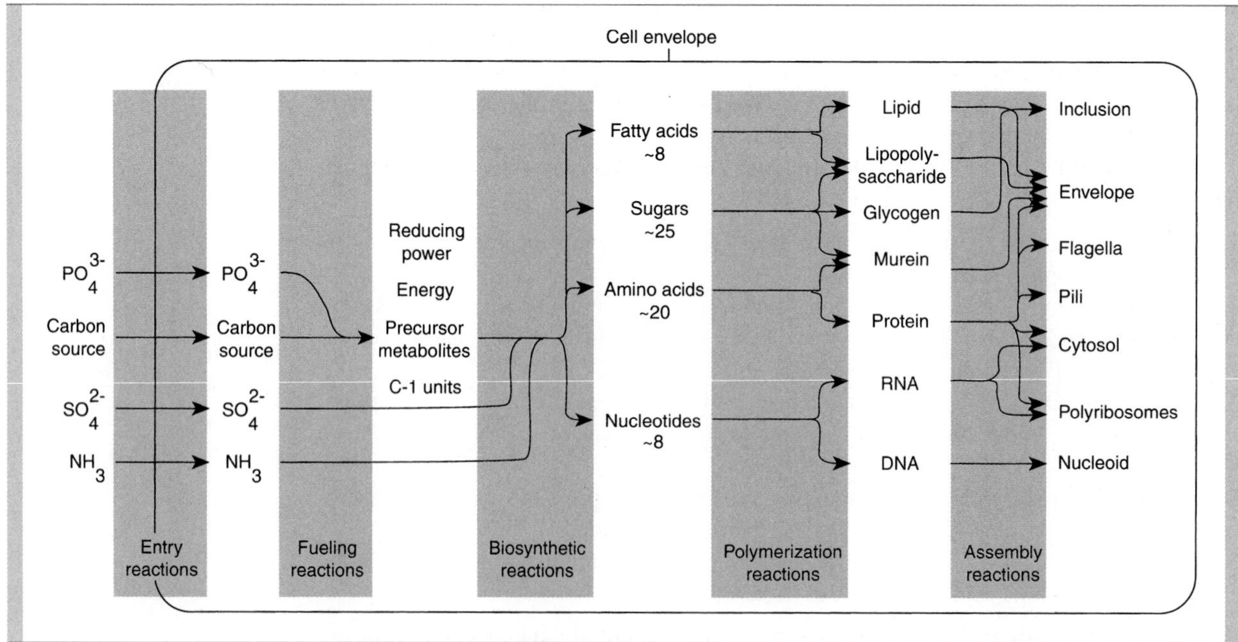

FIGURE 3–1
General pattern of metabolism leading to the synthesis of a bacterial cell from glucose.

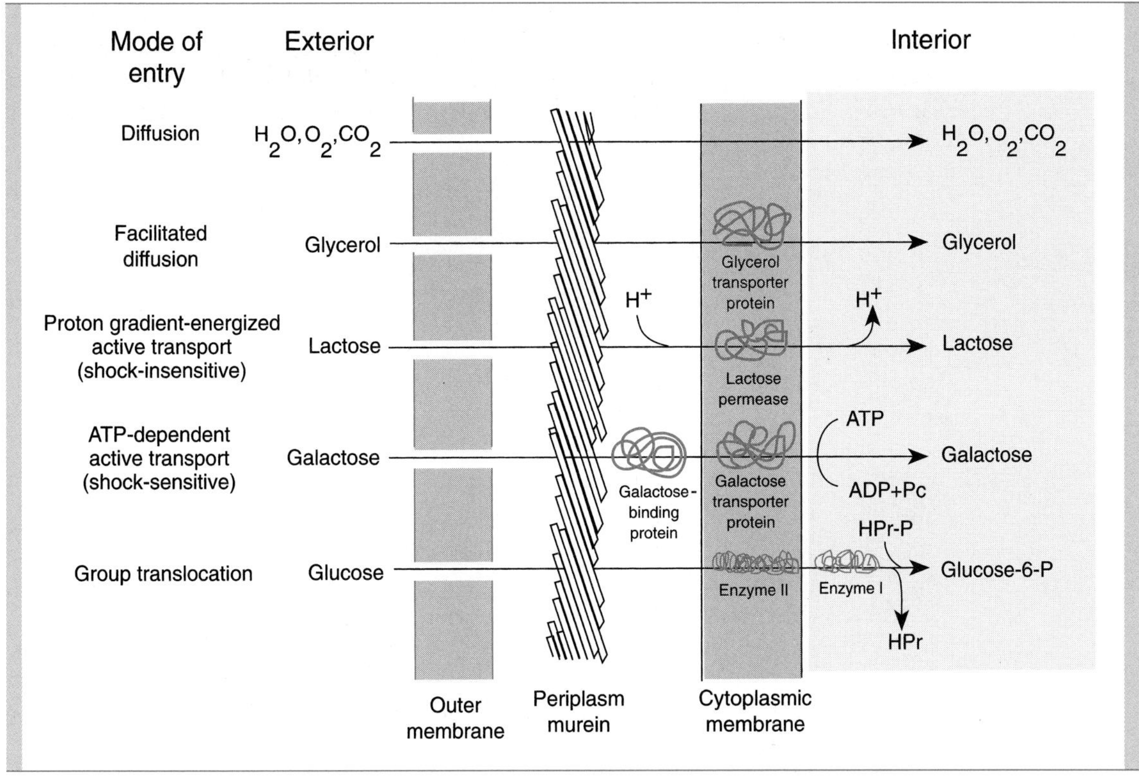

FIGURE 3–2
Schematic representation of the various modes of carbohydrate transport by *Escherichia coli.* Facilitated diffusion is demonstrated by glycerol transport; proton gradient-energized transport, by lactose uptake; shock-sensitive ATP-dependent transport, by galactose uptake; and group translocation, by glucose uptake.

the cell membrane. Shock-sensitive systems couple the transport across the cell membrane with the hydrolysis of ATP.

The other type of active transport involves only cell membrane components (and hence is **shock insensitive**) and is distinctive in that solute transport is coupled to the simultaneous passage of protons (H^+) through the membrane. The energy for this type of active transport is therefore derived not from ATP hydrolysis but from the proton gradient set up by electron transport within the energized cell membrane.

Shock-insensitive transport requires proton gradient energy

Finally, **group translocation** is an extremely common means of transport in the absence of oxygen. It involves the chemical conversion of the solute into another molecule as it is transported. The phosphotransferase system for sugar transport, which involves the phosphorylation of sugars such as glucose by specific enzymes, is a good example.

Group translocation involves chemical conversion of transported molecule

The transport of iron and other metal ions needed in small amounts for growth is special and of particular importance in virulence. There is little free Fe^{3+} in human blood or other body fluids, because it is sequestered by iron-binding proteins (eg, **transferrin** in blood and **lactoferrin** in secretions). Bacteria must have iron to grow, and their colonization of the human host requires capture of iron. Bacteria secrete **siderophores** (iron-specific chelators) to trap Fe^{3+}; the iron-containing chelator is then transported into the bacterium by specific active transport. One example of a siderophore is **aerobactin** (a citrate type of hydoxamate), another is **enterobactin** (a catechol). Some siderophores are produced as a result of enzymes encoded not in the bacterial genome, but in the genome of a plasmid, providing another example of the many ways in which plasmids are involved in virulence.

Iron is an essential nutrient but is sequestered by host Fe-binding proteins

Bacterial siderophores chelate iron and are actively transported into cell

Once inside the cell, sugar molecules or other sources of carbon and energy are metabolized by the Embden–Meyerhof glycolytic pathway, the pentose phosphate pathway, and the Krebs cycle to yield the carbon compounds needed for biosynthesis.

Central fueling pathways produce biosynthetic precursors

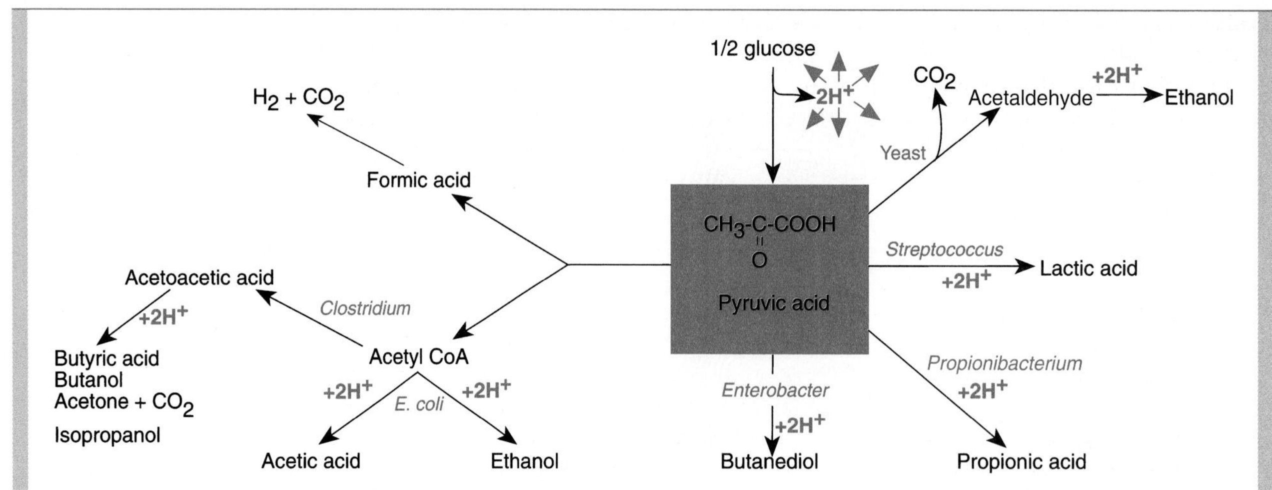

FIGURE 3–3

Some pathways of fermentation of sugars by various microorganisms. The protons (H^+) generated by the conversion of glucose to pyruvate by the Embden–Meyerhoff pathway are transferred to NAD. Oxidized NAD must be regenerated by reducing pyruvate and its derivatives.

Some bacteria have central fueling pathways (eg, the Entner–Doudoroff pathway) other than those familiar in mammalian metabolism.

Fermentation and respiration pathways each regenerate ATP and NAD^+

Working in concert, the central fueling pathways produce the 12 precursor metabolites. Connections to **fermentation** and **respiration** pathways allow the reoxidation of reduced coenzyme nicotinamide adenine dinucleotide (NADH) to NAD^+ and the generation of ATP. Bacteria make ATP by substrate phosphorylation in fermentation or by a combination of substrate phosphorylation and oxidative phosphorylation in respiration. (Photosynthetic bacteria are not important in medicine.)

Fermentation uses direct transfer of proton and electron to final organic receptor and produces organic acids and alcohols

It has low ATP-generating efficiency

Fermentation is the transfer of electrons and protons via NAD^+ directly to an organic acceptor. Pyruvate occupies a pivotal role in fermentation (Fig 3–3). Fermentation is an inefficient way to generate ATP, and consequently huge amounts of sugar must be fermented to satisfy the growth requirements of bacteria anaerobically. Large amounts of organic acids and alcohols are produced in fermentation. Which compounds are produced depends on the particular pathway of fermentation employed by a given species, and therefore the profile of fermentation products is a diagnostic aid in the clinical laboratory.

Respiration uses chain of electron carriers for which oxygen is usually but not always the terminal acceptor

Respiration involves fueling pathways in which substrate oxidation is coupled to the transport of electrons through a chain of carriers to some ultimate acceptor, which is frequently, but not always, molecular oxygen. Other inorganic (eg, nitrate) as well as organic compounds (eg, succinate) can serve as the final electron acceptor, and therefore many organisms that cannot ferment can live in the absence of oxygen (eg, *Pseudomonas aeruginosa* in the human colon).

Respiration is efficient energy producer

Respiration produces a proton-motive force that can generate ATP and power motility and active transport

Respiration is an efficient generator of ATP. Respiration in prokaryotes as in eukaryotes occurs by membrane-bound enzymes (quinones, cytochromes, and terminal oxidases), but in prokaryotes the cell membrane rather than mitochondrial membranes provide the physical site. The passage of electrons through the carriers is accompanied by the secretion from the cell of protons, generating an H^+ differential between the external surface of the cytosol membrane and the cell interior. This differential, called the **proton-motive force,** can then be used to (1) drive transport of solutes by the shock-insensitive systems of active transport (see above); (2) power the flagellar motors that rotate the filaments and result in cell motility in the case of motile species; and (3) generate ATP by coupling the phosphorylation of adenosine diphosphate (ADP) to the passage of protons inward through special channels in the cell membrane. The last pathway, facilitated by the enzyme anachronistically called **membrane ATPase,** can in fact function in either direction, coupling ADP phosphorylation to the inward passage of protons down the gradient or hydrolyzing ATP to accomplish the secretion of protons to establish a proton-motive force. The latter process explains how cells can generate a proton-motive force anaerobically (i.e., in the absence of electron transport).

In evolving to colonize every conceivable nook and cranny on this planet, bacteria have developed distinctive responses to oxygen. Bacteria are conveniently classified according to their fermentative and respiratory activities but much more generally by their overall response to the presence of oxygen. The response depends on their genetic ability to ferment or respire but also on their ability to protect themselves from the deleterious effects of oxygen.

Bacteria exhibit different characteristic responses to oxygen

Oxygen, though itself only mildly toxic, gives rise to at least two extremely reactive and toxic substances, **hydrogen peroxide** (H_2O_2) and the **superoxide anion** (O^{2-}). Peroxide is produced by reactions (catalyzed by flavoprotein oxidases) in which electrons and protons are transferred to O_2 as final acceptor. The superoxide radical is produced as an intermediate in most reactions that reduce molecular O_2. Superoxide is partially detoxified by an enzyme, **superoxide dismutase,** found in all organisms (prokaryotes and eukaryotes) that survive the presence of oxygen. Superoxide dismutase catalyzes the reaction

Aerobic metabolism produces peroxide and toxic oxygen radicals; aerobic growth is dependent on protective enzymes

Superoxide dismutase and peroxidase allow growth in air; their absence requires strict anaerobiosis

$$2O^{2-} + 2H^+ \rightarrow H_2O_2 + O_2.$$

Hydrogen peroxide is degraded by peroxidases by the reaction

$$H_2O_2 + H_2A \rightarrow 2H_2O + A$$

where A is any of a number of chemical groups (in the case in which H_2A is another molecule of H_2O_2, the reaction yields $2H_2O + O_2$, and the peroxidase is called catalase). Bacteria that lack the ability to make superoxide dismutase and catalase are exquisitely sensitive to the presence of molecular oxygen and, in general, must grow anaerobically using fermentation. Bacteria that possess these protective enzymes can grow in the presence of oxygen, but whether they use the oxygen in metabolism or not depends on their ability to respire. Whether these oxygen-resistant bacteria can grow anaerobically depends on their ability to ferment.

Organisms growing in air may or may not have a respiratory pathway

Various combinations of these two characteristics (oxygen resistance and the ability to use molecular oxygen as a final acceptor) are represented in different species of bacteria, resulting in the five general classes shown in Table 3–1. There are important pathogens within each class. Both the nature of the diseases they cause and the methods for cultivating and identifying these pathogens in the laboratory are dictated to a large extent by their response to oxygen. Many medically important bacteria classified as anaerobes (including those listed in Table 3–1) are in fact moderately aerotolerant, and may possess low levels of superoxide dismutases and peroxidases that provide some survival protection, if not the ability to grow.

Important pathogens are found among aerobes, anaerobes, facultatives, indifferents, and microaerophiles

Biosynthesis

Biosynthetic reactions form a network of pathways that lead from 12 precursor metabolites (provided by the fueling reactions) to the many amino acids, nucleotides, sugars, amino sugars, fatty acids, and other building blocks needed for macromolecules (see Fig 3–1). In addition to the carbon precursors, large quantities of reduced nicotinamide adenine dinucleotide phosphate (NADPH), ATP, amino nitrogen, and some source of sulfur are needed for biosynthesis of these building blocks. These pathways are similar in all species of living things, but bacterial species differ greatly as to which pathways they possess. Because all cells require the same building blocks, those that cannot be produced by a given cell must be obtained preformed from the environment. Nutritional requirements of bacteria, therefore, differ from species to species and serve as an important practical basis for laboratory identification.

Biosynthesis requires 12 precursor metabolites, energy, amino nitrogen, sulfur, and reducing power

Nutritional requirements differ depending on synthetic ability

Relatively few unique reactions in the domain of biosynthesis are present to form the basis for specific therapeutic attack on the microorganism rather than the host. The effectiveness of sulfonamides and trimethoprim is one of these exceptional situations; many

Only a few antimicrobics target biosynthetic processes

TABLE 3–1

Classification of Bacteria by Response to Oxygen

Type of Bacteria	Growth Response		Possession of Catalase and Superoxide Dismutase	Comment	Example
	Aerobic	Anaerobic			
Aerobe (strict aerobe)	+	–	+	Requires O_2; cannot ferment	*Mycobacterium tuberculosis* *Pseudomonas aeruginosa* *Bacillus subtilis*
Anaerobe (strict anaerobe)	–	+	–	Killed by O_2; ferments in absence of O_2	*Clostridium botulinum* *Bacteroides melaninogenicus*
Facultative	+	+	+	Respires with O_2; ferments in absence of O_2	*Escherichia coli* *Shigella dysenteriae* *Staphylococcus aureus*
Indifferent (aerotolerant anaerobe)	+	+	+	Ferments in presence or absence of O_2	*Streptococcus pneumoniae* *Streptococcus pyogenes*
Microaerophilic	(+)[a]	+	(+)[a]	Grows best at low O_2 concentration; can grow without O_2	*Campylobacter jejuni*

[a](+) indicates small amounts of growth or catalase and superoxide dismutase.

bacteria must synthesize folic acid rather than use it preformed from their environment, as human cells do, which renders these bacteria susceptible to agents that interfere with the biosynthesis of folic acid.

Polymerization Reactions

Unlike fueling and biosynthetic processes, polymerization reactions offer many targets for antimicrobic chemotherapy. The reason is simple: the bacterial machineries for replication, transcription, and translation differ from that in the human host cells.

Polymerization of DNA is called **replication.** From studies largely made in *E. coli,* DNA replication involves 12 or more proteins acting at a small number of sites (replication forks) where DNA is synthesized from activated building blocks (dATP, dGTP, dCTP, and TTP). Replication always begins at special sites on the chromosome called *oriC* in *E. coli* (for origin of replication) and then proceeds bidirectionally around the circular chromosome (Fig 3–4). Synthesis of DNA at each replication fork is termed **semiconservative** because each of the DNA chains serves as the template for the synthesis of its complement, and, therefore, one of the two chains of the new double-stranded molecule is conserved from the original chromosome. One of the two new strands must be synthesized in chemically the opposite direction of the other; this is accomplished by having each new strand made in short segments, 5′ to 3′, which are then ligated by one of the DNA-synthesizing enzymes (see Fig 3–4). Interestingly, an RNA primer is involved in getting each of these segments initiated. The two replication forks meet at the opposite side of the circle. The frequency of initiation of chromosome replication (and, therefore, the number of growing points) varies with cell growth rate; the chain elongation rate is rather constant at a given temperature independent of cell growth rate.

Bidirectional, semiconservative replication occurs at replication forks, involves RNA primers, and proceeds at a pace largely independent of growth rate

Some chemotherapeutic agents derive their selective toxicity for bacteria from the unique features of prokaryotic DNA replication. The synthetic quinolone compounds inhibit DNA gyrase, one of the many enzymes participating in DNA replication.

DNA gyrase inhibitors are selectively toxic for bacteria

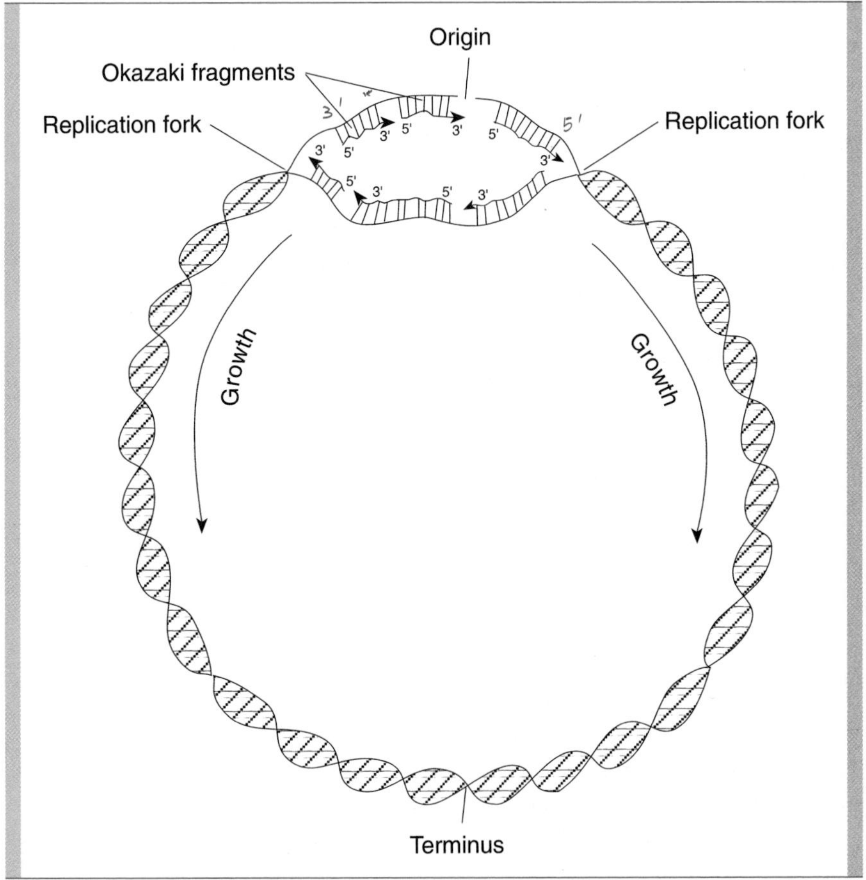

FIGURE 3–4
Schematic representation of DNA replication in bacteria. Shown is a portion of a replicating chromosome shortly after replication has begun at the origin. The newly polymerized strands of DNA are synthesized in the 5′ to 3′ direction (indicated by the arrows) using preexisting DNA strands as templates. The process creates two replication forks that travel in opposite directions until they meet on the opposite side of the chromosome.

A single RNA polymerase makes all forms of bacterial RNA

Transcription is the synthesis of RNA. Transcription in bacteria differs from that in eukaryotic cells in several ways. One difference is that all forms of bacterial RNA (mRNA, tRNA, and rRNA) are synthesized by the same enzyme, RNA polymerase. Like the several eukaryotic enzymes, the single bacterial RNA polymerase uses activated building blocks (ATP, GTP, CTP, and UTP) and synthesizes an RNA strand complementary to whichever strand of DNA is serving as template.

Bacterial mRNA needs no special transport to ribosomes

A second major difference is that bacterial mRNA need not be transported to the cytoplasm through a nuclear membrane, and hence no poly(A) cap is needed and no special means of transport exists. In fact, because each mRNA strand is directly accessible to ribosomes, binding of the latter to mRNA to form polysomes begins at an early stage in the synthesis of each mRNA molecule (Fig 3–5).

Bacteria constantly turn over their complement of mRNA

A third remarkable difference is that bacterial mRNA is synthesized, used, and degraded all in a matter of a few minutes. Although most bacteria have some long-lived species of mRNA, it is characteristic of bacterial cells to "wipe their [transcript] plate clean" every few minutes and make whatever new transcripts are called for by sensing the cell's environment.

σ Subunit recognizes promoters

RNA polymerase is a large, complicated molecule with a subunit structure of $\alpha 2\beta\beta'\sigma$. The σ subunit is the one that locates specific DNA sequences, called promoters, which precede all transcriptional units. More than one σ subunit, each designed to recognize a different set of related promoters, can associate with RNA polymerase, which provides a simple means to activate groups of related genes that cooperate in such cellular

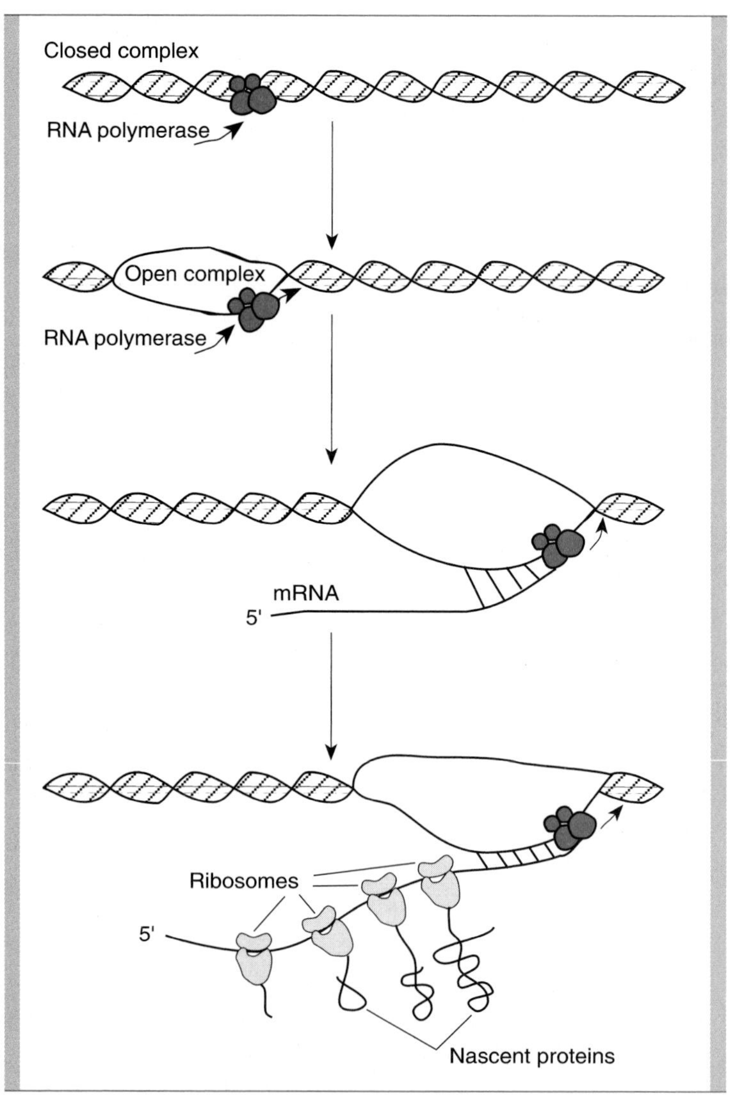

FIGURE 3–5
Schematic representation of the coupling of transcription and translation in bacteria.

processes as sporulation, nitrogen acquisition, heat shock stress response, and adaptation to nongrowth conditions.

As in eukaryotic cells, all stable RNA molecules are made from large precursor molecules that must be processed by nucleases and then extensively modified to produce the mature product (the tRNAs and rRNAs).

Bacterial RNA polymerase is the target of the **rifamycin** series of antimicrobics (including the semisynthetic compound **rifampin**). They block initiation of transcription. Other substances of biological origin block extension of RNA chains or inhibit transcription by binding to DNA. They have been of great value in molecular biological studies but are also toxic to human cells and thus are not used in human therapy.

Rifampin inhibits RNA polymerase

Translation is the name given to protein synthesis. Many antimicrobics derive their selective toxicity for bacteria from the unique features of the prokaryotic translation apparatus. In fact, protein synthesis is the target of a greater variety of antimicrobics than is any other metabolic process (see Chapter 13). Some agents inhibit the ribosomal large subunit (eg, **chloramphenicol** and **macrolides**), some the small subunit (eg, **tetracyclines** and **aminoglycosides**), and some aminoglycosides bind to both large and small subunits.

Many antibiotics act on bacterial translation machinery

Bacteria activate the 20-amino-acid building blocks of protein in the course of attaching them to specific transfer RNA molecules. The aminoacyl-tRNAs are brought to the ribosomes by soluble protein factors, and there the amino acids are polymerized into polypeptide chains according to the sequence of codons in the particular mRNA that is being translated. Having donated its amino acid, the tRNA is released from the ribosome to return for another aminoacylation cycle.

Amino acid residues are polymerized from specific tRNAs at the direction of mRNA

This description fits translation in eukaryotic as well as prokaryotic cells, but major differences do exist. The initiation of translation of a new polypeptide chain requires fewer proteins in bacteria. The ribosomes of bacteria are smaller and simpler in structure. Bacterial mRNA is largely polycistronic, that is, each mRNA molecule is the transcript of more than one gene (cistron) and therefore directs the synthesis of more than one polypeptide. No processing or transport of the mRNA is necessary. RNA polymerase makes mRNA at about 55 nucleotides per second (at 37°C), and ribosomes make polypeptide chains at about 18 amino acids per second. Therefore, not only does translation of each mRNA molecule occur simultaneously with transcription, but it occurs at the same linear rate (55 nucleotides per second/3 nucleotides per codon = 18 amino acids per second). This means that ribosomes are traveling along each mRNA molecule as fast as RNA polymerase makes it. This coupling plays a role in several aspects of regulation of gene expression unique to bacteria.

mRNA is polycistronic and requires no processing or transport

Translation of mRNA occurs simultaneously with transcription

These special features of translation in bacteria contribute to the streamlined efficiency of the process. The bacterial cytosol is packed with polyribosomes. Each ribosome functions near its maximal rate. Therefore, the faster the growth rate of the cell, the more ribosomes are needed for protein production. It can be estimated that during growth in rich media, more than half the mass of the *E. coli* cell consists of ribosomes and other parts of the translation machinery.

Bacteria synthesize proteins rapidly and efficiently

Other polymerization reactions involve synthesis of peptidoglycan, phospholipid, LPS, and capsular polysaccharide. All of these reactions involve activated building blocks that are polymerized or assembled within or on the exterior surface of the cytoplasmic membrane.

The entire process of synthesizing **peptidoglycan (murein),** which is completely absent from eukaryotic cells, offers many vulnerable attack points for antibiotics and other chemotherapeutic agents. Some of these are shown in Figure 3–6; others are described more fully in Chapter 13.

Uniqueness of wall offers many targets for antimicrobics

The synthesis of murein occurs in three compartments of the cell (see Fig 3–6).

1. In the cytosol a series of reactions leads to the synthesis, on a nucleotide carrier (UDP), of an *N*-acetylmuramic acid (NAM) residue bearing a pentapeptide (the tetrapeptide found in mature murein plus an additional terminal D-alanine).

NAM and attached peptide are synthesized in cytosol

2. This precursor is then attached, with the release of UMP, to a special, lipid-like carrier in the cell membrane called **bactoprenol** (or **undecaprenol**). Within the cell membrane *N*-acetylglucosamine (NAG) is added to the precursor, along with any amino

Precursor is added to bactoprenol carrier, and NAG and bridge amino acids are added in membrane

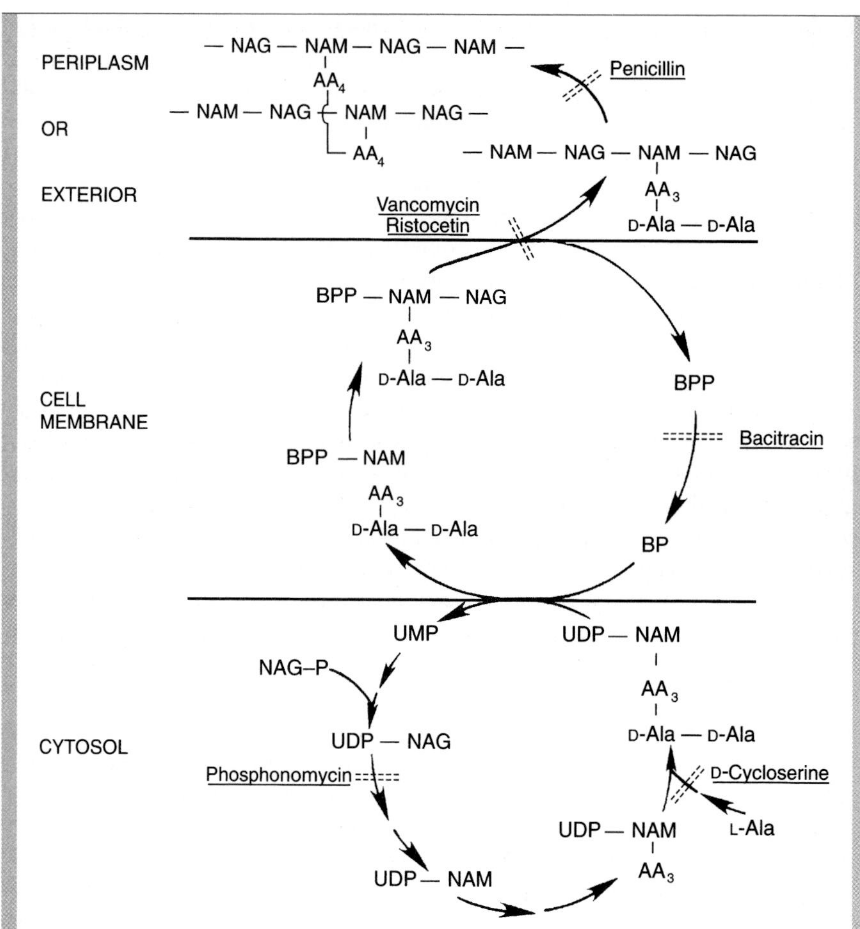

FIGURE 3–6
Schematic representation of murein synthesis with sites of action of some antibiotics. NAG, *N*-acetylglucosamine; NAM, *N*-acetylmuramic acid; BP and BPP, bactoprenol phosphate and bactoprenol pyrophosphate, respectively; AA_3, tripeptide residue that in *Escherichia coli* is L-alanyl-D-glutamyl-*m*-diaminopimelic acid; D-Ala and L-Ala, D-alanine and L-alanine, respectively; UMP and UDP, uridine mono- and diphosphate, respectively. Some of the arrows represent more than one chemical reaction. See the text for a description of this process.

acids that in this particular species will form the bridge between adjacent tetrapeptides. **Bacitracin** and **vancomycin** interfere with the function of bactoprenol as a carrier in polymerization and assembly reactions.

Glycan polymer and peptide cross-links are formed in periplasm or wall

PBPs are involved in assembly, expansion, and shaping of murein

3. Outside the cell membrane (in the periplasm of Gram-negative cells and the wall of Gram-positive cells), this disaccharide subunit is attached to the end of a growing glycan chain, and then cross-links between chains are formed by a transpeptidization using the energy transduced by the release of the terminal D-alanine—the extra amino acid on the tetrapeptide. Eventually, release from the carrier occurs. These transpeptidases, called **penicillin-binding proteins** (PBPs) for their property of combining with this antibiotic, are involved in forging, breaking, and reforging the peptide cross-links between glycan chains. This dynamic process is necessary to permit expansion of the murein sac during cellular growth, to shape the envelope, and to prepare for cell division. It is this process that goes awry in the presence of penicillin and related antimicrobics, the action of which can be broadly stated as preventing formation of stabilizing peptide cross-links.

Assembly Reactions and Protein Translocation

Guided assembly involves transport of components within cell

Self-assembly (eg, of ribosomes) can be mimicked in vitro

Assembly of cell structures occurs both by spontaneous aggregation (**self-assembly**) and by special, specific mechanisms (**guided assembly**). Some macromolecules are made at the sites of assembly (such as LPS in the outer membrane), and others must be transported to them (porin is made in the cytosol but ends up in the outer membrane). Self-assembly is illustrated by two cell structures that spontaneously assemble in a test tube from their component macromolecules: flagella and ribosomes. Important parts of envelope assembly include special mechanisms for the secretion of proteins, the use of

Bayer's zones of adhesion (see Chapter 2, Fig 2–9) to form the phospholipid/protein leaflets of the membranes, and the use of carrier molecules (eg, bactoprenol) to transport hydrophilic compounds within the lipid portions of the membrane.

Translocation of Proteins

A problem is posed by the difficulty of moving macromolecules out of the cell interior and into their proper place in the wall, outer membrane, and capsule. Proteins in their natural folded state present a hydrophilic surface that cannot be pushed through phospholipid membranes. These proteins may be part of the cell's assembly process, and are destined to reside within the membrane or wall of the cell, or in the case of Gram-negative cells to reside finally in either the periplasm or outer membrane. Moreover, many proteins are translocated through all layers of the cell envelope to the exterior environment. **Protein secretion** has become the general term to designate all these instances of translocation of proteins out of the cytosol (ie, whether the protein is to leave the cell or become part of the envelope), recognizing that all these events share the problem of passing a protein between hydrophilic and hydrophobic phases. An understanding of this complex process is beginning, and it turns out to have great relevance to bacterial virulence. Approximately 20% of the proteins of *E. coli* are estimated to reside in the envelope. Furthermore, many bacterial virulence factors are located on the surface of the cell, poised to interact with the cells and fluids of the mammalian host. Studies with *E. coli* and many other Gram-negative as well as Gram-positive bacteria have revealed a surprising number of mechanisms for protein translocation.

Proteins do not readily pass through membranes

Special mechanisms exist for protein translocation

Proteins destined for the wall, membranes, or periplasm are translocated by a **general secretory pathway (GSP),** which consists of cytosolic chaperones and an integral membrane **translocase** consisting of several proteins operating cooperatively. The role of the chaperones is to present the protein to be exported to the translocase, at which a special ATPase **"pusher"** is thought to physically drive the proteins through the membrane. Proteins of the GSP are products of what are called *sec* (secretory) genes, and the GSP is therefore also called the **Sec** pathway. Many, but not all, exported proteins are recognized by having a special **signal sequence** at their N-terminus; this peptide is cleaved off during translocation through the membrane by a **signal peptidase.** The translocation of some proteins occurs cotranslationally (ie, during their synthesis on a ribosome) before the polypeptide has a chance to fold. For some of these, the nascent polypeptide–ribosome complex is docked to the membrane by a **signal recognition particle,** similar to that in mammalian cells, consisting of a protein (Ffh) and a 4.5S RNA. For others, translocation occurs posttranslationally; the protein is completed and then may be escorted to the translocase by chaperone proteins. Some of these general aspects of protein translocation are shown in Figure 3–7.

The GSP or Sec system handles most protein translocation for cell assembly

Many components are products of *sec* genes

Chaperones, translocase proteins, and signal peptidase form the GSP

Many proteins are marked for translocation by being made with a signal sequence

Export of Proteins

In many cases, proteins are translocated completely through the entire envelope and into the surrounding media or tissue, or even directly into host cells. Secretion of toxins and other proteins contributes greatly to bacterial virulence, and occurs by several pathways, only some of which utilize components of the GSP. In Gram-negative species, secretion must translocate a protein across two membranes. In Gram-positive species, secretion is less complex and usually involves proteins marked by a signal sequence interacting with chaperones and translocases with general similarity to those of the GSP. Five pathways have been discovered in different Gram-negative pathogens that accomplish export of proteins into the environment (Fig 3–8). These pathways are important because many of the secreted proteins are toxins or other virulence factors.

Secretion is more complex in Gram-negative than Gram-positive cells

Type I secretion systems are Sec-independent (do not use the GSP), and consist of three proteins that form a transmembrane channel through which the secreted protein moves, driven by one of the proteins, an ATP-binding cassette (**ABC**) **transporter;** hence, these systems are sometimes called simply **ABC transporters.** In a single step,

Type I secretion is by relatively simple ABC transporter systems independent of the Sec system

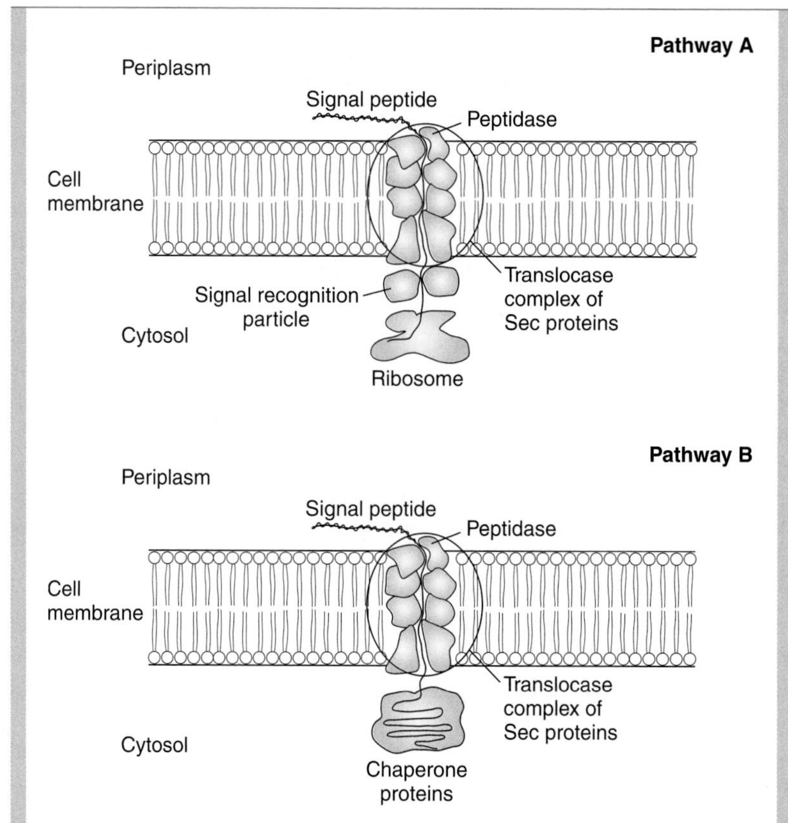

FIGURE 3–7
Translocation of proteins using the general secretory pathway (GSP). Pathway A depicts a protein being cotranslationally translocated, with the ribosome/polypeptide complex docked to the membrane by a signal recognition particle. Pathway B depicts a protein being posttranslationally translocated after protection in the cytosol by chaperone proteins.

the secreted protein, which normally lacks a classical signal sequence, passes from the cytosol to the external environment. The *E. coli* hemolysin is secreted in this manner.

Type II secretion is called two-step secretion; the first step occurs by GSP

Type II secretion systems, on the other hand, are Sec-dependent and use the traditional GSP to move a protein into the periplasm, but then in a second step, approximately 14 accessory protein molecules move the secreted protein across the outer membrane. This process is called **two-step secretion**. Like the type I systems, type II systems include an ATP-binding protein but also a peptidase to cleave a signal sequence from the secreted proteins, all of which have a signal sequence. These systems are common in such Gram-negative bacteria as *Klebsiella oxytoca, Vibrio cholerae, Pseudomonas aeruginosa,* and *E. coli*.

Type III secretion is called contact-dependent secretion and is Sec-independent

Type III secretion injects virulence proteins directly into human cells on contact

Type III systems, which are responsible for the secretion of many virulence factors in *Yersinia, Salmonella, Shigella,* and *Pseudomonas* species, involve as many as 20 protein components. One component is a chaperone specific for the given protein to be secreted, and another is an ATP-binding protein thought to energize the system. Type III systems are attracting intense study because they are responsible for **contact-dependent secretion,** in which secretion of virulence proteins is activated by contact with mammalian host cells, resulting in the direct injection of the secreted protein into the cytoplasm of the mammalian cell. Type III systems are Sec-independent.

Type IV secretion adapts a DNA-transfer system to proteins

Type IV systems are referred to as **conjugal transfer systems** because they were originally discovered as pathways by which DNA is conjugally transferred between bacterial cells or between a bacterial and a eukaryotic cell. They are used by the plant pathogen *Agrobacterium tumefaciens* to transfer oncogenic DNA and protein into plants, and a similar system is used by *Bordetella pertussis* to export pertussis (whooping cough) toxin. Genes similar to those responsible for this type of secretion in these organisms are found in the pathogenicity island of *Helicobacter pylori* and in *Legionella pneumophila*. Currently it is unclear whether the protein secretion by these systems requires the Sec machinery.

Type V secretion uses GSP for the first step; protein to be secreted accomplishes the second step

Type V secretion systems are two-step, Sec-dependent pathways. No helper protein is needed for translocation through the outer membrane; the transported protein itself accomplishes this feat. Hence, these systems are referred to as **autotransporters.** One

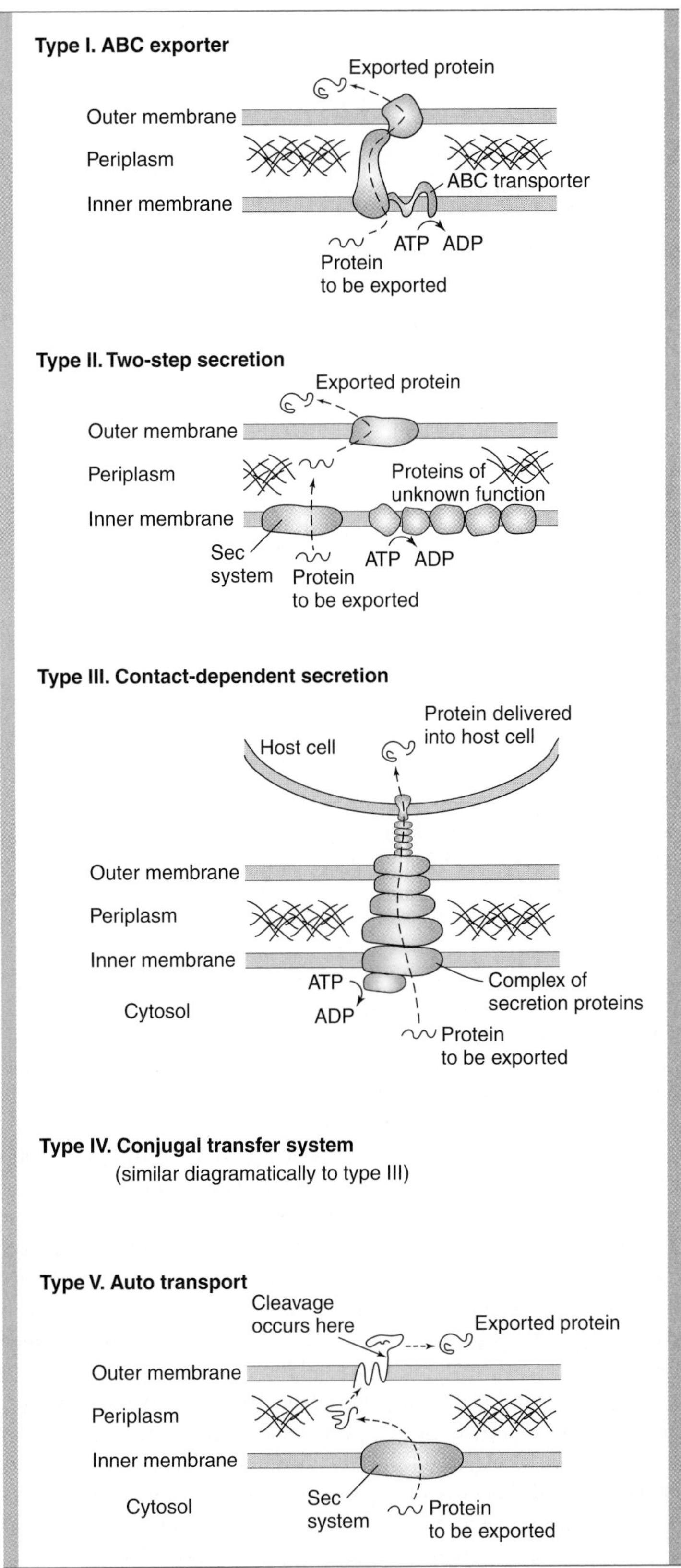

FIGURE 3–8
Simplified schematic diagrams that compare the main features of protein export by the five known pathways. (*Adapted from Harper JR, Silhavy TJ. Germ warfare: The mechanisms of virulence factor delivery. In: EA Groisman,* Principles of Bacterial Pathogenesis, *San Diego, CA: Academic Press; 2001, pp 43–74.*)

domain of the protein forms a channel in the outer membrane for the rest of the protein and then is cleaved off. These are the simplest of the Sec-dependent systems. A serine protease from *Serratia marcescens,* the important IgA proteases of *Haemophilus influenzae* and *Neisseria gonorrhoeae,* and the vacuolating cytotoxin VacA from *H. pylori* are each secreted as autotransporters.

Bacterial secretion and export offer potential targets for future design of chemotherapeutic agents.

Cell Division

Many genes are involved in cell division

Multiple replication forks allow faster cell division than chromosome replication

Bacteria multiply by binary fission. More than 30 genes in *E. coli* are known to be involved in the process that involves the polar separation of the daughter chromosomes, the formation of the cross-wall and envelope at the point of cell division, and ultimately the separation of the two newly formed cells. In rich medium at 37°C, the entire process is completed in 20 minutes in *E. coli* and many other pathogenic species. The most astounding aspect of this feat is that the replication of the chromosome in these cells takes approximately 40 minutes, largely independently of the nature of the medium. The trick of dividing faster than the chromosome can replicate is accomplished by a mechanism that triggers the start of a new round of replication before an earlier one has been completed. In other words, during rapid growth multiple pairs of replication forks are at work on a given chromosome, and a newborn cell inherits chromosomes that have already been partially replicated. Bacteria maintain a constant cell mass:DNA ratio, and because rapidly growing cells have extra DNA (due to the multiple replication forks), cell size obviously is related to growth rate; the faster bacteria grow, the larger is their average size.

Anucleate cells are produced unless division and replication are coordinated

Cell division must be precisely coordinated with the completion of a round of DNA replication, or nonviable offspring will be produced. This coordination does not just happen; it requires a special regulatory system. Mutants are known that are defective in this regulation; in some of them, cell division without chromosome replication and segregation leads to the formation of **minicells,** which are complete cells save for lacking DNA.

Division and morphology are distorted by many antimicrobics

The complexity of cell division would lead one to expect that it might be easily disrupted by chemotherapeutic agents, and this is the case. Nonlethal concentrations of antimicrobics that act, even indirectly, on the polymerization or assembly reactions of the cell wall cause the formation of bizarre and distorted cells. Long filaments can result from incomplete cell division in the case of rod-shaped bacteria such as *E. coli.* Such forms are frequently encountered in direct examination of specimens from patients treated with antimicrobics.

GROWTH OF BACTERIAL CULTURES

Pure cultures are produced by inoculating media with genetically identical cells

Growth on agar media yields visible colonies, each of which is a clone of cells if derived from a single cell

Colony size, form, and consistency are distinguishing features

Solutions of nutrients that support the growth of bacteria are called **media** (singular, **medium**), which can be solidified by the incorporation of agar. The introduction of live cells into liquid sterile media or onto the surface of solidified media is called **inoculation.** A population of bacterial cells is referred to as a **culture.** If the population is genetically homogeneous (ie, if all cells belong to the same strain of the same species), it is called a **pure culture.** Study of bacteria usually requires pure cultures, which can be obtained in several ways. The most common is to spread a very dilute suspension of a mixed culture on the surface of medium solidified with agar. Growth of individual cells deposited across the surface of solidified medium leads to visible mounds of bacterial mass called **colonies.** The cells in a colony are usually descended from a single original cell and, in this case, constitute a **clone.** There is little difference between a pure culture and a clone, except that a pure culture may have been produced by the original inoculation of several identical cells. Colonies of different species and strains show marked differences in size, form, and consistency resulting from differences in growth rates, surface properties of the organisms, and their response to the gradients of nutrients and metabolites that develop within the colony as it enlarges. This facilitates subculturing to pure cultures. The diagnostic application of these techniques is discussed in Chapter 15.

Growth of a liquid culture can be monitored by colony counts or turbidimetrically

Growth of a liquid bacterial culture can be monitored by removing samples at timed intervals and placing suitable dilutions in or on solidified medium to obtain a count of the number of colonies that develop. The count can be directly extrapolated to the number of viable units in the original sample (which, because certain bacteria clump or form chains, may not represent the number of bacterial cells). Growth can also be measured by determining the number of **total cells** in each sample. Direct count with a microscope is simple but tedious; more sensitive and accurate counts can be made with the aid of an electronic particle counter. More often, the turbidity of the culture is measured, because bacterial cultures above approximately 10^6 cells/mL are visibly turbid, and turbidity is proportional to the total mass of bacterial protoplasm present per milliliter. Turbidity is quickly and easily measured by means of a spectrophotometer.

The growth rate of a bacterial culture depends on three factors: the species of bacterium, the chemical composition of the medium, and the temperature. The time needed for a culture to double its mass or cell number is in the range of 30 to 60 minutes for most pathogenic bacteria in rich media. Some species can double in 20 minutes (*E. coli* and related organisms), and some (eg, some mycobacteria) take almost as long as mammalian cells, 20 hours. In general, the greater the variety of nutrients provided in the medium, the faster growth occurs. This superficially simple fact actually depends on the operation of metabolic regulatory devices of considerable sophistication, which, as we shall see in the next section, ensures that building blocks provided in the environment not be wastefully synthesized by the cells. For each bacterial species, there is a characteristic optimum temperature for growth, and a range, sometimes as broad as 40°, within which growth is possible. Most pathogens of warm-blooded creatures have a temperature optimum for growth near normal body temperature, 37°C; growth often occurs at room temperature, but slowly. Therefore, incubators set at 35 to 37°C are used for culture of most clinical specimens. Exceptions to this rule include some organisms causing superficial infections for which 30°C is more suitable. As a group, bacteria have the widest span of possible growth temperatures, extending over the entire range of liquid water, 0°C to 100°C. Bacteria that grow best at refrigerator temperatures are called **psychrophiles,** those that grow above 50°C are called **thermophiles;** in between are the **mesophiles,** including virtually all pathogens.

Some species can divide every 20 minutes, others much more slowly

Growth rate is dependent on nutrient availability, pH, and temperature

Pathogens are mesophiles

When first inoculated, liquid cultures of bacteria characteristically exhibit a **lag period** during which growth is not detectable. This is the first phase of what is called the **culture growth cycle** (Fig 3–9). During this lag, the cells are actually quite active in adjusting the levels of vital cellular constituents necessary for growth in the new medium. Eventually net growth can be detected, and after a brief period of **accelerating growth,** the culture enters a phase of constant, maximal growth rate, called the **exponential** or **logarithmic phase** of growth, during which the generation time is constant. During this phase, cell number, and total cell mass, and amount of any given component of the cells increase at the same exponential rate; such growth is called **balanced growth,** or **steady-state growth.** The full reproductive potential of bacteria is exhibited during this phase: one cell gives rise to 2 cells in 1 generation, to 8 cells after 3 generations, to 1024 cells after 10 generations, and to about 1 million cells in 20 generations. For a bacterial species

Following a lag period, liquid cultures exhibit exponential growth during which generation time is constant and reproductive capacity enormous

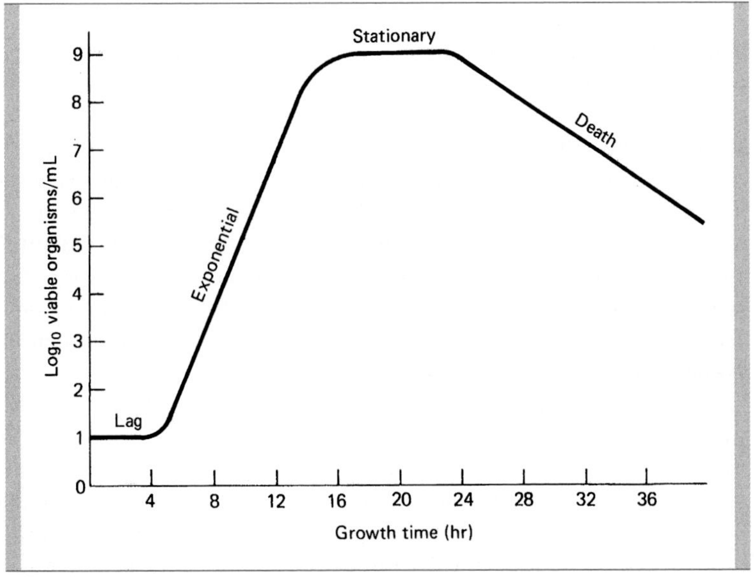

FIGURE 3–9
Phases of bacterial growth in liquid medium.

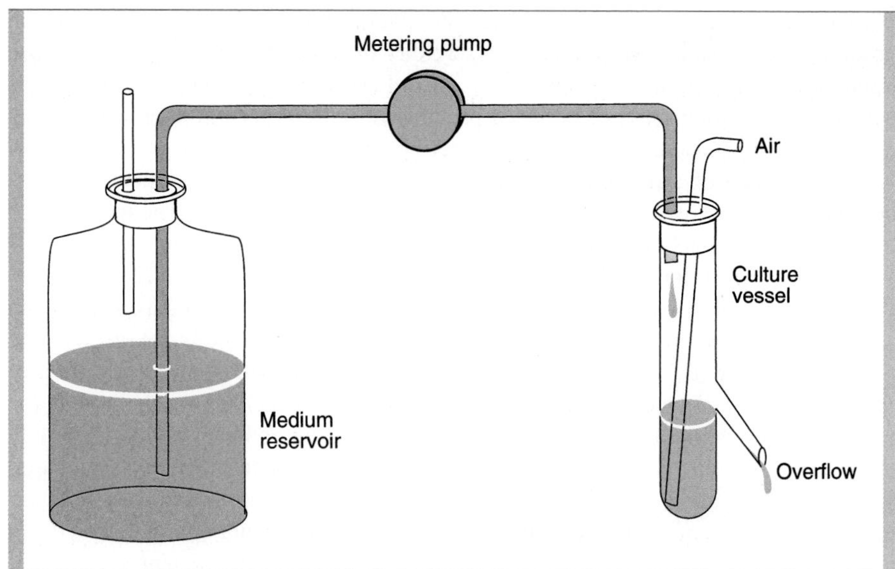

FIGURE 3–10
Schematic diagram of a chemostat. This continuous-culture device consists of a constant-volume growth chamber into which fresh sterile medium is fed at a constant rate by a pump.

with a generation time of 20 minutes, therefore, it takes less than 7 hours in the exponential phase of growth to produce a million cells from one.

Nutrient depletion or waste product accumulation terminates exponential growth

Cultures of some species die slowly after the stationary phase

By use of an equation for exponential growth, it can be demonstrated that 2 days of growth at this rate would be sufficient to generate a mass of bacteria equal to 500 times the mass of the earth. Fortunately, this never occurs, but not because the equation is faulty. Constant growth rate requires that there be no change in the supply of nutrients or the concentration of toxic by-products of metabolism (such as organic acids). This constancy can exist for only a short time (hours) in an ordinary culture vessel. Then growth becomes progressively limited (**decelerating phase**) and eventually stops (**stationary phase**). Cells in the stationary phase are different from those in the exponential phase. They are smaller, have a different complement of enzymes (to deal with survival during starvation), and have fewer ribosomes per unit mass. When an inoculum of such cells is placed into fresh medium, exponential growth cannot resume immediately, and hence the lag period is observed. Note that there is no lag phase if the inoculum consists of exponential-phase cells. Prolonged incubation of a stationary-phase culture leads to cell death for many bacterial species (such as the pneumococcus), although many (such as *E. coli*) are hardy enough to remain viable for days. During the **death phase** or **decline** of a culture, cell viability is lost by exponential kinetics as described in Chapter 11. As already noted, for those Gram-positive species that can sporulate, entry into the stationary phase usually triggers this event.

Continuous exponential growth can be maintained in a chemostat or a turbidostat

One way to maintain a culture in exponential, steady-state (balanced) growth for long periods is to use a device in which fresh medium is continuously added but the total volume of culture is held constant by an overflow tube. One such constant-volume device is called a **chemostat;** it operates by infusing fresh medium containing a limiting nutrient at a constant rate, and the growth rate of the cells is set by the flow rate (Fig 3–10). A similar constant-volume device is the **turbidostat;** it operates by the infusion of fresh medium by a pump controlled indirectly by the turbidity of the culture. Although such devices may sound artificial, they mimic many situations of interest to medical microbiologists. Most of the places in which bacteria live on and within our bodies, in health and disease, provide conditions more closely resembling those of nutrient-limited continuous-culture devices than of enclosed flasks.

BIOFILMS

Except for growth as colonies on agar-solidified media, bacterial cultures grown in a laboratory are smooth suspensions of individual cells dispersed in a liquid medium (see Chapter 15). In nature, whether in soil, in marine or riparian environments, or on the surface of physical agents, including medical prosthetic devices, bacteria grow as aggregated assemblies of cells. These **biofilms** frequently develop a multicellular arrangement that excludes antimicrobics and other toxic molecules and enhances the ability of the bacteria to capture nutrients. The full extent to which this phenomenon is related to infectious disease remains to be determined, but it is clear that adherence to cell and tissue surfaces is an attribute of most pathogens.

REGULATION AND ADAPTATION

Metabolic reactions must proceed in a coordinated fashion. It would not do to have them governed solely by the laws of "mass action" by which the concentrations of reactants and products determine the rate of reactions. Furthermore, it would not do to have rates of individual reactions set at some fixed levels. Bacteria can do little to control their environment, and any change in environment (eg, in temperature, pH, nutrient availability, osmolarity) would disrupt any preset synchronization or render it inappropriate. Bacteria must, therefore, not just coordinate reactions, but must do so in a flexible, adjustable manner to make growth possible in a changing environment. They accomplish this feat by many regulatory mechanisms, some of which operate to control **enzyme activity,** some to control **gene expression.**

Flexible coordination of metabolic reactions occurs by regulating both enzyme activity and gene expression

Control of Enzyme Activity

Although there are many examples of covalent modification of enzymes (eg, by phosphorylation, methylation, or acylation) to alter their activity, by far the most prevalent means by which bacterial cells modulate the flow of material through fueling and biosynthetic pathways is by changing the activity of **allosteric enzymes** through the reversible binding of low-molecular-weight metabolites **(ligands).** In fueling pathways it is common for AMP, ADP, and ATP to control the activity of enzymes by causing conformational changes of allosteric enzymes, usually located at critical branch points where pathways intersect. By this means, the flow of carbon from the major substrates through the various pathways is adjusted to be appropriate to the demands of biosynthesis. For example, the **energy charge** of the cell, defined as (ATP + 1/2 ADP)/(ATP + ADP + AMP), is kept very close to 0.85 under all conditions of growth and nongrowth. In biosynthetic pathways, it is common for the end product of the pathway to control the activity of the first enzyme in the pathway. This pattern, called **feedback inhibition** or **end-product inhibition,** ensures that each building block is made at exactly the rate it is being used for polymerization. It also ensures that building blocks supplied in the medium are not wastefully duplicated by synthesis. Because many biosynthetic pathways are branched and have multiple end products, special arrangements must be made to produce effective regulation. These include the production of multiple isofunctional enzymes for the controlled step, the design of allosteric enzymes that require the cumulative effect of all end products to be completely inhibited, and sequential inhibition of each subpathway by its last product (Fig 3–11).

Most metabolic pathways are controlled by allosteric enzymes

Fueling pathway enzymes are controlled by AMP, ADP, and ATP concentrations to maintain energy charge

Feedback inhibition controls biosynthetic pathways for both economy and efficiency

Control of Gene Expression

To a far greater extent than eukaryotic cells, bacteria regulate their metabolism by changing the amounts of different enzymes. This is accomplished chiefly by governing their rates of synthesis, that is, by controlling gene expression. This works rapidly for bacteria because of their speed of growth; shutting off the synthesis of a particular enzyme results in short order in the reduction of its cellular level due to dilution by the growth of the cell. Most importantly, bacterial mRNA is degraded rapidly. With an average half-life of 2 to 3 minutes at 37°C, the mRNA complement of the cell can be totally changed in a small fraction of a generation time. The synthesis of a given enzyme can therefore be rapidly turned on and just as rapidly turned off simply by changes in the rate of transcription of its gene.

Changes in transcription can rapidly change enzyme synthesis because of mRNA degradation

Most, although not all, of the regulation of gene expression occurs at or near the beginning of the process: the initiation of transcription. That is, gene expression is not

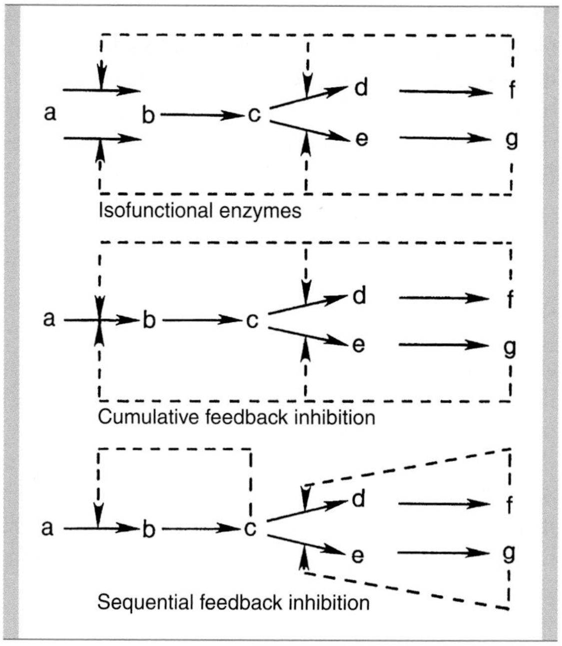

FIGURE 3–11
Patterns of end-product inhibition in branched biosynthesis pathways.

Much regulation operates at initiation of transcription

regulated by changing the rate of mRNA chain elongation; once started, transcription proceeds at a more or less constant rate. Regulation occurs by a decision of whether to initiate or not, or what amounts to the same thing, by setting the frequency of initiation.

Bacterial genes are organized as transcriptional units called operons, each of which contains one or more cistrons that encode polypeptides

A closer look at transcription is necessary to understand how it is controlled. Most of the genes we know about in bacteria are organized as **multicistronic operons.** A **cistron** is a segment of DNA encoding a polypeptide. An **operon** is the unit of transcription; the cistrons that it comprises are cotranscribed as a single mRNA. The structure of a typical operon (Fig 3–12) consists of a **promoter** region, an **operator** region, component cistrons, and a **terminator.** In the best-studied bacterium, *E. coli,* RNA polymerase, programmed by the major replaceable σ subunit, σ-70, recognizes the promoter region and binds to the DNA. Initially the binding is a closed complex, but this can be converted into an open complex in which the two strands of DNA are partially separated. Strand separation exposes the nucleotide bases and permits initiation of synthesis of a mRNA strand complementary to the sense strand of the DNA. In a simple case, transcription continues through the cistrons of the operon until the termination signal is reached. In some cases recognition of the termination signal requires another removable subunit of RNA polymerase, ρ. This process is shown in Figure 3–12.

RNA polymerase binds to the promoter of an operon and transcribes until it meets the terminator

Near the promoter in many operons is an operator to which a specific **regulator protein** or **transcription factor** can bind. In some cases the binding of this regulator blocks initiation; in such a case of negative control, the regulator is called a **repressor.** Repressors are allosteric proteins, and their binding to the operator depends on their conformation, which is determined by the binding of ligands that are called **corepressors** if their action permits binding of the repressor and **inducers** if their action prevents binding. In some cases, the regulator protein is required for initiation of transcription, and it is then called an **activator.** The functioning of both types of regulator proteins on transcription initiation is illustrated in Figure 3–13 using the regulation of the *lac* operon as an example. This operon encodes proteins necessary for the use of lactose as a carbon and energy source.

Activator and repressor proteins regulate transcription by binding to the operator region of operons

Some regulator proteins bend DNA on binding, and this can bring together what would otherwise be distant sites of the DNA. In this manner, proteins bound at sites called **enhancers** far upstream or downstream of a promoter can be brought into physical contact with RNA polymerase and influence its activity. One such DNA bender in ***E. coli*** is called the **integration host factor.**

Some proteins regulate transcription by binding to enhancers and bending DNA

Many regulator proteins are converted from inactive to active forms by covalent modification rather than by the allosteric binding of a ligand. Phosphorylation is by far the

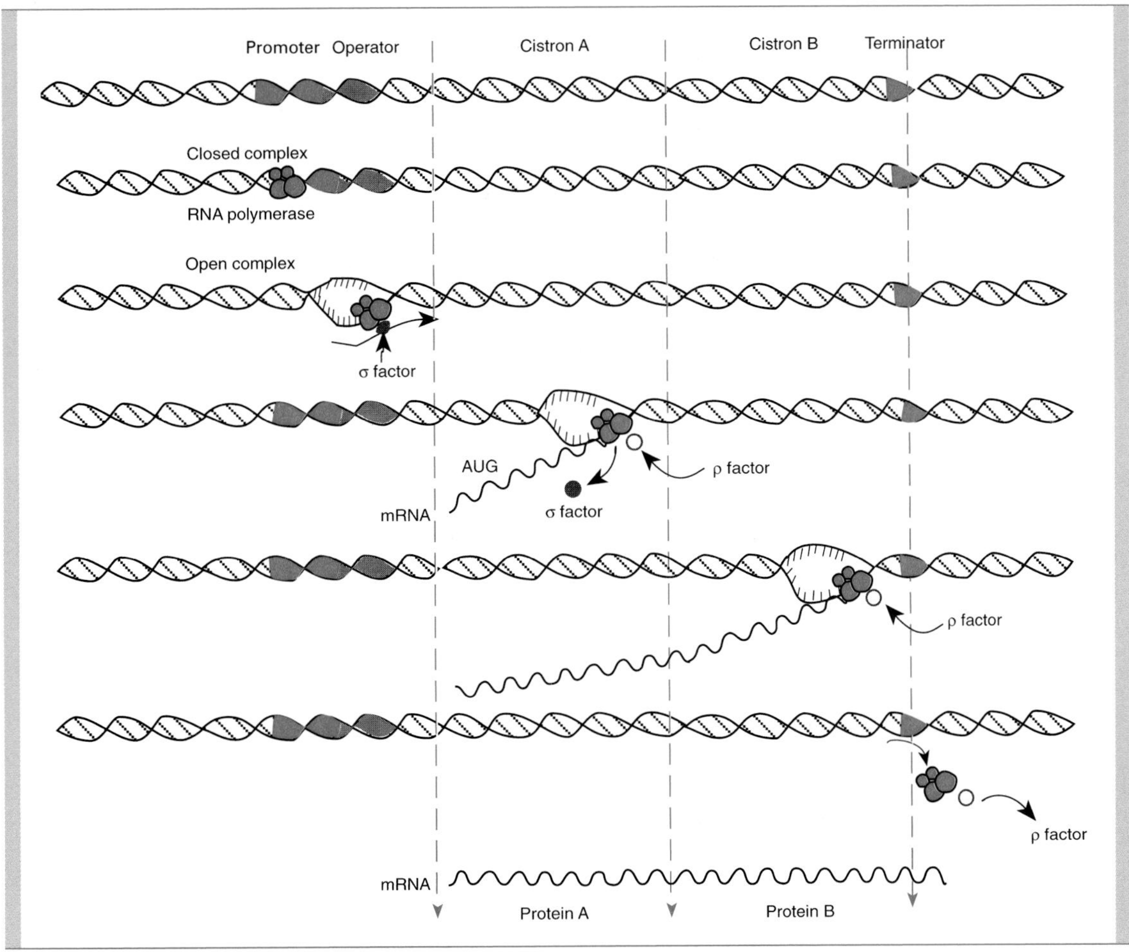

FIGURE 3–12
Control of transcription. Schematic representation of a bacterial operon and its transcription by RNA polymerase.

most common modifying event and operates in the widespread two-component **signal transduction** pathways described below under cell stress regulons.

Some regulators are controlled by phosphorylation

Once transcription is initiated it may continue uneventfully, but in some operons another site of control is quickly encountered. After transcription of a **leader region,** the RNA polymerase encounters a region known as an **attenuator.** Synthesis of mRNA is aborted at the attenuator; only a small percentage of the RNA polymerase molecules reaching the attenuator can successfully pass through it. However, the activity of the attenuator can be modified by a process that involves not a regulator protein but rather changes in the secondary structure of the mRNA. This regulatory process is illustrated in Figure 3–14 using the *his* operon, which encodes the enzymes necessary for the biosynthesis of the amino acid L-histidine, as an example. In enteric bacteria, attenuation is a common means of controlling biosynthetic operons. Note that it differs from the repression mechanism in that it requires no special regulatory gene or regulatory proteins.

Attenuation regulates some biosynthetic operons by controlling abortion of transcription early in the operon

There are many instances known in which groups of genes that are independently controlled as members of different operons must cooperate to accomplish some response to an environmental change. When such a group of genes is subject to the control of a common regulator, the group is called a **regulon.** One such regulon, or **global control system,** is catabolite repression. Its function is to prevent the cell from responding to the presence of alternative carbon sources when the environment already provides a more than adequate supply from the preferred substrate, glucose. This control is brought about as follows. Operons that encode catabolic enzymes (those responsible for initiating the use of carbon sources, such as lactose, maltose, arabinose, and other sugars and amino

Regulons are groups of unlinked operons controlled by a common regulator

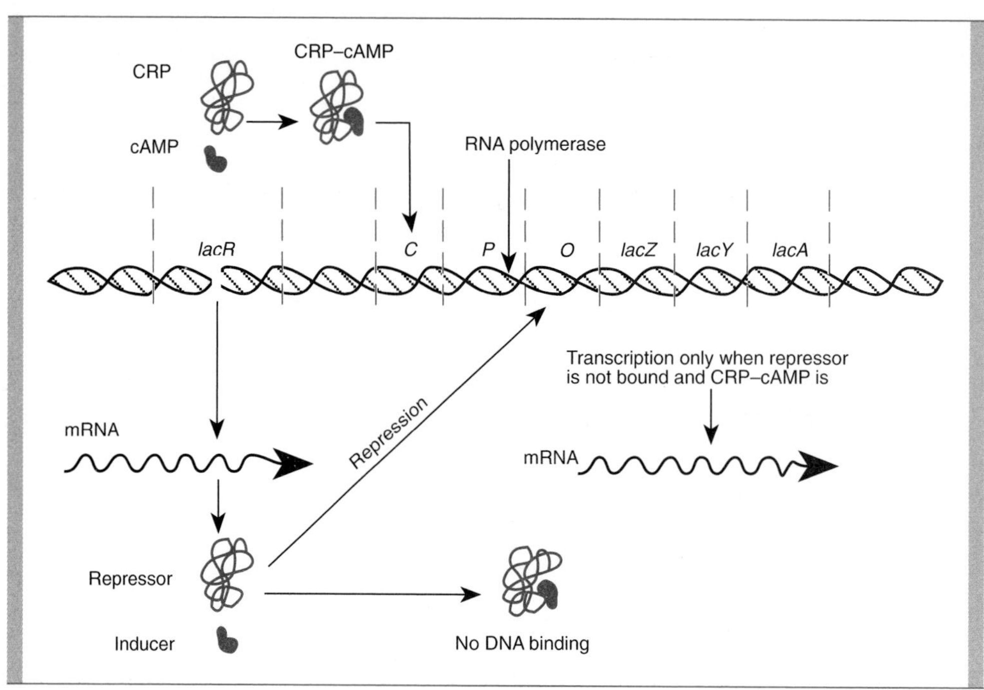

FIGURE 3–13
Schematic representation of the control of transcription initiation by repressor and activator proteins. The example chosen is the *lac* operon of *Escherichia coli. LacR* (or I), gene encoding the lac repressor protein; C, CAP region (binding site of cAMP receptor protein, or CRP); P, promoter region (binding site of RNA polymerase); O, operator region (binding site of repressor); *lacZ,* gene encoding ß-galactosidase; *lacY,* gene encoding permease for β-galactosides; *lacA,* gene encoding galactoside acetylase.

acids) have weak promoters that need help to promote high-level initiation of transcription by RNA polymerase. The help is supplied by a regulator protein called **catabolite activator protein** or **cAMP receptor protein** (CRP). This protein, if and only if cyclic AMP is bound to it, binds slightly upstream from the promoter and permits high-level expression if the operon is specifically induced (and the repressor has been removed by induction). Because cAMP levels are very low during growth on glucose or other favored substrates, there is insufficient cAMP–CRP complex to activate catabolic operons even if their inducers are present in the environment. As a result, the cells ignore the induction signal if they have an adequate supply of glucose.

Catabolite repression regulon ensures optimal use of preferred substrates

Finally, gene regulation in bacteria is accomplished by unique tactics so far discovered only in pathogens. These are included in the following section.

CELL SURVIVAL

Cell Stress Regulons

From studies with *E. coli,* it was learned that cells have many regulons involved in survival responses during difficult circumstances. The catabolite repression regulon just described is in essence a means by which the cell can optimize its synthesis of catabolic enzymes by making only those that contribute to growth. But this regulon can also be viewed as a survival device, helping the cell to respond to the nutritional stress of running out of glucose. If an alternative source of carbon is present in the environment, the cell can redirect its pattern of gene expression to make a suitable adjustment to the nutritional stress.

Bacteria have regulons that help cope with environmental stress

SOS system repairs damaged DNA and prevents multiplication during repair

Perhaps more obvious as a stress response is the **SOS system,** a set of 17 genes that are turned on when the cell suffers damage to its DNA. The products of these genes are

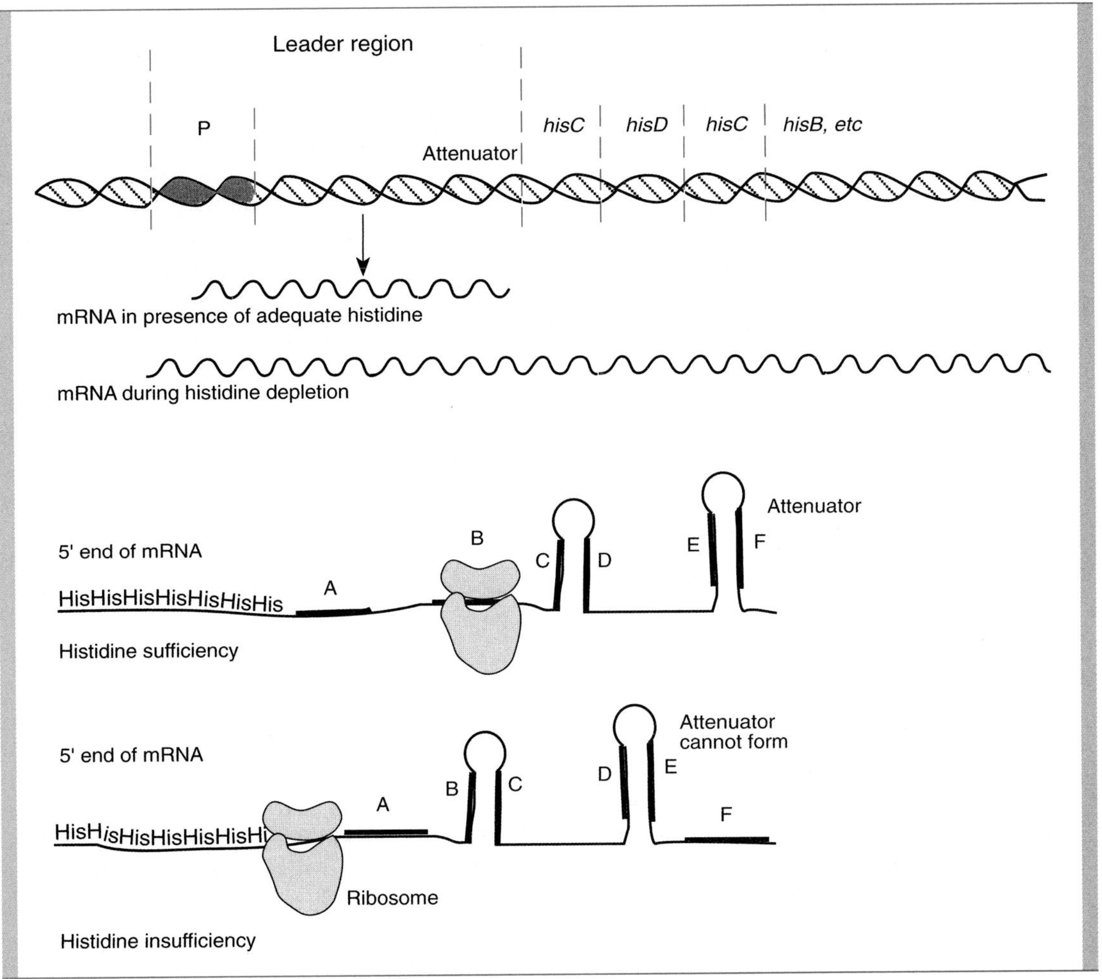

FIGURE 3–14
Schematic representation of the control of transcription by the process of attenuation. The example chosen is the *his* operon of *Escherichia coli.* How attenuation works is fascinating. The leader region is always transcribed and translated into a small oligopeptide. The peptide near the attenuator site has a string of seven *his* codons. Movement of the first ribosome coming behind the polymerase is drastically affected by the supply of charged *his* tRNA. If there is an adequate supply, the ribosome is not delayed, and an attenuator loop forms in the mRNA, causing transcription to terminate. With a shortage of histidine, the first ribosome gets hung up over the *his* codons, and the attenuator loop is not formed, because alternate loops form. As a result, transcription proceeds, the complete *his* mRNA is made, and the biosynthetic enzymes can be made in large quantities. The upper portion of the figure illustrates the difference in transcription of the *his* operon in histidine sufficiency and insufficiency; the lower two diagrams depict the molecular mechanism of attenuation.

involved in several processes that repair damaged DNA and prevent cell division during the repair.

Another prominent bacterial cell stress regulon is responsible for the **heat-shock response.** It encompasses some 20 genes, which are transcriptionally activated on an upward shift in temperature or on imposition of several kinds of chemical stress, including alcohol. In the case of *E. coli,* the heat-shock regulator protein is a special subunit of RNA polymerase, σ-32, which replaces the normal σ-70 subunit and locates the special promoters of the heat-shock genes. At least half of the heat-shock genes encode proteins that either are proteases or are **protein chaperones** that assist in the processing, maturation, or export of other proteins. It is thought that these chaperones and proteases are needed for normal protein processing at all temperatures but are required in higher amounts to counteract the

Heat-shock gene expression is enhanced at high temperature and allows cell survival

Some heat-shock genes encode protein chaperones

effects of high temperature on protein folding and protein–protein interactions. The bacterial chaperones are highly similar to their mammalian counterparts. For example, HtpG, DnaK, and GroEL of *E. coli* correspond to the mammalian hsp90, hsp70, and hsp60 families of chaperones, respectively. The precise involvement of the heat-shock response in infectious disease is still being explored, but it is striking that antibodies directed against bacterial heat-shock proteins constitute a major component of the serologic response of humans to infection or vaccine administration. Fever in humans can elevate body temperature sufficiently to induce the heat-shock response, and it is suspected that this response may affect the outcome of various infections. Also, some viruses both of bacteria and of humans use the heat-shock proteins of their host cells to promote their own replication.

Response to environment involves phosphorylation of a pair of specific signal transduction proteins, a protein kinase, and a response regulator

Other regulons deal with cell survival in the face of such stresses as osmotic shock, high or low pH, oxidation damage, presence of toxic metal ions, and restrictions for fundamental nutrients (phosphate, nitrogen, sulfur, and carbon). A large number of these responses involve teams of proteins that sense the environment, generate a signal, transmit that signal by protein–protein interactions, and activate the appropriate response regulon. In a striking number of cases, a response system includes a **protein kinase** that becomes phosphorylated by ATP on a particular conserved histidine residue in response to an environmental stimulus. This kinase is teamed with a second protein called a **phosphorylated response regulator.** The phosphate residue from the kinase is transferred to an aspartic acid residue of the response regulator, usually converting this protein into an activator of transcription of the appropriate genes. Members of these two families of **signal transduction proteins** share highly conserved domains throughout distantly related bacteria.

Endospores

Sporulation involves sequential activation of interrelated regulons resulting in production of a resistant endospore, capable later of germination

Two of the most elaborate bacterial survival responses involve the transition of growing cells into a form that can survive long periods without growth. In a few Gram-positive bacterial species, this involves **sporulation,** the production of an **endospore,** as we saw in Chapter 2. This process, extensively studied in a few species, involves cascades of RNA polymerase σ subunits, each sequentially activating several interrelated regulons that cooperate to produce the elaborately encased spore, which though metabolically inert and extremely resistant to environmental stress, is capable of germinating into a growing (vegetative) cell.

Stationary Phase Cells

Formation of a stationary phase cell involves activation of many regulons in a coordinated cascade

For all other bacteria, adaptation to a nongrowing state involves formation of a differentiated cell called the **stationary phase cell.** The product is certainly far different morphologically from an endospore, but a tough, resistant, and metabolically quiescent cell is produced that looks distinct from its growing counterpart. Its envelope is made tougher by many modification of its structure, its chromosome is aggregated, and its metabolism is adjusted to a maintenance mode. Producing this resistance involves a process surprisingly analogous to sporulation, because, as in sporulation, cascades of signals and responses involving the sequential activation of sets of genes appear to be involved. One of the many global regulators involved is RpoS, a σ subunit of RNA polymerase.

Motility and Chemotaxis

Flagellar motor uses proton-motive force energy

Motility in most bacterial species is the property of swimming by means of flagellar propulsion. The complex structure of a flagellum—its filament, hook, and basal body—was presented in Chapter 2. The helical filament functions as a propeller, the hook possibly as a universal joint, and the basal body with its rod and rings as a motor anchored in the envelope. The flagellar motors turn the filaments using energy directly from the electrochemical gradient (proton-motive force) of the cell membrane rather than from ATP. The filament can be rotated either clockwise or counterclockwise. Whatever the number of flagella on a cell and whatever their arrangement on the surface (polar, peritrichous, or lophotrichous), they are synchronized to rotate simultaneously in the same direction. Only counterclockwise rotation results in productive vectorial motion, called a **run.** Clockwise rotation of the flagella causes the cell to **tumble** in place. The flagella alternate between periods of clockwise and counterclockwise rotation according to an endogenous schedule. As a result, motile bacteria move in brief runs interrupted by periods of tumbling.

Direction of flagellar rotation determines a run or a tumble

Chemotaxis is directed movement toward chemical **attractants** and away from chemical **repellents.** It is accomplished by a remarkable molecular sensory system that possesses many of the characteristics that wouid be expected of behavioral systems in higher animals, including memory and adaptation. Beside the genes of the flagellar proteins (called *fla,* for flagella) more than 30 genes (called *mot,* for motility, and *che,* for chemotaxis) encode the proteins that make this system work: receptors, signalers, transducers, tumble regulators, and motors.

Multiple genes are required for chemotaxis

Whether a cell is moving toward an attractant or away from a repellent, chemotaxis is achieved by **biased random walks.** These result from alterations in the frequency of tumbling. When a cell is, by chance, progressing toward an attractant, tumbling is suppressed and the run is long; if it is swimming away, tumbling occurs sooner and the run is brief. It is sheer chance in what direction a cell is pointed at the end of a tumble, but by regulating the frequency of tumbles in this manner, directed progress is made.

Changes in duration of runs and tumbles determine chemotactic response

The mechanism of chemotaxis is fairly well understood from work with *E. coli.* It is complex and can be summarized as follows. Binding of an attractant alters the endogenous routine schedule of runs and tumbles by interrupting a **phosphorylation cascade** and thus prolonging the run. Accommodation by a **methylation** system restores the endogenous schedule and resets the cell's sensitivity to the attractant to require a higher concentration to prolong the run. This constitutes a **molecular memory.** The bacterial cell senses a concentration gradient not by measuring a difference between the concentration at each end of the cell but by a molecular memory that enables it to compare the concentration now with what it was a short time ago. Escape from a repellent occurs in an analogous fashion.

Molecular memory recognizes change in attractant concentration and ensures progress toward it

Chemotaxis is both a survival device (for avoiding toxic substances) and a growth-promoting device (for finding food). It can also be a virulence factor in facilitating colonization of the human host by bacteria.

Chemotaxis serves survival, growth-promoting, and pathogenic roles

BACTERIAL VIRULENCE

Special Attributes of Pathogens

Most bacteria have the ability to grow and survive under harsh conditions. Yet of the many thousands of bacterial species, only a small percentage are associated with humans as part of the natural flora or as causative agents of disease. This fact generates the question central to medical microbiology from the very start: What makes a bacterium pathogenic? The answer is not simple, because it turns out that many properties are necessary for a bacterial cell to gain entrance to a human, evade its defense systems, and establish an infection. The structures and activities described in Chapter 2 and in this chapter bear directly on virulence attributes of bacteria. They include:

Virulence results from many specialized bacterial structures and activities

- Adherence to and penetration of host cell surfaces
- Evasion of phagocytic and immunologic attack
- Secretion of toxic proteins to weaken the host and promote spread of the pathogen
- Acquisition of nutrients, including iron, to permit growth within the host
- Survival under adverse conditions both within and outside the host and its macrophages

As we shall see in detail in the next chapter, the genes unique to pathogens are frequently found clustered in genetic segments within either plasmids or the bacterial chromosome, with interesting implications for the evolution of pathogenic bacteria. These subjects are examined in detail in Chapter 10.

Regulation of Virulence

Most bacterial pathogens must survive and grow in two very different circumstances—in the broad external environment and in or on the human host. Expressing the very

Virulence genes must be regulated

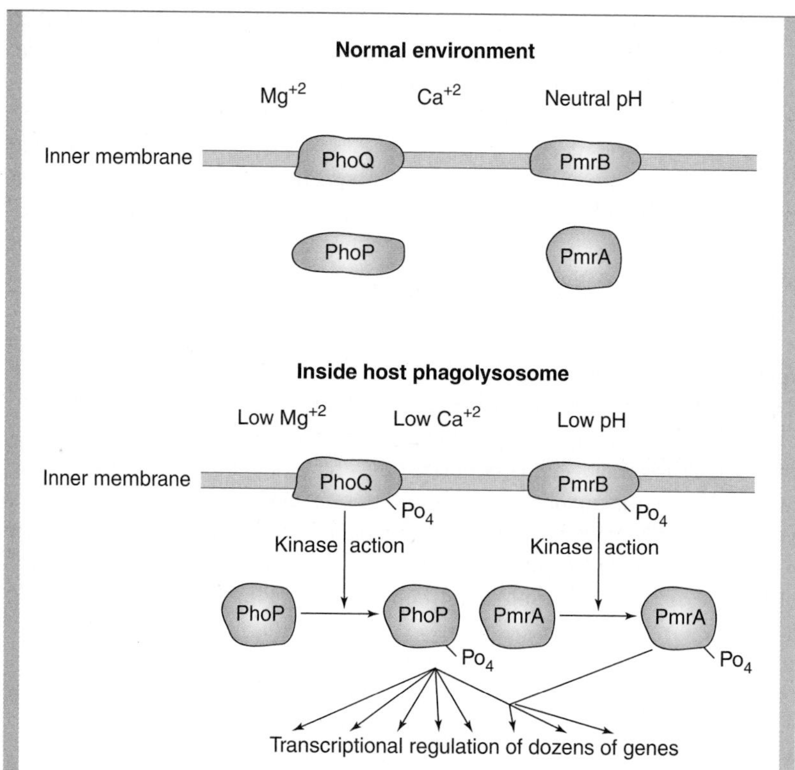

FIGURE 3–15
Schematic representation of regulation of virulence genes by the PhoP/PhoQ system of *Salmonella*. (*Adapted from Harper JR, Silhavy TJ. Germ warfare: The mechanisms of virulence factor delivery. In: EA Groisman,* Principles of Bacterial Pathogenesis, *San Diego, CA: Academic Press, 2001, pp 43–74.*)

many genes responsible for pathogenesis in the latter situation would be counterproductive, if not outright detrimental to growth and survival in nature, while failing to express them on encountering the host would commonly be fatal. To ensure their growth and survival in both circumstances, bacteria have evolved elaborate and effective mechanisms for regulation of virulence genes.

Many virulence genes are part of conventional response regulons

Virulence genes are commonly organized as regulons, and many of these share the attributes of general stress response regulons, described above. For example, many are regulated by classical two-component signal transcription systems in which environmental sensing is achieved by a sensor protein kinase, which relays information about the environment by phosphorylating its partner, a response regulator, which in turn acts to control transcription initiation of its gene set. Many dozens of these systems have been found in various pathogens. Here we examine one example, the **PhoP/PhoQ system,** which is essential to the virulence of *Salmonella* (Fig 3–15). PhoQ is a sensor protein kinase in the cell membrane, and PhoP is the response regulator to which it relates. PhoQ is sensitive to the concentration of magnesium ion in the periplasm of the *Salmonella* cell. With a normally adequate Mg^{2+} concentration, PhoQ is locked in an inactive state; however, when the concentration is very low, as happens when the *Salmonella* finds itself within the phagolysosome of human macrophages, PhoQ autophosphorylates one of its histidine residues. Phosphorylation of PhoP ensues, and this event activates it as a transcription regulator. The phosphorylated PhoP controls more than 40 genes. Some are induced, including those encoding an acid phosphatase, cation transporters, outer membrane proteins, and enzymes that modify LPS. Some are repressed, including some encoding proteins essential for epithelial cell invasion and others encoding components of a contact secretion system. The control network is complex, because some of the regulated genes are not directly controlled by PhoP, but by a second two-component response system, called PmrA/PmrB, which is responsive to low pH. The two systems, PhoP/PhoQ and PmrA/PmrB, act in cascade fashion to accomplish a rather intricate response. The induced proteins are believed to enable the cell to scavenge Mg^{2+} from its own LPS and to protect itself from the hostile environment of the phagolysosome; the repressed ones were useful in earlier stages of the infective process but now are superfluous. The *Salmonella* cell that finds itself in the phagolysosome of a macrophage has evolved a way to sense its situation and maximize its production of needed factors while dispensing with irrelevant ones.

An interesting principle has emerged from the study of bacterial luminescence and from the field of infectious diseases of plants. Researchers have discovered that several types of bacteria, including *Pseudomonas,* regulate the expression of genes in a cell density–dependent manner. That is, expression of certain genes occurred only when the population density of the bacteria reached a threshold level, called a **quorum.** Quorum sensing in some cases is achieved by secretion of a small, diffusible molecule (some are acyl-homoserine lactones) that is sensed by an envelope protein, triggering a regulatory response through a two-component signal transduction system. This **autoinduction** enables the bacteria to avoid "tipping their hand" and mounting an attack on the host before their numbers are sufficient to overwhelm the host's defenses. *Salmonella* are known to have a quorum-sensing protein, SdiA, that regulates at least one operon on a virulence plasmid in these cells. No evidence yet indicates the role of this regulation in *Salmonella* infection. Exploration of the possible role of quorum sensing in general in human disease is ongoing.

Some genes are autoinduced by cells after a critical population density, or quorum, is reached

Regulation of virulence gene expression is achieved also in a fashion totally unexpected from the study of metabolic gene regulation, namely by rearrangement of DNA. These instances do not involve mutations in the usual sense of the term, because the DNA alterations are readily reversible. Many well studied examples have generated the concept of a genetic switch, with an "on" and an "off" position determined by the inversion of a small segment of DNA adjacent to the regulated genes. Examples of this and related mechanisms dependent on DNA recombination are presented in Chapter 4.

Some virulence genes are controlled by genetic switches and other DNA rearrangements

ADDITIONAL READING

Groisman EA. *Principles of Bacterial Pathogenesis.* San Diego, CA: Academic Press; 2001. Chapter 2 (Harper JR, Silhavy TJ), Germ Warfare: The Mechanisms of Virulence Factor Delivery, presents details of protein export. Chapter 3 (Dorman CJ, Smith SGJ), Regulation of Virulence Gene Expression in Bacterial Pathogens, is a comprehensive description of the myriad of molecular mechanisms used by pathogens to regulate virulence genes.

Neidhardt FC, Ingraham JL, Schaechter M. *Physiology of the Bacterial Cell: A Molecular Approach.* Sunderland, MA: Sinauer Associates; 1990. Chapters 3 through 8 present bacterial metabolism and physiology in a manner similar to what was done here, but in more detail.

CHAPTER 4

Bacterial Genetics

FREDERICK C. NEIDHARDT

No aspect of the basic biology of the prokaryotic cell is so unfamiliar outside the community of microbiologists as the genetics of these essentially asexually reproducing cells. And yet, this subject has extremely important practical messages for clinicians and others interested in infectious disease. The genetic determinants of microbial properties and the rules that determine microbial evolution are of paramount importance to the treatment regimen for an individual patient as well as to thoughts about the origin and future course of the human–microbe interaction. This chapter explores the fundamentals of this area.

BACTERIAL VARIATION AND INHERITANCE

It was rather difficult to establish that many of the same rules of heredity apply to bacteria as to plants and animals. This may seem strange, because the most spectacular advances in molecular genetics have been achieved almost exclusively through work on *Escherichia coli* and its viruses. However, during the 1940s and early 1950s, serious experimental efforts were still being directed toward determining whether mutations in bacteria were random or specifically directed by the environment.

The difficulty of establishing the basis of heredity in bacteria grew out of their inherent properties and their manner of growth. First, because bacteria are **haploid,** the consequences of a mutation, even a recessive one, are immediately evident in the mutant cell. Because the generation time of bacteria is short, it does not take many hours for a mutant cell that has arisen by chance to become the dominant cell type in a culture under appropriate selective conditions. This can lead to the false conclusion that the environment has directed a genetic change. Second, as was noted in Chapter 3, bacteria, to a far greater extent than animals and plants, respond to change in their chemical and physical environment by altering their pattern of gene function, thereby taking on previously unexpressed properties. For example, *E. coli* cells make the enzymes for lactose metabolism only when grown with this sugar as carbon source. Superficially this might suggest that lactose changes the cell's **genotype** (its complement of genes), when instead it is only the **phenotype** (the characteristics actually displayed by the cell) that has been changed by the environment. Finally, even when rather exceptional technical measures are taken to ensure a pure culture, contamination can occasionally occur. With cultures containing more than one bacterial species, different conditions of growth can cause one or another species to predominate (by, for example, a million to one ratio), suggesting to the unwary observer that the characteristics of "the" bacterium under study are very unstable and dependent on the environment.

Mutations are rapidly expressed; mutants quickly predominate under selective conditions

Environment can influence phenotypic expression of genotype

Progress in bacterial genetics was rapid once it was recognized that mutation and selection can quickly change the makeup of a growing population and that bacterial cells inherit genes that may or may not be expressed depending on the environment. Even so, it

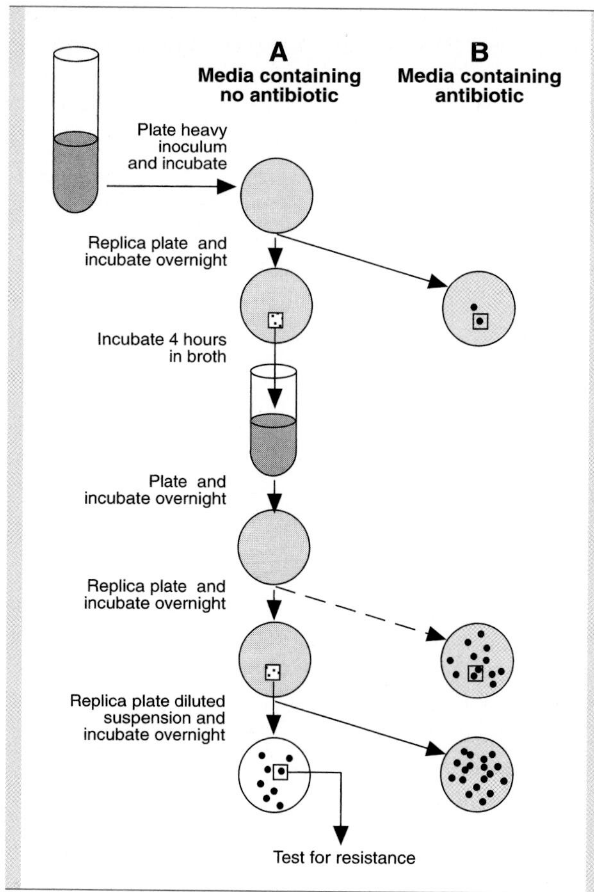

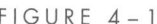

FIGURE 4–1
Lederberg technique for indirect selection of antimicrobic resistant mutants. Growth on plates in the left-hand column **(A)** is replicated to antimicrobic-containing plates in the right-hand column **(B)**. If resistant mutants arise in the absence of antimicrobic **(A)**, the position of colonies on antimicrobic-containing plates would indicate their position on the plates that do not contain antimicrobic. By selecting growth from this position and repeating the process with appropriate inoculum dilutions, resistant mutants that have never been exposed to the antimicrobic can be directly selected **(A)**.

Novel agents that transfer genes account for many puzzling genetic events

was not until the discovery in the 1980s of transposable genetic elements and insertion sequences (to be discussed later in this chapter) that certain examples of high-frequency variation, the so-called **phase transition,** could be satisfactorily explained within the framework of classic genetic principles.

Proof of randomness of mutation was important in clinical medicine

Several experiments were particularly important in establishing that mutations occur in nature as random events and are not guided by the environment. The most convincing introduced the technique of replica plating and was used to show how a population of cells totally resistant to an antimicrobic could be isolated from an initially sensitive population without ever exposing them to the toxic agent (Fig 4–1). This clarified the mechanism of an important clinical problem.

MUTATION AND REPAIR

The spontaneous development of mutations is a major factor in the evolution of bacteria. Mutations occur in nature at a low frequency, on the order of one mutation in every million cells for any one gene, but the large size of microbial populations ensures the presence of many mutants.

Kinds of Mutations

The several kinds of mutations all involve changes in nucleotide sequence

Mutations are heritable changes in the structure of genes. The normal, usually active, form of a gene is called the **wild-type allele;** the mutated, usually inactive, form is called the **mutant allele.** There are several kinds of mutations, based on the nature of the change in nucleotide sequence of the affected gene(s). **Replacements** involve the substitution of one base for another. **Microdeletions** and **microinsertions** involve the removal and addition, respectively, of a single nucleotide (and its complement in the opposite strand). **Insertions** involve the addition of many base pairs of nucleotides at a single site. **Deletions** remove a contiguous segment of many base pairs. **Inversions** change the direction of a segment of

DNA by splicing each strand of the segment into the complementary strand. **Duplications** produce a redundant segment of DNA, usually adjacent (tandem) to the original segment.

By recalling the nature of genes and how their nucleotide sequence directs the synthesis of proteins, one can understand the immediate consequence of each of these biochemical changes. If a replacement mutation in a codon changes the mRNA transcript to a different amino acid, it is called a **missense mutation** (eg, an AAG [lysine] to a GAG [glutamate]). The resulting protein may be enzymatically inactive or very sensitive to environmental conditions, such as temperature. If the replacement changes a codon specifying an amino acid to one specifying none, it is called a **nonsense mutation** (eg, a UAC [tyrosine] to UAA [STOP]), and the truncated product of the mutated gene is called a **nonsense fragment.** Microdeletions and microinsertions cause **frame shift mutations,** changes in the reading frame by which the ribosomes translate the mRNA from the mutated gene. Frame shifts usually result in polymerization of a stretch of incorrect amino acids until a nonsense codon is encountered, so the product is usually a truncated polypeptide fragment with an incorrect amino acid sequence at its N terminus. Deletion or insertion of a segment of base pairs from a gene shortens or lengthens the protein product if the number of base pairs deleted or inserted is divisible evenly by 3; otherwise it also brings about the consequence of a frame shift. Inversions of a small segment within a gene inactivate it; inverting larger segments may affect chiefly the genes at the points of inversion. Duplications, probably the most common of all mutations, serve an important role in the evolution of genes with new functions. Mutations are summarized in Table 4–1.

Changes in nucleotide sequence affect the synthesis of the protein products of genes

Many mutations, particularly if they occur near the end of a gene, prevent the expression of all genes downstream (away from the promoter) of the mutated gene. Such **polar mutations** are thought to exert their effect on neighboring genes by the termination of

Mutations may affect neighboring genes by termination of transcription

TABLE 4–1

Mutations

TYPE	CAUSATIVE AGENT	CONSEQUENCES
REPLACEMENT		
Transition: pyrimidine replaced by a pyrimidine or a purine by a purine	Base analogs, ultraviolet radiation, deaminating and alkylating agents, spontaneous	Transitions and transversions: if nonsense codon formed, truncated peptide; if missense codon formed, altered protein
Transversion: purine replaced by a pyrimidine or vice versa	Spontaneous	
DELETION		
Macrodeletion: large nucleotide segment deleted	HNO_2, radiation, bifunctional alkylating agents	Truncated peptide; other products possible, such as fusion peptides
Microdeletion: one or two nucleotides deleted	Same as macrodeletions	Frame shift, usually resulting in nonsense codon and truncated peptide
INSERTION		
Macroinsertion: large nucleotide segment inserted	Transposons or insertion sequence (IS) elements	Interrupted gene yielding truncated product
Microinsertion: one or two nucleotides inserted	Acridine	Frame shift, usually resulting in nonsense codon yielding a truncated product
INVERSION	IS or IS-like elements	Many possible effects

transcription of downstream genes when translation of the mRNA of the mutated gene is blocked by a nonsense codon.

Mutagens increase the natural frequency of mutation

There is a certain natural frequency of mutations brought about by errors in replication, but various environmental and biological agents can increase the frequency greatly. Different types of mutations are increased selectively by different agents, as listed in Table 4–1.

Common biological consequences of mutations include resistance to antimicrobics, nutritional requirements, and altered response to environment

Mutations in essential genes are not lethal if they are expressed only conditionally, as within a particular temperature range

Mutations may also be classified according to their biological consequences. Some mutations change the susceptibility of a cell to an antimicrobic or other toxic agent; these **resistance mutations** might, for example, affect the structure of certain cell proteins in such a way that the agent cannot enter the cell or cannot inactivate its normal target. Some mutations, called **auxotrophic mutations,** affect the production of a biosynthetic enzyme and result in a nutritional requirement of the mutant cell for the amino acid, nucleotide, vitamin, or other biosynthetic product it can no longer make for itself. The wild type from which the mutant was derived is said to be **prototrophic** for that nutrient. Some mutations affect a gene whose product is essential for growth and cannot be bypassed nutritionally; these are called **lethal mutations.** If the product of a mutated gene is active in some circumstances but inactive under others (eg, high or low temperature), the mutation is called **conditional** (meaning **conditionally expressed**). The most common kind of conditional mutation is one in which the protein product of the mutated gene is inactive at a normally physiologic temperature, but active at a higher or lower temperature; these are called **temperature-sensitive mutations.**

Reversion and Suppression of Mutations

Back mutations are rare because highly specific corrections are needed

Suppressor mutations reestablish original phenotype

A **reversion,** or **back mutation,** is the conversion of a mutated gene back to its original wild-type allele. True back mutation can occur but at a low frequency, because a very specific and improbable event is required. Much more commonly observed is the conversion of a mutant cell into one that is phenotypically identical to the original wild-type bacterium for the affected character but still retains the original mutation. These **suppressor** mutations can arise in several ways. Within the mutated codon a second mutation can create a new codon specifying the original amino acid. Alternatively, secondary mutations in other codons of the mutated gene can lead to a change in amino acid sequence that results in an active product despite the continued presence of the original amino acid error. Suppressing mutations can occur even in genes other than the one that was originally mutated. For example, when two proteins interact to perform a function, the mutant form of one may be active when combined with a mutant form of the other. Another example involves tRNA molecules, the translators of the genetic code, which can themselves be altered by mutation; it is possible for a mutant tRNA to "mistake" a mutant codon and insert the original correct amino acid, a case of two wrongs making a right.

Repair of DNA Damage

Several processes involving many genes operate to repair various sorts of damage to DNA

Many mutagenic agents directly alter the structure of DNA, and some are ubiquitous components of the environment (heat, sunlight, acid, oxidants, and alkylating agents). It is therefore not surprising to learn that bacteria have evolved multiple biochemical mechanisms for repairing damaged DNA. In *E. coli,* for example, more than 30 genes are known to be involved in DNA repair; many of these are members of the SOS response discussed in Chapter 3. Collectively these repair systems can remove thymine dimers produced by ultraviolet (UV) irradiation, can remove methyl or ethyl groups placed on guanine residues, can excise bases damaged by deamination or ring breakage and replace them with authentic residues, and can recognize and repair DNA depurinated by acid or heat. In large measure these repair systems use the fact that DNA is double stranded. Damage is recognized by the mispairing it causes, and the information on one strand is used to direct the proper repair of the damaged strand. Also, a proofreading process operates during DNA replication to detect any mismatch between each newly polymerized base and its mate in the template strand. Mismatches are excised to permit repolymerization with the properly matched nucleotide. Failures of this proofreading process can be detected and handled by an excision and resynthesis system similar to those that recognize and repair chemically damaged DNA.

One system bypasses DNA damaged by UV irradiation when repair has failed. It directs replication to proceed across a region badly damaged by the formation of thymine dimers. This **error-prone replication** is responsible for the mutations induced by UV light.

Some repair processes result in mutation

GENETIC EXCHANGE

Mutation and selection are important factors in bacterial evolution, but evolution proceeds far faster than it could by these processes alone. For instance, the probability that the process of random mutation alone can produce a cell that, let us say, requires five mutations for optimal growth in a new environment is extremely low. It is in fact the product of the individual mutation frequencies (eg, $10^{-6} \times 10^{-6} \times 10^{-6} \times 10^{-6} \times 10^{-6} = 10^{-30}$), and that essentially precludes a natural population from ever acquiring the new property in this manner. However, such alterations occur because organisms exchange genetic material, thereby permitting combinations of mutations to be collected in individual cells.

Evolution is speeded by exchange of genetic material

Despite the fact that bacteria reproduce exclusively asexually, the sharing of genetic information within and between related species is now recognized to be quite common and to occur in at least three fundamentally different ways. All three processes involve a one-way transfer of DNA from a **donor cell** to a **recipient cell.** The molecule of DNA introduced into the recipient is called the **exogenote** to distinguish it from the cell's own original chromosome, called the **endogenote.**

One-way passage of DNA from a donor to a recipient adds an exogenote to the recipient endogenote

One process of DNA transfer, called **transformation,** involves the release of DNA into the environment by the lysis of some cells, followed by the direct uptake of that DNA by the recipient cells. By another means of transfer, called **transduction,** the DNA is introduced into the recipient cell by a nonlethal virus that has grown on the donor cell. The third process, called **conjugation,** involves actual contact between donor and recipient cell during which DNA is transferred as part of a plasmid (an autonomously replicating, extrachromosomal molecule of circular double-stranded DNA); in conjugation, donor and recipient cells are referred to as male and female, respectively. The three means of gene transfer are summarized in Figure 4–2.

Transformation, transduction, and conjugation are the major processes of DNA transfer

Species of bacteria differ in their ability to transfer DNA, but all three mechanisms are distributed among both Gram-positive and Gram-negative species; however, only transformation is governed by bacterial chromosomal genes. Transduction is totally mediated by virus genes, and conjugation, by plasmid genes.

Transformation, transduction, and conjugation are mediated by chromosomal, viral, and plasmid genes, respectively

Transformation

Transformation was first demonstrated in 1928 by F. Griffith, a British public health officer, who showed that virulent, encapsulated *Streptococcus pneumoniae* (pneumococci) that had been killed by heat could confer on living, avirulent, nonencapsulated pneumococci the ability to make the polysaccharide capsule of the killed organisms and thus become virulent for mice. Subsequent work in 1944 by O. T. Avery, C. M. MacLeod, and M. McCarty at the Rockefeller Institute revealed that the "transforming factor" from the dead pneumococci was nothing other than DNA. This discovery had enormous impact on biology, because it was the first rigorous demonstration that DNA is the macromolecule in which genetic information is encoded. It opened the door to modern molecular genetics.

Studies on pneumococcal transformation led to identification of genetic material

The ability to take up DNA from the environment is called **competence,** and in many species of bacteria, it is encoded by chromosomal genes that become active under certain environmental conditions. In such species, transformation can occur readily and is said to be natural. Other species cannot enter the competent state but can be made permeable to DNA by treatment with agents that damage the cell envelope making an **artificial transformation** possible.

Genes encoding competence enable uptake of DNA; species lacking them must be made permeable

Natural transformation must be important in nature, judged by the variety of mechanisms that different bacteria have evolved to accomplish it. Two of the best-studied systems are those of the Gram-positive pneumococcus and a Gram-negative rod, *Haemophilus influenzae*. Pneumococcal cells secrete a protein **competence factor** that induces many of the cells of a culture to synthesize special proteins necessary for transformation, including an autolysin that exposes a cell membrane DNA-binding protein. Any DNA present in the medium is bound indiscriminately; even salmon sperm DNA can be bound and taken up as

Pneumoccal competence involves a nonspecific DNA-binding protein

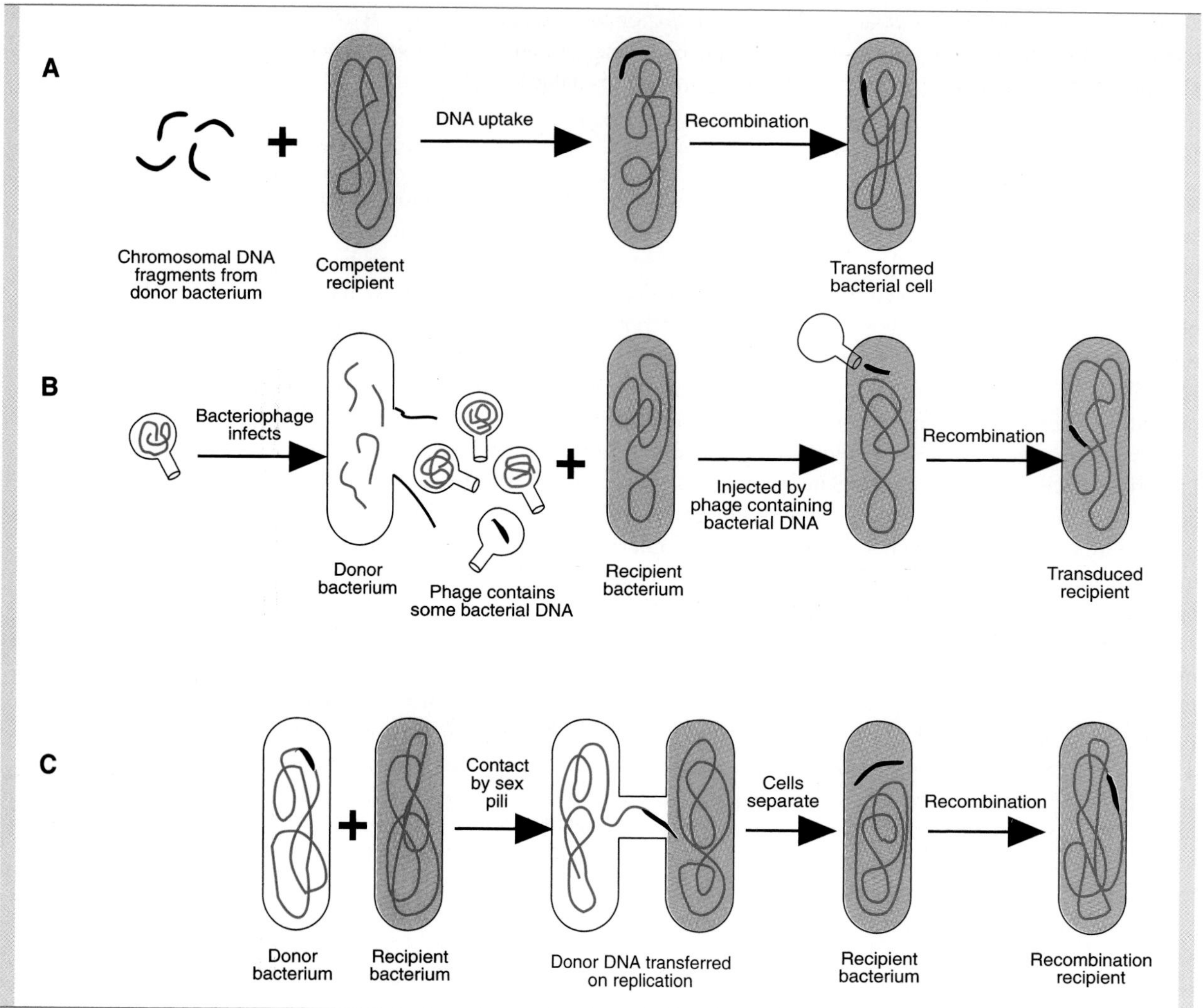

FIGURE 4–2
Chromosomal gene transfer mechanisms in bacteria. **A.** Transformation. **B.** Transduction. **C.** Conjugation.

readily as DNA from another pneumococcal cell. The surface-bound double-stranded DNA is cleaved into fragments of about 6 to 8 kilobases (kb). One strand is degraded by a nuclease, while the complementary strand of each fragment is taken up by a process that seems to be driven by the proton-motive force of the cell membrane (see Chapter 3). The fate of the internalized DNA fragment then depends on whether it shares homology (the same or similar in base sequence) with a portion of the recipient cell's DNA. If so, recombination can occur by a process described later, but heterologous DNA (no similarity to the endogenote) is degraded and causes no heritable change in the recipient.

All DNA is taken up, but heterologous DNA is degraded

Transformation in *H. influenzae* is somewhat different. There is no competence factor, and cells become competent merely by growth in an environment rich in nutrients. Only homologous DNA (ie, DNA from the same or a closely related species of *Haemophilus*) is taken up, and it is taken up in double-stranded form. The selectivity is brought about by the presence of a special membrane protein that binds to an 11-base pair (bp) sequence (5'-AAGTGCGGTCA-3') that occurs frequently in *Haemophilus* DNA and infrequently in other DNAs. Following binding to molecules of this protein, the homologous DNA is internalized by a mechanism that resembles membrane invagination, resulting in the temporary residence of the exogenote in cytosolic membrane vesicles. Although the DNA taken up is double stranded, only one of the two strands participates in the subsequent recombination with the endogenote.

H. influenzae endocytoses only homologous dsDNA, recognized by a characteristic 11-bp sequence

The common use of *E. coli* as a host cell in which to clone genes on hybrid plasmids (see Invertible DNA Segments and Recombinational Regulation of Gene Expression) depends on procedures involving treatment with salt and temperature shocks to bring about artificial transformation; this organism has no natural competence mechanism. In contrast, the pathogen, *Neisseria gonorrhoeae* regularly uses transformation to bring about changes in the antigenic nature of its pili, as described later in the section on recombination.

Transformation is common among many pathogens; artificial transformation enables use of *E. coli* for gene cloning

Transduction

Transduction is virus-mediated transfer of genetic information from donor to recipient cell. To understand transduction and its several mechanisms, it is necessary to preview the nature of bacterial viruses, a topic dealt with more extensively in Chapters 5, 6, and 7.

Viruses are capable of reproduction only inside living cells. Those that grow in bacteria are called **bacteriophages**, or simply **phages.** They are minimally composed of protein and nucleic acid, although some may have a very complex structure and composition. The individual virus particle or virion consists of a protein capsid enclosing genomic nucleic acid, which is either RNA or DNA, but never both. Virions infect sensitive cells by adsorbing to specific receptors on the cell surface and then, in the case of phages, injecting their DNA or RNA. Phages come in two functional varieties according to what happens after injection of the viral nucleic acid. **Virulent** (lytic) **phages** cause lysis of the host bacterium as a culmination of the synthesis of many new virions within the infected cell. **Temperate phages** may initiate a lytic growth process of this sort or can enter a quiescent form (called a **prophage**), in which the infected host cell is permitted to proceed about its business of growth and division but passes on to its descendants a prophage genome capable of being **induced** to produce phage in a process nearly identical to the growth of lytic phages. The bacterial cell that harbors a latent prophage is said to be a **lysogen** (capable of producing lytic phages), and its condition is referred to as **lysogeny**. Lysogens are immune to infection by virions of the type they harbor as prophage. Occasionally, lysogens are spontaneously induced and lysed by the phage and release mature virions (as many as 75 to 150 or more per cell) into the environment. When triggered by UV irradiation or certain chemicals, an entire population of lysogens are induced simultaneously to initiate reproduction of their latent virus followed by lysis of the host cells. Infection of a sensitive cell with the temperate phage can lead to either lysis or lysogeny. How this choice comes about is described in Chapter 7.

Phages are viruses of diverse structure and modes of replication

Virulent phages produce new virions in the host bacterial cell, usually lysing it

Temperate phages can either lyse a bacterial host cell or lysogenize it as a prophage

Prophage induction leads to virion production and cell lysis

The prophage of different temperate phages exists in one of two different states. In the first, the prophage DNA is physically integrated into a bacterial chromosome; in the second, it remains separate from the chromosome as an independently replicating, circularized, molecule of DNA. Prophages of this sort are in fact plasmids.

Some prophages integrate; others behave as plasmids

For the most part, transduction is mediated by temperate phage, and the two broad types of transduction result from the different physical forms of prophage and the different means by which the transducing virion is formed. These are termed **generalized transduction,** by which any bacterial gene stands an equal chance of being transduced to a recipient cell, and **specialized** or **restricted transduction,** by which only a few genes can be transduced.

Transduction, whether generalized or specialized, is mediated by temperate phage

Generalized Transduction

Some phages package DNA into their capsids in a nonspecific way, the headful mechanism, in which any DNA can be stuffed into the capsid head until it is full. (The head is the principal structure of the virion to which, in some cases, a tail is attached; see Chapter 5.) An endonuclease then trims off any projecting excess. If fragments of host cell DNA are around during the assembly of mature virions, they can become packaged in place of virus DNA, resulting in **pseudovirions.** Pseudovirions are the transducing agents. They can adsorb to sensitive cells and inject the DNA they contain as though it were viral DNA. The result is the introduction of donor DNA into the recipient cell.

In generalized transduction, pseudovirions inject a random piece of host DNA into a recipient

Any given gene has an equal probability of being transduced by this process. With the temperate phage P1 of *E. coli,* this probability is approximately one transduction event per 10^5 to 10^8 virions, because nearly 1 out of every 1000 phage particles made in a P1

Genes have low but equal probability of being transduced

lytic infection are pseudovirions, and the bacterial DNA fragments packaged are 1 to 2% of the length of the chromosome. Cotransduction of two bacterial genes by a single pseudovirion occurs only if they are located close together within this small length of the chromosome, and this fact facilitates mapping the position of a newly discovered gene.

Once injected into the host cell, the transduced DNA is lost by degradation unless it can recombine with the chromosome of the recipient cell, usually by homologous recombination (see below, Invertible DNA Segments and Recombinational Regulation of Gene Expression) in which both strands of the exogenote cross into and replace the homologous segment of the recipient's chromosome. However, sometimes the exogenote can persist without degradation by assuming a stable circular configuration.

Specialized Transduction

Specialized transduction involves imprecise excision of an integrated prophage

A few genes adjacent to the prophage are transferred to the recipient and cointegrated with prophage

It has been noted that the prophage of some phages is integrated into the lysogen's chromosome. This integration does not occur haphazardly but is restricted to usually one site, called the *att* (attachment) site. When a lysogen carrying such a prophage is induced to produce virions, excision of the viral genome from the bacterial chromosome occasionally (eg, in 1 of 10^5 to 10^6 lysogens) occurs imprecisely, resulting in a pickup of genes of the bacterium adjacent to the *att* site. The resulting virion may be infectious (if no essential phage genes are missing) or defective (if one or more essential genes are missing). In either case, adsorption to a sensitive cell and injection of the DNA can occur, and integration of the aberrant phage genome into the chromosome of the new host cell results in the formation of a lysogen containing a few genes that have been transduced as hitchhikers with the phage genome. Integration of the phage genome automatically accomplishes the recombinational event needed to guarantee reproduction of the transduced genes. Only genes that border the *att* site stand a chance of being transduced by this process, which is why it is called specialized or restricted transduction.

All virions produced by lysogenic transductants carry original transduced gene

Because the original pickup event is rare, the first transducing process is termed **low-frequency transduction;** however, when a lysogenic transductant is, in turn, induced to produce phage, all of the new virions carry the originally transduced bacterial gene. The resulting mixture of lysed cells and virions now brings about **high-frequency transduction** of the attached genes.

Specialized transduction has been valuable in gene cloning and sequencing

Bacterial geneticists have learned to move genes of interest near the phage integration site and thereby construct specialized transducing phages containing these genes. Such transducing phages are valuable aids to cloning and sequencing genes and to studying their function and regulation. Obviously a temperate phage that could form a prophage by integrating randomly at any site in the bacterial chromosome would be of special use. The temperate phage Mu of *E. coli* has this property.

Transduction is common in nature, important clinically, and useful in research

Although both generalized transduction and specialized transduction can be regarded as the result of errors in phage production, transfer of genes between bacterial cells by phage is a reasonably common phenomenon. It occurs at significant frequency in nature; for example, genes conferring antimicrobic resistance in staphylococci are often transduced from strain to strain in this way. The toxins responsible for the severe clinical symptoms of diphtheria and of cholera are encoded by genes transduced into *Corynebacterium diphtheriae* and *Vibrio cholerae,* respectively. Transduction is also used extensively as a tool in molecular biology research.

Conjugation

Conjugation is plasmid-encoded and requires cell contact

Conjugation is the transfer of genetic information from donor to recipient bacterial cell in a process that requires intimate cell contact; it has been likened to mating. By themselves, bacteria cannot conjugate. Only when a bacterial cell contains a self-transmissible **plasmid** (see below for definition) does DNA transfer occurs. In most cases, conjugation involves transfer only of plasmid DNA; transfer of chromosomal DNA is a rarer event, and is mediated by only a few plasmids. Plasmids are of enormous importance to medical microbiology. They are discussed in detail later in this chapter, but to understand conjugation we should introduce some of their features at this point.

Plasmids are autonomous extrachromosomal elements composed of circular double-stranded DNA; a few rare linear examples have been found. Plasmids are found in most species of Gram-positive and Gram-negative bacteria in most environments. Plasmids govern their own replication by means of special sequences and proteins. They replicate within the host cell (and only within the host cell) and are partitioned between the daughter cells at the time of cell division. In addition, many plasmids are able to bring about their own transfer from one cell to another by the products of a group of genes called ***tra*** (for transfer); such plasmids are called **conjugative plasmids.** Other plasmids, called **nonconjugative,** lack this ability. The *tra* genes, of which there may be dozens, encode the structures and enzymes that accomplish conjugation. One of these structures is a specialized pilus (see Chapter 2) called the **sex pilus,** which confers the ability to seize recipient cells on the plasmid-containing donor cells. Retraction of the pilus draws the donor and recipient cell into the intimate contact needed to form a conjugal bridge through which DNA can pass. One strand of the plasmid DNA is then enzymatically cleaved at a site called the **origin of transfer** (***oriT***), and the resulting 5' end of the strand is guided into the recipient cell by the action of various *tra*-encoded proteins (Fig 4–3). Both the introduced strand and the strand remaining behind in the donor cell direct the synthesis of their complementary strand in a process called **transfer replication,** resulting in complete copies in both donor and recipient cell. Finally, circularization of the double-stranded molecules occurs, the conjugation bridge is broken, and both cells can now function as donor cells.

Plasmids are ubiquitous in most bacterial species

Conjugative plasmids can transfer themselves through activity of *tra* genes

Transfer replication ensures retention of plasmid copy in donor

Conjugation is a highly evolved and efficient process. Suitable mixtures of donor and recipient cells can lead to nearly complete conversion of all the recipients into donor, plasmid-containing cells. Furthermore, although some conjugative plasmids can transfer themselves only between cells of the same or closely related species, others are quite promiscuous, promoting conjugation across a wide variety of (usually Gram-negative) species. Conjugation appears to be a carefully regulated process, normally kept in check by the production of a repressor encoded by one of the *tra* genes. Interestingly, nonconjugative plasmids that happen to inhabit a cell with a conjugative plasmid can under some circumstances be transferred due to the conjugation apparatus of the latter; this process is called **plasmid mobilization.** As the later discussion of plasmids shows, their conjugal properties have enormous implications in medicine.

Conjugation is efficient, well regulated, and may cross species lines

Nonconjugative plasmids can be transferred by plasmid mobilization

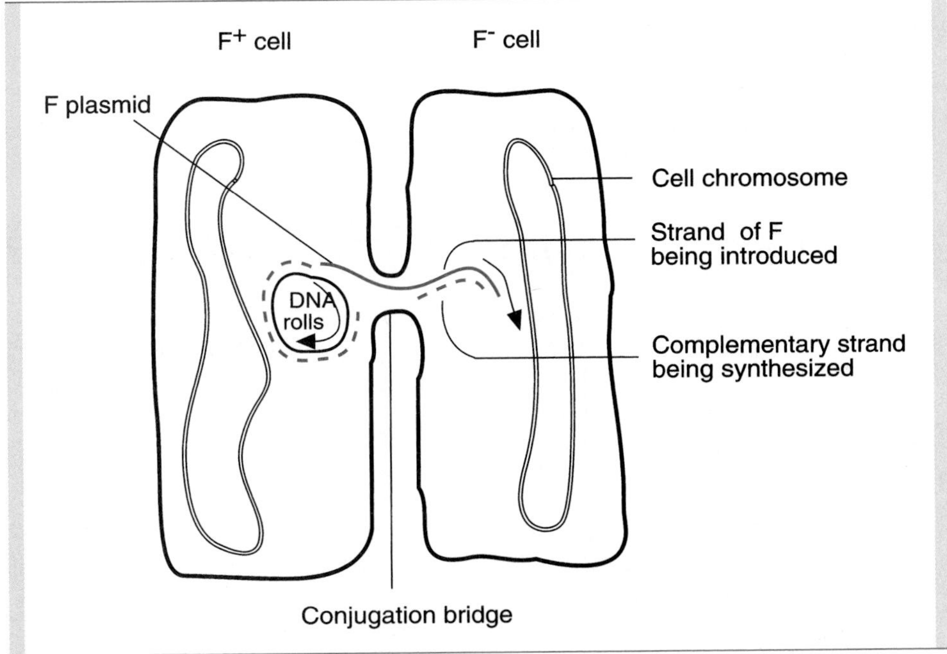

FIGURE 4–3
Bacterial conjugation resulting in the introduction of an F plasmid into an F^- cell by replicative transfer from an F^+ cell.

Conjugation in Gram-Negative Species

F factor is a conjugative plasmid that can transfer bacterial chromosome genes

After many inconclusive attempts by microbiologists to learn whether a sexual process of genetic exchange existed among bacteria, J. Lederberg and E. Tatum discovered conjugation in 1946. What they observed was a transfer of chromosomal genes between cells of two different strains of *E. coli.* Their discovery stimulated an intensive analysis of the mechanism, leading to the discovery of an agent, the **F factor** (for fertility factor), that conferred on cells the ability to transfer bacterial chromosome genes to recipient cells. Now it is recognized that the F factor is a conjugative plasmid, although an atypical one in several respects.

Rare integration of F into the bacterial chromosome leads to transfer of chromosomal genes during conjugation

The F plasmid is a normal conjugative plasmid in that it possesses many *tra* genes encoding a sex pilus (the **F-pilus**) as well as the ability to form a conjugation bridge, to initiate transfer replication, and to perform all the other steps of plasmid transfer. Thus, a cell harboring the F plasmid (an **F^+ cell**) can conjugate with a recipient **F^- cell,** and in the process the latter becomes F^+. The process is immediate and efficient because the F factor has lost autoregulation of the conjugation process. However, these properties do not explain how the F plasmid can bring about transfer of chromosomal genes, which is more closely related to another property of F—its ability to integrate at low frequency into the bacterial chromosome at seven or eight chromosomal sites, resulting in linearization of the plasmid DNA as part of the giant circular chromosomal molecule. A cell in which this integration event has occurred is designated a **high-frequency recombination** (Hfr) cell; it is only this spontaneous mutant in an F^- population that transfers donor chromosomal genes. When an Hfr cell encounters an F^- cell, conjugation occurs and the usual transfer replication is initiated at *oriT*, within the linear F segment. However, in this circumstance, breaking the integrated plasmid DNA at *oriT* results in the formation of a linear strand in which the entire bacterial chromosome lies between two portions of the F genome (Fig 4–4), and therefore the leading segment of F enters the F^- cell followed by bacterial genes one after the other. The conjugation bridge usually ruptures long before the entire bacterial chromosome can be introduced, resulting in the transfer of only one part of the F genome and a variable length of the bacterial chromosome. Thus, conjugation between an Hfr and an F^- cell leaves the recipient still F^-, but having received bacterial genes; the donor remains Hfr because it retains a copy of the chromosome with its integrated F genome. There are other fertility plasmids, but F remains the best studied.

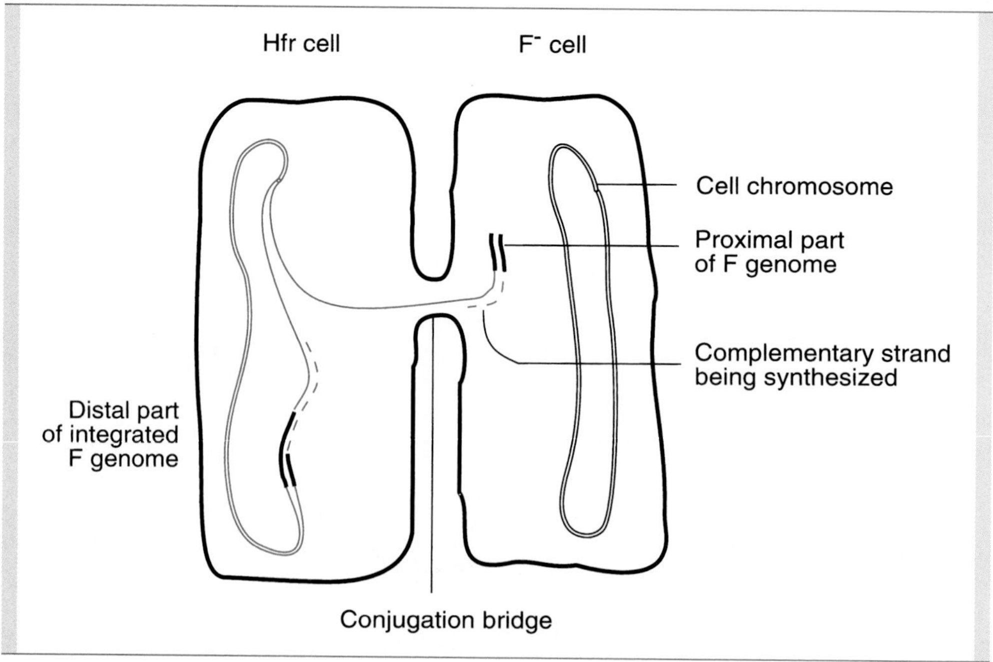

FIGURE 4–4
Bacterial conjugation resulting in the introduction of chromosomal genes and a portion of the F plasmid genome into an F^- cell by replicative transfer from a high-frequency recombination (Hfr) cell.

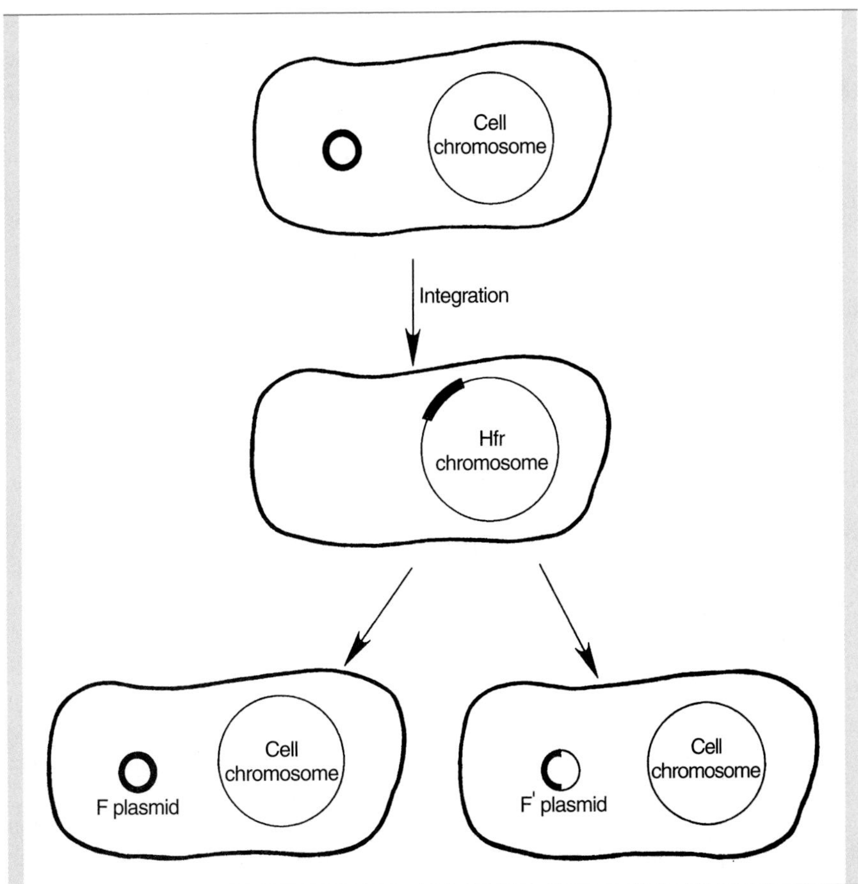

FIGURE 4–5
Integration of the F plasmid into a bacterial chromosome to form a high-frequency recombination (Hfr) chromosome, followed either by exact excision to reform the F plasmid or by inexact excision to form an F′ plasmid containing some bacterial chromosome genes.

There is an additional wrinkle to the transfer of chromosomal genes by conjugation in *E. coli*. It is a process termed **sexduction,** in which an F plasmid transfers from one cell to another a few bacterial chromosomal genes that it happens to contain. This comes about because the F genome in an Hfr cell can, at low frequency, excise itself from the chromosome and circularize into plasmid form. When this excision is imperfect, or involves recombinations with other insertion sites, segments of the bacterial chromosome can become included in the plasmid (Fig 4–5). When the resulting plasmid, called F′ to note its content of some bacterial DNA, is transmitted to recipient cells at high frequency by conjugation, the chromosomal genes are transferred as hitchhikers; this is the process of sexduction. By similar processes, segments of bacterial chromosomes can become incorporated into other plasmids, discussed later in this chapter, that confer resistance to antimicrobics.

Hybrid F′ plasmids can include segments of the bacterial chromosome and transfer them at high frequency to F^- cells during conjugation

Conjugation in Gram-Positive Species

Plasmids carrying genes encoding antimicrobic resistance, common pili and other adhesins, and some exotoxins are readily transferred by conjugation among Gram-positive bacteria in the natural environment as well as in the laboratory. However, conjugation involving chromosomal genes may differ between Gram-negative and Gram-positive species, as judged by its characteristics in two well-studied examples, *E. coli* and *Enterococcus faecalis.* Conjugation in *E. faecalis* is mediated by plasmids, but there is also an involvement of chromosomal genes in the process. Donor and recipient cells do not couple by means of a sex pilus but rather by the clumping of cells that contain a plasmid with those that do not. This clumping is the result of interaction between a proteinaceous **adhesin** on the surface of the donor (plasmid-containing) cell and a **receptor** on the surface of the recipient (plasmid-lacking) cell. Both types of cells make the receptor (possibly cell wall lipoteichoic acid), but only the plasmid-containing cell can make the adhesin, presumably because it is encoded by a plasmid gene. Interestingly, donor cells make the adhesin only when in the vicinity of recipient

E. faecalis coupling results from adhesin–receptor interaction

Plasmid-encoded *E. faecalis* adhesin is produced in response to recipient pheromone

cells because the recipients secrete small peptide **pheromones** that serve to notify the donor cells of the presence of recipients. Donor cells promptly make adhesin when they sense the pheromone. As a result, clumps are formed, and plasmid DNA is transferred across conjugation bridges into the recipient cells held in the clumps.

Some Gram-positive conjugal transfers may be mediated by DNA elements that are only transiently plasmids

In addition to enterococcal species, species of *Bacillus*, *Staphylococcus,* and *Clostridium* have been found to contain conjugative plasmids. Conjugative transfer of genes has also been observed in a number of Gram-positive species in the apparent absence of plasmid DNA. In several instances these transfers involve conjugative transposons (to be discussed later in this chapter), and it appears that a plasmid intermediate is formed, although only transiently.

Before continuing with our discussion of plasmids, we should complete the story of what happens to DNA introduced into recipient cells by any of the three transfer processes, transformation, transduction, and conjugation.

GENETIC RECOMBINATION

Exogenote may be degraded, circularized, or integrated into recipient chromosome

By whatever means an exogenote is conveyed into a recipient cell, its effect depends on what happens after transfer. There are basically three possible fates. The exogenote DNA may be degraded by a nuclease, in which case no heritable change is brought about. It may be stabilized by circularization and remain separate from the endogenote. In this case, if it is unable to replicate, it will be unilinearly inherited (eg, abortive transduction). If it is capable of self-replication, it will become established as an autonomous, inherited plasmid. The third possible fate is **recombination** between exogenote and endogenote, resulting in the formation of a partially hybrid chromosome with segments derived from each source. These possibilities are diagrammed in Figure 4–6.

In this section we examine the two principal processes by which recombinant chromosomes are formed following genetic transfer: homologous recombination and site-specific recombination. A third sort of recombinational process exists, called **illegitimate recombination,** because it does not obey the legitimate laws governing homologous

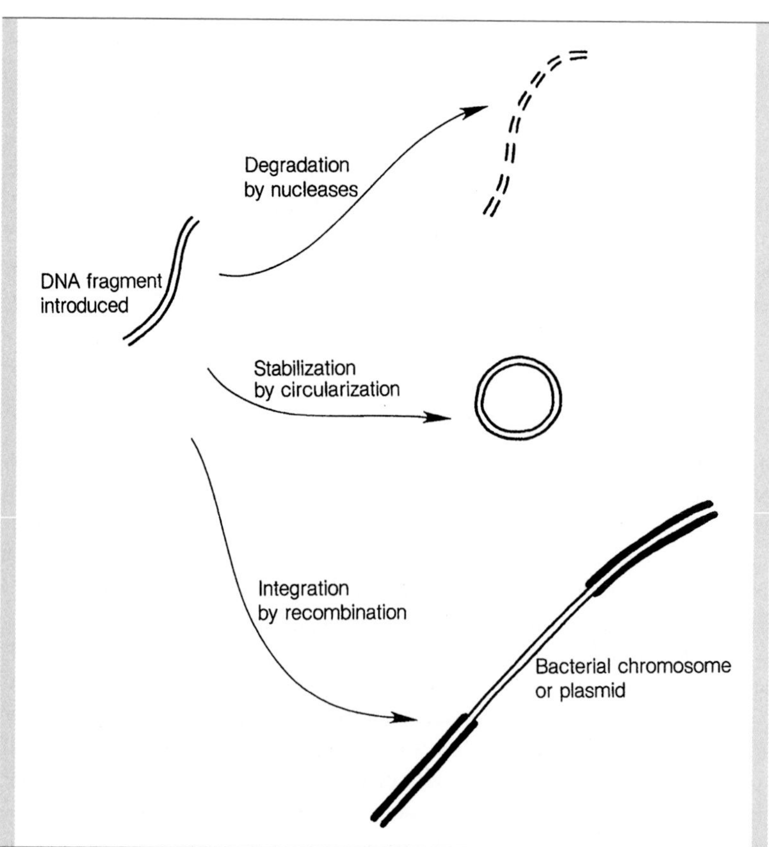

FIGURE 4–6
Possible fates of a DNA fragment after transfer into a bacterial cell.

and site-specific recombination. Little is known other than it results in some types of gene duplications and deletions, and this chapter shall say no more about it.

Homologous Recombination

One mechanism by which an exogenote can recombine with the bacterial chromosome is called **homologous recombination.** This term reflects one of the two requirements for this process: (1) the exogenote must possess reasonably large regions of nucleotide sequence identity or similarity to segments of the endogenote chromosome, because extensive base pairing must occur between strands of the two recombining molecules; and (2) the recipient cell must possess the genetic ability to make a set of enzymes that can bring about the covalent substitution of a segment of the exogenote for the homologous region of the endogenote. Not all the details are known, but the latter process includes breaking one strand of each recombining molecule at a time and pairing it with the unbroken, complementary strand of the other molecule. The ends of the broken strands are partially digested, then repaired and joined so that the rejoined strands are now continuous between the chromosomes. A protein known as RecA (recombination) controls the entire process. The same **breakage** and **reunion** process then links the second strand of each recombining DNA molecule. This **crossover** event repeated further down the chromosome results in the substitution of the exogenote segment between the two crossovers for the homologous segment of the endogenote. This process is schematically presented in a very simplified form in Figure 4–7. Homologous recombination is responsible for integration of DNA fragments transferred by generalized transduction, by plasmid-mediated conjugation, and by natural transformation.

Homologous recombination involves nucleotide similarity and specific enzymes such as RecA

Homologous recombination can follow generalized transduction, conjugation, or transformation

Site-Specific Recombination

The second major type of recombination is actually a group of separate mechanisms that are RecA independent, that rely on only limited DNA sequence similarity at the sites of crossover, and that are mediated by different sets of specialized enzymes designed to catalyze recombination of only certain DNA molecules. The name for this large group of mechanisms, **site-specific recombination,** reflects the fact that these recombinational events are restricted to specific sites on one or both of the recombining DNA molecules. The enzymes that bring about site-specific recombination operate not on the basis of

Site-specific recombination is RecA independent and requires enzymes that operate only on unique sequences

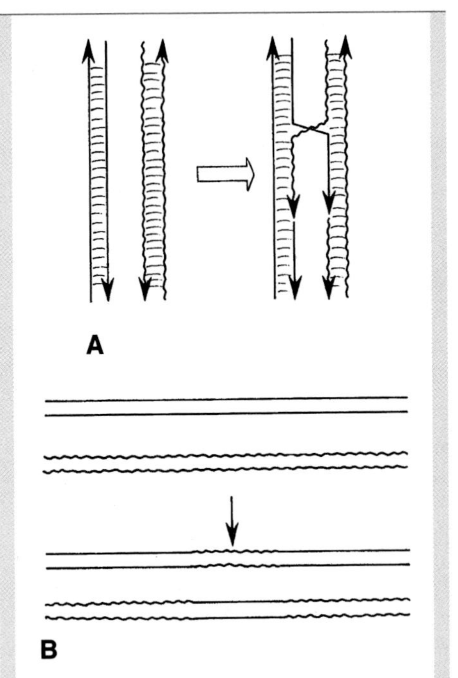

FIGURE 4–7
Homologous recombination. **A.** Central event in homologous recombination. Extensive base pairing between homologous regions of strands of two DNA molecules is illustrated. Events that accompany or follow this event include strand nicking, migration of the crossover point with partial digestion of the nicked strands, and resynthesis and ligation. Both strands of both recombining molecules must participate to effect a crossover event. **B.** Result of homologous recombination. Two crossover events are necessary to achieve the exchange of segments shown.

Enzymes are usually encoded by exogenote genes

DNA homology but on recognition of unique DNA sequences that form the borders of the specific sites. These enzymes are commonly encoded by genes on the exogenote.

Integration of many prophages occurs by site-specific recombination

One good example of site-specific recombination has already been shown. The integration of some phage genomes into the chromosome occurs only at one site on the bacterial chromosome and one site on the phage chromosome. It was noted briefly that some phages, notably phage Mu, differ in being able to integrate almost anywhere in the bacterial chromosome. Because the site of recombination (the crossover site) in the Mu genome is the same in all cases, this, too, is a case of site-specific recombination.

In addition to the special kind of recombination represented by prophage integration, a particular form of site-specific recombination occurs in other situations of enormous consequence to medical microbiology. These involve special genetic units called transposable elements, which have proven to be so important in the life of bacteria, particularly in their roles in the pathogenesis of infectious disease, that a separate section must be devoted to their description.

TRANSPOSABLE ELEMENTS

Transposable elements are genetic units that move within and between chromosomes and plasmids by means of specific transposases

Transposable elements are genetic units that are capable of mediating their own transfer from one chromosome to another, from one location to another on the same chromosome, or between chromosome and plasmid. This **transposition** relies on their ability to synthesize their own site-specific recombination enzymes, called **transposases.**

The three major kinds of transposable elements are **insertion sequence** elements; **transposons;** and certain prophages, such as Mu.

Insertion Sequence Elements

Insertion sequence (IS) elements are segments of DNA of approximately 1000 bp. They encode enzymes for site-specific recombination and have distinctive nucleotide sequences at their termini. Different IS elements have different termini, but, as illustrated in Figure 4–8, a given IS element has the same sequence of nucleotides at each end, but in an inverted order. Only genes involved in transposition (eg, one encoding a transposase) and in the regulation of its frequency are included in IS elements, and they are therefore the simplest transposable elements.

IS elements encode only proteins for their own transposition

Because IS elements contain only genes for transposition, their presence in a chromosome is not always easy to detect. However, if an IS element transposes to a new site that is within a gene, this insertion is actually a mutation that alters or destroys the activity of the gene. Because most IS elements contain a transcription termination signal, the insertion also eliminates transcription of any genes downstream in the same operon. This property of IS elements led to their first recognition. Reversion of insertion mutations can occur by deletion, but the frequency of deletion is 100- to 1000-fold lower than that of insertion.

Insertion of IS elements into a gene causes mutation

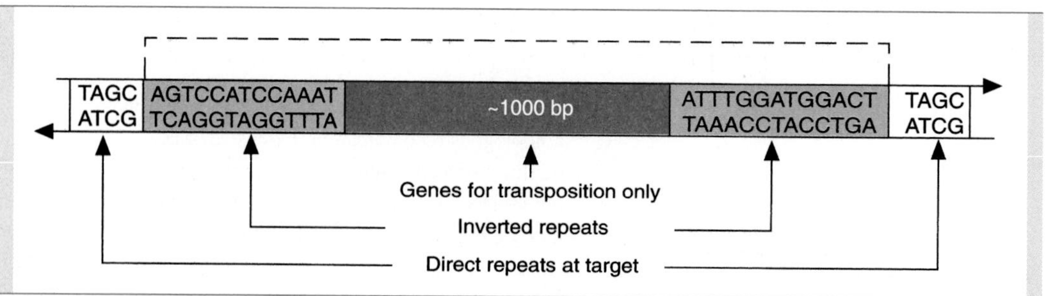

FIGURE 4–8

Structure of an insertion sequence (IS) element. The general features of bacterial IS elements are illustrated. As an example, IS2 has a total of 1327 bp, of which there are terminal inverted repeat sequences of 41 bp flanking the central region that encodes the one or two proteins required for transposition of IS2. A direct repeat of 5 bp was created at the site of insertion of the element. Approximately five IS2 elements are found in the chromosome of many strains of *Escherichia coli.*

Numerous IS elements reside naturally at different locations in *E. coli* chromosomes and in *E. coli* plasmids, and this has many consequences for the cell. Because their size is sufficient to permit strong base pairing between different copies of the same IS element, they can provide the basis for RecA-mediated homologous recombination. In this manner, the presence of particular IS elements in both the F plasmid and the bacterial chromosome provides a means for the formation of Hfr molecules by cointegration using IS sequence homology and the RecA system.

Base pairing between copies of IS elements can promote homologous recombination

Transposons

One of the major aspects of IS elements is that they are components of **transposons** (Tn elements), which are transposable segments of DNA containing genes beyond those needed for transposition. Transposons are as much as 10-fold larger than IS elements. One class, of which transposon Tn10 is a good example, are composite structures consisting of a central area of genes bordered by IS elements. The genes may code for such properties as antimicrobic resistance, substrate metabolism, or other functions. A generalized transposon structure of the Tn10 variety is shown in Figure 4–9.

Transposons encode functions beyond those needed for their own transposition

Some transposons are bordered by IS elements

Composite transposons of the Tn10 sort can translocate by what is called simple or **direct transposition,** in which the transposon is excised from its original location and inserted without replication into its new site. A second class, typified by transposon Tn3, has inverted repeat sequences rather than IS elements at its ends and encodes not only a transposase but also an enzyme called a **resolvase.** Transposition of Tn3 involves formation of a **cointegrate** of the two DNA molecules (or segments of the same molecule) involved in the transposition—that is, the one carrying the Tn3 and the one serving as the target. Replication of the transposon then occurs, and the resolvase separates (resolves) the cointegrate, restoring the two DNA molecules, each now with its own copy of Tn3. Transposition of this sort is called **replicative** or **duplicative transposition.**

Direct transposition moves the transposon from its original site to a new site

Replicative transposition leaves a copy of the transposon at its original site

Besides the primary insertion reaction, all transposable units promote other types of DNA rearrangements, including deletion of sequences adjacent to a transposon, inversion of DNA segments, fusion of separate plasmids within a cell, similar fusions that integrate plasmids with the cell chromosome, and repeated duplications that result in **amplification** of genes within transposons. All of these events have great significance for understanding the formation and spread of antimicrobic resistance through natural populations of pathogenic organisms. These subjects are discussed in the description of plasmids in the next section.

Transposons promote many changes in DNA

Some strains of streptococci harbor transposon-like, drug-resistance elements within their chromosome that are capable of mediating their own transfer to other cells by conjugation. One such **conjugative transposon** is Tn916, found originally in a strain of *E. faecalis*. This element, approximately 16 kb in size, contains a gene for tetracycline resistance. It and similar elements resemble transposons in many respects, including size, multiple target sites, ability to transfer from a chromosome to a plasmid, and ability to be removed from a plasmid or a chromosome by precise excision. What is unusual, however, is their ability to mediate their own intercellular transfer. It now appears that Tn916, and presumably similar elements, can form a transient plasmid-like structure as part of the process of conjugational transfer.

Conjugative transposons can mediate their own transfer between cells

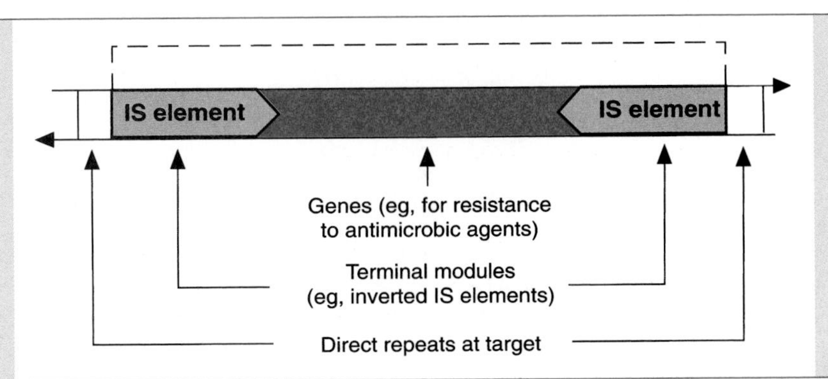

FIGURE 4–9
Structure of a composite transposon. The general features of bacterial transposons resembling Tn10 are illustrated. Tn10 has a total of 9500 bp. It consists of terminal direct-repeat IS10 elements flanking a central region that contains a gene for tetracycline resistance and genes needed for transposition.

The prophage of phage Mu is a transposon

The third type of transposable element is **transposable prophage,** such as that of bacteriophage Mu, which has the alternative of lytic growth or of lysogeny. During lysogeny, the prophage of Mu can insert virtually anywhere in the *E. coli* chromosome and later can transpose itself from one location to another. In fact, it is a transposon. When it integrates within a bacterial gene, it inactivates it in the same manner as any other transposable element. It was originally recognized as a virus that causes mutation, hence its name.

Invertible DNA Segments and Recombinational Regulation of Gene Expression

Phase variation can be brought about by a recombinational event

A fascinating aspect of DNA rearrangements brought about by genetic recombination is that the expression of some chromosomal genes important in virulence are actually controlled by recombinational events. All the known cases involve **phase variation** of surface antigens. In *N. gonorrhoeae,* the bacteria that causes gonorrhea (see Chapter 20), multiple genes encoding antigenically different pilin sequences exist throughout the chromosome. Many, called *pilS*, are silent because they lack effective promoters; some are only fragments of pilin sequences. These silent genes or gene fragments serve as a reservoir of antigenic variability; each can, wholly or in part, become inserted by RecA-dependent homologous recombination into an actively expressed gene (*pilE*), resulting in the synthesis of a new pilin. The entire process resembles the insertion of cassette tapes into a tape player and, therefore, is referred to as the **cassette mode** of gene regulation (Fig 4–10).

Invertible elements can act as a genetic switch

A different DNA rearrangement is responsible for the alternation of expression of antigenically distinct flagellins, H1 and H2, in *Salmonella* species. An **invertible element** of 995 bp lies between the two flagellin genes (Fig 4–11). The phase-2 encoding gene (B) lies in an operon that also encodes a repressor for the phase-1 encoding gene (C). The latter gene is, therefore, active only if the former operon is inactive. Activity of the phase-2 operon, which

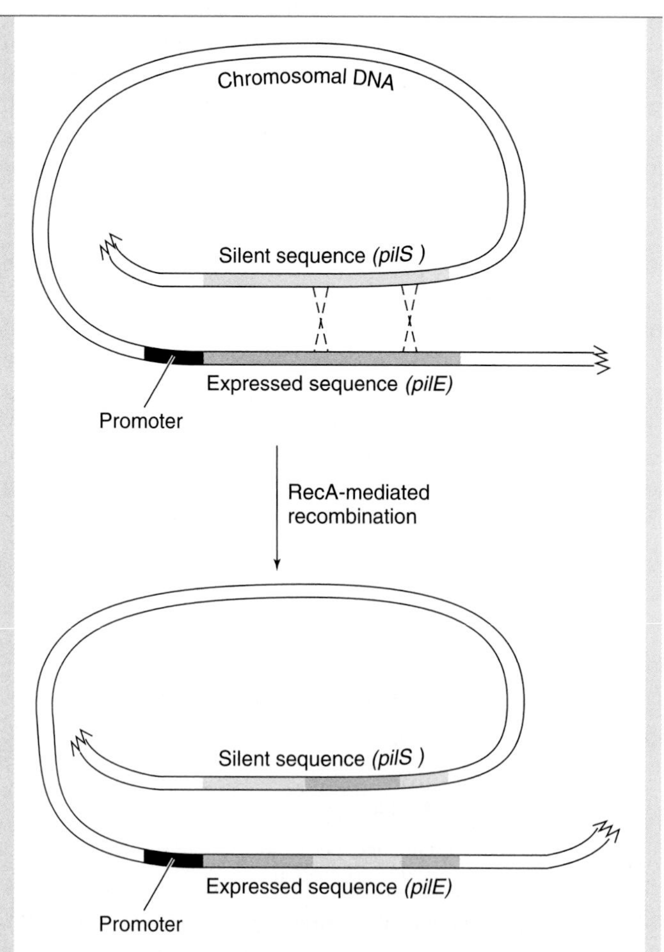

FIGURE 4–10
Schematic diagram illustrating phase variation of surface antigens in *Neisseria gonorrhoeae* by the cassette mode of gene regulation involving recombination at an expression site.

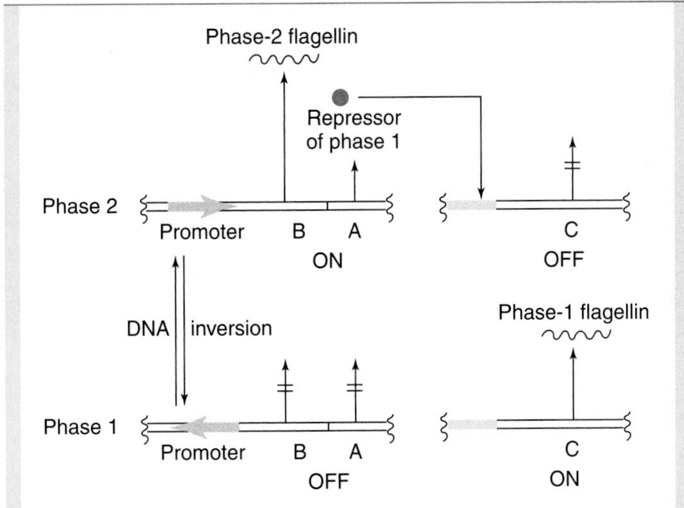

FIGURE 4–11
Schematic diagram illustrating alternate expression of flagellins in *Salmonella* by a genetic switch composed of an invertible element. (*Adapted from Macnab RM. Flagella and motility. In: Neidhardt FC, Curtiss R III, Ingraham JL, et al,* Escherichia coli and Salmonella: Cellular and Molecular Biology, Washington DC: ASM Press; 1966. pp 123–145.)

lacks its own promoter, depends on a promoter within the invertible element. In one orientation, this promoter can initiate transcription of the B gene; in the other orientation transcription, if it starts, proceeds in the opposite direction, and the B gene is silent, allowing the C gene to work. In this manner, excision of the invertible element and its reinsertion at the same site but in the opposite orientation lead to a shift from one flagellar form to the other (ie, to antigenic phase variation). The invertible element encodes its own site-specific **recombinase enzyme** that catalyzes the inversion in response to currently unknown signals. A similar situation exists in *E. coli,* where a 314-bp invertible segment containing a promoter controls transcription of the adjacent, promoter-less *fimA* gene. This gene encodes the structural protein for type 1 (common) pili, which function as an adhesin in mediating the binding of *E. coli* to eukaryotic cells, thereby aiding in the early stages of tissue colonization by these bacteria.

It is believed that antigenic variation mediated by these site-specific transpositional rearrangements provides a selective advantage to the bacteria in allowing invading populations to include individuals that can escape the developing immune response of the host and thus continue the infectious process. Similar strategies are used by some eukaryotic parasites of humans, notably the trypanosomes (see Chapter 54).

MORE ABOUT BACTERIAL PLASMIDS

One of the unanticipated features of microbial genetics has been the revelation that many virulence factors and much clinically significant resistance to antibiotics are the result of the activities not of bacterial chromosomal genes but of the accessory genomes present in plasmids. In a certain sense, the health professional treating infectious disease is frequently coping with autonomous self-replicating DNA molecules. Many of the properties of plasmids have already been touched on, but the information is now consolidated and considered in more detail.

General Properties and Varieties of Plasmids

We have already encountered plasmids in our consideration of conjugation. To recap, plasmids are ubiquitous extrachromosomal elements composed of double-stranded DNA that typically is circular (Fig 4–12). (Linear plasmids occur in medically relevant strains of *Borrelia*.) A single organism can harbor several distinct plasmids. Like the chromosome, they have the property of governing their own replication by means of special sequences and regulatory proteins, including a genetic region called *ori* (origin of replication) at which specific proteins initiate replication. Any DNA molecule that is self-reproducing, including all plasmids as well as the bacterial chromosome, is said to be a **replicon.**

Plasmids are replicons found in most bacterial species in nature

Plasmids vary greatly in size, in the mode of control of their replication, and in the number and kinds of genes they carry. Naturally occurring plasmids range from less than

Plasmids very greatly in size and control of replication

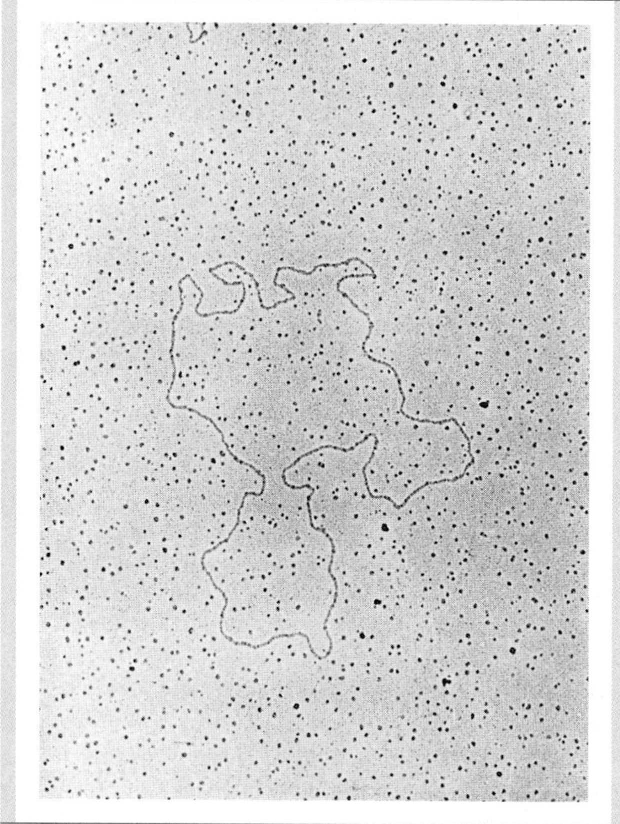

FIGURE 4–12
Electron micrograph of an R plasmid from *Escherichia coli*. The plasmid is 64 megadaltons and contains about 40 kilobase pairs. (*Courtesy of Dr. Jorge H. Crosa.*)

5 million to more than 100 million daltons, but even the largest are only a few percent of the size of the bacterial chromosome. The number of molecules of a given plasmid that is present in a cell, called the **copy number,** varies greatly among different plasmids, from only a few molecules per cell to dozens of molecules per cell. In general, small plasmids tend to be represented by more copies per cell.

Small plasmids are often present in multiple copies per cell

Conjugal transfer is an important property of those plasmids that possess the complex of *tra* genes, but even nonconjugative plasmids can transfer to some extent to other cells as a result of mobilization by conjugative plasmids. Some plasmids, again including the F factor, can replicate either autonomously or as a segment of DNA integrated into the chromosome. These are sometimes termed **episomes.** Certain prophages can exist as plasmids, but most plasmids are not viruses, because at no point of their life cycle do they exist as a free viral particle (**virion**). Most plasmids show little or no DNA homology with the chromosome and can, in this sense, be regarded as foreign to the cell.

Conjugative plasmids can facilitate transfer of nonconjugatives

Some plasmids, called episomes, can integrate and replicate with the chromosome

Most plasmids are nonhomologous with the host cell chromosome

Plasmids usually include a number of genes in addition to those required for their replication and transfer to other cells. The variety of cellular properties associated with plasmids is very great and includes fertility (the capacity for gene transfer by conjugation), production of toxins, production of pili and other adhesins, resistance to antimicrobics and other toxic chemicals, production of bacteriocins (toxic proteins that kill some other bacteria), production of siderophores for scavenging Fe^{3+}, and production of certain catabolic enzymes important in biodegradation of organic residues.

Bacterial adaptation to environment depends heavily on properties encoded by plasmids

Many plasmid genes promote survival and colonization and hence pathogenesis

On the other hand, plasmids can add a small metabolic burden to the cell, and in many cases, a slightly reduced growth rate results. Thus, under conditions of laboratory cultivation where the properties coded by the plasmid are not required, there is a tendency for **curing** of a strain to occur, because the progeny cells that have not acquired a plasmid (or have lost it) have a selective advantage during prolonged growth and subculture. Conversely, where the property conferred by the plasmid is advantageous (eg, in the presence of the antimicrobic to which the plasmid determines resistance), selective pressure favors the plasmid-carrying strain.

In absence of selection pressure for their properties, plasmids may be lost due to spontaneous curing

Although plasmids are central to infectious disease and have been studied for decades, their origin remains uncertain. They could possibly be descendants of bacterial viruses that evolved a sophisticated means of self-transfer by conjugation and then lost their unneeded protein capsid. Alternatively, they may have evolved as separated parts of a bacterial chromosome that could provide both the means for genetic exchange and a way to amplify certain genes of special value in a particular environment (eg, coding for an adhesin) or to dispense with them where they are superfluous.

Plasmids could have any of several theoretically possible origins

A great many bacterial plasmids are known. Some show similarity with each other in nucleotide sequence; thus, plasmids can be classified by their degree of apparent relatedness. Unrelated plasmids can coexist within a single cell, but closely related plasmids become segregated during cell division and eventually all but one are eliminated. For this reason, a group of closely related plasmids that exclude each other are referred to as an **incompatibility group.**

Cells may harbor more than one plasmid type provided they are unrelated to each other

R Plasmids

Plasmids that include genes conferring resistance to antimicrobics are of great significance to medicine. They are termed **R plasmids** or **R factors** (**resistance factors**). The genes responsible for resistance usually code for enzymes that inactivate antimicrobics or reduce the cell's permeability to them. In contrast, resistance conferred by chromosomal mutation usually involves modification of the target of the antimicrobics (eg, RNA polymerase or the ribosome).

Plasmids confer resistance by inactivating antimicrobics or reducing their entry

R plasmids occupy center stage in approaches to chemotherapy because of the constellation of properties they possess. Those of Gram-negative bacteria can be transmitted across species boundaries and, at lower frequency, even between genera. Many encode resistance to several antimicrobics and can thus spread multiple resistance through a diverse microbial population under selective pressure of only one of those agents to which they confer resistance. Nonpathogenic bacteria can serve as a natural reservoir of resistance determinants on plasmids that are available for spread to pathogens.

R plasmids can encode and transfer multiresistance

R plasmids evolve rapidly and can easily acquire additional resistance-determining genes from fusion with other plasmids or acquisition of transposons. Many have the capability of amplifying the number of copies of their resistance genes either by gene duplications within each plasmid or by increasing the number of plasmids (copy number) per cell. By these means resistance can be achieved to very high concentrations of the antimicrobic. One process of gene amplification is based on the ability of some conjugative plasmids to dissociate their components into two plasmids, one (called the **resistance transfer factor**) containing genes for replication and for transfer and another (called the **resistance** or **r determinant**) containing genes for replication and for resistance. Subsequent relaxed replication of the r determinant expands the cell's capacity to produce the resistance-conferring enzyme (Fig 4–13).

Resistance genes can be acquired by plasmids from transposons or through plasmid fusion

Resistance genes can be amplified by increasing copy number

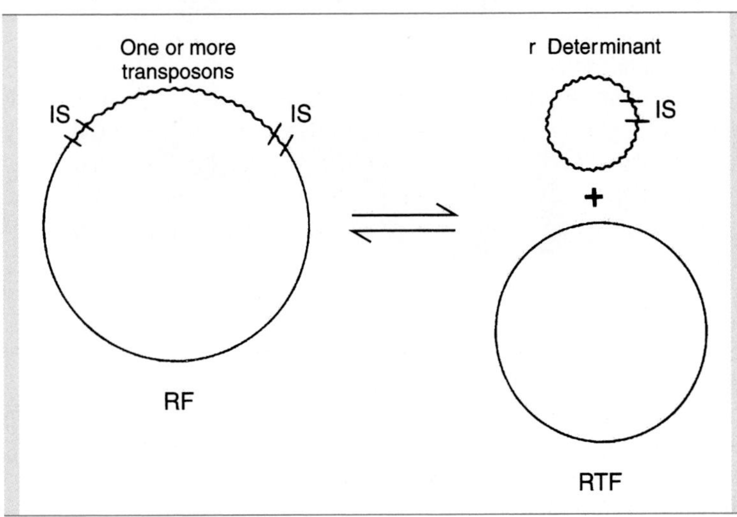

FIGURE 4–13
Structure and dissociation of an R-factor (RF) plasmid. The RF plasmid is shown with its two components: the r determinant, which contains one or more genes for antibiotic resistance (frequently present as transposons), and the resistance transfer factor (RTF), which contains the genes necessary for replication of the plasmid and its transfer to other cells. IS, insertion resistance.

Over the past three decades, many of the molecular feats of R plasmids have been explained on the basis of known genetic and evolutionary mechanisms. The discovery of transposable elements (insertion sequences and transposons) and their properties provides an explanation for many of these phenomena. Most plasmids, and all R factors, contain many IS elements and transposons. In fact, virtually all the resistance determinant genes on plasmids are present as transposons. As a result, these genes can be amplified by tandem duplications on the plasmid and can hop to other plasmids (or to the bacterial chromosome) in the same cell. Combined with the natural properties of many plasmids to transfer themselves by conjugation (even between dissimilar bacterial species), the rapid evolutionary development of multiple drug resistance plasmids and their spread through populations of pathogenic bacteria during the past three decades can be seen as a predictable result of natural selection resulting from the widespread and intensive use of antimicrobics in human and veterinary medicine (see Chapter 14).

Resistance spread is facilitated by transposition of plasmid genes for resistance

Widespread use of antimicrobics selects formation and spread of R plasmids

The properties of transposons can explain the present-day ubiquity and mobility of resistance genes but not their origin. Two facts help point to at least a direction in which to search for an answer. First, R plasmids carrying the genes encoding antimicrobic-inactivating enzymes have been found in bacterial cultures preserved by lyophilization (freeze-drying) since before the era of antimicrobic therapy; an accelerated evolutionary development need not be invoked. Second, the enzymes themselves are remarkably similar to those found in certain bacteria (*Streptomyces* spp) that produce many clinically useful antimicrobics. Perhaps a long time ago there was a cross-genus transfer of genetic information (by transformation?) that became stabilized on plasmids under the selection pressure of an antimicrobic released into the environment under natural conditions.

Resistance genes preexisted antimicrobic use in medicine

Detection of Plasmids

A number of physical, morphologic, and functional tests can be used to reveal the presence of plasmids in a bacterial population. The rapid transfer of characteristics, such as resistance to antimicrobics, from strain to strain or, alternatively, the rapid loss of such traits is a hallmark of plasmid-encoded characteristics. When several genetically distinct characteristics are transferred simultaneously in the laboratory into cells known not to have possessed them previously, the evidence is very strong that a plasmid is responsible. Plasmids, including nonconjugative plasmids and those coding for no presently known trait, can be

Plasmid involvement is implicated by rapid transfer of multiresistance

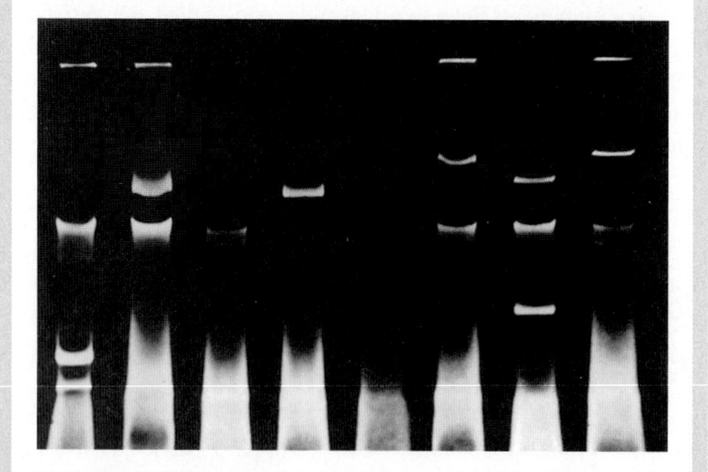

FIGURE 4–14

Agarose gel electrophoresis of various strains of staphylococci isolated from patients in a large metropolitan hospital. Each vertical lane displays the DNA of a separate isolate. The sharp bands visible in the upper half of most lanes are plasmids. The broad smear of DNA in the lower half is chromosomal DNA. The results illustrate the prevalence of multiple plasmids in freshly isolated bacterial strains. Most isolates contain more than one plasmid. (*Courtesy of Dr. D. R. Schaberg, University of Michigan.*)

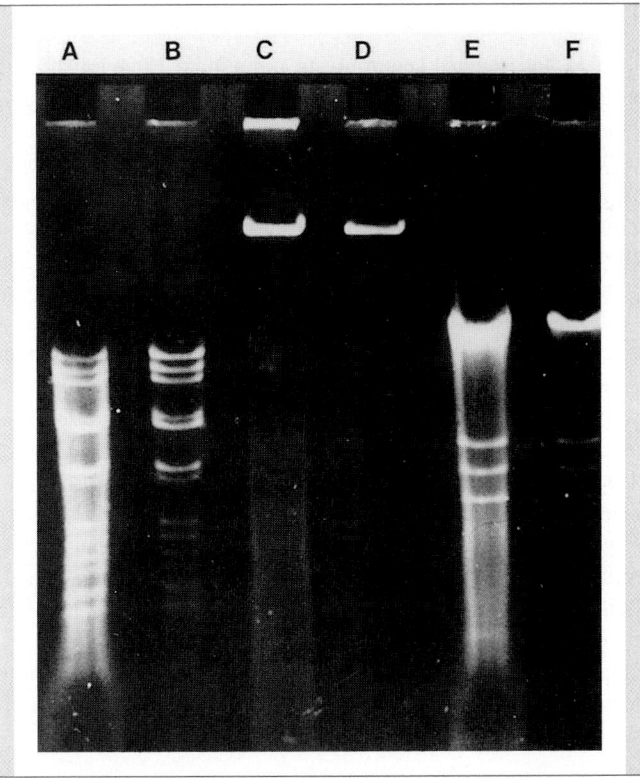

FIGURE 4–15
Use of agarose gel electrophoresis in molecular epidemiology. During an outbreak of bacteremia in infants in a neonatal intensive care unit, strains of *Klebsiella aerogenes* and *Enterobacter cloacae* were isolated that harbored R-factor plasmids of similar electrophoretic mobility and conferred resistance to some aminoglycosides, ampicillin, and chloramphenicol. To learn if an identical plasmid had established itself in both bacterial species, a restriction digest analysis was performed and the products were separated by electrophoresis. Lanes C and D display the intact plasmid DNA isolated from *K. aerogenes* and *E. cloacae,* respectively. Lanes A and B display the fragments produced by the action of the restriction enzyme *Bam*HI on the plasmids, and lanes E and F display the fragments produced by the restriction enzyme *Eco*RI. For each pair of treated samples, the plasmid DNA from *K. aerogenes* is on the left (ie, lanes A and E). The identical restriction patterns make it almost certain that the plasmids from the two bacterial species are identical, and raise the possibility that the epidemic itself was caused by the chance introduction and spread of this R plasmid. (*Kindly provided by Dr. D. R. Schaberg, University of Michigan.*)

demonstrated directly by agarose gel electrophoresis. These methods and their diagnostic application are discussed in Chapter 15. Electron microscopy can also be used to visualize plasmids, to measure the length of their DNA, and to see the forms they take on hybridization to other nucleic acid molecules (see Fig 4–12).

Plasmid DNAs are separable electrophoretically

Bacterial plasmids, including R factors, have become valuable markers for comparing closely related strains of bacteria in epidemiologic studies. In outbreaks, spread of an epidemic strain can sometimes be followed more easily and more accurately by monitoring the profile of plasmids carried in strains isolated from different patients than by using traditional typing methods (Fig 4–14). This approach is particularly useful in studying outbreaks of nosocomial (hospital-acquired) infections. Likewise, the spread of an R plasmid between different species can be followed by showing that they carry an identical plasmid conferring the same pattern of antimicrobic resistance. The plasmid comparison can be carried one step further in specificity by cutting the plasmid DNA with specific restriction endonucleases (see next section) and examining the resulting fragments by agarose gel electrophoresis (Fig 4–15). Variations of this procedure enable even the spread of specific genes among a variety of plasmids to be detected.

Tracing plasmids is valuable in the epidemiology of disease outbreaks

Endonuclease digestion is useful in comparing plasmids

BACTERIAL CLASSIFICATION

Bacteria are classified into genera and species according to a binomial Linnean scheme similar to that used for higher organisms. For example, in the case of *Staphylococcus aureus, Staphylococcus* is the name of the **genus** and *aureus* is the **species** designation. Some genera with common characteristics are further grouped into **families.** However, bacterial classification has posed many problems. Morphologic descriptors are not as abundant as in higher plants and animals, there is little readily interpreted fossil record to help establish phylogeny, and there is no elaborate developmental process (ontogeny) to recapitulate the evolutionary path from ancestral forms (phylogeny). These problems are minor compared with others: bacteria mutate and evolve rapidly, they reproduce asexually, and they exchange genetic material over wide boundaries. The single most important test of species, the ability of individuals within a species to reproduce sexually by mating and exchanging genetic material, cannot be applied to bacteria. As a result, bacterial taxonomy developed pragmatically by determining multiple characteristics and weighting them according to which seemed most fundamental; for example, shape, spore formation, Gram reaction, aerobic or anaerobic growth, and temperature for growth were given special weighting in defining genera. Such properties as ability to ferment particular carbohydrates, production of specific enzymes and toxins, and antigenic composition of cell surface components were often used in defining species. As presented in Chapter 15, such properties and their weighting continue to be of central importance in identification of unknown isolates in the clinical laboratory, and the use of determinative keys is based on the concept of such weighted characteristics. These approaches are much less sound in establishing taxonomic relationships based on phylogenetic principles.

Weighted classification schemes are more valuable for identification than for taxonomy

New Taxonomic Methods

The recognition that sound taxonomy ought to be based on the genetic similarity of organisms and to reflect their phylogenetic **relatedness** has led in recent years to the use of new methods and new principles in taxonomy. The first approach was to apply **Adansonian** or **numeric taxonomy,** which gives equal weighting to a large number of independent characteristics and allocates bacteria to groups according to the proportion of shared characteristics as determined statistically. Theoretically, a significant correspondence of a large number of phenotypic characteristics could be considered to reflect genetic relatedness.

Degrees of genetic similarity are important for sound taxonomy

A more direct approach available in recent years involves analysis of chromosomal DNA. Analysis can be somewhat crude, such as the overall ratio of A–T to G–C base pairs; differences of greater than 10% in G–C content are taken to indicate unrelatedness, but closely similar content does not imply relatedness. Closer relationships can be assessed by determining base sequence similarity, as by DNA–DNA hybridization, in which single strands of DNA from one organism are allowed to anneal with single strands of another. Some clinical laboratory tests have been devised based on the ability of DNA from a reference strain to undergo homologous recombination with DNA from an unknown isolate (see Chapter 15). However, overwhelmingly the molecular genetic technique that is introducing the greatest change in infectious disease diagnosis is the comparison of nucleotide sequences of genes highly conserved in evolution, such as 16 S ribosomal RNA genes. So successful have been the deductions of phylogenetic relatedness based on these sequences that the absence of a fossil record is now regarded as insignificant. Part of the excitement in this field is that the use of polymerase chain reaction to amplify the DNA of cells has made it possible to identify even infectious organisms that cannot be cultivated in the laboratory.

Phylogentic relationships are assuming greater significance as the result of DNA sequence analysis

Genomic Approaches to Virulence

The most startling recent advance in medical microbiology is indicated by the fact that in the few years since the printing of the previous edition of this book, the complete nucleotide sequences of the genomes of several dozen medically significant bacteria have been determined. Furthermore, advances in the technology of DNA sequencing promise the rapid determination of many more genomes in the next few years. It is difficult to overstate the significance of the present situation. First, comparison of virulent with nonvirulent species of closely related bacteria is providing means to identify virulence genes, that is, genes responsible for the disease-producing capability of these bacteria. Second, thanks to the sequence information, the products of these genes can readily be produced and studied, and mutants can be prepared for genetic and functional analysis. Among the genes being discovered in this way are many organisms of hitherto unknown virulence, providing new information about the many molecular processes involved in pathogenesis. Third, new information on virulence factors and how they work is suggesting new, rational design of therapeutic and prophylactic agents to replace our current overreliance on natural antimicrobics and their chemical derivatives.

Finally, detailed genomic analysis of pathogens involves suggesting pathways of the evolution of important human and animal pathogens. Already, molecular genetic studies have uncovered the existence of pathogenicity islands (PAIs) within genomes—that is, groups of adjacent genes that encode functions important for colonization, invasion, avoidance of host defenses, and production of tissue damage. These PAIs exist not only within the chromosome of pathogens but also within the plasmids that assist in conferring virulence properties on the bacteria. As described in Chapter 10, analysis of PAIs provides important clues to the origin of these gene clusters and to their transmission between species. This should be a fertile area for understanding the evolution of pathogens.

Genome sequences will greatly accelerate studies on infectious disease processes, their evolution, and their successful management

POPULATION GENETICS OF PATHOGENS

One of the discoveries to come from the application of molecular diagnostic tools to infectious diseases is the clonal nature of many infectious diseases. That is, over long periods and large geographic distances, the organisms of a given species isolated from clinical samples tend to be so similar in chromosomal genetic makeup (and in their plasmid profiles) that one is forced to envision that a clone of bacteria descended from a relatively recent common ancestor is responsible for all or most of the disease incidence. This evidence comes partly from studies of **plasmid profiles,** but mostly it is a conclusion drawn by examining the specific alleles of various genes present in a population of cells using the technique of **multilocus enzyme electrophoresis.** Differences in electrophoretic migration are used to detect subtle differences in amino acid sequence in a battery of two to three dozen different enzymes. The results have been striking. For example, isolates of *Bordetella pertussis* from the United States represent a single clone, whereas in Japan there is a slightly different clone. Another study has determined that only 11 multilocus genotypes (clones) of *Neisseria meningitidis* have been responsible for the major epidemics of serogroup A organisms worldwide over the past 60 years. These discoveries provide an entirely new method for study of the epidemiology of infectious disease.

Natural populations of many pathogens are proving to have a clonal structure

In some cases single clones are responsible for geographically widespread disease

ADDITIONAL READING

Finlay BB, Falkow S. Common themes in microbial pathogenicity revisited. *Microbiol Mol Biol Rev* 1997;61:136–169. An interesting and highly readable account of the major contemporary themes in microbial pathogenicity.

PART II

BIOLOGY OF VIRUSES

CHAPTER 5

Viral Structure

JAMES J. CHAMPOUX

A virus is a set of genes, composed of either DNA or RNA, packaged in a protein-containing coat. The resulting particle is called a **virion.** Viruses that infect humans are considered along with the general class of animal viruses; viruses that infect bacteria are referred to as bacteriophages, or phages for short. Virus reproduction requires that a virus particle infect a cell and program the cellular machinery to synthesize the constituents required for the assembly of new virions. Thus, a virus is considered an intracellular parasite. The infected host cell may produce hundreds to hundreds of thousands of new virions and usually dies. Tissue damage as a result of cell death accounts for the pathology of many viral diseases in humans. In some cases, the infected cells survive, resulting in persistent virus production and a chronic infection that can remain asymptomatic, produce a chronic disease state, or lead to relapse of an infection.

A virus is an intracellular parasite composed of DNA or RNA and a protein coat

In some circumstances, a virus fails to reproduce itself and instead enters a latent state (called **lysogeny** in the case of bacteriophages), from which there is the potential for reactivation at a later time. A possible consequence of the presence of viral genes in a latent state is a new genotype for the cell. Some determinants of bacterial virulence and some malignancies of animal cells are examples of the genetic effects of latent viruses. Apparently vertebrates have had to coexist with viruses for a long time because they have evolved the special nonspecific interferon system, which operates in conjunction with the highly specific immune system to combat virus infections.

Instead of reproducing, the virus may enter a latent state from which it can later be activated

In the discussion to follow, the biological and genetic bases for these phenomena are presented; three themes are emphasized.

1. Different viruses can have very different genetic structures, and this diversity is reflected in their replicative strategies.
2. Because of their small size, viruses have achieved a very high degree of genetic economy.
3. Viruses depend to a great extent on host cell functions and, therefore, are difficult to combat medically. They do exhibit unique steps in their replicative cycles that are potential targets for antiviral therapy.

VIRION SIZE AND DESIGN

Viruses are approximately 100- to 1000-fold smaller than the cells they infect. The smallest viruses (parvoviruses) are approximately 20 nm in diameter (1 nm = 10^{-9} m), whereas the largest animal viruses (poxviruses) have a diameter of approximately 300 nm

Viral size ranges from 20 to 300 nm

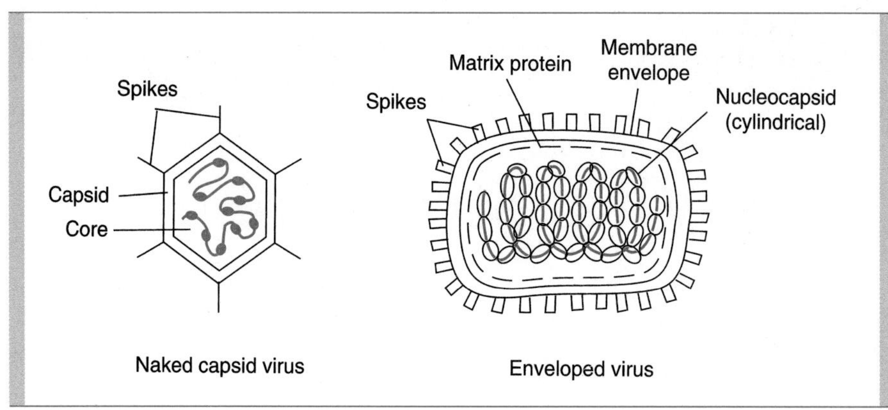

FIGURE 5–1
Schematic drawing of two basic types of virions.

and overlap the size of the smallest bacterial cells (*Chlamydia* and *Mycoplasma*). Therefore, viruses generally pass through filters designed to trap bacteria, and this property can, in principle, be used as evidence of a viral etiology.

Naked capsid viruses have a nucleic acid genome within a protein shell

Enveloped viruses have a nucleocapsid of nucleic acid complexed to protein

Viruses often have surface protrusions

The basic design of all viruses places the nucleic acid genome on the inside of a protein shell called a **capsid.** Some animal viruses are further packaged into a lipid membrane, or **envelope,** which is usually acquired from the cytoplasmic membrane of the infected cell during egress from the cell. Viruses that are not enveloped have a defined external capsid and are referred to as **naked capsid viruses.** The genomes of enveloped viruses form a protein complex and a structure called a **nucleocapsid,** which is often surrounded by a matrix protein that serves as a bridge between the nucleocapsid and the inside of the viral membrane. Protein or glycoprotein structures called **spikes,** which often protrude from the surface of virus particles, are involved in the initial contact with cells. These basic design features are illustrated schematically in Figure 5–1 as well as in the electron micrographs in Figures 5–2 and 5–3.

Two basic shapes: cylindrical and spherical

The protein shell forming the capsid or the nucleocapsid assumes one of two basic shapes: cylindrical or spherical. Some of the more complex bacteriophages combine these two basic shapes. Examples of these three structural categories can be seen in the electron micrographs in Figure 5–2.

Outer shell is protective and aids in entry and packaging

The capsid or envelope of viruses functions (1) to protect the nucleic acid genome from damage during the extracellular passage of the virus from one cell to another, (2) to aid in the process of entry into the cell, and (3) in some cases to package enzymes essential for the early steps of the infection process.

Nucleic acid must be condensed during virion assembly

In general, the nucleic acid genome of a virus is hundreds of times longer than the longest dimension of the complete virion. It follows that the viral genome must be extensively condensed during the process of virion assembly. For naked capsid viruses, this condensation is achieved by the association of the nucleic acid with basic proteins to form what is called the **core** of the virus (see Fig 5–1). The core proteins are usually encoded by the virus, but in the case of some DNA-containing animal viruses, the basic proteins are histones scavenged from the host cell. For enveloped viruses, the formation of the nucleocapsid serves to condense the nucleic acid genome.

Plant viroids are infectious RNA molecules

Prions may cause spongiform encephalopathies

Two classes of infectious agents exist that are structurally simpler than viruses. **Viroids** are infectious circular RNA molecules that lack protein shells; they are responsible for a variety of plant diseases. Hepatitis delta, an infectious agent sometimes found in association with hepatitis B virus, appears to share many properties with the viroids. **Prions,** which apparently lack any genes and are composed only of protein, are agents that appear to be responsible for some transmissible and inherited spongiform encephalopathies such as scrapie in sheep; bovine spongiform encephalopathy in cattle; and kuru, Creutzfeldt-Jakob disease, and Gerstmann-Sträussler-Scheinker syndrome in humans.

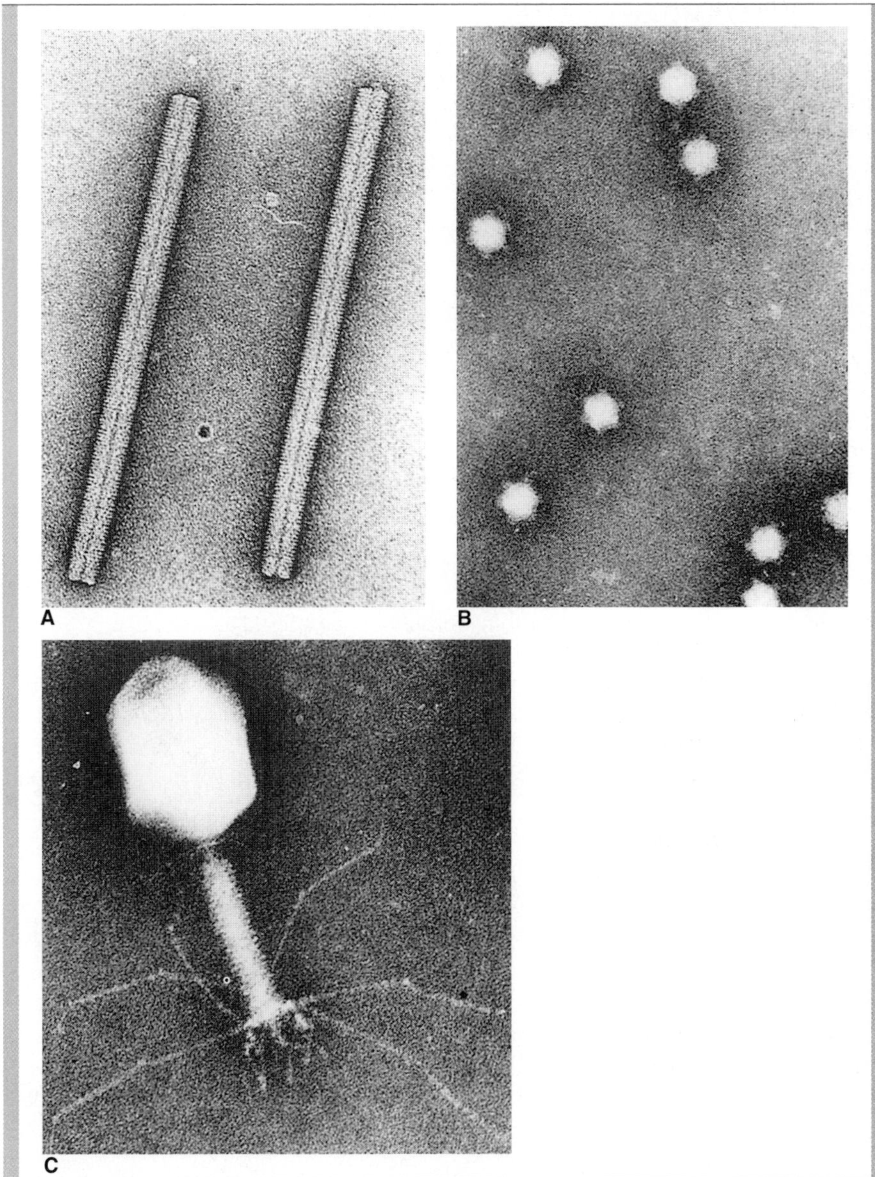

FIGURE 5–2
Three basic virus designs:
A. Tobacco mosaic virus.
B. Bacteriophage ϕX174.
C. Bacteriophage T4. (*Kindly provided by Dr. Robley C. Williams.*)

GENOME STRUCTURE

Structural diversity among the viruses is most obvious when the makeup of viral genomes is considered. Genomes can be made of RNA or DNA and be either double stranded or single stranded. For viruses with single-stranded genomes, the nucleic acid can be either of the same polarity (indicated by a +) or of a different polarity (−) from that of the viral mRNA produced during infection. In the case of adeno-associated viruses, the particles are a mixture: about half contain (+)DNA; the other half contain (−)DNA. The arenaviruses and bunyaviruses are unusual in having an RNA genome, part of which has the same polarity as the mRNA and part of which is complementary to the corresponding mRNA.

DNA or RNA genomes may be single or double stranded

Both linear and circular genomes are known. Whereas the genomes of most viruses are composed of a single nucleic acid molecule, in some cases several pieces of nucleic acid constitute the complete genome. Such viruses are said to have **segmented** genomes. One virus class (retroviruses) carries two identical copies of its genome and is therefore diploid. A few viral genomes (picornaviruses, hepatitis B virus, and adenoviruses) contain covalently attached protein on the ends of the DNA or RNA chains that are remnants of the replication process.

Genomes may be linear or circular

Some genomes are segmented

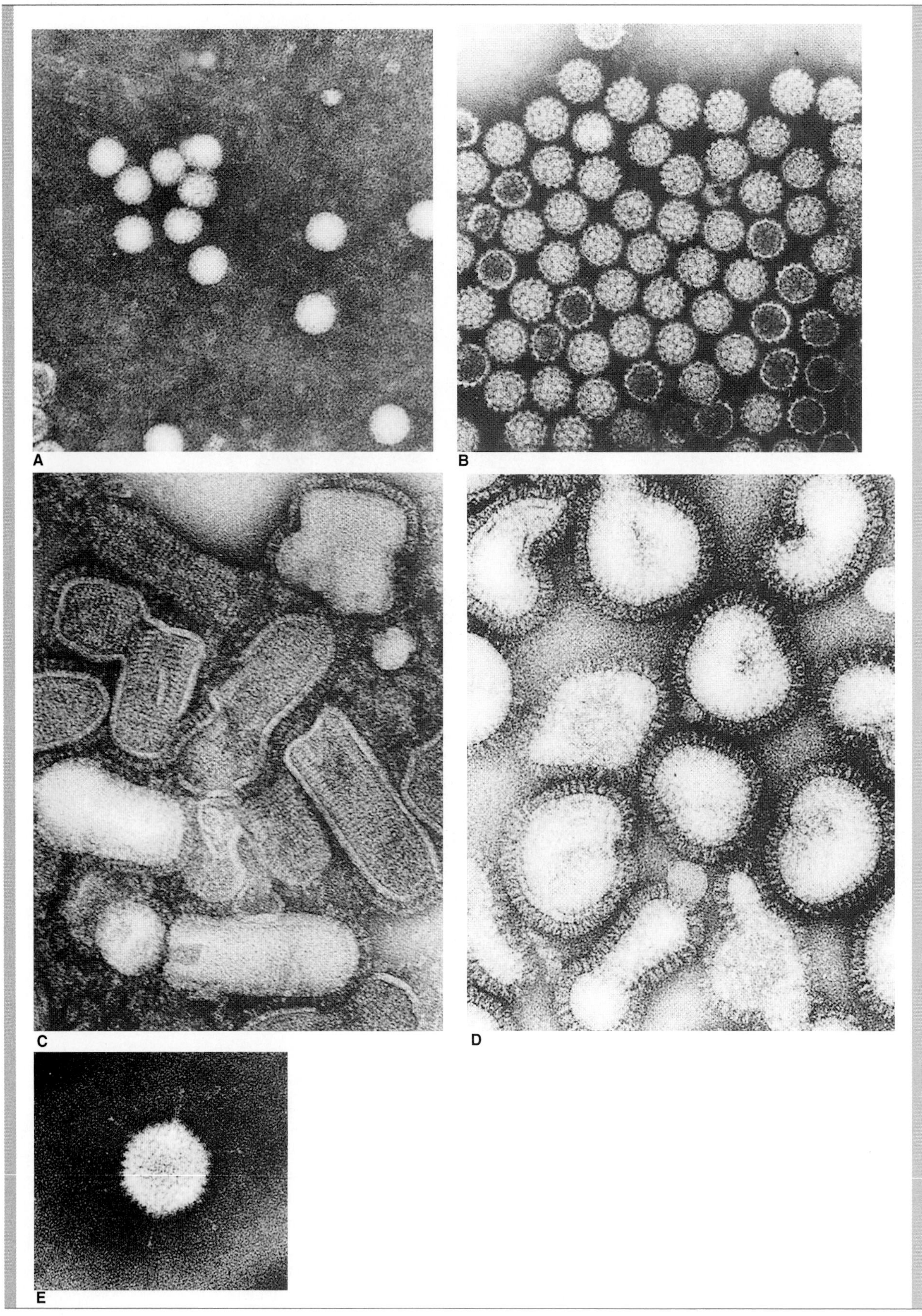

FIGURE 5–3

Representative animal viruses: **A.** Poliovirus. **B.** Simian virus 40. **C.** Vesicular stomatitis virus. **D.** Influenza virus. **E.** Adenovirus. (*Kindly provided by Dr. Robley C. Williams.*)

CAPSID STRUCTURE

Subunit Structure of Capsids

The capsids or nucleocapsids of all viruses are composed of many copies of one or at most several different kinds of protein subunits. This fact follows from two fundamental considerations. First, all viruses code for their own capsid proteins, and even if the entire coding capacity of the genome were to be used to specify a single giant capsid protein, the protein would not be large enough to enclose the nucleic acid genome. Thus, multiple protein copies are needed, and, in fact, the simplest spherical virus contains 60 identical protein subunits. Second, viruses are such highly symmetric structures that it is not uncommon to visualize naked capsid viruses in the electron microscope as a crystalline array (eg, simian virus 40 in Fig 5–3B). The simplest way to construct a regular symmetrical structure out of irregular protein subunits is to follow the rules of crystallography and form an aggregate involving many identical copies of the subunits, where each subunit bears the same relationship to its neighbors as every other subunit.

Capsids and nucleocapsids are composed of multiple copies of protein molecule(s) in crystalline array

The presence of many identical protein subunits in viral capsids or the existence of many identical spikes in the membrane of enveloped viruses has important implications for adsorption, hemagglutination, and recognition of viruses by neutralizing antibodies (see Chapter 6).

Cylindrical Architecture

A cylindrical shape is the simplest structure for a capsid or a nucleocapsid. The first virus to be crystallized and studied in structural detail was a plant pathogen, tobacco mosaic virus (TMV) (see Fig 5–2A). The capsid of TMV is shaped like a rod or a cylinder, with the RNA genome wound in a helix inside it. The capsid is composed of multiple copies of a single kind of protein subunit arranged in a close-packed helix, which places every subunit in the same microenvironment. Because of the helical arrangement of the subunits, viruses that have this type of design are often said to have helical symmetry. Although less is known about the architecture of animal viruses with helical symmetry, it is likely their structures follow the same general pattern as TMV. Thus, the nucleocapsids of influenza, measles, mumps, rabies, and poxviruses (Table 5–1) are probably constructed with a helical arrangement of protein subunits in close association with the nucleic acid genome.

Cylindrical viruses have capsid protein molecules arranged in a helix

Spherical Architecture

The construction of a spherically shaped virus similarly involves the packing together of many identical subunits, but in this case the subunits are placed on the surface of a geometric solid called an **icosahedron.** An icosahedron has 12 vertices, 30 sides, and 20 triangular faces (Fig 5–4). Because the icosahedron belongs to the symmetry group that crystallographers refer to as cubic, spherically shaped viruses are said to have cubic symmetry. (Note that the term **cubic,** as used in this context, has nothing to do with the more familiar shape called the cube.)

Spherical viruses exhibit icosahedral symmetry

When viewed in the electron microscope, many naked capsid viruses and some nucleocapsids appear as spherical particles with a surface topology that makes it appear that they are constructed of identical ball-shaped subunits (see Fig 5–3B and E). These visible structures are referred to as **morphological subunits,** or **capsomeres.** A capsomere is generally composed of either five or six individual protein molecules, each one referred to as a **structural subunit,** or **protomer.** In the simplest virus with cubic symmetry, five protomers are placed at each one of the 12 vertices of the icosahedron as shown in Figure 5–4 to form a capsomere called a **pentamer.** In this case, the capsid is composed of 12 pentamers, or a total of 60 protomers. It should be noted that as in the case of helical symmetry, this arrangement places every protomer in the same microenvironment as every other protomer.

Capsomeres are surface structures composed of five or six protein molecules

To accommodate the larger cavity required by viruses with large genomes, the capsids contain many more protomers. These viruses are based on a variation of the basic icosahedron in which the construction involves a mixture of pentamers and hexamers instead of only pentamers. A detailed description of this higher level of virus structure is beyond the scope of this text.

TABLE 5-1

Classification of RNA Animal Viruses

Family	Virion Structure	Genome Structure and Molecular Weight	Representative Members
Hepatitis δ	Cubic, enveloped	ss circular (−) (6×10^5)	Human hepatitis δ virus
Picornaviruses	Cubic, naked	ss linear (+) ($2-3 \times 10^6$); protein attached	Human enteroviruses: poliovirus, coxsackievirus, echovirus; rhinoviruses; bovine foot-and-mouth disease virus; hepatitis A
Arenaviruses	Helical, enveloped	2 ss linear segments (+/−) (3×10^6)	Lassa virus; lymphocytic choriomeningitis virus of mice
Caliciviruses	Cubic, naked	ss linear (+) (2.6×10^6)	Vesicular exanthema virus, Norwalk-like viruses of humans
Rhabdoviruses	Helical, enveloped	ss linear (−) ($3-4 \times 10^6$)	Rabies virus; bovine vesicular stomatitis virus
Retroviruses	Cubic, enveloped	ss linear (+), diploid ($3-4 \times 10^6$)	RNA tumor viruses of mice, birds, and cats; visna virus of sheep; human immunodeficiency viruses (human T-cell leukemia and acquired immunodeficiency syndrome)
Togaviruses	Cubic, enveloped	ss linear (+) (4×10^6)	Alphaviruses: Sindbis virus and Semliki Forest virus; flaviviruses: dengue virus and yellow fever virus; rubella virus; mucosal disease virus
Orthomyxoviruses	Helical, enveloped	8 ss linear segments (−) (5×10^6)	Type A, B, and C influenza viruses of humans, swine, and horses
Coronaviruses	Helical, enveloped	ss linear (+) ($5-6 \times 10^6$)	Respiratory viruses of humans; calf diarrhea virus; swine enteric virus; mouse hepatitis virus
Filoviruses	Helical, enveloped	ss linear (−) (5×10^6)	Marburg and Ebola viruses
Bunyaviruses	Helical, enveloped	3 ss linear segments (+/−) (6×10^6)	Rift Valley fever virus; bunyamwera virus; hantavirus
Paramyxoviruses	Helical, enveloped	ss linear (−) ($6-8 \times 10^6$)	Mumps; measles; Newcastle disease virus; canine distemper virus
Reoviruses	Cubic, naked	10 ds linear segments (15×10^6)	Human reoviruses; orbiviruses; Colorado tick fever virus; African horse sickness virus; human rotaviruses

Abbreviations: ss, single stranded; ds, double stranded.

Special Surface Structures

Surface structures are important in adsorption and penetration

Many viruses have structures that protrude from the surface of the virion. In virtually every case these structures are important for the two earliest steps of infection, adsorption and penetration. The most dramatic example of such a structure is the tail of some bacteriophages (see Fig 5–2C), which, as described in Chapter 6, acts as a channel for the transfer of the genome into the cell. Other examples of surface structures include the spikes of adenovirus (see Fig 5–3E) and the glycoprotein spikes found in the membrane of enveloped viruses (see influenza virus in Fig 5–3D). Even viruses without obvious

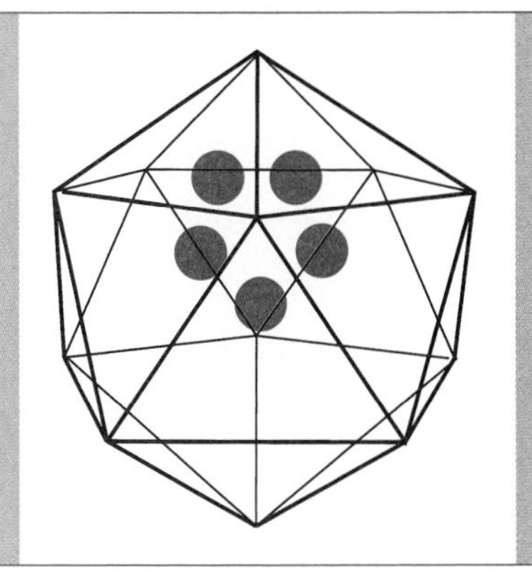

FIGURE 5–4
Diagram of an icosahedron showing 12 vertices, 20 faces, and 30 sides. The colored balls indicate the position of protomers forming a pentamer on the icosahedron.

surface extensions probably contain short projections, which, like the more obvious spikes, are involved in the specific binding of the virus to the cell surface (see Chapter 6).

Classification of Viruses

Tables 5–1 and 5–2 present a classification scheme for animal viruses that is based solely on their structure. The viruses are arranged in order of increasing genome size. It is important to bear in mind that phylogenetic relationships cannot be inferred from this taxonomic scheme. The tables should not be memorized, but instead used as a reference guide to virus structure. In general, viruses with similar structures exhibit similar replication strategies as is discussed in Chapter 6.

TABLE 5–2

Classification of DNA Animal Viruses

Family	Virion Structure	Genome Structure and Molecular Weight	Representative Members
Parvoviruses	Cubic, naked	ss linear ($1–2 \times 10^6$)	Minute virus of mice; adeno-associated viruses
Hepatitis B	Cubic, enveloped	ds circular (2×10^6), gap in one strand; protein attached	Hepatitis B virus of humans, woodchuck hepatitis virus
Papovaviruses	Cubic, naked	ds circular ($3–5 \times 10^6$)	Papillomaviruses, polyomavirus (mouse), SV40 (monkey)
Adenoviruses	Cubic, naked	ds linear ($20–25 \times 10^6$); protein attached	Human and animal respiratory disease viruses
Herpesviruses	Cubic, enveloped	ds linear ($80–130 \times 10^6$)	Herpes simplex virus types 1 and 2; varicella–zoster virus; cytomegalovirus; Epstein–Barr virus; human herpesvirus 6, human herpesvirus 8 (Kaposi's sarcoma)
Poxviruses	Helical, enveloped	ds linear ($160–200 \times 10^6$)	Smallpox; vaccinia; molluscum contagiosum; fibroma and myxoma viruses of rabbits

Abbreviations: ss, single stranded; ds, double stranded.

TABLE 5–3

Some Important Bacteriophages

Bacteriophage	Host	Genome Structure and Molecular Weight	Comments
MS2	*Escherichia coli*	ss linear RNA (1.2×10^6)	Lytic
Filamentous (M13, fd)	*Escherichia coli*	ss circular DNA (2.1×10^6)	No cell death
ϕX174	*Escherichia coli*	ss circular DNA (1.8×10^6)	Lytic
β	*Corynebacterium diphtheriae*	ds linear DNA (23×10^6)	Temperate, codes for diphtheria toxin
λ	*Escherichia coli*	ds linear DNA (31×10^6)	Temperate
T4	*Escherichia coli*	ds linear DNA (108×10^6)	Lytic

Abbreviations: ss, single stranded; ds, double stranded.

Representative and important bacteriophages are listed along with their properties in Table 5–3. In the chapters to follow the properties of the well-studied temperate bacteriophage, λ, are described to illustrate the replicative strategies of the more medically important, but less well-studied, β phage of *Corynebacterium diphtheriae.*

CHAPTER 6

Viral Multiplication

JAMES J. CHAMPOUX

A virus multiplication cycle is typically divided into the following discrete phases: (1) adsorption to the host cell, (2) penetration or entry, (3) uncoating to release the genome, (4) virion component production, (5) assembly, and (6) release from the cell. This series of events, sometimes with slight variations, describes what is called the **productive** or **lytic response;** however, this is not the only possible outcome of a virus infection. Some viruses can also enter into a very different kind of relationship with the host cell in which no new virus is produced, the cell survives and divides, and the viral genetic material persists indefinitely in a latent state. This outcome of an infection is referred to as the **nonproductive response.** The nonproductive response is called **lysogeny** in the case of bacteriophages and under some circumstances may be associated with **oncogenic transformation** by animal viruses. (This use of the term transformation is to be distinguished from DNA transformation of bacteria discussed in Chapter 4.)

Viral infections may be productive or nonproductive

Some animal viruses can cause oncogenic transformation

The outcome of an infection depends on the particular virus–host combination and on other factors such as the extracellular environment, multiplicity of infection, and physiology and developmental state of the cell. Those viruses that can enter only into a productive relationship are called **lytic** or **virulent viruses.** Viruses that can establish either a productive or a nonproductive relationship with their host cells are referred to as **temperate viruses.** Some temperate viruses can be reactivated or "induced" to leave the latent state and enter into the productive response. Whether induction occurs depends on the particular virus–host combination, the physiology of the cell, and the presence of extracellular stimuli.

Temperate viruses can either replicate or enter a latent state

The remainder of this chapter is concerned with the details of the steps of the lytic response. In Chapter 7, the topics of lysogeny and oncogenic transformation are considered.

GROWTH AND ASSAY OF VIRUSES

Viruses are generally propagated in the laboratory by mixing the virus and susceptible cells together and incubating the infected cells until lysis occurs. After lysis, the cells and cell debris are removed by a brief centrifugation and the resulting supernatant is called a **lysate.**

The growth of animal viruses requires that the host cells be cultivated in the laboratory. To prepare cells for growth in vitro, a tissue is removed from an animal and the cells are disaggregated using the proteolytic enzyme trypsin. The cell suspension is seeded into a plastic petri dish in a medium containing a complex mixture of amino acids, vitamins, minerals, and sugars. In addition to these nutritional factors, the growth of animal cells requires components present in animal serum. This method of growing cells is referred to as **tissue culture,** and the initial cell population is called a **primary culture.** The cells attach to the bottom of the plastic dish and remain attached as they divide and eventually cover the surface of the dish. When the culture becomes crowded, the cells generally

Viruses are cultivated in cell cultures derived from animal tissues cease dividing and enter a resting state. Propagation can be continued by removing the cells from the primary culture plate using trypsin and reseeding a new plate.

Permanent cell lines are useful for growing viruses

Cells taken from a normal (as opposed to cancerous) tissue cannot usually be propagated in this manner indefinitely. Eventually most of the cells die; a few may survive, and these survivors often develop into a permanent cell line. Such cell lines are very useful as host cells for isolating and assaying viruses in the laboratory, but they rarely bear much resemblance to the tissue from which they originated. When cells are taken from a tumor and cultivated in vitro, they display a very different set of growth properties, including long-term survival, reflecting their tumor phenotype (see Chapter 7).

Cytopathic effects are characteristic for individual viruses

When a virus is propagated in tissue culture cells, the cellular changes induced by the virus, which usually culminate in cell death, are often characteristic of a particular virus and are referred to as the **cytopathic effect** of the virus (see Chapter 15).

Viruses are quantitated by a plaque assay

Viruses are quantitated by a method called the plaque assay (see Plaque Assay under Quantitation of Viruses for a detailed description of the method). Briefly, viruses are mixed with cells on a petri plate such that each infectious particle gives rise to a zone of lysed or dead cells called a **plaque.** From the number of plaques on the plate, the titer of infectious particles in the lysate is calculated. Virus titers are expressed as the number of plaque-forming units per milliliter (pfu/mL).

ONE-STEP GROWTH EXPERIMENT

One-step growth experiments are useful in the study of infections

To describe an infection in temporal and quantitative terms it is useful to perform a one-step growth experiment (Fig 6–1). The objective in such an experiment is to infect every cell in a culture so that the whole population proceeds through the infection process in a synchronous fashion. The ratio of infecting plaque-forming units to cells is called the multiplicity of infection (MOI). By infecting at a high MOI (eg, 10 as in Fig 6–1), one can be certain that every cell is infected.

Shortly after infection, a virus loses its identity (eclipse phase)

Infectious virus reappears at end of eclipse phase inside the cell

The time course and efficiency of adsorption can be followed by the loss of infectious virus from the medium after removal of the cells (solid line in Fig 6–1). In the example shown, adsorption takes about a half-hour and all but 1% of the virus is adsorbed. If samples of the culture containing the infected cells are treated so as to break open the cells prior to assaying for virus (broken line in Fig 6–1), it can be observed that infectious virus initially disappears, because no infectious particles are detectable above the background of unadsorbed virus. The period of infection in which no infectious viruses are found inside the cell is called the **eclipse phase** and emphasizes that the original virions lose their infectivity soon after entry. Infectivity is lost because, as is discussed later, the virus particles are dismantled as a prelude to their reproduction. Later, infectious virus

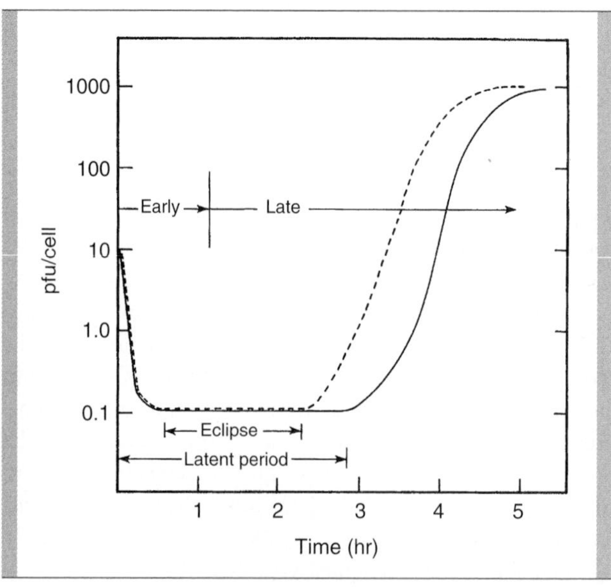

FIGURE 6–1
One-step growth experiment. pfu, plaque-forming units.

particles rapidly reappear in increasing numbers and are detected inside the cell prior to their release into the environment (see Fig 6–1). The length of time from the beginning of infection until progeny virions are found outside the cells is referred to as the **latent period.** Latent periods range from 20 minutes to hours for bacteriophages and from a few hours to many days for animal viruses.

The time in the infection at which genome replication begins is typically used to divide the infection operationally into early and late phases. Early viral gene expression is largely restricted to the production of those proteins required for genome replication; later, the proteins synthesized are primarily those necessary for construction of the new virus particles.

Proteins for replication are produced early and those for construction of virions are produced late

The average number of plaque-forming units released per infected cell is called the burst size for the infection. In the example shown, the burst size is about 1000. Burst sizes range from less than 10 for some relatively inefficient infections to millions for some highly virulent viruses.

ADSORPTION

The first step in every viral infection is the attachment or adsorption of the infecting particle to the surface of the cell. A prerequisite for this interaction is a collision between the virion and the cell. Viruses do not have any capacity for locomotion, and so the collision event is simply a random process determined by diffusion. Therefore, like any bimolecular reaction, the rate of adsorption is determined by the concentrations of both the virions and the cells.

Only a small fraction of the collisions between a virus and its host cell lead to a successful infection, because adsorption is a highly specific reaction that involves protein molecules on the surface of the virion called **virion attachment proteins** and certain molecules on the surface of the cell called **receptors.** Typically there are 10^4 to 10^5 receptors on the cell surface. Receptors for some bacteriophages are found on pili, although the majority adsorb to receptors found on the bacterial cell wall. Receptors for animal viruses are usually glycoproteins located in the plasma membrane of the cell. Table 6–1 lists

Adsorption involves virion attachment proteins and cell surface receptor proteins

TABLE 6–1

Examples of Viral Receptors

Virus	Receptor	Cellular Function
Influenza A	Sialic acid	Glycoprotein
Reoviruses	Sialic acid	Glycoprotein
	EGF receptor	Signaling
Adenoviruses	Integrins	Binding to extracellular matrix
Epstein–Barr	CR2	Complement receptor
Herpes simplex	Heparan sulfate	Glycoprotein
Human herpes 7	CD4	Immunoglobulin superfamily
HIV	CD4	Immunoglobulin superfamily
	CXCR4 and CCR5	Chemokine receptors
Human coronavirus	Aminopeptidase N	Protease
Human rhinoviruses	ICAM-1	Immunoglobulin superfamily
Measles	CD46	Complement regulation
Poliovirus	PVR	Immunoglobulin superfamily
Rabies	Acetylcholine receptor	Signaling
SV40	MHC I	Immunoglobulin superfamily
Vaccinia	EGF receptor	Signaling

Abbreviations: EGF, endothelial growth factor; HIV, human immunodeficiency virus; ICAM, intercellular adhesion molecule; MHC, major histocompatibility complex; PVR, poliovirus receptor.

some of the receptors that have been identified for medically important viruses. It appears that viruses have evolved to make use of a wide variety of surface molecules as receptors, which are normally signaling devices or immune system components. Any attempts to design agents that block viral infections by binding to the receptors must consider the possibility that the loss of the normal cellular function associated with the receptors would have serious consequences for the host organism.

For some viruses, two different surface molecules, called **coreceptors,** are involved in adsorption. Although CD4 was originally thought to be the sole receptor for human immunodeficiency virus type 1 (HIV-1), the discovery of a family of coreceptors that normally function as chemokine receptors may explain why natural resistance against the virus is found in individuals with variant forms of these signaling molecules. Receptors for some animal viruses are also found on red blood cells of certain species and are responsible for the phenomena of hemagglutination and hemadsorption discussed later.

Viral spikes and phage tails carry attachment proteins

Virion attachment proteins are often associated with conspicuous features on the surface of the virion. For example, the virion attachment proteins for the bacteriophages with tails are located at the very end of the tails or the tail fibers (Fig 6–2). Likewise, the spikes found on adenoviruses (Fig 5–3E) and on virtually all of the enveloped animal viruses contain the virion attachment proteins.

In some cases, a region of the capsid protein serves the function of the attachment protein. For polioviruses, rhinoviruses, and probably other picornaviruses, the region on the capsid that binds to the receptor is found at the bottom of a cleft or trough that is too narrow to allow access to antibodies. This particular arrangement is clearly advantageous to the virus because it precludes the production of antibodies that might directly block receptor recognition.

Adsorption is enhanced by presence of multiple attachment and receptor proteins

The repeating subunit structure of capsids and the multiplicity of spikes on enveloped viruses are probably important in determining the strength of the binding of the virus to the cell. The binding between a single virion attachment protein and a single receptor protein is relatively weak, but the combination of many such interactions leads to a strong association between the virion and the cell. The fluid nature of the animal cell membrane may facilitate the movement of receptor proteins to allow the clustering that is necessary for these multiple interactions.

Differences in host range and tissue tropism are due to presence or absence of receptors

A particular kind of virus is capable of infecting only a limited spectrum of cell types called its **host range.** Thus, although a few viruses can infect cells from different species, most viruses are limited to a single species. For example, dogs do not contract measles, and humans do not contract distemper. In many cases, animal viruses infect only a particular subset of the cells found in their host organism. Clearly this kind of tissue tropism is an important determinant of viral pathogenesis. In most cases studied, the specific host range of a virus and its associated tissue tropism are determined at the level of the binding between the cell receptors and virion attachment proteins. Thus, these two protein components must possess complementary surfaces that fit together in much the same way as a substrate fits into the active site of an enzyme. It follows that adsorption occurs only in that fraction of collisions that lead to successful binding between receptors and attachment proteins and that the inability of a virus to infect a cell type is usually due to the absence of the appropriate receptors on the

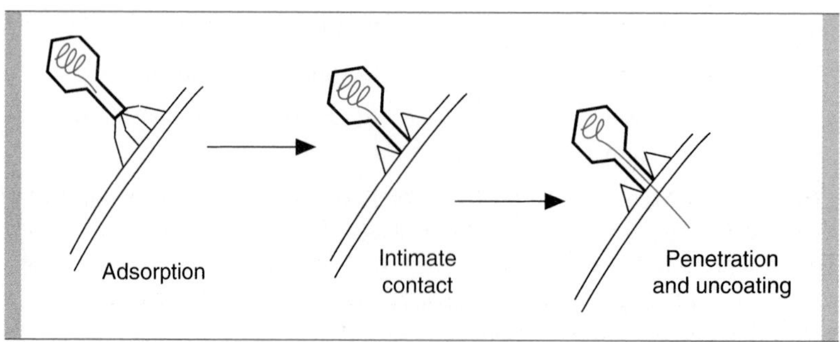

FIGURE 6–2
Bacteriophage entry.

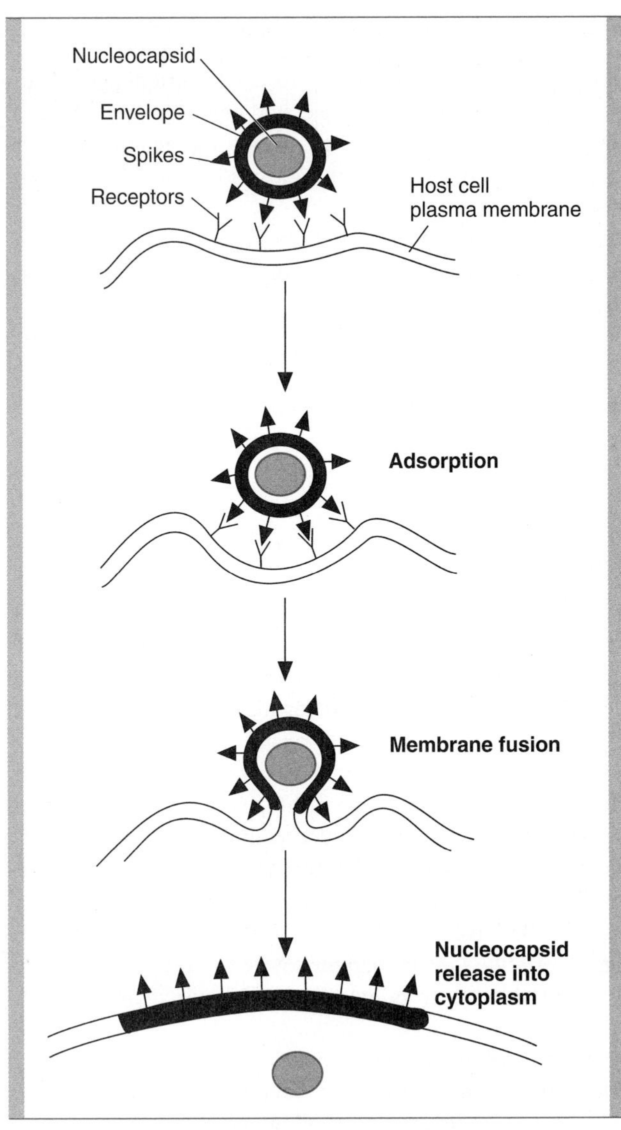

FIGURE 6–3
Entry by direct fusion.

cell. The exquisite specificity of these interactions is well illustrated by the case of a particular mouse reovirus. It has been found that the tissue tropism, and therefore, the resultant pathology, are altered by a point mutation that changes a single amino acid in the virion attachment protein. A few cases are known in which the host range of a virus is determined at a step after adsorption and penetration, but these are the exceptions rather than the rule.

Once a virus particle has penetrated to the inside of a cell, it is essentially hidden from the host immune system. Thus, if protection from a virus infection is to be accomplished at the level of antibody binding to the virions, it must occur before adsorption and prevent the virus from attaching to and penetrating the cell. It is therefore not surprising that most neutralizing antibodies, whether acquired as a result of natural infection or vaccination, are specific for virion attachment proteins.

Neutralizing antibodies are often specific for attachment proteins

ENTRY AND UNCOATING

The disappearance of infectious virus during the eclipse phase is a direct consequence of the fact that viruses are dismantled prior to being replicated. As is discussed later, the uncoating step may be simultaneous with entry or may occur in a series of steps. Ultimately the nucleocapsid or core structure must be transported to the site or compartment in the cell where transcription and replication will occur.

Viruses are dismantled before being replicated

The Bacteriophage Strategy

Bacteriophage capsids are shed and only the viral genome enters the host cell

The processes of penetration and uncoating are simultaneous for all bacteriophages. Thus, the viral capsids are shed at the surface, and only the nucleic acid genome enters the cell. In some cases, a small number of virion proteins may accompany the genome into the cell, but these are probably tightly associated with the nucleic acid or are essential enzymes needed to initiate the infection.

Tailed phages attach by tail fibers and DNA is injected through the tail

Bacteriophages with tails have evolved these special appendages to facilitate the entry of the genome into the cell. The process of penetration and uncoating for bacteriophage T4 is shown schematically in Figure 6–2. The tail fibers extending from the end of the tail are responsible for the attachment of the virion to the cell wall, and, in the next step, the end of the tail itself makes intimate contact with the cell surface. Finally the DNA of the virus is injected from the head directly into the cell through the hollow tail structure. The process has been likened to the action of a syringe, but the energetics and the nature of the orifice in the cell surface through which the DNA travels are poorly understood.

Enveloped Animal Viruses

There are two basic mechanisms for the entry of an enveloped animal virus into the cell. Both mechanisms involve fusion of the viral envelope with a cellular membrane, and the end result in both cases is the release of the free nucleocapsid into the cytoplasm. What distinguishes the two mechanisms is the nature of the cellular membrane that fuses with the viral envelope.

Some enveloped viruses enter cells by direct fusion of plasma membrane and envelope

Paramyxoviruses (eg, measles), some retroviruses (eg, HIV-1), and herpesviruses enter by a process called **direct fusion** (see Fig 6–3). The envelopes of these viruses contain protein spikes that promote fusion of the viral membrane with the plasma membrane of the cell, releasing the nucleocapsid directly into the cytoplasm. Because the viral envelope becomes incorporated into the plasma membrane of the infected cell and still possesses its fusion proteins, infected cells have a tendency to fuse with other uninfected cells. Cell–cell fusion is a hallmark of infections by paramyxoviruses and HIV-1 and can be important in the pathology of diseases such as measles and acquired immunodeficiency syndrome (AIDS).

The mechanism for the entry of most of the remaining enveloped animal viruses, such as orthomyxoviruses (eg, influenza viruses), togaviruses (eg, rubella virus), rhabdoviruses (eg, rabies), and coronaviruses, is shown in Figure 6–4. Following adsorption, the virus particles are taken up by a cellular mechanism called **receptor-mediated endocytosis,** which is normally responsible for internalizing growth factors, hormones, and some nutrients. When it involves viruses, the process is referred to as **viropexis.**

Other enveloped and naked viruses are taken in by receptor-mediated endocytosis (viropexis)

In viropexis, the adsorbed virions become surrounded by the plasma membrane in a reaction that is probably facilitated by the multiplicity of virion attachment proteins on the surface of the particle. Pinching off of the cellular membrane by fusion encloses the virion in a cytoplasmic vesicle termed the **endosomal vesicle.** The nucleocapsid is now surrounded by two membranes, the original viral envelope and the newly acquired endosomal membrane. The surface receptors are subsequently recycled back to the plasma membrane, and the endosomal vesicle is acidified by a normal cellular process. The low pH of the endosome leads to a conformational change in a viral spike protein, which results in the fusion of the two membranes and release of the nucleocapsid into the cytoplasm. In some cases, the contents of the endosomal vesicle may be transferred to a lysosome prior to the fusion step that releases the nucleocapsid.

Naked Capsid Animal Viruses

Acidified endosome releases nucleocapsid to cytoplasm

Naked capsid viruses, such as poliovirus, reovirus, and adenovirus, also appear to enter the cell by viropexis. However, in this case, the virus cannot escape the endosomal vesicle by membrane fusion as described earlier for enveloped viruses. For poliovirus it appears that the viral capsid proteins in the low-pH environment of the endosome expose hydrophobic domains. This process results in the binding of the virions to the membrane and release of

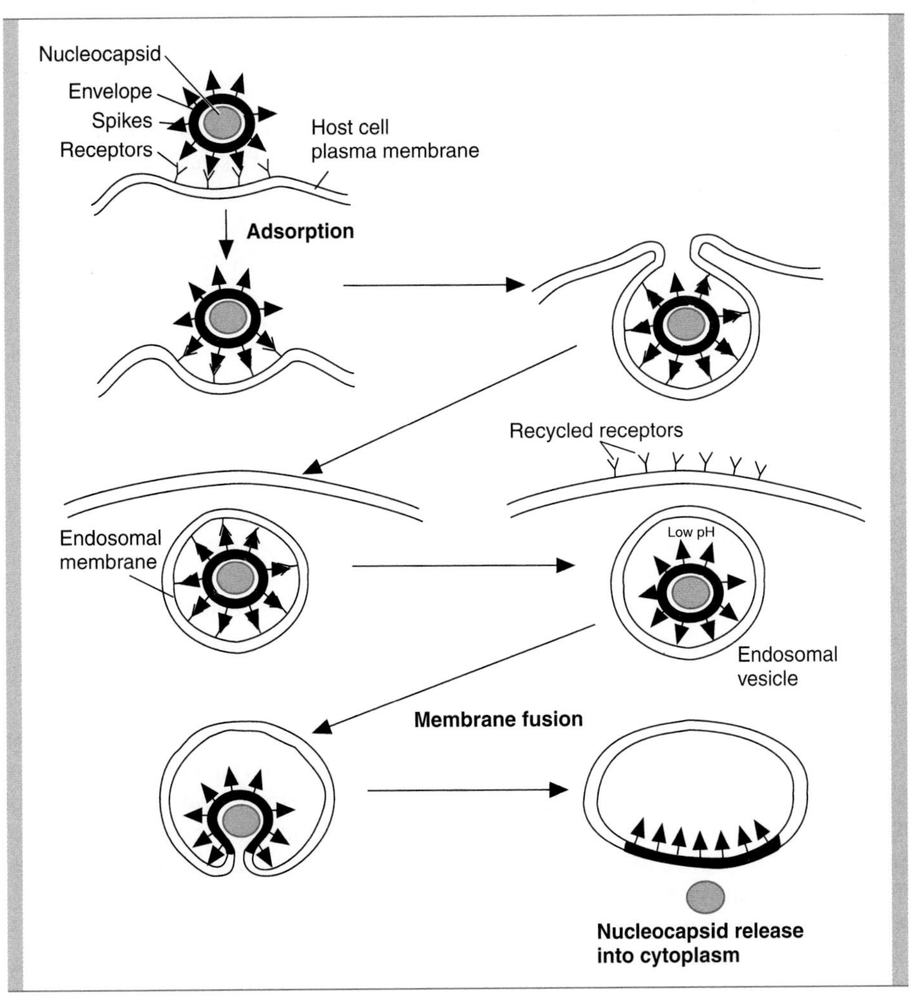

FIGURE 6–4
Viropexis.

the nucleic acid genome into the cytoplasm. In other cases the virions may escape into the cytoplasm by simply promoting the lysis of the vesicle. This step is a potential target of antiviral chemotherapy, and some drugs have been developed that bind to the capsids of picornaviruses and prevent the release of the virus particles from the endosome.

Virions may escape endosome by dissolution of the vesicles

Reovirus is unusual in that prior to release into the cytoplasm, the contents of the endosome are transferred to a lysosome where the lysosomal proteases strip away part of the capsid proteins and activate virion-associated enzymes required for transcription.

Fate of Intracellular Particles

Even in the relatively simple bacterial cell, there is evidence that the entering nucleic acid must be directed to a particular cellular locus to initiate the infection process. **Pilot proteins** have been described that accompany the phage genome into the bacterial cell and serve the function of "piloting" the nucleic acid to a particular target, such as a membrane site where transcription and replication are to occur.

The ultimate fate of internalized animal virus particles depends on the particular virus and on the cellular compartment where replication occurs. Most RNA viruses with the exception of influenza viruses and the retroviruses replicate in the cytoplasm, the immediate site of entry. Retroviruses, influenza viruses, and all the DNA viruses except the poxviruses must move from the cytoplasm to the nucleus to replicate. The larger DNA viruses, such as herpesviruses and adenoviruses, must uncoat to the level of cores prior to entry into the nucleus. The smaller DNA viruses, such as the parvoviruses and the papovaviruses, enter the nucleus intact through the nuclear pores and subsequently uncoat inside. The largest of the animal viruses, the poxviruses, carry out their entire replicative cycle in the cytoplasm of the infected cell.

Most RNA viruses replicate in cytoplasm

Influenza viruses, retroviruses, and DNA viruses except poxviruses replicate in the nucleus

THE PROBLEMS OF PRODUCING mRNA

From Genome to mRNA

Virus-specified mRNAs direct synthesis of viral proteins

An essential step in every virus infection is the production of virus-specific mRNAs that program the cellular ribosomes to synthesize viral proteins. Besides the structural proteins of the virion, viruses must direct the synthesis of enzymes and other specialized proteins required for genome replication, gene expression, and virus assembly and release. The production of the first viral mRNAs at the beginning of the infection is a crucial step in the takeover of the cell by the virus.

Most DNA virus mRNAs are synthesized by host polymerase

(+)-strand RNA virus genome serves as mRNA

For some viruses, the presentation of mRNA to the cellular ribosomes poses no problems. Thus, the genomes of most DNA viruses are transcribed by the host DNA-dependent RNA polymerase to yield the viral mRNAs. The (+)-strand RNA viruses, such as the picornaviruses, the togaviruses, and the coronaviruses, possess genomes that can be used directly as mRNAs and are translated (at least partially, as discussed later) immediately on entry into the cytoplasm of the cell.

Other RNA viruses synthesize and package transcription enzymes to produce initial mRNAs

However, for many viruses, the production of mRNA starting from the genome is not so straightforward. The fact that poxviruses replicate in the cytoplasm means that the cellular RNA polymerase is not available to transcribe the DNA genome. Moreover, no cellular machinery exists that can use either single-stranded or double-stranded RNA as a template to synthesize mRNA. Therefore, the poxviruses and those viruses that utilize an RNA template to make mRNAs must provide their own transcription machinery to produce the viral mRNAs at the beginning of the infection process. This feat is accomplished by synthesizing the transcriptases in the later stages of viral development in the previous host cell and packaging the enzymes into the virions, where they remain associated with the genome as the virus enters the new cell and uncoats. In general, the presence of a transcriptase in virions is indicative that the host cell is unable to use the viral genome as mRNA or as a template to synthesize mRNA. At later times in the infection, any special enzymatic machinery required by the virus and not initially present in the cell, can be supplied among the proteins translated from the first mRNA molecules.

There are a variety of pathways for synthesis of mRNA by different virus groups

The pathways for the synthesis of mRNA by the major virus groups are summarized in Figure 6–5 and related to the structure of viral genomes. The polarity of mRNA is designated as (+) and the polarity of polynucleotide chains complementary to mRNA as (−). The black arrows denote synthetic steps for which host cells provide the required enzymes, whereas the colored arrows indicate synthetic steps that must be carried out by virus-encoded enzymes. Several additional points should be emphasized. The parvoviruses and some phages have single-stranded DNA genomes. Although the RNA polymerase of the cell requires double-stranded DNA as a template, these viruses need not

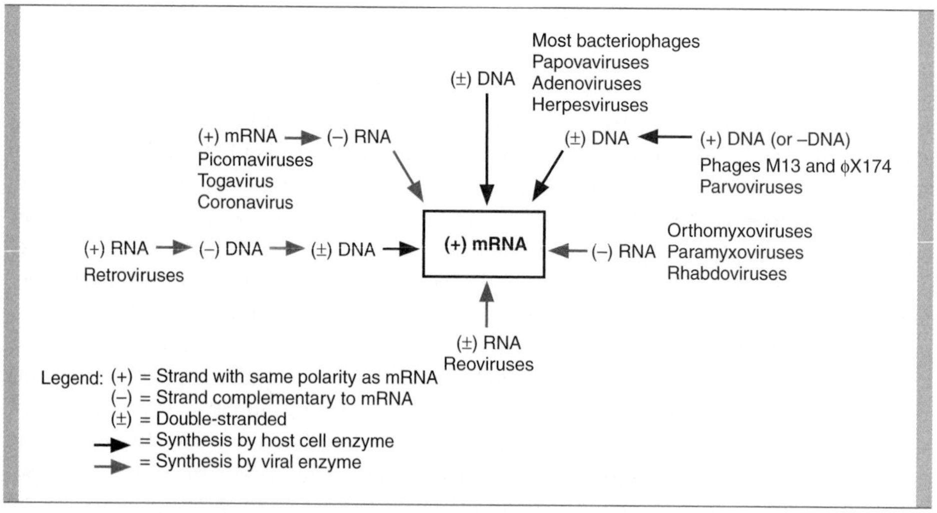

(±) DNA
Most bacteriophages
Papovaviruses
Adenoviruses
Herpesviruses

(+) mRNA → (−) RNA
Picornaviruses
Togavirus
Coronavirus

(±) DNA ← (+) DNA (or −DNA)
Phages M13 and ϕX174
Parvoviruses

(+) RNA → (−) DNA → (±) DNA → **(+) mRNA** ← (−) RNA
Retroviruses

Orthomyxoviruses
Paramyxoviruses
Rhabdoviruses

(±) RNA
Reoviruses

Legend: (+) = Strand with same polarity as mRNA
(−) = Strand complementary to mRNA
(±) = Double-stranded
→ = Synthesis by host cell enzyme
→ = Synthesis by viral enzyme

FIGURE 6–5

Pathways of mRNA synthesis for major virus groups.

carry special enzymes in their virions because host cell DNA polymerases can convert the genomes into double-stranded DNA. Note that the production of more mRNA by the picornaviruses and similar (+)-strand RNA viruses requires the synthesis of an intermediate (−)-strand RNA template. The enzyme required for this process is produced by translation of the genome RNA early in infection.

The retroviruses are a special class of (+)-strand RNA viruses. Although their genomes are the same polarity as mRNA and could in principle serve as mRNAs early after infection, their replication scheme apparently precludes this. Instead, the RNA genomes of these viruses are copied into (−)DNA strands by an enzyme carried within the virion called **reverse transcriptase.** The (−)DNA strands are subsequently converted by the same enzyme to double-stranded DNA in a reaction that requires the degradation of the original genomic RNA by the RNase H activity of the reverse transcriptase. The DNA product of reverse transcription is integrated into the host cell DNA and ultimately transcribed by the host RNA polymerase to complete the replication cycle as well as produce viral mRNA. For example, the replication of the hepatitis B DNA genome is mechanistically similar to that of a retrovirus. Thus, the viral DNA is transcribed to produce a single-stranded RNA, which in turn is reverse transcribed to produce the progeny viral DNA that is encapsidated into virions.

Retroviral RNA is copied to DNA by virion reverse transcriptase; host RNA polymerase transcribes DNA into more RNA

The Monocistronic mRNA Rule in Animal Cells

The ribosome requires input of information in the form of mRNA. For a viral mRNA to be recognized by the ribosome, its production must conform to the rules of structure that govern the synthesis of the cellular mRNAs. Prokaryotic mRNA is relatively simple and can be polycistronic, which means it can contain the information for several proteins. Each cistron or coding region is translated independently beginning from its own ribosome binding site.

Prokaryotic mRNAs can be polycistronic

Eukaryotic mRNAs are structurally more complex, containing special 5′-cap and 3′-poly(A) attachments. In addition, their synthesis often involves removal of internal sequences by a process called **splicing.** Most importantly, virtually all eukaryotic mRNAs are monocistronic. Accordingly, eukaryotic translation is initiated by the binding of a ribosome to the 5′-cap, followed by movement of the ribosome along the DNA until the first AUG initiation codon is encountered. The corollary to this first AUG rule is that eukaryotic ribosomes, unlike prokaryotic ribosomes, generally cannot initiate translation at internal sites on a mRNA. To conform to the monocistronic mRNA, most animal viruses produce mRNAs that are translated to yield only a single polypeptide chain following initiation near the 5′ end of the mRNA.

Animal virus mRNAs are almost always monocistronic

Because most DNA animal viruses replicate in the nucleus, they adhere to the monocistronic mRNA rule either by having a promoter precede each gene or by programming the transcription of precursor RNAs that are processed by nuclear splicing enzymes into monocistronic mRNAs. The virion transcriptase of the cytoplasmic poxviruses apparently must synthesize monocistronic mRNAs by initiation of transcription in front of each gene.

RNA-containing animal viruses have evolved three different strategies to circumvent or conform to the monocistronic mRNA rule. The simplest strategy involves having a segmented genome. For the most part, each genome segment of the orthomyxoviruses and the reoviruses corresponds to a single gene; therefore, the mRNA transcribed from a given segment constitutes a monocistronic mRNA. Unlike most RNA viruses, the orthomyxovirus virus influenza A replicates in the nucleus, and some of its monocistronic mRNAs are produced by splicing of precursor RNAs by host cell enzymes. Moreover, orthomyxoviruses use small 5′ RNA fragments derived from host cell pre-mRNAs found in the nucleus to prime the synthesis of their own mRNAs.

Some RNA viruses have segmented genomes

A second solution to the monocistronic mRNA rule is very similar to the strategy employed by cells and the DNA viruses. The paramyxoviruses, togaviruses, rhabdoviruses, filoviruses, bunyaviruses, arenaviruses, and coronaviruses synthesize monocistronic mRNAs by initiating the synthesis of each mRNA at the beginning of a gene. In most cases, the transcriptase terminates mRNA synthesis at the end of the gene so that each message corresponds to a single gene. For coronaviruses, RNA synthesis initiates at the beginning of each

Some viruses make monocistronic RNAs by initiating synthesis at the start of each gene

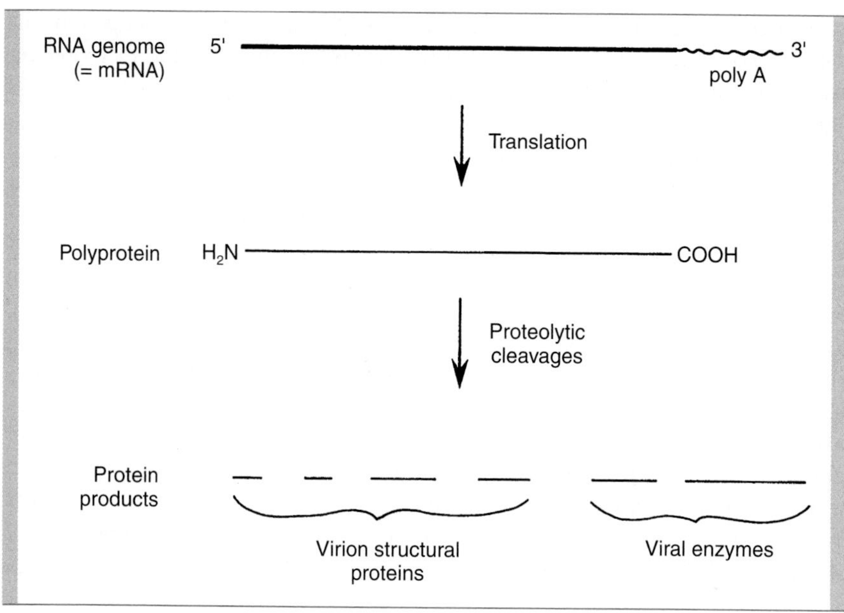

FIGURE 6–6
Poliovirus gene expression.

gene and continues to the end of the genome so that a nested set of mRNAs is produced. However, each mRNA is functionally monocistronic and is translated to produce only the protein encoded near its 5′ end.

Picornaviruses make a polyprotein that is proteolytically cleaved later

The picornaviruses have evolved yet a third strategy to deal with the monocistronic mRNA requirement (Fig 6–6). The (+)-strand genome contains just a single ribosome binding site near the 5′ end. It is translated into one long polypeptide chain called a **polyprotein,** which is subsequently broken into the final set of protein products by a series of proteolytic cleavages. Most of the required protease activities reside within the polyprotein itself.

Several viruses use more than one of these strategies to conform to the monocistronic mRNA rule. For example, retroviruses, togaviruses, arenaviruses, and bunyaviruses synthesize multiple mRNAs, each one coding for a polyprotein that is subsequently cleaved into the individual protein molecules.

GENOME REPLICATION

DNA Viruses

Cells obviously contain the enzymes and accessory proteins required for the replication of DNA. In bacteria these proteins are present continuously, whereas in the eukaryotic cell they are present only during the S phase of the cell cycle, and they are restricted to the nucleus. The extent to which viruses use the cell replication machinery depends on their protein-coding potential and thus on the size of their genome.

The smallest DNA viruses depend exclusively on host DNA replication machinery

The largest DNA viruses code for enzymes important for DNA replication

The smallest of the DNA viruses, the parvoviruses, are so completely dependent on host machinery that they require the infected cells to be dividing so that a normal S phase will occur and replicate the viral DNA along with the cellular DNA. At the other end of the spectrum are the large DNA viruses, which are relatively independent of cellular functions. The largest bacteriophages such as T4 degrade the host cell chromosome early in infection and replace all of the host replication machinery with virus-specified proteins. The largest animal viruses, the poxviruses, are similarly independent of the host. Because they replicate in the cytoplasm, they must code for virtually all of the enzymes and other proteins required for replicating their DNA.

The remainder of the DNA viruses are only partially dependent on host machinery. For example, bacteriophages ϕX174 and λ code for proteins that direct the initiation of DNA synthesis to the viral origin. However, the actual synthesis of DNA occurs by the complex of cellular enzymes responsible for replication of the *Escherichia coli* DNA. Similarly the small DNA animal viruses, such as the papovaviruses, code for a protein that is involved in the initiation of synthesis at the origin, but the remainder of the replication process is carried out by host machinery. The somewhat more complex adenoviruses and herpesviruses, in addition to providing origin-specific proteins, also code for their own DNA polymerases and other accessory proteins required for DNA replication.

Herpesvirus-encoded DNA polymerase is a target of chemotherapy (eg, acyclovir)

The fact that the herpesviruses code for their own DNA polymerase has important implications for the treatment of infections by these viruses and illustrates a central principle of antiviral chemotherapy. Certain antiviral drugs (adenine arabinoside and 5′-iododeoxyuridine) have been found to be effective against herpesvirus infections (see Chapter 38); they are sufficiently similar to natural substrates that the virally encoded DNA polymerase mistakenly incorporates them into viral DNA, resulting in an inhibition of subsequent DNA synthesis. The host cell enzyme is more discriminating and fails to use the analogs in the synthesis of cellular DNA; thus, the drugs do not kill uninfected cells. The same principle applies to the chain-terminating drugs such as zidovudine (AZT) and dideoxyinosine (ddI) that target the HIV-1 reverse transcriptase. Similarly, the antiviral drugs acyclovir (acycloguanosine) and ganciclovir preferentially kill herpesvirus-infected cells because the viral nucleoside kinases, unlike the cellular counterparts, phosphorylate the nucleoside analog, converting it to a form that inhibits further DNA synthesis when DNA polymerases incorporate it into DNA. In principle, any viral process that is distinct from a normal cellular process is a potential target for antiviral drugs. As more becomes known about the details of viral replication, more drugs will become available that are targeted to these unique viral processes.

Viral processes that are distinct from normal cellular processes are potential targets for antiviral drugs

As noted earlier, with the exception of the poxviruses, all of the DNA animal viruses are at least partially dependent on host cell machinery for the replication of their genomes. However, unlike the parvoviruses, the other DNA viruses do not need to infect dividing cells for a productive infection to ensue. Instead, all of these viruses code for a protein expressed early in infection that induces an unscheduled cycle of cellular DNA replication (S phase). In this way, these viruses ensure that the infected cell makes all of the machinery required for the replication of their own DNA. It is noteworthy that all of the DNA viruses except the parvoviruses are capable, in some circumstances, of transforming a normal cell into a cancer cell (see Chapter 7). This correlation suggests that the unlimited proliferative capacity of the cancer cells may be due to the continual synthesis of the viral protein(s) responsible for inducing the unscheduled S phase in a normal infection. The fact that these DNA viruses can induce oncogenic transformation of cell types that are nonpermissive for viral multiplication may simply be an accident related to the need to induce cellular enzymes required for DNA replication during the lytic infection.

All DNA viruses except parvoviruses can transform host cells

All DNA polymerases, including those encoded by viruses, synthesize DNA chains by the successive addition of nucleotides onto the 3′ end of the new DNA strand. Moreover, all DNA polymerases require a primer terminus containing a free 3′-hydroxyl to initiate the synthesis of a DNA chain. In cellular replication, a temporary primer is provided in the form of a short RNA molecule. This primer RNA is synthesized by an RNA polymerase, and after elongation by the DNA polymerase it is removed. With circular chromosomes, such as those found in bacteria and many viruses, the unidirectional chain growth and primer requirement of the DNA polymerase pose no structural problems for replication. However, as illustrated in Figure 6–7, when a replication fork encounters the end of a linear DNA molecule, one of the new chains (heavy lines) cannot be completed at its 5′ end, because there exists no means of starting the DNA portion of the chain exactly at the end of the template DNA. Thus, after the RNA primer is removed, the new chain is incomplete at its 5′ end. This constraint on the completion of DNA chains on a linear template is called the **end problem** in DNA replication. Some eukaryotic cells add short repetitive sequences to chromosome ends using an enzyme called telomerase to prevent the shortening of the DNA with each successive round of replication.

Replication of linear viral DNAs must solve the end problem

Several viruses are faced with the end problem during replication of their linear genomes, but none use the cellular telomerase to synthesize DNA ends. It is beyond the scope of this text to detail all of the strategies viruses have evolved to deal with the end problem, but it is worth mentioning some of the structural features found in linear viral genomes whose presence is related to solutions of the end problem. These structures are diagrammed schematically in Figure 6–8. The linear double-stranded genome of

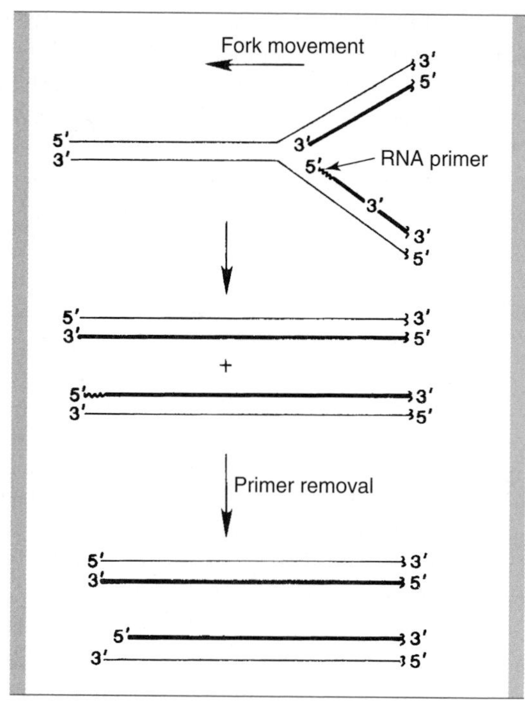

FIGURE 6–7
The end problem in DNA replication.

bacteriophage λ possesses 12-bp single-stranded extensions that are complementary in sequence to each other and thus called **cohesive ends.** Very early after entry into the cell, the two ends pair up to convert the linear genome into a circular molecule to avoid the end problem in replication. The linear double-stranded adenovirus genome contains a protein molecule covalently attached to the 5′ end of both strands. These proteins provide the primers required to initiate the synthesis of the DNA chains during replication, circumventing the need for RNA primers and thus solving the end problem in replication. The single-stranded parvovirus genome contains a self-complementary sequence at the 3′ end that causes the molecule to fold into a hairpin, making it self-priming for DNA replication. The poxviruses contain linear double-stranded genomes in which the ends are continuous. With the parvovirus and poxvirus genomes, the solutions to the end problem create additional problems that must be solved to produce replication products that are identical to the starting genomes.

RNA Viruses

RNA viruses must encode their own transcriptases

Because nuclear functions are primarily designed for DNA metabolism, RNA animal viruses generally replicate in the cytoplasm. Moreover, cells do not have RNA polymerases that can copy RNA templates. Therefore, RNA viruses not only need to code for transcriptases, as discussed earlier, but also must provide the replicases required to duplicate the genome RNA. Furthermore, except in the cases of the RNA phage and the

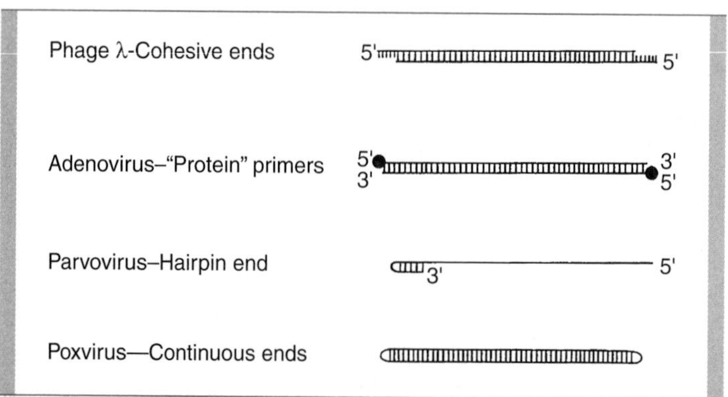

FIGURE 6–8
Some solutions to the end problem.

picornaviruses, where transcription and replication are synonymous, the RNA viruses must temporally and functionally separate replication from transcription. This requirement is especially apparent for the rhabdoviruses, paramyxoviruses, togaviruses, and coronaviruses, where a complete genome, or complementary copy of the genome, is transcribed into a set of small monocistronic mRNAs early in infection. After replication begins, these same templates are used to synthesize full-length strands for replication.

Two mechanisms exist to separate the process of replication from transcription. First, in some cases, transcription is restricted to subviral particles and involves a transcriptase transported into the cell within the virion. Second, in other cases, the replication process involves either a functionally distinct RNA polymerase or depends on the presence of some other viral-specific accessory protein that directs the synthesis of full-length copies of the template rather than the shorter monocistronic mRNAs. In the case of the reoviruses, the switch from transcription to replication appears to involve the synthesis of a replicase that converts the (+)mRNAs synthesized early in infection to the double-stranded genome segments.

Transcription and replication must be separated for most RNA viruses

Viral RNA polymerases, like DNA polymerases, synthesize chains in only one direction; however, in general, RNA polymerases can initiate the synthesis of new chains without primers. Thus, there is no obvious end problem in RNA replication. There is one exception to this general rule. The picornaviruses contain a protein that is covalently attached to the 5′ end of the genome, called Vpg. This protein is present on the viral RNA because it is involved in the priming of new RNA viral genomes during the infection, similar to the process described earlier for adenoviruses.

Picornaviruses use a protein to prime RNA synthesis

ASSEMBLY OF NAKED CAPSID VIRUSES AND NUCLEOCAPSIDS

The process of enclosing the viral genome in a protein capsid is called assembly or **encapsidation.** Four general principles govern the construction of capsids and nucleocapsids. First, the process generally involves self-assembly of the component parts. Second, assembly is stepwise and ordered. Third, individual protein structural subunits or protomers are usually preformed into capsomeres in preparation for the final assembly process. Fourth, assembly often initiates at a particular locus on the genome called a **packaging site.**

Capsids and nucleocapsids self-assemble from preformed capsomeres

Viruses With Helical Symmetry

The assembly of the cylindrically shaped tobacco mosaic virus (TMV) has been extensively studied and provides a model for the construction of helical capsids and nucleocapsids. For TMV, doughnut-shaped disks containing a number of individual structural subunits are preformed and added stepwise to the growing structure. Elongation occurs in both directions from a specific packaging site on the single-stranded viral RNA (Fig 6–9). The addition of

Tobacco mosaic virus is a model for the construction of viral components

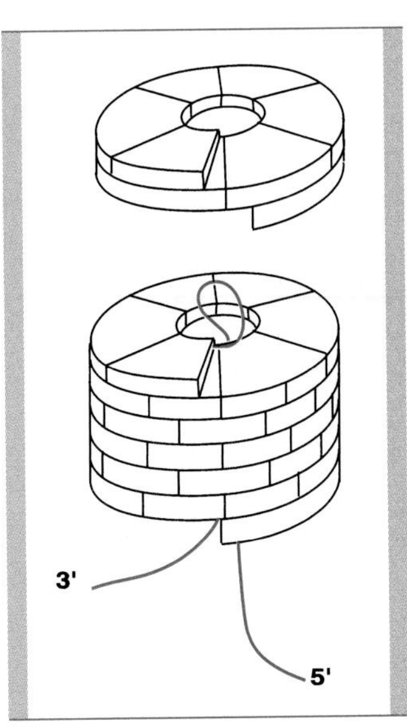

FIGURE 6–9
Tobacco mosaic virus assembly.

each disk involves an interaction between the protein subunits of the disk and the genome RNA. The nature of this interaction is such that the assembly process ceases when the ends of the RNA are reached. The structural subunits as well as the RNA trace out a helical path in the final virus particle.

The basic design features worked out for TMV probably apply in general to the assembly of the nucleocapsids of enveloped viruses. Thus, it is likely that the individual protein subunits are intimately associated with the RNA and that the nucleoprotein complexes are assembled by the stepwise addition of protein subunits or complexes of subunits. For influenza and the other helical viruses with segmented genomes, the various genome segments are assembled into nucleocapsids independently and then brought together during virion assembly by a mechanism that is as yet poorly understood. It is notable that virtually all of the animal RNA viruses with helical symmetry are enveloped.

Viruses with Cubic Symmetry

Icosahedral capsids are generally preassembled, and the genomes are threaded in

For both phage and animal viruses, icosahedral capsids are generally preassembled and the nucleic acid genomes, usually complexed with condensing proteins, are threaded into the empty structures. Construction of the hollow capsids appears to occur by a self-assembly process, sometimes aided by other proteins. The stepwise assembly of components involves the initial aggregation of structural subunits into pentamers and hexamers, followed by the condensation of these capsomeres to form the empty capsid. In some cases, it appears that a small complex of capsid proteins associates specifically with the viral genome and nucleates the assembly of the complete capsid around the genome.

Phage heads, tails, and tail fibers are synthesized separately and then assembled

The morphogenesis of a complex bacteriophage such as T4 involves the prefabrication of each of the major substructures by a separate pathway, followed by the ordered and sequential construction of the final particle from its component parts (Fig 6–10). An intermediate in the assembly of a bacteriophage head is an empty structure containing an internal protein network that is removed prior to insertion of the nucleic acid. The constituents of this network are often appropriately referred to as **scaffolding proteins,** which apparently provide the lattice necessary to hold the capsomeres in position during the early stages of head assembly.

Some phage DNA is replicated to produce concatemers

For many DNA bacteriophages and the herpesviruses, the products of replication are long linear DNA molecules called **concatemers,** which are made up of tandem head-to-tail repeats of genome-size units. During the threading of the DNA into the preformed capsids, these concatemers are cleaved by virus-encoded nucleases to generate genome-size pieces.

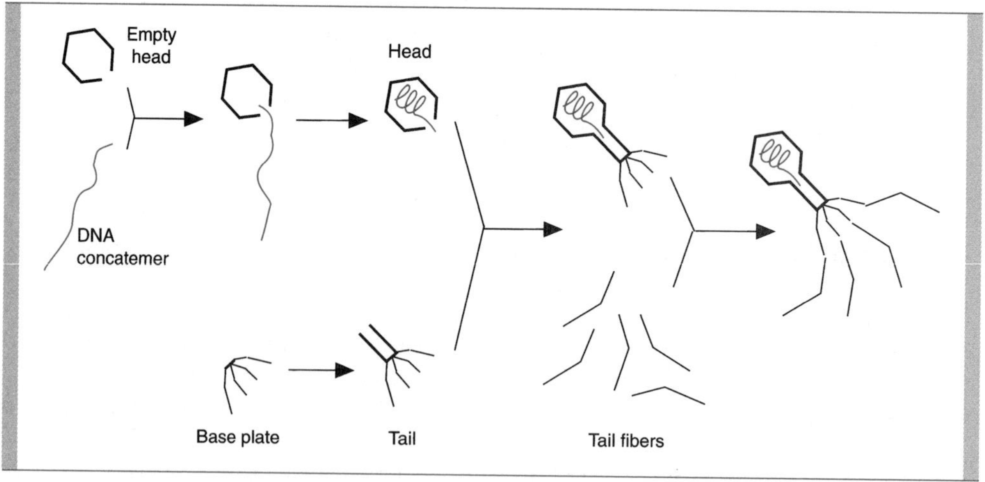

FIGURE 6–10
Assembly of bacteriophage T4.

There are two mechanisms for determining the correct sites for nuclease cleavage during packaging of a concatemer. Bacteriophage λ and the herpesviruses typify one type of mechanism in which the enzyme that makes the cuts is a sequence-specific nuclease. The enzyme sits poised at the orifice of the capsid as the DNA is being threaded into the capsid, and just before the specific cut site enters, the DNA is cleaved. For bacteriophage λ, the breaks are made in opposite strands, 12 bp apart, to generate the cohesive ends. Bacteriophages T4 and P1 are examples of bacterial viruses that illustrate the second mechanism. For these phages, the nuclease does not recognize a particular DNA sequence, but instead cuts the concatemer when the capsid is full. Because the head of the bacteriophage can accommodate slightly more than one genome equivalent of DNA and packaging can begin anywhere on the DNA, the "headful" mechanism produces genomes that are terminally redundant (the same sequence is found at both ends) and circularly permuted. The nonspecific packaging with respect to DNA sequence explains why bacteriophage P1 is capable of incorporating host DNA into phage particles, thereby promoting generalized transduction (see Chapter 4). Bacteriophage T4 does not carry out generalized transduction, because the bacterial DNA is completely degraded to nucleotides early in infection.

Mechanisms for cutting phage DNA during packaging involve site-specific nucleases or headful cleavage

Host DNA may be incorporated by the headful mechanism, and generalized transduction results

RELEASE

Bacteriophages

Most bacteriophages escape from the infected cell by coding for one or more enzymes synthesized late in the latent phase that causes the lysis of the cell. The enzymes are either lysozymes or peptidases that weaken the cell wall by cleaving specific bonds in the peptidoglycan layer. The damaged cells burst as a result of osmotic pressure.

Phages encode lysozyme or peptidases that lyse bacterial cell walls

Animal Viruses

CELL DEATH

Nearly all productively infected cells die (see below for exceptions), presumably because the viral genetic program is dominant and precludes the continuation of normal cell functions required for survival. In many cases, direct viral interference with normal cellular metabolic processes leads to cell death. For example, picornaviruses shut off host protein synthesis soon after infection, and many DNA animal viruses interfere with normal cell cycle controls. In many cases, the end result of such insults is a triggering of a cellular stress response called programmed cell death or **apoptosis.** Some viruses are known to code for proteins that block or delay apoptosis, probably to stave off cell death until the virus replication cycle has been completed. Ultimately, the cell lysis that accompanies cell death is responsible for the release of naked capsid viruses into the environment.

Naked capsid viruses lacking specific lysis mechanisms are released with cell death

Some viruses block or delay apoptosis to allow completion of the virus replication cycle

BUDDING

With the exception of the poxviruses, all enveloped animal viruses acquire their membrane by budding either through the plasma membrane or, in the case of herpesviruses, through the membrane of an exocytic vesicle. Thus, for these viruses, release from the cell is coupled to the final stage of virion assembly. How the herpesviruses ultimately escape from the cell when the membrane of the exocytic vesicle fuses with the plasma membrane. The poxviruses appear to program the synthesis of their own outer membrane. How the poxvirus envelope is assembled on the nucleocapsid is not known.

The membrane changes that accompany budding appear to be just the reverse of the entry process described before for those viruses that enter by direct fusion (compare Fig 6–3 and Fig 6–11). The region of the cellular membrane where budding is to occur

Most enveloped viruses acquire an envelope during release by budding

Poxviruses synthesize their own envelopes

The membrane site for budding first acquires virus-specified spikes and matrix protein

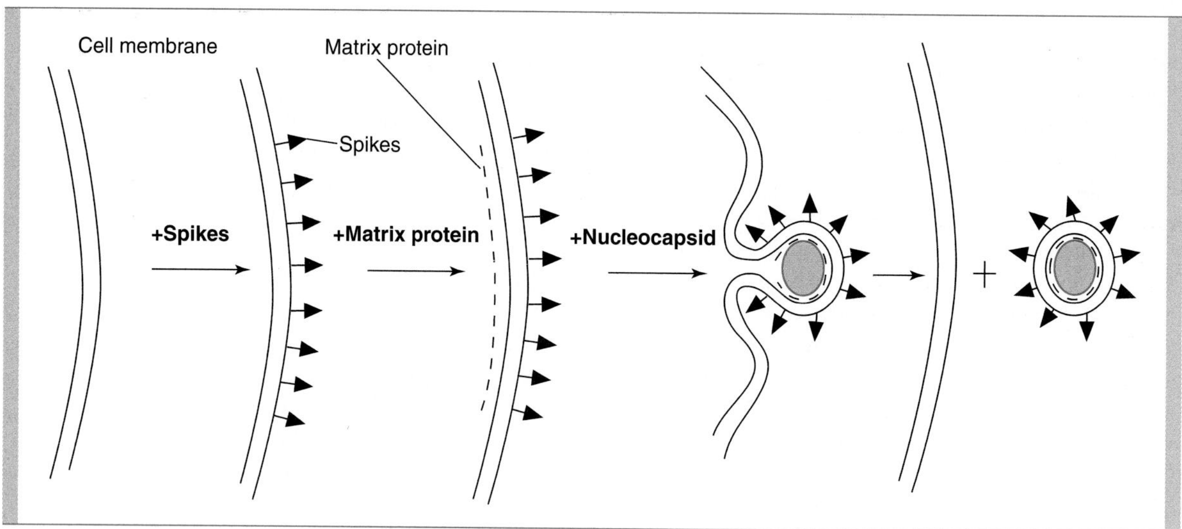

FIGURE 6–11
Viral release by budding.

acquires a cluster of viral glycoprotein spikes. These proteins are synthesized by the pathway that normally delivers cellular membrane proteins to the surface of the cell by way of the Golgi apparatus. At the site of the glycoprotein cluster, the inside of the membrane becomes coated with a virion structural protein called the **matrix** or **M protein.** The accumulation of the matrix protein at the proper location is probably facilitated by the presence of a binding site for the matrix protein on the cytoplasmic side of the transmembrane glycoprotein spike. The matrix protein attracts the completed nucleocapsid that triggers the envelopment process leading to the release of the completed particle to the outside (see Fig 6–11).

For viruses that bud, it is important to note that the plasma membrane of the infected cell contains virus-specific glycoproteins that represent foreign antigens. This means that infected cells become targets for the immune system. In fact, cytotoxic T lymphocytes that recognize these antigens can be a significant factor in combating a virus infection.

The budding process rarely causes cell death

Most retroviruses (except HIV) reproduce without cell death

The process of viral budding usually does not lead directly to cell death because the plasma membrane can be repaired following budding. It is likely that cell death for most enveloped viruses, as for naked capsid viruses, is related to the loss of normal cellular functions required for survival or as a result of apoptosis. Unlike most retroviruses that do not kill the host cell, HIV-1 is cytotoxic. Although the mechanism of HIV-1 cell killing is not entirely understood, factors such as the accumulation of viral DNA in the cytoplasm, the toxic effects of certain viral proteins, alterations in plasma membrane permeability, and cell–cell fusion, are believed to contribute to the cytotoxic potential of the virus.

CELL SURVIVAL

Filamentous phages assemble during extrusion without damaging cells

For retroviruses (except HIV-1 and other lentiviruses) and the filamentous bacteriophages, virus reproduction and cell survival are compatible. Retroviruses convert their RNA genome into double-stranded DNA, which integrates into a host cell chromosome and is transcribed just like any other cellular gene (see Chapter 42). Thus, the impact on cellular metabolism is minimal. Moreover, the virus buds through the plasma membrane without any permanent damage to the cell.

Because the filamentous phages are naked capsid viruses, cell survival is even more remarkable. In this case, the helical capsid is assembled onto the condensed single-stranded DNA genome as the structure is being extruded through both the membrane and the cell wall of the bacterium. How the cell escapes permanent damage in this case is unknown. As with the retroviruses, the infected cell continues to produce virus indefinitely.

QUANTITATION OF VIRUSES

Hemagglutination Assay

For some animal viruses, red blood cells from one or more animal species contain receptors for the virion attachment proteins. Because the receptors and attachment proteins are present in multiple copies on the cells and virions, respectively, an excess of virus particles coats the cells and causes them to aggregate. This aggregation phenomenon was first discovered with influenza virus and is called **hemagglutination.** The virion attachment protein on the influenza virion is appropriately called the **hemagglutinin.** Furthermore, the presence of the hemagglutinin in the plasma membrane of the infected cell means that the cells as well as the virions will bind the red blood cells. This reaction, called **hemadsorption,** is a useful indicator of infection by certain viruses (see Chapter 15).

Virion and infected cell attachment proteins also bind red blood cells

Hemagglutination can be used to estimate the titer of virus particles in a virus-containing sample. Serially diluted samples of the virus preparation are mixed with a constant amount of red blood cells, and the mixture is allowed to settle in a test tube. Agglutinated red blood cells settle to the bottom to form a thin, dispersed layer. If there is insufficient virus to agglutinate the red blood cells, they will settle to the bottom of the tube and form a tight pellet. The difference is easily scored visually and the endpoint of the agglutination is used as a relative measure of the virus concentration in the sample.

Plaque Assay

The plaque assay is a method for determining the titer of infectious virions in a virus preparation or lysate. The sample is diluted serially and an aliquot of each dilution is added to a vast excess of susceptible host cells. For an animal virus, the host cells are usually attached to the bottom of a plastic petri dish; for bacterial cells, adsorption is typically carried out in a cell suspension. In both cases the cells are then immersed in a semisolid medium such as agar, which prevents the released virions from spreading throughout the entire cell population. Thus the virus released from the initial and subsequent rounds of infection can only invade the cells in the immediate vicinity of the initial infected cell on the plate. The end result is an easily visible clearing of dead cells at each of the sites on the plate where one of the original infected cells was located. The clearing is called a **plaque** (Fig 6–12). Visualization

Plaque assay: dilutions of virus are added to excess cells immobilized in agar

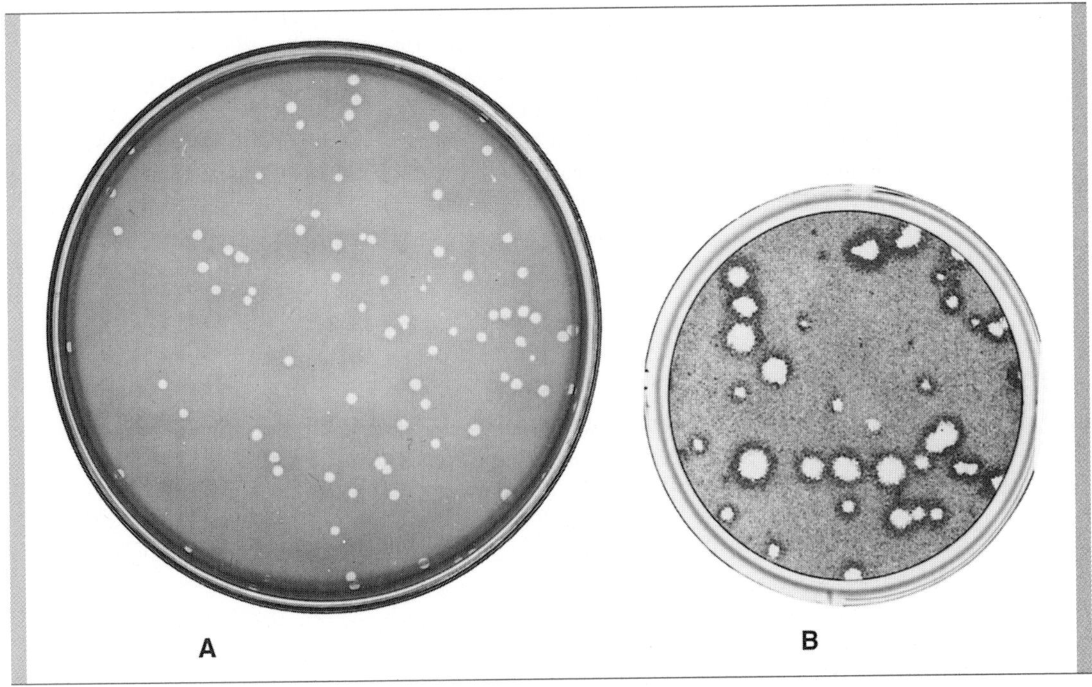

FIGURE 6–12
Plaque assays: **A.** Bacteriophage λ. **B.** Adenovirus.

Replicated virus infects only neighboring cells, producing countable plaques

in the case of animal cells usually requires staining the cells. By counting the number of plaques and correcting for the dilution factor, the virus titer in the original sample can be calculated. The titer is usually expressed as the number of plaque-forming units per milliliter (pfu/mL).

INTERFERONS

Interferons are chemokines produced by virally infected cells that inhibit virus production in other cells

Interferons are not virus specific

Interferons are host-encoded proteins that provide the first line of defense against viral infections. They belong to the class of molecules called **chemokines,** which are proteins or glycoproteins that are involved in cell-to-cell communication. Virus infection of all types of cells stimulates the production and secretion of either interferon α or interferon β, which acts on other cells to induce what is called the **antiviral state.** Unlike immunity, the interferons are not specific to a particular kind of virus; however, interferons usually act only on cells of the same species. Other agents stimulate the production of interferon γ by lymphoid cells. In this case, interferon appears to play an important role in the immune system independent of any role as an antiviral protein (see Chapter 10).

Interferons are produced in response to accumulation of double-stranded RNA during viral synthesis

The signal that leads to the production of interferon by an infected cell appears to be double-stranded RNA. This conclusion is based on the observation that treatment of cells with purified double-stranded RNA or synthetic double-stranded ribopolymers results in the secretion of interferon. Although the mechanisms are largely unclear and probably vary from one virus to another, viral infections in general lead to the accumulation of significant levels of double-stranded RNA in the cell.

Interferons inhibit viral protein synthesis by inducing cellular enzymes that require double-stranded RNA

All protein synthesis is inhibited but only in infected cells

Changes in the synthesis of a large number of cellular proteins are characteristic of the antiviral state induced by interferon. However, the cells exhibit only minimal changes in their metabolic or growth properties. The machinery to inhibit virus production is mobilized only on infection. Interferon has multiple effects on cells, but only three systems have been extensively studied. The first system involves a protein called Mx that is induced by interferon and specifically blocks influenza infections by interfering with viral transcription. The second system involves the upregulation of protein kinase that is dependent on double-stranded RNA and PKR which phosphorylates and thereby inactivates one of the subunits of an initiation factor (eIF-2) necessary for protein synthesis. In some cases, viruses have evolved quite specific mechanisms to block the action of this protein kinase. The third system involves the induction of an enzyme called 2′,5′-oligoadenylate synthetase, which synthesizes chains of 2′,5′-oligo(A) up to 10 residues in length. In turn, the 2′,5′-oligo(A) activates a constitutive ribonuclease, called RNase L, that degrades mRNA. The activities of both PKR and 2′,5′-oligo(A) synthetase require the presence of double-stranded RNA, the intracellular signal that an infection is occurring. This requirement prevents interferon from having an adverse effect on protein synthesis in uninfected cells. In these latter two cases, viral infection of a cell that has been exposed to interferon results in a general inhibition of protein synthesis, leading to cell death and no virus production. A cell that was destined to die anyway from a viral infection is sacrificed for the benefit of the entire organism.

ADDITIONAL READING

Knipe DM, Howley PM, eds. *Fields Virology.* 4th ed. Philadelphia: Lippincott Williams & Wilkins; 2001. A current and comprehensive overview of animal viruses.

White DO, Fenner FJ, eds. *Medical Virology.* 4th ed. San Diego: Academic Press; 1994. A good overview of medical aspects of virology.

CHAPTER 7

Viral Genetics

JAMES J. CHAMPOUX

In the typical lytic infection described in Chapter 6, viruses invade a host cell and usurp the machinery of the cell for their own reproduction. The end result is usually cell death with the release of large numbers of new infectious virus particles, most of which are phenotypically identical to the original invading virus. This apparent homogeneity is deceptive.

This chapter considers the methods whereby viral genomes change by mutation and recombination and examines the medical consequences of some of these changes. In addition, it also discusses the methods used by temperate viruses to enter, maintain, and sometimes leave the latent state. Furthermore, it examines in some detail the means by which both bacterial and animal cells can be permanently changed by viral latency.

MECHANISMS OF GENETIC CHANGE

For DNA bacteriophages, the ratio of infectious particles to total particles usually approaches a value of one. Such is not the case for animal viruses. Typically fewer than 1% of the particles derived from a cell infected with an animal virus are infectious in other cells as determined by a plaque assay. Although some of this discrepancy may be attributable to inefficiencies in the assay procedures, it is clear that many defective particles are being produced. In part, this production of defective particles arises because the mutation rates for animal viruses are unusually high and because many infections occur at high multiplicities, where defective genomes are complemented by nondefective viruses and therefore propagated.

Most of the animal virus particles from an infected cell are defective

Mutation

Many DNA viruses use the host DNA synthesis machinery for replicating their genomes. Therefore, they benefit from the built-in proofreading and other error-correcting mechanisms used by the cell. However, the largest animal viruses (adenoviruses, herpesviruses, and poxviruses) code for their own DNA polymerases, and these enzymes are not as effective at proofreading as the cellular polymerases. The resulting higher error rates in DNA replication endow the viruses with the potential for a high rate of evolution, but they are also partially responsible for the high frequency of defective viral particles.

The replication of RNA viruses is characterized by even higher error rates because viral RNA polymerases do not possess any proofreading capabilities. The result is that error rates for RNA viruses commonly approach one mistake for every 2500 to 10,000 nucleotides polymerized. Such a high misincorporation rate means that even for the smallest RNA viruses, virtually every round of replication introduces one or more nucleotide changes somewhere in the genome. If it is assumed that errors are introduced at random, most of the members of a clone (eg, in a plaque) are genetically different from all other members of the clone. The resulting mixture of different genome sequences for a particular RNA virus has been referred to as a **quasispecies** to emphasize that the level of genetic variation is much greater than what normally exists in a species.

High error rates for RNA viruses produce genetically heterogeneous populations

Because of the redundancy in the genetic code, some mutations are silent and are not reflected in changes at the protein level, but many occur in essential genes and contribute to the large number of defective particles found for RNA animal viruses. The concept of genetic stability takes on a new meaning in view of these considerations, and the RNA virus population as a whole maintains some degree of homogeneity only because of the high degree of fitness exhibited by a subset of the possible genome sequences. Thus, strong selective forces continually operate on a population to eliminate most mutants that fail to compete with the few very successful members of the population. However, any time the environment changes (eg, appearance of neutralizing antibodies), a new subset of the population is selected and maintained as long as the selective forces remain constant.

High mutation rates permit adaptation to changed conditions

Mutations are responsible for antigenic drift in influenza viruses

The high mutation rates found for RNA viruses endow them with a genetic plasticity that leads readily to the occurrence of genetic variants and permits rapid adaptation to new environmental conditions. The large number of serotypes of the rhinoviruses causing the common cold, for instance, likely reflect the potential to vary by mutation. Although rapid genetic change occurs for most if not all viruses, no medically important RNA virus has exhibited this phenomenon as conspicuously as influenza virus. Point mutations accumulate in the influenza genes coding for the two envelope proteins (hemagglutinin and neuraminidase), resulting in changes in the antigenic structure of the virions. These changes lead to new variants not recognized by the immune system of previously infected individuals. This phenomenon is called **antigenic drift** (see Chapter 33). Apparently, those domains of the two envelope proteins that are most important for immune recognition are not essential for virus reproduction and, as a result, can tolerate amino acid changes leading to antigenic variation. This feature may distinguish influenza from other human RNA viruses that possess the same high mutation rates, but do not exhibit such high rates of antigenic drift. Antigenic drift in epidemic influenza viruses from year to year requires continual updating of the strains used to produce immunizing vaccines.

Retroviruses use two error-prone polymerases for replication

The retroviruses likewise show high rates of variation because they depend for their replication on two different polymerases, both of which are error prone. In the first step of the replication cycle, the reverse transcriptase that copies the RNA genome into double-stranded DNA lacks a proofreading capability. Once the viral DNA has integrated into the chromosome of the host cell, the DNA is transcribed by the host RNA polymerase II, which similarly is incapable of proofreading. Accordingly, the retroviruses, including human immunodeficiency virus type 1 (HIV-1), the causative agent of acquired immunodeficiency syndrome (AIDS), exhibit a high rate of mutation. This property gives them the ability to evolve rapidly in response to changing conditions in the infected host.

HIV-1 antigenic variation makes vaccine development difficult

Retroviruses that exhibit high rates of antigenic variation such as HIV-1 pose particularly difficult problems for the development of effective vaccines. Attempts are being made to identify conserved, and therefore presumably essential, domains of the envelope proteins for these viruses, which might be useful in developing a genetically engineered vaccine.

Von Magnus Phenomenon and Defective Interfering Particles

Defective interfering particles accumulate at high multiplicities of infection

In early studies with influenza virus, it was noted that serial passage of virus stocks at high multiplicities of infection led to a steady decline of infectious titer with each passage. At the same time, the titer of noninfectious particles increased. As is discussed below, the noninfectious genomes interfere with the replication of the infectious virus and so are called **defective interfering (DI) particles.** Later, these observations were extended to include virtually all DNA as well as RNA animal viruses. The phenomenon is now named after von Magnus, who described the initial observations with influenza virus.

A combination of two separate events lead to this phenomenon. First, deletion mutations occur at a significant frequency for all viruses. For DNA viruses, the mechanisms are not well understood, but deletions presumably occur as a result of mistakes in replication or by nonhomologous recombination. The basis for the occurrence of deletions in RNA viruses is better understood. All RNA replicases have a tendency to dissociate from the template RNA but remain bound to the end of the growing RNA chain. By reassociating with the same or a different template at a different location, the replicase "finishes" replication, but in the process creates a shorter or longer RNA molecule. A subset of these variants possess the proper signals for initiating RNA synthesis and continue replicating. Because the deletion variants in the population require less time to complete a replication cycle, they eventually predominate and constitute the DI particles.

Deletions result from mistakes in replication, recombination, or the dissociation–reassociation of replicases

Second, as their name implies, the DI particles interfere with the replication of nondefective particles. Interference occurs because the DI particles successfully compete with the nondefective genomes for a limited supply of replication enzymes. The virions released at the end of the infection are therefore enriched for the DI particles. With each successive infection, the DI particles can predominate over the normal particles as long as the multiplicity of infection is high enough so that every cell is infected with at least one normal infectious particle. If this condition is satisfied, then the normal particle can complement any defects in the DI particles and provide all of the viral proteins required for the infection. Eventually, however, as serial passage is continued, the multiplicity of infectious particles drops below one, and the majority of the cells are infected only with DI particles. When this happens the proportion of DI particles in the progeny virus decreases.

Defective interfering particles compete with infectious particles for replication enzymes

In good laboratory practice, virus stocks are passaged at high dilutions to avoid the problem of the emergence of high titers of DI particles. Nevertheless, the presence of DI particles is a major contributor to the low fraction of infectious virions found in all virus stocks.

Recombination

Besides mutation, genetic recombination between related viruses is a major source of genomic variation. Bacterial cells as well as the nuclei of animal cells contain the enzymes necessary for homologous recombination of DNA. Thus, it is not surprising that recombinants arise from mixed infections involving two different strains of the same type of DNA virus. The larger bacteriophages such as λ and T4 code for their own recombination enzymes, a fact that attests to the importance of recombination in the life cycles and possibly the evolution of these viruses. The fact that recombination has also been observed for cytoplasmic poxviruses suggests that they too code for their own recombination enzymes.

Homologous recombination is common in DNA viruses

As far as is known, cells do not possess the machinery to recombine RNA molecules. However, recombination among at least some RNA viruses has been observed by two different mechanisms. The first, which is unique to the viruses with segmented genomes (orthomyxoviruses and reoviruses), involves reassortment of segments during a mixed infection involving two different viral strains. Recombinant progeny viruses that differ from either parent can be accounted for by the formation of new combinations of the genomic segments that are free to mix with each other at some time during the infection. Reassortment of this type occurring during infections of the same cell by human and certain animal influenza viruses is believed to account for the occasional drastic change in the antigenicity of the human influenza A virus. These dramatic changes, called **antigenic shifts**, produce strains to which much of the human population lacks immunity and, thus, can have enormous epidemiologic and clinical consequences (see Chapter 33).

Recombination for viruses with segmented RNA genomes involves reassortment of segments

Segment reassortment in mixed infections probably accounts for antigenic shifts in influenza virus

The second mechanism of RNA virus recombination is exemplified by the genetic recombination between different forms of poliovirus. Because the poliovirus RNA genome is not segmented, reassortment cannot be invoked as the basis for the observed recombinants. In this case, it appears that recombination occurs during replication by a "copy choice" type of mechanism. During RNA synthesis, the replicase dissociates from one template and resumes copying a second template at the exact place where it left off on the first. The end result is a progeny RNA genome containing information from two different input RNA molecules. Strand switching during replication, therefore, generates a recombinant virus. Although this is not frequently observed, it is likely that most of the RNA animal viruses are capable of this type of recombination.

Poliovirus replicase switches templates to generate recombinants

A "copy choice" mechanism has also been invoked to explain a high rate of recombination observed with retroviruses. Early after infection, the reverse transcriptase within

The diploid nature of retroviruses permits template switching and recombination during DNA synthesis

Occasional incorporation of host mRNA into retroviral particles may produce oncogenic variants

the virion synthesizes a DNA copy of the RNA genome by a process called reverse transcription. In the course of reverse transcription, the enzyme is required to "jump" between two sites on the RNA genome (see Chapter 42). This propensity to switch templates apparently explains how the enzyme generates recombinant viruses. Because reverse transcription takes place in subviral particles, free mixing of RNA templates brought into the cell in different virus particles is not permitted. However, retroviruses are diploid, because each particle carries two copies of the genome. This arrangement appears to be a situation ready-made for template switching during DNA synthesis and most likely accounts for retroviral recombination.

Occasionally, retroviruses package a cellular mRNA into the virion instead of a second RNA genome. This arrangement can lead to copy choice recombination between the viral genome and a cellular mRNA. The end result is sometimes the incorporation of a cellular gene into the viral genome. This mechanism is believed to account for the production of highly oncogenic retroviruses containing modified cellular genes (see below).

THE LATENT STATE

The latent state involves infection of a cell with little or no virus production

Latent virus may be silent, change cell phenotype, or be induced to enter the lytic cycle

Temperate viruses can infect a cell and enter a latent state that is characterized by little or no virus production. The viral DNA genome is replicated and segregated along with the cellular DNA when the cell divides. There exist two possible states for the latent viral genome. It can exist extrachromosomally like a bacterial plasmid, or it can become integrated into the chromosome like the bacterial F factor in the formation of a high-frequency recombination (HFR) strain (see Chapter 4). Because the latent genome is usually capable of reactivation and entry into the lytic cycle, it is called a **provirus** or, in the case of bacteriophages, a **prophage.** In many cases, viral latency goes undetected; however, limited expression of proviral genes can occasionally endow the cell with a new set of properties. For instance, lysogeny can lead to the production of virulence-determining toxins in some bacteria (lysogenic conversion) and latency by an animal virus may produce oncogenic transformation.

LYSOGENY

E. coli phage λ may be lytic or latent

When λ is integrated, the only active gene encodes a repressor for the other phage genes

Inactivation of repressor causes induction and virus production

Infection of an *Escherichia coli* cell by bacteriophage λ can have two possible outcomes. A portion of the cells (as many as 90%) enters the lytic cycle and produces more phage. The remainder of the cells enter the latent state by forming stable lysogens. The proportion of the population that lyses depends on as yet undefined factors including the nutritional and physiologic state of the bacteria. In the lysogenic state, the phage DNA is physically inserted into the bacterial chromosome (see below) and thus replicates when the bacterial DNA replicates. Lambda can thus replicate either extrachromosomally as in the lytic cycle or as a part of the bacterial chromosome in lysogeny. The only phage gene that remains active in a lysogen is the gene that codes for a repressor protein that turns off expression of all of the prophage genes except its own. This means that the lysogenic state can persist as long as the bacterial strain survives. Environmental insults such as exposure to ultraviolet light or mutagens, cause inactivation of the repressor, resulting in induction of the lysogen. The prophage DNA is excised from the bacterial chromosome, and a lytic cycle ensues.

Latent genomes can exist extrachromosomally or can be integrated

Once established, perpetuation of the lysogenic state requires a mechanism to ensure that copies of the phage genes are faithfully passed on to both daughter cells during cell division. Integration of the λ genome into the *E. coli* chromosome guarantees its replication and successful segregation during cell division. In bacteriophage P1 lysogens, the viral genome exists extrachromosomally as an autonomous single-copy plasmid. Its replication is tightly coupled to chromosomal replication and the two replicated copies are precisely partitioned along with the cellular chromosomes to daughter cells during cell division.

Phage λ integrates by site-specific recombination

Because of its mechanistic importance and relevance to lysogenic conversion and phage transduction (see Chapter 4), λ integration and the reverse reaction called excision are described in some detail. Bacteriophage λ integrates by a site-specific, reciprocal recombination event as outlined in Figure 7–1. There exist unique sequences on both the phage and

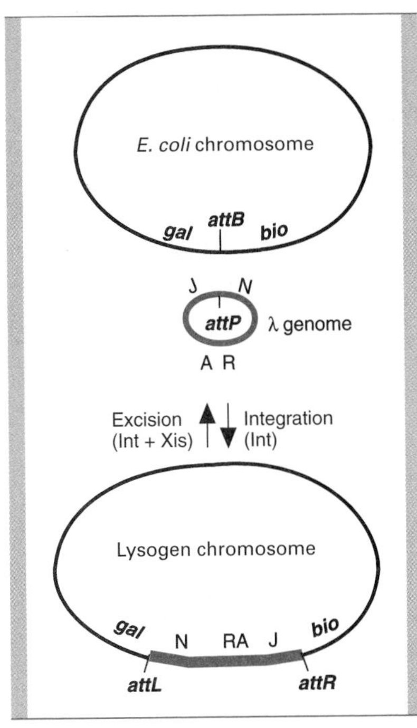

FIGURE 7–1
λ integration and excision. A, J, N, and R show the locations of some λ genes on the λ genome; *gal* and *bio* represent the *Escherichia coli* galactose and biotin operons, respectively.

bacterial chromosomes called attachment sites where the crossover occurs. The phage attachment site is called *attP* and the bacterial site, which is found on the *E. coli* chromosome between the galactose and biotin operons, is called *attB.* The recombination reaction is catalyzed by the phage-encoded integrase protein (Int) in conjunction with two host proteins and occurs by a highly concerted reaction that requires no new DNA synthesis.

Excision of the phage genome after induction of a lysogen is just the reverse of integration, except that excision requires, in addition to the Int protein, a second phage protein called Xis. In this case the combined activities of these two proteins catalyze site-specific recombination between the two attachment sites that flank the prophage DNA, *attL* and *attR* (see Fig 7–1). Early after infection, when integration is to occur in those cells destined to become lysogens, synthesis of the Xis protein is blocked. Otherwise, the integrated prophage DNA would excise soon after integration and stable lysogeny would be impossible. However, after induction of a lysogen, both the integrase and the Xis proteins are synthesized and catalyze the excision event that releases the prophage DNA from the chromosome.

Excision after λ induction involves recombination at junctions between host DNA and prophage

At a very low frequency, excision involves sites other than the *attL* and *attR* borders of the prophage and results in the linking of bacterial genes to the phage genome. Thus, if a site to the left of the bacterial *gal* genes recombines with a site within the λ genome (to the left of the J gene, otherwise the excised genome is too large to be packaged), then the resulting phage can transduce the genes for galactose metabolism to another cell (see Chapter 4). Similarly, transducing particles can be formed that carry the genes involved in biotin biosynthesis. Because only those cellular genes adjacent to the attachment site can be acquired by an aberrant excision event, this process is called **specialized transduction** to distinguish it from generalized transduction, in which virtually any bacterial gene can be transferred by a headful packaging mechanism (see Chapters 4 and 6).

Specialized transduction occurs because excision occasionally includes genes adjacent to the phage genome

Occasionally, one or more phage genes, in addition to the gene coding for the repressor protein, are expressed in the lysogenic state. If the expressed protein confers a new phenotypic property on the cell, then it is said that lysogenic conversion has occurred. Diphtheria, scarlet fever, and botulism are all caused by toxins produced by bacteria that have been "converted" by a temperate bacteriophage. In each case, the gene that codes for the toxin protein resides in the phage DNA and is expressed along with the repressor gene in the lysogenic state. It remains a mystery as to how these toxin genes were acquired by the phage; it is speculated that they may have been picked up by a mechanism similar to specialized transduction.

Lysogenic conversion results from expression of a prophage gene that alters cell phenotype

Several bacterial exotoxins are encoded in temperate phages

MALIGNANT TRANSFORMATION

Malignant cells fail to respond to signals controlling the growth and location of normal cells

A tumor is an abnormal growth of cells. Tumors are classified as benign or malignant, depending on whether they remain localized or have a tendency to invade or spread by metastasis. Therefore, malignant cells have at least two defects. They fail to respond to controlling signals that normally limit the growth of nonmalignant cells, and they fail to recognize their neighbors and remain in their proper location. When grown in tissue culture in the laboratory, these tumor cells exhibit a series of properties that correlate with the uncontrolled growth potential associated with the tumor in the organism.

1. They have altered cell morphology.
2. They fail to grow in the organized patterns found for normal cells.
3. They grow to much higher cell densities than do normal cells under conditions of unlimited nutrients; therefore, they appear unable to enter the resting G_0 state.
4. They have lower nutritional and serum requirements than normal cells.
5. They have the capacity to divide in suspension, whereas normal cells require an anchoring substrate and grow only on surfaces (eg, glass or plastic).
6. They are usually able to grow indefinitely in cell culture.

Malignant transformation of cells in culture can be accomplished by most DNA viruses and some retroviruses

Many DNA animal viruses and some representatives of the retroviruses can convert normal cultured cells into cells that possess the properties listed above. This process is called **malignant transformation.** In addition to the listed properties, viral transformation usually, but not always, endows the cells with the capacity to form a tumor when introduced into the appropriate animal. Although the original use of the term **transformation** referred to the changes occurring in cells grown in the laboratory, current usage often includes the initial events in the animal that lead to the development of a tumor. In recent years, it has become increasingly clear that some but not all of these viruses also cause cancers in the host species from which they were isolated.

Transformation by DNA Animal Viruses

Some oncogenic viruses cause tumors in their natural hosts

The oncogenic potential of animal DNA viruses is summarized in Table 7–1. All known DNA animal viruses, except parvoviruses, are capable of causing aberrant cell proliferation under some conditions. For some viruses, transformation or tumor formation has been observed only in species other than the natural host. Apparently infections of cells

TABLE 7–1

Oncogenicity of DNA Viruses

Virus or Virus Group	Tumors in Natural Host[a]	Tumors in Other Species[b]	Transform Cells in Tissue Culture
Parvoviruses (rat, mouse, human)	No	No	No
Animal polyomaviruses (polyoma, simian virus 40)	No	Yes	Yes
Human polyomaviruses (JC, BK)	No	Yes	Yes
Papillomaviruses (human, rabbit)	Yes, often benign	?	Yes
Human hepatitis B virus	Yes	?	No
Human adenoviruses	No	Yes	Yes
Human herpesviruses	Yes	Yes	Yes
Poxviruses (human, rabbit)	Occasionally, usually benign	Yes	No

[a] "Yes" means that at least one member of the group is oncogenic.
[b] Test usually done in newborns of immunosuppressed hosts.

from the natural host are so cytocidal that no survivors remain to be transformed. In addition, some viruses have been implicated in human or animal tumors without any indication that they can transform cells in culture.

In nearly all cases that have been characterized, viral transformation is the result of the continual expression of one or more viral genes that are directly responsible for the loss of growth control. Two targets have been identified that appear to be critical for the transforming potential of these viruses. Adenoviruses, papilloma viruses, and simian virus 40 all code for either one or two proteins that interact with the tumor suppressor proteins known as p53 and Rb (for retinoblastoma protein) to block their normal function which is to exert a tight control over cell cycle progression. The end result is endless cell cycling and uncontrolled growth.

In many respects, transformation is analogous to lysogenic conversion and requires that the viral genes be incorporated into the cell as inheritable elements. Incorporation usually involves integration into the chromosome (eg, papovaviruses, adenoviruses, and retroviruses), although the DNAs of some papillomaviruses and some herpesviruses are found in transformed cells as extrachromosomal plasmids. Unlike some of the temperate bacteriophages that code for the enzymes necessary for integration, papovaviruses and adenoviruses integrate by nonhomologous recombination using enzymes present in the host cell. The recombination event is therefore nonspecific, both with respect to the viral DNA and with respect to the chromosomal locus at which insertion occurs. It follows that for transformation to be successful, the insertional recombination must not disrupt a viral gene required for transformation. In summary, two events appear to be necessary for viral transformation: a persistent association of viral genes with the cell and the expression of certain viral "transforming" proteins.

Transformation by DNA viruses is analogous to lysogenic conversion

Transformation by Retroviruses

Two features of the replicative cycle of retroviruses are related to the oncogenic potential of this class of viruses. First, most retroviruses do not kill the host cell, but instead set up a permanent infection with continual virus production. Second, a DNA copy of the RNA genome is integrated into the host cell DNA by a virally encoded integrase (IN); however, unlike bacteriophage λ integration, a linear form of the viral DNA, rather than a circular form, is the substrate for integration. Furthermore, unlike λ, there does not appear to be a specific site in the cell DNA where integration occurs.

Most retroviruses produce virions without causing host cell death

A DNA copy of the retroviral genome is integrated, but not at a specific site

Retroviruses are known to transform cells by three different mechanisms. First, many animal retroviruses have acquired transforming genes called **oncogenes.** More than 30 such oncogenes have now been found since the original oncogene was identified in Rous sarcoma virus (called v-*src*, where the v stands for viral). Because normal cells possess homologs of these genes called **protooncogenes** (eg, c-*src*, where c stands for cellular), it is generally thought that viral oncogenes originated from host DNA. It is possible they were picked up by "copy choice" recombination involving packaged cellular mRNAs as previously described. Because these transforming viruses carry cellular genes, they are sometimes referred to as **transducing** retroviruses. Most of the viral oncogenes have suffered one or more mutations that make them different from the cellular protooncogenes. These changes presumably alter the protein products so that they cause transformation. Although the mechanisms of oncogenesis are not completely understood, it appears that transformation results from inappropriate production of an abnormal protein that interferes with normal signaling processes within the cell. Uncontrolled cell proliferation is the result. Because tumor formation by retroviruses carrying an oncogene is efficient and rapid, these viruses are often referred to as **acute transforming viruses.** Although common in some animal species, this mechanism has not yet been recognized as a cause of any human cancers.

Retroviruses may carry transforming oncogenes

Oncogenes encode a protein that interferes with cell signaling

The second mechanism is called **insertional mutagenesis** and is not dependent on continued production of a viral gene product. Instead, the presence of the viral promoter or enhancer is sufficient to cause the inappropriate expression of a cellular gene residing in the immediate vicinity of the integrated provirus. This mechanism was first recognized in avian B-cell lymphomas caused by an avian leukosis virus, a disease characterized by a very long latent period. Tumor cells from different individuals were found to have a copy

Insertional mutagenesis causes inappropriate expression of a protooncogene adjacent to integrated viral genome

of the provirus integrated at the same place in the cellular DNA. The site of the provirus insertion was found to be next to a cellular protooncogene called c-*myc*. The *myc* gene had previously been identified as a viral oncogene called v-*myc*. In this case, transformation occurs not because the c-*myc* gene is altered by mutation but because the viral promoter adjacent to the gene turns on its expression continuously and the gene product is overproduced. The disease has a long latent period; because, although the birds are viremic from early life, the probability of an integration occurring next to the c-*myc* gene is very low. Once such an integration event does occur, however, cell proliferation is rapid and a tumor develops. No human tumors are known for certain to result from insertional mutagenesis caused by a retrovirus; however, human cancers are known where a chromosome translocation has placed an active cellular promoter next to a cellular protooncogene (Burkitt's lymphoma and chronic myelogenous leukemia).

Human T-cell leukemia is caused by transactivating factor encoded in integrated HTLV-1

Transactivating factor turns on cellular genes, causing cell proliferation

The third mechanism was revealed by the discovery of the first human retrovirus. The virus, human T-cell lymphotropic virus type 1 (HTLV-1), is the causative agent of adult T-cell leukemia. HTLV-1 sequences are found integrated in the DNA of the leukemic cells and all the tumor cells from a particular individual have the proviral DNA in the same location. This observation indicates that the tumor is a clone derived from a single cell; however, the sites of integration in tumors from different individuals are different. Thus, HTLV-1 does not cause malignancy by promoter insertion near a particular cellular gene. Instead, the virus has a gene called *tax* that codes for a protein that acts in trans (ie, on other genes in the same cell) to not only promote maximal transcription of the proviral DNA, but also to transcriptionally activate an array of cellular genes. The resulting cellular proteins cooperate to cause uncontrolled cell proliferation. The *tax* gene is therefore different from the oncogenes of the acute transforming retroviruses in that it is a viral gene rather than a gene derived from a cellular protooncogene. HTLV-1 is commonly described as a **transactivating** retrovirus.

ADDITIONAL READING

Natanson N. *Viral Pathogenesis and Immunity*. Philadelphia: Lippincott Williams & Wilkins; 2002. This readable, concise book covers viral pathogenesis, virus–host interactions, and host responses to infection. Specific topics include virulence, persistence, and oncogenesis.

PART III

Host-Parasite Interactions

CHAPTER 8

Immune Response to Infection

JOHN J. MARCHALONIS

Many innate defenses protect us from potential pathogens, including structural barriers and cells and molecules of the innate immune system such as phagocytes and acute phase proteins (also called inflammation), which are considered in Chapter 10. The **adaptive immune response** of vertebrates differs from these in that it is a specific, inducible, and anticipatory defense mechanism that allows the discrimination between self and nonself. The concept of immunity on which the science of immunology is built begins with ancient observations, such as Thucydides' description of the plague of Athens in 430 BC in which individuals who were infected and survived were not susceptible to infection by the same pathogen. A specific contemporary definition of the immune response is that it is a complex and precisely regulated inducible defense mechanism that allows the specific discrimination between self and nonself. The immune system requires for its function the presence of antigen-specific lymphocytes of two major types, thymus-derived lymphocytes (T cells) and bone marrow–derived lymphocytes (B cells), and it builds on the more primitive defense mechanisms of the **innate immune system** such as phagocytosis, while using mediators of cell communication termed **cytokines** to facilitate regulation of the complex system. Another characteristic that defines the immune response of mammals is that it is anticipatory; a process of combinatorial gene rearrangement generates an array of T and B cells with the aggregate populations comprising hundreds of millions of individual lymphocytes, each expressing a different receptor specificity in advance of any challenge. This preexisting readiness allows the production of circulating antibodies to the foreign challenge as well as the generation of the T-cell receptors that initiates the specific immune process leading to the elaboration of specific effector T lymphocytes (eg, helpers or killers).

Immunity discriminates between self and nonself

Specific mechanisms are inducible

One of the major recent successes of immunology has been eradication by vaccination of historic scourges such as smallpox. In addition to defense against infection, the immune system is important in normal developmental processes, aging, maintenance of internal homeostasis, and surveillance against neoplasms. This chapter presents an overview of major features of the immune system that are relevant to medical microbiology and infectious diseases. It is also intended to allow readers who have not yet studied immunology to understand the details of host–parasite interactions and immune responses to specific infections that are given elsewhere in the text. A listing of current immunology texts is provided at the end of the chapter.

Immune system is important for developmental processes and defense against infectious disease

The adaptive immune response differs from the innate or constitutive mechanisms in two major respects. The first is that the response is inducible; that is, the challenge to a healthy individual by a bacterium, virus, or other foreign (nonself) matter initiates a process

TABLE 8–1

Cells Involved in the Immune System

Cell	Function	Specific Receptors for Antigen	Characteristic Cell Surface Marker	Special Characteristics
B cells	Production of antibody Present antigen to T cells	Surface immunoglobulin (IgM_m, IgD_m)	Fc and complement C3d receptors; MHC class II	Differentiate into plasma cells (major antibody producers)
T cells Helpers (T_H)	Stimulate B cells by providing specific and nonspecific (cytokine) signals for activation and differentiation Activate macrophages by cytokines	α/β Tcr	CD3+, CD4+, CD8−	Activation is restricted by MHC class II Can be classified into two types: T_H1 activates macrophages, makes interferon γ, T_H2 activates B cells, makes IL-4
Cytotoxic (T_C)	Lyse antigen-expressing cells such as virally infected cells or allografts	α/β Tcr	CD3+, CD4−, CD8+	Restricted by MHC class I
Suppressors (T_S)	Downregulate cellular or humoral immunity	α/β Tcr, other variant Tcr	Can be CD3+ or CD3−; usually CD4−, CD8+	
Regulatory T cell (T_{REG})	Suppresses T cell–mediated inflammation	α/β Tcr	CD4+, CD25+	Diminishes autoimmunity
Natural killer (NK) cells	Spontaneous lysis of tumor cells, antibody-dependent cellular cytotoxicity	Inhibitory (KIR); activating (eg, NKG2D)	Fc receptor for IgG	KIR recognize MHC class I
NK T cells	Amplify both cell-mediated and humoral immunity	α/β Tcr	CD4+	Express a restricted subset of Vα
Macrophages (monocytes)	Phagocytosis, secretion of cytokines to activate T cells (eg, IL-1) or other accessory cells such as neutrophils	None but can be "armed" by antibodies binding to Fc receptors	Macrophage surface antigens	Express surface receptors for the activated third component of complement (C3), kill ingested bacteria by oxidative bursts
Polymorphonuclear leukocytes (neutrophils, eosinophils)	Phagocytosis killing	None but can be "armed" by antibodies		Protective in parasitic infections, but adverse side effects such as granuloma formation can occur

Abbreviations: Tcr, T-cell receptor; MHC, major histocompatibility complex.

leading to the production of circulating proteins called **antibodies** that recognize and bind the invading pathogen in a specific manner. A second challenge by the same pathogen results in an accelerated immune response (secondary or anamnestic) that can confer greater protection on the host in a manner specific for that pathogen (eg, vaccination against measles protects against measles but not against polio).

Antibodies are inducible proteins that recognize and bind to invaders

The second major definitive characteristic of the human immune response is that it is anticipatory; that is, because of the combinatorial generation of the recognition repertoire, it has the potential to respond to pathogens not yet encountered in evolutionary history. This striking feature of the immune response results from the large number of genes specifying individual antibody combining sites for antigen and from a genetic recombination mechanism that allows us to form millions of potential antibody combining sites. Each antigen-specific lymphocyte (T or B) expresses a single receptor, and the cells are thus clonally restricted. In 1959, Sir MacFarlane Burnet predicted **clonal restriction** and **selection** by antigen, thus providing the intellectual foundation of modern immunology. The system is also endowed with the property of memory, so that reexposure to the inciting agent in the future usually brings about an enhanced response. Another crucial property of the combinational system is that it can be come **tolerant** or nonreactive to self based on contact during early development. Immune defenses against infectious organisms involve both the innate and adaptive systems, with emphasis on different aspects for individual pathogens.

Enormous capacity for diversity derives from clonal selection

Immune system has memory

THE IMMUNORESPONSIVE CELLS

The function of the immune system requires antigen-specific lymphocytes of two major types (Table 8–1) and cytokines. **T cells** are thymus-derived lymphocytes and **B cells** are bone marrow–derived lymphocytes. **Cytokines** are secreted polypeptides that modulate the functions of cells (Table 8–2). Those produced by mononuclear cells (ie, lymphocytes and mononuclear phagocytic cells) are called **interleukins.** These regulate the growth and differentiation of lymphocytes and hematopoietic stem cells and the interactions among T cells, B cells, and monocytes in the elaboration of an immune response (see later discussion).

T cells, B cells, and mononuclear cells secrete peptides

T cells are responsible for (1) the initiation and modulation of immune responses (including B-cell responses); (2) cell-mediated immune processes that involve direct damage to antigen-bearing tissue or blood cells (eg, virally infected host cells); and (3) stimulation and enhancement of the nonspecific immune functions of the host (eg, the inflammatory reaction and antimicrobial activity of phagocytes). T cells are classified by the presence of the surface molecules called **CD4** and **CD8,** which in turn are related to functional activities classified as helper, suppressor, or cytotoxic.

T cells initiate and modulate immune responses and act directly

TABLE 8–2

Biological Properties of Some Characterized Cytokines

PROPERTY	IFN-α	IFN-β	IFN-γ	IL-1α	IL-1β	IL-2	IL-3	IL-4	IL-5	IL-10
Mitogenesis			+	+	+	+	+	+	+	+
Effect on macrophages	+	+	+			+		+		+
B-cell activation			+	+	+			+	+	
B-cell proliferation	+	+	+	+	+	+	+	+	?	
B-cell differentiation	+		+	+	+	+	+	+	?	+
Ig isotype selection								IgE: IgG1	IgA	+
T-cell activation				+	+	+		+		
T-cell proliferation	+			+	+	+		+		+
T-cell differentiation						+		+		
Pyrogenic	+	+	+	+	+	+				

B cells are responsible for humoral immunity

T and B cells are widely distributed

B cells are responsible for humoral immunity through antibody production. Individual B cells have antibody of a single specificity on their surface that can bind directly to foreign antigens. B cells can also differentiate into plasma cells, which produce a soluble antibody that can circulate in blood and body fluids independent of cells. T and B cells are found throughout the body, particularly in the bone marrow; specialized areas of the lymph nodes and spleen; lymphoid structures adjacent to the alimentary and respiratory tracts (eg, Peyer's patches and adenoids); and subepithelial tissues of the internal organs. They are continually replaced, and there is considerable circulation of B and T cells between the different areas of the body through the lymphatic and blood vascular circulations.

ANTIGENS AND EPITOPES

Antigens stimulate and react with antibody

Epitopes fit to the combining site of T-cell receptors and antibodies

An **antigen** is a substance (usually foreign) that reacts with antibody and may stimulate an immune response when presented in an effective fashion. A large structure such as a protein, virus, or bacterium contains many subregions that are the actual antigenic determinants, or **epitopes.** These epitopes can consist of peptides, carbohydrates, or particular lipids of the correct size and three-dimensional configuration to fill the combining site of an antibody molecule or a T-cell receptor (Fig 8–1). Approximately six amino acids or monosaccharide units provide a correctly sized epitope. Much of our knowledge of the combining sites of antibodies and their specificities was determined by immunizing animals experimentally with small organic molecules called **haptens.** Some of the best examples of these are substituted phenols, such as 2,4-dinitrophenol, which themselves do not induce the production of antibodies but must be coupled to a **carrier molecule** to be immunogenic. The term **immunogen** is a synonym for antigen, but it is sometimes restricted to those antigens able to elicit an immune response as distinguished from the ability to react only with antibodies and with T-cell receptors.

B cells multiply and produce antibody

A foreign antigen entering a human host may by chance encounter a B cell whose surface antibody is able to bind it. This interaction stimulates the B cell to multiply, differentiate, and produce more surface and soluble antibody of the same specificity. Eventually, the process leads to production of enough antibody to bind more of the antigen. This mechanism is most likely to operate with antigens such as polysaccharides that have repeating subunits, thus improving the chance that exposed epitopes are recognized.

Protein antigens must be processed first

Large, complex antigens such as proteins and viruses must be processed before their epitopes can be effectively recognized by the immune system. This processing takes place in macrophages or specialized epithelial cells found in the skin and lymphoid organs,

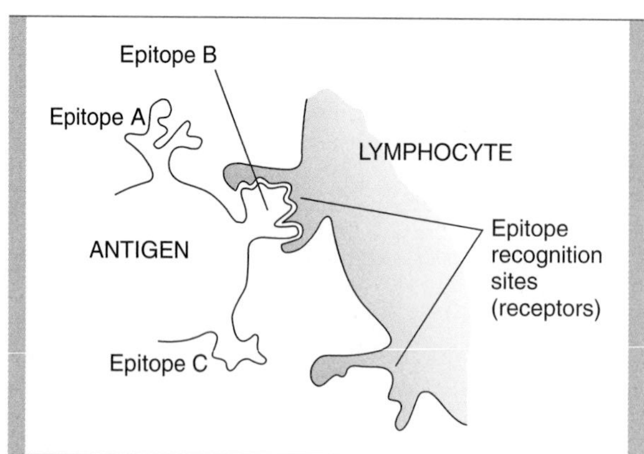

FIGURE 8–1
Schematic of epitope recognition by an immunoresponsive lymphocyte. Epitope B on the antigen binds to a complementary recognition site on the surface of the immunoresponsive cell. Antigens may have multiple different epitopes, but an immunoresponsive lymphocyte has receptors of only one specificity. In most cases, epitopes are recognized on the surface of macrophages that have processed the antigen. The receptor for antigens on B cells is the combining site of the surface immunoglobulin.

where they are adjacent to other immunoresponsive cells. The ingested antigen is degraded to peptides of 10 to 20 amino acids that are presented by major histocompatibility (MHC) products on the host cell surface to be recognized by T cells.

BASIS OF IMMUNOLOGIC SPECIFICITY

The intellectual framework for understanding the mechanisms of immunologic specificity was laid down by the theory of **clonal selection.** It is now generally accepted that human lymphocyte populations, both B and T cells, show a great heterogeneity inasmuch as different cells possess surface receptors, which differ from each other with respect to combining site. This is shown in Figure 8–2 for B cells. In the actual process, great heterogeneity in the immune response even to particular antigens is observed. Particular domains termed **hypervariable regions** provide the actual amino acid residues that confer individual specificity. In the role of B cells in antibody production, there would be a differentiation from the lymphocytes to the plasma cells, and shifts of types of antibody would occur, depending on secondary stimulation and regulatory cytokines.

Clonal selection provides diversity in amino acid residues

With the elimination of antigen, the majority of the clone of immunoreactive lymphocytes is lost over time by normal cell replacement. However, the speed with which antigen is lost is very variable and depends on such factors as excretion and enzymatic breakdown. Some polysaccharide antigens and bacterial cell wall peptidoglycans are so resistant to host enzymatic breakdown that they can persist for years, whereas many protein antigens are rapidly metabolized. Fortunately, the immune system has a recall

Some antigens persist for years

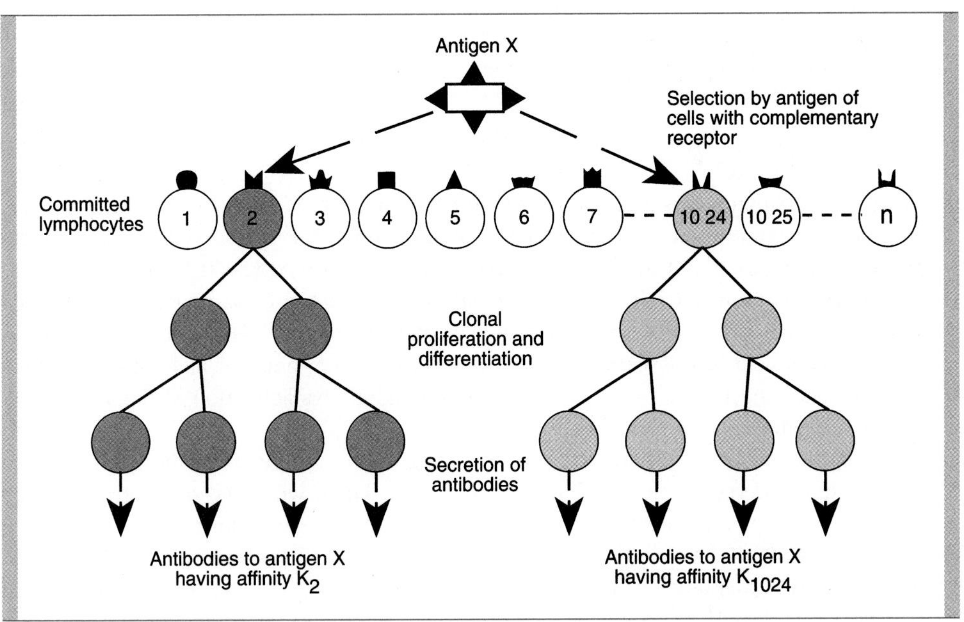

FIGURE 8–2
Diagram of the cellular events involved in the clonal selection of specifically reactive B lymphocytes by antigen. Clonal selection of T lymphocytes could be depicted by a comparable scheme, but T cells do not secrete antibodies and the antigen would be presented in association with molecules of the major histocompatibility complex. Each B cell is numbered to show that it represents an individual clone. The schematic representation of the surface immunoglobulin receptors indicates that these have distinct combining sites. The combining sites are formed by interaction of V_H and V_L domains, and the cell-to-cell distinction in receptor specificity results from essentially a random genetic process. If a particular antigen, designated X here, enters the system, it can bind specifically, albeit with different affinities, to two of the cells shown here. If there are proper antigen presentation and interplay of cytokines involved in activation in differentiation, the recognition of antigen by the surface immunoglobulin receptor results in clonal proliferation and differentiation of those cells recognizing the antigen. In this case, antibodies representing two types of combining sites are generated.

Memory cells survive to provide recall ability

ability in the case of protein antigens, because certain cells in the clone, termed **memory cells,** survive long periods and probably slowly replicate to maintain a core population with the capacity to expand very rapidly if the antigen (or the same epitope on another antigen) is encountered again.

Secondary response is rapid and greater than primary response

Vaccines stimulate secondary responses

Memory cells may be either T or B cells and are probably variants within the original clone having recognition sites with higher specific affinity for the relevant antigenic determinant and, thus, greater immunologic efficiency. As a consequence, the response to a second encounter with an antigen is more rapid than the first and quantitatively greater in its effect. It is referred to as a secondary response, in contrast to the initial primary response. Memory cells and the secondary response phenomenon account for the prolonged or lifelong immunity that follows many infections (eg, measles), and the secondary response is exploited in scheduling doses of various vaccines to obtain the maximum and most long-lived immunity.

THE T-CELL RESPONSE

The major roles of T cells in the immune response are:

1. Recognition of peptide epitopes presented by MHC molecules on cell surfaces. This is followed by activation and clonal expansion of T cells in the case of epitopes associated with class II MHC molecules.
2. Production of lymphokines that act as intercellular signals and mediate the activation and modulation of various aspects of the immune response and of nonspecific host defenses.
3. Direct killing of foreign cells, of host cells bearing foreign surface antigens along with class I MHC molecules (eg, some virally infected cells), and of some immunologically recognized tumor cells.

Antigen-Specific Receptors of T Cells

α/β and γ/δ T-cell receptors are associated with CD3 complex

There are two major types of T-cell receptors in humans. More than 90% of T cells in adult spleen, lymph nodes, and peripheral blood express the α/β receptor, which is depicted in Figure 8–3. A small subset (usually 5%) of T cells express the γ/δ receptor. The γ/δ receptor is more prevalent on fetal T cells, has a limited capacity for diversity, and shows an association with responses to mycobacterial infections. Both the α/β and γ/δ T-cell receptors occur in association with the CD3 complex, a set of at least five distinct proteins that is necessary for signal transduction and allows activation of the T cells following recognition of antigen.

MHC presents processed peptides to the T-cell receptor

MHC class II are only on lymphocytes and macrophages

A particular set of cell surface proteins specified by the genes of the MHC plays a major role in the recognition of antigens by T cells. These were first discovered through transplantation experiments, where it was found that they were major markers recognized in graft rejection. Subsequently, a strong association between susceptibility to disease and particular MHC markers was found. The MHC contains sets of genes that are designated as class I and class II determinants. These loci are highly polymorphic, and within populations, association with particular MHC markers correlates with the capacity to respond to particular antigens. Recent studies have shown that peptide determinants produced by proteolytic degradation of proteins by antigen-presenting accessory cells bind to MHC products, which then present the peptide antigen to the α/β T-cell receptor. Human class I molecules (HLA-A, HLA-B, and HLA-C) are expressed on virtually all cells of the body, whereas class II molecules (HLA-DR) are restricted to lymphocytes and macrophages, including important antigen-presenting cells such as dendritic cells.

CD4 and CD8 surface markers vary on T cells

Cytotoxic T cells recognize antigen on MHC class I molecules and express the CD8 marker. By contrast, cells bearing the γ/δ antigen-specific T-cell receptor (Tcr) lack both CD4 and CD8. Figure 8–3 shows a membrane form of antibody expressed on B cells as a comparison with the α/β antigen-specific receptor of T cells. α/β T-cell receptors have not been found to any degree in serum and exist predominantly as cell surface recognition molecules. The affinity of T-cell receptors for antigen is low, and the role of MHC presentation of antigen is most probably to compensate for the low affinity.

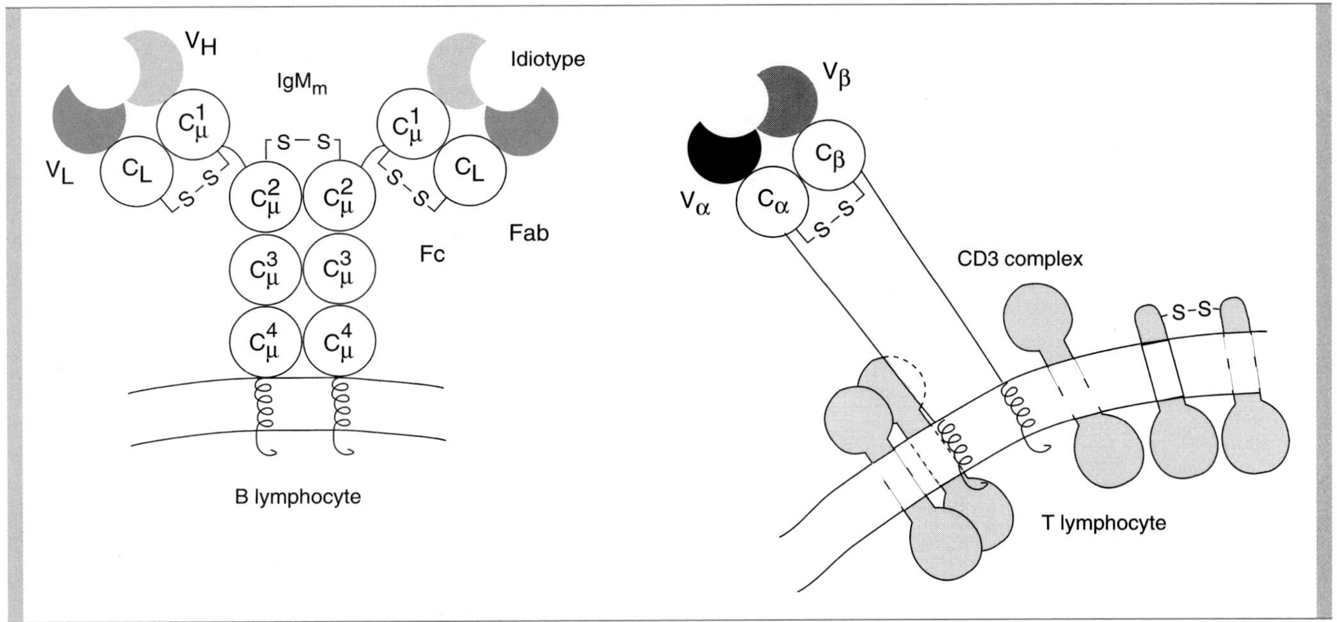

FIGURE 8–3
Comparison of the membrane IgM receptor of primary B cells with the α/β T-cell receptor of helper, cytolytic, and delayed-type hypersensitivity T cells. The IgM_m molecule is a monomer consisting of two μ chains and two light chains, in contrast with the pentamer shown in Figure 8–6. The locations of the combining sites for antigen and the idiotypic marker are depicted. An additional difference between the serum form and the membrane form is the presence of a helical transmembrane region at the C-terminal end of the membrane receptor. In overall form, the α/β T-cell receptor is a disulfide-bonded heterodimer that resembles a single Fab fragment of immunoglobulin. In addition, it has an elongated stretch comparable to a hinge that terminates in a membrane-spanning helical region.

Specific T-cell help is initiated by the binding of α/β Tcr to antigen presented by MHC class II molecules. Most of the details of antigen presentation have been established using protein antigens, with an emphasis on virally infected cells so that the general principles apply to specific cytolytic cells as well. These proteins are digested into peptides by phagocytic cells (sometimes referred to as accessory cells), with certain peptides bound in a peptide-binding cleft within the MHC molecules intracellularly. These peptide–MHC complexes are then expressed on the cell surface, where the peptide epitope can be presented to the low-affinity antigen combining site of the α/β Tcr on T cells of compatible MHC type.

Peptides digested in phagocytes are presented to T cells

The initial specificity of cytotoxic T cells is, likewise, impacted by the α/β Tcr, but the MHC restriction involves class I molecules. In humans, the vast majority of circulating T cells bear the α/β Tcr. The CD3 surface marker comprises at least five distinct proteins involved in forming a membrane activation complex in association with the Tcr. The γ/δ Tcr is the first to appear in fetal development, but it constitutes less than 5% of T cells in the adult. Like the α/β Tcr, it occurs in association with CD3. γ/δ Tcr-bearing T cells are cytotoxic but do not show MHC restriction.

Surface CD3 associates with Tcr

Other cellular phenomena can be nonspecific in the sense that neither antigen-specific antibodies nor T-cell receptors are involved. These include natural killer (NK) cells and armed or activated macrophages such as mast cells, basophils and eosinophils, and macrophages. Activated macrophages produce substances toxic to intracellular pathogens, including reactive nitrogen and oxygen intermediates that can kill the organisms. NK cells are cells related to lymphocytes that are present in the absence of antigenic stimulation that recognize and kill particular types of turnor cells. NK cells recognize MHC class I through inhibitory receptors and lyse cells such as tumors that lack the MHC markers. Two major types of NK cells have been described: NK cells and NKT cells. The first type are usually large and granular and kill certain tumors and also function in innate immunity to viruses

NK cells do not require antigen stimulation

Innate viral immunity is related to NK cells

and intracellular pathogens. NKT cells express the α/β Tcr but with only one Vα gene product, have T-cell markers, and are secreted by T_H1 (interferon-γ, or IFN-γ) and T_H2-type (interleukin-4, or IL-4) cytokines.

Cytotoxic T cells are antigen-specific killer cells

Antigen-specific sensitized killer cells are induced by specific sensitization with the target antigen. The cytotoxic T cells are activated by the presence of processed antigen and cytokines by a MHC-compatible antigen-presenting cell and show a subsequent MHC restriction in their capacity to destroy target cells. Cytotoxic T cells use the α/β T-cell receptor in recognition of peptide I MHC antigens. Cells with delayed-type hypersensitivity also are antigen-specific T cells that can be generated in the absence of circulating antibodies. An example of delayed-type hypersensitivity is skin sensitization with small organic molecules, such as the quinone produced by poison ivy.

CD4+ Helper T Lymphocytes

T_H cells are stimulated by MHC II presented antigen

IL-1 then IL-2 are secreted

B-cell differentiation is triggered

Helper T cells (T_H cells) are stimulated by antigen in the context of MHC class II presentation and are further marked by the presence of the CD4 cell surface antigen. If T cells are of the proper MHC background to recognize the antigen specifically, T-cell activation occurs in the presence of IL-1. The antigen–MHC complex presented to a specific T cell by the macrophage is the specific signal that induces the T cell to become activated and divide. The secretion of IL-2, following stimulation by IL-1, promotes the division of T cells following contact with antigens. The activated T_H cell presents both antigen and regulatory cytokines to the B cells, orchestrating the scheme of B cell differentiation from small lymphocytes to plasma cells producing antibodies of various types. The ability of particular B cells or T cells to respond to stimulation by individual cytokines is dependent on the presence of surface receptors for those cytokines.

Cytokines regulate physiologic processes

Role of T_H1 and T_H2 varies with antibody, cells, and infectious agents

Table 8–2 outlines the biological properties of some characterized cytokines. Cytokines can be involved in general physiologic or aphysiologic processes such as the induction of fever, mitogenesis or division of lymphocytes, and the stimulation of phagocytic cells. Other cytokines are involved in regulating activation of specific subsets of lymphocytes, and some have an extremely specific function in regulating the immunoglobulin isotypes expressed. The immune response is a complex but precisely regulated defense system in which specific recognition is imparted by antibodies, B-cell immunoglobulin receptors, and T-cell receptors, and activation and differentiation are dependent on a regulatory cascade of cell–cell communication molecules. The functional roles of cytokines produced by subsets of CD4+ helper cells; T_H1 and T_H2, are essential for the discrimination between antibody formation (T_H2) and inflammatory cell-mediated immunity (T_H1) and, consequently, for the severity of autoimmune disease (T_H1), the capacity to reject tumors (T_H1), the immune resistance to viruses and intracellular parasites (T_H1), the resistance to helminth worms (T_H2), the susceptibility to viruses and intracellular parasites (T_H2), and susceptibility to allergic disorders (T_H2).

HIV binds to CD4 molecule

The critical significance of CD4+ helper cells to the body is shown by the catastrophic effects of acquired immunodeficiency syndrome (AIDS), in which the human immunodeficiency virus (HIV) binds to the CD4 molecule, enters the cell, and interferes with its function or destroys it. As a result, the body becomes susceptible to a wide variety of bacterial, viral, protozoal, and fungal infections, both through loss of preexisting immunity and through failure to mount an effective immune response to newly acquired pathogens.

CD8+ Cytotoxic T Lymphocytes

CD8+ lymphocytes react with MHC I

Eliminate virally infected cells

CD8+ cytotoxic T lymphocytes are a second class of effector T cells. They are lethal to cells expressing the epitope against which they are directed when the epitope is in conjunction with class I MHC molecules. They too have specific epitope recognition sites, but they are characterized by the CD8 cell surface marker; thus, they are referred to as CD8+ cytotoxic T cells. These cells recognize the association of antigenic epitopes with class I MHC molecules on a wide variety of cells of the body. However, this recognition does not itself lead to the necessary clonal expansion of CD8 cells, which also requires the lymphokine IL-2 to be produced by activated CD4+ lymphocytes. In the case of virally infected cells, cytotoxic CD8+ cells prevent viral production and release by eliminating the host cell before viral synthesis or assembly is complete.

CD8+ Suppressor T Cells

Suppressor T lymphocytes also carrying the CD8 marker and epitope recognition sites are involved in modulating and terminating the immunologic activities of both T and B cells, thus avoiding excessive or needlessly prolonged responses that could interfere with other immunologic activities. It is known that the suppression they produce may be antigen specific or it may be polyclonal (ie, affecting general immunologic responses irrespective of the inciting antigen). The mechanisms of suppression and control are less well defined than are the activities of CD4+ helper cells. In AIDS, the proportion of CD8+ suppressor cells relative to CD4+ helper T cells is substantially increased, because CD8+ lymphocytes are not attacked by HIV. This imbalance, in addition to the depletion of CD4+ helper cells, may contribute to the immunosuppression that is characteristic of the disease.

Suppressor T cells modulate T- and B-cell activities

Spared by HIV

Regulatory T Cells

Regulatory T cells are CD4+, Tcr α,β+ T cells that also express the CD25 marker. They suppress T_H1-type mediated inflammatory responses, particularly destructive autoimmunity.

Autoimmunity is suppressed

Response to Superantigens

A group of antigens have been termed **superantigens** because they stimulate a much larger number of T cells than would be predicted based on the generation of combining site diversity through clonal selection. Superantigens activate 3 to 30% of T cells in unstimulated animals. The action of superantigens is based on their ability to bind directly to MHC proteins and to particular Vβ regions of the T-cell receptor (see Fig 8–3) without involving the antigen combining site. Individual superantigens recognize exposed portions defined by framework residues that are common to the structure of one or more Vβ regions. Any T cells bearing those Vβ sites may be directly stimulated. A variety of microbial products have been identified as superantigens. An example in which the pyrogenic exotoxins of *Staphylococcus aureus* and group A streptococci act as superantigens is **toxic shock syndrome** (see Chapters 16 and 17).

Superantigens bind directly to MHC proteins and Tcr Vβ region

Higher proportion of T cells are stimulated

CELL-MEDIATED IMMUNITY

Cell-mediated immunity is most dramatically expressed as a response to obligate or facultative intracellular pathogens. These include certain slow-growing bacteria, such as the mycobacteria, against which antibody responses are ineffective. In experimental infections, cell-mediated immunity can be passively transferred from one animal to another by T lymphocytes but not by serum. (In contrast, short-term, antibody-mediated [B-cell] immunity can be passively transferred with serum.) The mechanisms of cell-mediated immunity are complex and involve a number of cytokines with amplifying feedback mechanisms for their production. The initial processing of antigen is accompanied by sufficient IL-1 production by the macrophages to stimulate activation of the antigen-recognizing CD4+ (helper) cell. Lymphokine feedback from the CD4+ T cells to macrophages further increases IL-1 production. IL-2 produced by the CD4+ T cells facilitates their clonal expansion and activates CD8+ (cytotoxic) T lymphocytes. Other lymphokines from CD4+ T cells chemotactically attract macrophages to the site of infection, hold them there, and activate them to greatly enhance microbicidal activity. The sum of the individual and collaborative activities of T cells, macrophages, and their products is a progressive mobilization of a range of nonspecific host defenses to the site of infection and greatly enhanced macrophage activity. In the case of viruses, IFN-γ inhibits replication, and CD8+ cytotoxic lymphocytes destroy their cellular habitat, leaving already assembled virions accessible to circulating antibody. The interplay among cells of the innate immune system, including monocytes, macrophages, and dendritic cells; the essential elements of specific immune system, T cells (particularly T_H1 and T_H2 cells), B cells, and antibodies; and the regulatory roles of proinflammatory (eg, IL-2, IFN-γ)

Of primary importance with intracellular pathogens

Helper and cytotoxic T lymphocytes interact

Macrophages are mobilized and enhanced

and anti-inflammatory (eg, IL-4, IL-6) cytokines in adaptive resistance to particular types of pathogenic organisms will be considered below.

With certain infections in which reaction to protein antigens is particularly strong (eg, in the response to *Mycobacterium tuberculosis*), the cell-mediated responses are of such magnitude that they become major deleterious factors in the disease process itself. This is called delayed-type hypersensitivity, because reexposure of the host to the antigen that elicited the immune response produces a maximum hypersensitive reaction only after a day or two, when mobilization of immune lymphocytes and of phagocytic macrophages is at its peak.

Prolonged cell-mediated immune response may cause injury

B CELLS AND ANTIBODY RESPONSES

B lymphocytes are the cells responsible for antibody responses. They develop from precursor cells in the yolk sac and fetal liver before birth and thereafter in the bone marrow before migrating to other lymphoid tissues. Each mature cell of this series carries a specific epitope recognition site on its surface—the antigen-recognizing (variable) region of antibody that will be produced subsequently by its progeny. In the process of antibody formation, B lymphocytes, following stimulation by antigen, divide and differentiate into plasma cells, which are end cells adapted for secretion of large amounts of antibodies. In addition to their essential role in antibody production, B cells can present antigen to T cells.

B cells carry epitope recognition sites on their surface

Stimulated cells differentiate to form plasma cells

There are two broad types of antigens. **T-independent antigens** are those that do not require help by T cells to stimulate B-cell antibody production, and **T-dependent antigens** are those that are dependent on collaboration between helper T cells and B cells to initiate the process of antibody production. T-independent antigens are generally limited to large polymeric molecules such as carbohydrates with repeating sugar epitopes. Antibodies are particularly effective and essential to the protective immune response to the polysaccharide capsule of *Streptococcus pneumoniae,* because these bacteria would not otherwise be bound and ingested by phagocytes. Killing of the bacteria is initiated by the specific binding of antibodies to the surface polysaccharides, and it is carried out by either the binding of complement to the antibody on the bacterial surface or by the binding of Fc receptors on phagocytic cells to the bound antibody, thus facilitating ingestion and intracellular killing. Immunologic reactivity to such polysaccharides usually develops much more slowly after birth than do the T-dependent responses, and memory cells do not result from the clonal B-cell expansion. This delay in responsiveness probably contributes to the increased susceptibility to some bacterial infections in early life. Most common antigens, particularly proteins, require T-cell help by CD4+ cells for antibody production to occur. Following stimulation by antigen processed and presented by macrophages, T cells can become helper cells collaborating with B cells, antigen-specific cytotoxic T cells capable of killing tumor cells, suppressor T cells downregulating the immune system, or T cells mediating delayed-type hypersensitivity. Table 8–1 lists major cells in the immune response and their antigen-specific and nonspecific functions.

T-cell independent responses require only polysaccharide antigen and B cells

T-cell dependent responses require helper T cells

T-independent responses develop more slowly from birth

Following challenge with foreign antigen, there is a lag period of 4 to 6 days before antibody can be detected in serum. This period reflects the events involved in the recognition of the antigen, its processing, and the specific activation of the cells of the immune system. The first event is the clearance of antigen from the circulation by what is essentially a metabolic process in which the antigen is recognized in a nonspecific sense and ingested. The vast preponderance of antigen ends up in circulating phagocytes or in stationary macrophages such as the Kupffer cells in the liver. The macrophages process the antigen so that immunogenic moieties can be presented to T cells (Fig 8–4). IL-4, IL-5, and IL-6, in addition to specific presentation of antigen, cause the B cells to produce immunoglobulins and also are involved in class switches. The antibody-forming system is a learning system that responds to challenge by foreign molecules by producing large amounts of specific antibody. In addition, the affinity of its binding to the specifically recognized antigen often increases with time or secondary challenge.

Antigen processing causes delay in antibody response

Learning system increases affinity with time or secondary challenge

Antibodies

Antibodies belong to the **immunoglobulin** family of proteins, which occur in quantity in serum and on the surfaces of B cells. The basic structure of an immunoglobulin is illustrated

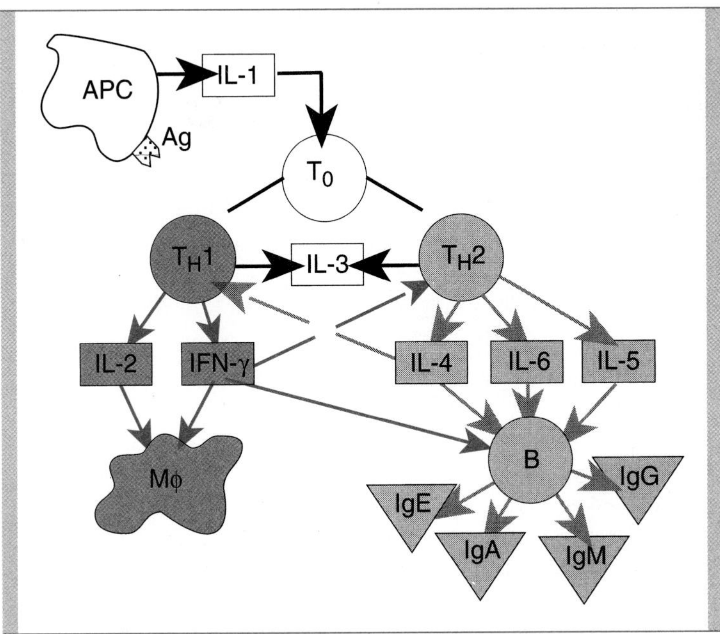

FIGURE 8–4
Simplified diagram illustrating events of helper T-cell activation leading to either cellular immunity of the delayed-type hypersensitive type (T_H1 cells) or antibody production (T_H2) involving stimulation of B cells by specific and nonspecific (cytokine) means. The cytokine interleukin-2 (IL-2) plays a major role in causing T-cell mitogenesis and also in the activation of macrophages. This is abbreviated as an antigen-presenting cell (APC), which presents both processed antigen (Ag) to antigen-specific T cells and a stimulatory cytokine (IL-1) that causes the stimulated T cell to differentiate into one of two broad types of T cells; termed T_H1 and T_H2 here. The T_H1 cells produce IL-2 and IL-3 and interferon-γ and can stimulate macrophages, T_H2 cells, and B cells. The T_H2 cells produce IL-3, -4, -5, and -6 and carry out a major role as helpers in activating B cells.

in Figure 8–5, which depicts an IgG molecule. Immunoglobulins have a basic tetrameric structure consisting of two light polypeptide chains and two heavy chains usually associated as light/heavy pairs by disulfide bonds. The two light/heavy pairs are covalently associated by disulfide bonds to form the tetramer. There are two types of light chains, κ chains and λ chains, which are the products of distinct genetic loci. The class or isotype of the immunoglobulin is defined by the type of heavy chain expressed. In this IgG molecule, the heavy chains are termed γ chains and have characteristic sequences and antigenic markers. IgG immunoglobulins can have either κ or λ chains associated with the γ, but only one type of light chain would be present in the intact molecule. That is, an individual IgG molecule would be either $\gamma2\kappa2$, or $\gamma2\lambda2$; mixed molecules do not occur. This diagram illustrates other basic structural features of the molecule. The basic building block of immunoglobulins is a domain of approximately 110 amino acids containing an internal disulfide bond stabilizing the structure. **Domains** are compact, tightly folded structures having a characteristic "immunoglobulin fold." The light chains contain two domains: a variable domain and a constant domain. The γ heavy chain contains four domains: V_H, $C_\gamma1$, $C_\gamma2$, and $C_\gamma3$.

Immunoglobulins have tetrameric structure combining light chains and heavy chains

Isotypes are defined by type of heavy chain

Antibodies carry out two broad sets of functions: the recognition function is the property of the combining site for antigen, and the effector functions are mediated by the constant regions of the heavy chains. Antibodies combine with foreign antigens, but the actual destruction or removal of antigen requires the interaction of portions of the Fc fragment with other molecules such as complement components or with effector cells, which then engulf the recognized cell or particle.

Antibodies have recognition and effector functions

The combining site for antigen (antigen binding site) is formed by interaction of the **variable domains** of the heavy chain and the light chain. The IgG molecule has two such combining sites. Immunoglobulin in the serum of normal individuals occurs as a large pool of individual molecules, each of which has a unique sequence and a defined combining

Combining site is idiotype

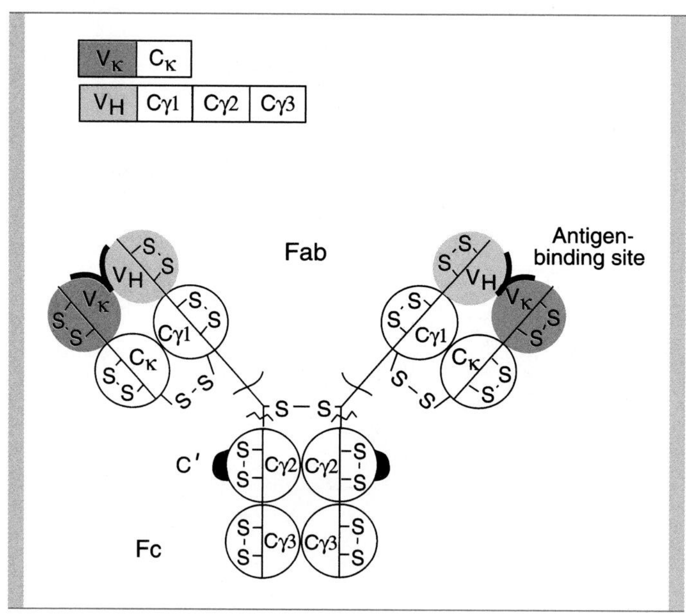

FIGURE 8–5
Schematic representation of an IgG immunoglobulin molecule. This model illustrates the domain structure of immunoglobulin light and heavy chains in a stick model form (top) and as compact, circular domains (bottom). Two combining sites for antigen are present, and these are formed by interaction between the V_H and V_K domains of the molecule. The binding site for complement (C′) is shown to be located in the Cγ2 domain. The region of the heavy chain where no domain structure is shown is the "hinge" region. This region is the site of cleavage of the proteolytic enzymes papain and pepsin. The Fc fragment produced by proteolysis contains the binding site for complement and is crystallizable. The Fab fragment contains the variable regions and binds antigen.

site. The defined combining site of an immunoglobulin has been termed an **idiotype.** The idiotype is a combining site-related antigenic marker that defines individual immunoglobulins. Other types of antigenic markers of immunoglobulins define classes or isotypes. These occur on the constant regions of light chains, where they define the κ and λ isotypes. Heavy chains have C_H markers identifying μ, γ, δ, α and ε isotypes. These markers are found in all normal individuals. The third general type of immunoglobulin antigenic determinant is termed **allotypic.** These markers may be found on the light chains (eg, the KM determinant of human κ chains) or heavy chains (eg, the GM markers of human IgG) and define genetic markers that behave as Mendelian alleles in the human population. Allotypic markers are usually associated with constant regions but have been reported for the variable domains of heavy chains as well.

Allotype markers are in light or heavy chains

Another structural feature of immunoglobulins that merits consideration is the fact that proteolytic digestion of the IgG molecule by the enzyme papain can cleave the structure into two defined regions. As illustrated in Figure 8–5, two **antigen-binding** or **Fab** fragments are generated, and a single **constant** or **Fc** fragment is produced. The cleavage occurs in the so-called hinge region, which is a relatively loose stretch of polypeptide connecting the Fab domains to the $C_\gamma 2$ domain. The tight domain structures themselves are relatively resistant to proteolysis. The positions of the intradomain disulfides are indicated (S-S bonds). The intrachain disulfide bonds connecting the C_κ and $C_\gamma 1$ are also indicated, as is the location of the S-S bonds linking the two heavy chains. This basic structure, although using different heavy chains, occurs in all five of the major human immunoglobulin classes, but the number of subunits and the overall arrangement can vary. For example, Figure 8–6 gives a schematic representation of a serum IgM immunoglobulin. This molecule, which was originally called immune macroglobulin because of its large size (approximate mass of 900,000 daltons), consists of five subunits of the form of the typical IgG. The light chains can be either κ or λ, but the type of heavy chain defining the IgM class is termed the μ chain. The molecule occurs as a cyclic pentamer, and a J or joining

Fab is antigen-binding region

IgM has five subunits

IgA is a monomer or dimer

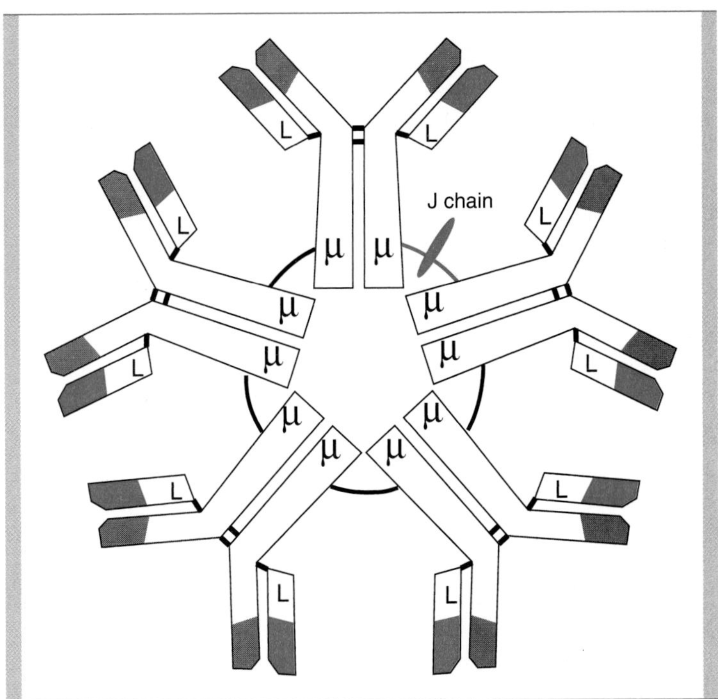

FIGURE 8–6
A planar projection model of serum IgM showing the structure as a cyclic pentamer held together by disulfide bonds. One joining (J) chain is associated with the pentamer. Approximately 10% of the mass of the μ chain consists of carbohydrate, which is associated with the constant region of the heavy chain.

chain is also associated with the intact structure. When IgM is present on B cells where it serves as a primary receptor for antigen, it is present as a monomer. Other immunoglobulins showing a difference in arrangement from the typical IgG model are the IgA immunoglobulins. In serum these can occur as a monomer, but they can also occur in dimers where the joining chain is required to stabilize the dimer. IgA molecules present in the gut (secretory IgA) occur as dimers where both the J chain and an additional polypeptide, termed the **secretory component,** are present in the complex.

Functional Properties of Immunoglobulins

Immunoglobulin G Antibody

Immunoglobulin G is the most abundant immunoglobulin in health and provides the most extensive and long-lived antibody response to the various microbial and other antigens that are encountered throughout the life span of the individual. Although at least four subclasses of IgG have been characterized, they are grouped together for the purpose of this chapter. The IgG molecule is bivalent, with two identical and specific combining sites. The rest of the molecule is the constant (Fc) region, which does not vary with differences in specificity of combining sites of different antibody molecules. The constant region has specific sites for binding to phagocytic cells and for reaction with the first component of complement. These sites are made available when the variable region of the antibody molecule has reacted with specific antigen.

Bivalent molecule with specific combining site and constant region

Constant region binds phagocytes

Immunoglobulin G antibody is characteristically formed in large amounts during the secondary response to an antigenic stimulus and usually follows production of IgM (see below) in the course of a viral or bacterial infection. Memory cells are programmed for rapid IgG response when another antigenic stimulus of the same type occurs later. Immunoglobulin G antibodies are the most significant antibody class for neutralizing soluble antigens (eg, exotoxins) and viruses. They act by blocking the sites on the antigenic molecule or virus that determine attachment to cell receptors. IgG also enhances phagocytosis of particulate antigens such as bacteria, because the exposed Fc sites of antibody that is bound to the antigen have a specific affinity for receptors on the surface of phagocytic cells. As described later, the third component of complement also mediates attachment to phagocytes. Enhancement of phagocytosis by antibody, complement, or both is referred to as **opsonization.** Accelerated IgG responses from memory cell expansion frequently

Antibodies produced during secondary response neutralize toxins and viruses

Binding may block attachment receptor

Opsonization enhances phagocytosis

confer lifelong immunity when directed against microbial antigens that are determinants of virulence. There is active transport of the IgG molecule across the placental barrier, which allows maternal protective antibody to pass and, thus, provides passive immune protection to the fetus and newborn pending development of a mature immune system. It is the only immunoglobulin class known to be placentally transferred. The half-life of passively transferred IgG within the same species is approximately 1 month, and thus the infant is protected during a particularly vulnerable period of life.

Immunoglobulin M Antibody

Effective agglutinating antibody

Binds complement at multiple sites

Monomers of IgM constitute the specific epitope recognition sites on B cells that ultimately give rise to plasma cells producing one or another of the different immunoglobulin classes of antibody. Because of its multiple specific combining sites, IgM is particularly effective in agglutinating particles carrying epitopes against which it is directed. It also contains multiple sites for binding the first component of complement. These sites become available once the IgM molecule has reacted with antigen. IgM is particularly active in bringing about complement-mediated cytolytic damage to foreign antigen-bearing cells. It is not, itself, an opsonizing antibody because its Fc portion is not recognized by phagocytes. Opsonization occurs through its activation of the complement pathway; this process is discussed later in the chapter.

Earliest antibody after antigenic stimulation

Does not cross placental barrier

Immunoglobulin M is usually the earliest antibody to appear after an antigenic stimulus, but it tends to decline rapidly and is often succeeded by IgG production from the same clone of cells. It is primarily intravascular and does not cross the placental barrier to the fetus (in contrast to IgG). Thus, the presence of specific IgM against a potentially infecting agent in the blood of a neonate is a priori evidence of active infection rather than of passively acquired antibody from the mother. Antibody response to certain antigens, including the lipopolysaccharide O antigen of Gram-negative bacteria, is characteristically IgM. Some universally occurring antibodies (natural antibodies), such as those directed against blood group antigens, are also of the IgM class.

Immunoglobulin A Antibody

Secretory antibody is produced at mucosal surfaces

Secretory piece combines molecules and resists proteolysis

Immunoglobulin A has a special role as a major determinant of so-called local immunity in protecting epithelial surfaces from colonization and infection. Certain B cells in lymphoid tissues adjacent to or draining surface epithelia of the intestines, respiratory tract, and genitourinary tract are encoded for specific IgA production. After antigenic stimulus, the clone expands locally and some of the IgA-producing cells also migrate to other viscera and secretory glands. At the epithelia, two IgA molecules combine with another protein, termed the **secretory piece,** which is present on the surface of local epithelial cells. The complex, then termed **secretory IgA** (sIgA), passes through the cells into the mucous layer on the epithelial surface or into glandular secretions where it exerts its protective effect. The secretory piece not only mediates secretion but also protects the molecule against proteolysis by enzymes such as those present in the intestinal tract.

Interferes with attachment of microbes to mucosal surfaces

The major role of sIgA is to prevent attachment of antigen-carrying particles to receptors on mucous membrane epithelia. Thus, in the case of bacteria and viruses, it reacts with surface antigens that mediate adhesion and colonization and prevents the establishment of local infection or invasion of the subepithelial tissues. It can agglutinate particles but has no Fc domain for activating the classic complement pathway; however, it can activate the alternative pathway (see below). Reaction of IgA with antigen within the mucous membrane initiates an inflammatory reaction that helps mobilize other immunoglobulin and cellular defenses to the site of invasion. IgA response to an antigen is shorter lived than the IgG response.

Immunoglobulin E Antibody

Bound to mast cells and basophils

Immunoglobulin E is a monomer consisting of two light chains (either κ or λ) and two heavy chains. It is normally present in very small amounts in serum, and most IgE is bound firmly by its Fc portion to tissue mast cells and basophils, which are major producers of histamine. When IgE bound to mast cells reacts with specific antigen, the mast cells degranulate and release histamine and other factors that mediate an inflammatory reaction with dilation of the capillaries, exudation of plasma components, and attraction of neutrophils and eosinophils to the site. Thus, IgE contributes to a rapid second line of defense if surface-protective mechanisms are breached. IgE also plays a significant indirect role in the immune response to a number of helminthic (worm) infections because of attraction of eosinophils to the site at which it reacts with antigen. The eosinophils bind to the Fc portions of IgG molecules that have reacted with surface antigens of the parasite and help bring about its destruction. Certain types of allergies, to be discussed later in this chapter, are due to excessive production of IgE with specificity for a foreign protein. The pharmacologic effects of histamine and the other vasoactive mediators released from mast cells largely account for the symptoms of the disorder.

Important in parasitic infections

Allergies linked to IgE

Immunoglobulin D Antibody

Immunoglobulin D antibody consists of two light chains and two heavy chains. It is highly susceptible to proteolytic enzymes in the tissues and is found only in very low concentrations in serum. Its role is not fully understood, although, as indicated earlier, it is present on the surface of unstimulated B cells and may serve as a receptor for antigen. The chain composition, size, and some major biological properties of the separate classes of immunoglobulins are summarized in Table 8–3.

May be an antigen receptor

TABLE 8–3

Structural and Biological Properties of Human Immunoglobulins

	IgG	IgA	IgM	IgD	IgE
Heavy chain class	γ ($\gamma1$, $\gamma2$, $\gamma3$, $\gamma4$)	α ($\alpha1$, $\alpha2$)	μ	δ	ε
Light chain class	κ or λ	κ or λ	κ or λ	κ or λ	κ or λ
Molecular formula	$\gamma2\kappa2$, or $\gamma2\lambda2$	$\alpha2\kappa2$ or $\alpha2\lambda2$; ($\alpha2\kappa2$) SC-J or ($\alpha2\lambda2$) SC-J (mucosal form)	$(\mu2\kappa2)_5$J or $(\mu2\lambda2)_5$J or $\mu2\kappa2_m$ or $\mu2\lambda2_m$ (B-cell membrane)	$\delta2\kappa2_m$ or $\delta2\lambda2_m$	$\varepsilon2\kappa2$ or $\varepsilon2\lambda2$
Approximate mass	150,000	160,000 400,000	900,000 memb. 180,000	180,000	190,000
Serum concentration (mg/mL)	10	2	1.2	0.03	trace
Complement fixation (classic)	+	0	+++	0	0
Placental transfer	+	0	0	0	0
Reaginic activity	?	0	0	0	+++
Lysis of bacteria	+	+	+++	?	?
Antiviral activity	+	+++	+	?	?
B-cell receptor for antigen	+ (memory)	+ (memory)	+ (primary)	+ (primary)	+ (memory)

Antibody Production

The major events characterizing the general phenomenon of antibody production are illustrated in Figure 8–7 and summarized as follows: Initial contact with a new antigen (primary stimulus) evokes the so-called **primary response,** which is characterized by a lag phase of approximately 1 week between the challenge and the detection of circulating antibodies. In general, the length of the lag phase depends on the immunogenicity of the stimulating antigen and the sensitivity of the detection system for the antibodies produced. **Immunogenicity,** or the capacity to generate an immune response, is contingent on the state of the antigen when injected, the immunologic status of the animal, and the use of adjuvants or nonspecific amplifiers of immune reactivity. Once antibody is detected in serum, the levels rise exponentially to attain a maximal steady state in about 3 weeks. These levels then decline gradually with time if no further antigenic stimulation is given. The major antibodies synthesized in the primary immune response are the immune macroglobulins (IgM class). In the latter phase of the primary response, IgG antibodies arise, and these molecules eventually predominate. This transition is termed the IgM/IgG switch. Following a secondary or booster injection of the same antigen, the lag time between the immunization and the appearance of antibody is shortened, the rate of exponential increase to the maximum steady-state level is more rapid, and the steady-state level itself is higher, representing a larger amount of antibody. Another key factor of the **secondary response** is that the antibodies formed are predominantly of the IgG class. In addition to higher levels of antibody, the secondary IgG antibodies are often better antibodies in the sense that there has been a maturation in affinity of the combining sites so that the secondary antibodies are more effective at binding the antigen than were the IgM and initial IgG molecules produced. This process of affinity maturation results from a process of somatic mutation ongoing during the response.

After a lag phase, the primary response lasts for weeks and then declines

IgM response switches to IgG

Secondary response is primarily IgG

The preceding description of primary and secondary immune responses represents the idealized case that would be expected in normal individuals. Figure 8–8 illustrates the detailed sequence of IgG, IgM, and IgA antibodies to poliovirus that appears in the serum of a child who was immunized with three doses of attenuated live poliovirus. The inactivated virus was given at monthly intervals to a newborn beginning at 2 months of age. The contributions of serum IgM, IgG, and IgA antibodies are individually depicted. The overall capacity of the serum to neutralize the poliovirus is first detectable about 1 week following the primary immunization and reaches a plateau after the second immunization. The IgM antibody peaks at 1 week and gradually declines during the course of vaccination. Primary IgG plateaus at approximately 2 weeks and increases with the secondary booster injection. IgA appears later than either IgM or IgG and is enhanced by secondary and tertiary boosts. It should be emphasized that in developing vaccines, the quantity or

IgG, IgM, and IgA responses occur during immunization

Quantity may not predict biologic effect

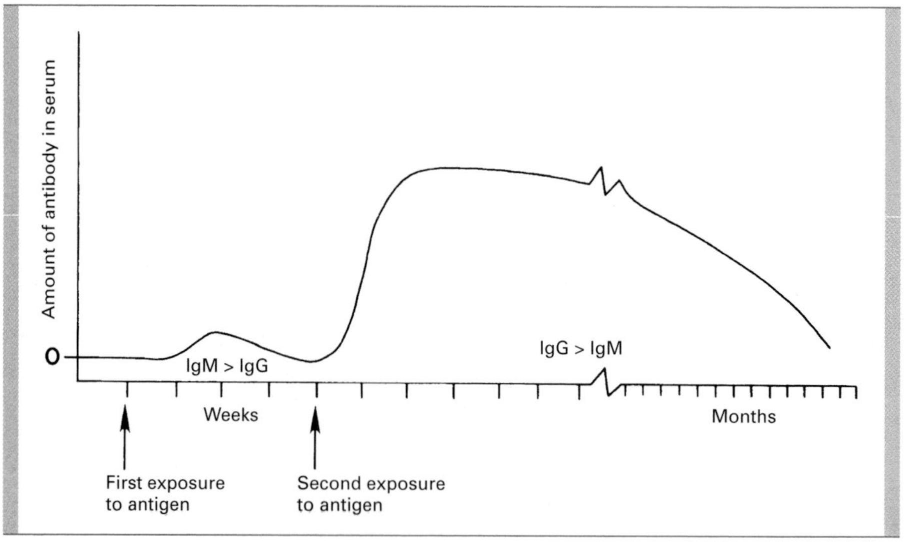

FIGURE 8–7
Primary and secondary immunologic responses. The response to first inoculation of antigen becomes apparent in a week to 10 days. It is small, predominantly of IgM class, and declines rapidly. Activation of memory cells by a second inoculation leads to a much greater, more rapid, and more long-lived IgG response.

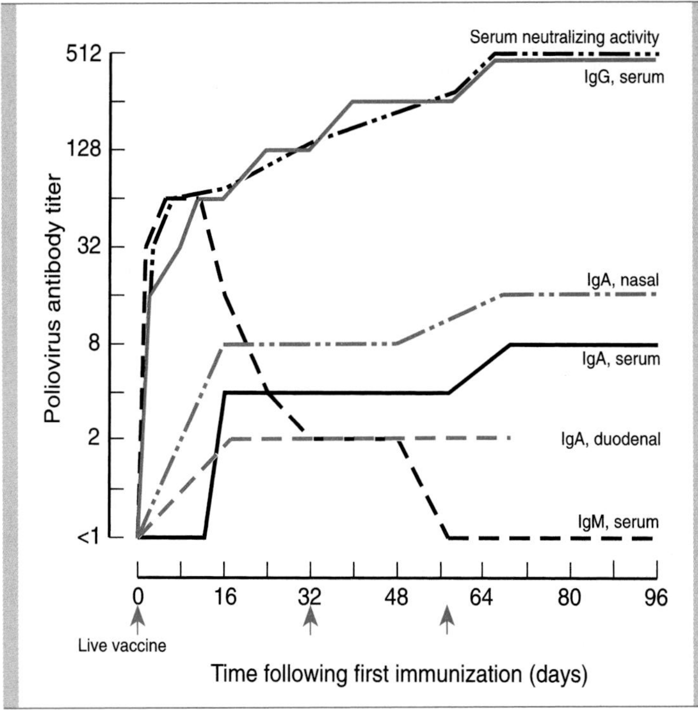

FIGURE 8–8
Detailed sequence of IgG, IgM, and IgA antibodies to poliovirus in serum and secretions of an infant immunized with live attenuated poliovirus. *(Based on Ogra PL, et al.* N Engl J Med *1968;279:893–900.)*

class of antibody produced is secondary to the biological effect. In the polio example, the serum IgA antibody is probably less important than that produced at the mucosal surfaces of the gut where it can block virus attachment.

Antibody-Mediated Immunity

Antibodies provide immunity to infection and disease in a variety of ways:

1. They can neutralize the infectivity of a virus, the toxicity of an exotoxin molecule, or the ability of a bacterium to colonize. This is usually brought about by reaction between the antibody and an epitope that is required for attachment of the organism or toxin to a target host cell. IgA and IgG antibodies are particularly significant in neutralizing activity.
2. Antibodies can inhibit essential nutrient assimilation by some bacteria. This occurs when a specific antigenic site or protein is involved in transport of the essential nutrient into the cell. For example, some iron-binding siderophores (see Chapter 3) are antigenic, and antibody against them can prevent assimilation of the iron that is essential for growth.
3. Immunoglobulin G antibody can promote phagocytosis of extracellular bacteria by combining with capsules or other surface antigens that otherwise inhibit ingestion of the organism by phagocytes. When antigen–antibody reactions occur, the attachment sites for phagocytes on the Fc regions of the antibodies are exposed, the organism is bound to the phagocyte, and ingestion occurs. The significance of such opsonization is that many bacteria and some viruses are rapidly destroyed within the phagocytic cell.
4. Antigen–antibody reactions involving IgG and IgM activate the classic pathway of the complement cascade, which is described later. Complement components enhance a wide range of nonspecific host defense mechanisms, synergize antibody-mediated opsonization, and lead to lysis of many Gram-negative bacteria with which antibody has reacted. A similar event occurs with blood and tissue cells carrying surface antigens recognized as foreign.
5. Antibodies that recognize foreign antigens on the surface of a host cell, such as a virally infected cell, react with them and can mediate destruction of the cell by the process of antibody-dependent cell-mediated cytotoxicity (ADCC).

In ADCC, the antibodies bind to the cells through their Fc portions that attach to cell surface receptors specific for the Fc regions of particular IgG classes. These are termed Fc receptors (FcR). For example, the human monocyte–macrophage has a plasma membrane receptor that recognizes both IgG1 and IgG3 subclasses through a binding site on the C_g3 domain. Eosinophils have a low-affinity FcR for IgE, which is much lower than that of mast cells. If the antibody is bound by its Fc piece, the Fab regions are free to bind antigen to initiate ADCC in the case of monocytes or polymorphs or an allergic response when IgE molecules on mast cells are cross-linked by binding to the antigen (allergen). A variety of clinical problems arise from this antibody-mediated cytotoxicity, including transfusion reactions; autoimmune hemolytic anemias; and the autoimmune disease myasthenia gravis, in which antibodies are directed at the acetylcholine receptor in the motor end plate.

Fc portions bind to cells in ADCC

Fab binding of antigen triggers cytotoxicity

THE COMPLEMENT SYSTEM

The complement system plays a critical adjunctive role to the specific immune system. Complement consists of 20 major distinct components and several other precursors. It is a highly complex system, and for the purposes of this chapter, we will focus on only nine major components. Some of the components are proenzymes, and all are present in the plasma of healthy individuals. When the complement system is triggered, a cascade of reactions occurs that activates the different components in a fixed sequence. Several of these activated components have differing and important effects in defense against infection. Components of complement are designated by numbers, which, unfortunately for the student, reflect the order in which they were first described rather than the sequence in which they are activated. There is no immunologic specificity in complement activation or in its effects, although specific antigen–antibody reactions are major initiators of activation, and some complement components enhance the effects of antigen–antibody interactions, for instance, in opsonization.

Multiple components reacting in cascade fashion when triggered

No immunologic specificity is involved

Essential for lysis of bacteria by antibody

Classic Complement Pathway

The classic complement pathway is summarized in Figure 8–9. It is initiated by antigen–antibody reactions involving IgM or IgG. These reactions expose specific sites on the Fc portion of immunoglobulin molecules that bind and activate the C1 component of complement. C1 then activates C4 and C2, and this complex splits C3 into two components, C3a and C3b. C3a liberates histamine and other vasoactive mediators from mast cells and stimulates the respiratory burst of phagocytes, thus increasing their microbicidal power. C3b binds to the membrane of microorganisms or to such cells as tumor cells or red cells and to specific sites on Fc portions of IgM and IgG. Polymorphonuclear neutrophils (PMNs) and macrophages have receptors for C3b, which thus serves as an opsonin for microorganisms. The opsonic process is markedly enhanced when specific antibody has reacted with the organism.

Antigen antibody reaction exposes complement binding sites

C3b has receptors for phagocytes

C3b, in association with activated C4 and C2, continues the cascade by splitting C5 into two components, C5a and C5b. C5a stimulates release of histamine and other vasoactive mediators from mast cells, is a chemotactic factor for PMNs, and enhances their metabolic antimicrobial activity. C5b binds to the membrane of cells on which an antigen–antibody reaction has occurred and initiates activation of the terminal components C6 to C9. Insertion of the complex C5b, C6, C7, C8, C9 into the cell membrane produces functional holes and leads to the osmotic lysis of eukaryotic cells against which the antibody was directed. Some Gram-negative bacteria are similarly affected when there is an antibody response to accessible sites on the outer membrane. In this case, lysis (bacteriolysis) requires also the activity of lysozyme from phagocytes to break down the peptidoglycan layer of the cell wall.

C5a is chemotactic for PMNs

Complete complex creates membrane holes

Alternative Pathway

The alternative pathway is more primitive than the classic pathway and does not require the presence of antibody. Instead, C3 can be activated by certain nonimmunologic stimuli. These include endotoxin, other bacterial cell wall components, aggregated IgA, and feedback from activation of the classic pathway. The alternative pathway is shown with the

Antibody not required for activation

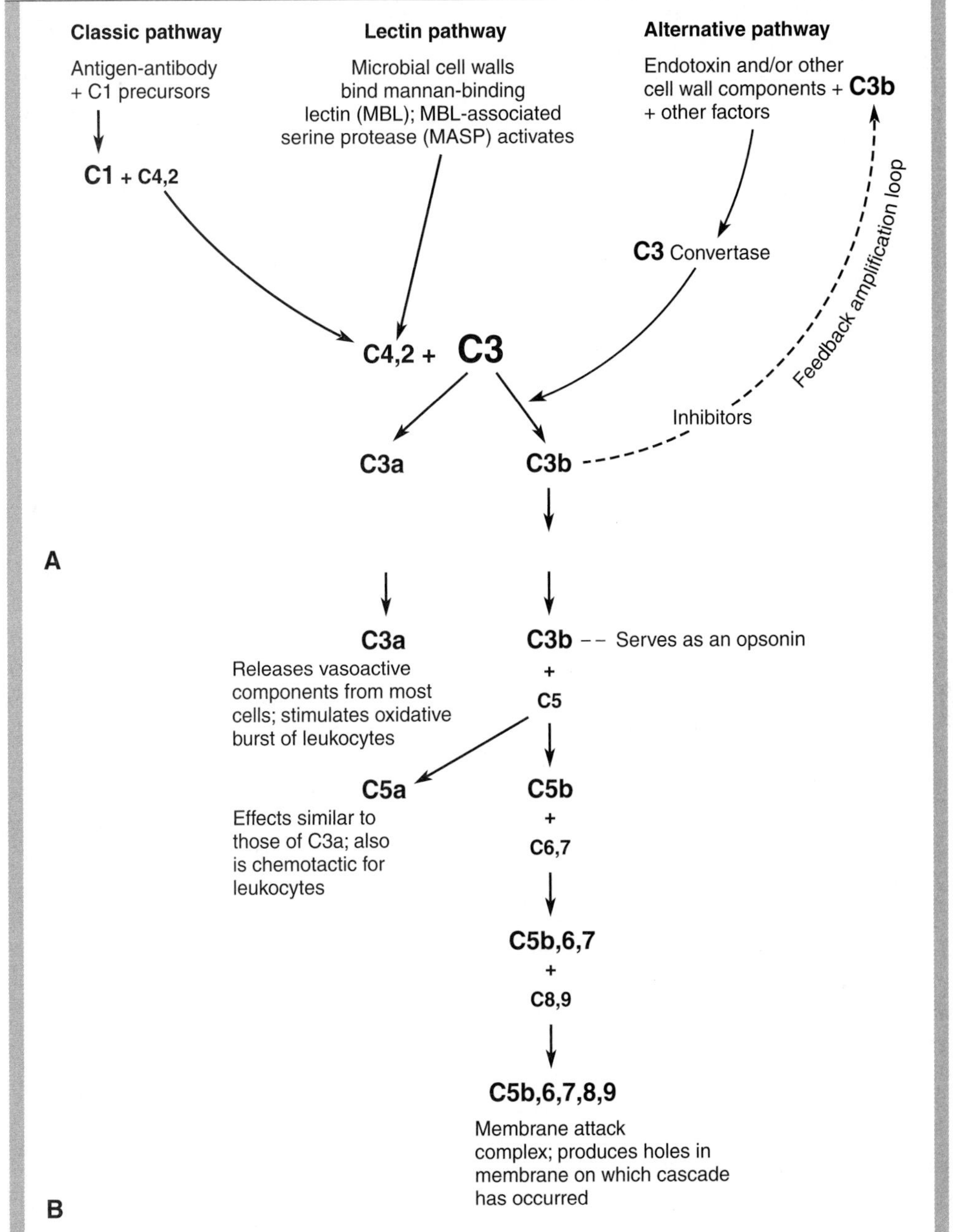

FIGURE 8–9
Schematic of the complement system. **A.** Pathways for activation of C3. (*Note:* Both pathways converge at C3.) **B.** Subsequent cascade and biological effects. Activated components are shown in bold type.

classic pathway in Figure 8–9. It produces the same inflammatory mediators (C3a, C5a) and increased phagocytic activity that result from activation of the classic pathway, but it is not as efficient in cell lysis, because direction of complement components to the cell membrane by antibody is not involved. This pathway is particularly important in early response to infection. Another non–antibody-mediated means of activating the complement system is based on the building of the mannose-binding lectin to pathogens via their carbohydrate-rich external surfaces and activation of serine esterases that act at the level of C4 in the cascade. Inherited deficiencies in complement components are often associated with increased susceptibility to bacterial infections. Most noticeable is the association of recurrent or unusually severe infections due to *Neisseria* (see Chapter 20) and individual complement component deficiencies (usually of C5, C6, C7, or C8).

Important early response

Cell lysis is less efficient

ADVERSE EFFECTS OF IMMUNOLOGIC REACTIONS AND HYPERSENSITIVITY

Multiple classes of hypersensitivity reactions occur in combinations

Immunologic reactions in the body may result in excessive responses, sometimes far beyond those needed to remove or neutralize microbial pathogens or molecules contributing to disease. Such responses are classified as hypersensitivity reactions if they cause marked physiologic changes or tissue damage or exacerbate disease processes. Four distinct classes of hypersensitivity are recognized, but these do not occur in isolation, and injury often results from a combination of the reactions. In each case they represent an extension of a normal defense mechanism. The immune response in practice is very potent and leads to deleterious consequences for the host if it is in operation too long. The antigen-specific portion of the humoral or T-cell reactions constitutes only a small fraction of the overall response and amplification by complement components that can stimulate phagocytic cells and the release of cytokines; these can cause a general recruitment of lymphocytes, monocytes, and polymorphonuclear cells, leading to a cascade of inflammation and prolonged disease. The aspects of hypersensitivity are overexpressions of the beneficial immune responses that act inappropriately. The normal immune basis of the four types of hypersensitivity are described below and included in Tables 8–1 and 8–4. Types I, II, and III hypersensitivity are mediated by antibody; type IV (delayed-type) hypersensitivity is carried out by antigen-specific T cells assisted by macrophages.

Anaphylactic (Type I) Hypersensitivity

IgE activities liberate vasoactive mediators from mast cells

Bronchospasm and muscle contraction are life-threatening

Type I hypersensitivity, also called **anaphylaxis,** is represented by the allergic reactions that occur immediately following contact with the sensitizing antigen (allergen). IgE antibodies are bound to Fc receptors on the surface of mast cells (Fig 8–10). If a multivalent antigen binds to the cell-bound IgE molecules, it cross-links them, with the result that the mast cell degranulates, releasing a variety of pharmacologically active mediators. Among the prominent mediators released following binding of the allergen is histamine, which increases capillary permeability and causes bronchoconstriction. Preformed mediators such as the anticoagulant heparin, complement 3 convertase, and a group of compounds involved in chemotaxis of eosinophils, neutrophils, and platelet activation are also released by degranulation. Slow reactive substances involved in bronchoconstriction and

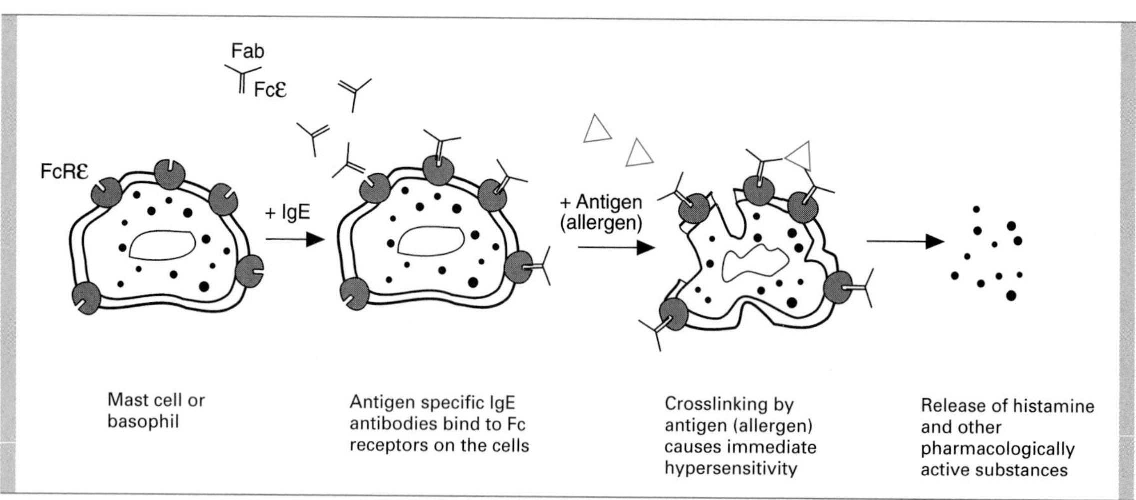

FIGURE 8–10
Diagram outlining the sequence of events in the anaphylactic (allergic) hypersensitive response (type 1) in which IgE antibodies arm mast cells by binding to Fc receptors (FcR) and the response is triggered by cross-linking of these by antigen. Comparable diagrams can be drawn for the arming of macrophages or polymorphonuclear leukocytes by IgG immunoglobulins adhering via their Fc receptors. In these reactions, the Fab arms of the bound antibodies are free to bind antigen specifically, and this binding initiates cellular events leading to sensitized phagocytosis and destruction or, in this case, the release of destructive pharmacologically active substances.

TABLE 8–4

Effector Cells in Cell-Mediated Immunity

Cell	Function	Special Properties
Specific helper T (T_H) cells	MHC class II–restricted help to B cells (T_H2), or in activation of macrophages (T_H1); distinct cytokines are used in the two processes	T_H cells use α/β Tcr; T_H2 cells can activate eosinophils as well as B cells through IL-5; T_H1 cells can activate NK cells through IL-12, and macrophages through IL-2 and IFN-γ, T_H2 cells can communicate either positively or negatively with one another via cytokines
Specific cytotoxic T (T_C) cells	MHC class I–restricted specific killing; use endogenous α/β Tcr	Can kill multiple targets sequentially; have major role in eliminating virally infected target cells
Specific suppressor T (T_S) cells	Antigen specific; involves "suppressor inducer" T cells (CD4), which generate "suppressor effector"; T_S cells can be antigen specific or idiotype specific; some aspects of the interactions are MHC restricted	"Infectious tolerance" (ie, transfer of T_S cells transfers antigen-specific immunosuppression)
Regulatory T cells	Antigen specific	CD4+, CD25+, suppress inflammation
"K cells," macrophages, polymorphonuclear cells	Antibody-dependent cell-mediated cytotoxicity (ADCC)	Bind IgG via Fc receptors; IgG acts as an antigen-specific opsonin on these cells
Natural killer (NK) cells	Occur in unchallenged animals; can kill a variety of tumors and virus-infected or embryonic cells in vitro without expression of classic Tcr or bound antibody	Are large, granular lymphocytes; do not phagocytize target cells but kill by release of toxins
NK T cells	Tcr α/β but restricted Vα	CD4+ T cells produce cytokines that stimulate T_H1 (IF-α) and T_H2 (IL-4) responses

chemotaxis are also produced, as are prostaglandins and thromboxanes, which are implicated in bronchospasm, muscle contraction, and platelet aggregation. Thus, the specific binding of an allergen to the combining site of its antibody can result in a potent release of compounds, leading to painful and life-threatening consequences for the allergic individual. Despite the suffering that hypersensitivity to common allergens such as pollen, bee stings, house dust, and cat dander brings to a large percentage of people, there are possible beneficial consequences of binding of allergen by IgE. These include situations in which ADCC by monocytes and eosinophils may provide protection against parasites such as schistosomes (a trematode worm) and trypanosomes (a protozoan).

When hypersensitivity is very marked, or antigen is introduced systemically, mast cells throughout the body degranulate, and systemic anaphylaxis results with constriction of the bronchi, edema of the larynx and other tissues, vascular collapse, and sometimes death. A generalized anaphylactic reaction rarely if ever occurs as a manifestation of an infection but may occur following parenteral inoculation of an antigen to which the individual has been sensitized (eg, bee sting venom). It may also occur in individuals who have been sensitized to a low-molecular-weight hapten that binds to a tissue protein and becomes antigenic because of the size of the complex. An IgE response to hapten epitopes can then lead to anaphylactic-type hypersensitivity if the epitope is again encountered. A penicillin degradation product has this property, and occasionally, individuals develop severe anaphylactic reactions to penicillins, although this complication is very rare.

Mast cells throughout the body may degranulate

Systemic anaphylaxis may occur with low-molecular-weight haptens

Rapid therapeutic intervention is critical in systemic anaphylaxis. It includes parenteral administration of epinephrine, which reverses the major manifestations of the syndrome by producing bronchodilation, vasoconstriction, and increased blood pressure. Tracheostomy or intubation may be needed to overcome respiratory obstruction due to laryngeal edema.

Epinephrine reverses anaphylaxis

Antibody-Mediated (Type II) Hypersensitivity

Type II hypersensitivity is an inappropriate elaboration of antibody-dependent cytotoxicity that occurs when antibody binds to antigens on host cells, leading to phagocytosis, killer cell activity, or complement-mediated lysis. Antibody directed against cell surface or tissue antigens results in the fixation of complement such that a variety of effector cells become involved. The cells to which the antibody is specifically bound, as well as the surrounding tissues, are damaged because of the inflammatory amplification. Such mechanisms appear to be responsible for the tissue damage of rheumatic fever following a streptococcal infection or some clinical manifestations of viral diseases, such as group B coxsackievirus infection (see Chapter 36). These phenomena may involve not only antibodies but also cytotoxic T cells. It should be recalled that humoral antibodies are required to arm macrophages, and PMNs are needed to bind cellular antigens in ADCC and to serve as opsonins that facilitate ingestion with eventual intracellular destruction of target cells by macrophages.

Host cells are damaged when targeted antigen is bound to cell surface

Reactions may follow infections

Immune Complex (Type III) Hypersensitivity

When IgG is mixed in appropriate proportions with multivalent antigen molecules (ie, bearing multiple epitopes), aggregates containing a lattice of many antigen and antibody molecules forms. With appropriate concentrations of the two reactants, a macroscopic precipitate can develop (see Chapter 15). A similar situation applies to IgM, which is multivalent. When the epitope is present on the surface of a larger particle, such as a bacterium or red blood cell, the particles can be cross-linked by antibody, and microscopic or macroscopic agglutination results. These phenomena can occur in vivo when sufficient amounts of specific antibody and of free antigen from an infecting microorganism react locally or in the bloodstream to form an antigen–antibody lattice; the size of the immune complex depends on the relative properties of the two reactants. Large immune complexes are phagocytosed and usually broken down within the phagocyte. However, smaller complexes are deposited in small blood vessels and capillaries through which they do not pass, activate the complement system, and thus produce an acute inflammatory response mediated largely by C3a and C5a. This results in the manifestations of vasculitis. Phagocytes attracted chemotactically to the site release hydrolytic enzymes, and the sum of these effects is acute tissue damage, which can become chronic depending on the survival of the antigen or on whether it is continually replaced. Acute glomerulonephritis following certain streptococcal infections is an example of an immune complex disease in which glomeruli of the kidney are damaged by the complexes, resulting in various manifestations of renal impairment. Inflammatory skin lesions can result from deposition of immune complexes in the cutaneous blood vessels in patients with infective endocarditis. Deposition in joints, the pericardium, or the pleura produces arthritis, pericarditis, and pleuritis or pleurisy, respectively.

Cross-linking forms lattice of antigen and antibody

Small complexes reach capillaries

Complement deposition attracts phagocytes

A systemic form of immune complex disease, termed **serum sickness,** can follow the injection of foreign antigen. An example is the therapeutic use of diphtheria antitoxin that has been produced in horses. About 10 days after inoculation, sufficient antibody against

Antitoxins can form immune complexes

horse proteins has been produced to form immune complexes made up of human antibody reacting against horse serum protein (including horse immunoglobulins). These complexes are deposited in various organs, resulting in a syndrome of arthritis, nephritis, rash, urticaria, and fever. The disease usually resolves as the foreign antigen concentration decreases through immune clearance and catabolism of the antigen(s).

Delayed-Type (Type IV) Hypersensitivity

The fourth type of hypersensitivity is termed, **delayed-type hypersensitivity.** Unlike types I, II, and III, this process cannot be transferred from one animal to another by serum alone. However, it can be transferred by antigen-specific T lymphocytes. All are initiated by the function of antigen-specific T cells, which then recruit effector cells into the area of recognition of the antigen. Unlike the forms of "immediate" hypersensitivity that can be transferred by antibody, delayed-type hypersensitivity requires days to weeks to express full reactivity. In all of these, the initial reaction is the induction and function of antigen-specific T cells that bear α/β T-cell receptors and have been generated in response to antigenic challenge. The time course depends on the involvement of other cells and the properties of the infectious agent involved.

Requires T lymphocyte transfer

Four major types of delayed-type hypersensitivity are all part of the same process differing in site, mechanism of challenge, and timing. The shortest is the Jones–Mote phenomenon, in which the site of antigen injection is infiltrated by basophils, and the skin swelling is maximal 24 hours after antigen injection. This type of hypersensitivity can be raised to soluble antigens, and the reactivity disappears following the appearance of antibody. Contact and tuberculin-type hypersensitivity show maximal reactivity at 48 to 72 hours. Contact sensitivity is observed in response to sensitization with common antigens such as chemicals found in rubber or the small organic compounds produced by poison ivy and poison oak. It is predominantly an epidermal reaction, in contrast to the tuberculin-type hypersensitivity, which is a dermal reaction. The cell that presents antigen for contact sensitization is the Langerhans cell, a dendritic antigen-presenting cell carrying MHC class II antigens. Tuberculin-type hypersensitivity is manifested by individuals who have been sensitized with lipoprotein antigens derived from the tubercle bacillus. Twenty-four hours after intradermal injection of tuberculin, an antigen derived from *Mycobacterium tuberculosis,* there is intense infiltration by lymphocytes, which reaches a maximum in 2 to 3 days.

Contact sensitivity is from chemicals

Tuberculin hypersensitivity is from sensitization by lipoprotein from tubercle bacillus

Probably the most clinically important form of type IV sensitivity is the granuloma, an organized inflammatory lesion that requires at least 14 days to develop. These result from the long-term continuation of the stimulation of effector cells by cytokines produced in initial antigen-specific T-cell response. Granulomatous lesions are a major part of the disease process in chronic diseases caused by bacteria (tuberculosis), fungi (histoplasmosis), and parasites (schistosomiasis).

Long-term stimulation is required for granuloma

TOLERANCE

As discussed earlier, induced cellular and antibody responses follow challenge with antigens that are normally foreign; however, immunization may not only induce the enhanced reactivities described but may also lead to a diminished reactivity known as **tolerance.** When specifically diminished reactivity is induced by treatment with large doses of antigen, the phenomenon is referred to as **immune paralysis.** Because the immune system is based on a random generation of combining sites directed against molecular configurations, there is in principle no reason why the immune response cannot react with self components. When it does, autoimmune diseases such as rheumatoid arthritis, systemic lupus erythematosus, and others may result. However, it is now known that normal healthy individuals express detectable levels of autoantibodies against a variety of self components. A regulatory function for these autoantibodies in the maintenance of homeostasis is suggested by the fact that aged red cells are removed from human circulation by a natural mechanism in which normally occurring IgG autoantibodies specific for a modified membrane component (senescent cell antigen) bind to the cells, leading to their

Diminished reactivity prevents pathologic reactivity to self antigens

Autoantibodies may have homeostatic functions

removal by phagocytic cells. Nevertheless, the generation of tolerance or the inability to react against self is a fundamental part of the process of development in vertebrates, which results essentially from the removal or inactivation of T cells in the thymus that can react to self antigens.

B-cell tolerance also occurs

Parallel tolerization procedures for B cells occur, but currently a number of mechanisms now must be proposed for maintenance of nonreactivity to self. Antigen-specific T cells may be either deleted by contact with antigen (clonal abortion) or inactivated without being destroyed. In addition, suppressor T cells that downregulate the specific immune response may be generated that either shut off the antigen-specific helper T cells or are directed toward combining sites of B-cell antibodies. Antigen-specific B cells may be deleted or inactivated or rendered insensitive to secondary stimulation by cytokines. These central effects operate at the level of antigen-specific T or B cells.

Tolerance may be disturbed by quantitative or cross-reactive mechanisms

Both experimentally induced tolerance and innate tolerance can be broken down in two general ways. First, if a large amount of antigen is needed to maintain tolerance, immunity can be generated if the level of antigen falls below the required tolerogenic level. A second way of breaking of tolerance is immunization with a cross-reactive antigen. Two clinically well-known examples of the capacity of cross-reactive antigens to break normal self tolerance are (1) the induction of experimental allergic encephalomyelitis in an animal by the injection of heterologous brain tissue homogenates in emulsified adjuvant and (2) the capacity of infections with group A streptococci to cause rheumatic fever because of a cross-reaction between bacterial antigens and myocardial tissue. The concept of tolerance is critical to much of modem medicine because of increasing interest in autoimmune diseases, which can be considered to result from a failure or breakdown of tolerance.

FUNCTIONAL INTEGRATION OF THE IMMUNE SYSTEM IN RESPONSE TO INFECTIOUS ORGANISMS

Viral proteins induce T_H1 responses and cytokines

B cells and macrophages are activated later

T_H1 is effective against intracellular parasites

The innate immune system involves phagocytic cells such as monocytes, macrophages and dendritic cells, and cytokines such as interleukin-1 that are generated following activation of phagocytic cells by binding of bacterial lipopolysaccharide to surface receptors. Once the innate system is activated, the cytokines it produces and the peptide antigens presented to T cells serve to activate and condition the response of the specific adaptive system (Fig 8–11). The upper half of the figure illustrates how activation of the antigen-presenting cell (monocyte, macrophage, or dendritic cell) can stimulate NK cells, CD8+ cytotoxic T cells, or T_H1 type CD4+ cells. The T_H1 cells are induced by presentation of peptides derived from antigens such as a viral coat protein presented to the α/β T-cell receptor of an unstimulated T cell with the activation and transformation process mediated by IL-12 and IFN-α. Once the T_H1 cell is specifically activated, the process can lead to the activation of B cells to make IgM or IgG but, more importantly, to activate macrophages to act in an inflammatory manner. T_H1 type cell-mediated immunity is particularly effective against intracellular parasites but has the drawback of increasing the severity of autoimmune diseases.

T_H2 responses activate B cells and immunoglobulins

Protective against helminth worm infections

The lower half of (Figure 8–11) illustrates the activation of T_H2 type helper cells via the mediation of the cytokine IL-6 and the production of IL-4 to drive the differentiation pathway. The specificity for antigen is maintained by presentation of peptide antigen via MHC of the antigen presenting cell to the α/β T-cell receptor of the unstimulated helper T cell. A separate type of NK cell, one that is CD4+ and expresses a restricted Tcr Vα is involved in this process. T_H2 type immunity is most prominent in the activation of B cells, allowing the generating of IgM, IgG, IgA, and IgE. Antibodies are valuable in the protective immune response to many bacteria and also in maintaining protection against viruses. Most notably, the T_H2 response is host protective in infections by gastrointestinal helminth worms such as schistostomes, where production of specific IgE antibody bound to macrophages, basophils, or acinophils appears to confer protection. On the other hand, T_H2 type immunity in antibodies appear to offer little protection against retroviruses, including HIV. IgE production to allergens produced by dust mites or ragweed may lead to serious clinical consequences of allergic responses.

The above scheme depicting the critical role of the polarization of helper T cell type and function in resistance to certain diseases and in the exacerbation of others is not yet

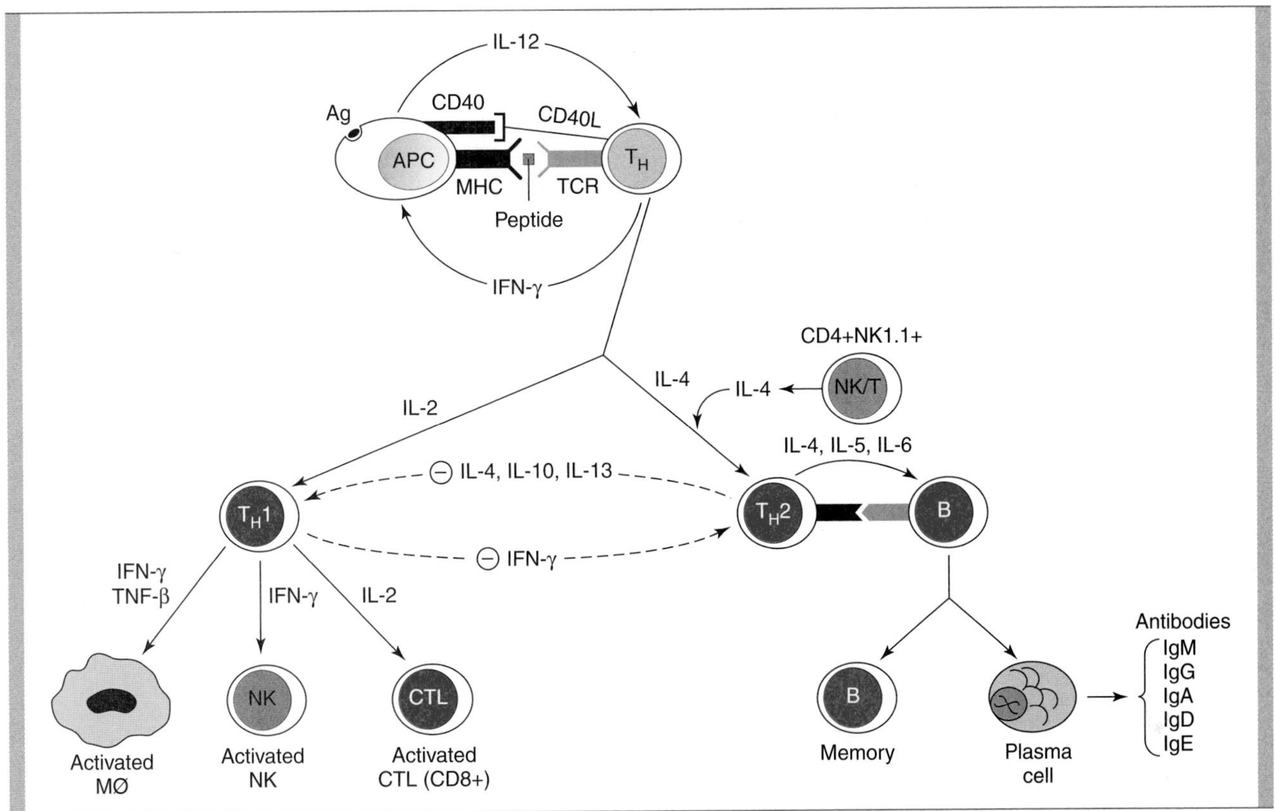

FIGURE 8–11
Diagram of T_H1 and T_H2 cells in the generation of cell-mediated immunity or antibody production. *Abbreviations*: AG, antigen; APC, antigen-presenting cell; B, B cells; CTL, cytotoxic T lymphocyte; CD, cell surface determinant; IFN, interferons; IL, interleukins; MHC, major histocompatibility complex; MΦ, macrophage; NK, natural killer cell; NK/T, natural killer cell related to T cells; TCR, T cell receptor; T_H, helper T cells.

completely established. It has been sufficiently documented to make it a worthwhile overall conceptual framework in which to place infectious diseases caused by distinct types of pathogens, autoimmune diseases, immunity to tumors, and allergy. The difficulty is that there is no such thing as a pure T_H1 or T_H2 response; rather, there is a balance between the two types of effector T cells as manifested by levels of cytokines. In the most simple case, bacteria coated with polysaccharides that protect them from ingestion by phagocytes are readily attacked by antibodies. Furthermore, antibodies of the IgM class against these polysaccharides can be generated in the relative absence of T-cell help. Nonetheless, T_H2 type cytokines are required for activation and differentiation of the B cells and their differentiation into antibody-secreting plasma cells. Recently, it has also been shown that natural antibodies to viruses are protective in experimental infections of mice. *S. pneumoniae* are extracellular pathogens that enter the lungs and colonize the space in the alveoli, where their multiplication causes tissue damage and inflammation that can impair breathing. Antibodies to these organisms enable them to be phagocytized and also to be killed by activation of the complement cascade following binding of the antibody. By contrast, *Leishmania* is an intracellular parasite that proliferates within macrophages inside vesicles called endosomes. Thus, the parasites are protected from attack by antibodies. T_H1 type immunity plays a major role in their destruction because the infected macrophages can break down the organisms into peptides that are then presented by MHC class II molecules to the receptor on CD4+ cells. The T cells then become activated by interaction of the accessory CD28 molecule on the T cell with the B7 molecule on the macrophage. The activated T_H1 type cells now secrete cytokines such as IFN-γ that induce the macrophage to produce tumor necrosis factor and nitric oxide that kill the parasites within the cells. Viruses are intracellular parasites that replicate within the nucleus or within the cytoplasm. Both the

T_H1 and T_H2 responses are balanced, not pure

Antipolysaccharide antibodies facilitate complement deposition and phagocytosis

T_H1-stimulated cytokines cause intracellular killing

production of cytotoxic CD8+ T cells and T_H1 type inflammation are protective against virus infections. Cytotoxic T cells are induced by the presentation of viral peptides by MHC class I molecules, as opposed to helper cell reactivity, that involves that presentation of antigenic class II MHC.

Strong cell-mediated immunity and T_H1 in leprosy lead to resolution

T_H2 responses are associated with bacterial proliferation

Leprosy appears to be a human disease for which the elaboration of a T_H1 type response is essential for cure, but the elaboration of T_H2 type responses is harmful to the infected person. There are two polar forms of clinical presentation of leprosy. Tuberculoid leprosy is characterized by a strong cell-mediated immune response to the causative organism, *Mycobacterium leprae*. This cell-mediated T_H1 type immune response kills the mycobacteria but at the price of immune-mediated tissue damage to the host. Lepromatous leprosy, the other extreme of the clinical spectrum, is characterized by a pronounced antibody response in the virtual absence of a cellular response against the bacterial pathogen. This situation results in extensive bacterial loads and ultimately in the death of the patient. Analyses of messenger RNA in lesions of the two types of leprosy indicate that T_H1 type cytokines predominate in the tuberculoid form and T_H2 cytokines are the major types generated in lepromatous leprosy. In parallel, T_H1 immunity is more effective in the response to *Mycobacterium tuberculosis* than are antibodies.

T_H2 responses clear intestinal worms

A vigorous T_H2 type response is required for the clearance of infections with gastrointestinal helminths. There is convincing evidence that T_H2 type responses are required for the explusion of gastrointestinal parasites, but the exact mechanisms by which the T_H2 type cells mediate the protective responses are unknown. The cytokine IL-4 induces the production of IgG1 (in mice) and IgE, generation of mast cells in the intestinal mucosa, increased contractility of the intestine smooth musculature, and reduced intestinal fluid uptake. IL-5 is induced by infection with intestinal nematodes (roundworms), and this cytokine promotes the production and activation of eosinophils. Although the production of IgE and its binding to mast cells and basophils in producing allergic responses is generally considered destructive, recent evidence suggests that important eosinophils and these allergy-type reactions may be mediating immunity against extraintestinal helminth larvae, including those of schistomes (parasitic flatworms).

Antigen Surrogates

Antibody protein can induce antibodies directed against Fab and epitope recognition sites

A recently developed approach has the potential to allow the use of antibodies as antigen surrogates in immunization. Antibodies are themselves antigenic in animal species to which they are foreign. The antiantibodies that can be produced include some with specificity for unique epitope-reacting portions of the Fab variable region of the antibody against which they are directed as well as for epitope-recognizing sites on immunoresponsive B cells. These are termed **anti-idiotypic antibodies** and have the same three-dimensional geometry as would the epitope molecule. Monoclonal antibodies that have this structure can be selected and produced in large amounts and may then act as antigens for the production of specific antibodies against the epitope of interest. Immunization with such anti-idiotype antibodies has promise for producing specific immunity against critical antigens that are impossible or uneconomical to produce in bulk. At present, there are many problems to overcome before such procedures could begin to be applied to humans.

ADDITIONAL READING

Abbas AK, Lichtman AH, Pober JS. *Cellular and Molecular Immunology*. Philadelphia: WB Saunders; 2000. A detailed survey of immunologic mechanisms.

Eisen HN. *General Immunology*. Philadelphia: JB Lippincott; 1990. A comprehensive presentation of cellular and molecular immunologic mechanisms.

Janeway CA, Travers P, Walport M, Capra JD. *Immunobiology,* 4th ed. New York: Current Biology Publications; 1999. A detailed survey of contemporary immunology.

Paul WE. *Fundamental Immunology,* 4th ed. New York: Lippincott-Raven Press; 1999. A comprehensive, detailed, multiauthored volume.

CHAPTER 9

Normal Microbial Flora

KENNETH J. RYAN

The term **normal flora** is used to describe microorganisms that are frequently found in various body sites in normal, healthy individuals. The constituents and numbers of the flora vary in different areas and sometimes at different ages and physiologic states. They comprise microorganisms whose morphologic, physiologic, and genetic properties allow them to colonize and multiply under the conditions that exist in particular sites, to coexist with other colonizing organisms, and to inhibit competing intruders. Thus, each accessible area of the body presents a particular ecologic niche, colonization of which requires a particular set of properties of the invading microbe. The number of organisms in the flora is estimated to exceed the number of cells in the body by a factor of 10.

Organisms of the normal flora may have a symbiotic relationship that benefits the host or may simply live as commensals with a neutral relationship to the host. A parasitic relationship that injures the host would not be considered "normal," but in most instances not enough is known about the organism–host interactions to make such distinctions. Like houseguests, the members of the normal flora may stay for highly variable periods. **Residents** are strains that have an established niche at one of the many body sites, which they occupy indefinitely. **Transients** are acquired from the environment and establish themselves briefly but tend to be excluded by competition from residents or by the host's innate or immune defense mechanisms. The term **carrier state** is used when potentially pathogenic organisms are involved, although its implication of risk is not always justified. For example, *Streptococcus pneumoniae,* a cause of pneumonia, and *Neisseria meningitidis,* a cause of meningitis, may be isolated from the throat of 5 to 40% of healthy people. Whether these bacteria represent transient flora, resident flora, or carrier state is largely semantic. The possibility that their presence could be the prelude to disease is impossible to determine simply by culture of a normal flora site.

Flora may stay for short or extended periods

If pathogens are involved the relationship is called the carrier state

It is important for students of medical microbiology and infectious disease to understand the role of the normal flora, because of its significance both as a defense mechanism against infection and as a source of potentially pathogenic organisms. English poet W. H. Auden understood the desired state of balance between host and microbial flora when he wrote:

Balance is the desired state

Build colonies: I will supply
adequate warmth and moisture,
the sebum and lipids you need,
on condition you never
do me annoy with your presence,
but behave as good guests should,
not rioting into acne
or athlete's-foot or a boil.

FROM AUDEN WH,
Epistle to a Godson

It is also important to know its sites and composition to avoid interpretive confusion between normal flora species and pathogens when interpreting laboratory culture results.

ORIGIN OF THE NORMAL FLORA

Initial flora is acquired during and immediately after birth

The healthy fetus is sterile until the birth membranes rupture. During and after birth, the infant is exposed to the flora of the mother's genital tract, to the skin and respiratory flora of those handling it, and to organisms in the environment. During the infant's first few days of life, the flora reflects chance exposure to organisms that can colonize particular sites in the absence of competitors. Subsequently, as the infant is exposed to a broader range of organisms, those best adapted to colonize particular sites become predominant. Thereafter, the flora generally resembles that of other individuals in the same age group and cultural milieu.

FACTORS DETERMINING THE NATURE OF THE NORMAL FLORA

Physiologic conditions such as local pH influence colonization

Adherence factors counteract mechanical flushing

Ability to compete for nutrients is an advantage

Local physiologic and ecologic conditions determine the nature of the flora. These conditions are sometimes highly complex, differing from site to site, and sometimes vary with age. Conditions include the amounts and types of nutrients available, pH, oxidation–reduction potentials, and resistance to local antibacterial substances such as bile and lysozyme. Many bacteria have adhesin-mediated affinity for receptors on specific types of epithelial cells, which facilitates colonization and multiplication while avoiding removal by the flushing effects of surface fluids and peristalsis. Various microbial interactions also determine their relative prevalence in the flora. These interactions include competition for nutrients, inhibition by the metabolic products of other organisms (eg, by hydrogen peroxide or volatile fatty acids), and production of antibiotics and bacteriocins.

NORMAL FLORA AT DIFFERENT SITES

The total normal flora of the body probably contains more than 1000 distinct species of microorganisms. The major members known to be important in preventing or causing disease as well as those that may be confused with etiologic agents of local infections are summarized in Table 9–1, and most are described in greater detail in subsequent chapters. The student should not attempt to memorize unfamiliar names at this point.

Blood, Body Fluids, and Tissues

Tissues and body fluids such as blood are sterile in health

Transient bacteremia can result from trauma

In health, the blood, body fluids, and tissues are sterile. Occasional organisms may be displaced across epithelial barriers as a result of trauma (including physiologic trauma such as heavy chewing) or during childbirth; they may be briefly recoverable from the bloodstream before they are filtered out in the pulmonary capillaries or removed by cells of the reticuloendothelial system. Such transient bacteremia may be the source of infection when structures such as damaged heart valves and foreign bodies (prostheses) are in the bloodstream.

Skin

Propionibacteria and staphylococci are dominant bacteria

Skin flora is not easily removed

Conjunctiva resembles skin

The skin plays host to an abundant flora that varies somewhat according to the number and activity of sebaceous and sweat glands. The flora is most abundant on moist skin areas (axillae, perineum, and between toes). Staphylococci and members of the genus *Propionibacterium* occur all over the skin, and facultative diphtheroids (corynebacteria) are found in moist areas. Propionibacteria are slim, anaerobic, or microaerophilic Gram-positive rods that grow in subsurface sebum and break down skin lipids to fatty acids. Thus, they are most numerous in the ducts of hair follicles and of the sebaceous glands that drain into them. Even with antiseptic scrubbing it is difficult to eliminate bacteria from skin sites, particularly those bearing pilosebaceous units. Organisms of the skin flora are resistant to the bactericidal effects of skin lipids and fatty acids, which inhibit or kill many extraneous bacteria. The conjunctivae have a very scanty flora derived from the skin flora. The low bacterial count is maintained by the high lysozyme content of lachrymal secretions and by the flushing effect of tears.

TABLE 9–1

Predominant and Potentially Pathogenic Flora of Various Body Sites

	Flora	
Body Site	Potential Pathogens (Carrier)	Low Virulence (Resident)
Blood	None	None[a]
Tissues	None	None
Skin	*Staphylococcus aureus*	*Propionibacterium, Corynebacterium* (diphtheroids), coagulase-negative staphylococci
Mouth	*Candida albicans*	*Neisseria* spp., viridans streptococci, *Moraxella, Peptostreptococcus*
Nasopharynx	*Streptococcus pneumoniae, Neisseria meningitidis, Haemophilus influenzae,* group A streptococci, *Staphylococcus aureus* (anterior nares)	*Neisseria* spp., viridans streptococci, *Moraxella, Peptostreptococcus*
Stomach	None	Streptococci, *Peptostreptococcus,* others from mouth
Small intestine	None	Scanty, variable
Colon		
Breastfeeding infant	None	*Bifidobacterium, Lactobacillus*
Adult	*Bacteroides fragilis, Escherichia coli, Pseudomonas, Candida, Clostridium (C. perfringens, C. difficile)*	*Bifidobacterium, Lactobacillus, Bacteroides, Fusobacterium,* Enterobacteriaceae, *Enterococcus, Clostridium*
Vagina		
Prepubertal and Postmenopausal	*C. albicans*	Diphtheroids, staphylococci, Enterobacteriaceae
Childbearing	Group B streptococci, *C. albicans*	*Lactobacillus,* streptococci

[a]Organisms such as viridans streptococci may be transiently present following disruption of a mucosal site.

Intestinal Tract

The **mouth** and **pharynx** contain large numbers of facultative and strict anaerobes. Different species of streptococci predominate on the buccal and tongue mucosa because of different specific adherence characteristics. Gram-negative diplococci of the genera *Neisseria* and *Moraxella* make up the balance of the most commonly isolated facultative organisms. Strict anaerobes and microaerophilic organisms of the oral cavity have their niches in the depths of the gingival crevices surrounding the teeth and in sites such as tonsillar crypts, where anaerobic conditions can develop readily. Anaerobic members of the normal flora are major contributors to the etiology of dental caries and periodontal disease (see Chapter 62).

Oropharynx has streptococci and *Neisseria*

The total number of organisms in the oral cavity is very high, and it varies from site to site. Saliva usually contains a mixed flora of about 10^8 organisms per milliliter, derived mostly from the various epithelial colonization sites. The stomach contains few, if any, resident organisms in health because of the lethal action of gastric hydrochloric acid and peptic enzymes on bacteria. The small intestine has a scanty resident flora, except in the lower ileum, where it begins to resemble that of the colon.

Stomach and small bowel have few residents

Small intestinal flora is scanty but increases toward lower ileum

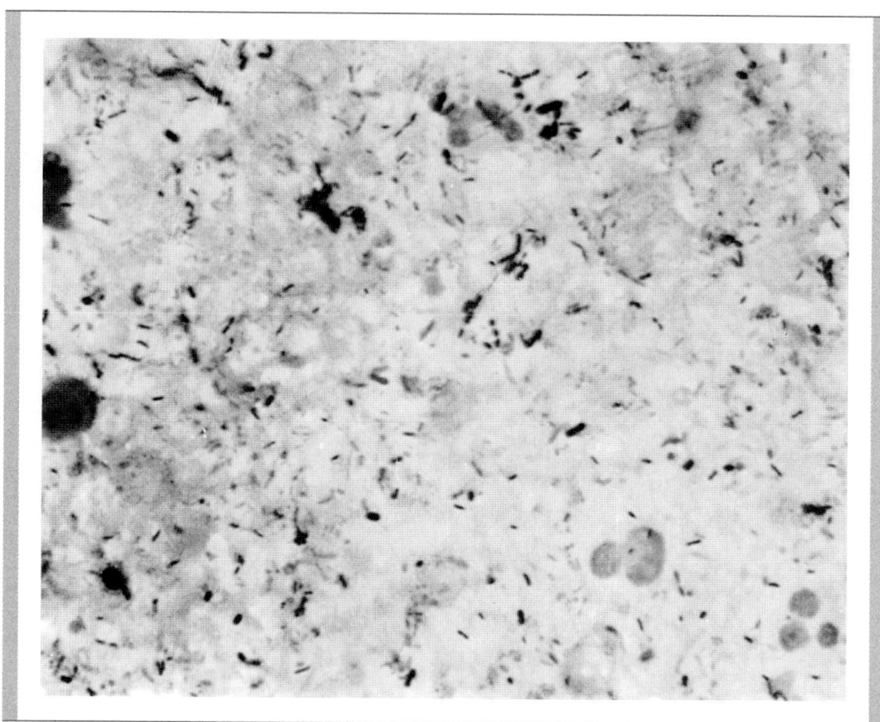

FIGURE 9–1
Smear of feces, showing great diversity of microorganisms.

Adult colonic flora is abundant and predominantly anaerobic

Diet affects species composition

The colon carries the most prolific flora in the body (Fig 9–1). In the adult, feces are 25% or more bacteria by weight (about 10^{10} organisms per gram). More than 90% are anaerobes, predominantly members of the genera *Bacteroides, Fusobacterium, Bifidobacterium,* and *Clostridium*. The remainder of the flora is composed of facultative organisms such as *Escherichia coli,* enterococci, yeasts, and numerous other species. There are considerable differences in adult flora depending on the diet of the host. Those whose diets include substantial amounts of meat have more *Bacteroides* and other anaerobic Gram-negative rods in their stools than those on a predominantly vegetable or fish diet.

Bifidobacteria are predominant flora of breastfed infants

Bottle-fed infants have a flora similar to that of weaned infants

The fecal flora of breastfed infants differs from that of adults, with anaerobic Gram-positive rods of the genus *Bifidobacterium* constituting as much as 99% of the total. Human milk is high in lactose and low in protein and phosphate, and its buffering capacity is poor compared with that of cow's milk. These conditions select for bifidobacteria, which ferment lactose to yield acetic acid and grow optimally under the acidic conditions (pH 5–5.5) that they produce in the stool. Infants who are fed cow's milk, which has a greater buffering capacity, tend to have less acidic stools and a flora more similar to that found in the colon of the weaned infant or the adult. These findings also apply to infants fed some artificial formulas.

Respiratory Tract

S. aureus is carried in anterior nares

Nasopharynx is often a site of carriage of potential pathogens

The external 1 cm of the anterior nares is lined with squamous epithelium. The nares have a flora similar to that of the skin except that it is the primary site of carriage of a pathogen, *Staphylococcus aureus*. About 25 to 30% of healthy people carry this organism as either resident or transient flora at any given time. The organism may spread to other skin sites or colonize the perineum; it can be disseminated by hand-to-nose contact, by desquamation of the epithelium, or by droplet spread during upper respiratory infection. The nasopharynx has a flora similar to that of the mouth; however, it is often the site of carriage of potentially pathogenic organisms such as pneumococci, meningococci, and *Haemophilus* species.

Lower tract is protected by mucociliary action

The respiratory tract below the level of the larynx is protected in health by the action of the epithelial cilia and by the movement of the mucociliary blanket; thus, only transient inhaled organisms are encountered in the trachea and larger bronchi. The accessory sinuses are normally sterile and are protected in a similar fashion, as is the middle ear by the epithelium of the eustachian tubes.

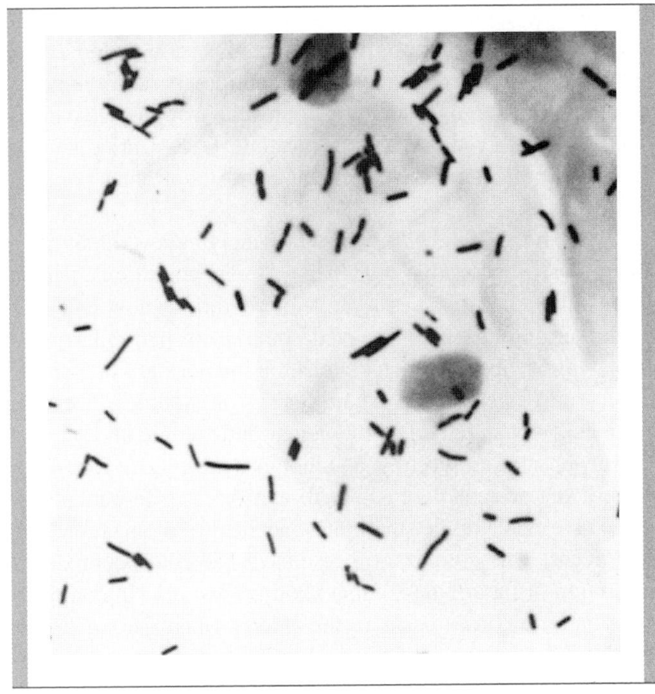

FIGURE 9–2
Smear of normal adult vagina, showing predominant large elongated lactobacilli and squamous epithelial cells.

Genitourinary Tract

The urinary tract is sterile in health above the distal 1 cm of the urethra, which has a scanty flora derived from the perineum. Thus, in health the urine in the bladder, ureters, and renal pelvis is sterile. The vagina has a flora that varies according to hormonal influences at different ages. Before puberty and after menopause, it is mixed, nonspecific, relatively scanty, and contains organisms derived from the flora of the skin and colon. During the childbearing years, it is composed predominantly of anaerobic and microaerophilic members of the genus *Lactobacillus,* with smaller numbers of anaerobic Gram-negative rods, Gram-positive cocci, and yeasts that can survive under the acidic conditions produced by the lactobacilli. These conditions develop because glycogen is deposited in vaginal epithelial cells under the influence of estrogenic hormones and metabolized to lactic acid by lactobacilli. This process results in a vaginal pH of 4 to 5, which is optimal for growth and survival of the lactobacilli, but inhibits many other organisms. The consistency of the lactobacillary adult flora is seen in Gram-stained preparations of vaginal smears (Fig 9–2).

Bladder and upper urinary tract are sterile

Hormonal changes affect the vaginal flora

Use of epithelial glycogen by lactobacilli produces low pH

ROLE OF THE NORMAL FLORA IN DISEASE

Many species among the normal flora are opportunists in that they can cause infection if they reach protected areas of the body in sufficient numbers or if local or general host defense mechanisms are compromised. For example, certain strains of *E. coli* can reach the urinary bladder by ascending the urethra and cause acute urinary tract infection, usually in sexually active women. Perforation of the colon from a ruptured diverticulum or a penetrating abdominal wound releases feces into the peritoneal cavity; this fecal contamination may be followed by peritonitis, caused primarily by facultative members of the flora, and by intraabdominal abscesses, caused primarily by Gram-negative anaerobes. Viridans streptococci from the oral cavity may reach the bloodstream as a result of physiologic trauma or injury (eg, tooth extraction) and colonize a previously damaged heart valve, initiating bacterial endocarditis (see Chapter 68). These and other diseases, such as actinomycosis, result from displacement of normal flora into body cavities or tissues.

Flora that reach sterile sites may cause disease

Mouth flora may reach heart valves by transient bacteremia

Reduced specific immunologic responses, defects in phagocytic activity, and weakening of epithelial barriers by vitamin deficiencies can all result in local invasion and disease by normal floral organisms. This source accounts for many infections in patients whose defenses are compromised by disease (eg, diabetes, lymphoma, and leukemia) or

Compromised defense systems increase the opportunity for invasion

Mouth flora plays a major role in dental caries

by cytotoxic chemotherapy for cancer. One specific local infection of this type is Vincent's angina of the oral mucosa, a local invasion and ulceration apparently caused by the combined action of oral spirochetes and members of the genus *Fusobacterium*. Death after lethal radiation exposure usually results from massive invasion by normal floral organisms, particularly those of the intestinal tract. Caries and periodontal disease are both caused by organisms that are members of the normal flora. They are considered in detail in Chapter 62.

Nonspecific "toxic" effects of colonic flora are postulated

Early in the 20th century, it was widely believed that the normal flora of the large intestine was responsible for many "toxic conditions," including rheumatoid arthritis, degenerative diseases, and a range of conditions now recognized as psychosomatic. Ritualistic purging and colonic lavage flourished, particularly at expensive mineral spas. At the height of this misdirected attack on the normal flora, some London patients were even subjected to colectomy as a cure for thyroid nodules. These notions persist in the form of the alleged beneficial effect of enemas and colonic lavages.

Blind-loop overgrowth may cause fat malabsorption and B_{12} deficiency

Colonization of jejunum occurs in tropical sprue

However, more recently, attention has again been focused on the less specific contributions of the normal flora to health and disease. In patients with large or multiple blind-ended diverticula in the small intestine, heavy colonization by the anaerobic intestinal flora may occur. This colonization results in bacterial deconjugation of bile salts needed for absorption of fat and fat-soluble vitamins and also in competition for vitamin B_{12}. Similar situations sometimes occur in the elderly when the small intestine is invaded by colonic flora. If the primary cause cannot be eliminated surgically, these conditions can be ameliorated with antibiotic therapy and fat-soluble vitamin supplements. An analogous situation occurs in tropical sprue, in which secondary colonization of the jejunum by facultative Gram-negative enteric bacteria leads to fat malabsorption and vitamin B_{12} and folic acid deficiencies. It has been postulated that the higher colon cancer rates in those consuming Western as opposed to Asian diets may be a result of greater production by members of the normal flora of carcinogens such as nitrosamines and bile acid derivatives.

Ammonia production and bypass lead to hepatic encephalopathy

Under certain conditions, a "toxemia" can result from the action of the normal colonic flora. In severe hepatic cirrhosis, the portal circulation may be partially diverted to the systemic circulation. The detoxification by the liver of ammonia produced by bacterial action on protein residues is bypassed, and severe dysfunctions of the central nervous system (hepatic encephalopathy) can result. This problem can be ameliorated with a strict low-protein diet.

BENEFICIAL EFFECTS OF THE NORMAL FLORA

Priming of Immune System

Sterile animals have little immunity to microbial infection

Low exposure correlates with asthma risk

Organisms of the normal flora play an important role in the development of immunologic competence. Animals delivered and raised under completely aseptic conditions ("sterile" or gnotobiotic animals) have a poorly developed reticuloendothelial system, low serum levels of immunoglobulins, and none of the antibodies to normal floral antigens that often cross-react with those of pathogenic organisms and confer a degree of protection against them. There is evidence of immunologic differences between children who are raised under usual conditions and those that minimize the exposure to diverse flora. Some studies have found a higher incidence of asthma in the more isolated children.

Exclusionary Effect

Breastfeeding and a bifidobacterial flora have a protective effect

Lactobacillus vaginal flora can protect against fomite-transmitted gonorrhea

The normal flora produces conditions that tend to block the establishment of extraneous pathogens and their ability to infect the host. The bifidobacteria in the colon of the breast-fed infant produce an environment inimical to colonization by enteric pathogens; this protective effect is aided by ingested maternal IgA. Breastfeeding has clearly been shown to help protect the infant from enteric bacterial infection. The normal vaginal flora has a similar protective effect. Before the introduction of antibiotic therapy, researchers found that synthetic estrogen therapy controlled institutional outbreaks of fomite-transmitted gonococcal vulvovaginitis in prepubertal girls. This treatment led to glycogen deposition in the vaginal epithelium and establishment of a protective lactobacillary flora. The possible hazard of such therapy in this population was not then recognized.

Antibiotic therapy, particularly with broad-spectrum agents, may so alter the normal flora of the gastrointestinal tract that antibiotic-resistant organisms multiply in the relative ecologic vacuum, sometimes causing significant infections, particularly in immunocompromised patients. The pathogenic yeast *Candida albicans,* a minor component of the normal flora, may multiply dramatically and cause superficial fungal infections in the mouth, vagina, or anal area. Pseudomembranous colitis results from overproliferation of a toxin-producing anaerobe, *Clostridium difficile,* which has a selective advantage in the presence of antibiotic therapy. It may be resistant to several antibiotics that act on other members of the colonic flora, allowing *C. difficile* to increase from a minor to a major component. Its toxins cause diarrhea and direct damage to the colonic epithelium.

Antibiotic therapy may provide a competitive advantage for pathogens

The exclusionary effect of the flora in health has been demonstrated in numerous experiments on gnotobiotic and antibiotic-treated animals. For example, *C. albicans* attaches to oral epithelial cells of germ-free rats; however, prior colonization with certain viridans streptococci that attach to similar epithelial cells prevents establishment of *C. albicans*. In another experiment, the infecting oral dose for mice of streptomycin-resistant *Salmonella* was approximately 10^5 organisms in untreated animals. Oral streptomycin treatment, which inhibits many members of the normal flora, reduced the infecting dose by approximately 1000-fold.

Exclusionary effect makes entrance of pathogens more difficult

Production of Essential Nutrients

In ruminants, the action of the extensive anaerobic flora in the rumen is essential to the nutrition of the animal. The flora digests cellulose to usable form and provides many vitamins, including 70% of the animal's vitamin B requirements. In humans, members of the vitamin B group and vitamin K are produced by the normal flora; however, except for vitamin K the amounts available or absorbed are small compared with those in a well-balanced diet. Bacterial vitamin production is reduced during broad-spectrum antibiotic therapy, and supplementation with vitamin B complex is indicated in malnourished individuals.

Some vitamins are produced by members of the normal flora

MANIPULATION OF THE NORMAL FLORA

Attempts to manipulate the normal flora have often been fruitless and have sometimes been dangerous. Exclusion of the normal flora has been effective in patients whose immunologic defenses are massively compromised (eg, following the whole-body irradiation used in bone marrow transplantation). Significant effects require the use of antimicrobics, sterilization of food and supplies, air filtration, and strict aseptic nursing procedures. These conditions substantially reduce the risk of infection during highly vulnerable periods.

Efforts to control which organisms make up the flora have been more problematic. During nursery outbreaks of *S. aureus* infections in the 1950s, deliberate colonization of an infant's nares with *S. aureus* 502A, a strain of low virulence, was attempted as a control measure. This approach was based on the hope that it would exclude more virulent strains of *S. aureus*. Unfortunately, some infections occurred with the 502A strain.

One area where there has been some success in promoting colonization with "good" flora is with lactobacilli in the intestinal tract. Elie Metchnikoff originally suggested that the longevity of Bulgarian peasants was attributable to their consumption of large amounts of yogurt; the live lactobacilli in the yogurt presumably replaced the colonic flora to the general benefit of their health. This notion persists today in the alleged benefit of natural (unpasteurized) yogurt, which contains live lactobacilli. Although we now know that lactobacillary replacement of the flora of the adult colon does not take place so easily, there have been some successes with capsules containing lyophilized bacteria. In some studies, administration of preparations containing a particular strain of *Lactobacillus* (*L. rhamnosus* strain GG, LGG) has reduced the duration of rotavirus diarrhea in children and prevented relapses of antibiotic-associated diarrhea caused by *C. difficile*. LGG suppositories have also been used to prevent recurrent vaginitis caused by the yeast *C. albicans* with mixed results. A better understanding of the relationship between virulence and the extremely complex interactions of the normal flora is needed for the rational deployment of "good" flora to our benefit.

ADDITIONAL READING

Alvarez-Olmos MI, Oberhelman RA. Probiotic agents and infectious diseases: A modern perspective on a traditional therapy. *Clin Infect Dis* 2001;32:1567–1576. This review gives a critical analysis of the effectiveness of using "good" flora to prevent or treat disease.

Ball TM, Castro-Rodriguez JA, Griffith KA, Holberg CJ, Martinez FD, Wright AL. Siblings, day-care attendance, and the risk of asthma and wheezing during childhood. *N Engl J Med* 2000;343:538–543. This study suggests on epidemiologic grounds that failure to prime the immune system by exposure to the flora of other individuals is associated with an increased risk for asthma.

Rosebury T. *Life on Man*. New York: Berkeley; 1970. A delightful, wry, and instructive paperback. Highly recommended for recreational reading.

CHAPTER 10

Host-Parasite Relationships

STANLEY FALKOW

Infectious diseases have been the major causes of human death and suffering throughout history. Indeed, infectious diseases remain the leading cause of death throughout a world in which most of the population does not have the luxury of living long enough to succumb to the chronic diseases of aging. The major factors that have influenced the emergence of infectious diseases as the leading cause of morbidity and mortality historically are discussed below.

EMERGENCE OF INFECTIOUS DISEASE

The presence of human populations is large enough to sustain and amplify parasites, thus contributing to increased disease. Humans have lived in communities large enough to perpetuate parasites only for about 10,000 years, barely a blink of the eye in the time frame of evolution. Thus, many of the human diseases that have been predominant historically probably did not exist in early humans. Many of the well-known infectious diseases of humans are very recent in the evolutionary sense. For example, the great Black Death of the 14th century, just 700 years ago, led to the death of approximately one third to one half of the known human population. The effects of plague on the human population are still largely unknown. In terms of the evolution of the human gene pool, those that died were likely as important as those that survived. It has been suggested that the resistance of some Caucasian populations to the recent scourge of human immunodeficiency virus (HIV) may actually reflect the genetic consequences of survival from some infectious disease prevalent 20 generations ago. However, some diseases such as treponematosis, mycobacterial infection, infections caused by some protozoans and worms, and diseases caused by herpesviruses, likely afflicted early humans because of their latency and their tendency to reactivate over long periods of time.

Growth and changers in human populations may influence prevalence

Poverty, with its crowding, unsanitary conditions, and often malnutrition, leads to an increased susceptibility to infection and disease. War, famine, civil unrest, and, of course, epidemic disease lead to a breakdown in public infrastructure and the increased incidence of infectious diseases.

Poverty → disease

War → disease

In the history of human civilization, one of the most important facets of the evolution of human infectious diseases was the domestication of animals, which began about 12,000 years ago. There is good cause to think many of the best-known epidemic diseases evolved from animal species and only became adapted to humans rather recently. We are still in an evolutionary dynamic with our large and small parasites; the relationship between humans and the microbes they are heir to has not stopped evolving. Perhaps it

Animal domestication is important

never will. While microbes have evolutionary flexibility, humans try to meet the onslaught of infection with genes that are essentially still those of primitive hunter-gatherers. The actual large-scale domestication of animals has slowed, and it has been replaced by the encroachment of human populations into the domain of animal, insect, and marine species all over the globe. It is little wonder that our deliberate destruction of predators and the outgrowth of human populations into previously virgin land with its attendant destruction of habitat lead to the emergence of "new" diseases such as Lyme disease; Legionnaires' disease; and likely, acquired immunodeficiency syndrome (AIDS).

THE OUTCOME OF INFECTION

Infectious diseases are complex. They involve much more than growth of microbes or parasitic animals in the body. The factors that determine the initiation, development, and outcome of an infection involve a series of complex and shifting interactions between the invading organism and the host, which can vary with different infecting organisms. These interactions include the following:

Multiple steps influence the outcome

1. The organism's ability to breach host barriers and to evade destruction by innate local and tissue host defenses.
2. The organism's biochemical tactics to replicate, to spread, to establish infection, and to cause disease.
3. The microbe's ability to transmit to a new susceptible host.
4. The body's innate and adaptive immunologic ability to control and eliminate the invading parasite.

Broad principles apply

Despite the complexity of interactions between different parasites and hosts, several components of pathogenic processes and principles have broad application to infectious diseases and are described in this chapter. Details of individual organisms and diseases are given in subsequent chapters. Basic mechanisms of specific immune responses are discussed in Chapter 8 and are not recapitulated here. In considering this topic, it is essential to bear in mind that the ability of an organism to infect or to cause disease depends on the susceptibility of the host. There are remarkable species differences in host susceptibility to many infections. For example, dogs do not get measles, nor do humans get canine distemper, although the causative viruses are closely related.

WHAT IS A PATHOGEN?

Humans live in a world filled with microbes

Most microbes are beneficial, not harmful

In medicine, we define a pathogen as any microorganism capable of causing disease. The emphasis is on disease, not the microorganism. However, from the microbial standpoint, being pathogenic is a strategy for survival and simply one more remarkable example of the extraordinary diversity of the microbial world. Humans, including physicians, probably spend too little time reflecting on the fact that we are home to a myriad of other living creatures. From mouth to anus, from head to toe, every millimeter of our cells that is exposed to the outside world has a rich biological diversity. From the mites that inhabit the eyebrows of many of us to the seething cauldron of over 600 species of bacteria that inhabit our large bowel, we are a veritable garden of microorganisms. Most of these microorganisms are not only innocuous but play a useful, if unseen, role. Not only do they provide us with protection against the few harmful microorganisms that we encounter each day, but they also give us some vitamins and nutrients and help digest our food. We have harbored them so long in our evolution that they are even a necessary part of the developmental pathways required for the maturation of our intestinal mucosa and our innate local immune system.

Commensals exist in mutual comfort

Most human microbes are **commensal;** that is, they eat from the same table that we do. These microbes are constant companions and often depend on humans for their existence. Although humans do not appear to be absolutely dependent on microbes for life (at least the cultivatable ones we know), we exist more comfortably with microbes than without them. We also encounter transient microbes, which are just passing through or on us, so to speak. Some commensal transient species may be **opportunistic pathogens.** These organisms can cause disease only if one or more of the usual defense mechanisms humans have evolved to restrict microorganisms from their usually sterile internal organs and tissue are breached by accident, by intent (eg, surgery), or by an underlying metabolic or an infectious disorder (eg, AIDS). Nevertheless, a small group of microorganisms often causes infection and overt disease in seemingly normal individuals. These are the **primary pathogens** such as the common cold virus, the mumps virus, the typhoid bacillus, gonococcus, the tubercle bacillus, and the treponema of syphilis. Each organism is adapted exclusively to humans; other pathogens such as *Salmonella typhimurium,* a common cause of human food poisoning, can cause disease both in humans and other animals, birds, and even reptiles.

Opportunists can cause disease under certain circumstances

Pathogens regularly cause overt disease

What is the difference between a commensal, an opportunist, and a primary pathogen? All of these organisms can cause disease under the proper circumstances. One distinction to make between an opportunistic pathogen and a primary pathogen is on the basis of the essentiality of the host for the long-term survival of a microbe. Long-term survival in a primary pathogen is absolutely dependent on its ability to replicate and to be transmitted in a particular host; however, this is not necessarily the case for a number of the opportunistic pathogens that infect humans. The major distinction that emerges is that primary pathogens have evolved the genetic ability to breach human cellular and anatomic barriers that ordinarily restrict or destroy commensal and transient microorganisms. Thus, pathogens can inherently cause damage to cells to gain access by force to a new unique niche that provides them with less competition from other microorganisms, as well as a ready new source of nutrients. For microorganisms that inhabit mammals as an essential component of their survival tactic, success can be measured by the capacity to multiply sufficiently to be maintained or be transmitted to a new susceptible host. This is true for commensal and pathogen alike. However, if the pathogen gains a new niche free of competition and rich in nutrients, it also faces a more hostile environment designed by evolution to restrict microbial entry and, indeed, to destroy any intruders that dare to enter these protected regions. Thus, pathogens have not only acquired the capacity to breach cellular barriers, they also have, by necessity, learned to circumvent, exploit, subvert, and even manipulate our normal cellular mechanisms to their own selfish need to multiply at our expense.

Pathogens must move on to another host

The strategy for survival of a pathogen requires infection (persistence, usually by multiplication on or within another living organism). Disease (ie, the overt clinical signs and symptoms of damage that occur in a host as a result of its interaction with an infectious agent) may not be an inevitable outcome of the host-parasite interaction. Rather, the requirement for a microbial infection is sufficient multiplication by the pathogen to secure its establishment within the host by transient or long-term colonization or to bring about its successful transmission to a new susceptible host. Thus, many (or most) common infections are inapparent and asymptomatic. Symptoms of disease can reflect part of the microbe's strategy for survival within the host. For example, coughing promotes the transmission of the tubercle bacillus and influenza virus, and diarrhea spreads enteric viruses, protozoa, and bacteria.

Features of disease may be linked to transmission

Physicians often use the terms virulent and pathogenic interchangeably. Originally, **virulence** was used as a comparison of pathogenicity in the quantitative sense, and this use of the term is still preferred. For example, the bacterial species *Haemophilus influenzae* is a common inhabitant of the upper respiratory tract of humans. Members of this species regularly cause middle-ear infection and sinusitis in children and bronchitis in smokers, but one variety of *H. influenzae* (those with capsule type b) can cause systemic disease (meningitis and epiglottitis). All *H. influenzae* are pathogenic, but *H. influenzae* type b is more virulent.

Virulence expresses degrees of pathogenicity

CHANGES IN MICROBIAL PATHOGENICITY

Many of the major public health crises of the past two decades have been infectious in origin. If we examine them closely, many can be seen to be a natural consequence of human behavior and progress. For example, Legionnaires' disease can be traced to subtle differences in human behavior and social convention. *Legionella pneumophila* is widely

Human progress may enhance spread of some diseases

found in nature as an infectious agent of predatory protozoa and is normally found in potable water supplies throughout the world. But showers and other widespread aerosolization technology (eg, spray devices for produce in supermarkets) can introduce the bacteria into the alveolus of the lung. *Legionella* finds a new niche in the human phagocytic macrophage instead of its usual protozoan hosts *Acanthamoeba* or *Hartmannella.* The microbe is programmed to replicate, and the consequence is characterized as a new or emerging infectious disease. Women in our society asked for more absorbent tampons to achieve more social freedom and unwittingly, American commerce supplied a product that helped select for certain strains of staphylococcus. Another new emerging disease, toxic shock syndrome (TSS) was recognized and caused near panic.

Aerosols spread *Legionella*

TSS is linked to tampons

These examples are not meant to turn our attention away from the pathogenic traits of the disease-causing microbes, but it seems true, on reflection, that humans, with their technology and social behavior, have played a significant role in providing pathogenic microbes with new venues for their wares. Food poisoning by *Escherichia coli* O157:H7, *Campylobacter,* and *Salmonella* arise as much from food technology and modern food distribution networks than from any fundamental change in the virulence properties of the bacteria in question. HIV, Hantavirus, and Lyme disease seem likely to be a consequence of the encroachment of humans on previously undisturbed ecological niches and the increased likelihood of human contact with animal species and their carried microorganisms. In the case of HIV, the expansion of rapid travel throughout the globe magnified this consequence. No part of our planet is more than 3 days away by air travel, a fact known and feared by all public health officials.

E. coli O157:H7 is spread by food processing

Today, physicians deal more and more with opportunists because our population is getting older, and the practice of medicine keeps individuals alive longer by surgical procedures and powerful drugs that affect the immune status. As a consequence, in the Western world, microorganisms that a scant 40 years ago were considered harmless commensals or environmental isolates are now feared opportunistic pathogens. Many of the primary pathogens such as measles virus are controlled now by immunization. One view is that infectious diseases are under control. Another view is that the host–parasite relationship is still in a dynamic state. Just as many people die of infection as did 40 years ago; they just die later and because of different infectious agents. It is important to understand that for most of the world, the "classic" pathogens of history such as malaria, the tubercle and leprosy bacillus, and the cholera vibrio, together with newcomers such as HIV, are the leading causes of human misery and death.

Opportunists attack vulnerable populations

Classic pathogens are dominant in most of the world

TOWARD A GENETIC AND MOLECULAR DEFINITION OF PATHOGENICITY

The classic investigation of pathogenicity has been based on linking natural disease in humans with experimental infection produced by the same organism. The analysis of bacterial virulence determinants usually was the result of the comparative analysis of different clinical isolates of the same species that were either virulent or avirulent in a particular model system. This led to speculation about the potential role of a number of microbial traits as virulence determinants.

Comparison of strains of varying virulence is classic approach

This comparative approach now has given way to mutational analysis within a single or limited number of strains of a pathogenic species. The goal is to obtain a single, defined genetic change that alters a single virulence property and affects the pathogenesis of infection or the ability of the organism to cause pathology in an appropriate model system. The advances in microbial genetics, DNA biochemistry, and molecular biology have made it possible to apply a kind of molecular Koch's postulates to the analysis of virulence traits.

1. The phenotype or property under investigation should be associated significantly more often with pathogenic strains of a species than with nonpathogenic strains.
2. Specific inactivation of the gene or genes of interest associated with the suspected virulence trait should lead to a measurable decrease in virulence.
3. Restoration of pathogenicity or full virulence should accompany replacement of the mutated allele with the original wild-type gene.

Genetic manipulation can inactivate and restore virulence

This simplistic goal is not always possible because it is dependent on a suitable infection model in which to test a microorganism. The ideal model can be infected by a natural route using numbers analogous to those seen in human infection and can duplicate the relevant pathology observed in the natural host. Except for other primates, such models do not exist for pathogens that are restricted to humans. For example, it is still difficult to assess the role of IgA1 protease in the pathogenicity of *Neisseria gonorrhoeae,* because the enzyme works only on human IgA1 and the microorganism is an exclusive human pathogen.

Strict human pathogens are more difficult to study

Despite these technical limitations, there has been a revolution over the past decade in understanding of the basic pathogenic mechanisms and how microbes bring about infection and disease. The use of transgenic animals, reconstituted human immune systems in rodents, and the extension of cell and organ culture methods to the study of infectious agents will lead to greater understanding of the pathogenesis of infectious diseases. In parallel, new methods to visualize living microbes in tissue and to monitor genetic activity through "reporter molecules" will permit the monitoring of microbes in infected tissue in real time. The full genomic sequence of most pathogenic microbial species will be completed within the coming decade. This information, coupled with contemporary technology of DNA arrays and the parallel knowledge about the human genome, soon will allow examination of the expression of every bacterial gene and a representative expression of host genes in both experimental infection models and in samples obtained from infected patients. This knowledge will continue to impact how infectious diseases are diagnosed, treated and prevented in the not-too-distant future.

Transgenic animals allow monitoring of virulence determinants

ATTRIBUTES OF MICROBIAL PATHOGENICITY

Whether a microbe is a primary or opportunistic pathogen, it must be able to enter a host; find a unique niche; avoid, circumvent or subvert normal host defenses; and multiply. To be successful, a primary pathogen also must be transmitted to a new susceptible host or establish themselves in the host for an extended period of time and eventually be transmitted.

Entry

Like all other living organisms, humans must maintain contact with the environment to see, breathe, ingest food, reproduce, and eliminate wastes. Consequently, each of the portals in the body that communicates with the outside world becomes a potential site of microbial entry. Human and other animal hosts have various protective mechanisms to prevent microbial entry (Table 10–1). A simple, although relatively efficient, mechanical barrier to microbial invasion is provided by intact epithelium, the most effective of which is the stratified squamous epithelium of the skin with its superficial cornified anucleate layers. Organisms can gain access to the underlying tissues only by breaks or by way of hair follicles, sebaceous glands, and sweat glands that traverse the stratified layers. The surface of the skin continuously desquamates and thus tends to shed contaminating organisms. The skin also inhibits the growth of most extraneous microorganisms because of low moisture, low pH, and the presence of substances with antibacterial activity.

Microbes gain access from the environment

Skin is a major protective barrier

A viscous mucus covering protects the epithelium lining the respiratory tract, the gastrointestinal tract, and urogenital system secreted by goblet cells. Microorganisms become trapped in the mucus layer and may be swept away before they reach the epithelial cell surface. Secretory IgA (sIgA) secreted into the mucus and other secreted antimicrobials such as lysozyme and lactoferrin aid this cleansing process. Ciliated epithelial cells constantly move the mucus away from the lower respiratory tract. In the respiratory tract, particles larger than 5 μm are trapped in this fashion. The epithelium of the intestinal tract below the esophagus is a less efficient mechanical barrier than the skin, but there are other effective defense mechanisms. The high level of hydrochloric acid and gastric enzymes in the normal stomach kill many ingested bacteria. Others are susceptible to pancreatic digestive enzymes or to the detergent effect of bile salts. Similarly, the multilayered transitional epithelium of the urinary tract uses the flushing effect of urine and its relatively low pH as additional defense mechanisms to limit microbial entry and growth.

Secretions coat mucosal epithelium

Acids and enzymes aid in cleansing

TABLE 10–1

Nonspecific Defenses Against Colonization with Pathogens

Site	Mechanical Barrier	Ciliated Epithelium	Competition by Normal Flora	Mucus	sIgA	Lymphoid Follicles	Low pH	Flushing Effects of Contents	Peristalsis	Special Factors
Skin	+++	–	+	–	–	–	++	–	–	Fatty acids from action of normal flora on sebum
Conjunctiva	++	–	–	–	+	–	–	+++	–	Lysozyme
Oropharynx	+++	–	+++	–	+	Yes	–	++	–	
Upper respiratory tract	++	+	+++	++	++	Yes	–	+	–	Turbinate baffles
Middle ear and paranasal sinuses[a]	++	+++	–	++	?	–	–	+	–	
Lower respiratory tract[a]	++	+++	–	++	++	Yes	–	–	–	Mucociliary escalator, alveolar macrophages; cough reflex
Stomach	++	–	–	++	–	–	+++	+	+	Production of hydrochloric acid
Intestinal tract	++	–	+++	+++	+++	Yes	–	+	+++	Bile; digestive enzymes
Vagina	+++	–	+++	+	+	–	+++	–	–	Lactobacillary flora ferments epithelial glycogen
Urinary tract[a]	++	–	–	–	+	–	+	+++	–	

Abbreviations: +, ++, +++ = relative importance in defense at each site; – = unimportant.

[a] Sterile in health.

Urinary tract infections are much more common in women than men because the short urethra in females allows easier passage of organisms to the bladder; such infections in women are often associated with sexual intercourse.

Pathogenic organisms have evolved mechanisms to capitalize on each of these human sites of environmental contact as points of entry. Removal of the epithelial barrier and normal host cell functions makes human into the victims of opportunists. One natural method of bypassing the skin is direct inoculation by insect bites; several organisms use this route, including the plague bacillus *Yersinia pestis* and the malarial parasite. These microorganisms, which must spend part of their lives in remarkably different environments than their mammalian hosts, have adapted mechanisms for survival. Another means in the modern world of bypassing the skin is through the deliberate inoculation used by drug addicts who suffer from a particular constellation of infectious disease agents as a result.

Pathogens are adapted to mucosal environments

Insect injection allows pathogens to bypass barriers

We still know very little about the microbial factors essential to ensure infectious transmission from host to host. Obviously, microbes adapted to life in humans have evolved to take advantage of existing avenues of contact between their hosts. Dissemination by aerosol is common, but success is more than just random chance; the parasite must design itself for the rigors of atmospheric drying and other environmental factors. The virus of the common cold must exist on inanimate objects (fomites) waiting for a hand to touch and carry them to the conjunctiva or nasopharynx. The burden on an enteric pathogen that follows the fecal–oral route is substantial: feces, mouth to stomach to small bowel to large bowel and back to the cold cruel world in stool. Thus, bacteria causing enteric infection are exposed to extremes of temperature, pH, bile salts, digestive enzymes, and a myriad of competing microorganisms. Sexually transmitted pathogens ordinarily are delivered by direct inoculation onto mucosal surfaces. This microbial strategy avoids life in the external environment but is not without its own set of special requirements to overcome changing pH, mucus obstruction, anatomic barriers, local antibodies, and phagocytic cells.

Environmental survival facilitates host-to-host transmission

Sexual transmission is direct

All of the factors in the initial encounter of the host with the parasite can be assessed to some degree by measuring the infectious dose of the organism. How many organisms must be given a host to ensure infection in some proportion of the individuals? The measure of the infectious dose-50 (ID_{50}) for several pathogens is shown in Table 10–2. It is a simple measurement of a very complex interaction. Moreover, it is somewhat misleading, as the endpoint is disease in human volunteers or death (a rigorous endpoint) in animal experiments.

Infection is dose-related

Adherence: The Search for a Unique Niche

The first major interaction between a pathogenic microorganism and its host entails attachment to an eukaryotic cell surface. In its simplest form, adherence requires the participation of two factors: a receptor on the host cell and an **adhesin** on the invading microbe. Most viruses attach specifically to sites on target cells through an envelope protein. For example, the influenza viruses attach specifically to neuraminic acid–containing

Molecular adhesins attach to surface receptors on host cells

TABLE 10–2

Dose of Microorganisms Required to Produce Infection in Human Volunteers

MICROBE	ROUTE	DISEASE-PRODUCING DOSE
Rhinovirus	Pharynx	200
Salmonella typhi	Oral	10^5
Shigella spp.	Oral	10–1000
Vibrio cholerae	Oral	10^8
V. cholerae	Oral + HCO_3^-	10^4
Mycobacterium tuberculosis	Inhalation	1–10

glycoprotein receptors on the surface of respiratory cells before penetrating to the interior of the cell. Bacteria, like viruses, generally have protein structures on their surface that recognize either a protein or a carbohydrate moiety on the host cell surface. Finding the correct host cell surface in many cases appears to be a probability event related to the infectious dose. Because the mucosal surface is constantly bathed by a moving fluid layer, it is not surprising that many bacteria that infect the bladder or gastrointestinal tract are motile, and some (such as the typhoid bacillus) may use chemotaxis (see Chapter 3) to home in on the correct host cell surface. Some bacteria use mucolytic enzymes to reach epithelial surfaces.

Some bacterial adherence may involve hydrophobic interruptions between nonpolar groups present on the microbe and host cell. Alternatively, one can envision cationic bridging between cells. Such interactions lack the specificity seen in most host–pathogen interactions. Rather, pathogens most often employ highly specific receptor-ligand binding. In the last decade, it has become clear that most pathogenic microorganisms have more than a single mechanism of host cell attachment, which is not just a redundant feature. More often it reflects that pathogenic microbes require different types of adherence factors depending on their location and the types of host cells they may encounter. Thus, bacteria may employ one set of adhesins at the epithelial surface but respond with a different set when they encounter cells of the immune system. Finally, not all adhesins are essential virulence factors; they may play a role in survival outside of a host or add to the biology of the microbe outside of its pathogenic lifestyle.

Many pathogens have multiple attachment mechanisms

Bacterial adhesins can be divided into two major groups: pili (fimbriae) and nonpilus adhesins (afimbrial adhesins). The pili of many Gram-negative bacteria bind directly to sugar residues that are part of glycolipids or glycoproteins on host cells or act as a protein scaffold to which another more specific adhesive protein is affixed. One of the major features among diverse pili is conservation of the molecular machinery needed for pilus biogenesis and assembly onto the bacterial surface. One of the best-studied examples of pilus assembly is P-pili (pyelonephritis-associated pili), which are encoded by *pap* genes. *E. coli* strains that express P-pili are associated with pyelonephritis, which arises from urinary tract colonization and subsequent infection of the kidney. It is thought that P-pili are essential adhesins in this disease process. The *pap* operon is a useful paradigm, because it contains many conserved features found among various pilus operons. Two molecules guide newly synthesized pilus components to the bacterial surface. The major subunit of the pilus rod is PapA, which is anchored in the bacterial outer membrane by PapH. At the distal end of the pilus rod is the tip fibrillum, composed of PapE, and the actual tip adhesin, PapG, which mediates attachment to the host cell surface. Two other proteins, PapF and PapK, are involved in tip fibrillum synthesis. Although the host receptor varies for different bacterial pili, the general concepts provided by studying the P pilus operon are conserved in many other pilus systems, and components are often interchangeable. Homologous sequences to *pap* genes also have been found in genes involved in bacterial capsule and lipopolysaccharide biosynthesis.

Pili are major bacterial adhesins

P-pili are specific for urinary epithelium

Components are regulated by an operon

Although many pili look alike morphologically, there are at least five general classes in various Gram-negative bacteria that recognize different entities on the host cell surface. Thus, although *pap*-like sequences are common throughout Gram-negative adhesins, other families of pili use alternative biogenesis and assembly machinery to form a pilus. One such group, type IV pili, is found in diverse Gram-negative organisms, including the causal agents of gonorrhea and cholera. Type IV pili subunits contain specific features, including a conserved, unusual amino-terminal sequence that lacks a classic leader sequence and, instead, generally utilizes a specific leader peptidase that removes a short, basic peptide sequence. Several possess methylated amino termini on their pilin molecules and usually contain pairs of cysteines that are involved in intrachain, disulfide bond formation near their carboxyl termini; however, analogous to the P-pilus tip adhesin, a separate tip protein may function as a tip adhesin for type IV pili. The host receptor that a pathogenicity-associated adhesin recognizes probably determines the tissue specificity for that adhesin and bacterial colonization or persistence; of course, other factors also may make a contribution. The location of the adhesin at the distal tip of pili ensures adhesin exposure to potential host receptors. Alterations in the pilus subunit can also affect

Gram-negative bacteria have five types of pili

Receptor determines tissue specificity

adherence levels, and antigenic variation in the actual structural pilin protein can be an important source of antigenic diversity for the pathogen.

The pilus model of attachment is the best-known means of bacterial attachment to a host cell surface; however, nonpilin adhesins have been demonstrated in a number of bacterial species. These are often specific outer membrane proteins that form an intimate contact between the bacterial surface and the surface of the host cell. Several of these are intriguing because they resemble or "mimic" eukaryotic sequences that mediate cell–cell adhesion and adherence to the extracellular matrix. Similar classes of molecules thought to mediate adherence in the Gram-positive bacteria are surface fibrils composed of proteins and lipoteichoic acid. For example, streptococci causing pharyngitis, express an M protein–lipoteichoic acid structure believed to mediate attachment to the prevalent host cell protein, fibronectin.

Outer membrane proteins may be adhesins

Bacterial capsular polysaccharide also may mediate adherence to host cells or play an important role in binding layers of bacteria to others immediately adherent to the epithelial surface. These bacterial biofilms not only can coat the mucosal surface but play an important role in the bacterial colonization of the inert materials used as catheters.

Polysaccharide capsules and biofilms stick to surfaces

Some organisms excrete an enzyme IgA protease, which cleaves human IgA1 in the hinge region to release the Fc portion from the Fab fragment. This enzyme might play an important role in establishing microbial species at the mucosal surface, as bacteria that cleave IgA can bind the antigen-binding domain of the immunoglobulin. This is one of several cases of molecular mimicry where bacteria (and probably viruses as well) can coat themselves with a secreted host cell product. This provides a microorganism with two advantages. First, microbes use these secreted products as a bridge to adhere to cell receptors that ordinarily bind these secreted products. Second, by binding a host cell product on its surface, the microbe disguises itself from the host cell immune system.

Proteases cleave IgA

Unlike bacteria, viruses generally only have one major adhesin that they use to attach to the host cell surface and to gain entry into the cytoplasm. Otherwise, both bacteria and viruses share the same strategy: a protein structure that recognizes a specific receptor. Host cell receptors do not exist for the sole use of infectious agents; they generally are associated with important cellular functions. The adhesive molecule on the microorganism has been selected to take advantage of the host cell's biological function(s). In this way, the adhesin provides the microbe with a unique niche where the infectious agent has the greatest chance to achieve success. Presumably, a pathogen's success can be measured by the extent of multiplication subsequent to entry. Adherence is important not only during the initial encounter between the pathogen and its host but also throughout the infection cycle.

Viral adhesins exploit host cell functions

Strategy for Survival: Avoid, Circumvent, Subvert, or Manipulate Normal Host Cell Defenses

Once a pathogenic species reaches its unique niche, it may face formidable host defense mechanisms including dangerous phagocytic cells. Such a site may be devoid of a normal heavy commensal bacterial burden precisely because it contains added defense measures not found at the usual mucosal sites. The ways by which microbes avoid, circumvent, or even subvert or manipulate such host barriers are relatively unique for each species, although certain common pathogenic tactics have begun to be appreciated. We now know that bacterial pathogenicity is a multifaceted process that can be likened to a symphony in which each part contributes to a common theme. Yet, even though pathogenic species sometimes use genetic homologs and exhibit similar tactics to outwit host defenses, each pathogen has evolved a unique style of survival—a pathogenic signature.

Getting into Cells

Many pathogenic bacteria are content to fight their way to the mucosal surface, adhere, nullify local host defense factors, and multiply. However, adherence to a cellular surface may only be the first step in other infections. Some pathogenic microbes are capable of entering into and surviving within eukaryotic cells. Some organisms direct their uptake

Some pathogens enter mucosal cells or phagocytes

into host cells that are not normally phagocytic, including epithelial cells lining mucosal surfaces and endothelial cells lining blood vessels. Invasion may provide a means for a microorganism to breach host epithelial barriers. Presumably, this invasion tactic ensures a protected cellular niche for the microbe to replicate or persist. Alternatively, phagocytic cells, such as macrophages, may internalize organisms actively by several mechanisms. Pathogens that survive and replicate within phagocytic cells possess additional mechanisms that enhance their survival. Even quite different organisms can employ mechanistically similar invasion strategies.

Viruses and some bacteria must replicate in cells

Some replicate in cytosol, and others in host cell membranes

Intracellular growth and replication is an essential step for all viruses. Bacterial entry into host cells is usually divided into two broad groups. Bacteria that, like viruses, are obligate intracellular pathogens, include the typhus group *(Rickettsia)* and the trachoma group *(Chlamydia).* Other microbes such as the typhoid–paratyphoid group *(Salmonella),* the dysentery group *(Shigella),* the Legionnaires' disease bacillus *(Legionella),* and the tubercle bacillus *(Mycobacterium)* are classified as facultative intracellular pathogens and can grow as free-living cells in the environment as well as within host cells. Whereas some pathogens do whatever they can to avoid phagocytosis, these virulent facultative intracellular organisms establish themselves and replicate within the intracellular environment of phagocytes. All of these bacteria are taken up by host cells through a specific receptor-mediated, often bacterial-directed, phagocytic event. The entering bacteria initially are seen within a membrane-bound, host-vesicular structure. Yet, both the facultative and obligate bacterial pathogens can be further classified with respect to the mechanism by which they replicate intracellularly. Thus, *Shigella* and some *Rickettsia* lyse the phagosome and multiply in the nutrient-rich safe haven of the host cell cytosol. In contrast, *Salmonella, Chlamydia, Legionella,* and *Mycobacterium* remain enclosed in a host cell–derived membrane for their entire intracellular life and modulate their environment to suit their own purposes. They survive and replicate intracellularly within a host cell vacuole by thwarting the normal host cell trafficking pattern to avoid becoming fused to the hydrolytically active components of lysosomes.

Generally, invasive organisms adhere to host cells by one or more adhesins but employ a class of molecules, called **invasins,** that either direct bacterial entry into cells or provide an intimate direct contact between the bacterial surface and the host cell plasma membrane. In both cases, invasins are the first step in mediating direct interaction between one or more bacterial products and host cell molecules. Invasins are adhesins in their own right, but obviously not all adhesins (such as the pili mentioned earlier) mediate entry into host cells. Invasins usually trigger or activate signals in the host cell that directly or indirectly mediate and facilitate specific membrane–membrane interaction and, in some cases, bacterial entry. For example, enteropathogenic *E. coli* and *Helicobacter pylori,* the causative agent of peptic ulcer, use contact-dependent secretory systems to actually insert bacterial proteins into the host cell membrane. This is the first step in a cascade of events that triggers a massive redeployment of host cell cytoskeletal elements. The bacteria in question do not enter the host cell but remain tightly affixed to the host cell. The molecular manipulation by the bacteria leads to a microenvironment that is essential for bacterial persistence and proliferation. The host suffers from diarrhea in one case or an inflamed gastric mucosa in the other, an unfortunate consequence for many infected hosts. Likewise, some other bacteria do not enter host cells. The typhoid bacillus and the etiologic agent of dysentery adhere intimately to the host cell surface, and, in a contact-dependent manner, directly "inject" bacterial proteins into the host cell cytoplasm, which induces a cataclysmic rearrangement of host cell actin that envelops the bacteria by a process that resembles normal macropinocytosis. Thus, ultimately, host cell cytoskeletal components and normal cellular mechanisms are exploited by bacteria to their own end. The specific tactics used by different microbes are discussed in subsequent chapters.

Invasin proteins direct entry

Proteins are inserted by contact secretion

Cell signal systems are triggered

Phospholipase digestion facilitates cytosol entry

Following cell entry, the invading bacterium immediately is localized within a membrane-bound vacuole inside the host cell. As noted, the invading pathogen organism may or may not escape this vacuole, depending on the pathogen and its strategy for survival. A small number of bacterial species appear to forcibly enter directly into host cells by a local enzymatic digestion of the host cell membrane following adherence to the cell surface. One such pathogen, *Rickettsia prowazekii,* produces phospholipases that appear to degrade the host wall localized beneath the adherent organisms, thereby enabling the pathogen to enter directly into the cytoplasm. How the bacterium controls the enzymatic degradation to prevent host cell lysis and how the host cell reseals its membrane after invasion remain uncharacterized.

Invasin binding sites can be members of the integrin family, a family of integral membrane glycoproteins mediating cell–cell and cell–extracellular matrix interactions. Integrins include the receptors for fibronectin, collagen, laminin, vitronectin, and the complement binding receptor of phagocytes. Integrins are linked to the actin microfilament system through a variety of molecules, including talin, vinculin, and α-actinin. Thus, the binding of a microbe to an integrin or integrin-like molecule on the host surface may trigger a host cell signal that causes actin filaments to link to the membrane-bound receptor, which then generates the force necessary for parasite uptake. Understanding the cell biology of microbial invasion is still in its early stages, but once again it is important to emphasize that pathogenic microbes most often gain entry into the host cell by altering or exploiting normal host cell mechanisms.

Integrins can be receptors and links to cytoskeleton

Some viruses are internalized in much the same way. For example, rhinoviruses of the common cold use membrane-bound glycoprotein intercellular adhesion molecule 1 (ICAM-1) as a receptor. ICAM-1 is also a ligand of certain integrins. More often, as already discussed, virus particles are taken up by the receptor-mediated endocytosis mechanism (see Chapter 6), which is normally responsible for internalizing hormones, growth factors, and some important nutrients.

Avoiding Intracellular Pitfalls

Intracellular pathogens enjoy a number of advantages. Besides avoiding the host immune system, intracellular localization places pathogens in an environment potentially rich in nutrients and devoid of competing microorganisms. Intracellular life is not free of difficulty. Viruses that enter by fusion are “dumped” directly into the cytoplasm where they may begin the replicative cycle. Bacteria or viruses internalized through the reorganization of the cytoskeleton find themselves in a membrane-bound vesicle in an acidic environment and may be destined for fusion with potentially degradative lysosomes. Some viruses respond to the acidic environment by changing conformation, binding to the endosomal membrane, and releasing their nucleic acid into the cytoplasm. Bacteria such as *Shigella,* the cause of bacillary dysentery, and *Listeria monocytogenes,* a causative agent of meningitis and sepsis in the very young or very old, elaborate an enzyme that dissolves away the surrounding membrane and permits the bacterium to replicate within the relative safety of the cytoplasm. Other organisms, such as the typhoid bacillus and the tubercle bacillus, apparently tolerate the initial endosome–lysosome fusion event; however, most recent evidence suggests that they then modify this intracellular compartment into a privileged niche in which they can replicate optimally. *Mycobacterium* somehow inhibit the acidification of the phagosome. Still other organisms, for example, the protozoan *Toxoplasma gondii,* inhibit the acidification of the endosomal vesicle and this, in turn, inhibits lysosomal fusion. The common theme again is that the microorganism has found a way to circumvent or to exploit host cell factors to suit its own purpose.

Intracellular site is free of competition, immune system

Resistance to degradative enzymes is needed

Establishment: Overcoming the Host’s Immune System

Once a microorganism has breached the surface epithelial barrier, it is subject to a series of nonspecific and specific processes designed to remove, inhibit, or destroy it. These defenses are complex, dynamic, and interactive. Microorganisms that reach the subepithelial tissues are immediately exposed to the intercellular tissue fluids, which have defined properties that inhibit multiplication of many bacteria. For example, most tissues contain lysozyme in sufficient concentrations to disrupt the cell wall of some Gram-positive bacteria. Other less well-defined inhibitors from leukocytes and platelets have also been described. Tissue fluid itself is a suboptimal growth medium for most bacteria and deficient in free iron. Iron is essential for bacterial growth, but it is sequestered by the body’s iron-binding proteins such as transferrin and lactoferrin and is inaccessible to organisms that do not themselves produce siderophores (see Chapter 3). Virtually all pathogenic species come equipped with a means to extract the essential iron they need from the host's iron-sequestering defenses.

Subepithelial environment is different

Iron sources are important for the pathogen

Apoptosis may be induced

If an organism proceeds beyond the initial physical and biochemical barriers, it may meet strategically placed phagocytic cells of the monocyte/macrophage lineage whose function is to engulf, internalize, and destroy large particulate matter, including infectious agents. Examples of such resident phagocytic cells include the alveolar macrophages, liver Kupffer cells, brain microglial cells, lymph node and splenic macrophages, kidney mesangial cells, and synovial A cells. As noted above, many pathogens are facultative intracellular parasites that actually seek out, enter, and replicate within these phagocytic defenders. One of the most common tactics of these pathogens is to induce programmed cell death (apoptosis). This clever microbial tactic not only inactivates the killing potential of the phagocyte but also reduces the number of defenders available to inhibit other bacterial invaders. The invading bacteria that induce apoptosis obtain the added benefit that death by apoptosis nullifies the normal cellular signaling processes of cytokine and chemokine signaling of necrotic death. Hence, the myriads of microbes that infect humans and make up their normal flora are held at bay by our innate and adaptive immune mechanisms. Pathogenic bacteria, almost by definition, can overcome these biochemical and cellular shields after they breach the mucosal barrier.

Not all pathogens can deactivate the host's early warning system, inflammation. Inflammation is a normal host response to a traumatic or infectious injury. When many microorganisms multiply in the tissues, the usual result is an inflammatory response, which has several immediate defensive effects. It increases tissue fluid flow from the bloodstream to the lymphatic circulation and brings phagocytes, complement, and any existing antibody to the site of infection. Macrophage-derived interleukin-1 (IL-1) and tumor necrosis factor (TNF) stimulates or enhances these processes. The increased lymphatic drainage serves to bring microbes or their antigens into contact with the cells in the local lymph nodes that mediate the development of specific immune responses. Microorganisms that escape from a local lesion into the lymphatic circulation or bloodstream are rapidly cleared by reticuloendothelial cells or arrested in the small pulmonary capillaries and then ingested by phagocytic cells. This process is so efficient that when a million organisms are injected into a vein of a rabbit, few, if any, are recoverable in cultures of blood taken 15 minutes after injection, although the ultimate result of such clearance may not be a cure. The end results are the classic inflammatory manifestations of **swelling** (tumor), vasodilatation of surface vessels with **erythema** (rubor), **heat** (calor) from increased skin temperature, **pain** (dolor) from increased pressure and tissue damage, and **loss of function** because of reflex nerve inhibition or the pain caused by movement.

Cytokines induce inflammation

Tissues may be injured by PMNs

Function of fever is unknown

Fever, a frequent concomitant of inflammation, is mediated primarily by IL-1 and TNF released by macrophages. The value of fever is not completely clear; however, it increases the effectiveness of several processes involved in phagocytosis and microbial killing and frequently reduces the multiplication or replication rate of bacteria or viruses. Taken together, these host cell factors serve to produce an environment that is highly hostile to most organisms and also is hostile to adjacent normal tissue. Lysosomal enzymes, including collagenase and elastase, when released from polymorphonuclear neutrophils (PMNs) damage tissues and contribute to the enhancement of the inflammatory process; however, failure of the phagocytes to clear bacteria results in continued release of toxic products from the inflammatory exudate, which can be as damaging to the host as released bacterial virulence products. Ultimately, phagocytes kill almost all bacteria. When the invading microorganisms (or their surviving antigenic material) cannot be degraded or are resistant to removal or degradation, T cells accumulate and release lymphokines. This leads to the aggregation and proliferation of macrophages and the characteristic appearance of a nodular mass called a **granuloma,** which consists of multinucleate giant cells, epithelioid cells, and activated macrophages. Granulomas are characteristic of infections caused by the tubercle bacillus *Mycobacterium tuberculosis* and other facultative intracellular parasites.

VIRULENCE FACTORS: TOXINS

The successful pathogen must survive and multiply in the face of these formidable host defenses. Microbial virulence factors that permit the establishment of the pathogen in the hostile host environment are essential. If these factors are lost, the capacity to infect the host or become transmitted successfully goes with them. Not surprisingly, these virulence factors are also the target(s) in the design of vaccines. The following sections provide a general overview of the classes of bacterial virulence factors that permit them to overcome host defenses. No pathogen possesses all of the classes of virulence factors, nor are all virulence factors absolutely essential for a pathogen to reach its goal of sufficient multiplication to establish itself in the host or to be transmitted to a new susceptible host.

Exotoxins

A number of microorganisms synthesize protein molecules that are toxic to their hosts and are secreted into their environment or are found associated with the microbial surface. These exotoxins usually possess some degree of host cell specificity, which is dictated by the nature of the binding of one or more toxin components to a specific host cell receptor. The distribution of host cell receptors often dictates the degree and the breadth of the toxicity. Bacterial exotoxins, whether synthesized by Gram-positive or Gram-negative bacteria, fall into two broad classes, each of which represents a general pathogenic theme common to many bacterial species.

Secreted into their environment

A–B Exotoxins

The best known pathogenic exotoxin theme is represented by the A–B exotoxins. These toxins are divisible into two general domains. One, the B subunit, is associated with the binding specificity of the molecule to the host cell. Generally speaking, the B region binds to a specific host cell surface glycoprotein or glycolipid. The other, subunit A, is the catalytic domain, which enzymatically attacks a susceptible host function or structure. The actual biochemical structure of exotoxins varies. In some cases (diphtheria toxin), the single B subunit of the toxin is linked through a disulfide bond to the A subunit. In other cases (pertussis toxin), multiple B subunits may join with a single A enzymatic subunit. In any event, following attachment of the B domain to the host cell surface, the A domain is transported by direct fusion or by endocytosis into the host cell. Many of the most potent A–B bacterial toxins are ADP-ribosylating enzymes. Some of these affect the protein-synthesizing apparatus of the cell (diphtheria toxin, *Pseudomonas* exotoxin); others affect the cytoskeleton (*Clostridium botulinum* toxin C2) or the normal signal transduction activities of the host (*Bordetella pertussis* and *Vibrio cholerae*). It is notable that the major natural substrates of the toxin ADP-ribosyltransferases are guanine nucleotide-binding proteins (G proteins), which are involved in signal transduction in eukaryotic cells. In a very simplistic way, one can think that the ADP-ribosylating toxins are all geared to interrupt the biochemical lines of communication within and between host cells. An understanding of bacterial toxins, therefore, sheds as much light on the intimate details of normal animal cell regulation as it does on bacterial pathogenicity.

B unit binds to cell receptor

A is enzymatically active

Several bacterial toxins have been examined in exquisite detail at the biochemical level. The crystal structures of several have been "solved." In many cases, the precise amino acids making up the catalytic site of the toxin are so well known that a single amino acid substitution can be made that is sufficient to detoxify the molecule. These **toxoids** are the basis for new generations of vaccines. Given this level of biochemical sophistication, it is somewhat disconcerting to realize that the actual role of bacterial toxins in microbial pathogenicity has not been clarified. A number of the most fearsome human diseases are the result of intoxication by secreted bacterial toxins. Human disease as a consequence of an accidental contamination of a wound with the tetanus bacillus or the accidental ingestion of food contaminated with botulinum toxin is an individual human disaster, but it does not necessarily reveal the actual role of the toxin in the biology of *Clostridium tetani* or *Clostridium botulinum.* These organisms are not primary pathogens of humans, although their toxins presumably have evolved to play some role in their

Single amino acid substitutions may render inactive

Role of the toxin for the organism is unknown

interaction with other eukaryotic life forms. Nontoxigenic variants of tetanus or the botulinum bacterium are totally avirulent for humans.

Some toxigenic microbes are highly adapted to humans including *Corynebacterium diphtheriae* (diphtheria), and *B. pertussis* (whooping cough). Others such as *V. cholerae* are very toxic to humans but have a reservoir, presumably on or in a marine animal. For these A–B toxins, we understand the biochemical basis for toxigenicity and the indispensability of the toxins for the pathogenicity of the microorganism. We even understand that if we immunize individuals against these toxins, we can prevent disease. What we do not fully understand is the role of the toxin in the biology of the microorganism. The toxin cannot be so potent that it rapidly kills all of the hosts that are infected. Toxins may represent the principal determinant of bacterial virulence in some species but may not be the principal determinant of infectivity; however, it seems likely that toxins play a role in the establishment of the organism in the early phases of infection or they are elaborated only if the organism "senses" danger. Thus, *V. cholerae* devoid of cholera toxin does not colonize susceptible animals as well as toxigenic organisms, nor is it as efficiently transmitted. It is possible that the effects of cholera toxin, the induced net secretion of water and electrolytes into the lumen of the bowel, make conditions right for cholera replication. On the other hand, nontoxigenic *C. diphtheriae* and *B. pertussis* can still colonize humans and be transmitted, although not as well as their toxigenic parents.

Immunization against toxin can prevent disease

Currently, molecular cloning techniques, coupled with appropriate infection models, are leading to the elucidation of the roles of some toxins in the pathogenesis of infections. Not all toxins are essential for pathogenicity. For example, *Shigella dysenteriae* produces a very potent cytotoxin called Shiga toxin. Nontoxigenic variants of this organism are still pathogenic but are not as virulent. The high death rates associated with toxigenic *S. dysenteriae* appear to be associated with damage done to the colonic vasculature by Shiga toxin.

Toxin may not be essential for disease

Ras Inhibitors and Other Toxins Affecting Host Cell Trafficking and Signal Transduction Pathways

The A–B toxin paradigm focused on the fact that a variety of distinct toxins harbored by a variety of distinct pathogens attached the ADP-ribose moiety from NAD to a preferred target molecule, generally a G protein that bound and hydrolyzed GTP. However, the B (binding) specificity of the toxins varies considerably. Thus, seemingly identical catalytic properties of toxin molecules have different effects in a host animal because the toxin binds to a different receptor molecule in the host. For example, the most potent neurotoxins known produced by the clostridia causing botulism and tetanus target four proteins (syntaxin, VAMP/synaptobrevin 1 and 2, and snap-25) that are involved in the docking of host cell vesicles and are involved with the release of neurotransmitters. Yet, each toxin is delivered differently and preferentially binds to different cell types when introduced into humans by accidental oral ingestion or by introduction by contaminated soil. Because these toxins were recognized to be introduced into host cells and functioned intracellularly, they became a favored reagent of cell biologists to investigate the normal biology of mammalian cells.

G protein is a common target

Binding may be to multiple receptors

Some toxins, such as botulinum toxin, are used in medicine to relieve the effects of some nerve disorders. The recognition that many toxins are internalized in a membrane-bound vesicle from which the catalytically active A part has to escape into the cytoplasm led to the investigation of binding specificity within the toxin itself. In this vein, the A subunit of cholera toxin has a C-terminal motif that provides retention of the molecule in the endoplasmic reticulum; similar binding motifs are found in other toxic molecules. In recent years, the capacity of invading bacteria and other parasites to undermine the host cell biology with such exquisite sensitivity has become a hallmark of research into bacterial pathogenicity. Ten years ago, we scarcely dreamed that the study of bacterial toxins would provide such a wealth of information about human biology. The most avid medical microbiologists did not think that such a diversity of bacterial toxins were yet to be discovered. For example, a number of bacterial toxins have been recognized that modifies proteins of the Ras superfamily, particularly the Rho subfamily. Some bacteria ADP-ribosylate Rho A, B, and C at a specific asparagine residue. Others, such as the bacterium *Clostridium difficile,* a commensal that can cause severe diarrhea in patients whose flora has been

Toxins interact with cell organelles and Ras proteins

suppressed by antibiotic therapy, glycosylate (add a glucose moiety) to their target and attack all members of the Rho subfamily (Rho, Rac, and CDC-42). Still others, such as the dermonecrotic toxin of the whooping cough bacillus, deamidate a glutamine residue in the Rho protein, changing it to glutamic acid, which, in the end, causes large-scale cytoskeletal rearrangements.

Membrane-Active Exotoxin

While the A–B exotoxins and the toxins described thus far are, strictly speaking, intracellular toxins, a plethora of other bacterial toxins are described in the medical literature. Most of these are not well characterized, although many of them act directly on the surface of host cells to lyse or to kill them. They may facilitate penetration of host epithelial or endothelial barriers, and some toxins can kill white cells or paralyze the local immune system. Many bacteria elaborate substances that cause hemolysis of erythrocytes, and this property has been postulated to be an important virulence trait. In fact, some bacterial hemolysins are representative of general classes of bacterial exotoxins (the cytotoxins) that kill host cells by disrupting the host cell membrane. Moreover, hemolysins may liberate necessary growth factors such as iron for the invading microorganisms.

Red blood cells, white blood cells, and epithelial cells are penetrated

Among Gram-negative bacteria, a surprising number of these cytotoxins are members of a single family called the RTX (repeats in toxin) group based on a recurrent theme of a nine-amino-acid tandem duplication. RTX toxins are calcium-dependent proteins that act by creating pores in eukaryotic membranes, which may cause cellular death or at least a perturbation in host cell function. Such toxins are thought to be particularly effective against phagocytic cells. Other exotoxins contribute to the capacity of an organism to invade and spread. The lecithinase α-toxin of *Clostridium perfringens,* for example, disrupts the membranes of a wide variety of host cells, including the leukocytes that might otherwise destroy the organism, and produces the necrotic anaerobic environment in which it can multiply.

RTX toxins create membrane pores

Hydrolytic Enzymes and Nontoxic Toxins of Type III Secretion Systems

Many bacteria produce one or more enzymes that are nontoxic per se but facilitate tissue invasion or help protect the organism against the body's defense mechanisms. For example, various bacteria produce collagenase or hyaluronidase or convert serum plasminogen to plasmin, which has fibrinolytic activity. Although the evidence is not conclusive, it is reasonable to assume that these substances facilitate spread of infection. Some bacteria also produce deoxyribonuclease, elastase, and many other biologically active enzymes, but their function in the disease process or in providing nutrients for the invaders is uncertain. All are proteins and have most of the characteristics of exotoxin, except specific toxicity. Although many such factors have been thought to be involved in bacterial virulence, formal proof that they may contribute to pathogenicity has not been obtained in many cases.

Secreted proteins may facilitate other aspects of virulence

In the past 5 years there has been a growing recognition that many Gram-negative bacteria have blocks of genes called pathogenicity islands (PAIs) (see below), which are composed of a secretory pathway that delivers virulence factors into the cytoplasm of host cells. Several of these were described earlier when considering *Salmonella* invasion. The difference between these molecules and the classical bacterial toxins is that these virulence molecules are not in and of themselves toxic but they induce host cellular damage like apoptosis. These factors are described in considerable detail in the chapter that describes *Salmonella, Shigella,* and *Yersinia* (see Chapter 21).

Cellular changes are induced

Superantigens: Exotoxins That Interfere With the Immune Response

It has become clear in recent years some microbial exotoxins have a direct effect on cells of the immune system and this interaction leads to many of the symptoms of disease. Thus, the enterotoxins causing staphylococcal food poisoning, the group A streptococcal exotoxin A responsible for scarlet fever, and the TSS exotoxin responsible for the staphylococcal toxic shock syndrome interact directly with the T-cell receptor. The effect of this interaction is dramatic. Cytokines such as IL-1 and TNF are produced, which leads to their familiar effects systemically and to local skin and gastrointestinal effects (depending on the toxin and its site of action). In addition, after binding to class II major histocompatibility complex (MHC) molecules on antigen-presenting cells, these exotoxins act as polyclonal stimulators of T cells so that a significant proportion of all T cells respond by dividing and releasing cytokines. This eventually leads to immunosuppression for reasons that are not totally clear. When trying to assess these findings from the standpoint of bacterial pathogenicity, it is important to divorce the disease entity seen in ill patients from the potential role of these toxins in the normal life of the microorganism.

Bind directly to T-cell receptor

Cytokines are released from large proportion of T cells

For example, staphylococcal food poisoning is an intoxication and does not involve infection by living microbes but rather the ingestion of the products produced by staphylococci in improperly handled food. The toxins that cause such food poisoning are resistant to digestive enzymes. Staphylococcal enterotoxins are also resistant to boiling, so that disease may follow ingestion of contaminated foods in which the organism has already been killed. What then is the role of the toxin in the normal biology of the microbe? Although the complete answer to this question is unknown, it seems likely that the toxins would play a role in the interaction of the microorganism with local host defenses in its preferred human niche, on the skin and the mucosal surface. Here, at the microscopic level, the capacity to neutralize the antigen-presenting cells in the microcosm of the pores of the skin is clearly more important than the induction of vast systemic symptoms. Not all staphylococci carry the enterotoxin genes. Indeed, enterotoxin genes may be carried on plasmids or bacterial viruses. Perhaps, the staphylococci that carry such "superantigens" have an advantage over their competing brethren. Such questions need to be answered at the experimental level. We must examine the determinants of bacterial pathogenicity with an eye to their role in the biology of the microbe, as well as from the view that they play an essential role in relatively rare cases of overt disease.

Ingestion of preformed toxin is a cause of food poisoning

Superantigens are not restricted simply to bacterial toxins of Gram-positive bacteria. Increasingly, they are reported as potential factors in the pathogenesis of viral infection and in a number of other bacteria. Moreover, polyclonal activation of other immune cells is seen, as in the activation of B cells by the Epstein–Barr virus. Hence, the interaction of microbial products directly with cells of the immune system that leads to immunosuppression may be a common theme of microbial pathogenicity.

Endotoxin

In many infections caused by Gram-negative organisms, the endotoxin (see Chapter 2) of the outer membrane is a significant component of the disease process. Recall that endotoxin is a lipopolysaccharide and that the lipid portion (lipid A) is the toxic portion. The conserved polysaccharide core and the variable O-polysaccharide side chains of endotoxin are responsible for the antigenic diversity seen among enteric bacterial species. The major characteristics of endotoxin are contrasted with those of exotoxin in Table 10–3. As noted earlier, endotoxin is a major cue to the human innate defense system that bacterial multiplication is taking place in the tissues. Endotoxin in nanogram amounts causes fever in humans through release of IL-1 and TNF from macrophages. In larger amounts, whether on intact Gram-negative organisms or cell wall fragments, it produces dramatic physiologic effects associated with inflammation. These include hypotension, lowered polymorphonuclear leukocyte and platelet counts from increased margination of these cells to the walls of the small vessels, hemorrhage, and sometimes disseminated intravascular coagulation from activation of clotting factors. Rapid and irreversible shock may follow passage of endotoxin into the bloodstream. This syndrome is seen when materials that have become heavily contaminated are injected intravenously or when a severe local infection leads to massive bacteremia. The role of endotoxin in more chronic disease processes is less clear, but some manifestations of typhoid fever and meningococcal septicemia, for example, are fully compatible with the known effects of endotoxin in humans. It should be noted that endotoxins are considerably less active than many

Located in Gram-negative outer membrane

Lipid A is most toxic

Shock syndrome may be fatal

TABLE 10–3

Differential Characteristics of Endotoxins and Exotoxins

CHARACTERISTIC	ENDOTOXINS	EXOTOXINS
Chemical nature	Lipopolysaccharide (lipid A component)	Protein
Part of Gram-negative cell outer membrane	Yes	No
Most from Gram-positive bacteria	No	Yes
Usually extracellular	No	Yes
Phage or plasmid coded	No	Many
Antigenic	Weakly	Yes
Can be converted to toxoid	No	Many
Neutralized by antibody	Weakly	Yes
Differing pharmacologic specificities	No	Yes
Stable to boiling[a]	Yes	No

[a] Enterotoxin of *Staphylococcus aureus* withstands boiling.

exotoxins, incompletely neutralized by antibody against their carbohydrate component, and stable even to autoclaving. The latter characteristic is important, because materials for intravenous administration that have become contaminated with Gram-negative organisms are not detoxified by sterilization.

Gram-positive bacteria do not contain endotoxin but they release peptidoglycan fragments and other cell wall determinants that act to "alarm" the host to the presence of bacteria in the tissues. The same cytokines are released and the same physiologic cascade is seen.

AVOIDING THE HOST IMMUNE SYSTEM

The host immune system evolved in large part because of the selective pressure of microbial attack. To be successful, microbial pathogens must escape this system at least long enough to be transmitted to a new susceptible host or to take up residence within the host in a way that is compatible with mutual coexistence.

Serum Resistance

Many bacteria that come into contact with human complement can be destroyed by opsonization or by direct lysis of the bacterial membrane by complement complexes. Some can avoid this fate by a process called serum resistance. Pathogenic *Salmonella* possess a lipopolysaccharide inhibiting the C5b–9 complement complex from attacking the hydrophobic domains of the bacterial outer membrane. Other bacteria employ different mechanisms, but the end result is the same. These organisms can persist in an environment that is rapidly lethal for nonpathogens.

Complement interference allows persistence

Antiphagocytic Activity

A fundamental requirement for many pathogenic bacteria is escape from phagocytosis by macrophages and polymorphonuclear leukocytes. It seems likely that the ability to avoid phagocytosis was an early necessity for microorganisms following the evolution of predatory protozoans. Some bacteria such as the causative agent of Legionnaires' disease, *Legionella pneumophila,* learned how to replicate in free-living amoebae following phagocytosis and used them as part of their life cycle. *Legionella* uses similar mechanisms to outwit human macrophages. In this one example, it can be seen that pathogenicity in some microorganisms evolved from a very early time in their development.

Avoiding phagocytosis is big advantage

The most common bacterial means to avoid phagocytosis is an antiphagocytic capsule. The significance of the bacterial capsule can hardly be overemphasized. Almost all principal pathogens that cause pneumonia and meningitis have antiphagocytic polysaccharide capsules. Nonencapsulated variants of these organisms are usually avirulent. In many cases, it has been found that the capsule of pathogens prevents complement deposition on the bacterial cell surface. Thus, the capsule prevents nonimmune opsonization and confers resistance to phagocytosis. As noted earlier, along with encapsulation, a common factor of many organisms that cause pneumonia and meningitis is the elaboration of an enzyme that specifically cleaves human IgA1 molecules. IgA proteases are found in the pathogenic *Neisseria, Haemophilus influenzae* type b (Hib), and *Streptococcus pneumoniae.* The combination of a capsule to avoid opsonization and/or an enzyme that cleaves an important class of secretory antibody is a potent stratagem to avoid phagocytosis.

Capsules block complement deposition

The group A streptococcal M protein is another example of a bacterial surface product employed by the organism to escape opsonization and phagocytosis. In part, this is a reflection of the ability of M protein to bind fibrinogen and its breakdown product fibrin to the bacterial surface. This sterically hinders complement access and prevents opsonization. There are many other examples. The principle is clear. If microorganisms can inhibit phagocytosis, they can often gain the upper hand long enough to replicate sufficiently to establish themselves in the host or become transmitted to a new host. It is important to understand that these encapsulated pathogens are often carried asymptomatically in the normal flora (see Table 9–1). The capsule is important for the organism to establish itself in the nasopharynx.

Surface proteins block complement and bind fibrinogen

The host responds to its initial encounter with the encapsulated organism by elaborating anticapsular antibodies that opsonize and permit efficient phagocytosis and destruction of the microorganism in subsequent encounters. Thus, the initial interaction between an encapsulated microbe and its host usually has two outcomes. First, the host becomes asymptomatically colonized, and, second, the colonization is an immunizing event for the host. The host is protected against serious systemic infection by the organism, but this immunity may not affect the capacity of the organism to live happily on a mucosal surface. Epidemiologic investigations show that serious disease caused by encapsulated pathogens when it occurs does so shortly after a susceptible individual encounters the microorganism for the first time. This scenario contrasts with the idea that carriers of microorganisms come down with the disease at some time in the future. If a microorganism meets a host with a compromised immune system or some short-term deficit in its defense systems, then the organism's capacity for replication can overwhelm the host defense mechanisms and cause serious disease. Once colonization and immunity have been established, the steady state is a satisfactory host–parasite relationship. For example, the outcome of encounters with *Neisseria meningitidis* in military recruits followed for colonization and anticapsular antibody throughout training camp has been demonstrated. Disease developed only in those entering the camp lacking both specific antibody and nasopharyngeal colonization with the *N. meningitidis* serogroup responsible for a subsequent meningitis outbreak. Unaffected recruits either had a "successful" encounter followed by development of antibody or already had protective antibody, presumably from a similar experience earlier in life.

Opsonizing antibody reverses effect of capsule

Disease occurs in period of absent immune response

Cutting Lines of Communication

Pathogens such as *Yersinia* and *Salmonella* have evolved means to neutralize phagocytes directly by using the equivalent of eukaryotic signal transduction molecules. Pathogenic *Yersinia* synthesize tyrosine phosphatase molecules and serine kinase molecules and introduce them into the cytoplasm of macrophages, which leads to a complete loss in the capacity of these cells either to phagocytose microorganisms or to signal other components of the host immune system by cytokine release. Likewise, both *Salmonella* and *Yersinia* inject bacterial proteins into the cytoplasm of host cells that directly induce apoptosis or disrupt cellular function. As noted earlier, microbial mimicry can have the same effect by concealing the microorganism under a shroud of host proteins; however, the strategy of directly interfering with host cell function by use of an alternative enzyme

Secreted proteins alter phagocyte function

or modifying and activating existing host cell effectors has been discovered to be a more common pathogenic strategy for the invading microbe than previously realized. This helps resolve the mystery that bacteria not known to produce toxins nonetheless cause cellular toxicity.

Antigenic Variation

Another method by which microorganisms avoid host immune responses is by varying surface antigens. *N. gonorrhoeae* displays an endless array of pili and outer membrane proteins to the host immune system. The organism has learned to preserve its binding specificity but to vary endlessly the molecular scaffolding on which the functional units are placed. The host "sees" a bewildering array of new epitopes, whereas the critical regions of the molecule remain hidden from immune surveillance. Of course, among the viruses, antigenic variation is also a common theme; the best known example is the influenza virus. It is instructive that in both the bacterial example and the viral example, recombination mechanisms act to bring together novel sequences of genetic material. A number of microorganisms known for their antigenic diversity such as those of the genus *Borrelia,* which causes relapsing fever, and the group A streptococci also use homologous recombination of DNA from repeated sequences to generate the diversity in size and sequence observed in their principal immunodominant antigens.

Alteration in surface epitopes confounds immune surveillance

INADVERTENT TISSUE DAMAGE FROM IMMUNE REACTIONS DIRECTED AGAINST INVADING BACTERIA

Tissue damage and the manifestations of disease may also result from interaction between the host's immune mechanisms and the invading organism or its products. Reactions between high concentrations of antibody, soluble microbial antigens, and complement can deposit immune complexes in tissues and cause acute inflammatory reactions and immune complex disease. In poststreptococcal acute glomerulonephritis, for example, the complexes are sequestered in the glomeruli of the kidney, with serious interference in renal function from the resulting tissue reaction. Sometimes, antibody produced against microbial antigens can cross-react with certain host tissues and initiate an autoimmune process. Such cross-reaction is almost certainly the explanation for poststreptococcal rheumatic fever, and it may be involved in some of the lesions of tertiary syphilis. Some viruses have been shown to have small peptide sequences that are occasionally shared by host tissues. Thus, a virus-induced immune response may also generate antibodies that react with shared determinants on host cells, such as in the heart.

Immune reactions may injure or cross-react with host tissue

In some other infections, the pathologic and clinical features are due largely to delayed-type hypersensitivity reactions to the organism or its products. Such reactions are particularly significant in tuberculosis and other mycobacterial infections. The mycobacteria possess no significant toxins, and in the absence of delayed hypersensitivity, their multiplication elicits little more than a mild inflammatory response. The development of delayed-type, cell-mediated hypersensitivity to their major proteins leads to dramatic pathologic manifestations, which in tuberculosis comprise a chronic granulomatous response around infected foci with massive infiltration of macrophages and lymphocytes followed by central devascularization and necrosis. Rupture of a necrotic area into a bronchus leads to the typical pulmonary cavity of the disease; rupture into a blood vessel can produce extensive dissemination or massive bleeding from the lung. Injection of tuberculoprotein into an animal with an established tuberculous lesion can lead to acute exacerbation and sometimes death. Thus, the body's defense mechanisms are themselves contributing to the severity of the disease process.

Continued delayed-type hypersensitivity causes injury

Granuloma is typical manifestation

These examples illustrate processes that are probably involved to varying degrees in the pathology and course of most infections. Immune reactions are essential to the control of infectious diseases; however, they are potentially damaging to the host, particularly when large amounts of antigens are involved and the host response is unusually active. It is likely that some pathogenic bacteria have deliberately modified the nature of the host immune response so that the effects are directed away from direct antimicrobial factors.

By the same token, the misdirected immune response may provide a needed niche for the invading microbe to complete its mission of survival.

DISEASE AND TRANSMISSIBILITY

Host survival facilitates pathogen survival

Lethal disease is probably an inadvertent and even unfavorable outcome of infection from the standpoint of a microorganism. Pathogens that are highly adapted to their host usually spare the majority of their victims. In many cases, it is to the advantage of the microbe to cause some degree of illness that may aid its transmission. In other cases, the interplay between the microbe and the host is subclinical resolution; there may be damage but no disease. Indeed, many of the most severe infectious diseases occur when a microorganism adapted to a nonhuman environment finds itself inadvertently in a human host. The probability of disease is a reflection of the microbial design to live and multiply within a host balanced against the host's capacity to control and limit bacterial proliferation. For certain microorganisms, such as *Streptococcus pyogenes,* contact with susceptible hosts that possess normal host defense systems renders a certain proportion clinically ill. In contrast, normal individuals usually shrug off *Proteus* and *Serratia* species. How different the outcome of this interaction when the host is compromised!

For microbes exclusively adapted to humans, transmissibility is the key to continued survival. For many organisms, this entails microbial persistence in the host and in the environment. A stable pathogen population must retain its viability outside of its preferred niche and still be capable of infection when it next encounters a susceptible host. We are still rather ignorant of the microbial factors at play that ensure their transmissibility from host to host. These conditions are difficult to recapitulate experimentally. However, the use of bacteria carrying sensitive reporter molecules will likely permit a better view of transmissibility.

COROLLARIES OF MICROBIAL PATHOGENICITY

As noted, all parasitic microorganisms need to enter a host, find a unique niche, overcome local defenses, replicate, and be transmitted to a new host. Other factors have become apparent because of these pathogenic attributes. Some are more applicable to bacteria and fungi than to viruses and the larger parasites. The general principles are likely to be true for all pathogens.

Successful pathogens have created a balanced adaptation to the host

1. **Pathogenic microorganisms adapt to changes in the host's biological and social behavior.** Imagine the profound changes in the host–parasite relationship that must have occurred when humanoids began to live in communities and began to husband animals. The older diseases such as tuberculosis remained, but the increase in population density meant that "new" epidemic diseases could evolve. In recent times, we have seen new diseases emerge. Diseases such as TSS, Legionnaires' disease, and nosocomial infections are a reflection, in part, of human progress. We need to remind ourselves that we live in a balanced relationship with microorganisms on this planet. Microorganisms will take advantage of any selective benefit that is made available to them to replicate and to establish themselves in a new niche. The advent of the birth control pill and the replacement of barrier contraception led to an enormous increase in sexually transmitted diseases. As humans increasingly impinge on other forms of life that have been largely isolated from human populations, there has been an increase in "new" infectious diseases such as Lyme disease, and quite probably, AIDS. As we have become more efficient at food production and mass global distribution, there has been an increase, rather than a decrease, in food-borne infection and disease. One need no longer go to an esoteric place in the world to acquire traveler's diarrhea, it can be readily acquired on imported food now at the corner food market!
2. **Pathogens are clonal.** Bacteria are haploid, as are viruses and some fungi. Consequently, there cannot be a helter-skelter amalgam of genes brought about by promiscuous genetic exchange. If this were so, there would be no bacterial specialization and all would possess a consensus chromosomal sequence. Thus, most bacteria (and

TABLE 10–4

Proportion of Certain Infectious Diseases Caused by Common Bacterial Clonal Types

Species	Total Number of Clonal Types Identified	Number of Clonal Types Commonly Isolated from Cases of Disease	Percentage of Disease Due to Common Clonal Types
Bordetella pertussis	2	2	100
Haemophilus influenzae type b			
North America	104	6	81
Europe	60	3	78
Legionella pneumophila			
Global	50	5	52
Wadsworth VA Hospital	10	1	86
Shigella sonnei	1	1	100

Modified from Mandell GL, Bennett JE, Dolin R. Principles and Practice of Infectious Diseases, *5th ed. New York: Churchill Livingstone; 2002, with permission.*

viruses) have some degree of built-in reproductive isolation, except for members of their own or very closely related species (members of the same gene pool). In this way, diversity within the species through mutation can be maximized (usually by transformation or transduction), while conserving useful gene sequences. The end result of husbanding of important genes during evolution is that at any given time in the world, many bacterial and viral pathogens are representatives of a single or, more often, a relatively few clonal types that have become widespread for the (evolutionary) moment. Thus, all the strains of the typhoid bacillus that have been studied since humans learned to culture them belong to two basic clonal types (Table 10–4). When microbes establish a unique niche, they protect their selective advantage.

Useful genes are preserved by clonality

However, the bacterial gene pool must be expanded. Indeed, how could microorganisms have become pathogens in the first place or adapt to new potential niches? Bacteria have remarkable ways of expanding their genetic diversity, but they do so in a way that is consistent with their haploid lifestyle. From this corollary follows the next.

3. **Pathogens often carry essential virulence determinants on mobile genetic elements.** It is now well established that many of the essential determinants of pathogenicity are actually replicated as part of an extrachromosomal element or as additions to the bacterial chromosome (Table 10–5). If haploid organisms must limit their genetic interactions to preserve their individuality, it is not surprising that new genes with important new attributes are found on genetic elements that do not disrupt the organization of the bacterial chromosome. The interchange of plasmids and bacterial viruses among bacteria, coupled with transpositional (illegitimate) recombination between the extrachromosomal element and the chromosome, provides a means for microorganisms to exploit new genes in a haploid world. It is of some note that pathogenic determinants not found associated with a plasmid or a phage are often seen as duplicated genes or associated with transposon-like structures.

Virulence determinants are often extrachromosomal and transmissible

While it was clear for some time that mobile genetic elements played an essential role in the evolution of pathogenicity, only recently, with the advent of new DNA sequencing methods, have we learned that large blocks of genes found on the bacterial chromosome are associated with pathogenicity. These blocks of genes have been given the name pathogenicity islands (PAIs) to describe unique chromosomal regions found exclusively associated with virulence. It is now generally believed that parts of a plasmid associated with virulence are likely PAIs as well. PAIs most often occupy large genomic areas of 10 to 200 or more kilobases. However, certain bacterial strains also carry insertions of smaller

Multiple pathogenicity genes are present in PAIs

TABLE 10–5

Examples of Plasmid and Phage-Encoded Virulence Determinants

ORGANISM	VIRULENCE FACTOR	BIOLOGICAL FUNCTION
Plasmid-encoded		
Enterotoxigenic *Escherichia coli*	Heat-labile, heat-stable enterotoxins (LT, ST)	Activation of adenyl/guanylcyclase in the small bowel, which leads to diarrhea
	CFA/I and CFA/II	Adherence/colonization factors
Salmonella spp.	Serum resistance and intracellular survival	Invasion of reticuloendothelial system
Shigella spp. and enteroinvasive *E.coli*	Gene products involved in invasion	Induces internalization by intestinal epithelial cells
Yersinia spp.	Adherence factors and gene products involved in invasion	Attachment/invasion
Bacillus anthracis	Edema factor, lethal factor, and protective antigen	Edema factor has adenylcyclase activity
Staphylococcus aureus	Exfoliative toxin	Causes toxic epidermal necrolysis
Clostridium tetani	Tetanus neurotoxin	Blocks the release of inhibitory neurotransmitter; which leads to muscle spasms
Phage-encoded		
Corynebacterium diphtheriae	Diphtheria toxin	Inhibition of eukaryotic protein synthesis
Streptococcus pyogenes	Erythrogenic toxin	Rash of scarlet fever
Clostridium botulinum	Neurotoxin	Blocks synaptic acetylcholine release, which leads to flaccid paralysis
Enterohemorrhagic *E. coli*	Shiga-like toxin	Inhibition of eukaryotic protein synthesis

Modified from Mandell GL, Bennett JE, Dolin R. Principles and Practice of Infectious Diseases, *5th ed. New York: Churchill Livingstone; 2002, with permission.*

pieces of DNA with the attributes of PAIs, but they are only 1 to 10 kilobases in size and are referred to by some as pathogenicity islets. All of the available data are consistent with the idea that horizontal gene transfer likely is mediated by phage or plasmids acquired these large (and small) DNA sequences. However, the PAIs described thus far are not mobile in themselves. There is an eerie quality about the composition of many PAIs in the sense that they have a very different guanine + cytosine content and codon usage as compared to the rest of the genome. The fact PAIs are so often associated with tRNA genes suggests that gene transfer from a foreign species is the likely origin. (In many prokaryotic and eukaryotic species, tRNA genes often act as the site of integration of foreign DNA.) Many PAIs have strikingly similar homologs in bacteria that are pathogenic for plants and animals and range from obligate intracellular parasites such as *Chlamydia* to free-living environmental opportunistic pathogens such as *Pseudomonas aeruginosa.*

PAIs are organized blocks of genes that appear to come from an unrelated organism

In a bacterial genus that contains both pathogenic and nonpathogenic species, the attributes of pathogenicity are encoded on sequences that do not have any counterpart in the nonpathogen. It seems unlikely that pathogenicity arose as a result of long adaptation of an initially nonpathogenic organism to a more parasitic, host-dependent lifestyle. It is more likely that organisms inherited new gene sequences, often in a large block, that provided them with the capacity to establish themselves more efficiently in a host or to exploit some new niche within the host.

TABLE 10–6

Examples of Bacterial Virulence Regulatory Systems

Organism	Regulatory Gene(s)	Environmental Stimuli	Regulated Functions
Escherichia coli	*drd*X	Temperature	Pyelonephritis-associated pili
	fur	Iron concentration	Shiga-like toxin, siderophores
Bordetella pertussis	*bvg*AS	Temperature, ionic conditions, nicotinic acid	Pertussis toxin, filamentous hemagglutinin, adenylate cyclase, others
Vibrio cholerae	*tox*R	Temperature, osmolarity, pH, amino acids	Cholera toxin, pili, outer membrane proteins
Yersinia spp.	*lcr* loci	Temperature, calcium	Outer membrane proteins
	*vir*F	Temperature	Adherence, invasiveness
Shigella spp.	*vir*R	Temperature	Invasiveness
Salmonella typhimurium	*pag* genes	pH	Virulence, macrophage survival
Staphylococcus aureus	*agr*	pH	α-, β-hemolysins; toxic shock syndrome toxin 1, protein A

Modified from Mandell GL, Bennett JE, Dolin R. Principles and Practice of Infectious Diseases, *5th ed. New York: Churchill Livingstone; 2002, with permission.*

4. **Bacteria and other pathogens use elaborate means to modulate their free-living life from their parasitic life.** Bacteria, fungi, and larger parasites have evolved signal transduction networks using environmental clues such as temperature, iron concentration, and calcium flux to turn on genes important for pathogenicity (Table 10–6). It was puzzling to consider how a microorganism that makes potent toxins in the laboratory could possibly spare any host it infected. It became clearer when we learned that toxin biosynthesis by the microbe is tightly regulated together with other genes to be activated only in particular sets of circumstances. Only in selective circumstances are genes involved in pathogenicity used and then often sparingly. The organism's reaction to the host need only be sufficient to establish itself and replicate.

Regulatory systems sense temperature and ions

CONCLUSION

Host-parasite interactions are wonderfully complex and have evolved in a manner that has tended to produce a more balanced state of parasitism between well-established species and the microorganisms with which they frequently come into contact. In this chapter, the components of these interactions have been discussed separately, but it is important to recognize the dynamic and shifting nature of their role in determining the course and outcome of an infection. As you review the microbial tactics for survival and the ensuing host response to acute infection and its consequences, it is important to see that systemic symptoms of many viral and bacterial infections—fever, malaise, and anorexia—are the same because they reflect a basic innate host response to a foreign intruder. The diversity of mechanisms by which a host controls infection can be particularly appreciated if one recognizes that they are all intimately interrelated. Many of the infected patients you will aid during your career will not have inherited defects in their host defense matrix, but they will have disease-associated deficiencies. Increasingly, cytotoxic chemotherapy, radiotherapy, and other forms of medical intervention bring about physician-induced deficits in their innate and adaptive immune systems. For example, because of their tumors or treatment, cancer patients often have a variety of interrelated defects and mucosal disruptions increasing the risk of infection. The single most important of these is neutropenia (usually defined as an absolute granulocyte count of $500/mm^3$ or less). It is no wonder that the presenting symptom in tumors of the bowel may be sepsis or bacterial endocarditis. During the natural progression of malignancy and as a consequence of its current therapy, infection remains as the major cause of morbidity and mortality.

The above examples suffice, but the significant point is the importance of normal defense mechanisms. It is more important to preserve and augment the normal host defenses of a patient in many circumstances than to use the newest "wonder drug." We can also be fully confident that an understanding of the molecular basis of microbial pathogenesis will provide considerable information about the biology of the pathogens, the host-parasite relationship, human (and other) host-specific defense mechanisms, and, ultimately, ways to prevent infection and disease. Finally, from this brief overview of the properties of pathogenic bacteria, it is important to never underestimate the capacity of these small creatures to persist and survive in human society.

ADDITIONAL READING

Salyers AA, Whitt DD. *Bacterial Pathogenesis: A Molecular Approach.* 2nd ed. Washington, D.C.: American Society for Microbiology; 2002. This modern text beautifully discusses topics from the clinical to the molecular level.

PART IV

SPREAD AND CONTROL OF INFECTION

CHAPTER 11

Sterilization and Disinfection

KENNETH J. RYAN

From the time of debates about the germ theory of disease, killing microbes before they reach patients has been a major strategy for preventing infection. In fact, Ignaz Semmelweiss successfully applied disinfection principles decades before bacteria were first isolated (see Chapter 72). This chapter discusses the most important methods used for this purpose in modern medical practice. Understanding how they work is of increasing importance in an environment that includes immunocompromised patients, transplantation, indwelling devices, and acquired immunodeficiency syndrome (AIDS).

DEFINITIONS

Death/killing as it relates to microbial organisms is defined in terms of how we detect them in culture. Operationally, it is a loss of ability to multiply under any known conditions. This is complicated by the fact that organisms that appear to be irreversibly inactivated may sometimes recover when appropriately treated. For example, ultraviolet (UV) irradiation of bacteria can result in the formation of thymine dimers in the DNA with loss of ability to replicate. A period of exposure to visible light may then activate an enzyme that breaks the dimers and restores viability by a process known as photoreactivation. Mechanisms also exist for repair of the damage without light. Such considerations are of great significance in the preparation of safe vaccines from inactivated virulent organisms.

Absence of growth does not necessarily indicate sterility

Sterilization is complete killing, or removal, of all living organisms from a particular location or material. It can be accomplished by incineration, nondestructive heat treatment, certain gases, exposure to ionizing radiation, some liquid chemicals, and filtration.

Sterilization is killing of all living forms

Pasteurization is the use of heat at a temperature sufficient to inactivate important pathogenic organisms in liquids such as water or milk but at a temperature below that needed to ensure sterilization. For example, heating milk at a temperature of 74°C for 3 to 5 seconds or 62°C for 30 minutes kills the vegetative forms of most pathogenic bacteria that may be present without altering its quality. Obviously, spores are not killed at these temperatures.

Pasteurization uses heat to kill vegetative forms of bacteria

Disinfection is the destruction of pathogenic microorganisms by processes that fail to meet the criteria for sterilization. Pasteurization is a form of disinfection, but the term is most commonly applied to the use of liquid chemical agents known as disinfectants, which usually have some degree of selectivity. Bacterial spores, organisms with waxy coats (eg, mycobacteria), and some viruses may show considerable resistance to the common disinfectants. **Antiseptics** are disinfectant agents that can be used on body surfaces such as the skin or vaginal tract to reduce the numbers of normal flora and pathogenic

Disinfection uses chemical agents to kill pathogens with varying efficiency

contaminants. They have lower toxicity than disinfectants used environmentally but are usually less active in killing vegetative organisms. **Sanitization** is a less precise term with a meaning somewhere between disinfection and cleanliness. It is used primarily in housekeeping and food preparation contexts.

Spores are particularly resistant

Asepsis describes processes designed to prevent microorganisms from reaching a protected environment. It is applied in many procedures used in the operating room, in the preparation of therapeutic agents, and in technical manipulations in the microbiology laboratory. An essential component of aseptic techniques is the sterilization of all materials and equipment used. Asepsis is more fully discussed in Chapter 72.

Asepsis applies sterilization and disinfection to create a protective environment

MICROBIAL KILLING

Killing of bacteria by heat, radiation, or chemicals is usually exponential with time; that is, a fixed proportion of survivors are killed during each time increment. Thus, if 90% of a population of bacteria are killed during each 5 minutes of exposure to a weak solution of a disinfectant, a starting population of 10^6/mL is reduced to 10^5/mL after 5 minutes, to 10^3/mL after 15 minutes, and theoretically to 1 organism (10^0)/mL after 30 minutes. Exponential killing corresponds to a first-order reaction or a "single-hit" hypothesis in which the lethal change involves a single target in the organism, and the probability of this change is constant with time. Thus, plots of the logarithm of the number of survivors against time are linear (Fig 11–1A); however, the slope of the curve varies with the effectiveness of the killing process, which is influenced by the nature of the organism, lethal agent, concentration (in the case of disinfectants), and temperature. In general, the rate of killing increases exponentially with arithmetic increases in temperature or in concentrations of disinfectant.

Bacterial killing follows exponential kinetics

An important consequence of exponential killing with most sterilization processes is that sterility is not an absolute term, but must be expressed as a probability. Thus, to continue the example given previously, the chance of a single survivor in 1 mL is theoretically 10^{-1} after 35 minutes. If a chance of 10^{-9} were the maximum acceptable risk for a single surviving organism in a 1-mL sample (eg, of a therapeutic agent), the procedure would require continuation for a total of 75 minutes.

Achieving sterility is a matter of probability

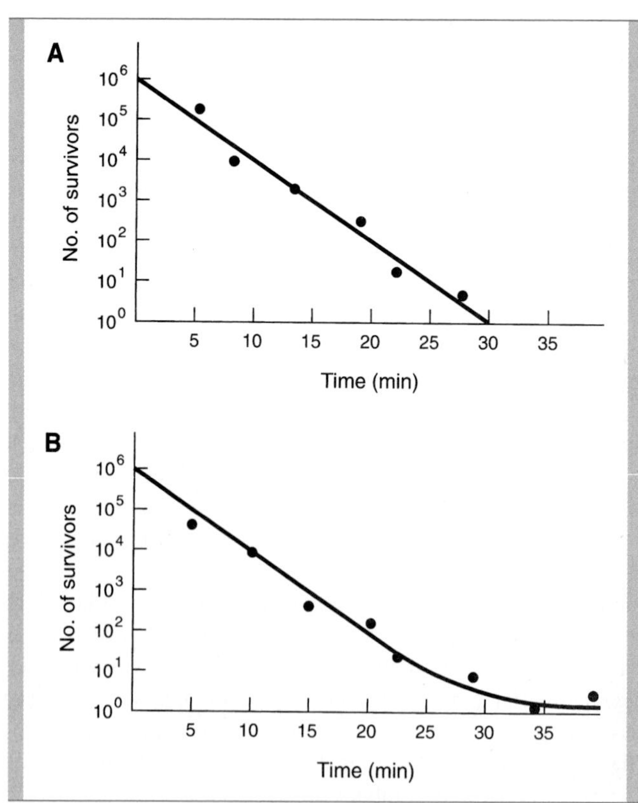

FIGURE 11–1
Kinetics of bacterial killing.
A. Exponential killing is shown as a function of population size and time. **B.** Deviation from linearity, as with a mixed population, extends the time.

A simple single-hit curve often does not express the kinetics of killing adequately. In the case of some bacterial endospores, a brief period (activation) may elapse before exponential killing by heat begins. If multiple targets are involved, the experimental curve will deviate from linearity. More significant is the fact that microbial populations may include a small proportion of more resistant mutants or of organisms in a physiologic state that confers greater resistance to inactivation. In these cases, the later stages of the curve are flattened (Fig 11–1B), and extrapolations from the exponential phase of killing may seriously underestimate the time needed for a high probability of achieving complete sterility. In practice, materials that come into contact with tissues are sterilized under conditions that allow a very wide margin of safety, and the effectiveness of inactivation of organisms in vaccines is tested directly with large volumes and multiple samples before a product is made available for use.

Heterogeneous microbial subpopulations may extend the killing kinetics

STERILIZATION

The availability of reliable methods of sterilization has made possible the major developments in surgery and intrusive medical techniques that have helped to revolutionize medicine over the past century. Furthermore, sterilization procedures form the basis of many food preservation procedures, particularly in the canning industry. The various modes of sterilization described in the text are summarized in Table 11–1.

TABLE 11–1

Methods of Disinfection and Sterilization

METHOD	ACTIVITY LEVEL	SPECTRUM	USES/COMMENTS
Heat			
Autoclave	Sterilizing	All	General
Boiling	High	Most pathogens, some spores	General
Pasteurization	Intermediate	Vegetative bacteria	Beverages, plastic hospital equipment
Ethylene oxide gas	Sterilizing	All	Potentially explosive; aeration required
Radiation			
Ultraviolet	Sterilizing	All	Poor penetration
Ionizing	Sterilizing	All	General, food
Chemicals			
Alcohol	Intermediate	Vegetative bacteria, fungi, some viruses	
Hydrogen peroxide	High	Viruses, vegetative bacteria, fungi	Contact lenses; inactivated by organic matter
Chlorine	High	Viruses, vegetative bacteria, fungi	Water; inactivated by organic matter
Iodophors	Intermediate	Viruses, vegetative bacteria,[a] fungi	Skin disinfection; inactivated by organic matter
Phenolics	Intermediate	Some viruses, vegetative bacteria, fungi	Handwashing
Glutaraldehyde	High	All	Endoscopes, other equipment
Quaternary ammonium compounds	Low	Most bacteria and fungi, lipophilic viruses	General cleaning; inactivated by organic matter

[a]Variable results with *Mycobacterium tuberculosis*.

Heat

Incineration is rapid and effective

Dry heat requires 160°C for 2 hours to kill

The simplest method of sterilization is to expose the surface to be sterilized to a naked flame, as is done with the wire loop used in microbiology laboratories. It can be used equally effectively for emergency sterilization of a knife blade or a needle. Of course, disposable material is rapidly and effectively decontaminated by incineration. Carbonization of organic material and destruction of microorganisms, including spores, occur after exposure to dry heat of 160°C for 2 hours in a sterilizing oven. This method is applicable to metals, glassware, and some heat-resistant oils and waxes that are immiscible in water and cannot, therefore, be sterilized in the autoclave. A major use of the dry heat sterilizing oven is in preparation of laboratory glassware.

Moisture allows for rapid denaturation of protein

Boiling water fails to kill bacterial spores

Moist heat in the form of water or steam is far more rapid and effective in sterilization than dry heat, because reactive water molecules denature protein irreversibly by disrupting hydrogen bonds between peptide groups at relatively low temperatures. Most vegetative bacteria of importance in human disease are killed within a few minutes at 70°C or less, although many bacterial spores (see Chapter 2) can resist boiling for prolonged periods. For applications requiring sterility the use of boiling water has been replaced by the autoclave, which when properly used ensures sterility by killing all forms of microorganisms.

Autoclave creates increased temperature of steam under pressure

Steam displaces air from the autoclave

Killing rate increases logarithmically with arithmetic increase in temperature

In effect, the **autoclave** is a sophisticated pressure cooker (Fig 11–2). In its simplest form, it consists of a chamber in which the air can be replaced with pure saturated steam under pressure. Air is removed either by evacuation of the chamber before filling it with steam or by displacement through a valve at the bottom of the autoclave, which remains open until all air has drained out. The latter, which is termed a **downward displacement autoclave,** capitalizes on the heaviness of air compared with saturated steam. When the air has been removed, the temperature in the chamber is proportional to the pressure of the steam; autoclaves are usually operated at 121°C, which is achieved with a pressure of 15 pounds per square inch. Under these conditions, spores directly exposed are killed in less than 5 minutes, although the normal sterilization time is 10 to 15 minutes to account for variation in the ability of steam to penetrate different materials and to allow a wide margin of safety. The velocity of killing increases logarithmically with arithmetic increases in temperature, so a steam temperature of 121°C is vastly more effective than 100°C. For example, the spores of *Clostridium botulinum,* the cause of botulism, may survive 5 hours of boiling, but can be killed in 4 minutes at 121°C in the autoclave.

Condensation and latent heat increase effectiveness of autoclave

The use of saturated steam in the autoclave has other advantages. Latent heat equivalent to 539 cal/g condensed steam is immediately liberated on condensation on the cooler surfaces of the load to be sterilized. The temperature of the load is thus raised very rapidly to that of the steam. Condensation also permits rapid steam penetration of porous materials such as surgical drapes by producing a relative negative pressure at the surface, which allows more steam to enter immediately. Autoclaves can thus be used for sterilizing any

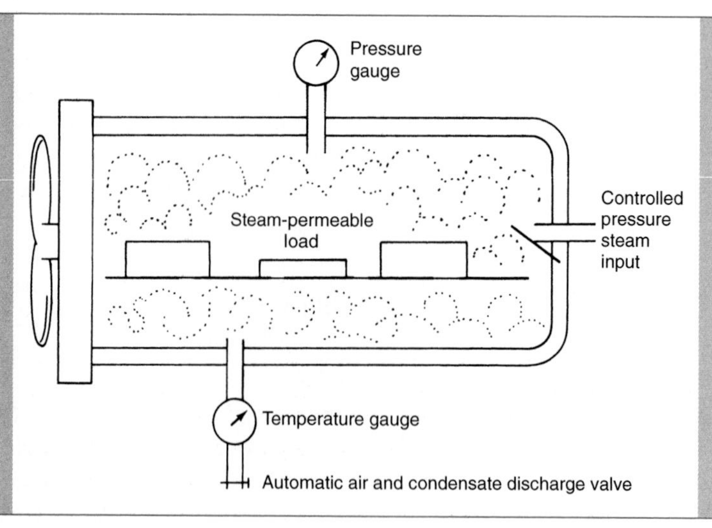

FIGURE 11–2
Simple form of downward displacement autoclave.

materials that are not damaged by heat and moisture, such as heat-stable liquids, swabs, most instruments, culture media, and rubber gloves.

It is essential that those who use autoclaves understand the principles involved. Their effectiveness depends on absence of air, pure saturated steam, and access of steam to the material to be sterilized. Pressure per se plays no role in sterilization other than to ensure the increased temperature of the steam. Failure can result from attempting to sterilize the interior of materials that are impermeable to steam or the contents of sealed containers. Under these conditions, a dry heat temperature of 121°C is obtained, which may be insufficient to kill even vegetative organisms. Large volumes of liquids require longer sterilization times than normal loads, because their temperature must reach 121°C before timing begins. When sealed containers of liquids are sterilized, it is essential that the autoclave cool without being opened or evacuated; otherwise, the containers may explode as the external pressure falls in relation to that within.

Access of pure saturated steam is required for sterilization

Impermeable or large volume materials present special problems

"Flash" autoclaves, which are widely used in operating rooms, often use saturated steam at a temperature of 134°C for 3 minutes. Air and steam are removed mechanically before and after the sterilization cycle so that metal instruments may be available rapidly. Quality control of autoclaves depends primarily on ensuring that the appropriate temperature for the pressure used is achieved and that packing and timing are correct. Biological and chemical indicators of the correct conditions are available and are inserted from time to time in the loads.

Flash autoclaves use 134°C for 3 minutes

Gas

A number of articles, particularly certain plastics and lensed instruments that are damaged or destroyed by autoclaving, can be sterilized with gases. **Ethylene oxide** is an inflammable and potentially explosive gas. It is an alkylating agent that inactivates microorganisms by replacing labile hydrogen atoms on hydroxyl, carboxy, or sulfhydryl groups, particularly of guanine and adenine in DNA. Ethylene oxide sterilizers resemble autoclaves and expose the load to 10% ethylene oxide in carbon dioxide at 50 to 60°C under controlled conditions of humidity. Exposure times are usually about 4 to 6 hours and must be followed by a prolonged period of aeration to allow the gas to diffuse out of substances that have absorbed it. Aeration is essential, because absorbed gas can cause damage to tissues or skin. Ethylene oxide is a mutagen, and special precautions are now taken to ensure that it is properly vented outside of working spaces. Used under properly controlled conditions, ethylene oxide is an effective sterilizing agent for heat-labile devices such as artificial heart valves that cannot be treated at the temperature of the autoclave. Other alkylating such as **formaldehyde** vapor can be used without pressure to decontaminate larger areas such as rooms, and oxidizing agents (hydrogen peroxide, ozone) have selective use.

Ethylene oxide sterilization is used for heat-labile materials

Aeration needed after ethylene oxide sterilization

Formaldehyde and oxidizing agents are useful in sterilization

Ultraviolet Light and Ionizing Radiation

Ultraviolet (UV) light in the wavelength range 240 to 280 nm is absorbed by nucleic acids and causes genetic damage, including the formation of the thymine dimers discussed previously. The practical value of UV sterilization is limited by its poor ability to penetrate. Apart from the experimental use of UV light as a mutagen, its main application has been in irradiation of air in the vicinity of critical hospital sites and as an aid in the decontamination of laboratory facilities used for handling particularly hazardous organisms. In these situations, single exposed organisms are rapidly inactivated. It must be remembered that UV light can cause skin and eye damage, and workers exposed to it must be appropriately protected.

UV light causes direct damage to DNA

Use of UV light is limited by penetration and safety

Ionizing radiation carries far greater energy than UV light. It, too, causes direct damage to DNA and produces toxic free radicals and hydrogen peroxide from water within the microbial cells. Cathode rays and gamma rays from cobalt-60 are widely used in industrial processes, including the sterilization of many disposable surgical supplies such as gloves, plastic syringes, specimen containers, some foodstuffs, and the like, because they can be packaged before exposure to the penetrating radiation. Ionizing irradiation does not always result in the physical disintegration of killed microbes. As a result, plasticware sterilized in this way may carry significant numbers of dead but stainable

Ionizing radiation damages DNA

Use for surgical supplies, food

Killed organisms may remain morphologically intact and stainable

bacteria. This has occasionally caused confusion when it has involved containers used to collect normally sterile body fluids such as cerebrospinal fluid. The dead bacterial bodies may produce a "false-positive" Gram-stained smear and result in inappropriate administration of antibiotics. Recent foodborne outbreaks (*Escherichia coli*) and bioterrorism (anthrax) have increased the use of ionizing radiation.

DISINFECTION

Physical Methods

Filtration

Membrane filters remove bacteria by mechanical and electrostatic mechanisms

Both live and dead microorganisms can be removed from liquids by positive- or negative-pressure filtration. Membrane filters, usually composed of cellulose esters (eg, cellulose acetate), are available commercially with pore sizes of 0.005 to 1 μm. For removal of bacteria, a pore size of 0.2 μm is effective because filters act not only mechanically but by electrostatic adsorption of particles to their surface. Filtration is used for disinfection of large volumes of fluid, especially those containing heat-labile components such as serum. For microorganisms larger than the pore size filtration "sterilizes" these liquids. It is not considered effective for removing viruses.

Pasteurization

Kills vegetative bacteria but not spores

Used for foods and fragile medical equipment

Pasteurization involves exposure of liquids to temperatures in the range 55 to 75°C to remove all vegetative bacteria of significance in human disease. Spores are unaffected by the pasteurization process. Pasteurization is used commercially to render milk safe and extend its storage quality. With the outbreaks of infection due to contamination with enterohemorrhagic *E. coli* (see Chapter 21), this has been extended (reluctantly) to fruit drinks. To the dismay of some of his compatriots, Pasteur proposed application of the process to winemaking to prevent microbial spoilage and vinegarization. Pasteurization in water at 70°C for 30 minutes has been effective and inexpensive when used to render inhalation therapy equipment free of organisms that may otherwise multiply in mucus and humidifying water.

Microwaves

Microwaves kill by generating heat

The use of microwaves in the form of microwave ovens or specially designed units is another method for disinfection. These systems are not under pressure, but they but can achieve temperatures near boiling if moisture is present. In some situations, they are being used as a practical alternative to incineration for disinfection of hospital waste. These procedures cannot be considered sterilization only because the most heat-resistant spores may survive the process.

Chemical Methods

Most agents are general protoplasmic poisons

Disinfectants are variably inactivated by organic material

Given access and sufficient time, chemical disinfectants cause the death of pathogenic vegetative bacteria. Most of these substances are general protoplasmic poisons and are not currently used in the treatment of infections other than very superficial lesions, having been replaced by antimicrobics (see Chapter 13). Some disinfectants such as the quaternary ammonium compounds, alcohol, and the iodophors reduce the superficial flora and can eliminate contaminating pathogenic bacteria from the skin surface. Other agents such as the phenolics are valuable only for treating inanimate surfaces or for rendering contaminated materials safe. All are bound and inactivated to varying degrees by protein and dirt, and they lose considerable activity when applied to other than clean surfaces. Their activity increases exponentially with increases in temperature, but the relationship between increases in concentration and killing effectiveness is complex and varies for each compound. Optimal in-use concentrations have been established for all available disinfectants. The major groups of compounds currently used are briefly discussed next.

Chemical disinfectants are classified on the basis of their ability to sterilize. High-level disinfectants kill all agents except the most resistant of bacterial spores. Intermediate-level disinfectants kill all agents but not spores. Low-level disinfectants are active against most vegetative bacteria and lipid-enveloped viruses.

Activity against spores and viruses varies

Alcohol

The alcohols are protein denaturants that rapidly kill vegetative bacteria when applied as aqueous solutions in the range 70 to 95% alcohol. They are inactive against bacterial spores and many viruses. Solutions of 100% alcohol dehydrate organisms rapidly but fail to kill, because the lethal process requires water molecules. Ethanol (70–90%) and isopropyl alcohol (90–95%) are widely used as skin decontaminants before simple invasive procedures such as venipuncture. Their effect is not instantaneous, and the traditional alcohol wipe, particularly when followed by a vein-probing finger, is more symbolic than effective, because insufficient time is given for significant killing. Isopropyl alcohol has largely replaced ethanol in hospital use because it is somewhat more active and is not subject to diversion to housestaff parties.

Alcohols require water for maximum effectiveness

Action of alcohol is slow

Halogens

Iodine is an effective disinfectant that acts by iodinating or oxidizing essential components of the microbial cell. Its original use was as a tincture of 2% iodine in 50% alcohol, which kills more rapidly and effectively than alcohol alone. This preparation has the disadvantage of sometimes causing hypersensitivity reactions and of staining materials with which it comes into contact. Tincture of iodine has now been largely replaced by preparations in which iodine is combined with carriers (povidone) or nonionic detergents. These agents, termed **iodophors,** gradually release small amounts of iodine. They cause less skin staining and dehydration than tinctures and are widely used in preparation of skin before surgery. Although iodophors are less allergenic than inorganic iodine preparations, they should not be used on patients with a history of iodine sensitivity.

Tincture of iodine in alcohol is effective

Iodophors combine iodine with detergents

Chlorine is a highly effective oxidizing agent, which accounts for its lethality to microbes. It exists as hypochlorous acid in aqueous solutions that dissociate to yield free chlorine over a wide pH range, particularly under slightly acidic conditions. In concentrations of less than one part per million, chlorine is lethal within seconds to most vegetative bacteria, and it inactivates most viruses; this efficacy accounts for its use in rendering supplies of drinking water safe and in chlorination of water in swimming pools. Chlorine reacts rapidly with protein and many other organic compounds, and its activity is lost quickly in the presence of organic material. This property, combined with its toxicity, renders it ineffective on body surfaces; however, it is the agent of choice for decontaminating surfaces and glassware that have been contaminated with viruses or spores of pathogenic bacteria. For these purposes it is usually applied as a 5% solution called **hypochlorite.**

Chlorine oxidative action is rapid

Activity is reduced by organic matter

The use of chlorination to disinfect water supplies has proved insufficient in some hospitals because of the relative resistance of *Legionella pneumophila* to the usual concentrations of chlorine. Some institutions have been forced to augment chlorination with systems that add copper and silver ions to the water.

Legionella may resist chlorine

Hydrogen Peroxide

Hydrogen peroxide is a powerful oxidizing agent that attacks membrane lipids and other cell components. Although it acts rapidly against many bacteria and viruses, it kills bacteria that produce catalase and spores less rapidly. Hydrogen peroxide has been useful in disinfecting items such as contact lenses that are not susceptible to its corrosive effect.

Hydrogen peroxide oxidizes cell components

Surface-Active Compounds

Surfactants are compounds with hydrophobic and hydrophilic groups that attach to and solubilize various compounds or alter their properties. Anionic detergents such as soaps are highly effective cleansers but have little direct antibacterial effect, probably because their charge is similar to that of most microorganisms. Cationic detergents, particularly the **quaternary ammonium compounds** ("quats") such as benzalkonium chloride, are highly bactericidal in the absence of contaminating organic matter. Their hydrophobic and lipophilic groups react with the lipid of the cell membrane of the bacteria, alter the membrane's surface properties and its permeability, and lead to loss of essential cell components and death. These compounds have little toxicity to skin and mucous membranes and, thus, have been used widely for their antibacterial effects in a concentration of 0.1%. They are inactive against spores and most viruses. "Quats" in much higher concentrations than those used in medicine (eg, 5–10%) can be used for sanitizing surfaces.

Hydrophobic and hydrophilic groups of surfactants act on lipids of bacterial membranes

Little activity against viruses

The greatest care is needed in the use of quats because they adsorb to most surfaces with which they come into contact, such as cotton, cork, and even dust. As a result, their concentration may be lowered to a point at which certain bacteria, particularly *Pseudomonas aeruginosa,* can grow in the quat solutions and then cause serious infections. Many instances have been recorded of severe infections resulting from contamination of ophthalmic preparations or of solutions used for treating skin before transcutaneous procedures. It should also be remembered that cationic detergents are totally neutralized by anionic compounds. Thus, the antibacterial effect of quaternary ammonium compounds is inactivated by soap. Because of these problems, quats have been replaced by other antiseptics and disinfectants for most purposes.

"Quats" adsorbed to surfaces may become contaminated with bacteria

Cationic detergents are neutralized by soaps

Phenolics

Phenol, one of the first effective disinfectants, was the primary agent employed by Lister in his antiseptic surgical procedure, which preceded the development of aseptic surgery. It is a potent protein denaturant and bactericidal agent. Substitutions in the ring structure of phenol have substantially improved activity and have provided a range of phenols and cresols that are the most effective environmental decontaminants available for use in hospital hygiene. Concern about their release into the environment in hospital waste and sewage has created some pressure to limit their use. This is another of the classic environmental dilemmas of our society: a compound that reduces the risk of disease for one group may raise it for another. Phenolics are less "quenched" by protein than are most other disinfectants, have a detergent-like effect on the cell membrane, and are often formulated with soaps to increase their cleansing property. They are too toxic to skin and tissues to be used as antiseptics, although brief exposures can be tolerated. They are the active ingredient in many mouthwash and sore throat preparations.

Relatively stable to protein

Environmental contamination with phenols and cresols limits use

Two diphenyl compounds, hexachlorophene and chlorhexidine, have been extensively used as skin disinfectants. **Hexachlorophene** is primarily bacteriostatic. Incorporated into a soap, it builds up on the surface of skin epithelial cells over 1 to 2 days of use to produce a steady inhibitory effect on skin flora and Gram-positive contaminants, as long as its use is continued. It was a major factor in controlling outbreaks of severe staphylococcal infections in nurseries during the 1950s and 1960s, but cutaneous absorption was found to produce neurotoxic effects in some premature infants. When it was applied in excessive concentrations, similar problems occurred in older children. It is now a prescription drug.

Skin binding of hexachlorophene enhances effectiveness for staphylococci

Absortion through skin limits use

Chlorhexidine has replaced hexachlorophene as a routine hand and skin disinfectant and for other topical applications. It has greater bactericidal activity than hexachlorophene without its toxicity but shares with hexachlorophene the ability to bind to the skin and produce a persistent antibacterial effect. It acts by altering membrane permeability of both Gram-positive and -negative bacteria. It is cationic and, thus, its action is neutralized by soaps and anionic detergents.

Chlorhexidine also binds to skin but is less toxic

Glutaraldehyde and Formaldehyde

Glutaraldehyde and formaldehyde are alkylating agents highly lethal to essentially all microorganisms. Formaldehyde gas is irritative, allergenic, and unpleasant, properties that limit its use as a solution or gas. Glutaraldehyde is an effective high-level disinfecting agent for apparatus that cannot be heat treated, such as some lensed instruments and equipment for respiratory therapy. Formaldehyde vapor, an effective environmental decontaminant under conditions of high humidity, is sometimes used to decontaminate laboratory rooms that have been accidentally and extensively contaminated with pathogenic bacteria, including those such as the anthrax bacillus that form resistant spores. Such rooms are sealed for processing and thoroughly aired before reoccupancy.

Glutaraldehyde is useful for decontamination of equipment

Some risk of infection exists in all health care settings. Hospitalized patients are particularly vulnerable and the hospital environment is complex. The proper matching of the principles and procedures described here to general and specialized situations together with aseptic practices can markedly reduce the risks. The building of such systems is generally referred to as infection control and is discussed further in Chapter 72.

ADDITIONAL READING

Block SS. *Disinfection, Sterilization, and Preservation.* 5th ed. Philadelphia: Lippincott Williams & Wilkins; 2001. A standard reference source that contains detailed information.

Widmer AF, Frei R. Decontamination, disinfection, and sterilization. In: Murray PR, ed: *Manual of Clinical Microbiology.* 7th ed. Washington, DC: American Society for Microbiology; 1999. A good account of the practical use of disinfectants, including the meeting of regulatory standards.

CHAPTER 12

Epidemiology of Infectious Diseases

W. LAWRENCE DREW

Epidemiology, the study of the distribution of determinants of disease and injury in human populations, is a discipline that includes both infectious and noninfectious diseases. Most epidemiologic studies of infectious diseases have concentrated on the factors that influence acquisition and spread, because this knowledge is essential for developing methods of prevention and control. Historically, epidemiologic studies and the application of the knowledge gained from them have been central to the control of the great epidemic diseases, such as cholera, plague, smallpox, yellow fever, and typhus.

An understanding of the principles of epidemiology and the spread of disease is essential to all medical personnel, whether their work is with the individual patient or with the community. Most infections must be evaluated in their epidemiologic setting; for example, what infections, especially viral, are currently prevalent in the community? Has the patient recently traveled to an area of special disease prevalence? Is there a possibility of nosocomial infection from recent hospitalization? What is the risk to the patient's family, schoolmates, and work or social contacts?

The recent recognition of emerging infectious diseases has heightened appreciation of the importance of epidemiologic information. A few examples of these newly identified infections are cryptosporidiosis, hantavirus pulmonary syndrome and *Escherichia coli* O157:H7 disease. In addition, some well-known pathogens have assumed new epidemiologic importance by virtue of acquired antimicrobial resistance (eg, penicillin-resistant pneumococci, vancomycin-resistant enterococci, and multiresistant *Mycobacterium tuberculosis*).

Factors that increase the emergence or reemergence of various pathogens include:

- Population movements and the intrusion of humans and domestic animals into new habitats, particularly tropical forests
- Deforestation, with development of new farmlands and exposure of farmers and domestic animals to new arthropods and primary pathogens
- Irrigation, especially primitive irrigation systems, which fail to control arthropods and enteric organisms
- Uncontrolled urbanization, with vector populations breeding in stagnant water
- Increased long-distance air travel, with contact or transport of arthropod vectors and primary pathogens

SOURCES AND COMMUNICABILITY

Infectious diseases of humans may be caused by exclusively human pathogens, such as *Shigella;* by environmental organisms, such as *Legionella pneumophila;* or by organisms that have their primary reservoir in animals, such as *Salmonella*.

Noncommunicable infections are those that are not transmitted from human to human and include (1) infections derived from the patient's normal flora, such as peritonitis after rupture of the appendix; (2) infections caused by the ingestion of preformed toxins, such as botulism; and (3) infections caused by certain organisms found in the environment, such as clostridial gas gangrene. Some zoonotic infections (diseases transmitted from animals to humans) such as rabies and brucellosis are not transmitted between humans, but others such as plague may be at certain stages. Noncommunicable infections may still occur as common-source outbreaks, such as food poisoning from an enterotoxin-producing *Staphylococcus aureus*–contaminated chicken salad or multiple cases of pneumonia from extensive dissemination of *Legionella* through an air-conditioning system. Because these diseases are not transmissible to others, they do not lead to secondary spread.

Noncommunicable infections are not spread from person to person but can occur as common-source outbreaks

Communicable infections require that an organism be able to leave the body in a form that is directly infectious or is able to become so after development in a suitable environment. The respiratory spread of the influenza virus is an example of direct communicability. In contrast, the malarial parasite requires a developmental cycle in a biting mosquito before it can infect another human. Communicable infections can be **endemic,** which implies that the disease is present at a low but fairly constant level, or **epidemic,** which involves a level of infection above that usually found in a community or population. Communicable infections that are widespread in a region, sometimes worldwide, and have high attack rates are termed **pandemic.**

Endemic = constant presence

Epidemic = localized outbreak

Pandemic = widespread regional or global epidemic

INFECTION AND DISEASE

An important consideration in the study of the epidemiology of communicable organisms is the distinction between infection and disease. **Infection** involves multiplication of the organism in or on the host and may not be apparent, for example, during the incubation period or latent when little or no replication is occurring (eg, with herpesviruses). **Disease** represents a clinically apparent response by or injury to the host as a result of infection. With many communicable microorganisms, infection is much more common than disease, and apparently healthy infected individuals play an important role in disease propagation. Inapparent infections are termed **subclinical,** and the individual is sometimes referred to as a **carrier.** The latter term is also applied to situations in which an infectious agent establishes itself as part of a patient's flora or causes low-grade chronic disease after an acute infection. For example, the clinically inapparent presence of *S. aureus* in the anterior nares is termed **carriage,** as is a chronic gallbladder infection with *Salmonella* serotype Typhi that can follow an attack of typhoid fever and result in fecal excretion of the organism for years.

With some infectious diseases, such as measles, infection is invariably accompanied by clinical manifestations of the disease itself. These manifestations facilitate epidemiologic control, because the existence and extent of infection in a community are readily apparent. Organisms associated with long incubation periods or high frequencies of subclinical infection such as human immunodeficiency virus (HIV) or hepatitis B virus may propagate and spread in a population for long periods before the extent of the problem is recognized. This makes epidemiologic control more difficult.

Infection can result in little or no illness

Carriers can be asymptomatic, but infectious to others

INCUBATION PERIOD AND COMMUNICABILITY

The **incubation period** is the time between exposure to the organism and appearance of the first symptoms of the disease. Generally, organisms that multiply rapidly and produce local infections, such as gonorrhea and influenza, are associated with short incubation periods (eg, 2–4 days). Diseases such as typhoid fever, which depend on hematogenous

Incubation periods range from a few days to several months

spread and multiplication of the organism in distant target organs to produce symptoms, often have longer incubation periods (eg, 10 days to 3 weeks). Some diseases have even more prolonged incubation periods because of slow passage of the infecting organism to the target organ, as in rabies, or slow growth of the organism, as in tuberculosis. Incubation periods for one agent may also vary widely depending on route of acquisition and infecting dose; for example, the incubation period of hepatitis B virus infection may vary from a few weeks to several months.

Communicability of a disease in which the organism is shed in secretions may occur primarily during the incubation period. In other infections, the disease course is short but the organisms can be excreted from the host for extended periods. In yet other cases, the symptoms are related to host immune response rather than the organism's action, and thus the disease process may extend far beyond the period in which the etiologic agent can be isolated or spread. Some viruses can integrate into the host genome or survive by replicating very slowly in the presence of an immune response. Such dormancy or latency is exemplified by the herpesviruses, and the organism may emerge long after the original infection and potentially infect others.

Transmission to others can occur before illness onset

The inherent infectivity and virulence of a microorganism are also important determinants of attack rates of disease in a community. In general, organisms of high infectivity spread more easily and those of greater virulence are more likely to cause disease than subclinical infection. The infecting dose of an organism also varies with different organisms and thus influences the chance of infection and development of disease.

ROUTES OF TRANSMISSION

Various transmissible infections may be acquired from others by direct contact, by aerosol transmission of infectious secretions, or indirectly through contaminated inanimate objects or materials. Some, such as malaria, involve an animate insect vector. These routes of spread are often referred to as **horizontal transmission,** in contrast to **vertical transmission** from mother to fetus. The major horizontal routes of transmission of infectious diseases are summarized in Table 12–1 and discussed next.

Horizontal transmission = direct or indirect person-to-person

Vertical transmission = mother to fetus

Respiratory Spread

Many infections are transmitted by the respiratory route, often by aerosolization of respiratory secretions with subsequent inhalation by others. The efficiency of this process depends in part on the extent and method of propulsion of discharges from the mouth and nose, the size of the aerosol droplets, and the resistance of the infectious agent to desiccation and inactivation by ultraviolet light. In still air, a particle 100 μm in diameter requires only seconds to fall the height of a room; a 10-μm particle remains airborne for about 20 minutes, smaller particles even longer. When inhaled, particles with a diameter of 6 μm or greater are usually trapped by the mucosa of the nasal turbinates, whereas particles of 0.6 to 5.0 μm attach to mucous sites at various levels along the upper and lower respiratory tract and may initiate infection. These "droplet nuclei" are most important in transmitting many respiratory pathogens (eg, *M. tuberculosis*). Respiratory secretions are often transferred on hands or inanimate objects (fomites) and may reach the respiratory tract of others in this way. For example, spread of the common cold may involve transfer of infectious secretions from nose to hand by the infected individual, with transfer to others by hand-to-hand contact and then from hand to nose by the unsuspecting victim.

Droplet nuclei are usually less than 6 μm in size

Salivary Spread

Some infections, such as herpes simplex and infectious mononucleosis, can be transferred directly by contact with infectious saliva through kissing. Transmission of infectious secretions by direct contact with the nasal mucosa or conjunctiva often accounts for the rapid dissemination of agents such as respiratory syncytial virus and adenovirus. The risk of spread in these instances can be reduced by simple hygienic measures, such as handwashing.

Handwashing is especially important

TABLE 12–1

Common Routes of Transmission[a]

Route of Exit	Route of Transmission	Example
Respiratory	Aerosol droplet inhalation	Influenza virus; tuberculosis
	Nose or mouth → hand or object → nose	Common cold (rhinovirus)
Salivary	Direct salivary transfer (eg, kissing)	Oral–labial herpes; infectious mononucleosis, cytomegalovirus
	Animal bite	Rabies
Gastrointestinal	Stool → hand → mouth and/or stool → object → mouth	Enterovirus infection; hepatitis A
	Stool → water or food → mouth	Salmonellosis; shigellosis
Skin	Skin discharge → air → respiratory tract	Varicella, poxvirus infection
	Skin to skin	Human papilloma virus (warts); syphilis
Blood	Transfusion or needle prick	Hepatitis B; cytomegalovirus infection; malaria; AIDS
	Insect bite	Malaria; relapsing fever
Genital secretions	Urethral or cervical secretions	Gonorrhea; herpes simplex; *Chlamydia* infection
	Semen	Cytomegalovirus infection
Urine	Urine → hand → catheter	Hospital-acquired urinary tract infection
Eye	Conjunctival	Adenovirus
Zoonotic	Animal bite	Rabies
	Contact with carcasses	Tularemia
	Arthropod	Plague; Rocky Mountain spotted fever; Lyme disease

[a] The examples cited are incomplete, and in some cases more than one route of transmission exists.

Fecal–Oral Spread

Fecal–oral spread involves direct or finger-to-mouth spread, the use of human feces as a fertilizer, or fecal contamination of food or water. Food handlers who are infected with an organism transmissible by this route constitute a special hazard, especially when their personal hygienic practices are inadequate. Some viruses disseminated by the fecal–oral route infect and multiply in cells of the oropharynx and then disseminate to other body sites to cause infection. However, organisms that are spread in this way commonly multiply in the intestinal tract and may cause intestinal infections. They must therefore be able to resist the acid in the stomach, the bile, and the gastric and small-intestinal enzymes. Many bacteria and enveloped viruses are rapidly killed by these conditions, but members of the Enterobacteriaceae and unenveloped viral intestinal pathogens (eg, enteroviruses) are more likely to survive. Even with these organisms, the infecting dose in patients with reduced or absent gastric hydrochloric acid is often much smaller than in those with normal stomach acidity.

Reduced gastric hydrochloric acid can facilitate enteric infections

Skin-to-Skin Transfer

Skin-to-skin transfer occurs with a variety of infections in which the skin is the portal of entry, such as the spirochete of syphilis (*Treponema pallidum*), strains of group A streptococci that cause impetigo, and the dermatophyte fungi that cause ringworm and athlete's foot. In most cases, an inapparent break in the epithelium is probably involved in infection. Other diseases may be spread through fomites such as shared towels and inadequately cleansed shower and bath floors. Skin-to-skin transfer usually occurs through abrasions of the epidermis, which may be unnoticed.

Syphilis, ringworm, and impetigo are examples of skin-to-skin transfer

Bloodborne Transmission

Bloodborne transmission through insect vectors requires a period of multiplication or alteration within an insect vector before the organism can infect another human host. Such is the case with the mosquito and the malarial parasite. Direct transmission from human to human through blood has become increasingly important in modern medicine because of the use of blood transfusions and blood products and the increased self-administration of illicit drugs by intravenous or subcutaneous routes, using shared nonsterile equipment. Hepatitis B and C viruses as well as HIV were frequently transmitted in this way prior to the institution of blood screening tests.

Parenteral drug abuse is a major risk factor

Genital Transmission

Disease transmission through the genital tract has emerged as one of the most common infectious problems and reflects changing social and sexual mores. Spread can occur between sexual partners or from the mother to the infant at birth. A major factor in these infections has been the persistence, high rates of asymptomatic carriage, and frequency of recurrence of organisms such as *Chlamydia trachomatis*, cytomegalovirus (CMV), herpes simplex virus, and *Neisseria gonorrhoeae*.

Asymptomatic carriage and recurrence are common

Eye-to-Eye Transmission

Infections of the conjunctiva may occur in epidemic or endemic form. Epidemics of adenovirus and *Haemophilus* conjunctivitis may occur and are highly contagious. The major endemic disease is trachoma, caused by *Chlamydia,* which remains a frequent cause of blindness in developing countries. These diseases may be spread by direct contact via ophthalmologic equipment or by secretions passed manually or through fomites such as towels.

Fomites, unsterile ophthalmologic instruments are associated with transmission

Zoonotic Transmission

Zoonotic infections are those spread from animals, where they have their natural reservoir, to humans. Some zoonotic infections, such as rabies are directly contracted from the bite of the infected animal, while other are transmitted by vectors, especially arthropods (eg, ticks, mosquitoes). Many infections contracted by humans from animals are dead-ended in humans, while others may be transferred between humans once the disease is established in a population. Plague, for example, has a natural reservoir in rodents. Human infections contracted from the bites of rodent fleas may produce pneumonia, which may then spread to other humans by the respiratory droplet route.

Zoonotic = animals to humans

Vertical Transmission

Certain diseases can spread from the mother to the fetus through the placental barrier. This mode of transmission involves organisms such as rubella virus that can be present in the mother's bloodstream and may occur at different stages of pregnancy with different organisms. Another form of transmission from mother to infant occurs by contact during birth with organisms such as group B streptococci, *C. trachomatis,* and *N. gonorrhoeae,* which colonize the vagina. Herpes simplex virus and CMV can spread by both vertical methods as it may be present in blood or may colonize the cervix. CMV may also be transmitted by breast milk, a third mechanism of vertical transmission.

Vertical transmission can occur transplacentally, during birth, or through breast milk

EPIDEMICS

The characterization of epidemics and their recognition in a community involve several quantitative measures and some specific epidemiologic definitions. **Infectivity,** in epidemiologic terms, equates to attack rate and is measured as the frequency with which an infection is transmitted when there is contact between the agent and a susceptible individual. The **disease index** of an infection can be expressed as the number of persons who develop the disease divided by the total number infected. The **virulence** of an agent can be estimated as the number of fatal or severe cases per the total number of cases. **Incidence,** the number of new cases of a disease within a specified period, is described as a rate in which the number of cases is the numerator and the number of people in the population under surveillance is the denominator. This is usually normalized to reflect a percentage of the population that is affected. **Prevalence,** which can also be described as a rate, is primarily used to indicate the total number of cases existing in a population at risk at a point in time.

Incidence and prevalence rates are usually expressed as number of cases per 100, 1000, or 100,000 population

The prerequisites for propagation of an epidemic from person to person are a sufficient degree of infectivity to allow the organism to spread, sufficient virulence for an increased incidence of disease to become apparent, and sufficient level of susceptibility in the host population to permit transmission and amplification of the infecting organism. Thus, the extent of an epidemic and its degree of severity are determined by complex interactions between parasite and host. Host factors such as age, genetic predisposition, and immune status can dramatically influence the manifestations of an infectious disease. Together with differences in infecting dose, these factors are largely responsible for the wide spectrum of disease manifestations that may be seen during an epidemic.

Interaction between host and parasite determines extent

The effect of age can be quite dramatic. For example, in an epidemic of measles in an isolated population in 1846, the attack rate for all ages averaged 75%; however, mortality was 90 times higher in children less than 1 year of age (28%) than in those 1 to 40 years of age (0.3%). Conversely, in one outbreak of poliomyelitis, the attack rate of paralytic polio was 4% in children 0 to 4 years of age and 20 to 40% in those 5 to 50 years of age. Sex may be a factor in disease manifestations; for example, the likelihood of becoming a chronic carrier of hepatitis B is twice as high for males as for females.

Attack rates and disease severity can vary widely by age

Prior exposure of a population to an organism may alter immune status and the frequency of acquisition, severity of clinical disease, and duration of an epidemic. For example, measles is highly infectious and attacks most susceptible members of an exposed population. However, infection gives solid lifelong immunity. Thus, in unimmunized populations in which the disease is maintained in endemic form, epidemics occur at about 3-year intervals when a sufficient number of nonimmune hosts has been born to permit rapid transmission between them. When a sufficient immune population is reestablished, epidemic spread is blocked and the disease again becomes endemic. When immunity is short-lived or incomplete, epidemics can continue for decades if the mode of transmission is unchecked, which accounts for the present epidemic of gonorrhea.

Immune status of a population influences epidemic behavior

Prolonged and extensive exposure to a pathogen during previous generations selects for a higher degree of innate genetic immunity in a population. For example, extensive exposure of Western urbanized populations to tuberculosis during the 18th and 19th centuries conferred a degree of resistance greater than that among the progeny of rural or geographically isolated populations. The disease spread rapidly and in severe form, for example, when it was first encountered by Native Americans. An even more dramatic example concerns the resistance to the most serious form of malaria that is conferred on peoples of West African descent by the sickle-celled trait (see Chapter 52). These instances are clear cases of natural selection, a process that accounts for many differences in racial immunity.

Immunity in population influences spread

Occasionally, an epidemic arises from an organism against which immunity is essentially absent in a population and that is either of enhanced virulence or appears to be of enhanced virulence because of the lack of immunity. When such an organism is highly infectious, the disease it causes may become pandemic and worldwide. A prime example of this situation is the appearance of a new major antigenic variant of influenza A virus against which there is little if any cross-immunity from recent epidemics with other

Sudden appearance of "new" agents can result in pandemic spread

strains. The 1918–1919 pandemic of influenza was responsible for more deaths than World War I (about 20 million). Subsequent but less serious pandemics have occurred at intervals because of the development of strains of influenza virus with major antigenic shifts (see Chapter 32). Another example, acquired immunodeficiency syndrome (AIDS), illustrates the same principles but also reflects changes in human ecologic and social behavior.

A major feature of serious epidemic diseases is their frequent association with poverty, malnutrition, disaster, and war. The association is multifactorial and includes overcrowding, contaminated food and water, an increase in arthropods that parasitize humans, and the reduced immunity that can accompany severe malnutrition or certain types of chronic stress. Overcrowding and understaffing in day-care centers or institutes for the mentally impaired can similarly be associated with epidemics of infections.

Social and ecological factors determine aspects of epidemic diseases

In recent years, increasing attention has been given to hospital (nosocomial) epidemics of infection. Hospitals are not immune to the epidemic diseases that occur in the community; and outbreaks result from the association of infected patients or persons with those who are unusually susceptible because of chronic disease, immunosuppressive therapy, or the use of bladder, intratracheal, or intravascular catheters and tubes. Control depends on the techniques of medical personnel, hospital hygiene, and effective surveillance. This topic is considered in greater detail in Chapter 72.

Nosocomial = hospital-acquired

CONTROL OF EPIDEMICS

The first principle of control is recognition of the existence of an epidemic. This recognition is sometimes immediate because of the high incidence of disease, but often the evidence is obtained from ongoing surveillance activities, such as routine disease reports to health departments and records of school and work absenteeism. The causative agent must be identified and studies to determine route of transmission (eg, food poisoning) must be initiated.

Surveillance is the key to recognition of an epidemic

Measures must then be adopted to control the spread and development of further infection. These methods include (1) blocking the route of transmission if possible (eg, improved food hygiene or arthropod control); (2) identifying, treating, and, if necessary, isolating infected individuals and carriers; (3) raising the level of immunity in the uninfected population by immunization; (4) making selective use of chemoprophylaxis for subjects or populations at particular risk of infection, as in epidemics of meningococcal infection; and (5) correcting conditions such as overcrowding or contaminated water supplies that have led to the epidemic or facilitated transfer.

Control measures can vary widely

GENERAL PRINCIPLES OF IMMUNIZATION

Immunization is the most effective method to provide individual and community protection against many epidemic diseases. Immunization can be active, with stimulation of the body's immune mechanisms through administration of a vaccine, or passive, through administration of plasma or globulin containing preformed antibody to the agent desired. Active immunization with living attenuated organisms generally results in a subclinical or mild illness that duplicates to a limited extent the disease to be prevented. Live vaccines generally provide both local and durable humoral immunity. Killed or subunit vaccines such as influenza vaccine and tetanus toxoid provide immunogenicity without infectivity. They generally involve a larger amount of antigen than live vaccines and must be administered parenterally with two or more spaced injections and subsequent boosters to elicit and maintain a satisfactory antibody level. Immunity usually develops more rapidly with live vaccines, but serious overt disease from the vaccine itself can occur in patients whose immune responses are suppressed. Live attenuated virus vaccines are generally contraindicated in pregnancy because of the risk of infection and damage to developing fetus. Recent developments in molecular biology and protein chemistry have brought greater sophistication to the identification and purification of specific immunizing antigens and epitopes and to the preparation and purification of specific antibodies for passive protection. Thus, immunization is being applied to a broader range of infections.

Prophylaxis or therapy of some infections can be accomplished or aided by passive immunization. This procedure involves administration of preformed antibody obtained from humans, derived from animals actively immunized to the agent, or produced by hybridoma techniques. Animal antisera induce immune responses to their globulins that result in clearance of the passively transferred antibody within about 10 days and carry the risk of hypersensitivity reactions such as serum sickness and anaphylaxis. Human antibodies are less immunogenic and are detectable in the circulation for several weeks after administration. Two types of human antibody preparations are generally available. Immune serum globulin (gamma globulin) is the immunoglobulin G fraction of plasma from a large group of donors that contains antibody to many infectious agents. Hyperimmune globulins are purified antibody preparations from the blood of subjects with high titers of antibody to a specific disease that have resulted from natural exposure or immunization; hepatitis B immune globulin, rabies immune globulin, and human tetanus immune globulin are examples. Details of the use of these globulins can be obtained from the chapters that discuss the diseases in question. Passive antibody is most effective when given early in the incubation period.

Passive immunization has a temporary effect

ADDITIONAL READING

American Academy of Pediatrics. Report of the Committee on Infectious Diseases. *Red Book 2000,* 25th ed. Elk Grove Village, IL: American Academy of Pediatrics; 2000. This manual is published every 3 years, with periodic interim updates as necessary. A comprehensive resource on immunization recommendations, it contains much other information regarding the epidemiology and control of infectious diseases.

Gladwell M. The Dead Zone. *The New Yorker* 1997; Sept 29:52–56. A fascinating lay person's account of an attempt to define the cause of the influenza pandemic of 1918.

Ryan ET, Kain KC. Health advice and immunization for travelers. *N Engl J Med* 2000;342:1716–1725. This review includes consideration of noninfectious as well as infectious risks for travelers and ways to minimize them.

US Department of Health and Human Services. Health Information for International Travel, 2001–2002. www.cdc.gov/travel/yb/index.htm. This reference is the most timely and up-to-date source for travel recommendations, including updates on infectious outbreaks around the world.

US Public Health Service. Impact of vaccines universally recommended for children, 1990–1998. *MMWR* 2000;48:243–248. This report summarizes the dramatic effects on infectious diseases by routine immunization in the last decade of the 20th century.

CHAPTER 13

Antibacterial and Antiviral Agents

KENNETH J. RYAN AND W. LAWRENCE DREW

The ability to direct therapy specifically at a disease-causing infectious agent is unique to the management of infectious diseases. Its initial success depends on exploiting differences between our own makeup and metabolism and that of the microorganism in question. The mode of action of antimicrobials on bacteria and viruses is the focus of this chapter. The continued success of antibacterial and antiviral agents depends on whether the organisms to which the agent was originally directed develop resistance. Resistance to antibacterial agents is the subject of Chapter 14. Specific information about pathogenic organisms can be found in later chapters; a complete guide to the treatment of infectious diseases is beyond the scope of this book.

Natural materials with some activity against microbes were used in folk medicine in earlier times, such as the bark of the cinchona tree (containing quinine) in the treatment of malaria. Rational approaches to chemotherapy began with Ehrlich's development of arsenical compounds for the treatment of syphilis early in the 20th century. Many years then elapsed before the next major development, which was the discovery of the therapeutic effectiveness of a sulfonamide (prontosil rubrum) by Domagk in 1935. Penicillin, which had been discovered in 1929 by Fleming, could not be adequately purified at that time; however, this was accomplished later, and penicillin was produced in sufficient quantities so that Florey and his colleagues could demonstrate its clinical effectiveness in the early 1940s. The first antiviral agent, methisazone, was a derivative of sulfonamides shown to be active against pox viruses. Numerous new antimicrobial agents have been discovered or developed, and many have found their way into clinical practice.

Sulfonamides and penicillin were the first effective antibacterial agents

ANTIBACTERIAL THERAPY

GENERAL CONSIDERATIONS

Clinically effective antimicrobial agents all exhibit selective toxicity toward the parasite rather than the host, a characteristic that differentiates them from the disinfectants (see Chapter 11). In most cases, selective toxicity is explained by action on microbial processes or structures that differ from those of mammalian cells. For example, some agents act on bacterial cell wall synthesis, and others on functions of the 70 S bacterial

Ideally, selective toxicity is based on the ability of an antimicrobial agent to attack a target present in bacteria but not humans

ribosome but not the 80 S eukaryotic ribosome. Some antimicrobial agents, such as penicillin, are essentially nontoxic to the host, unless hypersensitivity has developed. For others, such as the aminoglycosides, the effective therapeutic dose is relatively close to the toxic dose; as a result, control of dosage and blood level must be much more precise.

Definitions

- **Antibiotic**—antimicrobials of microbial origin, most of which are produced by fungi or by bacteria of the genus *Streptomyces.*
- **Antimicrobial, antimicrobic**—any substance with sufficient antimicrobial activity that it can be used in the treatment of infectious diseases.
- **Bactericidal**—an antimicrobial that not only inhibits growth but is lethal to bacteria.
- **Bacteriostatic**—an antimicrobial that inhibits growth but does not kill the organisms.
- **Chemotherapeutic**—a broad term that encompasses antibiotics, antimicrobials, and drugs used in the treatment of cancer. In the context of infectious diseases, it implies the agent is not an antibiotic.
- **Minimal inhibitory concentration (MIC)**—a laboratory term that defines the lowest concentration (μg/mL) able to inhibit growth of the microorganism.
- **Resistant**—organisms that are not inhibited by clinically achievable concentrations of a antimicrobial agent.
- **Sensitive**—term applied to microorganisms indicating that they will be inhibited by concentrations of the antimicrobic that can be achieved clinically.
- **Spectrum**—an expression of the categories of microorganisms against which an antimicrobial is typically active. A narrow-spectrum agent has activity against only a few organisms. A broad-spectrum agent has activity against organisms of diverse types (eg, Gram-positive and Gram-negative bacteria).
- **Susceptible**—term applied to microorganisms indicating that they will be inhibited by concentrations of the antimicrobic that can be achieved clinically.

Sources of Antimicrobial Agents

Antibiotics are synthesized by molds or bacteria

Production in quantity is by industrial fermentation

There are several sources of antimicrobial agents. The antibiotics are of biological origin and probably play an important part in microbial ecology in the natural environment. Penicillin, for example, is produced by several molds of the genus *Penicillium,* and the prototype cephalosporin antibiotics were derived from other molds. The largest source of naturally occurring antibiotics is the genus *Streptomyces,* the members of which are Gram-positive, branching bacteria found in soils and freshwater sediments. Streptomycin, the tetracyclines, chloramphenicol, erythromycin, and many other antibiotics were discovered by screening large numbers of *Streptomyces* isolates from different parts of the world. Antibiotics are mass produced by techniques derived from the procedures of the fermentation industry.

Chemicals with antibacterial activity are discovered by chance or as the result of screening programs

Chemically synthesized antimicrobial agents were initially discovered among compounds synthesized for other purposes and tested for their therapeutic effectiveness in animals. The sulfonamides, for example, were discovered as a result of routine screening of aniline dyes. More recently, active compounds have been synthesized with structures tailored to be effective inhibitors or competitors of known metabolic pathways. Trimethoprim, which inhibits dihydrofolate reductase, is an excellent example.

Naturally occurring antimicrobics can be chemically modified

A third source of antimicrobial agents is molecular manipulation of previously discovered antibiotics or chemotherapeutics to broaden their range and degree of activity against microorganisms or to improve their pharmacologic characteristics. Examples include the development of penicillinase-resistant and broad-spectrum penicillins, as well as a large range of aminoglycosides and cephalosporins of increasing activity, spectrum, and resistance to inactivating enzymes.

Spectrum of Action

Spectrum is the range of bacteria against which the agent is typically active

The **spectrum** of activity of each antimicrobic describes the genera and species against which it is typically active. For the most common antimicrobics and bacteria, these are shown in Table 13-1. Spectra overlap but are usually characteristic for each broad class of

TABLE 13-1

Usual Susceptibility Patterns of Common Bacteria to Some Commonly Used Bacteriostatic and Bactericidal Antimicrobial Agents

Antimicrobic	Bactericidal	Bacteriostatic	*Staphylococcus aureus*	*Enterococci*	*Other Streptococci*	*Neisseria*	*Haemophilus*	*Legionella*	*Mycoplasma*	*Escherichia coli*	*Proteus mirabilis*	*Other Proteus spp*	*Klebsiella*	*Enterobacter*	*Serratia*	*Pseudomonas aeruginosa*	*Bacteroides fragilis*	*Other Gram-negative Anaerobes*	*Clostridium*	*Rickettsia*	*Chlamydia*	
Benzyl penicillin	+		1 ◕	C ◍◔	1 ◔	1 ◔	◍◔	●	●	●	◍	●	●	●	●	●	●	1 ◔	1 ○	●	●	Narrow-spectrum agents
Penicillinase-resistant penicillins	+		1 ◔	●	2 ◔	●	●	●	●	●	●	●	●	●	●	●	●	●	●	●	●	
Erythromycin	±	+	2 ◔	2 ◔	2 ◔	◔		1 ○	1 ○	●	●	●	●	●	●	●	–	–	–	–	2 ○	
Clindamycin	±	+	2 ◔	–	◔	●	●	–	–	●	●	●	●	●	●	●	◔	◔	◔	–	–	
Vancomycin	+		2 ◔	1 ◔	2 ○	●	●	●	●	●	●	●	●	●	●	●	–	–	1 ○	–	–	
Ampicillin	+		2 ◕	1 ◔	2 ◔	1 ◔	1 ◔	●	●	1 ◔	1 ◔	●	●	●	●	●	●	–	1 ○	●	●	Broad-spectrum agents
Piperacillin	+		–	○	○	–	◔	●	●	–	1 ○	1 ◔	1 ◔	1 ◔	1 ◔	1 ◔	2 ◔	1 ○	–	●	●	
Cephalothin	+		2 ◔	●	2 ◔	–	●	●	●	◔	○	●	◔	●	●	●	●	◔	◔	●	●	
Cefotetan	+		–	●	1 ○	1 ○	–	●	●	1 ○	1 ○	1 ○	1 ○	●	◔	●	2 ◔	○	–	●	●	
Ceftazidime	+		–	–	–	–	○	●	●	1 ○	1 ○	1 ○	1 ○	2 ◔	2 ◔	◔	◔	–	–	●	●	
Imipenem	+		2 ○	2 ○	2 ○	1 ○	1 ○	–	●	1 ○	1 ○	1 ○	1 ○	1 ○	1 ○	1 ◔	1 ○	1 ○	1 ○	–	–	
Aztreonam	+		●	●	●	1 ○	1 ○	–	●	1 ◔	1 ◔	1 ○	1 ○	◔	1 ◔	1 ◔	●	●	●	–	–	
Gentamicin	+		◔	C ●	●	–	–	●	–	1 ◔	1 ○	1 ○	1 ◔	1 ◔	1 ◔	1 ◔	●	●	●	–	–	
Amikacin	+		◔	C ●	●	–	–	●	–	1 ◔	1 ○	1 ○	1 ◔	1 ◔	1 ◔	1 ◔	●	●	●	–	–	
Tetracycline		+	◔	●	◕	◔	○	2 ○	1 ○	◔	●	●	◔	◔	◕	●	◕	◔	◔	1 ○	1 ○	
Chloramphenicol		+	◔	◔	◔	◔	◔	2 ●	–	◔	◔	◔	◔	◔	◕	●	1 ◔	2 ○	–	1 ○	–	
Ciprofloxacin	+		◔	◍	◍	2 ○	–	–	●	1 ◔	1 ○	1 ○	1 ○	1 ○	1 ○	2 ◔	●	●	–	–	◍	
Sulfamethoxazole + trimethoprim	±	+	–	–	–	–	1 ◔	–	–	1 ◔	◔	◔	◔	◔	◔	●	◔	–	–	–	3 –	

Proportions of susceptible and resistant strains: ○, 100% susceptible ◔, 25% resistant ●, 100% resistant ◍, intermediate susceptibility.

Abbreviations: – = no present indication for therapy or insufficient data 1 = antimicrobic of choice for susceptible strains 2 = second-line agent
3 = *c. trachomatis*-sensitive, *c. psittaci*-resistant C = useful in combinations of a ß-lactam and an aminoglycoside

antimicrobic. Some antibacterial antimicrobics are known as **narrow-spectrum agents;** for example, benzyl penicillin is highly active against many Gram-positive and Gram-negative cocci but has little activity against enteric Gram-negative bacilli. Chloramphenicol, tetracycline, and the cephalosporins, on the other hand, are **broad-spectrum agents** that inhibit a wide range of Gram-positive and Gram-negative bacteria, including some obligate

Broad-spectrum agents inhibit both Gram-positive and Gram-negative species

intracellular organisms. When resistance develops in an initially sensitive genus or species, that species is still considered within the spectrum even when the resistant subpopulation is significant. For example, the spectrum of benzyl penicillin is considered to include *Staphylococcus aureus,* although more than 80% of strains now are penicillin resistant.

SELECTED ANTIBACTERIAL ANTIMICROBICS

Various aspects of the major antimicrobics are now considered in more detail, with emphasis on their modes of action and spectrum. Resistance is mentioned here in the context of spectrum, with mechanisms of resistance covered in Chapter 14. Details on specific antimicrobic use, dosage, and toxicity should be sought in one of the specialized texts or handbooks written for that purpose.

Antimicrobics That Act on Cell Wall Synthesis

Cross-linking of peptidoglycan is the target of β-lactams and glycopeptides

The peptidoglycan (murein sac) component of the bacterial cell wall gives it its shape and rigidity. This giant molecule is formed by weaving the linear glycans *N*-acetylglucosamine and *N*-acetylmuramic acid into a basket-like structure. Mature peptidoglycan is held together by cross-linking of short peptide side chains hanging off the long glycan molecules. This cross-linking process is the target of two of the most important groups of antimicrobics, the β-lactams and the glycopeptides (vancomycin and teicoplanin) (Fig 13–1). Peptidoglycan is unique to bacteria and its synthesis is described in more detail in Chapter 2.

β-Lactam Antimicrobics

A β-lactam ring is part of the structure of all β-lactam antimicrobics

The β-lactam antimicrobics comprise the penicillins, cephalosporins, carbapenems, and monobactams. Their name derives from the presence of a β-lactam ring in their structure; this ring is essential for antibacterial activity. Penicillin, the first member of this class, was derived from molds of the genus *Penicillium,* and later natural β-lactams were derived from both molds and bacteria of the genus *Streptomyces.* Today it is possible to synthesize β-lactams, but most are derived from semisynthetic processes involving the chemical modification of the products of fermentation.

Interfere with peptidoglycan cross-linking by binding to transpeptidases called PBPs

The β-lactam antimicrobics interfere with the transpeptidation reactions that seal the peptide crosslinks between glycan chains. They do so by interference with the action of the transpeptidase enzymes which carry out this cross-linking. These targets of all the β-lactams are commonly called penicillin-binding proteins (PBPs), reflecting the stereochemical nature of their interference, which was first described in experiments with penicillin. Several distinct PBPs occur in any one strain, are usually species specific, and vary in the avidity of their binding to different β-lactam antimicrobics.

Penicillins, cephalosporins, monobactams, and carbapenems differ in terms of the structures fused to the β-lactam ring

The β-lactams are classified by chemical structure (Fig 13–2). They may have one β-lactam ring (monobactams), or a β-lactam ring fused to a five-member penem ring (penicillins, carbapenems), or a six-member cephem ring (cephalosporins). Within these major groups, differences in the side chain(s) attached to the single or double ring can have a significant effect on the pharmacologic properties and spectrum of any β-lactam. The pharmacologic properties include resistance to gastric acid, which allows oral administration, and their pattern of distribution into body compartments (eg, blood, cerebrospinal fluid, joints). The features that alter the spectrum include permeability into the bacterial cell, affinity for PBPs, and vulnerability to the various bacterial mechanisms of resistance.

β-Lactam antimicrobics kill growing bacteria killed by lysing weakened cell walls

β-Lactam antimicrobics are usually highly bactericidal, but only to growing bacteria synthesizing new cell walls. Killing involves attenuation and disruption of the developing peptidoglycan "corset," liberation or activation of autolytic enzymes that further disrupt weakened areas of the wall, and finally osmotic lysis from passage of water through the cytoplasmic membrane to the hypertonic interior of the cell. As might be anticipated, cell wall–deficient organisms, such as *Mycoplasma,* are not susceptible to β-lactam antimicrobics.

Penicillins Penicillins differ primarily in their spectrum of activity against Gram-negative bacteria and resistance to staphylococcal penicillinase. This penicillinase is one

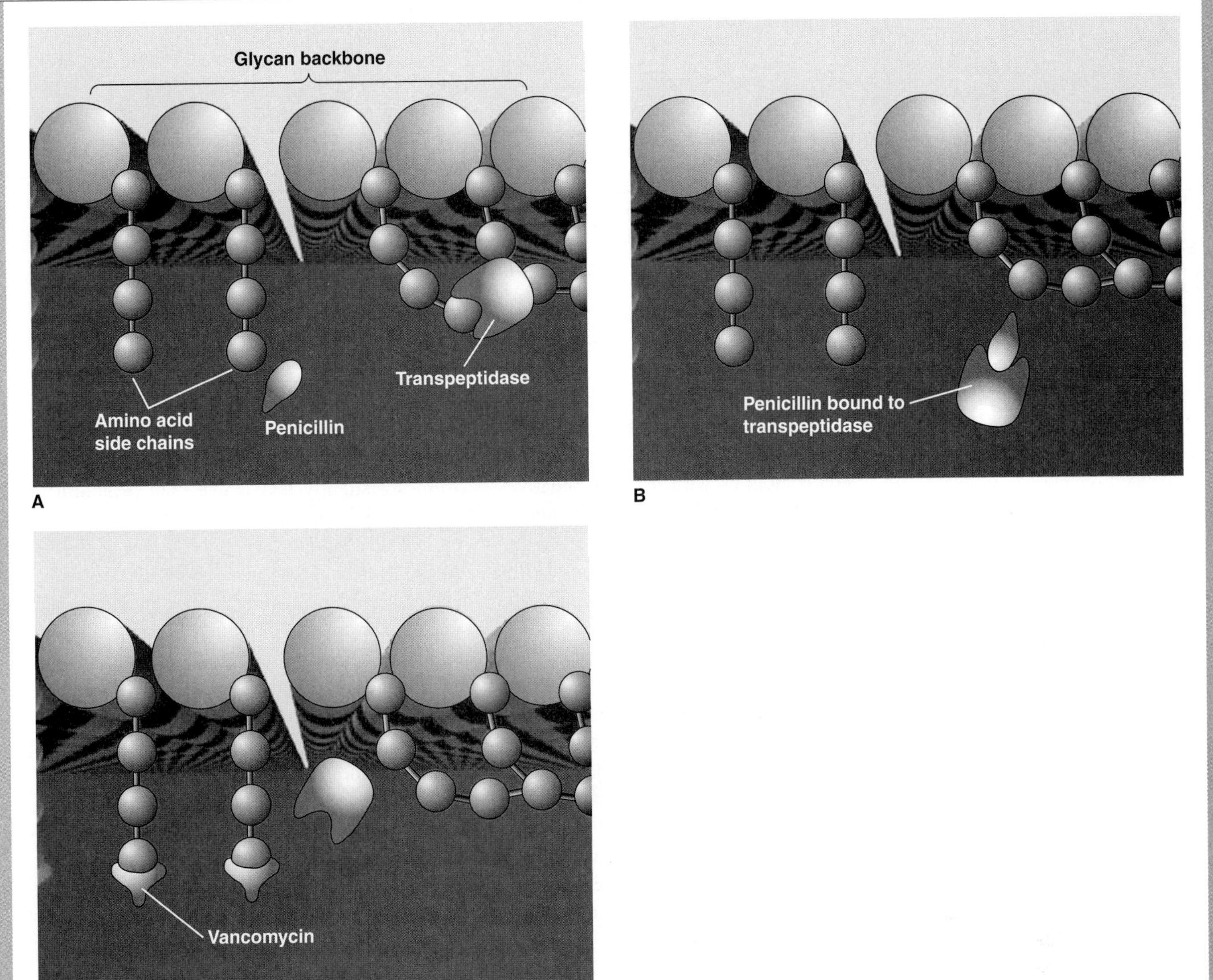

FIGURE 13–1
Action of antimicrobics on peptidoglycan synthesis. The glucan backbone and the amino acid side chains of peptidoglycan are shown. The transpeptidase enzyme catalyzes the cross-linking of the amino acid side chains. Penicillin and other β-lactams bind to the transpeptidase, preventing it from carrying out its function. Vancomycin binds directly to the amino acids, preventing the binding of transpeptidase.

of a family of bacterial enzymes called β-lactamases that inactivate β-lactam antimicrobics (see Chapter 14). **Penicillin G** is active primarily against Gram-positive organisms, Gram-negative cocci, and some spirochetes, including the spirochete of syphilis. They have little action against most Gram-negative bacilli, because the outer membrane prevents passage of these antibiotics to their sites of action on cell wall synthesis. Penicillin G is the least toxic and least expensive of all the penicillins. Its modification as penicillin V confers acid stability, so it can be given orally.

Resistance to staphylococcal and Gram-negative β-lactamases determines spectrum

Penetration of outer membrane is often limited

The penicillinase-resistant penicillins **(methicillin, nafcillin, oxacillin)** also have narrow spectra, but are active against penicillinase-producing *S. aureus*. The broader spectrum penicillins owe their expanded activity to the ability to traverse the outer membrane of some Gram-negative bacteria. Some, such as ampicillin, have excellent activity against a range of Gram-negative pathogens but not *P. aeruginosa,* an important opportunistic pathogen.

Broad-spectrum penicillins penetrate the outer membrane of some Gram-negative bacteria

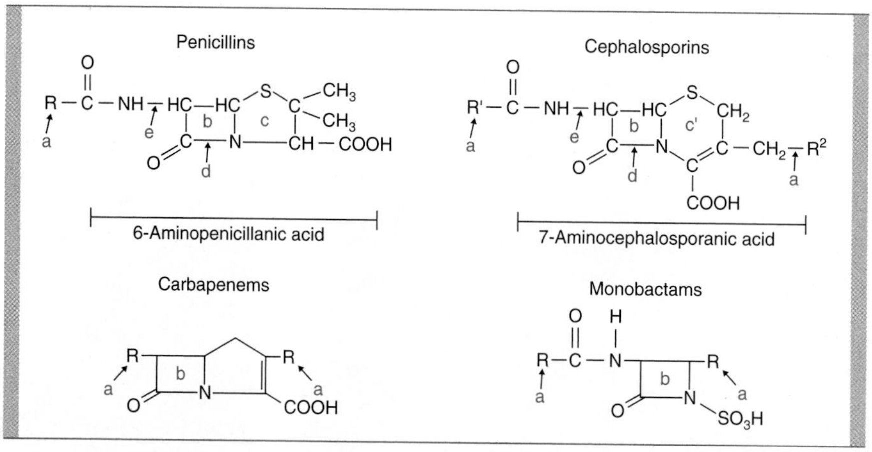

Penicillins

6-Aminopenicillanic acid

Cephalosporins

7-Aminocephalosporanic acid

Carbapenems

Monobactams

FIGURE 13–2
Basic structure of β-lactam antibiotics. a, Different side chains determine degree of activity, spectrum, pharmacologic properties, resistance to β-lactamases; b, β-lactam ring; c, thiazolidine ring; c′ dihydrothiazine ring; d, site of action of β-lactamases; e, site of action of amidase.

Some penicillins are inactivated by staphylococcal penicillinase

Others, such as **carbenicillin** and **ticarcillin,** are active against *Pseudomonas* when given in high dosage but are less active than ampicillin against some other Gram-negative organisms. The penicillins with a Gram-negative spectrum are slightly less active than penicillin G against Gram-positive organisms and are inactivated by staphylococcal penicillinase.

Cephalosporins are penicillinase resistant

Shifting between first- and third-generation cephalosporins gives a wider Gram-negative spectrum

Second- and third-generation cephalosporins have less activity against Gram-positive bacteria

Cephalosporins The structure of the cephalosporins confers resistance to hydrolysis by staphylococcal penicillinase and to the β-lactamases of groups of Gram-negative bacilli, which vary with each cephalosporin. The cephalosporins are classified by generation—first, second, third, or fourth. The "generation" term relates to historical breakthroughs in expanding their spectrum through modification of the side chains. In general, a cephalosporin of a higher generation has a wider spectrum, in some instances, more quantitative activity (lower minimum inhibitory concentration; MIC) against Gram-negative bacteria. As the Gram-negative spectrum increases, these agents typically lose some of their potency (higher MIC) against Gram-positive bacteria.

First-generation cephalosporins inhibit Gram-positive bacteria and a few Enterobacteriaceae

The first-generation cephalosporins **cefazolin** and **cephalexin** have a spectrum of activity against Gram-positive organisms that resembles that of the penicillinase-resistant penicillins, and in addition, they are active against some of the Enterobacteriaceae (see Table 13–1). These agents continue to have therapeutic value because of their high activity against Gram-positive organisms and because a broader spectrum may be unnecessary.

Second-generation cephalosporins are also active against anaerobes

Second-generation cephalosporins **cefoxitin** and **cefaclor** are resistant to β-lactamases of some Gram-negative organisms that inactivate first-generation compounds. Of particular importance is their expanded activity against Enterobacteriaceae species and against anaerobes such as *Bacteroides fragilis*.

Third-generation cephalosporins have increasing potency against Gram-negative organisms

Ceftriaxone and cefotaxime are preferred for meningitis

Ceftazidime is used for *Pseudomonas*

Third-generation cephalosporins, such as **ceftriaxone, cefotaxime,** and **ceftazidime,** have an even wider spectrum; they are active against Gram-negative organisms, often at MICs that are 10- to 100-fold lower than first-generation compounds. Of these three agents, only ceftazidime is consistently active against *P. aeruginosa.* The potency, broad spectrum, and low toxicity of the third-generation cephalosporins have made them the preferred agents in life-threatening infections in which the causative organism has not yet been isolated. Selection depends on the clinical circumstances. For example, ceftriaxone or cefotaxime is preferred for childhood meningitis because it has the highest activity against the three major causes, *Neisseria meningitidis, Streptococcus pneumoniae,* and *Haemophilus influenzae.* For a febrile bone marrow transplant patient, ceftazidime might be chosen because of the prospect of *P. aeruginosa* involvement.

Fourth-generation cephalosporins have enhanced ability to penetrate outer membrane

Fourth-generation cephalosporins have enhanced ability to cross the outer membrane of Gram-negative bacteria as well as resistance to many Gram-negative β-lactamases. Compounds such as **cefepime** have activity against an even wider spectrum of Enterobacteriaceae as well as *P. aeruginosa.* These cephalosporins retain the high affinity of third-generation drugs and activity against *Neisseria* and *H. influenzae.*

Carbapenems The carbapenems **imipenem** and **meropenem** have the broadest spectrum of all β-lactam antibiotics. This fact appears to be due to the combination of easy penetration of Gram-negative and Gram-positive bacterial cells and high level of resistance to β-lactamases. Both agents are active against streptococci, more active than cephalosporins against staphylococci, and highly active against both β-lactamase-positive and -negative strains of gonococci and *H. influenzae*. In addition, they are as active as third-generation cephalosporins against Gram-negative rods, and effective against obligate anaerobes. Imipenem is rapidly hydrolyzed by a renal tubular dehydropeptidase-1; therefore, it is administered together with an inhibitor of this enzyme (cilastatin), which greatly improves its urine levels and other pharmacokinetic characteristics. Meropenem is not significantly degraded by dehydropeptidase-1 and does not require coadministration of cilastatin.

Carbapenems are very broad spectrum

Monobactams **Aztreonam,** the first monobactam licensed in the United States, has a spectrum limited to aerobic and facultatively anaerobic Gram-negative bacteria, including Enterobacteriaceae, *P. aeruginosa, Haemophilus,* and *Neisseria*. Monobactams have poor affinity for the PBPs of Gram-positive organisms and anaerobes and thus little activity against them, but they are highly resistant to hydrolysis by β-lactamases of Gram-negative bacilli. Anaerobic superinfections and major distortions of the bowel flora are less common with aztreonam therapy than with other broad-spectrum β-lactam antimicrobics, presumably because aztreonam does not produce a general suppression of gut anaerobes.

Activity is primarily against Gram-negatives

β-Lactamase Inhibitors A number of β-lactams with little or no antimicrobic activity are capable of binding irreversibly to β-lactamase enzymes and, in the process, rendering them inactive. Three such compounds, **clavulanic acid, sulbactam,** and **tazobactam,** are referred to as suicide inhibitors, because they must first be hydrolyzed by a β-lactamase before becoming effective inactivators of the enzyme. They are highly effective against staphylococcal penicillinases and broad-spectrum β-lactamases; however, their ability to inhibit cephalosporinases is significantly less. Combinations of one of these inhibitors with an appropriate β-lactam antimicrobic protects the therapeutic agent from destruction by many β-lactamases and significantly enhances its spectrum. Four such combinations are now available in the United States: amoxicillin/clavulanate, ticarcillin/clavulanate, ampicillin/sulbactam, and piperacillin/tazobactam. Bacteria that produce chromosomally encoded inducible cephalosporinases are not susceptible to these combinations. Whether these combinations offer therapeutic or economic advantages compared with the β-lactamase–stable antibiotics now available remains to be determined.

β-lactamase inhibitors are β-lactams that bind β-lactamases

Other β-lactams are enhanced in the presence of β-lactamase inhibitors

Clinical Use The β-lactam antibiotics are usually the drugs of choice for infections by susceptible organisms because of their low toxicity and bactericidal action. They have also proved of great value in the prophylaxis of many infections. They are excreted by the kidney and achieve very high urinary levels. Penicillins reach the cerebrospinal fluid when the meninges are inflamed and are effective in the treatment of meningitis, but first- and second-generation cephalosporins are not. In contrast, the third-generation cephalosporins penetrate much better and have become the agents of choice in the treatment of undiagnosed meningitis and meningitis caused by most Gram-negative organisms.

Low toxicity favors use of all β-lactams

Glycopeptide Antimicrobics

Two agents, **vancomycin** and **teicoplanin,** belong to this group. Each of these antimicrobics inhibit assembly of the linear peptidoglycan molecule by binding directly to the terminal amino acids of the peptide side chains. The effect is the same as with β-lactams, prevention of peptidoglycan cross-linking. Both agents are bactericidal, but are primarily active only against Gram-positive bacteria. Their main use has been against multiresistant Gram-positive infections including those caused by strains of staphylococci that are resistant to the penicillinase-resistant penicillins and cephalosporins. Neither agent is absorbed by mouth, although both have been used orally to treat *Clostridium difficile* infections of the bowel (see Chapter 19).

Glycopeptide antimicrobics bind directly to amino acid side chains

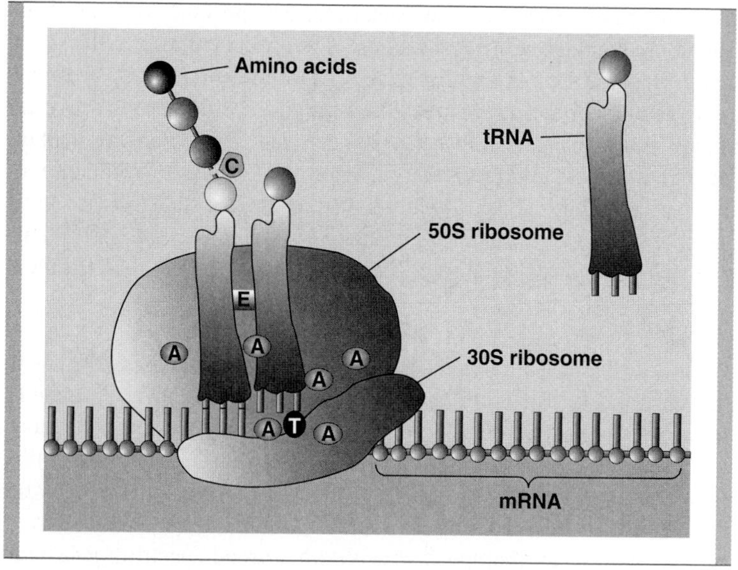

FIGURE 13–3
Action of antimicrobics on protein synthesis. Aminoglycosides (A) bind to multiple sites on both the 30S and 50S ribosomes in a manner that prevents the tRNA from forming initiation complexes. Tetracyclines (T) act in a similar manner, binding only to the 30S ribosomes. Chloramphenicol (C) blocks formation of the peptide bond between the amino acids. Erythromycin (E) and macrolides block the translocation of tRNA from the acceptor to the donor side on the ribosome.

Inhibitors of Protein Synthesis (Fig 13–3)

Aminoglycosides

Aminoglycosides must be transported into cell by oxidative metabolism

Not active against anaerobes

All members of the aminoglycoside group of antimicrobics have a six-member aminocyclitol ring with attached amino sugars. The individual agents differ in terms of the exact ring structure and the number and nature of the amino sugar residues. Aminoglycosides are active against a wide range of bacteria, but only those organisms that are able to transport them into the cell by a mechanism that involves oxidative phosphorylation. Thus, they have little or no activity against strict anaerobes or facultative organisms that metabolize only fermentatively (eg, streptococci). It appears highly probable that aminoglycoside activity against facultative organisms is similarly reduced in vivo when the oxidation–reduction potential is low.

Ribosome binding disrupts initiation complexes

Newer agents bind to multiple sites

Once inside bacterial cells, aminoglycosides inhibit protein synthesis by binding to the bacterial ribosomes either directly or by involving other proteins. This binding destabilizes the ribosomes, blocks initiation complexes, and thus prevents elongation of polypeptide chains. The agents may also cause distortion of the site of attachment of mRNA, mistranslation of codons, and failure to produce the correct amino acid sequence in proteins. The first aminoglycoside, streptomycin, is bound to the 30S ribosomal subunit, but the newer and more active aminoglycosides bind to multiple sites on both 30S and 50S subunits. This gives the newer agents broader spectrum and less susceptibility to resistance due to binding site mutation.

No entry into human cells

Eukaryotic ribosomes are resistant to aminoglycosides, and the antimicrobics are not actively transported into eukaryotic cells. These properties account for their selective toxicity and also explain their ineffectiveness against intracellular bacteria such as *Rickettsia* and *Chlamydia*.

Spectum includes *P. aeruginosa*

Gentamicin and **tobramycin** are the major aminoglycosides; they have an extended spectrum, which includes staphylococci; Enterobacteriaceae; and of particular importance, *P. aeruginosa.* **Streptomycin** and **amikacin** are now primarily used in combination with other antimicrobics in the therapy of tuberculosis and other mycobacterial diseases. **Neomycin,** the most toxic aminoglycoside, is used in topical preparations and as an oral preparation before certain types of intestinal surgery, because it is poorly absorbed.

Renal and vestibular toxicity must be monitored

All of the aminoglycosides are toxic to the vestibular and auditory branches of the eighth cranial nerve to varying degrees; this damage can lead to complete and irreversible loss of hearing and balance. These agents may also be toxic to the kidneys. It is often essential to monitor blood levels during therapy to ensure adequate yet nontoxic doses, especially when renal impairment diminishes excretion of the drug. For example, blood levels of gentamicin should be below 10 μg/mL to avoid nephrotoxicity, but many strains of *P. aeruginosa* require 2 to 4 μg/mL for inhibition.

The clinical value of the aminoglycosides is a consequence of their rapid bactericidal effect, their broad spectrum, the slow development of resistance to the agents now most often used, and their action against *Pseudomonas* strains that resist many other antimicrobics. They cause fewer disturbances of the normal flora than most other broad-spectrum antimicrobics, probably because of their lack of activity against the predominantly anaerobic flora of the bowel, and because they are only used parenterally for systemic infections. The β-lactam antibiotics often act synergistically with the aminoglycosides, most likely because their action on the cell wall facilitates aminoglycoside penetration into the bacterial cell. This effect is most pronounced with organisms such as streptococci and enterococci, which lack the metabolic pathways required to transport aminoglycosides to their interior.

Broad spectrum and slow development of resistance enhance use

Often combined with β-lactam antimicrobics

Tetracyclines

Tetracyclines are composed of four fused benzene rings. Substitutions on these rings provide differences in pharmacologic features of the major members of the group, **tetracycline, minocycline,** and **doxycycline.** The tetracyclines inhibit protein synthesis by binding to the 30S ribosomal subunit at a point that blocks attachment of aminoacyl-tRNA to the acceptor site on the mRNA ribosome complex. Unlike the aminoglycosides, their effect is reversible; they are bacteriostatic rather than bactericidal.

Tetracyclines block tRNA attachment

Activity is bacteriostatic

The tetracyclines are broad-spectrum agents with a range of activity that encompasses most common pathogenic species, including Gram-positive and Gram-negative rods and cocci and both aerobes and anaerobes. They are active against cell wall–deficient organisms, such as *Mycoplasma* and spheroplasts, and against some obligate intracellular bacteria, including members of the genera *Rickettsia* and *Chlamydia*. Differences in spectrum of activity between members of the group are relatively minor. Acquired resistance to one generally confers resistance to all.

Broad spectrum includes some intracellular bacteria

The tetracyclines are absorbed orally. In practice, they are divided into those agents that generate blood levels for only a few hours and those that are longer-acting (minocycline and doxycycline), which can be administered less often. The tetracyclines are chelated by divalent cations, and their absorption and activity are reduced. Thus, they should not be taken with dairy products or many antacid preparations. Tetracyclines are excreted in the bile and urine in active form.

Orally absorbed but chelated by some foods

The tetracyclines have a strong affinity for developing bone and teeth, to which they give a yellowish color, and they are avoided in children up to 8 years of age. Common complications of tetracycline therapy are gastrointestinal disturbance due to alteration of the normal flora, predisposing to superinfection with tetracycline-resistant organisms and vaginal or oral candidiasis (thrush) due to the opportunistic yeast *Candida albicans*.

Dental staining limits use in children

Chloramphenicol

Chloramphenicol has a simple nitrobenzene ring structure that can now be mass produced by chemical synthesis. It influences protein synthesis by binding to the 50S ribosomal subunit and blocking the action of peptidyl transferase, which prevents formation of the peptide bond essential for extension of the peptide chain. Its action is reversible in most susceptible species; thus, it is bacteriostatic. It has little effect on eukaryotic ribosomes, which explains its selective toxicity.

Chloramphenicol blocks peptidyl transferase

A broad-spectrum antibiotic, chloramphenicol, like tetracycline, has a wide range of activity against both aerobic and anaerobic species (see Table 13–1). Chloramphenicol is readily adsorbed from the upper gastrointestinal tract and diffuses readily into most body compartments, including the cerebrospinal fluid. It also permeates readily into mammalian cells and is active against obligate intracellular pathogens such as *Rickettsia* and *Chlamydia*.

Diffusion into body fluid compartments occurs readily

The major drawback to this inexpensive, broad-spectrum antimicrobial with almost ideal pharmacologic features is a rare but serious toxicity. Between 1 in 50,000 and 1 in 200,000 patients treated with even low doses of chloramphenicol have an idiosyncratic

Marrow suppression and aplastic anemia are serious toxicities

reaction that results in aplastic anemia. The condition is irreversible and, before the advent of bone marrow transplantation, it was universally fatal. In high doses, chloramphenicol also causes a reversible depression of the bone marrow and, in neonates, abdominal, circulatory, and respiratory dysfunction. The inability of the immature infant liver to conjugate and excrete chloramphenicol aggravates this latter condition.

Use is sharply restricted

Chloramphenicol use is now restricted to treatment of rickettsial or ehrlichial infections in which tetracyclines cannot be used because of hypersensitivity or pregnancy. Its central nervous system (CNS) penetration and activity against anaerobes continue to lend support to its use in brain abscess. In some developing countries, chloramphenicol use is more extensive because of its low cost and proven efficacy in diseases such as typhoid fever and bacterial meningitis.

Macrolides

Ribosomal binding blocks translocation

The macrolides, **erythromycin, azithromycin,** and **clarithromycin,** differ in the exact composition of a large 14- or 15-member ring structure. They affect protein synthesis at the ribosomal level by binding to the 50S subunit and blocking the translocation reaction. Their effect is primarily bacteriostatic. Macrolides, which are concentrated in phagocytes and other cells, are effective against some intracellular pathogens.

Erythromycin is active against Gram-positives and *Legionella*

Erythromycin, the first and still the most commonly used macrolide, has a spectrum of activity that includes most of the pathogenic Gram-positive bacteria and some Gram-negative organisms. The Gram-negative spectrum includes *Neisseria, Bordetella, Campylobacter,* and *Legionella,* but not the Enterobacteriaceae. Erythromycin is also effective against *Chlamydia* and *Mycoplasma.*

Azithromycin and clarithromycin have enhanced Gram-negative spectrum

Bacteria that have developed resistance to erythromycin are usually resistant to the newer macrolides azithromycin and clarithromycin as well. These newer agents have the same spectrum as erythromycin, with some significant additions. Azithromycin has quantitatively greater activity (lower MICs) against most of the same Gram-negative bacteria. Clarithromycin is the most active of the three against both Gram-positive and Gram-negative pathogens. Clarithromycin is also active against mycobacteria. In addition, both azithromycin and clarithromycin have demonstrated efficacy against *Borrelia burgdorferi,* the causal agent of Lyme disease and the protozoan parasite *Toxoplasma gondii,* which causes toxoplasmosis.

Clindamycin

Spectrum is similar to macrolides with addition of anaerobes

Clindamycin is chemically unrelated to the macrolides but has a similar mode of action and spectrum. It has greater activity than the macrolides against Gram-negative anaerobes, including the important *Bacteroides fragilis* group. Although clindamycin is a perfectly adequate substitute for a macrolide in many situations, its primary use is in instances where anaerobes are or may be involved.

Oxazolidinones

Activity against Gram-positive bacteria resistant to other agents

Linezolid is the most widely used of a new class of antibiotics that act by binding to the bacterial 50S ribosome. The exact mechanism is not known, but it does not involve peptide elongation or termination of translation. Oxazolidinones are clinically useful in pneumonia and other soft tissue infections, particularly those caused by resistant strains of staphylococci, pneumococci, and enterococci.

Streptogramins

Useful against vancomycin-resistant enterococci

Quinupristin and dalfopristin are used in a fixed combination known as **quinupristin-dalfopristin** in a synergistic ratio. They inhibit protein synthesis by binding to different sites on the 50S bacterial ribosome; quinupristin inhibits peptide chain elongation, and dalfopristin interferes with peptidyl transferase. Their clinical use thus far has been limited to treatment of vancomycin-resistant enterococci.

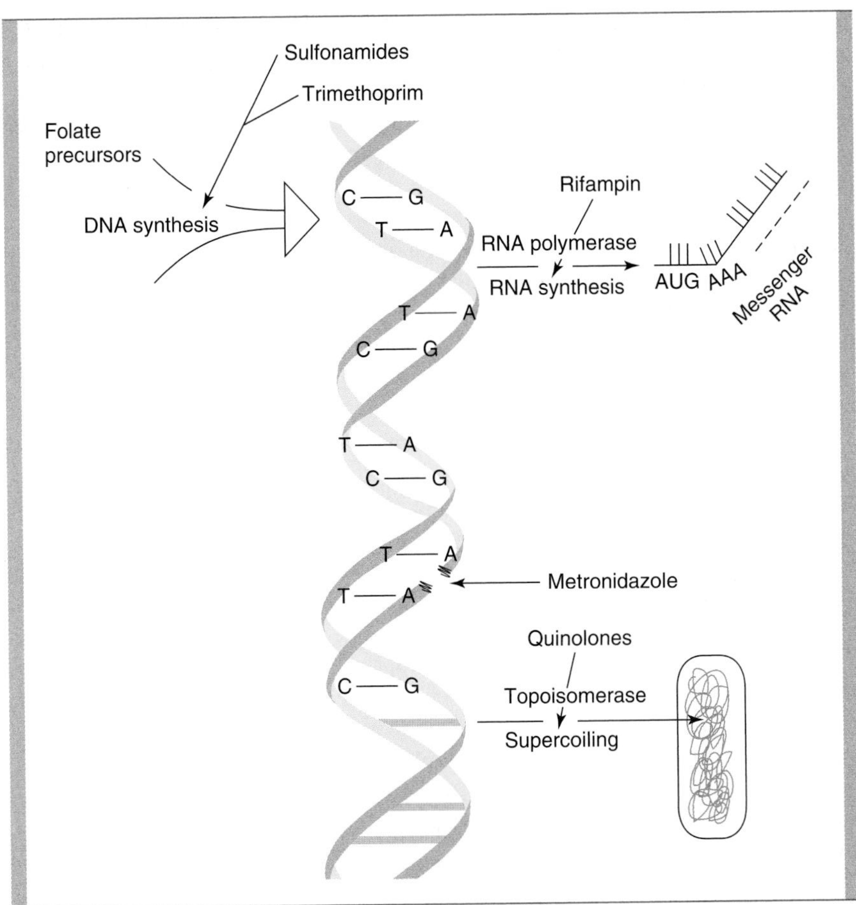

FIGURE 13–4
Diagrammatic representation of antimicrobials acting on nucleic acids. Sulfonamides block the folate precursors of DNA synthesis, metronidazole inflicts breaks in the DNA itself, rifampin inhibits the synthesis of RNA from DNA by inhibiting RNA polymerase, and quinolones inhibit DNA topoisomerase and thus prevent the supercoiling required for the DNA to "fit" inside the bacterial cell.

Inhibitors of Nucleic Acid Synthesis (Fig 13–4)

Quinolones

The quinolones have a nucleus of two fused six-member rings that when substituted with fluorine become fluoroquinolones, which are now the dominant quinolones for treatment of bacterial infections. Among the fluoroquinolones, **ciprofloxacin, norfloxacin,** and **ofloxacin,** the addition of a piperazine ring and its methylation alter the activity and pharmacologic properties of the individual compound. The primary target of all quinolones is DNA topoisomerase (gyrase), the enzyme responsible for nicking, supercoiling, and sealing bacterial DNA during replication. Bacterial topoisomerases have four subunits, one or more of which are inhibited by the particular quinolone. The enhanced activity and lower frequency of resistance seen with the fluoroquinolones is attributed to binding at multiple sites on the enzyme. This greatly reduces the chance a single mutation can lead to resistance, which was a problem with the first quinolone, nalidixic acid, a single-binding site agent.

Fluorinated derivatives are now dominant

Inhibition of topoisomerase blocks supercoiling

The fluoroquinolones are highly active and bactericidal against a wide range of aerobes and facultative anaerobes. However, streptococci and *Mycoplasma* are only marginally susceptible, and anaerobes are generally resistant. Ofloxacin has significant activity against *Chlamydia,* whereas ciprofloxacin is particularly useful against *P. aeruginosa.* Fluoroquinolones has several favorable pharmacologic properties in addition to their broad spectrum. These include oral administration, low protein binding, good distribution to all body compartments, penetration of phagocytes, and a prolonged serum half-life that allows once- or twice-a-day dosing. Norfloxacin and ciprofloxacin are excreted by hepatic and renal routes, resulting in high drug concentrations in the bile and urine. Ofloxacin is excreted primarily by the kidney.

Fluoroquinolones have a broad spectrum, including *Pseudomonas*

Well distributed after oral administration

Folate Inhibitors

Agents that interfere with synthesis of folic acid by bacteria have selective toxicity because mammalian cells are unable to accomplish this feat and use preformed folate

Bacteria must synthesize folate that humans acquire in their diet

from dietary sources. Folic acid is derived from *para*-aminobenzoic acid (PABA), glutamate, and a pteridine unit. In its reduced form, it is an essential coenzyme for the transport of one-carbon compounds in the synthesis of purines, thymidine, some amino acids, and, thus, indirectly of nucleic acids and proteins. The major inhibitors of the folate pathway are the sulfonamides, trimethoprim, *para*-aminosalicylic acid, and the sulfones.

Competition with PABA disrupts nucleic acids

Sulfonamides Sulfonamides are structural analogs of PABA and compete with it for the enzyme (dihydropteroate synthetase) that combines PABA and pteridine in the initial stage of folate synthesis. This blockage has multiple effects on the bacterial cells; the most important of these is disruption of nucleic acid synthesis. The effect is bacteriostatic, and the addition of PABA to a medium that contains sulfonamide neutralizes the inhibitory effect and allows growth to resume.

Major use is urinary tract infections

When introduced in the 1940s, sulfonamides had a very broad spectrum (staphylococci, streptococci, many Gram-negative bacteria) but resistance developed quickly, and this has restricted their use for systemic infections. Now their primary use is for uncomplicated urinary tract infections caused by members of the Enterobacteriaceae, particularly *Escherichia coli.* Sulfonamides are convenient for this purpose because they are inexpensive, well absorbed by the oral route, and excreted in high levels in the urine.

Dihydrofolate reductase inhibition is synergistic with sulfonamides

Trimethoprim-Sulfamethoxazole Trimethoprim acts on the folate synthesis pathway but at a point after sulfonamides. It competitively inhibits the activity of bacterial dihydrofolate reductase, which catalyzes the conversion of folate to its reduced active coenzyme form. When combined with sulfamethoxazole, a sulfonamide, trimethoprim leads to a two-stage blockade of the folate pathway, which often results in synergistic bacteriostatic or bactericidal effects. This quality is exploited in therapeutic preparations that combine both agents in a fixed proportion designed to yield optimum synergy.

Activity against common bacteria and some fungi

Trimethoprim-sulfamethoxazole (TMP-SMX) has a much broader and stable spectrum than either of its components alone; this includes most of the common pathogens, whether they are Gram-positive or Gram-negative, cocci or bacilli. Anaerobes and *P. aeruginosa* are exceptions. It is also active against some uncommon agents such as *Nocardia*. TMP-SMX is widely and effectively used in the treatment of urinary tract infections, otitis media, sinusitis, prostatitis, and infectious diarrhea, and it the agent of choice for pneumonia caused by *Pneumocystis carinii,* a fungus.

Metronidazole

Metronidazole is a nitroimidazole, a family of compounds with activity against bacteria, fungi, and parasites. The antibacterial action requires reduction of the nitro group under anaerobic conditions, which explains the limitation of its activity to bacteria that prefer anaerobic or at least microaerophilic growth conditions. The reduction products act on the cell at multiple points; the most lethal of these effects is induction of breaks in DNA strands.

Action requires anaerobic conditions

Metronidazole is active against a wide range of anaerobes, including *Bacteroides fragilis*. Clinically, it is useful for any infection in which anaerobes may be involved. Because these infections are typically polymicrobial, a second antimicrobial (eg, β-lactam) is usually added to cover aerobic and facultative bacteria.

Rifampin

Blocking of RNA synthesis occurs by binding to polymerase

Rifampin binds to the β-subunit of DNA-dependent RNA polymerase, which prevents the initiation of RNA synthesis. This agent is active against most Gram-positive bacteria and selected Gram-negative organisms, including *Neisseria* and *Haemophilus* but not members of the Enterobacteriaceae. The most clinically useful property of rifampin is its antimycobacterial activity, which includes *Mycobacterium tuberculosis* and the other species that most commonly infect humans. Because resistance by mutation of the polymerase readily occurs, rifampin is combined with other agents in the treatment of active infections. It is used alone for chemoprophylaxis.

Antimicrobics Acting on the Outer and Cytoplasmic Membranes

The polypeptide antimicrobics **polymyxin B** and **colistin** have a cationic detergent-like effect. They bind to the cell membranes of susceptible Gram-negative bacteria and alter their permeability, resulting in loss of essential cytoplasmic components and bacterial death. These agents react to a lesser extent with cell membranes of the host, resulting in nephrotoxicity and neurotoxicity. Their spectrum is essentially Gram-negative; they act against *P. aeruginosa* and other Gram-negative rods. Although these antimicrobics were used for systemic treatment in the past, their use is now limited to topical applications. They have an advantage; resistance to them rarely develops.

Binding to cytoplasmic membrane occurs

Other Agents

Several other effective antimicrobics are in use almost exclusively for a single infectious agent or types of infections such as tuberculosis, urinary tract infections, and anaerobic infections. Where appropriate, these agents will be discussed in the relevant chapter. It is beyond the scope and intent of this book to provide comprehensive coverage of all available agents.

ANTIVIRAL THERAPY

GENERAL CONSIDERATIONS

Viruses are comprised of either DNA or RNA, a protein coat (capsid) and, in many, a lipid or lipoprotein envelope. The nucleic acid codes for enzymes involved in replication and for several structural proteins. Viruses use molecules (eg, amino acids, purines, pyrimidines) supplied by the cell and cellular structures (eg, ribosomes) for synthetic functions. Thus, one of the challenges in the development of antiviral agents is identification of the steps in viral replication that are unique to the virus and not used by the normal cell. Among the unique viral events are attachment, penetration, uncoating, RNA-directed DNA synthesis (reverse transcription), and assembly and release of the intact virion. Each of these steps may have complex elements with the potential for inhibition. For example, assembly of some virus particles requires a unique viral enzyme, protease, and this has led to the development of protease inhibitors.

Events in the cell unique to viral replication are the target

In some cases, antivirals do not selectively inhibit a unique replicative event but inhibit DNA polymerase. Inhibitors of this enzyme take advantage of the fact that the virus is synthesizing nucleic acids more rapidly than the cell, so there is relatively greater inhibition of viral than cellular DNA. In many acute viral infections, especially respiratory ones, the bulk of viral replication has already occurred when symptoms are beginning to appear. Initiating antiviral therapy at this stage is unlikely to make a major impact on the illness. For these viruses, immuno- or chemoprophylaxis, rather than therapy, is a more logical approach. However, many other viral infections are characterized by ongoing viral replication and do benefit from viral inhibition, such as human immunodeficiency virus (HIV) infection and chronic hepatitis B and C.

DNA polymerase is often inhibited

The principal antiviral agents in current use are discussed according to their modes of action. Their features are summarized in Table 13–2.

SELECTED ANTIVIRAL AGENTS

Inhibitors of Attachment

Attachment to a cell receptor is a virus-specific event. Antibody can bind to extracellular virus and prevent this attachment. However, although therapy with antibody is useful in prophylaxis, it has been minimally effective in treatment.

TABLE 13–2

Summary of Antiviral Agents

Mechanism of Action	Antiviral Agent	Viral Spectrum[a]
Inhibition of viral uncoating, penetration		
	Amantadine	Flu A
	Rimantadine	Flu A
Neuraminidase inhibition		
	Oseltamivir	Flu A, Flu B
	Zanamivir	Flu A, Flu B
Inhibition of viral DNA polymerase		
	Acyclovir	HSV, VZV
	Famciclovir	HSV, VZV
	Penciclovir	HSV
	Valacyclovir	HSV, VZV
	Ganciclovir	CMV, HSV, VZV
	Foscarnet	CMV, resistant HSV
	Cidofovir	CMV
	Trifluridine	HSV, VZV
Inhibition of viral reverse transcriptase		
	Zidovudine	HIV
	Dideoxyinosine	HIV
	Dideoxycytidine	HIV
	Stavudine	HIV
	Lamivudine	HIV, HBV[b]
	Nevirapine	HIV
	Delavirdine	HIV
	Efavirenz	HIV
Inhibition of viral protease		
	Saquinavir	HIV
	Indinavir	HIV
	Ritonavir	HIV
	Nelfinavir	HIV
	Lopinavir	HIV
Inhibition of viral protein synthesis		
	Interferon α	HBV, HCV, HPV
Inhibition of viral RNA polymerase		
	Ribavirin	RSV, HCV,[b] Lassa fever
Antisense inhibition of viral mRNA synthesis		
	Fomivirsen	CMV

[a] Flu A, influenza A; Flu B, influenza B; HSV, herpes simplex viruses; VZV, varicella-zoster virus; CMV, cytomegalovirus; HIV, human immunodeficiency virus; HBV, hepatitis B virus; HCV, hepatitis C virus; RSV, respiratory syncytial virus; HPV, human papillomavirus.

[b] Used in combination with interferon.

Inhibitors of Cell Penetration and Uncoating

Rimantadine differs from **amantadine** by the substitution of a methyl group for a hydrogen ion. These two amines inhibit several early steps in viral replication, including viral uncoating. They are extremely selective, with activity against only influenza A. In addition, they are effective in preventing influenza but are less useful in treatment of this viral infection due in part to the brief period of viral replication.

Amantadine and rimantadine are symmetrical amines, or acyclics, that inhibit early steps in replication

Effective only against influenza A viruses

Pharmacology and Toxicity

Both amantadine and rimantadine are available only as oral preparations. The pharmacokinetics of the two agents is quite different. Amantadine is excreted by the kidney without being metabolized and its dose must be decreased in patients with impaired renal function. In contrast, rimantadine is metabolized by the liver and then excreted in the kidney and dosage adjustment for renal failure is not necessary.

Amantadine is excreted by the kidney

Rimantadine is metabolized by the liver

Treatment

In healthy adults or children, amantadine and rimantadine show a slight but statistically significant improvement in symptoms compared to placebos or antipyretics. It has been assumed but not proved that these drugs are efficacious for treatment of influenza in elderly or other high-risk patients who may have more severe influenza. Influenza A strains resistant to these agents may appear rapidly in patients treated for clinical illness. Such strains can spread to patients receiving the drug prophylactically and can impair its efficacy as a preventive.

Viral resistance can appear rapidly

Prophylaxis

The acyclics amantadine and rimantadine are approximately 70% effective in preventing influenza A illness when given daily during influenza outbreaks. Although illness is prevented or diminished, patients may still develop evidence of infection (ie, antibody), which is desirable because this antibody may provide some protection against future influenza A infection. These agents may be given alone or with vaccine. In the latter case, they may be given only until vaccine-induced antibody develops (eg, approximately 2 weeks) or they may be continued if a vaccine response is expected to be poor or marginal.

Useful in prophylaxis of influenza A

Neuraminidase Inhibitors

Oseltamivir and **zanamivir** are new antivirals that selectively inhibit the neuraminidase of influenza A and B viruses. The neuraminidase cleaves terminal sialic acid from glycoconjugates and plays a role in the release of virus from infected cells. Zanamivir was the first approved neuraminidase inhibitor. It is given by oral inhalation using a specially designed device. Oseltamivir phosphate is the oral prodrug of oseltamivir, a drug comparable to zanamivir in antineuraminidase activity.

Treatment with either oseltamivir and zanamivir reduces influenza symptoms and shortens the course of illness by 1 to 1.5 days. The activity of these compounds against both influenza A and B offers an advantage over amantadine and rimantadine, which are active only against influenza A.

Neuraminidase inhibitors are effective in treatment and prophylaxis of influenza A and B viruses

Inhibitors of Nucleic Acid Synthesis

At present, most antiviral agents are nucleoside analogs that are active against virus-specific nucleic acid polymerases or transcriptases and have much less activity against analogous host enzymes. Some of these agents serve as nucleic acid chain terminators after incorporation into nucleic acids.

Idoxuridine and Trifluorothymidine

Idoxuridine (5-iodo-2′-deoxyuridine, IUdR) is a halogenated pyrimidine that blocks nucleic acid synthesis by being incorporated into DNA in place of thymidine and producing a nonfunctional molecule (ie, by terminating synthesis of the nucleic acid chain). It is phosphorylated by thymidine kinase to the active compound. Unfortunately, it inhibits both viral and cellular DNA synthesis, and the resulting host toxicity precludes systemic administration in humans. Idoxuridine can be used topically as effective treatment of herpetic infection of the cornea (keratitis). **Trifluorothymidine,** a related pyrimidine analog, is effective in treating herpetic corneal infections, including those that fail to respond to IUdR. It has largely replaced idoxuridine.

Idoxuridine and trifluorothymidine block DNA synthesis

Acyclovir

This antiviral agent differs from the nucleoside guanosine by having an acyclic (hydroxyethoxymethyl) side chain. Acyclovir is unique in that it must be phosphorylated by thymidine kinase to be active, and this phosphorylation occurs only in cells infected by certain herpesviruses. Therefore, the compound is essentially nontoxic, because it is not phosphorylated or activated in uninfected host cells. Viral thymidine kinase catalyzes the phosphorylation of acyclovir to a monophosphate. From that point, host cell enzymes complete the progression to the diphosphate and finally the triphosphate.

Activity of acyclovir against herpesviruses directly correlates with the capacity of the virus to induce a thymidine kinase. Herpes simplex virus types 1 and 2 (HSV-1 and HSV-2) are the most active thymidine kinase inducers and are the most readily inhibited by acyclovir. Cytomegalovirus (CMV) induces little or no thymidine kinase and is not inhibited. Varicella-zoster and Epstein-Barr viruses are between these two extremes in terms of both thymidine kinase induction and acyclovir susceptibility.

Acyclovir is effective against herpesviruses that induce thymidine kinase

Acyclovir triphosphate inhibits viral replication by competing with guanosine triphosphate and inhibiting the function of the virally encoded DNA polymerase. The selectivity and minimal toxicity of acyclovir is aided by its 100-fold or greater affinity for viral DNA polymerase than for cellular DNA polymerase. A second mechanism of viral inhibition results from incorporation of acyclovir triphosphate into the growing viral DNA chain. This causes termination of chain growth, because there is no 3′-hydroxy group on the acyclovir molecule to provide attachment sites for additional nucleotides. Resistant strains of HSV have been recovered from immunocompromised patients, including patients with acquired immunodeficiency syndrome (AIDS), and in most instances, resistance results from mutations in the viral thymidine kinase gene, rendering it inactive in phosphorylation. Resistance may also result from mutations in the viral DNA polymerase. Resistant virus has rarely, if ever, been recovered from immunocompetent patients, even after years of drug exposure.

Inhibits viral DNA polymerase and terminates viral DNA chain growth

Pharmacology and Toxicity Acyclovir is available in three forms: topical, oral, and parenteral. Topical acyclovir is rarely used. The oral form has low bioavailability (approximately 10%) but achieves concentrations in blood that inhibit HSV and to a lesser extent varicella-zoster virus (VZV). Intravenous acyclovir is used for serious HSV infection (eg, congenital), encephalitis, and VZV infection in immunocompromised patients. Because acyclovir is excreted by the kidney, the dosage must be reduced in patients with renal failure. CNS and renal toxicity have been reported in patients treated with prolonged high intravenous doses. Acyclovir is remarkably free of bone marrow toxicity, even in patients with hematopoietic disorders.

Inhibits herpes viruses in blood

Treatment and Prophylaxis Acyclovir is effective in the treatment of primary HSV mucocutaneous infections or for severe recurrences in immunocompromised patients. The agent is also useful in neonatal infectious herpes encephalitis, and it is also recommended for VZV infection in immunocompromised patients and varicella in older children or adults. Acyclovir is beneficial against herpes zoster in elderly patients or any patient with eye involvement. In patients with frequent severe genital herpes, the oral form is effective in preventing recurrences. Because it does not eliminate the virus from the host, it must be taken daily to be effective. Acyclovir is minimally effective in the treatment of recurrent genital or labial herpes in otherwise healthy individuals.

Effective against herpes and zoster

Valacyclovir, Famciclovir, and Penciclovir

Valacyclovir is a prodrug of acyclovir that is better absorbed and therefore can be used in lower and less frequent dosage. Once absorbed, it becomes acyclovir. It is currently approved for use in HSV and VZV infections in immunocompetent adult patients. Dosage adjustment is necessary in patients with impaired renal function.

Famciclovir is similar to acyclovir in its structure and requirement for phosphorylation but differs slightly in its mode of action. After absorption, the agent is converted to penciclovir, the active moiety, which is also a competitive inhibitor of a guanosine triphosphate. However, it does not irreversibly terminate DNA replication. Famciclovir is currently approved for treatment of HSV and VZV infections. **Penciclovir,** itself, is approved for topical treatment of recurrent herpes labialis.

Agents that are similar to or become acyclovir after absorption are available

Ganciclovir

Ganciclovir (DHPG), a nucleoside analog of guanosine, differs from acyclovir by a single carboxyl side chain. This structural change confers approximately 50 times more activity against CMV. Acyclovir has low activity against CMV, because it is not well phosphorylated in CMV-infected cells due to the absence of the gene for thymidine kinase in CMV. However, ganciclovir is active against CMV and does not require thymidine kinase for phosphorylation. Instead, another viral-encoded phosphorylating enzyme (UL97) is present in CMV-infected cells that is capable of phosphorylating ganciclovir and converting it to the monophosphate. Then cellular enzymes convert it to the active compound, ganciclovir triphosphate, which inhibits the viral DNA polymerase.

Ganciclovir does not require viral thymidine kinase for phosphorylation

Oral ganciclovir is available but is inferior to the intravenous form. Oral valganciclovir, a prodrug of ganciclovir, has improved bioavailability and is equivalent to the intravenous form. Toxicity frequently limits therapy. Neutropenia, which is usually reversible, may occur early but often develops during later therapy. Discontinuation of therapy is necessary in patients whose neutrophils do not increase during dosage reduction or in response to cytokines. Thrombocytopenia (platelet count $<20,000/mm^3$) occurs in approximately 15% of patients.

Neutropenia and thrombocytopenia limit use

Clinical Use Administration of ganciclovir is indicated for the treatment of active CMV infection in immunocompromised patients, but other herpesviruses (particularly HSV-1, HSV-2, and VZV) are also susceptible. Because AIDS patients with severe CMV infection frequently have concurrent illnesses caused by other herpesviruses, treatment with ganciclovir may benefit associated HSV and VZV infections.

Resistance After several months of continuous ganciclovir therapy for treatment of CMV, between 5 and 10% of AIDS patients excrete resistant strains of CMV. In virtually all isolates, there is a mutation in the phosphorylating gene, and in a lesser number there may also be a mutation in the viral DNA polymerase. The great majority of these strains remains sensitive to foscarnet, which may be used as alternate therapy. If only a UL97 mutation is present, the strains remain susceptible to cidofovir; however, most of the strains with a ganciclovir-induced mutation in DNA polymerase are cross-resistant to cidofovir. Many clinicians tend to assume that when a patient with CMV retinitis has progression of the disease during treatment, viral resistance has developed. Progression of CMV disease during treatment is probably the result of many factors, only one of which is the susceptibility of the CMV strain to the drug. Blood and tissue concentrations of ganciclovir, penetration of ganciclovir into the retinal tissue, and the host immune response probably play important roles in determining when clinical progression of CMV disease occurs. Ganciclovir resistance is beginning to be noted in transplant recipients, especially those requiring prolonged treatment.

CMV mutant resistance increases with continuous therapy

Inhibitor of Viral RNA Synthesis: Ribavirin

Ribavirin is another analog of the nucleoside guanosine. Unlike acyclovir, which replaces the ribose moiety with an hydroxymethyl acyclic side chain, ribavirin differs from guanosine in that the base ring is incomplete and open. Like other purine nucleoside analogs, ribavirin must be phosphorylated to mono-, di-, and triphosphate forms. It is active against a broad range of viruses in vitro, but its in vivo activity is limited. The mechanism of the antiviral effect of ribavirin is not as clear as that of acyclovir. The triphosphate is an inhibitor of RNA polymerase and it also depletes cellular stores of guanine by inhibiting inosine monophosphate dehydrogenase, an enzyme important in the synthetic pathway of guanosine. Still another mode of action is by decreasing synthesis of the mRNA 5′ cap because of interference with both guanylation and methylation of the nucleic acid base.

Ribavirin has several modes of action

Aerosol administration enables ribavirin to reach concentrations in respiratory secretions up to ten times greater than necessary to inhibit viral replication and substantially higher than those achieved with oral administration. Problems encountered with aerosolized ribavirin include precipitation of the agent in tubing used for administration and exposure of health care personnel.

Ribavirin is somewhat beneficial if given early by aerosol to infants who are infected with respiratory syncytial virus. Oral and intravenous forms have been used for patients with Lassa fever, although studies have been limited. In a recent trial of hantavirus treatment, ribavirin was ineffective. The oral form has limited activity against hepatitis C as monotherapy but provides additional benefit when combined with interferon alpha. A reversible anemia has been associated with oral administration of ribavirin.

Ribavirin is active against respiratory syncytial virus, Lassa fever virus, and hepatitis C

Inhibitors of HIV

Nucleoside Reverse Transcriptase Inhibitors

Azidothymidine Azidothymidine (AZT), a nucleoside analog of thymidine, inhibits the reverse transcriptase of HIV. As with other nucleosides, AZT must be phosphorylated; host cell enzymes carry out the process. The basis for the relatively selective therapeutic effect of AZT is that HIV reverse transcriptase is more than 100 times more sensitive to AZT than is host cell DNA polymerase. Nonetheless, toxicity frequently occurs.

AZT was the first useful treatment for HIV infection but now is recommended for use only in combination with other inhibitors of HIV replication (eg, lamivudine and protease inhibitors). Toxicity includes malaise, nausea, and bone marrow toxicity. All hematopoietic components may be depressed but usually reverse with discontinuation of the drug or dose reduction. Resistance is associated with one or more mutations in the HIV reverse transcriptase gene.

AZT is now used only in combination therapy

Didanosine and Zalcitabine Didanosine (ddI, dideoxyinosine) and zalcitabine (ddC, dideoxycytidine) are nucleoside analogs that inhibit HIV replication. Following intracellular phosphorylation by host enzymes to their active triphosphate form, they block viral replication by inhibiting viral reverse transcriptase, like zidovudine. Serious adverse effects of treatment include peripheral neuropathy with either ddI or ddC, and pancreatitis with ddI; both conditions are dose related. Dose reduction is required for impaired renal function. As with other anti-HIV drugs, these agents should be used only in combination with one or two other anti-HIV drugs to limit the development of resistance and to enhance antiviral effect.

ddI and ddC are always used in combination with other anti-HIV drugs

Stavudine Stavudine (D4T) is another nucleoside analog that inhibits HIV replication. D4T is phosphorylated by cellular enzymes to an active triphosphate form that interferes with viral reverse transcriptase, and it also terminates the growth of the chain of viral nucleic acid. D4T is well absorbed and has a high bioavailability. Adverse effects include headache, nausea and vomiting, asthenia, confusion, and elevated serum transaminase and creatinine kinase. A painful sensory peripheral neuropathy that appears to be dose related has also been noted. Dose reduction is required for impaired renal function. D4T should be used only in combination with other anti-HIV agents.

D4T is a reverse transcriptase inhibitor that also terminates chain growth

Lamivudine Lamivudine (3TC), another reverse transcriptase inhibitor, is a comparatively safe and usually well-tolerated agent and is used in combination with AZT or other

3TC suppresses development of AZT resistance

nucleoside analogs. AZT and 3TC have a unique interaction; 3TC suppresses the development and persistence of AZT resistance mutations. When combined with interferon alpha, 3TC is also useful for treating hepatitis B.

Non-Nucleoside Reverse Transcriptase Inhibitors (NNRTIs)

Compounds that are not nucleoside analogs also inhibit HIV reverse transcriptase. Several compounds, e.g., nevirapine, delavirdine, and efavirenz, have been evaluated alone or in combination with other nucleosides. These compounds are very active against HIV-1, do not require cellular enzymes to be phosphorylated, and bind to essentially the same site on reverse transcriptase. They are active against both AZT-resistant and AZT-sensitive isolates. In addition, most of these compounds do not inhibit human DNA polymerase and are not cytotoxic at concentrations required for effective antiviral activity; therefore, they are relatively nontoxic. Unfortunately, drug resistance readily emerges with even single passage of virus in the presence of drug in vitro and in vivo. Thus, NNRTIs should only be used in combination regimens with other drugs active against HIV.

NNRTIs are often active against AZT-resistant strains

Rapid development of drug resistance occur when NNRTIs are used alone

Protease Inhibitors

The newest agents that inhibit HIV are the protease inhibitors. These agents block the action of the viral-encoded enzyme protease, which cleaves polyproteins to produce structural proteins. Inhibition of this enzyme leads to blockage of viral assembly and release. The protease inhibitors are potent suppressors of HIV replication in vitro and in vivo, particularly when combined with other antiretroviral agents.

In late 1995, **saquinavir** was the first protease inhibitor to receive approval. **Ritonavir, indinavir,** and **nelfinavir** are other potent protease inhibitors that have since been released. These drugs may cause hepatotoxicity and all agents inhibit P450, resulting in important drug interactions. Because drug resistance develops to all protease inhibitors, they should not be used alone without other anti-HIV drugs.

Protease inhibitors block viral-encoded proteases

Used in combination with other anti-HIV drugs

Nucleotide Analogs: Cidofovir

In recent years a new series of antiviral compounds, the nucleotide analogs, have been developed. The best known example of this class of compounds is **cidofovir.** This compound mimics a monophosphorylated nucleotide by having a phosphonate group attached to the molecule. This appears to the cell as a nucleoside monophosphate, or nucleotide, and cellular enzymes then add two phosphate groups to generate the active compound. In this form, the drug inhibits both viral and cellular nucleic acid polymerases but selectivity is provided by its higher affinity for the viral enzyme.

Nucleotide analogs do not require phosphorylation, or activation, by a viral-encoded enzyme and remain active against viruses that are resistant due to mutations in codons for these enzymes. Resistance can develop with mutations in the viral DNA polymerase, UL54. An additional feature of cidofovir is a very prolonged half-life, due to slow clearance by the kidneys.

Cidofovir inhibits viral DNA polymerase

Cidofovir is approved for intravenous therapy of CMV retinitis, and maintenance treatment may be given as infrequently as every 2 weeks. Nephrotoxicity is a serious complication of cidofovir treatment, and patients must be monitored carefully for evidence of renal impairment.

Other Antiviral Agents

Foscarnet

Foscarnet, also known as phosphonoformate, is a pyrophosphate analog that inhibits viral DNA polymerase by blocking the pyrophosphate-binding site of the viral DNA polymerase and preventing cleavage of pyrophosphate from deoxyadenosine triphosphate. This action is relatively selective; CMV DNA polymerase is inhibited at concentrations less than 1% of that required to inhibit cellular DNA polymerase. Unlike such nucleosides as acyclovir and ganciclovir, foscarnet does not require phosphorylation to be an active inhibitor of viral DNA polymerases. This biochemical fact becomes especially important with regard to viral resistance, because the principal mode of viral resistance to nucleoside analogs is a mutation that eliminates phosphorylation of the drug in virus-infected cells. Thus, foscarnet can usually be used to treat patients with ganciclovir-resistant CMV and acyclovir-resistant HSV. Excretion is entirely renal without a hepatic component, and dosage must be decreased in patients with impaired renal function.

Foscarnet inhibits viral DNA polymerases

Effective against resistant CMV and HSV

Interferons

Recombinant DNA techniques allow large-scale production

Interferons inhibit viral protein synthesis

Interferons are host cell–encoded proteins synthesized in response to double-stranded RNA that circulate to protect uninfected cells by inhibiting viral protein synthesis. Ironically, interferons harvested in tissue culture were the first antiviral agents, but their clinical activity was disappointing. Recombinant DNA techniques now allow relatively inexpensive large-scale production of interferons by bacteria and yeasts.

Interferon alpha is combined with ribavirin to treat chronic hepatitis C

Interferon alpha is beneficial in the treatment of chronic active hepatitis B and C infection, although its efficacy is often transient. Combinations of interferon alpha with 3TC, famciclovir, and other nucleosides are being evaluated for treatment of hepatitis B. Interferon alpha is given for 6 to 12 months to treat chronic hepatitis C disease, and combination with ribavirin usually produces improved results. Topical interferon application is beneficial in the treatment of human papilloma virus infections. Interferons cause symptomatic systemic toxicity, (eg, fever, malaise), partly because of their effect on host cell protein synthesis.

Fomivirsen

Fomivirsen inhibits CMV mRNA

Fomivirsen, the first antisense compound to be approved for use in human infection, is a synthetic oligonucleotide, complementary to and presumably inhibiting a coding sequence in CMV messenger RNA (mRNA). The major immediate early transcriptional unit of CMV encodes several proteins responsible for regulation of viral gene expression. Presumably, fomivirsen inhibits production of these proteins. In this agent, oligonucleotide phosphorothioate linkages replace the usual nucleases. Fomivirsen, which exhibits greater antiviral activity than ganciclovir on a molar basis, is approved for the local (intravitreal) therapy of CMV retinitis in patients who have failed other therapies.

ANTIVIRAL RESISTANCE

Herpesviruses often develop resistance by mutations in phosphorylation

Viral genomes and their replication, as well as the mechanisms of action of the available antiviral agents, have been intensively studied. Accordingly, an understanding of resistance to antiviral drugs has evolved; investigation of resistance mechanisms has shed light on the function of specific viral genes. For example, it has become clear that a common mechanism of resistance to nucleosides (eg, acyclovir, ganciclovir) by herpesviruses are mutations in the viral-induced enzyme responsible for phosphorylating the nucleoside. For herpes simplex virus, this is thymidine kinase, and for CMV, this gene is designated UL97.

Genetic alterations (ie, mutations or deletions) are the basis for antiviral resistance. The likelihood of resistant mutants results from at least four functions:

1. **Rate of viral replication.** Herpesviruses, especially CMV and VZV do not replicate as rapidly as HIV and hepatitis B and C. Higher rates of replication are associated with higher rates of spontaneous mutations.
2. **Selective pressure of the drug.** The selective pressure increases the probability of mutations to the point that virus replication is substantially reduced.
3. **Rate of viral mutations.** In addition to viral replication, the rate of mutations differs among different viruses. In general, single-stranded RNA viruses (eg, HIV, influenza) have more rapid rates of mutation than double-stranded DNA viruses (eg, herpesviruses).

4. **Rates of mutation in differing viral genes.** For example, within the herpesviruses, the genes for phosphorylating nucleosides (eg, UL97) are more susceptible to mutation than the viral DNA polymerase.
   Resistance to antivirals may be detected in several ways:

   - **Phenotypic.** This is the traditional method of growing virus in tissue culture in medium containing increasing concentrations of an antiviral agent. The concentration of the agent that reduces viral replication by 50% is the end point; it is referred to as the inhibitory concentration (IC_{50}). The IC_{50} of resistant virus is higher than that of susceptible virus. The degree of viral replication is obtained by counting viral plaques (ie, equivalent to viral "colonies") or by measuring viral antigen or nucleic acid concentration. Unfortunately, phenotypic assays are very time-consuming, requiring days to weeks for completion. IC_{50} values increase as the percent of the viral population with the mutation increases.

Phenotypic resistance is detected by in vitro methods

   - **Genotypic.** When the exact mutation or deletion responsible for antiviral resistance is known, it is possible to sequence the viral gene or detect it with restriction enzyme patterns. These tests are rapid but require knowledge of the expected mutation, and they do not provide quantitation of the percent of the viral population harboring the mutation. If only 1 or 5% of the population has the mutation, this result may not be clinically significant when compared to a virus population that is 90% mutated.

Genotypic = molecular detection of expected mutation

   - **Viral quantitation in response to treatment.** Various methods of quantitating virus (eg, culture, polymerase chain reaction, antigen assay) provide a means of assessing the decline of viral titer in response to treatment with an antiviral agent. These assays are rapid and do not require knowledge of the expected mutation. If no decline occurs despite adequate dosage and compliance, viral resistance may be responsible. Likewise, if viral titer initially decreases but subsequently recurs and/or increases, then resistance may have developed.

No reduction or increase in patient's viral burden suggests development of resistant mutants

ADDITIONAL READING

Balfour HH Jr. Antiviral drugs. *N Engl J Med* 1999;340:1255–1268. An excellent review of antivirals other than those used to treat HIV infections.

Hardman JG, Limbird LE, eds. *Goodman and Gilman's The Pharmacological Basis of Therapeutics.* 10th ed. New York: McGraw-Hill; 2001. A standard reference text with excellent sections on antibiotics and chemotherapy.

Mandell GL, Bennett JE, Dolin R, eds. *Mandell, Douglas, and Bennett's Principles and Practice of Infectious Diseases,* 5th ed. Philadelphia: Churchill Livingstone; 2002. This reference work discusses the mechanisms and clinical use of each antimicrobic in an individual chapter.

CHAPTER 14

Antimicrobial Resistance

KENNETH J. RYAN

The continuing success of antimicrobial therapy depends on keeping ahead of the ability of the microorganisms to develop resistance to antimicrobics. At times, resistance seems to occur at a rate equal to that of the development of new antimicrobics. The nature of resistance and the mechanisms bacteria use to achieve it are the subject of this chapter. The ways in which resistance affect medical practice and the way in which laboratory tests are used to guide clinicians through the uncertainties of modern treatment are also considered.

SUSCEPTIBILITY AND RESISTANCE

Deciding whether any bacterium should be considered susceptible or resistant to any antimicrobic involves an integrated assessment of in vitro activity, pharmacologic characteristics, and clinical evaluation. Any agent approved for clinical use has demonstrated in vitro its potential to inhibit the growth of some target group of bacteria at concentrations that can be achieved with acceptable risks of toxicity. That is, the minimal inhibitory concentration (MIC) can be comfortably exceeded by doses tolerated by the patient. Use of the antimicrobic in animal models and then human infections must have also demonstrated a therapeutic response. Because the influence of antimicrobics on the natural history of different categories of infection (eg, pneumonia, meningitis, diarrhea) varies, extensive clinical trials must include both a range of bacterial species and infected sites. These studies are important to determine whether what should work actually does work and, if so, to define the parameters of success and failure.

MICs must be below achievable blood levels

Clinical experience must validate in vitro data

Once these factors are established, the routine selection of therapy can be based on known or expected characteristics of organisms and pharmacologic features of antimicrobics. With regard to organisms, use of the term **susceptible** (sensitive) implies that their MIC is at a concentration attainable in the blood or other appropriate body fluid (eg, urine) using the usually recommended doses. **Resistant,** the converse of susceptible, implies that the MIC is not exceeded by normally attainable levels. As in all biological systems, the MIC of some organisms lies in between the susceptible and resistant levels. Borderline strains are called **intermediate, moderately sensitive,** or **moderately resistant,** depending on the exact values and conventions of the reporting system. Antimicrobics may be used to treat these organisms but at increased doses, perhaps to reach body compartments where pathogens are concentrated. For example, nontoxic antimicrobics such as the penicillins and cephalosporins can be administered in massive doses and may thereby inhibit some pathogens that would normally be considered resistant in vitro.

Susceptible bacteria are inhibited at achievable nontoxic levels, resistant strains are not

Borderline isolates are called intermediate

Furthermore, in urinary infections, urine levels of some antimicrobics may be very high, and organisms that are seemingly resistant in vitro may be eliminated.

Pharmacologic properties such as absorption, distribution, and metabolism affect the usefulness of antimicrobics

Important pharmacologic characteristics of antimicrobics include dosage as well as the routes and frequency of administration. Other characteristics include whether the agents are absorbed from the upper gastrointestinal tract, whether they are excreted and concentrated in active form in the urine, whether they can pass into cells, whether and how rapidly they are metabolized, and the duration of effective antimicrobial levels in blood and tissues. Most agents are bound to some extent to serum albumin, and the protein-bound form is usually unavailable for antimicrobial action. The amount of free to bound antibiotic can be expressed as an equilibrium constant, which varies for different antibiotics. In general, high degrees of binding lead to more prolonged but lower serum levels of an active antimicrobic after a single dose.

LABORATORY CONTROL OF ANTIMICROBIAL THERAPY

Bacteria are tested against antimicrobics over a range of concentrations

A unique feature of laboratory testing in microbiology is that the susceptibility of the isolate of an individual patient can be tested against a battery of potential antimicrobics. These tests are built around the common theme of placing the organism in the presence of varying concentrations of the antimicrobic in order to determine the MIC. The methods used are standardized, including a measured inoculum of the bacteria and the growth conditions (eg, medium, incubation, time).

Final selection of therapy considers susceptibility, pharmacology, and clinical experience

Bactericidal action is required for infections such as endocarditis

In selecting therapy, the results of laboratory tests cannot be considered by themselves, but must be examined with information about the clinical pharmacology of the agent, the cause of the disease, the site of infection, and the pathology of the lesion. These factors must all be taken into account when selecting the appropriate antimicrobic from those to which the organism has been reported as susceptible. If the agent cannot reach the site of infection, it will be ineffective. For example, the agent must reach the subarachnoid space and cerebrospinal fluid in the case of meningitis. Similarly, therapy may be ineffective for an infection that has resulted in abscess formation unless the abscess is surgically drained. In some instances (eg, bacterial endocarditis, agranulocytosis), it is necessary to use a bactericidal agent. Previous clinical experience is also critical. In typhoid fever, for instance, chloramphenicol is effective and aminoglycosides are not, even though the typhoid bacillus may be susceptible to both in vitro. This finding appears to result from the failure of aminoglycosides to achieve adequate concentrations inside infected cells.

Dilution Tests

MIC is the lowest concentration that inhibits growth

Dilution tests determine the MIC directly by using serial dilutions of the antimicrobic in broth that span a clinically significant range of concentrations. The dilutions are prepared in tubes or microdilution wells, and by convention, they are doubled using a base of 1 μg/mL (0.25, 0.5, 1, 2, 4, 8, and so on). The bacterial inoculum is adjusted to a concentration of 10^5 to 10^6 bacteria/mL and added to the broth. After incubation overnight (or other defined time), the tubes are examined for turbidity produced by bacterial growth. The first tube in which visible growth is absent (clear) is the MIC for that organism (Fig 14–1).

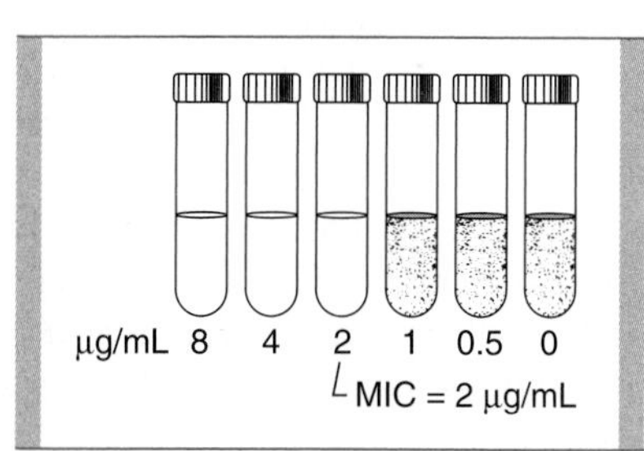

FIGURE 14–1
Broth dilution susceptibility test. The stippled tubes represent turbidity produced by bacterial growth. The MIC is 2 μg/mL.

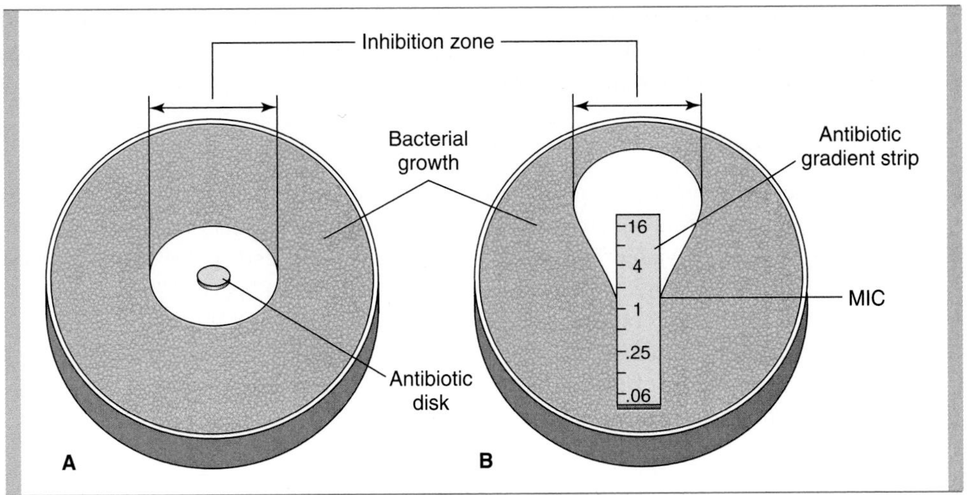

FIGURE 14–2
Diffusion tests. **A.** Disk diffusion. The diameter of the zone of growth inhibition around a disk of fixed antimicrobial content is inversely proportional to the minimum inhibitory concentration (MIC) for that antimicrobic. The larger the zone, the lower the MIC. **B.** The E test. A strip containing a gradient of antimicrobial content creates an elliptical zone of inhibition. The conditions are empirically adjusted so that the MIC is marked where the growth intersects the strip.

Diffusion Tests

In diffusion testing, the inoculum is seeded onto the surface of an agar plate, and filter paper disks containing defined amounts of antimicrobics are applied. While the plates are incubating, the antimicrobic diffuses into the medium to produce a circular gradient around the disk. After incubation overnight, the size of the zone of growth inhibition around the disk (Fig 14–2A) can be used as an indirect measure of the MIC of the organism. It is also influenced by the growth rate of the organism, the diffusibility of the antimicrobic, and some technical factors. In the United States, a standardized diffusion procedure accounts for these factors and includes recommendations for interpretation. The diameters of the zones of inhibition obtained with the various antibiotics are converted to "susceptible," "moderately susceptible," and "resistant" categories by referring to a table. This method is convenient and flexible for rapidly growing aerobic and facultative bacteria such as the Enterobacteriaceae, *Pseudomonas,* and staphylococci. Another diffusion procedure uses gradient strips to produce elliptical zones that can be directly correlated with the MIC. This method, the E test (Fig 14–2B), can also be applied to slow-growing, fastidious, and anaerobic bacteria.

Antimicrobic diffuses into agar from disks to produce a circular concentration gradient/24

The diameter of the inhibition zone around the disk is a measure of the MIC

Automated Tests

Instruments are now available that carry out rapid, automated variants of the broth dilution test. In these systems the bacteria are incubated with the antimicrobic in specialized modules that are read automatically every 15 to 30 minutes. The multiple readings and the increased sensitivity of determining endpoints by turbidimetric or fluorometric analysis makes it possible to generate MICs in as little as 4 hours. In laboratories with sufficient volume, these methods are no more expensive than manual methods, and the rapid results have enhanced potential to influence clinical outcome, particularly when interfaced with computerized hospital information systems.

Automated tests read endpoints of broth dilution tests in a few hours

Molecular Testing

The molecular techniques of nucleic acid hybridization, sequencing, and amplification (see Chapter 15) have been applied to the detection and study of resistance. The basic strategy is to detect the resistance gene rather than measure the phenotypic expression of resistance. These methods offer the prospect of automation and rapid results, but as with

Molecular methods detect resistance genes

most molecular methods, are not yet practical for routine use. Their application will also have to take consideration of the fact that they will be limited to known genes and that phenotypic expression is the "bottom line."

Bactericidal Testing

Quantitation of the bactericidal effect determines the MBC

The above methods do not distinguish between inhibitory and bactericidal activity. To do so requires quantitative subculture of the clear tubes in the broth dilution test and comparison of the number of viable bacteria at the beginning and end of the test. The least amount required to kill a predetermined portion of the inoculum (usually 99.9%) is called the **minimal bactericidal concentration (MBC).** Direct bactericidal testing is important in the initial characterization and clinical evaluation of antimicrobics but is rarely needed in individual cases. Most of the antimicrobics used for acute and life-threatening infections (eg, β-lactams, aminoglycosides) act by bactericidal mechanisms.

Antimicrobial Assays

Pharmacologic monitoring is necessary in some situations

For antimicrobics with toxicity near the therapeutic range, monitoring the concentration in the serum or other appropriate body fluid is sometimes necessary. Therapeutic monitoring may also be required when the patient's pharmacologic handling of the agent is unpredictable, as in renal failure. A variety of biologic, immunoassay, and chemical procedures have been developed for this purpose.

BACTERIAL RESISTANCE TO ANTIMICROBICS

Resistance has eroded the effectiveness of many agents

The seemingly perfect nature of antimicrobics, originally hailed as "wonder drugs," has been steadily eroded by the appearance of strains resistant to their action. This resistance may be inherent to the organism or appear in a previously susceptible species by mutation or the acquisition of new genes. The mechanisms by which bacteria develop resistance and how this resistance is spread are of great interest for the continued use of current agents and to develop strategies for the development of new antimicrobics. The following sections discuss the biochemical mechanisms of resistance, how resistance is genetically controlled, and how resistant strains survive and spread in our society. How these features relate to the antimicrobic groups is summarized in Table 14–1 and further discussed in the chapters on specific bacteria (see Chapters 16 to 32).

Resistance and virulence are separate properties

Antimicrobial resistance has survival value for the organism, and its expression in the medical setting requires that virulence be retained despite the change that mediates resistance. There are no direct connections between resistance and virulence. Resistant bacteria may have increased opportunities to produce disease, but the disease is the same as that produced by the susceptible bacteria's counterpart.

Mechanisms of Resistance

The major mechanisms of bacterial resistance are (1) accumulation barriers to an antimicrobic due to impermeability or active efflux; (2) alterations of an antimicrobic target, which render it insusceptible; and (3) inactivation of an antimicrobic by an enzyme produced by the microorganism. Changes in metabolic pathways can also translate into resistance in a few antimicrobic–organism combinations.

Accumulation Barriers (Fig 14–3)

Cell wall and outer membrane are barriers to antimicrobics

Outer membrane protein porins restrict access to interior

An effective antimicrobic must enter the bacterial cell and achieve concentrations sufficient to act on its target. The cell wall, particularly the outer membrane, of Gram-negative bacteria presents a formidable barrier for access to the interior of the cell. Outer membrane protein porin channels may allow penetration depending on the size, charge, degree of hydrophobicity, or general molecular configuration of the molecule. This is a major reason for inherent resistance to antimicrobics, but these transport characteristics may change even in typically susceptible species due to mutations in the porin proteins.

TABLE 14–1

Features of Bacterial Resistance to Antimicrobial Agents

	Mechanism[a]			Emerging Resistance[b]
Antimicrobic	Altered Accumulation (AA)	Altered Target (AT)	Enzymatic Inactivation (EI)	(Organism/Antimicrobic/Mechanism)
β-lactams	Variable outer membrane[c] penetration	Mutant and new PBPs	β-lactamases	*Staphylococus aureus*/penicillin/EI *S. aureus*/methicillin/AT *Streptococcus pneumoniae*/penicillin/AT *Haemophilus influenzae*/ampicillin/AT, EI *Neisseria gonorrhoeae*/penicillin/AT, EI *Pseudomonas aeruginosa*/ceftazidime/AA *Klebsiella, Enterobacter*/third-generation cephalosporins/EI
Glycopeptides	–	Amino acid substitution	–	*Enterococcus*/vancomycin/AT *S. aureus*/vancomycin (rare)
Aminoglycosides	Oxidative transport required	Ribosomal binding site mutations	Adenylases, acetylases, phosphorylases	*Klebsiella, Enterobacter*/gentamicin/EI *P. aeruginosa*/gentamicin/AA
Macrolides, clindamycin	Minimal outer membrane[c] penetration, efflux pump	Methylation of rRNA	Phosphotransferase, esterase	*Bacteroides fragilis*/clindamycin/AT *S. aureus*/erythromycin/AT
Chloramphenicol	–	–	Acetyltransferase	*Salmonella*/chloramphenicol/EI
Tetracycline	Efflux pump	New protein protects ribosome site	–	
Fluoroquinolones	Efflux pump, permeability mutation	Mutant topoisomerase	–	*Escherichia coli*/ciprofloxacin/AT *P. aeruginosa*/ciprofloxacin/AT
Rifampin	–	Mutant RNA polymerase	–	*Mycobacterium tuberculosis*[d]/rifampin/AT *Neisseria meningitidis*/rifampin/AT
Folate inhibitors	–	New dihydropteroate synthetase, altered dihydrofolate reductase	–	Enterobacteriaceae/sulfonamides/AT

[a] Only primary mechanisms of resistance are listed.
[b] A highly selective list of resistance emergence that has altered or threatens a major clinical use of the agent.
[c] Outer membrane of Gram-negative bacteria.
[d] See Chapter 28.
Abbreviations: PBP, penicillin-binding protein.

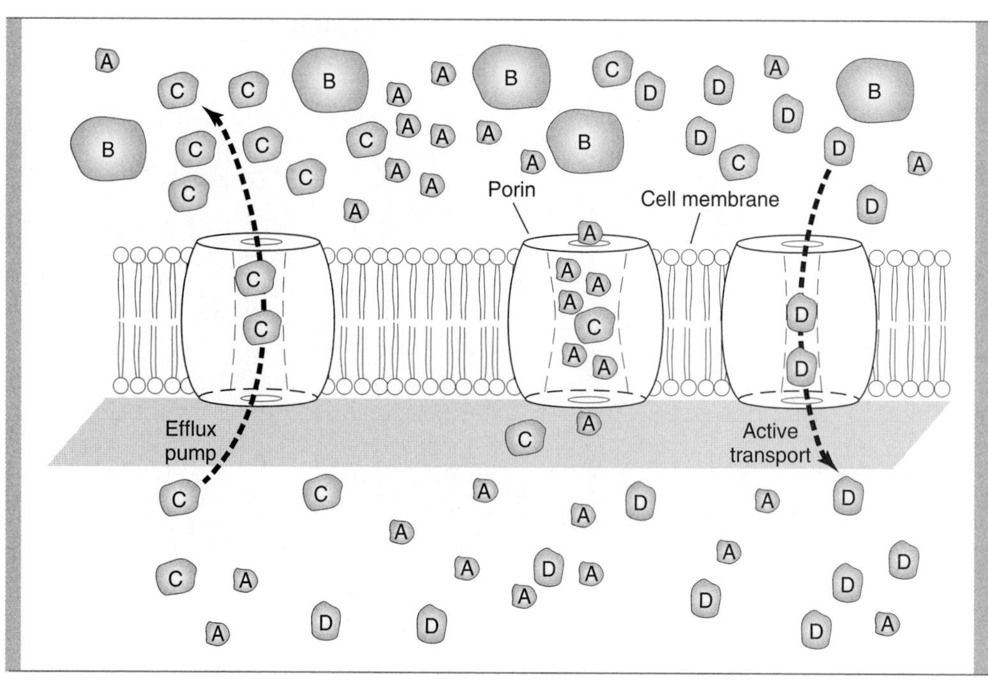

FIGURE 14–3
Diagrammatic representation of accumulation barrier resistance. A, B, C, and D molecules are external to the cell wall. A molecules pass through and remain inside the cell, B molecules are unable to pass because they cannot fit through any of the channels, C molecules pass through but are pushed back out by an efflux pump, and D molecules must be pulled through the wall by active transport.

For example, strains of *Pseudomonas aeruginosa* commonly develop resistance to imipenem due to loss of the outer membrane protein most important in its penetration.

Drugs are actively transported in and out of cells

As mentioned above, some antimicrobics must be actively transported into the cell. Bacteria such as streptococci, enterococci, and anaerobes, which lack the necessary oxidative pathways for transport of aminoglycosides, are resistant. Conversely, some antimicrobics are actively transported out of the cell. A number of bacterial species have energy-dependent efflux mechanisms that pump either tetracyclines or fluoroquinolones from the cell.

Altered Target (Fig 14–4)

Binding affinity for enzymes and ribosomes can change

Once in the cell, antimicrobics act by binding and inactivating their target, which is typically a crucial enzyme or ribosomal site. If the target is altered in a way that decreases its affinity for the antimicrobic, the inhibitory effect will be proportionately decreased. Substitution of a single amino acid at a certain location in a protein can alter its binding to the antimicrobic without affecting its function in the bacterial cell.

Multiple binding sites reduces chances for resistance

If an alteration at a single site of the target does not render it susceptible to the antimicrobic, mutation to resistance can occur in a single step, even during therapy. This occurred with the early aminoglycosides (streptomycin), which bound to a single ribosomal site, and the first quinolone (nalidixic acid), which attached to only one of the four topoisomerase subunits. Newer agents in each class bind at multiple sites on their target, making mutation to resistance statistically improbable.

PBPs are altered transpeptidases

One of the most important examples of altered target involves the β-lactam family and the peptidoglycan transpeptidase penicillin-binding proteins (PBPs) on which they act. In widely divergent Gram-positive and Gram-negative species, changes in one or more of these proteins have been correlated with decreased susceptibility to multiple β-lactams. These alterations were initially detected as changes in electrophoretic migration of one or more PBPs using radiolabeled penicillin (hence the origin of the term PBP). These changes have now been traced to point mutations, substitutions of amino acid sequences, and even synthesis of a new enzyme.

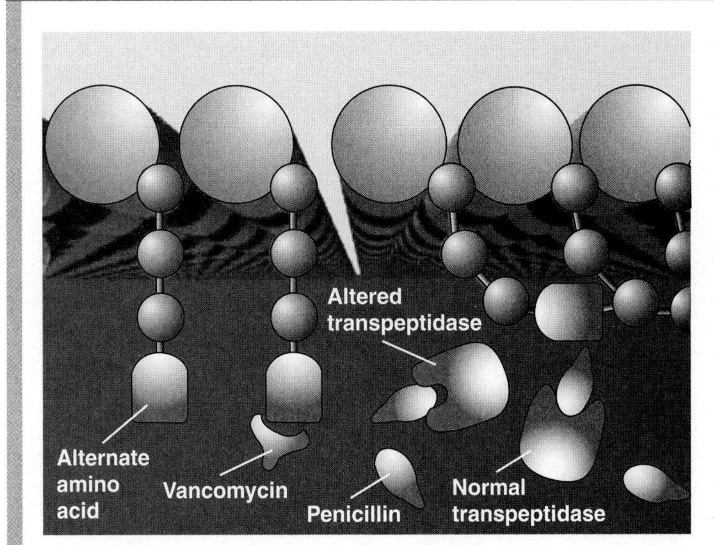

FIGURE 14–4
Altered target resistance. (For a diagrammatic representation of peptidoglycan synthesis, see Figure 13–1.) A normal transpeptidase is inactivated by penicillin, but penicillin no longer attaches to those with altered binding sites. The transpeptidase is still able to carry out its cross-linking function so the β-lactam is no longer effective. Here, vancomycin is no longer able to bind to its usual site, because another amino acid with a different shape has been substituted.

Because the altered binding is not absolute, decreases in susceptibility are incremental and often small. Wild-type pneumococci and gonococci are inhibited by 0.06 μg/mL of penicillin, while those with altered PBPs have MICs of 0.1 to 8.0 μg/mL. At the lower end, these MICs still appear to be within therapeutic range but are associated with treatment failures, even when dosage is increased. Altered PBPs generally affect all β-lactams. Although the exact MICs vary, a strain with a 10-fold decrease in susceptibility to penicillin has decreased susceptibility to cephalosporins to about the same degree.

Altered PBPs have reduced affinity for β-lactams

Penicillins and cephalosporins are affected to the same degree

PBP alterations are the prime reason for emergence of penicillin-resistant pneumococci and methicillin-resistant *Staphylococcus aureus* (MRSA). They are one of multiple mechanisms of resistance for a variety of other bacteria including enterococci, gonococci, *Haemophilus influenzae,* and many other Gram-positive and Gram-negative species.

Pneumococci and MRSA have altered PBPs

Alteration of the target does not require mutation and can occur by the action of a new enzyme produced by the bacteria. Vancomycin-resistant enterococci have enzyme systems that substitute an amino acid in the terminal position of the peptidoglycan side chain (alanyl lysine for alanyl alanine). Vancomycin does not bind to the alternate amino acid, and these strains are resistant. Resistance to sulfonamides and trimethoprim occurs by acquisition of new enzymes with low affinity for these agents but still allows bacterial cells to carry out their respective functions in the folate synthesis pathway.

New enzymes can alter bacterial targets

Clindamycin resistance involves an enzyme that methylates ribosomal RNA, preventing attachment. This modification also confers resistance to erythromycin and other macrolides, because they share binding sites. Interestingly, induction with erythromycin leads to clindamycin resistance, although the reverse is unusual.

Mutation or acquisition of a new enzyme is possible

Enzymatic Inactivation (Fig 14–5)

Enzymatic inactivation of the invading antimicrobic is the most powerful and robust of the resistance mechanisms. Literally hundreds of distinct enzymes produced by resistant bacteria may inactivate the antimicrobic in the cell, in the periplasmic space, or outside the cell. They may act on the antimicrobic molecule by disrupting its structure or by catalyzing a reaction that chemically modifies it.

Enzymes may disrupt or chemically modify antimicrobics

β-Lactamases β-Lactamase is a general term referring to any one of hundreds of bacterial enzymes able to break open the β-lactam ring and inactivate various members of the β-lactam group. The first was discovered when penicillin-resistant strains of *S. aureus* emerged and were found to inactivate penicillin in vitro. The enzyme was called penicillinase, but with expansion of the β-lactam family and concomitant resistance, it has become clear that the situation is quite complex. Each β-lactamase is a distinct enzyme with its own physical characteristics and substrate profile. For example, the

Enzymes break open the β-lactam ring

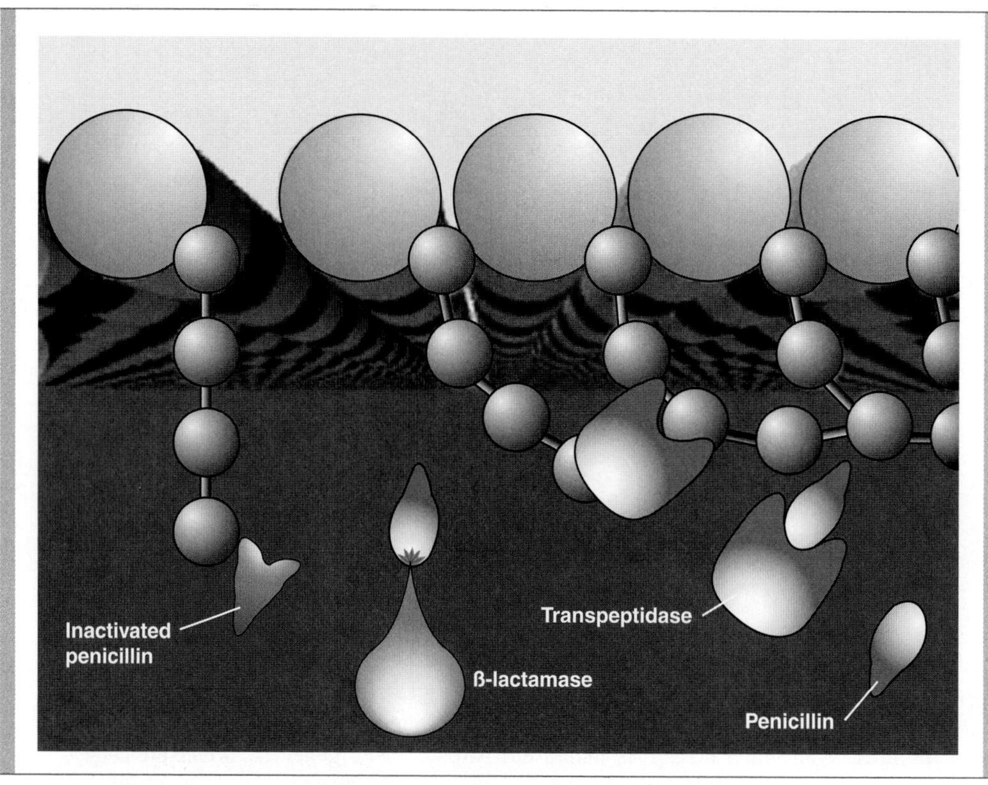

FIGURE 14–5
Enzymatic inactivation resistance. (For a diagrammatic representation of peptidoglycan synthesis, see Figure 13–1.) The bacterium is producing a β-lactamase enzyme, which destroys penicillin by breaking open the β-lactam ring. If the penicillin can reach the transpeptidase, it can still inactivate it; the more β-lactamase produced, the higher the level of resistance.

β-Lactamases have variable activity against β-lactam substrates

original staphylococcal penicillinase is also active against ampicillin but not against methicillin or any cephalosporin. β-Lactamases produced by *Escherichia coli* may add cephalosporinase activity but vary in their potency against individual first-, second-, third-, and fourth-generation cephalosporins. Some β-lactamases are bound by clavulanic acid, and others are not.

To keep track of the β-lactamase identifiers (eg, TEM-1, TEM-2, OXA, SVH), classification schemes have been created based on molecular structure, substrate profile, and inducibility (ie, whether enzymes are inducible or produced constitutively). A consideration of β-lactamase classification is beyond the scope of this book, but some discussion of the major types is useful. Gram-positive β-lactamases are exoenzymes with little activity against cephalosporins or the antistaphylococcal penicillins (methicillin, oxacillin). They are bound by β-lactamase inhibitors such as clavulanic acid. Gram-negative enzymes act in the periplasmic space and may have penicillinase and/or cephalosporinase activity. They may or may not be inhibited by clavulanic acid. Many of the Gram-negative β-lactamases are constitutively produced at very low levels but can be induced to high levels by exposure to a β-lactam agent. A newer class, called extended-spectrum β-lactamases (ESBLs) because their range includes multiple cephalosporins, is particularly worrisome. The laboratory detection of ESBLs is complex because they are inducible enzymes, and the conditions for induction may not be met in the susceptibility test.

May be exoenzymes or act in periplasmic space

ESBLs have broad activity against cephalosporins

Bacteria that produce β-lactamases typically demonstrate high-level resistance with MICs far outside the therapeutic range. Even weak β-lactamase producers are considered resistant because the outcome of susceptibility tests (and presumably infected sites) is strongly influenced by the number of bacteria present. Rapid direct tests for β-lactamase can provide this information in a few minutes.

Weak β-lactamase producers are still considered resistant

Modifying Enzymes The most common cause of acquired bacterial resistance to aminoglycosides is through production of one or more of over 50 enzymes that acetylate, adenylate, or phosphorylate hydroxyl or amino groups on the aminoglycoside molecule. The modifications take place in the cytosol or in close association with the cytoplasmic membrane. The resistance conveyed by these actions is usually high level; the chemically modified aminoglycoside no longer binds to the ribosome. As with the β-lactamases, the aminoglycoside-modifying enzymes represent a large and diverse group of bacterial proteins, each with its characteristic properties and substrate profile. Inactivating enzymes have been described for a number of other antimicrobics. Most of these act by chemically modifying the antimicrobic molecule in a manner similar to the aminoglycoside-modifying enzymes. The most clinically significant enzymes convey resistance to erythromycin (esterase, phosphotransferase) and chloramphenicol (acetyltransferase).

Chemically modified aminoglycosides do not bind to ribosomes

Genetics of Resistance

Intrinsic Resistance

For any antimicrobic, there are bacterial species that are typically within its spectrum and those which are not. The resistance of the latter group is referred to as **intrinsic** or **chromosomal** to reflect its inherent nature. The resistant species have features such as permeability barriers, a lack of susceptibility of the cell wall, or ribosomal targets that make them inherently insusceptible. Some species constitutively produce low levels of inactivating enzymes, particularly the β-lactamases of Gram-negative bacteria. The chromosomal genes encoding these β-lactamases may be under repressor control and subject to induction by certain β-lactam antimicrobics. This leads to increased production of β-lactamase, which usually results in resistance not only to the inducer but other β-lactams to which the organism would otherwise be susceptible. Many of the ESBLs operate in this manner.

Permeability barriers or enzyme production may be intrinsic

Inducible enzymes may have broad spectrum

Acquired Resistance

When an initially susceptible species develops resistance, such acquired resistance can be mutational or derived from another organism by the acquisition of new genes using one of the mechanisms of genetic exchange described in Chapter 4. Of these, conjugation and transposition are the most important and often work in tandem.

Mutational Resistance Acquired resistance may occur when there is a crucial mutation in the target of the antimicrobic or in proteins related to access to the target (ie, permeability). Mutations in regulatory proteins can also lead to resistance. Mutations take place at a regular but low frequency and are expressed only if they are not associated with other effects that are disadvantageous to the bacterial cell. Mutational resistance can emerge in a single step or evolve slowly requiring multiple mutations before clinically significant resistance is achieved. Single-step mutational resistance is most likely when the antimicrobic binds to a single site on its target. Resistance can also emerge rapidly when it is related to gene regulation, such as mutational derepression of a chromosomally encoded cephalosporinase. A slow, progressive resistance evolving over years, even decades, is typical for β-lactam resistance related to altered PBPs.

Mutations in structural or regulatory genes can confer resistance

Mutations are usually low-frequency

Plasmids and Conjugation The transfer of plasmids by conjugation was the first discovered mechanism for acquisition of new resistance genes, and it continues to be the most important. Resistance genes on plasmids (R plasmids) can determine resistance to one antimicrobic or to several that act by different mechanisms. After conjugation, the resistance genes may remain on a recircularized plasmid or less often become integrated into the chromosome by recombination. Of course, resistance is not the only concern of plasmids. A single cell may contain more than one distinct plasmid and/or multiple copies of the same plasmid. Although most resistance mechanisms have been linked to plasmids in one species or another, plasmid distribution among the bacterial pathogens is by no means uniform. The compatibility systems that maintain plasmids from one bacteria cell generation to the next are complex. Some species of bacteria are more likely than others

Plasmid conjugation allows multidrug resistance

Species may carry multiple or no plasmids

to contain plasmids at all. For example, *Neisseria gonorrhoeae* typically has multiple plasmids, whereas closely related *Neisseria meningitidis* rarely has any.

Conjugation genes and host range enhance plasmid spread

Plasmids are most likely to be transferred to another strain if they are conjugative, that is, if the resistance plasmid also contains the genes mediating conjugation. Another factor in the spread of plasmids is their host range. Some plasmids can be transferred only to closely related strains; others can be transferred to a broad range of species in and beyond their own genus. A conjugative plasmid with a broad host range has great potential to spread any resistance genes it carries.

Transposons resistance genes move between chromosomes and plasmids

Transposition and conjugation combine for resistance spread

Transposons and Transposition Transposons containing resistance genes can move from plasmid to plasmid or between plasmid and chromosome. Many of the resistance genes carried on plasmids are transposon insertions which can be carried along with the rest of the plasmid genome to another strain by conjugation. Once there, the transposon is free to remain in the original plasmid, insert in a new plasmid, insert in the chromosome, or any combination of these (Fig 14–6). Theoretically, plasmids can accomplish the same events by recombination, but the nature of the transposition process is such that it is much more likely to result in the transfer of an intact gene. Transposons also have a variable host range which in general is even broader than plasmids. Together, conjugation and transposition provide extremely efficient means for spreading resistance genes.

Transduction is limited by specificity of bacteriophages

Importance of transformation is unknown

Other Genetic Mechanisms Although the transfer of resistance genes by transduction has been demonstrated in the laboratory, its association to clinically significant resistance has been uncommon. Transduction of imipenem resistance by wild-type bacteriophages carried by *P. aeruginosa* to other strains of the same bacteria is a recent example. Because of the high specificity of bacteriophages, transduction is typically limited to bacteria of the same species. Transformation is the most common way genes are manipulated in the laboratory, but detecting its occurrence in the clinical situation is particularly difficult. Plasmids are readily isolated and characterized, and transposons have flanking insertion sequences to flag their presence, but there is little to mark the uptake of naked DNA. Molecular epidemiologic studies suggest that the spread of PBP mutations in *Streptococcus pneumoniae* is due to transformation, and there may be many more examples awaiting discovery.

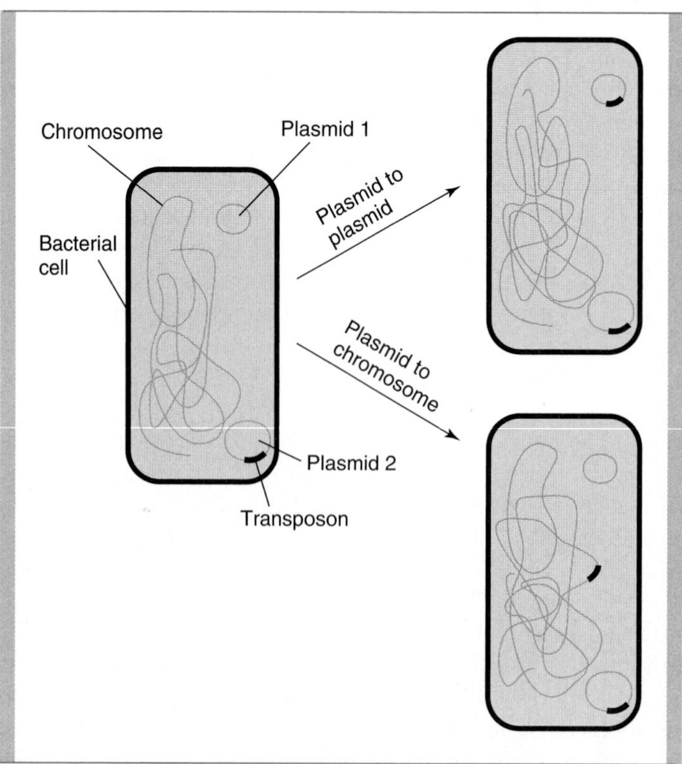

FIGURE 14–6
Plasmids and transposons. When passed to the next generation, transposons incorporated in plasmids may be inserted in another plasmid or in the chromosome.

Epidemiology of Resistance

The laws of evolution dictate that sooner or later microorganisms will develop resistance to any antimicrobic to which they are exposed. Since the start of the "antibiotic era," each new antimicrobic has tended to go through a remarkably similar sequence. When an agent is first introduced, its spectrum of activity seems almost completely predictable; some species are naturally resistant, and others are susceptible, with few exceptions. With clinical use, resistant strains of previously susceptible species begin to appear and become increasingly common.

Clinical use is followed by resistance

In some situations, resistance develops rapidly; in other cases it takes years, even decades. For example, when penicillin was first introduced in 1944, all strains of *S. aureus* appeared to be fully susceptible to this antimicrobic. By 1950, less than one third of isolates remained susceptible. Currently, that figure has now declined below 15%. On the other hand, the discovery of *Haemophilus influenzae* strains resistant to ampicillin did not occur until ampicillin had been used heavily for more than a decade. Penicillin was the primary treatment for pneumonia and meningitis caused by *S. pneumoniae* for 30 years before resistance emerged. Enteric Gram-negative rods rapidly developed resistance to antimicrobics such as ampicillin, cephalosporins, tetracycline, chloramphenicol, and aminoglycosides, with many strains becoming resistant to as many as 15 agents. Fortunately, these developments have not been universal. The spirochete of syphilis and the group A streptococcus have thus far retained their susceptibility to penicillin.

Predominant susceptibility can turn to resistance

Resistance may emerge after decades of use

Some pathogens remain universally susceptible

Origin of Resistant Strains

Resistant strains may exist prior to the introduction of an antimicrobic but at a frequency so small they are unlikely to be detected. For example, penicillinase-producing *S. aureus* have been found in culture collections that proceeded the development and use of this antibiotic. Under the selective pressure provided by use of any antimicrobic, preexisting resistant clones are likely to increase and, if they are virulent, spread.

Preexisting strains are selected by antimicrobial use

The origin of plasmid-carried determinants of resistance remains somewhat obscure. Some may have played a role in nature by protecting the organism from antimicrobics produced by another organism or even for protection of the cell from its own antibiotic. Plasmids and transposons carrying resistance genes have little, if any, adverse influence on the capacity of most organisms to survive, infect, and spread.

Plasmid carriage may have survival value

Enhancement and Spread of Resistance

The central factors involved in the increasing incidence of resistance are the selective effect of the use of antimicrobics, the spread of infection in human populations, and the ability of plasmids to cross species and even generic lines. Therapeutic or prophylactic use of antimicrobics, particularly those with a broad spectrum of activity, produces a relative ecologic vacuum in sites with a normal flora or on lesions prone to infection and allows resistant organisms to colonize or infect with less competition from others. Treatment with a single antimicrobic may select for strains that are also resistant to many other agents. Thus, chemotherapy can both enhance the opportunity for acquiring resistant strains from other sources and increase their numbers in the body. The amplifying effect of antimicrobial therapy on resistance is also apparent with the transfer of resistance plasmids to previously susceptible strains. This effect has been most clearly demonstrated in the lower intestinal tract, where the antimicrobic may reduce the flora and also produce an increased oxidation–reduction potential that favors plasmid transfer.

Antimicrobial use creates an ecologic vacuum

Broad-spectrum effects are greatest

Plasmids amplify availability of resistance genes

As an example, consider a male patient harboring a strain of *E. coli* carrying a plasmid with genes encoding resistance to tetracycline, ampicillin, chloramphenicol, and the sulfonamides as a very small part of his facultative intestinal flora. He develops an infection with *Shigella dysenteriae* that is susceptible to all of these antimicrobics and is treated with tetracycline. Most of the normal flora and the *Shigella* are inhibited, but the resistant *E. coli* increases because its multiplication is not impeded and competition is removed. Plasmid transfer occurs between the resistant *E. coli* and some surviving

Benign *E. coli* can transfer multiple resistance genes to virulent *Shigella* in the intestine

Shigella, which then multiply, causing a relapse of the disease with a strain that is now multiresistant. Any endemic or epidemic spread of dysentery from this patient to others will now be with the multiresistant *Shigella* strain, and its ability to infect will be enhanced if the recipient is on prophylaxis or therapy with any of the four antimicrobics to which it is resistant.

Antimicrobics in animal feeds increase the resistant population

Outbreaks have been traced from patients back to farms

The use of antimicrobics added to animal feeds for their growth-promoting effects represents a major source of resistant strains. Cattle or poultry that consume feed supplemented with antimicrobics rapidly develop a resistant enteric flora that spreads throughout the herd. Resistance is largely plasmid determined and has been shown capable of spreading to the flora of those living in close proximity to cattle-rearing farms. The links to human disease have been established, particularly for bacteria where these animals are the direct reservoir for human infection. For example, the techniques of molecular epidemiology have allowed the tracing of resistance plasmids involved in outbreaks of *Salmonella* gastroenteritis from the contaminated food back to the food processing plant and then to the originating farm. As a consequence, many countries have banned or controlled addition to animal feeds of antimicrobics that are useful for systemic therapy in humans. The United States has not yet taken any action because of opposition by business forces in the animal husbandry industry that fear lost profits.

Control of Resistance

In the past, numerous examples in the literature showed that the extent of resistance in a hospital directly reflects the extent of usage of an antimicrobic, and that withdrawal or control can lead to rapid reduction of the incidence of resistance. Although this is more difficult to demonstrate in the community setting, experience and our understanding of the mechanisms and spread of resistance indicate that certain principles can help keep the problem under control:

1. Use antimicrobics conservatively and specifically in therapy.
2. Use an adequate dosage and duration of therapy to eliminate the infecting organism and reduce the risk of selecting resistant variants.
3. Select antimicrobics according to the proved or anticipated known susceptibility of the infecting strain whenever possible.
4. Use narrow-spectrum rather than broad-spectrum antimicrobics when the specific etiology of an infection is known, if possible.
5. Use antimicrobic combinations when they are known to prevent emergence of resistant mutants.
6. Use antimicrobics prophylactically only in situations in which it has been proven valuable and for the shortest possible time to avoid selection of a resistant flora.
7. Avoid environmental contamination with antimicrobics.
8. Rigidly apply careful, aseptic and handwashing procedures to help prevent spread of resistant organisms.
9. Use containment isolation procedures for patients infected with resistant organisms that pose a threat to others, and use protective precautions for those who are highly susceptible.
10. Epidemiologically monitor resistant organisms or resistance determinants in an institution and apply enhanced control measures if a problem develops.
11. Restrict the use of therapeutically valuable antimicrobics for nonmedical purposes.

Selection and Administration of Antibacterial Antimicrobics

Antimicrobics are effective along with other treatments

This topic is largely beyond the scope of this book, but a few principles merit emphasis. Most bacterial infections are now potentially curable by chemotherapy alone or its use as an adjunct to surgical or other treatment. However, the plethora of antimicrobics available to physicians makes selection of the most appropriate agent(s) particularly challenging. Although the clinical indications for use vary widely, they usually fit into one of three categories: empiric, specific, or prophylactic.

Empiric Therapy

The first decisions on selection of antimicrobic(s) are based on the physician's assessment of the probable microbial etiology of the patient's infection. The variables involved are the subject of much of this book and include the site of infection (eg, throat, lung, urine) and epidemiologic factors such as age, season, geography, and predisposing conditions. A mental list of probable etiologies must then be matched with their probable antimicrobial susceptibilities as shown in Table 13–1. Specific local "batting averages" for each antimicrobic against the common organisms are available from hospital laboratories and infection control committees. Many astute clinicians carry statistics concerning bacterial effectiveness in a pocket.

Probable etiology and susceptibility statistics guide initial selection

This process may be as simple as selecting penicillin to treat a patient with suspected group A streptococcal pharyngitis, or as complex as resorting to a cocktail of broad-spectrum antibacterial, antifungal, and antiviral agents to treat a febrile patient who has had a bone marrow transplant. In general, the risks of broad-spectrum treatment (superinfection, overgrowth) become more tolerable as the severity of the infection increases. When the risk of not "covering" an improbable pathogen is death, it is difficult to be selective. This treatment selection based on clinical criteria alone must be coupled with appropriated diagnostic steps (see Chapter 15) to determine the etiology, so the empiric therapy can be converted to specific therapy as quickly as possible.

Narrow versus broad spectrum is influenced by clinical severity

Specific Therapy

Specific antimicrobial therapy is directed at the known agent of infection, usually a single species. It is unique to infectious diseases and is made possible by isolation and identification of the microorganism from the patient. In the case of bacterial diseases, it can even be made specific to the patient's own isolate by the use of antimicrobial susceptibility tests. The ideal goal of specific therapy is to attack the infecting organism and nothing else—to be the mythical "silver bullet." As the results of Gram smears, cultures, and susceptibility tests are gathered from the laboratory, unnecessary antimicrobics can be discontinued and the spectrum of therapy narrowed as much as possible. For example, a patient with suspect staphylococcal or streptococcal infection might be empirically started on a cephalosporin to cover both possibilities. The isolation of a *S. aureus* susceptible to a cephalosporin and oxacillin but resistant to penicillin requires reassessment of that regimen. Even though the cephalosporin is active, the oxacillin is the better choice, because its narrower spectrum carries less risk of complications for the patient and reduces the selective pressure for emergence of resistance.

Isolation of the causative agent allows narrowing of spectrum

Susceptibility tests provide final guide

In general, the best specific therapy is a single antimicrobic, but there are exceptions. Two or more antimicrobics acting by different mechanisms may be combined to reduce the possibility that mutations to resistance can be expressed. This is particularly true for chronic infections such as tuberculosis, in which the microbial load is high and the treatment period is long. For example, if a lesion contains 10^9 organisms, and the frequency of resistant mutants is 10^{-6}, the chance of relapse by selection of a resistant mutant is significant. Adding a second drug with the same mutation rate but a different mechanism requires a double mutant for expression of the resistance in the patient. Because the chance of this event is to 10^{-12}, the addition of a second antimicrobic should prevent development of resistance during therapy.

Pharmacologic combinations reduce the chances that resistant mutants are expressed

Another indication for antimicrobial combinations is the desire to achieve a greatly enhanced biologic effect called **synergism.** For example, relatively low concentrations of a β-lactam and an aminoglycoside may be bactericidal for *Enterococcus faecalis* when combined, but neither agent is lethal at clinically achievable levels. This occurs because inhibition of cell wall synthesis by penicillin allows passage of the aminoglycoside to its ribosomal target in the cell. Unfortunately, combinations may also be **antagonistic**. This happens when the action of one antimicrobic partially prevents the second from expressing its activity. Examples include certain combinations of bacteriostatic antimicrobics with a β-lactam antimicrobic, such as penicillin. Penicillin exerts its bacterial effect only on dividing cells, and inhibition of growth by a bacteriostatic antimicrobic may prevent

Combinations may be synergistic

Combination of a bacteriostatic agent and a β-lactam may be antagonistic the lethal activity of penicillin. Although specific therapy is the ideal, it is not always possible. Any degree of uncertainty about the etiologic diagnosis will broaden the therapeutic coverage, and in some instances an etiologic diagnosis may not even be attempted. Empirical treatment of acute otitis media usually stands, because reaching the middle ear to culture the specific etiology is judged to carry more risk and discomfort for the patient.

Prophylaxis

Prophylaxis risks enhancing spread

Administration during procedures is most effective

The use of antimicrobics to prevent infection is a tempting but potentially hazardous endeavor. The risk for the individual patient is infection with a different, more resistant organism. The risks for the population are in increasing the pressure for the selection and spread of resistance. After many years of experience, the indications for antimicrobial prophylaxis have now been narrowed to a limited number of situations in which antimicrobics have been shown to decrease transmission during a period of high risk. Prophylaxis can reduce the risk of endogenous infection associated with certain surgical and dental procedures if given during the procedure (a few hours at most). The transmission of highly infectious bacteria to close contacts can also be reduced by prophylaxis. This has been effective for some pathogens spread by the respiratory route, such as the etiologic agents of meningitis, whooping cough, and plague. One of the outstanding successes of antimicrobial prophylaxis is the reduction of group B streptococcal sepsis and meningitis in neonates. In this instance, prophylactic penicillin is administered during labor to mothers with demonstrated vaginal group B streptococcal colonization.

ADDITIONAL READING

Bradford PA. Extended-spectrum β-lactamases in the 21st century: Characterization, epidemiology, and detection of this important resistance threat. *Clin Microbiol Rev* 2001;14:933–951. This article addresses the difficulty in detecting the most potent family of inactivating enzymes.

Fluit AC, Maarten Visser MR, Schmitz FJ. Molecular detection of antimicrobial resistance. *Clin Microbiol Rev* 2001;14:836–871. This review focuses on the new molecular detection of resistance genes, and it also includes concise summaries of resistance mechanisms.

Zinner SH, Wise R, Moellering RC Jr, eds. Maximizing antimicrobial efficacy/minimizing antimicrobial resistance: A paradigm for the new millennium. *Clin Infect Dis* 2001;33(Suppl 3):S107–S235. The proceedings of a symposium held at the American Academy of Arts and Sciences address the broad issues of resistance such as overuse and strategies to reduce resistance in the population at large.

CHAPTER 15

Principles of Laboratory Diagnosis of Infectious Diseases

KENNETH J. RYAN AND C. GEORGE RAY

The diagnosis of a microbial infection begins with an assessment of clinical and epidemiologic features, leading to the formulation of a diagnostic hypothesis. Anatomic localization of the infection with the aid of physical and radiologic findings (for example, right lower lobe pneumonia, subphrenic abscess) is usually included. This clinical diagnosis suggests a number of possible etiologic agents based on knowledge of infectious syndromes and their courses (see Chapters 59 through 72). The specific cause is then established by the application of methods described in this chapter. A combination of science and art on the part of both the clinician and laboratory worker is required: The clinician must select the appropriate tests and specimens to be processed and, where appropriate, suggest the suspected etiologic agents to the laboratory. The laboratory worker must use those methods that will demonstrate the probable agents, and be prepared to explore other possibilities suggested by the clinical situation or findings of the laboratory examinations. The best results are obtained when communication between the clinic and laboratory is maximal.

The general approaches to laboratory diagnosis vary with different microorganisms and infectious diseases. However, the types of methods are usually some combination of direct microscopic examinations, culture, antigen detection, and antibody detection (serology). Newer approaches involving direct detection of genomic components are also important, although few have become practical enough for routine use. In this chapter, these principles will be considered, with emphasis on their application to the diagnosis of diseases caused by bacteria and viruses. Most of the approaches to be described can also be applied, with certain variations, to the diagnosis of diseases caused by fungi and parasites. All of these begin with some kind of specimen collected from the patient.

Microscopic, culture, antigen, and antibody detection are classic methods

Genomic approaches are being developed

THE SPECIMEN

The primary connection between the clinical encounter and diagnostic laboratory is the specimen submitted for processing. If it is not appropriately chosen and/or collected, no degree of laboratory skill will rectify the error. Failure at the level of specimen collection is the most common reason for failure to establish an etiologic diagnosis, or worse, for suggesting a wrong diagnosis. In the case of bacterial infections, the primary problem lies in distinguishing resident or contaminating normal floral organisms from those causing the infection. The three specimen categories illustrated in Figure 15–1 and discussed below are covered more specifically in Chapters 59 to 72.

Quality of the specimen is crucial

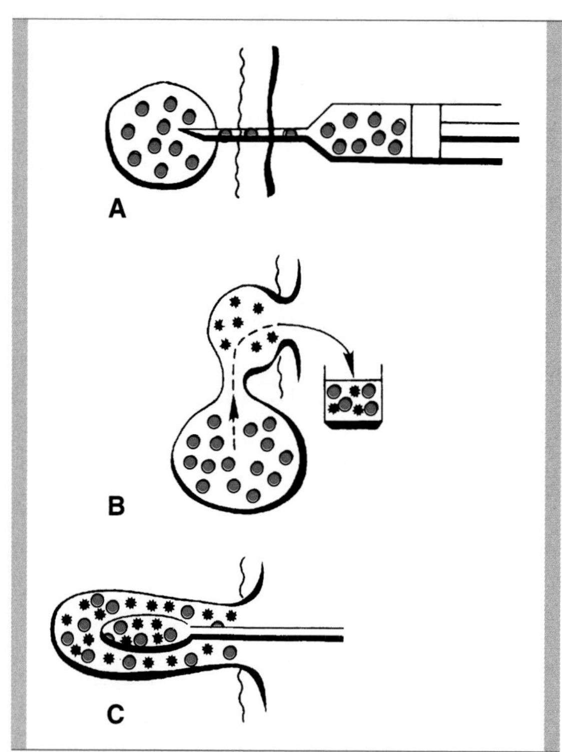

FIGURE 15–1
Specimens for the diagnosis of infection. **A.** Direct specimen. The pathogen (●) is localized in an otherwise sterile site, and a barrier such as the skin must be passed to sample it. This may be done surgically or by needle aspiration as shown. The specimen collected contains only the pathogen. Examples: deep abscess, cerebrospinal fluid. **B.** Indirect sample. The pathogen is localized as in A but must pass through a site containing normal flora (✱) in order to be collected. The specimen contains the pathogen but is contaminated with the nonpathogenic flora. The degree of contamination is often related to the skill with which the normal floral site was "bypassed" in specimen collection. Examples: expectorated sputum, voided urine. **C.** Sample from site with normal flora. The pathogen and nonpathogenic flora are mixed at the site of infection. Both are collected and the nonpathogen is either inhibited by the use of selective culture methods or discounted in interpretation of culture results. Examples: throat, stool.

Direct Tissue or Fluid Samples

Direct samples give highest quality and risk

Direct specimens (Fig 15–1A) are collected from normally sterile tissues (lung, liver) and body fluids (cerebrospinal fluid, blood). The methods range from needle aspiration of an abscess to surgical biopsy. In general, such collections require the direct involvement of a physician and may carry some risk for the patient. The results are always useful, because positive findings are diagnostic and negative findings can exclude infection at the suspected site.

Indirect Samples

Bypassing the normal flora requires extra effort

Results require interpretive evaluation of contamination

Indirect samples (Fig 15–1B) are specimens of inflammatory exudates (expectorated sputum, voided urine) that have passed through sites known to be colonized with normal flora. The site of origin is usually sterile in healthy persons; however, some assessment of the probability of contamination with normal flora during collection is necessary before these specimens can be reliably interpreted. This assessment requires knowledge of the potential contaminating flora (see Chapter 9) as well as the probable pathogens to be sought. Indirect samples are usually more convenient for both physician and patient, but carry a higher risk of misinterpretation. For some specimens, such as expectorated sputum, guidelines to assess specimen quality have been developed by correlation of clinical and microbiologic findings (see Chapter 64).

Samples from Normal Flora Sites

Frequently the primary site of infection is in an area known to be colonized with many organisms (pharynx and large intestine) (Fig 15–1C). In such instances, examinations are selectively made for organisms known to cause infection that are not normally found at the infected site. For example, *Salmonella, Shigella,* and *Campylobacter* may be specifically sought in a stool specimen because they are known to cause diarrhea. It is neither practical nor relevant to describe the other stool flora.

Strict pathogens can be specifically sought

Specimens for Viral Diagnosis

The selection of specimens for viral diagnosis is easier because there is essentially little normal viral flora to confuse interpretation. This allows selection guided by knowledge of which sites are most likely to yield the suspected etiologic agent. For example, enteroviruses are the most common viruses involved in acute infection of the central nervous system. Specimens that might be expected to yield these agents on culture include throat, stool, and cerebrospinal fluid.

Lack of normal viral flora simplifies interpretation

Specimen Collection and Transport

The **sterile swab** is the most convenient and most commonly used tool for specimen collection; however, it provides the poorest conditions for survival and can only absorb a small volume of inflammatory exudate. The worst possible specimen is a dried-out swab; the best is a collection of 5 to 10 mL or more of the infected fluid or tissue. The volume is important because infecting organisms present in small numbers may not be detected in a small sample.

Swabs limit volume and survival

Specimens should be transported to the laboratory as soon after collection as possible, because some microorganisms survive only briefly outside the body. For example, unless special **transport media** are used, isolation rates of the organism that causes gonorrhea (*Neisseria gonorrhoeae*) are decreased when processing is delayed beyond a few minutes. Likewise, many respiratory viruses survive poorly outside the body. On the other hand, some bacteria survive well and may even multiply after the specimen is collected. The growth of enteric Gram-negative rods in specimens awaiting culture may in fact compromise specimen interpretation and interfere with the isolation of more fastidious organisms. Significant changes are associated with delays of more than 3 to 4 hours.

Viability may be lost if specimen is delayed

Various transport media have been developed to minimize the effects of the delay between specimen collection and laboratory processing. In general, they are buffered fluid or semisolid media containing minimal nutrients and are designed to prevent drying, maintain a neutral pH, and minimize bacterial growth. Other features may be required to meet special requirements, such as an oxygen-free atmosphere for obligate anaerobes.

Transport media stabilize conditions and prevent drying

DIRECT EXAMINATION

Of the infectious agents discussed in this book, only some of the parasites are large enough to be seen with the naked eye. Bacteria can be seen clearly with the light microscope when appropriate methods are used; individual viruses can be seen only with the electron microscope, although aggregates of viral particles in cells (viral inclusions) may be seen by light microscopy. Various stains are used to visualize and differentiate microorganisms in smears and histologic sections.

All but some parasites require microscopy for visualization

Light Microscopy

Direct examination of stained or unstained preparations by **light (bright field) microscopy** (Fig 15–2A) is particularly useful for detection of bacteria. Even the smallest bacteria (0.15 μm wide) can be visualized, although some require special lighting techniques. As the resolution limit of the light microscope is near 0.2 μm, the optics must be ideal if organisms are to be seen clearly by direct microscopy. These conditions may be achieved with a 100× oil immersion objective, a 5 to 10× eyepiece, and optimal lighting.

Bacteria are visible if optics are maximized

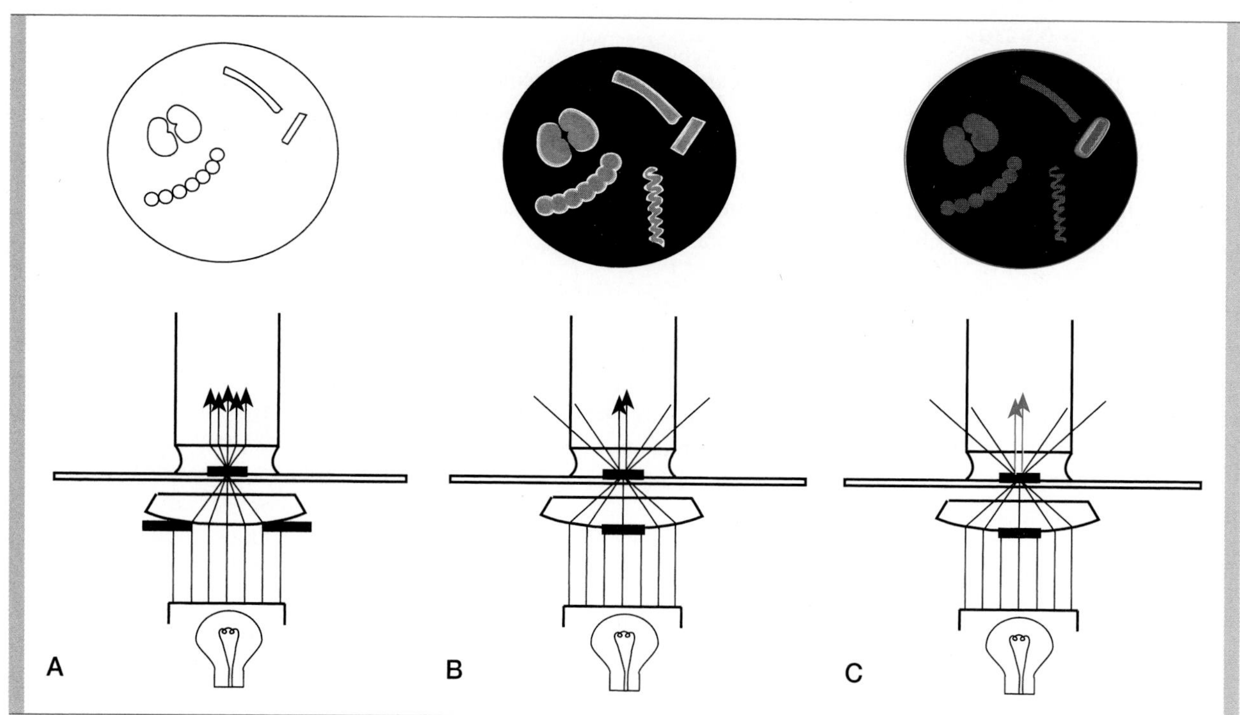

FIGURE 15–2
Bright-field, darkfield, and fluorescence microscopy. **A.** Bright-field illumination properly aligned. The purpose is to focus light directly on the preparation for optimal visualization against a bright background. **B.** In darkfield illumination, a black background is created by blocking the central light. Peripheral light is focused so that it will be collected by the objective only when it is reflected from the surfaces of particles (eg, bacteria). The microscopic field shows bright halos around some bacteria and reveals a spirochete too thin to be seen with bright-field illumination. **C.** Fluorescence microscopy is similar to darkfield microscopy, except the light source is ultraviolet and the organisms are stained with fluorescent compounds. The incident light generates light of a different wavelength, which is seen as a halo (colored in this illustration) around only the organism tagged with fluorescent compounds. For the most common fluorescent compound, the light is green.

Unstained bacteria are too transparent to see directly, although their presence can be indicated by the voids they create when suspended in particulate matter such as India ink.

Bacteria must be stained

Bacteria may be stained by a wide variety of dyes, including methylene blue, crystal violet, carbol-fuchsin (red), and safranin (red). The two most important methods, the Gram and acid-fast techniques, employ staining, decolorization, and counterstaining in a manner that helps to classify as well as stain the organism.

The Gram Stain

Gram-positive bacteria retain purple iodine-dye complexes

Gram-negative bacteria do not retain complexes when decolorized

The differential staining procedure described in 1884 by the Danish physician Hans Christian Gram has proved one of the most useful in microbiology and medicine. The procedure (Fig 15–3) involves the application of a solution of iodine in potassium iodide to cells previously stained with an acridine dye such as crystal violet. This treatment produces a mordanting action in which purple insoluble complexes are formed with ribonuclear protein in the cell. The difference between Gram-positive and Gram-negative bacteria is in the permeability of the cell wall to these complexes on treatment with mixtures of acetone and alcohol solvents. This extracts the purple iodine–dye complexes from Gram-negative cells, whereas Gram-positive bacteria retain them. An intact cell wall is necessary for a positive reaction, and Gram-positive bacteria may fail to retain the stain if the organisms are old, dead, or damaged by antimicrobial agents. No similar conditions cause a Gram-negative organism to appear Gram positive. The stain is completed by the addition of red counterstain such as safranin, which is taken up by bacteria that have been

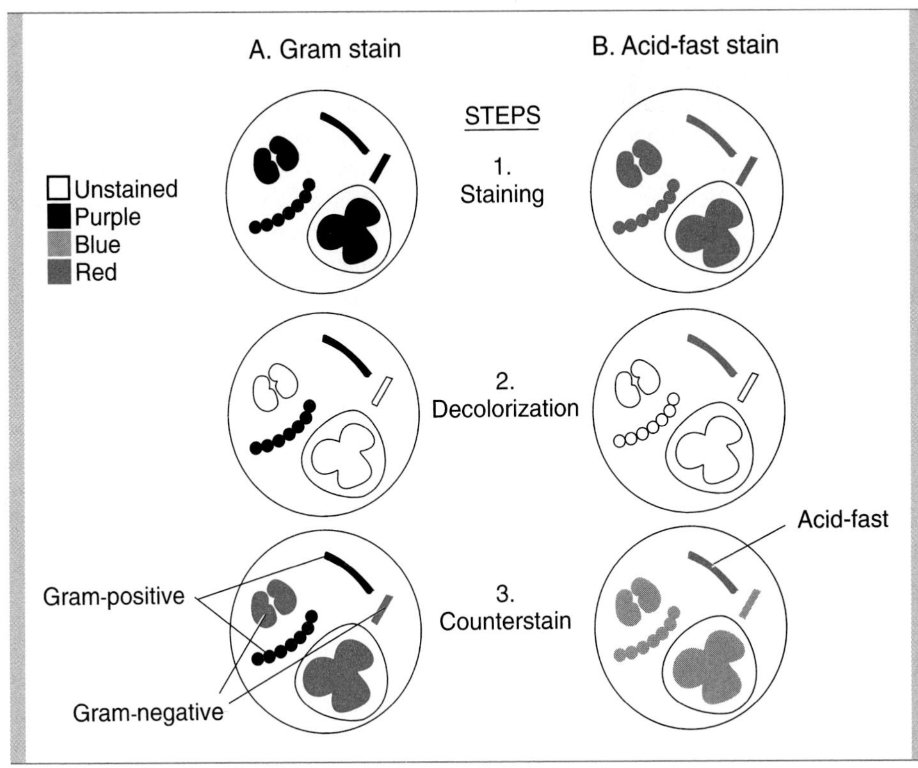

FIGURE 15-3
The Gram and acid-fast stains. Four bacteria and a PMN are shown at each stage. All are initially stained purple by the crystal violet and iodine of the Gram stain (A1) and red by the carbol fuchsin of the acid-fast stain (B1). Following decolorization, Gram-positive and acid-fast organisms retain their original stain. Others are unstained (A2, B2). The safranin of the Gram counterstain stains the Gram-negative bacteria and makes the background red (A3), and the methylene blue leaves a blue background for the contrasting red acid-fast bacillus (B3).

decolorized. Thus, cells stained purple are Gram positive, and those stained red are Gram negative. As indicated in Chapter 2, Gram positivity and negativity correspond to major structural differences in the cell wall.

When the Gram stain is applied to clinical specimens, the purple or red bacteria are seen against a Gram-negative (red) background of leukocytes, exudate, and debris. Retention of the purple dye in tissue or fluid elements, such as the nuclei of polymorphonuclear leukocytes, is an indication that the smear has been inadequately decolorized. In smears of uneven thickness, judgments on the Gram reaction can be made only in well-decolorized areas.

Properly decolorized background should be red

In many bacterial infections, the etiologic agents are readily seen on stained Gram smears of pus or fluids. This information, combined with the clinical findings, may guide the management of infection before culture results are available. Interpretation requires considerable experience and knowledge of probable causes, of their morphology and Gram reaction, and of any organisms normally present in health at the infected site.

Gram reaction plus morphology guide clinical decisions

The Acid-Fast Stain

Acid fastness is a property of the mycobacteria (eg, *Mycobacterium tuberculosis*) and related organisms. Acid-fast organisms generally stain very poorly with dyes, including those used in the Gram stain. However, they can be stained by prolonged application of more concentrated dyes, and staining is facilitated by heat treatment. Their unique feature is that once stained, acid-fast bacteria resist decolorization by concentrations of mineral acids and ethanol that remove the same dyes from other bacteria. This combination of weak initial staining and strong retention once stained is probably related to the high lipid content of the mycobacterial cell wall. Acid-fast stains are completed with a counterstain to provide a contrasting background for viewing the stained bacteria (see Fig 15-3).

Acid-fast bacteria take stains poorly

Once stained retain it strongly

In the acid-fast procedure, the slide is flooded with carbol-fuchsin (red) and decolorized with hydrochloric acid in alcohol. When counterstained with methylene blue, acid-fast organisms appear red against a blue background. A variant is the **fluorochrome stain,** which uses a fluorescent dye, (auramine, or an auramine-rhodamine mixture) followed by decolorization with acid-alcohol. Acid-fast organisms retain the fluorescent stain, which allows their visualization by fluorescence microscopy.

There are multiple variants of the acid-fast stain

Darkfield and Fluorescence Microscopy

Darkfield creates a halo around organisms too thin to see by bright-field

Fluorescent stains convert darkfield to fluorescence microscopy

Some bacteria, such as *Treponema pallidum*, the cause of syphilis, are too thin to be visualized with the usual bright-field illumination. They can be seen by use of the dark-field technique. With this method, a condenser focuses light diagonally on the specimen in such a way that only light reflected from particulate matter such as bacteria reaches the eyepiece (Fig 15–2B). The angles of incident and reflected light are such that the organisms are surrounded by a bright halo against a black background. This type of illumination is also used in other microscopic techniques, in which a high light contrast is desired, and for observation of fluorescence. Fluorescent compounds, when excited by incident light of one wavelength, emit light of a longer wavelength and thus a different color. When the fluorescent compound is conjugated with an antibody as a probe for detection of a specific antigen, the technique is called **immunofluorescence,** or fluorescent antibody microscopy. The appearance is the same as in darkfield microscopy except that the halo is the emitted color of the fluorescent compound (Fig 15–2C). For improved safety, most modern fluorescence microscopy systems direct the incident light through the objective from above (epifluorescence).

Electron Microscopy

Viruses are visible only by electron microscopy

Electron microscopy demonstrates structures by transmission of an electron beam and has 10 to 1000 times the resolving power of light microscopic methods. For practical reasons its diagnostic application is limited to virology, where due to the resolution possible at high magnification it offers results not possible by any other method. Using negative staining techniques, direct examination of fluids and tissues from affected body sites enables visualization of viral particles. In some instances, electron microscopy has been the primary means of discovery of viruses that do not grow in the usual cell culture systems.

CULTURE

Growth and identification of the infecting agent in vitro is usually the most sensitive and specific means of diagnosis and is thus the method most commonly used. Most bacteria and fungi can be grown in a variety of artificial media, but strict intracellular microorganisms (eg, *Chlamydia*, *Rickettsia*, and human and animal viruses) can be isolated only in cultures of living eukaryotic cells.

Isolation and Identification of Bacteria

Bacteria grow in soup-like media

Almost all medically important bacteria can be cultivated outside the host in artificial culture media. A single bacterium placed in the proper culture conditions will multiply to quantities sufficient to be seen by the naked eye. Bacteriologic media are soup-like recipes prepared from digests of animal or vegetable protein supplemented with nutrients such as glucose, yeast extract, serum, or blood, to meet the metabolic requirements of the organism. Their chemical composition is complex, and their success depends on matching the nutritional requirements of most heterotrophic living things.

Large numbers of bacteria in broth produce turbidity

Agar is a convenient gelling agent for solid media

Growth in media prepared in the fluid state (broths) is apparent when bacterial numbers are sufficient to produce turbidity or macroscopic clumps. Turbidity results from reflection of transmitted light by the bacteria; depending on the size of the organism, more than 10^6 bacteria per milliliter of broth are usually required. Most bacteria grow diffusely, but strictly aerobic bacteria may grow as a film on the surface of the broth, and other bacteria grow as a sediment. The addition of a gelling agent to a broth medium allows its preparation in solid form as plates in Petri dishes. The universal gelling agent for diagnostic bacteriology is **agar,** a polysaccharide extracted from certain types of seaweed. Agar has the convenient property of becoming liquid at about 95°C but not returning to the solid state as a gel until cooled to less than 50°C. This allows the addition of a heat-labile substance, such as blood, to the medium before it sets. At the temperatures used in the diagnostic laboratory (37°C or lower), broth–agar exists as a smooth, solid, nutrient gel. This medium, usually termed "agar," may be qualified with a description of any supplement (eg, blood agar).

Separation of bacteria may be accomplished by using a sterile wire loop to spread a small sample over the surface of an agar plate in a structured pattern called **plate streaking.** Bacteria that are well separated from others grow as isolated colonies, often reaching 2 to 3 mm in diameter after overnight incubation. For diagnostic work, growth of bacteria on solid media has advantages over the use of broth cultures. It allows isolation of bacteria in pure culture (Fig 15–4), because a colony well separated from others can be assumed to arise from a single organism or an organism cluster (colony-forming unit). Colonies vary greatly in size, shape, texture, color, and other features. For example, colonies of organisms possessing large polysaccharide capsules are usually mucoid; those of organisms that fail to separate after division are frequently granular. Colonies from different species or genera often differ substantially, whereas those derived from the same strain are usually consistent. Differences in **colonial morphology** are very useful for separating bacteria in mixtures and as clues to their identity. Some examples of colonial morphology are shown in Figure 15–5.

Bacteria may be separated in isolated colonies on agar plates

Colonies may have consistent and characteristic features

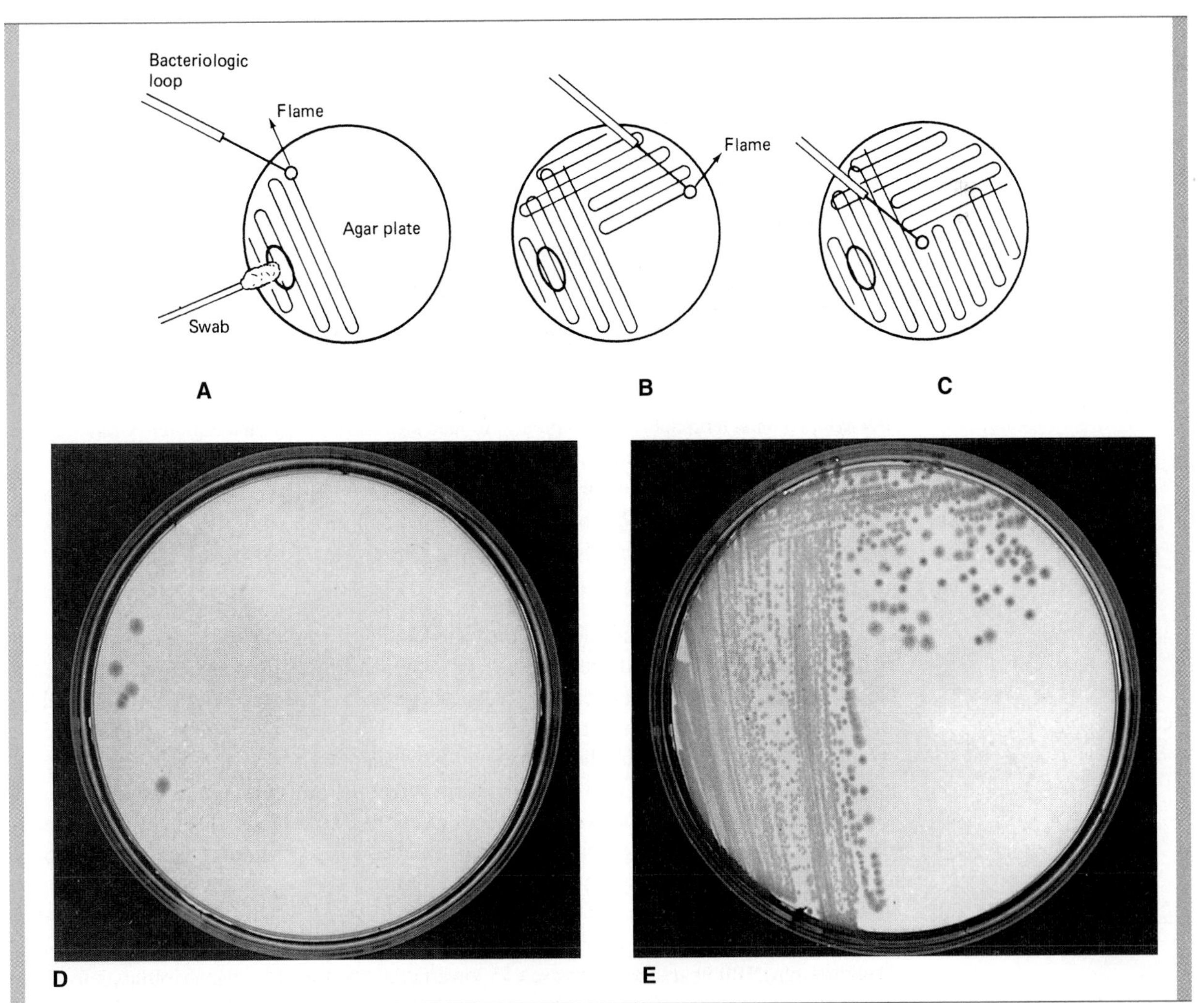

FIGURE 15–4

Bacteriologic plate streaking. Plate streaking is essentially a dilution procedure. **A.** The specimen is placed on the plate with a swab, loop, or pipette, and evenly spread over approximately one fourth of the plate surface with a sterilized bacteriologic loop. **B.** The loop is flamed to remove residual bacteria. A secondary streak is made, overlapping the primary streak initially but finishing independently. **C.** The process is repeated in a tertiary streak. **D.** and **E.** Two plates streaked in a similar manner. **D.** Only a few bacteria grew. **E.** A large number of bacteria grew. However, isolated colonies were produced for further study in each case.

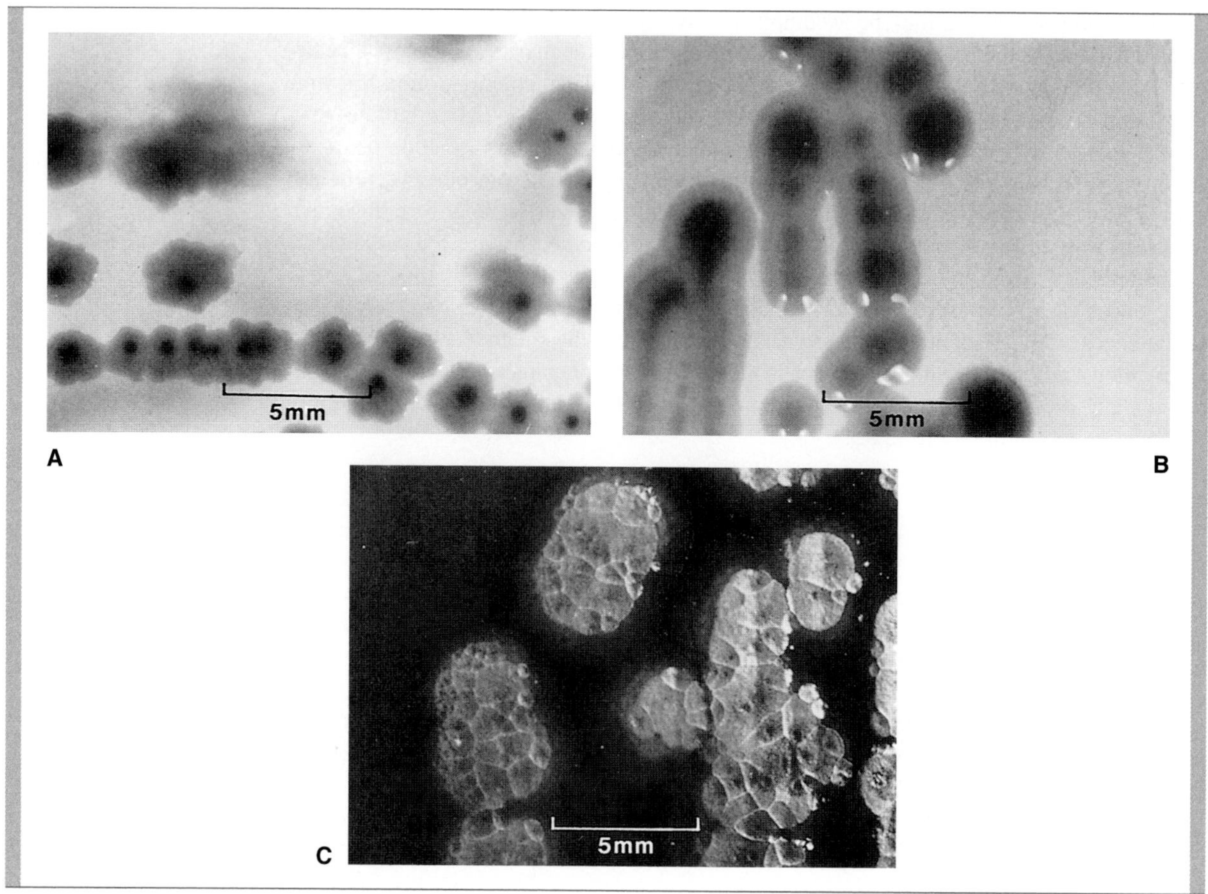

FIGURE 15–5
Bacterial colonial morphology. The colonies formed on agar plates by three different Gram-negative bacilli are shown at the same magnification. Each is typical for its species but variations are common. **A.** *Escherichia coli* colonies are flat with an irregular scalloped edge. **B.** *Klebsiella pneumoniae* colonies with a smooth entire edge and a raised glistening surface. **C.** *Pseudomonas aeruginosa* colonies with an irregular reflective surface, suggesting hammered metal.

Optical, chemical, and electrical methods can detect growth

New methods that do not depend on visual changes in the growth medium or colony formation are also used to detect bacterial growth in culture. These techniques include optical, chemical, and electrical changes in the medium, produced by the growing numbers of bacterial cells or their metabolic products. Many of these methods are more sensitive than classical techniques and thus can detect growth hours, or even days, earlier than classical methods. Some have also been engineered for instrumentation and automation. For example, one fully automated system that detects bacterial metabolism fluorometrically can complete a bacterial identification and antimicrobial susceptibility test in 2 to 4 hours.

Bacteriologic Media

Over the past 100 years, countless media have been developed by bacteriologists to aid in the isolation and identification of medically important bacteria. Only a few have found their way into routine use in clinical laboratories. These may be classified as nutrient, selective, or indicator media.

Media are prepared from animal or plant products

Nutrient Media The nutrient component of a medium is designed to satisfy the growth requirements of bacteria to permit isolation and propagation. For medical purposes, the ideal medium would allow rapid growth of all bacteria. No such medium exists; however, several suffice for good growth of most medically important bacteria. These media are prepared with enzymatic or acid digests of animal or plant products such as muscle, milk, or beans.

The digest reduces the native protein to a mixture of polypeptides and amino acids that also includes trace metals, coenzymes, and various undefined growth factors. For example, one common broth contains a pancreatic digest of casein (milk curd) and a papaic digest of soybean meal. To this nutrient base, salts, vitamins, or body fluids such as serum may be added to provide pathogens with the conditions needed for optimum growth.

Selective Media Selective media are used when specific pathogenic organisms are sought in sites with an extensive normal flora (eg, *N. gonorrhoeae* in specimens from the uterine cervix or rectum). In these cases, other bacteria may overgrow the suspected etiologic species in simple nutrient media, either because the pathogen grows more slowly or because it is present in much smaller numbers. Selective media usually contain dyes, other chemical additives, or antimicrobics at concentrations designed to inhibit contaminating flora but not the suspected pathogen.

Unwanted organisms are inhibited with chemicals or antimicrobics

Indicator Media Indicator media contain substances designed to demonstrate biochemical or other features characteristic of specific pathogens or organism groups. The addition to the medium of one or more carbohydrates and a **pH indicator** is frequently used. A color change in a colony indicates the presence of acid products and thus of fermentation or oxidation of the carbohydrate by the organism. Other indicator media may enhance the production of a **pigment** or other changes useful for early recognition of certain bacteria. The addition of red blood cells (RBCs) to plates allows the **hemolysis** produced by some organisms to be used as a differential feature (see Chapter 16). In practice, nutrient, selective, and indicator properties are often combined to various degrees in the same medium. It is possible to include an indicator system in a highly nutrient medium and also make it selective by adding appropriate antimicrobics. Some examples of culture media commonly used in diagnostic bacteriology are listed in Appendix 15–1, and more details of their constitution and application are provided in Appendix 15–2.

Metabolic properties of bacteria are demonstrated by substrate and indicator systems

Atmospheric Conditions

Aerobic Once inoculated, cultures of most aerobic bacteria are placed in an incubator with temperature maintained at 35 to 37°C. Slightly higher or lower temperatures are used occasionally to selectively favor a certain organism or organism group. Most bacteria that are not obligate anaerobes will grow in air; however, CO_2 is required by some and enhances the growth of others. Incubators that maintain a 2 to 5% concentration of CO_2 in air are frequently used for primary isolation, because this level is not harmful to any bacteria and improves isolation of some. A simpler method is the candle jar, in which a lighted candle is allowed to burn to extinction in a sealed jar containing plates. This method adds 1 to 2% CO_2 to the atmosphere.

Incubation temperature and atmosphere vary with organism

Anaerobic Strictly anaerobic bacteria will not grow under the conditions described previously, and many will die if exposed to atmospheric oxygen or high oxidation–reduction potentials. Most medically important anaerobes will grow in the depths of liquid or semisolid media containing any of a variety of **reducing agents,** such as cysteine, thioglycollate, ascorbic acid, or even iron filings. An anaerobic environment for incubation of plates can be achieved by replacing air with a gas mixture containing hydrogen, CO_2, and nitrogen and allowing the hydrogen to react with residual oxygen on a catalyst to form water. A convenient commercial system accomplishes this chemically in a packet to which water is added before the jar is sealed. Specimens suspected to contain significant anaerobes should be processed under conditions designed to minimize exposure to atmospheric oxygen at all stages.

Anaerobes require reducing conditions and protection from oxygen

Clinical Bacteriology Systems

Routine laboratory systems for processing specimens from various sites are needed because no single medium or atmosphere is ideal for all bacteria. Combinations of broth and solid-plated media and aerobic, CO_2, and anaerobic incubation must be matched to

Routine systems are designed to detect the most common organisms

TABLE 15–1

Routine Use of Gram Smear and Isolation Systems for Selected Clinical Specimens[a]

Medium (Incubation)	Specimen							
	Blood	Cerebrospinal Fluid	Wound, Pus	Genital, Cervix	Throat	Sputum	Urine	Stool
Gram smear		×	×	×		×	×	
Soybean–casein digest broth (CO_2)	×	×	×					
Selenite F broth (air)								×
Blood agar (CO_2)		×	×	×		×	×	
Blood agar (anaerobic)			×		×[b]			
MacConkey agar (air)			×	×		×	×	×
Chocolate agar (CO_2)		×	×	×		×		
Martin–Lewis agar (CO_2)				×				
Hektoen agar (air)								×
Campylobacter agar (CO_2, 42°C)[c]								×

[a] The added sensitivty of a nutrient broth is used only when contamination by normal flora is unlikely. Exact media and isolation systems may vary between laboratories.

[b] Anaerobic incubation used to enhance hemolysis by β-hemolytic streptococci.

[c] Incubation in a reduced oxygen atmosphere.

the organisms expected at any particular site or clinical circumstance. Examples of such routines are shown in Table 15–1. In general, it is not practical to routinely include specialized media for isolation of rare organisms such as *Corynebacterium diphtheriae.* For detection of these and other uncommon organisms, the laboratory must be specifically informed of their possible presence by the physician. Appropriate media and special procedures can then be included.

Bacterial Identification

Extent of identification is linked to medical relevance

Once growth is detected in any medium, the process of identification begins. Identification involves the use of methods to obtain pure cultures from single colonies, followed by tests designed to characterize and identify the isolate. The exact tests and their sequences vary with different groups of organisms, and the taxonomic level (genus, species, subspecies, and so on) of identification needed varies according to the medical usefulness of the information. In some cases, only a general description or the exclusion of particular organisms is important. For example, a report of "mixed oral flora" in a sputum specimen or "no *N. gonorrhoeae*" in a cervical specimen may provide all of the information needed.

Features Used to Classify Bacteria

Growth under various conditions has differential value

Cultural Characteristics Cultural characteristics include the demonstration of properties such as unique nutritional requirements, pigment production, and the ability to grow in the presence of certain substances (sodium chloride, bile) or on certain media (MacConkey, nutrient agar). Demonstration of the ability to grow at a particular temperature or to cause hemolysis on blood agar plates is also used.

Biochemical reactions analyzed by tables and computers give identification probability

Biochemical Characteristics The ability to attack various substrates or to produce particular metabolic products has broad application to the identification of bacteria. The most common properties examined are listed in Appendix 15–3. Biochemical and cultural tests for bacterial identification are analyzed by reference to tables that show the reaction patterns characteristic for individual species. In fact, advances in computer analysis have now been applied to identification of many bacterial and fungal groups. These systems use the same biochemical principles along with computerized databases to determine the most probable identification from the observed test pattern.

Toxin Production and Pathogenicity Direct evidence of virulence in laboratory animals is rarely needed to confirm a clinical diagnosis. In some diseases caused by production of a specific toxin, the toxin may be detected in vitro through cell cultures or immunologic methods. Neutralization of the toxic effect with specific antitoxin is the usual approach to identify the toxin.

Detection of specific toxin may define disease

Antigenic Structure As discussed in Chapter 2, bacteria possess many antigens, such as capsular polysaccharides, flagellar proteins, and several cell wall components. Serology involves the use of antibodies of known specificity to detect antigens present on whole bacteria or free in bacterial extracts (soluble antigens). The methods used for demonstrating antigen–antibody reactions are discussed in a later section.

Antigenic structures of organism demonstrated with antisera

Genomic Structure Nucleic acid sequence relatedness as determined by homology comparisons have become a primary determinant of taxonomic decisions. They are discussed later in the section on nucleic acid methods.

Isolation and Identification of Viruses

Cell and Organ Culture

Living cell cultures that can support their replication are the primary means of isolating pathogenic viruses. The cells are derived from a tissue source by outgrowth of cells from a tissue fragment (explant) or by dispersal with proteolytic agents such as trypsin. They are allowed to grow in nutrient media on a glass or plastic surface until a confluent layer one cell thick (monolayer) is achieved. In some circumstances, a tissue fragment with a specialized function (eg, fetal trachea with ciliated epithelial cells) is cultivated in vitro and used for viral detection. This procedure is known as organ culture.

Cell cultures derived from human or animal tissues are used to isolate viruses

Three basic types of cell culture monolayers are used in diagnostic virology. The **primary cell culture,** in which all cells have a normal chromosome count (diploid), is derived from the initial growth of cells from a tissue source. Redispersal and regrowth produces a **secondary cell culture,** which usually retains characteristics similar to those of the primary culture (diploid chromosome count and virus susceptibility). Monkey and human embryonic kidney cell cultures are examples of commonly used primary and secondary cell cultures.

Monkey kidney is used in primary and secondary culture

Further dispersal and regrowth of secondary cell cultures usually leads to one of two outcomes: the cells eventually die, or they undergo spontaneous transformation, in which the growth characteristics change, the chromosome count varies (haploid or heteroploid), and the susceptibility to virus infection differs from that of the original. These cell cultures have characteristics of "immortality"; that is, they can be redispersed and regrown many times (serial cell culture passage). They can also be derived from cancerous tissue cells or produced by exposure to mutagenic agents in vitro. Such cultures are commonly called **cell lines.** A common cell line in diagnostic use is the *Hep*-2, derived from a human epithelial carcinoma. A third type of culture is often termed a **cell strain.** This culture consists of diploid cells, commonly fibroblastic, that can be redispersed and regrown a finite number of times; usually 30 to 40 cell culture passages can be made before the strain dies out or spontaneously transforms. Human embryonic tonsil and lung fibroblasts are common cell strains in routine diagnostic use.

Primary cultures either die out or transform

Cell strains regrow a limited number of times

Cells from cancerous tissue may grow continuously

Detection of Viral Growth

Viral growth in susceptible cell cultures can be detected in several ways. The most common effect is seen with lytic or cytopathic viruses; as they replicate in cells, they produce alterations in cellular morphology (or cell death) that can be observed directly by light microscopy under low magnification (30× or 100×). This **cytopathic effect (CPE)**

Viral CPE is due to morphologic changes or cell death

CPE is characteristic for some viruses

varies with different viruses in different cell cultures. For example, enteroviruses often produce cell rounding, pleomorphism, and eventual cell death in various culture systems, whereas measles and respiratory syncytial viruses cause fusion of cells to produce multinucleated giant cells (syncytia). The microscopic appearance of some normal cell cultures and the CPE produced in them by different viruses are illustrated in Figure 15–6.

Hemadsorption or interference marks cells that may not show CPE

Other viruses may be detected in cell culture by their ability to produce **hemagglutinins.** These hemagglutinins may be present on the infected cell membranes, as well as in the culture media, as a result of release of free, hemagglutinating virions from the cells. Addition of erythrocytes to the infected cell culture results in their adherence to the cell surfaces, a phenomenon known as **hemadsorption.** Another method of viral detection in cell culture is by **interference.** In this situation, the virus that infects the susceptible cell culture produces no CPE or hemagglutinin, but can be detected by "challenging" the cell culture with a different virus that normally produces a characteristic CPE. The second, or challenge, virus fails to infect the cell culture because of interference by the first virus, which is thus detected. This method is obviously cumbersome, but has been applied to the detection of rubella virus in certain cell cultures.

EBV and HIV antigens are expressed on lymphocytes

Immunologic or genomic probes detect incomplete viruses

For some agents, such as Epstein–Barr virus (EBV) or human immunodeficiency virus (HIV), even more novel approaches may be applied. Both EBV and HIV can replicate in vitro in suspension cultures of normal human lymphocytes such as those derived from neonatal cord blood. Their presence may be determined in several ways; for example, EBV-infected B lymphocytes and HIV-infected T lymphocytes will express virus-specified antigens and viral DNA or RNA, which can be detected with immunologic or genomic probes. In addition, HIV reverse transcriptase can be detected in cell culture by specific assay methods. Immunologic and nucleic acid probes (see below) can also be used to detect virus in clinical specimens or in situations where only incomplete, noninfective virus replication has occurred in vivo or in vitro. An example is the use of in situ cytohybridization, whereby specific labeled nucleic acid probes are used to detect and localize papillomavirus genomes in tissues where neither infectious virus nor its antigens can be detected.

In Vivo Isolation Methods

Embryonated eggs and animals are required for isolation of some viruses

In vivo methods for isolation are also sometimes necessary. The embryonated hen's egg is still used for the initial isolation and propagation of influenza A virus. Virus-containing material is inoculated on the appropriate egg membrane, and the egg is incubated to permit viral replication and recognition. Animal inoculation is still used for detecting some viruses. The usual animal host for viral isolation is the mouse; suckling mice in the first 48 hours of life are especially susceptible to many viruses. Evidence for viral replication is based on the development of illness, manifested by such signs as paralysis, convulsions, poor feeding, or death. The nature of the infecting virus can be further elucidated by histologic and immunofluorescent examination of tissues or by detection of specific antibody responses. Many arboviruses and rabies virus are detected in this system.

Specimen preparation is required

Time to detection varies from days to weeks

Viral isolation from a suspect case involves a number of steps. First, the viruses believed most likely to be involved in the illness are considered, and appropriate specimens are collected. Centrifugation or filtration and addition of antimicrobics are frequently required with respiratory or fecal specimens to remove organic matter, cellular debris, bacteria, and fungi, which can interfere with viral isolation. The specimens are then inoculated into the appropriate cell culture systems. The time between inoculation and initial detection of viral effects varies; however, for most viruses positive cultures are usually apparent within 5 days of collection. With proper collection methods and application of the diagnostic tools discussed later, many infections can even be detected within hours. On the other hand, some viruses may require culture for a month or more before they can be detected.

Viral Identification

Nature of CPE and cell cultures affected may suggest virus

On isolation, a virus can usually be tentatively identified to the family or genus level by its cultural characteristics (eg, type of CPE produced). Confirmation and further identification may require enhancement of viral growth to produce adequate quantities for testing. This

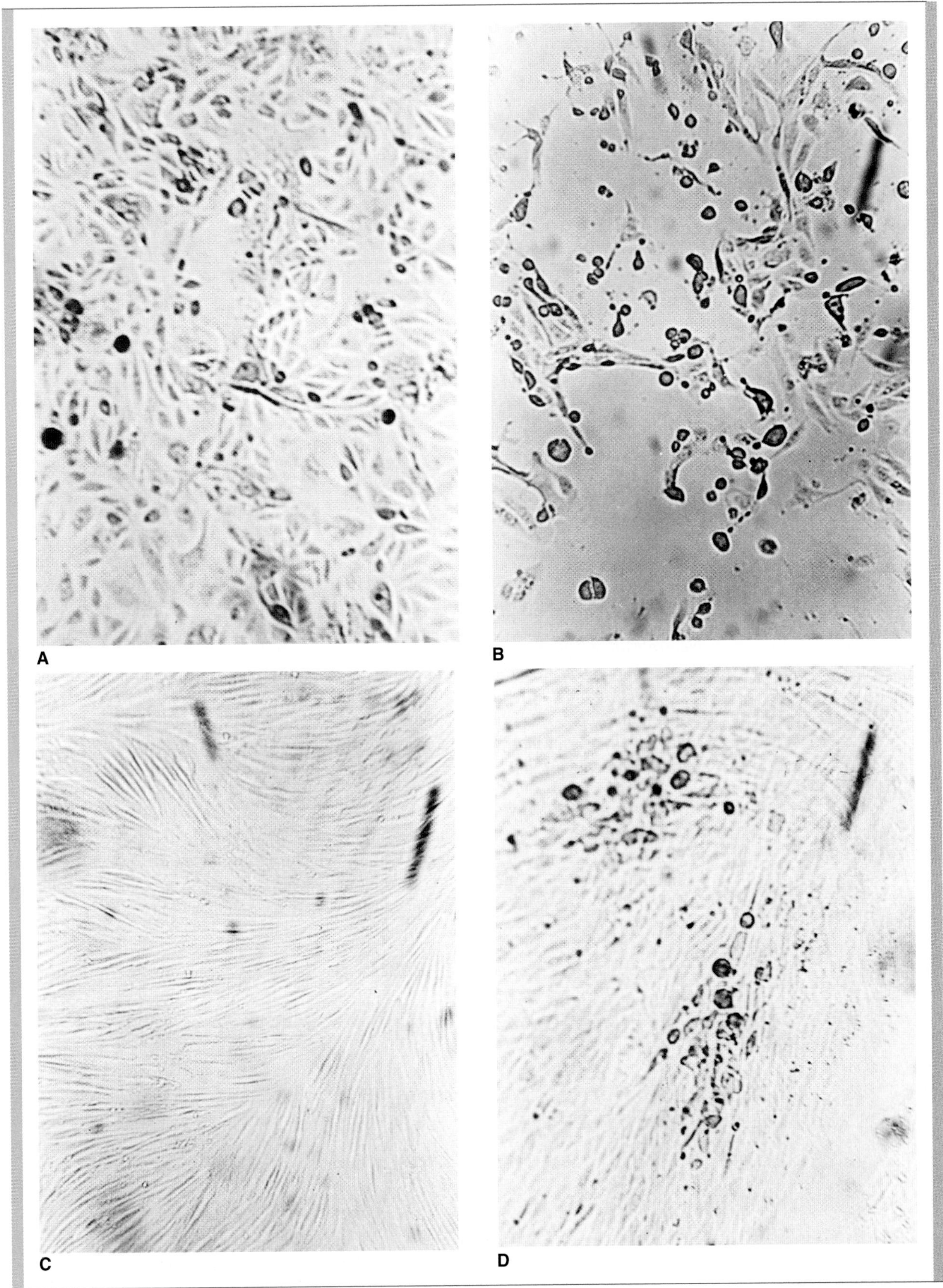

FIGURE 15–6

A. Normal monkey kidney cell culture monolayer. **B.** Enterovirus cytopathic effect in a monkey kidney cell monolayer. Note cell lysis and monolayer destruction. **C.** Normal human diploid fibroblast cell monolayer. **D.** Cytomegalovirus cytopathic effect in human diploid cell monolayer. Note rounded, swollen cells in a focal area. (A–D × 40.)

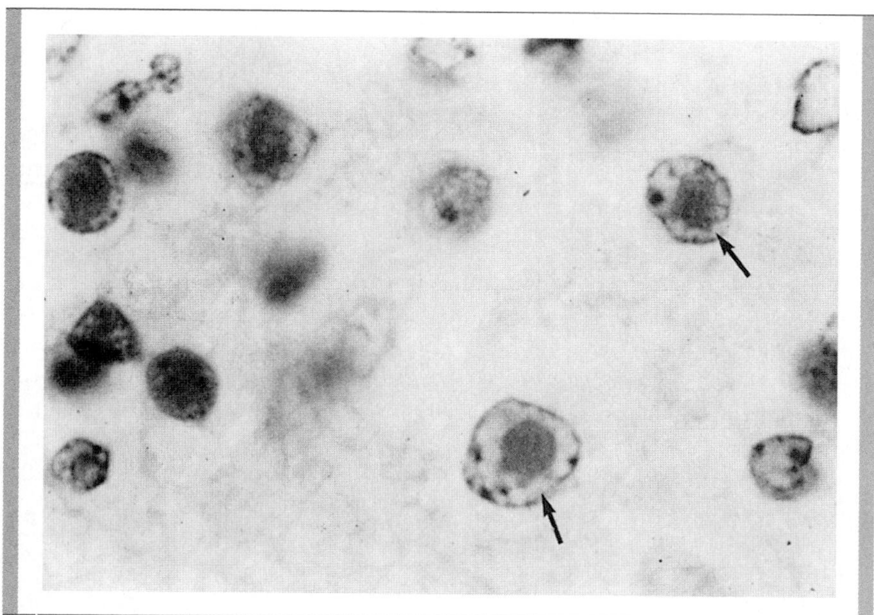

FIGURE 15–7
Brain biopsy from a patient with herpes simplex encephalitis. Arrows indicate infected neuronal nuclei with marginated chromatin and typical intranuclear inclusions. The cytoplasmic membranes are not clearly seen in this preparation (hematoxylin–eosin stain; × 400).

result may be achieved by inoculation of the original isolate into fresh culture systems (viral passage) to amplify replication of the virus, as well as improve its adaptation to growth in the in vitro system.

Neutralization of biologic effect with specific antisera confirms identification

Neutralization and Serologic Detection Of the several ways to identify the isolate, the most common is to neutralize its infectivity by mixing it with specific antibody to known viruses before inoculation into cultures. The inhibition of the expected viral effects on the cell culture such as CPE or hemagglutination is then evidence for that virus. As in bacteriology, demonstration of specific viral antigens is a useful way to identify many agents. Immunofluorescence and enzyme immunoassay (EIA) are the most common methods.

Inclusions and giant cells suggest viruses

Cytology and Histology In some instances, viruses will produce specific cytologic changes in infected host tissues that aid in diagnosis. Examples include specific intranuclear inclusions (herpes, Fig 15–7); cytoplasmic inclusions; and cell fusion, which results in multinucleated epithelial giant cells (chickenpox, Fig 15–8). Although such findings are useful when seen, their overall diagnostic sensitivity and specificity are usually considerably less than those of the other methods discussed.

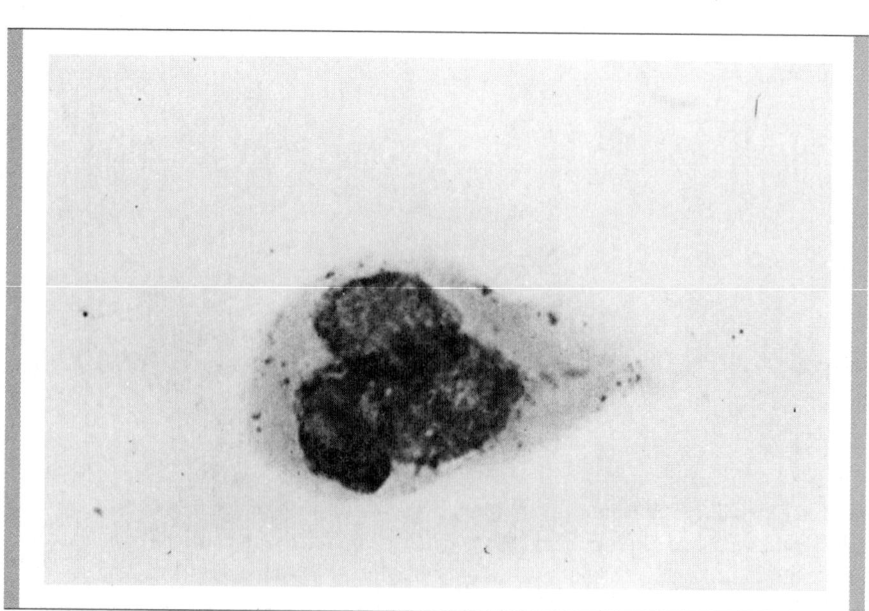

FIGURE 15–8
Multinucleated epithelial cells from a vesicle scraping of a patient with chickenpox. Cell fusion of this type can be seen with both varicella-zoster and herpes simplex infections (Wright's stain; × 400).

Electron Microscopy When virions are present in sufficient numbers, they may be further characterized by specific agglutination of viral particles on mixture with type-specific antiserum. This technique, immune electron microscopy, can be used to identify viral antigens specifically or to detect antibody in serum using viral particles of known antigenicity.

Immune electron microscopy shows agglutinated viral particles

Some viruses (eg, human rotaviruses, hepatitis A and B viruses) grow poorly or not at all in the laboratory culture systems currently available. However, they can be efficiently detected by immunologic or molecular methods, to be described later in this chapter.

Not all viruses grow in culture

IMMUNOLOGIC SYSTEMS

Diagnostic microbiology makes great use of the specificity of the binding between antigen and antibody. Antisera of known specificity are used to detect their homologous antigen in cultures, or more recently, directly in body fluids. Conversely, known antigen preparations are used to detect circulating antibodies as evidence of a current or previous infection with that agent. Many methods are in use to demonstrate the antigen–antibody binding. The greatly improved specificity of **monoclonal antibodies** has had a major impact on the quality of methods where they have been applied. Before discussing their application to diagnosis, the principles involved in the most important methods will now be discussed.

Antisera detect viral antigens

Viral antigens detect immune response

Methods for Detecting an Antigen–Antibody Reaction

Precipitation

When antigen and antibody combine in the proper proportions, a visible precipitate is formed (Fig 15–9A). Optimum antigen–antibody ratios can be produced by allowing one to diffuse into the other, most commonly through an agar matrix **(immunodiffusion).**

Both the speed and the sensitivity of immunodiffusion are improved by CIE

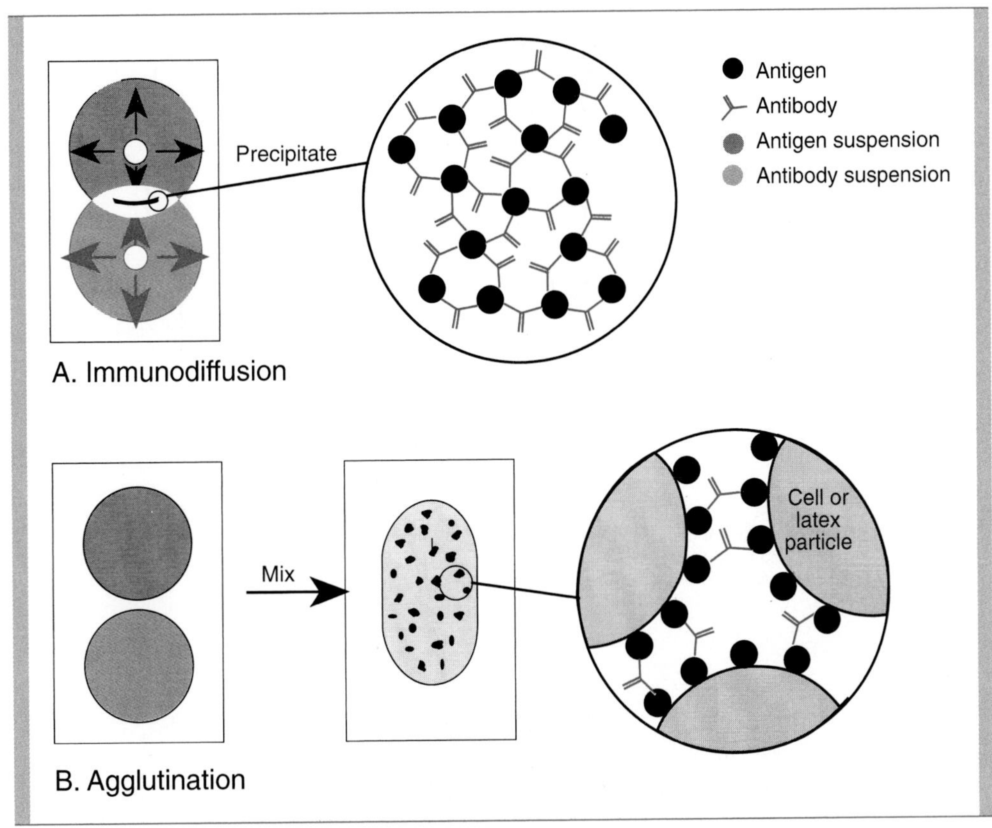

FIGURE 15–9
Immunodiffusion and agglutination. **A.** In immunodiffusion the antigen and antibody diffuse through a support matrix (eg, agarose). Where they reach optimal proportions a precipitin line is formed by the antigen–antibody complex. **B.** In agglutination the antigen–antibody reaction can be seen because one is on the surface of a relatively large particle. In the figure, the antigen is bound to the particle, but the reaction could be reversed.

Antigen–antibody precipitates demonstrated by immunodiffusion and CIE

In the immunodiffusion procedure, wells are cut in the agar and filled with antigen and antibody. One or more precipitin lines may be formed between the antigen and antibody wells; depending on the number of different antigen–antibody reactions occurring. **Counterimmunoelectrophoresis** (CIE) is immunodiffusion carried out in an electrophoretic field. The net effect is that antigen and antibody are rapidly brought together in the space between the wells to form a precipitin line.

Agglutination

RBCs and latex particles coated with antigen or antibody enhance demonstration

Simple mixing on slide causes agglutination

The amount of antigen or antibody necessary to produce a visible immunologic reaction can be reduced if either is on the surface of a relatively large particle. This condition can be produced by fixing soluble antigens or antibody onto the surface of RBCs or microscopic latex particles (Fig 15–9B). Whole bacteria are large enough to serve as the particle if the antigen is present on the microbial surface. The relative proportions of antigen and antibody thus become less critical, and antigen–antibody reactions are detectable by agglutination when immune serum and particulate antigen, or particle-associated antibody and soluble antigen, are mixed on a slide. The process is termed bacterial agglutination, passive hemagglutination, or latex agglutination depending on the nature of the sensitized particle.

Neutralization

Bacterium, virus, or toxin are mixed with antibody prior to addition to test system

Neutralization as commonly used takes some observable function of the agent, such as cytopathic effect of viruses or the action of a bacterial toxin, and neutralizes it. This is usually done by first reacting the agent with antibody, and then placing the antigen–antibody mixture into the test system. The steps involved are illustrated in Figure 15–10. In viral

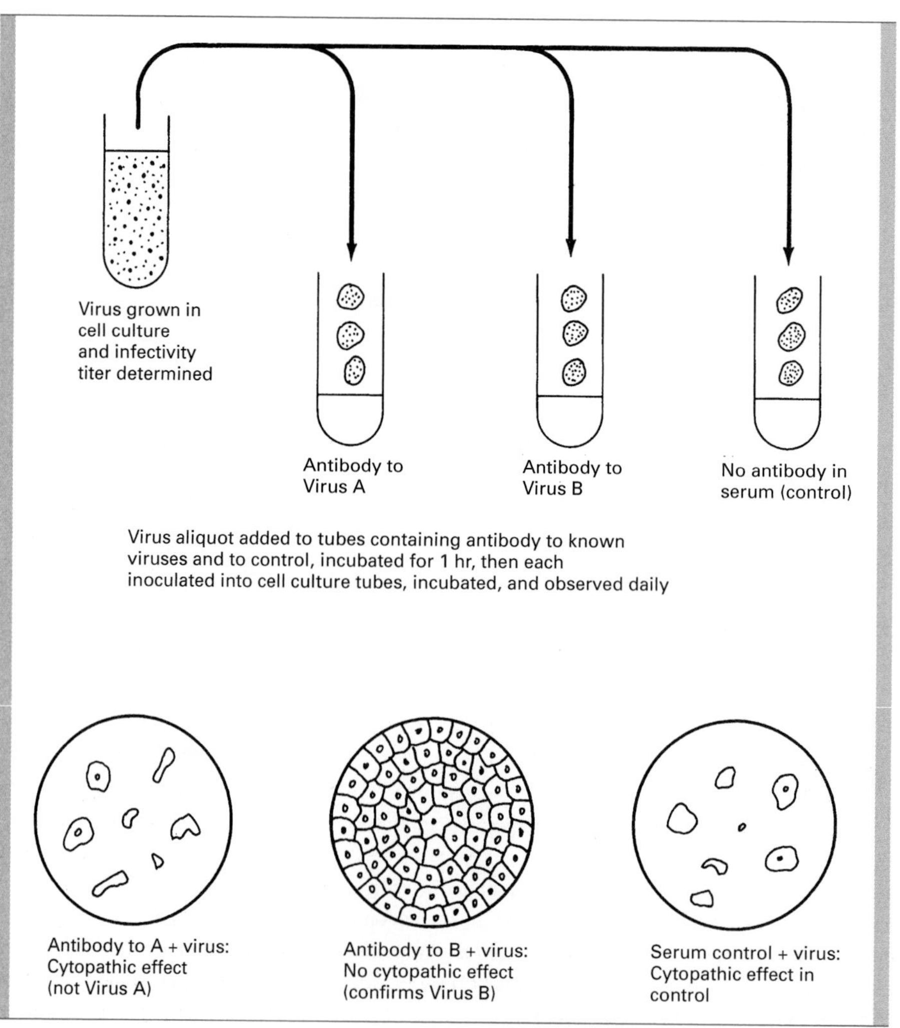

FIGURE 15–10
Identification of a virus isolate (cytopathic virus) as "Virus B."

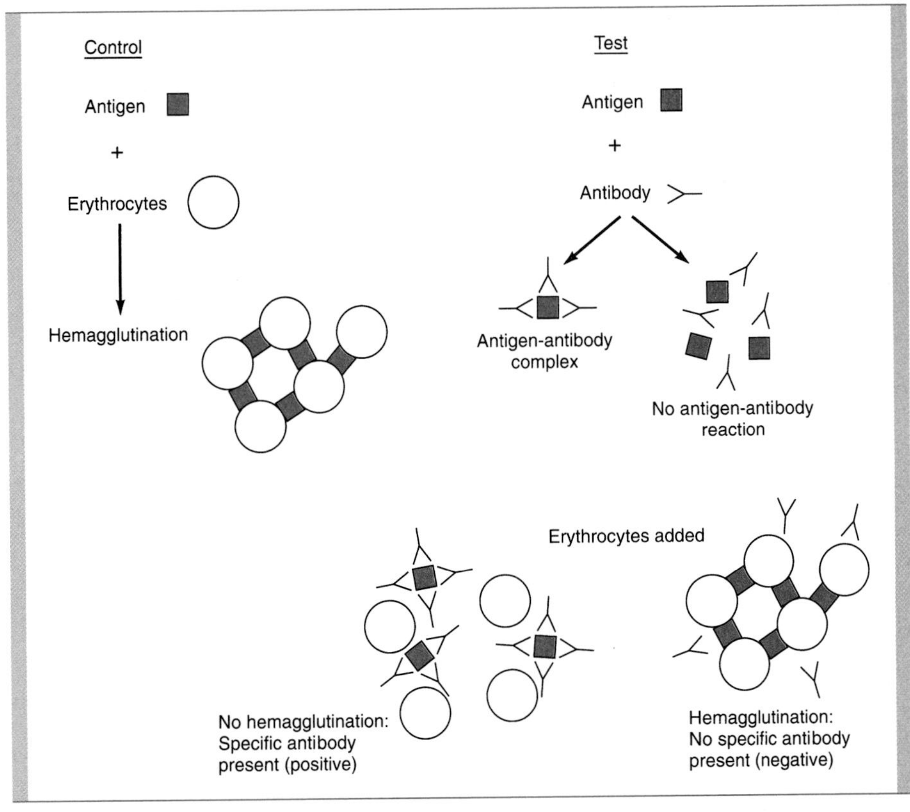

FIGURE 15–11
Hemagglutination inhibition for antibody detection (used when antigen agglutinates erythrocytes).

neutralization, a single antibody molecule can bind to surface components of the extracellular virus and interfere with one of the initial events of the viral multiplication cycle (adsorption, penetration, or uncoating). Some bacterial and viral agents directly bind to RBCs (hemagglutination). Neutralization of this reaction by antibody blocking of the receptor is called hemagglutination inhibition (Fig 15–11).

Complement Fixation

Complement fixation assays depend on two properties of complement. The first is fixation (inactivation) of complement on formation of antigen–antibody complexes. The second is the ability of bound complement to cause hemolysis of sheep (RBCs coated with anti-sheep RBC antibody (sensitized RBCs). Complement fixation assays are performed in two stages: The test system reacts the antigen and antibody in the presence of complement; the indicator system, which contains the sensitized RBCs, detects residual complement. Hemolysis indicates that complement was present in the indicator system and therefore that antigen–antibody complexes were not formed in the test system. Primarily used to detect and quantitate antibody, complement fixation is gradually being replaced by simpler methods.

Action of complement on RBCs is used as indicator system

Labeling Methods

Detection of antigen–antibody binding may be enhanced by attaching a label to one (usually the antibody) and detecting the label after removal of unbound reagents. The label may be a fluorescent dye (immunofluorescence), a radioisotope **(radioimmunoassay,** or **RIA),** or an enzyme **(enzyme immunoassay,** or **EIA**). The presence or quantitation of antigen–antibody binding is measured by fluorescence, radioactivity, or the chemical reaction catalyzed by the enzyme.

Labeling antibody allows detection of fluorescence, radioactivity, or enzyme

Immunofluorescence The most common labeling method in diagnostic microbiology is immunofluorescence (Fig 15–12), in which antibody labeled with a fluorescent dye, usually **fluorescein isothiocyanate (FITC)**, is applied to a slide of material that may contain

Light halo enhances microscopic visualization

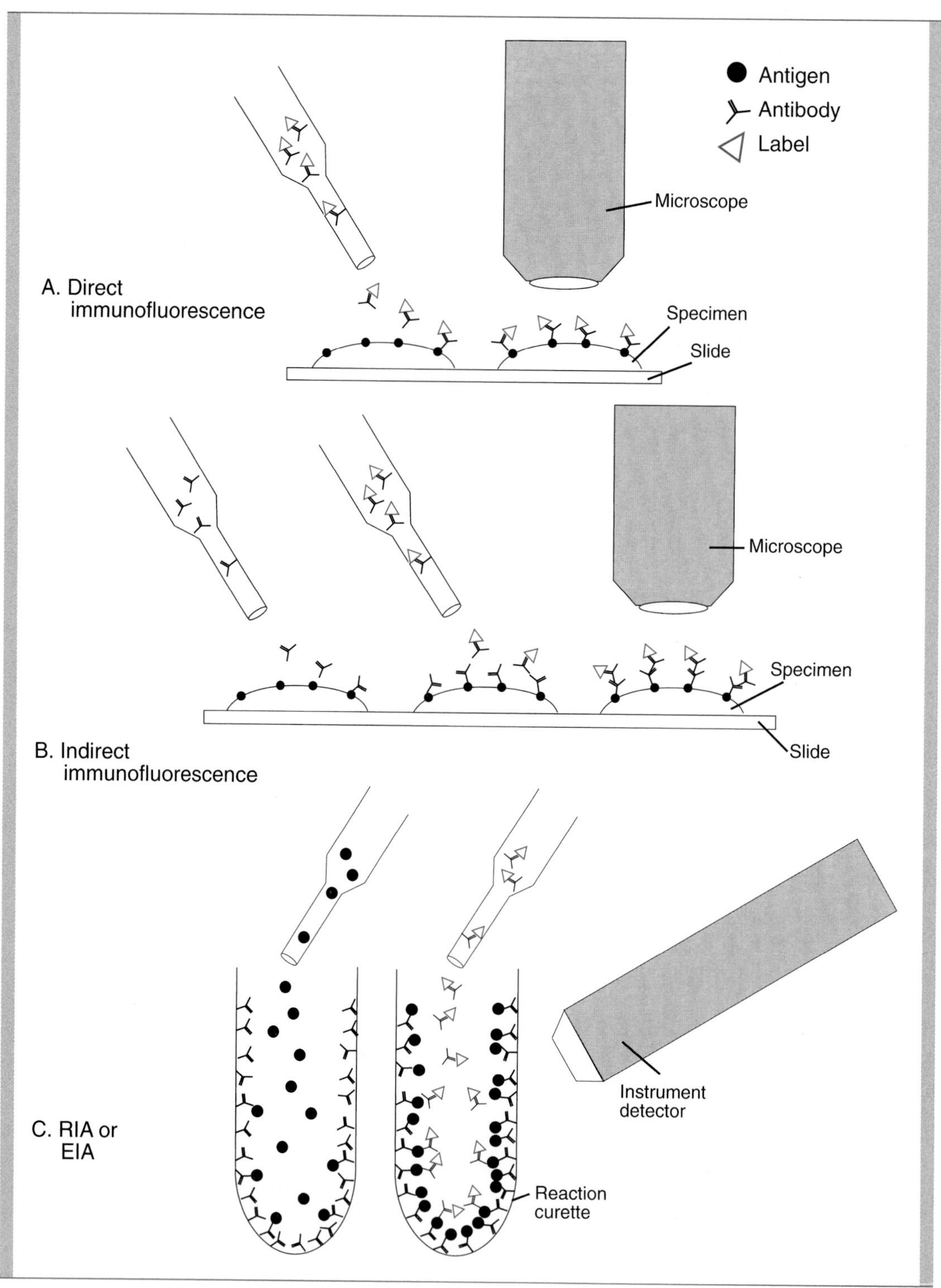

FIGURE 15–12

Labeling methods. **A.** In direct immunofluorescence the fluorescent compound is bound to the specific antibody and can be visualized as shown in Figure 15–2C. **B.** Indirect immunofluorescence has an extra step because the specific antibody is unlabeled. Its binding is detected by a second labeled antiglobulin antibody. **C.** A liquid phase immunoassay is shown. The antigen is "sandwiched" between an antibody bound to the tube and the labeled antibody. If the label is radioactive this is called radioimmunoassay (RIA), and if it is an enzyme it is called enzyme immunoassay (EIA). Many variations are possible.

the antigen sought. Under fluorescence microscopy, binding of the labeled antibody can be detected as a bright green halo surrounding bacterium, or in the case of viruses, as a fluorescent clump or on an infected cell. The method is called "direct" if the FITC is conjugated directly to the antibody with the desired specificity. In "indirect" immunofluorescence the specific antibody is not labeled, but its binding to an antigen is detected in an additional step using an FITC-labeled anti-immunoglobulin antibody that will bind to the specific antibody. Choice between the two approaches involves purely technical considerations.

Indirect methods use a second antibody

Radioimmunoassay (RIA) and Enzyme Immunoassay (EIA) The labels used in RIA and EIA are more suitable for liquid phase assays and are particularly used in virology. They are also used in direct and indirect methods and many other ingenious variations such as the "sandwich" methods, so called because the antigen of interest is "trapped" between two antibodies (Fig 15–12C). These extremely sensitive techniques will be discussed further with regard to antibody detection.

Liquid phase RIA and EIA methods have many variants

Serologic Classification

For most important antigens of diagnostic significance, antisera are commercially available. The most common test methods for bacteria are agglutination and immunofluorescence; and for viruses, neutralization. In most cases these methods subclassify organisms below the species level and thus are primarily of value for epidemiologic and research purposes. The terms "serotype" or "serogroup" are used together with numbers, letters, or Roman numerals with no apparent logic other than historical precedent. For a few genera the most fundamental taxonomic differentiation is serologic. This is the case with the streptococci (see Chapter 17), where an existing classification based on biochemical and cultural characteristics was superseded because a serologic classification scheme developed by Rebecca Lancefield correlated better with disease.

Antigenic systems classify below the species level

Serologic classification is primarily of epidemiologic value

Before these techniques can be applied to the diagnosis of specific infectious diseases, considerable study of the causative agent(s) is required. Antigen–antibody systems may vary in complexity from a single epitope to scores of epitopes on several macromolecular antigens whose chemical nature may or may not be known. The cause of the original 1976 outbreak of Legionnaires' disease (caused by *Legionella pneumophila*; see Chapter 26) was proven through the development of immune reagents that detected the bacteria in tissue and antibodies directed against the bacteria in the serum of patients. Now, more than 25 years later, there are more than a dozen serotypes and many additional species, each requiring specific immunologic reagents for antigen or antibody detection for diagnosis.

Proof of etiologic relationship depends on antigen detection

Antibody Detection (Serology)

During infection—whether viral, bacterial, fungal, or parasitic—the host usually responds with the formation of antibodies, which can be detected by modification of any of the methods used for antigen detection. The formation of antibodies and their time course depends on the antigenic stimulation provided by the infection. The precise patterns vary depending on the antigens used, classes of antibody detected, and method. An example of temporal patterns of development and increase and decline in specific antiviral antibodies measured by different tests is illustrated in Figure 15–13. These responses can be used to detect evidence of recent or past infection. The test methods do not inherently indicate immunoglobulin class but can be modified to do so, usually by pretreatment of the serum to remove IgG to differentiate the IgM and IgG responses. Several basic principles must be emphasized:

Antibodies are formed in response to infection

Antibodies may indicate current, recent, or past infection

1. In an acute infection, the antibodies usually appear early in the illness, and then rise sharply over the next 10 to 21 days. Thus, a serum sample collected shortly after the onset of illness (acute serum) and another collected 2 to 3 weeks later (convalescent serum) can be compared quantitatively for changes in specific antibody content.
2. Antibodies can be quantitated by several means. The most common method is to dilute the serum serially in appropriate media and determine the maximal dilution that will still yield detectable antibody in the test system (eg, serum dilutions of 1:4, 1:8, and 1:16). The highest dilution that retains specific activity is called the antibody titer.

Paired specimens are compared

Titer is the highest serum dilution demonstrating activity

Seroconversion or fourfold rise in titer most conclusive

3. The interpretation of significant antibody responses (evidence of specific, recent infection) is most reliable when definite evidence of seroconversion is demonstrated; that is, detectable specific antibody is absent from the acute serum (or preillness serum, if available) but present in the convalescent serum. Alternatively, a fourfold or greater increase in antibody titer supports a diagnosis of recent infection; for example, an acute serum titer of 1:4 or less and a convalescent serum titer of 1:16 or greater would be considered significant.

Single titers may be useful in some circumstances

IgM responses indicate acute infection

4. In instances in which the average antibody titers of a population to a specific agent are known, a single convalescent antibody titer significantly greater than the expected mean may be used as supportive or presumptive evidence of recent infection. However, this finding is considerably less valuable than those obtained by comparing responses of acute and convalescent serum samples. An alternative and somewhat more complex method of serodiagnosis is to determine which major immunoglobulin subclass constitutes the major proportion of the specific antibodies. In primary infections, the IgM-specific response is often dominant during the first days or weeks after onset but is replaced progressively by IgG-specific antibodies; thus, by 1 to 6 months after infection, the predominant antibodies belong to the IgG subclass. Consequently, serum containing a high titer of antibodies of the IgM subclass would suggest a recent, primary infection.

Experience with systems and temporal relationships aids interpretation

The immunologic methods used to identify bacterial or viral antigens are applied to serologic diagnosis by simply reversing the detection system: that is, using a known rather than an unknown antigen to detect the presence of an antibody. The methods of serologic diagnosis to be used are selected on the basis of their convenience and applicability to the antigen in question. As shown in Figure 15–13, the temporal relationships of antibody response to infection vary according to the method used. Of the methods for measuring antigen–antibody interaction discussed previously, those now used most frequently for serologic diagnosis are agglutination, RIA, and EIA (see Figs 15–9 and 15–11).

Western Blot

Western blot confirms specificity of antibodies for protein components of the agent (eg, HIV)

The Western blot immunoassay is another technique that is now commonly employed to detect and confirm the specificity of antibodies to a variety of epitopes. Its greatest use has been in the diagnosis of HIV infections (see Chapter 42), in which virions are electrophoresed in a polyacrylamide gel to separate the protein and glycoprotein components

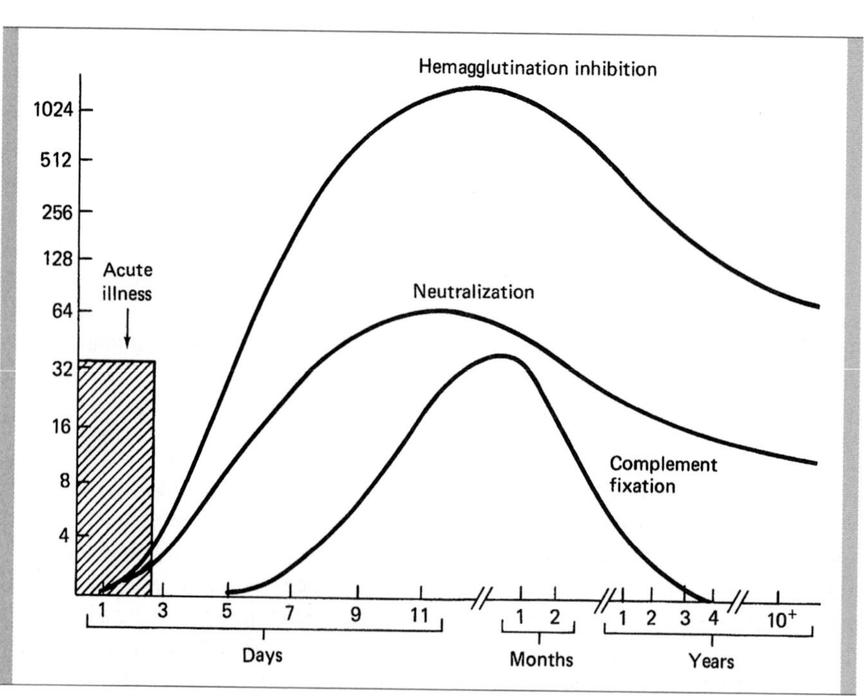

FIGURE 15–13
Examples of patterns of antibody responses to an acute infection, measured by three different methods.

and then transferred onto nitrocellulose. This is then incubated with patient serum, and antibody to the different viral components is detected by using an antihuman globulin IgG antibody conjugated with an enzyme label.

Antigen Detection

Theoretically, any of the methods described for detecting antigen–antibody interactions can be applied directly to clinical specimens. The most common of these is immunofluorescence, in which antigen is detected on the surface of the organism or in cells present in the infected secretion. The greatest success with this approach has been in respiratory infections where a nasopharyngeal, throat washing, sputum, or bronchoalveolar lavage specimen may contain bacteria or viral aggregates in sufficient amount to be seen microscopically. Although the fluorescent tag makes it easier to find organisms, these methods are generally not as sensitive as culture. With some genera and species, the immunofluorescent detection of antigens in clinical material provides the most rapid means of diagnosis, as with *Legionella* and respiratory syncytial virus.

Immunofluorescence detects agents in respiratory secretions

Another approach is to detect free antigen released by the organism into body fluids. This offers the possibility of bypassing direct examination, culture, and identification tests to achieve a diagnosis. Success requires a highly specific antibody, a sensitive detection method, and the presence of the homologous antigen in an accessible body fluid. The latter is an important limitation, because not all organisms release free antigen in the course of infection. At present, diagnosis by antigen detection is limited to some bacteria and fungi with polysaccharide capsules (eg, *Haemophilus influenzae*), *Chlamydia*, and to certain viruses. The techniques of agglutination with antibody bound to latex particles, CIE, RIA, and EIA are used to detect free antigen in serum, urine, cerebrospinal fluid, and joint fluid. Live organisms are not required for antigen detection, and these tests may still be positive when the causative organism has been eliminated by antimicrobial therapy. The procedures can yield results within an hour or two, sometimes within a few minutes. This feature is attractive for office practice, because it allows diagnostic decisions to be made during the patient's visit. A number of commercial products detect group A streptococci in sore throats with over 90% sensitivity; however, because these tests are less sensitive than culture, negative results must be confirmed by culture.

Soluble antigens may be detected in body fluids

Rapid detection can replace culture

NUCLEIC ACID ANALYSIS

Analysis of the DNA or RNA of microorganisms is the basis of newer taxonomic studies and increasingly applied to diagnostic and epidemiologic work. It is also possible to use cloned or synthesized nucleic acid probes to detect genes or smaller nucleotide sequences specific for a variety of bacterial, viral, and other infectious agents. As with antigen–antibody reactions, a variety of methods have been developed for analysis of nucleic acids. Those relevant to the study of infectious diseases are briefly summarized below. The student is referred to textbooks of molecular biology for more complete coverage. DNA is a hardy molecule that will withstand fairly harsh chemical treatment. RNA is more fragile, primarily because it is readily digested by the RNAse enzymes commonly found in biologic systems. The extraction process for bacteria and fungi involves breaking open the cells, precipitating the protein, and extracting the nucleic acid with ethanol. Viral procedures are similar except that much of the separation and concentration may be accomplished by ultracentrifugation.

DNA is extracted from bacteria and fungi

Viral DNA and RNA are concentrated by ultracentrifugation

Methods of Nucleic Acid Analysis

Agarose Gel Electrophoresis

Nucleic acids may be separated in an electrophoretic field in an **agarose** (highly purified agar) gel. The speed of migration depends on size, with the smaller molecules moving faster and appearing at the bottom (end) of the gel. This method is able to separate DNA fragments in the range of 0.1 to 50 kilobases, which is far below the size of bacterial genomes but includes some naturally occurring genetic elements such as bacterial plasmids (Fig 15–14). A variant of agarose gel electrophoresis, **pulsed field electrophoresis**, alternates the orientation of electrical field in a fashion that allows resolution of much larger DNA fragments.

Agarose gel electrophoresis separates DNA fragments or plasmids based on size

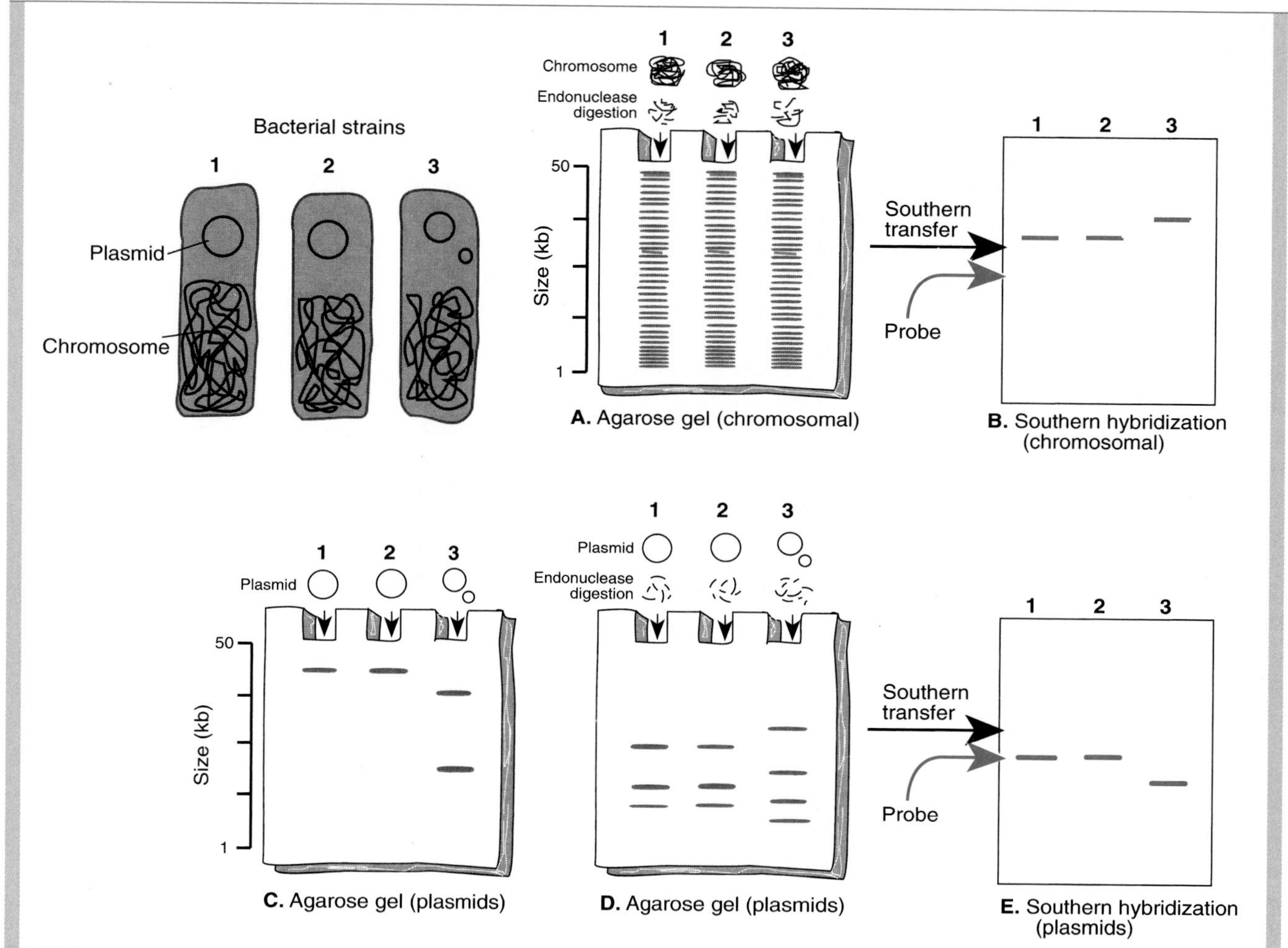

FIGURE 15–14
Molecular diagnostic methods. Three bacterial strains of the same species are shown each with chromosome and plasmid(s). **A.** The chromosomal DNA of each strain is isolated, digested with a restriction endonuclease, and separated by agarose gel electrophoresis. An almost continuous range of fragment sizes is generated for each strain, making them difficult to distinguish. **B.** The restriction fragments in A are transferred to a membrane (Southern transfer) and hybridized with a probe. The probe binds to a single fragment from each strain, but the larger size of the fragment from strain 3 indicates variation in restriction sites and thus a genomic difference between it and strains 1 and 2. **C.** Plasmids from each strain are isolated and separated in the same manner as A. The results show a plasmid of the same size from 1 and 2. Strain 3 has two plasmids each of a different size than strains 1 and 2. **D.** The same plasmids are restriction digested prior to electrophoresis. The plasmids from strains 1 and 2 show three fragments of identical size, proving they are identical. The plasmids of strain 3 appear unrelated. **E.** The fragments in D are transferred and reacted with a probe. The positive result with the largest of the strain 1 and 2 fragments confirms their relatedness. The positive hybridization with one of the strain 3 fragments suggests that it contains at least some DNA that is homologous to the plasmid from strains 1 and 2.

Restriction Endonuclease Digestion

Restriction endonuclease digestion refines electrophoretic analysis of DNA

Restriction endonucleases are enzymes that recognize specific nucleotide sequences in DNA molecules and digest (cut) them at all sites at which the sequence appears. A large number of these enzymes have been isolated from bacterial strains and are commercially available together with information on the sequences they recognize. While the four- to eight-base pair sequences recognized by these endonucleases are not unique to any one organism, their spacing along the chromosome or other genomic structure may be. The

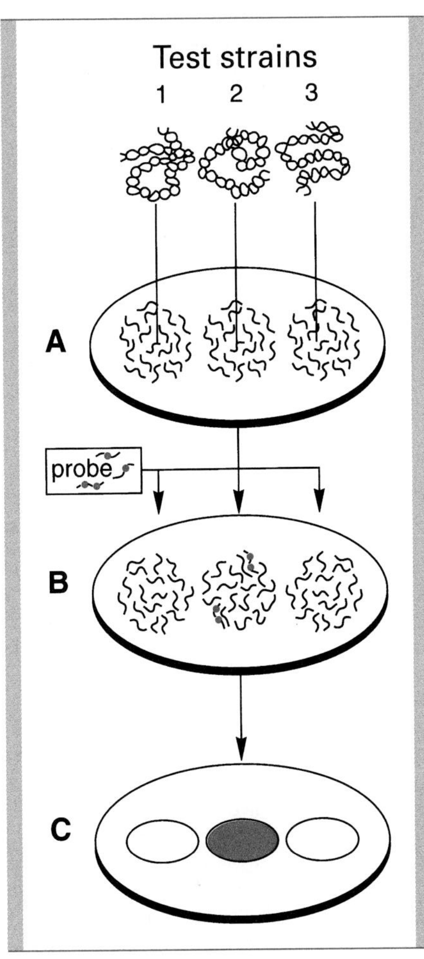

FIGURE 15–15
DNA probe detection. **A.** Chromosomal and/or plasmid DNA from three unknown strains is fragmented, denatured, and bound to filters. **B.** The probe (⤴) is a small DNA fragment labeled with a radioactive or other marker. It is allowed to react with the single-stranded test DNAs on the filter and binds wherever homologous sequences are found. **C.** Probe that has hybridized with test DNA is detected on the filter by an appropriate test for the marker. Test strain 2 contains sequences homologous to the probe and thus gives a positive reaction.

size of fragments generated by endonuclease digestion of DNA molecules may be compared by agarose gel electrophoresis (Fig 15–15).

DNA Hybridization

If the DNA double helix is opened, leaving single-stranded (denatured) DNA, the nucleotide bases are exposed and thus available to interact with other single-stranded nucleic acid molecules. If complementary sequences of a second DNA molecule are brought into physical contact with the first, they will hybridize to it, forming a new double-stranded molecule in that area. A variety of methods are in use that allow hybridization to take place between two or more nucleic acid molecules. The reaction mixtures vary from tiny probes to the entire genome of an organism. Most immobilize the single-stranded target DNA on a membrane to prevent it from rehybridizing with its own complementary strand, but liquid phase assays have also been developed. A variant in which the DNA is separated by agarose gel electrophoresis before binding to the membrane is called **Southern hybridization.**

DNA hybridization methods allow DNA from different sources to combine

Polymerase Chain Reaction

The polymerase chain reaction (PCR) is an amplification technique that allows the detection and selective replication of a targeted portion of the genome. The technique uses special DNA polymerases that through alternate changes in test conditions such as temperature can be manipulated to initiate replication in either the 3′ or 5′ direction. The specificity is provided by primers that recognize a pair of unique sites on the chromosome so that the DNA between them can be replicated by repetitive cycling of the test conditions. Because each newly synthesized fragment can serve as the template for its own replication, the amount of DNA doubles exponentially with each cycle (Fig 15–16).

PCR amplifies targeted segments of the genome

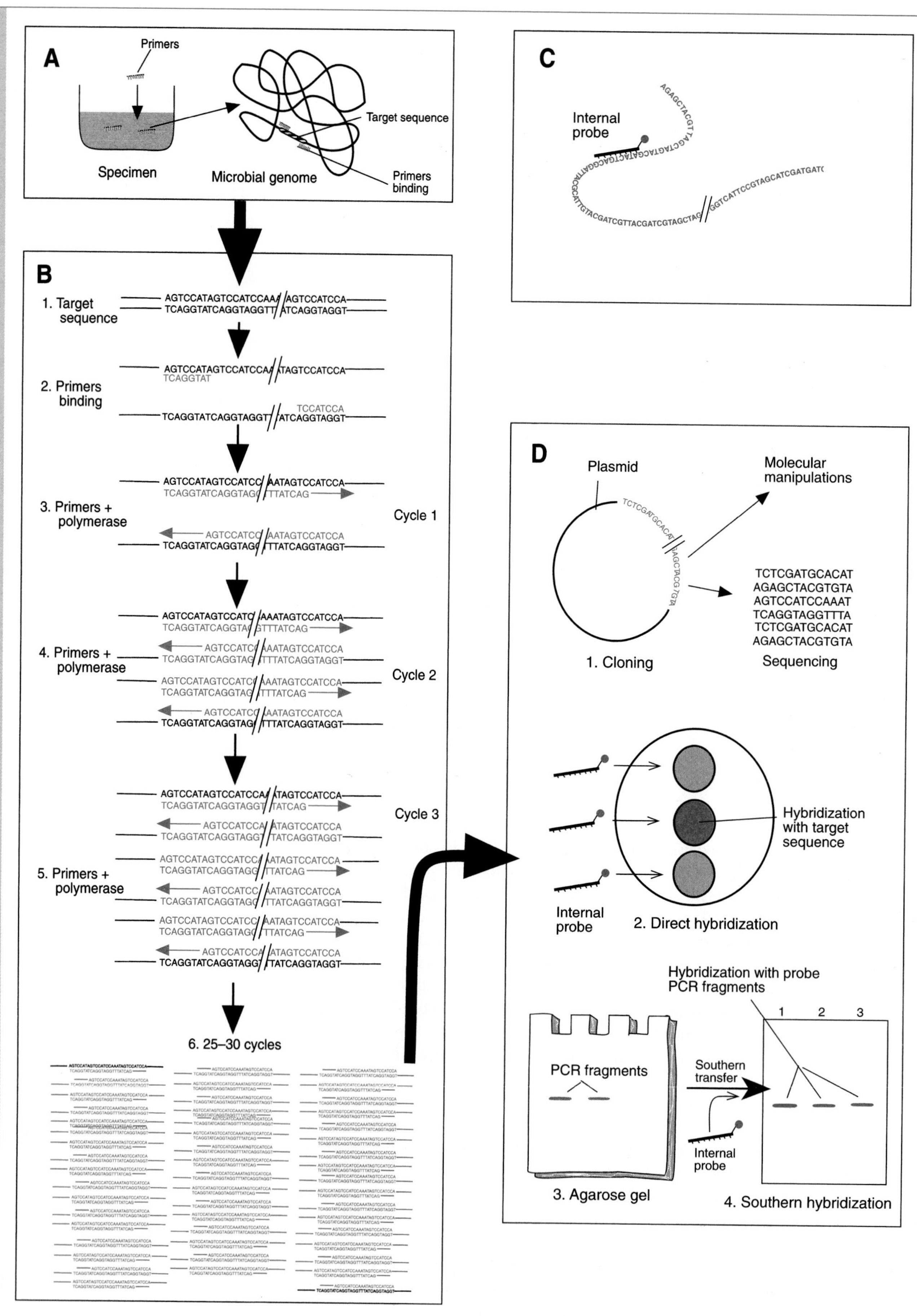
A
Primers
Target sequence
Specimen
Microbial genome
Primers binding
B
1. Target sequence
2. Primers binding
3. Primers + polymerase
Cycle 1
4. Primers + polymerase
Cycle 2
5. Primers + polymerase
Cycle 3
6. 25–30 cycles
C
Internal probe
D
Plasmid
Molecular manipulations
TCTCGATGCACAT
AGAGCTACGTGTA
AGTCCATCCAAAT
TCAGGTAGGTTTA
TCTCGATGCACAT
AGAGCTACGTGTA
1. Cloning
Sequencing
Hybridization with target sequence
Internal probe
2. Direct hybridization
Hybridization with probe PCR fragments
PCR fragments
Southern transfer
Internal probe
3. Agarose gel
4. Southern hybridization

Nucleic Acid Sequence Analysis

For some time, it has been possible to chemically determine the exact nucleotide sequence of genomic segments or cloned genes. Published sequences are systematically entered into computer databases such as GenBank and are widely available for analysis by computer software designed to solve a wide variety of problems. Conversely, given the known sequence, short segments of DNA can be synthesized for use as probes or primers. It is even possible to compare a sequenced gene or putative probe against all known sequences using the computer, an "experiment" that would be impossible in the laboratory.

Nucleic acid sequence data is available in computerized formats

Application of Nucleic Acid Methods to Infectious Diseases

Bacterial and Viral Genomic Sizing

The only intact genetic elements of infectious agents that are small enough to be directly detected and sized by agarose gel electrophoresis are bacterial plasmids. Not all bacterial species typically harbor plasmids, but those that do may carry one or a number of plasmids ranging in size from less than 1 to over 50 kilobases. This diversity makes the presence or absence, number, and sizes of plasmids of considerable value in differentiating strains for epidemiologic purposes. Because plasmids are not stable components of the bacterial genome, plasmid analysis also has the element of a timely "snapshot" of the circumstances of a disease outbreak. The specificity of these results can be improved by digesting the plasmids with restriction endonucleases prior to electrophoresis. Two plasmids of the same size from different strains may not be the same, but if an identical pattern of fragments is generated from the digestion, they almost certainly are. These principles are illustrated Figure 15–14 and their application to an outbreak is shown in Figures 4–12 and 4–13.

Number and size of plasmids differentiates strains

Endonuclease digestion of plasmids refines their comparison

Because of their larger size, the chromosomes of bacteria must be digested with endonucleases to resolve them on gels. For viruses the outcome is much like that with plasmids, depending on the genomic size and the endonuclease used. Digested bacterial chromosomes can be compared in this manner, but the number of fragments is very large and the patterns complex. The combined use of endonucleases, which make infrequent cuts, and pulsed-field electrophoresis can produce a comparison comparable to that possible with plasmids. This approach is also used for analysis of the multiple chromosomes of fungi and parasites.

Bacterial chromosomes must be digested prior to electrophoresis

---

FIGURE 15–16

Diagnostic applications of the polymerase chain reaction (PCR). **A.** A clinical specimen (eg, pus, tissue) contains DNA from many sources as well as the chromosome of the organism of interest. If the DNA strands are separated (denatured), the PCR primers can bind to their target sequences in the specimen itself. **B.** Amplification of the target sequence by PCR. (1) The target sequence is shown in its native state. (2) The DNA is denatured, allowing the primers to bind where they find the homologous sequence. (3) In the presence of the special DNA polymerase, new DNA is synthesized from both strands in the region between the primers. (4 to 6) Additional cycles are added by temperature control of the polymerase with each new sequence acting as the template for another. The DNA doubles with each cycle. After 25 to 30 cycles enough DNA is present to analyze diagnostically. **C.** Internal probe. The amplified target sequence is shown. A probe can be designed to bind to a sequence located between (internal to) the primers. **D.** Analysis of PCR amplified DNA. (1) The amplified sequence can be cloned into a plasmid vector. In this form, a variety of molecular manipulations or sequencing may be carried out. (2) Direct hybridizations usually make use of an internal probe. The example shows three specimens, each of which went through steps **A** and **B**. Following amplification each was bound to a separate spot on a filter (dot blot). The filter is then reacted with the internal probe to detect the PCR-amplified DNA. The result shows that only the middle specimen contained the target sequence. (3) The amplified DNA may be detected directly by agarose gel electrophoresis. The example shows detection of amplified fragments in two of three lanes on the gel. (4) The sensitivity of detection may be increased by use of the internal probe following Southern transfer. The example shows detection of a third fragment of the same size that was not seen on the original gel because the amount of DNA was too small.

DNA Probes

Probes may be cloned or synthesized from known sequences

A "probe" is a fragment of DNA that has been cloned or otherwise recovered from a genomic or plasmid source. It may contain a gene of known function or simply sequences empirically found to be useful for the application in question. In some cases, the probe is synthesized as a single chain of nucleotides (oligonucleotide probe) from known sequence data. The probes are labeled with a radioisotope or other marker and used in hybridization reactions either to detect the homologous sequences in unknown specimens (see Fig 15–15) or to further refine gel electrophoresis findings (see Fig 15–14). In the latter instance, Southern hybridizations are used to retain knowledge of the size of fragments involved. For example, the information that the same gene is present in each of two strains but in different size restriction fragments is evidence for a genomic difference between the two strains (Fig 15–14B).

Probes can detect DNA of pathogen directly in clinical specimens

The diagnostic use of DNA probes is to detect or identify microorganisms by hybridization of the probe to homologous sequences in DNA extracted from the entire organism. A number of probes have been developed that will quickly and reliably identify organisms already isolated in culture. The application of probes for detection of infectious agents directly in clinical specimens such as blood, urine, and sputum is more difficult, because most of the systems developed to date are not as sensitive as culture and are more expensive. However, this approach offers the potential for rapid diagnosis and the detection of characteristics not possible by routine methods. For example, a bacterial toxin gene probe can demonstrate both the presence of the related organism and its toxigenicity without the need for culture.

Applications of Polymerase Chain Reaction (PCR)

PCR combined with probes gives the greatest sensitivity

The amplification power of the PCR offers a solution for the sensitivity problems inherent in the direct application of probes (Fig 15–16). Although the nucleic acid segment amplified by PCR can be seen directly on a gel, the greatest sensitivity and specificity are achieved when probe hybridization is carried out following PCR. This approach has been successful for a wide range of infectious agents and awaits only further resolution of practical problems for wider use.

PCR from tissue allows study of organisms that cannot be cultured

Another creative use of PCR has been in the study of infectious agents seen in tissue but not grown in culture. PCR primers derived from sequences known to be highly conserved among bacteria, such as ribosomal RNA, have been applied to tissue specimens. The amplification produces enough DNA to clone and sequence. This sequence can then be compared with sequences published for other organisms using computers. Thus, taxonomic relationships can be inferred for an organism that has never been isolated.

Ribotyping

Ribotyping refines comparison of chromosomal endonuclease digestion patterns

Ribotyping also makes use of the conserved nature of bacterial ribosomal RNA and of the ability of RNA to hybridize to DNA under certain conditions. Labeled ribosomal RNA of one organism can be hybridized with restriction endonuclease–digested chromosomal DNA of another. In this case, ribosomal RNA is being used as a massive probe of restriction fragments separated by electrophoresis. Hybridization to multiple fragments is common, but if the organisms are genetically different, the restriction fragments, which contain the ribosomal RNA sequences, will vary in size. The pattern of bands produced by epidemiologically related strains can then be compared side by side.

Genomic Analysis

Percent DNA homology is now a primary tool for taxonomic comparisons

DNA homology techniques hybridize the total genomic DNA of one organism to that of another in a manner demonstrated in Figure 15–17. The relatedness of strains can be expressed as a percent homology. Strains related at the species level should show homology in the 60 to 90% range, whereas strains with increasing taxonomic divergence show progressively less homology. These findings are now a major factor in decisions on the

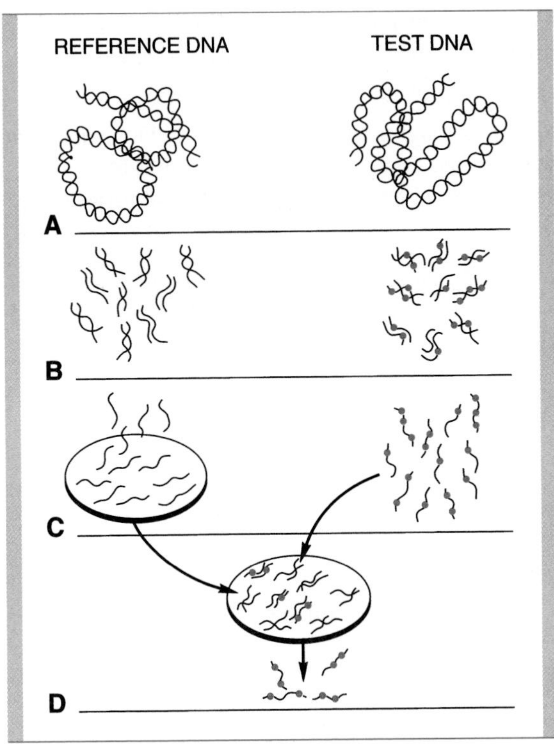

FIGURE 15–17

DNA–DNA homology. **A.** Double-stranded chromosomal DNA from a test strain is to be compared with a reference strain of the same or another species. **B.** Both DNAs are fragmented and denatured. The test DNA is labeled (⌐) with a radioisotope or some other marker. **C.** The denatured (single-stranded) reference DNA is bound to a support matrix such as a nitrocellulose or nylon filter, thus leaving the nucleotide bases available for pairing. **D.** The labeled test DNA is reacted with the material on the filter allowing homologous sequences to pair (hybridize) with the reference DNA. Nonhomologous DNA is washed away, and the amount of bound label measured. The percentage homology of the test to the reference DNA is determined from the ratio of bound to unbound label.

taxonomic classification of all microorganisms, allowing species, genus, and higher taxonomic groupings to be assessed by means that are not subject to the phenotypic variation inherent with classical methods. Sequence analysis of mutations in genes related to the action of drugs used in the treatment of AIDS can now be used to study and even predict emergence of drug resistance.

Drug resistance can be predicted by sequence analysis

SUMMARY

The application of some combination of the principles described in this chapter is appropriate to the diagnosis of any infectious disease. The usefulness of any individual method differs among infectious agents due to biologic variation and uneven study. In general, for agents that can be grown in vitro, culture remains the "gold standard" as both the most sensitive and specific method. Molecular methods have the potential to replace culture once they are more fully evaluated and cost effective.

ADDITIONAL READING

Cumulative Techniques and Procedures in Clinical Microbiology (CUMITECH). Washington, DC: American Society for Microbiology. CUMITECH is a series of 10- to 25-page pamphlets, each of which covers important topics related to diagnostic microbiology (eg, blood cultures, urinary tract infections, antimicrobial susceptibility testing). Each pamphlet is jointly written by at least three authors representing the clinical as well as the laboratory viewpoint and includes clinical, specimen collection, isolation, and identification recommendations for all agents pertinent to the topic.

Murray PR (ed). *Manual of Clinical Microbiology*, 7th ed. Washington, DC: American Society for Microbiology; 1999. A widely used comprehensive text written for pathologists and medical technologists includes clinical bacteriology, mycology, parasitology, and virology.

Relman DA, Schmidt TM, MacDermott RP, Falkow S. Identification of the uncultured bacillus of Whipple's disease. *N Engl J Med* 1992;327:293–301. A wonderful example of taxonomy using molecular methods alone.

APPENDIX 15–1. SOME MEDIA USED FOR ISOLATION OF BACTERIAL PATHOGENS

Medium	Uses
General-purpose Media	
Nutrient broths (eg, Soybean–Casein digest broth)	Most bacteria, particularly when used for blood culture
Thioglycolate broth	Anaerobes, facultative bacteria
Blood agar	Most bacteria (demonstrates hemolysis)
Chocolate agar	Most bacteria, including fastidious species (eg, *Haemophilus*)
Selective Media	
MacConkey agar	Nonfastidious Gram-negative rods
Hektoen-enteric agar	*Salmonella* and *Shigella*
Selenite F broth	*Salmonella* enrichment
Special-purpose Media	
Löwenstein–Jensen medium, Middlebrook agar	*Mycobacterium tuberculosis* and other mycobacteria (selective)
Martin–Lewis medium	*Neisseria gonorrhoeae* and *N. meningitidis* (selective)
Fletcher medium (semisolid)	Leptospira (nonselective)
Tinsdale agar	*Corynebacterium diphtheriae* (selective)
Charcoal agar	*Bordetella pertussis* (selective)
Buffered charcoal–yeast extract agar	*Legionella* species (nonselective)
Campylobacter blood agar	*Campylobacter jejuni* (selective)
Thiosulfate-citrate-bile-sucrose agar (TCBS)	*Vibrio cholerae* and *V. parahaemolyticus* (selective)

APPENDIX 15–2. CHARACTERISTICS OF COMMONLY USED BACTERIOLOGIC MEDIA

1. **Nutrient broths.** Some form of nutrient broth is used for culture of all direct tissue or fluid samples from sites that are normally sterile to obtain the maximum culture sensitivity. Selective or indicator agents are omitted to prevent inhibition of more fastidious organisms.
2. **Blood agar.** The addition of defibrinated blood to a nutrient agar base enhances the growth of some bacteria, such as streptococci. It often yields distinctive colonies and provides an indicator system for hemolysis. Two major types of hemolysis are seen:

β-hemolysis, a complete clearing of red cells from a zone surrounding the colony; and α-hemolysis, which is incomplete (that is, intact red cells are still present in the hemolytic zone), but shows a green color caused by hemoglobin breakdown products. The net effect is a hazy green zone extending 1 to 2 mm beyond the colony. A third type, α'-hemolysis, produces a hazy, incomplete hemolytic zone similar to that caused by α-hemolysis, but without the green coloration.

3. **Chocolate agar.** If blood is added to molten nutrient agar at about 80°C and maintained at this temperature, the red cells are gently lysed, hemoglobin products are released, and the medium turns a chocolate brown color. The nutrients released permit the growth of some fastidious organisms, such as *Haemophilus influenzae,* that fail to grow on blood or nutrient agars. This quality is particularly pronounced when the medium is further enriched with vitamin supplements. Given the same incubation conditions, any organism that grows on blood agar will also grow on chocolate agar.
4. **Martin–Lewis medium.** A variant of chocolate agar, Martin–Lewis medium is a solid medium selective for the pathogenic *Neisseria* (*N. gonorrhoeae* and *N. meningitidis*). Growth of most other bacteria and fungi in the genital or respiratory flora is inhibited by the addition of antimicrobics. One formulation includes vancomycin, colistin, trimethoprim, and anisomycin.
5. **MacConkey agar.** MacConkey agar is both a selective and an indicator medium for Gram-negative rods, particularly members of the family Enterobacteriaceae and the genus *Pseudomonas.* In addition to a peptone base, the medium contains bile salts, crystal violet, lactose, and neutral red as a pH indicator. The bile salts and crystal violet inhibit Gram-positive bacteria and the more fastidious Gram-negative organisms, such as *Neisseria* and *Pasteurella.* Gram-negative rods that grow and ferment lactose produce a red (acid) colony, often with a distinctive colonial morphology.
6. **Hektoen enteric agar.** The Hektoen medium is one of many highly selective media developed for the isolation of *Salmonella* and *Shigella* species from stool specimens. It has both selective and indicator properties. The medium contains a mixture of bile, thiosulfate, and citrate salts that inhibits not only Gram-positive bacteria, but members of the Enterobacteriaceae other than *Salmonella* and *Shigella* that appear among the normal flora of the colon. The inhibition is not absolute; recovery of *Escherichia coli* is reduced 1000- to 10,000-fold relative to that on nonselective media, but there is little effect on growth of *Salmonella* and *Shigella.* Carbohydrates and a pH indicator are also included to help to differentiate colonies of *Salmonella* and *Shigella* from those of other enteric Gram-negative rods.
7. **Anaerobic media.** In addition to meeting atmospheric requirements, isolation of some strictly anaerobic bacteria on blood agar is enhanced by reducing agents such as L-cysteine and by vitamin enrichment. Sodium thioglycolate, another reducing agent, is often used in broth media. Plate media are made selective for anaerobes by the addition of aminoglycoside antibiotics, which are active against many aerobic and facultative organisms but not against anaerobic bacteria. The use of selective media is particularly important with anaerobes because they grow slowly and are commonly mixed with facultative bacteria in infections.
8. **Highly selective media.** Media specific to the isolation of almost every important pathogen have been developed. Many will allow only a single species to grow from specimens with a rich normal flora (eg, stool). The most common of these media are listed in Appendix 15–1; they are discussed in greater detail in following chapters.

APPENDIX 15–3. COMMON BIOCHEMICAL TESTS FOR MICROBIAL IDENTIFICATION

1. **Carbohydrate breakdown.** The ability to produce acidic metabolic products, fermentatively or oxidatively, from a range of carbohydrates (eg, glucose, sucrose, and lactose) has been applied to the identification of most groups of bacteria. Such tests are crude and imperfect in defining mechanisms, but have proved useful for taxonomic purposes. More recently, gas chromatographic identification of specific

short-chain fatty acids produced by fermentation of glucose has proved useful in classifying many anaerobic bacteria.

2. **Catalase production.** The enzyme catalase catalyzes the conversion of hydrogen peroxide to water and oxygen. When a colony is placed in hydrogen peroxide, liberation of oxygen as gas bubbles can be seen. The test is particularly useful in differentiation of staphylococci (positive) from streptococci (negative), but also has taxonomic application to Gram-negative bacteria.
3. **Citrate utilization.** An agar medium that contains sodium citrate as the sole carbon source may be used to determine ability to use citrate. Bacteria that grow on this medium are termed **citrate positive.**
4. **Coagulase.** The enzyme coagulase acts with a plasma factor to convert fibrinogen to a fibrin clot. It is used to differentiate *Staphylococcus aureus* from other, less pathogenic staphylococci.
5. **Decarboxylases and deaminases.** The decarboxylation or deamination of the amino acids lysine, ornithine, and arginine is detected by the effect of the amino products on the pH of the reaction mixture or by the formation of colored products. These tests are used primarily with Gram-negative rods.
6. **Hydrogen sulfide.** The ability of some bacteria to produce H_2S from amino acids or other sulfur-containing compounds is helpful in taxonomic classification. The black color of the sulfide salts formed with heavy metals such as iron is the usual means of detection.
7. **Indole.** The indole reaction tests the ability of the organism to produce indole, a benzopyrrole, from tryptophan. Indole is detected by the formation of a red dye after addition of a benzaldehyde reagent. A spot test can be done in seconds using isolated colonies.
8. **Nitrate reduction.** Bacteria may reduce nitrates by several mechanisms. This ability is demonstrated by detection of the nitrites and/or nitrogen gas formed in the process.
9. **O-Nitrophenyl-β-D-galactoside (ONPG) breakdown.** The ONPG test is related to lactose fermentation. Organisms that possess the β-galactoside necessary for lactose fermentation but lack a permease necessary for lactose to enter the cell are ONPG positive and lactose negative.
10. **Oxidase production.** The oxidase tests detect the *c* component of the cytochrome–oxidase complex. The reagents used change from clear to colored when converted from the reduced to the oxidized state. The oxidase reaction is commonly demonstrated in a spot test, which can be done quickly from isolated colonies.
11. **Proteinase production.** Proteolytic activity is detected by growing the organism in the presence of substrates such as gelatin or coagulated egg.
12. **Urease production.** Urease hydrolyzes urea to yield two molecules of ammonia and one of CO_2. This reaction can be detected by the increase in medium pH caused by ammonia production. Urease-positive species vary in the amount of enzyme produced; bacteria can thus be designated as positive, weakly positive, or negative.
13. **Voges–Proskauer test.** The Voges–Proskauer test detects acetylmethylcarbinol (acetoin), an intermediate product in the butene glycol pathway of glucose fermentation.

PART V

PATHOGENIC BACTERIA

CHAPTER 23

Pseudomonas and Other Opportunistic Gram-negative Bacilli

CHAPTER 24

Haemophilus and *Bordetella*

CHAPTER 25

Mycoplasma and *Ureaplasma*

CHAPTER 26

Legionella

CHAPTER 27

Spirochetes

CHAPTER 28

Mycobacteria

CHAPTER 29

Actinomyces and *Nocardia*

CHAPTER 30

Chlamydia

CHAPTER 31

Rickettsia, Coxiella, Ehrlichia, and *Bartonella*

CHAPTER 32

Plague and Other Bacterial Zoonotic Diseases

CHAPTER 16

Staphylococci

KENNETH J. RYAN

Members of the genus *Staphylococcus* (staphylococci) are Gram-positive cocci that tend to be arranged in grape-like clusters. Worldwide, *Staphylococcus aureus* is one of the most common and virulent causes of acute purulent infections. Other species are common in the skin flora but produce lower grade disease, typically in association with some abridgment of the host defenses such as an indwelling catheter.

STAPHYLOCCOCI: GROUP CHARACTERISTICS

Although staphylococci have a marked tendency to form clusters (from the Greek staphyle, bunch of grapes), some single cells, pairs, and short chains are also seen. Staphylococci have a typical Gram-positive cell wall structure. Like all medically important cocci, they are nonflagellate, nonmotile, and non-spore-forming. Staphylococci grow best aerobically but are facultatively anaerobic. In contrast to streptococci, staphylococci produce catalase. More than one dozen species of staphylococci colonize humans; of these, three are of major medical importance: *S. aureus, S. epidermidis,* and *S. saprophyticus* (Table 16–1). The ability of *S. aureus* to form coagulase separates it from the other, less virulent species.

Staphylococci form clusters and are catalase positive

Coagulase distinguishes *S. aureus* from other species

Staphylococcus aureus

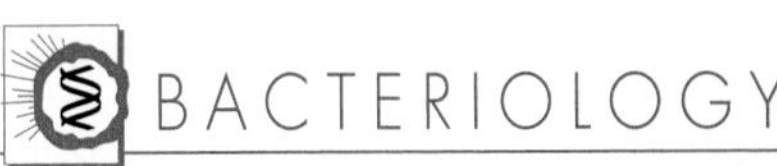

MORPHOLOGY AND STRUCTURE

In growing cultures, the cells of *S. aureus* are uniformly Gram-positive and regular in size, fitting together in clusters with the precision of pool balls. In older cultures, in resolving lesions, and in the presence of some antibiotics, the cells often become more variable in size, and many lose their Gram positivity.

The cell wall of *S. aureus* consists of a typical Gram-positive peptidoglycan (see Chapter 2) interspersed with molecules of a ribitol-teichoic acid, which is antigenic and

TABLE 16–1

Features of Human Staphylococci

Species	Coagulase	Common Habitat	Pathogenic Features: Catheter Colonization	Furuncles	Exotoxin Production
S. aureus	+	Anterior nares, perineum	+	+	+[b]
S. epidermidis	–	Anterior nares, skin	+[a]	–	–
S. saprophyticus[c]	–	Urinary tract	+	–	–
Others	–	Various	+[a]	–	–

[a] Some strains produce surface slime.
[b] Including exfoliatin pyrogenic and toxin superantigens.
[c] Species statistically associated with urinary infection in young women.

Protein A binds Fc portion of IgG

relatively specific for *S. aureus*. In most strains, the peptidoglycan of the cell wall is overlaid with surface proteins; one protein, protein A, is unique in that it binds the Fc portion of IgG molecules, leaving the antigen-reacting Fab portion directed externally. This phenomenon has been exploited in test systems for detecting free antigens (see Chapter 15). It probably contributes to the virulence of *S. aureus* by interfering with opsonization.

CHARACTERISTICS FOR IDENTIFICATION AND SUBTYPING

Colonies are white or golden and hemolytic

After overnight incubation on blood agar, *S. aureus* produces white colonies that tend to turn a buff-golden color with time, which is the basis of the species epithet *aureus* (golden). Most, but not all, strains show a rim of clear β-hemolysis surrounding the colony.

Coagulase produces a fibrin clot

Slide clumping factor correlates with coagulase

The most important test used to distinguish *S. aureus* from other staphylococci is the production of **coagulase,** which nonenzymatically binds to prothrombin, forming a complex that initiates the polymerization of fibrin. It is demonstrated by incubating staphylococci in plasma; this produces a fibrin clot within hours. A dense emulsion of *S. aureus* cells in water also clumps immediately on mixing with plasma due to direct binding of fibrinogen to a factor on the cell surface. This is the basis of a quick laboratory test called the slide clumping test, which has a high correlation with coagulase (95%). Commercial agglutination tests that correlate well with the coagulase test are also used.

Bacteriophage typing defines fingerprints for epidemiologic investigations

S. aureus isolates can be organized into broad groups, and individual strains can be "fingerprinted" for epidemiologic purposes by using bacteriophage typing. This procedure depends on differing susceptibilities of the organism to lysis by bacteriophages derived from lysogenic strains of *S. aureus*. Suspensions of the phages are dropped onto a plate seeded with the staphylococcal strain to be tested, and the plates are incubated. Lysis in the area of a drop indicates susceptibility to that phage (Fig 16–1). The phage type is simply a listing of the phages that gave a positive reaction (eg, 52/52A/80/81). Phage typing is a specialized procedure performed only in a few reference laboratories.

TOXINS AND BIOLOGICALLY ACTIVE EXTRACELLULAR ENZYMES

α-Toxin

α-Toxin inserts in lipid bilayer to form transmembrane pores

α-Toxin is a protein secreted by almost all strains of *S. aureus* but not by coagulase-negative staphylococci. It lyses cytoplasmic membranes by direct insertion into the lipid bilayer to form transmembrane pores (Fig 16–2). The resultant egress of vital molecules leads to cell death. This action is similar to other biologically active cytolysins such as streptolysin O (see Chapter 17), complement, and the effector proteins of cytotoxic T lymphocytes.

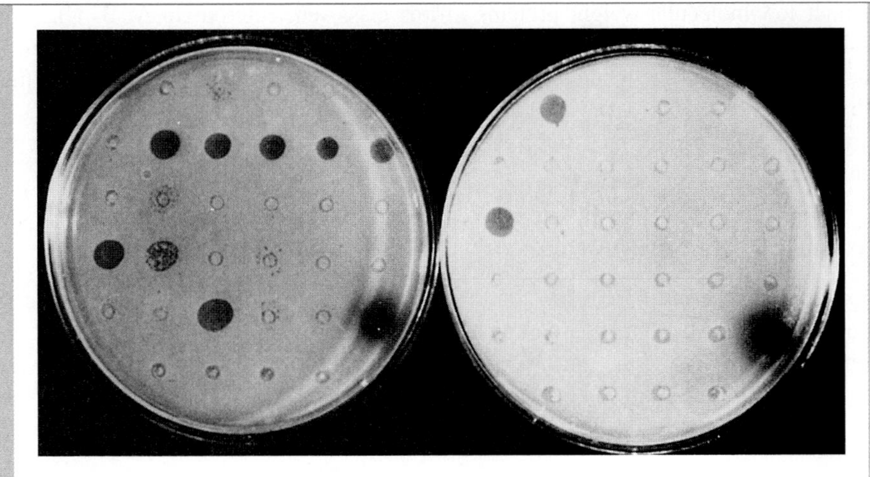

FIGURE 16–1
Bacteriophage typing of two strains of *Staphylococcus aureus:* results after overnight incubation. Lysis is indicated by absence of growth at the site of deposition of individual phages to which the strain is susceptible. The test shows that the two strains are not of common origin.

Exfoliatin

Exfoliatin causes intercellular splitting of the epidermis between the stratum spinosum and stratum granulosum, presumably by disruption of intercellular junctions. Two antigenic variants of exfoliatin are antigenic in humans, and circulating antibody confers immunity to their effects.

Exfoliatin splits intercellular junctions

Pyrogenic Toxin Superantigens

The pyrogenic toxin superantigens (PTSAgs) are a family of secreted proteins able to stimulate systemic effects due to absorption from the site where they are produced by multiplying staphylococci. An individual strain may produce one or more toxins but less than 10% of *S. aureus* strains produce any PTSAg. These toxins share physiochemical and biologic activity similarities with each other and PTSAgs produced by group A streptococci (see Chapter 17). As superantigens they are strongly mitogenic for T cells and do not require proteolytic processing prior to binding with class II major histocompatibility complex (MHC) molecules on antigen-presenting cells. They interact with class II MHC molecules outside the antigenic peptide groove, and are specific for the Vβ region of the T-cell receptor. Thus, T cells with the appropriate Vβ element may be directly activated by the toxin. This stimulates both T cells and macrophages to release massive amounts of cytokines, particularly tumor necrosis factor-α and interleukin-1. Other activities of these toxins are pyrogenicity and enhanced susceptibility to the lethal effects of endotoxin.

PTSAgs of group A streptococci are similar

PTSAgs bind MHC II without processing

Superantigens cause massive cytokine release

Staphylococcal Enterotoxins

The ability of *S. aureus* enterotoxins to stimulate gastrointestinal symptoms (primarily vomiting) in humans and animals has long been known. There are several antigenically

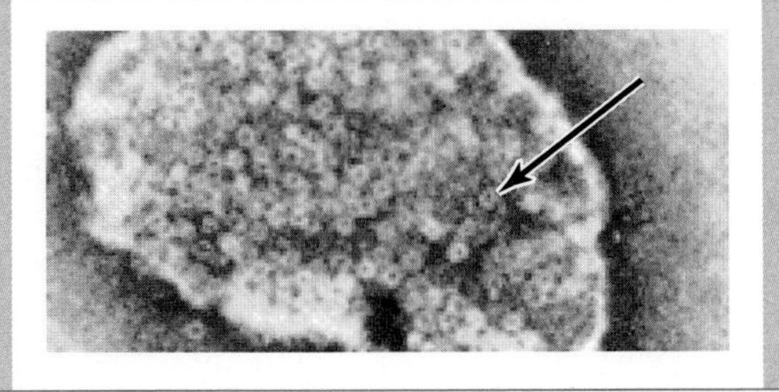

FIGURE 16–2
Staphylococcus aureus alpha toxin. A fragment of a rabbit erythrocyte lysed with alpha toxin is shown. Note the ring-shaped pores in the membrane created by insertion of the toxin. (From Bhadki S, Tranum-Jensen J. Alpha toxin of *Staphylococcus aureus. Microbiol Rev* 1991;55:733–751, with permission.)

Once formed, enterotoxins are stable to boiling and digestive enzymes

Vomiting is stimulated by neural mechanism

distinct low-molecular-weight proteins in this class (eg, enterotoxin A, B, C), some of which are encoded by temperate bacteriophages. Once formed, these toxins are quite stable, retaining activity even after boiling or exposure to gastric and jejunal enzymes. In addition to superantigen-mediated actions, they appear to act directly on neural receptors in the upper gastrointestinal tract, leading to stimulation of the vomiting center in the brain.

Toxic Shock Syndrome Toxin

TSST-1 has superantigen and direct effects

Toxic shock syndrome toxin-1 (TSST-1), the major cause of staphylococcal toxic shock syndrome, shares many properties with the staphylococcal enterotoxins and was, in fact, confused with one of them during the course of its discovery. It can stimulate the release of cytokines through the superantigen mechanism, but may also have direct toxic effects on endothelial cells. The latter action may lead to capillary leakage, hypotension, and shock.

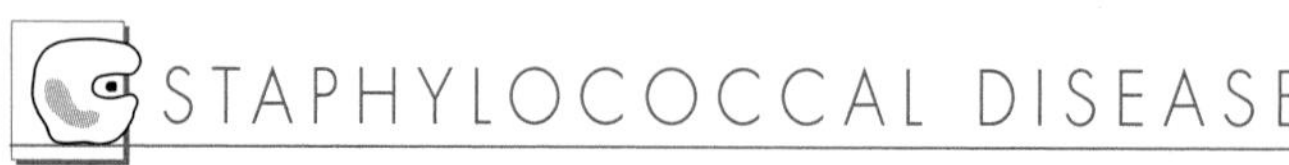

STAPHYLOCOCCAL DISEASE

CLINICAL CAPSULE

Infections produced by *S. aureus* are typified by acute, aggressive, locally destructive purulent lesions. The most familiar of these is the common boil, a painful lump in the skin that has a necrotic center and fibrous reactive shell. Infections in organs other than the skin such as the lung, kidney, or bone are also focal and destructive but have greater potential for extension within the organ and beyond to the blood and other organs. Such infections typically produce high fever, systemic toxicity, and may be fatal in only a few days. A subgroup of *S. aureus* infections has manifestations produced by secreted toxins that contribute to the primary infection. Symptoms include diarrhea, rash, skin desquamation, or multiorgan effects as in staphylococcal toxic shock syndrome (TSS). Ingestion of preformed staphylococcal enterotoxin causes a form of food poisoning in which vomiting begins in only a few hours.

EPIDEMIOLOGY

Anterior nares colonization is common

Strains with increased virulence cannot be distinguished

The basic human habitat of *S. aureus* is the anterior nares. About 30% of individuals carry the organism in this site at any given time, and rates among hospital personnel and patients may be much higher. Some nasal carriers and individuals with colonization at other sites such as the perineum may disseminate the organism extensively with desquamated epithelial cells, thus constituting a source of infection to others. The central problem in understanding the link between colonization and disease is that although we know some strains clearly have enhanced potential to produce disease, we have no way to predict which they are. Bacteriophage typing allows tracking of strains during an outbreak but by itself allows no conclusions about virulence.

Community infections are endogenous

S. aureus survives drying

Most *S. aureus* infections acquired in the community are autoinfections with strains that the subject has been carrying in the anterior nares, on the skin, or both. Community outbreaks are usually associated with poor hygiene and fomite transmission from individual to individual. Unlike many pathogenic vegetative organisms, *S. aureus* can survive long periods of drying; for example, recurrent skin infections can result from use of clothing contaminated with pus from a previous infection.

Hospital spread is on the hands of medical personnel

Hospital outbreaks caused by a single strain of *S. aureus* most commonly involve patients who have undergone surgical or other invasive procedures. The source of the outbreak may be a patient with an overt or inapparent staphylococcal infection (eg, decubitus ulcer) that is then spread directly to other patients on the hands of hospital personnel. A nasal or perineal carrier among medical, nursing, or other hospital personnel may also be the source of an outbreak, especially if carriage is heavy and numerous organisms are disseminated. The most hazardous source is a medical attendant who works despite having a staphylococcal lesion such as a boil. Hospital outbreaks of *S. aureus* infection can be self-perpetuating: infected patients and those who attend them frequently become carriers, and the total environmental load of the causative staphylococcus is increased. Bacteriophage typing and patterns of resistance to antimicrobics (antibiograms) are used as epidemiologic tools to detect carriers who may have initiated or contributed to continuation of the outbreak. The principles of control of epidemics in general and of hospital outbreaks are described in Chapters 12 and 72.

Outbreaks involve nasal carrier or worker with lesion

Phage typing and antibiograms are useful tools

Staphylococcal food poisoning has been an unhappy and embarrassing sequel to innumerable group picnics and wedding receptions in which gastronomic delicacies have been exposed to temperatures that allow bacterial multiplication. Characteristically, the food is moist and rich (eg, potato salad, creamy dishes). The food becomes contaminated by a preparer who is a nasal carrier or has a staphylococcal lesion. If the food is inadequately refrigerated, the staphylococci multiply and produce enterotoxin in the food. Because of the heat resistance of the toxin, toxicity persists even if the food is boiled before eating.

Enterotoxin is produced in rich foods before they are ingested

PATHOGENESIS

Primary Infection

The initial stages of colonization by *S. aureus* are mediated by a number of surface proteins, each of which binds to host elements in or covering tissues, body fluids, or foreign bodies such as catheters. Proteins that bind to fibronectin, fibrinogen, and collagen have been discovered, and others are under investigation. Mechanisms for bacterial extension beyond the surface are not clearly understood. Of the many potential virulence factors produced by *S. aureus,* none can be assigned the single or even primary role contributing to the ability of the bacteria to multiply and cause progressive lesions in tissues. In fact, *S. aureus* is generally of quite low infectivity unless trauma, foreign matter, or other local conditions provide access for initiation of infection. Experimentally, intradermal injection of up to 10^6 organisms is required to initiate a local lesion unless a suture or talcum powder is added with the bacteria.

Surface proteins bind to tissue elements such as fibronectin

Trauma and foreign matter lower infecting dose

Once beyond the mucosal or skin barrier, any mechanism that protects the organisms from phagocytosis may allow multiplication to continue long enough for products such as α-toxin to initiate local injury. One factor known to interfere with phagocytosis is surface protein A. Its binding to the Fc portion of IgG may compete with phagocytic cells for available IgG–Fc sites, thus effectively diminishing opsonization. Production of coagulase can retard migration of phagocytes to the site of infection, and even phagocytosed *S. aureus* may resist lysosomal killing. The acute inflammatory response continues, and the developing lesion has a marked tendency for localization, perhaps due to the fibrotic reaction to the α-toxin–mediated injury to host cells.

Resistance to phagocytosis allows α-toxin production

Protein A competes for IgG–Fc sites

The fate of the lesion depends on the ability of the host to localize the process, which differs depending on the tissue involved. In the skin, spontaneous resolution of the boil by granulation and fibrosis is the rule. In the lung, kidney, bone, and other organs, the process may continue to spread with satellite foci and involvement of broad areas. In all instances the action of the cytotoxins is highly destructive, creating cavities and massive necrosis with little respect to anatomic boundaries. In the worst cases, the staphylococci are not contained, spreading to the bloodstream and distant organs. Circulating staphylococci may also shed cell wall peptidoglycans, producing massive complement activation, leukopenia, thrombocytopenia, and a clinical syndrome of septic shock.

Destruction and spread are prominent

Peptidoglycan fragments may trigger shock

Toxin-mediated Disease

If the strain of *S. aureus* causing any of the effects described above also produces one or more of the exotoxins, those actions are added to those of the primary infection. The primary infection serves as a site for absorption of the toxin and need not be extensive or even clinically apparent for the toxic action to occur. In staphylococcal food poisoning, there is no infection at all. The contaminating bacteria produce pyrogenic exotoxin in the food that can initiate its enterotoxic action on the intestine within hours of its ingestion.

Preformed enterotoxin acts within hours

Exfoliative toxin causes blisters or scalded skin syndrome

The in vivo production of toxin takes at least a few days and may exert its effect locally or systemically. Exfoliative toxin-producing strains cause blisterlike separation of the epidermis by their action on intercellular junctions, which is most commonly localized to the site of skin infection. In staphylococcal scalded skin syndrome, absorbed toxin causes extensive epithelial desquamation at sites remote from the primary infection.

TSST-1–producing strain must colonize vagina

Menstruation and tampons enhance local toxin production

In staphylococcal TSS, the pyrogenic exotoxin TSST-1 is produced during the course of a staphylococcal infection with systemic disease as a result of absorption of toxin from the local site. Menstruation-associated TSS requires a combination of improbable events. Less than 5% of women carry *S. aureus* in their vaginal flora, and only one in five of these staphylococci have the potential to produce TSST-1. In the presence of such a strain, the combination of menstruation and high-absorbency tampon usage appear to provide growth conditions that enhance the production of TSST-1. Toxin absorbed from the vagina can then circulate to produce superantigen-mediated cytokine release and direct effects on the vasculature (Fig 16–3).

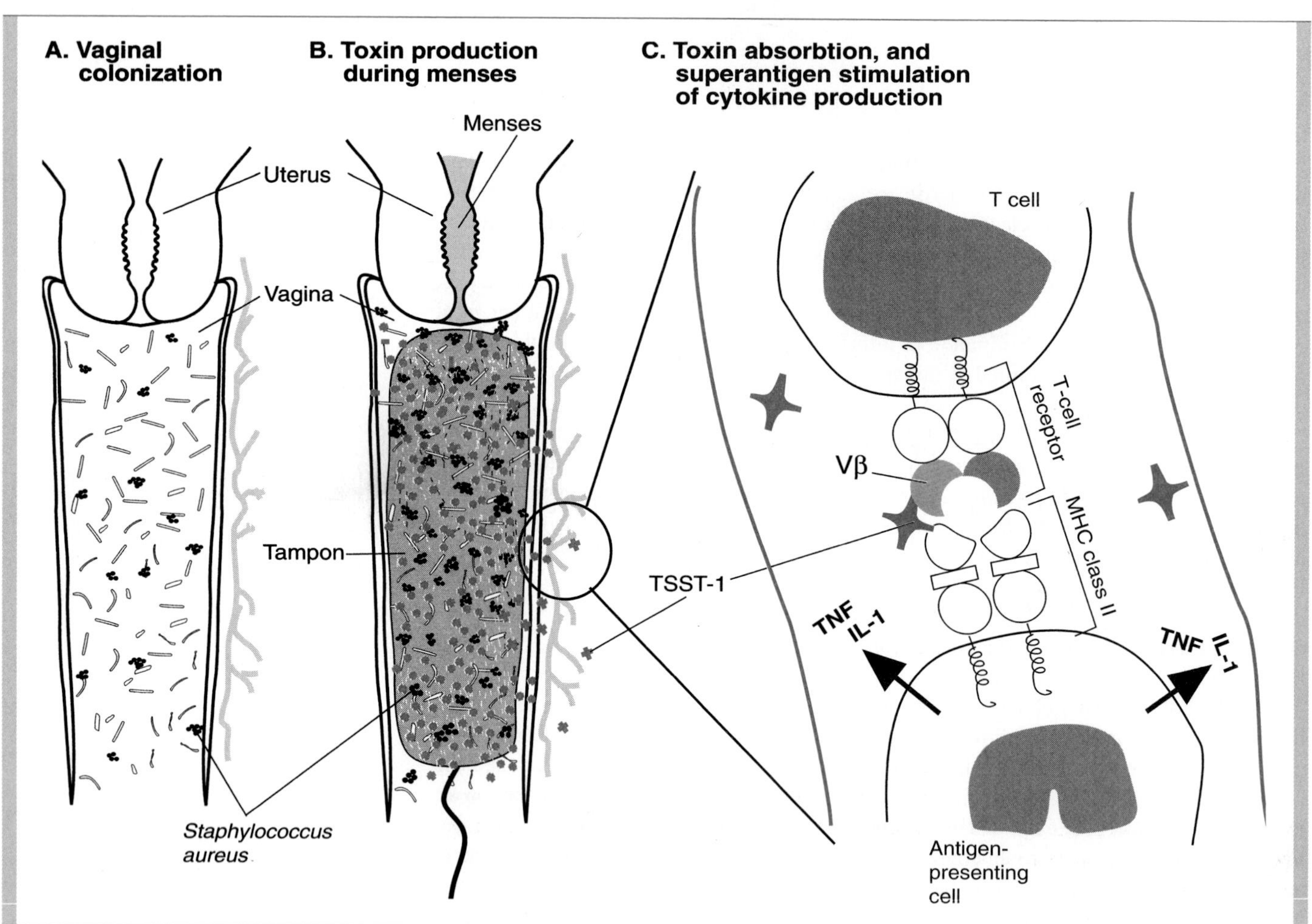

FIGURE 16–3

Pathogenesis of staphylococcal toxic shock syndrome. **A.** The vagina is colonized with normal flora and a strain of *Staphylococcus aureus* containing the TSST-1 gene. **B.** The conditions with tampon usage facilitate growth of the *S. aureus* and TSST-1 production. **C.** The toxin is absorbed from the vagina and circulates. The systemic effects may be due to the direct effect of the toxin or via cytokines released by the superantigen mechanism. The toxin is shown binding directly with the Vβ portion of the T-cell receptor and the class II major histocompatibility complex (MHC) receptor. This Vβ stimulation signals the production of cytokines such as interleukin-1 (IL-1) and tumor necrosis factor (TNF).

Some cases of full-blown staphylococcal TSS are associated with strains that do not produce TSST-1. This is particularly true of nonmenstrual cases. Other PTSAgs have been detected in these strains and have been shown to produce experimental toxic shock. TSS may be the result of in vivo production of any of the staphylococcal pyrogenic exotoxins, with TSST-1 simply the most common offender. The mechanisms by which the pyrogenic exotoxins produce the multiple renal, cutaneous, intestinal, and cardiovascular manifestations of TSS are not known.

Nonmenstrual TSS cases may have any PTSAg-producing strain

IMMUNITY

The natural history of staphylococcal infections indicates that immunity is of short duration and incomplete. Chronic furunculosis, for example, can recur over many years. The relative roles of humoral and cellular immune mechanisms are uncertain, and attempts to induce immunity artificially with various staphylococcal products have been disappointing at best. In menstruation-associated TSS, many patients have low or absent antibody levels to TSST-1 and often fail to mount a significant antibody response during the disease. Repeated attacks have been recorded, suggesting a genetic predisposition.

Immunity is poorly understood

Relapsing infections show little evidence of immunity

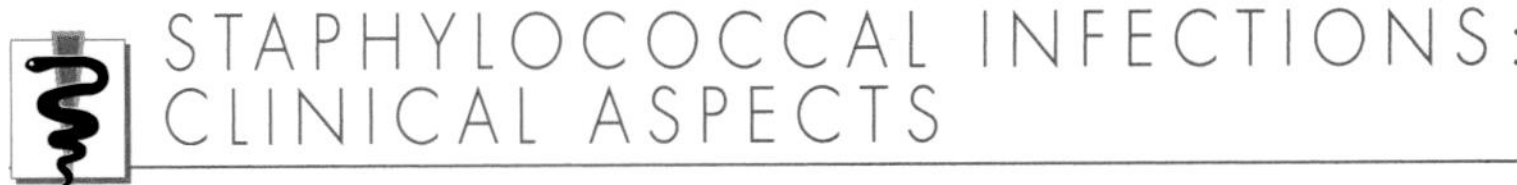

STAPHYLOCOCCAL INFECTIONS: CLINICAL ASPECTS

MANIFESTATIONS: PRIMARY INFECTION

Furuncle and Carbuncle

The furuncle or boil is a superficial skin infection that develops in a hair follicle, sebaceous gland, or sweat gland. Blockage of the gland duct with inspissation of its contents causes predisposition to infection. Furunculosis is often a complication of acne vulgaris. Infection at the base of the eyelash gives rise to the common stye. The infected patient is often a carrier of the offending *Staphylococcus,* usually in the anterior nares. The course of the infection is usually benign, and the infection resolves upon spontaneous drainage of pus. No surgical or antimicrobic treatment is needed. Infection can spread from a furuncle with the development of one or more abscesses in adjacent subcutaneous tissues. This lesion, known as a carbuncle, occurs most often on the back of the neck but may involve other skin sites. Carbuncles are serious lesions that may result in bloodstream invasion (bacteremia).

Focal lesions drain spontaneously

Boils develop in hair follicles

Multiple boils become a carbuncle

Chronic Furunculosis

Some individuals are subject to chronic furunculosis, in which repeated attacks of boils are caused by the same strain of *S. aureus.* There is little, if any, evidence of acquired immunity to the disease; indeed, delayed-type hypersensitivity to staphylococcal products appears responsible for much of the inflammation and necrosis that develops. Chronic staphylococcal disease may be associated with factors that depress host immunity, especially in patients with diabetes or congenital defects of polymorphonuclear leukocyte function. However, in most instances, predisposing disease other than acne is not present.

Links to immune dysfunction are limited

Impetigo

S. aureus is most often seen as a secondary invader in group A streptococcal pustular impetigo (see Chapter 17), but it can produce the skin pustules of impetigo on its own. Strains of *S. aureus* that produce exfoliatin cause a characteristic form called bullous impetigo, characterized by large blisters containing many staphylococci in the superficial layers of the skin. Bullous impetigo can be considered a localized form of scalded skin syndrome.

Exfoliatin-producing strains cause bullous impetigo

Deep Lesions

Acute osteomyelitis is primarily a *S. aureus* disease

Pneumonia and deep tissue lesions are highly destructive

Bacteremic spread and endocarditis are most common in drug abusers

S. aureus can cause a wide variety of infections of deep tissues by bacteremic spread from a skin lesion that may be unnoticed. These include infections of bones, joints, deep organs, and soft tissues, including surgical wounds. More than 90% of the cases of acute osteomyelitis in children are caused by *S. aureus*. Staphylococcal pneumonia is typically secondary to some other insult to the lung, such as influenza, aspiration, or pulmonary edema. At deep sites the organism has the same tendency to produce localized, destructive abscesses that it does in the skin. All too often the containment is less effective, and spread with multiple metastatic lesions occurs. Bacteremia and endocarditis can develop. All are serious infections that constitute acute medical emergencies. In all of these situations, diabetes, leukocyte defects, or general reduction of host defenses by alcoholism, malignancy, old age, or steroid or cytotoxic therapy can be predisposing factors. Severe *S. aureus* infections, including endocarditis, are particularly common in drug abusers using injection methods.

MANIFESTATIONS CAUSED BY STAPHYLOCOCCAL TOXINS

Scalded Skin Syndrome

Widespread desquamation in neonates is caused by exfoliatin-producing strains

Staphylococcal scalded skin syndrome results from the production of exfoliatin in a staphylococcal lesion, which can be quite minor (eg, conjunctivitis). Erythema and intraepidermal desquamation takes place at remote sites from which *S. aureus* cannot be isolated (Fig 16–4). The disease is most common in neonates and children less than 5 years of age. The face, axilla, and groin tend to be affected first, but the erythema, bullous formation, and subsequent desquamation of epithelial sheets can spread to all parts of the body. The disease occasionally occurs in adults, particularly those who are immunocompromised. Milder versions of what is probably the same disease are staphylococcal scarlet fever, in which erythema occurs without desquamation, and bullous impetigo, in which local desquamation occurs.

Toxic Shock Syndrome

Fever, vomiting, diarrhea, and muscle pain are early findings

Shock, renal and hepatic injury may follow

Toxic shock syndrome (TSS) was first described in children but came to public attention during the early 1980s, when hundreds of cases were reported in young women using intravaginal tampons. The disease is characterized by high fever, vomiting, diarrhea, sore throat, and muscle pain. Within 48 hours, it may progress to severe shock with evidence of renal and hepatic damage. A skin rash may develop, followed by desquamation at a deeper level than in scalded skin syndrome. Blood cultures are usually negative. The outbreak receded with the withdrawal of certain brands of highly absorbent tampons.

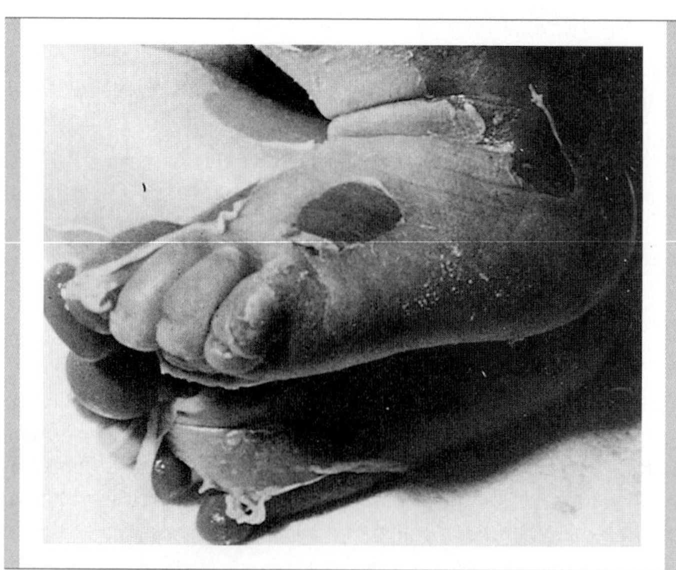

FIGURE 16–4
Staphylococcal scalded skin syndrome in a neonate. The focal staphylococcal infection was a breast abscess in the infant.

Staphylococcal Food Poisoning

Ingestion of staphylococcal enterotoxin contaminated food results in acute vomiting and diarrhea within 1 to 5 hours. There is prostration, but usually no fever. Recovery is rapid, except sometimes in the elderly and in those with another disease.

Vomiting is prominent without fever

DIAGNOSIS

Laboratory procedures to assist in diagnosis of staphylococcal infections are quite simple. Most acute, untreated lesions contain numerous polymorphonuclear leukocytes and large numbers of Gram-positive cocci in clusters. Staphylococci grow overnight on blood agar incubated aerobically. Catalase and coagulase tests performed directly from the colonies are sufficient for identification. Antibiotic susceptibility tests are indicated because of the emerging resistance of *S. aureus* to multiple antimicrobics, particularly methicillin and vancomycin.

Gram stain and culture are primary diagnostic methods

Deep staphylococcal infections such as osteomyelitis or deep abscesses present special diagnostic problems when the lesion cannot be directly aspirated or surgically sampled. Blood cultures are usually positive in conditions such as acute staphylococcal arthritis, osteomyelitis, and endocarditis but less often in localized infection such as deep abscesses.

Aspirates and blood cultures are necessary for deep infections

TREATMENT

Most boils and superficial staphylococcal abscesses resolve spontaneously without antimicrobial therapy. Those that are more extensive, deeper, or in vital organs require a combination of surgical drainage and antimicrobics for optimal outcome. Penicillins and cephalosporins are active against *S. aureus* cell wall peptidoglycan and vary in their susceptibility to inactivation by staphylococcal β-lactamases. Although penicillin G is the treatment of choice for susceptible strains, the penicillinase-resistant penicillins (methicillin, nafcillin, oxacillin) and first-generation cephalosporins are more commonly used because of resistance. For strains resistant to these agents or patients with β-lactam hypersensitivity, the alternatives are vancomycin, clindamycin, or erythromycin. Synergy between cell wall–active antibiotics and the aminoglycosides is present when the staphylococcus is sensitive to both types of agents. Such combinations are often used in severe systemic infections when effective and rapid bactericidal action is needed, particularly in compromised hosts.

Superficial lesions resolve spontaneously

Penicillinase-resistant β-lactams are used pending susceptibility tests

ANTIMICROBIAL RESISTANCE

When penicillin was introduced to the general public following World War II, virtually all strains of *S. aureus* were highly susceptible. Since then, the selection of preexisting strains able to produce a penicillinase has shifted these proportions to the point at which 80 to 90% of isolates are now penicillin resistant. The penicillinase is encoded by plasmid genes and acts by opening the β-lactam ring, making the drug unable to bind with its target.

Most strains of *S. aureus* are now penicillin resistant

Penicillinase production is plasmid mediated

Alterations in the β-lactam target, the peptidoglycan transpeptidases (often called penicillin-binding proteins, or PBPs), is the basis for resistance to methicillin. These methicillin-resistant *S. aureus* (MRSA) strains are also resistant to the other penicillinase-resistant penicillins such as oxacillin. The most common mechanism is the acquisition of a gene for a new transpeptidase, which has reduced affinity for β-lactam antibiotics, but is still able to carry out its enzymatic function of cross-linking peptidoglycan.

Methicillin-resistant strains produce new PBP

The frequency of MRSA has great geographic variation. Most American hospitals report MRSA rates of 5 to 25%, but outbreaks are increasing and resistance rates over 50% have been reported in other countries. There are some problems in detecting MRSA; resistant cells may represent only a small portion of the total population (heteroresistance). Tests are generally performed with methicillin or oxacillin under technical conditions that facilitate detection of the resistant subpopulation, and the results extrapolated to other relevant agents. For example, oxacillin resistance is considered proof of resistance to methicillin, nafcillin, dicloxacillin, and all cephalosporins. Vancomycin is often used to treat

MRSA rates are variable but increasing

MRSA detection requires special conditions

Vancomycin use for MRSA is threatened

serious infections with MRSA. The recent emergence of *S. aureus* with decreased susceptibility to vancomycin is of great concern, these strains are still very rare.

PREVENTION

In patients subject to recurrent infection, such as chronic furunculosis, preventive measures are aimed at controlling reinfection and, if possible, eliminating the carrier state. Clothes and bedding that may cause reinfection should be washed at a sufficiently high temperature to destroy staphylococci (70°C or higher) or dry-cleaned. In adults, the use of chlorhexidine or hexachlorophene soaps in showering and washing increases the bactericidal activity of the skin (see Chapter 11). In such individuals, or persons found to be a source of an outbreak, anterior nasal carriage can be reduced and often eliminated by the combination of nasal creams containing topical antimicrobics (eg, mupirocin, neomycin, and bacitracin) and oral therapy with antimicrobics that are concentrated within phagocytes and nasal secretions (eg, rifampin or ciprofloxacin). Attempts to reduce nasal carriage more generally among medical personnel in an institution are usually fruitless and encourage replacement of susceptible strains with multiresistant ones.

Antistaphylococcal soaps block infection

Elimination of nasal carriage is difficult

Chemoprophylaxis is effective in surgical procedures such as hip and cardiac valve replacements, in which infection with staphylococci can have devastating consequences. Methicillin, a cephalosporin, or vancomycin given during and shortly after surgery may reduce the chance for intraoperative infection while minimizing the risk for superinfection associated with longer periods of antibiotic administration.

Chemoprophylaxis during high-risk surgery is effective

Coagulase-Negative Staphylococci

S. epidermidis and a number of other species of coagulase-negative staphylococci are normal commensals of the skin, anterior nares, and ear canals of humans. Their large numbers and ubiquitous distribution result in frequent contamination of specimens collected from or through the skin, making these organisms among the most frequently isolated in the clinical laboratory. In the past, they were rarely the cause of significant infections, but with the increasing use of implanted catheters and prosthetic devices, they have emerged as important agents of hospital-acquired infections. Immunosuppressed or neutropenic patients and premature infants have been particularly affected.

Common colonizers of the skin

Commonly colonize implanted medical devices

Organisms may contaminate prosthetic devices during implantation, seed the device during a subsequent bacteremia, or gain access to the lumina of shunts and catheters when they are temporarily disconnected or manipulated. The outcome of the bacterial contamination is determined by the ability of the microbe to attach to the surface of the foreign body and to multiply there. Initial adherence is facilitated by the hydrophobic nature of the synthetic polymers used in medical devices and the natural hydrophobic nature of many coagulase-negative staphylococci. Following attachment, some strains produce a viscous extracellular polysaccharide **slime** or biofilm. This biofilm provides additional adhesion, completely covers the bacteria, and serves as a mechanical barrier to antimicrobial agents and host defense mechanisms; it is also believed to enhance nutrition of the microbes by functioning as an ion-exchange resin. Strains able to produce the polysaccharide biofilm are more likely to colonize intravenous catheters but have no known advantage in adherence to human tissues such as heart valves. The resistance of many coagulase-negative staphylococci to multiple antimicrobic agents contributes further to their persistence in the body. Infections are generally low grade, but unless controlled, they can proceed to serious tissue damage or a fatal outcome.

Polysaccharide slime production enhances attachment and survival

The interpretation of cultures that grow coagulase-negative staphylococci is fraught with difficulty. In most cases, the finding is attributable to skin contamination, although it can indicate infection when a patient has implanted devices, or has defenses that are otherwise compromised. The presence of at least moderate numbers of organisms or the

Most common skin contaminant in cultures

repeated isolation of a strain with the same antibiogram argues for infection over skin contamination. There is no phage-typing system for coagulase-negative staphylococci but a number of molecular procedures (see Chapter 15) have been used to compare isolates for epidemiologic purposes.

Repeated positives suggest infection

Most coagulase-negative staphylococci now encountered are resistant to penicillin, and many are also methicillin resistant. Resistance to multiple antimicrobics usually active against Gram-positive cocci, including vancomycin, is more common than with *S. aureus.* Eradication of coagulase-negative staphylococci from prosthetic devices and associated tissues with chemotherapy alone is very difficult unless the device is also removed.

Multiple antimicrobic resistance is common

ADDITIONAL READING

Chambers HF. Methicillin resistance in staphylococci: Molecular and biochemical basis and clinical implications. *Clin Microbiol Rev* 1997;10:781–791. The complex topic of staphylococcal heteroresistance and its detection is clearly explained in only seven pages. A discussion of alternate treatment strategies is also included.

Dinges MM, Orwin PM, Schlievert PM. Exotoxins of *Staphylococcus aureus. Clin Microbiol Rev* 2000;13:16–34. The structural biology and the role of the pyrogenic exotoxins in food poisoning and TSS are carefully but concisely explained. The locally acting toxins are also discussed.

Elek SD, Conan PE. The virulence of *Staphylococcus pyogenes* for man. A study of the problems of wound infections. *Br J Exp Pathol* 1957;38:573–586. A classic study of the factors influencing the development of staphylococcal wound infections in humans.

Lowry FD. *Staphylococcus aureus* infections. *N Engl J Med* 1998;339:520–532. A review that considers the epidemiologic, clinical, therapeutic, and pathogenesis of *S. aureus* infection. The pathogenesis discussion is particularly well-illustrated.

CHAPTER 17

Streptococci and Enterococci

KENNETH J. RYAN

Bacteria of the genus *Streptococcus* are Gram-positive cocci arranged in chains that form a significant portion of the indigenous microflora of the oropharynx. In addition to relatively harmless species, the genus includes three of the most important pathogens of humans. One is *S. pyogenes,* the cause of "strep throat," which can lead to rheumatic fever and heart disease; the ability of some strains to cause catastrophic deep tissue infections recently led British tabloids to give them the gory label "flesh-eating bacteria." Second is *S. agalactiae,* the most frequent cause of sepsis in newborns. Third is *S. pneumoniae,* a leading cause of pneumonia and meningitis in persons of all ages.

STREPTOCOCCI

Group Characteristics

MORPHOLOGY

Streptococci stain readily with common dyes, demonstrating coccal cells that are generally smaller and more ovoid in shape than staphylococci. They are usually arranged in chains with oval cells touching end to end, because they divide in one plane and tend to remain attached. Length may vary from a single pair to continuous chains of over 30 cells, depending on the species and growth conditions. Medically important streptococci are not acid fast, do not form spores, and are nonmotile. Some members form capsules composed of polysaccharide complexes or hyaluronic acid.

Oval cells arranged in chains end to end

CULTURAL AND BIOCHEMICAL CHARACTERISTICS

Streptococci grow best in enriched media under aerobic or anaerobic conditions (facultative). Growth of many strains is enhanced by the presence of carbon dioxide. Blood agar is preferred because it satisfies the growth requirements and also serves as an indicator for patterns of hemolysis. The colonies are small, ranging from pinpoint size to 2 mm in diameter, and they may be surrounded by a zone where the erythrocytes suspended in the agar have been hemolyzed. When this zone is clear, this state is called **β-hemolysis.**

β hemolysis is clear

α hemolysis is incomplete, with greening of blood agar

Catalase negative

When the result is hazy (incomplete hemolysis), with a green discoloration of the agar, it is called **α-hemolysis.** Streptococci are metabolically active, attacking a variety of carbohydrates, proteins, and amino acids. Glucose fermentation yields mostly lactic acid. In contrast to staphylococci, streptococci are catalase negative.

CLASSIFICATION

Lancefield antigens are cell wall carbohydrates

Presence of Lancefield antigens defines the pyogenic streptococci

At the turn of the 20th century, a classification based on hemolysis and biochemical tests was sufficient to associate some streptococcal species with infections in humans and animals. Rebecca Lancefield, who demonstrated carbohydrate antigens in cell-wall extracts of the β-hemolytic streptococci, put this taxonomy on a sounder basis. Her studies formed a classification by serogroups (eg, A, B, C), each of which is generally correlated with an established species. Later it was discovered that some nonhemolytic streptococci had the same cell wall antigens. Over the years it has become clear that possession of one of the Lancefield antigens defines a particularly virulent segment of the streptococcal genus regardless of hemolytic patterns. These are called the **pyogenic streptococci,** and in medical circles they are now better known by their Lancefield letter than the older species name. Pediatricians instantly recognize GBS as an acronym for group B streptococcus but may be confused by use of the proper name, *Streptococcus agalactiae* (Table 17–1).

Hemolysis is a practical guide to classification

Only pyogenic streptococci are β-hemolytic

For practical purposes, the type of hemolysis and certain biochemical reactions remain valuable for the initial recognition and presumptive classification of streptococci, and as an indication of what subsequent taxonomic tests to perform. Thus, β-hemolysis indicates that the strain has one of the Lancefield group antigens, but some Lancefield positive strains or groups may be α-hemolytic or even nonhemolytic. The streptococci will be considered as follows: (1) pyogenic streptococci (Lancefield groups); (2) pneumococci; (3) viridans and other streptococci (see Table 17–1).

Pyogenic Streptococci

Groups A and B streptococci are most common cause of disease

Of the many Lancefield groups, the ones most frequently isolated from humans are A, B, C, F, and G. Of these, groups A (*S. pyogenes)* and B (*S. agalactiae*) are the most frequent causes of serious disease. The group D carbohydrate is found in the genus *Enterococcus,* which used to be classified among the streptococci.

Pneumococci

Pneumococci have an antigenic polysaccharide capsule

This category contains a single species, *S. pneumoniae,* commonly called the pneumococcus. Its distinctive feature is the presence of a capsule composed of polysaccharide polymers that vary in antigenic specificity. More than 90 capsular immunotypes have been defined. Although the pneumococcal cell wall shares some common antigens with other streptococci, it does not possess any of the Lancefield group antigens. *S. pneumoniae* is α-hemolytic.

Viridans and Other Streptococci

Viridans and nonhemolytic species lack Lancefield antigens or capsules

Viridans streptococci are α-hemolytic and lack both the group carbohydrate antigens of the pyogenic streptococci and the capsular polysaccharides of the pneumococcus. The term encompasses several species, including *S. salivarius* and *S. mitis*. Viridans streptococci comprise members of the normal oral flora of humans. They rarely demonstrate invasive qualities. A variety of other streptococci may be encountered that lack the features of the pyogenic streptococci or pneumococci; they would be classified with the viridans group, except that they are not α-hemolytic. Such strains are usually assigned descriptive terms such as nonhemolytic streptococci or microaerophilic streptococci. They have been less thoroughly studied, but generally have the same biologic behavior as the viridans streptococci.

TABLE 17–1

Classification of Streptococci and Enterococci

Group/Species	Common Term	Hemolysis	Major Antigens/Structures: Lancefield Cell Wall	Major Antigens/Structures: Surface Protein	Major Antigens/Structures: Capsule	Virulence Factors	Disease
Streptococci							
Pyogenic							
Streptococcus pyogenes	Group A strep, GAS	β	A	M protein (80+)	Hyaluronic acid	M protein, leipoteichoic acid, streptococcal pyrogenic exotoxins, streptolysin O, streptokinase	Strep throat, impetigo, pyogenic infections, toxic shock, rheumatic fever, glomerulonephritis
S. agalactiae	Group B strep, GBS	β, –	B	–	Sialic acid (9)	Capsule	Neonatal sepsis, meningitis, pyogenic infections
S. equi		β	C	–	–	–	Pyogenic infections
S. bovis		–, α	D	–	–	–	Pyogenic infections
Other species		β, α, –	E-W	–	–	–	Pyogenic infections
Pneumococcus							
S. pneumoniae	Pneumococcus	α	–	Choline-binding protein	Polysaccharide (90+)	Capsule, pneumolysin, neuraminidase	Pneumonia, meningitis, otitis media, pyogenic infections
Viridans and Nonhemolytic							
S. sanguis		α	–	–	–	–	Low virulence, endocarditis
S. salivarius		α	–	–	–	–	Low virulence, endocarditis
S. mutans		α	–	–			Dental caries
Other species		α, –	–	–	–	–	Low virulence, endocarditis
Enterococci							
Enterococcus faecalis	Enterococcus	–, α	D	–	–	–	Urinary tract, pyogenic infections
E. faecium	Enterococcus	–, α	D	–	–	–	Urinary tract, pyogenic infections
Other species		–, α	D, –	–	–	–	Urinary tract, pyogenic infections

Group A Streptococci (*Streptococcus pyogenes*)

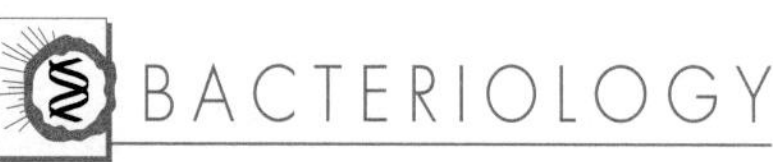

BACTERIOLOGY

MORPHOLOGY AND GROWTH

Streptolysin O or S cause β-hemolysis

Aerobically, only S is active

Group A streptococci typically appear in purulent lesions or broth cultures as spherical or ovoid cells in chains of short to medium length (4 to 10 cells). On blood agar plates, colonies are usually compact, small, and surrounded by a 2- to 3-mm zone of β hemolysis that is easily seen and sharply demarcated. β-hemolysis is caused by either of two hemolysins, **streptolysin S** and the oxygen-labile **streptolysin O,** both of which are produced by most group A strains. Strains that lack streptolysin S are β-hemolytic only under anaerobic conditions, because the remaining streptolysin O is not active in the presence of oxygen. This feature is of practical importance, because such strains would be missed if cultures were incubated only aerobically.

STRUCTURE

Wall contains group antigen with multiple surface molecules extending beyond

The structure of group A streptococci is illustrated in Figure 17–1. The cell wall is built on a peptidoglycan matrix that provides rigidity, as in other Gram-positive bacteria. Within this matrix lies the group carbohydrate antigen, which by definition is present in all group A

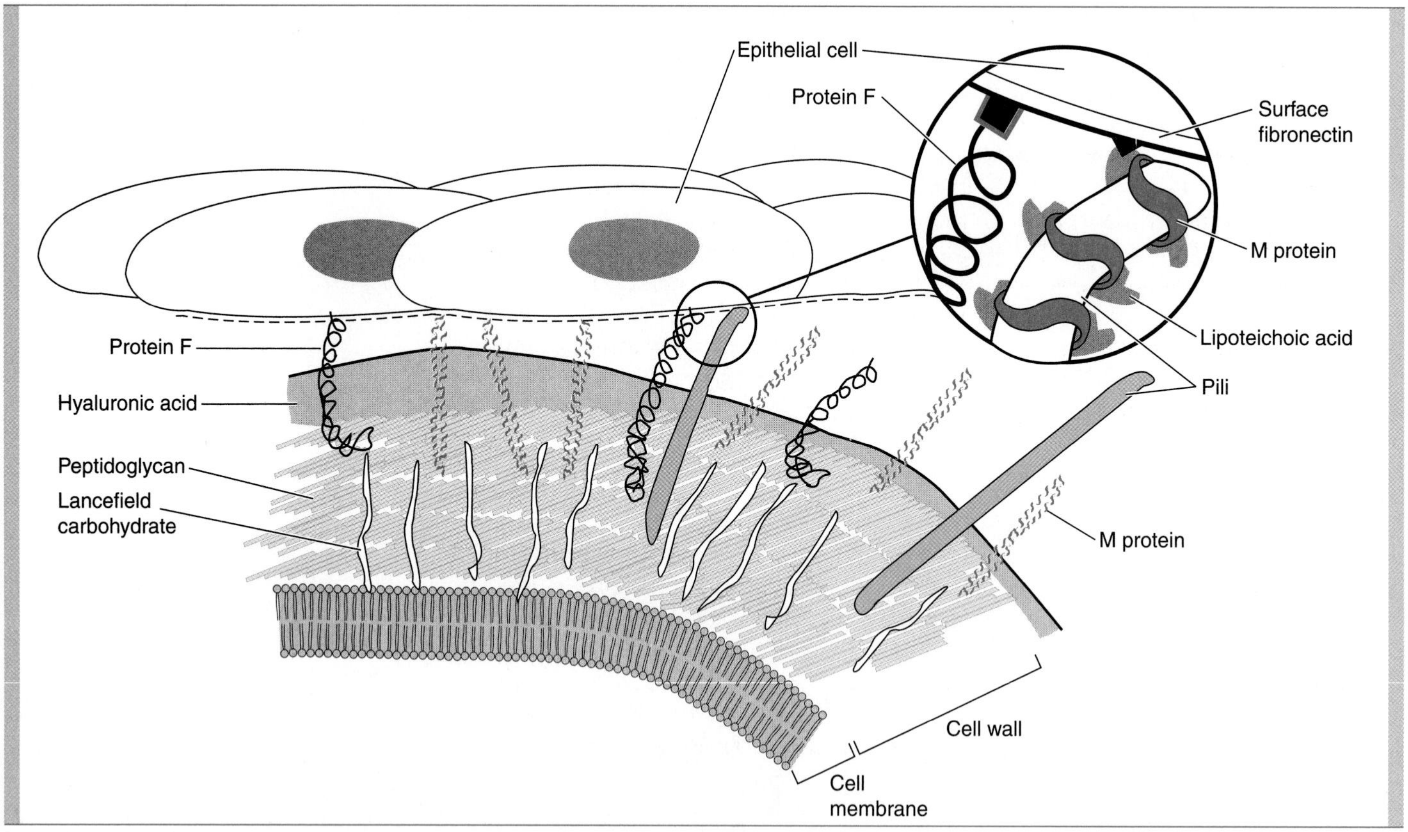

FIGURE 17–1

Antigenic structure of *S. pyogenes* and adhesion to an epithelial cell. The location of peptidoglycan and Lancefield carbohydrate antigen in the cell wall is shown in the diagram. M protein and lipoteichoic acid are associated with the cell surface and the pili. Lipoteichoic acid and protein F mediate binding to fibronectin on the host surface.

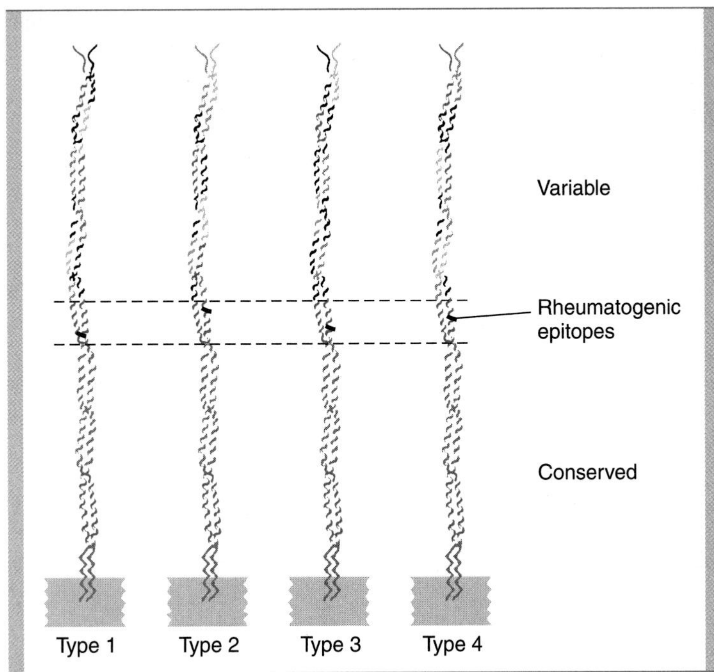

FIGURE 17–2
The coiled-coil structure of M protein is shown. The most variable parts of the molecule are oriented to the outside and provide the antiphagocytic effect and serologic specificity. The conserved portions are rooted in the cell wall. All four types contain epitopes which may stimulate the cross-reactive immune reactions seen in rheumatic fever.

streptococci. A number of other molecules such as M protein and lipoteichoic acid (LTA) are attached to the cell wall but extend beyond often in association with the hair-like pili. Group A streptococci are divided into more than 80 serotypes based on antigenic differences in the M protein. Some strains have an overlying nonantigenic hyaluronic acid capsule.

M Protein

The M protein itself is a fibrillar coiled-coil molecule (Fig 17–2) with structural homology to myosin. Its carboxy terminus is rooted in the peptidoglycan of the cell wall, and the amino-terminal regions extend out from the surface. The specificity of the more than 80 serotypes of M protein is determined by variations in the amino sequence of the amino-terminal portion of the molecule. Because of its location, this part of the M protein is also the most available to immune surveillance. The middle part of the molecule is less variable, and some carboxy terminal regions are conserved across many M types. There is increasing evidence that some the many known biologic functions of M protein can be assigned to specific domains of the molecule. This includes both antigenicity and the capacity to bind other molecules such as fibrinogen, serum factor H, and immunoglobulins.

Coiled-coil is similar to myosin

Antigenic variation and function differ in domains of the molecule

80+ M protein serotypes exist

Other Surface Molecules

A number of surface proteins have been described on the basis of their similarity with M protein or some unique binding capacity. Of these, a fibronectin binding **protein F** and **LTA** are both exposed on the streptococcal surface (see Fig 17–1) and may have a role in pathogenesis. An IgG binding protein has the capacity to bind the Fc portion of antibodies in much the same way as staphylococcal protein A. In principle, this could interfere with opsonization by creating a covering of antibody molecules on the streptococcal surface that are facing the "wrong way." Group A streptococci may have a **hyaluronic acid capsule,** which is a polymer containing repeating units of glucuronic acid and N-acetylglucosamine.

Protein F and LTA bind fibronectin

Hyaluronic acid capsule may be present

BIOLOGICALLY ACTIVE EXTRACELLULAR PRODUCTS

Streptolysin O

Streptolysin O is a general cytotoxin, lysing leukocytes, tissue cells, and platelets. The toxin inserts directly into the cell membrane of host cells, forming transmembrane pores in a manner similar to complement and staphylococcal α-toxin (see Chapter 16). Streptolysin

Streptolysin O is pore-forming and antigenic

O is antigenic and the quantitation of antibodies against it is the basis of a standard serologic test called antistreptolysin O (ASO).

Pyrogenic Exotoxins

SPEs are produced by some strains

SPEs are superantigens and some have enzymatic activity

The manifestations of classical **scarlet fever** have long been associated with the action of an erythrogenic toxin. This toxin is now included in a family of nine proteins called **streptococcal pyrogenic exotoxins (SPEs),** one of which is produced by approximately 10% of group A streptococci. The SPEs are identified by letters (eg, A, B, C) and are similar in structure and biological activity to the pyrogenic exotoxins produced by *Staphylococcus aureus*. They have multiple effects including fever, rash (scarlet fever), T-cell proliferation, B-lymphocyte suppression, and heightened sensitivity to endotoxin. At least some of these actions are due to cytokine release through the superantigen mechanism (see Chapter 8). SPE-B also has enzymatic activity cleaving elements of the extracellular matrix, including fibronectin and vitronectin.

Other Extracellular Products

C5a peptidase degrades complement

Streptokinase converts plasminogen to plasmin

Most strains of group A streptococci produce a number of other extracellular products including streptokinase, hyaluronidase, nucleases, and a **C5a peptidase**. The C5a peptidase is an enzyme that degrades complement component C5a, the main factor that attracts phagocytes to sites of complement deposition. The enzymatic actions of the others likely play some role in tissue injury or spread, but no specific roles have been defined. Some are antigenic and have been the basis of serologic tests. **Streptokinase** causes lysis of fibrin clots through conversion of plasminogen in normal plasma to the protease plasmin.

GROUP A STREPTOCOCCAL DISEASE

CLINICAL CAPSULE

Group A streptococci are the cause of "strep throat," an acute inflammation of the pharynx and tonsils that includes fever and painful swallowing. Skin and soft tissue infections range from the tiny skin pustules called impetigo to a severe toxic and invasive disease that can be fatal in a matter of days. In addition to acute infections, group A streptococci are responsible for inflammatory diseases that are not direct infections but represent states in which the immune response to streptococcal antigens causes injury to host tissues. Acute rheumatic fever (ARF) is a prolonged febrile inflammation of connective tissues, which recurs following each subsequent streptococcal pharyngitis. Repeated episodes cause permanent scarring of the heart valves. Acute glomerulonephritis is an insidious disease with hypertension, hematuria, proteinuria, and edema due to inflammation of the renal glomerulus.

EPIDEMIOLOGY

Pharyngitis

Most common bacterial cause of sore throat

Droplets spread over short distances from throat and nasal sites

Group A streptococci are the most common bacterial cause of pharyngitis in school-age children 5 to 15 years of age. Transmission is person to person from the large droplets produced by infected persons during coughing, sneezing, or even conversation. This droplet transmission is most efficient at the short distances (2 to 5 feet) at which social interactions commonly take place in families and schools, particularly in fall and winter months. Asymptomatic carriers (<1%) may also be the source particularly if colonized in the nose as well as the throat. Although group A streptococci survive for some time in dried secretions, environmental sources and fomites are not important means of spread. Unless the condition is treated, the organisms persist for 1 to 4 weeks after symptoms have disappeared.

Impetigo

Impetigo occurs when transient skin colonization with group A streptococci is combined with minor trauma such as insect bites. The tiny skin pustules are spread locally by scratching and to others by direct contact or shared fomites such as towels. Impetigo is most common in summer months when insects are biting and when the general level of hygiene is low. The M protein types of *S. pyogenes* most commonly associated with impetigo are different from those causing respiratory infection.

Skin colonization plus trauma leads to impetigo

Wound and Puerperal Infections

Group A streptococci, once a leading cause of postoperative wound and puerperal infections, retain this potential, but these conditions are now less common. As with staphylococci, transmission from patient to patient is by the hands of physicians or other medical attendants who fail to follow recommended handwashing practices. Organisms may be transferred from another patient or come from the health care workers themselves.

Hospital outbreaks are linked to carriers

Streptococcal Toxic Shock Syndrome

Since the late 1980s, a severe invasive form of group A streptococcal soft tissue infection appeared with increased frequency (5 to 10 cases/100,000) in the United States and other countries. Rapid progression to death in only a few days occurred in previously healthy persons, including Muppet creator Jim Henson (of Sesame Street fame). The outstanding features of these infections are their multiorgan involvement suggesting a toxin and rapid invasiveness with spread to the bloodstream and distant organs. The toxic features together with the discovery that almost all the isolates produce one of the SPEs have caused this syndrome to be labeled streptococcal toxic shock syndrome (STSS).

STSS may be fatal in healthy persons

Strains produce SPEs

Poststreptococcal Sequelae

The association between group A streptococci and the inflammatory disease acute rheumatic fever (ARF; see the text) is based on epidemiologic studies linking group A streptococcal pharyngitis, the clinical features of rheumatic fever, and heightened immune responses to streptococcal products. ARF does not follow skin or other nonrespiratory infection with group A streptococci. Although some M types may be more "rheumatogenic," it is generally believed that recurrences of ARF can be triggered by infection with any group A streptococcus. Injury to the heart caused by recurrences of ARF leads to **rheumatic heart disease,** a major cause of heart disease worldwide. Although ARF has declined in developed countries (<0.5 cases/1000), a resurgence in the form of small regional outbreaks in the United States began in the late 1980s. These outbreaks involved children of a higher socioeconomic status than previously associated with ARF and a shift in prevalent M types. The underlying basis of the resurgence is unknown.

ARF follows respiratory, not skin, infection

Rheumatic heart disease is produced by recurrent ARF

Poststreptococcal glomerulonephritis may follow either respiratory or cutaneous group A streptococcal infection and involves only certain "nephritogenic" strains. It is more common in temperate climates where insect bites lead to impetigo. The average latent period between infection and glomerulonephritis is 10 days from a respiratory infection, but generally about 3 weeks from a skin infection. Nephritogenic strains are limited to a few M types and seem to have declined in recent years.

Glomerulonephritis follows respiratory or skin infection

Only nephritogenic strains are involved

PATHOGENESIS

Acute Infections

As with other pathogens, adherence to mucosal surfaces is a crucial step in initiating disease. A dozen adhesins have been described that facilitate the ability of the group A streptococcus to adhere to epithelial cells of the nasopharynx and/or skin. Of these, the most important are M protein, LTA, and protein F. In the nasopharynx, all three appear to be involved in mediating attachment to the fatty acid–binding sites in the

Surface molecules binding to fibronectin is important first step

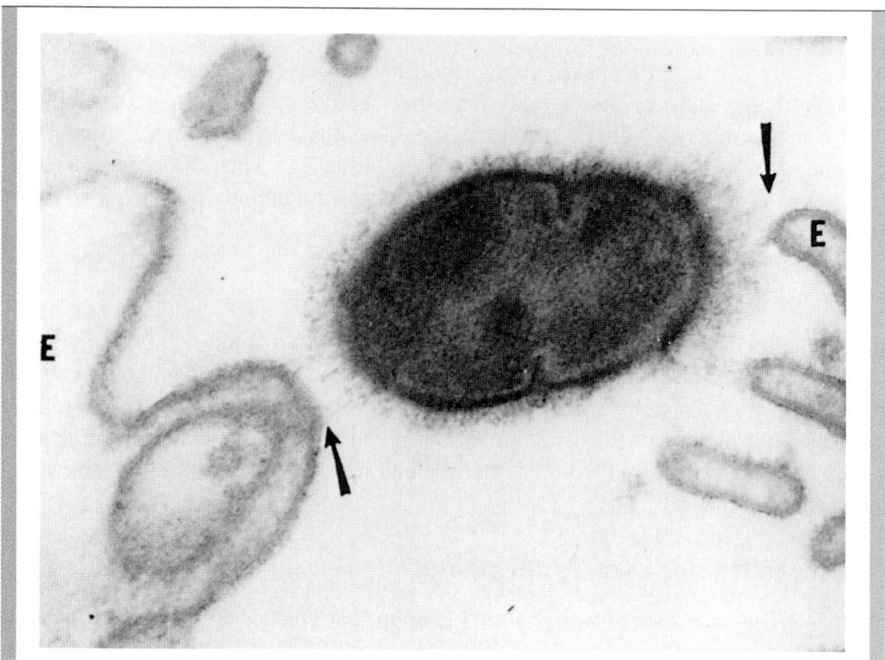

FIGURE 17–3
A group A β-hemolytic streptococcus is shown attaching to the cell membrane of a human oral epithelial cell (E). Note the hairlike pili (*arrows*), which mediate the attachment. As in Figure 16–1, both M protein and lipoteichoic acid are associated with the pili. (*Reproduced with permission from Beachey EH, Ofek I.* J Exp Med *1976;143:764. Figure 2.*)

M protein supports nasopharyngeal cell adherence

glycoprotein fibronectin covering the epithelial cell surface. The role of M protein is not direct but it appears to provide a scaffold for LTA, which is essential for it to reach its binding site (Fig 17–3).

M protein and protein F are involved in epidermis binding

Expression is environmentally regulated by O_2 and CO_2

On the other hand, M protein appears to be direct and dominant in binding to the skin through its ability to interact with subcorneal keratinocytes, the most numerous cell type in cutaneous tissue. This adherence takes place at domains of the M protein that bind to CD46 and possibly other receptors on the keratinocyte surface. Protein F is also involved primarily in adherence to antigen-presenting Langerhans cells. Expression of M protein and protein F is environmentally regulated in response to changing concentrations of O_2 and CO_2. Experimental evidence suggests that a high O_2 environment favors protein F and adherence to Langerhans cells, while an environment richer in CO_2 favors M protein synthesis and interaction with keratinocytes. This environmentally controlled sequential interaction of *S. pyogenes* with different types of host cells should play some mitigating role either in establishing the microbe or in altering the development of a normally protective host response.

Multiple factors are involved in invasion

Clinical evidence makes it clear that group A streptococci have the capacity to be highly invasive. The events following attachment that trigger invasion are only starting to be understood. It appears that M protein, protein F, and other fibronectin-binding proteins are required for invasion of nonprofessional phagocytes. This invasion involves integrin receptors and is accompanied by cytoskeleton rearrangements but the molecular events do not yet make a coherent story.

Antiphagocytic M protein binds fibrinogen and factor H

Surface C3b deposition is diminished

C5a peptidase blocks phagocyte chemotaxis

After the initial events of attachment and invasion, it appears that the concerted activity of the M protein, immunoglobulin-binding proteins, and the C5a peptidase play the key roles in allowing the streptococcal infection to continue. M protein plays an essential role in group A streptococcal resistance to phagocytosis. The antiphagocytic activity of M protein is related to the ability of domains of the molecule to bind fibrinogen and serum factor H. This leads to a diminished availability of alternative pathway generated complement component C3b for deposition on the streptococcal surface (Fig 17–4). In the presence of M type–specific antibody, classical pathway opsonophagocytosis proceeds, and the streptococci are rapidly killed. As a second antiphagocytic mechanism the C5a peptidase inactivates C5a and thus blocks chemotaxis of polymorphonuclear neutrophils (PMNs) and other phagocytes to the site of infection. Although the hyaluronic acid capsule contributes to resistance to phagocytosis, the mechanisms involved are unknown.

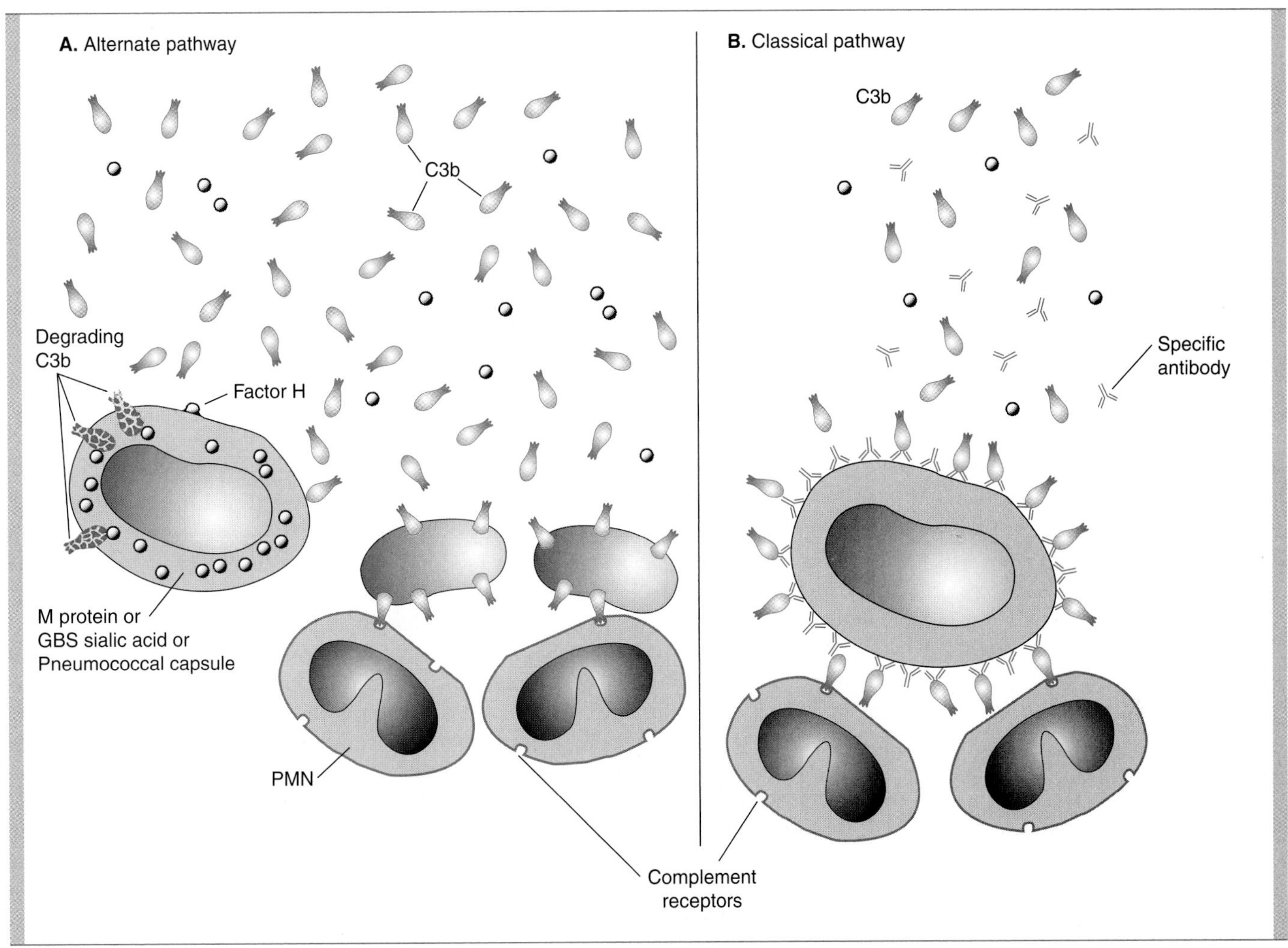

FIGURE 17–4

Streptococcal resistance to opsonophagocytosis. **A.** Alternate pathway. In the alternate complement pathway, C3b binds to the surface of bacteria, providing a recognition site for professional phagocytes and sometimes causing direct injury. Streptococci with special surface structures such as capsules or M protein are able to bind serum factor to their surface. This interferes with complement deposition by accelerating the breakdown of C3b. **B.** Classical pathway. Specific antibody binding to an antigen on the surface provides another binding cite for C3b. Phagocyte recognition may occur even if factor H is present.

The precise role of other bacterial factors in the pathogenesis of acute infection is uncertain, but the combined effect of streptokinase, DNAase, and hyaluronidase may prevent effective localization of the infection, while the streptolysins produce tissue injury and are toxic to phagocytic cells. If any of the SPEs are produced, they may contribute as well but their presence is not essential for acute infections. Antibodies against these components are formed in the course of streptococcal infection but are not known to be protective.

Other virulence factors contribute to spread and injury

In **streptococcal toxic shock syndrome (STSS),** as with staphylococcal toxic shock syndrome, the findings of shock, renal impairment, and diarrhea seem to be explained by the massive cytokine release stimulated by the superantigenicity of the SPEs. Exotoxin production, however, does not easily explain the enhanced invasiveness of group A streptococci, which is an added feature of STSS compared to its staphylococcal counterpart. The enzymatic activity of SPE-B has been linked to invasiveness, but strains with SPE-A and SPE-C are much more common in STSS than SPE-B. This syndrome may represent bacteriophage-mediated horizontal transfer of the SPE genes among recently emerged clones with enhanced invasive potential, a deadly combination. The basis of the enhanced invasiveness remains to be determined.

Superantigenicity of SPEs contributes to STSS

Invasive component is unexplained

Poststreptococcal Sequelae

Acute Rheumatic Fever (ARF)

ARF is an autoimmune state induced by streptococcal infection

Of the many theories advanced to explain the role of group A streptococci in ARF, an autoimmune mechanism related to antigenic similarities between streptococci and human tissue antigens has the most experimental support. Streptococcal pharyngitis patients who develop ARF have higher levels of antistreptococcal and autoreactive antibodies and T cells than those who do not. Some of these have been shown to react with both heart tissue and streptococcal antigens.

Antistreptococcal antibodies cross-react with heart sarcolemma

M protein epitopes differ from antiphagocytic domains

Antibodies to group A carbohydrate react with valves

The antigen stimulating these antibodies is most probably M protein, but the group A carbohydrate is also a possibility. The similarity between the structure of M protein and myosin is an obvious connection, and M protein fragments have been shown to stimulate antibodies that bind to human heart sarcolemma membranes. Immunochemical studies of M proteins from different M types are now directed at defining unique epitopes responsible for ARF and the extent to which they are shared between serotypes and strains. Domains of the M protein molecule responsible for the heart cross-reactivity have been identified, which differ from those responsible for the factor H and fibrinogen binding. Thus, the cross-reactive and antiphagocytic properties of M protein appear to reside in separate parts of the molecule (see Fig 17–2). Antibodies to the dominant epitope of the group A carbohydrate (N-acetylglucosamine) may play a role in injury to the valvular endothelium, but T cells stimulated by M protein have been seen in valves as well.

Cell-mediated immunity responses include cytotoxic lymphocytes

ARF patients also show enhanced cell-mediated immune responses to streptococcal antigens. Cytotoxic T lymphocytes may be stimulated by M protein, and cytotoxic lymphocytes have been observed in the blood of patients with ARF. A cellular reaction pattern consisting of lymphocytes and macrophages aggregated around fibrinoid deposits is found in human hearts. This lesion, called the **Aschoff body,** is considered characteristic of rheumatic carditis. Suggestions that M protein has superantigen properties must still be reconciled with the prolonged nature of the illness.

Alloantigens are associated with hyperreactivity to streptococci

Genetic factors are probably also important in ARF because only a small proportion of individuals infected with group A streptococci develop the disease. Attack rates have been highest among those of lower socioeconomic status and vary among those of different racial origins. The gene for an alloantigen found on the surface of B lymphocytes occurs among rheumatic fever patients at a frequency fourfold to fivefold greater than the general population. This further suggests a genetic predisposition to hyperreactivity to streptococcal products.

Acute Glomerulonephritis

Autoimmune reactions to M protein or streptokinase are implicated

The renal injury of acute glomerulonephritis is caused by deposition in the glomerulus of antigen–antibody complexes with complement activation and consequent inflammation. The M proteins of some nephritogenic strains have been shown to share antigenic determinants with glomeruli, which suggests an autoimmune mechanism similar to rheumatic fever. Streptokinase has also been implicated both through molecular mimicry and through its plasminogen activation capacity.

IMMUNITY

Type-specific IgG reverses antiphagocytic effect of M protein

Repeated infections and ARF are due to many M types

It has long been known that antibody directed against M protein is protective for subsequent group A streptococcal infections. This protection, however, is only for subsequent infection with strains of the same M type. This is called **type-specific immunity.** This protective IgG is directed against epitopes in the amino-terminal regions of the molecule and reverses the antiphagocytic effect of M protein. Streptococci opsonized with type-specific antibody bind complement C3b by the classical mechanism, facilitating phagocyte recognition (see Fig 17–4). There is evidence that mucosal IgA is also important in blocking adherence while the IgG is able to protect against invasion. Unfortunately, because there are over 80 M types, repeated infections with other M types occurs. Eventually, immunity to the common M types is acquired and infections become less common in adults. In ARF patients, it is the hyperreaction seen in each episode that produces the lesions associated with rheumatic heart disease.

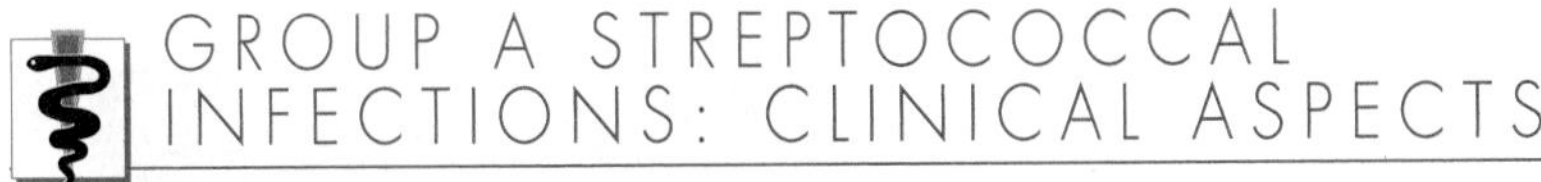

GROUP A STREPTOCOCCAL INFECTIONS: CLINICAL ASPECTS

MANIFESTATIONS

Streptococcal Pharyngitis

Although it may occur at any age, streptococcal pharyngitis is most frequent between the ages of 5 and 15 years. The illness is characterized by acute sore throat, malaise, fever, and headache. Infection typically involves the tonsillar pillars, uvula, and soft palate, which become red, swollen, and covered with a yellow-white exudate. The cervical lymph nodes that drain this area may also become swollen and tender. Group A streptococcal pharyngitis is usually self-limiting. Typically, the fever is gone by the third to fifth day, and other manifestations subside within 1 week. Occasionally the infection may spread locally to produce peritonsillar or retropharyngeal abscesses, otitis media, suppurative cervical adenitis, and acute sinusitis. Rarely, more extensive spread occurs, producing meningitis, pneumonia, or bacteremia with metastatic infection in distant organs. In the preantibiotic era, these suppurative complications were responsible for a mortality of 1 to 3% following acute streptococcal pharyngitis. Such complications are much less common now, and fatal infections are rare.

Strep throat syndrome overlaps with viral pharyngitis

Spread beyond the pharynx uncommon

Impetigo

The primary lesion of streptococcal impetigo is a small (up to 1 cm) vesicle surrounded by an area of erythema. The vesicle enlarges over a period of days, becomes pustular, and eventually breaks to form a yellow crust. The lesions usually appear in 2- to 5-year-old children on exposed body surfaces, typically the face and lower extremities. Multiple lesions may coalesce to form deeper ulcerated areas. Although *S. aureus* produces a clinically distinct bullous form of impetigo (see Chapter 16), it can also cause vesicular lesions resembling streptococcal impetigo. Both pathogens are isolated from some cases.

Exposed skin of 2- to 5-year-old children

Tiny pustules may combine to form ulcers

Erysipelas

Erysipelas is a distinct form of streptococcal infection of the skin and subcutaneous tissues, primarily affecting the dermis. It is characterized by a spreading area of erythema and edema with rapidly advancing, well-demarcated edges, pain, and systemic manifestations, including fever and lymphadenopathy. Infection usually occurs on the face (Fig 17–5), and a previous history of streptococcal sore throat is common.

Spreading erythema of dermal tissues

Puerperal Infection

Infection of the endometrium at or near delivery is a life-threatening form of group A streptococcal infection. Fortunately, it is now relatively rare, but in the 19th century, the clinical findings of "childbed fever" were characteristic and common enough to provide the first clues to the transmission of bacterial infections in hospitals (see Chapter 72). Other organisms can cause puerperal fever, but this form is the most likely to produce a rapidly progressive infection.

Group A streptococcus causes the most virulent form of puerperal fever

Disease Associated with Streptococcal Pyrogenic Exotoxins

Scarlet Fever

Infection with strains that elaborate any of the SPEs may superimpose the signs of scarlet fever on a patient with streptococcal pharyngitis. In scarlet fever, the buccal mucosa, temples, and cheeks are deep red, except for a pale area around the mouth and nose (circumoral pallor). Punctate hemorrhages appear on the hard and soft palates, and the tongue becomes covered with a yellow-white exudate through which the red papillae are prominent (strawberry tongue). A diffuse red "sandpaper" rash appears on the second day

Scarlet fever is strep throat with a characteristic rash

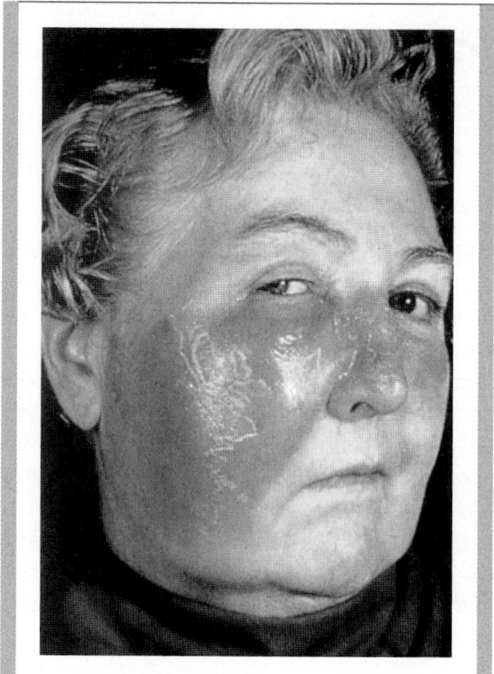

FIGURE 17–5
Streptococcal erysipelas. The diffuse erythema and swelling in the face of this woman are characteristic of group A streptococcal cellulitis at any site. *(Reproduced with permission from Connor DH, Chandler FW, Schwartz DQA, Manz HJ, Lack EE (eds).* Pathology of Infectious Diseases, *vol. 1. Stamford, CT: Appleton & Lange; 1997.*)

of illness, spreading from the upper chest to the trunk and extremities. Circulating antibody to the toxin neutralizes these effects. For unknown reasons, scarlet fever is both less frequent and less severe than early in the 20th century.

Streptococcal Toxic Shock Syndrome (STSS)

STSS is a rapidly progressive multisystem disease

Shock, azotemia, and bacteremia are common

STSS may begin at the site of any group A streptococcal infection even at the site of seemingly minor trauma. The systemic illness starts with vague myalgia, chills, and severe pain at the infected site. Most commonly, this is in the skin and soft tissues and leads to necrotizing fasciitis and myonecrosis. The striking nature of this progression when it involves the extremities is the basis of the label "flesh-eating bacteria." STSS continues with nausea, vomiting, and diarrhea followed by hypotension, shock, and organ failure. The outstanding laboratory findings are a lymphocytosis; impaired renal function (azotemia); and, in over half the cases, bacteremia. Some patients are in irreversible shock by the time they reach a medical facility. Many survivors have been left as multiple amputees as the result of metastatic spread of the streptococci.

Poststreptococcal Sequelae

Acute Rheumatic Fever (ARF)

ARF causes inflammation of connective tissue and endocardium

Infection with new M types triggers recurrences

Recurrences lead to heart valve damage

ARF is a nonsuppurative inflammatory disease characterized by fever, carditis, subcutaneous nodules, chorea, and migratory polyarthritis. Cardiac enlargement, valvular murmurs, and effusions are seen clinically and reflect endocardial, myocardial, and epicardial damage, which can lead to heart failure. Attacks typically begin 3 weeks (range, 1 to 5 weeks) after an attack of group A streptococcal pharyngitis, and in the absence of antiinflammatory therapy last 2 to 3 months. ARF also has a predilection for recurrence with subsequent streptococcal infections as new M types are encountered. The first attack usually occurs between the ages of 5 and 15 years. The risk of recurrent attacks after subsequent group A streptococcal infections continues into adult life and then decreases. Repeated attacks lead to progressive damage to the endocardium and heart valves, with scarring and valvular stenosis or incompetence (rheumatic heart disease).

Acute Glomerulonephritis

Poststreptococcal glomerulonephritis is primarily a disease of childhood that begins 1 to 4 weeks after streptococcal pharyngitis and 3 to 6 weeks after skin infection. It is characterized clinically by edema, hypertension, hematuria, proteinuria, and decreased serum complement levels. Pathologically, there are diffuse proliferative lesions of the glomeruli. The clinical course is usually benign, with spontaneous healing over weeks to months. Occasionally, a progressive course leads to renal failure and death.

Children develop a nephritis, which slowly resolves

DIAGNOSIS

Although these clinical features of streptococcal pharyngitis are fairly typical, there is enough overlap with viral pharyngitis that a culture of the posterior pharynx and tonsils is required for diagnosis. A direct Gram-stained smear of the throat is unhelpful because of the other streptococci in the pharyngeal flora, but smears from normally sterile sites usually demonstrate streptococci. Blood agar plates incubated anaerobically give the best yield because they favor the demonstration of β-hemolysis (see streptolysins, above). β-hemolytic colonies are identified by Lancefield grouping using immunofluorescence or agglutination methods. In smaller laboratories, an indirect method based on the exquisite susceptibility of group A strains to bacitracin and the relative resistance of strains of other groups may be used for presumptive separation of group A strains from the others (Table 17–2).

Throat culture followed by Lancefield grouping is definitive

Bacitracin susceptibility predicts group A

Detection of group A antigen extracted directly from throat swabs is now available in a wide variety of kits marketed for use in physicians' offices. These methods are rapid and specific, but most are only 90 to 95% sensitive compared to culture. Given the importance of the detection of group A streptococci in prevention of ARF (the reason physicians culture sore throats), missing even 5% of cases is not tolerable. Until direct antigen detection methods gain a higher sensitivity, negative results must be confirmed by culture before withholding treatment. Some of the newer antigen detection procedures are approaching a sensitivity that would allow their substitution for culture.

Direct detection of A antigen is rapid

Several serologic tests have been developed to aid in the diagnosis of poststreptococcal sequelae by providing evidence of a previous group A streptococcal infection. They

TABLE 17–2

Usual Hemolytic, Biochemical, and Cultural Reactions of Common Streptococci and Enterococci[a]

	Susceptibility to		Bile	Bile/Esculin	
	Bacitracin	Optochin	Solubility	Reaction[b]	PYR[c]
Streptococci					
β-Hemolytic					
Lancefield group A	+	–	–	–	+
Lancefield groups B, C, F, G	–	–	–	–	–
α-Hemolytic					
S. pneumoniae	–	+	+	–	–
Viridans group	–	–	–	–	–
Nonhemolytic	–	–	–	–	–
Enterococci	–	–	–	+	+

[a] All are tests commonly substituted for serologic identification in clinical laboratories.

[b] Tests for the ability to grow in bile and reduce esculin.

[c] PYR = pyrrolidonyl arylamidase test.

ASO antibodies document previous infection in suspect ARF

include the ASO, anti-DNAase B, and some tests that combine multiple antigens. High titers of ASO are usually found in sera of patients with rheumatic fever, so that test is used most widely.

TREATMENT

Group A streptococci remain susceptible to penicillin

Group A streptococci are highly susceptible to penicillin G, the antimicrobic of choice. Concentrations as low as 0.01 μg/mL have a bactericidal effect, and penicillin resistance is so far unknown. Numerous other antimicrobics are also active, including other penicillins, cephalosporins, tetracyclines, and macrolides, but not aminoglycosides.

Treatment of pharyngitis within 10 days prevents ARF

Patients allergic to penicillin are usually treated with erythromycin if the organisms are susceptible. Impetigo is often treated with erythromycin to cover the prospect of *S. aureus* involvement. Adequate treatment of streptococcal pharyngitis within 10 days of onset prevents rheumatic fever by removing the antigenic stimulus; its effect on the duration of the pharyngitis is less, because of the short course of the natural infection. Treatment does not prevent the development of acute glomerulonephritis.

PREVENTION

Prophylactic penicillin prevents ARF recurrences

Penicillin prophylaxis with long-acting preparations is used to prevent recurrences of ARF during the most susceptible ages (5 to 15 years). Patients with a history of rheumatic fever or known rheumatic heart disease receive antimicrobial prophylaxis while undergoing procedures known to cause transient bacteremia, such as dental extraction. Vaccines using epitopes of the M protein molecule, which would provide protection against acute infection without stimulating autoantibodies are in development. This is a sizable task given the large number of M protein serotypes.

Group B Streptococci (Streptococcus agalactiae)

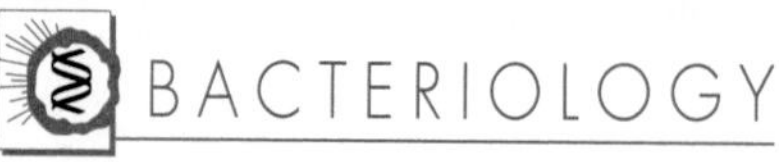

Nine capsular types contain sialic acid

Group B streptococci (GBS) produce short chains and diplococcal pairs of spherical or ovoid Gram-positive cells. Colonies are larger and β-hemolysis is less distinct than with group A streptococci and may even be absent. In addition to the Lancefield B antigen, GBS produce polysaccharide capsules of nine antigenic types (Ia, Ib, II through VIII) all of which contain sialic acid in the form of terminal side chain residues.

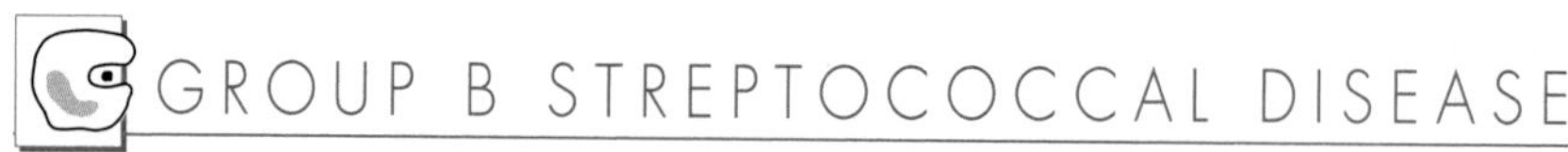

CLINICAL CAPSULE

The typical GBS case is a newborn in the first few days of life who is not doing well. Fever, lethargy, poor feeding, and respiratory distress are the most common features. Localizing findings are usually lacking, and the diagnosis is revealed only by isolation of GBS from blood or cerebrospinal fluid. The mortality rate is high even when appropriate antibiotics are used.

EPIDEMIOLOGY

Neonatal sepsis is acquired from mother's vaginal flora

GBS are the leading cause of sepsis and meningitis in the first few days of life. The organism is resident in the gastrointestinal tract, with secondary spread to other sites, the most important of which is the vagina. GBS can be found in the vaginal flora of 10 to 30% of women, and during pregnancy and delivery, these organisms may again access to the amniotic fluid or colonize the newborn as it passes through the birth canal. Judging from US surveillance data (1.8 cases/1000 live births), GBS produce disease in approximately 2% of these encounters. The risk is much higher when factors are present that decrease the infant's innate resistance (prematurity) or increase the chances of transmission (ruptured amniotic membranes). Some infants are healthy at birth but develop sepsis 1 to 3 months later. It is not known whether the organism in these "late-onset" cases was acquired from the mother, in the nursery, or in the community after leaving the hospital.

Ruptured membranes and prematurity increase risk

PATHOGENESIS

GBS disease requires the proper combination of organism and host factors. The GBS capsule is the major organism factor. The sialic acid moiety of the capsule has been shown to bind serum factor H, which in turn accelerates degradation of C3b before it can be effectively deposited on the surface of the organism. This makes alternate pathway–mediated mechanisms of opsonophagocytosis relatively ineffective (see Fig 17–4). Thus, complement-mediated phagocyte recognition requires specific antibody and the classical pathway. Newborns will have this antibody only if they receive it from their mother as transplacental IgG. Those who lack the protective "cover" of antibody specific to the type of GBS they encounter must rely on alternate pathway mechanisms, a situation in which the GBS has an advantage over less virulent organisms. GBS have also been shown to produce a peptidase that inactivates C5a, the major chemoattractant of PMNs. This may correlate with the observation that serious neonatal infections often show a paucity of infiltrating PMNs.

Capsule binds factor H

C3b deposition is disrupted

Transplacental IgG is protective

IMMUNITY

Antibody is protective against GBS disease, but as with group A streptococcal M protein, the antibody must be specific to the infecting type of GBS. Fortunately, there are only nine types and type III produces the majority of cases in the first week of life. Antibody is acquired by GBS infection, and specific IgG may be transmitted transplacentally to the fetus, providing protection in the perinatal period. In the presence of type-specific antibody, classical pathway C3b deposition, phagocyte recognition, and killing proceed normally.

Type-specific anticapsular antibody is protective

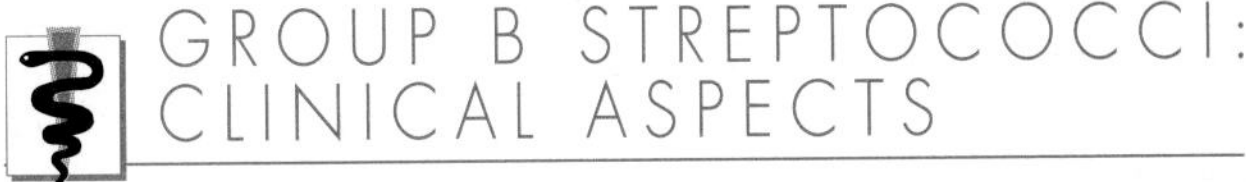

GROUP B STREPTOCOCCI: CLINICAL ASPECTS

MANIFESTATIONS

The clinical findings are nonspecific and similar to those found in other serious infections in the neonatal period (see Chapter 69). Respiratory distress, fever, lethargy, irritability, apnea, and hypotension are common. Fever is sometimes absent, and infants may even be hypothermic. Pneumonia is common, and meningitis is present in 5 to 10% of cases, but most infections have GBS circulating in the bloodstream without localizing findings. The onset is typically in the first few days of life, and signs of infection are present at birth in almost 50% of cases. The late-onset (1 to 3 month) cases have similar findings but are more likely to have meningitis and focal infections in the bones and joints. Even with appropriate and prompt treatment, the mortality rate for early onset GBS infection approaches 20%.

Nonspecific findings evolve to pneumonia and meningitis

First few days of life or months later

GBS infections in adults are uncommon and fall in two groups. The first are peripartum chorioamnionitis and bacteremia, the mother's side of the neonatal syndrome. Other infections include pneumonia and a variety of skin and soft tissue infections similar to those produced by other pyogenic streptococci. Although adult GBS infections may be serious, they are usually not fatal unless patients are immunocompromised. GBS are not associated with rheumatic fever or acute glomerulonephritis.

Maternal and other adult infections can be serious

DIAGNOSIS

Culture is only standard method

The laboratory diagnosis of GBS infection is by culture of blood, cerebrospinal fluid, or other appropriate specimen. Definitive identification involves serologic determination of the Lancefield group by the same methods used for group A streptococci. Methods for direct detection of GBS antigen in vaginal specimens have been evaluated, but their sensitivity is far too low for use in the diagnosis of neonatal infection.

TREATMENT

Combinations of β-lactam and aminoglycoside are used

GBS are susceptible to the same antimicrobics as group A organisms. Although penicillin is the treatment of choice, GBS are slightly less susceptible to β-lactams than other streptococci. For this reason neonatal infections are often initially treated with combinations of penicillin (or ampicillin) and an aminoglycoside. These combinations have been shown to accelerate killing of GBS in vitro.

PREVENTION

Intrapartum prophylaxis is protective

Third trimester vaginal culture and/or clinical factors determine risk

Vaccine is a prospect

Current strategies for prevention of neonatal GBS disease are focused on reducing contact of the infant with the organism. In colonized women, attempts to eradicate the carrier state have not been successful, but intrapartum antimicrobial prophylaxis with penicillin or ampicillin has been shown to reduce transmission and disease in high-risk populations. It is now recommended by expert obstetric and perinatology groups that all newborns at risk receive such prophylaxis, but there is debate about the practical aspects of determining risk. One approach is to screen all expectant mothers for vaginal GBS colonization in the third trimester and administer prophylaxis during labor to all found to be culture positive. This safe but expensive approach can be applied only to those who seek regular prenatal care. A second approach is to assign risk on clinical grounds (eg, prematurity, prolonged membrane rupture, fever), which is less expensive but will miss some colonized babies. There is evidence that prophylaxis is working. The incidence of early-onset neonatal GBS disease dropped 65% over a 5-year period when these strategies were being implemented. Prevention by immunization with purified GBS capsular polysaccharide has been shown to be feasible, and considerable effort is now being directed at development of a vaccine.

Other Pyogenic Streptococci

All are virulent but uncommon

None associated with immunologic sequelae

The other pyogenic streptococci occasionally produce various respiratory, skin, wound, soft tissue, and genital infections, which may resemble those caused by group A and B streptococci. Although a few food-borne outbreaks of pharyngitis have been linked to non–group A streptococci, their role as a cause of everyday sore throats is not established. These streptococci are susceptible to penicillin, and infections are managed in a manner similar to deep tissue infections caused by group A and B strains. None of the non–group A streptococci have been associated with poststreptococcal sequelae.

Streptococcus pneumoniae

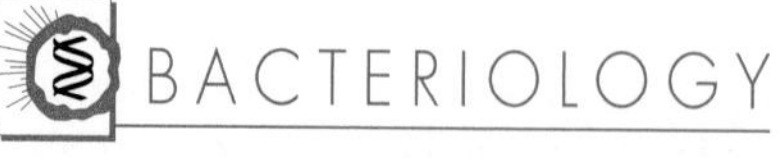

BACTERIOLOGY

MORPHOLOGY AND STRUCTURE

Capsule has 90+ serotypes

S. pneumoniae (pneumococci) are Gram-positive, oval cocci typically arranged end to end in pairs (diplococcus) giving the cells a bullet shape (Fig 17–6). The distinguishing structural feature of the pneumococcus is its capsule. All virulent strains have surface capsules,

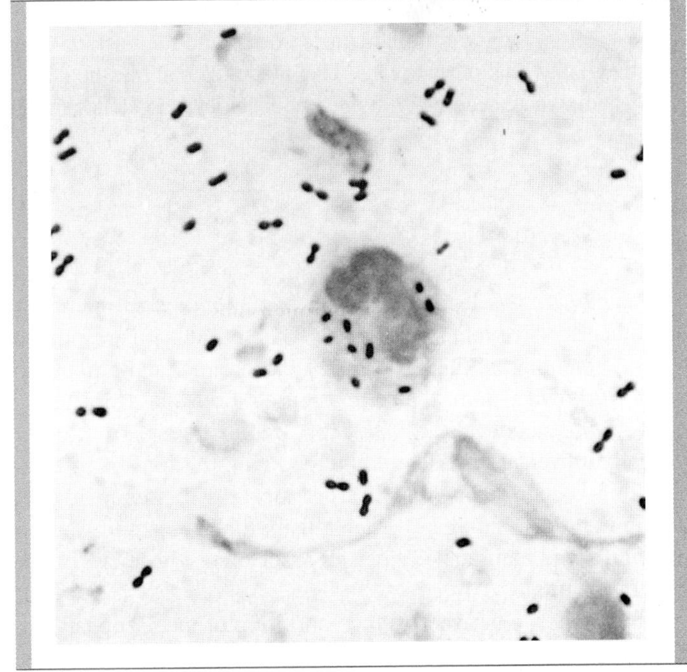

FIGURE 17–6
Streptococcus pneumoniae in sputum of patient with pneumonia. Note the marked tendency to form oval diplococci.

composed of high-molecular-weight polysaccharide polymers that are complex mixtures of monosaccharides, oligosaccharides, and sometimes other components. The exact makeup of the polymer is unique and distinctly antigenic for each of more than 90 serotypes. A number of pneumococcal surface proteins have been identified but their function is not known.

Pneumococcal cell wall structure is similar to other streptococci. Teichoic acid, LPA, and phosphocholine are rooted in the peptidoglycan extending outward into the capsule where they provide binding domains for a variety of surface proteins. At least one of these, a **choline binding protein,** is able to bind to both pneumococcal cell wall cholines and carbohydrates present on the surface of epithelial cells.

Choline binding protein attaches to cells

GROWTH

On blood agar, pneumococci produce round, glistening 0.5- to 2.0-mm colonies surrounded by a zone of α-hemolysis. Both colonies and broth cultures have a tendency to undergo autolysis due to their susceptibility to peroxides produced during growth and the action of **autolysins,** a family of pneumococcal enzymes that degrade peptidoglycan. Accelerating the autolytic process with bile salts is the basis of the bile solubility test that separates pneumococci from other α-hemolytic streptococci.

Colonies are α-hemolytic

EXTRACELLULAR PRODUCTS

All pneumococci produce **pneumolysin,** which is a member of the family of transmembrane pore-forming toxins that includes staphylococcal α toxin, *S. pyogenes* streptolysin O, and others. The pneumococcus does not secrete pneumolysin but it is released on lysis of the organisms augmented by autolysins. Pneumolysin has a number of other effects, including its ability to stimulate cytokines and disrupt the cilia of cultured human respiratory epithelial cells. Pneumococci also produce a **neuraminidase,** which cleaves sialic acid present in host mucin, glycolipids and glycoproteins.

Pneumolysin forms pores after release by autolysins

PNEUMOCOCCAL DISEASE

The most common form of infection with *S. pneumoniae* is pneumonia, which begins with fever and a shaking chill followed by signs that localize the disease to the lung. These include difficulty breathing and cough with production of purulent

CLINICAL CAPSULE

sputum, sometimes containing blood. The pneumonia typically fills part or all of a lobe of the lung with inflammatory cells, and the bacteria may spread to the bloodstream and thus other organs. The most important of the latter is the central nervous system, where seeding with pneumococci leads to acute purulent meningitis.

EPIDEMIOLOGY

Pneumonia is common

Young and old are most affected

S. pneumoniae is a leading cause of pneumonia, acute purulent meningitis, bacteremia, and other invasive infections. In the United States it is responsible for an estimated 3000 cases of meningitis, 50,000 cases of bacteremia, and 500,000 cases of pneumonia each year. Worldwide, more than 5 million children die every year from pneumococcal disease. *S. pneumoniae* is also the most frequent cause of otitis media (see Chapter 61), a virtually universal disease of childhood with millions of cases every year. Pneumococcal infections occur throughout life but are most common in the very young (<2 years) and in the old (>60 years). Alcoholism, diabetes mellitus, chronic renal disease, asplenia, and some malignancies are all associated with more frequent and serious pneumococcal infection.

Respiratory colonization is common

Microaerosols transmit person to person

Infections are derived from colonization of the nasopharynx, where pneumococci can be found in 5 to 40% of healthy persons depending on age, season, and other factors. The highest rates are among children in the winter. Respiratory secretions containing pneumococci may be transmitted from person to person by direct contact or from the microaerosols created by coughing and sneezing in close quarters. Such conditions are favored by crowded living conditions, particularly when colonized persons are mixed with susceptible ones, as in child care centers, recruitment barracks, and prisons. As with other bacterial pneumonias, viral respiratory infection and underlying chronic disease are important predisposing factors.

Some serotypes are more common

About 23 of the 90 pneumococcal serotypes produce disease more often than the others. There is also a variation in the age and geographic distribution of cases. These differences are presumably due to enhanced virulence factors in these types, but the specific reasons are not known. These features do not influence the medical management of individual cases but are important in devising prevention strategies such as immunization (see below).

PATHOGENESIS

Aspiration of colonizing bacteria starts the disease process

Impaired clearance mechanisms enhance susceptibility

Pneumococcal adherence to nasopharyngeal cells involves multiple factors. The primary relationship is the bridging effect of the choline binding protein's attachment to cell wall cholines and carbohydrates covering or exposed on the surface of host epithelial cells. This binding may be aided by the exposure of additional receptors by neuraminidase digestion or pneumolysin stimulated cytokine activation of host cells. Aspiration of respiratory secretions containing these pneumococci is the initial event leading to pneumonia. This must be a common event. Normally, aspirated organisms are cleared rapidly by the defense mechanisms of the lower respiratory tract, including the cough and epiglottic reflexes; the mucociliary "blanket;" and phagocytosis by alveolar macrophages. Host factors that impair the combined efficiency of these defenses can allow pneumococci to reach the alveoli and multiply there. These include chronic pulmonary diseases; damage to bronchial epithelium from smoking or air pollution; and respiratory dysfunction from alcoholic intoxication, narcotics, anesthesia, and trauma.

Capsule interferes with phagocytosis

Pneumolysin causes injury

When organisms reach the alveolus, the involvement of pneumococcal virulence factors appears to operate in two stages. The first stage is early in infection, when the surface capsule of intact organisms acts to block phagocytosis by complement inhibition. This allows the organisms to multiply and spread despite an acute inflammatory response. The second stage occurs when organisms begin to disintegrate and release a number of factors either synthesized by the pneumococcus or part of its structure, thus causing injury. These include pneumolysin, autolysin, and components of the cell wall.

Capsule

The polysaccharide capsule of *S. pneumoniae* is the major determinant of virulence. Unencapsulated mutants do not produce disease in humans or laboratory animals. Like the GBS capsule, pneumococcal polysaccharide interferes with effective deposition of complement on the organism's surface and thus phagocyte recognition and engulfment. This property is particularly important in the absence of specific antibody, when alternate pathway is the primary means for C3b mediated opsonization. The exact mechanism for interference with C3b deposition (see Fig 17–4) may differ in detail with that of GBS sialic acid and between the capsular polysaccharide polymers of individual pneumococcal serotypes. The net effect is that the complement fragments recognized by phagocyte receptors are not available on the surface of the organism. When antibody binds to the capsular polysaccharide, C3b generated by the classical pathway binds and opsonophagocytosis proceeds efficiently.

Unencapsulated pneumococci are avirulent

Alternate pathway C3b deposition blocked by capsule

Pneumolysin

Some of the clinical features seen in the course of pneumococcal infections are not explainable by the capsule alone. These include the dramatic abrupt onset, toxicity, fulminant course, and disseminated intravascular coagulation seen in some cases. Pneumolysin's toxicity for pulmonary endothelial cells and direct effect on cilia contributes to the disruption of the endothelial barrier and facilitates the access of pneumococci to the alveoli and eventually their spread beyond into the bloodstream. Pneumolysin also has direct effects on phagocytes and suppresses host inflammatory and immune functions. Injection of purified pneumolysin into the lung of rats causes all of the salient histologic hallmarks of pneumococcal pneumonia. Because pneumolysin is not actively secreted outside the bacterial cell, the action of the autolysins is required to release it.

Pneumolysin disrupts cells and cilia

Lysis required to release from bacterial cell

Other Virulence Determinants

Although the search for the host epithelial cell's adhesin has been unrewarding, it seems logical that one or more of the surface proteins attached to cell wall teichoic acid are involved. Pneumococcal surface protein A (PspA) is found in virtually all pneumococci and has been shown to interfere with complement deposition. In addition to its role in attachment, neuraminidase may have a role at other stages of disease. Peptidoglycan and teichoic acid components of the cell wall have been shown to stimulate inflammation and cerebral edema in experimental meningitis and may do so at other stages of infection. Along with pneumolysin, these may be responsible for the heightened acute inflammatory response seen in pneumococcal infection, which of itself may be destructive to the host.

PspA and neuraminidase act on cell surface

Peptidoglycan stimulates inflammation

The combined effects of pneumococcal and host factors produce a pneumonia, which progresses through a series of stages. Initial alveolar multiplication produces a profuse outpouring of serous edema fluid, which is then followed by an influx of polymorphonuclear leukocytes (PMNs) and erythrocytes (red blood cells; RBCs). By the second or third day of illness, the lung segment has increased three- to fourfold in weight through accumulation of this cellular, hemorrhagic fluid typically in a single lobe of the lung. In the consolidated alveoli, neutrophils predominate initially, but once actively growing pneumococci are no longer present, macrophages replace the granulocytes and resolution of the lesion ensues. A remarkable feature of pneumococcal pneumonia is the lack of structural damage to the lung, which usually leads to complete resolution on recovery.

PMNs and RBCs consolidate alveoli

Lesions resolve without structural damage

IMMUNITY

Immunity to *S. pneumoniae* infection is provided by antibody directed against the specific pneumococcal capsular type. When antibody binds to the capsular surface, C3b is deposited by classical pathway mechanisms, and phagocytosis can proceed. Because the number of serotypes is large, complete immunity through natural experience is not realistic, which is why pneumococcal infections occur throughout life. Infections are most often

Immunity is specific to capsular type

Antibody leads to classical pathway complement deposition

seen in the very young, when immunologic experience is minimal, and in the elderly, when immunity begins to wane and risk factors are more common. Antibodies to surface proteins and enzymes, including pneumolysin, are also formed in the course of disease, but their role in immunity is unknown.

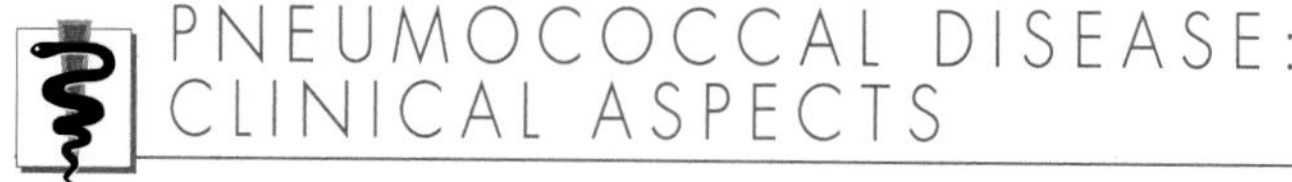

PNEUMOCOCCAL DISEASE: CLINICAL ASPECTS

MANIFESTATIONS

Pneumococcal Pneumonia

Shaking chill is followed by bloody sputum

Lung consolidation is typically lobar

Clinically, pneumococcal pneumonia begins abruptly with a shaking chill and high fever. Cough with production of sputum pink to rusty in color (indicating the presence of RBCs) and pleuritic chest pain are common. Physical findings usually indicate pulmonary consolidation. Children and young adults typically demonstrate a lobular or lobar consolidation on chest radiography, whereas older patients may show a less localized bronchial distribution of the infiltrates. Without therapy, sustained fever, pleuritic pain, and productive cough continue until a "crisis" occurs 5 to 10 days after onset of the disease. The crisis involves a sudden decrease in temperature and improvement in the patient's condition. It is associated with effective levels of opsonizing antibody reaching the lesion. Although infection may occur at any age, the incidence and mortality of pneumococcal pneumonia increase sharply after 50 years.

Pneumococcal Meningitis

Sequelae are slightly higher than other meningeal pathogens

S. pneumoniae is one of the three leading causes of bacterial meningitis. The signs and symptoms are similar to those produced by other bacteria (see Chapter 67). Acute purulent meningitis may follow pneumococcal pneumonia, infection at another site, or appear with no apparent antecedent infection. It may also develop after trauma involving the skull. The mortality and frequency of sequelae are slightly higher with pneumococcal meningitis than with other forms of pyogenic meningitis.

Other Infections

Sinusitis and otitis media are common

Pneumococci are common causes of sinusitis and otitis media (see Chapter 61). The latter frequently occurs in children in association with viral infection. Chronic infection of the mastoid or respiratory sinus sometimes extends to the subarachnoid space to cause meningitis. Pneumococci may also cause endocarditis, arthritis, and peritonitis, usually in association with bacteremia. Patients with ascites caused by diseases such as cirrhosis and nephritis may develop spontaneous pneumococcal peritonitis. Pneumococci do not cause pharyngitis or tonsillitis.

DIAGNOSIS

Sputum quality complicates diagnosis

Gram smears of material from sputum and other sites of pneumococcal infection typically show Gram-positive, lancet-shaped diplococci (see Fig 17–6). Sputum collection may be difficult, however, and specimens contaminated with respiratory flora are useless for diagnosis. Other types of lower respiratory specimens may be needed for diagnosis (see Chapters 15 and 64).

Optochin or bile solubility distinguish from viridans streptococci

S. pneumoniae grows well overnight on blood agar medium and is usually distinguished from viridans streptococci by susceptibility to the synthetic chemical ethylhydrocupreine (Optochin) or by a bile solubility (see Table 17–2). Bacteremia is common in pneumococcal pneumonia and meningitis, and blood cultures are valuable supplements to cultures of local fluids or exudates. Detection of pneumococcal capsular antigen in body fluids is possible but valuable primarily when cultures are negative.

TREATMENT

For decades pneumococci were uniformly susceptible to penicillin at concentrations below 0.1 μg/mL. In the late 1960s, this began to change, and strains with decreased susceptibility to all β-lactams began to emerge. These strains have penicillin minimal inhibitory concentrations (MICs) of 0.12 to 8.0 μg/mL and are associated with treatment failures in cases of pneumonia and meningitis. The resistance is not absolute and can be overcome with increased dosage depending on the MIC. The mechanism involves alterations in the β-lactam target, the transpeptidases that cross-link peptidoglycan in cell wall synthesis. Resistant strains have mutations in one or more of these transpeptidases, which cause decreased affinity for penicillin and other β-lactams. Penicillinase is not produced. Resistance to erythromycin is uncommon but more likely with penicillin-resistant strains.

Altered transpeptidases decrease penicillin susceptibility

Penicillin is still the antimicrobic of choice for susceptible strains but resistance rates now exceed 10% in most locales and may be greater than 30% in some areas. Penicillin-resistant strains may be treated with erythromycin, vancomycin, or quinolones, if susceptible. Despite the β-lactam cross resistance, high doses of third-generation cephalosporins have also been used in situations such as meningitis, where their added spectrum may be an advantage. The therapeutic response to treatment of pneumococcal pneumonia is often (but not always) dramatic. Reduction in fever, respiratory rate, and cough can occur in 12 to 24 hours but may occur gradually over several days. Chest radiography may yield normal results only after several weeks.

High doses of third-generation cephalosporins may overcome resistance

PREVENTION

A vaccine prepared from capsular polysaccharide extracted from the 23 most common serotypes of *S. pneumoniae* is available. This vaccine is presently recommended for patients who are particularly susceptible to pneumococcal infection because of advanced age, underlying disease, or immune status. As with other polysaccharide vaccines it is poorly immunogenic in infants. The newest vaccines follow the success of *Haemophilus influenzae* type b (see Chapter 24) by conjugating the polysaccharide to protein in order to stimulate T-cell dependent responses. This task is greatly complicated by the multiple serotype-specific polysaccharides involved in *S. pneumoniae* disease. A seven-valent conjugate vaccine is now available and recommended for use beginning at 2 months of age. The polysaccharide continues to be recommended beyond the age of 5 years.

23-valent polysaccharide vaccine is available

Protein conjugate vaccine is recommended for children

Viridans and Nonhemolytic Streptococci

The viridans group comprises all α-hemolytic streptococci that remain after the criteria for defining pyogenic streptococci and pneumococci have been applied. Characteristically members of the normal flora of the oral and nasopharyngeal cavities, they have the basic bacteriologic features of streptococci but lack the specific antigens, toxins, and virulence of the other groups. Although the viridans group includes many species (see Table 17–2), they are usually not completely identified in clinical practice because there is little difference among them in medical significance.

"Left over" α-hemolytic species are in respiratory flora

Although their virulence is very low, viridans strains can cause disease when they are protected from host defenses. The prime example is subacute bacterial endocarditis. In this disease, viridans streptococci reach previously damaged heart valves as a result of transient bacteremia associated with manipulations, such as tooth extraction, that disturb their usual habitat. Protected by fibrin and platelets, they multiply on the valve, causing local and systemic disease that is fatal if untreated. Extracellular production of glucans, complex polysaccharide polymers, may enhance their attachment to cardiac valves in a manner similar to the pathogenesis of dental caries by *S. mutans* (see Chapter 62). The clinical course of viridans streptococcal endocarditis is subacute, with slow progression over weeks or months (see Chapter 68). It is effectively treated with penicillin, but uniformly fatal if untreated.

Low virulence species may cause bacterial endocarditis

Glucan production enhances attachment

The disease is particularly associated with valves damaged by recurrent rheumatic fever. The decline in the occurrence of rheumatic heart disease has reduced the incidence of this particular type of endocarditis.

ENTEROCOCCI

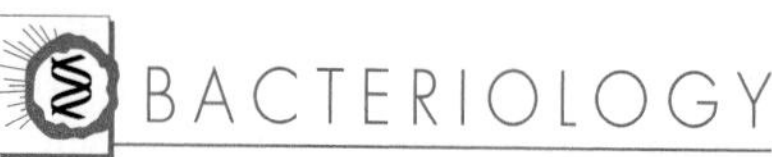

BACTERIOLOGY

Formerly called streptococci, enterococci possess group D antigen

Intestinal inhabitants resist action of bile salts

Until DNA homology studies dictated their separation into the genus *Enterococcus,* the enterococci were classified as streptococci. Indeed, the most common enterococcal species share the bacteriologic characteristics described above for pyogenic streptococci, including presence of the Lancefield group D antigen. The term enterococcus derives from their presence in the intestinal tract and the many biochemical and cultural features that reflect that habitat. These include the ability to grow in the presence of high concentrations of bile salts and sodium chloride. Most enterococci produce nonhemolytic or α-hemolytic colonies that are larger than those of most streptococci. *E. faecalis, E. faecium,* and several other species are recognized based on biochemical and cultural reactions, but enterococci are generally not speciated in the clinical laboratory.

ENTEROCOCCAL DISEASE

CLINICAL CAPSULE

Enterococci cause infection almost exclusively in hospitalized patients with significant compromise of their defenses. The primary sites are the urinary tract and soft tissue sites adjacent to the intestinal flora where enterococcal species are resident. The infections themselves are often low grade and have no unique clinical features.

EPIDEMIOLOGY

Endogenous infection is associated with medical procedures

Enterococci are part of the normal intestinal flora. Although they are capable of producing disease in many settings, the hospital environment is where a substantial increase has occurred in the last two decades. Patients with extensive abdominal surgery, indwelling devices, or who are undergoing procedures such as peritoneal dialysis are at greatest risk. Most infections are acquired from the endogenous flora but spread between patients has been documented. From 10 to 15% of all nosocomial urinary tract, intra-abdominal, and bloodstream infections are due to enterococci.

PATHOGENESIS

Virulence factors are not known

Enterococci are a significant cause of disease in specialized hospital settings, but they are not highly virulent. On their own, they do not produce fulminant disease and in wound and soft tissue infections are usually mixed with other members of the intestinal flora. Some have even doubted their significance when isolated with more virulent members of the Enterobacteriaceae (see Chapter 21) or *Bacteroides fragilis* (see Chapter 19). Although some surface proteins are candidate adhesins, no virulence factors have been discovered.

ENTEROCOCCAL DISEASE: CLINICAL ASPECTS

MANIFESTATIONS

UTIs and soft tissue infections are most common

Enterococci cause opportunistic urinary tract infections (UTIs) and occasionally wound and soft tissue infections, in much the same fashion as members of the Enterobacteriaceae.

Infections are often associated with urinary tract manipulations, malignancies, biliary tract disease, and gastrointestinal disorders. Vascular or peritoneal catheters are often points of entry. Respiratory tract infections are rare. There is sometimes an associated bacteremia, which can result in the development of endocarditis on previously damaged cardiac valves.

TREATMENT

The outstanding feature of the enterococci is their high and increasing levels of resistance to antimicrobial agents. Inherently relatively resistant to β-lactams and aminoglycosides, enterococci also have particularly efficient means of acquiring plasmid and transposon resistance genes from themselves and other species. All enterococci require 4 to 16 μg/mL of penicillin for inhibition due to decreased affinity of their penicillin-binding proteins for all β-lactams. Higher levels of resistance have been increasing, including the emergence of β-lactamase-producing strains, particularly in *E. faecalis*. The β-lactamase genes are identical to those in *Staphylococcus aureus*. Fortunately β-lactamase–producing strains have not yet become widely disseminated. Ampicillin remains the most consistently active agent against enterococci.

Inherent penicillin resistance is enhanced with β-lactamase emergence

Enterococci share with streptococci a relative resistance to aminoglycosides based on failure of the antimicrobic to be actively transported into the cell. Despite this, many strains of enterococci are inhibited and rapidly killed by combinations of low concentrations of penicillin and aminoglycosides. Under these conditions, the action of penicillin on the cell wall allows the aminoglycoside to enter the cell and act at its ribosomal site. Some strains show high level resistance to aminoglycosides based on mutations at the ribosomal binding site or the presence of aminoglycoside-inactivating enzymes. These strains do not demonstrate synergistic effects with penicillin.

Synergy between penicillin and aminoglycosides is based on access to ribosomes

Recently, resistance to vancomycin, the antibiotic most used for penicillin-resistant strains has emerged. Vancomycin resistance is due to a subtle change in peptidoglycan precursors, which are generated by ligases that modify the terminal amino acids of cross-linking acid side chains at the point at which β-lactams bind. The modifications decrease the binding affinity for penicillins 1000-fold without a detectable loss in peptidoglycan strength. Although hospitals vary, the average rate of resistance in enterococci isolated from intensive care units is around 20%. Enterococci are consistently resistant to sulfonamides and often resistant to tetracyclines, erythromycin, and cephalosporins.

Vancomycin resistance is emerging threat

Ligases modify peptidoglycan side chains

Penicillin or ampicillin remain the agents of choice for most UTIs and minor soft tissue infections. More severe infections, particularly endocarditis, are usually treated with combinations of a penicillin and aminoglycoside. If the strain fails to demonstrate penicillin–aminoglycoside synergism and/or is vancomycin resistant, some other combination guided by susceptibility testing must be selected.

Ampicillin or combinations of antimicrobics are used

ADDITIONAL READING

Cunningham MW. Pathogenesis of group A streptococcal infections. *Clin Microbiol Rev* 2000;13:470–511. This scholarly review pays particular attention to pyrogenic exotoxins and newly discovered virulence factors.

Jedrzejas MJ. Pneumococcal virulence factors: structure and function. *Microbiol Mol Biol Rev* 2001;65:187–207. This review makes it clear that there is much more to the pneumococcus than its capsule.

Lancefield RC: A serological differentiation of human and other groups of hemolytic streptococci. *J Exp Med* 1933;57:571–595. This classic study changed streptococcal classification.

Schuchat A. Epidemiology of group B streptococcal disease in the United States: Shifting paradigms. *Clin Microbiol Rev* 1998;11:497–513. In addition to a very complete coverage of GBS disease, this review describes and evaluates the various strategies for prevention.

Schuchat A. Group B streptococcal disease: From trials and tribulations to triumph and trepidation. *Clin Infect Dis* 2001;33:751–756. This published lecture by the author of the above review gives an update on the prevention of GBS disease.

Stollerman GH. Rheumatic fever in the 21st century. *Clin Infect Dis* 2001;33:806–814. This brief review reads like a personal conversation with this seasoned veteran of the field.

CHAPTER 18

Corynebacterium, Listeria, and *Bacillus*

KENNETH J. RYAN

This chapter includes a variety of highly pathogenic Gram-positive rods that are not currently common causes of human disease. Their medical importance lies in the lessons learned when they were more common, and the continued threat their existence poses. *Corynebacterium diphtheriae,* the cause of diphtheria, is a prototype for toxigenic disease. *Listeria monocytogenes* is a sporadic cause of meningitis and other infections in the fetus, newborn, and immunocompromised host. Occurrences in 2001 have served as a painful reminder that *Bacillus anthracis,* the cause of anthrax, is still the agent with the most potential for use in bioterrorism. The characteristics of these bacilli are presented in Table 18–1.

CORYNEBACTERIA

Corynebacteria (from the Greek koryne, club) are small and pleomorphic. The genus *Corynebacterium* includes many species of aerobic and facultative Gram-positive rods. The cells tend to have clubbed ends, and often remain attached after division, forming "Chinese letter" or palisade arrangements. Spores are not formed. Growth is generally best under aerobic conditions on media enriched with blood or other animal products, but many strains will grow anaerobically. Colonies on blood agar are typically small (1 to 2 mm), and most are nonhemolytic. Catalase is produced, and many strains form acid (usually lactic acid) through carbohydrate fermentation.

Pleomorphic club-shaped rods grow on blood agar

Corynebacterium diphtheriae

C. diphtheriae produces a powerful exotoxin that is responsible for diphtheria. Other corynebacteria are nonpathogenic commensal inhabitants of the pharynx, nasopharynx, distal urethra, and skin; they are collectively referred to as "diphtheroids." The species that have disease associations are included in Table 18–2.

C. diphtheriae produces exotoxin

Other corynebacteria are called diphtheroids

TABLE 18–1

Features of Aerobic Gram-Positive Bacilli

Organism	Capsule	Endospores	Motility	Toxins	Source	Disease
Corynebacterium diphtheriae	–	–	–	DT	Human cases, carriers	Diphtheria
Listeria monocytogenes	–	–	+	LLO	Food, animals	Meningitis, bacteremia
Bacillus						
B. anthracis	+	+	–	Exotoxin[a]	Imported animal products	Anthrax
B. cereus	–	+	+	Enterotoxin, pyogenic toxin	Ubiquitous	Food poisoning, opportunistic infection
Other species	–	+	+		Ubiquitous	

Abbreviations: DT, diphtheria toxin; LLO, listerolysin O.

[a] Exotoxin contains three components: lethal factor, protective antigen, and edema factor.

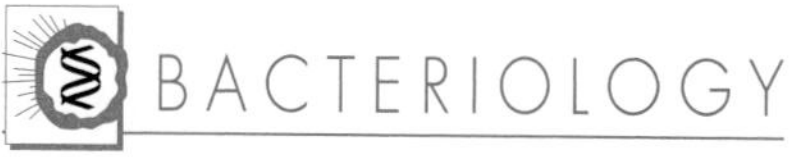

BACTERIOLOGY

C. diphtheriae can produce DT coded by lysogenic phage

C. diphtheriae are differentiated from other corynebacteria by the appearance of colonies on the selective media used for its isolation and a variety of biochemical reactions. Strains of *C. diphtheriae* may or may not produce **diphtheria toxin (DT)**. Those that do have the structural gene for DT acquired from the genome of a specific bacteriophage. Only strains that are lysogenic for these phages produce toxin.

TABLE 18–2

Other Aerobic and Facultative Gram-Positive Bacilli

Organism	Features	Epidemiology	Disease
Corynebacterium ulcerans	Closely related to *C. diphtheriae,* including ability to produce small amounts of DT	Similar to diphtheria, also infects animals	Pharyngitis
Corynebacterium jeikeium	Multiresistant, often susceptible only to vancomycin	Acquired from skin colonization	Bacteremia, IV catheter colonization
Erysipelothrix rhusiopathiae	Resembles corynebacteria and *Listeria*	Traumatic inoculation from animal and decaying organic matter	Erysipeloid, painful, slow-spreading, erythematous swelling of skin. Occupational disease of fishermen, butchers, and veterinarians
Lactobacillus spp.	Long, slender rods with squared ends, often chain end to end	Normal oral, gastrointestinal, and vaginal flora	No human infections *L. acidophilus* plays role in pathogenesis of dental caries
Propionibacterium	Resemble corynebacteria, anaerobes, or microaerophiles	Normal skin flora	Rare cause of bacterial endocarditis

Abbreviations: DT, diphtheria toxin; IV, intravenous.

DT is an A-B toxin that acts in the cytoplasm to inhibit protein synthesis irreversibly in a wide variety of eukaryotic cells (Fig 18–1). After binding mediated by the B subunit, both the A and B subunits enter the cell in a endocytotic vacuole. In the low pH of the vacuole, the toxin unfolds exposing sites that facilitate translocation of the A subunit from the phagosome to the cytosol. Separation is required for full activity of the A subunit on its target protein elongation factor 2 (EF-2), which transfers polypeptidyl-transfer RNA from acceptor to donor sites on the ribosome of the host cell. The specific action of the A subunit is to catalyze the transfer of the adenine ribose phosphate portion of nicotinamide adenine dinucleotide (NAD) to EF-2, an enzymatic reaction called **ADP-ribosylation.** This inactivates EF-2 and shuts off protein synthesis. The ADP-ribosylation leaves the toxin itself free to catalyze another reaction, making it possible for a single DT molecule to inhibit protein synthesis in a cell within a few hours. ADP-ribosylation is now known to be the enzymatic mechanism of action for a number of toxins including those that act on EF-2 (DT, *Pseudomonas aeruginosa* exotoxin A) and those with other target proteins (cholera toxin, *Escherichia coli* LT, pertussis toxin). *C. diphtheriae* itself is unaffected because it uses a protein other than EF-2 in protein synthesis.

A subunit enters the cytosol from a vacuole

EF-2 is inactivated by ADP-ribosylation

Transfer of tRNA and protein synthesis are stopped

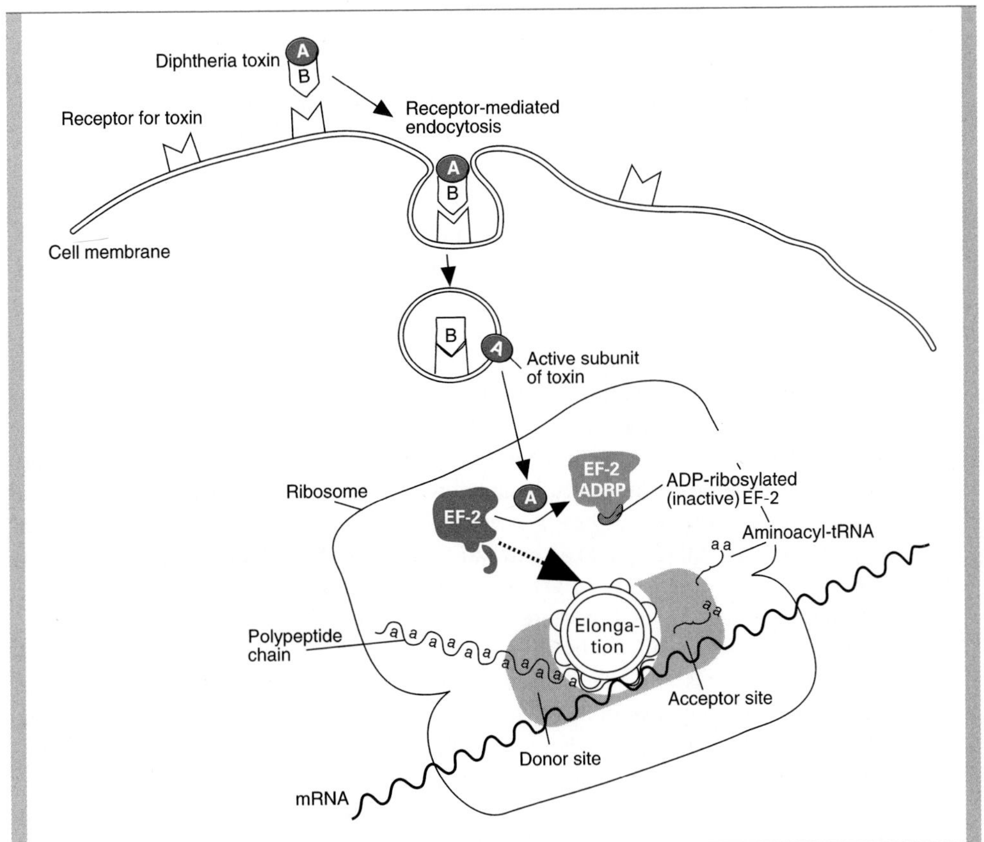

FIGURE 18–1
Action of diphtheria toxin. The toxin-binding (B) portion attaches to the cell membrane, and the complete molecule enters the cell. In the cell, the A subunit dissociates and catalyzes a reaction that ADP-ribosylates and thus inactivates elongation factor 2 (EF-2). This factor is essential for ribosomal reactions at the acceptor and donor sites, which transfer triplet code from messenger RNA (mRNA) to amino acid sequences via transfer RNA (tRNA). Inactivation of EF-2 stops building of the polypeptide chain.

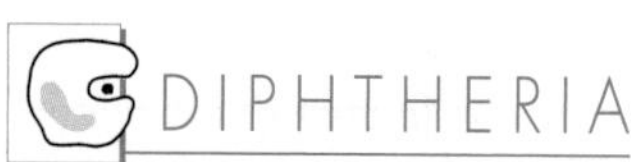

DIPHTHERIA

CLINICAL CAPSULE

Diphtheria is a disease caused by the local and systemic effects of diphtheria toxin, a potent inhibitor of protein synthesis. The local disease is a severe pharyngitis typically accompanied by a plaquelike pseudomembrane in the throat and trachea. The life-threatening aspects of diphtheria are due to the absorption of the toxin across the pharyngeal mucosa and its circulation in the bloodstream. Multiple organs are affected, but the most important is the heart, where the toxin produces an acute myocarditis.

EPIDEMIOLOGY

Transmitted by respiratory droplets

Most cases are in unimmunized transients

C. diphtheriae is transmitted by droplet spread, by direct contact with cutaneous infections, and, to a lesser extent, by fomites. Some subjects become convalescent pharyngeal or nasal carriers and continue to harbor the organism for weeks to months or even for a lifetime. Diphtheria is rare where immunization is widely used. In the United States, for example, fewer than 10 cases are now reported each year. These usually occur as small outbreaks in populations that have not received adequate immunization, such as migrant workers, transients, and those who refuse immunization on religious grounds. It has been more than 20 years since any outbreak exceeded 50 cases.

Outbreaks occur when immunization rates decrease

Diphtheria still occurs in developing countries and in those places where public health infrastructure has been disrupted. For example, in the former Soviet Union, where the annual number of diphtheria cases had been below 200, over 47,000 cases and 1700 deaths occurred between 1990 and 1995. This outbreak followed the introduction of diphtheria into a population where the immunization rate for children was not sufficiently high, adults were not given boosters, and the efforts at mass immunization early in the epidemic were inadequate.

PATHOGENESIS

A subunit inhibits protein synthesis

B-subunit binding determines cell susceptibility

C. diphtheriae has little invasive capacity, and diphtheria is due to the local and systemic effects of DT, a protein exotoxin with potent cytotoxic features. It inhibits protein synthesis in cell-free extracts of virtually all eukaryotic cells, from protozoa and yeasts to higher plants and humans. Its toxicity for intact cells varies among mammals and organs, primarily as a result of differences in toxin binding and uptake. In humans the B subunit binds to one of a common family of eukaryotic receptors that regulate cell growth and differentiation, thus exploiting a normal cell function.

Local effects produce pseudomembrane

Absorption of DT leads to myocarditis

The production of DT has both local and systemic effects. Locally, its action on epithelial cells leads to necrosis and inflammation, forming a pseudomembrane composed of a coagulum of fibrin, leukocytes, and cellular debris. The extent of the pseudomembrane varies from a local plaque to an extensive covering of much of the tracheobronchial tree. Absorption and circulation of DT allows binding throughout the body. Myocardial cells are most affected; eventually, acute myocarditis develops.

Iron concentration modulates toxin and other correlates of virulence

Nontoxigenic strains produce mild disease

The DT **tox gene** is regulated by a repressor protein (DtxR) in response to iron limitation. Toxin biosynthesis is greatest when the bacteria are grown at low iron concentrations. Iron seems to play a central role in the expression of virulence; the repressor also regulates a corynebacterial siderophore system and a number of other proteins. Nontoxigenic strains of *C. diphtheriae* can produce pharyngitis, but not the toxic manifestations of diphtheria. They can be converted to toxigenicity by lysogenization in vitro with phage, and this process can probably occur in vivo.

IMMUNITY

Antibodies neutralize toxin

Toxoid is formalin inactivated DT

Diphtheria toxin is antigenic, stimulating the production of protective antitoxin antibodies during natural infection. Formalin treatment of toxin produces **toxoid,** which retains the antigenicity but not the toxicity of native toxin and is used in immunization against the disease. It is clear that this process functionally inactivates fragment B. Whether it also inactivates fragment A or prevents its ability to dissociate from fragment B is not known. Molecular studies of the A subunit structure and action suggest that another approach to immunization may be through genetic engineering. For example, substitution of a single amino acid located in the NAD-binding site of the A subunit of DT can completely detoxify but retain the immunogenic specificity of the toxin. The membrane-translocation properties of the B subunit have also been used to transport other proteins into the cytosol by linking them to DT.

DIPHTHERIA: CLINICAL ASPECTS

MANIFESTATIONS

After an incubation period of 2 to 4 days, diphtheria usually presents as pharyngitis or tonsillitis. Typically, malaise, sore throat, and fever occur, and a patch of exudate or membrane develops on the tonsils, uvula, soft palate, or pharyngeal wall. The gray-white pseudomembrane adheres to the mucous membrane, and may extend from the oropharyngeal area down to the larynx and into the trachea. Associated cervical adenitis is common, and in severe cases cervical adenitis and edema produce a "bullneck" appearance. In uncomplicated cases, the infection gradually resolves, and the membrane is coughed up after 5 to 10 days.

Severe pharyngitis may have exudate or membrane

The complications and lethal effects of diphtheria are caused by respiratory obstruction or by the systemic effect of DT absorbed at the site of infection. Mechanical obstruction of the airway produced by the pseudomembrane, edema, and hemorrhage can be sudden and complete and can lead to suffocation, particularly if large sections of the membrane separate from the tracheal or laryngeal epithelial surface. The DT absorbed into the circulation causes injury to various organs, most seriously the heart. Diphtheritic myocarditis appears during the second or third week in severe cases of respiratory diphtheria. It is manifested by cardiac enlargement and weakness, arrhythmia, and congestive heart failure with dyspnea. Nervous system involvement appears later in the course of disease, most often involving paralysis of the soft palate, oculomotor (eye) muscles, or select muscle groups. The paralysis is reversible and is generally not serious unless the diaphragm is involved. The disease resolves with the formation of antitoxin antibody.

Pseudomembrane can block the airway

DT myocarditis may lead to congestive heart failure

C. diphtheriae may produce nonrespiratory infections, particularly of the skin. The characteristic lesion, which ranges from a simple pustule to a chronic, nonhealing ulcer, is most common in tropical and hot, arid regions. Cardiac and neurologic complications from these infections are infrequent, suggesting that the efficiency of toxin production or absorption is low compared to that in respiratory infections.

Cutaneous diphtheria produces ulcerative lesion

DIAGNOSIS

The initial diagnosis of diphtheria is entirely clinical. There are presently no rapid laboratory tests of sufficient value to influence the decision regarding antitoxin administration. Direct smears of infected areas of the throat are not reliable diagnostic tools. Definitive diagnosis is accomplished by isolating and identifying *C. diphtheriae* from the infected site and demonstrating its toxigenicity. Isolation is usually achieved with a selective medium containing potassium tellurite (eg, Tinsdale medium).

Primary diagnosis is clinical

Culture requires special medium

It should be recognized that while the diagnosis of diphtheria could be once be made and confirmed with great confidence, it is now more difficult because experience with the disease is rare. Most physicians have never seen a case of diphtheria, and most laboratories have never isolated the organism and do not even stock the required medium. Because routine throat culture procedures will not detect *C. diphtheriae,* the physician must advise the laboratory of the suspicion of diphtheria in advance. Generally, 2 days are required to exclude *C. diphtheriae* (ie, no colonies isolated on Tinsdale agar); however, more time is needed to complete identification and toxigenicity testing of a positive culture.

Laboratory must be notified of suspicion in advance

TREATMENT

Treatment of diphtheria is directed at neutralization of the toxin with concurrent elimination of the organism. The former is most critical and is accomplished by promptly administering a

Antitoxin therapy aimed at neutralizing free toxin

Erythromycin most effective antimicrobic therapy

diphtheria antitoxin that neutralizes free toxin, but it will have no effect on toxin already fixed to cells. *C. diphtheriae* is susceptible to a variety of antimicrobics, including penicillins, cephalosporins, erythromycin, and tetracycline. Of these, erythromycin has been the most effective. The complications of diphtheria are managed primarily by supportive measures.

PREVENTION

The mainstay of diphtheria prevention is immunization. The vaccine is highly effective. Three to four doses of diphtheria toxoid produce immunity by stimulating antitoxin production. The initial series is begun in the first year of life (see Chapter 12). Booster immunizations at 10-year intervals maintain immunity. Fully immunized individuals may become infected with *C. diphtheriae*, because the antibodies are directed only against the toxin, but the disease is mild. Serious infection and death occur only in unimmunized or incompletely immunized individuals. Immunization with DT toxoid prevents serious toxin-medicated disease.

LISTERIA MONOCYTOGENES

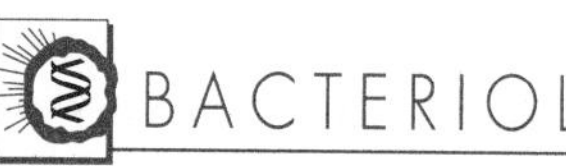

BACTERIOLOGY

Rods resemble corynebacteria

Colonies are β hemolytic

Listeria monocytogenes is a Gram-positive rod with some bacteriologic features that resemble those of both corynebacteria and streptococci. In stained smears of clinical and laboratory material, the organisms resemble diphtheroids. *Listeria* are not difficult to grow in culture, producing small, β-hemolytic colonies on blood agar. This species is able to grow slowly in the cold even at temperatures as low as 1°C. *Listeria* species are catalase positive, which distinguishes them from streptococci, and produce a characteristic tumbling motility in fluid media at 25°C that distinguishes them from corynebacteria.

Pathogenic serotypes have unique teichoic acid

Eleven *L. monocytogenes* serotypes are recognized based on flagellar and somatic surface antigens, but the majority of human cases are limited to only three serotypes (1/2a, 1/2b, 4b). These serotypes differ from other *Listeria* in elements of the chemical teichoic acid composition, a major component of their cell wall. The teichoic acid of serotype 4b, which accounts for almost all food-borne listeriosis outbreaks, is distinctive in that there are both galactose and glucose substituents in its *N*-acetylglucosamine.

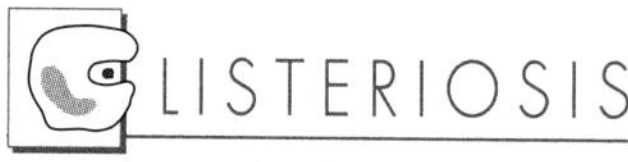

LISTERIOSIS

CLINICAL CAPSULE

Listeriosis is often an insidious infection in humans. Infection of the fetus or newborn may result in stillbirth or a fulminant neonatal sepsis. In most adults, there are usually only general manifestations, such as fever and malaise, associated with bacteremia.

EPIDEMIOLOGY

Reservoir is intestine of animals and humans

Food-borne transmission is from animal products

Members of *Listeria* are widespread among animals in nature, including those associated with our food supply (eg, fowl, ungulates). The human reservoir appears to be intestinal colonization, which various studies have shown to range from 2 to 12%. The importance of food-borne transmission of listeriosis was not recognized until the early 1980s. A widely publicized 1985 California outbreak involved consumption of Mexican-style soft cheese and included 86 cases and 29 deaths. Most of the cases were among mother–infant pairs. Dairy product outbreaks have been traced to post-pasteurization contamination or deviation from recommended time and temperature guidelines. An important feature of some epidemics has been the ability of *L. monocytogenes* to grow at refrigerator temperatures, allowing scant numbers to reach an infectious dose during storage. Heightened awareness has implicated many other foodstuffs, particularly those prepared from animal products in a ready-to-eat form such as sausages and delicatessen poultry items.

Cold growth enhances infectivity

L. monocytogenes may also be transmitted transplacentally to the fetus, presumably following hematogenous dissemination in the mother. It may also be transmitted to newborns in the birth canal in a manner similar to group B streptococci. Listeriosis is still not a reportable disease in the United States, but active surveillance studies indicate that it may account for more than 1000 cases and 200 deaths each year. Most cases occur at the extremes of life (eg, in infants less than 1 month of age or adults over 60 years of age).

Transplacental and birth canal transmission can occur

PATHOGENESIS

L. monocytogenes animal models have long been used for the study of cell-mediated immunity because of the ability of the organism to grow in nonimmune macrophages. An activated macrophage is needed to clear the infection, and in fact the concept of the activated macrophage that appears throughout this book owes much to the study of experimental *Listeria* infection. More recently, *Listeria* has generated great interest because of the mechanisms it uses to invade and survive in macrophages and efficiently spread among epithelial cells.

Grows in nonimmune macrophages

The first step in this process takes place when *L. monocytogenes* attaches to and is internalized into nonprofessional and professional phagocytes. These include enterocytes, fibroblasts, dendritic cells, hepatocytes, endothelial cells, M cells, and macrophages. Under the influence of a surface protein called **internalin,** *Listeria* causes a local reorganization of the cytoskeleton of the cell and stimulates its own entry in a membrane-bound vacuole. The invading bacteria rapidly escape into the host cell cytosol by elaborating **listeriolysin O** (LLO), which acts in a manner similar to streptolysin O and other pore-forming cytotoxins.

Surface internalin starts epithelial cell invasion

Enters cell in vacuole

LLO aids escape to cytosol

Once in the cytosol, *L. monocytogenes* continues to move through the cell by controlling the metabolism of the cell's actin filaments. This process is stimulated by other surface proteins (ActA, gelsolin), which control the actin polymerization so that actin monomers are sequentially concentrated directly behind the bacterium. The net effect is the appearance of a bacterial "tail" that is connected to the long actin filaments. The addition of new actin units to the tail propels the organisms through the cytosol like a comet through the evening sky (Fig 18–2). The motile *Listeria* eventually reach the edge of the cell where, instead of stopping, they protrude into the adjacent cell taking the original cell membrane along with them. When these pinch off, the organisms are surrounded by a

Actin polymerization forms motile comet tails

Protrudes into adjacent cell

LLO releases bacteria again

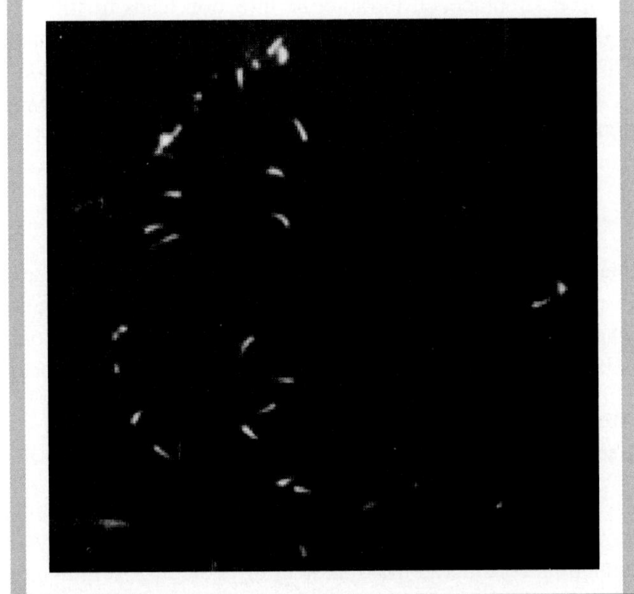

FIGURE 18–2
Intracellular movement of *Listeria monocytogenes. L. monocytogenes* cells are shown within infected cells in culture. The immunofluorescent stain used an antibody that binds to actin, demonstrating the comet-like actin "tails," which trail the bacteria as they move through the cell. (*From Niebuhr K, Chakraborty T, Rohde M, et al:* Infect Immun *1993;61:2793–2802, Figure 4a, with permission.*)

double set of host cell membranes that are dissolved by LLO and phospholipases, releasing the organisms to start the cycle again.

Cell-to-cell spread avoids the immune system

Multiple virulence factors are regulated together

This complex strategy allows *L. monocytogenes* to survive in macrophages by escaping the phagosome, and then to spread from epithelial cell to epithelial cell without exposure to the immune system. How does *Listeria* keeps its LLO from destroying the host cell membrane from the inside as the pore-forming toxins of other bacteria do from the outside? It appears that *L. monocytogenes* may be able to not only regulate the timely production of LLO but also to trigger its degradation by host cell proteolytic enzymes after it has left the endosome vacuole. LLO and several other genes, including those involved in actin rearrangement, are all part of a virulence regulon. The result is a surgically precise deployment of virulence factors.

IMMUNITY

Listeria-specific T-cell activation protects

Immunity to *Listeria* infection owes little to humoral and much to cell-mediated mechanisms. The generation of antigen-specific CD4+ and CD8+ T-cell subsets is required for the resolution of infection and the establishment of long-lived protection. Neutrophils play a role in early stages by lysing *Listeria* infected cells, but it is cytokine-activation that reverses the intracellular growth in macrophages. The importance of cellular immunity is emphasized by the increased frequency of listeriosis in those with its compromise due to disease such as acquired immunodeficiency syndrome (AIDS), immunosuppressive therapy, age, or pregnancy.

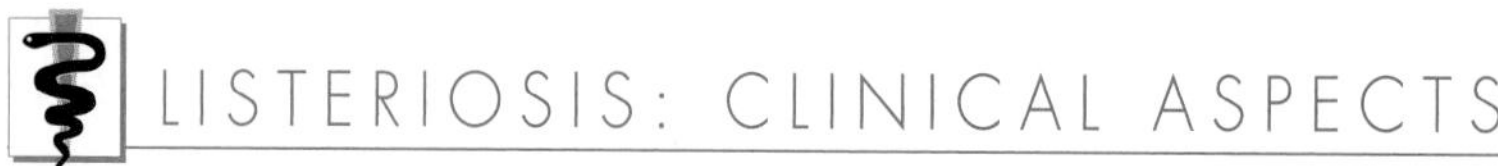

MANIFESTATIONS

Bacteremia is usually occult

Meningitis and encephalitis are produced

Listeriosis usually does not present clinically until there is disseminated infection. In foodborne outbreaks, sometimes gastrointestinal manifestations of primary infection such as nausea, abdominal pain, diarrhea, and fever occur. Disseminated infection in adults is usually occult, involving fever, malaise, and constitutional symptoms without an obvious focus. *L. monocytogenes* has a tropism for the central nervous system (CNS), including the brain parenchyma (encephalitis) and brainstem, but the meningitis it causes is not distinct from that associated with other leading bacterial pathogens (*Streptococcus pneumoniae, Neisseria meningitidis*).

Puerperal infection leads to stillbirth and dissemination

Incidence in AIDS is greatly increased

Neonatal and puerperal infections appear in settings similar to those of infections with group B streptococci. Intrauterine infection leads to stillbirth or a disseminated infection at or near birth. If the pathogen is acquired in the birth canal, the onset of disease is later. The risk of disease is increased in elderly and immunocompromised individuals as well as women in late pregnancy. The number of cases in AIDS patients has been estimated at 300 times the general population.

DIAGNOSIS

Blood and CSF culture reveals Gram-positive rods

Diagnosis of listeriosis is by culture of blood, cerebrospinal fluid (CSF), or focal lesions. In meningitis, CSF Gram stains are usually positive. The first indication that *Listeria* is involved is often the discovery that the β-hemolytic colonies subcultured from a blood culture bottle are Gram-positive rods rather than streptococci.

TREATMENT AND PREVENTION

Penicillins and TMP-SMX are effective

L. monocytogenes is susceptible to penicillin G, ampicillin, and trimethoprim/sulfamethoxazole, all of which have been used effectively. Ampicillin combined with gentamicin is considered the treatment of choice for fulminant cases. Intense surveillance to prevent the sale of *Listeria*-contaminated ready-to-eat meat products has led to a marked decrease in the incidence of new infections. There is no vaccine.

Bacillus

The genus *Bacillus* includes many species of aerobic or facultative, spore-forming, Gram-positive rods. With the exception of one species, *B. anthracis,* they are low-virulence saprophytes widespread in air, soil, water, dust, and animal products. *B. anthracis* causes the zoonosis anthrax, a disease of animals that is occasionally transmitted to humans.

The genus is made up of rod-shaped organisms that can vary from coccobacillary to rather long-chained filaments. Motile strains have peritrichous flagella. Formation of round or oval spores, which may be central, subterminal, or terminal depending on the species, is characteristic of the genus. *Bacillus* species are Gram positive; however, positivity is often lost, depending on the species and the age of the culture.

Gram-positive spore-forming rods

With *Bacillus,* growth is obtained with ordinary media incubated in air and is reduced or absent under anaerobic conditions. The bacteria are catalase positive and metabolically active. The spores survive boiling for varying periods and are sufficiently resistant to heat that those of one species are used as a biologic indicator of autoclave efficiency. Spores of *B. anthracis* survive in soil for decades.

Aerobic conditions preferred for growth

Heat-resistant spores survive boiling

Bacillus anthracis

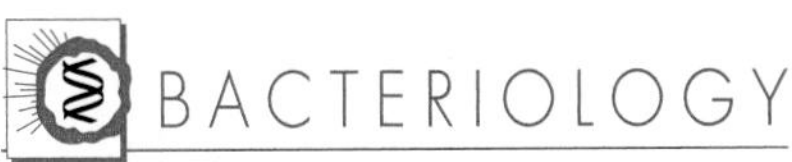

BACTERIOLOGY

B. anthracis has a tendency to form very long chains of rods and in culture is nonmotile and nonhemolytic; colonies are characterized by a rough, uneven surface with multiple curled extensions at the edge resembling a "Medusa head." *B. anthracis* has a D-glutamic acid polypeptide capsule of a single antigenic type that has antiphagocytic properties. The organism is also is a potent producer of one or more exotoxins, which although they have been given multiple names (lethal factor, edema factor, protective antigen), represent separate activities of a protein complex. In various combinations and configurations these proteins may exhibit binding, cytolytic, or enzymatic activity. One such combination exhibits adenylate cyclase activity similar to that seen in *Bordetella pertussis* (see Chapter 24).

Chained rods and "Medusa head" colonies are typical

Polypeptide capsule is antiphagocytic

Exotoxin complex has multiple actions

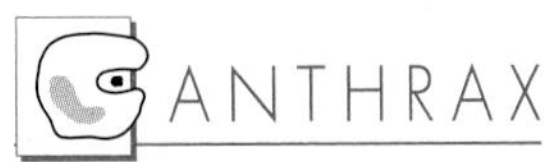

ANTHRAX

CLINICAL CAPSULE

Human anthrax is typically an ulcerative sore on an exposed part of the body. Constitutional symptoms are minimal, and the ulcer usually resolves without complications. If anthrax spores are inhaled, a fulminant pneumonia may lead to respiratory failure and death.

The isolation of *B. anthracis,* the proof of its relationship to anthrax infection, and the demonstration of immunity to the disease are among the most important events in the history of science and medicine. Robert Koch rose to fame in 1877 by growing the organism in artificial culture using pure culture techniques. He defined the stringent criteria needed

Pasteur produced animal vaccine with attenuated anthrax strain

to prove that the organism caused anthrax (Koch's postulates), then met them experimentally. Louis Pasteur made a convincing field demonstration at Pouilly-le-Fort to show that vaccination of sheep, goats, and cows with an attenuated strain of *B. anthracis* prevented anthrax. He was cheered and carried on the shoulders of the grateful farmers of the district, an experience now, unhappily, largely restricted to winning football coaches.

EPIDEMIOLOGY

Infection is through injection of spores derived from herbivores into the skin

Contaminated materials are imported from countries with animal anthrax

Anthrax is primarily a disease of herbivores such as horses, sheep, and cattle who acquire it from spores of *B. anthracis* contaminating their pastures. Humans become infected through contact with these animals or their products in a way that allows the spores to be inoculated through the skin, ingested, or inhaled. In the 1920s, more than 100 cases occurred annually in the United States among farmers, veterinarians, and meat handlers, but the control of animal anthrax in developed countries has made human cases rare. A few endemic foci persist in North America and have been the source of naturally acquired disease. Another source is animal products such as wool, hides, or bone meal fertilizer that have been imported from a country where animal anthrax is endemic.

Use for biological warfare is a continuing threat

Aerosols could spread pulmonary anthrax widely

Weapons-grade spores are specially treated

The real threat associated with anthrax comes from its continuing appeal to those bent on using it as an agent of biological warfare or terrorism. The long life, stability, and low mass of the dried spores make the prospect of someone producing a "cloud of death" leading to massive pulmonary anthrax a chilling reality. A 1979 episode resulting in more than 50 anthrax deaths in the former Soviet Union is now attributed to an accidental explosion at a biological warfare research facility that involved more than 20 pounds of anthrax spores. United Nations inspection teams in the Middle East recently uncovered facilities for the production of massive amounts of spores together with plans to create and spread infectious aerosols using missile warheads. The inhalation anthrax among postal workers following the September 11, 2001 terrorist attacks appears to have been due to the mailing of envelopes containing "weapons-grade" anthrax spores stolen from a biologic warfare research facility. Such spores had been treated to enhance their aerosolization and dissemination.

PATHOGENESIS

Antiphagocytic effect of D-glutamic acid capsule is required for virulence

Exotoxins have multiple activities

When spores of *B. anthracis* reach the rich environment of human tissues, they germinate and multiply in the vegetative state. The antiphagocytic properties of the capsule aid in survival, eventually allowing production of large enough amounts of the exotoxins to cause disease. The tripartite nature of the anthrax exotoxin complex must play an important role but the timing and relative importance of the components are not known. The adenylate cyclase activity is believed to correlate with the striking edema seen at infected sites.

IMMUNITY

Immune mechanisms are unknown

The specific mechanisms of immunity against *B. anthracis* are not known. Experimental evidence favors antibody directed against the toxin complex, but the relative role of the components of the toxin is not clear. The capsular glutamic acid is immunogenic but antibody against it is not protective.

ANTHRAX: CLINICAL ASPECTS

Initial papule evolves to malignant pustule

Cutaneous anthrax usually begins 2 to 5 days after inoculation of spores into an exposed part of the body, typically the forearm or hand. The initial lesion is an erythematous papule, which may be mistaken for an insect bite. This papule usually progresses through vesicular and ulcerative stages in 7 to 10 days to form a black eschar (scab) surrounded by edema. This lesion complex is known as the "malignant pustule," although it is neither malignant nor a pustule. Associated systemic symptoms are usually mild, and the lesion typically heals very slowly after the eschar separates. Less commonly, the disease progresses with massive local edema, toxemia, and bacteremia; it has a fatal outcome if untreated.

Pulmonary anthrax is contracted by inhalation of spores. Historically, this occurred when contaminated hides, hair, wool, and the like are handled in a confined space (woolsorter's disease) or following laboratory accidents. Today it is the form we would expect from the dissemination of a spore aerosol in biologic warfare. In the pulmonary syndrome, 1 to 5 days of nonspecific malaise, mild fever, and nonproductive cough lead to progressive respiratory distress and cyanosis. Massive spread to the bloodstream and CNS follow rapidly. Mediastinal edema was a prominent finding in the postal workers. If untreated, progression to a fatal outcome is usually very rapid once bacteremia has developed.

Pulmonary anthrax is acquired by inhaling spores

Fever and cough progress to cyanosis and death

DIAGNOSIS

Culture of skin lesions, sputum, blood, and CSF are the primary means of anthrax diagnosis. Given some suspicion on epidemiologic grounds, Gram stains of sputum or other biologic fluids showing large numbers of Gram-positive bacilli can indicate the diagnosis. In September of 2001, diagnosis of the first case in Florida was speeded by an infectious disease specialist who knew such rods were extremely rare in the spinal fluid. Such bacilli are also unusual in sputum.

B. anthracis and other *Bacillus* species are not difficult to grow. In fact, clinical laboratories frequently isolate the nonanthrax species as environmental contaminants. The saprophytic species are usually β-hemolytic and motile; these features can be used to exclude *B. anthracis.* Blood cultures are positive in most cases of pulmonary anthrax.

Smears with large Gram-positive rods are suggestive

Hemolysis and motility exclude *B. anthracis*

Sputum and blood cultures are positive in pneumonia

TREATMENT

Antimicrobial treatment has little effect on the course of cutaneous anthrax but does protect against dissemination. Almost all strains of *B. anthracis* are susceptible to penicillin, which remains the treatment of choice for all forms of anthrax. Doxycycline or ciprofloxacin are alternatives and are also recommended for chemoprophylaxis in the case of known or suspected exposure.

Penicillin is the recommended treatment

Ciprofloxacin or doxycycline is used for prophylaxis

PREVENTION

The most important preventive measures are those that eradicate animal anthrax and limit imports from endemic areas. Vaccines are also useful. Pasteur's vaccine used a live strain attenuated by repeated subculture that resulted in the loss of a plasmid encoding toxin production. A similar live vaccine is still effective for animals, but inactivated human vaccines have a less certain efficacy. The vaccine used by the US military is prepared from filtrates of a nonencapsulated *B. anthracis* strain that produces the protective antigen component of the toxin complex. Its acceptance is complicated by fears that the architects of biological warfare may have crafted strains for which this vaccine is not protective. Proof of the efficacy of the vaccine in humans is neither practical nor ethical.

Eradication of animal anthrax is most important

Live and inactivated vaccines are available but controversial

Other Bacillus Species

Bacillus spores are widespread in the environment, and isolation of one of the more than 20 *Bacillus* species other than *B. anthracis* from clinical material usually represents contamination of the specimen. Occasionally *B. cereus, B. subtilis,* and some other species produce genuine infections, including infections of the eye, soft tissues, and lung. Infection is usually associated with immunosuppression, trauma, an indwelling catheter, or contamination of complex equipment such as an artificial kidney. The relative resistance of *Bacillus* spores to disinfectants aids their survival in medical devices that cannot be heat sterilized.

Spores enhance survival in medical devices

B. cereus produces pyogenic toxin and enterotoxin

B. cereus deserves special mention. This species is most likely to cause opportunistic infection, which suggests a virulence intermediate between that of *B. anthracis* and the other species. A strain isolated from an abscess has been shown to produce a destructive pyogenic toxin. *B. cereus* can also cause food poisoning by means of enterotoxins. One enterotoxin acts by stimulating adenyl cyclase production and fluid excretion in the same manner as toxigenic *E. coli* and *Vibrio cholerae* (see Chapters 21 and 22).

ADDITIONAL READING

Aureli P, Fiorucci GC, Caroli D, Marchiaro G, Novara O, Leone L, Salmaso S. An outbreak of gastroenteritis associated with corn contaminated by *Listeria monocytogenes. N Engl J Med* 2000;342:1236–1241. This carefully studied outbreak in schools in adjacent Italian towns gives the best indication of the clinical findings in primary *Listeria* infection.

Dixon TC, Meselson M, Gillemin J, Hanna PC. Anthrax. *N Engl J Med* 1999; 341:815–826. This comprehensive review considers pathogenesis and clinical aspects.

Lorber B. Listeriosis. *Clin Infect Dis* 1997;24:1–11. A state-of-the-art review of the epidemiologic, clinical, and therapeutic aspects of the disease.

Mayer TA, et al. Clinical presentation of inhalation anthrax following bioterrorism exposure. *JAMA* 2001;286:2549–2553. This paper gives a detailed account of anthrax in two postal workers, including Gram stains, radiographs, and CT scans; these patients survived. (The paper that follows describes two fatal cases.)

McCloskey RV, Eller JJ, Green M, et al. The 1970 epidemic of diphtheria in San Antonio. *Ann Intern Med* 1970;75:495–503. A clear and informative description of a diphtheria outbreak is provided. The clinical features are given in detail, including color photographs of diphtheritic membranes.

Schlech WF, Lavigne PM, Bortolussi RA, et al. Epidemic listeriosis—evidence for transmission by food. *N Engl J Med* 1983;308:203–206. This epidemiologic study nicely traces events beginning on a Halifax farm to 34 cases of listeriosis. This outbreak was the first evidence that *Listeria* was a food-borne pathogen.

Southwick FS, Purich DL. Intracellular pathogenesis of listeriosis. *N Engl J Med* 1996;334:770–776. For a well-illustrated explanation of how *Listeria* uses the actin metabolism of the cell to make comet "tails," be sure to read this paper.

Vazquez-Boland JA, Kuhn M, Berche P, Chakraborty T, Dominguez-Bernal G, et al. *Listeria* pathogenesis and molecular virulence determinants. *Clin Microbiol Rev* 2001;14:584–640. This extensive review covers all topics from disease in animals to molecular genetics.

Vitek C, Warton M. Diphtheria in the former Soviet Union: Reemergence of a pandemic disease. *Emerg Infect Dis* 1998;4:539–550. A concise summary of the problems and attempted solutions to the major diphtheria outbreak of the last quarter century.

CHAPTER 19

Clostridium, *Peptostreptococcus*, *Bacteroides*, and Other Anaerobes

KENNETH J. RYAN

The bacteria discussed in this chapter are united by a common requirement for anaerobic conditions for growth. Organisms from multiple genera and all Gram stain categories are included. Most of them produce endogenous infections adjacent to the mucosal surfaces, where they are members of the normal flora. The clostridia form spores that allow them to produce diseases, such as tetanus and botulism, following environmental contamination of tissues or foods. Another anaerobic genus of bacteria, *Actinomyces*, is discussed in Chapter 29.

GENERAL FEATURES: ANAEROBES AND ANAEROBIC INFECTION

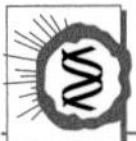

BACTERIOLOGY: ANAEROBIC BACTERIA

THE NATURE OF ANAEROBIOSIS

Anaerobes not only survive under anaerobic conditions, they require them to initiate and sustain growth. By definition, anaerobes fail to grow in the presence of 10% oxygen, but some are sensitive to oxygen concentrations as low as 0.5% and are killed by even brief exposures to air. However, **oxygen tolerance** is variable, and many organisms can survive in 2 to 8% oxygen, including most of the pathogenic species. The mechanisms involved are incompletely understood but clearly represent a continuum from species described as **aerotolerant** to those that require the culture medium to be prepared and stored under anaerobic conditions.

Anaerobes require low oxygen to initiate growth

Oxygen tolerance is a continuum

Anaerobes lack the cytochromes required to use oxygen as a terminal electron acceptor in energy-yielding reactions, and thus generate energy solely by fermentation (see Chapter 3). Some anaerobes will not grow unless the oxidation-reduction potential is

Low redox potential is required

extremely low (−300 mV), because critical enzymes must be in the reduced state to be active, aerobic conditions create a metabolic block.

Defense against oxygen products is lacking

Pathogens often have catalase and superoxide dismutase

Another element of anaerobiosis is the direct susceptibility of anaerobic bacteria to oxygen. For most aerobic and facultative bacteria, **catalase** and/or **superoxide dismutase** neutralize the toxicity of the oxygen products **hydrogen peroxide** and **superoxide** (see Chapter 3). Most anaerobes lack these enzymes and are injured when these oxygen products are formed in their microenvironment. As will be discussed below, some of the most virulent anaerobic pathogens are able to produce catalase or superoxide dismutase.

CLASSIFICATION

Biochemical, cultural, and molecular criteria define many species

The anaerobes indigenous to humans include almost every morphotype and hundreds of species. Typical biochemical and cultural tests are used for classification, although this is difficult because the growth requirements of each anaerobic species must be satisfied. Characterization of cellular fatty acids and metabolic products by chromatography has been useful for many anaerobic groups. Nucleic acid base composition and homology have been used extensively to rename older taxonomy. The genera most commonly associated with disease are shown in Table 19–1 and discussed below.

Anaerobic Cocci

Gram(+) = *Peptostreptococcus*

Gram(−) = *Veillonella*

Virtually all the medically important species of anaerobic Gram-positive cocci are now classified in a single genus, ***Peptostreptococcus.*** With Gram staining, these bacteria are most often seen as long chains of tiny cocci. ***Veillonella,*** a Gram-negative genus, deserves mention because of its potential for confusion with *Neisseria,* the only other Gram-negative coccus (see Chapter 20).

Clostridia

The clostridia are large, spore-forming, Gram-positive bacilli. Like their aerobic counterpart, *Bacillus,* clostridia have spores that are resistant to heat, desiccation, and disinfectants. They are able to survive for years in the environment and return to the vegetative form when placed in a favorable milieu. The shape of the cell and location of the spore varies with the species, but the spores themselves are rarely seen in clinical specimens.

Spores vary in shape and location

Hemolysin, neurotoxin, and enterotoxin production cause disease

The medically important clostridia are potent producers of one or more protein exotoxins. The histotoxic group including ***Clostridium perfringens*** and five other species (see Table 19–2) produces hemolysins at the site of acute infections that have lytic effects on a wide variety of cells. The neurotoxic group including ***C. tetani*** and ***C. botulinum*** produces neurotoxins that exert their effect at neural sites remote from the bacteria. ***C. difficile*** produces enterotoxins and disease in the intestinal tract. Many of the more than 80 other nontoxigenic clostridial species are also associated with disease.

TABLE 19–1

Usual Locations of Opportunistic Anaerobes

Organism	Gram Stain	Mouth or Pharynx	Intestine	Urogenital Tract	Skin
Peptostreptococcus	Positive cocci	+	+	+	–
Propionibacterium	Positive rods	–	–	–	+
Clostridium	Positive rods (large)	–	+	–	–
Bacteroides fragilis group	Negative rods (coccobacillary)	–	+	–	–
Fusobacterium	Negative rods (elongated)	+	+	–	–
Prevotella	Negative rods	+		+	–
Porphyromonas	Negative rods	+		+	

TABLE 19–2

Features of Pathogenic Anaerobes

Organism	Bacteriologic Features	Exotoxins	Source	Disease
Gram-positive cocci				
Peptostreptococcus			Mouth, intestine	Oropharyngeal infections, brain abscess
Gram-negative cocci				
Veillonella			Intestine	Rare opportunist
Gram-positive bacilli				
Clostridium perfringens	Spores	α-toxin, θ-toxin, enterotoxin	Intestine, environment, food	Cellulitis, gas gangrene, enterocolitis
Histotoxic species similar to *C. perfringens*[a]	Spores		Intestine, environment	Cellulitis, gas gangrene
C. tetani	Spores	Tetanospasmin	Environment	Tetanus
C. botulinum	Spores	Botulinum	Environment	Botulism
C. difficile	Spores	A enterotoxin, B cytotoxin	Intestine, environment (nosocomial)	Antibiotic-associated diarrhea, enterocolitis
Propionibacterium			Skin	Rare opportunist
Eubacterium			Intestine	Rare opportunist
Gram-negative bacilli				
Bacteroides fragilis[b]	Polysaccharide capsule	Enterotoxin	Intestine	Opportunist, abdominal abscess
Bacteroides species			Intestine	Opportunist
Fusobacterium			Mouth, intestine	Opportunist
Prevotella	Black pigment		Mouth, urogenital	Opportunist
Porphyromonas			Mouth, urogenital	Opportunist

[a] *C. histolyticum, C. noyyi, C. septicum,* and *C. sordellii.*

[b] The *Bacteroides fragilis* group includes *B. fragilis, B. distasonis, B. ovatus, B. vulgatus, B. thetaiotaomicron,* and six other species.

Nonsporulating Gram-positive Bacilli

Propionibacterium is a genus of small pleomorphic bacilli sometimes called anaerobic diphtheroids because of their morphologic resemblance to corynebacteria. They are among the most common bacteria in the normal flora of the skin. *Eubacterium* is a genus that includes long slender bacilli commonly found in the colonic flora. These organisms are occasionally isolated from infections in combination with other anaerobes but rarely produce disease on their own.

Members of the normal flora

Gram-negative Bacilli

Gram-negative, non–spore-forming bacilli are the most common bacteria isolated from anaerobic infections. In the past, most species were lumped into the genus *Bacteroides,* which still exists but now includes five other genera. Of these, *Fusobacterium, Porphyromonas,* and *Prevotella* are medically the most important. The *Bacteroides fragilis* group contains *B. fragilis* and 10 similar species noted for their virulence and production

Five genera are medically important

B. *fragilis* group produces β-lactamase and superoxide dismutase

of β-lactamases. (Species outside this group generally lack these features and are more similar to the other anaerobic Gram-negative bacilli.) *B. fragilis* is a relatively short Gram-negative bacillus with rounded ends sometimes giving a coccobacillary appearance. The lipopolysaccharide (LPS) in its outer membrane has a much lower lipid content and thus lower toxic activity than that of most other Gram-negative bacteria. Virtually all *B. fragilis* strains have a polysaccharide capsule and are relatively oxygen tolerant through production of superoxide dismutase. *Prevotella, Porphyromonas,* and *Fusobacterium* are distinguished by biochemical and other taxonomic features. *Prevotella melaninogenica* forms a black pigment in culture, and *Fusobacterium,* as its name suggests, is typically elongated and has tapered ends.

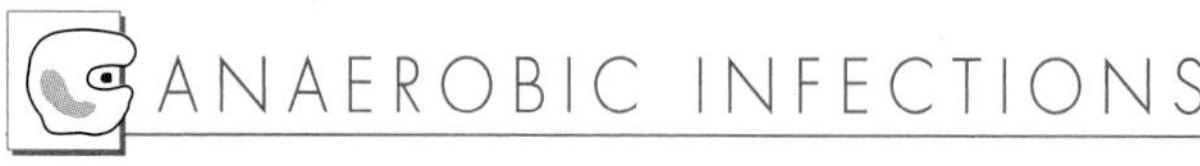

ANAEROBIC INFECTIONS

EPIDEMIOLOGY

Low redox normal flora sites are the origin of most infections

Spore-forming clostridia also come from the environment

Despite our constant immersion in air, anaerobes are able to colonize the many oxygen-deficient or oxygen-free microenvironments of the body. Often these are created by the presence of facultative organisms whose growth reduces oxygen and decreases the local oxidation-reduction potential. Such sites include the sebaceous glands of the skin, the gingival crevices of the gums, the lymphoid tissue of the throat, and the lumina of the intestinal and urogenital tracts. Except for infections with some environmental clostridia, anaerobic infections are almost always endogenous with the infective agent(s) derived from the patient's normal flora. The specific anaerobes involved are linked to their prevalence in the flora of the relevant sites as shown in Table 19–1. In addition to the presence of clostridia in the lower intestinal tract of humans and animals, their spores are widely distributed in the environment, particularly in soil exposed to animal excreta. The spores may contaminate any wound caused by a nonsterile object (eg, splinter, nail) or exposed directly to soil.

PATHOGENESIS

Anaerobes displaced from normal flora to deeper sites may cause disease

Trauma and host factors create the opportunity for infection

The anaerobic flora normally live in a harmless commensal relationship with the host. However, when displaced from their niche on the mucosal surface into normally sterile tissues these organisms may cause life-threatening infections. This can occur as the result of trauma (eg, gunshot, surgery), disease (eg, diverticulosis), or isolated events (eg, aspiration). Host factors such as malignancy or impaired blood supply increase the probability that the dislodged flora eventually produce an infection. The organisms involved are anaerobes normally found at the mucosal site adjacent to the infection. For example, *B. fragilis,* which is one of the most common species in the colonic flora, is the organism most frequently isolated from intra-abdominal abscesses.

Flora may be aspirated or displaced at a distance

Brain abscess typically involves anaerobic bacteria

The relationship between normal flora and site of infection may be indirect. For example, aspiration pneumonia, lung abscess, and empyema typically involve anaerobes found in the oropharyngeal flora. The brain is not a particularly anaerobic environment, but brain abscess is most often caused by these same oropharyngeal anaerobes. This presumably occurs by extension across the cribriform plate to the temporal lobe, the typical location of brain abscess. In contaminated open wounds, clostridia can come from the intestinal flora or from spores surviving in the environment.

Capsules and toxins are known for some anaerobes

Survival in oxidized conditions can be a virulence factor

While gaining access to tissue sites provides the opportunity, additional virulence factors are needed for anaerobes to produce infection. Some anaerobic pathogens produce disease even when present as a minor part of the displaced resident flora, and other common members of the normal flora rarely cause disease. Classical virulence factors such as toxins and capsules are known only for the toxigenic clostridia and *B. fragilis,* but a feature such as the ability to survive brief exposures to oxygenated environments can also be viewed as a virulence factor. Anaerobes found in human infections are far more likely to produce catalase and superoxide dismutase than their more

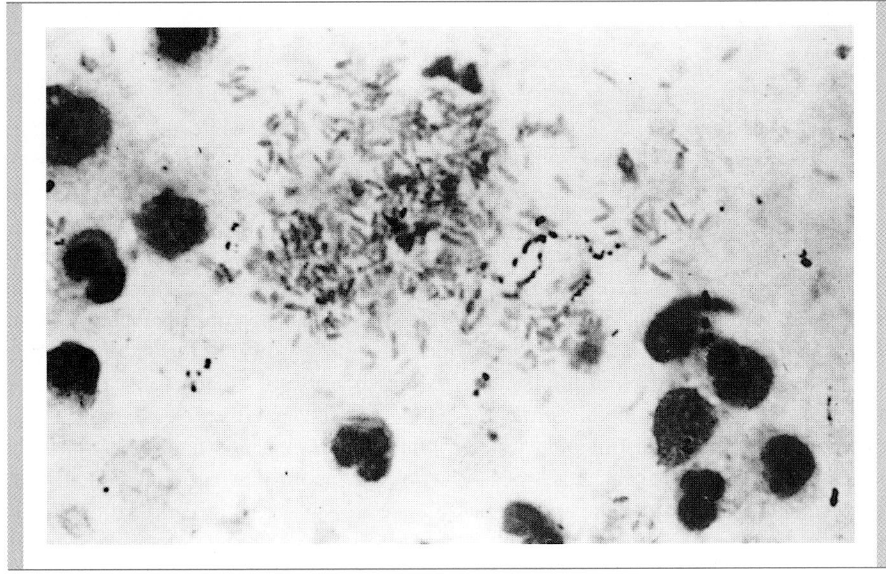

FIGURE 19–1
Gram smear of pus from an abdominal abscess showing polymorphonuclear leukocytes, large numbers of Gram-negative anaerobes and some peptostreptococci. (*Reproduced with permission of Schering Corporation, Kenilworth, NJ, the copyright owner. All rights reserved.*)

docile counterparts of the normal flora. Exquisitely oxygen-sensitive anaerobes are seldom involved, probably because they are injured by even the small amounts of oxygen dissolved in tissue fluids.

A related feature is the ability of the bacteria to create and control a reduced microenvironment, often with the apparent help of other bacteria. The great majority of anaerobic infections are mixed; that is, two or more anaerobes are present, often in combination with facultative bacteria such as *Escherichia coli* (Fig 19–1). In some cases the components of these mixtures are believed to synergize each other's growth either by providing growth factors or by lowering the oxidation-reduction potential. These conditions may have other advantages such as the inhibition of oxygen-dependent leukocyte bactericidal functions under the anaerobic conditions in the lesion. Anaerobes that produce specific toxins have a pathogenesis all their own, which will be discussed in the sections devoted to individual species.

Mixed infections may facilitate an anaerobic microenvironment

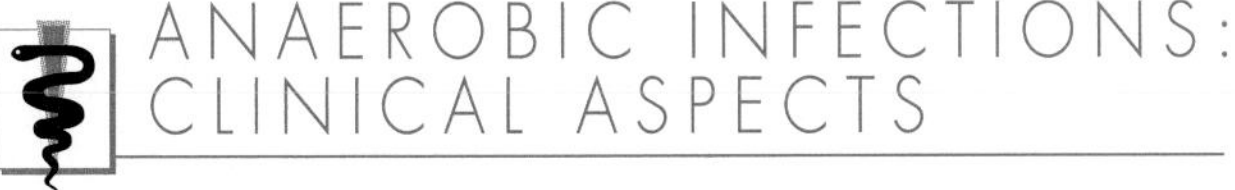

ANAEROBIC INFECTIONS: CLINICAL ASPECTS

MANIFESTATIONS

Bacteroides, Fusobacterium, and peptostreptococci, alone or together with other facultative or obligate anaerobes, are responsible for the overwhelming majority of localized abscesses within the cranium, thorax, peritoneum, liver, and female genital tract. As indicated earlier, the species involved relate to the pathogens present in the normal flora of the adjacent mucosal surface. Those derived from the oral flora also include dental infections and infections of human bites.

Abscesses are usually caused by *Bacteroides, Fusobacterium,* or peptostreptococci

In addition, anaerobes play causal roles in chronic sinusitis, chronic otitis media, aspiration pneumonia, bronchiectasis, cholecystitis, septic arthritis, osteomyelitis, decubitus ulcers, and soft tissue infections of patients with diabetes mellitus. Dissection of infection along fascial planes (necrotizing fasciitis) and thrombophlebitis are common complications. Foul-smelling pus and crepitation (gas in tissues) are signs associated with, but by no means exclusive to, anaerobic infections. As with other bacterial infections, they may spread beyond the local site and enter the bloodstream. The mortality rate of anaerobic bacteremias arising from nongenital sources is equivalent to the rates with bacteremias due to staphylococci or Enterobacteriaceae.

Foul-smelling pus suggests anaerobic infection

DIAGNOSIS

Specimens must be direct and protected from oxygen

The key to detection of anaerobes is a high quality specimen, preferably pus or fluid taken directly from the infected site. The specimen needs to be taken quickly to the microbiology laboratory and protected from oxygen exposure while on the way. Special anaerobic transport tubes may be used or any air from the syringe in which the specimen was collected may be expressed. Actually, a generous collection of pus serves as an adequate transport medium unless transport is delayed for hours.

Gram staining is particularly useful

Anaerobic incubation jar provides atmosphere

Selective media inhibit facultative bacteria

A direct Gram-stained smear of clinical material demonstrating Gram-negative and/or Gram-positive bacteria of various morphologies is highly suggestive, often even diagnostic of anaerobic infection. Because of the typically slow and complicated nature of anaerobic culture, the Gram stain often provides the most useful information for clinical decision-making. Isolation of the bacteria requires the use of an anaerobic incubation atmosphere and special media protected from oxygen exposure. Although elaborate systems are available for this purpose, the simple anaerobic jar is sufficient for isolation of the clinically significant anaerobes. The use of media that contain reducing agents (cysteine, thioglycollate) and growth factors needed by some species further facilitates isolation of anaerobes. The polymicrobial nature of most anaerobic infections requires the use of selective media to protect the slow growing anaerobes from being overgrown by hardier bacteria, particularly members of the Enterobacteriaceae. Antibiotics, particularly aminoglycosides to which all anaerobes are resistant, are frequently used. Once the bacteria are isolated, identification procedures including morphology, biochemical characterization, and metabolic end-product detection by gas chromatography may begin.

TREATMENT

Mixed infections and slow growth dictate empiric therapy

Abdominal infections require β-lactamase–resistant antimicrobics

As with most abscesses, drainage of the purulent material is the primary treatment, in association with appropriate chemotherapy. Antimicrobics alone may be ineffective because of failure to penetrate the site of infection. The selection of antimicrobics used is empiric to a degree; such infections typically involve mixed species, and cultural diagnosis is delayed by the slow growth and the time required to distinguish multiple species. In addition, antimicrobial susceptibility testing methods are slow and less standardized than they are for the rapidly growing bacteria. The usual approach involves selection of antimicrobics based on the expected susceptibility of the anaerobes known to produce infection at the site in question. For example, anaerobic organisms derived from the oral flora are often susceptible to penicillin, but infections below the diaphragm caused by fecal anaerobes such as *B. fragilis* are usually resistant to β-lactams. These latter infections are most likely to respond to clindamycin, metronidazole, or a cephalosporin such as cefoxitin, which is not inactivated by the β-lactamases produced by anaerobes.

CLOSTRIDIUM PERFRINGENS

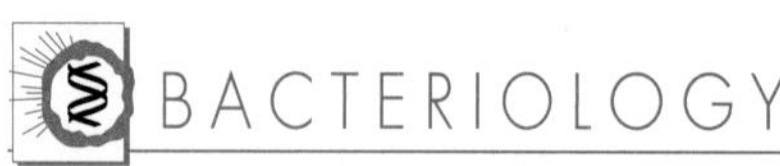

BACTERIOLOGY

Double zone of hemolysis is characteristic

C. perfringens is a large, Gram-positive, nonmotile rod with square ends. It grows overnight on blood agar medium under anaerobic conditions, producing colonies surrounded by a double zone of hemolysis (Fig 19–2). In broth containing fermentable carbohydrate, growth of *C. perfringens* is accompanied by the production of large amounts of hydrogen and carbon dioxide gas, which can also be produced in necrotic tissues; hence the term gas gangrene.

C. perfringens produces multiple exotoxins that have different pathogenic significance in different animal species and serve as the basis for classification of the five types (A to E). Type A is by far the most important in humans and is found consistently in the

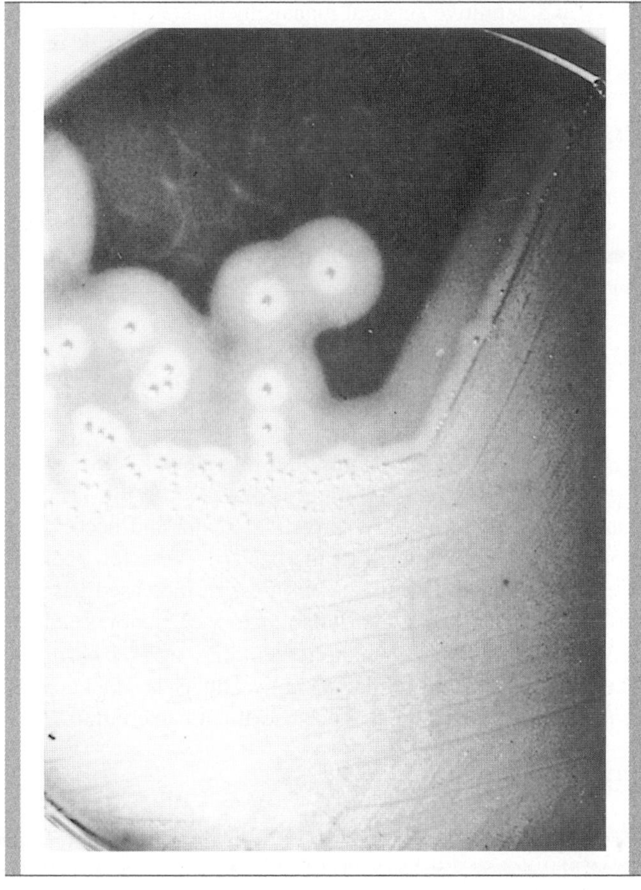

FIGURE 19–2
C. perfringens colonies on a blood agar plate showing double zone of hemolysis. The inner clear zone is caused by θ-toxin and the wider zone of incomplete hemolysis caused by α-toxin.

colon and often in soil. The most important exotoxin is the **α-toxin**, a phospholipase that hydrolyzes lecithin and sphingomyelin, thus disrupting the cell membranes of various host cells, including erythrocytes, leukocytes, and muscle cells. The **θ-toxin** alters capillary permeability and is toxic to heart muscle. This pore-forming toxin is closely related to streptolysin O (see Chapter 17). When the **enterotoxin** is attached to enterocyte membranes, it causes an increase in intracellular calcium and altered membrane permeability which leads to loss of cellular fluid and macromolecules.

Typing system is based on toxins

Phospholipase α-toxin, pore-forming θ-toxin, and enterotoxin cause disease

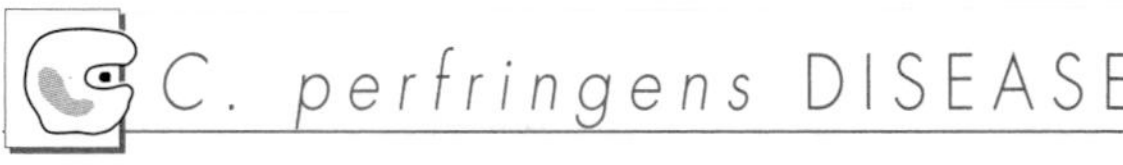

C. perfringens DISEASE

CLINICAL CAPSULE

C. perfringens produces a wide range of wound and soft tissue infections, many of which are no different from those caused by other opportunistic bacteria. The most dreaded of these, gas gangrene, begins as a wound infection but progresses to shock and death in a matter of hours. Another form of *C. perfringens*-caused disease, food poisoning, is characterized by diarrhea without fever or vomiting.

EPIDEMIOLOGY

Gas Gangrene

Gas gangrene develops in traumatic wounds with muscle damage when they are contaminated with dirt, clothing, or other foreign material containing *C. perfringens* or another species of histotoxic clostridia. The clostridia can come from the patient's own intestinal flora or spores in the environment. Compound fractures, bullet wounds, or the kind of trauma seen in wartime are prototypes for this infection. A significant delay between the

Spores from the host or environment contaminate wounds

Delays allow multiplication

injury and definitive surgical management is an additional requirement. These conditions are more likely to occur in peacetime in a hiking accident in a remote area rather than in an automobile accident on a freeway.

Clostridial Food Poisoning

C. perfringens can cause food poisoning if large numbers of an enterotoxin-producing strain are ingested. Outbreaks usually involve meat dishes such as stews, soups, or gravies. Clostridial food poisoning is one of the most common food-borne illnesses in developed countries.

PATHOGENESIS

Gas Gangrene

Low redox favors multiplication and toxin production

Toxins lead to shock

If the oxidation–reduction potential in a wound is sufficiently low, *C. perfringens* spores can germinate and can multiply, elaborating α-toxin. The process passes along the muscle bundles, producing rapidly spreading edema and necrosis as well as conditions that are more favorable for growth of the bacteria. Very few leukocytes are present in the myonecrotic tissue. As the disease progresses, increased vascular permeability and systemic absorption of the toxin and inflammatory mediators leads to shock. θ-toxin and oxygen deprivation due to the metabolic activities of *C. perfringens* are probable contributors. The basis for the profound systemic effects is not known, but toxin absorption seems probable, because fatal cases occur without bacteremia.

Clostridial Food Poisoning

Spores survive cooking

Vegetative cells produce enterotoxin

The spores of some *C. perfringens* strains are often particularly heat resistant and can withstand temperatures of 100°C for an hour or more. Thus, spores that survive initial cooking can convert to the vegetative form and multiply if food is not refrigerated or is rewarmed. After ingestion, the enterotoxin is released into the upper gastrointestinal tract, causing a fluid outpouring in which the ileum is most severely involved.

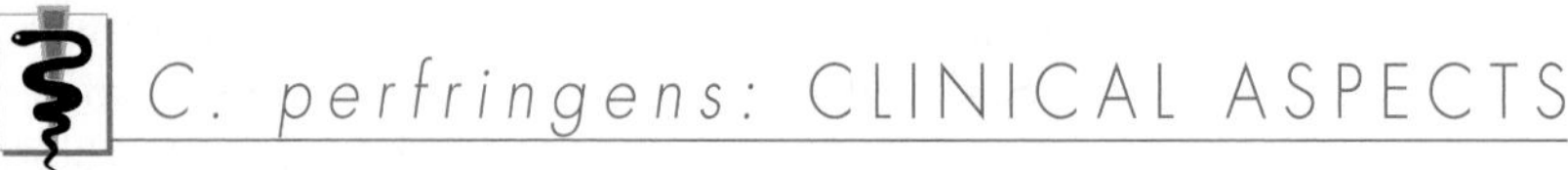

C. perfringens: CLINICAL ASPECTS

MANIFESTATIONS

Gas Gangrene

Wound pain evolves to edema and shock

Gas gangrene usually begins 1 to 4 days after the injury but may start within 10 hours. The earliest reported finding is severe pain at the site of the wound accompanied by a sense of heaviness or pressure. The disease then progresses rapidly with edema, tenderness, and pallor, which is followed by discoloration and hemorrhagic bullae. The gas is apparent as crepitance in the tissue, but this is a late sign. Systemic findings are those of shock with intravascular hemolysis, hypotension, and renal failure leading to coma and death. Patients are often remarkably alert until the terminal stages.

Anaerobic Cellulitis

Gas is more likely than in gas gangrene

Anaerobic cellulitis is a clostridial infection of wounds and surrounding subcutaneous tissue in which there is marked gas formation (more than in gas gangrene) but in which the pain, swelling, and toxicity of gas gangrene are absent. This condition is much less serious than gas gangrene and can be controlled with less rigorous methods.

Endometritis

Nonsterile abortion is greatest risk

If *C. perfringens* gains access to necrotic products of conception retained in the uterus, it may multiply and infect the endometrium. Necrosis of uterine tissue and septicemia with massive intravascular hemolysis due to α-toxin may then follow. Clostridial uterine infection occurred more commonly in the past, usually after an incomplete illegal abortion with inadequately sterilized instruments.

Food Poisoning

The incubation period of 8 to 24 hours is followed by nausea, abdominal pain, and diarrhea. There is no fever, and vomiting is rare. Spontaneous recovery usually occurs within 24 hours.

Diarrhea without fever or vomiting is most common

DIAGNOSIS

Diagnosis is based ultimately on clinical observations. Bacteriologic studies are adjunctive. It is quite common, for example, to isolate *C. perfringens* from contaminated wounds of patients who have no evidence of clostridial disease. The organism can also be isolated from the postpartum uterine cervix of healthy women or from those with only mild fever. Occasionally, *C. perfringens* is even isolated from blood cultures of patients who do not develop serious clostridial infection. In clostridial food poisoning, isolation of more than 10^5 *C. perfringens* per gram of ingested food in the absence of any other cause is usually sufficient to confirm the etiology of a characteristic food poisoning outbreak.

Isolation of clostridia alone is not sufficient

TREATMENT AND PREVENTION

Treatment of gas gangrene and endometritis must be initiated immediately because these conditions are almost always fatal if untreated. Excision of all devitalized tissue is of paramount importance, because it denies the organism the anaerobic conditions required for further multiplication and toxin production. This often entails wide resection of muscle groups, hysterectomy, and even amputation of limbs. Administration of massive doses of penicillin is an important adjunctive procedure. Because nonclostridial anaerobes and members of the Enterobacteriaceae frequently contaminate injury sites, clindamycin and broad-spectrum cephalosporins are often added to the antibiotic regimen. Placement of patients in a hyperbaric oxygen chamber, which increases the tissue level of dissolved oxygen, has been shown to slow the spread of disease, probably by inhibiting bacterial growth and toxin production and by neutralizing the activity of θ-toxin.

Surgical treatment is essential for gas gangrene and endometritis

Antibiotics and hyperbaric oxygen are useful

The most effective method for prevention of gas gangrene is the surgical debridement of traumatic injuries as soon as possible. Thorough cleansing, removal of dead tissue and foreign bodies, and drainage of hematoma limit organism multiplication and toxin production. Antimicrobic prophylaxis is indicated but cannot replace surgical debridement, because the antimicrobics may fail to reach the organism in devascularized tissues.

Debridement of dead tissue is best

Prevention involves good cooking hygiene and adequate refrigeration. There is growing evidence that enterotoxin-producing strains of *C. perfringens* may also be responsible for some cases of antimicrobic-induced diarrhea in a setting similar to *C. difficile.*

CLOSTRIDIUM TETANI

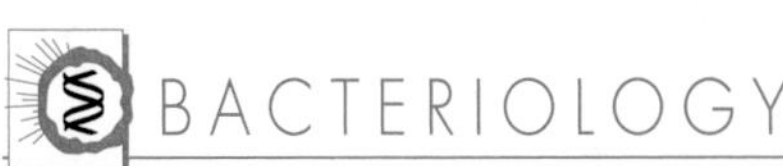

BACTERIOLOGY

C. tetani is a slim, Gram-positive rod, which may stain Gram negative in very young or old cultures. It forms spores readily in nature and in culture, yielding a typical round terminal spore that gives the organism a drumstick appearance before the residual vegetative cell disintegrates. The organism is flagellate and motile. *C. tetani* requires strict anaerobic conditions. Its identity is suggested by cultural and biochemical characteristics, but definite identification depends on demonstrating its neurotoxic exotoxin. *C. tetani* spores remain viable in soil or culture for many years. It is resistant to most disinfectants and withstands boiling for several minutes.

Gram-positive rods decolorize readily

The most important product of *C. tetani* is its neurotoxic exotoxin, **tetanospasmin** or tetanus toxin, a metalloproteinase that enzymatically degrades a protein required for

Toxin blocks release of inhibitory neurotransmitters

Formaldehyde treatment removes toxicity but retains antigenicity

docking of neurotransmitter vesicles at the appropriate site on presynaptic membranes. Loss of this function prevents release of neurotransmitters used by inhibitory afferent motor neurons. The effect is unopposed firing of the motor neurons, generating spasms. The toxin is heat labile, antigenic, readily neutralized by antitoxin, and rapidly destroyed by intestinal proteases. Treatment with formaldehyde yields a nontoxic product or **toxoid** that retains the antigenicity of toxin and thus stimulates production of antitoxin.

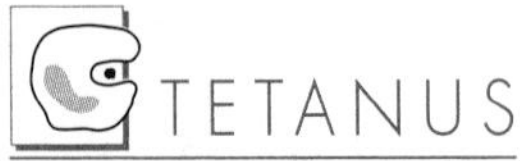

TETANUS

CLINICAL CAPSULE

The striking feature of tetanus is severe muscle spasms (or "lockjaw" when the jaw muscles are involved). This occurs despite minimal or no inflammation at the primary site of infection, which may be unnoticed even though the outcome is fatal. The disease is caused by in vivo production of a neurotoxin that acts centrally, not locally. Immunization with inactivated toxin, even after stepping on a rusty nail, prevents tetanus.

EPIDEMIOLOGY

Spores from environment germinate in wounds

Nonsterile technique can lead to tetanus

The spores of *C. tetani* exist in many soils, especially those that have been treated with manure, and the organism is sometimes found in the lower intestinal tract of humans and animals. The spores are introduced into wounds contaminated with soil or foreign bodies. The wounds are often quite small, (eg, a puncture wound with a splinter). In many developing countries, the majority of tetanus cases occur in recently delivered infants when the umbilical cord is severed or bandaged in a nonsterile manner. Similarly, tetanus may follow an unskilled abortion, scarification rituals, female circumcision, and even surgery performed with nonsterile instruments or dressings.

PATHOGENESIS

Trauma provides growth conditions

Tetanospasmin produced at the local site ascends through nerves to anterior horn

Blockage of reflex inhibition causes spasmodic contractions

The usual predisposing factor for tetanus is an area of very low oxidation–reduction potential in which tetanus spores can germinate, such as a large splinter, an area of necrosis from introduction of soil, or necrosis after injection of contaminated illicit drugs. Infection with facultative or other anaerobic organisms can contribute to the development of an appropriate anaerobic nidus for spore germination. Tetanus bacilli multiply locally and neither damage nor invade adjacent tissues. Tetanospasmin is elaborated at the site of infection and enters the presynaptic terminals of lower motor neurons, reaching the central nervous system (CNS) mainly by exploiting the retrograde axonal transport system in the nerves. In the spinal cord, it acts at the level of the anterior horn cells, where its blockage of postsynaptic inhibition of spinal motor reflexes produces spasmodic contractions of both protagonist and antagonist muscles. This process takes place initially in the area of the causative lesion but may extend up and down the spinal cord. Minor stimuli, such as a sound or a draft, can provoke generalized spasms.

TETANUS: CLINICAL ASPECTS

MANIFESTATIONS

The incubation period of the disease is from 4 days to several weeks. The shorter incubation period is usually associated with wounds in areas supplied by the cranial motor nerves, probably because of a shorter transmission route for the toxin to the CNS. In general, shorter incubation periods are associated with more severe disease.

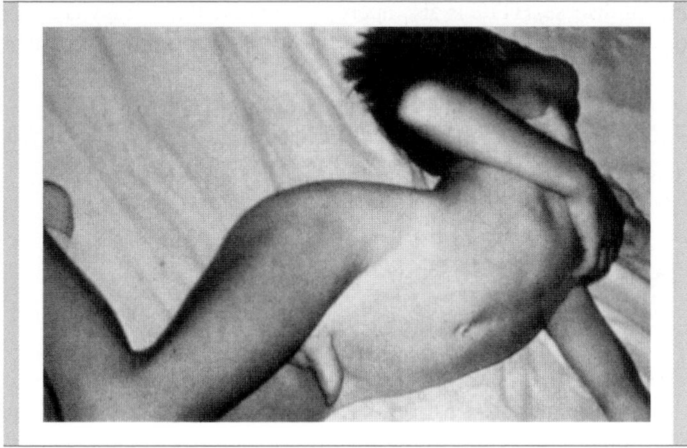

FIGURE 19–3
Generalized tetanus. This child shows opisthotonic posturing caused by spasm of the spinal musculature. (*Photo courtesy of Anastacio de Queiroz Sousa, MD, Universidade Federal do Ceara, Fortaleza, Brazil, and Martin Cetron, MD, Centers for Disease Control and Prevention, Atlanta.*)

The diagnosis is clinical; neither culture nor toxin testing are useful. Although tetanus may be localized to muscles innervated by nerves in the region of the infection, it is usually more generalized. The masseter muscles are often the first to be affected, resulting in inability to open the mouth properly **(trismus);** this effect accounts for the use of the term **lockjaw** to describe the disease. As other muscles become affected, intermittent spasms can become generalized to include muscles of respiration and swallowing. In extreme cases, massive contractions of the back muscles (opisthotonos) develop (Fig 19–3).

Incubation period varies with distance to CNS

Masseter muscle contraction causes lockjaw

Untreated patients with tetanus retain consciousness and are aware of their plight, in which small stimuli can trigger massive contractions. In fatal cases, death results from exhaustion and respiratory failure. Untreated, the mortality caused by the generalized disease varies from 15 to more than 60%, according to the lesion, incubation period, and age of the patient. Mortality is highest in neonates and in elderly patients.

Respiratory failure leads to death

TREATMENT

Specific treatment of tetanus involves neutralization of any unbound toxin with large doses of human tetanus immune globulin (HTIG), which is derived from the blood of volunteers hyperimmunized with toxoid. Most important in treatment are nonspecific supportive measures, including maintenance of a quiet dark environment, sedation, and provision of an adequate airway. Benzodiazepines are also used to indirectly antagonize the effects of the toxin. The value of antimicrobics is not clear. Because toxin binding is irreversible, recovery requires the generation of new axonal terminals.

Supportive treatment required until axons regenerate

PREVENTION

Routine active immunization with tetanus toxoid, combined with diphtheria toxoid and pertussis vaccine (DTaP) for primary immunization in childhood and DT for adults, can completely prevent the disease. It has reduced the incidence of tetanus in the United States to less than 50 reported cases per year. Five doses of DT are recommended, to be given at the ages of 2, 4, 6, and 18 months, and once again between the ages of 4 and 6 years. Thereafter a booster of adult-type tetanus diphtheria toxoid should be given every 10 years. Unfortunately, routine childhood immunization is not administratively and economically feasible in many less well-developed countries, where as many as a million cases of tetanus occur annually. In such settings, immunization efforts have been focused on pregnant women, because transplacental transfer of antibodies to the fetus also prevents the highly lethal neonatal tetanus.

Childhood toxoid immunization prevents disease

Boosters required every 10 years

Unimmunized subjects with tetanus-prone wounds should be given passive immunity with a prophylactic dose of HTIG as soon as possible. This immunization provides immediate protection. Those who have had a full primary series of immunizations and appropriate boosters are given toxoid for tetanus-prone wounds if they have not been immunized within the previous 10 years in the case of clean minor wounds or 5 years for more contaminated wounds. If immunization is incomplete or the wound has been neglected and poses a serious

Passive immunization used when immunization is neglected

risk of disease, HTIG is also appropriate. Penicillin therapy is a prophylactic adjunct in serious or neglected wounds but in no way alters the need for specific prophylaxis.

Clostridium botulinum

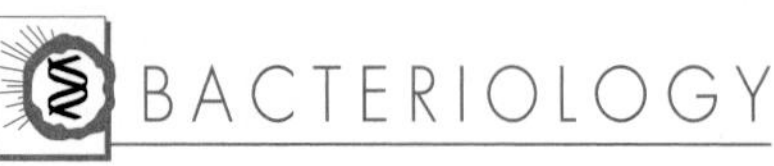

BACTERIOLOGY

C. botulinum is a large Gram-positive rod much like the rest of the clostridia. Its spores resist boiling for long periods, and moist heat at 121°C is required for certain destruction. Germination of spores and growth of *C. botulinum* can occur in a variety of alkaline or neutral foodstuffs when conditions are sufficiently anaerobic.

Cells germinating from spores produce neurotoxin in food

Blockage of synaptic acetylcholine release causes paralysis

The major characteristic of medical importance is that when *C. botulinum* grows under these anaerobic conditions, it elaborates a family of neurotoxins of extraordinary toxicity. **Botulinum toxin** is the most potent toxin known in nature, with an estimated lethal dose for humans of less than 1 μg. Like tetanospasmin, botulinum toxin is a metalloproteinase that acts on the presynaptic membranes at neuromuscular junctions. Once bound, it cleaves proteins involved in the release of acetylcholine at the synapse. The major effect of this blockage of acetylcholine release is paralysis of the motor system, but it also causes dysfunction of the autonomic nervous system.

Toxin is destroyed by boiling

C. botulinum is classified into multiple types (A to G) based on the antigenic specificity of the neurotoxins. All of the toxins are heat labile and destroyed rapidly at 100°C but are resistant to the enzymes of the gastrointestinal tract. If unheated toxin is ingested, it is readily absorbed and distributed in the bloodstream.

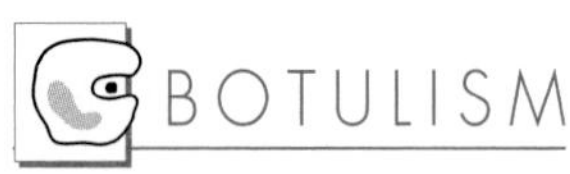

BOTULISM

CLINICAL CAPSULE

Botulism begins with cranial nerve palsies and develops into descending symmetrical motor paralysis, which may involve the respiratory muscles. No fever or other signs of infection occur. The time course depends on the amount of toxin present and whether it was ingested preformed in food or produced endogenously in the intestinal tract or a wound.

EPIDEMIOLOGY

Spores are widely distributed

Alkaline foods favor toxin production

Inadequately heated home-canned foods are most common source

Spores of *C. botulinum* are found in soil, pond, and lake sediments in many parts of the world, including the United States. If spores contaminate food, they may convert to the vegetative state, multiply, and produce toxin in storage under proper conditions. This may occur with no change in food taste, color, or odor. The alkaline conditions provided by vegetables, such as green beans, and mushrooms and fish support the growth of *C. botulinum,* and the acidic conditions provided by foods such as canned fruit do not support the growth of the bacterium. Botulism most often occurs after ingestion of home-canned products that have not been heated at temperatures sufficient to kill *C. botulinum* spores, although inadequately sterilized commercial fish products have also been implicated. Because the toxin is heat labile, food must be ingested uncooked or after insufficient cooking. Botulism often occurs in small family outbreaks in the case of home-prepared foods or less often as isolated cases connected to commercial products. Infant and wound botulism results when the toxin is produced endogenously, beginning with environmental spores that are either ingested or contaminate wounds.

PATHOGENESIS

Food-borne botulism is an intoxication, not an infection. The ingested preformed toxin is absorbed in the intestinal tract and reaches its neuromuscular junction target via the bloodstream. Once bound there, its inhibition of acetylcholine release causes paralysis due to lack of neuromuscular transmission. The specific disease manifestations depend on the specific nerves to which the circulating toxin binds. Cardiac arrhythmias and blood pressure instability are believed to be due to effects of the toxin on the autonomic nervous system. As with tetanus, the damage to the synapse once the toxin has bound is permanent and recovery requires the sprouting of the presynaptic axons and formation of new synapses.

Preformed toxin is readily absorbed

Acetylcholine block leads to paralysis and autonomic effects

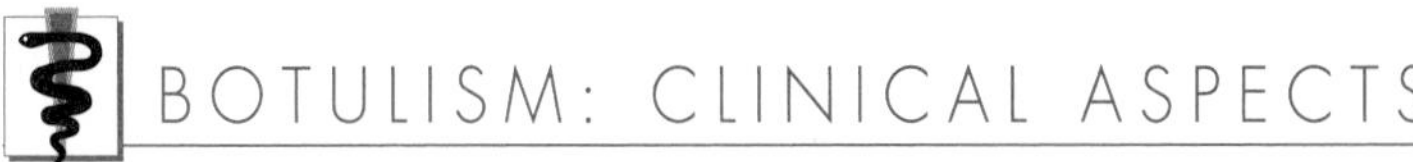

BOTULISM: CLINICAL ASPECTS

MANIFESTATIONS

Food-borne botulism usually starts 12 to 36 hours after ingestion of the toxin. The first signs are nausea, dry mouth, and, in some cases, diarrhea. Cranial nerve signs, including blurred vision, pupillary dilatation, and nystagmus, occur later. Symmetrical paralysis begins with the ocular, laryngeal, and respiratory muscles and spreads to the trunk and extremities. The most serious finding is complete respiratory paralysis. Mortality is 10 to 20%.

Blurred vision progresses to symmetrical paralysis

Infant Botulism

A syndrome associated with *C. botulinum* that occurs in infants between the ages of 3 weeks and 8 months is now the most commonly diagnosed form of botulism. The organism is apparently introduced on weaning or with dietary supplements, especially honey, and multiplies in the infant's colon, with absorption of small amounts of toxin. The infant shows constipation, poor muscle tone, lethargy, and feeding problems and may have ophthalmic and other paralyses similar to those in adult botulism. Infant botulism may mimic sudden infant death syndrome. The benefits of antitoxin and antimicrobic agents have not been clearly established.

Nonsterile honey introduces spores to intestine

Lethargy, poor feeding occur in addition to adult signs

Wound Botulism

Very rarely, wounds infected with other organisms may allow *C. botulinum* to grow. Wound botulism in parenteral users of cocaine and maxillary sinus botulism in intranasal users of cocaine has been reported. Disease similar to that from food poisoning may develop, or it may begin with weakness localized to the injured extremity. Botulism without an obvious food or wound source is occasionally reported in individuals beyond infancy. It is possible that some such cases result from ingestion of spores of *C. botulinum* with subsequent in vivo production of toxin in a manner similar to that in infant botulism.

Contaminated wounds of drug users are sites of toxin production

DIAGNOSIS

The toxin can be demonstrated in blood, intestinal contents, or remaining food, but these tests require inoculation of mice and are performed only in reference laboratories. *C. botulinum* may also be isolated from stool or from foodstuffs suspected of responsibility for botulism.

Toxin can be detected in some laboratories

TREATMENT AND PREVENTION

The availability of intensive supportive measures, particularly mechanical ventilation, is the single most important determinant of clinical outcome. With proper ventilatory support, mortality should be less then 10%. The administration of large doses of horse *C. botulinum* antitoxin is thought to be useful in neutralizing free toxin. Frequent hypersensitivity reactions related to the equine origin of this preparation makes it unsuitable for use in infants. Antimicrobial agents are given only to patients with wound botulism.

Supportive measures and antitoxin allow survival

Cooking food inactivates toxin

Adequate pressure cooking or autoclaving in the canning process kills spores, and heating food at 100°C for 10 minutes before eating destroys the toxin. Food from damaged cans or those that present evidence of positive inside pressure should not even be tasted because of the extreme toxicity of the *C. botulinum* toxin.

CLOSTRIDIUM DIFFICILE

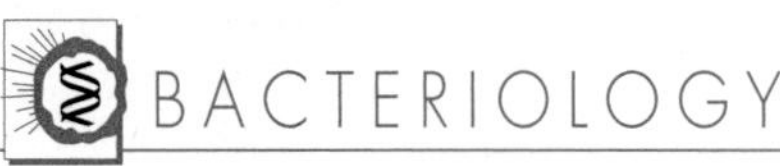

BACTERIOLOGY

A and B toxins disrupt cytoskeleton signal transduction

A is a enterotoxin

B is a cytotoxin

C. difficile is a Gram-positive rod that readily forms spores. Its early reputation for fastidious growth is responsible for its species epithet. Like the other clostridia described in this section, *C. difficile* has a most important medical feature: its ability to produce toxins. In this species, two distinct large polypeptide toxins, A and B, with similar structure (45% homology) are released during late growth phases of the vegetative organism, perhaps at the time of cell lysis. Both toxins act in the cytoplasm by disrupting proteins involved in signal transduction, particularly those involving the actin cytoskeleton. The A toxin causes cell rounding and the disruption of intercellular tight junctions followed by altered membrane permeability and fluid secretion. The net effect is that of an enterotoxin, although inflammation and cytoxic activity are also present. The B toxin lacks the enterotoxic properties of the A toxin but has cytotoxic potency at least 10 times higher. The two toxins appear to act synergistically by a mechanism yet to be determined.

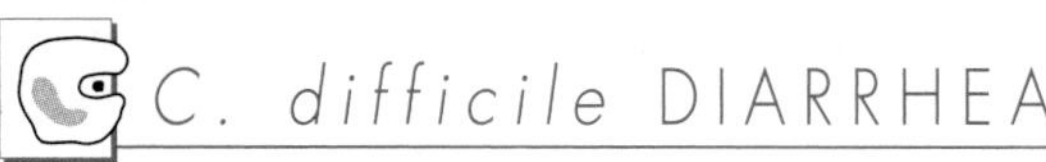

C. difficile DIARRHEA

CLINICAL CAPSULE

C. difficile is the most common cause of diarrhea that develops in association with the use of antimicrobial agents. The diarrhea ranges from a few days of intestinal fluid loss to life-threatening pseudomembranous colitis (PMC). This condition is associated with intense inflammation and the formation of a pseudomembrane composed of inflammatory debris on the mucosal surface.

EPIDEMIOLOGY

Source is endogenous or environmental

C. difficile is present in 2 to 5% of the general population, sometimes at higher rates among hospitalized persons and infants. More than two decades of the antibiotic era had elapsed before the medical importance of *C. difficile* was recognized through its association with antibiotic-associated diarrhea (AAD). Although infection is endogenous in most cases, hospital outbreaks have clearly established that the environment can be the source as well.

Frequent cause of AAD

Major cause of PMC

C. difficile is by no means the only cause of ADD, but it is the most common identifiable cause. In simple diarrhea following antimicrobial administration, this organism is responsible for approximately 30% of cases. As the disease progresses to colitis, the association is stronger, rising to 90% if PMC is present. Person-to-person transfer is very rare except in the instance of hospital-acquired *C. difficile* infections, where environmental or hand contamination leads to infection of another patient.

PATHOGENESIS

Antimicrobic effect on flora selects for *C. difficile*

When *C. difficile* becomes established in the colon of individuals with normal gut flora, few if any direct consequences result, probably because its numbers are dwarfed by the other flora. Alteration of the colonic flora with antimicrobics (particularly ampicillin,

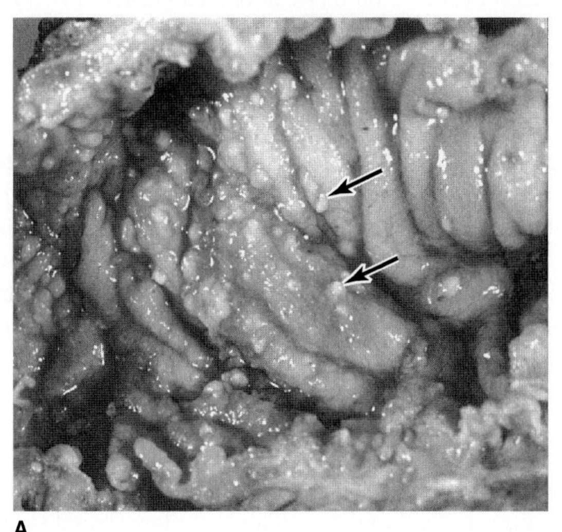

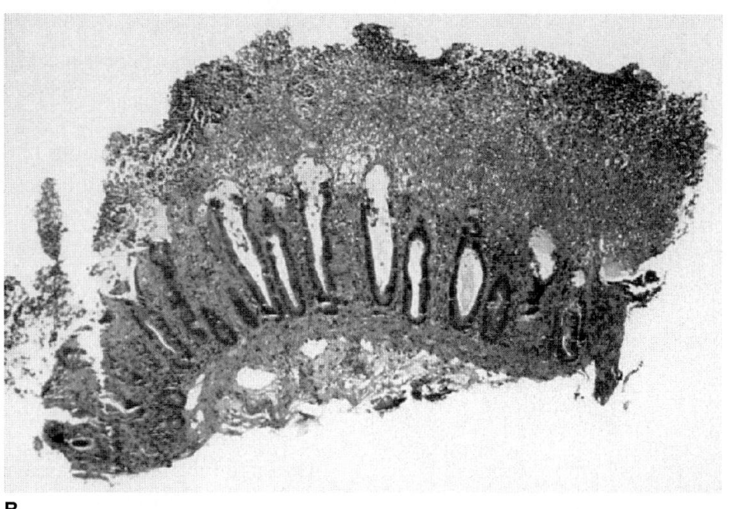

FIGURE 19-4
Clostridium difficile pseudomembranous colitis. The plaques (arrows) on the surface of the intestinal mucosa (A) are composed of inflammatory cells and platelets (B).

cephalosporins, and clindamycin) favors *C. difficile* in two ways. First, strains resistant to the antimicrobic can grow in its presence and assume a larger if not dominant position in the flora. Second, in an antimicrobial milieu, the readiness with which *C. difficile* forms spores may favor its survival over non–spore-forming bacteria. In either case, the minor niche of the species is improved to the point at which the effect of its toxins on the colonic mucosa becomes significant.

Increased numbers make toxin more effective

Although the vast majority of strains produce both toxins, the enterotoxic properties of the A toxin seem to dominate in watery diarrhea cases. In PMC, the colonic mucosa is studded with inflammatory plaques, which may coalesce into an overlying "pseudomembrane" composed of fibrin, leukocytes, and necrotic colonic cells (Fig. 19–4). This picture fits better with the action of the cytotoxic B toxin. It is intriguing that colonized newborn children, who lack the complex flora of adults, rarely suffer any clinical consequences even though toxin production can be demonstrated. The extent to which these differences are due to variability in toxin expression or intestinal receptors is unknown.

A enterotoxin stimulates watery diarrhea

B cytotoxin causes inflammation and pseudomembrane formation

IMMUNITY

Antibody against the A toxin is associated with resolution of disease in experimental animals. This feature and the inverse relationship between severity of disease and anti-A antibody both support the importance of humoral immunity in *C. difficile* diarrhea. Antibodies directed against the B toxin also appear to offer protection, but the relationship is less clear than with toxin A.

Antitoxin antibodies have protective effect

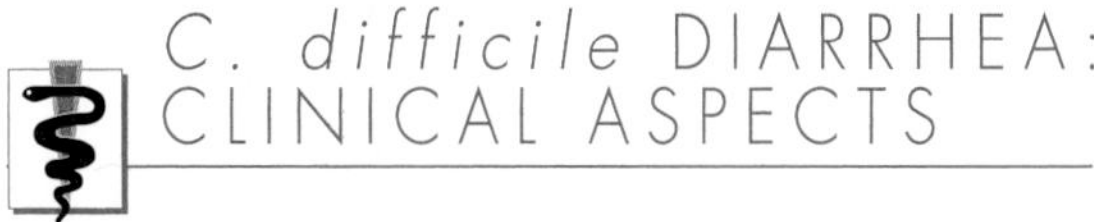

C. difficile DIARRHEA: CLINICAL ASPECTS

MANIFESTATIONS

Diarrhea is a frequent side effect of antimicrobic treatment. In *C. difficile*–caused diarrhea, the onset is usually 5 to 10 days into the antibiotic treatment, but the range is from the first day to weeks after cessation. The diarrhea may be mild and watery or bloody and accompanied by abdominal cramping, leukocytosis, and fever. In PMC, it progresses to a

Diarrhea ranges from mild to PMC

severe, occasionally lethal inflammation of the colon that can be demonstrated by endoscopic examination.

DIAGNOSIS

Stool toxin detection is the primary diagnostic tool

Although selective media have been developed for isolation of *C. difficile,* direct detection of toxins in the stool has largely replaced culture for diagnostic purposes. *C. difficile* is the only pathogen for which detection of its toxin has become routine. The standard toxin assay requires demonstration and neutralization of cytopathic effect in cell culture. Newer enzyme immunoassays, which demonstrate toxin A and/or B in stool, are slightly less sensitive but less expensive and thus more widely available. False-positive results (toxins found but not associated with disease) may occur, particularly among infants.

TREATMENT

Oral metronidazole or vancomycin reach bacteria in the intestine

Discontinuing the implicated antimicrobic usually results in the resolution of clinical symptoms. If patients are severely ill or fail to respond to drug withdrawal, they should receive metronidazole or vancomycin administered orally. The poor absorption of vancomycin is an advantage in this situation, but its use is now being restricted due to concern about its role in selecting resistant enterococci and other organisms. *C. difficile* is susceptible to the penicillins and cephalosporins in vitro, but they are ineffective because of access in the intestinal lumen and the hazard of destruction by β-lactamases produced by other bacteria. Relapses or reinfections requiring retreatment occur in as many as 20% of patients.

BACTEROIDES FRAGILIS

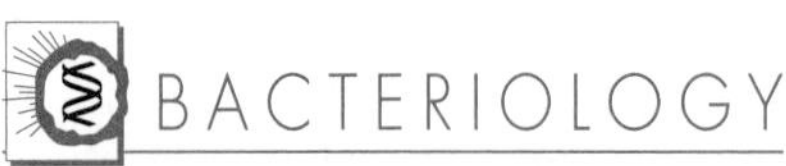

BACTERIOLOGY

Oxygen-tolerant species that produce superoxide dismutase

Polysaccharide capsule is present

The *B. fragilis* group constitute the most common opportunistic pathogens of the genus *Bacteroides*. These slim, pale-staining, capsulate, Gram-negative rods form colonies overnight on blood agar medium. The implication of fragility in the name is misleading, because they are actually among the hardier and more easily grown anaerobes. Most strains produce superoxide dismutase and are relatively tolerant to atmospheric oxygen. *B. fragilis* has surface pili and a capsule composed of a polymer of two polysaccharides. The LPS endotoxin in the *B. fragilis* outer membrane is less toxic than that of most other Gram-negative bacteria, possibly due to modification or absence of the lipid A portion.

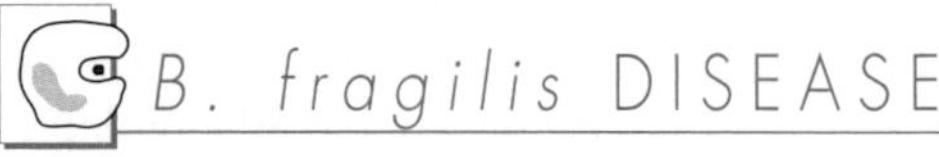

B. fragilis DISEASE

CLINICAL CAPSULE

Deep pain and tenderness anywhere below the diaphragm is typical of the onset of *B. fragilis* infection. Depending on the extent and spread of the intra-abdominal abscess, fever and widespread findings of an acute abdomen may also be seen.

EPIDEMIOLOGY

Endogenous infection mixed with other intestinal bacteria

Like the other Gram-negative anaerobes, *B. fragilis* infections are endogenous, originating in the patient's own intestinal flora. Although *B. fragilis* is among the most common of intestinal anaerobes, the frequent presence of this species in clinically significant infections is striking. It is typically mixed with other anaerobes and facultative bacteria. Human-to-human transmission is not known and seems unlikely.

PATHOGENESIS

The relative oxygen tolerance of *B. fragilis* probably plays a role in its virulence by aiding its survival in oxygenated tissues in the period between its displacement from the intestinal flora and the establishment of a reduced local microenvironment. Its pili have adhesive properties, and the polysaccharide capsule confers resistance to phagocytosis and inhibits macrophage migration. The most distinguishing pathogenic feature of the organism is its ability to cause abscess formation. This capsule experimentally stimulates abscess formation, even in the absence of live bacteria. This property is not found in the capsular polysaccharides of organisms such as *Streptococcus pneumoniae*. *B. fragilis* and other *Bacteroides* species produce a number of extracellular enzymes (collagenase, fibrinolysin, heparinase, hyaluronidase) that may also contribute to the formation of the abscess.

Pili and oxygen-tolerance aid initial stages

Capsule resists phagocytosis and stimulates abscess production

Some strains of *B. fragilis* produce an enterotoxin that causes enteric disease in animals, and in some studies they have been associated a self-limited, watery diarrhea in children. Because these enterotoxin-producing strains are found in up to 10% of healthy individuals, their pathogenic importance is still undetermined.

Diarrheal enterotoxin is possible

IMMUNITY

Although it has been demonstrated that antibody to capsular polysaccharide facilitates classical complement pathway killing, there is no evidence that this confers immunity to reinfection. In contrast, there is some evidence that cell-mediated immunity may be protective.

Cell-mediated immunity may be protective

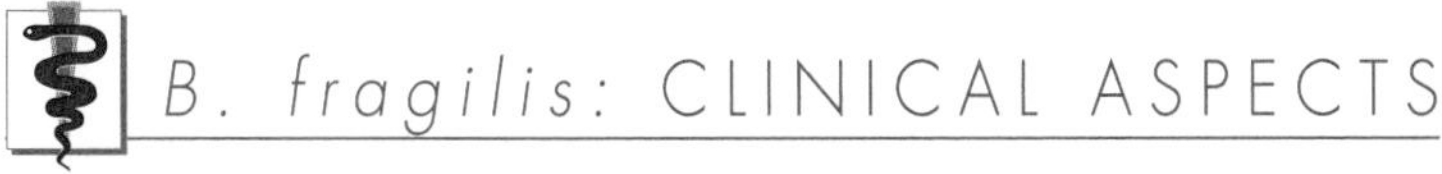

B. fragilis: CLINICAL ASPECTS

MANIFESTATIONS

Some event that displaces *B. fragilis* along with other members of the intestinal flora is required to initiate infection; there is no evidence the organism is invasive on its own. This mucosal break may be the result of trauma or other disease states such as diverticulitis.

The local effects of the developing abscess include abdominal pain and tenderness, often with a low-grade fever. The subsequent course depends on whether the abscess remains localized or ruptures through to other sites such as the peritoneal cavity. This may cause several other abscesses or peritonitis. The course of illness is strongly influenced by the other bacteria in the abscess, particularly members of the Enterobacteriaceae. Spread to the bloodstream is more common with *B. fragilis* than any other anaerobe.

Abdominal pain and fever may evolve to peritonitis

Abscesses combined with anaerobes and Enterobacteriaceae

TREATMENT

Drainage of abscesses and debridement of necrotic tissue are the mainstays of the treatment of *B. fragilis* infections, as with anaerobic infections in general. The accompanying antimicrobial therapy is complicated by the fact that abdominal *B. fragilis* isolates almost always produce a β-lactamase, which not only inactivates penicillin but other β-lactams, including many cephalosporins. Resistance to tetracycline is also common, but most strains are susceptible to chloramphenicol, clindamycin, and metronidazole. Among the β-lactams, cefoxitin and imipenem have been used effectively, as have combinations of a β-lactamase inhibitor (clavulanate, sulbactam) and a β-lactam (ampicillin, ticarcillin).

Cephalosporin resistant to β-lactamase is required

ADDITIONAL READING

Hatheway CL. Toxigenic clostridia. *Clin Microbiol Rev* 1990;3:66–98. A comprehensive review of the historical aspects, organism characteristics, clinical diseases, and toxins of 13 species of clostridia.

Kasper DL, Onderdonk AB. Introduction: International symposium on anaerobic bacteria and bacterial infections. *Rev Infect Dis* 1990;12:S121–S252. This supplemental issue is devoted to the scientific papers given at an international symposium held in Monte Carlo. It is a comprehensive and timely presentation of the microbiologic and structural aspects, pathogenesis, immune mechanisms, susceptibility testing, and management of infections caused by the obligate anaerobes.

Midura TF. Update: Infant botulism. *Clin Microbiol Rev* 1996;9:119–125. This comprehensive review of this puzzling disease puts environmental aspects in perspective.

Murdoch DA. Gram positive anaerobic cocci. *Clin Microbiol Rev* 1998;11:81–120. This review contains more detail about the species of *Peptostreptococcus* than most students need, but the summaries of clinical syndromes are concise and informative.

Mylonakis E, Ryan ET, Calderwood SB. *Clostridium difficile*–associated diarrhea. *Arch Intern Med* 2001;161:525–533. This well-illustrated review includes a complete discussion on the management of *C. difficile* diarrhea.

Schreiner MS, Field E, Ruddy R. Infant botulism: A review of 12 years' experience at the Children's Hospital of Philadelphia. *Pediatrics* 1991;87:159–165. A well-referenced update of this disease.

Weber JT, Hibbs RG Jr, Darwish A, et al. A massive outbreak of type E botulism associated with traditional salted fish in Cairo. *J Infect Dis* 1993;167:451–454. A good example of how botulism can be spread widely.

CHAPTER 20

Neisseria

KENNETH J. RYAN

Neisseria are Gram-negative diplococci. The genus contains two pathogenic and many commensal species, most of which are harmless inhabitants of the upper respiratory and alimentary tracts. The pathogenic species are *Neisseria meningitidis* (meningococcus), a major cause of meningitis and bacteremia, and *Neisseria gonorrhoeae* (gonococcus), the cause of gonorrhea.

NEISSERIA: GENERAL FEATURES

Neisseria are Gram-negative cocci that typically appear in pairs with the opposing sides flattened, imparting a "kidney bean" appearance. They are nonmotile, non-spore forming, and non-acid fast. Their cell walls are typical of Gram-negative bacteria, with a peptidoglycan layer and an outer membrane containing endotoxic glycolipid complexed with protein. The structural elements of *N. meningitidis* and *N. gonorrhoeae* are the same, except that the meningococcus has a polysaccharide capsule external to the cell wall.

Gram-negative diplococci are bean-shaped

Gonococci and meningococci require an aerobic atmosphere with added carbon dioxide and enriched medium for optimal growth. Gonococci grow more slowly and are more fastidious than meningococci, which can grow on routine blood agar. All *Neisseria* are oxidase positive. Species are defined by growth characteristics and patterns of carbohydrate fermentation. Reagents are also available to distinguish *N. gonorrhoeae* and *N. meningitidis* from the other *Neisseria* by immunologic methods such as slide agglutination and immunofluorescence.

Gonococci are more fastidious than meningococci

All *Neisseria* are oxidase positive

Both pathogenic species possess pili, which vary in their antigenic composition, and several classes of outer membrane proteins (OMPs), which also vary antigenically. Various classes of the pili and OMPs of gonococci and meningococci have been separately named, but the structure and functional features of some are similar to each other and to diverse pathogens such as *Pseudomonas aeruginosa* and *Bacteroides* (Table 20–1). The outer membrane of pathogenic *Neisseria* contains a variant of lipopolysaccharide (LPS) in which the side chains are shorter and lack the repeating polysaccharide units found in the LPS of most other Gram-negative bacteria. This short chain neisserial LPS is called lipooligosaccharide (LOS). The lipid A and core oligosaccharide are structurally and functionally similar to other Gram-negative LPS. The pili, OMPs, and LOS are antigenic and have been used in typing schemes.

Pili and OMPs are present in both species

Outer membrane LOS has short side chains

TABLE 20–1

Bacteriologic and Pathogenic Features of *Neisseria*

	Growth		Antigenic Structure						
					Outer Membrane Proteins				
Organism	Blood Agar	ML Agar[a]	Capsule	Pili	Adherence-Associated	Porins	Blocking AB-Associated[b]	Transmission	Disease
N. meningitidis	+	+	Polysaccharide (12 serogroups[c])	Class I,[d] II Antigenically diverse	Class 5 (4 variants)	PorA, PorB[e]	Class 4	Inhalation of respiratory droplets	Meningitis, septic shock
N. gonorrhoeae	−	+	None[f]	Antigenically diverse[d]	Protein II or Opa (12 variants)	Protein I (A and B)	Protein III	Sexual contact of mucosal surfaces	Urethritis, cervicitis, PID
Other *Neisseria* species	+	−	None	Present	Unknown	Unknown	Absent	Normal respiratory flora	None

Abbreviations: PID, pelvic inflammatory disease.

[a] Martin–Lewis or similar selective medium.

[b] Bind IgG in a way that interferes with bactericidal activity of antibodies directed at other antigens.

[c] A, B, C, H, I, K, L, X, Y, Z, 29E, W-135.

[d] Gonococcal and meningococcal class I are similar to each other and members of a class of bacterial pili with amino-terminal *N*-methylphenylalanine residues (*Bacteroides, Moraxella, Pseudomonas aeruginosa*).

[e] Two classes, similar to gonococcal protein I (A and B).

[f] LOS sialylation has some of the effects of a capsule (see text).

NEISSERIA MENINGITIDIS

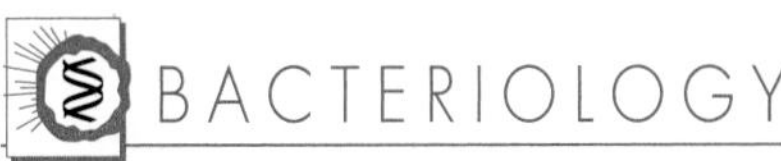

BACTERIOLOGY

Meningococci produce medium-sized smooth colonies on blood agar plates after overnight incubation. Carbon dioxide enhances growth, but is not required. Twelve serogroups have been defined on the basis of the antigenic specificity of a polysaccharide capsule. The most important disease-producing serogroups are A, B, C, W-135, and Y. In addition to the group polysaccharides, individual *N. meningitidis* strains may contain two distinct classes of pili and multiple classes of OMPs. Some OMPs, porins, and adherence proteins have structural and functional similarities to those found in gonococci (see Table 20–1). The function of other OMPs is unknown.

Serogroups are based on the polysaccharide capsule

Some OMPs are similar to gonococci

MENINGOCOCCAL DISEASE

CLINICAL CAPSULE

Meningococci are usually quiescent members of the nasopharyngeal flora but may produce fulminant infection of the bloodstream and/or central nervous system (CNS). There is little warning; localized infections that precede systemic spread are rarely recognized. The major disease is an acute, purulent meningitis with fever, headache, seizures, and mental signs secondary to inflammation and increased intracranial pressure. Even when the CNS is not involved, *N. meningitidis* infections have a marked tendency to be accompanied by rash, purpura, thrombocytopenia, and other manifestations associated with endotoxemia. This bacterium causes one of the few infections in which patients may progress from normal health to death in less than a day.

EPIDEMIOLOGY

Meningococci are found in the nasopharyngeal flora of approximately 10% of healthy individuals. Transmission occurs by inhalation of aerosolized respiratory droplets. Close, prolonged contact such as occurs in families and closed populations promotes transmission. The estimated attack rate among family members residing with an index case is 1000 times higher than in the general population; this fact is evidence of the contagious nature of meningococcal infection. Other factors that foster transmission are contact with a virulent strain and susceptibility (lack of protective antibody). Typical settings of larger outbreaks are schools, dormitories, and camps for military recruits. In these close living circumstances, *N. meningitidis* spreads readily among newly exposed individuals, but disease develops only in those who lack group-specific antibody.

Nasopharyngeal carrier rate is 10%

Spread in is by respiratory droplets

The annual incidence of meningococcal infections in the United States varies between 0.5 and 1.5 cases per 100,000 population. Most cases are in children under 6 years of age. They occur as isolated cases, as sporadic small epidemics, or in small family or closed-population (school or day-care center) outbreaks. B, C, and Y are the most common serogroups involved. Group A strains are generally rare but historically have a more ominous epidemiologic potential. For unknown reasons, group A meningococci have the capability to cause widespread epidemics sweeping through communities, even countries. In the past these have appeared in 8- to 12-year cycles. It has been more than 40 years since group A strains have been responsible for significant disease in the United States, although epidemics have occurred in Brazil, China, the Sudan, Kenya, and South Africa.

B, C, and Y are the most common serogroups

Group A strains can cause widespread epidemics

PATHOGENESIS

Meningococci range from carrier state to bacteremia

Pili attach to microvilli as prelude to invasion

The meningococcus is an exclusively human parasite; it can either exist as an apparently harmless member of the normal flora or produce acute disease. For most individuals, the carrier state is associated with acquisition of protective antibodies, but for some, spread from the nasopharynx to produce bacteremia, endotoxemia, and meningitis takes place too quickly for immunity to develop. Meningococci use pili for initial attachment to the microvilli of the nonciliated nasopharyngeal epithelium as a prelude to invasion. In the invasion process, the microvilli come in close contact with the bacteria, which then enter the cells in membrane-bound vesicles. Once inside meningococci quickly pass through the cytoplasm, exiting into the submucosa on the other side. In the process they damage the ciliated cells, possibly by direct release of endotoxin.

Proteins scavenge iron from transferrin

Polysaccharide capsules are antiphagocytic

LOS + sialic acid interferes with complement deposition

Once meningococci gain access to the submucosa, their ability to produce disease is enhanced by several factors that allow them to scavenge essential nutrients and evade the host immune response. One critical nutrient, iron, is supplied by *N. meningitidis* proteins, which are able to acquire it from the human iron transport protein transferrin. As with other encapsulated bacteria, the polysaccharide capsule enables meningococci to resist complement-mediated bactericidal activity and subsequent neutrophil phagocytosis. Meningococcal (and gonococcal) LPS/LOS also has features that facilitate evasion of host immune responses. Its chemical structure mimics sphingolipids found in the human brain enough for them to be recognized as self by the immune system. In addition, meningococci are able to incorporate sialic acid from host substrates as terminal substitutions of their LOS side chains. This sialyated LOS is able to downregulate complement deposition by binding serum factor H in a manner already described for streptococcal surface molecules such as group B streptococcal capsular sialic acid (see Chapter 17). The capsules of group B and C meningococci are also polymers of sialic acid.

Spread to blood and CNS produce systemic endotoxemia

LPS and peptidoglycan trigger cytokine release

Shedding outer membrane blebs hyperproduces LPS

The most serious manifestations of meningococcal disease are related to its spread to the bloodstream and, its namesake, the meninges. The exact mechanism of CNS invasion is unclear but is probably related to the level of the bacteremia. It occurs in the choroid plexus with its exceptionally high rate of blood flow. After CNS invasion, an intense subarachnoid space inflammatory response is generated, induced by the release of cell wall peptidoglycan fragments, LPS, and possibly other virulence factors causing the release of inflammatory cytokines. A prominent feature of meningococcal disease with or without CNS invasion is disseminated, potent, endotoxic activity (see Manifestations). When grown in culture, *N. meningitidis* readily releases endotoxin-containing blebs of its outer membrane from the cell surface as shown in Fig 20–1. It is not known whether this occurs in vivo, but the model of the meningococcus as a hyperproducer of LPS endotoxin certainly fits with its most serious disease manifestations.

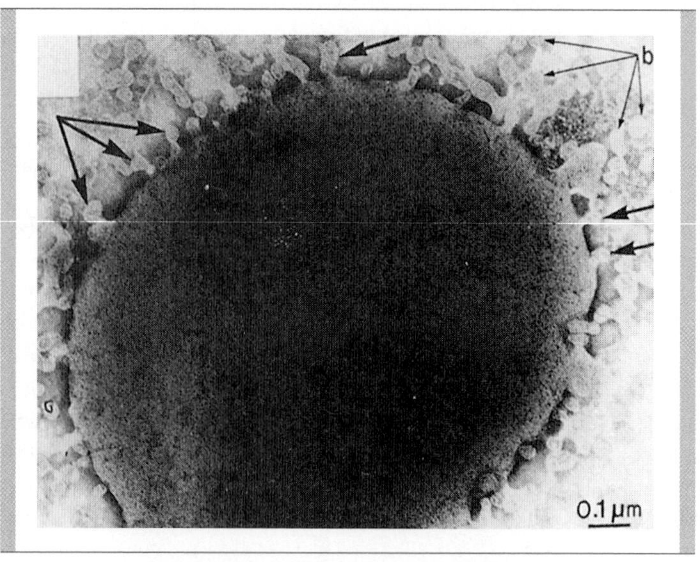

FIGURE 20–1
Neisseria meningitidis. Cell wall is shown shedding multiple "blebs" (*arrows*) containing lipopolysaccharide–endotoxin. Note the typical trilamellar Gram-negative cell wall structure in the wall and the blebs. (*Reprinted with permission from Devoe IW, Gilcrist JE.* J Exp Med *1973;138:1160, Figure 3.*)

IMMUNITY

Immunity to meningococcal infections is related to group-specific antipolysaccharide antibody, which is bactericidal and facilitates phagocytosis. The bactericidal activity is due to complement-mediated cell lysis via the classical complement pathway. Individuals with deficiencies in the terminal complement components have an enhanced risk for meningococcal disease but not for other polysaccharide capsule pathogens such as *Haemophilus influenzae* type b (see Chapter 24).

Group-specific anticapsular antibody is protective

Complement component deficiencies enhance risk

The peak incidence of serious infection is between 6 months and 2 years of age. This corresponds to the nadir in the prevalence of antibody in the general population, which is the time between loss of transplacental antibody and the appearance of naturally acquired antibody (Fig 20–2). By adult life, serum antibody to one or more meningococcal serogroups is usually present but an immune deficit to the other serogroups remains. Infections appear when populations carrying virulent strains mix with susceptible individuals lacking group-specific antibody.

Most common age of infection is 6–24 months

Absence of antibody correlates with susceptibility

Protective antibody is stimulated by infection and through the carrier state, which produces immunity within a few weeks. Natural immunization may not require colonization with every serogroup or even with *N. meningitidis,* because antibody may be produced in response to cross-reactive polysaccharides possessed by other *Neisseria* or even other genera. For example, *Escherichia coli* strains of a particular serotype (K1) have a polysaccharide capsule identical to that of the group B meningococcus. These *E. coli* also have enhanced potential to produce meningitis in neonates.

Infection, carrier state, or other polysaccharides may stimulate antibody

Purified capsular polysaccharides are immunogenic, generating T cell–independent immune responses in which IgG_2 is the predominant antibody. As with other polysaccharide immunogens, these responses are not strong, particularly in early childhood when there is a relative deficiency of IgG_2. The group B polysaccharide differs from that of the other groups in failing to stimulate bactericidal antibody at all. This is believed to be due

T cell–independent mechanisms are involved

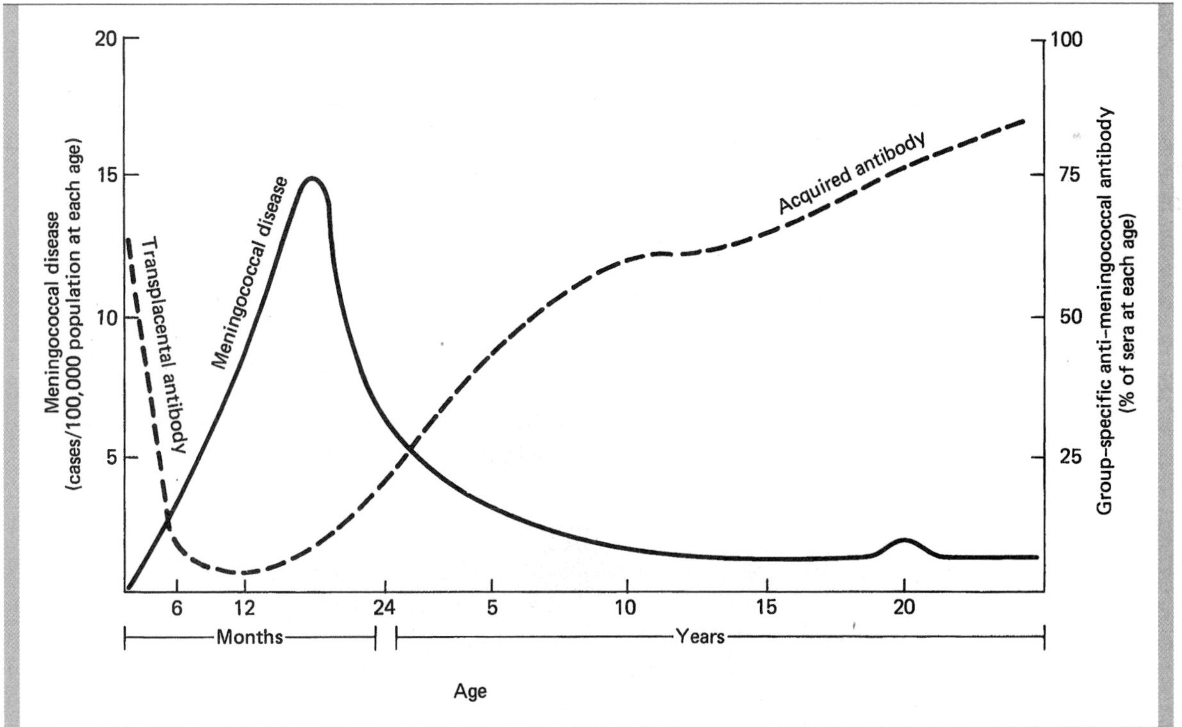

FIGURE 20–2
Immunity to the meningococcus. The inverse relationship between bactericidal meningococcal antibody and meningococcal disease is demonstrated. The "blip" in the disease curve around age 20 is attributable in part to military and other closed-population outbreaks. (*Adapted with permission from Goldschneider I, Gotschlich EC, Liu TY, Artenstein MS. Human immunity to the meningococcus I–V.* J Exp Med *1969;129:1307–1395.*)

Group B polysaccharide is not immunogenic

to the similarity of its sialic acid polymer to human brain antigens. That is, like the sialated LOS, it may be recognized as self by the immune system.

OMPs may be important in immunity

Exposed outer membrane proteins have also been shown to stimulate bactericidal antibody. Antibody directed against the porin PorA has demonstrated protection in animal models. PorA is present in the outer membrane of almost all meningococcal isolates but is subject to considerable antigenic variation.

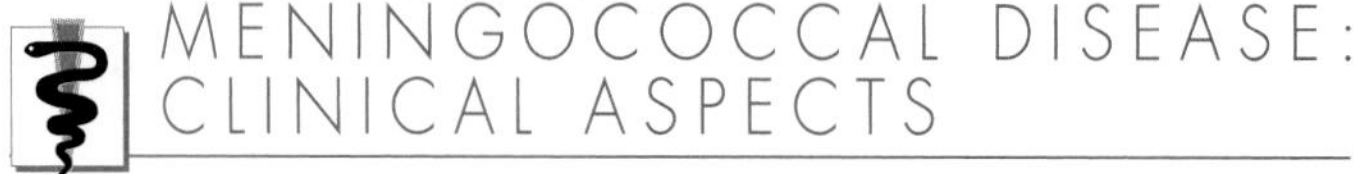

MENINGOCOCCAL DISEASE: CLINICAL ASPECTS

MANIFESTATIONS

Meningitis is most frequent infection

Meningococcemia and rash may progress to DIC

Systemic features resemble endotoxic shock

The most frequent form of meningococcal infection is acute purulent meningitis, with clinical and laboratory features similar to those of meningitis from other causes (see Chapter 67). A prominent feature of meningococcal meningitis is the appearance of scattered skin petechiae, which may evolve into ecchymoses or a diffuse petechial rash. These cutaneous manifestations are signs of the disseminated intravascular coagulation (DIC) syndrome that is part of the endotoxic shock brought on by meningococcal bacteremia (meningococcemia). Meningococcemia sometimes occurs without meningitis and may progress to fulminant DIC and shock with bilateral hemorrhagic destruction of the adrenal glands (Waterhouse–Friderichsen syndrome). However, the disease is not always fulminant, and some patients have only low-grade fever, arthritis, and skin lesions that develop slowly over a period of days to weeks. Meningococci are a rare cause of other infections such as pneumonia, but it is striking that localized infections are almost never recognized in advance of systemic disease.

DIAGNOSIS

Direct CSF Gram smears are diagnostic

Culture requires only blood agar

Direct Gram smears of cerebrospinal fluid (CSF) in meningitis usually demonstrate the typical bean-shaped, Gram-negative diplococci. Definitive diagnosis is by culture of CSF, blood, or skin lesions. Although *N. meningitidis* is reputed to be somewhat fragile, it requires no special handling for isolation from presumptively sterile sites such as blood and CSF. Growth is good on blood or chocolate agar after 18 hours of incubation. Speciation is based on carbohydrate degradation patterns or immunologic tests. Serogrouping may be performed by slide agglutination methods but has no immediate clinical importance.

TREATMENT

Penicillin resistance is still rare

Penicillin is the treatment of choice for meningococcal infections because of its antimeningococcal activity and good CSF penetration. Resistance mediated by both β-lactamase and altered penicillin-binding proteins (PBPs) has been reported but is still extremely rare. Third-generation cephalosporins such as cefotaxime are effective alternatives to penicillin.

PREVENTION

Rifampin is primary antimicrobic for chemoprophylaxis

Close contact with case is indication for prophylaxis

Until the development and spread of sulfonamide resistance in the 1960s, chemoprophylaxis with these agents was the primary means of preventing spread of meningococcal infections. Rifampin is now the primary chemoprophylactic agent, but ciprofloxacin has also been effective. Penicillin is not effective, probably because of inadequate penetration of the uninflamed nasopharyngeal mucosa. Selection of cases to receive prophylaxis is based on epidemiologic assessment. Risk is highest for siblings of the index case and declines with increasing age and less close contact. For example, an infant sibling sharing the same room as an affected individual would be at the highest risk. Typically, family members are given prophylaxis, but other adults are not. Common-sense exceptions, such as playmates and healthcare workers with very close contact (eg, mouth-to-mouth resuscitation), are made at the discretion of the physician. The presence or absence of nasopharyngeal carriage of *N. meningitidis* plays no role in this decision, because it does not accurately predict risk of disease.

Purified polysaccharide meningococcal vaccines have been shown to prevent group A and C disease in military and civilian populations, and a quadrivalent vaccine containing A, C, Y, and W-135 polysaccharides is now licensed for use in the United States. Meningococcal vaccines are currently used to control epidemics in populations at particular risk such as in military recruits and in those with unique predisposing factors such as complement deficiencies or asplenia. Routine immunization of children is not recommended.

A, C, Y, and W-135 polysaccharide vaccines are useful in high-risk populations

This reluctance for widespread use of meningococcal polysaccharide vaccines is ironic, because it was their development that led to the success of other vaccines made from capsular polysaccharides (see Additional Reading). Like other pure polysaccharides, these vaccines are ineffective in young children, because they stimulate immune responses that are underdeveloped in the first year of life (see Immunity).

Protein conjugate vaccines may enhance immunogenicity in children

With *H. influenzae* and now *Streptococcus pneumoniae,* this problem has been overcome by the development of polysaccharide–protein conjugate vaccines, which stimulate T cell–dependent responses (see Chapter 24). The protein conjugate approach, which is under investigation with *N. meningitidis,* faces a difficulty not shared by these other two pathogens—the failure of the group B polysaccharide to be immunogenic at all. If this is due to its similarity to human brain antigens, as suspected, it may not be overcome simply by protein conjugation. Group B causes one third of all disease, so no vaccine that omits it is likely to be completely successful. For this reason, other approaches such as the use of OMPs (eg, PorA) are being pursued. Genetically engineered vaccines based on the sequence of the entire group B meningococcal genome hold the promise of defining proteins that would immunize against all serogroups of *N. meningitidis.*

Nonimmunogenic serogroup B polysaccharide remains a problem

PorA and other OMPs are vaccine candidates

NEISSERIA GONORRHOEAE

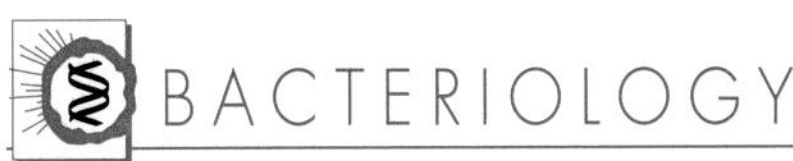

BACTERIOLOGY

N. gonorrhoeae grows well only on chocolate agar and on specialized medium enriched to ensure its growth. It requires carbon dioxide supplementation. Small, smooth, nonpigmented colonies appear after 18 to 24 hours and are well developed (2 to 4 mm) after 48 hours. Gonococci possess numerous pili that extend through and beyond the outer membrane (Fig 20–3), which are structurally similar to those of meningococci (see Table 20–1). In general, only fresh virulent isolates have pili.

Chocolate agar and CO_2 are required

Fresh isolates have pili

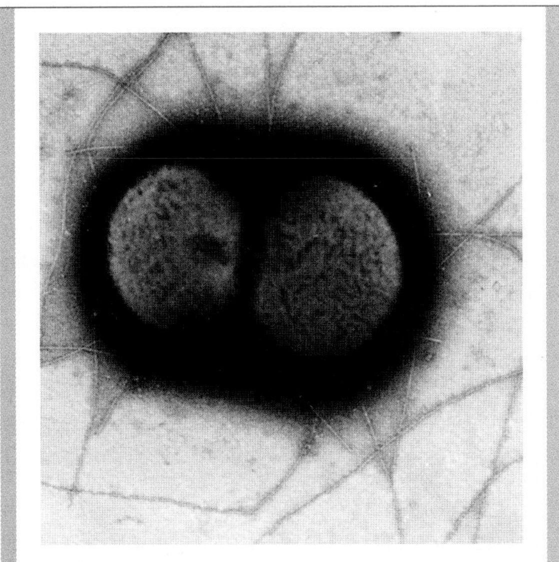

FIGURE 20–3
Neisseria gonorrhoeae. Surface pili are shown. These structures are associated with virulence and may mediate initial attachment to epithelial surfaces. (*Courtesy of Dr. John Swanson.*)

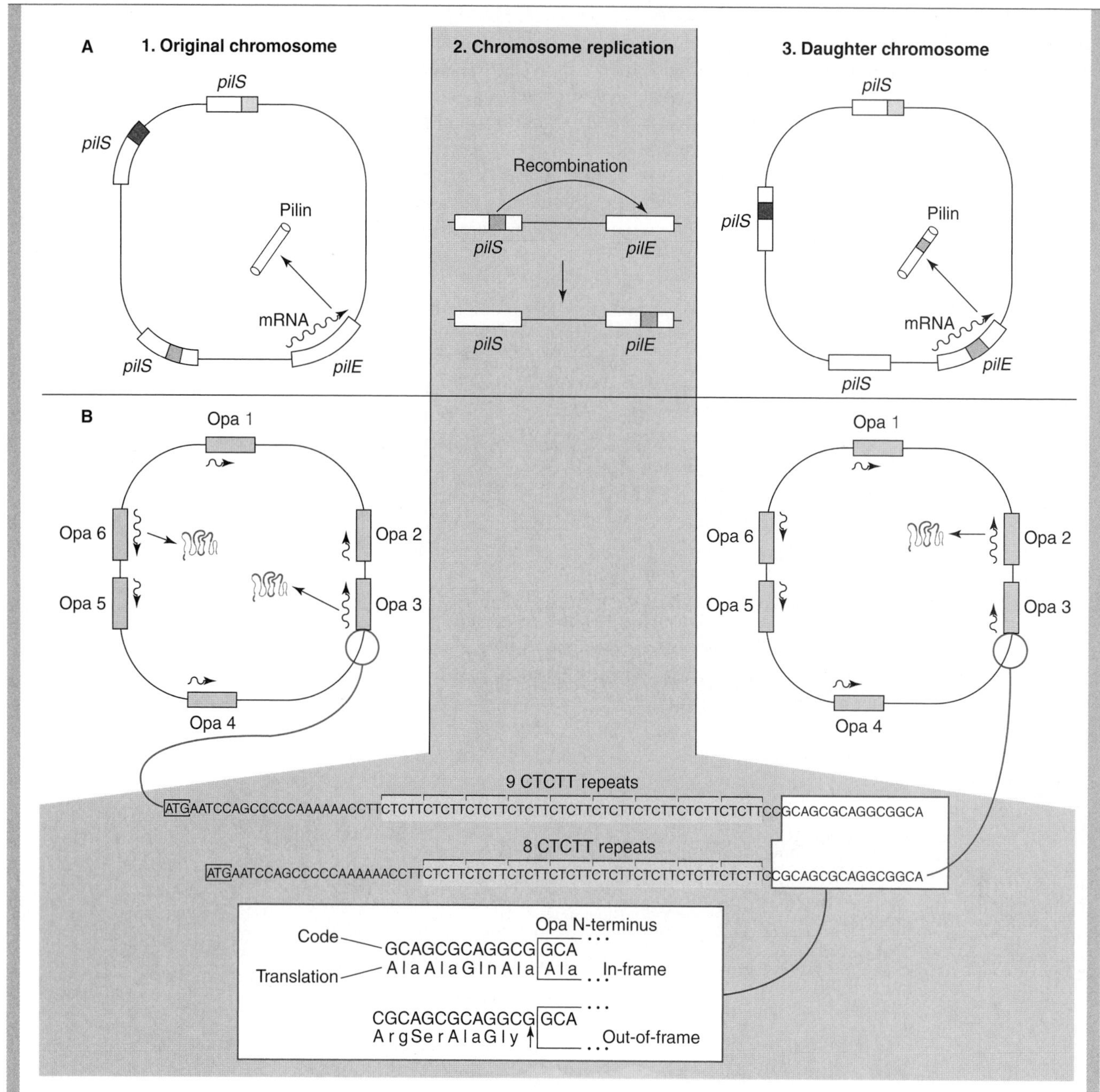

FIGURE 20–4

Antigenic variation of gonococci showing the mechanisms for change in the antigenic makeup of both pili and outer membrane Opa proteins. **A**. The chromosome contains multiple unlinked pilin genes, which are either expressing (*pilE*) or silent (*pilS*). The expressing gene is transcribing a mature pilin protein subunit. During chromosome replication, one of the *pilS* genes recombines with one of the *pilE* genes, donating some of its DNA. The new daughter chromosome now produces an antigenically different pilin based on transcription of the donated sequences into protein. **B.** The chromosome contains multiple Opa genes. Opa 3 and Opa 6 are "on" (producing protein), and the others are "off." During chromosome replication, replicative slippage in the leader peptide causes a five-base sequence (CTCTT) to be repeated variable numbers of times. Translation of the Opa will remain in-frame only if the number of added CTCTT nucleotides is evenly divisible by three. For the Opa gene in **B1**, the triplet code for alanine (GCA) is in-frame ($9 \times 5 = 45 \div 3 = 15$) but the **B3** it is out-of-frame.

The gonococcal outer membrane is composed of phospholipids, LPS, LOS, and several distinct OMPs. The OMPs include porins (proteins IA and IB) and adherence proteins known as Opa or protein II. Opa proteins are a set of at least 12 proteins that get their name from the opaque appearance they give to colonies as a result of adhesion between gonococcal cells. A variable number of the Opa proteins may be expressed at any one time.

LPS, LOS, and OMPs are in outer membrane

Opa proteins are adherence OMPs

ANTIGENIC VARIATION

N. gonorrhoeae and *N. meningitidis* are among several microorganisms whose surface structures are known to change antigenically from generation to generation during growth of a single strain. The mechanisms involved have been more extensively studied in gonococci but appear to be similar in both species. The antigenic structures of major interest are pili, Opa proteins, and LOS, for which there is evidence of antigenic variation both in vitro and in vivo. The genetic mechanisms involved are illustrated in Figure 20–4.

Pili, OMPs, and LOS vary in gonococci and meningococci

Gonococcal pili are antigenically variable to an extraordinary extent. There are multiple genetic mechanisms, but the most important one appears to be recombinational exchange between the multiple pilin genes present in the chromosome of every strain. Some of these genes are complete and able to express pilin (*pilE*). Others are not due to lack of an effective promoter and are thus silent (*pilS*). When recombination between expression and silent loci results in the donation of new sequences to an expression locus, the result can be expression of a pilin with changes in its amino acid composition and thus its antigenicity. The recombination could also involve exogenous DNA from another cell or strain, because gonococci naturally take up species-specific DNA by transformation. The process is complex, involving other genes that play a role in the assembly of pili and their functional characteristics, such as cellular adhesion. The numerous possible outcomes include no pilin subunits, pilin subunits unable to assemble, mature pili with altered functional characteristics, and fully functional pili with a new antigenic makeup.

Genes for pilin subunits may be expressive or silent

Recombination between multiple genes occurs

Outcome may be nonfunctional or antigenically altered pili

The multiple gonococcal Opa proteins are each encoded by separate genes scattered around the genome. Various combinations of these genes may be either "on" or "off" at any one time. It has been observed that this switching between different Opa proteins occurs at a high rate per cell per generation. Control of the switch is via the number of repeats of a pentameric sequence (CTCTT) within the leader peptide encoding region of the gene. These are created by replicative slippage—a kind of "stuttering" during transcription. The number of repeats of this sequence varies widely (7 to 28), and when it comes time for translation the number of repeats determines whether the gene will be in or out of frame to translate the protein (Figure 20–4, B). Thus, by virtue of a translational frame shift mechanism, each Opa gene has its own switch, which can change with every cell cycle.

Multiple Opa genes may be "on" or "off"

Translational frame shift controls the switch

Variation in gonococcal LOS has been observed in volunteer subjects challenged with intraurethral *N. gonorrhoeae,* but the genetic mechanism is unknown. Taken together, these multifactorial, antigenic variations of the gonococcal surface may serve the dual purposes of escape from immune surveillance and timely provision of the ligands required to bind to human cell receptors.

LOS also varies antigenically

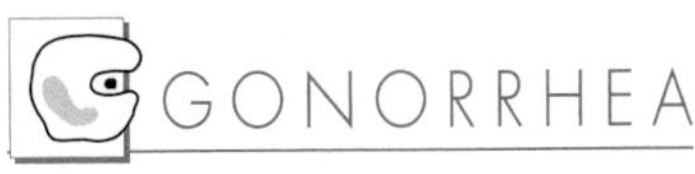

GONORRHEA

CLINICAL CAPSULE

In contrast to meningococcal disease, gonorrhea is primarily localized to mucosal surfaces with relatively infrequent spread to the bloodstream or deep tissues. Infection is sexually acquired by direct genital contact, and the primary manifestation is pain and purulent discharge at the infected site. In men, this is typically the urethra, and in women, the uterine cervix. Direct extension of the infection up the fallopian tubes produces fever and lower abdominal pain, a syndrome called pelvic inflammatory disease (PID). For women, sterility or ectopic pregnancy can be long-term consequences of gonorrhea.

EPIDEMIOLOGY

Rates among adolescents are very high and increasing

Inability to detect asymptomatic cases hampers control

Although official reports of gonorrhea in the United States, which represent approximately 50% of the true cases, have been declining for 20 years, the disease is still one of our greatest public health problems. The overall incidence is now 130 cases per 100,000 population, but the rates for adolescents are alarmingly high and increasing by 10% a year. The highest rates are in women between the ages of 15 and 19 years (761/100,000) and men between the ages of 20 and 24 years (564/100,000). No truly effective means of control is yet in sight. Our ability to stem the tide of changed sexual mores continues to be hampered by lack of an effective means to detect asymptomatic cases, resistance of *N. gonorrhoeae* to antibiotics (see Treatment), and, to some extent, lack of appreciation of the importance of this disease. The latter is evidenced by failure of patients to seek medical care and of physicians to report cases to public health authorities in order to protect the privacy of their patients. In the minds of too many, syphilis is dreaded and "unclean," whereas gonorrhea is only "the clap" ("clap" is from the archaic French clapoir, "a rabbit warren"; later, "a brothel").

Risk of sexual contact is up to 50%

Asymptomatic cases are highest in women

Nonsexual transmission is rare

The major reservoir for continued spread of gonorrhea is the asymptomatic patient. Screening programs and case contact studies have shown that almost 50% of infected women are asymptomatic or at least do not have symptoms usually associated with venereal infection. Most men (95%) have acute symptoms with infection. Many who are not treated become asymptomatic but remain infectious. Asymptomatic male and female patients can remain infectious for months. The attack rates for those engaging in genital intercourse with an infected patient are estimated to be 20 to 50%. The organism may also be transmitted by oral–genital contact or by rectal intercourse. When all of these factors operate in a sexually active population, it is easy to explain the high prevalence of gonorrhea. Although gonococci can survive for brief periods on toilet seats, nonsexual transmission is extremely rare. Fomite transmission of a purulent vulvovaginitis in prepubescent girls has been reported, but virtually all gonococci isolated from children can be traced to sexual abuse by an infected adult.

PATHOGENESIS

Attachment and Invasion

Pili and Opa proteins mediate attachment to nonciliated epithelium

Gonococci are not normal inhabitants of the respiratory or genital flora. When introduced onto a mucosal surface by sexual contact with an infected individual, adherence ligands such as pili, Opa proteins, and possibly LOS allow initial attachment of the bacteria to receptors (CD46, CD66) on nonciliated epithelial cells. Pili are the primary mediators of adherence to urethral and vaginal epithelium, nonciliated fallopian tube cells, sperm, and neutrophils. Opa proteins are involved in cervical and urethral epithelial cell adherence and in adhesion between gonococcal cells.

Invasion initiated by protein IA and Opa proteins

Bacteria pass to submucosa

Following attachment, gonococci invade epithelial cells. The microvilli surround the bacteria and appear to draw them into the host cell in the same manner as meningococci. This process is called **parasite-directed endocytosis** because it appears to be initiated by bacterial rather than host cell factors and involves cells which are not ordinarily phagocytic. Gonococcal OMPs such as protein IA and some of the Opa proteins appear to facilitate this process. Once inside, the bacteria transcytose the cell and exit through the basal membrane to enter the submucosa.

Survival in the Submucosa

Receptors scavenge iron

Sialated LOS acts like a capsule

Once in the submucosa, the bacteria must survive and resist innate host defenses as well as defenses that may have been acquired from previous infection. As with meningococci, receptors on the gonococcal surface enable the organisms to scavenge iron needed for growth from the human iron transport proteins transferrin and lactoferrin. Although gonococci lack the polysaccharide capsule of the meningococcus, they still have multiple mechanisms that protect them against serum complement and antibody. One of these, LOS sialyation, appears to provide a mechanism for blocking C3b deposition that is identical to that of the encapsulated bacteria. In a sense, the gonococci create their own "capsule" by incorporating host sialic acid into their LOS. Another mechanism for phenotypic serum resistance is the binding of antibodies to another class of OMPs found in both gonococci and meningococci (see Table 20–1). IgG bound to these OMPs appears to block the bactericidal activity of antibodies directed against other surface antigens such as protein I. Blocking antibodies have been found in patients with repeated gonococcal infection.

Some antibodies to OMPs have blocking effect on bactericidal activity

Even when phagocytes do encounter gonococci, surface factors such as pili and Opa proteins interfere with effective phagocytosis. The organisms are also able to defend against oxidative killing inside the phagocyte by upregulation of catalase production. Taken together, these factors provide ample evidence that killing by neutrophils is sufficiently retarded to allow prolonged survival of gonococci in mucosal and submucosal locations.

Phagocytosed gonococci resist killing

Spread and Dissemination

In contrast to meningococci, *N. gonorrhoeae* bacteria tend to remain localized to genital structures, causing inflammation and local injury, which no doubt facilitate their continued venereal transmission. Purulent exudates containing "sticky" clusters of gonococci held together by Opa proteins could be the primary infectious unit. Infection may spread to deeper structures by progressive extension to adjacent mucosal and glandular epithelial cells. These include the prostate and epididymis in men and the paracervical glands and the fallopian tubes in women. Spread to the fallopian tubes may be facilitated by pilus-mediated attachment to sperm and then to the microvilli of nonciliated fallopian tube cells. Injury to the fallopian epithelium seems to be mediated by LPS/LOS and fragments of gonococcal cell wall peptidoglycan. Gonococci are known to turn over their peptidoglycan rapidly during exponential growth, releasing peptidoglycan fragments into the local environment. Injury by this mechanism has been demonstrated in fallopian tube organ cultures and presumably may also operate at other sites.

Disease remains localized

Local spread is to epididymis and fallopian tubes

Peptidoglycan shedding causes local injury

In a small proportion of infection, organisms reach the bloodstream to produce disseminated gonococcal infection (DGI). When this happens, the systemic findings have their own pattern (see Manifestations) and seldom take on the endotoxic shock picture of meningococcemia. Although differences have been noted between *N. gonorrhoeae* strains that remain localized and those that produce DGI, their connection to pathogenesis is unknown. Both DGI and salpingitis tend to begin during or shortly after completion of menses. This may relate to changes in the cervical mucus and reflux into the fallopian tubes during menses.

DGI differs from meningococcal endotoxic shock

Reflux during menses may facilitate spread

Genetic Regulation of Virulence

Through all the stages of gonorrhea, gonococci are able to use a particularly rich variety of genetic mechanisms in deployment of the virulence factors described above at the right time. Some are regulatory responses to environmental cues, such as iron in relation to iron-binding proteins, while others involve the changes in the genome. Antigenic changes in both pili and Opa proteins have been demonstrated in human infection, including the isolation of antigenic variants from different sites in the same patient. These presumably take place by the recombinational and translational mechanisms (see Antigenic Variation) as the organisms replicate in the patient.

Regulation, recombination, and translational changes deploy virulence factors

IMMUNITY

The apparent lack of immunity to gonococcal infection has long been a mystery. Among sexually active persons with multiple partners, repeated infections are the rule rather than the exception. Both serum and secretory antibodies are generated during natural infection but the levels are generally low, even after repeated infections. Another aspect is that even when antibodies are formed, antigenic variation defeats their effectiveness and allows the gonococcus to escape immune surveillance. Antigenic variation of pili, Opa proteins, and LOS is particularly likely to be important. Outbreaks have been traced to a single strain that demonstrated multiple pilin variations and Opa types in repeated isolates from the same individual or from sexual partners. In experimental models, passive administration of antibody directed against one pilin type has been followed by emergence of new pilin variants. Changes in Opa proteins may also occur, as suggested by differences in its expression in mucosal versus tubal isolates. It appears that although some immunity to gonococcal infection is present, its effectiveness is compromised by the ability of the organism to change key structures during the course of infection.

Antibody response is weak

Gonococcus varies multiple structures to avoid immune surveillance

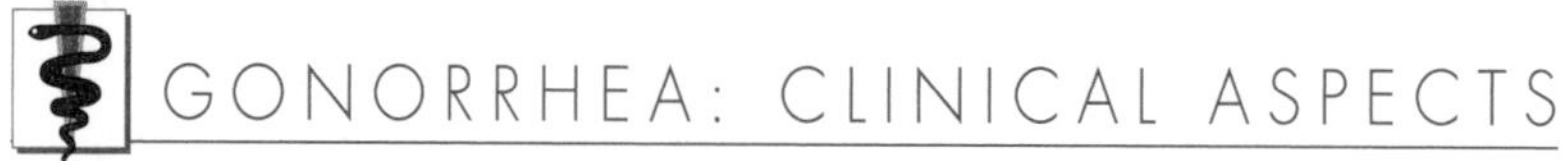

GONORRHEA: CLINICAL ASPECTS

MANIFESTATIONS

Genital Gonorrhea

In men, the primary site of infection is the urethra. Symptoms begin 2 to 7 days after infection and consist primarily of purulent urethral discharge and dysuria. Although uncommon, local extension can lead to epididymitis or prostatitis. The endocervix is the primary site in women, in whom symptoms include increased vaginal discharge, urinary frequency, dysuria, abdominal pain, and menstrual abnormalities. As mentioned previously, symptoms may be mild or absent in either sex, particularly women.

Urethritis and endocervicitis are primary infections

Other Local Infections

Rectal gonorrhea occurs after rectal intercourse or, in women, after contamination with infected vaginal secretions. This condition is generally asymptomatic but may cause tenesmus, discharge, and rectal bleeding. Pharyngeal gonorrhea is transmitted by oral–genital sex and, again, is usually asymptomatic. Sore throat and cervical adenitis may occur. Infection of other structures near primary infection sites, such as Bartholin's glands in women, may lead to abscess formation.

Rectal and pharyngeal infections relate to sexual practices

Inoculation of gonococci into the conjunctiva produces a severe, acute, purulent conjunctivitis. Although this infection may occur at any age, the most serious form is gonococcal ophthalmia neonatorum, a disease acquired by a newborn from an infected mother. The disease was formerly a common cause of blindness, which is now prevented by the use of prophylactic topical eye drops or ointment (silver nitrate, erythromycin, or tetracycline) at birth.

Transmission at birth causes ophthalmia neonatorum

Pelvic Inflammatory Disease (PID)

The clinical syndrome of PID develops in 10% to 20% of women with gonorrhea. The findings include fever, lower abdominal pain (usually bilateral), adnexal tenderness, and leukocytosis with or without signs of local infection. These features are caused by spread of organisms along the fallopian tubes to produce salpingitis and into the pelvic cavity to produce pelvic peritonitis and abscesses. PID is also known to develop when other genital pathogens ascend by the same route. These organisms include anaerobes and *Chlamydia trachomatis,* which may appear alone or mixed with gonococci. The most serious complications of PID are infertility and ectopic pregnancy secondary to scarring of the fallopian tubes.

Salpingitis and pelvic peritonitis cause scaring and infertility

Disseminated Gonococcal Infection (DGI)

Any of the local forms of gonorrhea or their extensions such as PID may lead to bacteremia. In the bacteremic phase, the primary features are fever; migratory polyarthralgia; and a petechial, maculopapular, or pustular rash. Some of these features may be immunologically mediated; gonococci are infrequently isolated from the skin or joints at this

Skin rash, arthralgia, and arthritis are associated with bacteremia

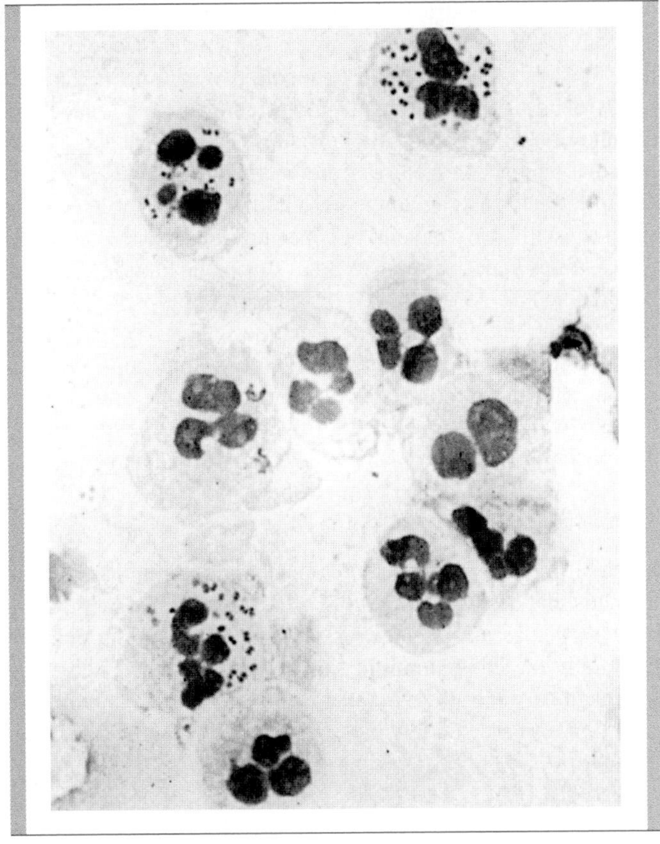

FIGURE 20–5
Gram smear of urethral exudate of an acute case of gonorrhea in a male. Note typical intracellular diplococci in polymorphonuclear leukocytes and the Gram-negative gonococci.

stage despite their presence in the blood. The bacteremia may lead to metastatic infections such as endocarditis and meningitis, but the most common is purulent arthritis. The arthritis typically follows the bacteremia and involves large joints such as elbows and knees. Gonococci are readily cultured from the pus.

Purulent arthritis involves large joints

DIAGNOSIS

Gram Smear

The presence of multiple pairs of bean-shaped, Gram-negative diplococci within a neutrophil is highly characteristic of gonorrhea when the smear is from a genital site (Fig 20–5). The direct Gram smear is more than 95% sensitive and specific in symptomatic men. Unfortunately, it is only 50 to 70% sensitive in women, and its specificity is complicated by the presence of other bacteria in the female genital flora that may have a similar morphology. Experience is required in reading smears, particularly in women. Although a positive Gram smear is generally accepted as diagnostic in men, it should not be used as the sole source for diagnosis when the findings are unexpected or have social (divorce) or legal (rape, child abuse) implications.

Direct smear is useful in men

Interfering flora complicates interpretation in women

Culture

Attention to detail is necessary for isolation of the gonococcus, because it is a fragile organism that is often mixed with hardier members of the normal flora. Success requires proper selection of culture sites, protection of specimens from environmental exposure, culture on appropriate media, and definitive laboratory identification. In men, the best specimen is urethral exudate or urethral scrapings (obtained with a loop or special swab). In women, cervical swabs are preferred over urethral or vaginal specimens. The highest diagnostic yield in women is with the combination of a cervical and an anal canal culture, because some patients with rectal gonorrhea have negative cervical cultures. Throat or rectal cultures in men are needed only if indicated by the patient's sexual practices.

Urethra and cervix are preferred culture sites

Transport media required unless plating is immediate

Selective medium inhibits competing flora

Swabs may be streaked directly onto culture medium or transmitted to the laboratory in a suitable transport medium if the delay is not more than 4 hours. Laboratory requests must specify the suspicion of gonorrhea, so that media that satisfy the nutritional requirements of the gonococcus and inhibit competing normal flora can be seeded. The most common medium is Martin–Lewis agar, an enriched selective chocolate agar. The exact formulation has changed over the years, but includes antimicrobics active against Gram-positive bacteria (vancomycin), Gram-negative bacteria (colistin, trimethoprim), and fungi (nystatin, anisomycin) at concentrations that do not inhibit *N. gonorrhoeae*.

Isolates are identified by fermentation or immunoassay

Colonies appear after 1 to 2 days of incubation in carbon dioxide at 35°C. They may be identified as *Neisseria* by demonstration of typical Gram stain morphology and a positive oxidase test. Classically, speciation is by carbohydrate degradation pattern, but this approach has been replaced by immunologic procedures (immunofluorescence, coagglutination, enzyme immunoassay) using monoclonal antibodies to unique antigens such as protein I. *Neisseria* species other than *N. gonorrhoeae* are unusual in genital specimens, but speciation is the only way to be certain of the diagnosis.

Direct Detection

DNA amplification methods are sensitive but expensive

Much effort has been directed at developing immunoassay and nucleic acid hybridization methods that detect gonococci in clinical specimens without culture. Such methods could have particular importance for screening populations where culture is impractical. Of these only the DNA amplification methods have the sensitivity to substitute for culture. The main barrier to their broader use is cost, which may be overcome by combining them with *Chlamydia* detection that targets the same clinical population.

Serology

No serologic test

Attempts to develop a serologic test for gonorrhea have not yet achieved the needed sensitivity and specificity. A test that would detect the disease in asymptomatic patients would be very useful in control of this disease.

TREATMENT

Compliance dictates treatment on first encounter

The treatment of gonorrhea, as with other sexually transmitted diseases, includes individual patient issues as well as public health concerns. Patients who do not complete a course of treatment once they begin to feel better present a risk of continued transmission and selection of resistant strains. For this reason, definitive treatment at the time of the initial visit has been the favored approach. For decades, this was easily accomplished with a single intramuscular injection of penicillin G.

PBP alterations cause incremental resistance

β-Lactamase–producing strains are highly resistant

Penicillin is no longer used, because of the development of two mechanisms of resistance. The first to be recognized was a slightly decreased susceptibility linked to altered PBPs. Over three decades, the minimum inhibitory concentrations (MICs) of altered PBP gonococci gradually increased (0.1 to more than 4.0 μg/mL), along with the dosage of the single injection favored for outpatient treatment. Eventually, the volume required to deliver the recommended dose began to exceed that which could be humanely administered, even injecting both buttocks. A second resistance mechanism, penicillinase production, first appeared in the Far East during the Viet Nam war and by the mid-1980s was endemic throughout the world. These strains produce a plasmid-encoded β-lactamase identical to that of members of the Enterobacteriaceae and have MICs that far exceed achievable therapeutic levels.

Ceftriaxone, quinolones, and azithromycin are recommended therapy

This situation has caused a shift in treatment of genital gonorrhea to third-generation cephalosporins, because of their resistance to the β-lactamases prevalent in gonococci. The recommended agents have high enough activity to still be used as single dose treatment either intramuscularly (ceftriaxone) or orally (cefixime). Other agents recommended for primary treatment include fluoroquinolones (ciprofloxacin or ofloxacin) and azithromycin. Doxycycline is also effective but must be given orally for 7 days. Doxycycline and azithromycin have the additional advantage of also being effective against

Chlamydia trachomatis (see Chapter 30), which may also be present in up to one third of gonorrhea cases. Resistance to quinolones is frequent enough to limit their use in some parts of the world. Azithromycin resistance is just beginning to be reported.

Quinolone and azithromycin resistance is still uncommon

PREVENTION

Methods to block direct mucosal contact (condoms) or inhibit the gonococcus (vaginal foams, douches) have been shown to provide protection against gonorrhea if used properly. The classic public health methods of case–contact tracing and treatment are important but difficult due to the size of the infected population. The availability of a good serologic test would greatly aid control, as it has for syphilis. The development of a gonococcal vaccine awaits further understanding of immunity and its relationship to the shifting target provided by the gonococcus.

Condoms should block transmission

Vaccine strategies await better understanding of immunity

ADDITIONAL READING

Goldschneider I, Gotschlich EC, Liu TY, Artenstein MS. Human immunity to the meningococcus I–V. *J Exp Med* 1969;129:1307–1395. This series of five classic papers from the Walter Reed Army Institute of Research define the basis of immunity to *Neisseria meningitidis* and lay out the steps which lead to the development of vaccines from the polysaccharide capsule.

Pizza M, Rappuoli R, et al [37 authors]. Identification of vaccine candidates against serogroup B meningococcus by whole-genome sequencing. *Science* 2000;287:1816–1820. This progress report is by an Italian group that is using an entirely genetic approach to development of meningococcal vaccines. The researchers derive their candidate proteins from the chromosome sequence—not the organism itself.

Van Deuren M, Brandtzaeg, Van der Meer, JMM. Update on meningococcal disease with emphasis on pathogenesis and clinical management. *Clin Microbiol Rev* 2000;13:144–166. This review presents a detailed but clear discussion of how the virulence factors of the meningococcus are translated into septic shock in the infected patient.

CHAPTER 21

Enterobacteriaceae

KENNETH J. RYAN

The Enterobacteriaceae are a large and diverse family of Gram-negative rods, members of which are both free-living and part of the indigenous flora of humans and animals. A few are adapted strictly to living in humans. The Enterobacteriaceae grow rapidly under aerobic or anaerobic conditions and are metabolically active. They are by far the most common cause of **urinary tract infections (UTIs),** and a limited number of species are also important etiologic agents of **diarrhea.** Spread to the bloodstream causes Gram-negative endotoxic shock, a dreaded and often fatal complication.

GENERAL CHARACTERISTICS

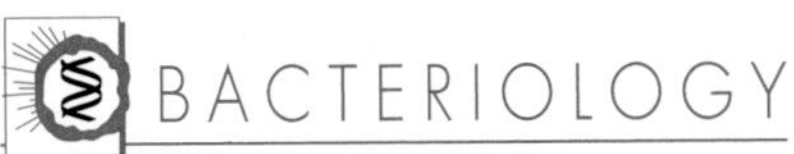

BACTERIOLOGY

MORPHOLOGY AND STRUCTURE

The Enterobacteriaceae are among the largest bacteria, measuring 2 to 4 μm in length and 0.4 to 0.6 μm in width, with parallel sides and rounded ends. Forms range from large coccobacilli to elongated, filamentous rods. The organisms do not form spores or demonstrate acid fastness.

Rods are large

The cell wall, cell membrane, and internal structures are morphologically similar for all Enterobacteriaceae, and follow the cell plan described in Chapter 2 for Gram-negative bacteria. Components of the cell wall and surface, which are antigenic, have been extensively studied in some genera and form the basis of systems dividing species into serotypes (Fig 21–1). The outer membrane lipopolysaccharide (LPS) is called the **O antigen.** Its antigenic specificity is determined by the composition of the sugars that form the long terminal polysaccharide side chains linked to the core polysaccharide and lipid A. Cell surface polysaccharides may form a well-defined capsule or an amorphous slime layer and are termed the **K antigen** (from the Danish Kapsel, capsule). Motile strains have protein peritrichous flagella, which extend well beyond the cell wall and are called the **H antigen.** Many of the Enterobacteriaceae have surface pili, which are antigenic proteins but not yet part of any formal typing scheme.

O = LPS

K = polysaccharide capsule

H = flagellar protein

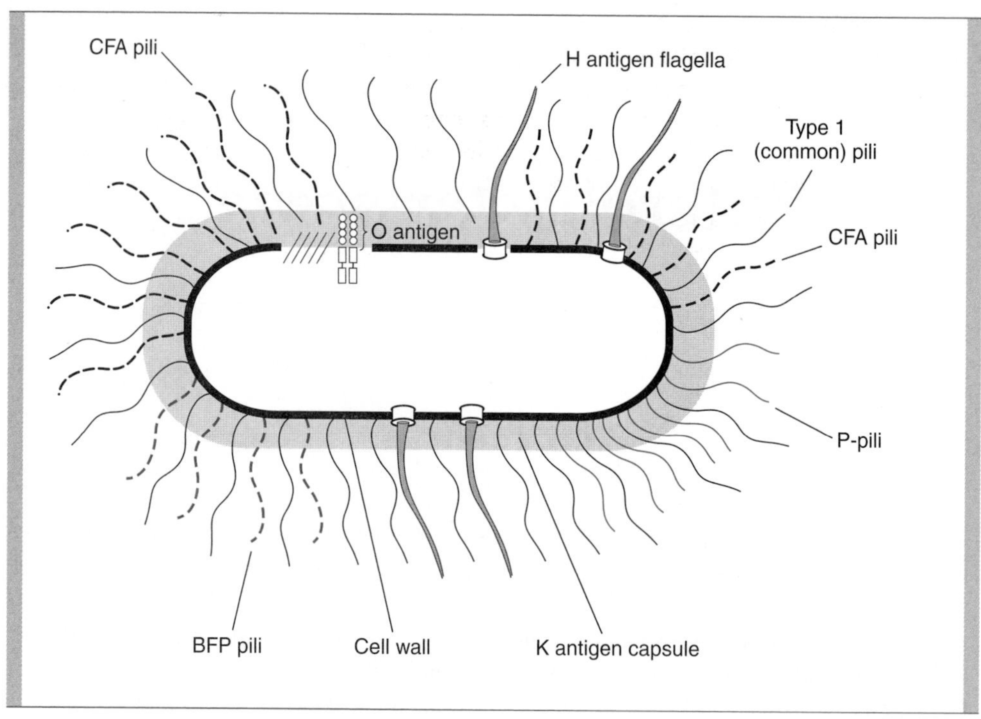

FIGURE 21–1
Antigenic structure of *Escherichia coli*. The O antigen is contained in the repeating polysaccharide units of the lipopolysaccharide (LPS) in the outer membrane of the cell wall. The H antigen is flagellar protein. The K antigen is the polysaccharide capsule present in some strains. Most *E. coli* have type 1 (common) hair-like pili extending from the surface. Some *E. coli* have specialized P, colonization factor antigens (CFAs), or bundle-forming pili (BFP), as well as type 1 pili.

GROWTH AND METABOLISM

Facultative growth is rapid

Enterobacteriaceae grow readily on simple media, often with only a single carbon energy source. Growth is rapid under both aerobic and anaerobic conditions, producing 2- to 5-mm colonies on agar media and diffuse turbidity in broth after 12 to 18 hours of incubation. All Enterobacteriaceae ferment glucose, reduce nitrates to nitrites, and are oxidase negative.

CLASSIFICATION

Biochemical characteristics establish species

Antigenic characters define serotypes within species

Genus and species designations are based on phenotypic characteristics, such as patterns of carbohydrate fermentation, and amino acid breakdown. The O, K, and H antigens are used to further divide some species into multiple **serotypes.** These types are expressed with letter and number of the specific antigen, such as *Escherichia coli* **O**157:**H**7, the cause of numerous food-borne outbreaks. These antigenic designations have been established only for the most important species and are limited to the structures at hand. For example, many species lack capsules and/or flagella. In recent years, DNA and RNA homology data have been used to validate these relationships and establish new ones. The genera containing the species most virulent for humans are *Escherichia, Shigella, Salmonella, Klebsiella,* and *Yersinia.* Other less common medically important genera are *Enterobacter, Serratia, Proteus, Morganella,* and *Providencia.*

TOXINS

All have LPS

In addition to the **LPS endotoxin** common to all Gram-negative bacteria, some Enterobacteriaceae also produce **protein exotoxins,** which act on host cells by damaging membranes, inhibiting protein synthesis, or altering metabolic pathways. The end result of these actions may be cell death (cytotoxin) or a physiologic alteration, the net effect of which depends on the function of the affected cell. For example, enterotoxins act on intestinal enterocytes, causing the net secretion of water and electrolytes into the gut to produce diarrhea. Although these toxins are most strongly associated with *E. coli, Shigella,* and *Yersinia,* others with the same or very similar actions have now been discovered in other species. When found in another species, the toxin may differ by a few amino acids in structure and in genetic regulation but has the same basic action on host cells. Details of these toxins are discussed below in relation to their prototype species.

Cytotoxins kill cells

Enterotoxins cause diarrhea

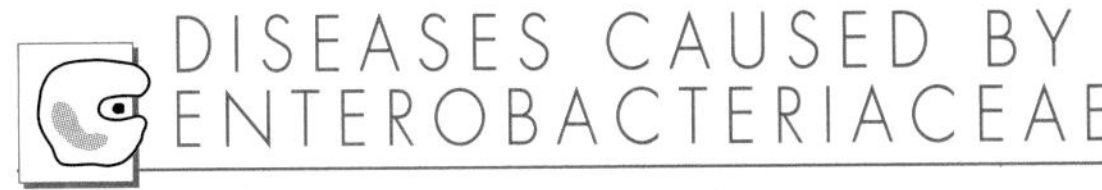

DISEASES CAUSED BY ENTEROBACTERIACEAE

EPIDEMIOLOGY

Most Enterobacteriaceae are primarily colonizers of the lower gastrointestinal tract of humans and animals. Many species survive readily in nature and live freely anywhere water and minimal energy sources are available. In humans, they are the major facultative components of the colonic bacterial flora and are also found in the female genital tract and as transient colonizers of the skin. Enterobacteriaceae are scant in the respiratory tract of healthy individuals; however, their numbers may increase in hospitalized patients with chronic debilitating diseases. *E. coli* is the most common species of Enterobacteriaceae found among the indigenous flora, followed by *Klebsiella, Proteus,* and *Enterobacter* species. *Salmonella* and *Shigella* species are not considered members of the normal flora, although carrier states can exist. *Shigella* and *Salmonella* serotype Typhi are strict human pathogens.

Present in nature and the intestinal tract

Shigella and *S. typhi* are found only in humans

PATHOGENESIS

Opportunistic Infections

Enterobacteriaceae are often poised to take advantage of their common presence in the environment and normal flora to produce disease when they gain access to normally sterile body sites. Surface structures such as pili are known to aid this process for some species and surely do for many others. Once in deeper tissues, their ability to persist and cause injury is little understood except for the action of LPS endotoxin and the species known to produce exotoxins or capsules. The prototype opportunistic infection is the UTI, in which Enterobacteriaceae gain access to the urinary bladder due to minor trauma or instrumentation. Strains able to adhere to uroepithelial cell can persist and multiply in the nutrient-rich urine, sometimes spreading through the ureters to the renal pelvis and kidney (pyelonephritis). Likewise, mucosal or skin trauma can allow access to soft tissues and aspiration to the lung when the relevant site is colonized with Enterobacteriaceae.

Colonization presents opportunity when defense barriers open

UTI follows access and adherence to bladder mucosa

Intestinal Infections

Salmonella, Shigella, Yersinia enterocolitica, and certain strains of *E. coli* are able to produce disease in the intestinal tract. These intestinal pathogens have invasive properties or virulence factors such as cytotoxins and enterotoxins, which correlate with the type of diarrhea they produce. In general, the invasive and cytotoxic strains produce an inflammatory diarrhea called **dysentery** with white blood cells (WBCs) and/or blood in the stool. The enterotoxin-producing strains cause a **watery diarrhea** in which fluid loss is the primary pathophysiologic feature. For a few species, the intestinal tract is the portal of entry, but the disease is systemic due to spread of bacteria to multiple organs. **Enteric (typhoid) fever** caused by *Salmonella* serotype Typhi is the prototype of this form of infection.

Cell destruction causes dysentery

Enterotoxins cause watery diarrhea

Enteric fever is a systemic illness

Regulation of Virulence

In addition to adherence pili, LPS, and exotoxins, the Enterobacteriaceae produce a myriad of other virulence factors in order to cause disease. Many of them are deployed in a

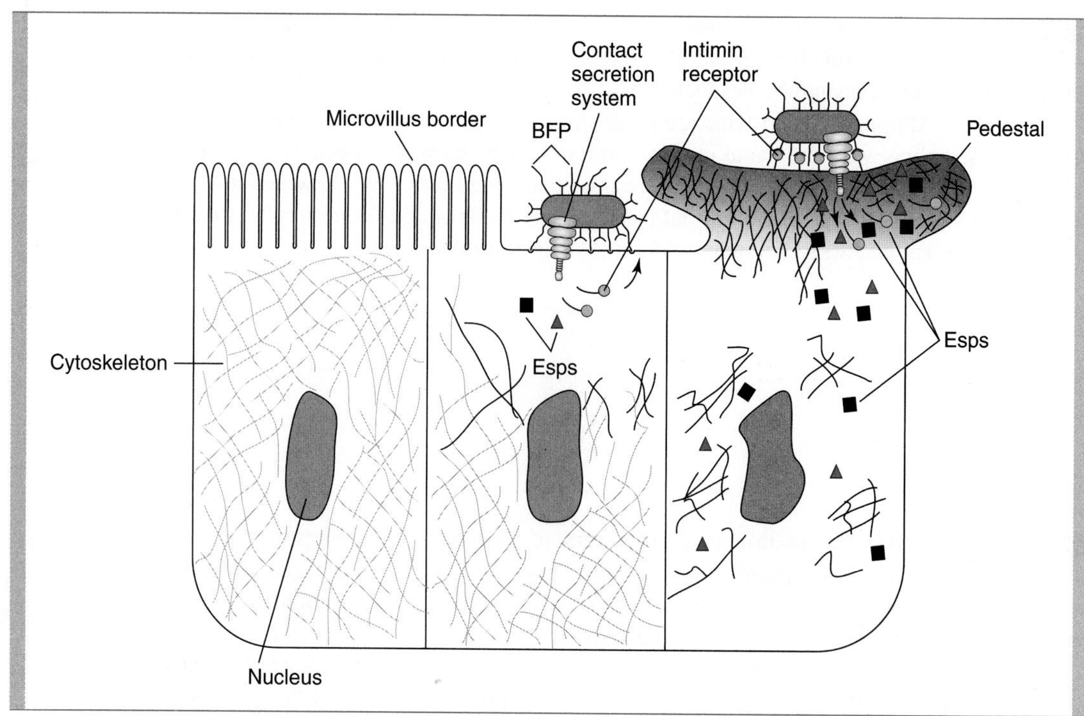

FIGURE 21–2
Enteropathic *Escherichia coli* (EPEC) contact secretion system. **Left.** An enterocyte is shown with a microvillus border and a delicate supporting cytoskeleton. **Middle.** An EPEC has attached to the cell surface by binding of the bundle-forming pili to receptors on the host cell surface. A contact secretion apparatus (see Figure 3–8) has been inserted into the cell and is exporting secretion proteins (Esps) into the cytoplasm. One of these is the receptor for intimin. **Right.** The intimin receptor has been inserted below the host cell membrane and is now mediating tight binding to the surface. The other Esps have disrupted multiple cellular functions, including the structure of the cytoskeleton. Cytoskeleton elements have been concentrated to form a pedestal cradling the EPEC.

complex and sequential fashion in response to environmental cues (temperature, iron, calcium) or as yet unknown factors.

Some bacteria have **contact secretion systems** (Fig 21–2) that target human cells by literally delivering a syringe-like injection of virulence factors into the cytoplasm of host cells.

Virulence genes are organized into gene clusters

Expression may be stimulated by environmental cues

PAIs contain DNA from another bacterium

The genes for these factors, located in the chromosome, plasmids, or both, are controlled by interactive regulators that seem to produce each virulence factor exactly when it is needed. The genes themselves are often organized into clusters that include the genes for the effector molecules as well as their regulatory proteins. This is particularly true for complex characteristics like invasiveness which involve multiple sequential steps. Some of these gene clusters are called **pathogenicity islands** (PAIs) because their overall genetic makeup is foreign enough to the rest of the genome of the organism that they appear to have been acquired from another bacterium in the genetically distant past. In particular, PAIs are associated with contact secretion systems where they contain the structural genes for the injection apparatus as well as the virulence factors injected.

IMMUNITY

Immunity is short-lived

Little is understood about immunity to the broad range of opportunistic infections caused by Enterobacteriaceae. Antibody directed against an LPS core antigen has been shown to provide a degree of protection against Gram-negative endotoxemia, but the diversity of antigens and virulence factors among the Enterobacteriaceae is too great to expect broad immunity. Immunity to intestinal infection is generally short-lived and will be discussed where it is relevant to specific intestinal pathogens.

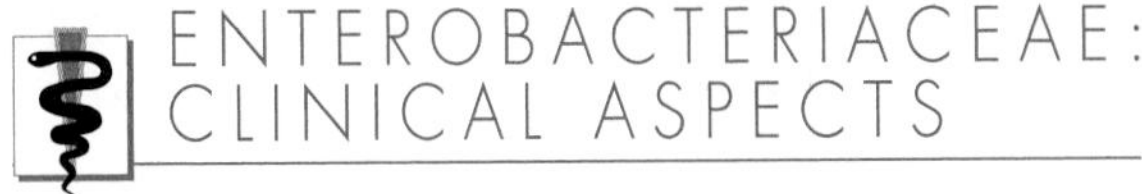

ENTEROBACTERIACEAE: CLINICAL ASPECTS

MANIFESTATIONS

The Enterobacteriaceae produce the widest variety of infections of any group of microbial agents, including two of the most common infectious states, UTI and acute diarrhea. UTIs are manifested by dysuria and urinary frequency when infection is limited to the bladder, with the addition of fever and flank pain when the infection spreads to the kidney. Enterobacteriaceae are by far the most common cause of UTIs, and the most common species involved is *E. coli.* The features of UTIs are discussed in more detail in Chapter 66.

UTI and acute diarrhea are most common

DIAGNOSIS

Culture is the primary method of diagnosis; all Enterobacteriaceae are readily isolated on routine media under almost any incubation conditions. Special indicator media such as MacConkey agar are commonly used in primary isolation to speed separation of the many species. For example, the common pathogens *E. coli* and *Klebsiella* typically ferment lactose rapidly, producing acid (pink) colonies on MacConkey agar, whereas the intestinal pathogens *Salmonella* and *Shigella* do not. Separation of the intestinal pathogens from all the other Enterobacteriaceae present in stool requires the use of highly selective media designed solely for this purpose. They will be discussed as they relate to individual pathogens.

Improved understanding of the genetic and molecular basis for virulence has led to the development of direct nucleic acid and immunodiagnostic techniques for direct detection of toxin, adhesin, or invasin genes in clinical material (eg, stool). These methods are still too expensive for use in clinical laboratories but are of extraordinary value in epidemiologic work and clinical research.

Culture on MacConkey agar demonstrates lactose fermentation

Selective media required for *Salmonella* and *Shigella* in stools

TREATMENT

Antimicrobial therapy is crucial to the outcome of infections with members of the Enterobacteriaceae. Unfortunately, combinations of chromosomal and plasmid-determined resistance (see Chapter 14) render them the most variable of all bacteria in susceptibility to antimicrobial agents. They are usually resistant to high concentrations of penicillin G, erythromycin, and clindamycin, but may be susceptible to the broader-spectrum β-lactams, aminoglycosides, tetracycline, chloramphenicol, sulfonamides, quinolones, nitrofurantoin, and the polypeptide antibiotics. Because the probability of resistance varies among genera and in different epidemiologic settings, the susceptibility of any individual strain must be determined by in vitro tests. Typical frequencies of resistance for some of the more common Enterobacteriaceae appear in Table 13–1.

Susceptibility to antimicrobials is highly variable

ESCHERICHIA COLI

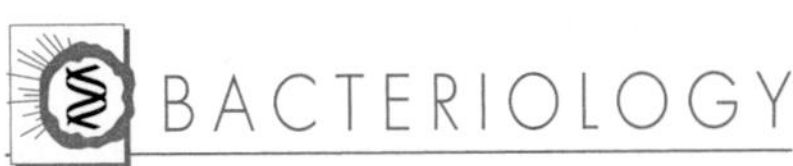

BACTERIOLOGY

CLASSIFICATION

Most strains of *E. coli* ferment lactose rapidly and produce indole. These and other biochemical reactions are sufficient to separate it from the other species. There are over 150 distinct O antigens and a large number of K and H antigens, all of which are designated

Hundreds of serotypes are possible

by number. The antigenic formula for serotypes is described by linking the letter (O, K, or H) and number of the antigens present (eg, **O**111:**K**76:**H**7).

PILI

Pili (also called fimbriae) are frequently present on the surface of *E. coli* strains. Research has shown that some of these structures play a role in virulence as mediators of attachment to human epithelial surfaces. Pili show marked tropism for different epithelial cell types, which is determined by the availability of their specific receptor on the host cell surface. Most *E. coli* express **type 1** (common) pili. Type 1 pili bind to the D-mannose residues commonly present on epithelial cell surfaces and thus mediate binding to a wide variety of cell types.

Type 1 pili bind mannose

More specialized pili are found in subpopulations of *E. coli.* **P pili** (also called Pap or Gal–Gal) bind to digalactoside (Gal–Gal) moieties present on certain mammalian cells, including uroepithelial cells and erythrocytes of the P blood group. Other pili bind to intestinal cells and have their own set of specificities. Those binding to human enterocytes are called **colonization factor antigens** (CFAs) or **bundle-forming pili** (BFP), depending on the pathogenic type of *E. coli* involved and possibly the cell type in the gastrointestinal tract. The specific binding receptors for the enterocyte binding pili are not known.

P pili bind uroepithelial cells

CFA and BFP pili bind enterocytes

The genetics of pilin expression is complex. The genes are organized into multicistronic clusters that encode structural pilin subunits and regulatory functions. Pili of different types may coexist on the same bacterium, and their expression may vary under different environmental conditions. Type 1 pilin expression can be turned "on" or "off" by inversion of a chromosomal DNA sequence containing the promoter responsible for initiating transcription of the pilin gene. Other genes control the orientation of this switch.

Type 1 has on–off switch

TOXINS

E. coli can produce every kind of toxin found among the Enterobacteriaceae. These include a pore-forming cytotoxin, inhibitors of protein synthesis, and a number of toxins that alter messenger pathways in host cells.

The **α-hemolysin** is a pore-forming cytotoxin that inserts into the plasma membrane of a wide range of host cells in a manner similar to streptolysin O (see Chapter 17) and *Staphylococcus aureus* α-toxin (see Chapter 16). The toxin causes leakage of cytoplasmic contents and eventually cell death.

α-hemolysin is pore-forming cytotoxin

Shiga toxin is named for the microbiologist who discovered *Shigella dysenteriae,* and this toxin was once believed to be limited to that species. It is now recognized to exist in at least two molecular forms released by multiple *E. coli* and *Shigella* strains on lysis of the bacteria. In the years following the discovery of this toxin, the term Shiga toxin was reserved for the original toxin, and others were called Shiga-like. In this discussion, the term Shiga toxin will be used for all the molecular variants that have the same mode of action. Shiga toxins are of the AB type. The B unit directs binding to a specific glycolipid receptor (Gb_3) present on eukaryotic cells and is internalized in an endocytotic vacuole. Inside the cell, the A subunit crosses the vacuolar membrane in the trans-Golgi network, exits to the cytoplasm, and enzymatically modifies 28S-ribosomal RNA of the 60S-ribosomal subunit by removing an adenine base. This prevents the elongation-factor-1–dependent binding of amino acyl tRNA to the ribosome blocking protein synthesis, leading to cell death.

Shiga toxin is produced by *Shigella* and *E. coli*

Inhibits protein synthesis by ribosomal binding

Labile toxin (LT) is also an AB toxin. Its name relates to the physical property of heat lability, which was important in its discovery, and contrasts with the heat-stable toxin described below. The B subunit binds to the cell membrane, and the A subunit catalyzes the ADP-ribosylation of a regulatory G protein located in the membrane of the intestinal epithelial cell. This inactivation of part of the G protein causes permanent activation of the membrane-associated adenylate cyclase system and a cascade of events, the net effect of which depends on the biological function of the stimulated cell. If the cell is an

LT ADP-ribosylates G protein

Adenylate cyclase stimulation is similar to cholera toxin

enterocyte, the result is the stimulation of chloride secretion out of the cell and the blockage of NaCl absorption. The net effect is the accumulation of water and electrolytes into the bowel lumen. The structure and biological effect of LT is very similar to cholera toxin, which is described in Chapter 22.

Stable toxin (ST) toxin is a small (17- to 18-amino acid) peptide that binds to a glycoprotein receptor, resulting in the activation of a membrane-bound guanylate cyclase. The subsequent increase in cyclic GMP concentration causes an LT-like net secretion of fluid and electrolytes into the bowel lumen.

ST stimulates guanylate cyclase

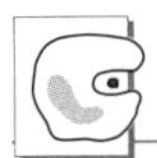

E. coli OPPORTUNISTIC INFECTIONS

URINARY TRACT INFECTION (UTI)

CLINICAL CAPSULE

The term UTI encompasses a range of infections from simple cystitis involving the bladder to full-blown infection of the entire urinary tract, including the renal pelvis and kidney (pyelonephritis). The primary feature of cystitis is frequent urination, which has a painful burning quality. In pyelonephritis, symptoms include fever, general malaise, and flank pain in addition to the frequent urination. Cystitis is usually self-limiting, but infection of the upper urinary tract carries a risk of spread to the bloodstream. It is the leading cause of Gram-negative sepsis and septic shock.

Epidemiology

E. coli accounts for more than 90% of the more than 7 million cases of cystitis and 250,000 of pyelonephritis estimated to occur in otherwise healthy individuals every year in the United States. UTIs are more common in women, 40% of whom have an episode in their lifetime, usually when they are sexually active. The reservoir for these infections is the patient's own intestinal *E. coli* flora, which contaminate the perineal and urethral area. In individuals with urinary tract obstruction or instrumentation, environment sources assume some importance.

Perineal flora is reservoir of common cystitis

Pathogenesis

Relatively minor trauma or the mechanical effect of sexual intercourse have been shown to allow bacteria access to the bladder. In most instances, these bacteria are purged by the flushing action of voiding. Factors that violate bladder integrity (urinary catheters) or that obstruct urine outflow (enlarged prostate) are also associated with infection. However, this cannot be the whole story; fewer than 10 *E. coli* serotypes account for the majority of UTI cases, and these UTI serotypes are not the dominant ones in the fecal flora.

Minor trauma admits *E. coli* to the bladder

The ability of uropathic *E. coli* (UPEC) to produce UTI is related to general virulence factors such as α-hemolysin, together with pili-mediated adherence to uroepithelial cells. The percentage of *E. coli* with P pili increases from 20% in the fecal flora to 70% in pyelonephritis isolates. Asymptomatic bacteriuria and cystitis isolates fall in between. The digalactoside receptor for P is present on uroepithelial cells, to which the bacteria bind avidly, particularly in the upper urinary tract. By aiding in periurethral colonization as the prelude to bladder access, type 1 pili are important as well. In addition, type 1 pili are essential for attachment to urinary epithelium in the urinary bladder where they appear to keep their invertible segment in the "on" position. They are not involved in pyelonephritis where P pili are more important. Antipilin antibody blocks adherence in experimental systems, suggesting that immunization could be an approach to UTI prevention. The pathogenic features that allow *E. coli* to play such a prominent role in this disease are illustrated in Figure 21–3.

P pili adhere to digalactoside receptor

Upper tract is favored by P pili

Type 1 pili are important in the bladder

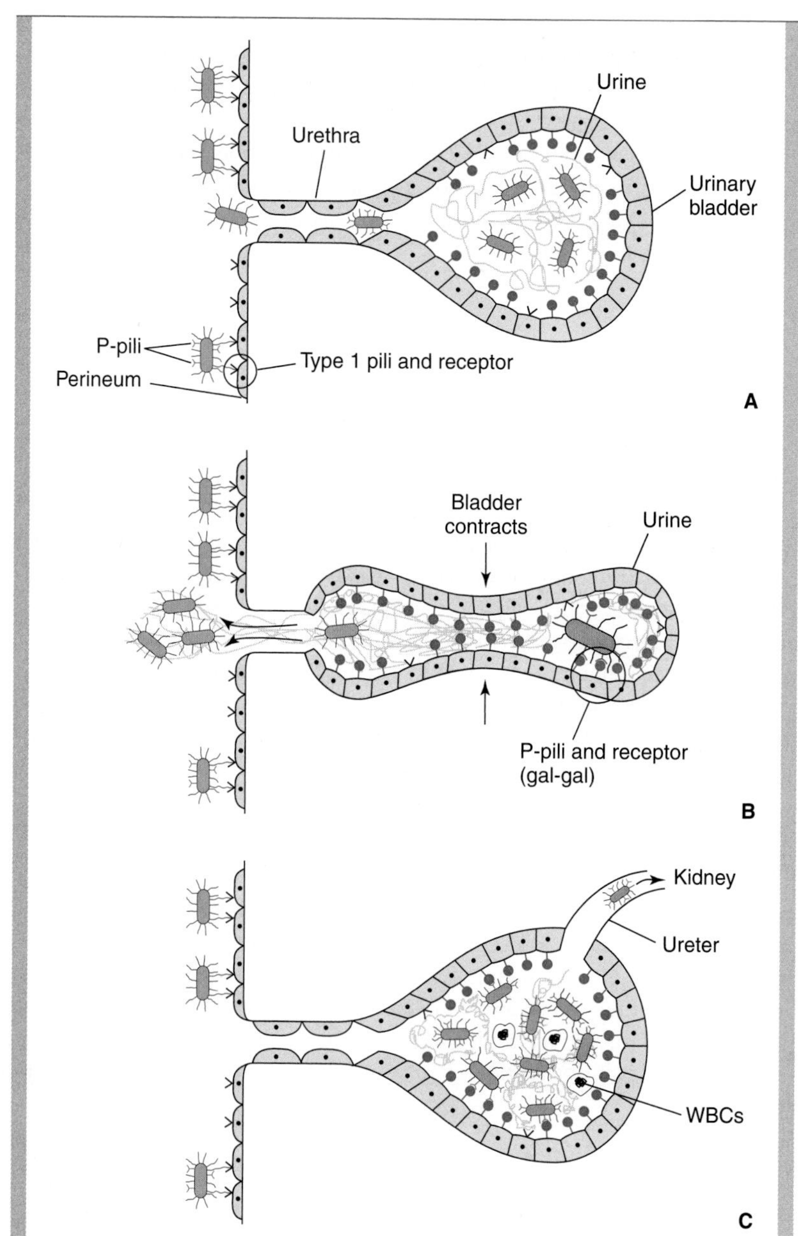

FIGURE 21–3
Urinary tract infection due to *Escherichia coli.* The urinary bladder, perineal mucosa, and short female urethra are shown. *E. coli* from the nearby rectal flora have colonized the perineum, utilizing binding by type 1 (common) pili. *E. coli* with P-pili are also present but are of no use at this site. **A.** A few *E. coli* have gained access to the bladder due to mechanical disruptions, such as sexual intercourse or instrumentation (catheters). Note that receptors for the P-pili not present on the perineal mucosa are found on the surface of bladder mucosal cells. **B.** During voiding, the bladder has expelled the *E. coli,* which only have type 1 pili. The P- pili–containing bacteria remain behind due to the strong binding to the P (gal-gal) receptor. **C.** The remaining *E. coli* have multiplied and are causing a urinary tract infection (cystitis) with inflammation and hemorrhage. In some cases, the bacteria ascend the ureter to cause pyelonephritis.

OTHER OPPORTUNISTIC INFECTIONS

Meningitis

Infection from vaginal flora such as group B streptococci

K1 capsular polysaccharide is identical to meningococcus

E. coli is one of the most common causes of neonatal meningitis, many features of which are similar to group B streptococcal disease (see Chapter 17). The pathogenesis involves vaginal *E. coli* colonization of the infant via ruptured amniotic membranes or during childbirth. Failure of protective maternal immunoglobulin M (IgM) antibodies to cross the placenta and the special susceptibility of newborns surely plays a role. Fully 75% of cases are caused by strains possessing the K1 capsular polysaccharide that contains sialic acid and is structurally identical to the group B polysaccharide of *Neisseria meningitidis,* another cause of meningitis. There is some evidence that these strains have a type of pili with the property of adherence to brain microvascular endothelial cells.

Non-UTI infections require some breach of defenses

With the exception of UTIs, extraintestinal *E. coli* infections are uncommon unless there is a significant breach in host defenses. Opportunistic infection may follow mechanical damage such as a ruptured intestinal diverticulum, trauma, or involve a generalized impairment of immune function. The virulence factors involved are likely the same as with UTI (eg, pili, α-hemolysin) but have been less specifically studied. Failure of local control of infection can lead to spread and eventually Gram-negative septic shock. A significant proportion of blood isolates have the K1 surface polysaccharide. The particular diseases that result depend on the sites involved and include many of the syndromes covered in Chapters 59 to 72.

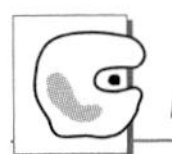

E. coli INTESTINAL INFECTIONS

CLINICAL CAPSULE

Diarrhea is the universal finding with *E. coli* strains that are able to cause intestinal disease. The nature of the diarrhea varies depending on the pathogenic mechanism. Enterotoxigenic and enteropathogenic strains produce a watery diarrhea, the enterohemorrhagic strains produce a bloody diarrhea, and the enteroinvasive strains may cause dysentery with blood and pus in the stool. The diarrhea is usually self-limiting after only 1 to 3 days. The enterohemorrhagic *E. coli* are an exception, with life-threatening manifestations outside the gastrointestinal tract due to Shiga toxin production.

Diarrhea-causing *E. coli* are conveniently classified according to their virulence properties as **enterotoxigenic (ETEC), enteropathogenic (EPEC), enteroinvasive (EIEC), enterohemorrhagic (EHEC),** or **enteroaggregative (EAEC).** Each group causes disease by a different mechanism, and the resulting syndromes usually differ clinically and epidemiologically. For example, human ETEC and EIEC strains infect only humans. Food and water contaminated with human waste and person-to-person contact are the principal means of infection. A summary of the pathogenesis of infection, clinical syndromes, and epidemiology of infection for each enteropathogen is shown in Table 21–1.

Multiple pathogenic mechanisms have their own epidemiologic and clinical features

ENTEROTOXIGENIC *E. coli* (ETEC)

Epidemiology

ETEC are the most important cause of traveler's diarrhea in visitors to developing countries. ETEC also produce diarrhea in infants native to these countries, where they are a leading cause of morbidity and mortality during the first 2 years of life. Repeated bouts of diarrhea caused by ETEC and other infectious agents are an important cause of growth retardation, malnutrition, and developmental delay in the third world countries where ETEC are endemic. ETEC disease is rare in industrialized nations.

Traveler's diarrhea affects children of developing countries

Transmission is by consumption of food and water contaminated by human cases or convalescent carriers. Uncooked foods such as salads or marinated meats and vegetables are associated with the greatest risk. Direct person-to-person transmission is unusual, because the infecting dose is high. Animals are not involved in ETEC disease.

Oral ingestion of uncooked foods requires high dose for disease

Pathogenesis

ETEC diarrhea is caused by strains of *E. coli* that produce LT and/or ST enterotoxins in the small intestine. Strains that elaborate both LT and ST cause more severe illness. Adherence to surface microvilli mediated by the CFA class of pili is essential for the efficient delivery of toxin to the target enterocytes. The genes encoding the ST, LT, and the CFA pili are borne in plasmids. A single plasmid can carry all three sets of genes. The bacteria remain on the surface, where the adenylate cyclase–stimulating action of the toxin(s) creates the flow of water and electrolytes from the enterocyte into the intestinal lumen. The mucosa becomes hyperemic but is not injured in the process. There is no invasion or inflammation.

LT and/or ST cause fluid outpouring in small intestine

CFA pili are required

TABLE 21–1

Characteristics of Pathogenic Enterobacteriaceae

		Virulence Factors							
		Surface							
	Diagnostic Antigens	Adherence	Capsule	Exotoxin(s)	Pathogenic Lesions	Secreted Proteins[a]	Genetics	Transmission	Disease
Escherichia coli	O, H, K								
Common	More than 150 types	Type 1[b] pili	K1	α-Hemolysin	Inflammation			Adjacent flora	Opportunistic
Uropathic UPEC		Type 1[b] P pili		α-Hemolysin	Inflammation			Fecal flora, ascending	Urinary tract
Enterotoxigenic (ETEC)		CFA pili		LT, ST	Hypersecretion		Plasmid (CFA, LT, ST)	Fecal–oral	Watery diarrhea (travelers)
Enteropathogenic (EPEC)		Bundle-forming pili, Intimin			A/E, small intestine	Esp	PAI	Fecal–oral	Watery diarrhea
Enteroinvasive (EIEC)					Invasion, inflammation, ulcers		Large plasmid, PAI	Fecal–oral	Dysentery
Enterohemorrhagic (EHEC)	0157;H7	Intimin		Shiga toxin	A/E, colon, hemorrhage	Esp	PAI	Fecal–oral direct, low dose, cattle	Bloody diarrhea, HUS
Enteraggregative (EAEC)					Adherent biofilm				Mucoid, watery diarrhea
Shigella	O serogroups								
S. dysenteriae	A(10 types)			Shiga toxin (A1 potent)	Invasion, inflammation, colonic ulcers	Ipa	Large plasmid, PAI	Fecal–oral, direct, low dose	Dysentery (severe), HUS
S. flexneri	B (6 types)			Shiga toxin (variable)	Invasion, inflammation, colonic ulcers	Ipa	Large plasmid, PAI	Fecal–oral, direct, low dose	Dysentery, HUS
S. boydii	C (15 types)			Shiga toxin (variable)	Invasion, inflammation, colonic ulcers	Ipa	Large plasmid, PAI	Fecal–oral, direct, low dose	Dysentery, HUS

S. sonnei	D			Shiga toxin (variable)	Invasion, inflammation, colonic ulcers	Ipa	Large plasmid, PAI	Fecal–oral, direct, low dose	Dysentery, HUS
Salmonella enterica	O, H_1, H_2, K								
Serotypes	More than 2000	Pili			Ruffles, invasion, inflammation	Inv, Spa, others	PAI	Fecal–oral, animals and humans	Gastroenteritis, sepsis
Typhi	O group D	Pili	Vi		Macrophage survival, RES growth	As in serotypes[c]	PAI	Fecal–oral, moderate dose, humans only	Enteric (typhoid) fever
Yersinia	O, H								
Y. pestis		Invasin	Protein	Protease, fibrinolysin	RES growth, bacteremia, pneumonia	Yop	PAI	Rats, flea bite, aerosol (human)	Plague
Y. pseudotuberculosis	10 types	Invasin			RES growth, microabscesses	Yop	PAI	Fecal–oral, animal	Mesenteric adenitis
Y. enterocolitica	More than 50 types	Invasin			RES growth, microabscesses	Yop	PAI	Fecal–oral, animals	Mesenteric adenitis, enteric fever
Klebsiella	70 capsular types	Pili	Polysaccharide					Adjacent flora	Opportunistic, pneumonia
Enterobacter								Adjacent flora	Opportunistic
Serratia								Adjacent flora	Opportunistic
Citrobacter								Adjacent flora	Opportunistic
Proteus								Adjacent flora	Opportunistic

Abbreviations: A/E, attaching and effacing lesion; CFA, colonizing factor antigen; Esp, *E. coli*–secreted protein; HUS, hemolytic uremic syndrome; lpa, invasion protein antigen; LT, labile toxin; PAI, pathogenicity island; RES, reticuloendothelial system; ST, stable toxin; Yop, *Yersinia* outer membrane protein.

[a] Delivered by type III secretion system.

[b] Bind to mannose.

[c] No animal model, presumed to be similar to *S. enterica* serotypes.

Immunity

sIgA to LT and CFAs may provide some protection

Although there can be more than one episode of diarrhea, infections with ETEC can stimulate immunity. Travelers from industrialized nations have a much higher attack rate than adults living in the endemic area. This natural immunity is presumably mediated by sIgA specific for LT and CFAs. The small ST peptides are nonimmunogenic. The disease is of very low incidence in breast-fed infants, underscoring the protective effect of maternal antibody and the importance of transmission by contaminated food and water.

ENTEROPATHOGENIC *E. coli* (EPEC)

Epidemiology

Nursery outbreaks and endemic diarrheas occur in developing world

EPEC strains were first identified as the cause of explosive outbreaks of diarrhea in hospital nurseries in the United States and Great Britain during the 1950s. The disease seems to have disappeared in industrialized nations, although it may be underestimated due to the difficulty of diagnosis. In developing countries throughout the world, EPEC account for up to 20% of diarrhea in bottle-fed infants younger than 1 year of age. The reservoir is infant cases and adult carriers with transmission by the fecal–oral route. Nursery outbreaks demonstrate the importance of spread by fomites, which suggests that the infecting dose for infants is low. Documented adult cases have usually been in circumstances where the number of organisms ingested was very large.

Pathogenesis

A/E lesions involve modification of cytoskeleton

Secretion system injects receptor for intimin of EPEC

EPEC initially attach to enterocytes using pili of the BFP type to form clustered microcolonies on the enterocyte cell surface. The lesion then progresses with effacement of the microvilli and changes in the cell morphology including the production of dramatic "pedestals" with the EPEC bacterium at their apex. The combination of these actions is called the **attachment and effacing (A/E)** lesion (Fig 21–4). The many steps involved in the formation of the A/E lesion are genetically controlled in a PAI, which includes the genes for the major attachment protein, **intimin,** and a contact secretion system. The secretion system injects at least five ***E. coli*** **secretion proteins (Esps)** into the host cell cytoplasm including, remarkably, the receptor for intimin. The other *E. coli* secretion proteins perturb intracellular signal transduction pathways, one effect of which is the induction of modifications in enterocyte cytoskeleton proteins (actin, talin). The cytoskeleton accumulates beneath the attached bacteria to form the pedestals and complete the A/E lesion. Exactly how this leads to diarrhea is not known, but the change from the normal microvillus border to the A/E must disrupt intestinal absorptive functions.

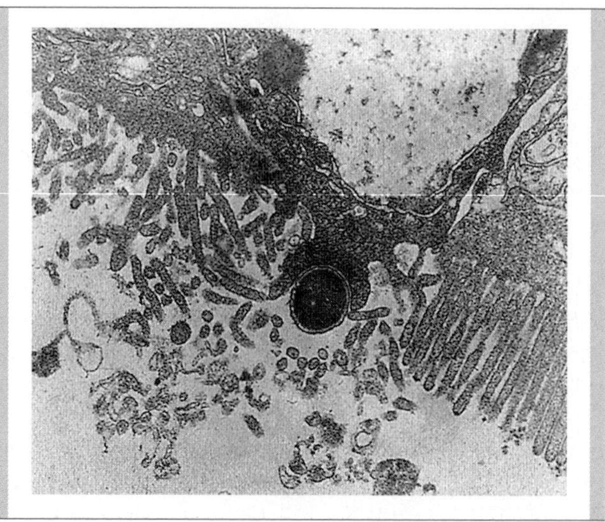

FIGURE 21–4
Enteropathogenic *Escherichia coli* (EPEC) attachment to epithelial cells. The EPEC are attaching to and effacing the microvilli on the epithelial cell surface. The cell's filamentous actin is rearranged at the attachment point

Immunity

In endemic areas, EPEC can be isolated often from the stool of asymptomatic adults, but unlike ETEC, these strains do not seem to cause traveler's diarrhea in individuals new to the area. This casts doubt on whether adults have acquired immunity or resistance based on physiologic factors.

Little evidence for immunity

ENTEROHEMORRHAGIC *E. coli* (EHEC)

Epidemiology

EHEC disease and the accompanying **hemolytic uremic syndrome (HUS)** are the result of consumption of products from animals colonized with EHEC strains. It is also clear from secondary cases in families during outbreaks that person-to-person transmission also occurs. This disease occurs more in developed rather than in developing countries.

Consumption of contaminated animal products is the main source

EHEC was first recognized in the early 1980s when outbreaks of HUS (hemolytic anemia, renal failure, and thrombocytopenia) were linked to a single *E. coli* serotype, O157:H7. Since then EHEC disease has emerged as an important cause of **bloody diarrhea** in industrialized nations and retained a remarkable but not exclusive relationship with the O157:H7 serotype, particularly in North America. Regional and national outbreaks associated with unpasteurized juices and hamburger have caught the attention of the public, the press, and the government.

Bloody diarrhea and HUS are linked to O157:H7

The emergence of EHEC is related to its virulence (see below), low infecting dose, common reservoir (cattle), and changes in the modern food processing industry that provide us with fresher meat (and bacteria). The low infecting dose, estimated at 100 to 200 organisms, is particularly important. This is a level where food need not come directly from the infected animal, only be contaminated by it. For example, large modern meat processing plants can mix EHEC from colonized cattle at one ranch into beef from hundreds of other farms and quickly ship it all over the country. Therefore, the worst outbreaks have been seen in countries with the most advanced food production systems. If the organisms are ground into hamburger, an infecting dose of EHEC may remain even after cooking if the meat is left rare in the middle. Unpasteurized milk carries an obvious risk but fruits and vegetables have also been the source for EHEC infection. In these instances the EHEC from the manure of cattle grazing nearby has contaminated these products in the field. The bacterial dose from a few "drop" apples (those picked up from the ground) included in a batch of cider has been enough to cause disease.

Low infecting dose facilitates transmission

Modern meat processing facilitates widespread outbreaks

Unpasteurized beverages are another risk

Pathogenesis

The distinguishing feature of the EHEC is the production of both Shiga toxins and the A/E lesions described above for EPEC. Another difference between EHEC and EPEC is that EHEC primarily attacks the colon while EPEC infects the small intestine. The multiple extraintestinal features such as HUS appear to be the result of circulating Shiga toxin. The interaction of EHEC with enterocytes is much the same as EPEC, except the EHEC strains do not form localized microcolonies on the mucosa. The outer membrane protein intimin mediates adherence and the contact secretion system injects the *E. coli* secretion proteins, which cause alterations in the host cytoskeleton. The genes for these properties are also found in a PAI.

Produce both Shiga toxin and A/E lesions

Circulating Shiga toxin leads to HUS

The A/E features alone are sufficient to cause nonbloody diarrhea. Shiga toxin production causes capillary thrombosis and inflammation of the colonic mucosa, leading to a hemorrhagic colitis. Although it has not been detected in the blood of human cases, Shiga toxin is presumed to be absorbed across the denuded intestinal mucosa. Circulating Shiga toxin binds to renal tissue where its glycoprotein receptor is particularly abundant, causing glomerular swelling and the deposition of fibrin and platelets in the microvasculature. How Shiga toxin causes hemolysis is less clear; perhaps the erythrocytes are simply damaged as they attempt to traverse the occluded capillaries. The strong association between EHEC disease and the O157:H7 serotype suggests that EHEC are more than just Shiga toxin–producing EPEC. The O157:H7 strains invariably have a large plasmid which may

Shiga toxin capillary thrombosis and inflammation have a hemorrhagic component

O157:H7 strains differ from EPEC in more than Shiga toxin

contain other virulence genes. Cases and outbreaks caused by Shiga toxin–producing *E. coli* of other serotypes may be on the rise and are common in some countries. How they differ from O157:H7 EPEC remains to be seen.

ENTEROINVASIVE *E. coli* (EIEC)

EIEC closely resemble *Shigella*

Virtually all aspects of EIEC disease are identical to *Shigella* (see below), which underscores the close relationship of the *Shigella* and *Escherichia* genera. Epidemiologically, EIEC infections are essentially restricted to children under 5 years of age living in developing nations. The occasional documented outbreaks in industrialized nations are usually linked to contaminated food or water. This lower incidence of person-to-person transmission correlates with the observation that the infecting dose for EIEC is higher than it is for *Shigella*. Humans are the only known reservoir.

ENTEROAGGREGATIVE *E. coli* (EAEC)

Adherence alone may create a biofilm

EAEC is associated with a protracted (>14 days) mucoid, watery diarrhea in infants and children in developing countries. The EAEC strains are defined on the basis of the pattern the bacteria make (eg, localized, diffuse, stacked) when adhering to cultured mammalian cells. Even though EAEC adheres tightly to the intestinal mucosa, the A/E lesions of the EPEC and EHEC are not present. The pathogenesis of diarrhea is not clearly understood but may involve the ability to form a mucus–bacteria biofilm on the intestinal surface. Inflammatory cells are not seen.

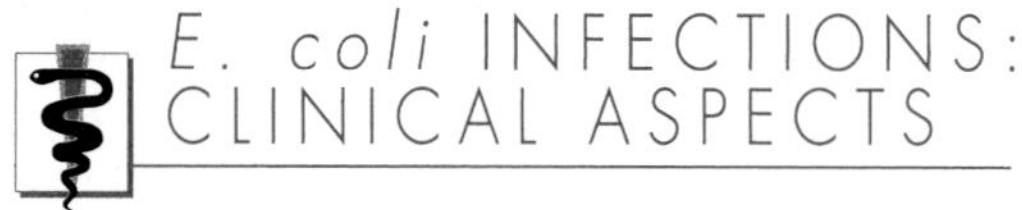

E. coli INFECTIONS: CLINICAL ASPECTS

MANIFESTATIONS

Opportunistic Infections

Dysuria and frequency are features of UTIs

The most common symptoms of *E. coli* UTI are dysuria and urinary frequency and do not differ significantly in character from those produced by the other less common Gram-negative urinary pathogens discussed in Chapter 66. If the infection ascends the ureters to produce pyelonephritis, fever and flank pain are common and bacteremia may develop. Although *E. coli* may have enhanced virulence in the production of pneumonia as well as soft tissue and other infections, no clinical features distinguish these cases from those caused by other members of the Enterobacteriaceae.

Intestinal Infections

ETEC and EPEC diarrhea is watery

EHEC diarrhea is bloody

Infections caused by all of the *E. coli* virulence types usually begin with a mild watery diarrhea starting 2 to 4 days after ingestion of an infectious dose. In most instances, the duration of diarrhea is limited to a few days, with the exception of EAEC diarrhea, which can last for weeks. With ETEC and EPEC, the diarrhea remains watery, but with EIEC and EHEC, a dysenteric illness follows. Some EPEC cases may also become chronic. EHEC disease begins like the others but often also includes vomiting. In 90% of cases this is followed in 1 to 2 days by intense abdominal pain and bloody diarrhea, but fever is not prominent. Some EHEC cases develop into a dysentery that is less severe than that seen in shigellosis. Colonoscopy reveals edema, hemorrhage, and pseudomembrane formation. Resolution usually takes place over a 3- to 10-day period, with few residual effects on the bowel mucosa.

HUS begins as oliguria and may progress to renal failure

HUS develops as a complication in about 10% of cases of EHEC hemorrhagic colitis, primarily in children under 10 years of age. The disease begins with oliguria, edema, and pallor, progressing to the triad of microangiopathic hemolytic anemia, thrombocytopenia, and renal failure. The systemic effects are often life-threatening, requiring transfusion and hemodialysis for survival. The mortality rate is 5%, and as many as 30% of those individuals who survive suffer sequelae such as renal impairment or hypertension.

DIAGNOSIS

Like the rest of the Enterobacteriaceae, *E. coli* is readily isolated in culture. For the diagnosis of intestinal disease, separating the virulent types discussed above from the numerous other *E. coli* strains commonly found in stool presents a special problem. A myriad of immunoassay and nucleic acid methods have been described that are able to detect the toxins and genes associated with virulence. These methods work but are still too expensive to be practical, especially in the developing countries where ETEC, EIEC, EPEC, and EAEC are prevalent. A screening test for EHEC takes advantage of the observation that the O157:H7 serotype typically fails to ferment sorbitol. Incorporating sorbitol in place of lactose in MacConkey agar provides an indicator medium from which suspect (colorless) colonies can be selected and then confirmed with O157 antisera. This procedure has become routine in areas where EHEC is endemic.

Methods to detect virulence factors are expensive

Sorbitol agar screens for O157:H7

TREATMENT

Because most *E. coli* diarrheas are mild and self-limiting, treatment is usually not an issue. When it is, rehydration and supportive measures are the mainstays of therapy, regardless of the causative agent. In the case of EHEC with hemorrhagic colitis and HUS, heroic supportive measures such as hemodialysis or hemapheresis may be required. Treatment with trimethoprim/sulfamethoxazole (TMP-SMX) or quinolones reduces the duration of diarrhea in ETEC, EIEC, and EPEC infection, but neither the course of hemorrhagic colitis nor the risk of HUS are altered by antimicrobial therapy. Because the risk of HUS may be increased by antimicrobial treatments, many physicians feel that treatment is not indicated. Antimotility agents are not helpful and are contraindicated when EIEC or EHEC might be the etiologic agent.

Antimicrobics may help all but EHEC

PREVENTION

Traveler's diarrhea is usually little more than an inconvenience. Because the infecting dose is high, the incidence of the disease can be greatly reduced by eating only cooked foods and peeled fruits, and drinking hot or carbonated beverages. Avoiding uncertain water, ice, salads, and raw vegetables is a wise precaution when traveling in developing countries. High-priced hotel accommodations have no protective effect. Chemoprophylaxis against traveler's diarrhea is not routinely recommended. TMP-SMX or ciprofloxacin have been recommended for a short-term (<2 weeks) for those at high risk for disease resulting from such chronic conditions as achlorhydria, gastric resection, prolonged use of H_2 blockers or antacids, and underlying immunosuppressive diseases.

Avoid uncooked foods

Chemoprophylaxis works for defined periods

These public health measures apply equally to EHEC, but here prevention is more difficult because the infecting dose is so low. Cooking hamburgers all the way through is sensible, but no one is recommending abstinence from salads when at home. Recent US recommendations for the irradiation of meats and the extension of pasteurization requirements to fruit juices are largely designed to stem the spread of EHEC.

Rare hamburgers carry risk for EHEC

SHIGELLA

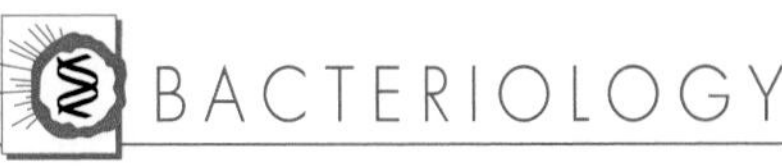

Shigella species are closely related to *E. coli*. Most fail to produce gas when fermenting glucose and do not ferment lactose. Their antigenic makeup has been characterized in a manner similar to *E. coli* with the exception that they lack flagella and thus H antigens.

All *Shigella* species are nonmotile. The genus is divided into four species which are defined by biochemical reactions and specific O antigens organized into serogroups. The species are *Shigella dysenteriae* (serogroup A), *Shigella flexneri* (serogroup B), *Shigella boydii* (serogroup C), and *Shigella sonnei* (serogroup D). All but *S. sonnei* are further subdivided into a total of 38 individual O antigen serotypes specified by numbers. *Shigella* is the prototype invasive bacterial pathogen. All species are able to invade and multiply inside a wide variety of epithelial cells, including their natural target, the enterocyte. *S. dysenteriae* type A1 (Shiga bacillus), the species that was first discovered, is the most potent producer of Shiga toxin. Other *Shigella* species produce various molecular forms of Shiga toxin.

O antigens and biochemicals define four species

Invasiveness and Shiga toxin production are virulence factors

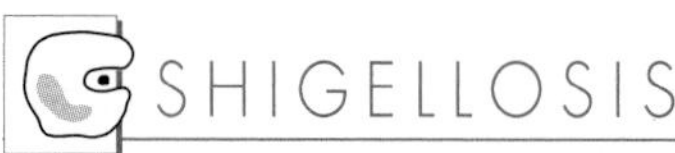

SHIGELLOSIS

CLINICAL CAPSULE

Shigella is the classic cause of dysentery, which is typically spread person-to-person under poor sanitary conditions. The illness begins as a watery diarrhea but evolves into an intense colitis with frequent small-volume stools that contain blood and pus. Despite the invasive properties of the causal organism, the infection usually does not spread outside the intestinal tract.

EPIDEMIOLOGY

Shigellosis is a strictly human disease with no animal reservoirs. In the United States, the number of reported cases has remained in the range of 8 to 12 cases per 100,000 population for over 30 years. Worldwide, it is consistently one of the most common causes of infectious diarrhea in both developed and developing countries, and it is estimated to cause 600,000 deaths per year. The organisms can be readily transmitted by the fecal–oral route through person-to-person contact or by contamination of food or water. This mode of spread is efficient; the infecting dose is less than 200 organisms in volunteer studies. The secondary attack rates among family members are as high as 40%.

Low infecting dose facilitates fecal–oral spread

Strictly human disease

The incidence and spread of shigellosis is directly related to personal and community sanitary practices. In developed countries, it is largely a pediatric disease. In countries where the sanitary infrastructure is inadequate and in institutions plagued by crowding and poor hygienic conditions the disease may be more widespread. Wartime and natural disasters create similar circumstances. The most common species are *S. sonnei* and *S. flexneri,* with *S. dysenteriae* largely limited to underdeveloped tropical areas. *S. dysenteriae,* type 1 produces the most severe disease, historically known as "bacillary dysentery." This condition has slowed the march of many an army; it was the leading cause of death in the notorious Andersonville prison camp during the American Civil War.

Personal and community sanitary practices determine incidence

Wars and disasters create outbreaks

PATHOGENESIS

Shigella, unlike *Vibrio cholerae* and most *Salmonella* species, is acid-resistant and survives passage through the stomach to reach the intestine. Once there, the fundamental pathogenic event is invasion of the human colonic mucosa. This triggers an intense acute inflammatory response with mucosal ulceration and abscess formation. Invasion and spread is a multistep process (Fig 21–5), which is the same in *Shigella* and EIEC.

Bacteria pass stomach acid and invade colon

Shigella initially crosses the mucosal membrane by entering the follicle-associated M cells of the intestine, which lack the highly organized brush borders of absorptive enterocytes. The *Shigella* adhere selectively to M cells and can transcytose through them into the underlying collection of phagocytic cells (Fig 21–6). Bacteria inside M cells and phagocytic macrophages are able to cause their demise by activating normal programmed cell death (apoptosis). Bacteria released from the M cell contact the basolateral side of

M cells are transcytosed

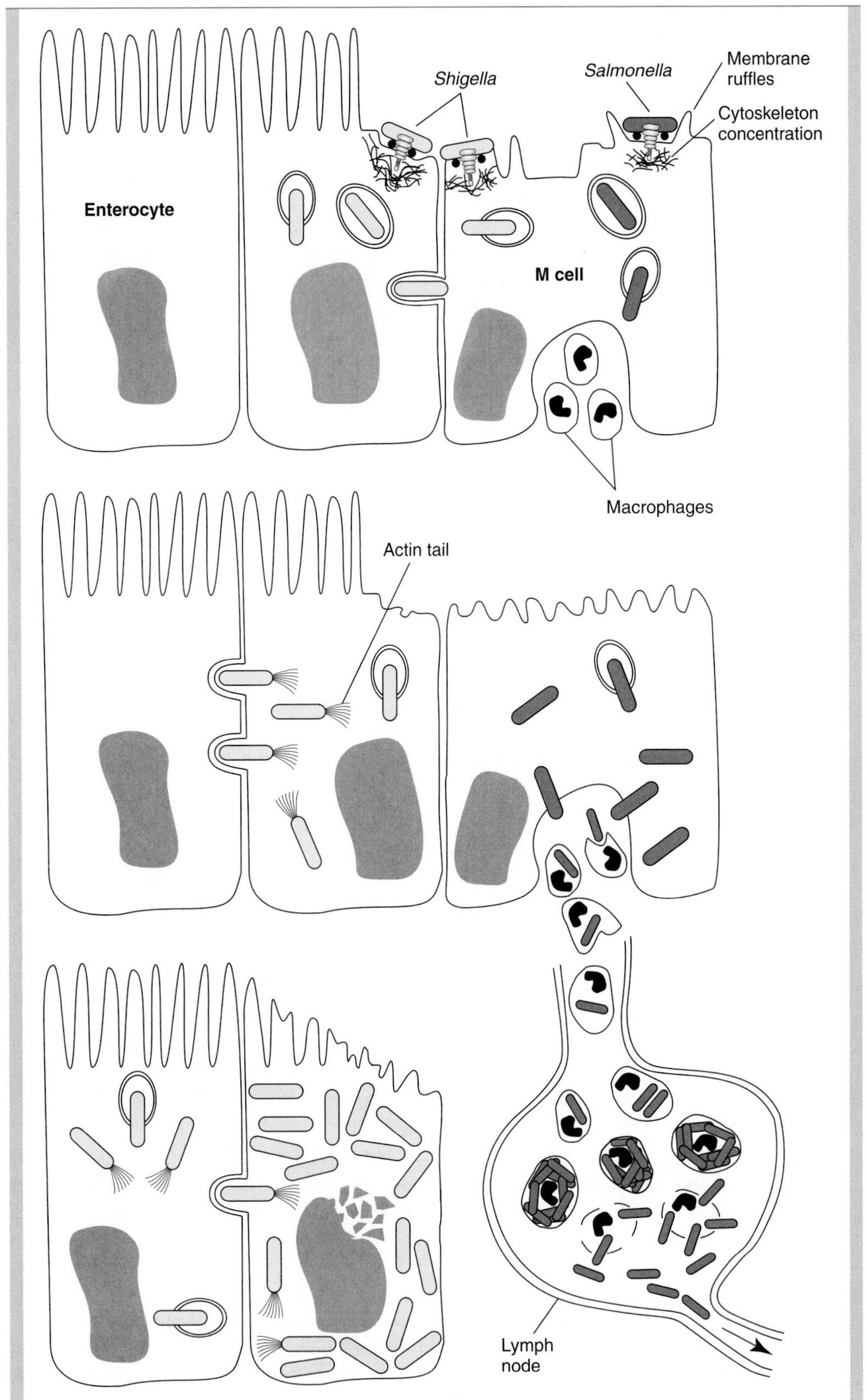

FIGURE 21–5

Invasion by *Shigella flexneri* and *Salmonella* serotype Typhi. The *Shigella* and *Salmonella* are shown invading the intestinal M cells but taking different paths after escaping the endocytotic vacuole. The *Shigella* multiplies in the cell and propels itself through the cytoplasm to invade adjacent cells, and the *Salmonella* passes through the cell to the submucosa, where it is taken up by macrophages. Serotype Typhi is able to multiply in the macrophages in the lymph node and other reticuloendothelial sites. Both organisms induce apoptosis in their host cells. In the case of *Shigella,* this produces a mucosal ulcer; in the case of Typhi, it leads to seeding of the bloodstream and typhoid fever.

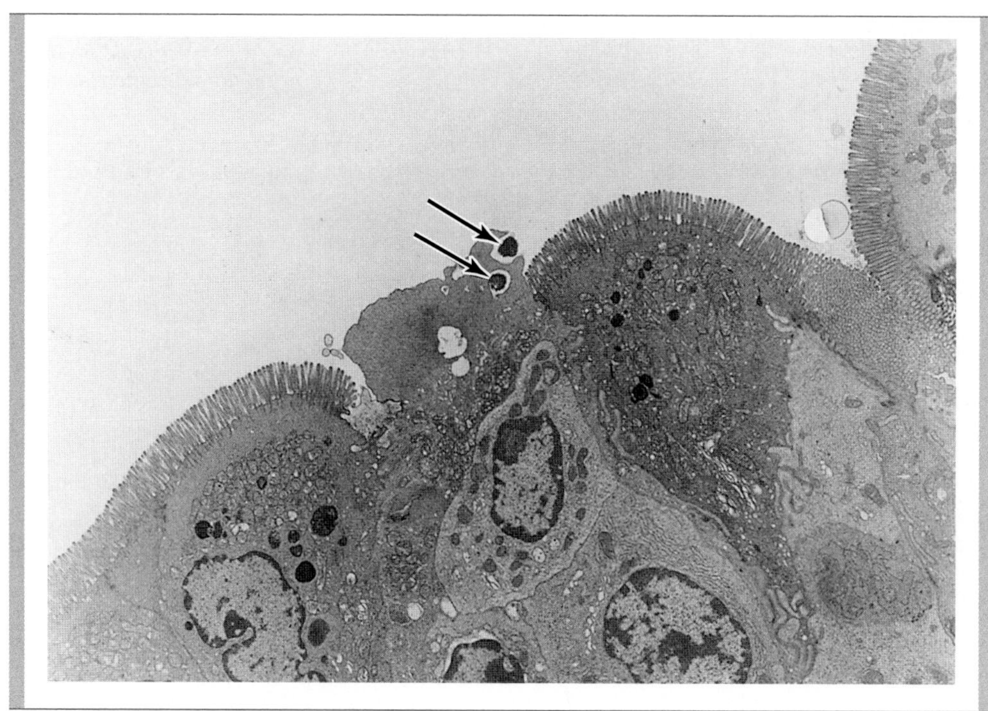

FIGURE 21–6
Salmonella entering an M cell. Two organisms (arrows) are seen attaching to the M cell surface. Note the contrast with the flanking enterocytes and the macrophage just below the M cell.

Injected Ipa proteins direct stages of enterocyte invasion

Cytoskeleton accumulation leads to endocytosis

enterocytes and initiate a multistep invasion process mediated by a set of **invasion plasmid antigens** (IpaA, IpaB, IpaC). On contact with the enterocyte, these antigens are injected by a contact secretion system and each has its individual action. These include cell attachment, cytoskeleton reorganization, actin polymerization, and induction of apoptosis. Rather than create A/E lesions as with EPEC and EHEC, this cytoskeleton modification process involves accumulation of filamentous actin underneath the host cell cytoplasmic membrane, inducing engulfment and internalization of the bacterium into the host cell by endocytosis.

Polymerization of cytoskeletal actin propels bacteria

Adjacent enterocytes are invaded directly

Double-membrane lysis restarts process

Shigella brought into cells are highly adapted to the intracellular environment and make unique use of it to continue the infection. Although initially the bacteria are surrounded by a phagocytic vacuole, they escape within 15 minutes and enter the cytoplasmic compartment of the host cell. Almost immediately, they orient in parallel with the filaments of the actin cytoskeleton of the cell and initiate a process in which they control polymerization of the monomers that make up the actin fibrils. This process creates an actin "tail" at one end of the microbe, which appears to propel it through the cytoplasm like a comet. This exploitation of the cytoskeletal apparatus allows nonmotile *Shigella* to not only replicate in the cell but to move efficiently through it. Eventually, the bacteria encounter the host cell membrane, much of which is adjacent to the neighboring enterocytes. At this point some *Shigella* rebound, but others push the membrane as much as 20 μm into the adjacent cell. This invasion of the neighboring enterocyte forms finger-like projections, which eventually pinch off, placing the bacterium within a new cell but surrounded by double membrane. The organisms then lyse both membranes and are released into the cytoplasm, free to begin the cycle anew.

Enterocyte invasion creates ulcers

Diarrhea + WBCs + RBCs = dysentery

The cell-by-cell extension of this process radially creates focal ulcers in the mucosa, particularly in the colon. The ulcers add a hemorrhagic component and allow *Shigella* to reach the lamina propria, where they evoke an intense acute inflammatory response. Extension of the infection beyond the lamina is unusual in healthy individuals. The diarrhea created by this process is almost purely inflammatory, consisting of small volume stools containing WBCs, RBCs, bacteria, and little else. This is classic dysentery.

Some *Shigella* produce Shiga toxin, which is not essential for disease, but does contribute to the severity of the illness. The original and most potent producer of Shiga toxin, *S. dysenteriae* type 1, is the only *Shigella* with a significant mortality rate among previously healthy individuals. This is probably due to systemic effects of the toxin, which can be the same as described above for the EHEC, including HUS. Enterotoxins have also been described that may be the basis of the watery diarrhea sometimes observed in the early phases.

Shiga toxin increases severity of disease

All virulent *Shigella* and EIEC carry a very large plasmid that has several genes essential for the attachment and entry process, including the Ipa genes. The characteristics of *Shigella* entry and interaction with cellular elements are very similar to those observed with *Listeria monocytogenes* (see Chapter 18), which is Gram-positive, motile, and prefers livestock to humans. Finding that such dissimilar bacteria use such similar tactics to infect their preferred host suggests that this represents a common thread in the selective pressures for a microbe to become a "successful" enteric pathogen.

Large plasmid containing Ipa genes is required for virulence

IMMUNITY

Shigella infection produces relatively short-lived immunity to reinfection with homologous serogroups. There is no consensus on the mechanisms involved.

Immunity is brief

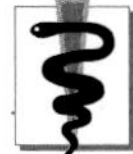

SHIGELLOSIS: CLINICAL ASPECTS

MANIFESTATIONS

Shigella organisms cause an acute inflammatory colitis and bloody diarrhea, which in the most characteristic state presents as a dysentery syndrome—a clinical triad consisting of cramps, painful straining to pass stools (tenesmus), and a frequent, small-volume, bloody, mucoid discharge. However, most clinical shigellosis due to *S. sonnei* in the United States is a watery diarrhea that is often indistinguishable from that of other bacterial or viral diarrheal illness. The disease usually begins with fever and systemic manifestations of malaise, anorexia, and sometimes myalgia. These nondescript symptoms are followed by the onset of watery diarrhea containing the large numbers of leukocytes detectable by light microscopy. The diarrhea may turn bloody with or without the other classical signs of dysentery. The manifestations may be more severe when *S. flexneri,* the species that predominates in the developing world, is involved and most severe with *S. dysenteriae* type 1 (Shiga bacillus). Although the vast majority of shigellosis cases resolve spontaneously after 2 to 5 days, the mortality in Shiga epidemics in Asia, Latin America, and Africa has been as high as 20%.

Watery diarrhea is followed by fever, bloody mucoid stools, and cramping

Mortality significant with *S. dysenteriae* type 1

Most infections are self-limiting

DIAGNOSIS

All *Shigella* species are readily isolated using selective media (e.g. Hektoen enteric agar) which are part of the routine stool culture in clinical laboratories. These media contain chemical additives empirically shown to inhibit facultative flora (eg, *E. coli, Klebsiella*), with relatively little effect on *Shigella* (or *Salmonella*). They also contain indicator systems which utilize typical biochemical reactions to mark suspect *Shigella* colonies among the other flora. Isolates are identified with further biochemical tests. Slide agglutination tests using O group specific antisera (A, B, C, D) confirm both the species and the *Shigella* genus.

Selective media are routinely used

O antigens confirm species

TREATMENT

Several antimicrobics have proved effective in the treatment of shigellosis. Because the disease is usually self-limiting, the beneficial effect of treatment is in shortening the illness and the period of excretion of organisms. Ampicillin was once the treatment of

Treatment may shorten illness and period of excretion

choice, but resistance rates of 5 to 50% have caused a shift to TMP-SMX in many areas. In recent years, quinolones and third-generation cephalosporins have been used in the face of resistance to other agents. Antispasmodic agents may aggravate the condition and are contraindicated in shigellosis and other invasive diarrheas.

Ampicillin resistance is common

PREVENTION

Standard sanitation practices such as sewage disposal and water chlorination are important in preventing the spread of shigellosis. In certain circumstances, insect control may also be important, because flies can serve as passive vectors when open sewage is present. Good individual sanitary practices, such as handwashing and proper cooking of food, are highly protective. Parenteral vaccines have proved disappointing, and current efforts are directed toward finding orally administered live vaccines that can stimulate mucosal IgA. Many strains, including attenuated *Shigella* mutants, *E. coli–Shigella* genetic hybrids, and *E. coli* with genes for some (but not all) the invasive (Ipa) proteins, are vaccine candidates. The general idea is to find a strain that will go through enough of the multistage process (see Pathogenesis) to stimulate an immune response but stop short of full penetration and spread.

Sanitation, insect control, handwashing, and cooking block transmission

Live attenuated vaccines are under investigation

SALMONELLA

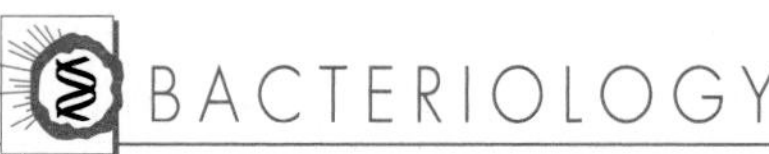

BACTERIOLOGY

More than any other genus, *Salmonella* has been a favorite of those who love to subdivide and apply names to biologic systems. At one time, there were over 2000 names for various members of this genus, often reflecting colorful aspects of place or circumstances of the original isolation (eg, *S. budapest, S. seminole, S. tamale, S. oysterbeds*). This has now been reduced to a single species, *Salmonella enterica,* with the previous species names relegated to the status of serotypes. All of this is made particularly robust by the fact that, in addition to a large number of the LPS O and some capsular K antigens, the flagellar H antigens of most *Salmonella* undergo phase variation. This adds the prospect of two sets of H antigens to the already complex system. As in *Shigella,* the specific O antigens are organized into serogroups (eg, A, B, . . . K, and so on) to which the two H and K (if present) antigen designations are appended to achieve the full antigenic formula. It is not difficult to understand why microbiologists, when confronted with a salmonella with the antigenic formula O:group B [1,4,12] H:I;1,2, still prefer to call it *Salmonella typhimurium.* The proper name for this organism is *Salmonella enterica* serotype Typhimurium, but indulging in the convenience of elevating the serotype to species status is still common.

Complexity of O, K, and H antigens leads to many serotypes

Historic names persist as serotypes of *S. enterica*

Another feature distinguishing *Salmonella* serotypes is their host range. Some are highly adapted to particular mammals or amphibians, and others infect a broad range of hosts. Of interest for medical microbiology are those that infect humans and other animals and those strictly adapted to humans and higher primates. *S. enterica* serotype Typhimurium is the prototype for the former and *S. enterica* serotype Typhi for the latter. In the following discussions, Typhi will be used for the strictly human species that produce enteric (typhoid) fever. Unless otherwise specified, *S. enterica* will be used for the serotypes that are able to infect animals or humans and typically cause gastroenteritis in the latter.

Salmonella species vary in preferred host

S. typhi infects only humans

Salmonellae possess multiple types of pili, one of which is morphologically and functionally similar to the *E. coli* type 1 pili, which bind D-mannose receptors on various eukaryotic cell types. Most strains are motile through the action of their flagella.

Pili and flagella are functional

SALMONELLA GASTROENTERITIS (*S. enterica*)

CLINICAL CAPSULE

The typical example of *Salmonella* "food poisoning" is the community picnic or bazaar, where volunteers prepare poultry, salads, and other potential culture media to be eaten later in the day. Because the refrigerators are filled with beer and soda, the food is left out in covered pans. A near physiologic incubation temperature is provided by the still-warm contents and the afternoon sun. This allows the organisms to enter logarithmic growth during the softball game. The bacteria usually produce no noticeable change in the food. One to two days after the feast, a significant portion of the revelers develop abdominal pain, nausea, vomiting, and diarrhea lasting for 3 or 4 days. An investigation points to a particular food such as potato salad or turkey dressing, which is found to have a correlation with both attack rate and severity of illness.

EPIDEMIOLOGY

S. enterica gastroenteritis is predominantly a disease of industrialized societies and improper food handling, which allows the transmission from the animal reservoir to humans. The infecting dose delivered in contaminated food is higher than with *Shigella*. Ingestion of 1000 or more *Salmonella* bacilli is required to cause illness, making direct human-to-human transmission difficult. Achlorhydric individuals or those taking antacids can be infected with considerably smaller inocula. Consistently, *Salmonella* are a leading cause of food-borne intestinal infection under conditions similar to those described in the above capsule.

Poultry products, including eggs infected transovarially, are most often implicated as the vehicle of infection of *Salmonella* gastroenteritis. Food preparation practices that allow achievement of an infecting dose by growth of the bacteria in the food prior to ingestion are most commonly involved. The incidence in the United States is approximately double that of *Shigella,* with 40,000 to 50,000 reported cases per year. This is believed to reflect only about 1 to 5% of the actual infections. The number of cases varies seasonally, with peak incidence in summer and fall.

Infecting dose is higher than *Shigella*

Poultry products are common source

The highest rates of infection are in children less than 5 years old, persons aged 20 to 30, and those older than 70. If one household member becomes infected, the probability that another will become infected approaches 60%. Nearly one third of all *Salmonella* epidemics occur in nursing homes, hospitals, mental health facilities, and other institutions. A recent increase in the popularity of raw milk has been associated with outbreaks of *Salmonella* (and *Campylobacter*) infection. Exotic pets such as turtles have also been the source of infection. Humans can also be the source of disease. Fully 5% of patients recovering from gastroenteritis still shed the organisms 20 weeks later. Chronic carriers who are food handlers are an important reservoir in the epidemiology of food-borne disease.

Outbreaks in institutions are common

Human carriers can be a source

In recent years, the epidemiology of salmonellosis has changed, and the number of multistate outbreaks has increased, often through the contamination of foodstuffs during large-scale production at a single plant. Efficient interstate and international distribution systems that deliver large amounts of the contaminated food over a wide area facilitate spread. Under these conditions, an attack rate as low as 0.5% can still produce many infections, because of the large number of individuals at risk. It is of concern that relatively small numbers of cases sprinkled over a massive area will be missed by local surveillance systems crippled by budgetary cutbacks.

Modern delivery systems can spread disease efficiently

PATHOGENESIS

Ingested *S. enterica* cells that pass the stomach acid and swim through the intestinal mucous layer eventually reach the enterocytes and M cells of the large and small bowel. Adherence is probably mediated by pili, but on initial contact of bacteria with M cells, the stimulation of membrane "ruffles" dramatically alters the normal architecture within minutes (Fig 21–7).

Adherence triggers surface ruffles

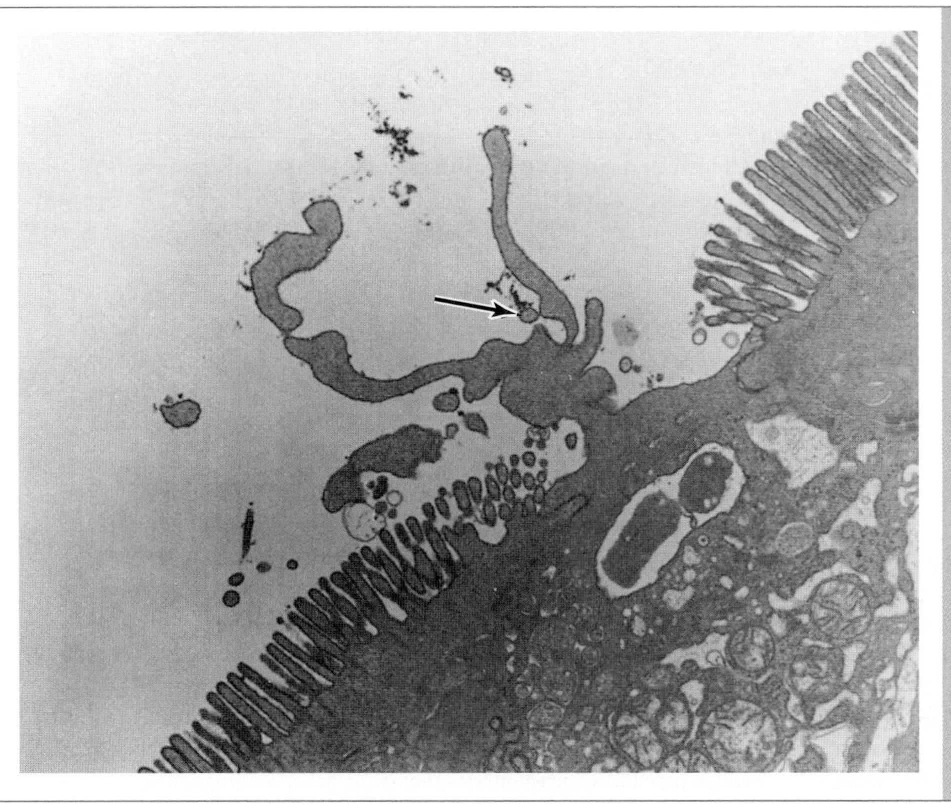

FIGURE 21–7
Salmonella membrane ruffles. These extensions of the plasma membrane are stimulated by the *Salmonella* (arrow) and are related to internalizing the bacteria.

Secretion system genes are in PAIs

These "ruffles" are specialized mammalian plasma membrane sites of filamentous actin cytoskeletal rearrangement normally induced by physiologic molecules such as growth factors. In the case of *Salmonella,* they are stimulated by one or more of a family of more than 12 proteins whose genes (invA, invB, spaP, spaQ) are located in at least two PAIs inserted into the *Salmonella* genome. The virulence factors coded by the genes in the PAIs are either components of the apparatus of a contact secretion system or the effector proteins it injects.

"Ruffles" create transcytosed vacuoles

Macrophage apoptosis aids survival

The "ruffles" seem to engulf the organism in an endocytotic vacuole and allow it to transcytose from the apical surface to the basolateral membrane. Once through the cell, the organisms enter the lamina propria, where they induce a profound inflammatory response. When taken up by macrophages, they are able to persist by inducing apoptosis of the phagocyte. Genes for macrophage survival are located in a second PAI. This process contrasts with *Shigella,* which escapes the endocytotic vacuole (and double vacuole) and prefers to invade adjacent enterocytes rather than move through to the submucosa.

Enterotoxin role is unclear

Invasion and inflammation cause diarrhea

Although some enterotoxins have been described in *Salmonella,* their role in diarrhea is unclear. The best estimate is that the invasion and transcytosis of enterocytes together with the associated increased vascular permeability and inflammatory response are enough to account for the diarrhea. The release of prostaglandins and chemotactic factors may trigger inflammation and biochemical changes in enterocytes. Although the process remains localized to the mucosa and submucosa with most *S. enterica* strains, some invade more deeply, reaching the bloodstream and distant organs. Some serotypes (eg, Choleraesuis) even invade so rapidly that they produce minimal diarrhea and are isolated more frequently from the blood than stool.

IMMUNITY

Immune mechanisms unclear

Evidence that both humoral and cell-mediated immune responses are stimulated by infection with *S. enterica* is ample. How these processes relate to immunity and control of the bacterial infection is largely unknown.

ENTERIC (TYPHOID) FEVER (*Salmonella serotype Typhi*)

CLINICAL CAPSULE

Typhoid is the fever of the phrase "she died of a fever," as in Victorian novels or the street ditty of sweet Molly Malone. Typhoid fever has a slow, insidious onset and if untreated, lasts for weeks. It ends either by a gradual resolution or in death due to complications (eg, rupture of the intestine or spleen). Family members may note only the extended fever, although physicians may observe a subtle rash or feel an enlarged spleen. Diarrhea may occur once or twice during the course but is not a consistent feature.

EPIDEMIOLOGY

Typhoid is a strictly human disease. Chronic carriers of serotype Typhi are the primary reservoir. Some patients become chronic carriers for years (hence the famous "typhoid Mary" Mallon), typically because of chronic infection of the gallbladder and the biliary tract when stones are present. All cases should be traced back to their human source. If a patient with typhoid has not traveled to an endemic area, the source must be a visitor or someone else who prepared food. The pathogen can be transmitted in the water supply in developing endemic areas or where defects in any system allow sewage from carriers to contaminate drinking water. Transmission is by the fecal–oral route. The infecting dose of 10^5 to 10^6 bacteria is intermediate between *Shigella* and most *S. enterica* and decreases in the presence of the capsular Vi antigen.

Cases are traceable to a human source

Fecal–oral transmission requires moderate dose

Typhoid fever is still an important cause of morbidity and mortality worldwide. In the United States and most other industrialized nations, it is mostly seen in travelers to endemic areas such as Latin America, Asia, and India. Visitors from these areas who are carriers are often the source of isolated cases. The decline in disease in industrialized nations largely reflects the availability of clean water supplies and improved disposal of fecal waste.

Prevalence is linked to sanitary infrastructure

PATHOGENESIS

As there is no animal model for the strictly human Typhi, the details of the cellular events are inferred from studies of Typhimurium, which in mice produces a disease similar to typhoid (thus the name). The invasion and killing of intestinal M cells and macrophages are presumed to follow the same pattern as *S. enterica.* Two differences are the surface polysaccharide Vi antigen and the extended multiplication of Typhi in macrophages. In the submucosa, the Vi antigen retards polymorphonuclear neutrophil (PMN) phagocytosis by interfering with complement deposition in a manner similar to other bacterial surface polysaccharides. This may favor uptake by macrophages where at least some Typhi cells establish a privileged niche. Like other serotypes of *Salmonella,* the typhoid bacteria remain within a membrane-bound vacuole and replicate, leading in many cases to macrophage death.

Typhi invades M cells and macrophages

Vi polysaccharide limits PMN phagocytosis

The primary difference between Typhi and the other serotypes is its prolonged intracellular survival in macrophages. This is due to the organism's ability to inhibit the oxidative metabolic burst and continue to multiply. As the bacteria proliferate in macrophages, they are carried through the lymphatic circulation to the mesenteric nodes, spleen, liver and bone marrow, all elements of the reticuloendothelial system (RES). At the RES sites, Typhi continues to multiply, infecting new host macrophages, but eventually the bacteria begin to spill into the bloodstream. This seeding of Gram-negative bacteria and their LPS endotoxin starts the fever, which increases and persists with the continuing bacteremia, sometimes resulting in infection of the urinary tract and other organs. Spread to the biliary tree leads to reinfection of the bowel. This cycle beginning and ending in the small intestine takes approximately 2 weeks to complete.

Inhibition of oxidative burst prolongs macrophage survival

RES sites seed the bloodstream and other organs

Endotoxin produces the fever

IMMUNITY

Immunity follows natural infection

The immune response to enteric fever is both humoral and cell mediated. In nonfatal cases, humoral antibody and activated macrophages eventually subdue the untreated infection over a period of about 3 weeks. Reinfection is rare unless the course was shortened by early administration of antimicrobics. Which antigens stimulate this immunity is not clearly understood. The Vi antigen is usually credited, but various surface proteins are also candidates.

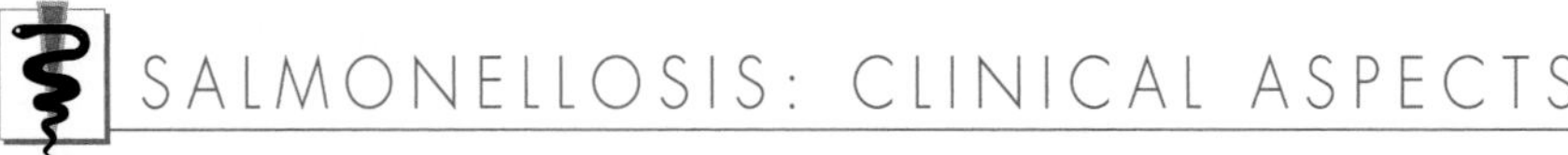

SALMONELLOSIS: CLINICAL ASPECTS

MANIFESTATIONS

S. enterica = gastroenteritis

Typhi = enteric fever

The clinical patterns of salmonellosis can be divided into gastroenteritis, bacteremia with and without focal extraintestinal infection, enteric fever, and the asymptomatic carrier state. Any *Salmonella* serotype can probably cause any of these clinical manifestations under appropriate conditions, but in practice the *S. enterica* serotypes are associated primarily with gastroenteritis. Typhi and a few related serotypes (Paratyphi) cause enteric fever.

Gastroenteritis

Diarrhea, vomiting, and cramps are common

Typically, the episode begins 24 to 48 hours after ingestion, with nausea and vomiting followed by, or concomitant with, abdominal cramps and diarrhea. Diarrhea persists as the predominant symptom for 3 to 4 days and usually resolves spontaneously within 7 days. Fever (39°C) is present in about 50% of the patients. The spectrum of disease ranges from a few loose stools to a severe dysentery-like syndrome.

Bacteremia and Metastatic Infection

Bacteremia is most common and severe in immunocompromised

Metastatic sites linked to previous injury particularly sickle-cell

The acute gastroenteritis caused by *S. enterica* can be associated with transient or persistent bacteremia. Frank sepsis is uncommon, except in those with a compromised cell-mediated immune system. *Salmonella* infection in patients with acquired immunodeficiency syndrome (AIDS) is common and often severe. Bacteremia occurs in 70% of these patients and can cause septic shock and death. Despite adequate antimicrobial coverage, relapses are frequent. Patients with lymphoproliferative disease, perhaps owing to T-cell defects similar to those in patients with AIDS, are also highly susceptible to disseminated salmonellosis. Metastatic spread by salmonellae is a significant risk when bacteremia occurs. These organisms have a unique ability to colonize sites of preexisting structural abnormality including atherosclerotic plaques, sites of malignancy, and the meninges (especially in infants). *Salmonella* infection of the bone typically involves the long bones; in particular, sites of trauma, sickle cell injury, and skeletal prosthesis are at risk.

Enteric Fever

Slowly increasing fever lasts for weeks

Diarrhea is intermittent or absent

Enteric fever is a multiorgan system *Salmonella* infection characterized by prolonged fever, sustained bacteremia, and profound involvement of the RES, particularly the mesenteric lymph nodes, liver, and spleen. The manifestations of typhoid (Fig 21–8) have been well documented in human volunteer studies conducted during vaccine trials. The mean incubation period is 13 days, and the first sign of disease is fever associated with a headache. The fever rises in a stepwise fashion over the next 72 hours. A relatively slow pulse is characteristic and out of phase with the elevated temperature. In untreated patients, the elevated temperature persists for weeks. A faint rash (rose spots) appears during the first few days on the abdomen and chest. Few in number, these spots are readily overlooked, especially in dark-skinned individuals. Many patients are constipated, although perhaps one third of patients have a mild diarrhea. As the untreated disease progresses, an increasing number of patients complain of diarrhea.

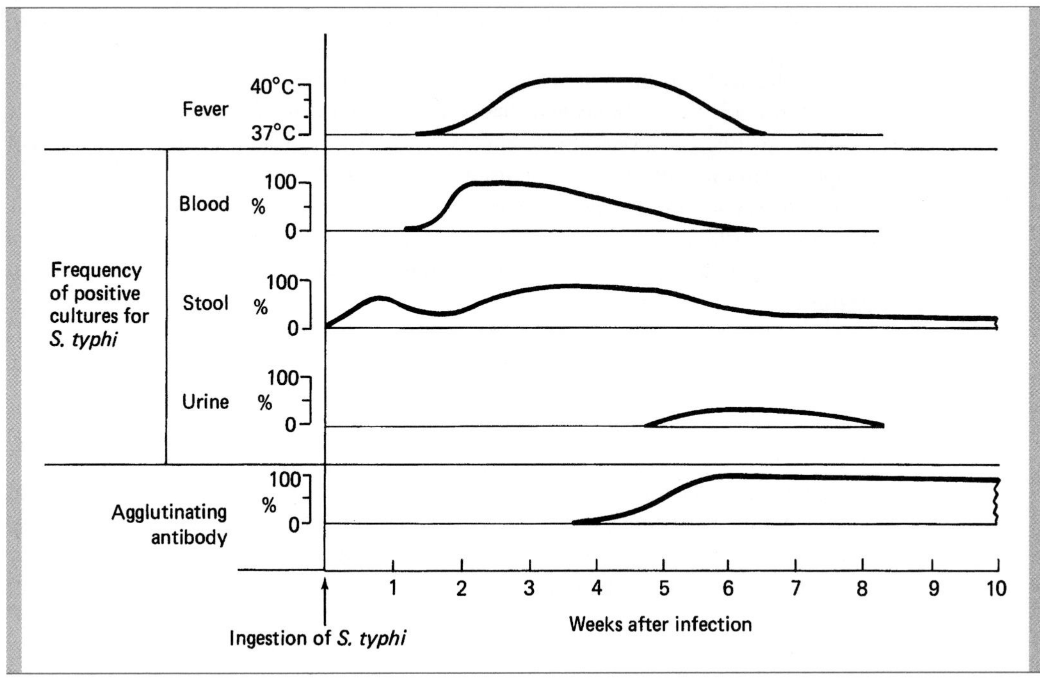

FIGURE 21–8
Natural history of enteric (typhoid) fever. The course of disease without antimicrobial therapy. Fever chart shows time course for typical patient. Culture and agglutinating antibody show timing and probability of positive results in a group of typhoid fever patients.

Obviously, chronic infection of the bloodstream is a serious disease, and the effects of endotoxin can lead to myocarditis, encephalopathy, or intravascular coagulation. Moreover, the persistent bacteremia can lead to infection at other sites. Of particular importance is the biliary tree, with reinfection of the intestinal tract and diarrhea late in the disease. UTI and metastatic lesions in bone, joint, liver, and meninges may also occur. However, the most important complication of typhoid fever is hemorrhage from perforations through the wall of the terminal ileum at the site of necrotic Peyer's patches or in the proximal colon. These occur in patients whose disease has been progressing for 2 weeks or more.

Biliary tree infection reseeds intestine

Urinary tract, bone, and joints are metastatic sites

DIAGNOSIS

Culture of *Salmonella* from the blood or feces is the primary diagnostic method. Early in the course of enteric fever, blood is far more likely to give a positive culture result than culture from any other site. The media used for stool culture are the same as those used for *Shigella.* Failure to ferment lactose and the production of hydrogen sulfides from sulfur-containing amino acids are characteristic features used to identify suspect colonies on the selective isolation media. Characteristics of biochemical tests are used to identify the genus, and O serogroup antisera are available in larger laboratories for confirmation. Typhi has a pattern of biochemical reactions which are sufficient to characterize it without reference to its serogroup (D). All isolates should be referred to public health laboratories for confirmation and epidemiologic tracing. Serologic tests are no longer used for diagnosis.

Stool and blood culture are routine

Typhi has characteristic features

TREATMENT

The primary therapeutic approach to *Salmonella* gastroenteritis is fluid and electrolyte replacement and the control of nausea and vomiting. Antibiotic therapy is usually not appropriate because it has a tendency to increase the duration and frequency of the carrier state. When used to eradicate the carrier state it meets with erratic success and usually fails in the presence of coexisting biliary tract disease. In patients with underlying risk

Antimicrobics are of limited use in gastroenteritis

factors, antimicrobial treatment is used as a prophylactic measure aimed at preventing systemic spread.

Typhoid responds to chemotherapy but resistance is common

Chloramphenicol was the first antibiotic to be used to treat typhoid in 1948, and it reduced the mortality from 20% to less than 2%. Although resistance has developed, it is still a preferred drug in developing countries because it is inexpensive. Ampicillin and trimethoprim–sulfonamide have been used successfully to treat infections caused by chloramphenicol-resistant strains. Newer cephalosporins (ceftriaxone) and quinolones (ciprofloxacin, norfloxacin) are also effective. With proper antimicrobial therapy, patients feel better in 24 to 48 hours, their temperature returns to normal in 3 to 5 days, and they are generally well in 10 to 14 days.

PREVENTION

Typhoid vaccines are only moderately effective

Sanitation and public health measures can eliminate Typhi

Typhoid vaccines have been available since before the turn of the century. An intramuscular killed whole bacterial vaccine was widely used by the military and in travelers but gave poor protection against exposure to large doses of organisms. Recently, a live oral vaccine containing an attenuated Typhi strain has been licensed. Probably as effective as the injectable vaccine, it protects as many as 70% of children in endemic areas. No human vaccine is available for the other *Salmonella* serotypes. When all is said and done, the provision of clean water supplies and the treatment of carriers will lead to the disappearance of typhoid. The importance of carriers and sanitation was emphasized by a 1973 typhoid outbreak among migrant workers in Florida. The source was traced to leakage of sewage into the water supply, failure of chlorination, and a chronic carrier.

YERSINIA

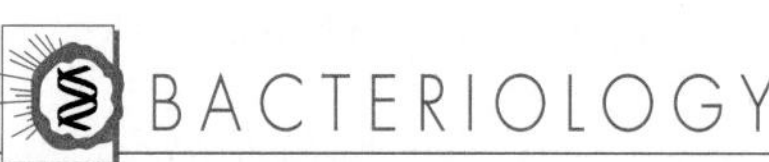

BACTERIOLOGY

Coccobacillary and grow at variable temperatures

Human pathogens are linked to animals

Morphologically, *Yersinia* tends to be coccobacillary and to retain staining at the ends of the cells (bipolar staining). In general, growth and metabolic characteristics are the same as those of other Enterobacteriaceae, although some strains grow more slowly or have optimal growth temperatures below 37°C. The genus includes 11 species, of which *Yersinia pestis, Yersinia pseudotuberculosis,* and *Yersinia enterocolitica* are the important pathogens for humans. *Yersinia pestis* is antigenically homogenous, but *Y. pseudotuberculosis* and *Y. enterocolitica* have multiple O and H antigens. *Yersinia* are primarily animal pathogens, with occasional transmission to humans through direct or indirect contact. *Y. pestis,* the cause of plague, is discussed primarily in Chapter 32, although features of its pathogenesis common to other *Yersinia* are included in this discussion.

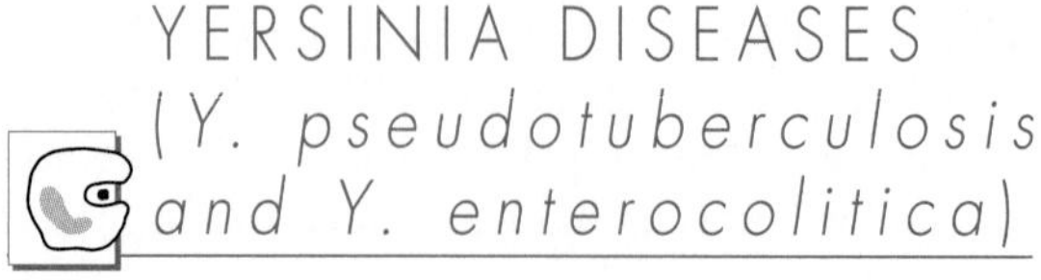

YERSINIA DISEASES (*Y. pseudotuberculosis* and *Y. enterocolitica*)

CLINICAL CAPSULE

Enteropathogenic species of *Yersinia* produce diseases associated with the gastrointestinal tract, ranging from simple gastroenteritis with diarrhea and vomiting to syndromes in which the primary features are abdominal pain and fever. *Yersinia* mesenteric adenitis can simulate acute appendicitis. *Y. enterocolitica* is one of the causes of the enteric fever syndrome.

EPIDEMIOLOGY

In animals, *Y. pseudotuberculosis* causes pseudotuberculosis, a disease characterized by lesions ranging from local necrosis to granulomatous inflammation in the lymph nodes, spleen, and liver. The portal of entry for humans is the gastrointestinal tract, presumably by consumption of contaminated food or water. In most cases animals, including wild animals, are the most likely source of infection, but the exact mode of transmission is unknown. Geographic variation in the frequency of *Y. enterocolitica* infections is marked. The highest rates have been reported from some Scandinavian and other European countries, with much lower rates in the United Kingdom and the United States. Low isolation rates may be partially attributable to the difficulty of growing *Y. enterocolitica* from stool specimens.

Transmitted by ingestion from animal source

Geographic variation is great

PATHOGENESIS

Enteropathogenic *Yersinia* entering the human host in contaminated food invade the M cells of the Peyer's patch. The invasive process and its effect on the host cell are driven by a large array of virulence factors that are deployed under complex genetic and environmental regulation. These proteins include **invasin,** which binds to integrins on the surface of host cells, and the ***Yersinia* outer membrane proteins (Yops),** which are the major effector proteins. The Yops are part of yet another contact secretion system that is deployed between the bacterial cell and host cell cytoplasm. When the Yops are injected into the host cell, they trigger cytotoxic events, including disruption of biochemical pathways (dephosphorylation, serine kinase), sensor functions, and the actin cytoskeleton.

Intestinal M cells are invaded

Secreted Yops disrupt cellular function

Some of the virulence factors produced by *Yersinia* are regulated in a system in which expression responds to either temperature or free calcium (Ca^{2+}) concentration. The physiologic temperature in a mammalian host is different from that in an insect or the environment, and the intracellular calcium concentration is markedly different from that of extracellular fluids. By sensing the environment, *Yersinia* is able to express or suppress virulence factors at different stages of the pathogenic process. The results seem timed to support the pathogenic strategy of *Yersinia,* which is to paralyze the phagocytic activity of defending macrophages and neutrophils and to nullify the host cellular immune response. The virulence determinants are encoded both on the bacterial chromosome and on a plasmid that contains genes for the secretion apparatus and the Yops. Another genetic component is a PAI, which is found only in the three pathogenic species and not the other *Yersinia.* The only known component of this PAI is an iron scavenging siderophore (yersiniabactin).

Ca^{2+} and temperature regulate virulence factor expression

Plasmid and PAI contain virulence genes

The biological outcome of this extraordinary multifactorial process is the enhanced capacity of the pathogenic *Yersinia* to enter and replicate within the RES and to delay the cellular immune response. This leads to the formation of microabscesses and destruction of the cytoarchitecture of Peyer's patches and the mesenteric lymph nodes. The systemic symptoms seen with dissemination can largely be attributed to the effects of endotoxin.

Spread leads to microabscesses in lymph nodes

Y. pestis is a specialized variant closely related to *Y. pseudotuberculosis.* Instead of entering the intestinal tract *Y. pestis* reaches the dermal lymphatics by the bite of an infected flea. It has it own adhesin similar to that of invasin and two plasmids not found in the enteropathogenic *Yersinia.* Unique virulence factors for *Y. pestis* include a capsular protein antigen with antiphagocytic properties, a plasminogen activator protease that promotes adherence to basement membranes, and a fibrinolysin that may play a survival role in the flea.

Y. pestis has capsule, plasminogen activator, and fibrinolysin

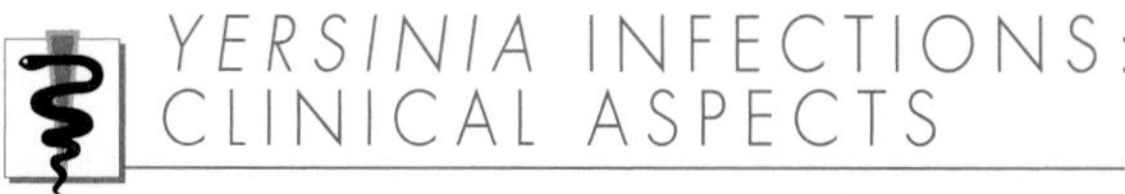

YERSINIA INFECTIONS: CLINICAL ASPECTS

Both *Y. enterocolitica* and *Y. pseudotuberculosis* cause acute mesenteric lymphadenitis, a syndrome involving fever and abdominal pain that often mimics acute appendicitis. *Y. enterocolitica* also produces a wider variety of manifestations. The most common of

Mesenteric lymphadenitis creates abdominal pain

Yersinia are not routinely sought in stools

these is an enterocolitis, which usually occurs in children. It is characterized by fever, diarrhea, and abdominal pain. It also causes enteric fever, terminal ileitis, and a polyarthritic syndrome associated with its diarrheal manifestations. Few laboratories in the United States routinely screen stools for *Yersinia,* because yield has been low and good selective media are not available.

Antimicrobics have variable effect

The role of antimicrobial therapy in the enteric *Yersinia* infections is uncertain, because they are usually self-limiting. *Y. pseudotuberculosis* is susceptible to ampicillin, cephalosporins, aminoglycosides, tetracyclines, and chloramphenicol, but *Y. enterocolitica* is usually resistant to penicillins and cephalosporins through the production of β-lactamases.

OTHER ENTEROBACTERIACEAE

All of the Enterobacteriaceae are capable of producing opportunistic infections of the type discussed above for *E. coli.* None are considered proven causes of enteric disease, although no doubt some will be in the future. The genera isolated in at least moderate frequency are discussed briefly below. There are many other less common species.

KLEBSIELLA

Polysaccharide capsule blocks complement deposition

The most distinctive bacteriologic features of the genus *Klebsiella* are the absence of motility and the presence of a polysaccharide capsule. This gives colonies a glistening, mucoid character and forms the basis of a serotyping system. Over 70 capsular types have been defined, including some that cross-react with those of other encapsulated pathogens, such as *Streptococcus pneumoniae* and *Haemophilus influenzae.* Limited studies suggest that the capsule interferes with complement activation in a way similar to the other encapsulated pathogens. Several types of pili are also present on the surface and probably aid in adherence to respiratory and urinary epithelium.

Often are multiresistant

K. pneumoniae, the most common species, is able to cause classic lobar pneumonia, a characteristic of other encapsulated bacteria. Most *Klebsiella* pneumonias are indistinguishable from those produced by other members of the Enterobacteriaceae. Of all the Enterobacteriaceae, *Klebsiella* species are now among the most resistant to antimicrobics.

ENTEROBACTER

Modest virulence but are linked to hospital contamination

Enterobacter species generally ferment lactose promptly and produce colonies similar to those of *Klebsiella,* although not as mucoid. A differential feature is motility by peritrichous flagella, which are generally present in *Enterobacter* species but uniformly absent in *Klebsiella. Enterobacter* species, which appear to be less virulent than *Klebsiella,* are usually found in mixed infections, in which their significance must be decided on clinical and epidemiologic grounds. Several hospital outbreaks traced to contaminated parenteral fluid solutions have implicated *Enterobacter* species. In addition to ampicillin, most isolates are resistant to first-generation cephalosporins, but may be susceptible to second- or third-generation cephalosporins; however, mutants derepressed for β-lactamase production occur at relatively high frequency and confer resistance to many cephalosporins.

SERRATIA

Red pigment and multiresistance are characteristic

Serratia strains ferment lactose slowly (3 to 4 days), if at all. Some produce distinctive brick-red colonies. Although less common, this genus produces the same range of opportunistic infections seen with the remainder of the Enterobacteriaceae. *Serratia* strains show consistent resistance to ampicillin and cephalothin, with the frequent addition of plasmid-determined resistance to many other antimicrobics, including the aminoglycosides.

Sporadic infections and nosocomial outbreaks with multiresistant strains have often been difficult to control.

CITROBACTER

The genus *Citrobacter,* although biochemically and serologically similar to *Salmonella,* is an uncommon cause of opportunistic infection; it does not cause enterocolitis or enteric fever. Like many other Enterobacteriaceae, *Citrobacter* strains may be present in the normal intestinal flora and cause opportunistic infections. Despite reports of association with diarrheal disease, present evidence does not indicate that *Citrobacter* should be considered an enteric pathogen. *C. freundii* has been associated with neonatal meningitis and brain abscess.

Opportunistic infection and brain abscess are uncommon

PROTEUS, PROVIDENCIA, AND *MORGANELLA*

Proteus, Morganella, and *Providencia* are also opportunistic pathogens found with varying frequencies in the normal intestinal flora. *Proteus mirabilis,* the most commonly isolated member of the group, is one of the most susceptible of the Enterobacteriaceae to the penicillins; this characteristic includes moderate susceptibility to penicillin G. Other Proteeae are regularly resistant to ampicillin and the cephalosporins. *Proteus mirabilis* and *Proteus vulgaris* share the ability to swarm over the surface of media, rather than remaining confined to discrete colonies. This characteristic makes them readily recognizable in the laboratory—often with dismay, because the spreading growth covers other organisms in the culture and thus delays their isolation. *Proteus* and *Morganella* differ from other Enterobacteriaceae in the production of a very potent urease, which aids their rapid identification. It also leads to production of urinary stones and produces alkalinity and an ammoniac odor to the urine. *Providencia* species do not produce urease, are the least frequently isolated, and are generally the most resistant of the group to antimicrobics.

Swarming is a feature of some species

Urease production is linked to urinary stones

ADDITIONAL READING

Darwin KH, Miller VI. Molecular basis of the interaction of *Salmonella* with the intestinal mucosa. *Clin Microbiol Rev* 1999;12:405–428. A well-illustrated review of how *Salmonella* enters and moves through cells. It includes a discussion of the regulation of virulence factors.

Goosney DL, Knoechel DG, Finlay BB. Enteropathogenic *E. coli, Salmonella,* and *Shigella:* Masters of host cell cytoskeleton exploitation. *Emerging Infect Dis* 1999;5:214–223. A concise synopsis that finds similarities among the three major enteropathogenic members of the Enterobacteriaceae.

Nataro JP, Kaper JB. Diarrheagenic *Escherichia coli. Clin Microbiol Rev* 1998;11:142–201. A very comprehensive review that includes pathogenesis and epidemiology as well as clinical aspects. Considerable attention is devoted to molecular diagnostics.

Schaechter M and The View From Here Group. *Escherichia coli* and *Salmonella* 2000: The View From Here. *Microbiol Mol Biol Rev* 2001;65:119–130. As suggested in the title, this is a broad, visionary view of these two pathogens, which extends beyond their medical importance.

CHAPTER 22

Vibrio, Campylobacter, and *Helicobacter*

KENNETH J. RYAN

This group includes *Vibrio cholerae,* the cause of cholera, one of the first proven infectious diseases, and two newcomers incriminated as pathogens in the past two decades (see Table 22–1). The peptic ulcer disease now known to be caused by *Helicobacter pylori* had been long accepted to be due to stress and disturbed gastric acid secretion. *Campylobacter jejuni* is one of the most common causes of diarrhea in virtually every country of the world. Cholera has undergone a resurgence in the last quarter of the 20th century, spreading from its historic Asiatic locale to the Americas, including the coastline of the United States.

VIBRIO

Vibrios are curved, Gram-negative rods commonly found in saltwater. Cells may be linked end to end, forming S shapes and spirals. They are highly motile with a single polar flagellum, non–spore forming, oxidase positive, and can grow under aerobic or anaerobic conditions. The cell envelope structure is similar to that of other Gram-negative bacteria. *Vibrio cholerae* is the prototype cause of a water-loss diarrhea called **cholera.** Other species causing diarrhea, wound infections, and, rarely, systemic infection are listed in Table 22–2.

Rapidly motile curved rods are found in seawater

Vibrio cholerae

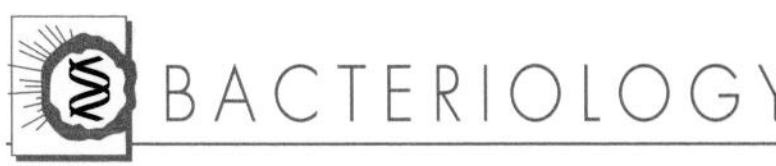

GROWTH AND STRUCTURE

V. cholerae has a low tolerance for acid, but grows under alkaline (pH 8.0 to 9.5) conditions that inhibit many other Gram-negative bacteria. It is distinguished from other vibrios by its biochemical reactions, lipopolysaccharide (LPS) O antigenic structure, and production of cholera toxin (CT). There are over 150 O antigen serotypes, only two of

TABLE 22–1

Features of *Vibrio, Campylobacter,* and *Helicobacter*[a]

Organism	Bacteriology: Growth	Bacteriology: Urease	Epidemiology	Pathogenesis	Disease
Vibrio cholerae	Facultative	–	Fecal–oral, water-borne, pandemics	Cholera toxin (Ace, Zot)	Watery diarrhea (cholera)
Campylobacter jejuni	Microaerophilic	–	Animals, unpasteurized dairy products	Unknown	Dysentery, watery diarrhea
Helicobacter pylori	Microaerophilic	+	Unknown	Vacuolating cytotoxin, urease	Chronic gastritis, ulcers, adenocarcinoma, lymphoma

[a]All are curved Gram-negative rods with similar morphology.

Abbreviations: Ace, accessory cholera enterotoxin; Zot, zona occludens toxin (loosens tight junctions).

TABLE 22–2

Features of Less Common *Vibrio* and *Campylobacter* Species

Organism	Features	Epidemiology	Disease
Vibrio			
V. mimicus	Closely related to *V. cholerae,* cholera-like enterotoxin	Ingestion of raw seafood	Watery diarrhea
V. parahaemolyticus	Produces bowel inflammation, enterotoxin unclear	Coastal seawater; ingesting raw seafood; outbreaks on cruise ships; common in Japan	Watery diarrhea, occasionally dysentery
V. vulnificus	Produces powerful siderophores which scavenge iron from host transferrin and lactoferrin	Coastal seawater, particularly when water temperatures rise; ingesting raw seafood or contamination of wound with seawater	Fulminant bacteremia following ingestion, cellulitis from wound contamination, high fatality in those with Fe^+ storage disease
V. alginolyticus		Wounds contaminated by seawater	Cellulitis
Campylobacter			
C. fetus	Fails to grow on selective medium used for *C. jejuni*	Cause of abortion in cattle and sheep	Bacteremia, thrombophlebitis
C. upsaliensis	Fails to grow on selective medium used for *C. jejuni*	Associated with dogs and cats	Diarrhea similar to *C. jejuni*
C. hyointestinalis		Enteritis in swine	Diarrhea in immunocompromised and homosexual men
C. lari		Associated with birds	Diarrhea, bacteremia in immunocompromised

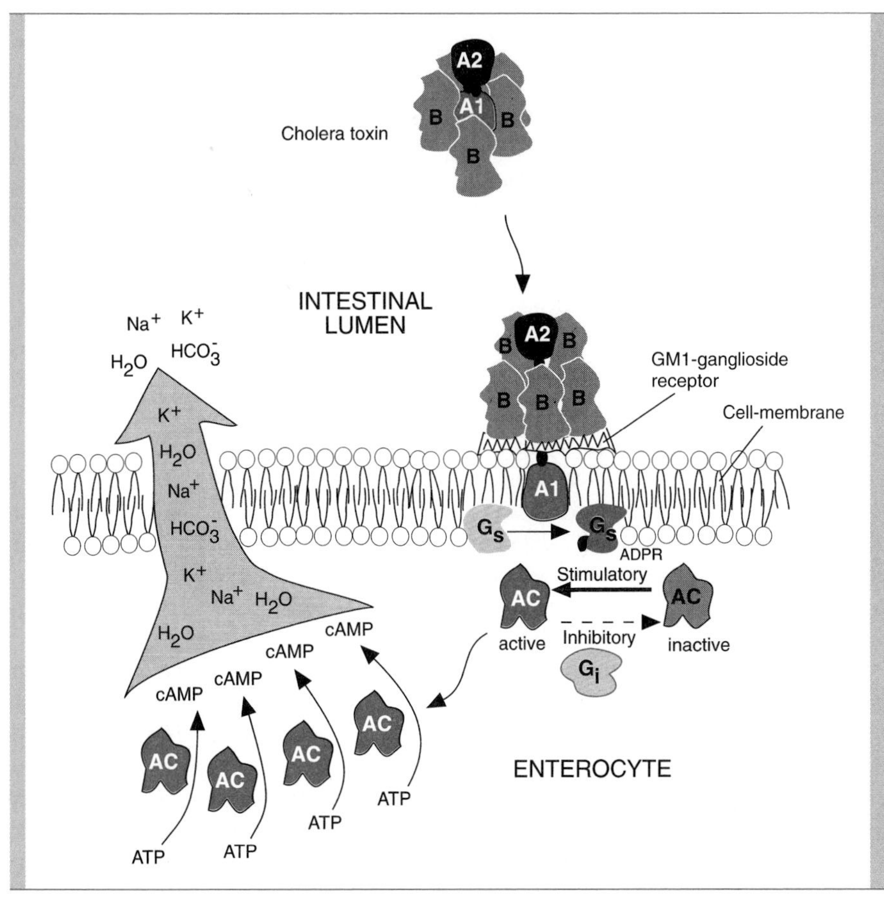

FIGURE 22–1
The action of cholera toxin. The complete toxin is shown binding to the GM1-ganglioside receptor on the cell membrane via the binding (B) subunits. The active portion (A1) of the A subunit catalyzes the ADP-ribosylation of the G_S (stimulatory) regulatory protein, "locking" it in the active state. Because the G_S protein acts to return adenylate cyclase from its inactive to active form, the net effect is persistent activation of adenylate cyclase. The increased adenylate cyclase activity results in accumulation of cyclic adenosine 3′,5′-monophosphate (cAMP) along the cell membrane. The cAMP causes the active secretion of sodium (Na^+), chloride (Cl^-), potassium (K^+), bicarbonate (HCO_3^-), and water out of the cell into the intestinal lumen.

which (O1 and O139) cause cholera. An O1 variant, *V. cholerae* biogroup El Tor is distinguished by biochemical reactions. O139 strains resemble O1 El Tor strains but possess a unique O antigen and have a polysaccharide capsule. *V. cholerae* possess long filamentous pili that form bundles on the bacterial surface and belong to a family of pili whose chemical structure is similar to those of the gonococcus, and a number of other bacterial pathogens. All strains capable of causing cholera produce a colonizing factor known as the toxin-coregulated pilus (TCP) because its expression is regulated together with CT.

Growth prefers alkaline over acid conditions

Cholera is limited to O1 and O139 serotypes

Serotype O139 is encapsulated

CHOLERA TOXIN

The structure and mechanism of action of CT has been studied extensively (Fig 22–1). CT is an A-B type ADP-ribosylating toxin. Its molecule is an aggregate of multiple polypeptide chains organized into two toxic subunits (A1, A2) and five binding (B) units. The B units bind to a GM1-ganglioside receptor found on the surface of many types of cells. Once bound, the A1 subunit is released from the toxin molecule by reduction of the disulfide bond that binds it to the A2 subunit, and it enters the cell by translocation. In the cell, it exerts its effect on the membrane-associated adenylate cyclase system at the basolateral membrane surface. The target of the toxic A1 subunit is a guanine nucleotide (G) protein, Gsα, that regulates activation of the adenylate cyclase system. CT catalyzes the ADP ribosylation of the G protein, rendering it unable to dissociate from the active adenylate cyclase complex. This causes persistent activation of intracellular adenylate cyclase, which in turn stimulates the conversion of adenosine triphosphate to cyclic adenosine 3′, 5′-monophosphate (cAMP). The net effect is excessive accumulation of cAMP at the cell membrane, which causes hypersecretion of chloride, potassium, bicarbonate, and associated water molecules out of the cell. Strains of *V. cholerae* other than the two epidemic serotypes may or may not produce CT.

B subunit receptor is a ganglioside on cell surface

A1 enters cytoplasm and ADP-ribosylates regulatory G protein

Adenylate cyclase becomes locked in active state

Hyperproduction of cAMP causes hypersecretion of water and electrolytes

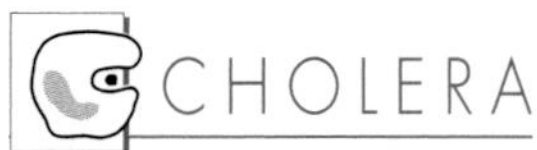

CHOLERA

CLINICAL CAPSULE

Cholera produces the most dramatic watery diarrhea known. Intestinal fluids pour out in voluminous bowel movements; this eventually leads to dehydration and electrolyte imbalance. These effects come from the action of cholera toxin secreted by *V. cholerae* in the bowel lumen. Despite the profound physiologic effects, there is no fever, inflammation, or direct injury to the bowel mucosa.

EPIDEMIOLOGY

Transmission is through untreated water supply

Incubation period is 2 days

Epidemic cholera is spread primarily by contaminated water under conditions of poor sanitation, particularly where sewage treatment is absent or defective. Even though convalescent human carriage is brief, if the numerous vibrios purged from the intestines of cases are able to reach the primary water supply, the conditions for spread are established. The short incubation period (2 days) ensures that organisms ingested by others quickly enter the epidemic cycle. Even so, modern travel makes imported cases possible. One man developed diarrhea in Florida after eating ceviche (marinated uncooked fish) just before departure from an airport in Ecuador.

Cholera is endemic in India and Africa

Pandemics span decades

Gulf Coast cases result from undercooked shellfish

Latin American epidemic is widespread

Cholera is endemic in the Indian subcontinent and Africa. Over the past two centuries, its spread beyond this historic locale to other parts of Asia, Indonesia, and Europe has been described in eight great pandemics, each lasting 5 to 25 years. The current pandemic has brought cholera to the Western Hemisphere for the first time since 1911. Sporadic cases in the United States first appeared in the early 1970s and were traced to inadequately cooked crabs and shrimp caught off the Gulf Coast of Louisiana and Texas. In 1991, Latin America was hit with epidemic cholera with cases reported from 21 countries from Peru to northern Mexico. In Peru alone, over 500,000 cases and 4500 deaths occurred in 2 years. The disease is now endemic, claiming thousands of lives every year. Virulent *V. cholerae* now lurks in coastal waters throughout the hemisphere and in the drinking water of locales with poor sanitation.

El Tor biotype dominated 20th century

New O139 serotype is spreading

The dominant strain of the 20th century was the El Tor biotype, first isolated from Mecca pilgrims at the El Tor quarantine camp in 1905. This strain survives slightly longer in nature and is more likely to produce subclinical cases of cholera, both of which facilitated its spread. In 1992, the first cholera cases due to a serotype other than O1 were detected in India and Bangladesh. The new serotype (O139 Bengal) is fully virulent with the additional threat of enhanced ability to produce disease in persons whose immunity is due to exposure to the old serotype. This development is important for the global spread of cholera and for the vaccine strategies designed to prevent it.

Dormant form in plankton may facilitate interepidemic survival

The triggering of epidemics and the interepidemic survival of *V. cholerae* in the environment is incompletely understood but may be linked to **crustaceans** and the **plankton** population. *V. cholerae* in a dormant state can be demonstrated by immunofluorescence in plankton, and epidemics follow plankton blooms. Otherwise the organism is fragile, surviving only a few days in the environment unless maintained longer in marine and freshwater crustaceans.

PATHOGENESIS

Large doses required to pass stomach acid barrier

Pili mediate epithelial adherence

CT-stimulated intestinal hypersecretion causes diarrhea

To produce disease, *V. cholerae* must reach the small intestine in sufficient numbers to multiply and colonize. In healthy people, ingestion of large numbers of bacteria is required to offset the acid barrier of the stomach. Colonization of the entire intestinal tract from the jejunum to the colon by *V. cholerae* requires organism adherence to the epithelial surface, most probably by surface pili. The outstanding feature of *V. cholerae* pathogenicity is the ability of virulent strains to secrete CT, which is responsible for the disease cholera. The water and electrolyte shift from the cell to the intestinal lumen is the fundamental cause of the watery diarrhea of cholera.

Fluid Loss

The fluid loss that results from the adenylate cyclase stimulation of cells depends on the balance between the amount of bacterial growth, toxin production, fluid secretion, and fluid absorption in the entire gastrointestinal tract. The outpouring of fluid and electrolytes is greatest in the small intestine, where the secretory capacity is high and absorptive capacity low. The diarrheal fluid can amount to many liters per day, with approximately the same sodium content as plasma but two to five times the potassium and bicarbonate concentrations. The result is dehydration (isotonic fluid loss), hypokalemia (potassium loss), and metabolic acidosis (bicarbonate loss). The intestinal mucosa remains unaltered except for some hyperemia, because *V. cholerae* does not invade or otherwise injure the enterocyte. Mutants lacking CT may still cause mild diarrhea due to recently discovered accessory toxins which cause fluid secretion or increase intestinal permeability.

Small intestine loses liters of fluid

K^+ and bicarbonate losses cause hypokalemia and acidosis

Intestinal mucosa is structurally unaffected; no invasion

Genetic Regulation of Virulence

The expression of the multiple virulence factors of *V. cholerae* is controlled in a complex but coordinated system involving environmental sensors and as many as 20 chromosomal genes divided between a pathogenicity island (PAI) containing CT and one containing TCP. The chief regulator is a transmembrane protein (ToxR) that "senses" environmental changes in pH, osmolarity, and temperature which convert it to an active form. In the active state, ToxR can directly turn on CT genes as well as activate transcription of a second regulatory protein, ToxT. ToxT can then activate transcriptional of virulence genes in both PAIs, including TCP, CT, and accessory toxins.

Regulatory system turns on CT and TCP in response to environmental changes

IMMUNITY

Nonspecific defenses such as gastric acidity, gut motility, and intestinal mucus are important in preventing colonization with *V. cholerae*. For example, in persons who lack gastric acidity (gastrectomy or achlorhydria from malnutrition), the attack rate of clinical cholera is higher. Natural infection provides long-lasting immunity. The immune state has been associated with IgG directed against the cell wall LPS and with the production of secretory IgA by lymphocytes in the subepithelial areas of the gastrointestinal tract. The precise protective mechanisms remain to be established.

Attack rate is higher with achlorhydria

Immunity is associated with sIgA

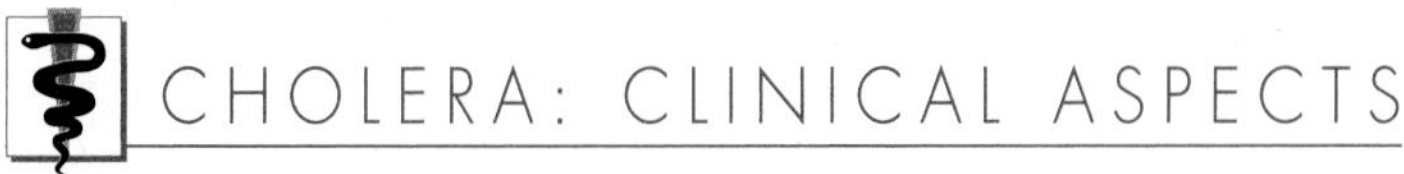

CHOLERA: CLINICAL ASPECTS

MANIFESTATIONS

Typical cholera has a rapid onset, beginning with abdominal fullness and discomfort, rushes of peristalsis, and loose stools. Vomiting may also occur. The stools quickly become watery, voluminous, almost odorless, and contain mucus flecks, giving it an appearance called **rice-water stools.** Neither white blood cells or blood are present in the stools, and the patient is afebrile. Clinical features of cholera result from the extensive fluid loss and electrolyte imbalance, which can lead to extreme dehydration, hypotension, and death within hours if untreated.

Extreme watery diarrhea causes large fluid loss

Dehydration and electrolyte imbalance are the major problems

DIAGNOSIS

The initial suspicion of cholera depends on recognition of the typical clinical features in an appropriate epidemiologic setting. A bacteriologic diagnosis is accomplished by isolation of *V. cholerae* from the stool. The organism grows on common clinical laboratory media such as blood agar and MacConkey agar, but its isolation is enhanced by the use of a selective medium (thiosulfate-citrate-bile salt-sucrose agar). Once isolated, the organism is readily identified by biochemical reactions. Outside cholera endemic areas, the

Stool culture using selective media is required

selective medium is not routinely used for stool cultures, so clinical laboratories must be alerted to the suspicion of cholera.

TREATMENT

Oral or intravenous fluid and electrolyte replacement is crucial

Antimicrobic therapy can reduce duration and severity

The outcome of cholera is dependent on balancing the diarrheal fluid and ionic losses with adequate fluid and electrolyte replacement. This is accomplished by oral and/or intravenous administration of solutions of glucose with near physiologic concentrations of sodium and chloride and higher than physiologic concentrations of potassium and bicarbonate. Exact formulas are available as dried packets to which a given volume of water is added. Oral replacement, particularly if begun early, is sufficient for all but the most severe cases and has substantially reduced the mortality from cholera. Antimicrobial therapy plays a secondary role to fluid replacement. Tetracyclines shorten the duration of diarrhea and magnitude of fluid loss. Trimethoprim–sulfamethoxazole and erythromycin are alternatives for use in children and pregnant women.

PREVENTION

Water sanitation and cooking shellfish prevent infection

Vaccines are disappointing

Epidemic cholera, a disease of poor sanitation, does not persist where treatment and disposal of human waste is adequate. Because good sanitary conditions do not exist in much of the world, secondary local measures such as boiling or chlorination of water during epidemics are required. The cases associated with crustaceans can be prevented by adequate cooking (10 minutes) and avoidance of recontamination from containers and surfaces. Vaccines prepared from whole cells, lipopolysaccharide, and CT B subunit have been disappointing, providing protection that is not long-lasting. Current interest includes live attenuated vaccine strains because of their potential to stimulate the local sIgA immune response.

Other Vibrios

V. parahaemolyticus in undercooked or raw seafood causes diarrhea

V. vulnificus sepsis and wound infections linked to raw oysters and iron overload

Species of *Vibrio* other than *V. cholerae* may still produce disease but are uncommon and typically restricted to seacoast locales. Most, such as *V. parahaemolyticus,* produce a diarrheal illness following ingestion of raw or inadequately cooked seafood. They do not produce cholera toxin, but some have been shown to produce their own enterotoxins. Of these, *V. vulnificus* stands out because it can produce a rapidly progressive cellulitis in wounds sustained in seawater and a bacteremic infection following ingestion of raw seafood. The latter has a high mortality rate and has been common enough in Florida to threaten the local oyster trade. *V. vulnificus* has also been shown to be a spectacular scavenger of host iron stores and produces particularly fulminant disease in persons with iron-overload states (eg, thalassemia, hemochromatosis). Features of the less common vibrios are included in Table 22–2.

CAMPYLOBACTER

Campylobacters are motile, curved, oxidase-positive, Gram-negative rods similar in morphology to vibrios. The cells have polar flagella and are often are attached at their ends giving pairs "S" shapes or a "seagull" appearance. More than a dozen *Campylobacter* species have been associated with human disease. Of these *C. jejuni,* and *C. coli* are by far the most common and similar enough to be considered as one. Some other *Campylobacter* species are potential causes of diarrhea, but only *C. jejuni* will be discussed here. The features of other species are summarized in Table 22–2.

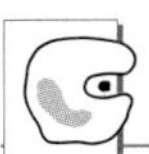

BACTERIOLOGY: *Campylobacter jejuni*

Before 1973, *C. jejuni* was not recognized as a cause of human disease. It was not until selective methods for its isolation were developed that it was recognized as one of the most common causes of infectious diarrhea. Like other campylobacters, *C. jejuni* grows well only on enriched media under microaerophilic conditions. That is, it requires oxygen at reduced tension (5–10%), presumably due to vulnerability of some of its enzyme systems to superoxides. Growth usually requires 2 to 4 days, sometimes as much as a week. *C. jejuni* has the structural components found in other Gram-negative bacteria (eg, outer membrane, LPS). In contrast to the vibrios, it does not break down carbohydrates, but uses amino acids and metabolic intermediates for energy.

Microaerophilic atmosphere is required for growth

CAMPYLOBACTER ENTERITIS

CLINICAL CAPSULE

C. jejuni infection typically begins with lower abdominal pain, which evolves into diarrhea over a matter of hours. The diarrhea may be watery or dysenteric, with blood and pus in the stool. Most patients are febrile. The illness resolves spontaneously after a few days to 1 week.

EPIDEMIOLOGY

It is humbling to consider how a pathogen as common as *C. jejuni* could have been missed for decades. Studies from many countries find *C. jejuni* in 4 to 30% of diarrheal stools, making it the leading cause of gastrointestinal infection in developed countries. Over 2 million cases occur each year in the United States, at a rate roughly double the second most common bacterial enteric pathogen, *Salmonella.* This high rate of disease is facilitated by the low infecting dose of *C. jejuni*—only a few hundred cells.

Causes diarrhea worldwide

Infecting dose is low

The primary reservoir is in animals and the bacteria are transmitted to humans by ingestion of contaminated food or by direct contact with pets. Campylobacters are commonly found in the normal gastrointestinal and genitourinary flora of warm-blooded animals, including sheep, cattle, chickens, wild birds, and many others. Domestic animals such as dogs may also carry the organisms and probably play a significant role in transmission to humans. The most common source of human infection is undercooked poultry, but outbreaks have been caused by contaminated rural water supplies and unpasteurized milk often consumed as a "natural" food. Sometimes a direct association can be made as with a sick household pet.

Reservoir is animals

Undercooked poultry and unpasteurized milk are major sources

PATHOGENESIS

Infection is established by oral ingestion, followed by colonization of the intestinal mucosa. The bacteria have been shown to adhere to endothelial cells and then enter cells in endocytotic vacuoles. Once inside, they move in association with the cell's microtubule structure, rather than the actin microfilaments associated with many other invasive bacteria. The search for enterotoxins associated with *C. jejuni* has thus far been unrewarding. A cytolethal distending toxin arrests cell division while the cytoplasm continues to grow, but how this leads to diarrhea remains to be established. All in all, the virulence determinants of this microorganism remain uncertain.

Intracellular movement is associated with microtubules

Cytolethal distending toxin is a candidate

There is an association between *C. jejuni* infection and the **Guillain-Barré syndrome,** an acute demyelinating neuropathy that is frequently preceded by an infection. Although *C. jejuni* is not the only antecedent to this syndrome, it is the most common of identifiable causes. Up to 40% of patients have culture or serologic evidence of *Campylobacter* infection at the time the neurologic symptoms occur. The mechanism is believed to involve antibody elicited by ganglioside-like structures in the *C. jejuni* LPS core

Guillain-Barré syndrome may follow infection

Antiganglioside antibodies cross-react with neural tissue

oligosaccharide that cross-react with similar molecules in the host peripheral nerve myelin. These antiganglioside antibodies are found in the serum of patients with Guillain-Barré syndrome motor neuropathies. This molecular mimicry is similar to the mechanism of rheumatic fever stimulated by the group A streptococcus (see Chapter 17).

IMMUNITY

Immune mechanisms are unclear

Acquired immunity following natural infection with *C. jejuni* has been demonstrated in volunteer studies, but the mechanisms involved are unknown. Antibodies are formed in the weeks following infection but decline rapidly thereafter. The high rate of *Campylobacter* infection in patients with acquired immunodeficiency syndrome suggests the importance of cellular immune mechanisms.

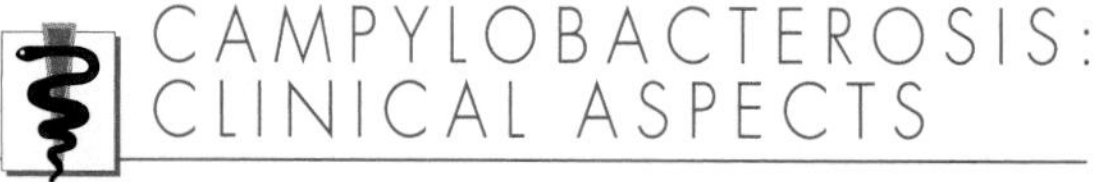

CAMPYLOBACTEROSIS: CLINICAL ASPECTS

MANIFESTATIONS AND DIAGNOSIS

Abdominal pain and dysentery are present

Selective medium is incubated in microaerophilic atmosphere

The illness typically begins 1 to 7 days after ingestion, with fever and lower abdominal pain that may be severe enough to mimic acute appendicitis. These are followed within hours by dysenteric stools that usually contain blood and pus. The illness is typically self-limiting after 3 to 5 days but may last 1 to 2 weeks. The diagnosis is confirmed by isolation of the organism from the stool. This requires a special medium made selective for *Campylobacter* by inclusion of antimicrobics that inhibit the normal facultative flora of the bowel. Plates must be incubated in a microaerophilic atmosphere that can now be conveniently generated in a sealed jar by hydration of commercial packs similar to those used for anaerobes.

TREATMENT

Erythromycin may shorten course

Since less than half of patients clearly benefit from antimicrobial therapy, cases are usually not treated unless the disease is severe or prolonged (>1 week). *C. jejuni* is typically susceptible to macrolides and fluoroquinolones but resistant to β-lactams. Erythromycin is considered the treatment of choice but must be given early for maximal effect. Fluoroquinolones are also effective, but resistance is becoming more common.

HELICOBACTER

Everything we once knew about ulcers was wrong

In 1983, a pair of Australian microbiologists suggested that gastritis and peptic ulcers were infectious diseases, contradicting long-held beliefs concerning their epidemiology, pathogenesis, and treatment. In the same year, the 10th edition of *Harrison's Principles of Internal Medicine* described peptic ulcers as due to an unfavorable balance between gastric acid–pepsin secretion and gastric or duodenal mucosal resistance. Underlying causes cited included genetic and lifestyle (smoking) as well as psychological factors (anxiety, stress). Treatment with bismuth salts, antacids, and inhibitors of acid secretion gave relief but not cure. Relapsing patients (50 to 80%) were subjected to surgical treatments (vagotomy, partial gastrectomy), which had their own set of complications (reflux, afferent loop syndrome, dumping syndrome). All of this was logical and supported by clinical observations and research studies. It was simply incorrect. The bacteria now called *Helicobacter* had been observed but dismissed because they were so common and its urease was once considered a secretory product of the stomach itself. The paper by Warren and Marshall (see Additional Reading) stimulated the reversal, which has led to cures using antimicrobics and new ideas linking *Helicobacter* infection to cancer. This experience has also left us with a sense that we can never be smug about what we "know" in medicine.

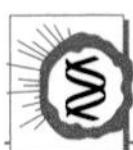 BACTERIOLOGY: *Helicobacter pylori*

H. pylori has morphologic and growth similarities to the campylobacters, with which they were originally classified. The cells are slender, curved rods with polar flagella. The cell wall structure is typical of other Gram-negative bacteria, although *Helicobacter* LPS may be less toxic than its enteric counterparts. Growth requires a microaerophilic atmosphere and is slow (3 to 5 days).

Features are similar to *Campylobacter* including microaerophilic requirement

A number of unique bacteriologic features have been found in *H. pylori.* The most distinctive is a **urease** whose action allows the organism to persist in low pH environments by the generation of ammonia. The urease is produced in amounts so great (6% of bacterial protein) that its action can be demonstrated within minutes of placing *H. pylori* in the presence of urea. Another secreted protein called the **vacuolating cytotoxin** (VacA) causes apoptosis in eukaryotic cells it enters generating multiple large cytoplasmic vacuoles. The vacuoles are felt to be generated by the toxin's formation of channels in lysosomal and endosomal membranes.

Urease raises pH rapidly

VacA injures lysosomal and endosomal membranes

Most *H. pylori* strains also contain a 30+ gene PAI, so called because the guanine + cytosine content of the PAI differs from the rest of the genome. This suggests the PAI is a genetic cassette acquired from some unknown organism in the distant past. Most of the PAI genes code for elements of a **contact secretion system,** which in other bacteria transfers DNA or proteins across the outer membrane to the extracellular space or into other cells. The cells receiving the products of these secretion systems include bacterial, plant, and epithelial cells. In *H. pylori,* the secretion system injects VacA and a protein *Cag*, also coded in the PAI, into epithelial cells. Once in the cell, *Cag* induces changes in multiple cellular proteins and has a strong association with virulence (see Pathogenesis).

PAI contains genes for *Cag* and contact secretions system

Cag induces changes inside host cell

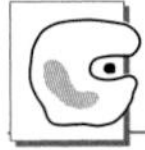 HELICOBACTER GASTRITIS

CLINICAL CAPSULE

Helicobacter infections are limited to the mucosa of the stomach, and most are asymptomatic even after many years. Burning pain in the upper abdomen, accompanied by nausea and sometimes vomiting, is a symptom of gastritis. Ulcers may cause additional symptoms, depending on their anatomic location. It is common for gastric and duodenal ulcers to be unrecognized by the patient until they cause frank bleeding or rupture.

EPIDEMIOLOGY

Infection with *H. pylori* causes what is perhaps the most prevalent disease in the world. The organism is found in the stomachs of 30 to 50% of adults in developed countries and it is almost universal in developing countries. The exact mode of transmission is not known, but is presumed to be person to person by the fecal–oral route or by contact with gastric secretions in some other way. Colonization increases progressively with age, and children are believed to be the major amplifiers of *H. pylori* in human populations. A declining prevalence in developed countries may be due to decreased transmission because of less crowding and frequent exposure to antimicrobics.

Infection is transmitted by human fecal or gastric secretions

Gastric colonization is prevalent worldwide

Once established, the same strain persists at least for decades, probably for life. Molecular epidemiologic analysis indicates the strains themselves have strong linkages to ethnic origins that can be traced back to the earliest known patterns of human migration. *H. pylori* has been called an "accidental tourist," which was established in the stomachs of

Colonization persists indefinitely

Ethnic links are strong

humans before migration began and remained bound to the original population as it dispersed from continent to continent over thousands of years.

H. pylori is the sole nondrug cause of gastritis and ulcers

Adenocarcinoma and lymphoma are preceded by infection

H. pylori is the most common cause of gastritis, gastric ulcer, and duodenal ulcer. In addition *Helicobacter* gastritis caused by Cag^{+} strains is acknowledged to be the antecedent cause of gastric adenocarcinoma, one of the most common causes of cancer death in the world. It is also linked to a gastric mucosa-associated lymphoid tissue (MALT) lymphoma, which is less common but shows the striking property of regressing with antimicrobial therapy. *H. pylori* recently gained the dubious distinction of being the first bacterium declared a class I carcinogen by the World Health Organization.

Other *Helicobacter* species occur in animals

H. pylori is exclusive to humans, but other species have been found in the stomachs of a wide range of animals, where they are also associated with gastritis. It is difficult to imagine the old "stress ulcer" theories surviving the discovery of a cheetah with *Helicobacter* gastritis. Speculation that domestic animals may serve as a reservoir for human infection has not been confirmed.

PATHOGENESIS

Urease ammonia production neutralizes acid

Motility facilitates surface microenvironment

In order to persist in the hostile environs of the stomach, *H. pylori* employs multiple mechanisms to adhere to the gastric mucosa and survive the acid milieu of the stomach. Motility provided by the flagella allows the organisms to swim to the less acid pH locale beneath the gastric mucus, where the urease further creates a more neutral microenvironment by ammonia production. At the mucosa, adherence is mediated by surface proteins, one of which binds to Lewis blood group antigens, often present on the surface of gastric epithelial cells.

VacA and *Cag* stimulate inflammation

H. pylori colonization is virtually always accompanied by a cellular infiltrate ranging from minimal mononuclear infiltration of the lamina propria to extensive inflammation with neutrophils, lymphocytes, and microabscess formation. This inflammation may be due to toxic effects of the urease or the VacA. The *Cag* protein may contribute by stimulation of cytokines (interleukin-8), and a neutrophil-activating protein (NAP) has been shown to recruit neutrophils to the gastric mucosa. Added together urease, *Cag*, and NAP provide ample explanation for the gastritis that is universal in *H. pylori* infection.

VacA directly induces cellular changes and death

Cag has strong association but uncertain role

A prolonged and aggressive inflammatory response could lead to epithelial cell death and ulcers, but other virulence factors play a more direct role. The chief of these is VacA, which is responsible for much of the epithelial cell erosion seen in human infection. The vacuolar degeneration it induces is readily visible histologically in gastric biopsies (Fig 22–2). The importance of *Cag* is clear from its epidemiologic association with ulcers, but its exact role is unclear. When *Cag* is transported into epithelial cells by the PAI secretion system, it induces an active reorganization of the cellular actin cytoskeleton and activation of multiple host cell proteins. How these changes are integrated to contribute to ulcer formation remains to be demonstrated.

Carcinogenic mechanisms are unknown

That decades of inflammation and assault by the virulence factors described above could eventually lead to cancer seems logical, but the specific mechanisms of carcinogenesis are unknown. *Cag* is a leading candidate. A curious paradox is that while Cag^{+} strains are associated with ulcers and adenocarcinoma of the lower stomach, they are associated with a decreased incidence of adenocarcinoma of the upper stomach (cardia) and esophagus. Dissection of the many actions *Cag* has within cells should shed light on these issues.

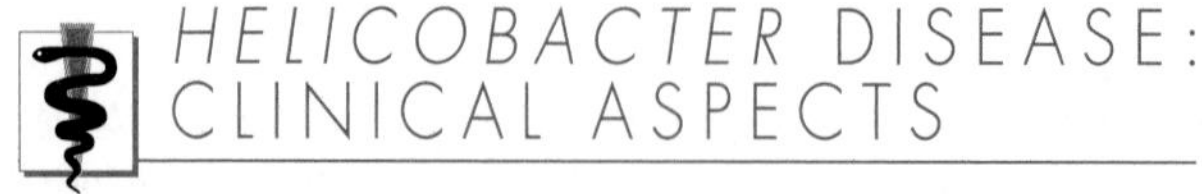

HELICOBACTER DISEASE: CLINICAL ASPECTS

MANIFESTATIONS

Epigastric pain and nausea are signs of gastritis

Primary infection with *H. pylori* is either silent or causes an illness with nausea and upper abdominal pain lasting up to 2 weeks. Years later, the findings of gastritis and peptic ulcer disease include nausea, anorexia, vomiting, epigastric pain, and even less specific symptoms

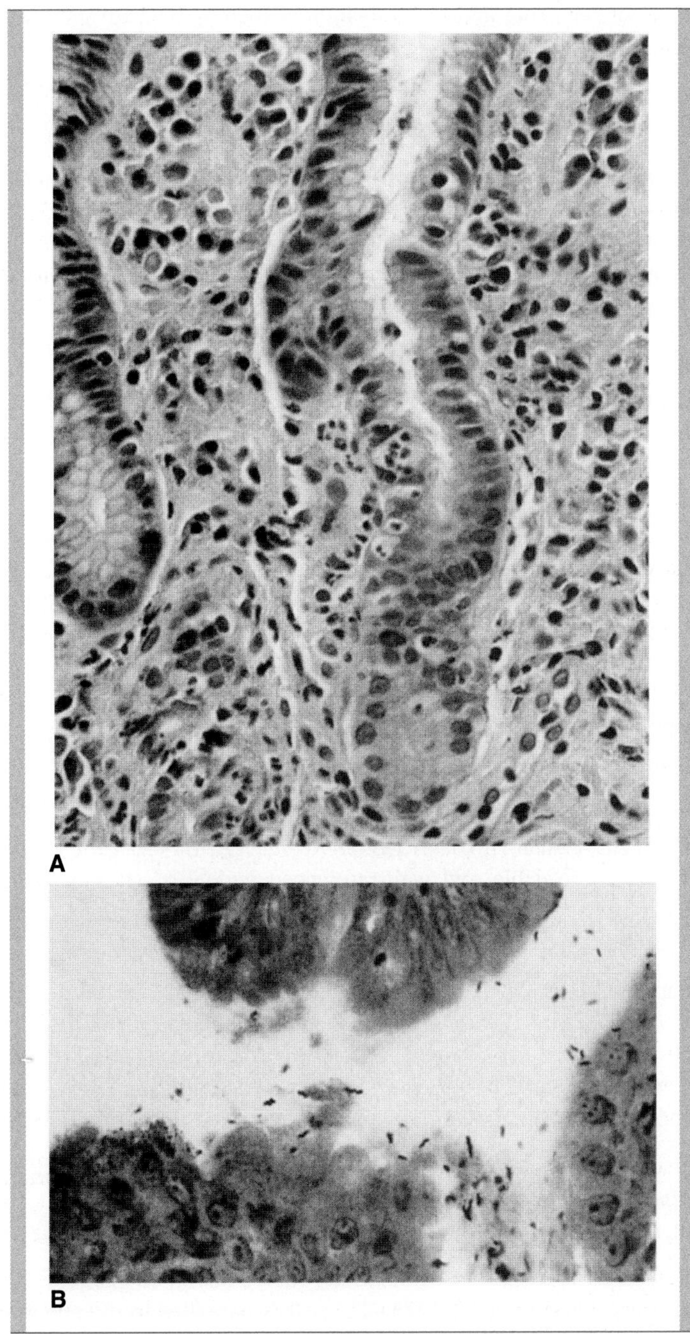

FIGURE 22–2
Helicobacter gastritis. **A.** Gastric mucosa shows infiltration of neutrophils and destruction of epithelial cells. **B.** High magnification shows curved bacilli. *(Reproduced with permission from Connor DH, Chandler FW, Schwartz DQA, Manz HJ, Lack EE (eds).* Pathology of Infectious Diseases, *vol. 1. Stamford, CT: Appleton & Lange; 1997.)*

such as belching. Many patients are asymptomatic for decades, even up to perforation of an ulcer. Perforation can lead to extensive bleeding and peritonitis due to the leakage of gastric contents into the peritoneal cavity.

DIAGNOSIS

The most sensitive means of diagnosis is endoscopic examination, with biopsy and culture of the gastric mucosa. The *H. pylori* urease is so potent its activity can be directly demonstrated in biopsies in less than an hour. Noninvasive methods include serology and a urea breath test. For the breath test, the patient ingests ^{13}C- or ^{14}C-labeled urea, from which the urease in the stomach produces products that appear as labeled CO_2 in the breath. A number of methods for detection of antibody directed against *H. pylori* are now available. Because IgG or IgA remain elevated as long as the infection persists, these tests are valuable

Urease detection is diagnostic

Serologic tests demonstrate chronic infection

both for screening and for evaluation of therapy. The advantage of direct detection of the organism is that culture is the most sensitive indicator of cure following therapy.

TREATMENT AND PREVENTION

Antimicrobics and bismuth salts achieve lasting cures

Regimen may be difficult to tolerate

H. pylori is susceptible to a wide variety of antimicrobial agents. Bismuth salts (eg, Pepto-Bismol), which in the past were believed to act by coating the stomach, also have antimicrobial activity. Cure rates approaching 95% have been achieved with various combinations of bismuth salts and two antibiotics. Metronidazole, tetracycline, clarithromycin, and amoxicillin have been effective. Relapse rates are low, particularly when acid secretion is also controlled with the use of a proton pump inhibitor. These combination regimens must be continued for at least 2 weeks and may be difficult for some patients to tolerate. Prevention of *H. pylori* disease awaits further understanding of transmission and immune mechanisms. Prophylactic treatment of asymptomatic persons colonized with *H. pylori* is not yet recommended.

ADDITIONAL READING

Blake PA, Allegra DT, Snyder JD, et al: Cholera—A possible endemic focus in the United States. *N Engl J Med* 1980;302:305–309. This study was the first to detail the epidemiologic features of cholera cases along the Gulf Coast of Louisiana.

Covacci A, Telford JL, Del Giudice G, Parsonnet J, Rappuoli R. *Helicobacter pylori* virulence and genetic geography. *Science* 1999;284:1328–1333. This paper provides an elegant argument for *H. pylori* as the most prevalent and ancient of infectious diseases.

Dunn BE, Cohen H, Blaser MJ. *Helicobacter pylori. J Clin Microbiol* 1997;10:720–741. This very readable and well-referenced review of all aspects of *Helicobacter* disease includes discussion of pathogenesis and treatment and some comments about animal helicobacters.

Farque SM, Albert, Mekalanos JJ: Epidemiology, genetics, and ecology of toxigenic *Vibrio cholerae. Microbiol Mol Biol Rev* 1998;62:1301–1314. This review mixes a discussion of the historic pandemics with a clear explanation of the complex regulation of virulence factors of *V. cholerae.* It concludes with some provocative ideas about how the cholera vibrio emerges from its mysterious environmental reservoir.

Nachamkin I, Alos BM, Ho T. *Campylobacter* species and Guillain-Barré syndrome. *Clin Microbiol Rev* 1998;11:555–567. This review gives a detailed examination of the molecular mimicry model for the connection between Guillain-Barré syndrome and *C. jejuni.*

Warren JR, Marshall B. Unidentified curved bacilli on gastric epithelium in active chronic gastritis. *Lancet* 1983;1:1273–1275. This paper led to the recognition of gastritis and ulcers as infectious diseases.

CHAPTER 23

Pseudomonas and Other Opportunistic Gram-negative Bacilli

KENNETH J. RYAN

A number of opportunistic Gram-negative rods of several genera not considered in other chapters are included here. With the exception of *Pseudomonas aeruginosa,* they rarely cause disease, and all are frequently encountered as contaminants and superficial colonizers. The significance of their isolation from clinical material thus depends on the circumstance and site of culture and on the clinical situation of the patient.

PSEUDOMONAS

There are a large number of *Pseudomonas* species, the most important of which is *P. aeruginosa.* The total number of infections produced by the other species is far lower than that produced by *P. aeruginosa* alone. *Pseudomonas* species are most frequently seen as colonizers and contaminants but are able to cause opportunistic infections. The assignment of species names has little clinical importance beyond differentiation from *P. aeruginosa.* Reports vary regarding the frequency of their isolation from cases of bacteremia, arthritis, abscesses, wounds, conjunctivitis, and urinary tract infections. In general, unless isolated in pure culture from a high-quality (direct) specimen, it is difficult to attach pathogenic significance to any of the miscellaneous *Pseudomonas* species.

P. aeruginosa most important

Other *Pseudomonas* species cause opportunistic infection

Pseudomonas aeruginosa

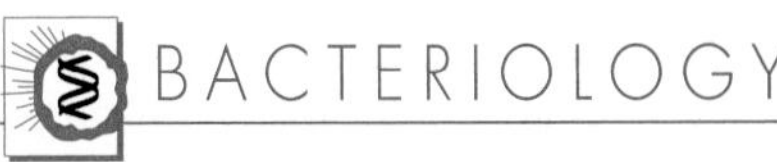

BACTERIOLOGY

Pseudomonas aeruginosa is an aerobic, motile, Gram-negative rod that is slimmer and more pale staining than members of the Enterobacteriaceae. Its most striking bacteriologic feature is the production of colorful water-soluble pigments. *P. aeruginosa* also

Pigment-producing rod is resistant to many antimicrobics

demonstrates the most consistent resistance to antimicrobics of all the medically important bacteria.

GROWTH AND METABOLISM

P. aeruginosa is sufficiently versatile in its growth and energy requirements to use simple molecules such as ammonia and carbon dioxide as sole nitrogen and carbon sources. Thus, it does not require enriched media for growth, and it can survive and multiply over a wide temperature range (20 to 42°C) in almost any environment, including one with a high salt content. The organism uses oxidative energy-producing mechanisms and has a high level of cytochrome oxidase (oxidase positive). Although an aerobic atmosphere is necessary for optimal growth and metabolism, most strains multiply slowly in an anaerobic environment if nitrate is present as an electron acceptor.

Grows aerobically with minimal requirements

Colonies are oxidase positive

Growth on all common isolation media is luxurious, and colonies have a delicate, fringed edge. Confluent growth often has a characteristic metallic sheen and emits an intense "fruity" odor. Hemolysis is usually produced on blood agar. The positive oxidase reaction of *P. aeruginosa* differentiates it from the Enterobacteriaceae, and its production of blue, yellow, or rust-colored pigments differentiates it from most other Gram-negative bacteria. The blue pigment, **pyocyanin,** is produced only by *P. aeruginosa*. **Fluorescin,** a yellow pigment that fluoresces under ultraviolet light, is produced by *P. aeruginosa* and other free-living less pathogenic *Pseudomonas* species. Pyocyanin and fluorescin combined produce a bright green color that diffuses throughout the medium.

Blue pyocyanin produced only by *P. aeruginosa*

Yellow fluorescin and pyocyanin combine for green color

STRUCTURE

Lipopolysaccharide (LPS) is present in the outer membrane, as are porin proteins, which differ from those of the Enterobacteriaceae in offering much less permeability to a wide range of molecules, including antibiotics. Pili composed of repeating monomers of the pilin structural subunit extend from the cell surface. A single polar flagellum rapidly propels the organism.

Outer membrane protein porins are relatively impermeable

A mucoid exopolysaccharide slime layer is present outside the cell wall in some strains. This layer is created by secretion of **alginate,** a copolymer of mannuronic and glucuronic acids. It is created by the action of several enzymes that effectively channel carbohydrate intermediates into the alginate polymer. All *P. aeruginosa* produce moderate amounts of alginate, but those with mutations in regulatory genes overproduce the polymer. These mutants appear as striking mucoid colonies in cultures from the respiratory tract of patients with cystic fibrosis.

Secreted alginate forms a slime layer

Overproduction is due to regulatory mutations

EXTRACELLULAR PRODUCTS

Most strains of *P. aeruginosa* produce multiple extracellular products, including **exotoxin A** and other enzymes with hemolytic, lecithinase, collagenase, or elastase activity. Exotoxin A enters cells via receptor-mediated endocytosis and is internalized into a low pH vesicle from which it translocates and reaches its target molecule, elongation factor 2 (EF-2). It catalyzes the inactivation of EF-2 by ADP-ribosylation, leading to shutdown of protein synthesis and cell death. Although this action is the same as diphtheria toxin, the two toxins are otherwise unrelated. Expression of exotoxin A is influenced by oxygen, temperature, and iron regulated genes.

Multiple extracellular enzymes are produced

Exotoxin A action is same as diphtheria toxin

Exoenzyme S ADP-ribosylates several intracellular proteins, including the cytoskeleton filament vimentin, and may also function as a surface-bound adhesin. The **elastase** acts on a variety of biologically important substrates, including elastin, human IgA and IgG, complement components, and some collagens. *P. aeruginosa* elastase shows homology with other proteases, including those produced by *Legionella pneumophila* and *Vibrio cholerae.*

Vimentin is ADP-ribosylated

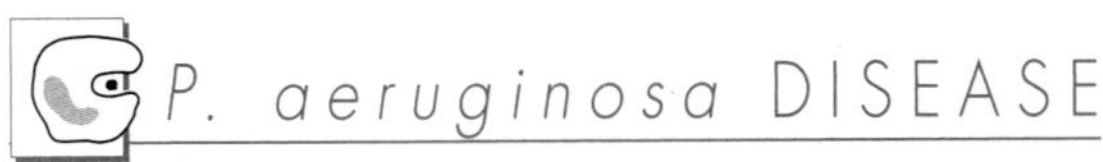

P. aeruginosa DISEASE

CLINICAL CAPSULE

P. aeruginosa produces infection at a wide range of pulmonary, urinary, and soft tissue sites, much like the opportunistic Enterobacteriaceae. The clinical manifestations of these infections reflect the organ system involved and are not unique for *Pseudomonas*. However, once established, infections are particularly virulent and difficult to treat. Affected patients almost always have some form of debilitation or compromise of immune defenses.

EPIDEMIOLOGY

The primary habitat of *P. aeruginosa* is the environment. It is found in water, soil, and various types of vegetation throughout the world. *P. aeruginosa* has been isolated from the throat and stool of 2 to 10% of healthy persons. Colonization rates may be higher in hospitalized patients. Infection with *P. aeruginosa,* rare in previously healthy persons, is one of the most important causes of invasive infection in hospitalized patients with serious underlying disease, such as leukemia, cystic fibrosis (CF), and extensive burns.

Primary habitat is environmental

Colonizes humans

The ability of *P. aeruginosa* to survive and proliferate in water with minimal nutrients can lead to heavy contamination of any nonsterile fluid, such as that in the humidifiers of respirators. Inhalation of aerosols from such sources can bypass the normal respiratory defense mechanisms and initiate pulmonary infection. Infections have resulted from the growth of *Pseudomonas* in medications, contact lens solutions, and even in some disinfectants. Sinks and faucet aerators may be heavily contaminated and serve as the environmental source for contamination of other items. The presence of *P. aeruginosa* in drinking water or food is not a cause for alarm. The risk lies in the proximity between items susceptible to contamination and patients uniquely predisposed to infection.

Multiplies in humidifiers, solutions, and medications

Risk for immunocompromised persons is high

P. aeruginosa is now the most common bacterial pathogen to complicate the management of patients with CF, an inherited defect in chloride ion transport that leads to a buildup of thick mucus in ducts and the tracheobronchial tree. In a high proportion of cases, the respiratory tract becomes colonized with *P. aeruginosa,* which, once established, becomes almost impossible to eradicate. This infection is a leading cause of morbidity and eventual death of these patients.

Respiratory colonization of CF patients becomes chronic

PATHOGENESIS

Although *P. aeruginosa* is an opportunistic pathogen, it is one of particular virulence. The organism usually requires a significant break in first-line defenses (such as a wound) or a route past them (such as a contaminated solution or intratracheal tube) to initiate infection. Attachment to epithelial cells is the first step in infection and is likely mediated by pili, flagella, and the extracellular polysaccharide slime. The receptors include sialic acid and N-acetylglucosamine borne by cell surface glycolipids. There is evidence that attachment is favored by loss of surface fibronectin, which explains in part the propensity for debilitated persons.

Needs break in first-line defenses

Pili, flagella, and slime mediate adherence

Once established, the virulence of *P. aeruginosa* involves multiple factors, particularly exotoxin A, exotoxin S, and elastase, which are directly injected into host cells by a specialized contact secretion system. The importance of exotoxin A is supported by studies in human and animals, which correlate its presence with a fatal outcome and antibody against it with survival. No diphtheria-like systemic effect of exotoxin has been demonstrated, but its cytotoxic action correlates with the primarily invasive and locally destructive lesions seen in *P. aeruginosa* infections.

Extracellular enzymes are injected by contact secretion system

Exotoxin A is cytotoxic and immunogenic

Exoenzyme S is associated with dissemination from burn wounds and with actions destructive to cells, including its action on the cytoskeleton. The many biologically important substrates of elastase argue for its importance, particularly its namesake, elastin. Elastin is found at some sites *P. aeruginosa* preferentially attacks, such as the lung and blood vessels. Hemorrhagic destruction, including the walls of blood vessels (Fig 23–1), is the histologic hallmark of *Pseudomonas* infection.

Elastin is attacked in lung and blood vessels

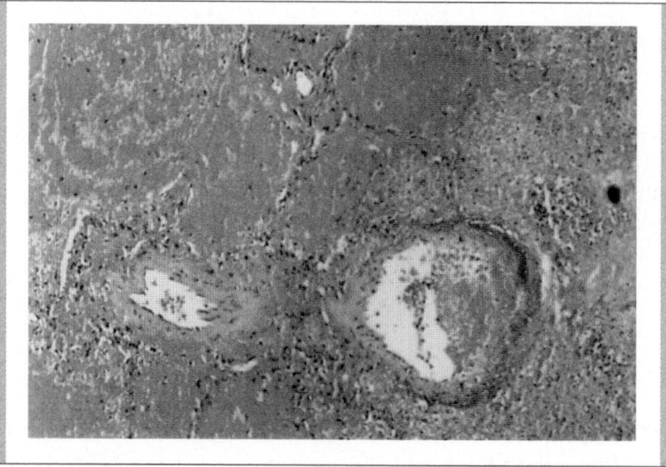

FIGURE 23–1
Pseudomonas aeruginosa pneumonia. This blood vessel in the lung of a fatal case is infected with *P. aeruginosa* and is undergoing destruction. A thrombus is forming in the lumen as well. (*Reproduced with permission from Connor DH, Chandler FW, Schwartz DQA, Manz HJ, Lack EE (eds).* Pathology of Infectious Diseases, *vol. 1. Stamford, CT: Appleton & Lange; 1997.*)

P. aeruginosa and Cystic Fibrosis (CF)

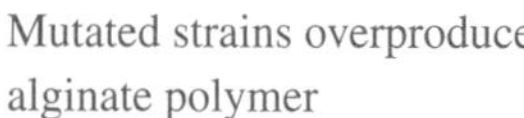

Mutated strains overproduce alginate polymer

Glycocalyx biofilm protects bacteria

P. aeruginosa is the most persistent of the infectious agents that complicate the course of CF. Initial colonization may be aided by the fact that cells from CF patients are less highly sialylated than normal epithelial cells, providing increased receptors for *P. aeruginosa* attachment. Defects in the epithelia of CF patients may also retard their clearing by desquamation. Once the bronchi are colonized, the organisms remain, forming a biofilm containing microcolonies of bacteria, which together are called a **glycocalyx.** The most striking feature of this association is the unique presence of strains with multiple mutations in regulatory genes that cause overproduction of the alginate polymer. These genes are activated by the high osmolarity of the thick CF secretions. The selective advantages of this biofilm include adhesion; inaccessibility of the immune system (complement, antibody, phagocytes); and interference with the access and action of antimicrobial agents.

Virulence Regulation

Multiple virulence factors are regulated by cell-to-cell signaling

The multiple virulence factors of *P. aeruginosa* are controlled by several regulatory pathways, some of which respond to environmental stimuli. In addition, some of the extracellular products, including exotoxin A and elastase, are regulated in an interactive way by cell-to-cell signaling. These signaling systems are able to monitor bacterial population density in a way that only initiates transcription of a virulence factor when certain population thresholds are reached. This could be valuable either as an economy measure or as a mechanism to withhold the onslaught of injury-producing molecules until the host has little time to respond.

IMMUNITY

Humoral and cellular immune responses both important

Human immunity to *Pseudomonas* infection is not well understood. Inferences from animal studies and clinical observations suggest that both humoral and cell mediated immunity are important. The strong propensity of *P. aeruginosa* to infect those with defective cell-mediated immunity indicates that these responses are particularly important.

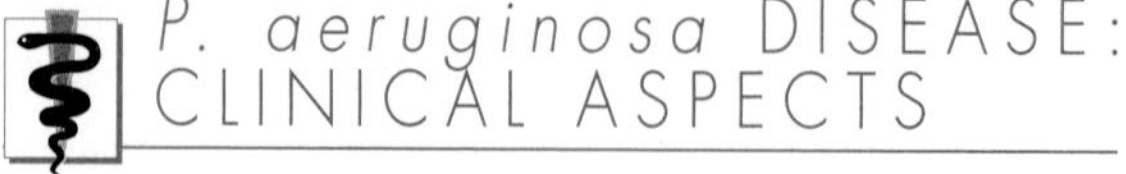

P. aeruginosa DISEASE: CLINICAL ASPECTS

MANIFESTATIONS

Infects burns and environmentally contaminated wounds

P. aeruginosa can produce any of the opportunistic extraintestinal infections caused by members of the Enterobacteriaceae. Burn, wound, urinary tract, skin, eye, ear, and respiratory infections all occur and may progress to bacteremia. *P. aeruginosa* is also one of the most common causes of infection in environmentally contaminated wounds (eg, osteomyelitis after compound fractures or nail puncture wounds of the foot).

P. aeruginosa pneumonia is a rapid, destructive, infection particularly in patients with granulocytopenia. It is associated with alveolar necrosis, vascular invasion, infarcts, and bacteremia. Pulmonary infection in CF patients is quite different; it is a chronic infection that alternates between a state of colonization and more overt bronchitis or pneumonia. Although the more aggressive features of *Pseudomonas* infection in the immunocompromised are not common, the infection is still serious enough to be a leading cause of death in CF patients.

Pneumonia is aggressive in the immunocompromised and chronic in CF

P. aeruginosa is also a common cause of otitis externa, including "swimmer's ear" and a rare but life-threatening "malignant" otitis externa seen in patients with diabetes. Folliculitis of the skin may follow soaking in inadequately decontaminated hot tubs that can become heavily contaminated with the organism. The organism can cause conjunctivitis, keratitis, or endophthalmitis when introduced into the eye by trauma or contaminated medication or contact lens solution. Keratitis can progress rapidly and destroy the cornea within 24 to 48 hours. In some cases of *P. aeruginosa* bacteremia, cutaneous papules develop that progress to black, necrotic ulcers. It is called **ecthyma gangrenosum** and is the result of direct invasion and destruction of blood vessel walls by the organism.

Common cause of otitis externa

Contamination of contact lenses leads to keratitis

Bacteremia may cause ecthyma gangrenosum

DIAGNOSIS

P. aeruginosa is readily grown in culture. The combination of characteristic oxidase positive colonies, pyocyanin production and the ability to grow at 42°C is sufficient to distinguish *P. aeruginosa* from other *Pseudomonas* species. No other diagnostic modalities are in routine use.

Pigments typically produced in culture

TREATMENT

Of the pathogenic bacteria, *P. aeruginosa* is the organism most consistently resistant to many antimicrobics. This is primarily due to the porins that restrict their entry to the periplasmic space. *P. aeruginosa* strains are regularly resistant to penicillin, ampicillin, cephalothin, tetracycline, chloramphenicol, sulfonamides, and the earlier aminoglycosides (streptomycin, kanamycin). Much effort has been directed toward the development of antimicrobics with anti-*Pseudomonas* activity. The newer aminoglycosides—gentamicin, tobramycin, and amikacin—are all active against most strains despite the presence of mutational and plasmid-mediated resistance. Carbenicillin and ticarcillin are active and can be given in high doses, but plasmid-mediated resistance and permeability mutations occur more frequently than with the aminoglycosides. The most prized feature of some of the third-generation cephalosporins (ceftazidime, cefepime, cefoperazone), carbapenems (imipenem, meropenem), and monobactams (aztreonam) is their activity against *Pseudomonas*. In general, urinary infections may be treated with a single drug, but more serious systemic *P. aeruginosa* infections are usually treated with a combination of an anti-*Pseudomonas* β-lactam antimicrobic and an aminoglycoside, particularly in neutropenic patients. Ciprofloxacin is also used in treatment of such cases. In all instances, susceptibility must be confirmed by in vitro tests.

Multiresistance is by restricting permeability

Mutational and plasmid mediated resistance occurs to penicillins and aminoglycosides

Third-generation cephalosporins are often active

The treatment of *P. aeruginosa* in CF presents special problems because most of the effective antimicrobics are only given intravenously. There is a reluctance to hospitalize in many patients, and oral agents are used instead. There is less experience with their efficacy under these conditions, and the chronic nature of CF is a set-up for development of resistance during therapy. This has already been seen with ciprofloxacin and aztreonam. Aerosolized tobramycin has also been used in some CF patients, with some evidence of clinical improvement.

Effective oral agents are scarce

PREVENTION

Vaccines are experimental

Vaccines incorporating somatic antigens from multiple *P. aeruginosa* serotypes have been developed and proved immunogenic in humans. The primary candidates for such preparations are patients with burn injuries, CF, or immunosuppression. Although some protection has been demonstrated, these preparations are still experimental.

BURKHOLDERIA

Melioidosis is a tropical pneumonia that relapses

B. cepacia is a nosocomial, CF pathogen

Burkholderia pseudomallei is a saprophyte in soil, ponds, rice paddies and vegetables located in Southeast Asia, the Philippines, Indonesia, and other tropical areas. Infection is acquired by direct inoculation or by inhalation of aerosols or dust containing the bacteria. The disease, **melioidosis,** is usually an acute pneumonia; however, it is sufficiently variable that subacute, chronic, and even relapsing infections may follow systemic spread. Some soldiers relapsed years after their return from Vietnam. The clinical and radiologic features may resemble tuberculosis. In fulminant cases, rapid respiratory failure may ensue and metastatic abscesses develop in the skin or other sites. Tetracycline, chloramphenicol, sulfonamides, and trimethoprim–sulfamethoxazole have been effective in therapy. *B. cepacia* is an opportunistic organism that has been found to contaminate reagents, disinfectants, and medical devices in much the same manner as *P. aeruginosa.* It has also complicated the course of CF but does not produce the mucoid colony type seen with *P. aeruginosa.*

ACINETOBACTER

Respiratory and urinary infection come from soil and water

The genus *Acinetobacter* comprises Gram-negative coccobacilli that occasionally appear sufficiently round on Gram smears to be confused with *Neisseria.* On primary isolation, they closely resemble the Enterobacteriaceae in growth pattern and colonial morphology but are distinguished by their failure to ferment carbohydrates or reduce nitrates. As with most of the organisms discussed in this chapter, the isolation of *Acinetobacter* from clinical material does not define infection, because they appear most frequently as skin and respiratory colonizers. They are most frequently found as contaminants of almost anything wet, including soaps and some disinfectant solutions. Pneumonia is the most common infection, followed by urinary tract and soft tissue infections. Nosocomial respiratory infections have been traced to contaminated inhalation therapy equipment, and bacteremia to infected intravenous catheters. Treatment is complicated by frequent resistance to penicillins, cephalosporins, and occasionally aminoglycosides.

MORAXELLA

Bronchitis and otitis come from respiratory flora

Moraxella is another genus of coccobacillary, Gram-negative rods that are usually paired end to end. Some species require enriched media, such as blood or chocolate agar. Their morphology, fastidious growth, and positive oxidase reaction can result in confusion with

Neisseria. This is particularly true for *M. catarrhalis*, which for many years was classified with *Neisseria*. More recently it was called *Branhamella catarrhalis*, and it is an occasional cause of otitis media and lower respiratory tract infection. Both infections relate to the presence of *M. catarrhalis* in the normal oropharyngeal flora. With the exception of *M. catarrhalis*, which frequently produces β-lactamase, *Moraxella* species are generally susceptible to penicillin.

AEROMONAS AND *PLESIOMONAS*

The genera *Aeromonas* and *Plesiomonas* have bacteriologic features similar to those of the Enterobacteriaceae, *Vibrio*, and *Pseudomonas*. They are aerobic and facultatively anaerobic, attack carbohydrates fermentatively, and demonstrate various other biochemical reactions. *Aeromonas* colonies are typically β-hemolytic. The major taxonomic resemblance to *Pseudomonas* is that both *Aeromonas* and *Plesiomonas* are oxidase positive with polar flagella. Their habitat is basically environmental (water and soil), but they can occasionally be found in the human intestinal tract.

Resemble other enteric bacteria

Aeromonas is an uncommon but highly virulent cause of wound infections acquired in fresh or saltwater. The onset can be as rapid as 8 hours after the injury and the cellulitis progresses rapidly to fasciitis, myonecrosis, and bacteremia in less than a day. *Aeromonas* is also the leading cause of infections associated with the use of leeches, due to its regular presence in the leech foregut. In addition to opportunistic infection, some evidence suggests an occasional role for *Aeromonas* in gastroenteritis through production of toxins with enterotoxic and cytotoxic properties. *Plesiomonas* is also associated with an enterotoxic diarrhea. These associations are not yet strong enough to justify attempts to routinely isolate *Aeromonas* and *Plesiomonas* from diarrheal stools. Resistance to penicillins and cephalosporins is common. Most strains show susceptibility to tetracycline, with variable susceptibility to aminoglycosides, including gentamicin.

Rapid cellulitis follows injury in water

Diarrheas relate to enterotoxin production

OTHER GRAM-NEGATIVE RODS

There are many other Gram-negative rods that rarely cause disease in humans. Some are members of the normal flora and others come from the environment. Because many of these do not ferment carbohydrates or react in many of the tests routinely used to characterize bacteria, their identification is frequently delayed as additional tests are tried or the organism is sent to a reference laboratory. The clinical significance of all these organisms is essentially the same; the clinician usually receives a report of a "nonfermenter" or another descriptive term and a susceptibility test result. The significance of the isolate is then determined on clinical grounds. The major characteristics of some of these organisms are shown in Table 23–1. The types of infection listed represent the most common among scattered case reports, and should not be interpreted as typical for each organism.

Rare species are interpreted on the basis of their clinical setting

Some Gram-negative bacilli fail to conform to any of the species currently recognized. If clinically important, such strains are sent to reference centers, such as the Centers for Disease Control and Prevention (CDC) in Atlanta, Georgia. Eventually, some are given designations such as "CDC group IIF," which may appear in clinical reports. Much later, a new genus and/or species name may be issued if agreement among taxonomists is sufficient.

Some bacteria remain unnamed for years

TABLE 23–1

Pseudomonas and other Opportunistic Gram-negative Rods

Species	Bacteriologic Features			Adherence	Virulence Factors	Epidemiology	Disease
	MacConkey Growth	CO_2 Required	Pigments				
Pseudomonas							
P. aeruginosa	+	–	Pyocyanin, fluorescin	Pili, flagella, alginate slime	Exotoxin A, exoenxyme S, elastase, alginate slime	Environmental, normal flora, mucosal breaks, nosocomial	Wounds, pneumonia, burns, otitis externa, cystic fibrosis
P. fluorescens	+	–	Fluorescin			Environmental	Opportunistic
Other species	+	–	Fluorescin			Environmental	Opportunistic
Stenotrophomonas maltophilia	+	–	–		Elastase	Environmental, mucosal breaks, water, nosocomial	Pneumonia, bacteremia
Acinetobacter	+	–	–		Capsule	Environmental, skin colonization, water, nosocomial	Respiratory, urinary catheter bacteremia
Burkholderia							
B. mallei	+	–	–			Contact with horses	Glanders
B. pseudomallei	+	–	–		Lethal toxin, dermonecrotic toxin	Environmental in Southeast Asia and tropical regions	Melioidosis
B. cepacia	+	–	–	Pili	Elastase	Environmental, mucosal breaks, water, nosocomial	Wounds, pneumonia, cystic fibrosis

Aeromonas	+	–	–		Enterotoxin, cytotoxin	Environmental, fresh and salt water, leeches, intestinal flora	Wounds, diarrhea
Plesiomonas	+	–	–		Enterotoxin	Water, seafood, soil	Diarrhea
Alkaligenes	+	–	–			Respiratory, intestinal flora	Blood, urine, wounds
Cardiobacterium	–	+	–			Nasopharyngeal, intestinal flora	Endocarditis
Chromobacterium	+	–	Violet			Water, soil, (tropical)	Cellulitis, bacteremia
Flavobacterium	–	–	Yellow			Environmental, nosocomial	Meningitis
Eikenella	–	+	–			Respiratory flora	Oropharyngeal abscess, draining sinuses
Actinobacillus	–	+	–			Respiratory flora, animals	Endocarditis, periodontal disease
Moraxella	–	–	–	Pili		Respiratory flora	Bronchitis, pneumonia

ADDITIONAL READING

Govan JRW, Deretic V. Microbial pathogenesis in cystic fibrosis: Mucoid *Pseudomonas aeruginosa* and *Burkholderia cepacia. Microbiol Rev* 1996;60:539–574. This review nicely covers the two Gram-negative rods that complicate the lives of those with cystic fibrosis.

Livermore DM. Multiple mechanisms of antimicrobial resistance in *Pseudomonas aeruginosa*: Our worst nightmare? *Clin Infect Dis* 2002;34:634–640. A review that illustrates the enormous capabilities of *P. aeruginosa* to develop resistance quickly.

Van Delden C, Iglewski BH. Cell to cell signaling and *Pseudomonas aeruginosa* infections. *Emerg Infect Dis* 1998;4:551–560. The complex way *P. aeruginosa* deploys its virulence factors is concisely explained and well illustrated.

CHAPTER 24

Haemophilus and *Bordetella*

KENNETH J. RYAN

Haemophilus and *Bordetella* are small, Gram-negative rods that tend to assume a coccobacillary shape. They are nonmotile, non–spore forming, with complex nutritional growth requirements for blood-containing media. Members of both genera contain species exclusively found in humans that cause respiratory infections. The major species are *Haemophilus influenzae,* a major cause of purulent meningitis and *Bordetella pertussis,* the cause of whooping cough.

HAEMOPHILUS

Haemophilus are among the smallest of bacteria. The curved ends of the short (1.0 to 1.5 μm) bacilli makes many appear nearly round, hence the term coccobacilli. The cell wall has a structure similar to that of other Gram-negative bacteria. *H. influenzae* may have a polysaccharide capsule, but other species of *Haemophilus* are not encapsulated.

Tiny Gram-negative coccobacilli

The cultivation of *Haemophilus* species requires the use of culture media enriched with blood or blood products (Greek "haema," blood, and "philos," loving) for optimal growth. This requirement is attributable to the need for exogenous hematin and/or nicotinamide adenine dinucleotide (NAD). These growth factors, also termed X factor (hematin) and V factor (NAD), are both present in erythrocytes. In culture media, optimal concentrations of X and, particularly, V factors are not available to *Haemophilus* from blood unless the red blood cells are lysed by gentle heat (chocolate agar) or digested and added separately as a supplement. Although erythrocytes are the only convenient source of hematin, the V factor is present in a variety of biologic sources and is produced by some other bacteria and yeasts. These conditions are responsible for the "satellite phenomenon," in which the bacteria form colonies on blood agar only in the vicinity of a colony of *Staphylococcus* that is producing V factor. The several species of *Haemophilus* are defined by their requirement for X and/or V factor, CO_2 dependence, and other cultural characteristics (Table 24–1).

All require hematin (X) and/or NAD (V)

Chocolate agar has X and V factors

Satellite formation around colonies of *S. aureus* is based on V factor

Species of *Haemophilus* other than *H. influenzae* have the same biology described below for the nonencapsulated strains of *H. influenzae*. Most of these other *Haemophilus* species have been reported to cause systemic illness, including pneumonia, meningitis, arthritis, endocarditis, and soft tissue infections. Such cases are even more rare than those in which nonencapsulated *H. influenzae* cause invasive disease.

Species other than *H. influenzae* are similar

TABLE 24–1

Features of *Haemophilus* and *Bordetella*

Species	Type	Growth Requirement	Capsule	Adherence Factors	Toxins	Epidemiology	Disease
Haemophilus							
H. influenzae	a–f	X and V	Polysaccharide	Pili	—	Normal flora, respiratory droplet spread	Meningitis, epiglottitis, arthritis, sepsis, otitis media
H. influenzae	—	X and V	—	HMW proteins, pili	—	Normal flora, respiratory droplet spread	Otitis media, bronchitis, sinusitis
H. ducreyi	—	X	—	Pili	Cytolethal distending toxin	Sexual contact	Chancroid
Other species[a]	—	X or V	—	—	—	Normal flora	Bronchitis
Bordetella							
B. pertussis	—	Nicotinamide[b]	—	Fha, PT, pertactin	PT, adenylate cyclase, tracheal cytotoxin	Strict pathogen, respiratory droplet spread	Whooping cough
B. parapertussis	—	Nicotinamide	—		—	Presumed similar to *B. pertussis*	Rhinitis, cough
B. bronchiseptica	—	Nicotinamide	—		—	Dogs, rabbits	Rhinitis, cough

Abbreviations: X factor, hematin; V factor, nicotinamide adenine dinucleotide (NAD); HMW, high-molecular-weight proteins (HMW1, HMW2); Fha, filamentous hemagglutinin; PT, pertussis toxin.

[a] *H. parainfluenzae, H. aphrophilus, H. hemolyticus.*

[b] Also requires additives to neutralize toxicity in standard media.

Haemophilus influenzae

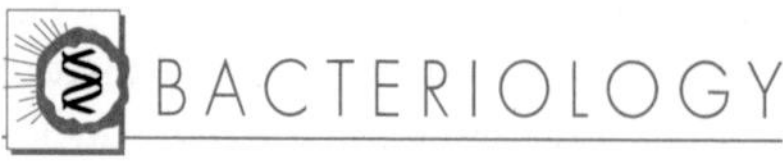

Six serotypes are based on capsular polysaccharide

Hib capsule is PRP

Nonencapsulated strains are less virulent

Haemophilus that meet the species requirements for *H. influenzae* may or may not have a capsule. Those that do are divided into six serotypes, designated a to f, based on the capsular polysaccharide antigen. The type b capsule is made up of a polymer of ribose, ribitol, and phosphate, called **polyribitol phosphate (PRP)**. These surface polysaccharides are strongly associated with virulence, particularly *H. influenzae* type b (Hib). The nonencapsulated, and thus nontypable, *H. influenzae* can be classified by a number of typing schemes based on outer membrane proteins and other factors. These protein systems can also be applied to capsulated *H. influenzae* but have no particular association with virulence.

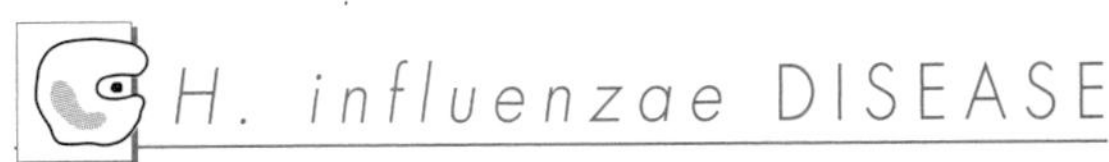

H. influenzae DISEASE

CLINICAL CAPSULE

Hib produces acute, life-threatening infections of the central nervous system, epiglottis, and soft tissues, primarily in children. Disease begins with fever and lethargy, and in the case of acute meningitis, can progress to coma and death in less than 1 day. In affluent countries, Hib disease has been controlled by immunization. *H. influenzae* also produces common but less fulminant infections of the bronchi, respiratory sinuses, and middle ear. The latter are usually associated with nonencapsulated strains.

EPIDEMIOLOGY

H. influenzae can be found in the normal nasopharyngeal flora of 20 to 80% of healthy persons, depending on age, season, and other factors. Most of these are nonencapsulated, but capsulated strains, including Hib, are not rare. Prior to the introduction of effective vaccines, approximately 1 in every 200 children developed invasive Hib disease by the age of 5 years. Meningitis is the most common form and most often attacks those under 2 years of age. Cases of epiglottitis and pneumonia tend to peak in the 2- to 5-year age range. Over 90% of these cases are due to the single serotype, Hib.

Nasopharyngeal colonization is common

Meningitis develops in children under 2 years of age

By the end of the first decade of universal immunization with the Hib protein conjugate vaccine in the United States (see Prevention), invasive disease rates have already declined by 99%. Now, invasive disease strikes only 1 in 100,000 children, and most of these cases are not caused by the type b serotype. Similar results have been seen in other countries, but Hib disease continues in those unable to afford the vaccine. Under the direction of the World Health Organization, government and philanthropic efforts are now underway to make this vaccine available to all children throughout the world.

Immunization has dramatically reduced disease

Countries that cannot afford vaccine are targeted

At one time *H. influenzae*–caused meningitis was believed to be an isolated endogenous infection, but reports of outbreaks in closed populations and careful epidemiologic studies of secondary spread in families have changed this view. The risk of serious infection for unimmunized children under 4 years of age living with an index case is more than 500-fold that for nonexposed children. This risk indicates a need for prophylaxis for contacts in the susceptible age group. Rifampin is currently recommended for this purpose.

Person-to person spread is blocked by vaccine or prophylaxis

PATHOGENESIS

Invasive Disease

For unknown reasons, *H. influenzae* strains commonly found in the normal flora of the nasopharynx occasionally invade into deeper tissues. Bacteremia then leads to spread to the central nervous system and metastatic infections at distant sites such as bones and joints. These events seem to take place within a short period (<3 days) after an encounter with a new virulent strain. Systemic spread is typical only for capsulated *H. influenzae* strains, and over 90% of invasive strains are type b. Even among Hib strains there are distinct clones, which account for about 80% of all invasive disease worldwide, and other clones, which are rarely associated with invasion.

Only capsulated strains are invasive

Limited number of Hib clones account for disease

The pathogenic mechanisms involved in Hib invasiveness remain to be fully understood. Attachment to respiratory epithelial cells is mediated by pili and other adhesins. There is some evidence to suggest that this is a complex regulatory cascade, coordinating capsular biosynthesis and adherence factors that act cooperatively in establishing the microbe within susceptible hosts. *H. influenzae* can be seen to invade between the cells of the respiratory epithelium, and for a time resides between and below them. Once past the mucosal barrier, the antiphagocytic capsule confers resistance to opsonophagocytosis in the same manner as it does with other encapsulated bacteria (*Streptococcus pneumoniae, Neisseria meningitidis*). Endotoxin in the cell wall is toxic to ciliated respiratory cells, but

Pili and other adhesins bind to epithelial cells

Invasion goes between cells

Capsule prevents phagocytosis

endotoxemia is not a prominent feature of *Haemophilus* infection to the extent that it is with *N. meningitidis. H. influenzae* produces no known exotoxins.

Localized Disease

Bacterial trapped in middle ear, sinuses, and bronchi produce localized infections

Most are noncapsulated strains

Adherence is related to surface proteins

Nonencapsulated *H. influenzae* produce disease under circumstances in which they are entrapped at a luminal site adjacent to the normal respiratory flora such as the middle ear, sinuses, or bronchi. This is usually associated with some compromise of normal clearing mechanisms, which is caused by a viral infection or structural damage. Consistent with their relative prevalence in the respiratory tract, nontypeable organisms account for more than 90% of localized *H. influenzae* disease, particularly otitis media, sinusitis, and exacerbations of chronic bronchitis. Nonencapsulated *H. influenzae* may have pili capable of promoting attachment to host cells, but they are relatively uncommon. However, a family of nonpilus, surface-exposed, high-molecular-weight proteins (eg, HMW1, HMW2) has been identified in nonencapsulated strains and have not been found in capsulated strains. These proteins also mediate adherence to epithelial cells, and some of them show homology with the filamentous hemagglutinin that plays an essential role in adherence of *Bordetella pertussis* to ciliated epithelial cells (see below).

IMMUNITY

Anticapsular antibody is bactericidal and protective

Hib infections occur at ages when antibody is absent

Immunity to Hib infections has long been associated with the presence of anticapsular (PRP) antibodies, which are bactericidal in the presence of complement. The infant is usually protected by passively acquired maternal antibody for the first few months of life. Thereafter the presence of actively acquired antibody increases with age; it is present in the serum of most children by 10 years of age. The peak incidence of Hib infections in unimmunized populations is 6 to 18 months of age, when serum antibody is least likely to be present. This inverse relationship between infection and serum antibody is similar to that for *N. meningitidis* (see Fig 20–2). The major difference is that substantial immunity is provided by antibody directed against a single type (Hib) rather than the multiple immunotypes of other bacteria. Thus, systemic *H. influenzae* infections (meningitis, epiglottitis, cellulitis) are rare in adults. When such infections develop, the immunologic deficit is the same as that with meningococci—lack of circulating antibody.

T cell–independent response to PRP is poor at < 18 months

Protein conjugate vaccine elicits T-cell response in infants

Like many polysaccharides, Hib PRP behaves as a T cell–independent antigen. B cells mount the primary response without significant involvement of helper T cells. Antibody responses from immunization with PRP are variable and typically poor at less than 18 months of age. Significant secondary responses from boosters are not elicited. Conjugation of PRP to protein dramatically improves the immunogenicity by eliciting the T-cell responses typical of protein antigens while preserving the specificity for PRP, even in infants.

H. influenzae DISEASE: CLINICAL ASPECTS

MANIFESTATIONS

Of the major acute Hib infections, meningitis accounts for just over 50% of cases. The remaining are distributed among pneumonia, epiglottitis, septicemia, cellulitis, and septic arthritis. Localized infections can be caused by capsulated strains including Hib, but most are noncapsulated *H. influenzae.*

Meningitis

Acute purulent meningitis may follow sinusitis or otitis media

Hib meningitis follows the same pattern as other causes of acute purulent bacterial meningitis (see Chapter 67). Meningitis is often preceded by signs and symptoms of an upper respiratory infection, such as pharyngitis, sinusitis or otitis media. Whether these represent a predisposing viral infection or early invasion by the organism is not known.

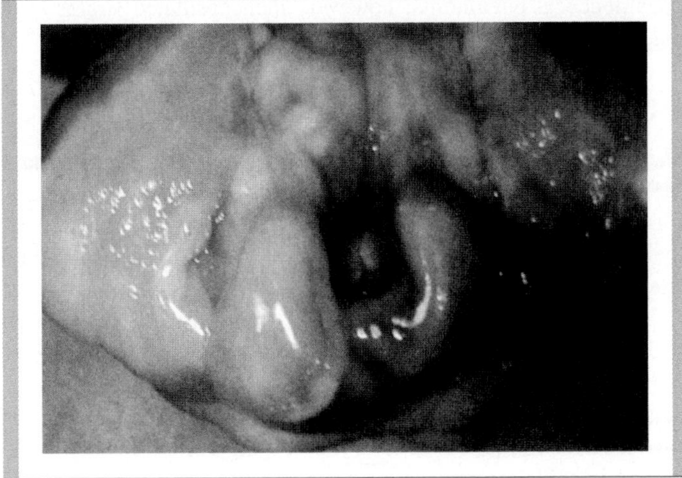

FIGURE 24–1
The swollen epiglottis characteristic of *Haemophilus influenzae* acute epiglottitis. (*Reproduced with permission from Connor DH, Chandler FW, Schwartz DQA, Manz HJ, Lack EE (eds).* Pathology of Infectious Diseases, *vol. 1. Stamford, CT: Appleton & Lange; 1997.*)

Just as often, meningitis is preceded by vague malaise, lethargy, irritability, and fever. Mortality is 3 to 6% despite appropriate therapy, and roughly one third of all survivors have significant neurologic sequelae.

Mortality and neurologic sequelae are significant

Acute Epiglottitis

Acute epiglottitis is a dramatic infection in which the inflamed epiglottis and surrounding tissues obstruct the airway. Hib is one of a number of causes. The onset is sudden, with fever, sore throat, hoarseness, an often muffled cough, and rapid progression to severe prostration within 24 hours. Affected children have air hunger, inspiratory stridor, and retraction of the soft parts of the chest with each inspiration. The hallmark of the disease is an inflamed, swollen, cherry-red epiglottis that protrudes into the airway (Fig 24–1) and can be visualized on lateral x-rays. As with meningitis, this infection is treated as a medical emergency, with prime emphasis on antimicrobics and maintenance of an airway (tracheostomy or endotracheal intubation). Manipulations, including routine examination or attempting to take a throat swab, can trigger a fatal laryngospasm and acute obstruction.

Cherry-red, swollen epiglottis, and stridor are hallmarks

Airway maintenance is needed

Cellulitis and Arthritis

A tender, reddish-blue swelling in the cheek or periorbital areas is the usual presentation of Hib cellulitis. Fever and a moderately toxic state are usually present, and the infection may follow an upper respiratory infection or otitis media. Joint infection begins with fever, irritability, and local signs of inflammation, often in a single large joint. *Haemophilus* arthritis is occasionally the cause of a more subtle set of findings, in which fever occurs without clear clinical evidence of joint involvement. Bacteremia is often present in both cellulitis and arthritis.

Cellulitis is usually facial

Large joints are involved

Other Infections

H. influenzae is an important cause of conjuctivitis, otitis media, and acute and chronic sinusitis. It is also one of several common respiratory organisms that can cause and exacerbate chronic bronchitis. Most of these infections are caused by nonencapsulated strains and usually remain localized without bacteremia. Disease may be acute or chronic, depending on the anatomic site and underlying pathology. For example, otitis media is acute and painful because of the small, closed space involved, but after antimicrobic therapy and reopening of the eustachian tube, the condition usually clears without sequelae. The association of *H. influenzae* with chronic bronchitis is more complex. There is evidence that *H. influenzae* and other bacteria play a role in inflammatory exacerbations, but a unique cause-and-effect relationship has been difficult to prove. The underlying cause of the bronchitis is usually related to chronic damage resulting from factors such as smoking. *Haemophilus* pneumonia may be caused by either encapsulated or nonencapsulated organisms. Encapsulated strains have been observed to produce a disease much like

Nonencapsulated strains are common in otitis media, sinusitis, and bronchitis

Pneumonia is linked to underlying damage

pneumococcal pneumonia; however, unencapsulated strains may also produce pneumonia, particularly in patients with chronic bronchitis.

DIAGNOSIS

Blood cultures are useful in systemic infections

Demonstrating X and V requirement defines species

The combination of clinical findings and a typical Gram smear is usually sufficient to make a presumptive diagnosis of *Haemophilus* infection. The tiny cells are usually of uniform shape except in cerebrospinal fluid, where some may be elongated to several times their usual length. The diagnosis must be confirmed by isolation of the organism from the site of infection or from the blood. Blood cultures are particularly useful in systemic *H. influenzae* infections, because it is often difficult to obtain an adequate specimen directly from the site of infection. Bacteriologically, small coccobacillary Gram-negative rods that grow on chocolate agar but not blood agar strongly suggest *Haemophilus*. Confirmation and speciation depends on demonstration of the requirement for X and V factors and/or biochemical tests. Serotyping is unnecessary for clinical purposes but important in epidemiologic and vaccine studies.

TREATMENT

Ampicillin-resistant strains produce β-lactamase

Third-generation cephalosporin is initial treatment

H. influenzae is often susceptible in vitro to ampicillin and amoxicillin, and usually susceptible to the newer cephalosporins, tetracycline, aminoglycosides, and sulfonamides. It is less susceptible to other penicillins and to erythromycin. Since the 1970s, the therapy of systemic infections has been complicated by the emergence of strains that produce a plasmid-mediated β-lactamase identical to that found in *Escherichia coli.* The frequency of resistant strains varies between 5 and 50% in different geographic areas. Ampicillin-resistant strains that do not produce β-lactamase also occur but are less common. Current practice is to start empiric therapy with a third-generation cephalosporin (eg, ceftriaxone, cefotaxime), which can be changed to ampicillin if susceptibility tests indicate that the infecting strain is susceptible.

PREVENTION

PRP vaccine missed peak age of disease

PRP conjugated to bacterial proteins stimulates T cells

Purified PRP vaccines became available in 1985; however, due to the typically poor immune response of infants to polysaccharide antigens, their use was limited to children 24 months of age and older. Because immunization at this age misses the group most susceptible to Hib invasive disease, a new vaccine strategy was needed that included improved stimulation of T cell–dependent immune responses in infants. To achieve this, three PRP-protein conjugate vaccines were developed using proteins derived from *Corynebacterium diphtheriae* (toxoid, CRM 197) or *N. meningitidis* (outer membrane protein). The first PRP–protein conjugate vaccines were licensed in 1989, and by late 1990, they were recommended for universal immunization beginning at 2 months of age. As illustrated in Figure 24–2, the impact has been dramatic (see Epidemiology). So far

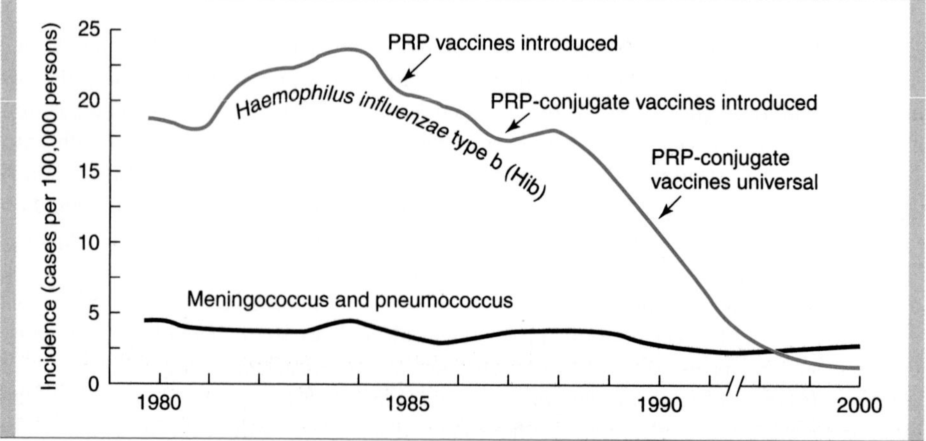

FIGURE 24–2
The recent decline in *Haemophilus influenzae* type b (Hib) meningitis and its association with the introduction of new vaccines.

this 99% reduction in what was the most common cause of childhood meningitis has not been accompanied by an increase in disease by either the non–type b strains or other causes of meningitis. An unexpected concomitant finding has been a dramatic drop in *H. influenzae* colonization rates in immunized populations.

Dramatic reduction in Hib disease has been sustained

Haemophilus ducreyi

H. ducreyi causes chancroid, a common cause of genital ulcer in Africa, Southeast Asia, India, and Latin America. Occasional outbreaks in North America have most often been associated with the exchange of sex for drugs or money. The typical lesion is a tender papule on the genitalia that develops into a painful ulcer with sharp margins. Satellite lesions may develop by autoinfection, and regional lymphadenitis is common. The incubation period is usually short (2 to 5 days). The lack of induration around the ulcer has caused the primary lesion to be called "soft chancre" to distinguish it from the primary syphilitic chancre, which is typically indurated and painless. The presence of open genital sores due to *H. ducreyi* enhances the risk of transmission of HIV either by providing a portal of entry or by the recruitment of CD4+ cells to the site. This may contribute to the heterosexual spread of acquired immunodeficiency syndrome (AIDS) on the African continent, where chancroid is common. Candidate *H. ducreyi* virulence factors include adhesive pili, resistance to phagocytosis, and complement-mediated killing. A seeming lack of immunity may be due to the action of a toxin (cytolethal distending toxin) on T cells.

Soft chancre is a genital ulcer with satellite lesions

May contribute to spread of AIDS in Africa

The specific diagnosis of *H. ducreyi* infection is difficult. Although the organism grows on chocolate agar, it does so slowly and other organisms present in the genital flora are apt to overgrow the plates. A special medium incorporates vancomycin as a selective agent, but few laboratories in the United States have it on hand. Chancroid is effectively treated with azithromycin, ceftriaxone, or erythromycin.

Culture is difficult

BORDETELLA

The genus *Bordetella* contains seven species. *B. pertussis* is by far the most important because it is the cause of classic pertussis (whooping cough). Nucleic acid homology and other analyses indicate that *B. parapertussis* and *B. bronchiseptica* are close enough to *B. pertussis* to be considered variants of the same species. *B. parapertussis* occasionally causes a disease similar to, but milder than, pertussis. This is probably because it does not produce pertussis toxin even though it has a silent copy of the toxin gene. The remainder of this section will focus solely on *B. pertussis*.

Species similar to *B. pertussis* do not cause classical whooping cough

Bordetella pertussis

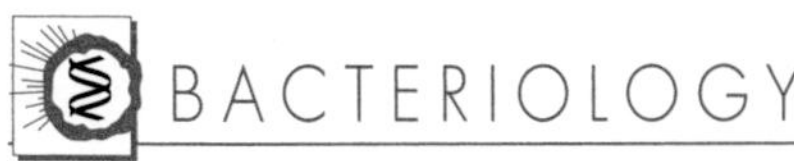

BACTERIOLOGY

GROWTH AND STRUCTURE

B. pertussis is a tiny (0.5 to 1.0 μm), Gram-negative coccobacillus morphologically much like *Haemophilus*. Growth requires a special medium supplemented with **nicotinamide** and other additives such as charcoal, which is thought to neutralize the effect of inhibitory

Coccobacilli are similar to *Haemophilus*

Nicotinamide required for slow growth

compounds present in standard bacteriologic media. Under the best conditions, growth is still slow, requiring 3 to 7 days for isolation. The organism is also very susceptible to environmental changes and survives only briefly outside the human respiratory tract.

Fha binds amino acid sequences found in host cells

Pili and pertactin are adhesins

The cell wall has the structure typical of Gram-negative bacteria, although the outer membrane lipopolysaccharide differs significantly in structure and biologic activity from that of the Enterobacteriaceae. The surface exhibits a rod-like protein called the **filamentous hemagglutinin (Fha)** because of its ability to bind to and agglutinate erythrocytes. Fha has strong adherence qualities, based on domains in its structure that interact with an amino acid sequence (arginine, glycine, aspartic acid) present in host integrins, epithelial cells, and macrophages. The organism surface also contains surface **pili** and the outer membrane includes a protein called **pertactin.**

EXTRACELLULAR PRODUCTS

Pertussis Toxin

A-B toxin ADP-ribosylates G protein

Adenylate cyclase and cell regulation are disrupted

Pertussis toxin (PT) is the major virulence factor of *B. pertussis*. It is an A-B toxin produced from a single operon as an enzymatic subunit and five distinct binding subunits that are assembled into the complete toxin on the bacterial surface. The binding subunits mediate attachment of the toxin to carbohydrate moieties on the host cell surface. The enzymatic subunit is then internalized and ADP-ribosylates a G-protein that affects adenylate cyclase activity. Unlike cholera toxin, which in essence keeps cyclase activity "turned on," pertussis toxin freezes the opposite side of the regulatory circuit and cripples the capacity of the host cell to inactivate cyclase activity. Other intracellular effector pathways are also disrupted by the G-protein modification. The binding subunits have a biologic effect on lymphocytes and other cells independent of the enzymatic function of the toxin.

Other Toxins

Bacterial adenylate cyclase disrupts immune cell function

Peptidoglycan fragments injure tracheal cells

Another potent toxin, an invasive **adenylate cyclase,** enters host cells and catalyzes the conversion of host cell ATP to cyclic AMP at levels far above what can be achieved by normal mechanisms. This enzyme is hemolytic and interferes with cellular signaling, chemotaxis, superoxide generation, and microbicidal function of immune effector cells, including polymorphonuclear leukocytes and monocytes. It can also induce programmed cell death (apoptosis). Remarkably, after the adenylate cyclase enters the cell, it requires activation by calmodulin, a eukaryotic Ca^{2+}-binding protein. Such activation of a bacterial enzyme by an intracellular mammalian protein is unusual, but is also seen with another bacterial adenylate cyclase, anthrax toxin (see Chapter 18). **Tracheal cytotoxin** is essentially fragments of cell-wall peptidoglycan (1,6-anhydromuramic acid-*N*-acetylglucosamine-tetrapeptide). The fragments are released by multiplying bacterial cells and cause the death of ciliated tracheal cells. This cytotoxin is similar, if not identical to, one produced by *Neisseria gonorrhoeae* (see Chapter 20).

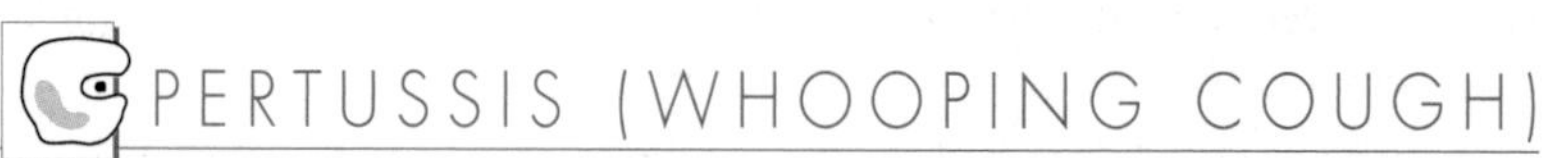

PERTUSSIS (WHOOPING COUGH)

CLINICAL CAPSULE

Pertussis is a prolonged illness caused by toxins produced by *B. pertussis* bacteria attached to the cilia of respiratory epithelial cells. It progresses in stages over many weeks beginning with a rhinorrhea (runny nose) that evolves into a persistent cough. The name "whooping cough" comes from children who exhibit an inspiratory "whoop" following an exhausting series of paroxysmal coughs.

EPIDEMIOLOGY

B. pertussis is spread by airborne droplet nuclei produced by patients in the early stages of illness. It is highly contagious, infecting 80 to 100% of exposed susceptible persons. Secondary spread in families, schools, and hospitals is rapid. Sporadic epidemics occur, but there is no strong seasonal pattern. *B. pertussis* is not found in animals and survives poorly in the environment. Asymptomatic carriers are very rarely found. However, infections in previously immunized adults have become an increasingly important reservoir, because the mild symptoms are often not recognized as any more than a "bad cold." Unwitting adults have served as the source for outbreaks in highly susceptible populations, such as infants in a newborn nursery. Mortality remains the highest in infants, with over 70% of fatal cases occurring in children under 1 year of age.

Highly contagious and spread by airborne droplet nuclei

Atypical, unrecognized disease in adults facilitates spread

After the introduction of immunization in the 1940s, the incidence of pertussis in the United States dropped from over 250,000 cases a year to well below one case per 100,000 population. Since the 1980s, a slow rise, augmented by epidemics every 3 to 4 years, has resulted. The 7796 cases reported in 1996 was a 30-year high. The greatest increase has been in the 10- to 20-year-age group. In general, pertussis has increased when immunization rates have fallen largely due to concerns about vaccine reactions. For example, when childhood immunization rates in England fell below 50% in 1981, pertussis cases rose dramatically. There were 47,000 cases in the first 9 months of 1982 alone.

Immunization reduces disease

Outbreaks correlate with incomplete immunization

PATHOGENESIS

B. pertussis is a strict human pathogen. When introduced into the respiratory tract, the organism has a remarkable tropism for ciliated bronchial epithelium attaching to the cilia themselves. This adherence is mediated by Fha, pili, pertactin, and the binding subunits of PT. Once attached, the bacteria immobilize the cilia and begin a sequence in which the ciliated cells are progressively destroyed and extruded from the epithelial border (Fig 24–3). This local injury is caused primarily by the action of the tracheal cytotoxin. This produces an epithelium devoid of the ciliary blanket, which moves foreign matter away from the lower airways. Persistent coughing is the clinical correlate of this deficit. Although considerable local inflammation and exudate are produced in the bronchi, *B. pertussis* does not directly invade the cells of the respiratory tract or spread to deeper tissue sites.

Only infects humans

Attachment to cilia provides site for toxin production

Mucosa becomes devoid of ciliated cells

Virulence Factors

In addition to the local effects on the bronchial epithelium, the virulence factors of *B. pertussis* contribute to the disease in many other ways. The combined action of PT and

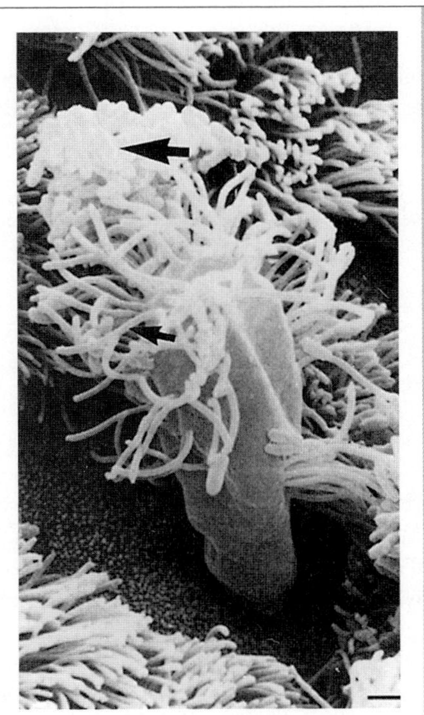

FIGURE 24–3
A tracheal organ culture 72 hours after infection with *Bordetella pertussis*. The organisms have attached to the cilia of some cells and killed them. These balloon-like cells with attached bacteria are extruded from the epithelium. The large arrow shows the *Bordetella* and the small arrow the cilia. Note the background of uninfected ciliated cells and denuded epithelium where nonciliated cells remain. (*Reproduced with permission from Muse KE, Collier AM, Baseman JB.* J Infect Dis *136:768–777. Figure 3, copyright 1977 by University of Chicago, publisher.*)

adenylate cyclase on neutrophils, macrophages, and lymphocytes creates paralysis and even death of these crucial effector cells of the immune system. Many of the systemic manifestations of the disease such as lymphocytosis, histamine sensitization, and insulin secretion are due to the action of circulating PT absorbed at the primary infection site. The specific biologic effect depends on how disruption of G-protein regulation by PT is manifested by the host cell type the toxin reaches. Pertussis is the result of a well-orchestrated delivery by *B. pertussis* of toxic and adhesive factors to host cells at local and distant sites to produce a disease that persists for many weeks.

PT and adenylate cyclase attack immune cells

Absorbed PT acts on multiple cell types

Genetic Regulation of Pathogenicity

How *B. pertussis* deploys its repertoire of virulence genes is a model for the control of bacterial pathogenicity (Fig 24–4). *B. pertussis* regulates the synthesis of PT, the invasive adenylate cyclase, Fha, pili, and many other genes through genetic loci that control the expression of at least 20 unlinked chromosomal genes at the transcriptional level. Expression is modulated by changes in specific environmental parameters, including temperature.

Multiple virulence genes respond to temperature and ionic changes

Transcriptional regulation is controlled by a two-compartment system, which involves a regulatory protein that spans the bacterial membrane (BvgS) and an activator protein in the cytoplasm (BvgA). The membrane protein has a periplasmic domain that responds to temperature or ionic changes. When the temperature changes from 25°C to 37°C, it autophosphorylates and subsequently donates a phosphate group to the cytoplasmic protein, allowing it to bind to DNA recognition sequences in the chromosome. There it promotes the transcription of its own gene and those located in an operon containing at least the Fha and pilin structural genes. Experimentally, Fha, pilin, and BvgA mRNA are produced at this point, followed about 6 hours later by PT and adenylate cyclase. This delay is believed to be due to the time required for the production of a second BvgS directed activator which then turns on these genes.

Virulence genes are activated in two-compartment model

Environmental factors trigger Fha, PT, and adenylate cyclase when needed

Thus, the induction of virulence factors in *B. pertussis* is sequential, with adhesin expression (Fha and pili) preceding expression of factors involved in tissue injury. The finely honed responses of *B. pertussis* virulence factors to changes in temperature and ionic conditions presumably play a role in the pathogenesis of infection and help the organism adapt in a stepwise fashion to the diverse local conditions within the human respiratory tract.

Adherence factors precede injury products

IMMUNITY

Although IgG antibodies are produced to PT, pili, and pertactin during the course of natural infection and by immunization, they are not long lasting and their role in immunity is not well understood. Naturally acquired immunity is not lifelong, although second attacks, when recognized, tend to be mild. The high susceptibility of newborns and infants before immunization may reflect a low level of antibody in adults and thus lack of passive transfer to the infant at birth.

IgG to virulence factors does not produce long-term immunity

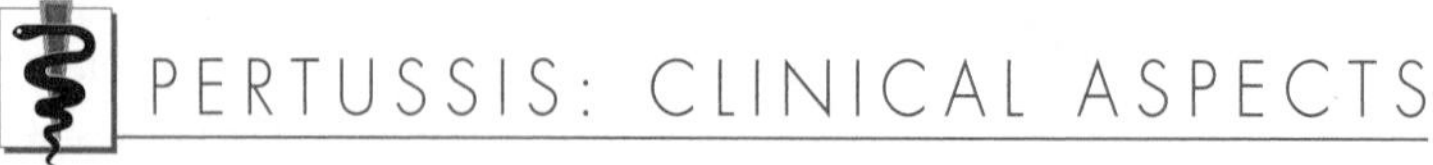

PERTUSSIS: CLINICAL ASPECTS

MANIFESTATIONS

After an incubation period of 7 to 10 days, pertussis follows a prolonged course consisting of three overlapping stages: (1) catarrhal, (2) paroxysmal, and (3) convalescent. In the catarrhal stage, the primary feature is a profuse and mucoid rhinorrhea that persists for 1 to 2 weeks. Nonspecific findings such as malaise, fever, sneezing, and anorexia may also be present. The disease is most communicable at this stage, because large numbers of organisms are present in the nasopharynx and the mucoid secretions.

Catarrhal phase is most communicable

The appearance of a persistent cough marks the transition from the catarrhal to the paroxysmal coughing stage. At this time, episodes of paroxysmal coughing occur up to

Paroxysmal coughing phase lasts for weeks

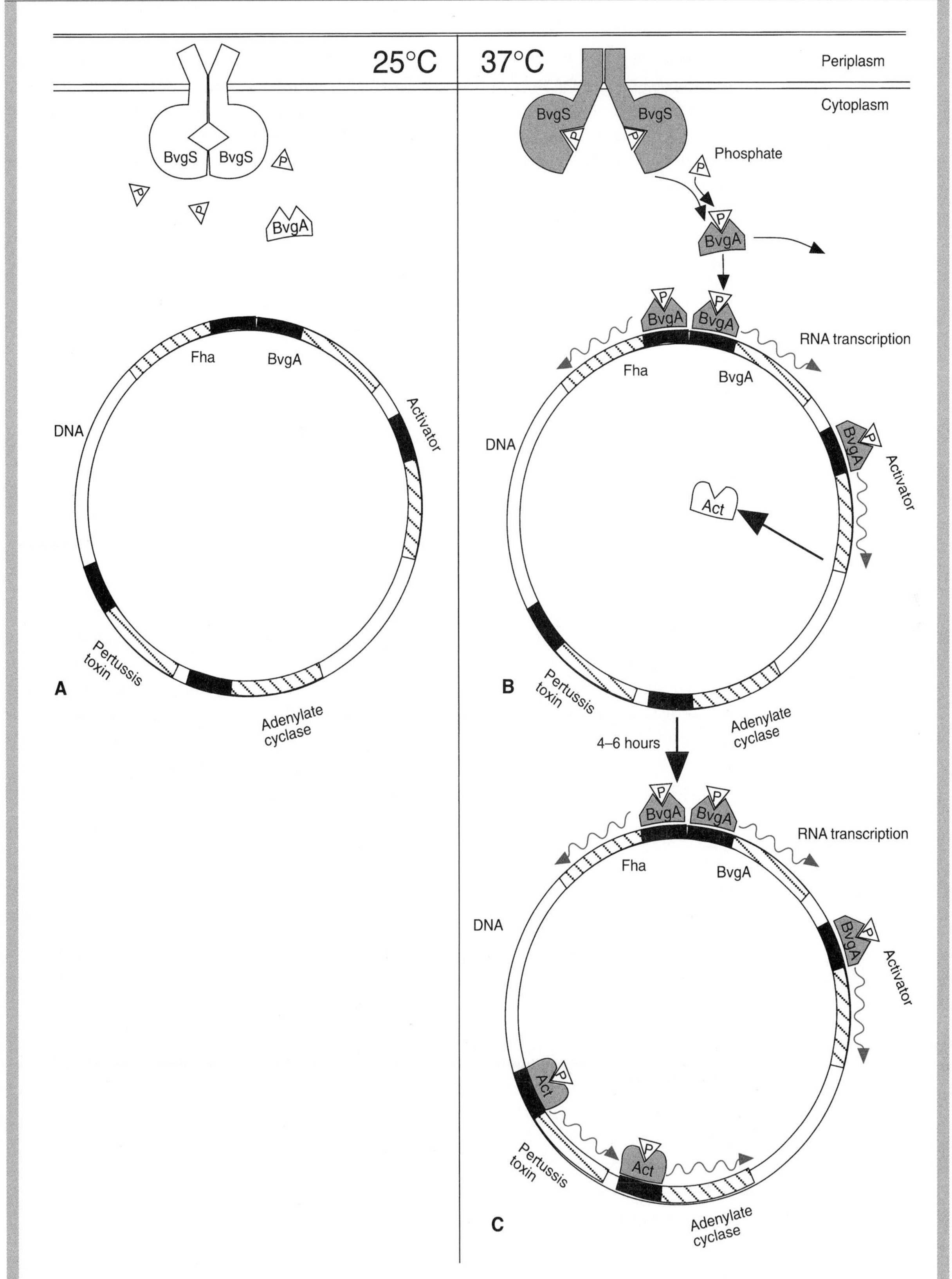

FIGURE 24–4

Regulation of *Bordetella pertussis* virulence factors. **A.** At 25°C the membrane-associated regulatory protein BvgS is inactive as are the genes for virulence factors filamentous hemagglutinin (Fha), pertussis toxin, and adenylate cyclase. **B.** At 37°C BvgS autophosphorylates and activates a cytoplasmic regulatory protein, BvgA, by phosphorylation. BvgA activates transcription of genes for production of BvgS, BvgA, Fha, and a postulated second regulator, Act. **C.** Hours later transcription of the pertussis toxin and adenylate cyclase is activated by Act. (*Adapted from Melton, AR, Weiss AA. Characterization of environmental regulators of* Bordetella pertussis. *Infect Immun 1993;61:807–815.*)

Inspiratory whoop and coughing may lead to apnea

Lymphocytosis is marked

50 times a day for 2 to 4 weeks. The characteristic inspiratory whoop follows a series of coughs as air is rapidly drawn through the narrowed glottis. Vomiting frequently follows the whoop. The combination of mucoid secretions, whooping cough, and vomiting produces a miserable, exhausted child barely able to breathe. Apnea may follow such episodes, particularly in infants. Marked lymphocytosis reaches its peak at this time, with absolute lymphocyte counts of up to 40,000/mm^3.

Convalescent phase is a gradual fading

During the 3- to 4-week convalescent stage, the frequency and severity of paroxysmal coughing and other features of the disease gradually fade. Partially immune persons and infants under 6 months of age may not show all the typical features of pertussis. Some evolution through the three stages is usually seen, but paroxysmal coughing and lymphocytosis may be absent.

Atelectasis and superinfection are major complications

The most common complication of pertussis is pneumonia caused by a superinfecting organism such as *S. pneumoniae*. Atelectasis is also common but may be recognized only by radiologic examination. Other complications, including convulsions and subconjunctival or cerebral bleeding, are related to the venous pressure effects of the paroxysmal coughing and the anoxia produced by inadequate ventilation and apneic spells.

DIAGNOSIS

Nasopharyngeal swab is plated on charcoal blood agar

Organisms are often gone by later paroxysmal phase

A clinical diagnosis of pertussis is best confirmed by isolation of *B. pertussis* from nasopharyngeal secretions or swabs. Throat swabs are not suitable, because the cilia to which the organism attaches are not found there. Specimens collected early in the course of disease (during the catarrhal or early paroxysmal stage) provide the greatest chance of successful isolation. Unfortunately, the diagnosis is frequently not considered until paroxysmal coughing has been present for some time, and the number of organisms has decreased significantly. The nasopharyngeal specimens are plated onto a special charcoal blood agar medium made selective by the addition of a cephalosporin. This allows the slow-growing *B. pertussis* to be isolated in the presence of more rapidly growing members of the normal upper respiratory flora. The characteristic colonies appear after 3 to 7 days of incubation and look like tiny drops of mercury. Immunologic methods (agglutination, immuofluorescence) are required for specific identification.

DFA allows rapid diagnosis

A direct immunofluorescent antibody (DFA) technique has been successfully applied to nasopharyngeal smears for rapid diagnosis of pertussis. DFA is particularly helpful in pertussis because of the many days required for culture results. Because the sensitivity and specificity of DFA can vary with the quality of the reagents, these results should always be confirmed by culture, if possible. Serologic and molecular diagnostic methods have been developed but are not widely used for clinical diagnosis.

TREATMENT

Erythromycin or clarithromycin are effective in catarrhal phase

Once the paroxysmal coughing stage has been reached, the treatment of pertussis is primarily supportive. Antimicrobial therapy is useful at earlier stages and for limiting spread to other susceptible individuals. Of a number of antimicrobics active in vitro against *B. pertussis,* erythromycin or clarithromycin are preferred because of their clinical effectiveness and relative lack of toxicity.

PREVENTION

Whole cell vaccine was effective but had side effects

Acellular vaccines are purified preparations

Active immunization is the primary method of preventing pertussis. The original vaccine, which produced a 99% reduction in disease, was prepared from inactivated whole cell suspensions and given together with diphtheria and tetanus toxoids as DTP. The undoubted efficacy of this vaccine was colored by a high rate of side effects due to the crude nature of the whole cell preparation. These included local inflammation, fever and, rarely, febrile seizures. Although permanent neurologic sequelae were never convincingly linked to pertussis immunization, there were those who argued that the vaccine was worse than the disease. This led to the development of acellular vaccines, guided by knowledge of the virulence factors involved in the pathogenesis of pertussis. One type of vaccine is made by purification of virulence factors from whole cell preparations followed by formaldehyde inactivation where appropriate. Another vaccine strategy is the production of recombinant components, genetically engineered to be immunogenic but nontoxic.

The multiple acellular vaccines licensed in the United States have different combinations of virulence factors. All contain PT toxoid and Fha and some add pertactin or pili (vaccine manufacturers use the term fimbriae). The efficacy of these vaccines has now been established and all have dramatically lower frequencies of side effects. They have been combined with diphtheria and tetanus toxoids as DTaP replacing the whole cell DTP. This vaccine is now recommended for the full primary immunization (2, 4, and 6 months) and boosters (15–18 months, 4–6 years). Additional boosters are recommended every 10 years after the last dose.

Vaccines include PT, Fha, and other virulence factors

DTaP has replaced DTP

ADDITIONAL READING

Bisgard KM, Kao A, Leake J, Strebel PM, Perkins BA, Wharton M. *Haemophilus influenzae* invasive disease in the United States, 1994–1995: Near disappearance of a vaccine-preventable childhood disease. *Emerg Infect Dis* 1998;4:229–237. This concise paper documents one of the most successful episodes in the history of immunization.

DeSerres G, Shadman R, Duval B, et al. Morbidity of pertussis in adolescents and adults. *J Infect Dis* 2000;182:174–179. A large group of patients was studied, showing that morbidity can be significant in age groups other than children, particularly in asthmatics, smokers, and older adults.

Fothergill LD, Wright J. Influenzal meningitis: The relation of age incidence to the bactericidal power of blood against the causal organism. *J Immunol* 1933;24:273–284. A classic study, the first to advance the currently accepted concepts of humoral immunity in *H. influenzae* disease.

Hewlett EL. Pertussis: Current concepts of pathogenesis and prevention. *Pediatr Infect Dis J* 1997;16:S78–S84. A concise summary of the role of *B. pertussis* virulence factors.

Muse KE, Collier AM, Baseman JB. Scanning electron microscopic study of hamster tracheal organ cultures infected with *Bordetella pertussis*. *J Infect Dis* 1977;136:768–777. The unique tropism of *B. pertussis* for ciliated cells and the subsequent destruction of those cells are shown experimentally and visually.

C H A P T E R 2 5

Mycoplasma and *Ureaplasma*

W. Lawrence Drew

Mycoplasma and *Ureaplasma* are unique microbes in that they lack a cell wall. They are ubiquitous in nature as the smallest of free-living microorganisms. Numerous *Mycoplasma* species have been isolated from animals and humans, but only three species have been associated with human disease (Table 25–1). *Mycoplasma pneumoniae* is a lower respiratory tract pathogen. *Mycoplasma hominis* and *Ureaplasma urealyticum* cause genitourinary tract infections.

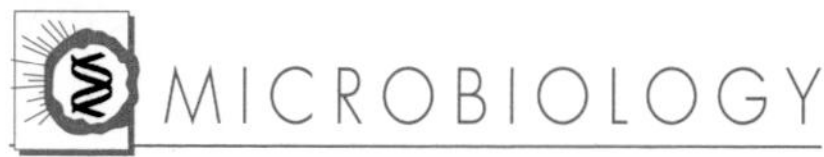

MICROBIOLOGY

The organisms have diameters of about 0.2 to 0.3 mm, but they are highly plastic and pleomorphic and may appear as coccoid bodies, filaments, and large multinucleoid forms. They do not have a cell wall and are bounded only by a single triple-layered membrane (Fig 25–1) that, unlike other bacteria, contains sterols. The sterols are not synthesized by the organism but are acquired as essential components from the medium or tissue in which the organism is growing. Lacking a cell wall, *Mycoplasma* and *Ureaplasma* stain poorly or not at all with the usual bacterial stains. Their double-stranded DNA genome is small, probably because of lack of genes encoding a complex cell wall. *M. pneumoniae* is an aerobe, but most other species are facultatively anaerobic. All grow slowly in enriched liquid culture medium and on special *Mycoplasma* agar to produce minute colonies only after several days of incubation. The center of the *M. pneumoniae* colony grows into the agar and appears denser, giving the appearance of an inverted "fried egg." Growth in culture is inhibited by specific antisera directed at the particular species. Colonies of *M. pneumoniae* bind red blood cells (RBCs) onto the surface of agar plate cultures (hemadsorption). This is due to binding by the mycoplasma to sialic acid–containing oligosaccharides present on the RBC surface.

No cell walls

Cell membrane contains sterols

Not stained well by common methods

Slow growth in specialized media

Hemadsorption is a feature of *M. pneumoniae*

TABLE 25–1

Pathogenic *Mycoplasma* and *Ureaplasma* Species of Humans

Organism	Site	Prevalence	Disease
M. pneumoniae	Upper and lower respiratory tract	Common	Primary atypical pneumonia
M. hominis	Genitourinary tract	Common	Postpartum fever; pelvic inflammatory disease
U. urealyticum	Genitourinary tract	Very common	Nongonococcal urethritis

MYCOPLASMA PNEUMONIAE

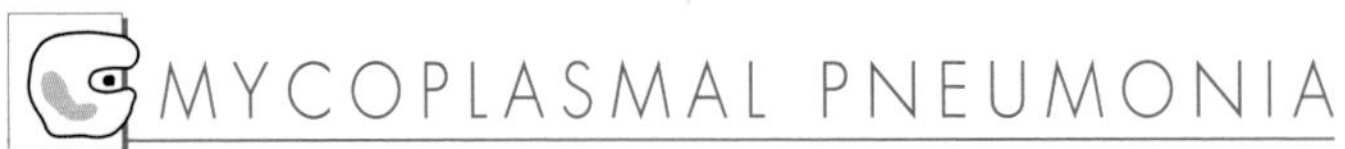

CLINICAL CAPSULE

M. pneumoniae produces a common form of pneumonia, which tends to occur in any season and has a predilection for younger individuals. The illness is characterized by a nonproductive cough, fever, and headache, with radiologic and clinical evidence of scattered areas of pneumonia. The course is almost always benign, but improvement is accelerated by treatment with non–cell wall–active antimicrobials.

EPIDEMIOLOGY

Infecting dose is very low

Found worldwide most often in teenagers

M. pneumoniae accounts for approximately 10% of all cases of pneumonia. Infection is acquired by droplet spread. Experimental challenges indicate that the human infectious dose is very low, possibly less than 100 colony-forming units. Endemic infections with *M. pneumoniae* occur worldwide, but they are especially prominent in temperate climates. Epidemics at 4- to 6-year intervals have been noted in both civilian and military populations. The most common age for symptomatic *M. pneumoniae* infection is between 5 and 15 years, and the disease accounts for more than one third of all cases of pneumonia

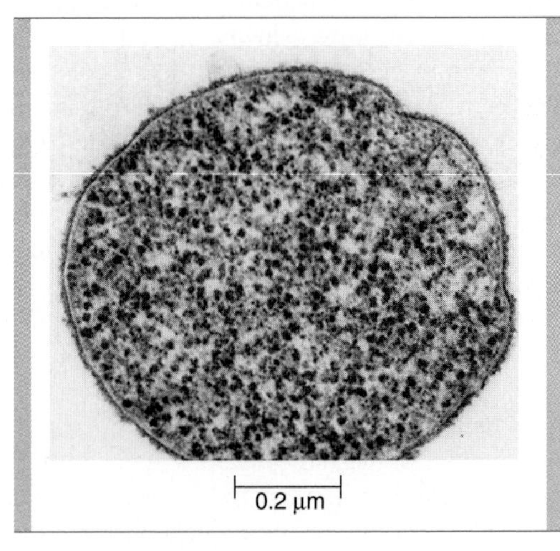

FIGURE 25–1
Electron micrograph of *Mycoplasma*. Note cytoplasmic membrane ribosomes and surface amorphous material with absence of cell wall. (*Courtesy of the late Dr. E. S. Boatman.*)

in teenagers, but is also seen in older persons. Infections in children less than 6 months of age are uncommon. The disease often appears as a sporadic, endemic illness in families or closed communities because its incubation period is relatively long (2 to 15 days) and because prolonged shedding in nasal secretions may cause infections to be spread over time. In families, attack rates in susceptible individuals approach 60%. Asymptomatic infections occur, but most studies have suggested that more than two thirds of infected cases develop some evidence of respiratory tract illness.

Outbreaks occur in families and closed communities

PATHOGENESIS

M. pneumoniae infection involves the trachea, bronchi, bronchioles, and peribronchial tissues, and may extend to the alveoli and alveolar walls. Initially, the organism attaches to the cilia and microvilli of the cells lining the bronchial epithelium. This attachment is mediated by a surface mycoplasmal cytadhesin (P1) protein that binds to complex oligosaccharides containing sialic acid found in the apical regions of bronchial epithelial cells. The oligosaccharide receptors are chemically similar to the I antigen on the surface of erythrocytes and are not found on the nonciliated goblet cells or mucus, to which *M. pneumoniae* does not bind. The organisms interfere with ciliary action and initiate a process that leads to desquamation of the involved mucosa and a subsequent inflammatory reaction and exudate. The inflammatory response is at first most pronounced in the bronchial and peribronchial tissue and is composed of lymphocytes, plasma cells, and macrophages, which may infiltrate and thicken the walls of the bronchioles and alveoli. Organisms are shed in upper respiratory secretions for 2 to 8 days before the onset of symptoms, and shedding continues for as long as 14 weeks after infection.

Adherence to bronchial epithelial cells is mediated by P1 protein

Interferes with ciliary action and leads to desquamation

IMMUNITY

Both local and systemic specific immune responses occur. Local IgA antibody is produced but disappears 2 to 4 weeks after the onset of the infection. Complement-fixing serum antibody titers reach a peak 2 to 4 weeks after infection and gradually disappear over 6 to 12 months. Nonspecific immune responses to the glycolipids of the outer membrane of the organism often also develop, which can be detrimental to the host. For example, cold hemagglutinins are IgM antibodies that react with the I antigen of human RBCs and are seen in about two thirds of symptomatic patients infected with *M. pneumoniae*.

Complement-fixing antibody titers peak at 2–4 weeks

Cold agglutinins are IgM

Immunity is not complete, and reinfection with *M. pneumoniae* is common. Clinical disease appears to be more severe in older than in younger children, which has led to the suggestion that many of the clinical manifestations of disease are the result of immune responses rather than invasion by the organism. High titers of cold agglutinations may be associated with hemolysis and Raynaud's phenomena. Antibodies may develop in response to an alteration of the I antigen by the organism or may represent cross-reacting antibodies.

Immunity is incomplete, and reinfection is common

MYCOPLASMAL PNEUMONIA: CLINICAL ASPECTS

MANIFESTATIONS

A mild tracheobronchitis with fever, cough, headache, and malaise is the most common syndrome associated with acute *M. pneumoniae* infection. The pneumonia is typically less severe than other bacterial pneumonias. It has been described as "walking" pneumonia, because most cases do not require hospitalization. The disease is of insidious onset, with fever, headache, and malaise for 2 to 4 days before the onset of respiratory symptoms. Pulmonary symptoms are generally limited to a non- or minimally productive cough. X-rays reveal a unilateral or patchy pneumonia, usually in a lower lobe, although multiple lobes are sometimes involved. Small pleural effusions are seen in up to 25% of cases.

"Walking" pneumonia has insidious onset

Cough is usual

Pharyngitis and otitis are also common

Pharyngitis with fever and sore throat may also occur. Nonpurulent otitis media or myringitis occurs concomitantly in approximately 15% of patients with *M. pneumoniae* pneumonitis. The presence of nonpurulent otitis media and lower respiratory illness in a teenager suggests *M. pneumoniae* infection.

DIAGNOSIS

Diagnosis is usually serologic

Single high complement fixation or IgM-specific antibody titer supports diagnosis

Clinical diagnosis of *M. pneumoniae* infection may be difficult because the manifestations overlap with those of bacterial and viral infections. Gram-stained sputum usually shows some mononuclear cells, but, because it lacks a cell wall, *M. pneumoniae* is not seen. The absence of organisms, however, may help to suggest the etiology. The organism can be isolated from throat swabs or sputum of infected patients using special culture media and methods, but because of its slow growth, isolation usually requires incubation for a week or longer. Thus, serologic tests rather than cultures are more commonly used for specific diagnosis. A fourfold rise of serum antibody titer in acute and convalescent sera indicates *M. pneumoniae* infection. The most widely used serologic method is complement fixation. With the relatively long incubation period and insidious onset of the disease, many patients already have high antibody titers at the time they are first seen. In these situations, a single high titer, such as a complement fixation titer greater than 1:128 or IgM-specific antibody (measured by enzyme immunoassay or immunofluorescence), indicates recent or current infection, because these antibodies are generally of short duration.

Cold agglutinins are nonspecific but helpful

Because more than two thirds of patients with symptomatic lower respiratory *M. pneumoniae* infection develop high titers of cold hemagglutinins, their demonstration can be useful in some clinical situations. It must be remembered that cold hemagglutinins are nonspecific and have been observed in adenovirus infections, infectious mononucleosis, and some other illnesses. The test is simple, however, and can be performed rapidly in any clinical laboratory. Direct detection of the organism in respiratory secretions has been attempted using immunoassay methods, DNA hybridization, and the polymerase chain reaction. These methods are not yet available for routine diagnosis.

TREATMENT

Erythromycin, tetracycline, clarithromycin, or azithromycin used in treatment

Erythromycin or tetracycline are the usual agents used for treatment of *M. pneumoniae* infections. They shorten the course of infection, although eradication from the nasopharynx may take much longer. Azithromycin and clarithromycin are comparable to erythromycin, but clindamycin is not effective. Most quinolones are also active.

MYCOPLASMA HOMINIS

Genitourinary inhabitant

Grows rapidly on specialized agar

Association with postpartum fever

M. hominis is a common inhabitant of the genitourinary tract. Although some strains grow on ordinary blood agar as nonhemolytic pinpoint colonies, the organism is best detected on *Mycoplasma* agar, on which it grows rapidly. *M. hominis* and *Ureaplasma* can be differentiated by demonstrating arginine breakdown by the former and urease activity by the latter. At least seven antigenic variants of *M. hominis* have been described. To date, the major clinical condition associated with *M. hominis* infection is postabortal or postpartum fever. *Mycoplasma hominis* is isolated from the blood of about 10% of women with this condition. Occasional infections of the central nervous system or joints also have been described, primarily in patients with antibody deficiency syndromes or premature infants.

Association with pelvic inflammatory disease

Resistant to erythromycin

The diseases appear to be self-limiting, although antibiotic therapy may decrease the duration of fever and hospitalization. Serologic studies and animal experiments have also indicated that pelvic inflammatory disease syndromes in women may be associated with *M. hominis* infection of the fallopian tubes. The organism is sensitive to tetracycline. In contrast to *U. urealyticum* and *M. pneumoniae, M. hominis* is resistant to erythromycin.

UREAPLASMA UREALYTICUM

The genus *Ureaplasma* contains a single species, *U. urealyticum*, of which some 14 serotypes have been described. *Ureaplasma* is distinguished from *Mycoplasma* by its production of urease. On special *Ureaplasma* agar media, colonies are small and circular and grow downward into the agar. In liquid media containing urea and phenol red, growth of *Ureaplasma* results in production of ammonia from the urea, with a resultant increase in pH and a change in color of the indicator.

Urease production marks the species

EPIDEMIOLOGY

The main reservoir of human strains of *U. urealyticum* is the genital tract of sexually active men and women; it is rarely found before puberty. Colonization, which probably results primarily from sexual contact, occurs in more than 80% of individuals who have had three or more sexual partners.

Most commonly acquired by sexual contact

MANIFESTATIONS

Because of the high colonization rate, it has been difficult to associate specific illness with *Ureaplasma*; however, studies suggest that approximately one half of cases of nongonococcal, nonchlamydial urethritis in men may be caused by *U. urealyticum.* In women, *Ureaplasma* has been shown to cause chorioamnionitis and postpartum fever. The organism has been isolated from 10% of women with the latter syndrome.

Association with urethritis in men

DIAGNOSIS AND TREATMENT

Men with nongonococcal urethritis should be treated since *Ureaplasma* infection may be involved. Tetracycline is the treatment of choice because it is also active against *Chlamydia*, but tetracycline-resistant strains of *Ureaplasma* have been reported that have been associated with recurrences of nongonococcal urethritis in men. In such cases, spectinomycin treatment or treatment with quinolone antimicrobics is also effective. Women with postpartum fever due to *U. urealyticum* may respond to tetracycline treatment.

Tetracyclines, spectinomycin, or quinolones are effective

ADDITIONAL READING

Taylor-Robinson D. Infections due to species of mycoplasma and ureaplasma: An update. *Clin Infect Dis* 1996;23:671–684. Excellent review by one of the "fathers" of the field.

Taylor-Robinson D, et al. Antibiotic susceptibilities of mycoplasma and treatment of mycoplasma infections. *J Antimicrob Chemother* 1997;40:622–630. Reviews the currently available agents for treatment of mycoplasma infections.

Waris ME, Toikka P, Saarinen T, et al. Diagnosis of *Mycoplasma pneumoniae* pneumonia in children. *J Clin Microbiol* 1998;36:3155–3159. This paper examines the pros and cons of various diagnostic tests.

CHAPTER 26

Legionella

KENNETH J. RYAN

Legionella is a genus of Gram-negative bacilli that take their name from the American Legion convention where they were first discovered. The species designation of the prime human pathogen, *Legionella pneumophila,* reflects its propensity to cause pneumonia. *Legionella* species are widespread in the environment.

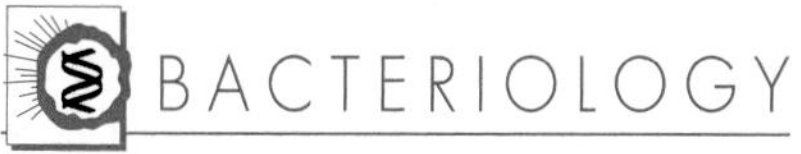

BACTERIOLOGY

MORPHOLOGY AND STRUCTURE

Legionella pneumophila is a thin (0.5 to 0.7 μm), pleomorphic, Gram-negative rod that may show elongated, filamentous forms up to 20 μm long. In clinical specimens, the organism stains poorly or not at all by Gram stain or the usual histologic stains; however, it can be demonstrated by certain silver impregnation methods (Dieterle stain) and by some simple stains that omit decolorization steps. Polar, subpolar, and lateral flagella may be present. Most species of *Legionella* are motile. Spores are not found.

Gram-negative rod that stains with difficulty

Structurally, *L. pneumophila* has features similar to those of Gram-negative bacteria with a typical outer membrane, thin peptidoglycan layer, and cytoplasmic membrane. The toxicity of *L. pneumophila* lipopolysaccharide (LPS) is significantly less than that of other Gram-negative bacteria such as *Neisseria* and the Enterobacteriaceae. This has been attributed to chemical makeup of the LPS side chains, which are a homopolymer of an unusual sugar (legionaminic acid), which renders the cell surface highly hydrophobic. It has been postulated that this hydrophobicity may promote adherence of bacterial cells to membranes or their concentration in aerosols.

LPS is less toxic than that of most Gram-negative species

Side chains are hydrophobic

GROWTH AND CLASSIFICATION

Legionella species fail to grow on common enriched bacteriologic media such as blood agar. This is due to unusual requirements for certain amino acids (L-cysteine), ferric ions, and slightly acidic conditions (optimal pH 6.9). Even when these requirements are met, growth under aerobic conditions is slow requiring 2 to 5 days to produce colonies that have a distinctive surface resembling ground glass.

Growth requires iron and low pH

Due to the difficulty in growing *Legionella* there are few phenotypic properties to use in its classification. It is possible to directly demonstrate some enzymatic actions (catalase, oxidase, β-lactamase), but the other cultural and metabolic taxonomic tests used to

Few phenotypic properties are demonstrable

Classification is based on antigenic structure and DNA homology

Multiple *L. pneumophila* serogroups and *Legionella* species exist

classify other bacteria cannot be applied to *Legionella*. Thus, the classification depends largely on antigenic features, chemical analysis, and nucleic acid homology comparisons.

L. pneumophila has 14 serogroups and there are more than 30 other *Legionella* species (eg, *L. bozemanii, L. dumoffii, L. micdadei*). The original Philadelphia strain (serogroup 1) is still the most common and a limited number of *L. pneumophila* serogroups (1 to 4) account for 80 to 90% of cases. Not all of the non–*L. pneumophila* species have been isolated from human infections.

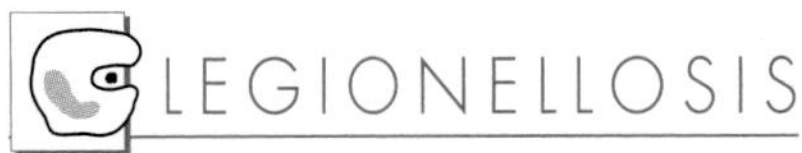

LEGIONELLOSIS

CLINICAL CAPSULE

Legionella are inhaled into the lung from an aquatic source in the environment. Once there, they produce a destructive pneumonia marked by headache, fever, chills, dry cough, and chest pain. Although there may be multiple foci in both lungs and extension to the pleura, spread outside the respiratory tree is very rare.

EPIDEMIOLOGY

1976 outbreak lead to discovery of new bacterium

Earlier outbreaks have been solved

The widely publicized outbreak of pneumonia among attendees of the 1976 American Legion convention in Philadelphia led to the isolation of a previously unrecognized infectious agent, *L. pneumophila*. The event was unique in medical history; for months the American public had entertained theories of its cause that ranged from sabotage to viroids, only to find that a Gram-negative rod that could not be stained or grown by the common methods was responsible. It was an outstanding example of the benefits of pursuing sound epidemiologic evidence until it is explained by equally sound microbiologic findings. We now know the disease had occurred for many years. Specific antibodies and organisms have been detected in material preserved from the 1950s, and a mysterious hospital outbreak in 1965 has been solved retrospectively.

Amoebas in fresh water habitat act as reservoir

Infections are associated with aerosols distributed by humidifying and cooling systems

In nature, *Legionella* species are ubiquitous in fresh water particularly in warm weather. In these sites they are also found as parasites of protozoa including numerous species of amoebae which appear to be the environmental reservoir. Transmission to humans is possible when the water supply of buildings becomes colonized and the system includes devices that create aerosols. Most outbreaks have occurred in or around large buildings such as hotels, factories, and hospitals involving cooling towers or some other part of the air-conditioning system. Some hospital outbreaks have implicated respiratory devices and potable water coming from parts of the hot water system such as faucets and shower heads. *Legionella* can persist in a water supply despite what appear to be adequate levels of chlorine particularly if the pipes contain abundant scale and/or dead end branches.

Person-to-person transmission or carriers are unknown

Disease rate among exposed is low

Person-to-person transmission has not been documented, and the organisms have not been isolated from healthy individuals. It is difficult to ascertain the overall incidence of *Legionella* infections; most information has been from outbreaks. Serologic surveys indicate that outbreaks constitute only a small part of the total cases, many of which currently go undetected. Estimates based on seroconversions suggest approximately 25,000 cases in the United States each year. Both serologic and environmental studies indicate that *Legionella* has low virulence for humans. The attack rate among those exposed is estimated at less than 5% and most serious cases are in immunocompromised persons.

PATHOGENESIS

Strong tropism for the lung

Necrotizing multifocal pneumonia with intracellular bacteria

L. pneumophila is striking in its propensity to attack the lung, producing a necrotizing multifocal pneumonia. Microscopically, the process involves the alveoli and terminal bronchioles, with relative sparing of the larger bronchioles and bronchi (Fig 26–1). The inflammatory exudate contains fibrin, polymorphonuclear neutrophils (PMNs), macro-

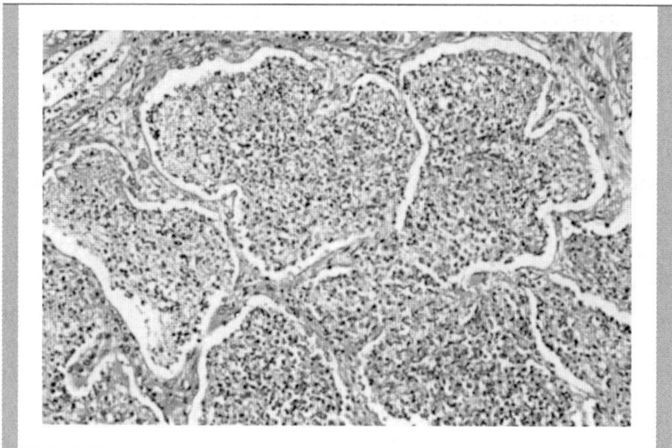

FIGURE 26–1
Legionella pneumonia. Note the filling of alveoli with exudate. Some of the alveolar septa are starting to degenerate. (*Reproduced with permission from Connor DH, Chandler FW, Schwartz DQA, Manz HJ, Lack EE (eds).* Pathology of Infectious Diseases, *vol. 1. Stamford, CT: Appleton & Lange; 1997.*)

phages, and erythrocytes. A striking feature is the preponderance of bacteria within phagocytes and the lytic destruction of inflammatory cells.

Facultative intracellular pathogen multiplies in alveolar macrophages

L. pneumophila is a facultative intracellular pathogen. Its pathogenicity depends on its ability to survive and multiply within cells of the monocyte–macrophage series. Inhaled *Legionella* bacteria reach the alveoli, where they enter alveolar macrophages utilizing

OMPs facilitate phagocyte entry to specialized vacuole

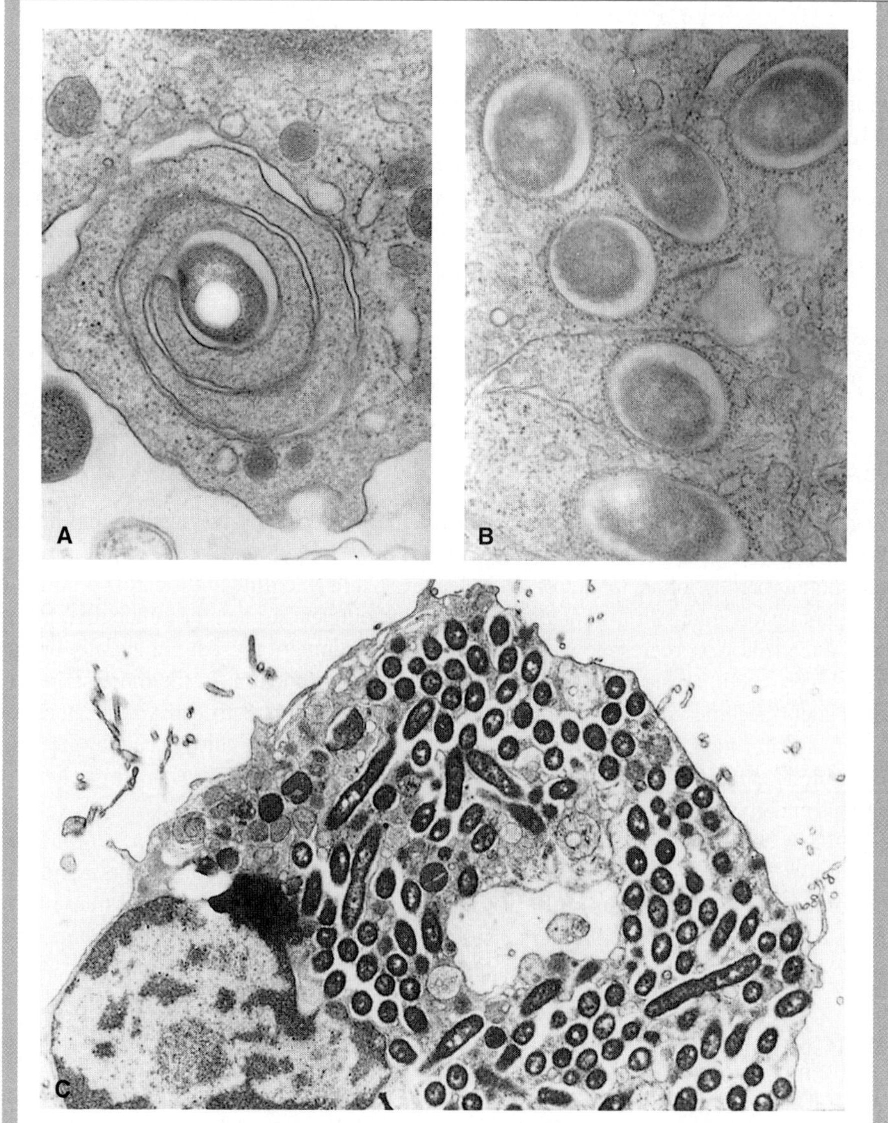

FIGURE 26–2
Multiplication of *Legionella pneumophila* in human macrophages. *Legionella pneumophila* enters the cell by coiling phagocytosis (**A**), and the phagosome created is lined by ribosomes and mitochondria (**B**). The bacteria multiply within the macrophages to reach very high numbers (**C**). (*Courtesy of Dr. Marcus Horwitz.*)

mechanisms involving multiple molecules. One outer membrane protein (OMP) binds C3, facilitating phagocyte recognition, and induces pores in the membrane of the macrophage. Another OMP called **macrophage invasion potentiator** (Mip) determines cell entry.

Secreted proteins block phagosomal fusion with lysosomes

Control of vesicular traffic creates replicative vacuole

Intracellular events are similar in amoeba

Inside the vacuole the bacteria continue to replicate by preventing phagosome-lysosome fusion and instead recruiting rough endoplasmic reticulum to the phagosome. The morphology of the replicative vacuole created is reflected in a process called **coiling phagocytosis** and is shown in Figure 26–2. *L. pneumophila* appears to accomplish this control of the phagocyte by use of a system that secretes proteins able to modulate host cell vesicle traffic. Other elements of the organism's intracellular success include its ability to extract iron from intracellular transferrin and a peptide toxin that inhibits activation of the oxidative killing mechanisms of PMNs. Thus, instead of being killed by the bactericidal mechanisms of phagocytes *L. pneumophila* multiplies freely. Death of cells is also related to induction of programmed cell death and formation of a pore-forming toxin. The progression of intracellular events in free-living amoebae is remarkably similar to that in human alveolar macrophages.

IMMUNITY

Cytokine activated macrophages limit intracellular growth

Antibody is less important

Just as intracellular multiplication is the key to *L. pneumophila* virulence, its inhibition by cell-mediated mechanisms appears to be the most important aspect of immunity. Whether *L. pneumophila* is able to interfere with development of these responses is not known, but hypoexpression of major histocompatibility complex class I and II molecules has been observed in phagosomes containing the organisms. In immunocompetent persons cytokine-activated macrophages eventually inhibit intracellular multiplication and limit growth of *Legionella*. Most progressive cases of Legionnaires' disease are in immunocompromised patients. The role of humoral immunity appears to be less important. In the presence of activated cellular immune responses antibody may play an ancillary role through enhancement of phagocytosis. It is unknown whether humans who have had Legionnaires' disease are immune to reinfection and disease.

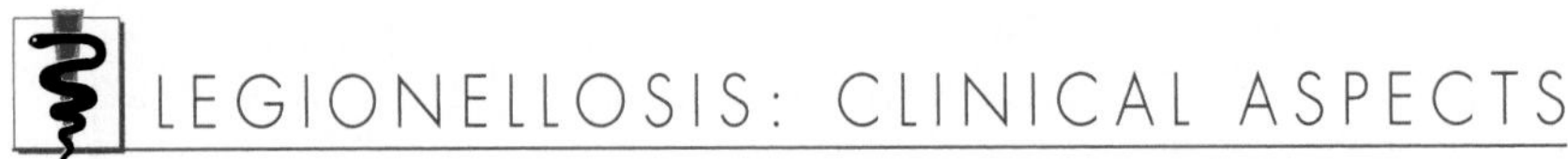

MANIFESTATIONS

Severe toxic pneumonia occurs in 5% of those exposed

Mortality is high among the immunocompromised

Pontiac fever may be hypersensitivity response

Legionnaires' disease is a severe toxic pneumonia that begins with myalgia and headache, followed by a rapidly rising fever. A dry cough may develop and later become productive, but sputum production is not a prominent feature. Chills, pleuritic chest pain, vomiting, diarrhea, confusion, and delirium may all be seen. Radiologically, patchy or interstitial infiltrates with a tendency to progress toward nodular consolidation are present unilaterally or bilaterally. Liver function tests often indicate some hepatic dysfunction. In the more serious cases the patient becomes progressively ill and toxic over the first 3 to 6 days, and the disease terminates in shock, respiratory failure, or both. The overall mortality is about 15%, but has been higher than 50% in some hospital outbreaks. It is particularly high in patients with serious underlying disease or suppression of cell-mediated immunity.

A less common form of disease called **Pontiac fever** (named for a 1968 Michigan outbreak), is a nonpneumonic illness with fever, myalgia, dry cough and a short incubation period (6 to 48 hours). Pontiac fever is a self-limiting illness and may represent a reaction to endotoxin or hypersensitivity to components of the *Legionella* or their protozoan hosts.

DIAGNOSIS

High-quality specimens are needed

The best means of diagnosis is direct fluorescent antibody (DFA) smears combined with culture of infected tissues. For this purpose, a high-quality specimen such as lung aspirates, bronchoalveolar lavage, or biopsies are preferred, because the organism may not be found in sputum. Typically, the Gram smear shows no bacteria, but the organisms are demonstrated by DFA using *L. pneumophila*–specific conjugates. These conjugates utilize monoclonal antibodies, which bind to all serotypes of *L. pneumophila* but not the non–*L. pneumophila* species. DFA is rapid, but it is positive in only 25 to 50% of culture-proved cases.

DFA is rapid but only 50% sensitive

Cultures must be made on buffered charcoal yeast extract (BCYE) agar medium that meets the growth requirements of *Legionella*. BCYE contains amino acids, vitamins, L-cysteine, ferric pyrophosphate, and charcoal to adsorb toxic fatty acids. It is buffered optimally for *Legionella* growth (pH 6.9). The isolation of large Gram-negative rods on BCYE after 2 to 5 days that have failed to grow on routine media (blood agar, chocolate agar), is presumptive evidence for *Legionella*. Diagnosis is confirmed by DFA staining of bacterial smears prepared from the colonies. BCYE also allows isolation of species of *Legionella* other than *L. pneumophila*.

Culture on BCYE is required for isolation

Cultures will isolate other species

The diagnosis of legionellosis can also be established by polymerase chain reaction (PCR) amplification of a rRNA gene common to all *Legionella* species or detection of antigen by immunoassay of urine. The antigenuria test was originally limited to *L. pneumophila* serogroup 1 but has been recently expanded to all *L. pneumophila* serogroups. Demonstrating a significant rise in serum antibody is used primarily for retrospective diagnosis and in epidemiologic studies. Diagnostic procedures for legionellosis are likely to be available only in reference facilities and the laboratories of hospitals treating immunocompromised patients. Even here, DFA and culture remain the mainstay until the newer methods prove cost-effective.

PCR detects rRNA gene

Antigenuria is detected by immunoassay

TREATMENT

The best information on antimicrobial therapy is still provided by the original Philadelphia outbreak. Because the etiology was completely obscure at the time, the cases were treated with many different regimens. Patients treated with erythromycin clearly did better than those given the penicillins, cephalosporins, or aminoglycosides. Subsequently, it was shown that most *Legionella* produce β-lactamases. In vitro susceptibility tests and animal studies have confirmed the activity of erythromycin and showed that tetracycline, rifampin, and the newer quinolones are also active. Although the other antimicrobics are sometimes used in combination, erythromycin and the newer macrolides (azithromycin, clarithromycin) remain the agents of choice.

Erythromycin is treatment of choice

Tetracycline, rifampin, and quinolones are alternatives

PREVENTION

The prevention of legionellosis involves minimizing production of aerosols in public places from water that may be contaminated with *Legionella*. Although outbreaks connected with large buildings have received the most attention, cases have been traced to sources as common as the mists used in supermarkets to make the vegetables look shiny and fresh. Prevention is complicated by the fact that, compared with other environmental bacteria, *Legionella* bacteria are relatively resistant to chlorine and heat. They have been isolated from hot water tanks held at over 50°C. Methods for decontaminating water systems are still under evaluation. Some outbreaks have been aborted by hyperchlorination, by correcting malfunctions in water systems, or by temporarily elevating the system temperature above 70°C. The installation of silver and copper ionization systems similar to those used in large swimming pools has been effective as a last resort in hospitals plagued with recalcitrant nosocomial legionellosis.

Preventing *Legionella* aerosols is primary goal

Heat, hyperchlorination, and metal ions may be needed in institutions

ADDITIONAL READING

Fraser DW, Tsai TR, Orenstein W, et al. Legionnaires' disease: Descriptions of an epidemic of pneumonia. *N Engl J Med* 1977;297:1189–1197.

McDade JE, Shepard CC, Fraser DW, et al. Legionnaires' disease: Isolation of a bacterium and demonstration of its role in other respiratory disease. *N Engl J Med*

1977;297:1197–1203. This study and the report by Fraser et al describe the 1976 outbreak at the Philadelphia American Legion convention and the methods that led to the discovery of the cause of this "new" disease. It makes good reading as an example of medical discovery and the requirements of proof.

Rohr U, Senger M, Selenka F, Turley R, Wilhelm M. Four years of experience with silver-copper ionization for control of *Legionella* in a German university hospital hot water plumbing system. *Clin Infect Dis* 1999;29:1507–1511. The paper illustrates the difficulty presented by the "colonization" of a hospital water supply by *Legionella.*

Stout JE, Yu VL. Legionellosis. *New Engl J Med* 1997;337:682–687. This concise review emphasizes clinical aspects.

CHAPTER 27

Spirochetes

KENNETH J. RYAN

Spirochetes generally refer to bacteria with a spiral morphology ranging from loose coils to a rigid corkscrew shape. The three medically important genera include the cause of syphilis, the ancient scourge of sexual indiscretion, and Lyme disease, a newly discovered consequence of an innocent walk in the woods (Table 27–1).

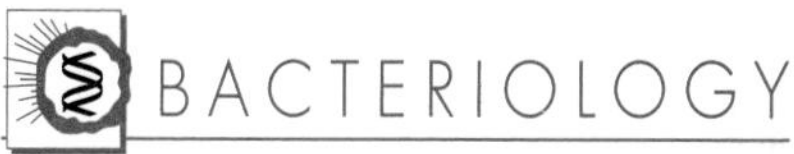

BACTERIOLOGY

MORPHOLOGY AND STRUCTURE

The spiral morphology of spirochetes is produced by a flexible, peptidoglycan cell wall around which several axial fibrils are wound. These fibrils have the structure of flagella and are referred to as **endoflagella** (Fig 27–1). The cell wall and endoflagella are completely covered by an outer bilayered membrane similar to the outer membrane of other Gram-negative bacteria. In some species, a hyaluronic acid slime layer forms around the exterior of the organism and may contribute to its virulence. Spirochetes are motile, exhibiting rotation and flexion; this motility is believed to result from movement of the endoflagellar filaments, although the mechanism is not clear.

Spiral structure is wound around endoflagella

Motility includes rotation and flexion

Many spirochetes are difficult to see by routine microscopy. Although they are Gram-negative, many either take stains poorly or are too thin (0.15 μm or less) to fall within the resolving power of the light microscope. Only darkfield microscopy, immunofluorescence, or special staining techniques that effectively increase their diameter can demonstrate these spirochetes. Other spirochetes such as *Borrelia* are larger and readily visible in stained preparations, even routine blood smears.

Many are thin and take stains poorly

Darkfield demonstrates spirochetes

GROWTH AND CLASSIFICATION

Parasitic spirochetes grow more slowly in vitro than most other disease-causing bacteria. Some species, including the causative agent of syphilis, have not been grown beyond a few generations in cell culture. Some are strict anaerobes, others require low concentrations of oxygen, and still others are aerobic. Compared to other bacterial groups the taxonomy of the spirochetes is underdeveloped. Because spirochetes are difficult to grow, they are difficult to study; thus, there are relatively few phenotypic properties on which to base a classification. The medically important genera *Treponema, Leptospira,* and *Borrelia* have been distinguished primarily by morphologic characters such as the nature of their spiral shape

Some have not been isolated in culture

May be aerobic or anaerobic

TABLE 27–1

Features of Spirochetal Diseases

Organism	Morphology	Transmission	Reservoir	Diagnosis: Microscopy	Diagnosis: Culture	Diagnosis: Serology	Disease
Treponema pallidum	Corkscrew spirals	Sexual, transplacental, transfusion	Humans	Darkfield of chancre or secondary lesions	None	VDRL, RPR, FTA-ABS, MHA-TP	Syphilis
Leptospira interrogans	Close spirals, hooked ends	Ingestion of contaminated water	Rodents, cattle, dogs	Not recommended[a]	Rarely performed[b]	MAT	Fever, meningitis, hepatitis
Borrelia recurrentis	Loose spirals	Lice	Humans	Giemsa or Wright stain of blood smear	Rarely performed[c]	None	Relapsing fever
Borrelia hermsii	Loose spirals	Ticks[d]	Rodents	Giemsa or Wright stain of blood smear	Rarely performed[c]	None	Relapsing fever
Borrelia burgdorferi	Loose spirals	Ticks[e]	White-footed mice, other rodents, (deer)[f]	Not recommended[a]	Rarely performed[c]	EIA + Western blot	Lyme disease

Abbreviations: FTA-ABS, fluorescent treponemal antibody; MAT, microagglutination test; MHA-TP, microhemagglutination test for *T. pallidum;* RPR, rapid plasma reagin; VDRL, Venereal Disease Research Laboratory.

[a] Organisms are small in number and rarely seen in clinical lesions.
[b] Culture of blood or urine in semisolid Fletcher's medium takes 1 to many weeks and is generally not available.
[c] Culture of blood in liquid Barbour–Stoener–Kelly medium takes 1 to many weeks and is generally not available.
[d] *Ornithodoros hermsi.*
[e] *Ixodes scapularis* in the eastern and central United States, *I. pacificus* in the western United States.
[f] Transmitting ticks mature on deer that are not actually a reservoir.

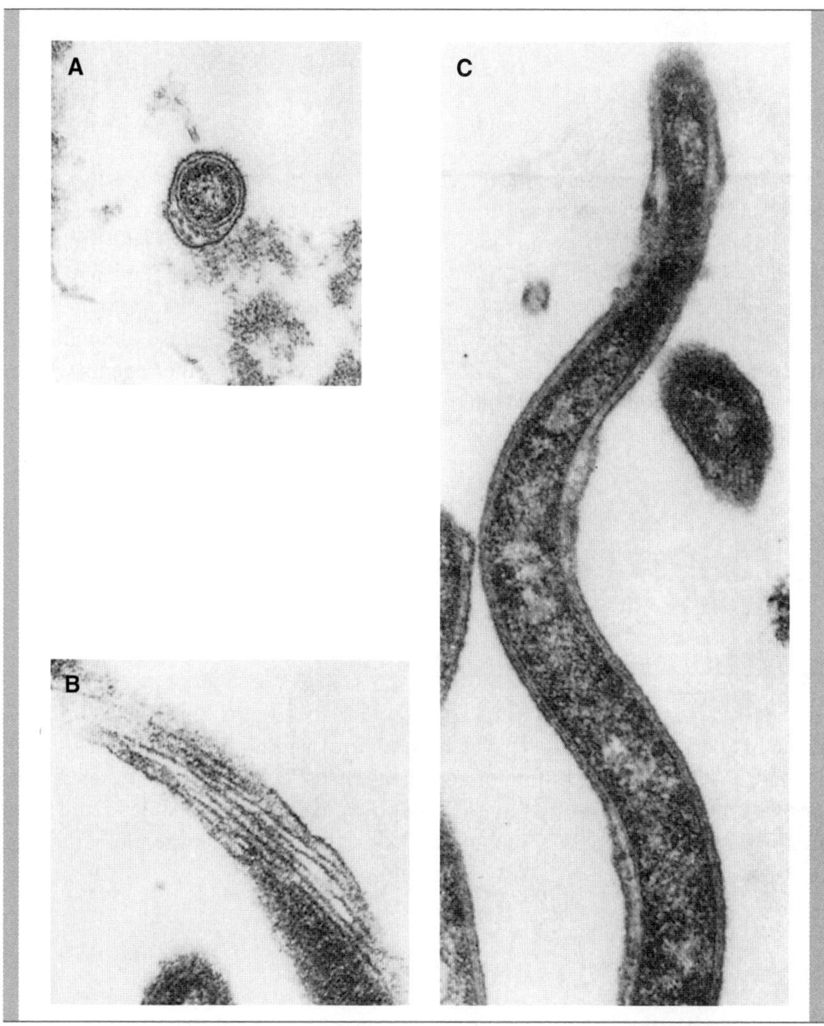

FIGURE 27–1
Spirochete of Lyme disease. Original magnification × 40,000. **A, B.** Note endoflagella. **C.** Note outer membrane. (*Reprinted with permission from Dr. Steere AC.* N Engl J Med *1983;308:736.*)

and the arrangement of flagella. Modern DNA homology and ribosomal RNA analyses have supported these groupings.

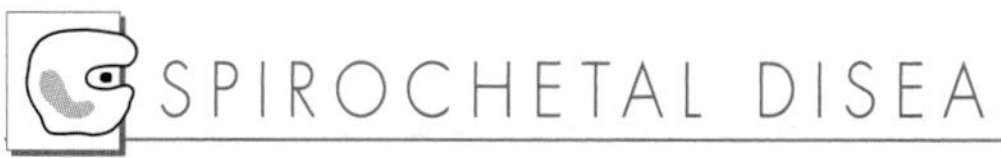

SPIROCHETAL DISEASES

Some spirochetes are free living; some are members of the normal flora of humans and animals. The oral cavity, particularly the dental crevice, harbors a number of species of the genera *Treponema* and *Borrelia* as part of its normal flora. Under unusual conditions these spirochetes together with anaerobes in the normal flora can cause necrotizing, ulcerative infection of the gums, oral cavity, or pharynx (Vincent's infection, trench mouth). The pathogenesis of these opportunistic infections is not understood but they are correlated with immunocompromise, severe malnutrition, and neglect of basic hygiene. The term "trench mouth" refers to the occurrence of these infections in troops under the appalling conditions that existed in the trenches during World War I.

Many are part of oropharyngeal flora

Overgrowth causes trench mouth

The major spirochetal diseases are caused by selected species of three genera which are not found in the normal flora, *Treponema (T. pallidum), Leptospira (L. interrogans),* and *Borrelia (B. recurrentis, B. hermsii,* and *B. burgdorferi).* Most *Borrelia* and *Leptospira* infections are zoonoses transmitted from wild and domestic animals. *T. pallidum* is a strict human pathogen transmitted by sexual contact. Some rare nonvenereal treponemal diseases are summarized in Appendix 27–1.

Diseases are zoonoses or venereal

TREPONEMA PALLIDUM

Syphilis represents an extended balance of parasitism and disease

T. pallidum is the causative agent of syphilis, a venereal disease first recognized in the 16th century as the "great pox" that rapidly spread through Europe in association with urbanization and military campaigns. Some argue that it was brought back from the New World by the sailors with Christopher Columbus. Its extended course and the protean, often dramatic nature of its findings (genital ulcer, ataxia, dementia, ruptured aorta) are due to a state of balanced parasitism which spans decades. The cause of syphilis is actually a subspecies (*T. pallidum* subsp. *pallidum*) closely related to other agents which cause rare nonvenereal treponematoses which are summarized in Appendix 27–1. *T. pallidum* is used here to indicate the *pallidum* subspecies.

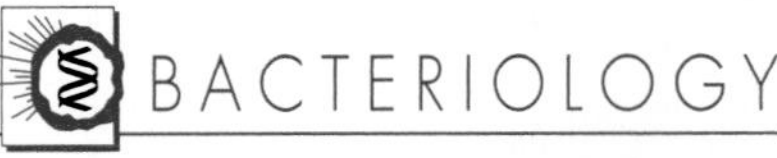

BACTERIOLOGY

MORPHOLOGY

Corkscrew spiral demonstrates characteristic motility and flexion

T. pallidum is a slim (0.15 μm) spirochete 5 to 15 μm long with regular spirals that resemble corkscrews with a wavelength (1 μm) and amplitude (0.3 μm). The organism is readily seen only by immunofluorescence, darkfield microscopy, or silver impregnation histologic techniques. Live *T. pallidum* cells show characteristic slow, rotating motility with sudden 90-degree angle flexion that suggests a gentleman quickly bowing at the waist.

GROWTH AND METABOLISM

Growth is limited and slow in cell culture

T. pallidum has not been grown in the absence of cultured mammalian cells. Although it prefers low oxygen tensions, it is not a strict anaerobe. With careful control of oxygen tension and pH, the organism has now been shown to multiply through several generations in primary cell culture, but is difficult to subculture. Growth is slow, with a mean generation time of about 30 hours. Information about its metabolic properties is limited because of the extreme difficulty in obtaining sufficient organisms for study. [In vivo growth is usually achieved by injection into rabbit testes—a source of antigens for specific antibody testing.]

Heat, drying, and disinfectants kill quickly

T. pallidum is extremely susceptible to any deviation from physiologic conditions. It dies rapidly on drying and is readily killed by a wide range of detergents and disinfectants. The lethal effect of even modest elevations of temperature (41° to 42°C) was the basis of fever therapy early in the last century. These fragile properties account for its almost exclusive transmission by direct contact.

ANTIGENIC STRUCTURE

Outer membrane and surface are relatively devoid of proteins

Many studies of *T. pallidum* suggest its surface is inert lacking proteins and other exposed antigens. The search for such structures has been hampered by the inability to grow the organism free of animals or cell culture. This not only makes potential antigens difficult to isolate and purify but also introduces the issues of whether a component has been derived from the host or the bacteria. The outer membrane of *T. pallidum* contains antigenic transmembrane proteins and lipoproteins but in quantities that are approximately 100-fold less than other Gram-negative bacteria such as *Escherichia coli.*

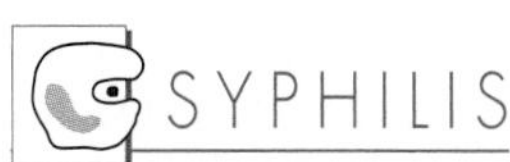

SYPHILIS

CLINICAL CAPSULE

Syphilis is typically acquired by the direct contact of mucous membranes during sexual intercourse. The disease begins with a lesion at the point of entry, usually a genital ulcer. After healing of the ulcer, the organisms spread systemically, and the disease returns weeks later as a generalized maculopapular rash called secondary syphilis. The disease then enters a second eclipse phase called latency. The latent infection may be cleared by the immune system or reappear as tertiary syphilis years to decades later. Tertiary syphilis is characterized by focal lesions whose locale determines the injury. Isolated foci in bone or liver may be unnoticed, but infection of the cardiovascular or nervous systems can be devastating. Progressive dementia or a ruptured aortic aneurysm are two of many fatal outcomes of untreated syphilis.

EPIDEMIOLOGY

T. pallidum is an exclusively human pathogen under natural conditions. In most cases, infection is acquired from direct sexual contact with an individual who has an active primary or secondary syphilitic lesion. Partner notification studies suggest transmission occurs in over 50% of sexual contacts where a lesion is present. Less commonly, the disease may be spread by nongenital contact with a lesion (eg, of the lip), sharing of needles by intravenous drug users, or transplacental transmission to the fetus within approximately the first 3 years of the maternal infection. Late disease is not infectious. Modern screening procedures have essentially eliminated blood transfusion as a source of the disease. Since 1990, the number of reported new cases of syphilis in the United States has been declining; levels are now below 40,000 per year. Approximately 20% of cases are primary or secondary syphilis; the remainder are latent or tertiary disease. Worldwide, syphilis remains a major public health problem, with an estimated 12 million new cases annually.

Transmission is by contact with mucosal surfaces or blood

Congenital infection is transplacental

Tertiary lesions are not transmitted

PATHOGENESIS

When certain strains of *T. pallidum* are inoculated into the skin, cornea, or testicle of animals lesions resembling primary syphilis can be produced, but there is no model for the other stages of disease. Because of our inability to grow the organism in culture, our knowledge of disease mechanisms is limited to the following extrapolations based on observations of human disease and experiments in animal models.

Experimental systems are limited

The spirochete reaches the subepithelial tissues through inapparent breaks in the skin or possibly by passage between the epithelial cells of mucous membranes, where it multiplies slowly with little initial tissue reaction. This may be due to the relative paucity of exposed antigens on the surface of the organism, but no specific reasons are known. As lesions develop, the basic pathologic finding is an endarteritis. The small arterioles show swelling and proliferation of their endothelial cells. This reduces or obstructs local blood supply, probably accounting for the necrotic ulceration of the primary lesion and subsequent destruction at other sites. Dense, granulomatous cuffs of lymphocytes, monocytes, and plasma cells surround the vessels. Although the primary lesion heals spontaneously the bacteria disseminate to other organs by way of local lymph nodes and the bloodstream.

Access is through mucosal breaks

Slow multiplication produces endarteritis, granulomas

Ulcer heals but spirochetes disseminate

For reasons that are not understood, syphilis is then silent until the disseminated secondary stage develops and then silent again with entry into latency. Although evasion of host defenses is clearly taking place, the mechanisms involved are unknown. The appearance of new epitopes in outer membrane proteins (OMPs) has been demonstrated during the course of experimental infections, but *T. pallidum* strains found in secondary lesions have not been demonstrated to differ antigenically from those in primary lesions. The organism has been observed to bind host proteins, immunoglobulins, and complement to its surface without sacrificing viability or motility. *T. pallidum* may be able to put on a host-like molecular "disguise" and thus avoid immune recognition.

Latent periods may be due to surface binding of host components

Injury is due to prolonged hypersensitivity responses

The inflammatory response to immune complexes, spirochetal lipoproteins, and complement in arteriolar walls accounts for some of the injury in syphilitic lesions. The granulomatous nature of the lesions in late syphilis is consistent with injury caused by delayed-type hypersensitivity responses prolonged by persistence of the spirochetes. In all of this, no toxins, virulence factors, or other molecules can yet be linked with specific features of syphilis.

IMMUNITY

Immunity develops slowly and incompletely

Clinical observations suggest an immune response in syphilis which is vigorous but slow and imperfect. Immunity to reinfection does not appear until early latency, and for at least one third of those infected the subsequent host response is successful in clearing most but not all of the treponemes.

Antibodies to OMP are associated with reinfection resistance

Development of cell-mediated immunity clears lesions

Variable T lymphocyte suppression may link to stages

The immune mechanisms involved are far from clear but appear to involve both humoral and cell-mediated responses. Resistance to reinfection is correlated with appearance of antitreponemal antibody which is able to immobilize and kill the organism. Exposed treponemal OMPs are the most probable target of these antibodies. Cell-mediated responses appear to be dominant in syphilitic lesions with T lymphocytes (CD4+ and CD8+) and macrophages the primary cell types present. Activated macrophages play a major role in the clearance of *T. pallidum* from early syphilis lesions. The relapsing course of primary and secondary syphilis may reflect shifts in the balance between developing cellular immunity and suppression of T lymphocytes. Syphilis in immunocompromised patients such as those with acquired immunodeficiency syndrome may present with unusually aggressive or atypical manifestations.

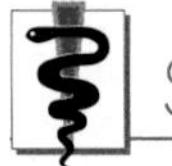

SYPHILIS: CLINICAL ASPECTS

MANIFESTATIONS

Primary Syphilis

Painless, indurated ulcer starts the disease

Heals spontaneously after weeks

The primary syphilitic lesion is a papule which evolves to an ulcer at the site of infection. This is usually the external genitalia or cervix but could be in the anal or oral area depending on the nature of sexual contact. The lesion becomes indurated and ulcerates but remains painless although slightly sensitive to touch. The fully developed ulcer with a firm base and raised margins is called the chancre (Fig 27–2). Firm, nonsuppurative, painless enlargement of the regional lymph nodes usually develops within 1 week of the primary lesion and may persist for months. The median incubation period from contact until appearance of the primary lesion is about 3 weeks (range 3 to 90 days). It heals spontaneously after 4 to 6 weeks.

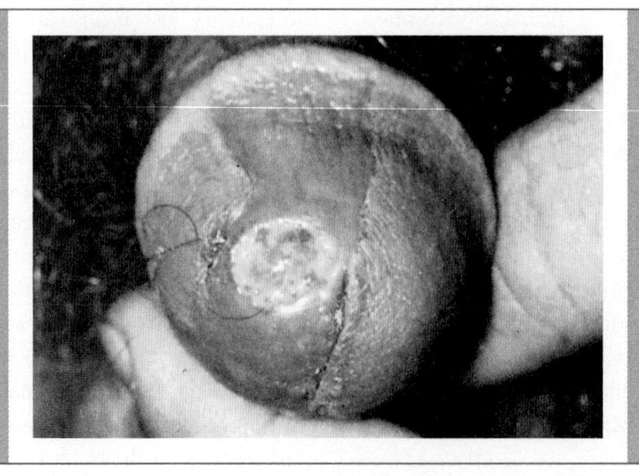

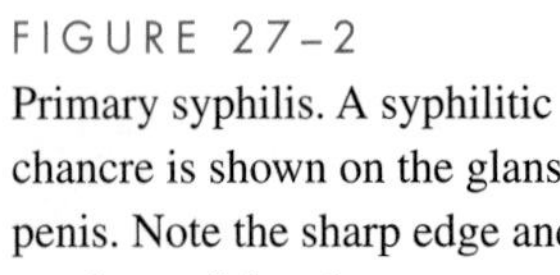

FIGURE 27–2
Primary syphilis. A syphilitic chancre is shown on the glans penis. Note the sharp edge and raw base of the ulcer.

Secondary Syphilis

Secondary or disseminated syphilis develops 2 to 8 weeks after the appearance of the chancre. The primary lesion has usually healed but may still be present. This most florid form of syphilis is characterized by a symmetric mucocutaneous maculopapular rash and generalized nontender lymph node enlargement with fever, malaise and other manifestations of systemic infection. Skin lesions are distributed on the trunk and extremities, often including the palms, soles, and face, and can mimic a variety of infectious and noninfectious skin eruptions. About one third of patients develop painless mucosal warty erosions called **condylomata lata.** These erosions usually develop in warm, moist sites such as the genitals and perineum. All the lesions of secondary syphilis are teeming with spirochetes and are highly infectious. They resolve spontaneously after a few days to many weeks, but the infection has resolved in only one third of patients. In the remaining two thirds of patients, the illness enters the latent state.

Lymphadenopathy and maculopapular rash are generalized

Spirochetes are abundant

Lesions resolve but disease continues in one third of patients

Latent Syphilis

Latent syphilis is by definition a stage where there are no clinical manifestations but continuing infection is evidenced by serologic tests. In the first few years latency may be interrupted by progressively less severe relapses of secondary syphilis. In late latent syphilis (>4 years) relapses cease, and patients become resistant to reinfection. Transmission to others is possible from relapsing secondary lesions and by transfusion or other contact with blood products. Mothers may transmit *T. pallidum* to their fetus throughout latency. About one third of untreated cases do not progress beyond this stage.

Secondary relapses interrupt latency

Blood-borne transmission risk continues

Tertiary Syphilis

Another one third of patients with untreated syphilis develop tertiary syphilis. The manifestations may appear as early as 5 years after infection but characteristically occur after 15 to 20 years. The manifestations depend on the body sites involved the most important of which are the nervous and cardiovascular systems.

Neurosyphilis is due to the damage produced by a mixture of meningovasculitis and degenerative parenchymal changes in virtually any part of the nervous system. The most common entity is a chronic meningitis with fever, headache, focal neurologic findings, and increased cells and protein in the cerebrospinal fluid (CSF). Cortical degeneration of the brain causes mental changes ranging from decreased memory to hallucinations or frank psychosis. In the spinal cord demyelination of the posterior columns, dorsal roots, and dorsal root ganglia produces a syndrome called tabes dorsalis which includes ataxia, wide-based gait, foot slap, and loss of the sensation. The most advanced central nervous system (CNS) findings include a combination of neurologic deficits and behavioral disturbances called **paresis,** which is also a mnemonic (**p**ersonality, **a**ffect, **r**eflexes, **e**yes, **se**nsorium, **i**ntellect, **s**peech) for the myriad of changes seen.

Chronic meningitis leads to degenerative changes, and psychosis

Demylination causes peripheral neuropathies

Syphilitic paresis has many signs

Cardiovascular syphilis is due to arteritis involving the vasa vasorum of the aorta causing a medial necrosis and loss of elastic fibers. The usual result is dilatation of the aorta and aortic valve ring. This in turn leads to aneurysms of the ascending and transverse segments of the aorta and/or aortic valve incompetence. The expanding aneurysm can produce pressure necrosis of adjacent structures or even rupture. A localized, granulomatous reaction to *T. pallidum* infection called a **gumma** may be found in skin, bones, joints, or other organ. Any clinical manifestations are related to the local destruction as with other mass-producing lesions, such as tumors.

Aortitis leads to aneurysm

Gummas are destructive, localized granulomas

Congenital Syphilis

Fetuses are susceptible to syphilis only after the fourth month of gestation, and adequate treatment of infected mothers before that time prevents fetal damage. Because active syphilitic infection is devastating to infants, routine serologic testing is performed in early pregnancy and should be repeated in the last trimester in women at high risk of acquiring syphilis. Untreated maternal infection may result in fetal loss or congenital syphilis, which is analogous to secondary syphilis in the adult. Although there may be

Rhinitis, rash, and bone changes are common

Serologic screening and treatment is preventative

no physical finding at all, the most common are rhinitis and a maculopapular rash. Bone involvement produces characteristic changes in the architecture of the entire skeletal system (saddle nose, saber shins). Anemia, thrombocytopenia, and liver failure are terminal events.

DIAGNOSIS

Microscopy

Darkfield requires experience and fluid from deep in lesion

May be negative due to small numbers

T. pallidum can be seen by darkfield microscopy in primary and secondary lesions, but the execution of this procedure requires experience and attention to detail. The suspect lesion must be cleaned and abraded to produce a serous transudate from below the surface of the ulcer base. This material can be captured in a capillary tube or placed directly on a microscope slide if a darkfield setup is close at hand. The microscopist must observe the corkscrew morphology and characteristic motility to make a diagnosis (Fig 27–3). A negative examination does not exclude syphilis, because to be readily seen, the fluid must contain thousands of treponemes per milliliter. Darkfield microscopy of oral and anal lesions is not recommended because of the risk of misinterpretation of other spirochetes present in the normal flora. Direct fluorescent antibody methods have been developed but are available only in certain centers.

Serologic Tests

Tests may or may not use treponemes

Most cases of syphilis are diagnosed serologically using serologic tests that detect antibodies directed at either lipid or specific treponemal antigens. The former are called nontreponemal tests, and the latter are referred to as treponemal tests. Their use in screening, diagnosis, and therapeutic evaluation of syphilis has been refined over many decades.

Nontreponemal Tests

Reagin antibody reacts with cardiolipin, a lipid complex

Antibody level peaks in secondary syphilis

Nonspecfic reactions linked to autoimmune diseases

Nontreponemal tests measure antibody directed against **cardiolipin,** a lipid complex so called because one component was originally extracted from beef heart. Anticardiolipin antibody is called **reagin,** and the tests which detect it depend on immune flocculation of cardiolipin in the presence of other lipids. The most common nontreponemal tests are the rapid plasma reagin (RPR) and the Venereal Disease Research Laboratory (VDRL). They become positive in the early stages of the primary lesion and, with the possible exception of some patients with advanced human immunodeficiency virus (HIV) infection, are uniformly positive during the secondary stage. They slowly wane in the later stages of the disease. In neurosyphilis, VDRL tests on CSF may be positive when the serum VDRL has reverted to negative. Nontreponemal tests are nonspecific; they may become positive in a variety of autoimmune diseases or in diseases involving substantial tissue or liver destruction, such as lupus erythematosus, viral hepatitis, infectious mononucleosis, and malaria. False-positive results can also occur occasionally in pregnancy and in patients with HIV infection.

Titer is used to follow therapy

Sensitivity and low cost make nontreponemal tests preferred for screening, but if positive, they must be confirmed by one of the more specific treponemal tests described below. They are also valuable for following treatment because the height of the antibody titer is directly related to activity of disease. With successful antibiotic therapy nontreponemal serologies slowly revert to negative.

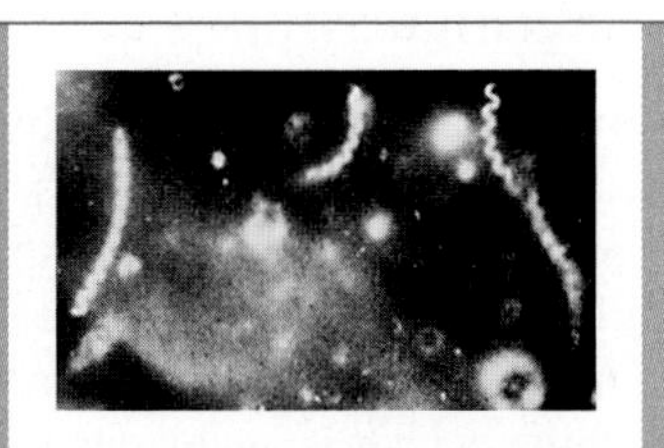

FIGURE 27–3
Treponema pallidum seen by darkfield microscopy. The darkfield method creates a bright halo around the corkscrew-shaped spirochetes.

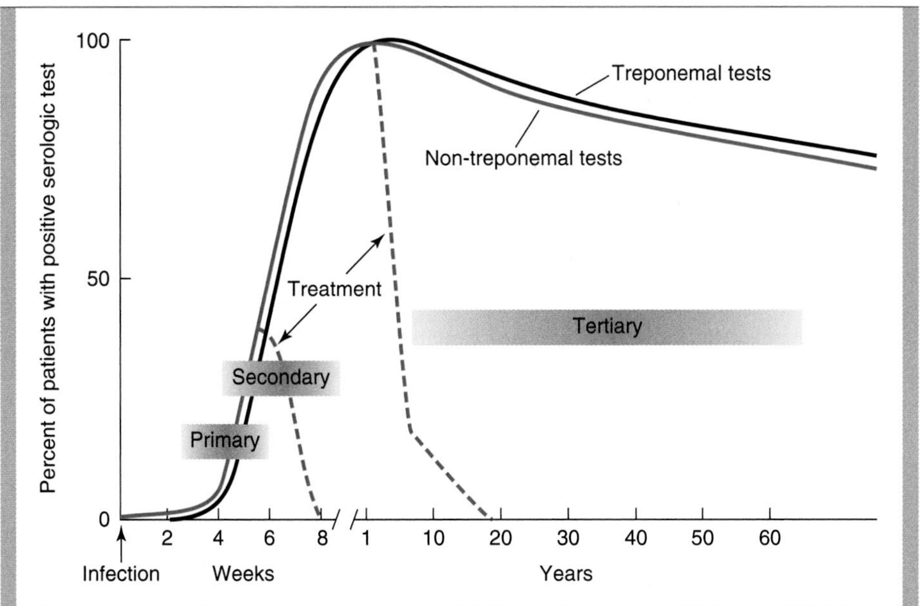

FIGURE 27–4
Treponemal and nontreponemal tests in syphilis. The time course of treated and untreated symphilis in relation to serologic tests is shown. The non-treponemal tests (VDRL, RPR) rise during primary syphilis and reach their peak in secondary syphilis. They slowly decline with advancing age. With treatment they revert to normal over a few weeks. The treponemal tests (FTA-ABS, MHA-TP) follow the same course but remain elevated even following successful treatment.

Treponemal Tests

Treponemal tests detect antibody specific to *T. pallidum* such as an indirect immunofluorescent procedure called the fluorescent treponemal antibody (FTA-ABS) which uses spirochetes fixed to slides. The "ABS" refers to an absorption step that removes nonspecific antispirochetal antibodies often found in normal serum. Another method, the microhemagglutination test for *T. pallidum* (MHA-TP), uses antigens attached to the surface of erythrocytes, which then agglutinate in the presence of specific antibody.

T. pallidum is used as the antigen

Treponemal tests are considerably more specific than the cardiolipin-based nontreponemal tests. Their primary role in diagnosis is to confirm positive RPR and VDRL results obtained in the evaluation of a patient suspect for syphilis or in screening programs. They are not useful for screening or following therapy because, once positive, they usually remain so for life. Thus, if nontreponemal tests can be thought of as the measure of active syphilis, treponemal tests are the indelible print of sin. The time course of serologic tests in the various stages of syphilis is illustrated in Figure 27–4. Until recently, it was believed that a negative treponemal test excluded the possibility of prior syphilis.

Positive result confirms RPR and VDRL

Remain positive for life

The use of serologic tests in the diagnosis of congenital syphilis is complicated by the presence of IgG antibodies in infants, who acquire it transplacentally from their mothers. If available, treponemal IgM tests are useful in establishing the presence of an acute infection in infants.

IgM is used to diagnose congenital syphilis

TREATMENT AND PREVENTION

T. pallidum remains exquisitely sensitive to penicillin, which is the preferred treatment in all stages. In primary, secondary, or latent syphilis persons hypersensitive to penicillin may be treated with tetracyclines, erythromycin, or cephalosporins. The efficacy of agents other than penicillin has not been established in tertiary or congenital syphilis. It is recommended that penicillin-hypersensitive patients with neurosyphilis or congenital syphilis be desensitized rather than use an alternate antimicrobial. Safe sex practices are as effective for prevention of syphilis as they are for other sexually transmitted diseases. Their use to prevent HIV infection probably accounts for much of the recent decline in new syphilis cases. The development of a vaccine awaits greater understanding of pathogenesis and immunity.

Penicillin is preferred

Safe sex blocks transmission

LEPTOSPIRA INTERROGANS

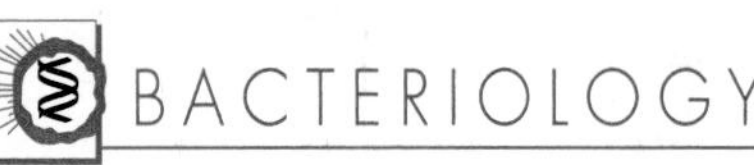

BACTERIOLOGY

Loose spirals seen in darkfield

L. interrogans is the member of the genus *Leptospira* that is pathogenic to humans and animals. There are other free-living species of *Leptospira*. This species is a slim (approximately 0.15 μm) spirochete 5 to 15 μm long, with a single axial filament; fine, closely wound spirals; and hooked ends. It is not visualized with the usual staining procedures, and detection is best accomplished using darkfield microscopy. It can be grown in aerobic culture using certain special enriched semisolid media.

Multiple serogroups have geographic associations

Survives in water

L. interrogans has multiple serogroups and over 200 serotypes, many of which were previously accorded species status (eg, *L. icterohaemorrhagiae, L. canicola, L. pomona*) based on geographic occurrence, differences in host species, and associated clinical syndromes. The distinction between serogroups and serotypes is of epidemiologic and epizoologic importance but has no clinical significance. *Leptospira interrogans* can survive days or weeks in some waters in the environment at a pH above 7.0. Acidic conditions, such as those that may be found in urine, rapidly kill the organism. It is highly sensitive to drying and to a wide range of disinfectants.

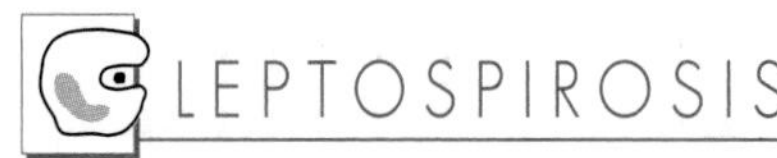

LEPTOSPIROSIS

CLINICAL CAPSULE

Leptospirosis is a systemic flu-like illness associated with water contaminated by animal urine. It begins with fever, nausea, vomiting, headache, abdominal pain, and severe myalgia. In severe cases, a second phase is characterized by impaired hepatic and renal function with jaundice, prostration, and circulatory collapse. The CNS is often involved, with stiff neck and inflammatory changes in the cerebrospinal fluid.

EPIDEMIOLOGY

Animals are reservoir

Water is transmission route

Leptospirosis is a worldwide disease of a variety of wild and domestic animals particularly rodents, cattle, and dogs. It is usually transmitted to humans through water contaminated with animal urine. Secondary human-to-human transmission occurs rarely. Individuals who are exposed to animals (eg, farmers, veterinarians, slaughterhouse employees) are at increased risk, although most clinical cases in North America are now associated with recreational exposure to contaminated water (eg, irrigation ditches or other bodies of water receiving farmland drainage). In tropical areas leptospirosis may account for up to 10% of hospital admission, particularly following rains or floods.

PATHOGENESIS AND IMMUNITY

Enters through small mucosal breaks

Blood and CNS spread is common

The organism gains entrance to the tissues through small skin breaks, the conjunctiva or, most commonly, through ingestion and the upper alimentary tract mucosa. The active motility of the hooked ends driven by periplasmic flagella may allow the organism to burrow into tissues. The organisms spread widely through the bloodstream to all parts of the body including the CSF. In animals they colonize the proximal renal tubule, from which they are shed into the urine, facilitating transmission to new hosts. The kidney is also a target organ in human disease causing tubular infection and interstitial nephritis.

Antibody may be part of disease

Clearing of the bacteremia is associated with the appearance of circulating antibody but little else is known of immune mechanisms. Antibody is also rising during the second phase of the disease which suggests an immunologic component to its pathogenesis. This is supported by absence of response to antimicrobics when given at this stage and failure usually to recover the organism from the CSF in cases of leptospiral meningitis.

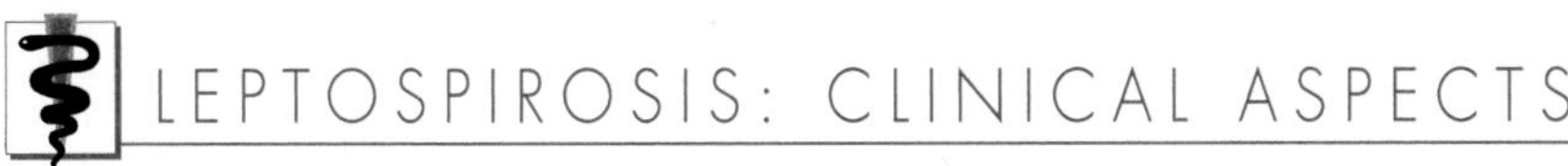

LEPTOSPIROSIS: CLINICAL ASPECTS

MANIFESTATIONS

Most infections are subclinical and detectable only serologically. After an incubation period of 7 to 13 days, an influenza-like febrile illness with fever, chills, headache, conjunctival suffusion, and muscle pain develops in persons who become ill. This disease is associated with bacteremia. Leptospires are also found in the CSF at this stage, but without clinical or cytologic evidence of meningitis. The fever often subsides after about a week coincident with the disappearance of the organisms from the blood but may recur with a variety of clinical manifestations depending partly on the serogroup involved. This second phase of the disease usually lasts 3 or more weeks and may present as an aseptic meningitis resembling viral meningitis (see Chapter 67) or as a more generalized illness with muscle aches, headache, rash, pretibial erythematous lesions, biochemical evidence of hepatic and renal involvement, or all of these. In its most severe form (Weil's disease), there is extensive vasculitis, jaundice, renal damage, and sometimes a hemorrhagic rash. The mortality in such cases may be as high as 10%.

Initial disease is flu-like

Meningitis and muscle aches last for weeks

Hemorrhagic rash is linked to fatal outcome

DIAGNOSIS

The diagnosis of leptospirosis is primarily serologic. Although the spirochetes could theoretically be detected, darkfield examination of body fluids is not recommended. The yield is very low and the chance for confusion with fibrin and debris is significant. Likewise, leptospires can be isolated from the blood, CSF, or urine, but culture is rarely attempted because the organisms take weeks to grow in a special medium which few laboratories bother to stock. The standard serologic test (microscopic agglutination) is also limited to reference laboratories. A simpler slide agglutination is less specific but may be suggestive of infection in the presence of a compatible clinical picture.

Serologic tests are limited to reference laboratories

TREATMENT

Penicillin, ampicillin, and erythromycin are effective for severe forms of leptospirosis. Tetracyclines (including doxycycline) are also recommended for milder disease. Third-generation cephalosporins and other antimicrobics are active in vitro but are not yet backed up by sufficient clinical experience.

Multiple antimicrobics are effective

PREVENTION

Vaccines are used in cattle and household pets to prevent the disease, and this has reduced its occurrence in humans. Doxycycline, given once weekly, prevents leptospirosis in individuals working in high-risk environments for short periods. Other measures include rodent control, drainage of waters known to be contaminated, and care on the part of those subject to occupational exposure to avoid ingestion or contamination with *L. interrogans*.

Rodent and water control are important

BORRELIA

More than 15 species of *Borrelia* have been associated with human disease, and other species are responsible for similar diseases in animals. *B. burgdorferi* is the cause of Lyme disease. Other members of the genus cause relapsing fever, an illness with intermittent fevers and

Relapsing fever and Lyme disease caused by different species

little else. The relapsing fevers differ in their specific vector and geographic distribution. The human body louse is the vector for *B. recurrentis,* but the remainder of the relapsing fevers are linked to several ticks and species of *Borrelia;* these are discussed together here as *B. hermsii,* the most common cause of relapsing fever in North America.

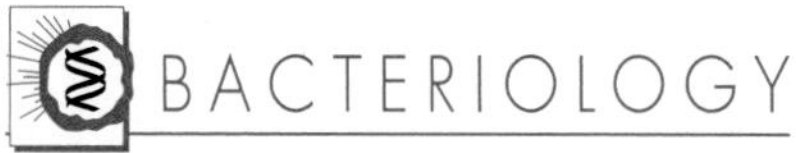

BACTERIOLOGY

MORPHOLOGY, STAINING, AND CULTURE

Loose, irregular spirals take common stains

Borrelia are long (10 to 30 μm), slender (0.2 to 0.5 μm) spirochetes containing multiple (7 to 20) axial flagella. In contrast to *Treponema* and *Leptospira,* its spirals form loose, irregular waves. The basic organizational structure of the cell and its motility conform to that of the other Gram negative spirochetes, but unlike the others, *Borrelia* are readily demonstrated by common staining methods like the Giemsa or Wright stains. *Borrelia* are microaerophilic and have been successfully grown in liquid or semisolid media containing N-acetylglucosamine and long-chain fatty acids.

ANTIGENIC STRUCTURE AND VARIATION

Surface proteins undergo antigenic variation

Recombination between linear plasmids leads to altered protein

The outer membrane of all *Borrelia* species contains abundant outer membrane proteins and lipoproteins. In some species these surface proteins have been observed to vary antigenically at a frequency too high to be explained by simple mutation. Experiments with *B. hermsii* have demonstrated up to 40 antigenically distinct variants of the same protein arising from a single cell. The genetic mechanism for this antigenic variation involves recombination between the distinctive linear plasmids found in many *Borrelia* species. Multiple copies of the genes for these proteins are present. Some genes express the protein while others are "silent" because they lack crucial promoter sequences. When structural sequences from a silent gene are transferred by recombination to an expressing gene on another plasmid, the protein expressed is altered in a which may make it antigenically different. This mechanism resembles that described for trypanosomes (see Chapter 54) and gonococcal pili (see Chapter 20).

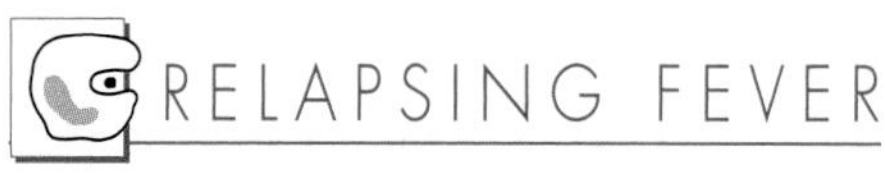

RELAPSING FEVER

CLINICAL CAPSULE

Relapsing fever is an illness with fever, headache, muscle pain, and weakness but no signs pointing to any organ system. It lasts about 1 week and returns a few days later. The relapses may continue for as many as four cycles. During each relapse, spirochetes are present in the bloodstream. The causative *Borrelia* species are transmitted to humans from ticks or body lice.

EPIDEMIOLOGY

Body lice or ticks transmit the spirochete

Relapsing fever occurs in two forms linked to the mode of transmission and the *Borrelia* species involved. The louse-borne form usually appears in epidemics, because of circumstances connected with body lice, whereas the tick-borne form does not. For this reason, the two forms are sometimes called epidemic (louse-borne) and endemic (tick-borne) relapsing fever. Here they will be identified simply by the insect involved.

Tick reservoir feeds on rodents and small animals

The occurrence and distribution of tick-borne relapsing fever are determined by the biology of the relevant tick species and its relationship to the primary *Borrelia* reservoir in rodents and other small animals (rabbits, birds, lizards). Ticks may remain infectious for several years even without feeding and transovarial passage to their progeny extends the infectious chain even further. Humans are infected when they accidentally enter this cycle and are bitten by an infected tick. The bite is painless and the feeding period is brief (<20 minutes). Because the ticks usually feed at night, cases are most often associated with overnight recreational forays into wild, wooded areas. The largest outbreak in the United States involved National Park employees and tourists who slept in tick- and rodent-infested cabins on the Northern Rim of the Grand Canyon.

Nighttime painless tick bite transmits bacteria

The epidemiologic conditions associated with louse-borne relapsing fever are much more exacting. The human body louse has no other host, infected lice live no more than 2 months, and there is no transovarial passage to progeny. *B. recurrentis* is the only species involved. Lice are infected from human blood but the spirochetes multiply in their hemolymph, not any of the feeding parts or excrement. This means they can infect another human only if the louse is crushed by scratching and the *Borrelia* reach a superficial wound or mucosal surface. Infected lice must be passed human to human for the disease to persist. These conditions are met by circumstances that combine overcrowding with extremely low levels of general hygiene. War, other kinds of social breakdown, and dire poverty are the prime associates. Currently, this variety of relapsing fever appears to be limited to east and central Africa and the Peruvian Andes.

Body lice infected from human blood

Lice must be transferred from human to human

PATHOGENESIS

The disease manifestations develop at times when thousands of spirochetes are circulating per milliliter of blood. The febrile illness has endotoxin-like features, but the exact mechanisms of disease are unknown. Between episodes the organisms disappear from the blood and are sequestered in internal organs only to reappear during relapses. The OMPs are antigenically different with each relapse. The relapsing cycles correlate with antibody production to the new protein followed by clearing followed by emergence of a new antigenic type.

Spirochetes appear in blood

Altered OMPs occur with relapse

IMMUNITY

Immunity to the disease is largely humoral and appears to involve lysis of the organism in the presence of complement. The disease is controlled when variants from the antigenic repertoire are no longer able to escape the immune response.

Antibody eventually controls disease

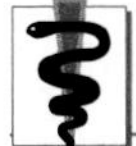

RELAPSING FEVER: CLINICAL ASPECTS

MANIFESTATIONS

After a mean incubation period of 7 days, massive spirochetemia develops, with high fever, rigors, severe headache, muscle pains, and weakness. The febrile period lasts about 1 week and terminates abruptly with the development of an adequate immune response. The disease relapses 2 to 4 days later, usually with less severity, but following the same general course. Tick-borne relapsing fever is usually limited to one or two relapses, but with louse-borne disease three or four may occur.

Fever, headache and muscle pain last 2–4 days

Louse-borne relapsing fever is more severe than tick-borne disease, possibly because of predisposing social conditions. Fatalities are rare in tick-borne disease but may be as high as 40% in untreated louse-borne fever. Fatal outcomes are due to myocarditis, cerebral hemorrhage, and hepatic failure.

Louse-borne is more severe

DIAGNOSIS

Diagnosis is readily made during the febrile period by Giemsa or Wright staining of blood smears. The appearance of the spirochete among the red cells is characteristic. Cultural and animal inoculation procedures are also used for recovery of the infecting organism. Serodiagnostic tests are unhelpful.

Blood smears demonstrate *Borrelia*

TREATMENT

Tetracycline and erythromycin are favored

The disease responds well to tetracycline or erythromycin therapy, and single-dose treatment with these agents can be effective. Jarisch–Herxheimer reactions are particularly common in the treatment of relapsing fever perhaps because of the height of the spirochetemia at the time of antibiotic administration.

PREVENTION

Attention to ticks and general hygiene are important

Prevention of tick-borne relapsing fever involves attention to deticking, insecticide treatment, and rodent control around habitations, such as mountain cabins, shown to be associated with infection. Control of louse-borne relapsing fever involves delousing, particularly dusting of clothing with appropriate insecticides. Ultimately, improved hygiene stops outbreaks and prevents further occurrences.

BORRELIA BURGDORFERI

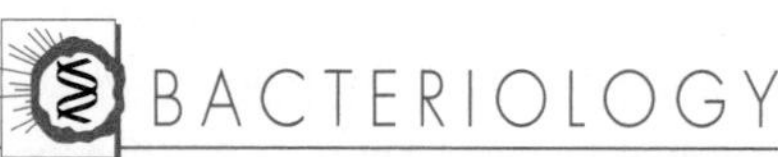

BACTERIOLOGY

Grows in microaerophilic atmosphere

Osps differ at stages of infection

B. burgdorferi is microaerophilic and can be grown with some difficulty in a specialized artificial culture medium. The doubling time under these conditions is long (8 to 24 hours), so growth for isolation takes many days to weeks. *B. burgdorferi* consists of at least 10 different subspecies (eg, *B. burgdorferi* sensu stricto, *B. afzelii, B.garini*), which differ in geographic distribution and some clinical manifestations. All will be referred to as *B. burgdorferi* here. As with other species of *Borrelia,* there are multiple classes of OMPs, many of which undergo antigenic variation. Recent studies have focused on a class called outer surface proteins (Osps), which have been linked to aspects of pathogenesis and immunity. Two of these, OspA and OspC, are differentially expressed depending on the stage of tick or mammalian infection.

LYME DISEASE

CLINICAL CAPSULE

Acute Lyme disease is characterized by fever, a migratory "bull's eye" skin rash, muscle and joint pains, often with evidence of meningeal irritation. In a chronic form evolving over several years meningoencephalitis, myocarditis, and a disabling recurrent arthritis may develop. *B. burgdorferi* is transmitted to humans by *Ixodes* ticks.

EPIDEMIOLOGY

Spirochetes are transmitted in tick–mouse–deer cycle

Ticks must feed on humans in the woods

B. burgdorferi exists in a complex cycle involving ticks, mice, and deer. Lyme disease occurs when the ticks feed on humans who enter their wooded habitat. The disease is endemic in several regions of the United States, Canada, and temperate Europe and Asia. Approximately 90% of the 10,000 to 15,000 cases reported each year in the United States occur in areas along the northeastern and mid-Atlantic seaboard, including Old Lyme, Connecticut, where the disease was first recognized. The majority of cases probably go unreported, particularly outside the primary endemic regions.

The primary reservoir of *B. burgdorferi* is rodents, particularly white-footed mice. Infection is transmitted by *Ixodes* ticks, whose complete life cycle involves rodents for the early stages and deer for adult maturation. In the spring, fertile female ticks, engorged from their blood meals, fall from their deer hosts to the ground and deposit their eggs. During the summer, the tick larvae seek out and obtain a blood meal from mice and the *B. burgdorferi* ingested by the larvae are maintained through the subsequent development stages of the tick. The following spring or summer, the small (1 to 2 mm) nymphs feed again on vertebrate hosts to obtain the blood required for maturation to adulthood. The engorged, satiated nymphs fall off their hosts and mature into adults by parasitizing available deer, thus completing a life cycle that has occupied a full 2 years. Vertebrates other than deer can be infected by both the adult and nymph stages of the tick, but human Lyme disease is acquired primarily from nymphs, because they are active at the time of year when humans are most likely to invade their ecosystem. Deer are essential to the mating and survival of the tick and thus the disease does not occur in areas in which deer are not abundant.

Ticks feed on mice and then deer

Adult and nymph stages can infect humans

No deer, no disease

PATHOGENESIS

Because Lyme disease is a recently discovered disease with a complex biology, it is not surprising that the pathogenic mechanisms in humans remain to be established clearly. Studies in ticks have shown changes in the antigenic makeup of *B. burgdorferi* as it migrates from the midgut and salivary glands and again after it reaches mammalian tissue. OspA is the major outer surface protein expressed when *B. burgdorferi* resides in ticks, but its expression diminishes during tick engorgement, while OspC increases, so that by the time of transmission to hosts, OspC predominates. Although OspC has been shown to stimulate protective antibody in animals, its role in disease is unknown.

OspA predominates in ticks

Shift to OspC is completed at vertebrate transmission

Some candidate adhesins of *B. burgdorferi* could be important in the early stages of human infection. These surface proteins and lipoproteins have been shown to mediate attachment to integrins, platelets, and collagen-associated elements of the extracellular matrix (ECM). Other molecules which bind plasmin to the spirochete surface may activate host proteolytic systems and facilitate spread through the ECM to adjacent tissues. It is known that the outer membrane of the spirochete contains proteins and a toxic lipopolysaccharide that differs from the usual Gram-negative endotoxin. The spirochetal peptidoglycan has inflammatory properties, survives considerable periods in tissues, and may contribute to arthritis when deposited in joint tissues.

Surface proteins bind to ECM

Lipopolysaccharide differs from other endotoxins

Peptidoglycan causes inflammation

Clinical investigations in patients with Lyme disease have noted modulation of immune responses, including inhibition of mononuclear and natural killer cell function, lymphocyte proliferation, and cytokine production. The ability of *B. burgdorferi* to downregulate deleterious immune responses could serve as a survival strategy or play a role in chronic disease. Chronic disease, particularly Lyme arthritis, has aspects of autoimmunity. One candidate cross-reactive autoantigen is OspA. The sera of individuals with Lyme arthritis but not other forms of arthritis react with epitopes present in OspA and with homologous epitopes in human leukocyte antigens (HLAs). A genetic basis for this linkage is suggested by the statistical association between chronic arthritis and certain HLA types. Such theories must be reconciled with the downregulation of OspA in mammalian infection and clarification of the role of many other candidate virulence factors.

Downregulation of immune function contributes to chronicity

Anti-OspA antibody has autoimmune activities

IMMUNITY

The immune response to *B. burgdorferi* infection develops slowly with IgM followed by IgG antibody over weeks to months. Although immune-mediated killing by the classical complement pathway has been demonstrated the molecular target is unknown. Host neutrophils and macrophages can phagocytose opsonized spirochetes and induce a metabolic burst leading to spirochetal death. OspC elicits protective immunity in rodents, but this protection is short lived and ineffective against challenge with heterologous *B. burgdorferi* isolates. Antigens capable of eliciting broadly protective immune responses have not been identified.

Target of protective antibody is unclear

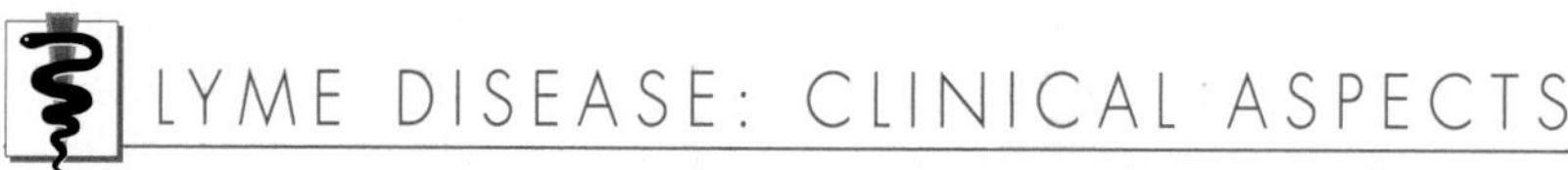

LYME DISEASE: CLINICAL ASPECTS

MANIFESTATIONS

Spreading lesion from bite site is most characteristic finding

Lyme borreliosis is a highly variable disease involving multiple body systems. It occurs in overlapping patterns that come and go at different times. The skin lesion spreading from the site of the tick bite is its most distinctive feature. Relapsing arthritis is the most persistent finding and the one most likely to become chronic. Lyme disease is rarely fatal, but if untreated, it is often a source of chronic ill health.

Erythema migrans and febrile aches mark acute disease

The primary lesion begins sometime in the first month after a tick bite, which is often unnoticed. A macule or papule appears at the site of the bite and expands to become an annular lesion with a raised, red border and central clearing forming a "bull's eye" pattern. As the bull's eye ring expands, the lesion known as **erythema migrans** forms. Along with the skin lesions fever, fatigue, myalgia, headache, joint pains, and mild neck stiffness are often present. Approximately 50% of untreated patients develop secondary skin lesions that closely resemble the primary one but are not at the site of the tick bite. In untreated patients, the skin lesions usually disappear over a period of weeks, but constitutional symptoms may persist for months.

Nerve palsies and cardiac findings appear later

Days, weeks, even months after the onset of the primary lesion, a second stage may develop in which involvement of the nervous or cardiovascular system may be superimposed. Neurologic abnormalities include a fluctuating meningitis, cranial nerve palsies, and peripheral neuropathy. Cardiac disease is usually limited to conduction abnormalities (atrioventricular block), but in some cases acute myocarditis can lead to cardiac enlargement. Both neurologic and cardiac abnormalities fluctuate in intensity but generally resolve completely in a matter of weeks.

Fluctuating arthritis may become chronic

Weeks to years after the onset of infection, arthritis marks the continuing state of the disease. It develops in almost two thirds of untreated patients. Typically, it too follows a fluctuating or intermittent course, generally involving the large joints, particularly the knees. The arthritis may become chronic with erosion of the bone and cartilage although the spirochetes are rarely demonstrable in the lesions. Less frequent chronic neurologic dysfunctions include subtle encephalitis affecting memory, mood, or sleep, and peripheral neuropathies.

DIAGNOSIS

Culture and PCR are not yet practical

Presently, the diagnosis of early Lyme disease is based on exposure and typical clinical findings. Although *B. burgdorferi* can be cultured from erythema migrans skin lesions, blood, joint fluid, and CSF, few laboratories stock the special medium required. The spirochetes are seldom detected on any kind of direct microscopic examination. Polymerase chain reaction (PCR) procedures able to detect *B. burgdorferi*–specific DNA sequences in body fluids have been developed but are expensive and not standardized for routine use.

Serologic tests are not diagnostic

With culture generally unavailable, the diagnosis in later stages of disease usually rests on the demonstration of circulating antibodies to *B. burgdorferi*. Despite considerable progress these tests still lack the sensitivity and specificity to be considered more than supportive of a clinical diagnosis. The current recommendation is to first perform a sensitive screening test (enzyme immunoassay or fluorescent antibody) followed by a more specific Western blot. Even with this two-step approach, patients in the early stages may be seronegative and cross-reactive antigens may cause false-positive results.

TREATMENT

Doxycycline and amoxicillin are the first-line antimicrobics for the treatment of early Lyme disease and arthritis. For individuals who cannot tolerate either of these agents, cefuroxime is a much more expensive alternative for oral therapy. Intravenous therapy with ceftriaxone or penicillin G is recommended for patients with neurologic involvement or cardiovascular findings such as atrioventricular heart block. The response to treatment is typically slow requiring the continuation of antimicrobics for 30 to 60 days.

Doxycycline and β-lactams are recommended

PREVENTION

The most useful preventive measures in endemic areas are the use of clothes that reduce the likelihood of the infected nymph reaching the legs or arms, careful search for nymphs after potential exposure, and removal of the tick by its head with tweezers. Duration of tick attachment to humans is also a factor in transmission; the risk is greatest when the tick has been feeding for at least 48 to 72 hours. Some insect repellents may provide added protection. The risk of Lyme disease following a random tick bite is too low to justify administration of antimicrobics prophylactically.

Preventing bites and removing ticks are important

A vaccine for Lyme disease composed of recombinant OspA is now licensed for use in the United States. Unlike typical vaccines directed at a molecule known to be important in human infection, the Lyme disease vaccine is designed to act in the feeding tick, not the human. As indicated above OspA is expressed by *B. burgdorferi* in tick infection but downregulated when the spirochetes enter mammalian tissues. The antibodies stimulated by OspA immunization are intended to reach the midgut of feeding ticks and mediate killing of spirochetes before transmission can occur. In addition, the spirochetes may retain enough OspA to render them susceptible to the antibody shortly after transmission. The vaccine has been shown to be protective with an efficacy of approximately 75%. Its widespread use is controversial, because the benefits depend on the relation between the morbidity and cost of complicated cases and the incidence of Lyme disease in any population. By some estimates, the incidence in even the highest risk areas in Connecticut and Massachusetts does not justify immunizing everyone.

Vaccine is directed against the feeding tick

Cost-effectiveness of immunization is unclear

ADDITIONAL READING

Centers for Disease Control and Prevention. Recommendations for the use of Lyme disease vaccine. *Morb Mortal Wkly Rep* 1999;48(RR-7):1–25. This supplement also includes a nice guide to the diagnosis of Lyme disease and a discussion of the cost-effectiveness from both the societal and payor perspective.

Horton JM, Blaser MJ. The spectrum of relapsing fever in the Rocky Mountains. *Arch Intern Med* 1985;145:871–875. This article analyzes the clinical manifestations, epidemiology, and treatment of 22 cases of tick-borne relapsing fever that occurred between 1944 and 1983 and describes in detail several of the later cases.

Levett PN. Leptospirosis. *Clin Microbiol Rev* 2001;14:296–326. This comprehensive review includes a good discussion of clinical and diagnostic features, with a nice figure that ties them together. The reader should not be dissuaded by the page count; almost half of the pages are for the reference list.

Shapiro ED, Gerber MA. Lyme disease. *Clin Infect Dis* 2000;31:533–542. This review emphasizes clinical and diagnostic features, including the complexities of interpreting serologic tests in immunized persons. There is also a short section on "Lyme anxiety."

Singh AE, Romanowski B. Syphilis: Review with emphasis on clinical, epidemiologic, and some biologic features. *Clin Microbiol Rev* 1999;12:187–209. This comprehensive review gives a detailed account of clinical findings, diagnosis, and treatment for all stages of syphilis without shortchanging pathogenesis.

Steere AC. Lyme disease. *N Engl J Med* 2001;345:115–123. An excellent review of all aspects of the disease, including clinical features, biology, and prevention. The same issue of this journal also presents a study of antibiotic prophylaxis (pages 79–84) and a well-reasoned editorial on prevention (pages 133–134).

APPENDIX 27–1

Nonvenereal Treponemes

Disease	Cause	Major Geographic Location	Primary Lesion	Secondary Lesions	Tertiary Lesions
Bejel	*T. pallidum,* subspecies *endemicum*[a]	Middle East; arid, hot areas	Oral cavity[b]	Oral mucosa	Rare; gummatous lessions of skin, periosteum, bone, and joint
Yaws	*T. pallidum,* subspecies *pertenue*	Humid, tropical belt	Skin, papillomatous	Systemic; resemble syphilis	Rare; gummatous lesions of skin, periosteum, bone, and joint[c]
Pinta	*T. carateum*	Central and South America	Skin, erythematous papule	Skin; merge into primary lesion; altered pigmentation	Areas of altered skin pigmentation and hyperkeratoses

[a] Probably a variant of that causing venereal syphilis.
[b] Often inapparent.
[c] Neurologic manifestations usually absent.

CHAPTER 28

Mycobacteria

JAMES J. PLORDE

> The Captain of all these men of death that came against him to take him away, was the consumption; for it was that that brought him down to the grave.
>
> JOHN BUNYAN
> *The Life and Death of Mr. Badman*

Mycobacterium is a genus of Gram-positive bacilli that demonstrate the staining characteristic of acid-fastness. Its most important species, *Mycobacterium tuberculosis,* is the etiologic agent of tuberculosis, the "consumption" referred to above. One of the oldest and most devastating of human afflictions, tuberculosis remains a leading cause of infectious disease deaths worldwide today. A second mycobacterium, *Mycobacterium leprae,* is the causative agent of leprosy. A large number of less pathogenic species collectively referred to as "atypical mycobacteria" or "nontuberculous mycobacteria," are assuming increasing importance as disease agents in immunocompromised patients, particularly those with acquired immunodeficiency syndrome (AIDS).

MYCOBACTERIUM: GENERAL CHARACTERISTICS

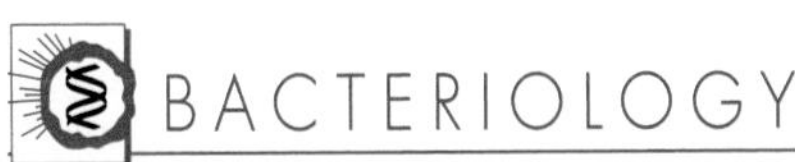

BACTERIOLOGY

MORPHOLOGY AND STRUCTURE

The mycobacteria are slim, Gram-positive bacilli (0.2–0.4 × 2–10 μm). They are nonmotile, obligate aerobes that do not form spores. The cell wall contains peptidoglycan similar to that of other Gram-positive organisms, except that it contains *N*-glycolylmuramic, rather than *N*-acetylmuramic, acid. Attached to peptidoglycan are a myriad of branched chain polysaccharides, proteins, and lipids. Of particular importance are long-chain fatty acids called mycolic acids. The **mycolic acids,** for which the *myco*bacteria are named, make up more than 60% of the total cell wall mass and are distinctive for each species. Other lipid components include mycosides, sulfolipids, and **lipoarabinomannan (LAM),** a complex molecule extending from the plasma membrane to the surface. LAM is structurally and functionally analogous to the lipopolysaccharide of Gram-negative bacteria. Porin and other proteins are found throughout the cell wall.

Cell wall has high lipid content

Mycolic acids and LAM are characteristic

The cell wall lipids make the cell surface hydrophobic, rendering mycobacteria resistant to staining with basic aniline dyes unless they are applied with heat or detergents, or for prolonged periods of time. Once stained, however, mycobacteria resist decolorization with a mixture of 3% hydrochloric acid and 95% ethanol. These properties are described as **acid fastness** or, more properly, acid–alcohol fastness, and the bacteria possessing them are called acid-fast bacilli. Details are described in Chapter 15. This characteristic allows mycobacteria to be readily distinguished from other genera by microscopic examination of smears stained with carbol fuchsin (Ziehl–Neelsen/Kinyoun techniques), or with the more recently introduced fluorochromes (auramine–rhodamine). Organisms stained with the latter reagents fluoresce brightly when viewed through an appropriate microscope, making the organisms more visually apparent and, thus, decreasing the time required for their detection.

Difficult to stain, but once stained, difficult to decolorize

Acid fastness distinguishes from most other bacteria

GROWTH

The most important pathogen, *M. tuberculosis,* shows enhanced growth in 10% carbon dioxide and at a pH of about 6.5 to 6.8. Nutritional requirements vary among species and range from the ability of some nonpathogens to multiply on the washers of water faucets to the strict intracellular parasitism of *M. leprae,* which does not grow in artificial media or cell culture. Mycobacteria grow more slowly than most human pathogenic bacteria because of their hydrophobic cell surface, which causes them to clump and inhibits permeability of nutrients into the cell. Addition of a surfactant (Tween 80) to cultures of *M. tuberculosis* wets the surface and leads to dispersed and more rapid growth.

Strict aerobes

Many species grow slowly

CLASSIFICATION

Until recently, mycobacterial classification has been based on a constellation of phenotypic characteristics, including nutritional and temperature requirements, growth rates, pigmentation of colonies grown in light or darkness, key biochemical tests, the cellular constellation of free fatty acids, and the range of pathogenicity in experimental animals. Some of the more important characteristics are summarized in Table 28–1. Increasingly, this classification system is yielding to molecular-based techniques. The identification of species-specific rRNA and DNA sequences has resulted in the revision and expansion of the older phenotype-based classification system, and the provision of an increasing array of species-specific DNA probes to clinical mycobacteriology laboratories.

Distinguished by cultural features, biochemical reactions, and pathogenicity

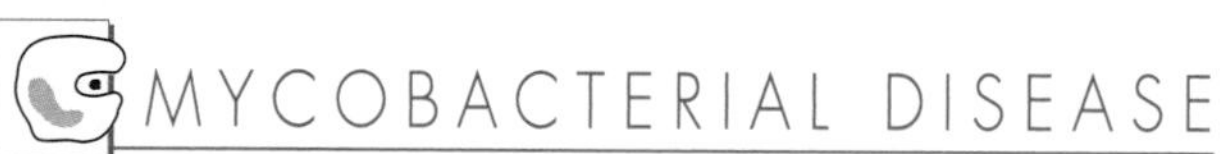

MYCOBACTERIAL DISEASE

Mycobacteria include a wide range of species pathogenic for humans and animals. Some, such as *M. tuberculosis,* occur exclusively in humans under natural conditions. Others, such as *Mycobacterium intracellulare,* can infect various hosts, including humans, but also exist in the free-living state. Most nonpathogenic species are widely distributed in the environment. Diseases caused by mycobacteria usually develop slowly, follow a chronic course, and elicit a granulomatous response. Infectivity of pathogenic species is quite high, but virulence for healthy humans is low. For example, disease following infection with *M. tuberculosis* is the exception rather than the rule.

Includes human and animal pathogens

Slowly progressive diseases

Mycobacteria do not produce classic exotoxins or endotoxins. Disease processes are thought to be the result of two related host responses. The first, a delayed-type hypersensitivity (DTH) reaction to mycobacterial proteins, results in the destruction of nonactivated macrophages containing multiplying organisms. It is detected by intradermal injections of purified proteins from the mycobacteria. The second, cell-mediated immunity (CMI) activates macrophages, enabling them to destroy mycobacteria contained

Lack exotoxins or endotoxins

TABLE 28–1

Mycobacteria of Major Clinical Importance[a]

	Characteristics								
Species	Reservoir	Virulence for Humans	Disease Caused	Case-to-Case Transmission	Growth Rate[b]	Optimum Growth Temperature	Pigment Production[c]	Substantial Niacin Production[d]	Virulence for Guinea Pigs[e]
M. tuberculosis	Human	+++	Tuberculosis	Yes	S	37	–	+	+
M. bovis	Animals	+++	Tuberculosis	Rare	S	37	–	–	+
Bacillus Calmette–Guérin	Artificial culture	±	Local lesion	Very rare	S	37	–	–	–
M. kansasii	Environmental	+	Tuberculosis-like	No	S	37	Photochromogen	–	–
M. scrofulaceum	Environmental	+	Usually lymphadenitis	No	S	37	Scotochromogen	–	–
M. avium-intracellulare	Environmental; birds	+	Tuberculosis-like	No	S	37	±	–	–
M. fortuitum	Environmental	±	Local abscess	No	F	37	±	–	Local abscess
M. marinum	Water; fish	±	Skin granuloma	No	S	30	Photochromogen	–	–
M. ulcerans	Probably environmental; tropical	+	Severe skin ulceration	No	S	30	–	–	–
M. leprae	Human	+++	Leprosy	Yes	NG	NG	NG	NG	–
M. smegmatis	Human, external urethral area	–	None	–	F	37	–	–	–

[a] Numerous nonpathogenic environmental mycobacteria exist and may contaminate human specimens.

[b] S = slow (colonies usually develop in 10 days or more); F = fast (colonies develop in 7 days or less); NG = not grown.

[c] Yellow–orange pigment. Photochromogen is pigment produced in light; scotochromogen is pigment produced in dark or light.

[d] Many other differential biochemical tests used, eg, nitrate reduction, catalase production, Tween 80 hydrolysis.

[e] Disease following subcutaneous injection of light inoculum (eg, 10^2 cells).

within their cytoplasm. The balance between these two responses determines the pathology and clinical response to a mycobacterial infection.

MYCOBACTERIUM TUBERCULOSIS

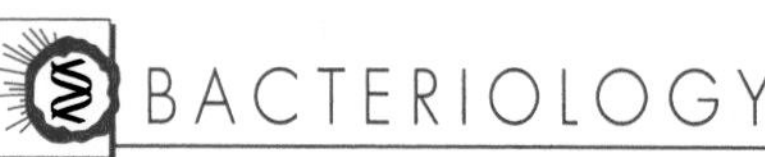

BACTERIOLOGY

M. tuberculosis is a slim, strongly acid–alcohol–fast rod. It frequently shows irregular beading in its staining, appearing as connected series of acid-fast granules (Fig 28–1). It grows at 37°C but not at room temperature, and it requires enriched or complex media for primary growth. Growth is enhanced by 5 to 10% carbon dioxide but is still very slow, with a mean generation time of 12 to 24 hours. The classic medium, Löwenstein–Jensen, contains homogenized egg in nutrient base with dyes to inhibit the growth of nonmycobacterial contaminants. The dry, rough, buff-colored colonies usually appear after 3 to 6 weeks of incubation. Mycobacterial growth is more rapid in two semisynthetic oleic acid–albumin media. Virulent strains grown in the latter demonstrate "cording" in which multiplying organisms remain attached in parallel bundles to form long intertwining cords or ropes. The major phenotypic tests for identification of *M. tuberculosis* are summarized in Table 28–1. Of particular importance is the ability of *M. tuberculosis* to produce large quantities of niacin, which is uncommon in other mycobacteria.

Growth requires rich medium and CO_2

Cording, biochemical tests distinguish from other mycobacteria

Due to its hydrophobic lipid surface, *M. tuberculosis* is unusually resistant to drying, to most common disinfectants, and to acids and alkalis. Tubercle bacilli are sensitive to heat, including pasteurization, and individual organisms in droplet nuclei are susceptible to inactivation by ultraviolet light.

Unusual resistance to drying and disinfectants but not to heat

As with other mycobacteria, the *M. tuberculosis* cell wall structure is dominated by mycolic acids and LAM. Its antigenic makeup includes many protein and polysaccharide antigens of which tuberculin is the most studied. It consists of heat-stable proteins liberated into liquid culture media. A purified protein derivative (PPD) of tuberculin is used for skin testing for hypersensitivity and is standardized in tuberculin units according to skin test activity.

PPD contains mix of tuberculin proteins

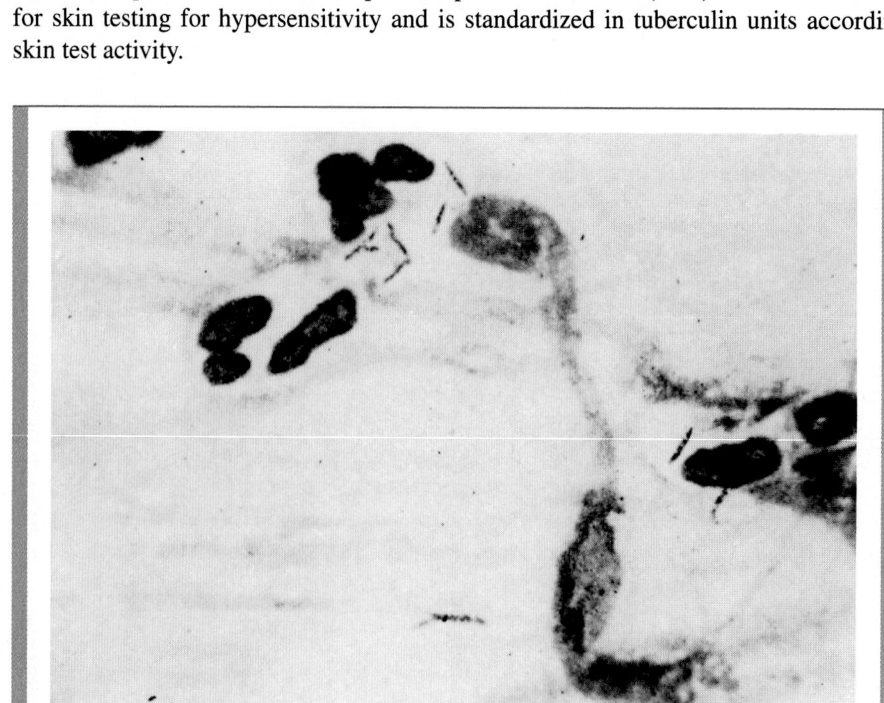

FIGURE 28–1
Mycobacterium tuberculosis in sputum stained by Ziehl–Neelsen technique. The mycobacteria retain the red carbol fuchsin through the decolorization step. The cells, background, and any other organisms stain with methylene blue counterstain.

TUBERCULOSIS

CLINICAL CAPSULE

Tuberculosis is a systemic infection manifested only by evidence of an immune response in most exposed individuals. In some infected persons, the disease either progresses or, more commonly, reactivates after an asymptomatic period (years). The most common reactivation form is a chronic pneumonia with fever, cough, bloody sputum, and weight loss. Spread outside of the lung also occurs and is particularly devastating when it reaches the central nervous system. The natural history follows a course of chronic wasting to death aptly called "consumption" in the past.

EPIDEMIOLOGY

A recognized disease of antiquity, tuberculosis first reached epidemic proportions in the western world during the major periods of urbanization in the 18th and 19th centuries. Mortality reached 200 to 700 per 100,000 population each year, accounting for 20 to 30% of all deaths in urban centers and winning tuberculosis the appellation of the "white plague." Morbidity was many times higher. The disease has had major sociologic components, flourishing with ignorance, poverty, overcrowding, and poor hygiene, particularly during the social disruptions of war and economic depression. Under these conditions, the poor are the major victims, but all sectors of society are at risk. Chopin, Paganini, Rousseau, Goethe, Chekhov, Thoreau, Keats, Elizabeth Barrett Browning, and the Brontës, to name but a few, were all lost to tuberculosis in their intellectual prime. With knowledge of the cause and transmission of the disease and the development of effective antimicrobial agents, tuberculosis was increasingly brought under control in developed countries. Unfortunately, mortality and morbidity remain at 19th-century levels in many developing countries despite extensive national and international control programs.

Infection of 18th and 19th centuries

Attack rates still high in many developing countries

The great majority of tuberculous infections are contracted by inhalation of droplet nuclei carrying the causative organism. Humans may also be infected through the gastrointestinal tract following the ingestion of milk from tuberculous cows (now uncommon due to pasteurization) or, rarely, through abraded skin. It has been estimated that a single cough can generate as many as 3000 infected droplet nuclei and that less than 10 bacilli may initiate a pulmonary infection in a susceptible individual. The likelihood of acquiring infection thus relates to the numbers of organisms in the sputum of an open case of the disease, the frequency and efficiency of the coughs, the closeness of contact, and the adequacy of ventilation in the contact area. Epidemiologic data indicate that large doses or prolonged exposure to smaller infecting doses is usually needed to initiate infection in humans. In some closed environments, such as a submarine or a crowded nursing home, a single open case of pulmonary tuberculosis can infect the majority of nonimmune individuals sharing sleeping accommodations.

Most infections are by respiratory route

Repeated coughing generates infectious dose into air

Poor ventilation increases risk

In the past, an animal variant (*Mycobacterium bovis*) was transmitted by drinking milk from infected herds. This disease has been largely eliminated by eradication programs and milk pasteurization.

The decline in mortality and occurrence of the disease in the United States over the last century is shown in Figure 28–2. Between 1953 to 1985 the number of new tuberculosis cases per annum fell from 84,304 to 22,201. By the mid-1980s, it was estimated that only 4 to 5% of American citizens, and less than 1% of American children, demonstrated positive tuberculin skin tests. However, the decline was not uniform throughout the American populace, and case rates among nonwhites and the urban poor remained significantly higher than the national average. As the incidence of infection in the United States and other developed countries decreased, there was also a major shift in the age of tuberculosis patients. Most were over 50 years of age and represented cases in which an old primary lesion, quiescent for decades, became reactivated. The grandfather who has developed "chronic bronchitis" is a classic source of infection to children.

Overall decline masks increases in some subpopulations

Reactivation among older persons

In 1985, the steady decline in reports of new tuberculosis cases and deaths in the United States ceased, and, in the ensuing 7 years, new cases increased by nearly 20%.

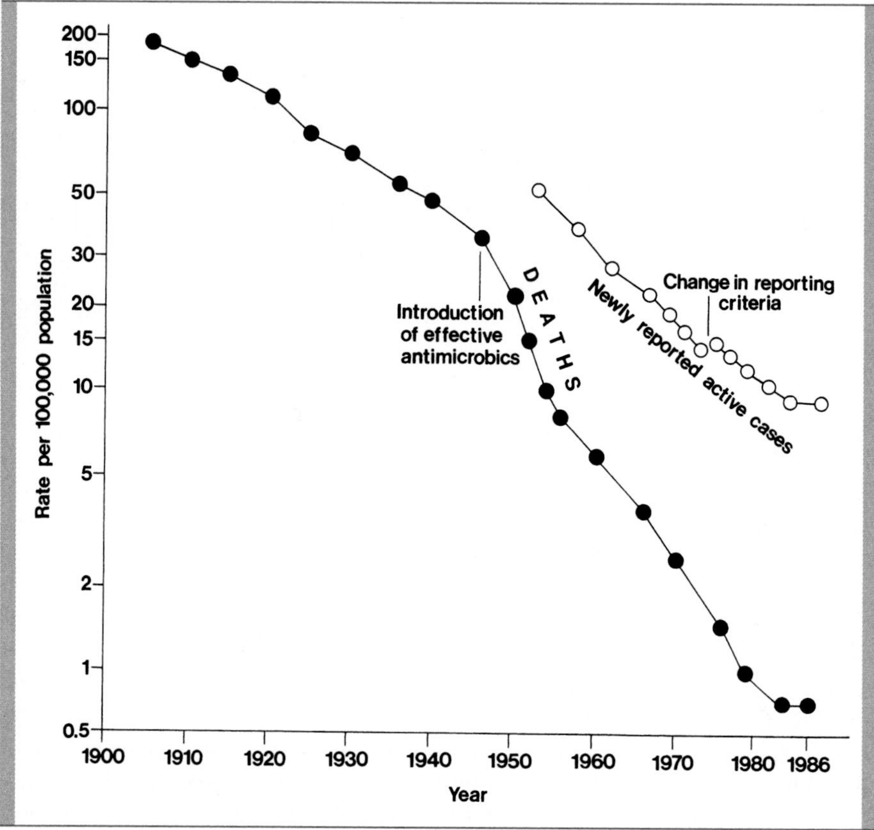

FIGURE 28–2
Morbidity and mortality of tuberculosis in the United States, 1900–1986.

Immigrants, impoverished, homeless, AIDS patients, and drug abusers

This change has been attributed to a significant decrease in the funding for tuberculosis control programs; spread of multiresistant strains of *M. tuberculosis;* increased immigration from tuberculosis-endemic areas of the world; social and economic changes that contributed to a burgeoning of incarcerated intravenous drug users and homeless populations; and, finally, to the AIDS epidemic. It is estimated that patients with latent tuberculosis increase their risk of reactivation disease by factors of 200 to 300 with the development of a human immunodeficiency virus (HIV) coinfection. The per annum reactivation rate of such individuals is estimated at 8%.

Rates increasing in children

Accompanying the increase in reactivation tuberculosis among high-risk US populations was an increase in the transmission of *M. tuberculosis*. Annual tuberculin skin conversions among intravenous drug abusers and the number of cases of tuberculosis among children under 5 years of age increased significantly between 1987 and 1990. Single-source epidemics involve school children and a teacher with unrecognized pulmonary tuberculosis, homeless shelters, nursing homes, and medical personnel exposed to patients with unrecognized tuberculosis. Since 1992, a reinvigorated public health effort in the United States has, again, led to a declining number of individuals with active tuberculosis, reaching a new low of 18,361 in 1998. This represents a rate of 6.8/100,000 population, still well short of the nation's interim goal of 3.5/100,000 for the year 2000 and 1/100,000 for the year 2010.

Resistance to antimicrobics increasing

Globally, the situation is more ominous. It is estimated that one third of the world's population is infected with *M. tuberculosis;* 30 million people have active disease, an additional 8 million develop new disease yearly, and 2 to 3 million die annually of this "captain of death." As a result, tuberculosis is the leading cause of death from an infectious disease worldwide. It is thought responsible for 6% of all deaths and 26% of avoidable adult deaths. Particularly concerning for the future control of tuberculosis worldwide is the marked susceptibility of patients with AIDS and the growing resistance of *M. tuberculosis* to the currently available antimicrobic agents. Because 40% of all new cases of tuberculosis in the United States are among foreign-born individuals, the elimination of this disease in the United States will be impossible without a substantial reduction in the global burden of tuberculosis.

PATHOGENESIS

Primary Infection

Primary tuberculosis is the response to the initial infection in an individual not previously infected and sensitized to tuberculoprotein. Inhaled droplet nuclei containing small numbers of tubercle bacilli are deposited in the peripheral respiratory alveoli, most frequently those of the well-ventilated middle and lower lobes. Here they are engulfed by **nonspecifically activated** alveolar macrophages. The ability of these cells to destroy ingested organisms depends significantly on their inherent microbicidal capacity. If the alveolar macrophages are unable to destroy ingested mycobacteria, they continue to multiply until the macrophage bursts. The released organisms are subsequently ingested by inactivated blood macrophages that, together with T cells, are attracted to the lung by chemotactic factors.

Inhaled organisms multiply in alveolar macrophages

The ingested mycobacteria continue to multiply intracellularly without damage to their host cell. Some of the bacterial-laden macrophages are transported through lymphatic channels to the hilar lymph nodes draining the infected site. From there, they may disseminate through blood and lymphatic systems to a number of tissues, including the liver, spleen, kidney, bone, brain, meninges, and apices or other parts of the lung. The inflammatory reaction in the seeded tissues is usually minor, and the signs and symptoms of infection are absent. However, the primary site of infection and some enlarged hilar lymph nodes can often be detected radiologically. In infants and immunocompromised adults, hematogenous dissemination of organisms may occasionally produce a life-threatening meningitis.

Low reactivity to the organism allows multiplication and dissemination to lymph nodes and bloodstream

Morphologically, the resulting tubercle is a microscopic granuloma comprised of some multinucleated giant cells formed by the fusion of several macrophages (Langhans cells), many epithelioid cells (activated macrophages), and a surrounding collar of lymphocytes (Fig 28–3) and fibroblasts. When many bacteria are present and there is a high degree of hypersensitivity, enzymes, reactive oxygen intermediates, and reactive nitrogen intermediates are released by dying macrophages and lead to necrosis of the center of the granuloma, which is termed caseous because of the cheesy, semisolid character of the gross lesion.

The tubercle includes activated macrophages and other cell types

Caseation occurs with high levels of antigen and hypersensitivity

Primary infections are usually handled well by the host. Bacterial multiplication ceases. Most microscopic lesions heal by fibrosis, and the organisms in them slowly die. In others, especially those in well-oxygenated tissues such as the subapical areas of the lung, renal

Organisms remain viable for long periods

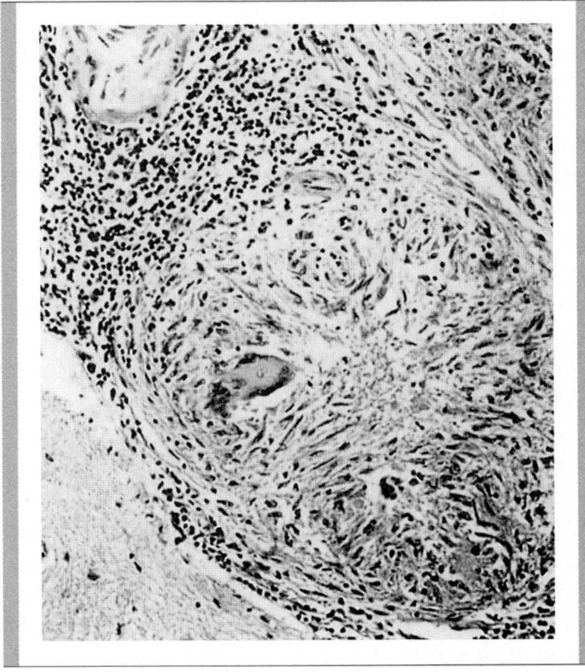

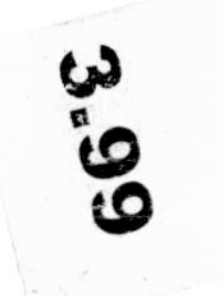

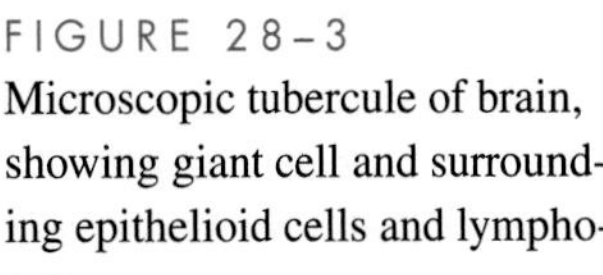

FIGURE 28–3
Microscopic tubercule of brain, showing giant cell and surrounding epithelioid cells and lymphocytes.

cortex and vertebral bodies, the tubercle bacilli remain viable for long periods and serve as a potential source of reactivation many months or years later if host defenses weaken.

Reactivation (Adult) Tuberculosis

Discharge of caseous material forms pulmonary cavities

Reactivation usually occurs in body areas of relatively high oxygen tension and low lymphatic drainage, most often in the apex of the lung. The lesions show spreading, coalescing tubercles with numerous tubercle bacilli, and large areas of caseous necrosis. Necrosis often involves the wall of a small bronchus from which the necrotic material is discharged, resulting in a pulmonary cavity and bronchial spread. Frequently, small blood vessels are also eroded. The chronic fever and weight loss may be mediated in part by macrophage-derived tumor necrosis factor.

Virulence Mechanisms

Ability to multiply in macrophages is central to virulence

Lipids modulate cytokines and inhibit killing

The basis for *M. tuberculosis* virulence is largely unknown. It produces no exotoxins, and both the intact cell and cellular components are remarkably innocuous to humans and experimental animals not previously sensitized to tuberculin. Cell wall components such as LAM have been implicated in binding to alveolar macrophages, utilizing surface fibronectin, mannose, or complement receptors (CR1, CR3). Once inside, multiple factors contribute to survival and continued multiplication. A number of genes have been identified that are linked to virulence by enhancing survival in the macrophage or by influencing the physical and chemical conditions (low pH, high lactic acid, high CO_2) present in developing lesions, but their function remains unknown. Mycolic acids, sulfolipids, LAM, and proteins have been shown to disrupt phagosome–lysosome interactions and interfere with oxidative killing. LAM has also been shown to modulate cytokine production and downregulate other aspects of T-cell function including antigen presentation.

IMMUNITY

Innate immunity is high and genetically variable

Humans generally have a rather high innate immunity to development of disease. This was tragically illustrated in the Lübeck disaster of 1926 where infants were administered *M. tuberculosis* instead of an intended vaccine strain. Despite the large dose, only 76 of 249 died and most of the others developed only minor lesions. Approximately 10% of immunocompetent persons infected with *M. tuberculosis* will develop active disease any time in their life. There is epidemiologic and historic evidence for differences in the immunity in certain population groups and between identical and nonidentical twins.

DTH and CMI develop in 2–6 weeks

Mycobacterial antigens are presented by infected macrophages

Cytokines mediate destruction and further inflammation

DTH to tuberculoprotein and CMI to *M. tuberculosis* develop 2 to 6 weeks after primary infection. The subsequent course of the infection depends on the balance between these two defensive mechanisms. DTH, through the mediation of natural killer cells, destroys the inactivated macrophages as well as the surrounding tissues, releasing still viable mycobacteria into an area of necrosis unsuitable for bacterial multiplication. CMI develops when competent T lymphocytes recognize mycobacterial antigen complexes on the surface of *M. tuberculosis*–containing macrophages. In the presence of macrophage-produced interleukin-1, the activated lymphocytes respond to the presented antigens with the elaboration of several cytokines. Some of these proteins attract circulating monocytes. Others, including interferon-γ and possibly tumor necrosis factor-α, activate local tissue macrophages and the recruited monocytes to enhanced destruction of ingested mycobacteria, resulting in a slowing or discontinuation of intracellular bacterial growth. Nitrous oxide or other reactive nitrogen intermediates probably mediate the destruction of the mycobacteria. Another cytokine, interleukin-2, induces clonal expansion of the activated lymphocytes, thus amplifying the host's immunologic response. Still others stimulate accumulation of fibroblasts and deposition of collagen, which help wall off the area of infection and prevent further dissemination.

Immunity is cell mediated but incomplete

Acquired immunity is cell mediated but incomplete. Both helper–inducer (CD4+) and cytotoxic (CD8+) T lymphocytes are involved. Two to three weeks after infection, macrophages are activated at the site of infection by a network of pro- and anti-inflammatory cytokines and chemokines from antigen-stimulated CD4+ T lymphocytes, macrophages, and dendritic cells. This interaction between *M. tuberculosis* and the host is what eventually limits its multiplication and spread. Cytotoxic T cells release bacilli from inactivated phagocytic cells and allow them to be ingested and handled by the activated macrophages. The concomitant DTH to tuberculoprotein plays an important part in immunity to reinfection by mobilizing immune cells and macrophages to the site of deposition of tubercle bacilli. In the past, it was believed that reinfection from external sources was extremely rare, but it is now clear that loss of hypersensitivity and CMI can occur over time and that reinfection can develop into clinical tuberculosis.

CD4+ and CD8+ T lymphocytes are involved

DTH enhances immunity to reinfection

The role of DTH in immunity of established tuberculosis is complex, because high degrees of sensitivity can precipitate caseous necrosis and lead to spread of the disease. The importance of CMI and hypersensitivity in modulating the course of tuberculosis is, perhaps, most dramatically illustrated in patients with AIDS. Those with minimal impairment of cellular immune responses develop typical tubercles containing relatively few bacilli. Those with advanced impairment demonstrate abundant acid-fast bacilli without epithelioid cell accumulation or associated tissue necrosis.

Hypersensitivity can precipitate caseation and spread in established disease

Lesions in AIDS patients related to degree of immunosuppression

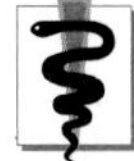

TUBERCULOSIS: CLINICAL ASPECTS

MANIFESTATIONS

Primary Tuberculosis

Primary tuberculosis is either asymptomatic or manifest only by fever and malaise. Radiographs may show infiltrates in the mid-zones of the lung and enlarged draining lymph nodes in the area around the hilum. When these lymph nodes fibrose and sometimes calcify, they produce a characteristic picture (Ghon complex) on radiograph. In approximately 5% of patients, the primary disease is not controlled and merges into the reactivation type of tuberculosis, or it disseminates to many organs to produce active miliary tuberculosis. The latter may result from a necrotic tubercle eroding into a small blood vessel.

Mid-lung infiltrates and adenopathy are produced

Primary infection may progress to reactivation or miliary tuberculosis

Reactivation Tuberculosis

Approximately 10% of those recovering from a primary infection develop clinical disease sometime during their lifetime. In Western countries, reactivation of previous quiescent lesions occurs most often after the age of 50 and is more common in men. Reactivation is associated with a period of immunosuppression precipitated by malnutrition, alcoholism, diabetes, old age, and a dramatic change in the individual's life, such as loss of a spouse. In areas in which the disease is more common, reactivation tuberculosis is more frequently seen in young adults experiencing the immunosuppression that accompanies puberty and pregnancy. Recently, reactivation and progressive primary tuberculosis among younger adults have increased as a complication of AIDS.

Reactivation is most common in older men

Predisposing factors include underlying disease and life events

Cough is the universal symptom. It is initially dry, but as the disease progresses sputum is produced, which even later is mixed with blood (hemoptysis). Fever, malaise, fatigue, sweating, and weight loss all progress with continuing disease. Radiographically, infiltrates appearing in the apices of the lung coalesce to form cavities with progressive destruction of lung tissue. Less commonly, reactivation tuberculosis can also occur in other organs, such as the kidneys, bones, lymph nodes, brain, meninges, bone marrow, and bowel. Disease at these sites ranges from a localized tumor-like granuloma (tuberculoma) to a fatal chronic meningitis. Untreated, the progressive cough, fever, and weight loss of pulmonary tuberculosis creates an internally consuming fire that usually takes 2 to 5 years to cause death. The course in AIDS and other CMI-compromised patients is more rapid.

Cough is universal

Cavities form in lung apices

Multiple organs are involved

DIAGNOSIS

Tuberculin Test

The tuberculin skin test measures DTH to tuberculoprotein. PPD is standardized biologically against an international reference preparation, and its activity expressed in

PPD test measures hypersensitivity to tuberculoprotein

tuberculin units (TU). Most initial skin tests employ 5 TU (intermediate strength). When an unusually high degree of hypersensitivity or eye or skin tuberculosis is suspected, then 1 TU (first strength) or less is used initially to avoid the risk of an excessive reaction locally or at the site of a mycobacterial lesion.

PPD test interpreted by area of induration

Positive PPD indicates past or current infection

The test most commonly performed involves intradermal injection that is read 48 to 72 hours later. An area of measured induration of 10 mm or more accompanied by erythema constitutes a positive reaction, although smaller areas of induration and erythema indicate a lesser degree of sensitization to mycobacterial proteins. No induration indicates a negative reaction. A positive PPD test indicates that the individual has been infected at some time with *M. tuberculosis* or with a strongly cross-reacting mycobacterium of another species. It carries no implication about the activity of the infection, which may have been simply a primary complex contracted 20 years previously.

Anergy may develop with therapy or disease affecting CMI

A negative PPD test in a healthy individual indicates that he or she has not been infected with *M. tuberculosis,* is in the prehypersensitive stage of a primary infection, or has finally lost tuberculin sensitivity along with disappearance of antigen from an old primary complex. Patients with severe disseminated disease, those on steroid or immunosuppressive drugs, or those with certain other diseases such as AIDS and measles, may also become anergic. They lose their tuberculin hypersensitivity and become more susceptible to the disease. Induration below the 10-mm diameter criterion for positivity indicates low-level sensitization, which may be attributable to *M. tuberculosis* infection or to a cross-reacting mycobacterial infection.

Clinical value of skin test depends on prevalence of reactivity in population

The clinical value of the PPD test depends on the occurrence of primary infection in different age groups. Now, primary infection is sufficiently uncommon in much of the Western world that a negative test is frequently important in excluding tuberculosis. A positive test in infancy or childhood has significance in diagnosis and can often be used to trace a household or school source of infection. Epidemiologic surveys of tuberculin reactivity indicate trends in the incidence of infection and constitute the simplest way of monitoring the effectiveness of control measures.

Laboratory Diagnosis

Mycobacteria are detected in direct smears of clinical material

Contaminating mycobacteria may yield "false" positives in some specimens

If present in sufficient numbers, acid-fast bacilli can be detected microscopically in direct smears of clinical specimens or in smears of material concentrated for culture (see below). Smears are stained by the Ziehl–Neelsen procedure or one of its modifications, including the fluorescence staining method. About 65% of culture-positive sputum samples yield positive smears from concentrated specimens. These procedures are not specific for *M. tuberculosis* because other mycobacteria may have a similar morphology and may be etiologic agents of disease, members of the normal flora, or external contaminants. Their significance depends on the specimen. Acid-fast bacilli in sputum are highly significant for mycobacterial infection. A clean-voided male urine specimen, on the other hand, is often contaminated with *Mycobacterium smegmatis* from the prepuce, and the finding of acid-fast bacilli does not per se indicate infection. Bronchoscopy equipment and nasotracheal tubes or their lubricants are prone to contamination with free-living mycobacteria, and false conclusions have been drawn from smears of such preparations. The polymerase chain reaction has been reported to be useful in the direct diagnosis of tuberculosis by a number of investigators. To date, none of these techniques are practical for routine use in the clinical laboratory.

Material contaminated with normal flora must be treated

Mucolytic agents used in sputum

NaOH used as antibacterial

Cultural confirmation of a tentative diagnosis of tuberculosis is thus essential, and the organism must be isolated for identification and susceptibility testing. Specimens from protected sites, such as cerebrospinal fluid, bone marrow, pleural fluid, and ureteric urine, can be seeded directly to culture media used for *M. tuberculosis* isolation. Those samples inevitably contaminated with normal flora, such as sputum, gastric aspirations (cultured when sputum is not available, for example, in young children), or voided urine, are treated with alkali, acid, or a detergent germicide under conditions that kill the normal flora but allow many mycobacteria to survive because of their resistance to these agents. The most commonly used treatment now employs *N*-acetylcysteine to dissolve mucus, combined with the antibacterial effect of a weak sodium hydroxide solution. The material is concentrated by centrifugation or filtration, neutralized or washed, and inoculated onto culture media.

Cultures on solid media usually take 3 weeks or longer to show visible colonies. Growth may be detected radiometrically in about half the time by using liquid oleic acid–albumin broth containing ^{14}C-labeled palmitic acid, which is metabolized by mycobacteria to liberate $^{14}CO_2$. The labeled CO_2 is detected in the space above the medium using an automated sampling procedure. Incorporation of a specific inhibitor of *M. tuberculosis* in a parallel vial increases the specificity of the test.

Traditional cultures take 3+ weeks; labeled substrate procedures are twice as fast

Whichever procedure is used, specific identification of an isolated mycobacterium is essential. It may be achieved with a number of cultural and biochemical tests, including those shown in Table 28–1, but the process usually takes several weeks. More rapid results can be obtained by high-resolution gas chromatographic analysis of fatty acids in mycobacterial colonies or by testing for homology between genetic probes of labeled mycobacterial DNA and ribosomal RNA extracted from the strain under test. Specific probes are now available commercially for detecting *M. tuberculosis* and the *Mycobacterium avium–intracellulare* complex.

Traditional speciation uses cultural and biochemical tests

DNA/RNA homology is useful

Susceptibility testing is important with newly diagnosed cases. When sufficient numbers of acid-fast bacilli are seen on direct smears, the treated clinical specimen can be seeded directly onto antimicrobic-containing media for susceptibility tests, thereby saving several weeks. If numbers are scanty, the initiation of tests must await primary isolation. More rapid test results can be obtained by incorporating antimicrobics into the medium used for radiometric detection of mycobacterial growth. These results show good concordance with conventional tests and are available 1 to 2 weeks earlier.

Susceptibility testing by conventional and labeled substrate procedures

TREATMENT

M. tuberculosis is susceptible to several effective antimicrobics (Table 28–2). Isoniazid, ethambutol, rifampin, pyrazinamide, streptomycin, and combinations of these agents constitute the primary drugs of choice for treatment of tuberculosis. All of these, except ethambutol, are bactericidal. Isoniazid and rifampin are active against both intra- and extracellular organisms, and pyrazinamide, a nicotinamide analog, acts at the acidic pH found within cells. Streptomycin does not penetrate into cells and is thus active only against extracellular organisms. *M. tuberculosis* is also susceptible to other drugs that may be used to replace those of the primary group if they are inappropriate because of resistance or drug toxicity. The fluoroquinolones, such as ciprofloxacin and ofloxacin, are active against *M. tuberculosis* and penetrate well into infected cells. Their role in the treatment of tuberculosis is under evaluation. Isoniazid and ethambutol act on the mycolic acid (isoniazid) and LAM (ethambutol) elements of mycobacterial cell wall synthesis. The molecular targets of the other agents have yet to be defined except for the general antibacterial agents (rifampin, streptomycin, fluoroquinolones) discussed in Chapter 13.

Multiple antimicrobics act intra- and extracellularly

Resistance or toxicity may limit some agents

TABLE 28–2

Antimicrobics Commonly Used in Treatment of Tuberculosis

First-Line Drug	Second-Line Drug[a]
Isoniazid	*para*-Aminosalicylic acid
Ethambutol	Ethionamide
Rifampin	Cycloserine
Pyrazinamide	Fluoroquinolones
Streptomycin	Kanamycin, etc

[a] Second-line drugs added to combinations if resistance or toxicity contraindicates first-line agent.

Combined therapy used to prevent resistance

Mutational resistance to antituberculous drugs occurs at frequencies of 10^{-7} to 10^{-10}. For example, mutation in a gene coding for a catalase-peroxidase enzyme causes failure of the conversion of isoniazid to its biologically active form. Such mutants often come to predominate and produce clinical relapse particularly when a single drug is used. Adequate, continuous treatment with two or three antituberculous drugs with different modes of action greatly reduces the probability a mutant will be expressed, because the chance of a doubly resistant mutant in a lesion's organism population is very low. The proportion of infections with strains resistant to first-line drugs varies between 5 and 15% but appears to be increasing in many locales, particularly among individuals who have been treated previously. Of particular concern is the establishment in the last decade of strains resistant to both isoniazid and rifampin, the mainstays of primary treatment. Susceptibility tests are required to guide drug selection.

Even "short" courses of treatment last 9 months

Resistance and HIV infection require lengthier treatment

Compliance a major problem

Treatment with multiple antimicrobics to which the organism is susceptible usually renders the patient noninfectious within 1 or 2 weeks, which has shifted the care of tuberculous patients from isolation hospitals and sanatoriums to the home or the general hospital. After an initial intense phase of systemic chemotherapy, treatment is usually continued with oral antimicrobics for several months. Until recently, therapy with two oral agents, isoniazid and ethambutol, was continued for a total of 18 to 24 months. Studies have now demonstrated that therapy can be shortened to 9 months when isoniazid and rifampin are used concomitantly and to 6 months when pyrazinamide is added as a third agent. In patients whose organisms display resistance to one or more of these drugs, and in those with HIV infection, a more prolonged treatment course is used. The effectiveness of chemotherapy on most forms of tuberculosis has been dramatic and has greatly reduced the need for surgical procedures such as pulmonary lobectomy. Failure of chemotherapy is often associated with lack of adherence to the regimen by the patient, the presence of resistant organisms, or both.

PREVENTION

Chemoprophylaxis may use single drug

Prophylactic chemotherapy, usually with isoniazid alone, is now used in situations in which known or suspected primary tuberculous infection poses the risk of clinical disease. Some indications for prophylaxis are summarized in Table 28–3. Isoniazid can be used alone in prophylaxis because the load of tubercle bacilli in a subclinical primary lesion is small in relation to that in reactivation tuberculosis, and experience has shown that the development of subsequent clinical disease from isoniazid-resistant strains selected by prophylaxis can be discounted. Unfortunately, isoniazid may cause a form of hepatitis, and the risk increases progressively after 20 years of age. Its use in older subjects involves balancing risk against potential benefit and requires monitoring with liver function tests.

BCG vaccine is a live attenuated derivative of *M. bovis*

Effectiveness of BCG is variable

At present, the bacillus Calmette-Guérin (BCG) vaccine (named for its originators, Calmette and Guérin) is the only available vaccine. It has been used for prophylaxis of tuberculosis in various countries since 1923; administration is usually intradermal. It is a live vaccine derived originally from a strain of *M. bovis* that was attenuated by repeated subculture. Since then, it has had a checkered history, with results in different controlled trials ranging from ineffectiveness to 80% protection. In most studies, however, it has substantially decreased the highly lethal miliary and meningeal forms of tuberculosis among young children. On the basis of these results, massive immunization campaigns sponsored by the World Health Organization have been organized in underdeveloped countries.

PPD conversion caused by BCG

BCG contraindicated for AIDS patients

BCG is used only in tuberculin-negative subjects. Successful vaccination leads to a minor local lesion, self-limiting multiplication of the organism locally and in draining lymphatic vessels, and development of tuberculin hypersensitivity. The latter results in loss of the PPD test as a diagnostic and epidemiologic tool, and when infection rates are low, as they are now in most Western countries, this loss may offset the possible immunity produced. In general, tuberculosis rates in the West have declined as rapidly in countries that have not used the BCG vaccine as in those that have adopted mass vaccination with its occasional complications. Its potential value in these countries is restricted to population groups at particular risk. Its role in developing countries remains a matter of some contention. The BCG vaccination is contraindicated for individuals in whom cell-mediated immune mechanisms are compromised, such as those infected with the HIV.

MYCOBACTERIUM LEPRAE

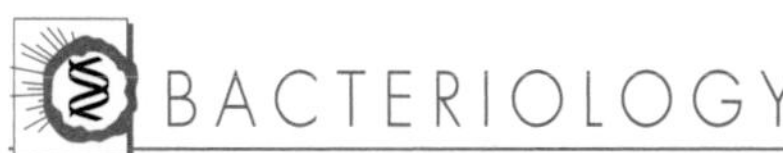

BACTERIOLOGY

Mycobacterium leprae, the cause of leprosy, is an acid-fast bacillus that has not been grown in artificial medium or tissue culture beyond, possibly, a few generations. However, it can be grown in the footpads of normal mice, in thymectomized irradiated mice, and in the armadillo, which may also be infected naturally. Its growth in animals is very slow, with an estimated doubling time of 12 to 14 days. Although lack of in vitro growth severely limits study of the organism, the structure and cell wall components appear to be similar to other mycobacteria. One mycoside, phenolic glycolipid I (PGL-1), is synthesized in large amounts and found only in *M. leprae*.

Fails to grow in culture

Slow growth in animals

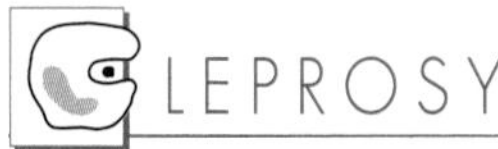

LEPROSY

CLINICAL CAPSULE

Leprosy is a chronic granulomatous disease of the peripheral nerves and superficial tissues, particularly the nasal mucosa. Disease ranges from slowly resolving anesthetic skin lesions to the disfiguring facial lesions responsible for the social stigma and ostracism of the individuals with leprosy (lepers).

EPIDEMIOLOGY

The exact mode of transmission is unknown but appears to be by generation of small droplets from the nasal secretions from cases of lepromatous leprosy. Traumatic inoculation through minor skin lesions or tattoos is also possible. The central reservoir is infected humans. The incubation period as estimated from clinical observations is generally 2 to 7 years but sometimes up to four decades. Very rarely, cases develop in nonendemic areas without known case contacts. The infectivity of *M. leprae* is low. Most new cases have had prolonged close contact with an infected individual. Biting insects may also be involved. Although virtually absent from North America and Europe, there are still an estimated 10 million infected persons in Asia, Africa, and Latin America. Immigration into Western countries from areas where the disease occurs has increased the numbers of cases seen.

Nasal droplets transmit infection

Rare in North America

PATHOGENESIS

M. leprae is an obligate intracellular parasite that must multiply in host cells to persist. In humans the preferred cells are macrophages and Schwann cells. PGL-1 and LAM have been implicated in the ability to survive and multiply in these cells. The organism may invade peripheral sensory nerves, resulting in patchy anesthesia. Few *M. leprae* are seen in tuberculoid lesions, which are granulomatous with extensive epithelioid cells, giant cells, and lymphocytic infiltration. In lepromatous multibacillary leprosy, CMI is deficient, and growth of *M. leprae* is, thus, relatively unimpeded. Histologically, lesions show dense infiltration with leprosy bacilli, and large numbers may reach the bloodstream.

Obligate intracellular parasite of macrophages and Schwann cells

IMMUNITY

Immunity to *M. leprae* is CMI mediated. The range of disease correlates with DTH responsiveness to lepromin, a skin test antigen derived from leprous tissue similar to tuberculin.

CMI determines extent of disease

Tuberculoid cases have minimal disease and positive skin tests. Lepromatous cases have progressive disease and negative skin tests. Other tests of CMI response to *M. leprae* correlate in the same way.

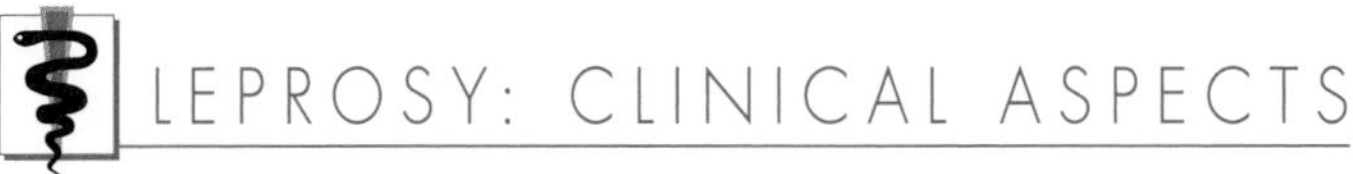

LEPROSY: CLINICAL ASPECTS

MANIFESTATIONS

Two major forms of the disease are recognized, tuberculoid and lepromatous. However, intermediate forms occur, and the first form may merge into the second.

Tuberculoid Leprosy

Skin and nerve involvement

Strong delayed hypersensitivity and CMI

Tuberculoid leprosy involves the development of macules or large, flattened plaques on the face, trunk, and limbs, with raised, erythematous edges and dry, pale, hairless centers. When the bacterium has invaded peripheral nerves, the lesions are anesthetic. The disease is indolent, with simultaneous evidence of slow progression and healing. Because of the small number of organisms present, this form of the disease is usually noncontagious.

Lepromatous Leprosy

Deficient CMI and anergy to lepromin

Many *M. leprae* in lesions

In lepromatous multibacillary leprosy, CMI is deficient, and patients are anergic to lepromin. Growth of *M. leprae* is, thus, relatively unimpeded. Histologically, lesions show dense infiltration with leprosy bacilli, and large numbers may reach the bloodstream. Skin lesions are extensive, symmetric, and diffuse, particularly on the face, with thickening of the looser skin of the lips, forehead, and ears, resulting in the classic leonine appearance. Damage may be severe, with loss of nasal bones and septum, sometimes of digits, and with testicular atrophy in men. The organism spreads systemically, with involvement of the reticuloendothelial system.

DIAGNOSIS

Acid-fast smears and biopsies are primary diagnostic methods

Laboratory diagnosis of lepromatous leprosy involves preparation of acid-fast stained scrapings of infected tissue, particularly nasal mucosa or ear lobes. Large numbers of acid-fast bacilli are seen. Tuberculoid leprosy is diagnosed clinically and by histologic appearance of full-thickness skin biopsies. PGL-1–based serologic tests have been evaluated for their usefulness in serodiagnosis. The specificity has been excellent, but the sensitivity for tuberculoid leprosy is still unsatisfactory. It is likely that suitable serologic tests will be available for this disease in the near future.

TREATMENT AND PREVENTION

Sulfones combined with rifampin primary treatment

Prevention requires early diagnosis and treatment of cases

Treatment has been revolutionized by the development of sulfones, such as dapsone, which blocks *para*-aminobenzoic acid metabolism in *M. leprae*. When combined with rifampin, dapsone usually controls or cures tuberculoid leprosy when given for 6 months. In lepromatous leprosy and multibacillary intermediate forms of the disease, a third agent (clofazimine) is added to help prevent the selection of resistant mutants, and treatment is continued at least 2 years. Prevention of leprosy involves recognition and treatment of infectious patients and early diagnosis of the disease in close contacts. Chemoprophylaxis with sulfones has been used for children in close contact with lepromatous cases. Immunization with BCG vaccine has been investigated, with varying results.

A possible diagnosis of leprosy elicits fear and distress in patients and contacts out of all proportion to its risks. Few clinicians in the United States have the experience to make such a diagnosis, and expert help should be sought from public health authorities before reaching this conclusion or indicating its possibility to the patient.

MYCOBACTERIA CAUSING TUBERCULOSIS-LIKE DISEASES

Mycobacteria causing diseases that often resemble tuberculosis are listed in Table 28–1. With the exception of *M. bovis,* they have become relatively more prominent as the incidence of tuberculosis has declined. All have known or suspected environmental reservoirs, and all the infections they cause appear to be acquired from these sources. Immunocompromised individuals or those with chronic pulmonary conditions or malignancies are more likely to develop disease. There is no evidence of case-to-case transmission. The organisms grow on the same media as *M. tuberculosis* but usually more rapidly. Colonies of some species produce yellow or orange pigment in the light (photochromogenic), and some in the light and dark (scotochromogenic). Species are distinguished by these characteristics and by biochemical reactions. Environmental mycobacteria that cause tuberculosis-like infections are usually more resistant than *M. tuberculosis* to some of the antimicrobics used in the treatment of mycobacterial diseases, and susceptibility testing is often needed as a guide to therapy.

Acquired from the environment; no case-to-case transmission

Some species are pigmented

Resistance common

Mycobacterium kansasii

Mycobacterium kansasii is a photochromogenic mycobacterium that usually forms yellow-pigmented colonies after about 2 weeks of incubation in the presence of light. In the United States, infection is most common in Illinois, Oklahoma, and Texas and tends to affect urban residents; it is uncommon in the Southeast. There is no evidence of case-to-case transmission, but the reservoir has yet to be identified. It causes about 3% of mycobacterial disease in the United States.

M. kansasii infections resemble tuberculosis and tend to be slowly progressive without treatment. Cavitary pulmonary disease, cervical lymphadenitis, and skin infections are most common, but disseminated infections also occur. They are an important cause of disease in patients with HIV infection and CD4+ T lymphocyte counts of less than 200 cells/μL; clinical features closely resemble tuberculosis in patients with AIDS. Hypersensitivity to proteins of *M. kansasii* develops and cross-reacts almost completely with that caused by tuberculosis. Positive PPD tests may thus result from clinical or subclinical *M. kansasii* infection. Prolonged combined chemotherapy with isoniazid, rifampin, and ethambutol is usually effective.

Resembles tuberculosis

Infection may cause PPD conversion

Mycobacterium avium–Intracellulare Complex

Mycobacterium avium–intracellulare complex is a group of related acid-fast organisms that grow only slightly faster than *M. tuberculosis* and can be divided into a number of serotypes. Among them are organisms that cause tuberculosis in birds (and sometimes swine) but rarely lead to disease in humans. Others may produce disease in mammals, including humans, but not in birds. They are found worldwide in soil and water and in infected animals. In the United States they are most common in the Southeast, Pacific Coast, and north central regions. They are second only to *M. tuberculosis* in significance and frequency of the diseases they cause.

M. avium-intracellulare complex associated with birds and mammals

Second only to *M. tuberculosis* as cause of disease in United States

The most common infection in humans is cavitary pulmonary disease, often superimposed on chronic bronchitis and emphysema. Most individuals infected are white men of 50 years of age or more. Cervical lymphadenitis, chronic osteomyelitis, and renal and skin infections also occur. The organisms in this group are substantially more resistant to antituberculous drugs than most other species, and treatment with the three or four agents

Wide range of diseases; most common are pulmonary

Relative resistance to antituberculous drugs

found to be most active often requires supplementation with surgery. About 20% of cases relapse within 5 years of treatment.

Disseminated infection is a common complication of AIDS

Organisms isolated from blood

Disseminated *M. avium–intracellulare* infections, once considered rare, are now the most common systemic bacterial infection in patients with AIDS. They usually develop when the patient's general clinical condition and CD4+ helper T lymphocyte concentrations are declining. Clinically, the patient experiences progressive weight loss and intermittent fever, chills, night sweats, and diarrhea. Histologically, granuloma formation is muted, and there are aggregates of foamy macrophages containing numerous intracellular acid-fast bacilli. The diagnosis is most readily made by blood culture, using a variety of specialized cultural techniques. Identification can be rapidly accomplished with the use of specific DNA probes. Response to chemotherapeutic agents is marginal, and the prognosis is grave.

Mycobacterium scrofulaceum

Granulomatous cervical lymphadenitis in children

Mycobacterium scrofulaceum is an acid-fast scotochromogen that occurs in the environment under moist conditions. It forms yellow colonies in the dark or light within 2 weeks, and it shares several features with the *M. avium–intracellulare* complex. *Mycobacterium scrofulaceum* is now one of the more common causes of granulomatous cervical lymphadenitis in young children. It derives its name from scrofula, an old descriptive term for tuberculous cervical lymphadenitis. The infection manifests as an indolent enlargement of one or more lymph nodes with little, if any, pain or constitutional signs. It may ulcerate or form a draining sinus to the surface. It does not cause PPD conversion. Treatment usually involves surgical excision.

MYCOBACTERIAL SOFT TISSUE INFECTIONS

Mycobacterium fortuitum Complex

Rapid growers cause abscesses and infections of prostheses

Mycobacterium fortuitum complex comprises free-living, rapidly growing, acid-fast bacilli that produce colonies within 3 days. Human infections are rare. Abscesses at injection sites in drug abusers are probably the most common lesions. Occasional secondary pulmonary infections develop. Some cases have been associated with implantation of foreign material (eg, breast prostheses, artificial heart valves). Except in the case of endocarditis, infections usually resolve spontaneously with removal of the prosthetic device.

Mycobacterium marinum

Cause of fish tuberculosis

Mycobacterium marinum causes tuberculosis in fish, is widely present in fresh and salt waters, and grows at 30°C but not at 37°C. It occurs in considerable numbers in the slime that forms on rocks or on rough walls of swimming pools and thrives in tropical fish aquariums. It can cause skin lesions in humans. Classically, a swimmer who abrades his or her elbows or forearms climbing out of a pool develops a superficial granulomatous lesion that finally ulcerates. It usually heals spontaneously after a few weeks but is sometimes chronic. The organism may be sensitive to tetracyclines as well as to some antituberculous drugs.

Mycobacterium ulcerans

Occurs in tropical areas

Severe, progressive ulcerations require surgical removal

Mycobacterium ulcerans is a much more serious cause of superficial infection. (Like *M. marinum, M. ulcerans* grows at 30°C but not at 37°C [see Table 28–1].) Cases usually occur in the tropics, most often in parts of Africa, New Guinea, and northern Australia, but have been seen elsewhere sporadically. Children are most often affected. The source of infection and mode of transmission are unknown. Infected individuals develop severe ulceration involving the skin and subcutaneous tissue that is often progressive unless treated effectively. Surgical excision and grafting are usually needed. Antimicrobic treatment is often unsuccessful.

ADDITIONAL READING

Advisory Council for the Elimination of Tuberculosis. Tuberculosis elimination revisited: Obstacles, opportunities, and a renewed commitment. *MMWR Morb Mortal Wkly Rep* 1999; 48(RR09);1–13. Review of the current status of tuberculosis in the United States, recognizing that additional diagnostic, therapeutic, and immunization tools will have to be developed to eradicate this disease.

Barnes PF, Bloch AB, Davidson PT, Snider DE Jr. Tuberculosis in patients with human immunodeficiency virus infection. *N Engl J Med* 1991;324:1644–1650. A recent review of the impact of one of humankind's newest scourges on one of its oldest.

Daniel TM. Antibody and antigen detection in the immunodiagnosis of tuberculosis. Why not? What more is needed? Where do we stand today? *J Infect Dis* 1988;158:678–680.

Dubos RJ, Dubos J. *The White Plague. Tuberculosis, Man, and Society*. Boston: Little, Brown; 1952. A scholarly and highly readable account of the history and impact of tuberculosis on Western culture.

Falkinham JO Jr. Epidemiology of infection by nontuberculous mycobacterium. *Clin Microbiol Rev* 1996;9:177–215.

Frieden TR, Sterling T, Pablos-Mendez A, Kilburn JO, Cauthen GM, Dooley SW. The emergence of drug-resistant tuberculosis in New York City. *N Engl J Med* 1993;328:521–526. A frightening look at the future.

Gaylord H, Brennan PJ. Leprosy and the leprosy bacillus. Recent developments in characterization of antigens and immunology of the disease. *Annu Rev Microbiol* 1987;41: 645–675.

Hastings RC, Gillis TP, Krahenbuhl JL, et al. Leprosy. *Clin Microbiol Rev* 1988; 1:330–348. The preceding two references are recent comprehensive reviews of this biblical disease, with an emphasis on its microbiology and immunology.

Interlied CB, Kemper CA, Bermudez LEM. The *Mycobacterium avium* complex. *Clin Microbiol Rev* 1993;6:266–310. A comprehensive review of all aspects of this increasingly important group including its role in AIDS patients.

Riley RL, Mills CC, O'Grady F, et al. Infectiousness of air from a tuberculosis ward. Ultraviolet irradiation of infected air: Comparative infectiousness of different patients. *Am Rev Resp Dis* 1962;85:511–525. This paper is the last in a series of "classic" studies exploring factors related to the aerial dissemination of tuberculosis. They demonstrated that infectivity varied greatly in different patients with similar pulmonary diseases, and that it decreased rapidly with the onset of chemotherapy. They also established that a patient with laryngeal tuberculosis was significantly more infectious than patients with cavitary pulmonary disease.

Schlossberg D (ed). *Tuberculosis and Nontuberculous Mycobacterial Infections,* 4th ed. Philadelphia: WB Saunders; 1999. A recent, excellent monograph covering all aspects of mycobacterial pathophysiology, pathogenesis, epidemiology, clinical manifestations, diagnosis, and treatment of mycobacterial infections.

Sepkowitz KA. How contagious is tuberculosis? *Clin Infect Dis* 1996;23:954–962. The author reviews and updates information on the contagiousness of pulmonary tuberculosis. This, in conjunction with Riley's articles, provides the most definitive information available.

Slutsker L, Castro KG, Ward JW, Dooley SW Jr. Epidemiology of extrapulmonary tuberculosis among persons with AIDS in the United States. *Clin Infect Dis* 1993; 16:513–518.

Tuberculosis Progress Report. *Lancet* 1999;353:995–1006. A compendium of articles on the worldwide status of tuberculosis, the impact of AIDS on its spread, and the implication of increasing antimicrobic resistance on its control.

van Crevel R, Ottenhoff THM, van der Meer JWM. Innate immunity to *Mycobacterium tuberculosis*. *Clin Microbiol Rev* 2002;15: 294–309. This review examines all aspects of the immune response to *M. tuberculosis* with particular emphasis on the roles of cytokines and chemokines.

Wolinsky E. Mycobacterial disease other than tuberculosis. *Clin Infect Dis* 1992; 15:1–12. A recent highly readable and comprehensive summary of the mycobacteria that have been termed "atypical" and of the clinical diseases they produce.

CHAPTER 29

Actinomyces and *Nocardia*

KENNETH J. RYAN

Actinomyces and *Nocardia* are Gram-positive rods characterized by filamentous, tree-like branching growth, which has caused them to be confused with fungi in the past. They are opportunists that can sometimes produce indolent, slowly progressive diseases. A related genus, *Streptomyces,* is of medical importance as a producer of many antibiotics, but it rarely causes infections. Important differential features of these groups and of the mycobacteria to which they are related are shown in Table 29–1.

ACTINOMYCES

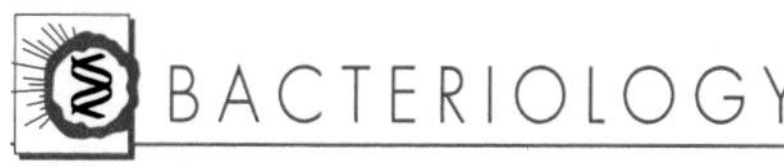

BACTERIOLOGY

Actinomyces are Gram-positive bacilli that grow slowly (4–10 days) under microaerophilic or strictly anaerobic conditions. The organisms typically appear as elongated Gram-positive rods that branch at acute angles and often show irregular staining. In pus the most characteristic form is the sulfur granule. This yellow–orange granule, named for its gross resemblance to a grain of sulfur, is a small colony (usually <0.3 mm) of intertwined branching *Actinomyces* filaments solidified with elements of tissue exudate.

Slow-growing anaerobic branching Gram-positive rods

Species of *Actinomyces* are distinguished on the basis of biochemical reactions, cultural features, and cell wall composition. Most human actinomycosis is caused by *Actinomyces israelii,* but other species have been isolated from typical actinomycotic lesions. *Propionibacterium propionicum* originally classified with the *Actinomyces,* can produce clinically similar disease. Other species of *Actinomyces* have been associated with dental and periodontal infections (see Chapter 62).

Most infections due to *A. israelii*

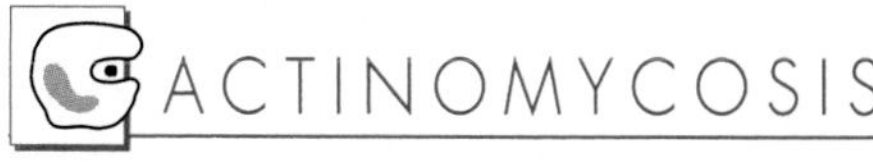

ACTINOMYCOSIS

CLINICAL CAPSULE

Actinomycosis is a chronic inflammatory condition originating in the tissues adjacent to mucosal surfaces. The lesions follow a slow burrowing course with considerable induration and draining sinuses eventually opening through the skin. The exact nature depends on the organs and structures involved.

TABLE 29-1

Features of Actinomycetes

Genus	Morphology	Acid Fastness	Growth	Source	Disease
Actinomyces	Branching bacilli	None	Anaerobic	Oral, intestinal endogenous flora	Chronic cellulitis, draining sinuses
Nocardia	Branching bacilli	Weak[a,b]	Aerobic	Soil	Pneumonia, skin pustules, brain abscess
Rhodococcus	Cocci to bacilli	Variable (weak[a])	Aerobic	Soil, horses[c]	Pneumonia
Streptomyces	Branching bacilli	None	Aerobic	Soil	Extremely rare[d]

[a] Modified stain, fast only to weak decolorizer (1% H_2SO_4).

[b] *N. asteroides* and *N. brasiliensis*; other species variable.

[c] *R. equi.*

[d] Nonpathogen but important producer of antibiotics.

Normal flora throughout gastrointestinal tract

Conditions for growth require displacement into tissues

Sinus tracts contain pus and sulfur granules

Actinomyces are normal inhabitants of some areas of the gastrointestinal tract of humans and animals from the oropharynx to the lower bowel. These species are highly adapted to mucosal surfaces and do not produce disease unless they transgress the epithelial barrier under conditions that produce a sufficiently low oxygen tension for their multiplication. Such conditions usually involve mechanical disruption of the mucosa with necrosis of deeper, normally sterile tissues (eg, following tooth extraction). Once initiated, growth occurs in microcolonies in the tissues and extends without regard to anatomic boundaries. The lesion is composed of inflammatory sinuses, which ultimately discharge to the surface. As the lesion enlarges, it becomes firm and indurated. Sulfur granules are present within the pus but are not numerous. Free *Actinomyces* or small branching units are rarely seen, although contaminating Gram-negative rods are common. As with other anaerobic infections (see Chapter 19) most cases are polymicrobial involving other flora from the mucosal site of origin.

No evidence of immunity

Human cases provide little evidence of immunity to *Actinomyces*. Once established, infections typically become chronic and resolve only with the aid of antimicrobic therapy. Antibodies can be detected in the course of infection but seem to reflect the antigenic stimulation of the ongoing infection rather than immunity. Infections with *Actinomyces* are endogenous, and case-to-case transmission does not appear to occur.

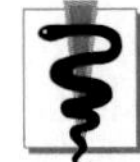

ACTINOMYCOSIS: CLINICAL ASPECTS

MANIFESTATIONS

Cervicofacial forms are linked to dental hygiene

Actinomycosis exists in several forms that differ according to the original site and circumstances of tissue invasion. Infection of the cervicofacial area, the most common site of actinomycosis (Fig 29–1), is usually related to poor dental hygiene, tooth extraction, or some other trauma to the mouth or jaw. Lesions in the submandibular region and the angle of the jaw give the face a swollen, indurated appearance.

Surgery, trauma, and intrauterine devices provide opportunity

Thoracic and abdominal actinomycoses are rare and follow aspiration or traumatic (including surgical) introduction of infected material leading to erosion through the pleura, chest, or abdominal wall. Diagnosis is usually delayed, because only vague or nonspecific symptoms are produced until a vital organ is eroded or obstructed. The firm, fibrous masses are often initially mistaken for a malignancy. Pelvic involvement as an extension from other sites also occurs occasionally. It is particularly difficult to distinguish

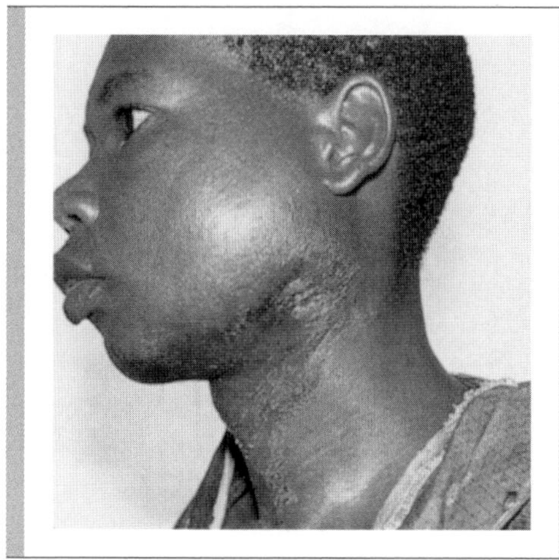

FIGURE 29–1
Cervicofacial actinomycosis. Note the "lumpy jaw" swelling and the draining sinuses at the angle of the jaw. *(Reproduced with permission from Connor DH, Chandler FW, Schwartz DQA, Manz HJ, Lack EE (eds).* Pathology of Infectious Diseases, *vol. 1 Stamford, CT: Appleton & Lange; 1997.)*

from other inflammatory conditions or malignancies. A more localized chronic endometritis, apparently caused by *Actinomyces*, has been associated with the use of intrauterine contraceptive devices.

DIAGNOSIS

A clinical diagnosis of actinomycosis is based on the nature of the lesion, the slowly progressive course, and a history of trauma or of a condition predisposing to mucosal invasion by *Actinomyces*. The etiologic diagnosis can be difficult to establish with certainty. Although the lesions may be extensive, the organisms in pus may be few and concentrated in sulfur granule microcolonies deep in the indurated tissue. The diagnosis is further complicated by heavy colonization of the moist draining sinuses with other bacteria, usually Gram-negative rods. This contamination not only causes confusion regarding the etiology but interferes with isolation of the slow-growing anaerobic *Actinomyces*. Material for direct smear and culture should include as much pus as possible to increase the chance of collecting the diagnostic sulfur granules.

Sinus drainage contains few *Actinomyces*

Drainage is often contaminated with other species

Sulfur granules crushed and stained show a dense, Gram-positive center with individual branching rods at the periphery (Fig 29–2). Granules should also be selected for culture, because material randomly taken from a draining sinus usually grows only superficial contaminants. Culture media and techniques are the same as those used for other anaerobes (see Chapters 15 and 19). Incubation must be prolonged, because some strains require 7 days or more to appear. Identification requires a variety of biochemical tests to differentiate *Actinomyces* from propionibacteria (anaerobic diphtheroids), which may show a tendency to form short branches in fluid culture.

Gram stains show branching rods

Anaerobic culture is required

Biopsies for culture and histopathology are useful, but it may be necessary to examine many sections and pieces of tissue before sulfur granule colonies of *Actinomyces* are found. The morphology of the sulfur granule in tissue is quite characteristic with routine hematoxylin and eosin (HE) or histologic Gram staining. With HE, the edge of the granule shows amorphous eosinophilic "clubs" formed from the tissue elements and containing the branching actinomycotic filaments.

Biopsy shows characteristic clubbed lesions

TREATMENT

Penicillin G is the treatment of choice for actinomycosis, although a number of other antimicrobics (tetracycline, erythromycin, clindamycin) are active in vitro and have shown some clinical effectiveness. High doses of penicillin must be used and therapy prolonged for 4 to 6 weeks or longer before any response is seen. Although slow, response to therapy is often striking given the degree of fibrosis and deformity caused by the infection. Because detection of the causative organism is difficult, many patients are treated empirically as a therapeutic trial based on clinical findings alone.

Penicillin may have to be used empirically

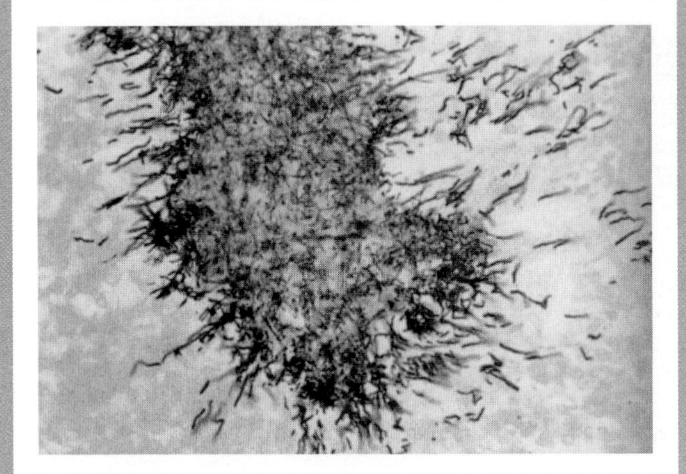

FIGURE 29–2
Sulfur granule. The bacteria are clearly seen to be Gram-positive and branching only at the edge. *(Reproduced with permission from Connor DH, Chandler FW, Schwartz DQA, Manz HJ, Lack EE (eds).* Pathology of Infectious Diseases, *vol. 1 Stamford, CT: Appleton & Lange; 1997.)*

Nocardia

BACTERIOLOGY

Beaded, branching Gram-positive rods are weakly acid fast

Nocardia species are Gram-positive, rod-shaped bacteria that show true branching both in culture and in stains from clinical lesions. The microscopic morphology is similar to that of *Actinomyces,* although *Nocardia* tend to fragment more readily and are found as shorter branched units throughout the lesion rather than concentrated in a few colonies or granules. Many strains take the Gram stain poorly, appearing "beaded" with alternating Gram-positive and Gram-negative sections of the same filament (Fig 29–3). The species most common in human infection (*N. asteroides* and *N. brasiliensis*) are weakly acid fast.

Grow on common media in 2–3 days

In contrast to *Actinomyces, Nocardia* species are strict aerobes. Growth typically appears on ordinary laboratory medium (blood agar) after 2 to 3 days incubation in air. Colonies initially have a dry, wrinkled, chalk-like appearance, are adherent to the agar, and eventually develop white to orange pigment. Speciation involves uncommon tests such as the decomposition amino acids and casein.

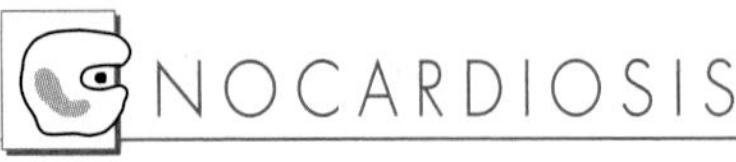

NOCARDIOSIS

CLINICAL CAPSULE

Nocardiosis occurs in two major forms. The pulmonary form is an acute bronchopneumonia with dyspnea, cough and sputum production. A cutaneous form produces localized pustules in areas of traumatic inoculation usually the exposed areas of the skin.

EPIDEMIOLOGY

Primary source is soil

Occurrence in the immunocompromised is increased

Nocardia species are ubiquitous in the environment, particularly in soil. In fact, fully developed colonies of *Nocardia* give off the aroma of wet dirt. The organisms have been isolated in small numbers from the respiratory tract of healthy persons, but are not considered members of the normal flora. The pulmonary form of disease follows inhalation of aerosolized bacteria, and the cutaneous form follows injection by a thorn prick or similar accident. The majority of pulmonary cases occur in patients with compromised immune systems due to underlying disease or the use of immunosuppressive therapy.

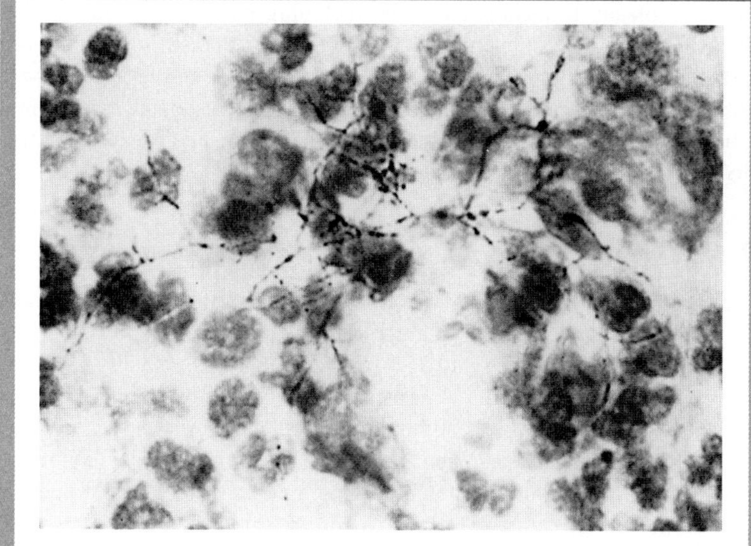

FIGURE 29–3
Nocardia in sputum. Note the filamentous bacteria forming treelike branches among the neutrophils. The beaded appearance of the rods is typical. (*Reprinted with permission of Schering Corporation, Kenilworth, NJ, the copyright owner. All rights reserved.*)

Transplant patients have been a prominent representative of the latter group. There is no case-to-case transmission.

PATHOGENESIS

Factors leading to disease following inhalation of *Nocardia* are poorly understood. Neutrophils are prominent in nocardial lesions but appear to be relatively ineffective. The bacteria have the ability to resist the microbicidal actions of phagocytes and may be related to disruption of phagosome acidification or resistance to the oxidative burst. No specific virulence factors are known. The primary lesions in the lung show acute inflammation, with suppuration and destruction of parenchyma. Multiple, confluent abscesses may occur. Unlike *Actinomyces* infections, there is little tendency toward fibrosis and localization. Dissemination to distant organs, particularly the brain, may occur. In the central nervous system (CNS), multifocal abscesses are often produced. The great majority of *Nocardia* pulmonary and brain infections are produced by *N. asteroides.*

Able to survive in phagocytes

Pulmonary infection is usually *N. asteroides*

CNS dissemination produces abscesses

Skin infections follow direct inoculation of *Nocardia.* This mechanism is usually associated with some kind of outdoor activity and with relatively minor trauma. The species is usually *N. brasiliensis*, which produces a superficial pustule at the site of inoculation. If *Nocardia* gain access to the subcutaneous tissues, lesions resembling actinomycosis may be produced, complete with draining sinuses and sulfur granules. This infection may occur with *Nocardia* species or related organisms such as *Actinomadura madurae* (formerly *Nocardia madurae*), a cause of the mycetoma syndrome (see Chapter 47).

Cutaneous infections follow minor trauma

IMMUNITY

There is evidence that effective T cell–mediated immunity is dominant in host defense against *Nocardia* infection. Increased resistance to experimental *Nocardia* infection in animals has been mediated by cytokine-activated macrophages, and activated macrophages have enhanced capacity to kill *Nocardia* that they have engulfed. Patients with impaired cell-mediated immune responses are at greatest risk for nocardiosis. There is little evidence for effective humoral immune responses.

Cell-mediated immunity mechanisms are dominant

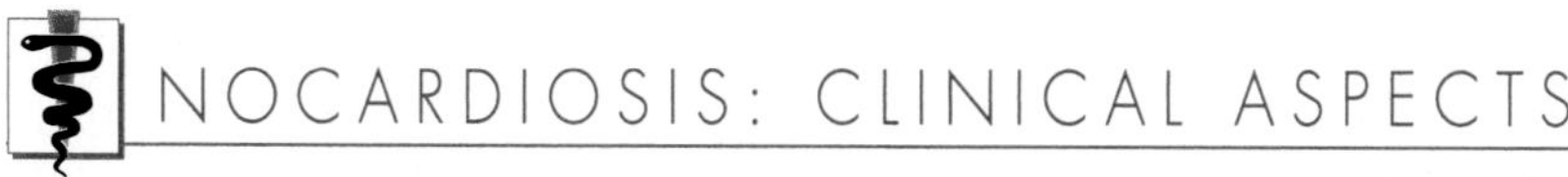

NOCARDIOSIS: CLINICAL ASPECTS

MANIFESTATIONS

Pulmonary infection is usually a confluent bronchopneumonia that may be acute, chronic, or relapsing. Production of cavities and extension to the pleura are common. Symptoms are those of any bronchopneumonia, including cough, dyspnea, and fever. The clinical signs of brain abscess depend on its exact location and size; the neurologic picture can be particularly confusing when multiple lesions are present. The combination of current or recent pneumonia and focal CNS signs is suggestive of *Nocardia* infection. The cutaneous syndrome typically involves a pustule, fever, and tender lymphadenitis in the regional lymph nodes.

Bronchopneumonia and cerebral abscess findings depend on localization

DIAGNOSIS

The diagnosis of *Nocardia* infection is much easier than that of actinomycosis, because the organisms are present in greater numbers throughout the lesions. Filaments of Gram-positive rods with primary and secondary branches can usually be found in sputum and are readily demonstrated in direct aspirates from skin or other purulent sites. Demonstration of acid-fastness, when combined with other observations, is diagnostic of *N. asteroides* or *N. brasiliensis*. The acid-fastness of *Nocardia* species is not as strong as that of mycobacteria. The staining method thus employs a decolorizing agent weaker than that used for the classic stain. Culture of *Nocardia* is not difficult, because the organisms grow on blood agar. It is still important to alert the laboratory to the possibility of nocardiosis, because the slow growth of *Nocardia* could cause it to be overgrown by the respiratory flora commonly found in sputum specimens. Specific identification can take weeks due the unconventional tests involved.

Gram stain is usually positive

Weak acid fastness is characteristic

Blood agar is sufficient for culture

TREATMENT

Nocardia are usually susceptible to sulfonamide, but relatively resistant to penicillin. The trimethoprim–sulfamethoxazole combination is the most widely used chemotherapeutic regimen. Technical difficulties in susceptibility testing have hampered the rational selection and study of other antimicrobics, but various reports support clinical activity of newer β-lactams (imipenem, ceftriaxone), minocycline, and aminoglycosides. Antituberculous agents and antifungal agents such as amphotericin B have no activity against *Nocardia*.

Sulfonamides are active

RHODOCOCCUS

Rhodococcus is a genus of aerobic actinomycetes with characteristics similar to those of *Nocardia.* Morphologically the rods vary from cocci to long, curved, clubbed forms. Some strains are acid-fast. *Rhodococcus* has recently been recognized as an opportunistic pathogen causing an aggressive pneumonia in severely immunocompromised patients, particularly those with acquired immunodeficiency syndrome. The organisms are found in the soil. One species, *Rhodococcus equi,* has an association with horses where it also causes pneumonia in foals. This species is a facultative intracellular pathogen of macrophages with features somewhat similar to those of *Legionella* and *Listeria*. Optimal treatment is unknown, although erythromycin, aminoglycosides, and some β-lactams show in vitro activity.

Morphology varies from cocci to rods

Pneumonia is associated with horses

ADDITIONAL READING

Lerner PI. Nocardiosis. *Clin Infect Dis* 1996;22:891–905.

Smego RA, Foglia G. Actinomycosis. *Clin Infect Dis* 1998;26:1255–1263.

Both these reviews are part of the “State-of-the-Art Clinical Article” series. They consider pathogenesis as well as clinical aspects and are well referenced.

CHAPTER 30

Chlamydia

W. LAWRENCE DREW

Members of the genus *Chlamydia* are obligate intracellular bacteria, which have all the elements of bacteria except a rigid cell wall. Of the three species causing disease in humans, *Chlamydia trachomatis* is the most common as a major cause of genital infection and conjunctivitis. A chronic form of *C. trachomatis* conjunctivitis, called trachoma, is the leading preventable cause of blindness in the world. *Chlamydia pneumoniae* and *Chlamydia psittaci* are respiratory pathogens. Our knowledge of biology and pathogenesis of these bacteria is based primarily on the study of *C. trachomatis*.

CHLAMYDIA TRACHOMATIS

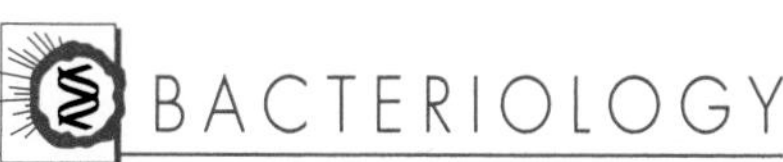

BACTERIOLOGY

MORPHOLOGY

C. trachomatis are round cells between 0.3 and 1 μm in diameter depending on the replicative stage (see below). The envelope surrounding the cells includes a trilaminar outer membrane that contains lipopolysaccharide and proteins similar to those of Gram-negative bacteria. A major difference is that chlamydiae lack the thin peptidoglycan layer between the two membranes. They are obligate intracellular parasites and have not been grown outside eukaryotic cells. The genome of is one of the smallest among prokaryotes and lacks genes for amino acid synthesis. *C. trachomatis* has ribosomes and is able to carry out the common energy producing pathways of other bacteria.

Envelope has no peptidoglycan layer between membranes

Obligate intracellular bacteria, which fail to grow in artificial media

DNA homology between *C. trachomatis, C. psittaci,* and *C. pneumoniae* is less than 30%, although rRNA sequence analysis suggests they share a common origin. The three species share a common group antigen. Their major differential features are shown in Table 30–1. Two biovars of *C. trachomatis* affect humans: trachoma and lymphogranuloma venereum (LGV). *C. trachomatis* has multiple outer membrane proteins that further divide the biovars into multiple serovars, or strains (Table 30–2).

REPLICATIVE CYCLE

The replicative cycle of chlamydiae is illustrated in Figure 30–1. It involves two forms of the organism: a small, hardy infectious form termed the elementary body (EB), and a larger fragile intracellular replicative form termed the reticulate body (RB). The major difference

Elementary body enters epithelial cells by endocytosis

TABLE 30–1

Major Differential Features of Chlamydia Species that Cause Human Disease

FEATURE	*C. TRACHOMATIS*	*C. PSITTACI*	*C. PNEUMONIAE*
Natural host	Humans	Birds; also livestock, cats	Humans
Disease	Conjunctivitis, pneumonia (infants), genital tract infections, lymphogranuloma venereum	Pneumonia, endocarditis	Bronchitis, pneumonia, ?atherosclerosis
Glycogen-containing inclusion bodies	Yes	No	No
Sulfonamide susceptibility	Yes	No	No

between the EB and the RB is the extent of cross-linking of the major outer membrane protein (MOMP); EB proteins are highly linked by disulfide bonds, and RBs less so. The EB is a metabolically inert form which neither expends energy nor synthesizes protein. The cycle begins when the EB attaches to unknown receptors on the plasma membrane of susceptible target cells (usually columnar or transitional epithelial cells). It then enters the cell in an endocytotic vacuole and begins the process of converting to the replicative RB. There is evidence that pinocytosis may also occur. Endosomes containing *C. trachomatis* EBs maintain a near neutral pH and fuse with each other but not with lysosomes. As the RBs increase in number, the endosomal membrane expands by fusing with lipids of the Golgi apparatus eventually forming a large inclusion body. After 24 to 72 hours, the process reverses and the RBs reorganize and condense to yield multiple EBs. The endosomal membrane then either disintegrates or fuses with the host cell membrane, releasing the EBs to infect adjacent cells. The metabolic changes that lead the EB to reorganize into the larger reticulate body are incompletely understood, but involve protein synthesis and modification of MOMPs between the monomeric and cross-linked state. *C. trachomatis* also inhibits apoptosis of epithelial cells, thus enabling completion of its replicative cycle.

Host cell metabolism used for growth and replication

Transiently inhibits apoptosis of infected cells

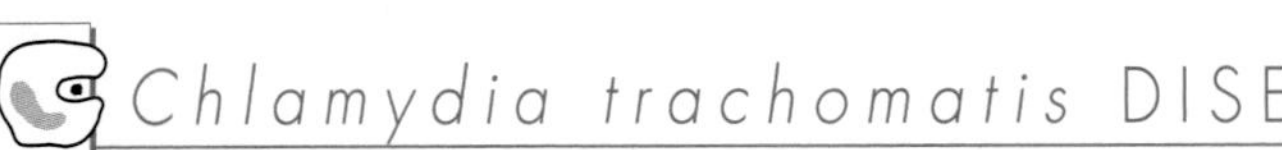

Chlamydia trachomatis DISEASES

CLINICAL CAPSULE

Ocular trachoma, with progressive inflammation and scarring leading to blindness, has been recognized since antiquity, but the role of *Chlamydiae* in conjunctivitis and pneumonia in young infants, and in a variety of genital infections was only clarified during the past 40 years. Like trachoma, the genital infections can persist or recur, with chronic sequelae.

TABLE 30–2

Epidemiologic Associations between Chlamydial Species, Serovars (Strains), and Diseases

SPECIES	SEROVARS (STRAINS)	MODES OF TRANSMISSION	DISEASES
C. trachomatis	A,B,Ba,C	Hand to eye, fomites, flies	Trachoma
	B,Ba,D–K	Sexual, intrapartum, hand to eye	Inclusion conjunctivitis; genital infection
	L_1,L_2,L_3	Sexual	Lymphogranuloma venereum
C. psittaci	Many	Aerosol	Psittacosis
C. pneumoniae	TWAR[a]	Human to human	Respiratory infection

[a] TW and AR were the laboratory designations for the first conjunctival and respiratory isolates, respectively.

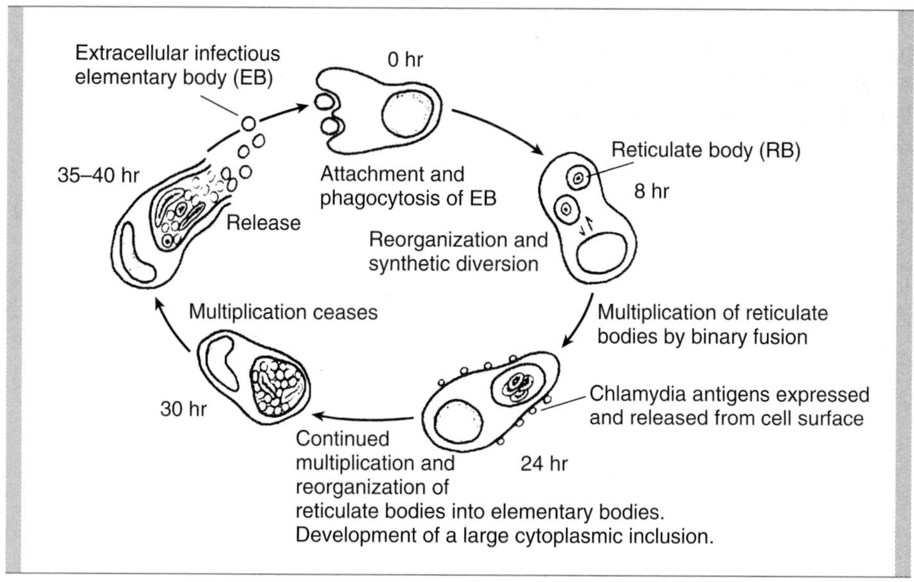

FIGURE 30–1
Reproduction cycle of *Chlamydia.*

EPIDEMIOLOGY

C. trachomatis causes disease in several sites, including the conjunctiva and genital tract. It is spread by secretions and is the most common sexually transmitted disease. In the United States over 700,000 cases are reported each year, which is twice the number for gonorrhea. Humans are the sole reservoir (see Table 30–1). Each of the major disease syndromes caused by chlamydiae are associated with several different strains (see Table 30–2). Inclusion conjunctivitis is seen among population groups in which the strains causing *C. trachomatis* genital infections are common. This disease is the most common form of neonatal conjunctivitis in the United States, occurring in 2 to 6% of newborn infants. The infection results from direct contact with infective cervical secretions of the mother at delivery.

Neonatal conjunctivitis contracted from maternal genital infection

High attack rate

Trachoma, a chronic follicular conjunctivitis, afflicts an estimated 500 million persons worldwide and has blinded millions, particularly in Africa. The disease is usually contracted in infancy or early childhood from the mother or other close contacts. Spread is by contact with infective human secretions, directly via hands to the eye, or via fomites transmitted on the feet of flies.

Fomites, fingers, and flies involved in transmission of trachoma

The prevalence of chlamydial urethral infection in US men and women ranges from 5% in the general population to 20% in those attending sexually transmitted disease clinics. Approximately one third of male sexual contacts of women with *C. trachomatis* cervicitis develop urethritis after an incubation period of 2 to 6 weeks. The proportion of men with mild to absent symptoms is higher than in gonorrhea. Nongonococcal urethritis is most commonly caused by *C. trachomatis* and less frequently by *Ureaplasma urealyticum*. Reinfection is common.

High rate of sexual transmission

PATHOGENESIS

Chlamydiae have a tropism for epithelial cells of the endocervix and upper genital tract of women, and the urethra, rectum and conjunctiva of both sexes. The LGV biovar can also enter through breaks in the skin or mucosa. Once infection is established, there is a release of proinflammatory cytokines such as interleukin-8 by infected epithelial cells. Chlamydial lipopolysaccharides probably also play an important role in initiation of the inflammatory process. This results in early tissue infiltration by polymorphonuclear leukocytes, later followed by lymphocytes, macrophages, plasma cells and eosinophils. If the infection progresses further (because of lack of treatment and/or failure of immune control), aggregates of lymphocytes and macrophages (lymphoid follicles) may form in the submucosa; these can progress to necrosis, followed by fibrosis and scarring.

Early release of proinflammatory cytokines

Later development of fibrosis and scarring

Persistent or recurrent infections cause chronic eye or genital sequelae

Autoimmunity may play an important role

The chronic sequelae of progressive inflammation with scarring that are seen in trachoma and some female genital tract infections are commonly due to persistent or recurrent infections, which may, in turn, be controlled by host cell immune responses. One theory is that this may result from molecular mimicry, involving epitopes found on the chlamydial 60-kd heat shock protein and also on human cells.

IMMUNITY

Immunity is short-lived

Secretory IgA and CD4+ lymphocytes may influence severity

C. trachomatis infections do not reliably result in protection against reinfection although there is evidence that secretory immunoglobulin A may confer at least some partial immunity against genital tract reinfection. Any strain-specific protection that may result is short-lived. Local production of antibody, along with CD4+ lymphocytes of the Th1 type that traffic to the genital mucosa may together play a role in mitigating most acute infections. This would at least partially explain why most untreated chlamydial genital tract infections are persistent, but often subclinical in character.

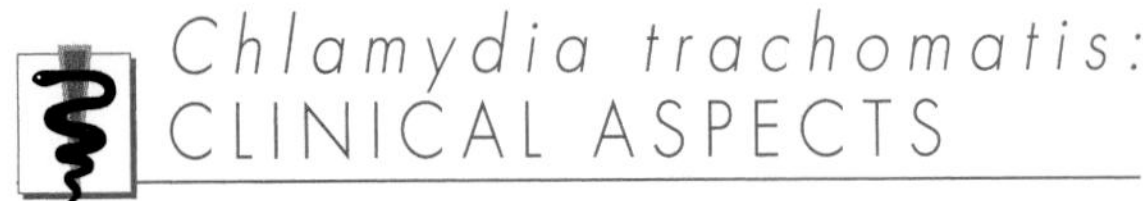

Chlamydia trachomatis: CLINICAL ASPECTS

MANIFESTATIONS

Eye Infections

Trachoma and inclusion conjunctivitis due to different serotypes

Trachoma and inclusion conjunctivitis are distinct diseases of the eye that have some overlap in their clinical manifestations. Trachoma, a chronic conjunctivitis caused by *C. trachomatis* strains A, B, Ba, and C, is usually seen in less developed countries and often leads to blindness. Inclusion conjunctivitis, an acute infection commonly caused by strains D to K, is usually not associated with chronicity or permanent eye damage. It occurs in newborns and adults worldwide.

Trachoma

Leading cause of blindness in some developing countries

Chronic inflammation of the eyelids and increased vascularization of the corneal conjunctiva are followed by severe corneal scarring and conjunctival deformities. Visual loss often occurs 15 to 20 years after the initial infection, due to repeated scarring of the cornea.

Inclusion Conjunctivitis

Smears or cultures from conjunctiva diagnostic

Inclusion conjunctivitis usually presents as an acute, copious, mucopurulent eye discharge 5 to 25 days after birth. Infection occurs in roughly two thirds of infants born vaginally to infected mothers, and one third of these become overtly ill. Inclusion conjunctivitis is clinically similar but less common in adults, and is usually associated with concomitant genital tract disease. Diagnosis can be made by demonstrating characteristic cytoplasmic inclusions in smears of conjunctival scrapings (Fig 30–2), by demonstration of antigen by direct immunofluorescence, or by culture from conjunctival swabs. Systemic therapy is preferred because the nasopharynx, rectum, and vagina may also be colonized and other forms of disease may develop, such as an infant pneumonia syndrome.

Genital Infections

Clinical spectrum is similar to *N. gonorrhoeae*

The clinical spectrum of sexually transmitted infections with *C. trachomatis* is similar to that of *Neisseria gonorrhoeae*. *C. trachomatis* can cause urethritis and epididymitis in men and cervicitis, salpingitis, and a urethral syndrome in women. In addition, three strains of *C. trachomatis* cause LGV, another sexually transmitted disease (see Table 30–2).

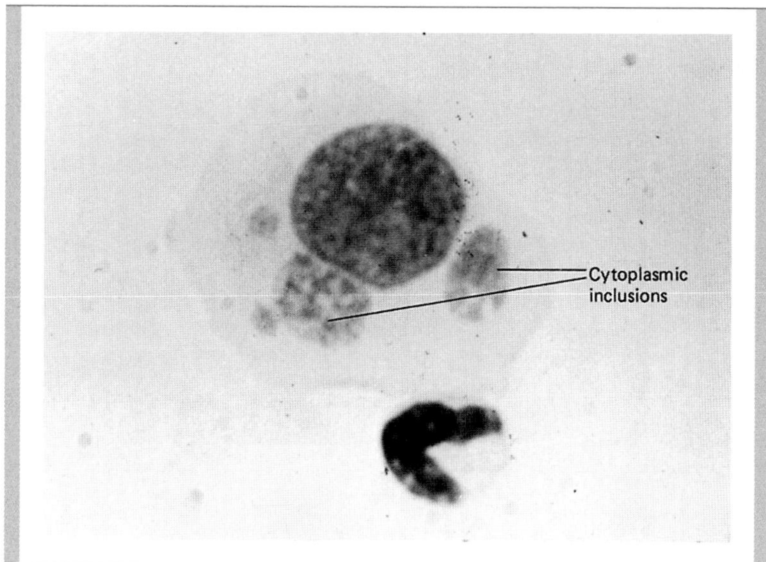

FIGURE 30–2
Chlamydia trachomatis cytoplasmic inclusion bodies in a conjunctival epithelial cell.

C. trachomatis urethritis is manifested by dysuria and a thin urethral discharge. Infections of the uterine cervix may produce vaginal discharge but are usually asymptomatic. Ascending infection in the form of salpingitis and pelvic inflammatory disease occurs in an estimated 5 to 30% of infected women. The scarring produced by chronic or repeated infection is an important cause of sterility and ectopic pregnancy.

Urethritis in men, but many asymptomatic

Salpingitis and pelvic inflammatory disease can cause permanent sequelae

More than 50% of all infants born to mothers excreting *C. trachomatis* during labor show evidence of infection during the first year of life. Most develop inclusion conjunctivitis (see earlier discussion), but 5 to 10% develop an infant pneumonia syndrome. *C. trachomatis* accounts for about one third to one half of all cases of interstitial pneumonia in infants. The illness usually develops between 6 weeks and 6 months of age and has a gradual onset. The child is usually afebrile, but develops difficulty in feeding, a characteristic staccato (pertussis-like) cough, and shortness of breath. The disease is rarely fatal but may be associated with decreased pulmonary function later in life.

Infant pneumonia syndrome has delayed, gradual onset

LGV is a sexually transmitted infection caused by *C. trachomatis* strains L_1, L_2, or L_3. It occurs principally in South America and Africa, although small outbreaks have recently occurred in North America. The clinical course is characterized by transient genital lesions followed by multilocular suppurative involvement of the inguinal lymph nodes. The primary genital lesion is usually a small painless ulcer or papule, which heals in a few days and may go unnoticed. The most common presenting complaint is inguinal adenopathy. Nodes are initially discrete, but as the disease progresses they become matted and suppurative (bubos). The skin over the node may be thinned, and multiple draining fistulas develop. Systemic symptoms such as fever, chills, headaches, arthralgia, and myalgia are common. Late complications include urethral or rectal strictures and perirectal abscesses and fistulas. In homosexual men, LGV strains can cause a hemorrhagic ulcerative proctitis. Lymph nodes may need to be aspirated to prevent rupture. A further consideration of genital tract infections is given in Chapter 70.

Papule and inguinal adenopathy

Abscesses, strictures, and fistulas with chronic infection

DIAGNOSIS

All direct *C. trachomatis* diagnostic tests require the collection of epithelial cells from the site of infection. Inflammatory cells are not useful and should be cleaned away as much as possible. For genital infections, cervical specimens are preferred in females and urethral scrapings in males. Eye infections require conjunctival scrapings.

Epithelial cells are required for detection

Isolation of *C. trachomatis* has been the "gold standard" for diagnosis. It is achieved in cell culture using idoxuridine- or cycloheximide-treated McCoy cells. Treatment of the cells with antimetabolites inhibits host cell replication but allows chlamydiae to use available cell nutrients for growth. After inoculation with samples and incubation for 3 to 7 days, the cells

Isolation requires special treatment of cell lines

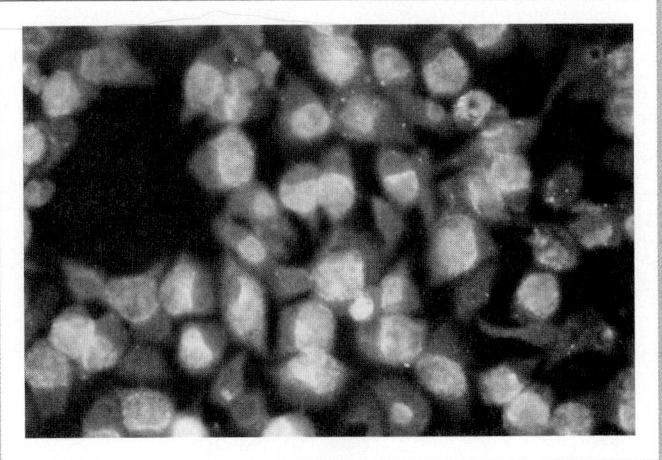

FIGURE 30–3
Chlamydia trachomatis cytoplasmic inclusions in tissue culture stained with fluorescein-labeled monoclonal antibodies. (*Reproduced with permission from Connor DH, Chandler FW, Schwartz DQA, Manz HJ, Lack EE (eds).* Pathology of Infectious Diseases, *vol. 1. Stamford, CT: Appleton & Lange; 1997.*)

C. trachomatis inclusions contain glycogen and are stainable with iodine

are stained with fluorescein-labeled monoclonal antibodies to detect intracytoplasmic chlamydiae (Fig 30–3). *C. trachomatis* reticulate bodies synthesize large amounts of glycogen, and the inclusion bodies in the cell thus stain reddish-brown with iodine. *C. psittaci* and *C. pneumoniae* inclusions do not contain glycogen.

LCR or PCR are most sensitive methods of noncultural diagnosis

A large number of procedures are now available for noncultural direct detection of *C. trachomatis* in clinical specimens. These include direct fluorescent antibody (DFA) methods using monoclonal antibodies directed against outer membrane proteins of elementary bodies in epithelial cells, enzyme immunoassays that detect chlamydial lipopolysaccharide, and assays for *C. trachomatis* DNA. These tests are faster, and, in the case of DNA assays, also more sensitive than culture. Ligase chain reaction (LCR) or polymerase chain reaction (PCR) are the most sensitive methods of diagnosis. The latter procedures can be used on urine samples, which are easier to obtain than cervical or urethral samples. This greatly aids the detection of chlamydial genital infections, especially in adolescents, and ultimately facilitates control of the spread of this sexually transmitted disease.

Serodiagnosis not helpful for most genital infections

Serodiagnostic methods have little use in diagnosis of chlamydial genital infection because of the difficulty of distinguishing current from previous infection. Detection of IgM antibodies against *C. trachomatis* is helpful in cases of infant pneumonitis. Chlamydial serology is also useful in the diagnosis of LGV, where a single high complement fixation antibody titer (>1:32) or a fourfold rise supports a presumptive diagnosis. The most satisfactory method for diagnosis of LGV is isolation of an LGV strain of *C. trachomatis* from aspirated bubos or tissue biopsies. In 80 to 90% of patients, the LGV complement fixation test is positive (titer > 1:64) shortly after the appearance of the bubo.

TREATMENT

Effective antimicrobics include erythromycin, azithromycin, and doxycycline

Strains of *C. trachomatis* are sensitive to tetracyclines, macrolides and related compounds, and some fluoroquinolones. Azithromycin is given as a single oral dose for non-LGV *C. trachomatis* infection. Erythromycin is used for pregnant women and infants because of the tooth staining that may result from tetracycline therapy and less experience with the newer agents. Doxycycline is an alternative for *C. trachomatis* and is the drug of choice for treating LGV.

Prevention of reinfection most important control measure

For trachoma, a single dose of azithromycin is now the treatment of choice, although a tetracycline for 14 days is an alternative. Corrective surgery may prevent blindness and is required for severe corneal and conjunctival scarring. Control of trachoma is directed toward prevention of continued reinfection during early childhood. Improvement in general hygienic practices is the most important factor in decreasing transmission of infection within families and, of course, one of the most difficult to implement on a broad scale.

PREVENTION

Prophylaxis for infants using topical erythromycin or silver nitrate on the conjunctiva has limited effectiveness for *Chlamydia,* because 15 to 25% of exposed infants still develop inclusion conjunctivitis. The primary approach to prevention of all forms of genital and infant *C. trachomatis* infection comprises detection of this infection in sexually active individuals and appropriate treatment, including infected women late in pregnancy. No vaccine is available or under development.

Primary approach is detection and treatment of infection in high-risk individuals

No vaccine available

CHLAMYDIA PSITTACI

EPIDEMIOLOGY

Human psittacosis (ornithosis) is a zoonotic pneumonia contracted through inhalation of respiratory secretions or dust from droppings of infected birds. It was initially described in psittacines, such as parrots and parakeets, but was subsequently shown to occur in a wide range of avian species, including turkeys. Human infections have also been linked to livestock and cat reservoirs. The disease is usually latent in its natural host but may become active, particularly with the stress of recent captivity or transport; *C. psittaci* is then excreted in large amounts.

Pneumonia contracted from birds

Psittacosis in humans is seen mainly as an occupational hazard of poultry workers and bird fanciers, particularly owners of psittacine birds. Reported cases of human psittacosis in the United States decreased during the 1950s, in association with the use of antimicrobials in poultry feeds and quarantine regulations for imported psittacine birds. Currently 100 to 200 cases are reported each year. Some strains of *C. psittaci* are highly contagious and pose a hazard for laboratory workers processing specimens for *C. psittaci* isolation.

Associated with poultry processing and captive psittacine birds

CLINICAL DISEASE AND TREATMENT

Psittacosis in humans is an acute infection of the lower respiratory tract, usually presenting with acute onset of fever, headache, malaise, muscle aches, dry hacking cough, and bilateral interstitial pneumonia. Occasionally, systemic complications such as myocarditis, encephalitis, endocarditis, and hepatitis may develop. The liver and spleen are often enlarged. The diagnosis of psittacosis should be suspected in any patient with acute onset of febrile lower respiratory illness who gives a history of close exposure to birds. Indeed, a history of bird exposure should be especially sought in patients who appear to have a bilateral pneumonia not proven to be caused by other agents. It must be remembered that spread can occur from both symptomatic and asymptomatic infections of birds. The specific diagnosis is usually made by demonstrating seroconversion, or a fourfold rise in the titer of complement-fixing or indirect fluorescent antibody to chlamydial group antigen. Although *C. psittaci* can be isolated from blood or sputum early in the disease, these methods are attempted only in specialized laboratories because of the risk of laboratory infection. Treatment with tetracycline or erythromycin is effective if given early in the course of illness.

Interstitial pneumonia is bilateral

Diagnosis is primarily serologic

Treatment with tetracycline or erythromycin

CHLAMYDIA PNEUMONIAE

C. pneumoniae has been shown to be a cause of "walking pneumonia" in adults worldwide. It is estimated that 10% of pneumonia and 5% of bronchitis cases are due to this agent. Epidemiologic evidence indicates that infection occurs throughout the year and is

Clinical manifestations are similar to *M. pneumoniae*

Possible role in atherosclerosis is proposed

Treatment is tetracycline or erythromycin

spread between humans by person to person contact. Unlike psittacosis, birds are not the reservoir. Outbreaks of community-acquired pneumonia caused by *C. pneumoniae* have been reported, as has apparent nosocomial spread. Reinfections occur, and clinically evident *C. pneumoniae* infection may be more evident in the elderly than in younger individuals. Most infections present as pharyngitis, lower respiratory tract disease, or both, and the clinical spectrum is similar to that of *Mycoplasma pneumoniae* infection. Pharyngitis or laryngitis may occur 1 to 3 weeks prior to bronchitis or pneumonia, and cough may persist for weeks. The diagnosis is established by serologic testing or culture, but these tests are not routinely available. Treatment with tetracycline or erythromycin is effective in ameliorating the signs and symptoms of *C. pneumoniae* infection. Currently, there is ongoing scientific interest in the potential role of persistent infection by *C. pneumoniae* in the pathogenesis of human vascular endothelial and intimal diseases, such as atherosclerosis.

ADDITIONAL READING

Buimer M, et al. Detection of *Chlamydia trachomatis* and *Neisseria gonorrhoeae* by ligase chain reaction–based assays with clinical specimens from various sites: Implications for diagnostic testing and screening. *J Clin Microbiol* 1996;34:2395–2400. A report of LCR and review of other tests for diagnosis.

Kuo CC, et al. *Chlamydia pneumoniae* (TWAR). *Clin Microbiol Rev* 1995;8:451–461. An excellent general review.

Schachter J. Biology of *Chlamydia trachomatis.* In Holmes KK et al (eds). *Sexually Transmitted Diseases,* 3rd ed. New York: McGraw Hill; 1999; pp. 391–405. A comprehensive review of the basic biology and pathogenesis of chlamydia.

Schnoles D, et al. Prevention of pelvic inflammatory disease by screening for cervical chlamydial infection. *N Engl J Med* 1997;334:1362–1366. Indicates the important role of *C. trachomatis* in producing pelvic inflammatory disease and infertility as well as the means to prevent these serious complications.

CHAPTER 31

Rickettsia, Coxiella, Ehrlichia, and *Bartonella*

W. LAWRENCE DREW

The terminology of the rickettsiae and rickettsiae-like organisms has been revised very recently. Rickettsiae are the causes of spotted fevers and typhus and related illnesses, but the cause of scrub typhus is now *Orientia tsutsugamushi*. Ehrlichia is a family distinct from true rickettsiae and has two medically important genera: *Ehrlichia* and *Anaplasma*. *Coxiella burnetii,* the cause of Q fever, is a bacterium which is no longer classified with the rickettsiae. All are Gram-negative bacilli, and all are strict intracellular pathogens. The reservoir is animals, and, except for Q fever, all are transmitted by arthropod vectors. The diseases are typically fevers, often with vasculitis. The most common infections are the various spotted fevers found throughout the world.

Obligate intracellular parasites

Bartonella is a genus of Gram-negative bacilli formerly classified with the rickettsiae. However, this is not a group of strict intracellular pathogens.

RICKETTSIA

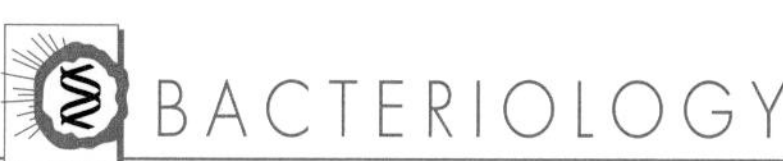

MORPHOLOGY AND STRUCTURE

Rickettsiae are small coccobacilli that often have a transverse septum between two bacilli, reflecting division by binary fission. They commonly measure no more than 0.3 to 0.5 μm. Although the Gram reaction is negative, they take the usual bacterial stains poorly and are better demonstrated by the Giemsa stain, particularly in infected cells. The ultrastructural morphology, which is similar to that of other Gram-negative bacteria, includes a Gram-negative type of cell envelope, ribosomes, and a nuclear body. Chemically, the cell wall contains lipopolysaccharide and at least two large proteins in the outer membrane, as well as peptidoglycan. The outer membrane proteins extend to the cell surface, where they are the most abundant protein present.

Small, Gram-negative coccobacilli stained best by Giemsa

Abundant outer membrane proteins at surface

GROWTH AND METABOLISM

Grow in cytoplasm following induced endocytosis

Growth slow compared to most bacteria

Spread involves actin polymerization

Rickettsia grow freely in the cytoplasm of eukaryotic cells to which they are highly adapted, in contrast to *Ehrlichia* and *Coxiella,* which replicate in cytoplasmic vacuoles. Rickettsiae can be grown only in living host cells such as cell cultures and embryonated eggs. Infection of the host cell begins by induction of an endocytic process, which is analogous to phagocytosis, but requires expenditure of energy by the rickettsiae. Penetration of infected cells appears to be facilitated by production of a rickettsial phospholipase. The organisms then escape the phagosome or endocytic vacuole to enter the cytoplasm, possibly aided by elaboration of the phospholipase. Recent studies indicate that intracellular and intercellular spread involves directional actin polymerization and use of the host cell cytoskeleton in a manner similar to *Listeria* (see Chapter 18) and *Shigella* (see Chapter 21). Intracytoplasmic growth eventually produces lysis of the cell. The estimated generation time of rickettsiae is much longer than that of bacteria such as *Escherichia coli* but more rapid than that of *Mycobacterium tuberculosis.*

Exogenous cofactors and ATP required for survival

Rapidly loses infectivity outside of host cell

The obligate intracellular parasitism of rickettsiae has several interesting features. Failure to survive outside the cell is apparently related to requirements for nucleotide cofactors (coenzyme A, nicotinamide adenine dinucleotide) and adenosine triphosphate (ATP). Outside the host cell, rickettsiae not only cease metabolic activity, but leak protein, nucleic acids, and essential small molecules. This instability leads to rapid loss of infectivity, because the penetration of another cell requires energy. In summary, rickettsiae have the metabolic capabilities of other bacteria, but must borrow some essential elements from host cells for adequate growth and, thus, do not survive well in the environment.

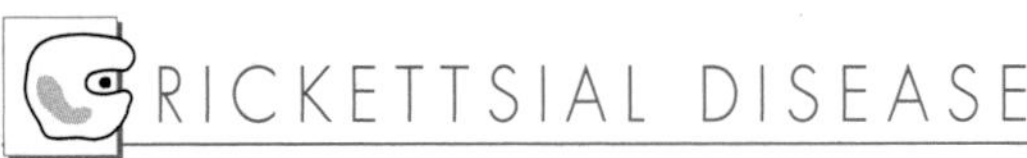

RICKETTSIAL DISEASE

CLINICAL CAPSULE

The classic example of rickettsial disease is epidemic typhus, but the most important rickettsiosis in the United States is Rocky Mountain spotted fever (RMSF). Both types of rickettsial disease are characterized by fever, rash, and myalgias/myositis. In RMSF, the rash appears first on the palms and soles, wrists, and ankles, and it migrates centripetally; in epidemic typhus, the rash begins on the trunk and spreads to the extremities, traveling in the opposite direction. Both diseases may be fatal as the result of severe vascular collapse. The vectors also differ; for RMSF, the vector is a tick, and for epidemic typhus, a louse.

EPIDEMIOLOGY AND PATHOGENESIS

Infect vascular endothelium with resultant vasculitis and thrombosis

Multiple vascular lesions, including adrenal glands

Most rickettsiae have animal reservoirs and are spread by insect vectors, which are prominent components of their life cycles (Table 31–1). Most rickettsial infections of humans result in clinical illness. Rickettsiae infect the vascular endothelium, and the primary pathologic lesion is a vasculitis in which rickettsiae multiply in the endothelial cells lining the small blood vessels. Focal areas of endothelial proliferation and perivascular infiltration leading to thrombosis and leakage of red blood cells into the surrounding tissues account for the rash and petechial lesions. Vascular lesions occur throughout the body, producing the systemic manifestations of the disease. They are obviously most apparent in skin but most serious in the adrenal glands. An endotoxin-like shock has been demonstrated in animals on injection of whole rickettsial cells, but the nature and role of any toxin in human disease are unknown.

DIAGNOSIS

In vitro cultivation is hazardous

Culture of rickettsiae is both difficult and hazardous. Their isolation in fertile eggs or cell cultures is generally attempted only in reference centers with special facilities and personnel experienced in handling the organisms. For this reason, serologic tests are the primary means of specific diagnosis. A number of test systems using specific rickettsial

TABLE 31–1

Examples of Pathogenic Rickettsiae

Disease	Organism	Most Common Geographic Distribution	Zoonotic Cycle	
			Vector	Reservoir
Spotted fever group Rocky Mountain spotted fever	*Rickettsia rickettsii*	North and South America	Tick	Rodents, dogs
Rickettsialpox	*Rickettsia akari*	United States former Soviet Union, Korea, Africa	Mite	Mouse
Mediterranean spotted fevers	*Rickettsia conorii*	Southern Mediterranean, Israel, Africa	Tick	Rodents, dogs
Typhus group epidemic	*Rickettsia prowazekii*	Africa, Asia, South America	Body louse	Humans[a]
Brill's	*Rickettsia prowazekii*	Worldwide[b]	None[c]	Humans
Murine	*Rickettsia typhi*	Worldwide (pockets)	Flea	Rodents
Scrub	*Orientia tsutsugamushi*	South Pacific, Asia	Mite	Rodents
Trench fever	*Bartonella quintana*[d]	Europe, Africa, Asia	Body louse	Humans
Q fever	*Coxiella burnetii*	Worldwide	None[e]	Sheep, cattle, goats
Cat scratch fever	*Bartonella henselae*[d]	Worldwide	None	Cats, dogs
Human ehrlichiosis	*Ehrlichia* (several species), *Anaplasma phagocytophilum*	Worldwide	Ticks	Dogs, deer, rodents

[a] An apparently identical organism has been isolated from flying squirrels in the United States.

[b] Related to immigration.

[c] Relapsing form of epidemic typhus.

[d] Related to *Rickettsia* but has been grown in artificial culture.

[e] Transmission by inhalation of infected aerosols.

antigens have been developed, of which the indirect fluorescent antibody (IFA) method is generally the most sensitive and specific. This test is usually available only in reference laboratories. For rapid diagnosis, examination of biopsies such as skin lesions by immunofluorescence or immunoenzyme methods to detect antigens can be used.

IFA method usually employed for serologic diagnosis

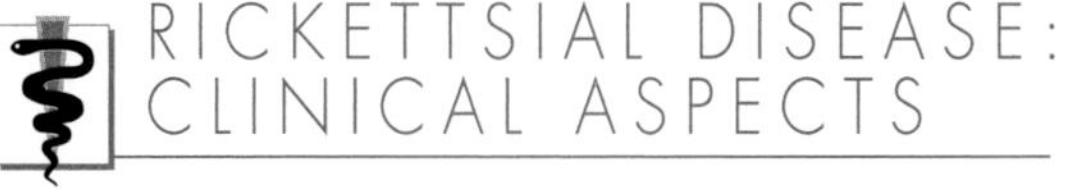

RICKETTSIAL DISEASE: CLINICAL ASPECTS

SPOTTED FEVER GROUP

The most important rickettsial disease in North America is RMSF, which is caused by *Rickettsia rickettsii.* A number of other spotted fever rickettsioses are found in other parts of the world (see Table 31–1); the name often reveals the locale (eg, Mediterranean spotted fever, Marseilles fever). They are caused by *Rickettsia conorii,* a species serologically related to, but distinct from, *R. rickettsii.* Another less severe spotted fever, rickettsialpox, also occurs in North America.

Many tick-borne rickettsioses occur throughout the world

Rocky Mountain Spotted Fever

RMSF is an acute febrile illness that occurs in association with residential and recreational exposure to wooded areas where infected ticks exist. The disease has a significant mortality (25%) if untreated.

Epidemiology

Ticks naturally infected

Transovarial spread perpetuates tick infection

R. rickettsii is primarily a parasite of ticks. In the western United States, the wood tick (*Dermacentor andersoni*) is the primary vector. In the East, the dog tick (*Dermacentor variabilis*) is the natural carrier and vector of the disease, and in the Southwest and Midwest, the vector is the Lone Star tick (*Amblyomma americanum*). *R. rickettsii* does not kill its arthropod host, so the parasite is passed through unending generations of ticks by transovarial spread. Adult females require a blood meal to lay eggs and thus may transmit the disease. Infected adult ticks have been shown to survive as long as 4 years without feeding.

Most cases in children

R. rickettsii is found in both North America and South America. The highest attack rates in the United States are in the central and mid-Atlantic states (Fig 31–1). The US incidence increased in the 1970s and early 1980s to more than 0.5 cases per 100,000 population but has since decreased to less than half that figure. More than two thirds of cases are in children less than 15 years of age. The illness is generally seen between April and September because of increased exposure to ticks. A history of tick bite can be elicited in approximately 70% of cases.

Manifestations

Incubation period 2–6 days after tick bite

The incubation period between the tick bite and the onset of illness is usually 2 to 6 days but may be as long as 2 weeks. Fever, headache, rash, toxicity, mental confusion, and myalgia are the major clinical features. The rash is the most characteristic feature of the illness. It usually develops on the second or third day of illness as small erythematous macules that rapidly become petechial. The lesions appear initially on the wrists and ankles and then spread up the extremities to the trunk in a few hours. A diagnostic feature of

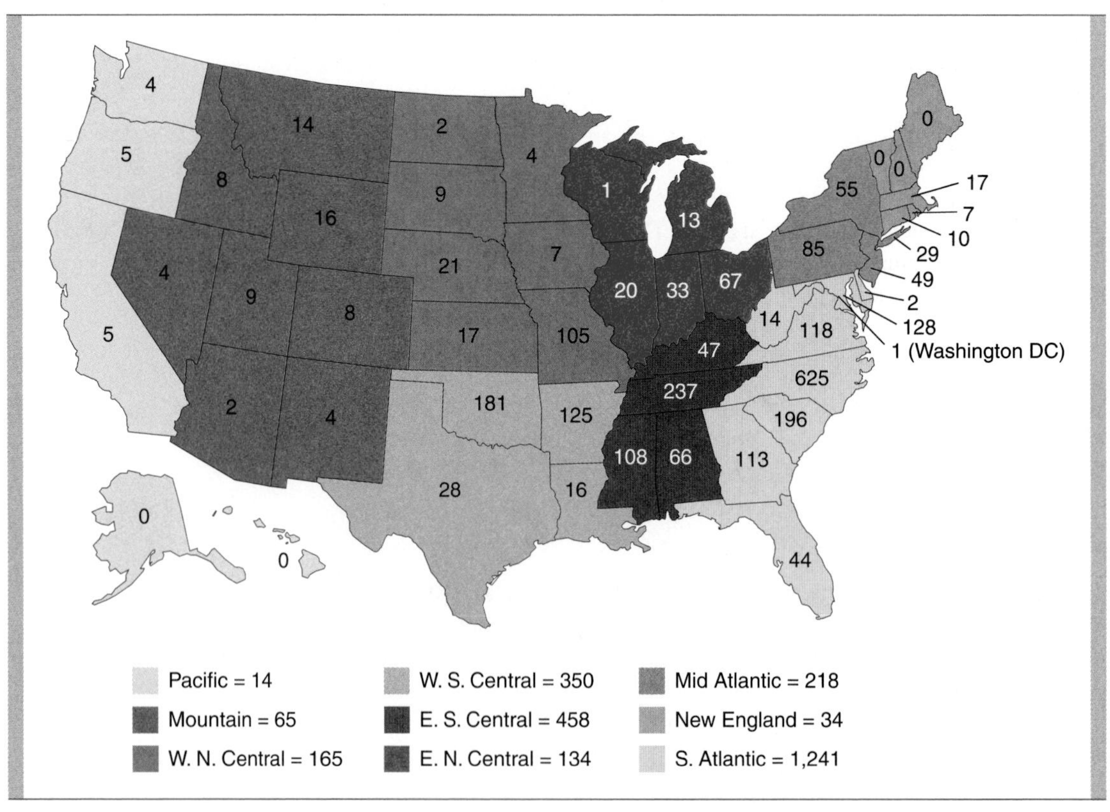

FIGURE 31–1

Rocky Mountain spotted fever. Number of cases in the United States in 1992. (*Reprinted with permission from Centers for Disease Control and Prevention. Summary of Notifiable Diseases, United States 1992.* MMWR Morb Mortal Wkly Rep *1993;41(55).*)

RMSF is the frequent appearance of the rash on the palms and soles, a finding not usually seen in maculopapular eruptions associated with viral infections. Muscle tenderness, especially in the gastrocnemius, is characteristic and may be extreme. If untreated, or in occasional cases despite therapy, complications such as disseminated intravascular coagulation, thrombocytopenia, encephalitis, vascular collapse, and renal and heart failure may ensue.

Rash spreads from extremities to trunk and often involves palms and soles

Diagnosis

Because serologic testing is the primary diagnostic approach, it is often difficult to establish the diagnosis of RMSF early in the course of illness. However, antibodies may appear by the sixth or seventh day of illness, and a fourfold rise in antibody titer between acute serum and convalescent serum establishes the diagnosis. Specific therapy must usually be started solely on the basis of clinical signs, symptoms, and epidemiologic considerations.

Rising antibody titers confirm diagnosis

Prompt initiation of therapy based on clinical and epidemiologic considerations

Treatment

Appropriate antibiotic therapy is highly effective if given during the first week of illness. If delayed into the second week or when pathologic processes such as disseminated intravascular coagulation are present, therapy is much less effective. The antibiotic of choice is doxycycline. Sulfonamides may worsen the disease process and are thus contraindicated. Before specific therapy became available, the mortality of RMSF was approximately 25%. Treatment has reduced this figure to between 5 and 7%. Death results primarily in patients in whom diagnosis and therapy are delayed into the second week of illness.

Treatment during first week most effective

Doxycycline is the treatment of choice

Prevention

The major means of preventing RMSF is avoidance or reduction of tick contact. Frequentineticking in tick-infested areas is important, because ticks generally must feed for 6 hours or longer before they can transmit the disease. Tick surveys in the Carolinas have shown infection in about 5% of samples. Killed vaccines prepared from infected ticks, or rickettsias grown in embryonated eggs and cell cultures have been developed. None is licensed for clinical use at present.

Frequent deticking, avoidance, and protective clothing important in prevention

Rickettsialpox

Rickettsialpox was first recognized in New York City in 1946. It is a benign rickettsial illness caused by *Rickettsia akari* and transmitted by a rodent mite. Distinguishing features of the disease include an eschar at the site of the bite and a vesicular rash. The house mouse and other semidomestic rodents are the primary reservoir. Humans acquire infection when the mite seeks an alternative host.

Benign disease transmitted by rodent mites

Rickettsialpox is a biphasic illness. The first phase is the local lesion at the bite, which starts as a papulovesicle and develops into a black eschar in 3 to 5 days. Fever and constitutional symptoms appear as the organism disseminates. The second phase of the disease is a diffuse rash similar to that of RMSF distributed randomly in the body, which, like the local lesion, becomes papulovesicular and develops into eschars. Rickettsialpox is self-limiting after 1 week, and no deaths have been reported. Tetracycline therapy shortens the course to 1 to 2 days.

Local eschar followed by fever and rash

Tetracycline therapy

TYPHUS GROUP

Epidemic Louse-Borne Typhus Fever

Primary louse-borne typhus fever is caused by *Rickettsia prowazekii,* which is transmitted to humans by the body louse. Historically, it has appeared during times of misery (war, famine) that create conditions favorable to human body lice (crowding, infrequent bathing). Although foci of endemic typhus are thought to persist in parts of Africa and Latin America, the number of reported cases has declined in recent decades. Most come

Severe louse-borne disease due to *R. prowazekii*

from a single country, Ethiopia, which has had more than its share of social upheaval. Epidemic typhus has not been seen in the United States for more than half a century. *R. prowazekii* has been recovered from flying squirrels and their ectoparasites in the southeastern United States, and a few human cases of sylvatic typhus have occurred in these areas.

Endemic foci in Africa

The chain of epidemic typhus infection starts with *R. prowazekii* circulating in a patient's blood during an acute febrile infection. The human body louse becomes infected during one of its frequent blood meals, and after 5 to 10 days of incubation, large numbers of rickettsiae appear in its feces. As the louse defecates while it feeds, the organisms can be rubbed into the louse bite wounds when the host scratches the site. Dried louse feces are also infectious through the mucous membranes of the eye or respiratory tract. The louse dies of its infection in 1 to 3 weeks, and the rickettsiae are not transmitted transovarially.

Infection involves feeding and defecation by louse

Fever, headache, and rash begin 1 to 2 weeks after the bite. A maculopapular rash appears first on the trunk and then spreads centrifugally to the extremities, a pattern opposite to that of RMSF. Headache, malaise, and myalgia are prominent components of the illness. Complications include myocarditis and central nervous system dysfunction. In untreated disease, the fatality rate increases with age from 10% to as high as 60%. Therapy with tetracycline or chloramphenicol is effective. Louse control is the best means of prevention and is particularly important in controlling epidemics. No effective vaccine is available.

Fever, headache, and rash with high mortality rate

Louse control is primary prevention

Recrudescent Typhus

Recrudescent typhus (**Brill's disease**) is a relapse of louse-borne typhus appearing 10 to 40 years after the primary attack. Factors triggering the relapse are unknown, but may involve fading immunity to rickettsiae that have remained dormant in reticuloendothelial cells. Recrudescent typhus is usually milder than the primary infection and is less often fatal, presumably because of partial immunity.

Less severe relapse of typhus after many years

Endemic Typhus

Endemic or murine typhus is caused by *Rickettsia typhi* and transmitted to humans by the rat flea (*Xenopsylla cheopis*). Human illness is incidental to the natural transmission of the disease among urban rodents, which serve as the reservoir. Only 30 to 60 cases of murine typhus are reported in the United States each year. Half of these typically occur along the Gulf Coast of Texas.

Transmitted by rat fleas

The pathogenesis is similar to that of louse-borne typhus but the history includes exposure to rats, rat fleas, or both. The flea defecates when it takes a blood meal, and the infected feces gain access through the bite wound. After an incubation period of 1 to 2 weeks, illness begins with headache, myalgia, and fever. The rash is maculopapular, not petechial; it starts on the trunk and then spreads to the extremities in a manner similar to typhus. Because of antigens shared by *R. typhi* and *R. prowazekii,* serologic tests may not separate the two diseases. In the untreated patient, fever may last 12 to 14 days. With tetracycline or chloramphenicol therapy, the course is reduced to 2 to 3 days. Mortality and complications are rare, even if the disease is untreated.

Resembles typhus but less severe

R. typhi shares antigens with *R. prowazekii*

Scrub Typhus

Scrub typhus is found in the southwest Pacific, Southeast Asia, and Japan. The causative organism is *Orientia tsutsugamushi,* a rickettsial organism. Mites that infest rodents are the reservoir and vectors, transmitting the rickettsiae to their own progeny via infected ova. Humans pick up the mites as they pass by low trees or brush. The mite larvae (chiggers) deposit rickettsiae as they feed.

Scrub typhus transmitted by rodent mite larvae (chiggers)

The typical initial lesion, a necrotic eschar at the site of the bite on the extremities, develops in only 50 to 80% of cases. Fever increases slowly over the first week, sometimes reaching 40.5°C. Headache, rash, and generalized lymphadenopathy follow later.

Local eschar followed by fever, headache, rash, and lymphadenopathy

The maculopapular rash, which appears after about 5 days, is more evanescent than that seen with louse-borne or murine typhus. Hepatosplenomegaly and conjunctivitis may also appear. Specific diagnosis requires demonstration of a serologic response using the IFA test. The prognosis is good with chloramphenicol or tetracycline therapy, but the mortality of untreated patients is as high as 30%.

Serologic diagnosis by IFA

Coxiella

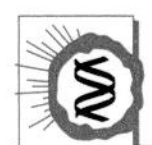

BACTERIOLOGY

Coxiella burnetii, the cause of **Q fever,** has morphologic features similar to those of rickettsiae but differs in DNA composition and a number of other features. Phase variation of surface polysaccharide in response to environmental conditions has been observed and linked to virulence. The organism is taken into host cells by a phagocytic process that in contrast to rickettsiae does not involve expenditure of energy by the parasite. It multiplies in the phagolysosome primarily because it is adapted to growth at low pH and resists lysosomal enzymes. *C. burnetii* is much more resistant to drying and other environmental conditions than rickettsiae, which substantially accounts for its ability to produce infection by the respiratory route.

Multiplies in phagolysosome

Resistant to drying

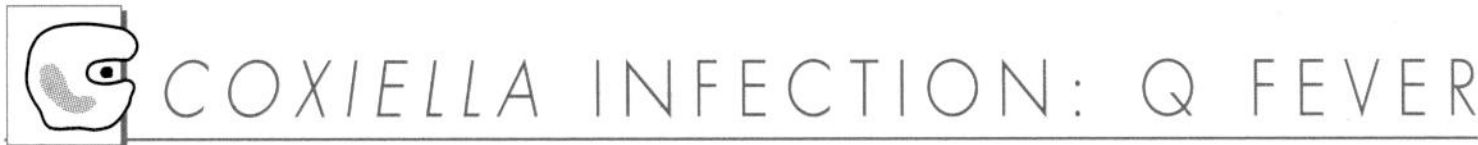

COXIELLA INFECTION: Q FEVER

Q fever is primarily a zoonosis transmitted from animals to humans by inhalation rather than by arthropod bite. Its distribution is worldwide among a wide range of mammals, of which cattle, sheep, and goats are most associated with transmission to humans. *C. burnetii* grows particularly well in placental tissue, attaining huge numbers (>10^{10} per gram), which at the time of parturition contaminate the soil and fomites, where it may survive for years. Q fever occurs in those individuals exposed to infected animals or their products, particularly workers involved with slaughtering. Another high-risk environment is animal research facilities that have not provided adequate protection for personnel. Infection in all of these circumstances is believed to result from inhalation, which may be at some distance from the site of generation of the infectious aerosols. Infection can also occur from ingestion of animal products such as unpasteurized milk.

Transmission usually by inhalation; occasionally by ingestion

Occupational exposure in abattoirs and research facilities

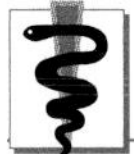

Q FEVER: CLINICAL ASPECTS

C. burnetii has an affinity for the reticuloendothelial system, but little is known of the pathology, because fatal cases are rare. As in livestock, most human infections are inapparent. When clinically evident, Q fever usually begins 9 to 20 days after inhalation, with abrupt onset of fever, chills, and headache. A mild, dry, hacking cough and patchy interstitial pneumonia may or may not be present. There is no rash. Hepatosplenomegaly and abnormal liver function tests are common. Complications such as myocarditis, pericarditis, and encephalitis are rare. Chronic infection is also rare but particularly important when it takes the form of endocarditis. There is evidence that the strains associated with endocarditis constitute an antigenic subgroup of *C. burnetii.*

Systemic infection without rash

Pneumonia and endocarditis may occur

Diagnosis is usually made by demonstrating high or rising titers of antibody to Q fever antigen by complement fixation, IFA, or enzyme immunoassay procedures. Although most infections resolve spontaneously, tetracycline therapy is believed to shorten the duration of fever and reduce the risk of chronic infection. Vaccines have been shown to stimulate antibodies, and some studies have suggested a protective effect for heavily exposed workers.

Diagnosis is serologic

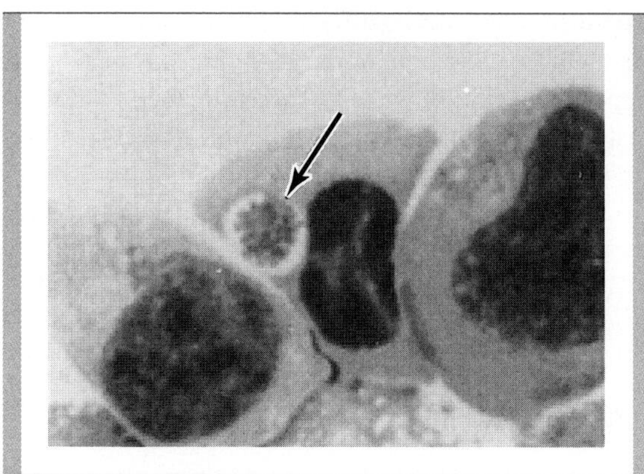

FIGURE 31–2
Mononuclear cell in the cerebrospinal fluid containing *Ehrlichia* intracytoplasmic inclusions (arrow). (*Reprinted with permission from Dunn BE, Monson TP, Dumler JS, et al. Identification of* Ehrlichia chaffeensis *morulae in cerebrospinal fluid mononuclear cells.* J Clin Microbiol *1992;30:2207–2210.*)

EHRLICHIA

The *Ehrlichia* genus includes several species of white blood cell (WBC)–associated bacteria that cause human disease. *Ehrlichia sennetsu,* the first species to be identified as a cause of human disease, is restricted to Japan and Malaysia. In the United States, two species are the principal causes of two diseases: (1) human monocytic ehrlichiosis (HME), which is due to *Ehrlichia chaffeensis;* and human granulocytic ehrlichiosis (HGE), which is due to *Anaplasma phagocytophilum. E. chaffeensis* infections tend to occur in the southeastern and lower midwestern United States, whereas the other infections tend to cluster in the northern states, with a distribution similar to Lyme disease (see Chapter 27). They were first reported to cause human disease in the 1950s. HGE is the predominant form of ehrlichiosis and is second only to Lyme disease as a tickborne infection in the United States. They are transmitted by deer or dog ticks. Both HME and HGE are clinically similar to RMSF, but rashes are less commonly seen. Still another species, *E. ewingii,* causes dog ehrlichiosis, which is occasionally contracted by humans.

Tickborne and WBC associated

On occasion, the diagnosis of ehrlichiosis may be suggested by observation of characteristic ehrlichial intracytoplasmic inclusions (morulae) in granulocytes (HGE) or mononuclear cells (HME) (Fig 31–2). Confirmation is usually made serologically by a fourfold or greater rise in IFA antibody or a titer greater than or equal to 1:64 to the specific antigen. These tests require the assistance of specialized laboratories. Another diagnostic test for detection of ehrlichia DNA is the polymerase chain reaction (PCR). Laboratory clues to human ehrlichiosis include a falling leukocyte count, thrombocytopenia, anemia, and impaired liver and renal function.

Intracytoplasmic inclusions (morulae) in monocytes or granulocytes

Doxycycline is the drug of choice for ehrlichiosis. The risk of infection can be reduced by avoiding wooded areas and tick bites.

Treatment is doxycycline

BARTONELLA

Bartonella species differ from rickettsiae in that they can be cultured on artificial media. By 16s ribosomal comparison they are actually more closely related to *Brucella* than to rickettsiae. *Bartonella quintana,* the best known species of this genus, causes **trench fever,** which has a worldwide distribution. The name derives from its prominence in the trenches of World War I. This disease has a reservoir in humans, and its vector is the body louse. Most cases are mild or subclinical. When symptomatic, the patient has sudden onset of chills, headache, relapsing fever, and a maculopapular rash on the trunk and abdomen. Illness can last for 14 to 30 days and the disease is suggested by a history of louse

B. quintana causes trench fever; it is also associated with alcoholism

contact. More recently, *B. quintana* bacteremia and endocarditis have been described in homeless alcoholic men in both France and the United States. The diagnosis can be made by culturing the organism on special agar medium or by demonstrating seroconversion.

Bartonella bacilliformis, a related organism, is the cause of acute Oroya fever and, in its chronic phase, verruga peruana. Infections with this agent are seen only in South America at intermediate altitudes, in keeping with the distribution of its sandfly vector.

Another species, *Bartonella henselae,* has been associated with a number of diseases, the most common of which is **cat scratch disease.** Cat scratch disease is a febrile lymphadenitis with systemic symptomatology that sometimes persists for weeks to months. Approximately 24,000 cases occur in the United States each year. The disease is thought to be transmitted by cat scratches or bites and perhaps by the bites of cat fleas. Manifestations may include skin rashes, conjunctivitis, encephalitis, and prolonged fever. Occasionally, retinitis, endocarditis, and granulomatous or suppurative hepatosplenic and osseous lesions have also been seen. *B. henselae* has been isolated directly from the blood of cats, although the latter do not appear ill. It can also be isolated from human blood, lymph nodes, and other materials using special media. Organisms can sometimes be directly demonstrated in infected tissues by using the Warthin–Starry silver impregnation stain. A serologic response to *B. henselae* antigens is the primary method of diagnosis. Azithromycin or erythromycin may reduce the duration of lymph node enlargement and symptoms.

Cat scratch disease is common in children

Persistent lymphadenitis is the usual finding

Bacillary angiomatosis, a proliferative disease of small blood vessels of the skin and viscera, seen in acquired immunodeficiency syndrome (AIDS) patients and other immunocompromised hosts, has been associated with *Bartonella* by molecular methods. The PCR (see Chapter 14) was used to amplify ribosomal RNA gene fragments directly from tissue samples. Sequence analysis of DNA transcribed from these fragments pointed to the *Bartonella* genus. Subsequently, both *B. henselae* and *B. quintana* have been isolated from AIDS patients with bacillary angiomatosis. Other conditions seen primarily in AIDS patients, such as peliosis hepatis and bacteremia with fever, have also been associated with *B. henselae. Bartonella* infections in AIDS and other immunosuppressed patients, as well as the bacteremia observed in alcoholic and homeless men, generally respond to prolonged courses of erythromycin. *Bartonella* endocarditis usually requires valve replacement as well.

AIDS and other immunocompromised states are associated with more severe, protracted infections

ADDITIONAL READING

Bakken JS, Dumier JS. Human granulocytic ehrlichiosis. *Clin Infect Dis* 2000;31:554–560. Reviews all aspects of this disease.

Bass JW, Vincent JM, Person DA. The expanding spectrum of *Bartonella* infections: II. Cat scratch disease. *Pediatr Infect Dis J* 1997;16:163–179. A historical and clinical review of *Bartonella* infections.

Jacobs RF, Schutze GE. Ehrlichiosis in children. *J Pediatr* 1997;131:184–192. An excellent treatise on both human granulocytic and monocytic forms.

Kelly DJ, Richards AL, Temenak J, et al. The past and present threat of rickettsial diseases to military medicine and international public health. *Clin Infect Dis* 2002;34:S145–S169. The authors present both historical and current perspectives on rickettsial diseases that are timely and highly informative.

La Scola B, Raoult D. Laboratory diagnosis of rickettsioses: Current approaches to diagnosis of old and new rickettsial diseases. *J Clin Microbiol* 1997;35:2715–2727. For those interested in learning more details of rickettsial diagnosis, this is an excellent review.

CHAPTER 32

Plague and Other Bacterial Zoonotic Diseases

KENNETH J. RYAN

Many bacterial, rickettsial, and viral diseases are classified as zoonoses, because they are acquired by humans either directly or indirectly from animals. This chapter considers bacteria causing four zoonotic infections that are not discussed in other chapters. All four species, *Brucella, Yersinia pestis, Francisella tularensis,* and *Pasteurella multocida,* are Gram-negative bacilli that are primarily animal pathogens. The diseases they cause, brucellosis, plague, tularemia, and pasteurellosis, are now rare in humans and develop only after unique animal contact. The full range of zoonoses considered in this and other chapters is shown in Table 32–1.

BRUCELLA

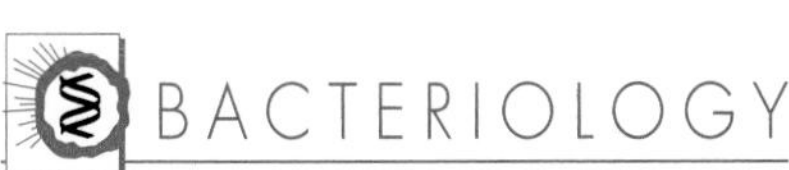

BACTERIOLOGY

Brucella species are small, coccobacillary, Gram-negative rods that morphologically resemble *Haemophilus* and *Bordetella.* They are nonmotile, non–acid fast, and non–spore forming. The cells have a typical Gram-negative structure and the outer membrane contains proteins and two major antigenic variants (A and M) whose relative proportion varies with species and growth conditions. Although DNA homology studies indicate that there is only a single species, medical microbiologists prefer to believe that there are six species, each of which is primarily associated with its own mammalian hosts. Of these, *Brucella melitensis* (sheep, goats), *Brucella abortus* (cattle), and *Brucella suis* (pigs) are the most important in human disease. Their growth is slow, requiring at least 2 to 3 days of aerobic incubation in enriched broth or on blood agar. All species produce catalase, oxidase, and urease, but do not ferment carbohydrates. They are differentiated by carbon dioxide requirements, hydrogen sulfide production, and susceptibility to dyes (thionin and basic fuchsin).

Coccobacilli resemble *Haemophilus*

Species are associated with different mammals

TABLE 32–1

Some Important Bacterial and Rickettsial Zoonotic Infections

Disease	Etiologic Agent	Usual Reservoir	Usual Mode of Transmission to Humans	Transmission Between Humans	Mode of Transmission Between Humans	Special Characteristics
Anthrax	*Bacillus anthracis*	Cattle, sheep, goats	Infected animals or products	No[a]		Resistant spores
Bovine tuberculosis	*Mycobacterium bovis*	Cattle	Milk	No[a]		
Brucellosis	*Brucella* spp.	Cattle, swine, goats	Milk, infected carcasses	No[a]		
Campylobacter infection	*C. jejuni*	Wild mammals, cattle, sheep, pets	Contaminated food and water	Yes	Fecal–oral	
Leptospirosis	*Leptospira* spp.	Cattle, rodents	Water contaminated with urine	No[a]		
Lyme disease	*Borrelia burgdorferi*	Deer, rodents	Ticks; transplacentally	No[a]		Relapsing disease
Pasteurellosis	*Pasteurella multocida*	Animal oral cavities	Bites, scratches	No[a]		
Plague	*Yersinia pestis*	Rodents	Fleas	Yes	Droplet (pneumonic) spread	Great epidemic potential
Other *Yersinia* infections	*Y. enterocolitica*, *Y. pseudotuberculosis*	Wild mammals, pigs, cattle, pets	Fecal–oral	Yes	Fecal–oral	
Relapsing fever	*Borrelia* spp.	Rodents, ticks	Ticks	Yes	Body louse[b]	Epidemic potential
Salmonellosis	*Salmonella* serotypes	Poultry, livestock	Contaminated food	Yes	Fecal contamination of food	
Rickettsial spotted fevers	*R. rickettsii*[c]	Rodents, ticks, mites	Ticks, mites	No[a]		
Murine typhus	*Rickettsia typhi*	Rodents	Fleas	No[a]		
Q fever	*Coxiella burnetii*	Cattle, sheep, goats	Contaminated dust and aerosols	No[a]		

[a] What never? No never. What *never*? Well, hardly ever! (W. S. Gilbert, "H.M.S. Pinafore").

[b] The relationship between tickborne relapsing fever and epidemic relapsing fever by the body louse remains uncertain.

[c] One of several etiologic agents.

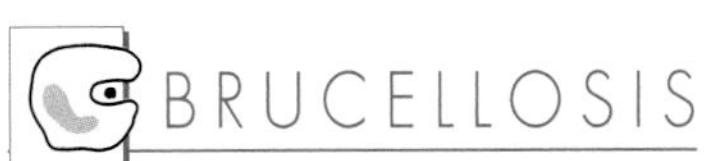

BRUCELLOSIS

CLINICAL CAPSULE

Brucellosis is a genitourinary infection of sheep, cattle, pigs, and other animals. Humans such as farmers, slaughterhouse workers, and veterinarians become infected directly by occupational contact or indirectly by consumption of contaminated animal products such as milk. In humans, brucellosis is a chronic illness characterized by fever, night sweats, and weight loss lasting weeks to months. Because the infection is localized in reticuloendothelial organs, there are few physical findings unless the liver or spleen become enlarged. When patients develop a cycling pattern of nocturnal fevers, the disease has been called undulant fever.

EPIDEMIOLOGY

Brucellosis, a chronic infection that persists for life in animals, is an important cause of abortion, sterility, and decreased milk production in cattle, goats, and hogs. It is spread among animals by direct contact with infected tissues and ingestion of contaminated feed and causes chronic infection of the mammary glands, uterus, placenta, seminal vesicles, and epididymis. Although the associations are not absolute, each species is linked to a different animal: *B. abortus* tends to infect cattle; *B. melitensis,* sheep and goats; and *B. suis,* pigs.

Causes abortion in cattle, goats, pigs

Humans acquire brucellosis by occupational exposure or consumption of unpasteurized dairy products. The bacteria may gain access through cuts in the skin, contact with mucous membranes, inhalation, or ingestion. In the United States, the number of cases has dropped steadily from a maximum of more than 6000 per year in the 1940s to the current level of less than 100 per year. Of these cases, 50 to 60% are in abattoir employees, government meat inspectors, veterinarians, and others who handle livestock or meat products. Consumption of unpasteurized dairy products, which accounts for 8 to 10% of infections, is the leading source in persons who have no connection with the meat processing or livestock industries. Some recent cases of this type have been associated with "health" foods. In the United States, the distribution of human cases of brucellosis includes virtually every state, but is concentrated in those with large livestock industries or proximity to Mexico (California, Texas). An outbreak of *B. melitensis* in Texas was traced to unpasteurized goat cheese brought in from Mexico.

Occupational disease for veterinarians

Unpasteurized dairy products and "health" foods are a risk

PATHOGENESIS

All *Brucella* species are facultative intracellular parasites of epithelial cells and professional phagocytes. After they penetrate the skin or mucous membranes, they enter and multiply in macrophages in the liver sinusoids, spleen, bone marrow, and other components of the reticuloendothelial system. Understanding the mechanisms for intracellular survival is incomplete but involves suppression of the myeloperoxidase system, inhibition of phagosome–lysosome fusion, and impairment of monocyte cytokine production. Thus, intracellular events in monocytes determine the outcome of a *Brucella* infection. In cows, sheep, pigs, and goats, erythritol, a four-carbon alcohol present in chorionic tissue, markedly stimulates growth of *Brucella.* This stimulation probably accounts for the tendency of the organism to locate in these sites. The human placenta does not contain erythritol.

Facultative intracellular pathogen multiplies in macrophages

Erythritol in animal placentas stimulates growth

If not controlled locally, infection progresses with the formation of small granulomas in the reticuloendothelial sites of bacterial multiplication and with release of bacteria back into the systemic circulation. These bacteremic episodes are largely responsible for the recurrent chills and fever of the clinical illness. These events resemble the pathogenesis of typhoid fever (see Chapter 21).

IMMUNITY

Although antibodies are formed in the course of brucellosis, there is little evidence they are protective. Control of disease is due to T cell–mediated cellular immune responses.

Immunity is T-cell mediated

Development of helper T cell–type responses and the production of cytokines (tumor necrosis factor-α, tumor necrosis factor-β, interleukin-1, interleukin-2) are associated with the elimination of *Brucella* from macrophages.

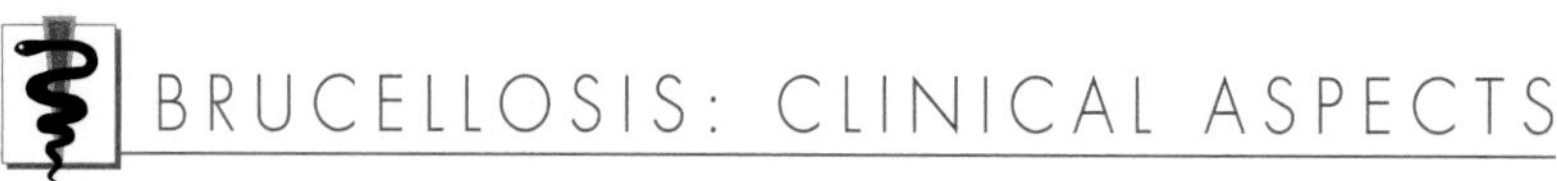

BRUCELLOSIS: CLINICAL ASPECTS

MANIFESTATIONS

Recurrent bacteremia comes from reticuloendothelial sites

Night sweats and periodic fever continue without obvious organ focus

Brucellosis starts with malaise, chills, and fever 7 to 21 days after infection. Drenching sweats in the late afternoon or evening are common, as are temperatures in the range of 39.4 to 40°C. The pattern of periodic nocturnal fever (undulant fever) typically continues for weeks, months, or even 1 to 2 years. Patients become chronically ill with associated body aches, headache, and anorexia. Weight loss of up to 20 kg may occur during prolonged illness. Despite these dramatic effects, physical findings and localizing signs are few. Less than 25% of patients show detectable enlargement of the reticuloendothelial organs, the primary site of infection. Of such findings, splenomegaly is most common, followed by lymphadenopathy and hepatomegaly. Occasionally, localized infection develops in the lung, bone, brain, heart, or genitourinary system. These cases usually lack the pronounced systemic symptoms of the typical illness.

DIAGNOSIS

Blood culture is primary method

Serologic tests may be useful

Definitive diagnosis requires isolation of *Brucella* from the blood or from biopsy specimens of the liver, bone marrow, or lymph nodes. Supplementation with carbon dioxide is needed for growth of *B. abortus.* The slow growth of some strains requires prolonged incubation of culture medium to achieve isolation. Blood cultures may require 2 to 4 weeks for growth, although most are positive in 2 to 5 days. The diagnosis is often made serologically but is subject to the same interpretive constraints as are all serologic tests. Antibodies that agglutinate suspensions of heat-killed organisms typically reach titers of 1:640 or more in acute disease. Lower titers may reflect previous disease or cross-reacting antibodies. Titers return to the normal range within a year of successful therapy.

TREATMENT AND PREVENTION

Tetracyclines are effective

Tetracyclines are the primary antimicrobics for the treatment of brucellosis. Doxycycline is preferred because of its pharmacologic characteristics. In seriously ill patients, streptomycin, gentamicin, or rifampin may be added. Although β-lactams are active in vitro, clinical response is poor, probably due to failure to reach the intracellular location of the bacteria. The therapeutic response is not rapid; 2 to 7 days may pass before patients become afebrile. Up to 10% of patients have relapses in the first 3 months after therapy.

Pasteurization is primary prevention

Prevention is primarily by measures that minimize occupational exposure and by the pasteurization of dairy products. Control of brucellosis in animals involves a combination of immunization with an attenuated strain of *B. abortus* and eradication of infected stock. No human vaccine is in use.

YERSINIA PESTIS

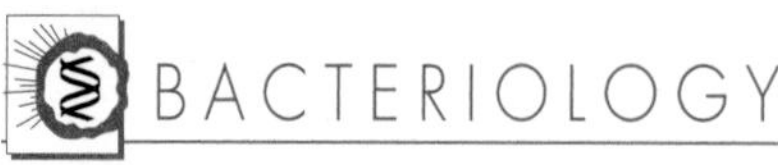

BACTERIOLOGY

Member of Enterobacteriaceae

Y. pestis is a nonmotile, non–spore-forming, Gram-negative bacillus with a tendency toward pleomorphism and bipolar staining. It is a member of the Enterobacteriaceae and is discussed in Chapter 21 with other members of the genus *Yersinia.* It shares features of the other *Yersinia* pathogenic for humans (*Y. pseudotuberculosis, Y. enterocolitica*), such as virulence plasmids and *Yersinia* outer membrane proteins (Yops). In addition, *Y. pestis* has two additional virulence plasmids, which code for a protein capsular antigen called F1 and enzymes with phospholipase, protease, and fibrinolytic activity. *Y. pestis* also has its own adhesin similar to the invasins of the other *Yersinia.*

Yops, protein capsule, and enzymes are present

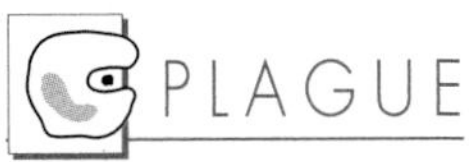

PLAGUE

CLINICAL CAPSULE

Plague, an infection of rodents transmitted to humans by the bite of infected fleas, is the most explosively virulent disease known. Most cases begin with a painful swollen lymph node (bubo) from which the bacteria rapidly spread to the bloodstream. Plague pneumonia (Black Death) is produced by seeding from the bloodstream or from another patient with pneumonia. All forms cause a toxic picture with shock and death within a few days. No other disease regularly kills previously healthy persons so rapidly.

EPIDEMIOLOGY

The term **plague** is often used generically to describe any explosive pandemic disease with high mortality. Medically, it refers only to infection caused by *Y. pestis,* and this application was justly earned, because *Y. pestis* was the cause of the most virulent epidemic plague of recorded human history, the Black Death of the Middle Ages. In the 14th century, the estimated population of Europe was 105 million; between 1346 and 1350, 25 million died of plague. Pandemics continued through the end of the 19th century and the early 20th century despite elaborate quarantine measures developed in response to the obvious communicability of the disease. Yersin isolated the etiologic agent in China in 1894 and named it after his mentor, Pasteur (*Pasteurella pestis*). The name was later changed to honor Yersin (*Yersinia pestis*).

Black Death continued into 20th century

Plague is a disease of rodents transmitted by the bite of rat fleas (*Xenopsylla cheopis)* that colonize them. It exists in two interrelated epidemiologic cycles, the **sylvatic** and the **urban** (Fig 32–1). Endemic transmission among wild rodents in the sylvatic (L. *sylvaticus,* belonging to or found in the woods) is the primary reservoir of plague. When infected rodents enter a city, circumstances for the urban cycle are created. Humans can enter the cycle from the bite of the flea in either environment. However, chances are greater in the urban setting.

Sylvatic transmission among rodents is primary reservoir

The plagues of the Middle Ages are examples of the urban cycle involving rats and humans. When food is scarce in the countryside, rats migrate to cities, which facilitates rat-to-rat transmission and brings the primary reservoir into closer contact with humans. When the number of nonimmune rats is sufficient, epizootic plague develops among them, with bacteremia and high mortality. Fleas feeding on the rats become infected, and the bacteria multiply in the intestinal tract of the fleas to numbers that eventually block the proventriculus. As an infected rat dies, its hungry fleas seek a new host, which is usually another rat but may be a human. The infected flea regurgitates *Y. pestis* from the proventriculus into the new bite wound. Therefore, the probability of transmission to humans is greatest when both rat population and rat mortality are high.

Rat migration to cities increases human risk

Fleas regurgitate into bite wounds

The bite of the flea is the first event in the development of a case of **bubonic plague,** which, even if serious enough to kill the patient, is not normally contagious to other humans. However, some patients with bubonic plague develop a secondary pneumonia by bacteremic spread to the lungs. This **pneumonic plague** is highly contagious person-to-person by the respiratory droplet route. It is not difficult to understand how rapid spread proceeds in conjunction with crowded unsanitary conditions and continued flea-to-human transmission. An urban plague epidemic is vividly described through the eyes of a physician in Albert Camus' novel *The Plague.*

Bubo is initial lesion

Bacteremia pneumonia is contagious

Although urban plague epidemics have been essentially eliminated by rat control and other public health measures, sylvatic transmission cycles persist in many parts of the world, including North America. These cycles involve nonurban mammals such as prairie

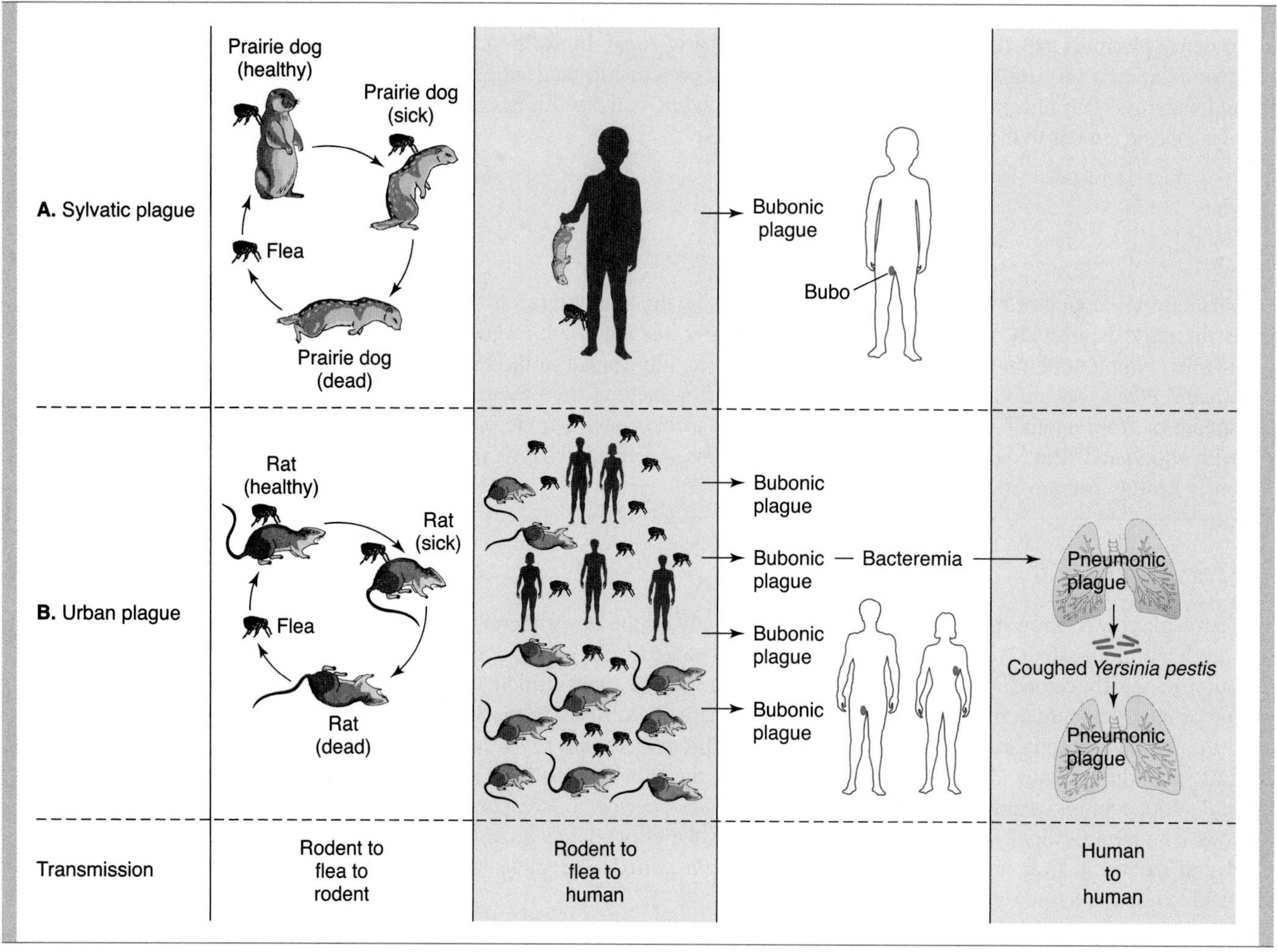

FIGURE 32–1

The epidemiology of plague. **A.** In the sylvatic cycle fleas leaving infected rodents, such as mice and prairie dogs, pass the infection to others in the population. Humans rarely contact these rodents but when they do, the flea bite transmits plague. **B.** In the urban cycle, masses of rats are in closer contact with humans and bites from infected fleas transmit the infection to many. In both cycles initial transmissions result in bubonic plague. Bacteremia with *Yersinia pestis* may infect the lungs to cause pneumonic plague. Pneumonic plague is transmitted human-to-human by the respiratory route without the involvement of fleas.

Nonepidemic disease is linked to animal contact

dogs, deer mice, rabbits, and wood rats. Transmission between them involves fleas. Coyotes or wolves may be infected by the same fleas or by ingestion of infected rodents. By their nature, the reservoir animals rarely come in contact with humans; when they do, however, the infected fleas they carry can transmit *Y. pestis.* The most common circumstance is a child exploring the outdoors who comes across a dead or dying prairie dog and pokes, carries, or touches it long enough to be bitten by the fleas leaving the animal. The result is a sporadic case of bubonic plague, which occasionally becomes pneumonic.

Most US cases are in western states

Pneumonia can be acquired from animals

Sylvatic plague, which exists in most continents, is common in Southeast Asia but is not found in Western Europe or Australia. In the United States, the primary enzootic areas are the semiarid plains of the western states. Infected animals and fleas have been detected from the Mexican border to the eastern half of Washington State. The geographic focus of human plague in the United States is in the "four corners" area where Arizona, New Mexico, Colorado, and Utah meet, but cases have occurred in California, west Texas, Idaho, and Montana. Most years, as many as 15 cases are reported, although this number rose to 30 to 40 in the mid-1980s. These variations are strongly related to changes in the size of the sylvatic reservoir. A fatal case of pneumonic plague reported in

1992 was linked to an infected domestic cat the patient had removed from the crawl space under a rural cabin in the endemic area.

PATHOGENESIS

The plague cycle begins when a rat flea feeds on a rodent infected with *Y. pestis.* Bacteria are taken with the blood meal and multiply in the infected flea. Some virulence factors such as the fibrinolysin and phospholipase are produced at the ambient temperature (20–28°C), where they may enhance the multiplication of *Y. pestis* in the flea and facilitate the agglutination that blocks the flea gut proventriculus. The flea, sensing starvation, feeds voraciously and eventually regurgitates blood and bacteria into the bite wound. If this wound is in a new uninfected host (rat or human), a new case is created.

Multiplication in flea foregut is aided by low temperature virulence factors

Once injected past the skin barrier by the flea, *Y. pestis* produces a new set of virulence factors as it senses the change from the temperature and ionic environment of the flea to that of the new host. These include the Yops and an array of other virulence factors discussed in Chapter 21, plus the F1 capsular protein and a plasminogen-activating protease. The F1 protein forms a gel-like capsule, which has antiphagocytic properties that allow the bacteria to persist and multiply in the submucosa. The organisms eventually reach the regional lymph nodes through the lymphatics, where they multiply rapidly and produce a hemorrhagic suppurative lymphadenitis known clinically as the **bubo.** Spread to the bloodstream quickly follows. The extreme systemic toxicity that develops with bacteremia appears to be due to lipopolysaccharide (LPS) endotoxin combined with the many actions of Yops, proteases, and other extracellular products. The bacteremia causes seeding of other organs, most notably the lungs, producing a necrotizing hemorrhagic pneumonia known as pneumonic plague.

New virulence factors are triggered by temperature and ionic shift

Capsular protein is antiphagocytic

Bubo progresses to bacteremia

LPS and other products produce shock

IMMUNITY

Recovery from bubonic plague appears to confer lasting immunity, but for obvious reasons the mechanisms in humans have not been extensively studied by modern immunologic methods. Animal studies suggest that antibody against the F1 capsular protein is protective by enhancing phagocytosis, but cell-mediated mechanisms are required for intracellular killing.

Anticapsular antibody may be protective

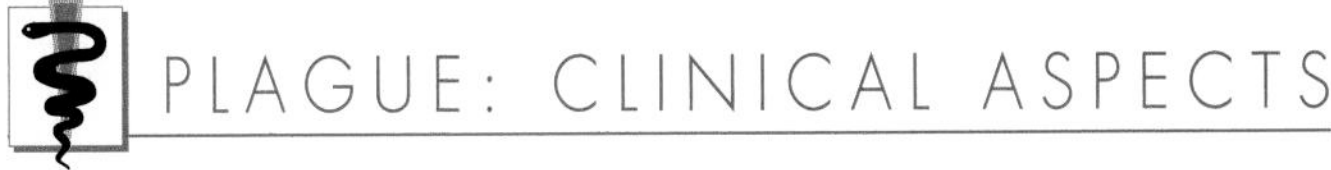

MANIFESTATIONS

The incubation period for bubonic plague is 2 to 7 days after the flea bite. Onset is marked by fever and the painful bubo, usually in the groin (**bubo** is from the Greek **boubon** for "groin") or, less often, in the axilla. Without treatment, 50 to 75% of patients progress to bacteremia and die in Gram-negative septic shock within hours or days of development of the bubo. About 5% of victims develop pneumonic plague with mucoid, then bloody sputum. Primary pneumonic plague has a shorter incubation period (2 to 3 days) and begins with only fever, malaise, and a feeling of tightness in the chest. Cough, production of sputum, dyspnea, and cyanosis develop later in the course. Death on the second or third day of illness is common, and there are no survivors without specific therapy. A terminal cyanosis seen with pneumonic plague is responsible for the term Black Death. Even today, plague pneumonia is almost always fatal if appropriate treatment is delayed more than a day from the onset.

Bubonic plague mortality is 50–75% in untreated cases

Pneumonic plague is fatal if untreated

Terminal cyanosis is the Black Death

DIAGNOSIS

Gram smears of aspirates from the bubo typically reveal bipolar-staining Gram-negative bacilli. An immunofluorescence technique is available in public health laboratories for

Immunofluorescent staining is rapid

immediate identification of smears or cultures. *Y. pestis* is readily isolated on the media used for other members of the Enterobacteriaceae (blood agar, MacConkey agar), although growth may require more than 24 hours of incubation. The appropriate specimens are bubo aspirate, blood, and sputum. Laboratories must be notified of the suspicion of plague to avoid delay in the bacteriologic diagnosis and to guard against laboratory infection.

Cultures grow on routine media

TREATMENT

Streptomycin is the treatment of choice for both bubonic and pneumonic plague, because its effectiveness has been proven. Tetracycline, chloramphenicol, and trimethoprim–sulfamethoxazole are alternatives. Timely treatment reduces the mortality of bubonic plague below 10%. Of the 31 human cases of plague reported in the United States in 1984, 6 (19%) died.

Streptomycin is primary treatment

PREVENTION

Urban plague has been prevented by rat control and general public health measures such as use of insecticides. Sylvatic plague is virtually impossible to eliminate because of the size and dispersion of the multiple rodent reservoirs. Disease can be prevented by avoidance of sick or dead rodents and rabbits. Eradication of fleas on domestic pets, which have been known to transport infected fleas from wild rodents to humans, is recommended in endemic areas. The continued presence of fully virulent plague in its sylvatic cycle poses a risk of extension to the urban cycle and epidemic disease in the event of major disaster or social breakdown. Chemoprophylaxis with tetracycline is recommended for those who have had close contact with a case of pneumonic plague. It is also used for the household contacts of a case of bubonic plague, because they may have had the same flea contact. A formalin-killed plague vaccine once used for those in high-risk occupations is no longer available.

Avoid sick or dead wild rodents

Tetracycline chemoprophylaxis is used for respiratory exposure

FRANCISELLA

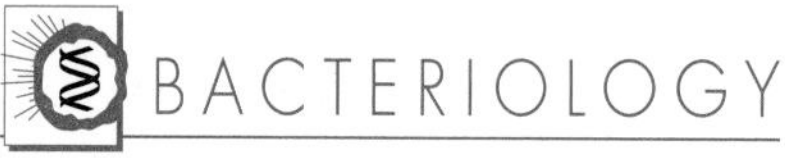

BACTERIOLOGY

Francisella tularensis is a small, facultative, coccobacillary, Gram-negative rod with much the same morphology as *Brucella.* It is one of the few bacterial species of medical importance that does not grow on the usual enriched media. This characteristic is due to a special requirement for sulfhydryl compounds, and growth occurs best on a cysteine–glucose blood agar medium incubated aerobically. On primary isolation, 2 to 10 days of incubation is required for appearance of the tiny transparent colonies. The species is antigenically homogeneous.

Gram-negative coccobacilli have requirement for –SH compounds

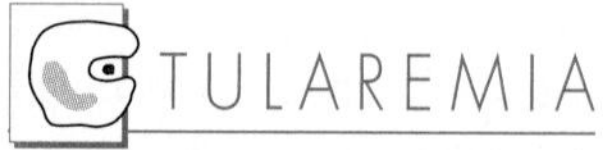

TULAREMIA

CLINICAL CAPSULE

Tularemia is a disease of wild mammals caused by *F. tularensis.* Humans become infected by direct contact with infected animals or through the bite of a vector (tick or deer fly). The illness is characterized by high fever and severe constitutional symptoms. The epidemiology of tularemia and many features of the clinical infection are similar to those of plague.

EPIDEMIOLOGY

Humans most often acquire *F. tularensis* by contact with an infected mammal or a bloodfeeding arthropod. Because the infecting dose is very low (<100 organisms), many routes of infection are possible. A tick bite or direct contact with minor skin abrasion are the most common mechanisms of infection. Many wild mammals can be infected, including squirrels, muskrats, beavers, and deer. A common history is that of skinning wild rabbits on a hunting trip. Inhalation may also lead to disease. In a recent outbreak of pulmonary tularemia on Cape Cod, experts believed that lawn mowing and brush cutting facilitated inhalation. Occasionally, the bite or scratch of a domestic dog or cat has been implicated when the animal has ingested or mouthed an infected wild mammal. Infected animals may not show signs of infection, because the organism is well adapted to its natural host. The usual vectors in animals are ticks and deer flies. Ticks may also serve as a reservoir of the organism by transovarial transmission to their offspring.

Infecting dose is low

Acquired by tick bites or directly from wild mammal

Tularemia is distributed throughout the Northern Hemisphere, although there are wide variations in specific regions. The highly virulent tick/rabbit-associated strains are common only in North America. In the United States 100 to 200 cases are reported each year half of which are in the lower Midwestern states (Arkansas, Missouri, Oklahoma). Tularemia is not found in the British Isles, Africa, South America, or Australia.

Distribution throughout Northern Hemisphere

PATHOGENESIS

Relatively little is known of the events that occur during the 2- to 5-day incubation period. A lesion often develops at the site of infection, which becomes ulcerated. The organism then infects the reticuloendothelial organs, often forming granulomas, and the disease may sometimes follow a chronic relapsing course. These properties suggest a facultative intracellular pathogen; multiplication within macrophages, hepatocytes, and endothelial cells has been demonstrated with *F. tularensis.* This intracellular survival has been attributed to failure of phagosome–lysosome fusion and phagosome acidification. Early bacteremic spread probably occurs, although it is rarely detected. Other areas of multiplication are characterized by necrosis or granuloma production, and a mixture of abscesses and caseating granulomas may be seen in the same organ.

Intracellular survival in macrophages by phagosome control

IMMUNITY

Naturally acquired infection appears to confer long-lasting immunity. Antibody titers remain elevated for many years, but cellular immunity plays the major role in resistance to reinfection. T cell–dependent reactions involving either CD4+ or CD8+ cell are detectable even before antibody responses.

Cell-mediated immunity is dominant

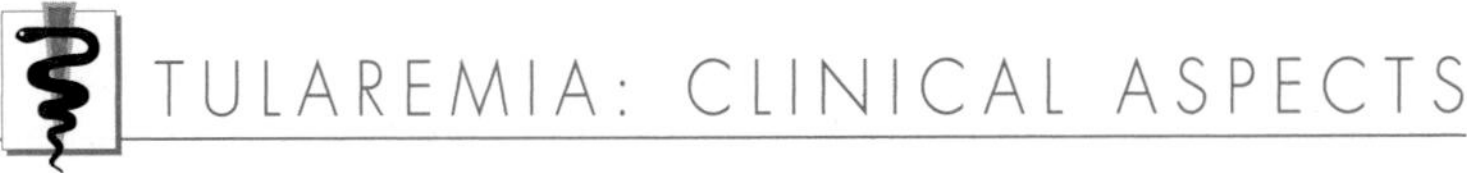

TULAREMIA: CLINICAL ASPECTS

MANIFESTATIONS

After an incubation period of 2 to 5 days, tularemia may follow a number of courses, depending on the site of inoculation and extent of spread. All begin with the acute onset of fever, chills, and malaise. In the ulceroglandular form, a local papule at the inoculation site becomes necrotic and ulcerative. Regional lymph nodes become swollen and painful. The oculoglandular form, which follows conjunctival inoculation, is similar except that the local lesion is a painful purulent conjunctivitis. Ingestion of large numbers of *F. tularensis* ($>10^8$) leads to typhoidal tularemia, with abdominal manifestations and a prolonged febrile course similar to that of typhoid fever. Inhalation of the organisms can result in pneumonic tularemia or a more generalized infection similar to the typhoidal form. Like plague pneumonia, tularemic pneumonia may also develop through seeding of the lungs by bacteremic

Ulceroglandular, oculoglandular, typhoidal, and pneumonic forms exist

spread of one of the other forms. Any form of tularemia may progress to a systemic infection with lesions in multiple organs.

Ulceroglandular has lowest mortality

Without treatment, mortality ranges from 5 to 30%, depending on the type of infection. Ulceroglandular tularemia, the most common form, generally carries the lowest risk of a fatal outcome. In the US surveillance study mentioned earlier, the mortality was 2%.

DIAGNOSIS

Special media are needed for culture

Serodiagnosis is most common

Because tularemia is uncommon and *F. tularensis* has unique growth requirements, the diagnosis is easily overlooked. Although some strains grow on chocolate agar, laboratories must be alerted to the suspicion of tularemia so that specialized media can be prepared and precautions taken against the considerable risk of laboratory infection. An immunofluorescent reagent is available in reference laboratories for use directly on smears from clinical material. Because of the difficulty and risk of cultural techniques, many cases are diagnosed by serologic tests. Agglutinating antibodies are usually present in titers of 1:40 by the second week of illness, increasing to 1:320 or greater after 3 to 4 weeks. Unless previous exposure is known, single high antibody titers are considered diagnostic.

TREATMENT AND PREVENTION

Aminoglycosides are effective

Streptomycin is the drug of choice in all forms of tularemia, although recent experience indicates that gentamicin may be just as effective. Tetracycline and chloramphenicol have also been effective, but relapses are more common than with streptomycin. Prevention mainly involves the use of rubber gloves and eye protection when handling potentially infected wild mammals. Prompt removal of ticks is also important. A live attenuated vaccine exists, but it is used only in laboratory workers and those individuals who cannot avoid contact with infected animals.

PASTEURELLA MULTOCIDA

Penicillin-sensitive, Gram-negative rods

Most common cause of infected animal bites or scratches

P. multocida, one of many species of *Pasteurella* in the respiratory flora of animals, is a cause of respiratory infection in some individuals. This small, coccobacillary, Gram-negative organism grows readily on blood agar but not on MacConkey agar. It is oxidase positive and ferments a variety of carbohydrates. Unlike most Gram-negative rods, *P. multocida* is susceptible to penicillin. Humans are usually infected by the bite or scratch of a domestic dog or cat. Infection develops at the site of the lesion, often within 24 hours. The typical infection is a diffuse cellulitis with a well-defined erythematous border. The diagnosis is made by culture of an aspirate of pus expressed from the lesion. Frequently, too few organisms are present to be seen on a direct Gram smear. *P. multocida* is by far the most common cause of an infected dog or cat bite. For unknown reasons, *P. multocida* is occasionally isolated from the sputum of patients with bronchiectasis. Infections are treated with penicillin.

ADDITIONAL READING

Butler T. *Yersinia* infections: Centennial of the discovery of the plague bacillus. *Clin Infect Dis* 1994;19:655–663. A very readable account of Yersin's life, his discoveries, and features of *Yersinia* infections.

Crook LD, Tempest B. Plague. A clinical review of 27 cases. *Arch Intern Med* 1992;152:1253–1256. A nice review of clinical aspects of plague cases seen between

1965 and 1989 at the Gallup, New Mexico, Indian Medical Center. Analysis of treatment outcomes is included.

LeVier K, Phillips RW, Grippe VK, Roop II RM, Walker GC. Similar requirements of a plant symbiont and a mammalian pathogen for prolonged intracellular survival. *Science* 2000;287:2492–2493. This article presents a fascinating bit of interdisciplinary scientific detective work in which *Rhizobium meliloti,* a plant pathogen, is found to use the same mechanisms for intracellular survival as *Brucella abortus.*

McNeill WH. *Plagues and Peoples.* New York: Anchor Press/Doubleday; 1976. An account of the impact of infectious diseases, including zoonoses, on the course of human history.

Perry RD, Fetherston JD. *Yersinia pestis*—etiologic agent of plague. *Clin Microbiol Rev* 1997;10:35–66. A comprehensive review of bacteriology, epidemiology, and pathogenesis.

Taylor JP, Istre GR, McChesney TC, Satalowich FT, Parker RL, McFarland LM. Epidemiologic characteristics of human tularemia in the southwest-central states, 1981–1987. *Am J Epidemiol* 1991;133:1032–1038. This study indicates tularemia is more common in the United States than most experts thought.

PART VI

Pathogenic Viruses

CHAPTER 37

Hepatitis Viruses

CHAPTER 38

Herpesviruses

CHAPTER 39

Viruses of Diarrhea

CHAPTER 40

Arthropod-Borne and Other Zoonotic Viruses

CHAPTER 41

Rabies

CHAPTER 42

Retroviruses, Human Immunodeficiency Virus, and Acquired Immunodeficiency Syndrome

CHAPTER 43

Papovaviruses

CHAPTER 44

Persistent Viral Infections of the Central Nervous System

CHAPTER 33

Influenza, Respiratory Syncytial Virus, Adenovirus, and Other Respiratory Viruses

C. GEORGE RAY

Respiratory disease accounts for an estimated 75 to 80% of all acute morbidity in the US population. Most of these illnesses (approximately 80%) are viral. If episodes not requiring medical attention are included, the overall average is three to four illnesses per year per person, although incidence varies inversely with age (the frequency is greater among young children). Seasonality is also a feature; incidence is lowest in the summer months and highest in the winter.

Respiratory viruses represented by diverse agents

The viruses that are major causes of acute respiratory disease (ARD) include influenza viruses, parainfluenza viruses, rhinoviruses, adenoviruses, respiratory syncytial virus (RSV), and respiratory coronaviruses. Reoviruses are of questionable importance but are also considered. Others, such as enterovirus and measles virus, can also cause respiratory symptoms but are discussed in other chapters.

Short incubation period

Transmission by droplet nuclei or hands

In addition to the ability to cause a variety of ARD syndromes, this somewhat heterogeneous group of viruses shares a relatively short incubation period (1–4 days) and a person-to-person mode of spread. Transmission is direct, by infective droplet nuclei, or indirect, by hand transfer of contaminated secretions to nasal or conjunctival epithelium. All of these agents are associated with an increased risk of bacterial superinfection of the damaged tissue of the respiratory tract, and all have a worldwide distribution.

INFLUENZA VIRUSES

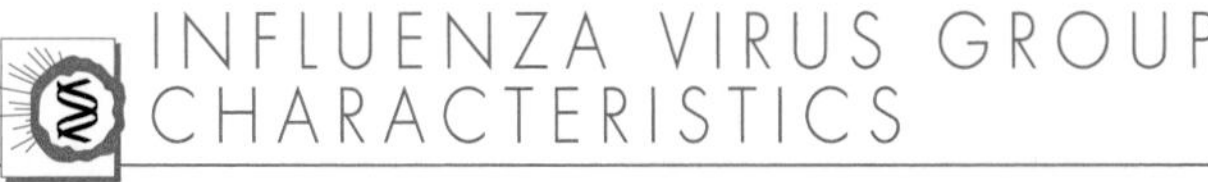

INFLUENZA VIRUS GROUP CHARACTERISTICS

Influenza viruses are members of the **orthomyxovirus** group, which are enveloped, pleomorphic, single-stranded RNA viruses. They are classified into three major serotypes, A, B, and C, based on different ribonucleoprotein antigens. Influenza A viruses are the

TABLE 33–1

Differences Among Influenza Viruses

Feature	Influenza A	Influenza B	Influenza C
Gene segments	8	8	7
Unique proteins	M2	NB	HEF
Host range	Humans, swine, avians, equines, marine mammals	Humans only	Humans, swine
Disease severity	Often severe	Occasionally severe	Usually mild
Epidemic potential	Extensive; epidemics and pandemics (antigenic drift and shift)	Outbreaks; occasional epidemics (antigenic drift only)	Limited outbreaks (antigenic drift only)

Orthomyxoviruses divided into types A, B, and C

Type A has greatest virulence and epidemic spread

most extensively studied of the three, and much of the following discussion is based on knowledge of this type. They generally cause more severe disease and more extensive epidemics than the other types; naturally infect a wide variety of species, including mammals and birds; and have a great tendency to undergo significant antigenic changes (Table 33–1). Influenza B viruses are more antigenically stable; are only known to naturally infect humans; and usually occur in more localized outbreaks. Influenza C viruses appear to be relatively minor causes of disease, affecting humans and pigs.

Enveloped RNA virus with segmented genome

Virus-specified hemagglutinin and neuraminidase spikes

Influenza A and B viruses each consist of a nucleocapsid containing eight segments of negative-sense, **single-stranded RNA,** which is enveloped in a glycolipid membrane derived from the host cell plasma membrane. The inner side of the envelope contains a layer of virus-specified protein (M1). Two virus-specified glycoproteins, hemagglutinin and neuraminidase, are embedded in the outer surface of the envelope and appear as "spikes" over the surface of the virion. Figure 33–1 illustrates the makeup of influenza A virus. Influenza B is somewhat similar but has a unique NB protein instead of M2. Influenza C differs from the others in that it possesses only seven RNA segments and has no neuraminidase, although it does possess other receptor-destroying capability (see below). In addition, the hemagglutinin of influenza C binds to a cell receptor different from that for types A and B.

The virus-specified glycoproteins are antigenic and have special functional importance to the virus. **Hemagglutinin** is so named because of its ability to agglutinate red

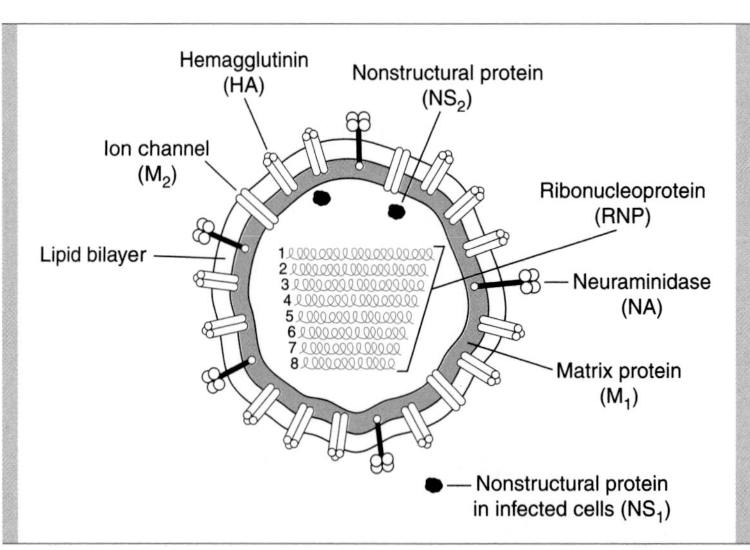

FIGURE 33–1
Diagrammatic view of influenza A virus. Three types of membrane proteins are inserted in the lipid bilayer: hemagglutinin (as trimer), neuraminidase (as tetramer), and M2 ion channel protein. The eight RNP segments each contain viral RNA surrounded by nucleoprotein and associated with RNA transcriptase.

blood cells from certain species (eg, chickens, guinea pigs) in vitro. Its major biological function is to serve as a point of attachment to *N*-acetylneuraminic (sialic) acid–only containing glycoprotein or glycolipid receptor sites on human respiratory cell surfaces, which is a critical first step in initiating infection of the cell.

Hemagglutinin acts in viral attachment

Neuraminidase is an antigenic hydrolytic enzyme that acts on the hemagglutinin receptors by splitting off their terminal neuraminic (sialic) acid. The result is destruction of receptor activity. Neuraminidase serves several functions. It may inactivate a free mucoprotein receptor substance in respiratory secretions that could otherwise bind to viral hemagglutinin and prevent access of the virus to the cell surface. It is important in fusion of the viral envelope with the host cell membrane as a prerequisite to viral entry. It also aids in the release of newly formed virus particles from infected cells, thus making them available to infect other cells. Type-specific antibodies to neuraminidase appear to inhibit the spread of virus in the infected host and to limit the amount of virus released from host cells.

Neuraminidase has role in envelope fusion and viral release

Nucleocapsid assembly takes place in the cell nucleus, but final virus assembly takes place at the plasma membrane. The ribonucleoproteins are enveloped by the plasma membrane, which by then contains hemagglutinin and neuraminidase. Virus "buds" are formed, and intact virions are released from the cell surface (see Chapter 6, Fig 6–11).

Nucleocapsid and virus assembly occur at different cell sites

Influenza A viruses were initially isolated in 1933 by intranasal inoculation of ferrets, which developed febrile respiratory illnesses. The viruses replicate in the amniotic sac of embryonated hen's eggs, where their presence can be detected by the hemagglutination test. Most strains can also be readily isolated in cell culture systems, such as primary monkey kidney cells. Some cause cytopathic effects in culture.

Viral isolation in eggs or cell cultures

The most efficient method of detection is demonstration of hemadsorption by adherence of erythrocytes to infected cells expressing hemagglutinin or by agglutination of erythrocytes by virus already released into the extracellular fluid. The virus can then be identified specifically by inhibition of these properties by addition of antibody directed specifically at the hemagglutinin. This method is called **hemadsorption inhibition** or **hemagglutination inhibition,** depending on whether the test is performed on infected cells or extracellular virus, respectively. Because the hemagglutinin is antigenic, hemagglutination inhibition tests can also be used to detect antibodies in infected subjects. Research has shown that antibody directed against specific hemagglutinin is highly effective in neutralizing the infectivity of the virus.

Hemadsorption and hemagglutination inhibition used to detect presence of virus

Antihemagglutinin antibodies detectable in serum

Influenza A

Influenza A is considered in detail because of its great clinical and epidemiologic importance.

The influenza A virion contains eight segments of single-stranded RNA with defined genetic responsibilities. These functions include coding for virus-specified proteins (see Fig 33–1; Table 33–2). A unique aspect of influenza A viruses is their ability to develop a wide variety of subtypes through the processes of mutation and whole-gene "swapping" between strains, called **reassortment.** Recombination, which occurs when new genes are assembled from sections of other genes, is thought to occur rarely, if at all. These processes result in antigenic changes called **drifts** and **shifts,** which are discussed shortly.

Influenza A genome in multiple segments

Mutability of virus produces antigenic changes

The 15 recognized subtypes of hemagglutinin and 9 neuraminidase subtypes known to exist among influenza A viruses that circulate in birds and mammals represent a reservoir of viral genes that can undergo reassortment, or "mixing" with human strains. Three hemagglutinins (H_1, H_2, and H_3) and two neuraminidases (N_1 and N_2) appear to be of greatest importance in human infections. These subtypes are designated according to the H and N antigens on their surface (eg, H_1N_1, H_3N_2). There may also be more subtle, but sometimes important, antigenic differences (drifts) within each subtype. These differences are designated according to the major representative virus to which they are most closely related antigenically, using the place of initial isolation, number of the isolate, and

Subtypes based on H and N antigens

Subtle changes known as antigenic drift

TABLE 33–2

Virus-coded Proteins of Influenza A

RNA Segment	Proteins	Function
1	PB2	RNA synthesis, ? virulence
2	PB1	RNA synthesis
3	PA	RNA synthesis
4	HA	Attachment
5	NP	RNA synthesis
6	NA	Virus release from infected cells
7	M1, M2	Matrix
8	NS1, NS2	Nonstructural; NS1 is interferon antagonist

year of detection. For example, two H_3N_2 strains that differ antigenically only slightly are A/Texas/1/77(H_3N_2) and A/Bangkok/1/79(H_3N_2).

Antigenic drift every few years with type A

Antigenic drifts within major subtypes can involve either H or N antigens, as well as the genes encoding nonstructural proteins, and may result from as little as a single mutation in the viral RNA. The mutant may come to predominate under selective immunologic pressures in the host population. Such drifts are frequent among influenza A viruses, occurring at least every few years and sometimes even during the course of a single epidemic. Drifts can also develop in influenza B viruses but at a considerably lower frequency.

Major antigenic shifts due to reassortment

New subtype may also develop mutations

In contrast to the frequently occurring mutations that cause antigenic drift among influenza A strains, major changes (>50%) in the nucleotide sequences of the H or N genes can occur suddenly and unpredictably. These are referred to as antigenic shifts. They almost certainly result from reassortment that can be readily reproduced in the laboratory. Simultaneously infecting a cell with two different influenza A subtypes yields progeny that contain antigens derived from either of the original viruses. For example, a cell infected simultaneously with influenza A (H_3N_2) and influenza A (H_1N_1) may produce a mixture of influenza viruses of the subtypes H_3N_2, H_1N_1, H_1N_2, and H_3N_1. When novel "new" epidemic strains emerge, they most likely have circulated into animal or avian reservoirs where they have undergone genetic reassortment (and sometimes also mutation), then readapted and spread to human hosts when a sufficient proportion of the population has little or no immunity to the "new" subtypes. A recent example was the appearance in Hong Kong in 1997 of human cases caused by an avian influenza A (H_5N_1). Studies indicated that all RNA segments were derived from an avian influenza A virus, but a single insert coding for several additional amino acids in the hemagglutinin protein facilitated cleavage by human cellular enzymes. In addition, a single amino acid substitution in the PB2 polymerase protein occurred. These two mutations together made the virus more virulent for humans; fortunately, human-to-human transmission was poor.

Major antigenic shifts correlate with epidemics

Major antigenic shifts, which occurred approximately every 8 to 10 years in the 20th century, often resulted in serious epidemics or pandemics among populations with little or no preexisting antibody to the new subtypes. Examples include the appearance of an H_1N_1 subtype in 1947, followed by an abrupt shift to an H_2N_2 strain in 1957, which caused the pandemic of Asian flu. A subsequent major shift in 1968 to an H_3N_2 subtype (the Hong Kong flu) led to another, but somewhat less severe epidemic. The Russian flu, which appeared in late 1977, was caused by an H_1N_1 subtype very similar to that which dominated between 1947 and 1957 (Table 33–3).

Minor antigenic drifts allow maintenance in population

The concepts of antigenic shift and drift in human influenza A virus infections can be approximately summarized as follows. Periodic shifts in the major antigenic components appear, usually resulting in major epidemics in populations with little or no immunologic

TABLE 33–3

Major Antigenic Shifts Associated with Influenza A Pandemics, 1947–1987

YEAR	SUBTYPE	PROTOTYPE STRAIN
1947	H_1N_1	A/FM1/47
1957	H_2N_2	A/Singapore/57
1968	H_3N_2	A/Hong Kong/68
1977	H_1N_1	A/USSR/77
1987	H_3N_2	No pandemic occurred; various strains circulating worldwide

experience with the subtype. As the population of susceptible individuals is exhausted (ie, subtype-specific immunity is acquired by increasing numbers of people), the subtype continues to circulate for a time, undergoing mutations with subtle antigenic drifts from season to season. This allows some degree of virus transmission to continue. Infectivity persists because subtype-specific immunity is not entirely protective against drifting strains; for example, an individual may have antibodies reasonably protective against influenza A/Texas/77(H_3N_2), yet be susceptible in succeeding years to reinfection by influenza A/Bangkok/79(H_3N_2). Eventually, however, the overall immunity of the population becomes sufficient to minimize the epidemic potential of the major subtype and its drifting strains. Unfortunately, the battle is never entirely won; the scene is set for the sudden and usually unpredictable appearance of an entirely new subtype that may not have circulated among humans for 20 years or more.

Individual variation is significant

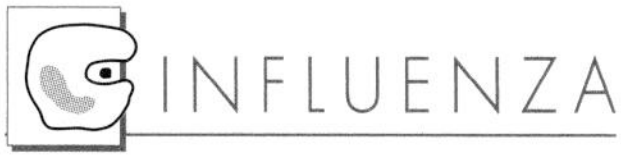

INFLUENZA

CLINICAL CAPSULE

Influenza virus types A and B typically cause more severe symptoms than influenza virus type C. The typical illness is characterized by an abrupt onset (over several hours) of fever, diffuse muscle aches and chills. This is followed within 12 to 36 hours by respiratory signs, such as rhinitis, cough, and respiratory distress. The acute phase usually lasts 3 to 5 days, but a complete return to normal activities may take 2 to 6 weeks. Serious complications, especially pneumonia, are common.

EPIDEMIOLOGY

Humans are the major hosts of the influenza viruses, and severe respiratory disease is the primary manifestation of infection. However, influenza A viruses closely related to those prevalent in humans circulate among many mammalian and avian species. As noted previously, some of these may undergo antigenic mutation or genetic recombination and emerge as new human epidemic strains.

Human, animal, and avian strains are similar

Characteristic influenza outbreaks have been described since the early 16th century, and outbreaks of varying severity have occurred nearly every year. Severe pandemics occurred in 1743, 1889–1890, 1918–1919 (the Spanish flu), and 1957 (the Asian flu). These episodes were associated with particularly high mortality; the Spanish flu was thought to have caused at least 20 million deaths. Usually, the elderly and persons of any age group with cardiac or pulmonary disease have the highest death rate.

Pandemic influenza may have high mortality

Direct droplet spread is the most common mode of transmission. Influenza infections in temperate climates tend to occur most frequently during midwinter months. Major epidemics of influenza A usually occur at 2- to 3-year intervals, and influenza

Seasonality favors winter months

Epidemic intervals usually a few years

Excess mortality or increased absenteeism are indictors of epidemics

B epidemics occur irregularly, usually every 4 to 5 years. The typical epidemic develops over a period of 3 to 6 weeks and can involve 10% of the population. Illness rates may exceed 30% among school-aged children, residents of closed institutions, and industrial groups. One major indicator of influenza virus activity is an abrupt rise in school or industrial absenteeism. In severe influenza A epidemics, the number of deaths reported in a given area of the country often exceeds the number expected for that period. This significant increase, referred to as **excess mortality,** is another indicator of severe, widespread illness. Influenza B rarely causes such severe epidemics.

PATHOGENESIS

Virus multiplies in respiratory epithelium

Synthetic blocks cause cilial damage and cell desquamation

Clearance mechanisms compromised

Influenza viruses have a predilection for the respiratory tract, and viremia is rarely detected. They multiply in ciliated respiratory epithelial cells, leading to functional and structural ciliary abnormalities. This is accompanied by a switch-off of protein and nucleic acid synthesis in the affected cells, the release of lysosomal hydrolytic enzymes, and desquamation of both ciliated and mucus-producing epithelial cells. Thus, there is substantial interference with the mechanical clearance mechanism of the respiratory tract. The process of programmed cell death (apoptosis) results in the cleavage of complement components, leading to localized inflammation. Early in infection, the primary chemotactic stimulus is directed toward mononuclear leukocytes, which constitute the major cellular inflammatory component. The respiratory epithelium may not be restored to normal for 2 to 10 weeks after the initial insult.

Viral toxicity causes inflammation

Phagocytic host defenses compromised

The virus particles are also toxic to tissues. This toxicity can be demonstrated by inoculating high concentrations of inactivated virions into mice, which produces acute inflammatory changes in the absence of viral penetration or replication within cells. Other host cell functions are also severely impaired, particularly during the acute phase of infection. These functions include chemotactic, phagocytic, and intracellular killing functions of polymorphonuclear leukocytes and perhaps of alveolar macrophage activity.

Damage creates susceptibility to bacterial invasion

Interferon and cytotoxic T-cell responses associated with recovery

The net result of these effects is that, on entry into the respiratory tract, the viruses cause cell damage, especially in the respiratory epithelium, which elicits an acute inflammatory response and impairs mechanical and cellular host responses. This damage renders the host highly susceptible to invasive bacterial **superinfection.** In vitro studies also suggest that bacterial pathogens such as staphylococci can more readily adhere to the surfaces of influenza virus-infected cells. Recovery from infection begins with interferon production, which limits further virus replication, and with rapid generation of natural killer cells. Shortly thereafter, class I major histocompatibility complex (MHC)–restricted cytotoxic T cells appear in large numbers to participate in the lysis of virus-infected cells and, thus, in initial control of the infection. This is followed by the appearance of local and humoral antibody along with an evolving, more durable cellular immunity. Finally, there is repair of tissue damage.

IMMUNITY

Antihemagglutinin antibody has protective effect

Antineuraminidase may limit viral spread

Although cell-mediated immune responses are undoubtedly important in influenza virus infections, humoral immunity has been investigated more extensively. Typically, patients respond to infection within a few days by producing antibodies directed toward the group ribonucleoprotein antigen, the hemagglutinin, and the neuraminidase. Peak antibody titer levels are usually reached within 2 weeks of onset and then gradually wane over the following months to varying low levels. Antibody to the ribonucleoprotein appears to confer little or no protection against reinfection. Antihemagglutinin antibody is considered the most protective; it has the ability to neutralize virus on reexposure. However, such immunity is relative, and quantitative differences in responsiveness exist between individuals. Furthermore, antigenic shifts and drifts often allow the virus to subvert the antibody response on subsequent exposures. Antibody to neuraminidase antigen is not as protective as antihemagglutinin antibody but plays a role in limiting virus spread within the host.

INFLUENZA: CLINICAL ASPECTS

MANIFESTATIONS

As stated previously, influenza A and B viruses tend to cause the most severe illnesses, whereas influenza C seems to occur infrequently and generally causes milder disease. The typical acute influenzal syndrome is described here.

The incubation period is brief, lasting an average of 2 days. Onset is usually abrupt, with symptoms developing over a few hours. These include fever, myalgia, headache, and occasionally shaking chills. Within 6 to 12 hours, the illness reaches its maximum severity, and a dry, nonproductive cough develops. The acute findings persist, sometimes with worsening cough, for 3 to 5 days, followed by gradual improvement. By about 1 week after onset, patients feel significantly better. However, fatigue, nonspecific weakness, and cough can remain frustrating lingering problems for an additional 2 to 6 weeks.

Short incubation period followed by acute disease with dry cough

Occasionally, patients develop a progressive infection that involves the tracheobronchial tree and lungs. In these situations, pneumonia, which can be lethal, is the result. Other unusual acute manifestations of influenza include central nervous system (CNS) dysfunction, myositis, and myocarditis. In infants and children, a serious complication known as Reye's syndrome may develop 2 to 12 days after onset of the infection. It is characterized by severe fatty infiltration of the liver and cerebral edema. This syndrome is associated not only with influenza viruses but with a wide variety of systemic viral illnesses. The risk is enhanced by exposure to salicylates, such as aspirin.

Progressive respiratory infection and pneumonia may be lethal

Reye's syndrome may follow

The most common and important complication of influenza virus infection is bacterial superinfection. Such infections usually involve the lung, but bacteremia with secondary seeding of distant sites can also occur. The superinfection, which can develop at any time in the acute or convalescent phase of the disease, is often heralded by an abrupt worsening of the patient's condition after initial stabilization. The bacteria most commonly involved include *Streptococcus pneumoniae, Haemophilus influenzae,* and *Staphylococcus aureus.*

Sudden worsening suggests bacterial superinfection

In summary, there are essentially three ways in which influenza may cause death:

- **Underlying disease with decompensation.** Individuals with limited cardiovascular or pulmonary reserves can be further compromised by any respiratory infection. Thus, the elderly and those of any age with underlying chronic cardiac or pulmonary disease are at particular risk.
- **Superinfection.** Superinfection can lead to bacterial pneumonia and occasionally disseminated bacterial infection.
- **Direct rapid progression.** Less commonly, progression of the viral infection can lead to overwhelming viral pneumonia with asphyxia.

DIAGNOSIS

During the acute phase of illness, influenza viruses can be readily isolated from respiratory tract specimens, such as nasopharyngeal and throat swabs. Most strains grow in primary monkey kidney cell cultures, and they can be detected by hemadsorption or hemagglutination. Rapid diagnosis of infection is possible by direct immunofluorescence or immunoenzymatic detection of viral antigen in epithelial cells or secretions from the respiratory tract. Serologic diagnosis is of considerable help epidemiologically and is usually made by demonstrating a fourfold or greater increase in hemagglutination inhibition antibody titers in acute and convalescent specimens collected 10 to 14 days apart.

Virus isolation detects virus

Rapid detection of antigen often used

Serodiagnosis is useful epidemiologically

TREATMENT

The two basic approaches to management of influenzal disease are symptomatic care and anticipation of potential complications, particularly bacterial superinfection. Once the diagnosis has been made, rest, adequate fluid intake, conservative use of analgesics for

Supportive therapy indicated

TABLE 33–4

Comparison of Antiviral Drugs for Influenza

Feature	Amantadine	Rimantadine	Zanamivir	Oseltamivir
Susceptible viruses	Influenza A only	Influenza A only	Influenza A and B	Influenza A and B
Emergent resistant strains	Yes	Yes	Not known	Not known
Administration	Oral	Oral	Inhalation	Oral

myalgia and headache, and antitussives for severe cough are commonly prescribed. It must be emphasized that nonprescription drugs must be used with caution. This applies particularly to drugs containing salicylates given to children, because the risk of Reye's syndrome must be considered.

Antibiotic prophylaxis does not prevent bacterial superinfection

Bacterial superinfection is often suggested by a rapid worsening of clinical symptoms after patients have initially stabilized. Antibiotic prophylaxis has not been shown to enhance or diminish the likelihood of superinfection but can increase the risk of acquisition of more resistant bacterial flora in the respiratory tract and make the superinfection more difficult to treat. Ideally, physicians should instruct patients regarding the natural history of the influenza virus infection and be prepared to respond to bacterial complications, if they occur, with specific diagnosis and therapy.

Antiviral therapy must begin early

When influenza A infection is proved or strongly suspected, 4 to 5 days of therapy with amantadine or rimantadine, two symmetric amines, may also be considered (Table 33–4). Such treatment has been shown to benefit some patients to a modest degree, as measured by reduction of number of days of confinement to bed, of fever, and of functional respiratory impairment. However, these effects have been observed only when the drug is administered early in the illness (within 12 to 24 hours of onset). The neuraminidase inhibitors (zanamivir or oseltamivir) have also proved beneficial, if begun early. They are also active against influenza B (see Table 33–4).

PREVENTION

Whole virus and "split" vaccines are protective but variable and of short duration

Annual revaccination against most current strains is necessary

Vaccination indicated for high-risk individuals

The best available method of control is by use of **killed viral vaccines** newly formulated each year to most closely match the influenza A and B antigenic subtypes currently causing infections. These inactivated vaccines may contain whole virions or "split" subunits composed primarily of hemagglutinin antigens. They are commonly used, in two doses given 1 month apart, to immunize children who may not have been immunized previously; among older children and adults, single annual doses are recommended just prior to influenza season. Vaccine efficacy is variable, and annual revaccination is necessary to ensure maximal protection. Used in this way, the virus vaccines may be 70 to 85% effective. It is recommended that vaccination be directed primarily toward the elderly, individuals of all ages who are at high risk (eg, those with chronic lung or heart disease), and their close contacts, including medical personnel and household members. Live attenuated vaccines that are administered by nose drops are also being evaluated, and show considerable promise for the future.

Amantadine or rimantadine prophylaxis effective short-term for influenza A only

Blocks virus uncoating and assembly

Studies have shown that both amantadine and rimantadine are effective in short-term (several weeks) oral prophylaxis of influenza A infections. They act by blocking the ion channel of the viral M2 protein, resulting in interference with the key role for M2 protein in early virus uncoating. Later virion assembly may also be affected. However, these agents have side effects and are recommended only for high-risk patients until vaccine-induced immunity can be achieved. A typical example of their use would be during an epidemic in which an elderly, potentially susceptible patient may become exposed to infection within a defined period. Oral prophylaxis may be initiated concurrently with administration of a vaccine containing the most current antigens and continued for 2 weeks. The immunogenic effect of the vaccine should ensure continued protection. It must be emphasized that these drugs have been proven effective for influenza A virus infections only; they are useless in the management and prevention of infections caused by other types of influenza or by any other respiratory virus. Unfortunately, virus resistance to both drugs can readily develop in vitro or in vivo. A single amino acid substitution in the transmembrane portion of the M2 protein is all that is necessary for this to occur.

Resistance from single amino acid substitution in M2 protein

Zanamivir and oseltamivir, approved for use in 1999, both act by blocking the enzymatically active neuraminidase glycoprotein present on the surfaces of influenza A and B viruses, thus limiting virus release from infected cells, and subsequent spread in the host. No viral resistance to these drugs has yet been noted (see Table 33–4).

Neuraminidase inhibitors are useful for influenza A and B

Respiratory Syncytial Virus

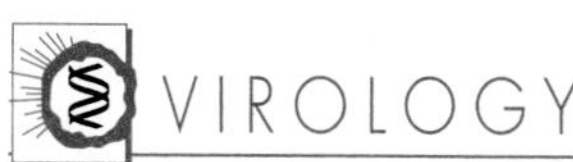

VIROLOGY

Respiratory syncytial virus (RSV) is classified as a pneumovirus within the paramyxovirus family. Its name is derived from its ability to produce cell fusion in tissue culture (syncytium formation). Unlike influenza or parainfluenza viruses, it possesses no hemagglutinin or neuraminidase. The RNA genome is nonsegmented, negative sense, and single stranded and codes for at least 10 different proteins. Among these are two matrix (M) proteins in the viral envelope. One forms the inner lining of the viral envelope; the function of the other is uncertain.

Pneumovirus causing syncytium formation in cell cultures

Enveloped RNA virus with unsegmented genome

The antigens on the surface spikes of the viral envelope include the G glycoprotein, which mediates virus attachment to host cell receptors, and the fusion (F) glycoprotein, which induces fusion of the viral envelope with the host cell surface to facilitate entry. F glycoprotein is also responsible for fusion of infected cells in cell cultures, leading to the appearance of multinucleated giant cells (syncytium formation). Antibodies directed at the F glycoprotein are more efficient than anti-G glycoprotein antibodies in neutralizing the virus in vitro.

Two glycoproteins mediate attachment and syncytium formation

At least two antigenic subgroups (A and B) of RSV are known to exist. This dimorphism is due primarily to differences in the G glycoprotein. The epidemiologic and biological significance of these variants is not yet certain; however, epidemiologic studies have suggested that group A infections tend to be more severe. RSV is the single most important etiologic agent in respiratory diseases of infancy, and it is the major cause of bronchiolitis and pneumonia among infants under 1 year of age.

RSV is most important respiratory virus in infants

RESPIRATORY SYNCYTIAL VIRUS DISEASE

CLINICAL CAPSULE

RSV primarily infects the bronchi, bronchioles, and alveoli of the lung. The illnesses clinically categorized as croup, bronchitis, bronchiolitis or pneumonia are extremely common in infants. The acute phase of cough, wheezing and respiratory distress lasts 1 to 3 weeks. The severity of respiratory involvement and the high prevalence during outbreaks both account for a large number of hospitalizations on pediatric units each year. Elderly or immunocompromised patients are also frequently susceptible and can be severely affected.

EPIDEMIOLOGY

Community outbreaks of RSV infection occur annually commencing at any time from late fall to early spring. The usual outbreak lasts 8 to 12 weeks and can involve nearly one half of all families with children. In the family setting, it appears that older siblings often introduce the virus into the home, and secondary infection rates can be almost 50%. The usual duration of virus shedding is 5 to 7 days; young infants, however, may shed virus for 9 to 20 days or longer.

High attack rate, introduced by older siblings

Nosocomial infection reduced by careful handwashing

Spread of RSV in the hospital setting is also a major problem. Control is difficult, but includes careful attention to handwashing between contacts with patients, isolation, and exclusion of personnel and visitors who have any form of respiratory illness. Masks are not effective in controlling nosocomial spread.

PATHOGENESIS

Confined to respiratory epithelium

RSV is spread to the upper respiratory tract by contact with infective secretions. Infection appears to be confined primarily to the respiratory epithelium, with progressive involvement of the middle and lower airways. Viremia occurs rarely. The direct effect of virus on respiratory tract epithelial cells is similar to that previously described for influenza viruses, and cytotoxic T cells appear to play a similar role in early control of the acute infection.

Enhanced disease in infants may have immunologic basis

Th_2 stimulated cytokines cause injury

The apparent enhanced severity of disease, particularly in very young infants, is not yet clearly understood but may have an immunologic basis. Factors that have been proposed to play a role include (1) qualitative or quantitative deficits in humoral or secretory antibody responses to critical virus-specified proteins, (2) formation of antigen–antibody complexes within the respiratory tract resulting in complement activation, or (3) excessive damage from inflammatory cytokines. Experimental evidence suggests that patients who respond to RSV infections with CD4+ cells that are predominantly of the T_H type 2 have more severe disease than those with predominant T_H type 1 responses. This is thought to be due to the inflammatory cytokines produced by T_H type 2 cells, including interleukin (IL)-4, IL-5, IL-6, IL-10, and IL-13.

Necrosis and inflammation plugs bronchioles and alveoli

The major pathologic findings are in the bronchi, bronchioles, and alveoli. These include necrosis of epithelial cells; interstitial mononuclear cell inflammatory infiltrates, which sometimes also involve the alveoli and alveolar ducts; and plugging of smaller airways with material containing mucus, necrotic cells, and fibrin (Fig 33–2). Multinucleated syncytial cells with intracytoplasmic inclusions are occasionally seen in the affected tracheobronchial epithelium.

IMMUNITY

Immunity to reinfection is brief

Infection results in IgG and IgA humoral and secretory antibody responses. However, immunity to reinfection is quite tenuous, as demonstrated by patients who have recovered from a primary acute episode and have become reinfected with disease of similar severity in the same or succeeding year. Illness severity appears to diminish with increasing age and successive reinfection.

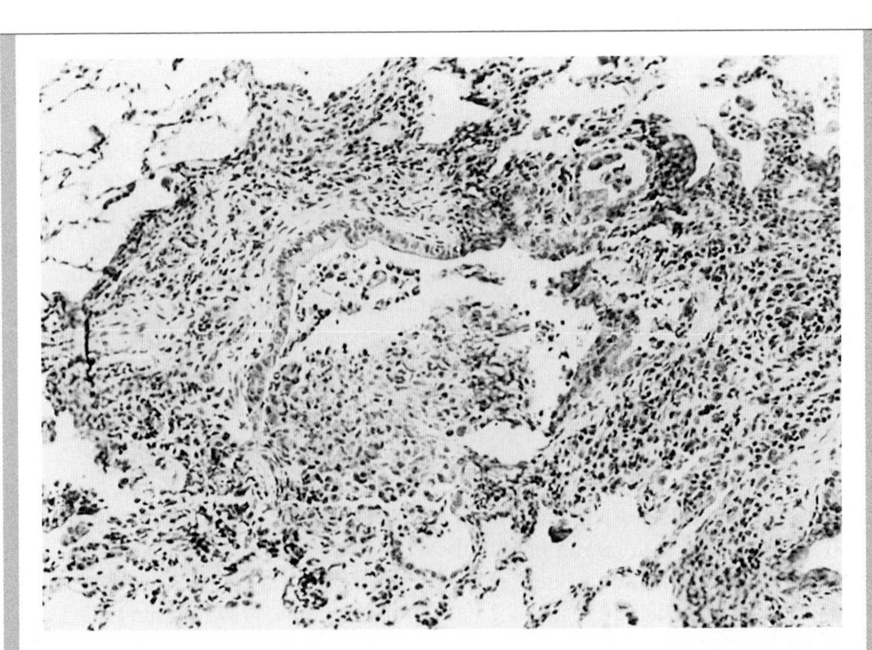

FIGURE 33–2
Photomicrograph illustrating the bronchiolar and surrounding interstitial inflammation in respiratory syncytial virus infection. (Original magnification ×100.)

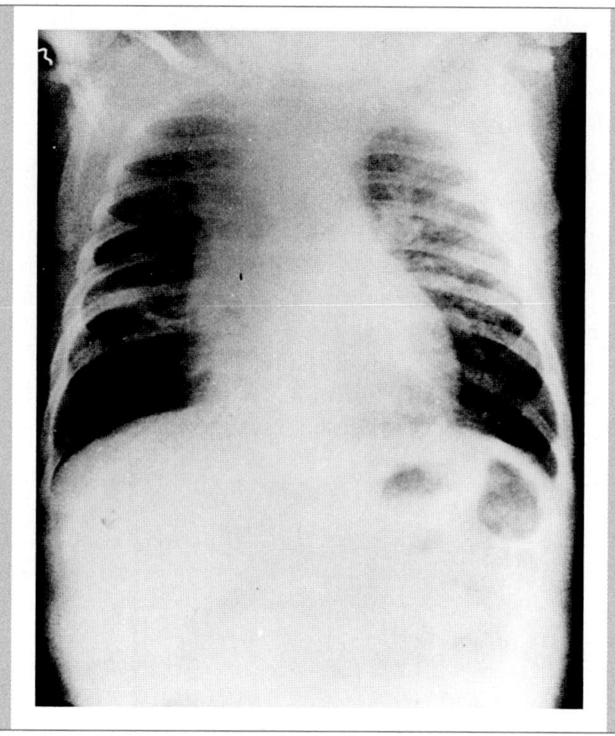

FIGURE 33–3
Chest radiograph of an infant with a severe case of respiratory syncytial virus pneumonia and bronchiolitis. Bilateral interstitial infiltrates, hyperexpansion of the lung, and right upper lobe atelectasis (arrow) are all present.

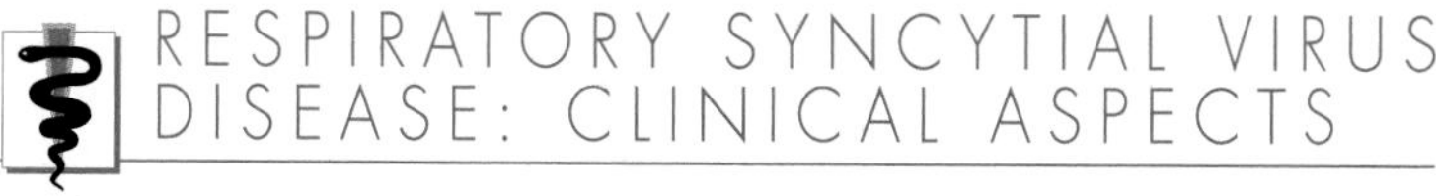

RESPIRATORY SYNCYTIAL VIRUS DISEASE: CLINICAL ASPECTS

MANIFESTATIONS

The usual incubation period is 2 to 4 days, followed by the onset of rhinitis; severity of illness progresses to a peak within 1 to 3 days. In infants, this peak usually takes the form of bronchiolitis and pneumonitis, with cough, wheezing, and respiratory distress. Clinical findings include **hyperexpansion** of the lungs, **hypoxemia** (low oxygenation of blood), and **hypercapnia** (carbon dioxide retention). Interstitial infiltrates, often with areas of pulmonary collapse, may be seen on chest radiography (Fig 33–3). Fever is variable. The duration of acute illness is often 10 to 14 days.

Infant bronchiolitis and pneumonitis lasts up to 2 weeks

The fatality rate among hospitalized infected infants is estimated to be 0.5 to 1%; however, this rises to 15% or greater in children receiving cancer chemotherapy, infants with congenital heart disease, and those with severe immunodeficiency. Infants with underlying chronic lung disease are also at high risk. Causes of death include respiratory failure, right-sided heart failure (cor pulmonale), and bacterial superinfection. Death has sometimes resulted from unnecessary procedures in patients in whom RSV infection was not considered. Bronchoscopy, lung biopsy, or overly aggressive therapy with corticosteroids and bronchodilators for presumed asthma can all pose a danger to such patients.

Mortality is highest with underlying disease

Older infants, children, and adults are also readily infected. The clinical illnesses in these groups are usually milder and include croup, tracheobronchitis, and upper respiratory infection (URI); however, elderly persons can experience severe morbidity. RSV can also cause acute flare-ups of chronic bronchitis and trigger acute wheezing episodes in asthmatic children.

Children and adults have milder illness

Can trigger wheezing in asthmatics

DIAGNOSIS

Rapid diagnosis of RSV infection can be made by immunofluorescence or immunoenzyme detection of viral antigen. The virus can also be isolated from the respiratory tract by prompt inoculation of specimens into cell cultures. Syncytial cytopathic effects

Virus isolation, immunofluorescence, or immunoassay detect RSV

develop over 2 to 7 days. Serodiagnosis may also be used but requires acute and convalescent sera and is less sensitive than antigen detection methods or culture.

TREATMENT AND PREVENTION

Supportive treatment is indicated

Treatment is directed primarily at the underlying pathophysiology and includes adequate oxygenation, ventilatory support when necessary, and close observation for complications such as bacterial superinfection and right-sided heart failure. Some studies suggest that ribavirin aerosol treatment may be effective in selected circumstances.

Monoclonal antibody and immune globulin used for prophylaxis

No vaccine is currently available. Attenuated live virus vaccines and immune globulin containing high antibody titers to RSV are also under active investigation; a high-titered monoclonal antibody against F protein has been used for prophylaxis in high-risk infants (those born prematurely or with chronic lung disease). This method requires monthly injections during the RSV season (usually 5 months) and is extremely expensive.

PARAINFLUENZA VIRUSES

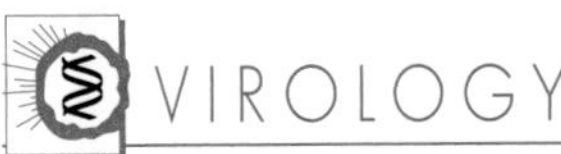

VIROLOGY

Enveloped paramyxoviruses have neuraminidase and hemagglutinin

Four serotypes are antigenically stable

There are four serotypes of parainfluenza viruses: parainfluenza 1, 2, 3, and 4. These enveloped viruses belong to the paramyxovirus group; contain nonsegmented, negative-sense, single-stranded RNA; and, like the influenza viruses, possess a neuraminidase and hemagglutinin. Their mode of spread and pathogenesis is similar to that of the influenza viruses. They differ from the influenza viruses in that RNA synthesis occurs in the cytoplasm rather than the nucleus. In addition, the antigenic makeup of the four serotypes is relatively stable, and significant antigenic shift or drift does not occur. Each serotype is considered separately.

PARAINFLUENZA DISEASE

Transient immunity

The parainfluenza viruses are important because of the serious diseases they can cause in infants and young children. Parainfluenza 1 and 3 are particularly common in this regard. Overall, the group is thought to be responsible for 15 to 20% of all nonbacterial respiratory diseases requiring hospitalization in infancy and childhood. Immunity to reinfection is transient; although repeated infections can occur in older children and adults, they are usually milder than the illnesses of infancy and early childhood.

PARAINFLUENZA DISEASE: CLINICAL ASPECTS

MANIFESTATIONS

The onset of illness may be abrupt, as in acute spasmodic croup, but usually begins as a mild URI with variable progression over 1 to 3 days to involvement of the middle or lower respiratory tract. Duration of acute illness can vary from 4 to 21 days but is usually 7 to 10 days.

Parainfluenza 1

Croup and tracheobronchitis are seen

Parainfluenza 1 is the major cause of acute croup (laryngotracheitis) in infants and young children but also causes less severe diseases such as mild upper respiratory illness (URI), pharyngitis, and tracheobronchitis in individuals of all ages. Outbreaks of infection tend to occur most frequently during the fall months.

Parainfluenza 2

Parainfluenza 2 is of slightly less significance than parainfluenza 1 or 3. It has been associated with croup, primarily in children, with mild URI, and occasionally with acute lower respiratory disease. As with parainfluenza 1, outbreaks usually occur during the fall months.

Croup is primary disease

Parainfluenza 3

Parainfluenza 3 is a major cause of severe lower respiratory disease in infants and young children. It often causes bronchitis, pneumonia, and croup in children less than 1 year of age. In older children and adults, it may cause URI or tracheobronchitis. Infections are common and can occur in any season; it is estimated that nearly one half of all children have been exposed to this virus by 1 year of age.

Produces severe lower respiratory disease in infants

Parainfluenza 4

Parainfluenza 4 is the least common of the group. It is generally associated with mild upper respiratory illness only.

Causes only URI

DIAGNOSIS, TREATMENT, AND PREVENTION

Specific diagnosis is based on virus isolation, usually in monkey kidney cell cultures, or on serology using hemagglutination inhibition, complement fixation, or neutralization assays on paired sera to detect a rising antibody titer. Immunofluorescence or immunoenzyme assays can also be used for rapid detection of antigen in respiratory epithelial cells. Currently, there is no method of control or specific therapy for these infections.

Laboratory diagnosis by isolation or antigen detection

Croup or URI are not treatable

ADENOVIRUSES

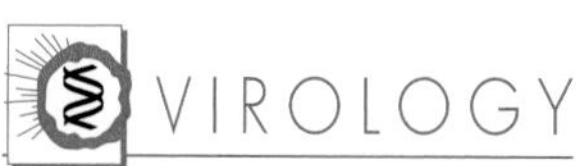

Of the almost 100 different serotypes of adenoviruses, 49 are known to affect humans. These viruses are naked and icosahedral and possess double-stranded DNA. Replication and assembly occur in the nucleus, and virions are released by cell destruction. All adenoviruses share a common group-specific, complement-fixing antigen associated with the hexon component of the viral capsid. Adenoviruses are characterized by their ubiquity and persistence in host tissues for periods ranging from a few days to several years. Their ability to produce infection without disease is illustrated by the frequent recovery of virus from tonsils or adenoids removed from healthy children (the group name is derived from its discovery in 1953 as a latent agent in many adenoid tissue specimens) and by prolonged intermittent shedding of virus from the pharynx and intestinal tract after initial infection.

Multiple serotypes of naked, double-stranded DNA viruses

Potential for prolonged infection without disease

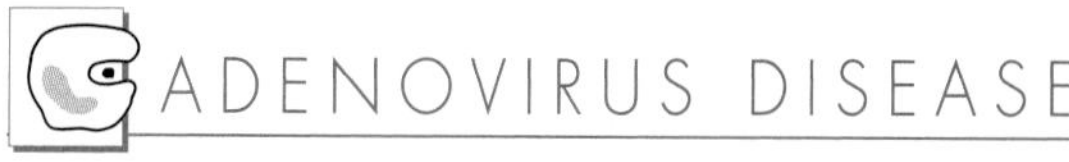

EPIDEMIOLOGY

Type 1 and 2 adenoviruses are highly endemic; type 5 is the next most common. Most primary infections with these viruses occur early in life and are spread by the respiratory or fecal–oral route. Overall, only about 45% of adenovirus infections result in disease. Their most significant contribution to acute illness is in children, particularly those under 2 years of age (approximately 10% of acute febrile illness). Adenoviruses are also major causes of acute respiratory disease in military recruits, usually by types 4 and 7.

Disease in children and military recruits is spread by respiratory or fecal–oral route

Swimming pool and medication-associated conjunctivitis occur in outbreaks

Infections caused by serotypes 1, 2, and 5 are generally most frequent during the first few years of life. All serotypes can occur during any season of the year but are encountered most frequently during late winter or early spring. Sharp outbreaks of disease caused by serotypes 3 and 7 have been traced to inadequately chlorinated swimming pools. Conjunctivitis is the illness most commonly associated with these episodes. Other outbreaks of conjunctivitis have been traced to physicians' offices and appear to have been spread by contaminated ophthalmic medications or diagnostic equipment.

PATHOGENESIS

Infects by droplet, oral route, or direct inoculation

Epithelial cell replication may be followed by viremic spread and remote disease

The adenoviruses usually enter the host by inhalation of droplet nuclei or by the oral route. Direct inoculation onto nasal or conjunctival mucosa by hands, contaminated towels, or ophthalmic medications may also occur. The virus replicates in epithelial cells, producing cell necrosis and inflammation. Viremia sometimes occurs and can result in spread to distant sites, such as the kidney, bladder, liver, lymphoid tissue (including mesenteric nodes), and, occasionally, the CNS. In the acute phase of infection, the distant sites may also show inflammation; for example, abdominal pain is occasionally seen with severe illnesses and is believed to result from mesenteric lymphadenitis caused by the viruses.

Integration of adenoviral DNA produces latency

After the acute phase of illness, the viruses may remain in tissues, particularly lymphoid structures such as tonsils, adenoids, and intestinal Peyer's patches, and become reactivated and shed without producing illness for 6 to 18 months thereafter. This reactivation is enhanced by stressful events (stress reactivation), such as infection by other agents. Integration of adenoviral DNA into the host cell genome has been shown to occur; this latent state can persist for years in tonsillar tissue and peripheral blood lymphocytes.

Penton projections are toxic to cells

Like the viruses described previously, adenoviruses have a primary pathology involving epithelial cell necrosis with a predominantly mononuclear inflammatory response. In some instances, smudgy intranuclear inclusions may be seen in infected cells (Fig 33–4). A potentially important pathogenic feature of the virion is the presence of pentons, which are located at each of the 12 corners of the icosahedron. These fiber-like projections with knob-like terminal structures are believed to bind to a cellular receptor that is similar or identical to the one for group B coxsackieviruses. The pentons also appear to be responsible for a toxic effect on cells, which manifests as clumping and detachment in vitro.

Proteins restrict cytotoxic T cells and enhance cytokine susceptibility

In addition, adenoviruses have developed other novel strategies to survive in the host yet produce deleterious effects. These include encoding a protein in its early E3 genomic region that binds class I MHC antigens in the endoplasmic reticulum, thus restricting their expression on the surface of infected cells and interfering with recognition and attack by cytotoxic T cells. This ability to evade immunosurveillance may be vital to establishment of latency. Another early protein (E1A) has been associated with increased susceptibility

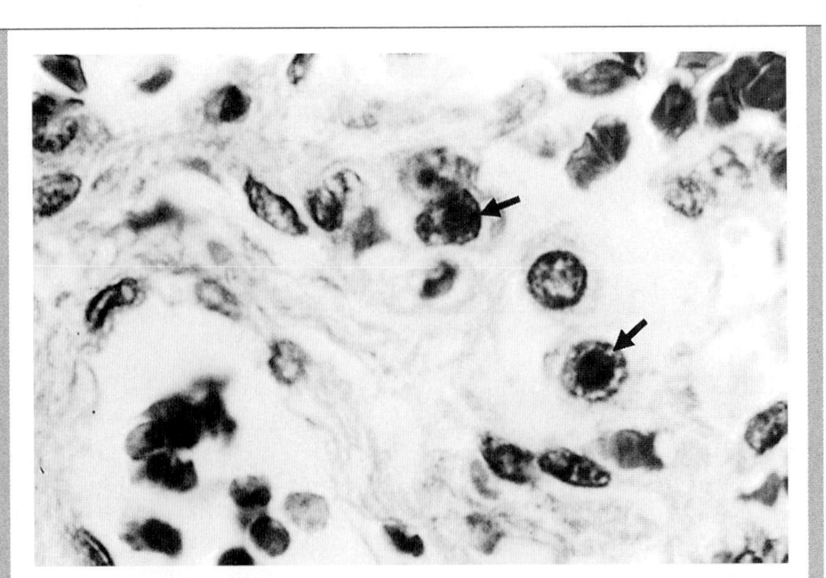

FIGURE 33–4
Lung tissue from a fatal case of adenovirus type 7 pneumonia. Large, smudgy intranuclear inclusions in alveolar epithelial cells (arrows), which are sometimes seen in adenovirus infections, are present. (Original magnification ×100.)

of epithelial cells to destruction by tumor necrosis factor and other cytokines. Other adenoviral proteins have been described that have a variety of effects on cell function and susceptibility to cytolysis. One of these, called the adenovirus death protein, is considered important for efficient lysis of infected cells and release of newly formed virions.

IMMUNITY

Immunity after infection is serotype specific and usually long lasting. In addition to type-specific immunity, group-specific complement-fixing antibodies appear in response to infection. These antibodies are useful indicators of infection, but do not specify the infecting serotype.

Immunity is type specific

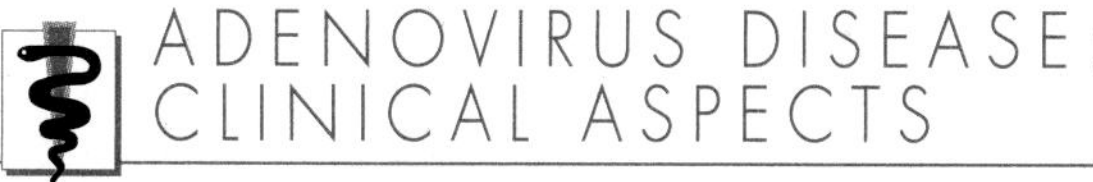

ADENOVIRUS DISEASE: CLINICAL ASPECTS

MANIFESTATIONS

The diversity of major syndromes and serotypes commonly associated with adenoviruses are summarized in Table 33–5. The acute respiratory syndromes vary in both clinical manifestations and severity. Symptoms include fever, rhinitis, pharyngitis, cough, and conjunctivitis. Adenoviruses are also common causes of nonstreptococcal exudative pharyngitis, particularly among children less than 3 years of age. Acute, and occasionally chronic, conjunctivitis and keratoconjunctivitis have been associated with several serotypes. More severe disease, such as laryngitis, croup, bronchiolitis, and pneumonia, may also occur. A syndrome of pharyngitis and conjunctivitis (pharyngoconjunctival fever) is classically associated with adenovirus infection. Adenoviruses can also cause acute hemorrhagic cystitis, in which hematuria and dysuria are prominent findings. Some serotypes are significant causes of gastroenteritis (see Chapter 39).

Multiple upper respiratory syndromes, conjunctivitis, and pharyngitis are common

More severe disease includes hemorrhagic cystitis

DIAGNOSIS

Many serotypes, other than those associated with acute gastroenteritis, can be readily isolated in heteroploid cell cultures. There is little difficulty in relating the virus detected to the illness in question when the isolate has been obtained from a site other than the upper respiratory or gastrointestinal tract (eg, lung biopsy, conjunctival swabs, urine). However, because of the known tendency for intermittent asymptomatic shedding into the oropharynx and feces, isolates from these latter sites must be interpreted more cautiously. Serologic testing of acute and convalescent sera may be necessary to confirm the relationship between the virus and the illness in question.

Viral isolation from oropharynx or feces may not mean disease

TABLE 33–5

Clinical Syndromes Associated with Adenovirus Infection

Syndrome	Common Serotypes[a]
Childhood febrile illness; pharyngoconjunctival fever	1, 2, **3**, 5, 7, **7a**
Pneumonia and other acute respiratory illnesses	1, 2, **3**, 5, 7, **7a**, **7b** (4 in military recruits)
Pertussis-like illness	1, 2, **3**, 5, **19**, 21
Conjunctivitis	2, 5, 7, 8, **19**, 21
Keratoconjunctivitis	**3**, 8, 9, **19**
Acute hemorrhagic cystitis	11
Acute gastroenteritis	40, 41

[a]Serotypes in **boldface** are those commonly associated with outbreaks.

TREATMENT AND PREVENTION

Live vaccine used in military

There is no specific therapy for infection. A live virus vaccine containing serotypes 4 and 7, enclosed in enteric-coated capsules and administered orally, has been used in military recruits. The viruses are released into the small intestine, where they produce an asymptomatic, nontransmissible infection. This vaccine has been found effective but is neither available nor recommended for civilian groups.

RHINOVIRUSES

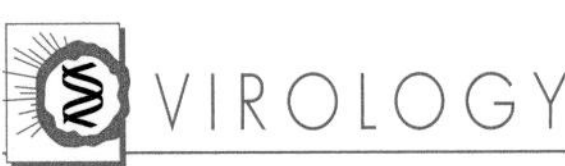

VIROLOGY

Small, naked RNA viruses include multiple serotypes

Optimum growth temperature is 33°C

Virus binds to ICAM intercellular adhesion molecule

The rhinovirus group comprises at least 115 accepted serotypes and more that are not yet classified. These picornaviruses are small (20 to 30 nm), naked particles containing single-stranded, positive-sense RNA. They are distinguished from enteroviruses by their acid lability and an optimum temperature of 33°C for in vitro replication. This temperature approximates that of the nasopharynx in the human host and may be a factor in the localization of pathologic findings at that site. Rhinoviruses are most consistently isolated in cultures of human diploid fibroblasts. The receptor for most rhinoviruses (and some coxsackieviruses) is glycoprotein intercellular adhesion molecule 1 (ICAM-1), a member of the immunoglobulin supergene family. ICAM-1 is best known for its role in immunologic cell adhesion; its ligand is lymphocyte function-associated antigen-1.

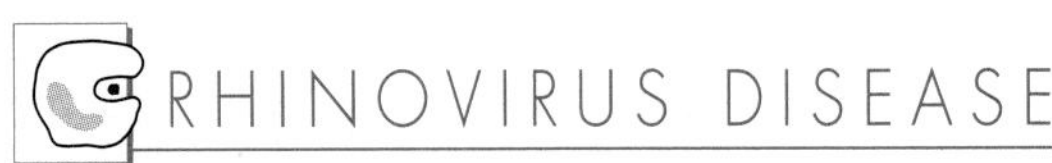

RHINOVIRUS DISEASE

Common cold viruses cause mild URI

Minimal cell injury is produced

Rhinoviruses are known as the common cold viruses. They represent the major causes of mild URI syndromes in all age groups, especially older children and adults. Lower respiratory tract disease caused by rhinoviruses is uncommon. The usual incubation period is 2 to 3 days, and acute symptoms commonly last 3 to 7 days. Interestingly, mucosal cell damage is minimal during the illness. Data suggest that activation and an increase in kinins, particularly bradykinin, may have a major role in the pathogenesis of increased secretions, vasodilation, and sore throat. Rhinovirus infections may be seen at any time of the year. Epidemic peaks tend to occur in the early fall or spring months.

RHINOVIRUS DISEASE: TREATMENT AND PREVENTION

Multiple serotypes make vaccine different

Pharmaceutical agents block attachment to ICAM

Currently there is no specific therapy and no methods of prevention with vaccines. Prospects for the development of an appropriate vaccine appear dim. The multiplicity of serotypes and their tendency to be type specific in the production of antibodies seem to demand the development of a multivalent vaccine, which would be extremely difficult to accomplish. However, recent studies have suggested that a monoclonal antibody directed at the virus receptor or the use of a recombinant soluble receptor (ICAM-1) might block attachment of rhinoviruses. Pleconaril, a capsid inhibitor that integrates into the viral capsid in the VP1 hydrophobic pocket of the virus, is another agent under study. This can block capsid attachment to cells and perhaps also affect viral uncoating after entry. In vitro, pleconaril shows broad activity against picornaviruses, including enteroviruses. It remains to be seen whether these observations can be translated into effective preventive or therapeutic applications. At present, the attitude toward these viruses is best summed up by Sir Christopher Andrewes, who suggested that we should accept these infections as "one of the stimulating risks of being mortal."

CORONAVIRUSES

Coronaviruses contain a single-stranded, positive-sense RNA genome, which is surrounded by an envelope that includes a lipid bilayer derived from intracellular rough endoplasmic reticulum and Golgi membranes of infected cells. Petal- or club-shaped spikes (peplomers) measuring approximately 13 nm project from the surface of the envelope, giving the appearance of a crown of thorns or a solar corona. The peplomers play an important role in inducing neutralizing and cellular immune responses. Like the rhinoviruses, coronaviruses are considered primary causes of the common cold. Based on serologic studies, it is estimated that they may cause as many as 5 to 10% of common colds in adults and a similar proportion of lower respiratory illnesses in children.

Enveloped RNA viruses

Disease similar to rhinoviruses

The number of serotypes is unknown. Two strains (229E and OC43) have been studied to some extent; it is clear that they can cause outbreaks similar to those of the rhinoviruses and that reinfection with the same serotype can occur. The cellular receptors for these strains are a cell surface metalloprotease and a sialic acid receptor similar to that bound by influenza C virus.

Metalloprotease and sialic acid receptors bind some strains

In late 2002, an illness called severe acute respiratory syndrome (SARS) appeared in China, spread throughout Asia, and is now found worldwide. The etiology has been identified as a previously undescribed coronavirus, with unusually high virulence for humans.

SARS is caused by a novel, new coronavirus

REOVIRUSES

The reoviruses (respiratory enteric orphans) are naked virions that contain segmented, double-stranded RNA and replicate in the cytoplasm of infected cells. They are ubiquitous and have been found in humans, simians, rodents, cattle, and a variety of other hosts. They have been studied in great detail as experimental models, revealing much basic knowledge about viral genetics and pathogenesis at the molecular level. Three serotypes are known to infect humans; however, their role and importance in human disease remain uncertain.

Association with human disease is uncertain

ADDITIONAL READING

Influenza Viruses

Cox NJ, Subbarao K. Influenza. *Lancet* 1999;354:1277–1282. An excellent explanatory review of influenza virology, epidemiology, and prevention.

Gubareva LV, Kaiser L, Hayden FG. Influenza virus neuraminidase inhibitors. *Lancet* 2000;355:827–835. An update of the field of antivirals for influenza viruses.

Hatta M, Gao P, Halfmann P, Kawaoka Y. Molecular basis for high virulence of Hong Kong H_5N_1 influenza A viruses. *Science* 2001;293:1840–1842. This report, along with the accompanying article and editorial, further clarifies the molecular reasons for development of "novel," dangerous influenza viruses.

Neuzil KM, Zhu Y, Griffin MR, et al. Burden of interpandemic influenza in children younger than 5 years: A 25-year prospective study. *J Infect Dis* 2002;185:147–152. Healthy young children are usually not routinely immunized against influenza. This report details the frequency and types of morbidity that can occur, suggesting a reevaluation of this general policy.

Subbarao K, Klimov A, Katz J, et al. Characterization of an avian influenza A (H_5N_1) virus isolated from a child with a fatal respiratory illness. *Science* 1998;279:393–396. This article helps explain how an influenza virus might cross species barriers with serious consequences.

Taubenberger JK, Reid AH, Krafft AE, et al. Initial genetic characterization of the 1918 "Spanish" influenza virus. *Science* 1997;275:1793–1976. Using a preserved lung tissue sample from a victim of the 1918 pandemic, the investigators were able to detect viral RNA sequences that indicate the virus belonged to subgroup of strains that infect humans and pigs.

Respiratory Syncytial Virus and Parainfluenza Viruses

Hall CB. Respiratory syncytial virus and parainfluenza virus. *N Engl J Med* 2001;344:1917–1928. This outstanding review further elucidates the nature of these viruses, their behavior, and what is currently known about their control.

Waris ME, Tsou C, Erdman DD, et al. Respiratory syncytial virus infection in BALB/c mice previously immunized with formalin-inactivated virus induces enhanced pulmonary inflammatory response with a predominant Th_2-like cytokine pattern. *J Virol* 1996;70:2852–2860. This study provides insight into the immunopathogenesis of respiratory syncytial virus and how vaccine-induced immunity can sometimes backfire.

Adenoviruses

Bergelson JM, Cunningham JA, Droguett G, et al. Isolation of a common receptor for coxsackie B viruses and adenoviruses 2 and 5. *Science* 1997;275:1320–1323. This article not only addresses fundamental questions about virus-cell interactions but is also relevant to the potential use of adenovirus vectors for gene therapy.

Tollefson AE, Scaria A, Hermiston TW, et al. The adenovirus death protein (E3-11.6K) is required at very late stages of infection for efficient cell lysis and release of adenovirus from infected cells. *J Virol* 1996;70:2296–2306. This and the next paper below illustrate the extraordinary ways in which adenoviruses can assure their ability to thrive and survive.

Rhinoviruses

Marlin SD, Staunton DE, Springer TA, et al. A soluble form of intercellular adhesion molecule-1 inhibits rhinovirus infection. *Nature* 1990;344:70–72. The experimental approach to defining the nature of a receptor and potential therapeutic applications is well illustrated.

Coronaviruses

Myint SH. Human coronaviruses: A brief review. *Med Virol* 1994;4:35–46. An apt review of the history of coronavirus discovery, our evolving knowledge and what remains to be learned.

Ksiazek TG, Erdman D, Goldsmith CS, et al. A novel coronavirus associated with severe acute respiratory syndrome. *N Engl J Med* 2003; 348:1947–1958. This, and accompanying articles in the same issue, are remarkable for the spread with which a previously unknown, highly virulent agent has become characterized clinically, epidemiologically, and biologically.

Reoviruses

Sharpe AH, Fields BN. Pathogenesis of viral infections: Basic concepts derived from the reovirus model. *N Engl J Med* 1985;312:486–497. A clearly presented review of the molecular basis of reovirus pathogenesis, with concepts that are relevant to our understanding of other viruses.

CHAPTER 34

Mumps Virus, Measles, Rubella, and Other Childhood Exanthems

C. GEORGE RAY

The major viruses to be described in this chapter (mumps, measles, rubella, and the human parvovirus B19) are genetically unrelated; however, they share several common epidemiologic characteristics: (1) distribution is worldwide, with a high incidence of infection in nonimmune individuals; (2) humans appear to be the sole reservoir of infection; and (3) person-to-person spread is primarily by the respiratory (aerosol) route.

The other disease discussed in this chapter, roseola infantum, is a common illness in early life.

MUMPS

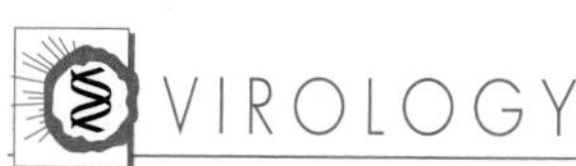

VIROLOGY

Mumps virus is a paramyxovirus, and only one antigenic type is known. Like fellow members of its genus, it contains single-stranded, negative-sense RNA surrounded by an envelope. There are two glycoproteins on the surface of the envelope; one mediates neuraminidase and hemagglutination activity, and the other is responsible for lipid membrane fusion to the host cell.

Enveloped single-stranded RNA virus with hemagglutinating and neuraminidase activity

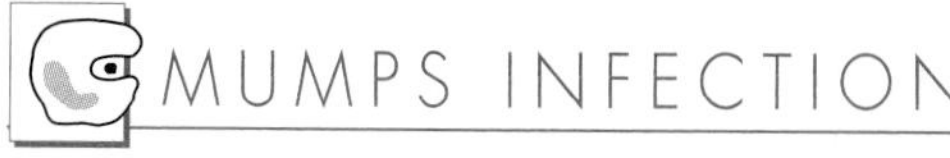

MUMPS INFECTION

CLINICAL CAPSULE

Before an effective vaccine against mumps was developed, the disease was a common childhood illness, commonly expressed as parotitis. It is also capable of causing aseptic meningitis, encephalitis, and (in adults) acute orchitis.

EPIDEMIOLOGY

High infectivity is present before and after onset of illness

The highest frequency of mumps infection is observed in the 5- to 15-year age group. Infection is rarely seen in the first year of life. Although about 85% of susceptible household contacts acquire infection, approximately 30 to 40% of these contacts do not develop clinical disease. The disease is communicable from approximately 7 days before until 9 days after onset of illness; however, virus has been recovered in urine for up to 14 days following onset. The highest incidence of infection is usually during the late winter and spring months, but it can occur during any season.

PATHOGENESIS

Viremic phase follows local replication

Viruria is common

After initial entry into the respiratory tract, the virus replicates locally. Replication is followed by viremic dissemination to target tissues such as the salivary glands and central nervous system (CNS). It is also possible that before development of immune responses, a secondary phase of viremia may result from virus replication in target tissues (eg, initial parotid involvement with later spread to other organs). Viruria is common, probably as a result of direct spread from the blood into the urine, as well as active viral replication in the kidney. The tissue response is that of cell necrosis and inflammation, with predominantly mononuclear cell infiltration. In the salivary glands, swelling and desquamation of necrotic epithelial lining cells, accompanied by interstitial inflammation and edema, may be seen within dilated ducts.

IMMUNITY

Neutralizing antibody is protective

As in most viral infections, the early antibody response is predominantly with IgM, which is replaced gradually over several weeks by specific IgG antibody. The latter persists for a lifetime but can often be detected only by specific neutralization assays. Immunity is associated with the presence of neutralizing antibody. The role of cellular immune responses is not clear, but they may contribute both to the pathogenesis of the acute disease and to recovery from infection. After primary infection, immunity to reinfection is virtually always permanent.

MUMPS: CLINICAL ASPECTS

MANIFESTATIONS

Incubation period is 12–29 days

Parotitis is unilateral or bilateral

After an incubation period of 12 to 29 days (average, 16 to 18 days), the typical case is characterized by fever and swelling with tenderness of the salivary glands, especially the parotid glands. Swelling may be unilateral or bilateral and persists for 7 to 10 days. Several complications can occur, usually within 1 to 3 weeks of onset of illness. All appear to be a direct result of virus spread to other sites and illustrate the extensive tissue tropism of mumps.

Complications, which can occur without parotitis, include infection of the following:

1. Meninges: Approximately 10% of all infected patients develop meningitis. It is usually mild, but can be confused with bacterial meningitis. In about one third of these cases, associated or preceding evidence of parotitis is absent.
2. Brain: Encephalitis is occasionally severe.
3. Spinal cord and peripheral nerves: Transverse myelitis and polyneuritis are rare.
4. Pancreas: Pancreatitis is suggested by abdominal pain and vomiting.
5. Testes: Orchitis is estimated to occur in 10 to 20% of infected men. Although subsequent sterility is a concern, it appears that this outcome is quite rare.
6. Ovaries: Oophoritis is an unusual, usually benign inflammation of the ovarian glands.

Other rare and transient complications include myocarditis, nephritis, arthritis, thyroiditis, thrombocytopenic purpura, mastitis, and pneumonia. Most complications usually resolve without sequelae within 2 to 3 weeks. However, occasional permanent effects have been noted, particularly in cases of severe CNS infection, in which sensorineural hearing loss and other impairment can occur.

DIAGNOSIS

Mumps virus can be readily isolated early in the illness from the saliva, pharynx, and other affected sites, such as the cerebrospinal fluid (CSF). The urine is also an excellent source for virus isolation. Mumps virus grows well in primary monolayer cell cultures derived from monkey kidney, producing syncytial giant cells and viral hemagglutinin. Rapid diagnosis can be made by direct detection of viral antigen in pharyngeal cells or urine sediment.

Cell culture of saliva, throat, CSF, and urine

The usual serologic tests are enzyme immunoassay (EIA) and indirect immunofluorescence to detect IgM- and IgG-specific antibody responses. Other serologic tests are also available, such as complement fixation, hemagglutination inhibition, and neutralization. Of these, the neutralization test is the most sensitive for detection of immunity to infection.

Viral antigen detected by immunofluorescence and EIA

EIA serology detects IgM and IgG

PREVENTION

No specific therapy is available. Since 1967, a live attenuated vaccine that is safe and highly effective has been available. As a result of its routine use, infections in the United States are now exceedingly rare. The vaccine is produced by serial propagation of virus in chick embryo cell cultures. It is commonly combined with measles and rubella vaccines (MMR) and given as a single injection at 12 to 15 months of age. A second dose of MMR is recommended at 4 to 6 years of age; those who have missed the second dose should receive it no later than 11 to 12 years of age. A single dose causes seroconversion in more than 95% of recipients. Duration of immunity, especially if the two-dose regimen is followed, appears to be more than 25 years and may be lifelong.

Live vaccine given at 12–15 months of age

MEASLES

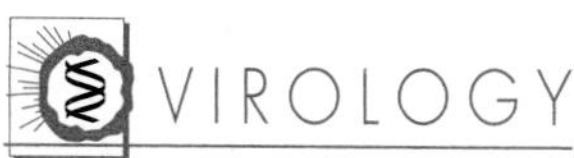

VIROLOGY

The measles virus is classified in the paramyxovirus family, genus *Morbillivirus.* It contains linear, negative-sense, single-stranded RNA, which encodes at least six virion structural proteins. Of these, three are in the envelope, comprising a matrix (M) protein that plays a key role in viral assembly and two types of glycoprotein projections (peplomers). One of the projections is a hemagglutinin (H), which mediates adsorption to cell surfaces; the other (F) mediates cell fusion, hemolysis, and viral entry into the cell. No neuraminidase activity is present. The receptor for measles virus is CD46 (membrane cofactor protein), a regulator of complement activation. Only a single serotype restricted to human infection is recognized; however, subtle antigenic and genetic variations among wild type measles strains do occur. These variations can be determined by sequencing analyses, enabling more precise epidemiologic tracking of outbreaks and their origins. Such ongoing molecular surveillance is also extremely important in determining whether significant antigenic drifts evolve over time.

Enveloped single-stranded RNA virus has hemagglutinating and fusion glycoproteins

CD46 is cell receptor

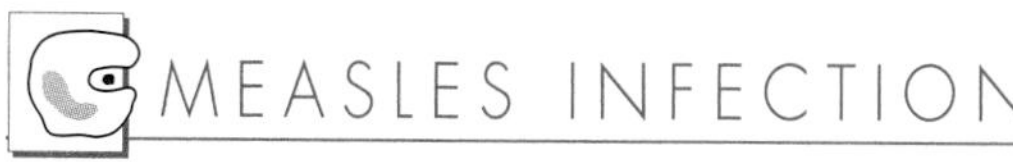

MEASLES INFECTION

CLINICAL CAPSULE

Measles infections often produce severe illness in children, associated with high fever, widespread rash, and transient immunosuppression. This condition remains a major cause of mortality among children in developing countries.

EPIDEMIOLOGY

Although a childhood disease, infections in young adults is important in transmission

Dramatic (99%) decrease recently in United States

The highest attack rates have been in children, usually sparing infants less than 6 months of age because of passively acquired antibody; however, a shift in age-specific attack rates to greater involvement of adolescents and young adults was observed in the United States in the 1980s. A marked decline in measles in the United States during the early 1990s may reflect decreased transmission as increased immunization coverage takes effect. However, in developing countries an estimated 1 million children still die from this disease each year.

Epidemics occur in unimmunized groups

Epidemics tend to occur during the winter and spring and increasingly are limited to one dose vaccine failures or groups who do not accept immunizations. The infection rate among exposed susceptible subjects in a classroom or household setting is estimated at 85%, and more than 95% of those infected become ill. The period of communicability is estimated to be 3 to 5 days before appearance of the rash to 4 days afterward.

PATHOGENESIS

Respiratory cell multiplication disrupts cytoskeleton

Viremia disseminates to multiple sites

After implantation in the upper respiratory tract, viral replication proceeds in the respiratory mucosal epithelium. The effect within individual respiratory cells is profound. Even though measles does not directly restrict host cell metabolism, susceptible cells are damaged or destroyed by virtue of the intense viral replicative activity and the promotion of cell fusion with formation of syncytia. This results in disruption of the cellular cytoskeleton, chromosomal disorganization, and the appearance of inclusion bodies within the nucleus and cytoplasm. Replication is followed by viremic and lymphatic dissemination throughout the host to distant sites, including lymphoid tissues, bone marrow, abdominal viscera, and skin. Virus can be demonstrated in the blood during the first week after illness onset, and viruria persists for up to 4 days after the appearance of rash.

T and B lymphocytes are infected

Leukocyte function is impaired

Susceptibility to bacterial superinfections enhanced

During the viremic phase, measles virus infects T and B lymphocytes, circulating monocytes, and polymorphonuclear leukocytes without producing cytolysis. Profound depression of cell-mediated immunity occurs during the acute phase of illness and persists for several weeks thereafter. This is believed to be a result of virus-induced downregulation of interleukin-12 production by monocytes and macrophages. The effect on B lymphocytes has been shown to suppress immunoglobulin synthesis; in addition, generation of natural killer cell activity appears to be impaired. There is also evidence that the capability of polymorphonuclear leukocytes to generate oxygen radicals is diminished, perhaps directly by the virus or by activated suppressor T cells. This may further explain the enhanced susceptibility to bacterial superinfections. Virion components can be detected in biopsy specimens of Koplik's spots and vascular endothelial cells in the areas of skin rash.

Vasculitis, giant cells, and inclusions are seen

In addition to necrosis and inflammatory changes in the respiratory tract epithelium, several other features of measles virus infection are noteworthy. The skin lesions show vasculitis characterized by vascular dilation, edema, and perivascular mononuclear cell infiltrates. The lymphoid tissues show hyperplastic changes, and large multinucleated reticuloendothelial giant cells are often observed (Warthin–Finkeldey cells). Some of the giant cells contain intracytoplasmic and intranuclear inclusions. Similarly involved giant epithelial cells can be found in a variety of mucosal sites, the respiratory tract, skin, and urinary sediment.

Encephalitis lesions due to cytotoxic T-cell activity

The major findings in measles encephalitis include areas of edema, scattered petechial hemorrhages, perivascular mononuclear cell infiltrates, and necrosis of neurons. In most cases, perivenous demyelination in the CNS is also observed. The pathogenesis is thought to be related to infiltration by cytotoxic (CD8+) T cells, which react with myelin-forming or virus-infected brain cells.

IMMUNITY

Lifelong immunity associated with neutralizing antibody

Cell-mediated immune responses to other antigens may be acutely depressed during measles infection and persist for several months. There is evidence that measles virus-specific cell-mediated immunity developing early in infection plays a role in mediating some of the features of disease, such as the rash, and is necessary to promote recovery from the illness.

Antibodies to the virus appear in the first few days of illness, peak in 2 to 3 weeks, and then persist at low levels. Immunity to reinfection is lifelong and is associated with the presence of neutralizing antibody. In patients with defects in cell-mediated immunity, including those with severe protein–calorie malnutrition, infection is prolonged, tissue involvement is more severe, and complications such as progressive viral pneumonia are common.

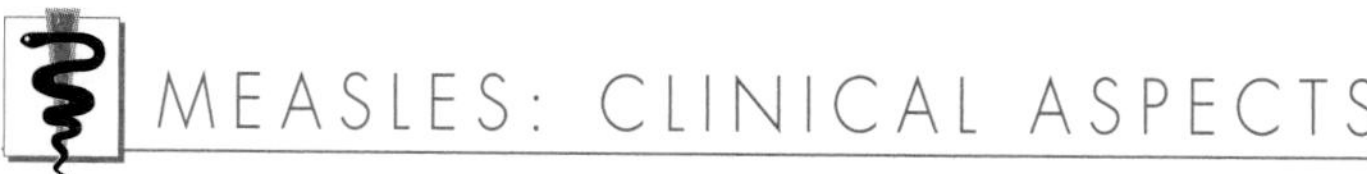

MANIFESTATIONS

Common synonyms for measles include **rubeola,** 5-day measles, and hard measles. The incubation period ranges from 7 to 18 days. A typical illness usually begins 9 to 11 days after exposure, with cough, coryza, conjunctivitis, and fever. One to three days after onset, pinpoint gray–white spots surrounded by erythema (grains-of-salt appearance) appear on mucous membranes. This sign, called **Koplik's spots,** is usually most noticeable over the buccal mucosa opposite the molar teeth and persists for 1 to 2 days. Within a day of the appearance of Koplik's spots, the typical measles rash begins, first on the head, then on the trunk and extremities. The rash is maculopapular and semiconfluent; it persists for 3 to 5 days before fading. Fever and severe systemic symptoms gradually diminish as the rash progresses to the extremities. Lymphadenopathy is also common, with particularly noticeable involvement of the cervical nodes.

Incubation period is 7–18 days

Koplik's spots appear on mucous membranes

Rash spreads from head to trunk and extremities

Measles can be very severe, especially in immunocompromised or malnourished patients. Death can result from overwhelming viral infection of the host, with extensive involvement of the respiratory tract and other viscera. In some developing countries, mortality rates of 15 to 25% have been recorded.

Complications

Bacterial superinfection, the most common complication, occurs in 5 to 15% of all cases. Such infections include acute otitis media, mastoiditis, sinusitis, pneumonia, and sepsis. Clinical signs of encephalitis develop in 1 of 500 to 1000 cases. This condition usually occurs 3 to 14 days after onset of illness and can be extremely severe. The mortality in measles encephalitis is approximately 15%, and permanent neurologic damage among survivors is estimated at 25%. Acute thrombocytopenic purpura may also develop during the acute phase of measles, leading to bleeding episodes. Abdominal pain and acute appendicitis can occur secondary to inflammation and swelling of lymphoid tissue.

Bacterial superinfection is common

Encephalitis can be severe

Thrombocytopenic purpura and bleeding occur in acute phase

Subacute Sclerosing Panencephalitis

Subacute sclerosing panencephalitis is a rare, progressive neurologic disease of children, which usually begins 2 to 10 years after a measles infection. It is characterized by insidious onset of personality change, poor school performance, progressive intellectual deterioration, development of myoclonic jerks (periodic muscle spasms), and motor dysfunctions such as spasticity, tremors, loss of coordination, and ocular abnormalities, including blindness. Neurologic and intellectual deterioration generally progress over 6 to 12 months, with children eventually becoming bedridden and stuporous. Dysfunctions of the autonomic nervous system, such as difficulty with temperature regulation, may develop. Progressive inanition, superinfection, and metabolic imbalances eventually lead to death. Most of the pathologic features of the disease are localized to the CNS and retina. Both the gray and the white matter of the brain are involved, the most noteworthy feature being the presence of intranuclear and intracytoplasmic inclusions in oligodendroglial and neuronal cells.

Neurologic deterioration is progressive in children

Inclusions seen in neuronal cells

The disease is a result of chronic wild measles virus infection of the CNS. Studies have shown that patients have a variety of patterns of missing measles virus structural proteins in brain tissue. Thus, any of several defects in viral gene expression may prevent normal viral assembly, allowing persistence of defective virus at an intracellular site with failure of immune eradication.

Chronic measles virus infection

Incomplete measles virus is present in brain tissue

Rarely, a similar progressive, degenerative neurologic disorder may be related to persistent rubella virus infection of the CNS. This condition is seen most often in adolescents who have had congenital rubella syndrome. Rubella virus has been isolated from brain tissue in these patients, again using cocultivation techniques.

Incidence declined after introduction of measles vaccine

The incidence of subacute sclerosing panencephalitis is approximately one per 100,000 measles cases. Its occurrence in the United States has decreased markedly over the past 25 years with the widespread use of live measles vaccine. At present, there is no accepted effective therapy for subacute sclerosing panencephalitis.

DIAGNOSIS

Rapid diagnosis is possible by immunofluorescence

The typical measles infection can often be diagnosed on the basis of clinical findings, but laboratory confirmation is necessary. Virus isolation from the oropharynx or urine is usually most productive in the first 5 days of illness. Measles grows on a variety of cell cultures, producing multinucleated giant cells similar to those observed in infected host tissues. If rapid diagnosis is desired, measles antigen may be identified in urinary sediment or pharyngeal cells by direct fluorescent antibody methods. Serologic diagnosis may involve complement fixation, hemagglutination inhibition, EIA, or indirect fluorescent antibody methods.

TREATMENT

No specific therapy is available other than supportive measures and close observation for the development of complications such as bacterial superinfection. Intravenous ribavirin has been suggested for patients with severe measles pneumonia, but no controlled studies have been performed.

PREVENTION

Live, attenuated vaccine is highly immunogenic

Vaccination is contraindicated in pregnant and immunocompromised individuals

Passive protection is appropriate for immunocompromised

Live, attenuated measles vaccine is available and highly immunogenic, most commonly administered as MMR. To ensure effective immunization, the vaccine should be administered to infants at 12 to 15 months of age with a second dose at 4 to 6 or 11 to 12 years of age. Immunity induced by the vaccine may be lifelong. Because the vaccine consists of live virus, it should not be administered to immunocompromised patients and it is not recommended for pregnant women. Exceptions to these guidelines include susceptible human immunodeficiency virus–infected persons. Exposed susceptible patients who are immunologically compromised (including small infants) may be given immune serum globulin intramuscularly. This treatment can modify or prevent disease if given within 6 days of exposure, but protection is transient.

RUBELLA

Rubella was considered a mild, benign exanthem of childhood until 1941, when the Australian ophthalmologist Sir Norman Gregg described the profound defects that could be induced in the fetus as a result of maternal infection. Since 1962, when the virus was first isolated, knowledge regarding its extreme medical importance and biological characteristics has increased rapidly.

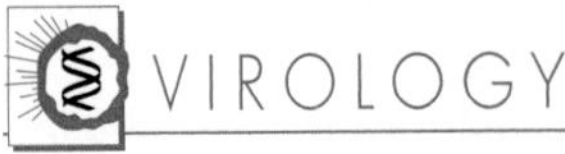

Enveloped togavirus contains single-stranded RNA

Rubella virus is classified as a member of the togavirus family. It is enveloped and contains single-stranded, positive-sense RNA. There is only one serotype, and no extrahuman reservoirs are known to exist. The virus can agglutinate some types of red blood cells, such as those obtained from 1-day-old chicks and trypsin-treated human type O cells.

RUBELLA INFECTION

CLINICAL CAPSULE

Infections by rubella virus are often mild, or even asymptomatic. The major concerns are the profound effects on developing fetuses, resulting in multiple congenital malformations.

EPIDEMIOLOGY

Infections are usually observed during the winter and spring months. In contrast to measles, which has a high clinical attack rate among exposed susceptible individuals, only 30 to 60% of rubella-infected susceptible persons develop clinically apparent disease. A major focus of concern is susceptible women of childbearing age, who carry a risk of exposure during pregnancy. Patients with primary acquired infections are contagious from 7 days before to 7 days after the onset of rash; congenitally infected infants may spread the virus to others for 6 months or longer after birth.

Virus has high infectivity but low virulence

Childbearing women are the major concern

PATHOGENESIS

In acquired infection, the virus enters the host through the upper respiratory tract, replicates, and then spreads by the bloodstream to distant sites, including lymphoid tissues, skin, and organs. Viremia in these infections has been detected for as long as 8 days before to 2 days after onset of the rash, and virus shedding from the oropharynx can be detected up to 8 days after onset (Fig 34–1). Cellular immune responses and circulating virus–antibody immune complexes are thought to play a role in mediating the inflammatory responses to infection, such as rash and arthritis.

Cellular immune responses and virus–antibody complexes mediate arthritis and rash

Congenital infection occurs as a result of maternal viremia that leads to placental infection and then transplacental spread to the fetus. Once fetal infection occurs, it persists chronically. Such persistence is probably related to an inability to eliminate the virus by immune or interferon-mediated mechanisms. There is too little inflammatory change in the fetal tissues to explain the pathogenesis of the congenital defects. Possibilities include placental and fetal vasculitis with compromise of fetal oxygenation, chronic viral infection of cells leading to impaired mitosis, cellular necrosis, and induction of chromosomal breakage. Any or all of these factors may operate at a critical stage of organogenesis to induce permanent defects. Viral persistence with circulating virus–antibody immune

Transmission to fetus by viremia

Fetal infection becomes chronic

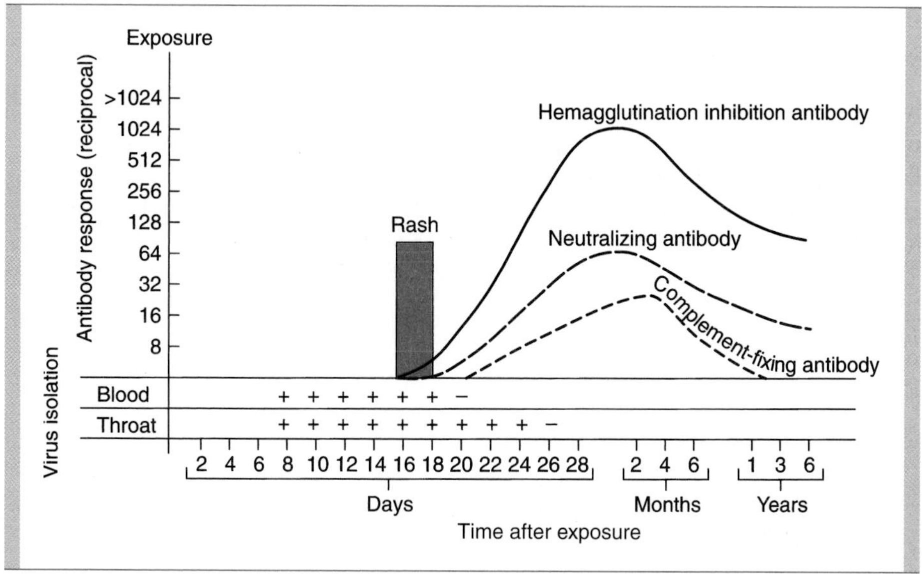

FIGURE 34–1
Antibody response and viral isolation in a typical case of acquired rubella.

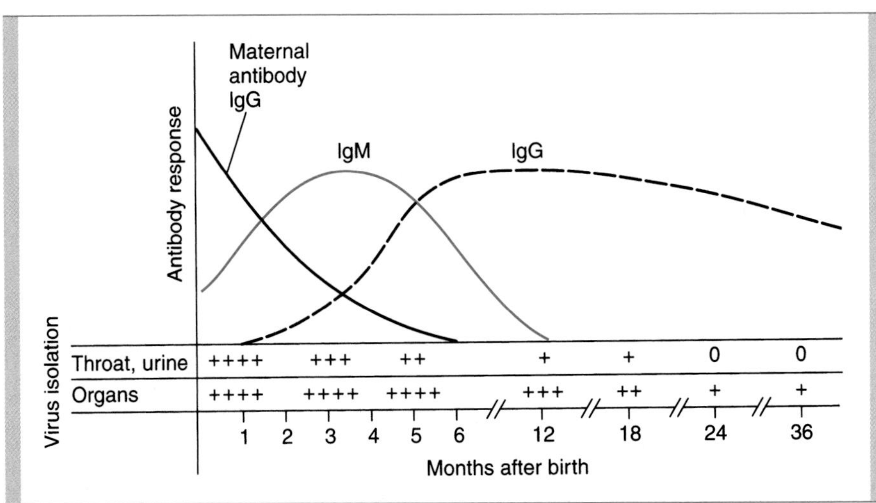

FIGURE 34–2
Persistence of rubella virus and antibody in congenitally infected infants.

complexes may evoke inflammatory changes postnatally and produce continuing tissue damage.

Infection and virus shedding continue long after birth

Virus persists despite antibody

After birth, affected infants continue to excrete the virus in the throat, urine, and intestinal tract (Fig 34–2). Virus may be isolated from virtually all tissues in the first few weeks of life. Shedding of virus in the throat and urine, which persists for at least 6 months in most cases, has been known to continue for 30 months. Virus has also been isolated from lens tissue removed 3 to 4 years later. These observations underscore the fact that such infants are important reservoirs in perpetuating virus transmission. The prolonged virus shedding is somewhat puzzling; it does not represent a typical example of immunologic tolerance. The affected infants are usually able to produce circulating IgM and IgG antibodies to the virus (see Fig 34–2), although antibodies may decrease to undetectable levels after 3 to 4 years. Many infants show evidence of depressed rubella virus-specific cell-mediated immunity during the first year of life.

PATHOLOGY

Fetal disease includes multiple malformations

Because postnatally acquired disease is usually mild, little is known about its pathology. Mononuclear cell inflammatory changes can be observed in tissues, and viral antigen can be detected in the same sites (eg, skin and synovial fluid). Congenital infections are characterized primarily by the various malformations. Necrosis of tissues such as myocardium and vascular endothelium may also be seen, and quantitative studies suggest a decrease in cell quantity in affected organs. In severe cases, normal calcium deposition in the metaphyses of long bones is delayed, sometimes referred to as a "celery stalk" appearance on a radiograph.

IMMUNITY

Lasting immunity is associated with IgG and IgA

After infection the serum antibody titer rises, reaching a peak within 2 to 3 weeks of onset. Natural infection also results in the production of specific secretory IgA antibodies in the respiratory tract. Immunity to disease is nearly always lifelong; however, reexposure can lead to transient respiratory tract infection, with an anamnestic rise in IgG and secretory IgA antibodies, but without resultant viremia or illness.

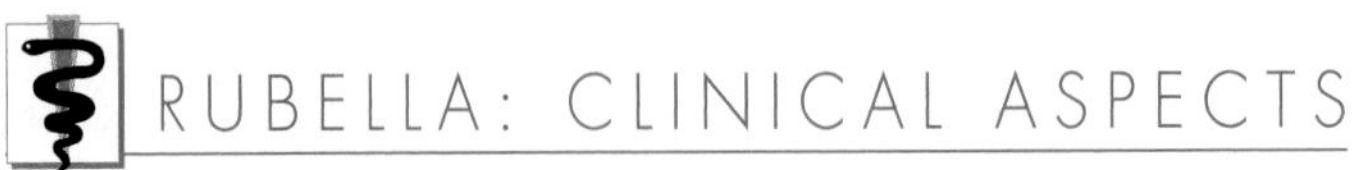

MANIFESTATIONS

Rubella is commonly known as **German measles** or 3-day measles. The incubation period for acquired infection is 14 to 21 days (average, 16 days). Illness is generally very mild, consisting primarily of low-grade fever, upper respiratory symptoms, and lymphadenopathy, which is most prominent in the posterior cervical and postauricular areas. A macular rash often follows within a day of onset and lasts 1 to 3 days. This rash, which is often quite faint, is usually most prominent over the head, neck, and trunk. Petechial lesions may also be seen over the soft palate during the acute phase. The most common complication is arthralgia or overt arthritis, which may affect the joints of the fingers, wrists, elbows, knees, and ankles. The joint problems, which occur most frequently in women, rarely last longer than a few days to 3 weeks. Other, rarer complications include thrombocytopenic purpura and encephalitis.

Illness is mild with lymphadenopathy and macular rash

Arthralgia and arthritis is common in women

The major significance of rubella is not the acute illness but the risk of fetal damage in pregnant women, particularly when they contract either symptomatic or subclinical primary infection during the first trimester. The risk of fetal malformation and chronic fetal infection, which is estimated to be as high as 80% if infection occurs in the first 2 weeks of gestation, decreases to 6 to 10% by the 14th week. The overall risk during the first trimester is estimated at 20 to 30%.

Clinical manifestations of congenital rubella syndrome vary, but may include any combination of the following major findings: cardiac defects, commonly patent ductus arteriosus and pulmonary valvular stenosis; eye defects such as cataracts, chorioretinitis, glaucoma, coloboma, cloudy cornea, and microphthalmia; sensorineural deafness; enlargement of liver and spleen; thrombocytopenia; and intrauterine growth restriction. Other findings include CNS defects such as microcephaly, mental retardation, and encephalitis; anemia; transient immunodeficiency; interstitial pneumonia; and intravascular coagulation; hepatitis; rash; and other congenital malformations. Late complications of congenital rubella syndrome have also been described, including an increased risk of diabetes mellitus, chronic thyroiditis, and occasionally the development of a progressive subacute panencephalitis in the second decade of life. Some congenitally infected infants may appear entirely normal at birth, and sequelae such as hearing or learning deficits may not become apparent until months later. The spectrum of defects thus varies from subtle to severe.

High risk for fetal damage with infection in first trimester

Lesions of congenital rubella include multiple body systems

DIAGNOSIS

Because of the rather nonspecific nature of the illness, a diagnosis of rubella cannot be made on clinical grounds alone. More than 30 other viral agents, which are discussed later in this chapter, can produce a similar illness. Confirmation of the diagnosis requires laboratory studies. The virus may be isolated from respiratory secretions in the acute phase (and from urine, tissues, and feces in congenitally infected infants) by inoculation into a variety of cell cultures, or detected by reverse transcriptase polymerase chain reaction. Serologic diagnosis is most commonly used in acquired infections; paired acute and convalescent samples collected 10 to 21 days apart are used. Hemagglutination inhibition, indirect immunofluorescence, EIA, and other tests are available.

Acquired infections are diagnosed serologically

Determination of IgM-specific antibody is sometimes useful to ascertain whether an infection occurred in the past several months; it has also been used in the diagnosis of congenital infections. Unfortunately, there are certain pitfalls in interpreting this test. Some individuals (<5%) with acquired infections may have persistent elevations of IgM-specific antibodies for 200 days or more afterward, and some congenitally infected infants do not produce detectable IgM-specific antibodies.

IgM tests can help detect congenital infections

TREATMENT AND PREVENTION

Other than supportive measures, there is no specific therapy for either the acquired or the congenital infection.

Since 1969, a live attenuated rubella vaccine has been available for routine immunization. As a result of the widespread use of the vaccine in the United States, the number of cases of rubella has declined dramatically. From 1990 through 1999, the median number of cases reported annually was only 232. The current vaccine virus, grown in human diploid fibroblast cell cultures (RA 27/3), has been shown to be highly effective.

Live attenuated rubella vaccine is indicated for children and hospital workers

It causes seroconversion in approximately 95% of recipients. Routine immunization is now recommended for infants after the first year of life and for other individuals with no history of immunization and lack of immunity by serologic testing. Target groups include female adolescents and hospital personnel in high-risk settings. The vaccine is contraindicated in many immunocompromised patients and in pregnancy. To date, more than 200 instances of accidental vaccination of susceptible pregnant women have been reported, with no clinically apparent adverse effects on the fetus; however, it is strongly recommended that immunization be avoided in this setting and that nonpregnant women avoid conception for at least 3 months after receiving the vaccine. Vaccine-induced immunity may be lifelong. Studies to date indicate that the duration of protection is at least 16 years.

Vaccine does not produce defects in fetus

Vaccine-induced immunity may be lifelong

Parvovirus B19 Infections

Parvoviruses are very small (18 to 26 nm), naked virions that contain a linear single-stranded DNA molecule. Diseases caused by parvoviruses have been recognized among nonhuman hosts for a number of years. Notable among these are canine parvovirus and feline panleukopenia virus, which produce particularly severe infections among puppies and kittens, respectively. These do not appear to cross species barriers. The human parvovirus B19 has been well described, but its origin is not yet known.

Small naked, single-stranded DNA viruses

Parvovirus B19 encodes three capsid proteins (VP1, VP2, and VP3). The virus can be grown in primary cultures of human bone marrow cells, fetal liver cells, hematopoietic progenitor cells generated from peripheral blood, and a megakaryocytic leukemia cell line. The major cellular receptor for the virus is globoside (also known as blood group P antigen, which is commonly found on erythroid progenitors, erythroblasts, megakaryocytes, and endothelial cells). All represent potential targets for disease production. A primary site of replication appears to be the nucleus of an immature cell in the erythrocyte lineage. Such infected cells then cease to proliferate, resulting in an impairment of normal erythrocyte development.

The clinical consequences of this effect on erythrocytes are generally trivial, unless patients are already compromised by a chronic hemolytic process, such as sickle cell disease or thalassemia, in which maximal erythropoiesis is continually needed to counterbalance increased destruction of circulating erythrocytes. Primary infection by parvovirus B19 in such individuals often produces an acute, severe, sometimes fatal anemia manifested as a rapid fall in red blood cell counts and hemoglobin. Patients may present initially with no clinical symptoms other than fever, and is commonly referred to as **aplastic crisis.** Immunocompromised patients such as those with acquired immunodeficiency syndrome sometimes have difficulty clearing the virus and develop persistent anemia with reticulocytopenia. Parvovirus B19 has also been occasionally implicated as a cause of persistent bone marrow failure and an acute hemophagocytic syndrome.

Replicates in erythroid precursor nuclei

Globoside is virus receptor

Endothelial cells and megakaryocytes can also be affected

Aplastic crisis develops in patients with chronic hemolytic anemias

Erythema infectiosum (also referred to as fifth disease or academy rash) is a more common disease that is clearly attributable to parvovirus B19. After an incubation period of 4 to 12 days, a mild illness appears, characterized by fever, malaise, headache, myalgia, and itching in varying degrees. A confluent, indurated rash appears on the face, giving a "slapped-cheek" appearance. The rash spreads in a day or two to other areas, particularly exposed surfaces such as the arms and legs, where it is usually macular and reticular (lace-like). During the acute phase, generalized lymphadenopathy or splenomegaly may be seen, along with a mild leukopenia and anemia.

The illness lasts 1 to 2 weeks, but rash may recur for periods of 2 to 4 weeks thereafter, exacerbated by heat, sunlight, exercise, or emotional stress. Arthralgia sometimes persists or recurs for weeks to months, particularly in adolescent or adult females. Overt arthritis or vasculitis have also been reported in some individuals. Serious complications,

Erythema infectiosum is usually mild "slapped cheek" rash

such as hepatitis, thrombocytopenia, nephritis or encephalitis are rare. However, like rubella, active transplacental transmission of parvovirus B19 can occur during primary infections in the first 20 weeks of pregnancy, sometimes resulting in stillbirth of fetuses that are profoundly anemic. The progress can be so severe that hypoxic damage to the heart, liver, and other tissues leads to extensive edema (hydrops fetalis). The frequency of such adverse outcomes is as yet undetermined.

Fetal infection is occasionally severe

Fetal anemia leads to hydrops fetalis

It is important to be aware that erythema infectiosum is extremely variable in its clinical manifestations; even the "classic" presentation can be mimicked by other agents, such as rubella and echoviruses. Before a firm diagnosis is made on clinical grounds, especially during outbreaks, it is wise to exclude the possibility of atypical rubella infection.

Epidemiologic evidence suggests that spread of the virus is primarily by the respiratory route, and high transmission rates occur in households. Outbreaks tend to be small and localized, particularly during the spring months, with the highest rates among children and young adults. Seroepidemiologic studies have demonstrated evidence of past infection in 30 to 60% of adults. Viremia usually lasts 7 to 12 days but can persist for months in some individuals. It can be detected by specific DNA probe or polymerase chain reaction (PCR) methods. Alternatively, the presence of IgM-specific antibody late in the acute phase or during convalescence strongly supports the diagnosis.

Detection requires DNA probe or PCR

IgM-specific antibody supports diagnosis

ROSEOLA INFANTUM (EXANTHEM SUBITUM)

Roseola infantum is a common illness observed in infants and children 6 months to 4 years of age. Its alternative name, exanthem subitum, means "sudden rash." Roseola has more than one cause: the most common is human herpesvirus type 6 and, less frequently, human herpesvirus type 7 (see Chapter 38). Several other agents, including adenoviruses, coxsackieviruses, and echoviruses, have occasionally been noted to cause similar manifestations. The illness is characterized by abrupt onset of high fever, sometimes accompanied by brief, generalized convulsions and leukopenia. After 3 to 5 days, the fever diminishes rapidly, followed in a few hours by a faint, transient, macular rash.

Associated with human herpesvirus type 6 or type 7

OTHER CAUSES OF RUBELLA-LIKE RASHES

In addition to erythema infectiosum, diseases caused by numerous other agents can mimic rubella. These include at least 17 echoviruses, 9 coxsackieviruses, several adenoviral serotypes, arboviruses such as dengue, Epstein–Barr virus, scarlet fever, and toxic drug eruptions. Because of the wide variety of diagnostic possibilities, it is not possible to diagnose or rule out rubella confidently on clinical grounds alone. Therefore, a specific diagnosis requires specific laboratory studies. Because rubella is an infection with such significant impact on the fetus, serologic study to rule out the possibility is mandatory if the diagnosis is suspected during early pregnancy.

ADDITIONAL READING

Mumps

Cheek JE, Baron R, Atlas H, et al. Mumps outbreak in a highly vaccinated school population. *Arch Pediatr Adolesc Med* 1995;149:774–778. An illustration of the importance of monitoring and implementing immunization programs.

Measles

Atabani SF, Syrnes AA, Jay A, et al. Natural measles causes prolonged suppression of interleukin-12 production. *J Infect Dis* 2001;184:1–9. An article that provides insight into the immunopathogenesis of measles virus infections.

Rota JS, Rota PA, Redd SB, et al. Genetic analysis of measles viruses isolated in the United States, 1995–1996. *J Infect Dis* 1998;177:204–208. This article illustrates how molecular epidemiologic studies can be used to monitor virus spread in populations and determine antigenic drift.

Rubella

Miller E, Cradock-Watson JE, Pollock TM. Consequences of confirmed maternal rubella at successive stages of pregnancy. *Lancet* 1982;2:781–784. A precise analysis of the risks of infection at various times during gestation.

Reef SE, Frey TK, Theall K, et al. The changing epidemiology of rubella in the 1990s. *JAMA* 2002;287:464–472. This report and the accompanying editorial highlight the profound impact resulting from widespread immunization and examine the barriers to ultimate eradication.

Parvovirus B19

Harel L, Straussberg R, Rudich H, et al. Raynaud's phenomenon as a manifestation of parvovirus B19 infection: Case reports and review of parvovirus B19 rheumatic and vasculitic syndromes. *Clin Infect Dis* 2000;30:500–503. An article that provides further insight into pathogenesis.

Heegaard ED, Hornsleth A. Parvovirus: The expanding spectrum of disease. *Acta Paediatr* 1995;84:109–117. The history of parvovirus B19, along with the broad spectrum of disease expression, is reviewed.

CHAPTER 35

Poxviruses

C. GEORGE RAY

The poxvirus family includes viruses that infect birds, mammals, and even insects. The agents most important in human disease are variola (smallpox), vaccinia, molluscum contagiosum, orf, cowpox, and pseudocowpox (Table 35–1).

POXVIRUSES: GROUP CHARACTERISTICS

Poxviruses are large, brick-shaped or ovoid, double-stranded DNA-carrying virions (Fig 35–1) measuring approximately 100 × 200 × 300 nm. Their structure is complex, and replication occurs in the cytoplasm of infected cells. They possess an envelope, which is not acquired by budding and not essential for infectivity.

Double-stranded DNA

Replication in cytoplasm

VARIOLA (SMALLPOX)

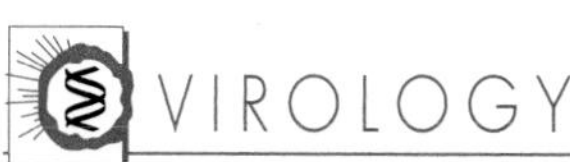

VIROLOGY

Two virus types are known: variola major and variola minor (alastrim). Although the viruses are indistinguishable antigenically, their fatality rates differ considerably (<1% for variola minor, 3–35% for variola major). They are also difficult to distinguish in the laboratory; however, variola major has slightly greater virulence in embryonated hen's eggs.

Variola major and minor are difficult to distinguish

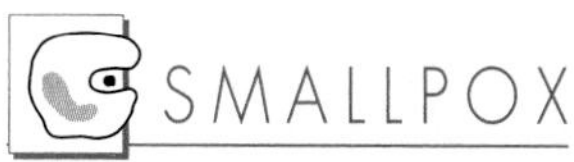

SMALLPOX

CLINICAL CAPSULE

Smallpox is an acute infection in which the dominant feature is a uniform papulovesicular rash that evolves to pustules over 1 to 2 weeks. The potential for spread and mortality is significant, particularly in a nonimmune population.

TABLE 35–1

Poxviridae that Affect Humans

GENERA	DISEASES
Orthopoxvirus	Variola Vaccinia Cowpox[a] Monkeypox[a]
Parapoxvirus	Bovine papular stomatitis[a] Orf[a] Pseudocowpox[a]
Molluscipoxvirus	Molluscum contagiosum
Yatapoxvirus	Tanapox[a] Yatapox[a]

[a] Viruses that have nonhuman reservoirs but can cause disease in humans (usually mild and localized).

Person-to-person communicability by respiratory droplets and fomites is high

Smallpox has played a significant role in world history with respect to both the serious epidemics recorded since antiquity and the sometimes dangerous measures taken to prevent infection. Smallpox virus is highly contagious and can survive well in the extracellular environment. Acquisition of infection by infected saliva droplets or by exposure to skin lesions, contaminated articles, and fomites has been well documented.

WHO eradication campaign based on lack of nonhuman reservoir and asymptomatic cases

Immunization and case tracing led to success in 1980

In 1967, the World Health Organization (WHO) launched an ambitious program aimed at eradication of smallpox. This goal was considered realistic for two major reasons: (1) no extrahuman reservoir of the virus was known to exist, and (2) asymptomatic carriage apparently did not occur. The basic approach included intensive surveillance for clinical cases of smallpox, prompt quarantine of such patients and their contacts, and immunization of contacts with vaccinia virus (vaccination) to prevent further spread. A tremendous amount of effort was involved, but the results were astonishing: the last recorded case of naturally acquired smallpox occurred in Somalia in 1977. Global eradication of smallpox was confirmed in 1979 and accepted by the WHO in May 1980. Since then, the virus has been solely secured in two WHO-restricted laboratories: one at the United States Centers for Disease Control and Prevention (CDC) in Atlanta, Georgia, and the other at a similar facility in Moscow, Russia.

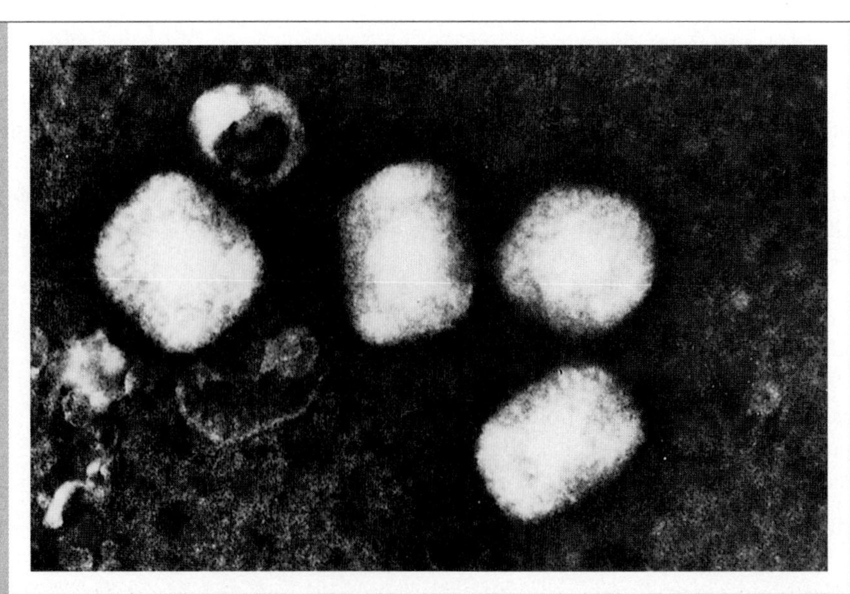

FIGURE 35–1
Electron microscopic appearance of a poxvirus (vaccinia). (Negative stain; original magnification × 60,000.) (*Courtesy of Dr. Claire M. Payne.*)

Unfortunately, the dramatic world events that occurred in 2001 have raised the chilling possibility that clandestine virus stocks may exist elsewhere and could be effectively used for major bioterrorist attacks. Reasons for such concern include (1) known high infectivity among humans; (2) high susceptibility among populations (routine vaccination against smallpox ended in 1972, and current vaccine supplies are limited); (3) risk that health care providers may not promptly recognize and respond to early cases; and (4) absence of specific antiviral treatment. A response plan and guidelines for such threats is posted on a CDC website **(www.cdc.gov/nip/smallpox)** and is updated at regular intervals.

Potential bioterrorist weapon

No proven antiviral treatment

Continuing surveillance also includes studies of poxviruses of animals (eg, buffalopox, monkeypox) that are antigenically somewhat similar to smallpox. Some virologists remain legitimately concerned that an animal poxvirus, such as monkeypox, could mutate to become highly virulent to humans—a further reminder that complacency could be dangerous.

Animal poxviruses could be a future threat

PATHOGENESIS

The orthopoxviruses as a group cause a dramatic effect on host cell macromolecular function, leading to a switch from cellular to viral protein synthesis, changes in cell membrane permeability and cytolysis. Eosinophilic inclusions, called **Guarnieri's bodies,** can be seen in the cytoplasm. Multiple viral proteins, such as complement regulatory protein and other factors that can interfere with induction or activities of multiple host mononuclear cell cytokines, are also synthesized; this serves to impair the host defenses that are important in early control of infection.

Profound effect on host cell protein synthesis

Viral proteins undermine host defenses

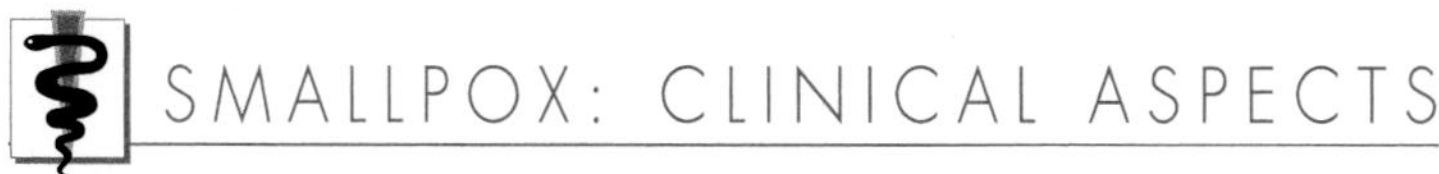

SMALLPOX: CLINICAL ASPECTS

MANIFESTATIONS AND DIAGNOSIS

The incubation period of smallpox is usually 12 to 14 days, although in occasional fulminating cases it can be as short as 4 to 5 days. The typical onset is abrupt, with fever, chills, and myalgia, followed by a rash 3 to 4 days later. The rash evolves to firm papulovesicles that become pustular over 10 to 12 days, then crust and slowly heal. Only a single crop of lesions (all in the same stage of evolution) develop; these lesions are most prominent over the head and extremities (Fig 35–2). Some cases are fulminant, with a hemorrhagic rash ("sledgehammer" smallpox). Death can result from the overwhelming primary viral infection or from bacterial superinfection. Diagnostic methods utilize vesicular scrapings, and include culture, electron microscopy, gel diffusion, and polymerase chain reaction.

Single-stage rash

Vesicular scrapings used for diagnosis

PREVENTION

The first major step toward modern prevention and subsequent eradication of smallpox can be credited to Edward Jenner, who noted that milkmaids who develop mild cowpox lesions on their hands appeared immune to smallpox. In 1798, he published evidence indicating that purposeful inoculation of individuals with cowpox material could protect them against subsequent infection by smallpox. The concept of vaccination gradually evolved, with the modern use of live vaccinia virus, a poxvirus of uncertain origin to be discussed later, which produced specific immunity.

Jenner vaccinated with cowpox

VACCINIA

Vaccinia virus is serologically related to smallpox, although its exact origin is unknown. Some virologists believe it is a recombinant virus derived from smallpox and cowpox, and others suggest it originated from a poxvirus of horses. The virus is usually propagated by

Origin is unknown

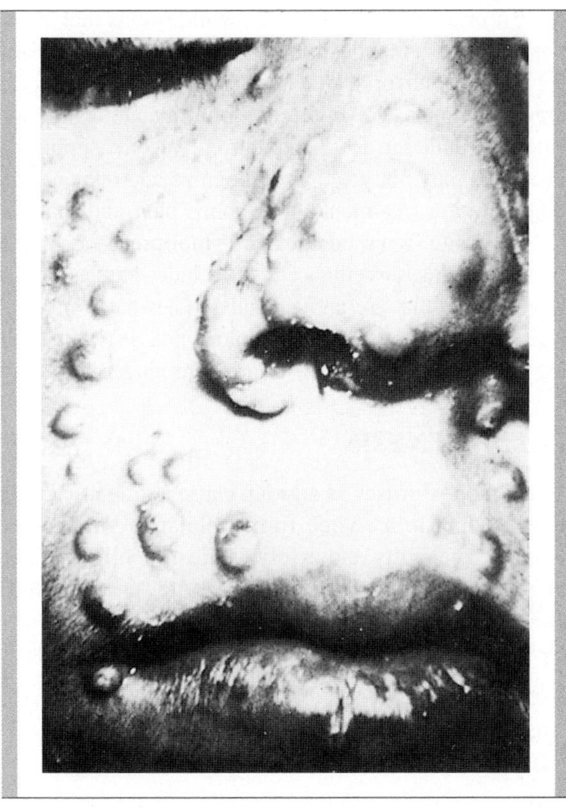

FIGURE 35–2
Closeup of facial lesions of smallpox during the first week of the illness.

Vaccination produces strong local reactions

Severe reactions seen in immunocompromised

Immunity wanes after 3 years

dermal inoculation of calves, and the resultant vesicle fluid ("lymph") is lyophilized and used as a live virus vaccine in humans. The vaccine is inoculated into the epidermis and produces a localized lesion, which indicates successful immunization. The lesion becomes vesicular, then pustular, followed by crusting and healing over 10 to 14 days. The local reaction is sometimes severe and accompanied by systemic symptoms such as fever, rash, and lymphadenopathy. Patients who are immunocompromised may experience severe reactions, such as progressive vaccinia. Vaccinia-produced immunity to smallpox wanes rapidly after 3 years, and the duration of long-term immunity beyond that time is uncertain.

Vaccinia of interest as mechanism for delivering the immunogenic proteins of other viruses

There has been a resurgence of scientific interest in vaccinia as a possible vector for active immunization against other diseases, such as hepatitis B, herpes simplex, and even human immunodeficiency virus. It has been shown that gene sequences coding for specific immunogenic proteins of other viruses can be inserted into the vaccinia virus genome, with subsequent expression as the virus replicates. For example, a recombinant vaccinia strain carrying the gene sequence for hepatitis B surface antigen (HbsAg) can infect cells, lead to production of HbsAg, and stimulate an antibody response to it. Theoretically, gene sequences coding for a variety of antigens could be packaged in a single viable vaccinia virus, thus allowing simultaneous active immunization against multiple agents. It has been suggested that use of other poxviruses of animal or avian orgin, such as canarypox, may be even safer, yet effective vectors for use in humans. Whether such approaches become routinely applicable to clinical medicine remains to be seen.

MOLLUSCUM CONTAGIOSUM

Transmission is direct skin-to-skin

Molluscum contagiosum is a benign, cutaneous poxvirus disease of humans, spread by direct contact with infected cells. It is usually acquired by inoculation into minute skin abrasions; events that commonly lead to transmission include "roughhousing" in shower rooms and swimming pools, sharing of towels, and sexual contact.

After an incubation period of 2 to 8 weeks, nodular, pale, firm (pearl-like) lesions usually 2 to 10 mm in diameter develop in the epidermis. These lesions are painless and umbilicated in appearance. A cheesy material may be expressed from the pore at the center of each lesion. Local trauma may cause spread of lesions in the involved skin area. The lesions are not associated with systemic symptoms, and they disappear in 2 to 12 months without treatment. Specific treatment, if desired, is usually by curettage or careful removal of the central core by expression with forceps.

Painless lesions express cheesy material

Pathologic findings, which are limited to the epidermis, include hyperplasia, ballooning degeneration, and acanthosis. The diagnosis, made on clinical grounds, can be confirmed by demonstration of large, eosinophilic cytoplasmic inclusions (molluscum bodies) in the affected superficial epithelial cells.

Molluscum bodies in cytoplasm are diagnostic

ORF

Orf is an old Saxon term for a human infection caused by a parapoxvirus of sheep and goats. Synonyms for the infection in animals include contagious pustular dermatitis, ecthyma contagiosum, pustular ecthyma, and "scabby mouth." Humans usually acquire the infection by close contact with infected animals and accidental inoculation through cuts or abrasions on the hand or wrist. The typical skin lesion is solitary; it begins as a vesicle and then evolves into a nodular mass that later develops central necrosis. Regional lymphadenopathy sometimes develops. Dissemination is rare. The average duration of the lesion is 35 days, followed by complete resolution. The diagnosis is usually made on the basis of clinical appearance and occupational history. Serologic confirmation or electron microscopy of the lesion can be performed but is rarely necessary.

Vesicular skin lesions seen in sheep- or goat-herders

MILKER'S NODULES AND COWPOX

Milker's nodules (pseudocowpox) is a cutaneous parapoxvirus disease of cattle, distinct from cowpox, that can cause local skin infections similar to orf in exposed humans. Healing of the skin lesions may take 4 to 8 weeks. There is no cross-immunity to cowpox. Cowpox is now very rare in the United States. It produces a vesicular eruption on the udders of cows and similar, usually localized, vesicular skin lesions in humans who are accidentally exposed.

Localized infection acquired by direct contact with bovines

ADDITIONAL READING

Barquet N, Domingo P. Smallpox: The triumph over the most terrible of the ministers of death. *Ann Intern Med* 1997;127:635–642. This first-rate account of the history, science, and successful eradication of this agent is highly recommended.

Breman JG, Henderson DA: Diagnosis and management of smallpox. *N Engl J Med* 2002;346:1300–1308. This updated review and accompanying articles in the same issue highlight the resurgence in concern that smallpox may return as a threat to humanity.

Cadoz M, Strady A, Meignier B, et al. Immunization with canarypox virus expressing rabies glycoprotein. *Lancet* 1992;339:1429–1432. A nonhuman poxvirus that undergoes only abortive replication in mammalian cells is exploited as a potentially safe vector for immunization. The editorial on pages 1448–1449 is also worthwhile reading.

Cohen J. Is an old virus up to new tricks? *Science* 1997;277:312–313. This article is a vivid reminder that although one scourge may have been eradicated, others may be capable of taking its place.

CHAPTER 36

Enteroviruses

C. GEORGE RAY

Enteroviruses constitute a major subgroup of small RNA viruses (picornaviruses) that readily infect the intestinal tract. The enteroviruses of humans and animals are ubiquitous and have been found worldwide. Their name is derived from their ability to infect intestinal tract epithelial and lymphoid tissues and to be shed into the feces. They include the polioviruses, coxsackieviruses, echoviruses, and more recently discovered agents that are simply designated enteroviruses.

These viruses, which have many characteristics in common, are first considered as a group. Some of the special features of important serotypes will be discussed in more detail later in this chapter.

ENTEROVIRUSES: GROUP CHARACTERISTICS

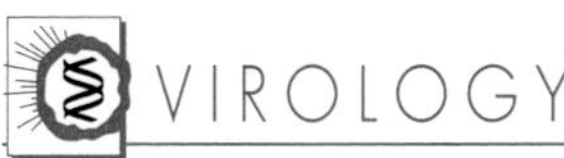

MORPHOLOGY AND BIOLOGICAL FEATURES

As a group, the enteroviruses are extremely small (22 to 30 nm in diameter), naked virions with icosahedral symmetry. They possess single-stranded, positive-sense RNA and a capsid formed from 60 copies of four nonglycosylated proteins (VP1, VP2, VP3, VP4). Replication and assembly occurs exclusively in the cellular cytoplasm; one infectious cycle can occur within 6 to 7 hours. This results in cessation of host cell protein synthesis and cell lysis with release of new infectious progeny.

Small, single-stranded RNA viruses

Replication and assembly takes place in cytoplasm

Unlike rhinoviruses, which are also members of the picornavirus family, enteroviruses are quite resistant to an acid pH (as low as 3.0). This feature undoubtedly helps ensure their survival during passage through the stomach to the intestines. Enteroviruses are also resistant to many common disinfectants such as 70% alcohol, substituted phenolics, ether, and various detergents that readily inactivate most enveloped viruses. Chemical agents, such as 0.3% formaldehyde or free residual chlorine at 0.3 to 0.5 ppm, are effective; however, if sufficient extraneous organic debris is present, the virus can be protected and survive long periods.

Resistant to acid, detergents, and many disinfectants

Formaldehyde and hypochlorite are active against enteroviruses

Some of the enterovirus serotypes share common antigens, but there are no significant serologic relationships between the major classes listed in Table 36–1. Genetic variation within specific strains occurs, and mutants that exhibit antigenic drift and altered tropism for specific cell types are now recognized. Polioviruses, which have been most extensively

Antigenic mutations and drifts occur

TABLE 36–1

Human Enteroviruses

Class	Number of Serotypes[a]
Poliovirus	3
Coxsackievirus	
Group A	23
Group B	6
Echovirus	28
Enterovirus	4

[a] More recently discovered enteroviruses, which have overlapping biological characteristics, are identified numerically (types 68–71). Two of the original 30 numbered echovirus serotypes have been reclassified; however, the remaining retain their original serotype number (eg, echovirus 30).

Antibody to surface proteins neutralize infectivity

studied as enterovirus prototypes, are known to have epitopes on three surface structural proteins (VP1, VP2, and VP3) that induce type-specific neutralizing antibodies. This appears to be generally the case for all enteroviruses; definitive identification of isolates usually requires neutralization tests.

GROWTH IN THE LABORATORY

Growth of some in primate cell cultures

Coxsackie A and B viruses have different effects on newborn mice

Most enteroviruses can be isolated in primate (human or simian) cell cultures and show characteristic cytopathic effects. Some strains, particularly several coxsackievirus A serotypes, are more readily detected by inoculation of newborn mice. In fact, the newborn mouse is one basis for originally classifying group A and B coxsackieviruses. Group A coxsackieviruses cause primarily a widespread, inflammatory, necrotic effect on skeletal muscle, leading to flaccid paralysis and death. Similar inoculation of group B coxsackieviruses causes encephalitis, resulting in spasticity and occasionally convulsions. Echoviruses and polioviruses rarely have an adverse effect on mice, unless special adaptation procedures are first employed. The higher-numbered enteroviruses (types 68–71), which have overlapping, variable growth and host characteristics, have been classified separately.

ENTEROVIRUS DISEASE

CLINICAL CAPSULE

Enterovirus infections can produce a great diversity of clinical disease. Some cause paralytic disease that may persist permanently (a typical feature of polioviruses), acute inflammation of the meninges with or without involvement of cerebral or spinal tissues, or sepsis-like illnesses in newborn infants. Inflammatory effects at other sites, such as the lungs, pleura, heart, and skin, have been also observed, often without concomitant or preceding central nervous system (CNS) involvement. Occasionally, infections may result in chronic, active disease processes.

EPIDEMIOLOGY

Animals are not involved in human disease

Humans are the major natural host for the polioviruses, coxsackieviruses, and echoviruses. There are enteroviruses of other animals with limited host ranges that do not appear to extend to humans. Conversely, viruses thought to be identical or related to human enteroviruses have been isolated from dogs and cats. Whether these agents cause disease in such animals is debatable, and there is no evidence of spread from animals to humans.

The enteroviruses have a worldwide distribution, and asymptomatic infection is common. The proportion of infected individuals who develop illness varies from 2 to 100%, depending on the serotype or strain involved and the age of the patient. Secondary infections in households are common and range as high as 40 to 70%, depending on factors such as family size, crowding, and sanitary conditions.

Proportion of asymptomatic infections varies with strain

In some years, certain serotypes emerge as dominant epidemic strains; they then may wane, only to reappear in epidemic fashion years later. For example, echovirus 16 was a major cause of outbreaks in the eastern United States in 1951 and 1974. Coxsackievirus B1 was common in 1963; echovirus 9 in 1962, 1965, 1968, and 1969; and echovirus 30 in 1968 and 1969. The emergence of dominant serotypes is quite unpredictable from year to year. All enteroviruses show a seasonal predilection in temperate climates; epidemics are usually observed during the summer and fall months. In subtropical and tropical climates, the transmission may occur year-round.

Dominant epidemic stains come and go

Strong prevalence in summer and fall

Direct or indirect fecal–oral transmission is considered the most common mode of spread. After infection, the virus persists in the oropharynx for 1 to 4 weeks, and it can be shed in the feces for 1 to 18 weeks. Thus, sewage-contaminated water, fecally contaminated foods, or passive transmission by insect vectors (flies, cockroaches) may occasionally be the source of infection. More commonly, however, spread is directly from person to person. This mode of transmission is suggested by the high infection rates seen among young children, whose hygienic practices tend to be less than optimal, and in crowded households. Approximately two thirds of all isolates are from children 9 years of age or younger.

Person-to-person fecal–oral transmission correlates with predominance in children

Incubation periods vary, but relatively short intervals (2 to 10 days) are frequent. Often, illness is seen concurrently in more than one family member, and the clinical features vary within the household.

Incubation periods are typically short

PATHOGENESIS

Initial binding of an enterovirus to the cell surface is commonly between an attachment protein in a "canyon" configuration on the virion surface and cell receptors belonging to the immunoglobulin gene superfamily. These receptors map to chromosome 19. A different receptor, belonging to the integrin group of adhesion molecules, has been identified for at least one echovirus serotype. Following attachment, the virion is enveloped by the cell membrane, and its RNA is released into the cellular cytoplasm where it binds to ribosomes and commences protein synthesis. Newly synthesized virions are released by lysis to spread to the other cells.

Initial attachment binds viral surface protein to cell surface receptors

Host receptor may relate to immunoglobulin or integrin families

After primary replication in epithelial cells and lymphoid tissues in the upper respiratory and gastrointestinal tracts, viremic spread to other sites can occur. Potential target organs vary according to the virus strain and its tropism, but may include the CNS, heart, vascular endothelium, liver, pancreas, lungs, gonads, skeletal muscles, synovial tissues, skin, and mucous membranes. Histopathologic findings include cell necrosis and mononuclear cell inflammatory infiltrates; in the CNS, the inflammatory cells are localized most prominently in perivascular sites. The initial tissue damage is thought to result from the lytic cycle of virus replication; secondary spread to other sites may ensue. Viremia is usually undetectable by the time symptoms appear, and termination of virus replication appears to correlate with the appearance of circulating neutralizing antibody, interferon, and mononuclear cell infiltration of infected tissue. The early dominant antibody response is with immunoglobulin M (IgM), which usually wanes 6 to 12 weeks after onset to be replaced progressively by increased IgG-specific antibodies. The important role of antibodies in termination of infection, demonstrated in mouse models of group B coxsackievirus infections, is supported by the observation of persistent echovirus and poliovirus replication in patients with antibody deficiency diseases.

Initial replication in epithelial and lymphoid cells is followed by viremic spread

Injury by cell lysis localized in perivascular sites

Antibody response terminates replication

Although initial acute tissue damage may be caused by the lytic effects of the virus on the cell, the secondary sequelae may be immunologically mediated. Enterovirus-caused poliomyelitis, disseminated disease of the newborn, aseptic meningitis, encephalitis, and acute respiratory illnesses, thought to represent primary lytic infections, can usually be identified through routine methods of virus isolation and determination of specific

In addition to lytic effects of virus there are probable immunopathologic manifestations

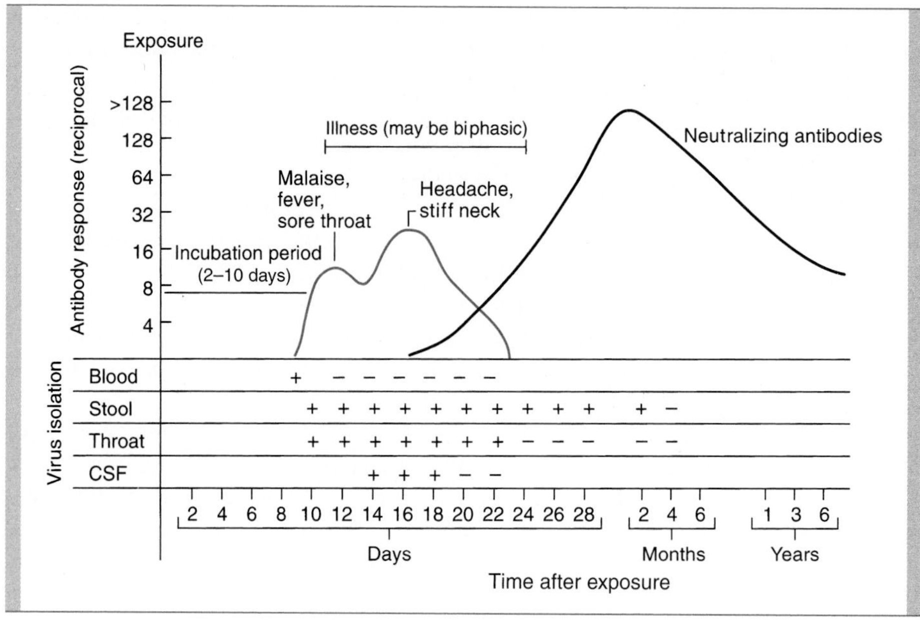

FIGURE 36–1
Antibody response and viral isolation from various sites in a typical case of enteroviral infection.

antibody titer changes. On the other hand, syndromes such as myopericarditis, nephritis, and myositis have been associated with enteroviruses primarily because of serologic and epidemiologic evidence. In many of these cases, viral isolation is the exception rather than the rule. The pathogenesis of these latter infections is not clear; however, observations suggest that the acute infectious phase of the virus may be mild or subclinical and often subsides by the time clinical illness becomes evident. Illness may represent a host immunologic response to tissue injury by the virus or to viral or virus-induced antigens that persist in the affected tissues. In experimental group B coxsackievirus myocarditis, mononuclear inflammatory cells (monocytes, natural killer lymphocytes) seem to play a greater role than antibody in termination of infection, and the persistence of inflammation after disappearance of detectable infectious virus or viral antigen appears to be mediated by cytotoxic T lymphocytes. Experimental findings have led to another hypothesis regarding pathogenic mechanisms, called **molecular mimicry.** This is best conceptualized as a form of virus-induced autoimmune response. It is known that small peptide sequences on viral epitopes can sometimes be shared by host tissues. Thus, an immune response produced by the virus may also generate antibodies or cytotoxic cross-reactive effector lymphocytes that recognize shared determinants located on host cells. For example, a monoclonal antibody directed against a neutralizing site of a group B coxsackievirus has also been shown to react strongly with normal myocardial cells.

Disease may follow the acute infection

Coxsackie B myocarditis may involve virus-induced cross reacting antibody

IMMUNITY

Infection by a specific serotype in an immunologically normal host is followed by a humoral antibody response, which can often be detected by neutralization methods for many years thereafter (Fig 36–1). There is relative immunity to reinfection by the same serotype; however, reinfection has been reported, usually resulting in subclinical infection or mild illness.

Immunity is serotype specific

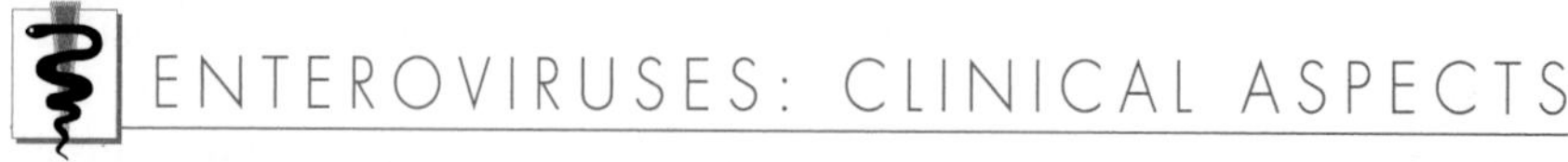

ENTEROVIRUSES: CLINICAL ASPECTS

DIAGNOSIS

In acute enterovirus-caused syndromes, diagnosis is most readily established by virus isolation from throat swabs, stool or rectal swabs, body fluids, and occasionally tissues.

Viremia is usually undetectable by the time symptoms appear. When there is CNS involvement, cerebrospinal fluid (CSF) cultures taken during the acute phase of the disease may be positive in 10 to 85% of cases (except in poliovirus infections, in which virus recovery from this site is rare), depending on the stage of illness and the viral serotype involved. Direct isolation of virus from affected tissues or body fluids in enclosed spaces (eg, pleural, joint, pericardial, or CSF) usually confirms the diagnosis. Isolation of an enterovirus from the throat is highly suggestive of an etiologic association; the virus is usually detectable at this site for only 2 days to 2 weeks after infection. Isolation of virus from fecal specimens only must be interpreted more cautiously; asymptomatic shedding from the bowel may persist for as long as 4 months (see Fig 36–1). The polymerase chain reaction with reverse transcription and complementary DNA amplification (RT-PCR) can also be used to detect enteroviral RNA sequences in tissues and body fluids, thus greatly enhancing diagnostic sensitivity and speed.

Viral isolation from pharynx or closed space is significant

Prolonged shedding in stool

RT-PCR enhances diagnostic sensitivity

The diagnosis may be further supported by fourfold or greater neutralizing antibody titer changes between paired acute and convalescent serum samples. However, this method is often expensive and cumbersome, requiring careful selection of serotypes for use in antigens. Quantitative interpretations of antibody titers on single serum samples are rarely helpful, because of the wide range of titers to different serotypes that can be found among healthy individuals.

Serodiagnosis is usually impractical

TREATMENT AND PREVENTION

None of the currently available, approved antiviral agents has been shown effective in treatment or prophylaxis of enterovirus infections; however, the antipicornaviral drug, pleconaril (see Chapter 33) is currently being studied. Treatment is symptomatic and supportive. Vaccines for the prevention of poliovirus infections are discussed later in this chapter. Although proper disposal of feces and careful personal hygiene are recommended, the usual quarantine or isolation measures are relatively ineffective in controlling the spread of enteroviruses in the family or community.

Hygenic factors make prevention of spread difficult

Enteroviruses: Specific Groups

Polioviruses

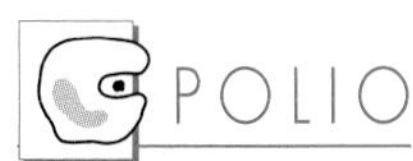

POLIO

EPIDEMIOLOGY

Worldwide, the most important enteroviruses are the three poliovirus serotypes (types 1, 2, and 3). They first emerged as important causes of disease in developed temperate zone countries during the latter part of the 19th century, and they have become increasingly important elsewhere as living conditions improve in developing countries. This somewhat paradoxical situation is related to the fact that the risk of paralytic disease resulting from infection increases with age. Improvement of sanitary conditions tends to impede spread of the viruses; thus, individuals may become infected not in early infancy but later in life, when paralysis is more likely to occur.

Risk of paralysis from infection increases with age

PATHOGENESIS

The particular tropism of polioviruses for the CNS, which they usually reach by passage across the blood–CNS barrier, is perhaps favored by reflex dilatation of capillaries supplying the affected motor centers of the anterior horn of the brainstem or spinal cord. An

CNS tropism by blood or peripheral nerves

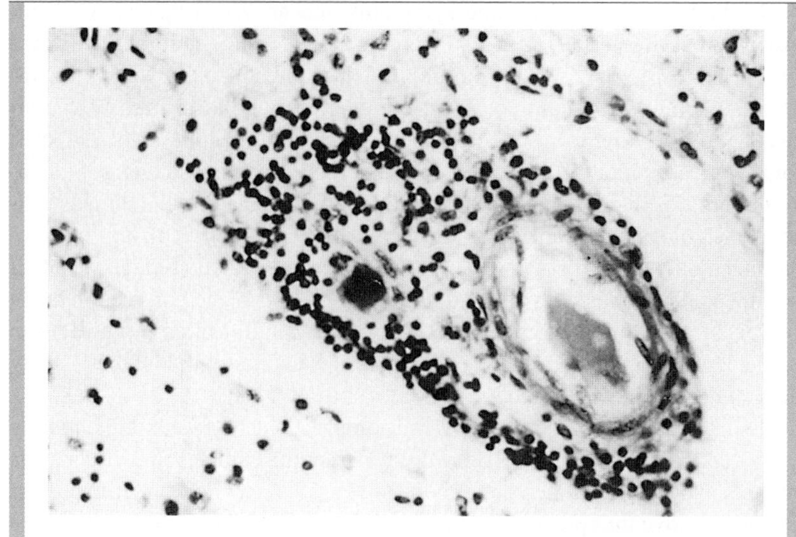

FIGURE 36–2
Section of spinal cord from a fatal case of poliomyelitis, demonstrating perivenous mononuclear cell inflammatory reaction. (*Courtesy of Dr. Peter C. Johnson.*)

Motor neuron cells destroyed

alternate pathway is via the axons or perineural sheaths of peripheral nerves. Motor neurons are particularly vulnerable to infection and variable degrees of neuronal destruction. The histopathologic findings in the brainstem and spinal cord include necrosis of neuronal cells and perivascular "cuffing" by infiltration with mononuclear cells, primarily lymphocytes (Fig 36–2).

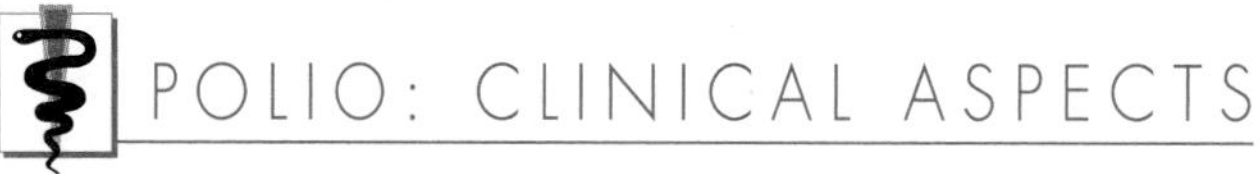

POLIO: CLINICAL ASPECTS

MANIFESTATIONS

Subclinical and abortive poliomyelitis common

Aseptic meningitis recovers rapidly

Paralytic poliomyelitis manifests flaccid paralysis without sensory loss

Recovery of function up to 6 months

Most infections (perhaps 90%) are either completely subclinical or so mild that they do not come to attention. When disease does result, the incubation period ranges from 4 to 35 days, but is usually between 7 and 14 days. Three types of disease can be observed. Abortive poliomyelitis is a nonspecific febrile illness of 2- to 3-day duration with no signs of CNS localization. Aseptic meningitis (nonparalytic poliomyelitis) is characterized by signs of meningeal irritation (stiff neck, pain, and stiffness in the back) in addition to the signs of abortive poliomyelitis; recovery is rapid and complete, usually within a few days. Paralytic poliomyelitis, occurs in less than 2% of infections. It is the major possible outcome of infection and is often preceded by a period of minor illness, sometimes with two or three symptom-free days intervening. There are signs of meningeal irritation, but the hallmark of paralytic poliomyelitis is asymmetric flaccid paralysis, with no significant sensory loss. The extent of involvement varies greatly from case to case; however, in its most serious forms, all four limbs may be completely paralyzed or the brainstem may be attacked, with paralysis of the cranial nerves and muscles of respiration (bulbar polio). The maximum extent of involvement is evident within a few days of first paralysis. Thereafter, as temporarily damaged neurons regain their function, recovery begins and may continue for as long as 6 months; paralysis persisting after this time is permanent.

PREVENTION

Two types of poliovirus vaccines are currently licensed in the United States: inactivated polio vaccine and live oral attenuated virus vaccine. Each contains all three viral serotypes.

Inactivated polio vaccine (IPV) was introduced in 1955; its use was associated with a dramatic decline in paralytic cases (Fig 36–3). Vaccination is by subcutaneous injection. Primary vaccination with three doses of the present enhanced-potency IPV (two doses 6–8 weeks apart and the third 8–12 months later) produces antibody responses in more

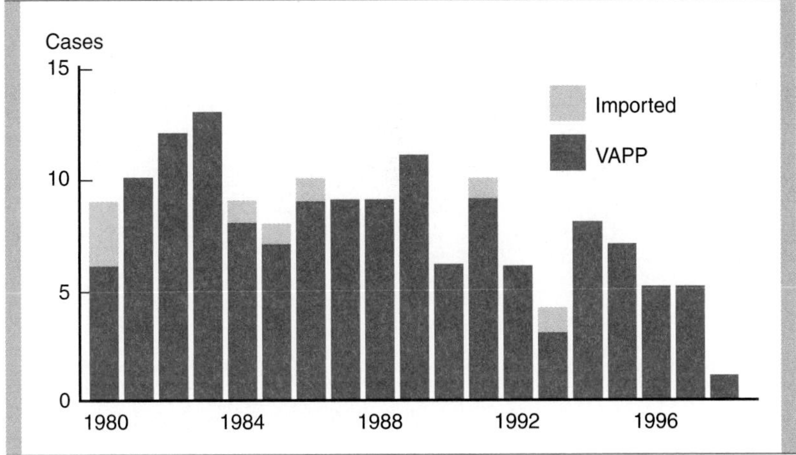

FIGURE 36–3
Total number of reported paralytic poliomyelitis cases and number of reported vaccine-associated cases (VAPP)—United States, 1950–1999. (*From the Centers for Disease Control and Prevention, 2000.*)

than 98% of recipients. The current product is considered quite safe, with no significant deleterious side effects. Inactivated (Salk) vaccine is used in many countries

Live (Sabin) vaccine is given orally (OPV)

Oral polio vaccine (OPV) is composed of live, attenuated viruses that have undergone serial passage in cell cultures from humans and subhuman primates. It was first licensed in the United States in 1963. The vaccine is given orally as a primary series of three doses (the first two doses usually 6–8 weeks apart and the third 8–12 months later) and produces antibodies to all three serotypes in more than 95% of recipients; these antibodies persist for several years. As with IPV, recall boosters are recommended to maintain adequate antibody levels. Like wild poliovirus, OPV viruses infect and replicate in the oropharynx and intestinal tract and can be spread to other persons.

Vaccine virus replicates and can spread

Vaccine-associated poliomyelitis is a remote risk with OPV

One disadvantage of OPV is the remote risk of vaccine-associated paralytic disease in some recipients or their household contacts, including immunocompromised persons. The incidence of vaccine-associated paralytic poliomyelitis is estimated at approximately 1 per 2.4 million doses distributed. Since the end of 1999, exclusive use of IPV has been recommended for all routine immunizations in the United States. OPV is recommended only in special circumstances (eg, an unvaccinated child who will be traveling in less than 4 weeks to an endemic area).

IPV is currently preferred

No cases of paralytic poliomyelitis attributed to indigenously acquired wild poliovirus have occurred in the United States since 1979, and the last case in the Western Hemisphere occurred in 1991. Nevertheless, it must be kept in mind that importation of these strains can readily occur from endemic areas in developing nations. Once introduced into a community, the virus can spread rapidly among susceptible individuals. Thus, continuing immunization programs are of utmost importance in preventing spread of this disease. In 1988, the World Health Organization resolved to eradicate polio from the world by the year 2000. Thus far, progress toward that goal has been hampered by political strife and severe poverty in many underdeveloped nations in Africa, Asia and the Middle East.

Coxsackieviruses and Echoviruses

EPIDEMIOLOGY

Often do not affect motor neurons

The coxsackieviruses and echoviruses are widespread throughout the world. Their epidemiology and pathogenesis are much the same as those of the polioviruses. Unlike polioviruses, they have a greater tendency to affect the meninges and occasionally the cerebrum, but only a few affect anterior horn cells.

The consequences of infection with these agents are highly variable and related only in part to virus subgroup and serotype. Up to 60% of infections are subclinical. The main

TABLE 36–2

Clinical Syndromes and Commonly Associated Enterovirus Serotypes[a]

Syndrome	Coxsackievirus Group A	Coxsackievirus Group B	Echovirus and Enterovirus (E)
Aseptic meningitis, encephalitis	2, 4, 7, **9,** 10	1, **2, 3, 4, 5**	**4, 6, 9, 11, 16, 30,** E70, E71
Muscle weakness and paralysis (poliomyelitis-like disease)	7, **9**	2, 3, 4, 5	2, 4, 6, 9, 11, 18, 30, **E71**
Cerebellar ataxia	2, 4, **9**	3, 4	4, 6, 9
Exanthems and enanthems	**4, 5, 6, 9, 10, 16**	2, 3, 4, 5	**2, 4, 5, 6, 9, 11, 16, 18, 25**
Pericarditis, myocarditis	4, 16	**2, 3, 4, 5**	1, 6, 8, 9, 19
Epidemic myalgia (pleurodynia), orchitis	9	1, **2, 3, 4, 5**	1, 6, 9,
Respiratory	9, 16, **21,** 24	1, 3, 4, 5	**4, 9, 11,** 20, 25
Conjunctivitis	**24**	1, 5	7, **E70**
Generalized disease (infants)	–	1, **2, 3, 4, 5**	3, 6, 9, 11, 14, 17, 19

[a] Serotypes most commonly associated with syndrome are in **boldface.**

Most infections subclinical

Wide range of clinical manifestations

interest in these agents stems from their ability to cause more serious illness, which becomes most evident during epidemics of infection with a particular agent. Inapparent infection is common. Illness manifestations vary from mild to lethal. Table 36–2 lists the major syndromes and serotypes commonly associated with each. However, considerable overlap occurs, and one should not be surprised if an enteroviral serotype found in connection with a specific syndrome differs from that most often encountered.

MANIFESTATIONS

Aseptic meningitis most common syndrome

Aseptic meningitis is the most frequently recognized clinical illness associated with enterovirus infections. This syndrome can be mild and self-limiting, lasting 5 to 14 days; however, it is sometimes accompanied by encephalitis, which can lead to permanent neurologic sequelae.

Myocarditis often associated with group B coxsackieviruses

Acute inflammation of the heart muscle (myocarditis), its covering membranes (pericarditis), or both can be caused by a variety of viral agents. Group B coxsackieviruses are the most commonly implicated enteroviruses. Such infections are usually self-limiting but may be fatal in the acute phase (arrhythmia or heart failure) or progress to chronic dilated myocardiopathy.

Exanthems can mimic other diseases

Herpangina infection of palate and tonsils

The exanthems are often not associated with CNS inflammation. They can resemble rubella, roseola infantum, or adenoviral macular or maculopapular exanthems but may also appear as vesicular or hemangioma-like lesions. One interesting syndrome is hand-foot-and-mouth disease, which usually affects children and is characterized by a vesicular eruption over the extremities and the oral cavity. Coxsackie virus A16 is most commonly implicated, but others, such as enterovirus 71, can cause a similar illness. Herpangina is an enanthematous (mucous membrane–affecting) febrile disease in which small vesicles or white papules (lymphonodules) surrounded by a red halo are seen over the posterior palate, pharynx, and tonsillar areas. This mild, self-limiting (1 to 2 week) illness has usually been associated with infection by several different group A coxsackievirus serotypes.

Epidemic myalgia, with pleuritic pain

Epidemic myalgia (pleurodynia or Bornholm disease) is characterized by fever and sudden onset of intense upper abdominal or thoracic pain. The pain may be aggravated by movement, such as breathing or coughing, and can persist as long as 14 days. Group B coxsackieviruses are often implicated.

Generalized disease of the newborn is a disseminated, often lethal enteroviral infection characterized by pathologic changes in the heart, brain, liver, and other organs.

It is apparent from Table 36–2 that the spectrum of disease produced by these viruses is enormous and that many other illnesses may also result from infections by this subgroup. Epidemics of acute hemorrhagic keratoconjunctivitis associated with enterovirus 70 and localized outbreaks of disease resembling paralytic poliomyelitis caused by enterovirus 71 infection have been described. In addition, there is evidence that certain enteroviruses, particularly group B coxsackievirus serotypes, may sometimes participate in the pathogenesis of insulin-dependent diabetes mellitus, acute arthritis, polymyositis, and idiopathic acute nephritis. Further investigations are required to establish whether such associations are significant.

ADDITIONAL READING

Cochi SL, Hull HF, Sutter RW, et al. Commentary: The unfolding story of global poliomyelitis eradication. *J Infect Dis* 1997;175:S1–3. This commentary and the papers that follow outline the remarkable strategies for global eradication and why they are expected to succeed.

Ho M, Chen E-R, Hsu K-H, et al. An epidemic of enterovirus 71 infection in Taiwan. *N Engl J Med* 1999;341:929–935. In 1998, a widespread epidemic of enterovirus 71 affected more than 100,000 persons in Taiwan. This report details the epidemiologic and often severe clinical features.

Rotbart HA. Enteroviral infectious of the central nervous system. *Clin Infect Dis* 1995;20:971–981. This paper describes the molecular pathogenesis, clinical diseases and diagnosis of enteroviral infections.

Starlin R, Reed N, Leeman B, et al. Acute flaccid paralysis syndrome associated with echovirus 19, managed with pleconaril and intravenous immunoglobulin. *Clin Infect Dis* 2001;33:730–732. This report describes the rationale for attempting newer treatments for severe enteroviral infections.

CHAPTER 37

Hepatitis Viruses

W. LAWRENCE DREW

The causes of hepatitis are varied and include viruses, bacteria, and protozoa, as well as drugs and toxins (eg, isoniazid, carbon tetrachloride, and ethanol). The clinical symptoms and course of acute viral hepatitis can be similar, regardless of etiology, and determination of a specific cause depends primarily on the use of laboratory tests. Hepatitis may be caused by at least five different viruses whose major characteristics are summarized in Table 37–1. *Non-A, non-B hepatitis* is a term previously used to identify cases of hepatitis not due to hepatitis A or B. With the discovery of the hepatitis viruses C, E, and G, virtually all the viral etiologies of non-A, non-B disease can be specifically identified. Other viruses, such as Epstein–Barr virus and cytomegalovirus, can also cause inflammation of the liver, but hepatitis is not the primary disease caused by them. Yellow fever is associated with hepatitis but is now uncommon.

HEPATITIS A

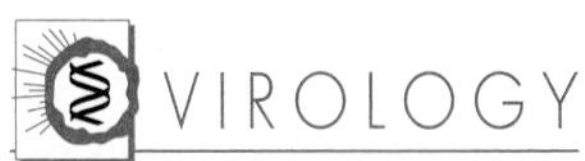

VIROLOGY

Hepatitis A virus is an unenveloped, single-stranded RNA virus with cubic symmetry and a diameter of 27 nm (Fig 37–1). The virus resists inactivation and is stable at –20°C with low pH. These properties are similar to those of picornaviruses, and hepatitis A virus has now been classified in a separate genus of picornaviruses as a hepatovirus. There is only one serotype of hepatitis A virus. The virus has been successfully cultivated in primary marmoset liver cell cultures and in fetal rhesus monkey kidney cell cultures.

Only one serotype

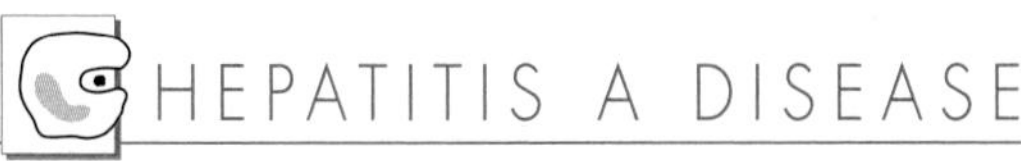

HEPATITIS A DISEASE

CLINICAL CAPSULE

Hepatitis A virus is the cause of what was formerly termed infectious hepatitis or short-incubation hepatitis. This virus is spread by the fecal–oral route, and outbreaks may be associated with contaminated food or water. The illness is subclinical in up to one half of infected adults. When symptomatic, there is usually fever and jaundice. Although fatal disease may occur, self-limited illness is the rule. Chronic hepatitis A rarely if ever occurs.

TABLE 37–1

Comparison of A, B, D (Delta), C, and E Hepatitis

FEATURE	A	B	D	C[a]	E
Virus type	Single-stranded RNA	Double-stranded DNA	Single-stranded RNA	RNA	RNA
Percent of viral hepatitis	50	41	<1	5	<1
Incubation period (days)	15–45 (mean, 25)	7–160 (mean, 60–90)	28–45	15–160 (mean, 50)	?
Onset	Usually sudden	Usually slow	Variable	Insidious	?
Age preference	Children, young adults	All ages	All ages	All ages	Young adult
Transmission					
Fecal–oral	+++	±	±	–	+++
Sexual	+	++	++	+	+?
Transfusion	–	++	+++	+++	–
Severity	Usually mild	Moderate	Often severe	Mild	Variable
Chronicity (%)	None	10	50–70	>50%	None
Carrier state	None	Yes	Yes	Yes	?
Immune serum globulin protective	Yes	Yes[b]	Yes[c]	Uncertain	?

Abbreviation: Plus and minus signs indicate relative frequencies.

[a] Many individuals with hepatitis C virus are also infected with the hepatitis G virus, which is similar to hepatitis C.

[b] Hyperimmune globulin more protective.

[c] Prevention of hepatitis B prevents hepatitis D.

EPIDEMIOLOGY

No chronic carriage

Humans appear to be the major natural hosts of hepatitis A virus. Several other primates (including chimpanzees and marmosets) are susceptible to experimental infection, and natural infections of these animals may occur. The major mode of spread of hepatitis A is fecal–oral. Inoculation of infectious material intramuscularly can produce disease; transmission through blood transfusion, although possible, is not an important means of spread. While most cases of hepatitis A are not linked to a single contaminated source and occur sporadically, outbreaks have been described. The disease is common under conditions of crowding, and it occurs at high frequency in mental hospitals, schools for the retarded, and day-care centers. A chronic carrier state has not been observed with hepatitis A; perpetuation of the virus in nature presumably depends on sporadic subclinical infections and

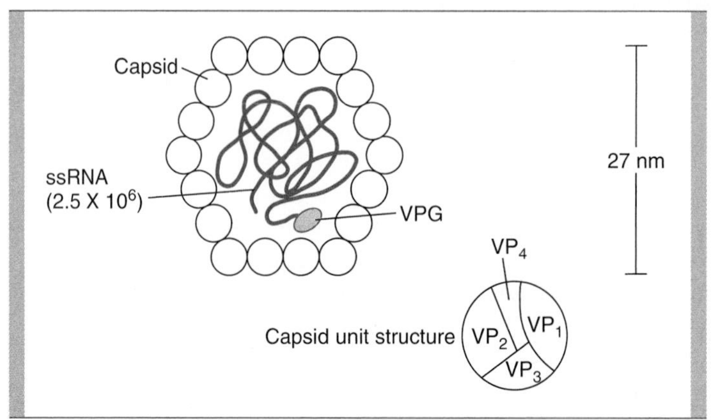

FIGURE 37–1
Diagram of the proposed structure of the hepatitis A virus. The protein capsid is made up of four viral polypeptides (VP_1 to VP_4). Inside the capsid is a single-stranded (ss) molecule of RNA (molecular weight 2.5 + 106), which has a genomic viral protein (VPG) on the 5′ end. (*Reprinted with permission of Dr. J. H. Hoofnagle and of Abbot Laboratories, Diagnostic Division, North Chicago, Illinois.*)

person-to-person transmission. Outbreaks of hepatitis A have been linked to the ingestion of undercooked seafood, usually shellfish from waters contaminated with human feces. Common-source outbreaks related to other foods, including vegetables as well as contaminated drinking water, have also been reported.

Hepatitis A is widespread but seroepidemiologic studies have shown marked variation in infection rates among various population groups. For example, rates are higher among those of lower socioeconomic status and among male homosexuals. Less than 50% of the general population of the United States now has serologic evidence of prior hepatitis A virus infection, and rates have been decreasing since 1970, apparently because of better sanitation and less crowding. In contrast, more than 90% of the adult population in many developing countries shows evidence of previous hepatitis A infection. The risk of clinically evident disease is much higher in infected adults than in children; travelers from developed countries who enter endemic areas are particularly susceptible. Patients are most contagious in the 1 to 2 weeks prior to the onset of clinical disease.

Subclinical infection is common in children

PATHOGENESIS

The virus is believed to replicate initially in the enteric mucosa. It can be demonstrated in feces by electron microscopy for 10 to 14 days before onset of disease. In most patients with symptoms of the disease, virus is no longer found in fecal specimens. Multiplication in the intestines is followed by a period of viremia with spread to the liver. The response to replication in the liver consists of lymphoid cell infiltration, necrosis of liver parenchymal cells, and proliferation of Kupffer cells. The extent of necrosis often coincides with the severity of disease. A variable degree of biliary stasis may be present. Detectable levels of IgG antibody to hepatitis A virus persist indefinitely in serum, and patients with anti–hepatitis A virus antibodies are immune to reinfection. Although virus-specific IgA has been demonstrated in stool, secretory immunity has not been shown to be important for hepatitis A.

Contagion is greatest 10–14 days before symptoms appear

IgG-specific antibody is protective

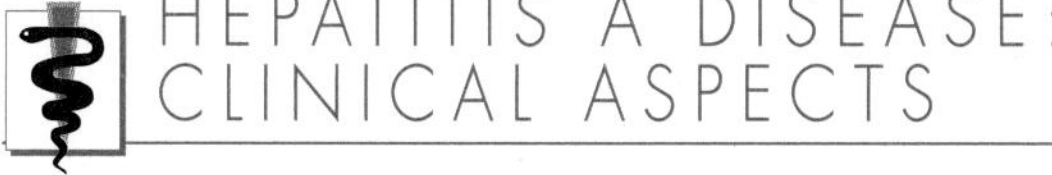

HEPATITIS A DISEASE: CLINICAL ASPECTS

MANIFESTATIONS

In hepatitis A virus infection, an incubation period of 10 to 50 days (mean, 25 days) is usually followed by the onset of fever; anorexia (poor appetite); nausea; pain in the right upper abdominal quadrant; and, within several days, jaundice. Dark urine and clay-colored stools may be noticed by the patient 1 to 5 days before the onset of clinical jaundice. The liver is enlarged and tender, and serum aminotransferase and bilirubin levels are elevated as a result of hepatic inflammation and damage. Recovery occurs in days to weeks.

Fever, anorexia, and jaundice are common

Many persons who have serologic evidence of acute hepatitis A infection are asymptomatic or only mildly ill, without jaundice (anicteric hepatitis A). The infection-to-disease ratio is dependent on age; it may be as high as 20:1 in children and approximately 4:1 in older adults. Almost all cases (99%) of hepatitis A are self-limiting. Chronic hepatitis such as that seen with hepatitis B is very rare. In rare cases, fulminant fatal hepatitis associated with extensive liver necrosis may occur (~0.1%).

Chronic infection is rare

DIAGNOSIS

Antibody to hepatitis A virus can be detected during early illness, and most patients with symptoms or signs of acute hepatitis A already have detectable antibody in serum. Early antibody responses are predominantly IgM, which can be detected for several weeks or months. During convalescence, antibody of the IgG class predominates. The best method for documentation of acute hepatitis A virus infection is the demonstration of high titers of virus-specific IgM antibody in serum drawn during the acute phase of illness. Because IgG antibody persists indefinitely, its demonstration in a single serum sample is not

IgM-specific antibody denotes acute infection

indicative of recent infection; a rise in titer between acute and convalescent sera must be documented. Immune electron microscopic identification of the virus in fecal specimens and isolation of the virus in cell cultures remain research tools.

TREATMENT AND PREVENTION

There is no specific treatment for patients with acute hepatitis A. Supportive measures include adequate nutrition and rest. Avoidance of exposure to contaminated food or water are important measures to reduce the risk of hepatitis A infection.

Passive Immunization

Immune serum globulin provides temporary protection

Passive (ie, antibody) prophylaxis for hepatitis A has been available for many years. Immune serum globulin (ISG), manufactured from pools of plasma from large segments of the general population, is protective if given before or during the incubation period of the disease. It has been shown to be about 80 to 90% effective in preventing clinically apparent type A hepatitis. In some cases, infection occurs but disease is ameliorated; that is, patients develop anicteric, usually asymptomatic, hepatitis A. At present, ISG should be administered to household contacts of hepatitis A patients and those known to have eaten uncooked foods prepared or handled by an infected individual. Once clinical symptoms have appeared, the host is already producing antibody, and administration of ISG is not indicated. Persons from areas of low endemicity traveling to areas with high infection rates may receive ISG before departure and at 3- to 4-month intervals as long as potential heavy exposure continues, but active immunization is preferable (see below).

Active Immunization

Inactivated virus vaccine confers long-term protection

For hepatitis A, live attenuated vaccines have been evaluated but have demonstrated poor immunogenicity and have not been effective when given orally. Formalin-killed vaccines induce antibody titers similar to those of wild-virus infection and are almost 100% protective. Use of this vaccine is preferable to passive prophylaxis for those with prolonged or repeated exposure to hepatitis A.

HEPATITIS B

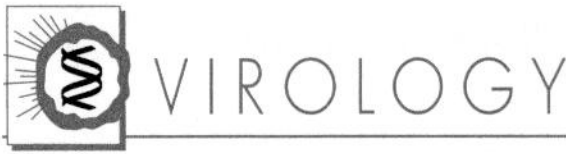

STRUCTURE

Enveloped DNA virus

Hepatitis B virus is an enveloped DNA virus belonging to the family Hepadnaviridae. It is unrelated to any other human virus; however, related hepatotropic agents have been identified in woodchucks, ground squirrels, and kangaroos. A schematic of the hepatitis B virus is illustrated in Figure 37–2. The complete virion is a 42-nm, spherical particle that consists of an envelope around a 27-nm core. The core comprises a nucleocapsid that contains the DNA genome.

Smallest known human DNA virus

The viral genome consists of partially double-stranded DNA with a short, single-stranded piece. It comprises 3200 nucleotides, making it the smallest DNA virus known. Closely associated with the viral DNA is a DNA polymerase. Other components of the core are a hepatitis B core antigen (HBcAg) and the hepatitis B e antigen (HBeAg), which is a low-molecular-weight glycoprotein.

HBsAg is produced in great abundance

The envelope of the virus contains the hepatitis B surface antigen (HBsAg), which is composed of one major and two other proteins. Antigenically there exist a group-specific determinant, termed *a,* and a number of subtypes that are important in epidemiologic typing, but not in immunity, because there is antigenic cross-reactivity and cross-protection

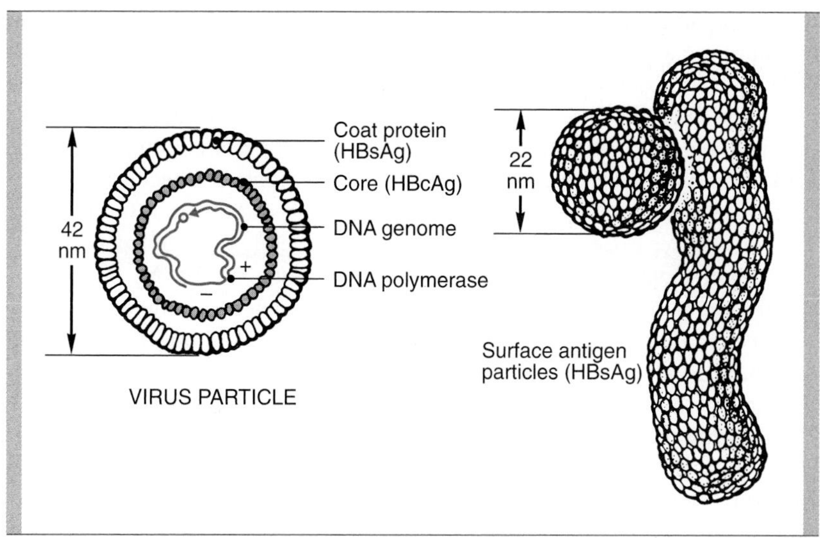

FIGURE 37–2
Schematic diagram of hepatitis B virion. The 42-nm particle is the "Dane particle" or the hepatitis B virus. The 22-nm particles are the filamentous and circular forms of hepatitis B surface antigen (HbsAg) or protein coat.

between subtypes. Aggregates of HBsAg are often found in great abundance in serum during infection. They may assume spherical or filamentous shapes with a mean diameter of 22 nm and may contain portions of the nucleocapsid (see Fig 37–2). Hepatitis B DNA can also be detected in serum and is an indication that infectious virions are present there. In infected liver tissue, evidence of HBcAg, HBeAg, and hepatitis B DNA is found in the nuclei of infected hepatocytes, whereas HBsAg is found in cytoplasm.

Found in cytoplasm of infected hepatocytes

REPLICATION CYCLE

The replication of hepatitis B virus involves a reverse transcription step, and, as such, is unique among DNA viruses. The double-stranded DNA is organized as two strands. One, a short strand, is associated with the viral DNA polymerase and is of positive polarity. The complete or long strand is complementary and thus of negative polarity. In viral replication, full-length positive viral RNA transcripts are inserted into maturing core particles late in the replicative cycle. These mRNA strands form a template for a reverse transcription step in which negatively stranded DNA is synthesized. The RNA template strands are then degraded by ribonuclease activity. A positive-stranded DNA is then synthesized, although this is not completed prior to virus maturation and release and thus results in the variable-length short positive DNA strands found in the virions.

Unique replication using a reverse transcriptase step

Despite extensive attempts, hepatitis B virus has not been propagated in the laboratory. Humans appear to be the major host; however, as with hepatitis A, infection of subhuman primates has been accomplished experimentally.

Humans are the major hosts

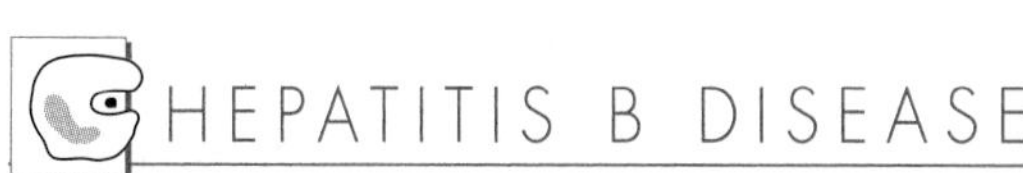

HEPATITIS B DISEASE

CLINICAL CAPSULE

Hepatitis B virus is the cause of what was formerly known as "serum hepatitis." This name was used to distinguish it from "infectious hepatitis" and reflected the association of this form of hepatitis with needle use or blood transfusion. Hepatitis B is usually an asymptomatic or limited illness with fever and jaundice for days to weeks. It becomes chronic in up to 10% of patients and may lead to cirrhosis or hepatocellular carcinoma.

EPIDEMIOLOGY

Hepatitis B infection is found worldwide, with prevalence rates varying markedly between countries. Chronic carriers constitute the main reservoir of infection: in some

Chronic carriers are common in the Far East

countries particularly in the far East, as many as 5 to 15% of all persons carry the virus and most are asymptomatic. About 10% of patients with human immunodeficiency virus (HIV) infection are chronic carriers of hepatitis B.

In the United States, it is estimated that 1.5 million people are infected with hepatitis B and that 300,000 new cases occur annually. About 300 of these patients die of acute fulminant hepatitis, and 5–10% of infected patients become chronic hepatitis B virus carriers. As many as 4000 people die yearly of hepatitis B–related cirrhosis, and 1000 die of hepatocellular carcinoma. Approximately 50% of infections in the United States are sexually transmitted, and the prevalence of HBsAg in serum is higher in certain populations, such as male homosexuals, patients on hemodialysis or immunosuppressive therapy, patients with Down's syndrome, and injection drug users. Routine screening of blood donors for HBsAg has markedly decreased the incidence of post-transfusion hepatitis B. Multiple-pool blood products still cause occasional cases. Exposure to hepatitis viruses from direct contact with blood or other body fluids, probably through needlestick injuries, has resulted in a higher risk of hepatitis B in medical personnel. Attack rates are also high in spouses and sexual partners of infected patients.

Needlestick transmission is a risk for health care workers

Hepatitis B infection of infants does not appear to be transplacentally transmitted to the fetus in utero but is acquired during the birth process by the swallowing of infected blood or fluids or through abrasions. The rate of virus acquisition is high (up to 90%) in infants born to mothers with acute hepatitis B infection or carrying HBsAg and HBeAg. Most infants do not develop clinical disease; however, infection in the neonatal period is associated with failure to produce antibody to HbsAg, allowing chronic carriage to occur in nearly 100% with perpetuation of transmission in the family setting.

Vertical transmission usually occurs during birth process

Hepatocellular carcinoma has been strongly associated with persistent carriage of hepatitis B virus by serologic tests and by detection of viral nucleic acid sequences integrated in tumor cell genomes. In many parts of Africa and Asia, primary liver cancer accounts for 20 to 30% of all types of malignancies, but in North and South America and Europe, only 1 to 2%. The estimated risk of developing the malignancy for persons with chronic hepatitis B is increased between 10- to more than 300-fold in different populations.

Strong association between chronic infection and hepatocellular carcinoma

PATHOGENESIS

In the past, hepatitis B was known as posttransfusion hepatitis or as hepatitis associated with the use of illicit parenteral drugs (serum hepatitis). However, over the past few years it has become clear that the major mode of acquisition is through close personal contact with body fluids of infected individuals. HBsAg has been found in most body fluids, including saliva, semen, and cervical secretions. Under experimental conditions, as little as 0.0001 mL of infectious blood has produced infection. Transmission is therefore possible by vehicles such as inadequately sterilized hypodermic needles or instruments used in tattooing and ear piercing.

Virus found in blood, saliva, and semen

The factors determining the different clinical manifestations of acute hepatitis B are largely unknown; however, some appear to involve immunologic responses of the host. The serum sickness–like rash and arthritis that may precede the development of symptoms and jaundice appear to be related to circulating immune complexes that activate the complement system. Antibody to HBsAg is protective and associated with resolution of the disease. Cellular immunity also may be important in the host response, because patients with depressed T-lymphocyte function have a high frequency of chronic infection with the hepatitis B virus. Antibody to the HBcAg, which appears during infection, is present in chronic carriers with persistent hepatitis B virion production and does not appear to be protective.

Antibody to HBsAg is protective

The morphologic lesions of acute hepatitis B resemble those of other hepatitis viruses. In chronic active hepatitis B, the continued presence of inflammatory foci of infection results in necrosis of hepatocytes, collapse of the reticular framework of the liver, and progressive fibrosis. The increasing fibrosis can result in the syndrome of post-necrotic hepatic cirrhosis.

Chronic infection leads to progressive fibrosis and cirrhosis

Integrated hepatitis B viral DNA can be found in nearly all hepatocellular carcinomas. The virus has not been shown to possess a transforming gene but may well activate a cellular oncogene. It is also possible that the virus does not play such a direct molecular role in oncogenicity, because the natural history of chronic hepatitis B infection involves cycles of damage or death of liver cells interspersed with periods of intense regenerative hyperplasia. This significantly increases the opportunity for spontaneous mutational changes that may activate cellular oncogenes. Whatever the mechanism, the association between chronic viral infection and hepatocellular carcinoma is clear, and liver cancer is a major cause of disease and death in countries in which chronic hepatitis B infection is common. The proven success of combined active and passive immunization in aborting hepatitis B infection in infancy or childhood makes hepatocellular carcinoma of the liver a potentially preventable disease.

Mechanism of hepatocellular carcinoma development is not clearly known

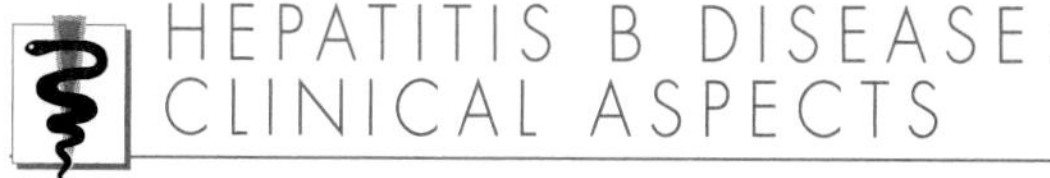

HEPATITIS B DISEASE: CLINICAL ASPECTS

MANIFESTATIONS

The clinical picture of hepatitis B is highly variable. The incubation period may be as brief as 7 days or as long as 160 days (mean, approximately 10 weeks). Acute hepatitis B is usually manifested by the gradual onset of fatigue, loss of appetite, nausea and pain, and fullness in the right upper abdominal quadrant. Early in the course of disease, pain and swelling of the joints and occasional frank arthritis may occur. Some patients develop a rash. With increasing involvement of the liver, there is increasing cholestasis and, hence, clay-colored stools, darkening of the urine, and jaundice. Symptoms may persist for several months before finally resolving.

Average incubation period is 10 weeks; range 7–160 days

In general, the symptoms associated with acute hepatitis B are more severe and more prolonged than those of hepatitis A; however, anicteric disease and asymptomatic infection occur. The infection-to-disease ratio, which varies according to age and method of acquisition, has been estimated to be approximately 6:1 or 7:1. Fulminant hepatitis, leading to extensive liver necrosis and death, develops in less than 1% of cases. One important difference between hepatitis A and hepatitis B is the development of chronic hepatitis. This occurs in approximately 10% of all patients with hepatitis B infection, but the risk is much higher for newborns (~100%), children (50%) and the immunocompromised. Chronic infection is associated with ongoing replication of virus in the liver and usually with the presence of HBsAg in serum. Chronic hepatitis may lead to cirrhosis, liver failure, or hepatocellular carcinoma, in up to 25% of patients.

Chronic hepatitis is most common with infection in early infancy or childhood

DIAGNOSIS

The nomenclature of hepatitis B antigens and antibodies is shown in Table 37–2 and the sequence of their appearance in Figure 37–3. During the acute episode of disease, when there is active viral replication, large amounts of HBsAg and hepatitis B virus DNA can be detected in the serum, as can fully developed virions and high levels of DNA polymerase and HBeAg. Although HBcAg is also present, antibody against it invariably occurs and prevents its detection. With resolution of acute hepatitis B, HBsAg and HBeAg disappear from serum with the development of antibodies (anti-HBs and anti-HBe) against them. The development of anti-HBs is associated with elimination of infection and protection against reinfection. Anti-HBc is detected early in the course of disease and persists in serum for years. It is an excellent epidemiologic marker of infection, but is not protective. The laboratory diagnosis of acute hepatitis B is best made by demonstrating the IgM antibody to hepatitis B core antigen in serum. Almost all patients who develop jaundice are anti-HBc IgM positive at the time of clinical presentation. HBsAg may also be detected in serum. Past infection with hepatitis B is best determined by detecting IgG anti-HBc, anti-HBs, or both.

Appearance of anti-HBs signals elimination of infection

Acute infection associated with appearance of anti-HBc IgM

TABLE 37–2

Nomenclature for Hepatitis B Virus Antigens and Antibodies

ABBREVIATION	DESCRIPTION
HBV	Hepatitis B virus; 42-nm double-stranded DNA virus; Dane particle
HBsAg	Hepatitis B surface antigen; found on surface of virus; formed in excess and seen in serum as 22-nm spherical and tubular particles; four subdeterminants (*adw, ayw, adr,* and *ayr*) identified
HBcAg	Core antigen (nucleocapsid core); found in nucleus of infected hepatocytes by immunofluorescence
HBeAg	Glycoprotein; associated with the core antigen; used epidemiologically as marker of potential infectivity; seen only when HBsAg is also present
Anti-HBs	Antibody to HBsAg; correlated with protection against and/or resolution of disease; used as marker of past infection or vaccination
Anti-HBc	Antibody to HBcAg; seen in acute infection and chronic carriers; anti-HBc IgM used as indicator of acute infection; anti-HBc IgG used as marker of past or chronic infection; apparently not important in disease resolution; does not develop in response to vaccine
Anti-HBe	Antibody to HBeAg

Chronic infection associated with HBsAg persistence and no development of anti-HBs

In patients with chronic hepatitis B, evidence of viral persistence can be found in serum (Figure 37–4). HBsAg can be detected throughout the active disease process and anti-HBs does not develop, which probably accounts for the chronicity of the disease. However, anti-HBc is detected. Two types of chronic hepatitis can be distinguished. In one, HBsAg is detected but not HBeAg; these patients usually show minimal evidence of liver dysfunction. In the other, both antigens are found; the process is more active, with continued hepatic damage that may result in cirrhosis. Chronic infection with hepatitis B is best detected by persistence of HBsAg in blood for more than 6 to 12 months.

TREATMENT

There is no specific treatment for acute hepatitis B. A high-calorie diet is desirable. Corticosteroid therapy has no value in uncomplicated acute viral hepatitis, and recent

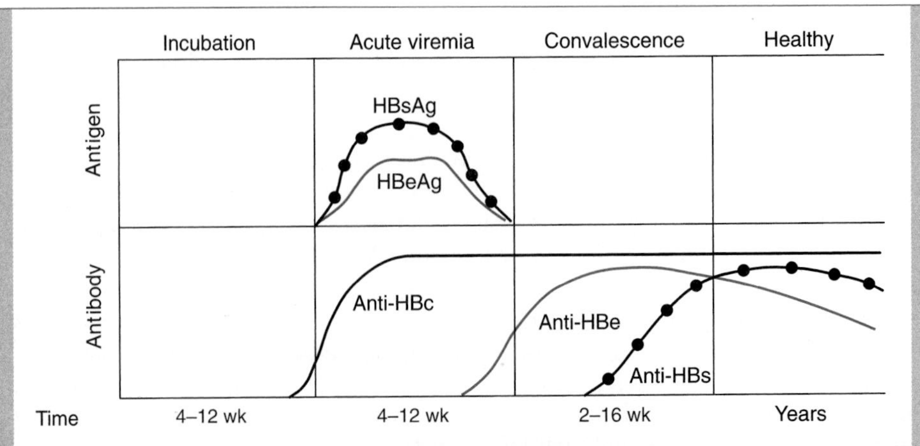

FIGURE 37–3
Sequence of appearance of viral antigens and antibodies in acute self-limiting cases of hepatitis B. HBsAg, hepatitis B surface antigen; HBeAg, hepatitis B e antigen; anti-HBc, antibody to hepatitis B core antigen; anti-HBe, antibody to HBeAg; anti-HBs, antibody to HBsAg.

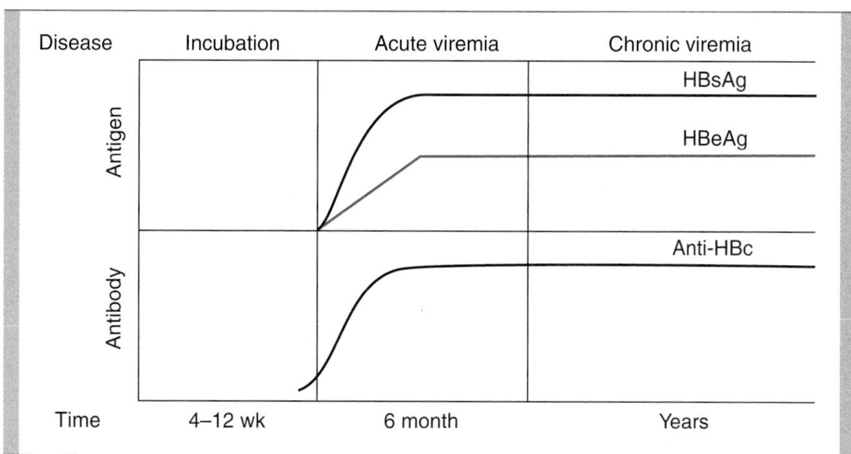

FIGURE 37–4
Sequence of appearance of viral antigens and antibodies in chronic active hepatitis B. HBsAg, hepatitis B surface antigen; HBeAg, hepatitis B e antigen; anti-HBc, antibody to hepatitis B core antigen; Antibodies to HBsAg and HBeAg not detected.

studies suggest that it may increase the severity of chronic hepatitis caused by hepatitis B virus. For chronic hepatitis B diseases, interferon alpha 10 million units three times weekly for 4 months provides long-term benefit in a minority (~33%) of patients, usually those who already demonstrate an acute immune response with low serum viral DNA levels. Lamivudine (3TC), a potent inhibitor of HIV is also active versus hepatitis B virus both in vitro and in initial clinical trials, but resistance to this agent develops in about 25% of patients after 12 months of therapy. Adefovir, a nucleotide analog of adenosine monophosphate, is newly approved for the treatment of chronic hepatitis B. Treatment should be considered for patients exhibiting chronic hepatitis B for more than 6 months with detectable serum levels of HBsAg, HBcAg, and hepatitis B DNA.

No specific treatment for acute infection

Interferon alpha lamivudine and adefovir are of benefit.

PREVENTION

Safe sex practices and avoidance of needlestick injuries or injection drug use are approaches to diminishing the risk of hepatitis B infection. Both active prophylaxis and passive prophylaxis of hepatitis B infection can be accomplished. Most preparations of ISG contain only moderate levels of anti-HBs; however, specific hepatitis B immune globulin (HBIG) with high titers of hepatitis B antibody is now available. HBIG is prepared from sera of subjects who have high titers of antibody to HBsAg but are free of the antigen itself. Administration of HBIG soon after exposure to the virus greatly reduces the development of symptomatic disease. Postexposure prophylaxis with HBIG should be followed by active immunization with vaccine. Inactivated hepatitis B vaccines have been available for several years. The first was developed by purification and inactivation of HBsAg from the blood of chronic carriers, but this is no longer in use. The current vaccine is a recombinant product derived from HBAg grown in yeast. Excellent protection has been shown in studies on homosexual men and medical personnel. These groups and others, such as laboratory workers and injection drug users who come into contact with blood or other potentially infected materials, should receive hepatitis B vaccine as the preferred method of preexposure prophylaxis. Recently, immunization of all children has been recommended.

Postexposure treatment with HBIG temporarily reduces risk

Recombinant vaccine recommended for children and high-risk persons

A combination of active and passive immunization is the most effective approach to prevent neonatal acquisition and the development of chronic carriage in the neonate. Most hospitals recommend routine screening of pregnant women for the presence of HBsAg. Infants born to those who are positive should receive HBIG in the delivery room followed by three doses of hepatitis B vaccine beginning 24 hours after birth. A similar combination of passive and active immunization is used for unimmunized persons who have been exposed by needlestick or similar injuries. The procedure varies depending on the hepatitis B status of the "donor" case linked to the injury.

Combination of HBIG and vaccine significantly reduces vertical transmission

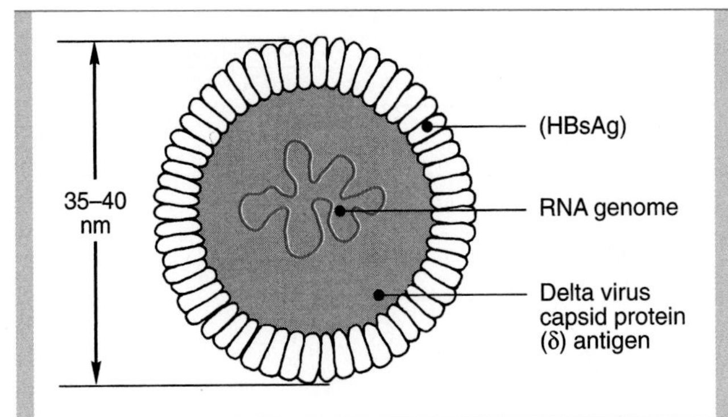

FIGURE 37–5
Schematic of delta hepatitis virus. Note outer layer derived from hepatitis B surface antigen (HBsAg).

Delta Hepatitis (Hepatitis D)

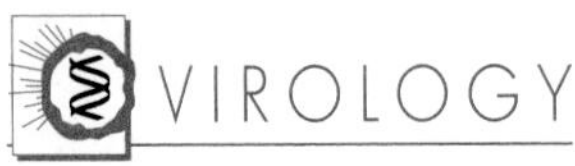

VIROLOGY

Hepatitis D is found only in hepatitis B–infected persons

Virus uses HBsAg for assembly

Delta hepatitis is caused by the hepatitis D virus. This small single-stranded RNA virus requires the presence of hepatitis B surface antigens for its transmission and is thus found only in persons with acute or chronic hepatitis B infection. Strategies directed at preventing hepatitis B are also effective in preventing delta hepatitis. The method of replication of hepatitis D viral RNA is not clear. Associated with the RNA are proteins of 27 and 29 kilodaltons that constitute the delta antigen. This protein–RNA complex is surrounded by HBsAg (Fig 37–5). Thus, although the delta virus produces its own antigens, it co-opts the HBsAg in assembling its coat.

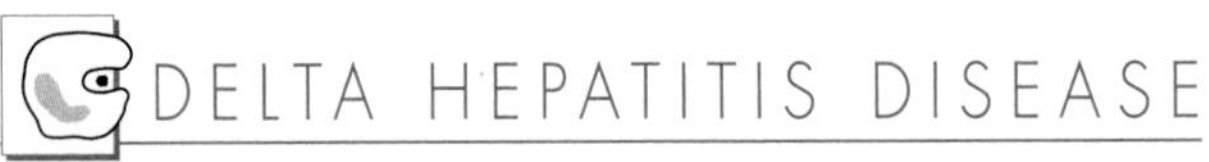

DELTA HEPATITIS DISEASE

Greatest risk is among injection drug abusers

Delta hepatitis is most prevalent in groups at high risk of hepatitis B. Injection drug users are those at greatest risk in the western parts of the world, and as many as 50% of such individuals may have IgG antibody to the delta virus antigen. Other risks include dialysis. Nonparenteral and vertical transmission can also occur.

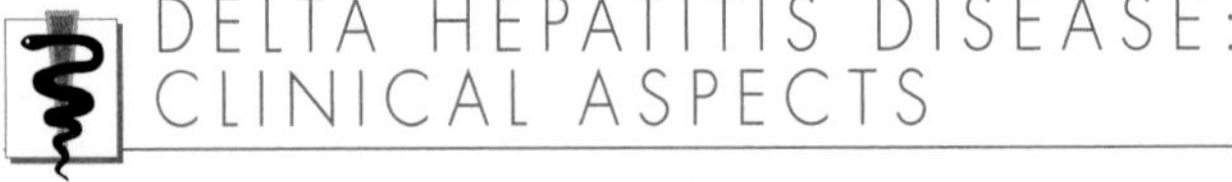

DELTA HEPATITIS DISEASE: CLINICAL ASPECTS

MANIFESTATIONS

Simultaneous hepatitis B and D infections cause more severe disease

Two major types of delta infection have been noted: simultaneous delta and hepatitis B infection or delta superinfection in those with chronic hepatitis B. Simultaneous infection with both delta and hepatitis B results in clinical hepatitis that is indistinguishable from acute hepatitis A or B; however, fulminant hepatitis is much more common than with hepatitis B virus alone. Persons with chronic hepatitis B who acquire infection with hepatitis D suffer relapses of jaundice and have a high likelihood of developing chronic cirrhosis. Epidemics of delta infection have occurred in populations with a high incidence of chronic hepatitis B and have resulted in rapidly progressive liver disease, causing death in up to 20% of infected persons.

DIAGNOSIS

Diagnosis is made most commonly by demonstrating IgM or IgG antibodies, or both, to the delta antigen in serum. IgM antibodies appear within 3 weeks of infection and persist for several weeks. IgG antibodies persist for years.

Diagnosis is by detection of antibodies

TREATMENT AND PREVENTION

Response to treatment with interferon alpha in patients with delta hepatitis (and hepatitis B) is less than in those with hepatitis B alone. Recommended doses are higher and may produce sustained improvement in only 15–25% of patients.

Because the capsid of delta hepatitis is HBsAg, measures aimed at limiting the transmission of hepatitis B (eg, vaccination, blood screening) prevent the transmission of delta hepatitis. Individuals infected with hepatitis B or D should not donate blood, organ, tissues, or semen. Safe sex should be practiced unless there is only a single sex partner who is already infected. Methods of reducing transmission include decreased use of contaminated needles and syringes by injection drug users and use of needle safety devices by health care workers.

Major for prevention of hepatitis B also prevent hepatitis

Hepatitis C

It is now known that a large number of hepatitis cases are due to an RNA virus termed hepatitis C virus. Its existence and role in the etiology of hepatitis was identified by preparing numerous complementary DNA clones from the presumed RNA virus in infectious serum. Peptides encoded by these clones were then tested for reaction with sera from cases of hepatitis and one was found to be highly specific, providing a basis for a serologic test.

Cause identified by molecular cloning techniques

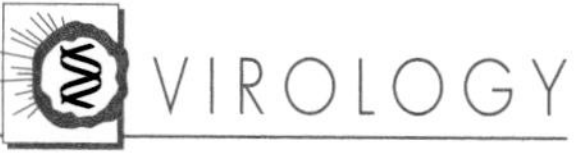

VIROLOGY

Hepatitis C virus is an RNA virus in the flavivirus (eg, yellow fever, dengue) family. It has a very simple genome, consisting of just three structural and five nonstructural genes. There are at least six major genotypes, with multiple subtypes. The genotypes have different geographic distributions and may be associated with differing severity of disease as well as response to therapy.

RNA virus, with six major genotypes

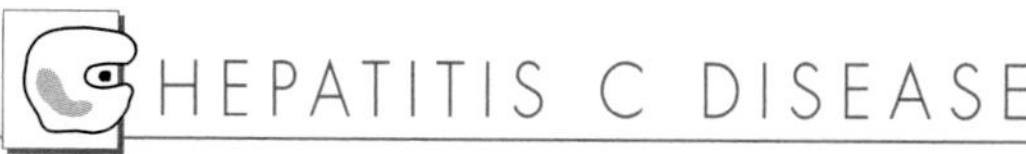

HEPATITIS C DISEASE

CLINICAL CAPSULE

Hepatitis C is an insidious disease in that it does not usually cause a clinically evident acute illness. Instead, its first manifestation (in 25% of those infected) may be the presence of smoldering chronic hepatitis that may ultimately lead to liver failure. Its transmission is less well understood than for hepatitis A, B, and D. Hepatitis C was the major cause of posttransfusion hepatitis until a serologic test for screening blood donors was developed.

The transmission of hepatitis C by blood is well documented: indeed, until screening blood for transfusions was introduced, it caused the great majority of cases of posttransfusion hepatitis. Hepatitis C may be sexually transmitted but to a much lesser degree than hepatitis B. Needle sharing accounts for up to 40% of cases. In the United States, 3.5 million

Major transmission was from blood and blood products but is now from “needle sharing”

people (1.8%) have antibody to hepatitis C. Screening of donor blood for antibody has reduced posttransfusion hepatitis by 80–90%. Since the 1980s, outbreaks of hepatitis C have been associated with IVIG. To reduce this risk, all US-licensed IGIV products now have additional viral inactivation steps included in the manufacturing process. Furthermore, all immunoglobulin products (including intramuscular immunoglobulin products that have not been associated with hepatitis C) that lack viral inactivation steps are now excluded if hepatitis C virus is detected by polymerase chain reaction (PCR). Other individuals considered at risk for hepatitis C are chronic hemodialysis patients and spouses.

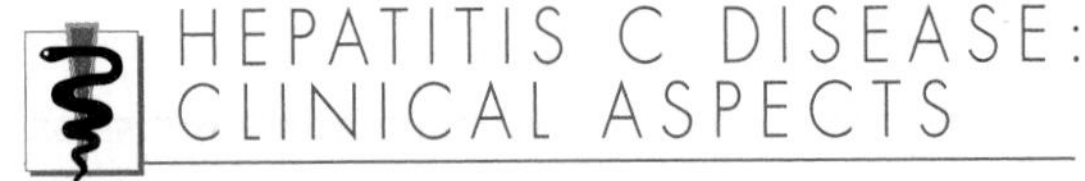

HEPATITIS C DISEASE: CLINICAL ASPECTS

MANIFESTATIONS

Acute illness usually not apparent

Chronic infection is common

The incubation period of hepatitis C averages 6–12 weeks. The infection is usually asymptomatic or mild and anicteric but results in a chronic carrier state in up to 85% of adults of patients. The average time from infection to the development of chronic hepatitis is 10–18 years. Cirrhosis and hepatocellular carcinoma are late sequelae of chronic hepatitis. Chronic hepatitis tends to wax and wane, is often asymptomatic, and may be associated with either elevated or normal alanine aminotransferase (ALT) values in serum. Chronic hepatitis C is the leading cause of liver transplantation in the United States.

DIAGNOSIS

Antibody responses are usually delayed

Hepatitis C RNA can be detected and quantitated by PCR

Antigens of hepatitis C are not detectable in blood, so diagnostic tests attempt to demonstrate antibody. Unfortunately, the antibody responses in acute disease remain negative for 1 to 3 weeks after clinical onset and may never become positive in up to 20% of patients with acute, resolving disease. Current tests measure antibodies to multiple hepatitis C antigens by either enzyme immunoassay or immunoblot testing. Even with these newer assays, IgG antibody to hepatitis C may not develop for up to 4 months, making the serodiagnosis of acute hepatitis C difficult. Quantitative assays of hepatitis C RNA may be used for diagnosis, estimating prognosis, predicting interferon responsiveness, and monitoring therapy, but there is not a very good correlation between viral load and histology.

TREATMENT AND PREVENTION

Combination therapy can benefit some persons with chronic infection

Immune globulin may not be protective; no vaccine exists

Combination therapy with interferon alpha and ribavirin is the current treatment of choice for patients with evidence of hepatitis due to hepatitis C. Criteria for initiating treatment are controversial, but most physicians would treat with abnormal liver histology and elevated liver enzymes. Responses are better in patients with genotypes other than 1 and those with low initial titers of viral RNA. Corticosteroids are not beneficial. Avoidance of injection drug use and screening of blood products are important preventive measures. It is not clear whether prophylactic ISG protects against hepatitis C. In addition, it is questionable whether a vaccine will be effective; patients may be reinfected by wild-type virus.

HEPATITIS E

Hepatitis E is the cause of another form of hepatitis that is spread by the fecal–oral route and therefore resembles hepatitis A. Hepatitis E virus is an RNA virus that is similar to but distinct from caliciviruses. The viral particles in stool are spherical, 27 to 34 nm in size, and unenveloped and exhibit spikes on their surface. Like hepatitis A, infection with this virus is frequently subclinical. When symptomatic, it causes only acute disease that may fulminate, especially in pregnant women. In endemic, developing areas, it has the highest attack rate in young adults, and infection is usually associated with contaminated drinking water. It does not appear to spread from person to person. Most cases have been identified in developing countries with poor sanitation (eg, in Asia, Africa, and the Indian subcontinent), and recurrent epidemics have been described in these areas. Rarely have cases been identified in the United States, and these have been in visitors or immigrants from endemic areas. The incubation period is approximately 40 days. The diagnosis may be confirmed by demonstrating the presence of specific IgM antibody. It is likely but unproven that ISG provides protection; no treatment is available. Liver transplant may be the only recourse in seriously ill patients.

Hepatitis E spreads similarly to hepatitis A

Usually associated with contaminated drinking water

HEPATITIS G

Although hepatitis C virus is a major cause of hepatitis, additional etiologic agent(s) continue to be sought. In 1995, hepatitis G, a newly discovered agent, was identified in sera from two different patients. Hepatitis G is an RNA virus similar to hepatitis C and members of the flavivirus family. An antibody assay can detect past, but not present, infection, and detection of acute infection with hepatitis G requires a PCR assay for viral RNA in serum. Up to 2% of volunteer blood donors are seropositive for hepatitis G RNA, which is a blood-borne virus. In addition to being closely related to hepatitis C, data suggest that the majority of patients infected by hepatitis C are also infected by hepatitis G. Given this association, it has been difficult to ascertain the contribution of hepatitis G to clinical disease. Patients infected with both viruses do not appear to have worse disease than those infected by hepatitis C virus only. Currently, there is no useful serologic test and no therapy is established.

RNA virus similar to hepatitis C

Role in human disease is currently uncertain

ADDITIONAL READING

Defranchis R, Meucci G, Vecchi M, et al. The natural history of asymptomatic hepatitis B. *Ann Intern Med* 1993;118:191–194. A follow-up of HbsAg-positive blood donors to determine the incidence and severity of chronic hepatitis B.

Johnson Y, Lau N, Wright TL. Molecular virology and pathogenesis of hepatitis B. *Lancet* 1993;342:1335–1339. This short review covers details of molecular structure and replication of the hepatitis B virus.

Jonas MM, Kelley DA, Mizerski J, et al. Clinical trial of lamivudine in children with chronic hepatitis B. *N Engl J Med* 2002;346:1706–1713. This large collaborative study demonstrated a modest but significant benefit with 52 weeks of treatment. The commentary on pages 1682–1683 by Lok is also well worth reading.

Lauer GM, Walker BD. Hepatitis C virus infections. *N Engl J Med* 2001;345:41–52. An exceptionally well-illustrated review of the problem, including pathogenesis and treatment.

Werzberger A, et al. A controlled trial of a formalin-inactivated hepatitis A vaccine in healthy children. *N Engl J Med* 1992;327:453–457. The inactivated purified hepatitis A vaccine is well tolerated, and a single dose is highly protective against clinically apparent hepatitis A.

CHAPTER 38

Herpesviruses

W. LAWRENCE DREW

The herpesvirus group, of the family Herpesviridae, comprises large, enveloped, double-stranded DNA viruses found in both animals and humans. They are ubiquitous and produce infections ranging from painful skin ulcers to chickenpox to encephalitis. Eight members of the family infect humans: two herpes simplex viruses (HSV-1 and HSV-2), cytomegalovirus (CMV), varicella–zoster virus (VZV), Epstein–Barr virus (EBV), human herpesvirus-6 (HHV-6), and the recently discovered human herpesvirus types 7 and 8 (HHV-7, HHV-8; Table 38–1). In addition a simian herpesvirus, herpes B virus, has occasionally caused human disease.

Large, enveloped double-stranded DNA viruses

GROUP CHARACTERISTICS

VIROLOGY

All herpesviruses are morphologically similar, with an overall size of 180 to 200 nm. The DNA core is up to 75 nm in diameter and is surrounded by an icosahedral capsid. Over the capsid is a protein-filled region called the tegument. The outside of the viral particle is covered by a lipoprotein envelope derived from the nuclear membrane of the infected host cell. The envelope contains at least nine glycoproteins that protrude beyond it as spike-like structures. The viral genome is large, up to 240 kbp of DNA, which code for approximately 75 viral proteins. This large genome is necessary, because herpesviruses frequently infect nondividing cells and must therefore provide their own enzymes necessary for DNA synthesis. Despite the morphologic similarity between herpesviruses, there are substantial differences in their genomic sequences and, in turn, their structural glycoproteins and polypeptides. Antigenic analysis is an important means for differentiation among herpesviruses despite some cross-reactions (eg, between HSV and VZV).

Morphology similar among herpesviruses but genomic sequences differ

Can infect nondividing cells

Based on certain virologic similarities, the herpes viruses may be divided into three subfamilies α, β, and γ. Herpes simplex 1 and 2, as well as varicella-zoster viruses, are in the subfamily; cytomegalovirus, HHV-6, and HHV-7 are in the β subfamily while EBV and HHV-8 are in the γ subfamily.

Cell tropisms for the individual viruses vary significantly. Herpes simplex virus has the widest range; it replicates in numerous animal and human host cells, although it affects only humans in nature. VZV infects only primates and is best grown in cells of human origin, although some laboratory-adapted strains can grow in primate cell lines. Human CMV replicates well only in human diploid fibroblast cell lines. EBV does not replicate in most

Herpes simplex has widest range of cell tropism

TABLE 38–1

Human Herpesviruses

Designation	Common Name	Disease
HHV-1	Herpes simplex virus-1	Oral (fever blisters), ocular lesions, encephalitis
HHV-2	Herpes simplex virus-2	Genital, anal lesions Severe neonatal infections, meningitis
HHV-3	Varicella–zoster virus	Chickenpox (primary infection) Shingles (reactivation)
HHV-4	Epstein–Barr virus	Infectious mononucleosis (primary infection) Tumors, including B-cell tumors (Burkitt's lymphoma, immunoblastic lymphomas of the immunosuppressed) Nasopharyngeal carcinoma, some T-cell tumors
HHV-5	Cytomegalovirus	Mononucleosis Severe congenital infection Infections in immunocompromised (gastroenteritis, retinitis, pneumonia)
HHV-6	Human herpesvirus-6	Roseola in infants (primary infection) Infections in allograft recipients (pneumonia, marrow failure)
HHV-7	Human herpesvirus-7	Some cases of roseola (primary infection)
HHV-8	Kaposi's sarcoma–associated herpesvirus (KSHV), human herpesvirus-8	Tumors, including Kaposi's sarcoma Some B-cell lymphomas

commonly used cell culture systems but can be grown in continuous human or primate lymphoblastoid cell cultures. Human HSV-6 grows only in lymphocyte cell cultures.

Viral latency and disease reactivation typical for all herpesviruses

Characteristically, all of these agents produce an initial infection followed by a period of latent infection in which the genome of the virus is present in cells, but infectious virus is not recovered. During latent infection of cells, viral DNA is maintained as an episome (not integrated), with limited expression of specific virus genes required for the maintenance of latency. Reactivation of virus due to complex host–virus interactions may then result in recurrent disease. For example, immunocompromised patients, especially those with altered cellular immunity, have frequent reactivations of herpesviruses that can lead to clinically severe disease.

Replication

Three classes of mRNAs produced

The replication of HSV is representative of all herpesviruses. The glycoproteins in the HSV envelope interact with cellular receptors to result in fusion with the cell membrane. Fusion delivers the capsid and DNA case into the cytoplasm, where it migrates to the nucleus, and the genome is circularized. Transcription of the large, complex genome is sequentially regulated in a cascade fashion. Three distinct classes of mRNAs are made: (1) immediate early (IE) mRNAs are synthesized 2 to 4 hours postinfection, which code for proteins initiating and regulating virus transcription; (2) early (E) mRNAs, which code for further nonstructural proteins involved in DNA replication and minor structural proteins; and (3) late (L) mRNAs (ie, 12 to 15 hours postinfection), which code for major structural proteins. The early (E) proteins include thymidine kinase and a DNA polymerase, which are distinct from host cell enzymes and are therefore important targets of antiviral chemotherapy. Gene expression is coordinated (ie, synthesis of early gene products turns off IE products and initiates genome replication); some of the late structural proteins are produced independently of genome replication, whereas others are only produced after replication. The pattern of viral DNA replication is complex, resulting in the formation of high-molecular-weight DNA concatemers. Genomic concatemers are cleaved and packaged into preassembled capsids in the nucleus.

Coordinated gene expression

The envelope is acquired from the inner lamella of the nuclear membrane. Budding occurs at the inner nuclear membranes, and virions then enter the cytoplasm to be released through the endoplasmic reticulum. HSV infection appears to be a "wasteful" process: only 25% of viral DNA/protein produced is incorporated into virions. The rest accumulates in the cell, which eventually dies. Moreover, the ratio of incomplete to complete viral particles is approximately 1000 to 1. Most herpesviruses shut down host cell metabolism and ultimately cause cell death, except for CMV, which actually stimulates cellular synthesis of nucleic acids and proteins.

Most herpesviruses, except CMV, shut down host cell metabolism

Herpes Simplex Virus

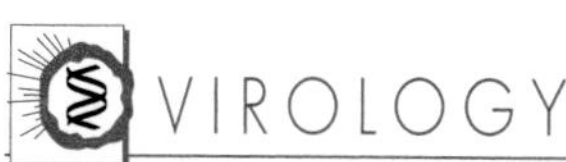

VIROLOGY

Two distinct epidemiologic and antigenic types of HSV exist (HSV-1 and HSV-2). The DNA genomes of both are linear, double-stranded molecules containing approximately 160 kbp. Their nucleic acids demonstrate approximately 50% base sequence homology, which is considerably greater than that shown between these viruses and other herpesviruses. HSV-1 and HSV-2 share antigens in almost all their surface glycoproteins and other structural polypeptides, but differences in glycoprotein gB enable them to be distinguished (ie, HSV-1 has gB1 and HSV-2 has gB2). Numerous strains of both HSV-1 and HSV-2 exist. In fact, by restriction endonuclease analysis of the viral genome, most strains of either HSV-1 or HSV-2 are found to differ somewhat, except in epidemiologically related cases such as mother–infant and sexual partners.

HSV-1 and HSV-2 are distinct epidemiologically, antigenically, and by DNA homology

Individual strains differ by restriction endonuclease techniques

HERPES SIMPLEX DISEASE

CLINICAL CAPSULE

HSV is one of the best known of all viruses, given its frequency of infection and its propensity to cause recurrent ulcers in areas of the skin and mucous membranes. The two types differ in their predilection for causing lesions "above the waist" (HSV-1) or "below the waist" (HSV-2). As with all herpesviruses, herpes simplex persists in a latent form and reactivates to cause viral excretion and/or disease.

EPIDEMIOLOGY

Herpes simplex viruses are distributed worldwide. There are no known animal vectors, and humans appear to be the only natural reservoir. Direct contact with infected secretions is the principal mode of spread. Seroepidemiologic studies indicate that the prevalence of HSV antibody varies according to the age and socioeconomic status of the population studied. In most developing countries, 90% of the population have HSV-1 antibody by the

No animal reservoirs

High seroprevalence among humans, which increases with age

age of 30. In the United States, HSV-1 antibody is currently found in approximately 60 to 70% of adult middle-class populations; among lower socioeconomic groups, however, the percentage is higher.

Infection with HSV-2 linked to sexual activity

Detection of HSV-2 antibody before puberty is unusual. The virus is associated with sexual activity, and direct sexual transmission is the major mode of spread. Approximately 15 to 30% of sexually active adults in Western industrialized countries have HSV-2 antibody. The virus can be isolated from the cervix and urethra of approximately 5 to 12% of adults attending sexually transmitted disease clinics; many of these patients are asymptomatic or have small, unnoticed lesions on penile or vulvar skin. Asymptomatic shedding accounts for transmission from a partner who has no active genital lesions and often no history of genital herpes. Genital herpes is not a reportable disease in the United States, but it is estimated that more than 1,000,000 new cases occur per year.

PATHOGENESIS

Acute Infections

Infection produces inflammation and giant cells

Virus can infect and spread in axons and ganglia

Pathologic changes during acute infections consist of development of multinucleated giant cells (Fig 38–1), ballooning degeneration of epithelial cells, focal necrosis, eosinophilic intranuclear inclusion bodies, and an inflammatory response characterized by an initial polymorphonuclear neutrophil (PMN) infiltrate and a subsequent mononuclear cell infiltrate. The virus can spread intra- or interneuronally or through supporting cellular networks of an axon or nerve, resulting in latent infection of sensory and autonomic nerve ganglia. Spread of virus can occur by cell-to-cell transfer and can therefore be unaffected by circulating immune globulin.

Latent Infection

No synthesis of early or late viral polypeptides in latent infection

In humans, latent infection by HSV-1 has been demonstrated by cocultivation techniques in trigeminal, superior cervical, and vagal nerve ganglia, and occasionally in the S2–S3 dorsal sensory nerve root ganglia. Latent HSV-2 infection has been demonstrated in the sacral (S2–S3) region. Latent infection of nervous tissue by HSV does not result in the death of the cell; however, the exact mechanism of viral genome interaction with the cell is incompletely understood. Several copies of the HSV viral genomes are in each latently infected neuronal cell. They exist in a circular form, and transcription of only a small portion of the viral genome occurs. Because latent infection does not appear to require synthesis of early or late viral polypeptides, antiviral drugs directed at the thymidine kinase enzymes or viral DNA polymerase do not eradicate the virus in its latent state.

Reactivation can be precipitated by sun exposure, fever, or trauma

Reactivation of virus from latently infected ganglionic cells with subsequent release of infectious virions appears to account for most recurrences of both genital and orolabial infections. The mechanisms by which latent infection is reactivated are unknown. Precipitating factors that are known to initiate reactivation of herpes simplex include; exposure to ultraviolet light, fever and trauma (eg, oral intubation).

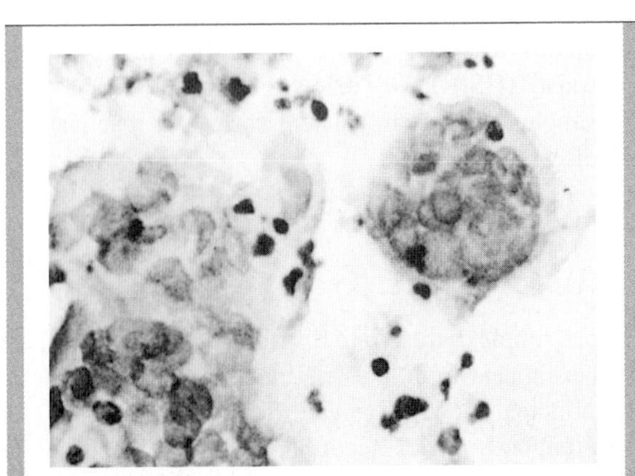

FIGURE 38–1
Multinucleated giant cells from herpes simplex virus lesion.

IMMUNITY

Host factors have a major effect on clinical manifestations of HSV infection. Many episodes of HSV infection are either asymptomatic or mildly symptomatic. Initial symptomatic clinical episodes of the disease are more severe than recurrent episodes, probably because of the presence of anti-HSV antibodies and immune lymphocytes in persons with recurrent infections. Prior infection with HSV-1 may protect against or shorten the duration of symptoms and lesions from subsequent infection with HSV-2 due to some degree of cross protection.

Some cross-protection between HSV-1 and HSV-2

Both cellular and humoral immune responses are important in immunity to HSV. Neutralizing antibodies directed against HSV envelope glycoproteins appear to be important in preventing exogenous reinfection. Antibody-dependent cellular cytotoxicity (ADCC) may be important in limiting early spread of HSV. By the second week after infection, cytotoxic T lymphocytes can be detected that are able to destroy HSV-infected cells prior to completion of the replication cycle. Conversely, in immunosuppressed patients, especially those with depressed cell-mediated immunity, reactivation of HSV may be associated with prolonged viral excretion and persistence of lesions.

ADCC may limit early spread of HSV; cytotoxic T lymphocytes destroy HSV-infected cells

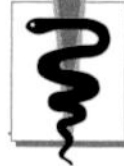

HERPES SIMPLEX: CLINICAL ASPECTS

MANIFESTATIONS

Herpes Simplex Type 1

Infection with HSV-1 is usually "above the waist." It consists characteristically of grouped or single vesicular lesions that become pustular and coalesce to form single or multiple ulcers. On dry surfaces, these ulcers scab before healing; on mucosal surfaces, they reepithelialize directly. Herpes simplex virus can be isolated from almost all ulcerative lesions, but the titer of virus decreases as the lesions evolve. Infections generally involve ectoderm (skin, mouth, conjunctiva, nervous system).

Vesicular lesions become pustular and then ulcerate

Primary infection with HSV-1 is often asymptomatic. When symptomatic, typically in children, it appears most frequently as gingivostomatitis, with fever and ulcerative lesions involving the buccal mucosa, tongue, gums, and pharynx. The lesions are quite painful, and the acute illness usually lasts 5 to 12 days. After this initial infection, HSV may become latent within sensory nerve root ganglia of the trigeminal nerve.

Primary infections often asymptomatic

Lesions usually recur on a specific area of the lip and the immediate adjacent skin; these lesions are referred to as mucocutaneous and are commonly called "cold sores" or "fever blisters." Because reactivation is usually from a single latent source, these lesions are typically unilateral. Their recurrence may be signaled by premonitory tingling or burning in the area. Systemic complaints are unusual, and the episode generally lasts approximately 7 days. It should be noted that HSV may be reactivated and excreted into the saliva with no apparent mucosal lesions present. Herpes simplex virus has been isolated from saliva in 5 to 8% of children and 1 to 2% of adults who were asymptomatic at the time.

Recurrent cold sores usually unilateral

Virus in saliva with asymptomatic reactivation

Herpes simplex virus sometimes infects the finger or nail area. This infection, termed **herpetic whitlow,** usually results from the inoculation of infected secretions through a small cut in the skin. Painful vesicular lesions of the finger develop and pustulate; they are often mistaken for bacterial infection and mistreated accordingly.

Herpetic whitlow mimics bacterial paronychia

Herpes simplex virus infection of the eye is one of the most common causes of corneal damage and blindness in the developed world. Infections usually involve the conjunctiva and cornea, and characteristic dendritic ulcerations are produced. With recurrence of disease, there may be deeper involvement with corneal scarring. Occasionally, there may be extension into deeper structures of the eye, especially if topical steroids are used.

Herpetic corneal and conjunctival infection can cause blindness

Encephalitis may rarely result from HSV-1 infection. Most cases occur in adults with high levels of anti–HSV-1 antibody, suggesting reactivation of latent virus in the trigeminal nerve root ganglion and extension of productive (lytic) infection into the temporoparietal

Herpes encephalitis may be reactivation

area of the brain. Primary HSV infection with neurotropic spread of the virus from peripheral sites up the olfactory bulb into the brain may also result in parenchymal brain infection.

Encephalitis typically localized to temporal lobe

Rapid diagnosis allows antiviral therapy

Classically, HSV encephalitis affects one temporal lobe, leading to focal neurologic signs and cerebral edema. If untreated, mortality is 70%. Clinically, the disease can resemble brain abscess, tumor, or intracerebral hemorrhage. Rapid diagnosis by the polymerase chain reaction (PCR) has replaced brain biopsy as the diagnostic test. Intravenous acyclovir can reduce the morbidity and mortality of the disease, especially if treatment is initiated early.

Herpes Simplex Type 2

HSV-2 associated with genital infections

Genital herpes is an important sexually transmitted disease. Both HSV-1 and HSV-2 can cause genital disease, and the symptoms and signs of acute infection are similar for both viruses. Seventy percent of first episodes of genital HSV infection in the United States are caused by HSV-2, and genital HSV-2 disease is also more likely to recur than genital HSV-1 infection. Ninety percent of HSV-2 antibody–positive patients have never had a clinically evident genital HSV episode. In many instances, the first clinical episode is years after primary infection.

Primary Genital Herpes Infection

Multiple painful vesicopustular lesions

Systemic symptoms and adenopathy common

For the relatively few individuals who develop clinically evident primary genital HSV disease, the mean incubation period from sexual contact to onset of lesions is 5 days. Lesions begin as small erythematous papules that soon form vesicles and then pustules (Fig 38–2). Within 3 to 5 days, the vesiculopustular lesions break to form painful coalesced ulcers that subsequently dry; some form crusts and heal without scarring. With primary disease, the genital lesions are usually multiple (mean number, 20), bilateral, and extensive. The urethra and cervix are also infected frequently, with discrete or coalesced ulcers on the exocervix. Bilateral enlarged tender inguinal lymph nodes are usually present and may persist for weeks to months. About one third of patients show systemic symptoms such as fever, malaise, and myalgia, and approximately 1% develop aseptic meningitis with neck rigidity and severe headache. First episodes of disease last an average of 12 days.

Recurrent Genital Herpes Infection

Prodromal paresthesias and shorter duration

In contrast to primary infection, recurrent genital herpes is a disease of shorter duration, usually localized in the genital region, and without systemic symptoms. A common symptom is prodromal paresthesias in the perineum, genitalia, or buttocks that occur 12 to 24 hours before the appearance of lesions. Recurrent genital herpes usually presents with grouped vesicular lesions in the external genital region. Local symptoms such as pain and itching are mild, lasting 4 to 5 days, and lesions usually last 2 to 5 days.

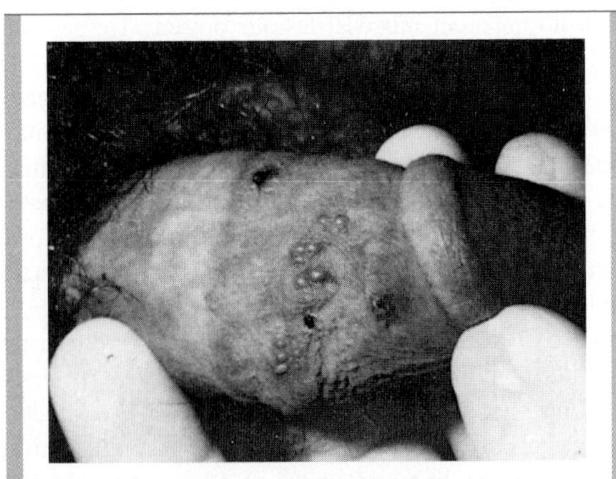

FIGURE 38–2
Multiple grouped vesicles of genital herpes.

At least 80% of patients with primary genital HSV-2 infection develop recurrent episodes of genital herpes within 12 months. In patients whose lesions recur, the median number of recurrences is four or five per year. They are not evenly spaced, and some patients experience a succession of monthly attacks followed by a period of quiescence. Over time, the number of recurrences decrease by a median of one-half to one recurrence per year. Most recurrences result from reactivation of virus from dorsal root ganglia. Rarely, recurrent infections may be due to reinfection with a different strain of HSV-2. Recurrent viral shedding from the genital tract may occur without clinically evident disease.

Recurrent episodes common; may involve shedding without lesions

Neonatal Herpes

Neonatal herpes usually results from transmission of virus during delivery through infected genital secretions from the mother. In utero infection, although possible, is uncommon. In most cases, severe neonatal herpes is associated with primary infection of a seronegative woman at or near the time of delivery. This results in an intense viral exposure of a seronegative infant during the birth process. The incidence rate of neonatal herpes simplex infection varies greatly among populations, but is estimated at approximately 1 per 2500 live births in the United States. Because a normal immune response is absent in the neonate born to a mother with recent primary infection, neonatal HSV infection is an extremely severe disease with an overall mortality of approximately 60%, and neurologic sequelae are high in those who survive. Manifestations vary. Some infants show disseminated vesicular lesions with a widespread internal organ involvement and necrosis of the liver and adrenal glands, and others have involvement of the central nervous system only, with listlessness and seizures.

Usually transmitted from mother at birth

High mortality if disseminated

DIAGNOSIS

Herpes simplex viruses are best cultured by isolation in a variety of other cell lines inoculated with infected secretions or lesions. The cytopathic effects of HSV can usually be demonstrated 24 to 48 hours after inoculation of the culture. Isolates of HSV-1 and HSV-2 can be differentiated by staining virus-infected cells with type-specific monoclonal antibodies to the two types. A direct smear prepared from the base of a suspected lesion and stained by either the Giemsa or Papanicolaou method may show intranuclear inclusions or multinucleated giant cells typical of herpes (Tzanck test), but this is less sensitive than viral culture and not specific; similar changes can be seen in cells infected with VZV. Enzyme immunoassays and immunofluorescence are rapid and relatively sensitive assays for direct detection of herpes antigen in lesions. Although early versions of these noncultural tests lacked sensitivity, more recent procedures have correlations with culture that approach 90%. Serology should not be used to diagnose active HSV infections, such as those affecting the genital or central nervous systems; frequently there is no change in antibody titer when reactivation occurs. Serology can be useful in detecting those with asymptomatic HSV-2 infection. PCR on cerebrospinal fluid (CSF) is the best test to diagnose HSV encephalitis. Restriction endonuclease digests can also be used to define epidemiologic relationships; that is, strains acquired between sexual partners or through mother–infant transmission.

Grow rapidly in many cell culture systems

HSV-1 and HSV-2 distinguished by type-specific monoclonal antibodies

Enzyme immunoassay, immunofluorescence, and PCR all used for rapid diagnosis

TREATMENT

Several antiviral drugs that inhibit HSV have been developed. The most effective and commonly used is the nucleoside analog acyclovir, which is converted by a viral enzyme (thymidine kinase) to a monophosphate and then by cellular enzymes to the triphosphate form, which is a potent inhibitor of the viral DNA polymerase. Acyclovir significantly decreases the duration of primary infection and has a lesser but definite effect on recurrent mucocutaneous HSV infections. If taken daily, it can also suppress recurrences of genital and oral–labial HSV. In its intravenous form, it is effective in reducing mortality of HSV encephalitis and neonatal herpes. Acyclovir-resistant HSV has been recovered from immunocompromised patients with persistent lesions, especially those with acquired immunodeficiency syndrome (AIDS). Foscarnet is active against acyclovir-resistant HSV. In 1996, the U.S. Food and Drug Administration approved both valacyclovir and famciclovir for the treatment of recurrent genital HSV. Valacyclovir is a prodrug of acyclovir with better bioavailability (54% as opposed to 15–20%). It is rapidly converted to acyclovir and, in every characteristic except absorption, it is identical to the parent compound. Valacyclovir is not more effective than acyclovir but can be given in lower dose and less frequently (500 mg twice daily). Famciclovir is the prodrug of another guanosine nucleoside analog, penciclovir. The bioavailability of penciclovir is also high (77%). After conversion, penciclovir must be phosphorylated, just like acyclovir. Penciclovir has a much longer tissue half-life than acyclovir and can be given as 125 mg twice daily for treatment of recurrent genital HSV. Valacyclovir and famciclovir are now also approved for chronic suppression of recurrent genital HSV. No antiviral agents have been developed that decrease the long-term risk of subsequent reactivation of disease.

Acyclovir or prodrugs can decrease duration of acute and recurrent disease

PREVENTION

Avoiding contact with individuals with lesions reduces the risk of spread; however, virus may be shed asymptomatically and transmitted from the saliva, urethra, and cervix by individuals with no evident lesions. Safe sex practices should reduce transmission. Although acyclovir has never been shown to reduce asymptomatic shedding from the genital tract, studies are in progress to determine whether oral antivirals can actually diminish transmission. Because of the high morbidity and mortality of neonatal infection, special attention must be paid to preventing transmission during delivery. Where active HSV lesions are present on maternal tissues, caesarean section may be used to minimize contact of the infant with infected maternal genital secretions, but caesarean section may not be effective if rupture of the membranes precedes delivery by more than several hours.

Caesarean section may be performed to avoid neonatal infection

VARICELLA–ZOSTER VIRUS

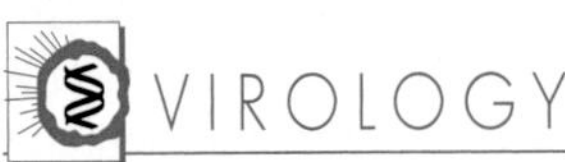

Varicella–zoster virus (VZV) has the same general structure as herpes simplex but contains its own envelope glycoproteins and other structures. Cellular features of infected cells such as multinucleated giant cells and intranuclear eosinophilic inclusion bodies are similar to those of HSV. VZV is more difficult to isolate in cell culture than HSV and grows best but slowly in human diploid fibroblast cells. The virus has a marked tendency to remain attached to the membrane of the host cell with less release of virions into fluids.

Slower growth and narrower range of infected cell types

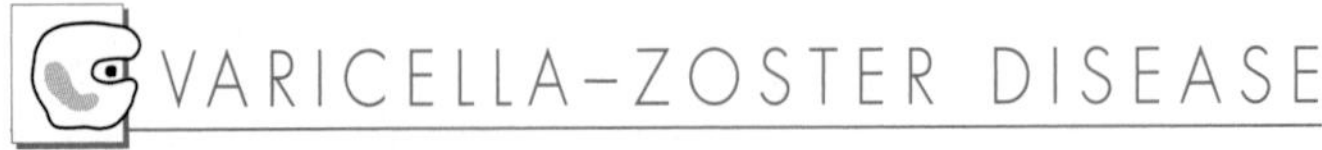

CLINICAL CAPSULE

VZV causes two diseases, chickenpox (varicella) and shingles (zoster). The former usually occurs in children, the latter in the elderly. In the intervening years, the virus remains latent in neural ganglia but activates due to waning cellular immunity. Almost 90% of the US population is infected with VZV by the age of 10 years, and the virus is spread primarily by respiratory secretions.

EPIDEMIOLOGY

VZV infection is ubiquitous. In temperate climates, nearly all persons contract chickenpox before they reach adulthood, and 90% of cases occur before the age of 10 years. In contrast, the mean age at infection in tropical countries is over 20 years, and the seroprevalence at age 70 may be only 50%. The virus is highly contagious, with attack rates among susceptible contacts of 75%. Varicella occurs most frequently during the winter and spring months. The incubation period is 11 to 21 days. The major mode of transmission is respiratory, although direct contact with vesicular or pustular lesions may result in transmission. Communicability is greatest 24 to 48 hours before the onset of rash and lasts 3 to 4 days into the rash. Virus is rarely isolated from crusted lesions.

Chickenpox acquired by respiratory route, usually before adulthood

Communicability greatest before rash onset

PATHOGENESIS

Respiratory spread leads to infection of the contact patient's upper respiratory tract followed by replication in regional lymph nodes and primary viremia. The latter results in infection of the reticuloendothelial system and a subsequent secondary viremia associated with T lymphocytes. Following secondary viremia, there is infection of the skin and finally a host immune response.

Secondary viremia results in skin lesions

The relationship between zoster and varicella was first described by Von Bokay in 1892, when he observed several instances of varicella in households after the introduction of a case of zoster. On the basis of these epidemiologic observations, he proposed that zoster and varicella were different clinical manifestations of a single agent. The cultivation of VZV in vitro by Weller in 1954 confirmed Von Bokay's hypothesis: the viruses isolated from chickenpox and from zoster (or shingles) are identical. Latency of VZV occurs in sensory ganglia, as shown by in situ hybridization methods in dorsal root ganglia of adults many years after varicella infection. Herpes zoster (shingles) occurs when latent varicella zoster virus reactivates and multiplies within a sensory ganglion and then travels back down the sensory nerve to the skin. The rash of herpes zoster is generally confined to the area of the skin (ie, dermatome) innervated by the sensory ganglion in which reactivation occurs (Fig 38–3).

Varicella virus latent in sensory ganglion cells; reactivation produces zoster

IMMUNITY

Both humoral immunity and cell-mediated immunity are important factors in determining the frequency of reinfection and reactivation of varicella–zoster. Circulating antibody prevents reinfection, and cell-mediated immunity appears to control reactivation. In patients with depressed cell-mediated immune responses, especially those with bone marrow transplants, Hodgkin's disease, AIDS, and lymphoproliferative disorders, reactivation can occur, and VZV infections are more frequent and more severe.

Circulating antibody prevents reinfection; cell-mediated immunity controls reactivation

The increase in the incidence and severity of herpes zoster observed with increasing age in immunocompetent individuals is correlated with an age-related decrease in

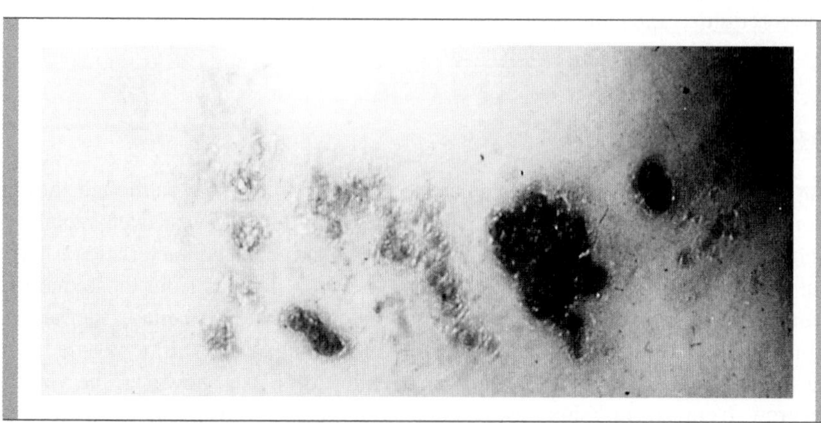

FIGURE 38–3
Herpes zoster lesion of the thorax. Note dermatomal distribution and presence of vesicles, pustules, and ulcerated and crusted lesions.

Aging associated with increasing risk of zoster

VZV-specific cellular immunity. Beginning in the fifth decade of life, there is a marked decline in cellular immunity to VZV, which can be measured by cutaneous delayed hypersensitivity as well as by a variety of in vitro assays. This occurs many years before there is any generalized decline in cellular immunity.

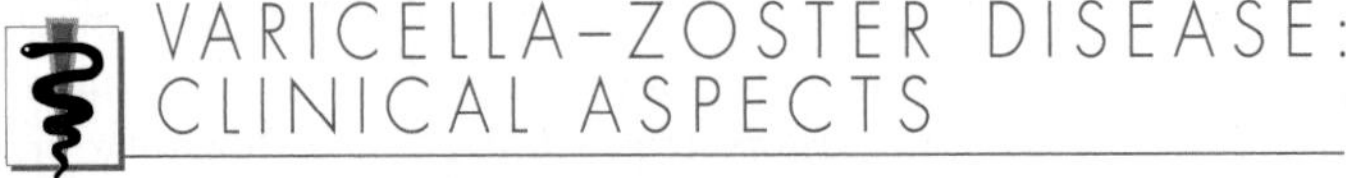

VARICELLA–ZOSTER DISEASE: CLINICAL ASPECTS

MANIFESTATIONS

Chickenpox lesions are widespread and pruritic

VZV produces a primary infection in normal children characterized by a generalized vesicular rash termed **chickenpox** or **varicella.** After clinical infection resolves, the virus persists for decades in the absence of clinical manifestation. Chickenpox lesions generally appear on the back of the head and ears, then spread centrifugally to the face, neck, trunk, and proximal extremities. Involvement of mucous membranes is common, and fever may occur early in the course of disease. Lesions appear in different stages of evolution; this characteristic is one of the major features used to differentiate varicella from smallpox, in which lesions are concentrated on the extremities and all had a similar appearance. Varicella lesions are pruritic (itchy), and the number of lesions may vary from 10 to several hundred.

Severe disease in immunocompromised patients

Immunocompromised children may develop progressive varicella, which is associated with prolonged viremia and visceral dissemination as well as pneumonia, encephalitis, hepatitis, and nephritis. Progressive varicella has an estimated mortality of approximately 20%. In thrombocytopenic patients, the lesions may be hemorrhagic. Susceptible adults are at higher risk (15×) for VZV pneumonia during chickenpox.

Reactivation to zoster most common in elderly

Follow sensory nerve distribution

Reactivation of VZV is associated with the disease herpes zoster (shingles). Although zoster is seen in patients of all ages, it increases in frequency with advancing age. Clinically, pain in a sensory nerve distribution may herald the onset of the eruption, which occurs several days to a week or two later. The vesicular eruption is usually unilateral, involving one to three dermatomes. New lesions may appear over the first 5 to 7 days. Multiple attacks of VZV infection are uncommon; if recurrent attacks of a vesicular eruption occur in one area of the body, HSV infection should be considered.

Postherpetic neuralgia after zoster

Dissemination with visceral infection in immunocompromised persons

The complications of VZV infection are varied and depend on age and host immune factors. Postherpetic neuralgia is a common complication of herpes zoster in elderly adults. It is characterized by persistence of pain in the dermatome for months to years after resolution of the lesions of zoster and appears to result from damage to the involved nerve root. Immunosuppressed patients may develop localized zoster followed by dissemination of virus with visceral infection, which resembles progressive varicella. Bacterial superinfection is also possible. Maternal varicella infection during early pregnancy can result in fetal embryopathy with skin scarring, limb hypoplasia, microcephaly, cataracts, chorioretinitis, and microphthalmia. Severe varicella can also occur in seronegative neonates, with mortality as high as 30%.

DIAGNOSIS

Diagnosis usually clinical

Rapid confirmation by immunofluorescent staining

Varicella or herpes zoster lesions can be diagnosed clinically, although they may occasionally be difficult to distinguish from those caused by HSV or even vaccinia smallpox. Scrapings of lesions may reveal multinucleated giant cells characteristic of herpesviruses, but cytologic examination does not distinguish HSV lesions from those due to VZV. For rapid viral diagnosis, the best procedure is to demonstrate varicella–zoster antigen in cells from lesions by immunofluorescent antibody staining. VZV can be isolated from vesicular fluid or cells inoculated onto human diploid fibroblasts; however, the virus is difficult to grow from zoster (shingles) lesions older than 5 days, and cytopathic effects are usually not seen for 5 to 9 days. PCR of CSF may be useful in the diagnosis of VZV encephalitis; culture is rarely positive.

TREATMENT

Acyclovir has been shown to reduce fever and skin lesions in patients with varicella, and its use is recommended in healthy patients over 18 years of age. There are insufficient data to justify universal treatment of all healthy children and teenagers with varicella. In immunosuppressed patients, controlled trials of acyclovir have been effective in reducing dissemination, and the use of this agent is definitely indicated. In addition, controlled trials of acyclovir have demonstrated effectiveness in the treatment of herpes zoster in immunocompromised patients. Acyclovir may be used to treat herpes zoster in immunocompetent adults, but it appears to have only a modest impact on the development of post-herpetic neuralgia, the most important complication of zoster. Treatment should be started within 3 days of the onset of zoster. VZV is less susceptible than HSV to acyclovir, so the dosage for treatment is substantially higher. Famciclovir or valacyclovir are more convenient and may be more effective.

Acyclovir or related prodrug therapy of immunocompromised patients

PREVENTION

High-titer immune globulin administered within 96 hours of exposure is useful in preventing infection or ameliorating disease in patients at risk for severe primary infection (eg, immunosuppressed children who are household or play contacts of patients with varicella or zoster). Once skin lesions have occurred, high-titer immune globulin has not proved useful in ameliorating disease or preventing dissemination. Immune globulin is not indicated for the treatment or prevention of reactivation (ie, zoster or shingles). In nonimmunosuppressed children, varicella is a relatively mild disease, and passive immunization is not indicated.

Passive immunization for immunocompromised

A live vaccine developed by a group of Japanese workers appears to be effective in both immunosuppressed and immunocompetent persons and is now recommended for routine use after 12 months of age in healthy children (Table 38–2). In immunocompromised patients who are susceptible to varicella, chickenpox can be extremely serious, even fatal. In these patients, the live vaccine appears to be protective although it is not approved for this use in the United States. The vaccine is being used routinely in immunocompetent seronegative adults, especially those at occupational risk, such as health care workers, and it can even be helpful if given to a seronegative, immunocompetent adult shortly after exposure. Varicella is a highly contagious disease, and rigid isolation precautions must be instituted in all hospitalized cases.

Live vaccine is safe and effective

Need for isolation of cases in hospital

TABLE 38–2

Properties of the Live Attenuated Varicella Vaccine (Oka)

- Rarely causes rash (5% in healthy children, mild)
- One dose induces antibody, which persists for >10 years in >90% of healthy children. Two doses are required for adults
- Induces cell-mediated immunity
- Lack of contact infection in most cases
- Induces long-term protective immunity
- Prevents disease when administered up to 3 days after exposure (postexposure prophylaxis)
- Incidence of herpes zoster in vaccinated children with leukemia is lower than in comparable children infected naturally with wild-type virus
- >90% protection vs. household exposure of healthy children

CYTOMEGALOVIRUS

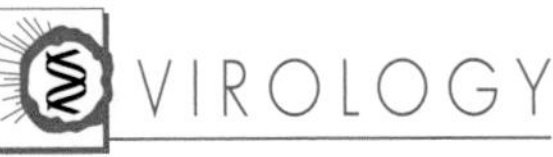

Nuclear and perinuclear cytoplasmic inclusions and cell enlargement

Human cytomegalovirus (CMV) possesses the largest genome of the herpesviruses (~240 kbp), and its replication, although slow, is similar to HSV with the sequential appearance of immediate early, early and late gene products. In addition to nuclear inclusions ("owl eye cells"), CMV produces perinuclear cytoplasmic inclusions and enlargement of the cell (cytomegaly), a property that gives the virus its name. Based on genomic and phenotypic heterogeneity, innumerable strains of CMV exist, and restriction endonuclease analysis of viral DNA has been useful for distinguishing strains epidemiologically. Antigenic variations have been observed but are not of clinical importance.

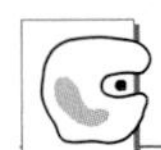

CYTOMEGALOVIRUS DISEASE

CLINICAL CAPSULE

CMV differs from HSV and VZV by not causing skin disease, but CMV is similar in its ability to establish latent infection. CMV produces visceral disease, including a mononucleosis syndrome in otherwise healthy individuals. Its major contribution to human misery is a high rate of congenital infection (1% of all infants; 40,000 in the United States per year), most of whom are asymptomatic; however, some 20% may have neurologic impairment. CMV is also an important cause of morbidity and mortality in immunocompromised patients with either primary or reactivation disease.

EPIDEMIOLOGY

High infection rates in early childhood and early adulthood

Present in urine, saliva, semen, and cervical secretions

CMV is ubiquitous, and in developed countries approximately 50% of adults have developed antibody. Age-specific prevalence rates show that approximately 10 to 15% of children are infected by CMV during the first 5 years of life, after which the rate of new infections levels off. The rate subsequently increases by 1 to 2% per year during adulthood, probably through close personal contact, including sexual, with a virus-excreting person. CMV has been isolated from saliva, cervical secretions, semen, urine, and white blood cells for months to years following infection. Excretion of CMV is especially prolonged after congenital and perinatal infections, with 35% of infected infants excreting virus for as long as 5 years after birth. Transmission of infection in day-care centers has been shown to occur from asymptomatic excreters to other children and, in turn, to seronegative parents. By age 18 months, up to 80% of infants in a day-care center are infected and actively excreting virus in saliva and urine. Seroconversion rates in seronegative parents who have children attending day-care centers are approximately 20% per year. This increases to approximately 30% if the child is shedding virus and up to 40% if the child is also under 18 months of age. In contrast to day-care centers, there is no substantial evidence of spread of CMV infection to health care workers in the hospital.

Viral latency in leukocytes

Latent infection, which occurs in leukocytes and their precursors, accounts for transfusion transmission, but this route is relatively infrequent; only 1 to 2% of blood units are believed to be infectious. Organ donation may also transmit latent virus, which causes primary infection in CMV-seronegative recipients and reinfection in seropositive patients.

PATHOGENESIS

As previously mentioned, CMV infects epithelial cells and leukocytes and produces characteristic inclusions in the former. In vitro, CMV DNA can be demonstrated in monocytes showing no cytopathology, indicating a restricted growth potential in these cells. It is conjectured that these are the cells of latency for CMV.

CMV DNA in monocytes

CMV can cause disease by a variety of different mechanisms, including direct tissue damage and immunologic damage. While direct infection and damage of mucosal epithelial cells in the lung is a potential mechanism for pneumonia, animal models have suggested that immunologic destruction of the lung by the host immune response to CMV infection may be the major mechanism of viral disease in this tissue. This hypothesis is supported by the observation that the degree of viral infection in lung tissue cannot account for the severity of CMV pneumonia; likewise, the disease does not respond well to antiviral therapy. While cytolytic T-lymphocyte activity may contribute to lung pathology, cytokines released by these cells have also been implicated.

Immune-mediated tissue damage

IMMUNITY

Both humoral and cellular immune responses are important in CMV infections. In immunocompetent persons, clinical disease, if it occurs at all, results from primary infection, and reactivation with viral excretion in cervical excretions or semen is invariably subclinical. In immunocompromised patients, both primary infection and reactivation are much more likely to be symptomatic. Furthermore, CMV infection of monocytes results in dysfunction of these phagocytes in immunocompromised patients, which may increase predisposition to fungal and bacterial superinfection. When latently infected monocytes are in contact with activated T lymphocytes, the former are activated to differentiate into macrophages that produce infectious virus. These monocyte–T cell interactions may occur following transfusion or transplantation and may explain not only transmission of CMV but also activation of latent virus in the allograft recipient. Vascular endothelial cells may be other sites of CMV latency.

Vascular endothelial cells can be infected and support viral latency

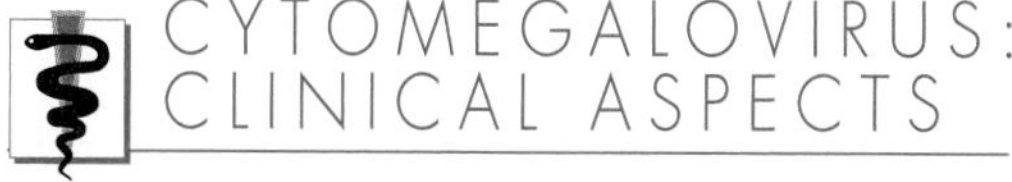

CYTOMEGALOVIRUS: CLINICAL ASPECTS

MANIFESTATIONS

Worldwide, 1% of infants excrete CMV in urine or nasopharynx at delivery as a result of infection in utero. On physical examination, 90% of these infants appear normal or asymptomatic; however, long-term follow-up has indicated that 10 to 20% go on to develop sensory nerve hearing loss, psychomotor mental retardation, or both. Infants with symptomatic illness (about 0.1% of all births) have a variety of congenital defects or other disorders, such as hepatosplenomegaly, jaundice, anemia, thrombocytopenia, low birth weight, microcephaly, and chorioretinitis. Almost all infants with clinically evident congenital CMV infection are born of mothers who experienced primary CMV infection during pregnancy. The apparent explanation is that these babies are exposed to virus in the absence of maternal antibody. It is estimated that one third of maternal primary infections are transmitted to the fetus and that fetal damage is most likely to occur in the first trimester. Congenital infection frequently also results from reactivation in the mother with spread to the fetus, but such infection rarely leads to congenital abnormalities since the mother also transmits antibody to the fetus.

Serious disease of fetus may develop with primary maternal infection

In contrast to the devastating findings with some congenital infections, neonatal infection acquired during or shortly after birth appears to be rarely associated with an adverse outcome. Most population-based studies have indicated that 10 to 15% of all mothers are excreting CMV from the cervix at delivery. Approximately one third to one half of all infants born to these mothers acquire infection. Almost all of these perinatally infected infants have no discernible illness unless the infant is premature or immunocompromised. CMV can also be efficiently transmitted from mother to child by breast milk, but these postpartum infections are also usually benign.

Perinatal infection asymptomatic or relatively benign

As with intrapartum acquisition of infection, most CMV infections during childhood and adulthood are totally asymptomatic. In healthy young adults, CMV may cause a mononucleosis-like syndrome. In immunosuppressed patients, both primary infection and reactivation may be severe. For example, in patients receiving bone marrow transplants, interstitial pneumonia caused by CMV is a leading cause of death (50–90% mortality) and in AIDS patients, CMV often disseminates to visceral organs, causing chorioretinitis, gastroenteritis, and neurologic disorders.

CMV pneumonia, visceral, and eye infections in immunocompromised patients

DIAGNOSIS

Laboratory diagnosis of CMV infection depends on (1) detecting CMV cytopathology, antigen, or DNA in infected tissues; (2) isolating the virus from tissue or secretions; or (3) demonstrating seroconversion. CMV can be grown readily in serially propagated diploid fibroblast cell lines. Demonstration of cytopathic effect generally requires 3 to 14 days, depending on the concentration of virus in the specimen and whether coverslip cultures in shell vials are used to speed detection. The presence of large inclusion-bearing cells in urine sediment may be detected in widespread CMV infection. This technique is insensitive, however, and provides positive results only when large quantities of virus are present in the urine. Culture of blood to detect viremia is now superseded by detection of CMV antigen in peripheral blood leukocytes or detection of CMV DNA in plasma or leukocytes. These procedures are more rapid and more sensitive than culture.

DNA detection by PCR or antigen detection useful to find viremia

Because of the high prevalence of asymptomatic carriers and the known tendency of CMV to persist weeks or months in infected individuals, it is frequently difficult to associate a specific disease entity with the isolation of the virus from a peripheral site. Thus, the isolation of CMV from urine of immunosuppressed patients with interstitial pneumonia does not constitute evidence of CMV as the cause of that illness. CMV pneumonia or gastrointestinal disease is best diagnosed by demonstrating CMV inclusions in biopsy tissue.

Histologic detection of inclusions in lung, gastrointestinal tissues is useful

The procedures listed below are recommended to facilitate the diagnosis of CMV infection in specific clinical settings:

1. Congenital infection. Virus culture or viral DNA assay positive at birth or within 1 to 2 weeks (to distinguish from natally or perinatally infected infants, who will not begin to excrete virus until 3 to 4 weeks after delivery).
2. Perinatal infection. Culture-negative specimens at birth but positive specimens at 4 weeks or more after birth suggest natal or early postnatal acquisition. Seronegative infants may acquire CMV from exogenous sources, e.g. blood transfusion.
3. CMV mononucleosis in nonimmunocompromised patients. Seroconversion and presence of IgM antibody specific for CMV are the best indicators of primary infection. Urine culture positivity supports the diagnosis of CMV infection but may reflect remote infection, because positivity may continue for months to years. A positive blood assay for CMV antigen or DNA, however, is diagnostic in this patient population.
4. Immunocompromised patients. Demonstration of virus by viral antigen, DNA, or culture in blood documents viremia. Demonstration of inclusions or viral antigen in diseased tissue (eg, lung, esophagus, or colon) establishes the presence of CMV infection but does not provide proof that CMV is the cause of disease unless other pathogens are excluded. Seroconversion is diagnostic but rarely occurs, especially in AIDS patients, because more than 95% of these patients are seropositive for CMV before infection with human immunodeficiency virus (HIV). CMV-specific IgM antibody may not be present in immunocompromised patients, especially during reactivation of virus. Conversely, in AIDS patients, this antibody frequently is present even when clinically important infection is absent.

TREATMENT

Ganciclovir, a nucleoside analog of acyclovir, has been shown to inhibit CMV replication; prevent CMV disease in AIDS patients and transplant recipients; and reduce the severity of some CMV syndromes, such as retinitis and gastrointestinal disease. Combining immune globulin with ganciclovir appears to reduce the very high mortality of CMV pneumonia in bone marrow transplant patients over that achieved with ganciclovir alone, but the prognosis for long-term survival of these patients remains poor. Foscarnet, a second approved drug for therapy of CMV disease, is equally efficacious. Its toxic effects are primarily renal, whereas ganciclovir is most apt to inhibit bone marrow function. Ganciclovir inhibits CMV DNA polymerase, like foscarnet, but the two drugs act on different sites, and cross resistance is rare. In 1996, a third drug, cidofovir, a nucleotide analog, was approved for therapy of retinitis; it is also nephrotoxic.

Ganciclovir used with immune globulin

PREVENTION

The use of blood from CMV-seronegative donors or blood that is treated to remove white cells decreases transfusion-associated CMV. Similarly, the disease can be avoided in seronegative transplant recipients by using organs from CMV-seronegative donors. Hyperimmune human anti-CMV globulin has been used to ameliorate CMV pneumonia associated with transplants. Safe sex practices including condom usage reduces transmission. CMV vaccines have been developed, and are being evaluated in clinical trials.

Use of CMV seronegative donors decreases risk

EPSTEIN–BARR VIRUS

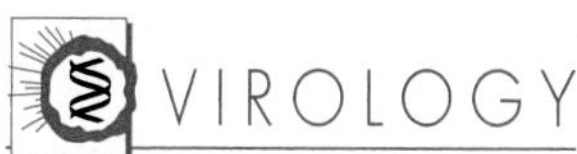

VIROLOGY

Epstein–Barr virus (EBV) is the etiologic agent of infectious mononucleosis and African Burkitt's lymphoma. Its complete nucleotide sequence of 172 kbp is smaller than other herpes viruses but has been thoroughly mapped. Although EBV is morphologically similar to the other herpesviruses, it can be cultured easily only in lymphoblastoid cell lines derived from B lymphocytes of humans and higher primates. In vivo, EBV is tropic for both human B lymphocytes and epithelial cells. The former is a nonproductive infection, while the latter is productive. The virus generally does not produce cytopathic effects or the characteristic intranuclear inclusions of other herpesvirus infections. After infection with EBV, lymphoblastoid cells containing viral genome can be cultivated continuously in vitro; they are thus transformed, or immortalized. Recent studies suggest that most of the viral DNA in transformed cells remains in a circular, nonintegrated form as an episome, while a lesser amount is integrated into the host cell genome. Viral antigen expression has been studied by immunofluorescent staining of transformed cell lines under various conditions. One group of proteins, called EBV nuclear antigens (EBNAs), appear in the nucleus prior to virus-directed protein synthesis. Viral capsid antigen (VCA) can be detected in cell lines that produce mature virions. Other cell lines, called nonproducers, contain no mature virions, but express certain virus-associated antigens called early antigens (EAs). The latter may be seen as diffuse (D) and as restricted (R) aggregates of staining.

Etiologic agent of infectious mononucleosis and certain lymphomas

Cultivated only in lymphoblastoid cell lines

EBNA, VCA, and EA represent stages of viral replication

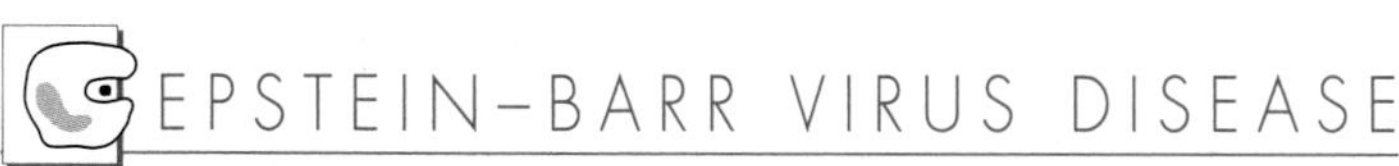

EPSTEIN-BARR VIRUS DISEASE

CLINICAL CAPSULE

Investigators discovered EBV in the course of their studies to determine the cause of Burkitt's lymphoma. Serologic studies later found that the virus was the cause of infectious mononucleosis. The greatest interest in EBV hinges on its role in malignant disease, including Burkitt's lymphoma, nasopharyngeal carcinoma, and lymphoproliferative disease of the immunocompromised.

EPIDEMIOLOGY

Widespread asymptomatic infection; disease most common in young adults

EBV can be cultured from saliva of 10 to 20% of healthy adults and is intermittently recovered from most seropositive individuals. It is of low contagiousness, and most cases of infectious mononucleosis are contracted after repeated contact between susceptible persons and those asymptomatically shedding the virus. Secondary attack rates of infectious mononucleosis are low (<10%), because most family or household contacts already have antibody to the agent (worldwide 90–95% of adults are seropositive). Infectious mononucleosis has also been transmitted by blood transfusions; most transfusion-associated mononucleosis syndromes, however, are attributable to CMV. In more highly developed countries and in individuals of higher socioeconomic status, EBV infection tends to be acquired later in life than in individuals from developing countries of lower socioeconomic status. When primary infection with EBV is delayed until the second decade of life or later, it is accompanied by symptoms of infectious mononucleosis in about 50% of cases.

At present, there appears to be many fewer variations of genomic strains among EBV isolates than other herpesviruses.

PATHOGENESIS

Infects B cells

Encodes proteins associated with immortalization of B cells

Although EBV initially infects epithelial cells, the hallmark of EBV disease is subsequent infection of B lymphocytes and polyclonal B lymphocyte activation with benign proliferation. The virus enters B lymphocytes by means of envelope glycoprotein binding to a surface receptor CD21, which is the receptor for the C36 component of complement; 18 to 24 hours later, EBV nuclear antigens are detectable within the nucleus of infected cells. Expression of the viral genome, which encodes at least two viral proteins, is associated with immortalization and proliferation of the cell. The EBV-infected B lymphocytes are polyclonally activated to produce immunoglobulin and express a lymphocyte-determined membrane antigen that is the target of host cellular immune responses to EBV-infected B lymphocytes. During the acute phase of infectious mononucleosis, up to 20% of circulating B lymphocytes demonstrate EBV antigens. After infection subsides, EBV can be isolated from only about 1% of such cells.

Lymphomas can develop in immunocompromised patients

EBV has been associated with several lymphoproliferative diseases, including African Burkitt's lymphoma, nasopharyngeal carcinoma, and lymphomas in immunocompromised patients. The factors that render the EBV infections oncogenic in these cases are obscure. The distribution of EBV infections in Africa has suggested an infectious cofactor, such as malaria, which may cause immunosuppression and predispose to EBV-related malignancy. In nasopharyngeal carcinoma, environmental carcinogens may create the precancerous lesion although genetic factors may also be operative. In vivo, EBV-associated lymphomas have been shown to be of both monoclonal and polyclonal origin. Chromosomal translocations in B cells are characteristic of Burkitt's lymphoma and involve specific breaks in chromosomes. These translocations lead to expression of oncogenes that may contribute to clonal activation and ultimately to malignancy. Some breakdown in immune surveillance also appears to play a role in the development of malignancy, because immunosuppressed patients are more prone to develop EBV associated B-cell lymphomas.

IMMUNITY

Suppressed cell-mediated immune responses in acute infection

Virus-induced infectious mononucleosis is associated with circulating antibodies against specific viral antigens, as well as against unrelated antigens found in sheep, horse, and some beef red blood cells. The latter, referred to as heterophile antibodies, are a heterogeneous group of predominantly IgM antibodies long known to correlate with episodes of infectious mononucleosis, and are commonly used as diagnostic tests for the disease. They do not cross-react with antibodies specific for EBV, and there is not good correlation between the heterophile antibody titer and the severity of illness. Cutaneous anergy and decreased cellular immune responses to mitogens and antigens are seen early in the course of mononucleosis. The "atypical" lymphocytosis associated with infectious mononucleosis is caused by an increase in the number of circulating T cells, which appear to be activated cells developed in response to the virus-infected B lymphocytes. With recovery from illness, the atypical lymphocytosis gradually resolves, and cell-mediated immune functions return to preinfection levels, although memory T cells maintain the capacity to limit proliferation of EBV-infected B cells. In rare cases, the initial EBV-induced proliferation of B cells is not contained, and EBV lymphoproliferative disease ensues. This syndrome is most often seen in immunocompromised organ transplant recipients.

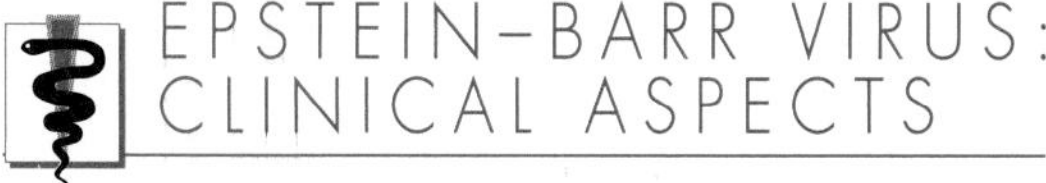

EPSTEIN–BARR VIRUS: CLINICAL ASPECTS

MANIFESTATIONS

Infectious Mononucleosis

Although most primary EBV infections are asymptomatic, clinically apparent infectious mononucleosis is characterized by fever, malaise, pharyngitis, tender lymphadenitis, and splenomegaly. These symptoms persist for days to weeks; they slowly resolve. Complications such as laryngeal obstruction, meningitis, encephalitis, hemolytic anemia, thrombocytopenia, or splenic rupture may occur in 1 to 5% of patients.

Primary infection asymptomatic or expressed as infectious mononucleosis

Lymphoproliferative Syndrome

Patients with primary or secondary immunodeficiency are susceptible to EBV-induced lymphoproliferative disease. For example, the incidence of these lymphomas is 1 to 2% following renal transplants and 5 to 9% following heart–lung transplants. The risk is greatest in patients experiencing primary EBV infection rather than reactivation. Most characteristic is persistent fever, lymphadenopathy, and hepatosplenopathy.

Lymphoproliferative disease occurs, especially in immunocompromised persons

Burkitt's Lymphoma

In sub-Saharan Africa, Burkitt's lymphoma is the most common malignancy in young children, with an incidence of 8 to 10 cases per 100,000 people per year. The risk is greatest in equatorial Africa, where there is a high incidence of malaria. Burkitt's lymphoma is thought to result from an early EBV infection that produces a large pool of infected B lymphocytes. Malarial infection may further increase the size of this pool and provide a constant antigenic challenge. Serologic screening for increased IgA antibody levels to both VCA and early EBV antigens can be used for early diagnostic purposes.

Tumors may involve cofactors

Translocation may lead to clonal activation

Nasopharyngeal Carcinoma

Nasopharyngeal carcinoma (NPC) is endemic in southern China, where it is responsible for approximately 25% of the mortality from cancer. The high incidence of NPC among the southern Chinese people suggests that genetic or environmental factors in addition to EBV may also be important in the pathogenesis of the disease.

Endemic NPC in southern China; suggests environmental or genetic cofactors

AIDS Patients

In AIDS patients, several distinct additional EBV-associated diseases may occur, including hairy leukoplakia of the tongue, interstitial lymphocytic pneumonia (especially in infants), and lymphoma.

DIAGNOSIS

Laboratory analysis of EBV infectious mononucleosis is usually documented by the demonstration of atypical lymphocytes, and heterophile antibodies, or positive EBV-specific serologic findings. Hematologic examination reveals a markedly raised lymphocyte and monocyte count with more than 10% atypical lymphocytes, called Downey cells (Fig 38–4). Atypical lymphocytes, although not specific for EBV, are present with the onset of symptoms and disappear with resolution of disease. Alterations in liver function tests may also occur, and enlargement of the liver and spleen is a frequent finding.

Atypical lymphocytosis common in acute infection

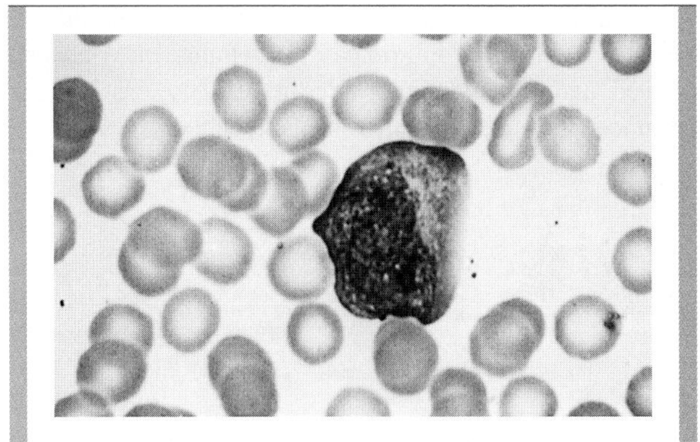

FIGURE 38–4
Atypical lymphocyte (Downey cell) in blood smear from a patient with infectious mononucleosis. Note indented cell membrane.

Heterophile antibodies nonspecific but appear early

Although not specific for EBV, tests for heterophile antibodies are used most commonly for diagnosis of infectious mononucleosis. In commercial kits, animal erythrocytes are used in simple slide agglutination methods, which incorporate absorptions to remove cross-reacting antibodies that may develop in other illnesses, such as serum sickness. The infectious mononucleosis heterophile antibody is absorbed by sheep erythrocytes but not by a guinea pig kidney cells. Heterophile antibodies can usually be demonstrated by the end of the first week of illness but may occasionally be delayed until the third or fourth week. They may persist many months.

IgM antibody to VCA suggest acute, primary infection

Approximately 5 to 15% of EBV-induced cases of infectious mononucleosis in adults and a much greater proportion in young children and infants fail to induce detectable levels of heterophile antibodies. In these cases, the EBV-specific serologic tests summarized in Table 38–3 may be used to establish the diagnosis. The panel to be tested includes antibodies to VCA, which rise quickly and persist for life. Antibodies to EBNAs rise later in

TABLE 38–3

Epstein–Barr Virus-Specific Antibodies

Antibody Specificity	Time of Appearance in Infectious Mononucleosis	Duration	Comments
Viral capsid antigen (VCA)			
IgM	Early in illness	1–2 months	Indicator of primary infection
IgG	Early in illness	Lifelong	Standard EBV titer reported by most commercial and state labs; major utility is as a marker for prior infection in epidemiologic studies; if present in the absence of EBNA antibody, indicates current infection
EBNA IgG	3–6 weeks after onset	Lifelong	Late appearance of anti-EBNA IgG antibodies in IM makes absence or seroconversion a useful marker for primary infection; persists for life
Early antigen			
EA diffuse protein (EA-D)	Peaks 3–4 weeks after onset	3–6 months	Present in IM patients; IgA antibodies useful for prediction of NPC in high-risk populations
EA restricted (EA-R)	Several weeks after onset	Months to years	Present in higher titer in African Burkitt's lymphoma; may be useful as indicator of reactivation of EBV

Abbreviations: EA, early antigen; EBV, Epstein–Barr virus; IM, infectious mononucleosis; NPC, nasopharyngeal carcinoma; EBNA, EBV nuclear antigen.

disease (after about 1 month) and also persist in low titers for life. Thus, a high titer to VCA and no titer to EBNA suggests recent EBV infection, whereas antibody titers to both antigens are indicative of past infection. The presence of IgM antibody to VCA is theoretically diagnostic of acute, primary EBV infection, but low levels may occur during reactivation of EBV and cross-reactions with antigens of other herpesviruses occur. Persistent antibody to early antigens (anti-EA, -D, or -R) may be correlated with severe disease, nasopharyngeal carcinoma (anti-D), or African Burkitt's lymphoma (anti-R), but are not useful in diagnosing infectious mononucleosis. Isolation of EBV from clinical specimens is not practical, because it requires fresh human B cells or fetal lymphocytes obtained from cord blood.

Virus isolation is impractical for routine diagnosis

TREATMENT

Treatment of infectious mononucleosis is largely supportive. More than 95% of patients recover uneventfully. In a small percentage of patients, splenic rupture may occur; restriction of contact sports or heavy lifting during the acute illness is recommended. The DNA polymerase enzyme of EBV has been shown to be sensitive to acyclovir, and acyclovir can decrease the amount of replication of EBV in tissue culture and in vivo. Despite this antiviral activity, systemic acyclovir makes little or no impact on the clinical illness. Laryngeal obstruction should be treated with corticosteroids. Hairy leukoplakia in AIDS patients does respond to acyclovir treatment.

Treatment is supportive

PREVENTION

The occurrence of Burkitt's lymphoma and nasopharyngeal carcinoma in restricted geographic areas offers the possibility of prevention by immunization with virus-specific antigen(s). At present, this approach is under exploration. A subunit vaccine has proved effective in preventing the development of tumors in tamarind monkeys, which are highly susceptible to the oncogenic effects of the virus under experimental conditions.

Immunization of humans not available

HUMAN HERPESVIRUS-6

In 1986, a herpesvirus, now called human herpesvirus type-6 (HHV-6), was identified in cultures of peripheral blood lymphocytes from patients with lymphoproliferative diseases. The virus, which is genetically distinct but morphologically similar to other herpesviruses, replicates in lymphoid tissue, especially CD4+ T lymphocytes and has two distinct variants, A and B. HHV-6 is more closely related to CMV than to the other earlier known herpesviruses and is the β subfamily.

Replicates in CD4+ T lymphocytes

EPIDEMIOLOGY

HHV-6 is the most rapidly spread of the herpesviruses and is shed in the throats of 10% of babies by age 5 months, 70% by 12 months, and 30% of adults. Almost all of the population has antibody to this virus by the age of 5 years.

Infection common in infancy

MANIFESTATIONS

HHV-6 type B is the etiologic agent of exanthem subitum (roseola), and both types A and B can cause acute febrile illnesses with or without seizures or rashes. Exanthem subitum generally occurs in infants aged 6 months to 1 year. It is characterized by fever (usually about 39°C) for 3 days, followed by a faint maculopapular rash spreading from the trunk to the extremities, which begins during defervescence.

Associated with roseola in infants

HHV-6 also appears to reactivate in transplant recipients. It may contribute to graft rejection and clinical illnesses such as meningoencephalitis, pneumonia, and bone marrow suppression after bone marrow transplantation. The virus reactivates in other

Reactivation common in immunosuppression

immunocompromised patients including those with AIDS, lymphoma, and leukemia, but its clinical significance is not known.

Latent infection of T cells

Initially, it was thought that HHV-6 would grow only in freshly isolated B lymphocytes, and the virus was referred to as the human B lymphotropic virus. Now it is clear that the virus infects mainly T lymphocytes. HHV-6 establishes a latent infection in T cells but may be activated to a productive lytic infection by mitogenic stimulation. Resting lymphocytes and lymphocytes from normal immune individuals are resistant to HHV-6 infection. In vivo, HHV-6 replication is controlled by cell-mediated factors.

DIAGNOSIS

Primary infection can be documented serologically

PCR used to detect viremic infection

Primary virus infection can be documented by seroconversion. Active virus infection can be documented by culture, antigenemia, or DNA detection in the blood (by PCR). Because asymptomatic viremic reactivation is common, it is very difficult to use these tools to identify HHV-6 as the cause of febrile or other miscellaneous syndromes.

TREATMENT

No viral thymidine kinase

Definitive therapy has not been established, but HHV-6 appears to be susceptible in vitro to ganciclovir and foscarnet. It is less susceptible to acyclovir, because the virus has no thymidine kinase.

Human Herpesvirus-7

Originally isolated from CD4+ T lymphocytes

Can cause exanthem subitum (roseola)

Isolation of human herpesvirus-7 (HHV-7) was first reported in 1990. The virus was isolated from activated CD4+ T lymphocytes of a healthy individual. The CD4 molecule appears to be a receptor for virus attachment. HHV-7 is distinct from all other known human herpesviruses but is most closely related to HHV-6 and CMV and is in the β subfamily with these two viruses. Seroepidemiologic studies indicate that this virus usually does not infect children until after infancy but that nearly 90% of children are antibody positive by 3 years of age. As with HHV-6, this virus is frequently isolated from saliva, and close personal contact is the probable means of transmission. Also, like HHV-6, this virus may be a cause of exanthem subitum. The diagnosis of acute infection can be made by the demonstration of seroconversion. No treatment has been identified.

Human Herpesvirus-8

Human herpesvirus-8 (Kaposi's sarcoma–associated herpesvirus, or KSHV; HHV-8) was discovered in 1994 by identification of unique viral DNA sequences in Kaposi's sarcoma tissue obtained from an AIDS patient, using subtractive hybridization analysis. These specific DNA sequences are found in 95% or more of Kaposi's sarcoma tissues, both AIDS related and non-AIDS in African cases. KSHV DNA has also been detected in cells from lymphoproliferative diseases (eg, primary effusion lymphomas, associated with AIDS and multicentric Castleman's disease).

Associated with Kaposi's sarcoma

Recently, HHV-8 was isolated in culture, and when characterized, it seems most closely related to EBV. Like EBV, the virus preferentially infects B lymphocytes and it is also considered to be a gamma herpes virus. Epidemiologic and virologic studies suggest that it is a necessary but perhaps not sufficient cause of Kaposi's sarcoma and that other factors (eg, immunosuppression, genetic predisposition) are cofactors in the development of this malignancy. On average, seropositivity to HHV-8 precedes the development of

Kaposi's sarcoma by 3 years. The virus appears to be sexually transmitted, as suggested by a higher prevalence of antibody in promiscuous gay men than those who are not promiscuous, and by higher prevalence in gay men with HIV versus other HIV-positive risk groups, such as transfusion recipients and hemophiliacs. Specific and sensitive antibody assays are being developed, and antibody to HHV-8 appears to be relatively rare in the general population. It is difficult to assess the impact of antivirals, because Kaposi's sarcoma may improve with immune reconstitution. Interferon-α can be effective against Kaposi's sarcoma, but this may result from immune enhancement rather than any specific antiviral activity. Evidence of active viral replication in Kaposi's sarcoma is minimal, so there may not be an appropriate target for antivirals at the time that Kaposi's sarcoma becomes manifest.

Infects B lymphocytes

ADDITIONAL READING

Herpes Simplex Virus

Brown ZA, Selke S, Zeh J, et al. The acquisition of herpes simplex virus during pregnancy. *N Engl J Med* 1997;337:509–515. Acquisition of infection with seroconversion completed before labor does not appear to affect the outcome of pregnancy, but infection acquired near the time of labor is associated with an increased risk of severe neonatal herpes infection.

Wald A. Herpes. Transmission and viral shedding. *Dermatol Clin* 1998;16:795–797. Reviews data on asymptomatic shedding of HSV from the genital tract of HSV-2 antibody–positive patients and its impact on transmission.

Wald A, Carrell D, Remington M, et al. Two day regimen of acyclovir for treatment of recurrent genital herpes simplex virus type 2 infection. *Clin Infect Dis* 2002;34:944–948. Reviews current therapy of genital HSV infection and introduces an effective 2-day acyclovir treatment option.

Whitley RJ, Kimberlin DW, Roizman B. Herpes simplex viruses. *Clin Infect Dis* 1998;26:541–555. This is a well-referenced, thorough review of HSV-1 and HSV-2.

Varicella–Zoster Virus

Gnann JW Jr, Whitley RJ. Herpes zoster. *N Engl J Med* 2002;347:340–346. A well-illustrated, excellent review, including current management guidelines and antiviral and other treatments to prevent postherpetic neuralgia.

Cytomegalovirus

Boppana SB, Rivera LB, Fowler KB, et al. Intrauterine transmission of cytomegalovirus to infants of women with preconceptional immunity. *N Engl J Med* 2001;344:1366–1371. This article illustrates how reinfection during pregnancy with different CMV strains can lead to intrauterine transmission and also includes an excellent review of the literature.

Drew WL. Ganciclovir resistance: Matter of time and titre. *Lancet* 2000;356:609–610. An editorial review of CMV resistance in transplant recipients and the lessons learned in HIV-positive patients.

Nichols WG, Corey L, Gooley T, et al. High risk of death due to bacterial and fungal infection among cytomegalovirus (CMV)–seronegative recipients of stem cell transplants from seropositive donors: Evidence for indirect effects of primary CMV infection. *J Infect Dis* 2002;185:273–282. An excellent background review of the role of CMV in immunocompromised patients and analysis of the significant immunomodulatory effects of CMV infection in predisposing to serious nonviral disease.

Paya CV, Wilson JA, Espy MJ, et al. Preemptive use of oral ganciclovir to prevent cytomegalovirus infection in liver transplant patients: A randomized placebo-controlled trial.

J Infect Dis 2002;185:854–860. Outlines past and present approaches to detection of CMV viremia and preemptive treatment.

Epstein–Barr Virus

Cohen JI. Epstein–Barr virus infection. *N Engl J Med* 2000;343:481–492. Excellent review, with illustrations and reference.

Mitarnum W, Suwiwat S, Pradutkanchana J, et al. Epstein–Barr virus–associated peripheral T-cell and NK-cell proliferative disease/lymphoma: Clinicopathologic, serologic, and molecular analysis. *Am J Hematol* 2002;70:31–38. A comprehensive review of 100 patients with EBV-associated lymphoproliferative disease. Presents evidence for active replication of EBV in lymphocytes.

Human Herpesvirus-6

Caserta MT, Mock DJ, Dewhurst S. Human herpesvirus 6. *Clin Infect Dis* 2001;33: 829–833. This is a concise, well-referenced review.

Hall CB, Long CE, Schnabel KC, et al. Human herpesvirus-6 infections in children: A prospective study of complications and reactivation. *N Engl J Med* 1994;331:432–438. This report identifies the contribution of HHV-6 to febrile disease, seizures, and rash.

Human Herpesvirus-7

Caserta MT, Hall CB, Schnabel K, et al. Primary human herpesvirus 7 infection: A comparison of human herpesvirus 7 and human herpesvirus 6 infections in children. *J Pediatr* 1998;133:386–389. This paper covers the clinical and laboratory diagnostic issues encountered.

Human Herpesvirus-8

Ablashi DV, Chatlynne LG, Whitman JE Jr., Cesarman E. Spectrum of Kaposi's sarcoma-associated herpesvirus, or human herpesvirus 8, diseases. *Clin Microbiol Rev* 2002;15:439–464. Extensive review of the biology of KSHV and its potential for producing disease.

CHAPTER 39

Viruses of Diarrhea

C. George Ray

Acute diarrheal disease is an illness, usually of rapid evolution (within several hours), that lasts less than 3 weeks. In addition to the bacterial and protozoal agents responsible for approximately 20 to 25% of these cases, viruses are a significant cause of the balance. Rotaviruses, caliciviruses, astroviruses, and some adenoviruses are considered here. Unfortunately, investigations have been hampered because most of these viruses cannot be readily cultivated in the laboratory.

General Features

Until the 1970s, proof of viral causation of acute diarrhea was usually based on exclusion of known bacterial or protozoan pathogens and supported by feeding cell-free filtrates of diarrheal stools to volunteers in an attempt to reproduce the disease. As might be expected, the results of such experiments were variable, and the methods were impractical for routine laboratory diagnosis. One aspect of such infections that proved of great help was the frequent association with abundant excretion of virus particles during the acute phase of illness. Virion numbers in excess of 10^8 per gram of diarrheal stool are relatively common, allowing ready visualization with an electron microscope. Direct electron microscopy and immunoelectron microscopy have been frequently used to detect and identify the presumed causative viruses; the latter method can also be used to detect humoral antibody responses to infection. More recently, polymerase chain reactions (PCR) and enzyme immunoassays (EIA) have been increasingly used for diagnosis.

Viral diarrhea was a diagnosis of exclusion

Many viral particles seen in stool by electron microscopy

Confirmation by EIA or PCR is now possible

Detection of a specific virus in the stools of symptomatic patients is not sufficient to establish the role of the virus in causing disease. Other criteria to be fulfilled include the following: (1) establish that the virus is detected in ill patients significantly more frequently than in asymptomatic, appropriately matched controls and that virus shedding temporally correlates with symptoms; (2) demonstrate significant humoral or secretory antibody responses, or both, in patients shedding the virus; (3) reproduce the disease by experimental inoculation of nonimmune human or animal hosts (usually the most difficult criterion to fulfill); (4) exclude other known causes of diarrhea, such as bacteria, bacterial toxins, and protozoa. Using these criteria, four groups of viruses have been clearly established as important causes of gastrointestinal disease: rotaviruses, caliciviruses, astroviruses, and some adenovirus serotypes ("enteric" adenoviruses). Other viruses have also been implicated, but all of the preceding criteria have not been

Multiple criteria used for establishing etiologic relationship

Rotaviruses, caliciviruses, astroviruses, and adenoviruses are established

"Candidate" viruses meet some criteria

fulfilled; therefore, they are currently regarded as "candidate" causes of gastrointestinal disease.

Vomiting commonly follows short incubation period

The currently established viruses are listed in Table 39–1 and all have several features in common, including a tendency toward brief incubation periods; fecal–oral spread by direct or indirect routes; and production of vomiting, which generally precedes or accompanies the diarrhea. The last feature has influenced physicians to use the term **acute viral gastroenteritis** to describe the syndrome associated with these agents.

ROTAVIRUSES

Most common cause of winter gastroenteritis in children <2 years of age

The human intestinal rotaviruses were first found in 1973 by electron microscopic examination of duodenal biopsy specimens from infants with diarrhea. Since then, they have been found worldwide and are believed to account for 40 to 60% of cases of acute gastroenteritis occurring during the cooler months in infants and children less than

TABLE 39–1

Biological and Epidemiologic Characteristics of Viruses that Cause Diarrhea

SPECIAL FEATURES	ROTAVIRUS	CALICIVIRUS	ASTROVIRUS	ADENOVIRUS
BIOLOGICAL				
Nucleic acid	Double-stranded RNA	Single-stranded RNA	Single-stranded RNA	Double-stranded DNA
Diameter, shape	65–75 nm, naked, double-shelled capsid	27–38 nm, naked, round	28–38 nm, naked, star-shaped	70–90 nm, naked, icosahedral
Replication in cell culture	Usually incomplete	None	None	None or incomplete
Number of serotypes	4 important to humans	More than 4	5, perhaps more	Unknown
PATHOGENIC				
Site of infection	Duodenum, jejunum	Jejunum	Small intestine	Small intestine
Mechanism of immunity	Local intestinal IgA	Unknown	Unknown	Unknown
EPIDEMIOLOGIC				
Epidemicity	Epidemic or sporadic	Family and community outbreaks	Sporadic	Sporadic
Seasonality	Usually winter	None known	None known	None known
Ages primarily affected	Infants, children <2 y old	Older children and adults	Infants, children	Infants, children
Method of tr1ansmission	Fecal–oral	Fecal–oral; contaminated water and shellfish	Fecal–oral	Fecal–oral
Incubation period (days)	1–3	0.5–2	?1–2	8–10
Major diagnostic tests	EIA, EM[a]	EM, IEM, PCR	EM, PCR	EIA, EM

[a] *Abbreviations:* EM, electron microscopy; IEM, immunoelectron microscopy; EIA, enzyme immunoassay; PCR, polymerase chain reaction.

2 years of age. These viruses have been detected in intestinal contents and in tissues from the upper gastrointestinal tract.

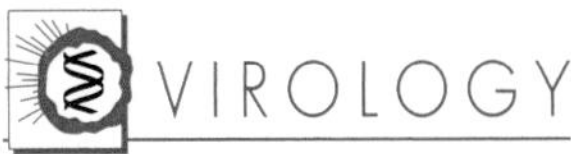

VIROLOGY

The rotaviruses belong to the family Reoviridae. They are naked, spherical particles 65 to 75 nm in diameter (smaller forms have also been described) with a genome containing 11 segments of double-stranded RNA and a double-shelled outer capsid; two segments encode proteins of the outer capsid (VP4 and VP7), which are targets for neutralizing antibodies. The name is derived from the Latin **rota** ("wheel") because of the outer capsid, which resembles a wheel attached by short spokes to the inner capsid and core (Fig 39–1). Three serogroups have been associated with disease in humans (groups A, B, and C). Four group A serotypes (1, 2, 3, and 4), based on VP7 type-specific antigens on the outer capsid, are of major epidemiologic importance. Rotaviruses can replicate in the cytoplasm of infected cell cultures in the laboratory but are difficult to propagate because the replicative cycle is usually incomplete, and mature, infectious virions are often not produced. However, successful propagation of human strains in vitro has been achieved in some instances.

Double-stranded RNA viruses are shaped like a wheel

Antigenic types are based on capsid proteins VP4 and VP7

Rotaviruses of animal origin are also highly prevalent and produce acute gastrointestinal disease in a variety of species. Very young animals, such as calves, suckling mice, piglets, and foals, are particularly susceptible. The animal rotaviruses can often replicate in cell cultures, and infection across species lines has been accomplished experimentally; however, there is no evidence that such interspecies spread occurs in nature (eg, animal rotaviruses are not known to affect humans and vice versa).

Animal rotaviruses produce diarrhea but interspecies spread not demonstrated in nature

One unique feature of rotaviruses is the ease with which the 11 RNA segments can undergo reassortment. This has enabled the development of live vaccines that combine genes from readily cultivated animal rotaviruses with human rotavirus genes that encode serotype-specific capsid proteins. For example, a current vaccine combines 10 RNA segments from a naturally attenuated rhesus monkey serotype 3 rotavirus with one human rotavirus genomic segment that encodes serotype 1, 2, and 4 VP7 neutralization specificities.

Reassortment of the 11 RNA segments readily occurs

Live vaccine accounts for variation

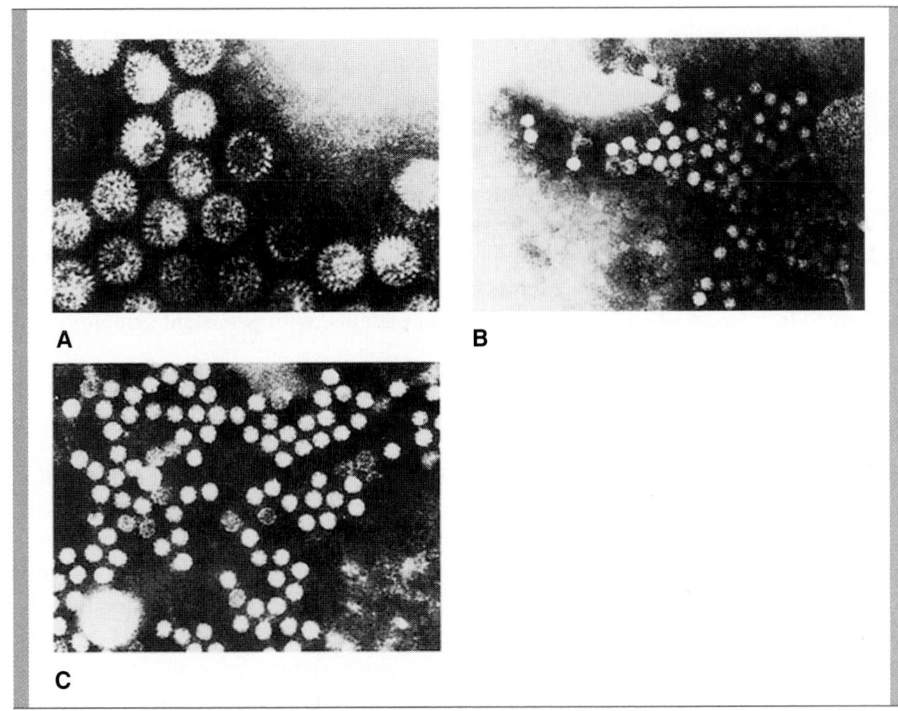

FIGURE 39–1
Viruses of diarrhea. **A.** Rotavirus. **B.** Calicivirus. **C.** Astrovirus. *(Courtesy of Claire M. Payne.)*

HUMAN ROTAVIRUS INFECTIONS

CLINICAL CAPSULE

Worldwide, an estimated one million infants die each year as a result of rotavirus diarrhea. Currently, in the United States, the total annual deaths now are thought to be less than 100, but these viruses are still major causes of severe illness and hospitalization in early life. Vomiting, abdominal cramps, and low-grade fever, followed by watery stools that usually do not contain mucus, blood, or pus, are all characteristic of the acute phase of illness, and can also be seen with infections due to caliciviruses, astroviruses and adenoviruses.

EPIDEMIOLOGY

Primarily infants and children in colder months

Outbreaks of rotavirus infection are common, particularly during the cooler months, among infants and children 1 to 24 months of age. Older children and adults can also be affected, but attack rates are usually much lower. Outbreaks among elderly, institutionalized patients have also been recognized.

Most older children and adults are immune

Although newborn infants can be readily infected with the virus, such infections often result in little or no clinical illness. This finding is illustrated by reported infection rates of 32 to 49% in some neonatal nurseries, but mild illness in only 8 to 28% of the infants. It is unclear whether this transient resistance to disease is a result of host maturation factors or transplacentally conferred immunity. Seroepidemiologic studies have been useful in demonstrating the ubiquity of these viruses and, perhaps, help to explain the age-specific attack rates. By the age of 4 years, more than 90% of individuals have humoral antibodies, suggesting a high rate of virus infection early in life.

PATHOGENESIS

Destroys villus cells of jejunum and duodenum

Absorptive surface is decreased

Enterotoxin-like effects are also present

Rotaviruses appear to localize primarily in the duodenum and proximal jejunum, causing destruction of villous epithelial cells with blunting (shortening) of villi and variable, usually mild, infiltrates of mononuclear and a few polymorphonuclear inflammatory cells within the villi. The gastric and colonic mucosa are unaffected; however, for unknown reasons, gastric emptying time is markedly delayed. The primary pathophysiologic effects are a decrease in absorptive surface in the small intestine and decreased production of brush border enzymes, such as the disaccharidases. The net result is a transient malabsorptive state, with defective handling of fats and sugars. It may take as long as 3 to 8 weeks to restore the normal histologic and functional integrity of the damaged mucosa. While the specific gene product associated with virulence is not yet known, some evidence suggests that one nonstructural protein, NSP4, may behave as an enterotoxin in a manner similar to the heat-labile enterotoxin (LT) of *Escherichia coli* and cholera toxin. This may further explain the excess fluid and electrolyte secretion in the acute phase of illness. Viral excretion usually lasts 2 to 12 days but can be greatly prolonged in malnourished or immunodeficient patients, with persistent symptoms.

IMMUNITY

Type-specific humoral and secretory IgA antibodies are protective

IgA and mucin glycoproteins confer protective role of breastfeeding

Patients with rotavirus infection respond with production of type-specific humoral antibodies that appear to last for years, perhaps a lifetime. In addition, type-specific secretory IgA (sIgA) antibodies are produced in the intestinal tract, and their presence seems to correlate best with immunity to reinfection. Breastfeeding also seems to play a protective role against rotavirus disease in young infants. Secretory IgA antibodies to rotaviruses appear in colostrum and continue to be secreted in breast milk for several months postpartum. Human breast milk mucin glycoproteins have also been shown to bind to rotaviruses, inhibiting their replication in vitro and in vivo.

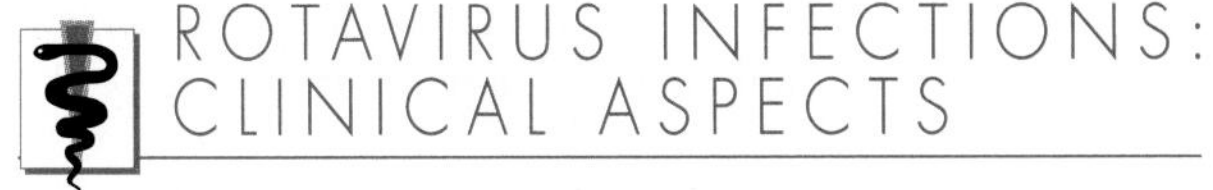

ROTAVIRUS INFECTIONS: CLINICAL ASPECTS

MANIFESTATIONS

After an incubation period of 1 to 3 days, there is usually an abrupt onset of vomiting, followed within hours by frequent, copious, watery, brown stools. In severe cases, the stools may become clear; the Japanese refer to the disease as **hakuri,** the "white stool diarrhea." Fever, usually low grade, is often present. Vomiting may persist for 1 to 3 days, and diarrhea for 4 to 8 days. The major complications result from severe dehydration, occasionally associated with hypernatremia.

This complication can lead to death, particularly in very small or malnourished infants

Short incubation period, vomiting, and watery diarrhea can lead to dehydration

DIAGNOSIS

Diagnosis of acute rotavirus infection is usually by detection of virus particles or antigen in the stools during the acute phase of illness. This can be accomplished by direct examination of the specimen by electron microscopy or, more conveniently, by immunologic detection of antigen with EIA methods (see Chapter 15).

Electron microscope or EIA detect virus

TREATMENT AND PREVENTION

There is no specific treatment. Vigorous replacement of fluids and electrolytes is required in severe cases and can be life-saving. The rotaviruses are highly infectious and can spread quickly in family and institutional settings. Control consists of rigorous hygienic measures, including careful hand washing and adequate disposal of enteric excretions. Live attenuated reassortant vaccines have been developed, as noted previously. The findings to date indicate that such an approach to control or amelioration of the natural infection is feasible. However, there remains some concern about safety, particularly with regard to reports of an increased risk of intussusception among recently immunized infants. Until this issue is resolved, vaccine will not be made available for routine use.

Live, attenuated, or recombinant vaccines are feasible

Intussuseption is vaccine safety concern

CALICIVIRUSES

Although the caliciviruses were the first to be clearly associated with outbreaks of gastroenteritis, considerably less is known about their biology than about that of the rotaviruses. They were first associated with an outbreak in Norwalk, Ohio, in 1968, and their role was confirmed by production of disease in volunteers fed fecal filtrates. The original virus was thus called the **Norwalk agent,** and similar viruses have been given names such as Hawaii agent, Montgomery County agent, Ditchling agent, and so on.

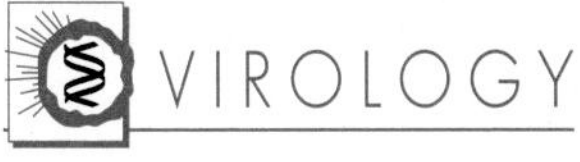

VIROLOGY

The viruses are small, naked, round RNA-containing particles 27 to 38 nm in diameter; their appearance is similar to that of the DNA-containing parvoviruses and hepatitis A virus (see Fig 39–1). They are classified as members of the Caliciviridae family. At present, two genera that cause diarrhea are recognized within this family: "Norwalk-like viruses" (sometimes referred to as "Noroviruses") and "Sapporo-like viruses." The viruses appear to be extremely hardy; their infectivity persists after exposure to acid, ether, and heat (60°C for 30 minutes). They have not been effectively propagated in cell or organ culture.

Small, round unenveloped RNA viruses are hardy

Two genera: "Norwalk-like" and "Sapporo-like"

At least four different serotypes have been demonstrated by immunoelectron microscopy with convalescent sera from affected patients. Knowledge of the antigenic

Several serotypes but not yet grown

characteristics and biology of these viruses has been seriously hampered by the current inability to grow them in the laboratory and by their lack of known pathogenicity for animals.

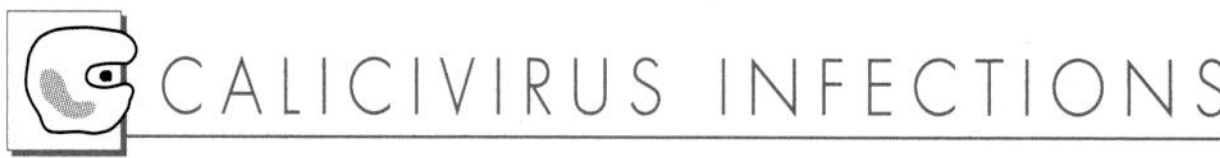

CALICIVIRUS INFECTIONS

EPIDEMIOLOGY

Sharp outbreaks include older children and adults

Transmission is by fecal–oral route

Sharp family and community outbreaks are common and can occur in any season. Unlike rotaviruses, caliciviruses are much more common causes of gastrointestinal illness in older children and adults. This difference in age-specific predilection is perhaps reflected in serosurveys, which have shown that the prevalence of antibodies rises slowly, reaching approximately 50% by the fifth decade of life, a striking contrast to the frequent acquisition of antibodies to rotaviruses early in life. Transmission is primarily fecal–oral; outbreaks have also been associated with consumption of contaminated water, uncooked shellfish, and other foods.

PATHOGENESIS

Enterotoxic features are not present

Both the pathogenesis and the pathology are similar to those described for rotaviruses, except that no enterotoxic features have yet been described for caliciviruses. The mucosal changes usually revert to normal within 2 weeks of onset of illness. Virus shedding in the feces generally lasts no more than 3 to 4 days.

IMMUNITY

Reinfection can occur with same serotypes

Patients and experimentally infected volunteers respond to infection with the production of humoral antibodies, which persist indefinitely; their role in protection from reinfection, however, appears minimal. Reinfection and illness with the same serotype occur, and the role of local antibody has not been well defined. It is possible that nonimmune or genetic factors are essential for protection.

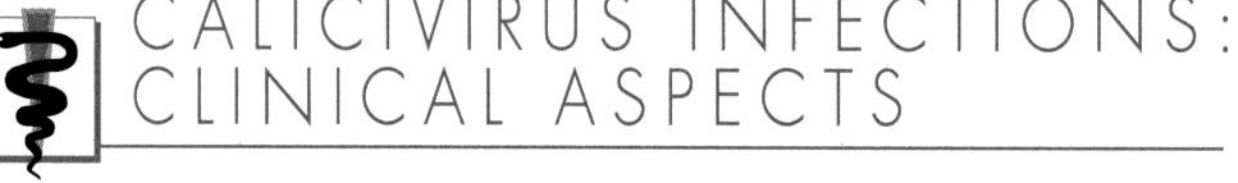

CALICIVIRUS INFECTIONS: CLINICAL ASPECTS

Clinical picture and diagnostic tests are similar to rotavirus

No treatment or vaccine exists

The incubation period is 10 to 51 hours, followed by abrupt onset of vomiting and diarrhea, a syndrome clinically indistinguishable from that caused by rotaviruses. Respiratory symptoms rarely coexist, and the duration of illness is relatively brief (usually 1–2 days). These viruses can be detected by electron microscopy or immunoelectron microscopy in stools during the acute phase of illness. In addition, EIA and PCR methods have been developed. As with rotavirus infection, there is no specific treatment other than fluid and electrolyte replacement. Prevention requires good hygienic measures.

ADENOVIRUSES, ASTROVIRUSES, AND "CANDIDATE" VIRUSES

Serotypes 40 and 41 are commonly found

Some **adenoviruses,** most of which are exceedingly difficult to cultivate in vitro (in contrast to those associated with respiratory diseases), are now recognized as significant intestinal pathogens. They may account for an estimated 5 to 15% of all viral gastroenteritis in young children. These include serotypes 40, 41, and perhaps 38.

Astroviruses have a shape that resembles a 5- or 6-pointed star (see Fig. 39–1). These have been known since 1975. In recent years astroviruses have been acknowledged as causes of often mild gastroenteritis outbreaks, primarily among toddlers, school children and elderly nursing home residents.

Illness is often, but not always, mild

Other agents associated with gastrointestinal diseases include coronavirus-like agents, toroviruses, and some group A coxsackieviruses (the latter primarily cause gastrointestinal symptoms in severely immunocompromised patients). This list may grow in the future; however, until more is learned about their biology, epidemiologic behavior, and impact on human health, they remain "candidate" viruses for now.

ADDITIONAL READING

Glass RI, Gentsch JR, Ivanoff B. New lessons for rotavirus vaccines. *Science* 1996; 272:46–48. This brief review provides excellent insight into the biology and importance of rotaviruses.

Kapikian AZ. Viral gastroenteritis. *JAMA* 1993;269:627–630. This prominent investigator presents a concise, well-referenced overview of the relative importance of these agents.

Lundgren O, Peregrin AT, Persson K, et al. Role of the enteric nervous system in the fluid and electrolyte secretion of rotavirus diarrhea. *Science* 2000;287:491–495. This report and the accompanying commentary on pp. 409–411 show how basic research can provide leads to new therapeutic approaches.

Murphy TV, Gargiullo PM, Massoudi MS, et al. Intussusception among infants given an oral rotavirus vaccine. *N Engl J Med* 2001;344:564–572. This large investigation well illustrates the reasons why close surveillance for vaccine-associated adverse events are so important.

CHAPTER 40

Arthropod-Borne and Other Zoonotic Viruses

C. GEORGE RAY

The zoonotic viruses comprise more than 400 agents, one or more of which occur in most parts of the world. Members of the group have their ultimate reservoirs in lower vertebrates or insects. They are from diverse taxonomic families of RNA viruses that primarily include the togaviruses, bunyaviruses, reoviruses, arenaviruses, and filoviruses. Their major morphologic and genetic features are summarized in Table 5–1. Certain DNA viruses (poxviruses) are also transmissible from animals to humans. These are considered in Chapter 35.

The zoonotic viruses discussed here are divided into two groups. The arboviruses are transmitted to humans by infected bloodsucking insects such as mosquitoes, ticks, and *Phlebotomus* flies (sandflies). The other zoonotic RNA viruses are generally believed to be transmitted by inhalation of infected animal excretions, by the conjunctival route, or occasionally by direct contact with infected animals. Rabies virus, which is commonly transmitted by animal bites, is discussed separately in Chapter 41.

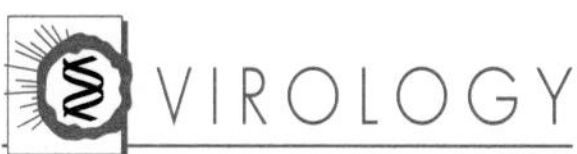

VIROLOGY

In most cases, the zoonotic viruses were first named after the place of initial isolation (eg, St. Louis encephalitis) or after the disease produced (eg, yellow fever). More recent studies have assigned the majority to families and genera on the basis of properties indicated in Table 5–1. The major characteristics of these families are summarized below.

Generally named after place of isolation

TOGAVIRUSES AND FLAVIVIRUSES

Togaviruses and flaviviruses are enveloped virions containing single-stranded, positive-sense RNA measuring 40 to 70 nm in external diameter. The envelope contains a hemagglutinin and lipoproteins. Virions mature by budding from cellular membranes. Replication can occur in cells of infected arthropods and vertebrate hosts. The *Alphavirus* and *Flavivirus* genera within these families include most arthropod-borne viruses. Each genus possesses its own unique primary structure of the RNA genome. Viruses within these genera are frequently serologically related to one another but not to others. Representatives are listed in Table 40–1.

Enveloped RNA viruses contain hemagglutinin and lipoproteins

TABLE 40–1

Selected Arboviruses of Major Importance to Humans

Genus and Member	Major Geographic Distribution	Primary Arthropod Vector	Usual Disease Expression
Togaviruses			
Alphavirus			
Western equine encephalitis	North America	Mosquito	Encephalitis
Eastern equine encephalitis	North America	Mosquito	Encephalitis
Venezuelan equine encephalitis	Central and South America	Mosquito	Encephalitis
Chikungunya	Africa and Asia	Mosquito	Febrile illness
Flaviviruses			
Flavivirus			
St. Louis encephalitis	North America	Mosquito	Encephalitis
Dengue	All tropical zones	Mosquito	Febrile illness or hemorrhagic fever
Yellow fever	Africa, South America, and Caribbean	Mosquito	Hepatic necrosis, hemorrhage
West Nile fever	Africa, Eastern Europe, Middle East, Asia, North America	Mosquito	Febrile illness or encephalitis
Murray Valley encephalitis	Australia	Mosquito	Encephalitis
Russian spring–summer encephalitis	Eastern Soviet Union and Central Europe	Tick	Encephalitis
Powassan	Canada	Tick	Encephalitis
Japanese B encephalitis	Japan, Korea, and Philippines	Mosquito	Encephalitis
Bunyaviruses			
Bunyavirus			
California	North America	Mosquito	Encephalitis
Bunyamwera	Africa	Mosquito	Febrile illness
Rift Valley fever	Africa	Mosquito	Febrile illness
Sandfly fever	Mediterranean	*Phlebotomus*	Febrile illness
Reoviruses			
Orbivirus			
Colorado tick fever	North America	Tick	Febrile illness

BUNYAVIRUSES

Spherical, enveloped RNA viruses mature by budding

Bunyaviruses are spherical, enveloped, single-stranded negative-sense RNA viruses approximately 90 to 100 nm in external diameter. They mature by budding into smooth-surfaced vesicles in or near the Golgi region of the infected cell. The major disease-causing bunyaviruses in North America are California virus and hantavirus.

REOVIRUSES

Unenveloped RNA viruses are prominent in North America

Reoviruses are spherical, unenveloped, double-stranded RNA viruses that measure about 80 nm in diameter with a segmented genome. The most important North American arbovirus of this family, which is a member of the genus *Coltivirus,* causes Colorado tick fever.

ARENAVIRUSES

The arenaviruses are enveloped, spherical or pleomorphic viruses containing single-stranded, negative-sense RNA in several segments and measuring 50 to 300 nm in diameter. They mature by budding from host cell cytoplasmic membranes and contain host cell ribosomes in their interior. These ribosomes confer a granular appearance to the viruses, hence their name (from the Latin **arenosus** for "sandy"). The most significant arenavirus infections in humans are the hemorrhagic fevers, including Lassa fever. The virus of lymphatic choriomeningitis is occasionally transmitted to humans from infected mice and other rodents.

Spherical, enveloped RNA contain host cell ribosomes

FILOVIRUSES

Filoviruses are enveloped, single-stranded, negative-sense RNA viruses. They are filamentous and highly pleomorphic, averaging 80 nm in diameter and 300 to 14,000 nm in length as they bud from the cell membrane. They are the cause of Marburg and Ebola fevers, two highly fatal hemorrhagic fevers.

Enveloped filamentous RNA viruses cause hemorrhagic fevers

ARBOVIRUSES

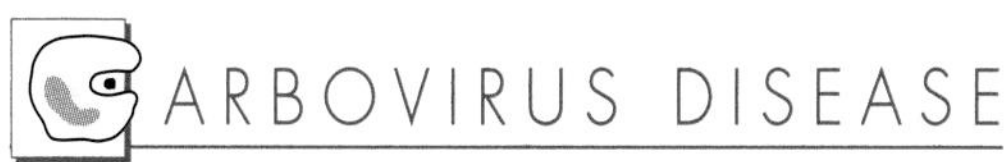

ARBOVIRUS DISEASE

CLINICAL CAPSULE

Some arboviruses cause severe inflammation of the brain (encephalitis) with damage or destruction of neural cells that may be fatal or lead to permanent neurologic damage in survivors. Others, such as dengue viruses, can produce illnesses that range from mild flu-like symptoms to overwhelming shock with widespread hemorrhage into tissues. Still another, yellow fever virus, primarily attacks liver cells, leading to extensive destruction and sometimes fatal liver failure.

EPIDEMIOLOGY

Arboviruses of major importance in human disease are listed in Table 40–1 with summaries of their geographic distribution, the arthropod vectors that transmit them, and the usual disease syndromes that can result from infection.

With the exception of urban dengue and urban yellow fever, in which the virus may simply be transmitted between humans and mosquitoes, other arboviral diseases involve nonhuman vertebrates. These are usually small mammals, birds, or, in the case of jungle yellow fever, monkeys. Infection is transmitted within the host species by arthropods (eg, mosquitoes or ticks) that become infected. In some cases, the infection can be maintained from generation to generation in the arthropod by transovarial transmission. Infection in the arthropod usually does not appear to harm the insect; however, a period of virus multiplication (termed **extrinsic incubation period**) is required to enhance the capacity to transmit infection to vertebrates by bite. The consequences of infection transmitted from the arthropod to susceptible vertebrate hosts are variable; some develop illness of varying severity with viremia, whereas others may have long-term viremia without clinical disease. Vertebrate hosts are then a source of further spread of the virus by amplification, in which noninfected arthropods feeding on viremic hosts acquire the virus, thereby increasing the risk of transmission.

Reservoirs are in nonhuman vertebrates

Sometimes maintained by vertical transmission in vector

Multiplication in vector is required

Transient viremia is a feature of many of these infections in hosts other than their reservoir; those affected, including humans and higher vertebrates (eg, horses and cattle),

Sustained viremia required for vertebrate host to be significant reservoir

are often referred to as blind-end hosts. In contrast, if viremia is sustained for longer periods (eg, weeks to months in a variety of togavirus, flavivirus, and bunyavirus infections of lower vertebrates), the vertebrate host becomes highly important as a reservoir for continuing transmission. Viremia may last a week or more in human dengue and yellow fever infections, and humans may then serve as a reservoir in urban disease.

Season-to-season survival has multiple mechanisms

Obviously, the usual arthropod vectors are rarely present during all seasons. The question then arises as to how the arboviruses survive between the time the vector disappears and the time it reappears in subsequent years. Several mechanisms can operate to sustain the virus between transmission periods (often referred to as **overwintering**): (1) sustained viremia in lower vertebrates such as small mammals, birds, and snakes, from which newly mature arthropods can be infected when taking a blood meal; (2) hibernation of infected adult arthropods that survive from one season to the next; and (3) transovarial transmission, whereby the infected female arthropod can transmit virus to its progeny.

The three basic cycles of arbovirus transmission are urban, sylvatic, and arthropod-sustained.

Urban

Urban cycle exists with dengue and yellow fever

As the term suggests, the urban cycle is favored by the presence of relatively large numbers of humans living in close proximity to arthropod (usually mosquito) species capable of virus transmission. The cycle is:

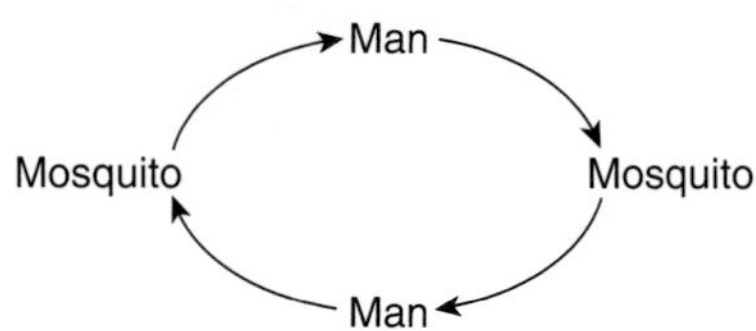

Examples of this cycle include urban dengue, urban yellow fever, and occasional urban outbreaks of St. Louis encephalitis.

Sylvatic

In the sylvatic cycle a single nonhuman vertebrate reservoir may be involved:

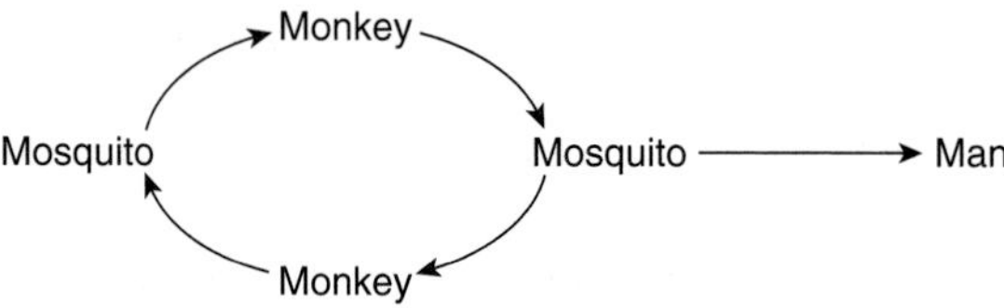

In this situation, the human, who becomes a tangential host through accidental intrusion into a zoonotic transmission cycle, is not important in maintaining the infection cycle. An example of this cycle is jungle yellow fever.

In other sylvatic cycles, multiple vertebrate reservoirs may be involved:

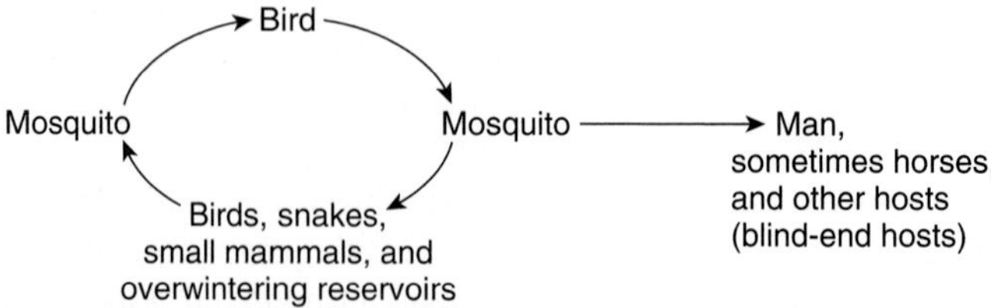

Sylvatic cycle occurs with many viruses

Humans are tangential hosts

Examples include western equine encephalitis, eastern equine encephalitis, and California viruses. In some situations, such as St. Louis encephalitis and yellow fever, the urban and sylvatic cycles may operate concurrently.

Arthropod-Sustained

Arthropods, especially ticks, may sustain the reservoir by transovarial transmission of virus to their progeny, with amplification of the cycle by spread to and from small mammals:

```
                        Tick ┐     ┌ Man          \
                         ↓   │     │ Cattle        )
Small mammals ⟺ Tick     ├──→{ Goats        /  ──────→  Man (via milk,
                         ↓   │     │ (Blind-end              an aberrant
                        Tick ┘     └  hosts)                 pathway)
```

Tick-borne encephalitis in Russia is transmitted by this cycle. In temperate climates such as the United States, arboviruses are major causes of disease during the summer and early fall months, the season of greatest activity of arthropod vectors (usually mosquitoes or ticks). When climatic conditions and ecologic circumstances (eg, swamps and ponds) are optimal for arthropod breeding and egg hatching, arbovirus amplification may begin.

Arthropod sustained by tick transovarial transmission

Weather, swamps, and ponds alter conditions

An example of amplification is provided by western equine encephalitis. When the mosquito vectors become abundant, the level of transmission among the basic reservoir hosts (birds and small mammals) increases, and the mosquitoes also turn to other susceptible species such as the domestic fowl. These hosts experience a rapidly developing asymptomatic viremia, which permits still more arthropods to become infected on biting. At this point, spread to blind-end hosts such as humans or horses and the development of clinical disease become likely. This occurrence depends on the accessibility of the host to the infected mosquito and on mosquito feeding preferences which, for unknown reasons, vary from one season to another.

Mosquito increases create risk for blind-end human infection

PATHOGENESIS

There are three major manifestations of arbovirus diseases in humans associated with different tropisms of various viruses for human organs, although overlap can occur. In some, the central nervous system (CNS) is primarily affected, leading to aseptic meningitis or meningoencephalitis. A second syndrome involves many major organ systems, with particular damage to the liver, as in yellow fever. The third is manifested by hemorrhagic fever, in which damage is particularly severe to the small blood vessels, with skin petechiae and intestinal and other hemorrhages.

CNS, visceral, and hemorrhagic fever are major syndromes

Infection of the human by a biting, infected arthropod is followed by viremia, which is apparently amplified by extensive virus replication in the reticuloendothelial system and vascular endothelium. After replication the virus becomes localized in various target organs, depending on its tropism, and illness results. The viruses produce cell necrosis with resultant inflammation which leads to fever in nearly all infections. If the major viral tropism is for the CNS, virus reaching this site by crossing the blood–brain barrier or along neural pathways can cause meningeal inflammation (aseptic meningitis) or neuronal dysfunction (encephalitis). The CNS pathology consists of meningeal and perivascular mononuclear cell infiltrates; degeneration of neurons with neuronophagia; and occasionally, destruction of the supporting structure of neurons.

After bite, viremia and viral tissue tropism define disease

In CNS, aseptic meningitis and encephalitis follow cell injury

In some infections, especially yellow fever, the liver is the primary target organ. Pathologic findings include hyaline necrosis of hepatocytes, which produces cytoplasmic eosinophilic masses called **Councilman bodies.** Degenerative changes in the renal tubules and myocardium may also be seen, as may microscopic hemorrhages throughout the brain. Hemorrhage is a major feature of yellow fever, largely because of the lack of liver-produced clotting factors as a result of liver necrosis.

Liver often the target, with necrosis of hepatocytes

Hemorrhagic fevers other than those related to primary hepatic destruction have a somewhat different pathogenesis which has been studied most extensively in dengue infections. In uncomplicated dengue fever, which is associated with a rash and influenza-like symptoms, there are changes in the small dermal blood vessels. These alterations include endothelial cell swelling and perivascular edema with mononuclear cell infiltration. More severe infection, as in dengue hemorrhagic fever, often complicated by shock, is characterized by perivascular edema and widespread effusions into serous cavities such as the pleura and hemorrhages

Dengue hemorrhagic fevers involve perivascular and endothelial injury

May progress to shock

from the upper respiratory and intestinal tracts. The spleen and lymph nodes show hyperplasia of lymphoid and plasma cell elements, and there is focal necrosis in the liver. The pathophysiology seems related to increased vascular permeability and disseminated intravascular coagulation, which is further complicated by liver and bone marrow dysfunction (eg, decreased platelet production, decreased production of liver-dependent clotting factors). The major vascular abnormalities may be provoked by circulating virus–antibody complexes (immune complexes) that mediate activation of complement and subsequent release of vasoactive amines. The precise reason for this phenomenon is not clear; it may be related to intrinsic virulence of the virus strains involved and to host susceptibility factors.

Lymphoid hyperplasia seen

Virus–antibody complexes may trigger complement activation

Two hypotheses are based on the existence of four distinct but antigenically related serotypes of dengue virus, any of which can generate group-specific cross-reacting antibodies that are not necessarily protective against other serotypes. One possibility is that preexisting group-specific antibody at a critical concentration serves as "enhancing" rather than neutralizing antibody. In the presence of enhancing antibody, virus–antibody complexes are more efficiently adsorbed to and engulfed by monocytes and macrophages. Subsequent replication leads to extensive spread throughout the host. Alternatively, or in concert with this, activation of previously sensitized T cells by viral antigen present on the surfaces of macrophages may result in release of cytokines, which mediate the development of shock and hemorrhage.

Cross reacting antibodies may enhance infection

IMMUNITY

The usual humoral responses (hemagglutination inhibition, complement fixation, neutralization, precipitation) in relation to onset of illness are illustrated in Figure 40–1. The rise in antibody titer generally correlates with recovery from infection. Neutralizing antibodies, which are the most serotype specific, generally persist many years after infection. The presence of IgM-specific antibodies indicates that primary infection likely occurred within the previous 2 months. Cellular and humoral immunity to reinfection are serotype specific and appear to be permanent.

Neutralizing antibodies protective and last for years

Immunity is serotype specific

ARBOVIRUS DISEASE: SPECIFIC ARBOVIRUSES

Western Equine Encephalitis

The agent that causes western equine encephalitis is prevalent in the central valley of California, eastern Washington (Yakima valley), Colorado, and Texas. It has also been responsible for outbreaks in midwestern states (Minnesota, Wisconsin, Illinois, Missouri, and Kansas) and as far east as New Jersey. Horses and humans represent blind-end hosts;

Human and equine illness

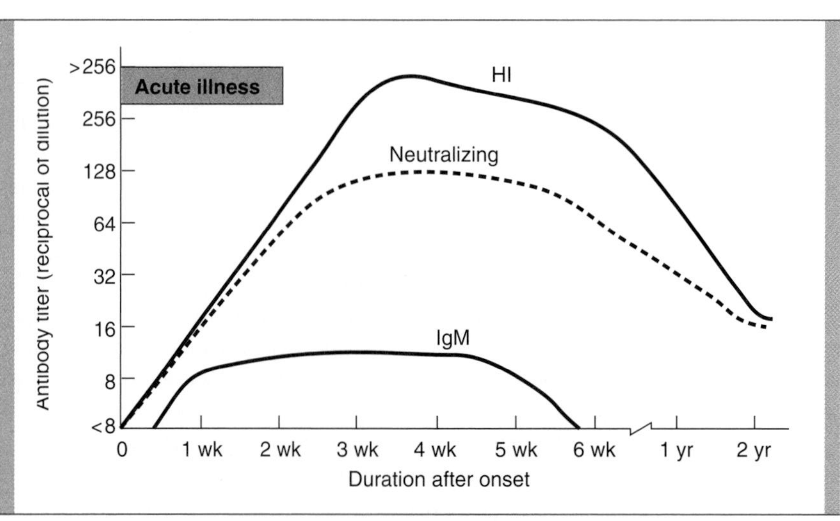

FIGURE 40–1
Typical patterns of antibody response after arbovirus infection. HI, hemagglutination inhibition antibodies; IgM, immunoglobulin M antibodies, begin to appear about 3 days after onset and disappear after about 6 weeks.

both are susceptible to infection and illness, commonly manifested as encephalitis. Although human infection in endemic areas is commonplace, overall only 1 of 1000 infections causes clinical symptoms. However, in young infants, 1 of every 25 infections may produce severe illness. The attack rates are therefore far higher in young infants than in other groups. The disease spectrum may range from mild, nonspecific febrile illness to aseptic meningitis or severe, overwhelming encephalitis. Mortality is estimated at 5% for cases of encephalitis. It is a very serious disease in infants less than 1 year of age; as many as 60% of survivors have permanent neurologic impairment.

Encephalitis is more likely in young infants

Eastern Equine Encephalitis

The eastern equine encephalitis virus is largely confined to the Atlantic Seaboard states from New England down the coasts of Central America and South America. The mosquito vector (principally *Culiseta melanura*) generally restricts its feeding to horses and birds, although occasional outbreaks among humans have occurred. The virus can cause severe encephalitis in horses and also in wild birds. The mortality among humans is estimated at 50% for individuals of all ages, and the incidence of severe sequelae among survivors is high.

New England to South America

Vector feeds on horses and birds

St. Louis Encephalitis

The St. Louis encephalitis virus is a major cause of arbovirus encephalitis in the United States. Its geographic distribution and major mosquito vector (*Culex tarsalis*) are similar to those of western equine encephalitis, but has been much more prevalent in eastern states and in Texas, Mississippi, and Florida. It infects but causes no disease in horses. The disease spectrum in humans is similar to that of western equine encephalitis, but the major morbidity and mortality, as well as the highest attack rates, are among adults more than 40 years of age. Infants and young children are relatively spared.

Distribution and disease is similar to western equine encephalitis

More disease seen in adults

West Nile Virus

During the summer of 1999 in the northeastern United States, human West Nile virus infections appeared for the first time in the Western Hemisphere. A subsequent outbreak occurred again in 2000. Together, these outbreaks resulted in 78 hospitalized patients and 9 deaths, mostly among the elderly. More widespread activity was observed in 2001 (66 human cases); then in 2002, a dramatic increase in virus spread was seen across the United States, with activity in 46 states and four Canadian provinces. There were at least 3600 human cases reported in the United States, with 212 deaths. Prior to 1999, outbreaks of human infections were primarily confined to eastern Africa, the Middle East, eastern Europe, west Asia and Australia.

First appeared in United States in 1999

The virus is antigenically related to St. Louis encephalitis and Japanese encephalitis. Transmission is from infected mosquitoes to birds, humans and horses, and clinical illness leading to death can result from infections in any of these hosts. Transmission among humans via blood transfusions, breast milk, or organ transplants is also possible. Crows are particularly affected; virus has been detected in dead crows found as far south as Florida, and more recently in the midwestern United States. Clinical illness in the United States has often included muscle weakness and flaccid paralysis, suggesting an axonal polyneuropathy in addition to encephalitis.

Dead crows often herald spread of virus in nature

Muscle weakness and flaccid paralysis can occur

California Virus

Although California virus was first isolated in that state, its major distribution in the United States has been in the Midwest; outbreaks due to the LaCrosse subtype are particularly prevalent in Wisconsin, Ohio, Minnesota, Indiana and West Virginia. In Wisconsin and Minnesota, California virus is considered the most important cause of encephalitis. However, studies elsewhere in North America and throughout the world, indicate that California virus or closely related agents are present nearly everywhere. The primary mosquito vector (*Aedes triseriatus*) is commonly encountered in suburban or rural environments. Unlike western equine, eastern equine, and St. Louis encephalitis viruses, the highest attack rates are seen in those aged 5 to 18 years. Infection is often characterized by abrupt onset of encephalitis, frequently with seizures.

Virus and vector common in suburban and rural areas

Highest attack rate in those aged 5 to 18 years

Yellow Fever

Widespread in tropical areas

Vector persists in United States

Geographically, yellow fever is distributed throughout the Caribbean and Central America, the Amazon valley in South America, and a broad central zone in Africa from the Atlantic Coast to the Sudan and Ethiopia. It continues to be a potential threat to the southeastern United States because of an urban vector (*Aedes aegypti*) in that area. The clinical disease is characterized by abrupt onset of fever, chills, headache, and hemorrhage. It may progress to severe vomiting (sometimes with gastric hemorrhage), bradycardia, jaundice, and shock. If the patient recovers from the acute episode, there are no long-term sequelae.

Dengue

Vector same as yellow fever

There are four related serotypes of dengue, any of which may exist concurrently in a given endemic area. These agents are widespread throughout the world, particularly in the Middle East, Africa, the Far East, and the Caribbean Islands, and they have invaded the United States in the past. The vector (*Aedes aegypti*) is the same as the domestic vector of yellow fever. The known transmission cycle is human–mosquito–human, although a sylvatic cycle involving monkeys may also exist.

Severe pain in back, muscles, and joints

The characteristic clinical illness usually results in fever, an erythematous rash, and severe pain in the back, head, muscles, and joints. Especially in the Far East (Philippines, Thailand, and India), the disease has periodically assumed a severe form characterized by shock, pleural effusion, and hemorrhage often followed by death.

Japanese B Encephalitis

Transmission is similar to St. Louis and western equine encephalitis

The flavivirus species that causes Japanese B encephalitis is prevalent on the eastern coast of Asia, on its offshore islands (Japan, Taiwan, and Indonesia), and in India. Its transmission cycle resembles that of the St. Louis encephalitis and western equine encephalitis viruses. A high proportion of human infections are subclinical, especially in children; when encephalitis does develop it is severe and often fatal.

Powassan Virus

Tick-borne but uncertain human importance

Powassan virus is the only known tick-borne *Flavivirus* species of North America. First isolated in Ontario from a fatal human case of encephalitis, it has been found in infected ticks in Ontario, British Columbia, and Colorado. Its significance to humans is not yet established; only a few patients with encephalitis proved to be caused by this agent have been described. However, serologic evidence suggests that the virus is prevalent in many areas of North America.

Colorado Tick Fever

Tick-borne throughout western United States

Most infections asymptomatic

The tick-borne *Orbivirus* species that causes Colorado tick fever has been found throughout the western United States, including Washington, Oregon, Colorado, and Idaho, and also Long Island. It is frequently found in *Dermacentor andersoni,* which are also vectors for *Rickettsia rickettsii.* The typical illness, which occurs 3 to 6 days after the tick bite, is characterized by a sudden onset with headache, muscle pains, fever, and occasionally encephalitis. Leukopenia is a consistent feature of infection. It is estimated that no more than one clinical illness occurs for every 100 infections with this agent.

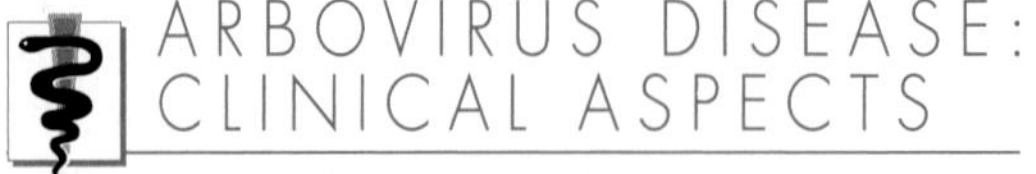

ARBOVIRUS DISEASE: CLINICAL ASPECTS

DIAGNOSIS

The arboviruses may be isolated in various culture systems including intracerebral inoculation of newborn mice, which often results in encephalitis and death. The viruses may be found in the blood (viremia) from a few days before onset of symptoms through the first 1 to 2 days of illness; attempts at isolation from the blood are generally useful only when viremia is prolonged, as in dengue, Colorado tick fever, and some of the hemorrhagic fevers. Virus is not present in the stool and is rarely found in the throat; viral recovery from cerebrospinal fluid (CSF) is also unusual. Virus can be detected in CSF or affected tissue by reverse transcriptase polymerase chain reaction, and sometimes by culture during the acute phase of illness. Specific diagnosis is usually accomplished by serologic techniques using acute and convalescent sera. Various tests have been used including hemagglutination inhibition, complement fixation, virus neutralization methods, and enzyme immunoassay. Early rapid presumptive diagnosis can sometimes be made by the detection of IgM-specific antibodies that often appear within a few days of onset (except in Colorado tick fever, where they may be delayed by 1 to 2 weeks), and persist 1 to 2 months.

Blood is best source but must be early in disease

Multiple serologic methods used

TREATMENT AND PREVENTION

There is generally no specific treatment for arboviral infections other than supportive care; ribavirin has been used on occasion, but controlled studies have not been reported to support or refute its effectiveness. Prevention is primarily avoidance of contact with potentially infected arthropods, a task that can be extremely difficult even with the use of adequate screening and insect repellents. In some settings, vector control can be accomplished by elimination of arthropod breeding sites (stagnant pools and the like) and sometimes by attempts to eradicate the arthropods with careful use of insecticides. Such measures have been highly effective in the control of urban yellow fever, in which elimination of urban breeding sites and other measures to eradicate the principal mosquito vector species (*Aedes aegypti*) have been used. Viruses maintained in complex sylvatic cycles are infinitely more difficult to control without risking major environmental disruption and inestimable expense.

Treatment is only supportive

Protection from bites and vector control are primary prevention

Vaccines are available for immunization of horses against western, eastern, and Venezuelan equine encephalitis virus infections, and the latter has also been used for some laboratory personnel who work with the virus. The only other arbovirus vaccine in general use for humans is a live attenuated yellow fever virus vaccine (17-D strain), which is used to protect rural populations exposed to the sylvatic cycle and international travelers to endemic areas. In fact, many countries in tropical Africa, Asia, and South America require proof of yellow fever vaccination before allowing travelers to enter.

Yellow fever vaccine is available

Other RNA Viruses of Zoonotic Origin

ARENAVIRUSES

A common feature of the arenaviruses is their zoonotic reservoir, particularly small rodents, in which they may be sustained for long periods. Primary infection (horizontal transmission) in mature rodents often results in disease and death, whereas intrauterine or perinatal infection (vertical transmission) usually leads to chronic lifelong viremia with persistent shedding of virus into the feces, urine, and respiratory secretions. Although chronically infected rodents are somewhat tolerant to the virus (ie, infection is persistent without causing illness), they produce antibodies, and evidence of deleterious effects can be found in older hosts, usually in the form of immune complex glomerulonephritis. The viruses are perpetuated by vertical transmission from infected mothers to their offspring. When environmental contact becomes close, spread from the rodent reservoir to humans (and, in some instances, subhuman primates) can occur via aerosols; through exposure to infective urine, feces, or tissues; or directly by rodent bites. This is in contrast to the arthropod spread of arboviruses.

Sustained in small rodent reservoirs

Vertical transmission in rodents

Spread to humans by aerosols and close contact

Arenaviruses Associated with Hemorrhagic Fevers

Person-to-person spread occurs by contact with body fluids

The agents of arenavirus hemorrhagic fevers are transmitted from infected rodents to humans in the manner described above, although person-to-person spread by contact with secretions and body fluids also occurs readily. The viruses in this group include the South American hemorrhagic fever agents (Junin virus, the cause of Argentinean hemorrhagic fever, and Machupo virus, the cause of Bolivian hemorrhagic fever) and Lassa virus, the cause of **Lassa fever** in West Africa.

All cause fever, shock, and hemorrhage

Hepatitis and myocarditis also occur with Lassa fever

High mortality and risk of further transmission

These viruses have pathogenic and pathologic features similar to those described for the arboviruses that cause hemorrhagic fevers; however, the mechanism involved in the coagulation abnormalities is not understood. All are characterized by fever, usually accompanied by hemorrhagic manifestations, shock, neurologic disturbances, and bradycardia. Lassa fever also frequently causes hepatitis, myocarditis, exudative pharyngitis, and acute deafness. The last deficit may persist after recovery. Mortality is estimated to be 10 to 50% for Lassa fever and 5 to 30% for the others. All are considered highly dangerous in terms of infectivity. Importation of cases to nonendemic areas has occurred, with significant risk of spread to medical and laboratory personnel.

Suggested by clinical findings and travel history

Diagnosis only in reference centers

Viremia may be prolonged

The diagnosis is suggested primarily by the recent travel history of the patient and the clinical syndromes. Although virus isolation and serologic diagnosis may be performed, these procedures should not be attempted in a hospital diagnostic laboratory. Any patient suspected of having such an infection should be immediately isolated and public health authorities notified. Because of the high risk of spread of infection from body fluids and excreta, even routine laboratory studies are best deferred until the diagnosis and proper disposition of specimens can be resolved. Viremia can persist 1 month, and virus shedding in the urine may continue more than 2 months after the onset of illness. Treatment is primarily supportive; however, intravenous ribavirin, if begun within 6 days of illness onset, has been shown to be helpful in Lassa fever.

Lymphocytic Choriomeningitis Virus

Transplacental infection in humans

Infection with lymphocytic choriomeningitis virus is particularly common in hamsters and mice. In the United States, most human illnesses have been traced to contact with rodent breeding colonies in research or pet supply centers and to pet hamsters in the home. The illness usually consists of fever, headache, and myalgia although meningitis or meningoencephalitis also occurs occasionally. Such CNS infections may persist as long as 3 months. There is also evidence that transplacental infection can occur in humans, resulting in fetal death, hydrocephalus, or chorioretinitis. No person-to-person transmission of infection has been documented.

Mice and hamsters in pet stores

Meningitis may persist for months

The diagnosis is suggested by a history of rodent contact. The virus may be isolated in the early stages of disease by cell culture or intracerebral inoculation of blood or CSF into weanling mice or young guinea pigs. Serologic testing of acute and convalescent sera is usually performed by indirect immunofluorescence.

FILOVIRUSES: MARBURG AND EBOLA VIRUSES

Initial cases transmitted from monkeys

The association of the Marburg virus with serious disease did not become apparent until 1967, when 26 cases of hemorrhagic fever occurred among persons in Germany and Yugoslavia who were handling a group of African monkeys imported from central Uganda. The agent was later identified as Marburg virus and was apparently transmitted by the infected monkeys. In 1975 the virus was associated with a similar disease in three travelers in South Africa, and in 1980 in Kenya.

Viruses differ antigenically

In 1976, severe outbreaks of hemorrhagic fever occurred in northern Zaire and southern Sudan, with case fatality rates from 50 to 90%. The illnesses were similar to those described for Marburg virus but were later shown to be caused by an antigenically different agent known as Ebola virus, named after a river in Zaire. More recently, another filovirus serologically related to Ebola virus was isolated from monkeys during an epizootic of simian hemorrhagic fever at a US quarantine facility. The reservoir was determined to be monkeys imported from the Philippines.

The reasons why these viruses can cause such fulminant, lethal hemorrhagic disease with shock in humans are not entirely clear. There is evidence that Marburg virus replicates in vascular endothelial cells, with subsequent necrosis. Other researchers have also shown that Ebola virus may exert its effects via a glycoprotein, synthesized in either a secreted or transmembrane form. The secreted glycoprotein interacts with neutrophils to inhibit early activation of the inflammatory response, while the transmembrane glycoprotein binds to endothelial cells. Ebola virus produces disease in humans and subhuman primates; onset is within 4 to 6 days of inoculation. The reservoir, although uncertain, is thought to be in small mammals, perhaps rodents. Serosurveys of humans residing in the areas where outbreaks have occurred suggest that human infections may be relatively common; as much as 7% of the survey group had antibodies, indicating past infection. In symptomatic infections, the mortality for both Marburg and Ebola viruses is extremely high (30 to 80%).

Reservoir may be small mammals

Mortality high in symptomatic infection

As with the arenavirus-associated hemorrhagic fevers, the diagnosis of infection by these agents is suggested by a similar syndrome and recent travel history. Person-to-person transmission similar to that described for Lassa fever occurs in Ebola virus infections and may be possible with Marburg virus. Diagnosis can be confirmed in a reference center by isolation of virus, as well as by serologic methods employing indirect immunofluorescence or EIA. However, as with the arenavirus-associated hemorrhagic fevers, utmost care in isolation precautions and prompt notification of public health authorities are mandatory for suspected cases before any diagnostic attempts are made. There is no specific therapy for the infections.

Diagnosis and precautions similar to arenavirus hemorrhagic fevers

HANTAVIRUSES

Hantavirus Hemorrhagic Fever

Korean hemorrhagic fever (KHF) is endemic to Korea and surrounding areas in the Far East. It is an important cause of hemorrhagic fever, often complicated by varying degrees of acute renal failure. In the 1950s, thousands of military personnel developed the disease during the Korean War. The first reported isolation of KHF was in 1978, when the antigen was detected in the lung tissues of wild rodents (*Apodemus* species) by indirect immunofluorescence using convalescent sera from affected patients. No illness was apparent in the rodents, suggesting a reservoir mechanism and mode of transmission similar to those described for the arenaviruses. Additional work indicated that the agent is a member of the family Bunyaviridae, and the generic designation of *Hantavirus* was given.

Causes of hemorrhagic fever during Korean War

Detected in lung of wild rodents

Evidence has accumulated indicating that other agents with close antigenic similarities to KHF virus are responsible for hemorrhagic–renal syndromes occurring throughout northern Eurasia, including Russia, Eastern Europe, Finland, and Scandinavia. These syndromes have been given a variety of names, including nephropathia epidemica. Methods similar to those used to detect KHF have detected nephropathia epidemica antigen in the lungs of small rodents (bank voles) in Finland.

Other viruses similar to KHF throughout northern Eurasia

Other *Hantavirus* Infections

It has been known for some time that rodents in the United States may be infected with a hantavirus, but no associated human disease was recognized. In early 1993, an outbreak of fulminant respiratory disease with high mortality (50 to 75%) occurred in the southwestern United States. This syndrome (hantavirus pulmonary syndrome, or HPS) has been related to at least three hantaviruses, of which Sin Nombre virus is the most common. Infections are associated with an increased population of infected mice in and around human habitations. Of the more than 30 documented HPS illnesses reported in 1993, 23 patients resided in rural areas of a region bordered by the states of Arizona, New Mexico, and Colorado; however, cases have also been reported from at least 19 other states. The virus is believed to be transmitted to humans most often by inhalation of infected rodent excreta, by the conjunctival route, or by direct contact with skin breaks. Human-to-human spread has not been encountered. Public health measures to inform inhabitants of routes of spread and to reduce the rodent population appear to have controlled the outbreak.

Hantavirus among rodents in United States

Southwestern US outbreak related to deer mice

Humans infected by inhalation of aerosolized excreta

No human-to-human transmission

Ribavirin may be useful

Treatment has involved aggressive respiratory support. Intravenous ribavirin appears to have been of benefit in Asian hantavirus infections; however, there are no data as yet regarding its efficacy against the US strains.

VESICULAR STOMATITIS VIRUS

A rhabdovirus, vesicular stomatitis virus, that causes outbreaks of disease in cattle, pigs, and horses can be transmitted between animals by arthropods. Human infection is acquired by contact with infected animals but is unusual; it consists of a self-limited febrile illness and occasional herpes-like eruptions over the lips and mucosa.

ADDITIONAL READING

Chen Y, Maguirre T, Hileman RE, et al. Dengue virus infectivity depends on envelope protein binding to target cell heparan sulfate. *Nature Med* 1997;3:866–871. This report illustrates how determining the nature of viral receptors facilitates understanding of viral pathogenesis and possible strategies for treatment.

Jahrling PB, Peters CJ. Lymphocytic choriomeningitis virus. A neglected pathogen of man. *Arch Pathol Lab Med* 1992;116:486–488. The history, unique biology, and clinical features of this virus are well summarized.

Johnson RT. Acute encephalitis. *Clinical Infect Dis* 1996;23:219–226. For the clinically curious, this article discusses the features of arbovirus encephalitides comparing them with other causes of brain inflammation.

Kautner I, Robinson MJ, Kuhnle U. Dengue virus infection: Epidemiology, pathogenesis, clinical presentation, diagnosis, and prevention. *J Pediatr* 1997;131:516–524. An excellent clinical review.

Khan AS, Khabbaz RF, Armstrong LR, et al. Hantavirus pulmonary syndrome: The first 100 U.S. cases. *J Infect Dis* 1996;173:1297–1303. A thorough review of the syndrome.

Martin AA, Gubler DJ. West Nile encephalitis: An emerging disease in the United States. *Clinical Infect Dis* 2001;33:1713–1719. A review of events that transpired and what might be expected in the future.

McCormick JB, King IJ, Webb PA, et al. Lassa fever. Effective therapy with ribavirin. *N Engl J Med* 1986;314:20–26. This article demonstrates approaches and difficulties encountered in evaluating a new drug for a serious disease.

McJunkin JE, Khan R, de los Reyes EC, et al. Treatment of severe LaCrosse encephalitis with intravenous ribavirin following diagnosis by brain biopsy. *Pediatrics* 1997;99:261–267. This intriguing case report illustrates how the laboratory can be used effectively in diagnosing and managing a serious disease.

Yang Z, Delgado R, Xu L, et al. Distinct cellular interactions of secreted and transmembrane Ebola virus glycoproteins. *Science* 1998;279:1034–1037. Insight is provided for how this virus may disarm host cell defenses and cause severe damage to the vascular endothelium.

CHAPTER 41

Rabies

W. LAWRENCE DREW

Rabies is an acute fatal viral illness of the central nervous system (CNS). The word rabies is derived from the Latin verb to rage, which suggests the appearance of the rabid patient. It can affect all mammals and is transmitted between them by infected secretions, most often by bite. It was first recognized more than 3000 years ago and has been the most feared of infectious diseases. It is said that Aristotle recognized that rabies could be spread by a rabid dog.

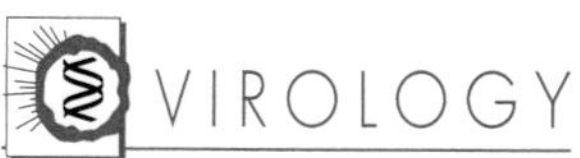

VIROLOGY

The rabies virus is a bullet-shaped, enveloped, single-stranded RNA virus of the rhabdovirus group (Fig 41–1). Other pathogens in this group include the vesicular stomatitis virus (see Chapter 40). Rabies virus is large, with dimensions of about 180 by 70 nm. Knob-like glycoprotein excrescences, which elicit neutralizing and hemagglutination-inhibiting antibodies, cover the surface of the virion. In the past, a single antigenically homogeneous virus was believed responsible for all rabies; however, differences in cell culture growth characteristics of isolates from different animal sources, some differences in virulence for experimental animals, and antigenic differences in surface glycoproteins have indicated strain heterogeneity among rabies virus isolates. These studies may help to explain some of the biological differences as well as the occasional case of "vaccine failure."

RNA virus is bullet-shaped

Strains from different sources are antigenically heterogeneous

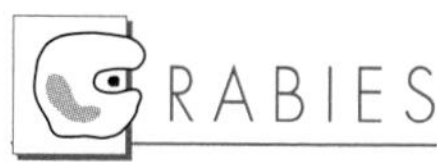

RABIES

CLINICAL CAPSULE

Rabies involves the development of severe neurologic symptoms and signs in a patient who was previously bitten by an animal. The neurologic abnormalities are very characteristic, with a relentlessly progressive excess of motor activity, agitation, hallucinations, and salivation. The patient appears to be foaming at the mouth and has severe throat contractions if swallowing is attempted. The neurologic abnormalities are explained by spread of the virus from the bite wound into the CNS and then centrifugally to the autonomic nervous system.

EPIDEMIOLOGY

Rabies exists in two epizootic forms, urban and sylvatic. The urban form is associated with unimmunized dogs or cats, and the sylvatic form occurs in wild skunks, foxes,

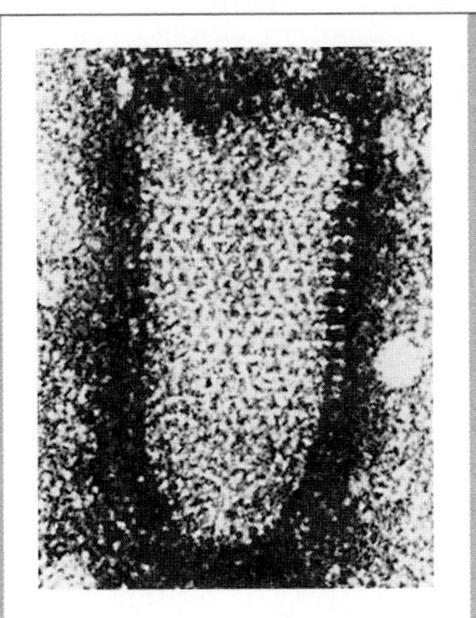

FIGURE 41–1
Rabies virus. (*Reprinted with permission from Dr. K. Hummular, from Hummuler K, Koprowski M, Wiktor TJ.* J Virol *1967;1:152–170.*)

wolves, raccoons, and bats but not rodents or rabbits. Introduction of an infected animal into a different geographic area can lead to infection of many new members of that species. For example, raccoon hunters apparently are to blame for the sudden appearance of raccoon strain rabies in West Virginia and Virginia in 1977. Prior to that time, the nearest cases of raccoon rabies were found several hundred miles away in South Carolina. The hunters are believed to have imported infected raccoons from another state. Since 1977, raccoon rabies has spread from West Virginia and Virginia to 12 northeastern states.

Risks to humans are from bites by infected carnivores, omnivores, and bats

Aerosol spread from exposure in bat caves

Human infection, or the much more common infection of cattle, is incidental, is blind-ended, and does not contribute to maintenance or transmission of the disease. In the United States, more than 75% of reported cases of rabies in animals occur among wildlife. Human exposures may be from wild animals or from unimmunized dogs or cats. In recent years, there has been a decrease of US cases to less than two per year, and bat exposure has been the source in almost all cases despite a resurgence of rabies in skunks and raccoons. An occasional case has resulted from aerosol exposure (eg, bat caves and no bite). Domestic animal bites are very important sources of rabies in developing countries because of lack of enforcement of animal immunization. Infection in domestic animals usually represents a spillover from infection in wildlife reservoirs. Human infection tends to occur where animal rabies is common and where there is a large population of unimmunized domestic animals. Worldwide, the occurrence of human rabies is estimated to be about 15,000 cases per year, with the highest attack rates in Southeast Asia, the Philippines, and the Indian subcontinent.

PATHOGENESIS

Replicates initially in muscle and then enters peripheral nervous system

Spreads to CNS gray matter

Negri bodies found in neurons

The essential first event in human or animal rabies infection is the inoculation of virus through the epidermis, usually as a result of an animal bite. Inhalation of heavily contaminated material, such as bat droppings, can also cause infection. Rabies virus first replicates in striated muscle tissue at the site of inoculation. Immunization at this time is presumed to prevent migration of the virus into neural tissues. In the absence of immunity, the virus then enters the peripheral nervous system at the neuromuscular junctions and spreads to the CNS, where it replicates exclusively within the gray matter. It then passes centrifugally along autonomic nerves to reach other tissues, including the salivary glands, adrenal medulla, kidneys, and lungs. Passage into the salivary glands in animals facilitates further transmission of the disease by infected saliva. The neuropathology of rabies resembles that of other viral diseases of the CNS, with infiltration of lymphocytes and plasma cells into CNS tissue and nerve cell destruction. The pathognomonic lesion is the Negri body (Fig 41-2), an eosinophilic cytoplasmic inclusion distributed throughout the brain, particularly in the hippocampus, cerebral cortex, cerebellum, and dorsal spinal ganglia.

Incubation period can be prolonged for months

The incubation period ranges from 10 days to a year, depending on the amount of virus introduced, the amount of tissue involved, the host immune mechanisms, the innervation of the site, and the distance the virus must travel from the site of inoculation

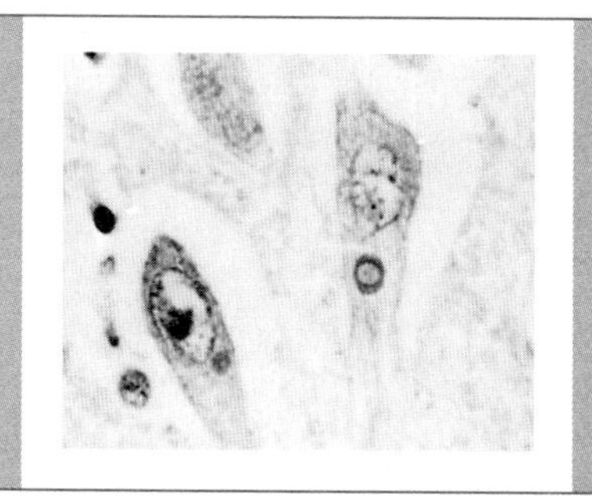

FIGURE 41–2
Negri body in cytoplasm of neuron.
(*Courtesy of Dr. Daniel P. Perl.*)

to the CNS. Thus, the incubation period is generally shorter with face wounds than with leg wounds. Immunization early in the incubation period frequently aborts the infection.

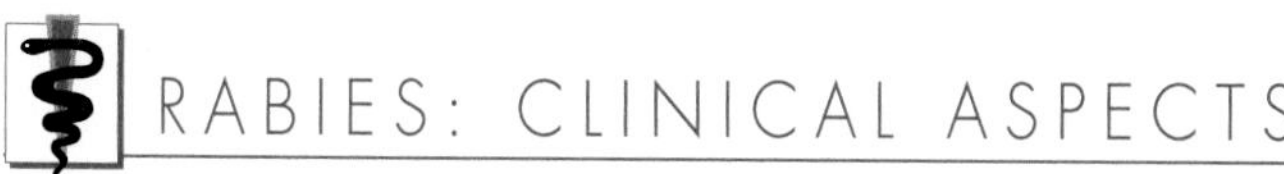

RABIES: CLINICAL ASPECTS

MANIFESTATIONS

Rabies in humans usually results from a bite by a rabid animal or contamination of a wound by its saliva. It presents as an acute, fulminant, fatal encephalitis; human survivors have been reported only occasionally. After an average incubation period of 20 to 90 days the disease begins as a nonspecific illness marked by fever, headache, malaise, nausea, and vomiting. Abnormal sensations at or around the site of viral inoculation occur frequently and probably reflect local nerve involvement. The onset of encephalitis is marked by periods of excess motor activity and agitation. Hallucinations, combativeness, muscle spasms, signs of meningeal irritation, seizures, and focal paralysis occur. Periods of mental dysfunction are interspersed with completely lucid periods; however, as the disease progresses, the patient lapses into coma. Autonomic nervous system involvement often results in increased salivation. Brainstem and cranial nerve dysfunction is characteristic, with double vision, facial palsies, and difficulty in swallowing. The combination of excess salivation and difficulty in swallowing produces the fearful picture of "foaming at the mouth." Hydrophobia, the painful, violent involuntary contractions of the diaphragm and accessory respiratory, pharyngeal, and laryngeal muscles initiated by swallowing liquids, is seen in about 50% of cases. Involvement of the respiratory center produces respiratory paralysis, the major cause of death. Occasionally rabies may appear as an ascending paralysis resembling Guillain–Barré syndrome. The median survival after onset of symptoms is 4 days, with a maximum of 20 days unless artificial supportive measures are instituted. Recovery is rare and has only been seen in partially immunized individuals.

Encephalitis common, sometimes with ascending paralysis

Almost uniformly fatal

DIAGNOSIS

The CSF of a rabies patient shows minimal to no abnormalities with some patients exhibiting a lymphocytic pleocytosis (5 to 30 cells/mm^3). The test of choice in a live patient is detection of rabies antigen by immunofluorescent stain of a nape of the neck biopsy. PCR of CSF or saliva may supplant the neck biopsy. Laboratory diagnosis of rabies in animals or deceased patients is accomplished by demonstration of virus in brain tissue. Viral antigen can be demonstrated rapidly by immunofluorescence procedures. Intracerebral inoculation of infected brain tissue or secretions into suckling mice results in death in 3 to 10 days. Histologic examination of their brain tissue shows Negri bodies in 80% of cases; electron microscopy may demonstrate both Negri bodies and rhabdovirus particles. Specific antibodies to rabies virus can be detected in serum but generally only late in the disease.

Virus or antigen detected in brain tissue

TREATMENT

Prevention is the mainstay of controlling human rabies. Intensive supportive care has resulted in two or three long-term survivals; despite the best modern medical care, however,

No specific treatment is available

the mortality still exceeds 90%. In addition, because of the infrequency of the disease, many cases die without definitive diagnosis. Human hyperimmune antirabies globulin, interferon, and vaccine do not alter the disease once symptoms have developed.

PREVENTION

Vaccine-induced antibody inhibits viral spread

In the late 1800s Pasteur, noting the long incubation period of rabies, suggested that a vaccine to induce an immune response before the development of disease might be useful in prevention. He apparently successfully vaccinated Joseph Meister, a boy severely bitten and exposed to rabies, with multiple injections of a crude vaccine made from dried spinal cord of rabies-infected rabbits. This treatment emerged as one of the best known and most noteworthy accomplishments in the annals of medicine. It is now believed that vaccination induces antibody that is either neutralizing or inhibits cell to cell spread of virus. Natural infection does not lead to an early immune response and limitation of viral migration, because the virus is replicating in muscle or neural tissue and lymphocytes do not access these sites. Cytotoxic T lymphocytes are also induced by vaccine and appear to be directed against an antigen of the virus.

High-risk individuals include veterinarians, spelunkers, laboratory workers

Currently, the prevention of rabies is divided into preexposure and postexposure prophylaxis. Preexposure prophylaxis is recommended for individuals at high risk of contact with rabies virus, such as veterinarians, spelunkers, laboratory workers, and animal handlers. The vaccine currently used in the United States for preexposure prophylaxis employs an attenuated rabies virus grown in human diploid cell culture and inactivated with β-propiolactone. Preexposure prophylaxis consists of two subcutaneous injections of vaccine given 1 month apart, followed by a booster dose several months later.

Careful history and studies of biting animal are important in decision-making

Postexposure prophylaxis requires careful evaluation and judgment. Every year more than one million Americans are bitten by animals, and in each instance a decision must be made whether to initiate postexposure rabies prophylaxis. The physician must consider (1) whether the individual came into physical contact with saliva or another substance likely to contain rabies virus; (2) whether there was significant wounding or abrasion; (3) whether rabies is known or suspected in the animal species and area associated with the exposure; (4) whether the bite was provoked or unprovoked (i.e., the circumstances surrounding the exposure); and (5) whether the animal is available for laboratory examination. Any wild animal or ill, unvaccinated, or stray domestic animal involved in a possible rabies exposure, such as an unprovoked bite, should be captured and killed. The head should be sent immediately to an appropriate laboratory, usually at the state health department, for search for rabies antigen by immunofluorescence. If examination of the brain by this technique is negative for rabies virus, it can be assumed that the saliva contains no virus and that the exposed person requires no treatment. If the test is positive, the patient should be given postexposure prophylaxis. It should be noted that rodents and rabbits are not important vectors of rabies virus.

Rabies immune globulin plus vaccine necessary in postexposure management

Postexposure prophylaxis is based on immediate, thorough washing of the wound with soap and water; passive immunization with hyperimmune globulin, of which at least half the dose should be instilled around the wound site; and active immunization with antirabies vaccine. With human diploid vaccine, five doses given on days 1, 3, 7, 14, and 28 are recommended. Physicians should always seek the advice of the local health department when the question of rabies prophylaxis arises.

ADDITIONAL READING

Advisory Committee on Immunization Practices (ACIP). Rabies prevention–United States 1999. *Morb Mortal Wkly Rep* 1999;48(RR-1):1-22. This report provides specific guidelines for rabies prophylaxis.

Fishbein DB, Robinson LE. Rabies. *N Engl J Med* 1993;329:1632–1638. A review of the epidemiology of rabies, including changes in animal reservoirs in differing geographical locations.

CHAPTER 42

Retroviruses, Human Immunodeficiency Virus, and Acquired Immunodeficiency Syndrome

JAMES J. CHAMPOUX AND W. LAWRENCE DREW

Retroviruses are enveloped, single-stranded plus-sense RNA viruses. They encode an enzyme called **reverse transcriptase** that converts the RNA genome into a double-stranded DNA copy that subsequently becomes integrated into the host cell DNA. Representatives of two major groups are considered in this chapter: the **oncoviruses** (*onco-*, "related to a tumor") and the **lentiviruses** (*lenti-*, "slow"). Like most enveloped viruses, all retroviruses are highly susceptible to factors that affect surface tension and are thus not transmissible through air, dust, or fomites under normal conditions, but instead intimate contact with the infecting source is required.

Enveloped RNA viruses that encode reverse transcriptase

Members of the oncovirus subgroup of retroviruses have long been associated with a variety of cancers in animals, including leukemias, lymphomas, and sarcomas, but until recent years had not been found to infect humans. The first human retrovirus, human T-cell leukemia virus type I (HTLV-1), was discovered in the late 1970s. It was shown to cause adult T-cell leukemia, a rare malignancy found only in Japan, Africa, and the Caribbean, although serologic evidence shows that the virus also occurs in the United States and has raised the possibility of an association with some chronic neurologic conditions. A relative of HTLV-1, HTLV-2, has been associated with a few rare cases of T-cell malignancies, including hairy cell leukemia, but its precise role in these diseases remains unclear.

Oncoviruses cause tumors in many animals

HTLV-1 and -2 associated with human leukemias

The most important disease resulting from a human retrovirus infection, **acquired immunodeficiency syndrome (AIDS),** is caused by either of two lentiviruses termed human immunodeficiency viruses types 1 and 2 (**HIV-1** and **HIV-2**). A devastating disease, for which there is no present cure, AIDS has spurred unprecedented research efforts to determine the nature and pathogenic mechanisms of the viruses in the hope of finding effective drugs and vaccines. Most of our present knowledge of HIV is derived from studies on HIV-1, which is the major cause of AIDS worldwide.

HIV-1 and -2 are lentiviruses that cause AIDS

Oncoviruses do not kill the cell they infect, but instead they continue to produce new virus indefinitely. This property, combined with the fact that they can transduce growth-promoting genes called **oncogenes** into a recipient cell, accounts in part for their

Oncoviruses usually not cytolytic; they transduce or activate oncogenes

ability to cause malignancies (see Chapter 7 and below). With lentivirus infections, the cell–virus relationship is quite different. Lentiviruses can apparently persist for long periods of time in a latent state without causing much cell killing, only to become highly cytolytic when the infected cells are subjected to certain stimuli. The prototype lentivirus is visna virus, which causes a slow degenerative neurologic disease in sheep. Like visna, HIV-1 can remain latent in the infected cell without serious effects, but when induced to replicate, high levels of virus are produced and the cell dies. Although HIV-1 can infect a variety of human cell types, its most drastic effects appear to result from destruction of the CD4+ subclass of T lymphocytes, which play a central role in the capacity of the host to mount effective and protective immunologic responses to a wide range of infections.

Lentiviruses can become cytopathic after latent period

HIV attacks and destroys CD4+ T lymphocytes

RETROVIRUSES

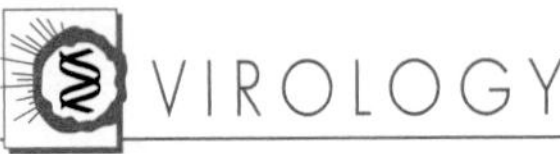

STRUCTURE

All retroviruses are remarkably similar in their basic composition. The structure of HIV-1 is depicted in Fig 42–1. The virion is about 100 nm in diameter, and because it contains two copies of the RNA genome, it is diploid. The RNA genome is coated with the nucleocapsid protein (NC), and the RNA–protein complexes are enclosed in a capsid (CA) composed of multiple subunits. Like all enveloped viruses, the membrane is acquired during budding from the host cell, but the surface (SU, also called gp120) and transmembrane (TM, also called gp41) glycoproteins found in the envelope are virally encoded. Between the capsid and the envelope is the matrix (MA) protein. In addition to the structural proteins shown in Fig 42–1, the virion core contains three virus-specific proteins that are essential for viral replication: reverse transcriptase (RT), protease (PR), and integrase (IN). The relationships between the viral genes found in all retroviruses (*gag, pol,* and *env*) and the proteins they encode are presented in Table 42–1. Some retroviruses, including HIV-1, encode additional regulatory and accessory proteins as will be described below.

Virion contains two single-stranded RNA molecules

Envelope acquired during budding contains two viral glycoproteins

LIFE CYCLE

Figure 42–2 depicts the life cycle of a typical retrovirus and serves to illustrate the many unique aspects of retroviral replication that could be potential targets of therapeutic intervention.

Viral Entry

The virions adsorb to cellular membrane receptors and enter the cell by direct fusion with the plasma membrane. For HIV-1, the virion attachment protein is the SU glycoprotein

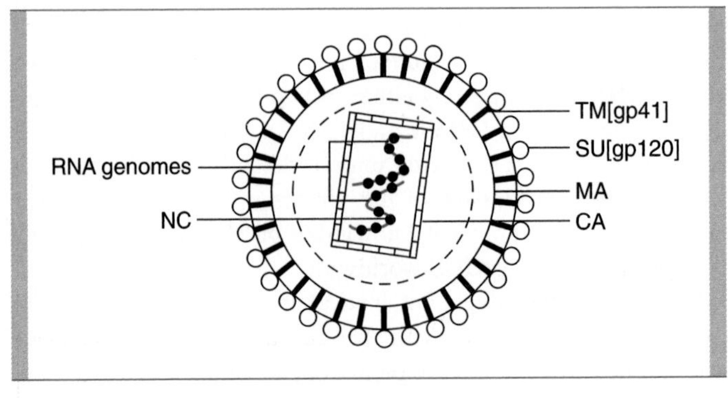

FIGURE 42–1
Structure of HIV particle. The two RNA molecules enclosed within the capsid (CA) are coated with the nucleocapsid protein (NC). The matrix protein (MA) lies just inside the membrane envelope. The envelope contains two membrane glycoproteins, gp41 and gp120, also called transmembrane protein (TM) and surface protein (SU), respectively.

TABLE 42–1

Major Retroviral Genes and Proteins

GENE[a]	PROTEIN PRODUCTS	FUNCTION
gag	Matrix (MA)	Structural
	Capsid (CA)	Structural
	Nucleocapsid (NC)	Structural
	Protease[b] (PR)	Protein processing
pol	Protease[b] (PR)	Protein processing
	Reverse transcriptase (RT)	DNA synthesis
	Integrase (IN)	Integration
env	Surface glycoprotein (SU)	Adsorption
	Transmembrane protein (TM)	Fusion of envelope with plasma membrane

[a] Each gene encodes a polyprotein that is subsequently processed by proteolysis to yield the individual proteins.
[b] The protease is encoded in either the *gag* gene or the *pol* gene, depending on the virus.

gp120, and the cellular receptor is the CD4 molecule with one of the chemokine receptors, CXCR4 or CCR5 acting as coreceptors. These receptors occur primarily in the plasma membrane of CD4+ T lymphocytes, cells of the monocyte–macrophage series, and some other target cells. Early in the infection of an individual, the viruses are often macrophage-tropic because they preferentially use the CCR5 coreceptor. The emergence of syncytia-forming variants that use the CXCR4 coreceptor and are T-cell tropic appears

HIV-1 surface (SU) glycoprotein gp120 attaches to CD4 cell and chemokine coreceptors

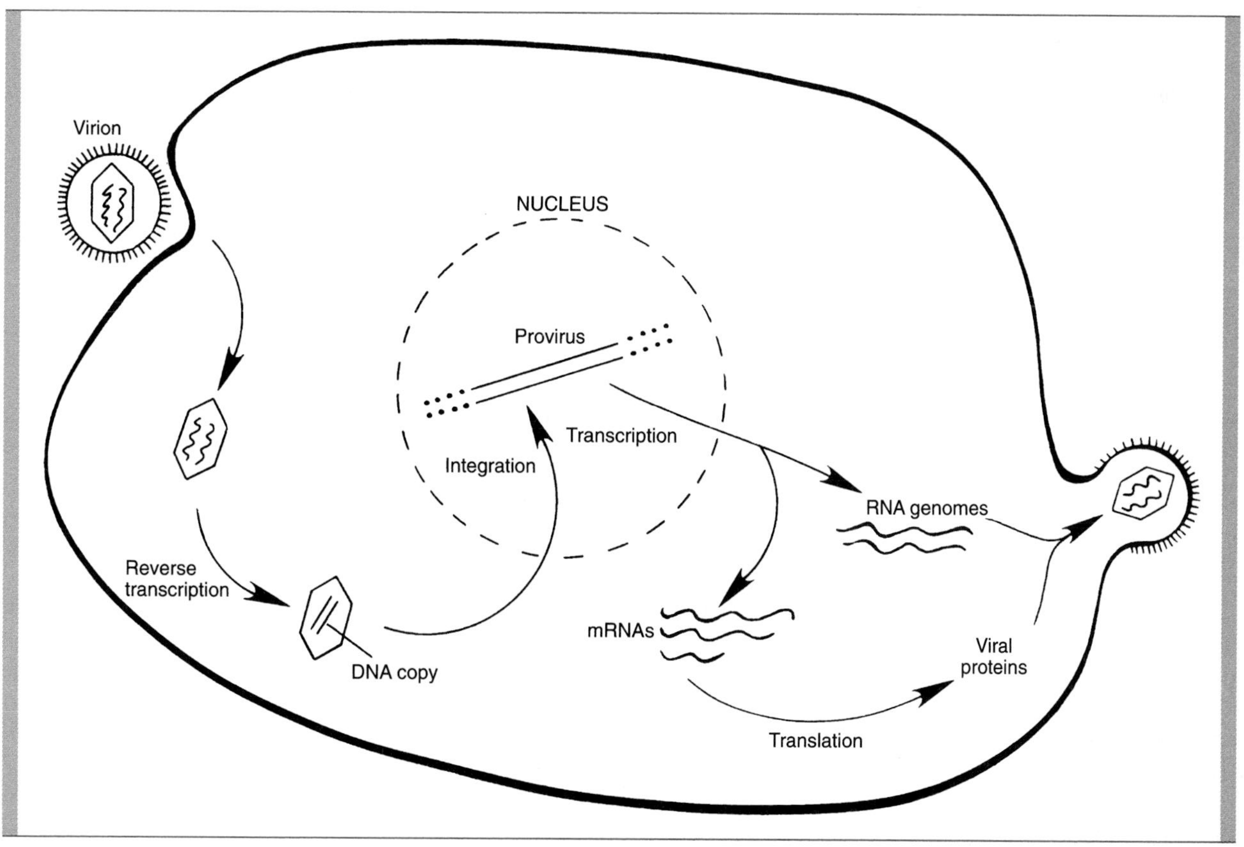

FIGURE 42–2
Retroviral life cycle.

Transmembrane (TM) gp41 protein mediates fusion of viral and cell membranes

to correlate with rapid advancement to AIDS. The HIV-1 transmembrane TM protein gp41 is responsible for fusion of the viral and cell membranes, leading to entry of the virion core complex into the cytoplasm of the cell.

Can infect cells without CD4 molecule

Fusion provides direct cell-to-cell transmission

HIV-1 can also infect cells such as fibroblasts and certain brain cells that lack the CD4 surface molecule, apparently because the chemokine receptors in combination with the fusion-inducing activity of the TM protein is sufficient in these cases to promote entry. Fusion activity may also play an important role in amplification of the effects of the virus infection, particularly during the later stages of the infection, because infected cells expressing viral glycoproteins in their membranes readily fuse with uninfected CD4+ T lymphocytes to form large syncytia. This process appears to provide a means for cell-to-cell transmission of the virus that bypasses the usual extracellular phase and may contribute to the overall depletion of CD4+ lymphocytes in an infected individual.

Viral RNA Replication

Reverse transcriptase copies RNA to double-stranded DNA

DNA integrates into host chromosome and replicates with the cell as a provirus

Among the RNA viruses, retroviral replication is unique. Soon after entry of the viral core into the cytoplasm of the infected cell, the RNA is copied into double-stranded DNA by reverse transcriptase, the virion-associated DNA polymerase. The overall process is referred to as **reverse transcription** and results in a linear DNA molecule that enters the nucleus and integrates more-or-less at random into a host cell chromosome. Once the viral genetic information has been converted to DNA and integrated, it essentially becomes part of the cellular genome. The viral genes, called the **provirus,** are therefore replicated and faithfully inherited as long as the infected cell continues to divide.

Provirus includes its own promoter and signals that control transcription by host RNA polymerase

Genomic RNA and spliced mRNAs are both produced: the latter encode envelope glycoproteins and regulatory proteins

HIV-1 can control extent of genomic or spliced mRNA production

Special sequences contained within the RNA are duplicated during the reverse transcription process so that the integrated provirus contains identical long terminal repeats (LTRs) at its ends. The LTR sequences contain the appropriate promoter, enhancer, and other signals required for transcription of the viral genes by the host RNA polymerase II. Transcription produces a full-length RNA genome and one or more spliced mRNAs. For the oncoviruses, the predominant spliced mRNA is translated to produce the envelope glycoproteins, but in HIV-1, a series of spliced mRNAs are produced that encode, in addition to the envelope proteins, a series of viral regulatory and accessory proteins. Unlike most retroviruses, HIV-1 and the other lentiviruses apparently exert considerable control over whether the primary transcripts are allocated to full-length RNA or are spliced to produce mRNAs (see below). With the exception of these regulatory and accessory proteins, all retroviral proteins are initially translated as polyproteins that are subsequently processed by proteolysis into the individual protein molecules. The enzyme responsible for most of these protein cleavages is the virus-specific protease (PR) that is encoded in either the *gag* gene or the *pol* gene, depending on the virus (see Table 42–1).

RNase H activity degrades original RNA genome

Integrase-catalyzed integration is random in host DNA

Integrated DNA is transcribed by host RNA polymerase

A simplified view of retroviral RNA replication is presented in Figure 42–3. In addition to DNA polymerase activity, the reverse transcriptase possesses an RNase H activity that is responsible for degrading the RNA portion of the DNA–RNA hybrid (+RNA/−DNA) produced in the first phase of reverse transcription. The immediate product of reverse transcription is a linear double-stranded DNA molecule that is flanked by the LTR sequences. The viral integrase (IN) catalyzes the integration of the linear DNA into host DNA. The integration process is highly specific with respect to the viral DNA, and two base pairs are generally lost from each end of the DNA. The choice of a target site for integration into the cellular DNA appears, however, to be nearly random. A short sequence of base pairs in the target DNA (four to six, depending on the virus) is duplicated during the integration process, and these repeat sequences immediately flank the integrated provirus. The replication process is completed by transcription of the proviral DNA by the host RNA polymerase II.

It should be noted that the scheme represented in Figure 42–3 also describes the replication cycle for hepatitis B virus (see Chapter 37). Instead of packaging the RNA form of the genome as occurs with retroviruses, hepatitis B virus packages the double-stranded DNA that is the immediate product of reverse transcription.

Of all the known retroviruses, HIV-1 possesses the most error-prone reverse transcriptase. The consequence of this high error rate is that each time the viral RNA is reverse

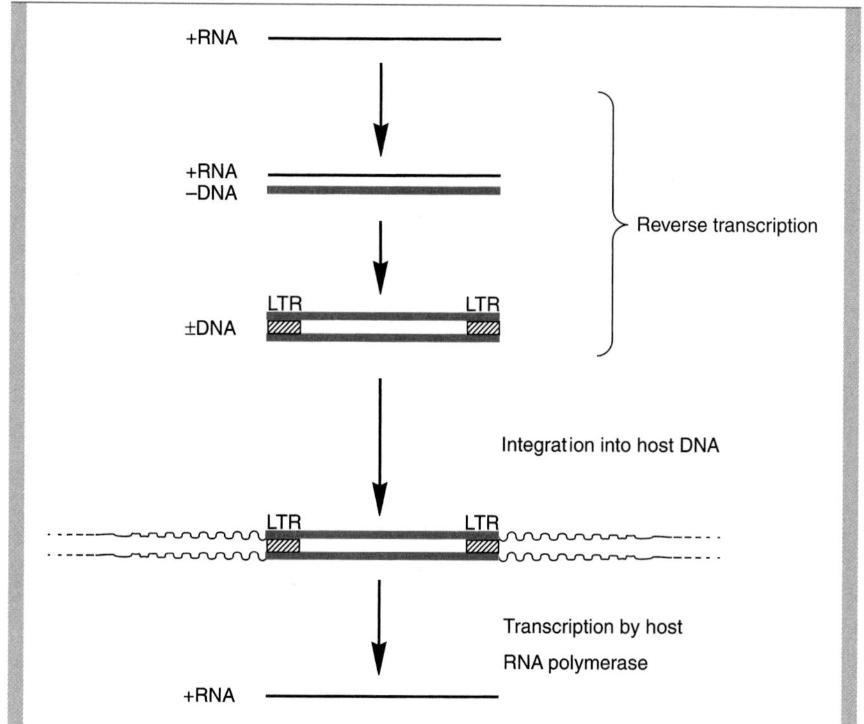

FIGURE 42–3
Retroviral RNA replication. LTR, long terminal repeat.

transcribed, one to two new mutations are introduced into the resulting DNA. Because the process of transcription of the integrated proviral DNA to produce new viral genomes is also error prone, mutant genomes accumulate rapidly over the course of an infection. The end result is a quasispecies that accounts for the many nucleotide differences observed between different isolates (even from the same infected individual) and for the variability of the SU envelope protein gp120. It may explain, in part, the failure of the immune system to control the infection and also the increases in viral virulence that appear to occur during the course of the infection.

HIV reverse transcriptase is error prone

Isolates from the same patient can differ in multiple properties

RETROVIRAL GENES

The organization of the genome of different types of retroviruses is shown in Figure 42–4 (see also Table 42–1). The order of the genes for a typical retrovirus is *gag–pol–env.* The *gag* (group-specific antigen) gene encodes the structural proteins of the virus and, in some cases, the protease. The *pol* (polymerase) gene encodes the reverse transcriptase, the integrase, and sometimes the protease. The *env* (envelope) gene encodes the two membrane glycoproteins found in the viral envelope. Not surprisingly, the SU protein (gp120 in HIV-1) is responsible for the host range of the virus and its antigenicity.

Genome is organized into *gag, pol,* and *env* genes

The genomes of acute transforming oncoviruses have a variety of structures, but one feature is common to nearly all of them: some viral genes are replaced by genes derived from their hosts that render them oncogenic (see below). In every case, the signals required for reverse transcription and for transcription of the provirus, which are located near the ends of the RNA, are retained in the infecting virus. In the example shown in Figure 42–4, the *pol* gene and parts of both the viral *gag* and *env* genes are deleted, but other configurations are possible. Such oncoviruses are defective and replicate only in the presence of a helper virus that can supply the missing functions.

Some retroviruses carry host genes rendering them oncogenic

Defective transforming oncogenic viruses require helper virus

A comparison of the genetic makeup of HIV-1 with that of a typical retrovirus (see Fig 42–4) reveals a larger number of genes and a much more complex organization. HIV-1 contains, in addition to the *gag, pol,* and *env* genes, an array of other genes (*tat, rev, nef, vif, vpr,* and *vpu*). Expression of these genes requires mRNA splicing, and all apparently encode proteins that serve regulatory or accessory roles during the infection (see below). HTLV-1 encodes the regulatory proteins, Tax and Rex, which are analogous to the HIV-1

HIV-1 has multiple regulatory genes

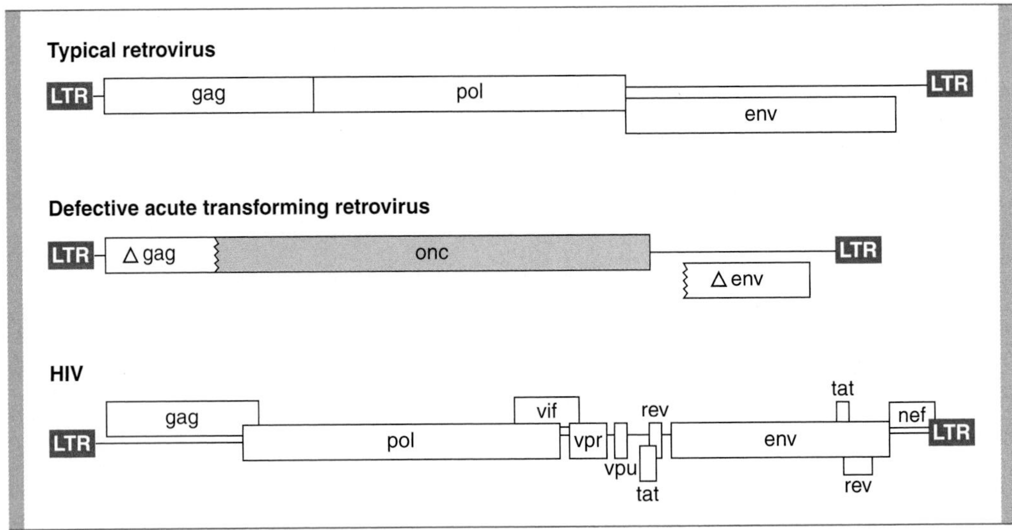

FIGURE 42–4
Maps of the integrated forms of various retroviral genomes are drawn with the genes and long terminal repeats (LTRs) shown as boxes. The vertical displacements of the boxes above and below the lines depict the different reading frames of the coding segments.

Tat and Rev proteins. The names of the genes that have been best characterized and the proteins and functions they determine are listed in Table 42–2.

TRANSFORMATION BY RETROVIRUSES

Oncogenic retroviruses appear to transform cells to an oncogenic state by three distinct mechanisms (see Chapter 7).

Noncytocidal viruses carrying cellular oncogenes can produce persistent transformation

First, the defective acute transforming viruses (see Fig 42–4) have acquired a cellular gene (thereafter called an **oncogene**) that when expressed in the infected cell results in loss of normal growth control. On infection, the transduced oncogene is expressed from the viral LTR promoter, resulting in a rapid and acute onset of malignant disease. Persistent transformation by oncogene transduction is possible only for those retroviruses that are not cytocidal. More than 30 different oncogenes have been identified in a variety of animal retroviruses, but no human retroviruses are known that transform by this mechanism.

Integration adjacent to cellular protooncogenes can activate them

The second mechanism is called **insertional mutagenesis.** Integration of a retrovirus in the vicinity of particular cellular genes can cause inappropriate expression of the gene, resulting in uncontrolled cell growth. These cellular genes are called

TABLE 42–2

HIV-1 Regulatory and Accessory Proteins

Gene	Protein	Function
tat	Tat	Transcriptional activator
rev	Rev	Promotes transport of unspliced mRNAs
nef	Nef	Downregulation of cellular CD4 and MHC I proteins
vpu	Vpu	Facilitate virus assembly and release
vpr	Vpr	Facilitates nuclear entry in nondividing cells
vif	Vif	Increases viral infectivity in certain cell types

Abbreviations: MHC, major histocompatibility complex.

protooncogenes, and insertional activation by the virus is apparently due to the close proximity of the integrated viral promoter or enhancer to the gene. Cancers that are caused by this mechanism have very long latent periods, because integration is random and only rarely occurs near a cellular protooncogene.

The causative agent of adult T-cell leukemia, HTLV-1, exemplifies the third mechanism. In this case, the integrated provirus in the leukemic cells from any one patient is found at a unique location on a particular chromosome. Thus, the tumors are probably monoclonal. The cancer is not the result of insertional activation, however, because the chromosomal location of the provirus is never the same in any two patients. Instead, transformation results from the continual expression of the viral *tax* gene (the HTLV-1 homolog of the HIV-1 *tat* gene; see Table 42–2). Apparently, the Tax protein not only can transactivate viral transcription in the same manner as Tat (see below), but Tax can also **transactivate** the expression of one or more cellular genes (possibly protooncogenes), resulting in malignant transformation.

HTLV-1 transforms by production of Tax, which activates cellular transforming genes

ROLES OF HIV-1 REGULATORY AND ACCESSORY PROTEINS

A unique feature of HIV-1 and other members of the lentivirus subfamily is the ability to produce a complex array of regulatory and accessory proteins that appear to be responsible for staging the infection, increasing the efficiency and yield of the infection, and in some cases contributing to viral latency. These proteins also appear to interact with cellular factors to modulate the infection differently in different host cells. The roles of the two HIV-1 regulatory genes, *tat* and *rev,* and the four accessory proteins, *nef, vpu, vpr,* and *vif,* are discussed below and summarized in Table 42–2. Although the four accessory proteins are dispensable in many cell culture systems, they appear to be important for the maximum pathogenic potential of the virus in infected individuals.

The products of the *tat* and *rev* regulatory genes are the Tat and Rev proteins, respectively. Both of these proteins have the effect of staging the infection, so that in the absence of abundant transcription of the proviral genome, only limited gene expression is possible. When the infected T-lymphocyte is stimulated, for example by antigen presentation, Tat and Rev play a positive role in promoting viral gene expression. In the absence of high levels of Tat, the host RNA polymerase initiates properly at the LTR promoter, but transcription is usually prematurely terminated leading to the production of short, dead-end transcripts. Tat is a transcriptional activator that acts at a sequence near the beginning of the viral mRNA, called TAR, to recruit cellular proteins to the transcribing RNA polymerase, resulting in a modification to the polymerase that prevents premature termination and allows complete transcription of the proviral genome.

Tat is transcriptional activator that promotes synthesis of full-length viral transcripts

The Rev protein acts at the level of mRNA splicing. Normally, unspliced cellular transcripts are retained in the nucleus and only fully spliced mRNAs are transported to the cytoplasm for translation. The only viral proteins that are made from fully spliced mRNAs are Tat, Rev, and Nef, and consequently only these proteins are found early after infection, when there is no mechanism to prevent complete splicing of pre-mRNAs. To express the Vif, Vpr, and Vpu proteins, and the Env polyprotein, which are all made from singly spliced transcripts, as well as the Gag and Pol polyproteins, which are translated from the unspliced genomic RNA, it is necessary to transport incompletely spliced RNAs to the cytoplasm. Transport of partially spliced transcripts is accomplished by Rev binding to a site on the viral RNA within the *env* gene called the Rev-responsive element (RRE). The RNA-bound Rev then interacts with normal cellular machinery responsible for protein export from the nucleus to mediate the movement of the RNA through the nuclear pore. By promoting translation of the virion structural proteins and some of the accessory proteins, Rev turns up late gene expression that leads directly to a high rate of virus production.

Rev promotes export of unspliced and partially spliced transcripts to cytoplasm

The Nef accessory protein enhances virus production and virion infectivity and also appears to interfere with immune recognition of infected cells. Nef causes the internalization and degradation of the CD4 protein, which likely contributes to virus release by preventing the formation of complexes between the cellular receptor and newly synthesized

Nef downregulates CD4 to promote virus release and also downregulates MHC I to interfere with immune recognition

virions. Nef also causes the downregulation of cell surface major histocompatibility complex (MHC) I molecules, which may prevent recognition of infected cells by cytotoxic T lymphocytes. In addition, virions produced in the absence of the Nef protein are at least partially blocked at some step prior to integration. The combination of these and perhaps other effects allows the Nef protein to play an essential pathogenic role in an infected individual.

Vpu targets CD4 destruction and virion release

The Vpu protein appears to play two separate roles during the late stages of infection. In the absence of Vpu, the Env protein forms complexes with CD4 in the endoplasmic reticulum and fails to reach the plasma membrane of the cell. One of the roles of Vpu is to target the destruction of CD4 in the endoplasmic reticulum to allow for incorporation of Env into newly synthesized virions. The second role of Vpu is to promote the release of virions from the infected cell by an unknown mechanism.

Vpr promotes transport of subviral particles into nucleus of nondividing cells

The Vpr protein is involved in promoting import of subviral particles into the nucleus after reverse transcription. Thus, the protein has little or no effect in proliferating T cells where nuclear access is ensured with each mitosis. However, successful infection of nondividing cells such as macrophages requires Vpr to allow the newly synthesized viral DNA to reach the nucleus and be integrated into the cellular DNA.

Vpu and Vif increase efficiency of infection and yield of virus

Vif (virion infectivity factor) increases the infectivity of HIV-1 in primary T cells and certain "nonpermissive" cells in culture. In the absence of Vif, the virus fails to complete reverse transcription in these cell types. "Permissive" cell lines infected by mutants defective in the *vif* gene produce normal yields of infectious virus. One possible explanation for this observation is that "permissive" cells contain a factor that can substitute for the missing Vif protein. Thus, one role of Vif may be to extend the host range of HIV-1 to cell types that would otherwise not be infected.

Acativation of CD4+ T lymphocytes increases virus production

Superimposed on this complex regulatory network is the fact that the viral promoter contains elements that are sensitive to specific cellular transcription factors. This observation may help explain why virus production in CD4+ T lymphocytes is greatly increased when the cells are activated. Clearly the outcome of an HIV-1 infection is determined by a complex interplay between a very large number of different factors.

ACQUIRED IMMUNODEFICIENCY SYNDROME (AIDS)

CLINICAL CAPSULE

The primary infection in AIDS ranges from asymptomatic to an infectious mononucleosis-like illness with up to a few weeks of fever, malaise, arthralgias, and rash. A long (years) asymptomatic period follows, after which the disease, AIDS, emerges. The progressive findings directly due to the virus are wasting, diarrhea, neurologic degeneration, and malignancies. The effect of the virus on the immune system causes an extensive array of viral, bacterial, fungal, and parasitic opportunistic infections whose findings are the same or worse than those seen in patients without AIDS.

EPIDEMIOLOGY

First recognized in male homosexuals, hemophiliacs, and drug abusers

The AIDS syndrome was first recognized in the United States in 1981, when it became apparent that an unusual number of rare skin cancers (Kaposi's sarcoma) and opportunistic infections were occurring among male homosexuals. These patients were found to have a marked reduction in CD4+ T lymphocytes and were subject to a wide range of opportunistic infections normally controlled by an intact immune system. The disease was found to progress relentlessly to a fatal outcome and was first identified in male homosexuals, hemophiliacs who were receiving blood-derived coagulation factors, and injection drug users.

Retrospective serologic studies with material saved from patients in various studies indicate that the disease was already occurring in Africa in the 1950s and in the United States in the 1970s. In 1985, HIV-2 was found to be endemic in parts of West Africa and to cause AIDS. To date, this virus has been relatively restricted geographically, although HIV-2 infections have occurred in the western hemisphere.

HIV-2 is endemic to West Africa

Transmission

The HIV virus is transmitted between humans in three ways: sexually, perinatally, and by exposure to contaminated blood or body fluids. The virus has been demonstrated in particularly high titers in semen and cervical secretions, and the majority of cases result from sexual contact. Infection is facilitated by breaks in epithelial surfaces, which provide direct access to the underlying tissues or bloodstream. The relative fragility of the rectal mucosa, together with large numbers of sexual contacts, are probable contributing factors to the predominance of the disease among promiscuous male homosexuals. Transmission appears to be more efficient from men to women, but the reverse is clearly documented. The probability of HIV transmission per unprotected sexual act is estimated at 0.0003 to 0.0015. The risk of perinatal transmission from an infected mother to her child has been estimated to range from 15 to 40%.

Transmission is sexual and by exposure to infective fluids

Perinatal transmission can readily occur

Growth of the virus in cell culture and identification of its antigens allowed development of effective test procedures for detecting HIV infection. These almost eliminated the risk of transmission by blood transfusion; testing of donors and the use of recombinant or specially treated coagulation factors have now virtually eliminated these sources of infection. Until serologic tests for the infection became available, in 1985, more than 10,000 cases of AIDS were probably acquired in the United States through blood transfusion, and about 80% of hemophiliacs treated with coagulation factors derived from pooled blood sources became infected. Transmission of infection by blood is now largely associated with sharing of needles and syringes by injecting drug users, and this has been an increasing source of the disease. In some areas of the world, the seroprevalence of HIV positivity among injecting drug users has been as high as 70%. It became apparent that heterosexual transmission could occur and that the infection could be transmitted from mother to infant either by intrauterine spread or during the birth process. It was also found that the disease had its greatest prevalence in parts of Africa, where the spread was predominantly heterosexual.

Testing of blood supply reduced risk

Intravenous drug abusers are at extremely high risk

Transmission of infection to health care workers after accidental sticks with potentially contaminated needles is very rare (considerably less than 1% of occurrences), presumably because the amount of infectious virus in the blood of infected cases is small and larger volumes or repeated exposures are needed for a significant chance of infection. Nevertheless, cases have occurred from both clinical and laboratory exposure, and extreme care in handling needles, sharps, and so on, is necessary. Transmission does not occur through day-to-day nonsexual contact with infected individuals or through insect vectors, because of the fragility of the virus and the need for direct mucosal or blood contact. It is of interest that the virus has been detected in saliva, tears, urine, and breast milk. With the possible exception of breast milk, these sources have not been shown to be infectious.

Accidental needlesticks among health care workers mandate extreme care in prevention

Shed in breast milk, where it may infect breastfeeding infants

Occurrence

As of December 2001, there have been 816,000 cases of AIDS in the United States, with 468,000 deaths. The highest prevalence rates of HIV infections have been in homosexual and bisexual males, intravenous drug users, prostitutes, and sexual partners of HIV-infected persons. In some areas of the United States, 40 to 60% of homosexual males attending sexually transmitted disease clinics were found to be infected. The epidemiology of HIV infection is changing in the United States as the pandemic evolves and as the modes of transmission become more generally understood. The numbers and proportions of heterosexually transmitted, drug abuse–related, and neonatal cases are increasing, particularly among the poor and disadvantaged racial minorities. Antibody rates in prostitutes may be as high as 40%, depending partly on the degree of associated intravenous drug abuse. Prevalence rates in the

Prevalence rates have shifted over time, with increasing cases among women and economically disadvantaged minority groups

heterosexual population, in general, are currently less than 1% but have been increasing. In 1985 in the United States, only 7% of AIDS cases were in women; by 2000 the percentage had risen to 25%. Approximately 2000 newborns per year are infected by HIV perinatally, but this number may be decreasing as more pregnant women receive antiretroviral therapy. The current distribution of AIDS cases is men who have sex with men (MSM) (40%), intravenous drug users (30%), heterosexual (25%) persons, and others (5%). Black patients now account for 50% of cases, exceeding the percentages in non-Hispanic white men.

Men and women nearly equally inffected in Africa and Asia

In contrast to the situation in the United States and Western Europe, heterosexual transmission is the primary route of transmission in Africa and Asia, where there is an approximately equal distribution of infection and disease between the sexes. This may be due to a high frequency in these areas of ulcerative genital lesions caused by other sexually transmitted diseases. These lesions facilitate passage of virus into the tissues of others during intercourse. In central and eastern Europe, where there is an emerging epidemic, the most common risk factor is intravenous drug use.

Increasingly widespread in Africa, South America, parts of Asia

AIDS has been reported in more than 150 countries. The disease continues to spread rapidly in Africa and South America. In sub-Saharan Africa alone, 25 million people are infected, and there are 4 million new cases per year. Until recently, the Far East had few cases, but now there is epidemic spread, especially in South and South East Asia (India, South China, Burma, Thailand, Cambodia, Viet Nam, and Malaysia). In China, there are more than 600,000 patients with AIDS, and the rate of new cases is increasing by more than 30% per year. HIV-2 infection is found primarily in West Africa and is spread by heterosexual transmission. Infection by this virus has, however, been reported in Europe in homosexual men, injection drug users, transfusion recipients, and hemophiliac men. For example, in Russia, there were 40,000 new cases of AIDS in 2000. In some countries in Africa, 25% of the population and up to 60% of women are HIV antibody–positive.

PATHOGENESIS

The pathogenesis of HIV-1 infection is very complex, but the following factors are likely to be important in the disease-causing process.

Infection

Major targets are CD4-bearing cells, but other cell types can also be infected

The initial target of HIV-1 is CD4 molecules, particularly on the surface of CD4+ helper T lymphocytes, monocytes, and macrophages. The virus can also infect other human cells expressing CD4, and a wide range of CD4 negative cells, including renal and gastrointestinal epithelium and brain astrocytes. The mechanism for infection of non–CD4-bearing cells is unknown but may involve other receptors or fusion with cells already infected with HIV. The virus replicates in macrophages, and these cells could serve as a reservoir for continued expansion of the infection to other cell types by cell-to-cell fusion, which allows the virus to spread without being exposed to neutralizing antibody. Infected macrophages may participate in breakdown of the blood–brain barrier, allowing enhanced exposure of the central nervous system (CNS). Although CNS and intestinal disturbances are a prominent part of fully developed AIDS, it is not clear whether they are a direct result of infection of these cells or mediated by cytokines from infected macrophages and T lymphocytes.

Rapid turnover of CD4+ cells during infection

Kinetic studies of changes in viral load with antiviral therapy demonstrated the half-life of HIV in plasma is 5 to 6 hours. In other words, more than 50% of the viral load measured on any given day has been produced in the past 24 hours. Because 99% of the viral load is produced by cells that were infected within the past 48 to 72 hours, cell turnover must be equally rapid. Indeed, when similar kinetic studies are performed on changes in CD4 cell counts, it is estimated that up to 1 billion CD4 cells are produced per day in response to the infection and that the half-life of these cells is only 1.6 days.

Latency

The long asymptomatic period following HIV infection (clinical latency) occurs despite active virus replication in the host. Several factors can terminate the long latent period of

HIV-1. Mutations occur during viral replication that appear to enhance induction of virulent forms of the virus, with increased cytopathic capacity and altered cell tropisms. Thus, the mutated forms of HIV-1 isolated from later stages of disease infect a broader range of cell types and grow more rapidly than those isolated in the asymptomatic period. Initially, it was believed that little or no viral replication occurred during this latent period, but studies of lymph nodes of individuals with early asymptomatic disease have shown intense immunologic reactions within the lymphoid tissue at early stages of disease. This implies that the immune system is capable of controlling the virus to some degree early in the course of disease, an ability that is later lost as the disease progresses over time.

Some immune control of virus during the latent period, but this is later lost

Recent studies of HIV infection have shown that the level of free virus in the plasma increases in direct relation to the stage of disease. Individuals with early-stage disease have less than 10 infectious virions/mL of plasma, whereas those in late-stage disease have between 100 and 1000 infectious virions/mL of plasma. These studies imply either that viral replication was increasing during later stages of disease due to more virulent mutations and/or the immune system had lost its ability to clear free virus as the disease progresses.

Level of plasma viremia directly correlates with disease progression

Immune Deficiency

The primary immune defect in AIDS results from the reduction in the numbers and effectiveness of CD4+ helper-inducer T lymphocytes, both in absolute numbers and relative to CD8+ suppressor T lymphocytes. This is due to direct killing of CD4+ T lymphocytes by the virus but may also involve other mechanisms as well. These include secondary killing of uninfected (bystander) cells during cell fusion, autoimmune processes that lead to the elimination of CD4+ T lymphocytes by opsonophagocytosis, and antibody-dependent cell-mediated cytotoxicity (ADCC) directed at gp120 expressed on the CD4+ cell surface. There are also functional defects in CD4+ T lymphocytes affecting lymphokine production and leading to inhibition of some macrophage functions.

Immune deficiency related to reduction in numbers and normal functions of CD4+ T lymphocytes

Effects on CD4+ T lymphocytes thus lead to a generalized failure of cell-mediated immune responses, but there is also an effect on antibody production due to polyclonal activation of B cells, possibly associated with other viral infections of these cells. This overwhelms the capacity of infected individuals to respond to specific antigens. The end result of these processes is a disturbance of immune balance that can give rise to malignancies as well as the susceptibility of AIDS patients to a range of opportunistic viral, fungal, and bacterial infections.

Inffected individuals are susceptible to other infections and malignancies

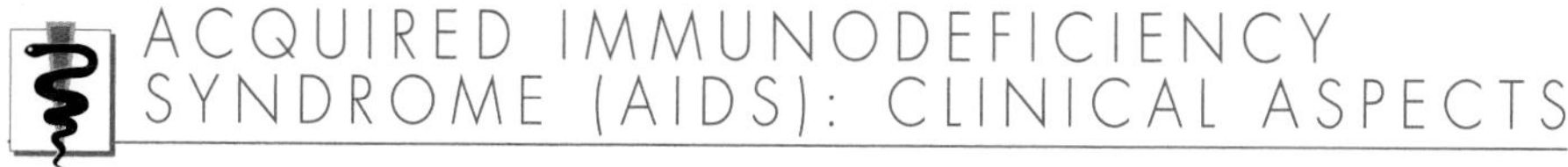

ACQUIRED IMMUNODEFICIENCY SYNDROME (AIDS): CLINICAL ASPECTS

MANIFESTATIONS

In 1993, the Centers for Disease Control and Prevention (CDC) definition of AIDS stated that all patients who are HIV antibody–positive and have CD4+ T-lymphocyte counts below 200/mm^3 or less than 14% of total T lymphocytes have the disease. The initial infection with HIV is usually asymptomatic, although in some cases a mononucleosis-like illness develops 2 to 4 weeks after infection and lasts about 2 to 6 weeks. This illness may exhibit any or all of the following: fever, malaise, lymphadenopathy, hepatosplenomegaly, arthralgias, and rash. Sometimes a mild aseptic meningitis is also present. Whether or not these early manifestations of infection occur, the virus persists and integrates into the genome of some host cells, and the individual is thus infected for life.

Infection is lifelong

The initial infection is followed by an asymptomatic period that, in most cases, continues for years before the disease becomes clinically apparent. During this time virus can be isolated from blood, semen, and the cervix. Approximately 50% of infected individuals develop significant disease within 10 years of infection, and the number continues to increase thereafter. It is expected that nearly all HIV-infected individuals eventually

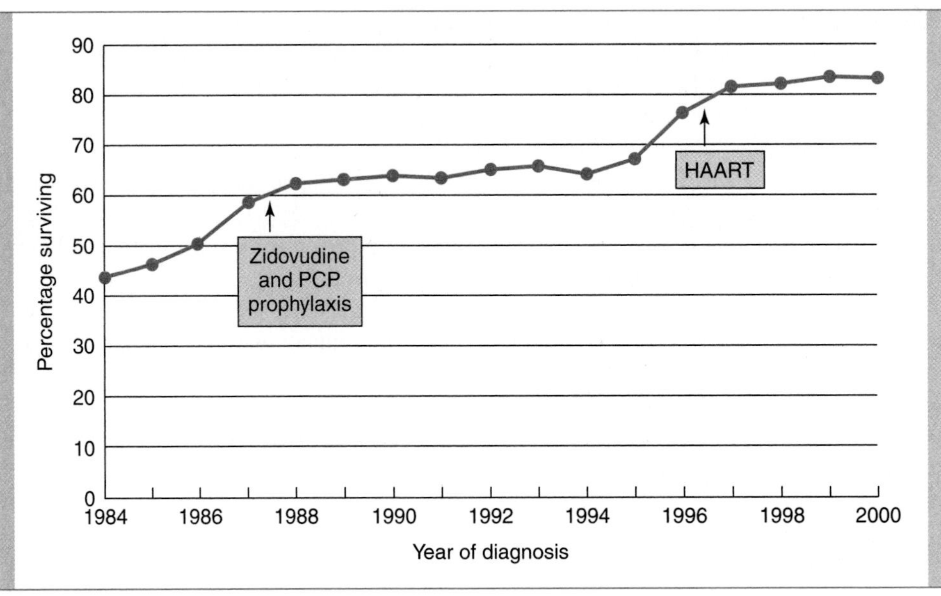

FIGURE 42–5

Proportion of AIDS patients surviving at least 1 year after diagnosis of their first AIDS-defining opportunistic illness, by year of diagnosis of opportunistic illness, 1984–2000, United States. HAART, highly active antiretroviral therapy; PCP *Pneumocystis carinii* pneumonia. (*From Centers for Disease Control and Prevention, National Center for HIV, STD, and TB Prevention, Divisions of HIV/AIDS Prevention. Surveillance Supplemental Report 2002, Vol 8, No 1.*)

develop some clinical aspects of this infection, although long-term (>1 years) nonprogressors are well documented. Approximately 5% of infected, untreated patients show no decrease in CD4 counts over a period of more than 10 years, but ultimately many of these individuals begin to progress. However, since the late 1990s, the increases in early diagnosis, combined with more aggressive, highly active antiretroviral therapy (HAART) in the United States, have shown promise in delaying progression of infection to death (Figs 42–5, 42–6).

Progression to AIDS is highly variable among individuals

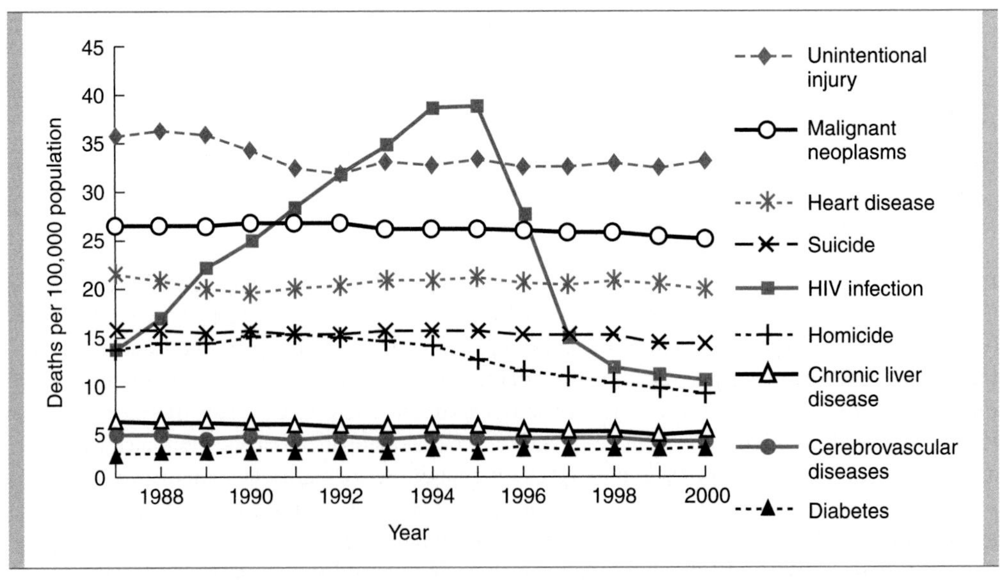

FIGURE 42–6

Death rates per 100,000 population from leading causes of death among persons 25–44 years old, United States, 1987–2000. (*From National Center for Health Statistics, National Vital Statistics System, 2002.*)

TABLE 42–3

Common Opportunistic Infections in Patients with AIDS

Common Opportunistic Infections in Patients with AIDS
PROTOZOAN
Pneumocystosis (*P. carinii* classification uncertain)
Toxoplasmosis
Isospora belli infection
Cryptosporidiosis
FUNGAL
Cryptococcosis
Candidiasis
Histoplasmosis (disseminated)
MYCOBACTERIAL
Disseminated tuberculosis (especially extrapulmonary)
Mycobacterium avium–intracellulare complex infections
VIRAL
Persistent mucocutaneous herpes simplex
Cytomegalovirus retinitis, gastrointestinal, or disseminated infection
Varicella–zoster, persistent or disseminated
Progressive multifocal leukoencephalopathy

As the disease progresses, the number of CD4+ T lymphocytes decline. There is increasing immunodeficiency, and opportunistic infections become more frequent, severe, and difficult to treat. One of the best markers of the severity of AIDS is the absolute number of CD4+ T lymphocytes. Those individuals with overt AIDS almost always have fewer than 400 CD4+ T lymphocytes/mm^3 of blood (normal = 800–1200/mm^3).

Individuals with overt AIDS usually have fewer than 400 CD4+ lymphocytes/mm^3

Patients with full-blown AIDS experience a wide spectrum of infections depending on the severity of their immune defect and on the opportunistic organisms in their normal flora or with which they come in contact (Table 42–3). Some clinical manifestations of AIDS may thus vary by locale. For example, disseminated histoplasmosis is a common complication in the Midwest of the United States, as disseminated toxoplasmosis is in France. These infections are uncommon in areas where the diseases are not endemic. The diversity and anatomic sites of infection vary between patients, and any one patient may have several infections. The most common infection is pneumocystosis, and approximately 50% of AIDS patients who do not receive prophylaxis for pneumocystosis develop *Pneumocystis carinii* pneumonia. In the past, about 25% of all AIDS patients developed Kaposi's sarcoma, but the number of cases has been falling in the United States despite increasing numbers of cases of AIDS. The apparent explanation is that Kaposi's sarcoma is due to a transmitted agent different from HIV, the Kaposi's sarcoma herpesvirus (KSHV); the spread of this organism has diminished as high-risk sexual behavior has decreased especially among homosexual men. Disease due to mycobacteria of the *Mycobacterium avium-intracellulare* complex is common, and AIDS patients are also highly susceptible to *Mycobacterium tuberculosis* infection. Oral thrush and esophagitis due to *Candida albicans* and meningitis due to *Cryptococcus* are commonly encountered fungal infections. Persistent progressive mucocutaneous herpes simplex and herpes zoster infections are common. CMV chorioretinitis is one of the most common opportunistic infections and may result in unilateral or bilateral blindness. Disseminated cytomegalovirus (CMV) infection is also seen and presents with fever and visceral (eg, gastrointestinal) organ involvement.

Pneumocystosis, candidiasis, mycobacteriosis, and CMV are common

CMV retinitis and mycobacterial dissemination usually occur with extremely low CD4+ counts

Specific opportunistic infections are associated with differing levels of CD4+ T-lymphocyte counts. For example, fungal and tuberculous pneumonia may occur with CD4+ T-lymphocyte counts of 200 to 500 cells/mm^3, whereas CMV and *M. avium-intracellulare* disease are seen almost exclusively in those whose counts are below 50 to 100 cells/mm^3.

As the duration of survival of AIDS patients became longer due to therapy with the earliest drugs, an increased number developed neurologic manifestations of the disease and lymphoid neoplasms, especially non-Hodgkin's lymphomas. HIV is a neurotropic virus and can be isolated from the cerebrospinal fluid of 50 to 70% of patients. CNS involvement may be asymptomatic, but many patients develop a subacute neurologic illness that produces clinical symptoms varying from mild cognitive dysfunction to severe dementia. Loss of complex cognitive function is usually the first sign of illness. Progression to severe memory loss, depression, seizures, and coma may ensue. Cerebral atrophy involving primarily cortical white matter can be demonstrated by computed tomography or magnetic resonance imaging. Histologically, focal vacuolation of the affected brain tissue with perivascular infiltration of macrophages is noted. Multinucleated giant cells with syncytium formation surround the perivascular infiltrates. Neurologic symptoms do not usually occur until CD4+ T-lymphocyte counts are below 200 cells/mm^3.

HIV is also neurotropic and can lead to dementia

The disease spectrum in Africa is similar in many respects to that in the Western world, but many more patients present with severe intractable wasting and diarrhea, known as *slim disease.* Tuberculosis is also more commonly encountered in AIDS patients in Africa, reflecting the higher incidence of the disease in the population in general. The 2-year mortality of AIDS, once the disease has been fully established, was initially 75%, with nearly all persons eventually dying of opportunistic infections or neoplasms. Recent advances in therapy have slowed progression of the disease. Combination therapy, with the inclusion of inhibitors of HIV protease, appears to be responsible for dramatic improvement in many patients, but toxicity or the development of resistance may limit their long-term usefulness. Progression of AIDS and the development of these neurologic manifestations have become less common with the advent of highly active antiretroviral therapy (HAART).

Aggressive antiviral therapy can slow progression or even result in clinical improvement

Toxicity or mutant resistance limit long-term drug usefulness

DIAGNOSIS

The diagnosis of AIDS is most commonly confirmed by demonstrating antibody to the virus or its components. Initial screening tests are performed using whole viral lysates as the target antigens in enzyme immunoassay (EIA) tests. These have a high level of sensitivity, but because false-positive results occur, all positive EIA tests must be confirmed. The confirmatory test is a Western blot analysis, which detects antibodies to specific viral proteins. In this procedure, viral proteins are separated by electrophoresis, transferred to nitrocellulose paper, and incubated with patient sera; antibody bound to the individual proteins is detected by enzyme-labeled anti–human globulin sera (Fig 42–7). Sera from infected patients have antibodies that react with the envelope glycoproteins, core proteins, or both. Tests made with HIV-1 detect antibody in 60 to 90% of patients infected by HIV-2.

EIA screens for antibody

Western blot used for confirmation

The combination of EIA and Western blot tests gives a high degree of specificity to test results, but antibody is not detectable by these procedures in the first 2 to 4 weeks after infection. During this period, the individual can still transmit the infection to others by sexual contact or blood donation. Closing this detection gap is particularly important for protection of blood products for transfusion. Although the virus can be grown during this time in mixed lymphocyte cell culture, the methods are impractical and may not be positive for up to 1 month. More practical approaches include nucleic acid–based assays such as the polymerase chain reaction (PCR) for plasma HIV RNA or DNA and the branched chain DNA (bDNA) assay. These are also useful in assessing the benefits of antiviral therapy, as well as in determining if infants born to seropositive mothers are infected or simply demonstrating passively transmitted transplacental antibody.

Viremia precedes appearance of antibody by 2 to 4 weeks

Quantitation of plasma HIV RNA plays an especially important part in management. For example, if a patient's HIV RNA copy number rises during therapy, or fails to fall to low levels (eg, $<$50 copies/mL), this signals that the antiviral efficacy of the drug regimen

PCR and bDNA testing used to quantitate plasma viremia and assess drug efficacy

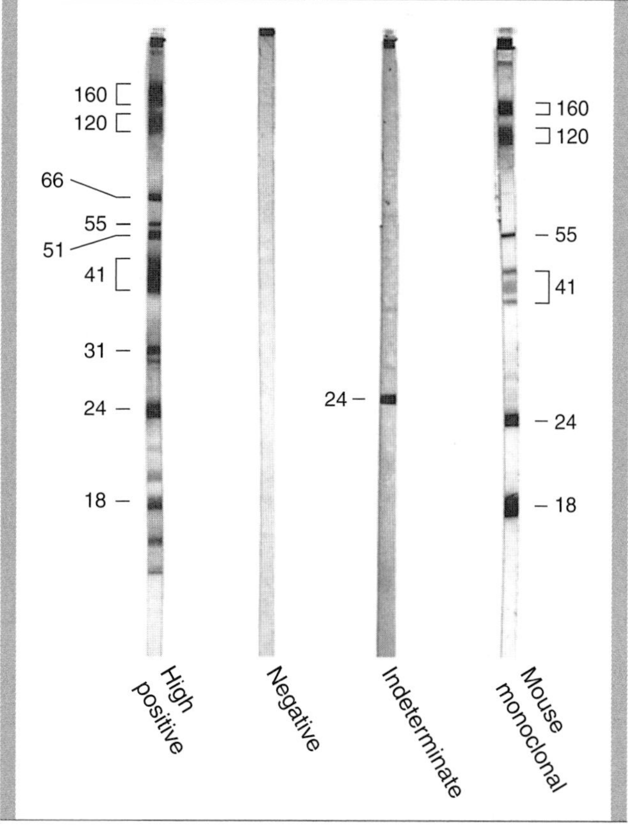

FIGURE 42–7
Western blot detection of HIV-1 antibodies. Note that the "high-positive" serum exhibits antibodies to the HIV-1 envelope glycoproteins of 160, 120 and 41 kilodaltons (kD), to the GAG (core) proteins of 24 and 18 kD, and to other HIV proteins (55 and 51 kD). The "indeterminate" serum exhibits antibody to only the GAG (core) 24-kD protein. The mouse monoclonal blot is a positive control and contains antibodies to key HIV antigens. A positive sample should exhibit antibodies to both envelope and GAG proteins or to both envelope proteins (41 and 120/160 kD).

is inadequate. The most likely explanation is mutational resistance that either preexisted or developed during treatment. Other explanations to be considered include patient noncompliance or inadequate dosing.

TREATMENT

Initially, only nucleoside inhibitors of HIV reverse transcriptase were available for therapy of HIV infection and they were used singly. Currently, there are at least 16 approved therapeutic agents that inhibit either of two essential viral enzymes: reverse transcriptase or protease. Other antiviral agents under development include those that can block viral entry into the cell, and others that may inhibit viral integrase activity. The characteristics of current representative anti-HIV agents are further summarized in Chapter 13. It is clear that various combinations of these agents are preferable to produce effective virologic and clinical responses.

Combinations of drugs used in treatment

Initiation of Treatment

Because viral replication proceeds at the phenomenal rate of approximately 10,000 new viruses per day, it seems most rational to begin treatment as soon as infection is detected. However, considerations of toxicity, resistance development, quality of life, cost, and patient wishes are extremely important additional determinants. Although these issues may cause debates regarding early intervention, there is a general consensus that combination therapy should be initiated when CD4+ count falls below 500/mm^3 or the plasma HIV viral load is more than 5000 copies/mm^3 of viral RNA.

Decision to treat aggressively is influenced by CD4+ count and viral load

Resistance

RNA viruses tend to have frequent mutations, and the genome of HIV is highly variable. This results in part from the extremely high turnover rate of virions per day. As a result, resistance to an antiviral is a regular and often rapid development. Use of antiviral therapies

Drug resistance is expected development with treatment

that maximally suppress HIV viral load appear to diminish the appearance of resistant virus.

Prophylaxis of opportunistic infections is especially important

In addition to the primary treatment of HIV, patients with CD4+ counts of less than 200/mm^3 should begin prophylactic regimens to prevent *P. carinii* pneumonia; when CD4+ counts are less than 75 to 100/mm^3 they should receive prophylaxis for mycobacterial and fungal infection.

PREVENTION

Education is the cornerstone of prevention

Screening for asymptomatic infection in pregnancy aids effective prophylaxis

The spread of AIDS has been facilitated by changing sexual mores, injection drug use, and, in some parts of the world, disruption of family and tribal units as a consequence of industrialization and urbanization. These factors are obviously not subject to rapid change. Immediate prevention must be based on education about the means of transmission and easy access to condoms and safe needles for those large numbers of people who continue to place themselves at risk. The epidemiologic and laboratory methods used to control foci of other major epidemic diseases pose particular problems in AIDS control at present. Quite apart from questions of potential discrimination against infected individuals and the calamitous effects of false-positive serologic test results, the sheer magnitude and cost of case finding and contact tracing at present limit this approach. Detection and treatment of HIV-infected pregnant women has also been shown to be effective in reducing perinatal infection.

Caesarian section, particularly elective rather than emergent, is also a preventive, as is the avoidance of breast feeding by HIV positive mothers. Much research is underway to develop vaccines against the virus, but the marked mutability of HIV greatly complicates this approach. Furthermore, passage of virus between fused cells and in syncytia protects it from antibody neutralization in established disease. The search continues for conserved epitopes of the surface glycopeptides that might provide possible antigenic targets. Antiviral treatment utilizing combinations of agents may prevent infection of accidentally exposed individuals (eg, health care workers). This therapy must be initiated within hours of an accident if it is to have any chance of success.

ADDITIONAL READING

Guidelines for using antiretroviral agents among HIV-infected adults and adolescents: Recommendations of the panel on clinical practices for the treatment of HIV. *MMWR* 2002;51:RR-7. Current guidelines and their rationale are periodically summarized. (Also available with updates on www.cdc.gov/mmwr.)

Levy JA. *HIV and the Pathogenesis of AIDS,* 2nd ed. Washington, D.C.: ASM Press; 1998. A current description of HIV and its pathogenic potential.

Mellors JW, Kingsley LA, Rinaldo CR Jr, et al. Quantitation of HIV-1 RNA in plasma predicts outcome after seroconversion. *Ann Intern Med* 1995;122:573–579. This illustrates how progression of HIV infection can be predicted based on viral load data.

CHAPTER 43

Papovaviruses

W. LAWRENCE DREW

The papovaviruses of medical interest include the papillomaviruses and polyomaviruses .

PAPILLOMAVIRUSES

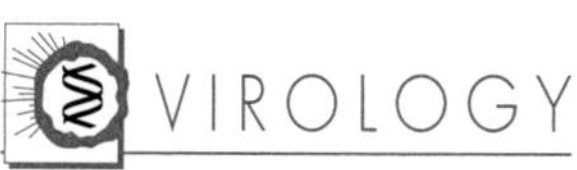

VIROLOGY

Papillomaviruses are small, unenveloped, double-stranded DNA viruses exhibiting cubic symmetry. About 55 nm in diameter, they cause epidermal papillomas and warts in a wide range of higher vertebrates. Different members of the group are generally species specific. For example, bovine and human papillomaviruses infect only the hosts reflected in their names. In some cases, tumors caused by these agents can become malignant and the role of these agents as causes of certain human cancers is being clarified. Papillomaviruses have not been grown in tissue culture, and most of the virologic information has derived from molecular studies.

Naked, double-stranded DNA viruses

Have not been grown in vitro

The genomes of many of the papillomaviruses have now been cloned and compared by restriction endonuclease and DNA homology procedures (see Chapters 4 and 15). These studies have shown a wide genomic diversity among papillomaviruses that infect different species and also among those that infect humans. This has led to the allocation of numbers for the different genotypes.

Great genomic diversity

PAPILLOMAVIRUS DISEASE

CLINICAL CAPSULE

More than 70 genotypes of human papillomaviruses (HPVs) have been identified in human specimens. Some of the genotypes are antigenically (phenotypically) different, and groups of genotypes are associated with specific lesions. HPVs have been identified in plantar warts; in flat and papillomatous warts of other skin areas; in juvenile laryngeal papillomas; and in a variety of genital hyperplastic epithelial lesions, including cervical, vulvar, and penile warts and papillomas. In addition, they are associated with premalignant (cervical intraepithelial neoplasia) and malignant disease (cervical cancer). Lesions comparable to those occurring in the cervix are now recognized in the anus, especially among men who have sex with men and are infected by human immunodeficiency virus, or HIV.

EPIDEMIOLOGY

Cutaneous nongenital warts usually occur in children and young adults; presumably immunity to the HPV genotypes causing these lesions develops and appears to provide protection. Twelve HPV genotypes have been identified in genital lesions of humans, and there are many apparently silent infections with these viruses. Cross immunity does not occur, and sequential infection with multiple genotypes does take place. The incidence of HPV infections has almost certainly been increasing, and they may now constitute the most common sexually transmitted disease. From 20 to 60% of adult women in the United States are infected with one or another of the genotypes. HPV types 6 and 11 are associated most commonly with benign genital warts in males and females and with some cellular dysplasias of the cervical epithelium, but these lesions rarely become malignant. They can be perinatally transmitted and cause infantile laryngeal papillomas. Types 16, 18, 31 and 45 may also cause warty lesions of the vulva, cervix, and penis. Infections with these viral types, especially 16, may progress to malignancy. Viral genomes of these four types are found in a proportion of markedly dysplastic uterine cervical cells, in carcinoma in situ, and in cells of frankly malignant lesions. Human papillomavirus infection is now considered to be a cause of the majority of carcinomas of the cervix. Papillomavirus infection of the anus is a clinical problem in homosexual men, especially those with acquired immunodeficiency syndrome (AIDS), and it appears to be related to the subsequent development of anal neoplasia in these individuals.

HPV types 6 and 11 common; rarely lead to malignancy

Types 16, 18, 31, and 45 associated with dysplasia and malignancy

PATHOGENESIS

Papillomaviruses have a predilection for infection at the junction of squamous and columnar epithelium (eg, in the cervix and anus). Papillomaviruses were the first DNA viruses linked to malignant changes. In the mid-1930s, Shope demonstrated that benign rabbit papillomas were due to filterable agents and could advance to become malignant squamous cell carcinomas. External cofactors, such as coal tar, could hasten this process. However, work on the biology and mechanism by which these agents foster malignant transformation has been impeded by the inability to cultivate papillomaviruses in vitro. Molecular probes to detect viral products in vivo indicate that replication and assembly of these viruses take place only in the differentiating layers of squamous epithelia, a situation that has not been reproduced in vitro.

Replication in squamous epithelium

The first evidence that HPVs could be associated with human malignant disease came from observations on epidermodysplasia verruciformis. This disease has a genetic basis that results in unusual susceptibility to HPV types 5 and 8, which produce multiple flat warts. About one third of affected patients develop squamous cell carcinoma from these lesions.

The mechanism of oncogenicity of HPV is less clear. Cells infected with genomes of several papillomaviruses can transform cells and produce tumors when injected into nude (T lymphocyte–deficient) mice. The viral genome exists as multiple copies of a circular episome within the nucleus of transformed cells but is not integrated into the cellular genome. This appears also to be the case with benign human lesions. In malignant tumors, part of the viral genome is found integrated into the cellular genome, but integration is not site specific. Both the integrated viral genome and the extrachromosomal form carry their own transforming genes. Host cells normally produce a protein that inhibits expression of papillomavirus transforming genes, but this can be inactivated by products of the virus and possibly by other infecting viruses, thus allowing malignant transformation to occur. HPV DNA is found in more than 95% of cervical carcinoma specimens when tested by polymerase chain reaction (PCR).

Viral genomes carry their own transforming genes

PAPILLOMAVIRUS: CLINICAL ASPECTS

MANIFESTATIONS

Cutaneous warts can vary from flat to deep plantar growths. Although they can persist for years, they ultimately spontaneously regress. Respiratory papillomatosis due most often to types 6 and 11 occurs as intraoral or laryngeal lesions. These tend to occur in infants as a result of natal exposure, or in full grown adults.

Oral or laryngeal papillomatosis in infants infected during delivery

External genital HPV infection occurs as exophytic genital warts (condyloma acuminata) caused most often by types 6 or 11. Lesions may increase in size to cauliflower-like appearance during pregnancy or immunosuppression. Genital HPV infection is most often benign, and many lesions reverse spontaneously. However they may become dysplastic and proceed through a continuum of cervical intraepithelial neoplasm to severe dysplasia and/or carcinoma in situ. The most common HPV in the malignant lesions is type 16, although this genotype, as well as the others, is most apt to cause lesions that regress spontaneously. Higher grade malignancy is most apt to occur in the cervix, but the rate of anal carcinoma related to HPV appears to be increasing, especially in AIDS patients.

Anal carcinoma due to HPV may be increasing

DIAGNOSIS

HPV does not grow in routine tissue culture, and antibody tests are rarely used. Papillomavirus infection leads to perinuclear cytoplasmic vacuolization and nuclear enlargement, referred to as poikilocytosis, in epithelial cells of the cervix or vagina. These changes can be seen in a routine Papanicolaou smear. The use of immunoassays to detect viral antigen and in situ hybridization or PCR to detect specific viral DNA in cervical swabs or tissue is more sensitive (Fig 43–1), but the clinical utility of detecting specific HPV types in clinical specimens remains to be determined. Detection of an abnormal cytology due to HPV should prompt colposcopy to assist in following or treating patients with abnormal lesions.

Poikilocytosis can be seen in cytologic specimens

Molecular methods to detect specific genotypes in biopsies of cervical swabs are available

TREATMENT AND PREVENTION

Current treatment of HPV is usually either cytotoxic or surgical. Among the topical cytotoxins are podophyllin, podophyllotoxin, 5-fluorouracil, and trichloroacetic acid.

Recurrences are common after topical treatment

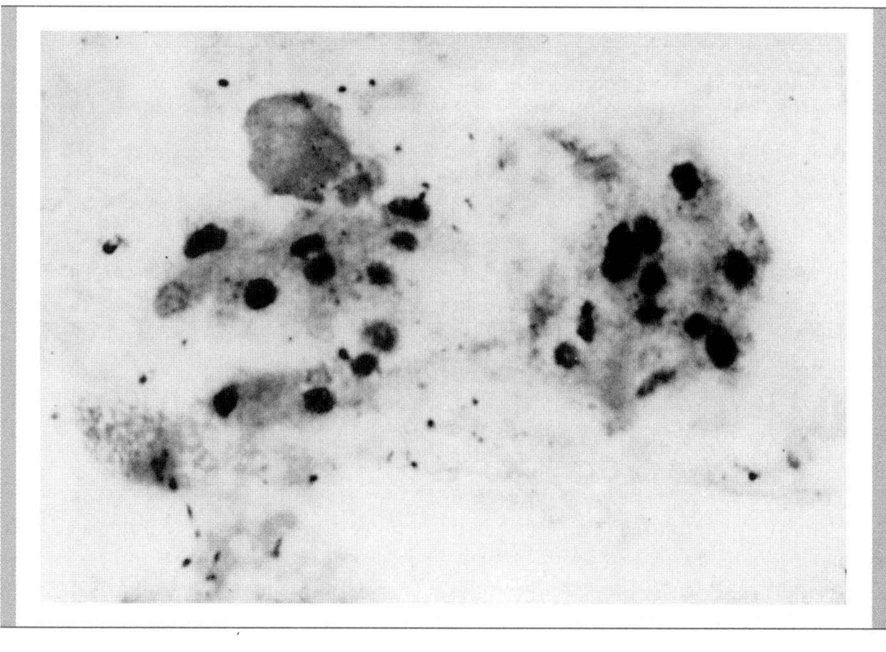

FIGURE 43–1
Human papillomavirus (HPV) type 16 DNA demonstrated in a cervical smear by in situ hybridization. The dark dots represent detection of HPV DNA sequences by the DNA probe.

Recurrences are common following cessation of treatment because of survival of virus in the basal layers of the epithelium. Systemic and local interferon therapy has shown some promise as a treatment, although lesions tend to recur after cessation of therapy. Cervical lesions may be treated with electrocautery.

Future prospects for prevention by vaccines

A recent large, prospective study of a HPV-16 virus-like-particle vaccine (an L1 polypeptide expressed in yeast) conducted among women 16 to 23 years of age indicated the potential for prevention of persistent infection, at least with this type, is high.

POLYOMAVIRUSES

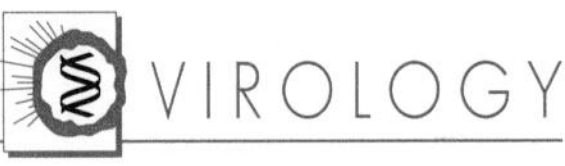

Naked DNA viruses

Can transform cells in vitro

The polyomaviruses include the JC virus (JCV) and BK virus (BKV) of humans and simian virus 40 (SV40) of monkeys. Polyomaviruses, like papillomaviruses, are members of the papovavirus family. They are also double-stranded, naked capsid DNA viruses and are widely distributed among various animal species, usually without causing apparent disease. However, they are able to transform cells of a variety of heterologous cell lines in culture.

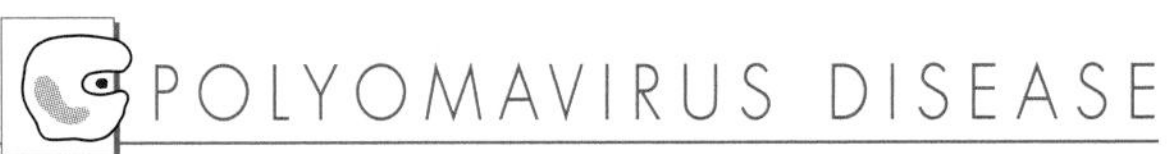

Clinical Capsule

Polyomaviruses are closely related to papillomaviruses but are not known to cause clinical disease in immunocompetent patients. They can cause progressive multifocal leukoencephalopathy (PML) and hemorrhagic cystitis/nephropathy in immunocompromised patients.

EPIDEMIOLOGY

Latency is common

Disease associated with immunocompromise

Approximately 80% of adults show serologic evidence of JCV and BKV infection with no known clinical manifestations, but the viruses remain latent and may reactivate and cause disease in immunocompromised patients. BKV is estimated to cause renal disease in 2 to 5% of renal transplant recipients.

PATHOGENESIS

Do not cause malignancies in their natural hosts

Polyomaviruses can produce malignant tumors in certain experimental animals but, interestingly, not in their natural hosts. For example, SV40 can produce lymphocytic leukemia and a variety of reticuloendothelial cell sarcomas in baby hamsters but is not oncogenic in its natural monkey host. Fortunately, even though it can transform some human cells in vitro, it fails to produce disease in humans, a fact that became apparent on follow-up of recipients of early batches of poliomyelitis vaccine produced in monkey kidney cell cultures that were contaminated with live SV40.

Interact with cells in a variety of ways

The reason polyomaviruses fail to produce tumors in their natural hosts is uncertain, but it may be due to the fact that the viruses are usually cytocidal under these conditions. From a biological point of view, the polyomaviruses are particularly useful models of oncogenicity because they can be readily studied in vitro and interact with cells in different ways. In some, they produce lytic infections and cell death with production of complete virions. In others, they integrate randomly into the cell genome and cause transformation by the expression of one or more of the viral genes. No human tumor has been shown to be caused by polyomaviruses.

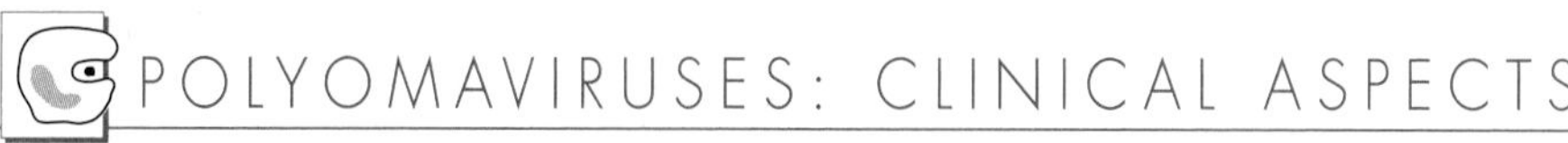

POLYOMAVIRUSES: CLINICAL ASPECTS

MANIFESTATIONS

Progressive Multifocal Leukoencephalopathy

PML is a rare, subacute, degenerative disease of the brain found primarily in adults with other chronic diseases, especially AIDS and reticuloendothelial malignancies, or those receiving immunosuppressive agents. The disease is characterized by the development of impaired memory, confusion, and disorientation, followed by a multiplicity of neurologic symptoms and signs that include hemiparesis, visual disturbances, incoordination, seizures, and visual abnormalities. PML is progressive, with death usually occurring 3 to 6 months after onset of symptoms. The incidence of PML has increased concomitantly with the AIDS epidemic.

PML is a degenerative, progressive brain disease

In PML, cerebrospinal fluid (CSF) findings are often normal, although some patients show a slight increase in lymphocytes, and protein levels may be elevated. Pathologically, foci of demyelination are found, surrounded by giant, bizarre astrocytes containing intranuclear inclusions. The demyelination is due to viral damage to oligodendroglial cells, which synthesize and maintain myelin. Abundant JCV particles can be seen in the brain by electron microscopy (Fig 43–2) and may be concentrated within the nuclei of oligodendrocytes. JCV DNA sequences have been demonstrated by PCR in the brain of patients without PML or demyelinating lesions, suggesting that the virus may be latent in the brain prior to immunosuppression. There is no specific treatment for PML, although reducing the immunosuppression, if possible, may have some clinical benefit.

JCV in cell nuclei, with demyelination

No specific treatment

Urinary Tract Infection

Infection of the urinary tract with JCV and BKV can be demonstrated frequently in immunocompromised patients but usually in those without symptoms or evidence of renal injury. BKV is associated with a hemorrhagic cystitis, particularly in bone marrow and renal transplant recipients. In addition, BKV is also the cause of a severe nephropathy and

BKV causes hemorrhagic cystitis and nephritis

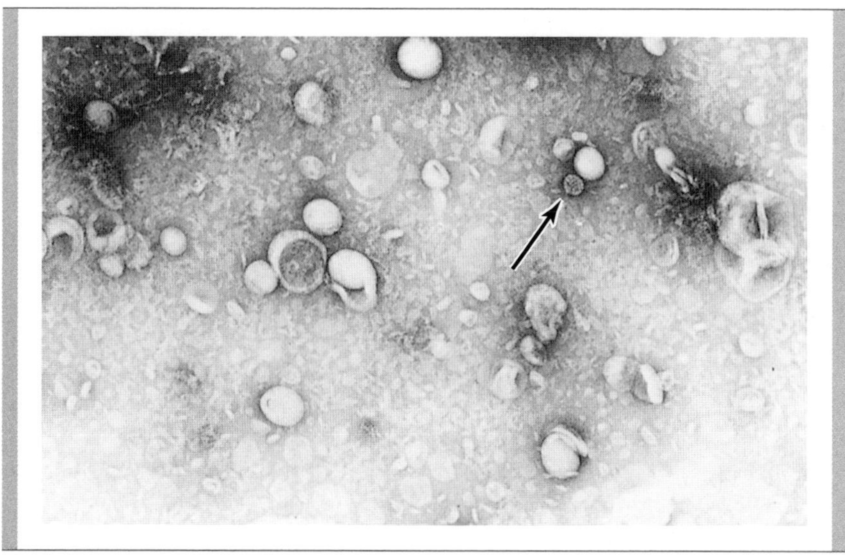

FIGURE 43–2
JC virus (arrow) among debris of cells from a brain biopsy of a case of progressive multifocal leukoencephalopathy. (*Reprinted with permission from Palmer E, Martin ML.* An Atlas of Mammalian Viruses. *Boca Raton, FL: CRC Press; 1982. Copyright 1982 by CRC Press, Inc.*)

vasculopathy that may lead to kidney loss in renal transplant recipients. The disease develops months after renal transplantation. Treatment consists of reducing immunosuppression, but as many as 50% of patients with this syndrome may require nephrectomy.

DIAGNOSIS

BKV can be isolated in cell culture

Both viruses can be detected by PCR

Urine from patients excreting these polyomaviruses may contain "decoy" cells similar to those from patients excreting cytomegalovirus. The nucleus of cytomegalovirus-infected cells is smaller with a larger halo effect, that is, a clear zone around the inclusion but within the nuclear membrane. The brain oligodendrocytes exhibit similar changes in patients with PML. BKV can be isolated by routine culture in diploid fibroblast or Vero monkey kidney cells, but nephropathy is preceded by plasma PCR positivity. At present, a kidney biopsy is required for definitive diagnosis. Viral antigens can be demonstrated in tissue by a variety of immunoassays. JCV DNA has been demonstrated in the brain of PML patients by PCR, and PCR of CSF is becoming the diagnostic test for PML.

ADDITIONAL READING

Bauer HM, Ting V, Greer CE, et al. Genital human papillomavirus infection in female university students as determined by a PCR-based method. *JAMA* 1991;265:472–477. Good report on the epidemiology of human papillomaviruses and means of diagnosis.

Koustky LA, Ault KA, Wheeler CM, et al. A controlled trial of a human papillomavirus type 16 vaccine. *N Engl J Med* 2002;347:1645–1651. This is a landmark trial, indicating it may indeed be possible to reduce the incidence of cervical cancer with vaccines. Administration of this HPV-16 vaccine reduced the incidence of both HPV-16 infection and HPV-16 related cervical intraepithelial neoplasia. Immunizing HPV-16-negative women may eventually reduce the incidence of cervical cancer.

Major EO, Ault GS. Progressive multifocal leukoencephalopathy: Clinical and laboratory observations in a viral induced demyelinating disease in the immunodeficient patient. *Curr Opin Neurol* 1995;8:184. An excellent review of papovavirus CNS disease.

Palefsky JM. Human papillomavirus infection among HIV-infected individuals. *Hematol Oncol Clin North Am* 1991;5:357–370. Provides guidelines for the management of cervical and anal neoplasia in HIV-infected persons.

Petrogiannis-Haliotis T, Sakoulas G, Kirby J, et al. BK-related polyomavirus vasculopathy in a renal transplant recipient. *N Engl J Med* 2001;345:1250–1255. This is an extremely well-executed case study, demonstrating current diagnostic approaches to human polyomavirus infections, and the virus tropism for vascular endothelial cells.

CHAPTER 44

Persistent Viral Infections of the Central Nervous System

W. Lawrence Drew

Evidence has accumulated during the past 30 years that a variety of progressive neurologic diseases in both animals and humans are caused by viral or other filterable agents that share some of the properties of viruses (Table 44–1). These illnesses have been termed "slow viral diseases" because of the protracted period between infection and the onset of disease as well as the prolonged course of the illness, but a better term is "persistent viral infection."

Progressive neurologic diseases

Most persistent viral infections involve well-differentiated cells, such as lymphocytes and neuronal cells. They can be classified as (1) diseases associated with "conventional" viral agents that possess nucleic acid genomes and protein capsids, induce immune responses, and can be grown in cell culture systems; and (2) diseases associated with "unconventional" viruses that are small, filterable infectious agents, known as "prions," which are transmissible to certain experimental animals, but that do not contain nucleic acids, do not appear to be associated with immune or inflammatory responses by the host and have not been cultivated in cell culture.

Include conventional viruses and unconventional agents

Do not produce immune or inflammatory responses

Persistence of conventional viruses can result from integration of viral nucleic acid into the host genome, mutations that interfere with or severely limit viral replication or antigenicity, failure of host immune systems to recognize virus or infected cells, or perhaps by encoding of the causative agent itself into the normal host cell genome.

Can be due to a variety of mechanisms

DISEASES ASSOCIATED WITH CONVENTIONAL AGENTS

The following conditions are the major persistent infections caused by conventional viral agents. They are summarized in Table 44–1.

Subacute Sclerosing Panencephalitis

Subacute sclerosing panencephalitis is considered in Chapter 34. It is a rare chronic measles virus infection of children that produces progressive neurologic disease characterized by an insidious onset of personality change, progressive intellectual deterioration, and both motor and autonomic nervous system dysfunctions.

Persistence of measles virus after acute childhood infection

TABLE 44–1

Conventional Viruses Causing Persistent Central Nervous System Infections

DISEASE	AGENT
Subacute sclerosing panencephalitis	Measles virus
Progressive panencephalitis following congenital rubella	Rubella virus
Progressive multifocal encephalopathy	Papovavirus (JC)
AIDS dementia complex	Human immunodeficiency virus
Persistent enterovirus infection of the immunodeficient	Enteroviruses

Abbreviations: AIDS, acquired immunodeficiency syndrome.

Progressive Postrubella Panencephalitis

Can be a late sequela of congenital rubella infection

Even more rarely, a degenerative neurologic disorder similar to subacute sclerosing panencephalitis may be related to persistent rubella virus infection of the central nervous system (CNS). This condition is seen most often in adolescents who have had the congenital rubella syndrome. Rubella virus has been isolated from brain tissue in these patients using cocultivation techniques.

Progressive Multifocal Leukoencephalopathy

Progressive neurologic disease of severely immunocompromised persons

Progressive multifocal leukoencephalopathy (PML) is a subacute, degenerative disease of the brain found primarily in adults with (1) immunosuppressive diseases, especially acquired immunodeficiency syndrome (AIDS) and reticuloendothelial malignancies; or (2) diseases requiring therapy with immunosuppressive agents. PML is due to a papovavirus and is considered in Chapter 43.

Persistent Enterovirus Infection

Associated with humoral immunodeficiencies

Temporary improvement with hyperimmune globulin

Persons with congenital or severe acquired immunodeficiency, especially those with agammaglobulinemia, may develop a chronic CNS infection due to an echovirus or other enterovirus. Headache, confusion, lethargy, seizures, and cerebrospinal fluid (CSF) pleocytosis are common manifestations. The virus can be isolated from the CSF. Clinical improvement may be achieved by the administration of human hyperimmune globulin to the infecting virus type. Relapse, however, occurs if therapy is discontinued, indicating persistence of virus despite the therapy.

AIDS Dementia Complex

Late stages of AIDS

Human immunodeficiency virus causes a persistent infection of the CNS in many patients with symptomatic AIDS. The clinical course may vary from a mild subacute illness to severe progressive dementia (see Chapter 42).

HUMAN DISEASES CAUSED BY UNCONVENTIONAL VIRAL AGENTS: SUBACUTE SPONGIFORM ENCEPHALOPATHIES

A group of progressive degenerative diseases of the CNS has been shown to be caused by infectious agents with unusual physical and chemical properties, which are now known as prions. The Nobel prize in Medicine for 1997 was awarded to Stanley Prusiner for his work in identifying the role of prions in disease. Prions cause bovine spongiform encephalopathy in cattle, scrapie in sheep, and five fatal CNS diseases in humans

TABLE 44–2

Unconventional Virus (Prion) Diseases[a]

HUMANS	ANIMALS (PRIMARY HOSTS)
Creutzfeldt-Jakob disease[b]	Scrapie (sheep)
Variant Creutzfeldt-Jakob disease	Transmissible mink encephalopathy (mink)
Gerstmann-Straüssler-Scheinker syndrome	Chronic wasting disease (mule deer, elk)
Kuru	Bovine spongiform encephalopathy (cows)[b]
Fatal familial insomnia	

[a] Subacute spongiform encephalopathies.
[b] Prion agents of variant Creutzfeldt-Jakob disease and bovine spongiform encephalopathy are identical.

(Table 44–2). Prions can be the etiologic agents of inherited, communicable, or sporadic diseases. The pathogenesis of these illnesses is not well understood, but the pathologic and clinical features are similar. Varying degrees of neuronal loss and astrocyte proliferation occur. The diseases are known as "spongiform" encephalopathies because of the vacuolar changes in the cortex and cerebellum. The incubation periods of these diseases are months to years, and their courses are protracted and inevitably fatal.

Prions affect animals and humans

Cause neuronal loss and spongiform changes in brain

A prion is defined as a "small proteinaceous infectious particle" that is not inactivated by procedures that destroy nucleic acids (Table 44–3). They are small with diameters of 5–100 nm or less, produce characteristic infections, and can remain viable even in formalinized brain tissue for many years. They are resistant to ionizing radiation, boiling, and many common disinfectants. Recognizable virions have not been found in tissues by electron microscopy, and the agents have not been grown in cell culture.

Infectious agents resist inactivation

Nucleic acids absent

A prion is composed of proteins encoded by a normal cellular gene. The protein, designated PrPc, is converted from a normal benign form into a disease-causing form by a change in conformation to a protein designated PrPsc (for the scrapie protein). Brain extracts from scrapie-infected animals contain PrPsc, which is not found in the brains of normal animals; PrPsc is the prion that is responsible for transmission and infection. The conformational change is also the way that prions multiply; that is, contact with PrPsc results in a conformational change of the normal host cell protein PrPc and the formation of additional PrPsc. Proliferation of PrPsc prions and the consequent pathology results from this process. During scrapie infection, prion protein may aggregate into birefringent rods

PrPc is encoded by a normal cellular gene

Conformational change to PrPsc results in disease and prion proliferation

TABLE 44–3

Biologic and Physical Properties of Prions

- Chronic progressive pathology without remission or recovery
- No inflammatory response
- No alteration in pathogenesis by immunosuppression or immunopotentiation
- Estimated diameter of 5–100 nm
- No virion-like structures visible by electron microscopy
- Replication to high titers in susceptible tissue
- Transmissible to experimental animals
- No interferon production or interference by conventional viruses
- Unusual resistance to ultraviolet irradiation, alcohol, formalin, boiling, proteases, and nucleases
- Can be inactivated by prolonged exposure to steam autoclaving or 1N or 2N NaOH

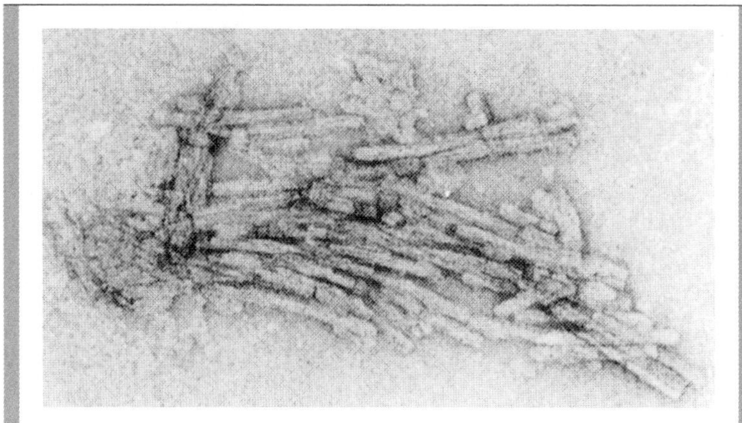

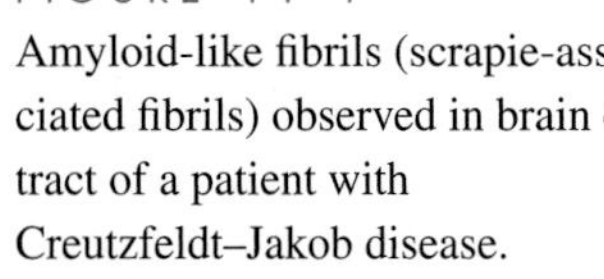

FIGURE 44–1
Amyloid-like fibrils (scrapie-associated fibrils) observed in brain extract of a patient with Creutzfeldt–Jakob disease. (*Reprinted with permission from Bockman JM, Kingsbury DT, McKinley MP, et al. Creutzfeldt–Jakob disease prion proteins in human brains.* N Engl J Med *1985;312:73–82.*)

and form filamentous structures termed scrapie-associated fibrils (Fig 44–1), which are found in membranes of scrapie-infected brain tissues.

Kuru

Women and children of the Fore people of New Guinea

Transmissible to primates

Associated with cannibalism

Kuru was a subacute, progressive neurologic disease of the Fore people of the Eastern Highlands of New Guinea. The disease was brought to the attention of the Western world by Gadjusek and Zigas in 1957. Although the illness was localized and decreasing in incidence, its study has thrown light on the transmissibility and infectious nature of similar encephalopathies. Epidemiologic studies indicated that kuru usually afflicted adult women, or children of either sex. The disease was rarely observed outside of the Fore region, and outsiders in the region did not contract the disease. The symptoms and signs were ataxia, hyperreflexia, and spasticity, which led to progressive dementia, starvation, and death. Pathologic examination revealed changes only in the CNS, with diffuse neuronal degeneration and spongiform changes of the cerebral cortex and basal ganglia. No inflammatory response was apparent. Inoculation of infectious brain tissue into primates produced a disease that caused similar neurologic symptoms and pathologic manifestations after an incubation period of approximately 40 months. Epidemiologic studies indicated that transmission of the disease in humans was associated with ingestion of a soup made from the brains of dead relatives and eaten in honor of the deceased. Clinical disease developed 4 to 20 years after exposure. Since the elimination of cannibalism from the Fore culture, kuru has disappeared.

Creutzfeldt–Jakob Disease

Progressive disease, usually occurring among elderly

Creutzfeldt–Jakob disease is a progressive, fatal illness of the CNS that is seen most frequently in the sixth and seventh decades of life. The initial clinical manifestations are a change in cerebral function, usually diagnosed initially as a psychiatric disorder. Forgetfulness and disorientation progress to overt dementia and the development of changes in gait, increased tone in the limbs, involuntary movement, and seizures. These manifestations resemble those of kuru. The disorder usually runs a course of 4–7 months, eventually leading to paralysis, wasting, pneumonia, and death.

Pathology identical to kuru

Transmission to animals

Creutzfeldt–Jakob disease is found worldwide, with an incidence of disease of one case per million per year. The mode of acquisition is unknown, but it occurs both sporadically (85%) and in a familial pattern (15%). Infection has also been transmitted by dura mater grafts, corneal transplants, by contact with contaminated electrodes or instruments used in neurosurgical procedures, and by pituitary-derived human growth hormone. The latter was responsible for more than 100 cases. The incubation period of the disease is approximately 3 to greater than 20 years.

The pathology of Creutzfeldt–Jakob disease is identical to that of kuru. It has been transmitted to chimpanzees, mice, and guinea pigs by inoculation of infected brain tissue, leukocytes, and certain organs. High levels of infectious agent have been found, especially in the brain, where they may reach 10^{-7} infectious doses per gram of brain tissue. Nonpercutaneous transmission of disease has not been observed, and there is no evidence of transmission by direct contact or airborne spread.

Brains from patients with Creutzfeldt–Jakob disease have the birefringent rods and fibrillar structures noted in scrapie (see Fig 44–1). Identification of PrPsc and antibodies directed against it may become a useful diagnostic adjunct to neuropathologic examination of brain tissue. Pathologic examination of brain tissue is the only definitive diagnostic test.

Scrapie-like structures seen in brain

There is no effective therapy for Creutzfeldt–Jakob disease, and all cases have been fatal. The small risk of nosocomial infection is related only to direct contact with infected tissue. Stereotactic neurosurgical equipment, especially that used in patients with undiagnosed dementia, should not be reused. In addition, organs from patients with undiagnosed neurologic disease should not be used for transplants. Growth hormone from human tissue has now been replaced by a recombinant genetically engineered product. The agent of Creutzfeldt–Jakob disease has not been transmitted to animals by inoculation of body secretions, and no increased risk of disease has been noted in family members or medical personnel caring for patients. Recommendations for disinfection of potentially infectious material include treatment for 1 hour with 2 N NaOH or by autoclaving at 132°C for 60–90 minutes. Others recommend even more extensive treatment such as combining these two procedures to ensure inactivation.

Nosocomial infections preventable by avoidance of potentially infectious materials, careful sterilization

Gerstmann-Straüssler-Scheinker Disease

Gerstmann-Straüssler-Scheinker disease is similar to Creutzfeldt–Jakob disease but occurs at a younger age (fourth to fifth decade). Cerebellar ataxia and paralysis are common, but dementia is less often seen. The disease evolves over several years. It was originally thought to be familial but also occurs sporadically, very rarely.

Gerstmann-Straüssler-Scheinker disease similar to Creutzfeldt–Jakob disease but evolves more slowly

Fatal Familial Insomnia

This is a recently recognized familial prion disease in which a syndrome of sleeping difficulty is followed by progressive dementia. It occurs in patients aged 35 to 61, culminating in death within 13 to 25 months. The infectious agent has been transmitted to experimental animals.

Sleeping difficulties progressing to dementia

Bovine Spongiform Encephalopathy ("Mad Cow Disease") and "Variant Creutzfeldt–Jakob Disease"

Bovine spongiform encephalopathy (BSE) was identified in 1986, after it began striking cows in the United Kingdom, causing them to become uncoordinated and unusually apprehensive. The source of the emerging epidemic was soon traced to a food supplement that included meat and bone meal from dead sheep. The methods for processing sheep carcasses had been changed in the late 1970s. Once they would have eliminated the "scrapie agent" in the supplement, but now they apparently did not.

To combat BSE, the British government banned the use of animal-derived feed supplements in 1988, and the epidemic among cattle, which peaked at nearly 40,000 cases in 1992, decreased to less than 4000 new cases in 1997. By February 2002, most European countries had reported cases of BSE but new infections have largely ceased as a result of imposing tight controls on cattle feed. The United States has been spared, as measured by over 19,000 cattle brain examinations. The incubation period in cattle was determined to be 2 to 8 years. In addition to the incoordination and apprehension, the cows exhibited hyperesthesia, hyperreflexia, muscle fasciculations, tremors, and weight loss. Autonomic dysfunction was frequently manifested as reduced rumination, bradycardia and other cardiac arrhythmias.

Source was meat and bone meal from sheep in cattle feed

Unfortunately, the prion that causes BSE survived the heat of cooking and was transmitted to humans who inadvertently consumed infected bovine neural tissue or bone marrow (both are sometimes found in processed meats, depending on the rendering procedures used). To date, over 100 humans with "variant Creutzfeldt–Jakob disease," have

Variant Creutzfeldt–Jakob disease apparently transmitted by infected bovine tissues to humans died in the United Kingdom. The cases frequently present in young adults as psychiatric problems progressing to neurologic changes and dementia, with death in an average of 14 months. It appears that destruction of diseased cattle and the changes in livestock feeds have prevented further cases.

ADDITIONAL READING

Almond J, Pattison J. Human BSE. *Nature* 1997;389:437–438. This article reviews evidence for transmission of BSE to humans, especially molecular identity of proteins from cattle and human brains.

Hill AF, Desbruslais M, Joiner S, et al. The same prion strain causes vCJD and BSE. *Nature* 1997;389:448–450. Summarizes evidence that the new variant Creutzfeldt–Jakob disease is caused by the same prion that causes BSE.

Johnson RT, Gibbs CJ Jr. Creutzfeldt-Jakob disease and related transmissible spongiform encephalopathies. *N Engl J Med* 1998;339:1994–2004. A review of prion-caused diseases, their clinical manifestations, and their diagnosis.

Prusiner SB. Molecular biology and pathogenesis of prion diseases. *Trends Biochem Sci* 1997;21:482–487. This article explains reproduction of prions and their neuropathologic potential.

PART VII

PATHOGENIC FUNGI

CHAPTER 45

Characteristics of Fungi

KENNETH J. RYAN

Fungi are a distinct class of microorganisms, most of which are free-living in nature where they function as decomposers in the energy cycle. Of the more than 200,000 known species, fewer than 200 have been reported to produce disease in humans. These diseases, the mycoses, have unique clinical and microbiologic features and are increasing in immunocompromised patients.

GENERAL NATURE OF FUNGI

Fungi are eukaryotes with a higher level of biological complexity than bacteria. They may be unicellular or may differentiate and become multicellular by the development of branching filaments. They reproduce sexually or asexually. The mycoses vary greatly in their manifestations but tend to be subacute to chronic with indolent, relapsing features. Acute disease, such as that produced by many viruses and bacteria, is uncommon with fungal infections.

Cell organization is eukaryotic

STRUCTURE

The fungal cell has typical eukaryotic features, including a nucleus with a nucleolus, nuclear membrane, and linear chromosomes. The cytoplasm contains an actin cytoskeleton and organelles, such as mitochondria and the Golgi apparatus. Fungal cells, which have a rigid cell wall external to the cytoplasmic membrane, differ from mammalian cells. The composition of that wall makes fungi different from bacteria and plants. Another important difference from mammalian cells involves the sterol makeup of the cytoplasmic membrane. In fungi, the dominant sterol is ergosterol; in mammalian cells, it is cholesterol. Fungi are usually in the haploid state, although diploid nuclei are formed through nuclear fusion in the process of sexual reproduction.

Presence of a nucleus, mitochondria, and endoplasmic reticulum

Ergosterol, not cholesterol, makes up cell membrane

The chemical structure of the cell wall in fungi is markedly different from that of bacterial cells in that it does not contain peptidoglycan, glycerol or ribitol teichoic acids, or lipopolysaccharide. In their place are the polysaccharides **mannan, glucan,** and **chitin** in close association with each other and with structural proteins (Fig 45–1).

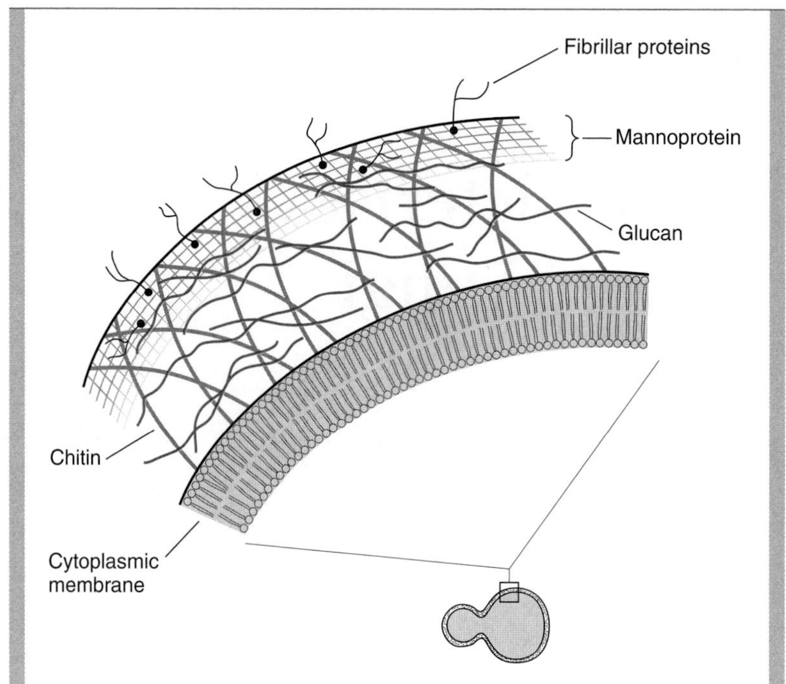

FIGURE 45–1
The fungal cell wall. The overlapping mannan, glucan, chitin, and protein elements are shown. Proteins complexed with the mannan (mannoproteins) extend beyond the cell wall

Cell wall mannan linked to surface proteins

Chitin and glucans give rigidity to cell wall

Mannoproteins are mannose-based polymers (mannan) found on the surface and in the structural matrix of the cell wall, where they are linked to protein. They are major determinants of serologic specificity because of variations in the composition and linkages of the polymer side chains. Glucans are glucosyl polymers, some of which form fibrils that increase the strength of the fungal cell wall, often in close association with chitin. Chitin is composed of long, unbranched chains of poly-*N*-acetylglucosamine. It is inert, insoluble, and rigid and provides structural support in a manner analogous to the chitin in crab shells or cellulose in plants. It is a major component of the cell wall of filamentous fungi. In yeasts, chitin appears to be of most importance in forming cross-septa and the channels through which nuclei pass from mother to daughter cells during cell division.

METABOLISM

Heterotrophic metabolism uses available organic matter

Photosynthetic mechanisms are lacking

Fungal metabolism is heterotrophic, requiring exogenous carbon for growth. Metabolic diversity is great, but most fungi grow with only an organic carbon source and ammonium or nitrate ions as a nitrogen source. In nature, nutrients for free-living fungi are derived from decaying organic matter. A major difference between fungi and plants is that fungi lack photosynthetic energy-producing mechanisms. Most are strict aerobes, although some can grow under anaerobic conditions. None are strict anaerobes.

REPRODUCTION

Asexual reproduction forms conidia by mitosis

Meiosis forms sexual spores in specialized structures

Fungi may reproduce by either asexual or sexual processes. Reproductive elements produced asexually are termed **conidia.** Those produced sexually are termed **spores** (e.g., ascospores, zygospores, basidiospores). Asexual reproduction involves mitotic division of the haploid nucleus and is associated with production by budding spore-like conidia or separation of hyphal elements. In sexual reproduction, the haploid nuclei of donor and recipient cells fuse to form a diploid nucleus, which may then divide by classical meiosis. Some of the four resulting haploid nuclei may be genetic recombinants and may undergo further division by mitosis. Highly complex specialized structures may be involved. Detailed study of this process in fungal species such as *Neurospora crassa* has been important in gaining an understanding of basic cellular genetic mechanisms.

FUNGAL MORPHOLOGY AND GROWTH

The size of fungi varies immensely. A single cell without transverse septa may range from bacterial size (2–4 μm) to a macroscopically visible structure. The morphologic forms of growth vary from colonies superficially resembling those of bacteria to some of the most complex, multicellular, colorful, and beautiful structures seen in nature. Mushrooms are an example and can be regarded as a complex organization of cells showing structural differentiation.

Vary from bacterial size to multicellular mushrooms

Mycology, the science devoted to the study of fungi, has many terms to describe the morphologic components that make up these structures. Fortunately, the terms and concepts that must be mastered can be limited by considering only the fungi of medical importance and accepting some simplification.

YEASTS AND MOLDS

Initial growth from a single cell may follow either of two courses, yeast or mold (Fig 45–2). The first and simplest is the formation of a bud, which extends out from a

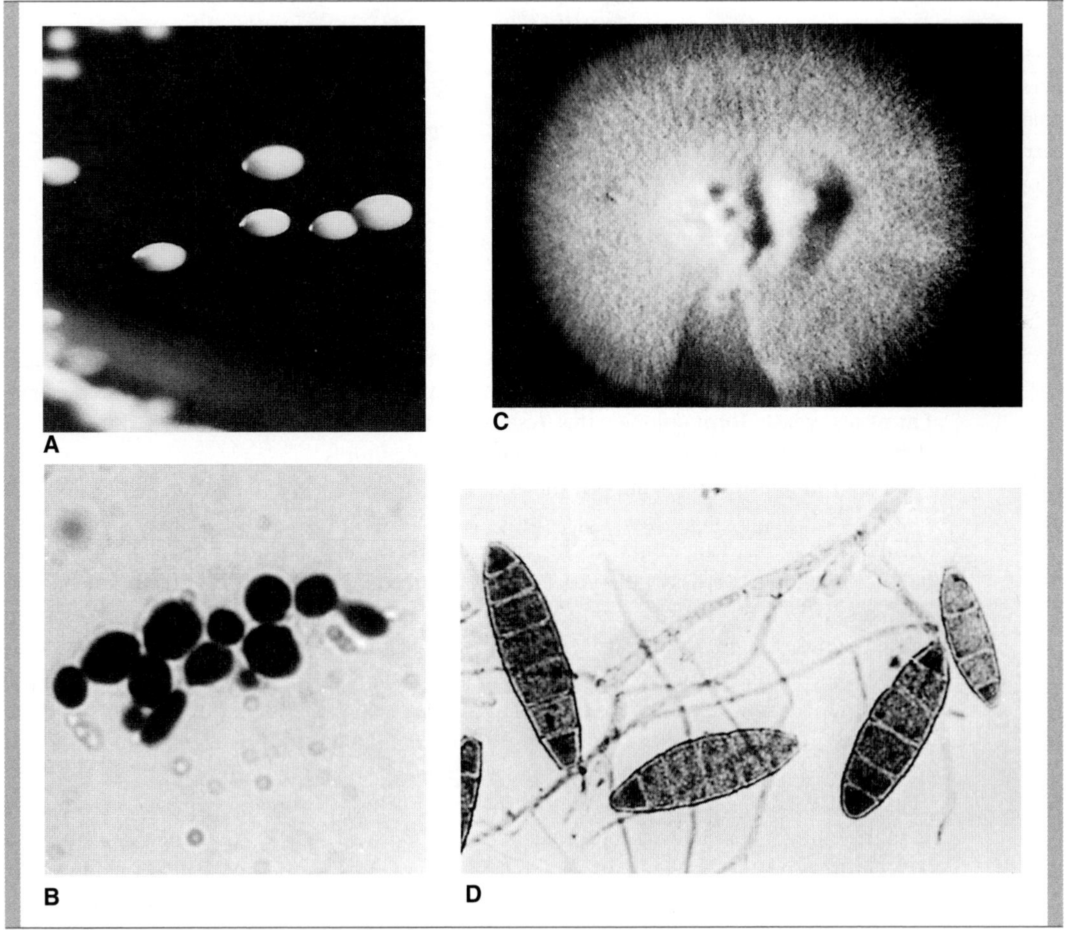

FIGURE 45–2
Yeast and mold forms of fungal growth. **A.** Yeasts form colonies similar to those of bacteria. **B.** Microscopically, they are large oval cells with occasional buds (blastoconidia). **C.** Molds form fuzzy, often pigmented colonies. **D.** Microscopically, molds are a complex of hyphae and associated conidia. (*Parts* C *and* D *reprinted with permission from Dr. E. S. Beneke and the Upjohn Company: Scope Publications, Human Mycoses.*)

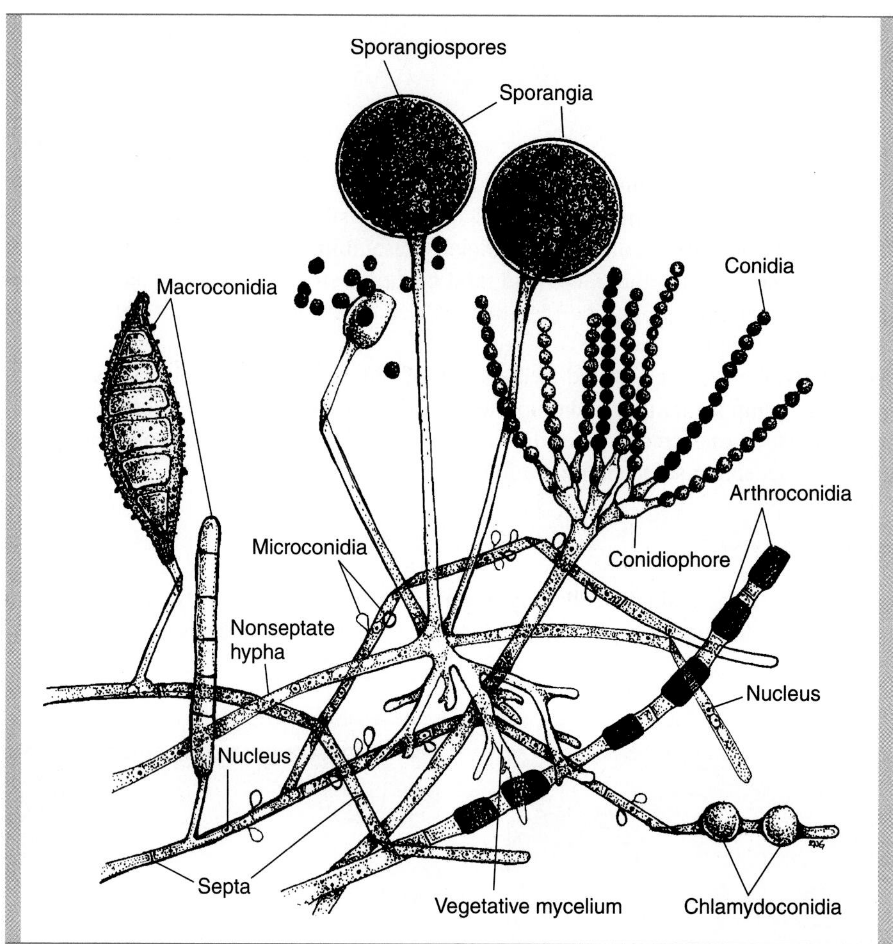

FIGURE 45–3
Mold forms. The tube-like hyphae constitute their basic structure. Examples of spores and conidia and of the structures that bear them are shown. They develop from the hyphal wall.

Yeasts produce blastoconidia by budding

round or oblong parent, constricts, and forms a new cell. These buds are called **blastoconidia** (see Fig 45–2), and fungi that reproduce in this manner are called **yeasts.** On plates, yeasts form colonies that resemble those of bacteria. In broth, yeasts produce diffuse turbidity or grow as sediments in unshaken cultures.

Molds produce septate or nonseptate hyphae

Vegetative mycelium acts as a root

Aerial mycelium bears reproductive conidia or spores

Pseudohyphae are less rigid

Fungi may also grow through the development of **hyphae** (singular, hypha), which are tube-like extensions of the cell with thick, parallel walls. As the hyphae extend, they form an intertwined mass called a **mycelium.** Most fungi form hyphal **septa** (singular, septum), which are cross-walls perpendicular to the cell walls that divide the hypha into subunits (Fig 45–3). These septa may not form complete walls and vary among species in the extent to which they restrict movement of organelles and nuclei. Some species are nonseptate; they form hyphae and mycelia as a single, continuous cell. In both septate and nonseptate hyphae, multiple nuclei are present, with free flow of cytoplasm along the hyphae or through pores in any septum. A portion of the mycelium (vegetative mycelium) usually grows into the medium or organic substrate (eg, soil) and functions like the roots of plants as a collector of nutrients and moisture. The more visible surface growth may assume a fluffy character as the mycelium becomes aerial. The hyphal walls are rigid enough to support this extensive, intertwining network, commonly called a **mold.** The aerial hyphae bear the reproductive structures of this class of fungi. Some fungi form structures called **pseudohyphae** (Fig 45–4), which differ from true hyphae in having recurring bud-like constrictions and less rigid cell walls.

Morphology of reproductive conidia and spores used for identification

The reproductive conidia and spores of the molds and the structures that bear them assume a great variety of sizes, shapes, and relationships to the parent hyphae, and the morphology and development of these structures are the primary basis of identification of medically important molds. The mycelial structure plays some role in identification,

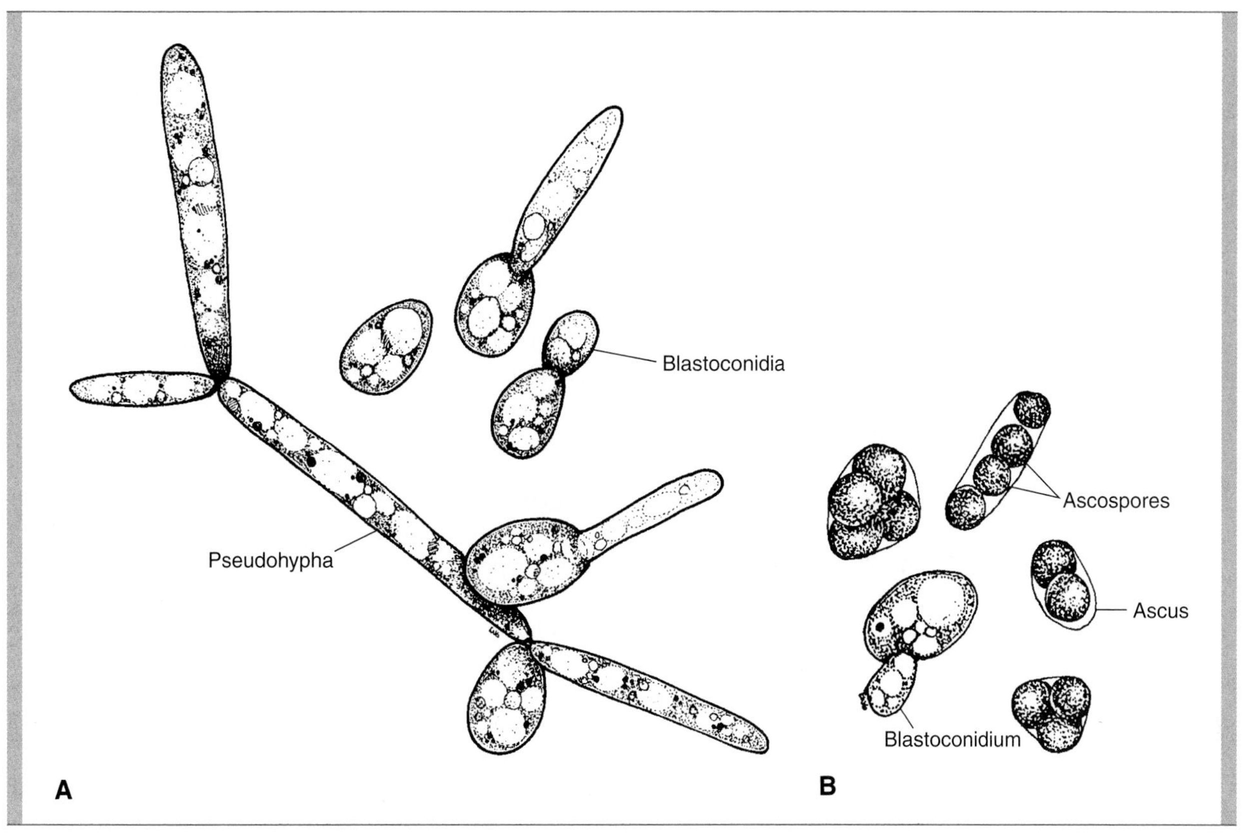

FIGURE 45–4
Yeast forms. **A.** Yeast reproduction is limited to the development of blastoconidia or longer extensions, pseudohyphae. **B.** Sexual reproduction leads to the formation of ascospores.

depending on whether the hyphae are septate or nonseptate, but differences are not sufficiently distinctive to identify or even suggest a fungal genus or species.

Exogenously formed conidia may arise directly from the hyphae or on a special stalk-like structure, the **conidiophore.** Occasionally, terms such as **macroconidia** and **microconidia** are used to indicate the size and complexity of these conidia. Conidia that develop within the hyphae are called either **chlamydoconidia** or **arthroconidia.** Chlamydoconidia become larger than the hypha itself; they are round, thick-walled structures that may be borne on the terminal end of the hypha or along its course. Arthroconidia conform more to the shape and size of the hyphal units but are thickened or otherwise differentiated. Arthroconidia may form a series of delicately attached conidia that break off and disseminate when disturbed. The most common sexual spore is termed an **ascospore.** Four or eight ascospores may be found in a sac-like structure, the **ascus.** The structures are illustrated in Figures 45–3 and 45–4.

Conidia and conidiophore arrangements determine names

Ascospores are borne in ascus sac

DIMORPHISM

In general, fungi grow either as yeasts or as molds; mold forms show the greatest diversity. Some species can grow in either a yeast or a mold phase, depending on environmental conditions. These species are known as **dimorphic fungi.** Several human pathogens demonstrate dimorphism; they grow in the mold form in their environmental reservoir and in culture at ambient temperatures, but convert to the yeast or some other form in infected tissue. For most, it is possible to manipulate the cultural conditions to demonstrate both yeast and mold phases in vitro. Yeast phase growth requires conditions similar to those of the parasitic in vivo environment, such as 35 to 37°C incubation and enriched

Dimorphic fungi grow as yeasts in tissue or molds in environment

Infectious conidia disseminate molds

medium. Mold growth requires minimal nutrients and ambient temperatures. The conidia produced in the mold phase may be infectious and serve to disseminate the fungus.

CLASSIFICATION

Although conidia are more readily observed, the major classification of fungi primarily depends on the nature of sexual spores and septation of hyphae as its differential characteristics. On this basis, fungi have been organized into four to six classes or phyla. A major problem of classifying the medically important fungi using these groups is that for most species, no sexual form has been demonstrated. This may be due to its loss during evolution or because the spores are so rarely produced that they have not been detected. One approach has been to give these fungi their own class (Deuteromycetes, or **fungi imperfecti**) and wait for the discovery of the sexual form to place it in one of the legitimate groups—the Ascomycetes, Basidiomycetes, or Zygomycetes. The application of molecular methods such as analysis of ribosomal RNA genes has allowed the placement of species pending discovery of the sexual forms. The medically important genera are shown in Table 45–1. Discovery of the sexual form may not bring immediate clarity from the student's standpoint; for instance, when the sexual stage of *Trichophyton mentagrophytes* was demonstrated, it was found to be identical to that of an already named ascomycete (*Arthroderma benhamiae*). Most medically important species are now assigned to the Ascomycetes and a few to the Basidiomycetes or Zygomycetes.

Taxonomy is based on sexual spores and septation of hyphae

Asexual form is unknown for most pathogens

rRNA genes are used for classification

The grouping of medically important fungi used in the following chapters is based on the types of tissues they parasitize and the diseases they produce, rather than on the principles of basic mycologic taxonomy. The **superficial** fungi, such as the dermatophytes, cause indolent lesions of the skin and its appendages, commonly known as ringworm and athlete's foot. The **subcutaneous** pathogens characteristically cause infection through the skin, followed by subcutaneous spread, lymphatic spread, or both. The **opportunistic** fungi are those found in the environment or in the normal flora that occasionally produce disease, usually in the compromised host. The **systemic** pathogens are the most virulent fungi and may cause serious progressive systemic disease in previously healthy persons. They are not members of the normal human flora. Although their major potential is to produce deep-seated visceral infections and systemic spread (systemic mycoses), they

Medical grouping organized by biological behavior in humans

Systemic fungi infect previously healthy persons

TABLE 45–1

Classification of Medically Important Fungi

Genus	Typical Growth	Septation[a]	Sexual Form	Phylum	Medical Classification
Aspergillus	Mold	+	?	Ascomycete	Opportunistic
Blastomyces	Dimorphic	+	?	Ascomycete	Systemic
Candida	Dimorphic	+	?	Ascomycete	Opportunistic
Coccidioides	Dimorphic	+	?	Ascomycete	Systemic
Cryptococcus	Yeast		+	Basidiomycete	Systemic
Epidermophyton	Mold	+	+	Ascomycete	Superficial
Histoplasma	Dimorphic	+	+	Ascomycete	Systemic
Microsporum	Mold	+	+	Ascomycete	Superficial
Mucor	Mold	–	+	Zygomycete	Opportunistic
Pneumocystis	Cysts[b]		?	Ascomycete	Opportunistic
Rhizopus	Mold	–	+	Zygomycete	Opportunistic
Sporothrix	Dimorphic	+	?	Ascomycete	Subcutaneous
Trichophyton	Mold	+	+	Ascomycete	Superficial

[a] For those that form hyphae.

[b] Tissue forms but does not grow in culture.

may also produce superficial infections as part of their disease spectrum or as the initiating event. The superficial mycoses do not spread to deeper tissues. As with all clinical classifications, overlaps and exceptions occur. In the end, the organism defines the disease, and it must be isolated or otherwise demonstrated.

EPIDEMIOLOGY

Most fungal infections arise from contact with an environmental reservoir or from the patient's own fungal flora. Some superficial mycoses can be transmitted from person to person by very close contact, such as sharing a comb with an individual who has scalp ringworm; others can be acquired from ringworm infections of animals. Other fungal infections are not communicable between humans or animals, and infected patients need not be isolated.

Infection is from environment or endogenous flora

Only dermatophyte infections are communicable

DIAGNOSIS

Because of their large size, fungi often demonstrate distinctive morphologic features on direct microscopic examination of infected pus, fluids, or tissues. The simplest method is to mix the specimen with a 10% solution of potassium hydroxide (KOH) preparation and place it under a coverslip. The strong alkali digests or clears the tissue elements (epithelial cells, leukocytes, debris) but not the rigid cell walls of both yeasts and molds. After digestion of the material, the fungi can be observed under the light microscope with or without staining (see Fig 47–1B). Some yeasts stain with common stains such as the Gram stain, to which they are usually positive. Direct examinations can be aided by the use of calcifluor white, a dye that binds to polysaccharides in cellulose and chitin. Under ultraviolet light, calcifluor white fluoresces, enhancing detection of fungi in fluids or tissue sections.

KOH digests tissue but not fungal wall

Some yeasts are Gram-positive

Calcifluor white enhances detection

Histopathologic examination of tissue biopsy specimens is widely used and shows the relationship of the organism to tissue elements and responses (blood vessels, phagocytes, granulomatous reactions). Most fungi can be seen in sections stained with the hematoxylin and eosin (H&E) method routinely used in histology laboratories (Fig 45–5). Specialized staining procedures such as the silver impregnation methods are frequently used because they stain almost all fungi strongly but only a few tissue components. The pathologist should be alerted to the suspicion of fungal infection when tissues are submitted, because special stains and searches for fungi are not made routinely.

Often visible in H&E preparations

Silver stains enhance detection

Fungi can be grown by methods similar to those used to isolate bacteria. Growth occurs readily on enriched bacteriologic media commonly used in clinical laboratories (eg, blood agar and chocolate agar). Many fungal cultures, however, require days to weeks of incubation for initial growth; bacteria present in the specimen grow more rapidly and may interfere with isolation of a slow-growing fungus. Therefore, the culture procedures of diagnostic mycology are designed to favor the growth of fungi over bacteria and to allow incubation to continue for a sufficient time to isolate slow-growing strains.

Growth in culture is simple but slow

Selective media allow isolation in the presence of bacteria

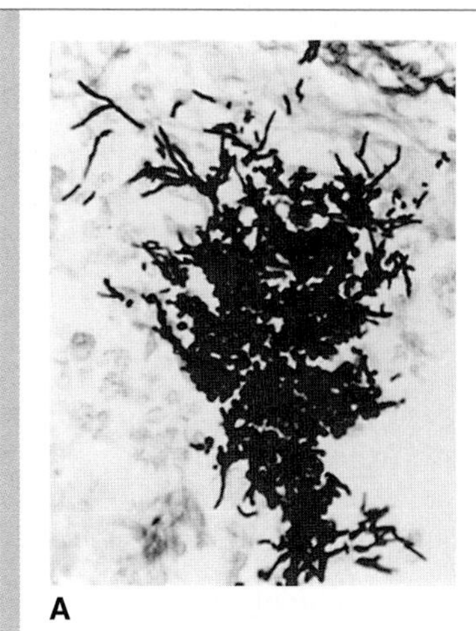

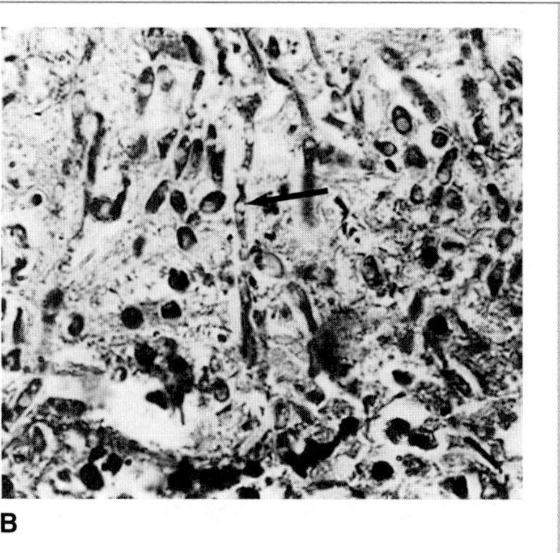

FIGURE 45–5
Direct examinations for fungi. **A.** Fungi such as *Candida albicans* are large enough to be demonstrated microscopically at low magnification. **B.** In histologic sections the invasive pseudohyphae (arrow) may be seen. (*Part* A *reproduced with permission from Dr. E. S. Beneke and the Upjohn Company: Scope Publications, Human Mycoses.*)

Sabouraud's agar optimal for fungi but poor for bacteria

The most commonly used medium for cultivating fungi is Sabouraud's agar, which contains only glucose and peptones as nutrients. Its pH is 5.6, which is optimal for growth of dermatophytes and satisfactory for growth of other fungi. Most bacteria associated with humans fail to grow or grow poorly on Sabouraud's agar.

Selective media make use of antimicrobics

Blood agar or another enriched bacteriologic agar medium is used when pure cultures would be expected. It is made selective for fungi by the addition of antibacterial antibiotics such as chloramphenicol and gentamicin. Cycloheximide, an antimicrobic that inhibits some saprophytic fungi, is sometimes added to Sabouraud's agar to prevent overgrowth of contaminating molds from the environment, particularly for skin cultures. Media containing these selective agents cannot be relied on exclusively because they can interfere with growth of some pathogenic fungi or because the "contaminant" may be producing an opportunistic infection. For example, cycloheximide inhibits *Cryptococcus neoformans,* and chloramphenicol may inhibit the yeast forms of some dimorphic fungi. Selective media are not needed for growing fungi from sterile sites such as cerebrospinal fluid or tissue biopsy specimens. In contrast to most parasitic bacteria, many fungi grow best at 25 to 30°C, and temperatures in this range are used for primary isolation. Paired cultures incubated at 30 and 35°C may be used to demonstrate dimorphism.

Cultures incubated at 30°C for primary isolation

Yeast identified biochemically

Once a fungus is isolated, identification procedures depend on whether it is a yeast or mold. Yeasts are identified by biochemical tests analogous to those used for bacteria, including some that are identical (eg, urease production). The ability to form pseudohyphae is also taxonomically useful among the yeasts.

Molds identified by morphology and culture features

Molds are most often identified by the morphology of their conidia and conidiophores. Other features such as the size, texture, and color of the colonies help characterize molds, but without demonstrating conidiation they are not sufficient for identification. The ease and speed with which various fungi produce conidia vary greatly. Minimal nutrition, moisture, good aeration, and ambient temperature favor development of conidia.

Lactophenol cotton blue stains mycelia, conidia, and spores

Microscopic fungal morphology is usually demonstrated by methods that allow in situ microscopic observation of the fragile asexual conidia and their shape and arrangement. Morphology may also be examined in fragments of growth teased free of a mold and examined moist in preparations containing a dye called lactophenol cotton blue. The dye stains the hyphae, conidia, and spores. Conidium production may not occur for days or weeks after the initial growth of the mold. It is somewhat like waiting for flowers to bloom, and it can be frustrating when the result has immediate clinical application.

Temperature variation demonstrates dimorphism

Exoantigen and DNA probes are more rapid

It is desirable, but not always possible, to demonstrate both the yeast and mold phases with dimorphic fungi. In some cases, this result can be achieved with parallel cultures at 30° and 35°C. The tissue form of *Coccidioides immitis* is not readily produced in vitro. An alternate approach has been developed for identification of some of the dimorphic systemic fungi, based on soluble antigens prepared from mycelial growth (exoantigens) and called the exoantigen test. When these exoantigens react with specific antibody in an immunodiffusion procedure, precipitin lines are formed between the unknown antigen and its homologous antibody. Results are usually available much more rapidly than are results of cultural tests. For a few fungi, DNA probes are available for rapid speciation.

Serologic tests are useful for systemic fungi

Serum antibodies directed against a variety of fungal antigens can be detected in patients infected with those agents. Except for some of the systemic pathogens, the sensitivity, specificity, or both, of these tests have not been sufficient to recommend them for use in diagnosis or therapeutic monitoring of fungal infections. The tests of value are discussed in sections on specific agents.

ADDITIONAL READING

Ajello L, Hay RJ (eds). Medical Mycology. Volume 4 in Collier L, Balows A, Sussman, M (eds). *Topley & Wilson's Microbiology and Microbial Infection.* London: Arnold, 1998. This classic British reference work now devotes an entire volume to fungi and fungal diseases beautifully written and illustrated by experts from both sides of the Atlantic.

Guarro J, Gené J, Stchigel AM. Developments in fungal taxonomy. *Clin Microbiol Rev* 1999;12:454–500. This review is a preview of what is ahead with the application of molecular methods to fungal taxonomy.

CHAPTER 46

Pathogenesis, Immunity, and Chemotherapy of Fungal Infections

KENNETH J. RYAN

We all have regular contact with fungi. They are so widely distributed in our environment that thousands of fungal spores are inhaled or ingested every day. Other species are so well adapted to humans that they are common members of the normal flora. Despite this ubiquity, clinically apparent systemic fungal infections are quite uncommon, even among persons living within the geographic habitat of the more pathogenic species. However, progressive systemic fungal infections pose some of the most difficult diagnostic and therapeutic problems in infectious disease, particularly among immunocompromised patients to whom they are a major threat. The purpose of this chapter is to give an overview of the pathogenesis and immunology of fungal infections and of the activity of antifungal agents. Details relating to specific fungi are given in Chapters 47 to 50.

GENERAL ASPECTS OF FUNGAL DISEASE

EPIDEMIOLOGY

Fungal infections are acquired from the environment or may be endogenous in the few instances where they are members of the normal flora. Inhalation of infectious conidia generated from molds growing in the environment is a common mechanism. Some of these molds are ubiquitous, whereas others are restricted to geographic areas whose climate favors their growth. In the latter case, disease can be acquired only in the endemic area. Some environmental fungi produce disease after they are accidentally injected past the skin barrier. The pathogenic fungi represent only a tiny fraction of those found in the environment. Endogenous infections are restricted to a few yeasts, primarily *Candida albicans*. These yeasts have the ability to colonize by adhering to host cells and, given the opportunity, invade deeper structures.

Environmental conidia are inhaled or injected

Endogenous yeasts may invade

PATHOGENESIS

Fungal pathogenesis is similar to bacteria

Most fungi are opportunists

Compared with bacterial, viral, and parasitic disease, less is known about the pathogenic mechanisms and virulence factors involved in fungal infections. Analogies with bacterial diseases come the closest because of the apparent importance of adherence to mucosal surfaces, invasiveness, extracellular products, and interaction with phagocytes. In general, the principles discussed in Chapter 10 apply to fungal infections. Most fungi are opportunists, producing serious disease only in individuals with impaired host defense systems. Only a few fungi are able to cause disease in previously healthy persons.

Adherence

Adherence is mediated by fungal adhesins and host cell receptors

Mannoprotein is an adhesin, and fibronectin a receptor

A number of fungal species, particularly the yeasts, are able to colonize the mucosal surfaces of the gastrointestinal and female genital tracts. It has been shown experimentally that the ability to adhere to buccal or vaginal epithelial cells is associated with colonization and virulence. Within the genus *Candida* (see Chapter 48), the species that adhere best to epithelial cells are those most frequently isolated from clinical infections. Adherence usually requires a surface adhesin on the microbe and a receptor on the epithelial cell. In the case of *C. albicans,* mannoprotein components extending from the cell wall have been implicated as the adhesin and fibronectin, and other components of the extracellular matrix as the receptor(s). A few binding mediators have been identified for other fungi, usually a surface mannoprotein.

Invasion

Traumatic injection is linked to trauma

Small conidia may pass airway defenses

Passing an initial surface barrier, whether skin, mucous membrane, or respiratory epithelium, is an important step for most successful pathogens. Some fungi are introduced through mechanical breaks. For example, *Sporothrix schenckii* infection typically follows a thorn prick or some other obvious trauma (see Chapter 47). Fungi that initially infect the lung must produce conidia small enough to be inhaled past the upper airway defenses. For example, arthroconidia of *Coccidioides immitis* (2 to 6 μm) can remain suspended in air for a considerable time and can reach the terminal bronchioles to initiate pulmonary coccidioidomycosis.

Invasion across mucosal barriers may involve enzymes

Triggered by temperature and possibly other cues, dimorphic fungi from the environment undergo a metabolic shift similar to the heat shock response and completely change their morphology and growth to a more invasive form. Invasion directly across mucosal barriers by the endogenous yeast *C. albicans* is similarly associated with a morphologic change, the formation of hyphae. The triggering mechanisms of this change are unknown, but the new form is able to penetrate and spread. Extracellular enzymes (eg, proteases, elastases) are associated with the hyphal form of *Candida* and with the invasive forms of many of the dimorphic and other pathogenic fungi. Although these enzymes must contribute to some aspect of invasion or spread, their precise role is unknown for any fungus.

Tissue Injury

No classic exotoxins are produced in vivo

Injury is due to inflammatory and immunologic responses

None of the extracellular products of opportunistic fungi or dimorphic pathogens have been shown to injure the host directly during infection in a manner analogous to bacterial toxins. Although the presence of necrosis and infarction in the tissues of patients with invasion by fungi such as *Aspergillus* suggests a toxic effect, direct evidence is lacking. A number of fungi do produce exotoxins, called **mycotoxins,** in the environment but not in vivo. The structural components of the cell do not cause effects similar to those of the endotoxin of Gram-negative bacteria, although mannan is known to circulate widely in the body. The injury caused by fungal infections seems to be due primarily to the inflammatory and immune responses that are stimulated by the prolonged presence of the fungus.

IMMUNITY

Phagocyte Interactions

There is considerable evidence that normal persons have a high level of natural resistance to most fungal infections. This is particularly true of opportunistic molds. An important component of this resistance is the ability of healthy neutrophils to kill hyphae of most fungi if they reach the tissues. A small number of species, all of which are dimorphic, are able to produce mild to severe disease in otherwise healthy individuals. In vitro studies have shown these fungi to be more resistant to killing by neutrophils than the opportunists. *C. albicans* is able to bind complement components in a way that interferes with phagocytosis.

Most fungi are readily killed by neutrophils

C. immitis, one of the best-studied species, has been shown to contain a component in the wall of its conidial (infective) phase that is antiphagocytic. As the hyphae convert to the spherule (tissue) phase, they also become resistant to phagocytic killing because of their size and surface characteristics. The tissue yeast form of *Histoplasma capsulatum* is resistant to phagocytic killing after ingestion and, in fact, multiplies within macrophages. These mechanisms of avoiding phagocytic killing appear to allow many dimorphic fungi to multiply sufficiently to produce an infection that can be controlled only by the immune response.

Tissue phases of dimorphic fungi resist phagocytic killing

Adaptive Immune Response

A recurrent theme with fungal infections is the importance of an intact immune response in preventing infection and progression of disease. Most fungi are incapable of producing even a mild infection in immunocompetent individuals.

A small number of species are able to cause clinically apparent infection that usually resolves once there is time for activation of normal immune responses. In most instances in which it has been investigated, the actions of neutrophils and T lymphocyte–mediated immune responses have been found to be of primary importance in this resolution. Progressive, debilitating, or life-threatening disease with these agents is commonly associated with depressed or absent cell-mediated immune responses, and the course of any fungal disease is worse in immunocompromised than previously healthy persons.

T cell–mediated responses of primary importance

Progressive fungal diseases occur in the immunocompromised

Humoral Immunity

Antibodies can be detected at some time during the course of almost all fungal infections, but for most there is little evidence that they contribute to immunity. The only encapsulated fungus, *Cryptococcus neoformans,* is one example of a fungus against which antibody plays a role in controlling infection. Although the polysaccharide capsule of *C. neoformans* has antiphagocytic properties similar to those of encapsulated bacterial pathogens (eg, *Streptococcus pneumoniae, Haemophilus influenzae*), it is less antigenic. Anticapsular antibody plays a role in resolving cryptococcal infection, but T cell–mediated responses are still dominant. Antibody also plays a role in control of *C. albicans* infections by enhancing fungus–phagocyte interactions, and this is probably true for other yeasts. In some other fungal infections, the lack of protective effect of antibody is striking. In coccidioidomycosis, for example, high titers of *C. immitis*–specific antibodies are associated with dissemination and a worsening clinical course.

Opsonizing antibody is effective in some yeast infections

Cellular Immunity

Considerable clinical and experimental evidence points toward the importance of cellular immunity in fungal infections. Most patients with severe systemic disease have neutropenia, defects in neutrophil function, or depressed T lymphocyte–mediated immune reactions. These can result from factors such as steroid treatment, leukemia, Hodgkin's disease, and acquired immunodeficiency syndrome. In other cases, an immunologic deficit can usually be demonstrated by absence of delayed-type hypersensitivity responses or by direct in vitro assays of T-cell responsiveness to the fungus in question. In

Systemic disease associated with deficiencies in neutrophils and T cell–mediated immunity

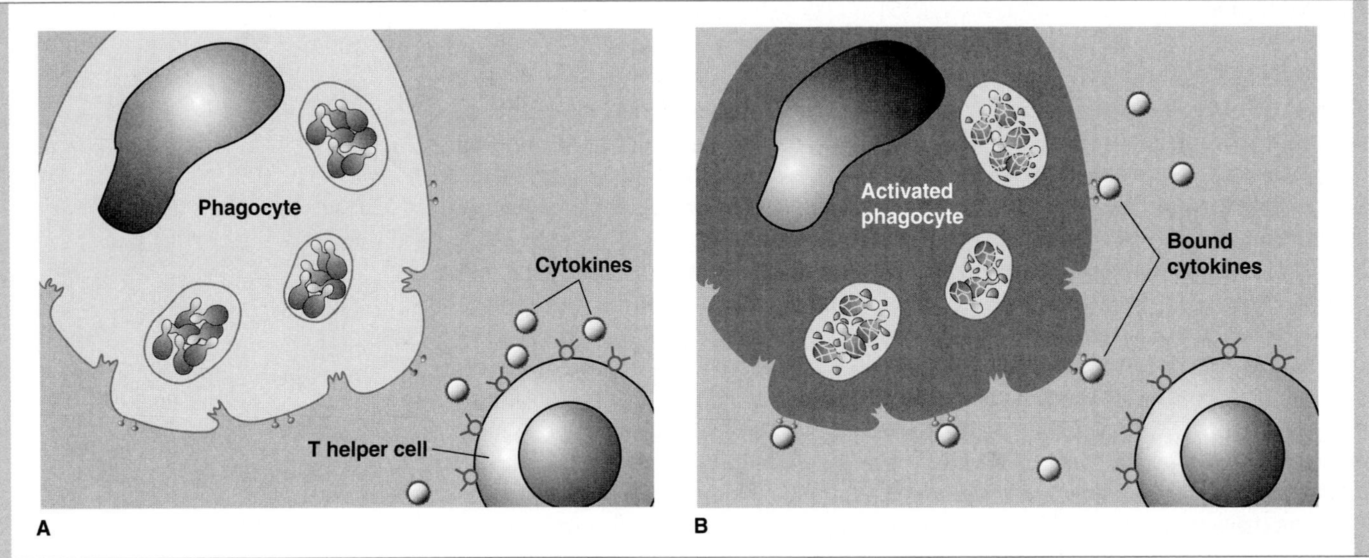

FIGURE 46–1
Cell-mediated immunity to fungal infections. **A.** Most pathogenic fungi are able to survive and multiply in phagocytes (**B**) until the phagocyte becomes specifically activated by cytokines from T cells. The growth is then restricted with development of cell-mediated immunity.

the latter case, it is possible that hyporesponsiveness is due at least in part to activation of suppressor cells or continued circulation of fungal antigen.

Fungi that escape neutrophils grow slowly in macrophages

Growth is restricted when macrophages activated by cytokines

Immune defects lead to progressive disease

Although not all fungi have been studied to the same degree, a unified picture emerging from clinical and experimental animal studies is illustrated in Figure 46–1. When hyphae or yeast cells of the fungus reach deep tissue sites, they are either killed by neutrophils or resist destruction by one of the antiphagocytic mechanisms described earlier. Surviving cells continue to grow slowly or, if they are dimorphic, convert to their yeast, hyphal, or spherule tissue phases. The growth of these invasive forms may be slowed but not killed by macrophages. In healthy persons, the extent of infection is small, and any symptoms are caused by the inflammatory response. Everything awaits the specific immune response. The turning point comes when the macrophages are activated by cytokine mediators produced by T lymphocytes that have interacted with the fungal antigen. Where they have been identified, these mediators, which are associated with helper T-cell responses, are those such as interleukin 2 or interferon-γ. The activated macrophages are then able to restrict the growth of the fungus, and the infection is controlled. Defects that disturb this cycle lead to progressive disease. To the extent that they are known, the specifics of these reactions are discussed in the following chapters.

ANTIFUNGAL CHEMOTHERAPY

Many antifungals are too toxic for use

Compared with antibacterial agents, relatively few antimicrobics are available for treatment of fungal infections. Many substances with antifungal activity have proved either to be unstable, to be toxic to humans, or to have undesirable pharmacologic characteristics, such as poor diffusion into tissues. Of the agents in current clinical use, none approaches the degree of selective toxicity that β-lactams provide for antibacterial therapy, but the newer azole compounds have significantly higher therapeutic activity and lower toxicity than earlier antifungal agents.

Fortunately, most fungal infections are self-limiting and require no chemotherapy. Superficial mycoses are often treated, but topical therapy can be used, thus limiting toxicity to the host. The remaining small group of deep mycoses that are uncontrolled by the host's immune system require the prolonged use of relatively toxic antifungals. This, combined with the fact that most of the patients have underlying immunosuppression, makes them the most difficult of all infectious diseases to treat successfully. The characteristics of currently used antifungal agents are discussed next and summarized in Table 46–1.

Treatment is most needed for dissemination in immunocompromised persons

ANTIFUNGAL ANTIMICROBICS THAT AFFECT MEMBRANE STEROLS

Polyenes

The polyenes **nystatin** and **amphotericin B** are lipophilic and bind to sterols in the cytoplasmic membrane of eukaryotic cells. Following binding, they form annular channels, which penetrate the membrane and lead to leakage of essential small molecules from the cytoplasm and cell death. The basis of their selective toxicity is their greater affinity for the sterols of fungal membranes, such as ergosterol, than the sterols of human cells. This difference is relative, because they also bind cholesterol in mammalian membranes, which creates the considerable toxicity that limits their use.

Sterol binding forms membrane channels

At physiologic pH, amphotericin B is insoluble in water and must be administered intravenously as a colloidal suspension. Amphotericin B is not absorbed from the gastrointestinal tract. Almost all fungi are susceptible to amphotericin B, and the development of resistance is too rare to be a consideration in its use. The major limitation to amphotericin B therapy is the toxicity created by its affinity for mammalian as well as fungal membranes. Infusion is commonly followed by chills, fever, headache, and dyspnea. The most serious toxic effect is renal dysfunction and is seen in virtually every patient receiving a therapeutic course. Experienced clinicians learn to titrate the dosage for each patient to minimize the nephrotoxic effects. For obvious reasons, use of amphotericin B is limited to progressive, life-threatening fungal infections. In these cases, despite its toxicity, it often remains the antifungal agent of choice. Preparations that complex amphotericin B with phospholipids to form liposomes have been used as a way to limit toxicity. The even greater toxicity of nystatin limits its use to topical preparations.

Insoluble compound must be infused in suspension

Active against most fungi

Therapy must be titrated against toxicity

Azoles

The azoles are a large family of synthetic organic compounds, which includes members with antibacterial, antifungal, and antiparasitic properties. The important antifungal azoles are the imidazole, **ketoconazole,** and the triazoles, **fluconazole** and **itraconazole.** Others are under development or evaluation. Their activity is based on inhibition of a cytochrome enzyme (P450 demethylase) responsible for conversion of lanosterol to ergosterol, the major component of the fungal cytoplasmic membrane. This leads to lanosterol accumulation and the formation of a defective cell membrane with altered permeability characteristics.

Enzyme inhibition is crucial for ergosterol synthesis

Ketoconazole was the first azole to be useful in systemic infections but is now being supplanted by either fluconazole or itraconazole for most systemic mycoses, including aspergillosis and candidiasis, for which ketoconazole was not effective. Ketoconazole and itraconazole are given orally, and fluconazole, either orally or intravenously. Although nausea, vomiting, and elevation of hepatic enzymes complicate the treatment of some patients, the azoles are much less toxic than amphotericin B. Endocrinologic defects can be a problem because of inhibition of conversion of lanosterol to cholesterol, a precursor of several hormones. Central nervous system penetration of ketoconazole is poor, which limits its effectiveness in systemic coccidioidomycosis and cryptococcosis, but fluconazole has been more effective. Currently, fluconazole and itraconazole are the primary alternates to amphotericin B for treatment of systemic fungal infections. Azoles are also effective for superficial and subcutaneous mycoses in which the initial therapy either fails or is not tolerated by the patient. Two other azoles, **clotrimazole** and **miconazole,** are used in over-the-counter topical preparations.

All are less toxic than amphotericin B

Fluconazole, itraconazole are most used

Voriconazole, a second-generation azole, inhibits both 14-α-sterol demethylase and 24-methylene dihydrolanosterol demethylation, providing a broader spectrum of activity

Voriconazole has broad-spectrum activity

TABLE 46–1

Features of Antifungal Agents

Agent	Mechanism of Action	Mechanism of Resistance	Route	Clinical Use
Polyenes				
Nystatin	Membrane disruption	Sterol modification	Topical	Most fungi
Amphotericin B	Membrane disruption	Sterol modification	Intravenous	Most fungi
Azoles				
Ketoconazole	Demethylase block of ergosterol synthesis	Active efflux, demethylase alteration, or overproduction[a]	Oral	*Candida, Cryptococcus,* dimorphic fungi[b]
Fluconazole	Demethylase block of ergosterol synthesis	Active efflux, demethylase alteration, or overproduction[a]	Oral, intravenous	*Candida, Cryptococcus,* dimorphic fungi
Itraconazole	Demethylase block of ergosterol synthesis	Active efflux, demethylase alteration, or overproduction[a]	Oral, intravenous	*Candida, Cryptococcus,* dimorphic fungi, invasive molds (*Aspergillus*)
Clotrimazole	Demethylase block of ergosterol synthesis	Unknown[c]	Topical	*Candida,* some other yeasts
Miconazole	Demethylase block of ergosterol synthesis	Unknown[c]	Topical	*Candida,* some other yeasts
Voriconazole	Demethylase block of ergosterol synthesis	Unknown[c]	Oral, intravenous	*Candida,* some other yeasts and molds
Allylamines				
Terbinafine	Squalene accumulation	?Active efflux	Oral	Dermatophytes, combined with azoles for *Candida, Aspergillus*
Naftifine	Squalene accumulation	Unknown	Topical	Dermatophytes
Flucytosine				
	RNA and DNA synthesis	Permease or modifying enzymes[d] absent or decreased	Oral	*Candida* and *Cryptococcus,* resistance emerges in monotherapy
Echinocandins				
Caspofungin	Block of glucan synthesis	Unknown	Intravenous	*Aspergillus, Candida*
Griseofulvin	Microtubule disruption	Unknown	Oral	Dermatophytes
Potassium iodide	Unknown	Unknown	Oral	*Sporothrix schenckii*
Tolnaftate	Unknown	Unknown	Oral	Dermatophytes

Abbreviation: 5FC, 5-flucytosine.

[a] Most work is with fluconazole and *Candida,* other azoles are to be assumed similar.

[b] Generally less absorbed and less active than fluconazole or itraconazole.

[c] Probably similar to other azoles, but resistance to the concentrations in topical preparations may differ.

[d] Cytosine deaminase and uracil phosphoribosyltransferase (the enzyme that forms 5-fluorodoxyuridine from 5FC).

against some yeasts and molds that are resistant to the other azoles. It can be given intravenously or orally.

Allylamines

The allylamines are a group of synthetic compounds that act by inhibition of an enzyme (squalene epoxidase) in the early stages of ergosterol synthesis. Their lethal effect is due to accumulation of squalene precursors rather than a deficiency of ergosterol. The allylamines include an oral agent, **terbinafine,** and a topical agent, **naftifine.** Both are used in the treatment of dermatophyte (ringworm) infections.

Cause squalene accumulation

ANTIFUNGALS THAT AFFECT NUCLEIC ACID SYNTHESIS

Flucytosine

5-Flucytosine (5FC), which was originally developed as an anticancer drug, is an antimetabolite analog of cytosine. It is a potent inhibitor of RNA, DNA, and ultimately protein synthesis. 5FC enters the cell aided by a permease, where it is converted to 5-fluorouracil by the action of cytosine deaminase. After further modification, 5FC is incorporated into what becomes defective RNA. Its effect on DNA synthesis is through its conversion to another metabolite (5-fluorodeoxyuridine), which is a potent inhibitor of thymidylate synthetase.

Enzymatically modified form makes defective RNA

Inhibits DNA synthesis

Flucytosine is well absorbed after oral administration. It is active against most clinically important yeasts, including *C. albicans* and *C. neoformans,* but has little activity against molds or dimorphic fungi. A significant limitation is the development of resistance that can occur by single-step mutation during therapy. Potential resistance limits flucytosine use to mild yeast infections or treatment in combination with amphotericin B for life-threatening systemic infections. Use in combination reduces the chance for expression of flucytosine resistance and allows a lower dose of amphotericin B to be used. In some instances, the combination is synergistic. The primary toxic effect of flucytosine is a reversible bone marrow suppression that can lead to neutropenia and thrombocytopenia. This effect is dose related and can be controlled by drug monitoring.

Active against yeasts but not molds

Resistance develops during therapy if used alone

ANTIFUNGALS THAT AFFECT CELL WALL SYNTHESIS

Given the unique chemical nature of the fungal cell wall, with its interwoven layers of mannan, mannoprotein, glucan, and chitin (see Chapter 45), it is disappointing that agents that act on any component of the cell wall have not yet made an impact in antifungal chemotherapy. The fungal equivalent of the β-lactam and glycopeptide inhibitors of bacterial peptidoglycan synthesis would be most welcome. One class of agents (echinocandins), which block glucan synthesis by inhibition of glucan synthetase, cause morphologic distortions and osmotic instability in yeast that are similar to the effect of β-lactams on bacteria. The first such agent to be licensed is **caspofungin,** which has good activity against *Candida* and *Aspergillus*. Another class of compounds (nikomycins), which disrupt chitin synthesis, are at an earlier stage of development.

Agents acting on glucan and chitin synthesis are emerging

OTHER ANTIFUNGAL AGENTS

Griseofulvin is a product of a species of the mold *Penicillium.* It is active only against the agents of superficial mycoses. Griseofulvin is actively taken up by susceptible fungi and acts on the microtubules and associated proteins that make up the mitotic spindle. It interferes with cell division and possibly other cell functions associated with microtubules. Griseofulvin is absorbed from the gastrointestinal tract after oral administration and concentrates in the keratinized layers of the skin. Clinical effectiveness has been demonstrated for all causes of dermatophyte infection, but the response is slow. Difficult cases may require 6 months of therapy to effect a cure.

Microtubule disruption interferes with cell division

Active against dermatophytes

Potassium iodide is the oldest known oral chemotherapeutic agent for a fungal infection. It is effective only for cutaneous sporotrichosis. Its activity is somewhat paradoxical, because the mold form of the etiologic agent, *Sporothrix schenckii,* can grow on medium containing 10% potassium iodide. The pathogenic yeast form of this dimorphic fungus appears to be susceptible to molecular iodine. **Tolnaftate** is a derivative of naphthiomate. It has activity against dermatophytes (see Chapter 47) but not against yeasts. It has been effective in topical treatment of dermatophytoses and is available in over-the-counter preparations.

Iodide inhibits *Sporothrix*

RESISTANCE TO ANTIFUNGAL AGENTS

Definition of Resistance

The concepts, definitions, and laboratory methods described in Chapter 14 for bacterial resistance are generally applicable to fungi. Quantitative susceptibility is measured by the minimal inhibitory concentration (MIC) under conditions that favor the growth of fungi. The diversity of growth rates and metabolic activity in the various fungi has made application of the MIC to therapy more difficult than in bacteria. The MICs performed in different types of fungal growth media can vary as much as 1000-fold. Although which medium is "right" cannot be determined, there has now been agreement on a standardized broth dilution method so experimental and clinical results can be reliably compared. Most of this work is with yeasts; molds are more difficult to work with and not suited to testing in broth. As with bacteria, fungi with MICs in the pharmacologically achievable range may or may not be clinically susceptible. Because of the variables cited above, high MICs do not predict resistance with the same certainty they do with bacteria. For these reasons, antifungal susceptibility testing is still considered investigational and not offered in hospital laboratories.

Concepts are similar to bacterial resistance

Laboratory methods are variable

Mechanisms of Resistance

The cell wall and cytoplasmic membrane present a barrier for antifungal agents to access the fungal interior. While this is generally considered a mechanism of innate resistance, there have been examples in which changes in membrane sterols appear to have restricted permeability to azoles. 5FC requires entry of a permease into the cell, and the absence of this enzyme is a significant mechanism of acquired resistance. Energy-requiring efflux pumps, which remove the drug from the cytoplasm, appear to be an even more important mechanism of resistance with the azoles. The efflux mechanism may confer resistance to multiple agents, and the mechanisms and genes involved are similar to the human P-glycoprotein pump associated with resistance to antineoplastic chemotherapeutics.

Alteration in membrane sterols restricts access

Efflux pumps remove drug from cytoplasm

Alterations in the target of the antifungal agent are an important means of acquired resistance. Although resistance to polyenes is rare, it has been traced to the appearance in the cytoplasmic membrane of sterols that have a decreased affinity for these agents. The production of cytochrome demethylases with lower affinity for azoles is also associated with resistance. Other mechanisms of resistance involve the absence or overproduction of crucial enzymes. Isolates resistant to 5FC lack either the permease or the cytosine deaminase that converts it to its active form. Resistance to both azoles and allylamines has been associated with overproduction of their target enzymes. It is surprising that enzymatic inactivation, the most potent bacterial resistance mechanism, is not important for any of the antifungals in current use.

Altered targets include membrane and enzymes

Overproduction of target enzymes negates effect

Inactivating enzymes are not produced

SELECTION OF ANTIFUNGALS

As with all chemotherapy, the selection of antifungal agents for treatment of superficial, subcutaneous, and systemic mycoses involves balancing probable efficacy against toxicity. The factors to be considered are (1) the threat of morbidity or mortality posed by the specific infection, (2) the immune status of the patient, (3) the toxicity of the antifungal, and (4) the probable activity of the antifungal agent against the fungus. In the case of superficial mycoses, the risks of appropriate therapy are small, and a number of topical agents may be tried. At the other extreme, an immunocompromised patient will most

Immune status dictates aggressiveness of therapy

Azoles with or without amphotericin B are the standard

likely be treated aggressively with systemic agents for proven or even suspected systemic fungal infection. Amphotericin B, despite its toxicity, is still the treatment of choice for almost all serious systemic fungal infections, but the newer azoles are often added. The most common regimen is an initial course of amphotericin B followed by one of the azoles.

ADDITIONAL READING

Calderone RA, Cihlar RL (eds). *Fungal Pathogenesis: Principles and Clinical Applications.* New York: Marcel Dekker; 2002. This volume is a collection of papers that gives the current status of advances in understanding of the pathogenesis and immune mechanisms of the major systemic and opportunistic pathogens.

Ghannoum MA, Rice LB. Antifungal agents: Mode of action, mechanisms of resistance, and correlation of these mechanisms with bacterial resistance. *Clin Microbiol Rev* 1999;12:501–517. This review focuses on mechanisms and includes interesting discussions of parallels with bacterial resistance (where they exist).

Kontoyiannis DP, Lewis RE. Antifungal drug resistance of pathogenic fungi. *Lancet* 2002;359:1135–1144. This concise review covers mechanisms of action and resistance and includes comprehensive tables on both topics.

Rex JH, Pfaller MA, Walsh TJ, et al. Antifungal susceptibility testing: Practical aspects and current challenges. *Clin Microbiol Rev* 2001;14:643–658. This review centers around the application of the method adopted as a standard in the United States but also discusses future methods (flow cytometry, biochemical tests) and the difficulty of testing molds.

CHAPTER 47

Dermatophytes, *Sporothrix*, and Other Superficial and Subcutaneous Fungi

KENNETH J. RYAN

The least invasive of fungi are the dermatophytes and other superficial fungi that are adapted to the keratinized outer layers of the skin. The subcutaneous fungi go a step further extending to the tissue beneath the skin but rarely invade deeper. Both are discussed here and summarized in Table 47–1.

SUPERFICIAL FUNGI

Dermatophytes

Dermatophytoses are superficial infections of the skin and its appendages, commonly known as ringworm, athlete's foot, and jock itch. They are caused by species of the genera *Microsporum, Trichophyton,* and *Epidermophyton,* which are collectively known as dermatophytes. These fungi are highly adapted to the nonliving, keratinized tissues of nails, hair, and the stratum corneum of the skin. The source of infection may be humans, animals, or the soil.

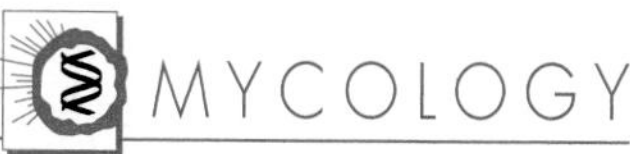

MYCOLOGY

Dermatophytes (literally, skin-plants) are molds that have been classified as Deuteromycetes (fungi imperfecti). The three genera of medical importance are *Epidermophyton, Microsporum,* and *Trichophyton,* which are separated primarily by the morphology of their macroconidia and presence of microconidia. The sexual forms have been discovered for many of the *Microsporum* and *Trichophyton* species and assigned to ascomycete

Form septate hyphae, macroconidia, and microconidia

TABLE 47–1

Agents of Superficial and Subcutaneous Mycoses

Fungus	Fungal Growth: In Lesion	Fungal Growth: In Culture (25°C)	Infection Site	Disease
Dermatophytes				
Microsporum canis	Septate hyphae	Mold	Hair,[a] skin	Ringworm
Microsporum audouini	Septate hyphae	Mold	Hair[a]	Ringworm
Microsporum gypseum	Septate hyphae	Mold	Hair, skin	Ringworm
Trichophyton tonsurans	Septate hyphae	Mold	Hair, skin, nails	Ringworm
Trichophyton rubrum	Septate hyphae	Mold	Hair, skin, nails	Ringworm
Trichophyton mentagrophytes	Septate hyphae	Mold	Hair, skin	Ringworm
Trichophyton violaceum	Septate hyphae	Mold	Hair, skin, nails	Ringworm
Epidermophyton floccosum	Septate hyphae	Mold	Skin	Ringworm
Other superficial fungi				
Malassezia furfur[b]	Yeast (mycelia)[c]	Yeast	Skin (pink to brown)[d]	Pityriasis (tinea) versicolor
Hortaea werneckii[e]	Septate hyphae, ellipsoidal cells	Yeast (mold)	Skin (brown–black)[d]	Tinea nigra
Trichosporon cutaneum	Septate hyphae	Mold	Hair (white)[b]	White piedra
Piedraia hortae	Septate hyphae	Mold, ascospores	Hair (black)[b]	Black piedra
Subcutaneous fungi				
Sporothrix schenckii	Cigar-shaped yeast (rare)	Mold	Subcutaneous, lymphatic spread	Sporotrichosis
Fonsecaea pedrosoi	Muriform body[f]	Mold	Wart-like foot lesions	Chromoblastomycosis
Phialophora verrucosa	Muriform body[f]	Mold	Wart-like foot lesions	Chromoblastomycosis
Cladophialophora (Cladosporium) carrionii	Muriform body[f]	Mold	Wart-like foot lesions	Chromoblastomycosis

[a] Specimens fluoresce under ultraviolet light.

[b] Previously known as *Pityrosporum orbiculare*.

[c] Denotes less frequent findings.

[d] Color of clinical lesions.

[e] Previously known as *Cladosporium werneckii*.

[f] Multicompartment yeast-like structure.

Epidermophyton, Microsporum, and *Trichophyton* are major genera

Grow best at 25°C

genera (*Arthroderma, Nannizzia*). Dermatophytes are still called by their previous names in the medical literature for reasons of familiarity and because identification procedures continue to be based on the characteristics of their conidia. Many species cause dermatophyte infections; the most common of these are shown in Table 47–1. They require a few days to a week or more to initiate growth. Most grow best at 25°C on Sabouraud's agar, which is usually used for culture. The hyphae are septate, and their conidia may be borne directly on the hyphae or on conidiophores. Small microconidia may or may not be formed; however, the larger and more distinctive macroconidia (Fig 47–1C) are usually the basis for identification.

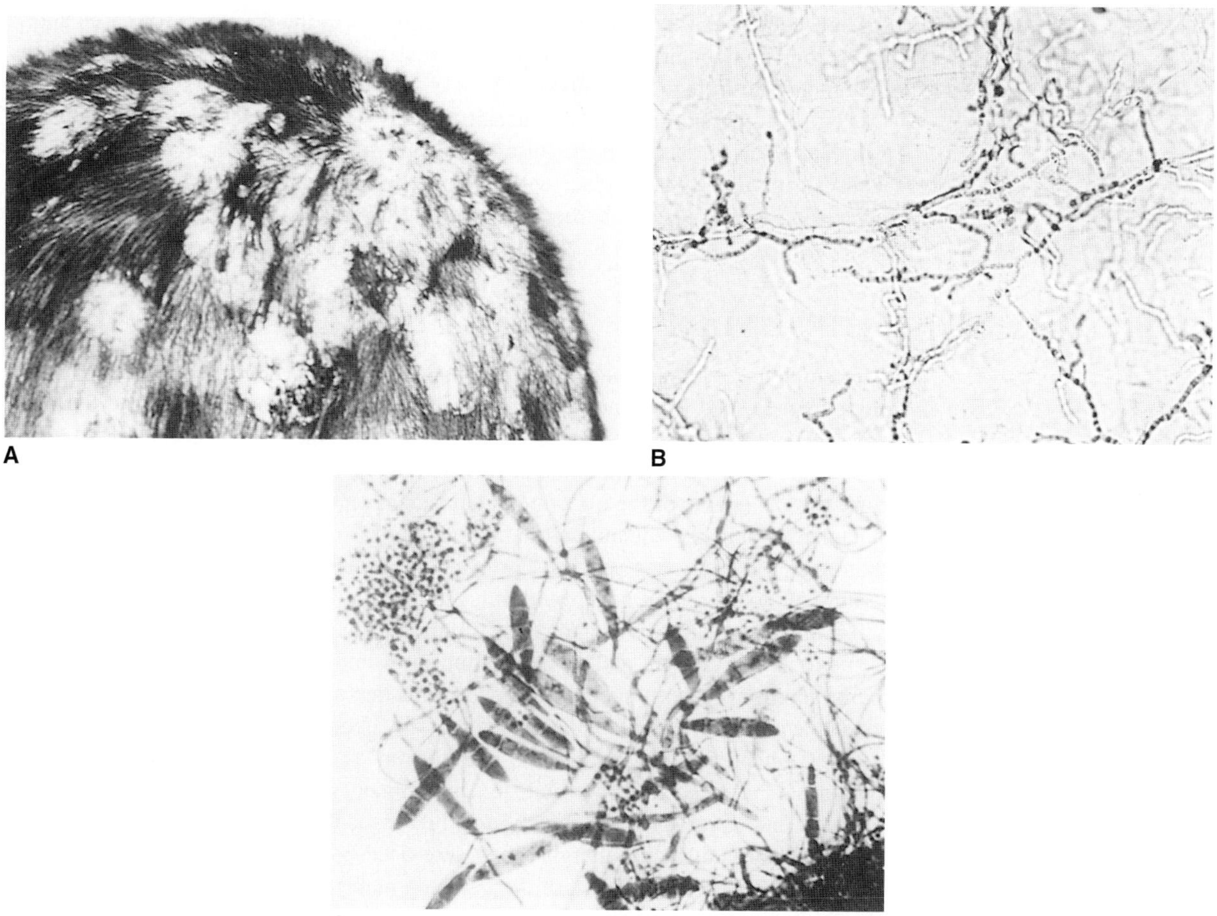

A B C

FIGURE 47–1
Dermatophyte infection of scalp (ringworm). **A.** Scalp lesions. Note the annular margination. **B.** Scrapings taken from the edge of the scalp lesion in KOH. Only the hyphal elements are visible. **C.** Culture. Hyphae, macroconidia, and microconidia are present. The macroconidia are characteristic of *Trichophyton*. (*Reprinted with permission from Dr. E. S. Beneke and the Upjohn Company: Scope Publications, Human Mycoses.*)

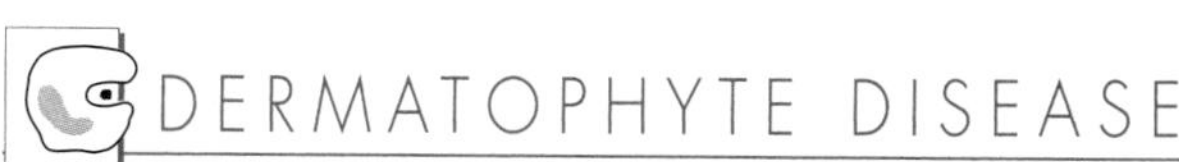

DERMATOPHYTE DISEASE

CLINICAL CAPSULE

Dermatophytoses are slowly progressive eruptions of the skin and its appendages which may be unsightly but are not painful or life threatening. The manifestations (and names) vary depending on the nature of the inflammatory response in the skin, but typically involve erythema, induration, itching, and scaling. The most familiar is "ringworm," which gets its name from the annular shape of creeping margin at the advancing edge of dermatophyte growth.

EPIDEMIOLOGY

There are both ecologic and geographic differences in the occurrence of the various dermatophyte species. Some are primarily adapted to the skin of humans, others to animals, and others to the environment. All may serve as the source for human infection. Many wild and domestic animals, including dogs and cats, are infected with certain dermatophyte

Reservoir may be human, animal, or soil

species and represent a large reservoir for infection of humans. There are large differences between temperate and tropical climates in the frequency of cases and isolations from nonhuman sources of the different species. Many of these differences are changing with shifts in population.

Transmission requires contact with intact or detached skin or hair

Human-to-human transmission usually requires close contact with an infected subject or infected person or animal, because dermatophytes are of low infectivity and virulence. Transmission usually takes place within families or in situations involving contact with detached skin or hair, such as barber shops and locker rooms. No special precautions beyond handwashing need be taken by the medical attendant after contact with an infected patient.

PATHOGENESIS

Initial infection is through minor skin breaks

Balance between fungal growth and skin desquamation determines outcome

Dermatophytoses begin when minor traumatic skin lesions come in contact with dermatophyte hyphae shed from another infection. Susceptibility may be enhanced by local factors such as the composition surface fatty acids. Once the stratum corneum is penetrated, the organism can proliferate in the keratinized layers of the skin aided by a variety of proteinases. The course of the infection is dependent on the anatomic location, moisture, the dynamics of skin growth and desquamation, the speed and extent of the inflammatory response, and the infecting species. For example, if the organisms grow very slowly in the stratum corneum, and turnover by desquamation of this layer is not retarded, the infection will probably be short-lived and cause minimal signs and symptoms. Inflammation tends to increase skin growth and desquamation rates and helps limit infection, whereas immunosuppressive agents such as corticosteroids decrease shedding of the keratinized layers and tend to prolong infection. Invasion of any deeper structures is extremely rare.

Poor inflammatory response leads to chronic infection

Most infections are self-limiting, but those in which fungal growth rates and desquamation are balanced and in which the inflammatory response is poor tend to become chronic. The lateral spread of infection and its associated inflammation produce the characteristic sharp advancing margins that were once believed to be the burrows of worms. This characteristic is the origin of the common name **ringworm** and the Latin term **tinea** (worm) that is often applied to the clinical forms of the disease (Fig 47–1A).

Hair shaft is penetrated and broken by hyphae

Infection may spread from skin to other keratinized structures, such as hair and nails, or may invade them primarily. The hair shaft is penetrated by hyphae, which extend as arthroconidia either exclusively within the shaft (endothrix) or both within and outside the shaft (ectothrix). The end result is damage to the hair shaft structure, which often breaks off. Loss of hair at the root and plugging of the hair follicle with fungal elements may result. Invasion of the nail bed causes a hyperkeratotic reaction, which dislodges or distorts the nail.

IMMUNITY

Delayed hypersensitivity responses occur

CMI responses are the most important

The great majority of dermatophyte infections pass through an inflammatory stage to spontaneous healing. Phagocytes are able to use oxidative pathways to kill the fungi both intracellularly and extracellularly. Little is known about the factors that mediate the host response in these self-limiting infections or whether they confer immunity to subsequent exposures. Antibodies may be formed during infection but play no known role in immunity. Most clinical and experimental evidence points to the importance of cell-mediated immunity (CMI), as with other fungal infections. The timing of the inflammatory response to infection correlates with appearance of delayed hypersensitivity, and resolution of infection is associated with the blastogenic T-lymphocyte responses. Enhanced desquamation with the inflammatory response helps remove infected skin.

Widespread infection is associated with T-lymphocyte defects and *T. rubrum*

Occasionally, dermatophyte infections become chronic and widespread. This progression has been related to both host and organism factors. Approximately half of these patients have underlying diseases affecting their immune responses or are receiving treatments that compromise T-lymphocyte function. These chronic infections are particularly associated with *Trichophyton rubrum,* to which both normal and immunocompromised persons appear to be hyporesponsive. Although a number of mechanisms have been proposed, how this organism is able to grow without stimulating much inflammation is unexplained.

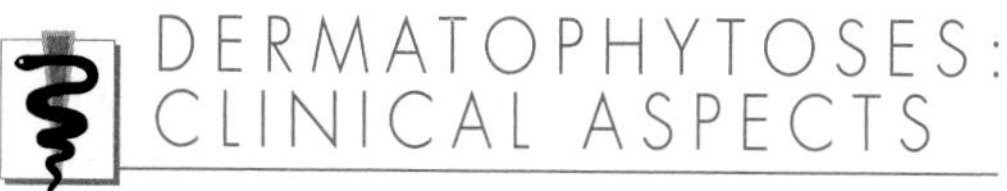

DERMATOPHYTOSES: CLINICAL ASPECTS

MANIFESTATIONS

Dermatophyte infections range from inapparent colonization to chronic progressive eruptions that last months or years, causing considerable discomfort and disfiguration. Dermatologists often give each infection its own "disease" name, for example, tinea capitis (scalp), tinea pedis (feet, athlete's foot), tinea manuum (hands), tinea cruris (groin), tinea barbae (beard, hair), and tinea unguium (nail beds). Skin infections not included in this anatomic list are called tinea corporis (body). There are some general clinical, etiologic, and epidemiologic differences between these syndromes, but there is also considerable overlap. The primary differences between etiologic agents that infect different sites are shown in Table 47–1.

Various skin sites are labeled as tinea "diseases"

Infection of hair begins with an erythematous papule around the hair shaft, which progresses to scaling of the scalp, discoloration, and eventually fracture of the shaft. Spread to adjacent hair follicles progresses in a ring-like fashion, leaving behind broken, discolored hairs and sometimes black dots where the hair is absent but the infection has gone into the follicle. The degree of inflammatory response markedly affects the clinical appearance and, in some cases, can cause constitutional symptoms. In most cases, symptoms beyond itching are minimal.

Hair infection leads to itching and hair loss

Skin lesions begin in a similar pattern and enlarge to form sharply delineated erythematous borders with skin of nearly normal appearance in the center. Multiple lesions can fuse to form unusual geometric patterns on the skin. Lesions may appear in any location, but are particularly common in moist, sweaty skin folds. Obesity and the wearing of tight apparel increase susceptibility to infection in the groin and beneath the breasts. Another form of infection, which involves scaling and splitting of the skin between the toes, is commonly known as athlete's foot. Moisture and maceration of the skin provide the mode of entry.

Skin infection favors moist areas and skin folds

Nail bed infections first cause discoloration of the subungual tissue, then hyperkeratosis and apparent discoloration of the nail plate by the underlying infection follow. Direct infection of the nail plate is uncommon. Progression of hyperkeratosis and associated inflammation cause disfigurement of the nail but few symptoms until the nail plate is so dislodged or distorted that it exposes or compresses adjacent soft tissue.

Hyperkeratosis can dislodge the nail bed

DIAGNOSIS

The goal of diagnostic procedures is to distinguish dermatophytoses from other causes of skin inflammation. Infections caused by bacteria, other fungi, and noninfectious disorders (psoriasis, contact dermatitis) may have similar features. The most important step is microscopic examination of material taken from lesions to detect the fungus. Potassium hydroxide (KOH) or calcifluor white preparations of scales scraped from the advancing edge of a dermatophyte lesion demonstrate septate hyphae (Fig 47–1B). Examination of infected hairs reveals hyphae and arthroconidia penetrating the hair shaft. Broken hairs give the best yield. Some species of dermatophyte fluoresce, and selection of hairs for examination can be aided by the use of an ultraviolet lamp (Wood's lamp).

KOH mounts of skin scrapings and infected hairs demonstrate hyphae

Some species fluoresce

The same material used for direct examination can be cultured for isolation of the offending dermatophyte. Mild infections with typical clinical findings and positive KOH preparations are often not cultured, because clinical management is not influenced significantly by the identity of the etiologic species. Clinically typical infections with negative KOH preparations require culture. The major reason for false-negative KOH results, however, is failure to collect the scrapings or hairs properly.

Culture is used when KOH preparations negative

TREATMENT AND PREVENTION

Many local skin infections resolve spontaneously without chemotherapy. Those that do not may be treated with topical tolnaftate, allylamines, or azoles. Nail bed and more extensive

Topical tolnaftate, allylamines, or azoles usually sufficient

Systemic griseofulvin, or azoles used in refractory cases

skin infections require systemic therapy with griseofulvin or itraconazole and terbinafine, often combined with topical therapy. Therapy must be continued over weeks to months, and relapses may occur. Keratolytic agents may be useful for reducing the size of hyperkeratotic lesions. Dermatophyte infections can usually be prevented simply by observing general hygienic measures. No specific preventive measures such as vaccines exist.

Other Superficial Mycoses

M. furfur requires lipids for growth

Pityriasis (tinea) versicolor occurs in tropical and temperate climates; it is characterized by discrete areas of hypopigmentation or hyperpigmentation associated with induration and scaling. Lesions are found on the trunk and arms; some assume pigments ranging from pink to yellow-brown, hence the term **versicolor.** Members of the genus *Malassezia,* of which *M. furfur* is the most common, are the cause; these organisms can be seen in skin scrapings as clusters of budding yeast cells mixed with hyphae. They grow in the yeast form in culture media enriched with lipids.

H. werneckii causes black lesions

Tinea nigra, another tropical infection, is characterized by brown to black macular lesions, usually on the palms or soles. There is little inflammation or scaling, and the infection is confined to the stratum corneum. The cause, *Hortaea werneckii,* is a black-pigmented fungus found in soil and other environmental sites. Scrapings of the lesion show brown–black-pigmented septate hyphae. In culture initial growth is in the yeast form, with slow development of hyphal elements.

Black or white piedra are infections of hair shaft

Piedra is an infection of the hair characterized by black or white nodules attached to the hair shaft. White piedra (caused by *Trichosporon cutaneum*) infects the shaft in hyphal forms, which fragment with occasional buds. Black piedra (caused by *Piedraia hortae*) shows branched hyphae and ascospores in sections of the hair.

Subcutaneous Fungi

Assignment of fungal organisms to the category of subcutaneous fungi is somewhat arbitrary, because fungal pathogens can produce many subcutaneous manifestations as part of their disease spectrum. Those considered here are introduced traumatically through the skin and involve mainly subcutaneous tissues, lymphatic vessels, and contiguous tissues. They rarely spread to distant organs. The diseases they cause include sporotrichosis, chromoblastomycosis, and mycetoma. Only sporotrichosis has a single specific etiologic agent, *Sporothrix schenckii.* Chromoblastomycosis and mycetoma are clinical syndromes with multiple fungal etiologies.

Sporothrix

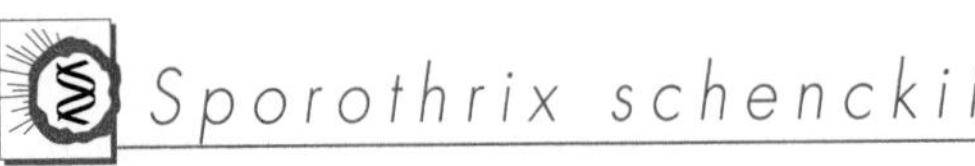

Sporothrix schenckii

Mold conidiophores convert to cigar-shaped yeast

S. schenckii is a dimorphic fungus that grows as a cigar-shaped, 3- to 5-mm yeast (Fig 47–2) in tissues and in culture at 37°C. In addition to the mannan, glucan, and chitin found in the cell wall of other fungi, the cell wall of *S. schenckii* contains a unique substance, L-rhamnose, in complexes with mannan. The mold, which grows in culture at 25°C, is presumably the infectious form in nature. The hyphae are thin and septate, producing clusters of conidia at the end of delicate conidiophores (see Fig 47–2B).

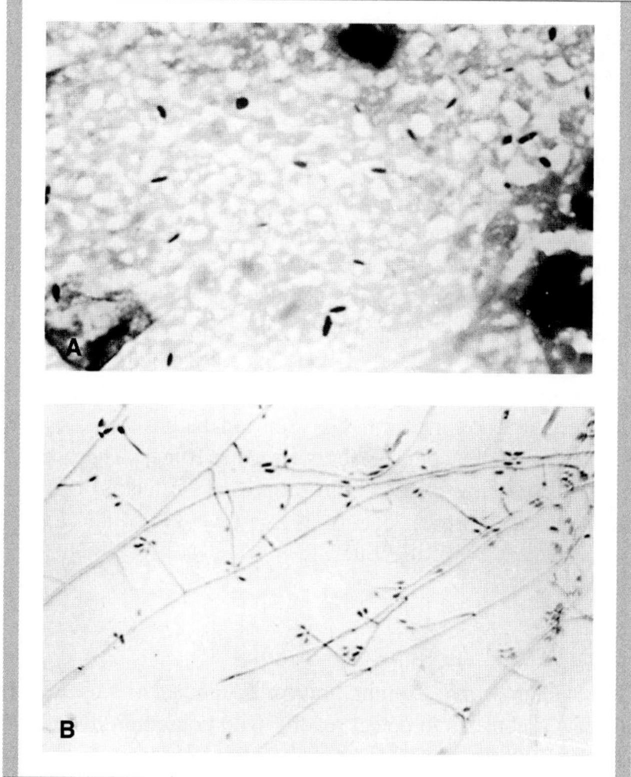

FIGURE 47–2
Sporothrix schenckii. **A.** The yeast form of *S. schenckii* is typically cigar-shaped but is rarely seen in human lesions. This smear is from infected mouse testis. **B.** Mold-phase cultures develop delicate hyphae and conidiophores bearing finger-like clusters of conidia. (*Reprinted with permission from Dr. E. S. Beneke and the Upjohn Company: Scope Publications, Human Mycoses.*)

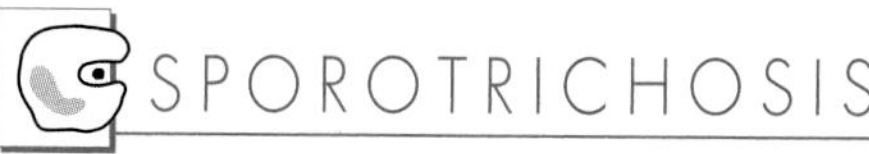

SPOROTRICHOSIS

EPIDEMIOLOGY

S. schenckii is a ubiquitous saprophyte particularly found in hay, moss, soil, and decaying vegetation, and on the surfaces of various plants. Infection is acquired by traumatic inoculation through the skin of material containing the organism. Exposure is largely occupational or related to hobbies. The skin of gardeners, farmers, and rural laborers is frequently traumatized by thorns or other material that may be contaminated with conidia of *S. schenckii.* An unusual outbreak of sporotrichosis involving nearly 3000 miners was traced to *S. schenckii* in the timbers used to support mine shafts. A 1988 outbreak covered 15 states and was traced to sphagnum moss. Infection is occasionally acquired by direct contact with infected pus or through the respiratory tract; these modes of infection, however, are much less common than the cutaneous route.

Soil saprophyte is introduced by trauma

Occupational disease of gardeners and farmers

Outbreaks involve wood and moss

PATHOGENESIS

Both the conidia and yeast cells of *S. schenckii* are able to bind to extracellular matrix proteins like fibronectin, laminin, and collagen. This may aid their survival in the early stages of infection. Local multiplication of the organism stimulates both acute pyogenic and granulomatous inflammatory reactions. Melanin production may provide resistance to oxidative killing. Proteinases similar to those seen in other fungal pathogens are present but no connection to virulence has been established. The infection spreads along lymphatic drainage routes and reproduces the original inflammatory lesions at intervals. The organisms are scanty in human lesions.

Surface binds to extracellular matrix

Melanin resists oxidative killing

IMMUNITY

The cellular response to *S. schenckii* is mixed. The increased frequency and greater severity of disseminated disease in patients with T-cell defects points to CMI as the primary immune mechanism. Antibody plays no known role in immunity.

CMI is primary immune mechanism

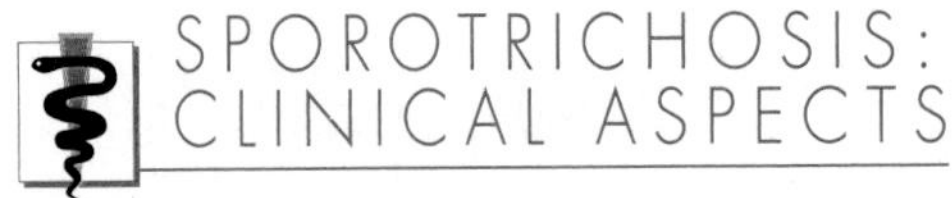

SPOROTRICHOSIS: CLINICAL ASPECTS

MANIFESTATIONS

Skin papule eventually ulcerates

Lymphatic involvement creates multiple lesions

A skin lesion begins as a painless papule that develops a few weeks to a few months after inoculation. Its location can usually be explained by occupational exposure; the hand is most often involved. The papule enlarges slowly and eventually ulcerates, leaving an open sore. Draining lymph channels are usually thickened, and pustular or firm nodular lesions may appear around the primary site of infection or at other sites along the lymphatic drainage route (Fig 47–3). Once ulcerated, lesions usually become chronic. Multiple ulcers often develop if the disease is untreated. Symptoms are those directly related to the local areas of infection. Constitutional signs and symptoms are unusual.

Deep infection is rare

Occasionally, spread occurs by other routes. The bones, eyes, lungs, and central nervous system are susceptible to progressive infection if the organisms reach these organs; such spread, however, occurs in less than 1% of all cases. Primary pulmonary sporotrichosis occurs but is also rare.

DIAGNOSIS

Direct microscopic examination for *S. schenckii* is usually unrewarding because there are too few organisms to detect readily with potassium hydroxide preparations. Even specially stained biopsy samples and serial sections are usually negative, although the presence of a histopathologic structure, the asteroid body, is suggestive. This structure is composed of *S. schenckii* yeast cells surrounded by amorphous eosinophilic "rays." Definitive diagnosis depends on culture of infected pus or tissue. The organism grows within 2 to 5 days on all media commonly used in medical mycology. Identification requires demonstration of the typical conidia and of dimorphism.

TREATMENT AND PREVENTION

Potassium iodide works for cutaneous fungi

Amphotericin or itraconazole required for progressive disease

Cutaneous sporotrichosis is effectively treated with a saturated solution potassium iodide (SSKI) administered orally. Systemic infections require the use of amphotericin B and/or azoles. Clinical experience with itraconazole has been excellent, and it may become the treatment of choice for all but cutaneous sporotrichosis. Eradication of the environmental reservoir of *S. schenckii* is not usually practical, although the mine outbreak mentioned previously was stopped by applying antifungal agents to the mine shaft timbers.

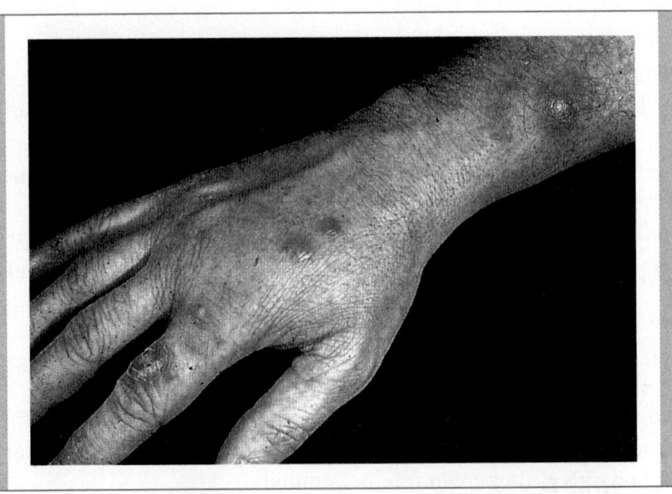

FIGURE 47–3
Sporotrichosis. This infection began on the finger and has started to spread up the arm, leaving satellite lesions behind. (*Reproduced with permission from Connor DH, Chandler FW, Schwartz DA, Manz HJ, Lack EE (eds).* Pathology of Infectious Disease, *Volume II. Stamford, CT: Appleton & Lange, 1997.*)

Chromoblastomycosis

Chromoblastomycosis is primarily a tropical disease caused by multiple species of *Fonsecaea, Phialophora,* and *Cladophialophora* (*Cladosporium*). The disease occurs typically on the foot or leg. It appears as papules that develop into scaly, wartlike structures, usually under the feet. Fully developed lesions have been likened to the tips of a cauliflower. Extension is by satellite lesions; it is slow and painless and does not involve the lymphatic vessels. The organisms are found in the soil of endemic areas, and most infections occur in individuals who work barefoot.

Multiple species produce wart-like pigmented lesions in tropics

The outstanding mycologic feature is the presence of brown-pigmented, thick-walled, multiseptate, 5- to 12-mm globose structures called muriform bodies on histologic section. Branching septate hyphae may also be demonstrated in KOH preparations of scrapings. Cultures grow as dark molds, but may take weeks to appear and longer for demonstration of characteristic conidia. Surgery and antifungal therapy have been used in chromoblastomycosis, but results in advanced disease are disappointing. Flucytosine or itraconazole have been the antifungal agents most frequently used.

Brown pigmented bodies are seen in tissues

Mycetoma

Mycetoma is a clinical term for an infection associated with trauma to the foot which causes inoculation of any of a dozen fungal species. Actinomycetes such as *Nocardia* may produce a similar disease. The usual clinical appearance is of massive induration with draining sinuses. Some of the fungi that cause mycetoma are geographically widespread; most cases, however, occur in the tropics, probably because the chronically damp, macerated skin of the feet that causes predisposition toward mycetoma occurs most often among those who go barefoot in the tropical environment. This finding is illustrated by the case of a college rower in Seattle who developed mycetoma; he was the only member of his shell who insisted on rowing barefoot. Once established, the treatment of mycetoma is difficult. No antimicrobic stands out as particularly helpful. The precise microbiologic features depend on the agent involved. Hyphae are usually present in tissue but may be difficult to demonstrate because of a tendency to form microcolonial granules.

Multiple species are involved

Trauma to bare feet injects the fungi

ADDITIONAL READING

Kauffman CA. Sporotrichosis. *Clin Infect Dis* 1999;29:231–237. A review emphasizing clinical aspects, including excellent photographs.

Weitzman I, Summerbell RC. The dermatophytes. *Clin Microbiol Rev* 1995;8:240–259. This review includes genetics and therapy in addition to classic mycology and all the "tinea" clinical descriptions.

CHAPTER 48

Candida, Aspergillus, and Other Opportunistic Fungi

KENNETH J. RYAN

The fungi considered in this chapter are usually found as members of the normal flora or as saprophytes in the environment. With breakdown of host defenses they can produce disease ranging from superficial skin or mucous membrane infections to systemic involvement of multiple organs. The most common opportunistic infections are caused by the yeast *Candida albicans,* a normal inhabitant of the gastrointestinal and genital floras, and a mold, *Aspergillus,* commonly found in the environment. The diseases caused by *Candida, Aspergillus,* and other opportunistic fungi are summarized in Table 48–1.

CANDIDA: GENERAL CHARACTERISTICS

Candida species grow as typical 4- to 6-μm, budding, round, or oval yeast cells (see Fig 45–1) under most conditions and at most temperatures. Under certain conditions, including those found in infection, they can form hyphae. Some species form chlamydoconidia in culture. *Candida* species identification is based on a combination of biochemical, enzymatic, and morphologic characteristics, such as carbohydrate assimilation; fermentation; and the ability to produce hyphae, germ tubes, and chlamydoconidia. Particular attention is given to the differentiation of *Candida albicans* from other species, because it is the most frequent cause of disease. It is also by far the best understood as to structure, metabolic activity, and pathogenesis.

Formation of hyphae and chlamydoconidia are distinguishing features

Carbohydrate assimilation and fermentation determine species

Most *Candida* species grow rapidly on Sabouraud's agar and on enriched bacteriologic media such as blood agar. Smooth, white, 2- to 4-mm colonies resembling those of staphylococci are produced on blood agar after overnight incubation. Aeration of cultures favors their isolation. The primary identification procedure involves presumptive differentiation of *C. albicans* from the more than 150 other *Candida* species with the germ tube test (see below). Germ tube–negative strains may be further identified biochemically or reported as "yeast not *C. albicans,*" depending on their apparent clinical significance.

Rapidly produce colonies resembling staphylococci

C. albicans produces germ tubes

TABLE 48–1

Agents of Opportunistic Mycoses

Organism	Growth: Tissue	Growth: Culture at 25°C	Growth: Culture at 37°C	Source	Infection
Candida	Yeast (hyphae)[a]	Yeast (hyphae)[a]	Yeast	Endogenous	Skin, mucous membranes, urinary, disseminated
Aspergillus	Hyphae (septate)	Mold	Mold	Environment	Lung, disseminated
Zygomycetes[b]	Hyphae (nonseptate)	Mold	Mold	Environment	Rhinocerebral, lung, disseminated

[a] Less common feature; pseudohyphae are produced as well.

[b] Such genera as *Absidia, Mucor,* and *Rhizopus*.

Candida albicans

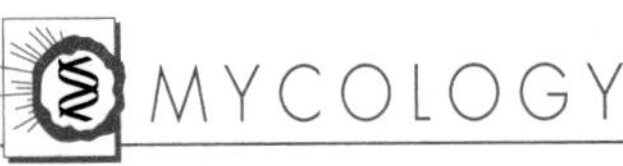

MYCOLOGY

Yeast, hyphae, and pseudohyphae are formed

Chlamydoconidia develop from hyphae in culture

C. albicans grows in multiple morphologic forms, most often as a yeast with budding by formation of blastoconidia. *C. albicans* is also able to form hyphae triggered by changes in conditions such as temperature, pH, and available nutrients. When observed in their initial stages when still attached to the yeast cell, these hyphae look like sprouts and are called germ tubes (Fig 48–1A). Other elongated forms with restrictions at intervals are called **pseudohyphae** because they lack the parallel walls and septation of the true hyphae. There is evidence that these three forms have distinct stimuli and genetic regulation, making *C. albicans* a polymorphic fungus. Unless otherwise specified, the term **hyphae** is used here to encompass both the true and pseudohyphal forms. The hyphal form also develops characteristic terminal thick-walled **chlamydoconidia** under certain cultural conditions (Fig 48–1B).

Cell wall includes surface mannoproteins

The *C. albicans* cell wall is made up of a mixture of the polysaccharides mannan, glucan, and chitin alone or in complexes with protein. A fibrillar outer layer extending to the surface contains a number of distinct mannoproteins. The exact composition of the cell wall and surface components varies under different growth and morphologic conditions.

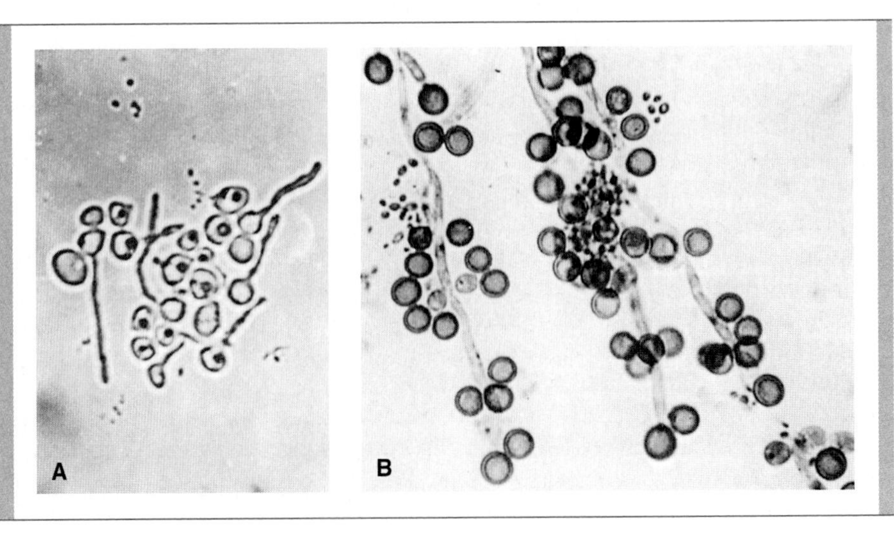

FIGURE 48–1
Candida albicans. **A.** When incubated at 37°C, *C. albicans* rapidly forms elongated hyphae called germ tubes. **B.** On specialized media, *C. albicans* forms thick-walled chlamydoconidia, which differentiate it from other *Candida* species. (*Reprinted with permission from Dr. E. S. Beneke and the Upjohn Company: Scope Publications, Human Mycoses.*)

CANDIDIASIS

CLINICAL CAPSULE

Candidiasis occurs in localized and disseminated forms. Localized disease is seen as erythema and white plaques in moist skin folds (diaper rash) or on mucosal surfaces (oral thrush). It may also cause the itching and thick white discharge of vulvovaginitis. Deep tissue and disseminated disease are limited almost exclusively to the immunocompromised. Diffuse pneumonia and urinary tract involvement are especially common.

EPIDEMIOLOGY

C. albicans is a common member of the oropharyngeal, gastrointestinal, and female genital flora. Infections are endogenous except in cases of direct mucosal contact with lesions in others (eg, through sexual intercourse). Although *C. albicans* is a common cause of nosocomial infections, the fungi are also derived more frequently from the patient's own flora than from cross-infection. Invasive procedures and indwelling devices may provide the portal of entry, and the number of available *Candida* may be enhanced by the used of antibacterial agents.

Infections are from endogenous flora

PATHOGENESIS

Because *C. albicans* is regularly present on mucosal surfaces, disease implies a change in the organism, the host, or both. The change from the yeast to the hyphal form is strongly associated with enhanced pathogenic potential of *C. albicans*. In histologic preparations, hyphae are seen only when *Candida* starts to invade, either superficially or in deep tissues (see Fig 45–4). This switch can be controlled in vitro by the manipulation of environmental conditions, but it is not known what triggers the change in human disease. What is known is that the morphologic change is also associated with the appearance of a number factors associated with tissue adherence and digestion.

Shift from yeast to hyphae is associated with invasion

Switch is controlled by environmental conditions

C. albicans hyphae have the capacity to form strong attachments to human epithelial cells. A mediator of this binding may be a surface **hyphal wall protein** (Hwp1), which is found only on the surface of germ tubes and hyphae. This protein has amino acid sequences similar to those in the substrates of mammalian keratinocyte transaminases, which form cross-links between squamous epithelial specific proteins. This novel pathogenic strategy makes use of host enzymes to bind the pathogen to epithelial cells. Other mannoproteins that have similarities to vertebrate integrins may also mediate binding to components of the **extracellular matrix** (ECM), such as fibronectin, collagen, and laminin. Hyphae also secrete proteinases and phospholipases that are able to digest epithelial cells and probably facilitate invasion (Figs 48–2 and 48–3). There is also evidence that *C. albicans* may be able to induce its own phagocytosis by endothelial cells. Taken together, these factors represent a rich armamentarium of virulence factors all seemingly linked to the change from yeast to hyphal growth.

Surface mannoproteins bind to keratinocytes and ECM

Host enzymes link Hwp to tissue

Hyphae produce proteinases

C. albicans has protein surface receptors that bind the C3 component of complement in a manner similar to that of the receptors on neutrophils. C3 bound to the candidal surface by these receptors is thus oriented in a fashion that makes it unavailable for opsonization. Enhanced production of these receptors under various conditions, for example, elevated glucose concentration, is associated with resistance to phagocytosis by neutrophils.

Receptors bind C3 in an antiopsonic manner

Factors that allow *C. albicans* to increase its relative proportion of the flora (antibacterial therapy), that compromise the general immune capacity of the host (leukopenia or corticosteroid therapy), or that interfere with T-lymphocyte function (acquired immunodeficiency syndrome; AIDS) are often associated with local and invasive infection. The

Antimicrobics and immunosuppression increase risk

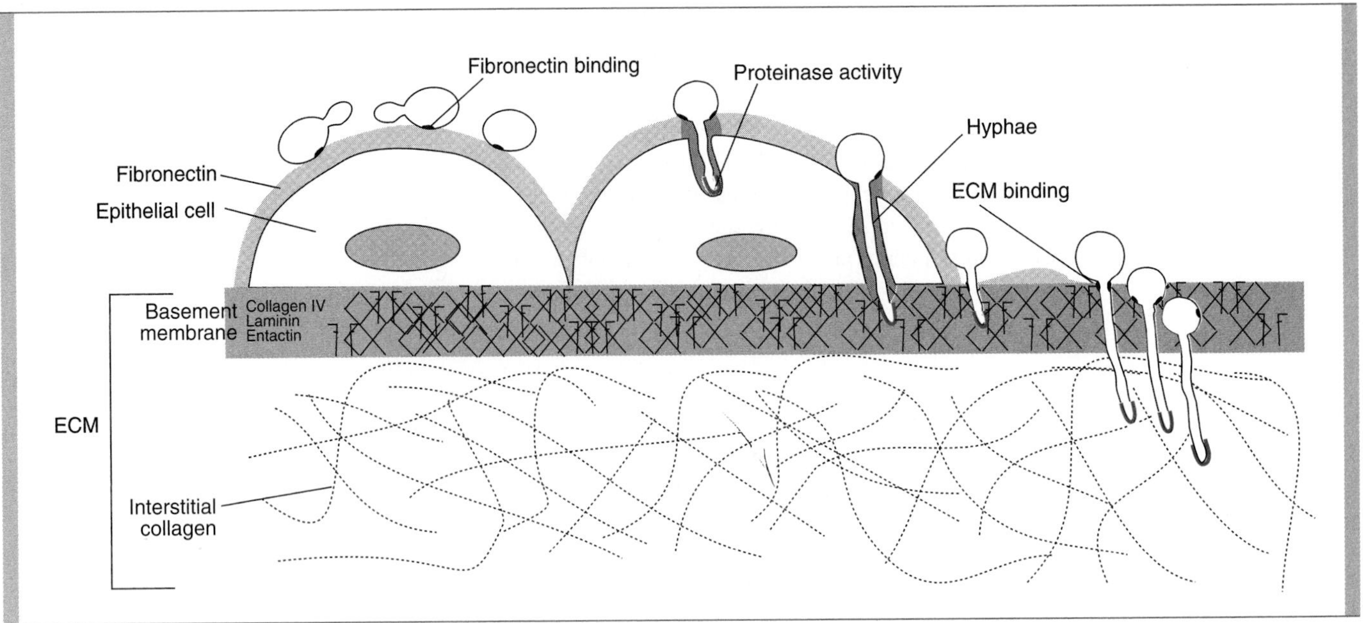

FIGURE 48–2
Pathogenesis of *Candida albicans* infections. Proposed mechanisms of *C. albicans* attachment and invasion are shown. Surface glucomannan receptor(s) on the yeast may bind to fibronectin covering the epithelial cell or to elements of the extracellular matrix (ECM) when the epithelial surface is lost or the *Candida* have invaded beyond it. Invasion is associated with formation of hyphae and production of proteinases, which may digest tissue elements.

Mechanical disruptions may provide access to ECM

disruptions of the mucosa associated with chronic disease and their treatments (indwelling devices, cancer chemotherapy) may enhance the invasion process by exposing *Candida* binding sites in the ECM. Diabetes mellitus also predisposes to *C. albicans* infection, possibly because of the known greater production of the surface mannoproteins in the presence of high glucose concentrations.

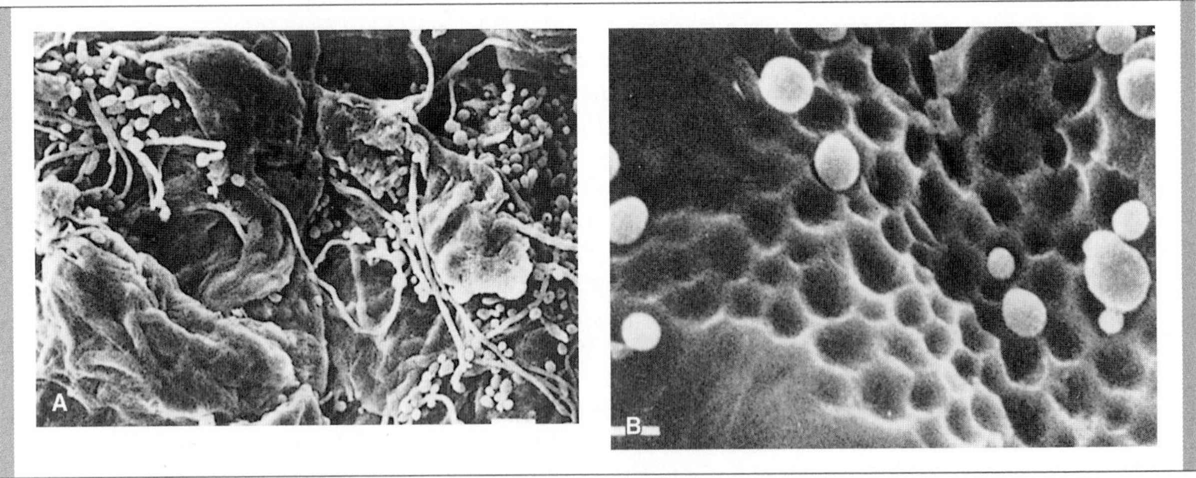

FIGURE 48–3
Invasiveness of *Candida albicans*. Two features of invasiveness are seen in these scanning electron micrographs taken from experiments with murine corneocytes. **A.** Both blastoconidia and mycelial elements are present. The mycelial elements spread over the surface and invade the cell cuticle. **B.** A *C. albicans* strain that produces a protease is seen producing cavity-like depressions in the cell surface. This action could play a role in invasion of the cell. (*Reprinted with permission of Thomas L. Ray and Candia D. Payne.* Infect Immun *1988;56:1945–1947, Figures 4,6B. Copyright American Society for Microbiology.*)

IMMUNITY

Both humoral immunity and cell-mediated immunity are important in defense against *Candida* infections. Neutrophils are the primary first-line defense. Yeast forms of *C. albicans* are readily phagocytosed and killed when opsonized by antibody and complement. In the absence of specific antibody, the process is less efficient, but a naturally occurring antimannan IgG is able to activate the classical complement pathway and facilitate the alternate pathway. Hyphal forms may be too large to be ingested by polymorphonuclear neutrophils (PMNs), but they can still kill the fungi by attaching to the hyphae and discharging metabolites generated by the oxidative metabolic burst. A deficit in neutrophils or neutrophilic function is the most common correlate of serious *C. albicans* infection.

Opsonized yeast forms are killed by PMNs

Antimannan IgG activates complement

The association of chronic mucocutaneous candidiasis (see below) with a number of T-lymphocyte immunodeficiencies emphasizes the importance of this arm of the immune system in defense against *Candida* infections. The increased frequency of oral and vaginal candidiasis in AIDS patients suggests that even superficial infections involve T-lymphocyte–mediated immune responses (cell-mediated immunity [CMI]). In animal studies, *Candida* cell wall mannan has been shown to play an immunoregulatory function by downregulating cell-mediated immune responses. A possible explanation for the association between AIDS and *Candida* infection is the upregulation of CD4 receptors on monocytes by *Candida* products. As with other fungi, cytokine activation of macrophages enhances their ability to kill *C. albicans*. A favorable outcome appears to require the proper balance between T_H1- and T_H2-mediated cytokine responses. The cytokines associated with T_H1 (interleukin-2 [IL-2], IL-12, interferon-γ, tumor necrosis factor-α) are correlated with enhanced resistance against infection where T_H2 responses (IL-4, IL-6, and IL-10) are associated with chronic disease.

Compromised CMI is associated with progressive infection

Candida mannan may downregulate CMI responses

Balance between T_H1 and T_H2 cytokines is necessary

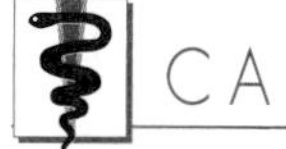

CANDIDIASIS: CLINICAL ASPECTS

MANIFESTATIONS

Superficial invasion of the mucous membranes by *C. albicans* produces a white, cheesy plaque that is loosely adherent to the mucosal surface. The lesion is usually painless, unless the plaque is torn away and the raw, weeping, invaded surface is exposed. Oral lesions, called **thrush,** occur on the tongue, palate, and other mucosal surfaces as single or multiple, ragged white patches. A similar infection in the vagina, vaginal candidiasis, produces a thick, curd-like discharge and itching of the vulva. Although most women have at least one episode of **vaginal candidiasis** in a lifetime, a small proportion suffer chronic, recurrent infections. No general or specific immune defect has yet been linked to this syndrome.

White mucosal plaque is called thrush

Vaginitis may be recurrent

C. albicans skin infections occur in crural folds and other areas in which wet, macerated skin surfaces are opposed. For example, one type of diaper rash is caused by *C. albicans*. Other infections of the skin folds and appendages occur in association with recurrent immersion in water (eg, dishwashers). The initial lesions are erythematous papules or confluent areas associated with tenderness, erythema, and fissures of the skin. Infection usually remains confined to the chronically irritated area, but may spread beyond it, particularly in infants.

Macerated skin is a common site

In rare persons with specific defects in T cell–mediated immune defense against *Candida,* a chronic, relapsing form of candidiasis known as **chronic mucocutaneous candidiasis** develops. Infections of the skin, hair, and mucocutaneous junctions fail to resolve with adequate therapy and management. There is considerable disfigurement and discomfort, particularly when the disease is accompanied by a granulomatous inflammatory response. Although lesions may become extensive, they usually do not disseminate. To some degree this disease may represent a clinical example of immunologic tolerance. Cutaneous anergy to *C. albicans* antigens is commonly seen in these patients and is often reversed during antifungal chemotherapy, suggesting that it is due to chronic antigen excess.

Chronic mucocutaneous candidiasis is associated with specific T-cell defects

Esophagitis and intestinal candidiasis are similar to thrush

Inflammatory patches similar to those in thrush may develop in the esophagus with or without associated oral candidiasis. Painful swallowing and substernal chest pain are the most common symptoms. Extensive ulcerations, deformity, and occasionally perforation of the esophagus may ensue. In immunocompromised patients, similar lesions may also develop in the stomach, together with deep ulcerative lesions of the small and large intestine.

Urinary tract infections are ascending or hematogenous

Endophthalmitis appears as white cotton on retina

Infection of the urinary tract via the hematogenous or ascending routes may produce cystitis, pyelonephritis, abscesses, or expanding fungus ball lesions in the renal pelvis. The clinical findings in disseminated infections of the kidneys, brain, and heart are generally not sufficiently characteristic to suggest *C. albicans* over the bacterial pathogens, which more commonly produce infection of deep organs. *Candida* **endophthalmitis** has the characteristic funduscopic appearance of a white cotton ball expanding on the retina or floating free in the vitreous humor. Endophthalmitis and infections of other eye structures can lead to blindness.

DIAGNOSIS

KOH and Gram smears of superficial lesions show yeast and hyphae

Lung involvement requires bronchoalveolar lavage

Superficial *C. albicans* infections provide ready access to diagnostic material. Exudate or epithelial scrapings examined by potassium hydroxide (KOH) preparations or Gram smear demonstrate abundant budding yeast cells; if associated hyphae are present, the infection is almost certainly caused by *C. albicans*. *C. albicans* is readily isolated from clinical specimens including blood if aerobic conditions are provided. Cultures from specimens such as sputum run the risk of contamination from the normal flora or a superficial mucous membrane lesion. A direct aspirate, biopsy, or bronchoalveolar lavage is often required to establish the diagnosis.

Endocarditis may require arterial cultures

Deep organ involvement is difficult to prove without a direct aspirate or biopsy. Even positive blood cultures must be interpreted with caution if they could represent colonization of intravenous catheters. *Candida* endocarditis represents a special diagnostic problem, because the yeasts seeding the blood from the valve may be filtered out in the capillary beds due to their large size. Arterial blood cultures may be required in this situation.

Immunodiagnostic procedures are not routine

Although many serologic tests have been developed for detection of *C. albicans* antibodies, none of the methods developed to date has the sensitivity or specificity needed for clinical diagnosis. Immunologic techniques for detection of circulating *Candida* cell components such as mannan show promise, but none are yet practical for clinical use.

TREATMENT

Topical nystatin or azoles for superficial lesions

Amphotericin B, flucytosine, and azoles for invasive disease

C. albicans is usually susceptible to amphotericin B, nystatin, flucytosine, and the azoles. Superficial infections are generally treated with topical nystatin or azole preparations. Measures to decrease moisture and chronic trauma are important adjuncts in treating *Candida* skin infections. Deeper *C. albicans* infections may resolve spontaneously with elimination or control of predisposing conditions. Removal of an infected catheter, control of diabetes, or an increase in peripheral leukocyte counts is often associated with recovery without antifungal therapy. Persistent relapsing or disseminated candidiasis is treated with amphotericin B, flucytosine, fluconazole, or combinations of amphotericin B with other drugs. Fluconazole has been the most effective treatment for chronic mucocutaneous candidiasis.

Other Candida Species

C. tropicalis is highly virulent

Species of *Candida* other than *C. albicans* produce infections in circumstances similar to those described previously, but do so less frequently. When contamination of an indwelling device is the portal of entry, the probability of infection by these other species increases. Little is known of the pathogenesis of these species with the exception of *Candida tropicalis*. Both experimental and clinical evidence indicate that *C. tropicalis* has virulence at least equal to that of *C. albicans*. *C. tropicalis* produces an extracellular proteinase similar to that of *C. albicans,* which may enhance its invasiveness.

Candida glabrata is another common species. This species is very small for a yeast (2- to 4-μm) and does not produce hyphae. It is a member of the normal gastrointestinal and genital flora. The most common infections are in the urinary tract, but deep tissue involvement and fungemia occur. The organisms are small enough to be confused with *Histoplasma capsulatum* in histologic preparations. Therapy is similar to that for *C. albicans* infections, although *C. glabrata* is more resistant to fluconazole.

C. glabrata is small for a yeast

Other species of *Candida,* which lack any distinguishing morphologic or clinical characteristics, may produce disease. Some of these fungi are inherently resistant to the antifungal azoles.

ASPERGILLUS

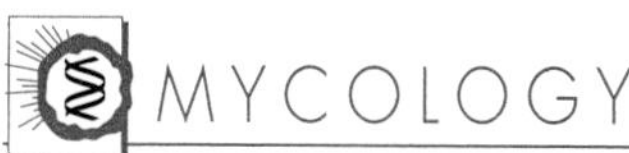

MYCOLOGY

Aspergillus species are rapidly growing molds with branching **septate hyphae** and characteristic arrangement of conidia on the conidiophore (Fig 48–4A). Fluffy colonies appear in 1 to 2 days and, by 5 days, may cover an entire plate with pigmented growth. Species are defined on the basis of differences in the structure of the **conidiophore** and the arrangement of the **conidia**. The most frequent in human infections are *Aspergillus fumigatus* and *Aspergillus flavus,* but others, such as *Aspergillus niger,* may be involved.

Species are based on arrangement of conidia on the conidiophore

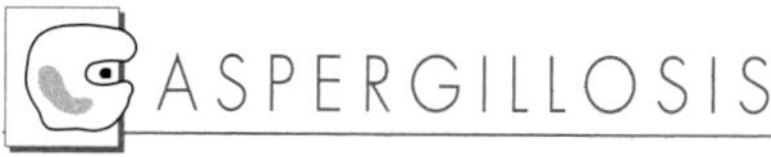

ASPERGILLOSIS

CLINICAL CAPSULE

Invasive aspergillosis is distinguished by its setting in immunocompromised individuals and its rapid progression to death. The typical patient is one with leukemia or under immunosuppression for a bone marrow transplant. The appearance of fever and a dry cough may be the only signs until pulmonary infiltrates are demonstrated radiologically. Until *Aspergillus* hyphae are demonstrated, almost any of the causes of pneumonia could be responsible.

EPIDEMIOLOGY

Aspergillus species are widely distributed in nature and found throughout the world. They seem to adapt to a wide range of environmental conditions, and the heat-resistant conidia provide a good mechanism for dispersal. Like bacteria spores, the conida survive well in the environment and their inhalation is the mode of infection. Hospital air and air ducts have received attention as sources of nosocomial *Aspergillus* isolates. Occasionally, construction, remodeling, or other kinds of major environmental disruption have been associated with increased frequency of *Aspergillus* contamination, colonization, or infection.

Conidia may be spread by construction projects

PATHOGENESIS

Aspergillus conidia are small enough to readily reach the alveoli when inhaled, but disease is rare in those without compromised defenses. Factors that aid the fungus in the initial stages are not known, but the ability of proteins on the surface of the conidia to bind fibrinogen and laminin probably contribute to adherence. Production of extracellular elastase, proteinases, and phospholipases has been associated with the more virulent species. The appearance of antibodies to these enzymes during and following invasive aspergillosis

Conidia bind to fibrinogen and laminin

Extracellular proteases may cause injury

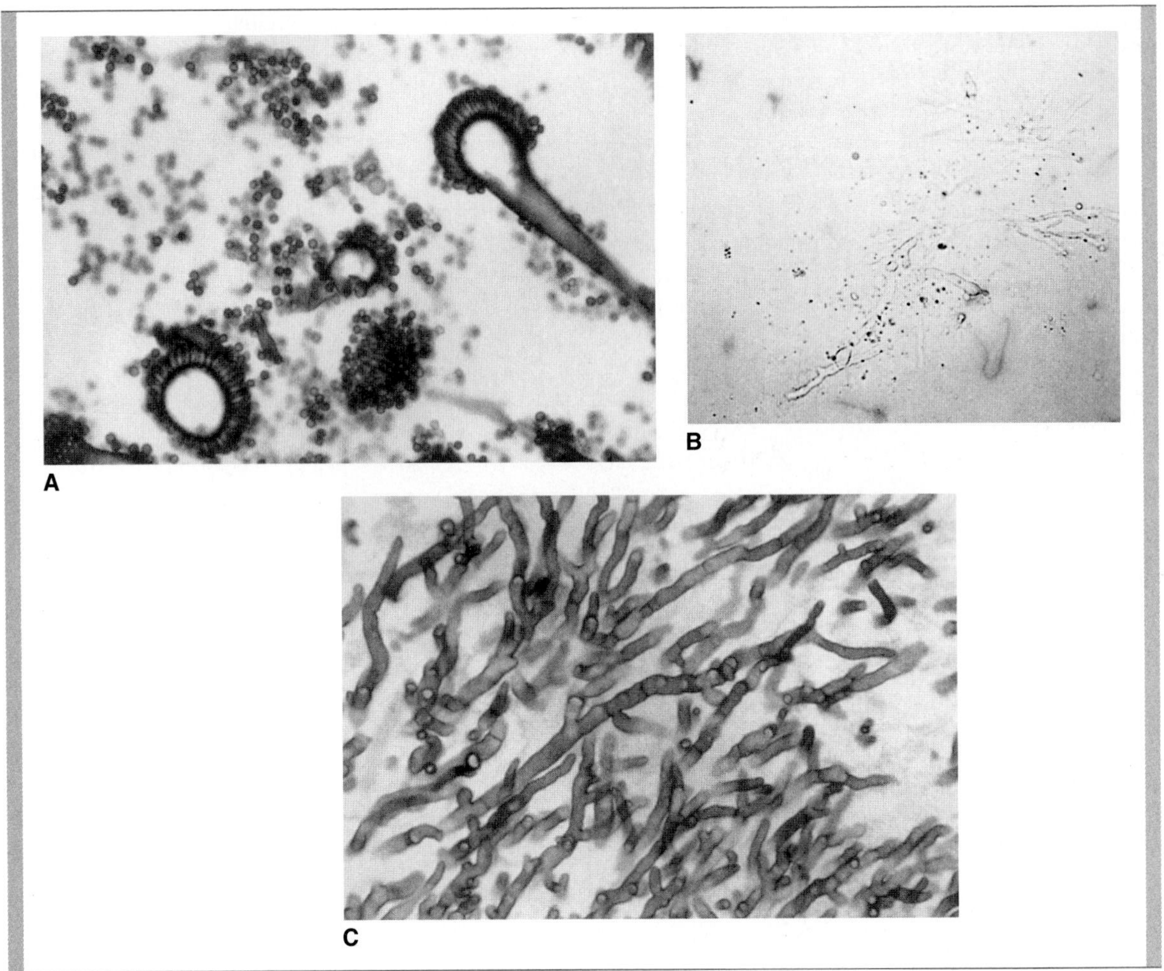

FIGURE 48–4
Aspergillus. **A.** This asexual conidium-forming structure is characteristic of *Aspergillus* species. The conidia are borne at the end of the finger-like extensions at the end of the conidiophore. These structures are rarely produced in vivo. **B.** This tissue aspirate mixed with KOH shows branching, septate hyphae. **C.** Histologic sections also show branching, septate hyphae, but because the conidia shown in **A** are not seen the findings are not diagnostic of *Aspergillus*. (*Reproduced with permission from Connor DH, Chandler FW, Schwartz DA, Manz HJ, Lack EE (eds).* Pathology of Infectious Disease, *Volume II. Stamford, CT: Appleton & Lange, 1997.*)

argues for their importance, but the pathogenic role of these enzymes remains to be demonstrated. Most species produce aflatoxins and other toxic secondary metabolites but their role in infection is also unknown.

IMMUNITY

Alveolar macrophages kill conidia, and PMNs attack hyphae

Macrophages, particularly pulmonary macrophages, are the first line of defense against inhaled *Aspergillus* conidia phagocytosing and killing them by nonoxidative mechanisms. For the conidia that survive and germinate, PMNs become the primary defense. They are able to attach to the growing hyphae, generate an oxidative burst, and secrete reactive oxygen intermediates. Little is known of adaptive immunity in humans. Antibodies are formed but their protective value is unknown. Although AIDS patients do develop *Aspergillus* infections, the association with T-cell deficiencies is not strong enough to draw conclusions about their importance.

ASPERGILLOSIS: CLINICAL ASPECTS

MANIFESTATIONS

Aspergillus can cause clinical allergies or occasional invasive infection. In both cases, the lung is the organ primarily involved. Allergic aspergillosis, which can be a mechanism of exacerbation in patients with asthma, is characterized by transient pulmonary infiltrates, eosinophilia, and a rise in *Aspergillus*-specific antibodies. These conditions follow direct inhalation of fungal elements or, more commonly, colonization of the respiratory tract. Areas of the bronchopulmonary tree with poor drainage because of underlying disease or anatomic abnormalities may serve as a site for growth of organisms and continuous seeding with antigen.

Allergic disease marked by eosinophilia and specific IgG

Invasive aspergillosis occurs in the settings of preexisting pulmonary disease (bronchiectasis, chronic bronchitis, asthma, tuberculosis) or immunosuppression. Colonization with *Aspergillus* can lead to invasion into the tissue by branching septate hyphae. In patients who already have a chronic pulmonary disease, mycelial masses can form a radiologically visible fungus ball (aspergilloma) within a preexisting cavity. Lung tissue invasion may penetrate blood vessels, causing hemoptysis or erosion into other structures with development of fistulas. Invasive disease outside the lung is rare unless patients are immunocompromised.

Highly invasive, including blood vessels

Fungus ball in cavities

An acute pneumonia may occur in severely immunocompromised patients, particularly those with phagocyte defects or depressed neutrophil counts due to immunosuppressive drugs. Multifocal pulmonary infiltrates expanding to consolidation are present with high fever. The prognosis is grave and dissemination to other organs common, which is not the case in immunocompetent hosts.

Pneumonia in immunocompromised host has grave prognosis

DIAGNOSIS

Aspergillus is relatively easy to isolate and identify. Its rapidly spreading mold growth and all too frequent contamination of cultures cause it to be regarded by microbiologists as a kind of weed. The diagnostic problem is distinguishing contamination and colonization with *Aspergillus* from invasive disease. The diagnosis cannot be made for certain without the use of lung aspiration, biopsy, or bronchoalveolar lavage. With material directly from the lesion, the presence of large, branching, septate hyphae (Fig 48–4B and 48–4C) and a positive culture are diagnostic. Occasionally, the complete fruiting bodies are produced in vivo, creating a striking and diagnostic histologic picture (see Fig 48–4A). Serologic methods have been developed to demonstrate *Aspergillus* antibodies. Although these tests may be helpful in suggesting allergic aspergillosis, they have little value in invasive disease because anti-*Aspergillus* antibody is common in healthy persons.

Direct aspirate or biopsy is required to distinguish colonization from invasion

Serodiagnosis is useful only for allergic disease

TREATMENT AND PREVENTION

Amphotericin B and itraconazole are the recommended antimicrobics for invasive aspergillosis. Neither can be considered particularly effective, because the mortality rate of invasive disease approaches 100%. In cases with pulmonary structural abnormalities and fungus balls, chemotherapy has little effect. Surgical removal of localized lesion is sometimes helpful, even in the brain. Construction of rooms with filtered air has been attempted to reduce exposure to environmental conidia.

Amphotericin B, itraconazole, and surgery are used for invasive disease

ZYGOMYCETES AND ZYGOMYCOSIS

Zygomycosis (mucormycosis) is the term applied to infection with any of a group of zygomycetes, the most common of which are *Absidia, Rhizopus,* and *Mucor*. These fungi are ubiquitous saprophytes in soil and are commonly found on bread and many other

Absidia, Rhizopus, and *Mucor* are soil saprophytes

Immunocompromised hosts with diabetes are infected

foodstuffs. They occasionally cause disease in persons with diabetes mellitus and in immunosuppressed patients receiving corticosteroid therapy. Diabetic acidosis has a particularly strong association with zygomycosis.

Pulmonary disease is similar to other fungi

Sinus infections erode straight to the brain

Pulmonary or rhinocerebral disease is acquired by inhalation of conidia. The pulmonary form has clinical findings similar to those of other fungal pneumonias; the rhinocerebral form, however, produces a dramatic clinical syndrome in which agents of zygomycosis show striking invasive capacity. They penetrate the mucosa of the nose, paranasal sinuses, or palate, often resulting in ulcerative lesions. Once beyond the mucosa, they progress through tissue, nerves, blood vessels, fascial planes, and often the vital structures at the base of the brain. The clinical syndrome begins with headache and may progress through orbital cellulitis and hemorrhage to cranial nerve palsy, vascular thrombosis, coma, and death in less than 2 weeks.

Large ribbons of nonseptate hyphae are seen in tissues

The pathologic cerebral and pulmonary findings are distinctive: the zygomycetes involved all show ribbon-like **nonseptate hyphae** in tissue which are so large their branch points can be difficult to visualize. Conidia are not seen. As with *Aspergillus,* tissue biopsies are necessary to demonstrate the invasive hyphae, unless they can be seen on scrapings from palatal or nasal ulcers. For reasons that are obscure, cultures are sometimes negative, even those from tissue containing characteristic hyphae. Therapy involves control of underlying disease, amphotericin B, and occasionally surgery.

ADDITIONAL READING

Denning DW. Invasive aspergillosis. *Clin Infect Dis* 1998;26:781–805. This review emphasizes the clinical aspects and illustrates them nicely.

Latge JP. *Aspergillus fumigatus* and aspergillosis. *Clin Microbiol Rev* 1999;12:310–350. A comprehensive review of mycologic and pathogenesis aspects, which also presents a nice view of diagnostic methods for the future.

Vazquez-Torrez A, Balish E. Macrophages in resistance to candidiasis. *Microbiol Mol Biol Rev* 1997;61:170–192. This review discusses all aspects of the immune response to *Candida* infection and their connection to the clinical forms of disease.

CHAPTER 49

Cryptococcus, *Histoplasma*, *Coccidioides*, and Other Systemic Fungal Pathogens

KENNETH J. RYAN

The fungi discussed in this group cause a variety of infections, each ranging in severity from subclinical to progressive, debilitating disease. Most species are dimorphic, growing in the infectious mold form in the environment but switching to a yeast form in tissues to produce infection. They differ from the opportunistic fungi in their ability to cause disease in previously healthy persons, but the most serious disease still occurs in immunocompromised individuals. With the exception of *Cryptococcus neoformans,* each of these species is restricted to a geographic niche corresponding to the environmental habitat of the mold form of the species. None are transmitted from human to human. The major features of the systemic pathogens are summarized in Table 49–1.

CRYPTOCOCCUS

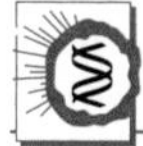

Cryptococcus neoformans

Cryptococcus neoformans (cryptococcus) is a yeast 4 to 6 μm in diameter that produces a characteristic **capsule** (Fig 49–1), extending the overall diameter to 25 μm or more. This capsule is unique among pathogenic fungi and is a complex polysaccharide polymer, the major component of which is **glucuronoxylomannan** (GXM). Capsule production varies by strain and with environmental conditions. It is repressed under environmental conditions and stimulated in the physiologic conditions found in tissues.

Yeasts produce large polysaccharide capsule in tissues

C. neoformans grows at 35 to 37°C on a variety of common media, including blood agar, chocolate agar, and Sabouraud's agar. Mucoid, bacteria-like colonies are produced

TABLE 49–1

Features of Systemic Fungal Pathogens

Organism	Growth: Culture at 25°C	Growth: Culture at 37°C	Growth: Tissue	Source	Primary Disease	Disseminated Disease
Cryptococcus neoformans	Encapsulated yeast	Encapsulated yeast	Encapsulated yeast	Environment, worldwide	Pneumonia	Chronic meningitis
Histoplasma capsulatum	Mold, tuberculate macroconidia[a]	Small yeast	Small intracellular yeast[b]	Environment, US Midwest[c]	Pneumonia, hilar adenopathy	RES enlargement
Blastomyces dermatitidis	Mold[a]	Yeast		Environment, US Midwest[c]	Pneumonia	Skin and bone lesions
Coccidioides immitis	Mold, arthroconidia	(Spherules)[d]	Spherules	Environment, Sonoran desert[c,e]	Valley fever	Pneumonia, meningitis, skin, bone
Paracoccidioides brasiliensis	Mold	Yeast, multiple blastoconidia		Environment, Latin America	Pneumonia	Mucocutaneous, RES

Abbreviations: RES, reticuloendothelial system (lymph nodes, liver, spleen, bone marrow).

[a] Micoconidia are formed but are not distinctive.

[b] Typically multiple yeast within macrophages.

[c] Ecologic "islands" are found throughout the Americas.

[d] It is difficult to grow the spherule phase in culture.

[e] In the United States includes parts of Arizona, California, Nevada, and western Texas.

Melanin and urease are produced in culture

in 2 to 3 days. In addition to the capsule, extracellular products include a urease enzyme and melanin pigment. The sexual state of *C. neoformans* places it in the Basidiomycetes, but this form has not been associated directly with disease.

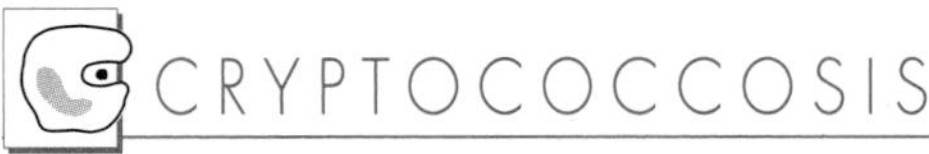

CRYPTOCOCCOSIS

CLINICAL CAPSULE

The primary disease caused by cryptococci is a chronic meningitis. The onset is slow, even insidious, with low-grade fever and headache progressing to altered mental state and seizures. In the cerebrospinal fluid (CSF) and in tissues, the inflammatory response is often remarkably muted. Most patients have some obvious form of immune compromise, although some show no demonstrable immune defect.

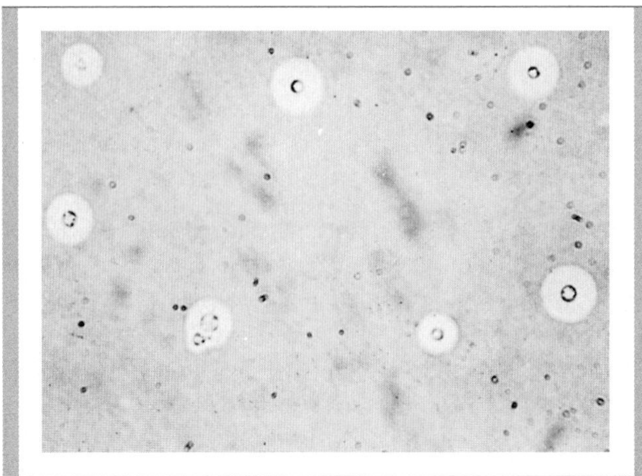

FIGURE 49–1
Cryptococcus neoformans. This India ink preparation was made by mixing cerebrospinal fluid containing cryptococci with India ink. The yeast cells can be seen within the clear space caused by the large polysaccharide capsule. (*Reprinted with permission from Dr. E. S. Beneke and the Upjohn Company: Scope Publications, Human Mycoses.*)

EPIDEMIOLOGY

C. neoformans is found throughout the world, particularly in soil contaminated with pigeon or other bird droppings. The birds themselves are not ill. The cryptococci in the soil produce few or no capsules, which makes them more readily aerosolized. Inhalation of yeast cells stirred up from these sites is the presumed mode of transmission. Cases appear sporadically, with no particular occupational predisposition, including pigeon fanciers or in those who work with the organism in the laboratory. Cryptococcosis in immunocompromised patients occurs primarily in those with defects in T-lymphocyte function, particularly acquired immunodeficiency syndrome (AIDS), or in those treated with immunosuppressive agents (eg, steroids). Cryptococcal disease is the most common fungal infection seen in AIDS. Case-to-case transmission has not been documented.

Reservoir is soil contaminated with bird droppings

Inhalation of unencapsulated yeasts starts infection

PATHOGENESIS

Following inhalation, the yeast begins to overproduce the polysaccharide capsule, which determines virulence. The capsule is antiphagocytic and has a number of other immunomodulating effects. The GXM is able to bind complement components while at the same time reducing the ability of polymorphonuclear neutrophils (PMNs) and macrophages to phagocytose and kill cryptococci. This may be due to the combination of the massive size of the capsule and the way in which it binds C3. There is also evidence that the capsule can interfere with antigen presentation and the development of T cell–mediated immune processes. This muting of the first lines of defense allows the organisms to multiply and eventually spread outside the lung. At this stage the organism has a strong affinity for the central nervous system (CNS), possibly due to its C3 binding and the relatively low levels of complement found there.

Antiphagocytic capsule is produced after inhalation

GXM binds C3 and interferes with antigen presentation

Cryptococci produce enough capsule that the GXM can be readily detected in the blood and other body fluids. This circulating polysaccharide is able to downregulate immune responses, particularly the development of protective T_H1-type mediators and suppression of the specific antibody response. These modulations may be either antigen specific or cause a general suppression of key immune functions, such as leukocyte migration. Cryptococci are also able to oxidize exogenous catecholamines to produce melanin, a process that may protect them from the oxidative injury of phagocytes.

Circulating antigen depresses humoral and cell-mediated immunity

Melanin production provides oxidative protection

Tissue reaction to *C. neoformans* varies from little or none to purulent or granulomatous. Many cases of pulmonary, cutaneous, and even meningeal cryptococcal infection show a remarkable paucity of inflammatory cells. This certainly fits for a fungus that not only blocks its own phagocytosis but is able to downregulate multiple aspects of the immune response.

Tissue reaction is often minimal

IMMUNITY

In immunocompetent persons, alternate pathway binding of complement by the capsule is probably sufficient for opsonophagocytosis. The capsule is not particularly antigenic, and anticryptococcal antibodies are not usually detected in the course of infection. When formed, the classical pathway can play a role in opsonization, but this mechanism is not believed to play a strong role in immunity. Anticryptococcal antibody and complement do not directly damage the organism but may be a key component in the development of cellular host defense mechanisms and the clearance of circulating antigen.

Alternate pathway is more important than classical

Animal studies and the strong clinical association of cryptococcosis with T-cell defects indicate that T lymphocyte–mediated immune responses are crucial to the outcome of infection. Cryptococci phagocytosed by macrophages may not be killed, and cytokine activation is needed to complete the clearing of the organisms. Patients with cryptococcosis who have no known immune defects often have subnormal cellular immune functions as measured by their lymphocyte-mediated responses to cryptococcal and other antigens. Clinical recovery in such cases is associated with return of cellular immune functions.

T-cell responses are crucial to outcome

Cell-mediated immunity may return with recovery

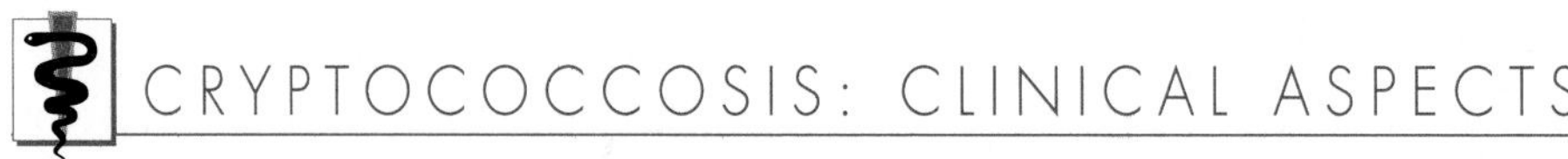

CRYPTOCOCCOSIS: CLINICAL ASPECTS

MANIFESTATIONS

Meningitis is insidious and chronic

Course is more rapid with AIDS

Meningitis is the most commonly recognized form of cryptococcal disease; it usually has a slow, insidious onset with relatively nonspecific findings until late in its course. Intermittent headache, irritability, dizziness, and difficulty with complex cerebral functions appear over weeks or months with no consistent pattern. Behavioral changes have been mistaken for psychoses. Fever is usually, but not invariably, present. Seizures, cranial nerve signs, and papilledema may appear later in the clinical course, as may dementia and decreased levels of consciousness. A more rapid course may be seen in AIDS patients, 5 to 15% of who become infected with *C. neoformans*.

Cryptococcal pneumonia is usually asymptomatic

Cryptococcal pneumonia is often asymptomatic or mild. Sputum production is minimal, and no findings are sufficiently specific to suggest the etiology. Skin and bone are the sites most frequently involved in disseminated disease; skin lesions are sometimes the presenting sign and are often remarkable for their lack of inflammation. The diagnosis is sometimes made when lesions are biopsied as suspected neoplasms.

DIAGNOSIS

Cells and glucose depression in CSF may be minimal

India ink prep is positive in 50% of cases

Typical cerebrospinal fluid (CSF) findings in cryptococcal meningitis are increased pressure, pleocytosis (usually $\geq$100 cells) with predominance of lymphocytes, and depression of glucose levels. In some cases, one or all of these findings may be absent, yet cryptococci are isolated on culture. Cryptococcal capsules are demonstrable in CSF in roughly 50% of cases by mixing centrifuged sediment with **India ink** and examining the mixture under the microscope (see Fig 49–1). Some experience is necessary to avoid confusion of lymphocytes with cryptococci. *C. neoformans* stains poorly or not at all with routine histologic stains; thus, it is easily missed unless special fungal stains are used.

Few cryptococci may be present in CSF

GXM is detectable in CSF and serum

In the isolation of *C. neoformans,* the volume of CSF sampled is important. The number of organisms present may be small enough to require a substantial volume of fluid (>30 mL) to yield a positive culture. If cryptococcosis is suspected and cultures are negative, detection of the GXM polysaccharide antigen in the CSF or serum by latex agglutination or enzyme immunoassay methods is recommended. These tests are very sensitive and specific, and their quantitation has prognostic significance. A rising antigen level indicates progression and a declining titer is a favorable sign.

TREATMENT

Amphotericin, fluconazole, and flucytosine used in combination

Amphotericin B (with or without flucytosine) or fluconazole is the usual treatment for systemic cryptococcal disease. Flucytosine use alone is limited by development of resistance during therapy. Although three fourths of persons with meningitis respond to treatment, a significant portion suffer relapses after antifungal therapy is stopped; many become chronic and require repeated courses of therapy. One half of those cured have some kind of residual neurologic damage.

HISTOPLASMA

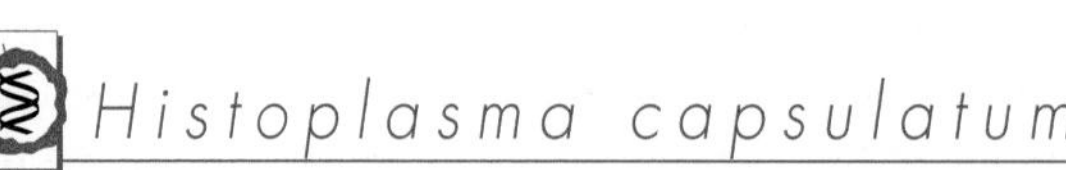

Histoplasma capsulatum

Histoplasma capsulatum is a dimorphic fungus that grows in the yeast phase in tissue (Fig 49–2A) and in cultures incubated at 37°C. The mold phase grows in cultures incubated at 22 to 25°C and as a saprophyte in soil. The yeast forms are small for fungi (2 to

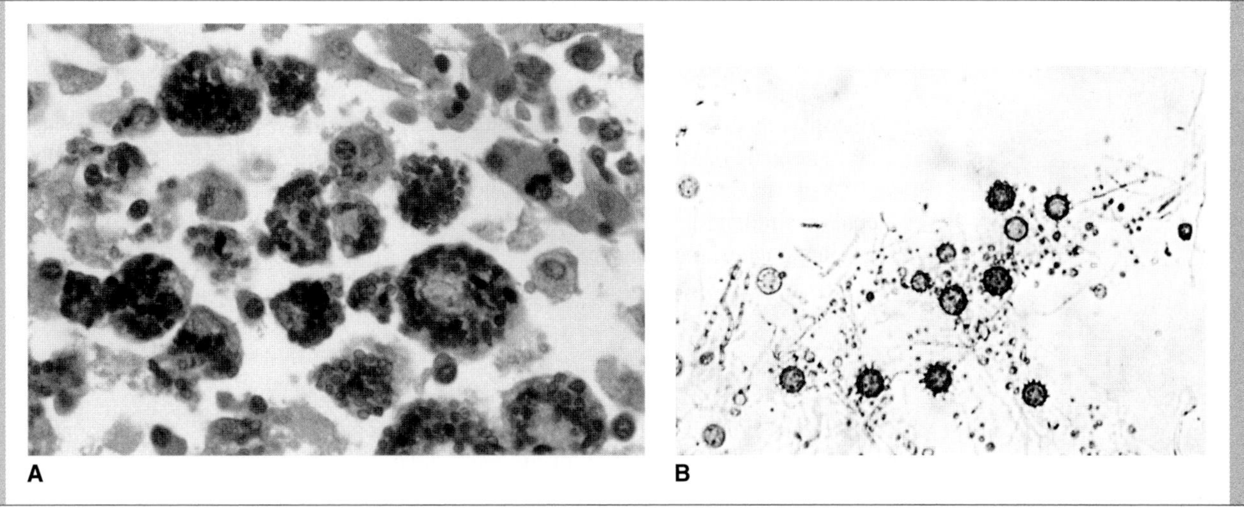

FIGURE 49–2
Histoplasma capsulatum. **A.** Multiple organisms are stuffed within the cytoplasm of alveolar macrophages in the lung. (*Reproduced with permission from Connor DH, Chandler FW, Schwartz DA, Manz HJ, Lack EE (eds).* Pathology of Infectious Disease, *Volume II. Stamford, CT: Appleton & Lange, 1997.*) **B.** The mold is shown with characteristic tuberculate macroconidia. (*Reprinted with permission from Dr. E. S. Beneke and the Upjohn Company: Scope Publications, Human Mycoses.*)

4 μm) and reproduce by budding (blastoconidia). The mycelia are septate and produce **microconidia** and macroconidia. The diagnostic structure is termed the **tuberculate macroconidium** because of its thick wall and radial, finger-like projections (see Fig 49–2B). Growth is obtained on blood agar, chocolate agar, and Sabouraud's agar, but may take many weeks. A sexual stage has now been discovered (*Ajellomyces capsulatum*), but the asexual name continues to be used in the medical literature. The designation *H. capsulatum* is actually a misnomer, because no capsules are formed. It comes from the halos seen around the yeasts in tissue sections, which are caused by a shrinkage artifact of routine histologic methods.

Small dimorphic fungus producing tuberculate macroconidia

Growth may take weeks

DIMORPHISM

The morphologic and physiologic events associated with conversion from the mold to the yeast phase of *H. capsulatum* have been extensively studied. They are understandably complex given the dramatic change of milieu encountered by the fungus when its mold conidia float from their soil habitat to the pulmonary alveoli. Conversion to the yeast phase is then triggered by the host temperature (37°C) and possibly by other aspects of the new environment. In vitro studies show that the earliest events in this shift from the mold to yeast form involve induction of the **heat shock response** and uncoupling of oxidative phosphorylation. These are followed by a shutdown of RNA synthesis, protein synthesis, and respiratory metabolism. The cells then pass through a metabolically inactive state, emerging with enhanced enzymatic capacities involving sulfhydryl compounds (eg, cysteine, cystine) that are exclusive to the yeast stage. In the yeast stage, there is recovery of mitochondrial activity and synthetic capacity, but a new constellation of oxidases, polymerases, proteins, cell wall glucans, and other compounds are present.

Shift from mold to yeast begins with heat shock response

Metabolic shift is toward sulfhydryl compounds in yeast form

Dimorphism in fungi is reversible, a feature that distinguishes it from developmental processes such as embryogenesis seen in higher eukaryotes. The importance of the conversion to virulence of *Histoplasma* is shown by animal studies using strains biochemically blocked from converting to the yeast phase. They neither produce disease nor persist in the host. To the extent known, these features are similar in the other dimorphic fungi.

Dimorphism is reversible and linked to virulence

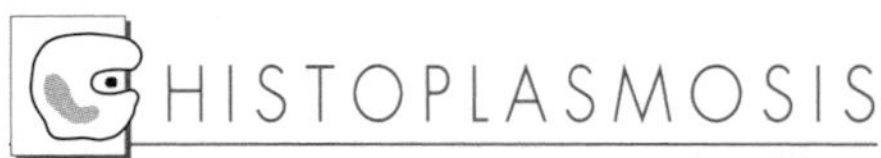

HISTOPLASMOSIS

CLINICAL CAPSULE

Histoplasmosis is limited to the endemic area, where the vast majority of cases are asymptomatic or show only a fever and cough. If affected individuals are seen by a physician, a pulmonary infiltrate and hilar adenopathy may or may not be evident on a radiograph. Progressive cases show extension in the lung or enlargement of lymph nodes, liver, and spleen.

EPIDEMIOLOGY

Microconidia are infectious

Mold grows in humid soil and bird droppings

Central US states have high prevalence

H. capsulatum grows in soil under humid climatic conditions, particularly soil containing bird or bat droppings. Inhalation of the mold microconidia, which are small enough (2 to 5 μm) to reach the terminal bronchioles and alveoli, is believed to be the mode of infection. The organism has a worldwide distribution but is particularly prevalent in certain temperate, subtropical, and tropical zones. In the United States, the greatest concentration by far is in the areas drained by the Ohio and Mississippi Rivers (see Fig 49–7). Over 50% of the residents of states in this area show evidence of previous infection, and in some locales, up to 90% of those have positive skin tests. Disturbances of bird roosts, bat caves, and soil have been associated with point source outbreaks. Persons in endemic areas whose employment (agriculture, construction) or avocation (spelunkers) brings them in contact with these sites are at increased risk. The infection is not transmitted from person to person. Disease is more common in men but there are no racial or ethnic differences in susceptibility.

PATHOGENESIS

Reticuloendothelial system is focus of infection

Grows in macrophages by controlling lysosomal pH

The hallmark of histoplasmosis is infection of the lymph nodes, spleen, bone marrow, and other elements of the reticuloendothelial system with intracellular growth in phagocytic macrophages. The initial infection is pulmonary, through inhalation of infectious conidia, which convert to the yeast form in the host. They attach to CD18 integrin receptors and are readily phagocytosed by macrophages and PMNs. Inside phagocytes, they continue to multiply in the cytoplasm, surviving the combined effects of the oxidative burst and phagolysosomal fusion. Key features in this survival are the ability of *H. capsulatum* to capture iron and calcium from the macrophage and to modulate phagolysosomal pH. The acidic pH required for optimal killing effect in the lysosome is elevated by *H. capsulatum* toward the neutral range (pH 6.0 to 6.5).

Lymphatic spread and reactivation are similar to tuberculosis

With continued growth, there is lymphatic spread and development of a primary lesion similar to that seen in tuberculosis (see Chapter 28). The extent of spread to the reticuloendothelial system within macrophages during primary infection is unknown, but such spread is presumed to occur. The vast majority of cases never advance beyond the primary stage, leaving only a calcified node as evidence of infection. Old lesions may reactivate in a small proportion of cases.

Granulomatous response seen in liver, spleen, and bone marrow

Pathologically, granulomatous inflammation with necrosis is prominent in pulmonary lesions, but *H. capsulatum* may be difficult to detect, even with special fungal stains. Extrapulmonary spread involves the reticuloendothelial system, with enlargement of the liver and spleen. Numerous organisms within macrophages may be found in these organs, in lymph nodes, or in bone marrow (see Fig 49–2A).

IMMUNITY

Histoplasmin skin test demonstrates delayed hypersensitivity

Infection with *H. capsulatum* is associated with the development of cell-mediated immunity, as demonstrated by a positive delayed hypersensitivity skin test to a mycelial antigen called **histoplasmin.** Infection is believed to confer long-lasting immunity, the most important component of which is CD4+ T lymphocyte mediated. In experimental infections, macrophages activated by T lymphocyte–derived cytokines are able to inhibit intracellular growth of *H. capsulatum* and thus control the disease. Neither B cells nor antibody have a significant influence on resistance to reinfection. Immunocompromised persons, particularly those with T lymphocyte–related defects, are unable to stop growth of the organism and tend to develop progressive, disseminated disease.

Immunity is derived from T-cell activation of macrophages

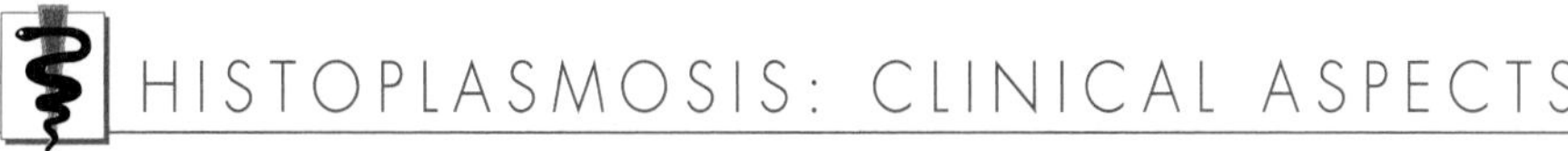

HISTOPLASMOSIS: CLINICAL ASPECTS

MANIFESTATIONS

Most cases of *H. capsulatum* infection are asymptomatic or show only fever and cough for a few days or weeks. Mediastinal lymphadenopathy and slight pulmonary infiltrates may be seen on x-rays. The histoplasmin skin test becomes positive after about 3 weeks. More severe cases may have chills, malaise, chest pain, and more extensive infiltrates, which usually resolve nonetheless. A residual nodule may continue to enlarge over a period of years, causing a differential diagnostic problem with pulmonary neoplasms. Progressive pulmonary disease occurs in a form similar to that of pulmonary tuberculosis, including the development of cavities, with sputum production, night sweats, and weight loss. The course is chronic and relapsing, lasting many months to years.

Most cases are asymptomatic or with fever and cough

Progressive pulmonary disease shows cavities and weight loss

Disseminated histoplasmosis generally appears as a febrile illness with enlargement of reticuloendothelial organs. The CNS, skin, gastrointestinal tract, and adrenal glands may also be involved. Painless ulcers on mucous membranes are a common finding. The course is typically chronic, with manifestations that depend on the organs involved. For example, chronic bilateral adrenal failure (Addison's disease) may develop when the adrenal glands are involved.

Dissemination involves reticuloendothelial organs, mucous membranes, and adrenal glands

DIAGNOSIS

In most forms of pulmonary histoplasmosis, the diagnostic yield of direct examinations or culture of sputum is low. In disseminated disease, blood culture or biopsy samples of a reticuloendothelial organ are the most likely to contain *Histoplasma*. Bone marrow culture has the highest yield. Because of their small size, the yeast cells are difficult to see in potassium hydroxide (KOH) preparations, and their morphology is not sufficiently distinctive to be diagnostic. Selective fungal stains such as methenamine silver demonstrate the organism but may not differentiate it from other yeasts. Hematoxylin and eosin (H&E)–stained tissue or Wright-stained bone marrow often demonstrates the organisms in their intracellular location in macrophages (see Fig 49–2). Specimens must be examined carefully under high magnification. Identification of culture isolates requires demonstration of the typical conidia and dimorphism. Demonstration of specific mycelial antigens by immunodiffusion (exoantigen test) may be used in place of dimorphism demonstration. Nucleic acid probes have been developed for culture identification.

Blood and bone marrow examination require special stains

Immunodiffusion and probes used with cultures

Antibodies can be detected during and following infection, but their usefulness in the endemic area is limited by false-negative results and cross-reactions in patients with blastomycosis. Rising antibody titers are suggestive of dissemination or relapse. The histoplasmin skin test is useful for epidemiologic studies but is not used for diagnosis or management of individual cases. Cultural isolation or clear histologic demonstration is necessary for a firm diagnosis. A circulating polysaccharide antigen has been demonstrated in serum and urine by enzyme immunoassay (EIA) in more than 90% of patients with disseminated disease.

Culture is required for firm diagnosis

EIA detects circulating antigen

TREATMENT

Primary infections and localized lung lesions usually resolve without treatment. Amphotericin B remains the treatment of choice, but its toxicity limits its use to cases of extensive disease such as progressive pulmonary and disseminated histoplasmosis. Itraconazole and ketoconazole have been effective for treatment and for suppression in AIDS patients with

Amphotericin B and itraconazole

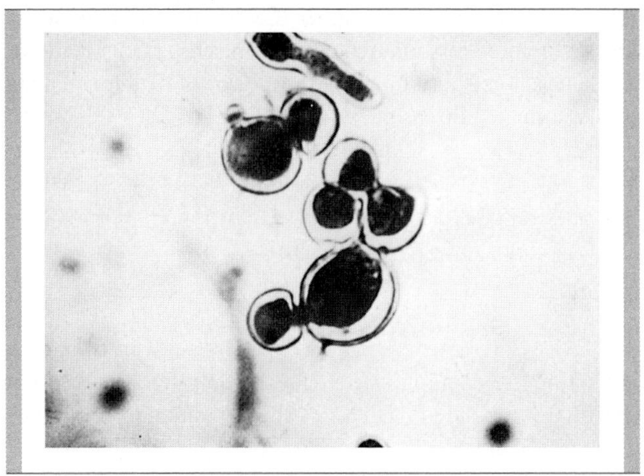

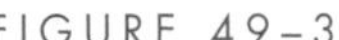

FIGURE 49–3
Blastomyces dermatitidis. Large thick-walled yeast cells are shown. Blastoconidia retain a broad attachment to the mother cell before separating. (*Reprinted with permission from Dr. E. S. Beneke and the Upjohn Company: Scope Publications, Human Mycoses.*)

histoplasmosis. In some cases amphotericin B treatment may be followed with a course of itraconazole.

BLASTOMYCES

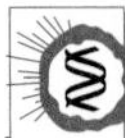

Blastomyces dermatitidis

Large yeast cells have broad-based buds

Mold has small oval conidia-like *Histoplasma*

Blastomyces dermatitidis is a dimorphic fungus with some characteristics similar to those of *Histoplasma*. Growth develops in the yeast phase in tissues and in cultures incubated at 37°C. The yeast cells are typically larger (8–15 mm) than those of *H. capsulatum,* with broad-based buds and a thick wall (Fig 49–3). The mold phase appears in culture at 25°C. Hyphae are septate and produce round to oval conidia sufficiently similar to the microconidia produced by *H. capsulatum* to cause confusion between the two in young cultures. Although older cultures may produce chlamydoconidia, *B. dermatitidis* produces no structure as distinctive as the tuberculate macroconidium of *Histoplasma*.

BLASTOMYCOSIS

CLINICAL CAPSULE

Most clinical features of blastomycosis are similar to histoplasmosis. Patients are asymptomatic or have only mild fever and cough unless the disease progresses outside the lung. Skin lesions are the most common manifestation of disseminated disease, not reticuloendothelial organ involvement.

EPIDEMIOLOGY

Geographic distribution is similar to *Histoplasma*

Cases of blastomycosis follow a geographic distribution and conditions for maturation of conidia in the soil, which are similar to that of histoplasmosis (see Fig 49–7). Most infections occur in the middle and eastern portions of North America, but cases have been reported worldwide. The lack of a specific skin test limits study of the endemic area.

PATHOGENESIS

Much less is known about blastomycosis than the more common systemic mycoses, such as histoplasmosis and coccidioidomycosis. The lower frequency of disseminated infections and the nonspecificity of skin and serologic tests are partly responsible for this lack of information. Much of what is believed to be true of blastomycosis is based on analogy with histoplasmosis.

The primary infection is pulmonary after inhalation of conidia, which develop in soil. Surface glucans and a glycoprotein adhesin (BAD1) have been identified, which bind the fungi to receptors on host cells, macrophages (CR3 and CD14), and the extracellular matrix. A mixed inflammatory response results, which ranges from neutrophil infiltration to well-organized granulomas with giant cells. The organisms grow in tissue as large yeasts with thick double walls with blastospores attached. A significant difference from *Histoplasma* is that the yeast cells are primarily extracellular rather than within macrophages. This may be due to their relatively large size, but there is little to suggest that *B. dermatitidis* shares the propensity for intracellular parasitism that is characteristic of *H. capsulatum*.

Surface adhesin binds to host cells

Large yeast are primarily outside cells

IMMUNITY

The principal host defense mechanisms against *B. dermatitidis* have not been clearly defined. The fungal cells activate the complement system by both the classical and alternate pathways, and antibodies directed against a glucan component of the cell wall have been identified. These antibodies decline as the infection resolves. As with other fungi, T lymphocyte–mediated responses appear to be the most important determinants of immunity. Macrophages activated with cytokines have enhanced capacity to kill *B. dermatitidis*.

Complement, antibody, and cell-mediated immunity are involved

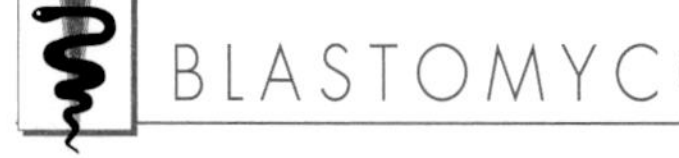

BLASTOMYCOSIS: CLINICAL ASPECTS

MANIFESTATIONS

Because mild cases are difficult to diagnose, most infections are recognized at advanced or disseminated stages of the disease. This problem was also posed by the other systemic mycoses before the development of sensitive and specific diagnostic procedures. Pulmonary infection is evidenced by cough, sputum production, chest pain, and fever. Hilar lymphadenopathy may be present, as may nodular pulmonary infiltrates with alveolar consolidation. The total picture may mimic a pulmonary tumor, tuberculosis, or some other mycosis. Skin lesions are common and were once considered a primary form of the disease. In contrast to histoplasmosis, lesions develop on exposed skin; mucous membrane infection is uncommon. Extensive necrosis and fibrosis may produce considerable disfigurement. Bone infection has features similar to those of other causes of chronic osteomyelitis. The urinary and genital tracts are the most commonly affected visceral sites; the prostate is especially prone to infection.

Pulmonary blastomycosis is similar to other mycoses

Skin lesions are on exposed surfaces

DIAGNOSIS

Direct demonstration of typical large yeasts with broad-based buds (blastoconidia) in KOH preparations is the most rapid means of diagnosis. Biopsy specimens also have a high yield, and the organisms are visible with either H&E or special fungal stains. *B. dermatitidis* grows on routine mycologic media, but culture may take as long as 4 weeks. Conidia are not particularly distinctive, and demonstration of dimorphism and typical yeast morphology is essential to avoid confusion with other fungi. The immunodiffusion test is particularly useful in differentiating cultures from *Histoplasma*. Serologic tests are available but may be negative in up to 50% of cases. Skin tests are no longer available.

KOH and biopsy show budding yeast

Culture takes weeks and conidia not distinctive

TREATMENT

Although amphotericin B is the preferred therapy, it is used only for progressive or disseminated disease. As with other systemic mycoses, response to treatment is slow, and relapse is common. Itraconazole, ketoconazole, and fluconazole have been effective in nonmeningeal

Amphotericin B and azoles are effective

cases and for suppression in AIDS. These azoles are considered alternatives to amphotericin in immunocompetent patients if the disease is not severe.

COCCIDIOIDES

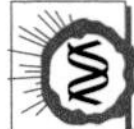

Coccidioides immitis

Dimorphism involves unique spherule

Spherules differentiate to form and release endospores

Coccidioides immitis is also a dimorphic fungus, but instead of a yeast phase, a large (12- to 100-μm), distinctive, round-walled **spherule** (Fig 49–4A and C) is produced in the invasive tissue form. This structure is unique among the pathogenic fungi. Its formation takes place in a process illustrated in Figure 49–5. Spherule development requires simultaneous invagination of the fungal membrane (plasmalemma) and production of new cell wall to form the large multicompartmental structure. The compartments differentiate into uninucleate structures called **endospores,** each with a thin wall layer. Multiple endospores develop within each spherule and the entire structure is surrounded by an extracellular matrix. The spherule eventually ruptures, releasing 200 to 300 endospores (Fig 49–6) each of which can differentiate into another spherule.

In alkaline soils and in culture, *C. immitis* grows only as a mold regardless of temperature. Growth becomes visible in 2 to 5 days. The hyphae are septate and produce

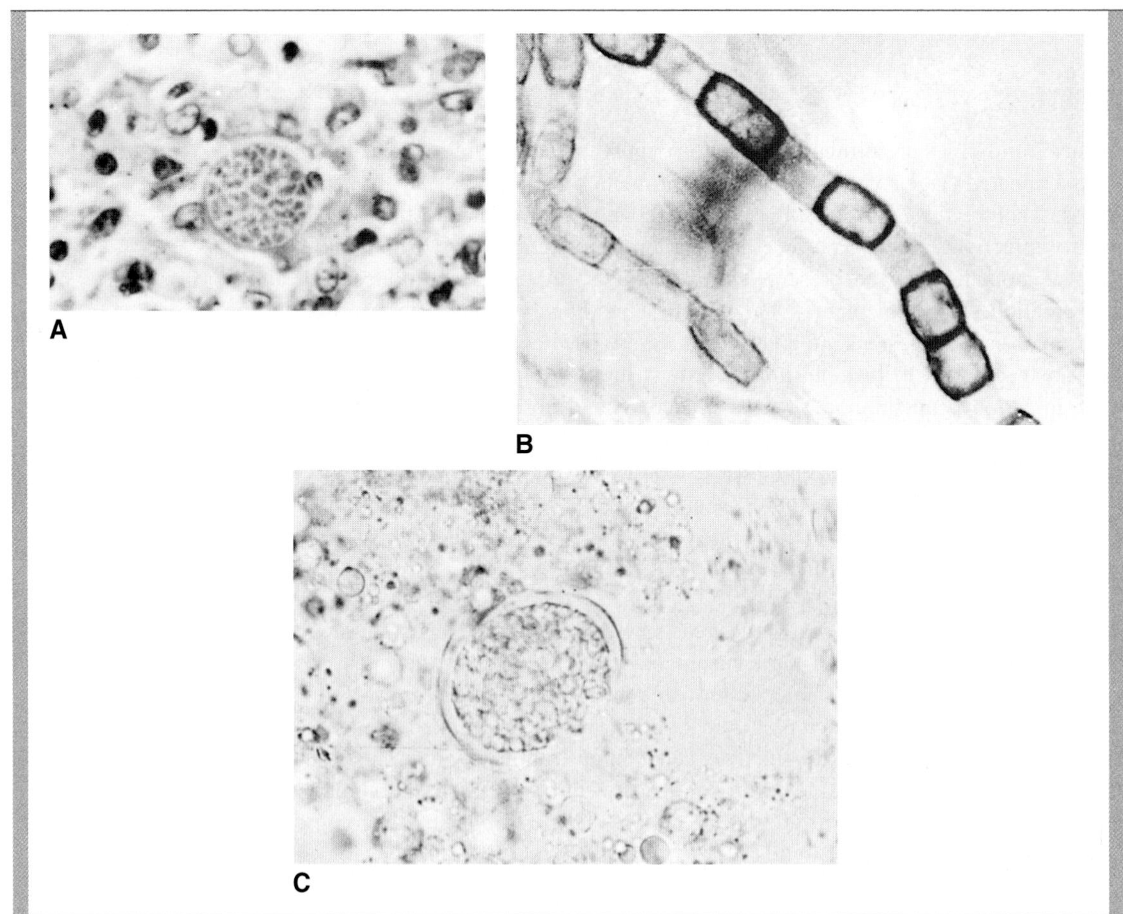

FIGURE 49–4

Coccidioides immitis. **A.** Tissue with thick-walled spherule containing multiple endospores. **B.** Mold phase with septate hyphae and arthroconidia. **C.** KOH preparation of sputum showing thick-walled spherule, which has just burst. (*Reprinted with permission from Dr. E. S. Beneke and the Upjohn Company: Scope Publications, Human Mycoses.*)

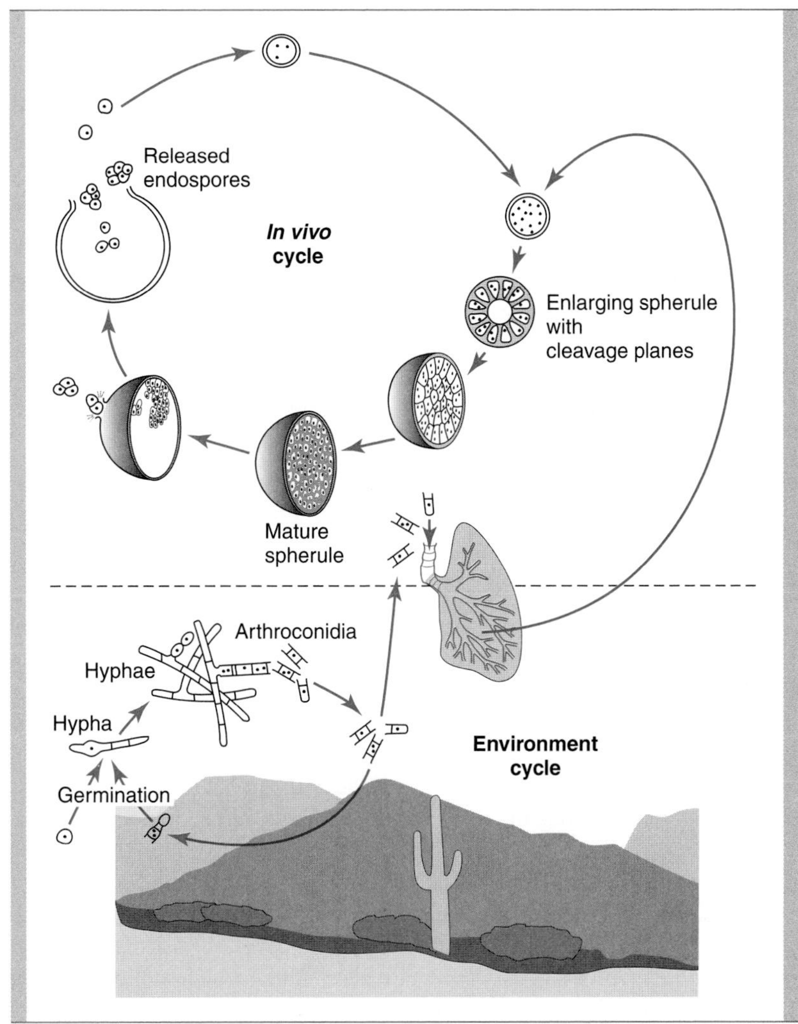

FIGURE 49–5
Life cycle of *Coccidioides immitis.* The nature cycle takes place in desert climates with modest rainfall. Hyphae differentiate into arthroconidia which break loose and may be suspended in the air. Soil disruptions and wind facilitate spread and the probability of inhalation into human lungs. In the human host environment in vivo differentiation produces cleavage planes and eventually huge spherules. The spherules rupture releasing endospores which can then repeat the in vivo cycle.

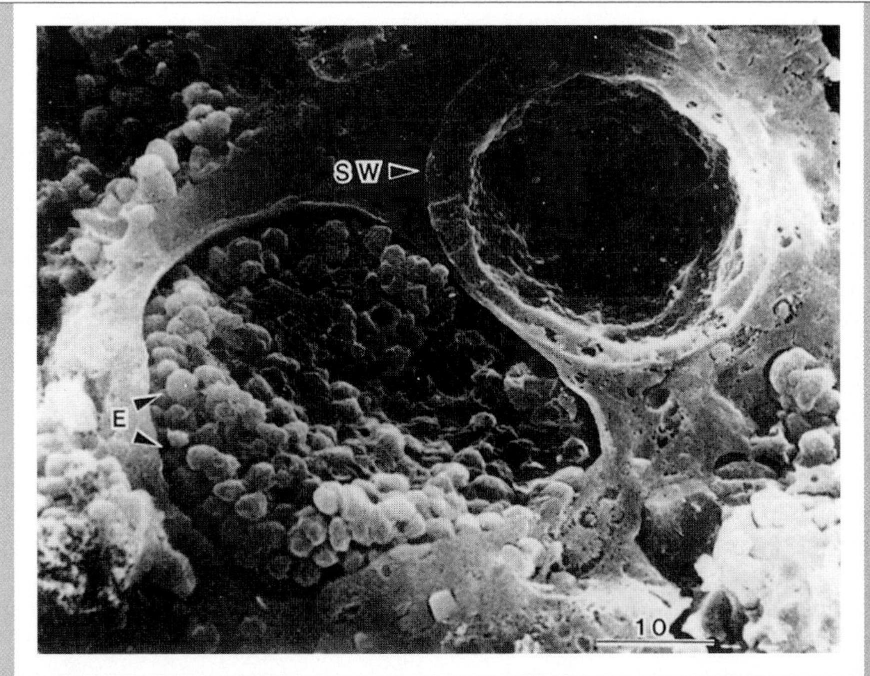

FIGURE 49–6
Coccidioides immitis. This electron micrograph of infected mouse lung shows a spherule filled with endospores (E) and one that has discharged its endospores into the surrounding tissue. Note the thickness of the spherule wall (SW). (*Reprinted with permission from Drutz DJ, Huppert M.* J Infect Dis *1983;147:379, Figure 7. Copyright University of Chicago Publisher.*)

Barrel-shaped arthroconidia are highly infectious

thick-walled, barrel-shaped **arthroconidia** (see Fig 49–4B), which are the infectious unit in nature and highly infectious when they develop in the laboratory. Spherules have been produced from arthroconidia in vitro under specialized conditions.

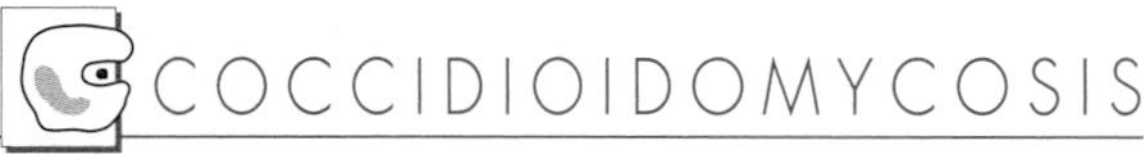

COCCIDIOIDOMYCOSIS

CLINICAL CAPSULE

Acute primary infection with *C. immitis* is either asymptomatic or presents as a complex called **valley fever** by residents of the endemic areas. Valley fever includes fever, malaise, dry cough, joint pains, and sometimes a rash. There are few physical or radiologic findings, but the illness persists for weeks. Disseminated disease involves lesions in the bones, joints, skin, and a progressive chronic meningitis.

EPIDEMIOLOGY

Geographically restricted to Sonoran desert

High proportion of locals have been infected

Coccidioidomycosis is the most geographically restricted of the systemic mycoses, because *C. immitis* grows only in the alkaline soil of semiarid climates known as the Lower Sonoran life zone (see Fig 49–7). These areas are characterized by hot, dry summers, mild winters with few freezes, and annual rainfall of about 10 inches during brief rainy seasons. Areas with these conditions are found scattered throughout the Americas, some as ecologic "islands." The primary endemic zones in the United States are in Arizona, Nevada, New Mexico, western Texas, and the arid parts of central and southern California. Persons living in the endemic areas are at high risk of infection, although disease is much less common. Positive skin test rates of 50 to 90% occur in longtime residents of highly endemic areas. Coccidioidomycosis is not transmissible from person to person.

Arthroconidia can be spread by dust storms

Rainfall pattern influences attack rate

Infection cannot be acquired without at least visiting an endemic area, although some interesting examples of the endemic zone itself paying a visit have been recorded. One such anecdote involves a gas station attendant with coccidioidomycosis whose only contact with an endemic area was changing a flat tire on a truck from California. In 1978, a storm originating in Bakersfield, California (endemic zone) carried a thick coat of dust all the way to San Francisco. This was followed by cases of coccidioidomycosis in persons who had never left the Bay Area. In 1992, a tenfold increase in disease in California followed an unusually wet winter in which the storms created a drought–rain–drought pattern just the right for growth of the mold (and wildflowers). When the Sonoran desert blooms, an arthroconidium "crop" is not far behind.

PATHOGENESIS

Arthroconidial wall resists phagocytosis

Spherules produce endospores with extracellular matrix

Inhaled arthroconidia are small enough (2 to 6 μm) to bypass the defenses of the upper tracheobronchial tree and lodge in the terminal bronchioles. Human monocytes can ingest and kill some arthroconidia on initial exposure, although the outer portion of the wall of the arthroconidium has antiphagocytic properties, which persist in the early stages of spherule development. Surviving arthroconidia convert to the spherule stage, which begins its slow growth to a size that makes effective phagocytosis difficult. Although PMNs are able to digest the spherule wall, their access appears to be restricted by the extracellular matrix surrounding it. The young endospores are released in packets that include the extracellular matrix derived from the parent spherule, which may protect them until they develop into new spherules.

Proteases and SOW may be linked to virulence

A number of proteases found in the conidial cell wall or in spherules have been proposed as *C. immitis* virulence factors. In addition to their role in the fungal life cycle, some of these enzymes attack host substrates such as collagen, elastin, and immunoglobulins, but no direct specific contribution to disease has been defined. Components of the spherule outer wall (SOW) have been linked to virulence in animals and to strong humoral and cellular immune responses in humans.

IMMUNITY

Lifelong immunity to coccidioidomycosis clearly develops in the vast majority of those who become infected. This immunity is associated with strong polymorphonuclear leukocyte and T lymphocyte–mediated responses to coccidioidal antigens. In most cases, a mixed inflammatory response is associated with early resolution of the infection and development of a positive delayed hypersensitivity skin test. Progressive disease is associated with weak or absent cellular immunity and skin test anergy. In most infected persons the infection is controlled after mild or inapparent illness. The disease progresses if cell-mediated immunity and consequent macrophage activation do not develop. Such immune deficits may be a result of disease (AIDS) or immunosuppressive therapy but may occur in persons with no other known cellular immune compromise.

Cell-mediated immunity is of prime importance

Progressive disease develops in patients with AIDS or defects in cell-mediated immunity

The central event appears to be the reaction to arthroconidia or to endospores released from ruptured spherules. Arthroconidia can be phagocytosed and killed by polymorphonuclear leukocytes even before an adaptive immune response is mounted. The handling of endospores requires the additional participation of macrophages that do not become maximally effective until activated by T lymphocyte–derived cytokines, particularly those produced by the T_H1 subsets. Prior to this, *C. immitis* endospores may be able to impair phagosome–lysosome fusion in the phagocyte.

Endospores must be destroyed by cytokine-activated macrophages

Humoral mechanisms are not known to play any role in immunity. In fact, *C. immitis* is resistant to complement-mediated killing, and levels of complement-fixing antibody are inversely related to the process of disease resolution. Persons with minimal objective indications of tissue involvement (eg, lesions, radiographs) have strong T-lymphocyte responses to *C. immitis* antigens and little if any detectable antibody. Those with disseminated disease and absent cellular immunity have high titers of antibody. Thus, the levels of antibody indicate the extent of antigenic stimulation with no known contribution to resolution of the infection.

Antibody production is inversely related to disease progress

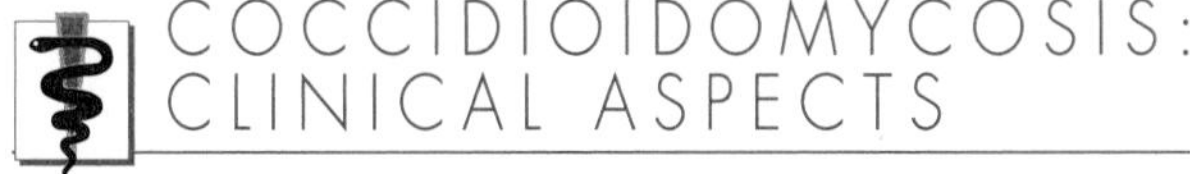

COCCIDIOIDOMYCOSIS: CLINICAL ASPECTS

MANIFESTATIONS

More than one half of those infected with *C. immitis* suffer no symptoms, or the disease is so mild that it cannot be recalled when skin test conversion is discovered. Others develop malaise, cough, chest pain, fever, and arthralgia 1 to 3 weeks after infection. This disease, which lasts 2 to 6 weeks, is known as **valley fever** by the local populations in the United States. Objective findings are few. The chest x-ray is usually clear or shows only hilar adenopathy. Erythema nodosum may develop midway through the course, particularly in women. In most cases, resolution is spontaneous but only after considerable discomfort and loss of productivity. In more than 90% of cases, there are no pulmonary residua. A small number of cases progress to a chronic pulmonary form characterized by cavity formation and a slow relapsing course that extends over years. Less than 1% of all primary infections disseminate to foci outside the lung.

Valley fever is usually asymptomatic and self-limiting

Erythema nodosum is common in women

Chronic and disseminated disease less than 1%

Disseminated disease is more common in men; in dark-skinned races, particularly Filipinos; and in AIDS patients and other immunosuppressed persons. Evidence of extrapulmonary infection almost always appears in the first year after infection. The most common sites are bones, joints, skin, and meninges. Coccidioidal meningitis develops slowly with gradually increasing headache, fever, neck stiffness, and other signs of meningeal irritation. The CSF findings are similar to those in tuberculosis and other fungal causes of meningitis, such as *C. neoformans*. Mononuclear cells predominate in the cell count, but substantial numbers of neutrophils are often present. If untreated, the disease is slowly progressive and fatal.

Racial orientation and immune status are risk factors for dissemination

Meningitis is chronic sign

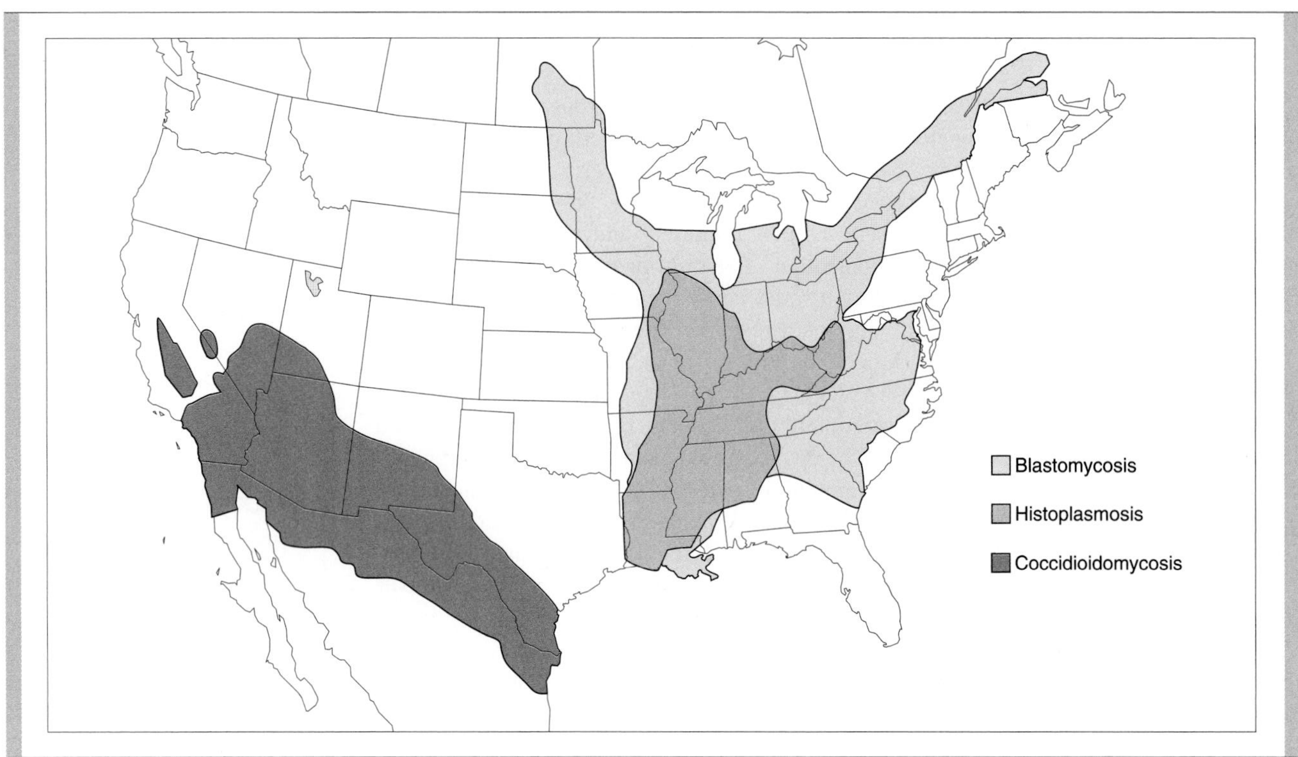

FIGURE 49–7
Geographic distribution of systemic fungal infections in the United States.

DIAGNOSIS

Direct examination for spherules is diagnostic

With enough persistence, direct examinations are usually rewarding. The thick-walled spherules are so large and characteristic (see Fig 49–4A and C) that they are difficult to miss in a KOH preparation or biopsy section. Skin and visceral lesions are most likely to demonstrate spherules; CSF is least likely. Spherules released into expectorated sputum are often small (10–15 mm) and immature without well-developed endospores. Spherules stain well in histologic sections with either H&E or special fungal stains.

Culture from CSF may be difficult

Substantial risk of laboratory infection with arthroconidia

Culture of *C. immitis* from sputum, visceral lesions, or skin lesions is not difficult, but must be undertaken only by those with experience and proper biohazard protection. Cultures of CSF are positive in less than half the cases of meningitis. Laboratories must be warned of the possibility of coccidioidomycosis to ensure diagnosis and avoid inadvertent laboratory infection. The latter is particularly significant outside the endemic areas, where routine precautions may not be in place. Identification requires observation of typical arthroconidia and demonstration of mycelial antigens using the exoantigen test or a gene probe.

Coccidioidin skin test remains positive for life

Precipitating IgM indicates acute infection

IgG detected by complement fixation quantitates disease

Skin and serologic tests are particularly useful in diagnosis and management of coccidioidomycosis. The coccidioidin skin test usually becomes positive 1 to 4 weeks after the onset of symptoms of primary infection and remains so for life. Although this skin test is generally believed to be useful in clinical diagnosis and management, it is currently not commercially available. Disseminated disease is frequently associated with anergy. One half to three quarters of patients with primary infection develop serum IgM precipitating antibody in the first 3 weeks of illness. These conditions persist for 2 to 4 months. IgG antibodies detected by complement fixation tests appear somewhat later in symptomatic infections. The amount and duration depend on the extent of disease. Antibodies disappear with resolution and persist with continuing infection. The height of the complement fixation titer is a measure of the extent of disease. The presence of complement-fixing antibody in the CSF is also important in the diagnosis of coccidioidal meningitis, because cultures are frequently negative. Precipitating and complement-fixing antibodies may be detected by classic methods or by more recently developed immunoassay procedures.

TREATMENT

Primary coccidioidomycosis is self-limiting, and no antifungal therapy is indicated. Progressive pulmonary disease and disseminated disease require the use of antifungal agents, usually amphotericin B. Ketoconazole has proved effective, but relapses are common. Fluconazole and itraconazole are also active against *C. immitis*. With the exception of fluconazole, none of these agents have significant penetration into the CNS. Amphotericin B is commonly given directly into the CSF for the treatment of *C. immitis* meningitis.

Amphotericin B in progressive disease

Azoles also active

PARACOCCIDIOIDES BRASILIENSIS

Paracoccidioides brasiliensis is the cause of paracoccidioidomycosis (South American blastomycosis), a disease limited to tropical and subtropical areas of Central and South America. The organism is a dimorphic fungus, the most noteworthy feature of which is the production of multiple blastoconidia from the same cell. Characteristic 5- to 40-μm cells covered with budding blastoconidia may be seen in tissue or in yeast-phase growth at 37°C. The disease manifests primarily as chronic mucocutaneous or cutaneous ulcers. The ulcers spread slowly and develop a granulomatous mulberry-like base. Regional lymph nodes, reticuloendothelial organs, and the lungs may also be involved.

Yeast with multiple blastoconidia are seen in ulcerative lesions

Little is known of the pathogenesis of the disease, although the route of infection is believed to be inhalation. Progression in experimental animals is associated with depressed T lymphocyte-mediated immune responses. The disease has a striking predilection for men, despite skin test evidence that subclinical cases occur at the same rate in both sexes. This may be related to the experimental observation that estrogens but not androgens inhibit conversion of mold-phase conidia to the yeast phase. Treatment is with sulfonamides, amphotericin B, and, more recently, the azole compounds.

Disease has a strong predilection for men

ADDITIONAL READING

Hogan LH, Klein BS, Levitz SM. Virulence factors of medically important fungi. *Clin Microbiol Rev* 1996;9:469–488. This review addresses aspects of pathogenesis and immunity completely but avoids excessive detail.

Practice guidelines for the management of systemic mycoses: The following four papers are were written by expert Mycoses Study Groups commissioned by the National Institute of Allergy and Infectious Diseases and the Infectious Diseases Society of America to define the management of cryptococcosis, histoplasmosis, blastomycosis, and coccidioidomycosis. Each begins with a concise summary of the disease and concludes with specific recommendations. They are definitive clinical summaries of each disease.

Chapman SW, Bradsher RW Jr, Campbell GD, Pappas PG, Kauffman CA. Practice guidelines for the management of patients with blastomycosis. *Clin Infect Dis* 2000;30: 679–683.

Galgiani JN, Ampel NM, Catanzaro A, Johnson RH, Stevens DA, Williams PL. Practice guideline for the treatment of coccidioidomycosis. *Clin Infect Dis* 2000;30:658–661.

Saag MS, Graybill RJ, Larsen RA, Pappas PG, Perfect JR, Powderly WG, Sobel JD, Dismukes WE. Practice guidelines for the management of cryptococcal disease. *Clin Infect Dis* 2000;30:710–718.

Smith CE, Saito MT, Simons SA. Pattern of 39,500 serologic tests in coccidioidomycosis. *JAMA* 1956;160:546–552. This study is the basis for the unique application of serologic tests to the diagnosis and prognosis of coccidioidomycosis.

Wheat J, Sarosi G, McKinsey, Hamill R, Bradsher R, Johnson P, Loyd J, Kauffman C. Practice guidelines for the management of patients with histoplasmosis. *Clin Infect Dis* 2000;30:688–695.

CHAPTER 50

Pneumocystis carinii

KENNETH J. RYAN

Pneumocystis carinii is the cause of a lethal pneumonia of immunocompromised persons, particularly those with AIDS. Its fungal nature is deduced from genomic studies; the organism has not been grown in culture.

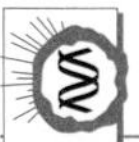

Pneumocystis carinii

To date, it has not been possible to cultivate *P. carinii.* Our knowledge of its nature rests on morphologic observations and the study of organisms purified from infected lungs. Until recently, *P. carinii* was believed to be a protozoan, and its "life cycle" was deduced from static images seen in infected tissues. The observed stages include a delicate 5- to 8-μm cystic structure within which elliptical subunits grow and repeat the cycle on rupture of the cyst. In parasitic parlance, these were called trophozoites, precysts, and cysts. The corresponding mycologic terms based on the same observations are spore, sporocyte, and spore case (Fig 50–1).

Life cycle is deduced from static images

Elliptical spores in sporocyte form spore case

The spherical sporocyte (precyst) is bounded by a cell wall and cytoplasmic membrane that enclose a nucleus and several mitochondria. As the precyst matures, the nuclei divide to form the eight spores (trophozoites) within the original structure to form the spore case (cyst). The spores have an eccentric nucleus, a nucleolus, and a single mitochondrion in the cytoplasm.

Eight spores each have nucleus and mitochondria

The confusion about the classification of *Pneumocystis* is understandable. The shape, nucleus, and reticular cytoplasm of the **spores** resemble protozoa, as does their aggregation into the cyst-like **spore case**. The cell wall lacks the rigidity typical of other fungi; however, biochemical elements of the fungal cell wall appear to be present. These include glucan and N-acetylglucosamine, the major subunit of chitin. The dominant sterol of the *P. carinii* cytoplasmic membrane is cholesterol, rather than the ergosterol characteristic of fungi. Other biochemical analyses, however, support the fungal nature such as the presence of elements of protein synthesis (elongation factor 3) that is unique to fungi. The fungal classification of *P. carinii* is most strongly supported by sequence analysis of the genes coding for ribosomal RNA, mitochondrial proteins, and major enzymes. These sequences show the closest homology with fungi and molecular phylogenic analysis, which places *Pneumocystis* near the ascomycetes.

Spores morphologically resemble protozoa

Cell wall is thin, but glucan and chitin elements are present

rRNA and mitochondrial gene sequences are homologous with fungi

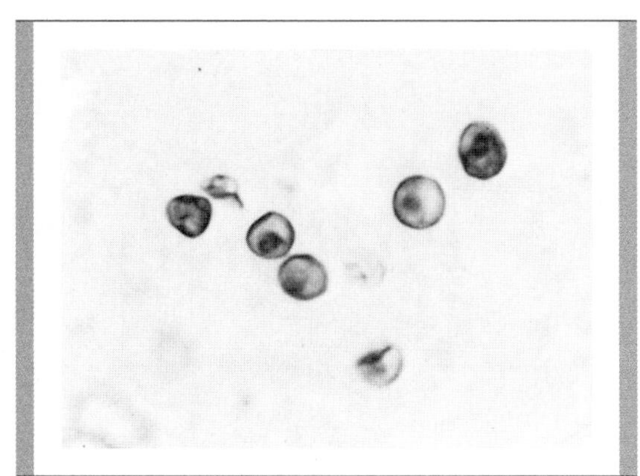

FIGURE 50–1
Sporocytes (cysts) of *Pneumocystis carinii* with developing spore nuclei.

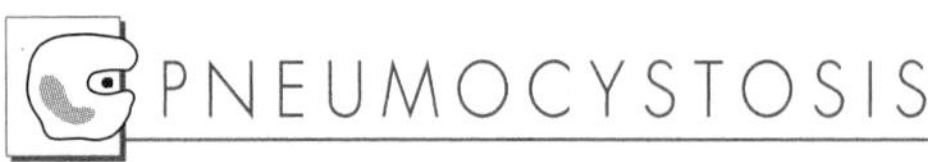

PNEUMOCYSTOSIS

CLINICAL CAPSULE

Pneumocystis pneumonia is insidious, beginning with mild fever or malaise in individuals whose immune system is compromised. Signs referable to the lung come later with nonproductive cough and shortness of breath. Radiographs reveal symmetrical alveolar pulmonary infiltrates, which spread from the hili. Progressive cyanosis, hypoxia, and asphyxia can lead to death in a 3- to 4-week period.

EPIDEMIOLOGY

Worldwide distribution in humans and animals

Antibodies are common

Airborne transmission is probable

Pulmonary infection with *P. carinii* occurs worldwide in humans and a broad spectrum of animal life. Exposure must be common; specific antibodies are present in nearly all children by the age of 4. The reservoir and mode of transmission remain unknown, but the view that the majority of *Pneumocystis carinii* pneumonia (PCP) cases represent reactivation of latent infection is no longer held. *P. carinii* is not found in the respiratory tract of asymptomatic persons, even among HIV-infected individuals, and the strains involved in second and third episodes are frequently antigenically different. Animal studies have shown that airborne transmission is possible, and the circumstances of hospital outbreaks point to active cases as a probable source.

PCP is a complication of immunodeficient states

AIDS patients are at high risk

Before the acquired immunodeficiency syndrome (AIDS) pandemic, PCP occurred sporadically among infants with congenital immunodeficiencies and in older children and adults as a complication of immunosuppressive therapy. Now AIDS has become the most common predisposing condition in the United States, and PCP is often the presenting manifestation of AIDS. In fact, prior to the development of effective chemoprophylactic regimens (see Treatment and Prevention), it was present in approximately half of all AIDS patients at the time of initial diagnosis. Eventually, most AIDS patients develop one or more bouts of PCP, often in conjunction with another opportunistic infection.

PATHOGENESIS

Low CD4 counts increase the risk in AIDS

P. carinii is an organism of low virulence that seldom produces disease in a host with normal T-lymphocyte function. In experimental animals, progressive infection can be initiated with starvation or corticosteroid administration, and in AIDS patients the risk of developing pneumocystosis increases dramatically once the CD4+ T lymphocyte count has fallen to 200 cells/mm^3 or below. Concurrent viral, bacterial, fungal, and protozoan infections are found frequently in human cases, suggesting that *P. carinii* may require the presence of another microbial agent for its multiplication.

Little is known about the early stages of disease. A **major surface glycoprotein** (MSG) abundant on the surface of *P. carinii* may act as an attachment ligand to several

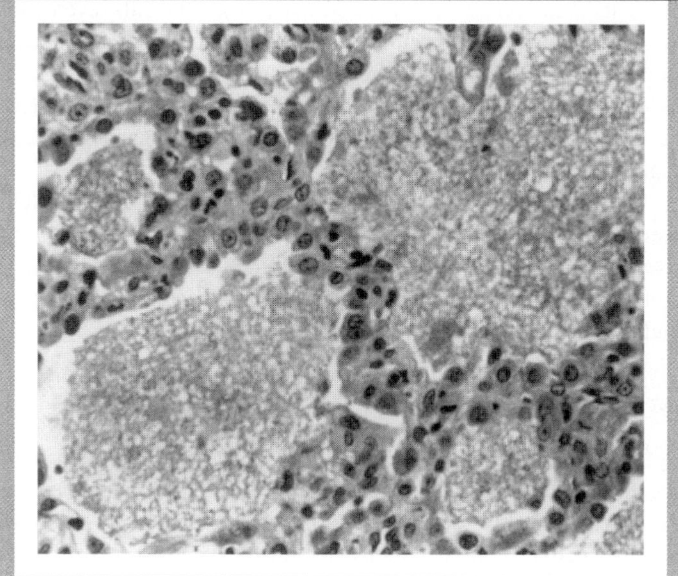

FIGURE 50–2
Lung biopsy specimen from *Pneumocystis carinii*–infected person, showing "foamy" contents of alveoli. (*Reproduced with permission from Connor DH, Chandler FW, Schwartz DA, Manz HJ, Lack EE (eds).* Pathology of Infectious Disease, *Volume II. Stamford, CT: Appleton & Lange, 1997.*)

host proteins, including fibronectin, vitronectin and surfactant proteins. MSG undergoes antigenic variation, which could aid in its persistence in human hosts. Histologically, PCP is characterized by alveoli filled with desquamated alveolar cells, monocytes, organisms, and fluid, producing a distinctive foamy, honeycombed appearance (Fig 50–2); hyaline membranes may be present, and round cell infiltrates may be visible in the septa. It has been suggested that *P. carinii* maintains an extracellular existence within alveoli obtaining essential nutrients from the alveolar fluid and lining cells.

MSG attaches to pneumocytes

Alveoli are filled with foamy exudate

IMMUNITY

The nature of the immunodeficiencies in patients with pneumocystosis points to the primacy of cell-mediated immunity (CMI) in resolution of infection with *P. carinii.* Alveolar macrophages are the first line of defense, with activated macrophages and CD4+ lymphocytes playing essential roles in the resolution of the infection. Activated macrophages release several cytotoxic factors, including O_2-derived radicals, reactive nitrogen intermediates, and cytokines (tumor necrosis factor-α, interleukin-2).

Activated macrophages and cytokines mediate CMI

Specific antibody responses to the MSG and other antigens appear in the course of pneumocystosis. A significant role for humoral immunity is suggested by the ability of MSG antibody to protect against experimental PCP in animals.

Antibody plays a role in protection

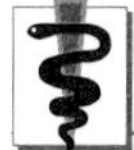

PNEUMOCYSTOSIS: CLINICAL ASPECTS

MANIFESTATIONS

In the immunocompromised host, the disease presents as a progressive, diffuse pneumonitis. Illness may begin after discontinuation or a decrease in the dose of corticosteroids or, in the case of acute lymphatic leukemia, during a period of remission. In infants and AIDS patients, onset is typically insidious, and the clinical course is 3 to 4 weeks in duration. Fever is mild or absent. In older individuals and patients who have previously been on high doses of corticosteroids, the onset is more abrupt, and the course is both febrile (38–40°C) and abbreviated. In both populations, the cardinal manifestations are progressive dyspnea and tachypnea; cyanosis and hypoxia eventually supervene. A nonproductive cough is present in 50% of all patients. Clinical signs of pneumonia are usually absent, despite the presence of infiltrates on x-ray. These infiltrates are alveolar in

Diffuse pneumonitis with insidious onset

Nonproductive cough, dyspnea, and cyanosis develop later

Alveolar infiltrates spread out from the hili

character and spread out symmetrically from the hili, eventually affecting most of the lung. Occasionally, unilateral infiltrates, coin lesions, lobar infiltrates, cavitary lesions, or spontaneous pneumothoraces are observed. Pleural effusions are uncommon. Clinical and radiographic abnormalities are generally accompanied by a decrease in arterial oxygen saturation, diffusion capacity of the lung, and vital capacity. Death occurs by progressive asphyxia.

Extrapulmonary lesions are seen in AIDS

Lesions outside the lung were rarely seen prior to the AIDS epidemic but are now seen with some regularity. The sites most often involved are lymph nodes, bone marrow, spleen, liver, eyes, thyroid, adrenal glands, gastrointestinal tract, and kidneys. The extrapulmonary clinical manifestations range from incidental autopsy findings to progressive multisystem disease.

DIAGNOSIS

Diagnostic yield from sputum is low

BAL is the best of the invasive procedures

Definite diagnosis depends on finding organisms of typical morphology in appropriate specimens. Because the pathologic process is alveolar rather than bronchial, the organisms are not readily seen in expectorated specimens such as sputum. The diagnostic yield is much better from specimens obtained by more invasive procedures. Of these, bronchoalveolar lavage (BAL) gives the best results with the least morbidity. Percutaneous needle aspiration of the lung, transbronchial biopsy, and open lung biopsy, although somewhat more sensitive techniques, are accompanied by more complications, including pneumothorax and hemothorax.

Silver and other stains readily demonstrate *P. carinii*

DFA is sensitive

P. carinii can be demonstrated by a wide variety of staining procedures. The standard stain is methenamine silver (Fig 50–3), but a direct fluorescent antibody (DFA) method, if available, is slightly more sensitive. Laboratories often perform a rapid stain (Wright, Giemsa, Papanicolaou) first and confirm by methenamine silver or DFA later. Methods developed for detection of *Pneumocystis* DNA in BAL and other specimens by polymerase chain reaction may soon be practical for clinical laboratories.

TREATMENT AND PREVENTION

TMP-SMX is treatment of choice

Treatment is extended in AIDS

The fixed combination of trimethoprim and sulfamethoxazole (TMP-SMX) is the treatment of choice for all forms of pneumocystosis. It is administered orally or intravenously for 14 to 21 days. Patients with AIDS receive the longer course because they start with a higher organism burden, respond more slowly, and suffer relapse more often. Unfortunately, AIDS patients have a high incidence of adverse effects to TMP-SMX, particularly the sulfonamide component. This requires the use of other antimicrobics (eg, clindamycin, primaquine, dapsone) alone or in combination with TMP. In hospitalized patients, two parenteral drugs, pentamidine and trimetrexate, are the major alternatives to TMP-SMX.

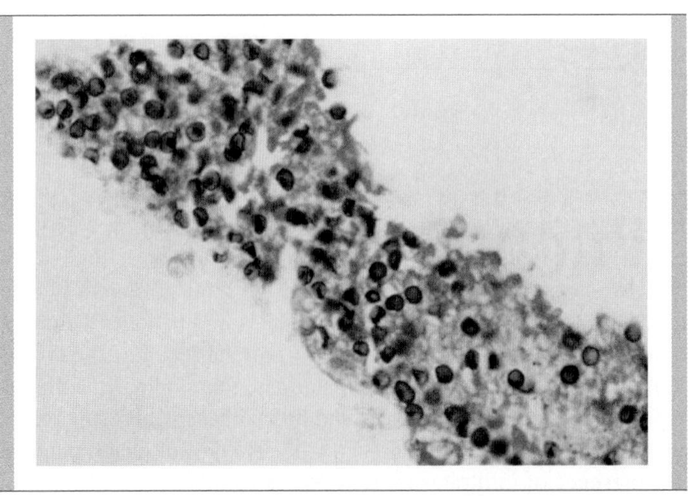

FIGURE 50–3
Multiple spherical and collapsed sporocytes (cysts) of *Pneumocystis carinii* stained by methenamine silver. Note the comma-shaped developing spores. (*Reproduced with permission from Connor DH, Chandler FW, Schwartz DA, Manz HJ, Lack EE (eds).* Pathology of Infectious Disease, *Volume II. Stamford, CT: Appleton & Lange, 1997.*)

Low-dose administration of TMP-SMX has been shown to significantly decrease the incidence of *P. carinii* pneumonia in high-risk patients and prevents relapse in AIDS patients. This chemoprophylaxis is indicated for patients who have CD4+ lymphocyte counts below 200/mm^3, unexplained fever, or a previous episode of PCP. Once begun, chemoprophylaxis is continued for life.

Chemoprophylaxis prevents PCP in high-risk groups

ADDITIONAL READING

Kovacs JA, Gill VJ, Meshnick S, Masur H. New insights into transmission, diagnosis, and drug treatment of *Pneumocystis carinii* pneumonia. *JAMA* 2001; 286:2450–2460. An excellent, concise review, which also points out that mutants may be emerging that are resistant to sulfa drugs and atovaquone.

PART VIII

PARASITES

CHAPTER 56

Tissue Nematodes

CHAPTER 57

Cestodes

CHAPTER 58

Trematodes

CHAPTER 51

Introduction to Pathogenic Parasites: Pathogenesis and Chemotherapy of Parasitic Diseases

JAMES J. PLORDE

This chapter provides an overview of parasitic diseases and of antiparasitic therapy. The student may find it valuable to reread it after studying the subsequent chapters in this section.

DEFINITION

Within the context of this section of the book, the term **parasite** refers to organisms belonging to one or two major taxonomic groups: protozoa and helminths. Protozoa are microscopic, single-celled eukaryotes superficially resembling yeasts in both size and simplicity. Helminths, in contrast, are macroscopic, multicellular worms possessing differentiated tissues and complex organ systems; they vary in length from a meter to less than a millimeter. The majority of both protozoa and helminths are free-living, play a significant role in the ecology of the planet, and seldom inconvenience the human race. The less common disease-producing species are typically obligate parasites, dependent on vertebrate hosts, arthropod hosts, or both for their survival. When their level of adaptation to a host is high, their presence typically produces little or no injury. Less complete adaptation leads to a more serious disturbance of the host and, occasionally, to death of both host and parasite.

Eukaryotic single-celled protozoa and multicellular macroscopic helminths

Most are free living

Disease-producing species usually obligate parasites

SIGNIFICANCE OF HUMAN PARASITIC INFECTIONS

The relative infrequency of parasitic infections in the temperate, highly sanitated societies of the industrialized world has sometimes led to the parochial view that knowledge of parasitology has little relevance for physicians practicing in these areas. The continuing presence of parasitic disease among the impoverished, immunocompromised, sexually active, and peripatetic segments of industrialized populations, however, means that most physicians will regularly encounter those pathogens. Parasitic diseases remain among the major causes of human misery and death in the world today and, as such, are important obstacles to the development of the economically less favored nations (Table 51–1).

Major cause of disease and death worldwide

Moreover, a number of recent medical, socioeconomic, and political phenomena have combined to produce a dramatic recrudescence of several parasitic diseases with important consequences to both the United States and the developing world.

Resistance of malarial parasites to chemotherapeutics

Resistance of insect vectors to insecticides

Recent increases in imported malaria

Currently, 2.5 billion people live in malarious areas, and of these, approximately 500 million are infected at any given time. Between 1 and 3 million people, predominately children, die of malaria each year. *Plasmodium falciparum,* the most deadly of the malarial organisms, has developed resistance to several categories of antimalarial agents, and resistant strains are now found throughout Southeast Asia, parts of the Indian subcontinent, southeast China, large areas of tropical America, and tropical Africa. Growing resistance of the mosquito vector of malaria to the less toxic and less expensive insecticides has resulted in a cutback of many malaria control programs. In countries such as India, Pakistan, and Sri Lanka, where eradication efforts had previously interrupted parasite transmission, the disease incidence has increased 100-fold in recent years. In tropical Africa, the intensity of transmission defies current control measures. Of direct interest to

TABLE 51–1

Prevalence of Parasitic Infections

Disease	Estimated Population Affected
Amebiasis	10% of world population
Annual deaths	40–110 thousand
Giardiasis	200 million
Malaria	400–490 million
Population at risk	2.5 billion
Annual deaths	2–3 million
Leishmaniasis	12 million
African trypanosomiasis	
Population at risk	50 million
New cases per year	100,000
Annual deaths	5000
American trypanosomiasis	24 million
Population at risk	65 million
New cases per year	60,000
Schistosomiasis	200 million
Population at risk	600 million
Annual deaths	0.5–1.0 million
Clonorchis and **opisthorchiasis**	13.5 million
Paragonimiasis	2.1 million
Fasciolopsiasis	10 million
Filiariasis	128 million
Onchocerciasis	18 million
Dracunculiasis	<100,000
Ascariasis	1.3 billion
Hookworm	1.3 billion
Trichuriasis	0.9 billion
Strongyloidiasis	35 million
Enterobius vermicularis	400 million
Cestodiasis	65 million

American physicians is the spillover of this phenomenon to the United States. Presently, approximately 1000 cases of imported malaria are reported annually.

Entamoeba spp. are intestinal protozoa that infect 10% of the world's population, including 2 to 3% in the United States. The majority of individuals are infected with the noninvasive *E. dispar.* The invasive *E. histolytica* produces amebiasis, a disease characterized by intestinal ulcers and liver abscesses. It is more commonly seen in the poorly sanitated areas of the world, but occurs in the United States as well, particularly in institutions for the mentally retarded and among migrant workers and some male homosexuals.

Amebic infections in 10% of world population

In the poor, rural areas of Latin America, *Trypanosoma cruzi* infects an estimated 16 million individuals annually, leaving many with the characteristic heart and gastrointestinal lesions of Chagas' disease. In Africa, from the Sahara Desert in the north to the Kalahari in the south, a related organism, *Trypanosoma brucei,* causes one of the most lethal of human infections, sleeping sickness. Animal strains of this same organism limit food supplies by making the raising of cattle economically unfeasible.

Trypanosomiasis produces disease and limits food supplies

Leishmaniasis, a disease produced by another intracellular protozoan, is found in parts of Europe, Asia, Africa, and Latin America. Clinical manifestations range from a self-limiting skin ulcer, known as oriental sore, through the mutilating mucocutaneous infection of espundia, to a highly lethal infection of the reticuloendothelial system (kala azar).

Leishmaniasis can cause cutaneous or disseminated disease

In 1947 Stoll, in an article entitled "This Wormy World," estimated that between the tropics of Cancer and Capricorn there were many more intestinal worm infections than people. The prevalence was judged to be far lower in temperate climates. Warren, however, recently estimated that 27% of the American population harbored worms. The most serious of the helminthic diseases, schistosomiasis, affects an estimated 200 million individuals in Africa, Asia, and the Americas. Individuals with heavy worm levels develop bladder, intestinal, and liver disease, which may ultimately result in death. Unfortunately, the disease is frequently spread as a consequence of rural development schemes. Irrigation projects in Egypt, the Sudan, Ghana, and Nigeria have significantly increased the incidence of the disease in these areas, often mitigating the economic gains of the development program itself.

Parasitic worm infections prevalent, may be spread by irrigation projects

Two closely related filarial worms, *Wuchereria bancrofti* and *Brugia malayi,* which are endemic in Asia and Africa, interfere with the flow of lymph and can produce grotesque swellings of the legs, arms, and genitals. Another filaria produces onchocerciasis (river blindness) in millions of Africans and Americans, leaving thousands blind.

Filariasis produces swellings

Toxoplasmosis, giardiasis, trichomoniasis, and pinworm infections are four cosmopolitan parasitic infections well known to American physicians. The first, a protozoan infection of cats, infects possibly one third of the world's human population. Although it is usually asymptomatic, infection acquired in utero may result in abortion, stillbirth, prematurity, or severe neurologic defects in the newborn. Asymptomatic infection acquired either before or after birth may subsequently produce visual impairment. Immunosuppressive therapy may reactivate latent infections, producing severe encephalitis.

Multiple parasitic diseases common in the United States

BIOLOGY, MORPHOLOGY, AND CLASSIFICATION

Protozoa

Morphology

Protozoa range in size from 2 to more than 100 μm. Their protoplasm consists of a true membrane-bound nucleus and cytoplasm. The former contains clumped or dispersed chromatin and a central nucleolus or **karyosome.** The shape, size, and distribution of these structures are useful in distinguishing protozoan species from one another.

The cytoplasm is frequently divided into an inner endoplasm and a thin outer ectoplasm. The granular **endoplasm** is concerned with nutrition and often contains food reserves, contractile vacuoles, and undigested particulate matter. The **ectoplasm** is organized into specialized organelles of locomotion. In some species, these organelles appear as blunt, dynamic extrusions known as pseudopods. In others, highly structured thread-like cilia or flagella arise from intracytoplasmic basal granules. Flagella are longer and less numerous than cilia and possess a structure and a mode of action distinct from those seen in prokaryotic organisms.

Endoplasm contains nutrients

Ectoplasm has organelles of locomotion

In some infections, parasite recovery is uncommon. Immunodiagnostic and nucleic acid hybridization techniques provide diagnostic alternatives for these situations. Although tests for circulating antibodies have long been available for a number of parasitic diseases, they have often lacked sensitivity and specificity. The replacement of crude, antigenically complex parasitic extracts with purified homologous antigens, together with the adaptation of highly reactive test systems, has significantly increased the sensitivity and specificity of such tests. Currently, reliable serologic procedures are available for amebiasis, cysticercosis, echinococciasis, paragonimiasis, schistosomiasis, strongyloidiasis, toxocariasis, toxoplasmosis, and trichinosis. More will undoubtedly follow in the near future.

Serologic tests available for some parasites

Techniques for the detection of parasitic antigens in blood, body fluids, tissues, and excreta also have been developed. Commercial immunofluorescent and immunosorbent kits for *Pneumocystis carinii* (pulmonary secretions), *T. vaginalis* (genitourinary fluids), and *E. histolytica, Giardia,* and *Cryptosporidium* (feces) are now commonly found in clinical laboratories. Less generally available are systems for the detection of malaria antigens in blood and *T. gondii* in tissue.

Antigen detection becoming available

DNA probes are available for the detection of *P. falciparum, T. cruzi, T. brucei, Onchocerca* species, and the etiologic agents of lymphatic filariasis. The probes for *P. falciparum* and lymphatic filariae have demonstrated sensitivities that match or exceed those of traditional techniques. The major limitations of DNA probes as diagnostic tools, relate to the technical aspects of the hybridization procedure which should soon be overcome.

Molecular methods for DNA detection being used with increasing frequency

CHEMOTHERAPY

The study and management of parasitic disease were seminal to the initiation of the chemotherapeutic era. Amazonian Indians first used quinine-containing extracts of cinchona tree bark to treat malarious patients more than 300 years ago. It was in the attempt to synthesize this same antimalarial compound that 19th-century German chemists discovered aniline dyes. The circle closed in the early years of this century when Ehrlich, while investigating the suitability of these dyes as protozoan stains, developed the concept that chemicals might be found that had the capacity to destroy microbial pathogens selectively without damage to the tissues of the human host. Although the most dramatic confirmation of that concept came with the introduction of arsenical compounds for the treatment of syphilis, his first successful chemotherapeutics were directed against protozoan agents. By 1930, chemically synthesized drugs had been marketed for the treatment of malaria, trypanosomiasis, and schistosomiasis.

Antiparasitic agents among first antimicrobics

The introduction and explosive increase in the number and variety of antimicrobic agents introduced in the latter three fourths of the 20th century forever changed the face of medicine. Unfortunately, however, few were effective against parasites because they share the eukaryotic characteristics of their hosts. With the resources of the pharmaceutical companies directed toward the development and introduction of antibacterial agents, work on antiparasitic agents lagged. Because of the lack of safer alternatives, chemotherapeutics synthesized in the preantibiotic era remained critical elements of the parasitologist's therapeutic armamentarium until very recently. Most required prolonged or parenteral administration, the effectiveness of many was restricted to particular disease stages, and the toxicity of a few mandated that use be limited to very severe or life-threatening conditions. With time, and at a pace much slower than that seen for the antibacterial agents, newer antiparasitic agents were developed that overcame many of these problems. Their numbers are still limited, and only recently has their safety and efficacy begun to match those of their antibacterial equivalents.

Newer antiparasitics have broader spectrum and are less toxic

Therapeutic Goals

The process of antiparasitic drug development and use has been shaped to a significant degree by the concentration of parasitic diseases in the impoverished areas of the world. Community-based public health measures aimed at interrupting pathogen transmission, such as provision of sanitary facilities and clean water supplies, are still often beyond the capacity of tightly constrained budgets, and the major burden of mitigating the impact of

Treatment programs difficult in underdeveloped economies

parasitic illnesses in endemic areas often falls on medical auxiliaries or village health workers who, operating in remote and relatively primitive conditions, must examine, diagnose, and treat sick patients with whom they have only fleeting contact. Given these limitations and the large numbers of the afflicted, optimal therapy requires drugs that are effective in a single dose, easily administered, safe enough to be dispensed with limited medical supervision, and sufficiently inexpensive to be widely used. Few such agents exist. Pharmaceutical companies, faced with the enormous costs of drug development and approval, have been reluctant to expend resources they are unlikely to recover. Until the international community provides the resources needed for the development of more suitable agents, the full potential of antiparasitic chemotherapy will not be realized.

Ideal agents would be inexpensive, of low toxicity, and effective in single doses; few of these exist

The practical aspects of antiparasitic therapy are illustrated in the principles governing the treatment of worm infections, which differ significantly from those applied to prokaryotic or protozoan infections. Helminths, with few exceptions, do not multiply within the human host, and severe infections thus require the repeated acquisition of infectious parasites. Interestingly, the intensity of infection or worm burden does not follow a normal distribution in human populations. Most infected individuals harbor fewer than a dozen adult worms; a small minority harbor very large worm numbers. Because there is a direct correlation between worm burden and clinical disease, only this minority suffers significant morbidity. Concentrating treatment on those few clinically ill patients moderates the medical impact of a helminthic disease on a community at a cost dramatically lower than that required for mass treatment. Moreover, it is usually unnecessary to eradicate all worms from treated patients; a significant decrease in the worm burden is adequate to alleviate clinical symptoms. This can often be accomplished with short, subcurative doses that further reduce cost and minimize the likelihood of drug toxicity. Because this approach can dramatically decrease the total community worm burden, the number of worm progeny shed into the environment is similarly reduced and the transmission of the disease slowed or, at times, eliminated.

For worms, treatment efforts should be concentrated on the most heavily parasitized individuals

Structure and Action

With few exceptions, antiparasitic agents have been synthesized de novo rather than developed from naturally occurring substances. Most are relatively simple and often contain benzene or other ring structures.

Most antiparasitics are synthetic

It is believed that the majority of antiprotozoan drugs interfere with nucleic acid synthesis or, less commonly, with carbohydrate metabolism. Anthelmintics, on the other hand, apparently act by compromising the worm's glycolytic pathways or neuromuscular function. In most cases, the parasite and host cells have functionally equivalent target sites. Differential toxicity is achieved by preferential uptake, metabolic alteration of the drug by the parasite, or differences in the susceptibility of functionally equivalent sites in parasite and host.

Differential toxicity based on uptake, metabolic factors

As has been the case for antibacterial agents, the impact of many antiparasitic agents has been compromised by the development of resistance in the parasite. This seems to have resulted from mutation and selection in the face of intensive, often prophylactic, drug use. The mechanisms responsible have been studied for only a few parasites, but appear to be related to reduced uptake of drug.

Acquired mutational resistance usually involves reduced uptake of drug

Drugs

Heavy Metals

Arsenic and antimonial compounds have been used since ancient times. They form stable complexes with sulfur compounds and probably exert their biological effects by binding to sulfhydryl groups. They are toxic to the host as well as to the parasite and have their greatest impact on cells that are most metabolically active such as neuronal, renal tubular, intestinal epithelial, and bone marrow stem cells. Their differential toxicity and therapeutic value are due to enhanced uptake by the parasite and its intense metabolic activity. Only one trivalent arsenical, melarsoprol* (Mel B), is now widely used. It is capable of

Arsenic and antimonial compounds inactivate —SH groups

Differential toxicity based on enhanced uptake by parasite

* Available from the Centers for Disease Control and Prevention Drug Service.

Melarsoprol is active against all stages of trypanosomiasis

penetrating the blood–brain barrier and is effective in all stages of trypanosomiasis. Because of its toxicity, it is employed only when less toxic agents have failed or the central nervous system is involved. The recently introduced less toxic trypanocides that penetrate the blood–brain barrier may soon replace this drug.

Antimonials used only for leishmanial infections

Antimonial agents are now restricted to the management of leishmanial infections. Two pentavalent compounds, sodium stibogluconate* (Pentostam) and meglumine antimoniate† (Glucantime), are used for all forms of leishmaniasis. In disseminated disease, prolonged therapy is usually required and relapses often occur. In localized cutaneous leishmaniasis, cure is usually achieved with a relatively brief course. Toxic side effects are similar to those of the arsenicals.

Antimalarial Quinolines

Quinine and quinoline analogs active against malaria

Cinchona bark was used in Europe for the treatment of fever as early as 1640. Only after Pelletier and Caventou isolated quinine from cinchona in 1820 did this alkaloid gain widespread acceptance as an antimalarial. Synthesis of new quinolines was stimulated by the interruption of quinine supplies during World Wars I and II and, after 1961, by the growing impact of drug-resistant falciparum malaria in several areas of the world. Among the most effective agents are those that share the double-ring structure of quinine.

Accumulate in parasitized cells and block DNA synthesis

Current analogs fall into three major groups: 4-aminoquinolines, 8-aminoquinolines, and 4-quinolinemethanols. Selective destruction of intracellular parasites results from accumulation of the quinolines by parasitized host cells. Most of these agents appear to block nucleic acid synthesis by intercalation into double-stranded DNA. However, the failure of the 4-quinolinemethanols to intercalate indicates that other mechanisms, perhaps inhibition of heme polymerase, with the build up of toxic hemoglobin metabolites within the malarial parasite, are involved.

Quinine, 4-aminoquinolines (eg, chloroquine), and 4-quinolinemethanols suppress malarial infection

8-Aminoquinolines (eg, primaquine) effect radical cure

Quinine, 4-aminoquinolines, and 4-quinolinemethanols are preferentially concentrated in parasitized erythrocytes and rapidly destroy the erythrocytic stage of the parasite that is responsible for the clinical manifestations of malaria. Thus, these agents can be used either prophylactically to suppress clinical illness should infection occur or therapeutically to terminate an acute attack. They do not concentrate in tissue cells, and thus organisms sequestered in exoerythrocytic sites, particularly the liver, survive and may later reestablish erythrocytic infection and produce a clinical relapse. The 8-aminoquinolines accumulate in tissue cells, destroy hepatic parasites, and effect a radical cure.

Primaquine has hematologic toxicity

Chloroquine phosphate, a 4-aminoquinoline, is the most widely used of the blood schizonticidal drugs. In the doses used for long-term malarial prophylaxis, it has proven remarkably free of untoward effects. Primaquine phosphate, the 8-aminoquinoline used to eradicate persistent hepatic parasites, has toxic effects related to its oxidant activity. Methemoglobinemia and hemolytic anemia are particularly frequent in patients with glucose-6-phosphate dehydrogenase deficiency, because they are unable to generate sufficient quantities of the reduced form of nicotinamide adenine dinucleotide to respond to this oxidant stress. Typically, the anemia is severe in patients of Mediterranean and Far Eastern ancestry and mild in black patients.

Quinine is active against many chloroquine-resistant malarial strains

Quinine is the most toxic of the quinolines and is currently used primarily to treat the strains of *P. falciparum* resistant to several blood schizonticidal agents that are spreading rapidly through Asia, Latin America, and Africa. Chloroquine resistance is the most frequent and worrisome, because suitable alternatives to this safe and highly effective agent are few. The mechanism of resistance is not clearly understood, but resistant organisms fail to accumulate chloroquine. Experimental reversal of resistance with calcium channel blockers suggests that the failure to accumulate this agent results from a rapid release mechanism. Quinidine, a less cardiotoxic optical isomer of quinine, is more readily available in the United States and is preferred to quinine when parenteral administration is required. Mefloquine, a more recently developed oral 4-quinolinemethanol, originally displayed a high level of activity against most chloroquine-resistant parasites; however, mefloquine-resistant

* Available from the Centers for Disease Control and Prevention Drug Service.

† Not available in the United States.

strains of *P. falciparum* are now widespread in Southeast Asia, and present, to a lesser degree, in South America. Resistant strains have recently been identified in Africa.

Phenanthrene methanols are not, in the strict sense, quinine analogs. Nevertheless, they are structurally similar to this group of agents and, together with them, were discovered to have antimalarial activity during the second World War. Halofantrine[†], the most effective of the group, has only recently become available. In vitro and in vivo studies demonstrated that it is an effective blood schizonticide against both sensitive and multidrug-resistant strains of *P. falciparum*. Its mechanism of action was originally thought to differ from that of quinine and mefloquine. Recently, mefloquine-resistant strains of *P. falciparum* have demonstrated decreased sensitivity to halofantrine, raising the possibility of cross-resistance between these two agents. Rarely, halofantrine has produced fatal heart arrhythmias, and it should not be given to patients with cardiac conduction abnormalities. It is otherwise well tolerated and appears to be free of teratogenicity. Oral absorption is both slow and erratic, reaching maximum concentrations in 5 to 7 hours; its half-life is relatively short (1 to 3 days). Clinical studies have demonstrated high failure rates when the drug is given in a single dose; cure rates with multiple-dose regimens, however, have been high.

Phenanthrene methanols active against multidrug-resistant malaria

Quinones

Atovaquone is a novel hydroxynaphthoquinone that shows promise in the treatment of malaria and toxoplasmosis. In the search for effective antimalarial agents during World War II, a number of hydroxynaphthoquinones were found to have antimalarial activity in experimental animals; however, all were rapidly metabolized in humans and proved ineffective in the treatment of malarious patients. In the 1980s a single hydroxynaphthoquinone, atovaquone, was found to be both highly effective in vitro against *P. falciparum* and metabolically stable in humans when administered orally. Its antiparasitic activity appears to result from the specific blockade of pyrimidine biosynthesis secondary to the inhibition of the parasite's mitochondrial electron transport chain at the ubiquinol–cytochrome c reductase region (complex III). Its long half-life (70 hours) and lack of serious adverse reactions suggested that it would be of great value in the treatment of malaria. Efficacy trials established its capacity to effect rapid clearance of parasitemia in patients with chloroquine-resistant falciparum malaria. Frequent parasitic recrudescences were eliminated when atovaquone was administered in combination with proguanil or tetracycline. Subsequently, this agent has shown to be effective for the treatment of toxoplasmosis in patients with acquired immunodeficiency syndrome (AIDS). Unlike other antitoxoplasma agents, atovaquone has been found to be active against *T. gondii* cysts as well as tachyzoites, suggesting this agent may produce radical cure. Supporting this is the infrequency with which cessation of atovaquone treatment of toxoplasmic cerebritis in AIDS patients has resulted in relapse. Relapse following atovaquone treatment of pneumocystosis in this same patient population appears similarly uncommon.

Atovaquone stable and active against malaria and toxoplasmosis

Folate Antagonists

Folic acid serves as a critical coenzyme for the synthesis of purines and ultimately DNA. In protozoa, as in bacteria, the active form of folic acid is produced in vivo by a simple two-step process. The first, the conversion of *para*-aminobenzoic acid to dihydrofolic acid, is blocked by sulfonamides. The second, the transformation of dihydro- to tetrahydrofolic acid, is inhibited by folic acid analogs (folate antagonists), which competitively inhibit dihydrofolate reductase. Used together with sulfonamides, folate antagonists are very effective inhibitors of protozoan growth.

Sulfonamide and folate antagonists inhibit protozoa

Trimethoprim, an inhibitor of dihydrofolate reductase, is used in combination with sulfamethoxazole to treat toxoplasmosis. Another folate antagonist, pyrimethamine, has a high affinity for sporozoan dihydrofolate reductase and has been particularly effective, when used with a sulfonamide, in the management of clinical malaria and toxoplasmosis.

Trimethoprim effective in *Toxoplasma* and *Pneumocystis* infections

[†] Not available in the United States.

In East Africa, a third folate antagonist, proguanil, is commonly taken in combination with chloroquine for malaria prophylaxis. Acquired protozoal resistance to folate antagonists is mutational and generally has been limited to particular species of malarial parasites.

Folate deficiency and sulfonamide toxicities occur

Folate antagonists may result in folate deficiency in individuals with limited folate reserves, such as newborns, pregnant women, and the malnourished. This is of great concern when large doses are used for prolonged periods, as in the treatment of acute toxoplasmosis. When folate antagonists are used with sulfonamides, the entire range of sulfonamide toxic effects may be seen. Patients with AIDS appear to suffer an unusually high incidence of toxic side effects to trimethoprim–sulfamethoxazole.

Qinghaosu (Artemisinin[†]*)*

Plant derivative active against malaria, amebas, and *Schistosoma*

Concentrated in parasitized erythrocytes

This natural extract of the plant *Artemisia annua* (qing hao, sweet wormwood) is a sesquiterpenelactone peroxide that is structurally distinct from all other known antiparasitic compounds. Extracts of qing hao were recommended for the treatment of fevers in China as early as AD 341; their specific antimalarial activity was defined in 1971. Although qinghaosu has also been shown to be active against the free-living ameba *Naegleria fowleria* and several trematodes, including *Schistosoma japonicum, Schistosoma mansoni,* and *Clonorchis sinensis,* its greatest impact to date has been in the treatment of malaria. Extensive investigations showed it to be schizonticidal for both chloroquine-sensitive and chloroquine-resistant strains of *P. falciparum*. Several derivatives, among them artemether[†] and artesunate, are significantly more active than the parent compound. All are concentrated in parasitized erythrocytes where they decompose, releasing free radicals, which are thought to be damaging to parasitic membranes. Artemisinin compounds act more rapidly than other antimalarial agents, stopping parasite development and preventing cytoadherence in falciparum malaria. Although depression of reticulocyte counts has been noted, these agents appear significantly less toxic than quinoline antimalarials. As there is some evidence that they may possess teratogenic properties, they should not be used in pregnancy. Importantly, they may be given orally, rectally (by suppository), and parenterally. Relapses can occur unless they are given for several days or combined with a second agent such as mefloquine or tetracycline.

Nitroimidazoles

Active against protozoa at low redox potential

Metronidazole, a nitroimidazole, was introduced in 1959 for the treatment of trichomoniasis. Subsequently, it was found to be effective in the management of giardiasis, amebiasis, and a variety of infections produced by obligate anaerobic bacteria. Energy metabolism in all of them depends on the presence of low-redox-potential compounds, such as ferredoxin, to serve as electron carriers. These compounds reduce the 5-nitro group of the imidazoles to produce intermediate products responsible for the death of the protozoal and bacterial cells, possibly by alkylation of DNA. Resistance, although uncommon, has been noted in strains of *T. vaginalis* lacking nitroreductase activity. Of greater concern is in vitro evidence of mutagenicity. Metronidazole is the drug of choice for trichomoniasis and invasive amebiasis. It is effective in giardiasis although not yet approved by the Food and Drug Administration for use in this infection. Tinidazole, a newer nitroimidazole not yet available in the United States, appears to be both a more effective and less mutagenic antiprotozoal agent. Its greater lipid solubility improves cerebrospinal fluid levels and in vitro activity.

Benzimidazoles

Broad-spectrum anthelmintics

As the name **benzimidazole** implies, the basic structure of these antiparasitic agents consists of linked imidazole and benzene rings. Unlike their antiprotozoal cousins discussed above, the benzimidazoles are broad-spectrum anthelmintic agents. The prototype drug,

[†] Not available in the United States.

thiabendazole, acts against both adult and larval nematodes and was shown to be useful in the management of cutaneous larva migrans, trichinosis, and most intestinal nematode infections soon after its introduction in the early 1960s. The mechanism by which it exerts its anthelmintic action is uncertain. It is known to inhibit fumarate reductase, an important mitochondrial enzyme of helminths. The primary mode of action, however, may derive from the known capacity of all benzimidazoles to inhibit the polymerization of tubulin, the eukaryotic cytoskeletal protein, as described for mebendazole below. Side effects are mild, related to the gastrointestinal tract or liver, and rapidly disappear with the discontinuation of the drug. Hypersensitivity reactions, induced either by the drug or by antigens released from the damaged parasite, may occur.

Inhibit helminth fumarate reductase

Mebendazole, a carbamate benzimidazole introduced in 1972, has a spectrum similar to that of thiabendazole, but also has been found to be effective against a number of cestodes, including *Taenia, Hymenolepsis,* and *Echinococcus*. It irreversibly blocks glucose uptake of both adult and larval worms, resulting in glycogen depletion, cessation of ATP formation, and paralysis or death. It does not appear to affect glucose metabolism in humans and is thought to exert its effect in worms by binding to tubulin, thus interfering with the assembly of cytoplasmic microtubules, structures essential to glucose uptake. Unlike thiabendazole, the drug is not well absorbed from the gastrointestinal tract and may owe part of its effectiveness against intestine-dwelling adult worms to its high concentrations in the gut. Toxicity is uncommon. Teratogenic effects have been observed in experimental animals; its use in infants and pregnant women is contraindicated.

Mebendazole blocks glucose uptake by adult and larval worms

Interferes with tubulin and cytoplasmic microtubules

Albendazole is a benzimidazole carbamate that has recently been made available in the United States. It has a somewhat broader spectrum than that of its close relative, mebendazole, being more active against *Strongyloides stercoralis* and several tissue nematodes. In addition to the vermicidal and larvicidal properties that it shares with other benzimidazoles, it is ovicidal, enhancing its effectiveness in tissue cestode infections such as echinococciasis and cysticercosis. Its activity against *Giardia,* one of the most common intestinal protozoa, makes it an appealing candidate for the treatment of polyparasitism. Although it shares the teratogenic potential of other benzimidazoles, it is otherwise extremely well tolerated. Single-dose therapy is effective in the management of many intestinal nematode infections.

Albendazole has broader spectrum

Avermectins

Avermectins are macrocyclic lactones produced as fermentation products of *Streptomyces avermitilis*. Structurally similar to the macrolide antibiotics, they are effective at extremely low concentration against a wide variety of nematodes and arthropods. The avermectins appear to induce neuromuscular paralysis by acting on a receptor of the parasites-peripheral neurotransmitter, gamma-aminobutyric acid (GABA). In mammals, GABA is confined to the central nervous system, and because the avermectins do not cross the blood–brain barrier in significant concentration, they do not appear to produce significant untoward effects in the mammalian host. Ivermectin, a derivative of avermectin B1, is currently the drug of choice for the treatment of onchocerciasis and is undergoing evaluation for the treatment of other human filarial infections. Its usefulness in other parasitic infections of humans remains to be established.

Antibiotics that influence nematode neurotransmitters

Activity against filariae

Praziquantel

Praziquantel, a heterocyclic pyrazinoisoquinoline, is an important new anthelmintic effective against a broad range of cestodes and trematodes, many of which had been poorly responsive to previously available agents. It is given in one to three doses. The drug is rapidly taken up by susceptible helminths, in which it appears to induce the loss of intracellular calcium, tetanic muscular contraction, and destruction of the tegument. The differential toxicity of this agent may be related to the inability of susceptible worms to metabolize the drug. Aside from transient, mild gastrointestinal symptoms, praziquantel appears remarkably free of side effects in humans. It is currently the drug of choice for the treatment of schistosomiasis, clonorchiasis, opisthorchiasis, and neurocysticercosis.

Causes loss of intracellular calcium in cestodes and trematodes

Safety of praziquantel allows use in mass therapy campaigns

TABLE 51–5

Miscellaneous Antiparasitic Agents

Compound	Drug Class	Route	Mechanism of Action	Clinical Use	Comments
Bithionol	Phenol	Oral	Uncouples phosphorylation	Paragonimiasis	Not commercially available in United States
Diethylcarbamazine	Piperazine	Oral	Neuromuscular paralysis	Filarial infections	Allergic reactions to filarial antigens
Diloxanide furoate	Acetanilide	Oral	Unknown	Intestinal amebiasis	Used only for asymptomatic carriers
Iodoquinol (diiodohydroxyquin)	Halogenated quinoline	Oral	Unknown	Intestinal amebiasis *Dientamoeba* infections	Related drug has caused optic atrophy
Nifurtimox	Nitrofuran	Oral	Alkylates DNA	Acute Chagas' disease	Toxicity Prolonged therapy Marginal effectiveness
Paromomycin	Aminoglycoside	Oral	Similar to other aminoglycosides	Intestinal cryptosporidiosis	Not absorbed Marginal effectiveness
Pentamidine	Diamidine	IV	Binds DNA	Leishmaniasis Trypanosomiasis	Toxic
Pyrantel pamoate	Tetrahydropyrimidine	Oral	Neuromuscular blockade; inhibits fumarate reductase	Pinworm infection, hookworm infection Ascariasis	Single-dose therapy
Spiramycin	Macrolide	Oral	Blocks protein synthesis	Toxoplasmosis	Used to treat pregnant women
Suramin	Sulfated naphthylamine	IV	Inhibits glycerophosphate oxidase and dehydrogenase	African trypanosomiasis Onchocerciasis	Not effective in central nervous system disease Renal toxicity

Abbreviation: IV, intravenous.

Good activity has been demonstrated against other common trematode and cestode infections. Its high level of safety suggests that it may well play a significant role in worldwide mass therapy campaigns.

Eflornithine[†] *(Difluoromethylornithine)*

Eflornithine is a specific, enzyme-activated, irreversible inhibitor of ornithine decarboxylase (ODC). In mammalian cells, decarboxylation of ornithine by ODC is a mandatory step in the synthesis of polyamines, compounds thought to play critical roles in cell division and differentiation. Originally developed as an antineoplastic agent, eflornithine proved ineffective in cancer chemotherapy trials. With the discovery that polyamines of *Trypanosoma* species were also synthesized from ornithine, eflornithine was successfully tested in the treatment of animal trypanosomiasis. Host survival was high and associated with decreases in parasitic polyamines and inhibition of nucleic acid synthesis. In the dosage required to treat trypanosomiasis, mammals tolerated the agent well, presumably because *T. brucei* is 100 times more sensitive to the effects of eflornithine than are mammalian cells. Eflornithine appears to be cytostatic and requires an intact host immune system for maximum effect.

Originally an anticancer drug

Active against trypanosomes

Other Antiparasitic Agents

A number of antiparasitic agents used in therapy, their properties, and their clinical uses are listed in Table 51–5.

CONTROL

The control of diseases spread by the fecal–oral route depends on the improvements in personal hygiene and sanitation that accompany general economic development. In contrast, efforts at preventing the spread of multihost parasites is usually focused on the simultaneous treatment of infected humans and control or elimination of the nonhuman host.

To be effective, such measures must be applied in a comprehensive and coordinated manner over large areas. Administrative problems, political imbroglios, development of resistance in parasites and intermediate hosts, technical difficulties, and funding shortages have, individually and together, limited the success of such efforts. A case in point was the failure of the worldwide malaria eradication effort launched by the World Health Organization in 1955. This has refocused attention on alternative control measures, including immunization. Until recently, the development of effective parasitic vaccines has been constrained by the complexities of their immunologic interactions with the human host. Monoclonal antibodies have helped identify antigens responsible for the induction of immunity to a number of parasitic infections, including malaria, leishmaniasis, and schistosomiasis. The subsequent cloning of the structural genes encoding such antigens has made a large-scale production of vaccine antigen feasible. It is further possible that the entire step of antigen production and purification could be bypassed by the use of synthetic peptide or anti-idiotype vaccines. All these approaches are currently being developed. Malaria vaccines are undergoing clinical trials.

Epidemiologic control in developing countries complex

Vaccines using antigens or synthesized peptides in development

ADDITIONAL READING

Armitage KB. Antiparasitic drugs and therapy. In: *Clinical Infectious Diseases,* Root RK, Waldvogel F, Corey L, et al. New York: Oxford University Press; 1999, pp 365–388. A recent, concise discussion of this subject.

Desowitz RS. *New Guinea Tapeworms and Jewish Grandmothers: Tales of Parasites and Peoples*. New York: Norton; 1981. A delightful look at the host–parasite relationship.

[†] Not available in the United States.

Drugs for parasitic infections. *Med Lett Drugs Ther* 2002;44:1–12. Concise guide to treatment of parasitic diseases, updated annually.

Horton RJ. Benzimidazole anthelmintics. *Parasitol Today* 1990;6:105–136. The best recent review of this important group of chemotherapeutic agents.

Liu LX, Weller PF. Antiparasitic drugs. *N Engl J Med* 1995;334:1178–1184. A concise review.

Maddison SE. Serodiagnosis of parasitic diseases. *Clin Microbiol Rev* 1991;4:457–469. A short but comprehensive review of current antibody and antigen detection procedures, use of monoclonal antibodies in serodiagnosis, molecular biological technology, and skin tests for parasitic diseases.

Markell EK, John DT, Krotoski WA. Parasites, parasitism, and host relations. In *Markell and Voge's Medical Parasitology,* 8th ed. Philadelphia: WB Saunders; 1999.

Stoll NR. This wormy world. *J Parasitol* 1947;33:1–18. This classic of quantitative helminth epidemiology has recently been updated by DAP Bundy (*Parasitol Today* 1997;13:407–408).

Warren KS (ed). *Immunology and Molecular Biology of Parasitic Infections.* 3rd ed. Boston: Blackwell Scientific; 1993. This relatively comprehensive monograph discusses general immune responses to parasitic infections as well as the immunity, immunopathology, immunodiagnosis, and molecular biology of specific parasitic diseases.

CHAPTER 52

Sporozoa

JAMES J. PLORDE

Sporozoa are a unique class of intracellular protozoa distinguished by their alternating cycles of sexual and asexual reproduction. Asexual multiplication occurs by a process of multiple fission termed schizogony. The nucleus of a trophozoite divides into several parts, forming a multinucleated schizont. Cytoplasm then condenses around each nuclear portion to form new daughter cells, or merozoites, which burst from their intracellular location to invade new host cells. After the completion of one or more of these asexual cycles, some merozoites differentiate into male and female gametocytes, initiating the cycle of sexual reproduction known as sporogony. The gametocytes mature and effect fertilization, forming a zygote. On encysting, the zygote is known as an oocyst. Sporozoites formed within the oocyst are released, penetrate host tissue cells, and begin another asexual cycle as trophozoites.

Intracellular protozoa with alternating sexual and asexual cycles

Two sporozoan infections, malaria and toxoplasmosis, are common diseases of humans; together, they affect more than one third of the world's population and kill or deform perhaps a million neonates and children each year. A third infection, cryptosporidiosis, has only recently been found to be an important cause of diarrhea, particularly in immunocompromised hosts.

Cause malaria, toxoplasmosis, and cryptosporidiosis

PLASMODIA

> Of all infectious diseases there is no doubt that malaria has caused the greatest harm to the greatest number.
>
> LADERMAN, 1975

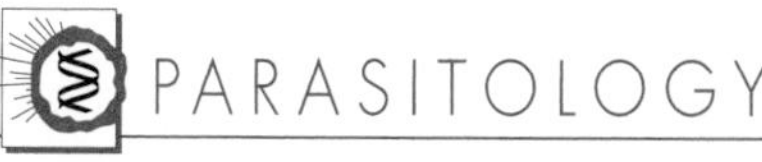

DEFINITION

The plasmodia are sporozoa in which the sexual and asexual cycles of reproduction are completed in different host species. The sexual phase occurs within the gut of mosquitoes. These arthropods subsequently transmit the parasite while feeding on a vertebrate host. Within the red blood cells (RBCs) of the vertebrate, the plasmodia reproduce asexually; they eventually burst from the erythrocyte and invade other uninvolved RBCs. This

Sexual phase in mosquito and asexual phase in humans

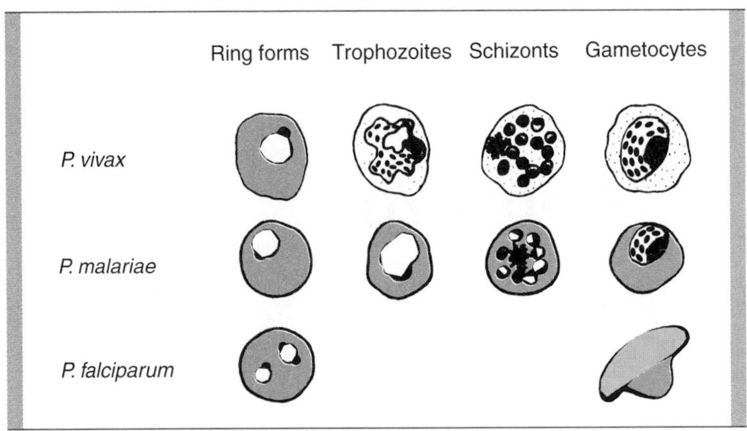

FIGURE 52–1
Examples of erythrocytic stages of malarial parasites. Note: Trophozoite and schizont forms of *Plasmodium falciparum* occur in visceral capillaries rather than in blood. Male and female gametophytes show distinctive morphologic differences.

Four species infect humans

event produces periodic fever and anemia in the host, a disease process known as malaria. Of the many species of plasmodia, four are known to infect humans and will be considered here: *Plasmodium vivax, P. ovale, P. malariae,* and *P. falciparum.*

MORPHOLOGY

Morphology of the parasite and the infected RBC vary by stage and species

The morphology of the stained intraerythrocytic parasites is shown in Figure 52–1. In stained smears, three characteristic features aid in the identification of plasmodia: red nuclear chromatin; blue cytoplasm; and brownish-black malarial pigment, or hemozoin, consisting largely of a hemoglobin degradation product, ferriprotoporphyrin IX. The change in the shape of the cytoplasm and the division of the chromatin at different stages of parasite development are obvious. Gametocytes can be differentiated from the asexual forms by their large size and lack of nuclear division. Some of the infected erythrocytes develop membrane invaginations or caveolae–vesicle complexes, which are thought to be responsible for the appearance of the pink Schüffner's dots or granules (see below).

Morphologic differences are the primary means of diagnosis

The appearance of each of the four species of plasmodia that infect humans is sufficiently different to allow their differentiation in stained smears. The parasitized erythrocyte in *P. vivax* and *P. ovale* infections is pale, enlarged, and contains numerous Schüffner's dots. All asexual stages (trophozoite, schizont, merozoite) may be seen simultaneously. Cells infected by *P. ovale* are elongated and frequently irregular or fimbriated in appearance. In *P. malariae* infections, the RBCs are not enlarged and contain no granules. The trophozoites often present as "band" forms, and the merozoites are arranged in rosettes around a clump of central pigment. In *P. falciparum* infections, the rings are very small and may contain two chromatin dots rather than one. There is often more than one parasite per cell, and parasites are frequently seen lying against the margin of the cell. Intracytoplasmic granules known as Maurer's dots may be present but are often cleft shaped and fewer in number than Schüffner's dots. Schizonts and merozoites are not present in the peripheral blood. Gametocytes are large and banana shaped. These characteristics are summarized in Table 52–1.

LIFE CYCLE OF MALARIAL PARASITES

Mosquito ingests gametocytes from blood of infected human

Sporozoites from oocyst reach mosquito salivary glands

Sporogony, or the sexual cycle, begins when a female mosquito of the genus *Anopheles* ingests circulating male and female gametocytes while feeding on a malarious human. In the gut of the mosquito, the gametocytes mature and effect fertilization. The resulting zygote penetrates the mosquito's gut wall, lodges beneath the basement membrane, and vacuolates to form an oocyst. Within this structure, thousands of sporozoites are formed. The enlarging cyst eventually ruptures, releasing the sporozoites into the body cavity of the mosquito. Some penetrate the salivary glands, rendering the mosquito infectious for humans. The time required for the completion of the cycle in mosquitoes varies from 1 to

TABLE 52–1

Differential Characteristics of *Plasmodium* Species

CHARACTERISTICS	*P. VIVAX*	*P. OVALE*	*P. MALARIAE*	*P. FALCIPARUM*
Erythrocyte				
Enlarged, pale	+	+	–	–
Oval, fimbriated	–	+	–	–
Schüffner's dots	+	+	–	–
Maurer's dots	–	–	–	+
Parasite				
All asexual stages seen	+	+	+	–
Band forms	–	–	+	–
Double infections	–	–	–	+
Double chromatin dots	–	–	–	+
Banana-shaped gametocytes	–	–	–	+

3 weeks, depending on the species of insect and parasite as well as on the ambient temperature and humidity.

Schizogony, the asexual cycle, occurs in the human and begins when the infected *Anopheles* takes a blood meal from another individual. Sporozoites from the mosquito's salivary glands are injected into the human's subcutaneous capillaries and circulate in the peripheral blood. Within 1 hour they attach to and invade liver cells (hepatocytes), a process thought to be mediated by a ligand present in the sporozoites' outer protein coat (circumsporozoite protein). In *P. vivax* and *P. ovale* infections, some of the sporozoites enter a dormant state immediately after cell invasion. The remaining sporozoites initiate exoerythrocytic schizogony, each producing about 2000 to 40,000 daughter cells, or merozoites. One to two weeks later, the infected hepatocytes rupture, releasing merozoites into the general circulation.

Humans infected by mosquito bite

Rapid infection of hepatocytes starts asexual cycle in humans

The erythrocytic phase of malaria starts with the attachment of a released hepatic merozoite to a specific receptor on the RBC surface. After attachment, the merozoite invaginates the cell membrane and is slowly endocytosed. The intracellular parasite initially appears as a ring-shaped trophozoite, which enlarges and becomes more active and irregular in outline. Within a few hours, nuclear division occurs, producing the multinucleated schizont. Cytoplasm eventually condenses around each nucleus of the schizont to form an intraerythrocytic cluster of 6 to 24 merozoite daughter cells. About 48 (*P. vivax, P. ovale,* and *P. falciparum*) to 72 (*P. malariae*) hours after initial invasion, infected erythrocytes rupture, releasing the merozoites and producing the first clinical manifestations of disease. The newly released daughter cells invade other RBCs, where most repeat the asexual cycle. Other daughter cells are transformed into sexual forms or gametocytes. These latter forms do not produce RBC lysis, and continue to circulate in the peripheral vasculature until ingested by an appropriate mosquito. The recurring asexual cycles continue, involving an ever-increasing number of erythrocytes until finally the development of host immunity brings the erythrocytic cycle to a close. The dormant hepatic sporozoites of *P. vivax* and *P. ovale* survive the host's immunologic attack, and may, after a latent period of months to years, resume intrahepatic multiplication. This leads to a second release of hepatic merozoites and the initiation of another erythrocytic cycle, a phenomenon known as relapse. The life cycle of malarial parasites is summarized in Figure 52–2.

Erythrocytic cycle begins with merozoite attachment to RBC receptor

Trophozoites multiply in RBC to form new merozoites

In 48–72 hours, RBCs rupture, releasing merozoites to infect new RBCs

Intrahepatic dormancy causes relapses with *P. vivax* and *P. ovale*

PHYSIOLOGY

Species of plasmodia differ significantly in their ability to invade subpopulations of erythrocytes; *P. vivax* and *P. ovale* attack only immature cells (reticulocytes), whereas *P.*

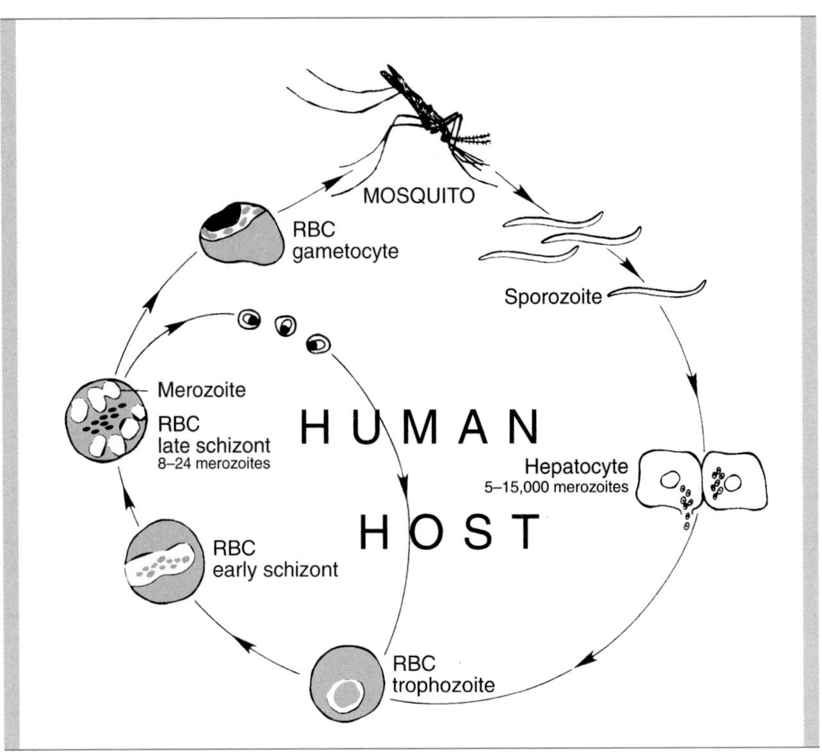

FIGURE 52–2
Life cycle of the malarial parasite. RBC = red blood cell.

malariae attacks only senescent cells. During infection with these species, therefore, no more than 1 to 2% of the cell population is involved. *P. falciparum,* in contrast, invades RBCs regardless of age and may produce very high levels of parasitemia and particularly serious disease. In part, these differences may be related to the known differences in the RBC receptor sites available to the individual *Plasmodium* species. In the case of *P. vivax,* the site is closely related to the Duffy blood group antigens (Fy^a and Fy^b). Duffy-negative individuals, who constitute the majority of people of West African ancestry, are therefore resistant to vivax malaria. RBC sialoglycoprotein, particularly glycoprotein A, has been implicated as the *P. falciparum* receptor site.

Parasites vary in ability to attack subpopulations of erythrocytes

RBC Duffy antigen and glycoprotein A are RBC receptors

Certain RBC abnormalities may also effect parasitism. The altered hemoglobin (hemoglobin S) associated with the sickle cell trait limits the intensity of the parasitemia caused by *P. falciparum,* and thereby provides a selective advantage to individuals who are heterozygous for the sickle cell gene. As a result, the sickle cell gene, which would otherwise be disadvantageous, is found at high frequency in populations living in malarious areas. Parasite growth appears to be retarded in RBCs heterozygous for hemoglobin S (SA) when they are exposed to conditions of reduced oxygen tension such as might be present in the visceral capillaries. Sickling may also render the erythrocyte more susceptible to phagocytosis or directly damage the parasite. A similar protective effect may be exerted by hemoglobins C, D, and E; thalassemias; and glucose-6-phosphate dehydrogenase (G6PD) or pyridoxal kinase deficiencies, because these abnormalities have also been found more frequently in malarious areas. The protection in these conditions may be related to the increased susceptibility of such RBCs to oxidant stress. In thalassemia, the protection may also be related in part to the production of fetal hemoglobin, which retards maturation of *P. falciparum,* as well as an increased binding of antibodies to modified parasitic antigens (neoantigens) presenting on the surface of the erythrocytes.

Sickle cell trait limits intensity of *P. falciparum* infection

Other hemoglobinopathies can also exert protection

Once invasion has occurred, malaria parasites may induce a number of changes in the erythrocytic membrane. These include alteration of its lipid concentration, modification of its osmotic properties, and incorporation of parasitic neoantigens, rendering the RBC susceptible to immunologic attack. *P. vivax* and *P. ovale* stimulate the production of caveolae–vesicle complexes, which are visualized as Schüffner's dots in stained smears. In *P. falciparum* infections, electron-dense elevated knobs or excrescences form on the RBC

Changes induced in erythrocyte membrane

Binding to endothelium may cause microinfarcts

surface. These produce a strain specific, high-molecular-weight adhesive protein (PfEMP1), which mediates binding to receptors on the endothelium of capillaries and postcapillary venules of the brain, placenta, and other organs, where they can produce obstruction and microinfarcts.

Malarial parasites generate energy by the anaerobic metabolism of glucose. They appear to satisfy their protein requirements by the degradation of hemoglobin within their acidic food vacuoles, resulting in the formation of the malarial pigment (hemozoin) mentioned previously. It has been estimated that the average plasmodium destroys between 25 and 75% of the hemoglobin of its host erythrocyte. Unlike their vertebrate hosts, malarial parasites synthesize folates de novo. As a result, antifolate antimicrobics such as pyrimethamine are effective antimalarial agents.

Malarial parasites metabolize anaerobically, synthesize their own folate

GROWTH IN THE LABORATORY

Continuous in vitro cultivation of plasmodia in human erythrocytes was first achieved in 1976. More recently, the successful in vitro completion of the entire sporogonic cycle, from ookinete to sporozoite, has been achieved. These twin developments provide new opportunities for studying the biology, immunology, and chemotherapy of human malaria. The most immediate impact of these advances has been on the introduction of methods for testing the sensitivity of *P. falciparum* to chemotherapeutic agents. Ultimately, these agents will play critical roles in the development of effective antimalarial vaccines.

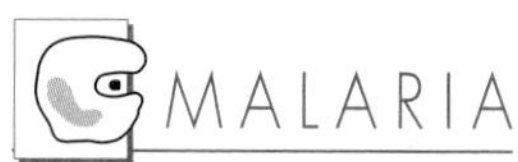

MALARIA

CLINICAL CAPSULE

Malaria is a febrile illness caused by a parasitic infection of human erythrocytes transmitted by the bite of a mosquito. The fevers are accompanied by headache, sweats, malaise, and typically appear in paroxysmal episodes lasting hours and recurring for weeks. Complications due to capillary blockade can be fatal, particularly in the brain.

EPIDEMIOLOGY

Malaria has a worldwide distribution between 45°N and 40°S latitude, generally at altitudes below 1800 m. *P. vivax* is the most widely distributed of the four species, and together with the uncommon *P. malariae,* is found primarily in temperate and subtropical areas. *P. falciparum* is the dominant organism of the tropics. *P. ovale* is rare and found principally in Africa.

Distribution in tropical areas worldwide

The intensity of malarial transmission in an endemic area depends on the density and feeding habits of suitable mosquito vectors and the prevalence of infected humans, who serve as parasite reservoirs. In hyperendemic areas (areas where more than half of the population is parasitemic), transmission is usually constant, and disease manifestations are moderated by the development of immunity. Mortality is largely restricted to infants and to nonimmune adults who migrate into the region. When the prevalence of disease is lower, transmission is typically intermittent. In this situation, solid immunity does not develop and the population suffers repeated, often seasonal, epidemics, the impact of which is shared by people of all ages.

Clinical manifestations muted with hyperendemicity

Presently, it is estimated that 2 billion people live in malaria endemic areas in 103 of the poorest countries of Africa, Asia, Latin America, and Oceania (Fig 52–3). Between 25 and 50% of these persons are thought to be carrying the malaria parasite at any given time. From 1 to 3 million individuals, primarily African children, die of this disease annually. A recent study concluded that the development of resistance to chloroquine, the single most widely used antimalarial agent, has increased mortality four- to eightfold. Although endemic malaria disappeared from the United States three decades ago,

Malaria kills 1–3 million annually; mostly children

Imported malaria may develop months after travel

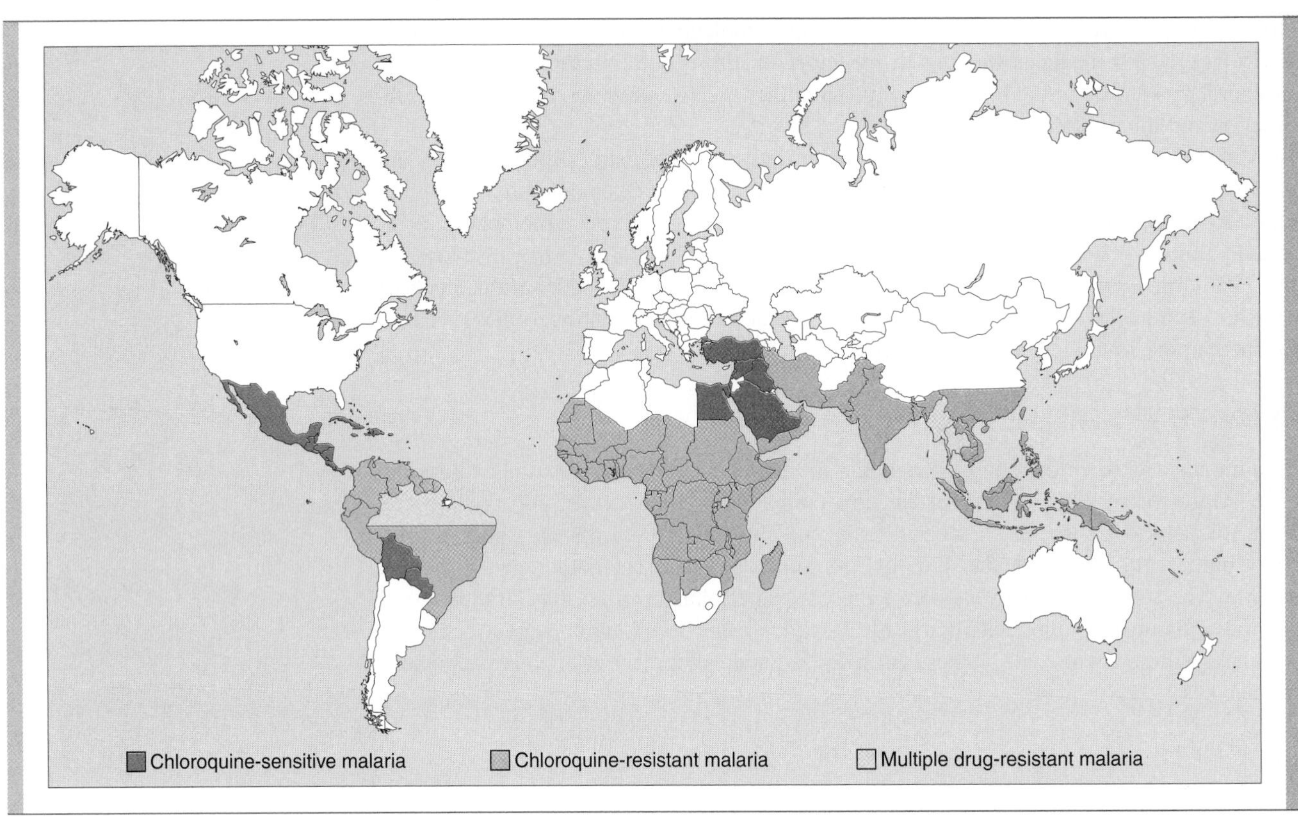

FIGURE 52–3
Distribution of malaria and drug-resistant *Plasmodium falciparum,* 1995. (*Data from the Centers for Disease Control and Prevention, Atlanta, Ga. From Mandell GL, Bennett JE, Dolin R (eds).* Mandell, Douglas, and Bennett's Principles and Practice of Infectious Diseases, *New York: Churchill Livingstone, 2002.*)

imported cases continue to be reported, and the recent worldwide resurgence of malaria combined with an increase in international travel has resulted in an increase in the number of US cases to approximately 1000 annually. Forty-five percent of patients with imported malaria have acquired the disease in Africa, 30% in Asia, and 10% in the Caribbean or Latin America. Fifty percent of recent infections have involved American travelers: nearly 60% of these acquired their infection in Africa. Clinical manifestations typically develop within 6 months of arrival of cases in the United States; however, one fourth of cases caused by *P. vivax* are delayed beyond that time. Approximately 40% of imported cases and almost all associated fatalities have been caused by the virulent *P. falciparum.* Tragically, most of these cases could have been prevented or successfully treated. Congenital malaria in infants born in the United States of mothers from malarious areas is occasionally observed. Infections transmitted by transfusions of whole blood, leukocytes, or platelets, or by organ transplantation are, fortunately, now unusual in this country due to the improved screening procedures of blood banks. Anopheline mosquitoes capable of transmitting malaria are present in the United States, and, rarely, malaria is transmitted from an imported case to individuals who have never traveled outside of the country.

PATHOGENESIS

The fever, anemia, circulatory changes, and immunopathologic phenomena characteristic of malaria are all the result of erythrocytic invasion by the plasmodia.

Fever

Fever, the hallmark of malaria, appears to be initiated by the process of RBC rupture that leads to the liberation of a new generation of merozoites (sporulation). To date, all attempts to detect the factor(s) mediating the fever have been unsuccessful. It is possible that parasite-derived pyrogens are released at the time of sporulation; alternatively, the fever might result from the release of interleukin-1 (IL-1) and/or tumor necrosis factor (TNF) from macrophages involved in the ingestion of parasitic or erythrocytic debris. Early in malaria, RBCs appear to be infected with malarial parasites at several different stages of development, each inducing sporulation at a different time. The resulting fever is irregular and hectic. Because temperatures in excess of 40°C destroy mature parasites, a single population eventually emerges, sporulation is synchronized, and fever occurs in distinct paroxysms at 48-hour or, in the case of *P. malariae,* 72-hour intervals. Periodicity is seldom seen in patients who are rapidly diagnosed and treated.

Fever associated with RBC rupture

Synchronization of sporulation causes cyclic fever

Anemia

Parasitized erythrocytes are phagocytosed by a stimulated reticuloendothelial system or are destroyed at the time of sporulation. At times, the anemia is disproportionate to the degree of parasitism. Depression of marrow function, sequestration of erythrocytes within the enlarging spleen, and accelerated clearance of nonparasitized cells all appear to contribute to the anemia. The mechanisms responsible for the latter are unclear. Intravascular hemolysis, although uncommon, may occur, particularly in falciparum malaria. When hemolysis is massive, hemoglobinuria develops, resulting in the production of dark urine. This process in conjunction with malaria is known as **blackwater fever.**

Destruction of normal and parasitized RBCs causes anemia

Massive intravascular hemolysis can occur

Circulatory Changes

The high fever results in significant vasodilatation. In falciparum malaria, vasodilatation leads to a decrease in the effective circulating blood volume and hypotension, which may be aggravated by other changes in the small vessels and capillaries. The intense parasitemias *P. falciparum* is capable of producing and the adhesion of infected RBCs to the endothelium of visceral capillaries can impair the microcirculation and precipitate tissue hypoxia, lactic acidosis, and hypoglycemia. Although all deep tissues are involved, the brain is the most intensely affected.

Blood flow decreased to vital organs

Cytokines

Elevated levels of IL-1 and TNF are consistently found in patients with malaria. Probably released at the time of sporulation, these proteins are certainly an essential part of the host's immune response to malaria (see below). By modulating the effects of endothelial cells, macrophages, monocytes, and neutrophils, they may play an important role in the destruction of the invading parasite. However, TNF levels increase with parasite density and high concentrations appear harmful. TNF has been shown to cause upregulation of endothelial adhesion molecules; high concentrations might precipitate cerebral malaria by increasing the sequestration of *P. falciparum*–parasitized erythrocytes in the cerebral vascular endothelium. Alternatively, excessive TNF levels might precipitate cerebral malaria by directly inducing hypoglycemia and lactic acidosis.

Elevated cytokine levels contribute to injury

Other Pathogenic Phenomena

Thrombocytopenia is common in malaria and appears to be related to both splenic pooling and a shortened platelet lifespan. Both direct parasitic invasion and immune mechanisms may be responsible. There may be an acute transient glomerulonephritis in falciparum malaria and progressive renal disease in chronic *P. malariae* malaria. These phenomena probably result from the host immune response, with deposition of immune complexes in the glomeruli.

Thrombocytopenia and nephritis common

IMMUNITY

Initial immune response limits parasite multiplication but does not eliminate infection (premunition)

Once infected, the host quickly mounts a species- and strain-specific immunologic response that typically limits parasite multiplication and moderates the clinical manifestations of disease, without eliminating the infection—a phenomenon referred to as **premunition.** A prolonged recovery period marked by recurrent exacerbations in both symptoms and number of erythrocytic parasites follows. With time, these recrudescences become less severe and less frequent, eventually stopping altogether.

Antibody-mediated immunity important

The exact mechanisms involved in this recovery are uncertain. In simian and probably in human malaria, recovery is known to require the presence of both T and B lymphocytes. It is probable that the T lymphocytes act partially through their helper effect on antibody production. Some authorities have suggested that they also play a direct role through lymphokine production by stimulating effector cells to release nonspecific factors capable of inhibiting intraerythrocytic multiplication. The B lymphocytes begin production of stage- and strain-specific antiplasmodial antibodies within the first 2 weeks of parasitemia. With the achievement of high levels of antibodies, the number of circulating parasites decreases. The infrequency with which malaria occurs in young infants has been attributed to the transplacental passage of such antibodies. It is uncertain whether they are directly lethal, act as opsonizing agents, or block merozoite invasion of RBCs.

Antigenic variation could play a role in persistence

Suppressor T lymphocytes in spleen may protect parasites

In simian malaria, the parasite can undergo antigenic variation and thereby escape the suppressive effect of the antibodies. This antigenic variation leads to cycles of recrudescent parasitemia but ultimately to production of specific antibodies to the variants, and cure. It seems probable that similar changes occur in humans, leading to the eventual disappearance of erythrocytic parasites. With *P. falciparum* and *P. malariae,* which have no persistent hepatic forms, this results in cure. With *P. falciparum,* the disease typically does not exceed 1 year, but with *P. malariae* the erythrocytic infection can be extremely persistent, lasting in one case up to 53 years. How erythrocytic parasites circulating in numbers too small to be detected on routine blood films escape immunologic destruction remains a puzzle. In a closely related simian malaria, splenectomy results in rapid cure, suggesting that suppressor T lymphocytes in the spleen may play a protective role. In infection with *P. vivax* and *P. ovale,* latent hepatic infection may result in the discharge of fresh merozoites into the bloodstream after the disappearance of erythrocytic forms. This phenomenon, known as relapse, is capable of maintaining infection for 3 to 5 years.

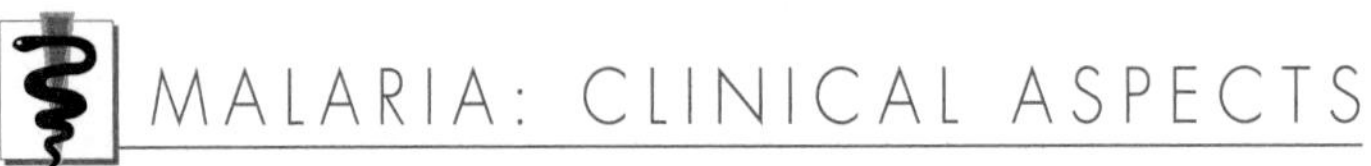

MALARIA: CLINICAL ASPECTS

MANIFESTATIONS

Incubation period prolonged by suppressant use

The incubation period between the bite of the mosquito and the onset of disease is approximately 2 weeks. With *P. malariae* and with strains of *P. vivax* in temperate climates, however, this period is often more prolonged. Individuals who contract malaria while taking antimalarial suppressants may not experience illness for many months. In the United States, the interval between entry into the country and onset of disease exceeds 1 month in 25% of *P. falciparum* infections and 6 months in a similar proportion of *P. vivax* cases.

Malarial paroxysm: cold, hot, wet stages

The clinical manifestations vary with the species of plasmodia but typically include chills, fever, splenomegaly, and anemia. The hallmark of disease is the malarial paroxysm. This manifestation begins with a cold stage, which persists for 20 to 60 minutes. During this time, the patient experiences continuous rigors and feels cold. With the consequent increase in body temperature, the rigors cease and vasodilatation commences, ushering in a hot stage. The temperature continues to rise for 3 to 8 hours, reaching a maximum of 40 to 41.7°C before it begins to fall. The wet stage consists of a decrease in fever and profuse sweating. It leaves the patient exhausted but otherwise well until the onset of the next paroxysm.

Typical paroxysms first appear in the second or third week of fever, when parasite sporulation becomes synchronized. In falciparum malaria, synchronization may never take place, and the fever may remain hectic and unpredictable. The first attack is often severe and may persist for weeks in the untreated patient. Eventually the paroxysms become less regular, less frequent, and less severe. Symptoms finally cease with the disappearance of the parasites from the blood.

Typical paroxysms after 2–3 weeks when sporulation is synchronized

In falciparum malaria, capillary blockage can lead to several serious complications. When the central nervous system is involved (cerebral malaria), the patient may develop delirium, convulsions, paralysis, coma, and rapid death. Acute pulmonary insufficiency frequently accompanies cerebral malaria, killing about 80% of those involved. When splanchnic capillaries are involved, the patient may experience vomiting, abdominal pain, and diarrhea with or without bloody stools. Jaundice and acute renal failure are also common in severe illness. These pernicious syndromes generally appear when the intensity of parasitemia exceeds 100,000 organisms per cubic millimeter of blood. Most deaths occur within 3 days.

Cerebral falciparum malaria often lethal

DIAGNOSIS

Malarial parasites can be demonstrated in stained smears of the peripheral blood in virtually all symptomatic patients. Typically, capillary or venous blood is used to prepare both thin and thick smears, which are stained with Wright or Giemsa stain and examined for the presence of erythrocytic parasites. Thick smears, in which erythrocytes are lysed with water before staining, concentrate the parasites and allow detection of very mild parasitemia. Nonetheless, it may be necessary to obtain several specimens before parasites are seen. Artifacts are numerous in thick smears, and correct interpretation requires experience. The morphologic differences among the four species of plasmodia allow their speciation on the stained smear by the skilled observer.

Thick and thin blood smears detect parasites

A number of attempts have been made to improve on the standard thin and thick smear. One such procedure involves acridine orange staining of centrifuged parasites in quantitative buffy coat (QBC) tubes. Although it is expensive, requires a fluorescence microscope, and permits less reliable parasite speciation, its rapidity and ease of use make it attractive to laboratories that are only occasionally called on to identify patients with malaria. Simple, specific card antigen detection procedures are now available. The most widely used test, ParaSight F, detects a protein (HRP2) excreted by *P. falciparum* within minutes. The test can be performed under field conditions and has a sensitivity more than 95%. A second rapid test, OptiMAL, detects parasite lactate dehydrogenase, and, unlike ParaSight F, can distinguish between *P. falciparum* and *P. vivax*. Serologic tests for malaria are offered at a few large reference laboratories but are used primarily for epidemiologic purposes. They are occasionally helpful in speciation and detection of otherwise occult infections. The recently completed sequencing of the malaria genome will lead to newer diagnostic methods.

Acridine orange stains and other rapid detection methods available

TREATMENT

The indications for treatment rest on two factors. The first is the infecting species of *Plasmodium,* and the second is the immune status of the afflicted patient. Falciparum malaria is potentially lethal in nonimmune individuals such as new immigrants or travelers to a malarious area and immunosuppressed indigenous individuals such as pregnant women. These individuals must be treated emergently.

The complete treatment of malaria requires the destruction of three parasitic forms: the erythrocytic schizont, the hepatic schizont, and the erythrocytic gametocyte. The first terminates the clinical attack, the second prevents relapse, and the third renders the patient noninfectious to *Anopheles* and thus breaks the cycle of transmission. Unfortunately, no single drug accomplishes all three goals. The present strategy of chemotherapy is shown in Table 52–2.

Need to destroy all forms of the parasite

Termination of Acute Attack

Several agents can destroy asexual erythrocytic parasites. Chloroquine, a 4-aminoquinoline, has been the most commonly used. It acts by inhibiting the degradation of hemoglobin,

TABLE 52–2

Chemotherapy of Malaria

Stage of Parasite	Clinical Goal	Drug
Erythrocytic schizont	Treat clinical attack	
	All species	Chloroquine
	CRFM	Quinine, antifolates, sulfonamides, artemisinin (regionally dependent)
	Suppress clinical attack	
	All species	Chloroquine
	CRFM	Antifolates, sulfonamides (regionally dependent)
Erythrocytic gametocyte	Prevent transmission	
	Relapsing malaria	Chloroquine
	Falciparum malaria	Primaquine, artemisinin
Hepatic schizont	Radical cure	
	Relapsing malaria	Primaquine
	Falciparum malaria	None required

Abbreviation: CRFM, chloroquine-resistant falciparum malaria.

Chloroquine inhibits hemoglobin degradation by parasite

Artemisinins prevent gametocyte development

thereby limiting the availability of amino acids necessary for growth. It has been suggested that the weak basic nature of chloroquine also acts to raise the pH of the food vacuoles of the parasite, inhibiting their acid proteases and effectiveness. When originally introduced, it was rapidly effective against all four species of plasmodia and, in the dosage used, free of serious side effects. However, chloroquine-resistant strains of *P. falciparum* are now widespread in Africa and Southeast Asia; they are also found, although less frequently, in other areas of Asia and in Central America and South America. Other schizonticidal agents include quinine/quinidine, antifolate–sulfonamide combinations, mefloquine, halofantrine, and the artemisinins. Except for the artemisinins, malaria resistance to all of the above agents is increasing. The artemisinins are also unique in their capacity to reduce transmission by preventing gametocyte development.

Strains of *P. malariae, P. ovale,* and *P. vivax* (except for some acquired in the South Pacific and South America) remain sensitive to chloroquine and may be treated with this agent. *P. vivax* infections acquired in New Guinea and Sumatra, however, should be assumed to be chloroquine-resistant and managed with mefloquine alone or in combination with other agents. *P. falciparum* has now become variably resistant to all drug groups except the artemisinin compounds (see Fig 52–3).

Resistance of chloroquine and other drugs now common with *P. falciparum*

Combination therapy may be necessary

There is a growing consensus that the most effective way to slow the further development of drug-resistant strains of *P. falciparum* is to use one of the artemisinins in combination with quinine/quinidine, antifolate–sulfonamide compounds, mefloquine, or halofantrine.

Radical Cure

Primaquine used to destroy hepatic schizonts of *P. vivax* and *P. ovale*

In *P. vivax* and *P. ovale* infections, hepatic schizonts persist and must be destroyed to prevent reseeding of circulating erythrocytes with consequent relapse. Primaquine, an 8-aminoquinaline, is used for this purpose. Some *P. vivax* infections acquired in Southeast Asia and New Guinea fail initial therapy due to relative resistance to this 8-aminoquinaline. Retreatment with a larger dose of primaquine is usually successful. Unfortunately, primaquine may induce hemolysis in patients with G6PD deficiency. Persons of Asian, African, and Mediterranean ancestry should thus be screened for this abnormality before treatment. Chloroquine destroys the gametocytes of *P. vivax, P. ovale,* and *P.*

malariae but not those of *P. falciparum*. Primaquine and artemisinins, however, are effective for this latter species.

PREVENTION

Personal Protection

In endemic areas, mosquito contact can be minimized with the use of house screens, insecticide bombs within rooms, and/or insecticide-impregnated mosquito netting around beds. Those who must be outside from dusk to dawn, the period of mosquito feeding, should apply insect repellent and wear clothing with long sleeves and pants. In addition, it is possible to suppress clinical manifestations of infection, should they occur, with a weekly dose of chloroquine. In areas where chloroquine-resistant strains are common, an alternative schizonticidal agent should be used. Mefloquine or doxycycline are usually preferred. The antifolate pyrimethamine plus a sulfonamide can be taken as well. However, use of this combination is occasionally accompanied by serious side effects, so it is recommended only when mefloquine- and doxycycline-resistant strains are present in the area, and then only for individuals residing in areas of intense transmission for prolonged periods of time. On leaving an endemic area, it is necessary to eradicate residual hepatic parasites with primaquine before discontinuing suppressive therapy.

Mosquito protection with screens and repellents

Chemoprophylaxis choice must consider resistance in area

General

Malaria control measures have been directed toward reducing the infected human and mosquito populations to below the critical level necessary for sustained transmission of disease. The techniques employed include those mentioned previously, treatment of febrile patients with effective antimalarial agents, chemical or physical disruption of mosquito breeding areas, and use of residual insecticide sprays. An active international cooperative program aimed at the eradication of malaria resulted in a dramatic decline in the incidence of the disease between 1956 and 1968. Eradication was not achieved, however, because mosquitoes became resistant to some of the chemical agents used, and today malaria still infects 200 to 300 million inhabitants of Africa, Latin America, and Asia. Tropical Africa alone accounts for 100 million of the afflicted and for most of the 1 to 3 million deaths that occur annually as a result of this disease. The long-term hope for progress in these areas now depends on the development of new technologies.

Reduce human reservoir and eradicate mosquitoes

Attempts at eradication have failed

Vaccines

Three advances in the last decade have produced the hope that an effective malaria vaccine might be within reach of medical science for the first time. The establishment of a continuous in vitro culture system provided the large quantities of parasite needed for antigenic analysis. Development of the hybridoma technique allowed the preparation of monoclonal antibodies with which antigens responsible for the induction of protective immunity could be identified. Finally, recombinant DNA procedures enabled scientists to clone and sequence the genes encoding such antigens, permitting the amino acid structure to be determined and peptide sequences suitable for vaccine development to be identified.

Peptide sequences for vaccine development being identified

As immunity to malaria is stage specific, the relative advantages and disadvantages of vaccines prepared against each of the plasmodial stages found in the human host (sporozoite, merozoite, and gametocyte) need to be considered. An effective sporozoite vaccine, by blocking the invasion of hepatocytes by mosquito-introduced sporozoites, would prevent the establishment of the infection within the host and, if widely administered, would interrupt parasite transmission within a community. However, to be effective, a sporozoite vaccine would have to prevent the invasion of all injected sporozoites. Theoretically, if even a single parasite reached and penetrated a liver cell, it would multiply intracellularly and later enter the bloodstream to invade erythrocytes. The patient could develop clinical disease and serve as a reservoir for subsequent transmission to others. A vaccine directed at the erythrocytic or merozoite stage, although preventing neither hepatic nor bloodstream infection, would limit the severity of the parasitemia

Sporozoite vaccine could help prevent initiation of infection

Combination vaccines may be necessary

and thus moderate or abort clinical manifestations of disease. Gametogenesis, and thus parasite transmission, would probably proceed unimpaired. Antibodies formed in response to a gametocyte vaccine might block the union of male and female gametes within the mosquito gut, interrupting parasite transmission. It would, however, neither prevent nor moderate malaria in the immunized patient. The limitations of each vaccine type has led some investigators to advocate the combination of all three in a single polyvalent preparation. Unfortunately, the results of field tests of a number of candidate vaccines have been disappointing.

TOXOPLASMA GONDII

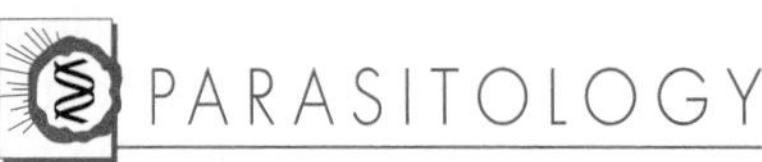

PARASITOLOGY

Asexual and sexual cycles in felines

Three forms of human disease

Like the plasmodia, *Toxoplasma gondii,* the cause of toxoplasmosis, is an obligate intracellular sporozoan. It differs from *Plasmodium* in that both sexual and asexual reproductive cycles occur within the gastrointestinal tract of felines, the definitive host. The disease is transmitted to other host species by the ingestion of oocysts passed in the feces of infected felines.

MORPHOLOGY

Spread to humans from felines via fecal–oral route

Tissue cysts killed by cooking as well as freezing and thawing

T. gondii was first demonstrated in 1908 in the gondi, an African rodent, by Nicolle and Marceaux. Its name, derived from the Greek toxo (arc), is based on the characteristic shape of the organism. All strains of this parasite appear to be closely related antigenically. The major morphologic forms of the parasite are the oocyst, trophozoite, and tissue cyst.

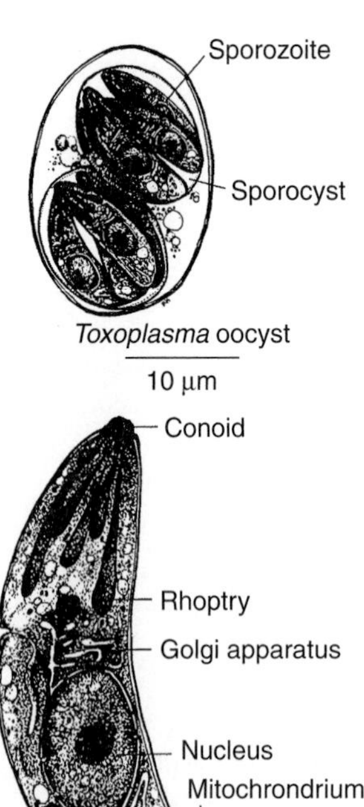

Toxoplasma oocyst

Toxoplasma tachyzoite (trophozoite)

Oocyst

The oocyst is ovoid, measures 10 to 12 μm in diameter, and possesses a thick wall that makes it resistant to most environmental challenges. It may be destroyed by heat in excess of 66°C and chemicals such as iodine and formalin. In its immature form, the center of the cyst lacks internal structure. With maturation two sporocysts appear, and later four sporozoites may be discerned within each sporocyst. Sporulation does not occur at temperatures below 4°C or above 37°C. This form is responsible for the spread of the parasites from felines to other warm-blooded animals via the fecal–oral route.

Tachyzoite (Trophozoite)

The term "trophozoite" is used in its broadest sense to refer to the asexual proliferative forms responsible for cell invasion and clinical disease. In different stages of the asexual cycle it is referred to by several other terms, including merozoite and tachyzoite. It is crescent or arc shaped, measures 3 by 7 μm, and can invade all nucleated cell types. Although tachyzoites are obligate intracellular organisms, they may survive extracellularly in a variety of body fluids for periods of hours to days. They cannot, however, survive the digestive activity of the stomach and therefore are not infective on ingestion.

Tissue Cysts

Cysts measure 10 to 200 μm in diameter. The contained organisms, referred to as bradyzoites, are similar to tachyzoites, but are smaller and divide more slowly. Tissue cysts are resistant to digestive enzymes, and like oocysts, are infectious to the animal that ingests them. They survive normal refrigerator temperatures but are killed by freezing and thawing and by normal cooking temperatures.

LIFE CYCLE

Definitive Host

Sexual reproduction of *T. gondii* occurs only in the intestinal tract of felines, most importantly in the domestic cat. Ingested parasites enter the epithelial cells of the ileum by mechanisms that remain poorly defined. Intracellularly, the trophozoites reside within a membrane-bound vacuole and undergo schizogony. With cell rupture, merozoites are released. The merozoites infect adjacent epithelial cells; they then repeat another asexual cycle or eventually differentiate into gametocytes, initiating sexual reproduction. Fusion of the mature male and female gametes leads to the formation of an oval, thick-walled oocyst that is then shed in the feces. In the typical infection, millions of these structures are released daily for 1 to 3 weeks. The oocysts are immature at the time of shedding and must complete sporulation in the external environment. In this process, two sporocysts, each containing four sporozoites, develop within each oocyst. The time required for sporulation varies from 1 day to 3 weeks, depending on the ambient temperature and moisture. Once mature, the resistant oocysts may remain viable and infectious for many years in soil.

Infection in cat ileal cells

Fusion of gametes leads to oocyst formation; shed in feces

Sporulate in external environment

Intermediate Hosts

After ingestion by a susceptible warm-blooded animal, sporozoites are released from the disrupted oocyst and enter macrophages. Within these cells, they are transported through the lymphohematogenous system to all organ systems. Continued intracellular schizogony results in macrophage rupture and release of new parasites, which may invade any adjacent nucleated host cell and continue the asexual cycle. With the development of host immunity, many of the parasites are destroyed. Within the cells of certain organs, particularly the brain, heart, and skeletal muscle, the trophozoites produce a membrane that surrounds and protects them: within this tissue cyst, multiplication continues at a more leisurely pace. Eventually, cysts that measure up to 200 μm in diameter and contain more than a thousand organisms are produced. These cysts persist intact for the life of the host or rupture, producing parasitologic relapse. If they are ingested by a carnivore, they survive the digestive enzymes and initiate infection in the new host.

Mature oocysts infect hosts orally

Released sporozoites invade macrophages

Cysts develop and can persist for life of host

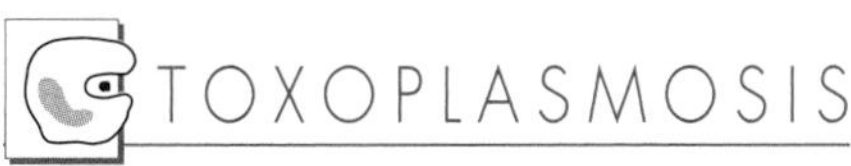

TOXOPLASMOSIS

CLINICAL CAPSULE

Toxoplasma can infect most warm-blooded animals, both domestic and wild; it is thus the most cosmopolitan of parasites. Approximately 50% of the human population of the United States has been infected. In the overwhelming majority of persons, infection is chronic, asymptomatic, and self-limiting. Clinical disease presents in three major forms: (1) self-limiting febrile lymphadenopathy, (2) highly lethal infection of immunocompromised patients, and (3) congenital infection of infants.

EPIDEMIOLOGY

Prevalence and Distribution

Toxoplasmosis is a cosmopolitan disease that occurs in almost all mammals and many birds. Human infections are found in every region of the globe; in general, the incidence is higher in the tropics and lower in cold and/or arid regions. In the United States, the prevalence of positive serologic evidence for the disease increases with age. By adulthood, approximately 50% of Americans can be shown to have circulating antibodies against *T. gondii.*

Worldwide distribution among mammals and birds

Transmission

Although it is known that humans may acquire toxoplasmosis in a variety of ways, data on their relative frequency are both meager and conflicting. It is likely that the route of transmission varies from population to population, and perhaps from age to age, within any given area. The most important transmission mechanisms are discussed below.

Ingestion of Oocysts

Increased hazard to children by close contact with contaminated areas

Felinophobes are inclined to the view that the deposition of oocysts in the feces of cats and their subsequent ingestion by the unsuspecting owner is the most frequent way in which humans acquire this important infection. Disease epidemics associated with exposure to infected cats have been reported. Unfortunately, data from studies relating the frequency of feline exposure to the prevalence of positive serologic tests are conflicting. Acutely infected cats shed oocysts for only a few weeks. It has been shown, however, that chronically infected felines can occasionally reshed oocysts, and prevalence studies have demonstrated that 1% of domestic cats excrete oocysts at any given time. The large number of these structures passed during active shedding and their prolonged survival in the external environment greatly enhance their chance of transmission. Particularly at risk are individuals such as children at play, who may come in close contact with areas likely to be contaminated with cat feces, and adults responsible for changing a cat's litter box. It is also possible that insects can mechanically transfer oocysts to human food.

Ingestion of Tissue Cysts

Cysts present in meat

Tissue cysts have been frequently demonstrated in meat produced for human consumption. They are most common in pork (25%) and mutton (10%) and less so in beef and chicken (<1%). Although such cysts are killed at normal (well-done) cooking temperatures, an impressive array of epidemiologic information links the handling and/or ingestion of raw or undercooked meat with serologic and, occasionally, clinical evidence of disease. Confounding these data is an Indian study that demonstrated no difference between meat eaters and vegetarians in the incidence of positive serologic tests.

Congenital

Transplacental transmission highest in third trimester

Approximately 1 of every 500 pregnant women acquires acute toxoplasmosis, and approximately 10 to 20% of the involved women become symptomatic. Regardless of the clinical status of the infected mother, the parasite involves the fetus in 33 to 50% of all acute maternal infections. The risk of transplacental transmission is independent of the clinical severity of the disease in the mother, but does correlate with the stage of gestation at which she is exposed. Fetal involvement occurs in 17% of first-trimester and 65% of third-trimester infections. Conversely, the earlier a fetal infection is acquired, the more severe it is likely to be. Overall, 20% of fetuses experienced severe consequences; a similar proportion develop mild disease. The remainder are asymptomatic.

Miscellaneous

Transmitted by transfusions and organ transplants

In addition to causing congenital infection, trophozoites have been responsible for disease transmission in a number of other situations, including laboratory accidents, transfusions of whole blood and leukocytes, and organ transplantation. Because trophozoites may survive for several hours in body fluids or exudates of acutely infected humans, it is possible for infection to occur after contact with such materials.

PATHOGENESIS AND IMMUNITY

Dissemination in immunosuppressed subjects

In the primary infection, the proliferation of trophozoites results in the death of involved host cells, stimulation of a mononuclear inflammatory reaction, and a parasite-specific secretory IgA response. In immunodeficient hosts, rapid organism proliferation continues, producing numerous widespread foci of tissue necrosis. The consequences are most serious in organs such as the brain, where the potential for cell regeneration is limited.

In normal hosts, however, acute infection is rapidly controlled with the development of humoral and cellular immunity. Extracellular parasites are destroyed, intracellular multiplication is hindered, and tissue cysts are formed. With the exception of lysis of extracellular parasites by antibody and complement, cell-mediated immunity appears to play the principal role in this process, mediated in part by IL-2, interferon-α, and cytotoxic T cells. Immunity appears to be lifelong, possibly because of survival of the parasite in the tissue cysts. The cysts, which are found most frequently in the brain, retina, heart and skeletal muscle, normally produce little or no tissue reaction. The suppression of cell-mediated immunity that accompanies serious illness, or the administration of immunosuppressive agents, may lead to the rupture of a cyst and the release of trophozoites. Their subsequent proliferation and the intense antibody reaction to their presence results in an acute exacerbation of the disease.

Immunity is primarily cell-mediated

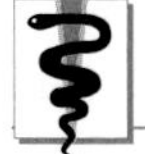

TOXOPLASMOSIS: CLINICAL ASPECTS

MANIFESTATIONS

In the vast majority of patients, infection with *T. gondii* is completely asymptomatic. Clinical manifestations, when they do appear, vary with the type of host involved. In general, they may be grouped into one of the three syndromes listed below.

Congenital Toxoplasmosis

Immune mechanisms are poorly developed in utero. As a result, a large proportion of fetal infections results in clinical illness. If the infection spreads to the central nervous system, the outcome is often catastrophic. Abortion and stillbirth are the most serious consequences. Liveborn children may demonstrate microcephaly, hydrocephaly, cerebral calcifications, convulsions, and psychomotor retardation. Disease of this severity is usually accompanied by evidence of visceral involvement, including fever, hepatitis, pneumonia, and skin rash. Infants infected later in prenatal development demonstrate milder disease. Many appear healthy at birth but develop epilepsy, retardation, or strabismus months or years later. Probably the most common delayed manifestation of congenital toxoplasmosis is chorioretinitis. This condition, which is thought to result from the reactivation of latent tissue cysts, typically presents during the second or third decade of life as recurrent bouts of eye pain and loss of visual acuity. The lesions are usually bilateral but focal. If the retinal macula is not involved, vision improves as the inflammation subsides. *T. gondii* accounts for 25% of all cases of granulomatous uveitis seen in the United States.

Infection in utero can produce malformations, chorioretinitis, and stillbirth

Normal Host

The most common clinical manifestation of toxoplasmosis acquired after birth is asymptomatic localized lymphadenopathy. The cervical nodes are most frequently involved, but nontender enlargement of other regional groups, including the retroperitoneal nodes, also occurs. At times, the adenopathy is accompanied by fever, sore throat, rash, hepatosplenomegaly, and atypical lymphocytosis, thus mimicking the clinical and laboratory manifestations of infectious mononucleosis. Occasionally the normal host develops severe visceral involvement, which may be manifested as meningoencephalitis, pneumonitis, myocarditis, or hepatitis. Chorioretinitis following postnatally acquired infection, although documented, is uncommon. Unlike congenitally acquired ocular disease, it occurs during midlife and is generally unilateral.

Fever and lymphadenopathy can mimic infectious mononucleosis

Immunocompromised Host

In the immunocompromised host, toxoplasmosis is a serious, often fatal disease. If primary infection is acquired while a patient is undergoing immunosuppressive therapy for malignancy or organ transplantation, widespread dissemination of the infection with necrotizing pneumonitis, myocarditis, and encephalitis may occur. More commonly, acute disease in this population results from the activation of chronic, latent infection by immunosuppressive therapy, or the acquisition of a concurrent immunosuppressive infection, particularly acquired immunodeficiency syndrome (AIDS). Encephalitis occurs in 50% of such cases and in more than 90% of fatal cases. Toxoplasmic encephalitis is particularly common in AIDS patients; it is seen in approximately 10% of those with circulating toxoplasma antibodies. As such, it is a major cause of morbidity and mortality in this patient population. Clinically, encephalitis may present as a meningoencephalitis, diffuse encephalopathy, or mass lesion.

Primary infection or reactivation of latent infections can produce severe, widespread disease

AIDS patients develop encephalitis

DIAGNOSIS

The diagnosis may be established by a variety of methods. In acute toxoplasmic lymphadenitis, the histologic appearance of the involved nodes is often pathognomonic. The trophozoite may be demonstrated in tissue with Wright or Giemsa stain. Electron microscopy and indirect fluorescent antibody techniques have also been used successfully on heart transplant or brain tissue obtained by biopsy. Although tissue cysts are selectively stained by periodic acid–Schiff, their presence is not indicative of acute disease. Isolation of the organism can be accomplished by inoculating blood or other body fluids into mice or tissue cultures. Inoculation of other tissues is not usually helpful, because a positive result may only reflect the presence of latent tissue cysts.

Demonstration of parasite in histopathologic specimens

Serologic procedures are the primary method of diagnosis. To establish the presence of acute infection, it is usual to demonstrate a fourfold rise in the IgG antibody titer between acute and convalescent serum specimens. Peak titers are often reached within 4 to 8 weeks, so the acute serum must be collected early in the course of illness. Of the many tests developed for the detection of IgG antibodies, the indirect hemagglutination test and the indirect fluorescent antibody test are those most frequently used; they both are sensitive and highly specific. With these tests, titers of 1:1000 or more are usually detected after an acute infection. These levels gradually fall but may remain high for many years.

Serodiagnosis is the primary approach

The detection of IgM antibodies provides a more rapid confirmation of acute infection. As detected by an indirect fluorescent antibody technique, these antibodies appear within the first week of infection, peak in 2 to 4 weeks, and quickly revert to negative. It also appears that IgM antibodies are produced after reactivation of latent disease. A single high titer (1:80 or more) therefore establishes the presence of acute infection or reactivation. Unfortunately, this test has been difficult to standardize, lacks sensitivity in neonates and immunocompromised (particularly AIDS) hosts, and is not widely available. Recently introduced enzyme immunoassays (EIA) for IgM antibody circumvent many of these difficulties, but still produce some false-positive results, and are not sufficiently sensitive in AIDS patients. A modification of the EIA procedure, the antibody-capture enzyme immunoassay, significantly improves both the sensitivity and specificity of the original procedure. Examination of urine and other body fluids for the presence of toxoplasma antigen, or DNA by the polymerase chain reaction, have been shown to be useful adjunctive tests in immunocompromised individuals; currently these procedures are not generally available to clinical laboratories.

Rising titers of IgG or detection of IgM suggest acute infection or reactivation

TREATMENT AND PREVENTION

Usually, patients do not require therapy unless symptoms are particularly severe and persistent or unless vital organs, such as the eye, are involved. Immunocompromised and pregnant women, however, should be treated if acute infection (or reactivation) is documented (Table 52–3). Routine serial serologic testing of such individuals would allow early detection of infected patients and enhance the prospects of a successful outcome. It is now clear that early treatment of acutely infected pregnant women significantly reduces the incidence of severe congenital infections and reduces the ratio of benign to subclinical forms in infants. At present, the most commonly used therapeutic regimen in the United States is the combination of pyrimethamine and sulfonamides. Unfortunately, the former

Spiramycin used to prevent congenital infection

TABLE 52–3

Indications for Treatment of Toxoplasmosis[a]

Serologic Criteria	Clinical Criteria
Elevated IgM titers	Potential laboratory acquired infection
Fourfold rise in IgG titers	Pregnant woman
Very high IgG titers (>1:1000)	Neonate
	Immunocompromised patient (including AIDS)
	Severe constitutional symptoms
	Vital organ involvement (including active chorioretinitis)

Abbreviation: Ig, immunoglobulin.

[a]Must satisfy one serologic plus one clinical criterion.

drug is teratogenic and should not be used in the first trimester of pregnancy; spiramycin, a cytostatic macrolide, is often substituted in this setting.

Although the pyrimethamine–sulfonamide combination is very effective against tachyzoites, it is inactive against the cyst forms. As both parasitic forms are present in patients with toxoplasmic encephalitis, recrudescence of illness generally follows completion of standard therapy in AIDS patients. This may be prevented by initiating chronic, low-dose suppressive therapy following the completion of the standard regimen. Atovaquone, a recently introduced hydroxynaphthoquinone, possesses activity against both tachyzoites and cysts. Its use, therefore, may result in radical cure of toxoplasma encephalitis, eliminating the need for chronic suppression.

Atovaquone is active against tachyzoites and cysts

Prevention should be directed primarily at pregnant women and immunologically compromised hosts. Hands should be carefully washed after handling uncooked meat. Cysts in meat can be destroyed by proper cooking (56°C for 15 min) or by freezing to –20°C. Cat feces should be avoided, particularly the changing of litter boxes.

Cryptosporidia

Cryptosporidia ("hidden-spore") are small parasites that can infect the intestinal tract of a wide range of mammals, including humans. Like other sporozoan parasites, they are obligate intracellular organisms that exhibit alternating cycles of sexual and asexual reproduction. As with *Toxoplasma,* both cycles are completed within the gastrointestinal tract of a single host. Long recognized as an important cause of diarrhea in animals, cryptosporidia were not identified as causes of human enteritis until 1976.

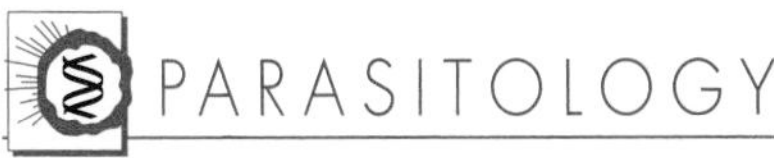

PARASITOLOGY

MORPHOLOGY

Regardless of animal host, all strains of this tiny (2 to 6 μm) parasite appear morphologically identical. Although all strains can reasonably be regarded as a single species, the one that infects humans and cattle is often referred to as *C. parvum*. The organisms appear as small spherical structures arranged in rows along the microvilli of the epithelial cells. They are readily stained with Giemsa and hematoxylin–eosin. Although they

Small spherical particles associated with microvilli

Oocysts are acid-fast

remain external to the cytoplasm of the intestinal epithelial cell, they are covered by a double membrane derived from the reflection, fusion, and attenuation of the microvilli, and are thus, by definition, intracellular organisms. Oocysts shed into the intestinal lumen mature to contain four sporozoites; their cell wall provides the unusual property of acid fastness, allowing them to be visualized with stains generally employed for mycobacteria.

LIFE CYCLE

Infective oocysts are excreted in the stool of the parasitized animal. Unlike those of *Toxoplasma,* cryptosporidia oocysts are fully mature and immediately infective on passage in the feces. Following ingestion by another animal, sporozoites are released from the oocyst and attach to the microvilli of the small bowel epithelial cells, where they are transformed into trophozoites. These divide asexually by multiple fission (schizogony) to form schizonts containing eight daughter cells known as type 1 merozoites. On release from the schizont, each daughter cell attaches itself to another epithelial cell, where it repeats the schizogony cycle, producing another generation of type 1 merozoites.

Mature, infective oocysts excreted in stools

Eventually, schizonts containing four type 2 merozoites are seen. Incapable of continued asexual reproduction, these develop into male (microgamete) and female (macrogamete) sexual forms. Following fertilization, the resulting zygote develops into an oocyst that is shed into the lumen of the bowel. The majority possess a thick protective cell wall that ensures their intact passage in the feces and survival in the external environment.

Protective cell wall ensures survival of oocysts

Approximately 20% fail to develop the thick protective wall. The cell membrane ruptures, releasing infective sporozoites directly into the intestinal lumen and initiating a new "autoinfective" cycle within the original host. In the normal host, the presence of innate or acquired immunity dampens both the cyclic production of type 1 merozoites and the formation of thin-walled oocysts, halting further parasite multiplication and terminating the acute infection. In the immunocompromised, both presumably continue, explaining why such individuals develop severe, persistent infections in the absence of external reinfection.

Some thin-walled oocysts can autoinfect

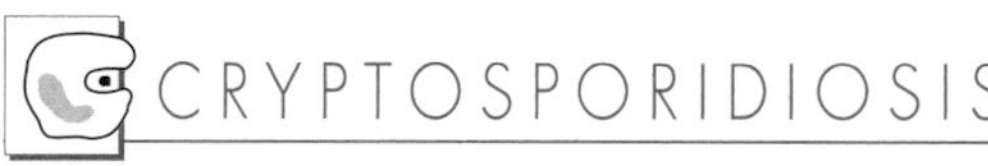

CLINICAL CAPSULE

Cryptosporidiosis is an intestinal illness acquired from domestic animals. The course includes profuse watery diarrhea, vomiting, and weight loss. Spontaneous complete recovery is the usual outcome.

EPIDEMIOLOGY

Cryptosporidiosis appears to involve most vertebrate groups. In all species, infection rates are highest among the young and immature. Experimental and epidemiologic data suggest that domestic animals constitute an important reservoir of disease in humans. However, outbreaks of human disease in day-care centers, hospitals, and urban family groups indicate that most human infections result from person-to-person transmission. In Western countries, between 1 and 4% of small children presenting to medical centers with gastroenteritis have been shown to harbor cryptosporidia oocysts. In third world countries, the rates have varied from 4 to 11%. In some outbreaks of diarrhea in day-care centers, the majority of attendees were found to have oocysts in their stool.

Animal reservoirs and person-to-person transmission both important

Infection rates in adults suffering from gastroenteritis is approximately one third of that reported in children; it has been highest in family members of infected children, medical personnel caring for patients with cryptosporidiosis, male homosexuals, and travelers to foreign countries. In the United States, the parasite has been identified in 15% of patients with AIDS and diarrhea; in Haiti and Africa, 50% of such individuals may be

Infection rates highest in young children

involved. Asymptomatic carriage is uncommon. Other enteric pathogens, particularly *Giardia lamblia,* are recovered from a significant minority of infected patients.

Because oocysts are found almost exclusively in stool, the principal transmission route is undoubtedly by direct fecal–oral spread. Transmission via contaminated water has been documented, and the hardy nature of the oocysts makes it likely that there is also indirect transmission via contaminated food and fomites.

Can be transmitted via contaminated water

PATHOGENESIS AND IMMUNITY

Although the jejunum is most heavily involved, cryptosporidia have been found throughout the gastrointestinal tract, particularly in immunocompromised subjects. Cryptosporidial cholecystitis is seen with some frequency in AIDS patients with enteritis. By light microscopy, bowel changes appear minimal, consisting of mild to moderate villous atrophy, crypt enlargement, and a mononuclear infiltrate of the lamina propria. The pathophysiology of the diarrhea is unknown, but its nature and intensity suggest that a cholera-like enterotoxin may be involved. The vital role played by the host's immune status in the pathogenesis of the disease is indicated by both the enhanced susceptibility of the young to infection and the prolonged severe clinical disease seen in immunocompromised patients. Indirect evidence suggests antibodies in the intestinal lumen exert a protective effect against initial *C. parvum* infection. Experimental animal studies indicate that CD4+ T lymphocytes and interferon play independent roles in the immunologic clearance of the parasite.

Minimal intestinal pathology

Prolonged disease in AIDS patients

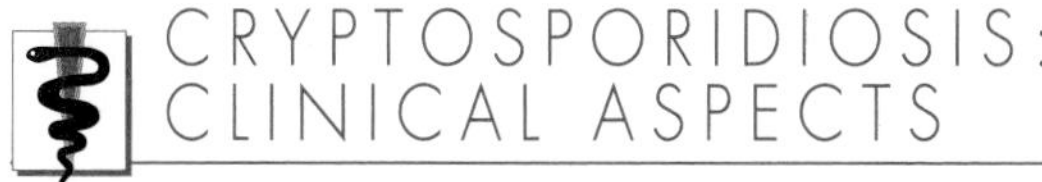

CRYPTOSPORIDIOSIS: CLINICAL ASPECTS

MANIFESTATIONS

Immunocompetent patients usually note the onset of explosive, profuse, watery diarrhea 1 to 2 weeks after exposure. Typically, the illness persists for 5 to 11 days and then rapidly abates. Occasionally, purging, accompanied by a mild malabsorption and weight loss, continues for up to 1 month. A few patients complain of nausea, anorexia, vomiting, and low-grade fever. Except for its shorter duration, more prominent abdominal pain, and relative lack of flatulence, the clinical manifestations of cryptosporidiosis closely resemble those produced by *G. lamblia*. Radiographic and endoscopic examinations of the gut are either normal or demonstrate mild, nonspecific abnormalities. Recovery is complete, and neither relapse nor reinfection has been reported.

Self-limiting diarrhea in normal hosts

Cryptosporidiosis has been described in patients with a broad range of immunodeficiencies, including childhood malnutrition in third world countries, AIDS, and congenital hypogammaglobulinemia, and in those resulting from cancer chemotherapy and immunosuppressive management of organ transplants. In such patients, cryptosporidiosis is usually indolent in onset and manifestations are similar to those seen in normal hosts, but the diarrhea is more severe. Fluid losses of up to 25 L/day have been described. Patients with biliary cryptosporidiosis present with typical manifestations of cholecystitis and cholangitis. Unless the immunologic defect is reversed, the disease usually persists for the duration of the patient's life. Weight loss is often prominent. The prognosis depends on the nature of the underlying immunologic abnormality; half of patients with AIDS die within 6 months. Although other intercurrent infections are usually the direct cause of death, malnutrition and complications of parenteral nutrition contribute.

DIAGNOSIS

The diagnosis of cryptosporidiosis is established by the recovery and identification of *Cryptosporidium* oocysts in a recently passed or preserved diarrheal stool. Oocyst excretion is most intense during the first week of illness, tapers during the second week, and generally stops with the cessation of diarrhea. Because cryptosporidia oocysts are one of

Detection of oocysts by acid-fast or immunofluorescent stains the few acid-fast particles found in feces, a definitive identification can be established with any one of the acid-fast staining procedures developed for mycobacteria. A direct immunofluorescence antibody stain using a monoclonal antibody to oocyst wall has been recently introduced that appears to be superior to acid-fast stains. When direct examinations are negative, concentration procedures are used and the concentrate restained. Immunofluorescence and EIAs for the detection of anticryptosporidial antibodies are now available.

TREATMENT AND PREVENTION

Specific treatment remains problematic

In the immunocompetent patient, the disease is self-limited and attempts at specific antiparasitic therapy are not warranted; rehydration may be required in small children. In the immunocompromised host, the severity and chronicity of the diarrhea warrants therapeutic intervention. Unfortunately, there is no uniformly effective anticryptosporidial agent available at this time. Paromomycin, a luminal antimicrobic, has been shown to reduce the intensity of diarrhea in some patients, and parenteral octreotide acetate, a somatostatin analog, has been useful in decreasing stool volumes. The only uniformly successful approach has been the reversal of underlying immunologic abnormalities. When appropriate, withdrawal of cancer chemotherapy agents or immunosuppressive drugs may result in a cure.

The stools of patients with cryptosporidiosis are infectious. Stool precautions should be instituted at the time the diagnosis is first suspected; for the immunosuppressed patient, this should be whenever diarrhea, regardless of presumed etiology, is first noted. This is particularly important in cancer chemotherapy and transplantation units, where spread of the disease from a symptomatic patient to other immunosuppressed patients can have life-threatening consequences.

ADDITIONAL READING

Bojang KA, et al. Efficacy of RTS,S/ASO2 malaria vaccine against *Plasmodium falciparum* infection in semi-immune adult men in The Gambia: a randomized trial. *Lancet* 2001;358:1927–1934.

Curtis CF, Lines JD. Should DDT be banned by international treaty? *Parasitol Today* 2000;16:119–121.

Denkers DY, Gassinelli RT. Regulation and function of T-cell–mediated immunity during *Toxoplasma gondii* infection. *Clin Microbiol Rev* 1998;11:569–588.

Foulin W, et al. Treatment of toxoplasmosis during pregnancy. *Am J Obstet Gynecol* 1999;189:410.

Frenkel JK, Ruiz A. Endemicity of toxoplasmosis in Costa Rica. Transmission between cats, soil, intermediate hosts and humans. *Am J Epidemiol* 1981;113:254–269. This article is the most comprehensive study on the role of cats in the transmission of toxoplasmosis. It suggests that humans are infected primarily from soil contaminated with cat feces, rather than direct contact.

Griffiths JK. Human cryptosporidiosis: epidemiology, transmission, clinical disease, treatment and diagnosis. *Adv Parasitol* 1998;40:37.

Guerin PJ, et al. Malaria: current status of control, diagnosis, treatment, and a proposed agenda for research and development. *Lancet (Infect Dis)* 2002;2:564–573. This article brings clarity, comprehensiveness, and brevity to one of the two or three greatest infectious disease scourges of mankind. It is a "must read" for anyone intent on exploring this disease.

Heyworth MF. Immunology of *Giardia* and *Cryptosporidium* infections. *J Infect Dis* 1992;166:465–472. A review of the immunology of these two important protozoa.

Krogstad DJ. Malaria as a reemerging disease. *Epidemiol Rev* 1996;18:77–89.

Luft BJ, Remington JS. Toxoplasmic encephalitis in AIDS. *Clin Infect Dis* 1995;15:211–222. A comprehensive review of an increasingly common presentation of toxoplasmosis.

Malaguamera L, Musumeci S. The immune response to *Plasmodium falciparum* malaria. *Lancet (Infectious Diseases)* 2002;2:472– 478. A concise review of recent developments.

Manabe YC, et al. Cryptosporidiosis in patients with AIDS: correlates of disease and survival. *Clin Infect Dis* 1998;27:536–542.

Newton P, White N. Malaria: new developments in treatment and prevention. *Annu Rev Med* 1999;50:179.

Phillips RS. Current status of malaria and potential for control. *Clin Microbiol Rev* 2001;14:208–226.

White NJ. Malaria pathophysiology. In *Malaria: Parasite Biology, Pathogenesis, Protection,* I Sherman (ed). Washington DC: ASM Press; 1998, pp 371–385.

Whitworth J, et al. Effect of HIV-1 and increasing suppression on malaria parasitology and clinical episodes in adults in rural Uganda: a cohort study. *Lancet* 2000;356: 1051–1056.

C H A P T E R 5 3

Rhizopods

JAMES J. PLORDE

Rhizopods, or amebas, are the most primitive of the protozoa. They multiply by simple binary fission and move by means of cytoplasmic organelles called pseudopodia. These projections of the relatively solid ectoplasm are formed by streaming of the inner, more liquid endoplasm. They move the ameba forward and, incidentally, engulf and internalize food sources found in its path. Most amebas, when faced with a hostile environment, can produce a chitinous, external wall that surrounds and protects them. These forms are referred to as cysts and may survive for prolonged periods under conditions that would rapidly destroy the motile trophozoite. The majority of amebas belong to free-living genera. They are widely distributed in nature, being found in literally all bodies of standing fresh water. Few free-living amebas produce human disease, although two genera, *Naegleria* and *Acanthamoeba,* have been implicated occasionally as causes of meningoencephalitis and keratitis.

Several genera of amebas, including *Entamoeba, Endolimax,* and *Iodamoeba,* are obligate parasites of the human alimentary tract and are passed as cysts from host to host by the fecal–oral route. Several are devoid of mitochondria, presumably because of the anaerobic conditions under which they exist in the colon. Only one, *Entamoeba histolytica,* regularly produces disease; it has been recently subdivided into two morphologically identical but genetically distinct species, an invasive pathogen that retains the species appellation "histolytica" and a commensal organism, now designated *E. dispar*. The two species can be differentiated by isoenzyme analysis, antibodies to surface antigens, and DNA markers.

ENTAMOEBA HISTOLYTICA

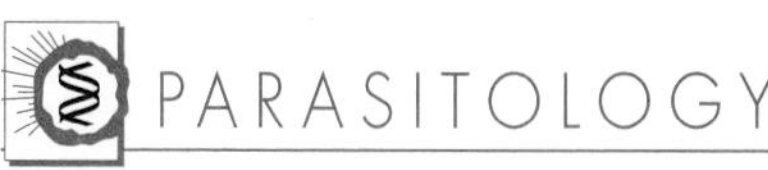

MORPHOLOGY AND PHYSIOLOGY

E. histolytica possesses both trophozoite and cyst forms. The trophozoites are microaerophilic, dwell in the lumen or wall of the colon, feed on bacteria and tissue cells, and multiply rapidly in the anaerobic environment of the gut. When diarrhea occurs, the trophozoites are passed unchanged in the liquid stool. Here they can be recognized by their size (12 to 20 μm in diameter); directional motility; granular, vacuolated

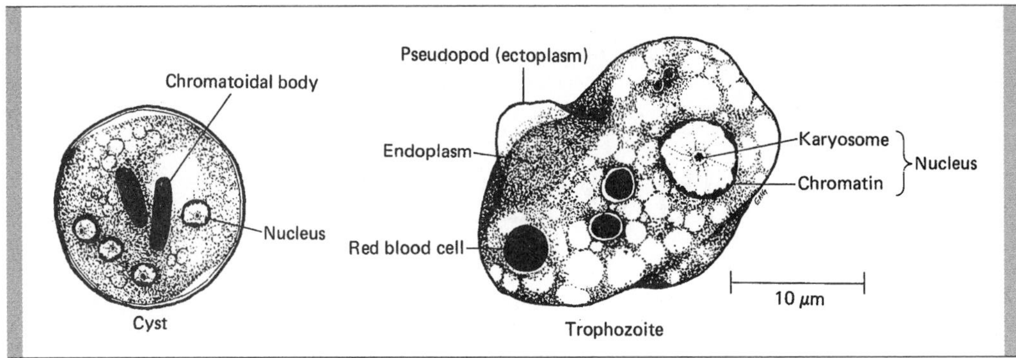

FIGURE 53–1
Entamoeba histolytica.

Trophozoites multiply rapidly in the gut

Cysts are hardy; can survive in chlorinated water supply

endoplasm; and sharply demarcated, clear ectoplasm with finger-like pseudopods. Invasive strains tend to be larger and may contain ingested erythrocytes within their cytoplasm (Fig 53–1). Appropriate stains reveal a 3- to 5-μm nucleus with a small central karyosome or nucleolus and fine regular granules evenly distributed around the nuclear membrane (peripheral chromatin). Electron microscopic studies demonstrate microfilaments, an external glycocalyx, and cytoplasmic projections thought to be important for attachment.

With normal stool transit time, trophozoites usually encyst before leaving the gut. Initially, a cyst contains a single nucleus, a glycogen vacuole, and one or more large, cigar-shaped ribosomal clusters known as chromatoid bodies. With maturation, the cyst becomes quadrinucleate, and the cytoplasmic inclusions are absorbed. In contrast to the fragile trophozoite, mature cysts can survive environmental temperatures up to 55°C, chlorine concentrations normally found in municipal water supplies, and normal levels of gastric acid. *E. histolytica* can be differentiated from the other amebas of the gut by its size, nuclear detail, and cytoplasmic inclusions (Table 53–1).

TABLE 53–1

Some Differential Characteristics of *Entamoeba* Species

CHARACTERISTICS	*E. HISTOLYTICA*	*E. HARTMANNI*	*E. COLI*
Trophozoites			
Cytoplasm	Differentiated[a]	Differentiated	Undifferentiated
Nucleus			
Peripheral chromatin	Fine	Fine	Coarse, irregular
Karyosome	Small, central	Small, central	Large, eccentric
Ingested particles			
Bacteria	No	—	Yes
Red blood cells	Yes	No	No
Size	>12 μm	<12 μm	>12 μm
Cysts			
Nuclei[b]	1–4	1–4	1–8
Chromatoid bodies	Rods	Rods	Splinters
Size	>10 μm	<10 μm	>10 μm

[a] Sharp differentiation between ectoplasm and endoplasm.

[b] Fine structure similar to that of trophozoites.

LIFE CYCLE

Humans are the principal hosts and reservoirs of *E. histolytica*. Transmission from person to person occurs when a parasite passed in the stool of one host is ingested by another. Because the trophozoites die rapidly in the external environment, successful passage is achieved only by the cyst. Human hosts may pass up to 45 million cysts daily. Although the average infective dose exceeds 1000 organisms, ingestion of a single cyst has been known to produce infection. After passage through the stomach, the cyst eventually reaches the distal small bowel. Here the cyst wall disintegrates, releasing the quadrinucleate parasite, which divides to form eight small trophozoites that are carried to the colon. Colonization is most intense in areas of fecal stasis such as the cecum and rectosigmoid but may be found throughout the large bowel.

Humans are the hosts and reservoir; fecal–oral transmission

LABORATORY GROWTH

Trophozoites are facultative anaerobes that require complex media for growth. Most require the addition of live bacteria for successful isolation. Sterile culture techniques (axenic) have been developed, however, and are essential for the preparation of the purified antigens required for serologic testing, zymodeme typing, and characterization of virulence factors. Such techniques are generally available only in research laboratories.

Facultative anaerobes

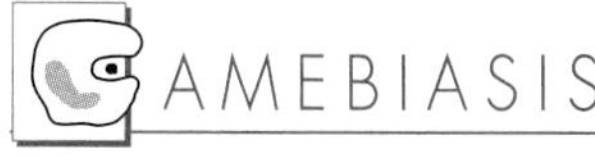

AMEBIASIS

CLINICAL CAPSULE

Amebiasis may be asymptomatic or produce intermittent diarrhea with abdominal pain. Invasion of the mucosa is typical and may spread to the liver, where an abscess is produced.

EPIDEMIOLOGY

E. histolytica infection rates are higher in warm climates, particularly in areas where the level of sanitation is low. Worldwide, this organism is thought to produce more deaths than any other parasite, except those that cause malaria and schistosomiasis. Reports of amebic liver abscess, for instance, emanate primarily from Mexico, western South America, South Asia, and West and South Africa. For reasons apparently unrelated to exposure, symptomatic illness is much less common in women and children than in men.

Worldwide infection; highest rates in warmer climates

Although stool surveys in the United States indicate that 1 to 5% of the population harbors *Entamoeba,* the vast majority of these are now known to be colonized with the nonpathogenic *E. dispar*. The incidence of invasive amebiasis in the United States decreased sharply over several decades, reaching a nadir in 1974. Since then, the numbers have increased steadily. It is now seen particularly in institutionalized individuals, Indian reservations, migrant labor camps, victims of acquired immunodeficiency syndrome (AIDS), and travelers to endemic areas.

Invasive disease rare in United States

Symptomatic amebiasis is usually sporadic, the result of direct person-to-person fecal–oral spread under conditions of poor personal hygiene. Venereal transmission is seen in male homosexuals, presumably the result of oral–anal sexual contact. Food- and water-borne spread occur, occasionally in epidemic form. Such outbreaks, however, are seldom as explosive as those produced by pathogenic intestinal bacteria. One outbreak of intestinal amebiasis was due to colonic irrigation at a chiropractic clinic.

Fecal–oral spread linked to poor hygiene

Food and water are other modes of transmission

PATHOGENESIS

A number of virulence factors have been identified in *E. histolytica*. In an experimental setting, invasiveness correlates well with endocytic capacity, the production of extracellular proteinases capable of activating complement and degrading collagen, the presence of a galactose-specific lectin apparently capable of mediating attachment of the organism to colonic mucosa, and perhaps most importantly, the capacity to lyse host cells on contact. The latter phenomenon is initiated by the galactose-specific lectin-mediated adherence of the trophozoite to a target cell. Following adherence, the ameba releases a pore-forming protein that polymerizes in the target cell membrane, forming large tubular lesions. Cytolysis rapidly follows.

Virulence determinants include lectin-mediated adherence to mucosa and capacity to lyse host cells

In most cases of infections, however, tissue damage is minimal, and the host remains symptom free, suggesting that host factors may modulate the invasiveness of virulent strains. These factors are still poorly understood, but changes in host resistance, the colonic milieu, or the parasite itself may amplify tissue damage and clinical manifestations. Protein malnutrition, high-carbohydrate diets, corticosteroid administration, childhood, and pregnancy all appear to render the host more susceptible to invasion. Certain colonic bacteria appear to enhance invasiveness, possibly by providing a more favorable redox potential for survival and multiplication or by facilitating the adherence of the parasite to colonic mucosa. Finally, it is known that the pathogenic strains in the tropics are more invasive than those isolated in temperate areas, possibly because poor sanitation results in more frequent passage through humans.

Most infected individuals symptom free

Colonic microflora may influence invasiveness

Virulence increased with passage through humans

PATHOLOGY

Amebas contact and lyse colonic epithelial cells, producing small mucosal ulcerations. There is little inflammatory response other than edema and hyperemia, and the mucosa between ulcers appears normal. Trophozoites are present in large numbers at the junction between necrotic and viable tissue. Once the lesion penetrates below the superficial epithelium, it meets the resistance of the colonic musculature and spreads laterally in the submucosa, producing a flask-like lesion with a narrow mucosal neck and a large submucosal body. It eventually compromises the blood supply of the overlying mucosa, resulting in sloughing and a large necrotic ulcer. Extensive ulceration leads to secondary bacterial infection, formation of granulation tissue, and fibrotic thickening of the colon. In approximately 1% of patients, the granulation tissue is organized into large, tumor-like masses known as amebomas. The major sites of involvement, in order of frequency, are the cecum, ascending colon, rectum, sigmoid, appendix, and terminal ileum. Amebas may also enter the portal circulation and be carried to the liver or, more rarely, to the lung, brain, or spleen. In these organs, liquefaction necrosis leads to the formation of abscess cavities.

Mucosal ulceration with little inflammatory response

Flask-like ulcers extend to submucosa

Amebomas and metastatic amebic abscesses in a few cases

IMMUNITY

Although *E. histolytica* elicits both humoral and cellular immune responses in humans, it is still not clear which, and to what degree, these responses are capable of modulating initial infection or thwarting reinfection. In endemic areas, the prevalence of gastrointestinal colonization increases with age, suggesting that the host is incapable of clearing *E. histolytica* from the gut. However, the relative infrequency with which populations living in these areas suffer repeated bouts of severe amebic colitis or liver abscess indicates that those who experience such infections have protection against recurrent disease.

Patients with invasive disease are known to produce high levels of circulating antibodies. Nevertheless, there is no correlation between the presence or concentration of such antibodies and protective immunity, possibly because pathogenic *E. histolytica* trophozoites have the capacity to aggregate and shed attached antibodies and are resistant to the lytic action of complement. The susceptibility to invasive amebiasis of malnourished populations, pregnant women, steroid-treated individuals, and AIDS patients indicates that cell-mediated immune mechanisms may be directly involved in the control of tissue invasion.

Immunity is incomplete and does not correlate with antibody response

Trophozoites shed antibody and resist complement lysis

Pathogenic *E. histolytica* strains produce a lectin-like substance that is mitogenic for lymphocytes. It has been suggested that this substance could stimulate viral replication of human immunodeficiency virus–infected lymphocytes as does another mitogen, phytohemagglutinin.

AMEBIASIS: CLINICAL ASPECTS

MANIFESTATIONS

Individuals who harbor *E. histolytica* are usually clinically well. In most cases, particularly in the temperate zones, the organism is avirulent, living in the bowel as a normal commensal inhabitant. Spontaneous disappearance of amebas, over a period of weeks to months, among such patients is common and perhaps universal. Serologic data, however, suggest that some asymptomatic carriers possess virulent strains and incur minimal tissue invasion. In this population, the infection may eventually progress to produce overt disease.

Relationship usually commensal

Diarrhea, flatulence, and cramping abdominal pain are the most frequent complaints of symptomatic patients. The diarrhea is intermittent, alternating with episodes of normality or constipation over a period of months to years. Typically, the stool consists of one to four loose to watery, foul-smelling passages that contain mucus and blood. Physical findings are limited to abdominal tenderness localized to the hepatic, ascending colonic, and cecal areas. Sigmoidoscopy reveals the typical ulcerations with normal intertwining mucosa.

Diarrhea, flatulence, and abdominal pain most common

Ulcerations with mucus and blood in stool occur in fulminant disease

Fulminating amebic dysentery is less common. It may occur spontaneously in debilitated or pregnant individuals or be precipitated by corticosteroid therapy. Its onset is often abrupt, with high fever, severe abdominal cramps, and profuse diarrhea. Most commonly, abscesses occur singly and are localized to the upper outer quadrant of the right lobe of the liver. This localization results in the development of point tenderness overlying the cavity and elevation of the right diaphragm. Liver function is usually well preserved. Isotopic or ultrasound scanning confirms the presence of the lesion. Needle aspiration results in the withdrawal of reddish-brown, odorless fluid free of bacteria and polymorphonuclear leukocytes; trophozoites may be demonstrated in the terminal portion of the aspirate.

Hepatic abscess may have acute or insidious onset

Approximately 5% of all patients with symptomatic amebiasis present with a liver abscess. Ironically, fewer than one half can recall significant diarrheal illness. Although *E. histolytica* can be demonstrated in the stools of 72% of patients with amebic liver abscess when a combination of serial microscopic examinations and culture is used, routine microscopic examination of the stool detects less than half of these. Complications relate to the extension of the abscess into surrounding tissue, producing pneumonia, empyema, or peritonitis. Extension of an abscess from the left lobe of the liver to the pericardium is the single most dangerous complication. It may produce rapid cardiac compression (tamponade) and death or, more commonly, a chronic pericardial disease that may be confused with congestive cardiomyopathy or tuberculous pericarditis.

Hepatic abscess may extend to other tissues

DIAGNOSIS

The microscopic diagnosis of intestinal amebiasis depends on the identification of the organism in stool or sigmoidoscopic aspirates. Because trophozoites appear predominantly in liquid stools or aspirates, a portion of such specimens should be fixed immediately to ensure preservation of these fragile organisms for stained preparations. The specimen may then be examined in wet mount for typical motility, concentrated to detect cysts, and stained for definitive identification. If trophozoites or cysts are seen, they must be carefully differentiated from those of the commensal parasites, particularly *E. hartmanni* and *E. coli* (see Table 53–1). *E. histolytica* trophozoites can be differentiated from those of *E. dispar* only by the presence of ingested erythrocytes in the former; the cysts appear identical.

Stools examined for trophozoites and cysts in stained or wet preparations

E. histolytica trophozoites ingest erythrocytes; *E. dispar* trophozoites do not

Recently, sensitive and specific stool antigen tests for *E. histolytica* have become commercially available; their value in the clinical diagnosis of amebiasis, when compared to microscopic examination, is now clear. Although cultural and polymerase chain reaction techniques are somewhat more sensitive, they are not widely available in most clinical laboratories.

Enzyme immunoassay and other methods can detect antigen in stool

The diagnosis of extraintestinal amebiasis is more difficult, because the parasite usually cannot be recovered from stool or tissue. Serologic tests are therefore of paramount importance. Typically, results are negative in asymptomatic patients, suggesting that tissue invasion is required for antibody production. Most patients with symptomatic intestinal disease and more than 90% with hepatic abscess have high levels of antiamebic antibodies. Unfortunately, these titers may persist for months to years after an acute infection, making the interpretation of a positive test difficult in endemic areas. At present, the indirect hemagglutination test and enzyme immunoassays using antigens derived from axenically grown organisms appear to be the most sensitive. Several rapid tests, including latex agglutination, agar diffusion, and counterimmunoelectrophoresis, are available to smaller laboratories.

Extraintestinal amebiasis usually demonstrates high antibody levels

TREATMENT

Treatment is directed toward relief of symptoms, blood and fluid replacement, and eradication of the organism. The need to eliminate the parasite in asymptomatic carriers remains uncertain. The drug of choice for eradication is metronidazole. It is effective against all forms of amebiasis, but should be combined with a second agent, such as diloxanide, to improve cure rates in intestinal disease and diminish the chance of recrudescent disease in hepatic amebiasis. Specific contraindications to the use of metronidazole are given in Chapter 54 in the section on trichomoniasis.

Metronidazole combined with other agents

PREVENTION

Because the disease is transmitted by the fecal–oral route, efforts should be directed toward sanitary disposal of human feces and improvement in personal hygienic practices. In the United States, this applies particularly to institutionalized patients and to camps for migrant farm workers. Male homosexuals should be made aware that certain sexual practices substantially increase their risk of amebiasis and other infections.

Naegleria and *Acanthamoeba* Infections

AMEBIC MENINGOENCEPHALITIS

Primary amebic meningoencephalitis is caused by free-living amebas belonging predominately to the *Naegleria* and *Acanthamoeba* genera. The disease produced by the former has been better defined; it affects children and young adults, appears to be acquired by swimming in fresh water, and is almost always fatal. *Acanthamoeba* meningoencephalitis is a subacute or chronic illness that also is usually fatal. *Naegleria* species are found in large numbers in shallow fresh water, particularly during warm weather. *Acanthamoeba* species are found in soil and in fresh and brackish water, and they have been recovered from the oropharynx of asymptomatic humans.

Meningoencephalitis due to free-living amebas

Warm weather and brackish water favor amebas

Approximately 140 cases of *Naegleria* meningoencephalitis have been reported, primarily in Great Britain, Belgium, Czechoslovakia, Australia, New Zealand, India, Nigeria, and the United States. Serologic studies suggest that inapparent infections are much more common. Most cases in the United States have occurred in the southeastern states. Characteristically, the patients have fallen ill during the summer after swimming or waterskiing in small, shallow, freshwater lakes. The Czechoslovakian cases followed swimming in a chlorinated indoor pool, and several have occurred after bathing in hot mineral water. A recent report from Africa suggests the disease may have been acquired by inhaling airborne cysts during the dry, windy season in the sub-Sahara.

Naegleria infections associated with freshwater swimming

Histologic evidence suggests that *Naegleria* traverses the nasal mucosa and the cribriform plate to the central nervous system. Here the organism produces a severe purulent, hemorrhagic inflammatory reaction that extends perivascularly from the

Passage to central nervous system across cribriform plate

olfactory bulbs to other regions of the brain. The infection is characterized by the rapid onset of severe bifrontal headache, seizures, and at times, abnormalities in taste or smell. The disease runs an inexorably downhill course to coma, ending fatally within a few days.

A careful examination of the cerebrospinal fluid often provides a presumptive diagnosis of *Naegleria* infection. The fluid is usually bloody and demonstrates an intense neutrophilic response. The protein level is elevated and the glucose level decreased. No bacteria can be demonstrated on stain or culture. Early examination of a wet mount preparation of unspun spinal fluid reveals typical trophozoites. Staining with specific fluorescent antibody confirms the identification. The organism can usually be isolated on agar plates seeded with a Gram-negative bacillus (to feed the amebas) or grown axenically in tissue culture. To date, there are reports of only four patients who have survived a *Naegleria* infection. All were diagnosed early; and treated with high-dose amphotericin B along with rifampin.

Purulent bloody cerebrospinal fluid containing *Naegleria* trophozoites

The epidemiology of *Acanthamoeba* encephalitis has not been clearly defined. Infections usually involve older, immunocompromised persons, and a history of freshwater swimming is generally absent. The ameba probably reaches the brain by hematogenous dissemination from an unknown primary site, possibly the respiratory tract, skin, or eye. Metastatic lesions have been reported. Histologically, *Acanthamoeba* infections produce a diffuse, necrotizing, granulomatous encephalitis, with frequent involvement of the midbrain. Both cysts and trophozoites can be found in the lesions. Cutaneous ulcers and hard nodules containing amebas have been detected in AIDS patients.

Acanthamoeba affects older immunocompromised persons

Granulomatous encephalitis with cysts and trophozoites

The clinical course of *Acanthamoeba* disease is more prolonged than that of *Naegleria* infection and occasionally ends in spontaneous recovery; the disease in immunocompromised hosts is invariably fatal. The spinal fluid usually demonstrates a mononuclear response. Amebas can occasionally be visualized in or cultured from the cerebrospinal fluid or biopsy specimens. Fluorescein-labeled antiserum is available from the Centers for Disease Control and Prevention. Definitive diagnosis is usually made histologically after death. *Acanthamoeba* species are sensitive to a variety of agents, but studies of clinical efficacy have not been performed.

More prolonged disease with occasional spontaneous recovery

OTHER *ACANTHAMOEBA* INFECTIONS

Skin lesions, uveitis, and corneal ulcerations have also been reported. The latter are serious, producing a chronic progressive ulcerative lesion that may result in blindness. Infection commonly follows mild corneal trauma; most recently reported cases have been in users of soft contact lenses. Clinically, severe ocular pain, a paracentral ring infiltrate of the cornea, and recurrent epithelial breakdown are helpful in distinguishing this entity from the more common herpes simplex keratitis. The diagnosis can be confirmed by demonstrating typical wrinkled, double-walled cysts in corneal biopsies or scrapings using wet mounts, stained smears, and/or fluorescent antibody techniques. Culture of corneal tissue and contact lenses is frequently successful when the laboratory is given time to prepare satisfactory media. Chemotherapy has generally been ineffective unless given very early in the course of infection. Although a combination of corneal transplantation and chemotherapy may be successful later in the course of the disease, enucleation of the eye may be necessary to cure advanced infections. The drugs of choice are propamidine and neomycin eyedrops administered alternately for a period of several months. Successful use of clotrimazole has been recently reported.

Corneal ulcerations associated with contact lens use

ADDITIONAL READING

Chesley AJ, Craig CF, Fishbein M, et al. Amebiasis outbreak in Chicago. Report of a special committee. *JAMA* 1934;102:369–372. A description of the best-known outbreak of amebiasis in the United States. Fourteen hundred clinical infections and 100 deaths resulted from an inadvertent connection between the water supply and sewage in two Chicago hotels.

Duma RJ, Helwig WB, Martinez AJ. Meningoencephalitis and brain abscess due to a free-living amoeba. *Ann Intern Med* 1978;88:468–473. A useful case report and discussion regarding the taxonomic criteria used to identify free-living amebas producing human disease.

Haque R, et al. Comparison of PCR, isoenzyme analysis and antigen detection for diagnosis of *Entamoeba histolytica* infection. *J Clin Microbiol* 1998;36:449.

Haque R, et al. The global problem of amebiasis: current status, research needs and opportunities for progress. *Rev Infect Dis* 1986;8:218–272. This series of five papers covers the status, epidemiology, pathogenesis, immunology, and diagnosis of amebiasis. It is the most comprehensive review of *E. histolytica* infections.

Moore MB, McCulley JP, Luckenbach M. *Acanthamoeba* keratitis associated with soft contact lenses. *Am J Ophthalmol* 1985;100:396–403. This report of three patients who developed *Acanthamoeba* keratitis discusses the relationship between use of contact lenses and this disease, reviews the literature, and discusses diagnostic and therapeutic approaches.

Petri WA, Singh W. Diagnosis and management of amebiasis. *Clin Infect Dis* 1999; 29:1117.

Sison JP, et al. Disseminated *Acanthamoeba* infection in patients with AIDS: case reports and review. *Clin Infect Dis* 1995;20:1207.

Spice WM, Acker JP. The amoeba enigma. *Parasitol Today* 1992;8:402–406. This brief paper clearly and concisely reviews the evidence for and against the presence of distinct pathogenic and nonpathogenic forms of *E. histolytica*.

CHAPTER 54

Flagellates

JAMES J. PLORDE

Like their amebic cousins, flagellate protozoa are widespread in nature, multiply by binary fission, and move about by means of cytoplasmic organelles of locomotion. Motility, however, is distinctly more vigorous among this group of organisms because of the efficiency of their locomotive apparatus, the flagellum. This organelle arises from an intracellular focus known as a blepharoplast, extends to the cell wall as a filamentous axoneme, and continues extracellularly as the free flagellum. In some species, the blepharoplast is paired with a second cytoplasmic structure known as a parabasal body. This structure is believed to be composed of modified mitochondria responsible for the control of flagellar movement. Both structures stain with nucleic acid stains, and they are known collectively as the kinetoplast.

In many flagellates the axoneme, before exiting from the cell, lifts a segment of external wall into a longitudinal fold. This undulating membrane is thrown into movement as the organism progresses, often imparting to it a characteristic rotary motion. The long, whip-like free flagella may be single or multiple. The number is distinctive for individual species. When more than one is present, each has its own associated blepharoplast and axoneme.

Although a number of flagellate genera parasitize humans, only four, *Trichomonas, Giardia, Leishmania,* and *Trypanosoma,* commonly induce disease. *Trichomonas* and *Giardia* are noninvasive organisms that inhabit the lumina of the genitourinary or gastrointestinal tract and are spread without benefit of an intermediate host. Disease is of low morbidity and cosmopolitan distribution. *Leishmania* and *Trypanosoma,* on the other hand, are invasive blood and tissue parasites that produce highly morbid, frequently lethal diseases. These hemoflagellates require an intermediate insect host for their transmission. As a result, their associated disease states are limited to the semitropical and tropical niches of these intermediate hosts.

NONINVASIVE LUMINAL FLAGELLATES

Luminal flagellates can be found in the mouth, vagina, or intestine of almost all vertebrates, and it is common for an animal host to harbor more than one species. Humans may serve as host and reservoir to eight species (Table 54–1), but only two cause disease. Of these, *Giardia lamblia* inhabits the intestinal tract, and *Trichomonas vaginalis* inhabits the vagina and genital tract.

Found in flora of vertebrates

TABLE 54–1

Luminal Flagellates Infecting Humans

Flagellate	Pathogenicity to Humans	Site
Giardia lamblia	+	Intestine
Dientamoeba fragilis	?	Intestine
Chilomastix mesnili	–	Intestine
Enteromonas hominis	–	Intestine
Retortamonas intestinalis	–	Intestine
Trichomonas hominis	–	Intestine
Trichomonas tenax	–	Mouth
Trichomonas vaginalis	+	Vagina

Morphology and rapid motility are distinctive

These organisms are elongated or oval in shape and typically measure 10 to 20 μm in length. They often possess a rudimentary cytostome (mouth aperture) and organelles such as sucking discs or axostyles, which help them maintain their intraluminal position. They are readily recognized in body fluid or excreta by their rapid motility, and some can be specifically identified in unstained preparations. All can be cultivated on artificial media.

May or may not have cyst stage

Some luminal flagellates, most notably *T. vaginalis,* possess only a trophozoite stage and are passed from host to host by direct physical contact. Most, including *G. lamblia,* possess both trophozoite and cyst forms. The latter, which is the infective form, is transmitted via the fecal–oral route. Human-to-human infection is thus found in populations where inadequate sanitation or poor personal hygiene favors spread.

Trichomonas vaginalis

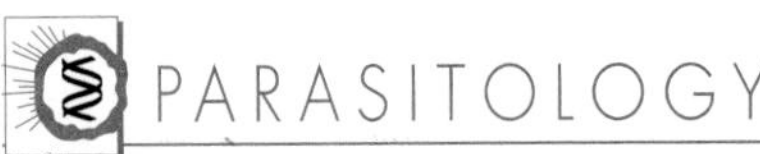

PARASITOLOGY

Three *Trichomonas* species have similar morphology

Three members of the genus *Trichomonas* parasitize humans (see Table 54–1), but only *T. vaginalis* is an established pathogen. The three species closely resemble one another morphologically, but confusion in identification is rare because of the specificity of their habitats.

Protruding axostyle may mediate attachment

The *T. vaginalis* trophozoite (Fig 54–1) is oval and typically measures 7 by 15 μm. Organisms up to twice this size are occasionally recovered from asymptomatic patients and from cultures. In stained preparations, a single, elongated nucleus and a small cytostome are observed anteriorly. Five flagella arise nearby. Four immediately exit the cell. The fifth bends back and runs posteriorly along the outer edge of an abbreviated undulating membrane. Lying along the base of this membrane is a cross-striated structure known as the costa. A conspicuous microtubule containing a supporting rod or axostyle bisects the trophozoite longitudinally and protrudes through its posterior end. It is thought that the pointed tip of this structure is useful for attachment, and it may be responsible for the tissue damage produced by the parasite. In unstained wet mounts, *T. vaginalis* is identified by its axostyle and jerky, nondirectional movements.

Cultivable in vitro

Lacks cyst form but survives a few hours outside host

The organism can be grown on artificial media under anaerobic conditions at pH 5.5 to 6.0. Soluble nutrients are absorbed across the cell membrane. Particulate material, including bacteria, leukocytes, and occasional erythrocytes, may be ingested through any area of the cell surface. A variety of carbohydrates are fermented by pathways similar to those of anaerobic bacteria. Although it lacks a cyst form, the trophozoite can survive outside of the human host for 1 to 2 hours on moist surfaces. In urine, semen, and water,

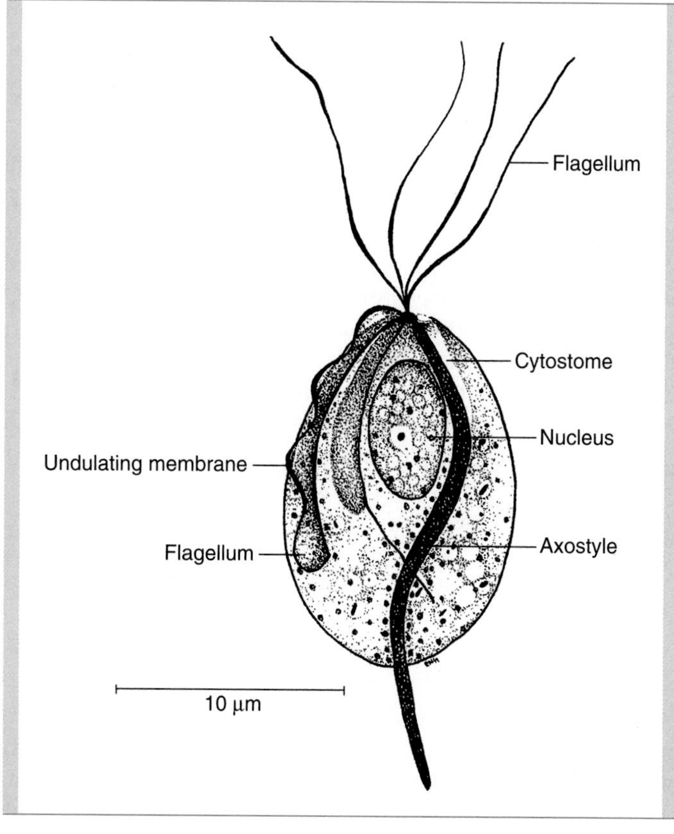

FIGURE 54–1
Trichomonas vaginalis.

it is viable for up to 24 hours, making it one of the most resistant of protozoan trophozoites. Attempts to infect laboratory animals have met with limited success.

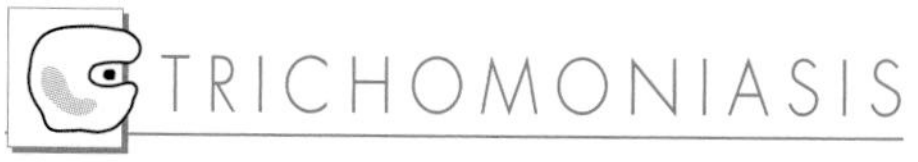

TRICHOMONIASIS

CLINICAL CAPSULE

Trichomoniasis is a sexually transmitted disease, which produces a vaginitis with pain, discharge, and dysuria. The infection fluctuates over weeks to months. Men are usually asymptomatic but may have urethritis or prostatitis.

EPIDEMIOLOGY

Trichomoniasis is a cosmopolitan disease usually transmitted by sexual intercourse. It is estimated that 3 million women in the United States and 180 million worldwide acquire this disease annually, and 25% of sexually active women become infected at some time during their lives; 30 to 70% of their male sexual partners are also parasitized, at least transiently. As would be expected, the likelihood of acquiring the disease correlates directly with the number of sexual contacts. Infection is rare in adult virgins, whereas rates as high as 70% are seen among prostitutes, sexual partners of infected patients, and individuals with other venereal diseases. In women, the peak incidence is between 16 and 35 years of age, but there is a relatively high prevalence in the 30- to 50-year age group.

Transmission usually sexual

Prevalence linked to sexual activity

Nonvenereal transmission is uncommon. Transfer of organisms on shared washcloths may explain, in part, the high frequency of infection seen among institutionalized women. Female neonates are occasionally noted to harbor *T. vaginalis,* presumably acquiring it during passage through the birth canal. High levels of maternal estrogen produce a transient decrease in the vaginal pH of the child, rendering it more susceptible to

Nonvenereal transmission uncommon

colonization. Within a few weeks, estrogen levels drop, the vagina assumes its premenarcheal state, and the parasite is eliminated.

PATHOGENESIS AND IMMUNITY

Parasite damages epithelial cells on contact

Direct contact of *T. vaginalis* with the squamous epithelium of the genitourinary tract results in destruction of the involved epithelial cells and the development of a neutrophilic inflammatory reaction and petechial hemorrhages. The precise pathogenesis of these changes is unknown. The organism is not invasive, and extracellular toxins have never been demonstrated. The expression of a 200-kd parasitic glycoprotein, however, has been found to correlate with clinical manifestations. Changes in the microbial, hormonal, and pH environment of the vagina as well as factors inherent to the infecting parasite are thought to modulate the severity of the pathologic changes. Although humoral, secretory, and cellular immune reactions can be demonstrated in most infected women, they are of little diagnostic help and do not appear to produce clinically significant immunity.

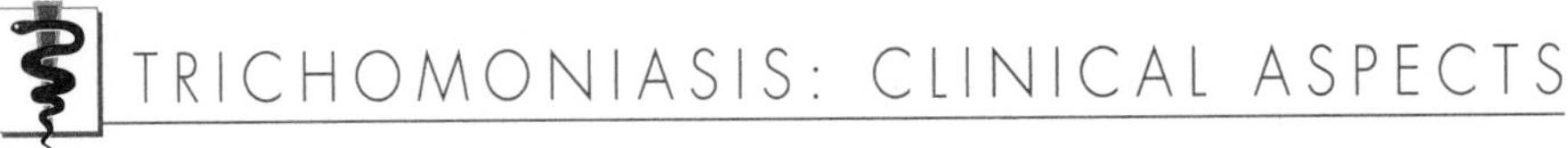

TRICHOMONIASIS: CLINICAL ASPECTS

MANIFESTATIONS

Chronic vaginitis lasting weeks to months

In women, *T. vaginalis* produces a persistent vaginitis. Although up to 50% are asymptomatic at the time of diagnosis, most develop clinical manifestations within 6 months. Approximately 75% develop a discharge, which is typically accompanied by vulvar itching or burning (50%), dyspareunia (50%), dysuria (50%), and a disagreeable odor (10%). Although fluctuating in intensity, symptoms usually persist for weeks or months. Commonly, manifestations worsen during menses and pregnancy. Eventually, the discharge subsides, even though the patient may continue to harbor the parasite. In symptomatic patients, physical examination reveals reddened vaginal and endocervical mucosa. In severe cases, petechial hemorrhages and extensive erosions are present. A red, granular, friable endocervix (strawberry cervix) is a characteristic but uncommon finding. An abundant discharge is generally seen pooled in the posterior vaginal fornix. Although classically described as thin, yellow, and frothy in character, the discharge more frequently lacks these characteristics. Recent studies have demonstrated that trichomoniasis both increases the risk of preterm birth and enhances susceptibility to human immunodeficiency virus (HIV) infections.

Urethral and prostatic infection in men usually asymptomatic

The urethra and prostate are the usual sites of infection in men; the seminal vesicles and epididymis may be involved on occasion. Infections are usually asymptomatic, possibly because of the efficiency with which the organisms are removed from the urogenital tract by voided urine. Symptomatic men complain of recurrent dysuria and scant, nonpurulent discharge. Acute purulent urethritis has been reported rarely. Trichomoniasis should be suspected in men presenting with nongonococcal urethritis, or a history of either prior trichomonal infection or recent exposure to trichomoniasis.

DIAGNOSIS

Wet mount examination for motile trophozoites sufficient in most symptomatic cases

The diagnosis of trichomoniasis rests on the detection and morphologic identification of the organism in the genital tract. Identification is accomplished most easily by examining a wet mount preparation for the presence of motile organisms. In women, a drop of vaginal discharge is the most appropriate specimen; in men, urethral exudate or urine sediment after prostate massage may be used. Although highly specific when positive, wet mounts have a sensitivity of only 50 to 60%. They are most likely to be negative in asymptomatic or mildly symptomatic patients and in women who have douched in the previous 24 hours. Giemsa- and Papanicolaou-stained smears provide little additional help. The recent introduction of a commercial system that allows direct, rapid microscopic examination without the need for daily sampling may ameliorate this situation. Direct immunofluorescent antibody staining has a sensitivity of 70 to 90%. Parasitic culture, while more sensitive, requires several days to complete and is frequently unavailable.

TREATMENT

Oral metronidazole is extremely effective in recommended dosage, curing more than 95% of all infections. It may be given as a single dose or over 7 days. Simultaneous treatment of sexual partners may minimize recurrent infections, particularly when single-dose therapy is used for the index case. Because of the disulfiram-like activity of metronidazole, alcohol consumption should be suspended during treatment. The drug should never be used during the first trimester of pregnancy because of its potential teratogenic activity. Use in the last two trimesters is unlikely to be hazardous but should be reserved for patients whose symptoms cannot be adequately controlled with local therapies. High-dose, long-term metronidazole treatment has been shown to be carcinogenic in rodents. No association with human malignancy has been described to date, and in the absence of a suitable alternative drug, metronidazole continues to be used.

Metronidazole cures 95% of cases

Giardia lamblia

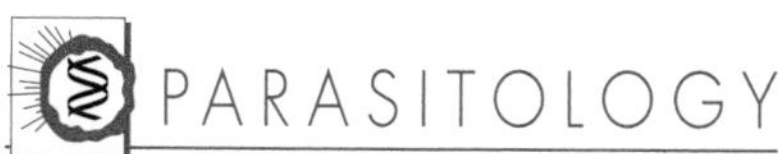

PARASITOLOGY

G. lamblia was first described by Anton von Leeuwenhoek 300 years ago when he examined his own diarrheal stool with one of the first primitive microscopes. It was not until the past several decades, however, that this cosmopolitan flagellate became widely regarded in the United States as a pathogen. Of the six other flagellated protozoans known to parasitize the alimentary tract of humans, only one, *Dientamoeba fragilis,* has been credibly associated with disease. Definitive confirmation or refutation of its pathogenicity will, it is hoped, not require the passage of another three centuries.

Unlike *T. vaginalis, Giardia* possesses both a trophozoite and a cyst form (Fig 54–2). It is a sting-ray–shaped trophozoite 9 to 21 μm in length, 5 to 15 μm in width, and 2 to 4 μm in thickness. When viewed from the top, the organism's two nuclei and central parabasal bodies give it the appearance of a face with two bespectacled eyes and a crooked mouth. Four pairs of flagella—anterior, lateral, ventral, and posterior—reinforce this

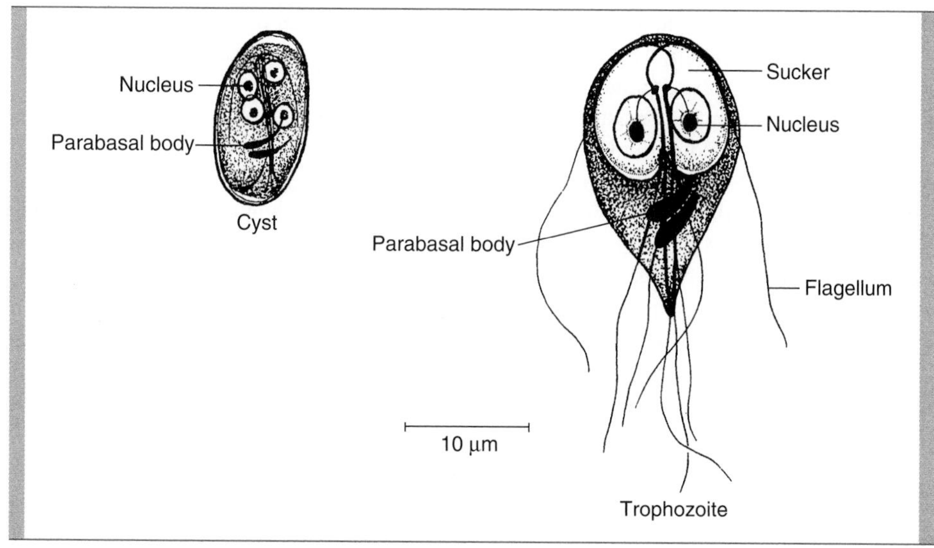

FIGURE 54–2
Giardia lamblia.

Trophozoite and cyst stages

Move about duodenum and jejunum with tumbling motility

image by suggesting the presence of hair and chin whiskers. These distinctive parasites reside in the duodenum and jejunum, where they thrive in the alkaline environment and absorb nutrients from the intestinal tract. They move about the unstirred mucous layer at the base of the microvilli with a peculiar tumbling or "falling leaf" motility or, with the aid of a large ventral sucker, attach themselves to the brush border of the intestinal epithelium. Unattached organisms may be carried by the fecal stream to the large intestine.

Cystic forms develop in colon

Resistant cysts transmitted from host to host

In the descending colon, if transit time allows, the flagella are retracted into cytoplasmic sheaths and a smooth, clear cyst wall is secreted. These forms are oval and somewhat smaller than the trophozoites. With maturation, the internal structures divide, producing a quadrinucleate organism harboring two sucking discs, four parabasal bodies, and eight axonemes (see Fig 54–2). When fixed and stained, the cytoplasm pulls away from the cyst wall in a characteristic fashion. The mature cysts, which are the infective form of the parasite, may survive in cold water for more than 2 months and are resistant to concentrations of chlorine generally used in municipal water systems. They are transmitted from host to host by the fecal–oral route. In the duodenum of a new host, the cytoplasm divides to produce two binucleate trophozoites.

Wide distribution in animal kingdom

Organisms of the genus *Giardia* are among the most widely distributed of intestinal protozoa; they are found in fish, amphibians, reptiles, birds, and mammals. At first, it was assumed that *Giardia* strains found in different animals were host specific; on this basis, some 40 different species were described. As it is now recognized that some strains can infect multiple animal hosts, the practice of assigning species status by the host from which the parasite was recovered is considered invalid. Unfortunately, there is still no general agreement on an alternate method of speciation. Three morphologically distinct groups of *Giardia* have been described on the basis of their central parabasal body morphology.

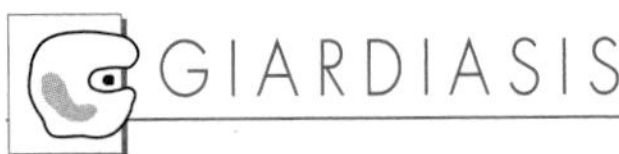

GIARDIASIS

CLINICAL CAPSULE

Giardiasis, an intestinal infection acquired from untreated water sources, is most often symptomatic. When disease occurs, it is in the form of a diarrhea lasting up to 4 weeks with foul-smelling, greasy stools. Abdominal pain, nausea, and vomiting are also present.

EPIDEMIOLOGY

Transmission facilitated by poor hygiene and IgA deficiency

High attack rates in day-care centers

Giardiasis frequent among male homosexuals

Giardiasis has a cosmopolitan distribution; its prevalence is highest in areas with poor sanitation and among populations unable to maintain adequate personal hygiene. In developing countries, infection rates may reach 25 to 30%; in the United States, *G. lamblia* is found in 4% of stools submitted for parasitologic examination, making it this country's most frequently identified intestinal parasite. All ages and economic groups are represented, but young children and young adults are preferentially involved. Children with immunoglobulin deficiencies are more likely to acquire the flagellate, possibly because of a deficiency in intestinal immunoglobulin A. Giardiasis is also common among attendees of day-care centers. Attack rates of over 90% have been seen in the ambulatory non–toilet-trained population (age, 1 to 2 years) of these institutions, suggesting direct person-to-person transmission of the parasite. The frequency with which secondary cases are seen among family contacts reinforces this probability. Undoubtedly, direct fecal spread is also responsible for the high infection rate among male homosexuals. In several recent studies, the prevalence of giardiasis and/or amebiasis in that population has ranged from 11 to 40% and is correlated closely with the number of oral–anal sexual contacts.

Water-borne and, less frequently, food-borne transmission of *G. lamblia* has also been documented, and probably accounts for the frequency with which American travelers to third world nations acquire infection. Unlike the typical bacterial diarrhea syndrome seen in travelers, the diarrhea begins late in the course of travel and may persist for several weeks. More than 20 water-borne outbreaks of giardiasis have also been reported in the United States. The sources have included untreated pond or stream water, sewage-contaminated municipal water supplies, and chlorinated but inadequately filtered water. In a few of these outbreaks, epidemiologic data have suggested that wild mammals, particularly beavers, served as the reservoir hosts. Domestic cats and dogs, which have recently been shown to have a high prevalence of *G. lamblia,* may also act as reservoirs for human infections.

Water- or food-borne traveler's diarrhea lasts for weeks

Beavers and other mammals possible sources

PATHOGENESIS

Disease manifestations appear related to intestinal malabsorption, particularly of fat and carbohydrates. Disaccharidase deficiency with lactose intolerance, altered levels of intestinal peptidases, and decreased vitamin B_{12} absorption have been demonstrated. The precise pathogenetic mechanisms responsible for these changes remain poorly understood. Mechanical blockade of the intestinal mucosa by large numbers of *Giardia,* damage to the brush border of the microvilli by the parasite's sucking disc, organism-induced deconjugation of bile salts, altered intestinal motility, accelerated turnover of mucosal epithelium, and mucosal invasion have all been suggested. None of these correlates well with clinical manifestations. Patients with severe malabsorption have jejunal colonization with enteric bacteria or yeasts, suggesting that these organisms may act synergistically with *Giardia.* Eradication of the associated microorganism, however, has not uniformly resulted in clinical improvement. Jejunal biopsies sometimes reveal a flattening of the microvilli and an inflammatory infiltrate, the severity of which correlates roughly with that of the clinical disease. Generally, both malabsorption and the jejunal lesions have been reversed with specific treatment. The demonstration of occasional trophozoites in the submucosa raises the possibility that these changes reflect T lymphocyte–mediated damage.

Basis for malabsorption and jejunal pathology remains uncertain

IMMUNITY

Susceptibility to giardiasis has been related to several factors, including strain virulence, inoculum size, achlorhydria or hypochlorhydria, and immunologic abnormalities. In one experimental study, humans were challenged with varying doses from as few as 10 cysts. They were uniformly parasitized when 100 or more were ingested. Several workers have noted the frequency with which giardiasis occurs in achlorhydric and hypochlorhydric individuals. Although reinfection is common, the frequent occurrence of giardiasis in patients with immunologic diseases, plus the rarity with which it is seen in older adults, suggests that protective immunity, albeit incomplete, does develop in humans. Animal studies have demonstrated that *Giardia*-specific, secretory IgA (sIgA) antibodies inhibit attachment of trophozoites to intestinal epithelium, perhaps by blocking parasite surface lectins. Moreover, antitrophozoite IgM or IgG antibodies, plus complement, are known to be capable of killing *Giardia* trophozoites.

Predisposing factors include hypochlorhydria and immunocompromise

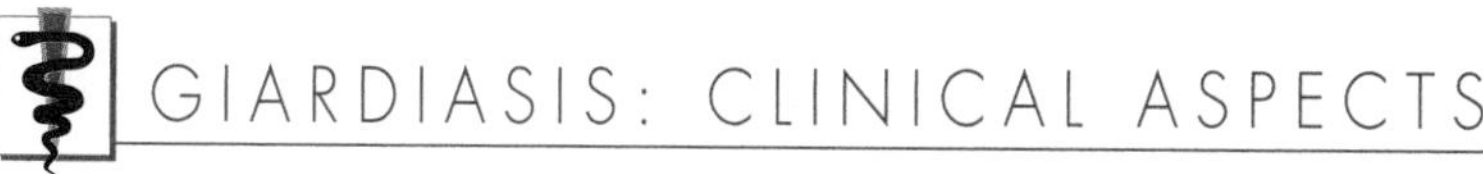

GIARDIASIS: CLINICAL ASPECTS

MANIFESTATIONS

In endemic situations, over two thirds of infected patients are asymptomatic. In acute outbreaks, this ratio of asymptomatic to symptomatic patients is usually reversed. When they do occur, symptoms begin 1 to 3 weeks after exposure; they typically include diarrhea, which is sudden in onset and explosive in character. The stool is foul smelling, greasy in appearance, and floats on water. It is devoid of blood or mucus. Upper abdominal cramping is common. Large quantities of intestinal gas produce abdominal distention, sulfuric eructations, and abundant flatus. Nausea, vomiting, and low-grade fever may be present. The acute illness generally resolves in 1 to 4 weeks; in children, however, it may persist for months, leading to significant malabsorption, weight loss, and malnutrition.

Subclinical infections common in endemic areas

Diarrhea, cramping, flatus, and greasy stools

In many adults, the acute phase is often followed by a subacute or chronic phase characterized by intermittent bouts of mushy stools, flatulence, and "heartburn" and weight loss that persist for weeks or months. At times, patients presenting in this fashion deny having experienced the acute syndrome described previously. In the majority, symptoms and organisms eventually disappear spontaneously. It is not uncommon for lactose intolerance to persist after eradication of the organisms. This condition may be confused with an ongoing infection, and the patient may be subjected to unnecessary treatment.

Subacute and chronic infections with weight loss in adults

Lactose intolerance may persist

DIAGNOSIS

The diagnosis is made by finding the cyst in formed stool or the trophozoite in diarrheal stools, duodenal secretions, or jejunal biopsy specimens. In acutely symptomatic patients, the parasite can usually be demonstrated by examining one to three stool specimens, providing appropriate concentration and staining procedures are used. In chronic cases, excretion of the organism is often intermittent, making parasitologic confirmation more difficult. Many of these patients can be diagnosed by examining specimens taken at weekly intervals over 4 to 5 weeks. Alternatively, duodenal secretions can be collected and examined for trophozoites in trichrome or Giemsa-stained preparations. There are now a number of reliable, commercially available, enzyme immunoassays (EIAs) for the direct detection of parasite antigen in stool. They appear to be as sensitive and specific as microscopic examinations. The organism can be grown in culture, but the methods are not currently adaptable to routine diagnostic work.

Demonstration of trophozoites and cysts in stool or duodenal aspirates diagnostic

EIAs detect *Giardia* antigen in stool

TREATMENT

Four drugs are currently available for the treatment of giardiasis in the United States: quinacrine hydrochloride, metronidazole, furazolidone, and paromomycin. Quinacrine and metronidazole are somewhat more effective (70 to 95%) and are preferred for patients capable of ingesting tablets. Furazolidone is used by pediatricians because of its availability as a liquid suspension, but it has the lowest cure rate. These three agents require 5 to 7 days of therapy. Tinidazole, an oral agent not yet available in the United States, is safe and effective in single-dose treatment. Because of the potential of giardiasis for person-to-person spread, it is important to examine and, if necessary, treat close physical contacts of the infected patient, including playmates at nursery school, household members, and sexual contacts. None of the aforementioned agents should be used in pregnant women because of their potential teratogenicity. Paromomycin, a nonabsorbed but somewhat less effective agent, may be used in this circumstance.

Several drugs available

Close contacts should be examined

PREVENTION

Hikers should avoid ingestion of untreated surface water, even in remote areas, because of the possibility of contamination by feces of infected animals. Adequate disinfection can be accomplished with halogen tablets yielding concentrations higher than that generally achieved in municipal water systems. The safety of the latter results from additional flocculation and filtration procedures.

Avoid drinking untreated surface water

BLOOD AND TISSUE FLAGELLATES

Two of the many genera of hemoflagellates are pathogenic to humans, *Leishmania* and *Trypanosoma.* They reside and reproduce within the gut of specific insect hosts. When these vectors feed on a susceptible mammal, the parasite penetrates the feeding site, invades the blood and/or tissue of the new host, and multiplies to produce disease. The life cycle is completed when a second insect ingests the infected mammalian blood or

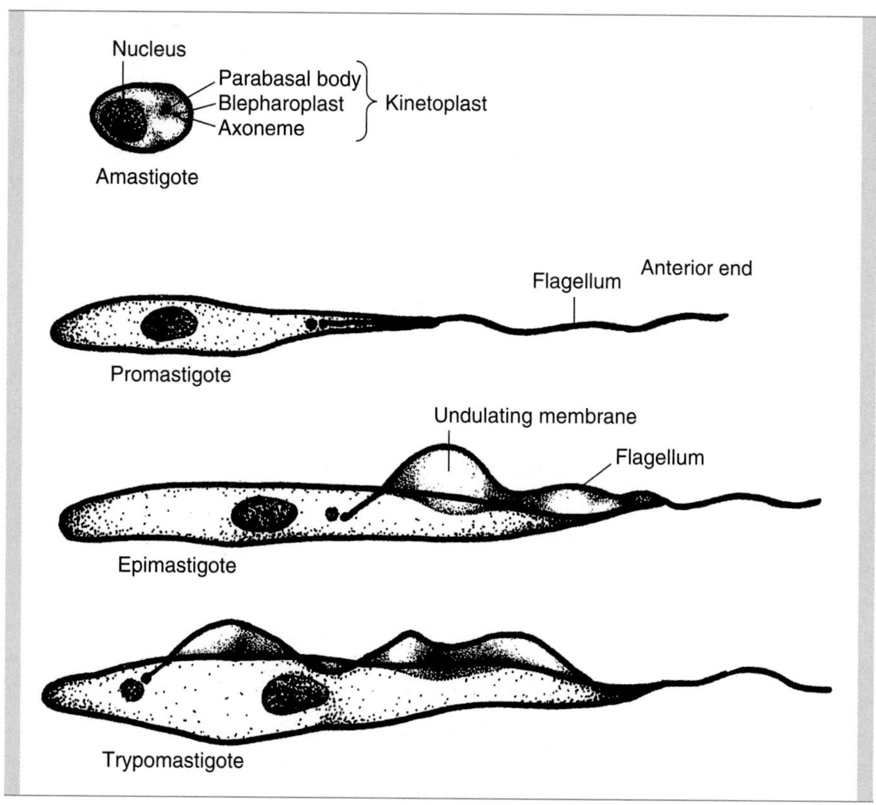

FIGURE 54–3
Stages in the life cycle of the hemoflagellates (Trypanosomidae).

tissue fluid. During the course of their passage through insect and vertebrate hosts, flagellates undergo developmental change. Within the gut of the insect (and in culture media), the organism assumes the promastigote (*Leishmania*) or epimastigote (*Trypanosoma*) form (Fig 54–3). These protozoa are motile, fusiform, and have a blunt posterior end and a pointed anterior from which a single flagellum projects. They measure 15 to 30 μm in length and 1.5 to 4.0 μm in width. In the promastigote, the kinetoplast is located in the anterior extremity and the flagellum exits from the cell immediately. The kinetoplast of the epimastigote, in contrast, is located centrally, just in front of the vesicular nucleus. The flagellum runs anteriorly in the free edge of an undulating membrane before passing out of the cell. In the mammalian host, hemoflagellates appear as trypomastigotes (*Trypanosoma*) or amastigotes (*Leishmania, T. cruzi*). The former circulate in the bloodstream and closely resemble the epimastigote form, except that the kinetoplast is in the posterior end of the parasite. The amastigote stage is found intracellularly. It is round or oval, measures 1.5 to 5.0 μm in diameter, and contains a clear nucleus with a central karyosome. Although it has a kinetoplast and an axoneme, there is no free flagellum.

Life cycle includes insect host stage

Promastigote and epimastigote forms in insects

Trypomastigote and amastigote forms in humans

The flagellated forms move in a spiral fashion, and all reproduce by longitudinal binary fission. The flagellum itself does not divide; rather, a second one is generated by one of the two daughter cells. The organisms use carbohydrate obtained from the body fluids of the host in aerobic respiration.

Leishmania

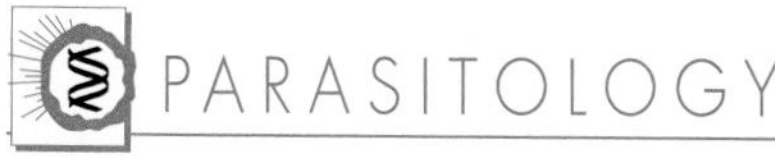

PARASITOLOGY

Leishmania species are obligate intracellular parasites of mammals. Several strains can infect humans; they are all morphologically similar, resulting in some confusion over their proper speciation. Definitive identification of these strains requires isoenzyme analysis, monoclonal antibodies, kinetoplast DNA buoyant densities, DNA hybridization, and DNA restriction endonuclease fragment analysis or chromosomal karyotyping using pulse-field electrophoresis. The many strains can be more simply placed in four major groups based on their serologic, biochemical, cultural, nosologic, and behavioral characteristics. For the sake of clarity, these groups will be discussed as individual species. Each, however, contains a variety of strains that have been accorded separate species or subspecies status by some authorities. The organisms can be propagated in hamsters and in a variety of commercially available liquid media.

Species morphologically similar; differ in molecular features

DISEASE TRANSMISSION

It is estimated that over 20 million people worldwide suffer from leishmaniasis and 1 to 2 million additional individuals acquire the infection annually. *Leishmania tropica* in the Old World and *L. mexicana* in the New World produce a localized cutaneous lesion or ulcer, known popularly as oriental sore and chiclero ulcer; *L. braziliensis* is the cause of American mucocutaneous leishmaniasis (espundia); and *L. donovani* is the etiologic agent of kala azar, a disseminated visceral disease.

Cutaneous ulcer or visceral infection (kala azar) the primary diseases

All four are transmitted by phlebotomine sandflies. These small, delicate, short-lived insects are found in animal burrows and crevices throughout the tropics and subtropics. At night, they feed on a wide range of mammalian hosts. Amastigotes ingested in the course of a meal assume the flagellated promastigote form, multiply within the gut, and eventually migrate to the buccal cavity. When the fly next feeds on a human or animal host, the buccal promastigotes are injected into the skin of the new host together with salivary peptides capable of inactivating host macrophages. Here, they activate complement by the classic (*L. donovani*) or alternative pathway and are opsonized with C3, which mediates attachment to the CR1 and CR3 complement receptors of macrophages. Following phagocytosis, the promastigotes lose their flagella and multiply as the rounded amastigote form within the phagolysosome. In stained smears, the parasites take on a distinctive appearance and have been termed Leishman–Donovan bodies. Intracellular survival is mediated by a surface lipophosphoglycan and an abundance of membrane-bound acid phosphatase, which inhibit the macrophage's oxidative burst and/or inactivate lysosomal enzymes. Continued multiplication leads to the rupture of the phagocyte and release of the daughter cells. Some may be taken up by a feeding sandfly; most invade neighboring mononuclear cells (Fig 54–4).

All four groups transmitted by nocturnally feeding sandflies

Complement activation mediates attachment to macrophages

Intracellular survival by inhibiting macrophage killing mechanisms

Amastigotes released from macrophages can infect feeding sandfly

Continuation of this cycle results in extensive histiocytic proliferation. The course of the disease at this point is determined by the species of parasite and the response of the host's T cells. CD4+ T cells of the T_H1 type secrete interferon-γ in response to leishmanial antigens. This, in turn, activates macrophages to kill intracellular amastigotes by the production of toxic nitric oxide. In the localized cutaneous forms of leishmaniasis, this immune response results in the development of a positive delayed skin (leishmanin) reaction, lymphocytic infiltration, reduction in the number of parasites, and, eventually,

In localized cutaneous disease, cellular immune responses produce spontaneous cure

Mucocutaneous metastases in *L. braziliensis* infections

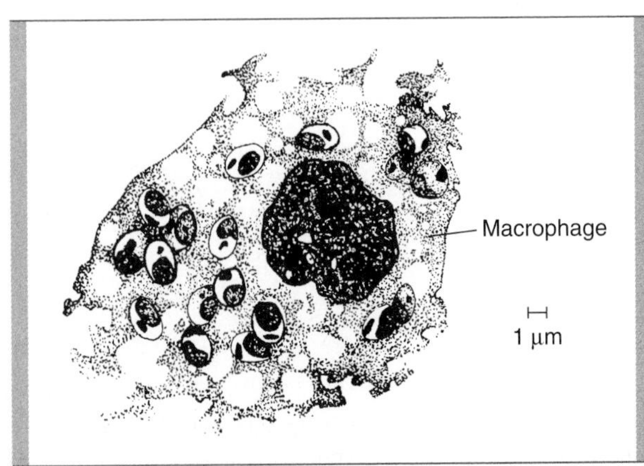

FIGURE 54–4
Leishmania within a mononuclear cell.

TABLE 54–2

Immune Response to Leishmaniasis

Human Disease	Parasite	Leishmanin Skin Test	Number of Lymphocytes	Number of Parasites	Prognosis	Humoral Antibody Titer
Localized skin ulcer (oriental sore, chiclero ulcer, uta)	*L. tropica* *L. mexicana*	Positive	Many	Few	Good	Low
Mucocutaneous lesions (espundia)	*L. braziliensis*	Positive	Many	Few	Poor	Low
Disseminated cutaneous						
Ethiopian	*L. tropica*[a]	Negative	Few	Many	Poor	High
American	*L. mexicana*[a]					
Disseminated visceral (kala azar)	*L. donovani*	Negative	Few	Many	Poor	High

[a] Different subspecies from those causing localized skin ulcers.

spontaneous disappearance of the primary skin lesion. In infections with *L. braziliensis,* this sequence may be followed weeks to months later by mucocutaneous metastases. These secondary lesions are highly destructive, presumably as a result of the host's hypersensitivity to parasitic antigens.

Some strains of *L. tropica* and *L. mexicana* fail to elicit an effective intracellular immune response in certain hosts. Such patients appear to have a selective suppressor T lymphocyte–mediated anergy to leishmanial antigens. Consequently, there is no infiltration of lymphocytes or decrease in the number of parasites. The skin test remains negative, and the skin lesions disseminate and become chronic (diffuse cutaneous leishmaniasis). In infections with *L. donovani,* there is a more dramatic inhibition of the T_H1 response. The leishmanial organisms are able to disseminate through the bloodstream to the visceral organs, possibly because of a relative resistance of *L. donovani* to the natural microbicidal properties of normal serum, and/or their ability to better survive at 37°C than strains of *Leishmania,* causing cutaneous lesions. Although dissemination is associated with the development of circulating antibodies, they do not appear to serve a protective function and may, via the production of immune complexes, be responsible for the development of glomerulonephritis. A simplified outline of the immune responses in different forms of leishmaniasis is presented in Table 54–2.

Lack of cellular immune response in disseminated and chronic infections

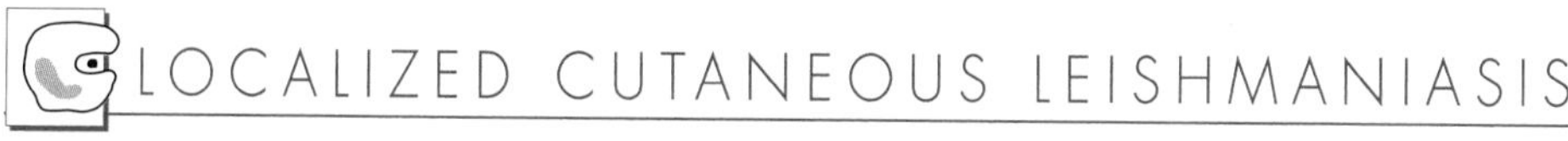

LOCALIZED CUTANEOUS LEISHMANIASIS

EPIDEMIOLOGY

The disease is a zoonotic infection of tropical and subtropical rodents. It is particularly common in areas of Central Asia, the Indian subcontinent, Middle East, Africa, the Mediterranean littoral, and Central and South America. In the latter area, *L. mexicana* infects several species of arboreal rodents. Humans become involved when they enter forested areas to harvest chicle for chewing gum and are bitten by infected sandflies. In the eastern hemisphere, the desert gerbil and other burrowing rodents serve as the reservoir hosts of *L. tropica.* Human infection occurs when rural inhabitants come in close contact with the burrows of these animals. In the Mediterranean area, southern Russia, and India, human disease involves urban dwellers, primarily children. In this setting, the domestic dog serves as the reservoir, although sandflies may also transmit *L. tropica* directly from human to human.

Geographic distribution related to human and rodent reservoirs

Canine reservoir in urban disease

LOCALIZED CUTANEOUS LEISHMANIASIS

MANIFESTATIONS

Chronic, self-limiting skin ulceration

Strain-specific immunity

Lesions usually appear on the extremities or face (the ear in cases of chiclero ulcer) weeks to months after the bite of the sandfly. They first appear as pruritic papules, often accompanied by regional lymphadenopathy. In a few months the papules ulcerate, producing painless craters with raised erythematous edges, sharp walls, and a granulating base. Satellite lesions may form around the edge of the primary sore and fuse with it. Multiple primary lesions are seen in some patients. Spontaneous healing occurs in 3 to 12 months, leaving a flat, depigmented scar. Occasionally the lesions fail to heal, particularly on the ears, leading to progressive destruction of the pinna. A permanent strain-specific immunity usually follows healing. Multiple, disseminated nonhealing lesions may be seen in patients with acquired immunodeficiency syndrome (AIDS).

TREATMENT

Demonstration of Leishman–Donovan bodies or culture from tissue biopsy

In endemic areas, the diagnosis is made on clinical grounds and confirmed by the demonstration of the organism in the advancing edge of the ulcer. Material collected by biopsy, curettage, or aspiration is smeared and/or sectioned, stained, and examined microscopically for the pathognomonic Leishman–Donovan bodies. Material should also be cultured in liquid media. The leishmanin skin test becomes positive early in the course of the disease and remains so for life. Recently, it has been demonstrated that small numbers of *Leishmania* may be detected in tissue by the polymerase chain reaction (PCR), and strains distinguished with probes to kinetoplast DNA. These techniques, although not widely available, permit direct, rapid, and specific diagnosis of all leishmanial infections.

Patients with small, cosmetically minor lesions that do not involve the mucous membrane may be carefully followed without treatment. Pentavalent antimonial agents and liposomal amphotericin B have proved to be effective chemotherapeutic agents for individuals with more consequential lesions. Recently, ketoconazole and itraconazole, alone or in combination with the previously mentioned agents, have been found to be effective in some forms of cutaneous leishmaniasis. Bacterial superinfections are treated with appropriate antibiotics. Prophylactic measures include the control of the sandfly vector by use of insect repellents and fine mesh screening on dwellings.

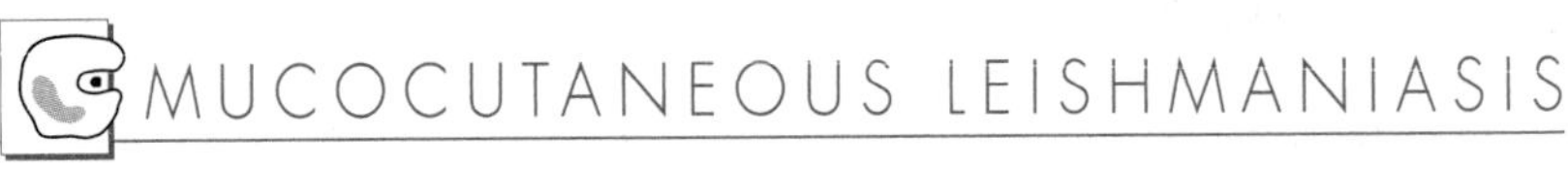

MUCOCUTANEOUS LEISHMANIASIS

EPIDEMIOLOGY

Rodent reservoir of *L. braziliensis*

L. braziliensis causes a natural infection in the large forest rodents of tropical Latin America. Sandflies transmit the infection to humans engaged in military activities, road builders opening jungle areas for new settlements, and others.

MUCOCUTANEOUS LEISHMANIASIS

MANIFESTATIONS

Primary lesion metastasizes to oral and nasal areas

A primary skin lesion similar to oriental sore develops 1 to 4 weeks after sandfly exposure. Occasionally it undergoes spontaneous healing. More commonly, it progressively enlarges, often producing large vegetating lesions. After a period of weeks to years, painful, destructive, metastatic mucosal lesions of the mouth, nose, and occasionally the perineum, appear in 2 to 50% of patients. Sometimes, decades pass and the primary lesion totally resolves before the metastases manifest themselves. Destruction of the nasal septum produces the characteristic tapir nose. Erosion of the hard palate and larynx may render the patient aphonic. In blacks, the lesions are often large, hypertrophic, polypoid masses that deform the lips and cheeks. Fever, anemia, weight loss, and secondary bacterial infections are common. Mucosal lesions caused by other *Leishmania* species may be seen following visceral dissemination in AIDS patients.

TREATMENT

The diagnosis is made by finding the organisms in the lesions as described for localized cutaneous leishmaniasis. Because the propensity to metastasize to mucocutaneous sites is specific to certain species and subspecies, precise identification of the responsible organism as described in the introduction is of clinical importance. The leishmanin skin test yields positive results, and most patients have detectable antibodies. As described for cutaneous leishmaniasis, it is now possible to provide a rapid, direct, species-specific diagnosis through the use of the PCR and probes to kinetoplast DNA.

Treatment is accomplished with the agents described later in the chapter for kala azar. Advanced lesions are often refractory, and relapse is common. Cured patients are immune to reinfection. Control measures, other than insect repellents and screening of dwellings, are impractical because of the sylvatic nature of the disease.

Detection of organisms as with cutaneous leishmaniasis

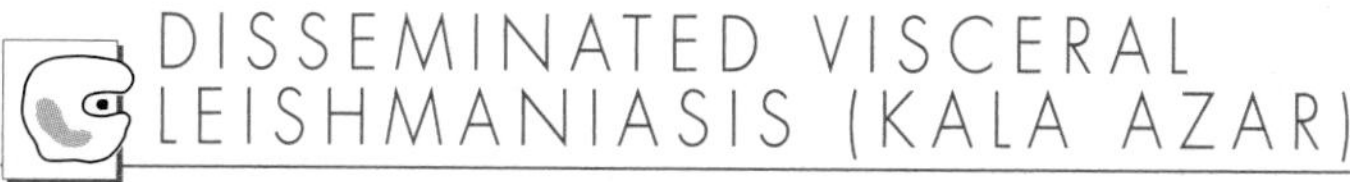

DISSEMINATED VISCERAL LEISHMANIASIS (KALA AZAR)

EPIDEMIOLOGY

Kala azar, which is caused by *L. donovani,* occurs in the tropical and subtropical areas of every continent except Australia. Its epidemiologic and clinical patterns vary from area to area. In Africa, rodents serve as the primary reservoir. Human cases occur sporadically, and the disease is often acute and highly lethal. In Eurasia and Latin America, the domestic dog is the most common reservoir. Human disease is endemic, primarily involves children, and runs a subacute to chronic course. In India, the human is the only known reservoir, and transmission is carried out by anthropophilic species of sandflies. The disease recurs in epidemic form at 20-year intervals, when a new cadre of nonimmune children and young adults appears in the community. There appears to be a high incidence of visceral leishmaniasis in patients with HIV infection. Presumably, HIV-induced immunosuppression either facilitates acquisition of the disease and/or allows reactivation of latent infection.

Marked geographic differences in reservoirs and disease severity

PATHOGENESIS

After the host is bitten by an infected sandfly, the parasites disseminate in the bloodstream and are taken up by the macrophages of the spleen, liver, bone marrow, lymph nodes, skin, and small intestine. Histiocytic proliferation in these organs produces enlargement with atrophy or replacement of the normal tissue.

Parasites invade macrophages of reticuloendothelial system

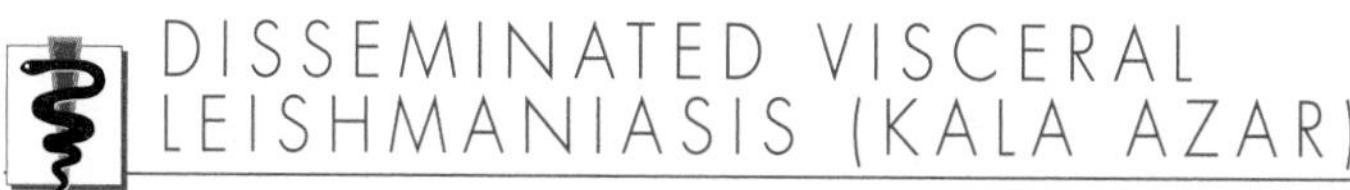

DISSEMINATED VISCERAL LEISHMANIASIS (KALA AZAR)

MANIFESTATIONS

The majority of infections are asymptomatic; these become symptomatic years later during periods of host immunocompromise. Symptomatic disease most commonly manifests itself 3 to 12 months after acquisition of the parasite. It is often mild and self-limited. A minority of infected individuals develop the classic manifestations of kala azar. Fever, which is usually present, may be abrupt or gradual in onset. It persists for 2 to 8 weeks and then disappears, only to reappear at irregular intervals during the course of the disease. A double-quotidian pattern (two fever spikes in a single day) is a characteristic but uncommon finding. Diarrhea and malabsorption are frequent in Indian cases, resulting in progressive weight loss and weakness. Physical findings include enlarged lymph nodes and liver, massively enlarged spleen, and edema. In light-skinned individuals, a grayish pigmentation of the face and hands is commonly seen, which gives the disease its name (kala azar, black disease). Anemia with resulting pallor and tachycardia are typical in advanced cases. Thrombocytopenia induces petechial formation and mucosal bleeding. The peripheral leukocyte count is usually less than 4000/mm^3; agranulocytosis with secondary bacterial infections contributes to lethality. Serum immunoglobulin G levels are enormously elevated but play no protective role. Circulating antigen–antibody complexes are present and are probably responsible for the glomerulonephritis seen so often in this disease.

Delayed onset; recurrent fever; chronic disease; diarrhea

Severe systemic manifestations

Immune complex glomerulonephritis

DIAGNOSIS AND TREATMENT

The diagnosis is made by demonstrating the presence of the organism in aspirates taken from the bone marrow, liver, spleen, or lymph nodes. In the Indian form of kala azar, *L. donovani* is also found in circulating monocytes. The specimens may be smeared, stained, and examined for the typical Leishman–Donovan bodies (amastigotes in mononuclear phagocytes) or cultured in artificial media and/or experimental animals. As described for cutaneous leishmaniasis, a limited number of reference laboratories can provide a rapid, direct, species-specific diagnosis through the use of the PCR and probes to kinetoplast DNA. Results of the leishmanin skin test are negative during active disease but become positive after successful therapy.

Demonstration of Leishman–Donovan bodies or culture

The mortality in untreated cases of kala azar is 75 to 90%. Treatment with pentavalent antimonial drugs lower this rate dramatically. Initial therapy, however, fails in up to 30% of African cases, and 15% of those that do respond eventually relapse. Resistant cases are treated with the more toxic pentamidine, amphotericin B, or liposomal amphotericin B. Allopurinol and interferon-γ have proven to be useful adjunctive therapies in resistant cases. Control measures are directed at the *Phlebotomus* vector, with the use of residual insecticides, and at the elimination of mammalian reservoirs by treating human cases and destroying infective dogs.

Up to 90% mortality without treatment

African Trypanosoma

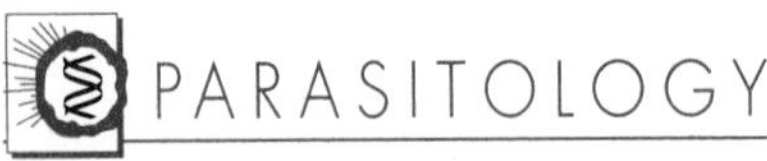

PARASITOLOGY

The trypanosomes that produce these diseases are morphologically and serologically identical. Accordingly, they are considered varieties of a single species, *Trypanosoma brucei*. The three subspecies, known as *T. brucei gambiense, T. brucei rhodesiense,* and *T. brucei brucei,* can be distinguished by their biologic characteristics, zymodeme types, mitochondrial morphology, and DNA hybridization patterns. All undergo similar developmental changes in the course of their passage between their insect and mammalian host. On ingestion by the tsetse fly (*Glossina* spp.), and after a period of multiplication in the midgut, they migrate to the insect's salivary glands and assume the epimastigote form. After a period of weeks they are transformed into metacyclic trypomastigotes, rendering them infectious to mammals. When the fly again takes a meal, the parasites are inoculated with the fly's saliva. In the mammalian host, they acquire a highly variable surface glycoprotein (VSG), multiply extracellularly, and eventually invade the bloodstream. During

Three recognized subspecies of *T. brucei*

Epimastigote and trypomastigote forms develop in tsetse fly

the initial stages of parasitemia, some trypomastigotes elongate to become graceful, slender organisms 30 μm or more in length and divide every 5 to 10 hours. For reasons apparently independent of the host's immune response, multiplication eventually slows. Some forms lose their flagella and assume a short, stumpy appearance. The latter forms have a more developed mitochondria and are thought to be particularly infective to the insect host. Near the end of the episode of parasitemia, both morphologic types may be seen in a single blood specimen. Individual strains of *T. brucei* can change the antigenic character of their glycoprotein coat in a sequential and, at times, predictable fashion. A single strain is capable of producing dozens, perhaps hundreds, of these variable antigen types, each of which is encoded in its own structural gene. The genetic repertoire seems to be strain specific. Expression of individual genes appears to be controlled by the sequential duplication and subsequent transfer of each gene (expression-linked copy) to one or more areas of the genome responsible for gene expression.

Infectious trypomastigote form injected into the bloodstream of mammalian host from fly's saliva

Antigenic variation of glycoprotein coat of trypomastigotes is due to shifting expression of preexisting genes

AFRICAN TRYPANOSOMIASIS (SLEEPING SICKNESS)

CLINICAL CAPSULE

African trypanosomiasis is a highly lethal meningoencephalitis transmitted to humans by bloodsucking flies of the genus *Glossina.* It occurs in two distinct clinical and epidemiologic forms: West African or Gambian sleeping sickness and East African or Rhodesian sleeping sickness. Nagana, a disease of cattle caused by a closely related trypanosome, renders over 10 million square kilometers of Central Africa unsuitable for animal husbandry.

EPIDEMIOLOGY

The tsetse fly, and consequently sleeping sickness, is confined to the central area of Africa by that continent's two great deserts, the Sahara in the north and the Kalahari in the south. Approximately 50 million people live in this area and 10,000 to 20,000 acquire sleeping sickness annually. Major outbreaks have been reported in several locations within the endemic area over the past two decades, due, in part, to the internecine wars in this area that have interrupted control programs. Although an estimated 20,000 Americans travel to endemic areas each year, less than two dozen cases of African trypanosomiasis have been diagnosed in Americans since 1967.

Tsetse fly confined to central Africa

Riverine tsetse flies found in the forest galleries that border the streams of West and Central Africa serve as the vectors of the Gambian disease. Although these flies are not exclusively anthropophilic, humans are thought to be the major reservoir of the parasite. The infection rate in humans is affected by proximity to water but seldom exceeds 2 to 3% in nonepidemic situations. Nevertheless, the extreme chronicity of the human disease ensures its continued transmission.

Humans major reservoir of West African sleeping sickness; chronicity ensures maintenance

Rhodesian sleeping sickness, in contrast, is transmitted by flies indigenous to the great savannas of East Africa that feed on the blood of the small antelope inhabiting these areas. The antelope serves as the major parasite reservoir, although human-to-human and cattle-to-human spread has been documented. Humans typically become infected only when they enter the savanna to hunt or to graze their domestic animals. Currently, Sudan is the only country where both the Gambian and Rhodesian forms of the disease are still found. At present, there is little evidence of coinfections with African trypanosomes and HIV, possibly because the former is primarily rural in distribution and the latter is concentrated in cities.

Savanna antelopes are reservoirs of East African trypanosomiasis; humans infected incidentally

PATHOGENESIS

Multiplication of the trypomastigotes at the inoculation site produces a localized inflammatory lesion. After the development of this chancre, organisms spread through

Local chancre at site of inoculation and lymphadenitis

Intermittent parasitemia with antigenic shifts

Parasites localize in blood vessels of heart and CNS with local vasculitis

lymphatic channels to the bloodstream, inducing a proliferative enlargement of the lymph nodes. The subsequent parasitemia is typically low grade and recurrent. As host antibodies (predominantly IgM) are produced to the surface antigen characteristic of a particular parasitemic wave, they bind to the organism, leading to its destruction by lysis and opsonization. The trypomastigotes disappear from the blood, reappearing 3 to 8 days later as new antigenic variants arise. The recurrences gradually become less regular and frequent but may persist for weeks to years before finally disappearing. During the course of the parasitemia, trypanosomes localize in the small blood vessels of the heart and central nervous system (CNS). This localization results in endothelial proliferation and a perivascular infiltration of plasma cells and lymphocytes. In the brain, hemorrhage and a demyelinating panencephalitis may follow.

High levels of IgM include specific and nonspecific antibodies

Immune complexes may cause anemia and vasculitis

The mechanism by which the trypanosomes elicit vasculitis is uncertain. The infection stimulates a massive, nonspecific polyclonal activation of B cells, the production of large quantities of immunoglobulin M (typically 8 to 16 times the normal limit) and the suppression of other immune responses. Most of this reaction represents specific protective antibodies that are ultimately responsible for the control of the parasitemia. Some, however, consists of nonspecific heterophile antibodies, antibodies to DNA, and rheumatoid factor. Antibody-induced destruction of trypanosomes releases invariant nuclear and cytoplasmic antigens with the production of circulating immune complexes. Many authorities believe that these complexes are largely responsible for the anemia and vasculitis seen in this disease.

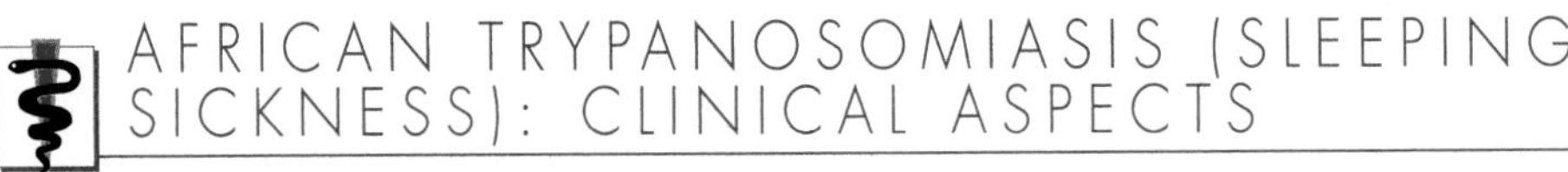

AFRICAN TRYPANOSOMIASIS (SLEEPING SICKNESS): CLINICAL ASPECTS

MANIFESTATIONS

Raised red papule on exposed surface

Parasitemic manifestations 2–3 weeks later

Late CNS involvement

The trypanosomal chancre appears 2 to 3 days after the bite of the tsetse fly as a raised, reddened nodule on one of the exposed surfaces of the body. With the onset of parasitemia 2 to 3 weeks later, the patient develops recurrent bouts of fever, tender lymphadenopathy, skin rash, headache, and impaired mentation. In the Rhodesian form of disease, myocarditis and CNS involvement begin within 3 to 6 weeks. Heart failure, convulsions, coma, and death follow in 6 to 9 months. Gambian sleeping sickness progresses more slowly. Bouts of fever often persist for years before CNS manifestations gradually appear. Spontaneous activity progressively diminishes, attention wavers, and the patient must be prodded to eat or talk. Speech grows indistinct, tremors develop, sphincter control is lost, and seizures with transient bouts of paralysis occur. In the terminal stage, the patient develops a lethal intercurrent infection or lapses into a final coma.

DIAGNOSIS

Trypomastigotes sought in lymph node aspirates, blood, and cerebrospinal fluid

Animal inoculation may be required in Rhodesian disease

A definitive diagnosis is made by microscopically examining lymph node aspirates, blood, or cerebrospinal fluid for the presence of trypomastigotes. Early in the disease, actively motile organisms can often be seen in a simple wet mount preparation coat smear; identification requires examination of an appropriately stained smear. If these tests prove negative, the blood can be centrifuged and the stained buffy coat examined. Inoculation of rats or mice can also prove helpful in diagnosing the Rhodesian disease. The patient may also be screened for elevated levels of IgM in the blood and spinal fluid or specific trypanosomal antibodies by a variety of techniques. A simple card agglutination test, which can be performed on finger-stick blood, can provide serologic confirmation within minutes. Subspecies-specific DNA probes may eventually prove useful for the identification of organisms in clinical specimens.

TREATMENT

Lumbar puncture must always be performed before initiation of therapy. If the specimen reveals evidence of CNS involvement, agents that penetrate the blood–brain barrier must be included. Unfortunately, the most effective agent of this type is a highly toxic arsenical, melarsoprol (Mel B). Although this agent occasionally produces a lethal hemorrhagic encephalopathy, the invariably fatal outcome of untreated CNS disease warrants its use. The ornithine decarboxylase inhibitor, eflornithine appears capable, when used alone, or together with suramin, of curing CNS disease caused by *T. brucei gambiense* without the serious side effects associated with melarsoprol. Unfortunately, it is very expensive and is only variably effective in *T. brucei rhodesiense* infections. If the CNS is not yet involved, less toxic agents, such as suramin, pentamidine, or eflornithine, can be used. In such cases, the cure rate is high and recovery complete.

Selection of drugs dependent on whether CNS is involved

Without CNS involvement, recovery often complete

PREVENTION

Although a variety of tsetse fly control measures, including the use of insecticides, deforestation, and the introduction of sterile males into the fly population, have been attempted, none has proved totally practicable. Similarly, eradication of disease reservoirs by the early detection and treatment of human cases and the destruction of wild game has had limited success. Attempts to develop effective vaccines are currently under way but are complicated by the antigenic variability of most trypomastigotes. A degree of personal protection can be achieved with insect repellents and protective clothing. Although prophylactic use of pentamidine was once advocated, enthusiasm for this treatment has waned.

Neither vector or reservoir control has been successful

American Trypanosoma

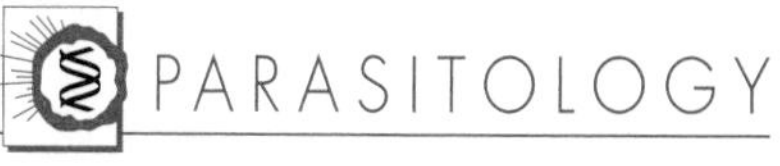

PARASITOLOGY

The trypomastigotes of *Trypanosoma cruzi* closely resemble those of *T. brucei,* and like them, disseminate from the site of inoculation to circulate in the peripheral blood of their mammalian hosts. Their developmental cycle, however, differs in several respects. Most significant, *T. cruzi* does not multiply extracellularly. The circulating trypomastigotes must invade tissue cells, lose their flagella, and assume the amastigote form before binary fission can occur. Continued multiplication leads to distention and eventual rupture of the tissue cell. Released parasites revert to trypomastigotes and regain the bloodstream. This new generation of trypomastigotes may invade other host cells, thus continuing the mammalian cycle. Alternatively, they may be ingested by a feeding reduviid and develop into epimastigotes within its midgut. On completion of the invertebrate cycle, the parasites migrate to the hindgut and are discharged as infectious trypomastigotes when the reduviid defecates in the process of taking another blood meal. This process can recur at each feeding for as long as 2 years. Infection in the new host is initiated when the trypomastigotes contaminate either the feeding site or the mucous membranes.

Mammalian cycle with nondividing extracellular trypomastigotes and dividing intracellular amastigotes

Invertebrate cycle produces trypomastigotes in bug

Reduviid bug may remain infectious for up to 2 years

T. cruzi comprises a number of strains, each with its own distinct geographic distribution, tissue preference, and virulence. They may be distinguished from one another with specific antisera and by differences in their isoenzyme and DNA restriction patterns. All are morphologically identical. In blood specimens, the trypomastigotes can be distinguished from those of *T. brucei* by their characteristic C or U shape, narrow undulating membrane, and large kinetoplast.

AMERICAN TRYPANOSOMIASIS (CHAGAS' DISEASE)

CLINICAL CAPSULE

American trypanosomiasis is a disease produced by *T. cruzi* and transmitted by true bugs of the family Reduviidae. Clinically, the infection presents as an acute febrile illness in children and a chronic heart or gastrointestinal malady in adults.

EPIDEMIOLOGY

Chagas' disease in South and Central America

"Kissing bug" feeds at night in rural areas

Chagas' disease affects 16 to 18 million people in a geographic area extending from Central America to southern Argentina, producing death in 50,000 annually. Within these areas, it is the leading cause of heart disease, accounting for one fourth of all deaths in the 25- to 44-year age group. Transmission occurs primarily in rural settings where the reduviid can find harborage in animal burrows and in the cracked walls and thatch of poorly constructed buildings. This large (3-cm), winged insect leaves its hiding place at night to feed on its sleeping hosts. Its predilection to bite near the eyes or lips have earned this pest the nicknames of "kissing bug" and "assassin bug." Most new infections in these areas occur in children. Infection can also be acquired in utero, and, less frequently, through breastfeeding.

Other wild and domestic animal reservoirs amplify transmission

In addition to humans, a number of wild and domestic animals, including rats, cats, dogs, opossums, and armadillos, serve as reservoirs. The close association of many of these hosts with human dwellings tends to amplify the incidence of disease in humans and the difficulty involved in its control.

Organ transplantation and transfusion-related infections are rapidly increasing problems in urban settings within endemic areas. Recrudescence of the latent infection is increasingly seen in immunosuppressed individuals, including patients with HIV infections. More effective blood bank screening provides hope that transmission of this disease will be substantially curtailed in the near future.

An estimated 50,000 infected Latin American immigrants are currently living in the United States. Because *T. cruzi* has been found in both vertebrate and invertebrate hosts in the southwestern United States, there is a possibility of sustained transmission of this organism within this country. Although serologic evidence suggests that the acquisition of human infection in this area is not uncommon, clinically apparent autochthonous cases have been rare. The majority of these acquired the infection through blood–blood transfusions.

PATHOGENESIS

Local chancre at site of inoculation

Entry to mesenchymal cells facilitated by fibronectin binding surface protein

Pore-forming protein aids escape from phagolysosome

Pseudocysts formed from cytoplasmic multiplication in host cells

Multiplication of the parasite at the portal of entry stimulates the accumulation of neutrophils, lymphocytes, and tissue fluid, resulting in the formation of a local chancre or chagoma. The subsequent dissemination of the organism with invasion of tissue cells produces a febrile illness that may persist for 1 to 3 months and result in widespread organ damage. Any nucleated host cell may be involved but those of mesenchymal origin, especially the heart, skeletal muscle, smooth muscle, and glial nerve cells, are particularly susceptible. Cell entry is facilitated by binding to host cell fibronectin; a 60-kd *T. cruzi* surface protein (penetrin) appears to promote adhesion. Following penetration, the trypomastigote escapes the phagolysosome via the production of a pore-forming protein, transforms to the amastigote form, and multiplies freely within the cytoplasm to produce a pseudocyst, a greatly enlarged and distorted host cell containing masses of organisms. With the rupture of the pseudocyst, many of the released parasites disintegrate, eliciting an intense inflammatory reaction with destruction of surrounding tissue. The development of an antibody-dependent, cell-mediated immune response leads to the eventual destruction of the *T. cruzi* parasites and the termination of the acute phase of illness.

Parasitic antigens released during this acute phase may bind to the surface of tissue cells, rendering them susceptible to destruction by the host's immune response. It has been suggested by some that this results in the production of antibodies that cross-react with host tissue, initiating a sustained autoimmune inflammatory reaction in the absence of systemic manifestation of illness. In the heart, this reaction leads to changes in coronary microvasculature, loss of muscle tissue, interstitial fibrosis, degenerative changes in the myocardial conduction system, and loss of intracardiac ganglia. In the digestive tract, loss of both ganglionic nerve cells and smooth muscle results in dilatation and loss of peristaltic movement, particularly of the esophagus and colon.

Damage to heart may have immune mechanism

Ganglionic and smooth muscle cells lost in digestive tract

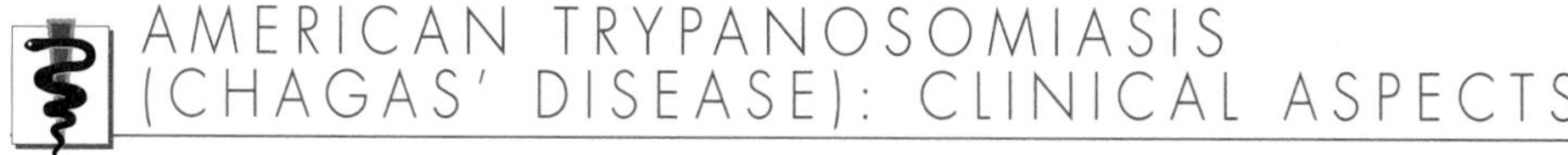

AMERICAN TRYPANOSOMIASIS (CHAGAS' DISEASE): CLINICAL ASPECTS

MANIFESTATIONS

Serologic studies suggest that only one third of newly infected individuals develop clinical illness. Acute manifestations, when they occur, are seen primarily in children. They begin with the appearance of the nodular, erythematous chagoma 1 to 3 weeks after the bite of the reduviid. If the eye served as a portal of entry, the patient will present with Romaña's sign: reddened eye, swollen lid, and enlarged preauricular lymph node. The onset of parasitemia is signaled by the development of a sustained fever; enlargement of the liver, spleen, and lymph nodes; signs of meningeal irritation; and the appearance of peripheral edema or a transient skin rash. In a small percentage of symptomatic patients, heart involvement results in tachycardia, electrocardiographic changes, and occasionally arrhythmia, enlargement, and congestive heart failure. Newborns may experience acute meningoencephalitis. Clinical manifestations persist for weeks to months. In 5 to 10% of untreated patients, severe myocardial involvement or meningoencephalitis leads to death.

Most infections asymptomatic; acute disease usually in children

Myocardial injury indicated by tachycardia and electrocardiographic changes

Chronic disease, the result of end-stage organ damage, is usually seen only in adulthood. Ironically, the majority of patients with late manifestations deny a history of acute illness. The most serious of the late manifestations is heart disease. Studies of asymptomatic, seropositive patients in endemic areas have shown that a significant proportion have cardiac abnormalities demonstrated by electrocardiographic, echocardiographic, or cineangiographic techniques, suggesting that Chagas' cardiomyopathy is a progressive, focal disease of the myocardium and conduction system, leading eventually to clinical disease. This may present as arrhythmia, thromboembolic events, heart block, enlargement with congestive heart failure, and cardiac arrest. In some areas of rural Latin America, as much as 10% of the adult population may show cardiac manifestations. In the United States, chagasic heart disease in immigrants is usually initially misdiagnosed as coronary artery disease or idiopathic dilated cardiomyopathy. Megaesophagus and megacolon, which are less devastating than the heart disease, are typically seen in more southern latitudes. This geographic variation in clinical manifestations is thought to be attributable to a difference in tissue tropism between individual strains of *T. cruzi.* Megaesophagus leads to difficulty in swallowing and regurgitation, particularly at night. Megacolon produces severe constipation with irregular passage of voluminous stools. *T. cruzi* brain abscess has been described in a small number of AIDS patients.

Chronic cardiomyopathy in adults leads to heart block and/or congestive heart failure

Dilatation of esophagus and colon seen in southern latitudes

DIAGNOSIS

The diagnosis of acute Chagas' disease rests on finding the trypomastigotes in the peripheral blood or buffy coat, and their morphologic identification as *T. cruzi.* The methods are similar to those described for diagnosis of African trypanosomiasis. If the results are negative, a laboratory-raised reduviid can be fed on the patient, then dissected and examined for the presence of parasites, a procedure known as xenodiagnosis. Alternatively, the blood may be cultured in a variety of artificial media or experimental animals. In the diagnosis of chronic disease, recovery of the organisms is the exception rather than the rule, and diagnosis depends on the clinical, epidemiologic, and immunodiagnostic findings.

Demonstration of trypomastigotes in peripheral blood

Xenodiagnosis involves allowing bugs to feed

Organisms difficult to recover in chronic disease

A variety of serologic tests are available; small numbers of false-positive results limit their usefulness, particularly when used as screening procedures in non-endemic areas. The recent production of specific recombinant proteins and synthetic peptides for use as antibody targets may improve the reliability of these procedures. PCR techniques for the amplification of trypomastigote DNA are available in a small number of research laboratories.

TREATMENT

Treatment may reduce acute disease

The role of treatment in Chagas' disease remains unsettled. Two agents, nifurtimox and benznidazole, effectively reduce the severity of acute disease but appear to be ineffective in chronic infections. Both drugs must be taken for prolonged periods of time, may cause serious side effects and do not always result in parasitologic cure. Allopurinol, a hypoxanthine oxidase inhibitor devoid of serious side effects, has recently been shown to be capable of suppressing parasitemia and reversing the serostatus of patients with acute disease. Additional studies to confirm these encouraging results are necessary.

PREVENTION

Control of reduviid bugs in rural homes most important measure

The reduviid vector can be controlled by applying residual insecticides to rural buildings at 2- or 3-month intervals. The addition of latex to the insecticide creates a colorless paint that prolongs activity. Fumigants can be used to prevent reinfection. Patching wall cracks, cementing floors, and moving debris and woodpiles away from human dwellings reduces the number of reduviids within the home. Transfusion-induced disease, a major problem in endemic areas, has been partially controlled by the addition of gentian violet to all blood packs before use or by screening potential donors serologically for Chagas' disease. The large number of infected immigrants now entering nonendemic countries presents an increasing risk of transfusion-mediated parasite transmission in these areas as well. Cases of acute Chagas' disease have been reported in the United States in immunosuppressed patients who received blood from donors unaware of their infection status; the resulting diseases were particularly fulminant. Immunodiagnostic tests for Chagas' disease are neither readily available nor sufficiently specific for use in nonendemic areas; prevention will probably require deferral of blood donations from persons who have recently immigrated from endemic areas. Immunoprophylaxis is not available at present.

ADDITIONAL READING

Adam RD. Biology of *Giardia lamblia. Clin Microbiol Rev* 2001;14:447–475. A detailed review of the biology and taxonomy of this pathogen, which leads the author to propose that the major strains infecting humans warrant separate species or subspecies designations.

Adler S. Darwin's illness. *Nature* (London) 1959;184:1102–1103. The author describes Charles Darwin's 40-year illness and offers convincing arguments that it represented Chagas' disease acquired during Darwin's round-the-world expedition on *H.M.S. Beagle.*

Berman JD. Human leishmaniasis: clinical, diagnostic and chemotherapeutic developments in the last 10 years. *Clin Infect Dis* 1997;24:684–703.

Burri C, Nkunku S, Merolle A, et al. Efficacy of new, concise schedule for melarsoprol in treatment of sleeping sickness caused by *Trypanosoma brucei gambiense*: a randomized trial. *Lancet* 2000;355:1419–1425.

Gardner TB, Hill DR. Treatment of giardiasis. *Clin Microbiol Rev* 2001;14:114–128. A recent update.

Legros D, et al. Treatment of human African trypanosomiasis—present situation and needs for research and development. *Lancet (Infect Dis)* 2002;2:437–440.

Leiby DA, Read EJ, Lenes BA, et al. Seroepidemiology of *Trypanosoma cruzi,* etiologic agent of Chagas' disease, in U.S. blood donors. *J Infect Dis* 1997;176:1047–1052.

Petrin D, Delgaty K, Bhatt R, Garber G. Clinical and microbiologic aspects of *Trichomonas vaginalis. Clin Microbiol Rev* 1998;11:300–317.

Prata A. Clinical and epidemiological aspects of Chagas disease. *Lancet (Infect Dis)* 2001;1:92–100. An excellent, brief current review of this fascinating, debilitating New World disease.

Warren KS (ed). *Immunology and Molecular Biology of Parasitic Infections,* 3rd ed. Boston: Blackwell Scientific; 1993. This relatively comprehensive monograph discusses general immune responses to parasitic infections as well as the immunity, immunopathology, immunodiagnosis, and molecular biology of specific parasitic diseases.

CHAPTER 55

Intestinal Nematodes

JAMES J. PLORDE

The intestinal nematodes have cylindric, fusiform bodies covered with a tough, acellular cuticle. Sandwiched between this integument and the body cavity are layers of muscle, longitudinal nerve trunks, and an excretory system. A tubular alimentary tract consisting of a mouth, esophagus, midgut, and anus runs from the anterior to the posterior extremity. Highly developed reproductive organs fill the remainder of the body cavity. The sexes are separate; the male worm is generally smaller than its mate. The female, which is extremely prolific, can produce thousands of offspring, generally in the form of eggs. Typically, the eggs must incubate or embryonate outside of the human host before they become infectious to another person; during this time, the embryo repeatedly segments, eventually developing into an adolescent form known as a larva. In some species of nematodes, offspring develop to the larval stage in the uterus of the worm. The duration and site of embryonation differ with each worm species and determine how it will be transmitted to the new host. In many cases, eggs of nematodes that dwell within the human gastrointestinal tract are carried to the environment in the feces and embryonate on the soil for a period of weeks before becoming infectious. The egg may then be ingested with contaminated food. In some species, the egg hatches outside of the host, releasing a larva capable of penetrating the skin of a person who comes in direct physical contact with it. Obviously, intestinal nematodes are principally found in areas where human feces are deposited indiscriminately or used for fertilizer.

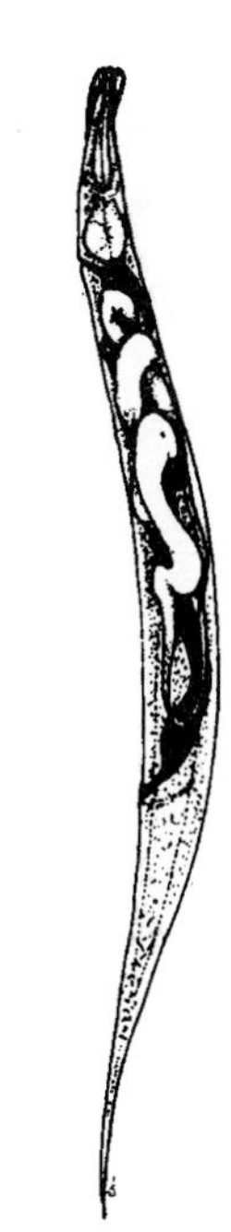

Nematode

Six intestinal nematodes commonly infect humans: *Enterobius vermicularis* (pinworm), *Trichuris trichiura* (whipworm), *Ascaris lumbricoides* (large roundworm), *Necator americanus* and *Ancylostoma duodenale* (hookworms), and *Strongyloides stercoralis.* Together they infect more than one fourth of the human race, producing embarrassment, discomfort, malnutrition, anemia, and occasionally death. Other closely related nematodes of animals that may occasionally infect humans are also listed in Table 55–1, but will not be discussed here.

Long survival in gut lumen

Worm load and repeated infection important to disease severity

The adults of each of the six nematodes listed previously can survive for months or years within the lumen of the gut. The severity of illness produced by each depends on the level of adaptation to the host it has achieved. Some species have a simple life cycle that can be completed without serious consequences to the host. Less well-adapted parasites, on the other hand, have more complex cycles, often requiring tissue invasion and/or production of enormous numbers of offspring to ensure their continued survival and dissemination. Within a given species, disease severity is related directly to the number of adult worms harbored by the host. The greater the worm load or worm burden, the more serious the consequences. Because nematodes do not multiply within the human, small worm loads may remain asymptomatic and undetected throughout the lifespan of the parasite. Repeated infections, however, progressively increase the worm burden and at some

TABLE 55–1

Intestinal Nematodes

Human Parasite	Animal Parasite	Human Disease
Enterobius vermicularis (pinworm)		Enterobiasis
Trichuris trichiura (whipworm)		Trichuriasis
	Capillaria philippinensis	Intestinal capillariasis
Ascaris lumbricoides (large roundworm)		Ascariasis
	Ascaris suum	Ascariasis
	Anisakis spp.	Anisakiasis
	Toxocara canis	Toxocariasis (visceral larva migrans)
	Toxocara cati	
Necator americanus (hookworm)		Hookworm disease
Ancylostoma duodenale (hookworm)	*Ancylostoma braziliense*	Cutaneous larva migrans
Strongyloides stercoralis		Strongyloidiasis

point induce symptomatic disease. Although humans can mount an immune response that will eventually lead to the expulsion of worms, it is slow to develop and incomplete. It is therefore the frequency and intensity of reinfection, more than the host's immune response, that determine the worm burden. This burden is seldom uniform within affected populations, but rather "aggregated" within subgroups related to their hygienic practices.

LIFE CYCLES

Enterobius vermicularis is the best adapted intestinal nematode

The life cycles of the intestinal nematodes are summarized in Table 55–2. *E. vermicularis* (pinworm), the best adapted of the intestinal nematodes, has the simplest life cycle. It feeds, grows, and copulates within the gut of its host before transiting the anus to deposit its eggs on the perineal skin. The eggs embryonate within hours and are subsequently transported to the same, or a new, host via fingers or dust. Following their inhalation or ingestion, the eggs are swallowed and hatch in the bowel lumen, completing the cycle. The only significant difference between this and the life cycle of *T. trichiura* (whipworm) is that the eggs of the latter are passed in the stool and must incubate on soil before becoming infectious. This relatively minor difference has profound epidemiologic ramifications, because *Trichuris* can be passed only in populations that practice indiscriminate defecation and live in climates suitable for the maturation of eggs in the soil.

Other nematodes have increasingly complex life cycles

S. stercoralis is least well adapted

A. lumbricoides is transmitted in a manner similar to *T. trichiura.* However, after hatching from the egg in the gut lumen, ascarid larvae penetrate the bowel wall and migrate through the host's liver and lung before returning, older and more sedentary, to the protective environment of the gut lumen. This maladaptive sojourn of juvenile worms through the host tissue is also seen in the life cycles of the hookworms and *S. stercoralis.* In contrast to *Ascaris,* however, the eggs of the latter two nematodes hatch shortly before or after they are passed in the stool of the original host, resulting in the seeding of the external environment with larval forms capable of penetrating human skin. Transmission is effected when a new host comes into physical contact with the contaminated soil. The adaptation of *S. stercoralis* is the least satisfactory of the intestinal nematodes and, in an evolutionary sense, appears to have occurred quite recently. In addition to the hookworm-like cycle described above, it has the twin capacities to complete its life cycle

TABLE 55–2

Life Cycles of Intestinal Nematodes

Parasite	Route of Infection	Migration in Body	Diagnostic Form	Site of Embryonation	Infective Form	Free-Living Cycle
Enterobius vermicularis	Mouth	Intestinal	Egg	Perineum	Egg	No
Trichuris trichiura	Mouth	Intestinal	Egg	Soil	Egg	No
Ascaris lumbricoides	Mouth	Pulmonary	Egg	Soil	Egg	No
Necator americanus[a]	Skin	Pulmonary	Egg	Soil	Filariform larvae	No
Stronglyoides stercoralis	Skin	Pulmonary	Rhabditiform larvae	Soil; intestine[b]	Filariform larvae	Yes

Reproduced with permission from Plorde JJ. In Isselbacher KJ, et al: *Harrison's Principles of Internal Medicine,* 9th ed. New York, McGraw-Hill, 1980, Table 206–3, p. 891.

[a]Also *Ancylostoma duodenale*.

[b]Intestine only in cases of autoinfection.

entirely within the body of the host or to survive in the external environment as a free-living soil organism.

PARASITES AND DISEASES

Enterobius

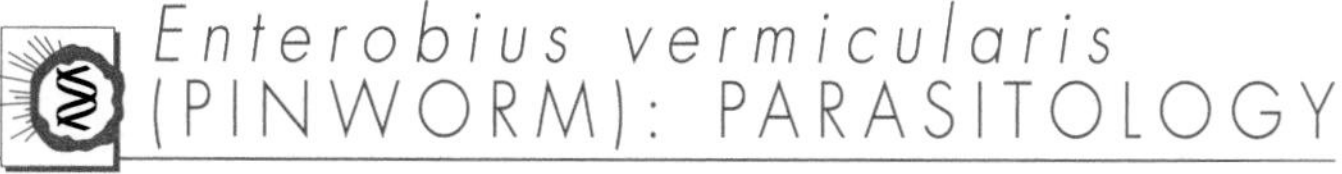

Enterobius vermicularis (PINWORM): PARASITOLOGY

The adult female is a 10-mm-long, cream-colored worm with a sharply pointed tail, characteristics that have given rise to the common name pinworm. Running longitudinally down both sides of the body are small ridges that widen anteriorly to fin-like alae. The seldom-seen male is smaller (3 mm) and possesses a ventrally curved tail and copulatory spicule. The clear, thin-shelled, ovoid eggs are flattened on one side and measure 25 by 50 μm (Fig 55–1).

Common name is pinworm

LIFE CYCLE

Adults inhabit cecum

The adult worms lie attached to the mucosa of the cecum. As its period of gravidity draws to a close, the female migrates down the colon, slips unobserved through the anal canal in the dark of the night, and deposits as many as 20,000 sticky eggs on the host's perianal skin, bedclothes, and linens. The eggs are near maturity at the time of deposition and become infectious shortly thereafter. Handling of bedclothes or scratching of the perianal area to relieve the associated itching results in adhesion of the eggs to the fingers and subsequent transfer to the oral cavity during eating or other finger–mouth maneuvers. Alternatively, the eggs may be shaken into the air (eg, during making of the bed), inhaled, and swallowed. The eggs subsequently hatch in the upper intestine and the larvae migrate

Female transits anus at night to deposit eggs on perineum

Eggs infectious to host and others shortly after deposition

Ingested eggs hatch and larvae mature to adults in intestine

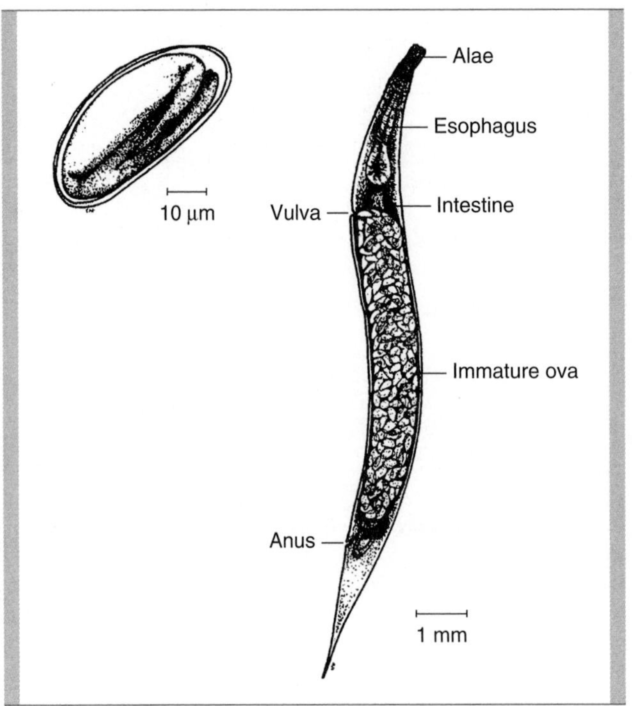

FIGURE 55–1
Female pinworm (*Enterobius vermicularis*) and embryonated egg.

to the cecum, maturing to adults and mating in the process. The entire adult-to-adult cycle is completed in 2 weeks.

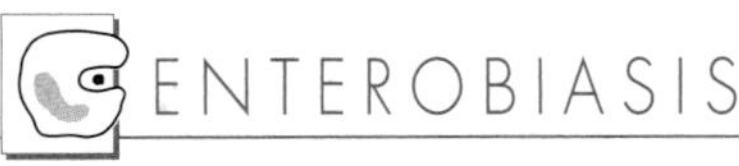

ENTEROBIASIS

EPIDEMIOLOGY

Infects 30–40 million in United States

The pinworm is the oldest and most widespread of the helminths. Eggs have been found in a 10,000-year-old coprolith, making this nematode the oldest demonstrated infectious agent of humans. It has been estimated to infect at least 200 million people, particularly children, worldwide, and 40 million in the United States alone. Despite evidence that its prevalence is now decreasing in the United States, in both that country and in western Europe it remains the single most common cause of human helminthiasis. Infection is more common among the young and poor, but may be found in any age or economic class.

Resistant infective eggs

The eggs are relatively resistant to desiccation and may remain viable in linens, bedclothes, or house dust for several days. Once infection is introduced into a household, other family members are rapidly infected.

PATHOGENESIS AND IMMUNITY

The adult worms produce no significant intestinal pathology and do not appear to induce protective immunity.

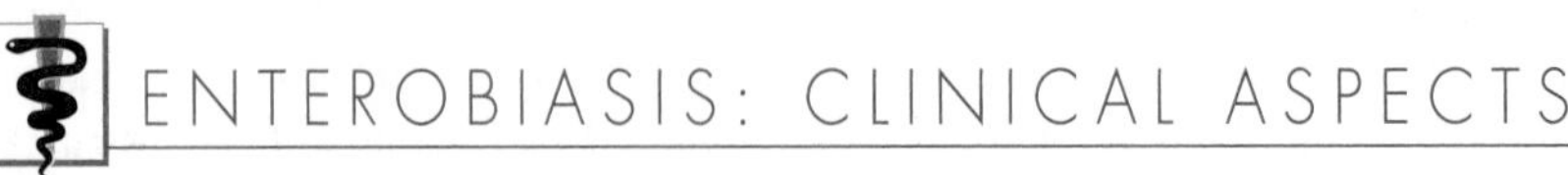

ENTEROBIASIS: CLINICAL ASPECTS

MANIFESTATIONS

E. vermicularis seldom produces serious disease. The most frequent symptom is pruritus ani (anal itching). This symptom is most severe at night and has been attributed to the migration of the gravid female. It may lead to irritability and other minor complaints. In severe infections, the intense itching may lead to scratching, excoriation, and secondary bacterial infection. In female patients, the worm may enter the genital tract, producing vaginitis, granulomatous endometritis, or even salpingitis. It has also been suggested that migrating worms might carry enteric bacteria into the urinary bladder in young women, inducing an acute bacterial infection of the urinary tract. Although this worm is frequently found in the lumen of the resected appendix, it is doubtful that it plays a causal role in appendicitis. Perhaps the most serious effect of this common infection is the psychic trauma suffered by the economically advantaged when they discover that they, too, are subject to intestinal worm infection.

Nocturnal pruritus ani

Occasional infection of female genitourinary tract

DIAGNOSIS

Eosinophilia is usually absent. The diagnosis is suggested by the clinical manifestations and confirmed by the recovery of the characteristic eggs from the anal mucosa. Identification is accomplished by applying the sticky side of cellophane tape to the mucocutaneous junction, then transferring the tape to a glass slide and examining the slide under the low-power lens of a microscope. Occasionally, the adult female is seen by a parent of an infected child or recovered with the cellophane tape procedure.

Anal cellophane tape test detects ova

TREATMENT AND PREVENTION

Several highly satisfactory agents, including pyrantel pamoate and mebendazole, are available for treatment. Many authorities believe that all members of a family or other cohabiting group should be treated simultaneously. In severe infections, retreatment after 2 weeks is recommended. Although cure rates are high, reinfection is extremely common. It need not be treated in the absence of symptoms.

All family members may need treatment

Reinfection common

Trichuris

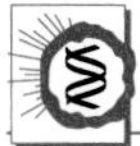

Trichuris trichiura (WHIPWORM): PARASITOLOGY

The adult whipworm is 30 to 50 mm in length. The anterior two thirds is thin and thread-like, whereas the posterior end is bulbous, giving the worm the appearance of a tiny whip. The tail of the male is coiled; that of the female is straight. The female produces 3000 to 10,000 oval eggs each day. They are of the same size as pinworm eggs but have a distinctive thick brown shell with translucent knobs on both ends (Fig 55–2).

Whipworm produces up to 10,000 eggs a day

LIFE CYCLE

Trichuris trichiura has a life cycle that differs from that of the pinworm only in its external phase. The adults live attached to the colonic mucosa by their thin anterior end. While retaining its position in the cecum, the gravid female releases its eggs into the lumen of the gut. These pass out of the body with the feces and, in poorly sanitated areas of the world, are deposited on soil. The eggs are immature at the time of passage and must incubate for at least 10 days (longer if soil conditions, temperature, and moisture are suboptimal) before they become fully embryonated and infectious. Once mature, they are picked up on the hands of children at play or of agricultural workers and passed to the mouth. In areas where human feces are used as fertilizer, raw fruits and vegetables may be contaminated and later ingested. Following ingestion, the eggs hatch in the duodenum, and the released larvae mature for approximately 1 month in the small bowel before migrating to their adult habitat in the cecum.

Adults inhabit cecum and release eggs to lumen

Eggs must mature in soil for 10 days

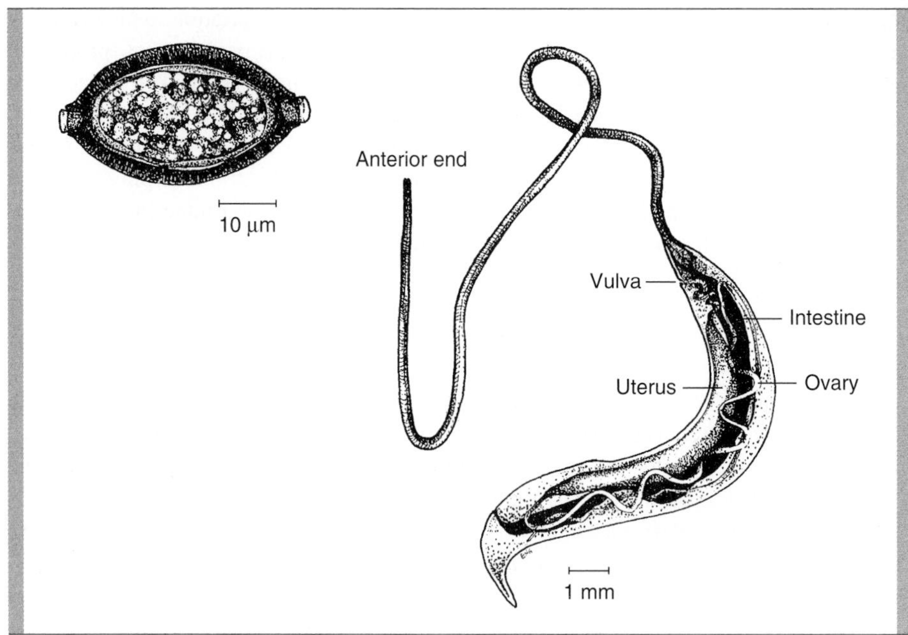

FIGURE 55–2
Female whipworm (*Trichuris trichiura*) and embryonated egg.

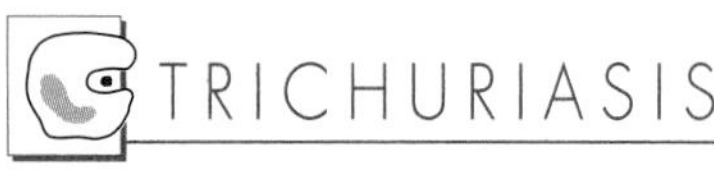

TRICHURIASIS

EPIDEMIOLOGY

Associated with defecation on soil and warm, humid climate

Adult worms live for years

Although it is less widespread than the pinworm, the whipworm is a cosmopolitan parasite, infecting approximately 1 billion people throughout the world. It is concentrated in areas where indiscriminate defecation and a warm, humid environment produce extensive seeding of soil with infectious eggs. In tropical climates, infection rates may be as high as 80%. Although the incidence is much lower in temperate climates, trichuriasis affects 2 million individuals throughout the rural areas of the southeastern United States. Here it occurs primarily in family and institutional clusters, presumably maintained by the poor sanitary habits of toddlers and the mentally retarded. Although the intensity of infection is generally low, adult worms may live 4 to 8 years.

PATHOGENESIS AND IMMUNITY

Local colonic ulceration provides entry point to bloodstream for bacteria

Attachment of adult worms to the colonic mucosa and their subsequent feeding activities produce localized ulceration and hemorrhage (0.005 mL blood per worm per day). The ulcers provide enteric bacteria with a portal of entry to the bloodstream, and occasionally a sustained bacteremia results. A decrease in the prevalence of trichuriasis in the postadolescent period and the demonstration of acquired immunity in experimental animal infections suggest that immunity may develop in naturally acquired human infections. An IgE-mediated immune mucosal response is demonstrable in humans, but is insufficient to cause appreciable parasite expulsion.

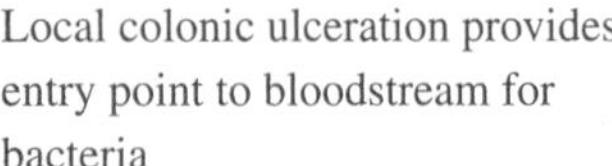

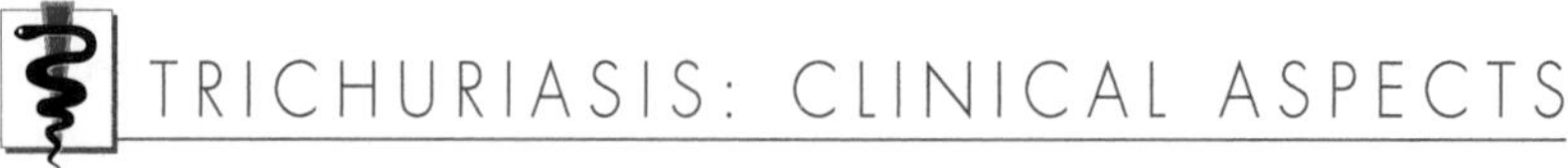

TRICHURIASIS: CLINICAL ASPECTS

MANIFESTATIONS

Light infections are asymptomatic. With moderate worm loads, damage to the intestinal mucosa may induce nausea, abdominal pain, diarrhea, and stunting of growth. Occasionally, a child may harbor 800 worms or more. In these situations, the entire colonic mucosa is parasitized, with significant mucosal damage, blood loss, and anemia. The shear force of the fecal stream on the bodies of the worms may produce prolapse of the colonic or rectal mucosa through the anus, particularly when the host is straining at defecation or during childbirth.

Colonic damage with abdominal pain and diarrhea

Colonic or rectal prolapse with heavy worm load

DIAGNOSIS

In light infections, stool concentration methods may be required to recover the eggs. Such procedures are almost never necessary in symptomatic infections, as they inevitably produce more than 10,000 eggs per gram of feces, a density readily detected by examining 1 to 2 mg of emulsified stool with the low-power lens of a microscope. A moderate eosinophilia is common in such infections.

Stools examined for characteristic eggs

TREATMENT AND PREVENTION

Infections should not be treated unless they are symptomatic. Mebendazole is the drug of choice; albendazole is thought to be equally effective. Although the cure rate is only 60 to 70%, more than 90% of the adult worms are usually expelled, rendering the patient asymptomatic. Prevention requires the improvement of sanitary facilities.

Ascaris

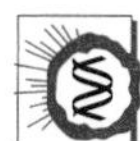

Ascaris lumbricoides: PARASITOLOGY

A. lumbricoides, a short-lived worm (6 to 18 months), is the largest and most common of the intestinal helminths. Measuring 15 to 40 cm in length, it dwarfs its fellow gut roundworms and brings an unexpected richness to our mental image of a parasite. Its firm, creamy cuticle and more pointed extremities differentiate it from the common earthworm, which it otherwise resembles in both size and external morphology. The male is slightly smaller than the female and possesses a curved tail with copulatory spicules. The female passes 200,000 eggs daily, whether or not she is fertilized. Eggs are elliptic in shape; measure 35 by 55 μm; and have a rough, mamillated, albuminous coat over their chitinous shells. They are highly resistant to environmental conditions and may remain viable for up to 6 years in mild climates (Fig 55–3).

Earthworm-sized roundworm produces elliptical eggs

Eggs viable up to 6 years

LIFE CYCLE

The adult ascarids live high in the small intestine, where they actively maintain themselves by dint of muscular activity. The eggs are deposited into the intestinal lumen and passed in the feces. Like those of *Trichuris,* the eggs must embryonate in soil, usually for a minimum of 3 weeks, before becoming infectious. The similarity to *Trichuris* ends, however, with the ingestion of the eggs by the host. After hatching, the larvae penetrate the intestinal mucosa and invade the portal venules. They are carried to the liver, where they are still small enough to squeeze through that organ's capillaries and exit in the hepatic vein. They are then carried to the right side of the heart and subsequently pumped out to the lung. In the course of this migration, the larvae increase in size. By the time they reach the pulmonary capillaries, they are too large to pass through to the left side of the heart. Finding their route blocked, they rupture into the alveolar spaces, are coughed up, and subsequently swallowed. After regaining access to the upper intestine, they complete their maturation and mate.

Adults inhabit small intestine

Eggs must mature for 3 weeks in soil

Larvae from ingested eggs enter bloodstream and pass through alveoli and via respiratory tract and esophagus to intestines

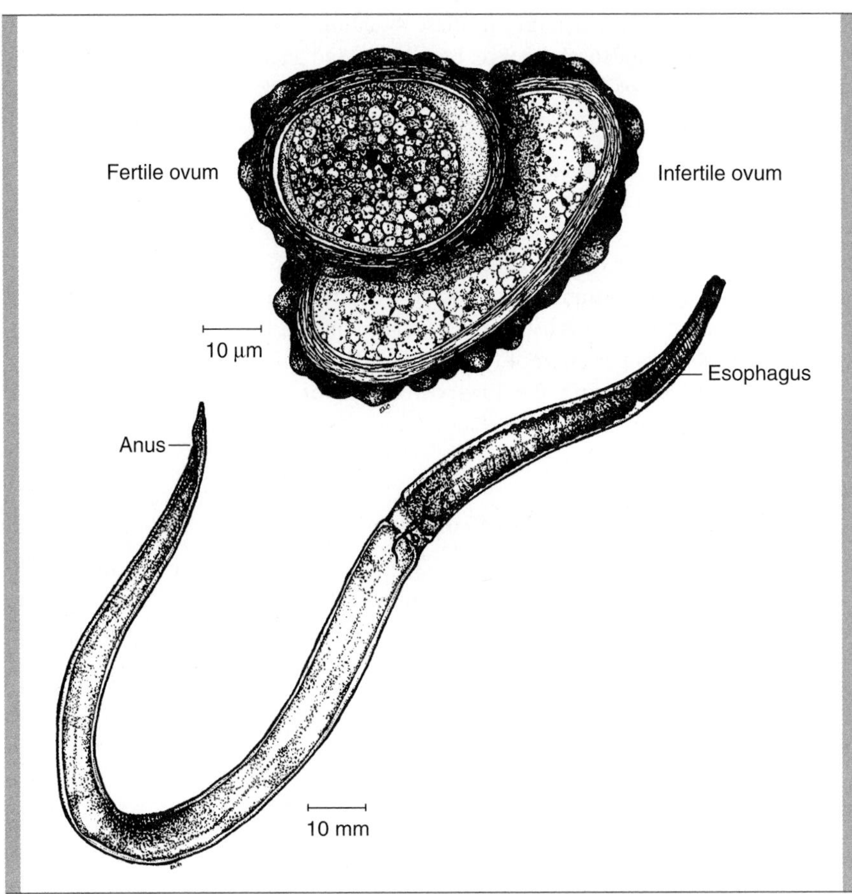

FIGURE 55–3
Female *Ascaris lumbricoides* worm and fertile and infertile egg.

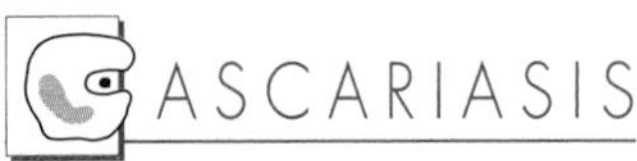

ASCARIASIS

EPIDEMIOLOGY

Epidemiology similar to that of *Trichuris*

More than 1 billion of the world's population, including 4 million Americans, are infected. Together they have been estimated to pass more than 25,000 tons of *Ascaris* eggs into the environment annually. Like trichuriasis, with which it is coextensive, ascariasis is a disease of warm climates and poor sanitation. It is maintained by small children who defecate indiscriminately in the immediate vicinity of the home and pick up infectious eggs on their hands during play. Geophagia may result in massive worm loads. The parasite may also be acquired through ingestion of egg-contaminated food by the host; in dry, windy climates, eggs may become airborne and be inhaled and swallowed. In tropical areas, the entire population may be involved; most worms, however, appear to be aggregated in a minority of the population, suggesting that some individuals are predisposed to heavy infections. Isolated infected family clusters are more common in temperature climates.

PATHOGENESIS AND IMMUNITY

Hypersensitive pulmonary reactions to larval migration

There is convincing evidence that ascariasis induces a protective immune response in the host. Moreover, the severity of pulmonary damage induced by the migration of larvae through the lung appears to be related in part to an immediate hypersensitivity reaction to larval antigens.

ASCARIASIS: CLINICAL ASPECTS

MANIFESTATIONS

Clinical manifestations may result from either the migration of the larvae through the lung or the presence of the adults in the intestinal lumen. Pulmonary involvement is usually seen in communities where transmission is seasonal; the severity of symptoms is related to the degree of hypersensitivity induced by previous infections and the intensity of the current exposure. Fever, cough, wheezing, and shortness of breath are common. Laboratory studies reveal eosinophilia, oxygen denaturation, and migratory pulmonary infiltrates. Death from respiratory failure has been noted occasionally.

Infections asymptomatic with small worm loads

Malabsorption and occasional obstruction produced with heavy worm loads

If the worm load is small, infections with adult worms may be completely asymptomatic. They come to clinical attention when the parasite is vomited up or passed in the stool. This situation is most likely during episodes of fever, which appear to stimulate the worms to increase motility. Most physicians who have worked in developing countries have had the disconcerting experience of observing an ascarid crawl out of a patient's mouth, nose, or ear during an otherwise uneventful evaluation of fever. Occasionally, an adult worm migrates to the appendix, bile duct, or pancreatic duct, causing obstruction and inflammation of the organ. Heavier worm loads may produce abdominal pain and malabsorption of fat, protein, carbohydrate, and vitamins. In marginally nourished children, growth may be retarded. Occasionally a bolus of worms may form and produce intestinal obstruction, particularly in children. Worm loads of 50 are not uncommon, and as many as 2000 worms have been recovered from a single child. In the United States, where worm loads tend to be modest, obstruction occurs in 2 per 1000 infected children per year. The mortality in these cases is 3%. Estimates of deaths from ascariasis range from 8000 to 100,000 annually worldwide.

DIAGNOSIS

Stool examination readily reveals characteristic eggs

The diagnosis is generally made by finding the characteristic eggs in the feces. The extreme productivity of the female ascarid generally makes this task an easy one, except when the atypical-appearing unfertilized eggs predominate. The pulmonary phase of ascariasis is diagnosed by the finding of larvae and eosinophils in the sputum.

TREATMENT AND PREVENTION

Albendazole, mebendazole and pyrantel pamoate are highly effective; the first two are preferred if *T. trichiura* is also present. Community-wide control of ascariasis can be achieved with mass therapy administered at 6-month intervals. Ultimately, control requires adequate sanitation facilities.

Hookworms

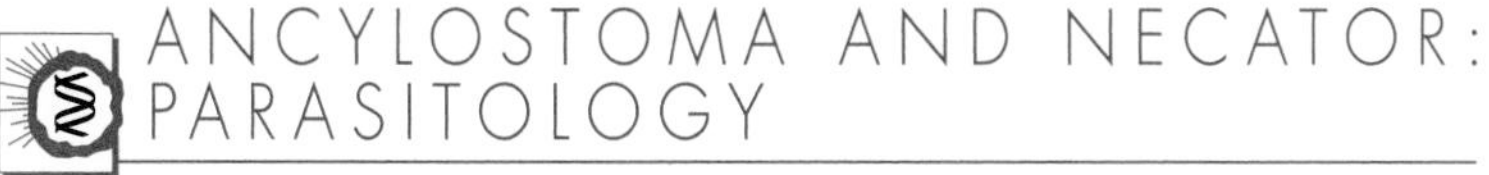

ANCYLOSTOMA AND NECATOR: PARASITOLOGY

Two species, *N. americanus* and *A. duodenale,* infect humans. Adults of both species are pinkish-white and measure about 10 mm in length (Fig 55–4). The head is often curved in a direction opposite that of the body, giving these worms the hooked appearance from which their common name is derived. The males have a unique fan-shaped copulatory bursa, rather than the curved, pointed tail common to the other intestinal nematodes. The

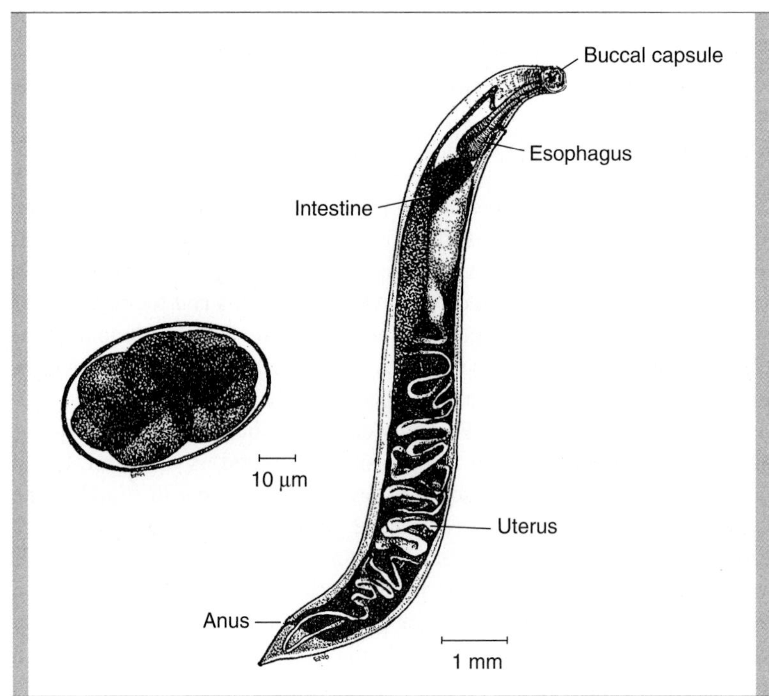

FIGURE 55–4
Female hookworm (*Necator americanus*) and egg.

N. americanus and *A. duodenale* infect humans

Species differentiated by morphology of oral cavity

two species can be readily differentiated by the morphology of their oral cavity. *A. duodenale,* the Old World hookworm, possesses four sharp toothlike structures, whereas *N. americanus,* the New World hookworm, has dorsal and ventral cutting plates. With the aid of these structures, the hookworms attach to the mucosa of the small bowel and suck blood. The fertilized female releases 10,000 to 20,000 eggs daily. They measure 40 by 60 μm, possess a thin shell, and are usually in the two- to four-cell stage when passed in the feces (see Fig 55–4).

LIFE CYCLE

In soil, eggs mature and release rhabditiform larvae that molt to produce infective filariform larvae

Filariform larvae penetrate skin and then follow same path as *Ascaris* larvae to gut

For all practical purposes, the life cycles of the two hookworms, *N. americanus* and *A. duodenale,* are identical. The eggs are passed in the feces at the 4- to 8-cell stage of development and, on reaching soil, hatch within 48 hours, releasing rhabditiform larvae. These move actively through the surface layers of soil, feeding on bacteria and debris. After doubling in size, they molt to become infective filariform larvae, which may survive in moist conditions without feeding, for up to 6 weeks. On contact with human skin, they penetrate the epidermis, reach the lymphohematogenous system, and are passively transported to the right side of the heart and onward to the lungs. Here they rupture into alveolar spaces and, like juvenile ascarids, are coughed up, swallowed, and pass into the small intestine, where they mature to adulthood. Larvae of *A. duodenale,* if swallowed, can survive passage through the stomach and develop into adult worms in the small intestine.

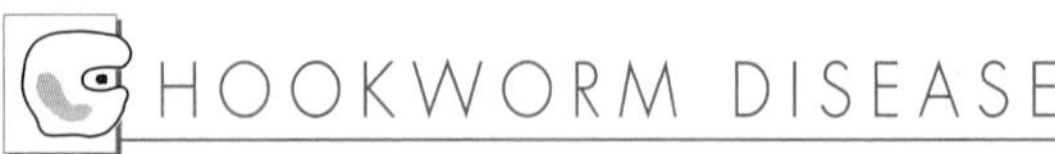

HOOKWORM DISEASE

EPIDEMIOLOGY

Hookworm infection is found worldwide between the latitudes of 45°N and 30°S. Transmission requires deposition of egg-containing feces on shady, well-drained soil; development of larvae under conditions of abundant rainfall and high temperatures (23 to 33°C); and direct contact of unprotected human skin with resulting filariform larvae. Infections become particularly intense in closed, densely populated communities, such as tea and coffee plantations. *N. americanus* is found in the tropical areas of South Asia, Africa, and America, as well as the southern United States, where it was introduced with the African slave trade. *A. duodenale* is seen in the Mediterranean basin, the Middle East, northern India, China, and Japan. It has been estimated that together these two worms extract over 7 million L of blood each day from 700 million individuals scattered around the globe, including 700,000 in the United States, leading to 50,000 to 60,000 deaths annually.

Larvae require hot, moist conditions

Limited to tropical areas and southern United States

PATHOGENESIS AND IMMUNITY

Each adult *A. duodenale* extracts 0.2 mL of blood daily and *N. americanus* 0.03 mL of blood. Additional blood loss may be related to the tendency of the worms to migrate within the intestine, leaving bleeding points at old sites of attachment. Because the adults may survive 2 to 14 years, the accumulated blood loss may be enormous. The infection elicits both a humoral antibody response and immediate hypersensitivity reaction in the host, but evidence that these moderate the infection is lacking. The peripheral and gut eosinophilia characteristic of this disease may play a role in the destruction of worms and/or modulation of the immediate hypersensitivity reaction.

Adult worms live in gut for years

Blood loss significant

Produce peripheral and gut eosinophilia

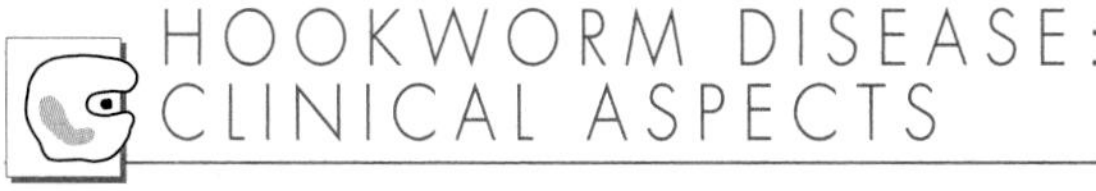

HOOKWORM DISEASE: CLINICAL ASPECTS

MANIFESTATIONS

In the overwhelming majority of infected patients, the worm burden is small and the infection asymptomatic. Clinical manifestations, when they do occur, may be related to the original penetration of the skin by the filariform larva, the migration of the larva through the lung, and/or the presence of the adult worm in the gut. Skin penetration may produce a pruritic erythematous rash and swelling, popularly known as ground itch. This manifestation is more common in infection with *N. americanus,* generally occurs between the toes, and may persist for several days. It is probably the result of prior sensitization to larval antigens.

Most infections asymptomatic depending on worm load

Pruritus at site of skin penetration

Pulmonary manifestations may mimic those seen in ascariasis, but are generally less frequent and less severe. In the gut, the adult worm may produce epigastric pain and abnormal peristalsis. The major manifestations, however—anemia and hypoalbuminemia—are the result of chronic blood loss. The severity of the anemia depends on the worm burden and intake of dietary iron. If iron intake exceeds iron loss resulting from hookworm infection, a normal hematocrit will be maintained. Commonly, however, dietary iron is ingested in a form that is poorly absorbed. As a result, severe anemia may develop over a period of months or years. In children, this condition may often precipitate heart failure or kwashiorkor. Mental, sexual, and physical development may be retarded.

Iron deficiency anemia caused by blood loss from intestinal worms

DIAGNOSIS

The diagnosis is made by examining direct or concentrated stool for the distinctive eggs. As they are nearly identical in the two species, precise identification of the causative worm is generally not attempted. Quantitative egg counts can permit accurate estimation of worm load. If the stool is allowed to stand too long before it is examined, the eggs may hatch, releasing rhabditiform larvae. These larvae closely resemble those of *S. stercoralis* and must be differentiated from them.

Eggs of both species look the same

TREATMENT AND PREVENTION

The anemia must be corrected. When it is mild or moderate, iron replacement is adequate. More severe anemia may require blood transfusions. The three most widely used anthelmintic agents, pyrantel pamoate, mebendazole and albendazole, are all highly effective. Prevention requires improved sanitation.

Strongyloides

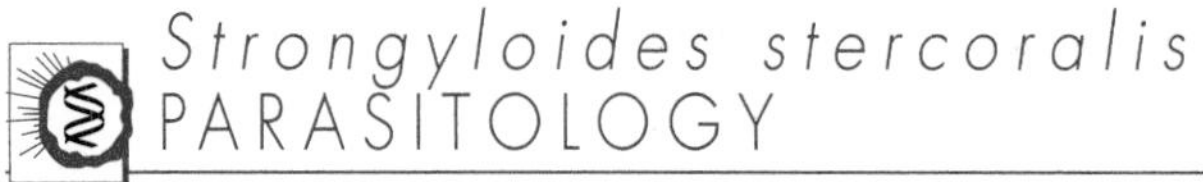

Strongyloides stercoralis: PARASITOLOGY

Larvae differ slightly from hookworm

S. stercoralis adults measure only 2 mm in length, making them the smallest of the intestinal nematodes. The male is seldom seen within the human host, leading some authorities to believe that the female can conceive parthenogenetically in this environment. Be that as it may, the gravid female penetrates the mucosa of the duodenum, where she deposits her eggs. In severe infections, the biliary and pancreatic ducts, the entire small bowel, and the colon may be involved. The eggs hatch quickly, releasing rhabditiform larvae that reenter the bowel lumen and are subsequently passed into the stool. These larvae, which measure about 16 by 200 μm, can be distinguished from the similar larval stage of the hookworms by their short buccal cavity and large genital primordium (Figs 55–5 and 55–6).

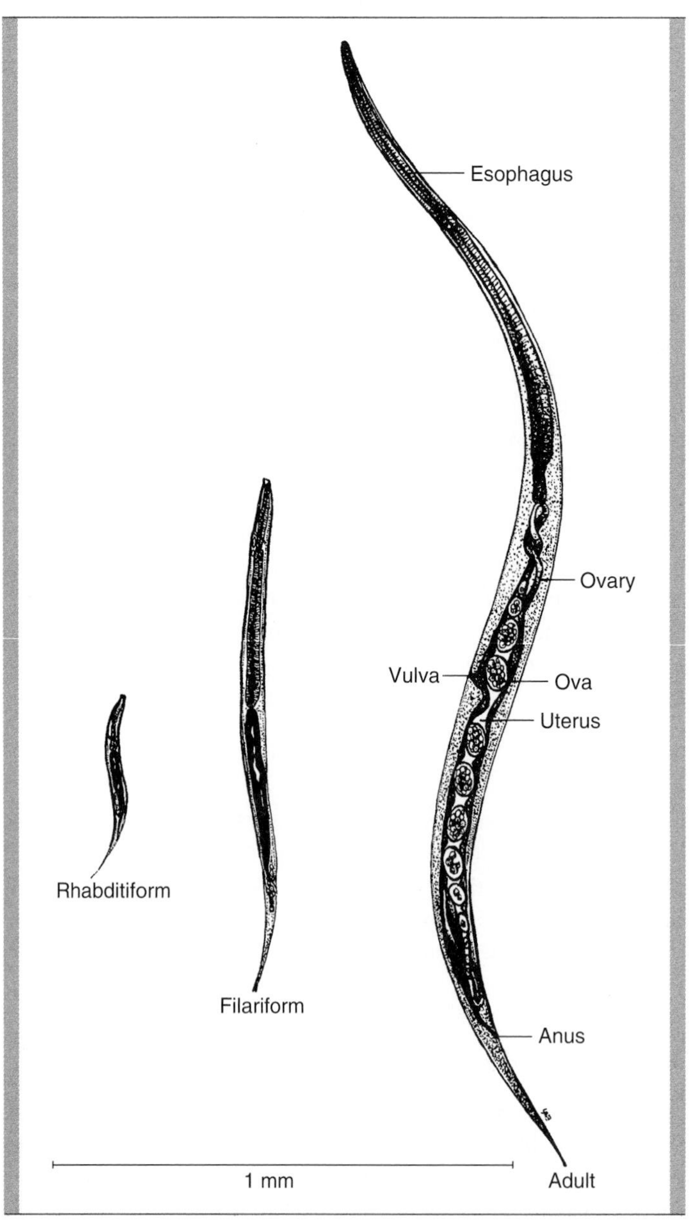

FIGURE 55–5
Strongyloides stercoralis worm and rhabditiform and filariform larvae.

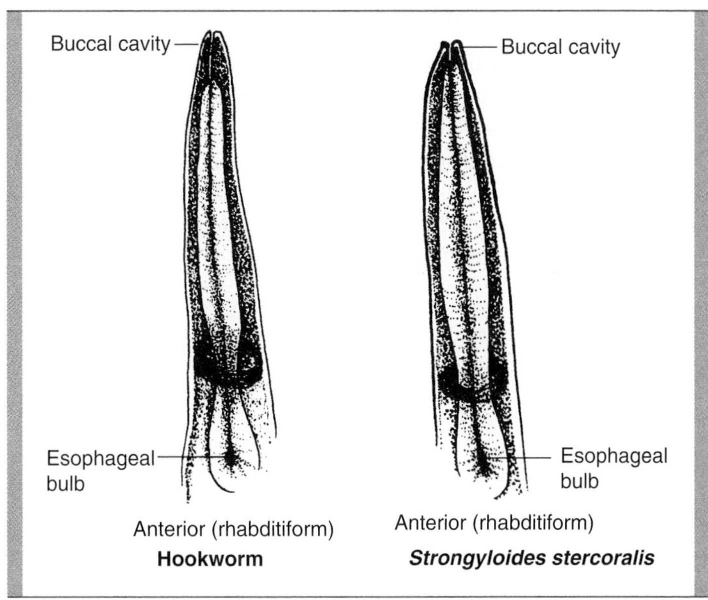

FIGURE 55–6
Anterior ends of hookworm and *Strongyloides stercoralis* rhabditiform larvae.

LIFE CYCLE

Three different life cycles have been described for this nematode. The first, or direct cycle, is similar to that observed with the hookworms. After rhabditiform larvae are passed in the stool, they molt on soil to become filariform larvae. Filariform larvae can penetrate human skin. After transport to the lung in the vascular system, they are coughed up, swallowed and then mature to adults in the small bowel. In the second, or autoinfective cycle, the rhabditiform larva's passage through the colon to the outside world is delayed by constipation or other factors, allowing it to transform into an infective filariform larva while still within the body of its host. This larva may then invade the internal mucosa (internal autoinfection) or perianal skin (external autoinfection) without an intervening soil phase. Thus, *S. stercoralis,* unlike any of the other intestinal nematodes, has the capacity to multiply within the body of the host. The worm burden may increase dramatically, and the infection persist indefinitely, without the need for reinfection from the environment, often with dire consequence to the host. In the third, or free-living cycle, the rhabditiform larvae, after passage in the stool and deposition on the soil, develop into free-living adult males and females. These adults may propagate through several generations of free-living worms before infective filariform larvae are again produced. This cycle creates a soil reservoir that may persist even without continued deposition of feces.

Primary cycle resembles hookworm except rhabditiform larvae develop in gut

Development of filariform stage in gut produces autoinfection

Adults can develop in soil, producing sustained life cycle

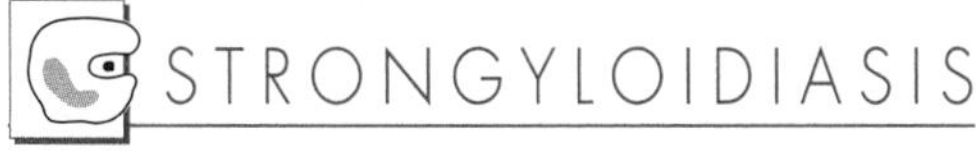

STRONGYLOIDIASIS

EPIDEMIOLOGY

The distribution of *S. stercoralis* parallels that of the hookworms, although it is less prevalent in all but tropical areas. It infects 90 million individuals worldwide, including 400,000 throughout the rural areas of Puerto Rico and the southeastern sections of the continental United States. Although, like hookworm infection, it is generally acquired by direct contact of skin with soil-dwelling larvae, infection may also follow ingestion of filariform-contaminated food. Transformation of the rhabditiform larvae to the filariform stage within the gut can result in seeding of the perianal area with infectious organisms. These larvae may be passed to another person through direct physical contact or autoinfect the original host. In debilitated and immunosuppressed patients, transformation to the filariform stage occurs within the gut itself, producing marked autoinfection or hyperinfection.

Distribution similar to hookworm but less common

Infection by ingestion of filariform larvae also occurs

PATHOGENESIS AND IMMUNITY

Damage to intestinal mucosa may cause malabsorptive syndrome

Immunosuppression enhances risk of autoinfection by accelerating larval development

Invasion of the intestinal epithelium may accelerate epithelial cell turnover, alter intestinal motility, and induce acute and chronic inflammatory lesions, ulcerations, and abscess formation, all of which may play a role in the malabsorptive syndrome that frequently characterizes clinical disease. Steroid- or malnutrition-related immunosuppression appears to accelerate the metamorphosis of rhabditiform to filariform larvae within the bowel lumen, enhancing the frequency and intensity of autoinfection. There is little evidence that protective immunity develops in the infected host.

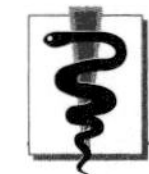

STRONGYLOIDIASIS: CLINICAL ASPECTS

MANIFESTATIONS

Pulmonary and intestinal manifestations can be similar to hookworm, ascaris infections

Patients with strongyloidiasis do not generally give a history of "ground itch." They do, however, manifest the pulmonary disease seen in both ascariasis and, less often, in hookworm infection. The intestinal infection itself is usually asymptomatic. With heavy worm loads, however, the patient may complain of epigastric pain and tenderness, often aggravated by intake of food. In fact, peptic ulcer-like pain associated with peripheral eosinophilia strongly suggests the diagnosis of strongyloidiasis. With widespread involvement of the intestinal mucosa, vomiting, diarrhea, paralytic ileus, and malabsorption may be seen.

External autoinfection causes lesions over buttocks and back

External autoinfection produces transient, raised, red, serpiginous lesions over the buttocks and lower back that reflect larval invasion of the perianal area. If the patient is not treated, these lesions may recur at irregular intervals over a period of decades; they are particularly common after recovery from a febrile illness. Over 25% of British and American servicemen imprisoned in Southeast Asia during World War II continued to demonstrate such lesions prior to diagnosis and treatment some 40 years after exposure.

Massive hyperinfection occurs in immunosuppressed but uncommon in AIDS

Massive hyperinfection may occur in immunosuppressed patients, especially in those receiving glucocorticoid therapy, producing severe enterocolitis and widespread dissemination of the larvae to extraintestinal organs, including the heart, lungs, and central nervous system. Inexplicably, this phenomenon has been unusual in acquired immunodeficiency syndrome (AIDS) patients, even in areas where strongyloidiasis is highly endemic. The larvae may carry enteric bacteria with them, producing Gram-negative bacteremia and occasionally Gram-negative meningitis that may result in death.

DIAGNOSIS

Rhabditiform larvae detected in stool or duodenal aspirates

The diagnosis is usually made by finding the rhabditiform larvae in the stool. Preferably, only fresh specimens should be examined to avoid the confusion induced by the hatching of hookworm eggs with the release of their look-alike larvae. The number of larvae passed in the stool varies from day to day, often requiring the examination of several specimens before the diagnosis of strongyloidiasis can be made. When absent from the stool, larvae may sometimes be found in duodenal aspirates or jejunal biopsy specimens. If the pulmonary system is involved, the sputum should be examined for the presence of larvae. Agar plate culture methods may recover organisms that go undetected by microscopic examination. Enzyme-linked immunosorbent assays for antibodies to excretory–secretory or somatic antigens are now available in reference laboratories.

TREATMENT AND PREVENTION

Treatment essential to prevent autoinfection cycle

All infected patients should be treated to prevent the buildup of the worm burden by autoinfection and the serious consequences of hyperinfection. The drugs of choice are ivermectin and thiabendazole. In hyperinfection syndromes, therapy must be extended for 1 week. The cure rate is significantly less than 100%, and stools should be checked after therapy to see if retreatment is indicated. Patients who have resided in an endemic area at some time in their lives should be examined for the presence of this parasite both before and during steroid treatment or immunosuppressive therapy. Medical personnel caring for patients with hyperinfection syndromes should wear gowns and gloves, because stool, saliva, vomitus, and body fluids may contain infectious filariform larvae.

Medical personnel can be infected with filariform larvae

ADDITIONAL READING

Chan MS. The global burden of intestinal nematode infections—fifty years on. *Parasitol Today* 1997;13:438. A much needed update to a classic survey of nematode infections worldwide.

Genta RM. Dysregulation of *Strongyloidiasis:* A new hypothesis. *Clin Microbiol Rev* 1992;5:345–355. A thorough, provocative, and iconoclastic review of the factors responsible for disseminated strongyloidiasis.

Prociv P. Immune responses in hookworm infections. *Clin Microbiol Rev* 2001;14:689–703.

Russell LJ. The pinworm, *Enterobius vermicularis. Prim Care* 1991;18:13–24. A comprehensive review of this common infection.

CHAPTER 56

Tissue Nematodes

JAMES J. PLORDE

The nematodes discussed in this chapter induce disease through their presence in the tissues and lymphohematogenous system of the human body. They are a heterogeneous group. Three of them, *Toxocara canis, Trichinella spiralis,* and *Ancylostoma braziliense,* are natural parasites of domestic and wild carnivores. Although capable of infecting humans, they cannot complete their life cycle in this host. Humans therefore serve only as injured bystanders, rather than major participants, in the life cycle of these parasites (Table 56–1).

The remaining four major nematodes, *Wuchereria bancrofti, Brugia malayi, Onchocerca volvulus,* and *Loa loa,* are members of a single superfamily (Filarioidea), and all use humans as their natural definitive host (see Table 56–1). The thin, thread-like adults live for years in the subcutaneous tissues and lymphatic vessels, where they discharge their live-born offspring or microfilariae. These progeny circulate in the blood or migrate in the subcutaneous tissues until they are ingested by a specific bloodsucking insect. Within this vector, they transform into filariform larvae capable of infecting another human when the invertebrate host again takes a blood meal.

The nematodes considered, diseases caused, and usual routes of infection in humans are listed in Table 56–1.

TOXOCARA

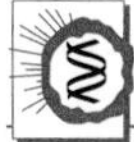

Toxocara canis: PARASITOLOGY

T. canis is a large, intestinal ascarid of canines, including dogs, foxes, and wolves. Each female worm discharges approximately 200,000 thick-shelled eggs daily into the fecal stream. After reaching the soil, these eggs embryonate for a minimum of 2 to 3 weeks. Thereafter, the eggs are infectious to both canines and humans and, in moist soil, may remain so for months to years. When ingested by a young dog, the larvae exit from the eggshell, penetrate the intestinal mucosa, and migrate through the liver and the right side of the heart to the lung. Here, like the offspring of *Ascaris lumbricoides,* they burst into the alveolar airspaces and are coughed up and swallowed; thereafter, they mature in the small bowel. In fully grown dogs, most of the migrating larvae pass through the pulmonary capillaries and reach the systemic circulation.

Cycle in canines resembles ascariasis in humans

Eggs embryonate 2–3 weeks in soil

TABLE 56–1

General Characteristics of Tissue Nematodes

Parasite	Disease	Usual Source of Human Infection
Toxocara canis	Toxocariasis (visceral larva migrans)	Ingestion of ova from canine stools
Trichinella spiralis	Trichinosis	Ingestion of improperly cooked pork
Ancylostoma braziliense	Cutaneous larva migrans	Soil contaminated with dog or cat feces
Major filarial worms		
Wuchereria bancrofti, Brugia malayi	Lymphatic filariasis (elephantiasis)	Mosquito
Onchocerca volvulus	Onchocerciasis (river blindness)	*Simulium* flies
Loa loa (eye worm)	Loiasis (Calabar swellings)	Deer flies

These larvae eventually are filtered out and encyst in the tissues. Hormonal changes and/or diminished immunity in the pregnant bitch stimulate the larvae to resume development, migrate across the placenta, and infect the unborn pups. Larvae may also pass to the newborn puppies in their mother's milk. Approximately 4 weeks after parturition, both the puppies and the lactating mother begin to pass large numbers of eggs in their stools. The mother may be superinfected by ingesting the newly passed eggs and can redevelop clinical symptoms.

Transplacentally infected puppies and infected lactating bitches excrete numerous ova

When humans ingest infectious eggs, the liberated larvae are small enough to pass through the pulmonary capillaries and reach the systemic circulation. Rarely does the organism break into the alveoli and reach the intestine to complete its maturation to adulthood. Larvae in the systemic circulation continue to grow. When their size exceeds the diameter of the vessel through which they are passing, they penetrate its wall and enter the tissue. The larvae induce a T_H2-type CD4+ response characterized by eosinophilia and IgE production.

Transmission to humans by ingestion of ova, and larvae invade tissues

TOXOCARIASIS

EPIDEMIOLOGY

T. canis is a cosmopolitan parasite. The infection rate in the 50 million dogs inhabiting the United States is very high; over 80% of puppies and 20% of older animals are involved. "Man's best friend" deposits more than 3500 tons of feces daily in the streets, yards, and parks of America, and there is a real health risk. In some areas, between 10 and 30% of soil samples taken from public parks have contained viable *Toxocara* eggs. Moreover, serologic surveys of humans indicate that approximately 4 to 20% of the population has ingested these eggs at some time. The incidence of infection appears to be higher in the southeastern sections of the United States; presumably the warm, humid climate prolongs survival of the eggs, thereby increasing exposure. Indeed, seroprevalence rates of more than 50% have been noted in some developing nations. The presence of puppies in the home increases the risk of infection. Clinical manifestations occur predominantly among children 1 to 6 years of age; many have a history of geophagia, suggesting that disease transmission results from direct ingestion of eggs in the soil. Most infections are subclinical, but the incidence of overt disease, although difficult to assess, is certainly underreported. Serious ocular infection by larvae is frequently seen by ophthalmologists.

Soil extensively contaminated with ova deposited by domestic animals

Children are most often infected

Infection much more common than disease, but disease underreported

TOXOCARIASIS: CLINICAL ASPECTS

MANIFESTATIONS

Larvae that reach the systemic circulation may invade any tissue of the body, where they can induce necrosis, bleeding, and the formation of eosinophilic granulomas and, subsequently, fibrosis. The liver, lungs, heart, skeletal muscle, brain, and eye are involved most frequently. The severity of clinical manifestations is related to the number and location of these lesions and the degree to which the host has become sensitized to larval antigens. Children with more intense infection may have fever and an enlarged, tender liver. Those who are seriously ill may develop a skin rash, an enlarged spleen, asthma, recurrent pulmonary infiltrates and abdominal pain, sleep and behavioral changes, focal neurologic defects, and convulsions. Illness often persists for weeks to months, a condition frequently referred to as visceral larva migrans. Death may result from respiratory failure, cardiac arrhythmia, or brain damage. In older children and adults, systemic manifestations are uncommon. Eye invasion by larvae (ocular larva migrans) is more common. Typically, unilateral strabismus (squint) or decreased visual acuity causes the patient to consult an ophthalmologist. Examination reveals granulomatous endophthalmitis, which is usually a reaction to a larva that is already dead; it is sometimes mistaken for malignant retinoblastoma, and an unnecessary enucleation is performed.

Any tissue invaded by larvae

Disease results from organ invasion and hypersensitivity

Ocular invasion produces granulomatous endophthalmitis

DIAGNOSIS

Stool examination is not helpful, because the parasite seldom reaches adulthood in humans. Definitive diagnosis requires demonstration of the larva in a liver biopsy specimen or at autopsy. A presumptive diagnosis may be made based on the clinical picture; eosinophilic leukocytosis; elevated levels of IgE; and on elevated antibody titers to blood group antigens, particularly the group A antigen. An enzyme immunoassay (EIA) using larval antigens has been developed, providing clinicians with a reasonably sensitive (75%) and specific (90%) serologic test. A Western blot procedure is somewhat more sensitive but is not widely available. Unfortunately, many patients with related ocular infections remain seronegative; some demonstrate elevated aqueous humor titers.

Tissue biopsy required for detection

Serodiagnosis using EIA reliable

TREATMENT AND PREVENTION

Corticosteroid treatment may be lifesaving if the patient has serious pulmonary, myocardial, or central nervous system involvement. Anthelmintic therapy with albendazole or mebendazole is generally administered, although the efficacy of these drugs remains uncertain. Prevention requires control of indiscriminate defecation by dogs and repeated worming of household pets. Worming must begin when the animal is 3 weeks of age and be repeated every 3 months during the first year of life and twice a year thereafter.

Corticosteroids helpful in serious disease

Worming of household pets important

TRICHINELLA

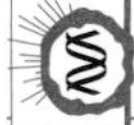

Trichinella spiralis: PARASITOLOGY

Adult *Trichinella* live in the duodenal and jejunal mucosa of flesh-eating animals throughout the world, particularly swine, rodents, bears, canines, felines, and marine mammals. Originally thought to be members of a single species, arctic, temperate, and tropical strains of *Trichinella* demonstrate significant epidemiologic and biologic differences and have

Intestinal parasite of many flesh-eating mammals

recently been reclassified into seven distinct species. Only two species, *T. spiralis* and the arctic species *T. nativa,* display a high level of pathogenicity for humans. This discussion focuses on the former, while highlighting the unique epidemiologic and clinical characteristics of the latter.

The tiny (1.5-mm) male copulates with his outsized (3.5-mm) mate and, apparently spent by the effort, dies. Within 1 week, the inseminated female begins to discharge offspring. Unlike those of most nematodes, these progeny undergo intrauterine embryonation and are released as second-stage larvae. The birthing continues for the next 4 to 16 weeks, resulting in the generation of some 1500 larvae, each measuring 6 by 100 μm.

Larvae reach striated muscle and encapsulate but are still viable

Eating infected flesh spreads the disease

From their submucosal position, the larvae find their way into the vascular system and pass from the right side of the heart through the pulmonary capillary bed to the systemic circulation, where they are distributed throughout the body. Larvae penetrating tissue other than skeletal muscle disintegrate and die. Those finding their way to striated muscle continue to grow, molt, and gradually encapsulate over a period of several weeks. Calcification of the cyst wall begins 6 to 18 months later, but the contained larvae may remain viable for 5 to 10 years. The muscles invaded most frequently include the extraocular muscles of the eye, the tongue, the deltoid, pectoral, and intercostal muscles, the diaphragm, and the gastrocnemius. If a second animal feeds on the infected flesh of the original host, the encysted larvae are freed by gastric digestion, penetrate the columnar epithelium of the intestine, and mature just above the lamina propria.

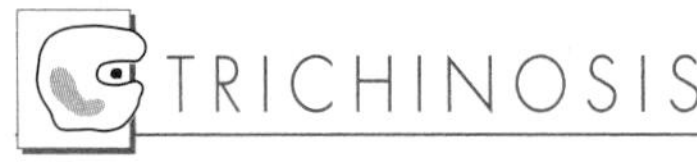

TRICHINOSIS

EPIDEMIOLOGY

Swine infected by eating rats or meat in garbage

Human infection most often from undercooked pork

Wild animals (eg, bear, walrus) also a risk

Trichinosis is widespread in carnivores. Among domestic animals, swine are most frequently involved. They acquire the infection by eating rats or garbage containing cyst-laden scraps of uncooked meat. Human infection, in turn, results largely from the consumption of improperly prepared pork products. In the United States, most outbreaks have been traced to ready-to-eat pork sausage prepared in the home or in small, unlicensed butcheries. Disease incidence is highest in Americans of Polish, German, and Italian descent, presumably because of their custom of producing and eating such sausage during holidays. Recent outbreaks have been reported among Indochinese refugees, apparently related to undercooking of fresh pork. Clusters have also followed feasts of wild pig in California and Hawaii. At present, nearly one third of human cases in the United States, particularly those in Alaska and other western states, have been attributed to consumption of the meat of wild animals, particularly bears. Outbreaks among Alaskan and Canadian Inuit populations have followed the ingestion of raw *T. nativa*–infected walrus meat. Several recent outbreaks in Europe have involved horse meat or wild boar. Each year, a few cases are acquired from ground beef intentionally but illegally adulterated with pork.

Prevalence declining due to cooking and freezing of pork

Human infections usually are subclinical

Human infections occur worldwide. In the United States, the prevalence of cysts found in the diaphragms of patients at autopsy has declined from 16.1 to 4.2% over a period of 30 years. This decline has been attributed to decreased consumption of pork and pork products; federal guidelines for the commercial preparation of such foodstuffs; the widespread practice of freezing pork, which kills all but arctic strains of *Trichinella*; and legislation requiring the thorough cooking of any meat scraps to be used as hog feed. Nevertheless, it is estimated that more than 1.5 million Americans carry live *Trichinella* in their musculature and that 150,000 to 300,000 acquire new infection annually. Fortunately, the overwhelming majority are asymptomatic, and only about 100 clinically recognized cases are reported annually to federal officials. In other areas of the world, infection is more commonly acquired from sylvatic sources, including wild boar, bush pigs, and warthogs.

PATHOGENESIS AND IMMUNITY

The pathologic lesions of trichinosis are related almost exclusively to the presence of larvae in the striated muscle, heart, and central nervous system. Invaded muscle cells enlarge, lose their cross-striations, and undergo a basophilic degeneration. Surrounding the involved area is an intense inflammatory reaction consisting of neutrophils, lymphocytes, and eosinophils. With the development of specific IgG and IgM antibodies, eosinophil-mediated destruction of circulating larvae begins, production of new larvae is slowed, and the expulsion of adult worms is hastened. A vasculitis demonstrated in some patients has been attributed to deposition of circulating immune complexes in the walls of the vessels.

Larvae in striated muscle, heart, and central nervous system

Acute inflammatory reaction with eosinophil-mediated destruction of larvae

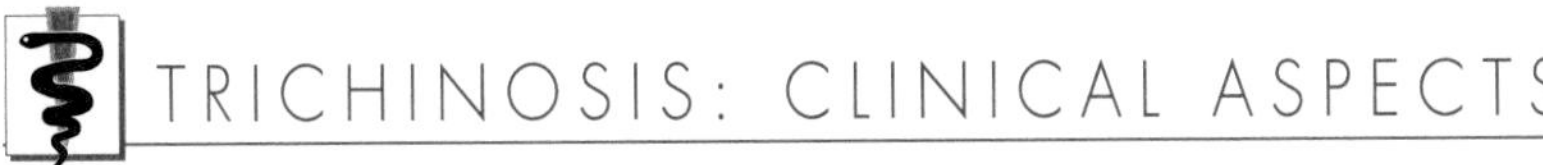

TRICHINOSIS: CLINICAL ASPECTS

MANIFESTATIONS

One or two days after the host has ingested tainted meat, the newly matured adults penetrate the intestinal mucosa, producing nausea, abdominal pain, and diarrhea. In mild infections, these symptoms may be overlooked, except in a careful retrospective analysis; in more serious infections, they may persist for several days and render the patient prostrate. Diarrhea persisting for a period of weeks has been characteristic of *T. nativa* outbreaks following ingestion of walrus meat by the Inuit population of northern Canada. Larval invasion of striated muscle begins approximately 1 week later and initiates the longer (6 weeks) and more characteristic phase of the disease. Patients in whom 10 or fewer larvae are deposited per gram of tissue are usually asymptomatic; those with 100 or more generally develop significant disease; and those with 1000 to 5000 have a very stormy course that occasionally ends in death. Fever, muscle pain, muscle tenderness, and weakness are the most prominent manifestations. Patients may also display eyelid swelling, a maculopapular skin rash, and small hemorrhages beneath the conjunctiva of the eye and the nails of the digits. Hemoptysis and pulmonary consolidation are common in severe infections. If there is myocardial involvement, electrocardiographic abnormalities, tachycardia, or congestive heart failure may be seen. Central nervous system invasion is marked by encephalitis, meningitis, and polyneuritis. Delirium, psychosis, paresis, and coma can follow.

Initial abdominal pain and diarrhea as adults penetrate

Symptoms depend on number and extent of larval muscle invasion

Severe complications include hemoptysis and heart failure

DIAGNOSIS

The most consistent abnormality is an eosinophilic leukocytosis during the second week of illness and persists for the remainder of the clinical course. Eosinophils typically range from 15 to 50% of the white cell count, and in some patients, this may induce extensive damage to the cardiac endothelium. In severe or terminal cases, the eosinophilia may disappear altogether. Serum levels of IgE and muscle enzymes are elevated in most clinically ill patients.

Eosinophilia up to 50% from second week on

There are a number of valuable serologic tests, including indirect fluorescent antibody, bentonite flocculation, and enzyme-linked immunosorbent assay. Significant antibody titers are generally absent before the third week of illness, but may then persist for years.

Antibody usually appears after 2 weeks and then persists

Biopsy of the deltoid or gastrocnemius muscles during the third week of illness often reveals encysted larvae.

Muscle biopsy reveals larvae

TREATMENT

Patients with severe edema, pulmonary manifestations, myocardial involvement, or central nervous system disease are treated with corticosteroids. The value of specific anthelmintic therapy remains controversial. The mortality of symptomatic patients is 1%, rising to 10% if the central nervous system is involved. Mebendazole and albendazole halt the production of new larvae, but in severe infection, the destruction of tissue larvae may provoke a hazardous hypersensitivity response in the host. This may be moderated with corticosteroids.

Corticosteroids used in severe cases

PREVENTION

Primary prevention involves thorough cooking

Control of trichinosis requires adherence to federal feeding regulations for pigs, and limiting contact between domestic pigs and wild animals, particularly rodents, who might be carry trichinella larvae in their tissues. Domestically, care should be taken to cook pork to an internal temperature of at least 76.6°C, freeze it at –15°C for 3 weeks, or thoroughly smoke it before it is ingested. *T. nativa* in the flesh of arctic animals may survive freezing for a year or more. All strains may survive apparently adequate cooking in microwave ovens due to the variability in the internal temperatures achieved.

CUTANEOUS LARVA MIGRANS

Caused usually by larvae of dog and cat hookworms

Filariform larvae penetrate and migrate in human skin

Cutaneous larva migrans, or creeping eruption, is an infection of the skin caused by the larvae of a number of animal and human parasites, most commonly the dog and cat hookworm *Ancylostoma braziliense.* Eggs discharged in the feces of infected animals and deposited on warm, moist, sandy soil develop filariform larvae capable of penetrating mammalian skin on contact. In the United States, parasite transmission is particularly common in the beach areas of the southern Atlantic and Gulf states.

Adult forms do not develop in humans

Although larvae do not develop further within humans, they may migrate within the skin for a period of weeks to months. Clinically, the patient notes a pruritic, raised, red, irregularly linear lesion 10 to 20 cm long. Skin excoriation from scratching enhances the likelihood of secondary bacterial infection. Half of infected patients develop Löffler's syndrome of transient, migratory pulmonary infiltrations associated with peripheral eosinophilia. The syndrome most probably reflects pulmonary migration of larvae. Larvae are rarely found in either sputum or skin biopsies, and the diagnosis must be established on clinical grounds.

The disease responds well to albendazole, ivermectin, or topical thiabendazole. Antihistamines and antibiotics may be helpful in controlling pruritus and secondary bacterial infection, respectively.

LYMPHATIC FILARIA

Lymphatic filariasis encompasses a group of diseases produced by certain members of the superfamily Filarioidea that inhabit the lymphatic system of humans. Their presence induces an acute inflammatory reaction, chronic lymphatic blockade, and in some cases, grotesque swellings of the extremities and genitalia known as elephantiasis.

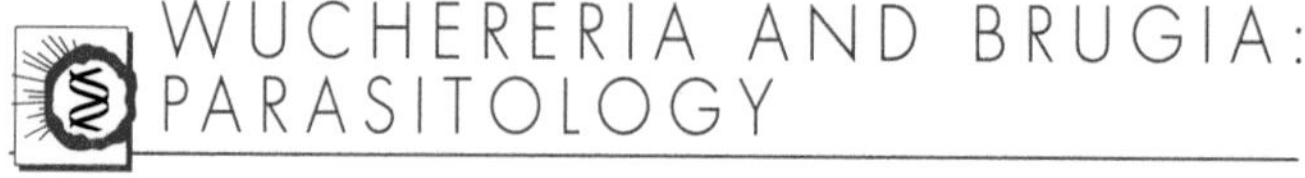

WUCHERERIA AND BRUGIA: PARASITOLOGY

Adult worms live in lymphatic vessels for a decade

Microfilariae develop from ova

The two agents most commonly responsible for lymphatic filariasis are *W. bancrofti* and *B. malayi.* Both are thread-like worms that lie coiled in the lymphatic vessels, male and female together, for the duration of their decade-long lifespan. The female *W. bancrofti* measures 100 mm in length, and the male 40 mm. *B. malayi* adults are approximately half these sizes. The gravid females produce large numbers of embryonated eggs. At oviposition, the embryos uncoil to their full length (200 to 300 μm) to become microfilariae. The shell of the egg elongates to accommodate the embryo and is retained as a thin, flexible sheath. Although the offspring of the two species resemble each other, they may be differentiated on

TABLE 56–2

Differentiation of Microfilariae

Parasite	Location	Sheath	Size (μm)	Nuclei of Tail	Periodicity
Wuchereria bancrofti	Blood	Yes	360	None	Usually nocturnal
Brugia malayi	Blood	Yes	220	Two	Nocturnal
Loa loa	Blood	Yes	275	Continuous	Diurnal
Onchocerca volvulus	Skin	No	300	None	None

the basis of length, staining characteristics, and internal structure (Table 56–2). The microfilariae eventually reach the blood. In most *W. bancrofti* and *B. malayi* infections, they accumulate in the pulmonary vessels during the day. At night, in response to changes in oxygen tension, they spill out into the peripheral circulation, where they are found in greatest numbers between 9 PM and 2 AM. A Polynesian strain of *W. bancrofti* displays a different periodicity, with the peak concentration of organisms occurring in the early evening. Periodicity has an important epidemiologic consequence, because it determines the species of mosquito to serve as vector and intermediate host. Within the thoracic muscles of the mosquito, microfilariae are transformed first into rhabditiform and then into filariform larvae. The latter actively penetrate the feeding site when the mosquito takes its next meal. Within the new host, the parasite migrates to the lymphatic vessels, undergoes a series of molts, and reaches adulthood in 6 to 12 months.

Microfilariae circulate in peripheral blood once each day

Mosquito is essential vector and intermediate host

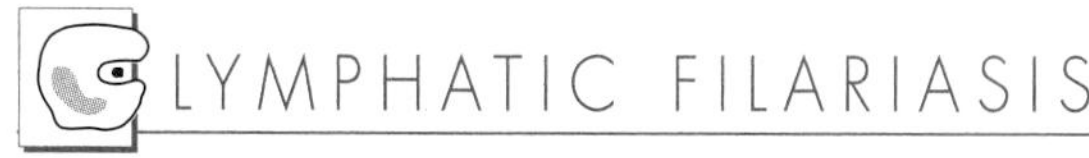

LYMPHATIC FILARIASIS

EPIDEMIOLOGY

Lymphatic filariasis currently infects about 120 million individuals in Africa, Latin America, the Pacific Islands, and Asia; more than 75% of these cases are concentrated in Asia. *W. bancrofti,* transmitted primarily by mosquitoes of the genera *Anopheles* or *Culex,* is the more cosmopolitan of the two species; it is found in patchy distribution throughout the poorly sanitated, densely crowded urban areas of all three continents. A small endemic focus once existed near Charleston, South Carolina, but died out in the 1920s. Moreover, some 15,000 *W. bancrofti* infections were acquired by American servicemen during World War II. The same infection has recently been found in approximately 7% of Haitian refugees to the United States.

Primarily in Asia and other tropical areas

B. malayi, transmitted by mosquitoes of the genus *Mansonia,* is confined to the rural coastal areas of Asia and the South Pacific. Strains with an unusual periodicity have been found in animals. Humans are the only known vertebrate hosts for most strains of *B. malayi* and for *W. bancrofti.* In the eastern Indonesian archipelago, a closely related species, *B. timori,* is transmitted by night-feeding anopheline mosquitoes.

Humans are the only vertebrate hosts for *Wuchereria*

PATHOLOGY AND PATHOGENESIS

Pathologic changes, which are confined primarily to the lymphatic system, can be divided into acute and chronic lesions. In acute disease, the presence of molting adolescent worms and dead or dying adults stimulates dilatation of the lymphatics, hyperplastic changes in the vessel endothelium, infiltration by lymphocytes, plasma cells, and eosinophils, and thrombus formation (ie, acute lymphangitis). These developments are followed by granuloma formation, fibrosis, and permanent lymphatic obstruction. Repeated infections eventually result in massive lymphatic blockade. The skin and subcutaneous tissues become edematous, thickened, and fibrotic. Dilated vessels may rupture, spilling lymph into the tissues or body cavities. Bacterial and fungal superinfections of the skin often supervene and contribute to tissue damage.

Lymphatic blockade with repeated infections

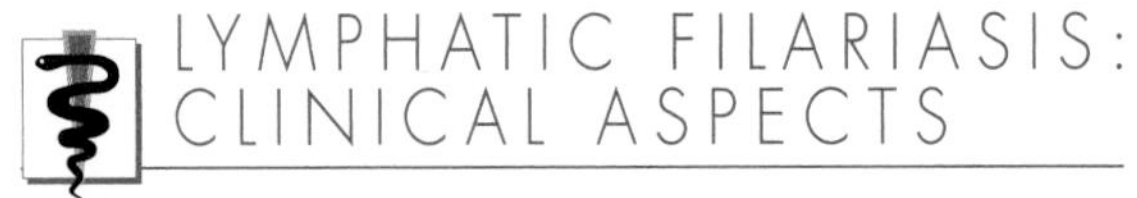

LYMPHATIC FILARIASIS: CLINICAL ASPECTS

MANIFESTATIONS

Individuals who enter endemic areas as adults and reside therein for months to years often present with acute lymphadenitis, urticaria, eosinophilia, and elevated serum IgE levels; they seldom go on to develop lymphatic obstruction. A significant proportion of indigenous populations present with asymptomatic microfilaremia. Some of these spontaneously clear their infection, and others go on to experience "filarial fevers" and lymphadenitis 8 to 12 months after exposure. The fever is typically low grade; in more serious cases, however, temperatures as high as 40°C, chills, muscle pains, and other systemic manifestations may be seen. Classically, the lymphadenitis is first noted in the femoral area as an enlarged, red, tender lump. The inflammation spreads centrifugally down the lymphatic channels of the leg. The vessels become enlarged and tender, the overlying skin red and edematous. In Bancroftian filariasis, the lymphatic vessels of the testicle, epididymis, and spermatic cord are frequently involved, producing a painful orchitis, epididymitis, and funiculitis; inflamed retroperitoneal vessels may simulate acute abdomen. Epitrochlear, axillary, and other lymphatic vessels are involved less frequently. The acute manifestations last a few days and resolve spontaneously, only to recur periodically over a period of weeks to months. With repeated infection, permanent lymphatic obstruction develops in the involved areas. Edema, ascites, pleural effusion, hydrocele, and joint effusion result. The lymphadenopathy persists and the palpably swollen lymphatic channels may rupture, producing an abscess or draining sinus. Rupture of intra-abdominal vessels may give rise to chylous ascites or urine. In patients heavily and repeatedly infected over a period of decades, elephantiasis may develop. Such patients may continue to experience acute inflammatory episodes.

Lymphadenitis, urticaria, and eosinophilia are early findings

Acute manifestations can recur

Elephantiasis may be end result

In southern India, Pakistan, Sri Lanka, Indonesia, Southeast Asia, and East Africa, an aberrant form of filariasis is seen. This form, termed tropical pulmonary eosinophilia, is characterized by an intense eosinophilia, elevated levels of IgE, high titers of filarial antibodies, the absence of microfilariae from the circulating blood, and a chronic clinical course marked by massive enlargement of the lymph nodes and spleen (children) or chronic cough, nocturnal bronchospasm, and pulmonary infiltrates (adults). Untreated, the disease may progress to pulmonary interstitial fibrosis. Microfilariae have been found in the tissues of such patients, and the clinical manifestations may be terminated with specific antifilarial treatment. It is believed that this syndrome is precipitated by the removal of circulating microfilariae by an IgG-dependent, cell-mediated immune reaction. Microfilariae are trapped in various tissue sites where they incite an eosinophilic inflammatory response, granuloma formation, and fibrosis.

For tropical eosinophilia syndrome, microfilaria not found in blood

DIAGNOSIS

Eosinophilia is usually present during the acute inflammatory episodes, but definitive diagnosis requires the presence of microfilaria in the blood or lymphatic, ascitic, or pleural fluid. They are sought in Giemsa- or Wright-stained thick and thin smears. The major distinguishing features of these and other microfilariae are listed in Table 56–2. Because the appearance of the microfilariae is usually periodic, specimen collection must be properly timed. If this procedure proves difficult, the patient may be challenged with the antifilarial agent diethylcarbamazine (DEC). This drug stimulates the migration of the microfilariae from the pulmonary to the systemic circulation and enhances the possibility of their recovery. If the parasitemia is scant, the specimen may be concentrated before it is examined. Once found, the microfilariae must be differentiated from those produced by other species of filariae. A number of serologic tests have been employed for the diagnosis of microfilaremic disease, but until recently they have lacked adequate sensitivity and specificity; even the more recent tests are of little diagnostic significance in individuals indigenous to the endemic area, because many people have experienced a prior filarial infection. Circulating

Eosinophilia during acute episodes

Search for microfilariae in the blood requires careful timing

filarial antigens can be found in most microfilaremic patients and also in some seropositive amicrofilaremic individuals. Antigen detection may thus prove to be a specific indicator of active disease. Tropical eosinophilia is diagnosed as described previously.

TREATMENT

DEC eliminates the microfilariae from the blood and kills or injures the adult worms, resulting in long-term suppression of the infection or parasitologic cure. Frequently the dying microfilariae stimulate an allergic reaction in the host. This response is occasionally severe, requiring the use of antihistamines and corticosteroids. The role of ivermectin in the treatment of lymphatic filariasis has not yet been established. Early studies have demonstrated a high level of effectiveness in clearing microfilaremia following the administration of a single dose. The tissue changes of elephantiasis are often irreversible, but the enlargement of the extremities may be ameliorated with pressure bandages or plastic surgery. Control programs combine mosquito control with mass treatment of the entire population.

Killing of microfilariae may stimulate allergic response

ONCHOCERCA

Onchocerciasis or river blindness, produced by the skin filaria *O. volvulus,* is characterized by subcutaneous nodules, thickened pruritic skin, and blindness.

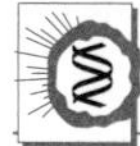

Onchocerca volvulus: PARASITOLOGY

The 40- to 60-cm thread-like female adults lie, together with their diminutive male partners, in coiled masses within fibrous subcutaneous and deep tissue nodules. The female gives birth to more than 2000 microfilariae each day of her 15-year lifespan. These progeny lose their sheaths soon after leaving the uterus, exit from the fibrous capsule, and migrate for up to 2 years in the subcutaneous tissues, skin, and eye. Ultimately they die or are ingested by black flies of the genus *Simulium,* which breed along the banks of turbulent, fast-moving streams. After transformation into filariform larvae, they are transmitted to another human host. There they molt repeatedly over 6 to 12 months before reaching adulthood and becoming encapsulated.

Adults in subcutaneous tissue, skin, and eye

Transmitted by *Simulium* fly

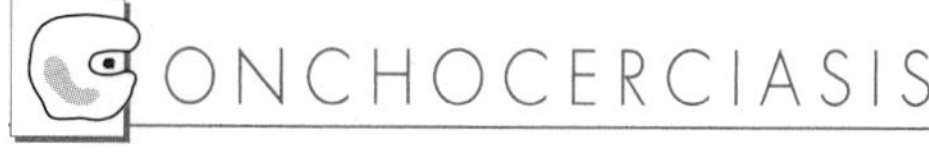

ONCHOCERCIASIS

EPIDEMIOLOGY

Onchocerciasis infects approximately 13 to 20 million persons, rendering 1 to 5% of them blind. The vast majority of the afflicted live in tropical Africa, over half of these in Nigeria and Congo. Foci of infection are also found in Yemen, Saudi Arabia, and Latin America from southern Mexico through the northern half of South America. It has been suggested that the disease was introduced into South America by West Africans enslaved and transported to the New World for the purpose of mining gold in the mountain streams of Venezuela and Colombia. The Central American foci date from Napoleon III's use of Sudanese troops to support his invasion of Mexico in 1862. The disease still persists on the high slopes of the Sierra, where coffee plantations lie along the rapidly flowing streams that serve as breeding places for *Simulium* species.

Most cases in tropical Africa

ONCHOCERCIASIS: CLINICAL ASPECTS

MANIFESTATIONS

Subcutaneous nodules may be multiple with hypersensitivity reaction to microfilariae

Important cause of blindness in affected areas

The subcutaneous nodules that harbor the adult worms can be located anywhere on the body, generally over bony prominences. In Mexico and Guatemala, where the fly vector typically bites the upper part of the body, they are concentrated on the head; in South America and Africa, they are found primarily on the trunk and legs. Although nodules may number in the hundreds, most infected individuals have less than 10. They are firm, freely movable, and measure 1 to 3 cm in diameter. Unless the nodule is located over a joint, pain and tenderness are unusual. Of greater consequence to the patient are the side effects of the presence of microfilariae in the tissues. An immediate hypersensitivity reaction to antigens released by dead or dying parasites results in acute and chronic inflammatory reaction. In the skin, this reaction is manifested as a papular or erysipelas-like rash with severe itching. In time, the skin thickens and lichenifies. As subepidermal elastic tissue is lost, wrinkles and large skin folds or hanging groins are formed. In parts of Africa, fibrosing, obstructive lymphadenitis may result in elephantiasis. Invasion of the eye, however, causes the most devastating lesions. Punctate keratitis, iritis, and chorioretinitis can lead to a decrease in visual acuity and, in time, total blindness. In Central America, eye lesions may be seen in up to 30% of infected patients. In certain communities in West Africa, 85% of the population has ocular lesions and 50% of the adult male population is blind.

DIAGNOSIS

Microfilariae seen in skin samples

The diagnosis is made by demonstrating the microfilariae in a thin skin snips taken from an involved area. When the eye is involved, the organism may sometimes be seen in the anterior chamber with the help of a slit lamp.

TREATMENT AND PREVENTION

Treatment may cause hypersensitivity reactions

Traditionally, DEC has been used to kill the microfilariae. Treatment was begun with very small doses to prevent rapid parasite destruction and the attendant allergic consequences. This consideration was particularly important when the eye was involved; a treatment-induced inflammatory reaction can damage it further. The newer microfilaremic agent, ivermectin, has been demonstrated to be more effective than DEC and does not appear to induce the severe allergic manifestations seen with the latter agent. Because it does not kill the adult worm, retreatment over a period of several years is necessary. No satisfactory methods of control have yet been developed. Application of insecticides to the vector's breeding waters must be sustained for decades to disrupt transmission permanently, because the parasite is so long-lived within humans. With the introduction of ivermectin, mass treatment or chemoprophylaxis is now possible.

There are no effective vaccines or chemoprophylactic agents. Annual mass distribution of ivermectin over a period of 10 to 15 years may interrupt the transmission cycle. A World Health Organization–funded *Simulium* larva control program utilizing aerial insecticides has succeeded in interrupting transmission of onchocerciasis in the savanna regions of West Africa.

LOA LOA

Loiasis is a filarial disease of West Africa produced by the eye worm, *Loa loa.* The long-lived adults migrate continuously through the subcutaneous tissues of humans at a maximum rate of about 1 cm/hr. During migration, they produce localized areas of allergic inflammation termed Calabar swellings. These egg-sized lesions persist for 2 to 3 days and may be accompanied by fever, itching, urticaria, and pain. At times, the adult worms may cross the eye subconjunctivally, producing intense tearing, pain, and alarm.

Adults migrate through subcutaneous tissues producing localized Calabar swellings

The female produces sheathed microfilariae, which are found in the bloodstream during daytime hours. Deer flies of the genus *Chrysops* serve as vectors.

The diagnosis is made by recovering the adult worm from the eye or by isolating the characteristic microfilariae from the blood or Calabar swellings. Eosinophilia is constant. DEC destroys both adults and microfilariae, but must be administered cautiously to avoid marked allergic reactions. Albendazole slowly decreases microfilarial levels without producing allergic reactions, possibly by preferential action on the adult worms.

Adult worm demonstrated in eye or microfilaria in blood or tissue

ADDITIONAL READING

Burnham G. Onchocerciasis. *Lancet* 1998;351:1341–1346.

Jelinek T, Maiwald H, Northdurft HD, et al. Cutaneous larva migrans in travelers: synopsis of histories, symptoms, and treatment of 98 patients. *Clin Infect Dis* 1994;19:1062.

Jongwutiwes S, et al. First outbreak of human trichinellosis caused be *Trichinella pseudospiralis. Clin Infect Dis* 1998;26:111.

Klion AD, Massougbodji A, Sadeler BC, et al. Loiasis in endemic and nonendemic populations: immunologically mediated differences in clinical presentation. *J Infect Dis* 1991;163:1318–1325. Authors note the differences in clinical presentation of loiasis in visitors to endemic areas and indigenous populations, and they relate this to differences in the modulation of the immune response to parasitic antigens.

MacLean JD, Viallet J, Law C, Staudt M. Trichinosis in the Canadian Arctic: report of five outbreaks and a new clinical syndrome. *J Infect Dis* 1989;160:513–520. Trichinosis, which appears to be both common and widespread in the Arctic, is characterized by a distinct clinical presentation in which gastrointestinal manifestations predominate.

Worley G, Green JA, Frothingham TE, et al. *Toxocara canis* infection. Clinical and epidemiological associations with seropositivity in kindergarten children. *J Infect Dis* 1984;149:591–597.

CHAPTER 57

Cestodes

JAMES J. PLORDE

Cestodes are long, ribbon-like helminths that have gained the common appellation of tapeworm from their superficial resemblance to sewing tape. Their appearance, number, and exaggerated reputation for inducing weight loss have made them the best known of the intestinal worms. Although improvements in sanitation have dramatically reduced their prevalence in the United States, they continue to inhabit the bowels of many of its citizens. In some parts of the world, indigenous populations take purgatives monthly to rid themselves of this, the largest and most repulsive of the intestinal parasites.

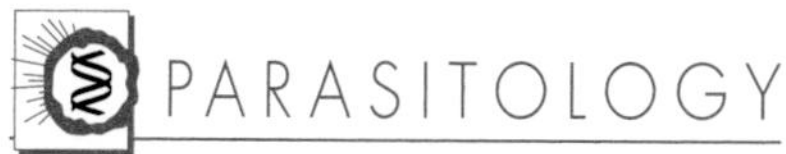

PARASITOLOGY

MORPHOLOGY

Without gut, food absorbed from host

Divided into scolex, neck, and segmented body parts

Each proglottid a hermaphroditic unit releasing eggs via rupture or through uterine pore

Like all helminths, tapeworms lack vascular and respiratory systems. In addition, they are devoid of both gut and body cavity. Food is absorbed across a complex cuticle, and the internal organs are embedded in a solid parenchyma. The adult is divided into three distinct parts: the "head" or scolex; a generative neck; and a long, segmented body, the strobila. The scolex typically measures less than 2 mm in diameter and is equipped with four muscular sucking discs used to attach the worm to the intestinal mucosa of its host. (In one genus, *Diphyllobothrium,* the discs are replaced by two grooves, or bothria.) As a further aid in attachment, the scolex of some species possesses a retractable protuberance, or rostellum, armed with a crown of chitinous hooks. Immediately posterior to the scolex is the neck from which individual segments, or proglottids, are generated one at a time to form the chain-like body. Each proglottid is a self-contained hermaphroditic reproductive unit joined to the remainder of the colony by a common cuticle, nerve trunks, and excretory canals. Its male and female gonads mature and effect fertilization as the segment is pushed farther and farther from the neck by the formation of new proglottids. When the segment reaches gravidity, it releases its eggs by rupturing, disintegrating, or passing them through its uterine pore. The eggs of the genus *Taenia* possess a solid shell and contain a fully developed, six-hooked (hexacanth) embryo. The eggs of *Diphyllobothrium latum,* in contrast, are immature at the time of deposition and possess a covered aperture, or operculum, through which the embryo exits once fully developed.

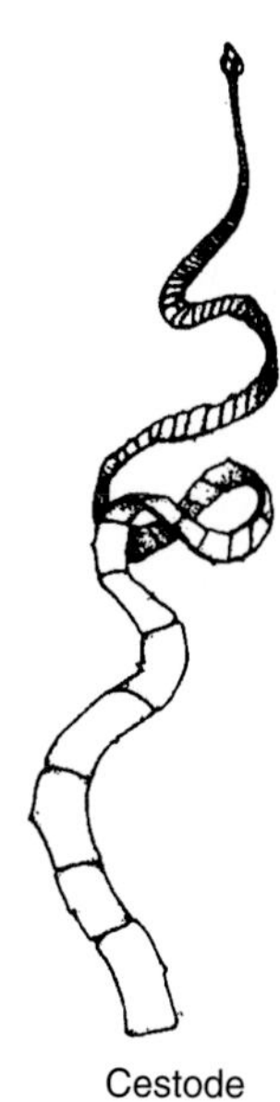
Cestode

LIFE CYCLE

With the exception of *Hymenolepis nana,* further development of all cestodes requires the passage of the larvae through one or more intermediate hosts. Eggs of the genus *Taenia*

TABLE 57–1

Intestinal and Tissue Tapeworms

Stage	*Diphyllobothrium latum*	*Taenia saginata*	*Taenia solium*	*Hymenolepis nana*	*Echinococcus granulosus*	*Echinococcus multilocularis*
Adult						
Definitive host	Humans, cats, dogs	Humans	Humans	Humans, rodents	Dogs, wolves	Foxes
Location	Gut lumen[a]	Gut lumen[a]	Gut lumen[a]	Gut lumen[a]	Gut lumen	Gut lumen
Length (m)	3–10	4–6	2–4	0.02–0.04	0.005	0.005
Attachment device	Grooves	Discs	Discs, hooklets	Discs, hooklets	Discs, hooklets	Discs, hooklets
Mature segment	Broad	Elongated	Elongated	Broad	Elongated	Elongated
Egg						
Maturation status	Nonembryonated	Embryonated	Embryonated	Embryonated	Embryonated	Embryonated
Distinguishing characteristics	Operculate	Radial striations	Radial striations	Polar filaments	Radial striations	Radial striations
Larval development in humans	No	No	Yes	Yes	Yes	Yes
Larva						
Intermediate host	Copepods, fishes	Cattle	Swine, humans	Humans, rodents	Herbivores, humans	Field mice, humans
Location	Tissue	Tissue	Tissue[a]	Gut mucosa[a]	Tissue[a]	Tissue[a]
Form	Procercoid (copepod) Plerocercoid (fish)	Cysticercus	Cysticercus	Cysticercoid	Hydatid cyst	Hydatid cyst

[a]Site of human infection.

Eggs of *Taenia* must be ingested by intermediate host

Infectious cysts of *Taenia* form in tissues of intermediate

Definitive host ingests cysts in flesh of intermediate hosts to yield adult intestinal worms

pass in the stool of their definitive host, reach the soil, and are ingested by the specific intermediate. They hatch within its gut, and the released embryos penetrate the intestinal mucosa, find their way through the lymphohematogenous system to the tissues, and encyst therein. From the germinal lining of this cyst, immature scolices or protoscolices are formed. A cyst with a single such structure is known as a cysticercus (or, in the case of *H. nana,* a cysticercoid); a cyst with multiple protoscolices is known as a coenurus. In some species of tapeworm, daughter cysts, each containing many protoscolices, are formed within the mother or hydatid cyst. The cycle for all is completed when the definitive host ingests the cyst-ridden flesh of the intermediate host. After digestion of the surrounding meat in the stomach, the cyst is freed, and the protoscolex everts to become a scolex. Following attachment to the mucosa, a new strobila is generated.

D. latum requires two intermediates—a copepod and a freshwater fish—to complete cycle

D. latum, whose eggs are immature on release, requires two intermediates to complete its larval development. The egg must reach fresh water before the operculum opens and a ciliated, free-swimming larva, or coracidium, is released. The coracidium is then ingested by the first intermediate host, a copepod, in which it is transformed into a larva (procercoid). When the copepod is, in turn, ingested by a freshwater fish, the larva penetrates the musculature of the fish to form an elongated and infectious larva, the plerocercoid. Life cycles and characteristics of important intestinal and tissue tapeworms infecting humans are summarized in Table 57–1.

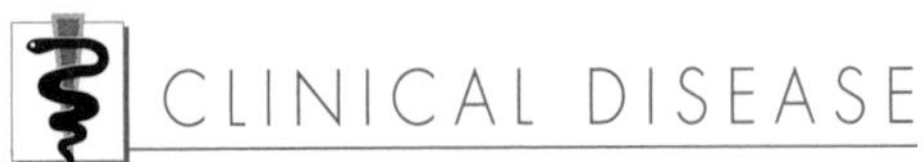

CLINICAL DISEASE

The clinical consequences of tapeworm infection in humans depend on whether the patient serves as the primary or the intermediate host. In the former case, the adult worm is confined to the lumen of the gut, and the consequences of the infection are typically minor. Taeniasis saginata and diphyllobothriasis are prime examples. In contrast, when the patient serves as the intermediate host (eg, for *E. granulosus*), larval development produces tissue invasion and frequently serious disease. The capacity of *H. nana* and *T. solium* to use humans as both primary and intermediate hosts is unique.

Clinical effects depend on whether humans are definitive hosts or intermediate hosts

BEEF TAPEWORM

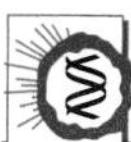

Taenia saginata: PARASITOLOGY

T. saginata inhabits the human jejunum, where it may live for up to 25 years and grow to a maximum length of 10 m. Its 1-mm scolex lacks hooklets but possesses the four sucking discs typical of most cestodes (Fig 57–1A). The creamy white strobila consists of 1000 to 2000 individual proglottids. The terminal segments are longer (20 mm) than they are wide (5 mm) and contain a large uterus with 15 to 20 lateral branches; these characteristics are useful in differentiating them from those of the closely related pork tapeworm, *T. solium.* When fully gravid, strings of 6 to 9 terminal proglottids, each containing approximately 100,000 eggs, break free from the remainder of the strobila. These muscular segments may crawl unassisted through the anal canal or be passed intact with the stool. Proglottids reaching the soil eventually disintegrate, releasing their distinctive eggs. These eggs are 30 to 40 μm in diameter, spherical, and possess a thick, radially striated shell (Fig 57–1B). In appropriate environments, the hexacanth embryo may survive for months. If ingested by cattle or certain other herbivores, the embryo is released, penetrates the intestinal wall, and is carried by the vascular system to the striated muscles of the tongue, diaphragm, and hindquarters. Here it is transformed into a white, ovoid (5 by 10 mm) cysticercus (*Cysticercus bovis*). When present in large numbers, cysticerci impart a spotted or "measly" appearance to the flesh. Humans are infected when they ingest inadequately cooked meat containing these larval forms.

T. saginata inhabits human jejunum

Gravid proglottids passed in stool

Eggs ingested by herbivore intermediates

Cysticerci in bovine striated muscle

Humans infected by eating inadequately cooked infected meat

BEEF TAPEWORM DISEASE

EPIDEMIOLOGY

In the United States, sanitary disposal of human feces and federal inspection of meat have nearly interrupted transmission of *T. saginata.* At present, less than 1% of examined carcasses are infected. Nevertheless, bovine cysticercosis is still a significant problem in the southwestern area of the country where cattle become infected in feedlots or while pastured on land irrigated with sewage or worked by infected laborers without access to sanitary facilities. Shipment of infected carcasses can result in human infection in other areas of the United States. In countries where sanitary facilities are less comprehensive and undercooked or raw beef is eaten, *T. saginata* is highly prevalent. Examples include Kenya, Ethiopia, the Middle East, Yugoslavia, and parts of the former Soviet Union and South America.

Indigenously acquired disease rare in United States

BEEF TAPEWORM DISEASE: CLINICAL ASPECTS

MANIFESTATIONS

Most infected patients are asymptomatic and become aware of the infection only through the spontaneous passage of proglottids. The proglottids may be observed on the surface

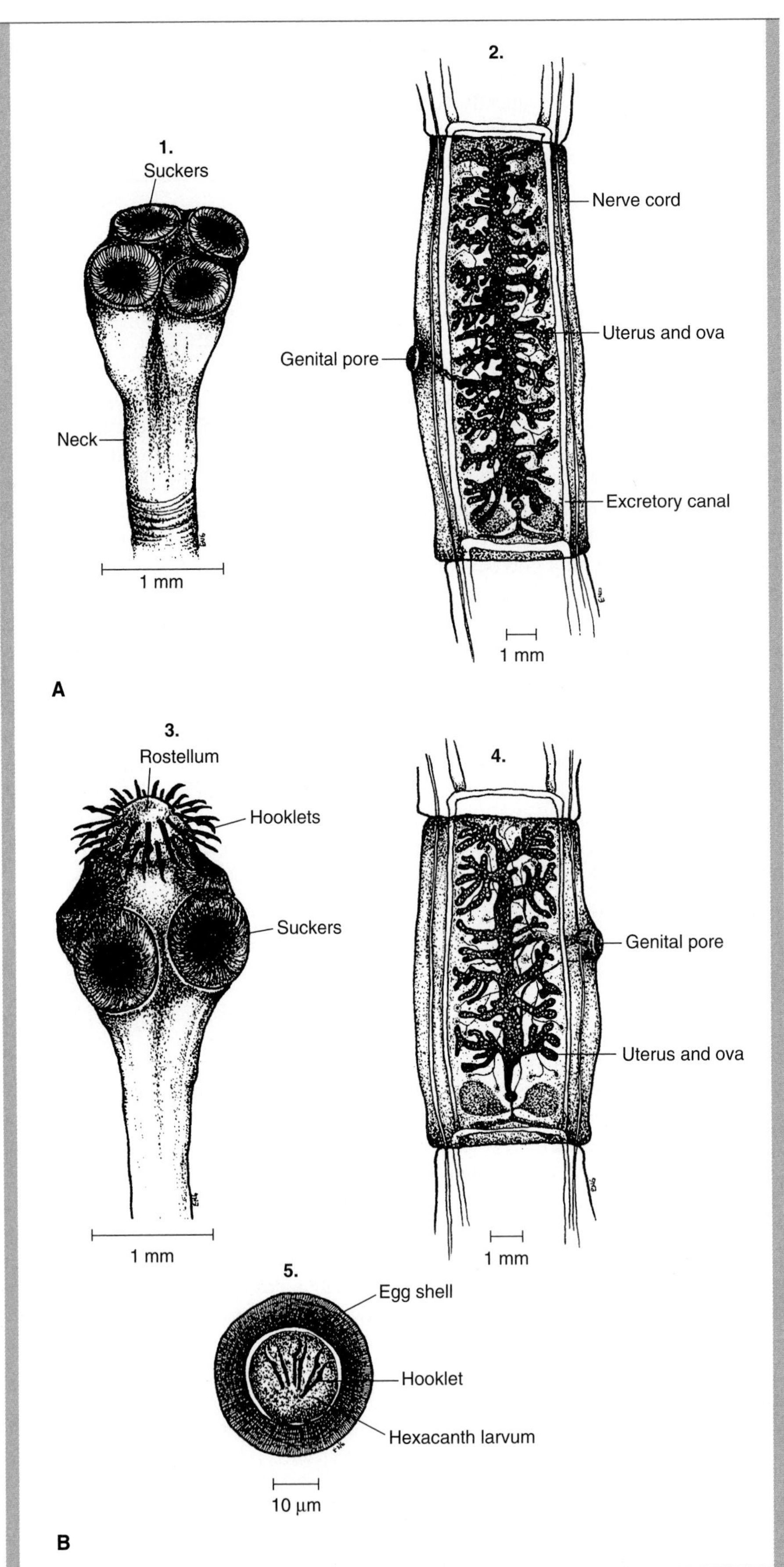

FIGURE 57–1
A. *Taenia saginata.* **B.** *Taenia solium.* (1, 3) Scolices; (2, 4) gravid proglottids; (5) ova (indistinguishable between species).

of the stool or appear in the underclothing or bed sheets of the alarmed host. Passage may occur very irregularly and can be precipitated by excessive alcohol consumption. Some patients report epigastric discomfort, nausea, irritability (particularly after passage of segments), diarrhea, and weight loss. Occasionally the proglottids may obstruct the appendix, biliary duct, or pancreatic duct.

Clinical symptoms usually mild

DIAGNOSIS

The diagnosis is made by finding eggs or proglottids in the stool. Eggs may also be distributed on the perianal area secondary to rupture of proglottids during anal passage. The adhesive cellophane tape technique described for pinworm can be used to recover them from this area. With this procedure, 85 to 95% of infections are detected, in contrast to only 50 to 75% by stool examination. Because the eggs of *T. solium* and *T. saginata* are morphologically identical, it is necessary to examine a proglottid to identify the species correctly.

Adhesive cellophane tape technique and stool examination detect eggs and proglottids

TREATMENT AND PREVENTION

The drugs of choice are praziquantel or niclosamide, which act directly on the worm. Both are highly effective in single-dose oral preparations. Ultimately, control is best effected through the sanitary disposal of human feces. Meat inspection is helpful; the cysticerci are readily visible. In areas where the infection is common, thorough cooking is the most practical method of control. Internal temperatures of 56°C or more for 5 minutes or longer destroy the cysticerci. Salting or freezing for 1 week at −15°C or less is also effective.

Sewage disposal, meat inspection, and adequate cooking

Pork Tapeworm

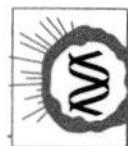

Taenia solium: PARASITOLOGY

Like the beef tapeworm, which it closely resembles, *T. solium* inhabits the human jejunum, where it may survive for decades. It can be distinguished from its close relative only by careful scrutiny of the scolex and proglottids; *T. solium* possesses a rostellum armed with a double row of hooklets (Fig 57–1B3). The strobila is generally smaller than that of *T. saginata,* seldom exceeding 5 m in length or containing more than 1000 proglottids. Gravid segments measure 6 by 12 mm and thus appear less elongated than those of the bovine parasite (Fig 57–1B4). Typically, the uterus has only eight to twelve lateral branches. Although the eggs appear morphologically identical to those of *T. saginata,* they are infective only to swine and, perhaps reflecting a genetic proximity we would prefer to overlook, humans. Both pigs and people become intermediate hosts when they ingest food contaminated with viable eggs. Some authorities have suggested that humans may be autoinfected when gravid proglottids are carried backward into the stomach during the act of vomiting, initiating the release of the contained eggs. It seems more likely that autoinfection results from the transport of the eggs from the perianal area to the mouth on contaminated fingers.

T. solium strobila shorter than in *T. saginata*

Eggs infective to swine and to humans

Regardless of the route, an egg reaching the stomach of an appropriate intermediate host hatches, releasing the hexacanth embryo. The embryo penetrates the intestinal wall and may be carried by the lymphohematogenous system to any of the tissues of the body. Here it develops into a 1 cm, white, opalescent cysticercus over 3 to 4 months. The cysticercus may remain viable for up to 5 years, eventually infecting humans when they ingest undercooked and "measly" flesh. The scolex everts, attaches itself to the mucosa, and develops into a new adult worm, thereby completing the cycle.

Tissue cysticerci develop in humans and swine

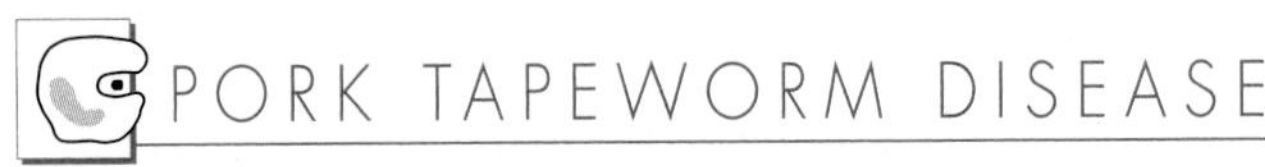

PORK TAPEWORM DISEASE

EPIDEMIOLOGY

T. solium rarely found in United States

Although infected swine are still occasionally found in the United States, most human disease is found in immigrants from endemic areas. Although this infection is widely distributed throughout the world, it is particularly common in south and southeast Asia, Africa, Latin America, and Eastern Europe.

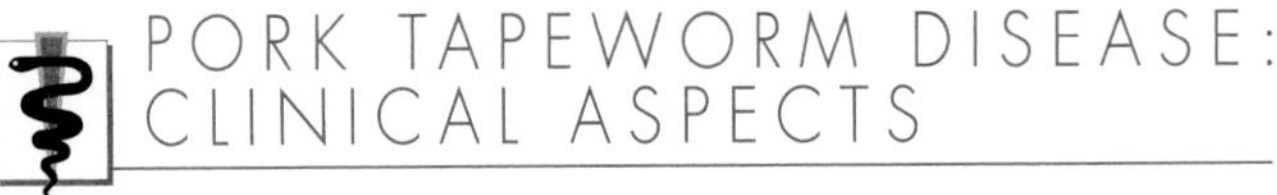

PORK TAPEWORM DISEASE: CLINICAL ASPECTS

MANIFESTATIONS

Major clinical manifestations caused by reaction to cysticerci

The signs and symptoms of infection with the adult worm are similar to those of taeniasis saginata. Clinical manifestations are totally different when humans serve as intermediate hosts. Cysticerci develop in the subcutaneous tissues, muscles, heart, lungs, liver, brain, and eye. As long as the number is small and the cysticerci remain viable, tissue reaction is moderate and the patient asymptomatic. The death of the larva, however, stimulates a marked inflammatory reaction, fever, muscle pains, and eosinophilia.

Meningoencephalitic syndrome with eosinophilia produced by CNS invasion

Multiple small cysts formed

Focal neurologic signs and epilepsy related to cysts

The most important and dramatic clinical presentation of cysticercosis results from lesions in the central nervous system (CNS). During the acute invasive stage, patients experience fever, headache, and eosinophilia. In heavy infections, a meningoencephalitic syndrome with cerebrospinal fluid (CSF) eosinophilic pleocytosis may be present. Established cysts can be found in the cerebrum, ventricles, subarachnoid space, spinal cord, or eye. Cerebral cysts are usually small, often measuring 2 cm or less in diameter; racemose lesions may be threefold larger. These parenchymal infections can induce focal neurologic abnormalities, personality changes, intellectual impairment and/or seizures; in many endemic areas, cysticercosis is the leading cause of epilepsy. Subarachnoid lesions and cysticerci located within the fourth ventricle may obstruct the flow of CSF, producing increased intracranial pressure with its associated headache, vomiting, visual disturbances, or psychiatric abnormalities. Multiple racemose lesions have a predilection for the basal cisterns, particularly in young women, from whence they rapidly spread around the base of the brain and cerebrum with catastrophic result. Spinal involvement produces cord compression or meningeal inflammation. Eye lesions incite pain and visual disturbances.

DIAGNOSIS

Presence of adult worm diagnosed from proglottids

Biopsy required for cysticerci

Infection with the adult worm is diagnosed as described for *T. saginata.* Cysticercosis is suspected when an individual who has been in an endemic area presents with neurologic manifestations or subcutaneous nodules. Roentgenograms of the soft tissues often reveal dead, calcified cysticerci. Viable lesions may be detected as low-density masses by computed tomography (CT) or magnetic resonance imaging (MRI). Brain cysticerci typically are 5 to 10 mm in diameter. Subarachnoid lesions are often larger, may be lobulated, and are often "isodense," making them difficult to visualize radiographically. The diagnosis is confirmed by demonstrating the larva in a biopsy sample of a subcutaneous nodule or specific antibodies in the circulating blood. Serum and CSF enzyme immunoassays and Western blot testing for specific anticysticercal antibodies have a sensitivity of 80 to 95%. The presence of IgG antibodies alone may reflect the presence of past or inactive disease.

TREATMENT AND PREVENTION

Infection with the adult worm is approached in the manner described for *T. saginata*. Because the mortality rate in patients with symptomatic neurocysticercosis approaches 50%, aggressive management is warranted. Patients with parenchymal lesions usually respond to prolonged treatment with praziquantel or albendazole. Concomitant corticosteroid administration helps minimize the inflammatory response to dying cysticerci. Intraventricular subarachnoid and eye lesions appear relatively refractory to chemotherapy; surgery, CSF shunts, and corticosteroids may help ameliorate symptoms.

Surgery occasionally needed for cysticercosis

FISH TAPEWORM

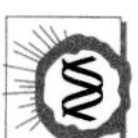

Diphyllobothrium latum: PARASITOLOGY

The adult *D. latum* attaches to the ileal mucosa with the aid of two sucking grooves (bothria) located in an elongated fusiform scolex (Fig 57–2). In lifespan and overall length, it resembles the *Taenia* species discussed previously. The 3000 to 4000 proglottids, however, are uniformly wider than they are long, accounting for this cestode's species designation as well as one of its common names, the broad tapeworm. The gravid segments contain a centrally positioned, rosette-shaped uterus unique among the tapeworms of humans. Unlike those of the *Taenia* species, ova are released through the uterine pore. Over 1 million oval (55 by 75 mm) operculate eggs are released daily into the stool (Fig 57–2B).

D. latum has broad proglottids

On reaching fresh water they hatch, releasing ciliated, free-swimming larvae or coracidia. If ingested within a few days by small freshwater crustaceans of the genera *Cyclops* or *Diaptomus,* they develop into procercoid larvae. When the crustacean is ingested by a freshwater or anadromous marine fish, the larvae migrate into the musculature of the fish and develop into infectious plerocercoid larvae. Humans are infected when they eat improperly prepared freshwater fish containing such forms.

Eggs release motile coracidia in water

Crustacean and fish intermediates; humans infected by ingesting inadequately cooked fish

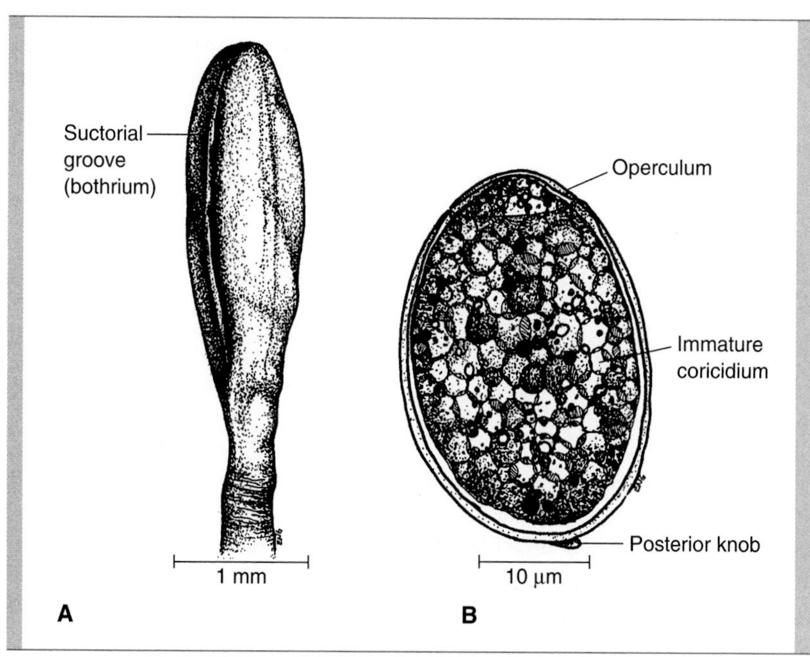

FIGURE 57–2
Diphyllobothrium latum.
A. Scolex. **B.** Ovum.

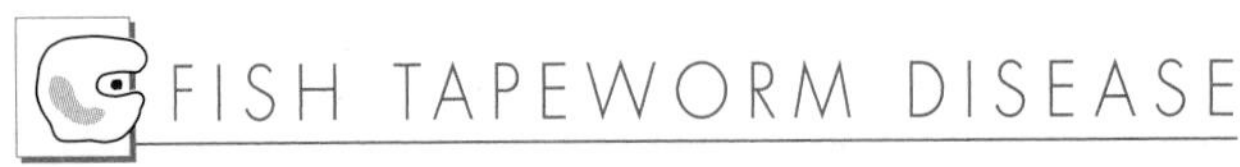

FISH TAPEWORM DISEASE

EPIDEMIOLOGY

Worldwide distribution

Worm found in Alaska, midwestern states, and Florida

Eating raw fish increases risk

Fish tapeworms are found wherever raw, pickled, or undercooked freshwater fish from fecally contaminated lakes and streams is eaten by humans. Other fish-eating mammals may also serve as reservoir hosts. Human infections have been described in the Baltic and Scandinavian countries, Russia, Switzerland, Italy, Japan, China, the South Pacific, Chile and Argentina. The worm, brought to North America by Scandinavian immigrants, is now found in Alaska, Canada, the midwestern states, California, and Florida. It was shown recently that infectious plerocercoid larvae may develop in anadromous salmon, and human cases have been traced to the ingestion of fish freshly taken from Alaskan waters. The increasing popularity of raw fish dishes such as Japanese sushi and sashimi may lead to increased prevalence of this disease in the United States. Among Ontario Indians, infection is acquired by eating fresh salted fish. Even when fish is appropriately cooked, individuals may become infected by sampling the flesh during the process of preparation.

FISH TAPEWORM DISEASE: CLINICAL ASPECTS

MANIFESTATIONS

Occasional intestinal obstruction

Vitamin B_{12} deficiency related to consumption by worm

Most infected patients are asymptomatic. On occasion, however, they have complained of epigastric pain, abdominal cramping, vomiting, and weight loss. Moreover, the presence of several adult worms within the gut has been known to precipitate intestinal or biliary obstruction. Forty percent of fish tapeworm carriers demonstrate low serum levels of vitamin B_{12}, apparently as a result of the competition between the host and the worm for ingested vitamin. Studies have shown that a worm located high in the jejunum may take up 80 to 100% of vitamin B_{12} given by mouth. Approximately 0.1 to 2% of patients develop macrocytic anemia. They tend to be elderly, to have impaired production of intrinsic factor, and to have worms located high in the jejunum. In many, folate absorption is also diminished. Lysolecithin, a tapeworm product, may also contribute to the anemia. Neurologic manifestations of vitamin B_{12} deficiency occur, sometimes in the absence of anemia. They include numbness, paresthesia, loss of vibration sense, and, rarely, optic atrophy with central scotoma.

DIAGNOSIS

Eggs demonstrated in stool

The diagnosis is established by finding the typical eggs in the stool. As *D. latum* produces large numbers of ova, identification is usually accomplished without the need for concentration techniques.

TREATMENT AND PREVENTION

Fish rendered noninfectious at $-10°C$ for 48 hours

Treatment is carried out as described for *T. saginata* infections. When anemia or neurologic manifestations are present, parenteral administration of vitamin B_{12} is also indicated. Personal protection can be accomplished by thorough cooking of all salmon and freshwater fish. Devotees of raw fish may choose to freeze their favorite dish at $-10°C$ for 48 hours before serving. Ultimately, control of diphyllobothriasis is accomplished only by prohibiting the discharge of untreated sewage into lakes and streams.

Echinococcus

Echinococcosis is a tissue infection of humans caused by larvae of *Echinococcus granulosus* and *E. multilocularis*. The former is a more common cause of human disease.

Echinococcus granulosus

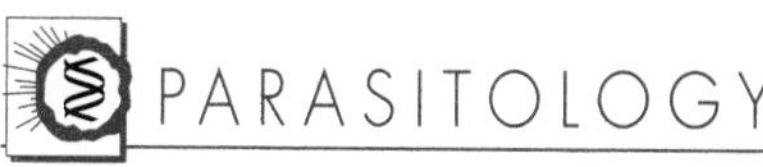

PARASITOLOGY

The adult *E. granulosus* inhabits the small bowel of dogs, wolves, and other canines, where it survives for a scant 12 months. The scolex, like that of the genus *Taenia,* possesses four sucking discs and a double row of hooklets. The entire strobila, however, measures only 5 mm in length and contains but three proglottids; one immature, one mature, and one gravid. The latter segment splits either before or after passage in the stool, releasing eggs that appear identical to those of *T. saginata* and *T. solium.* A number of mammals may serve as intermediates, including sheep, goats, camels, deer, caribou, moose, and, most important, humans. When one of these hosts ingests eggs, they hatch. The embryos penetrate the intestinal mucosa and are carried by the portal blood to the liver. Here, many are filtered out in the hepatic sinusoids. The rest traverse the liver and are carried to the lung, where most lodge. A few pass through the pulmonary capillaries, enter the systemic circulation, and are carried to the brain, heart, bones, kidneys, and other tissues. Many of the larvae are phagocytosed and destroyed. The survivors form a cyst wall composed of an external laminated cuticle and an internal germinal membrane. The cyst fills with fluid and slowly expands, reaching a diameter of 1 cm over 5 to 6 months. Secondary or daughter cysts form within the original hydatid. Within each of these daughter cysts, new protoscolices are produced from the germinal lining. Some break free, dropping to the bottom of the cyst to form hydatid sand. When hydatid-containing tissues of the intermediate host are ingested by a canine, thousands of scolices are released in the intestine to develop into adult worms.

Adult in small intestine of canines

Herbivores and humans serve as intermediates

Larvae penetrate to portal or systemic circulation

Cysts and daughter cysts develop in tissues

Cycle completed with ingestion of cysts by canine

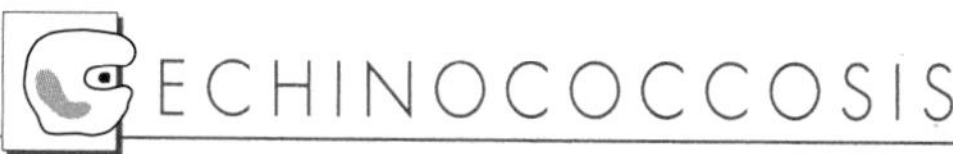

ECHINOCOCCOSIS

EPIDEMIOLOGY

There are two major epidemiologic forms of *E. granulosus*–induced echinococcosis, pastoral and sylvatic. The more common pastoral form has its highest incidence in Australia, New Zealand, South and East Africa, the Middle East, Central Europe, and South America, where domestic herbivores such as sheep, cattle, and camels are raised in close contact with dogs. Although approximately 200 human cases are reported each year in the United States, most were acquired elsewhere. Indigenous cases do occur, however, particularly among Basque sheep farmers in California, southwestern Native Americans, and some Utah shepherds. Animal husbandry practices that permit dogs to feed on the raw viscera of slaughtered sheep allow the cycle of transmission to continue. Shepherds become infected while handling or fondling their dogs. Eggs retained in the fur of these animals are picked up on the hands and later ingested. Sylvatic echinococcosis is found principally in Alaska and western Canada, where wolves act as the definitive host and

Pastoral infections maintained by allowing dogs to feed on sheep viscera

Hand-to-mouth infection of humans by dog contact

Sylvatic cycle in Alaska and western Canada

moose or caribou as the intermediate. In two counties in California, a second cycle involving deer and coyotes has been described. When hunters kill these wild deer and feed their offal to accompanying dogs, a pastoral cycle may be established.

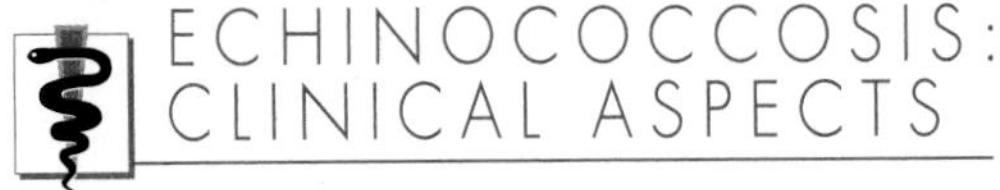

ECHINOCOCCOSIS: CLINICAL ASPECTS

MANIFESTATIONS

Disease caused by mechanical effects of cysts after many years

The enlarging *E. granulosis* cysts produce tissue damage by mechanical means. The clinical presentation depends on their number, site, and rate of growth. Typically, there is a latent period of 5 to 20 years between acquisition of infection and subsequent diagnosis. Intervals as long as 75 years have been reported occasionally.

Pulmonary cysts predominate in sylvatic disease, hepatic in pastoral

Cysts may attain large size

Rupture leads to hypersensitivity manifestations and dissemination

In sylvatic infections, two thirds of the cysts are found in the lung, the remainder in the liver. Most patients are asymptomatic when the lesion is discovered on routine chest x-ray or physical examination. Occasionally, the patient may present with hemoptysis, pain in the right upper quadrant of the abdomen, or a tender hepatic mass. Significant morbidity is uncommon, and death extremely rare. In the pastoral form of disease, 60% of the cysts are found in the liver, 25% in the lung. One fifth of all patients show involvement of multiple sites. The hydatid cysts, which grow more rapidly (0.25 to 1 cm/year) than the sylvatic lesions, may reach enormous size. Twenty percent eventually rupture, inducing fever, pruritus, urticaria, and, at times, anaphylactic shock and death. Release of thousands of scolices may lead to dissemination of the infection. Rupture of pulmonary lesions also induces cough, chest pain, and hemoptysis. Liver cysts may break through the diaphragm or rupture into the bile duct or peritoneal cavity. The majority, however, present as a tender, palpable hepatic mass. Intrabiliary extrusion of calcified cysts may mimic the signs of acute cholecystitis; complete obstruction results in jaundice. Bone cysts produce pathologic fractures, whereas lesions in the CNS are often manifest as blindness or epilepsy. Cardiac lesions have been associated with conduction disturbances, ventricular rupture, and embolic metastases. It has been suggested that circulating antigen–antibody complexes may be deposited in the kidney, initiating membranous glomerulonephritis.

DIAGNOSIS

Radiologic and scanning appearance characteristic

In *E. granulosis*–infected patients, chest x-rays reveal pulmonary lesions as slightly irregular, round masses of uniform density devoid of calcification. In contrast, more than one half of hepatic lesions display a smooth, calcific rim. CT, ultrasonography, and MRI may reveal either a simple fluid-filled cyst or daughter cysts with hydatid sand. Endoscopic retrograde cholangiography has been valuable for determining cyst location and possible communication with the biliary tree. Because of the potential for an anaphylactoid reaction and dissemination of infection, diagnostic aspiration has been considered contraindicated. Nevertheless, in the hands of some investigators, ultrasonically guided percutaneous drainage, followed by the introduction of ethanol to kill protoscoleces and germinal layer, has proven to be safe and useful, both diagnostically and therapeutically (see below). In patients with ruptured pulmonary cysts, scolices may be demonstrated in the sputum.

Serologic diagnosis important but needs improved sensitivity

In most cases, confirmation of the diagnosis requires serologic testing. Unfortunately, current procedures are not totally satisfactory. Indirect hemagglutination and latex agglutination tests are positive in 90% of patients with hepatic lesions and 60% of those with pulmonary hydatid cysts. When using hydatid cyst fluid or soluble scolex antigen, the presence of a precipitin line in the immunoelectrophoresis test appears to be more specific. An adaption of this test to an enzyme-linked immunoelectrodiffusion technique appears to provide a rapid, sensitive diagnostic test. Other serologic tests are in the process of evaluation. Polymerase chain reaction assay has been shown capable of detecting picogram quantities of *Echinococcus* genomic DNA in fine-needle biopsy material from patients with suspected echinococcosis.

TREATMENT AND PREVENTION

For years, the only definitive therapy available was surgical extirpation. Patients with pulmonary hydatid cysts of the sylvatic type and small calcified hepatic lesions underwent surgery only when they became symptomatic or the cysts increased dramatically in size over time. For other lesions, **P**ercutaneous **A**spiration, **I**nfusion of scolicidal and **R**easpiration (PAIR) can be utilized in lieu of surgery. Presently, it is recommended that high-dose albendazole be administered prior to, and for several weeks (or years in the case of *E. multilocularis* infection) after surgery and/or aspiration. Infected dogs should be wormed, and infected carcasses and offal burned or buried. Hands should be carefully washed after contact with potentially infected dogs.

Treatment may include careful aspiration with concomitant albendazole

Echinococcus multilocularis

E. multilocularis is found primarily in subarctic and arctic regions in North America, Europe, and Asia. The adult worms are found in the gut of foxes and, to a lesser extent, coyotes. Their larval forms find harborage in the tissues of mice and voles, the canines' rodent prey. Domestic dogs may acquire adult tapeworms by killing and ingesting these larval-infected sylvatic rodents. Humans are infected with larval forms through the ingestion of eggs passed in the feces of their domestic dogs or ingestion of egg-contaminated vegetation. Unlike the larval forms of *E. granulosis,* those of *E. multilocularis* bud externally, producing proliferative, multilocular cysts that slowly but progressively invade and destroy the affected organs and adjacent tissues.

Larvae bud externally; produce multilocular cysts

The clinical course in humans is characterized by epigastric pain; obstructive jaundice; and, less frequently, metastasis to the lung and brain, thus closely mimicking a hepatoma. Serologic tests are usually positive. Combined drug and surgical treatment often slows the progress of the disease and relieves symptoms. It is seldom curative.

ADDITIONAL READING

Bandres JC, White AC Jr, Samo T, et al. Extraparenchymal neurocysticercosis: Report of five cases and review of management. *Clin Infect Dis* 1992;15:799–811. A very good review of treatment of these refractory forms of neurocysticercosis.

Filice C, Di Perri G, Strosselli M, et al. Parasitologic findings in percutaneous drainage of human hydatid liver cysts. *J Infect Dis* 1990;161:1290–1295. Authors demonstrate that, when appropriately performed, diagnostic and therapeutic aspiration of echinococcal cysts is safe and effective.

Franchi C, et al. Long-term evaluation of patients with hydatidosis treated with benzimidazole carbamates. *Clin Infect Dis* 1999;29:304.

Khuroo MS, et al. Percutaneous drainage compared with surgery for hepatic hydatid cysts. *N Engl J Med* 1997;337:881.

Ruttenber AJ, Weniger BG, Sorvillo F, et al. Diphyllobothriasis associated with salmon consumption in Pacific Coast states. *Am J Trop Med Hyg* 1984;33:455–459.

Shantz PM, Kramer HJ. Larval cestode infections: cysticercosis and echinococcosis. *Curr Opin Infect Dis* 1995;8:32.

Schantz PM, Moore AC, Munoz JL, et al. Neurocysticercosis in an orthodox Jewish community in New York City. *N Engl J Med* 1992;327:692–701. An important paper that demonstrates that cysticercosis can be readily acquired from food-handlers infected with the adult tapeworm. Emigrants from countries endemic for *T. solium* infection should be screened for tapeworm infection before they are employed as housekeepers or food handlers.

White AC Jr. Neurocysticercosis: a major cause of neurologic disease worldwide. *Clin Infect Dis* 1997;24:101.

CHAPTER 58

Trematodes

JAMES J. PLORDE

Of the myriad relationships that have developed between helminths and humans over the millennia of our mutual existence, none has proved more destructive to our health and productivity than that forged with the indomitable flukes. Typically, the adults live for decades within human tissues and vascular systems, where they resist immunologic attack and produce progressive damage to vital organs. Morphologically, trematodes are bilaterally symmetric, vary in length from a few millimeters to several centimeters, and possess two deep suckers from which they derive their name ("body with holes"). One surrounds the oral cavity, and the other is located on the ventral surface of the worm. These organs are used for both attachment and locomotion; movement is effected in a characteristic inchworm fashion. The digestive tract begins at the oral sucker and continues as a muscular pharynx and esophagus before bifurcating to form bilateral ceca that end blindly near the posterior extremity of the worm. Undigested food is vomited out through the oral cavity. The excretory system consists of a number of hollow, ciliated flame cells that excrete waste products into interconnecting ducts terminating in a posterior excretory pore.

Persistent flukes move through tissue and vasculature with inchworm locomotion

The reproductive systems vary and serve as a means for dividing the trematodes into two major categories: the hermaphrodites and the schistosomes. The adult hermaphrodite contains both male and female gonads and produces operculate eggs. The schistosomes have separate sexes, and the fertilized female deposits only nonoperculated offspring. The two groups have similar life cycles. The major differential features are summarized in Table 58–1. Eggs are excreted from the human host and, if they reach fresh water, hatch to release ciliated larvae called miracidia. These larvae find and penetrate a snail host specific for the trematode species. In this intermediate host, they are transformed by a process of asexual reproduction into thousands of tail-bearing larvae or cercariae, which are released from the snail over a period of weeks and swim about vigorously in search of their next host. In the case of schistosomal cercariae, this host is the human. When they come in contact with the skin surface, they attach, discard their tails, and invade, thereby completing their life cycle. The cercariae of the hermaphroditic flukes encyst in or on an aquatic plant or animal, where they undergo a second transformation to become infective metacercariae. Their cycle is completed when the second intermediate host is ingested by a human.

Two types of reproductive systems

Snails release motile cercariae in water

Of the many trematodes that infect humans, only five are discussed: the blood flukes, all of which are members of the genus *Schistosoma* (*S. mansoni, S. haematobium,* and *S. japonicum*); and the lung (*Paragonimus* spp.) and liver (*Clonorchis sinensis*) flukes, which are hermaphroditic (Fig 58–1). Basic details of other hermaphroditic tissue and intestinal flukes are listed in Table 58–2.

Schistosoma cercariae infect humans through skin

Paragonimus and *Clonorchis* have second intermediate host

TABLE 58–1

General Characteristics of Trematodes

	Trematode Type	
Characteristic	Blood	Tissue/Intestinal
Genus	*Schistosoma*	*Paragonimus, Clonorchis, Opisthorchis, Fasciola*
Morphology		
Adult	Oral and ventral suckers Blind gastrointestinal tract Slender, worm-like	Oral and ventral suckers Blind gastrointestinal tract Flat, leaf-like
Egg	Nonoperculate	Operculate
Biology		
Sexes	Separate	Hermaphroditic
Intermediates	One	Two
Life span	Long	Long

FIGURE 58–1
Adult flukes and eggs.

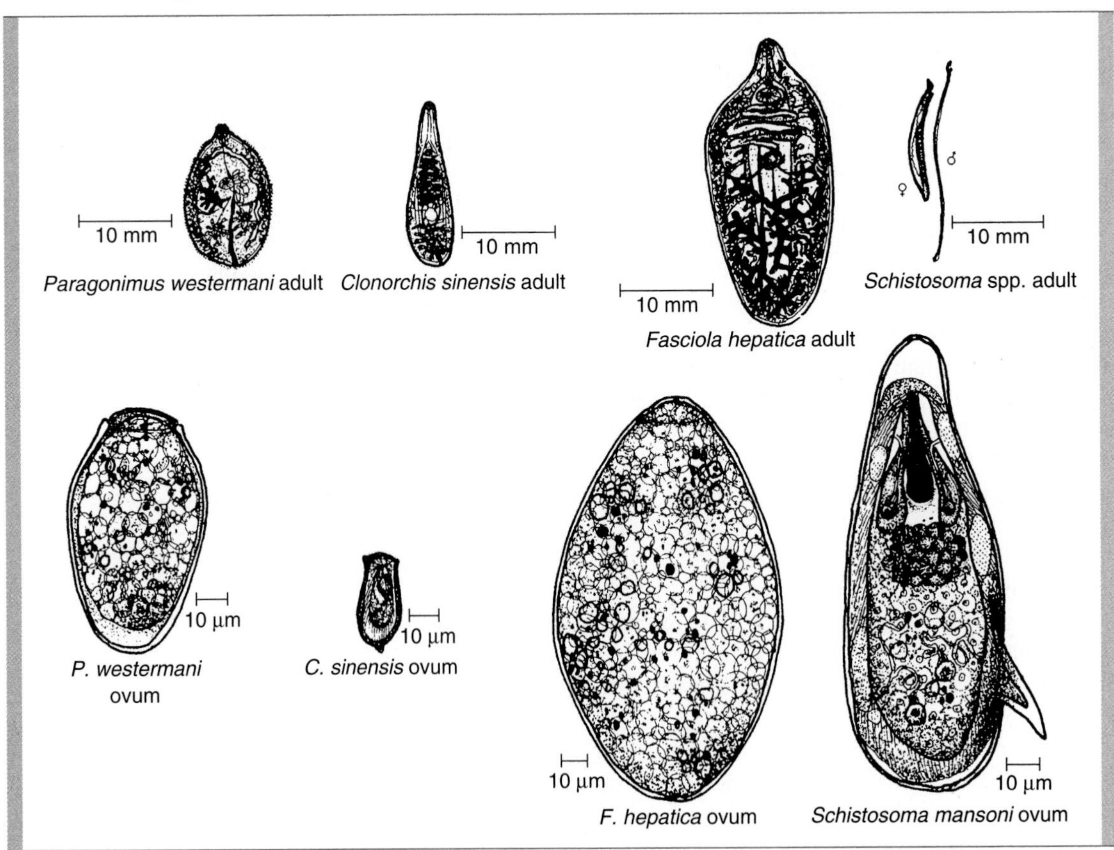

TABLE 58-2

Intestinal and Tissue Trematodes

	Paragonimus	*Clonorchis*	*Opisthorchis*	*Fasciola*	*Fasciolopsis*	*Heterophyes/ Metagonimus*
Distribution						
Geographic	Asia, Africa, Central America	Japan, China, Taiwan, Vietnam	Asia, Eastern Europe	Worldwide	East and Southeast Asia	Asia, former USSR, Mediterranean
Infected population (in millions)	3	20	4	–	10	–
Adult Worms						
Reservoir hosts	Domestic and wild animals	Cats, dogs	Domestic and wild animals	Sheep and other herbivores	Pigs	Fish-eating mammals
Location in body	Lungs, CNS	Biliary tract	Biliary tract	Biliary tract	Small intestine	Small intestine
Length (mm)	7–12	10–25	10	20–30	20–75	1–2
Life span (years)	4–6	20–30	20–30	10–15	0.5	1
Eggs						
Characteristics	Operculated	Operculated	Operculated	Operculated	Operculated	Operculated
Size (μm)	80–100	26–30	26–30	130–150	130–150	26–30
Location[a]	Sputum, stool	Bile, stool	Bile, stool	Bile, stool	Stool	Stool
Larvae						
First intermediate	Snail	Snail	Snail	Snail	Snail	Snail
Second intermediate	Freshwater crab and crayfish	Freshwater fish	Freshwater fish	Watercress and other aquatic plants	Water chestnut and other aquatic plants	Freshwater fish

Abbreviation: CNS = central nervous system.

[a] Diagnostic specimens.

Paragonimus

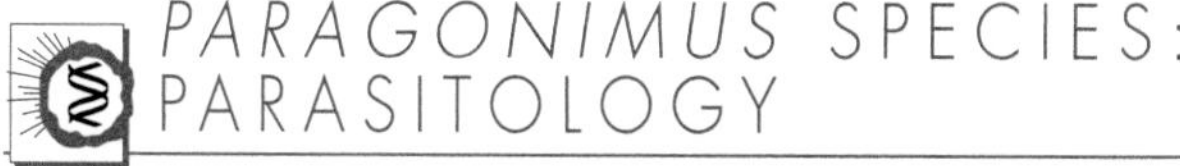

PARAGONIMUS SPECIES: PARASITOLOGY

Several *Paragonimus* species may infect humans. *P. westermani,* which is widely distributed in East Asia, is the species most frequently involved. The short, plump (10 by 5 mm), reddish-brown adults are characteristically found encapsulated in the pulmonary parenchyma of their definitive host. Here they deposit operculate, golden-brown eggs, which are distinguished from similar structures by their size (50 by 90 μm) and prominent periopercular shoulder. When the capsule erodes into a bronchiole, the eggs are coughed up and spat out or swallowed and passed in the stool. If they reach fresh water, they embryonate several weeks before the ciliated miracidia emerge through the open opercula. After invasion of an appropriate snail host, 3 to 5 months pass before cercariae are released. These larval forms invade the gills, musculature, and viscera of certain crayfish or freshwater crabs; over 6 to 8 weeks, the larval forms transform into metacercariae. When the raw or undercooked flesh of the second intermediate host is ingested by humans, the metacercariae encyst in the duodenum and burrow through the gut wall into the peritoneal cavity. The majority continue their migration through the diaphragm and reach maturity in the lungs 5 to 6 weeks later. Some organisms, however, are retained in the

Adults encapsulate in lung

Capsule erodes into bronchiole and eggs are coughed up; cycle continues if eggs reach water with susceptible snail

Crayfish and freshwater crabs are second intermediate hosts

Other carnivores are also definitive hosts

intestinal wall and mesentery or wander to other foci such as the liver, pancreas, kidney, skeletal muscle, or subcutaneous tissue. Young worms migrating through the neck and jugular foramen may encyst in the brain, the most common ectopic site. In addition to humans, other carnivores, including the rat, cat, dog, and pig, may serve as definitive hosts. Immature ectopic adults in the striated muscles of the pig may infect humans after ingestion of undercooked pork.

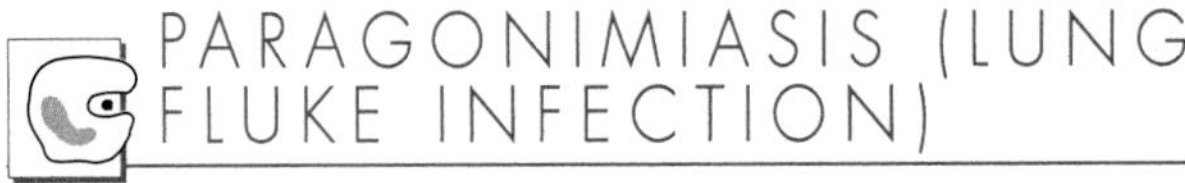

PARAGONIMIASIS (LUNG FLUKE INFECTION)

EPIDEMIOLOGY

Infected snails often found in mountain streams

Humans infected by ingesting infected crustaceans

Although most of the 5 million human infections are concentrated in the Far East (eg, Korea, Japan, China, Taiwan, the Philippines, and Indonesia), paragonimiasis has recently been described in India, Africa (*P. africanus*), and Latin America (*P. mexicanus*). *P. kellicotti,* a parasite of mink, is widely distributed in eastern Canada and the United States but rarely produces human infection. Approximately 1% of recent Indochinese immigrants to the United States are found to be infected with *P. westermani.* Infection of the snail host, which is typically found in small mountain streams located away from human habitation, is probably maintained by animal hosts other than humans. Human disease occurs when food shortages or local customs expose individuals to infected crabs. When these crustaceans are prepared for cooking, juice containing metacercariae may be left behind on the working surface and contaminate other foods subsequently prepared in the same area. Fresh crab juice, which is used for the treatment of infertility in Cameroon and of measles in Korea, may also transmit the disease. In the Far East, crabs are frequently eaten after they have been lightly salted, pickled, or immersed briefly in wine (drunken crab), practices that are seldom lethal to the metacercariae. Children living in endemic areas may be infected while handling or ingesting crabs during the course of play.

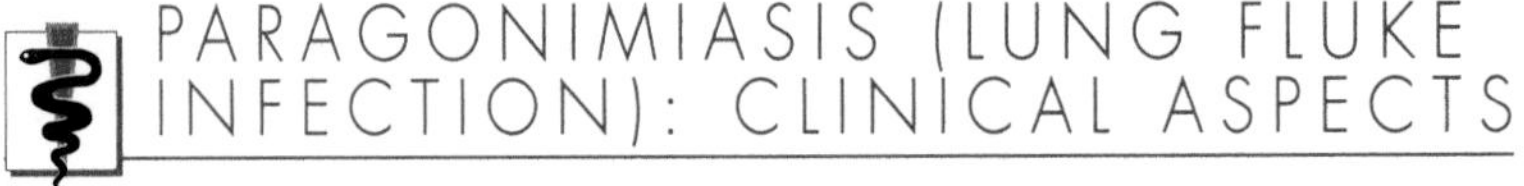

PARAGONIMIASIS (LUNG FLUKE INFECTION): CLINICAL ASPECTS

MANIFESTATIONS

Multiple lung cysts are formed

Secondary infection of ruptured cysts produces bronchitis

Chronic pulmonary abscess may resemble tuberculosis

The presence of the adult worms in the lung elicits an eosinophilic inflammatory reaction and, eventually, the formation of a 1- to 2-cm fibrous capsule that surrounds and encloses one or more parasites. The infected patient may harbor as many as 25 such lesions. With the onset of oviposition, the capsule swells and erodes into a bronchiole, resulting in expectoration of the brownish eggs, blood, and an inflammatory exudate. Secondary bacterial infection of the evacuated cysts is common, producing a clinical picture of chronic bronchitis or bronchiectasis. When cysts rupture into the pleural cavity, chest pain and effusion can result. Early in infection, chest x-rays demonstrate small segmental infiltrates; these are gradually replaced by round nodules that may cavitate. Eventually, cystic rings, fibrosis, and calcification occur, producing a picture closely resembling that of pulmonary tuberculosis. The confusion is compounded by the frequent coexistence of the two diseases.

Adult flukes in the intestine and mesentery produce pain, bloody diarrhea, and on occasion, palpable abdominal or cutaneous masses; the latter is characteristic of a second Chinese fluke, *P. skrjiabini.* In approximately 1% of cases in the Far East, more commonly in children, parasites lodge in the brain and produce a variety of neurologic manifestations, including epilepsy, paralysis, homonymous hemianopsia, optic atrophy, and papilledema.

DIAGNOSIS

Eggs are usually absent from the sputum during the first 3 months of overt infection; however, repeated examinations eventually demonstrate them in more than 75% of infected patients. When a pleural effusion is present, it should be checked for eggs. Stool examination is frequently helpful, particularly in children who swallow their expectorated sputum. Approximately 50% of patients with brain lesions demonstrate calcification on x-ray films of the skull. The cerebrospinal fluid in such cases shows elevated protein levels and eosinophilic leukocytosis. A diagnosis in these cases, however, often depends on the detection of circulating antibodies. Their presence usually correlates well with acute disease and disappears with successful therapy. Recently developed antigen detection techniques have been proven to be both highly sensitive and specific and may soon displace antibody detection procedures.

Eggs difficult to find in sputum, pleural fluid, and feces

Serodiagnosis, antigen detection procedures available

TREATMENT AND PREVENTION

The disease responds well to praziquantel or bithionol therapy. Control requires adequate cooking of shellfish before ingestion.

CLONORCHIS

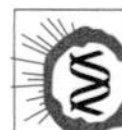

Clonorchis sinensis: PARASITOLOGY

Flukes of the genera *Fasciola, Opisthorchis,* and *Clonorchis* may all infect the human biliary tract and at times produce manifestations of ductal obstruction. *C. sinensis,* the Chinese liver fluke, is the most important and is discussed here (see Table 58–2). The small, slender (5 by 15 mm) adult survives up to 50 years in the biliary tract of its host by feasting on the rich mucosal secretions. A cone-shaped anterior pole, a large oral sucker, and a pair of deeply lobular testes arranged one behind the other in the posterior third of the worm distinguish it from other hepatic parasites. Approximately 2000 tiny (15 by 30 μm) ovoid eggs are discharged daily and find their way down the bile duct and into the fecal stream. The exquisite urn-shaped shells have a discernible shoulder at their opercular rim and a tiny knob on the broader posterior pole. On reaching fresh water, they are ingested by their intermediate snail host, transformed into cercariae, and released to penetrate the tissues of freshwater fish, in which they encyst to form metacercariae. If the latter host is ingested by a fish-eating mammal, the larvae are released in the duodenum, ascend the common bile duct, migrate to the second-order bile ducts, and mature to adulthood over 30 days.

Adults survive decades in biliary tract

Eggs discharged in bile ducts appear in feces

Snails are first intermediate host and fish second

Metacercariae from ingested fish migrate to biliary system

In addition to humans, rats, cats, dogs, and pigs may serve as definitive hosts.

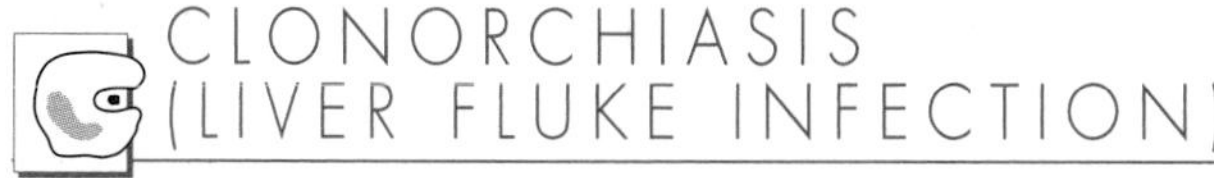

CLONORCHIASIS (LIVER FLUKE INFECTION)

EPIDEMIOLOGY

Clonorchiasis is endemic in the Far East, particularly in Korea, Japan, Taiwan, the Red River Valley of Vietnam, the Southern Chinese province of Kwantung, and Hong Kong. In previous years, parasite transmission was perpetuated by the practice of fertilizing commercial fish ponds with human feces. Recent improvements in the disposal of human waste have diminished acquisition of the disease in most countries. However, the

Endemic in Far East

Transmission to humans related to waste disposal

Ingestion of uncooked fish infects humans

extremely long lifespan of these worms is reflected in a much slower decrease in the overall infection rate. In some villages in southern China, the entire adult population is infected. A recent survey of stool specimens from immigrants from Hong Kong to Canada showed an infection rate of more than 15% overall and 23% in adults between 30 and 50 years of age. The disease is acquired by eating raw, frozen, dried, salted, smoked, or pickled fish. Commercial shipment of such products outside of the endemic area may result in the acquisition of worms far from their original source.

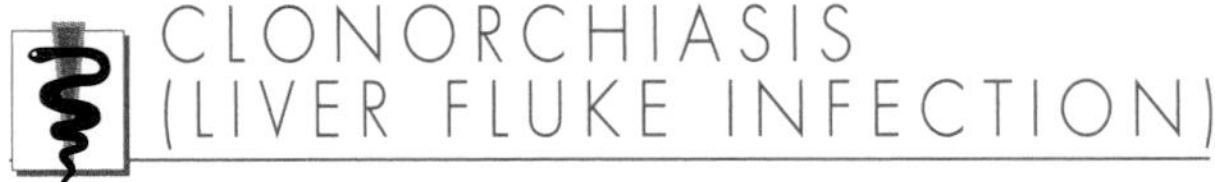

CLONORCHIASIS (LIVER FLUKE INFECTION)

MANIFESTATIONS

Light infection usually asymptomatic

Severe hepatic and biliary manifestations from heavy worm loads

Migration of the larvae from the duodenum to the bile duct may produce fever, chills, mild jaundice, eosinophilia, and liver enlargement. The adult worm induces epithelial hyperplasia, adenoma formation, and inflammation and fibrosis around the smaller bile ducts. In light infection, clinical disease seldom results. However, numerous reinfections may produce worm loads of 500 to 1000, resulting in the formation of bile stones and sometimes bile duct carcinoma in patients with severe, long-standing infections. Calculus formation is often accompanied by asymptomatic biliary carriage of *Salmonella typhi.* Dead worms may obstruct the common bile duct and induce secondary bacterial cholangitis, which may be accompanied by bacteremia, endotoxin shock, and hypoglycemia. Occasionally, adult worms are found in the pancreatic ducts, where they can produce ductal obstruction and acute pancreatitis.

DIAGNOSIS

Distinctive eggs present in feces and duodenal aspirates

Eosinophilia common in acute disease

Definitive diagnosis requires the recovery and identification of the distinctive egg from the stool or duodenal aspirates. In mild infections, repeated examinations may be required. Because most patients are asymptomatic, any individual with clinical manifestations of disease in whom *Clonorchis* eggs are found must be evaluated for the presence of other causes of illness. In acute symptomatic clonorchiasis, there is usually leukocytosis, eosinophilia, elevation of alkaline phosphatase levels, and abnormal computed tomography and ultrasonographic liver scans. Cholangiograms may reveal dilatation of the intrahepatic ducts, small filling defects compatible with the presence of adult worms, and occasionally cholangiocarcinoma.

TREATMENT AND PREVENTION

Praziquantel and albendazole have proven to be effective therapeutic agents. Prevention requires thorough cooking of freshwater fish and sanitary disposal of human feces.

SCHISTOSOMA

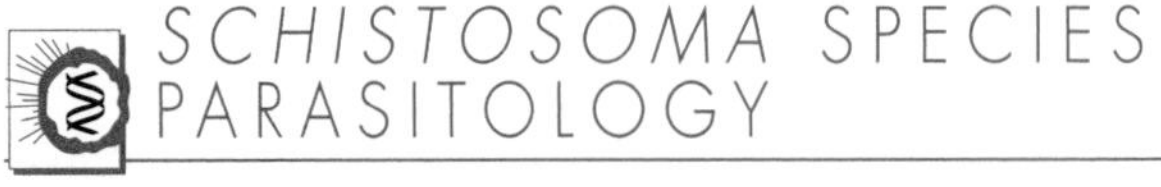

SCHISTOSOMA SPECIES: PARASITOLOGY

The schistosomes are a group of closely related flukes that inhabit the portal vascular system of a number of animals. Of the five species known to infect humans, three, *S. mansoni, S. haematobium,* and *S. japonicum,* are of primary importance. They infect 200 to

300 million individuals in Africa, the Middle East, Southeast Asia, the Caribbean and South America, and kill 1 million annually. The remaining two species are found in limited areas of West Africa (*S. intercalatum*) and Southeast Asia (*S. mekongi*), and will not be discussed in detail.

Inhabit portal vascular system

The adult worms can be distinguished from the hermaphroditic trematodes by the anterior location of their ventral sucker, by their cylindric bodies, and by their reproductive systems (ie, separate sexes). They are differentiated from one another only with difficulty. The 1- to 2-cm male possesses a deep ventral groove, or gynecophoral canal, in which it carries the longer, more slender female in lifelong copulatory embrace. After mating in the portal vein, the conjoined couple use their suckers to ascend the mesenteric vessels against the flow of blood. Guided by unknown stimuli, *S. japonicum* enters the superior mesenteric vein, eventually reaching the venous radicals of the small intestine and ascending colon; *S. mansoni* and *S. haematobium* are directed to the inferior mesenteric system. The destination of the former is the descending colon and rectum; the latter, however, passes through the hemorrhoidal plexus to the systemic venous system, ultimately coming to rest in the venous plexus of the bladder and other pelvic organs.

Different morphology and separate sexes

S. mansoni reaches colon and rectum and *S. haematobium* reaches veins of bladder and pelvic organs

On reaching the submucosal venules, the worms initiate oviposition. Each pair deposits 300 (*S. mansoni, S. haematobium*) to 3000 (*S. japonicum*) eggs daily for the remainder of its 4- to 35-year life span. Enzymes secreted by the enclosed miracidium diffuse through the shell and digest the surrounding tissue. Ova lying immediately adjacent to the mucosal surface rupture into the lumen of the bowel (*S. mansoni, S. japonicum*) or bladder (*S. haematobium*) and are passed to the outside in the excreta. Here, with appropriate techniques, they may be readily observed and differentiated. The eggs of *S. mansoni* are oval, possess a sharp lateral spine, and measure 60 by 140 μm. Those of *S. haematobium* differ primarily in the terminal location of their spine. The eggs of *S. japonicum,* in contrast, are more nearly circular, measuring 70 by 90 μm. A minute lateral spine can be visualized only with care.

Eggs deposited submucosally, rupture to lumina, and pass outside

When the eggs are deposited in fresh water, the miracidia hatch quickly. On finding a snail host appropriate for their species, they invade and are transformed over 1 to 2 months into thousands of forked-tailed cercariae. When released from the snail, these infectious larvae swim about vigorously for a few days. Cercariae coming in contact with human skin during this time attach, discard their tails, and penetrate. During a 1- to 3-day sojourn in the skin, the outer cercarial membrane is transformed from a trilaminar to a heptalaminar structure, an adaption that is thought to be critical to the survival of the parasite within the human body. The resulting schistosomula enter small venules and find their way through the right side of the heart to the lung. After a delay of several days, the parasites enter the systemic circulation and are distributed to the gut. Those surviving passage through the pulmonary and intestinal capillary beds return to the portal vein, where they mature to sexually active adults over 1 to 3 months.

In water eggs hatch to form miracidia, which invade snail

Cercariae from snail traverse human skin and vascular system

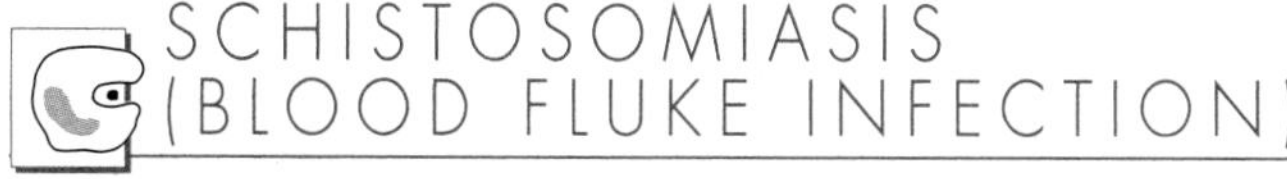

SCHISTOSOMIASIS (BLOOD FLUKE INFECTION)

EPIDEMIOLOGY

The widespread distribution and extensive morbidity of schistosomiasis makes it the single most important helminthic infection in the world today. Currently, more than 200 million individuals in 74 countries are infected. The continued presence of the parasite depends on the disposal of infected human excrement into fresh water, the availability of appropriate snail hosts, and the exposure of humans to water infected with cercariae. The construction of modern sanitation and water purification facilities would break this cycle of transmission but exceeds the economic resources of most endemic nations. Paradoxically, several massive land irrigation projects launched over the past two decades for the express purpose of speeding economic development have resulted in the dispersion of infected humans and snails to previously uninvolved areas. *S. mansoni,* the most

Most important of helminthic infections would be stopped by modern waste disposal

Spread to areas caused by new irrigation projects

widespread of the blood flukes, is the only one present in the Western Hemisphere. Originally thought to have been introduced by African slaves, it is now found in Venezuela, Brazil, Surinam, Puerto Rico, the Dominican Republic, St. Lucia, and several other Caribbean islands.

Geographic distribution varies with species and depends on presence of snail host

Because a suitable snail host is lacking, transmission does not occur within the continental United States; however, nearly half a million individuals residing there have acquired schistosomiasis elsewhere. Puerto Rican, Yemenite, and Southeast Asian populations are those predominantly involved. In the Eastern Hemisphere, the prevalence of *S. mansoni* infection is highest in the Nile Delta and the tropical section of Africa. Isolated foci are also found in East and South Africa, Yemen, Saudi Arabia, and Israel.

S. haematobium is largely confined to Africa and the Middle East, where its distribution overlaps that of *S. mansoni. Schistosoma japonicum* affects the agricultural populations of several Far Eastern countries, including Japan, China, the Philippines, and the Celebes. The closely related *S. mekongi* is found in the Mekong and Mun River valleys of Vietnam, Thailand, Cambodia, and Laos.

Age-related susceptibility with peak in second decade

Within endemic areas, there are wide variations in both infection rates and worm loads. In general, both peak in the second decade of life and then decrease with advancing age. This finding has been explained in part by changes in the intensity of water exposure and in part by the slow development of IgE-mediated immunity. Most infected patients carry fewer than 10 pairs of worms in the vascular system and, accordingly, lack clinical manifestations of disease. Individuals who develop much heavier loads as a result of repeated infections may experience serious morbidity or mortality. Patients with concomitant *S. mansoni* and human immunodeficiency virus infections excrete substantially fewer eggs in their stool.

PATHOGENESIS

There are three major clinicopathologic stages in schistosomiasis. The first stage is initiated by the penetration and migration of the schistosomula. The second or intermediate stage begins with oviposition and is associated with a complex of clinical manifestations. The third or chronic stage is characterized by granuloma formation and scarring around retained eggs.

IMMUNITY

Major manifestations from cell-mediated immune response to eggs

The major clinicopathologic manifestations of schistosomiasis result from the host's cell-mediated immune response to the presence of retained eggs. With time, the intensity of this reaction is muted; granulomas formed in the later stages of infection are smaller and less damaging than those formed early. The mechanisms responsible for this modulation are not fully understood. Present evidence suggests that both suppressor T lymphocyte activity and antibody blockade are involved. The correlation in humans between HLA types A1 and B5 and the development of hepatosplenomegaly suggests that the extent of the immunoregulation is influenced, at least in part, by the genetic background of the host.

Blocking antibodies and adsorption of host molecules provide antigenic disguise

Concomitant immunity prevents new infections

As evidenced by their prolonged survival, the adult worms are remarkably well tolerated by their hosts. In part, this tolerance may be attributable to the formation of IgG4 blocking antibodies early in the course of infection. Tolerance may also reflect the ability of the developing parasites to disguise themselves by adsorbing host molecules, including immunoglobulins, blood group glycolipids, and histocompatibility complex antigens. Nevertheless, as mentioned earlier, the prevalence and intensity of human infection begins to abate during adolescence, despite continuing exposure to infective cercariae. It has been suggested that schistosomula penetrating the skin after the primary infection are coated with specific antibody, bound to eosinophils, and destroyed before they can reach the portal system. Although protection is not complete, the 60 to 80% kill rate is highly effective in controlling the intensity of parasitism. This condition, in which adult worms from a primary infection can survive in a host resistant to reinfection, has been termed concomitant immunity. Eventually, production of blocking antibodies wanes and that of protective IgE antibodies active against adult worms increases, leading to a decrease in the host's total worm population.

SCHISTOSOMIASIS (BLOOD FLUKE INFECTION): CLINICAL ASPECTS

Early Stage

Within 24 hours of penetrating the skin, a large proportion of the schistosomula die. In *S. mansoni* and *S. haematobium* infections, immediate and delayed hypersensitivity to parasitic antigens results in an intensely pruritic papular skin rash that increases in severity with repeated exposures to cercariae. As the viable schistosomula begin their migration to the liver, the rash disappears and the patient experiences fever, headache, and abdominal pain for 1 to 2 weeks.

Local and systemic hypersensitivity reactions produce rash

Note: In the United States, cercariae of avian schistosomes can penetrate human skin and die, producing an intensely pruritic, transient rash known as "swimmers' itch." No further disease occurs.

Intermediate Stage

One to two months after primary exposure, patients with severe *S. mansoni* or *S. japonicum* infections may experience the onset of an acute febrile illness that bears a striking resemblance to serum sickness. The onset of oviposition leads to a state of relative antigen excess, the formation of soluble immune complexes, and the deposition of these in the tissues of the host. Indeed, high levels of such complexes have been demonstrated in the peripheral blood and correlate well with the severity of illness. In addition to the fever and chills, patients experience cough, urticaria, arthralgia, lymphadenopathy, splenomegaly, abdominal pain, and diarrhea. Sigmoidoscopic examination reveals an inflamed colonic mucosa and petechial hemorrhages; occasionally, patients with *S. japonicum* infection develop clinical manifestations of encephalitis. Typically, leukocytosis; marked peripheral eosinophilia; and elevated levels of IgM, IgG, and IgE immunoglobulins are present. This symptom complex is commonly termed the Katayama syndrome. It is more common and more severe in visitors to endemic areas in whom it may persist for 3 months or more, occasionally resulting in death.

Prolonged febrile period with circulating immune complexes

Intestinal inflammation and encephalitis occur acutely

Chronic Stage

Approximately one half of all deposited eggs reach the lumen of the bowel or bladder and are shed from the body. Those retained induce inflammation and scarring, initiating the final and most morbid phase of schistosomiasis. Soluble antigens excreted by the eggs stimulate the formation of T lymphocyte–mediated eosinophilic granulomas. Early in the infection, the inflammatory response is vigorous, producing lesions more than 100-fold larger than the inciting egg itself. Obstruction of blood flow is common. With time, the host's inflammatory response moderates, leading to a significant decrease in granuloma size. Fibroblasts stimulated by factors released by both retained eggs and the granulomas lay down scar tissue, rendering the earlier, granuloma-induced vascular obstruction permanent. As would be expected, the severity of tissue damage is directly related to the total number of eggs retained.

Inflammatory and fibrotic reactions to retained eggs cause chronic disease

In *S. haematobium* infection, the bladder mucosa becomes thickened, papillated, and ulcerated. Hematuria and dysuria result; repeated hemorrhages produce anemia. In severe infections the muscular layers of the bladder are involved, with loss of bladder capacity and contractibility. Vesicoureteral reflux, ureteral obstruction, and hydronephrosis may follow. Progressive obstruction leads to renal failure and uremia. Calcification of the bladder wall is occasionally seen, and approximately 10% of patients harbor urinary tract calculi. Secondary bacterial infections are common. Chronic *Salmonella* bacteriuria with recurrent bouts of bacteremia have been reported from Egypt. In the same country, bladder carcinoma is frequently seen as a late complication of disease.

S. haematobium produces bladder lesions with hemorrhage and obstruction

Chronic urinary carriage of *Salmonella* may cause bacteremia

In *S. mansoni* and *S. japonicum* infections, the bowel mucosa is congested, thickened, and ulcerated. Polyposis has been reported from Egypt but nowhere else. Patients experience abdominal pain, diarrhea, and blood in the stool. Eggs deposited in the larger intestinal veins may be carried by the portal blood flow back to the liver, where they lodge in the presinusoidal capillaries. The resulting inflammatory reaction leads to the development of periportal fibrosis and hepatic enlargement. The frequency and severity with which the liver is involved are genetically determined and associated with the human leukocyte antigen (HLA) type of the patient. In most cases, liver function is well preserved. Infected individuals who subsequently acquire hepatitis B or C viruses develop chronic active hepatitis more frequently than those free of schistosomes. The presinusoidal obstruction to blood flow can result in the serious manifestations of portal obstruction. Eggs carried around the liver in the portosystemic collateral vessels may lodge in the small pulmonary arterioles, where they produce interstitial scarring, pulmonary hypertension, and right ventricular failure. Immune complexes shunted to the systemic circulation may induce glomerulonephritis. Occasionally, eggs may be deposited in the central nervous system, where they may cause epilepsy or paraplegia.

Severity of liver involvement linked to HLA type

Hepatitis B or C superinfection may progress to chronic active hepatitis

Some differences between the clinical presentation of schistosomiasis mansoni and that of schistosomiasis japonicum have been noted. Manifestations of the latter disease typically occur earlier in the course of the infection and tend to be more severe. When involvement of the central nervous system develops, it is more likely to occur in the brain than the spinal cord. On the other hand, immune complex nephropathy and recurrent *Salmonella* bacteremia are more likely to be seen in hepatosplenic *S. mansoni* infections. The latter phenomenon is apparently related to the ability of *Salmonella* to parasitize the gut and integument of the adult fluke, providing a persistent bacterial focus within the portal system of the infected patient. This focus cannot be eradicated without treatment of the schistosomal infection.

Elimination of *Salmonella* focus requires eradication of parasite

DIAGNOSIS

Definitive diagnosis requires the recovery of the characteristic eggs in urine, stool, or biopsy specimens. In *S. haematobium* infections, eggs are most numerous in urine samples obtained at midday. When examination of the sediment yields negative results, eggs may sometimes be recovered by filtering the urine through a membrane filter. Cystoscopy with biopsy of the bladder mucosa may be required for the diagnosis of mild infection. Eggs of *S. mansoni* and *S. japonicum* are passed in the stool. Concentration techniques such as formalin–ether or gravity sedimentation are necessary when the ova are scanty. Results of rectal biopsy may be positive when those of repeated stool examinations are negative.

S. haematobium eggs found in urine

S. mansoni and *S. japonicum* eggs in stool; rectal biopsy

Because dead eggs may persist in tissue for a long time after the death of the adult worms, active infection is confirmed only if the eggs are shown to be viable. This confirmation may be obtained by observing the eggs microscopically for movement of flame cell cilia or by hatching them in water. Quantitation of egg output is useful in estimating the severity of infection and in following response to treatment.

Determination of egg viability and output useful

Conventional serologic tests detect circulating antibodies with sensitivities exceeding 90% but cannot distinguish active from inactive infection. Recently introduced enzyme immunoassay (EIA)–based reagent strip (dipstick) tests capable of detecting circulating, genus-specific, adult-worm **antigens** in blood and urine are rapid, simple and sensitive. They are particularly helpful in the diagnosis of the Katayama syndrome in individuals returning from endemic areas. Moreover, because antigen levels drop rapidly after successful therapy, these tests may prove helpful in distinguishing active from inactive disease.

EIA detection of antigens in blood and urine

TREATMENT

No specific therapy is available for the treatment of schistosomal dermatitis or the Katayama syndrome. Antihistamines and corticosteroids may be helpful in ameliorating their more severe manifestations. In the late stage of schistosomiasis, therapy is directed at interrupting egg deposition by killing or sterilizing the adult worms. Because the severity of clinical and pathologic manifestations is related to the intensity of infection, therapy of long-term residents of endemic areas is often reserved for patients with moderate or severe active infections.

Several anthelmintic agents may be used. Praziquantel, which is active against all three species of schistosomes, is the agent of choice. Unfortunately, several recent reports have suggested increased resistance to this single-dose oral agent in areas where it has been used in mass therapy programs. *S. mansoni* infections acquired in such areas may be treated with oxamniquine. Use of this agent is contraindicated in pregnancy.

Multiple anthelmintic drugs are used

PREVENTION

It has proved both difficult and expensive to control this deadly disease. Programs aimed at interrupting transmission of the parasite by the provision of pure water supplies and the sanitary disposal of human feces are often beyond the economic reach of the nations most seriously affected. Similarly, measures to deny snails access to newly irrigated lands are expensive. Chemical molluscicides have been shown effective in limited trials, but have been less successful when used over large areas for prolonged periods. Mass therapy of the infected human population has, until recently, been severely limited by the toxicity of effective agents. Newer agents, particularly praziquantel, has proven more suitable for this purpose. Nevertheless, discontinuation of mass therapy, in the absence of other control measures, can result in a rapid rebound of active disease. At present, programs that have incorporated all of these control measures have been the most successful.

Sanitary disposal of feces often limited by economic status

Molluscicides effective but large-scale application difficult

Currently, there is intense interest in developing a vaccine suitable for human use. A vaccine made from irradiated *S. bovis* cercariae, developed for cattle, appears to confer a significant degree of protection against infection. Although the use of a similar live vaccine would not be suitable for human populations, the success of the animal vaccine has provided clues to potential immunoprotective mechanisms in human schistosomiasis. Monoclonal antibodies have been used to identify a number of schistosomula and adult antigens thought to be capable of inducing protective immunity; the World Health Organization has selected six of these for further evaluation.

Vaccines under development

ADDITIONAL READING

Bergquist NR, Colley DG. Schistosomiasis vaccines. *Parasitol Today* 1998;14:99–104. Several companion articles in the same publication explore the current status of schistosomiasis vaccine development.

Capron A. Schistosomiasis: forty years' war on the worm. *Parasitol Today* 1998;14: 379–384. This is the opening article in a journal issue devoted exclusively to the control of schistosomiasis.

Hagen P. Reinfection, exposure and immunity in human schistosomiasis. *Parasitol Today* 1992;8:12–16. A brief, clear summary of a very complex topic.

Montenegro SML, et al. Cytokine production in acute versus chronic schistosomiasis: The cross-regulatory role of interferon-γ and interleukin-10 in the responses of peripheral blood mononuclear cells and splenocytes to parasite antigens. *J Infect Dis* 1999;179:1502.

Mostafa MH, Sheweita SA, O'Connor PJ. Relationship between schistosomiasis and bladder cancer. *Clin Microbiol Rev* 1999;12:97–111.

Yee B, et al. Pulmonary paragonimiasis in Southeastern Asians live in the Central San Joaquin valley. *West J Med* 1992;156:423–425.

PART IX

LOCAL AND SYSTEMIC INFECTIONS

CHAPTER 64

Middle and Lower Respiratory Tract Infections

CHAPTER 65

Enteric Infections and Food Poisoning

CHAPTER 66

Urinary Tract Infections

CHAPTER 67

Central Nervous System Infections

CHAPTER 68

Intravascular Infections, Bacteremia, and Endotoxemia

CHAPTER 69

Infections of the Fetus and Newborn

CHAPTER 70

Sexually Transmitted Diseases

CHAPTER 71

Infections in the Immunocompromised Patient

CHAPTER 72

Nosocomial Infections and Infection Control

CHAPTER 59

Skin and Wound Infections

KENNETH J. RYAN

SKIN INFECTIONS

Infections of the skin can result from microbial invasion from an external source or from organisms reaching the skin through the bloodstream as part of a systemic disease. Blood-borne involvement is evidenced by rashes in many viral and bacterial infections, such as measles and secondary syphilis, or may yield more chronic granulomatous skin lesions in blastomycosis, tuberculosis, and syphilis. Skin lesions remote from sites of infection can be produced by some bacterial toxins, such as the pyrogenic exotoxins of group A streptococci and *Staphylococcus aureus*. They can also result from immunologic responses to microbial antigens that have reached the skin. Thus, there are manifold skin manifestations of infections; however, this chapter will be restricted to the discussion of direct infections that may occur in the Western Hemisphere.

Skin lesions may be primary or the result of bacteremia

The skin is an organ system with multiple functions, including protection of the tissues from external microbial invasion. Its keratinized stratified epithelium prevents direct microbial invasion under normal conditions of surface temperature and humidity, and its normal flora, pH, and chemical defenses tend to inhibit colonization by many pathogens (see Chapters 9 and 10). However, the skin is subject to repeated minor traumas that are often unnoticed but that destroy its integrity and allow organisms to gain access to its deeper layers from the external environment. The surface is also penetrated by ducts of pilosebaceous units and sweat glands, and microbial invasion can occur along these routes, particularly if the ducts are obstructed.

Trauma and the appendages of the skin provide access

Infections in Hair Follicles, Sebaceous Glands, and Sweat Glands

Folliculitis

Folliculitis is a minor infection of the hair follicles and is usually caused by *S. aureus*. It is often associated with areas of friction and of sweat gland activity and is thus seen most frequently on the neck, face, axillae, and buttocks. Blockage of ducts with inspissated sebum, as in acne vulgaris, predisposes to the condition. Folliculitis can also be caused by *Pseudomonas aeruginosa,* and this form of the disease has become more common in recent years, with the popularity of hot tubs and whirlpool baths. Unless these facilities are thoroughly cleansed and adequately chlorinated, they can grow large numbers of pseudomonads at their normal operating temperatures, causing extensive folliculitis on areas of the body that have been immersed. The lesions subside rapidly when the insult is

Staphylococci and *Pseudomonas* infect hair follicles

discontinued. Occasionally, folliculitis may be caused by infection with *Candida albicans*. Such cases are particularly common in immunocompromised hosts.

Propionibacterium acnes contributes to inflammation of acne

Acne vulgaris also involves inflammation of hair follicles and associated sebaceous glands. The comedo of acne results from multiplication of *Propionibacterium acnes,* the predominant anaerobe of the normal skin, behind and within inspissated sebum. Organic acids produced by the organism are believed to stimulate an inflammatory response and thus contribute to the disease process. However, the primary cause of the disease is hormonal influences on sebum secretion that occur at puberty, and the disease usually resolves in early adult life.

Furuncles

Staphylococcal furuncles are skin abscesses that can spread

The furuncle is a small staphylococcal abscess that develops in the region of a hair follicle. Furuncles may be solitary or multiple and may constitute a troublesome recurrent disease. Spread of infection to the dermis and subcutaneous tissues can result in a more extensive multiloculated abscess, the **carbuncle.** These lesions and their treatment are considered in Chapter 16.

Treatment

Skin care and tetracycline may be used

Folliculitis and individual furuncles are normally treated locally by measures designed to establish drainage without the use of antibiotics. Chronic furunculosis may require attempts to eliminate nasal carriage of *S. aureus,* which is sometimes the source of the infection. Antimicrobics are not usually required unless surrounding cellulitis or carbuncles develops. Severe acne can often be treated effectively with topical drying agents. Prolonged administration of low oral doses of a tetracycline or macrolide is often effective, although the reason for the therapeutic response is uncertain.

Infections of Other Skin Layers

Minor or inapparent skin lesions serve as the route of infection in many localized skin infections and in some systemic diseases, such as syphilis and leptospirosis.

Infection of Keratinized Layers

Inflammatory response is important with dermatophytes

Cell-mediated immunity defects in chronic candidiasis

The only organisms that can use the keratin on cells, hairs, and nails are the dermatophyte fungi. The dermatophytes are particularly well adapted to these sites, cannot grow at 37°C, and fail to invade deeper layers. The clinical manifestations of these infections result from the inflammatory and delayed hypersensitivity responses of the host, and the desquamation induced by these processes is a major factor in the ultimate control of the infection by removing infected skin. In candidiasis, control involves cell-mediated immune mechanisms, and chronic *Candida* skin and nail infections are often associated with defects in cellular immunity.

Impetigo

Group A streptococci are primary cause

S. aureus may colonize or act as primary pathogen

Pyoderma, also termed impetigo, is a common, sometimes epidemic skin lesion. This disease is caused primarily by group A streptococci. The initial lesion is often a small vesicle that develops at the site of invasion and ruptures with superficial spread characterized by skin erosion and a serous exudate, which dries to produce a honey-colored crust. The exudate and crust contain numerous infecting streptococci. *S. aureus* may occasionally produce pustular impetigo or contaminate the lesions caused by streptococci. Epidemic impetigo is most common in childhood and under conditions of heat, humidity, poor hygiene, and overcrowding. The infection may be spread by fomites such as shared clothing and towels. It is sometimes caused by nephritogenic strains of *S. pyogenes,* particularly in the tropics, and acute glomerulonephritis may result. Rheumatic fever is not associated with streptococcal lesions of the skin.

Treatment is usually with penicillin or erythromycin and topical antimicrobics or skin antiseptics to limit spread.

Bullous impetigo is a distinct disease caused by strains of *S. aureus* that produce exfoliation. It is most common in small children, but may occur at any age. The infection is characterized by large serum-filled bullae (blisters) within the skin layers at the site of infection. Minor infections are treated topically; however, bullous impetigo in infants is a serious disease that usually requires systemic antimicrobic treatment. Epidemic spread may occur under conditions similar to those described for streptococcal impetigo.

Bullous impetigo is caused by exfoliation-producing *S. aureus*

Erysipelas

Erysipelas is a rapidly spreading infection of the deeper layers of the dermis that is almost always caused by group A streptococci. It is associated with edema of the skin; marked erythema; pain; and systemic manifestations of infection, including fever and lymphadenopathy. Because the infection is intradermal, the streptococci cannot usually be isolated from the skin surfaces. The disease can progress to septicemia or local necrosis of skin. It is serious and requires immediate treatment with penicillin or erythromycin.

Group A streptococcal erysipelas is a spreading cellulitis with risk of bacteremia

Cellulitis

Cellulitis is not a skin infection as such, but it can develop by extension from skin or wound infections. It usually presents as an acute inflammation of subcutaneous connective tissue with swelling and pain and often with marked constitutional signs and symptoms. It can be caused by many pathogenic bacteria, but *S. aureus* and group A streptococci are most common. *Haemophilus influenzae* type b is a cause in infants and children. Enteric Gram-negative rods, clostridia, and other anaerobes may also cause cellulitis as a complication of wound infections, particularly in immunocompromised hosts and individuals with uncontrolled diabetes.

Most often caused by pyogenic cocci or *H. influenzae* in children

Skin Ulcers and Granulomatous Lesions

Many acute and subacute skin infections are characterized by ulceration or a granulomatous response. Some are sexually transmitted and are discussed in Chapter 70. Others derive from systemic infection and are not direct infections of skin. A few examples of direct infections, which pose special diagnostic problems, are considered below. Herpes simplex virus can invade through the skin to produce a local vesicular lesion followed by ulceration. The lesion may then recur in the infected area. Primary herpetic lesions of the finger can mimic staphylococcal paronychia very closely, as well as produce lymphangitis and local lymph node enlargement with pain and fever.

Herpetic paronychia can mimic staphylococcal infections

Skin diphtheria, which remains common in some tropical areas, also occurred endemically among the transient population of the West Coast of the United States during the 1970s and early 1980s. The organism gains access through a wound or insect bite and causes chronic erosion and ulceration of the skin, sometimes with evidence of the systemic effects of diphtheria toxin.

Skin diphtheria is seen in transients

Mycobacterium marinum produces a self-limiting granuloma, usually of the forearms and knees. The organism usually enters through superficial abrasions from rocks or swimming pool walls. Infections with *M. ulcerans* are more serious and produce progressive ulceration, but are limited to tropical areas and do not occur in the United States or Europe. Several rare forms of necrotic spreading skin ulceration tend to develop in immunosuppressed hosts, in diabetics, and as complications of abdominal surgery. These lesions include bacterial synergistic gangrene, caused by mixtures of peptostreptococcus, *S. aureus,* and group A streptococci. Variants of these conditions produce extensive and spreading necrotic cellulitis. The major form of treatment is to excise the infected tissues widely and supplement such surgery with massive chemotherapy.

Mycobacterial species cause granulomas

Synergistic gangrene may require surgery

Several primary fungal diseases are associated with cutaneous ulceration or cellulitis, including mycetoma and chromoblastomycosis, which involve the feet, and sporotrichosis, in which ulceration often develops from infected subcutaneous lymph nodes and

Fungal and parasitic ulcerations are usually related to trauma

vessels. Likewise, some parasites directly infect and ulcerate the skin, as in cutaneous leishmaniasis and cutaneous amebiasis. These latter two diseases are not contracted in the United States.

WOUND INFECTIONS

Sources of infection include patient, environment, and infected persons

Wounds subject to infection can be surgical, traumatic, or physiologic. The latter include the endometrial surface, after separation of the placenta, and the umbilical stump in the neonate. Traumatic wounds comprise such diverse damage as deep cuts, compound fractures, frostbite necrosis, and thermal burns. Sources of infection include (1) the patient's own normal flora; (2) material from infected individuals or carriers that may reach the wound on fomites, hands, or through the air; and (3) pathogens from the environment that can contaminate the wound through soil, clothing, and other foreign material. Examples of such infections include contamination of a penetrating stab wound to the abdomen by colonic flora, contamination of a clean surgical wound in the operating room with *S. aureus* spread from the flora of a perineal carrier, and introduction of spores of *Clostridium tetani* into the tissues on a splinter.

Classification of Wounds

Wounds vary in risk of bacterial exposure

Surgical and traumatic wounds are classified according to the extent of potential contamination and thus, the risk of infection. These criteria carry important implications regarding surgical treatment and chemoprophylaxis. **Clean wounds** are surgical wounds made under aseptic conditions that do not traverse infected tissues or extend into sites with a normal flora. **Clean contaminated wounds** are operative wounds that extend into sites with a normal flora (except the colon) without known contamination. **Contaminated wounds** include fresh surgical and traumatic wounds with a major risk of contamination, such as incisions entering nonpurulent infected tissues. **Dirty and infected wounds** include old, infected traumatic wounds; wounds substantially contaminated with foreign material; and wounds contaminated with spillage from perforated viscera.

Infection rates in clean surgical wounds should be less than 1%, whereas untreated dirty wounds have a higher probability of infection. Similar considerations apply to the chance of infection developing in a placental site or on the umbilicus. A normal delivery without retained products will rarely be followed by endometrial infection. A prolonged delivery after rupture of the membranes with retained placental fragments poses an increased risk. In some rural cultures in Africa, soil is applied to the umbilical stump, and neonatal tetanus is common, whereas it is almost unknown in other cultures.

Factors Contributing to Wound Infection

Infectious risk increases with contaminating dose of organisms

Vascular integrity is important for defense

Various factors, in addition to those indicated previously, contribute to the probability of a wound becoming infected. The contaminating dose of microorganisms and their virulence can be critical and, other things being equal, the chance of infection developing increases progressively with the contaminating dose. The physical and physiologic condition of the wound also influences the probability of infection. Areas of necrosis, vascular strangulation from excessively tight sutures, hematomas, excessive edema, poor blood supply, and poor oxygenation all compromise normal defense mechanisms and substantially reduce the dose of organisms needed to initiate infection. Thus, removal of necrotic tissue and the surgeon's skill, gentleness, and attention to detail are major factors in preventing the development of infection.

Nutritional and immunologic status and inflammatory response of the host

The general health, nutritional status, and ability of patients to mount an inflammatory response are also major determinants of whether a wound infection develops. Infection rates are higher in the elderly, the obese, individuals with uncontrolled diabetes, and those on immunosuppressive or corticosteroid therapy. Nutritional deficiencies enhance the risk of infection, and new approaches to avoid protein–calorie malnutrition in patients with severe burns, for example, have led to substantial reductions in serious clinical infections.

There is strong evidence that the critical period determining whether contamination of surgical wounds proceeds to infection lies within the first 3 hours after contamination.

For this reason, prophylactic chemotherapy of some surgical wounds and procedures can be restricted to the operative and immediate perioperative period. There is general agreement that extending such prophylaxis beyond 24 hours increases the chance of complications without reducing the risk of infection.

First 3 hours is critical period for surgical wounds

Treatment and Prevention

Severe wound infections are almost always treated with a combination of surgical and chemotherapeutic approaches. Necrotic tissue and contaminated foreign bodies, such as sutures, must be removed, pockets of pus opened, and drainage established. This approach permits access of the appropriate antibiotics to viable tissues in which they can act. Epidemiologic approaches to the prevention of wound infection and the appropriate uses of chemoprophylaxis are considered in Chapter 13. There has been increasing interest in the possibilities of active or passive immunization against common Gram-negative antigens. Despite some encouraging experimental results, the clinical application of these findings to burns and severe trauma seems distant.

Chemoprophylaxis is mainstay

Immunization is not practical

ETIOLOGIC AGENTS

Some major causes of skin and wound infections are shown in Table 59–1. *S. aureus* remains the single most common cause of infection of clean surgical wounds; however, the number of infections caused by opportunistic Gram-negative organisms is increasing. This finding reflects the extension of surgical intervention to more patients whose defenses are compromised or who would have been unacceptable surgical risks before the introduction of new technical and therapeutic procedures. Severe invasive group A streptococcal infections with the toxic shock-like syndrome often begin with a simple skin or wound infection.

S. aureus and Gram-negative bacteria are most common

Streptococcal toxic shock begins with wound

Anaerobic Gram-negative wound infections have been reported increasingly in the last two decades or so as a result of the higher incidence of such infections in immunocompromised patients and better laboratory recognition. Most infecting organisms derive from normal floral sites and the majority are *Bacteroides,* often in combination with anaerobic Gram-positive cocci and facultative aerobic bacteria. They tend to be associated with necrosis, which may spread subcutaneously, and with thrombophlebitis, which may lead to bacteremia. Most postpartum uterine infections are now caused by Gram-negative anaerobes or anaerobic Gram-positive cocci; they can range from self-limiting infections to severe infections of the uterus with pelvic thrombophlebitis. Human bite wounds are particularly subject to anaerobic infections. In contrast, infected bites of domestic animals (dogs, cats) are almost always due to *Pasteurella multocida.*

Bacteroides and anaerobic Gram-positive coccal infections derived from patient's flora

Burns and areas of necrosis resulting from vascular stasis or insufficiency are subject to infection with the same organisms that predominate in postsurgical wound infections. However, *P. aeruginosa* causes particularly serious infections in burns, with loss of skin grafts and a high risk of septicemia and death. If the fluid electrolyte and nutritional deficiencies of a burned patient can be controlled, the greatest hazard to life is infection.

P. aeruginosa is a virulent cause of burn infections

Tetanus remains a threat to the unimmunized or inadequately immunized individual, particularly from heavy contamination of puncture wounds or introduction of foreign bodies such as splinters, soil, or clothing into the subcutaneous tissues. *C. tetani* never spreads beyond the site of the local lesion, and adequate circulating antibody from tetanus toxoid immunization will prevent the development of the disease. Gas gangrene (clostridial myositis) can develop within a few hours of traumatic injury and lead to rapid death. *C. perfringens* is the most common cause, and its α-toxin produces the spreading tissue damage and muscle death. Other aerobic and anaerobic bacteria are invariably present and sometimes play an important etiologic role. The disease is always associated with muscle trauma and necrosis, which provide the conditions for anaerobic multiplication. Compound fractures, gunshot wounds, and similar extensive injuries that allow entry of clostridial spores set the stage for the disease. Prevention involves surgically debriding all necrotic or potentially necrotic tissue as soon as possible and administering high-dose penicillin.

Tetanus is derived from the environment

Gas gangrene requires surgical intervention

TABLE 59–1

Major Causes of Skin and Wound Infections

SYNDROME	BACTERIA	FUNGI	OTHER
Impetigo	Group A streptococci *Staphylococcus aureus*		
Folliculitis	*Pseudomonas aeruginosa* *Staphylococcus aureus*	*Candida albicans*	
Acne	*Propionibacterium acne*		
Furuncle	*Staphylococcus aureus*		
Cellulitis	Group A streptococci[a] *Staphylococcus aureus* *Haemophilus influenzae*		
Intertrigo	*Staphylococcus aureus* Enterobacteriaceae	*Candida albicans*	
Chronic ulcers[b]	*Treponema pallidum* *Haemophilus ducreyi* *Corynebacterium diphtheriae* *Bacillus anthracis* *Nocardia* *Mycobacterium*	*Sporothrix*	Herpesvirus
Wounds			
Trauma	*Clostridium* Enterobacteriaceae *Pseudomonas aeruginosa*		
Surgical (clean)	*Staphylococcus aureus* Enterobacteriaceae Group A streptococci		
Surgical (dirty)[c]	*Staphylococcus aureus* Enterobacteriaceae Anaerobes		
Burns	*Pseudomonas aeruginosa* *Staphylococcus aureus* Enterobacteriaceae	*Candida albicans*	
Animal bites	*Pasteurella multocida*		

[a] Including "erysipelas," an infection primarily involving the deeper layers of the dermis.

[b] Usually begin as nodules or pustules.

[c] Etiology determined by the origin of the contaminating flora (eg, abdominal vs. gynecologic surgery).

ADDITIONAL READING

Bowler PG, Duerden BI, Armstrong DG. Wound microbiology and associated approaches to wound management. *Clin Microbiol Rev* 2001;14:244–269. This review emphasizes the surgical side of wound management and experimental study.

CHAPTER 60

Bone and Joint Infections

C. George Ray

Infections of bones and joints may exist separately or together. Both are most common in infancy and childhood. They are usually caused by blood-borne (hematogenous) spread to the infected site but can also result from local trauma with secondary infection. Sometimes there may be local spread from a contiguous soft tissue infection, often associated with the presence of a foreign body at the site of the primary wound.

The local effect of such infections can be devastating if they are inadequately treated, because inflammation and resultant tissue necrosis may produce irreparable damage. The presence of pus under pressure can compromise normal blood flow and even cause destruction of blood vessels with avascular necrosis of tissue. When this condition develops, a **sequestrum** can result, in which a part of the cartilage or bone becomes totally separated from its blood supply and cannot be incorporated into the healing process. In some patients, sequestrum formation can lead to a smoldering chronic infection with draining sinuses and loss of functional integrity. Normal growth of the affected site can be severely impaired in the infant or child, particularly when the epiphysis is involved. In the acute phase of infection, bacteremia may also cause sepsis and metastatic infections in sites such as the lungs and heart. The result may be fatal.

Sequestrum formation can lead to chronic infection with draining sinuses

Infection can cause growth impairment in children

Bacteremia and metastatic spread from bone and joint infections is common

OSTEOMYELITIS

The onset of acute hematogenous osteomyelitis is usually abrupt but can sometimes be quite insidious. It is classically characterized by localized pain, fever, and tenderness to palpation over the affected site. More than one bone or joint may be involved as a result of hematogenous spread to multiple sites. With progression, the classic signs of heat, redness, and swelling may develop. Laboratory findings often include leukocytosis and elevated acute-phase reactants, such as C-reactive protein and sedimentation rate. Osteomyelitis caused by a contiguous focus of infection is usually associated with the presence of local findings of soft tissue infection, such as skin abscesses and infected wounds.

Local pain and signs of inflammation

When osteomyelitis occurs in close proximity to a joint, septic arthritis may develop by direct spread through the epiphysis (usually in infants) or by lateral extension through the periosteum into the joint capsule. Such extension is particularly common in hip and elbow infections.

May come from contiguous focus

Extend to joints through epiphysis and adjacent periosteum

Common Etiologic Agents

The most common causes of acute osteomyelitis and those associated with special circumstances are shown in Table 60–1. It is clear that age plays a significant role in

TABLE 60–1

Common Causes of Acute Osteomyelitis

Situation	Usual Causative Organism
Age group	
Neonates (<1 mo)	*Staphylococcus aureus,* group B streptococci, Gram-negative rods (eg, *Escherichia coli, Klebsiella, Proteus, Pseudomonas*)
Older infants, children, adults	*S. aureus, S. pneumoniae, Kingella kingae*
Special problems	
Chronic hemolytic disorders (eg, sickle cell disease)	*S. aureus, S. pneumoniae, Salmonella* species
Infection after trauma or surgery	*S. aureus,* group A streptococci, Gram-negative aerobic or anaerobic bacteria
Infection after puncture wound of foot	*Pseudomonas aeruginosa, S. aureus*

Age-related etiologies, but staphylococcal osteomyelitis most common

influencing the relative frequency of the various infective agents, particularly in early infancy; however, most infections are caused by *Staphylococcus aureus.*

Chronic granulomatous osteomyelitis suggests mycobacteria or fungi

Low-grade smoldering infections may also occur with the organisms listed in Table 60–1; however, chronic granulomatous processes must also be considered, including tuberculosis, coccidioidomycosis, histoplasmosis, and blastomycosis. These latter infections usually result from systemic dissemination, and the lesions develop slowly over a period of months. Occasionally bone tumors or cysts and leukemia must also be considered in the differential diagnosis.

Diagnostic Approaches

The primary goals of diagnosis are to establish the existence of infection and to determine its cause. The following procedures are generally used:

1. Blood cultures, because many infections are associated with bacteremia.
2. Radionuclide scanning or magnetic resonance imaging to demonstrate evidence of localized infection.
3. Direct staining, culture, and histology of needle aspirates or biopsies of periosteum or bone.

Blood cultures, direct aspirates, and bone scans

X-rays may be normal in early stages of infection

4. X-rays of affected sites, which often appear normal in the early stages of infection. The first changes seen are swelling of surrounding soft tissues, followed by periosteal elevation. Demineralization of bone may not become apparent for 2 weeks or more after the onset of symptoms; calcification of the periosteum and surrounding soft tissues is usually delayed even longer.

Management Principles

Bactericidal antimicrobics continued for weeks

Surgery and prolonged therapy required for chronic osteomyelitis

In acute infections, early intervention is important. Management includes vigorous use of bactericidal antimicrobics, which must often be continued for several weeks to ensure a bacteriologic cure and prevent progression to chronic osteomyelitis. Surgical drainage is also essential if there is significant pressure from the localized, purulent process. In chronic osteomyelitis, sequestrum formation is frequent and sinuses may develop that drain the bone abscess to the skin surface. The infection is persistent, and treatment becomes extremely difficult. Such patients often require long-term antibiotic treatment (months to years) combined with surgical procedures to drain the abscesses and remove necrotic, infected tissues in an attempt to control infection while preserving the integrity of the affected bone.

SEPTIC ARTHRITIS

The usual clinical features of septic arthritis include onset of pain, which is often abrupt and accompanied by fever. Single or multiple joints may be involved. Tenderness and swelling of the affected joints and frequently other signs of local inflammation are present. Attempts to move the joints, either actively or passively, result in severe pain. In infants, the symptoms may be somewhat nonspecific; local swelling or excessive irritability with unwillingness to move the affected extremity (pseudoparalysis) may be the only clues to the diagnosis.

Pain on movement with swelling and fever

Common Etiologic Agents

The major causes of septic arthritis are listed in Table 60–2. Although *S. aureus* infection can occur at any age, there are some significant age-specific relationships to other bacterial causes. There is a high frequency of group B streptococcal infections in neonates, whereas in children between 1 month and 4 years of age, pneumococci are more likely to be involved. *Haemophilus influenzae* type b disease, which was once quite common in this age group, has been markedly diminished in the last decade; this is believed to be due to widespread use of an effective vaccine. *Neisseria gonorrhoeae* is implicated in most cases of septic arthritis in young adults. Subacute or chronic infective arthritis should prompt consideration of tuberculosis, Lyme disease, syphilis, and fungal infections such as coccidioidomycosis or *Candida.* Arthritis attributable to *Candida* is particularly likely in immunocompromised patients.

S. aureus appears at any age

Other pyogenic cocci are related to age and behavior

Tuberculous, spirochetal, and fungal arthritis have subacute or chronic course

Viruses and *Mycoplasma* can also cause acute arthritis in single or multiple joints. Such illnesses have been associated with rubella, hepatitis B, mumps, parvovirus B19, varicella, Epstein–Barr virus, coxsackievirus, and adenovirus infections, as well as with *M. pneumoniae* and *M. hominis.* These arthritides are usually self-limiting and rarely require specific therapy. Some bacterial infections of sites other than joints may be associated with noninfectious (reactive) arthritis, possibly resulting from deposition of circulating immune complexes and complement in synovial tissues, leading to inflammation. This has occurred with intestinal infections caused by *Yersinia enterocolitica, Campylobacter jejuni,* and some *Salmonella* species and also as a delayed sequela after successful treatment of sepsis due to *N. meningitidis* or *H. influenzae.*

Viral or *Mycoplasma* arthritis is usually self-limiting

Immune complexes from other sites may cause reactive arthritis

Noninfectious causes of arthritis must also be considered in the differential diagnosis. They can closely mimic septic arthritis. Examples include inflammatory collagen vascular disease such as rheumatoid arthritis, gout, traumatic arthritis, and degenerative arthritis.

TABLE 60–2

Common Causes of Septic Arthritis

AGE GROUP	USUAL CAUSATIVE ORGANISM
Neonate (<1 mo)	*Staphylococcus aureus,* group B streptococci, Gram-negative rods (eg, *Escherichia coli, Klebsiella, Proteus, Pseudomonas*)
1 mo–4 yr	*S. aureus,* group A streptococci, *Streptococcus pneumoniae, Neisseria meningitidis, Haemophilus influenzae* type b
4–16 yr	*S. aureus, Streptococcus pyogenes*
16–40 yr	*Neisseria gonorrhoeae, S. aureus*
>40 yr	*S. aureus*

TABLE 60–3

Findings in Synovial Fluid in Various Forms of Arthritis

Laboratory Test	Normal	Septic Bacterial Arthritis	Trauma, Degenerative Joint Disease	Rheumatoid Arthritis, Gout
Clarity and color	Clear	Opaque, yellow to green	Clear, yellow	Translucent, yellow; or opalescent
Viscosity	High	Variable	High	Low
White blood cells/mm^3	<200	25,000–100,000	200–2000	2000–20,000
Polymorphonuclear cells (%)	<25	>75	25–50	≥50
Glucose level (relative to simultaneous blood glucose level)	Nearly equal	<25%	Nearly equal	50–80%

Diagnostic Approaches

Blood culture is particularly useful

Needle aspiration of synovial fluid is used for analysis and culture

In acute cases, blood cultures are often useful because bacteremia may be present. The definitive diagnosis is established by examination of synovial fluid removed from the joint by needle aspiration (arthrocentesis). Because other noninfectious causes must be considered, it is important to analyze the chemical and cellular characteristics of the fluid in addition to performing a Gram stain and culture. Table 60–3 summarizes the major findings in synovial fluid in normal and various disease states. Septic bacterial arthritis is usually associated with grossly purulent fluid containing more than 25,000 white blood cells per cubic millimeter, predominantly polymorphonuclear cells. The glucose level in the synovial fluid is usually less than 25% of that in the blood.

Biopsy is especially useful in chronic cases

In viral, tuberculous, and fungal arthritis, as well as in partially treated bacterial arthritis, cell counts are usually lower, and mononuclear cells may constitute a greater proportion of the inflammatory cells. Occasionally, biopsy of the synovial membrane may be required to resolve the diagnosis. Histologic examination and culture of the tissue are particularly helpful in distinguishing granulomatous from rheumatoid disease.

Gonococci may be difficult to isolate from joint fluid

In most cases of acute septic arthritis, the blood culture and/or synovial fluid culture yields the specific etiologic agent. One major exception is *N. gonorrhoeae,* which can be difficult to isolate from these sources. When this organism is suspected, it is wise to include cultures of other sites of potential infection, such as the urethra, cervix, rectum, and pharynx, as well as skin lesions.

Management Principles

Drainage of hip infections often necessary

Prompt, vigorous, systemic antimicrobial therapy is required as soon as diagnostic tests suggest a bacterial cause. This treatment usually must be continued for 3 to 6 weeks, depending on the etiologic agent and the clinical response to therapy. Drainage of pus under pressure is also an important aspect of management. In cases of hip joint involvement, open surgical drainage is often necessary because collateral blood supply to the hip joint is relatively limited, and pus under pressure can lead to irreversible avascular necrosis of the tissues with permanent crippling. It is also difficult to evaluate the amount of pus that may be present because of the overlying muscles. Other joints can usually be managed by simple aspiration of pus whenever it reaccumulates significantly during the acute phase of infection.

CHAPTER 61

Eye, Ear, and Sinus Infections

C. GEORGE RAY

EYE INFECTIONS

Ocular infections can be divided into those that primarily involve the external structures—eyelids, conjunctiva, sclera, and cornea—and those that involve internal sites. The major defense mechanisms of the eye are the tears and the conjunctiva, as well as the mechanical cleansing that occurs with blinking of the eyelids. The tears contain secretory IgA and lysozyme, and the conjunctiva possesses numerous lymphocytes, plasma cells, neutrophils, and mast cells, which can respond quickly to infection by inflammation and production of antibody and cytokines. The internal eye is protected from external invasion primarily by the physical barrier imposed by the sclera and cornea. If these are breached (eg, by a penetrating injury or ulceration), infection becomes a possibility. In addition, infection may reach the internal eye via the blood-borne route to the retinal arteries and produce chorioretinitis and/or uveitis. Such infections are a particularly common problem in immunocompromised patients.

Defenses of the eye include tears, conjunctiva, and blinking

Tears have sIgA and lysozymes

Other causes of inflammation of the external or internal eye can involve autoimmune or allergic mechanisms, which may be provoked by infectious agents or diseases such as rheumatoid arthritis.

Autoimmune and allergic causes of inflammation

COMMON CLINICAL CONDITIONS

Blepharitis is an acute or chronic inflammatory disease of the eyelid margin. It can take the form of a localized inflammation in the external margin (hordeolum or stye) or a granulomatous reaction to infection and plugging of a sebaceous gland of the eyelid (chalazion).

Dacryocystitis is an inflammation of the lacrimal sac. It usually results from partial or complete obstruction within the sac or nasolacrimal duct, where bacteria may be trapped and initiate either an acute or a chronic infection.

Conjunctivitis is a term used to describe inflammation of the conjunctiva; it may extend to involve the eyelids, cornea (keratitis), or sclera (episcleritis). Extensive disease involving the conjunctiva and cornea is often called keratoconjunctivitis. Progressive keratitis can lead to ulceration, scarring, and blindness. **Ophthalmia neonatorum** is an acute, sometimes severe, conjunctivitis or keratoconjunctivitis of newborn infants.

Endophthalmitis is rare, but often leads to blindness even when treated aggressively. The term refers to infection of the aqueous or vitreous humor, usually by bacteria or fungi.

Uveitis consists of inflammation of the uveal tract—iris, ciliary body, and choroid. Although most inflammations of the iris and ciliary body (iridocyclitis) are not of infectious origin, some agents have been implicated. The acute disease may be associated with severe eye pain, redness, and photophobia; other cases may progress quite silently, with decreased visual acuity as the only symptom in the late stages. The most common infective involvement of the uveal tract is **chorioretinitis,** in which inflammatory infiltrates are seen in the retina; this infection can lead to destruction of the choroid and inflammation of the optic nerve (optic neuritis) and may extend into the vitreous humor to cause endophthalmitis. If the disease is not treated adequately, the end result can be blindness.

COMMON ETIOLOGIC AGENTS

Blepharitis often staphylococcal

Acute conjunctivitis: age-related etiologies

Chronic conjunctivitis: *C. trachomatis* and herpes simplex

The major infectious causes of various inflammatory diseases of the eye are listed in Table 61–1. *Staphylococcus aureus* is the principal offender in bacterial infections of the eyelid and cornea. *Haemophilus influenzae* and *Streptococcus pneumoniae* are common causes of acute bacterial conjunctivitis. In young infants, *Neisseria gonorrhoeae* and *Chlamydia trachomatis* are significant causes of external eye disease, contracted from the mother's birth canal, that must be diagnosed and treated promptly. Chronic conjunctivitis or keratoconjunctivitis at any age must also prompt consideration of *C. trachomatis* infection. Herpes simplex is also a major cause of chronic or recurrent conjunctivitis, especially in infections of the external structures, and specific therapy is available. Epidemic

TABLE 61–1

Major Infectious Causes of Eye Disease

Disease	Bacteria	Viruses	Fungi	Parasites
Blepharitis	*Staphylococcus aureus*			
Dacryocystitis	*Streptococcus pneumoniae, S. aureus*			
Conjunctivitis, keratitis, keratoconjunctivitis	*S. pneumoniae, Haemophilus influenzae, Haemophilus aegyptius, Streptococcus pyogenes, S. aureus, Chlamydia trachomatis, Neisseria gonorrhoeae, Neisseria meningitidis*	Adenoviruses, herpes simplex; measles, varicella–zoster	*Eusarium* species, *Aspergillus* species	*Acanthamoeba* (keratitis)
Ophthalmia neonatorum	*N. gonorrhoeae, Chlamydia trachomatis*	Herpes simplex		
Endophthalmitis	*S. aureus, Pseudomonas aeruginosa,* other Gram-negative organisms		*Candida* species, *Aspergillus* species	
Iridocyclitis	*Treponema pallidum*	Herpes simplex, varicella–zoster		
Chorioretinitis	*Mycobacterium tuberculosis*	Cytomegalovirus, herpes simplex, varicella–zoster	*Histoplasma capsulatum, Coccidioides immitis, Candida* species	*Toxoplasma gondii, Toxocara canis*

conjunctivitis or keratoconjunctivitis is most commonly associated with a variety of adenovirus serotypes. Outbreaks have been associated with inadequately chlorinated swimming pools, contaminated equipment or eyedrops in physicians' offices, and communal sharing of towels, which facilitates direct transmission.

Epidemic adenovirus conjunctivitis related to swimming pools and eyedrops

Chorioretinitis is frequently a manifestation of systemic disease (eg, histoplasmosis, tuberculosis) and congenital infections. It is particularly common in immunocompromised patients, who are liable to develop disseminated *Candida,* cytomegalovirus, or *Toxoplasma gondii* infections. Endophthalmitis may also result from blood-borne dissemination or by contiguous spread as a result of injury (eg, corneal ulcerations). In the latter situation, iatrogenic infection by agents such as *Pseudomonas* species can be induced by contaminated eye drops and ophthalmologic examination equipment.

Chorioretinitis usually linked to systemic disease, congenital infections, or immunocompromise

Endophthalmitis is from blood-borne or contiguous spread

Infection of the soft tissues surrounding the eye (periorbital or orbital cellulitis) is potentially severe and can spread to involve the functions of the eye itself. Major causes are *S. aureus, H. influenzae, Streptococcus pyogenes,* and *S. pneumoniae.*

DIAGNOSTIC APPROACHES

In external bacterial infections of the eye, etiologic diagnoses can usually be established by Gram stain and culture of surface material or, in the case of viral infections, by tissue culture. Conjunctival scrapings for *C. trachomatis* can be prepared for immunofluorescent or cytologic examination and for appropriate culture. Infections of internal sites pose a more difficult problem. Some, such as acute endophthalmitis, may require removal of infected aqueous humor for microbiologic studies. Infections involving the uveal tract may require indirect methods of diagnosis, such as serologic tests for toxoplasmosis and deep mycoses, blood cultures to demonstrate evidence of disseminated disease (eg, *Candida* sepsis), and efforts to demonstrate infection in other sites (eg, chest radiography and sputum culture to diagnose tuberculosis). Careful ophthalmologic examination using slit lamps and retinoscopy often helps suggest specific etiologic agents based on the morphology of the lesions observed.

Gram stain and cultures of surface scrapings

Most agents can be cultured

MANAGEMENT PRINCIPLES

Various topical antimicrobial agents have been used effectively in external eye infections of presumed or proved bacterial origin. In addition, topical antiviral treatment is available for herpes simplex infections but has not been proved efficacious for other viral diseases of the eye. Severe infections, whether external or internal, require specialized treatment that nearly always includes ophthalmologic consultation because they may threaten vision. Systemic infection associated with eye disease (eg, fungemia, tuberculosis) must be treated vigorously with appropriate antimicrobial agents.

Topical agents used for superficial bacterial and herpes simplex infections

Ophthalmologic consultation needed with severe or deep infection

EAR INFECTIONS

Most infections of the ear involve the external otic canal (otitis externa) or the middle ear cavity (otitis media), which contains the ossicles and is enclosed by bony structures and the tympanic membrane. Factors of importance in the pathogenesis of otitis externa include local trauma, furunculosis, foreign bodies, or excessive moisture, which can lead to maceration of the external ear epithelium (swimmer's ear). Occasionally, external otitis occurs as an extension of infection from the middle ear, with purulent drainage through a perforated tympanic membrane.

Otitis externa linked to ear canal trauma and excessive moisture

The eustachian tube, which vents the middle ear to the nasopharynx, appears to play a major role in predisposing patients to otitis media. The tube performs three functions: ventilation, protection, and clearance via mucociliary transport. Viral upper respiratory infections or allergic conditions can cause inflammation and edema in the eustachian tube or at its orifice. These developments disturb its functions, of which ventilation may be the most important. As ventilation is lost, oxygen is absorbed from the air in the middle ear cavity, producing negative pressure. This pressure in turn allows entry of potentially pathogenic bacteria from the nasopharynx into the middle ear, and failure to clear these normally can result in colonization and infection. Other factors that can lead to compromise of eustachian tube function include anatomic abnormalities, such as tissue hypertrophy or scarring around the orifice, muscular dysfunction associated with cleft palate, and lack of stiffness of the tube wall. The latter is common in infancy and early childhood and improves with age. It may explain in part why otitis media occurs most often in infants 6 to 18 months of age and then decreases in frequency as patency of the eustachian tube becomes established.

Viral infections and allergy predispose to otitis media

Microbes enter middle ear by the eustachian tube

Failure to clear leads to otitis media

MANIFESTATIONS

Otitis externa is characterized by inflammation of the ear canal, with purulent ear drainage. It can be quite painful, and cellulitis can extend into adjacent soft tissues. A common form is associated with swimming in water that may be contaminated with aerobic, Gram-negative organisms such as *Pseudomonas* species. "Malignant" otitis externa is a considerably more severe form of external ear canal infection that can progress to invasion of cartilage and adjacent bone, sometimes leading to cranial nerve palsy and death. It is seen most frequently in elderly patients with diabetes mellitus and in immunocompromised hosts of any age. *Pseudomonas aeruginosa* is the most common causative pathogen.

P. aeruginosa causes swimming pool and malignant otitis externa

Otitis media is arbitrarily classified as acute, chronic, or serous (secretory). Acute otitis media, nearly always caused by bacteria, is often a complication of acute viral upper respiratory illness. Fever, irritability, and acute pain are common, and otoscopic examination reveals bulging of the tympanic membrane, poor mobility, and obscuration of normal anatomic landmarks by fluid and inflammatory cells under pressure. In some cases, the tympanic membrane is also acutely inflamed, with blisters (bullae) on its external surface (myringitis). If treated inadequately, the infection can progress to involve adjacent structures such as the mastoid air cells (mastoiditis) or lead to perforation with spontaneous drainage through the tympanic membrane. Potential acute, suppurative sequelae include extension into the central nervous system (CNS) and sepsis.

Acute otitis media usually bacterial

Extension to deeper structures leads to mastoiditis and sometimes CNS involvement

Chronic otitis media is usually a result of acute infection that has not resolved adequately, either because of inadequate treatment in the acute phase or because of host factors that perpetuate the inflammatory process (eg, continued eustachian tube dysfunction, caused by allergic or anatomic factors or immunodeficiency). Sequelae include progressive destruction of middle ear structures and a significant risk of permanent hearing loss. Serous otitis media may represent either a form of chronic otitis media or allergy-related inflammation. It tends to be chronic, causing hearing deficits, and is associated with thick, usually nonpurulent secretions in the middle ear.

Chronic otitis media follows unresolved acute infections

COMMON ETIOLOGIC AGENTS

The usual causes of ear infections are listed in Table 61–2. *S. pneumoniae* is the single most common cause of acute otitis media after the first 3 months of life, accounting for 35 to 40% of all cases. *H. influenzae* is also common, particularly in patients less than 5 years of age. The majority of *H. influenzae* isolates from the middle ear are nontypeable; thus the current vaccine against type b strains would not be expected to markedly reduce the incidence of acute otitis media. Viruses and *Mycoplasma* are rare primary causes of acute or chronic otitis media; however, they predispose patients to superinfection by the bacterial agents.

S. pneumoniae most common cause

H. influenzae strains usually nontypeable

DIAGNOSTIC APPROACHES

The diagnosis is established on the basis of clinical examination. Tympanometry can be performed in suspected cases of otitis media to detect the presence of fluid in the middle ear and to assess tympanic membrane function. The specific etiology of otitis externa can

TABLE 61–2

Common Causes of Ear Infection

Disease	Cause
Otitis externa	*Pseudomonas aeruginosa* is common; occasionally *Proteus* species, *Escherichia coli,* and *Staphylococcus aureus;* bacteria found in otitis media may also be recovered if the process is secondary to middle ear infection with perforation and drainage through the tympanic membrane; fungi, such as *Aspergillus* species, are occasionally implicated
Acute otitis media	
<3 mo of age	*Streptococcus pneumoniae,* group B streptococci, *Haemophilus influenzae, Staphylococcus aureus, Pseudomonas aeruginosa,* and Gram-negative enteric bacteria
>3 mo of age	*Streptococcus pneumoniae* and *Haemophilus influenzae* are most common; others include *Streptococcus pyogenes, Moraxella catarrhalis,* and *Staphylococcus aureus*
Chronic otitis media	Mixed flora in 40% of cases cultured. Common organisms include *Pseudomonas aeruginosa, Haemophilus influenzae, Staphylococcus aureus, Proteus* species, *Klebsiella pneumoniae, Moraxella catarrhalis,* and Gram-positive as well as Gram-negative anaerobic bacteria
Serous otitis media	Same as chronic otitis media; however, many more of these effusions are sterile, with relatively few acute inflammatory cells

be determined by culture of the affected ear canal; however, one must keep in mind that surface contamination and normal skin flora may lead to mixed cultures, which can be confusing. In otitis media, the most precise diagnostic method is careful aspiration with a sterile needle through the tympanic membrane after decontamination of the external canal. Gram stain and culture of such aspirates is highly reliable; however, this procedure is generally reserved for cases in which etiologic possibilities are extremely varied, as in young infants, or when clinical response to the usual antimicrobial therapy has been inadequate. Respiratory tract cultures, such as those from the nasopharynx, cannot be relied on to provide an etiologic diagnosis.

External ear canal cultures often confusing

Middle ear aspirate cultures reliable but reserved for difficult cases

Respiratory tract cultures unhelpful

MANAGEMENT PRINCIPLES

Except in severe cases, otitis externa can usually be managed by gentle cleansing with topical solutions. The Gram-negative bacteria most commonly involved are often susceptible to an acidic environment, and otic solutions buffered to a low pH (3.0 or less), as with 0.25% acetic acid, are often effective. Various preparations are available, many of which also contain antimicrobics.

Otitis externa treated with topical agents

Acute otitis media requires antimicrobial therapy and careful follow-up to ensure that the disease has resolved. The choice of antimicrobic is usually empirical, designed specifically to cover the most likely bacterial pathogens, because direct aspiration for diagnostic purposes is usually unnecessary. In the usual case, these pathogens would be *S. pneumoniae* and *H. influenzae.* If there is extreme pressure with severe pain, drainage of middle ear exudates by careful incision of the tympanic membrane may be necessary. In patients with chronic or serous otitis media, management can be more complex, and it is often advisable to seek otolaryngologic consultation to determine further diagnostic procedures as well as to plan medical and possible surgical measures.

Antimicrobic therapy for otitis media directed at common agents for age group

Drainage may be required

SINUS INFECTIONS

The paranasal sinuses (ethmoid, frontal, and maxillary) all communicate with the nasal cavity. In healthy individuals, these sinuses are air-filled cavities lined with ciliated epithelium and are normally sterile. They are poorly developed in early life and, in contrast to otitis media, sinus infections are a rare problem in infancy. The pathogenesis of sinus infection can involve several factors, most of which act by producing obstruction or edema of the sinus opening, impeding normal drainage. Consequently, bacterial infection and inflammation of the mucosal lining tissues develop. Predisposing factors may be (1) local, such as upper respiratory infections producing edema of antral tissues, mucosal polyps, deviation of the nasal septum, enlarged adenoids, or a tumor or foreign body in the nasal cavity; or (2) systemic, such as allergy, cystic fibrosis, or immunodeficiency. Occasionally, maxillary sinusitis can result from extension of a maxillary dental infection.

Factors predisposing to sinusitis involve obstruction of drainage or extension from other sites

MANIFESTATIONS

Signs and symptoms vary according to which sinuses are affected and whether the illness is acute or chronic. Fever is sometimes present. In addition, nasal or postnasal discharge, daytime cough that may become worse at night, fetid breath, pain over the affected sinus, headache, and tenderness to percussion over the frontal or maxillary sinuses are all features that may appear in different combinations and suggest the diagnosis. Complications of sinusitis can include extension of infection to nearby soft tissues, such as the orbit, and occasionally spread, either directly or via vascular pathways, into the CNS.

Fever and tenderness in local area are common

COMMON ETIOLOGIC AGENTS

Table 61–3 summarizes the usual etiologies of sinus infections. Respiratory viruses are also occasional direct causes but are most important as predisposing factors to bacterial superinfection of inflamed sinuses and their antral openings. Together, *S. pneumoniae* and *H. influenzae* account for more than 60% of cases of acute sinusitis. Opportunistic, saprophytic fungi, such as *Mucor, Aspergillus,* and *Rhizopus* species, are being increasingly seen in compromised hosts, such as those with severe diabetes mellitus or immunodeficiency. These have a particular tendency to spread progressively to adjacent tissues and to the CNS and are very difficult to treat.

Opportunistic fungi are increasingly found in immunocompromised patients

DIAGNOSTIC APPROACHES

Radiographic studies of the sinuses confirms the diagnosis. If it becomes necessary to determine the specific infectious agent, fluid should be obtained directly from the affected sinus by needle puncture of the sinus wall or by catheterization of the sinus antrum after careful decontamination of the entry site. Gram smears and cultures are then made. Cultures of drainage from the antral orifices or nasal secretions are unreliable because of contaminating aerobic and anaerobic normal flora.

Gram stain and cultures of direct sinus aspirates most accurate

Cultures of sinus drainage unreliable

TABLE 61–3

Common Causes of Sinus Infection

Disease	Cause
Acute sinusitis	*Streptococcus pneumoniae* and *Haemophilus influenzae* are most common; also *Streptococcus pyogenes, Staphylococcus aureus,* and *Moraxella catarrhalis*
Chronic sinusitis	Same as for acute sinusitis; also Gram-negative enteric bacteria and anaerobic Gram-negative and Gram-positive bacteria; mixed aerobic and anaerobic infections are relatively common; opportunistic fungi may be found in compromised patients (eg, those with diabetes mellitus)

MANAGEMENT PRINCIPLES

In uncomplicated acute sinusitis, prompt antimicrobial therapy is initiated. The choice of antimicrobics is usually empirical, based on the most likely bacterial causes and their usual susceptibility. For example, amoxicillin is effective against most strains of *S. pneumoniae* and *H. influenzae.* Severe, complicated acute infections and chronic sinusitis often require otolaryngologic consultation. In such cases, it is often necessary to obtain cultures directly from the sinuses to select specific antimicrobial therapy, consider the need for surgical procedures to adequately remove the pus and inflammatory tissues, and correct any anatomic obstruction that may exist.

Antimicrobic choice is usually empirical in uncomplicated cases

Direct cultures may be required in severe, chronic cases

CHAPTER 62

Dental and Periodontal Infections

MURRAY R. ROBINOVITCH

Dental caries, chronic periodontitis, and the sequelae of these two diseases constitute the majority of oral and dental infections and the cause of tooth loss. In both, the source of the causative bacteria is the microbial plaque that forms on the teeth. Thus, although dental caries and chronic periodontitis are distinctly different, the prevention and/or halting of the progression of these diseases relies on the elimination of dental plaque from the tooth surfaces. In addition to causing caries and chronic periodontitis, the bacteria of dental plaque play a role in more aggressive forms of periodontitis and necrotizing periodontal diseases.

Dental plaque is a soft, adherent dental deposit that forms as a result of bacterial colonization of the tooth surface. It is rather insoluble, as well as adherent, and thus resists removal by water spray or mouth rinsing. Only more vigorous means such as tooth brushing and flossing between the teeth remove it. It consists almost entirely of bacterial cells (1.7×10^{11} cells/g wet weight).

Dental plaque is a deposit from bacterial colonization

Dental caries is the progressive destruction of the mineralized tissues of the tooth, primarily caused by the production of organic acids resulting from the glycolytic metabolic activity of plaque bacteria. The basic characteristic of the carious lesion is that it progresses inward from the tooth surface, either the enamel-coated crown or the cementum of the exposed root surface, involving the dentin and finally the pulp of the tooth (Fig 62–1). From there, infection can extend out into the periodontal tissues at the root apex or apices.

Caries produced by plaque bacteria

Plaque-induced periodontal disease encompasses two separate disease entities: gingivitis and chronic periodontitis. These diseases are believed to be related, in that gingivitis, although a reversible condition, is thought to be an early stage leading ultimately to chronic periodontitis in the susceptible subject. The term **gingivitis** is used when the inflammatory condition is limited to the marginal gingiva and bone resorption around the necks of teeth has not yet begun. **Chronic periodontitis** is used to connote the stage of chronic periodontal disease in which there is progressive loss of tooth support due to resorption of the alveolar bone and periodontal ligament. Periodontitis can also lead to periodontal abscess when the chronic inflammatory state around the necks of the teeth becomes acute at a specific location.

Chronic periodontal infection causes destruction of supporting tissues

Chronic periodontitis, formerly referred to as adult periodontitis, is responsible for most tooth loss in people greater than 35 to 40 years of age. The term chronic indicates that the disease progresses slowly and results in the progressive destruction of the supporting tissues of the tooth (periodontal ligament and alveolar bone) from the margins of the gingiva toward the apices of the roots of the teeth. Although the accumulative effects

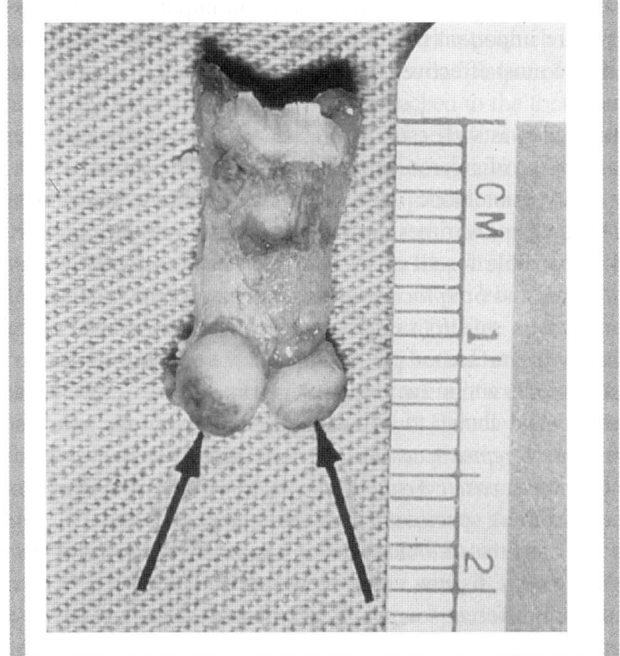

FIGURE 62–4
Periapical involvement of a premolar, resulting from the extension of infection through the root canals and into the periodontium at the root apices. In this case, chronic nonsuppurating lesions have formed at the apical ends of the two root canals (see arrows).

Extension to pulp and periapical locations complicate infections

More severe complications spread to bone or local fascia

The most common complications of dental caries are extension of the infection into the pulp chamber of the tooth (pulpitis), necrosis of the pulp, and extension of the infection through the root canals into the periapical area of the periodontal ligament. Periapical involvement may take the form of an acute inflammation (periapical abscess), a chronic nonsuppurating inflammation (periapical granuloma), or a chronic suppurating lesion that may drain into the mouth or onto the face via a sinus tract (Fig 62–4). A cyst may form within the chronic nonsuppurating lesion as a result of inflammatory stimulation of the epithelial rests normally found in the periodontal ligament. If the infectious agent is sufficiently virulent or host resistance is low, the infection may spread into the alveolar bone (osteomyelitis) or the fascial planes of the head and neck (cellulitis). Alternatively, it may ascend along the venous channels to cause septic thrombophlebitis. Because most carious lesions represent a mixed infection by the time cavities have developed, it is not surprising that most oral infections resulting from the extension of carious lesions are mixed and frequently include anaerobic organisms.

CHRONIC PERIODONTITIS

Subgingival plaque causes collagen loss

Both gingivitis and chronic periodontitis are now believed to be caused by certain bacteria in the dental plaque that lie in close proximity to the necks of the teeth and marginal gingival tissues. Thus, subgingival plaque found within the gingival crevice or the sulcus around the necks of the teeth is thought to house the etiologic agent(s). The characteristic histopathologic picture of gingivitis is of a marked inflammatory infiltrate of polymorphonuclear leukocytes, lymphocytes, and plasma cells in the connective tissue that lies immediately adjacent to the epithelium lining the gingival crevice and attached to the tooth. Collagen is lost from the inflamed connective tissue. There does not seem to be any direct invasion of the gingival tissues by large numbers of intact bacteria, at least in the early stages of the disease.

It has been proposed that tissue destruction is mediated by bacterial substances that pass through the epithelial barrier and cause either direct or indirect injury. Bacterial products that could cause direct injury to the tissues include toxins, such as endotoxin and leukotoxins, and enzymes, such as hyaluronidase and collagenase. Several mechanisms for indirect injury of the periodontal tissues have been proposed. These hypotheses include initiation of an unresolvable inflammatory response with excessive release of the lysosomal contents from polymorphonuclear leukocytes; activation of complement, which further magnifies the inflammatory response; and development of a host of humoral and cell-mediated immune responses, which can also magnify the inflammatory reaction as well as lead to tissue destruction. A complex pattern of interactions between various released chemokines and cytokines (eg, interleukins 1, 4, 5, 6, and 12; tumor necrosis factor-α; interferons-α and β; transforming growth factor-β; and prostaglandin E_2) and their target cells have been implicated in the modulation of the host response to the periodontal pathogens, some of which may lead to tissue destruction. Many oral bacteria have been found to contain potent polyclonal β-lymphocyte activators, leading some investigators to propose that periodontal pathogens release these substances into lesions. Polyclonal β-cell activation could promote an exaggeration of the inflammatory response and further tissue injury through enhanced antibody and cytokine production. Regardless of the mechanisms of tissue destruction, the true source of the disease, namely the causative bacteria, remains outside the gingival tissues in supra- and subgingival plaque and is therefore often resistant to the body's defense mechanisms. There is evidence that some bacteria do invade the gingival tissues, especially in the more aggressive forms of periodontitis, and this invasion may constitute a pathogenic mechanism. Nevertheless, the origin of these bacteria is the dental plaque, and so the disease continues to progress unless the dental plaque is removed and the involved tooth is kept plaque-free. If these measures are taken, chronic gingivitis can resolve completely and the tissues return to normal.

Tissue destruction mediated by bacterial products

Immunologic mediators play a role in tissue damage

Bacterial source of the disease is outside the affected tissues

As the disease progresses, a point may be reached at which the alveolar bone around the necks of the teeth is resorbed; the condition is then no longer termed gingivitis, but periodontitis. With resorption of the bone, the attachment of the periodontal ligament is lost and the gingival sulcus deepens into a periodontal pocket. Periodontitis is not considered to be a reversible disease in that the lost alveolar bone and periodontal ligament do not regenerate with cessation of the inflammation, even though further progression may be halted. If unchecked, bone resorption progresses to loosening of the tooth, which may ultimately be exfoliated. Figure 62–5 shows a case of advanced chronic periodontitis in which the gingival tissues are inflamed, gross deposits of plaque and calculus around the necks of the teeth are apparent, and the teeth have spread apart and extruded due to the major loss in their periodontal attachment. Occasionally, the neck of a periodontal pocket becomes constricted, the bacteria proliferate causing an acute inflammatory response in the occluded pocket, and a periodontal abscess results. This acute exacerbation requires drainage in the same way as abscesses elsewhere for the patient to obtain symptomatic relief.

With continued progress, periodontitis and bone resorption develop

Periodontal abscess may result

Gingivitis develops within 2 weeks in individuals who fail to practice effective tooth cleansing. It is not known whether particular species of plaque bacteria are responsible for gingival inflammation, but among those suspected of pathogenicity in the case of

Multiple organisms involved in chronic periodontitis

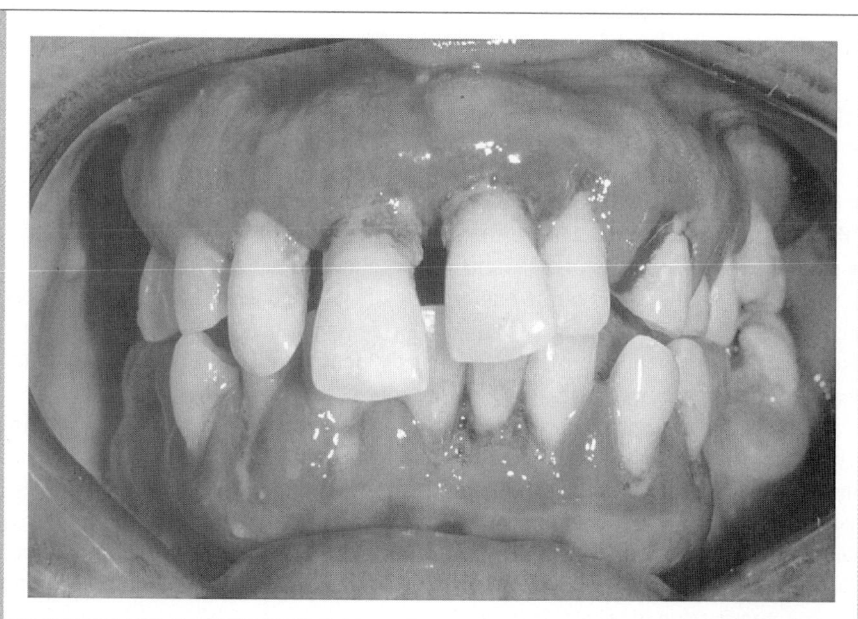

FIGURE 62–5
A patient exhibiting advanced chronic periodontitis as evidenced by marked recession, inflammation of the gingival tissues, and tooth mobility and separation. Note the presence of copious amounts of dental plaque and calculus (mineralized plaque) around the necks of the teeth.

chronic periodontitis are anaerobic Gram-negative rods (*Porphyromonas gingivalis, Prevotella intermedia, Bacteroides forsythus, Campylobacter rectus, Fusobacterium nucleatum*), *Peptostreptococcus micros, Eikenella corrodens,* and *Treponema denticola.* Many of these organisms produce periodontal disease in monoinfected animals. It has been suggested recently that the disease may be caused by the combined effects of two or more of these pathogens at a site, rather than there being only one species of microorganism responsible for the destructive lesion.

Acute juvenile periodontitis associated with *Actinobacillus*

There is some evidence that the causative agents in aggressive forms of periodontitis may differ from those associated with chronic marginal disease. In the condition known as localized aggressive periodontitis, a small capnophilic (carbon dioxide–requiring) Gram-negative rod (*Actinobacillus actinomycetemcomitans*) has been indicted based on studies of the flora of disease sites. A virulence factor found in those strains of *A. actinomycetemcomitans* that are associated with this disease is the production of a leukotoxin by the bacteria. In addition, it has been found that a significant proportion of patients with this condition demonstrate high serum antibody titers to *A. actinomycetemcomitans.* Also of interest is the fact that many of these patients have neutrophil chemotactic or phagocytic defects.

NECROTIZING PERIODONTAL DISEASES

Acute onset with painful ulcerative lesions

Fusospirochetal etiology together with other anaerobes

Necrotizing ulcerative gingivitis (previously called acute necrotizing ulcerative gingivitis, Vincent's infection, or trench mouth) and necrotizing ulcerative periodontitis represent a spectrum of acute inflammatory disease starting with destruction limited to the soft tissues (gingivitis) and extending to destruction of the alveolar bone and periodontal ligament (periodontitis). This disease spectrum is distinctly different from gingivitis–chronic periodontitis. It has an acute onset, frequently associated with periods of stress and poor oral hygiene. There is rapid ulceration of the interdental areas of the gingiva, resulting in destruction of the interdental papillae. The inflammatory condition initially confined to the gingival tissues can quickly extend into pathologic bone resorption. Unlike gingivitis and chronic periodontitis, acute necrotizing periodontal disease is painful. As the oral epithelium is destroyed, the causative bacteria come into direct contact with the underlying tissues and may invade them. Spirochetes and fusiform bacteria have been implicated; thus, the term fusospirochetal disease has been used to describe this infection, which can also be manifested as ulceration in other areas of the pharynx or oral cavity. *Prevotella intermedia* has also been found in high numbers in the lesions. Morphologic studies have shown that the spirochetes actually appear to invade the tissues. The disease may be treated with systemic antibiotics and topical antimicrobials for immediate relief of symptoms, but resolution is dependent on thorough professional cleaning of the teeth and institution of good home care. Further discussion of fusospirochetal disease is provided in Chapter 27.

DENTAL PLAQUE AND ORAL FLORA IN THE COMPROMISED PATIENT

Endocarditis from oral flora unless protected by prophylaxis

As it can be the source of transient bacteremia, dental plaque must be viewed as a hazard in the compromised patient. The best example is the patient with heart valve damage as a result of a congenital anomaly, rheumatic fever, or a heart prosthesis. If transient bacteremia develops, the blood-borne bacteria may form vegetative growths in the heart and cause bacterial endocarditis (see Chapter 68). Such patients should always be premedicated with prophylactic antibiotics before any dental procedure with the potential for causing a bacteremia is performed, including routine dental prophylaxis.

Severe opportunistic infections may develop in the immunocompromised patient

It has also been established that dental plaque organisms and other oral bacteria may give rise to serious systemic infections in patients whose host defense mechanisms are compromised. Patients who have undergone extensive radiation treatment of the jaw area, for example, are prone to develop osteomyelitis. Furthermore, one of the most frequent sources of fatal infections in leukemic patients is the oral cavity. Therefore, for these patients scrupulous home care and professional dental treatment are indicated prior to undergoing immunosuppressive therapies.

ADDITIONAL READING

The following references are authoritative reviews of caries and periodontal disease and new advances in understanding these conditions:

Newbrun E. *Cariology,* 3rd ed. Chicago: Quintessence Publishing; 1989.

Newman MG, Takei HH, Carranza FA (eds). *Carranza's Clinical Periodontology.* 9th ed. Philadelphia: WB Saunders; 2002.

Socransky SS, Haffajee AD (eds). Microbiology and immunology of periodontal diseases. In *Periodontology 2000,* vol 5. Copenhagen, Denmark: Munksgaard; 1994.

CHAPTER 63

Upper Respiratory Tract Infections and Stomatitis

C. GEORGE RAY

Upper respiratory infections usually involve the nasal cavity and pharynx, and most (more than 80%) are caused by viruses. Like middle and lower respiratory illnesses, the diseases of the upper respiratory tract are named according to the anatomic sites primarily involved. **Rhinitis** (or coryza) implies inflammation of the nasal mucosa, **pharyngitis** denotes pharyngeal infection, and **tonsillitis** indicates an inflammatory involvement of the tonsils. Because of the close proximity of these structures to one another, infections may simultaneously involve two or more sites (eg, rhinopharyngitis or tonsillopharyngitis). All such infections are grouped under the general term upper respiratory infections. **Stomatitis** is a term used to describe infections primarily localized to the mucous membranes of the oral cavity. These infections can sometimes also involve the tongue (**glossitis**) or the gingival and periodontal tissues (**gingivostomatitis** or acute necrotizing ulcerative gingivitis; see Chapter 62).

Most upper respiratory infections are caused by viruses

Other infections considered are peritonsillar abscess (quinsy), retrotonsillar abscess, and retropharyngeal abscess. These infections are the result of direct invasion from mucosal sites and localization in deeper tissues to produce inflammation and abscess formation.

CLINICAL FEATURES

Rhinitis is the most common manifestation of the common cold. It is characterized by variable fever, inflammatory edema of the nasal mucosa, and an increase in mucous secretions. The net result is varying degrees of nasal obstruction; the nasal discharge may be clear and watery at the onset of illness, becoming thick and sometimes purulent as the infection progresses over 5 to 10 days.

The common cold is characterized by rhinitis

Pharyngitis and **tonsillitis** are associated with pharyngeal pain (sore throat) and the clinical appearance of erythema and swelling of the affected tissues. There may be exudates, consisting of inflammatory cells overlying the mucous membrane, and petechial hemorrhages; the latter may be seen in viral infections but tend to be more prominent in bacterial infections. Viral infections, particularly herpes simplex, may also lead to the formation of vesicles in the mucosa, which quickly rupture to leave ulcers. Pharyngeal candidiasis can also erode the mucosa under the plaques of "thrush." On rare occasions, the local inflammation may be sufficiently severe to produce **pseudomembranes,** which

Inflammatory exudates and hemorrhages more common in bacterial infections

Vesicles and ulcerated lesions more common in viral disease

consist of necrotic tissue, inflammatory cells, and bacteria. This finding is particularly common in pharyngeal diphtheria, but may be mimicked by fusospirochetal infection (Vincent's angina) and sometimes by infectious mononucleosis. In acute tonsillitis or pharyngitis of any etiology, regional spread of the infecting agents with inflammation and tender swelling of the anterior cervical lymph nodes is also common.

Pharyngeal pseudomembranes in diphtheria

Stomatitis is inflammation of the oral cavity. Multiple ulcerative lesions of the oral mucosa, seen most frequently with severe primary herpes simplex infections, may extend to the tongue, lips, and face. In extreme cases, the pain may be so severe that the patient requires relief with topical anesthetics during the usual 9- to 12-day period of acute symptoms. *Candida* species can also invade oral surfaces to produce plaques identical to those of pharyngeal thrush. This infection is particularly common in young infants and immunocompromised individuals of any age.

Herpes and *Candida* most common causes of stomatitis

Aphthous stomatitis is a recurrent disease of the oral mucosa characterized by single or multiple painful ulcers with irregular margins, usually 2 to 10 mm in diameter. Healing usually occurs in a few days. The term commonly used to describe this condition is **canker sore.** The cause is unknown. It can easily be confused with recurrent herpes simplex lesions and, like herpes, tends to recur in relation to stress, menses, local trauma, and other nonspecific stimuli.

Aphthous stomatitis (canker sores) have unknown cause

A severe, gangrenous stomatitis that progresses beyond the mucous membranes to involve soft tissues, skin, and sometimes bone can complicate a variety of acute illnesses in patients who are severely debilitated and whose oral hygiene is poor. This infection, called **noma** or **cancrum oris,** is rarely seen in the United States. Typical cases occur among children with severe protein–calorie malnutrition or other immune compromise. Measles sometimes precipitates noma. Etiologic agents thought to be involved include *Fusobacterium* and *Bacteroides* species, as well as *Pseudomonas aeruginosa.* Milder forms of stomatitis are seen in a variety of other common viral infections. Examples include Koplik's spots in measles, buccal or palatal ulcers in chickenpox, and similar phenomena in some enteroviral infections such as hand, foot, and mouth disease.

Noma is an extensive stomatitis of debilitated persons

Mild stomatitis occurs with many viral infections

Peritonsillar or retrotonsillar abscesses are usually a complication of tonsillitis. They are manifested by local pain, and examination of the pharynx reveals tonsillar asymmetry with one tonsil usually displaced medially by the abscess. This infection is most common in children more than 5 years of age and in young adults. If not properly treated, the abscess may spread to adjacent structures. It can involve the jugular venous system, erode into branches of the carotid artery to cause acute hemorrhage, or rupture into the pharynx to produce severe aspiration pneumonia.

Tonsillar asymmetry a sign of peritonsillar abscess

Retropharyngeal or lateral pharyngeal abscesses occur most frequently in infants and children less than 5 years of age. They can result from pharyngitis or from accidental perforation of the pharyngeal wall by a foreign body. The infection is characterized by pain, inability or unwillingness to swallow, and, if the pharyngeal wall is displaced anteriorly near the palate, a change in phonation (nasal speech). The neck may be held in an extended position to relieve pain and maintain an open upper airway. Examination of the pharynx usually reveals anterior bulging of the pharyngeal wall; if this finding is not apparent, lateral x-rays of the neck may demonstrate a widening of the space between the cervical spine and the posterior pharyngeal wall. The complications of such abscesses are basically the same as those described for peritonsillar abscesses; in addition, the suppurative process can extend posteriorly to the cervical spine to produce osteomyelitis or inferiorly to cause acute mediastinitis.

Retropharyngal abscess causes anterior bulging of pharyngeal wall

In the immunocompromised patient, all of the various forms of stomatitis and pharyngitis described previously can be accentuated. Leukemia, agranulocytosis, chronic ulcerative colitis, congenital or acquired immunodeficiency (eg, AIDS), and treatment with cytotoxic or immunosuppressive drugs are commonly associated with such lesions. The marked damage to mucosal tissues that sometimes occurs can provide a portal of entry into deeper structures and then to the systemic circulation, creating a risk of bacterial or fungal sepsis. Conversely, oral lesions may also result from dissemination of infection from other remote sites. Examples include disseminated histoplasmosis and sepsis caused by *Pseudomonas* species.

Oral and pharyngeal lesions accentuated in immunocompromised hosts

May be portal of entry for systemic infection

TABLE 63–1

Major Infectious Causes of Upper Respiratory Disease

DISEASE	VIRUSES	BACTERIA AND FUNGI
Rhinitis	Rhinoviruses, adenoviruses, coronaviruses, parainfluenza viruses, influenza viruses, respiratory syncytial virus, some coxsackie A viruses	Rare
Pharyngitis or tonsillitis	Adenoviruses, parainfluenza viruses, influenza viruses, rhinoviruses, coxsackie A or B virus, herpes simplex virus, Epstein–Barr virus	Group A streptococcus (*S. pyogenes*) *Corynebacterium diphtheriae, Neisseria gonorrhoeae*
Stomatitis	Herpes simplex virus, some coxsackie A viruses	*Candida* species, *Fusobacterium* species, spirochetes
Peritonsillar or retropharyngeal abscess	None	Group A streptococcus (most common), oral anaerobes such as *Fusobacterium* species, *Staphylococcus aureus, Haemophilus influenzae* (usually in infants)

COMMON ETIOLOGIC AGENTS

Table 63–1 lists the more common causes of upper respiratory infections and stomatitis. Viral infections predominate. The most frequent bacterial cause to be considered is *S. pyogenes*. *Corynebacterium diphtheriae,* although rare in the United States, is a major pathogen that continues to cause infection in many other countries and must not be overlooked, particularly if clinical and epidemiologic findings suggest this possibility. *Neisseria gonorrhoeae,* isolated from adults with symptomatic pharyngitis in whom no other etiologic agent can be demonstrated, is now considered a pharyngeal pathogen that is usually transmitted by oral–genital contact. Occasionally, other bacteria have been implicated as causes of acute pharyngitis (eg, *Corynebacterium ulcerans, Arcanobacterium haemolyticum, Francisella tularensis,* and streptococci of groups B, C, and G). These are listed here for the sake of completeness but are not routinely sought except in unusual circumstances.

Viral infections predominate

S. pyogenes and *C. diphtheriae* are bacterial pathogens

Gonococcal pharyngitis occurs with oral–genital contact

In patients with purulent rhinitis, sinusitis should also be considered in the differential diagnosis (see Chapter 61). Unilateral and foul-smelling purulent discharge suggests the presence of a foreign body in the nose.

GENERAL DIAGNOSTIC APPROACHES

Although viruses cause the vast majority of upper respiratory infections, they are generally not amenable to specific therapy, and laboratory tests for viral infections are usually reserved for investigating outbreaks or in cases in which the illness seems unusually severe or atypical.

The primary diagnostic approach in pharyngitis and tonsillitis is to determine whether there is a bacterial cause requiring specific treatment. The only reliable method is to collect a throat swab for culture, taking care to thoroughly swab the tonsillar fauces as well as the posterior pharynx, and to include any purulent material from inflamed areas. Cultures are usually made only to detect the presence or absence of group A streptococci. Direct antigen tests for rapidly detecting *S. pyogenes* in throat swabs have gained popularity in recent years. These are usually enzyme immunoassay or latex agglutination–based methods. The most common limitation of such tests is lack of sensitivity; that is, false-negative results can occur.

Approach is to determine if there is a bacterial etiology by culture

Direct detection methods have false-negative results

For the laboratory diagnosis of diphtheria or pharyngeal gonorrhea, the clinical suspicion should be indicated to the laboratory so that specific cultures for *C. diphtheriae* or

N. gonorrhoeae may be made. *Candida* species, fusospirochetal bacteria, *Pseudomonas* species, and other Gram-negative organisms are often found in pharyngeal or oral specimens from healthy individuals as well as in certain infections. Their probable pathogenic significance in association with disease in these sites, largely based on the appearance of the lesions and the presence of the organisms in large numbers, can be supported by histologic demonstration of tissue invasion by the organisms. It is important to remember that other bacterial pathogens such as *Streptococcus pneumoniae, Staphylococcus aureus, Haemophilus influenzae,* and even *Neisseria meningitidis* may be present in the pharynx. These organisms are not primary etiologic agents in rhinitis, pharyngitis, and tonsillitis, and their presence in the throat does not implicate them as causes of the illnesses; they should instead be regarded as colonizers.

Evidence for pathogenic role of opportunists assessed by multiple means

Pathogens may be present in normal flora but not cause pharyngitis

The laboratory diagnosis of causes of peritonsillar and retropharyngeal abscesses is based on Gram staining and culture of purulent material obtained directly from the lesion, including anaerobic cultures.

GENERAL PRINCIPLES OF MANAGEMENT

Viral infections of the upper respiratory tract can only be treated symptomatically. If *S. pyogenes* is the cause, penicillin therapy is required; if the patient is allergic to penicillin, an alternative is chosen (eg, erythromycin or a cephalosporin). Such treatment prevents suppurative or toxigenic complications (eg, pharyngeal abscess, cervical adenitis, and scarlet fever) and the development of acute rheumatic fever. The latter, a serious complication, may occur in 1 to 3% of patients in certain population groups if they are not adequately treated. In addition, treatment of acute streptococcal infections can aid in reducing spread of the organisms to other persons.

Penicillins or cephalosporins necessary to treat *S. pyogenes* infections

Macrolides used in penicillin-allergic patients

C. diphtheriae infections involve more complex management, which includes antitoxin as well as antimicrobic treatment (see Chapter 18). Infections caused by *N. gonorrhoeae* are treated with appropriate antimicrobics (see Chapter 20). The management of stomatitis includes maintenance of adequate oral hygiene. If invasive *Candida* infection is present, topical and/or systemic antifungal therapy is sometimes necessary. Vincent's angina and other fusospirochetal infections are usually treated with systemic penicillin therapy as well as with appropriate dental and periodontal care. There is no specific, widely accepted treatment for aphthous stomatitis. Peritonsillar and retropharyngeal abscesses are treated aggressively with antimicrobics and often require surgical drainage, taking care to prevent accidental aspiration of the abscess contents into the lower respiratory tract.

Peritonsillar and retropharyngeal abscesses often require surgical drainage

CHAPTER 64

Middle and Lower Respiratory Tract Infections

C. George Ray and Kenneth J. Ryan

Middle Respiratory Tract Infection

For the purpose of this discussion, the middle respiratory tract is considered to comprise the epiglottis, surrounding aryepiglottic tissues, larynx, trachea, and bronchi. Inflammatory disease involving these sites may be localized (eg, **laryngitis**) or more widespread (eg, laryngotracheobronchitis). The majority of severe infections occur in infancy and childhood. Disease expression varies somewhat with age, partly because the diameters of the airways enlarge with maturation and because immunity to common infectious agents increases with age. For example, an adult with a viral infection of the larynx (laryngitis) who was exposed to the same virus in childhood has a relatively better immune response; in addition, the larger diameter of the larynx in the adult permits greater air flow in the presence of inflammation. An infant or child with the same infection in the same site can develop a much more severe illness, known as **croup,** which can lead to significant obstruction of air flow.

Most severe middle tract infections occur in infancy and childhood

CLINICAL FEATURES

Epiglottitis is often characterized by the abrupt onset of throat and neck pain, fever, and inspiratory stridor (difficulty in moving adequate amounts of air through the larynx). Because of the inflammation and edema in the epiglottis and other soft tissues above the vocal cords (supraglottic area), phonation becomes difficult (muffled phonation or aphonia), and the associated pain leads to difficulty in swallowing. If this disease is not treated promptly, death may result from acute airway obstruction.

Epiglottitis carries risk of acute airway obstruction

Laryngitis or its more severe form, croup, may have an abrupt onset (spasmodic croup) or develop more slowly over hours or a few days as a result of spread of infection from the upper respiratory tract. The illness is characterized by variable fever; inspiratory stridor; hoarse phonation; and a harsh, barking cough. In contrast to epiglottitis, the inflammation is localized to the subglottic laryngeal structures, including the vocal cords. It sometimes extends to the trachea (laryngotracheitis) and bronchi (laryngotracheobronchitis), where it is associated with a deeper, more severe cough that may provoke chest pain

Laryngitis and croup involve subglottic laryngeal structures and variable degrees of sputum production. When vocal cord inflammation is severe, transient aphonia may result.

Bronchitis involves larger airways

Bronchitis or **tracheobronchitis** may be a primary manifestation of infection or a result of spread from upper respiratory tissues. It is characterized by cough, variable fever, and sputum production, which is often clear at the onset but may become purulent as the illness persists. Auscultation of the chest with the stethoscope often reveals coarse bubbling rhonchi, which are a result of inflammation and increased fluid production in the larger airways.

Chronic bronchitis associated with smoking, air pollution, and other diseases

Nontypeable *H. influenzae* and *S. pneumoniae* found in exacerbations of chronic bronchitis

Chronic bronchitis is a result of long-standing damage to the bronchial epithelium. A common cause is cigarette smoking, but a variety of environmental pollutants, chronic infections (eg, tuberculosis), and defects that hinder normal clearance of tracheobronchial secretions and bacteria (eg, cystic fibrosis) can be responsible. Because of the lack of functional integrity of their large airways, such patients are susceptible to chronic infection with members of the oropharyngeal flora and to recurrent, acute flare-ups of symptoms when they become colonized and infected by viruses and bacteria, particularly *Streptococcus pneumoniae* and nontypeable *Haemophilus influenzae.* A vicious cycle of recurrent infection may evolve, leading to further damage and increasing susceptibility to pneumonia.

COMMON ETIOLOGIC AGENTS

Most subglottic middle airway infections are viral

With the exception of epiglottitis, acute diseases of the middle airway are usually caused by viral agents (Table 64–1). When acute airway obstruction is present, noninfectious possibilities, such as aspirated foreign bodies and acute laryngospasm or bronchospasm caused by anaphylaxis, must also be considered.

GENERAL DIAGNOSTIC APPROACHES

When a viral etiology is sought, the usual method of obtaining a specific diagnosis is by inoculation of cell cultures with material from the nasopharynx and throat. Acute and

TABLE 64–1

Major Causes of Acute Middle Respiratory Tract Disease

Syndrome	Viruses	Bacteria	Percentage Caused by Viruses
Epiglottitis	Rare	*Haemophilus influenzae, Streptococcus pneumoniae, Corynebacterium diphtheriae, Neisseria meningitidis*	10
Laryngitis and croup	Parainfluenza viruses, influenza viruses, adenoviruses; occasionally respiratory syncytial virus, rhinoviruses, coronaviruses, echoviruses	Rare	90
Laryngotracheitis and laryngotracheobronchitis	Same as for laryngitis and croup	*H. influenzae, Staphylococcus aureus*	90
Bronchitis	Parainfluenza viruses, influenza viruses, respiratory syncytial virus, adenoviruses, measles	*Bordetella pertussis, H. influenzae, Mycoplasma pneumoniae, Chlamydia pneumoniae*	80

convalescent sera can also be collected to determine antibody responses to the common respiratory viruses and *Mycoplasma pneumoniae.* In bacterial infections, the approaches noted below are valuable.

Epiglottitis

H. influenzae type b, once the most common cause of epiglottitis, produces an associated bacteremia in 85% of cases or more. Attempts to obtain cultures from the epiglottis or throat may provoke acute reflex airway obstruction in patients who have not undergone intubation to ensure proper ventilation; furthermore, the yield is lower than that of blood culture. In addition, other bacterial agents that cause epiglottitis can often be isolated from the blood. The exception is *Corynebacterium diphtheriae* infection, in which cultures of the nasopharynx or pharynx are required.

Incidence of bacteremia is high in epiglottitis

Laryngotracheitis and Laryngotracheobronchitis

Although most cases of laryngotracheitis and laryngotracheobronchitis have a viral etiology, a severe purulent process is seen occasionally. The latter is often referred to as acute **bacterial tracheitis,** and it can be rapidly fatal if not managed aggressively. Gram staining and culture of sputum, or better yet, of purulent secretions obtained by direct laryngoscopy, help establish the causative agent. Blood cultures are again useful in such cases when a bacterial etiology is suspected.

Bacterial tracheitis is best diagnosed by direct laryngoscopy specimens

Acute Bronchitis

A major bacteriologic consideration in acute bronchitis, especially in infants and preschool children, is *Bordetella pertussis.* Deep nasopharyngeal cultures plated on the appropriate media constitute the best specimens. Gram staining and examination of nasopharyngeal smears by direct fluorescent antibody methods are also useful adjuncts to establishing the diagnosis. When purulent sputum is produced, Gram staining and culture may be useful in suggesting other bacterial causes (see Table 64–1). Exceptions include *M. pneumoniae* and *Chlamydia pneumoniae* infections, which are usually diagnosed by serologic testing of acute and convalescent sera.

Nasopharyngeal specimens are appropriate for diagnosis of pertussis

Serodiagnosis commonly used for *M. pneumoniae* and *C. pneumoniae* infections

GENERAL PRINCIPLES OF MANAGEMENT

The primary initial concern is ensuring an adequate airway. It is particularly crucial in epiglottitis but can also become a major issue in laryngitis or laryngotracheobronchitis. Thus, some patients require placement of a rigid tube that provides communication between the tracheobronchial tree and the outside air (a nasotracheal tube or a surgically placed tracheostomy). Other adjunctive measures, such as highly humidified air and oxygen, may also provide relief in acute diseases involving the structures in and around the larynx. In proved or suspected bacterial infections, specific antimicrobic therapy is required; other treatment, such as antitoxin administration in diphtheria, may also be necessary.

Maintenance of airway patency required

Antimicrobic therapy for bacterial infections

LOWER RESPIRATORY TRACT INFECTION

Lower respiratory tract infection develops with invasion and disease of the lung, including the alveolar spaces and their supporting structure, the interstitium, and the terminal bronchioles. Bronchiolitis, an inflammatory process primarily affecting the small terminal airways in infants, is discussed extensively in Chapter 33. Infection may occur by extension of a middle respiratory tract infection, aspiration of pathogens past the upper airway defenses, or less commonly by hematogenous spread from a distant site such as an abscess or an infected heart valve. When infection develops through the respiratory tract, some compromise of the upper airway mechanisms for filtering or clearing inhaled

Infection can be by inhalation, aspiration, extension from middle tract, or blood-borne

infectious agents usually occurs. The most common are those that impair the epiglottic and cough reflexes, such as drugs, anesthesia, stroke, and alcohol abuse. Toxic inhalations and cigarette smoking may also interfere with the normal mucociliary action of the tracheobronchial tree. In healthy persons, the most common antecedent to lower respiratory infection is infection of the middle respiratory structures (usually viral), allowing an otherwise innocuous aspiration of oropharyngeal flora to reach the lower tract and progress to disease rather than undergo rapid clearance. Some small infectious particles can accomplish airborne passage through the middle airway and bypass mucociliary defenses; if they can survive or multiply in alveolar macrophages, they may produce a primary infection. Examples include arthroconidia of *Coccidioides immitis* and cells of *Mycobacterium tuberculosis* and *Bacillus anthracis*.

Infection through air passages is associated with compromised local clearance defenses

CLINICAL FEATURES

Acute Pneumonia

Acute pneumonia is an infection of the lung parenchyma that develops over hours to days and, if untreated, runs a natural course lasting days to weeks. The onset may be gradual, with malaise and slowly increasing fever, or sudden, as with the bed-shaking chill associated with the onset of pneumococcal pneumonia. The only early symptom referable to the lung may be cough, which is caused by bronchial irritation. In adults the cough becomes productive of **sputum,** which is purulent material generated in the alveoli and small air passages. In some cases the sputum may be blood streaked, rusty in color, or foul smelling. Labored or difficult breathing (dyspnea), rapid respiratory rate, and sometimes cyanosis are signs of increasing loss of alveolar air-exchange surface through spread of exudate. Chest pain from inflammatory involvement of the pleura is common. Physical signs on auscultation reflect the filling and eventual consolidation of alveoli by fluid and inflammatory cells.

Sputum is purulent material generated in the bronchi and alveoli

Fever, respiratory distress, and sputum production are signs of acute pneumonia

The radiologic pattern of inflammatory changes in the lung is very useful in the diagnosis of pneumonia and for clinical differentiation into likely etiologic categories. The most common pattern is patchy infiltrates related to multiple foci centering on small bronchi (bronchopneumonia), which may progress to a more uniform consolidation of one or more lobes (lobar pneumonia). A more delicate, diffuse, or "interstitial" pattern, which is also common, is particularly associated with viral pneumonia.

Radiologic changes confirm and refine diagnosis

Chronic Pneumonia

Chronic pneumonia has a slow insidious onset that develops over weeks to months and may last for weeks or even years. The initial symptoms are the same as those of acute pneumonia (fever, chills, and malaise), but they develop more slowly. Cough can develop early or late in the illness. As the disease progresses, appetite and weight loss, insomnia, and night sweats are common. Cough and sputum production may be the first indication of a vague constitutional illness referable to the lung. Bloody sputum (hemoptysis), dyspnea, and chest pain appear as the disease progresses. The physical findings and radiologic features can be similar to those of acute pneumonia, except that the diffuse interstitial infiltrates of viral pneumonia are uncommon. There may be parenchymal destruction and the formation of abscesses or cavities communicating with the bronchial tree. The clinical features of chronic pneumonia may be due to a number of infectious agents or noninfectious causes such as neoplasms, vasculitis, allergic conditions, infarction, radiation or toxic injury, and diseases of unknown etiology (eg, sarcoidosis).

Chronic pneumonia develops over weeks to months

Abscesses and cavities may develop

Chronic pneumonia may have noninfectious causes

Pleural effusion is the transudation of fluid into the pleural space in response to an inflammatory process in adjacent lung parenchyma. It may result from a wide variety of causes, both infectious and noninfectious. **Empyema** is a purulent infection of the pleural space that develops when the infectious agent gains access by contiguous spread from an infected lung through a bronchopleural fistula or, less often, by extension of an abdominal infection through the diaphragm. Symptoms are usually insidious and related to the primary infection until enough exudate is formed to produce symptoms referable to the chest wall or to compromise the function of the lung. The physical and radiologic findings are

Pleural effusions may be infectious or noninfectious

Empyema is a purulent infection of pleural space usually by extension of bacterial infection

characteristic, with dullness to percussion and localized opacities on x-ray. In contrast to noninfectious effusions, empyema is frequently loculated.

Lung Abscess

Lung abscess is usually a complication of acute or chronic pneumonia caused by organisms that can cause localized destruction of lung parenchyma. It may occur as part of a chronic process or as an extension of an acute, destructive pneumonia, often after aspiration of oral or gastric contents. The symptoms of lung abscess, which are usually not specific, resemble those of chronic pneumonia or an acute pneumonia that has failed to resolve. Persistent fever, cough, and the production of foul-smelling sputum are typical. Lung abscess can be diagnosed and localized with certainty only radiologically; it appears as a localized area of inflammation with single or multiple excavations or as a cavity with an air–fluid level. Multiple abscesses may develop as a result of blood-borne infection.

Lung abscess frequently follows aspiration pneumonia

Blood-borne infection may cause multiple abscesses

COMMON ETIOLOGIC AGENTS

The infectious agents that most frequently cause lower respiratory infection are listed in Table 64–2. The etiology of acute pneumonia is strongly dependent on age. More than 80% of pneumonias in infants and children are caused by viruses, whereas less than 10 to 20% of pneumonias in adults are viral. The reasons are probably the same as those indicated previously for middle respiratory tract infections. Influenza and other viruses,

Most pneumonias are viral in infants and children

Viral infections predispose to acute bacterial pneumonia

TABLE 64–2

Major Causes of Lower Respiratory Tract Infection

Syndrome	Viruses	Common Bacteria	Fungi	Other Agents
Acute pneumonia	Influenza,[a] parainfluenza, adenovirus, respiratory syncytial virus (infants)[a]	*Streptococcus pneumoniae, Staphylococcus aureus, Haemophilus influenzae,* Enterobacteriaceae, *Legionella,* mixed anaerobes (aspiration), *Pseudomonas aeruginosa*[b]	*Candida albicans*[b] *Aspergillus* species	*Mycoplasma pneumoniae, Pneumocystis carinii,*[b] *Chlamydia trachomatis* (infants), *Chlamydia pneumoniae*
Chronic pneumonia	Rare	*Mycobacterium tuberculosis,* other mycobacteria, *Nocardia*	*Coccidioides immitis,*[c] *Blastomyces dermatitidis,*[c] *Histoplasma capsulatum,*[c] *Cryptococcus neoformans*	*Paragonimus westermani*[c]
Lung abscess	None	Mixed anaerobes, *Actinomyces, Nocardia, S. aureus,*[d] Enterobacteriaceae,[d] *P. aeruginosa*[b,d]	*Aspergillus* species	*Entamoeba histolytica*
Empyema	None	Mixed anaerobes, *S. aureus,*[d] *S. pneumoniae,*[d] Enterobacteriaceae, *P. aeruginosa*[d]	Rare	

[a] Occurrence limited to seasonal epidemics.

[b] Primarily infects the immunologically compromised host.

[c] Geographically limited.

[d] Infection develops during or after acute pneumonia.

however, may provide the initial predisposition toward bacterial infection. Viruses are extremely rare as a cause of chronic as opposed to acute lower respiratory tract infections, although some symptoms of the acute infection, such as cough, may persist for weeks until the bronchial damage has healed. Influenza virus is noteworthy as a cause of acute life-threatening pneumonia, even in previously healthy young adults. Pneumonia caused by bacteria such as enteric Gram-negative rods, *Pseudomonas,* and *Legionella* is primarily limited to patients with serious debilitating underlying disease or as a complication of hospitalization and its procedures (nosocomial infection). At any age, the pneumococcus is the most common bacterial cause of acute pneumonia, and Gram-negative infections other than *Haemophilus* are rare in children unless they have cystic fibrosis or immunodeficiency. Acute and subacute pneumonia may be due to *Chlamydia; C. trachomatis* is almost exclusively limited to infants less than 7 months of age, whereas *C. pneumoniae* commonly affects school children and young adults, producing both bronchitis and pneumonia.

Gram-negative pneumonias occur in debilitated hosts

Pneumoccoccus is most common cause of acute bacterial pneumonia

Lung abscess and empyema follow infections with the more destructive organisms or aspiration of mixed anaerobic flora from the oropharynx. Several clinical clues can suggest some of the etiologic agents, given a typical clinical syndrome. For example, *Nocardia* and mycobacteria, which are strict aerobes, tend to produce upper lobe infiltrates, whereas aspiration pneumonia caused by anaerobes tends to develop in the most dependent parts of the lung. Textbooks on infectious disease should be consulted for further details regarding these features.

Lung abscess has different patterns

GENERAL DIAGNOSTIC APPROACHES

The degree of difficulty in establishing an etiologic diagnosis for a lower respiratory tract infection depends on the number of organisms produced in respiratory secretions, whether the causative species is normally found in the oropharyngeal flora, and how easily it is grown. In the presence of typical clinical findings, the isolation of influenza virus from the throat or of *M. tuberculosis* from sputum is sufficient for diagnosis of influenza or tuberculosis, because these organisms are not normally found in such sites. The same cannot be said for *S. pneumoniae* and most bacterial pathogens, because they may be found in the throat in a significant number of healthy persons (see Chapter 9).

Interpretation depends on whether agent is found in normal flora

The examination of expectorated sputum has been the primary means of diagnosing the causes of bacterial pneumonia, but this approach has several advantages and disadvantages. The advantages are ease of collection and absence of risk to the patient. The primary disadvantage is the confusion that results from contamination of the sputum with oropharyngeal flora in the process of expectoration and excessive contamination with saliva. Efforts have been unsuccessful to remove saliva from sputum by washing or to accomplish interpretive differentiation of infective from normal flora by quantitative culture as with urine specimens (see Chapter 66). The quality of a sputum sample can be enhanced by collection early in the morning (just after the patient arises), careful instruction of the patient, and occasionally by the use of saline aerosols (induced sputum) under the supervision of an inhalation therapy specialist. The worst results can be expected when the physician's only involvement is writing an order, which is then passed down the ward chain of command to an orderly, who directs the patient to put his "sputum" in a cup placed at the bedside.

Sputum collection has problems of quality and specificity

Contamination with oropharyngeal secretions is primary problem

Microscopic examination before culture of direct Gram smears of specimens alleged to be sputum has proved useful. Polymorphonuclear leukocytes and large numbers of a single morphologic type of organism are typical findings in sputum from patients with bacterial pneumonia. Squamous epithelial cells from the oropharynx and a mixed bacterial population are characteristic of saliva (Fig 64–1). Unfortunately, most specimens are a mixture of both, which makes interpretation more difficult. Studies have shown that more than 10 to 25 squamous epithelial cells per low-power microscopic field are evidence of excessive salivary contamination, and such specimens should not be cultured because the results may be misleading. Thus, the direct Gram smear is crucial to the use of expectorated sputum for diagnosis of acute bacterial pneumonia. The smear may be useful in the absence of cultural results, but cultures are useless without a Gram smear to assess specimen quality.

Microscopic characteristics of sputum can differentiate from saliva

Salivary specimens should not be cultured

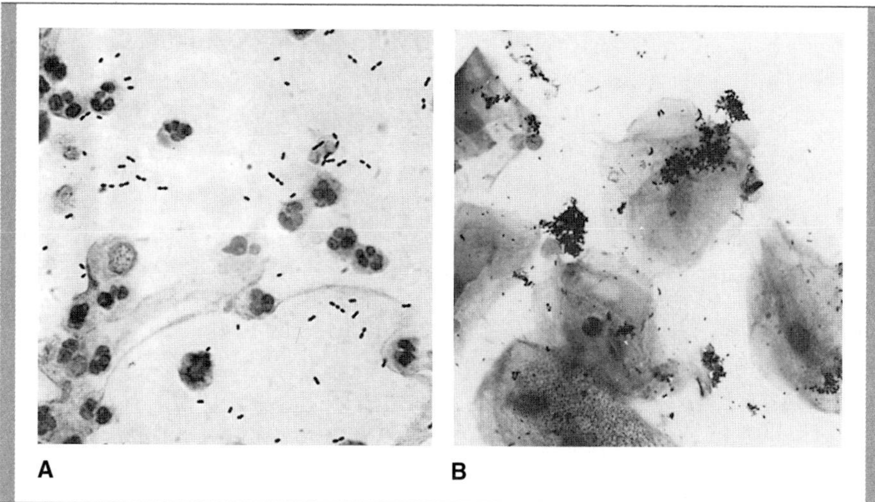

FIGURE 64–1
Comparison of findings in sputum and saliva. True sputum **(A)** should show an abundance of inflammatory cells and no squamous epithelial cells. In acute bacterial pneumonia, large numbers of a single organism are usually present. This Gram smear shows large numbers of polymorphonuclear leukocytes and *Streptococcus pneumoniae.* Saliva **(B)** typically contains squamous epithelial cells and a mixed bacterial population.

Another approach is to attempt a more direct collection from the lung using methods that bypass the oropharyngeal flora. This approach may be used in patients who are not producing sputum or in cases where analysis of expectorated sputum has been inconclusive. The major techniques include transtracheal aspiration, bronchoalveolar lavage (BAL), direct aspiration, and open biopsy. In transtracheal aspiration, an incision is made in the cricothyroid membrane and a catheter advanced deep into the tracheobronchial tree to aspirate sputum directly. This method is useful in diagnosis of both pneumonia and lung abscess. BAL is a modification of bronchoscopy in which the bronchi and alveoli are infused with saline, which is aspirated back through the bronchoscope.

Transtracheal and direct lung aspiration bypass oral flora

Specimens obtained by BAL have been increasingly useful for demonstration of organisms such as *Pneumocystis carinii* that were previously only seen in open lung biopsies. Because BAL involves initial passage of the instrument through the upper airway, interpretation must take into account the possibility of some contamination with oropharyngeal secretions. Aspirates taken through tracheostomies or endotracheal tubes are of almost no value, because these sites become colonized with Gram-negative bacteria within hours of their implantation. Direct aspiration through the chest wall can be used for diagnosis of pneumonia or empyema if the involved area can be well localized and is at the lung periphery. In some cases an open lung biopsy is the only way to obtain diagnostic material. Bacteremia may occur in acute pneumonia, particularly in its early stages. A blood culture should be part of the evaluation of every acute pneumonia. If positive, it can confirm or overrule a diagnosis based on expectorated sputum culture.

BAL washes material from deep in the lung

Blood culture is valuable in acute pneumonia

Once an appropriate specimen is obtained, diagnosis is usually readily made by culture using the methods described in Chapter 15 and in the sections on the individual etiologic agents. Only specimens collected by one of the invasive techniques should be used for anaerobic culture, because expectorated sputum is invariably contaminated with oropharyngeal anaerobes and results are meaningless.

Anaerobic infections cannot be diagnosed from expectorated sputum

GENERAL PRINCIPLES OF MANAGEMENT

The general principles of management of lower respiratory tract infections are similar to those of middle tract infections. Drainage or surgical measures are needed more often as adjuncts to antimicrobial therapy in cases of chronic pneumonia, lung abscess, and empyema. When bacterial infection is considered, empirical therapy is usually given until the results of cultures and antimicrobial susceptibility tests are available. Treatment may vary from penicillin alone for a previously healthy individual in whom the most reasonable nonviral possibility is *S. pneumoniae,* to multiple drugs for a debilitated or immunocompromised patient, in whom the possibilities are much broader.

CHAPTER 65

Enteric Infections and Food Poisoning

KENNETH J. RYAN

Acute infections of the gastrointestinal tract are among the most frequent of all illnesses, exceeded only by respiratory tract infections such as the common cold. Diarrhea is the most common manifestation of these infections; however, because it is usually self-limiting within hours or days, most of those afflicted do not seek medical care. Nonetheless, in the United States, gastrointestinal infection remains one of the three most common syndromes seen by physicians who practice general medicine. Worldwide, diarrheal disease remains one of the most important causes of morbidity and mortality among infants and children. It has been estimated that in Asia, Africa, and Latin America, depending on socioeconomic and nutritional factors, a child's chance of dying of a diarrheal illness before the age of 7 years can be as high as 50%. In developed countries, mortality is very much lower, but it is still significant. This chapter will summarize the known etiologies and epidemiologic circumstances of these infections, as well as diagnostic methods and some aspects of management. Chapters on the individual etiologic agents should be consulted for details.

Diarrheal diseases in developing countries cause death of children

CLINICAL FEATURES

The most prominent clinical features of gastrointestinal infections are fever, vomiting, abdominal pain, and diarrhea. Their presence varies with different diseases and different stages of infection. The occurrence of diarrhea is a central feature, and its presence and nature form the basis for classification of gastrointestinal infections into three major syndromes: watery diarrhea, dysentery, and enteric fever.

Watery Diarrhea

The most common form of gastrointestinal infection is the rapid development of frequent intestinal evacuations of a more or less fluid character known as diarrhea (derived from the Greek "dia," for "through," and "rhein," meaning to flow like a stream). Nausea, vomiting, fever, and abdominal pain may also be present, but the dominant feature is intestinal fluid loss. Diarrhea is produced by pathogenic mechanisms that attack the proximal small intestine, the portion of the bowel in which more than 90% of physiologic net fluid absorption occurs. The purest form of watery diarrhea is that produced by enterotoxin-secreting bacteria such as *Vibrio cholerae* and enterotoxigenic *Escherichia coli* (ETEC), which cause fluid loss without cellular injury. Other common pathogens that damage the epithelium, such as rotaviruses, also cause fluid loss, but are more likely to cause fever and vomiting as well. Most cases of watery diarrhea run an acute but brief

Fluid loss from proximal small intestine is the primary mechanism

(1 to 3 days) self-limiting course. Exceptions are those caused by *V. cholerae,* which usually produces a more severe illness, and those caused by *Giardia lamblia,* which produces a watery diarrhea that may last for weeks.

Dysentery

Inflammation, cytotoxins, or invasion produce pus and blood

Colon is primary location

Dysentery begins with the rapid onset of frequent intestinal evacuations, but the stools are of smaller volume than in watery diarrhea and contain blood and pus. If watery diarrhea is the "runs," dysentery is the "squirts." Fever, abdominal pain, cramps, and tenesmus are frequent complaints. Vomiting occurs less often. The focus of pathology is the colon. Organisms causing dysentery can produce inflammatory and/or destructive changes in the colonic mucosa either by direct invasion or by production of cytotoxins. This damage produces the pus and blood seen in the stools but does not result in substantial fluid loss because the absorptive and secretory capacity of the colon is much less than that of the small bowel. Dysenteric infections generally last longer than the common watery diarrheas, but most cases still resolve spontaneously in 2 to 7 days.

Enteric Fever

Systemic disease begins in the intestine

Focus often becomes lymphoid and reticuloendothelial invasion

Enteric fever is a systemic infection, the origin and focus of which are the gastrointestinal tract. The most prominent features are fever and abdominal pain, which develop gradually over a few days in contrast to the abrupt onset of the other syndromes. Diarrhea is usually present but may be mild and not appear until later in the course of the illness. The pathogenesis of enteric fever is more complex than that of watery diarrhea or dysentery. It generally involves penetration by the organism of the cells of the distal small bowel with subsequent spread outside the bowel to the biliary tract, liver, mesentery, or reticuloendothelial organs. Bacteremia is common, occasionally causing metastatic infection in other organs. Typhoid fever caused by *Salmonella enterica* serotype Typhi is the only infection for which these events have been well studied. Although it is usually self-limiting, enteric fever carries a significant risk of serious disease and significant mortality.

COMMON ETIOLOGIC AGENTS

Clinical syndromes overlap for specific etiologic agents

Great advances have been made in our understanding of gastrointestinal infections. Before the late 1960s, fewer than 20% of the infectious syndromes described above could be linked to a specific etiologic agent by any known diagnostic method regardless of cost. The organisms listed in Table 65–1 now account for 80 to 90% of cases, although diagnostic methods for all of them are not yet practical for clinical laboratories. The primary clinical syndrome listed for each agent in Table 65–1 should not be regarded as absolute because there are individual variations and overlap; some pathogens cause more than one syndrome. For example, *Shigella* infections frequently go through a brief watery diarrhea stage before localizing in the colon, and *Campylobacter* enteritis usually begins with fever, malaise, and abdominal pain, followed by dysentery. In any single case, the clinical findings may suggest a range of etiologic agents, but none is sufficiently specific to be diagnostic of any single organism.

EPIDEMIOLOGIC SETTING

Epidemiologic setting narrows the diagnostic possibilities

The epidemiologic setting of the infection is of great importance in assessing the relative probability of the infectious agents. When combined with clinical findings, the differential diagnosis can often be limited to two or three organisms. The major epidemiologic settings are (1) endemic infection, (2) epidemic infection, (3) traveler's diarrhea, (4) food poisoning, and (5) hospital-associated diarrhea.

Endemic Infections

High frequency in children is related to fecal–oral spread and lack of immunity

By definition, endemic diarrheas are those that occur sporadically in the usual living circumstances of the patient (from the Greek "endemos," dwelling in a place). Some organisms are endemic worldwide, whereas others are geographically limited. There are also seasonal variations and age-related attack rates within the endemic foci. In developed countries the most common causes of endemic gastrointestinal infections are rotaviruses, caliciviruses, *Campylobacter, Salmonella,* and *Shigella.* All are more common in infants and children because they are more prone to fecal–oral spread and because development of immunity is related to age. Rotaviruses account for 40 to 60% of diarrheal infections occurring during the cooler months in infants and children less than 2 years of age but are uncommon in older persons.

The geographically limited agents are common only in the areas listed (see Table 65–1). These distributions are not fixed, making it necessary to keep abreast of geographic changes in the distribution of established agents as well as the recognition of new ones. For example, cholera has long been limited to warm-climate river deltas in Asia, Africa, and the Middle East, but recently it has spread to South and Central America and the Gulf Coast of Louisiana and Texas.

Geographic distributions change

Epidemic Infections

Under certain epidemiologic conditions some of the organisms responsible for endemic infections can spread beyond the family unit to cause epidemics involving regional, national, and even international populations. The diarrheal diseases most frequently associated with epidemics are typhoid fever, cholera, and shigellosis. For all three, epidemics are related to the failure of basic public health sanitary measures. For example, *Salmonella* serotype Typhi and *Vibrio cholerae* may be spread for some distance through the water supply, a route blocked by modern sewage and water treatment practices. When these procedures are not employed or are interrupted by equipment failure or natural disasters (floods, earthquakes), these diseases can and do recur in epidemic form. Epidemics of shigellosis may be water-borne under the same conditions, but *Shigella* dysentery is more typically a disease "of wars and armies, and of crowds and movement."* The very low infecting dose of *Shigella* can make spreading through direct contact reach epidemic proportions when crowding and poor sanitary facilities are combined. *Giardia, Cryptosporidium,* and *E. coli* O157:H7 were the most frequent identified causes of recent waterborne epidemics in the United States.

Typhoid, cholera, and shigellosis spread where hygiene is poor or after major disasters

Although such epidemics are usually associated with the 19th century, it is clear that the potential remains. In the late 1970s large epidemics of both typhoid fever and shigellosis spread through Central and South America. In 1973 more than 200 cases of typhoid fever in Florida were associated with a defective chlorinator in the local water system. The current cholera epidemic claimed thousands of lives in South America in the last decade of the 20th century.

Most recent epidemic is cholera in South America

Traveler's Diarrhea

From 20% to 50% of travelers from developed countries who go to less developed countries experience a diarrheal illness in the first week that is usually brief but can be serious. The common names applied to this syndrome, such as "Delhi belly" and "Montezuma's revenge," reflect geographic associations and the cumulative frustration of those forced to spend part of their vacation next to the toilet rather than the swimming pool.

Visits to developing countries are frequently marred

The most extensive studies of traveler's diarrhea have involved travelers from the United States to Latin American countries, particularly Mexico. In nearly 50% of these cases, the diarrhea is caused by enterotoxigenic strains of *E. coli* acquired during travel. *Shigella* infections account for another 10 to 20%, and the remaining cases are attributable to various pathogens or unknown causes. Ingestion of uncooked or incompletely cooked foods is the most likely source of infection, but most epidemiologic studies have not shown specific food associations. An exception is the strong relationship between toxigenic *E. coli* diarrhea and the consumption of salads containing raw vegetables. "Don't drink the water" still seems like sound advice for travelers to countries where hygiene remains poor, but the adage is not well supported by studies relating infection to water or ice consumption.

ETEC is the predominant cause of traveler's diarrhea

Travelers should avoid salads and other uncooked foods

* Christie AB. *Infectious Disease, Epidemiology and Clinical Practice,* 2nd ed. New York: Churchill Livingstone; 1974, p 137.

TABLE 65–1

Features of Infectious Gastrointestinal Syndromes

Organism	Common Distribution	Clinical Syndrome	Pathogenic Mechanism	Stool Microscopy	Laboratory Diagnosis[a]: Culture: Stool[b]	Culture: Blood	Toxin in Stools	Serology: Antibody Detection	Serology: Antigen Detection
Salmonella serotypes	Worldwide	Dysentery	Mucosal invasion	PMNs	+	–	–	–	–
Salmonella serotype typhi	Tropical, developing countries	Enteric fever	Penetration, spread	Monocytes	+	+	–	+	–
Shigella spp.	Worldwide	Dysentery	Mucosal invasion, cytotoxin	PMNs, RBCs	+	–	–	–	–
Shigella dysenteriae (Shiga)	Tropical, developing countries	Dysentery	Mucosal invasion, cytotoxin	PMNs, RBCs	+	+	–	–	–
Campylobacter jejuni	Worldwide	Dysentery	Unknown	PMNs, RBCs	+	–	–	–	–
Escherichia coli (EIEC)	Worldwide	Dysentery	Mucosal invasion	PMNs, RBCs	+[c]	–	–	–	–
E. coli (ETEC)	Worldwide[d]	Dysentery	Enterotoxin(s)	–	+[c]	–	–	–	–
E. coli (EHEC)	Worldwide	Watery diarrhea	Cytotoxin	RBCs	+[c]	–	–	–	–
E. coli (EPEC)	Worldwide[d]	Watery diarrhea	Adherence	–	+[c]	–	–	–	–
Vibrio cholerae	Asia, Africa, Middle East, Central and South America, Louisiana, Texas	Watery diarrhea	Enterotoxin	–	+	–	–	–	–

Vibrio parahaemolyticus	Seacoast	Watery diarrhea	Unknown	−	+	−	−	−	−
Yersinia enterocolitica	Worldwide	Enteric fever[c]	Penetration, spread	−	+	+	−	−	−
Clostridium difficile	Worldwide	Dysentery	Cytotoxin, enterotoxin	−	+	−	+	−	−
Clostridium perfringens	Worldwide	Watery diarrhea	Enterotoxin	−	+	−	−	−	−
Bacillus cereus	Worldwide	Watery diarrhea	Enterotoxin	−	+	−	−	−	−
Rotavirus	Worldwide	Watery diarrhea	Mucosal destruction	Electron microscopy[f]	−	−	−	−	+
Caliciviruses	Worldwide	Watery diarrhea	Mucosal destruction	Electron microscopy[f]	−	−	−	−	−
Giardia lamblia	Worldwide	Watery diarrhea	Mucosal irritation	Flagellates, cysts	−	−	−	−	−
Entamoeba histolytica	Worldwide[d]	Dysentery	Mucosal invasion	Amebas, PMNs	−	−	−	+	−
Cryptosporidium	Worldwide	Watery diarrhea	?toxin	Acid-fast oocysts	−	−	−	−	−

Abbreviations: RBCs, red blood cells; PMNs, polymorphonuclear leukocytes; EIEC, enteroinvasive *E. coli;* ETEC, enterotoxigenic *E. coli;* EHEC, enterohemorrhagic *E. coli;* EPEC, enteropathogenic *E. coli.*

[a] Positive sign indicates procedure is useful and usually available in clinical laboratories.

[b] Which cultures are done routinely depends on the laboratory and/or physician's request.

[c] Organism may be isolated in culture, but demonstration of pathogenic potential (toxin production, etc.) is limited to specialized laboratories.

[d] Organism is more common in developing countries.

[e] Infection may also manifest watery diarrhea or dysentery.

[f] Appropriate methods may be available in only a limited number of laboratories.

Food Poisoning

Single-source outbreaks are becoming larger with modern food processing and distribution

Many gastrointestinal infections involve food as a vehicle of transmission. The term "food poisoning," however, is usually reserved for instances in which a single meal can be incriminated as the source. This situation typically arises when multiple cases of the same gastrointestinal syndrome develop at the same time among persons whose only common experience is a meal shared at a social event or restaurant. The probable etiologic agent can usually be assessed from knowledge of the incubation period, the food vehicle, and the clinical findings. Changes in the importation, processing, and distribution of foods have increased the complexity and potential for food-borne transmission of enteric pathogens. Outbreaks that in the past might have been limited, may now be widely distributed by fast-food chains or airline catering services.

Diseases from ingestion of preformed toxin have short incubation periods

The most common causes of food poisoning are shown in Table 65–2. Some are not infections but intoxications, caused by ingestion of a toxin produced by bacteria in the food before it was eaten. Intoxications have shorter incubation periods than infections and may involve extraintestinal symptoms (eg, the neurologic damage in botulism). Infectious food poisoning does not differ from endemic diarrheal infections caused by the same species. The length of the incubation period and the severity of the symptoms are generally related to the number of organisms ingested.

The epidemiologic circumstances of food poisoning vary with the etiologic agent but virtually always involve a breach in the recommended procedures for handling food. The organisms may be present as contaminants in raw food before cooking or introduced by a

TABLE 65–2

Clinical and Epidemiologic Features of Food Poisoning

Etiology	Percentage of Cases[a]	Typical Incubation Period	Primary Clinical Findings	Characteristic Foods
Intoxication[b]				
Bacillus cereus (vomiting toxin)	1–2	1–6 h	Vomiting, diarrhea	Rice, meat, vegetables
Clostridium botulinum	5–15	12–72 h	Neuromuscular paralysis	Improperly preserved vegetables, meat, fish
Staphylococcus aureus	5–25	2–4 h	Vomiting	Meats, custards, salads
Chemical[c]	20–25	0.1–48 h	Variable	Variable
Infections[d]				
Clostridium perfringens	5–15	9–15 h	Watery diarrhea	Meat, poultry
Salmonella	10–30	6–48 h	Dysentery	Poultry, eggs, meat
Shigella	2–5	12–48 h	Dysentery	Variable
Vibrio parahaemolyticus	1–2	10–24 h	Watery diarrhea	Shellfish
Trichinella spiralis	5–10	3–30 days	Fever, myalgia	Meat, especially pork
Hepatitis A	1–3	10–45 days	Hepatitis	Shellfish

[a] Based on documented outbreaks reported to the Centers for Disease Control and Prevention, Atlanta (variable from year to year).

[b] Disease caused by toxin in food at time of ingestion.

[c] Includes heavy metals, monosodium glutamate, mushrooms, and various toxins of nonmicrobial origin.

[d] Disease caused by infection after ingestion.

carrier or contaminated utensil involved in preparation. Causes of bacterial food poisoning include failure to kill the organisms by adequate cooking, almost always followed by a period of warming (incubation) long enough for the organisms to multiply to infectious numbers or, in the case of toxigenic disease, to produce sufficient toxin to cause disease. In 80 to 90% of investigated outbreaks of bacterial food poisoning, the most important contributing factor is the use of improper storage temperatures for the food. This factor may obtain in home-cooked meals as well as those prepared in restaurants, in schools, or at large social events such as community picnics.

Infection is associated with improper cooking and/or storage

The relative frequency of each etiologic agent and the foods most frequently involved are also shown in Table 65–2. This information is based on outbreaks investigated by public health agencies, but it is generally accepted that these represent the "tip of the iceberg" due to underreporting. Large outbreaks, restaurant-associated outbreaks, and outbreaks involving serious illness with hospitalization or death are more likely to be reported to health authorities than are mild diarrheas after a dinner party or airline meal. In recent years, of the 400 to 500 outbreaks (10,000 to 15,000 cases) reported each year in the United States, fewer than 200 are "solved." Food poisoning characterized by a short incubation period (eg *Staphylococcus aureus*) is more likely to be recognized because it can easily be associated with a specific meal and because the food itself may still be available for examination. There are also large geographic differences in reporting. For example, in 1979, New York City, in which 50% of the state population resides, reported 98% of New York state's food-borne outbreaks, and Connecticut reported more outbreaks than all of the southeastern states combined.

Reporting of outbreaks varies greatly

Sampling problems aside, the food poisoning syndromes listed in Table 65–2 are well recognized, with *Salmonella, Clostridium perfringens,* and *S. aureus* accounting for more than 70% of those for which a microbial etiology can be found. For bacterial infections such as *Salmonella* and *Shigella,* which are not normal members of the stool flora, establishing the diagnosis by isolating the causative organism is relatively easy. If the circumstances indicate *C. perfringens* or *S. aureus* food poisoning, investigation involves cultures of vomitus, stool from several cases, and the suspect food. In some cases, toxin detection is required to establish the etiology and source. Such investigations are best coordinated by public health authorities, who can also address the legal and community implications of the outbreak. For example, one investigation of *Salmonella* food poisoning led to the discovery that the owner of a restaurant was keeping and slaughtering chickens at the restaurant. Although this practice may have provided very fresh chicken, it guaranteed *Salmonella* contamination of the entire kitchen.

Determining the cause of microbial food poisoning is best done by public health authorities

Hospital-associated Diarrhea

The hospital environment should not allow spread of the usual causes of endemic intestinal infection. When such infection occurs, it can usually be traced to an employee who continues working while ill or to contaminated food prepared outside the hospital that is "smuggled" in by the patient's friends. Two special causes of hospital-associated diarrhea are caused by *E. coli* in infants and *Clostridium difficile* in patients treated with antimicrobial agents. Fortunately, *E. coli* outbreaks have become rare. *C. difficile* accounts for more than 90% of cases of a syndrome that ranges from mild diarrhea to fulminant pseudomembranous colitis during or after treatment with antibiotics. The responsible toxigenic *C. difficile* may be resident in the patient's intestinal flora before administration of antimicrobics or be acquired by spread from other patients in the hospital. Rotaviruses can also cause hospital outbreaks in infants.

E. coli, C. difficile, and rotaviruses can cause hospital outbreaks

GENERAL DIAGNOSTIC APPROACHES

Laboratory diagnostic procedures (summarized in Table 65–1) include microscopic examination, culture, toxin detection, and serologic procedures. The relative value of each is different for the various etiologies. The diagnostic approach therefore requires that the physician assess the clinical and epidemiologic features of the case, decide which organisms are potential causes, and provide this assessment to the laboratory so that appropriate procedures will be used.

Microscopic Examination

Stool microscopy demonstrates white blood cells and parasites

Electron microscopy detects rotaviruses

Microscopic examination is of value in the assessment of bacterial infections when they are positive. The presence of polymorphonuclear leukocytes or blood in the stool correlates with organisms that produce disease by invasion, but false-negative results are common. The leukocytes may be seen in unstained or methylene blue–stained wet mount preparations; the absence of fecal leukocytes, however, does not exclude invasive diarrhea. The observation and morphologic characterization of amebas and flagellates on wet or stained preparations are the primary means by which amebic (*Entamoeba histolytica*) and flagellate (*Giardia lamblia*) infections are diagnosed. Rotaviruses and other viruses of diarrhea cannot be grown in cell culture but can be detected by electron microscopy.

Culture

Blood cultures are positive in early stages of enteric fever

Stool culture requires selective media for common agents

Isolation of the etiologic agent is the primary means by which bacterial enteric infection is diagnosed. In enteric fever the organism is typically present in the blood in the early stages of disease. Blood cultures are, however, usually negative in watery diarrhea and dysenteric infections, and stool culture must be relied upon for diagnosis. Fortunately, several good selective media have been developed for both direct plating and enrichment culture, which allow isolation of the infecting organism in the presence of a predominant normal flora. Selective media are then used for the various enteric pathogens (see Chapter 15). Media routinely used may vary between clinical laboratories but should include those appropriate for *Salmonella, Shigella,* and *Campylobacter jejuni.* Diarrhea caused by *E. coli* is a special problem, because the methods that define the enterotoxigenic, invasive, or other pathogenic mechanisms are not yet practical for clinical laboratories.

Toxin Assay

Cell culture or antigen assays detect *C. difficile* toxin

The B cytotoxins of *C. difficile* can be detected by its cytopathic effect in a cell culture system. In most clinical cases, enough toxin is present for direct detection in a stool specimen. This assay is currently available only in reference laboratories. Methods that detect the *C. difficile* A and B toxins by latex agglutination are now in common use. The cost-benefit of various combinations of toxin detection methods is still controversial.

Antigen and Antibody Detection

Serology is generally ancillary

Antigen detection available for a rotaviruses

At present, antibody detection is useful in the diagnosis of amebic dysentery caused by *E. histolytica* and of typhoid fever. Both are considered ancillary to the primary diagnostic tests, which involve specific detection of the organism by microscopic and cultural methods. Reagents are commercially available for the detection of rotavirus antigen in stool by latex agglutination or enzyme immunoassay. These methods have a sensitivity roughly comparable to that of electron microscopy. Serologic methods have been described for many other causes of gastrointestinal infection but are not generally used because of lack of sensitivity, specificity, or availability of reagents.

OTHER CAUSES OF INTESTINAL INFECTION

Candidate agents await proof

Despite recent advances in defining the etiologies of enteric infections, there are surely more to be discovered. Organisms not listed in Table 65–1, such as *Aeromonas, Citrobacter,* and *Plesiomonas,* have occasionally been associated with intestinal infections, but the evidence for their enteropathogenicity is not yet strong enough to interpret their isolation from individual cases. At our present state of knowledge, it is not useful to attempt isolation of these organisms unless strong epidemiologic evidence, such as a foodborne outbreak, supports interpretation of the results.

GENERAL PRINCIPLES OF MANAGEMENT

In most gastrointestinal infections, the primary goal of treatment is relief of symptoms, with particular attention to maintaining fluid and electrolyte balance. The effects of common antidiarrheal medications such as subsalicylate-containing compounds (Pepto-Bismol) or antispasmodics (loperamide) are variable, depending on the etiology. In general, they may be helpful for the watery diarrhea caused by enterotoxins, but not for dysentery caused by mucosal invasion, and antispasmodics may be harmful in the latter instance. Antimicrobial agents are usually not indicated for self-limited watery diarrhea but are required for more severe dysenteric infections. Some enteric infections, such as typhoid fever, are always treated with antimicrobics. Prophylactic regimens for traveler's diarrhea have been effective if it is recognized they do not cover all potential causes. More information on therapy is given in the individual chapters, but texts on infectious diseases should be consulted for specific recommendations.

Maintenance of fluid and electrolyte balance always important

Antimicrobic therapy is primarily for invasive disease

ADDITIONAL READING

Guerrant RL, et al. Practice guidelines for the management of infectious diarrhea. *Clin Infect Dis* 2001;32:331–350. This consensus statement from the Infectious Disease Society of America gives clear algorithms for diagnosis and management of all the common situations.

Rendi-Wagner P, Kollaritsch H. Drug prophylaxis for travelers' diarrhea. *Clin Infect Dis* 2002;34:628–633. Here is the most recent advice to take along on "spring break."

CHAPTER 66

Urinary Tract Infections

KENNETH J. RYAN

Bacterial colonization of the urine within this tract **(bacteriuria)** is common and can, at times, result in microbial invasion of the tissues responsible for the manufacture, transport, and storage of urine. Infection of the upper urinary tract, consisting of the kidney and its pelvis, is known as **pyelonephritis.** Infection of the lower tract may involve the bladder **(cystitis),** urethra **(urethritis),** or prostate **(prostatitis),** the genital organ that surrounds and communicates with the first segment of the male urethra. Because all portions of the urinary tract are joined by a fluid medium, infection at any site may spread to involve other areas of the system.

EPIDEMIOLOGY

Urinary tract infection (UTI) is among the most common of diseases particularly among women. Prevalence is age and sex dependent. Approximately 1% of children, many of whom demonstrate functional or anatomic abnormalities of the urinary tract, develop infection during the neonatal period. It is estimated that 20% or more of the female population suffers some form of UTI in their lifetime. Infection in the male population remains uncommon through the fifth decade of life, when enlargement of the prostate begins to interfere with emptying of the bladder. In the elderly of both sexes, gynecologic or prostatic surgery, incontinence, instrumentation, and chronic urethral catheterization push UTI rates to 30 to 40%. A single bladder catheterization carries an infectious risk of 1%, and at least 10% of individuals with indwelling catheters become infected.

Young women are commonly infected

Prostate hypertrophy is linked to male disease

PATHOGENESIS

The urine produced in the kidney and delivered through the renal pelvis and ureters to the urinary bladder is sterile in health. Infection results when bacteria gain access to this environment and are able to persist. Access primarily follows an ascending route for bacteria that are resident or transient members of the perineal flora. These organisms are derived from the large intestinal flora, which is uncomfortably nearby. Conditions that create access are varied, but the most important is sexual intercourse, which has been shown to transiently displace bacteria into the bladder. This puts the female partner is at risk because of the short urethral distance. Other manipulations of the urethra carry risk as well, particularly medical ones such as catheterization. Bacteria may also reach the urinary tract from the bloodstream. This is obviously much less common, because it requires an uncontrolled infection at another site.

Bacteria ascend from perineal flora

Intercourse is common association

Catheters increase risk

For bacteria that reach the urinary tract, the major competing forces are the rich nutrient content of the urine itself and the flushing action of bladder voiding. Persistence is favored by host factors that interrupt or retard the urinary flow such as instrumentation, obstruction, or structural abnormalities. In youth, factors are congenital malformations, and with age these include changes that alter the mechanics of outflow, such as prostatic hypertrophy. Bacterial factors include the ability to adhere to the perineal and uroepithelial mucosa and to produce other classical virulence factors like exotoxins. These and other features of pathogenesis are discussed in Chapter 21; *Escherichia coli* is by far the most common and potent UTI pathogen. Urease-producing members of the genus *Proteus* are associated with urinary stones, which themselves are predisposing factors for infection.

Obstruction of urine flow increases risk

Bacterial adherence favors persistence

E. coli is virulence model

ETIOLOGIC AGENTS

Over 95% of UTIs are caused by a single bacterial species, and 90% of these are *E. coli.* Other Enterobacteriaceae, *Pseudomonas,* and Gram-positive bacteria become increasingly frequent with chronic, complicated, and hospitalized patients. Of the Gram-positive bacteria enterococci are the most important. *Staphylococcus saprophyticus,* a coagulase-negative staphylococcus, is now recognized as the etiology in a significant minority of symptomatic infections in young, sexually active women. Yeasts, particularly species of *Candida,* may be isolated from catheterized patients receiving antibacterial therapy and from diabetic individuals, but they seldom produce symptomatic disease.

Vast majority due to *E. coli*

Enterobacteriaceae and Gram-positive bacteria appear with complications

MANIFESTATIONS

The clinical manifestations of UTI are variable. Approximately 50% of infections do not produce recognizable illness and are discovered incidentally during a general medical examination. Infections in infants produce symptoms of a nonspecific nature, including fever, vomiting, and failure to thrive. Manifestations in older children and adults, when present, often suggest the diagnosis and sometimes the localization of the infection within the urinary tract.

Some cases are asymptomatic

Cystitis

The symptoms of cystitis are **dysuria** (painful urination), **frequency** (frequent voiding), and **urgency** (an imperative "call to toilet"). These findings are similar to those of urethritis caused by sexually transmitted agents. The cystitis complex is, in fact, produced by irritation of the mucosal surface of the urethra as well as the bladder. It is clinically distinguished from pure urethritis by a more acute onset, more severe symptoms, the presence of bacteriuria, and in approximately 50% of cases, hematuria. The urine is often cloudy and malodorous and occasionally frankly bloody. Cystitis patients also experience pain and tenderness in the suprapubic area. Fever and systemic manifestations of illness are usually absent unless the infection spreads to involve the kidney.

Urethral irritation differs from genital infections

Fever is usually absent

Pyelonephritis

The typical presentation of upper urinary infection consists of **flank pain** and **fever** that exceeds 38.3°C. These findings may be preceded or accompanied by manifestations of cystitis. Rigors, vomiting, diarrhea, and tachycardia are present in more severely ill patients. Physical examination reveals tenderness over the costovertebral areas of the back and, occasionally, evidence of septic shock. In the absence of obstruction, the clinical manifestations usually abate within a few days, leaving the kidneys functionally intact. It has been estimated, however, that 20 to 50% of pregnant women with acute pyelonephritis give birth to premature infants, one of the most serious consequences of UTI. In the presence of obstruction, a neurogenic bladder, or vesicoureteral reflux, clinical manifestations are more persistent, occasionally leading to necrosis of the renal papillae and progressive impairment of kidney function with chronic bacteriuria. If a renal calculus or necrotic renal papilla impacts in the ureter, severe flank pain with radiation to the groin occurs. The term chronic pyelonephritis is used to describe inflamed, scarred, contracted

Fever and flank pain mark upper tract disease

Prematurity is risk in pregnancy

Chronic pyelonephritis is not linked to UTI

kidneys often in association with compromised renal function. There is no known connection between UTI and chronic pyelonephritis.

Prostatitis

Infection of the prostate is typically manifested as pain in the lower back, perirectal area, and testicles. In acute infection, the pain may be severe and accompanied by high fever, chills, and the signs and symptoms of cystitis. Inflammatory swelling can lead to obstruction of the neighboring urethra and urinary retention. On rectal palpation, the prostate is boggy and exquisitely tender. Response to antibiotic therapy is good, but occasionally abscess formation, epididymitis, and seminal vesiculitis or chronic infection develop. Typically, acute prostatitis develops in young adults; however, it can also follow placement of an indwelling catheter in an older man. Patients with chronic prostatitis seldom give a history of an acute episode. Many are totally without symptoms; others experience low-grade pain and dysuria. Periodic spread of prostatic organisms to the urine in the bladder produces recurrent bouts of cystitis. In fact, chronic prostatitis is probably the major cause of recurrent bacteriuria in men. The etiologic agents are the same as in cystitis and pyelonephritis.

Back and perirectal pain are signs

Chronic disease a source for cystitis

DIAGNOSIS

Specimen Collection

The diagnosis of UTI is based on examination of the normally sterile urine for evidence of bacteria or an accompanying inflammatory reaction. Critical to this examination is the use of appropriate techniques for specimen collection. Urine is most easily obtained by spontaneous micturition. Unfortunately, voided urine is invariably contaminated with urethral flora and, in female patients, perineal and vaginal flora, which can confound the results of laboratory testing. Although the contaminants can never be completely eliminated, their quantity may be diminished by carefully cleansing the periurethrum before voiding and allowing the initial part of the stream to flush the urethra before collecting a specimen for examination. This **clean-voided midstream urine** collection procedure is preferred to catheterization for routine purposes because it avoids the risk of introducing organisms into the bladder. When the laboratory examination of such a specimen produces equivocal results or the patient cannot comply with the requirements of the clean-voided technique, catheterization or suprapubic aspiration from the distended bladder may be necessary.

Midstream collection intended to bypass contamination

Direct collections are confirmatory

For the diagnosis of prostatitis, urine is collected in three segments by interrupting a single bladder excavation. The first voiding is considered a urethral washout. The midstream specimen that follows is used to assess cystitis. The prostate is then massaged, and the final urine is a prostatic secretions washout. The quantitative culture results are then compared. In prostatitis, it is expected that the third specimen contains the largest numbers of the pathogen.

Prostatitis requires three-component voiding

Microscopic Examination

Approximately 90% of patients with acute symptomatic UTI have pyuria (that is, >10 white cells/mm^3 of urine). This finding is also common, however, in a number of noninfectious diseases. More specific is the presence of white cell casts, which occur primarily in patients with acute pyelonephritis. A more sensitive and specific microscopic procedure is a Gram-stained smear of uncentrifuged urine (Fig 66–1). The presence of at least one organism per oil-immersion field is almost always indicative of bacterial infection. The absence of white cells and bacteria in several fields makes the diagnosis of UTI unlikely. However, this finding does not rule it out, especially in young women with acute, symptomatic infection who may be infected with smaller numbers of organisms.

Pyruia suggests UTI but is not specific

Bacteria on unspun smear correlates with bacteriuria

Chemical Screening Tests

A number of nonmicroscopic urinary screening tests have been commercially marketed within the past several years. The most successful detects leukocyte esterase

Leukocyte esterase detects pyuria

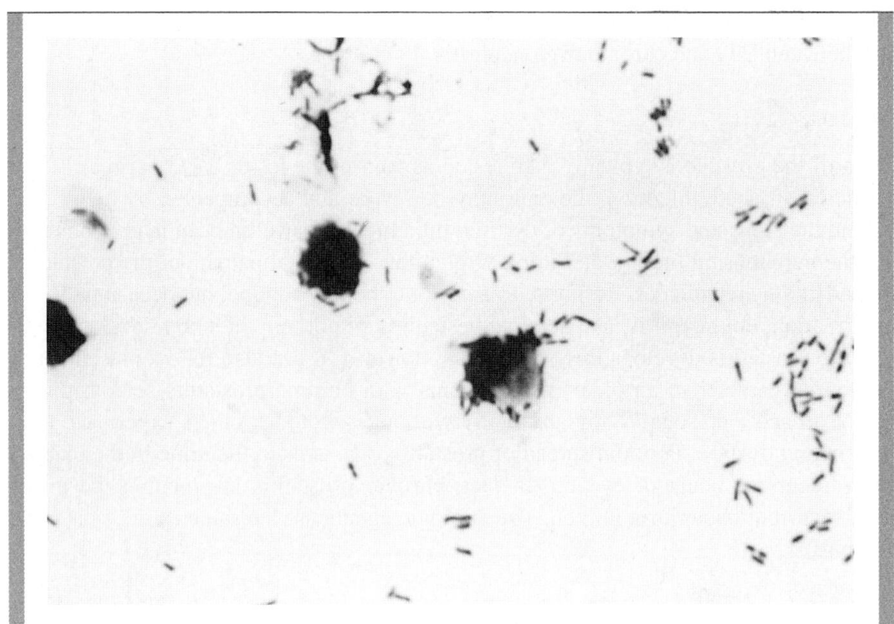

FIGURE 66–1
Gram stain of an uncentrifuged clean voided urine specimen from a patient with an acute *Escherichia coli* urinary tract infection. Some degenerating polymorphonuclear leukocytes and numerous Gram-negative rods are present.

from inflammatory cells and nitrite produced from urinary nitrates by bacterial metabolism. Although technically simpler, the sensitivity and specificity of these products are similar to that of microscopic examination. Like microscopic examination, they do not reliably detect bacteriuria below the level of 10^5 organisms/mL.

Urine Culture

>10^5 bacteria/mL is typical for UTI

Contaminants can be >10^5 bacteria/mL

Based on studies done half a century ago demonstrating that the number of bacteria in infected urine is large, quantitative bacteriology has been the gold diagnostic standard for UTI. Perhaps no number in medicine is better known or more slavishly adhered to than 10^5 bacteria/mL of urine. Above it is UTI, below it is contamination. We now know that it is possible to void more than 10^5 of contaminants and to have a genuine UTI with less than 10^5 bacteria as illustrated in Figure 66–2. Virtually no woman with sterile bladder

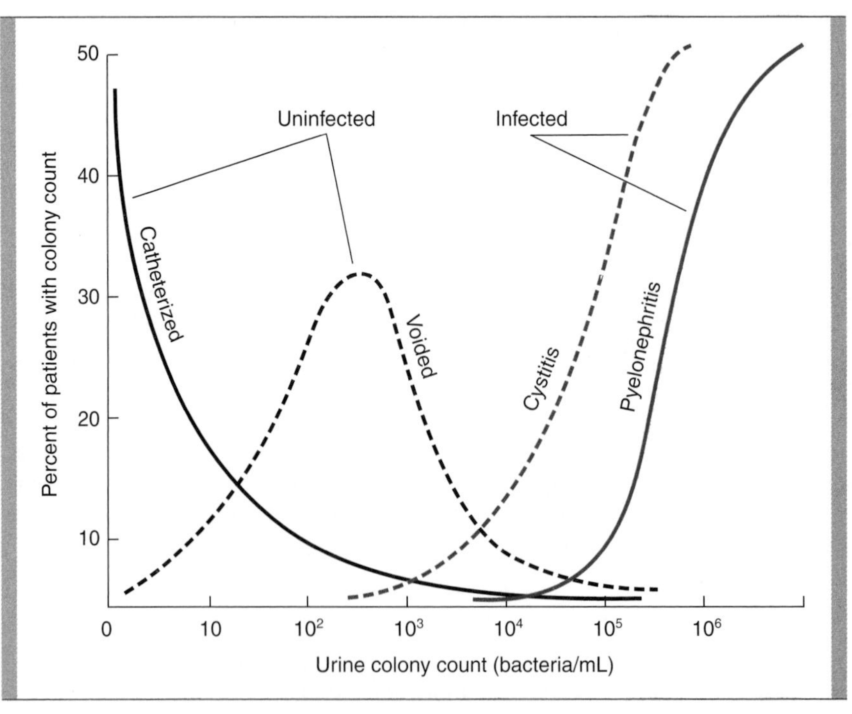

FIGURE 66–2
Quantitative urine culture. Bacteria are routinely quantitated in the range of 10 to >10^5. Uninfected persons may show bacteria in the urine due to contamination from the perineal flora. The number are small if the specimen is collected by catheterization but voided (midstream method) specimens contain larger numbers. Patients with pyelonephritis have very high numbers of bacteria but those with only cystitis often have numbers less than 10^5.

urine, as determined by suprapubic aspiration, can void a sterile specimen even with periurethral cleansing. Voided contaminants are most often mixtures of vaginal flora not associated with UTI such as lactobacilli, diphtheroids, and streptococci, but can include urinary pathogens. Conversely, we now know that bacterial counts in UTI represent a spectrum from 10^2 to more than 10^6 bacteria/mL. The lower counts are typical for simple cystitis and the high counts for pyelonephritis. Fully one third of women with UTI limited to the bladder demonstrate counts less than 10^5 bacteria/mL.

Bacterial counts may be $<10^5$ bacteria/mL in UTIs

Given the overlap, application of these findings to clinical practice requires linking the epidemiologic probability to the clinical findings. If a woman has symptoms of cystitis and a culture positive for a urinary pathogen, the probability she has a UTI is 90%, even if the count is as low as 10^3 bacteria/mL. If the woman is asymptomatic, the probability drops to 80% even if the count is more than 10^5/mL. In the latter case, the culture must be repeated before concluding that a UTI is present. Voiding more than 10^5 of the same contaminant twice in a row is unlikely. There is no reason to repeat positive cultures from symptomatic patients. Catheterized and suprapubic specimens may be accepted at face value, because they come directly from the bladder.

Presence of both pathogens and symptoms is diagnostic

Asymptomatic positives should be repeated

TREATMENT

The treatment of UTI is best guided by the results of cultures and antimicrobial susceptibility tests. In simple isolated instances of cystitis in a young woman, the etiology is often assumed to be *E. coli* and the antimicrobic selected empirically based on knowledge of the susceptibility of local strains. Sulfonamides and trimethoprim alone or in combination with sulfamethoxazole, a fluoroquinolone, and nitrofurantoin are the agents most commonly used. In most areas, the use of ampicillin is precluded by resistance rates exceeding 25%. For children and patients with risk factors or recurrent infections, empiric therapy should always be confirmed by culture and susceptibility testing. Likewise, the duration of therapy depends on the severity of the infection and the risk status of the patient. Success of treatment may be tested by a follow-up urine culture 1 to 2 weeks after therapy is completed.

Empiric treatment is common

Resistance limits ampicillin use

PREVENTION

Those with several symptomatic episodes annually may be helped with long-term, low-dose chemoprophylaxis. In women whose recurrences are related to sexual activity, administration of the chemoprophylactic agent may be limited to immediately after intercourse. Infected children, men, and those who experience UTI relapse should be investigated with intravenous pyelography to allow detection and correction of any factor causing predisposition to infection.

Chemoprophylaxis may be effective

ADDITIONAL READING

Kass EH. Asymptomatic infections of the urinary tract. *Trans Assoc Am Physicians* 1956;69:56–64. This paper, where the 10^5 bacteria/ mL value comes from, is one of the most cited papers in the medical literature. Many are not aware that the clear separation between UTIs and controls owes much to the fact that the specimens obtained in this study were catheterized, not voided.

Warren JW, Abrutyn E, Hebel JR, et al. Guidelines for antimicrobial treatment of uncomplicated acute bacterial cystitis and acute pyelonephritis in women. Infectious Diseases Society of America (IDSA). *Clin Infect Dis* 1999;29:745–758. This set of guidelines from the IDSA uses an evidence-based approach to the treatment of UTI.

CHAPTER 67

Central Nervous System Infections

C. George Ray

The cerebrum, cerebellum, brainstem, spinal cord, and their covering membranes (meninges) constitute the central nervous system (CNS). Because of the unique anatomic and physiologic features of the CNS, infections of this site can represent special challenges to the microbiologist and clinician. The CNS is encased in a rigid, bony vault, and it is highly vulnerable to the effects of inflammation and edema: its critical life-regulatory functions and the metabolic requirements to sustain these functions can also be easily disrupted by infection, with resultant local acidosis, hypoxia, and destruction of nerve cells. Thus, the effects of increased pressure, biochemical abnormalities, and tissue necrosis can be profound and sometimes irreversible. One specialized defense mechanism of the CNS is the blood–brain barrier, which serves to minimize passage of infectious agents and potentially toxic metabolites into the cerebrospinal fluid (CSF) and tissues, as well as to regulate the rate of transport of plasma proteins, glucose, and electrolytes. When CNS infection develops, however, this barrier also poses difficulties in control; some antimicrobial agents and host immune factors, such as immunoglobulins and complement, do not pass as readily from the blood to the site of infection as they do to other tissues.

Blood–brain barrier affects access of microbes, immune factors, and antimicrobics

Within the brain are the ventricles, which are cavities in which CSF is actively produced, primarily by specialized structures called the choroid plexuses. The CSF fills the lateral ventricles in each half of the brain, circulates into a central third ventricle, and then passes through the cerebral aqueduct to emerge through foramina at the brainstem. From cisterns at the base of the brain, the CSF circulates in the subarachnoid space over the entire CNS, including the spinal cord, to supply nutrients and serve as a hydraulic cushion for these tissues. It is reabsorbed primarily by the major venous system in the meninges. Obstruction of the normal flow of CSF in either the internal (ventricular) or external (subarachnoid) systems can result in increased intracranial pressure, because production of CSF by the choroid plexuses will continue within the ventricles. Such impairment of flow or normal reabsorption can occur as a result of inflammation or subsequent fibrosis, leading to dilatation of the ventricles, compression of brain tissue, and a condition known as **hydrocephalus.**

CSF continuously produced by choroid plexus

Obstruction of CSF flow or reabsorption causes hydrocephalus

ROUTES OF INFECTION

Most CNS infections appear to result from blood-borne spread; for example, bacteremia or viremia resulting from infection of tissue at a site remote from the CNS may result in penetration of the blood–brain barrier. Examples of infectious agents that commonly infect the CNS by this route are *Haemophilus influenzae, Neisseria meningitidis, Streptococcus pneumoniae, Mycobacterium tuberculosis,* and viruses such as enteroviruses and mumps (Tables 67–1 and 67–2). The initial source of infection leading to bloodstream invasion may be occult (eg, infection of reticuloendothelial tissues) or overt (eg, pneumonia, pharyngitis, skin abscess or cellulitis, or bacterial endocarditis). Occasionally, the route of infection is from a focus close to or contiguous with the CNS. These possible sources include middle ear infection (otitis media), mastoiditis, sinusitis, or pyogenic infections of the skin or bone. Infection may extend directly into the CNS, indirectly via venous pathways, or in the sheaths of cranial and spinal nerves.

Blood-borne spread most common access to CNS

Direct spread occurs from adjacent infected focus such as middle ear

In some cases, a contiguous or distant infectious focus may not be necessary to produce CNS infection. If an anatomic defect exists in the structures encasing the CNS, infectious agents may readily gain access to the vulnerable site and establish themselves. Such defects may be traumatically or surgically induced or result from congenital malformations. For example, fractures of the base of the skull may produce an opening between the CNS and the sinuses, nasal passages (defects in the cribriform plate), mastoid, or middle ear. All of these sites are contiguous with the upper respiratory tract, which enables a potentially pathogenic member of the respiratory flora to gain ready access to the CNS. Neurosurgical procedures also create transient communications between the external environment and the CNS that can be readily contaminated. This risk can be compounded when foreign bodies, such as shunts or external drainage tubes, must be left in place for the treatment of hydrocephalus. These foreign bodies, when colonized, can serve as chronic foci of infection. Congenital defects, such as meningomyeloceles or sinus tracts through the cranium or spine, may also be sources. The latter may be overlooked; the orifice of the sinus may be a small cleft on the skin surface, or occasionally it may open internally into the intestinal tract. Recurrent purulent meningitis or unusual pathogens in an otherwise healthy host should prompt a careful search for such defects.

Traumatic, surgical, or congenital lesions may give direct access

Implanted foreign bodies such as shunts increase risk

Perhaps the least common route of CNS infection is by intraneural pathways. Agents capable of intraneural spread to the CNS include rabies virus (presumably along peripheral sensory nerves), herpes simplex virus (often, but not exclusively, via the trigeminal nerve root or sacral nerves), polioviruses, and perhaps some togaviruses.

Intraneural pathways operate with a few viruses

Abscesses of the CNS deserve special mention. Although relatively uncommon compared with other CNS infections, they represent a special microbiologic and clinical problem. Such abscesses may be within the tissues of the CNS (eg, brain abscess; Fig 67–1) or localized in the subdural or epidural spaces. They sometimes develop as a complication

TABLE 67–1

Common Causes of Purulent Central Nervous System Infections

Age Group	Agent
Newborns (<1 mo old)	Group B streptococci (most common), *Escherichia coli, Listeria monocytogenes, Klebsiella* species, other enteric Gram-negative bacteria
Infants and children	*Streptococcus pneumoniae, Neisseria meningitidis, Haemophilus influenzae*
Adults	*S. pneumoniae, Neisseria meningitidis*
Special circumstances	
Meningitis or intracranial abscesses associated with trauma, neurosurgery, or intracranial foreign bodies	*Staphylococcus aureus, Staphylococcus epidermidis, S. pneumoniae;* anaerobic Gram-negative and Gram-positive bacteria; *Pseudomonas* species
Intracranial abscesses not associated with trauma or surgery	Microaerophilic or anaerobic streptococci, anaerobic Gram-negative bacteria (often mixed aerobic and anaerobic flora of upper respiratory tract origin)

TABLE 67–2

Primary Acute Viral Infections of the Central Nervous System

AGENT	MAJOR AGE GROUP AFFECTED	SEASONAL PREDOMINANCE
Enteroviruses	Infants, children	Summer–fall
Mumps	Children	Winter–spring
Herpes simplex		
Type 1	Adults	None
Type 2	Neonates, young adults	None
Arboviruses		
Western equine encephalitis	Infants, children	Summer–fall
St. Louis encephalitis	Adults >40 years	Summer–fall
California encephalitis	School-aged children	Summer–fall
Eastern equine encephalitis	Infants, children	Summer–fall
West Nile encephalitis	Adults	Summer–fall
Rabies	All ages	Summer–fall
Measles	Infants, children	Spring
Varicella–zoster	Infants, children	Spring
Lymphocytic choriomeningitis	Adults, children	None
Epstein–Barr virus	Children, young adults	None
Other (eg, myxoviruses, human immunodeficiency virus, cytomegaloviruses)	All ages	Variable

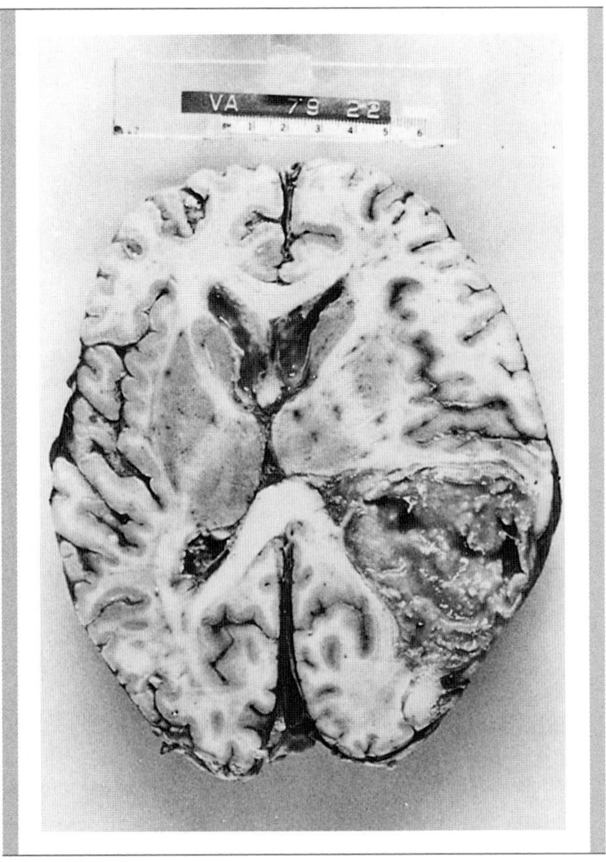

FIGURE 67–1
Coronal section of a brain demonstrating a poorly encapsulated abscess.

Abscesses present diagnostic problems and may localize in brain, at subdural or epidural sites

of pyogenic meningitis. More commonly, abscesses of the CNS result from embolization of bacteria or fungi from a distant focus, such as endocarditis or pyogenic lung abscess; extension from a contiguous focus of infection (eg, sinusitis or mastoiditis); or a complication of surgery or nonsurgical trauma.

CLINICAL FEATURES

Acute onset and progression with stiff neck and neurologic dysfunction

Usually fatal if untreated

Several terms commonly applied to CNS infections need to be understood. **Purulent meningitis** refers to infections of the meninges associated with a marked, acute inflammatory exudate and is usually caused by a bacterial infection. Such infections frequently involve the underlying CNS tissue to a variable degree, and often the ventricular system is also involved (ventriculitis). Most cases of purulent meningitis are acute in onset and progression and are characterized by fever, stiff neck, irritability, and varying degrees of neurologic dysfunction that, if untreated, usually progress to a fatal outcome. Large numbers of polymorphonuclear leukocytes are present in the CSF of established cases.

Granulomatous infections are chronic

Chronic meningitis has a more insidious onset, with progression of signs and symptoms over a period of weeks. This is usually caused by mycobacteria or fungi that produce granulomatous inflammatory changes, but occasionally protozoal agents are responsible (Table 67–3). The cellular response in the CSF reflects the chronic inflammatory nature of the disease.

Aseptic meningitis is commonly of viral etiology

Other causes include syphilis

Aseptic meningitis is a term used to describe a syndrome of meningeal inflammation associated mostly with an increase of cells (pleocytosis), primarily lymphocytes and other mononuclear cells in the CSF, and absence of readily cultivable bacteria or fungi. It is associated most commonly with viral infections and is often self-limiting. The syndrome can also occur in syphilis and some other spirochetal diseases, as a response to the presence of drugs or radiopaque substances in the CSF, or from tumors or bleeding involving the meninges or subarachnoid space. The primary site of inflammation is in the meninges without clinical evidence of involvement of the neural tissue. Such patients may have fever, headache, a stiff neck or back, nausea, and vomiting.

Encephalitis also implies a primary viral etiology; however, acute or chronic demyelinating diseases with or without inflammation must also be considered. This latter

TABLE 67–3

Other Causes of Central Nervous System Infections

Disease	Agent
Chronic granulomatous infection	*Mycobacterium tuberculosis*[a]
	Coccidioides immitis
	Cryptococcus neoformans
	Histoplasma capsulatum
Parasitic infection	
Protozoa	*Toxoplasma gondii*[b]
	Trypanosoma
	Acanthamoeba species
Nematodes	*Toxocara* species
	Trichinella spiralis
	Angiostrongylus cantonensis
Cestodes	*Taenia solium* (cysticercosis)
Other	*Leptospira* species
	Treponema pallidum
	Borrelia burgdorferi

[a] Tuberculous meningitis can appear as acute or chronically progressive disease.

[b] Toxoplasmosis of the central nervous system is usually seen in congenital infections or immunocompromised hosts.

group includes the postinfectious or allergic encephalomyelitis syndromes, in which the etiology and pathogenesis are not always clearly defined. Clinically, the diagnosis of encephalitis is applied to patients who may or may not show signs and CSF findings compatible with aseptic meningitis but also show objective evidence of CNS dysfunction (eg, seizures, paralysis, and disordered mentation). Many clinicians use the term **meningoencephalitis** to describe patients with both meningeal and encephalitic manifestations.

Viral and postinfectious etiology most common

Poliomyelitis refers to the selective destruction of anterior motor horn cells in the spinal cord and/or brainstem, which leads to weakness or paralysis of muscle groups and occasionally respiratory insufficiency. It is usually associated with aseptic meningitis, sometimes with encephalitis. The polioviruses are the major causes of this syndrome, although coxsackieviruses (primarily type A7) and other enteroviruses, such as enterovirus 71, have been implicated. The hallmark of poliomyelitis is asymmetric flaccid paralysis.

Viral destruction of anterior horn cells causes paralysis

Two other nervous system syndromes presumably associated with infection deserve brief mention. **Acute polyneuritis,** an inflammatory disease of the peripheral nervous system, is characterized by symmetric flaccid paralysis of muscles. In most cases, no specific etiology is found; some, however, have been associated with *Corynebacterium diphtheriae* toxin and infections by bacterial enteric pathogens, cytomegalovirus or Epstein–Barr virus. **Reye's syndrome** (encephalopathy with fatty infiltration of the viscera) is an acute, noninflammatory process, usually observed in childhood, in which cerebral edema, hepatic dysfunction, and hyperammonemia develop within 2 to 12 days after onset of a systemic viral infection. Although the influenza A and B and varicella–zoster viruses have been most frequently implicated in this syndrome, the precise pathogenesis is not yet known. Concomitant salicylate therapy is known to be a contributory factor.

Acute polyneuritis involves peripheral nervous system

Reye's syndrome precipitated by salicylate treatment of systemic viral infection

COMMON ETIOLOGIC AGENTS

The causes of CNS infections are numerous, as illustrated in Tables 67–1 through 67–3. Acute purulent meningitis is usually caused by one of three organisms: *H. influenzae* type b, *N. meningitidis,* or *S. pneumoniae*. The incidence of *H. influenzae* meningitis has now fallen sharply in the United States as a result of routine immunization. In neonatal infections, group B streptococci or *Escherichia coli* are most frequently implicated. However, many other bacteria can occasionally cause the disease if they gain access to the meninges.

Acute purulent meningitis caused by encapsulated pathogens

Of the viral causes of acute CNS disease, the categories most commonly encountered are the enteroviruses, human immunodeficiency virus, herpes simplex, Epstein–Barr virus, and arthropod-borne viruses. In the United States, enteroviruses account for the greatest proportion of infections. Viral CNS infections can be manifested clinically as aseptic meningitis, encephalitis, or poliomyelitis. The age of the patient and the season of occurrence help somewhat in predicting some of the agents that may be involved, (see Table 67–2); other epidemiologic, ecologic, and clinical factors associated with these infections are discussed in the individual chapters on specific virus groups.

Acute viral disease has a variety of manifestations

Seasonality and patient age important clues

Slow viral infections of the CNS, such as subacute sclerosing panencephalitis (due to measles or sometimes congenitally acquired rubella virus), acquired immunodeficiency syndrome encephalopathy, progressive multifocal leukoencephalopathy (due to JC polyomavirus), and Creutzfeldt–Jacob disease ("unconventional" viruses), are discussed in Chapters 34, 42, 43, and 44, respectively. Other important causes of CNS infections (see Table 67–3) that must not be overlooked include *Mycobacterium tuberculosis* and the deep mycoses (especially *Cryptococcus neoformans* and *Coccidioides immitis*). These chronic infections can be insidious in onset and mimic other processes, thus delaying consideration of the proper diagnosis.

Chronic meningitis is caused by slow-growing agents

Finally, there are noninfectious causes of CNS disease to be considered in the differential diagnosis. These include (1) metabolic disturbances, such as hypoglycemia, diabetic coma, and hepatic failure; (2) toxic conditions, such as those caused by bacterial toxins (diphtheria, tetanus, botulism), insect toxins (tick paralysis), poisons (lead), and drug abuse; (3) mass lesions, such as acute trauma, hematoma, and tumor; (4) vascular lesions, such as intracranial embolus, aneurysm, and subarachnoid hemorrhage; and (5) acute psychiatric episodes.

Noninfectious diseases may mimic infections

GENERAL DIAGNOSTIC APPROACHES

Lumbar puncture for pressure, cells, protein, and glucose in CSF

CSF glucose should be compared with simultaneous blood level

Except in unusual circumstances, in which severe increases in intracranial pressure make the procedure dangerous, a lumbar puncture is the first step in the workup of a patient with suspected CNS infection. The CSF pressure is determined at the time of the procedure, and CSF is removed for analysis of cells, protein, and glucose. Ideally, the glucose content of the peripheral blood is determined simultaneously for comparison with that in the CSF. Table 67–4 presents guidelines for interpretation of results of CSF analysis; these guidelines represent generalizations, however, and must not be considered as absolute findings in all cases. For example, although a patient with bacterial, mycobacterial, or fungal meningitis usually has a glucose level in the CSF of less than 40 mg/dL, or less than half the blood glucose level (hypoglycorrhachia), this finding may not be present in the early stages of infection. Viral infections of the CNS can occasionally produce low glucose values in the CSF; in addition, the early stages of viral infection may be associated with a preponderance of polymorphonuclear leukocytes. It is clearly important to recognize that viral CNS infections can exist with a negligible CSF cell count. This sometimes also occurs in the early stages of bacterial meningitis.

Viral and granulomatous infections often cause predominance of lymphocytes in CSF

Realizing the limitations, it is possible to make some general interpretations that are helpful in the diagnosis. Viral CNS infections are usually associated with a preponderance of lymphocytes, a normal glucose value, and a normal or moderately elevated protein level in the CSF. In contrast, acute bacterial meningitis usually causes a CSF pleocytosis consisting primarily of polymorphonuclear cells, a low glucose value, and a high protein level. Mycobacterial and fungal infections are more commonly associated with lymphocytosis (and sometimes moderate eosinophilia) in the CSF; like the acute bacterial infections, however, they tend to lower glucose and increase protein levels markedly.

Polymorphonuclear cells not often found in normal CSF

Normal values for CSF are also shown in Table 67–4. Polymorphonuclear cells are not usually seen in normal CSF, but as many as five lymphocytes/mm^3 may be found in healthy individuals. Neonatal CSF is considerably more difficult to interpret, because cell counts are often elevated in the absence of infection; glucose values, however, should be within the normal range.

Direct staining and culture are definitive diagnostic methods

Tests for free antigens useful in some circumstances

The other major procedures that must be performed on all CSF samples in which any infection is suspected include bacterial cultures and Gram staining. If the CSF is grossly purulent and the patient untreated, a Gram stain of the uncentrifuged CSF or of its centrifuged sediment frequently shows the infecting organism and indicates the specific diagnosis. According to the clinical indications and results of CSF cytology and chemistry, other microbiologic tests may be used, including viral cultures, special stains and cultures for fungi and mycobacteria, immunologic methods to detect fungal or bacterial antigens

TABLE 67–4

Findings of Cerebrospinal Fluid Analysis: Normal Versus Infection

CLINICAL SITUATION	LEUKOCYTES/mm^3	% POLYMORPHOUCLEARS	GLUCOSE (% OF BLOOD)	PROTEIN (mg/dL)
CHILDREN AND ADULTS				
Normal	0–5	0	≥60	≤30
Viral infection	2–2000 (80)[a]	≤50	≥60	30–80
Pyogenic bacterial infection	5–5000 (800)	≥60	≤45[b]	>60
[illegible]ulosis and mycoses	5–2000 (100)	≤50	≤45	>60
[illegible]				
[illegible]	0–32 (8)	≤60	≥60	20–170 (90)
[illegible])	0–29 (9)	≤60	≥60	65–150 (115)

[illegible]heses represent mean values.

(eg, latex agglutination for *Cryptococcus*), and polymerase chain reactions to detect viral or bacterial nucleic acids.

Tests on specimens other than CSF are selected on the basis of the clinical diagnostic possibilities. If acute bacterial meningitis is suspected, blood cultures should also be used to ensure the diagnosis. Viral cultures of the pharynx, stool, or rectal swabs may provide indirect evidence of CNS infection. In encephalitis, a biopsy specimen of the brain is sometimes obtained for culture, histology, and to demonstrate viral antigen or nucleic acid. Other studies may include acute and convalescent sera for viral serology and serologic tests to detect antibodies to certain fungi, such as *C. immitis*.

Culture of blood and other sites depend on suspected etiology

Biopsy and serology useful for some agents

Intracranial abscesses can often be detected with radiologic techniques, such as computerized tomography or magnetic resonance imaging. A definitive etiologic diagnosis is established by careful aerobic and anaerobic culture of the contents of the abscess.

Imaging methods useful to detect abscesses

GENERAL PRINCIPLES OF MANAGEMENT

In bacterial, mycobacterial, and fungal infections of the CNS, prompt and aggressive antimicrobial therapy is required. The duration of treatment varies from as little as 10 days for uncomplicated bacterial meningitis, to 12 months or longer for tuberculous meningitis, and to several years for some cases of fungal meningitis.

Antimicrobial therapy is administered immediately

In addition to antimicrobial therapy, correction of associated metabolic defects (acidosis, hypoxia, saline depletion, inappropriate antidiuretic hormone secretion) is necessary. Increased intracranial pressure as a result of vasogenic edema or hydrocephalus must be monitored and controlled accordingly; osmotic agents such as intravenous mannitol are often used to control acute cerebral edema, and neurosurgical shunting procedures may be needed to treat progressive hydrocephalus. Abscesses often require drainage. Except for those patients with herpes simplex encephalitis, who often respond to early treatment with antiviral agents, most viral infections of the CNS can only be managed supportively. This includes specific attention to the metabolic and respiratory problems that may develop in severe cases.

Correction of metabolic defects and raised intracranial pressure important

Viral infections are managed supportively

CHAPTER 68

Intravascular Infections, Bacteremia, and Endotoxemia

C. George Ray and Kenneth J. Ryan

In many cases the presence of circulating microorganisms in the blood is either a part of the natural history of the infectious disease or a reflection of serious, uncontrolled infection. Depending on the class of agent involved, this process is described as viremia, bacteremia, fungemia, or parasitemia. The terms **sepsis** and **septicemia** refer to the major clinical symptom complexes generally associated with bacteremia. The clinical findings may develop acutely, as in septic shock, or slowly, as in most forms of infective endocarditis. Viremia is usually a very early, even prodromal, event accompanied by fever, malaise, and other constitutional symptoms, such as muscle aches. With the exception of a few specific infections, the detection of viremia does not play a role in the diagnosis or management of viral infections. The presence of bacteremia defines some of the most serious and life-threatening situations in medical practice, and it has a marked impact on the management and outcome of bacterial infections. This chapter will focus on the causes and implications of bacteremia and, to a lesser extent, fungemia. Diseases in which parasitemia is a feature are covered in Chapters 51 to 54.

Sepsis refers to clinical findings

Onset can be insidious or dramatic

Bacteremia or fungemia may also result from microbial growth on the inner or outer surfaces of intravenous devices. Clinical manifestations may be minor initially, but may later become severe. Because the bloodstream is sterile in healthy individuals, bacteremia is considered potentially serious regardless of the symptoms present; however, transient bacteremia may occur when there is manipulation or trauma to a body site that has a normal flora. After such events, species indigenous to the site may appear briefly in the blood, but they are soon cleared. Such transient bacteremias usually have no immediate clinical significance, but they are important in the pathogenesis of infective endocarditis.

Bloodstream is sterile in health

Transient, benign bacteremia is common

INTRAVASCULAR INFECTION

Intracardiac infections (endocarditis) and those primarily involving veins (thrombophlebitis) or arteries (endarteritis) are usually caused by bacteria, although other agents including fungi and viruses have been occasionally implicated. This discussion will focus primarily on the bacterial causes, because they are the most frequent. Infections of the cardiovascular system are usually extremely serious and, if not promptly and adequately treated, can be fatal. They commonly produce a constant shedding of organisms into the

Primarily caused by bacteria

bloodstream that is often characterized by continuous, low-grade bacteremia (1 to 20 organisms/mL of blood) in untreated patients.

Infective Endocarditis

Sites of endocardial infection include prosthetic valves

The term **infective endocarditis** is preferable to the commonly used term **bacterial endocarditis,** simply because not all infections of the endocardial surface of the heart are caused by bacteria. Most infections occur on natural or prosthetic cardiac valves, but can also develop on septal defects, shunts (eg, patent ductus arteriosus), or the mural endocardium. Infections involving coarctation of the aorta are also classified as infective endocarditis because the clinical manifestations and complications are similar.

Pathogenesis

The pathogenesis of infective endocarditis involves several factors that, if concurrent, result in infection:

Hemodynamic effects of cardiac abnormalities create sites for attachment

1. The endothelium is altered to facilitate colonization by bacteria and deposition of platelets and fibrin. Most infections involve the mitral or aortic valves, which are particularly vulnerable when abnormalities such as valvular insufficiency, stenosis, intracardiac shunts (eg, ventricular septal defect), or direct trauma (eg, catheters) exist. The turbulence of intracardiac blood flow that results from such abnormalities can lead to further irregularities of the endothelial surfaces that facilitate platelet and fibrin deposition. These factors produce a potential nidus for colonization and infection.

Transient bacteremia with normal flora is the usual organism source

2. Transient bacteremia is common, but it is usually of no clinical importance. Often seen for a few minutes after a variety of dental procedures, it has also been shown to develop after normal childbirth and manipulations such as bronchoscopy, sigmoidoscopy, cystoscopy, and some surgical procedures. Even simple activities such as tooth brushing or chewing candy can cause such bacteremia. The organisms responsible for transient bacteremia are the common surface flora of the manipulated site such as viridans streptococci (oropharynx) and are usually of low virulence. Other, more virulent strains may also be involved, however; for example, intravenous drug abuse may lead to transient bacteremia with *Staphylococcus aureus* or a variety of Gram-negative aerobic and anaerobic bacteria. Whether or not the organisms causing bacteremia (or fungemia) are of high virulence, they can colonize and multiply in the heart if local endothelial changes are suitable.

Bacteria adhere and start development of vegetation

Embolization created by dislodged parts of vegetation

3. Circulating organisms adhere to the damaged surface, followed by complement activation, inflammation, fibrin, and platelet deposition and further endothelial damage at the site of colonization. The resulting entrapment of organisms in the thrombotic "mesh" of platelets, fibrin, and inflammatory cells leads to a mature vegetation, which protects the organisms from host humoral and phagocytic immune defenses, and to some extent from antimicrobial agents. As a result, the infection can be exceedingly difficult to treat. The vegetation can also create greater hemodynamic alterations in terms of obstruction to flow and increased turbulence. Parts of vegetations may break off and be deposited in smaller blood vessels (embolization) with resultant obstruction and secondary sites of infection. Emboli may be transported to the brain or coronary arteries, for example, with disastrous results.

Circulating immune complexes cause peripheral manifestations

Another phenomenon shown to contribute to the infective endocarditis syndrome is the development of circulating immune complexes of microbial antigen and antibody. These complexes can activate complement and contribute to many of the peripheral manifestations of the disease, including nephritis, arthritis, and cutaneous vascular lesions.

Rheumatoid factor and antinuclear antibodies contribute to pathogenesis

Frequently, there is a widespread stimulus to host cellular and humoral immunity, particularly if the infection continues for more than about 2 weeks. This condition is characterized by hyperglobulinemia, splenomegaly, and the occasional appearance of macrophages in the peripheral blood. Some patients develop circulating rheumatoid factor (IgM anti-IgG antibody), which may play a deleterious role by blocking IgG opsonic activity and causing microvascular damage. Antinuclear antibodies, which also appear occasionally, may contribute to the pathogenesis of the fever, arthralgia, and myalgia that is often seen.

In summary, infective endocarditis involves an initial complex of endothelial damage or abnormality, which facilitates colonization by organisms that may be circulating through the heart. This colonization, in turn, leads to the propagation of a vegetation, with its attendant local and systemic inflammatory, embolic, and immunologic complications.

Clinical Features

Infective endocarditis has often been classified by the progression of the untreated disease. **Acute endocarditis** is generally fulminant with high fever and toxicity, and death may occur in a few days or weeks. **Subacute endocarditis** progresses to death over weeks to months with low-grade fever, night sweats, weight loss, and vague constitutional complaints. The clinical course is substantially related to the virulence of the infecting organism; *S. aureus,* for example, usually produces acute disease, whereas infections by the otherwise avirulent viridans streptococci are more likely to be subacute. Before the advent of antimicrobial therapy, death was considered inevitable in all cases. Physical findings often include a new or changing heart murmur, splenomegaly, various skin lesions (petechiae, splinter hemorrhages, Osler's nodes, Janeway's lesions), and retinal lesions.

Acute, subacute, and chronic infective endocarditis determined by virulence of organism

Complications include the risk of congestive heart failure as a result of hemodynamic alterations, rupture of the chordae tendinea of the valves, or perforation of a valve. Abscesses of the myocardium or valve ring can also develop. Other complications relate to the immunologic and embolic phenomena that can occur. The kidney is commonly affected, and hematuria is a typical finding. Renal failure, presumably from immune complex glomerulonephritis, is possible. Left-sided endocarditis can readily lead to coronary artery embolization and "mycotic" aneurysms; the latter will be discussed later in this chapter. In addition, more distant emboli to the central nervous system can lead to cerebral infarction and infection. Right-sided endocarditis often causes embolization and infarction or infection in the lung.

Cardiac, embolic, and immunologically mediated complications lead to death without treatment

Etiologic Agents

Table 68–1 summarizes the most common causes of infective endocarditis. Alpha-hemolytic streptococci and enterococci are involved in just over 50% of the cases. In the so-called culture-negative group, infective endocarditis is diagnosed on clinical grounds, but cultures do not confirm the etiologic agent. This group of patients is difficult to treat, and the overall prognosis is considered poorer than when a specific etiology has been determined. Negative cultures may result from (1) prior antibiotic treatment; (2) fungal endocarditis with entrapment of these relatively large organisms in capillary beds; (3) fastidious, nutritionally deficient, or cell wall–deficient organisms that are difficult to isolate; (4) infection caused by

Streptococci are most common cause

TABLE 68–1

Common Etiologic Agents in Infective Endocarditis

Agent	Approximate Percentage of Cases
Viridans streptococci (several species)	30–40
Enterococci	5–18
Other streptococci	15–25
Staphylococcus aureus	15–40
Coagulase-negative staphylococci	4–30
Gram-negative bacilli	2–13
Fungi (eg, *Candida, Aspergillus*)	2–4

TABLE 68–2

Etiologic Agents More Commonly Observed in Special Circumstances

SITUATION	AGENT
Intravenous drug abuse	*Staphylococcus aureus;* enterococci; Enterobacteriaceae and *Pseudomonas;* fungi
Prosthetic valve infection	Coagulase-negative streptococci; *S. aureus;* Enterobacteriaceae and *Pseudomonas;* diphtheroids; *Candida* and *Aspergillus* spp.
Immunocompromise, chronic illness	Any of the above organisms

Many explanations for culture-negative endocarditis

obligate intracellular parasites, such as chlamydiae (*Chlamydia psittaci*), rickettsiae (*Coxiella burnetii*), *Rochalimaea* species, or viruses; (5) immunologic factors (eg, antibody acting on circulating organisms); or (6) subacute endocarditis involving the right side of the heart, in which the organisms are filtered out in the pulmonary capillaries.

Some special circumstances alter the relative etiologic possibilities, such as intravenous drug addiction, prosthetic valves, and immunocompromise. The major associations in these cases are summarized in Table 68–2.

General Diagnostic Approaches

Blood culture the most important diagnostic test

The diagnosis of infective endocarditis is usually suspected on clinical grounds; however, the most important diagnostic test for confirmation is the blood culture. In untreated cases, the organisms are generally present continuously in low numbers (1 to 20/mL) in the blood. If an adequate volume of blood is obtained, the first culture will be positive in over 95% of culturally confirmed cases. Most authorities recommend three cultures over 24 hours to ensure detection, and an additional three if the first set is negative. Multiple cultures yielding the same organism support the probability of an intravascular or intracardiac infection. In acute endocarditis, the urgency of early treatment may require collection of only two or three cultures within a few minutes so that antimicrobial therapy can begin.

Echocardiography defines vegetations

Cardiologic procedures such as transthoracic or transesophageal echocardiography can delineate the nature and size of the vegetations and progression of disease. They are also helpful in prediction of some complications such as embolization.

General Principles of Management

Bactericidal antimicrobics required because of protective effect of the vegetation

Antimicrobic combinations often used for synergistic effect

Because of the nature of the lesions and their pathogenesis, response to therapy may be slow and cure is sometimes difficult. Therefore, specific antimicrobial therapy must be aggressive, using agents that are bactericidal (rather than bacteriostatic) and can be given in amounts that achieve high continuous blood levels without causing toxicity to the patient. Treatment may involve a single antimicrobial if the organism is highly susceptible in vitro, or antimicrobial combinations if synergistic effects are possible (eg, a penicillin and an aminoglycoside for enterococcal endocarditis). Parenteral therapy is begun to produce adequate blood levels, and the patient may need to be monitored frequently to ensure antimicrobial activity in the serum sufficient to kill the organisms without causing unnecessary toxicity. Therapy is usually prolonged, lasting longer than 4 weeks in most cases. In some cases, surgery may be required to excise the diseased valve and replace it with a valvular prosthesis. The decision for surgery is sometimes difficult, requiring consultation with both a cardiologist and a surgeon.

Prophylaxis can prevent the development of endocarditis in persons with known congenital or acquired cardiac lesions that predispose to bacterial endocarditis. When they undergo procedures known to cause transient bacteremia (eg, dental manipulations or surgical procedures involving the upper respiratory, gastrointestinal, or genitourinary tracts), administration of high doses of antimicrobics is begun just before the procedure and continued for 6 to 12 hours thereafter. An example of prophylaxis is the case of a patient with rheumatic valvular disease who is planning to undergo dental work. The organism most likely to produce transient bacteremia would be a penicillin-sensitive member of the oral flora, especially viridans streptococci. Thus, an intramuscular dose of penicillin or ampicillin within 30 minutes before the procedure, followed by a high dose of intramuscular penicillin or oral amoxicillin 6 hours later, would be expected to afford protection. Several regimens similar to this approach are recommended, depending on the patient, the nature of the procedure, and the organisms that might be expected to be involved.

Antimicrobial prophylaxis indicated for those with cardiac abnormalities

Antimicrobial prophylaxis used with dental work

Mycotic Aneurysm

The term **mycotic aneurysm** is somewhat misleading, because it suggests infection by fungi. Originally used by Sir William Osler to describe the mushroom-shaped arterial aneurysm that can develop in patients with infective endocarditis, the term now applies to infection with any organism that causes inflammatory damage and weakening of an arterial wall with subsequent aneurysmal dilatation. This sequence can progress to rupture, with a fatal outcome.

Intra-arterial infection occurs at sites of vascular injury

Arterial infection can result from direct extension of an intracardiac infection or from septic microemboli from a cardiac focus, with seeding of vasa vasorum within the arterial wall. In addition to infective endocarditis, other predisposing factors include damaged arterial intima by atherosclerotic plaques, vascular thrombi, congenital malformations, trauma, or spread from a contiguous focus of infection directly into the artery. The clinical features vary according to the site of involvement. Common findings may include pain at the site of primary arterial supply (eg, back or abdominal pain in abdominal aortic infections) and fever. In many cases, the initial presentation is the result of a catastrophic hemorrhage, particularly intracerebral aneurysms. The etiologic agents, diagnosis, and management are similar to infective endocarditis.

Etiologic agents similar to those of infective endocarditis

Suppurative Thrombophlebitis

Suppurative (or septic) **thrombophlebitis** is an inflammation of a vein wall frequently associated with thrombosis and bacteremia. There are four basic forms: superficial, pelvic, intracranial venous sinus, and portal vein infection (pylephlebitis). With the steadily increasing use of intravenous catheters, the incidence of superficial thrombophlebitis has risen and represents a major complication in hospitalized patients.

Thrombotic site may become seeded with organisms from blood

The pathogenesis involves thrombus formation, which may result from trauma to the vein, extrinsic inflammation, hypercoagulable states, stasis of blood flow, or combinations of these factors. The thrombosed site is then seeded with organisms, and a focus of infection is established. In superficial thrombophlebitis, an intravenous cannula or catheter may cause local venous wall trauma, as well as serve as a foreign body nidus for thrombus formation. Infection develops if bacteria are introduced by intravenous fluid, local wound contamination, or bacteremic seeding from a remote infected site.

Intravenous catheter often associated with thrombophlebitis

Thrombophlebitis of pelvic, portal, or intracranial venous systems most often occurs as a result of direct extension of an infectious process from adjacent structures, or from venous and lymphatic pathways near sites of infection. For example, infections of intracranial venous sinuses usually result from orbital or sinus infections (causing cavernous sinus thrombophlebitis) or from infections of the mastoid and middle ear (causing lateral and sagittal sinus thrombophlebitis). Pelvic thrombophlebitis is a potential result of intrauterine infection (endometritis), particularly after pelvic surgery or 2 to 3 weeks after childbirth. Pelvic or intra-abdominal infections may also spread to the portal venous system to produce pylephlebitis.

Local infection may extend to veins

Clinical Features

Common features often include fever and inflammation over the infected vein. Pelvic or portal vein thrombophlebitis is usually associated with high fever, chills, nausea, vomiting,

TABLE 68–3

Common Etiologic Agents in Suppurative Thrombophlebitis

SITE	AGENT
Superficial veins (eg, saphenous, femoral, antecubital)	*Staphylococcus aureus;* Gram-negative aerobic bacilli
Pelvic veins, portal veins	*Bacteroides* spp.; microaerophilic or anaerobic streptococci; *Escherichia coli;* beta-hemolytic streptococci (group A or B)
Intracranial venous sinuses (cavernous, sagittal, lateral)	*Haemophilus influenzae, Streptococcus pneumoniae;* beta-hemolytic streptococcus (group A); anaerobic or microaerophilic streptococci; S. aureus

Signs and symptoms depend on anatomic site involved

and abdominal pain. Jaundice may develop in portal vein infections. Intracranial thrombophlebitis varies in its presentation. Headache, facial or orbital edema, and neurologic deficits are variably present; for example, cavernous sinus thrombophlebitis often causes palsies of the third through sixth cranial nerves. Complications include extension of suppurative infection into adjacent structures, further propagation of thrombi, bacteremia, and septic embolization. Embolization from pelvic or leg veins is to the lungs and pulmonary embolism with infarction may be the presenting manifestation of the remote infection.

Etiologic Agents

The major infectious causes of suppurative thrombophlebitis are outlined in Table 68–3. In superficial thrombophlebitis, which often follows intravenous therapy, organisms that are common nosocomial offenders predominate (*S. aureus,* Gram-negative aerobes). Deeper infections are more frequently caused by organisms that reside on adjacent mucous membranes (eg, *Bacteroides* species in intestinal and vaginal sites) or commonly infect adjacent sites (eg, *Haemophilus influenzae* and *S. pneumoniae* in acute otitis media and sinusitis).

General Diagnostic Approaches

Direct culture or blood culture is usually positive

The diagnosis is often suspected on clinical grounds and from associated events known to create predisposition to such infections (eg, surgery, presence of indwelling venous cannulas). Direct cultures of the infected site or blood cultures usually yield the infecting organism, because bacteremia is often present. Radiologic procedures, including scanning methods, may be necessary to localize the process and support the diagnosis. In some cases, surgical exploration is required, both for definitive treatment and to obtain specimens for cultures.

General Principles of Management

Antimicrobic therapy and removal of catheters

The choice of antimicrobial agents is based on culture and susceptibility test results, or in the absence of microbiologic data, the most likely possibilities listed in Table 68–3. Other important aspects of management include prompt removal of possible offending sources, such as intravenous catheters, vigorous treatment of adjacent infections, and sometimes surgical excision and drainage. Severe cases may also benefit from systemic anticoagulant therapy to prevent further propagation of thrombi and embolization.

Many cases are preventable. Unnecessary, long-term intravenous cannulation should be avoided. Whenever possible, it is better to use short needles such as "scalp vein" cannulas than venous catheters or plastic cannulas. Careful asepsis is essential with all

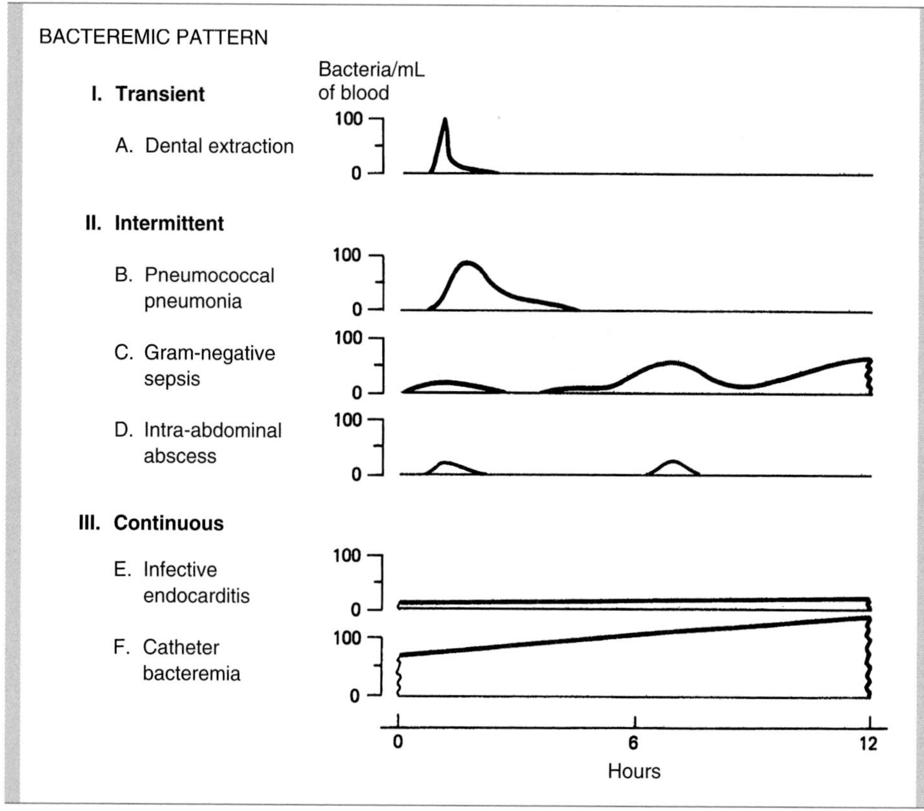

FIGURE 68–1
Patterns of bacteremia. The magnitude and timing of bacteremia for six typical patients (A–F) are depicted. These findings have implications for blood culture sampling plans. Cases such as A and B are detected only by cultures taken early in their course. Cases such as C and particularly D are more variable and more likely to be detected by cultures spaced over the time period shown. Continuous bacteremia (E and F) should be detected by any sampling plan. It could be confused with transient bacteremia on single blood cultures, because both are caused by organisms of low virulence (viridans streptococci, *Staphylococcus epidermidis*); in cases such as E and F, however, bacteremia is sustained, whereas cases of transient bacteremia yield multiple positive results only if they are collected at or near the same time.

intravenous procedures to prevent contamination of intravenous fluids, tubing, and the site of venous entry.

Intravenous Catheter Bacteremia

A variant of intravascular infection develops when a medical device such as an intravenous catheter or any of several types of monitoring devices placed in the bloodstream becomes colonized with microorganisms. The event itself does not have immediate clinical significance but, unlike transient bacteremia from manipulation of normal floral sites, the bacteremia continues. This persistence greatly increases the chances of secondary complications such as infective endocarditis and metastatic infection, depending on any underlying disease and the virulence of the organism involved.

Significant endocarditis and metastatic infection risk

The organisms involved are usually those found in the skin flora, such as *S. epidermidis, Corynebacterium jeikeium,* or *S. aureus.* In debilitated patients already on antimicrobial therapy, *Candida* species may be involved. Occasionally, the sources of contamination are the intravenous solutions themselves rather than the skin. In these cases, members of the Enterobacteriaceae, *Pseudomonas,* or other Gram-negative rods are more likely.

Skin flora most commonly involved

The clinical findings in catheter bacteremia are usually mild despite large numbers of organisms in the bloodstream (Fig 68–1). In addition to low-grade fever, signs of inflammation may or may not be present. Management includes removal of the contaminated catheter. Antimicrobial therapy alone often does not eradicate the organisms in the presence of a foreign body (the catheter).

Removal of contaminated catheter usually necessary

BACTEREMIA FROM EXTRAVASCULAR INFECTION

Although bacteremia is an integral feature of intravascular infection, most cases of clinically significant bacteremia are the result of overflow from an extravascular infection. In these cases, the organisms drained by the lymphatics or otherwise escaping from the infected focus reach the capillary and venous circulation through the lymphatic vessels. De-

Bacteremia may be high despite mild manifestations

pending on the magnitude of the infection and the degree of local control, these organisms may be filtered in the reticuloendothelial system or circulate more widely, producing bacteremia or fungemia. The process is dependent on the timing and interaction of multiple events and is thus much less predictable than intravascular infection. If the infection is extensive and uncontrolled, such as an overwhelming staphylococcal pneumonia, there may be hundreds or even thousands of organisms per milliliter of blood, a poor prognostic sign. An intra-abdominal abscess may only seed a few organisms intermittently until it is discovered and drained. Most infections that produce bacteremia fall between these extremes, with bloodstream invasion more common in the acute phases and intermittent at other times.

Bacteremia is more variable than with intravascular infection

The causative organisms and the frequencies with which they usually produce bacteremia (or fungemia) are listed in Table 68–4. There is considerable overlap, and the probability of bacteremia is dependent on the site as well as the organism. Any organism producing meningitis is likely to produce bacteremia at the same time. Infections with *H. influenzae* type b are usually bacteremic, whether the site is the meninges, epiglottis, or periorbital tissues. Meningitis caused by *S. pneumoniae* can be expected to be bacteremic, but only 20 to 30% of patients with pneumococcal pneumonia have positive blood cultures.

Frequently associated with severe infections such as meningitis

The most common sources of bacteremia are urinary tract infections, respiratory tract infections, and infections of skin or soft tissues, such as wound infections or cellulitis. The frequency with which any organism causes bacteremia is related to both its propensity to invade the bloodstream (see Table 68–4) and how often it produces infections. For example, cases of *Escherichia coli* bacteremia are common, attributable in part to the fact that *E. coli* is the most frequent cause of urinary tract infection.

Bacteremia is overflow from respiratory, urinary, wound, and other primary sites of infection

TABLE 68–4

Frequency of Detection of Bloodstream Invasion by Bacteria and Some Fungi during Significant Infections at Extravascular Sites

LARGE (>90%) PROPORTION OF CASES	
Haemophilus influenzae type b	*Brucella*[a]
Neisseria meningitidis	*Salmonella typhi*
Streptococcus pneumoniae (meningitis)	*Listeria*
VARIABLE (10–90%) DEPENDING ON STAGE AND SEVERITY OF INFECTION	
Beta-hemolytic streptococci	Enterobacteriaceae
S. pneumoniae	*Pseudomonas*
Staphylococcus aureus	*Bacteroides*
Neisseria gonorrhoeae	*Clostridium* (myositis and endometritis)
Leptospira[a]	Anaerobic cocci
Borrelia[a]	*Candida*
Acinetobacter	*Cryptococcus neoformans*[a]
Shigella dysenteriae	
SMALL (<10%) PROPORTION OF CASES	
Shigella (except *S. dysenteriae*)	*Pasteurella multocida*
Salmonella enteritidis	*Haemophilus*, nonencapsulated
Campylobacter jejuni[a]	
ISOLATION TOO RARE TO JUSTIFY ATTEMPT	
Vibrio (intestinal infections)	*Clostridium tetani*
Corynebacterium diphtheriae	*Clostridium botulinum*
Bordetella pertussis	*Clostridium difficile*
Mycobacterium[b]	*Legionella*[c]

[a] Isolation and/or demonstration requires special methods or prolonged incubation.

[b] *Mycobacterium avium-intracellulare* infections in AIDS patients often yield positive results.

[c] Infrequent isolation may be due to inadequate cultural methods.

SEPSIS AND SEPTIC SHOCK

Bacteremia is the presence of viable bacteria circulating in the blood. When signs and symptoms result, further terms are used to delineate the progression of potential consequences that may occur. Both Gram-negative and Gram-positive organisms can produce the same findings, as well as fungi, protozoa, and even some viruses.

Associated with bacteremic Gram-negative and Gram-positive infections

Sepsis is the suspicion (or proof) of infection and evidence of a systemic response to it (eg, tachycardia, tachypnea, hyperthermia, or hypothermia). The **sepsis syndrome** includes findings of sepsis plus evidence of altered organ perfusion. These can include reduction in urine output, mental status changes, systemic acidosis, and hypoxemia. If the process remains uncontrolled, there is subsequent progression to **septic shock** (development of hypotension); **refractory septic shock** (hypotension not responsive to standard fluid and pharmacologic treatment); and **multiorgan failure,** including major target organs such as the kidneys, lungs, and liver, and disseminated intravascular coagulation. Mortality is exceedingly high when patients develop refractory septic shock or multiorgan failure.

Sepsis syndrome progresses through shock to organ failure

The initial events in the sepsis syndrome appear to be vasodilatation with resultant decreased peripheral resistance and increased cardiac output. The patient is flushed and febrile. Capillary leakage and reduced blood volume follow, leading to a whole series of events identical to those seen in shock resulting from blood loss. These manifestations include vasoconstriction, reflex capillary dilatation, and local anoxic damage. Once this stage is reached, the patient may develop hypotension and hypothermia, and acidosis, hypoglycemia, and coagulation defects ensue with failure of highly perfused organs such as the lungs, kidneys, heart, brain, and liver.

Vasodilatation is followed by complex response

The mechanisms involved in development of septic shock have been studied extensively in experimental animals. Most of the features seen in humans can be produced with the lipopolysaccharide endotoxin of the Gram-negative cell wall, although there is some variation between animal species and with different preparations. The various events that occur are complex. They include (1) release of vasoactive substances such as histamine, serotonin, noradrenaline, and plasma kinins, which may cause arterial hypotension directly and facilitate coagulation abnormalities; (2) disturbances in temperature regulation, which may be due to direct central nervous system effects or, in the case of the early febrile response, mediated by interleukin 1 (IL-1) and tumor necrosis factor (TNF) released from macrophages; (3) complement activation and release of other inflammatory cytokines by macrophages (eg, IL-2, IL-6, IL-8, and interferon-gamma); (4) direct effects on vascular endothelial cell function and integrity; (5) depression of cardiac muscle contractility by TNF, myocardial depressant factor, and other less well-defined serum factors; and (6) impairment of the protein C anticoagulation pathway, resulting in disseminated intravascular coagulation. The resultant alterations in blood flow and capillary permeability lead to progressive organ dysfunction.

Endotoxin causes release of vasoactive substances

Cytokines, complement, and other mediators have physiologic effects

Early recognition of the problem is critical, and management obviously requires considerably more than antimicrobial therapy. Other primary therapeutic measures include maintenance of adequate tissue perfusion through careful fluid and electrolyte management and the use of vasoactive amines. There is also evidence that protein C replacement may ameliorate the coagulopathy.

Antimicrobic, fluid, and coagulation management are crucial

BLOOD CULTURE

The primary means for establishing a diagnosis of sepsis is by blood culture. The microbiologic principles involved are the same as with any culture. A sample of the patient's blood is obtained by aseptic venipuncture and cultured in an enriched broth or, after special processing, on plates. Growth is detected, and the organisms are isolated, identified, and tested for antimicrobial susceptibility. Because of the importance of blood cultures in the diagnosis and therapy of most bacterial and fungal infections, considerable attention must be paid to details of sampling if the prospects of obtaining a positive culture are to be maximized. The approach to blood culture must be tailored to the individual patient; no single procedure is best for all individuals. The important features are described below.

Importance of blood culture demands attention to details

Blood Culture Sampling

Venipuncture

Skin decontamination removes bulk of skin flora

Some anticoagulants have antimicrobial properties

Before venipuncture, the skin over the vein must be carefully disinfected to reduce the probability of contamination of the blood sample with skin bacteria. Although it is not possible to "sterilize" the skin, quantitative counts can be markedly reduced with a combination of 70% alcohol and an iodine-based antiseptic. Mechanical cleansing is as important as use of the antiseptic. Poor phlebotomy technique such as repalpating the vein after the preparation is related to introduction of contaminants. Blood is ideally drawn directly into a blood culture bottle or a sterile blood collection vacuum tube containing an anticoagulant free of antimicrobial properties. Sodium polyanethol sulfonate is currently preferred; other anticoagulants such as citrate and ethylenediaminetetraacetic acid have antibacterial activity. Blood should not be drawn through indwelling venous or arterial catheters unless it cannot be obtained by venipuncture.

Volume

Number of organisms in blood often <1 organism/mL

The number of organisms present in blood is often low (<1 organism/mL) and cannot be predicted in advance. Thus, small samples yield fewer positive cultures than larger ones. For example, as the volume sampled increases from 2 to 20 mL, the diagnostic yield increases by 30 to 50%. Samples of at least 10 mL should be collected from adult patients. The same principles apply with infants and young children, but the sample size must be reduced to take account of the smaller total blood volume of a child. Although it should be possible to obtain at least 1 mL, smaller volumes should still be cultured because bacteremia at levels of more than 1000 bacteria/mL is found in some infants.

Number

Two or three blood cultures usually adequate

If the volume is adequate, it is rarely necessary to collect more than two or three blood cultures to achieve a positive result. In intravascular infections (eg, infective endocarditis), a single blood culture is positive in more than 95% of cases. Studies of sequential blood cultures from bacteremic patients without endocarditis have yielded 80 to 90% positive results on the first culture, more than 90 to 95% with two cultures, and 99% in at least one of a series of three cultures.

Timing

Timing of intermittent bacteremia not predictable

Antimicrobic therapy may interfere with blood culture results

The best timing schedule for a series of two or three blood cultures is dependent on the bacteremic pattern of the underlying infection and the clinical urgency of initiating antimicrobial therapy. Figure 68–1 illustrates some typical bacteremic patterns that can be related to the probability of obtaining positive blood cultures. Transient bacteremia is usually not detected, because organisms are cleared before the appearance of any clinical findings suggesting sepsis. The continuous bacteremia of infective endocarditis is usually readily detected, and timing is not critical. Intermittent bacteremia presents the greatest challenge because fever spikes generally occur after, rather than during, the bacteremia. Little is known about the periodicity of bloodstream invasion, except that the bacteremia is more likely to be present and sustained in the early acute stages of infection. Closely spaced samples are less likely to detect the organism than those spaced an hour or more apart. In urgent situations, when antimicrobial therapy must be initiated, two or three samples should be collected at brief intervals and therapy begun as soon as possible. It is generally not useful to collect blood cultures while the patient is receiving antimicrobics unless none were collected before therapy or there is a change in the clinical course suggesting superinfection. The laboratory should be advised when such cultures are submitted, because it is sometimes possible to inactivate an antimicrobic, for example, with beta-lactamases.

Laboratory Processing

The basic blood culture procedure of incubating blood in an enriched broth is quite simple, but considerable effort must be expended to ensure detection of the broadest range of organisms in the least possible time. Daily examination of cultures for 1 week or more and a routine schedule of stains and/or subcultures of apparently negative cultures are required to detect organisms such as *H. influenzae* or *N. meningitidis,* which usually do not produce visual changes in the broth. Direct plating of blood onto blood or chocolate agar is accomplished in a system that concentrates the blood by centrifugation following lysis of the erythrocytes. This is particularly useful for bacterial quantification and rapid identification. Automated blood culture systems detect metabolic activity (primarily CO_2 generation) in broth culture for initial detection in place of the conventional visual and staining examinations. These systems detect growth sooner than conventional methods but still require subculture for confirmation, identification, and susceptibility testing.

Blood added to enriched broth

Automated and direct plating procedures now available

Isolation of fungi is favored by ensuring maximum aerobic conditions in direct plating systems and broth bottles. Conversely, anaerobes are recovered best when a highly reduced environment is provided for plates and broths. Some bacteria, such as *Leptospira,* are not isolated by routine blood culture procedures. The laboratory must be notified in advance so special media can be used.

Special cultural conditions required for yeasts and anaerobes

Because the blood is normally sterile, the interpretation of blood cultures growing a pathogenic organism is seldom a problem. The major problem is the differentiation of agents causing transient bacteremia and skin contamination from those opportunists associated with an intravascular or extravascular infection. Transient bacteremia is of short duration (see Fig 68–1), is associated with manipulation of or trauma to a site possessing a normal flora, and involves species indigenous to that site. Despite skin disinfection, 2 to 4% of venipunctures result in contamination of the culture with small numbers of cutaneous flora such as *S. epidermidis,* corynebacteria (diphtheroids), and propionibacteria. The presence of these organisms in blood cultures can be considered a result of skin contamination unless quantitative procedures indicate large numbers (>5 organisms/mL) or repeated cultures are positive for the same organism. These findings should suggest diseases such as infective endocarditis or catheter bacteremia.

Interpretation involves distinguishing infection from normal skin flora contamination

CHAPTER 69

Infections of the Fetus and Newborn

C. George Ray

The usual 10-month period from conception through birth and the first 4 weeks of extrauterine life is one of unusual susceptibility to infection but also a time at which special defenses acquired from the mother are operating.

1. During normal development, the fetus is in a protected intrauterine environment, with fetal membranes serving as a physical barrier to external infection and the placenta contributing, with maternal immunity, to protection against many blood-borne infections. Transplacental transmission of specific immunoglobulins, particularly of the IgG class (IgM does not normally cross the placental barrier), continues to provide some immunologic protection to the infant for weeks to months after birth, while cytokines from the mother can provide transient cell-mediated immune support. If the infant is breast-fed, specific immunoglobulins (predominantly of the IgA class) in maternal colostrum afford some protection against pathogens that involve or invade through the infant's gastrointestinal tract.

Fetus protected in intrauterine environment

Passive immunity is acquired from mother

2. On the other hand, the fetal immune system is immature, and there is relative suppression of maternal cell-mediated immunity as pregnancy progresses. These immune deficiencies serve an important biological purpose; they protect fetus and mother from activation of specific immunologic recognition and response mechanisms to differences in their histocompatibility locus antigens. If these processes did not occur normally, the fetus could be immunologically rejected by the mother or the fetal immune mechanisms activated to respond against maternal antigens in a form of "graft versus host" disease.

Fetal immune system immature and maternal cell-mediated immunity suppressed

3. Specific and nonspecific immune responses begin to develop in early fetal life, perhaps as early as 8 weeks' gestation; however, a nearly normal immunocompetent state is usually not achieved until the infant is more than 2 years of age. Deficiencies commonly seen in the early period include poor antibody response to polysaccharide antigens, decreased phagocytic capability and variability in intracellular killing of certain infectious agents, lower levels of complement components, and decreased opsonic capacity.

Specific deficiencies of neonate include poor T cell–independent responses

4. Cell growth and organ differentiation are at their highest rates in the fetal–neonatal period, making the host especially susceptible to permanent damage when an infectious process intervenes.

Infection may have teratogenic effects

The actual risk of infection and the types of pathogens encountered are influenced by a variety of interacting factors, including the state of maternal health and susceptibility to specific agents, adequacy of fetal and neonatal nutrition, integrity of fetal membranes, and degree of maturity at birth. This chapter outlines the major types of infection of concern to

Risk of infection influenced by fetal and maternal factors

those caring for the fetus and neonate and the general approaches to their diagnosis. Specific biological characteristics and aspects of prevention and treatment for each of the agents have been addressed in previous chapters.

DEFINITIONS

Infection can occur prenatally, natally, or postnatally

A number of terms are commonly used to describe the infections that can affect the fetus and newborn. **Prenatal** infections include those acquired by the mother and/or fetus at any time before birth. When fetal infection develops, it is usually blood-borne to the placenta with subsequent spread to the fetus (transplacental) or follows the ascending route from the vagina through torn or ruptured fetal membranes. **Natal,** or peripartum, infections are those acquired during delivery. They are often caused by agents in the maternal genital tract but occasionally result from organisms introduced from exogenous sources through attendants, fetal monitors, or other instruments. **Postnatal** infections, which constitute the remainder of the group, include all infections acquired after delivery throughout the newborn (or neonatal) period, defined as the first 4 weeks of life.

Congenital infections acquired prenatally or during delivery

Another commonly used term is **congenital** infection, which describes infection occurring at any time before or at birth (prenatal or natal). Consequently, the infection is usually still active in the newborn period and sometimes persists for months or years. **Perinatal** infection is often used to include a period extending from 20 to 28 weeks' gestation to 7 to 28 days after birth. The term will not be used in this chapter.

Prolonged rupture of membranes enhances risk of chorioamnionitis

Chorioamnionitis is an inflammatory response to infectious agents involving the chorionic and amniotic fetal membranes. It usually results from entry of pathogens from the vagina through tears or ruptures in the membranes, and it places the fetus at risk of direct exposure just before or at delivery. The risk of chorioamnionitis increases rapidly when membranes have been ruptured for longer than 12 hours before birth. When infection is by the blood-borne maternal route, there may be evidence of infection of the placenta, termed **placentitis. Endometritis** may be observed occasionally if the infection is an extension from a maternal pelvic focus along venous or lymphatic pathways. **Sepsis** is a term used to indicate a severe systemic bacterial infection associated with bacteremia.

COMMON ETIOLOGIC AGENTS

Rarity of some childhood infections in infancy related to exposure and passive immunity

S. aureus infections are typically postnatal

Table 69–1 lists the major pathogens affecting the fetus and newborn, according to the usual modes of acquisition. Some, such as *Mycobacterium tuberculosis* and *Plasmodium* species, are exceedingly rare, but require consideration in certain clinical and epidemiologic circumstances. It should also be noted that some pathogens that commonly affect older infants and children are quite rarely observed in newborns. This phenomenon is partially attributable to the protective effect of maternally derived immunity to organisms such as *Haemophilus influenzae* type b, *Streptococcus pneumoniae, Neisseria meningitidis,* and mumps and measles viruses but also reflects less opportunity for exposure to some agents early in life. Some organisms, such as *Staphylococcus aureus,* rarely cause prenatal or natal infections but commonly colonize in the postnatal period and most often cause disease after the first week of life.

First exposure is to pathogens in maternal genital flora

If one views the fetus as existing normally in a protected, "germ-free" intrauterine environment before emerging into a milieu of potential pathogens, it is easy to see how the newborn can be colonized with the first organisms encountered, some of which can cause disease. The external pathogenic flora initially acquired can include organisms frequently present in the maternal genital tract, such as group B streptococci and *Escherichia coli,* as well as less common *Neisseria gonorrhoeae, Listeria monocytogenes, Chlamydia trachomatis,* and herpes simplex virus, all of which are important causes of natal infection.

Human and environmental factors determine common neonatal infections

Postnatal infections may be late manifestations resulting from prenatal or natal colonization by pathogens such as those mentioned previously, but additional organisms may be acquired after birth. Particular risks include contamination of the nursery environment by a variety of Gram-negative bacteria, staphylococci, and some common viruses (see Table 69–1) and attendants who are infected with or carrying such organisms. The risks are increased if the infant is born prematurely or otherwise physically compromised, and

TABLE 69–1

Modes of Infection and Major Agents

Mode	Agents: Bacteria	Viruses	Other
Prenatal transplacental	*Listeria monocytogenes, Mycobacterium tuberculosis* (rare), *Treponema pallidum*	Rubella, cytomegalovirus, enteroviruses, Epstein–Barr virus, human immunodeficiency virus, parvovirus B19, lymphocytic choriomeningitis virus	*Toxoplasma gondii, Plasmodium* spp.
Ascending	Group B streptococci, *Escherichia coli, L. monocytogenes*	Cytomegalovirus, herpes simplex	*Chlamydia trachomatis, Mycoplasma hominis, Ureaplasma urealyticum*
Natal	Group B streptococci; *E. coli, L. monocytogenes, Neisseria gonorrhoeae*	Herpes simplex, cytomegalovirus, enteroviruses, hepatitis B, varicella–zoster, human immunodeficiency virus	*C. trachomatis*
Postnatal	E. coli, group B streptococci, *L. monocytogenes,* miscellaneous Gram-negative bacteria, *Staphylococcus aureus, Staphylococcus epidermidis, Clostridium tetani*	Cytomegalovirus, herpes simplex, enteroviruses, varicella–zoster, respiratory syncytial virus, influenza viruses, human immunodeficiency virus	

they are amplified by prolonged hospitalization and invasive procedures such as respiratory intubation, mechanical ventilation, and intravenous treatment, as well as by blood or blood product transfusions.

Prematurity, prolonged hospitalization, and invasive procedures increase risk

EFFECT OF PRENATAL INFECTION ON PREGNANCY AND INTRAUTERINE DEVELOPMENT

All of the agents indicated in Table 69–1 as causing prenatal infections have the potential of creating an adverse pregnancy outcome, either as a result of compromising the health of the mother or by directly affecting the fetus. The effect can be untimely termination of pregnancy resulting in abortion, stillbirth, or prematurity, as well as developmental defects and fetal malnutrition.

CLINICAL FEATURES, DIAGNOSIS, AND MANAGEMENT

Acute Bacterial Sepsis

When a physician first encounters a sick newborn, the primary concern is whether the illness represents sepsis and/or meningitis caused by bacteria. This determination is important, because treatment is both feasible and extremely urgent. Clinical disease apparent at birth or developing within the first 3 days of life (early onset) has usually been acquired prenatally. Mortality can exceed 70%, even with prompt treatment. Later onset of symptoms is commonly associated with natal or postnatal acquisition of pathogens; however, these infections can also be severe. If meningitis develops, the overall mortality, even with treatment, ranges from 10 to 25%, and permanent neurologic damage may occur in 30 to 50% of survivors. The two pathogens most commonly associated with neonatal sepsis and meningitis are group B streptococci and *E. coli.*

Early-onset neonatal infections may have 70% mortality

Group B streptococcal and *E. coli* sepsis and meningitis are most common

The diagnosis of neonatal infections is based first on clinical suspicion. There is sometimes a history of recent maternal febrile illness immediately before or at birth. Other suggestive features include fetal distress, prolonged rupture of membranes (>12 hours), foul-smelling amniotic fluid, and premature delivery. The first signs and symptoms of illness in the infant may be subtle and extremely variable, including respiratory distress, apneic episodes, cyanosis, irritability, unexplained jaundice, tachycardia, poor feeding, abdominal distention, and fever. Initial laboratory findings often include either leukocytosis, with an increased proportion of immature neutrophils, or leukopenia. The development of seizures, hypotension, or disseminated intravascular coagulation indicates a particularly grave prognosis.

Prematurity and prolonged rupture of membranes are risk factors

Clinical clues subtle in newborn

Diagnostic tests for suspected infections must be initiated as quickly as possible, followed by empirical antimicrobial therapy while waiting for culture results. The major tests include examination and culture of cerebrospinal fluid and blood culture. The antimicrobics initially chosen are those known to be effective against the pathogens most commonly encountered. They often include ampicillin for the streptococci (also useful for *L. monocytogenes*) and an aminoglycoside such as gentamicin for *E. coli.*

Blood and cerebrospinal fluid culture performed initially

Other Bacterial and Chlamydial Infections

Although *N. gonorrhoeae* and *C. trachomatis* are common natally acquired infections, they are usually not associated with sepsis. Both can produce a severe conjunctivitis in the newborn that requires prompt diagnosis and treatment. Gonococcal ophthalmia is usually apparent in the first 5 days after birth, whereas the onset of chlamydial conjunctivitis is frequently delayed until after the first week of life. Another significant illness associated with natally acquired *C. trachomatis* infection is infant pneumonia syndrome. The onset of respiratory symptoms is often delayed, with most cases occurring between 2 weeks and 6 months of age. This illness is also considered in Chapter 30.

C. trachomatis and gonococci produce severe conjunctivitis

Chlamydia infant pneumonia syndrome occurs in infants up to 6 months of age

Localized infections, such as cutaneous or subcutaneous abscesses, show a particular association with postnatally acquired *S. aureus* and occasionally with various Gram-negative bacteria. If the newborn is affected by a staphylococcal strain that produces exfoliative toxin, the local lesion may be relatively trivial in contrast to the more widespread effect of circulating toxin on the skin, which is termed **staphylococcal scalded skin syndrome.** Prompt treatment with an antistaphylococcal antimicrobial agent results in resolution of the disease within 2 weeks, usually with complete healing.

Postnatal infections by *S. aureus* may cause scalded skin syndrome

Syphilis

If prenatal infection by *Treponema pallidum* (congenital syphilis) is left untreated, the result can be long-term damage, often without apparent signs or symptoms in the newborn period. To minimize these risks, serologic screening is recommended for all pregnant women when first seen in early gestation and at delivery. In addition, serologic testing is recommended whenever clinical or epidemiologic circumstances suggest the possibility of exposure at any time during pregnancy. Prompt treatment of infected mothers during pregnancy, preferably with penicillin, markedly reduces the risk of fetal infection. Similar treatment is also effective for the infected infant.

Risk of congenital syphilis reduced by serologic screening and treatment during pregnancy

TORCH COMPLEX

When bacterial, spirochetal, and chlamydial infections have been reasonably excluded from consideration, other possibilities can best be remembered by the convenient acronym **TORCH** (**t**oxoplasmosis, **o**ther [viruses], **r**ubella, **c**ytomegalovirus, **h**erpes simplex). This term comprises major infections that can be particularly severe if acquired prenatally. There is often significant overlap of clinical manifestations associated with the various agents in the TORCH complex. Common features may include low birth weight, rash, jaundice, and hepatosplenomegaly. On the other hand, many newborn infants with TORCH infections can go undiagnosed, because the clinical signs may not appear until weeks, months, or even years later. For example, congenital cytomegalovirus infection may be manifested only as mild mental retardation and/or hearing loss that may not

Toxoplasma, rubella, cytomegalovirus, and herpes simplex are all common congenital pathogens

become apparent until after the first year of life. Toxoplasmosis also presents a dilemma. It is estimated that as many as 1 in 200 pregnancies in the United States is complicated by primary infection with *Toxoplasma gondii,* which is usually subclinical. Of these cases, approximately 30 to 40% result in fetal infection, but only 8 to 11% of the infected offspring demonstrate clinical symptoms in the newborn period. The remainder are at risk, however, and can ultimately develop neurologic deterioration and/or chorioretinitis, which may not be recognized until 5 or more years later. These observations only partially illustrate the importance of TORCH complex infections and our relative impotence in controlling many of them.

Clinical manifestations may be delayed for years

Of the array of miscellaneous agents grouped in the "other" category, three viruses deserve specific mention. If the mother has active infection with hepatitis B virus during pregnancy, the risk of natal or postnatal transmission to the infant is high (range, 20 to 80%, depending on the status of virus activity). Although it is unlikely that clinical disease will be apparent in the newborn period, it is important to promptly undertake specific measures to prevent infection in the infant when the mother is infected. They include administration of hepatitis B immune globulin immediately after birth as well as immunization of the infant with hepatitis B vaccine. The chance of maternal transmission of the human immunodeficiency virus (HIV), either transplacentally or natally, is estimated to be between 13 and 40%. Prenatal antiretroviral treatment of infected mothers can reduce this risk by 60 to 70%. Primary varicella is infrequent in pregnancy. If the mother develops varicella less than 5 days before or 2 days after delivery, however, the risk of severe neonatal varicella is significant, with a mortality of approximately 20%. It is recommended that the infant be given varicella–zoster immune globulin (or zoster immune globulin) immediately in an attempt to prevent or modify subsequent disease. Maternal zoster infections are not associated with a significant risk to the offspring, presumably because of adequate transplacental transmission of specific antibody.

Hepatitis B infection prevented by immune globulin and vaccine administration

HIV transmission reduced by prenatal antiviral treatment

Neonatal varicella from infected mother is severe if contracted perinatally

The approach to a suspected TORCH complex infection requires some thought in selection of appropriate tests. Table 69–2 summarizes the major clinical and historic features of specific agents and the diagnostic procedures that can be used. The following general comments should also be kept in mind:

1. Clinical and epidemiologic data are used as much as possible in ascertaining likely specific agents.
2. Probabilities must be weighed; for example, congenital cytomegalovirus infection is by far the most frequent TORCH complex agent encountered in the United States (>90% of all proved cases).
3. Potentially treatable infections must be considered first. If toxoplasmosis or herpes simplex is suggested by the historic and clinical findings, it may be controlled by prompt and aggressive therapy. Early identification and treatment of HIV-1 infections can significantly improve long-term prognosis in infants. Other infections, which are potentially preventable by early specific immunoglobulin therapy of the infant, include maternal varicella and hepatitis B infections. The remaining agents involved in the TORCH array are not amenable to specific therapy at present. Their importance lies more in long-term prognosis, planning of continuing care, and epidemiologic management.
4. Serologic testing, when indicated, should be performed on both infant and maternal sera collected at the same time to facilitate interpretation of specific antibody titer levels in the infant. This approach is based on the following principles: passive transplacental transmission of IgG antibodies occurs, but these maternal antibodies normally wane and disappear in the infant over 3 to 6 months. If the infant is actively infected, it usually produces its own specific antibodies to the agent, which then persist for much longer periods. Thus, a specific antibody titer in the infant's serum during the first month of life equal to or less than that of the mother may merely reflect passive transfer and does not support a diagnosis of active infection. On the other hand, if the infant's titer is significantly higher than the mother's (fourfold or greater) or rises progressively in serial samples obtained in later months, active infection by the agent in question is suggested.

Cytomegalovirus is most common congenital infection

Focus on treatable conditions

Comparison of infant and maternal antibody titers aids diagnosis

TABLE 69–2

TORCH Complex: Salient Features and Diagnostic Tests

Toxoplasmosis

Suggestive clinical findings: chorioretinitis (found in more than 90% of symptomatic neonatal cases); lymphadenopathy

Maternal history: usually negative; occasional cervical lymphadenopathy during pregnancy

Tests of choice: culture, PCR, specific maternal and infant antibody titers; follow-up titers may be helpful

Other Infections

The list of causes includes enteroviruses, hepatitis B, human immunodeficiency virus, varicella–zoster, Epstein–Barr virus, parvovirus B19, lymphocytic choriomeningitis virus, malaria, and tuberculosis. As the agents in this category most commonly encountered are the enteroviruses, the features summarized here pertain primarily to them.

Suggestive clinical findings: sepsis-like syndromes; meningitis; myocarditis (findings are variable)

Maternal history: fever common at or near parturition

Tests of choice: viral cultures of throat, rectum, and cerebrospinal fluid; rapid PCR analysis of cerebrospinal fluid and other body fluids

Rubella

Suggestive clinical findings: congenital malformations, often multiple. In severe cases, "celery stalking" of metaphyses of long bones may be seen in early radiographs (see also cytomegalovirus).

Maternal history: rubella-like illness or epidemiologic history of exposure in early pregnancy is common. If available, maternal serologic and immunization history can aid in supporting or refuting this diagnostic possibility.

Tests of choice: maternal and infant antibody titers, including IgM-specific antibody testing in the infant; serial determinations over 6 months may be of additional help

Cytomegalovirus

Suggestive clinical findings: none very specific in differentiating infection from most others in the group. Statistically, cytomegalovirus is the most common congenital infection encountered. In florid cases, early radiographs of the long bones may resemble those of congenital rubella (celery stalking).

Maternal history: usually none; occasionally, an account of a mononucleosis-like syndrome may be elicited

Tests of choice: urine culture (most sensitive test). If results are negative, this diagnosis is highly unlikely; if positive, the diagnosis is supported (especially if cultures are done in the first 3 weeks of life). With advancing age of the infant, however, positive cultures may require careful interpretation before an unequivocal diagnosis is made.

Herpes Simplex

Suggestive clinical findings: cutaneous vesicles and/or ocular or mucous membrane ulcerations; however, these lesions may not become apparent until other signs of illness have developed

Maternal history: up to 70% have no history of genital lesions or symptoms. Others may have a history of recent primary symptomatic infection. It is also important to ascertain whether genital lesions were known to exist in recent sexual partners.

Tests of choice: culture of lesions; immunofluorescent and cytologic studies may be available for rapid diagnosis. Throat, urine and cerebrospinal fluid culture, and rapid PCR testing of cerebrospinal fluid and blood are also helpful. Maternal cultures, if positive, may give indirect support regarding etiology.

Abbreviation: PCR, polymerase chain reaction.

Infant IgM-specific antibodies suggest active infection

In active congenital and neonatal infections, the infant's early responses often include IgM antibodies. Maternal IgM antibodies rarely cross the placental barrier, so specific IgM antibody determinations early in life may be useful for the diagnosis of congenital toxoplasma, rubella, and cytomegalovirus infections. However, both false-positive and false-negative results have been noted. The presence of rheumatoid factor has been a major cause of false-positive results. Tests with high specificity include solid-phase IgM assays with antihuman IgM as a "capture" antibody and enzyme-linked antibody markers.

Nonspecific tests, such as quantitation of total IgM or IgA or detection of rheumatoid factor, have limited or no usefulness. Negative results do not rule out infection, and positive results must be regarded cautiously.

5. In fetal and neonatal infections, such as those caused by HIV, specific antibody testing is not usually helpful in establishing a diagnosis in the first 15 to 18 months of life. Tests for p24 antigenemia, blood culture, or polymerase chain reaction methods for viral nucleic acid detection are preferred and may need to be serially repeated if initially negative.

Culture, PCR, and antigen detection are preferred for HIV diagnosis

CONCLUSION

Fetal and neonatal infections remain a highly significant and often frustrating challenge. They can be severe, and permanent sequelae are common. At the onset of infection, clinical signs and symptoms are often exceedingly subtle; thus, the physician must be quickly alerted to the infectious possibilities, particularly when specific treatment is available. Of all of these infections, the most preventable is rubella, and assurance of immunity before conception is a mandatory goal. Better control of the remainder may become possible in the future with newer bacterial and viral vaccines, better early diagnostic methods, and improved treatments.

CHAPTER 70

Sexually Transmitted Diseases

W. LAWRENCE DREW

With the emergence of acquired immunodeficiency syndrome (AIDS) in the 1980s, sexually transmitted diseases (STDs) received increased attention, although they have long been a major public health problem in all population groups and social strata. The most common agents are *Chlamydia trachomatis,* papillomavirus, herpes simplex virus, *Neisseria gonorrhoeae,* and the most worrisome, human immunodeficiency virus (HIV). Additional agents spread by sexual contact include hepatitis B, cytomegalovirus, syphilis, chancroid, and lymphogranuloma venereum. Table 70–1 lists the major sexually transmitted pathogens and the disease syndromes associated with them. These infections are discussed in detail in chapters related to the etiologic agents.

Depending on the pathogen, the disease produced may be local or systemic. For the localized STDs, due to chlamydia for example, the most common manifestations are inflammation (eg, urethritis, cervicitis), which may or may not be noticed by the patient. In some cases, deeper structures become involved when the infection spreads beyond the local site by direct extension (eg, epididymitis, salpingitis). As with other infectious diseases, some of these can gain access to the bloodstream and produce systemic symptoms and spread to other organs. The systemic STDs produce infection beyond the genital site as part of their basic pathogenesis (eg, HIV, hepatitis B, and syphilis); syphilis does and HIV and hepatitis B do not produce a local genital lesion. The most common clinical syndromes are discussed next.

Some STDs begin as localized infections; others are primarily systemic

GENITAL ULCERS

Single or multiple ulcerative lesions on the genitalia are one of the most common manifestations of STDs. Infection may begin as a papule or pustule and evolve into an ulcer. Table 70–2 lists the major features of genital ulcerations. The nature of the ulcer and whether it is painful are significant differential features. The ulcer (chancre) of syphilis is typically single, firm and indurated but painless, whereas genital herpes ulcers are often multiple and quite painful. The evaluation of genital ulcers usually focuses on the separation of genital herpes, the most common cause in industrialized nations, and syphilis from other causes. In the laboratory workup, it should be emphasized that direct microscopy and serologic tests may be negative at the time of presentation of the syphilitic chancre and that cultures for herpes simplex virus are usually positive from vesicular, pustular, or ulcerative lesions but may be negative from crusted areas. Chancroid caused by *Haemophilus ducreyi,* relatively rare in the developed world, may be suggested by direct microscopy but requires a special selective medium for culture. Granuloma inguinale, a disease also seen primarily in developing countries, is characterized by chronic, persistent genital papules or ulcers. It is

Pain and induration are major differential features

C. granulomatis shows encapsulated Gram-negative bacilli on smear

TABLE 70–1

Sexually Transmitted Agents and Diseases Caused

Agent	Disease or Syndrome
Bacteria	
Neisseria gonorrhoeae	Urethritis, cervicitis, proctitis, pharyngitis, conjunctivitis, endometritis, pelvic inflammatory disease, perihepatitis, bartholinitis, disseminated gonococcal infection
Chlamydia trachomatis	Nongonococcal urethritis, epididymitis, cervicitis, salpingitis, inclusion conjunctivitis, infant pneumonia, trachoma, lymphogranuloma venereum
Ureaplasma urealyticum	Nongonococcal urethritis
Treponema pallidum	Syphilis
Haemophilus ducreyi	Chancroid
Calymmatobacterium granulomatis	Granuloma inguinale
Viruses	
HIV	AIDS, AIDS-related complex (ARC), perinatal and congenital AIDS, aseptic meningitis, subacute neurologic syndromes, persistent generalized adenopathy, asymptomatic infection
Herpes simplex virus	Primary and recurrent genital herpes, aseptic meningitis, neonatal herpes
Papillomavirus	Condylomata accuminata, laryngeal papilloma of newborn, association with cervical carcinoma
Cytomegalovirus	Heterophil-negative infectious mononucleosis, congenital birth defects
Hepatitis B virus	Hepatitis B, acute and chronic infections
Molluscum contagiosum virus	Genital molluscum contagiosum
Protozoa	
Trichomonas vaginalis	Trichomonal vaginitis
Fungi	
Candida albicans	Vulvovaginitis, penile candidiasis
Ectoparasites	
Phthirus pubis	Pubic louse infestation
Sarcoptes scabiei	Scabies

Abbreviations: AIDS, acquired immunodeficiency syndrome; HIV, human immunodeficiency virus.

caused by *Calymmatobacterium granulomatis,* an encapsulated Gram-negative bacillus, which has not been grown in artificial medium. The diagnosis is usually made by examination of Wright- or Giemsa-stained impression smears from biopsy specimens that demonstrate clusters of encapsulated coccobacilli in the cytoplasm of mononuclear cells.

GENITAL WARTS

Many genotypes of papillomaviruses

Some types associated with carcinoma of the cervix

Genital warts may be caused by human papillomavirus (condyloma acuminatum) or *Treponema pallidum* (condyloma latum). There are over 70 genotypes of human papillomavirus (HPV), of which types 6, 11, 16, 18, and 32 are the predominant causes of genital warts. In women, HPV types 16, 18, and 31 are usually associated with flat or subclinical warts and are the viral types that may be associated with cervical dysplasias, carcinoma in situ, and invasive cervical cancer. Condylomata lata are painless mucosal warty erosions that develop in warm, moist sites such as the genitals and perineum in about one third of cases of secondary syphilis. Darkfield examinations are invariably positive as are both nontreponemal and treponemal serologic tests.

URETHRITIS

Urethritis usually manifests as dysuria, urethral discharge, or both. The discharge may be prominent enough to be the chief complaint or may have to be milked from the urethra.

TABLE 70–2

Causes of Genital Ulcerations

Disease	Type of Lesion	Type of Inguinal Adenopathy[a]	Diagnosis
Genital herpes	Multiple grouped vesicles to coalesced ulcers, painful	Tender, discrete, nonsuppurative	Culture, enzyme immunoassay
Chancroid	Tender, shallow, painful ulcer, not indurated ulcer	Suppurative	Culture
Syphilis	Nontender, indurated ulcer	Rubbery consistency	Darkfield exam, serology
Lymphogranuloma venereum	Painless, small ulcer or papule, usually healed at time of presentation	Discrete progressing to suppurative, draining fistulas	Culture, serology
Granuloma inguinale	Papular to nodular to ulcerative lesion(s), painless	"Pseudobubo" caused by induration of subcutaneous tissue in inguinal area	Giemsa stain of biopsy

[a]Involvement of inguinal lymph nodes.

The major causes of urethritis are *N. gonorrhoeae* and *C. trachomatis,* followed by *Ureaplasma urealyticum* and herpes simplex virus. Infection with more than one organism is common, particularly dual gonococcal and chlamydial infection. Up to 20% of cases have no established etiology but are probably infectious.

C. trachomatis and *N. gonorrhoeae* often coinfect

The diagnosis of gonorrhea is established primarily by culture, although direct examinations (Gram stain, DNA assays) may suffice in symptomatic patients. DNA-based assays are comparable to culture for screening. Newly developed nonculture techniques (eg, DNA amplification) are superior to culture for *C. trachomatis*, while culture is the most appropriate test for herpes simplex virus. Treatment depends on the etiologic agent and whether the disease has progressed beyond the local site. Empiric regimens are directed at the two most common causes, *N. gonorrhoeae* and *C. trachomatis.* In cases of gonorrhea, concurrent treatment for chlamydia is recommended, unless the latter has been specifically excluded. In general, the same approach is followed for epididymitis and cervicitis.

Culture and DNA-based assays available

Combined treatment often recommended

EPIDIDYMITIS

Unilateral swelling of the epididymis is a common clinical illness seen in sexually active men. It is usually quite painful, with fever and acute unilateral swelling of the testicle that is sometimes confused with testicular torsion. In the preantibiotic era, approximately 10 to 15% of untreated gonococcal infections resulted in epididymitis. In developed countries, the two most common causes of epididymitis are *N. gonorrhoeae* and *C. trachomatis,* especially in younger men. In men older than 35 and in homosexual men, Enterobacteriaceae and coagulase-negative staphylococci may also cause the disease, probably from reflux of infected urine into the epididymis. Treatment depends on demonstration of the etiologic agent in urethral specimens or epididymal aspirates (see treatment of urethritis for additional considerations).

Gonoccoccal and chlamydial infections more common in men 35 years and younger

Enterobacteriaceae and *S. epidermidis* more common in older men

CERVICITIS

Gonococcal, chlamydial, and herpes simplex virus infections most common

The microbial etiology of cervical infections is varied; *N. gonorrhoeae* and *C. trachomatis* cause endocervicitis, and herpes simplex virus can infect the stratified squamous epithelium of the ectocervix. The major clinical manifestation of cervicitis is a mucopurulent vaginal discharge. The cervix is friable and inflamed, and polymorphonuclear leukocytes are present in the exudate. Chlamydial, gonococcal, and viral cultures are needed to demonstrate the etiologic agent. Therapy depends on the etiologic agent involved (see treatment of urethritis for additional considerations).

VAGINITIS AND VAGINAL DISCHARGE

Pelvic examination helps define important infection sites

Symptomatic vaginal discharge may occur alone or accompany salpingitis, endometritis, and cervicitis. Evaluation includes pelvic examination, cervical cultures for *N. gonorrhoeae* and *C. trachomatis,* and microscopic examination of the discharge. Measurement of the pH of the discharge may also be helpful. Pelvic examination is valuable in determining whether uterine, adnexal, or cervical tenderness is present and whether the source of the discharge is the cervix or the vagina.

Candida vaginitis causes itching, thick discharge

Trichomonas infection produces foamy discharge

The clinical and laboratory findings vary with the etiologic agent. *Candida albicans* generally produces a vulvovaginitis associated with pruritus and erythema of the vulvar area and a discharge with the consistency of cottage cheese. Microscopic demonstration of yeast and pseudomycelia in a potassium hydroxide or Gram stain preparation of the exudate confirms the diagnosis. *Trichomonas vaginalis* typically produces a foamy, purulent vaginal discharge. The pH is variable (usually >5.0), and numerous polymorphonuclear cells and motile trichomonads are seen on wet mount examination.

Bacterial vaginosis a shift in flora with anaerobic overgrowth

KOH added to discharge produces a fishy smell (amines)

Clue cells are present, and lactobacilli are absent

Bacterial vaginosis (BV), previously termed "nonspecific vaginitis," is the most common form of vaginitis in women. BV is associated with overgrowth of multiple members of the vaginal anaerobic flora, genital mycoplasmas, and a small Gram-negative rod (*Gardnerella vaginalis*), once believed to be the sole cause of the disease. The vaginal discharge of BV is yellowish, homogenous, and adherent to the vaginal wall. The pH is greater than 5.0. Addition of KOH to the vaginal secretions produces a fishy smell as a result of volatilization of amines. The Gram stain shows a shift from the usual lactobacillary flora to one of many Gram-negative coccobacilli. Clue cells, which are vaginal epithelial cells heavily coated with *G. vaginalis,* may also be seen. Therapy depends on the etiologic agent.

PELVIC INFLAMMATORY DISEASE

Multiple etiologic agents; gonococcus predominant

Incidence higher with use of intrauterine devices

Clinical manifestations of pelvic inflammatory disease (PID) vary but generally include lower abdominal pain elicited by movement of the cervix or palpation of the adnexal or endometrial areas. About 50% of cases are caused by *N. gonorrhoeae.* Nongonococcal PID has a complex and sometimes polymicrobial etiology, including *C. trachomatis, Bacteroides,* anaerobic streptococci, and *Mycoplasma hominis* alone or in various combinations. In general, nongonococcal PID is milder than that associated with *N. gonorrhoeae* infection. The incidence of PID is five to ten times higher in women with intrauterine devices than in those not using this form of contraception. The diagnosis is established most reliably by culture of peritoneal aspirates from the vaginal cul-de-sac. Treatment of PID is complex because of the multiple etiologies and relative inaccessibility of the definitive diagnostic specimen.

LYMPHADENITIS

Generalized adenopathy in secondary syphilis

Inguinal lymphadenitis may be seen with several STDs, especially primary herpes simplex infection and lymphogranuloma venereum. The latter is caused by specific strains of *C. trachomatis.* It may begin as a small genital ulcer, which is frequently unnoticed. More often, the first evidence of lymphogranuloma venereum is a tender swollen inguinal lymphadenitis, which may suppurate and drain spontaneously if not treated. Primary syphilis may be associated with unilateral or bilateral inguinal lymph node enlargement, but these nodes are not usually tender. Secondary syphilis may be associated with generalized lymphadenopathy.

SYSTEMIC SYNDROMES

As indicated earlier, some STDs may manifest important pathology outside the genital tract, including diseases such as syphilis, hepatitis B, and AIDS whose most devastating consequences are at nongenital sites. These diseases can be highly complex, involving multiple organs and life-long illness. These organisms and diseases are best reviewed by referring back to the specific chapters that deal with each agent.

Most serious effects of syphilis, hepatitis B, and AIDS are outside of the genital tract

ADDITIONAL READING

Centers For Disease Control and Prevention. Sexually transmitted diseases treatment guidelines—2002. *MMWR Morb Mortal Wkly Rep* 2002;51(RR06):1–80. This is a thorough guide to the recognition and current treatment recommendations for all STDs.

CHAPTER 71

Infections in the Immunocompromised Patient

W. LAWRENCE DREW

Immunocompromised patients are those whose host defense mechanisms are impaired by an inherited deficit, disease, or treatment. The immunocompromised state increases the risk of infection with many of the common pathogens as well as with low-virulence organisms present in the normal flora or environment. The organisms involved are those most able to take advantage of situations such as disruption of the skin or mucosal barriers and the more specific immune defects, including (1) defects in the phagocytic response, (2) defects in the complement system, (3) defects in antibody-mediated immunity, (4) defects in cell-mediated immunity, and (5) loss of reticuloendothelial function. Each of these defects tends to be associated with infections caused by specific groups of organisms (Table 71–1). For example, neutropenia and disorders of phagocytosis are associated with infections by Gram-positive cocci, Enterobacteriaceae, *Pseudomonas,* and fungi. In contrast, patients with defects in cell-mediated immunity tend to have severe viral, parasitic, and fungal infections or disease caused by bacteria that can multiply intracellularly (eg, mycobacteria). Those with defects in antibody production, such as agammaglobulinemia, are prone to infection with encapsulated organisms such as *Streptococcus pneumoniae* and *Haemophilus influenzae* type b.

Different types of immunocompromise are associated with different infecting organisms

IMMUNE DEFICITS ASSOCIATED WITH INFECTION

Defects in Epithelial Barriers

Defects in mucosal barriers represent an important prelude to infection by allowing organisms that normally colonize the skin, gastrointestinal tract, or upper airway access to deeper more vulnerable tissues. Burns, extensive trauma, and decubitus ulcers remove the epithelial defense of the skin; however, less obvious factors, such as cytotoxic therapy, may cause damage to mucosal surfaces that predisposes to attachment and replication of potentially pathogenic organisms and can cause loss of host-clearing mechanisms (eg, ciliary function). Defects in intestinal mucosal barriers are often associated with infections caused by Gram-negative aerobic and anaerobic enteric bacteria from the gut flora. Staphylococcal, streptococcal, and pneumococcal infections of the lung are particularly likely when the respiratory epithelium is damaged, whereas *Pseudomonas aeruginosa* infections are a common feature of severe burns.

Breaks in skin or mucosa provide entry

TABLE 71–1

Infections in the Compromised Host

Type of Compromise	Example	Pathogen
↓ Leukocyte number or function	Myelocytic leukemias Chronic granulomatous disease Granulocytopenia Acidosis Burns	Extracellular bacteria[a] Opportunistic fungi
↓ Humoral immune response	Lymphocytic leukemias Multiple myeloma Nephrotic syndrome Antimetabolites Hypogammaglobulinemia AIDS	Encapsulated bacteria[b] Enteroviruses *Pneumocystis* *Giardia*[c]
↓ Complement components	Genetic deficiencies	Extracellular bacteria[a] *Neisseria*[d]
↓ Cellular immune response	AIDS Hodgkin's disease Transplantation Steroids Uremia Antimetabolites Malnutrition	*Pneumocystis* Intracellular bacteria[e] *Nocardia* *Candida* and fungi of systemic mycoses Viruses, especially herpesviruses Protozoa[f] *Strongyloides*
↓ Reticuloendothelial system function	Splenectomy Chronic hemolysis	*Pneumococcus* *Salmonella* *Listeria*

[a] Bacteria that are unable to multiply in phagocytes.

[b] For example, *Streptococcus pneumoniae* and *Haemophilus influenzae* type b.

[c] Associated with lgA deficiency.

[d] Associated with C5, C6, C7, and C8 deficiencies.

[e] Bacteria capable of multiplying in unactivated macrophage.

[f] Includes *Toxoplasma* and *Cryptosporidium*.

Defects in Number or Function of Phagocytes

When the natural barriers of the skin and mucosal surfaces are breached, the next major line of defense is the circulating phagocytes. To defend against infection, there must be an adequate number of these cells, and they must be able to move to the site of infection and ingest and kill invading organisms. Numerous defects in these processes have been described.

Neutropenia

Neutropenia <500/mm^3 associated with infection; <100/mm^3 with bloodstream spread

Although normal neutrophil granulocyte counts vary greatly according to the age, sex, and race of the patient, the usual value is 2500 to 7500 cells/mm^3 of blood in adults. Neutropenia may result from inherited or acquired diseases, malignancies, use of cytotoxic drugs, or adverse reactions to therapeutic agents such as chloramphenicol. If the absolute neutrophil count decreases to fewer than 500 cells/mm^3, the incidence of infections increases markedly, and counts below 100 cells/mm^3 are associated with bacteremia. Immunocompromised patients differ in their ability to tolerate profound neutropenia. For example, patients with acquired immunodeficiency syndrome (AIDS) may not experience bacteremia as frequently as patients receiving chemotherapy. This may reflect damage to mucous membranes from the chemotherapy in addition to the neutropenia. Severe neutropenia is accompanied most frequently by bacterial infections caused by the pyogenic Gram-positive cocci, Enterobacteriaceae, *P. aeruginosa,* and *H. influenzae.* Fungal infections with *Candida, Aspergillus,* or the Zygomycetes are also common.

Defects in Chemotaxis and Leukocytic Function

Defects in phagocytic defenses can be caused by multiple mechanisms that result in inadequate leukocyte chemotaxis or function (Table 71–2). Deficiencies of complement or immunoglobulins can decrease chemoattractants at the site of an infection, and certain metabolic diseases such as diabetes and uremia can alter the microenvironment of leukocytes to reduce their mobility and responsiveness to stimuli. This phenomenon has also been shown to occur in immune complex diseases such as lupus erythematosus. In each case, removal of the leukocyte to a normal environment restores its mobility and ability to respond chemotactically.

Diabetes and uremia can impair WBC function

Several genetic diseases produce specific defects in granulocyte bactericidal mechanisms that result in an immunocompromised host. Because they frequently diminish life span, these illnesses are usually seen in children. The most studied is chronic granulomatous disease, a group of inherited disorders of phagocytic cell superoxide production associated with frequent pyogenic infections, usually caused by catalase-positive organisms, such as *Staphylococcus aureus.* In Chédiak-Higashi disease, neutrophil lysosomes fail to fuse with the phagosome and the cells fail to destroy ingested organisms. These children also suffer recurrent infections with pyogenic organisms.

Chronic granulomatous disease due to lack of superoxide production

Chédiak-Higashi disease: failure of lysosome–phagosome fusion

The spectrum of infections in patients with phagocytic dysfunction is wide and includes repeated bouts of cellulitis, pharyngitis, perirectal and other abscesses, pneumonia, osteomyelitis, and bacteremia. Many pyogenic organisms other than staphylococci can be involved. Antimicrobic treatment given either therapeutically or prophylactically has helped greatly in the care of these patients, but they still suffer repeated bouts of infection that may ultimately prove fatal.

Prophylactic antimicrobics may be helpful

TABLE 71–2

Disorders of Phagocytosis and Intracellular Phagocytic Killing

Chemotactic Defects	**Ingestion**
Complement component deficiency	Actin–myosin dysfunction
Immunoglobulin deficiency	Drugs (colchicine, tetracycline, cyclophosphamide)
Intrinsic defects	Hyperosmolar states
"Lazy leukocytes"	Acute infections
Leukocyte adhesion disorders	
Burns	
Hyperimmunoglobulin E syndrome (Job's syndrome)	**Degranulation**
	Chédiak–Higashi syndrome
Collagen vascular disease	
Diabetes mellitus, uremia	**Killing**
	Lysosomal enzyme deficiency
Opsonization	Chronic granulomatous disease
Immunoglobulin deficiency	Glucose-6-phosphate dehydrogenase deficiency
Complement component deficiency	Drugs (phenylbutazone, chloramphenicol)
Interference by immune complexes (systemic lupus erythematosus)	
Sickle cell anemia	Glutathione reductase deficiency

Antibody Deficiency

Several congenital and acquired disorders can lead to inadequate synthesis of immunoglobulins as a result of deficiency or dysfunction of B lymphocytes. The most common and least serious is immunoglobulin A deficiency, which is associated with increased risk of gastrointestinal tract infection, especially with the parasite *Giardia lamblia.* Individuals with severe defects in IgG and IgM production (hypogammaglobulinemia or agammaglobulinemia) are prone to recurrent infections with encapsulated organisms such as *S. pneumoniae* or *H. influenzae,* which require opsonization for adequate phagocytosis. Sinusitis, otitis media, bacterial pneumonia, and bacteremia are the most common types of infection. Acquired deficiency in immunoglobulin production may occur in AIDS, multiple myeloma, non-Hodgkin's lymphoma, and certain types of chronic lymphocytic leukemia that involve monoclonal proliferation of one immunoglobulin-producing cell line and relative deficiencies of cells producing other antibodies. These patients are also prone to infections by systemically invasive organisms.

IgA deficiency is associated with giardiasis

IgM and IgG deficiencies associated with infection by encapsulated organisms

Repeated injections of immunoglobulins (immune serum globulin) may decrease the incidence and morbidity of infections in patients with hypo- or agammaglobulinemia. In those capable of some immune responses, the use of pneumococcal vaccine (Pneumovax) may provide a degree of protection against overwhelming infection with this organism.

Immune serum globulin or some vaccines are useful

Complement Deficiency

Defects of the complement system also predispose patients to many infections. Individuals with deficiencies in C3 are prone to infections with encapsulated organisms that require opsonization and to a range of infections similar to those seen in patients with hypogammaglobulinemia. Those with deficiencies in later components in the complement sequence are prone to develop recurrent bacteremia caused by *Neisseria meningitidis* or *Neisseria gonorrhoeae* if they are infected with these species. Patients with defects in the early complement components, C1, C2, or C4, have less of a problem than those with later complement pathway deficiencies, because they retain the ability to use the alternative complement pathway to activate C3 and hence C5 to C9.

Opsonization defects with C3 deficiency

Systemic *Neisseria* infection in C5–C8 deficiencies

Disorders in Cell-Mediated Immunity

Both congenital and acquired abnormalities of the cell-mediated immune system occur. Congenital abnormalities, which are uncommon, include thymic dysplasia syndrome, ataxia telangiectasia, and severe combined immunodeficiency (both T- and B-cell deficiency). AIDS, now the most important cause of acquired cellular immunodeficiency, causes a depletion of CD4+ T lymphocytes. Another common source of acquired defects is seen especially in transplant recipients due to treatment with immunosuppressive or cytotoxic agents that damage both macrophage precursors and T lymphocytes. Cytotoxic chemotherapy for cancer with cyclophosphamide and other antimetabolites has these effects and also inhibits humoral immune responses. Glucocorticoids can have multiple effects, causing neutropenia, lymphopenia, and monocytopenia through suppression of cell production, inhibition of mobilization of neutrophils to the site of inflammation, and interference with cell-mediated immune responses through alteration of the responsiveness of monocytes and macrophages to lymphokines. In addition, glucocorticoids impair the function of cells lining the mucosal surfaces, thus increasing the chance of microbial invasion by this route. Combinations of glucocorticosteroids and immunosuppressive drugs are essential in the treatment of certain diseases but are particularly likely to interfere with the ability of a patient to combat new or established infections.

CD4+ lymphocytes compromised in AIDS

Glucocorticoids have multiple effects on immune cell function

A detailed analysis of the infections associated with the different causes of cell-mediated and combined immune deficits is beyond the scope of this chapter. In general, defects in cell-mediated immunity are associated with increased susceptibility to infection with specific opportunistic pathogens, particularly facultative or obligate intracellular pathogens such as cytomegalovirus, fungi and mycobacteria (see Table 71–1). For example, infection with *Mycobacterium tuberculosis* and other mycobacteria in AIDS patients

Defective cell-mediated immunity associated with many infections by intracellular microbes and herpesviruses is an important clinical problem. Because of the wide range of potential infecting organisms, the sites of infection associated with defects in cell-mediated immunity are varied. These include superficial skin infections, lung infections, pharyngitis, otitis, sinusitis, bacteremia, retinitis, and abscesses. Simultaneous infections with multiple organisms are common.

CLINICAL SITUATIONS ASSOCIATED WITH INFECTION

Acquired Immunodeficiency Syndrome

The increasing worldwide prevalence and profound immunodeficiency of AIDS remains a major concern. Most patients die of human immunodeficiency virus infection per se or as a direct result of one of the opportunistic infections mentioned earlier. As a result of its importance, AIDS is discussed separately in Chapter 42.

AIDS is an extraordinary model of immunocompromise

Malignancies

Although some malignancies compromise the immune system directly, the chemotherapeutic agents used to treat them are the primary cause of immunosuppression. In particular, the periods of granulocytopenia between the administration of high-dose chemotherapy and recovery of granulocyte-producing function are associated with infection. The organisms most common during this vulnerable period are generally the same as among the general population; for example, *Staphylococcus aureus* and *Escherichia coli,* but other pathogens such as *P. aeruginosa* and *Candida albicans* are more prominent than in the immunocompetent individual. As discussed earlier, chemotherapy may also compromise cell-mediated immunity, in which case infections due to intracellular bacteria and viruses are common. Finally, chemotherapy may damage mucosa (oral, intestinal, vaginal, rectal), allowing ingress of bacteria, fungi or viruses.

Chemotherapy of malignancy commonly decreases granulocytes, and causes mucosal damage

Transplantation

Solid organ and bone marrow transplantations are among the most important advances in modern medicine. Their success depends to a great degree on the ability to control and manage the undesired aspects of the immunosuppressive regimens, primarily the susceptibility to infection as long as immunosuppression is used. The pattern of microorganisms varies with the type of transplant, as does the immunosuppressive therapy, but viruses are extremely important. Viruses of the herpesvirus family, such as herpes simplex, varicella–zoster, and cytomegalovirus are the most common, but respiratory syncytial virus and other respiratory viruses are also important. Bacteria associated with deficiencies in granulocytes and cell-mediated immunity are also involved; *Legionella* and *Nocardia* infections have been particularly prominent in kidney and heart transplant recipients and fungal infections are common. Recombinant granulocyte-macrophage colony-stimulating factor can accelerate the recovery of bone marrow myeloid elements in bone marrow transplant and some cancer chemotherapy patients, sometimes reducing the period of vulnerability.

Herpesviruses particularly common

Legionella and *Nocardia* in solid organ transplants

DIAGNOSIS

Clinical recognition and treatment of infections in the immunocompromised patient are often difficult, because the infection may be relatively silent due to impairment of the immune response. Laboratory diagnosis can also be difficult, because many of the organisms involved require special culture media and grow slowly (Table 71–3); others such as *Pneumocystis carinii* cannot be grown at all. The increased involvement of low-virulence organisms commonly found in the normal flora may make it difficult to distinguish colonization from infection. Thus, isolation of *C. albicans* from the urine or the pharynx does not prove that it is the cause of a concurrent renal abscess or pneumonitis. Diagnostic procedures such as biopsy of involved organs are often needed to identify the causative agent.

Diagnosis often requires aggressive procedures

TABLE 71-3

Agents Commonly Infecting Immunocompromised Patients

Agent	Decreased Phagocytosis	Complement Deficiencies	Hypo- or Agammaglobulinemia	Defects in Cell-Mediated Immunity
Bacteria				
Staphylococcus aureus and β-hemolytic streptococci	+++[a]	++	++	
Streptococcus pneumoniae	+++	+	+++	
Enterobacteriaceae	+++	+	+	
Pseudomonas aeruginosa	+++	++	+	
Haemophilus influenzae	+	+	+++	
Salmonella species	+	+		+++
Listeria monocytogenes				+++
Mycobacterium species				+++
Legionella				+++
Nocardia asteroides				+++
Neisseria species		++	+	
Fungi				
Candida species				
Systemic	++			
Chronic mucocutaneous				+++
Aspergillus species	+++			
Phycomyces species	+++			
Cryptococcus neoformans				+++
Coccidioides immitis				+++
Histoplasma capsulatum				+++
Pneumocystis carinii			++	+++
Viruses				
Herpes simplex			+	+++
Varicella–zoster			++	+++
Cytomegalovirus				+++
Epstein–Barr				+++
Papovaviruses				++
Respiratory syncytial virus				+++
Enteroviruses			+++	
Hepatitis B				+++
Influenza			+	+
Adenoviruses			+	+++
Parasites				
Giardia lamblia			++	+
Toxoplasma gondii				+++
Strongyloides stercoralis				+++
Cryptosporidium				+++

[a] Number of pluses indicates relative susceptibility to the organisms listed according to the immune deficits.

TREATMENT

Successful treatment of infections in the compromised host depends on recognition of the deficit, early diagnosis, and prompt intervention. This requires identification of the organisms most likely to be involved in the infection. The index of suspicion must be very high, because the signs and symptoms of infection that are seen in immunocompetent individuals may be lacking. For example, in neutropenia the clinical signs of infection (eg, abscess formation) may not be apparent when the patient is first seen because of lack of reaction to the disease. It is thus usually necessary to initiate antimicrobic treatment before results of culture and antibiotic susceptibility tests are available. Broad-spectrum antimicrobic coverage is used initially and replaced with narrower spectrum agents, when the etiologic agent and its susceptibility are known, to reduce the risk of superinfection. In general, bactericidal antimicrobics are needed to control infections when host defenses are inadequate, and with severe infections a combination of synergistic agents may be necessary to provide increased bactericidal action.

Early diagnosis and treatment particularly important

Bactericidal antimicrobics required

Patients with neutropenia have high rates of infection, and mortality may be as high as 20 to 30% if bacteremia develops. Therefore, short-term prophylactic antibiotic treatment has been advocated for neutropenic patients and can be effective in preventing infection until the neutrophil count improves. Selection of resistant organisms and "breakthrough" bacteremia as a result of overwhelming infection are major risks of these strategies in these susceptible patients, and the physician must be alert to the possibility of superinfection with other pathogens during treatment.

Careful use of antimicrobic prophylaxis during neutropenic periods

Neutropenia can be ameliorated by the use of cytokines (eg, granulocyte-colony stimulating factor). There is increasing attention to prevention of opportunistic infections in patients disposed to them. For example, patients undergoing bone marrow transplantation may receive prophylactic acyclovir or ganciclovir to prevent herpesvirus and cytomegalovirus infection. AIDS patients receive prophylactic trimethoprim–sulfamethoxazole to prevent *P. carinii* pneumonia as well as toxoplasmosis.

Antiviral, antifungal, and antiparasitic prophylaxis selectively used

ADDITIONAL READING

Dykewicz CA. Summary of the guidelines for preventing opportunistic infections among hematopoietic stem cell transplant recipients. *Clin Infect Dis* 2001;33:139–144. This nicely summarizes a much larger, joint report that is also referenced for readers seeking even greater detail.

Fishman JA, Rubin RH. Infection in organ-transplant recipients. *N Engl J Med* 1998;338:1741–1751. Review of infectious disease complications in solid organ transplant recipients.

CHAPTER 72

Nosocomial Infections and Infection Control

KENNETH J. RYAN

"Nosocomial" is a medical term for "hospital-associated." Nosocomial infections are complications that arise during at least 5% of all hospitalizations. The morbidity, mortality, and costs associated with these infections is preventable to a substantial degree. The purpose of hospital infection control is prevention of nosocomial infections by application of epidemiologic concepts and methods.

HISTORY: SEMMELWEIS AND CHILDBED FEVER

The shining example of the fundamental importance of epidemiology in detection and control of nosocomial infections is the work of Ignaz Semmelweis, which preceded the microbiologic discoveries of Pasteur and Koch by a decade. Semmelweis was assistant obstetrician at the Vienna General Hospital, where more than 7000 infants were delivered each year. Childbed fever (puerperal endometritis), which we now know is caused primarily by group A streptococci, was a major problem accounting for 600 to 800 maternal deaths per year. By careful review of hospital statistics between 1846 and 1849, Semmelweis clearly showed that the death rate in one of the two divisions of the hospital was 10 times that in the other. Division I, which had the high mortality, was the teaching unit in which all deliveries were by obstetricians and students. In division II, all deliveries were by midwives. No similar epidemic existed elsewhere in the city of Vienna, and mortality was very low in mothers delivering at home.

Childbed fever was associated with obstetricians on teaching unit

Midwife and home births had lower rates

Semmelweis postulated that the key difference between divisions I and II was participation of the physicians and students in autopsies. One or more cadavers were dissected daily, some from cases of childbed fever and other infections. Handwashing was perfunctory, and Semmelweis believed this allowed the transmission of "invisible cadaver particles" by direct contact between the mother and the physician's hands during examinations and delivery. In 1847, as a countermeasure, he required handwashing with a chlorine solution until the hands were slippery and the odor of the cadaver was gone. The results were dramatic. The full effect of the chlorine handwashing can be seen by comparing mortality in the two divisions for 1846 and 1848 (Table 72–1). The mortality in division I was reduced to that of division II, and both were below 2%.

Transmission from cadavers was suspected

Disinfectant handwashing reduced the infection rates

Unfortunately, because of his personality and failure to publish his work until 1860, Semmelweis' contribution was not generally appreciated in his lifetime. As his frustration mounted over lack of acceptance of his ideas, he became abusive and irrational, eventually alienating even his early supporters. Some believe that he also suffered from Alzheimer's disease. He died in an insane asylum in 1865, unaware that his concept of

TABLE 72–1

Childbed Fever at the Vienna General Hospital

	Division I (Teaching Unit)			Division II (Midwife Unit)		
Year	*Births*	*Maternal Deaths*	*Percentage*	*Births*	*Maternal Deaths*	*Percentage*
1846[a]	4010	459	11.4	3754	105	2.7
1848[b]	3556	45	1.3	3219	43	1.3

[a] No handwashing.

[b] First full year of chlorine handwashing.

spread via direct contact would later be recognized as the most important mechanism of nosocomial infection and that handwashing would remain the most important means of infection control in hospitals.

NOSOCOMIAL INFECTIONS AND THEIR SOURCES

Community infections are acquired before admission

Nosocomial infections are acquired in hospital

Infections occurring during any hospitalization are either community acquired or nosocomial. Community infections are those present or incubating at the time of hospital admission. All others are considered nosocomial. For example, a hospital case of chickenpox could be community acquired if it erupted on the fifth hospital day (incubating) or nosocomial if hospitalization was beyond the limits of the known incubation period (20 days). Infections appearing shortly after discharge (2 weeks) are considered nosocomial, although some could have been acquired at home. Infectious hazards are inherent to the hospital environment; it is there that the most seriously infected and most susceptible patients are housed and often cared for by the same staff.

Endogenous infections are part of hospital risk

The infectious agents responsible for nosocomial infections arise from various sources, including patients' own normal flora. In addition to any immunocompromising disease or therapy, the hospital may impose additional risks by treatments that breach the normal defense barriers. Surgery, urinary or intravenous catheters, and invasive diagnostic procedures all may provide normal flora with access to usually sterile sites. Infections in which the source of organisms is the hospital rather than the patient include those derived from hospital personnel, the environment, and medical equipment.

Hospital Personnel

Cross-infection is usually by direct contact

Infected medical attendants are particularly dangerous

Infection from carriers can transmit to patients

Physicians, nurses, students, therapists, and any others who come in contact with the patient may transmit infection. Transmission from one patient to another is called **cross-infection.** The vehicle of transmission is most often the inadequately washed hands of a medical attendant. Another source is the infected medical attendant. Many hospital outbreaks have been traced to hospital personnel, particularly physicians, who continue to care for patients despite an overt infection. Transmission is usually by direct contact, although airborne transmission is also possible. A third source is the person who is not ill but is carrying a virulent strain. For *Staphylococcus aureus* and group A streptococci, nasal carriage is most important, but sites such as the perineum and anus have also been involved in outbreaks. An occult carrier is less often the source of nosocomial infection than a physician covering up a boil or a nurse minimizing "the flu." The carrier is difficult to detect unless the epidemic strain has distinctive characteristics or the epidemiologic circumstances point to a single person.

Environment

Environmental contamination is relatively unimportant

The hospital air, walls, floors, linens, and the like are not sterile and thus could serve as a source of organisms causing nosocomial infections, but the importance of this route has generally been exaggerated. With the exception of the immediate vicinity of an infected individual or a carrier, transmission through the air or on fomites is much less important than that caused by personnel or equipment. Notable exceptions are when the environment becomes contaminated with *Mycobacterium tuberculosis* from a patient or *Legionella pneumophila* in the water supply. These events are most likely to result in disease when the organisms are numerous or the patient is particularly vulnerable (eg, after heart surgery or bone marrow transplant).

M. tuberculosis and *Legionella* are risks

Medical Devices

Much of the success of modern medicine is related to medical devices that support or monitor basic body functions. By their very nature, devices such as catheters and respirators carry a risk of nosocomial infection, because they bypass normal defense barriers, providing microorganisms access to normally sterile fluids and tissues. Most of the recognized causes are bacterial or fungal. The risk of infection is related to the degree of debilitation of the patient and various factors concerning the design and management of the device. Any device that crosses the skin or a mucosal barrier allows flora in the patient or environment to gain access to deeper sites around the outside surface. Possible access inside the device (eg, in the lumen) adds another and sometimes greater risk. In some devices, such as urinary catheters, contamination is avoidable; in others, such as respirators, complete sterility is either impossible or impractical to achieve.

Equipment that crosses epithelial barriers provides microbial access

The risk of contamination leading to infection is increased if organisms that gain access can multiply within the system. The availability of water, nutrients, and a suitable temperature largely determine which organism will survive and multiply. Many of the Gram-negative rods such as *Pseudomonas, Acinetobacter,* and members of the Enterobacteriaceae can multiply in an environment containing water and little else. Gram-positive bacteria generally require more physiologic conditions.

Conditions for bacterial growth increase risk

Even with proper growth conditions, many hours are required before contaminating organisms become numerous. Detailed studies of catheters and similar devices show the risk of infection begins to increase after 24 to 48 hours and is cumulative even if the device is changed or disinfected at intervals. It is thus important to discontinue transcutaneous procedures as soon as medically indicated. The medical devices most frequently associated with nosocomial infections are listed below. The infectious risk of others can be estimated from the principles discussed previously. New devices are constantly being introduced into medical care, occasionally without adequate consideration of their potential to cause nosocomial infection.

Transcutaneous and indwelling devices should be changed as soon as possible

Urinary Catheters

Urinary tract infection (UTI) accounts for 40 to 50% of all nosocomial infections, and at least 80% of these are associated with catheterization. The infectious risk of a single urinary catheterization has been estimated at 1%, and indwelling catheters carry a risk that may be as high as 10%. The major preventive measure is maintenance of a completely closed system through the use of valves and aspiration ports designed to prevent bacterial access to the inside of the catheter or collecting bag. Unfortunately, breaks in closed systems eventually occur if the system is in place for more than 30 days. The urine itself serves as an excellent culture medium once bacteria gain access. Although *Escherichia coli* is still a leading cause of nosocomial UTIs, other Enterobacteriaceae and *Pseudomonas* are more likely than in the community setting.

Closed urinary drainage systems are still violated

E. coli and other Gram-negative bacteria predominate

Vascular Catheters

Needles and plastic catheters placed in veins (or, less often, in arteries) for fluid administration, monitoring vital functions, or diagnostic procedures are a leading cause of nosocomial bacteremia. These sites should always be suspected as a source of organisms whenever blood cultures are positive with no apparent primary site for the bacteremia. Contamination at the insertion site is generally staphylococcal, with continued growth in the catheter tip. Organisms may gain access somewhere in the lines, valves, bags, or

Skin is primary source for intravenous contamination

bottles of intravenous solutions proximal to the insertion site. The latter circumstance usually involves Gram-negative rods. Preventive measures include aseptic insertion technique and appropriate care of the lines, including changes at regular intervals.

Respirators

Changing controls nebulizer contamination

Machines that assist or control respiration by pumping air directly into the trachea have a great potential for nosocomial pneumonia if the aerosol they deliver becomes contaminated. Bacterial growth is significant only in the parts of the system that contain water; in systems using nebulizers, bacteria can be suspended in water droplets small enough to reach the alveoli. The organisms involved include *Pseudomonas,* Enterobacteriaceae, and a wide variety of environmental bacteria such as *Acinetobacter.* The primary control measure is periodic changing and disinfection of the tubing, reservoirs, and nebulizer jets.

Blood and Blood Products

Risk of hepatitis B, hepatitis C, and HIV is related to blood manipulation

Screen is determined by institutional policy

Infections related to contact with blood and blood products are generally a risk for health care workers rather than patients. Manipulations ranging from phlebotomy and hemodialysis to surgery carry varying risk of blood containing an infectious agent reaching mucous membranes or skin of the health care worker. The major agents transmitted in this manner are hepatitis B, hepatitis C, and human immunodeficiency virus (HIV). Control requires meticulous attention to procedures that prevent direct contact with blood, such as the use of gloves, eyewear, and gowns. Cuts and needle sticks among health care workers carry a risk approaching 2%. Identification of hepatitis virus and HIV carriers is a part of a protective process that must be balanced by patient privacy considerations. Health care facilities all have established policies concerning serologic surveillance of patients and the procedures to follow (eg, testing, prophylaxis) when blood-related accidents occur. Similarly, products for transfusion undergo extensive screening in order to protect the recipient.

INFECTION CONTROL

Antisepsis attacks contaminating organisms

Asepsis prevents contamination

Infection control is the sum of all the means used to prevent nosocomial infections. Historically, such methods have been developed as an integral part of the study of infectious diseases, often serving as key elements in the proof of infectious etiology. Semmelweis' handwashing is the first example. Later in the 19th century, Joseph Lister achieved a dramatic reduction in surgical wound infections by infusion of a phenolic antiseptic into wounds. This local destruction of organisms was known as **antisepsis,** and it sometimes included liberal applications of disinfectants, including sprays to the environment. As it became recognized that contamination of wounds was not inevitable, the emphasis gradually shifted to preventing contact between microorganisms and susceptible sites, a concept called **asepsis.** Asepsis, which combines containment with the methods of sterilization and disinfection discussed in Chapter 11, is the central concept of infection control. The measures taken to achieve asepsis vary, depending on whether the circumstances and environment are most similar to the operating room, hospital ward, or outpatient clinic.

Asepsis

Operating Room

Sterile drapes and instruments prevent contact of organisms with wound

The surgical suite and operating room represent the most controlled and rigid application of aseptic principles. The procedure begins with the use of an antiseptic scrub of the skin over the operative site and the hands and forearms of all who will have contact with the patient. The use of sterile drapes, gowns, and instruments serves to prevent spread through direct contact, and caps and face masks reduce airborne spread from personnel to the wound. As all students learn the first time they scrub, even the manner of dressing and moving in the operating room are rigidly specified, and those involved assume a strict aseptic attitude as well as their masks and gowns. In some hospitals, the air entering the operating room is filter sterilized, but this practice is expensive and its value unproved. The level of bacteria in the air is generally more related to the number of persons and amount of movement in the operating room than to incoming air. The net effect of these procedures is to draw a sterile curtain around the operative site, thus minimizing contact with microorganisms. Surgical asepsis is also used in other areas where invasive special procedures such as cardiac catheterization are performed.

Airborne bacteria are associated with personnel in operating room

Hospital Ward

Although theoretically desirable, strict aseptic procedures as used in the operating room are impractical in the ward setting. Asepsis is practiced by the use of sterile needles, medications, dressings, and other items that could serve as transmission vehicles if contaminated. A "no touch" technique for examining wounds and changing dressings eliminates direct contact with any nonsterile item. Invasive procedures such as catheter insertion and lumbar punctures are performed under aseptic precautions similar to those used in the operating room. In all circumstances, handwashing between patient contacts is the single most important aseptic precaution.

Handwashing is the most important measure

Outpatient Clinic

The general, aseptic practices used on the hospital ward are also appropriate to the outpatient situation as preventive measures. The potential for cross-infection in the clinic or waiting room is obvious but has been little studied regarding preventive measures. Patients who may be infected should be segregated whenever possible using techniques similar to those of hospital ward isolation. The examining room may be used in a manner analogous to the private rooms on a hospital ward. Although this approach is difficult because of patient turnover, it should be attempted for infections that would require strict or respiratory isolation in the hospital.

Waiting areas present a risk

Isolation Procedures

Patients with infections pose special problems, because they may transmit their infections to other patients either directly or by contact with a staff member. This additional risk is managed by the techniques of isolation, which place barriers between the infected patient and others on the ward. Because not every infected patient presents with suspect signs and/or symptoms, some precaution should be taken with all patients. In the system recommended by the Centers for Disease Control and Prevention, these are called **standard precautions** and include the use of gowns and gloves when in contact with patient blood or secretions. These are particularly directed at protecting health care workers from HIV and hepatitis infection. For those with suspect or proven infection, additional precautions are taken, the nature of which is determined by the known mode of transmission of the organism. These **transmission-based precautions** are divided into those directed at airborne, droplet, and contact routes. The **airborne** transmission precautions are for infections known to be transmitted by extremely small (<5 μm) particles suspended in the air. This requires that the room air circulation be maintained with negative pressure relative to the surrounding area and be exhausted to the outside. Those entering the room must wear surgical masks, and in the case of tuberculosis, specially designed respirators. **Droplet** precautions are for infections where the organisms are suspended in larger droplets, which may be airborne, but generally do not travel more than 3 feet from the patient who generates them. These can be contained by the use of gowns, gloves, and masks when working close to the patient. **Contact** precautions are used for infections that require direct contact with organisms on or pass in secretions of the patient. Diarrheal infections are of special concern because of the extent to which they contaminate the environment. Details of the precautions and examples of the typical infectious agents are summarized in Table 72–2.

Standard precautions protect health care workers from HIV

Transmission precautions block airborne, droplet, and contact routes

TABLE 72–2

Precautions for Prevention of Nosocomial Infections

	Elements					
Precaution	Room	Handwashing[a]	Gloves	Gowns	Mask[b]	Typical Diseases
Standard		After removing gloves, between patients	Blood, fluid contact	Blood, fluid contact		All
Transmission-based						
Airborne	Private, negative pressure[c]	After removing gloves, between patients	Room entry	Room entry	Room entry or respirator[d]	Measles, chickenpox, tuberculosis[d]
Droplet	Private[e]	After removing gloves, between patients	Blood, fluid contact	Blood, fluid contact	Within 3 feet of patient	Meningococcal meningitis, pertussis, plague, group A streptococcus, adenovirus, influenza, rubella
Contact	Private[e]	After removing gloves, between patients	Room entry	Patient contact		Infectious diarrhea,[f] impetigo, *S. aureus* wounds, herpes, respiratory syncytial virus, parainfluenza virus, scabies

[a] Using a disinfectant soap.

[b] Standard surgical mask.

[c] Room pressure must be negative in relation to surrounding area and the circulation exhausted outside the building.

[d] For patients with diagnosed or suspect tuberculosis, a specially filtered respirator/mask must be worn.

[e] Door may be left open and patients with the same organism may share a room.

[f] Particularly *Clostridium difficile, Escherichia coli* O:157, *Shigella* and incontinent patient shedding rotavirus or hepatitis A.

Organization

Infection control programs determine and enforce policy

Modern hospitals are required to have formal infection control programs that include an infection control committee, epidemiology service, and educational activities. The infection control committee is composed of representatives of various medical, administrative, nursing, housekeeping, and support services. The committee establishes the institution's infection control procedures and regularly reviews information on the status of nosocomial infections in the hospital. When epidemiologic circumstances warrant it, the committee is empowered to take drastic action such as closing a hospital unit or suspending a physician's privileges.

Epidemiologic surveillance and outbreak investigation are required

The epidemiology service is the working arm of the infection control committee. Its functions are performed by one or more epidemiologists who usually have a nursing background. This work requires familiarity with clinical microbiology, epidemiology, infectious disease, and hospital procedures, as well as immense tact. The main activities are surveillance and outbreak investigation. Surveillance is the collection of data documenting the frequency and nature of nosocomial infections in the hospital to detect deviations from the institutional or national norms. Although routine microbiologic sampling of the hospital environment is of no value, programs to sample some of the medical devices known to be nosocomial hazards can be useful. On-the-spot investigation of potential outbreaks allows early implementation of preventive measures. This activity is probably the single most important function of the epidemiology service. Suspicion of an increased number of infections leads to an investigation to verify the facts, establish basic epidemiologic associations, and relate them to preventive measures. The primary concern is cross-infection, in which a virulent organism is being transmitted from patient to patient. Solution of the problem may require additional microbiologic investigations, such as bacteriophage typing of *S. aureus*.

PREVENTION

The prevention of nosocomial infections is contingent on basic and applied knowledge drawn from all parts of this book. Applied with common sense, these principles can both prevent disease and reduce the costs of medical care.

ADDITIONAL READING

Aitken C, Jeffries DJ. Nosocomial spread of viral diseases. *Clin Microbiol Rev* 2001;14:528–546. The viral component of nosocomial infections is often neglected. This review discusses viral agents by their route of transmission in the health care setting including the blood-borne viruses.

Fourth Decennial Conference on Healthcare-associated Infections. *Emerg Infect Dis* 2001;7:169–368. This special issue contains state-of-the-art articles on all the current topics in nosocomial infection. The cover reproduces a painting titled "Semmelweis: Defender of Motherhood."

Glossary

Glossary

The glossary is intended as an adjunct to the index for rapid reference. It includes words and phrases that have not been defined in the text or that have been defined but are used frequently in later chapters. Where a word has multiple uses, the one relevant to this text is emphasized.

The prefixes and suffixes in each alphabetical section include word elements used in combined form. The meaning of many words can be derived from the prefixes and suffixes and therefore have not been included in the glossary.

A-, An- Without.

Acanthosis Hyperplasia and thickening of prickle cell layer of skin.

Accessory sinuses Blind-ended cavities in bone draining into nasal cavity.

Achlorhydria Absence of hydrochloric acid in stomach.

Acid fast Describes an organism that resists acid decolorization after straining.

Acidosis Increased acidity of body fluid.

Aciduric Resistant to effects of acid.

Actin Major structural protein of the eukaryotic cell cytoskeleton.

Addison's disease Result of primary deficiency of production of adrenal hormones.

Adenocarcinoma Malignant tumor derived from glandular epithelium.

Adhesin Surface component of a microbe that binds to a cell receptor.

Adnexa (uterine) Fallopian tubes and ovaries.

Adrenal Important endocrine glands situated above the kidneys.

Aerobactin A hydroxamate siderophore produced by many bacteria.

Agammaglobulinemia Absence of immunoglobulins in the blood.

Agglutinate Clumping.

Agranulocytosis Failure of white blood cell production in bone marrow.

-algia Pain.

Allele Alternate forms of a gene at the same chromosomal locus.

Alloantigen An antigen that exists in alternate allelic forms.

Allosteric Property of a protein that leads to a change in conformation and function associated with attachment of a smaller effector molecule.

Alveoli (lung) Microscopic air sacs in lung.

Ameboma A local inflammatory mass caused by an amebal infection.

Amniotic fluid Fluid in amniotic sac surrounding the fetus.

Anaerobe Microorganism that multiplies only in the absence of oxygen.

Analog Structurally or functionally similar substance or property.

Anamnestic Enhanced immunological memory response on reexposure to antigen.

Anaphylaxis Immediate and severe antibody-mediated hypersensitivity reaction.

Anergic Absence of ability to respond to antigen.

Aneurysm Localized abnormal dilatation of blood vessel.

Anicteric Absence of clinical jaundice.

Anneal Subject to controlled heating and cooling to achieve a particular property.

Anorexia Loss of appetite.

Anoxia Lack of adequate oxygenation of blood or tissues.

Anterior horn cell Motor neuron in the anterior gray matter of the spinal cord.

Anthropo- Relationship to humans.
Antibiogram Pattern of in vitro susceptibilities to different antimicrobics.
Antibody An immunoglobulin molecule that interacts with the antigen that elicited its production.
Antigen A substance that elicits a specific immunological response or reacts with antibody in vitro. (See Immunogen *and* Hapten).
Antiserum Serum containing specific antibodies.
Antitoxin An antibody that neutralizes an exotoxin.
Antitussive Substance that helps control coughing.
Aphonia Loss of speech.
Aplastic anemia Failure of red cell production in bone marrow.
Apnea Temporary absence of breathing.
Aqueduct of Sylvius Canal connecting the third and fourth ventricles of the brain.
Arachidonic acid Precursor of prostaglandins.
Arachnoid The middle of three membranes that cover the brain and spinal cord (meninges).
Arrythmia Irregularity of heartbeat.
Arteriole Smallest artery leading to capillary.
Arthralgia Pain in a joint.
Arthro- Pertaining to joints.
Aryepiglottis Related to the epiglottis and the arytenoid cartilage.
Ascites Fluid in a peritoneal cavity.
Ascus A sac. In mycology, a specialized structure containing spores termed ascospores.
Asepsis Exclusion of pathogenic organisms.
Asphyxia Suffocation.
Astrocyte Connective tissue cell of the central nervous system.
Ataxia Disturbance of muscular coordination.
Ataxia telangiectasia Hereditary disorder causing ataxia and permanent dilatation of some blood vessels.
Atelectasis Collapse of part of lung.
Atherosclerosis Hardening of the arteries.
Atrophy Wasting.
Attenuated Reduced in virulence, (eg, organisms in a live vaccine).
Auto- Self, or arising from within.
Autochthonous flora Organism with intimate and permanent association with an epithelial surface.
Autoimmunity An immune response against the body's own tissues.
Autolysis Lysis of a cell by its own enzymes.
Autonomic Relates to involuntary nervous system controlling cardiac, vascular, intestinal, and other functions.
Auxo- Pertaining to growth.
Auxotroph Bacterial mutant that has lost the ability to synthesize an essential nutrient or metabolite.
Avascular Absence of blood vessels or blood supply.
Axenic Refers to pure cultures of a microorganism without presence of a contaminating or symbiotic organism.
Axon The extension of a neuron that conducts nerve impulses.

Bacteremia Bacteria in the blood.
Bacteriocins Proteins produced by one bacterium that kill another of the same or other species.
Bacteriophage Bacterial virus.
Bacteriostasis Inhibition of bacterial growth without killing.
Bacteriuria Bacteria in the urine.
Bartholin's glands Lubricating glands on either side of the vaginal opening.
Basophil Polymorphonuclear leucocyte with basophilic granules.
Basophilic Stains with a basic dye.
Biliary Pertaining to the bile and bile ducts.
Bilirubin A bile pigment.
Bio- Pertaining to life.
Biotype Subtype within a species characterized by physiologic properties.
-blast Precursor cell.
Bleb See Bulla.
Blepharal Pertaining to the eyelids.
Blepharo- Pertaining to the eyelid.
Blepharoplast Basal body of a cilium or flagellum.
Blood–brain barrier Functional barrier preventing passage of large molecules to the brain parenchyma.
Bolus Rounded mass that may obstruct (eg, fecal bolus) or a concentrated mass (eg, an antibiotic) given rapidly and intravenously.
Bothria Paired sucking grooves in the head of the fish tapeworm (*Diphyllobothrium*).
Brady- Slowing.
Bradycardia Unusually slow heartbeat.
Bronchial tree Bronchi and bronchioles that conduct gases to and from the lung alveoli.
Bronchiectasis Pathological dilatation of terminal bronchi.
Bronchiole Smallest subdivision of bronchial tree.
Broncho- Pertaining to the bronchial tree.
Bubo Swollen, inflamed, infected lymph node.
Buccal Pertaining to the cheek.
Bulla Blister or vesicle containing semipurulent fluid.
Bursa Sac filled with fluid (eg, protecting a joint or tendon).

Calculus Pathological stone (eg, renal or gallbladder calculus).
Calmodulin A protein present in eukaryotic cells that activates some essential enzymes when it has bound calcium.
Capillary The smallest blood vessel connecting the arterial and venous systems.
Capsid The outer protein coat of a virus that protects its nucleic acid.
Capsomeres Subunits of viral capsids.
Carbuncle A necrotic staphylococcal infection of skin and subcutaneous tissue that has spread from infected furuncles.
Carcinoma Malignant growth of epithelial cells.

Cardio- Pertaining to the heart.

Cardiolipin A phospholipid occurring naturally in mitochondrial membranes against which antibodies are formed in syphilitic infection.

Cardiomyopathy Disease of heart muscle.

Caseous Cheesy in consistency.

Catalase Enzyme that catalyzes the reduction of toxic hydrogen peroxide to oxygen and water.

Cell-mediated immunity Immune reactions in which T lymphocytes play the pivotal role.

Cellulitis Inflammation of subcutaneous tissue.

Cementum Layer of modified bone on tooth root.

Cerebrospinal fluid Fluid that fills spaces within and surrounding the central nervous system.

Cervical Pertaining to the neck or uterine cervix.

Cervix The constricted portion of an organ. Usually refers to the lower part of the uterus.

Chancre Sore or ulcer that develops at the site of an infection. Most often used to describe the primary syphilitic lesion.

Chelator Compound that binds metallic ions.

Chemoprophylaxis Use of antimicrobics to prevent infection.

Chemotaxis Attraction of a motile cell to a chemical.

Chitin Polysaccharide forming exoskeletons of some insects or cell walls of some fungi.

Cholangitis Inflammation of the bile ducts.

Chole- Pertaining to bile.

Cholecystitis Inflammation of the gallbladder.

Cholestasis Interruption of the flow of bile.

Cholinergic nerves Nerve fibers that release acetylcholine as a mediator at their effector terminals.

Chordae tendinae Small tendons that connect papillary muscles of the heart to the cusps of the atrioventricular valves.

Chorea Rapid purposeless involuntary movements.

Chorioallantoic membrane The outer membrane surrounding an avian embryo within the egg shell.

Chorionic membrane The outer extraembryonic membrane from which the placenta originates.

Chorioretinitis Inflammation of choroid and retina of the eye.

Choroid plexus Vascular invagination into the cerebral ventricles. Produces the cerebrospinal fluid.

Chromatin Complex of DNA and histones making up the chromosomes of eukaryotic cells.

Chronic granulomatous disease Genetic disorder causing absence of H_2O_2 production and myeloperoxidase activity of phagocytes. Results in repeated infections with catalase positive bacteria.

-cidal Killing.

CIE See Counterimmunoelectrophoresis.

Cilia Surface structures of some eukaryotic cells that beat rhythmically to move mucus over surfaces or confer motility on some single-celled organisms.

Cirrhosis Fibrosis and nodular regeneration of the liver with loss of function.

Cistron The smallest functional genetic unit. A gene.

Clone Identical progeny of a single cell, gene, or genes.

CMI See Cell-mediated immunity.

Co-agglutination Agglutination involving two organisms, one of which acts as an inert particle coated with specific antibody to the other.

Co-cultivation Process that can be used for unmasking latent virus by growing susceptible cells with those from affected tissue.

Coarctation Stricture or narrowing (eg, of the aorta).

Codon The three nucleotides encoding an amino acid or a chain termination signal.

Collagen Fibrous component of connective tissue.

Coloboma A defect of the eye.

Colostrum Initial secretion of the breast after delivery (contains antibodies and lymphocytes).

Comedo Blocked sebaceous duct with retention of sebum (blackhead).

Commensal Organism of the normal flora that has a symbiotic relationship with the host.

Complement A system of serum proteins that act in sequence to mediate inflammatory and some immune responses.

Condyloma acuminatum A wart-like infectious benign growth that occurs on the genitalia and in the anal canal.

Conidia Asexual fungal reproductive spore-like bodies.

Conidiophore Fungal structure that bears conidia.

Copepod Minute fresh water fleas that serve as intermediate hosts for some parasites.

Coprolith Stony, hard stool.

Coracidium The ciliated free swimming embryo of certain tapeworms.

Cornea Clear, anterior portion of the eyeball.

Cortex The outer layer of an organ.

Corticosteroid Steroid hormone from adrenal gland; some are anti-inflammatory.

Coryza Catarrhal rhinitis (eg, from the common cold).

Counterimmunoelectrophoresis A technique for increasing the sensitivity and speed of the immunodiffusion procedure by the application of an electrophoretic field (see Immunodiffusion).

Crepitation A crackling or rattling sound.

Cribriform plate Area of bone above nasal cavity through which pass the olfactory nerves.

Croup Manifestations of laryngeal obstruction from inflammation or other causes.

Crustacean Hard shelled invertebrates such as crabs, shrimp, and lobsters.

CSF *See* Cerebrospinal fluid.

Curare A plant extract that produces generalized paralysis by acting at neuromuscular junctions.

Cuticle Skin or surface layer.

Cyanosis Blue color of skin caused by lack of oxygen.

Cystic fibrosis Congenital disease of secreting glands affecting pancreas, respiratory tract, and sweat glands. Associated with viscid respiratory mucus and chronic respiratory infections.

Cysticercus Larval form of tapeworm enclosed in a cyst.
Cysto- Pertaining to the bladder.
Cystoscope Instrument for examining inside the urinary bladder.
Cyto- Pertaining to the cell.
Cytokine Hormone-like intercellular messenger molecule (eg, lymphokine and interleukin).
Cytology The study of cells rather than of tissues and organs.
Cytoplasm Cellular contents excluding the nucleus.
Cytosol Liquid portion of cytoplasm.
Cytosome The body of a cell apart from its nucleus.
Cytostome The mouth opening of certain ciliated protozoa.

Dalton Atomic mass unit that gives the same number as atomic weight.
Debridement Removing foreign matter and dead tissue.
Decubitus ulcer Pressure sore (bed sore).
Defensins A family of microbial, cationic, cystine rich polypeptides abundant in the azurophilic granules of polymorphonuclear leukocytes.
Demyelination Loss of nerve sheaths.
Dendritic Branched.
Dermatophyte Fungus that causes skin infections.
Dermis Skin connective tissue immediately below the epidermis.
Dermo- Pertaining to the skin.
Desquamation Loss of skin epithelial cells.
Dextran A polymer of D-glucose.
Dimorphism Occurring in two morphologic forms under different conditions.
Diploid Possessing two sets of chromosomes.
Disseminated intravascular coagulation (DIC) A clinical syndrome with multiple causes. Thrombocytopenia and complex coagulation abnormalities are prominent.
Diverticulum Blind-ended extrusion from a hollow organ.
Ductus arteriosus Fetal blood vessel connecting the pulmonary artery to the descending aorta.
Dys- Difficult or painful.
Dysentery Pain and frequent defecation resulting from inflammation of the colon or other intestines, with blood and pus in the stool.
Dyspareunia Difficult or painful intercourse.
Dysphagia Difficulty in swallowing.
Dysplasia Histological evidence of possible premalignant changes in cells.
Dyspnea Shortness of breath.
Dysuria Difficult or painful urination.

Ecchymosis A large area of hemorrhage into the skin, often a coalescence of petechiae.
Ecthyma Eroded, scabbed lesion of the skin.
Ecto- Outside or outer.
-ectomy Surgical removal of.
Ectopic pregnancy Fetal development outside the uterus (usually in the fallopian tubes).
Ectoplasm Clear layer of cytoplasm near the cell membrane of amebas.
Edema Excessive fluid in tissues.
EIA. See Enzyme immunoassay.
Elastosis Disorder of fibroelastic proteins.
Electrophoresis Procedure for separating charged particles by differences in their migration in an electric field.
ELISA Enzyme-linked immunosorbent assay (*See* Enzyme immunoassay).
Embolism Sudden blockage of an artery.
-emia Of the blood.
Emphysema (pulmonary) Irreversible enlargement of alveolar sacs of lung.
Empyema Pus in a body cavity (eg, pleural cavity).
Encephalitis Inflammation of brain tissue.
Endarteritis Inflammation of the inner coat of an artery or arteriole.
Endemic A disease that is continuously present at subepidemic levels in a particular region, locality, or group.
Endo- Within.
Endogenous Originating within an organism.
Endometrium Interior epithelial lining of the uterus.
Endonuclease Enzyme of a class that hydrolyzes internal bonds of DNA or RNA. Involved in synthesis and breakdown of nucleic acids.
Endophthalmitis Inflammation of interior tissues of the eye.
Endoplasm Central portion of cytoplasm of cell.
Endoplasmic reticulum Ramifying membranes within the cytoplasm of eukaryotic cells.
Endospore Bacterial spore.
Endotoxin lipid A toxic moiety of bacterial cell wall lipopolysaccharide.
Entactin Protein component of the extracellular matrix.
Enteric Pertaining to the intestinal tract.
Enteric fever Typhoid or similar systemic *Salmonella* or *Yersinia* infection.
Entero- Pertaining to intestines.
Enterobactin A phenolate siderophore produced by *E. coli* and some other enteric species of bacteria.
Enterochelin Synonym for Enterobactin.
Enucleation (ocular) Removal of an eye intact.
Enzootic Disease present at low levels at all times in an animal community.
Enzyme immunoassay A method for detecting antigen–antibody reactions by labeling one of the reagents with detectable enzyme.
Eosinophil Polymorphonuclear leucocyte with eosinophilic granules.
Epi- Upon or additional to.
Epicardium Outer lining of the heart.
Epidemic A disease that rapidly affects many people in a circumscribed period of time.
Epididymis Tubular structure attached to the testes in which spermatozoa mature.
Epigastrium Upper central region of the abdomen overlying the stomach.

Epiglottis Movable structure overlying and protecting the larynx.
Epiphysis Growing end of bone.
Episome Plasmid or viral DNA that can replicate extrachromosomally or can integrate into chromosome.
Epitope Structural part of an antigen that determines specificity of an antigen–antibody reaction (also called antigenic determinant).
Epitrochlear node Lymph node above inner side of elbow.
Erythema Red color caused by dilatation of blood vessels.
Erythema nodosum Red raised skin nodules usually on the legs. Usually a manifestation of a hypersensitivity reaction.
Erythro- Red.
Erythrocyte Red blood cell.
Eschar Necrotic scab-like area of skin.
Etiology Cause of a disease.
Eukaryote Organism comprising one or more cells containing true nuclei.
Eustachian tube Tube connecting the middle ear and the nasopharynx.
Exanthem Disease in which skin rashes are major manifestations.
Exocrine glands Glands excreting their products to skin, intestinal, respiratory, or genitourinary tracts.
Exotoxin Toxic protein liberated from a bacterial cell.

Facultative When describing bacteria without a qualification means ability to grow aerobically or anaerobically.
Fallopian tubes Tubes extending from ovaries to uterus.
Fascia Sheets of specialized connective tissue.
Fauces Area between the mouth and the pharynx. Bounded by the tonsils, soft palate, and base of tongue.
Febrile Having a raised temperature.
Felinophobe Cat hater.
Fibrin Insoluble protein of blood clots.
Fibrinogen Precursor of fibrin.
Fibroblast Specialized cell producing collagen and elastic connective tissue.
Fibronectin A glycoprotein widely distributed in connective tissue and coating cells at mucosal surfaces.
Fibrosis Formation of collagenous connective tissue.
Fimbriae Very fine fibrils on the surface of a bacterium analogous to the larger pili. Often referred to as pili.
Fistula An abnormal passage from a hollow organ (eg, intestine).
Flaccid Loose; absence of muscle tone.
Flagellum Organelle of motion of bacteria and some eukaryotic cells.
Fluke Flat parasitic worm (trematode).
Fluorochrome A fluorescent dye.
Follicle A small sac or cavity.
Folliculitis Usually describes localized inflammation of hair follicles without the purulence of furuncles.
Fomites Inanimate objects transmitting infectious agents.
Foramina Outlets to cavities.
Fulminant Rapid and severe development (eg, of an infection).
Fungemia Fungi in the bloodstream.
Funiculitis Inflammation a cord-like structure, usually the spermatic cord.
Furuncle Purulent infection of a hair follicle; a boil.
Fusiform Tapering at both ends.

Gametocyte Male or female sexual cell of the malarial parasite found in the blood of humans and transmissible to mosquitoes.
Ganglion Group of nerve cells outside the spinal cord.
Gangrene Death of tissue.
Gastro- pertaining to the stomach.
-genic arising from, origin.
Genital primordium First recognizable embryonic genital structure. Assists in distinguishing hookworm from *Strongyloides* larvae.
Genome The total gene complement of an organism.
Genotype The genetic constitution of an organism.
Geophagia Eating soil.
Giemsa stain A combination of basic and acidic dyes used to stain blood smears and to demonstrate some protozoa.
Gingival crevice Area between the tooth and the gums.
Gingivo- pertaining to the gums.
Glaucoma Excessive pressure in eyeball that can lead to blindness.
Glia Supporting cells of the central nervous system (neuroglia).
Glomerulus Microscopic organ of specialized capillaries in the kidney that filters waste products from the blood.
Glottis The sound-producing area of the larynx.
Glucans Polymers of glucose.
Gnotobiotic animals Animals reared under aseptic conditions which may either be sterile ("germ free") or in which defined microflora are introduced.
Gonads Ovaries or testes.
Granulocyte Polymorphonuclear leukocyte of the neutrophil, basophil, or eosinophil series.
Granuloma Chronic inflammatory lesion infiltrated with macrophages and lymphocytes and accompanied by fibroblast activity.
Gravid Pregnant.
Guillain-Barré syndrome Febrile polyneuritis with muscle weakness; may lead to paralysis.
Gumma Tertiary syphilitic granulomatous lesion, usually without demonstrable pirochetes.

Halophilic Preferring or requiring a high salt content (eg, for growth).
Haploid Half the number of chromosomes of eukaryotic tissue cells (see Meiosis) or number of chromosomes in asexual organisms.
Hapten A small molecule that can react with a specific antibody but does not elicit antibody production unless attached to a larger molecule.

Helminth A parasitic worm.

Hemagglutination Agglutination of erythrocytes.

Hematocrit Volume of erythrocytes in blood as a percentage of the total volume of blood (adult normal = 45%).

Hematogenous Derived from blood. Spread by the bloodstream.

Hematoma Extravasation of blood into the tissues causing a swelling.

Hematopoietic system Precursor cells that produce blood cells.

Hematoxylin–eosin stain Commonly used histological stain. Hematoxylin stains nuclei blue. Eosin is a red counter stain.

Hematuria Blood in the urine.

Hemianopsia Loss of vision in half the visual field.

Hemo-, Hema- Pertaining to blood.

Hemoglobulinemia Free hemoglobin in the blood.

Hemolysin A substance or enzyme causing lysis of erythrocytes.

Hemolysis Liberation of hemoglobin from red cells.

Hemolytic–uremic syndrome A syndrome that includes hemolytic anemia, thrombocytopenia, and evidence of renal disease.

Hemoptysis Coughing up of blood.

Hemothorax Blood in the pleural cavity of the chest.

Hepato- Pertaining to the liver.

Hepatocellular Pertaining to liver cells (hepatocytes).

Hepatocytes Liver cells.

Hepatoma Malignant tumor of liver cells.

Hetero- Of different origin.

Heterologous Derived from a different clone, strain, species or tissue.

Heterophil antibody Antibody reacting with an antigen other than that which elicited its production.

Heteroploid Eukaryotic cell with abnormal number of chromosomes.

Heterotroph An organism that requires organic carbon for nutrition.

Heterozygous Possessing different alleles at a particular genetic locus in a diploid cell.

Hexacanth A tapeworm embryo containing six pairs of hooklets.

Hexamer In virology, a capsomer comprising six subunits.

Hilar lymph nodes Nodes at the root of the lung.

Histiocyte Tissue macrophage.

Histocompatibility Antigens on tissue cells that are recognized by the host as self or foreign.

HIV-1 or -2 Abbreviation for human immunodeficiency viruses, the cause of AIDS.

Hodgkin's disease A malignant lymphoma initially affecting groups of lymph nodes.

Homeostasis Tendency to stability of conditions within a complex biological system.

Homonymous hemianopsia Blindness affecting the same half of the visual field in each eye.

Homozygous Possessing the same alleles at a particular genetic locus in a diploid cell.

Humoral Mediated by fluids. In immunology relates to antibody mediated immunity as opposed to cellular immunity.

Hyaline Clear and transparent.

Hyaluronic acid Acid mucopolysaccharide comprising the ground substance of connective tissue. Also found in synovial fluids.

Hybridization Process in which denatured, single stranded nucleic acids from different sources are annealed. Homologous sequences form double strands that can be detected and quantified.

Hybridoma A clone derived from fused cells of different origin (eg, from an antibody producing lymphocyte and a tumor cell).

Hydrocele Fluid accumulation within the scrotum.

Hydrocephalus Pathological accumulation of cerebrospinal fluid in the ventricles of brain.

Hydronephrosis Accumulation of urine in the renal pelvis due to obstruction of urinary flow. Associated with atrophy of the renal parenchyma.

Hyper- Greater than, above normal.

Hyperalimentation Intravenous administration of nutrients for treatment of actual or potential malnutrition.

Hyperammonemia Excessive amounts of ammonia in the blood.

Hyperbaric oxygen Oxygen under increased pressure relative to the atmosphere.

Hyperemia Increased blood flow to a tissue.

Hypernatremia Increased serum sodium.

Hyperplasia Increase in the number of cells in a tissue.

Hypersensitivity Exaggerated and harmful immune response to a normally innocuous antigenic stimulus.

Hypertension Elevated blood pressure.

Hypertonic Of higher osmotic pressure than fluid on the other side of a semipermeable membrane (eg, cell membrane).

Hypertrophy Enlargement of an organ due to increase in size of its cells. Note distinction from hyperplasia.

Hypha A fungal filament.

Hypo- Less than, below normal.

Hypochlorhydria Reduced hydrochloric acid in the stomach.

Hypoglycemia Blood sugar below normal levels.

Hypotension Low blood pressure.

Hypothalamus Portion of the brain that forms the floor and part of the lateral wall of the third ventricle.

Hypothermia Serious reduction in body temperature.

Hypoxia Decreased oxygen supply to the tissues.

Icosahedron A solid geometric shape having 12 vertices. Serves as the structural basis for many viruses.

Icteric Pertaining to jaundice.

Idiopathic Of unknown origin.

Ig Abbreviation for immunoglobulin antibodies. Classes include IgG, IgM, IgA, IgD, IgE, and sIgA.

Ileitis Inflammation of the lower ileum.
Ileum Portion of the small intestine between the jejunum and the cecum.
Immunocompromise Deficiency in some components of the body's immune mechanisms.
Immunocyte Cell of the lymphoid series that responds to an antigenic stimulus by producing antibodies or initiating cell mediated immune processes.
Immunodiffusion A procedure involving diffusion of antigen and antibody towards each other in a gel. A visible precipitate develops where optimal concentrations interact.
Immunofluorescence A serologic procedure using antibody labeled with a fluorescent dye that allows visible detection of sites of reaction with antigen.
Immunogen An antigen that induces an immune response.
Immunoglobulins Large class of glycoproteins that constitute the antibodies produced in response to antigenic stimuli.
Impetigo Superficial pustular skin infection.
In vitro Occurring in the test tube.
In vivo Occurring in the living animal.
Inclusion body A morphologically distinct intracellular mass of viruses or virus components.
Infarct Interference with the blood supply producing local death of tissue.
Integument Skin.
Integrins Family of transmembrane proteins of eukaryotic cells that interact with extracellular matrix and cytoskeleton proteins
Inter- Between.
Interferon Class of cytokine proteins. When produced by virally infected cells they inhibit viral replication in these and adjacent cells.
Interleukin Class of cytokine produced by macrophages or T cells that mediate immune responses.
Interstitial Spaces between the cells of a tissue.
Intertriginous Pertaining to area between folds of the skin.
Intima Inner lining of a blood vessel.
Intra- Within.
Intrapartum Occurring during the process of childbirth.
Intrathecal Within the membranes of the spinal cord.
Introitus An opening.
Isoantigen Normal substance present in one individual that may elicit an antibody response in another.
Isotonic Of the same osmotic pressure as a solution on the other side of a semipermeable membrane.
-itis inflammation.

Janeway's lesions Painless macular lesions of palms and soles seen in acute bacterial endocarditis.
Jejunum Portion of small intestine between duodenum and ileum.

Kaposi's sarcoma Multiple malignant vascular tumors. Occur most commonly as a complication of AIDS.
Karotype Size, structure, and organization of chromosomes within a cell.
Karyosome Area of chromatin concentration in a cell nucleus.
Keratin Major protein of the skin, hair, and nails.
Keratitis Inflammation of the cornea of the eye.
Kilobase Unit to describe the lengths of a nucleotide sequence. One kilobase = 1000 nucleotides.
Kinetoplast Structure at the base of a protozoal flagellum.
Kupffer cells Fixed phagocytic cells of the liver sinusoids. Part of the reticulo-endothelial system.
Kwashiorkor Condition caused by severe protein malnutrition in children.

Labia Structures of the external female genitalia.
Lactoferrin Iron-binding protein present in milk, other secretions, and granules of neutrophil leukocytes.
Lamina propria Connective tissue supporting the epithelial cells of a mucous membrane.
Laminin Major protein component of basal lamina.
Latex beads Used to adsorb soluble antigens. The treated beads agglutinate with specific antibody.
Leukemia Malignant tumor of white blood cells.
Leuko- White; relating to a leukocyte.
Leukocyte White blood cells including granulocytes, lymphocytes, and monocytes.
Leukocytosis Increased blood leukocyte count.
Leukopenia Abnormally low leukocyte count.
Leukotrienes Products of arachidonic acid that mediate inflammatory and allergic reactions.
Ligand One component of a complex involving the binding of molecules or structures.
Lipo- Relating to fats or lipids.
Lobar Related to a lobe of the lung.
Lophotrichous Describing several flagella at one or both ends of a bacillus.
Lumen Cavity within a tubular organ.
Lupus erythematosus (systemic) Autoimmune inflammatory disease of skin, joints, and other tissues.
Lymph Tissue fluid derived from the bloodstream and passing to the lymphatics.
Lymphadenitis Enlarged, inflamed lymph nodes.
Lymphangitis Inflammation of lymphatic vessels.
Lympho- Pertaining to the lymphatic system.
Lymphocytosis Increased blood lymphocyte count.
Lymphokine Cytokine produced by lymphocytes.
Lymphoma Tumor of lymphatic tissues.
Lymphoreticular Relating to the reticuloendothelial system.
Lysis Dissolution of cells.
Lysosome Intracellular granules of cells that contain hydrolytic digestive enzymes.
Lysozyme Enzyme that breaks down peptidoglycan.
-lytic Pertaining to lysis.

Macro- Large.
Macrocytic anemia Anemia characterized by large erythrocytes.

Macrophage Tissue phagocyte derived from blood mononuclear cells.

Macule A flat lesion of skin rash.

Masseter Major muscle controlling movement of the lower jaw.

Mast cell Connective tissue cell analogous to the blood basophil. Granules contain heparin, histamine, and other vasoactive mediators.

Mastitis Inflammation of the breast.

Mastoid Process of temporal bone behind the ear that contains air cells.

Matrix Extracellular substance of tissues.

Meatus Orifice.

Meckel's diverticulum Congenital diverticulum of the lower part of the ileum.

Mediastinum Mid-portion of the chest including heart, bronchial bifurcation, and esophagus.

Medulla The inner portion of an organ within the cortex.

Medulla oblongata Portion of central nervous system between the brain and spinal cord.

Mega- Large.

Megacolon Dilatation of the colon.

-megaly Enlargement, usually of an organ.

Meiosis Cellular division process yielding haploid gametes.

Meninges The membranes covering the brain and the spinal cord.

Meningomyelocele Malformation of vertebral column with protrusion of meninges.

Mentation Mental activity; thinking.

Merozoite A stage in the life cycle of a sporozoan parasite resulting from asexual division; a daughter cell.

Mesenchymal Derived from the embryonic mesoderm layer.

Mesentery Fold of peritoneum surrounding the intestinal tract and attaching it to the posterior abdominal wall.

Mesophile A microbe that grows best at temperatures of approximately those of the body.

Mesosome A complex invagination of the bacterial cell membrane.

Metastases Satellite tumors or infections spread through lymphatics or the bloodstream from a primary site.

-metry measure.

Micro- Small.

Microaerophilic Can grow only in less than the atmospheric concentration of oxygen, or anaerobically.

Microcephaly Small head with failure of development of the brain.

Microphthalmia Failure to develop normal sized eyes.

Microtubule Cylindrical cytoskeletal element of animal and plant cells.

Mitochondria Complex cytoplasmic organelles of eukaryotic cells involved in oxidative phosphorylation.

Mitogen Substance that increases the normal frequency of mutations.

Mitral valve Valve between the left atrium and ventricle of the heart.

Monoclonal Derived from a single cell.

Monocyte Large mononuclear phagocyte of the blood. Precursor of the macrophage.

Monolayer A single layer of cultured eukaryotic cells on a glass or plastic surface.

Monotrichous Possessing a single flagellum.

Mordant Substance that enhances the effect of a stain.

Morphology The shape, size, and form of an organism or cell.

Mucolytic Substance that dissolves mucus.

Multiple sclerosis Chronic disorder involving disseminated focal damage to nerve cells.

Mutagen Substance that increases the mutation rate of cells or organisms.

Myalgia Pain in the muscles.

Mycelium A mass of fungal hyphae.

Mycetoma A localized granuloma or lesion caused by a fungus.

Mycosis A fungal infection.

Myelin Component of the myelin sheath around the axon of a neuron that increases the conduction velocity of the nerve impulse.

Myelitis Inflammation of the spinal cord.

Myeloma Malignant tumor derived from bone marrow cells.

Myeloperoxidase Intracellular enzyme of professional phagocytes.

Myo- Pertaining to muscle.

Myocardium Heart muscle.

Myringitis Inflammation of the tympanic membrane of the ear.

Nares Interior of the nostrils.

Nasal turbinates Three scroll-like bony projections from the lateral wall of the nasal cavity (nasal conchae).

Nasolacrimal duct Duct draining the conjunctiva into the nasal cavity.

Necrosis Death of tissue.

Neo- New.

Neoplasm Tumor.

Nephrito- Pertaining to the kidney.

Nephritogenic Producing inflammation of the kidneys.

Neuro- Pertaining to the central nervous system or nerves.

Neuromotor synapses Connections between nerve endings and muscle.

Neurone Nerve and its nerve cell.

Neutropenia Reduced number of circulating neutrophil leukocytes.

Neutrophils Major class of polymorphonuclear phagocytic leukocytes.

NGU Nongonococcal urethritis.

Nidus Focus of infection, a cluster.

Noma A gangrenous condition spreading from the oral cavity to the skin; seen in undernourished children.

Nosocomial Acquired within a hospital.

Nucleocapsid The nucleic acid-protein complex found inside an enveloped virus.

Nucleoid The double stranded circular DNA genome of a bacterium.

Nucleolus Round body within a eukaryotic nucleus that is the site of synthesis of ribosomal RNA.

Occult Hidden, inapparent.

Olfactory Pertaining to the sense of smell.

Olfactory bulb Terminal enlarged portion of the olfactory tract from which the olfactory nerves emerge.

Oligo- Small, few.

Oligodendroglia Specialized connective tissue of the central nervous system.

Onco- Pertaining to tumors.

Oncogene Gene whose activation is associated with malignant change and progression.

Ontogeny Origin and course of development of an individual organism.

Operculum A lid or cover.

Operon Operator gene and the adjacent structural gene(s) that it controls.

Ophthalmia Severe inflammation of the eye.

Opisthotonos Severe spasm of back muscles leading to hyperextension of the spine.

Opportunist A microorganism that only causes disease when the body's defenses are compromised or bypassed.

Opsonin Antibody or complement component that facilitates phagocytosis when bound to a microorganism.

Orbit Skull cavity that contains the eyeball.

Orchitis Inflammation of a testis.

Organelles Membrane-bound cytoplasmic structures of eukaryotic cells (eg, mitochondria).

Organogenesis Formation of the organs of the body.

Oro- Pertaining to the mouth.

-oscopy Use of an instrument to see within a viscus or vessel.

Osler's nodes Skin papules, usually of hands and feet, seen in bacterial endocarditis.

Ossicles Small bones (eg, of hearing).

Osteo- Pertaining to bone.

Osteomyelitis Inflammation of bone marrow and adjacent bone.

Oto- Pertaining to the ear.

Oviparous Producing eggs from which the embryo is released outside the body.

Oxidase Oxidation-reduction enzyme that catalyzes transfer of electrons to molecular oxygen with formation of water.

Pan- All, throughout.

Pandemic Worldwide severe epidemic.

Panencephalitis Inflammation of all tissues of the brain.

Papilla Small nipple-like swelling.

Papilledema Edema of the optic nerve and adjacent retina.

Papilloma Warty tumor of the epithelium.

Papule Small, firm, elevated nodule on the skin.

Para- Beside, abnormal.

Parasite An organism that lives on and at the expense of another organism.

Parasitism Describes the relationship between parasite and host.

Parenchymal Substance of body organs in contrast to their covering.

Parenteral Administration by injection rather than by mouth.

Paresis Paralysis.

Paresthesias Disorders of sensation; tingling.

Paronychia Infection of nail fold.

Parotid glands Salivary glands beneath the cheek.

Parturition The process of giving birth.

Pathogenic Capable of causing disease.

Pathognomonic Diagnostic, distinctive.

-pathy denoting disease.

-penia decreased numbers.

Pentamer A polymer of viral capsid having five structural units.

Peptidoglycan High molecular weight cross-linked polymer forming the rigid structure of the bacterial cell wall.

Peptone Protein hydrolysed product used as a source of amino acids in bacterial culture media.

Peri- Around, covering.

Periapical Beside the root of a tooth.

Pericardium Membranous lining around the heart.

Perineum Area between vulva or scrotum and the anus.

Periodontal Area around the tooth including supporting tissues.

Perioplasm Area between the outer and cell membranes of a Gram-negative bacterium. Contains the peptidoglycan layer.

Periosteum Membrane around the bone.

Peristalsis Normal contractile waves of a hollow organ.

Peristome The mouth and surrounding areas of certain ciliated protozoa.

Peritrichous Presence of multiple flagella around a bacterial cell.

Permease A protein of the bacterial cell membrane transport system.

Petechiae Small ($<$3 mm) hemorrhages in the skin containing red blood cells or hemoglobin.

Peyer's patches Lymphoid follicles in the ileum.

Phage Common abbreviation for bacteriophage.

Phagocyte A cell that ingests foreign material.

Phagolysosome The digestive vacuole formed by fusion of the cell lysosomes with the phagocytic vacuole.

Phenotype The properties expressed by the complete genome under particular conditions.

Pheromone Hormone-like substance that elicits a favorable or attraction response in an individual of the same species.

-phobia fear of, repulsion.

Phonation Speech.

Photophobia Intolerance of light.

-phylia affection for.

Phylogeny Pertaining to the evolution of a species.

PID Pelvic inflammatory disease.

Pilo-sebaceous Unit of hair follicle and sebaceous gland.

Pilus Fibrillar structure on the surface of a bacterial cell.

Pinocytosis Uptake of fluids into a cell by a mechanism analogous to phagocytosis.

Plankton Minute free-floating organisms, vegetable and animal, which live in natural waters.

Plaque A patch or flat area. An area of lysis in fixed host cells by an infecting virus.

Plasma Noncellular component of whole blood.

Plasmid Extrachromosomal circular double stranded DNA molecule.

Plasmin Derived from plasminogen–dissolves fibrin.

Platelet Small anucleate cell involved in filling small holes in blood vessels and in clotting mechanisms.

Pleo- More.

Pleocytosis Increased number of cells in a particular area.

Pleomorphism Variation in shape and size.

Pleura Membrane covering the lungs and thoracic cavity enclosing the pleural space.

Pleurisy Inflammation of the pleura.

Pleuro- Relating to the pleura.

Pleurodynia Pain caused by inflammation or irritation of the pleura.

Pneumocyte, Type I Flat cell lining alveoli of lung which is involved in gas exchange.

Pneumocyte, Type II Rounded surfactant-producing cell in alveoli of the lung.

Pneumonitis Inflammation of the lung.

Pneumothorax Air in the pleural cavity.

Poly- Many, repeated.

Polyarthralgia Pain in several joints.

Polycistronic Encoding two or more proteins (eg, polycistronic mRNA).

Polyclonal activation Simultaneous activation of different antibody producing clones of lymphocytes.

Polymerase chain reaction Continuous enzyme-mediated amplification of a nucleotide sequence that allows its detection and analysis.

Polymorphonuclear Two or more lobes to the nucleus.

Polymyositis Inflammation of many muscles.

Polyneuritis Inflammation of many nerves.

Polyp A sessile benign or malignant tumor of a mucous membrane (usually of colon).

Polyposis Presence of many polyps.

Porin Protein of outer membrane pores of Gram-negative bacteria.

Portal venous system Veins carrying blood from the intestinal tract to the liver.

Premenarcheal Prepubertal years in the female (before onset of menses).

Prepuce Foreskin.

Pro- Before, a precursor.

Proctoscopy Use of an instrument to examine interior of the rectum.

Prodromal Initial symptoms before the characteristic manifestations of disease develop.

Proglottid One of the segments of the body of a tapeworm.

Prokaryote Organism lacking a true nucleus. Possesses a single chromosome.

Prophage Complete bacterial virus genome integrated in the chromosome.

Prophylaxis Measures or treatments designed to prevent disease.

Prostaglandins Derivatives of arachidonic acid that mediate a variety of biological reactions including inflammation.

Prostate gland Gland surrounding the male urethra that produces part of the seminal fluid.

Prosthesis Artificial replacement of a missing part of the body.

Proteinuria Protein in the urine indicating a renal abnormality.

Prothrombin Precursor of thrombin; thrombin activates the terminal blood clotting mechanism.

Protomer Protein subunit of a viral capsomere.

Protoplasm The viscid colloidal solution that makes up living matter.

Protoplast A Gram-positive bacterium that has lost its cell wall.

Prototroph Bacterial strains with complete synthetic pathways from which auxotrophs may be derived.

Protozoan A unicellular member of the animal kingdom.

Proventriculus An enlargement of the alimentary tract of an invertebrate that precedes the stomach.

Provirus Complete viral genome integrated into a eukaryotic genome.

Pruritus Itching.

Pseudo- False.

Pseudopod A pseudopodium. Moving extrusion of the cytoplasm of an amoeboid cell that brings about movement or ingestion of food particles.

Psychrophile A microorganism that grows best or exclusively at low temperatures.

Puerperal Following childbirth.

Purpura Multiple hemorrhages in the skin, mucous membrane, or other organs.

Pustule Pus in an infected hair follicle or sweat gland producing a visible inflammatory swelling.

Pyelonephritis Infection of the pelvis and tissues of the kidney.

Pylephlebitis Inflammation in the portal venous system.

Pyo- Producing pus.

Pyogenic Producing pus and pustular lesions.

Pyuria Pus in the urine.

Radioimmunoassay A method for detecting antigen-antibody reactions that uses a radioisotope as a readily detectable label.

Rales Crackling respiratory sounds heard with the stethoscope.

Receptor Component of the cell surface to which another substance or organism attaches specifically.

Redox potential Oxidation–reduction potential.
Reduviid A large winged "cone-nosed" insect.
Renal Pertaining to the kidney.
Repressor A regulatory protein that binds to an operator sequence and inhibits expression of the adjacent gene.
Reservoir of infection Natural habitat or source of an infecting organism.
Reticuloendothelial system System of phagocytic monocytes, particularly those in the spleen, bone marrow, and lymph nodes.
Retinoblastoma Malignant tumor of the retina.
Retrovirus RNA virus, the genome of which is transcribed into DNA by its reverse transcriptase.
Reverse transcriptase RNA-directed DNA polymerase.
Rhino- Pertaining to the nose.
Rhinorrhea Continuous discharge of watery mucus from the nose.
Rhonchi Coarse snoring or rattling respiratory sounds heard with a stethoscope.
RIA *See* Radioimmunoassay.
Romana's sign Unilateral ophthalmia, edema of the eyelids, and enlarged draining lymph nodes.
Rostellum Portion of tapeworm head that contains hooklets or other attachment organs.

Salpingitis Inflammation of the fallopian tubes.
Saprophyte Organism living on dead organic material in the environment.
Sarcoidosis Disease of unknown etiology characterized by granulomatous lesions of many tissues and organs.
Sarcolemma Membrane surrounding muscle fibers.
Schizogony Asexual reproduction in sporozoa producing merozoites by multiple nuclear fusion followed by cytoplasmic segregation.
Schizont The multinucleated stage of a sporozoan undergoing schizogony.
Sclera White part of the eyeball.
Scolex The attachment organ or head of a tapeworm.
-scopy Denotes use of an instrument for visual examination of a hollow viscus (eg., bronchoscopy).
Scotoma A blind spot in the visual field.
Sebaceous Relating to sebum and sebum production.
Sebum Waxy secretion of sebaceous glands.
Seminal vesicles Sacs in which semen is stored prior to ejaculation.
Sepsis A term often used synonymously with septicemia, but implies the presence of circulating infectious agents.
Septicemia Evidence of systemic disease associated with presence of organisms in the blood (*see* Bacteremia).
Sequelae Results occurring subsequent to an infection or other disease.
Sequestrum Necrotic bony fragment.
Seroconversion Development of antibodies in response to an infection.
Serodiagnosis Diagnosis of an infection by serologic procedures.
Serotonin Vasoconstricting amine usually derived from platelets
Serotype Subtype of species detectable with specific antisera.
Serpiginous Moving irregularly from one place to another, snake-like.
Serum Liquid part of blood separable after clotting.
Shunt Deviation of blood or other body fluids (eg, from artery to vein).
Sickle cell anemia Hereditary anemia associated with crescent-shaped erythrocytes resulting from an abnormal hemoglobin.
Siderophore Compound that binds iron.
Sigmoid colon Lower portion of the colon between descending colon and rectum.
Sinus A tract leading from an infected area or hollow viscus to the surface; a wide venous blood channel; accessory nasal sinuses that are blind sacs draining to the nasopharynx.
Sinusoid A wide thin-walled venous passage. Smaller than a sinus.
Slime layer Term sometimes used for polysaccharide surface components of bacteria that do not constitute a morphologic capsule.
Spasticity Excessive tone of muscles leading to awkward movement.
Spheroplast A circular, osmotically unstable, Gram-negative rod that has lost its peptidoglycan layer.
Sphincter Circular muscle controlling a natural orifice.
Splanchnic Pertaining to the viscera.
Spleno- Relating to the spleen.
Sporogony Sexual reproduction process in sporozoan parasites leading to formation of oocysts and sporozoites.
Sporozoite Motile, elongated, infective stage of sporogony.
Sprue A chronic form of intestinal malabsorption.
Squamous epithelium Composed of layers of flattened cells.
Stasis Stagnation or cessation of flow of body fluids.
Stenosis Reduction in diameter of a blood vessel or tubular organ.
Steroids Derivatives of cholesterol including hormones, some of which have anti-inflammatory effects.
Sterol Lipid-soluble steroid with long aliphatic side chains. Present in eukaryotic cell membranes as cholesterol or ergosterol.
Stevens-Johnson syndrome A serious allergic reaction, characterized by multiple blister-like lesions of skin and mucous membrane.
Stomatitis Inflammation of the mouth.
Strabismus Squint.
Stratum corneum Outer keratinized part of the skin.
Stridor Harsh respiratory sound due to partial respiratory obstruction.
Strobila Chain of segments making up the body of a tapeworm.
Sub- Below.

Subarachnoid Cerebrospinal fluid containing area between the middle (arachnoid) and inner (pia mater) layers of the meninges.

Subdural Between the outer (dura mater) and middle (arachnoid) layers of the meninges.

Submandibular Below the jaw.

Subphrenic Below the diaphragm.

Sulcus Groove.

Suppurative Producing pus.

Supra- Above.

Surfactant A substance that acts on a surface to reduce surface tension (eg, a detergent).

Sylvatic Pertaining to the woods. Commonly applied to nonurban plague whether occurring in wooded or prairie land.

Symbiont An organism living on or in close association with another.

Synapse A connection between neurons for nerve impulse transmission.

Syncytium A multinucleate mass of fused cells.

Syndrome Group of clinical manifestations characterizing a particular disease or condition.

Synergistic Enhanced rather than additive effect of two agents or processes acting together.

Synovium Lining membrane of a joint, tendon, or bursa.

T cells Thymus derived immunocytes: helper, suppressor, and cytotoxic T cells.

Tachy- Increased rate, swift.

Tachypnea Abnormally rapid rate of breathing.

Talin One of the proteins that connects integrins to the actin cytoskeleton of eukaryotic cells.

Tamponade (cardiac) Increased fluid or constriction around the heart leading to interference in cardiac function.

Tenesmus Ineffective and painful straining at stool or urination.

Tenosynovitis Inflammation of a tendon sheath.

Teratogenic Causing abnormalities of fetal development.

Thalassemia Hereditary hemolytic anemia resulting from abnormal hemoglobin synthesis.

Thermo- Pertaining to heat.

Thermophile Bacteria with an optimal growth temperature of over 50°C.

Thrombo- Pertaining to thrombosis.

Thrombocyte See platelet.

Thrombocytopenia Abnormally low platelet count.

Thrombophlebitis Inflammation of a vein with thrombosis; may release infected emboli.

Thrombus A blood clot developing in vivo.

Thymus A lymphoid organ located in the anterior upper portion of the mediastinum. The site of maturation of T cells.

Titer Highest dilution of an active substance (eg, antibody in serum) that still causes a discernible reaction (eg, an agglutination reaction).

Tracheo- Pertaining to the trachea.

Tracheostomy Surgically produced artificial air passage to the trachea.

Trans- Across.

Transcriptase DNA-directed RNA polymerase.

Transferrin Serum protein that binds and transports iron.

Transovarial Passage of infectious agents to progeny by way of the egg. Usually occurs in ticks and mites.

Transposon A DNA segment carrying one or more recognizable genes that can move between plasmid and between plasmid and chromosome in both directions.

Trimester Usually means a three-month period of pregnancy.

Trismus Spasm of the masseter muscle; lockjaw.

Trophozoite The motile feeding stage of a protozoan parasite.

Tropism Having an affinity for a particular organ, or moving towards or away from a particular stimulus.

Tubulin Protein subunit of microtubules.

Tumorigenesis The property of causing tumors.

Turgor pressure Osmotic pressure of the cellular contents.

Tympanic membrane Eardrum.

Ultrasonograph Picture of deep organs of the body derived from reflection of ultrasonic waves.

Uremia Toxic accumulation of nitrogenous metabolites due to renal insufficiency.

Ureter Tube carrying urine from the kidney to bladder.

Urethra Tube carrying urine from the bladder to the exterior.

-uria Pertaining to urine.

Uropathic Causing disease of the urinary tract.

Urticaria Local edema and itching of the skin.

Uvea Inner vascular coat of the eyeball, including the iris.

Uvula Small extension hanging from the back of the soft palate.

Vacuolate Forming small holes or vacuoles.

Vacuole Microscopic hole or cavity.

Vagotomy Surgical cutting of the vagus nerve.

Vasa vasorum Small blood vessels in walls of veins and arteries.

Vasculitis Inflammation of blood vessels.

Vaso- Pertaining to blood vessels.

Vector An aminate transmitter of disease (eg, an insect).

Venipuncture Insertion of a hypodermic needle into a vein—usually to draw blood.

Ventricle Fluid cavity (eg, chamber of the heart).

Vesicle Small fluid filled cavity (eg, a blister-like lesion of the skin).

Vesicoureteral junction Junction of ureter with the urinary bladder.

Vestibular function Function of the vestibular branch of the eighth cranial nerve concerned with the body's equilibrium.

Vinculin One of the proteins that connects integrins to the actin cytoskeleton of eukaryotic cells.

Viremia Presence of a virus in the bloodstream.

Virion A complete virus particle.

Viropexis Viral entry into the cell by phagocytosis.

Viruria Viruses in the urine.

Viscera Interior organs of the body (eg, the intestinal tract).

Vitreous humor The clear viscous fluid in the posterior chamber of the eye.

Vitronectin Protein component of extracellular matrix.

Viviparous Developing young within the body as opposed to oviparous.

Western blot Test for antibodies to specific proteins separated by gel electrophoresis.

Whitlow Abscess of the terminal pulp of the finger. Also paronychia.

Wright's stain Stain for blood cells that has similar properties to Giemsa stain.

Xenodiagnosis Recovery of a parasite by allowing an arthropod to feed on the patient and seeking the parasite in the arthropod.

Xerostomia Dry mouth from dysfunction of the salivary glands.

Zoonosis A disease transmittable to humans from an animal host or reservoir.

Zygote The cell that results from fusion of male and female gamete.

Zymodeme An isoenzyme typing pattern.

INDEX

INDEX

Page numbers followed by *t* and *f* indicate tables and figures, respectively. Page numbers in **boldface** indicate major discussions.

B

E

G

M

Q

R

S

T

U

V

W

X

Y

Z

A DICTIONARY

OF THE TARGUMIM, THE TALMUD BABLI AND YERUSHALMI, AND THE MIDRASHIC LITERATURE

COMPILED BY

MARCUS JASTROW, Ph. D. Litt. D.

WITH AN INDEX OF SCRIPTURAL QUOTATIONS

VOLUME I:

א—כ

PARDES PUBLISHING HOUSE, INC.
NEW YORK

PREFACE.

The literature embraced in this Dictionary covers a period of about one thousand years, and contains Hebrew and Aramaic elements in about equal proportions. The older Hebrew elements, which may conveniently be called the Mishnaic, and can in part be traced back to the first, if not to the second, century B. C. E., may be considered a continuation of the Biblical Hebrew—Biblical Hebrew tinged with Aramaisms. It is therefore apt to throw light, more directly than its successor, on many obscure words and passages in the Bible; nevertheless, the material for Biblical exegesis deposited in the later literature is an inexhaustible mine, which still awaits exploitation by sympathetic students. Besides the Mishnah and the Tosefta, the Mishnaic period embraces Sifra and Sifré, Mekhilta, and the older elements preserved in the Gemara, of which the prayers incidentally quoted are a very essential and interesting part.

The later Hebrew elements in the Gemara and in the Midrashim lead down to the fifth and the eighth century respectively, and to a larger degree than the earlier Hebrew sections are mixed with Aramaic elements, and with foreign words borrowed from the environment and reflecting foreign influences in language as well as in thought. The Aramaic portions of the literature under treatment comprise both the eastern and the western dialects.[1] Owing to the close mental exchange between the Palestinian and the Babylonian Jews, these dialects are often found inextricably interwoven, and cannot be distinguished lexicographically.

The subjects of this literature are as unlimited as are the interests of the human mind. Religion and ethics, exegesis and homiletics, jurisprudence and ceremonial laws, ritual and liturgy, philosophy and science, medicine and magics, astronomy and astrology, history and geography, commerce and trade, politics and social problems, all are represented there, and reflect the mental condition of the Jewish world in its seclusion from the outer world, as well as in its contact with the same whether in agreement or in opposition.

---

1 For these Aramaic elements the traditional (though admittedly incorrect) term Chaldaic (Ch., ch.) is retained in the Dictionary, wherever the designation is required for distinction from the corresponding Hebrew forms.

Owing to the vast range and the unique character of this literature, both as to mode of thinking and method of presentation, it was frequently necessary to stretch the limits of lexicography and illustrate the definitions by means of larger citations than would be necessary in a more familiar domain of thought. Especially was this the case with legal and with ethical subjects.

Archæological matters have often been elucidated by references to Greek and Roman customs and beliefs.

The condition of the texts, especially of the Talmud Yerushalmi and of some of the Midrashim, made textual criticism and emendations inevitable, but the dangers of arbitrariness and personal bias had to be guarded against. Happily there were, in most cases, parallels to be drawn upon for the establishment of a correct text, and where these auxiliaries failed, the author preferred erring on the conservative side to indulging in conjectural emendations. For the Babylonian Talmud Raphael Rabbinowicz's Variae Lectiones was an invaluable aid to the author.

The etymological method pursued in this Dictionary requires a somewhat fuller explanation than is ordinarily embodied in a preface.

The Jewish literature here spoken of is specifically indigenous, in which respect it is unlike the Syriac literature contemporary with it, which is mainly Christian, and as such was influenced, not only in thought but also in language, by the Greek and Latin tongues of the religious teachers of a people itself not free from foreign admixtures. Foreign influences came to Jewish literature merely through the ordinary channel of international intercourse. It is for this reason, if for no other, that the Jewish literature of post-Biblical days down to the ninth century may be called original. Hence it is natural to expect that, in extending the horizon of thought, it also extended its vocabulary on its own basis, employing the elements contained in its own treasury.

Starting from such premises, the investigator had to overhaul the laws regulating the derivation of words whose etymology or meaning is unknown from known Semitic roots; every word of strange appearance had to be examined on its merits both as to its meaning or meanings and as to its origin; the temptation offered by phonetic resemblances had to be resisted, and the laws of word-formation common to all other original languages as well as the environment in which a word appears had to be consulted before a conclusion could be reached. The foremost among these laws is that a word is imported into one language from another with the importation of the article it represents or of the idea it conveys. Unless these conditions of importation are apparent, the presumption should be in favor of the home market.

Take e. g. the word **סימטא** and its dialectic equivalent **איסמטא**, which means

[1] The attempt to make biliteral roots the basis for radical definitions of stems was found too cumbersome and too much subject to misunderstanding, and was therefore abandoned with the beginning of the third letter of the alphabet.

(a) a recess, an alley adjoining the market place to which the merchants retire for the transaction of business, also the trader's stand under the colonnade, and (b) an abscess, a carbuncle. The Latin *semita*, which since Musafia has been adopted as the origin of *simṭa*, offers hardly more than an assonance of consonants: a foot-path cannot, except by a great stretch, be forced into the meaning of a market stand; and what becomes of *simṭa* as *abscess*? But take the word as Semitic, and סמט, dialectically = שמט[1], offers itself readily, and as for the process of thought by which 'recess', 'nook', goes over into 'abscess' in medical language, we have a parallel in the Latin 'abscessus.' How much Latin medical nomenclature may have influenced the same association of ideas among the Jews is a theme of speculation for students of comparative philology or of the physiology of language.

A superficial glance at the vocabulary of this Dictionary will convince the reader that the example here given represents an extremely numerous class. The cases may not always be so plain, and the author is prepared for objections against his derivations in single instances, but the number of indisputable derivations from known Semitic roots remains large enough to justify the method pursued.

The problem becomes more complicated when both the meaning and the origin of words are unknown. Such is the case e. g. with the word אספרס in the phrase (Num. R. s. 4[20]) הופך אספירס ומשוור, he turned the *isperes* and leaped. Levy, guided by Musafia, resorts to σφυρόν, *ankle;* others suspect in it the name of a garment, σπεῖρος, a rare form for σπεῖρον. But the phrase itself and the context in which it appears indicate a native word, and this is found in the stem פ־ס, of which אספרס is an 'Ispeel' noun, that is to say, a noun formed from the enlarged stem ספ־ס. As פֶּרֶס or פַּרְסָה is the cloven foot, the latter being also applied to the human foot (Sifré Deuteronomy 2), so אִסְפֶּרֶס is the front part of the foot, where the toes begin to separate. The phrase quoted is to be translated, 'he (David) inverted the front part of his foot', i. e. stood on tiptoe, 'and leaped' (danced).

We meet with the same stem in the Aramaic, אספריסא. Referring to Lamentations III, 12, 'he has bent his bow and set me (literally: made me to stand) as a mark for the arrow', one Amora is recorded in the Midrash (Lamentations Rabbah a. l.) as having explained *kammaṭṭara laḥets* by כבורמא לאספריסא. Another is quoted as saying, 'like the pole of the archers (the Roman palus) at which all aim, but which remains standing.' What is בורמא? and what is אספריסא? The medieval Jewish commentators frankly admit their ignorance. Musafia, however, reads פרמא, maintaining that he had found it in some editions, and refers to Latin *parma*, explaining *isp'risa* as *sparus*, and translating, 'as the shield to the spear.' Ingenious, indeed! But on closer inspection this explanation is beset with intrinsic difficulties. To begin with, *parma* as shield does not appear in the Talmudic literature again, from which we may infer that it was not generally known to the Jews in their

---

1 In fact where Pesaḥim 50[b] has חגרי סימטא, Tosefta Biccurim end, in Mss. Erfurt and Vienna, reads חגרי שמיטה, which is obviously a corruption of שימטה, the pure Hebrew form for the Aramaic סימטא.

combats with the Romans. Furthermore, the *sparus* is a small hunting spear never used in battle to aim against the warrior's shield. As the entire passage in the Midrash quoted conveys the purpose of the interpreters to explain the Biblical text by means of a popular illustration, the Amora reported to have used this expression would have utterly missed his object, had he employed foreign and unfamiliar words, when he might have used plain words like כמגן לרומח, or their Aramaic equivalents. If, furthermore, it is taken into consideration that editio Buber of Lam. R., in agreement with the Arukh, reads רבנן דתמן אמרין for חד אמר, thus distinctly referring to Babylonian authorities, the supposition of foreign origin for בורמא and אספריסא falls to the ground.[1] But, on the other hand, take אספריסא as an 'Ispeel' noun of the stem פרס, and it means 'that which is to be cloven', i. e. the log, corresponding to the Hebrew בקעת. What is בורמא, or פרמא, again on the assumption that it is a home word? The root ברם like פרם means *to divide, to split*[2], and *burma* or rather *bor'ma* is 'the splitter', i. e. the wedge used to split the log. The Amora quoted in the Midrash therefore means to say that Israel, although the target of hostile attacks, is what the wedge is to the log: the wedge is struck, but the log is split. The other Amora quoted expresses the same idea by a different metaphor: 'as the pole of the arrows', and likewise a third, who lays stress on ריציבני, 'he caused me to stand', in the sense of enduring. An analogous expression to בורמא is פלגיסא (Pales of פלג), with which Targum renders the same Hebrew word (מטרה) that forms the subject of comment in the Midrash just referred to (I Samuel XX, 20).

The following lines are intended to give some specimens of such extension of roots, both Hebrew and Aramaic, as have not been recognized heretofore, or, if recognized, have not been applied to their full extent.

Ithpaal or Ithpeel nouns in Aramaean and Aramaicized Hebrew, and Hithpael nouns in Hebrew are too well known to require more than mere mention. Formations like השתחויה, אתכנע, אצטרכיא are recognized on their face. Except for the preconceived notions concerning the nature of the Talmudic vocabulary, it would seem no more than natural that the Mishnaic אצטלית or אסטלית (Yoma VII, 1) should be an enlargement of טלית, i. e. an Ithpaal noun of טלל, and אצטלית לבן merely a synonym of בגדי לבן in the same Mishnah, meaning 'covering', i. e. a suit of clothes, whereas the plainer form טלית is used for cloak or sheet. From among the vocables reclaimed for the Semitic store on the same principle, one more may be mentioned here. איצטמא or איסטמא is a derivative of צמם, and, as such, a phonetic and actual equivalent of the Biblical צַמָּה, and the meaning of the Hebrew word should be learned from its well-defined Aramaic representative: 'something which restrains the

---

1 That Arukh ed. Kohut and Buber in Lam. R. read אספריתא, with ת for ס, cannot be taken into consideration in view of the numerous evidences in favor of אספריסא.

2 Compare Targum I Chronicles V, 12, ברם מלכותא, 'a portion of the kingdom' and the particle ברם 'besides', and B'rakhoth 39a פרמינהו פרימי, 'he chopped them into pieces.'

flying locks' (Sabbath 57[b]), i. e. a hair-band worn, as we further learn from the discussion concerning *isṭ'ma,* under the hair net or cap. To uncover the צמה (Isaiah XLVII, 2) therefore means to throw off the matron's head-cover and appear as a slave. The variant אסט' for אצט' in these forms is a common phenomenon in Talmudic orthography.

In connection with this noun formation it may not be out of place to note that Ithpaal or Ithpeel nouns sometimes drop the initial Aleph, in which case they may resume the regular order of consonants, which is inverted in the verb. Thus מצדקא (M'naḥoth 41[a]) is formed from אצטדק, the Ithpaal of צדק, 'to justify one's self' (compare Genesis XLIV, 16), and means *justification, excuse.* Another מצדקא is formed from the root סדק, and means *split, breaking through, damage* (Baba Ḳamma 56[a]). מצהר (Giṭṭin 86[a]) is an Ithpeel noun of צהר (=זהר), and means *a shining white spot,* a suspicious symptom of leprosy; and, indeed, Alfasi reads צהר.[1] The Mandaic dialect offers analogies to these formations (see Noeldeke, Mand. Gramm. § 48, sq.).

The enlargement of stems by the prefix ש is well known in the Aramaic *Shafel,* but evidences of this same process are to be met with also in classical Hebrew. We have קוץ and שקץ, מוץ and שמץ, להב and שלהבת, and many more. More frequent is the use of the prefix ת for the formation of verbal nouns, as תְּפִלָּה, תְּרוּמָה, &c. Such verbal nouns may again become the basis for the formation of nominal verbs, as התפלל, 'to pray', which only by a stretch of the imagination can be explained as a plain Hithpael. So also הִתְרוֹעֵעַ, 'to shout' (Ps. LXV, 14; LX, 10; CVIII, 10), is to be taken as a derivative of תְּרוּעָה. The Talmudic Hebrew offers these formations in abundance, as הִתְחִיל from תְּחִלָּה, תָּרַם from תְּרוּמָה (see Abraham Geiger, Die Sprache der Mischnah, § 7).

On this principle of enlarged stems many words in this Dictionary have been regained from foreign origin for Semitic citizenship, e. g. תריס, 'shield', and its derivatives in Hebrew and Aramaic, שוכתא and שתך (see the Dictionary s. vv.).

The letter ס is an equivalent of ש in the Shafel forms in the later Hebrew as in the Aramaic; hence words like סרב, Piel סֵרֵב from רב; סרהב from רהב; סרגל from רגל; סרק, 'to be empty', from רק, and many more.

A further development of Safel stems consists in formations which for convenience' sake may be defined as 'Ispeel' nouns, of which the aforementioned אספירס and אספריסא may serve as examples.

The same letters, ש, ת, ס, and also ז, are used as intensive suffixes. The Biblical רטפש and פרשז have been explained by some as enlargements of רטף (= רטב) and פרש respectively. Be this as it may, the Talmudic Hebrew and the Aramaic possess such intensive suffixes. פרכס belongs to פרך, 'to crush, grind, scrape', and the various significations of this enlarged stem and its derivatives can easily be traced back to the fundamental meaning (see Dict. s. v. פרכס I and II). Only to

---

1 See Dictionary s. v. מצהר for an explanation of the misinterpretation which the word has suffered at the hands of commentators.

one derivative of פרכס reference may here be made. אפרכסת is 'the grinder', i. e. the hopper in the mill, and were it not for the tenacious prejudice in favor of foreign etymologies, no scholar would ever have thought of resorting for the original of *ăfarkheseth* to πρόχοος or ἅρπαξ, neither of which has any connection with the grinding process.[1]

For words with suffixed ז the reader is referred to אטליז and קטלוזא as specimens.

Enlargements by suffixed ד have been recognized in פרקד and אפרקיד. More frequent is the formation by prefixed ־ד, originally the demonstrative or relative pronoun. In the Dictionary these forms are designated as Difel, Dispeel, or Dithpeel nouns. The well-known דביתא in the form of ־ד דביתהו for 'the wife of' furnishes the key for the explanation of words like דמחמרא, דימחמ־א (Targum Isaiah XXIII, 13; XXX, 2, for Hebrew מפלה); דאיסקרתא, contracted דיסקרתא, an enlargement of קרתא, 'private town, settlement'; דישתקא and דיסתקא, a denominative of שקא, 'handle of an axe' (Syr. אסתקא and דסתקא); דיסתודר (Sabb. 48[a]), 'shreds of a turban' (Ms. M. סודר), and many more.

ל *as a formative suffix* appears in classical Hebrew, as כרמל, חרגל &c. (See Gesenius Thesaurus sub littera ל.) Of Talmudic Hebrew there may be mentioned here אַרְבֵּל, עַרְבֵּל (from ארב, ערב, *to knit, interlace*), meaning *sieve*, from which the verb אִרְבֵּל (רבל), *to sift.* Correspondingly the Aramaic ארבלא, ערבלא, is *sieve*, the verb ארבל, *to sift, shake*, ערבל, *to confound* (compare the metaphor in Amos IX, 9), and ערבלאין, *mixed multitude.*

It would have been superfluous to refer here to that well-known enlargement of stems by suffixed ל, were it not that even for so common a utensil as a sieve foreign languages have been ransacked, and *arb'la* or *'arb'la* has been found in the Latin cribellum. The enlarged stem ארבל finds a further extension in סרבל, for which verb and its derivatives the reader is referred to the Dictionary itself.

Reduplications of entire stems or of two letters of triliteral stems are well known. But there appear also reduplications of one letter employed for enlargement. גלגלתא=גוגלתא, דבדבא=דידבא, לשלשת=לשישית, which may be explained as contractions, find a counterpart in דשתנא, *thresher* or *grist-maker*, which is a reduplication of דוש or דשש.

These reduplications are especially remarkable for the transpositions of the radicals with which they are frequently connected. The stem געגע appears as a reduplication of געא, געה, in the sense of *lowing, roaring*, and figuratively of *longing for* and *howling against.* But it also occurs as a transposition of עגעג, a reduplication of עוג, with the meaning of *rolling around.* מלמל, from מלל, interchanges with למלם,

[1] This אפרכסת has nothing in common with ארפכס (ἅρπαξ=ὑδράρπαξ, ἁρπάγιον), 'the waterclock', which appears in Gen. R. s. 4. In Kelim XIV, 6, and XXX, 4, where a metal *harpax* and a glass *harpax* are respectively mentioned, the Arukh has preserved the correct reading ארפכס, where the editions have אפרכס. The latter reading has misled the commentators into identifying the word with אפרכסת, and it forced Maimonides, who realized the difficulty of a 'glass hopper', to assume the meaning of a hopper-shaped vessel, a funnel.

signifying *to talk against, murmur.* כַּסְכֵּס, apocopated כֶּסֶךְ, is a transposition of סכסך. שלשל interchanges with לשלש in the nouns שלשול and לשלשת, with their Aramaic equivalent לשלושתא, and in the contracted forms לשישית and שלשושית.[1]

It need scarcely be said that these outlines of Talmudic etymology by no means exhaust the subject. They have been given a place here for the purpose of showing the basis upon which the work has been constructed, and as a justification of the author's deviation from the views hitherto prevailing on the subject under consideration.

A few remarks on FOREIGN WORDS in the literature which for the sake of brevity is here called Talmudic, may not be out of place in this preface.

The intercourse between the Jews of the Talmudic ages with Greek and Latin speaking gentiles was not only that of trade and government, but also of thought and ideas. Along with the apostles and teachers of young Christianity, and even before their time, Jewish champions of religion and morality lectured in the private rooms of princes and princesses, noblemen and matrons. Instances of intimate association of prominent Jewish teachers with emperors, kings, philosophers, and scholars and their families are related in the Talmudic records in numbers large enough to account for the adoption of words like *philosophy, astrology, epilogue,* &c., not to speak of such terms as were borrowed by the Jews together with the objects or ideas which they represent. A footstool was called *hypopodion*, a tablet *pinax;* the profligate gourmand's emetic taken before meals, or rather between one stage of the banquet and the other, was called by its jocular name ἀποκοτταβίζειν (to play the cottabus), and adopted in the general medical sense; and so forth.

This accounts for the large number of Greek and Latin vocables in the so-called Jerusalem Talmud grown up under the Greco-Roman influences of the Cæsars, and more still in those Targumim and Midrashim which were compiled in the Byzantine empire. The Agadah, taking its illustrations from the daily environment, speaks of *Cæsar, Augustus, duces, polemarchi, legiones, matrona, schola,* &c., while in legal discussions the institutions of the governments, in so far as they influenced or superseded the Jewish law, had to be called by their foreign names. *Agoranomos* and *agronomia, angaria* and *parangaria, epimeletes, epitropos, bulé,* and innumerable other terms were embodied in the Jewish vocabulary, although not always dislodging their Hebrew or Aramaic equivalents.

Owing to copyists' mistakes and acoustic deficiencies of transmission in distant ages and countries in which these foreign words were but vaguely understood, the student has on this point to contend with a vast number of corruptions and glossators' guesses at interpretation. In most cases, however, these corruptions are recoverable through the medium of correct or differently corrupted parallels.

---

[1] See Jastrow, Transposed Stems, Drugulin, Leipzig 1891, and the Dictionary under the respective words.

אנדוכתרי (אנדכתרי, אונד׳, Giṭṭin 20[a]), not recognized by the commentators, and probably no longer understood by the Babylonian Rabbis, who received the word from Palestine together with the legal subject with which it is connected, fortunately finds a parallel in a worse copyist's corruption in the Jerusalem Talmud, namely הרנירק טיאניס (Yer. Giṭṭin IV, 45[d]), and both in אנטוקטא (Treatise Abadim, ed. Kirchheim, ch. IV). A combination of these corruptions together with an examination of the subject under discussion leads to *vindicta* or *vindicatio(-nis)* (see Révue des Études Juives, 1883, p. 150). It should be said, however, that this is one of the worst corruptions the author has met with.

Another class of corruptions owes its existence to the natural tendency to adapt foreign words to the organic peculiarities of the people. The people pronounced *Andrianos* or *Andrinos* more easily than *Hadrianos; unkeanos* was more congenial than *okeanos, agard'mos* and *agromos* are popular mutilations of *agoranomos;* גלגטיקא and כלכדיקא are organic transformations of *lectica;* although the correct forms Hadrianos, okeanos, &c. are by no means infrequent (see Collitz, The Aryan Name of the Tongue, in 'Oriental Studies', Boston, 1894, p. 201, note).

Otherwise the foreign consonants are transliterated as faithfully as can be expected with national organic peculiarities as different as the Aryan and the Semitic. Transpositions of *rd* and *dr*, frequent even in Hebrew or Aramaic homewords, or *sch* for *x (chs)*, need hardly surprise any one. Thus הרדולים and הרדבלא go side by side with אדרבלים, for *hydraulis;* סקימיון stands for *xenium;* דוכסוסטוס for *dyschistos*, and so forth.

As to vowels, the Greek η and the Latin ē are, as a rule, represented by י, the Greek οι by ו or וי, whereas the Greek ευ frequently appears as יו. The Greek υ and the Latin *u* keep their place as midway between vowels and consonants, so that they may be transcribed by י, ו, or ב. The last is especially the case in diphthongs, so that בולבטס is met with alongside of בולווטס, and בוליוטס for βουλεύτης.

Short vowels, except in cases of heavy accumulations of consonants, are most frequently ignored. This omission of vowels, congenial as it is to the Semitic spirit, means a loss of soul to the Aryan words, and offers difficulties not easily overcome.

The laws of transliteration of Greek and Latin loanwords are exhaustively treated in Samuel Krauss, „Griechische und Lateinische Lehnwörter in Talmud, &c." (Berlin, S. Calvary & Co., 1898). It is to be regretted that the proclivity to find Latin and Greek in words indisputably Semitic has led the author into a labyrinth of fatal errors.

Persian words are now and then encountered in the Talmud as remnants of the first period after the Babylonian exile, when the new Jewish commonwealth was organized under the Persian empire, and more still as modern arrivals of the time when Babylonia grew to be the centre of Jewish lore.

Arabic elements of direct importation, barring explicit linguistic references, came along with Arabic objects of trade, but there should be a considable reduction from the number hitherto accepted in Talmudic lexicography. The Hebrew and Aramaic of the Talmudic period had little to learn from a people which after the close of the Talmudic era became the world's teacher.

The difficulties besetting the study of Talmud and Midrash will be overcome in the degree in which modern scholars will take it up for philological and archæological purposes as adjuncts of those who are too much engrossed in its practical and doctrinal side to allow themselves time for what seems to them unessential. But even what has been heretofore rediscovered, as it were, thanks to the labors of Leopold Zunz, Samuel Loeb Rapaport, Heinrich Graetz, Zacharias Frankel, Michael Sachs, Solomon David Luzzatto, Abraham Geiger, M. Joel, Joseph Perles, Alexander Kohut, and a host of others, is enough to prove the marvellous familiarity of the Rabbis with the events, institutions, and views of life of the world outside and around their own peculiar civilization. What is more, we have been familiarized with the philosophical impartiality and sober superiority with which they appreciated what was laudable and reprehended what was objectionable in the intellectual and moral condition of the 'nations of the world', as they called the gentile world around them; kings and empires, nations and governments, public entertainments and social habits, they reviewed through the spy-glass of pure monotheism and stern morality.

In conclusion, the author begs to state his indebtedness to Jacob Levy's Targumic and Neo-Hebrew Dictionaries, where an amount of material far exceeding the vocabularies of the Arukh and Buxtorf's Lexicon Hebraicum et Chaldaicum is accumulated, which alone could have encouraged and enabled the author to undertake a task the mere preparation for which may well fill a lifetime.

Thanks are also rendered here for the munificent subventions which enabled the author to publish a work by its nature requiring great pecuniary sacrifices. To the list of subscribers mentioned on the title sheet of the first volume, the following should be added: Mr. Emanuel Lehman, Mr. Louis Stern, the Honorable Isidor Straus, the Honorable Oscar S. Straus, all of New York, and Judge Mayer Sulzberger of Philadelphia (additional subscription). It gives the author considerable pleasure to place among the subscriptions a gift of the school children of the Congregation Rodef Shalom of Philadelphia, on the occasion of the seventieth birthday of its Rabbi Emeritus.

The author also expresses his gratitude to the friends who have assisted him in the arduous task of proof reading, among whom special mention is due to Miss Henrietta Szold, of Baltimore. He also acknowledges his obligation to the Rev. Dr. S. Mendelsohn, of Wilmington, N. C., for the index of Scriptural citations appended to this work, a contribution which, the author is confident, will be welcomed by all Biblical students.

The religious sentiments inspiring the author at the completion of his labors of five and twenty years are too sacred to be sent abroad beyond the sanctuary of heart and home.

Philadelphia, May, 1903.

MARCUS JASTROW

Hebrew or Aramaic Abbreviations

in Talmud and Midrash, including abbreviations of the most frequently occurring names of Rabbis.

אברהם אבינו=א"א
אי אמרת=א"א
אי אפשר=א"א
אשת איש=א"א
אי אמרת בשלמא=אא"ב
אלא אם כן=אא"כ
איכא בינייהו=א"ב
אי בעית אימא=אב"א
איכא דאמרי=א"ד
אדם הראשון=אדה"ר
אי הכי=א"ה
אוה"ע=א"ה
(אומרים) אומר=או'
אומות העולם=אוה"ע
אחר כך=אח"כ
ארץ ישראל=א"י
אב"א=איב"א
אמן יהא שמיה רבה=א' יהש"ר
אם כן=א"כ
אמר, אמר להם, אמר לו=א"ל
אמרו לו, ליה &c.
אלהים=אל"ף למ"ד (in benedictions)
אלהינו מלך העולם=אמ"ה (in benedictions)
אי נמי=א"נ
את, את עצמה, את עצמו=א"ע
עצמן
אף על גב=אע"ג
אף על פי=אע"פ / אע"פי
אפילו=אפי'
אין צריך, אין צריכין &c.=א"צ
אמר קרא=א"ק
אשר קדשנו במצותיו וצונו=אקב"ו (in benedictions)
אמר רב, אמר רבי=א"ר
אתי שפיר=א"ש
אל תיקרי=א"ת
אם תימצי לומר=את"ל
בני אדם=ב"א
ברוך אתה יי'=בא"י (in benedictions)
בבא בתרא=ב"ב
בר בר=ב"ב
בר בר חנא=בב"ח
בית דין=ב"ד
במה דברים אמורים=בד"א
בית הלל=ב"ה
בית המקדש=ב"ה
בעל הבית=ב"ה
ברוך הוא=ב"ה
בית הלל אומרים=בה"א
בית הכנסת=בה"כ
בית הכסא=בה"כ
בית המדרש=בה"מ / בהמ"ד
ברכת המזון=בהמ"ז
בית המקדש=בהמ"ק
בין השמשות=בה"ש
בשר ודם=ב"ו / בו"ד
בן זכאי=ב"ז
בזמן הזה=בזה"ז
בעל חוב=ב"ח
בעלי חיים=ב"ח
בני ישראל=ב"י
בהמ"ק=ביהמ"ק
ברכת כהנים=ב"כ
בכל מקום=בכ"מ
בורא מיני מזונות=במ"מ (in benediction)
במה מצינו=במ"מ
בנותן טעם=בנ"ט
בעל הבית=בע"ה
בעל כרחו=בע"כ
בעל פה=בע"פ
בורא פרי=ב"פ (in benediction)
בורא פרי האדמה=בפה"א (in benediction)
בורא פרי העץ=בפה"ע (in benediction)
בפני נכתב ובפני=בפ"נ ובפ"נ
נחתם
בפני עצמו=בפ"ע
בר רב, בר רבי, בן רבי=ב"ר
ברכת המזון=ברהמ"ז
(בן רבי) ברבי שמעון=בר"ש
בית שמאי=ב"ש
בית שמאי אומרים=בש"א
בשם רבי, בשם רב=בש"ר
גזר דין=ג"ד / גז"ד
גזירה שוה=גז"ש
גמילות חסדים=ג"ח
גילוי עריות=ג"ע
גן עדן=ג"ע
גז"ש=ג"ש
דבר אחר=ד"א
דאמרי אינשי=דא"א
דברי הכל=ד"ה
דברי סופרים=ד"ס
דברי רבי=ד"ר
דברי, דבר תורה=ד"ת
יהוה, read אדני=ה'
הקב"ה=הב"ה
הכא במאי עסקינן=הב"ע
היכי דמי=ה"ד
הוא הדין=ה"ה
הדא הוא דכתיב=הה"ד
הרי זו, הרי זה=ה"ז
הוה להו, הוה ליה=ה"ל
הוה ליה למימר=הל"ל
הלכה למשה מסיני=הלמ"מ
הני מילי=ה"מ
היך מאי דאת אמר=המד"א
המוציא מחבירו עליו=המע"ה
הראיה
הכי נמי=ה"נ
ה"מ=הנ"מ
הכי קאמר=ה"ק / הק"א
הקדוש ברוך הוא=הקב"ה
ואין צריך לומר=ואצ"ל
ואם תאמר=וא"ת
וגומר=וגו'=&c.
וחד אמר=וח"א
וחכמים אומרים=וח"א / וחכ"א
ויש אומרים=וי"א
וכוליה, וכולו=וכו'=&c.
וכי תימא=וכ"ת
זו את זו, זה את זה=זא"ז
זכרונם, זכרונו) זכור לטוב=ז"ל
לברכה)
זה שאמר הכתוב=זש"ה
חד אמר=ח"א
חכ"א=ח"א
חול המועד=חה"מ
חס ושלום=ח"ו
חכמים אומרים=חכ"א
חוצה לארץ=ח"ל
ט"ו=*fifteen*
יש אומרים=י"א
יום הכפורים=י"ה / יה"כ
יהוה=יו"ד ה"א
י"ט=יו"ט
ידי חובתו=י"ח
שמונה עשרה=י"ח (benedictions)
יום טוב=י"ט
יהוה, read אדני=יי'
יצר הרע=יצה"ר
יצר טוב=יצ"ט
יהי רצון מלפניך=יר"מ (prayer)
כל אחד ואחד=כאו"א
כהן גדול=כ"ג
כדאמרי אינשי=כד"א / כדא"א
כ"ג=כה"ג
כי האי גונא=כה"ג
כנסת הגדולה=כה"ג
כמה וכמה=כו"כ
כל זמן=כ"ז
כל כך=כ"כ
כל מקום=כ"מ
כולי עלמא=כ"ע
כי פליגי=כ"פ
כל שכן=כ"ש
לישנא אחרינא=ל"א
לא היו דברים מעולם=להד"מ
לשון הקדש=לה"ק
לשון הרע=לה"ר
לא כל שכן=לכ"ש
למה לי=ל"ל
לא מיבעיא=ל"מ
(המוציא) לחם מן הארץ=למ"ה (benediction)
למה הדבר דומה=למה"ד

לעולם הבא=לעה"ב, לעוה"ב
לא צריכא=ל"צ
לא קשיא=ל"ק
לא שנו ,לא שנא=ל"ש
לא תעשה=ל"ת
מאי איכא למימר=מא"ל
מבעוד יום=מבע"י
מאן דאמר=מ"ד
(מה) מאי דאת אמר=מד"א
מדבר תורה=מד"ת
מנת"מ=מה"מ
מלאכי השרת=מה"ש
מן התורה=מה"ת
משא ומתן=מו"מ
מוצאי ,מוצאי שבת=מוצ"ש שבתות
מאי טעמא=מ"ט
משל למה הדבר דומה=מלה"ד
מצות לא תעשה=מל"ת
מכל מקום=מ"מ
מלך מלכי המלכים=ממ"ה
ממה נפשך=ממ"נ
מה נפשך=מ"נ
מנא הני מילי=מנה"מ
מר סבר=מ"ס
מצות עשה=מ"ע
מעשים טובים=מע"ט
מעשר ראשון=מע"ר
מעשר שני=מע"ש
מערב שבת=מע"ש
משה רבינו עליו השלום=מרע"ה
מוצ"ש=מ"ש
מאי שנא=מ"ש
מה שאין כן=משא"כ
משום הכי=מש"ה
מתן תורה=מ"ת

נוסחא אחרינא=נ"א (gloss)
נמי הכי=נ"ה (v. תנ"ה)
נותן טעם=נ"ט
נטילת ידים=נט"י, נ"י
נפקא מינה=נ"מ
סלקא דעתך=ס"ד
סלקא דעתך אמינא=סד"א
סבירא ליה ,סבר ליה=ס"ל
ספר תורה=ס"ת
עבודת,עובדי,עובד אלילים=ע"א
על אחת כמה וכמה=עאכ"ו
על גבי ,על גב=ע"ג
על דברי ,על דבר=ע"ד
עם הארץ=ע"ה
עליו השלום=ע"ה
עולם הבא=עה"ב
עולם הזה=עה"ז
עין הרע=עה"ר
עה"ב=עוה"ב
עה"ז=עוה"ז
עבודה זרה=ע"ז
על ידי=ע"י
ערב יום טוב=עיו"ט, עי"ט
עד כאן=ע"כ
על כורחו ,על כורחך=ע"כ &c.
עובד כוכבים ומזלות=עכו"ם, עבודת ,עובדי
על מנת=ע"מ
עובדי ,עובד עבודה זרה=עע"ז
על פי=ע"פ
עיין שם=ע"ש (glossator's note)
על שם=ע"ש
ערב שבת=ע"ש
פעם אחת=פ"א

צריכא למימר ,צריך לומר=צ"ל
(קאמר) קא אמר ליה=קא"ל
קדש הקדשים=קה"ק
קריאת התורה=קה"ת
קל וחומר=ק"ו, קו"ח
קיימא לן=קי"ל
(קמשמע) קא משמע לן=קמ"ל
קריאת שמע=ק"ש
רבנו ,רבן ,רבי ,רב=ר׳
ר׳ אלעזר ,ר׳ אליעזר=ר"א
ר׳ אליעזר בן יעקב=ראב"י
ר׳ אלעזר בן עזריה=ראב"ע
רבונו של עולם=רבש"ע
רבן גמליאל=ר"ג
ראש השנה=ר"ה
רב הונא=ר"ה
רה"ר=ר"ה
רשות היחיד=רה"י
רשות הרבים=רה"ר
רוח הקדש=רוה"ק
רב זירא=ר"ז
ראש חדש=ר"ח
ר׳ חנינא=ר"ח
ר׳ טרפון=ר"ט
ר׳ יוסי ,ר׳ יוחנן ,ר׳ יהושע=ר"י, ר׳ ישמעאל
רבן יוחנן בן זכאי=ריב"ז
ר׳ יהושע בן לוי=ריב"ל
ריש לקיש=ר"ל
ר׳ מאיר=ר"מ
רב נחמן ,ר׳ נחמיה=ר"נ
ר׳ עקיבא=ר"ע
רב פפא=ר"פ
רב ששת ,ר׳ שמעון=ר"ש
ר׳ שמעון בן אלעזר=רשב"א
רבן שמעון בן גמליאל=רשב"ג

רשב"ג אמר=רשבג"א
ר׳ שמעון בן יוחאי=ר"ש ב"י, רשב"י
ר׳ שמעון בן לקיש=ר"ש ב"ל, רשב"ל
ר׳ שמעון בן מנסיא=רשב"מ
שפיכות דמים=ש"ד
שפיר דמי=ש"ד
שהכל נהיה בדברו=שהנ"ב (in benediction)
שיר השירים=שה"ש
שומר חנם=ש"ח
שטר חוב=שט"ח
שמע מינה=ש"מ
שנאמר=שנ׳
שמונה עשרה=ש"ע (benedictions)
שוה פרוטה=ש"פ
שפיכות דמים=שפ"ד
שליח צבור=ש"צ, ש"ץ
שומר שכיר=ש"ש
שם שמים=ש"ש
שומע תפלה=ש"ת (benediction)
תה"מ=ת"ה
תפלת הדרך=ת"ה
תחיית המתים=תה"מ
תלמידי ,תלמיד חכם=ת"ח חכמים
תלמוד לומר=ת"ל
תניא נמי הכי=תנ"ה
תנא קמא=ת"ק
תנו רבנן=ת"ר
תא שמע=ת"ש
תקיעה שברים תקיעה=תש"ת
תלמוד תורה=ת"ת

List of Abbreviations.

a.=and.
a. e.=and elsewhere.
a. fr.=and frequently.
a. l.=ad locum.
a. v. fr.=and very frequently.
Ab.=Aboth (Mishnah).
Ab. d'R. N.=Aboth d'Rabbi Nathan (a late Talmudic treatise).
Ab. Zar.=Abodah Zarah (Talmud).
abbrev.=abbreviated or abbreviation.
add.=additamenta(Hosafah to Pesik.R.)
adj.=adjective.
adv.=adverb.
Ag.Hatt.=Agadoth hat-Torah (quoted in Rabbinowicz Variæ Lectiones).
Alf.=Alfasi (Hilkhoth Rabbenu Alfasi).
Am.=Amos.
Ar.=Arukh (Talmudic Lexicon by R. Nathan Romi).
Ar. Compl.=Arukh Completum ed. Alexander Kohut, Vienna 1878-85.
Arakh.=Arakhin (Talmud).
art.=article.
B. Bath.=Baba Bathra (Talmud), v. Kel.
b. h.=Biblical Hebrew.
B. Kam.=Baba Ḳamma (Talmud), v. Kel.
B. Mets.=Baba M'tsiʿa (Talmud), v. Kel.
B. N.=Beth Nathan (quoted in Rabbinowicz Variæ Lectiones).
Bab.=Babli (Babylonian Talmud).
Bart.=Bartenora, Bertinora (commentary to Mishnah).
beg.=beginning.
Beitr.=Beiträge zur Sprach- und Alterthumsforschung, by Michael Sachs, Berlin 1852—54, 2 vols, v. Berl. a. Hildesh.
Bekh.=B'khoroth (Talmud).
Ber.=B'rakhoth (Talmud).
Berl.=Berliner (editor of Targum Onkelos).
Berl. Beitr.=Berliner Beiträge zur Geographie und Ethnographie Babyloniens, Berlin 1884.
Bets.=Betsah (Talmud).
B'ḥuck.=B'ḥuḳḳothay (a pericope).
Bicc.=Biccurim, Bikkurim (Mishnah and Tosefta).
bot.=bottom of page.
B'resh.=B'reshith (name of a pericope).
B'shall.=B'shallaḥ (name of a pericope).
c.=common gender.

Cant.=Canticum (Song of Songs).
Cant. R.=Canticum Rabbah (Midrash Shir hash-Shirim or Hazitha).
ch. } Ch. } =Chaldaic.
Chron.=Chronicles, Book of.
cmp.=compare (mostly referring to association of ideas).
comment.=commentary or commentaries.
comp.=compound or composed.
contr.=contracted or contraction.
contrad.=contradistinguished.
corr.=correct.
corr. acc.=correct accordingly.
corrupt.=corruption.
Curt. Griech. Etym.=Curtius Griechische Etymologie.
Dan.=Daniel, Book of.
Darkhe-Mish.=Frankel, Hodegetica in Mishnam, Leipzig 1859 (Hebrew).
def.=defining or definition.
Del.=Delitzsch, Friedrich.
Del. Assyr. Handw.=Delitzsch Assyrisches Handwörterbuch, Leipzig 1896.
Del. Proleg.=Delitzsch Prolegomena eines neuen Hebräisch-Aramäischen Wörterbuchs &c.
Dem.=D'mai (Mishnah, Tosefta a. Y'rushalmi).
denom.=denominative.
Der. Er.=Derekh Erets (Ethics, a late Talmudic treatise, Rabbah [the great], Zuṭa [the small]).
Deut.=Deuteronomy, Book of.
Deut. R.=Deuteronomy Rabbah (Midrash Rabbah to Deut.).
diff. } differ. } =different interpretation or differently interpreted.
dimin.=diminutive.
Du.=Dual.
ed.=edition or editions (current editions, opposed to manuscripts or especially quoted editions).
Ed.=Eduyoth (Mishnah and Tosefta).
ellipt.=elliptically.
Erub.=Erubin (Talmud).
esp.=especially.
Esth.=Esther, Book of.
Esth. R.=Esther Rabbah (Midrash Rabbah to Esther).
Ex.=Exodus, Book of.
Ex. R.=Exodus Rabbah (Midrash Rabbah to Sh'moth).
expl.=explained.
explan.=explanation.
Ez.=Ezekiel, Book of.
Fl.=Fleisher, appendix to Levy's Targumic or Talmudic Lexicon.

foreg.=foregoing.
fr.=from.
freq.=frequently.
Fr.=Friedman (edition)
Frank.=Frankel, v. Darkhe, and M'bo.
Gem.=G'mara.
Gen.=Genesis, Book of.
gen. of=genitive of.
Gen. R.=Genesis Rabbah (Midrash Rabbah to B'reshith).
Ges. H. Dict.=Gesenius Hebrew Dictionary, 8th German edition.
Gitt.=Giṭṭin.
Gloss.=Glossary.
Hab.=Habakkuk, Book of.
Hag.=Haggai, Book of.
Ḥag.=Ḥăgigah (Talmud).
Ḥall.=Ḥallah (Mishnah, Tosefta and Y'rushalmi).
Hif.=Hifil.
Hildesh. Beitr.=Hildesheimer Beiträge zur Geographie Palestinas, Berlin 1886.
Hithpa.=Hithpaël.
Hithpo.=Hithpolel.
Hor.=Horayoth (Talmud).
Hos.=Hosea, Book of.
Ḥuck.=Ḥuḳḳath (a pericope).
Ḥull.=Ḥullin (Talmud).
intens.=intensive.
introd.=introduction (פתיחתא).
Is.=Isaiah, Book of.
Isp.=Ispeel.
Ithpa.=Ithpaal.
Ithpe.=Ithpeel.
Jer.=Jeremiah, Book of.
Jon.=Jonah.
Jos.=Josephus.
Josh.=Joshua, Book of.
Jud.=Judices, Book of Judges.
K.A.T. } KAT } =Keilinschriften und das Alte Testament by Schrader (second edition), Giessen 1883.
Kel.=Kelim (Mishnah and Tosefta, the latter divided into Baba Kamma, M'tsiʿa, and Bathra).
Ker.=K'rithoth (Talmud).
Keth.=K'thuboth (Talmud).
Kidd.=Ḳiddushin (Talmud).
Kil.=Kilayim (Mishnah, Tosefta and Talmud Y'rushalmi).
Kin.=Ḳinnim (Mishnah).
Koh.=Koheleth, Book of Ecclesiastes.
Koh. Ar. Compl.=Kohut in Aruch Completum.
Koh. R.=Koheleth Rabbah (Midrash Rabbah to Ecclesiastes).
l. c.=loco citato or locum citatum.
Lam.=Lamentations, Book of.

Lam. R.=Lamentations Rabbah (Midrash Rabbah to Lam.; Ekhah Rabbathi).
Lev.=Leviticus, Book of.
Lev. R.=Leviticus Rabbah (Midrash Rabbah to Leviticus, Vayyiḳra Rabbah).
M. Kat.=Moʿed Ḳaṭon (Talmud).
Maas. Sh.=Maʿăser Sheni (Mishnah, Tosefta, and Talmud Y'rushalmi).
Maasr.=Maʿasroth (Mishnah, Tosefta, and Talmud Y'rushalmi).
Macc.=Maccoth, Makkoth (Talmud).
Maim.=Maimonides.
Makhsh.=Makhshirin (Mishnah and Tosefta).
Mal.=Malachi, Book of.
marg. vers.=marginal version.
Mass.=Massekheth (Treatise).
Mat. K.=Matt'noth K'hunnah (commentary to Midrash Rabbah).
M'bo=Frankel, Introductio in Talmud Hierosolymitanum. Breslau 1870 (Hebrew).
Meg.=M'gillah (Talmud).
Meil.=M'ʿilah (Talmud).
Mekh.=M'khilta (a Midrash to portions of Exodus).
Men.=M'naḥoth (Talmud).
Mic.=Micah, Book of.
Midd.=Middoth (Mishnah).
Midr.=Midrash.
„ Sam.=Midrash Samuel.
„ Till.=Midrash Tillim (Midrash to Psalms, Shoḥer Ṭob).
Mikv.=Miḳvaoth (Mishnah and Tosefta).
Mish.=Mishnah.
„ N. or Nap.=Mishnah, editio Napolis.
„ Pes.=Mishnah, editio Pesaro.
Mishp.=Mishpaṭim (name of a pericope).
Ms.=Manuscript.
„ F.=Manuscript Florence.
„ H.= „ Hamburg.
„ K.= „ Karlsruhe.
„ M.= „ Munich.
„ O.= „ Oxford.
„ R.= „ Rome.
Mus.=Musafia (additamenta to Arukh).
Nah.=Nahum, Book of.
Naz.=Nazir (Talmud).
Neg.=N'gaʿim (Mishnah and Tosefta, also a subdivision in Sifra).
Neh.=Nehemiah, Book of.
Neub. Géogr.=Neubauer Géographie du Talmud, Paris 1868.
Ned.=N'darim (Talmud).
Nidd.=Niddah (Talmud).
Nif.=Nifal.

Nithpa.=Nithpaël.
Num.=Numeri, Book of (Numbers).
Num. R.=Numeri Rabbah (Midrash Rabbah to Numbers, B'midbar Rabbah).
Ob.=Obadiah, Book of.
Ohol.=Ohŏloth (Ahiloth, Mishnah and Tosefta).
onomatop.=onomatopoetic.
opin.=opinion.
opp.=opposed.
Orl.=ʿOrlah (Mishnah, Tosefta and Y'rushalmi).
oth.=other, another, others.
P. Sm.=Payne Smith, Thesaurus Syriacus.
Par.=Parah (Mishnah and Tosefta).
Par.=Parashah, referring to Sifra.
part.=participle.
Perl. Et. St.=Perles Etymologische Studien, Breslau 1871.
pers. pron.=personal pronoun.
Pes.=P'saḥim (Talmud).
Pesik.=P'siḳta d'R. Kahăna, ed. Buber.
„ R.=P'siḳta Rabbathi (ed. Friedman).
„ Zutr.=P'siḳta Zuṭrathi, ed. Buber.
Pfl.=Löw, Aramäische Pflanzennamen, Leipzig 1881.
phraseol.=phraseology.
Pi.=Piël.
pl.|
Pl.|=plural.
pr. n.=proper noun.
pr. n. f.=proper noun of a female person.
pr. n. m.=proper noun of a male person.
pr. n. pl.=proper noun of a place.
preced.=preceding.
„ art.=preceding article.
„ w.= „ word.
prep.=preposition.
prob.=probably.
pron.=pronoun.
prop.=properly.
prov.=a proverb.
Prov.=Proverbs, Book of.
Ps.=Psalms, Book of.
q. v.=quod vide.

r.=root or radix.
R.=Rab, Rabbi, or Rabbenu.
R. Hash.=Rosh hash-Shanah (Talmud).
R.S.=Rabbenu Shimshon (commentary to Mishnah).
Rabb. D. S.=Rabbinowicz Diḳduḳé Sof'rim (Variæ Lectiones &c., Munich 1867-84).
Rap.=Rapaport, ʿErekh Millin (Talmudic Cyclopedia, first and only volume).
ref.=referring, reference.
Ruth R.=Ruth Rabbah (Midrash Rabbah to Ruth).
S.=Sophocles, Greek Lexicon of the Roman and Byzantine Periods, Boston 1870.
s.=section (Parashah).
s. v.=sub voce.
Sabb.=Sabbath (Talmud).
Sam.=Samuel, Book of.
Schr.=Schrader, v. KAT.
Sef. Yets=Sefer Y'tsirah (Book of Creation, a Cabalistic work).
Shebi.=Sh'biith (Mishnah, Tosefta, and Y'rushalmi).
Shebu.=Sh'buoth (Talmud).
Shek.=Sh'kalim (Mishnah, Tosefta and Y'rushalmi, also a pericope in P'siḳta).
Sm. Ant.=Smith, Dictionary of Greek and Roman Antiquities, Third American Edition, New-York 1858.
S'maḥ.=S'maḥoth, Treatise (Abel Rabbathi).
Snh.=Sanhedrin (Talmud).
Sonc.=Soncino.
Sot.=Soṭah (Talmud).
sub.=subaudi.
Succ.=Succah (Talmud).
suppl.=supplement (Hosafah) to Pesikta Rabbathi.
Taan.=Taʿănith (Talmud).
Talm.=Talmud.
Tam.=Tamid (Talmud).
Tanḥ.=Midrash Tanḥuma.
„ ed. Bub.=Midrash Tanḥuma (enlarged), edited, from manuscripts, by Buber, Wilna 1885.

Targ.=Targum.
„ O.=Targum Onkelos.
„ Y.= „ Y'rushalmi (or Jonathan).
Targ. II=Targum Sheni (to Esther).
Tem.=T'murah (Talmud).
Ter.=T'rumoth (Mishnah, Tosefta and Y'rushalmi).
Toh.=Tohăroth (Mishnah and Tosefta).
Tosaf.=Tosafoth (Additamenta to Talmud Babli).
Tosef.=Tosefta.
„ ed. Zuck.=Tosefta editio Zuckermandel, Pasewalk 1881.
Treat.=Treatise (tractatus, Massekheth, one of the appendices to Talmud Babli).
Trnsf.=Transferred.
trnsp.=transposed or transposition.
Ukts.=ʿUḳtsin (Mishnah and Tosefta).
usu.=usually.
v.=vide.
Var.=Variant.
var. lect.=variatio lectionis.
Ven.=Venice.
vers.=version.
Vien.=Vienna.
w.=word.
Wil.=Wilna.
ws.=words.
Y.=Y'rushalmi (Palestinean Talmud).
Yad.=Yadayim (Mishnah and Tosefta).
Yalk.=Yalḳuṭ (Collectanea from Talmudim, Midrashim &c.).
Yeb.=Y'bamoth (Talmud).
Y'lamd.=Y'lamdenu (a lost book, corresponding to Tanḥuma, quoted in Arukh).
Zab.=Zabim (Mishnah and Tosefta).
Zakh.=Zakhor (a pericope in P'siḳta).
Zeb.=Z'baḥim (Talmud).
Zech.=Zechariah, Book of.
Zeph.=Zephaniah, Book of.
Zuck.=Zuckermandel, v. Tosef.
Zuckerm.=Zuckermann Talmudische Münzen und Gewichte, Breslau 1862.

By the designation (*Talmud*) are meant Mishnah, Tosefta and G'mara of Talmud Babli and, eventually, Talmud Y'rushalmi. By (Mishnah and Tosefta) or (Mishnah, Tosefta, and Y'rushalmi) is meant a Talmudic treatise in the collection of Mishnah &c., to which no discussions in either G'mara or respectively in the Babylonian are extant.

א׳

א *Aleph*, the first letter of the alphabet, interchanging with other gutturals, e. g. אבב, חבב, חבב, עבב; אליתא, עליתא &c.

א often used to form second roots of verbs ע״ע, e. g. אמם, טמם.

א frequ. prosthetic, e. g. אגודל, גודל, v. אַ־.

א sometimes inserted to replace a radical, as באגא= בגא, esp. in verbs ע״ו, as דָּאִיךְ fr. הוּךְ, קָאִים fr. קוּם &c.

א frequ. (in Talm. Y.) dropped in the beginning of words, e. g. אַבָּא=בָּא; אֲמַר=מַר.

א affixed to the end of Chald. nouns, corresponding to prefixed ה in Hebrew (status emphaticus), e. g. אָבָא= הָאָב.

א׳ as numeral letter, *one*, as אות א׳=אות אחת one letter. Sabb. 104[a]; a. fr. [Editions and Mss. vary, according to space, between the full numeral and the numeral letter, א׳ for אחד, אחת; ב׳ for שנים, שתים, שתי &c.]

אַ־, אֶ־, אִ־, אַי־, אָ־ &c. a prefix, 1) for the formation of nouns in Kal, Peel, Afel (Hifil) &c., e. g. אַסְפַּקְא, אִיס׳, אַפְּדָרָה, אַפְּטַרְתָּא &c.; 2) demonstrative, e. g. אִיהוּ=h. הוּא, אִנָּא, אִרְנָא &c.—3) euphonic (prosthetic) אַרְמָא=דְּמָא; אִית=h. יֵשׁ &c., esp. before foreign words beginning with two consonants, e. g. אַסְטְרַטִיגוֹס, אִיס׳= סְטְרַטִיגוֹס &c.

אַ־ a prefix (followed by Dagesh Forte)=עַל *upon, over*, e. g. אַמְּרָא = עַל מְרָא; even before gutturals, e. g. אַאַבְנָא.

אָאִין plur. of אל״ף q. v.

אאלר״ן, a fictitious word made up of each third letter in מנא מנא תקל ופרסין (Dan. V, 25). Snh. 22[a]; Cant. R. to III, 4 ממתו״ס וכ׳ the inscription on the wall was so arranged as to form words composed of its every first, every second and every third letter respectively.

אֲאָרָא, v. אוּאָרָא.

אַב־, אֶבִ־ a prefix of words of Greek origin answering to αὐ-, au-, e. g. אבטומטוס=αὐτόματος; or to εὐ, e. g. אבגינס=εὐγενής.

אָב I (Assyr. A-bu, Schr. K. A. T., p. 247) *Ab*, the fifth month of the Jewish calendar (of thirty days) beginning between the eighth of July and the seventh of August, and ending between the sixth of August and the fifth of September. R. Hash. I, 3, על אב וכ׳ for announcing the beginning of Ab messengers are sent out, for the sake of the fast. Ib. 18[b] ט׳ באב the ninth of Ab, anniversary of Temple destruction. Taan. IV, 6 משנכנס אב with the beginning of Ab. Ib. 29[b] לישתמיט מיניה באב let him try to be relieved of (the law-suit) in Ab. Meg. 5[b]; a. e.

אָב II m. (b. h.; אבה, cmp. אֵם), const. אֲבִי, אַב [embracer], *father, ancestor, progenitor; teacher; chief, leader; author, originator*. Ex. R. s. 46 end המגדל אב the educator is the real father. Lev. R. s. 1 אבי החכמה וכ׳, the father of all wisdom, . . the father of prophets. Y. Ned. V, 39[b]; a. fr.—אַב בית דין (abbr. אב״ד) president of the Court (Great Sanhedrin), next in dignity to the *Nassi*. Taan. II, 1; a. fr.—Metaph. *origin, cause*. Num. R. s. 10 (play on אֲבוֹי, Prov. XXIII, 29) א׳ אוי the cause of woe (sin).—אב מלאכה (for which also עיקר) *one of the chief labors forbidden on the Sabbath*, opp. תולדה a labor the prohibition of which is based on the ground of its being a species of the former, or derived from the former. Sabb. VII, 1 sq.; a. fr. — [Y. Sabb. II, 5[a], אב שלה, sub. מלאכה.]—אב הטומאה *one of the original or direct causes of levitical uncleanness*, opp. ולד (child) secondary cause. Toh. I, 5; a. fr.—א׳ הנזק v. *Pl.*—בנין א׳ *creation of a class*, i. e. a conclusion, by analogy, from a case explicitly stated in the bibl. law on all similar cases not specified in detail. Sifra introd.—Ib. K'doshim, end, ch. 11 (ref. to Lev. XX, 27) זה ב׳ א׳ לכל דמיהם בם this forms the rule for all cases in which the Bible uses the word *d'mēhem bam* (that the penalty is stoning to death); a. fr.; v. also בֵּית אב.—*Pl.* אָבוֹת, const. אֲבוֹת, 1) *fathers, ancestors, patriarchs* &c. Ber. 26[b] א׳ תקנום prayers have been instituted by the Patriarchs; a. fr.—אבות בתי דינין, v. supra. Hag. II, 2. —בת א׳ a woman *of noble descent*. Num. R. s. 1; a. e. —Metaph. *principal, chief* א׳ מלאכות, v. supra. א׳ הטומא׳ Kel. I, 1; v. supra.—א׳ נזיקין (sing. אב הנזק) the chief actionable injuries or damages, from which the subordinate are deduced (תולדות). B. Kam. I, 1; a. e.—2) *Aboth*, the first section of the Prayer of Benedictions (v. תְּפִלָּה), so called because it alludes to the Patriarchs.

R. Hash. IV, 5; a. fr.—3) *Aboth*, name of a treatise of the Mishnah, containing sayings of Talmudic authorities and belonging to the fourth section, נזיקין, of the Mishnah collection (משנוית); also styled פִּרְקֵי א׳ a. מַסֶּכֶת א׳. A similar collection of a later date is contained in Talmud Babli editions, named א׳ דרבי נתן *Aboth d'Rabbi Nathan*. [Y. Yoma VIII, 44[d] top אב בית נפש v. אֲבֵידָה.]

אָב II ch., v. אַבָּא.

אֵב, אִיב, (אוֹב) m. (b. h.; אבב) *swelling, spreading*, whence 1) *the young shoots of a tree*, opp. to the branches growing directly from the trunk. B. Kam. 81[a] אִיבוֹ שֶׁל אִילָן ed. (Ar. a. Ms. חובו, v. חוב II, cmp. Rashi a. l.). [Y. Erub. III, 21[a] top איבו; Y. Succ. II, 53[a] צידו.] —2) pl. אִיבִּין, אִבִּין *state of growth, development*. Hull. 58[a] *cascuta* which became wormy בְּאִבֶּיהָ during its growth. Ib. 127[b] figs which shrunk בְּאִבֵּיהֶן during development. Y. Sabb. VII, 10[c] bot. he who presses olives מֵאִבֵּיהֶן from where they grow (before they are ripe to be taken off). [Tosef. Maasr. I, 4 אִיבִּין אדומים, Var. אוּבִין, read אוֹגִין, v. אוֹג.] Ib. 5 they differ על האיבין concerning the plants in their growing state (between ripening [גמר] and blossoming [חנץ]; Var. אונין incorr.); cmp. רֵבָן. Ch. v. אִיבָּא I.

אַבָּא I, אָב ch.=h. אָב II. Targ. Gen. XVII, 4. Targ. O. ib. XLI, 43; a. fr.—Freq. אַבָּא (also in Hebr. phraseol.) *my father*. Snh. III, 2. B. Bath IX, 3; a. fr. Meg. 12[b] אהורירירה דא׳ my father's steward. א׳ אבי *my grandfather*. Ber. 10[a] bot.—Snh. 113[a] bot. א׳ אליהו father Elijah (sarcastically).—אֲבוּהַ דְּ־, אֲבוּי דְּ־ N.'s father. Ber. 18[b]; Y. B. Mets. IV, 9[c] top; a. fr.—א׳ רבה, א׳ סב *grandfather*. Targ. II, Esth. VII, 10. Yeb. 21[b].—Trnsf. *origin, source*. Sabb. 22[a] אֲבוּהוֹן דכולהון דם the source of all analogous cases is the law about blood (that you must cover it from a sense of propriety).—*Pl.* אֲבָהָן, אֲבָהָתָא Targ. Y. Deut. XXIV, 16. Targ. I Chr. I, 2; a. fr. Men. 53[a] בר א׳ of distinguished birth.—Kid. 83[a]; a. fr.—[אֲבָהֵי־ Targ. Prov. XIX, 14 Ms.; read with ed. Wil. אבהן; oth. ed. אבהו corr. acc.]

אַבָּא II, אַבָּה (וָוה, וָוא, בָּא, in Y.) pr. n. m. *Abba*, (*Ba, Va*), a frequent name. [Sometimes distinguished persons go by that name, being orig. a title (v. next w.) while their real names are dropped; v. esp. Ber. 18[b] בעינא א׳ I want Abba &c.] The most distinguished are 1) א׳ אריכא, v. רַב.—2) רַבָּא v. רב א׳.—3) (בר בא) א׳ בר אבהו Abba bar Abbahu (Ba), father of Samuel, an Amora.—4) א׳ בר רב הונא, in Bab. רַבָּה q. v.—5) א׳ מרי, contr. אבמרי *Abba Mari*, an Amora.—אבין, אבינא, contr. with ר׳ into רַבִּין, רַבִּינָא *Rabbin, Rabbina*.

אַבָּא III, *Abba* (father), a title of scholars (less than Rabbi), as Abba Saul, A. Yudan, etc.; cmp. foreg.

אַבָּא m. (אבב) 1) *thicket, woods, grove*. M. Kat. 12[b] א׳ בשלניא a forest in Sh'lanya. Keth. 79[a], v. זַרְדְּתָא. Snh. 39[b] (prov.) מיניה וביה א׳ נרזיל (לירזל) ביה נרגא (Ag. Hatt. בנרגא, v. Rabb. D. S. a. l. note) from the very woods shall it go into the hatchet (as a handle to strike the woods).—2) *fruit*, v. אִיבָּא.

עוּעִית, עַבְעָבִית, אַבְעָבִית, אֲבָאבִית (reduplic. of אב, עב, עו; v. עַוִּית) prop. *swelling, heaviness* (cmp. כאב), hence *disorder of the stomach, vomiting* (spasms); usu. in connection with חמה, *fever with vomiting*. Gen. R. s. 19 did you ever hear, this ass here that is driven out חמה עליה אבבית עליה Ar. (ed. corrup. צינה עליו כמה חכמים עליו) has fever, has vomiting (spasms)? Ib. s. 53 חמה ואכאבית. V. אֲבָאבִית.

אבאטיס, read אֲבָאטִיס.

אַבְאָשׁוּתָא f. (באש) *offence, displeasure*. Targ. Koh. VII, 3.

אָבַב (b. h.; √אב, cmp. עב, חב, גב, כב, קב &c., v. חָבַב I a. II; *to be thick, to be heavy, to press; to surround; to twist; to be warm, glow* etc. V. אבל, אבד, אבק, אבר, אבס, אבה &c.) *to be thick, to swell, break forth*; v. חבב a. חָבַב.

אֲבַב ch. same, *to grow, ripen*. Targ. Hos. IX, 10 מאבבא q. v.

אִבְבָא, v. אִיב׳.

אֶבְגִּינוֹס, אֶוְגִינוֹס, אֶוְגִינֵס m. (corr. -נֵיס—εὐγενής) *of noble descent*. Koh. R. beg.; a. fr. (Midr. Till. to Ps. I אבירנים; Cant. R. beg. איוגיטוס, corr. acc.). —*Pl.* Yalk. Ps. 863 שהוא אֶוְגֶנְסִין (read בן א׳) he is the son of nobles; Midr. Till. to Ps. CV בן גנסין (corr. acc.) cmp. גְּנִיס.

אֶבְגְּנִיסְטֵי (read אֶוְגֶינִיסְטָאטֵי, —סְטֵטֵי) m. pl. (εὐγενέστατοι) *most noble*. Ruth R. to I, 2. Midr. Sam. ch. I.

אבגרוטינה, v. אנג׳.

אָבַד (b. h.; √אב, v. אבב) *to be pressed, go around in despair* (v. Prov. XXXI, 6; Deut. XXVI, 6) *to be given up*, whence 1) *to be lost, perish; to be beyond recognition*. Sifré Deut. 301 (ref. to Deut. XXVI, 5) לא ירד . . . אלא לאובד (read לוֹבֵד or לְאַבּוֹד; Yalk. Deut. a. l. לאבדם prob. לְאַבְּדָן; Ms. Zer. Abr. 3 לְיַאֲבֵד) Jacob went to Aram with no hope but to perish (be a slave &c.). Ohol. XVII, 3 a field שא׳ בו קבר in which there is a grave that cannot be located. Keth. XIII, 7 אָבְדָה דרך וכ׳ the path to his field cannot be traced. Gen. R. s. 91 אבידה א׳ לנו we have lost something; a. fr.—2) *to lose*. Ib. ואנו שֶׁאָבַדְנוּ ר׳ ס׳ and we who have lost (mourn for) R. S.; a. fr.—Part. pass. אָבוּד *lost, irretrievable, perishing, decayed*. Keth. 108[a] על הא׳ on a contribution to the Temple which has been lost on the road. Y. Shebi. IX, 38[d] top מאיליהן הן אֲבוּדִין they perish of themselves (they decay naturally); a. fr.

Nif. נֶאֱבַד *to be lost, perish*. Keth. 104[a]; a. fr. Sifré Deut. 301 לְיַאֲבֵד, v. supra.

Pi. אִיבֵּד 1) *to waste, lose, forfeit, destroy*. Ned. 33[b] איבּ׳ את מעותיו he wasted his money, (cannot reclaim it). Keth. XIII, 6 אי׳ את זכותו he forfeited his claim. Ab. Zar. 55[a] אנו נְאַבֵּד וכ׳ shall we give up our honest dealing? Ib. IV, 7 יְאַבֵּד עולמו shall He destroy His world?

Hag. 3ᵃ ובקשתם לְאַבְּדָהּ ממני and you wanted to deprive me of it? Ib. 4ᵃ זה הַמְאַבֵּד א׳ וכ׳ one who destroys what is given to him.—א׳ עצמו לדעת *to commit suicide wilfully.* Gen. R. s. 82; a. fr.—2) *to drop from memory, to forget.* Aboth V, 12; a. e.

אֲבַד, אֲבַד ch. *to be lost.* Targ. I Sam. IX, 3; a. fr.—Snh. 111ᵃ; a. fr.—Y. Pes. IX, 37ᵃ כְּאָבִיד הוא it is to be looked upon as lost.

Pa. אַבֵּד *to destroy.* Targ. II Kings, XIX, 18; a. fr.

Af. אוֹבֵיד, אוֹבֵד 1)=*Pa.* Targ. Deut. XXVI, 5; a. fr. —Y. Kid. III, 64ᶜ bot. אובדתא חייך וכ׳ thou hast ruined this man's (my) life. Gen. R. s. 56 אובדת ליבך thou hast lost thy wits; a. fr.—2) *to be lost, to go to ruin.* Targ. Ps. XLI, 6; a. e.—Y. Hag. II, 77ᵇ ווי דמובדין alas for the lost (deceased)! Y. M. Kat. I, beg. 80ᵃ וויבדן and decay.

Ithpa. אִתְאַבַּד *to be lost.* Lev. R. s. 34 מִתְאַבְּדִין if they should be lost.—מִתְאֲבִיד=מִתְּבִיד Pes. 5ᵇ; a. e. [Lam. R., to IV, 21 לאיברא, read לאיעבדא, v. עֲבַד.]

אֲבֵד m. *perishable, irretrievable.* דבר הא׳ a business which cannot be postponed without irretrievable loss. M. Kat. 11ᵃ; a. fr.

אֲבַדָּא m. (אבד) *destruction.* Targ. Prov. XXVIII, 28.

אֲבֵדָה, v. אֲבֵ׳.

אֶבְדּוּמָא pr. n. m., v. אֶבְדִּימוֹס.

אבדומא, אבדומה, v. אברומא.

אבדימי, v. אֶבְדִּימוֹס.

אֲבַדּוֹן m. (b. h.; אבד) *perdition, hell.* Koh. R. to V, 8.

אֶבְדּוֹקוֹס pr. n. m. (Εὔτοκος) *Ebdocus* (Eutocus). Y. Meg. III, 74ᵃ bot. rendered in a secret political letter טוב ילד *Good-Child.* (Ed. קוס—, קין— corr. acc.)

אֶבְדִּימָא, v. next w.

אֶבְדִּימוֹס pr. n. m. (Εὔδημος) *Ebdimos, Eudemus.* Y. Keth. XI, 34ᵇ; mostly abbrev. אבדימא, אבדימי (corrupt. אבודמי, אבודמא, אבודמי), name of several *Amoraim*, the most prominent: Eb. of Zepphoris. Y. Ber. IV, 8ᵃ; a. fr. [V. Frankel Mebo, s. v.] V. וַרְדִּימוֹס.

אַבְדָּלָה h., **אַבְדַּלְתָּא** ch., f. (=הַבְדָּלָה; בדל) 1) *the act of distinguishing; separation.* Y. Ber. VIII, 12ᶜ top א׳ ודאי real separation.—2) *Habdalah*, a formula of prayer for the exit of the Sabbath or Holy Days. Ibid. beg. 11ᵈ. Pes. 113ᵃ; a. fr.—*Pl.* אַבְדָּלוֹת. Y. Ber. V, 9ᵇ bot. שבעה א׳ seven objects of distinction (mentioned in the Habdalah).

אַבְדָּן pr. n. m. *Abdan* (contr. of אבא יודן), an Amora of the first gener. Y. Ber. IV, 7ᶜ bot. (cmp. Gen. R. s. 10). Ber. 27ᵇ Ms. M. (ed. אבידן); a. e.

אוֹבְדָן, אָבְדָן m. (b. h. אבדן, אבד) *ruin, destruction.* Y. Dem. VII, 26ᵃ bot. אוֹ׳ אוכלין waste of eatables; a. fr.

אוֹבְדָנָא, אַבְדָנָא ch. same. Targ. Prov. XXVII, 20; a. e.

אֲבֵדְתָּא, v. אֲבֵ׳.

אבדתא, v. אֲבַרְתָּא.

אַבָּה pr. n. m. *Abbah;* father of Samuel; v. אַבָּא II.

אָבָה, v. אבי.

אַבָּהוּ pr. n. m. *Abbahu*, name of two Palestine *Amoraim*, one prob. of the first gener. Y. Ber. V, 8ᵈ bot; Y. Bicc. II, 64ᵈ top; the second a celebrated disciple of R. Yoḥannan, residing in Cæsarea. Y. Ber. II, 4ᵇ top. Succ. 48ᵇ; a. fr.—Babylonian *Amoraim* by that name. Sabb. 119ᵇ; Kid. 33ᵇ, father of Rabbah, v. רַבָּה. B. Kam. 117ᵇ, contemp. of R. Ashé, v. אַשֵׁי.

אבהונוס, אבהנוס Y. Kil. III, 31ᶜ Ar. (ed. אבחנס, read אַמְבָּטֵיס q. v. or אִיפּוֹבָּטֵיס (ἱπποβάτης) *stallion ass for mares.*

אֲבָהָתָא pl. of אַבָּא.

אבהתא, v. מְמְצִיא.

(אַיְבוּ) אִיבּוּ, אִבּוּ pr. n. m. *Ibbu* (Aïbu), all prob. forms of the same name, an Amora. Snh. 5ᵃ אבו Ar. ed. pr. (ed. אי׳, Ms. M. איי׳). Succ. 44ᵇ איי׳. Ruth R., Par. 2, beg. רבי אי׳. Num. R. s. 12. Y. Succ. II, 53ᵃ bot.; Pes. 4ᵃ, a. fr. איי׳. [אִבּוּ name of a bird, v. אִיבּוּ].

אִיבּוּב אַבּוּב m. (=אנב׳, נבב *to be hollow;* cmp. I ביב) *reed, flute; pipe, tube.* Arakh. II, 3 א׳ של קנה a reed flute, א׳ של נחושת brass flute. Kel. II, 3; Men. X, 4 א׳ של קלאים Ar. (ed. קליות) an iron tube for roasting grain.—א׳ רוֹעֶה (Var. אבובראה, אבוברואה) *shepherd's flute*, name of a plant (Eupatorium) used for medicinal purposes; v. חוּמְבְרִיא. Sabb. XIV, 3; ib. 109ᵇ; Y. ib. XIV, 14ᶜ.

אַבּוּבָא, אבוב ch. same. Yoma 20ᵇ (prov.) א׳ לחררי וכ׳ a flute is musical to nobles—give it to weavers, they will not accept it (fools criticise where sages admire). Succ. 50ᵇ.—*Pl.* אַבּוּבִין. Targ. Jerem. XLVIII, 36; a. fr.

אַבּוּב רוֹעֶה=אַבּוּבְרָאָה, v. foreg. h.

אַבּוּבְרָם pr. n. m. (=אבו אברם), בר א׳ *Bar Abbub'ram.* Hull. 38ᵃ.

אבוד, v. אִיבּוּד.

אבוד, v. אָבוּז.

אבודיינא, אַבּוּדְיָנָא pr. n. m. *Abbud'yana*, a gentile name (referring to idolatry). Git. 11ᵃ.

אבודמי, אֲבוּדְמָא, v. אֶבְדִּימוֹס.

אבוורנקי, אבוורנקא, v. אַבּוּרְנְקָא.

***אַבּוּז** m. (cmp. אבו; אֲבוּס, √אב) Euphem. for *buttocks, extremity.* Erub. 53ᵇ; v. אֲבוּז.

אֲבוֹי m. (b. h.; interj.=אוֹי) *woe! ah!* Num. R. s. 10 (ref. to Prov. XXIII, 29) האוי והא׳ the *woe* and the *ah.*

אֲבוּיָה pr. n. m. *Abuyah*, known as the father of Elisha, v. אֱלִישָׁע. Y. Ḥag. II, 77[b]; a. fr.

אבורין Y. Sabb. V, 8[b] bot. Ar., read אַטְּרִין or אַטְּרַיִן.

אִבּוּל I *mourning*, v. אֵיבוּל.

אִבּוּל II אֵיבוּל m. (יבל, cmp. יְבוּל) *the gate for carrying grain into the house, wagon-gate, gate-way. Pl.* אִיבּ׳, אִבּוּלִים. Tosef. B. Mets. XI, 10 אין חולקין את אי׳ וכ׳ ed. Zuck. (ed. הָאֵב׳) you dare not divide gate-ways between heirs unless there is the required space for each.

אִיבּוּלָא, אִבּוּלָא ch. same, esp. (corresp. to h. מבוא העיר) *city gate-way* which is opened for wagons &c.; *fortified place* where judges sit &c.; cmp. שַׁעַר.—M. Kat. 22[a] begin to count the days of mourning מבבא דא׳ from the time ye turn your faces from the city gate-way (to go home while the corpse is carried to the grave-yard). Keth. 17[a]; Meg. 29[a] when people form a lane מא׳ וכו׳ סיברא from the city gate-way to the burial place. [Ar. *house of mourning*, v. אִבּוּל I.] B. Bath. 58[a] bot. there was written אבבא דא׳ Ms. M. (ed. incorr. בא׳) over the gate of the town entrance (where court was held).—*Pl.* אִבּוּלֵי. Erub. 6[b]. Yoma 11[a]. Targ. Y. Deut. XXVIII, 52 אבוליכון (ed. Vien. אבול׳). Targ. Jer. L, 26 אִיבּוּלָהָא (h. text מאבסיה; v. Pesh. a. l.).

***אִבּוּלָאֵי** m. pl. (v. foreg.) *city-gate-guards, police.* Nid. 67[b] משום א׳ on account of the rude conduct of &c. [Rashi=אבולי dangerous, cavern-like entrances to the bath-house.]

אבולי, B. Bath 143[a], אאבולי read with Ms. M. אַבּוּלֵי ואסטרטיגר, v. בּוּלֵי II.

אבולין, v. אַבִּילִין.

אֲבוּן (אבין) pr. n. m. *Abbun*, an Amora. Y. Pes. IV, beg. 30[cd] (ר׳ א׳ בשם ר׳ אל׳; ר׳ אל׳ בשם ר׳ אבין); Y. Taan. I, 64[c]. Y. Shebu. VI, 37[a] bot.—V. בּוּן.

אֲבוּנָא, אֲבוּנָה, pr. n. m. *Abuna*, an Amora. Y. Shebi. II, 33[d]; a. fr.

אבונגרי, v. אַבְנְגַּר.

אֵבוּס, אֵיבוּס (אִיבּוּס?) m. (b. h.; אָב׳; אבס) 1) *feeding receptacle, bowl* for working men; *manger.* Ned. IV, 4.—Sabb. 140[b] אי׳ של כלי (Rashi אב׳) a real manger, opp. אי׳ של קרקע a piece of ground fenced in and used as manger.—2) *stall, stable.* Y. Shebu. VII, 37[d] top; VIII, beg. 38[b]. [Y. Ter. I, 40[b] אבוס read אֶבְיוֹם or אֶבְרִים.]—*Pl.* אֲבוּסִים. Y. Snh. 63[b] אֲבוּסֵיהֶן their stables. V. אֵיפּוּס.

אֲבוּקָא pr. n. m. *Abuka.* Yalk. Lam. 1001, v. אֲבִיקָה.

אֲבוּקָה f. (אבק, cmp. אבך, זבק; v. Sachs Beitr. I, p. 62; Naḥm. to Gen. XXXII, 25) [*bundle of twigs*], *torch* (with, or without של אור). Sot. 21[a] נזדמנה לו א׳ של אור a burning torch happened to come in his possession. Ber. 43[b] א׳ כשנים walking by torchlight is equal to two walking together (as regards protection from night-spirits).—*Pl.* אֲבוּקוֹת. Tosef. Succ. IV, 2 were dancing before them בא׳ with torches. Ib. 4 בשמונה א׳ של אור; Succ. 53[a] ח׳ א׳ של אור; Y. ib. V, 55[c] top א׳ של זהב (corr. acc. or read זֶפֶת?); Mish. ib. V, 4.

***אַבְרוּגְנָא, אַבּוּרְגָנָא** (Ar.) m. (=אַמְבּוּרְקְלוֹן q. v.; a Babyl. corrupt. of an imported Palestinean phrase) *bed-cover, ticking* (involucrum). *Pl.* אַבְרוּ׳, אַבּוּרְגָּנֵי. Erub. 62[a] בריאה במוהרקי וא׳ a lease of a court yard is called *sound* (legal and not merely a legal fiction), if connected with the privilege of placing in the yard chairs and seats, [Rashi, cmp. Mishnah;—מוהרקי, obviously a corruption for גוהרקי or גלופקרי, cmp. גמורקין.—Other explanations of our w., suggested by מוהרקי, v. s. v. מוד׳.]

אבורנקי, v. אַבְּנַר.

אבזייני, v. אַפּוֹזְיָינֵי.

אַבְזָקָה, אַבְזָקָא) אֲבוּקַת (אֲבִזְקָה f. (בזק) *breaking, crumbling, corrosion*, whence 1) *a foot-disease in animals* believed to arise from vermin in consequence of a stroke of lightning; 2) *moth-eaten condition of garments.* B. Mets. 78[b] (expl. הבריקה Mish.) אבוקת (Rashi אבזקא, Ms. M. אבוק, corr. ז for ו; cmp. Y. ib. VI, 11[a] top. s. v. בָּזָק) atrophy or paralysis of the feet. Ib. א׳ במילת׳ וכ׳ the moths are in the royal wardrobe.

אֲבִיזָרָא, אֲבִזְרָא m. (Arab. bazr, abzār, v. בזר, פזר) *anything used for seasoning, spices* &c.—Fig. *pl.* אֲבִזְרֵי, אֲבִיזְרֵי *requisites, appurtenances.* Snh. 74[b] אינהו וכל אבזרייהו they (the commands) and all appertaining thereto. Men. 73[b] עולה וכל אֲבִיזְרָהָא Ar. a. Rashi to Snh. l. c. (ed. חבירתא corr. acc.) the burnt-offering and &c.

אבחטס, v. אַמְפָּטִיס a. אבהוס.

אבטא, v. אַבְטֵי.

***אַבְטָא** m. (בטן; cmp. בטט, בוץ, בוט a. deriv.) *belly*, whence *leather wine-bag.* Ab. Zar. 34[b] א׳ דטייעי (Ar. אבטא) the travellers' wine-bag. [Y. Yeb. IV, 5[d], v. אֶפְטָא.] [אבטאות, v. אַבְטֵי.]

אבטר, v. אַבְטֵי.

אבטולוס, אבטולס, v. next w.

אַבְטוֹלְמוֹס pr. n. m. (prob. Πτολεμαῖος, or Εὐπτόλεμος=Εὐπόλεμος) *Abtolmos.* Erub. III, 4 (35[a]) ed. (Ms. M. אבטולס). Ib. 36[a]; Y. ib. 21[a] bot. אַבְטוֹלֵס (v. Rabb. D. S. Erub. l. c., notes). Ex. R. s. 21 אבטוליס (אבטלוס).—M. Kat. 18[a] אֲבִינוּל (prob. abbrev. of our w.), surnamed ספראה (v. Rabb. D. S. a. l.), an Amora.

אַבְטוֹמְטוּס m. (αὐτόματος) *self-moving, self-growing, spontaneous.* Midr. Till. to Ps. I, 5 האומרים א׳ הוא העולם Mus. (ed. טומטום, corr. acc.) who say the universe is a self-moving power (has no creator). [Better: אַבְטוֹמָטוֹן (αὐτόματον, S.) *chance.*]

***אַבְטוֹנְיוֹת** f. pl. (=אַבְטוֹנוֹמִיּוֹת; αὐτονομία; v. Sm. Ant. s. v. Autonomi) *cities enjoying their own laws, jurisdictions.* Y. Meg. I, 70ª bot. שני א׳ (read שְׁתֵּי). Y. B. Bath. III, 14ª top אבטני; Bekh. 55ª שני אבטילאות (corr. acc., Ar. אבטלאות, אבטליות). [Cmp. corruptions of אַגְרוֹנִימוֹס.]

אַבְטֵחַ, v. בְּטַח II.

אַבְטָחָה=הַבְטָחָה.

אַבְטֵי Tosef. Ohol. XIII, 3 (ed. Zuck. אבטוי) v. בְּטַח II.

אַבְטֵי, v. אַמְבְּטֵי.

***אבטיגא**, Var. חגה Sifré Deut. 80 (v. ed. Friedm. a. l. note 3), read טוֹגָא (toga) or טִיבְּרִינָא (τηβέννα) *Roman toga.*

***אַבְטִיוֹנָא** m. (ὀπτίων, optio; Perl. Et. St. p. 103; D. C. Lat. s. v.) *commissary, quartermaster in the Roman army.* Y. Sabb. VI, 8ᶜ bot. אתא א׳ וכ׳ a Roman quarterm. came and made him stand behind him (in the public convenience).

אֲבַטִּיחַ m. (b. h.; בטח, √בט *to swell;* cmp. אַבְטָא) *melon.* Maasr. I, 5.—*Pl.* אֲבַטִּיחִים. Ib. 4; a. fr.

אֲבַטִּיחָא ch. same.—Pl. אֲבַטִּיחַיָּא, אֲבַטִּיחִין. Targ. O. Num. XI, 5. Y. Snh. VII, end, 25ᵈ.

אבטילאות, v. אַבְטוֹנְיוֹת.

אַבְטִילוֹס abbr. of אַבְטוֹלְמוֹס.

אַבְטִינָס pr. n. m. *Abtinas.* בית א׳ Beth. Abt., name of a priestly family who had the secret for preparing the frank-incense for the Temple. Yoma III, 11; I, 5; a. e.

אַבְטָלָה f. (=הַבְטָלָה; בטל) *idleness, waste.* Y. Bets. V, 63ᵇ נר של א׳ a light burning to no purpose. Y. Shebi. VII, 37ᶜ top על הא׳ for the loss of time.

אַבְטַלְיוֹן pr. n. m. *Abtalion* (Greco-Romanized by Josephus Πολλίων, Pollio), name of a Chief Justice of the Sanhedrial court in the days of Hyrcan II and of Herod. Aboth I, 10; 11. Eduyoth I, 3. Yoma 71ᵇ; a. e.

אבטניות, v. אַבְטוֹנְיוֹת.

אָבָה, אָבִי (h. אָבָה, √אב *to press, surround, embrace,* v. אָבַב; cmp. אָוָה, חָפֵץ) *to be willing.* Targ. O. Deut. XXV, 7; a. fr.—[Targ. Prov. XXIX, 11, ed. Wil. מאבה, read מֵאֲבָה, v. מאך.]

אביא, v. אביה.

אָבִיב m. (b. h.; אבב) *early stage of ripening,* esp. of grains; *season of beginning barley-crop;* also *the offering of the first fruits* (on Passover). R. Hash. 21ª (ref. to Deut. XVI, 1) שמור א׳ וכ׳ observe the ripening of the equinoctial season that it be in the month of Nissan (rule for intercalation). Men. 84ª; a. fr.

אָבִיב, אֲבִיבָא (אֲבִיב, אֲבִיבָא) ch. same. Targ. O. Lev. II, 14; Ex. XIII, 4; a. e.—Snh. 11ᵇ; Y. ib. I, 18ᵈ top זימנא דא׳ וכ׳ the season of ripening has not yet come. [Y. Maasr. V, 52ª אביבא דפילא, read אַרְכּוּבָא.] — *Pl.* (adj.) אֲבִיבִין, אֲבִי׳. Targ. O. Ex. IX, 31 (ed. Berl. sing.).

אֲבֵדָה, אֲבִידָה f. (b. h. אֲבֵדָה; אבד) 1) *lost* or *missed object.* שומר א׳ the keeper of a lost object waiting for its owner to claim it B. Mets. 29ª; a. fr.—בעל א׳ the owner of the lost thing. Kid. 2ᵇ בעל א׳ מחזיר וכ׳ the owner hunts for what he has lost, i. e. man woos woman (allud. to Gen. II, 21); a. fr.—M. Kat. 25ᵇ בכו לאובדים ולא לא׳ Ms. M. (ed. בכו לאבילים) weep for the losers, but not for the lost (deceased). — 2) *loss, decrease.* אֲבֵידַת נפש decrease of physical strength. Yoma 74ᵇ.—(Y. ib. VIII, 44ᵈ top אב בית read אבידת).

אֲבִידָן m. (אבד; cacophemism for וַיְעְדָא q. v.), בֵּי א׳ (=בֵּי וַיְעֲדֵי) prop. *their place of ruin,* cacophemism for *meeting-place, gathering for idolatrous purposes and performances connected with idolatrous feasts* (games, &c.) which the Jews, under Hadrian, were forced to attend. Sabb. 152ª. Ab. Zar. 17ᵇ. — Transf. *meeting place of early Christians* where religious controversies used to be held. Sabb. 116ª ספרי דבי א׳ Christian writings. Ib. רב לא אזיל וכ׳ Rab would not attend a Be-Abedan, Samuel would.

אֲבִידַרְנָא pr. n. m. *Abidarna,* gentile friend of R. Yuda. Ab. Zar. 65ª top. [Ms. M. אבינדרא, Var. אבי דרבא; v. Rabb. D. S. a. l.]

אֲבִידְתָּא f. ch.=h. אֲבֵדָה. Targ. Ex. XXII, 8; a. e. B. Mets. 23ª; 27ᵇ; 28ᵇ.

אביה, אביא, v. אבזיירא a. אַסְרָא.

אַבְיוּ, בַּר א׳ pr. n. m. (Bar) *Abyu,* name of a renowned obituary poët. Yeb. 103ª; M. Kat. 25ᵇ בר אביו Ar. (ed. אובא, אבין, Ms. Var. אבו, איבו, v. Rabb. D. S a. l. note).

אֶבְיוֹן m. (b. h., אבי) *poor, distressed.* Lev. R. s. 34 (etymol.) he is called *ebyon,* שהוא מתאב לכל (Yalk. a. l. מתאוה) because he longs for everything. Gen. R. s. 71. B. Mets. 111ᵇ.

אֲבִיוֹנָה f. (b. h., אבי) *caper-tree,* or *caper-berry,* so called from the stimulating effects of its seed.—Pl. אֲבִיוֹנוֹת. Maasr. IV, 6; a. e.

אֲבִיוֹנָה f. pl. אֲבִיוֹנוֹת dial. for חֲבִיוֹנָה. Tosef. Kel. B. Kam. II, 2 (ed. Zuck. אביונות).

אֶבְיוֹנוּת f. (denom. of אֶבְיוֹן) *want, distress.* Midr. Till. to Ps. LXX, end.

***אֶבְיוֹנֵי**, בֵּי א׳ pr. n. pl. *Bê-Ebyonê* (Poor-House); Rashi. B. Kam. 117ª. [Ms. M. איביוני, Ms. F. אבוויני, Hal. G'dol. Ms. אכסני; v. Rabb. D. S. a. l.—Prob. a corrupt. of בֵּי זוינא, v. בְּזִוִינָא.]

אֲבִיזְרָא, v. אַבְזָרָא.

אַבַּיֵי pr. n. m. *Abbayi*, 1) a renowned Babyl. Amora (original name נַחְמָנִי). Keth. 65ª; a. fr.—2) Oth. Amoraim of that name. Ib. 94ª. Erub. 62ª.

אֲבָיֵי, v. אַבָּיָיה.

אבייא Y. Succ. II, 53ª, רב א׳ read אַבִּינָא.

אֲבָיָיה (**אֲבָיֵי**) f. (contr. of אבעיה; בעי) *prayer*. בר א׳ *reader, precentor*. Y. Pes. V, 32ᶜ bot.—Y. Taan. III, end, 67ª; Y. Sheb. I, 33ᵇ top אביי.

אביינוס, v. אֶבְנְיוּס.

אביך Y. Yeb. VII, 8ª bot א׳ אשקלון, read אַוִּיר; comp. Y. Shebi. VI, 36ᶜ.

אֲבֵיל *to mourn*, v. אֲבַל.

אֲבִיל, **אֲבִילָא**, v. אֲבֵל a. אֲבֵלָא.

אֲבִילָה f. 1)=אֵבֶל *mourning*. Lam. R. introd., (R. Abbahu 4); v. אֲבִינָה.—2) fem. of אָבֵל II.

אֲבִילוּתָא, **אֲבִילוּ** ch.=next w. Targ. Lam. II, 5; v. אֲבֵלוּ. — M. Kat. 20ᵇ א׳ נהיג באפה in her (thy wife's) presence observe mourning (when she is in mourning).

אֲבִילוּת f. (אבל) *mourning time*, *mourning ceremonies*. M. Kat. 20ª sq. א׳ שבעה the mourning time is seven days. Ib. 24ª אין א׳ בשבת no mourning ceremonies are to be observed on &c. Yeb. 43ᵇ א׳ חדשה recent (i. e. individual) mourning, in contrad. to א׳ ישנה mourning over Jerusalem. [Gen. R. s. 8 beg., some ed. אוביל—אברלות read אוביל—אברלות].

אֲבִילוּתָא, v. אֲבֵלוּ.

אֲבִילִין pr. n. pl. *Abelin*, *Abilena*, a district of Peræa (v. Graetz, Gesch. d. Jud. II, 2, p. 457). Lev. R. s. 17; Pesik. Vayhi, p. 66ª האבלין (corr. acc.); Pesik. R. s. XVIII (p. 88ᵇ ed. Friedm.) אובלים; Ruth R. to I, 5 אבילין. Tosef. Zeb. II, 3 ed. Zuck. אֵיבְלָיִים (Var. אובלים). Cmp. אָבוּל a. אָבֵל pr. n. pl.

אַבִּימִי pr. n. m. *Abbimi*, 1) a disciple of Rabbah. Shebu. 28ᵇ; Y. Ned. II, 37ᵇ; Y. Shebu. III, 34ᵈ top.—2) A. bar Tobi. Y. Naz. IX, beg., 57ᶜ.

אַבִּין pr. n. m. *Abbin*. Y. Bicc. II, beg., 64ᶜ, Rabbi A. Cmp. אָבוּן; v. אַבִּיי.

אַבִּינָא pr. n. m. *Abbina*, an Amora. Y. Pes. V, 32ᶜ; —Y. Ned. IV, beg. 38ᶜ (prob. Abbuna, as shortly before). [Y. Peah III, 17ᵈ bot. ביגא prob. the same.]—רב א׳ contr. רַבִּינָא q. v.

אביסנא Sabb. 151ᵇ, v. אַבְסָן.

***אֲבִיק** m. (בִּיק, v. בקק; comp. אָפִיק) *outlet*, esp. *a pot in the bath-tub to which a waste-pipe is attached*. Mikv. VI, 10.

אֲבֵיק, v. אֲבַק.

אֲבִיקָה pr. n. m. *Abikah*, a hero at the defence of Jerusalem. Pesik. R. s. 29—30, א׳ בן גבריתי (Yalk. Lam. 1001 אביקא בן גבתרי).

אביקלוס, v. אֶבְקוֹלָס.

אַבִּיר m. (b. h., אבר) *strong*, *mighty*, *eminent* (opp. קל light, of no influence); *noble*.—*Pl.* אַבִּירִים. R. Hash. 25ᵇ אביר שבא׳ the noblest of the nobility. Y. ib. II, 58ᵇ bot. אַבִּירֵי עולם (Babli ib. l. c. חֲמוּרֵי; Koh. R. to I, 4 גדולי) the world's noblest sons. [Esth. R. to II, 4, v. אַבִּירָם.]

אבירודימוס, v. וָרְדִּימוֹס.

אֲבִירָם pr. n. m. (b. h.) *Abiram*. Esth. R. to II, 4 ר׳ יהוש׳ בר א׳ (some ed. אבירים, Midr. Sam. ch. XIII בריה דר׳ בירוי).

אֲבִישְׁנָא, v. אַבְשׁוּנָא.

אֲבִית, א׳ ישימון pr. n. pl. *Abyath Y'shimon*, usu. בֵּית ה׳. Targ. Y. II, Num. XXI, 20.

אֶבְיָתָר (b. h.) pr. n. m. *Ebyathar*, an Amora. Git. 6ᵇ. Y. Ber. IX, 13ª.

אָבַךְ (b. h., √אב, cmp. אבק, עב) *to entangle*. *Hithp.* הִתְאַבֵּךְ *to blend* (of whirling smoke columns). Pesik. R. s. 29—30.

***אַבְּכָא** m. (Syr., P. Sm. 15; v. foreg., cmp. b. h. אָבַק) *the fighter*, whence *large cock*. Targ. Prov. XXX, 31; cmp. זַרְזִיר (Var. אַבְּבָא, Ms. אַבְּרָא).

אֲבָל (b. h.) 1) *indeed*, *yes*. Tosef. Erub. V (IV), 1 א׳ אמרו לו said they to him, *yes* (we admit). Erub. 30ᵇ top. Nid. 3ᵇ; a. e.—Gen. R. s. 91 לשון דרומית וכ׳ it is a South Palestine expression where *ăbal* means *bram*, v. בְּרַם.—2) *but, however*. Ber. VII, 1; a. v. fr.

אָבֵל I (b. h.) pr. n. pl. *Abel*, name of several towns; cmp. אֲבִילִין. Erub. 87ª ed. (Ms. M. בבל, corr. acc., Var. lect. v. Rabb. D. S. a. l. note).

אָבֵל II (b. h., √אב, v. אבב; cmp. אפל); [*dark*, cmp. קֹדֵר], *mourner*, esp. during seven days after burial. M. Kat. 14ᵇ; a. v. fr. — *Pl.* אֲבֵלִים, אֲבִילִים (אֲבִילִין). Keth. 8ᵇ; v. בְּרָכָה. Y. Ab. Zar. I, 39ᶜ bot. אֲבִילֵי גויים mourners among gentiles; a. fr.—Fem. אֲבֵלָה, אֲבִילָה. Y. Ber. IV, 8ª; Y. Taan. II, 65ᶜ bot.

אָבַל III (foreg.) *to mourn*. *Hithpa.* הִתְאַבֵּל, *Nithpa.* נִתְאַבֵּל *to observe mourning ceremonies*, *to be bound to mourn*, *be an* אָבֵל. M. Kat. 20ᵇ כל שמִתְאַבֵּל עליו מתא׳ עמו over whom one is bound to mourn, with him he must mourn, i. e. one must share in the mourning ceremonies of a relation at whose death he would have to observe mourning; a. fr.—Tanh. Sh'mini, 1 נתא׳. Pesik. Sos p. 148ᵇ; a. fr.

אֲבֵיל, **אֲבַל** ch. same. Targ. Lam. II, 8. *Ithpa.* אִתְאַבַּל (denom. of אֲבֵלָא) *to mourn*. Targ.

Gen. XXXVII, 34; a. fr.—Y. Ab. Zar. I, 39ᶜ top. v. אִימְרָא. Esth. R. beg. כד ילידת חוו מִתְאַבְּלִין when the Empress gave birth, they (the Jews) mourned (it being the Ninth of Ab). B. Kam. 59ᵇ את חשיבא לְאִתְאַבּוּלֵי וכ׳ ed. (Ms. R. לְאַבּוּלֵי, v. infra) art thou distinguished enough to wear mourning for Jerusalem?

*Pa. אַבֵּל, אֲבֵיל. Ib. מְאַבֵּילְנָא ed. (Ms. F. מאבלנא, v. Rabb. D. S. a. l., note 6) I wear mourning.

אֵבֶל m. (b. h., foreg.) *mourning*; cmp. אֲבֵילוּת. Y. M. Kat. III, 82ᵇ; a. fr.—*Pl.* אֲבֵילִים. M. Kat. 7ᵇ מי שתכפוהו אֲבֵילָיו he whom his mourning days overtook, i. e. a second case occurring before the mourning days of the first expired.—אֵבֶל רַבָּתִי *Ebel Rabbathi* (Great Mourning), name of a Talmudic treatise, also named euphemistically שְׂמָחוֹת *Rejoicings*.—[Chald. Targ. Gen. L, 11; v. אֶבְלָא.]

אֶבֶל, v. אוּבָל.

אֲבִילָא, אָבִיל, אֲבֵלָא ch.=h. אָבֵל. Targ. Koh. VII, 2; a. e.—Pl., אֲבִילַיָּא, אֲבֵלֵי, אֲבִילִין. Targ. Prov. XXXI, 6; a. e.—Y. M. Kat. III, 82ᵈ bot.; a. e.

אִיבְלָא, אֶבְלָה, אֶבְלָא ch.=h. אֵבֶל. Targ. Gen. L, 11 (Var. אִיבְלָא אֵבֶל). Ib. O. XXVII, 41; a. e. Targ. Y. II Lev. X, 19 אֲבֵילָא.—Gen. R. s. 27 (prov.) comes joy, rejoice; בשעת א׳ א׳ comes mourning, mourn.

אֶבְלוּ, אֲבִלוּ f.=אֲבֵילוּתָא. Targ. Y. II Deut. XXVI, 14.

אבלומוס Ar. ed. Koh., v. אבלוסמוס.

***אבלונים, אבלינים** (?) name of a *spring*. Gen. R. s. 33 (Snh. 108ᵃ בלועה דגדר). Cmp. אבילן, אובלן.

***אַבְלוּסְמוּס** (Ar. ed. Koh. אבלומוס) m. (αὔλισμος) *night-lodging in open air*. כלי א׳ *camping apparels* (leather covers etc.). Zeb. 94ᵃ Ar. (ed. אַבְסְלְוָא q. v.).

***אַבְלוּשֵׁי** m. pl. (בלש 2); cmp. פלש, a. b. h. פלס) *those who cut through* (cmp. בקע a. deriv.), whence *ground-diggers*. (Maim.). B. Mets. 77ᵃ א׳ דמחוזא Ar. Var. (ed. a. Ar. אב׳ q. v.; Ms. M. אוכלסי, Ms. R. אבלוזי) the ground-diggers (working men) of M.

אַבְלֶט pr. n. m. *Ablet*, a gentile scholar, Ab. Zar. 30ᵃ. Y. Sabb. III, 6ᵃ bot., Y. Bets. II, 61ᶜ.

***אבליג, אבליגה** pr. n. m. Pesik. R. s. 33 [Y. Naz. VII, 56ᵃ מגבילה; Y. Ber. III, 6ᵃ bot. גבילה].

***אַבְלִינָא** m. (ἐβέλινος=ἐβένινος S.) *ebony-wood*. Y'lamd. B'haal. מטות של א׳ (quot. in Ar., Tanh. a. Num. R. s. 14 only . . . מנורות) couches of ebony wood. [Jellin. Beth Hammidr. VI, 88, Nr. 53 אבלגא.]

***אַוְלָס, אַבְלָס** pr. n. pl. *Avlas*, in Cilicia, mentioned as one of the northern border places of the land of Israel. Targ. Y. I Num. XXXIV, 8 אב׳ דקילקאי; Y. II ibid. תחומא דאוו׳ דקל׳ (the district of) A. of the Cilicians. Tosef. Shebi. IV, 11 עילר רבתא ed. Zuck. (Var. אולס); Sifré Deut. 51 לולא רבתא; Yalk. Deut. 624 לילא רבתא; Y. Shebi. VI. 36ᶜ אילם רבתא. [Probably identical with Pylæ Ciliciæ, Πύλαι τῆς Κιλίκιας.] [Sifré Num. 131 סבטיא מאולם; Y. Snh. X, 28ᵈ סובתה מאולם S. of Ulam;- Bab. ib. 64ᵃ סבטא בן אלס(?).]

אֶבְמוּסוּס pr. n. m. (Εὔμουσος) *Eumusus*. Y. Meg. III, 74ᵃ bot., rendered in a secret letter טוב למיד well-learned; v. אֶבְדּוֹקוֹס.

אֶבְמָכוֹס pr. n. m. (Εὔμαχος) *Eumachus*, an Amora. Y. Snh. III, end, 21ᵈ.

אֶבֶן f. (b. h., √אב, comp. אבר, v. Ges. H. Dict. s. v.) *stone*. Sabb. 10ᵃ; Pes. 12ᵇ כזורק א׳ וכ׳ like throwing a stone into a leather bottle (has no effect, or is indigestible). Num. R. s. 22 (prov.) into a well out of which you drank אל תזורק בו א׳ cast no stone.—א׳ טובה *jewel*. B. Bath. 16ᵇ; a. fr. *Pl.* אֲבָנִים, const. אַבְנֵי. Gen. R. s. 68 אם מתאחות הן שלשה א׳ (read שלש) שנים עשרה א׳. Ib. if these three stones shall grow into one; a. fr.

Compounds and combinations: בית א׳ *Stone Chamoer*, name of a Temple compartment. Parah III, 1.—א׳ גלוין, v. בָּנָה (א׳ טוען, א׳ טוען) א׳ הטועים.—אֶבֶן *Stone of Losers* (Claims), a place in Jerusalem where lost and found things were deposited and claimed. Taan. III, 8; Y. ib. 66ᵈ bot.; B. Mets. 28ᵇ—א׳ המכר or א׳ המקח *auction place* (for slaves). Sifré Deut. 26. Sifra B'har ch. VII, s. 6. Yalk. Lev. 667 א׳ הלקח.—א׳ מסמא a stone used for closing a pit etc. Nid. 69ᵇ בא׳ מ׳ the corpse was put on a closing (immovable) stone; a. e.—א׳ קבועה *a stone rooted in the ground*, opp. תלושה. Y. Sotah IX, 23ᶜ top.—אבני חעדדה v. אדני.—א׳ שׁוֹאֶבֶת *magnetic stone, load-stone*. Snh. 107ᵇ; a. e.—א׳ הַשָּׁעוֹת *stone-dial*, Kel. XII, 4; a. e.—א׳ שְׁתִיָּה *foundation stone*, stone Sh'thiya which in the second Temple occupied the place of the Holy Arc. Yoma V, 2 (3); v. Gem. a. l.—אבנים תּוֹשָׁבוֹת *immigrant stones*, i. e. stones brought over from another ground. Tosef. Shebi. III, 4; cmp. Shebi. III, 7 a. Y. Gem. a. l.—א׳ תלושה v. sup. א׳ קבועה.—א׳ תקומה *preserving stone*, a stone believed to protect against abortion. Sabb. 66ᵃ.—[For other combinations see respective determinants.]

אַבְנָא, אֶבֶן ch. same. Targ. Gen. XXVIII, 18; a. fr.—Pl. אַבְנַיָּא, אַבְנֵי, אַבְנִין. Targ. Ex. XXVIII, 11; a. fr. Lev. R. s. 16; a. e.—א׳ דאבפא *weight-stones*, to prevent the sheaves being blown away. B. Bath. 69ᵃ.—א׳ דכוחלא *black marble stone*. Kid. 12ᵃ. [Targ. Prov. XXIII, 28, read with Ms. Luzz. וצארא בניא שברי and captures foolish sons.] [Y. B. Bath. II, 13ᶜ דייק אבן . . . corrupt a. defective.]

אֹבֶן m., only in Du. אָבְנַיִם (b. h., √בן, v. בֵּין, cmp. אֹפֶן) 1) *the potter's turning implement*.—2) *the passage of the embryo, vagina*. Ex R. s. 1 (etym.) מקום שהולד נפנה בו (some ed. נקנה incorr.) where the child turns (to come to light). [Oth. etym. v. ibid. a. Sot. 11ᵇ.]

אַבְנָא, v. אֶבֶן ch.

אבנגר Sabb. 109ᵇ, v. בנגר.

אַבְנֵט m. (b. h., בנט, √בט, cmp. בטן) *belt*. B. Kam. 94ᵇ. Yoma 6ᵃ; 12ᵃ; a. fr.—*Pl.* אַבְנֵטִים. Zeb. 18ᵃ.

אַבְנִימוֹס, נִימוֹס pr. n. m. *Abnimos*, *Nimos*, a gentile philosopher, friend of R. Meïr [prob. identical with the cynic philosopher *Oenomaus* of Gadara]. Gen. R. s. 65; a. e. א׳ הגרדי. Ḥag. 15[b] נ׳ הגרדי.

***אבניתא** Targ. Y. II Deut. XIV, 18, read with Y. I אֶכְמַתָא, v. אוּכ׳.

אוּבְנְתָא, אַבְנְתָא f. (בין) *understanding, speculation.* Meg. 24[b] בא׳ דל׳ תלי (Ms. M. באוב׳) it depends on the speculative faculty (not on the physical sight). Ab. Zar. 28[b] באי׳ דל׳ תלי (Ms. M. בליבא תליא, cmp. Tosaf. a. l.) an affection of the eye-sight is connected with (has influence on) the mental faculties; (oth. opin., cmp. אֹבֶן, *the fat surrounding the heart*).

אָבַס (b. h.; √אב, cmp. אפץ) *to stuff; to fatten, feed* (act. a. neut.) B. Mets 86[b] (expl. ăbusim, I Kings V, 3) שאוֹבְסִין אותן בע״כ which people fatten with force. Ib. שא׳ ועומדין וכ׳ that stand feeding as they please. Sabb. XXIV, 3 (155[b]) אין אוֹבסין וכ׳ you must not (on the Sabbath) stuff the camel; expl. ib. you must not make אֵבוּס בתוך וכ׳ a manger of her stomach (fill up to swelling); a. fr.—Part. pass. אָבוּס (=שור). Meg. 9[a], a. e. (one of the changes said to have been made by the authors of the Septuag.).

אַבַסְקַנְמָה (ἀβάσκαντα) *unbewitched! may no harm befall you!* Y. Ab. Zar. I, end, 40[b] א׳ לא אמר he did not say *abascanta*, but etc. Y. Ber. IV, 13[c] top (corr. acc.).

הֲבֵעַ=אַבֵּעַ, v. נבע.

אֲבַעְבּוּעִין m. pl. (ביע) *blains, pustules.* Targ. O. Ex. IX, 9 (Var. אֲבַעְבּוּעָן f. pl.).

אֲבַעַד, v. בְּעַד.

אוֹבְעָיָה, אֲבַעְיָה f. (בְּעָה) *search, begging, the appearance of the poor for their share in the crop. Pl.* אַבְעָיוֹת. Peah IV, 5 ג׳ אב׳ וכ׳ (Y. ed. IV, 3 אוּב׳) three times a day the poor would come (cmp. etym. Y. ib. 18[b] top). [Oth. comment. ref. to etym. in Y. l. c. a. Targ. Obad. v. 6: "the owner appears" &c.]

אֲבַצָּא m. (=אבּצּא, cmp. בעץ) *tin.* Targ. O. Num. XXXI, 22.

אָבָק m. (b. h.; v. אָבַק, cmp. עשן), (*thick, whirling*) *dust, powder.* Sabb. III, 3 אֲבַק דרכים the (heated) sand on the roads. Ḥull. 91[a]. Cant. R. to III, 6; a. fr.—א׳ הסופרים *the refuse of writing material*, or *the colored sand strewn over the writing.* Sabb. XII, 5 כתב במשקין וכ׳ if one writes (on the Sabb.) with a fluid or sap of fruits (instead of ink), or in the sand on roads or in the writer's powder.—Trnsf. (cmp. אָבַק) *connection, something akin to, shade of*, as א׳ לשון הרע a shade of slander; א׳ רבית a shade of usury; א׳ של שביעית an agricultural occupation indirectly related to those forbidden in the Sabbath year; v. infr.—*Pl.* אֲבָקוֹת. Tosef. Ab. Zar. I, 10 ארבע א׳ הן (ed. Zuck. אבקאות) the word *abak* in its figur. sense is applied to four things; cmp. B. Bath. 165[a]; B. Mets. 61[b]; 67[a]; Succ. 40[b].

אָבַק, *Pi.* אִבֵּק, אִיבֵּק (denom. of foreg.) *to cover with powder*, esp. plants, for fertilizing. Shebi. II, 2 מְאַבְּקִין (cmp. Y. Gem. a. l.). M. Kat. 3[a]. Y. Sabb. VII, 10[a] top.—Part. pass. מְאוּבָּק *powdered.* Y. Bicc. I, 63[d] bot. מאונקות (read מְאוּבָּ׳) grapes fertilized with powder. [Ar. "to remove the dust"(?)]

Hithpa. a. *Nithpa.* הִתְאַבֵּק, נִתְאַ׳ *to be covered*, or *cover one's self with dust.* Gen. R. s. 43.—Metaph. *to sit at one's feet as a disciple.* Aboth. I, 4.

אָבַק, אֲבִיק (√אב, עב, cmp. אבך, חבק) 1) *to entangle, twist, twine.* Men. 42[a] אביק להו מיבק (perh. אַבִּיק *Pa.*) he twined (the show-fringes) with loops.—2) (neut. v.) *to be attached to, cling to* (idolatry etc.). Snh. 64[a]; Ab. Zar. 14[b]. Ib. 17[a] א׳ בה טובא he was very deeply attached to sensuality.

אַבְקָא, אָבָק ch.=h. אָבָק. Targ. Ex. IX, 9; a. e.

אבק Tosef. Mikv. V, 7, read אָבִיק.

אַבְקָא, v. אָבָק ch.

אבקאות, v. אָבָק h.

אַבְקָה f. (b. h.; v. אָבָק) *spices, spice-box.* Fig. אַבְקַת רוֹכֵל (peddlar's spice-box) *a great scholar.* Cant. R. to III, 6 end.

אֶבְקוֹלֹס pr. n. m. (Εὔκολος) *Eucolus*, father of R. Zechariah. Git. 56[a]; Lam. R. to IV, 2. Tosef. Sabb. XVI (XVII), 6 (Var. אבטולס, אביקלוס). Cmp. אפיקולוס.

אבקת Men. 33[a], read אבקתא, v. next w.

אַבַקְתָא f. pl. (אָבַק) *loops, leather rings*, on bedsteads for the reception of cords; in door cases, for hanging doors in. Ned. 56[b]; Snh. 20[b]. דרגש בא׳ . . . . . a couch is called *dargesh*, when it is carried in and out (to be put up and taken apart) by means of loops (through which the cords are fastened); opp. *mittah*, v. בְּזִיוָנָא.—Men. 33[a], Erub. 11[b] ed. (Ms. M. אנקתא, v. Rabb. D. S. a. l. note), explain. היכר ציר 'an indication of hinges'.—Macc. 23[a] (*loops* in the punishing scourge).

אבר or יבר Hif. הוֹבִיר, v. בּוּר.

אָבַר (√אב, v. אבב; cmp. גבר, חבר) *to be bent, pressed, thick.*

Pi. אִבֵּר, אִיבֵּר 1) *to strengthen, harden* (cmp. אמץ). Snh. 109[b] (play on *Abiram*, Num. XVI, 1) שאי׳ לבו מ׳ וכ׳ Ms. M. (Rashi לִבּוֹ, ed. עצמו) he hardened his heart against repentance.—2) (denom. of אֵבֶר) *to measure wings, to define city limits, for Sabbath distances, in cases of wing-like projections beyond the line.* Erub. V, 1 כיצד מְאַבְּרִין (accord. to Rab's spelling, while Sam. read מְעַבְּרִין, v. Y. ib. 22[b], Bab. ib. 53[a]) how do we measure outskirts of a city in order to draw the Sabbath line?; v. etymol. definit. Y. a. Babl. ll. cc. a. Y. Ber. VII, 12[c] top.—3) (b. h. Hif.) *to soar, take wings.* Gen. R. s. 42 (play on *Shemeber*, Gen. XIV, 2) שמְּאַבֵּר וכ׳ Ar. s. v. שבאבר (ed. שהיה פורח) he took wings to fly and obtain wealth.

אֲבַר ch. Ithpe. אִתְאֲבַר (v. next w. a. foreg.) *to be winged, to soar.* Targ. Job XXXIX, 29.

אֵבֶר, (אֵיבֶר) m. (b. h. *wing*, v. אָבַר; cmp. כָּנָף, כַּף, כְּנָפָה) 1) *limb, part.*—א׳ מן החי a part cut off from a living animal. Ḥull. 101[b]; a. fr.—2) *membrum genitale.* Snh. 107[a]. Y. Keth. V, 30[b].—3) *town quarter, projecting outskirts* (v. אָבַר Pi. 2).—א׳ א׳ *limb by limb; piecemeal.* Sabb. 40[a]. Y. Yoma VI, 43[d] bot. Koh. R. to X, 15.—*Pl.* אֲבָרִים, אֵיבָרִים, אֵיבָרִין *limbs, parts* (of an animal). Shek. VII, 3 meat found אי׳ in entire limbs (opp. חתיכות cut slices). Sabb. 82[b] אינה מטמאה לא׳ Ms. M. (ed. אינה לא׳) does not make unclean when dismembered. Kel. XVIII, 9 (parts of a bedstead).—א׳ א׳ as sing. Ḥull. 11[b]. Treat. S'maḥ. II, 12.—Ber. I, 1 the fat וא׳ and other pieces of the daily offerings. Ohol. I, 8 רמ״ח א׳ 248 limbs (joints).—4) *balance of a load, ballast.* Sabb. 154[b], v. חֲבַר.—Ch. אֵיבְרָא.

אֲבָר m. (v. אָבַר; b. h. עֹפֶרֶת) *lead.* Snh. 52[a] פתילה של א׳ a string (bar) of lead. Ḥull. 8[a] א׳ מעיקרו lead directly from the mine (hot). Y. Sabb. VII, 10[b] bot. Kel. XIV, 5 הא׳ שבצד וכ׳ the lead hanging down from the neck of the animal (as ornament or mark). Git. 19[a]; Sabb. 104[b] כתבו בא׳ if he wrote the document with lead (solution); a. fr.

אֲבַר, אֲבָרָא (אַבְרָא) ch. same. Targ. Ex. XV, 10. Targ. Y. Lev. XX, 14; a. e.—Snh. 64[a] שדיוהו וכ׳ cast ye him into a kettle (of lead) וכסיוהו וכ׳ and cover him with lead (or heavy load; ed. שדיוה incorr.; Ms. M. omits דאברא; oth. var. v. Rabb. D. S. a. l.). Git. 19[a] בא׳ (writing) with lead pencil, במיא דא׳ with a solution of lead.

אֶבְרָא *limb*, v. אֵיבְרָא.

אִבְרָא, v. אֵיבְרָא.

***אַבְּרָא**, Targ. Prov. XXX, 31 Ms. *the cock*, cmp. אבר a. גבר; v. אַבְּבָא.

אַבְרַאי adv. (בר) *outside*, freq. with prefix מִ־, opp. אגואי. Ḥull. 130[a b] Ab. Zar. 2[b] למיתב מלכא מא׳ for the king to wait outside (of the court-room). R. Hash. 8[b] למיקם . . . א׳. Ber. 18[b] יתיב א׳ sat outside (of the gathering of the righteous in heaven). Cmp. בְּרָאֵי.

אברגני, אברוגני, Erub. 62[a], Var., v. אַבּוּרְגְּנָא.

אַבְרוּיֵ, v. בריי ch.

אַבְרוֹרֵי, אַבְרָוֹרֵי m. pl. (denom. of אבר, cmp. חבורורי) 1) (cmp. אָבַר Pi.) *wings* or *corners of city walls* (h. פִּנָּה), *pinnacles, mural turrets.* Sabb. 11[a] ed. (Ar. אברארי, read אבראורי; Ms. M. אַוְרָרֵי; Var. lect. v. Rabb. D. S. a. l. note) 2) (v., אֵבֶר a. חֲבַר) *balance, freight arranged for balancing, ballast.* B. Bath 24[b] אימור באברור׳ הוו מנחי Ms. M. (ed. באברו׳) I may say, the small kegs were placed among the large for balancing purposes.

אִבְרוֹטִי, v. אִבְרוֹסִי.

אברוכסים, v. ברייכסון.

אברומא, אבדומא f. *hash or brine of a certain fish* (Ἀβραμίς?). Succ. 18[a] (Ms. M. a. ed. אבר׳, v. Rabb. D. S. a. l.) [Rashi: *'a very small fish'.*]

***אִבְרוֹסִי** m. (prob. a. geogr. term) *ibrosi*, name of a species of olive of medium size, also called אֲגוּרִי q. v. Ber. 39[a] its name is not *egori*, אלא א׳ וכ׳ Ms. M. (ed. אברוטי, Ar. ed. Koh. אברוצי) but its original name is *ibrosi* or as some say סַבְרוֹסִי Ms. M. (ed. סמרוסי); Y. Bicc. I, 63[d] bot. אוורוס (אוורוס).

אברוקלון, v. אַסְתּוּרְקְלוֹן.

אַבְרוּרֵי, v. אַבְרָוֹרֵי.

***אַבְרוּשָׁן** m. (Pers. âfrôsah) *a dish of flour, honey, and oil;* a word in a marginal note in Ms. M. to Ber. 37[a], quoted in Ar. and in Rashi to 36[b] bot. (אברוש״די, corr. acc.), defining חביץ קדרה. V. Rabb. D. S. a. l.

***אבריות, אַבְרוֹת**, Tosef. Neg. VIII, 2, v. בְּרוֹת.

***אַבְרִזִין** m. pl. (בזא II, v. בְּרָזָא II; cmp. h. equiv. עֻבְצָה, עוּבְצָא) prop. *cutting, trimming*, hence *fur trimmed of its extremities (and pinked)*, in gen. *carriage-robe, cover* [R. Hai Gaon declares our w. to be Persian, v. Ar. ed. Koh. s. v., a. Fl. to Levy Targ. Dict. II, 579[b].] B. Kam. 66[b] מעיקרא קרו וכ׳ (Ms. M. אברזר) before its use was determined upon it was called *mishkha* (skin), and now (even before the trimming is done), it is called *ăbirzin* (fur, robe). V. קִיצוּיָ.

***אברייאה** *Pl.* fem. אַבְרָיְיתָא (v. בַּר II) lit. *outside places*, hence *villages, cottages.* Y. Ber. VI, 10[a] [Comment. *'to take refreshments'*, v. אֵיבְרָיָא.] [אברייאה Cant. R. to II, 14, read אִיפַּרְכַיָא, v. אִיפַּר.]

אַבְרִיקִין, Y. Sabb. XVI, 15[d], v. אַבְרָקִין.

אברית, v. אַבְרוֹת.

אַבְרֵךְ (Gen. XLI, 43) *Abhrekh*, a title; homiletically defined אָב בחכמה וַרךְ בשנים *father* in wisdom, *tender* in years. Gen. R. s. 90.

***אַבְרְנִי** m. (prob. fr. אָבַר; *well-winged*) name of a *bird*, prob. *sea-mew.* Yalk. Esth. 1054; (Esth. R. to III, 6 ציף).

***אַבְרְנִים** (?) (Pers., v. Fl. to Levy Talm. Dict. s. v., a. Lagarde Ges. Abh. vol. 23) *half-done meat.* Pes. 41[a] (explain. נָא Ex. XII, 9) כדאמרי פרסאי א׳ (Yalk. Ex. 197 כד׳ אינשי) as the Persians say *abarnim.* [כדאמרי פרסאי does not necessarily refer to the Persian language, cmp. דְּבִיר. Perh. our w. is a Hebrew expression known among Persian Jews, and a compound of אֵבֶר נִים (=נאים, נעים) *a tender piece.* Cmp. בְּנָאִים.]

אַבְרְנְסִי, v. אוּרְנוּס.

אברסקין, v. אוורקסין.

אַבְרְקִין, בְּרְקִין m. pl. (פרק=ברק; cmp. פקר=בקר, v. אפקרסין) *underclothes, inexpressibles, breeches* (cmp. Lat. bracæ, braccæ—of Oriental origin). Y. Sabb. XVI, 15^d שני א׳ Ar. (ed. Krot. אַבְרִיקִין; Bab. ib. 120^a וב׳ פרגד, Ms. M. פרגוד, Ar. פרגודין; Rashi *genouilliers*, a. German *Kniehosen*). Y'lamd. B'resh. quot. in Ar. (expl. פרישיחון Dan. III, 21) ב׳ הנהונות וכ׳ (fem.) the underclothes put around their loins.

אַבְרְתָא, אַבְרְתָה f. pl. (בריי, v. אִיבְרְיָיא, a. חַבְרָאָה) *hyssop* (used against indigestion &c.). Sabb. 128^a (explaining אֵזוֹב). Ib. 109^b אברתה (mentioning two species, one named אזוב=בר־הזמג, the other אזוב יון=בר־הזנג). Ab. Zar. 29^a Ms. M. a. Ar. (ed. אבדתא).

אַבִישׁוּנָא, אַבְשׁוּנָא m. (יבש=אבש) *something dried; parched* or *dried ears of grain*. Meg. 7^b; Ps. 39^b קמחא דא׳ flour of roasted ears. Ib. 40^a חצבא דאבשו׳ Ar. (ed. דאב׳) a basin wherein ears are roasted.

אַבְשִׁין, v. אוּבְשִׁין.

אָגָא (עָגָה) (Samar. אגה rendition of b. h. נקב; cmp. הָגָה) *to spell* (letters), *blaspheme, swear*. Snh. 101^b תנא (ו)בגבולין ובלשון אגא Ar. (ed. עגה), the Boraitha remarks (to ההוגה as in Mishn. a. l.) this (condemnation of one uttering the name of the Lord) refers to the country (not the Temple), and in the sense of Samaritan *aga* (swearing). Cmp. Y. Snh. X, 28^b top כגון אילין כותאי וכ׳ in a way as those Samaritans swear.

אגאלוגין, אגאליגין Gen. R. s. 28, beg., read אִרְלוּגִין.

אַגַּב (contr. of עַל=אל גב, cmp. אַ־) prop. *on the back, on top of*, hence, *upon, on the basis*; (logic.) *by dint of, on account of; by the way of*. Snh. 95^b א׳ אורחך while on thy road, i. e. *incidentally, occasionally*. Freq. א׳ אורחא, v. אוֹרְחָא.—B. Mets. 21^b א׳ דיקירי *because* they are heavy.—Ib. 11^b, a. fr. מטלטלין א׳ מקרקעי the sale of movable chattel made binding by dint of immovable property jointly sold; cmp. קַרְקַע.—Kid. 26^b א׳ אחך by means of somebody else (taking possession in behalf of the absent person). Ib. 27^a מי בעינן א׳ is it necessary that he must say, 'Acquire movable by dint of acquiring landed property'?—Pes. 113^a כל א׳ גבויא בעיא every claim the legality of which rests on some additional circumstance (e. g. a loan collectible only on producing the note of indebtedness) requires collection (cannot be considered actual property until collected).—Sabb. 116^a א׳ כתב הוא דקדוש the parchment is sacred only on account of the sacred character of what is written on it.— Shebu. 40^b, v. גַּדְדָא; a. fr.

אַגַּבָּא, v. גַּבָּא.

אגבאסטס, v. אָגוּסְטוֹס, end.

*****אַגְבִּין** m. (=אוּגְבִּין, h. גְּבִיעַ, גִּבְעוֹל) *calix* or *corolla* of flowers. Y. Kil. IX, 32^a top א׳ קסריר the *cissaros blossom* (v. Lat. Dict. s. v. *cissaros*, Gr. Dict. s. v. χρυσάνθεμον) "a woolly substance growing on stones at the Dead Sea, looking like gold, and being very soft; its name is כלך (χάλκη, κάλχη) and it resembles sheepwool".—(R. Ash. a. l. in Mishn.). Y. Sabb. II, 4^c top אגב׳ ק׳, corr. acc. [Var. lect. אנטין, אַצְוָא=אצבין?.—Sabb. 20^b, our w. appears as גושקרא, גשקרא, obviously a corruption of *cissaros;* Rashi ib. expl. 'the shell of the cocoon', prob. confounding with *chrysallis* which is likewise named from its gold color.]

אָגַד I (√אג, sec. r. of אוג, v. אוּגְרָא, cmp. חגר, אגר, עקד) 1) *to twine around, tie up; to close, forbid*. Succ. III, 1; a. fr.—Sabb. 60^a אוֹגֶדֶת בו וכ׳ Ar. (ed. אוגרת, Ms. M. חוגרת) she fastens her hair with it.—Pes. 87^a בנות ישראל שאוגדות וכ׳ ed. (Ms. M. שמגידות ... בחורות, v. Hif.) the maidens in Israel who forbid intimacy to their betrothed. Erub. 21^b ל׳ אאוגדות ed. (missing in Ms. M.).—2) (denom. of אֲגֻדָּה) *to form a union* or *faction*. Sifré Deut. 294, v. Nif. [B. Bath. 14^a לוחות אוגדות, v. אָגַר a. אָכַל.]

Nif. נֶאֱגַד *to be tied up, united* &c. Maasr. I, 5 ירק הנ׳ משיאגד vegetables ordinarily put up in bunches, are subject to tithes from the time they are tied. Y. Erub. III, 20^d top.—Sifré Deut. 296 שלא תאגוד עליך אגודה (read תֵּאָגֵד) no alliance (of the surrounding nations) shall be formed against thee.

Hif. הֶאֱגִיד, contr. הִגִּיד, part. מַגִּיד, מֵגִיד, *to tie up, fence in, forbid*. Erub. 21^b; Pes. 87^a Ms. M. (play on מגדים Cant. VII, 14) שמגידות וכ׳ who forbid &c., v. supra (Rashi: שֶׁמַּגִּידוֹת, v. נגד, who announce their menstruation); v. אָגַד II.

אָגַד I ch. same *to tie*. Part. pass. אָגִיד. Yeb. 39^b הא אֲגִידָא ביה is she not tied to him?, hence he *must* marry her.

אָגַד II (√גד, v. נגד a. גדל), Hif. הִגִּיד *to stretch, prolong, postpone*. Erub. 21^b; Pes. 87^a (Ar. s. v. גד, v. however אָגַד I) שמגידות וכ׳ who postpone (reserve) sexual intimacy for their husbands. Y. Keth. V, 29^d bot. אני מַגֶּדֶת וכ׳ I will extend (spend all the time of) my widowhood in my husband's house.

אֲגַד II ch. same; *to be lengthened*. Targ. Y. Ex. XIX, 13; Deut. XXX, 6. Denom. אוּגְדּוּתָא.

אגד III, אַגְדָּא m. (foreg.) *long staff*, whence 1) *crutch*. Targ. II Sam. III, 29 (some ed. אגר).—2) *pole* used as a yoke to carry burdens on the shoulder. B. Mets 83^a דדרי בא׳ Ar., Ms. H., Oxf. &c. (Ms. M. איגרא, ed. אגרא, v. Rabb. D. S. a. l. note) who carry a burden on a yoke. Bets. 30^a (v. Rabb. D. S. a. l. note 3); Sabb. 148^a Ms. M. marg. אגרתא! (v. Rabb. D. S. a. l. note 6). V. תְּגְדָא.

אֶגֶד (אִיגֶד) m. (אגד I) 1) *tie, knot*. Succ. 10^b, a. fr. צריך א׳ must be tied together. Ib. הותר אֶגְדוֹ if the tie of the Lulab became loosened. Erub. 101^b sq. בנינל באֶגְדוֹ (a. twice אִיגְ׳, Rabb. in D. S. a. l. באוגדו) when the door pin is handled by pulling the cord knotted to it.—2) *bunch*. Y. Ter. II, 41^b א׳ שנטמא a bunch of herbs that became unclean.—3) surgical *bandage*. Sabb. 53^a.

*****אִיגַד, אֱגַד** ch. same. Succ. 33^b א׳ מעלייתא וכ׳ (fem.!) it requires a substantial binding.

אַגְדָּא, v. אֲגַד III.

אַגָּדָה, or **אֲגָדָה** f. (נגד, נ absorbed or dropped=הַגָּדָה) *tale, story, lesson*, esp. *Agadah*, that class of Rabb. literature which explains the Bible *homiletically*, opp. to *Halakhah* or *legal interpretation* (שְׁמוּעָה, הֲלָכָה). M. Kat. 23ª שמ׳ וא׳ a legal tradition and an Agadah (homily). Y. Yeb. XII, 13ª. Y. B. Bath. VI, 15ᶜ מסורת א׳ היא it is a traditional Agadah.—Y. Git. IV, 45ᶜ ...מאן בא׳ דריק לך who among us can enter into what thy grandfather said?—בעל א׳ a lecturer on Agadah. Gen. R. s. 94; a. fr.—אֲגָדַת תלים the Agadah on Psalms. Ib. s. 33.—*Pl.* אֲגָדוֹת, אַגָּ׳. Lev. R. s. 22, beg.; a. fr.—Cmp. אֲגַדְתָּא.

אֲגֻדָּה, pl. אֲגֻדּוֹת Tosef. Makhsh. III, 8 ed. Zuck., v. אֲגוּדָּה.

אגדו, אגדון, v. אִגְּרוֹ.

אגדיס, v. הֲגְדָּס.

אֶגְדִּיקוֹס (אֶגְדִיקָס, popular corrupt. אנד׳, cmp. אַנְדִּיסְקֵר) m. (ecdicus=cognitor sive defensor civitatis, esp. in Asia Minor) *state's agent, syndic.* Gen. R. s. 12 א׳ ממונה על בריא שלה (ed. אנד׳; בית שלו, corr. acc.) when an ecdicus is in the country, he holds the authority over the public road (curator viæ, v. בְּיָא). Yalk. Ps. 794 (a. Ar.) אגר׳, corr. acc.—*Pl.* אֶגְדִּיקִין, אנ׳. Cant. R. to VII, 9 (ed. אנ׳).

אַגְדְּנָא m. (v. גְּדַד I a. גִּידָא, P. Sm. 23) *worm-wood* (Rashi: *horehound*). Ab. Zar. 29ª Ar. a. ed. (Ms. M. אוגרנא, with ר), in a prescription against asthma. Targ. Y. I Deut. XXIX, 17 אגר׳ (Var. אגד׳); ed. Vienna pl. אַגְדְּנַיָּא (אגר׳).

אַגַּדְתָּא f. ch. (=h. אֲגָדָה) 1) *Agadah, homiletic literature.* B. Kam. 60ᵇ opp. שמעתתא. Sotah 49ª יהא שמיה רבא דא׳ (abbr. יה״ש״ר) the *kaddish* (prayer) after lectures. Y. Sabb. XVI, 15ᶜ.—2) *the Haggadah*, i. e. *the recitations for the Passover night.* Ps. 115ᵇ א׳ והלילא Haggadah and Hallel. Ib. 116ᵇ מאן דאמר א׳ וכ׳ who recited the Hag. in the house of R. Joseph (who was blind)?

אֲגָה m. (אָגָה *to sting*, v. אָגָא, √חג=אג, v. חגג) *thorn, thorn-bush.* Y. Shebi. VII, 37ᵇ top.—*Pl.* אֲגִין. Y. Kil. V, 30ª bot.; v. הִיגָה.

אַגְוָאֵי adv. *inside, amid*, v. אַבְרָאֵי. Hull. 130ªᵇ. Cmp. גַּו.

אַגְוָגָא m. (אגג, v. אָגָה=h. חוֹגֵג q. v.) *cleft, fissure.* א׳ דמיא *cataract, water-falls* (issuing from a fissure). Lam. R. to I, 17 (play on *hogeg* ibid. Ps. XLII, 5) כהדין א׳ וכ׳ Ar. like the cataract that rests neither &c. [Ed. גגגנא].

אָגוּד m. (אגד I) *band.* Y. Sabb. VI, 8ª bot.; Y. Yeb. XII, 12ᵈ top א׳ מלבינקי a band (of bast) with which mala punica (pomegranates) are tied together.—*Pl.* אֲגוּדִים, const. אֲגוּדֵי. Peah VI, 10 א׳ חשום stalks of garlic plant used for tying bunches; [oth. opin. bunches of garlic on one stalk], opp. to אגודות tied bunches. [Tosef. ib. III, 8 אוגודי ed. Zuck., *piles* of garlic, v. אָגוֹר.] [Num. R. s. 4 beg. חשים אגודיהם, v. אָגוּדֵי.]

אֲגוּדָּה f. (b. h. אֲגֻדָּה, v. foreg.) 1) *bundle, bunch.* B. Mets. I, 8. Succ. 33ᵇ כא׳ של וכ׳ as a bunch of herbs is tied; a. fr.—2) *band, union; faction.* Lev. R. s. 30; Gen. R. s. 88 א׳ אחת one brotherhood.—*Pl.* אֲגוּדּוֹת. Peah VI, 10; v. foreg. Makhsh. VI, 2 א׳ של בית וכ׳ (herb) bunches which have been lying in the market houses; v. Tosef. ib. III, 8.—Yeb. 13ᵇ (ref. to תתגדדו Deut. XIV, 1) לא תעשו א׳ א׳ do not form yourselves into religious factions. Ber. 4ª א׳ א׳ in companies (amusing themselves).—3) בֵּית א׳ pr. n. of a family, *Beth-Aguddah.* Mass. Sof'rim IV, 1 ...של ב׳ א׳ the scribes of the family Beth-Ag.

אֲגוּדָל m. (=גּוּדָל) *thumb.* Yoma II, 1. Cant. R. to III, 6.

אֱגוֹז m. (b. h.) *nut.* Git. 64ᵇ (as signs of mental responsibility) א׳ ונוטלו if you throw a nut to it, and the child picks it up (at the same time throwing a pebble away); a. e.—*Pl.* אֱגוֹזִים, const. אֱגוֹזֵי. Orl. III, 8 נתפצעו הא׳ when the nuts are burst open. Ib. 7 אגוזי פרך crack-nuts (eatable); a. fr. [Tosef. Sabb. XIV (XV), 1 אגוז שבספינה ed. Zuck., read אוֹגְרָן, v. הוּגְרָן.] [For etymol. cmp. אָגַס.]

אֱגוֹזָא ch. same; also *nut-tree.* Keth. 77ᵇ גירדא דא׳ scrapings of the bark of a nut-tree; v. אזגא.—Cmp. אַמְגוּזָא, גּוֹזָא.

אֱגוֹזָה f. (v. אֱגוֹז) *nut-tree.* Cant. R. to VI, 11.

אגומרי, v. אָכְסִיגְרוֹן.

***אָגוּסְטוֹר** m. *Quæstor.* Gen. R. s. 12, v. אנגרטוס a. אָגוּסְטוּס, end.

אָגוֹמִין (ἄγωμεν, fr. ἄγω) *up! come on!* Gen. R. s. 78.

אָגוֹן m. (ἀγών) *assembly*, esp. *public games.* Y'lamd. Emor (quot. in Ar, missing in Tanh.) א׳ נעשה במדינה.

אגונה Tanh. Mishp. 1, read אֲגוּנָה.

אגוסטא, (אגוסטה) f. *Augusta*, title of a female member of the imperial family (of Rome), in gen. *princess* &c. Esth. R. to I, 9. [Tan'h. Vaëra 8, א׳, read ...מוס]

***אגוּסְטָאן, אגוּסְטַיין** m. (Augustanus, Augustianus) *a servant in a colonia Augustana*, (perhaps identical with Curialis or Decurio; cmp. Gibbon, ed. Milm. II, 142 sq., Amer. ed.). Snh. 26ª יכול לומר... טאן וכ׳ Ms. M. (Ms. C. a. F. יסטוון.. ed. אגוסטין, אגוסטין, corr. אגוסטירן) he may say (as an excuse for tilling in the Sabbath year), I am merely an imperial servant in the estate.

אגוסטולי, Gen. R. s. 1, v. אוּסְטְלִי.

אָגוּסְטוּס (אגושטוס) m. *Augustus*, title of the Roman emperor, in gen. *ruler, sovereign.* Y. Ber. IX, 12ᵈ bot. as one uses indiscriminately בסיליוס קיסר א׳

(βασιλεύς) Basileus, Cæsar, Augustus; Gen. R. s. 8 (corr. acc.). Ex. R. s. 23, beg.; a. fr.—[Gen. R. s. 12 א׳ במדינה ed. (Ar. אגבאסטס) read אֲגוּסְטוּר or אַגְבָּאִיסְטוּר v. אגוגטוס.]

אֲגוּסְטְיָאנֵי m. pl. *Augustiani*, a Prætorian legion entitled to proclaim the emperor. Esth. R. to I, 3, end דקומיני א׳ the Decumani (or Decimani) and the Aug.—Gen. R. s. 94 גאר׳ (corr. acc.); v. Sachs. Beitr. I, 113 sq.

אגוסטלא, v. next w.

***אֲגוּסְטָלִי** m. (Augustalis). *Præfectus Augustalis*, title of the prefect of Egypt. Gen. R. s. 1. ed. (Var. אגוסטולי, Ar. אגיסטלא).

אגוסתא Ex. R. s. 8 some ed., read אגוסטוס.

אֲגוּף m. (גפף I, גפס) 1) *sexual intercourse*. Y. Git. VII, 48[d] לשייר לו אֲגוּפָהּ to reserve to himself the right of embracing her; Y. B. Bath. VIII, 16[c] top גיפה.—2) *door-stop*, v. אֲגַף.—[אגוף v. אֲגַף.]

אֱגוֹר, אִיגּוֹר m. (אגר I) *heap, hill*. Tosef. Shebi. III, 3 ואגו׳ יוצא וכ׳ ed. Zuck. (Var. ואיגר) and a mound (of arable ground) rises out of it (the rock).—*Pl.* אִיגּ׳, אֱגוֹרִים; const. אִיגּוּרֵי. Tosef. Peah III, 8 אוגורי השום ed. Zuck. (Var. אגידי, אגודות, ed. אגודי, v. אֲגוּד) heaps of garlic on the field, not yet bunched.

אֱגוֹרָא I, אִיגּוֹרָא ch. same; esp. *heathen altar* (cmp. b. h. גַּל). Targ. Jud. VI, 25; a. fr.—*Pl.* אִיגּ׳, אֱגוֹרִין, אִיג׳, אֱגוֹרַיָּא. Targ. II Kings XXI, 3; a. fr.

אֲגוֹרָא II f. (ἀγορά) *market-place, court-session, court*. *Pl.* אֲגוֹרָאוֹת Git. 88[b] א׳ של נכרים (ed. אגוריאות corr. acc.) gentile courts.

***אֲגוֹרָה** f. (אגר) prop. *store-room*, hence *the compartments of the nut-shell*. *Pl.* אֲגוֹרוֹת. Pesik. R. s. 11 as the nut has ארבע א׳ four compartments (Yalk. Cant. 992 מגורות).

אֲגוֹרֵי inf. of אֲגַר—אגורי for אֲגִירֵי, v. אֲגִירָא.

אִיגּוּרִי, אֱגוֹרִי m. (v. אֲגוֹר, אֲגוֹרָה) *fit for storage, of good quality*. Kel. XVII, 8 the olive (as a size standard) . . . neither large nor small, but of medium size, זה א׳ which is the kind called *egori*. Ber. 39[a]; Y. Bicc. I, 63[d] (etymol. explan.); v. אַבְרוֹסִי. Yalk. Deut. 851 זית א׳. Gen. R. s. 91, end מור א׳ myrrh fit for storage. —*Pl.* אֱגוֹרִין Num. R. s. 4 beg. חטים אגודיהן, read אֱגוֹרִין הם are all storage wheat (opp. טרופת). Cmp. אגרו.

אגוריאות; v. אֲגוֹרָא II.

אגושטוס, תוס...., v. אֲגוּסְטוּס.

אגח, אֲגַח, v. גּוּחַ.

אגחותא, אֲגָחוּתָא (אֲגִיח׳) f. (נגח, גוח) *fighting*. Targ. Ps. CX, 3; a. e.

אגטין, Snh. 91[a], v. לֶגְטוֹן;—Y. Kil. IX, 32[a] v. אַגְבִּין.

אַגְטַרְגְטָא m. (καταῤῥάκτης, *cataracta*) *cataract, cascade*.—*Pl.* אַגְטַרְגְּטַיָּיא Y. M. Kat. I, beg. 80[b] אילין א׳ מה וכ׳ what is your opinion about those cascades?

אֲגִיָא, v. אוּגְיָא.

אֲגִיחַ, v. גּוּחַ.

אֲגִיחוּתָא, v. אֲגָחוּתָא.

אגין Tanh. Emor. 18, v. בַּאדִין.—Y. Sabb. II, 5[b] כפר א׳, read חֲנוּךְ=אֲנוּךְ Gen. R. s. 6.

***אַגֵּין** (denom. of אגן, אוגנא, Pa.) *to form disks or cakes* (of wax). Y. Sabb. VII, 10[b] bot. החן דא׳ גיר קררין he who forms cakes of wax dust (on a Sabbath).

אגינו Gen. R. s. 56, some ed. אנונו—a corrupt passage, prob. to be read: ששמר את גנו משבולת הנהר וחקקה את גן בני עמו.

אָגִיס m. *wife's brother* or *kindred, brother-in-law*, v. גִּיס. Snh. III, 7 ed. Y.; a. fr.

אגיסטון. אגיסמין v. אגוס׳.

אגיסטרין, v. אֶגְסְטֵרִין.

אֲגִיר, אֲגִירָא, (אַגִּירָא) אֲגִירָא m. (אֲגַר) *hired man, laborer*. Targ. Job VII, 1; 2; a. fr.—*Pl.* אֲגִירֵי. B. Mets. 76[b] sq. (interch. in ed. with. אגירר, corr. acc.).

***אגריסין**, m. pl., a corruption of a geographical term, perh. אפירוטין (Ἠπειρῶται) (steeds) *of Epyrus*. Targ. Jer. V, 8 (h. text מְשֻׁכָּרִים).

אגיש Lam. R. to I, 21; Pesik. Anokhi p. 138[b], v. גּוּשׁ I.

אגלא, אִיגָּלָא, אֶגְלָא m. (v. גַּל, גלל) *outside-door, city-gate*. —*Pl.* אִיגְּלֵי, אֶגְלֵי. B. Bath 8[a] הכל לאג׳ גפא Ar. (ed. לאג׳. all must contribute towards keeping the city gates in repair.; B. Mets. 108[a] (Ms. M. גַּלֵּי).

אגלוקי, v. גּוּאַלְקָא a. חֲבַר.

אֶגְלִים m. (b. h.; אגל, sec. r. of אוג, cmp. חוג, עוג) *rounded things, rain-drops*. Hag. 12[b] עלייית א׳ (allus. to Job XXXVIII, 28) the upper store in heavens containing the rains. [V. Var. lect. in Rabb. D. S. a. l. note 200.]

אגלין read אֶרְלוֹגִין.

אַגְלָפוּתָא f. (גלף) *engraving, setting*. Targ. Y. Ex. XXXI, 5.

אגלקי, v. גּוּאַלְקָא.

אָגַם I (h. עגם; √גם, v. גמם, גום) *to be bent*, whence *to be in grief*. Targ. Ps. CXIX, 28.

אָגַם II m. (b. h.; v. foreg. a. אַגְמוֹן) *anything bending and peeling*, whence 1) *leek*, or *leek-like plants*, opp. to שחת young grain &c. Kid. 62[b] this refers only to *shahath* אבל בא׳ לא but not to *ăgam*. Ib. מאי משמע דהאי א׳ לישנא דבוצלנא הוא (Ar. דבוצלא) what proof have you that *ăgam* in this case has the meaning of onion-plants? (Answ. ref. to אגמון Is. LVIII, 5).—2) (b. h.) *reed, reed-land* (juncetum), *dwelling places of wild beasts*, opp. שָׂדֶה cultivated land. Taan. 22[a].

אַגָּם m. (גמם) *a field which requires clearing in order to be made arable, uncleared ground containing roots of trees &c.* Ab. Zar. 38ª הַבְּ׳ את האור בא׳ set fire to an uncleared field. Y. ib. II, 44ᵈ bot. א׳ תמרים a field on which palms stood, the roots of which must be grubbed up.

אַגְמָא ch. same. Ab. Zar. 38ª לגלויי א׳ וכ׳ his intention was merely to clear the ground.

אַגְמָא m. ch. (גום, v. אֲגַם) *a depression, stagnant water, lake;* also *marshland, meadow.* B. Mets. 36ᵇ הבלא דא׳ the vapors of the meadow; a. fr. קטל קני בא׳ to cut reeds in the meadow=to be illiterate. Sabb. 95ª; Snh. 33ª.—*Pl.* אַגְמַיָּא, אֲגָמִין. Targ. Is. XXXV, 7; a. e.—אַגְמֵי. Sabb. 77ᵇ דייר בא׳ grazes in meadows.

אַגְמָא II pr. n. pl. *Agma,* in Babylon. B. Mets 86ª.—B. Bath. 127ª; Kid. 72ª אקרא דא׳ Akra d'Agma, v. אַקְרָא. Snh. 38ᵇ אקרא דא׳ (Ar. אגמא דיקורי; oth. var. v. Rabb. D. S. a. l. note).

אַגְמָה, עַגְמָה f. (v. אֲגַם I,) esp. (ע׳) אַגְמַת נפש *grief* of the soul. M. Kat. 14ᵇ; a. fr. Ms. M., s. Ar. א׳ (ed. ע).

אַגְמוֹן m. (b. h. אַגְמֹן; v. אֲגַם II) *reed, cane.*—בּ׳ל הא׳ *cane-bearer,* a subordinate executive officer. Y. Sot. IX, 24ᵇ top; a. e., v. זְמוֹרָה.

אַגְמוֹנָא, אגמון ch. same. Targ. Is. LVIII, 5.—Targ. Job. XL, 26 Ms. (ed. אוּנְקְלָא).

אֶגְמוֹן m.=חֶגְמוֹן. Sabb. 145ᵇ ed.

אַגְמוֹנָא, v. אַגְמוֹן ch.

אַגָּנָא, אַגָּנָא m. (b. h. אַגָּן, v. אוֹגֶן) *basin, kettle.* Sabb. 110ª א׳ דתיהלא a basin filled with cress. Ab. Zar. 31ª א׳ אפומא וכ׳ Ms. M. (ed. דפ׳) a basin-like vessel placed over the opening of the cask. Pes. 45ᵇ.—Ber. 22ª בא׳ דמיא in a bath tub.—*Pl.* אַגָּנִין, אַגָּנֵי, אַגָּ׳. Targ. Is. LXV, 11.—Pes. 30ᵇ א׳ דמחוזא the kneading basins of Maḥuza.—מֵישַׁר אַגָּנַיָּא pr. n. pl. Targ. Jud. IV, 11; Y. Meg. I, 70ª bot. אגניא דקדש, later name of בצענים *pools of Kadesh.* [B. Kam. 61ᵇ אגני דארעא Ms. R., *ponds of the field,* v. בְּאַגְנָא a. נְאַגְנָא.]

***אנגטוס, אגניטוס** (Var. v. infra) name of a Roman general in the days of R. Yoḥ. b. Zakkai, or of R. Gamliël, prob. a corrupt. of אגרינטוס *Quintus,* or אגריטוס *Quietus;* [Graetz: *Atticus,* v. Monatsschr. 1885 p. 17 sq.]. Sifré Deut. 351 אגניטוס. Y. Snh. I, 19ᵇ top אנגטוס; ib. ᶜ bot. אנטונינוס; ib. ᵈ top אנטיגנס. Num. R. s. 4 (קונגטיס) הונגטוס; Bekh. 5ª קונטרוקוס. [אגרינטוס, קורינטוס seem most probable.]

אגנטין Y. Ter. VII, 21ᵇ, v. ארגנטריא.

אגנייה, v. next. w.

***אַגְנִינָה** f. (agnina, sc. pellis) *lamb-skin.* Gen. R. s. 20 Mus. (ed. אגנייה).

אגניסטור, v. אנגיסטור.

אַגְנְתָא f. 1)=אַגָּנָא. Targ. II Esth. I, 2.—2) (גנן) *protection, guard.* Num. R. s. 12; Midr. Till. to Ps. XCI, 2 *maḥăsi* (Ps. l. c.) means אַגְנָתִי *my guard.*

אַגָּס (Tosef. עוּגָּס) m. (גוס, גסס to swell, v. גַּס III, cmp. תַּפּוּחַ) *pear, pear-tree.* [In oth. Semit. dial. except Syr., *plum,* Fl. to Levi Talm. Dict. s. v.] Y. Kil. I, 27ª bot.; Tosef. ib. 4. Ib. II, 15 (Var. עובש).—*Pl.* אַגָּסִים, אַגָּסִין (עוּגָּסִים). Y. Ter. XI, 47ᵈ bot. Kil. I, 4. Tosef. Shebi. VII, 16; a. fr. [Cmp. אֱגוֹז, esp. Cant. VI, 11, where the context points to *fruits* in gen. Cmp. חָבוּשׁ.]

אגסטון, v. אֲגוּסְטָאן.

אגסטרות Ar. s. v. קלסקה, read אִסְטַגְּיוֹת.

אַכְסִיטִירִין, אַגְסִיטְרִין m. (ἐξιτήριον S.) *farewell-address, bequest.* [Mostly corrupt.] Midr. Till. to Ps. LXXXIV. Ib. to Ps. LXXXVI, 1. Ib. to Ps. XXVII. Pesik. Aḥaré p. 175ªᵇ סקוטרים; Lev. R. s. 21 סקיטרים, read אקסיטרין (v. Buber to Pesik. l. c.).

אגע Koh. R. to III, 14, read פֶּגַע (Mat. K.).

אָגַף (sec. r. of גָּפַף, v. גּוּף) *to fill up a hole with pitch* &c. B. Kam. 105ª.

אֲגַף, אגוף m. (גּוּף I) *the moulding or eminence of the door frame against which the door shuts, door-stop* (esp. of door-ways in thick city walls &c. with reference to sacred limits in sacrificial law). Pes. VII, 12 מן הא׳ ולפנים וכ׳ the space of the wall inside the door-stop is subject to the laws which apply to the space enclosed by the wall. Ib. 85ᵇ א׳ עצמו the stop itself and the corresponding space. Y. ib. VII, 35ᵇ אגוף.

אֲגַף com. (v. foreg.=גַּף; cmp. b. h. אֲגַפִּים) 1) *wing, pinion. Pl.* אֲגַפִּים; *Du.* אֲגַפַּיִם. Neg. XIV, 1. Gen. R. s. 39; a. e.—2) *winged animals, poultry.* Succ. 42ª.—3) *arms, shoulders of a human being.* Y. Snh. VII, 24ᵇ bot. יכול יבלינו מבין הא׳ you might think the convict must be cut through at the arm-pits. Sabb. 129ª חברותיה נושאות וכ׳ her mates lift her by her arms.—4) *banks of* river &c. B. Kam. 61ª a rivulet which imparts שלל לַאֲגַפֶּיהָ booty (alluvium) to its banks. B. Bath. 99ᵇ שכלו א׳ whose embankments have disappeared (washed away).

אַגַּפָּא ch. same, *wing.* Gen. R. s. 75, beg. מנערא אַגַּפָּה וכ׳ shakes her wings to shake the ashes off. [Targ. Ezek. I, 14, prob. אַגְפָּא.]. [B. Bath. 8ª, v. גַּפָּא.]—*Pl.* אַגַּפַּיָּא, const. אַגַּפֵּי. Targ. Cant. V, 11. Cmp. גַּפָּא, גַּדְפָּא.

אֲגֻפָּה, v. חֲגָפָה.

אָגַר I (b. h., √גר, v. גרר) *to gather, collect.* Y. Yoma III, 41ª top (expl. *ăgartlé,* Ezr. I, 9). Y. Bicc. I, 63ᵈ bot. שהוא אוגר וכ׳ it stores up its oil, (does not let it trickle out), v. אֲגוֹרִי; Ber. 39ª שמני אָגוּר וכ׳ its oil remains stored up.—Y. Nid. III, beg. 50ᶜ top דם אָגוּר blood collected in one place.—Trnsf. *to store up thoughts, arguments.* Sifré Deut. 16 (play on *gêro* Deut. I, 16) זה שאוגר עליו דברים that means him who heaps arguments up against him (his opponent in litigation). Ex. R. s. 6 אגור שא׳ דברי

תורה (Var. שאִיגֵּר *Pi.*) he is called Agur (Prov. XXX, 1) because he collected words of the Law (stored up knowledge); Koh. R. beg. שֶׁאָגוּר בד״ת because he was stored (or *girded*, v. אָגַר II) with knowledge. Cant. R. to I, 1 end. [Sabb. 60ª אוגרת ed., v. אָגַד.]

Nif. נֶאֱגַר *to be gathered.* Num. R. s. 20 beg. (play on ויגר Num. XXII, 3) והן נֶאֱגָרִין לעריהם and they were gathered to their towns (for defence).

Hif. הוֹגִיר, *to store up.* Tosef. Dem. I, 10 המוגירות the store-keepers' places; v. מוֹגָרָה, מוֹגֶרֶת.

אֲגַר I ch. same; *Pa.* אַגַּר *to heap up.* Targ. Y. Deut. I, 16 דִּמְאַגַּר וכ׳ (ed. Vien. מְאַגַּר—) who heaps up litigations, v. foreg. [Targ. Ps. CIV, 7 למיגר Ms., v. נְגַד.]

אָגַר II (√אג, v. חגר). 1) *to gird, arm.* Midr. Prov. to XXX, 1 שא׳ חלציו who girded his loins for wisdom; Yalk. Prov. a. l. Part. pass. אָגוּר, v. אָגַר I. 2) *to halt,* whence part. f. אוֹגֶרֶת (sub. סַכִּין) a knife having indentations which catch the passing nail of the examiner. Hull. 17ᵇ.—*3) *to occupy space.* B. Bath 14ª (intercharging with אָכַל q. v.).

אֲגַר II (אֲגַר) (√אג, akin to חכר; v. foreg.) prop. *to tie,* whence *to hire, employ, rent.* Targ. Gen. XXX, 16; a. fr.—Koh. R. to IV, 6; Lev. R. s. 3 beg. (prov.) דא׳ גרנא וכ׳ he who rents one garden will eat birds; him who rents gardens, the birds will eat. Git. 73ª אגור מלחי they hired boatsmen. Snh. 73ª מֵיגַר אַגִּירֵי to hire help. Y. Taan. I, 64ᵇ bot. מיגר זנייתא hiring prostitutes. B. Mets. 79ª; a. fr.

Af. אוֹגַר 1) same. Targ. Y. Deut. XXIII, 5 (4).—B. Mets. 77ª (interch. with Pe.) אוגיר אגירי (אגירי) engages laborers.—2) *to rent out, lease.* Erub. 63ᵇ אוֹגַר לָן רשותך lease to us thy property. Y. Dem. VI, 25ᵇ top. Y. Taan. I, 64ᵇ bot. אוגרית חמרי I hired my ass out.

Ithpa. אִיתְּגַּר, *Ithpe.* אִתְּגַר (contr. of איתאגר) *to be hired, to work as a laborer.* Targ. O. Deut. XXIII, 25; a. e.—Yoma 20ᵇ (prov.) אי תגרת וכ׳ (combine into one w.) when thou hast hired thyself out to one, comb his wool (shrink from no labor).

אַגְרָא III, אַגְרָא I m. (foreg.) *rent, wages; reward, profit.* Targ. Gen. XV, 1; a. fr.—B. Mets. 63ᵇ א׳ נטר ליה compensation for waiting (giving time for delivery), i. e. advancing the money to the seller. Ib. 68ᵇ פלגא בא׳ כ׳ half profit or loss. Ib. 69ᵇ א׳ ופגרא payment for carrying freight, and indemnity to the boatsmen in case of wreck. Y. M. Kat. II, 81ᵇ top א׳ וקרנא profit and principal (cost-price).—Y. B. Mets. II, 8ᶜ top מא׳ כל הדין עלמא than all profit this world can offer.—2) *that which deserves reward, meritorious deed.* Ber. 6ᵇ א׳ דפירקא ריהטא the merit in attending a lecture lies in running [to it] (anxiety to hear it). [אַגְרָא, אֶגֶר *staff, pole,* v. אגד.]

אִגַּר, אִגָּרָא *roof;* **אִגַּרְתָּא** *letter,* v. אי׳.

אַגְרָא II pr. n. m. *Agra,* father-in-law of R. Abba; father of R. Y'hudah. Hull. 104ᵇ; 134ª. Nid. 53ª.

אגרדים v. next. w.

אֲגַרְדְּמִיס (freq. אגרדמים) m. (a corrupt. of ἀγοράνομος, v. אַגְרוֹנִימוֹס) *agoranomos,* corresponding to the Roman *ædilis, market commissioner, gauger,* &c. Ab. Zar. 58ª א׳ נכרי (כותי, Ms. V. גוי א׳) a gentile agoran.—B. Kam. 98ª א׳ טיייעא an Arabian agoran.—B. Bath. 89ª א׳ וכ׳ מעמידין Ar. (ed. מין—plur.) an agoran. may be appointed for superintending measures, but not for fixing the prices.—*Pl.* אֲגַרְדְּמִין B. Bath. l. c. (v. supra). [Pesik. Asser p. 96ª לא׳ שיצא (sing.) Ar. (ed. להגרונימוס read לא׳, cmp. Yalk. Ps. 729).]—אֲגַרְדְּמִים Sifra K'doshim ch. VIII; cmp. Y. B. Bath. V, 15ª bot. [Oth. corrupt. v. Pesik. l. c. note.]

אִגְּרוּ, אִיגְּרוּ f. (אגר I, Pi; cmp. אֲגוּרִי) *(grain) fit for storage, of superior quality.* Y. Maas. Sh. IV, beg. 54ᵈ מן הא׳ על השמיטה וכ׳ *T'rumah* may be taken from the stored-up wheat for the wheat which has to be quickly disposed of, or vice versa. Y. Peah. II, 17ª חצי אירגו וכ׳ (read איגרו). Y. Naz. V, 54ª שחתית ונמצאת אגרון (corr. acc.) from dark colored wheat (inferior), and found it was *igg'ru* (superior). [R. Simson to Peah II, 5 quotes אֲגוּרִי; El. W. in Sh'noth El. ibid. אֲגוּרָה.] [B. Bath. V, 6 has לבנה *white, pure* for our w.]

אגרוי, v. אוּגְדּוֹיְיקָנְטֵי.

אַגְרוֹמִי m. pl. (a corrupt. of אגרונומי, cmp. אגרדמיס a. next. art.) *costum-collectors,* (cmp. Sm. Ant. s. v. Agoranomos). Gen. R. s. 75 ed. (Ar. אירגמי).

אגרון, v. אִגְּרוּ.

אַגְרוֹנִימוֹן, v. next. w.

אַגְרוֹנִימוֹס (corr. אַגְרוֹנ׳), contr. אַגַּרְמוֹס m. (ἀγοράνομος) *agoranomos, market-commissioner;* v. אֲגַרְדְּמִיס a. אַגְרוֹמִי. Y. Dem. II, 22ᶜ top שהיה א׳ גדול the agor. was an influential man. Y. Ab. Zar. IV, 44ᵇ top. Lev. R. s. 1 אגרונימון (corr. acc.). Y. B. Bath. V, 15ª bot. אנג׳ (twice); a. fr.

אֶגְרוֹף m. (b. h., גרף; cmp. פּוּרְמִיזָא) *fist;* fig. *power, usurpation.* Kel. XVII, 12. Ex. R. s. 1.—בַּעַל א׳ *mighty, violent.* Y. Peah. VII, 20ᶜ top; v. infra.—Sot. 41ᵇ אגרופה של חנופה the power of sycophancy.—*Pl.* אֶגְרוֹפִין, אֶגְרוֹפִים. Kid. 76ᵇ בעלי א׳ וכ׳ the men of power of the house of David; Snh. 49ª. Pes. 53ᵇ בעל א׳ a strong, violent man (opp. גברא רבה a great man).

אַגְרוּפִינָא (גרופינא) pr. n. pl. *Agrippina,* one of the signal stations for announcing the New-Moon, prob. a tower or height near Cæsarea Philippi, enlarged by Agrippa II. R. Hash. II, 4 (22ᵇ) לא׳ . . מא׳ Ms. M. 2, Mish. Nap. (ed. לג׳ . . . מג׳; Y. ed. . . מְגְרִיפ׳); v. Rabb. D. S. a. l. note 4).

***אגרטין** Koh. R. to I, 18 read אֶגְרִיגְרוֹן or pl. אֶגְרִיגְרוֹנִין. Cmp. ארגסטירין.

אַגְרִיאוֹן, אַגְרִיוֹן m. (ἄγριος, neut. or. acc.) *wild* (opp. אִימֶרוֹן q. v.); *rough.* Gen. R. s. 77; Cant. R. to III, 6 כלב א׳. Num. R. s. 11 (refer. to Gen. III, 8) שומע

חקול א׳ after sinning, Adam heard the divine voice as a harsh one. Cant. R. to III, 7 (corr. acc.). Pesik. R. s. 15 ...בזעקה א׳ וכ׳ (leave out hebr. words as glosses to explain the Greek).

אגריסטיס, v. אַרְגֶּסְטֵיס.

אַגְרִיפָּא=next. w.

אַגְרִיפַּס pr. n. m. (Ἀγρίππας) *Agrippa*, 1) the last but one Herodian king of Judæa. Sot. VII, 8. Lev. R. s. 3; a. fr.—2) a captain of the former.—Ab. Zar. 55[a] אגריפא שר צבא של א׳ Ms. M. (v. Rashi a. l. a. Rabb. D. S. a. l. note).

אגריקוס, v. אֶגְדִּיקוֹס.

***אגרמא**, Y. Git. V, 47[b] דינר א׳, read דינרא גרדיינא, v. גּוֹרְדְּיָנֵר.

אגרנא, v. אַגְדְּנָא.

אֲגָרֵס, v. חֲגָדֵס.

אגרסטיס, v. אַרְגֶּסְטֵיס.

***אַגְרָפוֹס** m. (ἄγραφος) *unwritten*. Y. R. Hash. I, 57[a] bot. פרא בסיליאיס נימס א׳, cmp. Ar. h. v., a. s. v. בסיליאיס (ed. או נימוס או גריפוס) παρὰ βασιλέως ὁ νόμος ἄγραφος, for the king the law is unwritten (i. e. the king may disregard his own law). Lev. R. s. 35, beg. quot. in Ar. (missing in ed.).

***אִגְּרַת** pr. n. f. *Igrath*, name of the queen of demons Pes. 111[a] א׳ אולת (an incantation). Ib. 112[a]. Num. R s. 12. Cmp. נְגִירָא.

אִיגֶּרֶת, אִגֶּרֶת f. (b. h. אָגַר; א׳, נגר, *to join*, v. esp. Snh. 11[b]; ושלש איגרות וכ׳) *tablet, letter, brief, document*. Git. IX, 3 (formula of a letter of divorce) סֵפֶר ... ואי׳ ... וגט וכ׳. Ib. 85[b] ולא ....איגרת...אלא אגרת one must not write (in the letter of divorce) *egereth* with אי׳ which might mean *roof* (v. אִיגָּר), but &c. Keth. 64[a]; Y. Kid. I, 59[a] bot. א׳ מרד a document stating a wife's disobedience. Y. Meg. IV, 75[b] top; Y. Snh. I, 19[b] top א׳ ביקורת a document fixing the value of a property, v. אַבְרָנָה.—*Pl.* אִיגְּרוֹת, אִגְּרוֹת. M. Kat. III, 3 א׳ של רשות secular, social correspondence, opp. religious correspondence; cmp. Y. ib. 82[a] bot.; [commentaries: *documents of secular government*, v. רָשׁוּת]. Ib.; B. Mets. I, 8 א׳ שום א׳ מזון documents relating to legal assessment and to alimony.

אִגַּרְתָּא ch. same; v. אִיגַּרְתָּא.

אגש Lam. R. to I, 21; Pesik. Anokhi p. 138[b], v. גּוּשׁ.

אַד־ insep. conjunct. 1) (=עַד דְּ־; cmp. אַ־) prop. *until that*; *by the time that*; hence, *while, when*, in *the place of*. Hag. 5[a] אדזוטר when he was young.—Hull. 105[b], a. fr. אדהכי or אדהכי והכי *in the meanwhile*. Pes. 113[a] אדחלא אברעיך וכ׳ while the travelling dust is yet on thy knees, sell thy goods. Snh. 33[b] אדמוקדך יקיד while thy fire-place is lit. B. Mets. 81[a], a. fr. אדתני—ליתני וכ׳ in place of stating A let him state B, and A would be implied.—2) (=עַל דְּ־) *as regards —, in relation to* the statement &c. of—. Keth. 21[a] אדרבי דמיה on (the testimony) of one who was with him. B. Bath. 159[b], a. fr. קשיא דרבא אַדְּרָבָא there is a contradiction between (one opinion) of Raba and another opinion of Raba; B. Mets. 18[a] אַדְּרַבָּה .... of Rabbah (not to be confounded with אַדְּרַבָּא q. v.) Meg. 20[a] אַדְּיוֹם in relation to (the reading of the Book of Esther) in day-time.

אֵד m. (b. h., an apocopated form of אדיּ, cmp. זוּיִ, נאד, אדוּתא) *vapor, cloud*. Gen. R. s. 13 (homil. etym.). אד שהוא שובר אידן וכ׳ cloud is called *ēd* (destroyer) because it breaks the *ēd* (distress of scarcity) looked forward to by the speculators in the market. V. אֵיד.

אָדָא I, הָדָא f. (v. הָא) *this, that*. Y. Ber. III, end, 7[a], a. fr. הדא אמרת היא הדא היא א׳ this shows that this is like that, i. e. *all the same*. Y. Erub. IV, end, 22[a]; a. fr.

אַדָּא II (אִידָּא) pr. n. m. (v. אַדָּא IV) *Ada*, 1) name of several Amoraim; (v. Frankel Meb. Y. p. 61[b]). Y. Ter. X, 47[b] bot. Pes. 80[a]; a. fr.—Most prominent among them *R. Ada bar Ahăba* or Aḥăva. Y. Taan. III, end, 67[a]; Bab. ibid. 20[b]; a. fr.—2) A. דיילא, דיילא (attendant of scholars). B. Kam. 119[a]. Num. R. s. 9.—3) a slave. Kid. 70[b].

***אַדָּא III** בר א׳, v. בַּרְדָּא II, 2.

אַדָּא IV m. (b. h. צְדָה; cmp. b. h. עַד *prey*, a. אֵיד *destruction*) *fowler, one who puts up baits, snares* &c. for other people's doves. Snh. 25[a] (explain. *mafriḥe yonim*, Mishn.) ר׳—אמר א׳ Ms. M. a. Oxf., a. Ar. (ed. ארא; v. Rabb. D. S. a. l., a. Ar.) R—says, the Mishnah means a fowler (to be disqualified as witness &c.).

אדאני Sabb. 35[b], v. אָרוֹנֵי.

אדבאל Y. Maas. Sh. IV, 54[d] top, v. אַרְבֵּל I.

אֶדְבְּעָא, אֶדְבַּע f. (h. אֶצְבַּע) *finger*. Targ. Y. Num. XIX, 4; a. e.

אַדְדָא Ar., (אַדְרָא ed.) m. (√אד, v. אָדַר, cmp. חד, חדר, חדק &c.) *fish-bone* sticking in the throat. Sabb. 67[a] לא׳ וכ׳ against a fish-bone in the throat, say this spell. [For דר a. דר cmp. אודרא.]

אדדם Cant. R. to IV, 8, v. דדי ch.

אדהי, Y. Kil. IV, 29[b], bot., read אָדָא I (cmp. Y. Erub I, 19[c] bot. חדה וכ׳ a. corr. acc.)

אַדְהָכִי v. אַד־.

אַדְוָתָא, אֲדוּתָא, אדותא f. (Syr. דויתא דימא P. S. 933, דוע to sweat, drip; cmp. אֵד) prop. *sweat*, א׳ דימא *foam of the Sea*. B. Bath. 4[a]; Succ. 51[b] (Ms. M. אידותא) the Temple building of marble looks like a surging Sea (from a distance). Cmp. אוּדְיָתָא a. אֵוִי.

אַדוּכֵי, v. דּוּךְ.

אָדוֹם m., אֲדוּמָה f. (b. h. אָדֹם, אֲדָמָה; דם) *red*. Cant. R. to VII, 3, א׳ שושנה red rose (euphem. for menstruation).—פרה א׳ *red cow*, used for purification ceremonies

(Num. XIX). Ab. Zar. 24[a]; a. fr.—Lam. R. to IV, 5, v. קְלֹורִית.—*Pl.* אֲדוּמִּים, אֲדוּמּוֹת; Y. Succ. II, 53[d], v. אֲדַמְדָּם.—Gen. R. s. 89; a. fr.

אֱדוֹם (b. h. אָדֹם) 1) pr. n. m. *Edom*, surname of Esau, son of Isaac; mostly used as a nom. gentil. *Edomite, Edomite nation.*—2) fem. (sub. מלכות) *Rome, Roman government* (owing to the dependence of Herod on Rome). Ex. R. s. 35; a. fr. Ibid. מלכות א׳; a. fr. [In subsequent ages: *Christianity.*]

אֲדוֹמִי m. (b. h. אֲדֹמִי) *Edomite, Idumean.* Keth. 30[a] חייבי עשה מצרי וא׳ the laws of intermarriage with Egyptians and Edomites as implied in Deut. XXIII, 8.—Pes. III, 1 חומץ הא׳ Idumean vinegar; a. e.—Snh. 12[a] ולא חמרין א׳ חלו Ar. a. Ms. M. (later ed. under censorial influences ארמי. v. Rabb. D. S. a. l. note) and that Edomite (disguise for *Roman government*, v. foreg.) would not permit them.—Fem. אֲדוֹמִית.—*Pl.* אֲדוֹמִיּוֹת. Keth. 64[b] שעורין א׳ Idumean barley.

אָדוֹן m., const. אֲדוֹן (b. h.; דון) *lord, judge.* Hag. 3[b] אֲ׳ כל המעשים Lord of all creatures. Y. Kid. IV, beg. 65[b] (allud. to *Adon*, pr. n., Neh. VII, 61) אין דין אין א׳ there is no justice and no judge. Gen. R. s. 89 (play on *Kar*, Is. XXX, 23) קירי א׳ Kyri (κύριος) means Lord.

אֲדוֹנָה f. *mistress.* Gen. R. s. 89 נצטער יוסף עם אֲדוֹנָתוֹ Joseph suffered while being with his mistress. Ib. s. 98 (play on *ben porath* Gen. XLIX, 22) בן שהפר לא׳ וכ׳ the youth that broke (defeated the plans of) his mistress; the youth whom his mistress broke (having him put in prison). Ib. (play on *vay-mar'ruhu* Gen. ib. 23) בן שחמר וכ׳ the youth who made life bitter to his mistress (v. vers. Mat. K. a. l.).

אדוניא Tosef. Kel. B. Mets. VIII, 6, ed., v. אוּדְנָא III.

אדונקי, v. אדנקי.

אדור, v. אַדְרוּתָא.

אדורה, v. אֲדַר.

אֲדוּרֵי, אַדְּהוּרֵי m. pl. (הדר) *procession.* א׳ צלמא a procession in which an idol is carried. Y. Ab. Zar. III, 43[b] bot.; Y. Ber. II, 4[b] אה׳ צילמי׳; Y. Shek. II, end, 47[a] דארורא צילמא (read אדורי דצ׳); Midr. Sam. ch. XIX צלמא הורדוסיס(?).

אֲדוּתָא, v. אַדְוּוּתָא.

אֲדִי (=ידי, b. h. הדה) *to swing, throw, pitch.* Snh. 7[a]. v. גְּוִיזָא. B. Kam. 22[a]; Bets. 39[a] אַדְיֵיהּ אדויי he threw it off. B. Kam. 98[a] אדייה א׳ he pitched it out of his neighbor's hands.

אדיא Y. Maasr. I, 49[b], prob. אַרְזָא or אוּרְזָא; v. Y. Sabb. III, 6[b] top.

אדיבון read אִימִירוֹן.

אַדְיוּתָא f. (נדי=h. הַזָּאָה) *sprinkling* (for purification). Targ. Num. XIX, 13 (Var. אַדְיוּתָא; h. text נִדָּה). Targ. Ezek. XXXVI, 25 אַדְיוּתָא.

אֲדַיִין (=עֲדַיִין; עַד=אַד; הֵין=יִין a. h. עַד הֵנָּה) *until now*; whence, *still, yet; as yet.* Y. Ber. IV, 8[a] bot. וא׳ ארן את לזו art thou not yet up to this, i. e. dost thou not yet understand it? Y. Taan. II, 65[c] bot. א׳ את לזו. Y. Git. IX, end, 50[d] וא׳ את ליה art thou still at that point, i. e. dost thou still ask? Y. Peah I, 15[c]; Y. Kid. I, 61[b] top וא׳ לחצי וכ׳ and yet he has hardly come up to half the honor due to parents.

אֲדִיל, v. אֲדַל.

אֲדִילֵי m. pl., dialect. for אֲרִוּלֵי. B. Bath. 74[b], v אוּרְזִילָא.

אֲדִימָא m. ch. (=h. אָדוֹם) *red, full of sap, fresh.* Bets. 24[b], Rashi; v. however, חָדַם.

אֲדַיִן ch. (=h. אֱזַי, אָז; √ד־ה=ד״) *at that time, thereupon.* Dan. II, 15; 17; 19.—בֵּאדַ׳ *at the same time, forthwith.* Ibid. 14; 35.—מן א׳ *from that time.* Ezra V, 16.

אֲדִינָיא, v. אוּדְנָא III.

אֲדִיצוּתָא, v. אִידִיצוּתָא.

אוּדִיק, אֲדִיק, v. דִּיק.

אַדִּיר m. (b. h.; אָדַר); *distinguished, glorious, mighty.* —*Pl.* אַדִּירִים. Men. 53[a].

אַדִּירָא, אַדִּיר ch. same. Targ. O. Ex. XV, 6; a. fr.

***אֲדִירָא** m.=דִּיר, *rim, border.* Y. Sabb. III, 5[d] bot. leaned a vessel לא׳ דתנורא (Var. לאווירא) against the rim of a heated stove.

אֲדִישׁ, v. דוש ch.

אד״ך *Adakh*, substitute of תקל (Dan. V, 25) by permutation of letters called א״תב״ש q. v. Snh. 22[a]. Cant. R. to III, 4 אנם (corr. acc.).

אדכי, v. אוּרְבָא.

אַדְכָּרְתָּא, אַדְכָּרָה f. (דְּכַר) 1) *mention*, esp. *invocation of the Lord; Divine Name.* Y. Ber. IV, 8[a] top לכל חדא וחדא מנהון אדכרה for each benediction an invocation. R. Hash. 18[b] בטילת אדכרתא the use of the Divine Name in legal documents was abolished.—2) (=b. h. אַזְכָּרָה) *memorial offering.* Targ. O. Lev. II, 2; a. e.

אַדְכָּרוּתָא, אִדְכְּרוּ f. (v. foreg.) *remembrance, mention.* Targ. Ps. XXX, 5 Ms. רו...; ed. רות...

אַדְכַּרְתָּא, v. אַדְכָּרָה.

עֲדַל, אֲדִיל, אֲדַל m. (√אד, עד dial.=חד, גד; cmp. חַרְדָּל II, גִּרְגָּא I, גְּדָר) *garden-cress, summer-savory.* Tosef. Shebi. V, 11 (ed. Zuck. אדיל). Ukts. III, 4 ע׳. Y. Shebi. VII, 37[c] bot. ערל; ib. 37[b] bot. ערלה (corr. acc.)

אַדְלָקָה f. (=הַדְלָקָה) *lighting. Pl.* אַדְלָקוֹת. Y. Shebi. VII, beg. 37[b] מיני א׳ sorts of plants used for lighting purposes.

אֲדָם, v. חָדָם. [v. Rabb. D. S. to Ab. Zar. 38[b], Bets. 24[b], note.]

אָדַם (b. h.; √דם, v. דמם) [*to be viscous, thick, dark*] *to be red, grow red.*

Pi. אִדֵּם *to redden, make red.* Y. Sabb. VII, 10[c] top המאדם אודם he who produces a red spot (congestion of blood, on a Sabbath).

Hif. הֶאְדִּים 1) (b. h.) *to be, grow red.* Num. R. s. 9 (p. 231[b] ed. Amst.) מַאְדֶּמֶת (היתה) if she was red-faced. Hull. 53[b]; a. fr.—2) *to cause to blush, put to shame* (usu. הלבין). Num. R. s. 4 (p. 218[d] ed. Amst.) (play on טובד אדום).—*Part.* מַאְדִּים *the planet Mars.* Sabb. 156[a].—*Part. Hof.* מָאְדָּם, מְאוּדָּם. Y. Sabb. VII, 10[c] top מְאָדָּמִים dyed red.

אָדָם m. (b. h.) *man,* pr. n. m. *Adam,* frequ. א׳ הראשון (abbr. אה״ר). Gen. R. s. 17; a. fr.—ספרו של אה״ר, ספרא דאה״ר the (allegorical) book of Adam containing all generations and their leaders from beginning to resurrection, i. e. destinies of humanity. Ex. R. s. 40 beg. B. Mets. 85[b] bot.

אִדְמָא, אַדְמָא, אֲדָם m. ch. (=דָּמָא, דָּם) *blood.* Targ. I Chron. XXII, 7; a. e.—Y. Maas. Sh. V, 56[d] top מיגבלא אַדְמֵיה to mix its (the bird's) blood. Git. 47[a]; v. חזיII. *Pl.* אַדְמִין. Targ. I Chr. l. c.; a. e.

אֲדַמְדָּם m. (b. h.) *reddish.* Y. Succ. III, 53[d] איזהו א׳ שבאדומים which of the red colors is called *adamdam?* —Shebu. 6[a] *reddish leprosy* (Lev. XIII, 42); a. e.

אֲדַמְדְּמָנִי m. pl. (דמם) *lumps of dripping grapes.* Gen. R. s. 34, end אנא גבלין ליה א׳ we make for it a dough of &c., v. דְּמַדְמָנִיּוֹת, דַּבְדְּבָנִיּוֹת.

אֲדָמָה f. (b. h., prob. fr. דמם, cmp. foreg.; *thick and moist*) [earth], *clay.* Gen. R. s. 14 the potter takes sand (עפר) which is male (masc. gender) and clay (אדמה) which is female (fem. gender).—Sabb. VIII, 5 א׳ כחותם וכ׳ as much clay as is required for a seal on bag-knots. [For the meaning of the phonetic equivalents of our w. in other Semit. tongues, v. Ges. H. Dict. s. v.]

אֲדַמּוּמִית f. (אדם) *redness.* Hull. 87[b], a. e. כמראה א׳ reddish color.

אַדְמוֹן pr. n. m. *Admon,* one of the justices of the peace in Jerusalem. Keth. XIII, 1.—Ib. 105[a] א׳ בן גדאי.

אַדְמוֹנִי m. (b. h., אדם) *ruddy, gold-colored,* esp. with refer. to hair. Y. Ned. I, 36[d] bot.

אֲדָמִי pr. n. pl. *Adami* (Josh. XIX, 33). Y. Meg. I, 70[a] bot. וא׳ דמין *Adami* changes into *Damin.*

אַדְמְתָא, אֲדַמְתָא f. ch. (=h. אֲדָמָה) *earth.* Targ. O. Gen. II, 5; a. fr.

אֶדֶן m. (b. h., v. אודנא III; √דן, די) *base, pedestal. Pl.* אֲדָנִים. Y. Sabb. VII, 10[d] top; Babl. ib. 98[b]. Y. Shek. I, 45[d] bot.

אַדְנָא, אֶדֶן, v. אוּ׳.

אַדְנָא, v. אוּ׳.

* **אֲדַנְדְּקֵי** m. pl. (a Babyl. corrupt. of ἐθνάρχοι, v. P. Sm. 40) *chiefs of tribes.* Hull. 60[b]. א׳ שלהן אדנקא חמשה Ar. (ed. ארונקי, Mus. אדונקי) the six tribes had only five chiefs (v. Josh. XII, 3). Ib. כתוב א׳ וכ׳ record the word 'א in thy lecture notes (as a foreign word) and explain it.

אַדְנוּת f. (אָדוֹן) *lordship, authority.* Gen. R. s. 93; a. e.

אֲדֹנָי m. (b. h. plur. excellentiæ) *the Lord, Adonai.* Gen. R. s. 17; Koh. R. to VII, 23.

אַדְנֵי (אַבְנֵי), א׳ הַשָּׂדֶה m. pl. *name of a mythical animal, orangoutang*(?). Kil. VII, 5, defined Y. ibid. 31[c] bot. בר נש דטור *mountain-man,* brought forth by the mountain and drawing nourishment from the ground (cmp. Job V, 23). Koh. R. to VI, 11.

אדני, אדאני Sabb. 35[b], v. אֲרוֹנֵי.

אדני מריונים, read אַרְבֵּי בְּרֵיוֹנִים, v. בְּרִיוֹן a. אַרְבֵּי.

אָדַק (√אד, v. הדק, חדק) *to squeeze into, fasten.* Part. pass. אָדוּק, pl. אֲדוּקִים, אֲדוּקִין 1) *fastened to.* B. Bath. 77[b] בשאדוקין בו Ms. M. (ed. באד׳) when the mules are attached to the wagon; cmp. נבס a. נבק.—2) (cmp. אָחוּז, s. v. אחז) *holding fast.* B. Mets. 7[a b] sq.

אֲדַק ch. same, (neut. v.) *to be fastened, stick to.* Targ. Lam. IV, 8.—*Part. pass.* אֲדִיק, *attached, cleaving to.* Targ. Ps. XXII, 16 א׳ לי Ms. (ed. אדביק). Targ. Ex. XXVIII, 28; a. e.

Pa. אַדֵּק 1) *to fasten to, to cause to take hold.* Targ. Y. Deut. XXVIII, 21.—2) *to seize, take hold of.* Ibid. v. 45 ויאדקינכון (ed. Vien. a. oth. וירע׳ corr. ד for ר).

Ithpa. אִתְאַדַּק *to join, cling to.* Targ. Job. XLI, 9; 15 (Ms. מידבק).

אֶדֶק m. *clepsydra,* v. אֶרֶק.

* **ארקולאון, אדקולאון** Cant. R. to I, 11 לא׳ בן הדימה (Var. לאר׳ בן) a gloss inserted in the text, and which read לאו דוקא אלא כן הדימם 'not to be taken literally' (that the Divine Word kissed every Israelite &c.), 'but he made them so imagine'.

אָדַר (b. h., √אד; cmp. גד, חד, חד, חד in גדר, חדר, חדר) *to cut off, surround, isolate;* whence 1) (b. h.) *to distinguish.*—Den. אַדִּיר. 2) (Assyr. v. אָדַר) *to darken.*—3) **to strip.* cmp. עדר.—B. Kam. 11[a] (ref. to עד Ex. XXII, 12, v. עַד in H. Dict.) יביא אֲדוּרָה לב״ד Ar. (ed. עֲדוּדָה, v. עדד; Ms. ארורה, corr. acc.) let him bring the stripped (the remnants of the torn animal, skin &c.) before court for assessment of damages.

אֲדַר ch. same; v. אַדְרוֹנָא, אִדְּרָא, אִדְּרָא.

Pa. אַדַּר *to distinguish.* Snh. 63[b] (play on Adrammelekh II Kings XVI, 31) דא׳ ליה וכ׳ (the mule) that gives distinction to its owner when travelling.

אֲדָר (אֲדַר) m. (b. h., Assyr. *the cloudy;* v. Fred. Delitzsch, The Hebr. Lang. p. 15) *Adar,* the twelfth month of the Jewish calendar, containing twenty nine days, and varying between the eleventh of February and the twenty eighth of March. In leap years: א׳ רִאשׁוֹן *First Adar*, of thirty days duration between the thirty first of January and the tenth of March; א׳ שֵׁנִי *Second Adar*, of twenty-nine days, between the second of March and the eighth of April. Targ. II Esth. IX, 29; a. fr.—Meg. I, 4; a. fr.—*Pl.* אֲדָרִים, אֲדָרִין. R. Hash. 19ᵇ.

אִידְרָא, אִדְּרָא, אִידַר, אִדַּר m. (אדר, נדר v. אָדַר) *a place cut off, circle* (cmp. זִירָה), whence *threshing place, barn;* also *the grain piled up in the barn for threshing;* cmp. גּוֹרֶן. Targ. Hos. II, 11 בעידן א׳ at the season of its being piled up; a. fr.—Gen. R. s. 63 the shovel דאפיך אר׳ which upturns the grain in the barn (=prayer averting evil decrees). Ib. (play on אדרת Gen. XXV, 25) כקש מא׳ like chaff from the barn. Ruth R. to III, 3 להיכן אקימתא א׳ where didst thou put up the barn?—*Pl.* אִדְּרַיָּא, אִדְּרֵי &c. Dan. II, 35. Targ. I Sam. XXIII, 1; a. e. Cant. R. to VII, 3 (homilet. rendition of אגן הסהר Cant. l. c.) א׳ דאזהרה a rounded place (cmp. גורן, זירה) of enlightenment, i. e. hall of the Sanhedrin. [With א or ו rejected: בי דרי. Taan. 3ᵇ. B. Mets. 73ᵃ.]

אֲדַר I or **אֲדַר, אֲדְרָא I, אוּדְרָא** m. (v. אָדַר 3) *skin, hide, leather-bag.* Y. Maas. Sh. IV, 55ᶜ אדר תורתא hide of a cow. Ib. דתבנא (ברא) אדרא; Lam. R. to I, 1 (חד כותאי 2) אדר דתבן Ar. (ed. דור) a hide stuffed with straw. Y. Shebi. V, 36ᵃ top א׳ דאילין חכימא וכ׳ the leather of these bottles is distinguishable from the leather of those.—*Pl.* אוּדְרָיָתָא. Shebu. 29ᵇ תלוסר א׳ דתבנא Ar. (ed. אורזותא; Ms. F. אדידתא, v. Rashi a. l.) thirteen bagfuls of straw; Ned. 25ᵃ.

אֲדַר II h., **אֲדָרָא II** or **אֲדָרָא I** ch. m. (v. אָדַר) [*thick-leaved, dark*] 1) *a cedar species*, prob. *Spanish Juniper.* R. Hash. 23ᵃ מאי קדרוס (ם) אדרא Ms. M. (ed. קתרוס) what is *kedros* (κέδρος)? *Adara.* Snh. 108ᵇ what is *gofer?* רב אמר אדרא דבי ר׳ שילא אמר וכ׳ Ar. a Ms. Fl. (v. Rabb. D. S. a. l.); cmp. Gen. R. s. 31; Yalk. Gen. 51. —Bets. 15ᵇ יטע אדר וכ׳ let him plant an *edar* (allud. to *addir* &c., Ps. XCIII, 4); א״נ אדרא וכ׳ or *adara* as its (popular or Chald.) name is; as people say, it is called *adara* because it lasts for generations (א־דרא). Git. 69ᵇ אטרף א׳ leaves of ad. Ib. מיא דא׳ decoct thereof.—2) אֲדָרָא *fig-tree.* Targ. II, Esth. VII, 9 (to which perhaps belongs. Git. l. c.).

אַדְרָא II m. (v. אָדַר, cmp. Ges. H. Dict. s. v.) *flag* of a ship. B. Bath. 73ᵃ (for b. h. נֵס); Ms. M. אֲדָאֲרָא (v. Rabb. D. S. a. l.).

אדרא Sabb. 67ᵃ, v. אִדְּרָא.—אדרא B. Mets. 26ᵃ, read with Rashi אוּדְרָא v. אִדְּרָא.

אַדְּרַבָּה, אַדְּרַבָּא (contr. of על דרבה, v. אַדִּי) *turn to the stronger side*, whence as a dialectic term, *on the contrary.* Pes. 28ᵃ, a. fr. א׳ איפכא מסתברא on the contrary, the reverse stands to reason. Ib. 77ᵃ הוה אמינא א׳ I might have said, 'On the contrary' &c.; a. fr. [Not to be confounded with אִדְּרַבָּה, אִדְּרַבָּא, v. אֲדִי.]

אַדְרַבְלָא m. (ὑδραύλης, hydraula) *player on the hydraulis, organist.*—*Pl.* אַדְרַבְלִין. Gen. R. s. 50 א׳ וכרבלין וכ׳ there are organists and flute players in the land (or organs and cymbals, v. next w.), and such a land should be destroyed? [Comment.—Perh. to be read אַדְרִיבְלִין.] Ib. s. 23 (ארדיב׳) אדריבולין וכ׳, corr. acc.).

אַדְרַבְלִיס, אַדְרַבְלִיס (trnsp.) m. (ὕδραυλις) *water-organ.* Y. Succ. V, 55ᶜ bot. לא היה א׳ .עוגב זה ארד׳ Ib. וכ׳ there was no organ used in (the) Jerusalem (Temple) because it interferes with the sweetness (melody of the song).—*Pl.* אַדְרַבְלִין; v. foreg. Cmp. הרדולים.

אֲדַרְגָּזְרַיָּא m. pl. (v. Schr. K. A. T. p. 617 sq.; cmp. אדר a. גזר) *title of high officers.* Dan. III, 3. Cant. R. to VII, 9 א׳ איפרכיא *adarg.* means *governors.*

אַדְרוֹמָא pr. n. gent. *Adroma* (Southern) for b. h. תֵּימָא. Targ. I Chr. I, 30.

אַדְרוֹעָא=אֶדְרָעָא. Targ. Y. Num. VI, 19.

אַדְרוֹפִּיקוֹס m. (ὑδρωπικός) *suffering from dropsy.* Lev. R. s. 15 (var. corrup.); Yalk. Lev. 554. Ib. Job. 916 אֲנַדְר׳ (cmp. אדרוינוס a. אנד׳).

***אַדְרוּתָא** f. (אדר) *glory, distinction.* Ber. 56ᵇ top (oneirocritical play on *Adar*) בא׳ מִיתַת thou shalt die in glory. [Cmp. Y. Maas Sh. IV, end, 55ᶜ; Lam. R. to I, 1 (חד מתלמ׳).]

***אַדְרַזְדָּא** (=אזדרזדא; זרז) *diligently, quickly.* Ezra VII, 23.

אַדְרִיאָנוֹס=אַדְרִיָּינוּס. Tanh. B'resh. 7; a. fr.

אדריאנטין Deut. R. s. 1, interpret. נציבים (II Sam. VIII, 14) read אִסְטְרַטִיגִין, as Targ. a. l.

אַדְרִיאָס m. (Ἀδρίας) *Adriatic Sea.* Tanh. B'resh. 7 בין א׳ לאוקיינוס between the Adriatic Sea and the Mediterranean.

אַדְרִיבָא, אַדְרִיב, v. אַרְדָּב.

אדריבולין, v. אַדְרַבְלָא.

אדרוונמוס; v. אַנְדְּרוֹנִיטִיס a. אַדְרִיאַנְטוּס.

אַנְדְּרִיָּינוּס, אַדְרִיָּינוּס pr. n. m. *Hadrian*, the Roman emperor (117 to 138) under whom the insurrection of Bar Kokhba occurred; freq. mentioned with the imprecation שחיק עצמות. Deut. R. s. 3; a. fr. V. אַדְרִיאָנוּס.

אדרוינטיס, v. אַנְדְּרוֹנִיטִיס a. אַנְדְּרִיאַנְטוּס.

הַדְרִיָּינֵי, אַדְרִיָּינֵי m. *Hadrianic*, 1) of the town *Adria* or *Hadria* in Venetia. Ab. Zar. II, 3 חרס ה׳ (Y. Mish. a. Gem. א׳) earthen ware of Adria (forbidden for use on account of some unknown connection with idolatry, perh. suspected to have been used as wine vessels before they were offered for sale; v. infra).—2) *referring to Hadrian, Hadrianic.* Ib. 32ᵃ explain. חרס הד׳ 'earthen vessels soaked with wine, and distributed in pieces, by order of Hadrian, among the soldiers to be diluted with water for drinking'.—3) (genit. of Hadrianus) *Hadrian's* (followers). Lam. R. to I, 17, v. אספסיינוס.

אדריכולין Gen. R. s. 25, v. אַדְרִבְלָא.

אַדְרִיכוּתָא f. (דרך) *treading, stamping* the threshing floor. Targ. Jer. LI, 33.

אַדְרִיכַל, v. אַדְרִיכַל.

אדרינטוס Gen. R. s. 8 Ar., ed. אינדרגין, v. אַנְדְּרוֹגִינוֹס.

אֲדַרְכּוֹן, v. דַּרְכּוֹן.

אֲדַרְכִּיאָן, v. אֲדַרְכָּן.

אֲדַרְכַּל, v. אַדְרִיכַל.

אַדְרְכִּיאָן, אֲדַרְכָּן pr. n. m. (prob. corrupt. of אַרְטְבָן q. v.) *Adarkhan*, a Parthian ruler. Ab. Zar. 10[b] (Ms. כיון; oth. vers. אדרבך, v. Rabb. D. S. a. l.).—Esth. R. to I, 3 אדרכיאן.

אַדְרַכְתָּא f. (דְּרַךְ Af.) *tracing*; (law) 1) *legal permission to a creditor to trace the debtor's property for the purpose of having it seized, assessed, offered for public sale, and eventually delivered to him.* [Order of documents, acc. to B. Bath. 169[a], vers. of Maim. a. others: 1) אדרכתא; 2) טירפא the right of seizure of the debtor's property sold after the date of the loan (mortgage); 3) שומא record of the assessed value for which the creditor took possession;—acc. to vers. in ed. a. Mss. 1) טירפא right of seizure &c.; 2) א׳ authorization to seize the traced property, defining position &c.; 3) שומא.] B. Bath. 169[a]. B. Kam. 112[b]. B. Mets 16[b]. Ib. 35[b]. Keth. 104[b]. 2) *private authorization to collect or take possession of one's debt or deposit; assignment, transfer.* B. Kam. 70[a] Ms. M., Ar. (ed. אור׳); Shebu. 33[b] (ed. אור׳, v. Rabb. D. S. a. l.); Bekh. 49[a].

אַדְרַמֶּלֶךְ pr. n. m. (II Kings XVII, 31) *Adrammelekh*, name of an idol. Snh. 63[b] א׳ וכ׳ Adr. a. Anammelekh signify mule and horse; v. אֲדַר.

אֶדְרְעָא, אֶדְרַע f. (=h. אֶזְרוֹעַ, v. זְרוֹעַ) *arm.* Targ. Jer. XXXII, 21; a. fr.—Y. Ber. I, 4[c] top דאדרעיה the Tefillin of his arm. Koh. R. to XI, 2.—*Pl.* אֶדְרָעַיָּא. Targ. Job XXII, 9.—אֶדְרָעִין. Gen. R. s. 65.—V. דְּרַע III.

אֶדְרְעָיָא m. *of Edreï*, a town in Naftali (Josh. XIX, 37), another in Menasseh (Bashan, Num. XXI, 33; a. e.).—Y. Ber. V, 9[b] top; a. e.

אַדֶּרֶת f. (b. h.; אָדַר) 1) *cloak, cover.* Gen. R. s. 63 (ref. to Gen. XXV, 25) כולו ראוי לא׳ every one (of the Roman people) fit for the purple cloak (may become an emperor).—2) (homiletically, as if אַדֶּרֶת=ch. אִדְּרָא, אִדַּר) *the threshing floor, the store of grains.* Ib. כולו מפוזר ומפורד כא׳ entirely destined to be scattered (winnowed) like the grains, [שעתיד] לזורותו וכ׳ for the Lord will scatter him (Edom-Rome) like chaff &c. (ref. to Dan. II, 35).

אָדַשׁ, v. דוש ch.

אָהַב (b. h.; √חב; cmp. חבב) *to love.* Y. Ab. Zar. II beg. 40[c] אוֹהֲבָהּ her lover; a. fr. אוהב את חבריות *philanthropist.* Aboth I, 12; a. fr.—Part. pass. אָהוּב, f. אֲהוּבָה. Yeb. 23[a] א׳ בנשואיה beloved (worth loving) for her well chosen marriage. [Y. Ab. Zar. l. c. איחבתו read אוֹהַבְתּוֹ.]

Nif. נֶאֱהַב, *Hithpa.* הִתְאַהֵב *to be beloved, popular.* Lev. R. s. 32, beg., these blows (of persecution) had the effect לְהִתְאַהֵב וכ׳ to make me beloved of my Father in heaven. Yoma 86[a] שיהא ש״ש מִתְאַהֵב וכ׳ that the Divine Name may be beloved through thee (that thy doings may favorably reflect on thy religion).—

Pi. אִהֵב, *Hif.* הֶאֱהִיב *to make beloved, popular.* Tan. d'be El. I, 28 חתא מְאַהֵב ש״ש וכ׳ make the Divine Name &c. (v. supra).—*Part. Pu.* מְאוֹהָב *popular.* Yalk. Deut. 837. —Cant. R. to I, 1 לְהַאֲהִיבָן (לְאַהֲבָן) לקרבן וכ׳ to make them beloved (of God), draw them nigh (to God) &c. Ib. to V, 1. —Yalk. Cant. 981 הֶאֱהַבְנוּ לך עלמות הרבה we have made many maiden beloved of thee (converted them).

אֲהַבָא, const. אֲהַבַת ch.=next. w. Targ. Cant. VIII, 6.

אַהֲבָה I f. (b. h.; אהב) *love, friendship.* א׳ שהיא תלויה בדבר love dependent on something extraneous, i. e. sensual, selfish love. Aboth V, 16.—עשה מא׳ (or עבד) to do good (serve the Lord) from pure motives of love. Sot. 31[a]; Snh. 61[b]; a. fr.—

אַהֲבָה II (אַחֲוָא in Y.) pr. n. m. *Ahăbah, Ahava*, son of Zera, and father of R. Adda. R. Hash. 29[a]. Ab. Zar. 30[a]; a. fr. Y. Yeb. VIII, 9[bc].

אהדורי Y. Ber. II, 4[b], v. אַדּוּרֵי.

אהן Y. Ab. Zar. V, 45[a], read אָהֵן.

אהוליות, v. אָהֳלִית.

אהולין, v. אֹהֶל.

אהון, v. אָהֵן.

אֲהוּרְיָירָא, אֲהוּרְיָיר m. (horrearius, ὁρριάριος; v. Sm. Ant. s. v. Horreum) *store-keeper, steward.* [Comment.: fr. אָרְווָה, v. אוּרְיָא, *equerry.*] Meg. 12[b] בר אהורירייה דאבא thou, son of my father's steward. B. Mets. 85[a] (Ms. M. אהורירדה); Sabb. 113[b] אהורירדה (v. Rabb. D. S. a. l. note 4) א׳ דרבי Rabbi's house steward (manager).

אֲהוּרְמִין m. (Pers. Angra-Mainyus) *Ahriman*, the evil principle in the Zendavesta (Parsism); opp. הורמיז Ormuzd. Snh. 39[a] מפלגך לעילאי דהורמיז מפלגך לתתאי דאה׳ Ar. (ed. a. Mss. incorr., v. Rabb. D. S. a. l.; Tosef. a. l. Better vers. Ms. F. מפלגן *our* half) thy upper half belongs to Ormuzd, thy lower half to Ahriman. Ib. א״כ היכי שביק אהורמין להורמיז למעבר מיא בארעא (ed. corr. acc.) if this be so, why does Ahriman allow Ormuzd to let the water pass (through the former's dominion) to the ground?

אהיי Y. Shek. V, 48[d], read הָיי.

*__אָהִיל__ m (אהל) *staying under the same roof* with an unclean object. Naz. VII, 2 (49[b]) על אָהִילָן Talm. ed. (Mish. אָהֳלָן, v. אֹהֶל) upon staying with them under &c.

Ib. 53ª אֲהִילוֹ. [Sabb. 90ª Ms. M., v. אָהַל.].—*Pl.* f. אֲהִילוֹת the laws concerning *ahil*, whence *Ahiloth* (also אֳהָלוֹת), name of a treatise of the Mishnah (of Seder Tahăroth). Y. M. Kat. II, end, 81ᵇ there are things in the Order of Moēd קשיין מן א׳ וכ׳ more difficult than Ahiloth &c. —Hag. 14ª, a. fr. אהל׳. B. Mets. 86ª אהי׳.

אָהִיל, v. אָהַל.

אַהִילָא *tent;* v. אַהֲלָא.

אֲהִילַאי pr. n. m. *Ahilai.* Pes. 30ª.

אֲהִילָה f., pl. אֲהִילוֹת, v. אָהִיל.

אֲהִינָא f. *Ahina, a species of late and inferior dates* (cmp. אֲהִינְיָא). Hull. 46ᵇ lungs apparently so peeled as to resemble א׳ סומקא a red Ah. B. Mets. 113ᵇ א׳ מרירא a bitter Ah.—*Pl.* אֲהִינֵי. Tosef. Shebi. VII, 14; Pes. 53ª (m.!). Y. B. Kam. VI, 5ᵇ bot. כבשא דא׳ a preserve of A. Y. B. Bath. V, end, 15ᵇ כבשה דאהיני (corr. acc.), v. Ab. Zar. 38ᵇ א׳ שליקי.

אהיטו, v. foreg.

אָהַל (b. h.), *Pi.* אִיהֵל (deriv. of אֹהֶל) *to spread tent-like, to cover, shade, bend over* &c., usu. with refer. to levitical uncleanness arising from being under the same shelter with, or forming a shelter over, a corpse &c. Meïlah 17ª אי׳ על מקצתו if he bent over a portion (of the blood). Sabb. 17ª אי׳ צדו אחד וכ׳ he caused one side of his body *to overshadow* the grave.—[More freq.]

Hif. הֶאֱהִיל same. Ohol. III, 1; 3 sq. הא׳ על המת he formed a tent, i. e. spread himself, or bent, over a corpse. Ib. הבית מַאֲהִיל עליו the house forms a cover over part of it. Y. Sot. IX, 23ᶜ top; a. fr.

אֹהֶל, אוֹהֶל m. (b. h.; prob. √אה=או=אן, cmp. אַוְנָא) *tent, shelter.* Succ. 21ᵇ א׳ עראי a temporary dwelling. א׳ קבע a permanent dwelling.—Naz. 55ª א׳ זרוק a movable cover, e. g. a person carried in a vehicle over a grave, v. foreg.—B. Bath. 27ᵇ, a. fr. א׳ הטומאה something spread over an unclean object, e. g. a tree shading a corpse; v. foreg. Naz. VII, 2, v. אָהִיל.—*Pl.* אוֹהָלִים, אֹהָלִין (אֲהָלִין). Y. Sabb. XX, beg. 17ᶜ נטב א׳ to spread sheets over poles &c. (Tosef. ib. XII (XIII), 14, a. e. עשה א׳). Y. Erub. I, 19ᵈ א׳ בשיירה tents in a caravan, א׳ שבמחנה in a camp. Tosef. Kil. V, 25 אהלין ed. Zuck.

אָהָל (אוֹהָל) m. (Syr. אהלא P. Sm. 125; חל, הל, v. חלל, הלל, cmp. מוחל, מיחל) 1) *an alcalic plant,* used as *soap.* Sabb. 90ª; Nid. 62ª (counted among plants subject to the laws of the Sabbath year).—2) *a mineral substance* of the same use (in connection with נתר; v. however Maim. to Nid. IX, 6). Nid. l. c. והתניא חבורית והאהל; (Sabb. l. c. first time חול ed., Ms. M. אָהֵל; sec. time אהלא ed., Ms. M. אהיל). M. Kat. 17ᵇ; a. e. [The biblical אהלים a. אהלות have no connection of meaning with our w.]

אַהֲלָא ch.=h. אֹהֶל *tent, sheet.* Targ. Y. Num. XII, 12 (Var. אַהֲלָא, אַהִילָא). Bets. 30ᵇ קא סתר א׳ he breaks the tent up (by removing portions of the cover). Ib. 32ᵇ; a. fr.—*Pl.* אַהֲלֵי. Sabb. 137ᵇ אוסיפי א׳ extending the spread sheets (by opening a door or window over which they were spread).

אַהֲלָא, אוֹהֲלָא ch. 1)=h. אָהָל. Targ. Job. IX, 30 (h. text בור). Sabb. 90ª, v. אָהָל.—2) (=b. h. אהלים, אהלות?) *aloë* (used for medicinal purposes, v. Sm. Ant. s. v. Aloë). Ib. 110ᵇ א׳ תולנא; Git. 69ᵇ א׳ תולאנא purple-colored aloë.

אַהֲלוֹיָא m. (foreg.) *dealer in aloë* (prob. in b. h. אהלות, *perfumes*). *Pl.* אַהֲלוֹיֵי. Ned. 91ᵇ. B. Mets. 81ª.

אֲהָלוֹת, v. אָהִיל.

אַהֲלַיָּא, אוֹהֲלַיָּא pr. n. pl. *Oholaya* (tents) Eduy. VII, 4 אהו׳. Zeb. 25ᵇ אהו׳.

אֲהִילִית (אֲהוֹלִית) f. (אהל) *a group of tents, encampment;* only in *Pl.* אֲהִלִיּוֹת (=*castra*) *camps.* (Always in connection with בצוצריות or קסטרא fortifications). Cant. R. to II, 13. Yalk. Ps. 624 אהו׳. Lev. R. s. 1; a. e. [Cmp. גַּסְטְרָא a. בְּצוֹצְרִיּוֹת as to versions.]

אהמרא, v. אַחְמְרָא.

אָהֵן or אָהֵין, אָהוּן m. (הן=הָנָן, הָדֵן; √הן) 1) *this, that, he who.* Y. Ber. II, 4ᶜ bot. א׳ חזירא that swine. Ib. VI, 10ª bot. א׳ דמר he who says. Y. Yoma VI, 43ᵈ bot. כא׳ דתנינן as that (Mishnah) which we have been taught. Y. Shek. II, 47ª top א׳ דהכא the subject just quoted. Y. B. Mets. II, 8ᶜ אהין (אחון) לחן לי אהן מהו חשוב of what use is this to me? of what value is it to me?—Y. Shebu. III, 34ᵈ bot. וא׳ אפילו and this 'even'—i. e. why do you use the word 'even'?—a. fr.—2) *this place, where.* Y. Ber. IX, 13ᵇ top כל א׳ דאת אזיל wherever thou goest. *3) (adv. of time=על-הן, v. אי־) *thereupon, then.* Y. Taan. IV, 69ᵇ top אכלין ואהון וכ׳ eat ye and then drink.

אהנייתא Keth. 67ᵇ מקרבן אהנייתי, v. הֲנָיָיה ch.

אַהֲרֹן, אַהֲרוֹן pr. n. m. (b. h.) *Aaron;* the brother of Moses. Meg. 25ᵇ; a. fr.

אַהֲרוֹנִית f. (deriv. of foreg.) *of priestly parentage, Aaronide.* Erub. 53ᵇ נערה א׳ אהרונית (play on words) an Aaronide maiden, a second wife (in Ms. M. our w. is missing).

אַהֲרָן, v. אַהֲרֹן.

אוּ 1) prefix, esp. for verbal nouns, e. g. אודיצותא fr. דיין. 2) או, אוּ=εὐ-αὐ, v. אב.

אוֹ I (b. h.; אוה, v. Ges. H. Dict. s. v.) *or;* אי.. או *either.. or.* Shebu. 27ª או ... לחלק the word או in the Bible text is necessary as a disjunctif, (one *or* the other), contrad. from ו־ which is conjunctive (one *and* the other). Men. 91ª; או לדרשא the word או intimates something not explicitly stated in the text; a. fr.—*Pl.* אוין Shebu. 33ᵇ.—אוין, אוים, const. אוי־ *the word* או *in the biblical passages.* Y. ibid. IV, 35ᶜᵈ.

אוֹ ch. same. Targ. Ex. XXI, 20; a. e. Targ. Prov. VI, 28 Ms. (ed. אי).—Ber. 2ᵇ, v. דילמא; a. v. fr.

אוֹ II (ὁ) *the.* Y. R. Hash. I, 57[a] bot. (in a Greek sentence), v. אורפוס.

אוֹ m. (contr. of אֲחִי, אָחוּ v. חוּ, חִי) *he, that, this* (only in Y. Dial). [Y. Ber. II, 5[b] top או מקשי, read חוה מ׳; ed. Amst. בעי.] Y. B. Bath. III, 14[b] I was jesting באו גברא with that man. Y. Snh. XI, beg. 30[a] באו ד(א)מר with him who says—*Fem.* אי.—Y. Erub. III, 21[b] bot. אי אידא אי אידא it is all the same; v. אִידָא II.

אִוְּרָא (אִוֵּירָא) m. (אור; cmp. h. form צְוָּאר), only in א׳ דליבני *a pile of loose bricks with openings between,* opp. to solid wall. Bets. 31[b]; 36[a]; Erub. 34[b] Ms. Rash. (v. Rabb. D. S. a. l.; ed. אָוִירָא, cmp. אָוִירָא; Ar. אארא, derives fr. Pers.).

אוֹב *shoots,* v. אֵב.

אוֹב m. (b. h.; √אב or חב, v. אבב, חבאי) *cited ghost.* —בעל א׳ *necromancer.* Snh. 65[a]; a. fr.

אוֹב, אוֹבָא ch. same. Targ. Is. XXIX, 4; a. e.—א׳ טמיא necromancy over bones, sculls, also for *necromancer.* Targ. Y. I Deut. XVIII, 11. Ber. 59[a] א׳ כמיא כדיב וכ׳ the necromancer is a liar (necromancy is false), and his (its) words are lies. Sabb. 152[b] bot. (of the woman of En-Dor, I Sam. XXVIII, 7). [Yeb. 103[a] בר א׳, v. אָבִיו.]

אוּבְדָּן, אוּבְדָנָא, v. אָבְדָן, אָבְדָנָא.

אובינות, v. חֲבִיוֹנָה.

אוּבִיסוֹס, אֶפְסוֹס pr. n. pl. *Ephesus,* city of Ionia in Asia Minor. Targ. I Chr. I, 5 אוב׳ (var. lect.); Y. Meg. I, 71[b] bot. אוי׳ (rendit. of יוון); v. מַקְדוֹנְיָא.

אוּבַל, אֻבַל m. (v. יוּבַל) 1) *river.* Dan. VIII, 2; 3; 6. —2) as a pr. n. *Ubal* (The River). Gen. R. s. 16 (referring to Dan. l. c.) א׳ אויתנוין וכ׳ Ubal is the source of all the other rivers.

אוּבְלָא I=אֶבְלָא. Targ. Y. Gen. VII, 10; a. e.

אוּבְלָא II (אֻבְלָא, אוּבְּלָא) m. (יבל) *vessel made of willow twigs; basket,* or *perforated trough;* (as to shape v. Sm. Ant. s. v. *Călathus*). Bekh. 43[b], v. פְּרִלוֹן a. פְּרִילוֹן. Sab. 123[b]; Snh. 92[a], a. e. א׳ דקצרי Ar. (ed. אוב׳) the fuller's trough. Ib. 28[b] the father of the husband and the father of the wife are no more kinsmen אלא כי א׳ לדנא (ed. אכלא) than is a basket related to a barrel. [For אכלא, אבלא, איכלא cmp. פִּלְפְּלָה, פְּלִיל.]

אוּבְלִין, אוּבְלִים pr. n. pl. (v. אֲבִילִין) *Ub'lim, Ub'lin.* Erub. 12[a] top (var. v. Rabb. D. S. a. l. note 1). Hull. 55[b] אובלים (ed. אי׳).

אוּבַנְתָּא, v. אַבְנְתָּא.

אוּבְצָנָא m. (אבין, cmp. חֲבִין II, a. חבץ P. Sm. 1181 sq.) *heavy pressure, overload, prostration from heavy load.* Targ. Y. Num. XIX, 2.—B. Mets. 36[b] א׳ דחד the prostration from carriyng a load up hill. Ib. 78[a] מיתה מחמת א׳ died from fatigue. Sabb. 106[b]. [Ar. reads אוכצא, cmp. Syr. אכץ P. Sm. 190—corr. acc.]

אוּבְרִיזָא f., אוּבְרִיזִין, אוּבְרִיזוֹן m. (ὄβρυζον) *pure gold, unalloyed.* Targ. Ps. CXIX, 127; Targ. Prov. VIII, 19; a. e.

אֻבְשִׁין, אוּבְשִׁין m. pl. (b. h. בְּאֻשִׁים; cmp. אֻבְשׁוּנָא) *a species of inferior grapes.* Maasr. I, 2 הענבים והאו׳ משיבאישו Ar. (ed. Talm. B. משח׳ והאב׳; Talm. Y. והבאושין) grapes and *ubshin* are subject to tithes from the time they are called בְּאוּשָׁה q. v.—Y. Ter. VIII, 45[d] top ענבים ואו׳ וכ׳ grapes or ubshin for a sick person.

אוֹג m. (cmp. אֶגֶה; Syr. אוגא P. Sm. 53) (rhus coriaria), *red berry of the Venus' summachtree.* Peah I, 5. Dem. I, 1. Maasr. I, 2. Kel. XXVI, 3.—*Pl.* אוֹגִין. Tosef. Maas. I, 4 אובין אדומים (איבין, corr. acc.; cmp. Maasr. l. c. V. Löw Aram. Pfl. p. 44).

אוּגַד; v. אגד.

אוגדויר, v. next w.

אוגדויקונטא (ὀγδοήκοντα) *eighty.* Y. B. Bath. X, 17[c] (corrected text) שטר נפיק מר׳ הונה לר׳ שמי׳ אוגדויר מחיק קונטא לא מחיק. א״ר שמ׳לי לר׳ הונה פוק חזי עם החן אהן קונטא משמש. ומר עם טרויאקונטא. כי נפק אמר הדא בעי מתגרא תלתין אפסד עשרין. A bill of indebtedness passed from R. Huna (who could not decide or on whose decision the party would not rely) to R. Sh.—on which bill *ogdoë* was blurred (showing an erasure), and *conta* was clear. Said R. Sh. to R. H., Go and see what is the lowest numeral in Greek that *conta* is combined with. Said he, It is *triaconta* (thirty).—When the party had left, he said, That man intended to make thirty (by the erasure) and lost twenty (the original having been fifty, *penteconta*).

אוּגְדוֹר (זגדור) pr. n. pl. *Ogdor* (Zigdor) in Samaria. Y. Ab. Zar. V, 44[d]. Bab. ib. 31[a] זג׳ (Ms. M. זגרור).

אוּגְדוּתָא f. (אֲגַד II) *prolongation.* Targ. Y. Deut. XXX, 20, const. אוּגְדוּת (Var. אוּגְרוּת).

אוגורי, v. אֲגוּר end.

אוּגְיָא (אֻגְיָא) m. (אגר, sec. r. of איג, v. אָגַן; cmp. עוּגָה) *rounded off,* whence *a field* or *fields surrounded with a ridge or ditch.* Ned. 6[b]. Ber. 6[a] כי כסלא לא׳ like the ridge surrounding the field.

אוּגִיָּה f. (foreg.) *rounded ditch, hole dug around the grape-vine. Pl.* אוּגִיּוֹת M. Kat. I, 1 (Rashi to Ber. 6[a], Asheri to Ned. 6[b] expl. foreg. w.; ed. עוּגִיּוֹת).

אוּגֶן, חוּגֶן m. (אוג; v. foreg.) *border of a vessel, rim.* Hull. 25[a]; Tosef. Kel. B. Mets. II, 17 ח׳. *Hag.* 22[b] אוגנו its border. *Pl.* אוֹגְנִים, אוֹגְנִין, חו׳. Nid. 3[b]. Erub. 87[b] (banks). Kel. XXV, 6; a. e. [Hull. II, 9 (41[a]) אוגן של מים Ar., *a little pool,* ed. עוּגָה q. v.]

אוּנְגָא ch. (v. foreg.) something rounded basin, disk. Targ. Cant. VII, 3 א׳ דסיהרא the disk of the moon.—B. Mets. 69[b] א׳ דקירא (some ed. אוּנְגֵי pl., v. Rashi a. l., Ms. M. אֻגְּנֵי, v. אַגְּנָא) cake of wax. Cmp. אַגַּן.

אֻנְגְּנֵס, v. אֶבְגִּינוֹס.

אוּגַר Af. of אָגַר.

אוּגַר, אוּגְרָא m. (אָגַר, גָּדַר) heap of stones, stone-hill (h. גַּל). Targ. Y. Gen. XXXI, 46 (Bab. דְּגוֹרָא); a. fr. V. אֱגוֹרָא I.

אוגררי, read אוגדורי.

אוגרים, v. גָּרַם Af.

אוגרנא, v. אַגְּדְנָא.

אוּגֶרֶת f. a knife having notches, v. אֲגַר II.

אוּד m. (b. h., v. Ges. H. Dict. s. v.; cmp. אִיד) wooden poker. Bets. 33[a]; Sabb. 143[a].

אוּד, אוּדָא ch. same, also fire-brand. Targ. Am. IV, 11; a. e.—Pl. אוּדַיָּא, אוּדֵי. Targ. Is. VII, 4.—Snh. 93[a] (prov. concerning bad company) תרי א׳ וכ׳ two dry pieces of wood and a green one between &c.

אוֹדָאָה, אוֹדָאוּתָא, אוֹדוּתָא f. (ודי, Af. אודי) thanksgiving. Targ. Ps. XLV, 1 (var. אוֹדָאָתָא); a. e.

אוּדְרָא Ar. אוּדְרָא ed. m. (אדד, אדר, v. אֲדַר: Syr. אודדא; cmp. אַדְרָא, אֲדָרָא as to dial. var.) upholsterer's stuffing material, tow-cotton, wool. Sabb. 48[a] לאהדורי א׳ (Ms. M. אוּדְרֵי Pl.) to put the stuffing back into the mattress. Ib. 141[a] (Ms. M. אודרא); v. אֶשְׁרָשָׁא.—B. Bath. 58[a] חביתא דא׳ (Mss. דאודר׳) a vessel full of stuffings (enigmatical for bolsters). Ab. Zar. 28[b] א׳ דנדא וכ׳ (Ms. M. אודרא דנורא) tow cotton which has been dyed but not combed. B. Mets. 26[a]; a. fr.—Pl. אוּדְרֵי. Kid. 12[a] זוודא דאודרי (corr. acc.) a bundle of tow-cotton. [Cmp. עוּדְרָא, עוּדְרָא; also אִרְדָא a. אִירְדָן; v. Fuerst, H. Dict. lit. ר.]

אוּדְיָא f. (ידי, אדי; cmp. funda=sling and purse) purse. B. Mets. 28[b] א׳ דדינרי (ed. אוּדְיָא) a purse of denars.

אודיאר, Toh. VII, 7, v. אוֹרְיָיר.

אודייא, v. אוּדְיָא.

אודיין, read אוֹרְיָין.

אוּדְיָינֵי f. (ידי, נדי) whatever appertains to irrigation, sprinkling arrangements; hence the field cistern with its purtenances. B. Bath. 144[a] (Ms. אֻדְיָנֵי, אִידְרֵי; v. Rashi a. l.) if a father left nothing אלא א׳ וכ׳ but a sprinkling business, what is earned with it belongs to all heirs alike. Ib. שאני א׳ דלנטירותא וכ׳ it is different with a sprinkling business, since all the attendance it requires, is watching (which minors can do just as well as adults). [Tossaf. ib Var. אידווני, watching pedestal, fr. דוי q. v. Cmp. however אוּדְנָא III.—M. Kat. 21[a], read אוּדְיָינֵי.]

*__אוּדְיִיתָא__ I f. pl. (v. foreg.) irrigated fields. Targ. Jer. XXXI, 40 Ar. ed. pr. (ed. אֲרִיתָא q. v. ed. Ven. אֲדִיתָא).

*__אוּדְיִיתָא__ II f. (דוי, v. אַדְווּתָא) attendant, or superintendent of the vapor bath; cmp. אֲזֵי.—Y. Shebi. VIII, 38[a] זוסימי א׳ Zosime, the superintendent &c.

אוּדִיצוּתָא f. (דיץ) joy. Targ. Ps. LI, 10 (ed. Vien. אֲדִי׳).

אוּדִיקוּתָא f. prop. outlook (v. דְּיק) hence pr. n. pl. Odikutha (h. צִיץ). Targ. II Chron. XX, 16.

אוֹדִיתָא f. (ודי) confession, esp. document stating a debtor's admission of his indebtedness in presence of witnesses. Snh. 29[b].

אוֹדֶם m. (אדם) red substance, fleshy substance [cmp. אָדָם, אֲדָמָה; b. h. אֹדֶם rubin]. Y. Kil. VIII, 31[c] bot. הא׳ מן האשה from the mother the embryo receives the substance for forming skin, flesh, and blood; opp. לוֹבֶן white, sticky substance. Nid. 32[b] למעוטי אדם מא׳ to exempt man from being unclean from a red (blood) discharge, opp. to לובן white gonorrhoeic discharge.

אוּדְנָא, אוּדֶן, אוּדַן, אוּדֶן I f. ch. (=h. אֹזֶן, v. Ges. H. Dict. s. v.; √אדר, v. אֲדַר) ear. Targ. Is. LXIV, 3. Targ. Ps. XVIII, 45 אוּדְנִין (ed. Vien. אוּדְנִין?, Ms. אוזן). Targ. Ex. XXIX, 20; a. fr.—Y. Sabb. VI, 8[c] bot. טב לא׳ good for ear-ache; v. Bab. ib. 67[a]; a. fr.—Pl. אוּדְנִין, אוּדְנִין, אוּדְנַיָּא, אוּדְנֵי. Targ. Deut. XXIX, 3; a. fr. (also אֻדְנִין).—Snh. 106[a]. Y. Maas. Sh. IV, 55[b] bot.; Lam. R. to I, 1 (חד כותאר 1), v. next w.

אוּדְנָא II f. (from its shape, v. foreg. a. P. Sm. 40) 1) leather-bottle, jar (a liquid measure). Pl. אוּדְנִין. Y. Maas. Sh. IV, 55[b] bot. (to one who had dreamt he had four udnin=ears, v. foreg.) מלוי את תרתי אֻדְנָךְ ותרתי אודנוי דגרבא thou shalt have wine enough to fill thy own two udnin (wine jars), and two udnin (measures) of a garba (v. גַּרְבָּא I) besides.—2) (Syr. אוזנא, זונא P. Sm. 49, 1061) bath-tub. Ber. 22[a] was sitting בא׳ דמיא Ar. (ed. באגנא, Ms. Beth. Nath. באוזנא) in a tub filled with an udna of water. Sabb. 157[b] א׳ דמיא . . . Ar. (ed. באוזנא, Ms. M. אַבְּנָא) by a bath-tub.

אוּדְנָא III, אֲדִינָא (f.?) (=h. אֶדֶן; cmp. b. h. הֲדֹם; √דנא, דא; cmp. דוּךְ) foot-stool, camp-chair, folding stool. Targ. Jer. XLIII, 10 אודניה Ar. (ed. אפדניה).—Pl. אוּדְנַיָּא, אֲדִינַיָּא. Targ. II Est. I, 2 תרתין אודנוי (תרין?) the double footstool of king Solomon. Tosef. Kel. B. Mets. VIII, 6 מִטָּה וישן וכ׳ (not מיטה) when it bends in (under the weight) but one can sleep on it; if it was originally so made, כמאה (not כהורה) it is unclean מפני שהיא כאו׳ ed. Zuck. (Var. אדרניא, ed. אדוניא) because it is made like a double footstool.

אוּדְרָא, v. אוּדְרָא, a. אֲדַר I.

*__אוּדְרָךְ__ m. (דרך) a crushing tool, pestle, pounding club. Targ. Prov. XXVII, 22 ed. Buxt. (better, like oth. ed. אוּדְקָךְ).

אָוָה, v. אוי.

אוֹהֵל, אוֹהֲלָא, אוֹהַלְיָיא, אוֹהֵל, v. 'אהל.

אוֹהֲרָא (הוֹהֲרָא) m. (=חוחרא, redupl. of חרר Ar.) *net-work*, esp. *loose fisher's net*, contrad. to אִירְזְלָא. Y. M. Kat. III, 81[b] top 'הו.—*Pl.* אוֹהֲרֵי. M. Kat. 11[a] למיגדל א' (Alf. אוחרי) to plait nets. Git. 60[b] bot.

אֶוְגְּנִיסְטֵאטֵי, v. אבגניסטי.

אָוָז m. (√אוז, v. אֱוַשׁ; cmp. Syr. וזא, a. וזוז *bombum edit*, P. Sm. 1060) [the noisy], *goose*. Ber. 57[a] הרואה א' וכ' he who sees a goose in his dream, may hope for wisdom (with ref. to Prov. I, 20, 'wisdom cries' &c.). Y. B. Kam. V, end 5[a] אֲוַוז ים וא' יישוב וכ' the water goose (bernicle) and the domestic goose are two diff. species (כלאים); Y. Kil. VIII, 31[c] bot. א' עם א' מדבר וכ' the (domestic) goose and the goose of the steppes (wild g.); א' עם א' הים the domestic and the water goose; B. Kam. 55[a] א' וא' הבר (Ms. M. marg. אֲוַוז בית וא' בר) the domestic and the wild g.; Bekh. 8[a].

אַוְזָא or **אֲוָזָא** ch. same. Git. 86[a].—בר א' *duck*. Bets. 33[a]. *Pl.* אֲוָזֵי, אֲוָוזִין. Targ. II Esth. III, 8. Pes. 114[a]. B. Bath. 73[b]. Hull. 56[b] הנהו א' דידן וכ' our (Babylonian) geese are considered as water fowls.

אֲוֹל, אוּלָא, אֲוַל, v. אֱוַל.

אוּלָם, אוּלָס, v. אֲבְלָס.

אֹוֶן, v. אָוֶן.

אוּנָא, אֲוָנָא, אוּנָא, v. אִינָא a. אוּדְנָא II.

אֲוַנְכָּר, v. אֲוַנְכָּר.

אֶוְסוֹס, v. אוֹבִיסוֹס.

אוּקִי, v. אוקיי.

***אֲוָרָא** m.; pl. אֲוָרֵי (אֲוַר dial. for עבר, v. Nœld. Mand. Gr. p. 48 sq.; v. Ar. s. v. where עיברים=אוברים [not אובדים as in ed. Koh.] is twice used to account for the etymol. of our w.) *crossers of rivers, travelers*. בֵּי א' 1) *crossing, ford*. B. Mets. 103[b] אריסא עביד בי א' Ar. (ed. בי יאורי; Ms. H. בי אוריא, marg. יאורי) the tenant must entertain the crossings (of the dykes, ed. *the channels*) in the farm. M. Kat. 28[b] רהיט ונפיל בי א' ואמברי יזיפתא יזיף Ar. (ed. ונפיל אמברא ויזיפתא וכ' . . ., Ms. M. . . ונפיל בר זוירא אמברא, v. Rabb. D. S. a. l. note) one runs and rushes to the ford, and on the ferry he makes a loan (to pay the ferry-man; allegory of man's carelessness in providing for the life to come).—2) *among the crossing passengers*. Ib. (according to a second interpretation, v. Ar. s. v.) one runs and rushes among those ready to cross (mortals) &c. Cmp. עִיבְרָא B. Bath. 91[a] bot.

אֲוַרְדִּימָס, v. וַרְדִימוֹס.

אוורוס, v. אַבְרוֹסִי.

***אַוְרַקְסִין, אברסקין** m. pl. (cmp. אפקרסין, a. אַבְרָקִין) *trowsers*. Targ. Y. I, a. II Ex. XXVIII. 42; ib. I, Ex. XXXIX, 28 אוורקסי. Ib. Lev. VI, 3 (ed. Vien. אורקטין, II אברסקין). Ib. XVI, 4. [For וו=פ v. אֻוְשַׁר.]

אֲוַרְשִׁנָא Ar. (ed. אוּרְשִׁינָה) m. name of a *mythical bird, Phœnix*. Snh. 108[b].

אוּוְשׁ, v. אֱנַשׁ.

אֶפְשַׁר=אֻוְשַׁר, אֻוְשַׁר. Targ. Y. I, Gen. XVIII, 2; 17; a. e.

אוּתִיאוֹס, אֶוְתִּיּוֹס (אותיום) (εὐθέως) *forthwith, immediately after*. Nid. II, 2 (14[a]) נמצא על שלה א' Ar. (ed. אותיום, corr. acc.) if a stain is found on her bedclothes immediately after (the coïtion). Ib. 12[b]; 14[b] איזהו שיעור אוו' Ar. ed. Koh. (ed. וסת, ווסת, corr. acc.) what is the interval designated by *evthios*? Y. Nid. II, 49[d] bot. repeatedly הֶיוּתִיאוֹס or 'הֶיוּ.

אווּתנטייה, v. אוותנטיא.

***אֵיתָן, אֲוּתָן** m. (=h. אֵיתָן, r. אית) *full, proud, bright*. Targ. Job XXXI, 26 Ms. (ed. זִיוְתָן).—*Pl.* אֵיתְנַיָּא Ib. IX, 13 (ed. Buxt. a. oth. גִּיוְתָנַיָּא)

אוּתְּנְטֵי, v. אֲוּתֶנְטִין.

אֲוְתֶנְטְיָיה, אוּתָ', אֲוּתֶנְטְיָא f. (αὐθεντία) *origin, reality*; v. next w.—עיקר א' the *very reality, virtuality*. Gen. R. s. 25 עיקר א' וכ' the real famine was destined to be in the days of Saul. Cant. R. to I, 1 עיקר א' וכ' the real, authentic, among the several names of Solomon &c. Koh. R. to I, 1 'אית (corr. acc.). Num. R. s. 10 אוותינטיה (corr. acc.).

אֲוּתֶנְטֵי, (אפתנטי) m. (αὐθέντης) *originator, author*. Gen. R. s. 16 פרת א' של וכ' the Euphrates is the originator (ultimate source) of the rivers (mentioned Gen. II, 10 sq.).—*Pl.* m. אֲוּתֶנְטִין. Y'lamd. to Num. XI, 16 (quot. in Ar. s. v. אמתנטין) כנגד אפת' של ישראל וכ' (corr. 'אוו) corresponding to the number of the originators of Israel, for with seventy souls &c.—Fem. אֲוּתֶנְטִיּוֹת, אֲוּתֶנְטְיָאוֹת. Pesik. Sh'kal. p. 16[b] אומות א' (seventy) original nations.

***אוּזְיָא (אוּסְיָא)** f. (√אז, v. אֲזַד; cmp. קְצָה) *a piece, part, uzya*, a market term for a certain portion (quarter &c.) of meat. Bets. 29[a] in Pumb. they call it א' ופלגא א' Ms. M. (ed. ופלגו א' corr. acc.; Var. אוסיא) an uzya and half an uzya.

אוּזִילָא, v. אוּרְזִילָא.

אוּזִילְתָּא, v. אִיזְלָא.

***אוּזִינְקָא** m. (=אונו; נזק, v. אַנְזִיקָא) (*compensation for*) *loss, expense* of money and time. B. Bath. 6[b] שקול א' וכ' (Ms. R. עבדיה כוליה ויהיבנא לך א') take compensation and do thou the work (do thou it all, and I shall pay &c.).

אוּזְלָא, אוּזַלְתָּא, v. אִיזְלָא.

*אוּזְמָרָאוֹת f. pl. (זמר, יום; comp. זָמָם, צמם) *knots, fringes* (in the weaver's work). Tosef. Kel. B. Bath. ch. V, end 'שְׁיָרֵי .... והא the remnants &c. and the fringes (cut off for finishing).

אוּזְמֵל, v. אִיזְמֵל.

אוּזֶן, v. אֹזֶן.

אוּזְנָא, v. אוּדְנָא.

*אוּזְנִיּוֹת, **אֻזְנִיּוֹת** f. (?) pl. (=חוניות, v. חָזְרוֹן 2, a. חָזִיז; cmp. חֲבִיוֹנוֹת=אֲבִיוֹנוֹת) *lichen-dishes*. Tosef. Shebi. VII, 13. [El. Wil. emends אחיני=אחינוּת whereas the context intimates a vegetable.]

אוּזְפוּתָא f. (יזף) *loan*. Targ. Y. Deut. XV, 2.

*(אוזפידה), **אוּזְפֵי** m. pl. (=זיפין, v. זִיף) *a species of bees, wasps*. Targ. Y. Lev. XI, 20.

אוזרד, v. עוּזְרָד a. חֲזִרְדָּ.

*אוּחֲדָנָא m. (אחז=אחד) *possession, power* (h. חֹסֶן). Targ. Prov. XXVII, 24 (ed. corrupt אוחרנא; ed. Walt. אַחְסָנָא).

אוּחֲדְתָּא f. (v. foreg.) prop. *locking up*, hence, *trap, snare*. Targ. Job. XVIII, 10.

אוּחֲדְתָּא (אוּחֲדְתָּא) f. (b. h. חִידָה; v. חוד II) *enigma, epigram*. Targ. Ps. XLIX, 5 (Ms. אחדותא).

אוֹחַיִין m. pl. (b. h. אֹחִים) *howling animals, owls* &c. Targ. Is. XIII, 21.

אוּחְרֵי, v. אֲחוֹרֵי.

אוּחֲרָיָא c. (אחר) *last, outmost*. Targ. Y. II. Lev. XIX, 9; v. אוּמָן.

אוּחֲרָן, אוּחֲרָנָא, אוּחֲרַנְתָּא, v. אָחֳרָן.

אוּטָבוּתָא f. (יטב) *doing good, propriety*. Targ. Koh. IV, 4.

אוטימוס, v. אַטְּמוֹס.

אוטיפיטא, v. אַנְטִיפִיטָא.

אוּטֶם m. (אטם) 1) *obstruction; something closed, plugged up*. Hull. 47[b] א' בריאה Ar. (ed. אָטוּם) an obstruction in the lungs, a spot imperviable to air when blown up. Ohol. VI, 5 we regard the levitical uncleanness between the rafters 'כאילו הוא א as if it was locked up (and could not affect what is in the house).—2) *substructure* (filled with earth), *foundation*. Mid. IV, 6. Par. III, 6.

אוטם Tosef. Kil. III, 14 ed. Zuck., v. אִיטָן.

אוטנס Ab. Zar. 39[a], v. אַטּוּנָס.

אוטפוטא Koh. R. to XI, 1, read אנטיפיטא.

אָוָה I, אוֹי (b. h., √אב=או, cmp. אָבָה), *Pi.* אִיוָּה *to desire, covet*. Snh. 63[a] 'איוו אלוהות וכ (Ab. Zar. 53[b] לאלוהות; v. Rabb. D. S. a. l. note 8) they had a desire for many deities. Denom. תַּאֲוָה. Cmp. אוּת.

Hithpa. הִתְאַוָּה (b. h.), *Nithpa.* נִתְאַוָּה (denom. of תַּאֲוָה) *to desire, to be seized with a desire*. Num. R. s. 10 (play on יהאדם Prov. XXIII, 31) the drunken man 'יִתְאַוֶּה לדם וכ will covet blood (forbidden intercourse). Gen. R. s. 51. Ex. R. s. 24, end.—Num. R. s. 2 'התחילו מִתְאַוִּים וכ they began to express a desire for standards (in imitation of the angelic hosts). Ib. divide them into standards כמו שנִתְאַווּ as they desired.

אָוָה II, אוי (b. h., √אח, cmp. הא; v. חָוָה, a. Ges. H. Dict. s. v. אָוָה III) *to point, mark*. Denom. אוֹת II, תְּאוּ, תַּאֲוָה.

Hithpa. הִתְאַוָּה (denom. of תַּאֲוָה, תְּאוּ) *to mark, to mark out*. Koh. R. to XII, 7 התחיל מִתְאַוֶּה תאוים he began to put up marks.

אוֹי m. (v. אוי I) [pressure] *woe, sorrow*. Gen. R. s. 46 בי לא אוי there is no (cause for) woe with me. Num. R. s. 10 (play on ἄβοy, Prov. XXIII, 29) אב אוי father of woe.—2) interj. *woe! alas!* Kel. XVII, 16; a. v. fr.

אוּיָא I, אִוְיָא m. (v. חִוְיָא) *serpent*. Gen. R. s. 26 'בגלילא וכ in Galilee they call *hivya, ivya*.

אוּיָא II, אִוְיָא pr. n. m. (v. foreg.) *Ivya*, a Babyl. Amora. B. Bath. 19[a] R. Hiya son of R. Iv.—Men. 78[a]; a. e.

אויים, אויין pl. of אוֹי I.

אֱוִילָא, v. אֱוִיל.

אוֹיִים, אוֹיִם (?) an interjection (cmp. εὐαν, εὖα) *ho! hallo!* Y. Hag. II, 78[a] top; Snh. VI, 23[c] bot. א' א' 'פתחון לי וכ ho, ho! Open, for I am one of yours.

אֲוִיר, אֲוִיר m. (אור; cmp. רוּחַ a. רֶוַח); *space* corresp. to חָלָל, esp. 1) *open, empty space, blank*. Ohol. IV, 1 a tower 'שעומד בא standing isolated. Ib. XVIII, 10 אוירה של חצר the open space in the court-yard.—B. Bath. 163[a].—2) (cmp. b. h. מְאוּרָה) *hollow, cavity of a vessel*. Kel. II, 1 'מיטמאין ומטמאין בא become unclean and make unclean by contact with the hollow (of the vessel).—Yeb. 67[b] נפק לא' העולם came forth into the lighted space of the world, i. e. was born; a. fr.—3) (cmp. ἀήρ, aër) *air, atmosphere, climate, weather*. Num. R. s. 14 'הא' שממנו וכ (as one of the elements of nature) out of which the wind was made.—Gen. R. s. 34 א' יפה *fine weather*; a. fr. —*Pl.* אֲוִירִין *blank spaces in writings*. B. Bath. 163[a].— אֲוִירוֹת *climates*. Gen. R. s. 34 'ברית נחלקה לא a covenant has been made in favor of climates, i. e. God has implanted in man a love of his native soil even in bad climates.

אֲוִירָא, אֲוִיר, אֲוִירָא, אַוִּירָא ch. same. 1) *empty space, air*. Targ. Y. Ex. XIX, 17; a. fr.—Git. 20[b] א' דמגילתא the blank in a scroll (margin &c.). Men. 35[a] 'חזי א to face the inside of the T'fillin.—2) *air, weather*. Pes. 30[b] 'שליט בהו א the air strikes them. Y. R. Hash. II, 58[a] bot. 'מעונן א cloudy weather; a. fr.—3) *pile of bricks with openings between*, v. אַאֲרָא.

אוורא Y. M. Kat. I, 80[b] bot., v. אַיְרָא.

אֲוִירְטָא m. (averta, ἀβερτή) *knapsack*.—*Pl.* אֲוִירְטִין. Tosef. Kel. B. Bath. IV, 10.

*אֲוִירְיָא pr. n. pl. *Avirya*. Shebu. 24[b] (v. Rab. D. S. a.).

אוּכְחוּתָא, אוֹכַחְתָּא f. (יכח) *reproof.* Targ. Y. I, Deut. I, 1; a. e.

אוּכְמָא *eight,* v. אֻכְמָא.

***אוּכְּיִיפָא** m. (כוף) *bending, suppression.* Esth. R. to I, 1[b] (ref. to Lam. III, 13 בני אשפתו, the quotation being omitted by clerical error), [read] ר׳ ברכי׳ ורבנן ר׳ ברכי׳ אמר בני אוּכְּיִיפִיה ורבנן אמרי בני אמורייה. בני אוכייפיה שהוו מרוצין וכ׳ *B'ne Ashpatho* means 'the children of his pressure' &c., v. אֲמוּרְיָא.

אוכל Pes. 53[a] של א׳, read אָבֵל; v. Tosef. Shebi. VII, 15.

אוֹכֶל m. (b. h. אָכַל; אכל) *food, edible.* Bets. I, 8 בורר א׳ ואוֹכֵל (Y. ed. בורר אוכל אוכל) he selects singly what is edible and eats immediately; a. fr.—א׳ נפש the necessary food for the day. Meg. I, 5 אלא א׳ נ׳ בלבד except the preparation of food (cooking &c., permitted on Holy Days, Ex. XII, 16).—*Pl.* אוֹכָלִים, אוֹכָלִין *food, eatables.* Ber. 50[b]; a. fr. Ab. Zar. 52[b] תקרובת ע״ז של א׳ an idolatrous offering consisting of edibles; Y. ib. IV, 43[d] אֹכָ׳.

אוּכְלָא I ch. 1) same. Targ. Ps. LXXVIII, 18 (Ms. מֵיכְלָא).—Yoma 80[b] כל אכשורי א׳ א׳ הוא whatever is used for seasoning food, is considered as food.—2) *the digested food found in the entrails, excrements,* cmp. רעי.—Targ. Lev. I, 16; a. e.—3) *an eye-disease, itching* (cmp. חוּרְשָׁא). Ab. Zar. 28[b] תחלת א׳ the incipiency of &c., סוף א׳ last stage (near recovery).

אוּכְלָא II m. (כול=אכל) prop. *measure,* hence (cmp. כַּיְלָא) 1) *a certain measure, Ukhla,* (basket); cmp. כְּלָה.—Y. Sot. I, 17[a] תומן וחצי ת׳ וא׳ one Tuman (one eighth of a kab), and half a T. and one Ukhla; cmp. עוּכְלָא.—2) *basket,* v. אוּכְלָא II.

אוּכְלָה, v. אָכְלָה.

אוּכְלוּזָא (perh. fr. r. כלז, cmp. Arab. kalaza, *collegit,* a. כרז, קלס; v. Ges. H. Dict. s. v. כרש; var. forms: אֻכְלוֹזָא, כְּלוֹזָא, אוּכְלְסָא, אוּכְלוּסָא; h. form only in pl. אוּכְלוּסִין, const. (אוּכְלְסִין, אוּכְלוּסֵי) *levy of troops* or *forced laborers* (corresp. to h. צָבָא). Targ. I Chr. XI, 6; XX, 1.—B. Bath. 8[a]; B. Mets. 108[a] נפקי בא׳ (Ms. M. כלוזא) they have to go out themselves to do public labors (not permitted to hire substitutes). Ib. לאו בני א׳ וכ׳ are exempt from the levy. Ber. 58[a]; Yeb. 76[b] יצא בא׳ went out with the army; [strike out ודרש בא׳ Ber. l. c., v. Rabb. D. S. a. l. note 40]; a. fr.—*Pl.* אוּכְלְסִין, אוּכְלוּסִין, אוּכְלוּזִין (v. supra). Targ. I Chr. XII, 22; a. fr.—Tosef. Ber. VII (VI), 2 אוכלסין. Ber. 58[a]; אוּכְלוּסֵי ישראל a Jewish army. Y. Ber. IX, 13[c] top.; Y. Snh. X, 29[b] top. . . . אוכלוסייא ד the armies of students; a. fr.—Cmp. אֻכְלוֹשֵׁי. [Y. Ber. IX, 13[a]; Midr. Till. to Ps. IV, v. אִסְפּוֹלֵי].

אוּכָּם, אוּכְּמָא, אוּכָּמָא m. **אוּכַּמְתָּא, אוּכָּמְתָּא** f. (אכם) *black, dark-complected, freckled, ungainly.* Targ. Lev. XIII, 31; a. fr.—Pes. 88[a].—M. Kat. 9[b] הוה ליה ברתא א׳ Ms. M. (ed. our w. omitted) had an ungainly (freckled) daughter; Sabb. 80[b]. Git. 67[b] הרנגולתא אוּכַּמְתִּי a black (checkered?) hen. Ib. 68[a] אוכמא בחיורא a black spot on a white skin. *Pl.* masc. אוּכְּמִין, אוּכָּמֵי, אוּכָּמַיָּא, אוּכְמַיָּא. Targ. Jer. VIII, 21; a. e.—Hull. 46[b] א׳ א׳ covered with black spots.—Fem. אֻכָּמָתָא Sabb. 129[a]. Ib. 20[b] אוכמוותא Ar. (ed. אוכמתא) the black (greenish) moss on ships or puddles.

אוּכְמָא, m. **אוּכְמְתָא** f. (foreg.) *black color, darkness; distress.* Targ. Y. Lev. XXII, 22. Targ. Lam. IV, 8.

אוּכְמוּתָא f. same. Targ. Koh. XI, 10 dark hair, youth.

אוכמנא, v. אוּסְמָנָא.

אוּכְּמְתָּא, אוכמתא, אוכמתא, v. אוּכְּמָא, אוּכָּמָא.

***אוּכַּמְתִּי,** v. אוּכְּמָא.

אוּכָּף, אִיכּוּף c. (אכף) *saddle.* Kel. XXIII, 1; 2; a. e.—Y. Sabb. V, 7[b] bot. או׳ a. אי׳.—Y. Erub. I, 19[b] bot. בין או׳ לאי׳; Bab. ib. 16[a] או׳ לאו׳. Sabb. 53[a].—*Pl.* אוּכָּפוֹת, אִיכּוּפִין. Erub. 15[b] ed. (Ar. אִכּוּפִין). Y. Erub. l. c.

אוּכָּפָא ch. same. B. Mets. 27[b]. B. Kam. 92[b] (prov.) חברא קרייך חמרא א׳ וכ׳ if thy neighbor calls thee an ass, put a saddle on. Erub. 27[a] גבא דא׳ the upper part of the saddle (Ar., besides other var., גברא דא׳ man's figure on the upper part of the saddle) used as a handle by the rider.

אוכפייה Esth. R. to I, 1[b] בני או׳ (אוכ׳), v. אוּכְּיִיפָא.

אוכצנא, v. אוּכְצָנָא.

אוּל, אֱוִיל (אֱוּל), אֱוִילָא m. (אול *to circle,* v. חול, עול, cmp. עוֹלָם, תְּחִלָּה) *beginning, early season.* Targ. Hos. IX, 10; a. e.—מן א׳ from the beginning (of the world). Targ. Job. XX, 4; a. fr.—לאויל *to (its) previous condition.* Targ. Ez. XVI, 55 (some ed. לְאוּלְהֵן). Cmp. אלל.

אוּלְבָּנָא m., pl. אוּלְבָּנִין (denom. of לְבוּנְתָא) *unguent made of incense.* Targ. Cant. IV, 11; (h. text לבנון, LXX ἀρώματα, as if לְבֹנִין).

***אוֹלָר** m. (ילד, ולד) *a tool for hollowing out and cutting the writing reed* (scalprum), *a sort of pen-knife.* Tosef. Kel. B. Bath. end. Kel. XII, 8 אולר (corr. acc.; v. Ar. ed. Koh. s. v.).

אוֹלוֹ־ (ὅλο-) a prefix, sometimes separately printed, *whole, entirely of.* Pesik. Vay. B'yom p. 4[b] א׳ מרגליטין trimmed all over with pearls. Lev. R. s. 32, end אילו כורסין (corr. acc.) all gold, v. אוֹלוֹכְרוּסוֹן.

אולוגלוגין, v. אִילוּגִין.

אולוהתא Y. Taan. III, 66[c] top, read מוּלְיוּתָא, v. מוּלָא *mule.*

אולוכורסין, v. next w.

אוֹלוֹכְרוּסוֹן m. (ὁλόχρυσον) *all gold.* Lev. R. s. 32 (variously corrupted, v. אוֹלוֹ־.—Ar. אולון כרוסא); Cant. R. to IV, 7 (corr. acc.).

אוֹלוֹן, v. foreg.

אוֹלוֹסֵירִיקָא m. (ὁλοσήρικος) *all silk.*—*Pl.* אוֹלוֹסֵירִיקִין, mostly אוֹלוֹסֵירִיקִין *pure-silken garments.*

Koh. R. to I, 7. Y. Sabb. VI, 8[b] bot.. Yalk. Prov. 935.—[Koh. R. l. c. second time some ed. אולוסתיקין, corr. acc.]

אוּלוּסְרִיקָא, אולוסתיקין, v. foreg.

אולורין, v. אוֹלָיָיר.

אוליאוס, v. אֵילְיָאוֹס.

אוֹלְיָאר, אוֹלְיָיר m. (olearius, ὀλεάριος S.) *keeper of clothes at the baths.* Y. Maas. Sh. I, 52[d] top סימני הנתונות לא׳ tokens (in place of small change) given to the olearius; cmp. Tosef. Maas. Sh. I, 4.—Pesik. R. s. 22; a. e.—*Pl.* אוֹלְיָירִין, אוֹלְיָארִין. Tosef. Kel. B. Mets. II, 12 מגררות של אוּלָרְרִין ed. Zuck. (oth. ed. אולו׳ corr. acc.) the brushes (strigils) of the bathing attendants. Sabb. 147[b]. Y. Ber. II, 4[c] top; cmp. Pesik. R. l. c.; a. e. V. אוֹרְיָיר. [Sabb. 144[a] כלים הא׳, Nid. 20[a] האולרירין . . . , v. אוֹלָרִין.]

אולירין, v. foreg. a. אוֹלָרִין.

אוּלָּלָא, v. אֲלָלָא.

אוּלָם I m. (b. h.; v. אלם; cmp. Assyr. אלם *in front of, opposite*, Schr. K. A. T. glossary, a. b. h. conj. אוּלָם) *entrance, hall*, esp. *Ulam*, the hall leading to the interior of the Temple. Mid. IV, 7; a. e.

אולם II pr. n. pl. (v. foreg., Οὐλαμμοῦς Euseb. Onom.; Neub. Géogr. p. 18; 261) 1) *Ulam* (Porta) a place in Gilead, and one in Galilee. Y. Snh. X, 28[d].—2) in Cilicia; v. אַבְלָס.

אוּלָמָא, אוּלְמָא ch. אוּלָם I. Targ. I Kings VII, 6; a. fr.—Targ. II Chr. III, 4 אולם, Var. אוּלְמָנָא.—*Pl.* אוּלָמַיָּא. Targ. Ez. XL, 22; a. e.

אוּלְמָא m. (אֲלַם) *strength, strong side.* Sabb. 134[a] מא׳ לקוטנא from the thick to the thinner side.—Nid. 8[a], a. fr. מאי אוּלְמֵיהּ wherein does his (its) strength consist, i. e. why is this opinion preferable to &c.?

אוּלְמָנָא, v. אוּלָמָא.

אולפין, v. next w.

אוּלְפָּנָא, אוּלְפָּן m. (אלף, ילף) *custom, training, instruction; the Law.* Targ. Y. Gen. XXXIII, 14. Targ. Is. XXXII, 6; a. fr.—Y. R. Hash. IV, beg. 59[b] for it is impossible for one to go through his Bible lesson דלא א׳ (read בלא; cmp. Ḥag. 3[a] בלא חדוש) without some instructive observation. Y. Meg. I, 71[d] top דלא מן א׳ not according to the Law. Gen. R. s. 80 וא׳ קבל Mat. Keh. (ed. ואולפין קביל) and has he received traditions from teachers? Lev. R. s. 19 אולפני מה נהיר באפר how my learning shines in my face! Y. Ber. VI, 10[c] bot. נישבוק אולפנה וכ׳ let us drop discussion and return to the Mishnah. [Erub. 67[a] bot. משמיה דא׳, read with Ms. M. דְאִלְפָא.]—בר א׳ a scholar of traditional law. Lev. R. s. 3, beg.—*Pl.* אוּלְפָּנַיָּיא *instructive narratives, stories.* Y. Kid. 61[b]; Y. Peah I, 15[c] bot.

אוּלְצָנָא, אוּלְצָן m. (אלץ) *distress*, esp. *famine.* Targ. Job V, 11; a. e.

אולר, v. אוֹלָר.

***אולרויא** Y. Sabb. VI, 8[b] bot., read קוֹרוֹלָרְיָיא m. pl. (pl. of corollarium) *gilt*, or *silvered wreaths*, a rendition of צניפות (Is. III, 23); v. bibl. quot. ibid., a. Targ. Is. l. c.

אוֹלָרִין or אוֹלָרְיָין m. pl. (pl. of aularis or aularius =aulicus, D. C. Lat.) *belonging to the royal court, court-*, only in connect. with כלים or בגדים. Sabb. 114[a] בגדי הא׳ Ms. M. (ed. כלים האולרירין); Nid. 20[a] כלים האולרין court clothes, including white cloaks (גלימי), and red home or table dresses (פתורי, לבושי); v. Luebk. Alterth. s. v. Kleidung; Becker Gallus, ed. Gœll I, 16. Cmp. חִימוּצְתָא a. בּוּרְדִּיקָא.

אוּם f. (אֵם; cmp. שׁוּם, שֵׁם) 1) *mother.* Y. Yeb. XI, 11[d] top. א׳ זכר the mother of the male side, father-in-law's mother; א׳ נקבה mother-in-law's mother.—2) *substance, bulk*, as *the cluster of olives* (contrad. to leaves); *the starting point* of leprosy. Toh. IX, 8 אם היה נוגע בא׳ if the reptile touched the cluster. Neg. I, 5 הלכה לה הא׳ the original leprosy has disappeared.—3) *womb.* Lev. R. s. 14 end, Ar. (ed. אֵם).

***אוּמָּא** f. ch. (v. foreg.) *the leaven, flour used for leaven.* Pes. 42[a] קומניתא דא׳ (Ms. O. דנהמא) the decay of the flour-substance; v. כּוּתָּח. [V. also אוּנָא end.]

אוּמָּא *nation*, v. אוּמְּתָא.

הוֹמָאָה, אוֹמָתָא, אוֹמָאָה f. (ימי, Af. אוֹמֵי) *the act of administering an oath, swearing, imprecation.* Targ. Y. Lev. V, 1; 4.—*Targ. Y. II, Deut. XXVII, 15 פתחו הוֹמָהוֹם וכ׳ (Var. פומהום, ed. Vien. קתחו corr. acc.) they opened their imprecation with a blessing.

אוּמְד m. (אָמַד) *estimate, guess, measuring by mere sight, approximate assessment; medical opinion* as to the nature of injuries. Men. 54[b] ניטלת בא׳ may be set apart (for the priest) by estimating (without measuring) the quantity. Snh. IV, 5 מא׳ ומשמועה from mere supposition or hear-say. Ib. 78[b] אין א׳ אחר א׳ the first estimate (medical opinion declaring an inflicted injury fatal) cannot be upset by a second more favorable opinion (if erroneously formed under the resemblance of recovery); v. אָמַד.—Ib. א׳ האמצעי the (second) opinion intermediate between the first opinion and the actual fatal result.

אוּמְדוֹת f. same, adv. *by guess-work.* Y. Taan. IV, 68[c] top שלא . . . דן א׳ that one must not judge from mere guess (appearance). Aboth I, 16 אל תרבה לעשר א׳ in giving tithes do not give (even) too much by guessing (but measure accurately).

אוּמְדָנָא m. ch.=h. אוּמְד. B. Kam. 41[a]; a. fr.—*Pl.* אוּמְדָּנֵי Snh. 78[b].

אוּמָּה f. (b. h. אֻמָּה; אמם to join, v. אֵם) *people, nation, government.* Ab. Zar. 18[a] א׳ זו this (Roman) government; a. fr.—*Pl.* אוּמּוֹת *nations; gentiles* (contrad. to

Israel); freq. א׳ העולם (abbr. או״ח, א״ה). Gen. R. s. 39 שבעים א׳ the seventy nations (in the Noachidic genealogy), v. אֶוְיתַּנְטִין. Ab. Zar. 3ᵇ באין אוה״ע וכ׳ the gentiles shall come and be converted; a. fr.—דיני א׳ (freq. עכ״ום, גוי) gentile (not Israelitish) law. Y. Kid. I, 58ᵇ bot.; a. fr.—

*אוּמוֹלוֹגְיָיא f. (ὁμολογία) [agreement, admission] receipt, discharge. [This meaning of ὁμολογία as receipt cannot be proven from Greek literature; cmp. however, Sm. Dict. Ant. s. v. Acceptilatio.] Y. M. Kat. III, 82ᵃ bot., explaining שוברים (v. שׁוֹבֵר, receipt) אימולוגים (corr. acc., De Lara אומולוגין pl. m. fr. ὁμόλογον). Y. Keth. IX, end, 33ᶜ (ולית ליה לרב =) ולית רב אי׳ is it Rab's opinion that the divorced woman is not bound to write a receipt (for her dowry)?

אמלוגין, אומולוגין Pesik. R. s. 44, read אִרְלוֹגִין, v. ed. Friedm. p. 183ᵃ.

אומוניאה, read אֲגְמוּנְיָאָה, v. הֶגְמוֹנְיָא.

אוֹמִי Af. of יָמִי.

אומיקטרון, v. אימ׳.

אוּמְלָל m. (b. h. אֻמְלַל; v. מלל) broken down, crushed, low.—Pl. אוּמְלָלִים. Snh. 66ᵃ (ref. to Lev. XIX, 14) בא׳ שבעמך וכ׳ here the Bible speaks of the lowest among thy people (not נשיא בעמך as Ex. XXII, 27). [Ms. M. a. Ar. בְּמִילְלִין.]

אוֹמֶן m. (ימן, אמן) prop. straight line, leader, hence (agric.) the border-bed, outmost furrow. Peah IV, 5. B. Mets. VII, 4. Ned. IV, 4 (41ᵇ) לא יעשה עמו בא׳ he must not work with him together in the border bed.—Pl. אוֹמָנִיּוֹת, [fr. אוֹמָנִית, sub. ערוגה, f.]. B. Mets. 89ᵇ.

אוּמָן, אוּמָנָא ch. same. Targ. Y. I Lev. XIX, 9 (h. text פאה); Targ. Y. II ib. אי מן (read אוֹמָן). Ib. v. 27 Ar. (ed. צדדי), XXI, 5 (of the beard, h. text פאת זקנך).

אוּמָּן m. (b. h. אָמָן; ימן, אמן) skilled, artist, artisan, professional cook, architect &c. Ab. Zar. 34ᵇ מורייס א׳ brine prepared by a professional manufacturer and dealer. Gen. R. s. 1 מדעת א׳ after the plan of an architect. Pesik. R. s. 11 שאינו א׳ וכ׳ who is not skilled in climbing up.; a. fr.—Pl. אוּמָּנִין Ber. 16ᵃ; a. fr.

אוּמָּן, אוּמָּנָא (אוּמָּנָה) ch. same. Targ. Is. XXI, 10 (adj.). Targ. Ex. XXVI, 1; a. e.—Snh. 29ᵃ (prov.) שב שני וכ׳ seven years a famine may last, but the artisan's gate it will not cross. Sabb. 133ᵇ האי א׳ the surgeon (who circumcises). B. Mets. 97ᵃ טבחא וא׳ the butcher and the surgeon (of the community).—Pl. אוּמָּנַיָּא, אוּמָּנִין. Targ. I Chr. IX, 30. Targ. II Kings XXIV, 14; a. e. Y. Ber. IV, 13ᵃ top, as one uses promiscuously the words אומנין בניין וכ׳ (read אומנין) artisans, builders, architects.

אוֹמָנָא front bed, v. אוֹמֶן.

אוּמָנָה, v. אוּמָּן ch.

אוּמָנוּ, v. אוּמָנוּתָא.

אומנון, v. אוּמָּן.

אומנוס, read אֲמָנוֹס, v. אֲמָנָה II.

אוּמָּנוּת f. (v. אוּמָּן) 1) skill, handicraft, trade. Kid. IV, 14.—בעל א׳ mechanic. Hull. 54ᵇ.—בן אומנותו one's fellow-tradesman, competitor. Gen. R. s. 32, beg.—Ber. 43ᵇ כל אחד ואחד יָפָה לו וכ׳ to each man the Lord made his trade appear nice. Y. Succ. V, end, 55ᵈ (play on be-ĕmunatham I Chron. IX, 22) באומנותם through their skill; a. fr.—2) the workmanship (or its equivalent) to be furnished the (Roman) government. B. Bath. IX, 4. Y. Dem. VI, end, 26ᵃ; Tosef. Dem. VI, 4; cmp. אוֹצָר.—Pl. אוּמָּנִיּוֹת. Gen. R. s. 24. Num. R. s. 15 קורא א׳ invited people by trades (each day another trade); Tanh. B'haăl., 3 קורא בכל יום א׳.—Trnsf. arts, devices. Ex. R. s. 47, end כל הצדיקים באו בא׳ all the righteous (in their pleas and prayers) came with devices before the Lord (as Abraham prayed in behalf of fifty, forty &c.).

אוּמָּנוּ, אוּמָּנוּתָא ch. same. Targ. O. Ex. XXXV, 33; a. e.—Macc. 8ᵇ; a. e.—Koh. R. to III, 9 מאי מהנו אומנה באוּמָּנוּתֵיהּ what does the artist profit by his skill? Y. Git. V, 47ᵇ bot. יחבין בניהון לא׳ indenture their children as apprentices; Y. B. Bath. X, 17ᶜ bot. לאומנתה (corr. acc.). Sabb. 103ᵃ חזי א׳ וכ׳ sees a mechanical contrivance on a Sabbath and learns it. Y. Keth. IV, 28ᵈ אמנותא (corr acc.), v. טְרִיקְלִין.—Pl. אוּמָּנְוָתָא, אוּמָּנָוָן; אוּמָּנְוָן. Targ. Ex. l. c. Targ. II Esth VI, 12; a. fr. [Y. Ber. IV, 13ᵃ top, v. אוּמָּן.]

אוּמָנִית, pl. אוּמָנִיּוֹת, v. אוֹמֶן.

אומפירטור, v. אִמְפְּרָטוֹר.

אוּמְצָא com. (אמץ) a thick piece of meat, a piece which can be eaten raw after pressing &c. Sabb. 128ᵃ חזי לא׳ fit to be eaten raw. Hull. 44ᵇ א׳ מעלייתא a fine piece &c.; a. fr.—Pl. אוּמְצֵי. Git. 69ᵃ שב א׳ seven pieces.

אוּמְרִית f. fringe, border, v. אִמְרָה h.

אוּמָּא, אוּמָּתָא, אוּמַּת f. ch.=h. אומה people. Targ. Y. Deut. XXIX, 12; a. e. Midr. Prov. to XXX, 28; a. e.—Pl. אוּמִּין. Targ. Y. Gen. XXV, 3. Gen. R. s. 61. אוּמֵּי; אוּמַּיָּא, אוּמַּיָּא. Targ. Ps. CXVII, 1.—Midr. Till. to Ps. IX, 6 שנאיהון דא׳ those hated by the nations.—Sabb. 32ᵃ.—אוּמָּתָא, אוּמָאתָא. Targ. Prov. XXIV, 24.

אוּמָּתָא oath, v. אוּמָּאָה.

אָוֶן, אָוֶן m. (b. h.; √עו=אי to curve, be curved, hollow; to press, be pressed; v. אור, אוגיא &c.; comp. עב, גב, גו, חב, חו) 1) oppression, wrong (=עָוֹן)—2) falsehood, vanity (=הֶבֶל). א׳ גִלְּיוֹן a cacophemistic adaptation of εὐαγγέλιον (v. גליון). Sabb. 116ᵃ bot. (after לסכונה, omitted in ed.) ר׳ מאיר א׳ ג׳ ר׳ יוחנן קרי ליה עון גליון (Rashi Ms. ר׳ מאיר, v. Rabb. D. S. a. l. note) R. Meïr called the gospel falsehood of blank paper (or of revelation), R. Yoh. called it sin of &c. [Ib. several times און ג׳ or עון גליון in Ms. a. older editions, for אוריתא אחריתי &c. in recent ed., v. Rabb. D. S. a. l.]

און m. (b. h.; √או, v. foreg.; cmp. חזקה, חַיִל, חבל, a. next w.) *possession*, *power*. Tosef. Ab. Zar. III, 16 (IV, beg.) כתב לו אונו if he (the seller of the slave) wrote to him (gave him in writing) the liberty of his disposal of himself, i. e. that the slave, if he should run away from the buyer, would not be claimed by him who sold him; Git. 43ᵇ כתב עליו אונו (read אליו or לו). Ib. מאי אונו what means 'his own possession'? Ans. He wrote to him this, 'If thou run away from him (the purchaser), I have nothing to do with thee. Ib. 85ᵇ.—[Y. B. Mets. I, end, 8ᵃ; Y. Kid. I, 60ᶜ אונו, v. אוֹנִי.] V. אוֹנָה.

אַוָנָא, אַוְוָנָא, אוּוְנָא, אַיְנָא I, m. (v. foreg. ws.; cmp. מָעוֹן, עוֹנָה, a. חוּג, חָנָה, גנן) [circle], *night-lodging*, *station* for travellers (v. Sm. Ant. s. v. Mansio). Naz. 7ᵃ כל אוו׳ וא׳ every station. B. Mets. 79ᵇ; Ab. Zar. 65ᵃ מא׳ לא׳ from station to station.—Deut. R. s. 6 she dared to bring disorder into אונא של מלך (read אוונא or אַוְונָה, v. infra) the royal head quarters. *Pl.* אַוְונָיָין, אַוְונִין. Targ. Is. X, 32 (ed. Vien. אַוְנִין). [Sabb. 157ᵇ אוונא, v. אוּדְנָא II.] [Comment. use h. forms אַוְונָה, pl. אַוְונוֹת.]

אַוָנָא II, אַוְונָא pr. n. pl. (v. foreg.) *Avana*, on the Tigris. Kid. 71ᵇ אכברא וא׳ Ar. ed. Koh (oth. ed. Ar. אכבדא); Talm. ed. בגדא ואוונא [Var. בגדת] Okhbara and Avana as bordertowns of Babylonia (v. De Sacy Chrest. Ar. I, p. 358 sq.; Koh. in Ar. s. v.).

***אונא**, נקיס א׳ pr. n. m. *Nakis Una*(?), a gentile name. Git. 11ᵃ.

אוּנָא f. (contr. of אוּדְנָא, cmp. however אֹזֶן) 1) *ear*, v. pl.—2) *handle* of a vessel. Git. 69ᵇ. Sabb. 108ᵃ top.—3) *lobe* of a lung. Ḥull. 59ᵇ; a. fr.—*Pl.* אוּנֵי. Ib. 38ᵃ אזוזי א׳ moving the ears (as a sign of life in the last stages). Yeb. 60ᵇ מפיקנא ... מאוניך we shall get R... out of thy ears, i. e. we shall make thee give up thy authority (a threat of excommunication). Gen. R. s. 45 אוניך דחמר thy ears are those of an ass.—Ḥull. 47ᵃ ח׳ אוני וכ׳ the lungs have five lobes; a. fr. [Later Rabb. literature uses אוּמָא, v. אוּם, for the large lump from which the lobes branch off.] V. אוּנִין.

אוֹנָאָה f. (ינה; cmp. חוֹנָאָה) 1) *oppression*, *wrong*. B. Mets. 58ᵇ גדולה אוֹנָאַת דברים מא׳ ממון the wrong you do by means of words (wounding one's feelings) is worse than that by pecuniary imposition. Ib. 59ᵃ לעולם יהא .... באוֹנָאַת אשתו וכ׳ one should always be on his guard not to wound his wife's feeling, for as her tears are frequent אוֹנָאָתָהּ מרובה so is her sense of wrong (sensibility) deep.—2) (law) *imposition*, *overreaching*, *fraudulent representation* (which invalidates the transaction or requires redress); hence, *redress in case of overreaching*. Y. B. Mets. IV, 9ᵈ top, a. fr. whoever concludes a bargain במנת שאין לו א׳ וכ׳ with the provision that no legal redress shall be resorted to, is notwithstanding entitled to redress.—*Denomin. Verb* (אוֹנָה), Hithpa. הִתְאוֹנָה *to be imposed upon*, *to feel one's self overreached*. Y. B. Mets. IV, 9ᵈ top. בשעה שהמוכר מִתְאוֹנֶה וכ׳ if the seller sues for undue advantage taken of him, he has the privilege of redress, provided the advantage amounts to one fifth or more of the price charged; if the buyer sues &c. [In Babli the denomin. verb is אִינָּה, v. אני.]

אוֹנָאוּתָא, v. אוֹנָאִיתָא.

אונאר, v. אוֹסָאר.

***אוֹנָאוּתָא, אוֹנָאִיתָא** f. ch.=h. אוֹנָאָה, *oppression*, *tyranny*. Targ. Ps. LXXIV, 20 (ed. Ven. אוֹנאוּתָא; h. text נָאוֹת!). V. אוֹנָיָתָא.

אונדפא, אונדפי, v. אַנְדִּיפֵי.

אוֹנָה I *to oppress*, v. אני, and אוֹנָאָה.

אוֹנָה II f. (v. אוֹן) *possession*, *title of possession*, *deed*. Gen. R. s. 79 (ref. to the letters יה in קשׂיטה Gen. XXXIII, 19) יו״ד ה״א כותב הא׳ וכ׳ *Yod He* (i. e. the Lord) writes the deed; the Lord bears witness to the deed.—*Pl.* אוֹנוֹת. B. Bath. 52ᵃ א׳ ושטרות וכ׳ deeds of purchase and other documents were issued in his name.

אוֹנוּ, v. אוֹנִי I.

אוֹנוֹ (b. h.) pr. n. pl. *Ono*, W. N. W. of Jerusalem. Cant. R. to II, 2; Lam. R. to I, 17. Snh. 11ᵇ ארש א׳ Ms. M. (ed. אוני); a. fr. V. אוֹנִי II.

אונוס, v. אוֹנִיס.

אוֹנוֹס, א׳ קְטַמִּין (v. אֲנִקְטְמִין; ὄνος) *the pulley of the crippled*. Y. Sabb. VI, 8ᶜ. (Var. הונים.).

אונטוס (ὄντως) *really! verily!* Lev. R. s. 33, explain. הצדא (Dan. III, 14); (Ar. אנטוס, some ed. אונטיס, corr. acc.); Num. R. s. 15 אנטוס (Tanh. Noah 11 האמת).

אונטלית Tosef. Kel. B. Bath. IV, 6 ed. Zuck., ed. אצטלוס, Var. אצטלי׳ prob. אִצְטְלִית q. v.

אוֹנָה, אוני, v. אוֹנָאָה.

אוֹנִי I (אונו) אונית f.=אוֹנָה, cmp. אוֹנִיתָא. [The phonetic coïncidence with ὠνή produced the peculiar use of our w. in connection with Greek terms, in the Palest. literature.] Gen. R. s. 2 beg. בא׳ אחת ובטימי וכ׳ in one bill of sale and for the same price. Y. Pes. IV, 31ᵇ bot. מיסתיוסיס בא׳ הוא וכ׳ (read מיסתוס׳) it is a lease with a title of possession (for the term), and is (for the time being) an acquisition like a purchase. Y. Kid. I, 60ᶜ (אונו a. אוני); a. e.—*Pl.* אוֹנִיוֹת. Gen. R. s. 84, end כמה א׳ וכ׳ how many deeds were written for him (how many times was he sold)?, cmp. אוֹן. [Midr. Till. to Ps. CIV, 24; Pesik. Rosh. Hash. p. 151ᵃ, v. אוֹנָה.]

אוֹנִי II בית א׳ pr. n. pl. (*Beth*) *Oni* in Palestine, prob. identic with אוֹנוֹ. Tosef. Shebi. VII, 14 פגי בית א׳ (ed. Zuckerm. בֵּיתְיָינֵי, בֵּיתְיָאנֵי, Var. ביתיני) the unripe grapes of B. O. (Beth Yanai).—Y. Git. IV, 46ᵃ א׳ אסור וכ׳ if a slave fled to Oni, he must not be extradited (because O. is a Palestinean place). V. הִינִי 3.

אוּנְיָא, אוּנְיָיא; אֲנְיָיא, אוּנְיָיא m. (prob.) *of Oni*, v. foreg., or pr. n. m. *Onya* (=Onias?). Y. Orl. I, 61[a] top; Y. Sabb. I, 3[c]; ib.[d] אניא R. Joshua Onia, an Amora.

אוּנְיאוּתָא, v. אוּנָאַתָא.

אוּנְיָה f. (=אוֹנָאָה; cmp. Ezek. XLVI, 18) prop. *oppression, wrong*, hence *confiscation, dispossession. Pl.* אוּנְיוֹת. Midr. Till. to Ps. CIV, 24 (play on *oniyoth* ibid.) אלו הא׳ וכ׳ those are the oppressive measures which they inflict upon Israel, which they order to be written out eveny day. *Pesik. R. Hash. p. 151[a]; Yalk. Jer. 312 חוֹנִיוֹת וזמיות confiscations and fines (Yalk. Gen. 121; Lev. R. s. 29, a. e. ארנוניות, v. Buber Pesik. l. c. note).

אוּנְיָיא, v. אוּנְיָא.

אוּנְיָיקִי, בית א׳ pr. n. pl. *Beth-Unyaki, Bithynia*, in Asia Minor (cmp. Neub. Géogr. pp. 262; 422). Yoma 10[a] תובל זה בית א׳ (Ms. M. אונקר indistinct; oth. Var., v. Rabb. D. S. a. l. note) *Tubal* means B. Ab. Zar. II, 4 (29[b]) cheese of בית א׳ (Ms. M. אונקר, אוניקר, Mish. Nap. ותינייקי, v. Rabb. D. S. a. l.). Tosef. Shebi. V, 9 הוניקי (ed. Zuck. גבינת ב׳ ה׳ read גבינה ובית הוניקי); Tosef. Ab. Zar. IV, 13 בית הוניקי (Var. הוניקאי). Cmp. אַנְיָקָא a. וְתַנְיָה.

***אוּנִין** m. pl. (prob. pl. of אוּנָא *ear*) *bundles of wet flax*. Sabb. I, 6. Y. Shebi. V, 36[a] bot.; a. e. [Rashi a. Tosaf. to Succ. 12[b] אונץ as a plur., v. Rabb. D. S. a. l.; cmp. אָנִיץ.]

אוּנִיס (אונוס) m. (אנס) *tyrannus, lord, ruler*. Targ. Y. Ex. II, 16; XVIII, 1.

אוּנִיתָא f. ch.=h. אוֹנָה *title of possession, deed*. Y. Taan. IV, 69[a] וחוו משלחין א׳ וכ׳ they would send the (forged) deed of sale to the steward; Lam. R. to II, 2 (corr. acc.).

אוֹנָיְתָא or **אוֹנִיתָא** f. ch.=h. אוֹנָאָה *oppression, wrong*. B. Bath. 22[a] א׳ דמלכא וכ׳ the wrong inflicted on the king of Edom. Lev. R. s. 33, beg. (ref. to Amos VII, 7, v. אֲנָךְ I) על שורא דא׳ upon the wall of (i. e. watching over) the wrongs (in sale and purchase); cmp. B. Mets. 59[a].

***אוּנְכִּין** read קוּנְכִּין m. pl. (κόγχη, concha) *purple shells*. Targ. Y. Num. XXXIII, 8; cmp. קוֹנְכָּר.

אונכלי Tosef. Shebu. VI, 4 ed. Zuck., v. אַמְפְּלֵי.

אֲוַנְכְּרֵי, אֲוַנְכְּרֵי m. pl. (prob. a nom. gentil., from a trading station named אונכר, a compound of אוונא [a. אַכָּר?]; cmp. אֲוָנָא) *Avankreans* (?), *traders*. Succ. 30[b]. [Ar. identifies our w. with אַבְנְגָּר which is not in agreement with the context.]

אוּנֵן, v. אָנַן.

אונכא Deut. R. s. 6, read אֲוָנָא.

אונכיות Lev. R. s. 23, v. אֲוֹנָא.

אוֹנֶס m. (אָנַס) *compulsion, force; unavoidable interference, accident*. Git. 30[a], a. e. אין א׳ בגיטין the plea of unavoidable interference cannot be raised in letters of divorce (to which a condition is attached). Y. M. Kat. III, 81[d] bot., a. e. מחמת אוֹנְסוֹ through no fault of his. —*Pl.* אוֹנָסִין, אוֹנָסִים. Ned. III, 1, a. e. נדרי א׳ vows on conditions unavoidably unfulfilled.

אוֹנֶס m. ch. (v. foreg.) *wrong, oppression*. Targ. Is. LVIII, 9; 13 מלין דא׳ offensive (violent) words (h. text אָוֶן, cmp. אוֹנָאָה).

אוּנְסָא m. ch. (=h. אוֹנֶס, v. foreg.) *force, wrong, robbery; accident*. Targ. Y. Gen. XXXI, 12; a. fr.— Git. 34[a]. אי משום א׳ shall we take into consideration the possibility of an unavoidable accident?—*Pl.* אוּנְסַיָּא. Ned. 27[b] א׳ דמיגלרא (read דמיגליר, Rashi אונסא) accidents which may be foreseen.

אוּנְסָא m., pl. אוּנְסִין=אֲנוּסָא.

***אונסין**, פרק א׳ a corrupt. of פְּרוֹקוֹנֵיסוֹס pr. n. pl. *Proconnesus*, in Mysia, renowned for its marble. Esth. R. to I, 6.

אַנְפִּיל, אוּנְפִּיל m. (נפל) *a wooden vessel for the reception of refuse, remnants of victuals* &c. Tosef. Kel. B. Mets. V, 10. Cmp. next w.

אוּנְפְּלִי, אוּנְפְּלָא, v. אַמְפְּלֵי.

אוּנְקָא I עוּנְקָא m. (ענק) *neck, meat from the neck*. Sabb. 140[b] א׳ ed. (Ar. ע׳; Ms. M. עוזקא). Ber. 44[b] ע׳ ed. (Ms. M. א׳).

אוּנְקָא II m. *hook*, v. אוּנְקִי a. אוּנְקְלִי.

אוּנְקוּלִין, v. אוּנְקְלִי.

אונקוס m. (ὄγκος) 1) *bulk, pile;* (in philosophy) *a primitive body*. Tanh. T'rum. 11 א׳ של מים the body of water; א׳ של אש (some ed. אונקוס). 2) *trouble, difficulty, painstaking*. Gen. R. s. 12 (ref. to Neh. IX, 6 sq.) כל הא׳ הזה וכ׳ (ed. אונקים, corr. acc.) what is all this painstaking (creating the universe &c.) for? Ans. Because 'thou art the Lord who hast chosen Abraham' i. e. for the sake of establishing religion on earth; cmp. Midr. Till. to Ps. CIV, 18.

אוּנְקִי, אוּנְקָא f. (v. אוּנְקָא I, a. אוּנְקְלִי I) 1) *neck-shaped, hook, grapple.—Pl.* אוּנְקִיּוֹת (אוּנְקָאוֹת). Kel. XII, 2 (Var. in Mish. ed. אוּנְקְלִיּוֹת). Tosef. ib. B. Mets. II, 4 (disting. from אוּנְקְלָאוֹת).—[2) for אונקיא, v. next w.]

אוּנְקְיָא f. (uncia, οὐγκία) 1) *ounce*, one twelfth of a litra. Gen. R. s. 17 א׳ של כסף an ounce of silver. Lam. R. to I, 1 נסבון מן אונקא (הדיר) (corr. acc.) they bought ounce-wise (pepper).—2) trnsf. *a trifle, particle*. Y. Taan. IV, 68[c] top there is not a generation in which there is not (to be atoned for through suffering) אונקי אחת וכ׳ (read אונקיא אחת) a particle of the sin of the calf-worship. Ex. R. s. 43, beg. אוקיא (corr. acc.). Gen. R. s. 29; Yalk. Gen. 47; Job. 908 (play on אי נקי Job. XXII, 30) א׳ אחת היתה וכ׳ only an ounce (of merit) did Noah possess; v. ארנוניתא.—*Pl.* אוּנְקִיּוֹת. Gen. R. s. 79, end (play on the letters of קְשִׂיטָה Gen. XXXIII, 19) בְּמֵאָה אוּנְקִיּוֹת .. סְלָעִים .. טְלָאִים, for one hundred (ק) ounces (of gold) &c. V. אוּקְיָא.

אונקיינוס, v. אוֹקְיָינוֹס.

אונקילוסיא, v. אַנְקְלָסְיָא.

אונקים, v. אוּנְקוֹס.

אוּנְקַל, v. אוּנְקְלֵי II.

אוּנְקְלָא ch.=h. אוּנְקְלֵי I, *hook*, &c. Targ. Job. XL, 26.—*Pl.* אוּנְקְלִין. Targ. Y. Ex. XXVII, 10. Lev. (ed. ווי). Targ. Ez. XL, 43 עוּנְקְלִין (עֲנִקְלִין).—Fem. pl. אוּנְקְלָוָון. Targ. Y. Lev. X, 5. Targ. Esth. I, 6.—Targ. Y. II Ex. XXVI, 37 אַנְקְלָוָותְהוֹן their hooks.

אוּנְקְלָאוֹת plur. of אוּנְקְלֵי I.

אוּנְקְלָה, v. אוּנְקְלֵי II.

אַנְקְלוֹס, אוּנְקְלוֹס pr. n. m. (Ocellus?) *Onk'los*, the alleged translator of the Pentateuch into Chaldaic, freq. surnamed הַגֵּר the proselyte; often identified with ***Aquila***, the alleged author of a Greek translation of the Bible; v. עֲקִילַס. Cmp. Meg. 3ª; Ab. Zar. 11ª, with Tanh. Mishp. 5. Cant. R. to I, 11 אלקולאון q. v.

אונקלוסיא, v. אַנְקְלָסְיָא.

אוּנְקְלֵי I, אַנְקְלֵי f. (אנק, with ל format.;=אוּנְקֵי; corresp. to b. h. לוּלֵי; Greek adapt. ἀγκολη, LXX Ex. XXVI, 10; cmp. אוּנִי as to contact of the two languages) prop. *little* (*camel's*) *neck*, hence 1) *hook*, *rack*. Kel. XII, 2 א׳ של כתפין Ar. (ed. אונקליות; אונקלין with adject. in the sing., corr. acc.) the carriers' hook attached to their yoke, pole &c. Ib. א׳ של דרגש the hook of the bedstead (used for fastening the girths to the posts); של נקליטין the rack of the bed-curtain, v. נַקְלִיטִין. Ib. 3 א׳ שבכותלים hook attached to walls.—T'bul Yom IV, 6 ואנ׳ שלחם קיימת and the hook (attached to the now broken yoke) remained unimpaired; a. fr.—*Pl.* אוּנְקְלָאוֹת, אֻנְקְ׳, אוּנְקְלִיּוֹת (אונקלין). Tam. III, 5; Mid. III, 5; a. fr.—Kel. l. c.; Tosef. ib. B. Mets. II, 4; v. אוּנְקֵי.—2) [cmp. ἀγκαλίς in S.] *the load carried on the hook*, *the farmer's load of sheaves or bunches*; cmp. בלונקר. Tosef. Maas. Sh. IV, 10. כל הא׳ the whole load. [Ib. 11 אונקלי, אונקולין, read with ed. Zuck. ארנפולי].—3) Trnsf. (medic.) *bent cartilage*, esp. *the cartilage* (cart. ensiformis) *at the end of the sternum which, being bent inside, presses on the stomach and creates nausea* &c. Ab. Zar. 29ª מצלין א׳ וכ׳ you are permitted to lift the cartilage on the Sabbath (by means of a bandage &c.). Ib. מאי א׳ וכ׳ what *unklay* is meant? Ans. the cartilage in front of the heart; v. אִיסְתּוֹמְכָא.

אוּנְקְלֵי II, אוּנְקַל, נַקְלָה, נִיקְלֵי f. (קל, נקל, cmp. esp. II Sam. VI, 20 to 22) *the light garment*, whence, a name for the *easy dress* worn in the house and, under the cloak, in the street, but in which it was unbecoming to appear in public. [Cmp. II Sam. l. c. a. Num. R. s. 4; a. e.] Y. Yoma VI, 43ᵈ top נקלה, אוּנְקְלָה, for which Men. 109ᵇ אונקלי. Snh. 82ª he took off the point of his spear והניחה באונקלו (some ed. לי—) and put it (hiding it) in his undergarment. M. Kat. 24ª אָבֵל מטייל בא׳ וכ׳ (Ms. M. מטייל אָבֵל) a mourner may walk on the Sabbath within the limits of his house (garden &c.) in the easy dress (showing the rent on account of a death in the family; Rashi). Sabb. 120ª (garments to be saved from fire on a Sabbath) אונקלי; Y. ib. XVI, 15ᵈ top ניקלי.—Meg. IV, 8 (24ᵇ) בית א׳; (read as) Y. ib. a. Mss. בית יד א׳ the sleeve of his under-dress. [Tosef. Maas. Sh. IV, 11, v. foreg. 2.]

אונקלמוס, v. אִרְקוּמוּס.

אונקלסיא, v. אַנְקְלָסְיָא.

אוס Ar. ed. pr., Ms. אוּם q. v.

אוּסָאֵי m. pl., prob. מוּסָאֵי, name of a tribe. Targ. Ps. CXX, 5, v. אוסיא (some ed. אונאי).

אוסטולין Midr. Sam. ch. XI, v. אִסְטְלֵי.

אֻוסְיָא, אֻוסֵי (or אוּ׳) m. pl. (√אף soft. into או; cmp. אַף, אֲנַף; also אֶפֶס) *nose, nostrils*. Sabb. 67ª ואאוסי דגוריתא and on the nostrils of the young lioness. B. Bath. 73ᵇ דסליק עליה באוסיה אכלה טינא ומית Ms. R. (ed. דיתבא ליה אכלה טינא באוס׳, Ms. M. אבלה, Ar. ed. Koh. incorr., v. Rabb. D. S. a. l.) into whose nostrils a 'mud-eater' (worm) entered, and the fish died. Pes. 112ª ידא אאוסיא וכ׳ (Ms. M. a. Ar. אפנא) putting the hand to the nose is a step to fear (indicating anxiety). Hull. 67ᵇ ועיילי באוסייה and they (the worms) creep into its nostrils.

אוסי, v. אוּסְיָא.

אוסיא Pes. 111ª, v. אסיא.

אוסיא Targ. I Chr. Chr. I, 5; a. e. read with ed. Rahmer מוּסְיָא; cmp. Yoma 10ª; Y. Meg. I, 71ᵇ bot. (h. text מֶשֶׁךְ). [Targ. Y. II Gen. X, 2 אנסייא; Gen. R. s. 37 אוסנא (misplaced); corr. acc.]

אוּסְיָא f. a. *certain portion of meat*, v. אוּזְיָא.

אוּסְיָא (אוסי) f. (οὐσία) *substance*, (landed) *property, farm, estate*. Gen. R. s. 49 אוסי (corr. acc.).—Num. R. s. 23 שפחות מן א׳ וכ׳ maid-servants from another estate. Y. Taan. IV, 69ª; Lam. R. to II, 2 א׳ (corr. acc.). Lev. R. s. 34.—*Pl.* אוּסִיּוֹת. Ex. R. s. 20. Ch. pl. אוּסְיָאן, אוּסְיָיאן. Lev. R. s. 3, beg. he likes to be called מרי אס׳ (corr. acc.) lord of many estates; Koh. R. to IV, 6 אוסייאס (corr. acc.).

אוסיניסי Y. Ab. Zar. V, end, 45ᵇ דא׳, read דאניסטיסי, v. דְּנִיסְטֵיס.

אוסיתא Gen. R. s. 14, end, Ar. ed. pr., read אופיתא.

אוסכולי, v. אִיסְכּ׳.

אוּסְמָנָא m., pl. **אוּסְמָנַיָּא** (חָסַם=אסם II) [the glistening.] surname of an Egyptian tribe. Targ. Ps. LXVIII, 32 (Var. חוּסְמְנַיָּא, a. אוּכְמָנָא *the dark.*). Cmp. LXX χασμωνιειμ, for כסלחים; Gen. X, 14; v. Fürst. H. Dict. s. v. כסלח; Ges. H. Dict. s. v. חשם.

אוּסְנָא, v. אָסְנָא.

אוֹסֶף m. (b. h. אֹסֶף, אסף) *gathering in.* Snh. 94^b, v. חֲסִיל.

אוּסְפְּלִידָא, v. אִסְפְּלִידָא.

אוּסְקַנִּיתָא, סְקוּנִיתָא f. (נסק; cmp. מַסְקָנָא) *ascending, landing.* גמלא דא׳ *landing board.* Snh. 67^b וקם אג׳ דא׳ Ar. (ed. וקם ג׳ דוסקי׳ read with Rashi דסקי׳, Ms. M. אוסקניתא, oth. var. v. Rabb. D. S. a. l.) and he found himself standing on a landing board (ed. and there stood before him &c.).

אוּף I (=אַף) *too, also.* (Yer. Dial.). Targ. Y. Num. XVI, 13; a. fr.—Y. Dem. I, beg. 21^c א׳ הכא here too.

אוּף II m. *nature*, v. אוֹפִי.

אוּפֵי, אוּפְיֵי f. pl. (=כָּפִּי Dan. IV, 9; cmp. b. h. עָנָף, a. אִיבָּא, אִנְבָּא) *branches*, esp. *dry twigs, spray-wood.* Ber. 44^b א׳ פרסייתא twigs of Persian trees. Hull. 105^a פכבא דא׳ Ar. (ed. אופיי) a bundle of twigs. B. Mets. 30^b. Git. 61^a שדר אופיי (Ar. אופי) threw twigs down (which he cut off), and dates fell off (v. Tossaf. a. l.).

אוֹפִי f. (אוֹף m.) (b. h. אַפַּיִם; v. אַפָּא; cmp. אוּף I) *face, looks*, whence, *nature, disposition, ways* &c. Y. Shek. I, 45^d אין אתה יכול לעמוד על א׳ של וכ׳ You cannot understand the nature of that people. Lev. R. s. 30 אופו של דוד Ar. ed. Koh. (ed. pr. איפי, ed. אפו) David's ways. Y'lamd. Vaëthh. (quot. in Ar.) 'who is that nation' שהיא יודעת אופו של אלוהיה Ar. ed. Koh. (oth. ed. אופי) that knows the ways of her God (what he desires &c.); v. Yalk. Deut. 825.—Gen. R. s. 14 end נשמה זו הא׳ *n'shamah* (breath, soul) means the disposition, character, as people say חאופיתא טבא the good nature!

אוּפְיָא (חוּפְיָא) f. (אוף; v. אנף; b. h. אָפַע) *what is blown off, foam, froth.* Ab. Zara 26^a כי א׳ דימא Ms. M. (ed. דנהרא, v. Rabb. D. S. a. l., a. Ar. ed. Koh. s. v. אפי) as the foam of the Sea [river]; (Ar. *as logs on the river*, v. אוּפְתָּא, אוֹפִי). Ib. 70^b חזית נקיטנא א׳ (Var. חופיא, ח׳, v. Rabb. D. S. a. l. note 20) she took the froth off. Hull. 105^b א׳ (Ar. ח׳).

***אוֹפְיוֹן** m. (ὄπιον) *poppy-juice, opium.* Y. Ab. Zar. II, 40^d top אחן א׳ סכנה an opium drink (prepared by a gentile) is dangerous.

אוּפִיטָא, v. אַנְטִיפִיטָא.

אוּפְיֵי *twigs*, v. אוֹפִי.

אוּפִיכָא (אוּפְכָּרְיָא f.) (אפך) *destruction, ruin* Lam. R. to III, 13 (expl. בני אשפתו ibid., v. אַשְׁפָּה) בני אופיכיה (Var. אוּפְכָּרִיה) the children of those he laid in ruins; v. אִימְרִיָּא. [Differ. in Esth. R. to I, 1^b, v. אוּפְרִיפָא a. אֲמוֹרְיָא.]

אופילין Tosef. Ter. II, 4, v. אֲפִילִים.

***אופימשט׳, אופימטטאמא**, read אוּפוֹמְנִימָאטָא m. pl. (ὑπομνήματα) *public records, acts.* Ex. R. s. 28 a king wanted לעשות א׳ חוץ וכ׳ to pass acts without consulting the lieutenant-governor (hyparch).

אוֹפִיקִילִין m. pl. (officialis, ὀφφικιάλιος) *subordinate officials, constables.* Y'lamd. Balak (quot. in Ar. s. v. בלש) א׳ ed. Koh. Ib. שלח אפיקלין (corr. acc.) he sent constables (for her son).

אוֹפִיתָא f. ch. (=h. אוֹפִי) *nature, disposition.* Gen. R. s. 14, end, v. אוֹפִי.

אופכי, אופכין, v. אַפּוּכִי.

אוֹפֶל m. (b. h. אֹפֶל) *darkness.* Gen. R. s. 89, beg. v. אֲפֵילָה.

אוֹפָן m. (b. h.; אפן, $\sqrt{}$ פן, v. פנה) 1) *wheel.*—2) (with ref. to Ezek. I, 15) pr. n. *Ofan*, name of an angel. Hag. 13^b.—*Pl.* אוֹפַנִּים. Ib. 12^b. R. Hash. 24^b.—[In liturgic literature אופנים and איפן are used as the names of a section of the morning prayers; v. אוֹפַנָּא.]

אוֹפֶן m. (b. h. אֹפֶן; v. foreg.) *turn, method, plan.* [In later Hebr.: *method of interpretation*=פָּנִים.]—*Pl.* אוֹפָנִים; *Du.* אוֹפְנַיִם. Ruth. R. s. 2, beg. You will soon find out אופניים שלחם וכ׳ (Yalk. Josh. 7 אופנים) their plans (strategic movements). Ab. d'R. Nath. (ed. Taussig, N'veh Shal. p. 12) על אופניו in its proper way.

אוֹפַנָּא ch.=h. אוֹפָן.—*Pl.* אוֹפַנַּיָּא. Targ. Ezek. X, 13. —אוֹפַנַּיָּה *that section of the morning prayers beginning with v'hāofannim* and describing the angelic praises. Y. Ber. V, 9^c bot.

אוֹפְנָא ch.=אוֹפֶן. *turn, interpretation, qualification.* Y. Dem. VI: 25^b bot. א׳ לית לון א׳ לית לסתמא we do not recognize an interpretation (of an agreement, so as to say, נעשה כאומר וכ׳ 'it means as though they had said—'); no qualification is admissible for an unqualified agreement.

אוּפְסַיִם m. du. (cmp. אֶפֶס—, a. פַּס, פִּסָּה) *palms of the hand.* Mekh. B'shall. Vayissa, s. 3, to Ex. XVI, 12 the Mannah came down על האו׳ וכ׳ on the hands of the Lord, as if it were to say, the Lord held forth &c. [In some ed. אוּפְסִין.]

אוּפְסִין m. pl., v. foreg.

אופסנון, v. אַפְסוּנִין.

אוּפְתָּא f. (v. אוֹפִי) prop. *the large central branch*, hence *trunk, stalk.* Succ. 32^a ואימא א׳ may I not say (as you insist on the palm-branch being *kafuth*, tied, joined) that I must use the stalk?—Hull. 47^b lungs resembling לא׳ a trunk (in color, touch &c.). Ib. 16^a וי״ו דכתיב אא׳ a Vav written on a trunk (being broken on account of the rough surface=*idle-talk*).

אוּפְתִּיק, אוּפְתֵּק=חֲפִתִּק.

אוּץ (b. h.; √אוּ, v. אוּר I; cmp. אָפַץ; v. חוּץ a. חָצָה) *to be pressed* (*to press, hurry*).—Part. אוֹצֵה, pl. אוֹצִין (as from אצה, v. חוּץ, חוּל) *squeezed in*. Tosef. Kel. B. Mets. IX, 5 א׳ חבור (Var. חוּצִין) when they are squeezed in (tight), they are considered as connected for levitical purposes.

אוּצְבַּתָא, v. אֶצְבְּעָא a. אֶצְבַּע.

אוּצְיָא, v. אֶצְיָא.

אוּצְטוּלִין read אִיצְטוֹלִין, v. אִסְטְלָא.

אוּצֶן, v. חוּצָן.

אוֹצָר m. (b. h.; אצר) *store-house, magazine; provision; hoarded up treasure*. B. Bath 58[a]; Git. 67[a], v. בָּלָם a. בֶּלֶם. Ab. Zar. 40[b]; v. חֲפַתִּק; a. fr.—Esp. *treasury, the* (*Roman*) *government's treasury department* where taxes in kind and money had to be paid. Y. Dem. VI, end, 26[a] ושקול על ידי לא׳ and pay for me in the treasury-department. Tosef. Dem. VI, 4 ושקול תחהיר מן הא׳ (read אל הא׳). Ib. 8 ושוקל לא׳ ed. Zuck. (ed. incorr. ואוצר). Ib. 4 פוטרינר מן הא׳ get me a release from the treasury-dep. —Y. Dem. l. c. פרשינר מן הא׳ (read פוטריני). Ab. Zar. 71[a] מן הא׳, לא׳, Ms. M. (ed. עוצר); cmp. אָצַר.—*Pl.* אוֹצָרוֹת. B. Bath. 11[a] גנזו א׳ Ms. (ed. א׳ omitted); v. גָּנַז.—Hag. 12[b] אוֹצָרוֹת שלג וכ׳ the stores of snow &c. (in the heavens); a. fr. V. א׳ רוח, אֹצָרוֹת.

אוֹצְרָא ch. same. Targ. Jerem. XXXVIII, 11; a. fr.—*Pl.* אוֹצְרִין, אוֹצְרַיָּא. Targ. Gen. XLI, 56; a. e.

אוּקוּמִינִי, v. אִיקוּמֵינִי.

אוּקוּנִים read אִיקוֹנִין, v. אִיקוֹן.

אוּקְטוֹרְיָא, אוּקְטֹר׳, v. אַקְט׳.

אוּקִי=אוֹקִים, v. קוּם.

אוּקְ, v. אוּקִיי.

***אוּקְיָא** f.=אוּנְקְיָא [?] Ex. R. s. 43, beg.—[*Pl.* אוּקִיֵּי. Ber. 44[b] משיתא א׳ סולתא, Ar. s. v. גלגל I, 'than six ounces of fine flour'.—Ed. קייסי; Ms. M. omits the entire sentence.]

אוּקְיָאנוֹס, v. אוֹקְיָינוֹס.

***אוּקִיי** (Muss. אוּקִי) Cant. R. to VII, 8, read אוֹקְיָינוֹס. כמין א׳ inundating like an Ocean tide; v. טִלְנִס.

אוֹקְיָאנוֹס, אוֹקְיָנוֹס, אוֹקְיָינוֹס m. (Ὠκέανος) *Ocean*, mostly *Mediterranean Sea*. Targ. Y. Gen. I, 7; a. e.—Y. Hall. IV, 60[a] bot.; a. fr.—Tanh. Haye 3, and so is א׳ ים המת the Okeanos called the Sea of (covering) the dead. [Var. אוקי׳, אנק׳.]

אוֹקִים Af. of קוּם ch.

אוֹקִימוּתָא f. (קוּם) *raising*, [*rising*]. Targ. Ps. CXXXIX, 2 [prob. אוֹקָמוּתָא].

אוּקִינִין, read אִיקוֹנִין.

אוּקְצָא, v. עוּקְצָא.

אוּר I (b. h.; √אוּ, v. אוּר II; cmp. חָבַר, חוּר, a. sec. r. אָרַר) *to perforate, break through, shine*.—Denom. אָיִר, מְאוּרָה &c.

Nif. נֵאוֹר *to be broken through, grow light*. Y. Ber. I, 2[c] משיאור המזרח from the time the Eastern horizon is broken through, grows light.

Hif. הֵאִיר 1) (neut. v.) *to break through, shine*. Y. ib. III, 6[c] bot. open thy lips וְיָאִירוּ דבריך and let thy words come forth, speak out boldly. Yoma III, 1 ה׳ פני כל וכ׳ it has grown light all over the Eastern horizon.—פנים מְאִירוֹת *bright countenance*. Num. R. s. 11; a. e.—2) (act. v.) *to enlighten, brighten, make shine*. Y. M. Kat. III, 83[b] ה׳ עיניו וכ׳ (the teacher had opened his (Samuel's) eyes &c. B. Mets. 33[a]. Num. R. l. c. Ib. מְאִירִים את המזבח (fr. Mal. I, 10) making the altar bright (with fire), feeding the fire on the altar. Yoma 73[b], v. אוּר.

אוּר ch. same. Part. pass. נְאוֹר *clear*. Targ. Prov. IV, 25 נְאָרָן, נְאוֹרָן, v. חֲוַר.

אוֹר II m. (b. h.; foreg.) *breaking forth* (cmp. Is. LVIII, 8) whence 1) *break of day, light, day; fire*; trnsf. *rise, glory, power, happiness*. Ber. 2[b] ביאת אורו the entrance of his day-break (dawn of his eighth day; Tosaf. a. l. *the sunset* of his seventh day). Y. Pes. I, beg. 27[a] א׳ החמה sun-light. Ib. א׳ הנר candle light. Keth. 111[b] א׳ תורה light of the Law. B. Bath. 4[a] אורו של עולם intellectual light of the wold (a great man; the Law). Num. R. s. 15 אור של מעלן the celestial fire (believed to be the source of all light and fire); a. v. fr. 2) (breaking in of night) *twilight, evening*. Pes. I, 1 א׳ לארבעה וכ׳ on the evening (eve) of the fourteenth day of Nissan; v. discussion ibid. 2[a] sq., about the meaning of our w. R. Hash. 22[b]; Snh. 70[b] לא׳ עיבורו the evening following the eventual intercalation, i. e. the evening from the thirtieth of the past to the first of the beginning month.—3) (homil.=אוֹרָה II) *rue*. Gen. R. s. 20 in the Pentat. of R. M. it read כתנות אור וכ׳ (in place of עור Gen. III, 21) this alludes to the garments of Adam resembling the rue, wide below and narrow above; Ar. (Rashi diff.).

אוּר I m. (b. h.; foreg.) prop. *light, flame*; esp. *Pl.* אוּרִים ותומים *the Urim and Tummim* in the High-priest's breast-plate. Yoma 73[b] א׳ שמאירים את דבריהם they are called *Urim* because they give their decisions in a clear way (not ambiguous as the oracles); cmp. Y. ib. VII, end, 44[c]. Sot. IX, 12. Y. Kid. IV, beg. 65[b].

***אוּר II** m. (=עוּר q. v.) *chaff*. Y. Ab. Zar. II. 40[d] א׳ דשערין chaff of barley; (Y. Sabb. XIV, 14[d] עור דסערין).

אוּרָא I ch.=אוּר, *Pl.* אוּרַיָּא *the Urim*. Targ. Num. XXVII, 21; a. e.

***אוּרָא II** m. (h. עוֹר) *skin*. Y. Ned. III beg. 37[d] אוריה (read אוּדְרֵיהּ?, v. אֶדֶר I); v. however Y. Shebu. III, 34[d].

אוֹרָאָה f. ch.=הוֹרָאָה *teaching, decision.* Targ. Ez. VII, 26; a. e.

אוּרְבָּא, אַרְבָּא m. (ערב, ארב *to braid, interlace* &c.); pl. אוּרְבֵּי, אַרְבֵּי *meshes, void spaces, intervals.* Sabb. 50[b] בִּינֵי אוּ׳ ed. (Ar. ארבי, Var. אַרְבֵּי, v. אַרְבָּא I; אדבי, v. Ar. ed. Koh. s. v. ארבי, note) between the meshes or void spaces between the bricks. Git. 69[b]. B. Bath. 3[a] (Ms. ירבי, oth. Var. v. Rabb. D. S. a. l. note).

אוּרְבִּינָא m. (ארב, v. foreg., cmp. סבך, סכך) *brier, nettle* or a similar plant (corresp. to h. סרפד). Targ. II, Esth. II, 7 (Ar. ארבנא).

אוּרְבָּנָא, pl. אוּרְבָּנֵי m. (v. foreg.; cmp. עֲרָבָה) *bulrushes.* Sabb. 101[a] קְנֵי ואו׳ (some ed. ואר׳) reeds and bulrushes. Snh. 82[b] בֵּין קְנֵי לְאו׳ וכ׳ what has Sh'vilnai (a woman) to do between the reeds and the bulrushes? (prov. for suspicious movements of women). B. Bath. 6[a], v. צְרִיפָא.

***אוּרְבָּנִין** m. pl. (v. foreg.) name of a *seasoning reed.* Erub. 34[b].

אורדי Kid. 12[a], זוודא דא׳, read דאוּדְּרֵי or דאוּדְרֵי, v. אוּדְרָא.

***אוּרְדְּיָא,** Keth. 67[a] שַׁקֵי דא׳ (Ms. אדוריא, ed. רוּדְיָא) prob. pr. n. pl. *Urdaya, Rodaya,* [or identical with foreg. w.?].

אוּרְדִּילָאֵי, v. אַרְדִּילָיָא.

***אוּרְדְּךָ** m. (=אוּדְּךָ, דוך) *crushing tool, pestle.* Targ. Prov. XXVII, 22 some ed. (oth. אוּרְדְּךָ q. v.). [The entire verse is corrupted, combining the traditional vers. with one from which LXX is translated.]

אוּרְדְּעָה f. (v. עוּרְדְּעָן, and its hebr. phonet. equival. צְפַרְדֵּעַ) *frog.* Koh. R. to V, 8. Lev. R. s. 22 (אוּרְדְּעָן fem.).

אורדען, v. foreg.

אוּרְדְּעָנָה f. (v. foreg.) *a disease of the tongue, rana (frog).* Y. Sabb. XIV, 14[d] top.

אוֹרָה I f. (b. h.=אוֹר) *light, sun.* Y. Pes. II, 29[a] כְּאוֹרָה כא׳ clear as the sun. Zeb. 19[b], a. e. לא׳ *at daybreak.* Gen. R. s. 3 beg.; a. fr.—Chald. Adv. לְבָאוֹרָה *at first sight, apparently.* Keth. 54[a] לבא׳ כשמואל רהיטא apparently it would run (agree) with Samuel, כִּי מְעַיְּינַתְּ וכ׳ but when you consider &c.

אוֹרָה II f.; pl. אוֹרוֹת (b. h. אֹרֹת, II Kings IV, 39; prob. fr. אָרָה) *herbs,* esp. *rocket.* Yoma 18[b], expl. גַּרְגִּיר (etymol. שמאירות וכ׳; cmp. Plin. XX, 13 quot. in Löw Aram. Pfl. p. 93). [Gen. R. s. 20 אוֹר *rue;* v. אוֹר II, 3.]

אוֹרֶה part. of אָרָה, v. ארי.

אוֹרוורין, v. אוֹרְדִּיר.

אוֹרוֹת, v. אוֹרָיָא II a. אָרָה.

אוֹרְוָותָא, v. אוֹרָיָא II ch., a. אֵוֶר I.

אורולוגין, v. אוֹרְלוֹגִין.

***אורוסטי,** a corrupt., prob. רוֹסָאטוֹן, m. (ῥοσᾶτον, rosatum) *vin-aux-roses, rose-wine.* Y. Shebi. VII, beg. 37[b] א׳ שרי (Mas. אירויסטו) rose-wine is permitted in the Sabbath year.

אורורין, v. אוֹרְדִּיר.

אוֹרֶז m. (cmp. ὄρυζα, b. h. r. ארז *to be hard*) *rice.* Ber. 37[a]; a. fr.—Pes. 35[a] (opinions as to its classification with ref. to Passover laws). Cmp. אֶרֶז.

אוֹרִיזָא, אַרוּזָא, אוֹרְזָא ch. same. Targ. Y. Num. XV, 19 אוּרז׳.—Y. Sabb. III, 6[b] top אורז׳. Pes. 50[b] ארז׳ (Ms. M. אורז; ib. 51[a] top ארזא, corr. acc.). Ib. 114[b] ארוזא.

אוּרְזִילָא, אוּרְזְלָא m. (אזל with anorg. ר; Syr. עוזלא) 1) *a slender young animal,* esp. *the young of the gazelle* or any similar animal (Reëm). Targ. Cant. II, 9 א׳ דאיילא (h. text עֹפֶר). Zeb. 113[b] א׳ דרימא בת יומא (read בר); B. Bath. 73[b] (corr. as Zeb. l. c.; v. Rabb. D. S. a. l. note) a young antilope one day old. Num. R. s. 11; Cant. R. to II, 9; Pesik. R. s. 15 א׳ דאיילתא (עוּרְזִילְיהוֹן וכ׳ pl.) young deer.—*Pl.* אוּרְזִילִין, אוּר׳, אַרְזִלֵי. Targ. Cant. IV, 5; VII, 4. B. Bath. 74[b] ארזלי דימא (Ms. M. אידלי) sea-gazelles.—[2) *hammock,* v. אַרְזִלָא.]

אוּרְזָנִייָא, אוּרְזָנָיָה m. pl. (אורזא) *a rice dish* (prepared with wine). [Oth. opin. *cedar-fruits; millet.*] Y. Maas. Sh. II, beg. 53[b]. Y. Yoma VIII, 45[a] top; Y. Shebu. III, 34[b] bot. אורזריה (corr. acc.).

אוֹרֵחַ, אוֹרַח m. (b. h. אֹרֵחַ; ארח) *wayfarer,* esp. *guest.* Ber. 58[a]; a. fr.—Euphem. *menstruation.* Nid. 16[a] (cmp. Gen. XVIII, 11 *oraḥ*). Lev. R. s. 4.—*Pl.* אוֹרְחִים, אוֹרְחִין.—הכנסת א׳ the invitation of guests, *hospitality.* Sabb. 127[a]; a. fr.

אוֹרַח, אוֹרְחָא, אָרְחָא c.=h. אֹרַח, *road, path, way.* Targ. Jud. V, 6; a. fr.—א׳ ארעא (h. דרך ארץ) *custom.* Ab. Zar. 2[b]; a. fr.—א׳ דמילתא a usual incident. Git. 29[a]; a. fr.—אגב אורחיה, אגב אורחך &c. on thy road (his road &c.), i. e. *by the way, occasionally, incidentally.* Ber. 2[a]. Snh. 95[b]; a. fr.—Gen. R. s. 100 על א׳ for the journey (death). Targ. Y. II, Gen. XXXV, 9 ארחא דעלמא the way of the world (death).—*Pl.* אָרְחָתָא, אוֹרְחָן, אָרְחָן. Targ. Jud. l. c. Targ. Y. II Gen. XLIX, 17; a. e.—Snh. 109[a] יהביה אוֹרְחָתָה לְגַנָּבַיָּה (missing in Ms. M., v. Rabb. D. S. a. l. note) thou hast shown the thieves the ways (of stealing).—[אוֹרְחָא, אָרְחָא *guest,* v. אָרְחָא.]

אוּרִי pr. n. m. (b. h.) *Uri,* an Amora. Y. Ber. II, beg. 4[a] ר׳ חונה ר׳ א׳ R. Huna in the name of R. U.

אוֹרִי Af. of ירי.

אוֹרָיָא *teaching,* v. אוֹרָיְיָא.

אוּרְיָא, אוּרְיָה I, אוּרִית f. (v. אוּר a. אוּרְתָא) *evening horizon, Sun-set, West,* v. מערבא. B. Bath. 25ᵃ מאי אוריה ed. (Ar. אוריא) why is it called *Urya?* אויר יה (Var. אור) divine air (divine light=Palestine). Kid. 12ᵇ הא איכא סהדי באוריא Ar. (ed. אדידית, emend. in Tossaf. אורית), [read with ב"ח: הא אמרי איכא וכ׳] but people say, there are witnesses in the West &c. Cmp. אֶסְתָּן.

אוּרְיָא, אוּרְיָה II, אוּרִייָא f. (b. h. אֻרְוָה q. v.; ארי, אָרָה) *pile of plucked plants, stalk, shed containing feed* (dist. fr. אוֹצָר granary).—*Pl.* אוּרְיָאוֹת, אוּרְיָי׳ (אוּרְיוֹת). Tosef. Maasr. II, 20 ed. Zuck. (Var. אורויות); ib. Erub. VI (V), 4; Erub. 55ᵇ Ar. (ed. אורויות, אורוות, v. Rabb. D. S. a. l. note). [In bibl. h. אֻרְוָה *crib, stable* q. v.]

אוּרְיָא, אוּרְוָוא ch. (=b. h. אֻרְוָה) *crib; stable.* Targ. Is. I, 3 (h. text אֵבוּס q. v.).—Snh. 98ᵇ סוסיא באורייה.... a horse is placed at his (the ox's) crib., i. e. Israel is displaced and other nations feed on his soil.—M. Kat. 10ᵇ למבני א׳ to build a stable (during the festive week). [Targ. II Esth. VI, 10; 11 אוּרְנָא, read אוּרְיָא *stable.*]—*Pl.* אֻרְוָותָא, אוּרְוָותָא, אוּרְיָן (אוּרְיָיתָא). Targ. II Chr. IX, 25; I Kings V, 6. Targ. II Esth. l. c. (אוּרְיָיתָא prob. sing.); a. e.

אוּרְיָא or אוּרְיָיא III m. (horreum, pl. horrea, ὡρεῖον, ὥριον; v. Sm. Ant. s. v.) *store-house, store* (of all kinds). Tanh. B'resh. 7 וכל א׳ שלי בתוכה all my stores are in that ship.—*Pl.* אוּרְיָאֵי (ch. form). Targ. I Chr. XXI, 13. —אוּרְיָיאוֹת (h. form). Targ. II Chr. XXXII, 28 (h. text מסכנות). V. אוּרְיָיר, אֲהוּרְיָיר.

אוּרִיאֵל pr. n. *Uriël,* name of an angel. Targ. Y. Deut. XXXIV, 6.—Num. R. s. 2.

אוּרְיָאן, v. אוּרְיָין I.

אוּרְיָה I, II, v. אוּרְיָא.

אוּרְיָה, v. אוּרְיָיא.

אוּרְיוֹן, v. אוּרְיָין II.

אוּרְיָזָא, v. אוּרְזָא.

אוּרְיָיא, v. אוּרְיָא II h. a. ch.

אוֹרָיָיא, אוֹרָיְיתָא (אוֹרָיְתָא), (אוֹרְיָא, אוֹרְיְתָא, אוֹרַיְתָא) f. (ירי, Af. אוֹרִי=h. תּוֹרָה) 1) *instruction, the Law, Bible-verse.* Targ. Lev. VI, 7; a. fr. —מילה דא׳ (=דברי תורה) *religious discourse, lesson, remarks* &c. Y. B. Bath. VIII, 16ᵃ אורייא; Y. Taan. III, 66ᶜ bot. ויתא.... —Y. Snh. I, 18ᶜ אפלגינון במילי דא׳ he entertained them with religious discussions. Y. Hor. III, beg. 47ᵃ עתיד לך מילה דא׳ be prepared for a religious discourse. Y. Shek. III, 47ᶜ top מאי א׳ חדתא שמעת what novel interpretation hast thou heard? Y. Yeb. II, 4ᵃ top מן הדא אורייה from what verse?—Taan. 4ᵃ מרתח׳ ..... א׳ ליה it is the zeal of study that makes him warm (excited). Kid. 71ᵇ אורייתין כשר׳ my instruction is acceptable, but my daughters are not desired. Sabb. 116ᵇ א׳ דמשה the Mosaic dispensation (opp. א׳ אחריתי the new dispensation, v. אָוֶן).—דְּאוֹרַיְיתָא (sub. הלכה=h. מן התורה) *an enactment founded on the Bible text,* opp. דרבנן. Succ. 44ᵃ לולב דא׳ Lulab, the law concerning which is Biblical &c.; a. fr.—מִדְּאוֹרַיְיתָא, adv. *biblically, according to the Biblical law,* opp. מדרבנן. Pes. 10ᵃ; a. fr.—2) *the Torah, the scroll containing the Pentateuch,* used at divine service. Y. Yoma VII, 44ᵇ top כד היא חדא אוריא when you have no more than one scroll. Y. Meg. IV, 75ᵇ bot.; Y. Sot. VII, end, 22ᵃ כד חזרא אורייה (corr. as Y. Yoma l. c.). Ib. תמן מייבלין א—תא וכ׳ *there* (in Babylon) the Torah is carried to the Resh Galutha.—בר אוריא *a scholar, man of learning.* Yoma 78ᵃ. Ḥag. 14ᵃ אריא (corr. acc.); v. next w.

אוּרְיָין, אוּרְיָאן m. same; 1) the Law. Sabb. 31ᵇ. Ib. 88ᵃ א׳ תליתאי the threefold law (Pentat., Proph., Hagiogr.). —2) *scholarship, authority to teach and judge.* Ber. 12ᵃ בר אוריאן ed. (Ms. M. אוריא); v. foreg. w.—[3) **authority, office.* Gen. R. s. 50 בית אוריין ed. (Ar. מיתורין, Lev. R. s. 26 מתורין) *place of office.* V. מְתוּרִין.]

אוּרְיָין II, אוּרְיוֹן (v. foreg.) pr. n. m. *Oryan, Oryon.* Esth. R. beg. אבא א׳, Abba O. (cmp. אַבָּא). Y. Sabb. X, 12ᵈ top יצחק בר אוריין.

***אוּרְיָינִי** f. (v. foreg. ws.) *officer's or teacher's chair.* M. Kat. 21ᵇ; 27ᵃ א׳ גדולה Ms. M. (v. Rabb. D. S. a. l.; ed. אוד׳) a high (teacher's) chair. V. אִידְרִינִי.

אוּרְיָיר m. (horrearius, ὡρειάριος, v. אוּרְיָא, אֲהוּרְיָיר) *store-keeper,* used in the sense of אוֹלְיָיר. Y. B. Bath. IV, beg. 14ᶜ מקום הא׳ (Tosef. ibid. III, 3 בית האולירין) the clothes-keeper's room.—*Pl.* אוּרְיָירִין. Y. l. c. אורוי׳ אורורין (corr. acc.) Toh. VIII, 7 אודיארין (corr. acc.; Tosef. ib. VII, 8 אולי־אריך).

אוּרְיָירָא ch. same.—*Pl.* אוּרְיָירַיָּא. Targ. I Chr. XXVII, 25; XXVI, 22 (ed. Rahm. אוריד׳, corr. acc.; Var. אוּרְיָרַיָּא, h. text על אוצרות).

אוּרַיְיתָא, v. אוֹרָיְיא.

אוּרִית, v. אוּרְיָא I.

אוֹרַיְתָא, v. אוֹרָיְיא.

אוּרִיכוּת, v. אֲרִכּוּת.

אוּרִיכוּתָא, v. אוֹרְכוּתָא.

אוֹרֶךְ m. (b. h. אֹרֶךְ, ארך) *length, lengthiness.* Midr. Sam. ch. XIII, וכל הא׳ הזה למה and why all this lengthiness (of speech).

אוּרְכָּא ch. same, *length.* Targ. O. Gen. VI, 15 [Constr. אוֹרֶךְ Targ. Y. Ex. XXVI, 13; Targ. O. ib., corr. acc.]—Sabb. 140ᵇ טונא כי טונא וא׳ וכ׳ a load (of twigs) is a load, and the length goes in the bargain (the price is the same).

אוּרִיכוּתָא, אוֹרְכוּתָא f. (=אֲרִיכוּת) 1) *length* (of life). Targ. Ps. XCI, 16; a. e.—2) *waiting, hope.*

Ibid. XXXIX, 8; a. e.—3) *tarrying*. Targ. Y. Deut. II, 31.

***אוּרְכָנִיס** pr. n. m. *Urkhanes*. Y. Yeb. VIII, 8[d] bot. (allusion to a case concerning the child of a certain U., otherwise unknown).

אורכתא B. Kam. 70[a]; Shebu. 33[b], v. אַדְרַכְתָּא 2).

אורלוגין, אוֹרְלוֹגִין m. (ὡρολόγιον) *horologe, time-piece*. Y. R. Hash. I, 57[b] top. Pesik. R. s. 15; a. e.

אוֹרֶן, v. אֹרֶן.

אוֹרֶן, אוֹרְנָא ch.=h. אֹרֶן. Targ. Is. XL, 20; XLIV, 14.

***אַבְרָנוּס, אַוְרָנוּס** m. pl. אַבְרָ׳, אַיְרָנְסֵי (ῥάμνος, rhamnus) *a kind of prickly shrubs*, used for medical purposes and carried in lengthy bundles (v. D. C. Gr. s. v., a. Sm. Ant. s. v.). Sabb. 91[b] אי׳ ed. (Ms. M. אב׳; Ar. ארנסי). [As to בר ,יר for aspirate r, v. Lidd. a. Scott, Gr. Lex, 7th ed. s. lit. P.]

אורסיקין, אורסקין, v. אוורקסין.

אוֹרְעָא m., **אוֹרְעוּתָא** f. (ארע) *meeting*. לא׳ with suff. of pers. pron., *to meet—, against—*. Targ. Prov. VII, 10 (ed. Vien. לִקְּר׳); 15. Targ. Ps. XXXV, 3 לְאוֹרְעוּת.

אוֹרְעֵי, v. next w.

אוֹרְעִיתָא f. (ארע; corresp. to h. צִרְעָה) *wasp, hornet* (collect.). Targ. Y. Ex. XXIII, 28; a. e.—*Pl.* אוֹרְעָיָיתָא. Targ. Y. Deut. I, 44; a. e.—אוֹרְעֵי, אוֹרְעָיָה. Targ. Y. Lev. XI, 20 ed. pr. (corr. vowel signs; later ed. איזפיה). Y. Sabb. I, 3[b] bot. הילכתא דסוסיא וכ׳ the mite in the horse's carcass turns into hornets. [Cmp. same ideas among the Greek, Sachs Beitr. II, 92; Nican Ther. 741.]

אורשינא, v. אַוְרַשְׁנָא.

אוּרְתָא f. (v. אור 2) *evening, night*. Pes. 2[ab] אור א׳ the *or* of the Mishn. means *evening*. Ber. 3[b]; a. fr.—Y. Sot. I, 17[b] top, v. בְּרַת.

אוּשׁ, אַוּוֹשׁ, אַוֵּשׁ, *Pa.* אַוֵּישׁ (√ אוּ, v. אָוָה; cmp. אִיהּ, אבב, אוסר, אופר, אפף, אנק) 1) *to blow vehemently, make noise, shout*. B. Mets. 86[a] נשב זיקא וא׳ וכ׳ the wind blew and howled between the branches. Ber. 50[a] אידדי דאוושו וכ׳ because all shouted, the prayer was not heard. Ib. אוושו כ״ע ברכו they all shouted *'bar'khu'*.—Erub. 97[b] אוושא מילתא the thing grows loud, becomes known. Hull. 46[b] ריאה דא׳ lungs which give out a sound when blown up (indicating perforation). Ber. 58[a] כי קא אוושא (Ms. M. שמעו קל א׳) when shouting was heard.—2) *to swell, to be large, fulsome, lengthy* (in wording). R. Hash. 35[a] משום דאוושי ברכות (Ms. M. קרא׳ . . . .) because the benedictions are numerous and lengthy. Ned. 2[b] הלין משום דא׳ וכ׳ because the last named propositions are lengthy, he explained first what he had commenced with.

אוּשׁ I (v. foreg; cmp. אִישׁ ,יֵשׁ) *to be strong, exist*. *Nithpol.* נִתְאוֹשֵׁשׁ *to be confirmed*. Gen. R. s. 67; s. 78 והיכן נ׳ בידן when were the blessings made sure &c. Cmp. אָשַׁשׁ.

אוּשׁ II m. (אשש 2, cmp. foreg.) pl. אוּשִׁין *foundations*. B. Kam. 50[a] חופר לא׳ digs excavations for supporting walls.

אוּשָׁא, אֻשָּׁא, (אַוְשָׁא) ch. same, also *fortification*. Targ. Cant. VIII, 9.—*Pl.* אוּשַׁיָּא. [Ezra IV, 12; a. e.]. Targ. I Kings VII, 7; VI, 16; a. e. [Targ. Mic. I, 6 ed. Ven. אֻשָּׁהָא her foundations. Targ. Y. Ex. IX, 18 אוּשׁתא (corr. אֻ׳)]. [Not to be conf. with אשיתא.]

אוּשָׁא pr. n. pl. *Uhsa*, in Galilee; freq. the scene of rabbin. synods and enactments during and after the Hadrianic persecutions. Keth. 50[a] מרה דשמעתא דא׳ master of the traditions of U. (in whose name they are quoted). [Ib. קאי באיבלוסא דא׳, read בהילכתא engaged in teaching the laws passed at U.] R. Hash. 31[b]; a. fr.

אוּשְׁוָותָא, v. אֻשִׁיתָא.

אוּשְׁטוּתָא f. (ושט) *stretching forth, obtaining.—* אוֹשָׁטוּת ידא *acquisition, business*. Targ. Deut. XII, 7; a. e.

אוּשְׁיָיתָא, v. אֻשִׁיתָא.

***אַשְׁפִּי, אוּשְׁפִּי** a word in a charm formula, supposed to mean *day*. Sabb. 67[b] אוֹ׳ Ar. (ed. אש׳, Ms. M. אושקי). Cmp. Tosef. Sabb. VII (VIII), 1.

אוּשְׁכָּף, v. אַשְׁכָּף.

אוּשְׁכָּפָא m. ch. (=h. אַשְׁכָּף; שכף, √ כף, cmp. אוּכָּף) *worker in leather, saddler, shoemaker*. Git. 68[b].—*Pl.* אוּשְׁכָּפֵי. Sabb. 112[a] the travellers' sandals דקטרי א׳ which the shoemakers knot (tightly). Ib. 104[b] חרתא דא׳ the blacking used by shoemakers. Ib. 123[b] חרבא דא׳ the leather dressers' knife. Pes. 42[b] פרורא דא׳ the shoemakers' paste. Ib. 113[b].

אוּשְׁלָא=חוּשְׁלָא.

אוּשְׁלַיָא Targ. I Chr. I, 20, v. אֻשְׁלָא.

אוֹשַׁעְיָא (in Y. הוֹשַׁעְיָא q. v.) pr. n. m. *Oshāya*, 1) freq. surnamed רַבָּא (the elder), an Amora of the first generation, redactor of Tosefta. Yeb. 18[b]; a. fr.—2) one mentioned as a wool-washer. Y. B. Kam. end.

אוּשְׁפּוּיכָא, v. אוּשְׁפִּיזָא.

אוּשְׁפּוּזִיכְנָא, v. אוּשְׁפִּיזְכָנָא.

אושפזתי, v. אושפרתי.

אוּשְׁפִּיז m. (נשף, with ז format; cmp. אבליז) *night's lodging, inn.*—*Pl.* אוּשְׁפִּיזִין. בעלי א׳ *innkeepers*. Tosef. Maas. Sh. I, 13; Meg. 26[a]. [Mand. שפיזא, v. Nœld. Mand. Gr. p. 51.]

אוּשְׁפִּיזָא ch. same. Git. 44[b] אית ליה א׳ וכ׳ he has a lodging place in Palestine, (is an occasional resident), opp. ביתא permanent home. Meg. 26[a]; Yoma 12[a] it is customary to leave empty jars and hides of slaughtered animals באושפיזיה (ל) in one's inn. Zeb. 61[b] א׳ הוה נקט (Ms. M. נקיטא . . . אוּשְׁפִּיזָא, v. אושפיזכן; v. Rabb. D. S. a. l.) וכ׳ the Divine fire took up its abode now here and now there. Erub. 53[b] שאיל בא׳ (Rashi בעייל בענייך, read ניה . . . . אושפיזכני, v. Rabb. D. S. a. l. note 80) inquired after the character of an inn (of his landlord). Ib. (enigmatic inquiry that the landlord might not overhear it) גבר פים דיך חי מה טיבו Ar. (v. Rabb. l. c., note 90)=איש-פי-ז-נא our inn—what is its character?

אוּשְׁפִּיזִיכְנָא, אוּשְׁפִּיזִכְתָּא, v. אושפיזכ׳.

אוּשְׁפִּיזְכָן m. (Denom. of אושפיז=אושפיזך, with locat. ךְ, cmp. הָא, הָךְ) *innkeeper, landlord, host.* Meg. 26[a]; Yoma 12[a]; Sot. 37[a]; Zeb. 54[a] נעשה א׳ וכ׳ Benjamin became the host of the Divine Presence (the Temple being partly situated in his territory).

אוּשְׁפִּיזְכָנָא, אוּשְׁפִּיזִיכְנָא ch. same. Zeb. 18[b] בר אושפיזכניה (Ms. M. only אוּשְׁפִּיזִכְנֵיהּ) (the son of) his host. Snh. 7[b] bot. Yoma 78[a] פיזכנה . . . . Ms. M. (ed. נין . . . . .). Bets. 4[a]; a. fr.—Erub. 53[b], v. אוּשְׁפִּיזָא. —Fem. אוּשְׁפִּיזִכְתָּא *hostess.* Ber. 18[b] ed. Ms. M. (בת אושפיזכניה).

***אוּשְׁפַּרְתִּי** pr. n. f. (?) *Ushparti.* Taan. 24[b] Ms. (ed. אושפז׳, v. Rabb. D. S. a. l. note, a. Var. lect. ibid.).

אוּשְׁקְקָא, v. אִשְׁקְקָא.

אוֹשֶׁר, v. אִיּוֹשֵׁר.

אוּת I or **אוֹת** (b. h.; √אח, v. אוי I; cmp. אתא, אַת, אתר, a. אָתָה; v. also Ges. H. Dict. s. v.) *to join, fit.*

Nif. נֵיאוֹת, נָאוֹת (b. h.) *to be suited, pleased,* whence *to be gratified, to enjoy.* Y. Ber. III, 6[c] top ראה את עצמו נ׳ וכ׳ he dreamt he felt sexual gratification; Y. Yoma VII, 44[d] bot.; Y. Taan. I, 64[c] bot.—Y. Bets. I, 61[a] כל שנֵאותין בו בי״ט whatever you are permitted to make use of on Holy Days.—*Fut.* יֵאוֹת. Ber. VIII, 6 עד שיֵאוֹתוּ לאורו until being near enough to enjoy its light. Y. Ab. Zar. I, 39[c] top, a. e., differences as to spelling יֵאוֹתוּ or יֵעוֹתוּ.—Denom. נוֹי, נָאוֶה, נָאֶה, הֲנָאָה.

אוֹת II c. (b. h.; v. אִיי, אָוָה II; תְּאוֹ) 1) *mark, sign, emblem; test, signal, military ensign.* Ḥag. 16[a] (play on ואתה Deut. XXXIII, 2; cmp. foreg.) אות הוא וכ׳ He is the ensign among his myriad; v. דּוּגְמָא. M. Kat. 25[b] אל תזניחנו בא׳ וכ׳ forsake us not in the symbolic trial of bitter waters. (in our trials). *Pl.* אוֹתוֹת. Kil. IX, 10 א׳ הגרדין וכ׳ the marks which the weavers &c. put on goods in their charge. B. Kam. 119[b] you must not buy from the dyer לא א׳ ולא דוגמות either *tests* (pieces cut off to test the color) or samples (as specimens of color).—2) *letter, writing, symbol.* B. Bath. 15[a] אות אחת one letter. Sabb. 103[a]; a. fr.—*Pl.* אוֹתִיּוֹת (fr. אוֹתוּת or אוֹתִית). Kid. 30[a] סופרים כל הא׳ וכ׳ recorded (or counted) all the letters of the Torah. Snh. X, 1 השם באותיותיו the Divine Name with the letters in which it is written (Jehovah). Kid. 71[a] שם בן ארבע א׳ the quadriliteral Name; cmp. שֵׁם.—Lev. R. s. 26, beg. ח׳ א׳ eight letters. Sabb. XII. 3; a. fr.—Trnsf. *notes, documents.* Tosef. Kid. I, 7; B. Bath. 75[b]; a. e.

אוֹת III (b. h., v. אֵת) only with pronominal suffix 1) indicating the objective case, אוֹתִי *me,* אוֹתְךָ *thee,* &c. —2) with pronom. suffix of third person, for emphasizing the subject, אוֹתוֹ *he himself, this one, the same, he who* &c. Gen. R. s. 2, beg. ישב לו א׳ וכ׳ the latter now sat there confounded &c. Y. Git. VI, 47[d] באותו ענין on this very subject (divorce). Sabb. 13[b] זכור אותו האיש וכ׳ may that man be remembered for good. Ber. V, 3 באוֹתָהּ שעה in that hour; a. fr.—אותו מקום euphem. for *pudenda.* Nid. 47[b]. Git. 69[b]; a. e.—אותו ואת בנו *the law concerning the killing of the young with its mother on the same day* (Lev. XXII, 28). Ḥull. V, 1; a. fr.—*Pl.* אוֹתָן. Y. Meg. IV, 74[d] top א׳ שבפה those laws delivered orally. Keth. 4[a] כל א׳ הימים all those days; a. fr. [In later writings אותו האיש is freq. used for Jesus of Nazareth.

אוֹתְבוּתָא f. (יתב) *sitting down, sitting.* Targ. Ps. CXXXIX, 2.

אותוניך, Cant. R. to III, 11, read איקונין as Ex. R. s. 35, end.

***אוּתְיָא** f. *night-bird, owl.* Targ. Y. Lev. XI, 18 (Targ. O. ib. בותא q. v.; Targ. Y. Deut. XIV, 16 צַדְיָא). [Perh. corrupt. of בָּאוּתָא v. בָּאוּת.]

אוֹתְיוֹס, אותיום, v. אֶוְוּתִיאוֹס.

אותיכייה, v. אֲוֻתֵּקָנְיָא.

אותניתיה Y. Snh. II, 20[c] bot. read פִּיתְנִיתֵיהּ, v. פִּיתְנִיתָא.

אָזָא *to kindle,* v. אֲזֵי.

***אַזָּא** or **אֲזָא** m. *sea-eagle* (cmp. עוזא). Targ. Y. Deut. XIV, 12 Ar. (ed. בר גיזא, בר גזא; h. text עזניה).

אזביון, v. אֵזוֹב.

***אֲזָגָא** m. *glass* (v. זְגָגָא). Keth. 77[b] גירדא דא׳ Ar. parings of glass (ed. אגוזא).

אִזְגַּד, אִזְגַּדָּא, v. אִיזְ׳.

אזגור, v. אִיזְגָּדָר.

אזד־ Ithpe. prefix of verbs with prim. lit. ז as אזדוג fr. זוג &c.

אֲזַד (=אזז √ אז; cmp. אזל I; גז, חז, עז, חצד &c.) *to be cut off; to go apart, be gone.* Sabb. 34[b]; a. fr. ואזדו לטעמייהו they differ (cmp. פלג), each following his own principle (or consistent with opinions elsewhere expressed). Ned. 41[a] שיתא אזדו (Rashi אזלו ליה) six of them are gone (escaped his memory). Bets. 10[b] אזדו לעלמא disappeared (Ms. M. אזלו; 11[a] אזלו). Meïl. 17[b] נפק אזדא Ar. (read אזד, ed. אזל) he went out and away. V. אֲזַל.

אָזְדָא f. (foreg.) [*it is*] *decreed* (cmp. גְּזֵרָה). Dan. II, 5.—B. Mets. 116[b] if the landlord said, I let you *this* loft (as it is) א׳ it is a (divine) decree, i. e. it is the tenant's misfortune that the loft fell in, and he has no claims. V. Ges. H. Dict. s. v.

אֻזְדְּעוּעָא, v. next w.

אֻזְדַּעְזְעוּתָא f. (זוּע) *shaking, trembling.* Targ. Job. XII, 5 Ms. (ed. אזדעזעא, const. עת . . .).

אִזְדְּקִפוּתָא, אִזְדַּקְפוּתָא f. (*Ithpe.* or *Ithpa.* of זְקַף) *rising.* Targ. Job. XIII, 11. Ib. XLI, 17 Ms. Var., v. מספיא.

אָזְהוּ, v. אֵיזֶה.

אַזְהָרָא, v. אַזְהַרְתָּא.

אַזְהָרָה f. (זהר) 1) *forewarning, prohibition,* esp. *the explicit prohibition ('thou shalt not') in the Bible,* required for punishing trespassers. Y. Peah I, 16[a] top א׳ ללה״ר a biblical admonition against calumny. Num. R. s. 7 (play on *zara* Num. XI, 20) והי׳ לכם לא׳ it shall be a warning to you. Yeb. 3[b] א׳ שמענו וכ׳ we learn here the legal prohibition, whence do we derive the penalty? a. fr.—*Pl.* אַזְהָרוֹת. Kerith. III, 10; a. fr.—2) *enlightenment.* Cant. R. to VII, 3, v. אֹהַר.

אַזְהָרָא, אַזְהַרְתָּא ch. as foreg. 1. Shebu. 20[b] ואַזְהַרְתֵּיה מה׳ and the legal prohibition concerning it, is to be derived from this verse.—*Pl.* אַזְהָרָן. Y. Yoma VIII, 45[a] תלת א׳ three prohibitory verses.

אֵיזוֹב, אֵזוֹב m. (b. h.; זוב) *hyssop.* Neg. XIV, 6 א׳ יון (Ar. אזוביון) Greek hyssop. Sabb. XIV, 3 (109[b]) איזוביון, איזוביון (read two words, Ms. O., v. Rabb. D. S. a. l. note 4); a. fr.—*Pl.* אֵזוֹבִים M. Kat. 25[b] אֵזוֹבֵי קִיר the hyssop (moss) on the wall (common humanity); v. אֶרֶז.

אֵיזוֹבָא, אֵזוֹבָא ch. same. Targ. Ex. XII, 22; a. e.

אֵיזוֹר, אֵזוֹר c. (b. h.; אזר) *girdle, belt.* M. Kat. 14[a] אֵיזוֹרוֹ וכ׳ his girdle (around his house-gown) testifies for him (that he has no more than the shirt he is washing). Tosef. Shebu. V, 12 sq.; a. e.—*Pl.* אֵיז׳, אֵזוֹרִים. Gen. R. s. 100 אֵזוֹרֵי מתניהם וכ׳ they loosened the girdles of their loins (in mourning sympathy). [Ch. זרזו.]

אֵיזוֹרָא, אֵזוֹרָא ch. same. Sot. I, 17[b] top איזורי ואיזוריה דברי וכ׳ my belt, and my son's belt and that of his father in law; Num. R. s. 9 (p. 232[b] ed. Amst.); Y. Peah VII, 20[a] bot. (corr. acc.); cmp. Midr. Sam. ch. XIII.

אֲזָא, אֲזֵי (=אֲזַי, v. אזדקתא a. זִיק) *to heat* (*make steam*). Dan. III, 19; 22.—Targ. Is. XXXIII, 4 יֵאזֵן (Regia איזין) and they shall heat (baths, ovens) therewith (h. text מַשַּׁק=מַשְׁקֵ), v. זִיקְתָא; (cmp. Ezek. XXXIX, 9). Ib. XLIV, 15 (for baking); a. e.—Y. Ter. VIII, end, 46[c] a bath house דאזיה וכ׳ which he had heated for seven days. Koh. R. to II, 8; a. e. דהוון אָזֵין בהון that entertained the fires in them.—Lev. R. s. 28, end ועל בוניה וקנחיה (read ואַזְיֵיה Pa.) and he (Haman) went and made him sweat and cleansed him (with the scraper).

Ithpe. אִתְּזִי (contr. of אתאזי) *to be heated.* Gen. R. s. 63 קלוון אנא דיתְּזוּן וכ׳ I command that the bath-houses be heated. Ib. אזלון ואִתְּזוּן they went off, and the bath-houses were heated (some ed. דִּיתְחַמּוּן a. אִתְחַמּוּן).

אָזִיל, v. אֲזַל.

אֲזִינָא m., pl. אֲזִינִין (זין) *weapons,* בית א׳ *receptacle of weapons, quiver.* Targ. Jer. V, 16. Targ. Is. XLIX, 2 (ed. Ven. אָזִינִין). V. Targ. to Deut. XXIII, 14 אָזֵנֶךָ.

***אַזִּיק** (Af. of אזק, v. חזק, זקק, עזק) *to tie up.* Koh. R. to VIII, 1 א׳ לרישי I have to tie up my head. (Yalk. Koh. 977 דחיק, Vers. אדיק; Y. Pes. X, 37[c] חזיק רישיה his head was tied; cmp. Ned. 49[b].)

אַזְכָּרָה f. (b. h.;=הַזְכָּרָה, זכר) 1) *remembrance, mention* (of Div. Name), *recitation* (of prayer); *reference.* Y. Ber. V, 9[b] א׳ שהיא מריוח the reference to rain (in the second section of the eighteen benedictions) which is an expression of satisfaction (plenty), opp. שאלה, the prayer for rain (in the ninth benediction) which is an expression of anxiety.—Y. Meg. III, 74[b] top שתהא אַזְכָּרָתָן קודם וכ׳ that the recitation (of the events commemorated on Purim) precede the celebration thereof.—2) (v. אַדְכָּרָה) *the Divine Name, Tetragrammaton.* Num. R. s. 2, beg. the students מראים את הא׳ וכ׳ point out the Div. Name with their fingers; Cant. R. to II, 4 מדלג על הא׳ skips the Div. Name in recitation of lessons.—*Pl.* אַזְכָּרוֹת. Yoma 8[a] שיש בהן א׳ הרבה in which the Div. N. frequently occurs. Y. Ber. III, 6[c].—Y. Sabb. XVI, 15[c] bot.; Bab. ibid. 116[a] קודר אזכרותיהן you must cut out the Div. N. occurring in them (the heretic writings). Y. Taan. II, 65[c] top י״ח א׳ וכ׳ eighteen times that the Tetragrammaton appears in the Psalm *Habu* (XXIX). Num. R. s. 2, beg.; a. fr.

אֲזִיל, אֲזַל, I אֲזַל (b. h. אָזַל; √אז; v. אזר) *to be gone, to leave; to go.* Targ. Gen. XXXII, 1. *Imper.* אֵיזִיל, אֱזֵיל. Targ. O. Num. XXII, 20; a. fr.—Y. Snh. X, 28[b] איזיל חמי וכ׳ go, show thy face &c. Ib. לינה בֵּיזֵל . . . . דנא בייזל וכ׳ I will not go . . . for if I did go &c. Sabb. 116[a] א׳ כתב א׳ וכ׳ after the writing is gone, the sacredness of the scroll is gone (after the scroll has become unfit for sacred use, the material has lost its sacred character). Y. Dem. III, 23[b] bot. הא אזלא טיבלא וכ׳ that man's load would soon be gone (if each were permitted to take a chip). Y. Ber. VIII, 12[a] הא אזלא ההיא דרב וכ׳ is the decision of Rab and Samuel gone (to be disregarded)? Y. Snh. X, 28[a] bot. הא א׳ הדא וכ׳ (ed. Krot. חדא) is that which was received from (is the tradition of) . . . to be disregarded? Y. Yeb. VIII, 9[c] bot. הא אזלא היא וכ׳ (ed. Krot. אזלא, corr. acc.; for היא read הדא or ההיא).—Trnsf. *to depart life, die.* Y. Hag. II, 77[d] bot. this one committed a sin וא׳ בה and died in it, and the other &c. M. Kat. 28[b] ווי לאזלא woe, for the departed one! Y. Keth. XII, 35[a] top אזיל *to die,* contrad. to אתי to *resurrect.*—Imperat. usu. אזיל–זיל.—Hull. 11[b] זיל בתר רובא follow the majority of cases; a. fr.

אָזַל II (=טוּל; v. Ezek. XXVII, 19; √זל) *to spin, weave.* B. Mets. 24[b] קיבורא דאזלי ביה אזלויי a skein which the net-weavers had used; v. זוּל II. Denom. אַרְזְלָא, a. next w.

אַזְלוּיָא m. (foreg.) *weaver.* *Pl.* אַזְלוּיֵי. B. Mets. 24[b] (some ed. אזלוי corr. acc.), v. foreg.

***אָזְלַיָא** m. pl. (=נזל) *running waters, waves.* Targ. O. Ex. XV, 8 (Var. אָזְלַיָא; Y. נָזְלַיָא).

אזמאזמא, v. אִיזְמָא.

אזמורד, v. אִזְמַרַגַד.

אִזְמֵל, v. אִיזְמֵל.

אִזְמַרַגַד, אִזְמַרַגְדָא, אִזְמַרַגְדִין (אִזְמַרַגְזִין), אִזְמַרַגְדִין m. (σμάραγδος, σμαράγδιον) *emerald,* a jewel (also *colored crystal;* v. זמרגד a. זמרגדין). Targ. Job. XLII, 13. Targ. O. Ex. XXVIII, 18 (Targ. Y. ib. אִזְמוֹרַד); a. e. Ex. R. s. 38, end אִסְמַרַגְדִין.

אָזֵן Targ. Is. XXXIII, 4, third pers. pl. of אָזָא, v. אָזֵי.

אֹזֶן, אוֹזֶן m. (b. h.; √אז *to be pointed, cut,* cmp. חז, גז. v. אוּדְנָא) 1) *ear.* B. Kam. 79[b] א׳ של מַטָּה human ear, opp. Divine perception. Y. Sabb. I, 3[b] top; a. fr.—2) *handle.* Cant. R. beg. ולא הו׳ לה א׳ וכ׳ but had no handle and could not be carried; a. fr.—*Du.* אָזְנַיִם 1) *ears.* Lev. R. s. 32, beg. א׳ לדרך the road has ears (be on your guard in speaking); a. fr.—2) *handles.* Kel. IV, 3, v. גיסטרא; a. fr.—3) אָזְנַיִם or בנות א׳ *swollen glands of the throat* (Rashi). Ab. Zar. 28[b] א׳; Y. ib. II, 40[d] top; Y. Sabb. XIV, 14[d] top בנות א׳.

אָזְנִיּוֹת, v. אוּזְנִיּוֹת.

אָזַר (b. h.; √זר, cmp. זרז, אֶזְרוֹעַ) *to put around, girdle; to strengthen.*

Hithpa. הִתְאַזֵּר *to gird, strengthen one's self.* Ber. 16[b] וְתִתְאַזֵּר וכ׳ and gird thyself with thy mercy.

אֶזְרָח m. (b. h.; זרע=זרח) [*planted*], *native, citizen.* Succ. 28[a] א׳ זה א׳ if it read *ezraḥ* (Lev. XXIII, 42), it would mean every native (man or woman); a. fr.—*Pl.* אֶזְרָחִים. Sifra Emor, end.—Fem. אֶזְרָחִית, pl. אֶזְרָחִיּוֹת. Succ. l. c.

אֶזְרְעָא f. (b. h. אֶזְרוֹעַ) *arm.* Targ. Y. II. Num. XXXI, 50; v. זְרוֹעַ.

***אִיזְ׳, אִזְתְּוּדָא** m. (זווד) *attachment, handle.* *Pl.* אִזְתְּוּדֵי. Targ. Y. Ex. XXV, 12 ed. Vien. (oth. ed. אזתוור׳; ib. XXXVII, 3 אסתוור׳, v. Ibn Ezra comment. a. l.).

אָח I m. (b. h.; אחה; cmp. אָב) *brother, kinsman; fellow, equal, fellow-believer* &c. Meg. 11[a] (play on *ăhashverosh,* Ahasverus) אָחִיו שֶׁל רֹאשׁ וכ׳ a brother (in cruelty) to the chief tyrant (Nebucadn.); a. fr.—*Pl.* אַחִים, אַחִין. Gen. R. s. 89, beg. (play on *āḥu,* Gen. XLI, 2) in years of plenty הבריות נעשין א׳ וכ׳ people are brotherly to each other. Ib. s. 99 אחים דפחתא וכ׳ brothers to the degraded woman (Dinah), ... but not to Joseph; a. fr.—Cant. R. to VIII, 1 שני אחים *brother and sister.*

אָחָא, אַחָא, אַחָא, אַח ch. same. Targ. fr.—*Pl.* אַחִין. Targ. Gen. XIII, 8; a. e.—אַחֵי Yeb. 65[b].—Y. Yoma VI. 43[d] אַחִינָן *our brothers.*

אָח II interj. 1) (b. h.) exclamation of sorrow, *Oh!* Meg. 11[a] (play on *ăhashverosh;* v. אָח I) א׳ לראשו woe upon his head. Snh. 102[b] (play on *Ahab* אח־אב) א׳ לשמי׳ a subject of grief to the Lord, and father (friend) of idolatry.—2 (=Syr.) exclamation of joy, *Ah!* Targ. Is. XLIV, 16 (h. הֶאָח).

אָחָא, אַחָא 1) *brother;* v. אַח.—2) pr. n. m. *Aha.* Arakh. 22[b]; Keth. 88[a], surnamed שר הבירה superintendent of the palace. Y. Ber. II, 5[a] R. A. surnamed Roba; a. many others. Y. Taan. II, 65[a] bot.; a. v. fr.

אַחַאי pr. n. m. *Ahai.* Hull. 59[b].

אַחְבָּא, אַחְבָא m. (contr. of אחי אבא) *father's brother, uncle.* Targ. Jer. XXXII, 7 אַחְבּוּךְ thy uncle. Targ. O. Lev. X, 4 (Ms. I a. III אח אבוהי; Targ. Y. חביבא q. v.); a. e. Yeb. 21[b] Ar. s. v. אחבא בי (ed. בי דודי).

אֶחָד m., אַחַת f. (b. h.; v. next w., a. חד) *one.* [Freq. represented by א׳.] Kid. 50[b], a. fr. בבת אחת *simultaneously,* v. בַּת III. Peah III, 3 המחליק מאחת יד וכ׳ (Ms. M. בא׳) he who takes out onions with a unity of hand, i. e. all of them for one purpose. Ber. 61[b], a. fr. על אחת כמה וכמה (abbr. עאכ״ו) how much against one, i. e. *how much the more.*—אחד .... אחד *both ... as well as.* Tem. I, 1 א׳ האנשים וכ׳ both, men as well as women. Y. Keth. V, 29[d] top אחת זו ואחת זו the one as well as the other; a. fr.—כְּאֶחָד, כְּאַחַת *at the same time.* Tosef. Neg. I, 11; sq. Sot. 8[a]; a. fr.—Yoma I, 7 והפג אחת and cool thyself *for once, for a change,* v. חֲדַת.—*Pl.* אֲחָדִים 1) *singular, unique.* Yalk. Gen. 62 (ref. to דברים אחדים Gen. XI, 1) they spoke words א׳ על שני against two only ones (ref. to אחד Ezek. XXXIII, 24 a. Deut. VI, 4) [corr. acc. Gen. R. s. 38].—2) (cmp. אָחַד) *closed up, mysterious.* Gen. R. l. c. (Yalk. l. c. אֲחוּדִים v. next w.).

אָחַד (sec. r. of חוּד, v. חוּד I) *to join, close.* *Part. pass.* אָחוּד, *pl.* אֲחוּדִים 1) *closed up, mysterious.* Yalk. Gen. 62, v. foreg.—2) *joined, united.* Gen. R. s. 38 (ref. to Gen. XI, 1, v. foreg.) דברים א׳ common goods, communism.

אָחַד, *Pa.* אַחֵיד, אַחֵד ch. (v. foreg.) 1) (corresp. to h. סגר a. תפש; cmp. h. אחז) 1) *to close* (the door), *to lock up; to seize, capture.* Targ. Is. XXII, 22 אַחֵיד. Ib. יֵיחוּד יֵיחוּד (fut.).—Targ. Deut. XXI, 19 יַאֲ=יְחַדוּן (Pa.; Var. יֵאח׳=יַחְדוּן Pe.). Targ. Am. III, 5; a. fr.—Snh. 26[a] bot., a. e. אחדיה לדשא locked the door. Pes. 111[b] אחדא

לֵיהּ רוּחָא a spirit (demon, disease) seizes him.—*Part. pass.* אֲחִיד a) *locked up.* Targ. Josh. VI, 1; a. e.—b) (v. אָחַז, s. v. אֲחִיז) *holding.* Targ. Am. II, 15; a. fr.—*Part. pass. Pa.* מְאַחַד *locked up, hidden.* Targ. Job. XXVI, 9. 2) *to devote,* v. אֲחִיד.

Af. אוֹחַד *to seize.* Targ. Ps. LXXIII, 23.

Ithpa. אִתְאַחַד, אִתְּחַד, *Ithpe.* אִתְאֲחִיד 1) *to be seized.* Targ. Ez. XIX, 4; a. fr.—2) *to be locked up, joined.* Targ. Is. XXIV, 10 אֶת אחידו . . . (read איתאחידו). Ib. LIX, 10 Rashi (ed. אתא חד corr. acc.). Targ. Job XLI, 9 (8); a. e. —אִתְּחִיד. Hull. 52[b] א׳ דשא the door was locked.

אַחְדָא f. (v. foreg.) 1) *bolt.* Targ. Prov. XVIII, 19 (read ...ד א׳ ד (חיך.—2) *shutting up.* אַחְדַת רחמי shutting up of the womb, barrenness. Ibid. XXX, 16.

אַחַדְבּוֹי (contr. of אחד־דאבא; v. אחבא) pr. n. m. *Aḥadboy,* an Amora. Hull. 113[b]; a. e.

אַחֲה, v. אחי.

אַחְוָה, אַחְוָא m. (=b. h. אָחוּ, v. Ges. H. Dict. s. v.) [green], *meadow-grass, reed.* Targ. O. Gen. XLI, 2.

אַחוּדְתָּא f. (אֲחַד)=אַחוּזְתָּא *possession.* Targ. O. Num. XXVII, 7; a. e.

אַחֲוָה f. (b. h.; denom. of אָח) 1) *brotherhood, brotherly love, friendship.* Snh. 58[b] בא׳ among brothers and sisters. Gen. R. s. 89 (play on *aḥu,* Gen. XLI, 2) in days of plenty there is אהבה וא׳ love and friendship.—Lev. R. s. 2; a. fr.—Trnsf. בא׳ *jointly.* Sabb. 20[a] (explain. אָח Jer. XXXVI, 23) עצים שנדלקין בא׳ Ar., Ms. Oxf. (v. Rabb. D. S. a. l. note, ed. באחונא cler. error) wood kindled all together [perh. with *reeds?* v. next w.].—2) (law) *status of consanguinity.* B. Kam. 88[a] a slave שאין לו א׳ who has no legal status of consanguinity.

אַחֲוָה ch., v. אַחְוָא.

אַחֲוָוא pr. n. m., v. אַחֲבָה II.

אחווינא, v. אַחְוָנָא.

אחווִיתָא, v. אַחְוִיתָא.

אַחְוָנָא m. (v. אַחְוָא) 1) *meadow-grass, grass* (as fodder). Y. Ber. VI, 10[a], bot.—2) *willow-twigs* used for kindling, *kindling wood.* Sabb. 20[a] (explain. אָח Jer. XXXVI, 23; v. אַחֲוָה 1, end) אַחְוָנָא (Var. אַחֲוָנָא) willow-fire. Ib. one cried מאן בעי א׳ וכ׳ who wants *Aḥvana?*, and it was found he had willow twigs for sale.—3) *willow-bast.* Ib. 20[b] explaining אִירָן; Ms. M. (ed. אחוינא, אחוורנא).

אֲחוּזָה f. (b. h. אֲחֻזָּה; אחז) *possession, inheritance.* Y. Kid. I 60[c] top; a. e. Y. Hall. IV, 60[b]. [Ib. אחוזה עצמה וכ׳ strike out the entire sentence.]. Hull. 75[a] אחוזת עינים, v. אֲחִיזָה.

אֲחוּזְתָּא ch. same. Targ. Ps. II, 8 Ms. (ed. אחודתא).

אַחְוָיָה f. (חוי) *telling, interpretation.* Dan. V, 12.

אַחְוָיְתָא, אַחֲוָיְתָא f. (v. foreg.) *instruction.* Targ. Ps. XLIX, 5; a. fr.

אֲחוֹכֵי inf. of אַחוֹךְ, v. חוך a. אֲחִיךְ.

אחום, v. אַחִים (כפר).

אַחְוָנָא, v. אַחְוָנָא.

אַחְוָנַיָּא m. pl. (Syr. חחוניתא, v. חוֹחָא, a. Löw Aram. Pfl. p. 149) *plums.* Y. Ber. VI, 10[b] bot. (Bab. ib. 39[a] דורמסקין).

אַחְוָנִיתָא, אַחְוָנַיְיתָא f. (v. foreg.) *a dish of plums.* Y. Ber. VI, 10[c] top.

אָחוֹר m. (b. h.; v. חור a. חרר) 1) *back, hind-part, buttock.* Bekh. 8[a]; Gen. R. s. 20, beg.—Du. אֲחוֹרַיִים (Ar. אחורים). Pes. 17[b], a. fr. א׳ ותוך the back (outside) and the inside of a vessel.—Y. Yoma V, 42[c] top אֲחוֹרָיו לקדש his back turned to the sanctuary.—Y. Pes. VI, 33[a] bot., a. fr. מֵאֲחוֹרֵי (prepos.) *behind.*—לַאֲחוֹרֵי, אֲחוֹרֵי same. Ber. 61[a]; a. fr.—2) *last.* Ib. (ref. to Ps. CXXXIX, 5) א׳ למעשה וכ׳ the last of all things created; Lev. R. s. 14 א׳ לכל המעשים.—3) *farthest back, earliest.* Ib. א׳ זה יום ראשון *aḥor* (Ps. l. c.) means the first day.

אֲחוֹרָא (אֲחֹרָא) ch. same. לאחורא *backward.* Targ. Gen. XLIX, 17; a. fr.—*Pl.* אֲחוֹרִין, const. אֲחוֹרֵי. Targ. Ps. LXXVIII, 66 (buttocks).—אֲחוֹרֵי *behind, after.* Y. R. Hash. II, 58[b] top מן אחורוי behind him; a. fr. V. חוֹרֵי. [Targ. Y. Lev. XIX, 26, v. חֲרוֹרָא.]

אוֹחְרֵי, אֲחוֹרֵי f. (=h. אַחֶרֶת) *another, something else.* Y. Shebu. IV, 35[d] top איתא אר׳ another woman (wife). Y. Ber. IX, 13[a] bot. שיטה אר׳ another method, Lev. R. s. 14, beg. אמר אר׳ said differently. Y. Meg. II, 74[a] top אחר׳ another (scroll). Gen. R. s. 76 אחר׳ another (word, in reply). [Targ. אוֹחְרֵי. Targ. Gen. XXVI, 21; a. fr.]—[Dan. II, 39; VII, 5; 6; אָחֳרִי.] V. חוֹרֵי.

אָחוֹת f. (b. h.; אחת, v. אָח I) *sister.* Yeb. I, 1; a. fr. —Hull. 114[a] (of animals).—*Pl.* אֲחָיוֹת. Yeb. III. 1; a. e.

אָחַז (b. h.; sec. r. of חוז, cmp. אחד) 1) *to press, seize, hold, keep; to befall.* Snh. 27[b] אוֹחֲזִין מעשה וכ׳ holding in their hands the doing of their fathers, i. e. following their father's example. Bekh. 33[b] אֲחָזוֹ דם he had an attack of congestion. Y. Pes. I, 28[b] אֲחוּזַת הדם the animal attacked with congestion. Y. Sabb. XIV, 14[c] bot. אֲחָזָתוֹ עין a pain in the eye seized him. Ib. XIX, end, 17[b] אחזתו חמה fever overtook him; a. fr.—אָחַז בְּ־ *to have a hold of.*—B. Mets. I, 1. Y. Yoma II, 39[c] top; a. fr.—Part. pass. אָחוּז *holding fast, having a firm hold.* Ex. R. s. 46 (v. אָחַד).—2) א׳ את העינים *to capture the eyesight, to delude by optical deception.* Snh. 65[b]; a. e.

Nif. נֶאֱחַז *to be seized.* Y. Taan. II, 65[d] top; a. e.

**Hif.* הֶאֱחִיז *to distribute split wood (kindling chips) in the gaps of a large pile, to ignite with kindling wood.* Sabb. I, 11 (19[b] sq.) וּמַאֲחִיזִין ed. (Mss., Ar. a. Y. ib. beg. 4[c] ומחזין, ed. Ven. ומחזיקין); v. חָזָה.

אחזונת, v. חַזְיוֹן 2).

אחי, אָחָה (√חו, cmp. חבב) *to unite.* Part. pass. אָחוּי *united.* Num. R. s. 13, beg. שיהיו אֲחוּיִים אצלו they shall be united with him (around his table).

Pi. אִיחָה *to join; to sew together* (with fine stitches); cmp. חוּט; חוּט I. Gen. R. s. 39 beg. אברהם שא׳ את וכ׳ Abraham who united all mankind into a brotherhood (by the belief in one God), כזה שהוא מְאַחֶה וכ׳ like one who sews &c., v. infra. Ex. R. s. 40, end.—Esp. *to mend, by stitching, the rent of the garment torn in mourning.* M. Kat. 22ᵇ; a. fr. Ib. 26ᵃ לְאַחוֹתָן to stitch them together.

Hithpa. a. *Nithpa.* הִתְאַחָה, נִתְאַחָה 1) *to be joined; to be stitched together.* Num. R. s. 13, beg. (play on אחויה Cant. V, 1) נִתְאַחוּ לי וכ׳ they were joined to me (I joined them) in the captivity. Gen. R. s. 68 מִתְאַחוֹת, v. אֶבֶן. M. Kat. 26ᵃ אין מתאחין must not be stitched together.—2) *to be joined by grafting, to grow together.* Y. Kil. I, 27ᵃ top חן נתא׳ וכ׳ they (the two seeds) combine. Y. Shebi. II, end, 34ᵃ bot. Y. Orl. I, 61ᵃ bot.

אחי ch., *Pa.* אַחֵי as foreg. *Pi.* Targ. Koh. III, 7 לאחאה to sew together.

אֲחִיד 1) part. pass. of אֲחַד q. v.—2) (=h. מְיוּחָד, v. יחד) *singled out, devoted, betrothed.* Targ. O. Lev. XIX, 20. Targ. Ps. CXIV, 2. Targ. Cant. VI, 9.

אֲחִידָה I (אחד) *taking possession, capture.* Meg. 6ᵃ חיו קורין אותו אֲחִידַת מגדל צור Ms. (ed. שיר, Ar. שר) they recorded the act (of taking the place afterwards called Cæsarea) as the capture of Migdal Tsor.

אֲחִידָה II f. (h. חִידָה) *enigma.*—*Pl.* אֲחִידָן Dan. V, 12.

אֲחִיָּה (b. h.) pr. n. m. *Aḥiyah,* several men of various periods. 1) Shek. V, 1 א׳ על חנסכים A. superintendent of the Temple libations (wines, oils).—2) Ber. 63ᵇ A., a Babylonian scholar opposing Palestine authorities.—3) רבי אחייה R. A., a Tannai. M. Kat. 20ᵃ; a. e. Ibid.ᵇ ר׳ חייא לחוד וכ׳ R. Ḥiya (although a Chald. abbreviation of Aḥiyah) and R. A. are two different persons.

אַחֲוֹות pl. of אָחוֹת.

אַחְיוּתָא f. (חיי) *reanimation, resurrection.* Targ. Hos. VI, 2 ... אַחְיוּת resurrection of &c.; a. e.

אַחַי pr. n. m. *Aḥai* (v. אַחַאי). Kid. 22ᵇ.

אֲחִיַּת, v. אֲחִיָּה.

אַחִיךְ *to laugh,* v. חוּךְ.

אַחִילוּ f. (חִיל) *chills and fever, trembling.* Git. 70ᵃ (explained, as 'fire of the bones'). Ber. 32ᵃ (play on ויחל Ex. XXXII, 11). [Ib. 12ᵇ אחילו Af. of חול II.]

אַחִים, כְּפַר א׳ pr. n. pl. *K'far Aḥim.* Men. 85ᵃ. Tosef. ib. IX, 2 אחים.

אֲחִינִית f., pl. אֲחִינִיּוֹת (prob. to be read אַחְוָנִיּוֹת, v. אַחְוָנַיָּא) *plums.* Y. Dem. II, 22ᵈ top.

***אַחְלָה** f. (חלל) *defilement* of a priest's daughter, v. חֲלָלָה. Snh. 66ᵇ אם תחלת אַחְלָתָהּ וכ׳ if her first defilement occurred in whoredom (not in wedlock with one degraded).

***אַחְמִיתָא** f. (cmp. h. חֵמֶת) *pot, closed vessel. Pl.* אַחְמִיתָן. Targ. Esth. I, 4.

אַחְמַר m. (חמר) *ruby,* name of a jewel in the Highpriest's breast-plate. Targ. Cant. V, 14; v. סַמְקָן.

אחמרא, אַחְמְרָא m., Ar., v. חוּמְרָא III.

אַחְמְתָא pr. n. pl. *Aḥm'tha, Ecbatana,* capital of Media. Ezra VI, 2, v. חַמְדָּן; v. Schr. K. A. T. p. 378.

אח"ס, אח״ס בט״ע, a formula representing a permutation of letters wherein the first (א) interchanges with the eighth (ח) and with the fifteenth (ס); the second (ב) with the ninth (ט) and with the sixteenth (ע), &c. Sabb. 104ᵃ אני חָס עליהם מפני שֶׁבָּטְנוּ=אח״ס בט״ע גי״ק בגוּף I shall spare them because they resisted sensual temptations; v. גִּיק.

אחסנתא, אַחְסְנָא f. (חסן) *property, inheritance.* Targ. Lev. XIV, 34; a. e.—B. Bath. 133ᵇ מַעֲבִירֵי א׳ who unlawfully pass an inheritance from one hand to another.

אָחַר (b. h.; denom. of אָחוֹר) 1) *to be behind,* v. *Pi.* —2) (euphem.) *to cover* (of camels). B. Bath. 93ᵃ; Shebu. 34ᵃ; Snh. 37ᵇ (Ms. M. B. Bath. l. c. יחיר). Tosef. B. Kam. III, 6 אוֹחֵיר.

Pi. אִחֵר, אֵחַר, אִיחֵר *to tarry, hesitate; to set behind.* Pes. IX, 9 אם אֵחַרְתִּי if I should be late. Y. Yoma III, 40ᶜ top א׳ בו מעשה the text orders a later action after it. Y. Ned. X, 42ᵃᵇ א׳ בעמידה he tarried in standing, i. e. was the last to sit down. Gen. R. s. 81, beg. א׳ אדם את נדרו if one procrastinates the fulfillment of his vow; a. fr.

Pu. (and *Hof.*) הוּאֲחַר, אוּחַר *to be postponed, be done late, be placed later.* Y. Yoma III, 40ᶜ top בכלל מאוחר חיה would belong to things to be done later. Ib. יוּאֲחַר וכ׳ let it be done later than &c.—אין מוקדם ומאוחר בתורה there is no 'earlier' or 'later' (no chronological order) in the events or laws of the Scripture. Pes. 6ᵇ; a. e.; Y. Sot. VIII, 22ᵈ מוּאֲחַר.—Shebi. X, 5, a. fr. מאוחר (a document) *postdated,* opp. מוקדם antedated. B. Mets. V, 10 רבית מְאוּחֶרֶת postpaid interests.

אַחַר ch. same. 1) *to be behind.* 2) **to cover.* Targ. Jer. V, 8 (of steeds, h. text מיוזנים; some ed. ד for. ר).

Pa. as foreg. *Pi., to tarry; to retard.* Targ. O. Gen. XXXIV, 19; a. fr. Sabb. 119ᵃ אחריו take ye a later meal (on Sabbaths).

Af. אוֹחַר same. Targ. II Sam. XX, 5; a. fr.—[Targ. Prov. XXIII, 30 מְאַחֲרִין, מְאַחֲרִין Part. Af. or Pa. of יחר= מאחר, מוחר.]

**Ithpe.* אִתְאַחַר, contr. אִתַּחַר to *be delayed.* Targ. Y. I Deut. I, 2; cmp. however ib. v. 6, v. אָרַח.

אַחַר (b. h.; v. foreg.), pl. constr. אַחֲרֵי *after, behind*. Gen. R. s. 44 wherever the Bible uses the preposition *aḥarê* סמוך, it means *in connection with*, אחר מופלג while *aḥar* means without connection (*later on*). Yoma 6ª א׳ אחר after 'after', i. e. some time after the act, opp. חד אחר one 'after', immediately, v. אֶוְתְּרוֹס.—לְאַחֲרֶיהָ, לְאַחֲרָיו after it, as concluding, opp. לפניו, לפניה מֵאַחֲרֶיהָ, מֵאַחֲרָיו introductory (prayer).—Ber. I, 4 אחת לא׳ one benediction after the Sh'ma. Ib. III, 4 לאחריו (prayer) after meal; a. fr.—כִּלְאַחַר יד as if doing a thing with the back of the hand, i. e. in a manner different from the usual way of doing it. Sabb. 153ᵇ; a. fr.—מֵאַחַר 1) (conj. followed by ־ש or ־ד) *after, since, whereas, because*. Hull. 29ª מא׳ ששנינו after it has once been stated in the Mishnah . . . . . why was it necessary (?) &c. Ib.ᵇ ומאחר דאפי׳ וכ׳ and since it is not even rabbinically unfit, why &c.; a. fr.—2) a legal term, *meaḥar*, the presumption of the truth of one's statement, *because* he might have pleaded more profitably, if he had been inclined to lie. Y. Shebu. VI, 36ᵈ bot. אין אומרים בממון מא׳ מאחר וכ׳ in money matters we do not apply the principle of *meaḥer*, so as to say that because he might have said 'thou hast not lent me anything', he may say, 'thou didst lend me, but I paid half of it' (and his plea must be accepted without an oath); v. מִיגּוֹ s. v. גּוֹ.—אַחֲרֶיךָ *thy successor*. Y. Kil. IX, 32ᶜ top יהודה בני א׳ וכ׳ my son Judah shall succeed thee, none else (is worthy). Keth. 95ᵇ my property I bequeath to thee ואַחֲרֶיךָ לפ׳ and after thee it shall go over to . . .—אַחַר כָּךְ (abbrev. אח״כ) *afterwards, subsequently*. Pes. X, 2; a. v. fr.

אַחֵר m. (b. h.; v. foreg. a. חוֹרִי) [back of,] *another, the other, stranger*. דבר א׳ (abbr. ד״א) 1) *another thing, another explanation*. Snh. IV, 5; a. v. fr. in Midr.—2) euphem. for *idolatry, swine* &c., v. דָּבָר. 3) *Aḥer*, [apostate,] byname of Elisha ben Abuyah. Ḥag. 14ᵇ; a.e. —*Pl.* אֲחֵרִים *others*; 1) freq. in Mishn. for anonymous authorities differing in opinion, א׳ אומרים, v. Hor. 13ᵇ אסיקו לר׳ מאיר א׳ R. Meïr is quoted under the word *aḥerim*.—2) freq. for *strangers, gentiles*. Snh. 52ᵇ אשת א׳ the wife of a non-Israelite. B. Mets. 111ᵇ; a. fr.—Fem. אַחֶרֶת. Yoma I, 1 אשה א׳ a second (additional) wife; a. fr.—Snh. 104ª זאת ועוד א׳ this and something besides (shall happen).

אַחְרָא, אָחֳרָא v. אָחוֹרָא.

אַחְרָיו, אַחֲרָאִי m. (foreg. wds.) prop. *designated to step behind, substitute*; hence, *he who* (or *that which*) *is gone back to, obligated, pledged; surety, guarantor*.—*Pl.* אַחֲרָאִים, אַחֲרָיִין. Dem. III, 5 אין אנו א׳ וכ׳ we are not responsible for deceivers. Pes. IX, 9 אינן אחראין זה לזה they are not responsible to one another (need not care for each other). Y. Keth. VIII, end, 32ᵇ, a. fr. כל נכסיו א׳ all his landed property is pledged for &c.

אַחֲרוֹן m., אַחֲרוֹנָה f. (אַחֲרוֹנִית f. noun) *other, next, last*. Meg. 21ᵇ; a. fr. א׳ the last of those called up to read from the Torah.—*Pl.* אַחֲרוֹנִים m., אַחֲרוֹנוֹת f.—מים א׳ the washing of hands after meals before grace, opp. מים ראשונים washing before meals. Ber. 53ᵇ; a. fr.—דורות א׳ or only אחרונים the latter (present) generation, opp. ראשונים ancients. Yoma 9ᵇ; a. fr.—Ber. 13ª צרות א׳ וכ׳ the latter (present) troubles bring the former into oblivion.—(ברכות) א׳ the three last sections in the Prayer of Benedictions. Ibid. 34ª; a. fr.—Erub. 53ᵇ אַחֲרוֹנִית *second wife*; v. אַחֲרוֹנִית.—בָּאַחֲרוֹנָה (adv.) *last*. B.Kam. 8ª; a. e.

אַחֲרֵי v. אָחוֹרֵי.

אַחֲרָיוּת f. (v. אַחֲרָאִי) *surety*, esp. *mortgaged property*, or *property which may be resorted to in case of non-payment* (even if sold).—נכסים שיש להן א׳ property from which debts may eventually be collected (landed property), נ׳ שאין להם א׳ property which cannot be resorted to (movable property). Kid. I, 5; a. fr.—B. Mets. III, 11 חייב באחריותן is responsible for them (if lost). Men. 109ª; a. fr.—א׳ נכסים an obligation for which property is pledged. Keth. 34ᵇ; a. fr.—Ib. 51ᵇ, a. e. documents שאין בהן א׳ נ׳ in which the clause pledging property is omitted. Ib.ª; a. e. א׳ טעות סופר הוא the omission of the clause pledging property is considered as the scribe's mistake (hence has no legal consequences). B. Mets. 14ª, a. e. ראובן שמכר . . . בא׳ if R. sold to S. a field with surety (guaranteeing the title).

אַחֲרָיוּתָא f. (=h. אַחֲרִית) *future*. Targ. Y. II Deut. XXXII, 29; a. e.

אַחֲרָיִי v. אַחֲרָאִי.

אַחֲרָיָא m. *another, the other, later, last*. Y. Pes. I, end, 28ᵇ ר׳ יושוע א׳ the other (last named) R. Josh.—Y. Ber. II, 5ᵇ top פירקא א׳ last chapter.—*Pl.* אַחֲרָיִין. Y. Ter. VIII, 45ᵈ bot. א׳ ומיתון those (drinking) later, drank and died.—אַחֲרַיָּיא. Y. Meg. III, 74ᵇ bot. תומנתי פסוקייא א׳ the last eight verses.—Fem. אַחֲרַיְתָא, אַחֲרָיְתָא. Y. Taan. I, beg. 63ᶜ. Y. Shebu. III, 34ᵈ בא׳ in the last one.—Targ. Prov. V, 20 אחריתא *stranger*.—Ib. XXV, 8, a. fr. בא׳ *at last, in the end*.—*Pl.* אַחֲרָיָתָא. Ib. XXIV, 14 Ms. (ed. sing.).

אַחֲרָנָא m. *another*. Hull. 12ª אינש א׳ another man. Bets. 28ª מידי א׳ something different.—לישנא א׳ (abbr. ל״א) another version. Pes. 97ᵇ, a. fr.—*Pl.* אַחֲרָנֵי. Yeb. 45ª; a. fr. Cmp. אָחֳרָן.

אַחֲרִית f. (b. h.) *future, end*. Y. Meg. III, 74ª bot.

אַחֲרִיתָא v. אַחֲרָיְתָא s. v. אַחֲרָיָא.

אַחֲרִיתִי ch.=h. אַחֶרֶת *another, something besides*. Erub. 23ª מילתא א׳ another subject. Pes. 50ª; a. fr.

אָחֳרָן, אוֹחֲרָן, אוֹחֲרָנָא m. ch.=h. אַחֲרוֹן. Targ. Ex. XX, 3; a. fr.—Fem. אָחֳרָנִיתָא, אוֹחֲרָנִית, אוֹחֲרָנְתָא. Targ. O. ib. XXI, 10 (another, additional wife). Ibid. Gen. XVII, 21.—Lam. R. to IV, 2.—B. Bath. 16ª אחרניתא a stranger (not his own wife).—*Pl.* אוֹחֲרָנִין, אָחֳרָנִין. Targ. O. Gen. XLI, 3; a. e. אָחֳרָנְיָיאתָא. Cant. R. to IV, 12.—[Targ. Y. Gen. XXXV, 8 בכותא אוחרן a repetition of weeping, v. אַלּוֹן II.]

אֲחָרַת v. אַחַר.

אֲחַשְׁדַּרְפְּנַיָּא, ־נִין .... m. pl. (h. ־נים .....) *satraps, Persian governors.* Dan. III, 2; a. e.—Cant. R. to VII, 9.

אֲחַת v. אֶחָד.

אֲחָת (אֲחַת), אֲחָתָא f. ch.=h. אָחוֹת. Targ. Jer. XXII, 18; a. fr.—Pes. 4[a]; a. fr.—*Pl.* אַחְוָותָא. Targ. Job. I, 4 (ed. אַחְוָ׳); a. e.—Yeb. 32[b]. Sabb. 13[a]. Yeb. 66[a] top (*twin sisters*).

אטב״ח, א״ט *Atbaḥ*, a formula of combination or interchange of two letters the numerical sum of which is either ten (e. g. א״ט=1+9; ב״ח=2+8) or *one hundred* (e. g. צ״י=10+90; כ״פ=20+80=100), whereby ה and נ, remain isolated or substitute each other. Ex. R. s. 15 (allusion to הֵן Num. XXIII, 9).—Succ. 52[b] באטב״ח (של ר׳ חייא) קורין כ׳ לסהדה מנון in the Atbaḥ (of R. Ḥiya) *sahadah* finds a substitute in *manon* (v. Prov. XXIX, 21).

אִתָּא m. (אתט, cmp. חטט=b. h. אֵת, pl. אִתִּים), pl. אִתִּין *plough-shares.* Y. Sabb. VI, 8[b] bot. (expl. לְאִתִּים (Is. II, 4) לְאִ׳ (Ar. by cler. err. אבורין).

אַטָּא, Af. אַיְיטֵי, v. יְטָא, יְטַי.

אַטְבָּא (אַטְבְּעָא) m. (טבע, v. טַבַּעַת) *ring, hook, clasp.* Men. 32[a] א׳ דסיפרי clasp for fastening the leaves of books while reading.—*Pl.* אַטְבֵּי (אַטְבְּעֵי). Sabb. 98[a] Ar. אטבי (ed. באטבער אטבער, some ed. בא׳ בטבער, corr. acc., Ms. M. only בטבער, margin אטבי; v. Rabb. D. S. a. l.). Num. R. s. 6 (in Hebr. diction) א׳ של ברזל iron clasps (to fasten the boards on the wagon).

אט״בח v. א״ט.

אַטְבְּעָא v. אַטְבָּא.

אָטָד m. (b. h.; √אט, v. אִטָּא) *thorn.* Gen. R. s. 100. Sot. 13[a].—Y. Ned. VI, end 40[a] מדבר הא׳ the desert of *Atad.*—*Pl.* אֲטָדִין. Shebi. VII, 5; a. e. [V. Sm. Ant. s. v. Carduus.]

אָטַד, אָטְדָא ch. same. Targ. Gen. L, 10.—Targ. Ps. LVIII, 10. Ms. (ed. אַטְדָא); a. e.—*Pl.* אַטְדִין. Targ. O. Gen. III, 18. (Y. אַטְטִין). Targ. Hos. X, 8 (some ed. אטטין).

אַטוּ (abbrev. of אמטול, v. אַמְטוּ) 1) *on account of, because of, for the sake of* (h. בגלל). קנסו שוגג א׳ מזיד they fined the inadvertent transgressor for the sake of the wilful one (in order to prevent wilful sin). Git. 53[b]; a. fr.—2) (in questions expressing *surprise, indignation*) *is it because? do you mean to say?* Ib. 7[a] א׳ אנא לא ידענא do I not know it myself? Ib. 30[b] א׳ ברשיעי עסקינן is it with wicked men we have to deal? (i. e. shall we presume deliberate sin?); a. v. fr.

אֲטוּנָא, אַטּוּנָא m. (cmp. b. h. אֵטוּן; prob. fr. טוה *to spin*; for oth. etym. v. Ges. H. Dict. s. v. אטן) *rope, chord.* Targ. Josh. II, 15. Targ. Job. XXX, 11 (ed. give all var. combined, v. שׁוֹשַׁלְתָּא).—R. Hash. 23[a] א׳ דכיתנא (some ed. אטוני pl.) flaxrope.—*Pl.* אַטּוּנִין, אַטּוּנַיָּא (אַט׳). Targ. I Kings XX, 31; a. fr. [Tosef. Maasr. III, 8 אטונין ed., ed. Zuck. עטרנין, Var. אטרנין q. v.]

טוּנָס, אַטוּנָס m. (cmp. θύννος; v. Sm. Ant. s. v.) *tunny-fish.* Hull. 66[b]; Ab. Zar. 39[a] Ms. M. (ed. אוט׳). Tosef. Hull. III (IV), 27 אַנְתִּינִים ed. Zuck. (Var. אַנְתִּינוֹס). Ib. Kel. B. Mets. II, 17 ליטול בטונס; (read as) Hull. 25[a] לחטיהו בטו׳ to polish a vessel with the skin of a tunny. *Cant. R. to I, 7 במה מיני אונס וכ׳ (read אטו׳; Ex. R. s. 2 מזונות) how many kinds of tunny fish hast thou prepared for the lying-in among them? V. אכספטיאס.

אטורנגא Keth. 61[a] bot., v. אַבְוַנְגַּר.

אַטְמָא v. אַדְּדָא.

***אטימס** Hall. IV, 11 (12) Ar., Ms. M.; ed. Talm. Y. בן א׳, Mishn. אנטינוס; Tem. 21[a] Ar., ed. בן אַנְטִיגְנוֹס, q. v.

אטימריים, v. אירנים.

אֵיטִימוֹס, אֲטִימוֹס m. (ἕτοιμος) *present, ready.* Targ. Y. Num. XI, 26; a. fr.—Gen. R. s. 48 it does not read עומד (standing) but נצב (placed on his post), i. e. אט׳ ready (to proceed). Cant. R. to II, 9 אי׳. Gen. R. s. 100.

אטימטון v. אֲטִימִיטוֹן.

אֲטִימִיטָא v. next w.

אֲטִימִיטוֹן m. (neut., or accus. of ἀτίμητος (something) *invaluable, priceless.* Y. Peah I, 15[d] bot. חד מרגלי טבא א׳ (read חדא) a pearl worth a priceless treasure. Gen. R. s. 35 end מרגלית אטימטון. *Ruth R. next to I, 18 מילא דאריסטופרטא read מרגליתא אטימיטא an invaluable pearl.

אטימיסיאה v. next w.

אִיטִ׳, אֲטִימָסִיאָה f. (ἑτοιμασία) *well secured and supplied station.* Num. R. s. 16, end.

***(עטניך) עַטְנִיךְ, אַטוּנִיךְ** m. pl. (a contr. of נטע; אטעינין) *herbs selected for planting purposes.* Tosef. Maasr. III, 8 אטר׳ ed. Zuck. (Var. עטר׳; ed. אטו׳). Y. ib. V, beg. 51[c] עטנין. Cmp. שְׁתִילִין; שְׁתַל.

***אַטִּיפָא** m. (נטף, cmp. נִיטָף) *drop-like cavity in the cheese.* *Pl.* אַטִּיפֵי. Ab. Zar. 35[b] בינֵי א׳ Ar. (ed. אַטְפֵי) between the holes.

אַטֵּל Af. of נְטַל.

אִיטְ׳, אִטְלוּלָא m. (טְלַל) *jest.* Erub. 68[b] חוכא וא׳ derision and jest (Ar. a. Ms. Oxf. טְלוּלָא).

אַטְלוּתָא f., const. אַטְלוּת (נטל) *throwing, casting.* א׳ אבנין stoning to death. Targ. Y. Ex. XXI, 17; a. e.

אַמְלִיוֹן, אַמַלְיָא, v. אִימְלְיָא.

אִימְלִיס, אַמְלֵס, אִימְלִיז, אַמְלִיז m. (מלל, with format. ז or ס; cmp. אוּשְׁפִּיז; v. מְלַל II, מְלַל I, II) *a number of booths* put up for a *mercantile fair*, or for *popular entertainments;* whence (cmp. חָנוּת) *shops, bazaar* (v. esp. Gen. R. s. 79, quot. bel.). Ḥull. 91ᵇ א׳ של אמאוס the fair of Emmaus. Pesik. Asser p. 98ᵇ. Arakh. VI, 5 (24ᵃ) אם מכהינין אותה לארכלס if they delay the sale for the market day; a. fr.—*Pl.* אַמְלְסִין &c. Gen. R. s. 79 (ref. to ויחן 'and he encamped'=made a חנות Gen. XXXIII, 18) Jacob was the first מעמיד א׳ Ar. (ed. also חמלסין, v. חֶמְלֵים) to put up stores and sell cheap; [Koh. R. to X, 8; Est. R. to I, 9, sing., some ed. אַהְלִים, אִיהְלִים (!)]. Cmp. אִסְטֵל, עֲמַלֵּיז &c. [Tosef. Ḥull. I, 7 באמלס read בְּאַמְלֵק by *throwing;* cmp. Ḥull. 12ᵇ זרק סכין וכ׳.] V. אִיטְלִסִית.

אמליט, v. אַהֲלֵיט.

אַמְלֵס, אַמְלִיס, v. אַמְלִיז.

***אַמְלֵק** m. (v. next w.) *throw, thrust.* Tosef. Ḥull. I, 7; v. אַמְלֵיז end.

אמלקותא f. (מלק) *being thrown.* Targ. Job. III, 4 בְּאַמְלְקוּתֵיה (Var. אִימְלְ׳) on his being thrown.

אָמַם (b. h.; sec. r. of טמם) *to obstruct, close, fill up.* Part. pass. אָמוּם, f. אֲמוּמָה 1) *filled up, solid.* Zeb. 61ᵇ א׳ באדמה filled up with earth, opp. חָלוּל. Ḥull. 47ᵇ בריאה v. אוֹמֵם. Y. B. Bath. II, 13ᶜ top כותל א׳ a solid wall.—2) (cmp. מוּמְמוּם) *stumped, shapeless.* Nid. 24ᵃ גוף א׳ the stump of a human body (of the embryo). Ib. את שגולגלתו א׳ an embryo whose scull is a shapeless lump (no scull discernible). Y. ib. III, 50ᵈ top.—*Trnsf.* Snh. 44ᵇ אוֹמֵם עונות he locks up the sins (makes them invisible, cmp. טָמַן); v. אִימְמוֹן.

אַמְמָא (אִימְמָא) m. (v. foreg.) *something solid,* whence *the solid part, flank.* Targ. II, Esth. I, 2.—B. Mets. 23ᵇ אי דדפנא אי דא׳ Ar. (ed. או דא׳, אי, v. Rabb. D. S. a. l. note 3) whether from the ribs or from the flank. Ḥull. 42ᵇ בוקא דא׳ the thickest part of the flank (the thigh, hip).—B. Bath. 73ᵇ חדא דלי א׳ one (goose) lifted up its thigh (leg).—*Pl.* אַמְמֵי. Hull 8ᵃ א׳ דקייבי לקורבנא solid pieces (roast) intended for a present. Sabb. 49ᵃ.—אַמְמְתָא. Snh. 59ᵇ ed. (Ms. אַמְמְהָתָא). Lam. R. to I, 1 (רבתי) אַמְמָאְתָא.—Ḥull. 97ᵇ הנהו אַמְמְהָתָא those solid pieces of the thigh. Erub. 57ᵇ א׳ דשורא ed. (Ms. אטמאתא) flanks (projecting parts) of a wall. V. אִימְמָא.

אמנס, אמנם, אמנים Esth. R. to I, 14, read אֲנוֹנִים, v. אֲנוֹנָא.

אַמְפָּא v. אַמְרְפָא.

***אמקמיא**, prob. אַמַקְמִין or אַמַקְמֵי m. pl. (ἄτακτοι) *undisciplined, irregular troops.* Pesik. Ekhah p. 122ᵇ (explaining: 'thy princes are rebels' Is. I, 23) אדוניך מרדינים דהוו מזיינין א׳ 'thy lords are rebels'—for they equipped irregulars. [This seems to be the proper version restored from Ar. a. Var.; v. Pesik. l. c. note 75.]

אִימֵּר, אִמֵּר m. (b. h. אִמֵּר, v. Hebr. Dict.), sub. יד ימינו *one whose right hand is tied up* or *unfit for labor; left-handed.* Sabb. 103ᵃ א׳ יד. Men. 37ᵃ only א׳. Toset. Bekh. V, 8 א׳ בין בידיו וכ׳; Bekh. 45ᵇ א׳ בין ביד וכ׳ one either left-handed or left-legged (v. Rashi a. l.).

אַמְרְבּוּלִיס pr. n. pl. *Tripolis,* on the coast of Phœnicia. Y. Sabb. III, 6ᶜ top; (Bab. ib. 45ᵇ *Sidon*).

אִימְרוּגָא, אַמְרוּגָא m. (v. אֶתְרוּגָא) *orange* (tree, a. fruit). Targ. Cant. II, 3 (h. text תפוח, some ed. אֶתְ׳). Y. Ab. Zar. II, 41ᵃ bot.

אַמְרוֹן v. אִימְרוֹן.

אַמְרִיתָא, אַמְרִי f. (נטר; cmp. חֲמָרִי a. טְרִיה) prop. *something preserved,* hence *dough preserved, vermicelli.* Y. Ḥall. I, 57ᵈ bot. as I intend making אצוותי א׳ my dough into vermicelli. Y. Bets. I, 60ᵈ הדא אטריתא וכ׳ to make verm. (on Holy Days), if for drying them, it is forbidden &c.

אַמְרְכוֹנָא pr. n. pl. *Trachonitis,* a district east of Gaulanitis. Targ. Y. II, Deut. III, 14 (h. Argob). V. טרכונא.

אַמְרְפָא, אַמְרַף m. (=טְרַפָּא, h. טָרָף) *leaf.* Git. 69ᵇ (collect.).—*Pl.* אַמְרְפֵי, אַמְרְפִין. Targ. Ps. I, 3. B. Mets. 114ᵇ (Var. טרפי, v. Rabb. D. S. a. l.).

אִיר־ prefix, v. אַר־.

אִי I fem. of אַי q. v.

אִי II, אִי I (=אִין; h. אִם; cmp. אוֹ) 1) *if, whether.* Targ. Cant. VII, 13; a. e.—Ber. 2ᵃ, a. fr. אי הכי (abbrev. א״ה) if this be so (introducing an argument against one's opinion).—R. Hash. 3ᵃ כי משמש וכ׳ *khi* has four meanings, אי *if,* &c.—אי נמי (abbrev. א״נ) a) if you choose, it may also be said; *or.* B. Mets. 98ᵃ; a. fr.—b) *even if,* v. נְמִי. Ḥull. 12ᵃ א״נ דילמא וכ׳ (Rashi א״נ שבע ארניש וכ׳) even if somebody else overheard it; a. fr.—אי אמרת בשלמא (abbr. א״ב=אא״ב בעלמא אי אמרת) I grant, if you were to say .... הייני then would be right what &c.; v. בשלמא. Yoma 17ᵇ; a. fr.—אי .... אי *whether ... or.* Targ. Koh. XI, 6. B. Mets. 98ᵃ; a. fr.—2) adv. of interrogation, v. אִין II. Targ. Job XI, 2 Ms. (ed. אין).

אִי III (=h. אִין) *not.* Git. IV, 5 אי אפשר it is impossible. Keth. XII, 3 אי אפשי I want not; a. fr.

אִי IV (abbr. of אִית, as ליה=לי) *there is.* Y. Snh. VI, 23ᵇ bot. אי בי וכ׳ there is in me (the possibility of) doing, i. e. I can do it. Ib. כה אי וכ׳ what is it thou canst do? (v. Y. Ḥag. II, 78ᵃ top).

אִי II (b. h. אִי) Interj. *Eh! Oh! Woe!* Targ. Y. II, Lev. XXVI, 29.—Taan. 7ᵃ אי חכמה וכ׳ Oh, for such a brilliant mind in such an ugly vessel (body)! R. Hash. 19ᵃ אי שמים Oh heavens!; a. fr. Y. Shek. V, end, 49ᵇ אי לי שאני וכ׳ woe unto me, that I thus see thee! Y. Yeb. XIII, 14ᵃ top; a. fr. [Babli, usually אוֹי.]

אִי III (אִיר) h. a. ch. (b. h. אִי, אַיֵּה) *where? what? how?*—אי מנך *whence?* Targ. Josh. II, 4; a. e.—Hebr. אי זה (often אֵיזֶה, אֵיזֶה in one word) *who? which?* Y. Kil. VIII, beg. 31[b] לאי זה דבר נאמר with regard to what (in what way, sense) has it been said? Y. Shebi. I, beg. 33[a] ואי זה זה and which (ploughing time) is this?; a. v. fr.—Y. Peah III, 17[c] top ואיר דינו מירוג (=אירדין) and what is the meaning of *merog?* Kerith. 6[b] לאיר מיצרך צרכי what need is there (of the others)? Cmp. אֵיזֶה; בֵּיצַד; אֵימָתַי.

אֵיב v. אֵב.

אִיבָּא I, אִבָּא m. (cmp. אֵב) *growth, fruit.* Targ. Gen. IV, 3; a. e.; v. אִנְבָּא.

אִיבָא II, אִיבָּא m.=אַבָּא *father.* Targ. Y. Num. XXX, 4; a. fr.

***אִיבָּא=אִיבְּבָא** I, pl. אִיבְבַיָּא. Targ. I Kings VI, 38 (ed. Vien. אִבְבַיָּא).

אֵיבָה f. (b. h.; אֵיב, $\sqrt{}$ אוב or אב, cmp. אֲבָבִית, אֵוֶן, עָוֶן) 1) *enmity, hostility, grudge.* Snh. III, 5 an enemy is he who has not spoken to his neighbor for three days באי׳ in his grudge; a. fr.—משום (מפני) א׳ for the sake of preventing ill-feeling. Y. Dem. IV, 24[a]; a. fr.—2) *aversion, disgust, loss of attraction.* Y. Yoma VIII, 44[d] bot. חכלה מפני א׳ the bride (is permitted to wash her face on the Day of Atone.) that she may not lose her attraction.

אִיבּוֹ, אִבּוֹ (אִיבּוֹ) f. (אנב, $\sqrt{}$ אב. cmp. אבל) *[black]*, name of a bird (h. אֲנָפָה) *vulture* or *kite.* Targ. O. Lev. XI, 19; Deut. XIV, 18 (Targ. Y. אוכמתא). [Targ. Y. I, II Deut. XIV, 13; 14, gloss to v. 18; confounded with v. 13—h. text אַיָּה.]—איבו pr. n. m., v. אבו.

אִיבּוּד m. (אבד) *ruin, destruction.* Ab. Zar. 33[a] אזיל לא׳ is wasted. Hull. 11[b] משום א׳ נשמה to prevent loss of life (to save the convict). Bets. 22[a] אִבּוּד ממון pecuniary loss; a. fr.

אִיבּוּל I m. (אבל) *mourning;* v. אֲבֵילוּת. Yeb. IV, 10; a. e.

אִיבּוּל II, **אִיבּוּלָא** ch., v. אִבּ׳.

אֵיבוּס v. אֵבוּס.

***כפר א׳, אִיבּוּס**, v. אָמוּס.

אִיבּוּס m. (אָבַס) *stuffing, forcing food down the animal's throat.* Erub. 20[b] (first time) והא אי׳ כמאן וכ׳ in stuffing, is it not as if taking a vessel in hand &c.? [Second time והא א׳ כמאן וכ׳ omitted in Ms. M.]

***אִיבְּוּרְיָיתָה, אִיבְּוּרְיָיתָא** f. pl. (prob. contr. of איבעיר׳; בער), א׳ דוהרא *lamp-lighters*, hand-maids who attended to the lights. Y. Yoma III, beg. 40[b]; Y. R. Hash. II, beg. 57[d] R . . . . handled things forbidden to handle on the Sabbath על פום א׳ דו׳ (Y. R. Hash. l. c., insert שום) on the lamplighters' declaring that night had set in (חשיכה מוצאי שבת). [The context proves that our w. designates a person or persons.]

אֶבְלָא=אִיבְלָא. Targ. O. Gen. L, 10; a. e. ed. Berl., oth. ed. אֶבְלָא.

אִיבְלַיִים, v. אֵבִילִן.

אִיבָּעוּת (=אִי בָּעֵית, v. בעי) *if thou so desirest; or.* א׳ איכא—וא׳ איכא (abbr. אב״א) if you choose, I may say ... or if you prefer (another solution) I may say ... Yoma 28[b]; a. fr.

אֵיבֶר, pl. אֵיבָרִין, אֵיבָרִים, v. אֵבֶר.

אִיבְרָא, אֵב׳ ch. (=foreg.) 1) *limb.* Targ. Job. II, 4 (Ms. אִיבְרָא). Yoma 25[b].—Trnsf. *arm, wing, pinion.* Sabb. 90[b] א׳ דשמאלא left arm.—*Pl.* אִיבְרִין, אִיבְרַיָּא. Targ. Lev. I, 8, a. e. *(pieces).* Targ. Ezek. XVII, 3; Deut. XXXII, 11 (wings).—2) *membrum genitale.* Targ. Y. Gen. XIV, 2; I ibid. XLIX, 24.—[B. Mets. 84[a], v. אִיבְרָיָה.]

-אִיבְרָא (אבר *to be strong*) *indeed, to be sure.* Hull. 59[b] א׳ חזינא ליה indeed, I should like to see him. Git. 56[b] top א׳ מלכא את indeed, thou art a sovereign.

***אִיבְרְיָאתָא** f. pl. (v. next w.) *enough for a meal in the household.* Erub. 82[b] תרתי רִיפָתָא א׳ Ms. M. (ed. איברייתא, Asheri, ed. Ven. כבריתא, v. Rabb. D. S. a. l. note) two large loaves of the household (or of mourners' meals). [Rashi, expl. our w. as loaves of *drivers of oxen*, appears to have had before him the vers. of Ms. M. and to derive our w. from ברא, v. בַּר I a. אָפַר.]

***אִיבְרָיָה** f. (ברי, v. הוּבְרָיָא) *a meal.* B. Mets. 84[a] א׳ דר׳ וכ׳ one meal of R. Ismael &c. (v. Rabb. D. S. to איברייאתא, Erub. 82[b], note 1); cmp. Pesik. B'shall. p. 90[b] sq., a. Ber. 44[a]). [Some read אִיבְרָיָה v. אִיבְרָא 2).]

איברוו Y. M. Kat. III, 82[b] bot. read אִיפְּרָיו; v. אִיפַּר. [V. however, אִיבְרְיָאתָא end.]

איברייא Y. M. Kat. III, end, 83[d], v. הוּבְרָיָא.

אִיגֶד, v. אֶגֶד.

אִיגוֹרָא, אִיגוּר v. אגור a. אֲגוֹרָא.

אִיגָּרָא=אִיגּוּרָא. Targ. Zeph. I, 5 (pl.) איגוריא (ed. Vien. אֶגּוּ׳).

אִיגוֹרֵי v. אֲגוֹרֵי.

אִיגְיָאה f. (αἰγεία, sub. δορά) *goat-skin.* Gen. R. s. 20, end..

אִיגְלָא v. אִגְלָא.

אִיגַּר (II אגר) *[vaulted] roof.* Arakh. 32[a]; Meg. 5[b] שור א׳ a city line formed by joining roofs, opp. חוֹמָה.—

אִיגְּרָא, אִיגָרָא, אִגָּרָא (also איג׳ with Dagesh) const. אִיגַּר same. Targ. Prov. XXI, 9; a. fr.—Ruth. R. to

I, 17 (Par. 3) איגר פלטין roof of the palace. Git. 85[b] (Rashi איגרת, corr. acc.), v. אִגָּרָה.—*Pl.* אִיגָּרַיָּא, אִיגָּרִין; איגרי. Targ. II Kings XIX, 26; a. e.—Y. Pes. VII, 35[b] (Cant. R. to II, 14 אברייאה, corr. acc.); v. זִירָא I. Lam. R. introd. (R. Yoḥ. 1) ולא׳ סלקין and they ascend the roofs. Pes. 111[b] דבי א׳ those (demons) dwelling on roofs.

אִיגְּרָא *letter*, v. אִיגַּרְתָּא.

אַגְרוֹנִימוֹס=אִיגְרָאנָאמוֹן q. v.

אִיגֶּרֶת, v. אִגֶּרֶת.

אִיגַּרְתָּא, אִגַּ׳ f. אִיגְּרָא m. (=h. אִגֶּרֶת) *letter* &c. Targ. II Kings V. 5; a. fr.—Y. Ned. X, end, 42[b], a. e. א׳ דאיקר letter of honor, recommendation. Sabb. 115[a]; a. fr.—B. Mets. 83[b]; Snh. 82[a]; 96[a] (prov.) קריינא דא׳ איהו ליהוי פרוונקא let him who composed the letter be himself its carrier.—*Pl.* (of אִיגְּרָא) אִיגְּרִין. Targ. Y. II Num. XXII, 7 אִגַּ׳.—Targ. Is. XXXIX, 1.—אִיגְּרָן, אִיגְּרָאן, אִיגַּרְתָּא, אִיגַּרְתָּתָא. Targ. I Kings XXI, 9; a. fr.—Y. Keth. II, 26[b] bot. Y. Ned. VI, 40[a] bot. Y. Snh. I, 19[a] top.

אֵיד m. (b. h.; עוּד, אוּד, cmp. עֵת, אִידָּנָא) *turn, due day*, whence 1) *evil fate, reverses*. Gen. R. s. 13, v. אֵד. —2) *anniversary, idolatrous festival*. Ab. Zar. 7[b] יום אֵידָם the very day of their festival.—*Pl.* אֵידִים. Ib. I, 2, a. fr. (של נכרים) אֵידֵיהֶן. Ib. 2[a]; Y. Erub. V, beg. 22[a] (controversy as to spelling with א׳ or with ע). [As to cacophemistic designation, cmp. אבידן &c.]

אִידָא I, עִידָא, עִדָּא ch. same. Targ. Esth. I, 3. Targ. Prov. VII, 20.

אֵידָא II, v. אִידִּין a. חֵידָא.

אִידָא I, אִידָא f. (=ידא; v. אִי־) *hand* (only in Targ. Y.). Targ. Y. Deut. IX, 26; a. fr.—*Pl.* אִידַיָּא, אִידַיָּא, אִידֵי. Targ. Ps. XXIV, 4; a. fr.

אִידָא II f. (=אִי דָא, v. אִי a. דָא) *this, the same*. Y. Erub. III, 21[b] bot. א׳ אי א׳ אי חדא אמרה this proves this is this, this is that, i. e. it is the same. [Ib. חדא חדא היא חדא.]

אִידְּרָא *wool*, v. אוּדְרָא, a. אִדְרָא.

אידור m. (ὕδωρ) *water*. Succ. 35[a]; v. הידור.

אידוּתָא v. אַדְוּתָא.

אִידֵּי־ pl. of אִידַךְ.

אִידִית, אִידִי pr. n. m. *Idi, Idith*, an Amora. Y. Yoma VII, beg. 44[a]. Snh. 38[b]; a. e.

אֵידִין m., **אֵידָא אֵידָא (אֵיידִי) אֵידָנָא** f. (h. אֵיזֶה, אֵיזוֹ) 1) *who now? what now? which now?* (*quisnam, quidnam*). Targ. I Sam. VI, 20. Targ. Jer. II, 10; a. fr.—Tam. 32[a] א׳ מתקרי חכים who is to be called wise? Lam. R. to I, 1 (4 חד מאת׳) אחמי לי אידא וכ׳ show me now which of these is from a white goat &c. Y. Pes. II, 28[c] top ואיידא אמר דא what (passage) now says this (is this derived from)? Y. Sot. V, 20[c] bot. ואיידי חובתא עבדית and what is the sin I have committed? Lam. R. to III, 7 באידנא אסטרטא וכ׳ by which road did you come? 2) (ellipt.) *what do you want?* Y. B. Kam. V, beg. 4[d], v. חֵידָא.

אִידְיָנֵי, v. אוּד׳.

אִידִית, v. אִידִי.

אִידָךְ m. a. fem. (=הָדָךְ, with אי prosth.) *this, that*, freq. *the other, another*. Yeb. 62[a]; a. fr. תניא א׳ another (author or Boraitha) teaches. Ib. 22[b] בא׳ קרא in another verse. B. Mets. 98[b] וא׳ לא ידענא and as to the other (cow), I don't know; a. fr.—*Pl.* אִידֵי.—א׳ וא׳ these and those, i. e. *both*. Yeb. 8[a]; a. fr.

אִידְכְּרוּ v. אִדְּכְּרוּ.

***אִידָן** m. (אדר, v. אוּדְרָא) *tow-cotton*, &c., esp. *bast twisted for a wick*. Sabb. II, 1, expl. in Babli (20[b]) אחוריגא, v. אַחֲוָנָא 3), in Y. (4[c]) ערדניתא.

אִידָנָא v. אִידִין.

אִידָּנָא, אִידְּנָא m. (=עִדָּן, עִידָּנָא; עוד, אוד) *time*.— הָאִידְּנָא *this time, now, to-day*. Targ. Y. Deut. I, 6 (usu. with ע).—Yeb. 62[a] לילא דהא׳ this night. Yoma 19[b] הא׳ יומא וכ׳ to-day is the Day of Atone. Ber. 4[a] כי הא׳ at this very time (hour). Kid. 71[b] והא׳ דאיכא רמאי but now-a-days when there are deceivers; a. fr.

אִידְּרָא, אִידָּר v. אִדָּר.

***אידרוטירון**, read

***אִידְרוֹמִילוֹן** m. (ὑδρόμηλον) *a cider of quince jelly*. Y. Shebi. III, beg. 37[b].

אִנְדְּרוֹנָא, אִינְדְּרוֹנָא, אִידְּרוֹנָא, אִידְּרוֹן m. (אדר; Assyr. *idrânu*, v. Fred. Del. Hebr. Lang. p. 24; cmp. חֶדֶר) *an enclosure, chamber*, esp. *dark alcove, bedroom*. Targ. Job XXXVII, 9. Meg. 26[b] איד׳ דהוה וכ׳ a room where the corpse was placed before burial. B. Bath. 7[a] השתא משוית לי איד׳ ed. (Ms. M. וחשתא אינד׳) now thou makest my (formerly open) compartment a lightless alcove. Hull. 52[b]; a. e.—Men. 38[b] (fem.) א׳ מעלייתא a fine room. B. Kam. 85[b], v. חַרְזַק. Taan. 25[a] עיילא לאיר׳ she went up to the bed-room.

אִידְּרוֹנָה=preced.

אִידְּרֵי v. הִדְּרֵי II.

אִדְרְעָא=אִידְרְעָא.

***אִידרתר**, Koh. R. to IV, 7 זו אידרתר של מלאך המות (Var. in Y'dê Mosheh a. l. של א״ח), a corruption of a mutilated clause, part of which is to be found in Deut. R. s. 2 where Prov. XXIV, 21 is reprehended and Solomon is made to emend it with Koh. IV, 8 יש אחד ואין שני.

The passage restored would probably read: זו יראה את ר׳ בנו ומלך עם וג׳. אמר ר׳ אחא כעס הקב״ה . . . . חזר ופירש את הדבר יש אחד ואין שני וכ׳.

***אידתיקרימא** Y. Dem. V, 24[d], a corruption; prob. אִינוֹקְפִילְיָא m. pl. (οἰνοκάπηλοι) *keepers of wine-shops*, opp. שפייא; q. v.

אַיָּה pr. n. m. *Ayah*. Git. 35[a] א׳ מרי A. Mari, surname of one Aha b. Hidya.

אִיהָא (v. next w. a. הָא) *that, the same*. Targ. Ruth I, 16.

אִיהוּ, איהוא m., אִיהִי f. (=הוּ, הִי, v. אִ־) *he, himself; she, herself*. Targ. Y. Lev. V, 3. Targ. Esth. I, 1; a. v. fr.—Gen. R. s. 49 יסב א׳ וכ׳ let himself take ashes; a. fr.—*Pl.* אִינְהוּ m., אִינְהִי f.; נִינְהוּ, נִיהוּ; אִינוּן, אִינְךְ m., אִינִין f. (contr. אִנּוּן, אִנִּין); very freq.—Y. Bicc. II, end, 65[b] אילין מרדן=דינון אמירן. Y. Meg. I, 71[a] top אינון אינון are there only these (differences between the Sabbath and Festivals)?

אִיהִי I, v. foreg.

***אִיהִי** II, (האי) א׳ דַקִּירָא pr. n. pl. *Ihi Dakkira, Is*, a city on the W. banks of the Euphrates, and upon a little river of the same name; (v. Rapap. Er. Mill. p. 33, a. Sm. Class. Dict. s. v. Is). Kid. 72[a]. א׳ ד׳ (Ar. האי־). B. Bath. 24[a] Ms. R. א׳ דקי׳ (ed. האי דקרא, v. Rabb. D. S. a. l.). Ber. 59[b] (v. Rabb. D. a. l.).

אַיּוֹ pr. n. m. *Ayo*, a scholar. Bets. 37[b]; a. fr.

אִיּוֹב (b. h.) pr. n. m. *Job*, the personage after whom the Biblical book (ספר א׳) *the Book of Job* is named. B. Bath. 14[b]; 15[a] sq. Y. Sot. V, end, 20[cd]. Nid. 52[ab]; a. fr.

איוונטיאות Yalk. Ex. 376, read אוותנטאות, v. אַוְתֶּנְטֵי.

אִיוְיָא, v. אִוְיָא.

אִיוּל, אייול, v. אַיִל 2).

אִיזָא, pl. אִיזַיָּא m. (אזז, cmp. גוזא, חזרין, אוד) *prickly twigs*. Y. Maas. Sh. IV, 55[b] bot. (to one who dreamt that people ran before him—meaning power) דאת מייתי א׳ וכ׳ thou wilt carry prickly twigs and everybody will run away from thee. [V. Lam. R. quot. s. v. גְּבַב.]

אִיזוֹבְיָין, v. אֵזוֹב.

אִיזְגַּד, אִיזְגַּדָּא (Targ. Y. עִזְגַּד, עִזְגַּד) m. (contr. of אזדגדרא, ג softened into א or ע, cmp. אדרזדא, אזד; also זעוע, s. v. זעוע; מודעוע=מודנדן; Massorah אִסְגַּד־, אִסְגַּד־, Ispe. of גזר; Berl. Targ. O. II, pp. 63, 68; cmp. Mand. אשגאנדא, Nöld. Mand. Gr. lithog. table; v. גזז, גזר) *runner*. Targ. Y. Gen. XLIX, 21 ע׳ קליל a light runner; a. e. In gen. *messenger*. *Pl.* אִיזְגַּדִּין, אִיזְגַּדַיָּא, עִזְ׳, עִזְ׳, אִיסְ׳. Targ. Is. XVIII, 2; a. v. fr.

אִיזְגַּדֵּר pr. n. m. (for איזדגרד) *Yesdigerd, Yezdjird*, a Persian King. Zeb. 19[a] top. Keth. 61[a] bot. אזגוד (corr. acc.).

***אִיזְגָּרָא** m., pl. אִיזְגָּרִין (גרר, v. אָגוֹר; prefix איז־, cmp. אִיזְמֵל a. אִיזְגַּד) *mounds*. Gen. R. s. 74 בחקל דאית ביה א׳ וכ׳ in a field in which there are mounds (behind which people may hide) talk no secrets. [Muss. incorr. ד for ר.]

אִיזְדְּקַר v. זְקַר.

אֵיזֶה, אֵיזוֹ, אֵיזֶ׳, אֵיזוּ m., **אֵיזוֹ** f. (b. h. אֵי זֶה=אֵיזֶה, אֵי זוּ, אֵיזֶה הוּא) *who? what? which?* Ab. IV, 1 איזהו חכם who is wise?; a. v. fr.—באיזה צד in what manner, v. כֵּיצַד. [Chald. אֵידָא, אֵידֵין.]

אֵיזוּ, v. foreg., a. אֵיזִי.

אֵיזוֹב, אֵיזוֹבָא, v. אֵזֹ׳.

אִיזִי, אִיזוּ (v. אֵיזֶה=b. h. אֵיפוֹא, אֵפֹה, אֵפוֹ) *now, then, pray*. Yoma 30[b] אודו לי א׳ (miss. in Mss., Ms. M. 2 זו) admit then at least. B. Mets. 70[a] אימא לי איזו tell me now; a. e. V. הֵידֵין.

אִיזְלָא, אוזְלָא m., **אוזַלְתָּא** f. (אָזַל II) *web, net, &c.* Hull. 51[b] א׳ ומקרבי קיטרי a net in which the knots are close. Erub. 28[b] אוזלתא דאיכרי Ms. M. (ed. אוזלתא, Ar. איזולתא) the twist (of bunches) of the farmer.—*Pl.* אִיזְלֵי. M. Kat. 11[a]. Git. 60[b] אִיזְלֵי; v. אוּהֲרָא.—Erub. 8[a] פסק ליה א׳ לסורא באי׳ (ed. Sonc. אי׳) he separated the court-yards of Sura with nets (*hurdles, matting*).

אִיזְמָא m., v. חִיזְמָא. Tosef. Kil. I, 11 ed. Zuck. (ed. corrupt אזמאזמא).

אִיזְמֵל, אִיזְ׳ (אוזְמֵל) אִיזְמֵיל m. h. a. ch. (זבל √מל; cmp. b. h. סכל; cmp. אִיזְגָּרָא) *cutting tool, knife*, esp. *surgeon's knife*. Targ. Job XVI, 9; a. e.—Hull. 31[a] א׳ שיש לו קרנים a knife which has hornlike projections as ornaments. Y. Sabb. XIX, beg. 16[d] אנשון מייתי א׳ they had forgotten to bring the knife (for circumcision). Ex. R. s. 26 man מכה באי׳ וכ׳ wounds with a knife (operating) and heals &c. *Pl.* Chald. אִזְמְלַיָּא; אִזְמְלָוָן (f.). Targ. Is. XLIV, 13. Targ. Josh. V, 2.

איזמר, Y. Shebi. IV, 35[a], v. זְמַר I.

אִיזְקְפָה (איזקפא), v. אסקופה.

אִיזְתוּדָא, v. אִזְ׳.

אִיחוּי m. (אחי, Pi.) *the act of stitching together seam*, esp. with ref. to the rent of garments in mourning. Y. M. Kat. III, 83[b] top; a. e.—M. Kat. 26[b] א׳ אלכסנדרי Alexandrian (invisible) seam.

אִיחוּר m. (אחר, Pi.) *delay, detention*. Y. Meg. III, 74[b] top.

אִיחוּרָא ch. same. Targ. Ps. LXXXIX, 52, const. אִיחוּר.

*אִיחְטָא m. (Ithp. of חטא) *one in the habit of sinning.* Y. Taan. I, 64ª top הוה א׳ בלישניה was foul-mouthed; v. Arakh. 15ᵇ.

אִיטָא, אִיטָה I (ἦτα) *the letter* (η) of the Greek Alphabet, the numerical value of which is *eight;* used in the way of a phonetic play (ἤτω, or ἰτά as though an adj. verbale of ἰέναι) to indicate *going* or *death.* Gen. R. s. 14, beg. (proving that a seven months' child can live, while an eight months' child cannot) מדידכון אנא ממטי לכון זיט״א אפ״טא, איט״א אוכ״טא from your own (Greek) language I will prove it to you, '*Live* (ζήτω) *seven, Go, eight*' (ζ=ἕπτα, η=ὄκτω). Y. Yeb. IV, 5ᵈ top; Tanh. B'midbar 18 (corr. acc.); Ibid. (ed. Buber) 21.

אִיטָאלְיָא, v. אִיטַלְיָא.

אִיטָה I, v. אִיטָא.

*אִיטָה II (Syr. איטא, εἶτα) *and so* (indignantly). Y. Snh. I, 18ᵈ top א׳ עבדתני וכ׳ how thou hast been the cause of my putting rabbis to shame!

אִיטִימוֹס v. אֶטִימוֹס.

אִיטוּמִיסִיה, v. אֶטִימ׳.

אִיטְלוּלָא v. אִטְל׳.

אִיטַלְיָה, אִיטַלְיָא pr. n. pl. *Italy,* esp. the southern part of the peninsula, called Magna Graecia. Meg. 6ᵇ ed. Ven. (omitt. in later ed.) א׳ של יון זה כרך גדול של רומי וכ׳ (Ms. M. שברומי v. Rabb. D. S. a. l.) Greek Italy, that means the great city of Rome &c. Gen. R. s. 37 beg. Ib. s. 67 איטאליה.—Targ. Ezek. XXVII, 7; a. e.—Targ. I Chr. I, 7 אִיטַלְיוֹן.

אִיטְלֵיס, אִיטְלֵיז, v. אַטְלֵיז.

אִיטְלִיסִית f. (v. אַטְלֵיז) *station. Pl.* אִיטְלִיסִיּוֹת. Tanh. Masé 11; ib. (ed. Buber אִיטְלַסִיּוֹת); v. אִסְטַל׳.

אִיטַלְקוּתָא, v. אִטַלְקוּתָא.

אִיטַלְקִי m., אִיטַלְקִית f. (v. אִיטַלְיָא) *Italian.* Kid. I, 1 א׳ איסר הא׳ *As Italicus,* Italian as. Snh. VIII, 2 באיטלקי Y. ed. (Bab. הא׳, corr. acc.); Lev. R. s. 37 באיטלקית in Italian measure. Y. Sabb. XVIII, beg. 16ᶜ; a. e.

אִיטֻם Lam. R. to I, 1 (העיר), הא׳ read הָאִיטְמָא v. הִירִיטְ׳.

אִיטְמָא m. (אטם) 1)=אַטְמָא.—2) *obstruction, dam.* Kid. 70ᵇ.

אִיטְמוֹן pr. n. m. *Itmon,* surname of the angel Gabriel (*coverer of sin*). Snh. 44ᵇ; v. אָטַם.

אִיטָן, m. (אטט; cmp. חטט, a. אֶטָט) *calamus,* a reed used for writing (cmp. b. h. עֵט). Tosef. Kil. III, 14 Var. ed. Zuck. (text אוטם, prob. אִיטִים). Y. Kil. V, end, 30ª חיטין. V. חִיטְנֵי.

*אִיטָנִי f. (foreg.) *pencil, tube.* Sot. 48ᵇ א׳ של אבר (Y. Sot. IX, 24ᵇ bot. a. Ar. טני) a leaden tube (Rashi=גּוּבְתָא). V. טָנִי.

אִיטַּר v. אִטֵּר.

אִיטְרָא B. Mets. 39ᵇ; B. Bath. 29ᵇ Ms. M., v. עִיטְרָא.

אִיטְרוֹן, אִיטְרוֹן m. (נטר, cmp. טוּרְנָא) *watchman, officer.* Targ. Is. IX, 13; XIX, 15.

אִיטְרְטְלִין read אִיסְטְרַטִילָטִין, v. אִסְטְרַטִילָטָא.

אִיר v. אֵר III.

אִייבוּ, v. אַבּוּ.

אִיידָא, אִיידִי, v. אִידַּךְ.

אִיידִי (contr. of על ידי; v. אַי) 1) *by the way of, through.* Sabb. 109ᵇ א׳ פומיה through his mouth.—Naz. 2ª א׳ בהמה through the instrumentality of the animal; a. fr.—2) (conj.) *because, since as.* א׳ דתני .... תני נמי as the compiler had to state this, he incidentally mentions also the other. Kid. 65ª; a. fr.

אִיזָן Snh. 106ª, v. זְנֵי.

אַיְיכַל Af. of אֲכַל.

אַיִל, אִילָא &c., v. איל׳.

אִילֵּךְ (=אי הלוך) *where are those?, which?.* Y. Ber. II, 5ᵇ א׳ רבנן which rabbis?

אַיִּים, Pi. of אָיַם.

אַיִּין, Pi. of אָיַן.

אִיכוּנִי (cmp. חֲיוּנוּ) *is it he?* Cant. R. to V, 16 א׳ בריך is this thy son?

אִיינטפ׳, איינטבלינית read אִסְפְּלָנִית.

*אִיינִיס, אִיינִים Y. Dem. VII, 26ᵇ, R. S. to Dem. VII, 3 אטימוס, אטימורי׳, prob. אֶטוֹנוֹס m. (ἄτονος) *languid, feeble.*

אִיָּיר m. (אור; cmp. b. h. זִיו) *Iyar,* the second month of the Hebrew calendar, of twenty nine days, varying betw. the tenth of April and the eighth of June. R. Hash. 3ª; a. fr. [V. Schrader K. A. T. glossary.]

*אִייְרָא f. (אור; cmp. יְאֹר esp. Job XXVIII, 10; v. H. Dict. s. v.) *channel, duct.* Y. M. Kat. I, 80ᵇ bot. א׳ דציפורין וכ׳ the duct of Zepph. was damaged during the festive week.

אִיירִי v. אֵרִי, אֲרָא.

אִיירִינוֹן m. (εἰρίνεον, εἰρινοῦν, neut.) *woolen.* Esth. R. to I, 6 (ref. to Aquila's translation).

אִיַּשַּׁר v. אַשַּׁר.

אֵיךְ *as, how.* Targ. Prov. XX, 20; a. fr.

אֵיכָא (=אֵי a. כָּא) *where now?* (ubinam). Targ. O. Gen. XXXVII, 16 (ed. Berl.); a. e., v. אֵיכָן a. הֵיכָא.

אִיכָּא (contr. of אִית־כָּא) 1) *there is, there are (sunt qui).* א׳ דאמרי (abbrev. א״ד.) some say. Hull. 3ᵇ; a. fr. א׳ בינייהו they differ in this &c. Ib. 4ᵃ; a. fr.— מאי א׳ למימר what is there to say? how can it be explained? what can you reply? Ib. 12ᵃ top; a. fr.—*2) *he who.* Targ. Prov. XIX, 7. [Prob. to be read אִיְנָא.]

אֵיכְדֵין *how then! how!* Targ. O. Deut. I, 12; a. e.; v. אֵיכָא.

אֵיכָה (b. h.=אֵי־כֹה) 1) *oh how! oh!* Gen. R. s. 19; a. fr.—2) *Ekhah*, name of the Book of Lamentations, also מגילת א׳.—א׳ רבתי *Ekhah Rabbathi (Lam. R.)*, Midrash Rabboth on Lamentations.

אִיכּוּ 1) (=אִי כּוּ) *if now; oh that.* Bets. 4ᵇ top א׳ השתא אשתלאי if I (had given my decision forthwith) I should have made a mistake. Yeb. 46ᵃ.—Snh. 107ᵃ א׳ זממא וכ׳ oh that a muzzle had been put on my enemy's (euphem. for *my*) mouth! i. e. oh that I never had said this!—2) pr. n. f. *Ikhu.* Taan. 35ᵃ what is thy name? She said, Ikhu.—Said he א׳ נמטו כשוריך oh that thy joists were sufficiently long!

אִיכּוּל m. (אכל) *consumption, combustion.* Y. Ber. IV, 7ᵇ top, a. e. א׳ איברים the consumption on the altar of the pieces of the daily offering; v. אֵבֶר. [V. עִיכּוּל.]

אִיכּוּמָא m. (אכם) *black color, something black.* Y. Sabb. II, 4ᵈ א׳ החן black naphta.

אִיכּוּף v. אוּכָּף.

אֵיכָן, אֵיכָּן (אֵי־כָּאן, v. אֵי־כָא) *where?* also relat. *where*, &c. Targ. Gen. XXXVII, 16. Y. Ber. I, 3ᵇ bot. א׳ יצאת בת קול where did that divine voice come forth? Ib. III, 6ᵃ bot. מא׳ ללמוד one from whom to learn. Ib. IV, 7ᵃ מא׳ למדו וכ׳ whence did they derive the obligation of three prayers?—עד א׳ how far? how long? Y. Peah VIII, beg. 20ᵈ. Cant. R. to VI, 4; a. e. [In Babli הֵיכָן q. v.]

איכספיה, איכספות Esth. R. to I, 1ᵇ בני א׳ (Var. אוב׳), v. אוּסְפְּיָא.

אִיכְּפַת v. אִכְפַּת.

אִכָּר, אִיכָּר m. (b. h., אכר, √כר, cmp. כָּפַר) *husbandman, farm-laborer.* Arakh. VI, 3 (23ᵇ) אם היה א׳ (Mish. אכ׳) if he is a husbandman; a. e.—*Pl.* אִיכָּרִים. Y. M. Kat. III, 82ᵇ bot. איבריו (read אִיכָּרָיו) his farm-hands. [V. איבריו.]

אִכָּ׳, אִיכָּרָא ch. same. Targ. Is. XXI, 10; a. e.—*Pl.* אִיכָּרֵי, אִיכָּרַיָּא, אִיכָּרִין. Targ. Jer. XXXI, 23; a. e.—Erub. 28ᵇ, v. אִיזְלָא.—*Denom. אִיכָּרָיְיתָא f. pl. Erub. 82ᵇ רפתא א׳ *farmer's loaves;* v., however, אִיבְּרַיְיתָא.

איכרום v. אִכְּ׳.

אִיכָּרַיְיתָא v. אִיכָּרָא.

***אֵיל, אֱיָל, אִיל** m. (b. h.; אול) *superiority, patronage, arbitration;* v. Midr. Till. to Ps. LXXXVIII, 5. Ib. to Ps. CIV, 29 (ref. to Is. LVII, 19 *peace, peace* &c.) אילולי (אֱיָלוֹ) אֱיָלוֹ של וכ׳ but for the peace-making arbitration of the Lord &c

אַיִל, אַיִל m. (b. h.; אול) 1) *ram (the strong).* B. Kam. 65ᵇ if one stole טלה ונעשה א׳ a lamb and it grew to be a ram. Ib. א׳ בן יומו קרוי א׳ a ram one day old is called a ram (*ayil* is used in a general sense, irrespective of age). R. Hash. 16ᵃ; a. fr.—[*Pl.* אֵלִים. Tosef. R. Hash. III (II), 3 (Var. יעלים).]—*2) א׳ קמצא [perh. אֵיַל q. v.] *a species of locusts.* Eduy. VIII, 4; Pes. 16ᵃ; Ab. Zar. 37ᵃ אייל ed. (Ms. M. איריל), v. קָמָר.

אַיָּל m. (b. h.; prob. fr. עול=אול, cmp. Var. lect. of אַיֶּלֶת II; cmp. אלל) [*the climber*], *hart.* Hull. 28ᵃ; a. e.

אֵילָא, אֵילָא ch.=h. אַיִל 1); trnsf. 1) *beak of a ship* (a beam to which the head of a ram was attached), *prow.* Ned. 50ᵃ.—2) *projection from a lateral wall, buttress,* &c. Targ. Ezek. XL, 48; a. e. (Var. אִלָּא).—*3) (cmp. אַיִל 2) name of a *worm* or *mite* in grapes. Sabb. 90ᵃ איל (Rashi a. Ms. Oxf. איר׳).

אַיְלָא, אַיְלָא, אַיָּלָא ch.=h. אַיָּל. Targ. O. Deut. XIV, 5; a. fr.—Bekh. 7ᵇ.—*Pl.* אַיָּלִין, אַיְלַיָּא, אַיְרֵי. Targ. Y. Deut. l. c. (ed. Vien. ואִילָּן) Targ. Lam. I, 6.

אִילָא pr. n. m. *Ila* 1); a Tannai. Bekh. IV, 5 (29ᵃ), a medical expert כא׳ ביבנה like I. in Yabneh'.—2) an Amora. Yoma 73ᵇ; a. fr. [Other forms אילעא, אילא, חילא; v. Frankel M'bo p. 75ᵇ.]

אִילָא v. אֶלָּא. Y. Shebu. I, 33ᵇ bot. לא מסתברא דא׳ v. חִילּוּפָא.

אילאסריך v. אִילְצְרָא.

אֵילָהּ v. אֱלָהּ.

אַיָּלָה, אַיָּלָה, אַיֶּלֶת f. (b. h. אַיֶּלֶת; v. אַיִל) 1) *hind, roe.* B. Bath. 16ᵇ top א׳ רחמה צר the hind has a narrow womb (vagina).—2) mostly אילת השחר *the first rays* (climber) *of the morning dawn*; cmp. Yoma 29ᵃ. Y. Ber. I, 2ᶜ; a. fr.; (cmp. Gen. XIX, 15 השחר עלה).

אִילָהִין, v. אֱלָ׳.

אִילוּ v. אִלּוּ.

אילו, Pesik. R. s. 17 א׳ פילוס v. אִילְוּפוֹלִים.

אִלּוּ, אִילּוּ (late b. h.=אִן לוּ; cmp. Ez. III, 6) *if* (oh that!). Targ. Ez. l. c.; a. fr.—Gen. R. s. 12 א׳ היו.... היתה נאה if the pillars had been higher, it would have looked better; a. fr.—וא׳ *but if (considering), whereas.* Ber. 20ᵃ; a. fr.—וא׳ ר׳ whereas R. Yudah &c.—א׳ .... וא׳ *while ...., in this case on the contrary.* Ib. 37ᵃ א׳.... וא׳ וכ׳ דא׳ במעשה for while over pot-dishes we say the benediction &c., here, in our case we say—; a. fr. Y. Shebu. I, 33ᵇ top

—אי׳ מי ש׳ in the case of one who .....—כְּאִלּוּ, כְּאִילּוּ, contr. כִּילּוּ as if, as though. Y. Maas. Sh. V, 56[d] bot. כא׳ לפניו שינה as if the Lord were, so to say, asleep, when Israel is in trouble; a. v. fr.—Y. Kil. IV, end, 29[d] כילו.

אֱלוֹגִין, אִילוֹגִין m. (elogium) *record, bill of indictment, sentence stating the crime, verdict.* Ex.R. s. 15 שאעביר אי׳ שלכם I may set aside (cancel) your verdict. Ib. s. 31 אל׳. [Corr. acc. Num. R. s. 16 אלוגין; Gen. R. s. 28, beg. אגאלוגין; Lam. R. to I, 14 אנלוגין, אולוגלוגין Ar.; Midr. Till. to Ps. I, 5 אגלין; Pesik. R. s. 44 אמלוגין, אבלגין.]

אילווא Git. 69[b], v. אַלְוָא.

אִילְוָיוּתָא f. (לוי) *(lamentation at) funeral escorts.* Targ. Job. III, 7 Ms. (ed. אִלְוִיתָא; h. text לִוְיָתָן).

אֱלוּל=אִילוּל. Targ. Y. Num. XIV, 37.

אִל׳, אִילוּלֵי, אִילוּלָא 1) (b. h. אִילּוּ לֹא=לוּלֵי, ch. אִילּוּ לָא) *were it not, but for* (followed by h. שֶׁ־, ch. דְּ־, or by a noun without a verb; v. אִלְמָלֵא). Targ. Y. Deut. I, 1; a. e.—Mekh. B'shall., Amalek 1 א׳ שאמר משה but for Moses, who said &c; a. fr.—2) (followed by a verb without ש־ or ד־=אִילוּלָא h. אִילּוּ) *if indeed, if.* Targ. Koh. VI, 6. Targ. Esth. VII, 4; a. e.—*3) *oh that!* Num. R. s. 2, beg. א׳ הוא מדגיל וכ׳ oh that He would allow His love to be a banner over me! [אלואי as in preceding lines?]—*4) *whether.* Targ. Cant. VI, 11 א׳ פשן וכ׳ whether the sages among them increase &c.

אִילוּלְפוֹן, אִילוּלֵיפוֹן (=preced. with פון=h. פֶּן) *if not perchance, but for.* Targ. Y. Gen. XXXI, 42; a. fr. (in some ed. in two words אילולי פון).

אַיְלוֹנִית, אַיְלוֹנִית f. (prob. fr. אַיִל; cmp. זָכָר a. דְּכַר) *(the man-like) barren, wombless, incapable of conception.* Keth. 11[a] (etymol. from אַיִל) איי׳ דוכרינת *aylonith* means ram-like. Nid. V, 9 (47[b]); a. fr.

אילוסיס, v. אֶלְסִיס.

אילוסריקא, v. אוֹלוֹסֵירִיקָא.

אִילוּפִיסָה* pr. n. m. (prob. ὑελέψης *glass*-smelter) *Ilofisa.* Y. Ter. I, 40[c] top.

אילטוס, v. אַלְסִיס.

אִלְיָא, אִילְיָא, אִלְיָא (אִלְיָה) m. (אִלִּי, ילל, v. ילל; cmp. אֱלִי Joel I, 8) *mourning, lamentation, dirge.* Targ. II Sam. I, 17; II Chron. XXXV, 25; a. fr.—Y. Sot. VII, 21[c] top; Meg. 1, 71[b] bot. סורסי לאיליא Syriac is adapted for dirges; Esth. R. to I, 22 פרסי לאליה (corr. acc.).

אִילְיוֹס, אִילְיָאוֹס* m. (ἥλιος) *Sun.* Ex. R. s. 15. [The words from סנדריאוס to אורח are a marginal gloss, prob. to be emended: (אלכ)סנדרוס איוס איליאו׳ הוה שמו והשמש וכ׳ Ἀλέξανδρος υἱὸς Ἡλίου (Alexander the son of Helios) was his name, and the Sun is called a hero &c.]

אִילְיָן, v. אִלָּ׳.

אִלְיוֹ׳, אִילְיוּפוֹלִיס pr. n. pl. (Ἡλιόπολις) *Heliopolis,* in lower Egypt. Pesik. Vayhi p. 63[b] Ar. (ed. פוליס); Pesik. R. s. 17 אילו פוליס (corr. acc.)

(אִלֵּ׳) אִילֵימָא (=אִי if, and לֵימָא=לֵימַר) prop. *if to say,* hence a dialectic term in debate, *you do not mean to say,* or *shall I say?* B. Mets. 12[b] א׳ כשחייב מודה shall I say (it means) when the debtor concedes (his indebtedness)? Kid. 74[a] א׳ אהייא וכ׳ what does it refer to? You cannot say it refers to ..... Sabb. 150[b] (some ed. אל׳). Yoma 52[b]; a. v. fr.

אִילֵימָא I *unless, but for;* v. אִלְמָא.

אִילֵימָא II *mute,* v. אִלְמָא.

אִילֵין, v. אִילֵּין.

אילין Tosef. Kil. V, 26, ed. Zuck. קלא אילן, v. קלא אילן.

אִילָךְ, v. אִילָּא.

אִילֵּין (אִלֵּין, אִילֵּין) com. pl. (h. אֵלֶּה, אֵלּוּ) *these, those.* Targ. Jud. XX, 17; a. e.—Y. Ber. V, 9[c] top א׳ דמתרגמין those who translate; a. v. fr.—Y. Erub. III, 20[d] top אילין אינון insert באי׳, what are those (names mentioned)?

אִילִיס, v. אֶלִיס.

אִילֵיתָא, v. אַלְוִיתָא.

אִילֵךְ, אִילֵךְ (ch. a. h.; cmp. אִילֵּין) *hither, thither.* Targ. Y. Num. XXII, 4.—מכאן וא׳ (מכן) from now and further on, i. e. *after that.* Targ. Esth. II, 14. Ber. I, 2; a. fr.—Men. 28[b] אחד א׳ ואחד א׳ one in this, another in that direction. Erub. 55[b]. [Diff. from. אֵלֵךְ.] V. הִילֵךְ.

אֵילָם pr. n. *Elam.* Y. Kid. IV, 65[d] top; v. עֵילָם.

אִילֵם *mute,* v. אִלֵּם.

אִילְמָא ch. same, v. אִלְמָא.

אִילְמְנָא, v. אַלְמְנָא.

אִילָן m. (cmp. b. h. אֵלוֹן *oak,* v. אֵלָה) *tree.* Shebi. I, 1, a. e. שדה הא׳ a field containing at least three trees within a distance of a S'ah (v. סְאָה). Ib. 3 א׳ סרק bearing no edible fruit, opp. א׳ מאכל.—Pes. 112[a] (prov.) אם בקשת וכ׳ if you desire to be strangled, be hanged on a large tree, (if you must refer to an authority, select a good one).—*Pl.* אִילָנוֹת, const. אִילָנֵי. Shebi. I, 2. Gen. R. s. 16; a. fr.

אִלָ׳, אִילָנָא, אִילָן ch. same. Targ. Gen. I, 11; a. fr.—Ab. Zar. 50[b], v. ברי ch.—*Pl.* אִילָנִין, אִילָנַיָּא, אִלָ׳, אִילָנֵי, אִילָנַיָּא. Targ. Gen. II, 5; a. fr.—Lev. R. s. 12 א׳ (insert פירוחן) מתקריין וכ׳ fruits are named after the trees. B. Bath. 16[b]; a. fr.—Lev. R. s. 5 א׳ דסדום, v. אמבוניא.—[קלא א׳, חלא א׳, v. s. קְלָא a. חְלָא respectively.]

אִילֵס, v. אֶלִּיס.

אִילְסְרִין, v. אִלְצְרִין.

אִילְפָא I, אִלְפָא f. (ילף, אלף; Assyr. êlippu) *ship, raft.* Targ. Jon. I, 3; a. e.—Lev. R. s. 12, beg. א׳ בהדא like the ship tossed about on high sea. Koh. R. to III, 2 (prov.) at the time thou tiest thy Lulab (for the Feast of Booths) קטר אלפך tie thy ship (cease navigation). Ab. Zar. 10[b] ווי לה לאי׳ א׳ וכ׳ woe to the ship which leaves without having paid its toll (of a convert who died before circumcision).—Trnsf. *the body of a chicken (chest-bone resembling a ship).* Lam. R. to I, 1 נסבית הדין אי׳ וכ׳ (רבתי) I took for myself this ship (of the chicken), for in a ship I came &c.—*Pl.* אִילְפַיָּא. Targ. Ps. CIV, 26; a. e.

אִילְפָא II pr. n. m. *Ilfa,* an Amora. Taan. 21[a]; a. fr. [In. Talm. Y. חילפיי]. R. Hash. 17[b] אילְפָי וא״ל א׳ *Ilfay* or, some say, *Ilfa* (v. Rabb. D. S. a. l.)

אִילְפַי, v. preced.

אִילְפֵס, אִילְקְטִי, אִילְקַט, v. אִלְ׳.

אַיֶּלֶת I, v. אַיָּלָה.

אַיֶּלֶת II, אֵיְלַת pr. n. pl. (*not bibl.* אַיֶּלֶת) *Ayeleth,* one day's journey south of Jerusalem. Maas. Sh. V, 2; Bets. 5[a] עלת ed. (Ms. M. איילת); R. Hash. 31[b] אילת ed. (Ms. M. עֲיֶלֶת; Ms. L. עלת corr. into עיר׳; Ms. 2 עגלת; v. Rabb. D. S. a. l. note). [Bets. a. R. Hash. l. c. read מן הדרום for מן הצפון a. vice versa.] Cmp. אַיָּל.

אַיַּלְתָּא, אַיַּלְתָּא, אַיַּלְתָּא f. (h. אַיָּלָה) *hind, roe.* Targ. Jer. XIV, 5; a. e. Cant. R. to II, 9; a. e.—א׳ דשחרא (v. אַיָּלָה) *morning dawn.* Y. Ber. I, 2[c]; a. e.—*Pl.* אַיַּלְתָא, אַיַּלְתָּא, אַיַּלְתָּא. Targ. Ps. XXIX, 9; a. e.

אָיַם (√אי, v. אֵיבָה) *to feel aversion, fright.* Denomin. אֵימָה.

Pi. אִיֵּים (denom. of אימה; with על) *to impress with awe, forewarn* (witnesses). R. Hash. 20[a] מְאַיְּימִין על העדים we may try to intimidate &c. Yoma 4[b] לְאַיֵּים עליו to impress him. Sot. I, 4; a. e.

אִימָא, v. אֵמָא.

אִימָא I *distaff,* v. אִימָּה II.

אִימָא II, אִמָּא, אִימָּה f. ch. (=h. אֵם) 1) *mother,* frequ. *my mother*; v. אַבָּא. Targ. Gen. III, 20; a. fr.—Ber. 18[b] אימא לה לא׳ tell my mother; a. fr.—א׳ זקינה *grandmother.* Meg. 27[b].—2) trnsf. *the flesh of a stone fruit.* Sabb. 143[a] חזירן אגב אִימָן may be handled on account of the flesh (with which they were surrounded when Sabbath came).—*Pl.* אִימְּהָתָא, אִמְּהָתָא. Targ. Jer. XVI, 3; esp. *the arch-mothers* of the Israel. nation. Targ. Y. Ex. XVII, 9; a. e.—Kid. 82[a] א׳ דינוקי the mothers of school children. [V. also אִימָּה II.]

אִימָּא III pr. n. f. [or *title*; cmp. אַבָּא]. *Imma.* Y. Git. I, 43[c]; Shebi VI, 36[c] top א׳ שלום Imma (Mother) Shalom.

אִימָּאוּס, v. אֶמָּאוּס.

אִימָּה I *mother,* v. אִימָּא II.

אִימָּה II f. (אמם, √אם *to gather*; cmp. אוּמָּה a. עמם I in Ges. H. Dict.) *distaff.* Kel. XI, 6 (Ar. אימא, Var. עִימָּא).

אֵימָה f. (b. h.; אָיַם) *fear, awe.* Num. R. s. 9; Y. Sot. I, beg. 16[b] אלא בתוך דבר של אמה (read אימה) but from a solemn conversation (v., however, Maim. Sotah IV, 18 a. comment.). R. Hash. 17[a]; a. fr.—*Pl.* אֵימוֹת. Sabb. 77[b] חמש א׳ הן there are five sorts of fear. [Tanḥ. Tsav 2 אימת שירוף (אימות), v. אִימּוּס.]

אִימָּהוֹת, v. אֵם.

אימהן, v. אִימְּתָן.

אימולוגים, v. אומולוגייא.

אימום, v. אִמּוּם. [Tosef. Kid. IV, 8 באימום read בבִּימוּס.]

אימונים Koh. R. to VII, 11, v. אֶמָּאוּס.

אימוס Sabb. 141[b], v. אִמּוּם.

***אִימּוּס** m. (contr. of מיאוס=אֶמְאוּס; מאס) *disfiguration.* א׳ שירוף *one disfigured by burns.* Cant. R. to VII, 9 ונעשה א׳ ש׳ and he (Nebucadn.) became &c. [Tanḥ. Tsav. 2 (ed. Buber 3) ונעשה אֵימַת שירוף עליו and the fright (repulsiveness) of a burned face was put upon him. Midr. Till. to Ps. XXII אמבירוס, read אֶמְפּוּרוֹס, ἔμπυρος, *fire-scathed.*]

אִימּוּר, v. אֲמַר.

אֵימוּרִין, אֲמוּרִים, אֵימוּרִים I m. pl. (אמר, v. Ges. H. Dict. s. v.; cmp. Deut. XXVI, 17 sq.) *devoted objects, sacrifices.* Succ. 55[b] אֵמוּרֵי תרגלים וכ׳ (Mish. ib. אֵיבֵ׳) are not the festive Emurim (v. infra) the Lord's, i. e. to be offered on the altar? Answ. כה שאמור ברגלים *Emuré* &c. means, whatever is consecrated as offering for festivals.—Esp. *Emurim, Emurin, those portions of sacrifices offered on the altar.* Pes. 71[a] אֵימוּרֵי חגיגה וכ׳ the Emurim of the pilgrim's feast offering. Zeb. II, 2; a. fr.

אִימוּרִים, אִימוּרִין, אֲמוּ׳ II m. pl. (ימר, מור) *exchange* (cmp. חלופין as to pl.). בני א׳ *hostages* in place of their parents. Lam. R. to III, 13 ed. (Ar. אימרריא q. v.). V. also אמוריא.

אִימּוּרִין, v. preced. ws.

***אִימְּתִין** m. pl. (=אימת׳, play on מִיטָּה and אמיטתא) *those who go to bed with the setting in of darkness* (a witty expression made up in oppos. to שיחרין, v. שְׁחַר). Ex. R. s. 47 למדו תורה דא׳ learn the teachings of those who rested well by night (as better fitted to teach).

***אימיקנטרון, אי׳** Koh. R. to II, 17, prob. a. corruption of מקטרג *a malicious informer.*

***אִימִירָא** f. (ἡμέρα) *day.* Y. Ab. Zar. I, 39ᶜ top, they lament over it מילנר אי׳, μέλαινα ἡμέρα, oh, the black (luckless) day! V. Macrob. Sat. I, 15 *dies atri.*

אִימִירוֹן m. (ἥμερον, neut. or accus.) *tame, soft, gentle* (opp. אַגְרִיאוֹן q. v.). Gen. R. s. 77 end נמירון (corr. acc.). Num. R. s. 11; Pesik. Haḥod. p. 44ᵇ אי׳ מכון; Pesik. R. s. 15 אימירון; Cant. R. to III, 7 אדריבון (corr. acc.). Midr. Sam. ch. XVII (for אגריון read אימירון, for נימירון read אגריון).

***אִימְלָא** m. (=h. מְעִיל; contr. of אימעלא; cmp. מִילְתָא) *cloak.* *Pl.* אִימְלִין. Targ. Ez. XXVII, 24.

אִימָמָא m. (v. אִיר) *day time.* Y. Ber. III, 6ᵈ top; a. e. Y. Ab. Zar. I, 39ᶜ top א׳ ארך the day growing longer.

אימן Tosef. Kel. B. Bath. II, 6 read אִימּוּם.

אִימַן, v. אָמַן.

הַמְנוּן=אִימְנוּן.

אימְמריר, read אימריר׳, v. אִימוּרִים II a. אִימְרְרָיָא.

אִימְצִי, v. מְצִי.

אֵימַר m. ch. (=h. אֵמֶר) *speech, utterance.* Targ. Num. XXIV, 3; a. e.—*Pl.* אִימְרַיָּא. Targ. Prov. IV, 5 Ms. (ed. מֵאֲמָרֵי); a. e.

אִימַר, אִימְרוּ, אִימְרִיא (אימראו) *to retract,* v. מרר ch.

אִימַר, אִימְרָא, אִמַּר, אִמְּרָא (אִימְרָה) m. (אמר, √אם, v. אִמֵּם; cmp. נִמְרָא, חוּמְרָא, צִמַּר) 1) [*thick, heavy,*] *lamb.* Targ. Gen. XXX, 32; a. fr.—Ned. I, 3 'this be as forbidden to me כאימרא (Y. ib. I, end, 37ᵃ כאימרה) as *the* lamb'—כאימר תמידא that means, 'as the lamb of the daily offering'. Lam. R. introd. (R. Josh. 2) דהוה נכיס אמ׳ וכ׳ who slaughters a lamb and augurs from its liver. Erub. 53ᵇ (deriding the Galilean dialect) a Galilean cried אמר למאן וכ׳ who wants *amar?* (indistinctly pronouncing the vowels, as well as the guttural sound of א), when they said to him . . . ., חמר למירכב או חמר למשתי עמר למילבש או אימר לאיתכסאה (for var. lect., v. Rabb. D. S. a. l. note 10) do you mean *ḥamâr* (an ass) to ride on, or *ḥămar* (wine) to drink, or *ămar* (wool) for putting on, or *immar* (lamb) for slaughtering?; a. fr.—*Pl.* אִימְרִין, אִימְרַיָּא, אִימְרַיָּה, אִמְ׳, אִמְּ׳. Ezra VII, 9; a. e.—Targ. Ex. XXIX, 38; XII, 5; a. e.—Y. Snh. I, 18ᵈ top אי׳ רכיכין the lambs (of the spring) are yet tender (in a letter announcing the intercalation of a month); Bab. ib. 11ᵇ א׳ עדקין (not ער׳; v. Tosef. ib. II, 6); a. e.—Fem. אִימַּרְתָּא *ewe.* Targ. Lev. V, 6; a. e.—Hull. 51ᵃ. Gen. R. s. 44 end, the sow (Rome) pastures with twenty (young ones), ואי׳ ולא בחד and the ewe (Sarah) not even with one.— 2) (cmp. חוּמְרָא) *knot, bandage* on wounds. Snh. 98ᵃ כולהו שרי ואסרי אר׳ וכ׳ Ar. (in ed. a. Ms. our w. omitted) all of them untie their bandages all at once and tie them up all at once, but he attends to one at a time.—3) *fringe, border.* Targ. Ps. CXXXIII, 2. Targ. Y. Ex. XXVI, 4 (Var. אִימְרָא). V. next w.—4)* pr. n. pl. כפר א׳ *K'far Imra* (Lamb-ville). Y. Taan. IV, 69ᵃ bot.; (Lam. R. to II, 2 נמרא).

אִימְרָה (אימרא) h. f. (v. preced.) 1) *fringe, border, skirt; trnsf. the bordered garment,* (toga prætexta), *state garment.* Taan. 11ᵇ; Ab. Zar. 34ᵃ חלוק לבן שאין בו אימרא a white plain frock without border (without official distinction; cmp. toga pura). Y. Kil. IX, 32ᵃ top; Tosef. ib. V, 19 א׳ (ה)מפורסמת a conspicuous border garment. Y. Kid. IV, beg. 65ᵇ (play on אִמֵּר Ezra II, 59) פירסמו וכ׳ they made themselves as conspicuous as the border on the frock. Sabb. 105ᵃ; Tosef. ib. XII (XIII), 1. —Y. Yoma I, 38ᵈ top; Y. Meg. I, 72ᵃ bot. אִימְרַת חלוקי the skirt of my frock; a. fr.—[Lam. R. to II, 17 explain. אֶמְרָתוֹ ib., פורפירא, v. בוּץ.] *Pl.* (of אוּמְרִית) אוּמְרִיּוֹת. Neg. XI, 10. Y. M. Kat. I, 80ᵈ bot.; v. זוּג.—2) trnsf. *object of distinction, decoration* (play on הֶאֱמִירְךָ II); cmp. חֲטִיבָה. Mekh. B'shall., Shirah, s. 3 (ref. to האמיר Deut. XXVI, 17) עשאני וכ׳ He made me (His) decoration (chosen people) &c.; Yalk. Ex. 244 אֲמִירָה.

***אִימְרְרָיָא** m. (מרי, v. next w.) *rebellion.* Lam. R. to III, 13 (rendering בני אשפתו ibid. 'the children of those thrown down' (into the dung, conquered), Rab explains 'the children of his destruction' (v. אוֹפִיכָא, בני אִימְרְרְיֵיה the children of rebellion against him. (Editions vary, אימריה, רריא . . . ., אמורים &c., v. אִימּוּרִים II). [Esth. R. to I, 1ᵇ, independently interpreted, v. אוּפִּירְיָא a. אֲמוּרְיָא.]

***אִימְרְנָא** m. (=h. מְרוֹן; v. אִימַּר a. preced.) *rebellion.* בני א׳ *rebels.* R. Hash. 18ᵃ (translating בני מרון Mish.) (all creatures pass before the Lord for receiving their decrees) כבני א׳ like rebels (after surrender brought before a court martial; cmp. Midr. Till. to Ps. XVII, 1, s. v. אפיפסין, a. Y. R. Hash. I, 57ᵇ). [Rashi אמרנא=Syr. אֲמַרְנָא 'like young lambs passing singly to be marked for tithes'.]

אִימַּרְתָּא 1) *ewe,* v. אִימַּר.—2) pr. n. f. *Immarta.* Snh. 52ᵇ Im. daughter of Tali (prob. pseudonyms).

אֵימָת, אֵימָתַי (b. h. מָתַי; v. אֵי) *when?* Hull. 17ᵃ.— Ber. I, 1, a. fr. מאימתי from what time (of the day)? Shebi. I, 1, a. fr. עד אימתי; ib. II, 1 עד אימת how long (until when)?

אֵימַת ch. 1) *whenever, when.* Targ. Y. Lev. XXIII, 42; a. e. Y. B. Kam. III, 3ᵈ top אי׳ דמתיבון וכ׳ when they quote the Mishnah in support of &c. Ab. Zar. 53ᵇ כל אי׳ דבעינא לה whenever I desire it. Nid. 66ᵃ.—2) also אֵימָתַי (אימתי) *when?* Targ. Job. VII, 4.—לא׳ *for what time? until what time?* Targ. O. Ex. VIII, 5; a. e.

אֵימְתָא ch.=h. אֵימָה. Targ. O. Ex. XV, 16; a. e.— B. Kam. 28ᵃ; a. e.

אִימְתַי, אִימַתַּי, v. אִימַת, אִימַּת.

אִימְתָן, אִימְתָנָא, אִימָ׳ m. (denom. of אימתא) 1) *fear-inspiring, powerful.* Targ. Jud. III, 30.—*Pl.* אִימְתָנִין, אִימְתָנֵי, אִימָ׳. Targ. Hab. I, 7. Targ. Gen. XIV, 5 (Y. II, אמתניא, h. text אֵימִים).—2) *timid.* Y. Meg. III, 74[a] bot. ספרא הוה אימתן וכ׳ (ed. Krot. אימהן, corr. acc.) the school-master was a timid man and but for R. Abbahu that passed by, he would not have cleared the children out of the premises of the Synagogue. [Hebr. form, v. אֵמְתָן.]

אָיַן, *Pi.* אַיֵּין (=צַיֵּין, v. next w.) *to look upon, investigate.* B. Bath. 115[a] (play on אין) אַיֵּין עליו Ar. (ed. עַיֵּין) investigate his family relations. Kid. 4[a].

אַיִן I m. (√אוי; cmp. אֹון, עַיִן) [b. h. *naught*], *something rounded, decorative.* Koh. R. to III, 12 expl. as נוי, ref. to the shape of the human buttock, v. אַפִּיפְיוֹן.

אַיִן II, אָיִן (b. h. אַי; Nun emphat; cmp. אָן) *where?* (only with pref. מ or ל). לְאַ׳ *whither?* מֵאַ׳ *whence?* Y. Snh. X, 28[d] bot; Y. Hag. II, 77[a] bot. מא׳ ולא׳ whence and whither?—Aboth III, 1. Gen. R. s. 2 מא׳ הרגלים whence art thou coming? i. e. where hast thou been staying?—Y. Snh. X, 28[b] top הוה לו מא׳ ללמוד he had (a precedent) to learn from.—Contr. of מִנַּיִן: מִבֵּין אין, v. מִן.

אֵין (b. h.; constr. of אַיִן I) *nothing, not.* Ber. 5[a] אין עיף אלא וכ׳ *uf* (flight, Job V, 7) means nothing else but &c.; a. v. fr.—אֵינִי, אֵינֶנִּי *not I* &c. אֵינִי יודע I do not know; do I not know? B. Mets. 97[b]; a. fr. Ber. l. c. but the Holy One . . . אֵינוֹ כן is not so; a. fr.—אינו דין is it not a legitimate conclusion?, whence *so much the more.* Y. Naz. VI, 55[a]; a. v. fr.— . . מניין . . אין לי אלא from this I could only prove . . . ., whence, however, will you deduct . . .? Hull. 65[b]; a. fr. [Y. Git. IX, end, 50[d] אפי׳ כתב אינו read סימנו.]

אִין I or **אִין** (Syr.=הֵין, הִין) *yes, indeed.* Keth. 65[a] השתא א׳ וכ׳ now,—yes, but not before. B. Mets. 98[a] חדא א׳ בעידן וכ׳ as regards the one (cow)—well, she died &c.; a. fr.—אין הוי=אִינִי *is it really so? indeed?*, i. e. it cannot be. Hull. 96[b] א׳ והאמר it cannot be so; for did not R. . . . say &c.? M. Kat. 20[a]; a. v. fr.

אִין II, אֵן (h. אם) 1) *if, whether.* Targ. Ps. VII, 4; a. e. [Apocopated: אִי q. v.]—אין תימר (h. אם תאמר) if thou wilt say (argue). Y. Macc. II, 31[d] bot.; a. fr.—אין כדון (h. אם כן הוא) if this is (be) the case. Y. Naz. VI, 54[d] bot.—Lam. R. introd. end אן את יתיב וכ׳ if thou remainest here, or &c. Koh. R. to X, 5 אן אתת ענתה וכ׳ if the (my dying) time comes first, what of it? and if &c. —2) adv. of interrogation, introducing the alternative, *or.* Targ. Job VI, 6; a. e.

אִינָא c. (cmp. אִינְהוּ), followed by ד־, *he who.* Targ. Prov. XI, 26; a. e. (also אִנָּא ed.).

אִינָב m. (=b. h. עֵנָב q. v.) *berry, an excrescence on the eye.* Tosef. Bekh. IV, 2. [Mish. ib. VI, 2 עִינְבָּב. Talm. ed. 38[ab] עצב (corr. acc.).]

אִינְבָּא, v. אִנְבָּא.

***אִינְגַּד (נגד)** *prolong! go further!* Git. 58[a] א׳ פוסתא וכ׳ go one page and a half further, (and you will find it). [Rashi: *a little*=אִי־נְגַד, v. אִי III.]

אינגורין, v. אֶנְגָּרוֹן.

אִינְדְּרָא m.=next w.—*Pl.* with suffix of third pers. sing. אִינְדְּרוֹי. Targ. Ps. CIV, 3 Ms. (ed. אכסדרוי). [The verse is variously corrupted and defective.]

אִינְדְּרוֹנָא, v. אִידְרוֹן.

אינדרטין, v. אַנְדְּרוֹנִיטִיס.

אִינְהוּ, אִינְהִי, v. אִיהוּ.

אִינוּ Y. Git. IX, end, 50[d] אפי׳ כתב א׳, read סִימָנוֹ, v. Bab. ib. 87[b].

אִינוּמִילִין (אִינוּמְלִין) (וינו׳, אי־נוּ׳) m. (οἰνόμελι) *wine mixed with honey.* Sabb. XX, 2 (139[b]) אי׳ Ar. (ed. אנ׳, var. in Mss. יינומילין, וינמי׳, v. Rabb. D. S. a. l. note 20). Ab. Zar. 30[a] defined as a mixture of wine, honey and pepper. Ter. XI, 1 יינומלין Ar. (ed. יינומלים; Ms. M. אנ׳, read אינו׳). Y. Sabb. XIV, 14[c] top יינומילין.

אִינוּן, אִינּוּן pl. of אִיהוּ, אִיהִי.

***אינוניתא,** Gen. R. s. 29 ר׳ חנינא א׳, a corruption of איניניא or אניניא, dialect.=חנינא; cmp. Frankel M'bo p. 64[b] א׳ בן סיסיי with p. 88[a] ח׳ בר סיסיי. [Our w. omitted in Yalk. Gen. 47, Job 908.]

***אִינַחְתָּא** f. (אנח) *sigh, grief.* Targ. II Esth. III, 3. V. אֲנָחְתָּא.

אינטפלונית, אינ׳ Tosef. Kil. V, 25, read with ed. Zuck. אִיסְפְּלָנִית.

אִינִי 1)=אִין אֵנִי, v. אֵין.—2) אִין הִי, v. אִין I.

אִינִי pr. n. m. *Ini,* an Amora; cmp. אִינְיָנִי. Cant. R. to VIII, 11. [Koh. R. to IX, 10 איבו.]

אִינִיבָא, v. אִנְבָּא.

אִינְיָא pr. n. m. (cmp. אִינִי) *Inya.* Y. Git. I, 43[d] (Y. B. Bath. 16[c] חייה). V. next w.

אִינְיָנִי, אִינְיָנִי (אִינִינְיָא) pr. n. m. *Inyani,* an Amora. Y. Yoma III, 40[c]; a. e. Y. [Maas. Sh. IV, 55[a] bot. איניא, seems to be a different person, v. preced. w. a. Frankel M'bo p. 64[b].] V. אינוניתא.

אִינִין, v. אִינּוּן.

אִינִישׁ, v. אֱנָשׁ.

אִינָךְ 1) *those,* v. אִיהוּ.—2) *onyx,* v. אֶנֶךְ.

אִינְמִרִינוֹן, אִינְמוּרִינוֹן m. (a contraction of ἔλαιον μύρρινον; cmp. אינגרון as to נ for ל) *unguent scented* *with Arabian myrtle.* Cant. R. to IV, 14. [Muss. οἶνος μυρίνης; but the context requires an unguent.]

אִינְפּוֹלֵי, v. אַמְפְּלֵי.

אִינְקָא m. (ינק) *suckling* (infant or animal); cmp. יַנְקָא. Targ. II Esth. I, 2 א׳ די דהבא a suckling (kid?) of gold (lying, on the third step, opposite נמרא [not נשרא] the panther; ref. to Is. XI, 6). *Pl.* אֶנְקִין (אֶנְקְתָא). Ib. (end) א׳ בכיין the sucklings were crying.

אַנְקוּרָא, אִינְקוּרָא m. (נקר) *a bird with traces of bites or wounds on its legs; [black bird with white spots on its head*, quot. in Rashi; to be read אינקידר?]. —*Pl.* אִינְקוּרֵי, אַנְ׳. Hull. 57ᵃ.

אִינְקְלַסִיא, v. אִנְקְלֻסִיא.

אִינִישׁ, אִינָשׁ (אֱינָשׁ, אִינָשָׁא), אֵינָשׁ, אִינָשָׁא, אֱנָשׁ m. (אנש, sec. r. of אוש; h. אֱנוֹשׁ, אִישׁ) *being*, esp. *human being* Dan. II, 10, a. fr. אנש.—Ib. VII, 13 בר א׳ son of man (in Talm. freq. בר נש). Targ. O. Lev. XIII, 2; a. fr.—Y. Snh. VIII, 25ᵃ bot., a. fr. כאי׳ דמר as if one says. Y. Ber. VIII, 12ᵃ bot. אֱנָשָׁא רבא a great man. Shebu. 22ᵇ; a. fr.—*Pl.* אִינָשִׁין, const. אִינָשֵׁי. Targ. O. Gen. VI, 4; a. e.—אִינָשֵׁי, אִינְשִׁין. Targ. Y. ibid.; a. e.—In Talm. mostly אִינָשֵׁי *people.* B. Kam. 92ᵇ אמרי א׳ (text רבנן, corr. acc.). Snh. 95ᵇ היינו דאמרי א׳ (abbr. הדא״א) this is what people say, it is a common saying (proverb). Ibid. 10;ᵃ; a. v. fr.—Git. 45ᵃ אִינָשִׁין (our people?).

אִנְתִּימְרוֹס, אנת׳ pr. n. m. prob. a corrupt. for אַנְטִיפַּטְרוֹס *Antipater.* Targ. II, Esth. III, 1.

אִס־, אִיס־, אַס־ a prefix for the formation of (verbal) nouns (Ispeel nouns), affecting the first radical in the same way as the prefix of the Hithpa. or Ithpe.; e. g. from סגר, אִסְטְגִירוֹת (pl.) *rims;* from שור=סור *to walk, stride*, אִיסְתְּוָרָא *ankle*, &c. Before dentals איס and אס interchange with אִיצ־ and אַצ־. [Words not found under איס־ must be looked for under אס־ and *vice versa.*]

***אִיס (אס)** m. (υἱός) *son.* Ex. R. s. 15, v. אִילִיאוֹס.

אִיסָא pr. n. m. *Isa*, an Amora, disciple of R. Yohanan. Y. Ter. I, 40ᶜ top. V. אִיסִי.

אִיסְגִּינְמִירִין, אִיסְגִּנְטִירִין, v. אסגנטירין.

אִיסָדָא m. *Pl.* אִיסָדֵי (v. סרא, סדיא) *head-side, pillow.* Targ. Gen. XXVIII, 11; a. e.—Ber. 56ᵃ אאיסדן by our head-side.—[Ib. בי סדיא *pillow.*]

אִיסוֹ f.=אַסוֹ.

אִיסוּדָא, אִסוּדָא, אֶסוּדָא, pl. אִיסוּדֵי m.=יְסוֹדָא. Targ. O. Num. V, 17 ed. Berl.

***אִיסוֹפּוֹלִיטִיָּיא (אסְפַלְטִייא)** f. (ἰσοπολιτεία) *civic rights granted to strangers, isopolity* (v. Sm. Ant. s. v. Civitas). Pesik. R. s. 15 עבדות וגרות בארץ לא להם ועינו אותם ארבע מאות שנה אפילו [על] א׳ שלהם Ar. s. v. פלטריא II (ed. איספטלים, איספטלים, corr. acc.) 'slavery and stranger's condition' (indicated Gen. XV, 13) were in a land not theirs (in Egypt), but, 'and they shall afflict them four hundred years' refers even to their isopolity (in Canaan, from the birth of Isaac); Cant. R. to II, 17 באיספטלידה.... (corr. as above.). Gen. R. s. 44; Yalk. Gen. 77 לאספטיא..... (corr. as above.). Pesik. Hahod. p. 47ᵇ note 96.

אִיסּוּר m. (אסר) 1) *imprisonment.* Ber. 28ᵇ אין אִיסּוּרוֹ א׳ עולם the imprisonment which he decrees is not everlasting (as he may die and his successor may relieve me). 2)*(=אָסִיר), pl. אִיסּוּרִין *prisoners.* Ex. R. s. 30 he burst the prison open והוציא האיס׳ (ib. also האַסִּרִין) and set the prisoners free [prob. to be read אסירין].

אִיסּוּר I pr. n. m. *Issur;* 1) a proselyte. Ab. Zar. 70ᵃ. B. Bath. 149ᵃ.—2) an expert on coins. B. Kam. 99ᵇ bot.

אִיסּוּר II, אִסּוּר m. (אסר; cmp. b. h. אֱסָר, a. אִיסָר) 1) *band, chain;* trnsf. *social circle.* Succ. 45ᵇ (ref. to Ps. CXVIII, 27) כל העושה א׳ לחג וכ׳ he who creates a circle for the festival with eating and drinking, i. e. social pleasures. [Oth. explan.: he who makes an *addition* to the number of festive days;—hence the popular name of אסרו חג for the day following the festivals.]—2) *prohibition, interdict;* also *the forbidden object.* Y. Ber. I, 3ᵇ bot. דברי תורה יש בהן א׳ וכ׳ the Biblical law contains prohibitions and permissions.—א׳ ערוה *an obstacle to marriage by the existing laws of incest*, e. g. a man prevented from performing a levirate marriage because his late brother's wife is his own wife's sister; &c.—א׳ מצוה *a marriage* (or sexual connection) *permitted in the Torah but forbidden by Rabbinical enactment*;—so called because obedience to the Rabbis is a meritorious act (מצוה); א׳ קדושה *marriage restrictions* incumbent *on priests* on account of their sacred office; (another opinion inverts the last two definitions). Yeb. II, 3 (20ᵃ).—אין א׳ חל על א׳ one prohibition can take no legal hold where another prohibition already exists; i. e. you can punish, or impose sacrificial expiation, only for the first one; e. g. if you eat the meat of an unclean animal which, besides, has not been slaughtered according to ritual (נבלה). Ib. 13ᵇ; a. fr.—Exceptions to this principle (adopted by most authorities) are when the acceding act is: 1) א׳ כולל *a more comprehensive prohibition*, i. e. *having a wider range of prohibited objects*; e. g. the law imposing abstinence from food on the Day of Atonement includes food in general, i. e. food otherwise allowed as well as food forbidden at all times; א׳ מוסיף *a more extensive prohibition*, i. e. *having a wider range of persons concerned;* e. g. the sister of A's wife is forbidden to him (אחות אשתו) but not to his brothers. If, afterwards, his brother B. marries that sister of A.'s wife, she is forbidden in marriage (after B.'s death) to *all* the brothers as a brother's wife, and to A. both as his own living wife's sister and as his late brother's wife (אשת אח);—3) א׳ בת אחת *a coincidental prohibition*, i. e. two prohibitions *taking effect at the same moment*, e. g. the Day of Atonement coinciding with the Sabbath day, in which case the restrictions connected with each take effect at the same time (night-fall); 4) א׳ חָמוּר *a heavier prohibition*, i. e. a prohibition *imposing larger restrictions*, e. g. the law prohibiting *any* profitable use of a thing (א׳ הנאה), compared to the lighter prohibition, א׳ קַל, not to eat or drink a thing (v. infra). Yeb. 32ᵇ sq; Shebu. 24ᵃᵇ; Ḥull. 101ᵃ sq; Kerith. 14ᵇ.—א׳ תורה *a Biblical prohibitory law;* א׳ דרבנן *a Rabbinical prohibitory enactment.*—א׳ לאו *a prohibition expressed in the Law by a plain* (לא) 'thou shalt not', without defining the penalty, in which case the latter consists of thirty nine lashes (v. מַלְקוּת).—א׳ כרת *a prohibition to which the Bible attaches the penalty of excision* (by the hand of God).—א׳ מיתה a prohibition the transgression of which the Bible punishes with death (execution).—א׳ אכילה *the law not to eat* (meat boiled with milk); א׳ הנאה *not to make any use* (of it, as selling &c.); א׳ בישול *not to boil* (meat with milk). Ḥull. 115ᵇ; a. fr.—א׳ במות, v. בָּמָה.—*Pl.* אִיסּוּרִין. Ḥull. 98ᵃ sq. כל א׳ שבתורה (בטלין) בששים all things Biblically forbidden are neutralized if mixed with a quantity sixty times as large; ib. במאה—in a quantity one hundred times as large; a. fr.

אֱסוּרָא, אִסּוּרָא, אִיסוּרָא I, אִיסּוּרָא ch. 1) as the preced. 1), *band.* Targ. Ezek. III, 25.—*Pl.* אִיסּוּרִין. Targ. ib. XVI, 4 (bandages).—2) as the preced. 2). Ḥull. 9ᵇ; a. fr.—B. Bath. 92ᵇ כי אזלינן בתר רובא בא׳ בממונא לא we follow the majority principle (that a doubtful thing is presumed to have the legal status of the majority of its class) only in *ritual questions*, but not in civil law.—עבד א׳ to commit a crime, euphem. for *prostitution*, &c. Ab. Zar. 18ᵃ. Git. 38ᵃ.—*Pl.* אִיסּוּרֵי, אִיסּוּרֵי. Sabb. 60ᵇ שרי א׳ בבלאי a Babylonian permitter of forbidden things (R. Ḥiya).—Nid. 24ᵇ, a. fr. הלכתא כרב בא׳ Rab is the adopted authority in ritual law. [Kid. 12ᵃ זיל איסורי &c. read אַיסְרֵי; v. אִיסָר.]

אִיסּוּרָא II m. (יסר) *chastisement. Pl.* אִיסּוּרִין. Targ. Koh. III, 10. Targ. Jer. XXX, 11 (Var. יסורין).

אֱסוּרְיָא, pl. אֱסוּרְיָיתָא, v. אֱסוּרְיָיתָא.

אִיסְט־, v. אִיס־. For words under איסט־ not found here below, v. אסט־, איצט־, אצט־.

אִיסְטְבָא, אִיסְטְוָא, אִיס׳, אִיצ׳, אִסְ׳, אִצְ׳ [also ה—, a. with one י] m. (Ispe. noun of סבב, סב=h. סבב; q. v., b. h. מֵסַב; v. אִיסְ־) *a surrounding, attachment*, whence 1) *balcony, colonnade, portico* (also *an independent colonnade*), esp. הָא׳ the Itst'ba (Ist'ba) *the Temple portico.* Pes. I, 5 (11ᵇ) על גג האיצ׳ Ms. M. (Bab. ed. incorr. גב, Var. אִסְטְוָה, v. Rabb. D. S. a. l. note). Ib. 13ᵇ one recited על גב on top (inside) . . . ., say על גג הא׳ on the roof of the Its. (so as to expose it to public view). Y. Sabb. I, 2ᵈ bot. איסטוה וכ׳; Bab. 7ᵃ איצ׳ שלפני העמודים a balcony in front of the columns (projecting into the street, used as a stand for dealers, v. אִיסְטְב). Ib. דוקא א׳ דלא ניחא תשמישיה Ms. M. (ed. א׳ הוא דלא) only the colonnade the use of which for passers by is not convenient. Num. R. s. 12 two columns of silver which were placed in front of the Ark כמין איסטויה (Cant. R. to I, 11 אִיסְטְוִוין pl.) forming a kind of balcony; Y. Sot. VIII, 22ᶜ תנם לא׳ allow the surplus of three handbreadths (over the space occupied by the Tablets) for the balcony.—Yoma 49ᵃ דעביד מעשה אסטווה Ar. (ed. איצ׳) they (the laymen) served only the purpose of a portico (holding the bowls up to view, v. Pes. I, 5, but not handing them to the altar).—Y. Succ. V, 55ᵃ bot., v. דִּיפְלִי.—2) (cmp. הֵסֵב, הַסִּיבָּה) *something to recline on; couch, seat.* Kid. 70ᵃ, (to one using the high-toned קפיטא q. v.) א׳ דאמרי אינשי call it itst'ba as the people do.—M. Kat. 10ᵇ למבני א׳ Ar. a. ed. (Var. as Yoma l. c.) to build a temporary *banqueting place* for guests during the festive week, cmp. אַבְּרִינְקָא, (Rashi: *stone building*, Ms. Rashi כסא).—*Pl.* אִיצְטְבָאוֹת (h. form). Ex. R. s. 31 (basilicas).—אִיצְטְבֵי (Chald. form). Pes. 65ᵇ דמסגי אא׳ they (the priests) walked alongside the walls on balconies (projecting boards made for them that they should not tread on the blood); Y. ib. V, 32ᶜ bot. מְטְעִיָּיתָא. V. מִסְטָוָה.

***אִיסְטַגְלִילִית** f. (Ispe. of סגלל; r. סגל; cmp. סגלגל a. b. h. אֶשְׁכּוֹל) *cluster, a crowded band.* Ber. 51ᵃ א׳ של מלאכים וכ׳ Ms. Beth Nath. (Ar. אִסְטַלְגָנִית, ed. אִיסְתַּלְגָנִית, transpose איסטגל׳, Ms. M. איסטלתנות read אִיסְתַּלְתָּלִית fr. תִּלְתֵּל; v. Rabb. D. S. a. l.) a cluster of angels of destruction.

אִיסְטַגְנִינוּת, אִיסְטַגְנִין, v. אִסְטַ׳.

אִיסטדומוטא, v. אִסְטְרִיפּוֹמְפָּא.

אִיסְטַדְיָה, אִיסְטַדְיָא &c., v. אִיצְטַ׳ a. אִסְטַרְיָא.

אִיסטדין, v. אִיצְטַדִין a. אִסְטַרִין.

אִיסְטְדִירָא, v. אִיסְטְרִידָא.

אִיסְטַהַר pr. n. f. (r. זהר=סהר) *Istahar* (beauty). Yalk. Gen. 44 (a legendary personage).

אִיסְטְוָה, אִיסְטְוָא I, v. אִיסְטְבָא.

אִיסְטְוָא II, אִס׳ (m.?) (Isp. noun of סוי; cmp. b. h. סוּת, מַסְוֶה) *cover, blanket, (coarse) cloak.* Y. Maas. Sh. IV, 55ᵇ א׳ דהדין גברא אית ביה—מרקען (ed. Krot. בָּה . . . מקרען . . . *rents*) this man's (thy) blanket has twelve patches (Lam. R. to I, 1 חד כיתאר, 1 has מרדעא).

אִיסְטְוָוה v. supra.

אִיסְטְוָונָא m. (v. אִיסְטְבָא) *a balcony* (h. עֹמֶד, עַמּוּד). Targ. II Kings XI, 14; II Chron. XXXIV, 31, a. e. בֵּיה . . . . the balcony (of his palace).

אִיסְטְוָונִית, אִיצ׳, אִס׳, אִצ׳ (v. אִיסְטְבָא) *a system of colonnades, colonnade with double rows, basilica* (v. Sm. Ant. s. v. Basilica). Pes. 13ᵇ א׳ היתה נקראת (the itst'ba of the Temple being of double rows) was called *ist'vanith*, v. סְטָיו, אִסְטְיו. Ohol. XVIII, 9 (ed. . . . נִיּוֹת pl.). Tosef. Sabb. I, 4; a. fr.—*Pl.* אִיסְטְוָונִיּוֹת. Ohol. l. c., v. supra.—Tanḥ. Mishp. 14 (ed. Bub. 6 איסטונין corr. acc.). Tosef. Oh. XVIII, 12 אִיסְטְוָנוֹת (prob. incorr.).

אִיסְטְווֹרָא, v. אִיסְתְּ׳.

אִיסְטְוִיט, v. סוּט ch.

אִיסְמוֹלִין, אִיסְמוֹלִי, v. אִסְטְלִי.

אִיסְטְוָנוֹת, v. אִיסְטְוָנִית.

איסטופימא, v. אֶטְרִימְיטוֹן.

***אִיסְטַטְיוֹן (אישטטיון)** m. (στατίων, statio, v. Harper's Lat. Dict. 1882 s. v. Statio II, B, 4) *seat of the fiscal officers in the Roman provinces*, also *the staff of officers*. Gen. R. s. 66 (play on *Shulamith* Cant. VII, 1) the people of Israel שמשלמת אִיסְטַטְיוֹנוֹ של עולם וכ׳ that preserves the (divine) government of the world complete (filling the vacancies) both in this world &c. Cant. R. to l. c. איסטטיונרון, read אִיסְטַטְיוֹנָרִין (stationarii) the number of officers (of the divine government). Cmp. צַדִּיק. V. סַטְטְיוֹנֵר.

איסטטיונרון, v. אִיסְטַטְיוֹן.

אִיסְטַטִית, v. אִסְטְנִית.

***אִיסְטְטָנִית** f. (Ispa. of סטן) *querulous*.—*Pl.* אִיסְטְטָנִיּוֹת. Gen. R. s. 45. [Deut. R. s. 6 אִיסְטְסוֹנִיּוֹת; אִיסְטְסָנִיּוֹת; Ar. סְטִיסְיָאגוֹת, denom. of סוּסְיָא, סִיס, *scratching like a bird*; v. Gen. R. l. c. quot. s. v. חָמַס, a. Hull. 62ᵃ s. v. סְנוּנִית.] V. אִסְטָנִית.

אִיסְטִיב, אִס׳ m. (Isp. n. of סב in סבב; cmp. b. h. מוּסַב, מֵסַב) *an extension around the house* (gen. with a stone bench) *used as workshop or dealer's shop, portico, colonnade* (cmp. מִסְטוֹבָא). Y. B. Bath. II, beg. 13ᵇ top, R.—drove a pastry dealer מא׳ לא׳ from portico to portico (it being private ground). Ib. III, end, 14ᵇ a window שהיא פתוחה לא׳ וכ׳ opening towards a porch is made only for letting light in. V. אִיסְטְבָא.

אִיסְטִיו, אִס׳ m. (v. preced., a. אִיסְטְבָא) *colonnade*. Y. Succ. V, 55ᵃ bot.; Y. Taan. III, 66ᵈ bot.; v. סְטָיו.

איסטיוט, v. סוּט.

איסטיוות Y. Ab. Zar. II, 42ᵃ bot., v. אִסְטְגִיּוֹת.

אִיסְטִימִית, v. אִסְטָנִית.

אִיסְטְיָיא pr. n. m. *Istya*. Y. Yeb. I, 2ᶜ.

***איסטילין** Midr. Sam. ch. XI, v. אִסְטְלִי.

איסטיס, איסטית Ex. R. s. 15, read אִיסְטִיב; cmp. Tanḥ. Hayé, 3 ארצטבא.

(סְטִיס) אִסְטִיס, אִיסְטִיס f. (ἰσάτις, isatis tinctoria) *a plant producing a deep blue dye, woad*. Shebi. VII, 1. Y. ib. 37ᵇ אסטים (corr. acc.). B. Kam. 101ᵇ אס׳ Ar. (ed. סטים, סטרם; corr. acc.). Meg. IV, 7; a. fr.

איסטיסית, v. אִסְטָנִית.

איסטירטיגוס Midr. Till. to Ps. XVII, beg. כמין א׳ read אִיסְפַּרְגּוֹס, v. סְפַרְגּוֹס. [V. אִסְטְרַטִיגוֹס.]

איסטי״ת Ex. R. s. 15, read אִיסְטִיב, v. איסטיס.

אִיסְטְמָא, אִצְטְמָא f. 1) (h. צָמָּה; Ispe. of √צם) *something restraining* (the hair from flying), *band, chaplet* (of woolen and other stuff). Sabb. 57ᵇ (Ms. M. אצ׳); v. בִּזְיוּנָא. Tosef. ib. IV, 7, Kil. V, 26.—2) *steel*, v. אִסְטְמָא.

***איסטמאה** Ms. M. איסטמי מייתי, Ar. אסטמיתיה, Ms. O. איסתמתיה, some ed. איסטמה, a word in a charm formula (apparently a fictitious denom. of סמי). Sabb. 67ᵃ.

איסטנינותיא, v. אִיסְטַפְנִינֵי.

אִיסְטְנִיס m. *delicate*, v. אִיסְתְּנִיס.

אִיסְטְסָנִית, אִיסְטְסוֹנִית, v. אִיסְטְסָנִית.

איסטפנין, v. next w.

(אִיסְתַּפְנִינֵי) אִיסְטַפְנִינֵי, אִיסְטַפְלִינִין m. pl. (σταφυλῖνος, οι, Syr. אסטפלינין P. Sm. 301, prob. of Semit. orig., rad. טבל) *a kind of carrot, parsnip*. Y. Maasr. II, end, 50ᵃ bot. Y. Hall. IV, 60ᵃ top אִיסְתַּ׳. Ib. אִיסְטַפְנִינוֹתָא read אִיסְטַפְנִינְיתֵיה his parsnip. Y. Kil. I, 27ᵃ bot. אסטפלינון R. Sims. to Kil. I, 4 (ed. corrupt). Tosef. Ukts. I, 1 אסטפנין.

אִיסְטְרָא, v. אִיסְתְּרָא.

אִיסְטְרוֹבִּיל, אִיסְטְרוֹבְּלָא, אִס׳, אִצְ׳, אִיצְ׳ m. (στρόβιλος) 1) *cone*, also *kernel of the stone pine*, (nux pinea).—*Pl.* אִיסְטְרוֹבִּילִין, אִיסְטְרוֹבְלִין &c. Ab. Zar. I, 5 (13ᵇ sq.); defined ibid. *fruit of the cedar* (stone pine); a. fr. Pesik. R. s. 10 אסטרובלית (read —לִים or —לוֹת).—2) (v. Sm. Ant. s. v. Mola) *the cone* or *lower millstone* (which is immovable, hence included in the sale of the house). B. Bath. IV, 3. Zabim IV, 2.—*Pl.* אִסְטְרוֹבְלִין, אִיסְטְרוֹבִילֵי &c. Gen. R. s. 28; a. e. Keth. 69ᵃ Ar. (ed. more correctly בל . . . . ., sing.).

אִיסְטְרוֹבִילוֹס pr. n. m. *Istrobilos* (v. preced.; but prob. a corrupt. of אֲרִיסְטוֹבוּלוֹס). Y. Kil. IX, 32ᶜ bot. (Y. Keth. XII, 35ᵇ איסטריבוליא, corr. acc.).

אִיסְטְרוֹגֵי m. pl., a. corrupt. of אִיסְטְרַטִיגֵי, v. אִסְטְ׳.

איסטרולוגוס and deriv., v. אִסְ׳. [Koh. R. to I, 14, read לוֹגִיסְטֵס.]

איסטרטטי Cant. R. to VII, 9, defining גבריא Dan. III, 2, read אִיסְטְרַטִילָטֵי, v. אִסְ׳.

איסטריא, Men. 103ᵇ, v. אִסְטְרַטְיָא a. אִסְטַרְיָא.

איסטריבוליא, v. אִיסְטְרוֹבִילוֹס.

***(אִיסְטְרִידָא (אִיסטדירא, אִיסְתְּ׳, אִצְטְ׳** m. (Ispe. of סרד, cmp. סְרִיד, סְרָדָא &c.) *net-work*, esp.

rigging, sail-yard, sails. [If the vers. אִסְתְּדִירָא, אִיסְטְדִירָא, v. Rabb. D. S. to Sabb. 111[b] note 2, be correct, it must be derived from סדר; cmp. b. h. סְדֵרָה, סְדרוֹן.] Sabb. 111[b] קטרא דקטרי באי׳ the loop which they make when attaching the sail to the rigging. Ib. ודאי׳ גופה and the (permanent) knots in the rigging or ropes.

איסטריפומטא, v. אִסְטְרוּפוּמָטָא.

***אִיסְטַרְכִין** m. pl. (Ispe. of סרך; cmp. b. h. שָׂרוֹךְ) *plaited chords*, as a collect. noun fem. *a girdle of strips of cloth* (used by washers). Y. B. Kam. X, end, 7[c] הוה עביד ליה חדא א׳ וכ׳ used to make for himself one girdle of one kind of wool (so as not to be suspected of using strips of the cloths given him for washing).

אִיסִי pr. n. m. *Isi*, abbr. of Joseph (v. Yoma 52[b] הוא יוסף הוא א׳), esp. known: I. b. Y'hudah, an Amora; (v. Frankel M'bo, p. 100[b]). Ḥull. 115[b]; a. fr.

איסיפקאות, v. אִסְקָפָא.

אִיסְכּוֹלִי, v. אִסְ׳.

אִסְ׳, אִיסְכּוֹלַסְטִיקָא m. (σχολαστικός, *scholasticus;* S.; D. C.) *scholasticus=causidicus, advocate, pleader.* Y. Ber. IV, 7[d]; cmp. Gen. R. s. 64, end, אסקולסטיקא דאיריותא Ar. (trnsp. ב a. ק; ed. איבלוסטקיא; corr. acc.) pleader in behalf of the Jewish law.—*Pl.* אִיסְכּוֹלַסְטִיקִי. Cant. R. to VII, 9 איסכליסקי, corr. acc.—אִיסְכּוֹלַסְטִיקִין. Ex. R. s. 43 בקתדרה של אסב׳ (corr. acc., כי mistaken for ט) like the pulpit of the scholastici. [Also written סְכּוֹ׳.]

איסכופיה pr. n. pl. א׳ דשילה *Iskufia, near Shiloh.* Y. Meg. I, 72[d] top, expl. תאנת שלה Josh. XVI, 6 (σκοπιά; cmp. Zeb. 118[b], as quot. in Yalk. Deut. 881).

איסכלא, v. אַסְכ׳ a. אִסְ׳.

איסכלוסקי, v. אִיסְכּוֹלַסְטִיקָא.

***איסמטא** f. (=סְמִטָא q. v.; סמט=שמט) *recess of the market place, alley.* Y. Ber. III, 6[c] bot.

***איסניא** Gen. R. s. 37, v. איסיא.

איספו, Tanḥ. T'rumah, 9 א׳ נרמוז, v. אִיסְפֶּנְדְּמְנוֹס.

איספוטיקוס read אִיפְּטִיקוֹס.

איספוסין, v. אִיפּוּסִין.

איספטיא, איספמ״יה, איספמלי״ה. v. אִיסוֹפּוֹלִיטִירָא.

איספטר, v. אִסְפָּתֵי.

איספי Tanḥ. T'rumah, 9, v. איספו.

איספיטין Yalk. Ps. 808, v. אִיסְפְּרִידִין.

***איספיסריאון, קומיס א׳,** Lev. R. s. 5, read אוֹפְּסְרִיאוֹ (ὀψαρίου)=*comes annonæ;* v. D. C. s. v. Comes.

אִיסְפְּלָנִית(א). איספליטון, אִיסְפְּלִידָא.

אִיסְפְּמִיָא, v. אִסְפְּ׳.

אִיסְפֶּנְדְּמְנוֹס m. (σφενδάμνος) *maple-tree.* Tanḥ. T'rumah, 9 איספי נרמוז ed. (Ar. אספינדמין; corr. acc.) *Tidhar* (Is. LX, 13) means &c.

***אִיסְפָּקָא** m. (ספק) prop. *feeder, supplier*, hence *vessel in which wine is put on the table* (amphora). Targ. O. Ex. XVI, 33 Ar. (ed. צלוחית). Git. 14[a]. Cmp. זֶפֶק.

איספקאות, v. אִסְקָפָא.

סְפִיקְלָטוֹר, אִיסְפִּקְלָטוֹר m. (speculator, spiculator) *arm-bearer*, esp. *guardsman* of the Roman Emperor; mostly *executioner, torturer* (v. D. C. s. v.). Sabb. 108[a]. Num. R. s. 19. Lev. R. s. 26 סְפ׳. Lam. R. to II, 1. V. סְפִיקוּלָא.

סְפוּקְלָטוֹרָא, אִיסְפַּקְלָטוֹרָא ch. same. *Pl.* ־רַיָא, ־רֵי ... Targ. II Esth. V, 2. Targ. Y. Gen. XXXVII, 36.

אִיסְפַּקְלַרְיָא, v. אִסְפְּ׳.

***איספקסיטין**, read אוֹפְּסַרְטִיטֵיס m. (ὀψαρτυτής) *cook.* Esth. R. to I, 14, read הא׳ של כולם (ממיכן=*preparing*).

איספקרפסטי, v. אִסְקְפְּסְטֵי.

אִיסְפָּרָגוֹס. אַסְפָּ׳ m. (ἀσπάραγος) 1) *asparagus*, also *shoots of cabbage*, like asparagus in form. Ned. VI, 10 if one vows abstinence from cabbage אסור בא׳ he is forbidden to eat asparagus (the latter being considered a species of the genus 'cabbage'). Tosef. Dem. IV, 5 לקוב את הא׳ שבו to cut off the stalks thereon (and throw the remainder away).—2) *asparagus, a beverage* of wine or beer with asparagus. Ber. 51[a]. Pes. 110[b]. Kid. 70[a] א׳ דקריוה רב׳ aspar. as the educated call (the morning drink). [Yalk. Gen. 34 איספרגים read אִיסְפְּרָגִים (σφραγίς) *seal*, v. סְפְרָגִים.]

אִיסְפַּרְגַּל (אספרלג) m. (Arab. safar-gel) *ispargal*, name of a fruit (called Persea, Περσαία), *plum;* others: *quince.*—*Pl.* אִיסְפַּרְגְּלִין. Y. Maasr. I, 48[d] bot.; Y. Kil. I, 27[a], explain. פרסיין=persæa. V. Löw Pfl. pp. 144, 289, a. Sm. Ant. s. v. *Perseæ.*

אִיסְפַּרְמְקִי (איספרקמי), v. אִסְפְּ׳.

איספרנמין, Tanḥ. ed. Bub. T'rumah. 9, v. אִיסְפֶּנְדְּמְנוֹס.

אִיסְפַּתְרִין, v. אִסְ׳.

אִיסַק pr. n. m. *Isak.* B. Mets. 39[b] Mari ben I. (v. Rabb. D. S. a. l.); Keth. 27[b].

איסקבמירוי, v. איסקרימורי.

אִיסְקוּדְרֵי, v. איסקונדרי.

***(אִיסְקוּזִית) אִיסְקוּזוּת** f. (Isp. of קוז-קוין; cmp. קְזוּזִית) *cutting*, trnsf. *fat. ..oom;* cmp. גְּזֵרָה. Esth. R.

to I, 14 (Ar. ed. Koh. ...יה). [Levy Talm. Dict. s. v. אִסְקוֹזוֹת, quotes הוו א׳ .... מיזוקנות, pl.]

איסקומדרי, v. next w.

סְקוּנְדְּרֵי, אִסְק׳, אִיסְקוּנְדְּרֵי m. pl. (Pers. iskodâr, ἀσκάνδης, σαγγάνδης, ἀστάδης; v. Perles Et. St. p. 113) prop. *despatch-bearers*, name of a game, *a kind of chess.* Kidd. 21ᵇ באר׳ אכללתו Ar. (Var. Ar. בסק׳; ed. איסקומדרי) you must have played at *iskundrê* (instead of studying). Shebu. 29ᵃ דילמא איס׳ וכ׳ (Ms. M. איסקודרי) perhaps he gave them checkers (tokens in game) and passed them for Zuzê. Ned. 25ᵃ. Cmp. איסקרנדה.

אִיסְקוּפָּא, אִיסְקוּפְּתָא, אִיסְקוּפָּה, v. אִסְק׳.

אִיסְקוֹרְטְיָא f. (scortea) *leather-coat.* Ned. 55ᵇ. V. סְקוֹרְטְיָא.

אִיסְקְרְיָא, v. אִסְקְרְיָא.

איסקריטורי, read אִיסְקְרֵיטָרֵי m. pl. (σηκρητάριοι, secretarii) *the sovereign's private secretaries* (Asecretis, v. D. C. Gr. a. Lat. s. v.). Y. Keth. XII, 35ᵇ; Y. Kil. IX, 32ᶜ איסקבטירוי (corr. acc.).

אִיסְקְרִיטִין, אִיסְקְרִיטֵי, v. אִסְק׳.

***איסקרנדה** m. (corrupt. of אִיסְקוּדְּרָא, Pers. iskodâr; Koh. Ar.; v. אִיסְקוּנְדְּרֵי) *courier.* Y. Ab. Zar. I, 39ᵈ top יהב הרהין וכ׳ he gave two pounds of pepper to a courier (to go to Tyre), and he (the courier) went up and found &c.

אִיסַר m. (contr. of איסהר, cmp. איסתירא, an adapt. of assarius=as) *As*, a Roman coin, usu. $1/24$ of a Denar (v. Zuckerm. Talm. Gew. p. 22 sq.), called א׳ האיטלקי *Italian As.* Kidd. I, 1; a. fr.—Y. ibid. I, 58ᵈ הא׳ אחד מכ״ד וכ׳ the As is $1/24$ of the silver Denar.—Trnsf. *coin.* Taan. 19ᵇ מדלית א׳ because there was a scarcity of coin.—*Pl.* אִיסְרִין. Y. Maas. Sh. IV, 55ᵇ top.—*Chald.* Kidd. 12ᵃ איסורי read אִיסְרֵי. [Gen. R. s. 42 א׳ לשם אלסר the Assar received its name from Elasar (Gen. XIV, 1), comment.; v. however next w.]

אִיסָּר m. (b. h. אֱסָר, אִסָּר) prop. *band*, hence *vow of abstinence*, (cmp. איסור). Y. Ned. I, beg. 36ᶜ.—*Pl.* אִיסָּרוֹת, אִיסָּרִין, אֱסָרִין. Ibid. אין לוקין על הא׳ the punishment of lashes is not applied for breaking vows. Y. Yeb. XIII, 13ᵈ אסורוה (corr. acc.). Y. Ned. I, 36ᵈ top. [אִיסַר *prisoner*, v. אִיסּוּר.] [Gen. R. s. 42 א׳ לשם אלסר bands (chains) forged for Elasar, v. preced.]

אִיסַר ch. same; 1) *band, chain. Pl.* אֱיסָרִין. Targ. Jud. XV, 14.—2) *vow.* Targ. O. Num. XXX, 3 (Y. אִיסְרָא); a. e.—*Pl.* אֱסָרִין, אֱסָרֵי. Targ. O. Num. XXX, 5; a. e.—[Targ. Ps. II, 3 אֱסָרָתָא (some ed. אֲסָרוּ׳), v. next w.]

אִיסְרָא I 1) m., v. preced.—2) אִיסְרָא, אֱסָרָא, אֱסַרְתָּא; f. *bundle, bunch, sheaf.* Targ. Y. Num. XIX, 18. Targ. O. Gen. XXXVII, 7; a. e.—*Pl.* אֱסָרִין, אֱסָרָתָא. Ibid. (ed. also אסרא, אסרתא). אֱסָרָתָא Targ. Ps. II, 3 (some ed. אֲסָרוּ׳) *chains;* v. preced.

אִיסְרָא II m. (v. סר) *prince, angel, genius.* Pes. 111ᵇ א׳ דמזוני וכ׳ (Ms. M. שדא, read שרא; v. Rabb. D. S. a. l.) the genius appointed over sustenance is named *Cleanliness.* Ib. א׳ דעניותא וכ׳ (in Ms. our w. omitted) the genius of want is named *Filth.* Yoma 77ᵃ א׳ דפרסי Ms. M. (ed. שרא, in a passage omitted in many editions, v. Rabb. D. S. a. l.) the genius of the Persians (Pharsees).

אִיסְרָטָא m. (strata) *street*, v. אִסְרָטָא.

***אִיסְרָטָה** f. same. Y. B. Bath. VIII, 16ᶜ top אינה היא א׳ that is not the proper way (=לא זו הדרך), i. e. it is inconsistent that the same formula should be illegal in the case of a letter of divorce, and legal in the case of a donation. Y. Gitt. VII, 48ᵈ אינה איסרתה (corr. acc., and supplement acc. to Y. B. Bath. l. c.).

***איסרטוס** Y. B. Mets. II, 8ᶜ מאילין דא׳, read הָאַנְדְּרֶסְטִירֵי, v. דֵּינִיסְטֵיס.

***אִיסְרָטִין** m. pl. (=אסטרטין, pl. of στρατός) *band* or *body of men.* Gen. R. s. 87 א׳ של נואפים (Ar. אסרטיון) bands of adulterers; א׳ של רוצחים bands of murderers; (Yalk. Gen. 145 איסטר׳).

איסרקא, v. אִסְרָטָא.

אִיסַרְתָּא, v. אִיסְרָא I.

איסרתה Y. Gitt. VII, 48ᵈ, v. אִיסְרָטָה.

אִיסְתְּוִירָא, אִיסְטְווּרָא, אִיסְתְּוִירָא, אִיסְתְּווּרָא m. (Ithpe. or Ispe. of שְׁוַר=סְוַר *to leap, stride;* b. h. אֲשׁוּר; cmp. אִסְפָּרֵס) *ankle, foot-step.* Targ. Job XXIII, 11; a. e. Yeb. 103ᵃ; Arakh. 19ᵇ הא׳ אי׳ עד ארעא נחית (Ar. אסתור׳) what is called *ist'vira* (*ankle*, in an anatomical sense) goes down to the ground (the entire length of the foot from the ankle). Men. 33ᵃ, דעבידא כי אי׳ a door turning horizontally like the foot from the ankle.—*Pl.* אִיסְתְּוָורִין, ... אֲתוּרֵי Targ. Koh. XII, 5; a. fr. Cmp. אֲתוּרֵי.

***איסתוננסין** Y. Maas. Sh. V, 56ᵇ top תלת׳ א׳ וכ׳, read תלתא סִיטוֹנִיסִין (pl. of σιτώνης) three *corn-dealers* upon whose estimates he redeemed the second tithes.

אִיסְתְּוֵרָא, v. אִיסְתְּוִירָא.

אִיצְטְרָא, אִיסְטְרָא, אִסְ׳, אִיסְתִּירָא m. (contr. of אסתהרא &c., r. צהר, סהר; cmp. אִסְתַּהַר a. אִיסַר) 1) *a silver coin*, (with זוזא or פשיטא, or sub. זוזא &c.) equal to a common (provincial) *Sela*, or *half a Zuz.* Keth. 64ᵃ; Gitt. 45ᵇ, v. טרפעיקא. B. Mets. 102ᵇ. Bekh. 49ᵇ א׳ סורסיא Syriac Istira (v. Zuckerm. Talm. Münz. p. 27). Kidd. 11ᵇ.—*Pl.* אִיסְתִּירֵי Gitt. 14ᵃ א׳ זוזי. Hull. 44ᵇ א׳ פשיטי.—Ib. 105ᵃ. 2) *Hebr. pl.* אִיצְטְרָאוֹת. Tosef. Shek. II, 4 א׳ של זהב (Var. אִיסְטְרָאוֹת) *gold coins* (*staters*). Y. ib. III, 47ᶜ איצטלי (corr. acc.). [Targ. II Esth. II, 7 כוכב נגהא, a gloss to זונית איסתירא, v. אִסְתַּהַר, confounding our w. with ἀστήρ.]

אִיסְתַּלְגִּינִית, איסתלגנית, v. אִיסְטְגְלִילִית.

אִיסְתָּנָא, v. אִסְ׳.

אִיסְתַּנְדְּרָא, v. אִסְטַנְדְּרָא.

אִיסְתְּנִיס, אִיסְטְנִיס, אִסְ׳ m. (ניס, Saf. סניס, Ithpe. אִיסְתּ׳, Ispe. אִיסְט׳; cmp. אִיתְנְיס; cmp. אֶשְׁתְּכוֹדַע as to Ishtafel) *of feeble health, delicate, fastidious in diet.* Yoma III, 5 איסת׳ Ms. a. Ar. (v. Rabb. D. S. a. l., note 10; Bab. ed. mostly איסט׳). Pes. 108ª. Snh. 100ᵇ (opp. דעתו יפה not choicy); a. fr.—*Pl.* אִיסְתְּנִיסִים &c. Gen. R. s. 11 Ar. (ed. איסט׳). Lam. R. to IV, 2 סיה . . . . (read סִים . . . .).—*Chald.* Targ. Job VI, 7 ed. אסת׳ (Ms. אסט׳). [Cmp. b. h. נָסַס, ch. נְסִיס.]

אִיסְתְּנִיסִיה, איסט׳, v. preced.

אִיסְתַּפְנִינִי, v. אִיסְט׳.

אִיסְתְּרוֹקָנִית, v. אִסְ׳.

אִיסְתְּרְתִיגִין read איסטרט׳, v. אִסְטְרָטֵיג a. foll.

איפאנימא Yalk. Ex. 167, v. אִיפִּטִימְיָא.

אֵיפָה I Sifra Sh'mini ch. VII, Par. 6, v. חֵיפָה II.

***אֵיפָה II** f. (cmp. אוֹפִי) *character, disposition, temper.* Ex. R. s. 40 (play on אֵיפֹה Job XXXVIII, 4) הא׳ שלך וכ׳ where was thy predestined temper suspended? (on which limb of Adam's head, hair &c.?, v. preceding passage ibid.). Ib. אֵיפָתְךָ.

אֵיפָה III f. (b. h.; אפה) [batch], *Ephah*, a dry measure. Sifré Deut. 294, both a small as well as a large Ephah קרויה א׳ is named Ephah.—Men. 45ᵇ top אֵיפָתָן the Ephah belonging to the sacrifices; a. fr.—*Pl.* אֵיפוֹת. Ibid.

***איפוטונקריק**, Pesik. R. s. 26, א׳ הינטין; ed. Lemb. אפיטונטריק לינטין, ed. Friedm. לינטין, read מִפַּלְטִין טְרִיקְלִין וְקִיטוֹן than the palace (with) triclinium and bed-chamber wherein I dwell.

איפוטיקוס, v. איפטיקוס.

אִיפוֹכִי, v. אַפּוֹ׳.

אִיפוֹלִין, v. אֲפּוֹלִים.

אִיפוּמָא m. (v. פּוּמָא) *mouth, orifice*, esp. *sky-light* (impluvium). Erub. 100ª דהוה סליק בא׳ Ms. M. (ed. והוה) (a palm-tree) which grew up through the impluvium. Kidd. 81ª. Hull. 51ª.

איפוממא, v. next w.

***איפומנימא** (Mus.), **איפוממא, איפמנימא, איפומג׳** &c. (read: אִיפִּיטִימְיָא) m. pl. (ἐπιτίμια, τά) *the imposed penalty, sentence.* Deut. R. s. 2; Yalk. Gen. 77; Ex. 167. [Mus. reads נקרית sing. fem.=ἐπιτιμία.]

***אֵיפוּס** m. (אפס, √אֵת, cmp. אֵבוּס) *fodder, feed.* *Pl.* אֵיפוּסִין. Midr. Till. to Ps. LXXVIII, 52 אין מתקנין איפוּסֵיהֶן . . . their feed is not prepared for them; (Ex. R. s. 24, in a passage otherwise miscopied, אפוטיקון).

אִיפוּפוֹדִין, v. אַפּוֹ׳.

איפופורין, v. אֲפּוּפּוֹדִין, אִפּוּפְסִין a. אַפִּיפְיוֹן.

***אֶיפוֹפֵי** *ĕfofé*, a disguise of *ĕlohê* (אֱלֹהֵי); cmp. אֲלַקֵי, אֶשְׁקוֹקָה. Y. Ned. XI, 42ᶜ top, how did you swear? He said, 'I swore Efofé Yisrael' (for, *By the God of Israel*), 'I will not enter my house'. He replied, (you said) *Efofe Yisrael*, ולא עללה לביתיך (not עללה) and on that account you would not enter your house?

איפופסים, איפופסין, איפופסים, איפופיס, v. אפופסין.

אִיפוּרִיא, read אוֹ׳, v. אָפּוּרְיָא.

אִיפוּרְיָיא, v. אַפַּרְיָין.

***אִיפּוֹתוֹרוֹס** f. (ἱπποθόρος, sub. νόμος, שירה) *a tune played to mares on being covered.* Cant. R. to I, 9 (being asked why they rushed into the water, the horses said) א׳ נעשית לכם בים (ed. אפ׳, איפיטיסים, איפיטיסים corr. acc.) a hippothoros is prepared for you in the Sea (a satire on Egyptian lasciviousness).

אִיפְטָא, אֶפְטָא (ἑπτά) *seven.* Gen. R. s. 14, beg.; a. e. V. אִיטָא.

אִיפַּטְיָא, אִיפַּטִיאָה (אִפַּטְיָא) f. (ὑπατεία) prop. *Roman consulship, consulate*, in gen. *era*, dating from accession to government or an other important event. Lev. R. s. 36 נמנה בא׳ של מלכים (Ahaz) was counted under the era of kings (under whom Isaiah prophesied). Num. R. beg. איזה יום—יאיזה א׳ what day, month, year and era (from the exodus from Egypt.). Pesik. Baḥod. p. 104ª הוו מונין א׳ וכ׳ count ye a new era from my son's redemption. Ib. Haḥod. p. 52ᵇ sq. he wrote her marriage contract וכתב לה א׳ in which he stated the era of his government.

אִיפַּטִיקוֹס (incorr. אפיט׳, ארפט׳) m. (ὑπατικός) *consularis, Emperor's delegate, viceroy.* Mekh. B'shall. Amalek, 2, א׳ מבטל וכ׳ the Hypaticus annuls it over his (the Hegemon's) hand (ignoring his authority).—*Pl.* אִיפַּטִיקִין. Tanḥ. (ed. Bub.), Vayesheb 2 אפסיקין (corr. acc., v. note 4). V. היפטיקוס.

איפיטיקוס, v. preced.

אִיפְּכָא f. (אפך) *the reverse, opposite.* Bekh. 5ª, a. fr. אנן א׳ מתנינן לה our version is the reverse. Hull. 20ᵇ, a. fr. אדרבא א׳ מסתברא, v. אַדְּרַבָּא. R. Hash. 20ª; a. v. fr.

איפליקתא, v. אַפִּיקִלְטָא.

אִיפַּסְטְלִין (אִפִּיצְטְלִין Mus.) m. pl. (pastilli) *lozenges, pills of sugar.* Cant. R. to I, 2. V. פסטילוס, פִּיצְטְלִין; cmp. Yalk. Cant. 981.

איפסטקין, v. אַפְּסְטְ׳.

אִיפְסַר, v. אַפְּסַר.

איפקינון, v. אַנְפְּקִינוֹן.

אִיפְקַרְסִין, v. אַפְּ׳.

אִיפְרָא, v. אַפְרָא.

אִיפְרָא pr. n. f. *Ifra.* Zeb. 116ᵇ I. Ormuzd, mother of king Shapur; B. Bath. 8ª bot; Taan. 24ᵇ; Nid. 20ᵇ אִפ׳.

אִיפַּרְוֹן, v. אַפַּרְוֹרִין.

***איפרומוס**, Midr. Sam. s. 5 א׳ מ׳שלו היה read הפירוטות . . . היו (v. פְּרוּטָה, esp. Pes. 50ᵇ) he (Nebucadnezar) had to pay the writer's fees (for the change of בר אלהין into מלאביה Dan. III, 25; 28), i. e. had to suffer for it; v. אימוס. Cant. R. to VII, 9 פריטין משלי היו read פרוטין.

אִיפַּרְכָא, אִיפַּרְכָה, אֶפַּרְכָא, אֶפַּרְכוֹס m. (ὕπαρχος, ἔπαρχος) *prefect of a province or town; governor, lieutenant.* Gen. R. s. 11; a. v. fr.—*Pl.* אִיפַּרְכִין, אַפַּרְכֵי, אִיפַּרְכַיָא, אִפ׳. Targ. Y. Num. XI, 26. Targ. Esth. I, 3; a. e.—Shebu. 6ᵇ; a. fr.

אִיפַּרְכוֹס, v. preced.

אִיפַּרְכוּסָיא f. (deriv. of preced.)=next w.

אִיפַּרְכִי, אִיפַּרְכְיָא, אִפ׳ f. (ἐπαρχία) *prefecture, province, town-government.* Gen. R. s. 39; a. fr. [In Targ. also אִיפַּרְכָיוּתָא.]—*Pl.* אִיפַּרְכִיוֹת, אִפ׳. Gen. R. s. 89; a. e. [Targ. Lam. I, 1 אַפַּרְכְיָא, read אִיפַּרְכַיָא. Targ. Y. II, Deut. III, 11 אפרכיון, read בֵּי אַרְכִיוָן.] [Midr. Sam. ch. VII, לא׳ (Var. לאפר׳), v. אַפַּנְיֵר.]

אִיפַּרְכָיוּתָא, v. preced.

***אִיפַּרְסַן** (Ithpe. denom. of פּוּרְסָן) *he was taxed* (by Roman officials), i. e. his property was seized for taxes. Y. Kidd. III, 64ª top א׳ לוי Levy's property &c.

איפרפוס, v. אַפּוֹפְסִין.

אִיפֶּשׁ, אִיפְשַׁר, v. אֶפֶּשׁ a. אֶפְשַׁר.

איפתוסים, איפתיסיס, v. אִיפִּיתוּרוֹס.

אִיצָא I m. (איץ) *ozier, prickly twigs.* Gitt. 69ᵇ א׳ דטיבא וכ׳ (Ar. אִצָּא) green twigs with which the river is dammed in (figur. for diarrhœa stopped). Cmp. חוּצָא.

אִיצָא II, **אִיצְצָא** m., **אִיצַצְתָּא** f. (אצץ, איץ) 1) *squeezing, pressure.* Yeb. 121ᵇ top, אגב איצצא מזקי (Ar. איצא) on account of the pressure (which the falling person exercises on the serpents in the pit) they injure him. Sabb. 144ᵇ דאתי בתר איצצא Ar. (ed. איצצתא; Ms. M. אִיצִיצָא) (the juice) which oozes out of the grapes through the pressure of their non weight. M. Kat. 11ª salted fish made fit for immediate use אגב א׳ by squeezing (and washing) out the salt.—*Pl.* אִיצְצֵי. Ib. שיתין א׳ sixty times pressed and washed.—2) trnsf. *depression, depreciation* in the market; [oth. opin. *deterioration* of quality]. Keth. 100ᵇ אע״ג דנפל ביה איצצתא (read דנפלא; Ar. דהוי ביה איצא, Rashi איצצא) though there is a risk *of depreciation* (on account of large supply for the festive season) [or *of getting sour*].

איצבתא, אִיצַבְתִּי, v. אֶצְבְּתִי.

אִיצְטַדְיָא f. (צדי, v. next w.) 1) *destruction.*—2) (cacophem.) *theatre;* v. אִצְטַדְיָא.

אִיצְטַדִּין f. (orig. m. pl., Ithp. of צדי q. v.; sub. שדה &c.) 1) *a place full of ruins.* Y. Erub. II, 22ᵇ את ריאה את הא׳ כילי וכ׳ you look upon the debris near Tiberias as &c. (cmp. אלסים).—*Pl. איצטדיינין. B. Bath. 103ᵇ א׳ מהו if the stones in the field are debris, how is it? [Comment. diff.]—2) cacophemism for *theatre* (a *place of destruction*). [The prevailing versions are אצטרין, אסטרין q. v.]

איצטוראן Tosef. B. Kam. VI, 28, read אצטבא or אצטווא.

אִיצְטְנִיסִית, v. אִסְטְנִית.

איצטרי Yeb. 17ª, v. צרי.

אִיצִיָיתָא, v. אֲצִירָא.

***אִיצְרָא** m. (אֲצַר q. v.) *what is pressed out, juice.* Gitt. 69ᵇ (Ar. עצרא).

אִיצְרוֹלוֹגִין, v. אַסְטְרוֹלוֹגוֹס.

***אִיקָא** m. (עיק=איק; cmp. Lat. ambire, b. h. סבב) *stallion-goat, buck.* Sabb. 152ª א׳ שליפא וכ׳ Ar. (ed. עיקרא, עקירא, Ms. Oxf. עיקר, Ag. Hatt. עקר, v. Rabb. D. S. a. l. note 40) a goat, if castrated, sells for eight &c. [V. Sachs Beitr. II, 131 sq.]

איקוביטון, v. אִק׳.

***איקומימא**, Lev. R. s. 5, v. דאיקוטטא.

איקומונוס=אִיקוֹנוֹמוֹס.

אִיקוּמֵינֵי f. (οἰκουμένη) *the inhabited earth.* Koh. R. VI, 3 אוקי׳ (corr. acc.); Gen. R. s. 32 יקו׳ (corr. acc.) (play on *y'kum* Gen. VII, 4).

איקמנוס, v. אִיקוֹנוֹמוֹס.

אִיקוֹן, אִיקוֹנָא, (אִק׳) c. (εἰκών) *likeness, portrait, iconic statue.* Targ. Y. Gen. V, 3.—*Pl.* h. אִיקוֹנִין, אִיקוֹנוֹת; ch. אִיקוֹנְיָא, אִיקוֹנָתָא. Ex. R. s. 30 (של מלך) א׳ emperor's *statues;* a. fr.—Y. Ab. Zar. III, beg. 42ᵇ איקוניות, איקוניות read אִיקוֹנוֹת. Ib. 42ᶜ top; a. e. V. אִיקוֹנִין. [Midr. Till. to Pss. XV, XVII, v. אִיקוֹנְיָא.]

אִיקוֹנוֹמוֹס m. (οἰκόνομος) *steward, town-clerk* (a slave). Y. B. Mets. IX, beg. 12ª. Y. B. Bath. IV, 14ᶜ bot. איקומנוס (corr. acc.). B. Bath. 68ᵇ אנקולמוס, אינקלמוס, אונק׳, אנקל׳ (popul. corrupt.).

***אִיקוֹנִיָא** I (pl. of εἰκόνιον) *statuary.* Midr. Till. to Ps. XV (ref. to Is. XXXI, 9, applied to the Roman empire or emperor) 'his rock' זה א׳ this means the statues with the likenesses of the emperors (v. Sm. Ant. s. v. Statuary).

***אִיקוֹנִיָא** II or **אִיקוּנְיָא** f. (pl. as a collect. noun) (denom. of אִיקוֹן) *a procession in which portable images are carried.* Midr. Till. to Ps. XVII א׳ של מלאכים וכ׳ a procession of angels passes before man and they cry, Make room לאיקונית של וכ׳ (read לְאִקוֹנִין or לְאִיקוֹנוֹת; Yalk. Ps. 670; Deut. R. s. 4 לְאִיקוֹנִין) for the images of the Lord (man being created in the image of God). Deut. R. l. c. אי׳ מהלכת (corr. acc.).

אִיקוֹנִיָה, v. preced.

אִיקוֹנִים read אִיקוֹנִין.

אִיקוֹנִין (אקונין) f. (εἰκόνιον) *picture, image;* Targ. Y. Gen. IV, 5 *features* (pl.); a. fr.—Ex. R. s. 15. Deut. R. s. 4, v. אִיקוֹנְיָא II; a. fr.—Esp. זיו א׳ the brightness of expression, *features.*—Gen. R. s. 53; a. fr.—Ex. R. s. 35 א׳ נאה (sub. זיו) *fine appearance;* Cant. R. to III, 11 אותונין (corr. acc.).—*Pl.* v. אִיקוֹן.

אִיקְלִימָא, v. אֶקְ׳.

אִיקְלִין, Y. Ab. Zar. II, 41ᵈ, read with some ed. איקרין, v. אִיקָר.

אִיקְלַס Ithpe. of קְלַס.

אִיקָנוֹס m. (ἱκανός) 1) *worthy, fit; wealthy.* Yalk. Job 919.—2) *sufficient,* v. אֶקְסְיוֹס.

אִיקָרָא, אִיקָר m. (=h. יְקָר, v. איר׳) *honor, glory.*—Targ. Prov. XI, 16; a. fr.—Y. Ber. I, 2ᵈ איקרי וכ׳ my honor counts for nothing before the honor of my Maker. Ib. II, 4ᵇ מה את פליג ליה א׳ (not אתפליג) what honor dost thou pay it (by passing by)?; Y. Shek. II, 47ª top.—Y. Peah VIII, 21ᵇ bot. פרנסה דא׳ an honorable livelihood. Y. Hag. I, 76ᵈ top איגרא דא׳, v. אִיגְּרָא.—*Pl.* אִיקְרִין *presents, greetings.* Y. Ab. Zar. II, 41ᵈ (some ed. איקלין).

אִירָא m. (אור, cmp. חור) *white substance, undyed wool* or *cotton.* Sabb. 11ᵇ; (Tosef. ib. I, 8 missing). Ib. 79ª דוגמא לא׳ a sample color for the wool (given to the dyer).—*Pl.* אִירִין. B. Kam. 119ᵇ, the remnants of wool in the hands of the dyer. [R. Hanan. reads אִידָא q. v.] [Tosef. Kel. B. Bath. I, 4 אִירָה; Kel. XXI, 1 עִירָה.]

***אִירוֹנִית, (אִרוֹנִית), חִירוֹנִית, חִרוֹנִית, עִירוֹנִית, (עָרְנִית)** f. (v. preced.) *made of white clay, unburned and flat clay-dish,* a kind of tray extemporized for immediate use in the field.—*Pl.* אִירוֹנִיּוֹת &c. Eduy. II, 5 לפסין אי׳ ed. (Ms. אלפסין ארנ׳, Mish. Nap. ארו׳). Y. Sabb. XI, 13ª ארו׳. Bets. 32ª חירו׳ Ms. M. (ed. חר׳) expl. =עיר׳ Ms. M. (ed. ער׳)=צעי חקלייתא field-dishes. [Rashi; from עיר *used in country towns*(!), hence *coarse, unfinished.*].

אִירוּס I, אֶרוּס m. (supposed to be=ἶρις) *Erus,* a lily with an aromatic root. Kil. V, 8, expl. Y. ib. 30ª bot. אִירְסִיָּה (pl. of אִירְסָא, v. P. Sm. s. v.). Tosef. ib. III, 13. Ohol. VIII, 1.

אִירוּס II, אֶרוּס m. (prob. from its use, v. ארס a. deriv.) *erus,* a musical instrument used at weddings and funerals, *drum, taboret.* Sot. IX, 14 גזרו—על האר׳ the use of the *erus* at weddings was interdicted; v. expl. Bab. ib. 49ᵇ; Y. ib. 24ᶜ top. Kel. XV, 6 הא׳ (used at funerals).

אִירוּסִין, v. אֵרוּסִין.

אִירוּעַ m. (ארע) *meeting, festive gathering.* Targ. Y. Num. XXIX, 35 (=h. מִקְרָא).

אִירְיָא, אִירְיָא, v. אַרְיָא.

אֶרִימוֹן, v. אֶרְמוֹן.

אֶרִימִיאָה f. (ἐρημία) *desert, desolation.* Koh. R. beg. (play on *Jeremiah*).

אִירָם, Y. Maasr. V, 52ª, read אִירָס.

אִירְסָא, אִירֶס, v. אֶרֶס.

אִירְסִיָּה, v. אִירוּס I.

אִירַע, v. אֲרַע, אָרַע.

אִישׁ m. (b. h.; אוש, cmp. יֵשׁ, v. אֱינָשׁ) *being, man; husband; lord.*—א׳ ירושלים a native or citizen of Jerusalem. Aboth I, 4; a. fr.—Yoma I, 7 אִישִׁי כה״ג my lord the High-priest. Sot. 17ª א׳ ואשה husband and wife; a. fr.—*Pl.* אֲנָשִׁים, v. אֱנוֹשׁ.

אִישָׁא *fire,* v. אֶשָּׁא.

אִישְׁבּוֹרָן, v. אֶשְׁבּוֹרָן.

אִישֶּׁה m. (b. h. אִשֶּׁה, v. אֵשׁ) *burnt-offering.*—*Pl.* אִישִּׁים, אִשִּׁי׳. Ned. 13ª. Zeb. V, 4 כליל לא׳ altogether to be burnt; a. fr.

אֲשׁוּן, אִישׁוּן m. constr. (v. אֱשֶׁן a. b. h. אִישׁוּן) *essence, exact time, season.* Targ. Y. Gen. XVIII, 5. Ib. XXVIII, 10; a. fr. (in Targ. Y.).—*Pl.* אֲשׁוּנֵי, אִשּׁוּנֵי. Targ. Y. Lev. XV, 25; Deut. XXXI, 10. Cmp. אֵיתָן.

אִישּׁוּר m. 1) (v. אָשַׁר, *Pi.* 2) *praise, adoration.* Cant. R. to VIII, 11 אישורך היא it is thy praise. Y. Succ. III, 54ª top, with ten var. expressions of praise are the psalms headed באי׳ with the word *ashré,* &c.—2) (v. אָשַׁר *Pi.* 1) *legal attestation.* Y. B. Mets. I, 8ª bot; v. אַשְׁרָא. [Some ed. אִישַׁר.]

אִישׁוּת f. (v. אִישׁ) *matrimony, marital state.* Ab. Zar. 36[b] דאורייתא א׳ דרך חתנות biblically intermarriage with gentiles is forbidden only in the way of legal marriage (opp. concubinage, &c.). Y. Kidd. I, 59[c] bot. שִׁפְחוּת אחר א׳ servitude after marriage, i. e. a father selling his daughter after she had been married and had returned to her parental home in widowhood &c. Yeb. 76[a], a. fr. לשום א׳ with the intention of establishing a matrimonial relation.

אישות Y. Erub. II, 20[a] קנים א׳, v. חִיצָה II.

אִישׁוּת *mole,* v. אֲשׁוּת.

אִישְׁטַמְיוֹן, v. אִיסְטַ׳.

אִישְׁפָּה, v. אַשְׁפָּה.

אישפותי, v. אוּשְׁפִּיזִי.

אִישְׁפַּת, pl. אִישְׁפַּתּוֹת, v. אַשְׁ׳.

אִישְׁקָקָא, אִישְׁקָק, v. אַשְׁ׳.

אַיְשַׁר, אַיְישַׁר, אִישַׁר (Af. of אֲשַׁר) *good luck!* Y. Shebi. IV, 35[b] what means 'we salute them'? Ans. (Saying) אי׳ good luck. Ib. אי׳. Y. Taan. I, 64[b] bot.; a. e.

אִישֵּׁר, *Pi.* of אָשַׁר.—אִישֵּׁר, v. אִישּׁוּר.

אִישַׁת, v. חִישָׁה.

אֶשָּׁתָא *fire,* v. אֶשָּׁא.

אִישְׁתָּא, אֶשְׁתָּא m., **אֶשְׁתָּה** f. (=שִׁיתָּא) *six.* Targ. I Chr. XII, 24; a. e.—Y. Sot. VIII, 22[c] bot. אמתא א׳ a cubit has six handbreadths. Y. Snh. I, end, 19[d] חד מן א׳ *one sixth.* Ib. X, 28[b] top אש׳ ירחין six months.—*Pl.* אֶשְׁתִּין *sixty.* Targ. Y. II, Num. XII, 16. Cmp. אֶשְׁתָּא.

***אִישְׁתַּטִּית** pr. n. pl. or river *Ishtattith.* Hull. 95[a] bot. מברא דאי׳ the ford of I.

אִישְׁתִּי *he drank;* v. שְׁתִי.

אישתתא, אִישְׁתִּיתָא, v. אֶשְׁתִּיתָא.

אִישְׁתְּמוֹדַע, v. אִשְׁ׳.

אִית־ formative prefix, v. אִתְ־. [Words not found here below, will be found under אִתְ־.]

אִית, אִיתָא (h. יֵשׁ; אית, cmp. אִישׁ, אֵת, יַת &c.) prop. *being, existence,* hence *there is, are; est qui* &c. Targ. Gen. XVIII, 24; a. fr.—Y. Ber. VI, end, 10[d] א׳ תנייה תני וכ׳ one Tannai reads.... R. Hash. 11[b], a. fr. כדאיתא as it is, i. e. as stated.—אית לי *I have, I hold* (the opinion).—Snh. 90[a], a. fr. מר כדאית ליה וכ׳ the one in accordance with the opinion he holds, and the other &c.—B. Mets. 5[a], a. fr. . . . . אם איתא לדר׳ if the opinion of R. . . . . has (had) any substance, i. e. if we must adopt his authority.—Yoma 41[a] מאי א׳ לך למימר what hast thou to reply?—B. Mets. 3[a] מאי א׳ לי גבי וכ׳ what have I to do with the hired man?—Yeb. 116[a] כי איתנכו בש׳ when ye are in Shili &c.—Compounds אית־כא, contr. אִיכָּא; לא איתא contr. לֵיתָא. [אִיתַי, אִיתַאי, *my existence, I am*=h. עוֹדִי. Targ. Ps. CIV, 33; a. e.] Cmp. אִיתַי.

אִיתָא come!, Imp. of אֲתָא.

אִתְּ׳, אִיתְּתָא, אִיתְּתָה, אִיתְּתָא f. (cmp. אִית a. אִישׁ;= h. אִשָּׁה; cmp. אִנְתְּתָא) *woman, wife.* Targ. Gen. II, 22; a. fr.—Y. Maasr. V, end, 52[a] חדא איתא a certain woman. Y. Taan. I, 64[b] bot. איתתה. Y. Ber. II, 5[c] bot. איתתיה דאבוהי his father's wife, step-mother (fig. for Babylon); a. fr.

אִיתוּ, אִתּוּ, אִנְתּוּ, אִיתוּ f. (preced.)=h. אִישׁוּת *matrimony;* לא׳ *in matrimony, as wife.* Targ. Gen. XII, 19; a. fr.

אִיתוּ *come ye!,* Imper. of אֲתָא.—[Pes. 50[a] איתו אנן, v. אִיתַי.]

אִיתוֹדָאָה, אִתּ׳ f. (אִתְוַדָּאָה=,ודי) *confession* of sin. Targ. Hos. XIV, 3.

***אִיתַי, אִיתַּיי** (pl. of אית) *there is, there are.* Dan. II, 10; a. fr.—Y. Shebi. X, 39[c] ל׳ יום לא איתיי (Y. Macc. I, 31[a] איתי . . . .) a loan on thirty days does not exist, i. e. does not come within the rule whereby a creditor may secure collection by announcing legal action before the Sabbath year limitation takes effect.—*Pes. 50[a] כי חיכי דאיתו אנן איתינן וכ׳ (read דאיתי or דאיתינן; Ms. M. אתינן; diff. vers. v. Rabb. D. S. a. l.) as we are esteemed *here* (in this world) so are we *there* (in the world of the beatified).

אִיתַי pr. n. m. *Ithi.* Kerith. 24[a].

***אִיתְּ׳, אִיתְּיַטְרוֹן, אִיתִּיַטְרוֹן** m. (v. תִּיאַטְרוֹן) *theatre.* Targ. Ezek. XXVII, 6 (ed. Vien. אִתִּיבְרוֹן).

אִיתִימָא (=אִית, אִיתֵי a. אֵימָא) *some say.*—שמואל וא׳ ר׳ יוחנן Samuel or, as some say, R. Johan. Bets. 6[a]; a. fr. [Diff. fr. ואי תימא.]

איתומוס, read אֶנְטִימוּס.

אִיתִינַן, v. אִיתַי and אִית.

אִתְּ׳, אִתְכָּלָא, אִיתְכָּלָא (const. אִיתְכַּל) m.=h. אֶשְׁכֹּל (q. v.) *bunch of grapes.* Targ. Num. XIII, 24; a. e.—*Pl.* אִיתְכָּלַיָּיא, אִתְכָּ׳, אִיתְכָּלִין. Targ. I Sam. XXV, 18; a. e.—Trnsf. *scholars,* opp. עילייא (leaves), the untutored. Hull. 92[a] ליבעו רחמי וכ׳ let the grapes pray for the leaves (the scholars for the untutored); for but for the leaves, the grapes could not exist. V. אֶשְׁכֹּל.

אִיתְלִיס, v. אַבְלִיז end.

***אִיתָם** m. (יָתוֹם; v. אִיד) *orphan.* Targ. Ps. X, 14; Job XXXI, 17 Ms. (ed. יתום).

אִיתְמַל, אִיתְמַלֵי, אִתְמוֹל=h. אֶתְמוֹל *yesterday.* Targ. Ex. IV, 10; a. e.—Erub. 15[a]; a. e.

אֵיתָן, אֵתָן m. (b. h.; אית; cmp. אית, עות, אִישׁוֹן, אֵשֶׁן) 1) *essence, permanent* or *normal condition.* Nidd. 48[b] חזר לאֵיתָנוֹ obtained again its normal condition. Sot. 36[b] שבה קשתו לא׳ his membrum resumed its normal condition. (Cmp. Ex. XIV, 27).—2) adj. *essential, strong.* R. Hash. 11[a] א׳ לישנא דתקיפי *ethan* means *strong.*—*Pl.* אֵיתָנִים. Ib. אֵיתָנֵי עולם the mighty of the world (patriarchs). Gen. R. s. 98 (play on *ăthono* Gen. XLIX, 11) בנים אֵתָנִים וכ׳ mighty sons (heroes) are destined to descend from him. —3) pr. n. river *Ethan.* Succ. 18[a] (Ms. M. נתן); a. e.

איתנטמייה Koh. R. beg., v. אַוְתֶּנְטְיָא.

אִיתְנִיס, אִתְנָס, אִתְנַס (=אתנסס, אתנסים, v. נסס; or Ithpe. of נוס or ניס) *to be taken sick.* Sabb. 145[b] אִיתְנַסִּי (Ms. M. אִיתְנַיִּסִי, אִיתְנַיִּיס *Ithpa.*) I should have grown sick; (Ms. Oxf. אִיסתכני I should have been in danger). Git. 56[a] אִתְנִיסָא (or אִתְנְיִסָה) she grew sick (from aversion), fainted. Cmp. אִיסְתְּנִיס. [אִתְאֲנִיס=אִיתְנִיס, v. אֲנַס.]

אִיתְנְכוּ, אִיתְנָן, v. אִית.

אִיתקוּטְלָא, v. אִסְקוּטְלָא I.

אִיתְתָא, v. אִיתָּא.

אַךְ I (b. h., נכי) *only, but.* Pes. 5[a] אך חלק the word *akh* (Ex. XII, 15 'but on the first [preceding] day') intimates a division of the day between two categories as to the laws concerning that day. Kerith 7[a]; a. fr.—*Pl.* אַכִּין (אַכִּים) *the word akh in the Biblical texts.* Y. Ber. IX, 14[b] bot., a. e. א׳ ורקין מיעוטין the *akh* and the *rak* intimate limiting qualifications.

אַךְ II m. (v. אֲנַךְ 2) *affliction, calamity.* B. Mets. 59[b]; v. חֲכַךְ. Gen. R. s. 32, end; Tanh. Noah 9, ed. Bub. 3, cmp. preced.

***אַךְ III**=אֵיךְ, only with חדא *together.* Targ. Prov. XXII, 18 (ed. Vien. אֵיךְ).

אַכְאָבִית f. (כאב) *fever connected with pains,* וזמה וא׳, a. vers. for אֲבַאֲבִית; q. v.

אַכָאטִיס m. (ἀχάτης) *agate.* Ex. R. s. 38, end (ed. אבאטים corr. acc.).

אַכְּבָא, v. אֲבְבָא.

אכבדא, אַכְבְּרָא pr. n. pl. *Okhbara.* Kidd. 71[b] Ar. (ed. בגדא, בגדת); v. אֲוָנָא II.

אַכְדֵן=אִיכְדֵין.

אכדרור, Targ. Ps. CIV, 3 Ms., read אִינְדְּרוֹר or אַכְסַדְרוֹר; v. אִינְדְּרָא.

אכוור Y. Succ. V, 55[b] bot. read מַכְוֶה.

אַכְוורְנְקִי · אַכְוּרְנְקָא, v. אַכְוָר׳.

***אַכוּז, עֲכוּז** m. (כוז, v. כוּז) [hollow, arched pitcher], euphem. for *buttocks* or *extremity* (*testicles* &c.). Bekh. VI, 6 (40[a]) ע׳. Erub. 53[b] (question as to spelling) א׳ or ע׳? (Ms. M. אכוז, עכוז, Rashi אבוז, עבוז; v. Rabb. D. S. a. l. note). V. P. Sm. s. v. כוז 1691 sq. V. הֶרְגֵּז, אֲבוּז.

אַכוּזָא ch. (v. preced.)=כּוּזָא. Taan. 20[b] Ms. M., ed. כוזא.

כפר א׳, אַכּוּם pr. n. pl. *K'far Iccum.* Y. Snh. X, 29[c] (Bab. ib. 110[b] כ׳ עַכּוֹ; Joseph. B. J. II, 20, 6 Καφαρεκχώ); Tanh. (ed. Bub.) B'resh. 25 עכו (Var. איכים); Hull. 55[b] עִיכּוּם; Y. Sot. VII, 21[c] bot. אמים (corr. acc.; Bab. ib. 37[b] עכו).

אַכְוָר׳, כְּוָאנְגָּר, אַכְנְגָּר, אַכְוְנְגָּר m. (Pers. Kh[w]angar, Kh[w]algar, Fl.) *table-steward, seneschal.* Keth. 61[a] כו׳ Ar. (ed. אטורנגא read אַכְוַנְגְּרָא; Var. in Ar. כונדקא, corr. acc.).—*Pl.* אַכְוַנְגְּרֵי. M. Kat. 12[a] (Ar. אכו׳, ed. אבו׳, corr. acc., Ms. M. אכוורנ׳, cmp. Rabb. D. S. a. l., a. vol. VIII, p. 75). [Pes. 40[b] Ms. M. בירדיקאי, ed. בורדקי, Ar. כוורדקי, prob. corrupt. of our w.]

כּוּרְנָק, אַכְוּרְנְקִי, אַכְוּרְנְקָא m. (v. preced.; Pers. *Khorengah,* Arab. *Khawarnak,* Fl.) *dining place, dining hall in the garden.* Targ. Y. Deut. XXXII, 50, א׳ .... קי דמלכיא a royal banqueting hall (put up for the wedding). Taan. 14[b]; Meg. 5[b] (distinguishing between בנין, erection of a building, and נטיעה, putting up a temporary structure), what is meant by 'putting up a tent of joy?'—זה הנוטע אב׳ של מלכים Ms. M. (Ar. כ׳; ed. אב׳, corr. acc.) it means one putting up a regal banqueting tent (for his son's wedding). Erub. 25[b] אב׳ וכ׳ (ed. אב׳) the Resh Galutha was to have a banquet (on a Sabbath) in his garden.

***אכזוויא** Targ. I Chr. I, 7 ed. Rahm.; Targ. Y. Gen. X, 4 אכזיא, v. אֲכְזָיָא.

אַכְזִיב pr. n. pl. (b. h.) *Achzib* (Ecdippa, Ecdippon), a sea-town in Northern Palestine. Y. Shebi. V, 36[b] bot. he who travels מעכו לא׳ (Git. 7[b]; Tosef. Oh. XVIII, 14 מעכו לכזיב) from Acco (Ptolemais) to Ach. (Chezib).

אַכְזָר, v. אַכְזָרִי. Denom. *Nithpa.* נִתְאַכְזֵר *to show one's self merciless.* Num. R. s. 8.

אכזראה, אַכְזְרָא m. (=b. h. אַכְזָר) *cruel.* Targ. Job XLI, 2 (1); a. e.—Lam. R. introd. (R. Joh. 1) קטילא א׳ merciless slaughter.—*Pl.* אַכְזְרָאִין. Targ. Deut. XXXII, 33. Targ. J. II ibid. אַכְזוֹרָאֵי.

אַכְזָרִי m., **אַכְזָרִית** f. (b. h., r. כזר) *cruel, merciless;* also *strictly just.* Koh. R. to VII, 16; a. e. B. Bath. 16[a] bot.—*Pl.* אַכְזָרִים, אַכְזְרִיִּים; fem. אַכְזָרִיּוֹת. Pesik. R. s. 44. Num. R. s. 8. [Ib. s. 9 מדת אכזרית, read אַכְזְרִיּוּת.]

אַכְזְרִיאֵל, v. אַבְרְזִיאֵל.

אַכְזְרִיּוּת f. (b. h.) *cruelty, severity; strict justice.* Succ. 14[a]; Num. R. s. 10 (p. 239, ed. Amst.) מדת א׳ the divine justice. Ib. s. 9, v. אַכְזָרִי.—Esth. R. to I, 15 שלא כדת אלא בא׳ not according to law but with cruelty.

אַכְזָרִית, v. אַכְזָרִי.

אכטא, Ab. Zar. 34ᵇ Ar., v. אַבְטָא.

אכטא, אָכְטָא, אוֹכְטָא (ὀκτώ) *eight*. Gen. R. s. 14 beg.; a. e.; v. אִיבָא. Tanḥ. (ed. Bub.) B'midb. 21 אקטו.

אכייא, אֲכָיָא, אֲכָיָה pr. n. pl. *Achaia*, the Roman province including Peloponnesus and northern Greece, south of Thessaly. Targ. I Chr. I, 7 אכזוויא (Var. אירבלין); Targ. Y. Gen. X, 4 אכזיא; Y. Meg. I, 71ᵇ bot. אכיא (Gen. R. s. 37 אירבליא), (for b. h. פְּתִים). [Sifré Num. 131 אביא, v. אסיא.]

אֲכִילָה f. (b. h.; אכל) *eating, food, meal, dish*. Y. Sabb. I, 4ᵃ top, a. e. אֲכִילַת בן דרוסא (דור׳, דרוסאר) the food Ben D'rosa used to eat, i. e. *third done*. Yoma 80ᵇ א׳ גסה excessive meal. Ib. 81ᵃ, a. fr. א׳ בכזית wherever אכל (to eat) is mentioned in the Bible text, the size of an olive is meant. Y. Sot. III, 19ᵇ top אכילת מזבח the consumption (of sacrifices) on the altar. Zeb. 31ᵇ; a. fr. א׳ פרס, v. פְּרָס. Kil. II, 10, v. אָכְלָה II.—*Pl.* אֲכִילוֹת. Pes. 78ᵃ. Gen. R. s. 86, beg. (play on אוכיל Hos. XI, 4) א׳ חרבה (some ed. אבילות—אוביל corr. acc.) *purveyances*.

אֲכִילְתָא ch. same. Targ. I Kings XIX, 8 (ed. Vien. אֲכִילְתָא).

*__אָכִים__ m. (אכם) *black (wine)*. Y. Gitt. VII, beg. 48ᶜ א׳ גו סמיק, v. סמיק; (Y. Ter. I, 40ᵇ אבוס read our w. or אִיפוּמָא=אָפוּם); cmp. Gitt. 67ᵇ.

אָכֵן, אָכֵין (v. כֵּן) *thus, in this manner*. Y. Ber. III, 6ᵃ א׳ בר נש וכ׳ is it thus man deals with his neighbor? Y. Keth. II, 26ᶜ bot. אתמול אמרת א׳ וכ׳ yesterday thou saidst so, and to-day thou sayest *otherwise*; a. fr. V. הָכֵין.

אכיס Af. of כסס.

אכיסן, v. לַאֲכִיסִין.

*__אַכְּכָא__ m. (אכך, cmp. כַּכָּא) *ground* or *pounded drug, poultice*. Targ. Job XXX, 24, Var. for אספלנרתא.

אככמה Targ. Prov. VII, 10, read אַסְכְּבָא.

אָכַל (b. h.; √ אך *to rub*, cmp. אָנַךְ) 1) *to gnaw, eat, consume*. Inf. in Y. freq. לֶאֱכוֹל=לוֹכַל. Ber. I, 1; a. v. fr.—2) trnsf. *to absorb, occupy, take away*. Y. Shebu. VII, 38ᵃ בשרבית אוֹכֶלֶת בו when interests gnaw on (absorb) the property. Y. Erub. IV, 21ᵈ bot. ד׳ אמות אוֹכְלוֹת וכ׳ four cubits entering into the area of Tiberias. Num. R. s. 4 כמה לוחות אוֹכְלוֹת how much space did the tablets occupy &c.? B. Bath. 14ᵃ (interchanging with אוגרות, Var. אוגדות, v. Rabb. D. S. a. l. note 5, 6).—3) (euphem.) *to sleep with*. Keth. V, 9, differ. of opin. ib. 65ᵇ; Y. ib. 30ᵇ top a. bot.

Nif. נֶאֱכַל *to be eaten* &c. Zeb. I, 3; Ber. I, 1; a. fr.

Pi. אִיכֵּל *to consume, burn*. Tam. I, 4 הַמְאוּכָּלוֹת הפנימיות (Talm. ed. חמער׳) the thoroughly lighted coals in the centre; Y. Yoma II, 39ᶜ.

Hif. הֶאֱכִיל *to give to eat, cause to eat*. Keth. V, 3 היבם אינו מַאֲכִיל וכ׳ the Yabam does not transfer the privilege of eating T'rumah to his sister-in-law. Kidd. 31ᵃ יש מאכיל וכ׳ one may feed his father on pheasants &c.; a. fr.

Hithpa. a. *Nithpa.* נִתְאַכֵּל, הִתְאַכֵּל 1) *to be consumed, burnt up, digested*. Ber. VIII, 7 כדי שיִּתְאַכֵּל וכ׳ Ar. (ed. שיתעכ׳) until the food is digested (or absorbed) in his bowels. Tam. II, 1; a. e.—2) *to be worn off, spent*. Snh. VI, 12 Y. ed. נתא׳ הבשר (Mish. 6 נתע׳) when the flesh of the corpse was gone. Cant. R. to IV, 4 שלא נתא׳ אחד מהן none of them was worn off. Kidd. 59ᵃ נתא׳ המעות the money was spent; a. e.

אֲכַל, אֲכַל I ch. 1) same.—Inf. מֵיכַל, מֵיכוּל. Targ. Gen. II, 16; a. fr.—Y. Ter. VIII, 46ᵃ כד אתון מיכלון when they came and were about eating; ib. (more corr.) אתון מיכל; a. fr.—2) with קרצי prop. *to eat (the bread of) destruction, eat the informer's bread*, hence *to inform against*. Dan. III, 8; VI, 25.—Targ. Ps. XV, 3; a. fr.—Gitt. 56ᵃ איכול בחו קר׳; Lam. R. to IV, 2 איכול קרצהון I will inform against them.

Af. אוֹכֵל, אַיְכֵל *to give to eat, to support*. Y. Ter. X, 47ᵇ bot. אוכלה ליה he gave it to him to eat. Gen. R. s. 48, end (read:) אוכליה אשקיה לוי hast thou given (thy guest) to eat? to drink? do escort him, i. e. perform thy duties fully. Y. Kidd. I, 61ᵇ הוה מייכל לאבוי וכ׳ fed his father on &c.; a. fr.

Ithpe. אִתְאֲכִיל, אִתְאֲכִיל, אִתְאַכַּל *to be eaten, consumed*. Targ. Ps. LXVIII, 23; a. fr. Tanḥ. Emor, 6 ומה דהבא מִתְאֲכִיל וכ׳; Lev. R. s. 27 ומה זה וכ׳ what is this? do they eat gold &c.? Kidd. 59ᵃ קא מתאכלי were eaten up (spent). [אכלי Af. of כלי *to cry*, v. כלי.]

אֲכַל II (sec. r. of כול) *to measure*. Ned. 51ᵃ איכיל לי מר please measure for me. Ruth R. introd. 2 .... הא סאה הקום אכול (read סאתה קום) here is the bag and here the measure, get up and fill it; v. כול.

אֲכַל, v. אוֹכֵל.

אַכְלָא m. (אכל) *eater*. Targ. Jud. XIV, 14.

אַכְלָאִין, Targ. Ps. CIV, 21 Ms., ed. אכלין, v. כְּלִי *to cry*.

אַכְלְבָא m. (כלב; v. Ges. H. Dict. s. v.; cmp. כְּלוּב, כְּלִיבָה; Var. lect. אַבְלְבָא, v. infra) *shed, store-room*. B. Mets. 63ᵇ חיטי .... באַכְלְבָאי (v. Var. lect. in Rabb. D. S. a. l.; Mss. a. Ar. אכלבא) would my wheat have gone to ruin in my granary? Taan. 24ᵃ (v. Rabb. D. S. a. l.).—*Pl.* אַכְלְבֵי. Gitt. 56ᵃ א׳ וכ׳ ... שיתין א׳ ...אכלבא one shed of wheat requires sixty sheds of wood (for baking). B. Mets. 72ᵇ חיטי דא׳ (Ms. M. באכלבי, v. Rabb. D. S. a. l.) wheat stored in granaries &c.

אָכְלָה I f., אכל א׳ טִינָא) *mud-eater*, name of a parasitic worm in fishes. B. Bath. 73ᵇ (Ms. M. אכל׳ טינא; oth. var., v. Rabb. D. S. a. l. note).

אָכְלָה II, **אוֹכְלָה** f. (אָכַל 2) *occupied space*. Kil. II, 10 Y. ed. אָכְלַת הגפן (Mish. ed. אֲכִילַת; Y. Gem. 28ᵃ אוֹכְלָה) the soil occupied by the vine roots, א׳ הקבר the ground needed for the formation of the cave, i. e. as far as the roots &c. extend.

אַכְלוֹנָא, v. אוּכְלוֹסָא.

אַכְלוֹנַס, v. קְלוֹנַס.

*__אַכְלוֹשֵׁי__ m. pl. (v. אוּכְלוֹסָא) *public laborers, working men.* B. Mets. 77ª; v., however, אַבְלוֹשֵׁי.

אַכְלֵי *to cry,* Af. of כְּלֵי. Targ. Ps. CIV, 24 אַכְלִין, some ed., read אֲכָלִין.

אַכְלְיוּתָא f. (v. preced.) *noise, cry.* Targ. Job IV, 10; a. e.

אכלים Y. Ab. Zar. IV, 43ᵈ, v. אוּכֶל.

אַכְלָן m. (אָכַל) *a greedy eater.* Y. Maasr. III, 50ᵈ bot.

אכלסין, v. אַלְכְּסִין.

אָכַם (√כם; cmp. חם) *to be sun-burnt, black, dark-colored. Nithpa. to be blackened.* נִתְאַכֵּם. Sot. 15ᵇ נִתְאַכְּמוּ פניו the outside of the pot grew black (Var. נתפחמו).

*__אִכְמַר__ (=חכ', onomatop.; cmp. חכך *Pi.*) *to cough.* Kidd. 81ᵇ top. א׳ שדא ביה כיחו he coughed, and threw his phlegm into the cup. [Perh. כסא א׳ a *black, dirty* cup?]

אָכֵן, v. אָכֵין.

אַכְנְגַר, v. אַדְנְגַר.

אכנס Tosef. Ḥull. III (IV), 27, v. אכספטיאס.

*__אַכְסָא__ m. *mad.* (?) Gitt. 69ª (a word in a charm formula). Cmp. אַכְתְּנָא.

אכסגרון, v. אַכְסִיגָרוֹן.

אַכְסַדְרָא, אַכְסְדְרָא, אַכְסַדְרָה f. (ἐξέδρα, exedra) (Greek) *a covered place in front of the house;* (Roman) *recess, parlor, hall for conversations and discussions.* Targ. Jud. III, 23. [*Pl.* Targ. Ps. CIV, 3, v. אִינְדְּרָא.] B. Bath. 11ᵇ א׳ דבי רב the hall of the school house (philosophers' exedra, v. Sm. Ant. s. v.), contrad. to א׳ רומיירתא (Ms. Oxf. דרומיתא, v. Rabb. D. S. a. l. note 10) Roman exedra (open but surrounded by a railing). Ib. 25ᵃᵇ עולם לא׳ וכ׳ the world resembles an exedra the northernmost side of which is not covered (מסוכבת Ms. M., ed. מסובבת not surrounded); a. fr.— *Pl.* אַכְסַדְרָאוֹת. Tam. 28ᵇ א׳ של בנין exedras forming, or belonging to, a structure (opp. to open exedra with plants).

אֶכְסוֹרְיָה f. (ἐξορία) *exile, banishment.* Lev. R. s. 18 אכסר׳ (Ar. כסוריא) (corr. acc.).

אכסר Tosef. Kel. B. Kam. VII, 4 א׳ קמטרא, read with R. S. to Kel. X, 1 עָה [אַךְ] כִּסוּי קִמטרא also the lid of a chest.

אַכְסִיגָרוֹן m. (ὀξύγαρον, oxygarum) *a sauce of vinegar and garum;* in gen. *a sauce of all kinds of vegetables.* Ber. 35ᵇ bot. Ms. M. (ed. אנס׳); Yoma 76ª; Shebu. 23ª. Tosef. Bets. II, 16. Y. Shebi. VIII, 38ª top אַקְסַר׳; Tosef. Ter. IX, 10; ib. Shebi. VI, 3 סְקַרִיגְרוֹן.—*Pl.* אַכְסִיגְרִיּוֹת, abbrev. סְפָרִיּוֹת *vegetable sauces, vegetables used for oxygarum.* Shebi. IX, 5 ed. (Var. סגרדות ,סנדיות ,סגריות, Ms. M. הנרדיוה); Tosef. ib. VII, 13 אגוטרר read אֲגְזוּגָרִין; Sifra B'har Par. II ch. 3 סנדרריות (Rabad סנדיות; corr. acc.). [Koh. R. to XI, 9 ארגסטירין read אוּגְסְיגָרִין.]

אכסיומא f. (ἀξίωμα) *request, petition.* Midr. Till. to Ps. VI, end אחרים מקבלים אכ׳ וכ׳ (corr. אכ׳) others receive the petition presented to him אני איני מבקש אלא שתהא מקבל) אנסיומין שלי (corr. acc., insert שאתה הקבל) I only ask that thou mayest receive my petition thyself. Ib. to Ps. CII אל תתן א׳ שלי בתוכה (read שלו); [the entire passage is obscure and seems out of place].

אכסיוס, אכסיוס Gen. R. s. 46, v. אַקְסִיוֹס.

אכסיטורין, read אֶכְסִיטֵירִין, v. אֶגְסִיטֵרִין.

אכסילין Tosef. Kil. V, 26, Var. of כלִיסִים, v. אכסלי.

אכסיריה, v. אֶכְסוֹרְיָה.

*__אַכְסַלְגָס, אַכְסִילְגוֹס__ m. (ξυληγός) *wood-carrier, forester.* Men. 97ª כלי א׳ common wooden vessels; Ḥag. 26ᵇ כלי אכסלגס Ar. (ed. אכסלגים Ms. M. אבלוגסין corr. acc.).— Zeb. 94ª כלי אַכְסַלְגְּיָא (Ms. M. אכסלמוס) forester's apparel (leather covers &c.); v. אַבְלוּסְמוֹס.

אַכְסַלְגְיָא f. (ξυληγία) *foresting;* v. preced.

אכסלגים, אַכְסַלְגָס, v. אַכְסִילְגוֹס.

*__אכסלי, אכסלית__, Tosef. Kil. V, 26 (ed. Zuck. כלִיסִים חגרגים, Var. כליסים, אכסילין) prob. כלים אַכְסִילִינִין (ξύλινος) *cotton clothes.*

*__אַכְסֵן__ (denom. of אַכְסְנַי II) *to harbor a guest. Nithpa.* נִתְאַכְסֵן *to be received; to lodge with.* Midr. Till. to Ps. CXVI.

אכסנא I, אַכְסְנָא, אַכְסַן m. (transpos. of אסכנא, v. סְפָא; h. מָנוֹר) *weaver's pin.* Targ. Jud. XVI, 13; 14; a. fr.—*Sabb. 151ᵇ אפי׳ מליא כא׳ דגרדאי Ms. Oxf. a. Ar. (ed. כאביסנא; Ms. M. מלי אכסניא וגרדאי) even if the painting stick is as thick (with paint) as a weaver's pin.

*__אַכְסַן__ II, pl. אַכְסְנִים, v. next art.

אַכְסְנָא II, read:

אַכְסְנַי, אכסנאי or **אַכְסְנַאי** m. (deriv. of אַכְסַנְיָא) *stranger, guest, lodger;* also (ξένος) *hired soldier.* Y. Erub. II, end 20ᵇ יֵעָשֶׂה כא׳ let him be considered as a stranger (transient lodger). Tosef. Shebi. V, 21 אכסנא some ed. (ed. Zuck. אַכְסְנָיִין pl.) *soldier,* v. אַכְסַנְיָא 3).— Arakh. 16ᵇ א׳ דאקראי an occasional guest. Ib. א׳ פוגם ונפגם a traveller (constantly changing his lodging place) discredits others a. himself; a. fr.—*Pl.* אַכְסְנָיִין (v. supra),

אַכְסְנַיִן Lev. R. s. 27.—אַכְסְנַאי, אַכְסַנְיָא, אַכְסְנַי. Targ. Y. II Gen. XLVII, 21 א׳ גּ׳לולאי exiled strangers. Gen. R. s. 50 א׳ חב לאילין give these travellers &c.—*אַכְסְנִים. Num. R. s. 10 (p. 239ᶜ ed. Amst.) מנהג הא׳ custom of hospitality [prob. אכסניא].

***אַכְסַנְדְּרִיָּה, אַכְסַנְדְּרְיָא** f. (v. אלכסנדריה) *an Alexandrian merchantman* (Alexandria navis); trnsf. *a high mast* (satyrically for *cross, gallows*). Targ. II, Esth. VII, 10 the son of Hamdatha wants to ascend לא׳ דבר פנדירא (Ms. לְאַלְכְּס׳) the mast of the son of Pandira (is to be hanged). Neg. XII, 1 באכסנדריא (marginal vers. in Mishn. edit., text אסקריא, Var. אסדא, אסכריא q. v.) in the *rigging*.

אַכְסַנְיָא f. (ξενία) 1) *hospitality, lodging*. Ex. R. s. 35 א׳ נעשו וכ׳ (Pes. 118ᵇ, corr. acc) they were a lodging place to my children in Egypt (they offered hospitality to &c.).—בעל א׳ *host*. Pesik. R. s. 11; cmp. אוּשְׁפִּיזְכָן.—B. Mets. 85ᵃ תורה מחזרת על א׳ שלה scholarship likes to come around to its inn again (to be hereditary in the family); a. fr.—2) (=בעלת א׳) *hostess*. B. Mets. 87ᵃ one must inquire בא׳ שלו after the health of his hostess.—3) *quarter given to troops on march* or *to transient poor men; also the passing troop*, or *the passing poor*; (individ.) *beggar*. Targ. Job XXXI, 32; a. e.—B. Bath. 11ᵇ א׳ לפי בני אדם the quartering (of soldiers takes place) in proportion to the number of inmates (of each house). Dem. III, 1; v. Y. ib. 23ᵇ top. Tosef. Shebi. V, 21 אין מאכילין אכסניין וכ׳ ed. Zuck. (Var. את אכסניא) you are not allowed to give.... to soldiers quartered with you. Y. Ber. IX, 13ᵇ חחן א׳ עלובתא this poor beggar. Ib. א׳ עלו׳ poor beggars. Lev. R. s. 34. Lam. R. to I, 1 (חד מירוי) בר נש א׳ a poor man.—4) *a gathering of scholars entertained by the hospitable of the place*. Y. Ber. IV, 8ᵇ top נפיק לא׳ leaving for the scholars' meeting. Bab. ib. 63ᵇ פתח בכבוד א׳ opened his speech in honor of hospitality to scholars.

אַכְסַנְיָאוּת, אַכְסַנְיוּת f. (v. preced.) 1) *stranger's condition, exile*. Sot. 36ᵇ.—2) *soldier's pay*. Mekh. B'shall. Shirah 4; Yalk. Ex. 246; a. e. (interchanging with אפסניא q. v.).

***אכסניי, א׳ פרכא** m. (read אכסנפרוכא Xenoparochus) *one who provides for strangers* or *soldiers, quartermaster*. Y. B. Kam. III, 3ᶜ top החן א׳ פ׳ . . . . שרי למיחשדוניה וכ׳ (read למישחדוניה) it is permissible to bribe the quartermaster (to let you off) before the Romans enter (the place), but not after that (when one man's release from quartering duty is a direct injury to the other inhabitants).

***אכספטייס, אכספטיאס**, Hull. 66ᵇ, Ab. Zar. 39ᵃ אקונס ואפונס . . . וא׳ (v. Var. lect. Rabb. D. S. a. l.), Tosef. Hull. III (IV), 27 קולייס ופולמוס כספתיאס אכונס וכ׳, restore (א)קולייס ופילמוס (א)כסיפיאס (כסיפיס) ואתניאס (ואתנייס) וכ׳ κολίας, πήλαμυς, ξίφιας, ἀθνίας, names of fishes (v. Greek Dict.) *Colias, Pelamys, Xiphias, Athnias* and *Thunny*; v. אֲכוּנָס.

אכסרא Tosef. Ohol. XVIII, 5, v. אסכריא a. אכסנדריא. —[V. also next w.]

אַכְסָרָה f. (used as adverb; a comp. of אך a. סרח *less or more*, v. כּבר) *in a lump, on measuring by sight*. Dem. II, 5 (Ms. M. אסכרא); Y. ib. III, 23ᶜ מוכרן א׳ he sells them in a lump (as many as there may be). Maas. Sh. IV, 2. Sifra B'hukk. Par. 4, ch. X; a. e.

אֲכַף, אֵכַף ch. (b. h. אֶכֶף, √כף, v. כפף), denomin. of אוּכָף, *to ride on a saddled ass*. Nid. 14ᵃ הא דמיכף וכ׳ Ar. (ed. מְאַכַּף=דמכף Pa.) in the one case it means that he rides on a saddled ass. [מיכף Snh. 36ᵃ, v. כוף.]

אַכְפָּא m. (v. preced.) 1) *load, weight*. B. Bath. 69ᵃ אבני דא׳ stones to weight the sheaves down to protect them from the wind.—2) *a contrivance to carry loads*, as a *hand-barrow* or *hand-basket*. Sabb. 66ᵇ חמרא דא׳, v. אַנְקְמְמִין. Bets. 30ᵃ (var. אכיתפא *on the shoulder*, v. Rabb. D. S. a. l.).

אִכְפָּה, v. next w.

אִכְפַּת, אִיכְפַּת (אִיכְּפָה) f. (אכף; cmp. b. h. אֶכֶף) *burden, care, solicitude*, followed by ל- of the person concerned. Targ. I Chr. XXI, 13 אִיכְפַּת.—Y. Sot. V, 20ᵇ top וביתא מאי אכפה ליה what concern is the Temple to him? Taan. 25ᵃ מאי א׳ לך why should that trouble thee? B. Mets. 40ᵃ וכי מאי א׳ וכ׳ what do the mice care whether &c. Koh. R. to IV, 1 זה מה א׳ ליה what concern is it to this one (if the other sinned), i. e. why should he suffer for it?; a. fr. Pesik. R. s. 10, beg. א׳ להם will people care for them (miss them)? Git. 62ᵃ מכפת לא אכפת ליה should he not care for it? Cmp. כפת.

אִכְּרָא, אִכָּר, v. אי׳.

אַכְרְגָא, v. כְּרָגָא.

אַכְרוּב m. (=כְּרוּב q. v.) *cabbage*. Y. Sabb. III, 5ᵈ top. Num. R. s. 7.—Y. Bets. V, 63ᵃ קולסי א׳ cabbage heads.

***אֲכָ׳, אִי׳, אֲכְרוּם** m. (קרם=כרם; √כר) *covering, coating*. א׳ אוכמין בקדרא a coating of blackness like a pot. Targ. Jer. VIII, 21 (h. text קדר). Targ. Joel II, 6; Nah. II, 11 (h. text פארור). Cmp. קְרוּם.

***אכרוע** Y. Maasr. I, 48ᵈ top, read אַכְרוּב; cmp. קֶלַח.

אַכְרָזָה f. h.=ch. אַכְרַזְתָּא. Y. Meg. IV, 75ᵇ top, expl. אִגֶּרֶת, v. אגרת בקורה; Y. Keth. XI, 34ᶜ; Y. Snh. I, 19ᵇ top.

אַכְרְזִיאֵל pr. n. [*the herald of God*], *Akhr'ziel*, an angel. Yalk. Deut. 940. Deut. R. s. 11 אכזרי׳ (corr. acc.)

אַכְרַזְתָּא f. (=h. הַכְרָזָה; כרז) *proclamation announcing public sale*, whence, *auction*, cmp. אֲגָרַת.—B. Mets. 35ᵇ יומי א׳ time appointed for public sale. Keth. 100ᵇ נכסי דא׳ property sold at auction. Ib. for capitation-tax &c. we sell בלא א׳ without previous announcement; a. fr.

אכרמוניא Midr. Till. to Ps. XIX, 5, Yalk. ib. ברטניא pr. n., prob. a corrupt. of איי ברינניא *Britannic Isles*.

אַכְרָעְתָּא f. (כרע) prop. *balancing*, hence *balances, scales, weighing.* Pesik. B'shall. p. 82ᵃ בא׳ דאברעין וכ׳ in the way they weighed, they were weighed. [Cmp. Buber l. c. note 43.]

אַכְשָׁרוּתָא f. (כְּשֵׁר) *propriety, proper use.* Targ. Koh. X, 10.

אַכַּתִּי (contr. of עַד כְּעַנְתָּא הִי) a scholastic term in Talm. Bab., *still, even now, yet.* Meg. 2ᵃ וא׳ מבעי ליה וכ׳ and still the plural form is needed. Yoma 27ᵃ; a. fr.—מִדְּאַכַּתִּי *since*, up to that time. R. Hash. 10ᵇ.

***אַכְתָּנָא** m. (אכת, v. P. Sm. 191; cmp. אכסא, כבס, כבסה, צבן) *venomous, vindictive.* Targ. Prov. XII, 28 Ms. Luzz. (v. Pesh., a. LXX b. c.); [some ed. אבחתנא, v. בְּהַת; עַוְתָנָא; h. text נתיבה אל וכ׳!]

***אַכְתַּר** m. (v. preced.; ר format., cmp. סביקר) *greenish, blighted.* Y. Dem. II, beg. 22ᵇ is there no rice in Hulta? א׳ הוא it is greenish.

***אַכְתְּרִיאֵל** m. (כתר) [divine crown], pr. n. *Akhtriel*, a divine surname (attribute). Ber. 7ᵃ.

אלב״ם, א״ל *Albam*, a formula of permutation of letters wherein the first interchanges with the twelfth, the second with the thirteenth, &c. Num. R. s. 18 טבאל באלב״ם רמלא *Tabel* in *Albam* reads *Ramla.* Sabb. 104ᵃ.

-אַל a prefix, =עַל; e. g. אֲלְהוּסְפְּרָאוֹת (=על האיצרות) *appointed over treasures,* v. אַ-.

אַל (b. h.) *not, no* (according to Talmud a milder form of prohibition than לֹא; v. Y. Pes. VI, 33ᵇ). Aboth I, 3.—אל תקרי (abbr. א״ת), v. אֶלָּא. Taan. 11ᵃ א׳ יראה וכ׳ shall not live to see &c.; a. v. fr.

אֶל (b. h.; איל *to turn*) prep. *to, toward.—Pl.*, with prefix מ a. suffix of pers. pron., *of itself, of my (his &c.) own accord, on my (his &c.) authority.* Yoma 5ᵇ לא מֵאֵלַי not on my own authority. Orlah I, 2 העולה מֵאֵלָיו growing spontaneously.—Y. Peah VII, 20ᵇ bot. its sacred character מֵאֵלָיו למדו they did derive from itself (i. e. from the wording of the law itself).—Hence מְמֵילָא, v. מֵילָא.

אֵל m. (b. h.; v. אלל) *God.* Shebu. 35ᵃ divine names which dare not be erased are *El* &c. Taan. 6ᵇ bot.; a. fr.

אֶלָא *buttress*, v. אִירְלָא.

אֱלָא I *to lament*, v. אלי.

אֱלָא II m. *club, bat.* Targ. Cant. VIII, 5; v. אַלְּתָא.

אֶלָּא (אִלָּא) (contr. of אִם לֹא=אִן לָא) 1) *if not; except, but, only.* Targ. O. Ex. XV, 11 לית א׳ את none but thou, none besides thee; a. e.—Ber. V, 1 אין עומדין.... א׳ וכ׳ one must stand up for prayer in no other disposition but that of humility.—Snh. 4ᵃ לא נהן א׳ שלשה he did only three times. Ber. I, 1 ולא זו בלבד (אמרו) א׳ וכ׳ and not only in this case they said so, but wherever &c. Ib. 5ᵃ אל תקרי תְּלַמְּדֶנּוּ א׳ תְּלַמְּדֶנּוּ read not *th'lamm'dennu* (thou instructest him) but *th'lamm'dēnu* (thou teachest us); a. v. fr.—2) (ellipt.) (you cannot say anything except . . .) *but,* a logical inference excluding all other explanations &c. Ib. 30ᵇ א׳ לא שנא but (the conclusion is proven) there is no difference. Ib. א׳ אמר ר׳ but, said R . . . . we may derive it &c.; a. fr.

אלאופטרא, read קְלָאו׳, v. קלפטרא.

אַלְבִּינָה, אַלְבִּינָא (אלב *to cut;* cmp. חֵלֶב, חלף, חִילְפָא &c.) *a bundle of shoots, broom.* Y. Meg. II, 73ᵃ (for b. h. מַטְאֲטֵא).

אַלְבָּנָא m. (v. preced.) *young shoot of the palm-tree, thin pointed branch. Pl.* אַלְבָּנִין, אַלְבָּנַיָּא. Cant. R. to VII, 9 the palm . . . has no less מן תלת אילנין אלבנין (strike out אילנין) than three new (cutting) shoots. Ib. in our place they call לאלבניא סנסניה the young shoots *sans'naya* (h. סנסנים). [Num. R. s. 3, beg., in Hebr. diction, אִנְבִּינִין, fr. אנב, cmp. אֵב; prob. to be read אַלְבּוּנִין.]

אֶלְגָּבִישׁ m. (b. h., cmp. גביש Job XXVIII, 18, a. Targ. a. l.) *hail, hailstone* (crystal). Ber. 54ᵇ (playful etymol. על גב איש).

אַלְגּוּמַיָּא m. pl. (=b. h. אַלְגּוּמִּים) name of *a tree.* Targ. II Chr. II, 7 (8). [Ib. IX, 10; 11 אלמוגייא, reading the h. text as in I Kings X, 11.] V. אַלְמוּג.

אלגוסין Tosef. Maasr. III, 14 Var. ed. Zuck., v. גְּרִיס.

אלדי, אלדים=אלהי, אלהים, v. אֱלוֹהַּ.

אָלָה *to curse,* v. אלי.

אָלָה f. (b. h.; אלה, √אל *to point,* cmp. ארר a. חרה) *imprecation, curse.* Sot. II, 5 (17ᵃ); a. fr.—*Pl.* אָלוֹת. Ib. a. e.

אֵלֶּה c. pl. (b. h.; v. preced.) *these, those* (cmp. הרי). Ex. R. s. 30 *v'elleh* (and this) adds to the preceding (continues), *elleh* (these) restricts. V. אֵלּוּ.

אֵלָה f. (b. h.; v. preced. ws.) *terebinth.* Shebi. VII, 5.

אלה Sabb. 90ᵃ Ar., v. אִירְלָא 3.

אַלָּה f. (b. h. Josh. XXIV, 26; v. אַלְּתָא) [pointed, prominent] 1) *lance, fork.* Kel. XVI, 8 חפוי הא׳, v. חִפּוּי. Pes. 57ᵃ אוי לי מֵאַלָּתָן woe to me (I am afraid) of their fork (weapon). Sabb. VI, 3 (63ᵃ) ed. (Ms. אלא); Y. ibid. 8ᵇ (expl. דוריקרן).—2) *sign-pole,* used in the barn as a mark. Ib; Y. Maasr. I, 49ᵃ bot.; Tosef. Ter. III, 11 משינעקר הא׳ (ed. Zuck. משיתעשר, corr. acc.) as soon as the sign-pole (fork) is removed (indicating that the grain is ready for use and priestly gifts).

אֱלָהּ, אֱלָהָא, אִילָה m. ch. (=h. אֱלוֹהַּ) *God.* Dan. III, 28; a. fr.—Targ. O. Deut. XXXIII, 26; a. fr.—Lev. R. s. 5, end את אלה רב Ar. (ed. אלוה). Y. B. Mets. II, א׳

אלהחון דיהודאי the God of the Jews. Y. Snh. X, 28[b].—*Pl.* (also plur. majest.) אֱלָהִין. Dan. II, 11; a. e.—אֱלָהַיָּא. Jer. X, 11. Targ. Ps. CXXXVI, 2 אלהי אלהיא the God of gods. [Gen. R. s. 26 כומריא גנבו א׳ וכ׳ (read אלהין) when priests rob—who would swear by their god?] Ib. (ref. to Gen. VI, 2).—Lev. R. s. 33 ....אֱלָהַיָּא תמן קריין there (in Rome) they call their kings *gods*.

אֱלֹהוּת, אֱלָהוּת f. (v. preced.) *Deity, divinity.* Gen. R. s. 46 שאין העולם—כדי לאלוהותי the universe and what it contains, are but inadequate manifestations of his divinity; a. e. Ib. s. 66 ויתן לך אלוהותו (some ed.) may he impart to thee his divine power; v. next w.—אֱלוֹהוּת, v. אֱלוֹהַּ.

אֱלָהוּתָא ch. same. Targ. Cant. VIII, 1; a. e. Gen. R. s. 66 Ar. (v. preced.).

אֱלֹהִים, v. אֱלוֹהַּ.

אִילָהֵין, אִלָּהֵין (=אלא הן) *but that, unless, except, only.* Targ. Gen. XXXII, 27; a. fr.—את א׳ *even only,* i. e. *so much the more* (or *less*), *not to say.* Targ. I Kings VIII, 27; II Kings V, 13. V. לָהֵן; cmp. אֶלָּא.

אִילּוּ, אֵלּוּ c. pl. (b. h. אֵלֶּה, q. v.) 1) *these, the following.* B. Mets. II, 1; a. v. fr.—א׳ וא׳ *both.* Zeb. V, 2; a. v. fr. *[2) (interrog.) *which?* Pesik. R. s. 29 (—30, ed. Friedm. p. 138[b]) לאילו נאמין in which of them shall we trust? Pesik. Naḥămu p. 127[b] sq.; Yalk. Is. 307 לאי זה, לאיזו.]

אִלּוּ, v. אִילּוּ.

אֲלוּ (=אֲרוּ, v. אֲלוּ) *behold.* Dan. II, 31; a. e.

אַלְוָא m. (ἀλόη, prob. of Semit. orig.) *the impissated juice of aloes,* used as a purgative. Git. 69[b] Ar. (ed. אילווא).

אֶלְוָאוֹן, v. אקסילאליאין.

חֲלַוַי, הֲלַוַאי, לְוַאי, אֲלַוַּי, אַלְוַאי (b. h. לוּ) *oh that!* Targ. Y. II Num. XXIII, 10; a. e. Targ. Ex. XVI, 3, a. fr. (לוי).—Targ. Y. ib. XXXII, 30 (h. text אולי) —Num. R. s. 2. Gen. R. s. 9; a. fr. *[Targ. Y. II Num. XXIV, 23 אַלְוַוי, Y. I וַי, *woe!*]

אַלְוָה m., pl. אַלְוִים (v. אַלְוָא) *aloe-wood.* Y. Keth. VII, end, 31[d]; Gen. R. s. 15, v. אַלְמוּג. V. also אַלְוֶוין.

אֱלוֹהַּ m. (b. h.; v. אֵל) *God. Pl. majest.* אֱלֹהִים, cmp. אֵל.—חאלהים by God! Sabb. 145[a]; a. fr. [ד is freq. substituted for ה as אלדים, ידוד, אלדי esp. in Targ. Y. ed. Sab.] אלקים, ch. אלקא, adopted in order to avoid uttering the divine name. B. Kam. 106[a]; cmp. אלעיקי, איפופי &c. —*Pl.* אֱלוֹהוֹת 1) *deities, powers.* Y. Ber. IX, beg. 12[d]. Lev. R. s. 4.—2) *biblical verses containing the word El, Elohim* &c. Y. R. Hash. IV, 59[c].

אֱלוֹהוּת, v. אֱלָהוּת.

אֱלוֹהוֹת, v. אֱלוֹהַּ.

אַלְוָה, אַלְוָא, v. אַלְוָה, אַלְוָא.

אַלְוַאי, v. אַלְוַאי.

אַלְוִים (אלווס Ar.), v. אַלְוָה.

אַלְוָוין (עַלְוָאין, עַלְוַיִּים) m. pl. (v. אַלְוָא) *the herbaceous plant aloe,* a kind of cress. Y. Shebi. IV, 35[b] bot.; Tosef. ib. I, end (ed. Zuck. עלוא׳, oth. ed. עלוין, עלוין) ומקיימין את הא׳ וכ׳ you may (in the Sabbath year) let the aloe grow on the top of the roof, but you must not water it.

אַלְוְויתָא, אַלְוָיתָא f. ch. (=h. לְוָיָה) *escort, reception on arriving and leaving.* Y. Maasr. II, 49[d] other people דלית אלוויתיה שכיחא לון (read תא ....) who do not frequently meet with a reception (an offer of refreshments &c.). Ib. דאל=)הַלְוְויָתֵיה וכ׳) who may fairly expect a reception. Cmp. אַרְבָּעוּתָא.

אלוונתית, v. אֱלוּנְתִית II.

אלווס Ar. read אַלְוִים.

אַלְוָתָא B. Bath. 73[a], v. אִבְּתָא a. אַבָּתָא.

אֱלוּל m. (b. h.) *Elul,* the sixth month of the Hebrew calendar, containing twenty nine days, varying between the seventh of August and the second of October. R. Hash. I, 1. Ib. 19[b]; a. fr. Y. Shek. III, beg. 47[b] bot. בני א׳ animals born in Elul. Targ. Y. Num. XIV, 37 אילול. Targ. II Esth. III, 7.

אלולגין, אלולננון, Tosef. Kel. B. Bath. VI, 9 read אַנְלוּגִין.

אֱלוּלִי m. (denom. of אֱלוּל) *born in Elul. Pl.* אֱלוּלִיִּים, אֱלוּלִיִּין. Y. Shek. III, beg. 47[b]; a. e.

אִלּוּלֵי, אִלּוּלָפוֹן, אִלּוּלֵיפוֹן, v. אִילּ׳.

אַלּוּם m. (אלם; אל√, cmp. חלם, חלב &c.) *a mucilaginous plant* (cmp. Lat. Alum), prob. *Silphium,* a kind of *Laserpitium* or *Asafœtida.* T'bul Yom I, 5 (Var. in Ar. אילוב, הלום). Cmp. אֶלֶל.

אֲלוּמָא m. ch.=next w. 2).—*Pl.* אֲלוּמַיָּא. Targ. Ruth II, 7; 15.

אֲלוּמָה f. (b. h. אֲלֻמָּה; אלם) 1) *binding, making sheaves.* Peah VI, 9 (10) ... נתנה לא׳ grain stalks intended for binding sheaves *thereof* (but not for binding the latter into bundles of sheaves עֹמֶר, Maim.)—[For binding sheaves *therewith* R. S.].—2) *sheaf.* Ex. R. s. 31.—*Pl.* אֲלוּמוֹת. B. Mets. 22[b] sq. *large sheaves,* opp. כריכות.

אַלּוֹן I m. (b. h.; v. אֵלָה) *oak.*—*Pl.* אַלּוֹנִים. Gen. R. s. 15 א׳ בלוטין the bibl. *allonim* means *b'lutin,* v. בָּלוּט. [Ib. אלמוגים א׳ read אַלְוִים, v. אַלְוָה, [אַלְמוּג]. R. Hash. 23[a] א׳ בוטמי, v. בּוּטְמָא; B. Bath. 80[b] א׳ בוטני, v. בּוּטְנָא. [Gen. R. s. 60 (play on *hallazeh* Gen. XXIV, 6) א׳ זה he is an oak (of fine appearance); Rashi refers to next w.]

אַלוֹן II m. (ἄλλος; acc.) another. Gen. R. s. 81 in Greek allon means אַחֵר; Pesik. Zakh. p. 24ᵃ א׳ תרי (read אַחֵר) another (one more).

אֲלוּנְטִית I (אֲלוּנְתִית) (interchanging with לוּנְטִית q. v.) f. (לוּט, to cover, wrap, cmp. I Sam. XX, 10, a. לאט in H. Dict.; נ inserted) wrapping cloth, sheet, bathing clothes. Sabb. 40ᵇ מיחם אדם אלונט׳ (Ms. M. אלונת׳, Tosef. ib. III (IV), 7 אלונתת) one may warm a sheet on the Sabbath to put it on the stomach; Y. Sabb. XIX, 17ᵃ bot. [Gen. R. s. 80 to put on a wound, prob. next w.]—Sabb. 147ᵇ (Ms. M. always אלונת׳, Ar. לונט׳). Men. 72ᵃ.—Y. Erub. VIII, 25ᵇ top.—Pl. אֲלוּנְטִיאוֹת Sabb. XXII, 5 (147ᵃ). Ib. 147ᵇ בעשר אלונטית (read טִיאוֹת . . ., or טִיּוֹת . . .). Tosef. ib. XVI (XVII), 15 אֲלוּנְטָאוֹת (Var. אֲלֻנְטִיאוֹת, לְנְטִיאוֹת). Ib. 17 אנלונטאות (Var. אלונטיאות).

אֲלוּנְטִית II, corr. אֲלוּנְתִית (אֲלִנְתִית) f., אֲלִינְתִין m. (a corrupt. of οἰνάνθη, οἰνάνθινος, œnanthe, œnanthinus; cmp. אניגרון as to נ a. ל) made of the grape (or leaves) of wild vine (œnanthe), whence 1) an aromatic water. Y. Ber. VI, 10ᵈ he who sprinkles אלינת׳ œnanthe.—2) an unguent. Y. ib. I, 3ᵃ top סכין אלונ׳ וכ׳ (corr. acc.) you may oint a sick person with œn. on the Sabbath. Y. Sabb. XIV, 14ᶜ bot. אלינתין. Y. Shebi. VII, beg. 37ᵇ יצאת א׳ . . . לתְּפִילִין (read תית . . . .) except œn. which is only for children (after circumcision).—3) a wine (vinum œnanthinum), used esp. after bathing. Ab. Zar. 30ᵃ (expl. as a mixture of old wine, pure water and balsam); Sabb. 140ᵃ אלונט׳ ed. (Ms. M. אלונת׳). Ḥull. 6ᵃ wine to be put לתוך הא׳ into a mixture called ălunțith; Tosef. Dem. I, 24. Y. Bets. I, 60ᵈ top.

אלוניסתין, v. אֲלִנְסְטִי.

אֲלוּנְכָא m. (=לוּנְכָא q. v.) spear-head, javelin. Pl. אֲלוּנְכֵי. Git. 70ᵃ בא׳ דפרסאי (Ar. בלונכי) with Persian (poisoned) javelins.

אַלוּנְקִי, v. אַלְנְקִי.

אֲלוּנְתִית, v. אֲלוּנְטִית.

אלוסטרוס, v. אַלָּס.

אַלּוּף m. (b. h.; אלף) prince, chief. Gen. R. s. 20 beg. אלופו של עולם the world's chief (Aleph, i. e. Adam).

אָלוּשׁ pr. n. pl. (b. h.) Alush, one of the stations of the Israelites on their journey to Kanaan. Yoma 10ᵃ. Gen. R. s. 48 (play on lushi, Gen. XVIII, 6). Y. Bets. II, beg. 61ᵃ.

אלות Pesik. R. s. 22 כ״ד א׳, read בוּלָאוֹת, v. בּוּלֵי.

אַלְוָתָא f. (v. אַלְוָא) a piece of aloe-wood. Bets. 33ᵇ; v. אַלְתָא.

אֲלוּתָא, v. אִלְיְתָא a. אַלְתָא.

*__אלמיכסיא, אלמיכסיה, אלמיכסיא__, Gen. R. s. 8 א׳ שלך Ar., ed. תכסיס א׳ שלך . . ., Yalk. Ps. 834 תכסיס אלתמסין, prob. אַלְכְּבַסְסִין (v. אַל- a. כַּבְסִיס) chief of the court-ceremonies (i. e. the angel of Truth); Rashi: seal (?).

אֶלָטִין (ἐλάτη) fir-trees. Tanh. T'rum. 9 ברוש א׳ Bibl. b'rosh means firs.

*__טירנון, אלטינון__, a corruption of יַאנְטִינוֹן for יַאנְתִינוֹן m. (ἰάνθινον, Aquila Ex. XXV, 5) violet-colored. Koh. R. to I, 9 אלט׳; Y. Sabb. II, 4ᵈ (expl. bibl. תחש as a color לטש צבעו, v. Ges. H. Dict. s. v. תַּחַשׁ). [Esth. R. to I, 6 טירנון (Var. סירנון) read יקרנטינון].

אלי I, אָלָה (b. h. √אל, v. אָלָה; cmp. נקב, הָגָה &c.) to curse. Sifré Num. 18 (ref. to Num. XVIII, 21) לאלה שיהו אָלִין בה וכ׳ 'as a curse' means that people shall curse by her (pointing to her), 'may happen unto thee what happened to . . . . .'.

אלי II, אֲלָא (=ילל, v. אִילְיָא) to lament, wail. Targ. II Sam. I, 17; a. e.

Pa. אַלָּא same. Targ. Jud. XI, 40 לְאַלָּאָה (some ed. לְאַלָּאָה).

אֱלִי mourning, v. אִלְיְתָא and אַלִיתָא.

אַלְיָא, אֱלְיָא, v. אִילְיָא.

אליאס read אִילְיָאוֹס q. v.

אַלִּיבָּא (=עַל-לִב=אַל-לִב) according to the opinion, in the sense of. B. Kam. 13ᵃ, a. fr. א׳ דמאן in whose sense? in accordance with whom? Sot. 21ᵃ א׳ דהלכתא in accord. with the adopted decision. Sabb. 28ᵇ, a. v. fr. א׳ דר׳ in the sense, developing the opinion, of R.—.

אַלְיָה f. (b. h.; לוי; v. infra) attachment, whence 1) (cmp. זָנָב, גּוּנְבָא) tail, fat-tail. Ab. Zar. 25ᵃ (ref. to I Sam. IX, 24) what means v'healeha (and that which is upon [or by] it)? שוק וא׳ that means the leg (with thigh) and the fat-tail. מאי והעליה וכ׳ and why is it called 'and that which is upon it'? Because the leg is near the fat-tail (back). Ḥull. 117ᵃ; a. fr.—כלפי א׳ (Ar. s. v. כלפי; ed. כלפי לְיָיא, Mss. לְיָא) towards the tail! i. e. just the reverse!, reverse it. Pes. 5ᵇ; Sabb. 93ᵇ; Ab. Zar. 75ᵃ; a. fr. [Rashi: כלפי לייא where are you turning to?]—2) ear-lap. Keth. 5ᵇ.

אֵלִיָּהוּ (b. h.) pr. n. m. Eliyahu, Elijah, the great prophet in the days of Ahab, freq. represented, in Talmud and Midrashim, as intervening in behalf of the pious and punishing wrong-doers, and expected, in the Messianic days, to clear up doubts and prepare the heavenly kingdom; cmp. Mal. III, 23.—Ber. 58ᵃ, a. fr. אתא א׳ אידמי ליה וכ׳ E. came and appeared to him in the disguise of &c. Gen. R. s. 33, a. fr. אתא א׳ זכור לטוב E., whose memory be blessed, came &c. B. Mets. I, 8 (37ᵃ), a. fr. יהא מונח עד שיבוא א׳ let it be deposited until E. shall come (and decide to whom it belongs, i. e. an indefinite time until the matter be cleared up). Men. 45ᵃ; a. fr.—סֵדֶר אֵלִיָּהוּ Seder Eliyahu, name of a lost Talmudic treatise, divided into Seder Eliyahu Rabba (Large) and S. E. Zuta (Small). Keth. 106ᵃ (of legendary origin).

אֱלִיהוּא pr. n. m. (b. h.) Elihu, one of Job's friends. Y. Sot. V, end, 20ᵈ. Yalk. Job 919. B. Bath. 15ᵇ.

אֶלְיְהוֹעֵינַי, אֶלְיוֹעֵנַי (b. h.) pr. n. m. *Elioenai*, a highpriest. Par. III, 5.

אַלְיוֹן m. (√ליי, v. אַלְיָה) *thumb, great toe. Pl.* אַלְיוֹנִים. Pesik. R. s. 31 אַלְיוֹנֵי ידיהם their thumbs; Midr. Till. to Ps. CXXXVII. 4; Yalk. a. l.

אַלְיוֹן, אַלְיוֹנָא, אִיל׳ ch. same. Targ. Ex. XXIX, 20; a. e.—Git. 69ᵃ טופרא דאַלְיוֹנָא (Rashi אליונא, corr. acc.) the nail of the thumb.—*Pl.* אַלְיוֹנַיָּא. Targ. Ps. CXXXVII, 4 קטעו לואר אַלְיוֹנֵיהוֹן בככיהון (missing in some ed.) the Levites cut their thumbs off with their teeth; v. quot. in preced.

אליוסטון, v. אֲלִיַּסְטוֹן.

אֶלְיוֹעֵינַי, v. אֶלְיְהוֹ׳.

אֶלְיוּפוּלִיס, v. אִיל׳.

אֲלִיוּתָא f. (אלי II) *wail, eulogy.* Targ. Job III, 7; v. אִילְיוּתָא.

אֶלְיוּתְרוֹפוּלִיס pr. n. pl. (Ἐλευθερόπολις) *Eleutheropolis* (Freetown), an Idumean town corresponding to *Hori* (Gen. XIV, 6). Gen. R. s. 42 (ed. corrup. מכרופ׳) read with Ar. את החורי א׳ ולמה קורא אותה א׳ שברוו אותה ויצאו להן לחירות . . . they selected it for their residence and made themselves independent.

אַלִיחְרוֹק pr. n. *Allihrok*, name of an Egyptian eparchy or nomos, prob. *Heracleotes.* Targ. Y. Gen. X, 6; I Chr. I, 8 (h. text פוט), ed. Rahm. אליחרק (Var. אליחרק).

אֲלִיטָא, v. חֲלִיטָא III.

אֲלִיָּוה, v. אִילְיָא.

אֲלִיַּסְטוֹן, v. אֲלִיַּסְטוֹן.

אֲלִית, אֲלִיַּת f. (אלי II) *female wailer.* Kel. XVI, 7 רביעית של א׳ the wailer's musical instrument. Ib. XV, 6. —Ch. אֲלִיתָא q. v.

אֱלִיל m. (אלל *to roll*, sec. r. of איל; cmp. חול a. גִּלּוּלִים) 1) (cacophem.) *idol.* Ab. Zar. IV, 3 (Talm. ed. ע״ז); a. e.—*Pl.* אֱלִילִים. עבודת א׳ (abbr. ע״א) *idolatry;* also *idol* (cmp. יִרְאָה). Snh. 97ᵇ. Yoma 9ᵇ; a. fr.—2) *offal of meat, v.* אֱלָל.

אֱלִיל ch. same.—*Pl.* אֱלִילַיָּא. Targ. Y. Lev. I, 2.

אֱלִיל (=יְלִיל) *to lament.* Targ. Is. XV, 4 (XIV, 31); Joel I, 11.

אַלִּיל Pa. of אֲלַל.

אַלִּילָא m. (v. preced.) *spy.*—*Pl.* אַלִּילֵי. Targ. Gen. XLII, 9; a. e. (ed. Berl. אָלֵי׳).

אֵלִים, 1) בֵּית א׳ pr. n. pl. *Beth-Elim*, near Mount Tabor. Gen. R. s. 99 beg. Mekh. Yithro s. 5 (אלהים).—2) אֵלִים pl. of אַיִל q. v.

אִלִּים, v. אִלֵּם.

אַלִּים, אַלִּימָא m., **אַלִּימָא** f. (אלם) *strong, influential; violent.* Targ. Y. Gen. XXV, 23; a. e.—Git. 60ᵇ, a. fr. כל דא׳ גבר whoever is in power wins (right of possession in cases in which the judge is unable to decide). Hull. 39ᵇ אינש אלמא a powerful man (defying the law).—Keth. 14ᵃ א׳ ליה בריא to him the positive assertion is the stronger argument.—*Pl.* אַלִּימֵי Hull. 76ᵃ *thick* (sinews). Kid. 59ᵃ באגא דא׳ a village community of violent men.—Fem. Kidd. 44ᵇ מי א׳ כיד אביה is she as strong, has she the same authority as her father has? B. Mets. 34ᵃ מי א׳ ממתניתין is (the Boraitha) stronger (less pliable) than our Mishnah?—Hull. 48ᵇ אַלִּימְתָּא the strong, thick (pin).—*Pl.* אַלִּימָתָא. Yeb. 43ᵃ א׳ strong, thick combs.

אַלִּימָא, v. preced.

אִילִּימָא I, אִילּוּמָא 1) (=אִין *if;* לָא=לִי *not;* מא *quidem, somehow*) *unless, but for* (followed by ש־; cmp. אִלְמָלֵא 1). Num. R. s. 18, end אי׳ כִּי ..... שמעמ׳ וכ׳ but for the sticky substance in the nose intercepting the evil smell.—2) (=אִילּוּ־מָא if somehow) *if* (ruling the verb without mediation of a relative; cmp. אִלְמָלֵא 2). Ib. א׳ היפשת וכ׳ if (the harsh ringing sound) should take a permanent hold of his ear, it would be bound up (with his body, sub. בלבו as in Tanh. Hukkath 1, where our w. is substituted by אִלְמָלֵא).—3) v. אִילִּימָא.

אַלִּימָא II, אִיל׳ (אֲלִימָא) m. 1) *mute*, v. אִלְמָא. Targ. Y. Ex. IV, 11.—*2) *thick*, v. אַלִּים. Hull. 76ᵇ.

אַלִּימוּתָא, אַלְמוּתָא f. (אֲלַם 1) *strength, force.* Targ. Job XXX, 21. Targ. Y. Ex. XXV, 2. Cmp. אוּלְמָא.

אִלִּימְנָא m. (אֲלַם 3) *mute.* Targ. Ps. XXXVIII, 14 Ms. (ed. אִילְמָנָא).

אַלִּימְתָּא, v. אַלִּים.

אֲלִינְתִּין, אֲלִינְתִּית, v. אֲלוּנְטִית.

***אֲלִיס, אֲלִיס (אִילִיס)** m., only in pl. אֲלִיסִים, אֲלִיסִין &c. (אלס, cmp. אלין in Hebr. Dict. a. רסס, רציץ) *ruins, debris.* Lev. R. s. 19 (referring to Amos VI, 11) הדין רסיסה אית מיניה אל׳ (read רסיסא) of what is demolished by making breaches, there remain ruins, והדין בקיעא לית מיניה אי׳ while of what is demolished by chopping, no ruins remain; Koh. R. to X, 18 (corr. acc.); Cant. R. to IV, 14. Cmp. בִּיזָא and אִלְסִים.

אַלִּיס, v. אֲלַס.

אֲלִיַּסְטוֹן, אֲלַיְיסְטוֹן, הֲלַיְיסְטוֹן m. (ἡλιαστός, acc., fr. ἡλιάζω, v. Gr. Dict.) *a luscious wine* (vinum dulce) for which the grapes were to be dried in the sun for three days, after which they were gathered and trodden on the fourth during the full fervor of the midday heat (Sm. Ant. s. v. *Vinum;* Columella XII, 27). Men. VIII, 6 אליסטון Mish. (Ar. ed. Koh. אלייס׳, Talm. ed. 86ᵇ הלי׳, הליסטיון). B. Bath. 97ᵇ אלייסטון Ar. (Var.

a. ed. הירליסטון; Ms. והלאסטון, והירליסטריון; v. Rabb. D. S. a. l.). Tosef. Men. IX, 9 (from which B. Bath. l. c. is quoted) אליסטון.

אֱלִיעֶזֶר pr. n. m. *Eliezer*, 1) servant of Abraham. Gen. R. s. 44; a. fr. 2) several Tanaim: a) E. ben Hyrcanus; E. b. Jacob, E. bar Zadok, disciples of R. Johanan b. Zaccai of the second gener.—b) E. b. Judah, E. b. Matathias; E. b. Ḥisma, of the third gener.—c) E. hak-Kappar, a late member of the fifth gener.

אֱלִיף, v. אֱלַף.

אליפיס, Y. Shebi. IV, 35[c] top, read אִלְפְּסִים.

***אֶלִיקָה** m. (ἕλιξ, acc. . . κα) *wind-lass* for launching ships. Y. Sabb. VII, 10[c] top, read: ההן דמגפר אעין למני וחבלין לא׳ he who pitches wood for vessels or ropes for a wind-lass.

***אֲלֵיקִי, אַלְעִיקִי** (a disguise of אלהים for the purpose of avoiding the utterance of the divine name, cmp. אֱלֹהַּ) *by God! forsooth* (ironically). Pesik. Baḥod. p. 104[a] אלי׳ אני חובע בה Ar. (ed. אל אחא, Ms. Oxf. אליקי אילי) forsooth, I shall propose to her, i. e. do you believe I shall &c.? Cant. R. to I, 4 אלעי׳ אני נותן וכ׳ forsooth (do you believe) I shall give &c. [V. Pesik. l. c. note 81.]

אֶלְיָקִים (b. h.) pr. n. m. *Eliakim*. Ab. Zar. 58[a] R. El. attendant of Rabba.

אלירא read אִלְּרִיָא.

אֱלִישָׁע pr. n. m. *Elisha*, 1) the prophet. Ber. 10[b]. Gen. R. s. 25; a. e.—2) E. ben Abuyah, surnamed אַחֵר, q. v. Aboth. IV, 20. M. Kat. 20[a].—3) one E. surnamed בעל כנפים 'winged'. Sabb. 49[a]; 130[a]. Y. Ber. II, 4[c] bot.

בֵּי אֱלִישָׁפָט, v. בֵּלְשָׁפָט.

אֲלִיַּת, v. אַלְיָית.

אֲלִיתָא f. ch.=h. אַלְיָית *wailing woman*. *Pl.* אֲלִיָתָא. Targ. Jer. IX, 16 (17) ed. Ven. אֲלִיָתָן, ed. Vien. אֲלִיָתָא.

***אֲלִיתָא** f.=אַלְיוּתָא. Gen. R. s. 15, end; Pesik. Ron. p. 142[b] א׳ ובכיתא wailing and weeping; v. אֲלִיתָא.

אַלְיְתָא (אֲלִיתָא) f. ch.=h. אַלְיָה, *fat-tail*. Targ. Ex. XXIX, 22; a. e.—Ḥull. 127[a] בשמתא נרש .... ואליתיה excommunicated be Narash with its fat, skin and tail, i. e. all its inhabitants.

אֲלִיתָא or **אַלְיְתָא** f. (cmp. אֵלָה, אֵלוֹן &c.) 1) *fig-tree* (of a certain species).—בְּרַת א׳ name of a fig species. Gen. R. s. 15, end ברת א׳ וכ׳ Ar. (ed. אלי) it is called *brqth alitha* (daughter of mourning, v. אֲלִיָתָא), because it has brought wailing and weeping into the world (as the fruit of the tree of knowledge).—2) *wood of the fig-tree*, used as kindling wood on the altar (h. form אַלְיְתָה). Tam. II, 4 (Mish. תא . . ., Talm. 29[a] תה . . . .). Yoma 24[b], Y. ib. II, 39[c] top.—*Pl.* אַלְיתוֹת. Par. III, 9.

***אֲלִיתָא, עֲלִיתָא** f. (pronunc. and meaning doubtful) *Illitha*, something supposed to render fire-proof or extinguish the fire. Snh. 108[b] יש לנו דבר אחד וא׳ שמה Ar. (ed. 'וע) we have something, its name is Ill. [perhaps to be read דבר אחר a (female) idol]; Yalk. Job 906 'עיל, Ms. עלוונה]. [B. Bath. 73[a] ומחינן ליה באלי׳ Ar. Var. s. v. אלתא, ed. אַלְּתָא, Rashi אַלְוָתָא, Ms. Oxf. ואית לן אלוותא pl. of אַלְּתָא. The use of the masc. gend. in connection with the word, makes the passage appear spurious.]

אַלִיְתָה, pl. אַלְיתוֹת, v. אַלְּתָא.

אֱלָךְ=אִילֵּךְ. Dan. III, 12; 13.

אֲלַכְּסָא, לִיכְּסָה pr. n. m. *Alaxa, Lixah*, abbrev. of Alexander. Y. Keth. V, beg. 29[c] R. Al.—Ib. IX, 33[b] א׳ אמר לו ר׳ מנא (read לר׳ מנא); Y. Shebu. VII, 38[a] bot. לִיכְּסָה וכ׳ name of a gentile judge.

אֲלַכְסוֹן (=לוכסן, λοξός; cmp. howev. ἀλλάξ) 1)(adv.) *athwart, crosswise*. Tosef. Kel. B. Mets. VIII, 5 two feet &c. of a bed cut off א׳ crosswise; (Kel. XVIII, 5 לוכסן).—2) אֲלַכְסוֹן, ch. form אֲלַכְסוֹנָא m. *diagonal line, diameter*. B. Bath. 101[b]; Succ. 8[a] כל אמתא .... באלכסונה a figure of one square cubit has a diagonal line of $1^2/_5$ cubits (approximately). Men. 35[a]; Meg. 24[b] must be square בתפרן ובאֲלַכְסוֹנָן both as to their seams (not warped) and as to the measure of their diagonal lines. Erub. 59[c] מידת העיר ואלכסונה Ms. K. (ed. 'בא, v. Rashi a. l.) the measure of the circumference of the town plus its diameter. B. Bath. 99[a] ודילמא בא׳ הוו קיימי perhaps the Cherubim in the Sanctuary were placed across the room; a. fr.

אֲלַכְסִין, אֲלַכְסַנְדְּרִין m. pl. (v. אֲלַכְּסָא) *Alexandrians*, name of a *nut*, prob. *a species of pistachio*. Ab. Zar. 14[a] אלכסין ed. (Ms. M. אלכסנדרין, Ar. אכלסין). Cmp. אִלְסְרִין.

אֲלֶכְּסַנְדְּרָא pr. n. m. *Alexander*. Y. Dem. II, 22[c] top, (an Amora of a place called Tsadoka). Cant. R. to IV, 12; v. אֲלֶכְּסַנְדְּרוֹס.

אֲלֶכְּסַנְדְּרוֹס, אֲלַכְּ׳ pr. n. m. *Alexander*. 1) A. the Great, מוקדון the Macedonian. Targ. Cant. VI, 8; Targ. II, Esth. I, 2.—Tam. 31[b]; a. fr.—2) name of a judge and of a robber. Y. Ber. IX, 13[b] top (for אלכסנדריאה ib. read our w.).

אֲלֶכְּסַנְדְּרִי m. 1) *Alexandrian*. Sifra B'ḥukk. chap. V, Lulianus the Alex.—2) pr. n. m. *Alexandri*, an Amora. Y. R. Hash. IV, 59[c] bot; a. e.—Cant. R. to IV, 2 דרא .... (corr. acc.).—3) v. אֲלַכְסִין.—*Pl.* אֲלֶכְּסַנְדְּרִיִּים; fem. אֲלֶכְּסַנְדְּרִיּוֹת. Men. 100[a] *Alexandrians*. Ib. 28[b] כוסות א׳ (Yalk. Ex. 369 ריות....) Alexandrian cups (lengthy and narrow). Tosef. Meg. III (II), 6 בה"כ של א׳ a Synagogue built by Alexandrians in Jerusalem.

אֲלֶכְּסַנְדְּרִיָא, אֲלֶכְּסַנְדְּרִיאָה, אֲלַכְּ׳ pr. n. pl. *Alexandria*, in Egypt. Targ. Ez. XXX, 15; a. e.—Y. Ḥag.

II, 77[d]; a. fr.—Kel. XV, 1, v. next w.—Midr. Till. to Ps. XIX, a ship coming 'בא' .V. אַכְסַנְדְּרְיָא.

אַלֶכְּסַנְדְּרִית f. *Alexandrian.* Kel. XV, 1 'ספינה א Mish. ed. (Talm. ed. ס' אלכסנדריא) Alexandrian ship, i. e. Sea ship with water reservoirs. Sabb. 90[a], a. e. 'נתר א Alex. nitron. Tosef. Nid. IV, 17 Cleopatra 'מלכת א (ed. Zuck. ־ים—) Egyptian queen.—*Pl.* אֲלֶכְּסַנְדְּרִיּוֹת, v. אֲלֶכְסַנְדְּרִי.

אָלַל (sec. r. of אוּל, v. אֵוַל; cmp. עלל) 1) *to circle. Pi.* אִילֵּל *to go around; to espy, track.* Cant. R. beg. (play on תורה a. תוּר) אחר ד"ת אִילַּלְתָּ thou didst search after the words of the Law. Pesik. R. s. 47 *ḥafar* (Job XXXIX, 29) לשון מְאַלֵּל has the meaning of espying (ed. incorr. ילל, v. ed. Friedm. p. 190[b]).—[2) *to point out;* 3) *to tie around; to be strong;* v. אֵל, אלי I, אֵלָה, אִילָן &c., a. אלם.]

אֲלַל, *Pa.* אַלֵּיל ch. same. Targ. Num. XIII, 2; a. fr.—Deriv. אֲלִילָא, מְאַלְּלָא.

אָלָל h., אֲלַל ch. m. (b. h. אֱלִל Job XIII, 4; v. אֱלִיל; cmp. חלל) *soft, lax object,* whence *fatty substance, offal of meat.* Targ. Job. l. c.—Ḥull. IX, 1 (Gem. 121[a], diff. of opin. as to what kind of offal is meant in the Mish., v. מַרְהֶקָא). Ib. 'החא חמכונס the offal gathered (as a ball). Zeb. III, 4.—Toh. I, 4 אֱלִיל. Meil. 7[a] 'א' כיון דלית ביה וכ *ălal,* because there is no substantial value in it. Zeb. 35[a] 'פיגל בא if one had an inappropriate thought about *ălal* of fowls (which is fit to eat).

אַלְלָא or **אוּלְלָא** m. (אֲלַל; cmp. b. h. דָּרַךְ) *treading the wine or olive press; quantity put into the press at a time.* B. Mets. 105[a] 'בא ..... חא באתרא Ar. (ed. 'אוּ) the one Rabbi treats of a place where they ordinarily put one *khor* (measure) into the press at a time, &c. Esth. R. to I, 2 (referring to Esth. l. c., and Neh. XIII, 15 'in those days'; play on *al'la* a. *al'lay;* v. next w.) 'א 'ווי וכ *'wine pressing'* (on Sabbath, Neh. l. c.) and 'woe' (persecution as punishment) were those days marked for.

אַלְלַי (b. h.; v. אלי II, ילל) *woe.* Lev. R. s. 17, a. e.; v. next w. Tanḥ. Aḥaré 2, אלילים (corr. acc.); ed. Bub. 3.

אַלְלַיָא m. pl. (v. preced.) *woe-makers,* a word coined for playing on הוֹלְלִים (Ps. LXXV, 5, a. e.). Lev. R. s. 20; a. e.; v. ווּיְנַיָא for correct vers.

אָלַם (b. h.; √אל, v. אָלַל) 1) [to surround]; *to connect, tie* (cmp. חגר. אסר); intr. *to be tied up, excluded, lonely, mute;* v. אוּלָם, אֲלְמָנָה, אַלְמוֹן II, אִלֵּם.—2) *to grow, be strong,* v. אֵלֶם. Cmp. אַלְמוֹן I. [Cmp. אֵלֶם Ps. LVIII, 2, LXX *ἄρα,* a. v. אוּלָם I.]

אֲלַם ch., intr. אֲלֵים (אַלֵּים *Pa.,* עלים) (v. preced.) 1) *to be* or *grow strong, to grow.* Targ. I Chr. XXII, 12 (13) אֱלַם (h. text אֱמָץ, Var. עילם). Targ. O. Deut. XXXI, 6; 7; 23 ed. Vien. 'א (ed. Berl. 'ע, v. Berl. Targ. O. II, p. 59).—B. Bath. 124[a]; 135[b] (he left them) 'דיקלא וא a slender palm-tree and it grew thick.—2) *to tie,* v. אֲלוּמָא.—3) *to be mute;* v. Ithp.

Pa. אַלֵּים 1) *to be strong,* v. supra.—2) *to strengthen, support.* Targ. II Chr. XI, 17; a. e. Part. pass. f. מְאַלְּמָא *resolved, insisting upon.* Targ. Ruth I, 18 (h. text מתאמצת).—B. Kam. 90[a] 'אַלְּמוּהָ רבנן וכ the Rabbis fortified the husband's right (gave him superior privileges). Kidd. 43[a] אַלּוּמֵי קא מְאַלְּמִינָא למילתיה (Rashi אַלְּמוּהָ) we (the court) give him privileges.—3) *to overpower.* Sabb. 156[b] אַלְּמֵיה יצריה his appetite overwhelmed him.

Ithpa. אִתְאַלַּם 1) *to make one's self strong, to summon strength.* Targ. Job XXXVI, 19.—2) *to become mute, be silenced.* Targ. Ps. XXXIX, 10. Targ. Koh. XII, 6. [Targ. Ps. XC, 10 מִתְאַלְּמִין (for h. text רָהְבָּם?). [Targ. Job VI, 6 Ms. Vers. מִתְאַלַּם (?), h. text חלמות!.]

אִלֵּם, אִילֵּם m. (b. h.; v. אָלַם 1) cmp. חֵרֵשׁ) *mute, unable to speak,* also *ignorant.* Ter. I, 6; a. fr.—Ruth. R. to IV, 1 (ref. to *almoni,* Ruth. l. c.) 'א' הוה מד"ת he was unable to speak of (excluded from) the Law (ignorant).—*Pl.* 'אִילְ' אִלְּמִין אִלְּמִים. Snh. 71[a]; 100[a].—Fem. אִלֶּמֶת, 'אִילְ. Num. R. s. 9. Ḥull. 79[a]. Sot. 10[b] 'אי; a. e.

אֲלוּמָא, אִילֵימָא, אִילְמָא, אַלְמָא ch. same. Targ. Ex. IV, 11.—*Pl.* אִילְמֵי &c. Ḥag. 3[a]; Yalk. Ex. 356; Deut. 440. [Ḥull. 76[b] חד אילימא, v. אֲלִימָא II, 2.]

אַלְמָא *strong,* v. אֲלִימָא.

אַלְמָא m. (cmp. b. h. אֻלָם, v. אָלַם) *confirmation;* (dial. term) *consequently.* Pes. 2[b] 'א' אור וכ consequently *ôr* means day-light. Sabb. 151[a]; a. fr.

אַלְמָה, אַלְמָא (=על למה) *why?, wherefore?* Erub. 3[a] 'אלמא אמר וכ why did R... say &c.?—Yoma 2[b] 'אלמה לא ניבעי וכ why should separation not be required &c.?; a. fr.

אַלְמוֹג m. (b. h. עצי אלמגים, 'ע' אלגומים) 1) *red coral.* Tosef. Kel. B. Mets. III, 13; Kel. XIII, 6; Sabb. 59[b]; Y. ib. VI, 8[b] top.—2) pl. אַלְמוּגִים, אַלְמוּגִין *a species of cedar-tree,* prob. *coral-wood* (v. infra as to various opinions). R. Hash. 23[a]; B. Bath. 80[b] sq. 'א' כסיתא *almugim* is coral (apparently a confusion of *coral* and *coral-wood*). Y. Keth. VII, end, 31[d] 'א' אלוים *alm.* is the aloe-wood (agallochum); (Gen. R. s. 15 beg. אלווס Ar., ed. אלווים, אלונים corr. acc.). Pesik. R. s. 33 (ref. to II Chr. II, 7 a. I Kings X, 12); v. גלומי.

אַלְמוּגָא, pl. אַלְמוּגַיָּא, אַלְמוּגִין ch. same. Targ. I Kings X, 11; 12. II Chr. IX, 10; 11.

אַלְמוֹן I m. (v. אלם) *a cedar species, oak* [or *terebinth*]. *Pl.* אַלְמוֹנִים. R. Hash. 23[a]; B. Bath. 80[b]; v. בְּלוּט a. בּוּטְמָא.

אַלְמוֹן II m. (b. h. אַלְמָן, v. אלם) [*tied up, secluded;* cmp. Targ. I Sam. XXI, 3 טמיר for h. אלמני] *widower.* Keth. 7[b]; a. fr.

אַלְמוֹנִי m. (b. h. אַלְמֹנִי *unnamed, unknown,* v. preced.) pr. n. m. *Almoni.* Ruth R. to IV, 1 'פלוני א' וכ the man's name was Ploni Almoni. Cmp. אִלֵּם.

אלמיג Tosef. Kel. B. Mets. III, 13 read אַלְמוֹג.

אַלְמִין* m. (prob. corrupt., for לִימִין λιμήν) *harbor.* Y. Succ. II, beg. 52[d] 'בנהונה בא when the ship lies in port.

אַלְמָלֵא, אַלְמָלֵי, אִילְ׳ 1) (=אִילוּ־מָא־לָא) *if in any way not, if not, but for* (usu. without verb or followed by שֶׁ־ or דְּ־; cmp. אִלֵּימָאI, 1). Snh. 49ᵃ א׳ דוד וכ׳ but for David (studying the Law), Joab could wage no war. Meg. 12ᵇ א׳ אגרות וכ׳ but for the previous letters. Tanh. Hukkath 1 (ed. Bub. 1 אם לא); a. fr.—2) (=אִילוּ־מָא־לָא: cmp. אִלֵּימָאI, 2) *if indeed.* Meg. 24ᵇ אלמלי אתה לוי [Ms. M. אלמלא לוי אתה) if thou wert a Levite. Keth. 33ᵇ אלמלא נגדוה וכ׳ if they had lashed Hananiah &c. Sabb. 118ᵇ; a. fr. [A differentiation of spelling which may have existed for the two opposite meanings of our w., is untraceable; v. Lowe, Pesachim, p. 28.] Cmp. אִילּוּלֵי.

אַלְמֵן (deriv. of next w.) *to reduce to widowhood, bereave, desert.* Pes. 49ᵃ וּמְאַלְמֵן את אשתו will be forced to desert his wife (to leave his home).—*Nithpa.* נִתְאַלְמְנָה *to become a widow.* Y. Keth. II, beg. 26ᵃ (Mishn. ed., a. Talm. Bab. נִתְאַרְמְלָה, v. אַרְמֵל).

אַלְמָנָה f. (b. h.; v. אַלְמוֹן) *widow.* Keth. I, 1; 2, v. אֲרוּסִין. Kidd. 75ᵃ אַלְמְנַת עיסה the widow of one of spurious descent; v. עִיסָּה; a. fr. Trnsf. דלת א׳ a *frameless* door (or *made of one piece*). Erub. 101ᵃ; v. גַּשְׁמָה.—Denom.

אַלְמָנוּת f. (b. h.) *widowhood.* B. Bath. VI, 4 בית א׳ (98ᵇ; Ms. M. אַרְמְלוּת) a house in which to live in case of widowhood. Yeb. 45ᵃ; a. e. Y. Keth. V, 29ᵈ bot. הרי אני מרגדת אַלְמְנוּתִי, v. אָגַדII.

אלנטיאות, v. אֲלוּנְטִית I.

אֲלוּנִיסְתִּין, אֲלַנְסְטִי (read אלי׳ ἑλληνιστί) *Hellenic, in Greek.* Tanh. Tsav, 2 [a gloss] לשון א׳ קטבך קטאב״א in Greek *katab'kha* (Hos. XIII, 14) means κατάβα *descend;* v. Yalk. Jer. 333. Y. Sot. VII, beg. 21ᵇ שמע קלון קריין שמע אלונ׳ heard them read the *Sh'ma* in Greek.

***אֲלוּנְקֵי, אֲלַנְקֵי** f. pl. (=על־ענקא *on the neck*) *poles used to carry burdens on the shoulder of two or more persons* (v. Sm. Ant. s. v. *Falangæ, phalangæ,* which is of Semitic origin). Bets. 25ᵇ what means 'provided no carrying on shoulders takes place'? Ans. באלנקי .... Ar., Ms. M. (ed. באלו׳) by means of *alanke* (phalangæ). Ib. למיפק אאלו׳ ed. (Ms. באל׳) to be taken out &c. (carried in a sedan chair through which poles are put). Ib. Am. and Mar Zut. allowed themselves to be carried on shoulders of men בשבתא דריגלא באלנ׳ Ar., Ms. M. (ed. our w. absent) on a Sabbath during the festive week on phalangæ (to the lecture room). V. בְּלוּנְקֵי.

אֲלַס, *Pa.* אַלֵּס, אַלֵּיס (contr. of אלעס, v. לעס) *to craunch, bite.* B. Kam. 84ᵃ. Git. 70ᵃ.

אָלָס pr. n. m. *Alas* (Valens; v. וָולָס) 1) an Amora. Y. Kil. I, 27ᵃ top.—2) (?) Snh. 64ᵃ Sabta son of A.; v. אַבְלַס.

אֶלָס, אֲלַס pr. n. *Hellas* (=Græcia Magna). [That Italian places are meant in quot. below, is obvious from Targ. Ezek. XXVII, 7, v. אִיטַלְיָא.] Targ. Y. I Gen. X, 4 א׳ וטרסס (h. text אלישה ותרשיש) Hellas and Taras (Tarentum, v. טַרְסִיס); Targ. Y. II ib.; Y. Meg. I, 71ᵇ bot. אלסטרסס; Gen. R. s. 37, beg. אלוסטרוס, אלסיט׳ (corr. acc.). [Targ. Y. a. Midr. reflect geograph. a. ethnograph. conditions and notions of their own days.]

***אִלְסִיס, אֱלִיסִיס (אילוסיס)** [the final ס freq. read ם in ed., as אֱלִיסִים &c.] f. (v. אָלִים) pr. n. pl. *Ilsis* &c. (grottoes near Tiberias; v. Jos. B. J. II, 20, 6) *ruins* of fortified caves. Koh. R. to III, 9 אלס׳. Y. Shebi. IV, 35ᶜ top אליפים; Gen. R. s. 34 אילטרם; Ruth. R. to I, 17 אילוסים (או׳); Yalk. Ezek. 351 אלפסס; cmp. בְּטִירָא a. אִרְצְטַהְרִין.

אַלְסְרִין, v. אִלְצְרִין.

אֶלְעָזָר, לְעָזָר pr. n. m. *Elazar.* 1) E. b. Poïra, counsellor of John Hyrcanus. Kidd. 66ᵃ.—2) Several Tanaim: a) E. b. Azariah; E. b. Arakh. of the second generation; b) E. b. P'rata; E. of Modim, of the third gener.—c) E. b. Jacob; E. b. Shamua; E. b. Simon (bar Yohai); E. b. R. Yose the Galilean, of the fourth gener.—3) Several Amoraim: a) E. b. Antigonus; E. b. R. Yannai, of the second gener. Y. Ber. V, 9ᵇ bot.; a. e.—b) E. bar Abina. Ib. I, 3ᶜ bot.—c) R. Lazar or E. (in Babli E. b. P'dath) one of the most renowned Amoraim of the third gener. Erub. 65ᵇ; a. v. fr.

אֶלְעִיקֵי, v. אֱלִיקֵי.

אֶלֶף (b. h.) *thousand. Du.* אַלְפַּיִם.—*Pl.* אֲלָפִים.—א׳ אלפים *a million.* Gen. R. s. 8 שני א׳; a. fr.—Ex. R. s. 5 אַלְפַּיִם *two thousand* (men); a. e.

אַלְפָא, אֲלַף, אֲלַףI ch. same. Targ. O. Ex. XXXVIII, 25 אַלַּף ed. Berl. (Y. אלפא); a. fr.—Snh. 95ᵇ חד א׳ one thousand. Bekh. 8ᵇ מאה א׳ זוזי one hundred thousand zuz; a. fr.—*Pl.* אַלְפַּיָּא, אַלְפִין. Targ. Ex. XXXVIII, 26; a. fr. Targ. I Sam. XVIII, 8; a. fr.—Y. Dem. VII, 26ᵇ bot.; a. fr.

אֲלַףII, אֲלֵיף (יְלֵיף) (h. אָלַף, √לף *to join, be joined*) *to become used; to learn, study, train one's self.*—אֲלִיף *accustomed, used to.* Targ. I Sam. XVII, 39. Targ. O. Num. XXII, 30.—Targ. Deut. V, 1; a. fr. (v. also יְלַף).—Cant. R. to II, 2 צבי רבי דיילף would you like to study? B. Bath. 111ᵇ top גוד לית דין צבי למילף take me away from here, this man has no desire to learn (but only to argue). Taan. 4ᵃ man is bound לְמֵילַף נפשיה בניחותא [prob. לְמַלְּפָה, v. infra] to train himself to be gentle; a. fr.

Pa. אַלֵּף, אַלֵּיף *to train, teach.* Targ. Ps. XVIII, 35 מַלֵּיף (=מְאַלֵּף). Targ. Prov. XI, 25; a. fr.—Koh. to IX, 10 thou didst emigrate למילף for the sake of studying, והוא גלי לְאַלָּפָא but he emigrated for the sake of teaching. Y. Dem. I, 22ᵃ top ולא כן אַלְּפָן רבי (not אִיל׳) did you not teach us thus?—א׳ זכו׳, v. infra.

Af. אוֹלֵף as *Pa.* Lev. R. s. 30 מוֹלִיף (מַלֵּיף) עלי זכו offers arguments in my favor.

Ithpa. אִתְאַלַּף *to exercise, practice, exert one's self.* Targ. Is. II, 4; XXVI, 9.

אל״ף *Alef*, the first letter of the Alphabet. Y. Snh. I, 18[a] bot.; a. fr. Y. Yeb. IV, 6[a] כל שהוא בה״י רבה באל״ף רבא (referring to *harbah arbeh* Gen. III, 16) the embryo that counts *harbah* with Hé, (the numerical value being 212—days), will grow; that which counts *arbeh* with Alef (i. e. 208 days, or less than seven months) will lie down (die); (cmp. הַרְבָּה for differ. versions).—B. Bath. 168[b] א׳ בית וכ׳ mere Alef Beth (arbitrary words). Gen. R. s. 1 הא׳ קרא תגר the Alef complained.—Y. Sabb. XVI, 15[c] top א׳ בי״ת אחד one of the alphabetical acrostics (chapters) of Lamentations.—*Pl.* אלפ״ין. Sabb.103[b]. Ex. R. s. 38; a. e.—אָאִין. Y. Ber. II, 4[d] bot. they pronounce עיינין א׳ Ayins like Alefs.—[Sabb. 103[b] אלף אלף דאאזרך וכ׳ ed. (Ms. M. omits דאאזרך) they differ as to one who wrote on the Sabbath two such letters as Alef, Alef (of *ăazzerkha* Is. XLV, 5) being merely vowels; v. בגלטורי.]

אלפ״א 1) ch. *Alfa*=Alef. Cant. R. beg. the poet כד עביד א׳ בית״א when writing alphabetical acrostics. Lam. R. introd. (R. Ḥama b. Ḥ.) מן תלתא תלתא פסוקי בא׳ בית״א belonging to the alphab. acrostics (in Lamentations) of three verses for each letter.; a. fr.—2) (ἄλφα) *Alpha*, the first letter of the Greek Alphabet. Shek. III, 2. Men. VIII, 1 א׳ לסולה best quality of flour. Ib. 6.

אַלְפָא, v. אַלְף I.

אַלְפָא *ship*, v. אִילְפָא.

אַלְפַבֵּטְרִין m. pl. (ἀλφαβητάριον) *alphabetic acrostics, songs*. Ruth R. to III, 13 (ed. אלפנטרין, אלפבתרין, corr. acc.).

אַלְפְבֵּיתָא m., pl. אַלְפְבֵּיתִין same. Koh. R. to I, 13; v. אלפ״א.

אלפבתרין, אלפנטרין, v. אלפבטרין.

אִילְפֵּס, אִלְפָּס c. (=לְפָס q. v.) *a tightly covered pot, stew-pot*, contrad. to קדירה a boiling pot. Ned. 51[a] a dish goes first in a pot קודם שיורד לאי׳ before it is put in a stew-pot for steaming. Y. Hall. I, 58[a] top.—Pes. 37[a] מעשה אי׳ *stew*.—Gen. R. s. 1, end כא׳ וכיסויו as a pot with its lid.—*Pl.* אִלְפָּסִין. Bets. 32[a], v. אירונית.

***אַלְסָרִין, אִלְצָרִין** m. pl. (Syr. אלסרא P. Sm. 155; 212; an abbrev. of אלכסנדרין, v. אַלַכְּסִין) *a species of pistachio* (tree or fruit). Y. Dem. II, beg. 22[b]; Y. Maasr. I, 48[d] bot. אלצ׳.—Tosef. ib. I, 1 אילס׳. Ib. III, 14 אִילָאסָרִין ed. Zuck. (Var. אליסין).

***אלקולאין, אלקולאון** Cant. R. to I, 11 שלמד א׳ בדעתו של הקב״ה, a corruption; read: שלמד אונקלס (עקילס) בן אחותו של הדריינוס; cmp. Tanḥ. Mishp. 5. [The entire clause seems to be a gloss.]

***אַלְקוּם** (b. h.) a symbolized pr. n.: *No-Standing*. Y. R. Hash. I, 57[a] bot. ומלך א׳ עמו but the King (the Lord)—no standing (on his decrees) is with him; he desires not to insist upon his decrees (but permits repentance to set them aside).

אלקטו, אִילקט, אלקט, v. next w.

אִילְ׳, אִלְקְטִי f. (ἑλικτή, sub. κλῖμαξ; v. also חִילְקְטִי) *winding staircase*. Tosef. Erub. VIII, 11 (V, end) five compartments הפתוחות לא׳ ed. Zuck. (ed. אלקט) opening towards a common winding staircase. Ib. ואסורין בהילקטי ed. Zuck. (ed. באלקטון, Var. בדיאלקטו corr. acc.) and are forbidden the use of &c.

אִלְקְטִית f., pl. אִלְקְטִיּוֹת (לקט, v. חֵילָקֵט) *stack of grain, shed for stacks* in the field. [Comment. fr. קייט summer.] Maasr. III, 7 the stores in הבורגנין והא׳ (Ms. M. אלנקטיות) turrets and sheds in the field are exempt from tithes (until brought home).

אלקא, אֱלָקִים=אֱלָהָא, אֱלֹהִים, v. אֱלוֹהַּ.

אלקים Pesik. R. s. 21, ed. Fr. p. 108[a], read ולוּקְיוֹס, v. פִּיוּס.

אַרְקַבְטָא, אַרְקַפְטָא, אַלְקַפְטָא m. (ἀργαπέτης, ארגבטא, Palm. inscript., Zeitschr. der Deutsch. Morgenl. Ges. XVIII, 89—90; Syr. ארזבד, Pers. arzabedes; v. Perl. Et. St. p. 105) *Arkafta*, a high dignitary in Persia. Targ. Y. Gen. XLI, 44 (ed. Vienna אַלְקַפְטָא); a. e.—Shebu. 6[b] אלקפ׳. Y. ib. I, 32[d] bot. ארקב׳. Y. Ber. II, 5[a] top Ar. (ed. בסא . . . , corr. acc.).—Zeb. 96[b] (prov.) ארקפ׳ נקטן ביד ריח׳ אתי ליה ליד Ms. M. (ed. . . . אלקפתא נקטן ריחא) the Ark. took us by the hand, and the scent came into the hand (undue pride of accidental acquaintances.

אלקפרין, v. אַקְלַפְּרִין.

אַלְקַפְתָּא=אַלְקַפְטָא.

אִילָ׳, אִלָרִיָא f. (ἱλάρια) *day of rejoicing*, both private and public; esp. *days of public rejoicings appointed by a new emperor, consisting of games, masquerades* &c. Pesik. Sh'mini p. 193[b] while the King is engaged בא׳ שלו וכ׳ in his hilaria, ask of him what you need. Cant. R. to IV, 4 לא היו עומדין באלירא וכ׳ (corr. acc.) (at Mount Sinai) they did not stand (as) in hilaria, but in awe, trembling &c.

***אלריא** *a disease;* prob. a corruption of אִילְיָרִיא (εἰλεός, ileus) *iliac passion, spasm of the abdominal muscles connected with vomiting*. Git. 70[a] מי שב אחזהו א׳ Ar. (ed. דלריא as in the sentence following).

אַלְתָּא, אֲלָתָא (אַלוּתָא) f. ch. (=h. אַלָּה) *post, pole, door-post*. Targ. Josh. XXIV, 26 (ed. Vien. I אילנא).—*Pl.* (of אלותא) אַלְוָתָא. Targ. Is. VI, 4 אַלְוַיָּה (ed. Vien. אֶרְלְוָות.) B. Bath. 73[a] ומחינן ליה באלותא Rashi (ed., sing. אלותא) and we struck it with clubs; v., however, אִלִיתָא. Bets. 33[b] ויהיב לן א׳ א׳ and gave us each several branches (Rashi), v., however, אַלְוָתָא.

אַלְתּוּסְבַּרְאוֹת m. (על=אַל, a. תוס׳, v. תּוּסְבַּרָא; cmp. 1 Chron. XXVII, 25); v. אַל־) *comes thesaurorum, chief-treasurer*. Midr. Till. to Ps. XV *magor* (his resort, stores) that is א׳ שלו his (the Roman Emperor's) chief treasurer (or plur. treasurers).

אִלְתִּית f. *Iltith*, name of a large fish (prob. from its place, v. חוּלְתָּא). Makhsh. VI, 3 (Mish. ed. אלתית). Tosef. Kel. B. Mets. V, 7.

אַלְתַּר (=עַל־אֲתַר) *on the spot, forthwith*, always with -לְ. Gitt. III, 3 (Mish. Talm. Y. על אתר). R. Hash. 6ᵃ; a. v. fr. (in Hebr. phraseol.).

אִם (b. h.; cmp. אוֹ a. אִי) 1) *if, when*. Mekh. Yithro, end כל א׳ שבתורה רשות every *Im* (If) in the Torah refers to voluntary actions (which you may or may not do) except three &c. Y. Gitt. VII, 48ᵈ בגין דאמר א׳ because he said, *If* (I die), i. e. conditional divorce. Succ. 53ᵃ א׳ אני כאן when I am here; a. fr.—2) *whether*. Yoma III, 1; a. fr.—א׳ . . . א׳ *whether . . . or*. Y. Pes. VI, beg. 33ᵃ א׳ פסח וכ׳ whether or not the Passover ceremonies supersede the Sabbath; a. fr. [Ib. אם יש הוחלת read אפשר יש וכ׳, as before.]—אִם כֵּן (abbrev. א״כ) *if this be so*. Ber. I, 1; a. fr.—אֶלָּא אִם כֵּן (abbr. אא״כ) *only when indeed, not until, unless*. Keth. 76ᵃ; a. fr.

אֵם f. (b. h.; אמה, אמם, √אם; *to press, embrace, join, support, lead*; v. אמן, אמר, אמץ &c.; cmp. אָב) 1) *mother*, freq.=*my mother*. Sabb. 134ᵃ; a. fr.—Y. M. Kat. III, beg. 81ᶜ הניח חק אמו left his mother's lap (Palestine).—Num. R. s. 10 (ref. to *immo* Prov. XXXI, 1) אמו זו . . . התורה וכ׳ 'his mother' that means the Law which trained Solomon and which is called a mother of those studying it, as you read (Prov. II, 3; text אִם is read אֵם *ēm*).—2) *womb, mouth of the womb*. Hull. III, 2 (54ᵃ) ניטלה האם וכ׳ if the mouth of the womb is absent, cut out. Bekh. IV, 4 (28ᵇ).—Trnsf. *legitimate existence, authority*. Succ. 6ᵇ, a. fr. יש א׳ למסורת the traditional Scripture text (letters without vowels) is authoritative in Biblical interpretation, opp. יש א׳ למקרא the traditional reading (vowels) must guide us, e. g. בחלב (Ex. XXIII, 19) may be read בַּחֵלֶב as the traditional vocalization, or בְּחֵלֶב *in the fat of*.—*Pl.* אִמָּהוֹת, אִימָּהוֹת. Kidd. IV, 4 her genealogy must be traced back ארבע א׳ to the mothers of four generations (on each side) which is eight mothers. Y. Snh. II, 20ᵇ bot. they are not אֲמָהוֹת אלא אִימָּהוֹת maid-servants but mothers (of the nation).—Trnsf. א׳ של בצלים *seed-onions*. Peah III, 4. Erub. 29ᵃ; a. e.—Ch. אִימָּא. [Koh. R. to XII, 7 א׳ דבצלי׳, v. אַמָּה.]

אִמָּא, v. אִימָּא.

אַמָּא *cubit*, v. אַמְּתָא.

אַמָּא I, **אַמָּא** f.=h. אָמָה. Targ. O. Deut. XXIII, 18; v. אַמְּתָא.

אַמָּא II, **אֲמַר**, fut. יֵימָא, imper. אֵימָא (√אם *to join*, v. אמר) *to say, speak, think*. Targ. Y. Gen. XXXIII, 10.—Freq. in Talmud.—אפילו תימא even if you will say, i. e. it may come right even if you assume that &c. Succ. 13ᵇ; a. fr.—לֵימָא, מִי נֵימָא (מי), or לימא must it be said, *does it mean to say?* Ib.; a. fr.—וכי תימא (ואי) and if you should object. Ib.; a. fr.—אלא אימא but rather say, i. e. the correct version is. Ib.; a. fr.—אימא סיפא now read the second clause, i. e. how will you understand &c.? Ber. 21ᵇ; a. fr.—אֵימָא I might think. Ib.; a. fr.—הוה אמינא I might have thought, I might have been led to believe. Erub. 74ᵇ מאי הוה א׳ what might I have been led to believe?; a. fr.—נימא כוותיה let him express his opinion in agreement with his authority, i. e. why does he not say so expressly? Taan. 3ᵃ; a. fr.—Pes. 7ᵇ היכי נימא what else should he say? נימא לבול should he use the expression *lamol?*—Gitt. 47ᵇ, a. fr. ס״ד אמינא it may occur to you to think; v. דַּעְתָּא. Yoma 85ᵇ אי הואי התם הוה אמינא had I been there, I should have said.—קאמינא=קא אמינא I say, speak of, v. קָא. Gitt. 47ᵇ; a. fr.

אִימָּאוּס, אַמָּאוּס pr. n. pl. (Ἐμμαοῦς, Ἀμμαοῦς, hellenized form of חמה, חמתה) *Emmaus, Ammaus*, a town in the plain of Judæa (or Philistæa), renowned, in Talmudic days, for its warm springs and luxurious life. Koh. R. to VII, 7, a. e. [Ib. 11 אימונים prob. אימאוס.] Cmp. דימסית. [Other forms: עמאום, עמיס, עמאוס, אמאום.] For other places by that name, v. Neub. Géogr. p. 100.]

אַמַּאי (=אַמָּה=עַל מַאי) *wherefore? why?* א׳ לא *why not?* Sabb. 48ᵃ. Erub. 70ᵃ; a. v. fr.

אַמַּאן (=עַל מַאן) *to whom?*, v. אַ־ and מאן.

אַמְבּוּהָא, אַמְבּוּהָ m. (Pers. anbûh, Perl. Et. St. p. 18; cmp., however, מבוא עם Ezek. XXXIII, 31) *crowd, escort*. Yoma 87ᵃ; Snh. 7ᵇ. Succ. 55ᵃ.

אַמְבּוֹל m., *pl.* אַמְבּוֹלִין (=עִינְבּוֹל; ענב) *little grape*, i. e. *clapper* in the bell. Y. Sabb. VI, beg. 7ᵈ עשה להן אמבולי (corr. acc.) he put clappers in. V. אִנְבּוֹל.

***אמבוניא**, Lev. R. s. 5 על א׳ דסדום Ar. (ed. by cler. error ארלניא) read אַמְבַּטְיָא *towers, battlements*; v. אַנְבָּטֵר.

אַמְבּוּרְקְלוֹן, אַמְבּוּרִיקְלוֹן m. **אַנְבּוּרְקְרָא** f. (ἐμβούρικλον, imburuclum, corrupt. of involucrum, D. C. s. v.) *wrapper, cover, bundle*. Y. B. Mets. IV, beg. 9ᶜ המחליף א . . . ין בא׳ Ar. (read ון . . . . .; ed. אברוקלון, באמבירוקלון, corr. acc.) if one exchanges one bundle for another; cmp. ציבור ibid.—*Pl.* אַנְבּוּרְקְרָאוֹת. B. Kam. 114ᵇ ed. (Ar. אנבקראות, Ms. M. אגבו׳, v. Rabb. D. S. a. l. note).

אַמְבְּטִי, אַמְבַּטָה f. (v. next w.) *bottom*. Gen. R. s. 68, v. דִּיוּטֵי.

אַבְטִי, אַמְבְּטִי f. (√בט, v. אַבְטָא; מ inserted) *bath-tub, bathing reservoir*. Ned. IV, 4 (Var. ־ביא . . .). Hag. 15ᵃ אב׳ Ar. (ed. אמב׳); a. fr.—*Pl.* אַמְבַּטְאוֹת, אַמְבַּטְיוֹת (אמבטיאות). Y. Sabb. III, 6ᵃ.—Bab. ib. 40ᵃ אמבט׳ (Ar. אבטאות); Tosef. ib. III (IV), 3, ed. Zuck. אבטאות (Var. אמבטאות) baths in large cities with ambulatories (v. Sm. Ant. s. v. *Baths*). [Y. Pes. III, beg. 29ᵈ א׳ של בצק (?), prob. a corruption.] Cmp. בִּיבָה II.

***אַמְבָּטֵיס** m. (ἀναβάτης, contr. ἀμβάτης) prop. *rider, traveller* on horseback &c.; hence (sub. חמור) *an ass used for marching* through the desert alongside of (and sometimes tied to) the camel. Y. Sabb. v, 7[b] top מהו א׳ what is an *ambates?* חֲמַר סלק the ass of the traveller (from Egypt to Asia). Y. Kel. VIII, 31[c] אבהנים, אבחנס (corr. acc.). V. לִיבְּדְקוֹס.

אַמְבַּטִיתָא f. (deriv. of אמבטי) *water of the bath-tub, waste of the bath-tub.* Y. Sabb. VIII, 11[c] (גו) החן דמשזג א׳ וכ׳ he who washes (his anus) in &c., is liable to a disease of the rectum.

***אמבירוס**, read אֶמְפִּירוֹס m. (ἔμπυρος) *fire-scathed.* Midr. Till. to Ps. XXII, v. אִימוּס.

אַמְבְּרָא m. (cmp. עַבּוּרָא; מ׳ inserted) *crop, store.* Keth. 105[a] smelt at (was an expert of) א׳ דחמרא (Rashi, pl.) wine stores.—*Pl.* אַמְבְּרֵי. Gitt. 56[a] קלנהו·לחנהו א׳ וכ׳ set fire to all those stores of wheat and barley.

אַמְגּוּזָא m. (=אגוזא, v. foreg.) *nut.* Sabb. 109[b] מא׳ אליבא וכ׳ from eating a nut on an empty stomach. Men. 35[a] כי א׳ in the shape of a nut; a. e.—*Pl.* אַמְגּוּזֵי. Hull. 59[a]. B. Mets. 60[a].

אַמְגּוּשָׁא m. (h. מְגוּשׁ) *magus, magian,* a Persian priest and interpreter of dreams; *magician, sorcerer.* Targ. Y. I Ex. VII, 15; VIII, 16.—B. Beth. 58[a]. Yoma 35[a] (Hull. 62[b]) פרוה א׳ Parvah is the name of a Persian magus after whom the cell in the Temple was named.—Sabb. 75[a] רב ושמואל א׳ Var. (read אַמְגּוּשְׁתָא).—*Pl.* אַמְגּוּשֵׁי. Snh. 98[a] אי בטלי יהירי בטלי א׳ when (in Israel) the haughty shall cease to exist, the magians (among the Persians) shall cease.

אַמְגּוּשִׁי m. (v. preced.) *a follower of magianism, believer in sorcery.* M. Kat. 18[a].

אַמְגּוּשְׁתָא f. (deriv. of preced. ws.) *magianism, magian practices.* Sabb. 75[a] רב ושמואל א׳ Ms. M. (ed. מגושתא, Var. אמגישא) as to magianism Rab and Samuel differ, one declaring it to be sorcery, the other—blasphemy.

***אַמְגֵּיירְתֵּיהּ** *referring to (the blood) which made him a proselyte* (circumcision). Y. Ab. Zar. II, 41[a] top ולא הוון אלא א׳ his visions as to bloodshed had reference only to that (blood) which made him &c.; v. גּוּר.

אָמַד (√מד; v. מָדַד) *to form an approximate estimate, to guess; to appraise, judge, deliver an expert's opinion.* Erub. 58[b] אוֹמְדוֹ וכ׳ he forms an approximate estimate of the height of the hill, and passes on. Snh. 78[b] אֲמָדוּהוּ למיתה they (the experts) declared his injuries to be fatal; (Y. ib. IX, 27[a] bot., also עמד׳) א׳ לחיים the opinion was that he would recover; a. fr.—Hull. 51[a] אמדה נפשה the animal before taking a leap measures its strength.

Hif. הֶאֱמִיד same. Gen. R. s. 64 שהאמידו אותה they had appraised it (the field,—as to how much it would yield). V. אוֹמֶד.

אֲמַד ch. same. Bekh. 61[a] לחכי אמדתיך I guessed this was thy intention. Keth. 68[a] הא דאמידניה in the one case it means that we have formed an opinion about him (know whether he is stingy or liberal).—*Part. pass.* אָמִיד. Arakh. 20[a] הא א׳ וקאי he stands appraised, he has been valued before this.—Hence אָמִיד *believed to be wealthy.* B. Kam. 62[a] אִינִישׁ א׳. Keth. 85[b] ידענא ביה דלא א׳ I know he is not rich. B. Bath. 8[b].—Ib. 52[a] אם אֲמִידָא לך if you believe her to be wealthy. V. אוּמְדָּנָא.

***אַמִּידְלָא, אַמַּדְלָא** m. (=על מדלא, על מיד׳; דלי; cmp. דָּלִית) *watchman's lodge on top of trees.* Sabb. 155[a] דרגא דא׳ Ar., Ms. M. (ed. דְּמַדְלָא) ladder for climbing up to the lodge.

אמדלאי a word in a charm formula. Sabb. 67[a] Ms. M. a. Ar. (ed. אמרלאי).

***אַמְּדְרוֹמָה**=אִי מִדָּ׳ *or from Daromah.* Y. Hor. III, end, 48[c].

אַמָּה f. (b. h.; אמם, v. אֵם) 1) *fore-arm, arm.* Sot. 12[b]; Ex. R. s. 1 אמתה חד אמר ידה the word אמתה (Ex. II, 5)—one says it means אַמָּתָהּ, her arm, the other says it means אֲמָתָהּ, her maid-servant (v. אָמָה).—Lam. R. introd. (R. Josh. 2) א׳ דבצלי׳ an arm (direction-post) &c.; v. בְּצַל; Koh. R. to XII, 7 אַמַּת (בית) השחי—אם the arm up to the axilla, *arm-pit,* name of an opening in a Temple door; v. however, infra. 4).—2) *cubit,* a measure equal to the distance from the elbow to the tip of the middle-finger. Keth. 5[b]; Men. 11[a] זו א׳ this one (the middle-finger) is used for defining the cubit measure. Kel. XVII, 10 אַמַּת הבנין וכ׳ the standard cubit of the Temple proportions was six, that of the vessels five hand-breadths. Sabb. 31[a] א׳ הבנין the builder's cubit (instrument).—א׳ על א׳ square-cubit. Yoma 31[a]; a. e.—Zeb. 62[b] א׳ גדומה (גרומה); Y. Yoma IV, 41[c] bot. גמידה a reduced cubit; v. גָּדַם; also called א׳ בת ששה עצבות a cubit of six hand-breadths pressed together (sorrowing), opp. to א׳ (בת ששה) שוחקות a cubit of six wide-spread (laughing) hand-breadths. Erub. 3[b]. Y. Shek. VI, end, 50[b].—Gen. R. s. 31 (א׳) תביקין Theban (Egypt.) cubit(?). B. Bath. 99[b] אמה בית השלחין land for digging a dyke of one cubit's width; א׳ בית הקילון (Var. קלון, סילון) land for a creek or pond for watering cattle and washing clothes, of one cubit's width. —3) (=אצבע) *membrum virile.* Sabb. 108[b]. Nid. 13[a] sq. B. Kam. 19[b].—4) prop. *river-arm,* hence *canal, dyke, sewer.* Peah II, 2 אַמַּת המים.—Yoma V, 6 אלו ואלו מתערבין בא׳ the blood of both was mixed in the sewer; Tam. III, 6; B. Mets. 33[a]; Y. Hor. III, 48[b] top אמת (בית) השחי a sewer in the Temple called *the duct of the arm-pit* (from its shape; v. Grætz Monatsschr. 1880, p. 289; [emendation שית unnecessary]; v. supra.—*Pl.* אַמּוֹת *cubits.* Kel. XVII, 10; a. fr.

אָמָה f. (b. h.; v. אֵם; cmp. preced.) *hand-maid.* Sot. 12[b], v. preced.; a. e.—*Pl.* אֲמָהוֹת. Y. Snh. II, 20[b] bot.; v. אֵם; a. e.

אַמְהָתָא, אַמְתָא, אֲמָתָא ch. same. Targ. Job XXXI, 13. Targ. Gen. XVI, 1; a. fr.—Y. M. Kat. III, 81[d]. —Meg. 18[a]; a. fr.—Erub. 53[b].—*Pl.* אַמְהָתָא; אַמְהָן. Targ. Gen. XX, 17; a. fr.

אַמְהוּ f. ch.=next w. Targ. O. Ex. XXI, 7 a. e. (Concrete: *servant.*); cmp. אִיתוּ.

אֲמָהוּת f. (אָמָה) *servitude of a maid, servile condition.* Mekh. Mishp., sect. 3 קידוש אחר א׳ the father's privilege of giving away his daughter in marriage is valid even after having hired her out as a servant.

אִמְהָתָא, אַמְהָתָא, v. אַמְהָא.

אַמְהָתָא, pl. of אַמְהָא.

***אֲמוּדַאי**, with בַּר m. *diver.* R. Hash. 23ᵃ; B. Bath. 74ᵇ Ms. a. Ar. (ed. בר אמוראי).

אמודין Y. Snh. IX, 27ᵃ, read אוּמְדִין, pl. of אוּמְד.

אִימוּם, אִמּוּם m. (=אמאום, denom. of אֵם) *model, form, shoe-maker's last,* &c. Kel. XXVI, 4; XXIII, 1.—Ib. XVI, 7 הא׳ של גודלי וכ׳ the block of the cap-makers; של עושי וכ׳ א׳ of dressmakers. Sabb. 141ᵇ Ms. M. (ed. אימוס, corr. acc.); a. fr.

אָמוֹן I m. (b. h.; אמן) *artist;* (homilet.) a)=אוֹמֵן, *tutor;* b)=אָמוּן *nursed (well-covered); guarded;* c)=next w., *metropolis,* (great). Gen. R. s. 1.

אָמוֹן II pr. n. pl. 1) (b. h. נוא א׳) *No-Amon* (Thebes) in Egypt. Gen. R. s. 1 (*=Alexandria, the metropolis*).—[*2) A., near Tyre. Y. Dem. II, 22ᵈ top; Tosef. Shebi. IV, 9 עמק.]

אֱמוּנָה f. (b. h.; אמן) *firmness, faith, honesty, surety.* B. Bath. X, 8, a. e. לא על אֱמוּנָתוֹ הלוהו at the time he extended the loan, he did so not because he was relying on his (the friend's) surety. Ib. שכן על א׳ וכ׳ for in this case he did &c. Ab. Zar. 55ᵃ אנו נאבד את אֱמוּנָתֵנוּ shall we abandon our honesty? Ḥull. 133ᵇ אין א׳ בכותים Samaritans are (usually) not trusted. Tam. 28ᵃ א׳ יתירה scrupulous honesty. V. אֲמָנָה.

***כְּפַר א׳ אָמוּס**, Y. Sot. VII, 21ᶜ bot., v. אִבּוּם.

אָמוֹרָא m. (אמר) 1) *speaker, lecturer, interpreter;* esp. *Amora,* one who, in lengthy popular discourses, expounds what the lecturer (Tanna, v. תַּנָּא) says before him in brief and in a low voice; often called מְתוּרְגְּמָן. Ex. R. s. 8, end כשם שהדורש .... והא׳ וכ׳ as the lecturer sits ... and the Amora speaks in his presence.—Snh. 7ᵇ קום עליה בא׳ stand by him as an expounder. Taan. 8ᵃ, a. fr. אוקים .... א׳ עליה ודרש S. ... placed an Amora by his side and lectured. Sot. 40ᵃ ואמר אֲמוֹרֵיה חד טעמא and his Amora gave a different reason. Ḥull. 15ᵃ do people listen to the Tanna? לא׳ צייתי they listen to the Amora.—2) in a particular sense אָמוֹרָא, *Amora* (*Amoraïm*), that class of Talmudic authorities who lived after the final redaction of the Mishnah, and whose discussions on the opinions of the *Tannaïm* or authors of the *Mishnah* and *Boraitha,* are deposited in the *Guemara,* thus adding a second element to the development of the oral law, called *Talmud.*—*Pl.* אָמוֹרִין. Y. Ber. I, 2ᶜ top, a. e. תרי א׳ two Amoraïm differ, for which Babli usually: ... אָמוֹרָאֵי נינהו ואליבא two Amoras differ in their relation (or conception) of the opinion of ... Shebu. 40ᵇ; a. fr.

אֲמוֹרָאָה m. (=preced.) *teacher.* Targ. Job III, 17.—*Pl.* אֲמוֹרָאִין. Targ. Y. I, Num. XXI, 29.

אֱמוֹרָאָה ch. (=h. אֱמוֹרִי) *Emorite.* Targ. Gen. XV, 16; a. fr.—Keth. 112ᵃ בר א׳.—*Pl.* אֱמוֹרָאֵי. Targ. Ex. III, 8; a. fr.—פרק א׳ *the chapter treating of idolatrous practices* (v. אֱמוֹרִי). Sabb. 67ᵃ, (v. Tosef. Sabb. ch. VII, sq.).

בר א׳, אמוראי, v. אמודאי.

אֱמוֹרִי m. (b. h.) *Emorite; Emorean.* Gen. R. s. 41 none among the nations are קשה מא׳ more obstinate than the Em.—Trnsf. *Emorean, superstitious, heathenlike.* דרכי הא׳ *superstitious practices.* Sabb. 67ᵃ, a. fr. אין בו משום דרכי הא׳ is not to be looked upon (not forbidden) as an imitation of &c.; יש בו משום דרכי הא׳ it is forbidden because it has the appearance of superstitious practices.

***אֲמוֹרְיָא** m. (ימר, מור) *exchange.* Esth. R. to 1, 1ᵇ, בְּנֵי אֲמוֹרְיֵיה his hostages; v. אוּפְרִיפָא for corr. vers.

אֱמוֹרִים, v. אֵימוּרִים.

אַמְטוּ (abbrev. of next w.) *on account of, for the sake of.* Ber. 56ᵃ bot. א׳ זוזא וכ׳ for the sake of thy *zuz* (which has been refused, v. Ms. M. in Rabb. D. S. a. l.) shall the wardrobe of the king go to ruin? Lev. R. s. 27 א׳ בעירא כ׳ for the sake of the tender cattle.—א׳ הכי, א׳ להכי *therefore.* Naz. 25ᵃ. B. Kam. 71ᵃᵇ (Ms. H. אמטול הכי); a. fr. V. אָמְטוּ.

אַמְטוּל (=על מטול; טלל, טול) *for the protection of,* whence (=h. בִּגְלַל, בְּעַד) *for the sake of, on account of* &c. Targ. Y. Lev. IX, 7; a. fr. V. מְטוּל and preced. w.

אַמְטוּלְתָא=preced., only with suffix of personal pronoun. Targ. Y. Lev. IX, 7 לְךָ .... =h. בעדך. Targ. Job I, 10 לְהֵיה ... around him (protecting him). Targ. Ps. VII, 8 אַמְטוּלְתָהּא for her sake; a. e.—Keth. 67ᵇ אַמְטוּלְתֵיה for his sake.

אמטי, v. אַמְטוּ.

אַמְטִיתָא f. (מטי Af.) *balances, scales.* Pesik. B'shall. p. 82ᵃ; v. אַבְרַנְתָא.

אַמְטְלִית־ אַמְטְל, v. אַמְטוּל.

אַמְטְתָא, v. אֲמִיטְתָא.

אָמִי, v. אָמָא.

אָמֵים, Af. of מוּם.

אמיטון, v. אַמִּיַנְטוֹן.

אמיטליא Tosef. Maasr. III, 6 ed. Zuck., v. הֶמְטְלְיָא.

עֲמִיטְתָא, אַמְטְתָא, אֲמִיטְתָא f. (עמט, אמט; √אם, עם, v. אָמַם; cmp. חוּמְצָא I) *darkness, dense cloud, mist.* Targ. Deut. IV, 11. Targ. II Chr. VI, 1, ed. Beck. עמ׳; a. e.—Gen. R. s. 44 (transl. עֲלָטָה).

אֲמִינְטוֹן, אֲמִיַּנְטוֹן m. (ἀμίαντος, ἀμίαντον) *amiant*, a variety of asbestos from which the reputed asbestos linen was spun, which was cleansed by being thrown into the fire. Cant. R. to IV, 11; Pesik. B'shall. p. 92ª. [Deut. R. s. 7, end אסיטון; Midr. Till. to Ps. XXIII, 2 חסיטון; Yalk. Deut. 850 אמיטון; corr. acc.]—Deriv. המיינטון, read הַמְּיַנְּטֵן *he who cleanses the amiant*. Y. Sabb. VII, 10ᶜ top.

אֲמִילְתָא Snh. 44ª Ar., v. מִילְּתָא.

אֲמִינְטוֹן, v. אֲמִיַּנְטוֹן.

אֲמִיר, אֲמִיר (part. pass. of אֲמַר) *told, proclaimed, commanded.* Targ. Mic. V, 1. Targ. Mal. I, 6; a. fr.

אֲמִירָה I f. (אמר I) 1) *speaking, speech.* Gen. R. s. 5, beg. לא א׳ לא דיבור no (power of) speech or word; a. fr.—הא א׳ this is speech, i. e. *this is right.* Y. Snh. IV, 22ᵇ top; VI, beg. 23ᵇ. Y. B. Kam. IX, beg. 6ᵈ (contracted) הא׳ same.—2) *the word amar* (אמר) *in the Scripture text.* Y. Snh. VII, 25ᵇ bot. נאמר כאן א׳ וכ׳ here *amar* is used &c.; as well as *amar* here indicates that the word is considered a deed &c.; a. e.—3) *dedication* (cmp. אִימּוּרִים. Kidd. I, 6 אֲמִירָתוֹ לגבוה וכ׳ dedication to the Lord (by word of mouth) is equal to what delivery is in private transactions.—*Pl.* אֲמִירוֹת mostly in the sense of 2). Num. R. s. 14, end א׳ וצִיוּויים texts in which *amar* and *tsivvah* occur; a. fr.

אֲמִירָה II f. (v. preced. 3); cmp. Ps. IV, 5; XCVI, 10; Is. III, 10) 1) *proclamation, receiving homage.* Ex. R. s. 29 when a human king יוצא לא׳ וכ׳ comes forth for a reception of homage, he comes forth singly (not with his army).—2) *distinction, ornament.* Yalk. Ex. 244, v. אִימְּרָה.

אֲמִיתָא, חֲמִיתָא f. (אמם, חמם) *ammi, Bishop's weed* (v. Löw Pflzn. p. 260; Rashi=מינתא *mint*). Tosef. Sabb. XIV (XV), 13 א׳ (Var. ח׳). Sabb. 128ª; 140ª, v. נִינְיָא. Tosef. Kil. III, 12, Var. (ed. Zuck. חמיטא).

אֲמִיתָךְ, v. אֱמֶת.

אֲמִיתִּי m. (אמת) *true, truthful.* Y. Ber. VII, 11ᶜ. Gen. R. s. 70 do ye not admit יעקב א׳ that Jacob was truthful? Ib. s. 78. [In later Hebrew: *real.*]

אַמֵּךְ Af. of מוּךְ or מְכָא.

***אמכותי** Koh. R. to VI, 1 או חד א׳ וכ׳ prob. to be read או חד מְפִיחֵיה או חד מעקיצֵיה וכ׳ either one bites him (v. נְכַת) or one stings him—what benefit has he (the keeper of the obnoxious beasts) of them?

אמלוגין, v. אִילוֹגִין.

אֲמְלַל or **אֲמֻלָל**, v. אוּמְלָל.

אֲמַלְּתָא, v. הִימַלְּתָא.

מַלְתְּרָא, אֲמַלְתְּרָא f. (μέλαθρον) *main-beam of the ceiling, ceiling; beam projecting outside the house, cornice.* Erub. 3ª (differ. opinions as to the meaning of our w.).—*Pl.* מַלְתְּרָאוֹת, אֲמַלְתְּרָאוֹת. Erub. l. c. א׳. Midd. III, 7 מ׳.

אָמַם, עָמַם (b. h. עמם; √אם, עם to be pressed, dark; cmp. אֵם; חמם a. deriv.; v. אמיטתא) *to grow dim,* (in b. h. also *to obscure, excel;* v. infra). Sabb. 77ᵇ; Ber. 53ᵇ; Pes. 75ᵇ גחלים אוֹמְמוֹת (or עוֹמְמוֹת) dying coals (question as to spelling decided in favor of ע by reference to Ezek. XXXI, 8 'the cedars did not *obscure* him, i. e. excel his beauty).

אָמַן (b. h.; √אם, v. אֵם; cmp. אַמָּה) *to arrange in lines, array.* Ukts. II, 5 nuts שֶׁאֲמָנָן which one arranged (Var. Ar. שחמרן which one piled).—Denom. אוּמָּן *expert, skilful,* whence

Pi. אִימֵּן, אִמֵּן *to make skilful, to train.* Sabb. 103ª מְאַמֵּן את ידו he trains his hand (practicing). V. next w.

אָמַן I (√אם, v. אֵם; cmp. preced.) *to be strong, enduring;* (act. v. אָמַן *to support,* v. II Kings XVIII, 16 אֹמְנוֹת).—*Pi.* אִימֵּן, אִמֵּן *to support; trnsf. to confirm, verify, approve.* Tosef. Ter. I, 4 it is not the minor that made it T'rumah אלא אביו שֶׁאִימֵּן אחריו Var. (ed. Zuck. שאומן) but his father who confirmed his act (=ib. קיים על ידו); Y. ib. 40ᵇ א׳ על ידו. Ib.ᶜ top מְאַמֵּין.

Nif. נֶאֱמַן (b. h.) 1) part. נֶאֱמָן m., נֶאֱמֶנֶת f. *approved, trustworthy, reliable.* Peah VIII, 2 נֶאֱמָנִים על וכ׳ (the poor) may be relied upon concerning garnered fruit &c., i. e. if they declare the fruits to be the poor man's share, they are exempt from tithes. Keth. I, 6 נאמנת her statement is acted upon as true. Ab. Zar. 16ᵇ נ׳ עלי הדיין my judge is a reliable witness concerning me, i. e. I appeal to thy own judgment that I could not have engaged in such follies.—Dem. II, 2 if one resolves להיות נ׳ to be one of the reliable (conscientious in giving tithes); a. fr.—2) *to be confirmed.* Y. Sot. II, 18ᵇ top אמן יֵאָמְנוּ הדברים Amen means, May the words (of the oath) be fulfilled.

Hif. הֶאֱמִין (b. h.) *to declare trustworthy, to trust, believe in.* Dem. VII, 1 והוא אינו מַאֲמִינוֹ but he (the invited guest) trusts him not in tithe affairs. Ib. 3; a. fr.—Ab. Zar. 16ᵇ הואיל וְהֶאֱמַנְתַּנִי עליך ed. Pes., En Yak. (v. Rabb. D. S. a. l. note; ed. הָאֳמַנְתִּי *Hof.*; since thou didst declare me a reliable witness unto thyself (appealing to my judgment), v. supra; [Ms. M. האמנת עלי thou reliedst on me]. Ch., v. הֵימַן.

אָמֵן II m. (b. h.; v. preced.) *firm, straight,* whence 1) *Amen!, true! so may it be!* Shebu. 36ª א׳ בו שבועה וכ׳ in *Amen* is implied an oath, a promise, and a prayer for fulfillment. Ab. Zar. 65ª; a. fr.—2) fem., *the response Amen.* Ber. 47ª א׳ חטופה an Amen hastily pronounced (*'men*); א׳ קטופה an Amen cut short (*ame-*); א׳ יתומה an orphan Amen, the responder not having heard the benediction to which the Amen refers; Tosef. Meg. IV (III), 27.

אֲמָנָה f. (b. h.; v. preced.) 1) *faith, trust.* B. Bath. 48ᵇ; Keth. 19ᵇ if witnesses say א׳ היו דברינו our statement (over our signatures as to having seen the loan handed over) was a matter of trust (that the negotiation would be consummated afterwards). Ib. שטר א׳ a bill of indebtedness signed on trust (that the loan would be consummated subsequently). B. Mets. 63[a] א׳ בפירות advanced payment at present prices for future delivery; א׳ בדמים with the option of paying the difference. Gen. R. s. 100 end, שמר א׳ to deal in good faith with. Tosef. B. Bath. V, 8 אֲמָנַת המדות honesty in measures. B. Mets. 49[a] מחוסרי א׳ (the way of) those lacking honesty (unfair dealing); Bekh. 13[b] מחוסר א׳; a. fr.—2) *faith in Providence.* Mekh. B'shall. s. 6, v. הָאֲמָנָה. Sot. 48[b] אנשי א׳ men of faith, trusting in God; ib. קטני א׳ wanting in faith; Gen. R. s. 32 מחוסר א׳ same; a. fr. Cmp. הָאֲמָנָה, אֱמוּנָה.

אֲמָנָה II pr. n. 1) (b. h.) *Amanah, Abanah* (Banas), a river crossing the city of Damascus. Targ. II Kings V, 12.—2) אֲמָנָה, אֲמָנוֹס (אמנס), אֲמָנוֹן *Amanah,* hellenized *Amanos, Amanon* &c. (Banias), a mountain range forming the northern limits of the Holy Land. Tosef. Ter. II, 12 אמנוס (Var. אמנון, סמנון). Ib. Ḥall. II, 11 אמנוס (Var. אמנון). Git. 8[a] ...ון (Ar. אמנים, סמנים); Y. Ḥall. IV, 60[a] bot. אמנס (ref. to אמנה Cant. IV, 8). Shebi. VI, 1; Hall. IV, 8 (Ms. M. ...ם); Ex. R. s. 23. V. טַוְרוֹס.

אֲמָנוֹס, אֲמָנוֹן, v. preced.

אמנותא Y. Keth. IV, 28[d] top, v. אוּמְנוּתָא.

אמנם, v. אֲמָנָה II.

אמפוטמא, v. אמפומטא.

אַמְפּוּלֵי, v. אֲמִפְּלֵי.

***איפומטא, אמפוטמא, אמפומטא** Pesik. B'shall. p. 86[b], Yalk. Sam. 152, corrupt. of אִסְטְרוֹפוֹמָּא, or אִסְטְרוֹפוֹטָא q. v.

***אמפומיות, אמפיביות**, Pirké d'Rabbi Eliez. ch. XLII חלונות א׳ Ar. (in ed. our w. omitted); read אוֹפִּסְרָנִיּוֹת (denom. of אֲפִּסְרִין q. v.) *glass-windows.*

אמפורטור, v. אִמְפְּרָטוֹר.

***אֶמְפּוֹרִין, אַמְפּוֹרִין** m. pl. (ἔμποροι) *travelers, traders.* Targ. Y. I Gen. XXV, 3 (a gloss to preceding חגרין; Targ. Y. II inserts אומנין for לְטוּשִׁם; h. text אַשּׁוּרִים). Ib. XLVI, 23 (h. text חשים). [Gen. R. s. 61, quoting Targ. Gen. XXV, 3, reads לופרין!]

אִנְפְּלָ׳, אִנְפְּי׳, אִמְפְּלְיָא, אִמְפִּילְיָא f. (pl. of ἐμπίλιον, impilia) (pair of) *felt-shoes,* in gen. *shoes, socks.* Kel. XXVII, 6. Yeb. XII, 1. Ib. 102[b] א׳ של בגד cloth-shoes; א׳ של עור leather-covered shoes; a. fr.—*Pl.* אִנְפִּילָאוֹת, אִנְפִּילָן, אִמְפִּילָיוֹת, אִנְפְּלָ׳ *pairs of &c.* Sabb. 120[a]; Y. ib. XVI, 15[d] שתי א׳ two pairs &c. Gen. R. s. 61. Yeb. 102[b].

אִינְפּוּלֵי, אַנְפְּלֵי, אַמְפּוּלֵי, אֲמִפְּלֵי f. (נֶפֶל; cmp. אוּנְקְלֵי as to form) *the merchant's money-chest into which receipts are dropped through a slit.* Shebu. VII, 6 (45[a]) אמפלי Mish. Nap. (Ar. אמפו׳, ed. אינ׳; Y. אנ׳; v. Rabb. D. S. a. l. note 10). Tosef. Maas. Sh. IV, 11 ed. Zuck. ארנפו׳ (ed. אונקלי, אונקולין). Ib. Shebu. VI, 4 אונכלי ed. Zuck. (corr. acc.; oth. ed. אוּנְקְלָא). Cmp. אוּנְפֵּל.

אִמְפְּרָטוֹר m. (imperator) *commander, Roman Emperor.* Lam. R. to I, 5 ביבי דומינו א׳ Ar. (ed. וביבא מארי אפלטור, v. בִּיבֵי) be saluted, my lord, the Emperor. Tanḥ. Mikkets, 9 אמפירטיר, אונפירטיר (corr. acc.)

אָמַץ (b. h.; √אם, cmp. אמם, חמץ) *to press, harden.* אוֹמְצֵי חלב hard-hearted. Tosef. Sot. XIV, 7; v. infra.

Pi. אִימֵּץ, אִמֵּץ 1) *to make strong, to strengthen.* Y. Taan. III, 66[d] all shall be מְאַמְּצִין כחך strengthening thy power (assist thee). Snh. 44[b] מאמץ עצמו וכ׳ who concentrates his energies for prayer.—2) *to press, close; to make impervious.* Sot. 47[b] מְאַמְּצֵי הלב those who close their hearts, the hard-hearted; v. supra. [Sabb. XXIII, 5 מאמצין את המת Y. ed. (Mish. מעמ׳, Bab. 151[b] מעצמין, Ms. M. מעמ׳) *to close* the eyes of a deceased person. Tosef. ib. XVII (XVIII), 19 לְעַמֵּץ ed. Zuck. (Var. לאַמֵּץ). Sabb. 77[b] מעמצין או מאמצין וכ׳ is *m'amm'tsin* (l. c.) spelt with ע or with א? Answer by ref. to עוצם Is. XXXIII, 15 (!).] V. אוּמְצָא.

Hithpa. הִתְאַמֵּץ *to be closed.* Tosef. l. c. מִתְאַמְּצוֹת מאליהן they will be closed of themselves.

אֶמְצַע m. (v. מִצַּע; √מץ; cmp. b. h. תָּוֶךְ, תּוֹךְ, חֲבָבִים) [*lying in a press*], whence—בא׳ *in the centre, between two extremes.* Y. Ḥag. II, 77[a] bot. יהלך בא׳ he must walk between the extremes. B. Mets. 70[b] יד הנכרי בא׳; Y. Ab. Zar. I, 40[a] top אצבע הגוי בא׳ the hand [finger] of the gentile is between, i. e. he has a share in it; a. fr.—2) *common fund, estate.* B. Bath. X, 7 השבח לא׳ the profit belongs to the common fund. Ib. IX, 3 השביחו לא׳ they improved for the common fund, i. e. the profit must be equally divided. Ib. 144[b] מן הא׳ from the estate; a. fr. Cmp. מִצַּע, בֵּיסְיָין.—[Also in Ch. Targ. Job II, 8 (Ms. מצע) Targ. Y. II, Num. XXII, 24 בא׳ *between.*]

אֶמְצָעוּת f. (v. preced.) *centre.* Y. Snh. I, 18[a] bot. מ״ם באמצעיתה the Mem is in the middle of the alphabet.

אֶמְצָעִי m., **אֶמְצָעִית** f. (preced.) *central, middle.*— Erub. V, 2 הא׳ the intermediate village, opp. חיצונים; a. fr.— Shebi. III, 4 הא ... יח the central part of the field, lying in the middle. Kil. IV, 8; a. fr.—*Pl.* אֶמְצָעִיִּים, אֶמְצָעִיִּין m.; אֶמְצָעִיּוֹת f. Y. Peah II, 17[a] top; a. e.—Y. Ber. II, 4[d] bot. הא׳ (sub. ברכות) the intermediate (central) sections of the benedictions (between the first three and the last three). Kil. V, 2 הא׳ the central garden beds; a. fr.

אֶמְצָעִי m., **אֶמְצָעִיתָא** f. ch. same, also as a noun. Y. B. Kam. IV, 4[b] top I was present ... ובא׳ ... ברישא at the discussion on the first, the last, and of the intermediate clause (or case). Ber. 3[a]; a. e.

אָמַר I (b. h.; √אם, v. אֵם; cmp. חמר, עמר) (a) *to join, knot; to be knotted, thick;* b) *to heap up;* c) transf. *to join words, compose,* cmp. דבר; d) *to contract, bargain, exchange.* [As to Assyr. *to see,* cmp. חמא.]) 1) *to speak, think, say, relate* &c. ... א׳ ר׳ ... ר׳ Rabbi .... related in the name of R. ... Ber. 3[b]; a. v. fr.—Part. pass. אָמוּר *expression.* Yoma 70[b], a. fr. היא הא׳ וכ׳ it is the same

expression (*'one ram'*) used here and in the Book of Numbers. Sifré Deut. s. 334, a. fr. אֱמוֹר מעתה say from now, i. e. from this draw the conclusion. Gen. R. s. 39 תאמר שחבירה וכ׳ (usu. שמא תאמר) will you say (is it possible), this castle has no commander?—במה דברים אֲמוּרִים (abbr. בד״א) in what case are these words said? i. e. *this applies only.* Ḥull. 3ᵃ; a. fr.—זאת אוֹמֶרֶת this tells, i. e. *this proves.* Ber. 11ᵇ; a. fr.—אָמְרוּ it is said, told &c.; v. next w.—Inf. לֵאמֹר=לוֹמַר. Ḥag. 14ᵇ; a. fr.—2) *to vow, devote.* (לגבוה) אָמוּר devoted to the Lord. Succ. 55ᵇ; v. אֲמִירָה I, 3, a. אֲמוּרִים.

Nif. נֶאֱמַר (b. h.) *to be said, to read* ... נא׳ כאן... ונ׳ לחלן we read *here* .... and we read *there* ... (the same expression is used here and there in the Scriptural text). Ber. 9ᵃ; a. v. fr.—שֶׁנֶּאֱמַר (abbr. שנא׳, שנ׳) for it is said in the Scriptures (as evidence in favor of an opinion). Snh. X, 1; a. v. fr.; also כמה שנ׳ (כמו) as it is said.—מִשּׁוּם שנ׳ because it is said in the Scriptures, i. e. you may possibly be misled by a certain expression to think ...., therefore another term is used in its stead in an analogous case, or added to the ambiguous word; v. שׁוּם.

אֲמַר, אֲמַר ch. 1) as preced. 1). Targ. Gen. I, 3; a. v. fr.—א׳ מר above you quoted an authority, or, it has been stated. Ber. 2ᵃ; a. fr.—א׳ קרא the Scripture says. Ib. 13ᵃ; a. fr.—Y. Orl. III, end, 63ᵇ, a. fr. ... אמרונה בשם (in Bab. heb. אֲמָרוּהָ) they said it in behalf of ... i. e. as a tradition.—Y. Ber. I, 2ᵈ מילתיה אמרה his word (statement, opinion &c.) proves.—זאת אומרת=הדא אמרה; v. preced.—אָמְרֵי (h. אָמְרוּ) *they say, it is said.* Sabb. 19ᵃ אמרו עליו על ... ואמרי לה וכ׳ it is told about R. ...., and another relation refers this to R.—; a. fr.—קאמר, קאמרי &c.=קא אמר &c. Ḥull. 85ᵃ; a. fr.—מנא תימרא whence dost thou prove? Sabb. 23ᵃ; a. fr.—*Inf.* מֵימַר, מֵימְרָא. סבר למ׳, סבר מ׳ originally he was of the opinion. Y. Sabb. VI, 8ᶜ top; Keth. 87ᵇ; a. v. fr.—לְמֵימְרָא *does this mean to say?* Sabb. 15ᵇ; a. fr. .... לא אמרן אלא ... אבל this has been said, i. e. this applies only to a case .... but if .... Ber. 43ᵇ; a. fr.—כְּלוֹמַר *as if saying, meaning to say, viz;* v. כְּלוֹ.—Y. Kil. IV, 32ᶜ bot. אימורין לבני וכ׳ say ye to &c.—אֵימוֹר מאי אִיכָּא למימר, v. אִיכָּא; Answ. say .... Sabb. 6ᵃ; a. fr.—Hor. 13ᵃ א׳ כולה who orders every thing (as an etymol. of אֲמַרְכָּל).—2) *to praise, proclaim.* Targ. Is. VIII, 13; a. fr.—Part. pass. אָמִיר q. v.

Ithpe. אִתְּאֲמַר, contr. אִתְּמַר, אִתְּ׳ *it is said, taught.* Targ. Job XXXIV, 31.—Y. Yoma V, end, 43ᵃ אתאמרת, contr. אִתְּמְרַת it has been said with refer. to the opinion of ....—אִתְּ׳, אִתְּמַר *it has been said* (*above*); *we have been taught.* Succ. 15ᵃ; a. fr.

Ithpa. אִתְּאַמַּר same. Targ. Gen. XXII, 14; a. e.

אָמַר II (b. h.; √אם, v. אָמַר I, a) *to be thick, strong.*

Hif. הֶאֱמִיר 1) *to thrive; to boast, vaunt, be oppressive* (cmp. Ps. XCIV, 4). Sot. IX, 15 (49ᵇ) יוקר יַאֲמִיר the nobility shall be oppressive (Snh. 97ᵃ יִעַוֵּת; Der. Er. Zut. X יעוות; Cant. R. to II, 13 הווה).—*[2) (denom. of מריא *to fatten.* Sabb. XXIV, 3 (155ᵇ) Bab. מַאֲמִירִין, Ms. Oxf., Mish. a. Y. מַמְרִין, מַמְרִים, v. מרר.]

אֶמֶר, v. אִימַר a. אִמְרָה.

אִמַּר *lamb,* v. אִימַּר.

אִמְרָה f. (b. h.; אמר) *speech.* *Gen. R. s. 42 play on *Amraphel,* א׳ אפילה (quot. in Ar. s. v. אספרון) obscure speech (ed. שהיתה אֲמִירָתוֹ אפ׳).—*Pl.* אֲמָרוֹת, constr. אִמְרוֹת. Pesik. Parah, p. 30ᵇ (*promises*); Tanh. Ḥukk. 4. Pesik. R. s. 14.

אַמְרֵי Af. of מרי.

אמריו, v. אמוריא a. איכריסא.

***אַמַרְכָּל, אֲמַרְכּוֹל (אַמ׳)**; in Y. Dial. מַרְכָּל, מַרְכּוֹל m. (=מלכל; fr. מלך; ר for ל for euphony) *counsellor, officer* &c. Targ. Is. XXII, 23 (h. text יתד, LXX ἄρχοντα). Targ. Y. Num. I, 6 sq. (corresponding to ראש בית אב, נשיא, פקיד &c.; O. ib. III, 32 אֲמַרְכְּלָא); a. fr.—Esp. *Amarkal,* one of the seven Temple trustees superintending the cashiers. Tosef. Shek. II, 15 (etymol. מר על חכל mastering all, v. מַר; cmp. Hor. 13ᵃ אמר כולא). Y. ib. V, 49ᵃ; a. fr.—*Pl.* (h.) אֲמַרְכָּלִים, אֲמַרְכָּלִין (ch.) אֲמַרְכְּלַיָּא, אֲמַרְכּוֹלִין &c. Targ. II Kings XXII, 4 (h. text שומרי הסף); a. fr.—Shek. V, 2. Tosef. l. c.; Y. l. c. (=פקידים II Chr. XXXI, 13); a. e. V. מלך a. deriv.

אמרלאי, v. אמדלאר.

אַמְרָפֶל (b. h.) pr. n. m. *Amraphel,* King of Shin'ar; v. אִמְרָה.

אֶמֶשׁ m. (b. h.; √אם; cmp. אמיטתא) 1) *twilight, evening, nightfall.* Pesik. Vayhi p. 63ᵇ; Pesik. R. s. 17 מא׳ (ו)עד חצות from nightfall to midnight.—2) (adv.) *this evening, last night.* Meg. 3ᵃ, a. e. א׳ ביטלתם וכ׳ this evening you neglected the evening offering.—Snh. 40ᵇ א׳ הרגו last night he killed him. B. Mets. 60ᵃ שמרים של א׳ dregs of last night (yesterday), opp. to היום; a. fr.

אֱמֶת f. (b. h.;=אמנת; אמן) *truth, faith, reality.* Y. Snh. XI, 30ᶜ top לחם א׳ bread of truth, unfeigned hospitality. Gen. R. s. 96 חסד של א׳ true (unselfish) charity. Y. Meg. I, 70ᵃ top כַּאֲמִיתָהּ של תורה as the Law itself, i.e. as though the Scroll of Esther were the Pentateuch. Y. Shebu. VI, 37ᵃ top אֲמִיתָן של דברים the truth of &c. Num. R. s. 12 א׳ של תורה וכ׳ the truth of the Law is a weapon (of protection) to its owner.—בא׳ אמרו in fact they said that &c. Sabb. I, 3; a. fr.—B. Mets. 60ᵃ, a. e. כל בא׳ אמרו הלכה היא wherever an opinion is introduced with the words 'In fact they said' it means to say that it is an established legal rule. Y. Sabb. I, 3ᵇ bot., a. e. כ״מ ששנו בא׳ וכ׳ wherever the Mishnah says, 'In fact', it indicates a rule dating from Moses on Ṣinai, i. e. an ancient tradition; v. Frank. Darké p. 286.—הא׳ *indeed?* Tanh. Noah, 10 (ed. Bub. 15, corr. acc.); v. אוֹנְטוֹס.

אַמְתָא f. ch.=h. אַמָּה. 1) *cubit.* Targ. Ex. XXV, 10; a. fr.—Y. Sot. VIII, 22ᶜ bot. א׳ אישתא a cubit has six hand-breadths; a. fr.—2) *membrum virile*. M. Kat. 17ª טרקיה אאַמְתֵיה stung him on his membrum.—3) trnsf. *enclosure; protection* (cmp. חוֹמָה). א׳ דריחיא enclosure of the millstones, mill. Ber. 18ᵇ.—*Pl.* אַמִּין (fr. אַמָּא). Targ. Ezek. XL, 5; a. fr. אַמָּהָתָא. Hull. 59ᵇ תשע א׳ nine cubits.

אַמְתָא *hand-maid*, v. אַמְהָא.

אֲמָתוֹת f. pl. *the use of the word* אֲמַת־. Ber. 31ᵇ שלש א׳ three times אֲמַת־ (I Sam. I, 11; Ms. M. אֲמָהוֹת).

אַמְתְלָא (Y. מַתְלָא) m. (cmp. h. משל) *something tangible* (=דבר שיש בו ממש); *plausible reason for correcting or retracting an evidence*. Keth. 22ª אם נתנה א׳ וכ׳ if she offers a reasonable explanation of her contradictory statements, her second one is accepted. Gitt. IX, 9 ובלבד שלא יהא שם א׳ provided no reasonable explanation is offered to show how the report may have arisen by mistake; a. fr. V. מַתְלָא.

אֲמַתְלַאי pr. n. f. *Amathlai*, legendary name of Abraham's mother (א׳ בת כרנבו), and of Haman's mother (א׳ בת עורביתא). B. Bath. 91ª.

אֶמְתָן m. (denom. of אֵימָה; י absorbed by preceding א; cmp. next w.) *one who rules through fear, tyrannical*. *Pl.* אֶמְתָּנִין. Der. Er. II, beg.; cmp. R. Hash. 17ª. V. אֵימְתָן.

אֶמְתָנִי f. ch. (v. preced.) *fear-inspiring, powerful*. Dan. VII, 7 (quot. Gen. R. s. 44 אימ׳; Ex. R. s. 25 אימתני; Lev. R. s. 13 אימ׳ a. אמ׳; Yalk. Gen. 77; Lev. 536 אמ׳). [Ges. H. Dict. אֶמְתְּנִי, not found in editions, fr. מתן *to be strong*; cmp., however, אֶמְתָן a. אֵימְתָן.] [Edit. Letteris, Berl. 5644 a. m., אֵימְתָנִי.]

אֶן *if*, v. אִין.

אָן (b. h.) *where?* לְאָן *whither*. Ab. III, 1.

אָן, אַן ch. same; (interrog.) *where?* Targ. Gen. IV, 9; a. e.—Y. Yoma VIII, 44ᵈ bot. אן מן הדה (read מן אן . .) wherefrom this? i. e. where is your authority? Y. Yeb. XII, 12ᵈ bot. החן סבא לְאָן ליך of what use is this old man to thee?; a. e.—(relat.) *where, wherever*. Lev. R. s. 27 beg. א׳ את יהיב וכ׳ (Yalk. Ps. 727 הן) wherever thou givest, thou givest abundantly.

אָנָּא (b. h.) *oh! I pray*. Succ. III, 9. Yoma VI, 2.

אֲנָא, emph. אֲנָנָא ch.=h. אֲנִי, *I*. הא אנא contr. הָאנָא. Targ. O. Gen. XXII, 7; a. fr.—Hull. 2ᵇ א׳ וכ׳ as to myself &c. Y. Taan. IV, 68ᵈ bot. דאנא משלים וכ׳ that I myself should surrender the country.—*Pl.* אֲנַן *we*. Targ. Y. Gen. XLIII, 8; a. e.—Ber. 49ᵇ נחזי א׳ let us see; a. fr.—אֲנַחְנָא, נַחְנָא. Targ. O. Gen. l. c.; a. fr.—

אִנָּא, 1) v. אִירָא.—*2)=אִן אֲנָא *if I*.

אִנְבָּא I=אִיבָּא I, *fruit, produce*. Dan. IV, 9.—Targ. Job XXXI, 12; a. e.

אִנְבָּא II, אִירְבָּא f. (=עִרְבָּא) [berries], *eggs of lice. nits*. Naz. 39ª. Taan. 22ᵇ מתחזי ליה כר אנ׳ Ar. (Ms. M. ומחזו כי אינ׳, ed. מתחזיר אירבא) looked as small as &c.; v. רינבא.

אַנְבַּג, אַנְבְּגָא, אַנְפַּק, אַנְפְּקָא m. (v. נַבְגָא; whence ἄμβιχος, ἄμβιξ, ambiga) *a small cup; a measure* containing one fourth of a Log. B. Bath. 58ᵇ on the gates of ... it is written, אנבג אנפק וכ׳ (Ms. differ. order) Anbag, Anpak a. Antal (as the same measures). Kid. 70ª לישתי מר אנבגא will you take a cup (of wine &c.)? [Popular pronunciation: *anpak*.] Sabb. 109ᵇ אנפקא; a. e.

אִנְבּוֹל m. (=עִרְבּוֹל, v. אִמְבּוֹל) *clapper of a bell*.—*Pl.* ....ין, אִנְבּוֹלִים Zeb. 88ᵇ Ar. (ed. ערנבלין). Tosef. Kel. B. Mets. I, 13 עשה לה האנבילים ed. Zuck. (read לחם אנבולים...) if he put clappers in. Ib. אנבילהן (corr. acc.).

אִנְבּוֹנִין, v. אִלְבְּנָא.

אִנְבּוּרְקְרָאוֹת, v. אִמְבּוּרְקְלוֹן.

אַנְבְּטִי f. (נבט;=b. h. מצפה) *observatory, watch-tower, battlement*. *Pl.* אַנְבְּטָאוֹת. Ex. R. s. 12 the hailstones formed א׳ א׳ lines of battlements; (Midr. Till. to Ps. LXXVIII כותל). V. אמבוניא.

*****אַנְבְּטֵי** m. pl. (v. preced.) *platforms or elevations erected for public spectacles*. Yalk. Esth. 1058 all the people shall go out להדין א׳ (read לחנהו א׳; Lev. R. s. 28, end לחון פרטי, corr. acc.) to the spectacular elevations, for a Jew (Mordecai) is to be hanged. V. אמבוניא.

אנביל, v. אִנְבּוֹל.

אנבין, v. אַגְבִין.

אנבקראות, v. אִמְבּוּרְקְלוֹן.

אנגמוס, v. אנגיטוס.

*****אנגיטוס** Yalk. Ps. 794; אגוסטוס Gen. R. s. 12, א׳ במדינה (Ar. אגבאסטס) read אַגְוִיסְטוֹר (אגב׳) m. (quæstor, κυαίστωρ) *quæstor provincialis, assistant of the consul*. א׳ . . . ביא שלו (read שלה) the quæstor in the province is appointed over its roads, v. בִּיָא.

אנגיטירין, v. אַרְגַּנְטְרְיָא.

אנגימריס Y. Ter. VIII, 46ᶜ top, read אַרְגְּנְטִיס.

אנגיסטור read אֲנֻגִּיסְטִיר m. (ὀνυχίστηρ=ὀνυχιστήριον) *knife* or *scissors for cutting nails*. Tosef. Kel. B. Mets. III, 12 (ed. Zuck. אגניסטר corr. acc.). Nid. 17ª גנוסטרי; M. Kat. 18ª גנוסטרא (Ms. M. גנוסטרי, v. Ar. s. v. גנסטר).

אַנְגְּלַיָּא, אַנְגְּלֵי m. pl. (ἄγγελοι, v. Perles Et. St. p. 113) *messengers, angels*. Targ. Job XV, 15; a. e.

אנגלין, v. אַגְלְגִין.

*****אַנְגְּרָא** (read אַנְגּוּרָא?) pr. n. pl. *Ancyra*, a city of Galatia in Asia Minor. B. Mets. 46ᵇ דינרי אניאקא ואנגרא Ms. M. (ed. אנקא ואניגרא, Var. אַנְיְקָא, נִיקְא; v. Rabb. D. S. a. l. note, Ar. Compl. ed. Koh. s. v. אנגרא) the Bithynian and the Ancyrean Denars, one of which was repealed by the central Government, the other by the local authority. V. אַנְיָאקָא. [Ancyra prob. of Semitic origin, v. נִיגְרָא a. אַפְּגָרָא.]

אַנְגַּרְוְטָא, אַנְגַּרְבַּטִּים m. (ἀγγαρευτής, ἀγγαρευτάς) *commissioner* or *superintendent of forced public labor;* v. אַנְגַּרְיָא. Pesik. B'shall. 92[b] אתמני א' (for Var. v. Bub., note) was appointed angareutes.

***אנגרומינא, אנגרוטינה, אבג׳,** Gen. R. s. 64 והלך א', prob. to be read אַנְגַּרְיָא זו . . . , as in Esth. R. introd. [B. Bath. 8[a]; Ned. 62[b] אַרְנוֹנָא.]

אנגרון, v. אֶפִּרְגָּרוֹן.

אַנְגַּרְיָא f. (ἀγγαρεία, angaria) *forced labor, service,* esp. *seizure for public services* or *works.* Y. Ber. I, 2[d] bot. איתצדית בא' וכ' I was pressed into service to carry myrtles &c. B. Mets. VI, 3 (78[a]) נעשית א' (the ass) was seized for public service. Ib. 78[b] בא' חוזרת in the case that the animal pressed into service is sent back again. Lev. R. s. 12 שמעון א' במדינתא they heard that seizure for public service was to take place in the country. Esth. R. introd. והלך זו א' hălakh (Ezra IV, 13) means *angaria* (v. אנגרומינא). Snh. 101[b]; a. fr.—*Pl.* אַנְגַּרְיוֹת. Lev. R. s. 23 אע"פ שהן נגבין . . . . וא' though annonæ and angariæ are collected from them. Yalk. Esth. 1051 א' של נשים levies of women (for the king).—Trnsf. בא' as a forced labor, *reluctantly.* Midr. Till. Ps. CXII.—Pesik. R. s. 21 שלא באנגרים (corr. acc.) not as a forced labor.

אנגרים, אנגריס v. preced.

אנגרכמים, v. אַנְגַּרְבַּטִּים.

אַנְגַּרְמוֹס corrupt. of אַגְרוֹנִימוֹס.

אנדוכתרי, v. אנדכ'.

***אַנְדִּיסְקֵי** m. pl. (a Babylonian adoption of *ecdicus,* v. אנדיקוס, אגדיקוס) *syndics, state-officials.* B. Bath. 55[a] אבל אצלוהו א' וכ' Ar. (ed. omit אצלוהו) but if the syndics exempted him from taxes, it is like a divine grant.

אַנְדִּיפָא m., אַנְדִּיפָה f., v. next w.

***אַנְטִיפֵי, אַנְדִּיפֵי** m. pl. (b. h. נְטִיפוֹת; נטף or נדף) *locks* or *ringlets falling from the temples.* Sabb. VIII, 4 כדי לעשות א' enough toilet material to make side curls (Mish. Pes. אנטיפי, Nap. אנטפי, Talm. אונד'). Ib. 80[b] מאי כלכול ומאי א' what locks are meant by *kilkul,* and what by *andifê?* Answ. the upper and the lower &c. Ib. אמר ר' יצחק דבי ר' אמי אנדיפה וכ' Ms. M. (ed. . . . אלא אמר ר' אמר . . . אַנְדִּיפָא) R. Isaac of the school of . . . . (in reciting that Mishnah) used the word *andifah* (in the sing.) upon which R. . . . asked 'Will a person waste his money' (i. e. of what use is the material for one curl so as to make a person guilty of a transgression when carrying it on the Sabbath)? Ib. מאי אנדיפא אפותא by *andifa* (in the sing.) is meant the lock on the forehead. Ib. מחתיה באַנְדִּיפֵיה וכ' Ms. M. (ed. incorr. באנדיפי) it stung him on his forehead and he died. [Rashi:=דיופי!]

אַנְדִּיקָס, אַנְדִּיקוֹס m., a popular corrupt. of *ecdicus,* v. אֶגְדִּיקוֹס a. אַנְדִּיסְקֵי.

***אנדיתיקוס** m. pl. Esth. R. to I, 12, a corruption; according to the sense it may have been קַטָאדִיקִין (κατάδικοι) *convicts.*

***אונדכתרי, אנדוכתרי, אנדכתרי,** a corruption of אִינְדִּיקְטָא or אֵיוִנְדִּיקְטָא f. (vindicta, Gr. form βινδίκτα, οὐινδίκτα) *manumission of a slave by declaration before court* (v. Sm. Ant. s. vv. Manumissio and Pileus). Gitt. 20[a] but does not go free בכתב שע"ג כיפה וא' (ought to have read בכיפה וא', v. infra) by referring to his wearing a freedman's cap or to a *vindicta;* Y. ib. IV, 45[d] בכפה והרנירק מיאניס (read ובוינדיקטא); Treat. Abadim ch. III (ed. Kirchh.) יוצא באנטוקטא (corr. acc.). [Commentators to Gitt. l. c., misled by בכתב שע"ג וכ', guess at embroideries &c. V. Révue des Etudes Juives 1883, Nr. 13, p. 150.]

אנדנא Ab. Zar. 29[a], some ed.; v. אַגְדָּנָא.

בַּר א', אַנְדְּרַאי pr. n. m. *Bar Andrai* (Andrew). Y. Keth. IX, 33[a] top אילין דבר א' those of the family of B. A. (who were very rich). V. אַנְדְּרַיי.

אַנְדְּרוֹגִינוֹס m. (ἀνδρόγυνος) *hermaphrodite.* Bicc. I, 5; a. fr.

אנדרואנטיא, read אַנְדְּרִיאַנְטוֹס.

***אנדרולומוסיא** (read אַנְדְּרוֹלֵמְסְיָא, אַנְדְּרוֹלֵמְסִיָה), f. (popular pronunc. of ἀνδρολημψία=ἀνδροληψία; cmp. λῆμψις for λῆψις) *seizure of men,* a Greek right of reprisals (v. Sm. Ant. s. v.), in gen. *punishment of men regardless of guilt or innocence.* Gen. R. s. 26 א' באה וכ' an androlepsia comes which kills the good and the bad; Lev. R. s. 23; Num. R. s. 9; Y. Sot. I, 17[a] top.—Num. R. s. 5 in case of a rebellion עוש' בה א' the king orders an androlepsia. [Gen. R. s. 32 דרולמוסיא; Pesik. Vayhi, p. 67[a]; Tanh. Bo, 4; Pesik. R. s. 17 דורמסיאות, דורמיים', דורמסיות (corr. acc.); cmp. Pesik. R. suppl., ed. Fr. p. 197[a].]

אנדרולינאי Yeb. 115[b], read דוד בר נהילאי as Asheri Gitt. ch. IV, to p. 34[b].

אנדרומוסיא, אַנְדְּרוֹלֵמְסִיָה, v. אנדרולומוסיא.

אַנְדְּרוֹנָא, v. אִידְּרוֹן.

***אַנְדְּרוֹנִיטִין, אַנְדְּרוֹנִימִיס** f. (ἀνδρωνῖτις) *banqueting hall, royal reception hall.* Gen. R. s. 8 אדריינטים אני עושה אותה Ar. ed. Koh. (ed. אינדרטין; corr. acc.) I shall make it into (use the vacant ground for the erection of) a banqueting hall. [The context forbids the identification of our w. with אַנְדְּרִיאַנְטוֹס.]

אַנְדְּרוֹפִיקוֹס, v. אִדְּרוֹפ'.

אַנְדְּרָטָא m. (a. contract. of ἀνδριάς,—άντος) *statue,* also *portable bust, image.* Targ. Esth. III, 2—5 (some ed. pl., incorr.). R. Hash. 24[b] a synagogue דאוקימו בה א׳ Ms. M. (ed. הוח בה א׳) in which they placed a bust (of a Persian king). Snh. 62[b]; a. fr.—*Pl.* אַנְדְּרָטַיָּא, אַנְדְּרָטֵי. Ab. Zar. 40[b] א׳ של מלכים royal (imperial) busts. M. Kat. 25[b] אתעקרו כל א׳ Ms. M. (ed. אתקציצו) all royal statues were overthrown. Y. Ab. Zar. III, 42[c] top. [Gen. R. s. 8 אינדרטין, v. אַנְדְּרוֹנִיטִים.]

*אנדרטין f., Tosef. Kel. B. Mets. IV, 8, prob. אוֹדוֹנְטוֹטֵר (ὀδοντωτή, sub. ξύστρα) *a teethed strigil;* cmp. Kel. XIV, 3 מגררה.

אַנְדְּרִיאַנְטוֹס m. (ἀνδριάς—άντος) *statue*, v. אַנְדְּרָטָא. Ex. R. s. 27 נפלה . . . . של אנדרואנטיא (read נפלטה) (לתוך ידו של א׳) it escaped into the hand of a (royal) statue; (v. ibid. ישבה על איקונין של מלך). Tanh. P'kudé, 4 אדריונטוס (corr. acc.); Ex. R. s. 51. [Gen. R. s. 8 אינדרטין, v. אַנְדְּרוֹנִיטִים; v. Ar. s. v. אדרינטים.]

אַנְדְּרֵיי pr. n. m. (Ἀνδρέας) *Andray.* Y. Meg. IV, 75[b]; cmp. אַנְדְּרַאי.

אַנְדְּרִיינוֹס, v. אַדְרִיָּינוֹס. Ex. R. s. 51.

אנדריינטוס, v. אַנְדְּרוֹנִיטִים, a. אַנְדְּרִיאַנְטוֹס.

אנדרכטוס, v. אַנְגַּרְבִּטִים.

אנדרמוסיה Ar., v. אנדרולומוסיא.

*אַנְדְּרַפְתָּא, אַנְדְּרַפְטָא m. (prob. Pers.) *Indrafta*, name of two species of birds, one called *Shabur And.*, and permitted, the other *Peruz And.*, and forbidden. Hull. 62[b].

אָנֶה, v. אנו.

אַנְהוֹרֵי f. (Inf. Af. of נהר used as a verbal noun) *lighting, illumination.* Targ. Ex. XXXV, 14; a. e.

אַנְהָרוּתָא f. same, also *enlightenment.* Targ. Num. IV, 16. Targ. Y. Gen. II, 7.

אֲנוּ pl. of. אֲנִי.

אָנוֹךְ (Coptic ânokh) *I.* Pesik. R. s. 21; Yalk. Ex. 286 (in Egyptian) אנכי א׳ *Anokhi* is Anokh. Esth. R. to I, 22 לשון יחנך (corr. acc.).

אֲנוֹמְלִין, אֲנוֹמִילִין, v. אִינוֹמִילִין.

אִנּוּן, pl. of אִיהוּ.

אַנּוֹנָה, אַנּוֹנָא f. (annona) prop. *annual produce*, hence *ration*, or *portions of provision granted to courtiers as salaries or pensions.* Gen. R. s. 47 the king מעלה לו א׳ raised an *annona* in his behalf, i. e. granted him a pension. Ib. s. 87 אני חותכת א׳ שלך Ar. (ed. פרנסה) I shall cut down (reduce) thy pension; a. fr.—*Pl.* אַנּוֹנוֹת, אַנּוֹנִיּוֹת. Ex. R. s. 41 אנונית (corr. acc.). Lev. R. s. 23 נגבין אונניות (corr. acc.) annonæ are collected from them. Ib. s. 10 אַנּוֹנִים Ar. (ed. אַנּוֹנָס annonas, acc. pl., incorr. ed. אנינוס). [Cant. R. to I, 7 read אֲטוּנָס.] Cmp. אַרְנוֹנָא, אַרְנוֹן.

אנונים, אנונית, אנונס, v. preced.

אָנִיסָא (אוֹנְסָא) אָנוֹסָא m. (אנס) *violent man, oppressor.* Targ. Koh. VII, 7 (h. text עוֹשֶׁק).—*Pl.* אָנוֹסִין, אָנוֹסַיָּא (אנו׳). Targ. Jer. VI, 6 ed. Ven. I אנו׳ (ed. Vien. אוֹנְסִין, oth. ed. אנו׳). Targ. Is. XXI, 2; V, 7, a. e. Cmp. אַנָּס.

אנוקי, read אֲנִיקֵי, v. אַנִּיקָא.

אֱנוֹשׁ m. (b. h.; v. אינש) [being], *man.*—*Pl.* (of איש) אֲנָשִׁים, const. אַנְשֵׁי. Ex. R. s. 25; a. fr.—א׳ כנסת הגדולה (abbr. אכה״ג) *the Men of the Great Assembly, Synagoga Magna*, a religious and judicial authority said to have been established by Ezra. Aboth I, 1; a. fr.; cmp. כנסת.—א׳ בית אב(ות) the division on duty of priests having charge of the services of the day; א׳ משמר the division of priests alternately on duty during one week; א׳ מעמד the division (of Israelites) assisting the priests on duty, by prayers &c. on the platform (מעמד) and divided in parties corresponding to the priestly divisions. Taan. II, 6; 7; a. fr.

*אָנוּשׁ m. (b. h.; v. preced. a. איש) *strong, severe, overwhelming.* Num. R. s. 7 (ref. to Is. XVII, 11) א׳ לשון גבר *anush* has the meaning of *strong;* Lev. R. s. 18.

*אַנְזִיקָא m. (נזק) *injury, loss.* Targ. Esth. VII, 4 the adversary is (of) no value or gain בא׳ דמלכא against the King's loss. [Levy Targ. Dict. reads אוניקא expense(?), v. אוּזִינְקָא.]

אָנַח (b. h.; cmp. אנק) *to press. Hithpa.* הִתְאַנַּח *to sigh.* Ber. 59[a], v. next w. Yalk. Ex. 391 מִתְאַנֵּחַ על כבודו וכ׳ is anxious for the honor of the Lord &c.

אֲנַח ch., *Peil* אֲנִיחַ, *Ithpa.* אִתְאַנַּח same. Targ. Lam. I, 4; 11.—Targ. Is. XXIV, 7; a. e. Contr. אִתְּנַח. Targ. O. Ex. II, 23 late ed.—*Ithpe.* אִיתְּנַח, אִתְּ׳. Ber. 58[b]. Ib. 59[a] אִתְנְחִיד מתנח Ms. M. (ed. אנחה מִתְאַנַּח) he sighs.—Pesik. R. s. 18, end; Pesik. Haom. p. 72[a] שרי מיתנח he began to sigh.

אֲנָחָה f. (b. h.; preced.) *sigh, grief.* Ber. 58[b]; a. e.

אַנְחוּתָא I f. (נחת, נחי) *layer.* Targ. Y. Ex. XVI, 13; 14.

נְחוּתָא (אַנְחוּתָא II, נְחוּתָה (אַנְחוּתָה f. (v. preced.) *tray, board.* Nidd. 7[a] אנ׳ (Ar. a. T'bul Yom IV, 2 נ׳). Gitt. 62[a]; Tosef. Kel. B. Mets. VI, 7 אנחותא.

אֲנַחְנוּ, אֲנַחְנָא pl. of אֲנָא, אֲנִי.

אַנְחָתָא f. (נוח; cmp. אַנְחוּתָא) *rest.* בית א׳ *rest for beams.* Targ. I Kings VI, 4.

אַנְחָתָא f. pl. (אנח) *sighs.* Targ. Lam. I, 22.

בית א׳, אַנְטְבִילָא pr. n. *Beth Ant'bila*, name of a Jerusalem family. Y. Peah VIII, 21[a] bot. Tosef. Peah IV, 11 נבלטא ed. Zuck., אנטיבלאי &c. (Var. גלבטא, גבטלא).

אנמג׳, אנמד׳, v. אנמ׳.

***הִינְדְּבִי, אַנְטוּבִּין** m. (ἐντύβιον, Arab. hindeb, prob. fr. נדב to flow, curl, cmp. אַנְדִּיפִי) endive. Y. Kil. I, 27ᵃ top אנטוכין (corr. acc.). Pes. 39ᵃ הינדבי (Rashi הִינְדְּבִי, Ms. הנדבי).

אַנְטוּכָאֵי, v. next w.

אַנְטְיוֹכִי, אַנְטוּכִי m. (v. next w.) *Antiochian, native of Antiochia, resident of A.* Gitt. 44ᵇ אנטו׳; Tosef. Ab. Zar. III (IV), 18; Y. Gitt. IV, 46ᵃ top אנטי׳.—*Pl.* ch. אַנְטוּכָאֵי. Targ. Y. Gen. X, 18 (ed. אנטכאי, אנטוכיא corr. acc.; h. text חֲמָתִי).

אַנְטְיוֹכְיָאה, אַנְטוּכִיאָה, אַנְטוּכְיָה, אַנְטוּכְיָא pr. n. (Ἀντιόχεια) 1) *Antioch*, surnamed Epidaphnes, the capital of Syria founded by Seleucus Nicator, situated on the Orontes. Targ. Y. Num. XIII, 21; a. e. (Hamath in Bible).—Keth. 67ᵃ. Gitt. 44ᵇ; a. fr.—Y. Shek. VI, 50ᵃ bot. דפני של א׳ Daphne near Ant.; Lev. R. s. 19 כייא . . .—2) *the country* or *district of Ant., Antiochene.* Y. Dem. II, 22ᵈ top; Y. Nidd. III, 48ᵃ bot.; a. e.; v. חוֹלָה, חֲמַת a. חוּלְתָא.

אנטוכין, v. אַנְטוּבִּין.

אַנְטוֹלִי pr. n. m. (Ἀνατόλιος) *Antoli.* Y. Dem. V, 24ᵈ bot.

אַנְטוֹלִינוּס, v. next w.

אַנְטוֹנִינוּס pr. n. m. *Antoninus,* 1) a Roman emperor freq. mentioned as a friend of R. Judah Han-Nassi, and supposed to be Ant. Alexander Severus (Graetz) or Ant. Marcus Aurelius (Rap. a. oth.). Ab. Zar. 10ᵃ א׳ בר אסוירוס Severus son of A.; Ib.ᵇ A. son of Severus. —Y. Meg. I, 72ᵇ bot. אית מילין וכ׳ there is one report that A. embraced the Jewish religion, another &c.—Y. Snh. X, 29ᶜ אנטונ׳ a. אנטולי׳; cmp. Y. Kil. IX, 32ᵇ top.—Koh. R. to IX, 10 אנטלימוס וכ׳ (corr. acc.)—2) א׳ זעירא A. junior, grandson of the former. Ibid. to X, 5.—[3) (?) a Roman general mentioned in conversation with R. Joh. b. Zaccai; v. אגניטוס.]

אָנְטוֹס, v. אוֹנְטוֹס.

אנטוסאי, v. אנתוסאי.

אנטוקטא, v. אנדכתרי.

אַנְטִיגְנוֹס, אַנְטִיגְנֹס pr. n. m. (Ἀντίγονος) *Antigonus,* 1) A. of Sokho, disciple of Simon the Just. Aboth I, 3.—2) Bets. 34ᵃ, a. fr. R. Elazar son of A.—Tem. 21ᵃ ed. (Ar. אטיטס). [Y. Snh. I, 19ᵈ, v. אגנ׳טוס.]

אַנְטִיגְרָפִין f. (ἀντιγραφή) 1) (=ἀντίγραφον) *duplicate.* Targ. Esth. III, 14 Mus. (ed. דיוגמא); Esth. R. to ibid. (explain. פתשגן ib.).—2) *answer to a letter.* Gen. R. s. 67 הב לי א׳ Ar. (ed. אנטיגרפא, corr. פי . . . .) give me an answer (to the emperor's letter). Ib. הן א׳ where is the answer?

אַנְטִידִיקוֹס m. (ἀντίδικος) *opponent in a suit,* in gen. *adversary.* Gen. R. s. 82.—Ib. s. 100 אנטידרוקוס (corr. acc.); Pesik. Naḥa'mu p. 126ᵃ; a. fr.—*Pl.* אַנְטִידִיקִין *parties to a suit.* Deut. R. s. 5 האנטדריקון (corr. acc.).

אַנְטְיוֹכוּס (אַנְטְיוֹכָס) pr. n. m. *Antiochos* (III) of Syria. Targ. II Esth. I, 2. Gen. R. s. 23; a. e.

אַנְטְיוֹכִיאָה, אַנְטְיוֹכִי, v. אנטוכ׳.

אַנְטְיוֹכָס, v. אַנְטְיוֹכוּס.

***אנטיניא, אנטיניה,** corruptions; read אִימַטְיָא m. pl. (pl. of ἱμάτιον) *blankets used at the bath* which may also serve as cloaks (v. Sm. Ant. s. v. Pallium). Y. Kil. IX, 32ᵃ bot.; Y. M. Kat. III, 82ᵃ (explain. the sort of בלנרי in question).

אנטיירדס, read אַנְטִיךוּס.

***אַנְטִיכִי** f. (ἀγγοθήκη, ἐγγυθήκη, lat. mutilat. incitega) *a receptacle for vessels, a stand for hanging in kettles, tripods* &c. Sabb. III, 4 (41ᵃ); Gem. ib. one opin., בי כירי *antichi* (in the Mishnah) means a vessel suspended between fire places (heated bricks); another opin., בי דודי a metal vessel suspended within a caldron-like vessel, the vacant space beneath being filled with coals. Ib. (in evidence of the latter opin.) א׳ אע״פ שהיא גרופה וכ׳ Ms. M. (ed. אע״פ שגרופה וקטומה) an *antichi,* even when cleaned of coals &c. Y. Sabb. III, 6ᵃ bot. Tosef. Bets. III, 20. Y. ib. I, 60ᶜ bot. כהדא א׳ נפלת וכ׳ as in the case of an *antichi* which fell &c.—*M. Kat. 28ᵇ (in a funeral dirge) גוד גרמא מככא ונמטי מיא לא׳ take the bone (pin) out of the jaw (the base in which the vessel is suspended) and let water be put into the *antichi,* i. e. body and soul are now separated, the latter being the vessel going back to the (divine) spring; cmp. Koh. XII, 6 sq.; [Ms. M. מכבא . . . . לאנטוכיא . . . ., v. Rabb. D. S a. l. note.]

אַנְטִיכְרִיסִיס f. (ἀντίχρησις) *an agreement allowing the creditor the use of a pledged object* (in place of interest on the loan). Y. B. Mets. VI, end, 11ᵃ הדא א׳ ריבית הוא antichresis is considered usury.

אַנְטִילַיָּא, אַנְטִילָא, v. אַנְטְלְיָא.

אנטימטון, v. אַטִימְטוֹן.

אַנְטִינוּס pr. n. m. (Ἀντίνους) *Antinous;* v. אטינס.

אנטינייא Y. M. Kat. III, 82ᵃ, v. אנטיניה.

אנטיפותא=אַנְטִיפּוּטָא.

אנטיפטרוס, read אנטיפטריס.

אנטיפטרין, v. after next w.

אַנְטִיפַּטְרִיס, אַנְטִיפַּטְרָס (אנטיפרס) pr. n. pl. *Antipatris,* a town north-north-west of Jerusalem, founded by Herod the Great and named after his father. Gitt. VII, 7 (76ᵃ) (the second ט freq. dropped). Y. B. Mets. VII, end, 11ᶜ. Y. Taan. IV, 69ᵇ top פריס . . . .; a. fr. Tosef. Gitt. VII (V), 9 אנטיפרוס, פנרוס . . ., (corr. acc.)

אַנְטִיפַּטְרִית f. (preced.) *of Antipatris, Antipatridic.* Sabb. 90[a] נתר א׳ Ms. M. (ed. אנפנטרין, Ar. אנטיפטרין); Nidd. 62[a] אנטפטרית Antip. nitrum.

אַנְטִיפַּטְרֵס, v. אנטיפטריס.

אַנְטִיפֵּי, v. אַנְדִּיפֵּי.

אַנְטִיפִּיטָא, אַנְטִיפּוּתָא, אַנְטִיפִּיטָה, אַנְטִיפִּיטָא .... m. (corrupt. of אַנְתוּפָּטָא ἀνθύπατος) *proconsul* (residing in Cæsarea). Y. Meg. III, 74[a]; Y. Ber. V, 9[a] top; Koh. R. to III, 6. [Ib. to XI, 1 אנטפיטר, אוטפיטא and var. corrupt. in var. ed.]

אנטיפרוס, אנטיפריס, אנטיפרס, v. אַנְטִיפַּטְרִיס.

אַנְטִיפָּתָא, v. אַנְטִיפִּיטָא.

אַנְטִיקֵיסַר m. (Ἀντι-Καίσαρος) *Pro-Cæsar,* the highest dignitary next to the Emperor; in gen. *vice-roy.* Gen. R. s. 53; s. 85, end (also אנטקיס׳).

אַנְטִיקִירוֹס, v. אֲפִּיקֵירוֹס.

אנטירוקוס, אנטירריקון, v. אַנְטִידִּיקוֹס.

אַנְטִירִידִינָאֵי m. pl., v. אַנְטַרְדּוּס.

אנטכנון, v. אִסְטַכְטוֹן.

אַנְטָל m. (נטל) *Antal,* one fourth of a Log (liquid measure). B. Bath. 58[b]; v. נַטְלָא. V. אַנְטְלַיָא.

*__אֶנְטְלֵר__ m. (ἐντολεύς) *procurator, mandatary.* Y. Snh. II, beg. 19[d] וימנה לו א׳ (ed. incorr. לֵיה אנטלר) let him appoint a mandatary. Ib. וא׳ בשבועה can the mandatary take an oath for his client?

אַנְטִילַיָּא, אַנְטְלַיָא m. pl. (of אנטל; from which Greek ἄντλος, ἄντλον &c. and our w. ἄντλεια, antlia) *baling out bilge-water, pump* (with wheels and buckets). Ruth R. to II, 19 גלגל אנטר׳; Lev. R. s. 34 אנטל׳ (ed. אנטרלא, corr. acc.) the pumping wheel. Tosef. Makhsh. III, 4 מפני א׳ שלהן on account of their baling machine (besprinkling the wheat). Ib. Mikv. IV, 2 אנטליא.

אנטלימוס, v. אַנְטוֹנִינוֹס.

אנטלר, v. אֶנְטְלֵר.

*__אנטנה__ Mass. Tsits. (ed. Kirchh. p. 22) perh. *Antoniana,* a cloak; v. אבטינא.

*__אנטניא__ Midr. Till. Ps. XV, beg., perh. מוֹנִיטִין or מוֹנִיטַיָּא (monetæ) *mints;* cmp. אַלְתּוּסְבָרָאוֹת.

אנטנינוס, v. אַנְטוֹנ׳.

אַנְטִפַּטְרִית, v. אַנְטִיפּ׳.

אַנְטַרְדָּס, אַנְטַרְדּוּס pr. n. pl. (Ἀντάραδος) *Antaradus,* a Syrian town opposite the Isle of Aradus. Y. Bets. III, 62[a] top. Y. Sabb. I, 4[a] bot. אנטיירים (corr. acc.).—Cmp. טַנְתוּרְדִּיָּא.—Deriv. אַנְטְרִידִינָאֵי *inhabitants of Ant.* Targ. Y. II, Gen. X, 18.

אנטרי Pesik. R. s. 24, p. 122[b] ed. Friedm. מטרילין בא׳, v. אסלטין.

אַנְטְרִידִינָאֵי, v. אַנְטַרְדּוּס.

אנטרין Y. Sabb. VII, 10[a] bot. משקע בא׳, v. באנטרין.

אנטריס, prob. corrupt. of אַנְטִיפַּטְרִיס q. v. Y. Gitt. IV, 46[a] שרי א׳ if a slave escaped to A., he may be extradited; v. אוני II.

אנה, אני (=b. h. ינה, sec. r. of און, cmp. אָנַן a. b. h. ענה); *Pi.* אִינָּה (אָנָּה) *to press, wrong, oppress; to impose, overreach in dealing,* v. אוֹנָאָה. B. Mets. 59[b] המאנה את הגר he who wounds a stranger's (proselyte's) feeling. Ib. 49[b] תן לי מה שאִינִיתָנִי return to me the amount with which thou hast overreached me. Ib. 50[a] top מה שאניתני (Ms. R. 1 שנתאונֵּתָנִי, v. infra). Ib. 51[a] שאניתני (Ms. M. שֶׁאֲנַנְתָּנִי, fr. אָנַן; Mish. IV, 2 שאוניתני, v. אוֹנָאָה, Ms. R. 1 שהוניתני, v. הוֹנָאָה, Ms. R. 2 שאונתני, v. Rabb. D. S. a. l. note).

Nithpa. נִתְאַנָּה *to be overreached.* Ib. 49[b] מי נ׳ which of them has been overreached? Ib. 50[b] מי שנ׳ (Ms. M. מִתְאוֹנֶה); a. fr. [Nithpol. of אנן, נִתְאוֹנֵן, v. supra.] [In. Y. אוֹנָה, v. אוֹנָאָה.]

אֲנִי (b. h.; demonstr. אן, v. אָנֹכִי) *I.* Succ. 53[a]; a. v. fr.—[Ib. IV, 5 אני והו (Y. והוא), reverential transcription of אנא יהוה, to avoid the utterance of the Tetragrammaton.]—*Pl.* אָנוּ. Keth. I, 6; a. fr.

אֲנִיָא, v. אוֹנְיָא.

אֲנִייקָא, אֲנִיאקָא pr. n. pl. (v. אוֹנִיקִי) an abbreviation of בית אוניקי, *Bithynia,* a district of Asia Minor. B. Mets. 46[b] דינר א׳ the Denars issued in Bithynia; v. אַנְגְּרָא for var. lect.

אניגורין, v. אֲנִיגָרוֹן.

אַנִּיגְרָא pr. n. pl. v. אַנְגְּרָא; cmp. next w.

אַנִּיגְרָא m. (=על ניגרא *by the creek*) *shore;* v. נִיגְרָא, נִגְרָא. B. Mets. 107[b]; a. e.

אניגרון Pes. 112[b], a word in a charm formula against thirst (var. lect. Rabb. D. S. a. l.), prob.=next w.

אֲנִיגָרוֹן (אניגורין) m. (ἐλαιόγαρον, נ corrupt. for ל) *a sauce of oil and garum* (to which wine is sometimes added). Ber. 35[b] sq. א׳ מיא וכ׳ *elaiogaron* contains the juice of beets; oxygaron the sauce of all kinds of boiled vegetables. Yoma 76[a]. Shebu. 23[a] ודילמא ע״י א׳ perhaps if used as an admixture to *elaiogarum*? Tosef. Bets. II, 16 א׳ ואכסיגרון ועליהן וכ׳ (Y. Bets. II, end, 61[d] ארגגורין ובתובן וכ׳, corr. acc.; cmp. Rashi to Shebu. l. c.). Tosef. Ter. IX, 10; 12; Shebi. VI, 3. Koh. R. to I, 18 אגרטין (corr. acc.).

אֲנִיָא, v. אוֹנְיָא.

אֲנִייקָא, v. אַנְיָאקָא.

***אנים** Y. M. Kat. III, 83c bot., read אניא, contr. of אחניא, v. חני.

אֲנִין, אָנִין, v. אָנַן, אֲנַן.

אֲנִינָה f. (אָנַן) *grief, retired mourning*, esp. the status of the mourner between death and burial of a kinsman, contrad. to אֲבֵילוּת, אֲבֵילָה. Lam. R. introd. (R. Abbahu 4) א׳ מבפנים *ăninah* is indoor (retired) grief. Y. Hor. III, 48a top ארוזהו א׳ וכ׳ what is *ăninah?*—The time from death to &c. Y. Pes. VII, 35a top אֲנִינַת לילה תורה observance of ăninah by night is biblical. Gen. R. s. 85 he is named *Onan* שהביא א׳ לעצמו because he brought mourning over his early death.

אֲנִינוּת f. same. Kidd. 80b; a. fr. in Babli.

אֲנִינוּתָא ch. same. Targ. Lam. II, 5; a. e.

אֲנִינְקָא, v. אֲנַנְקָא a. אֲנִיקָא.

אָנִיסָא, v. אָנוּסָא.

אֲנִיסָא m. (אנס) *oppression, ill-gotten wealth*. Targ. Is. I, 13; a. e.

אֲנִיסוּתָא f. (preced.) *oppression*. Targ. Koh. V, 7; a. e.

אֲנִיסִין m. pl. (v. נִיסוֹס; νῆσος) *islands*. Tosef. Ter. II, 12; Ḥall. II, 11; (also נסין a. נירסין; Y. Shebi. VI, 36d נירסים; Gitt. 8a נסין).

אֲנִיסְכָּא com. (v. נִיסְכָּא) *made of cast metal*, opp. ארוקתא of wrought or stretched metal. Sabb. 59b דא׳ כ״ע וכ׳ (Rashi ed. דניסכא) as to those made of cast metal there is no difference of opinion. Ib. א׳ עיקר (prob. to be read מיקר, v. Ms. M.) what is made of cast metal is more precious (original).

***אניפונים** Targ. II Esth. I, 2 read אֶפִּיפָנֵיס pr. n. m. (*Antiochus*) *Epiphanes*, King of Syria.

אָנִיץ Af. of נוץ.

עֲנִיץ, אֲנִיץ m. (ענץ, אנץ, sec. r. of עוץ, אוץ) [*tight bundle*], only in pl. const. (צְ) אֲנִיצֵי פשתן *flax-stalks after they are soaked, beaten and baked*. B. Mets. II, 1 (21a). Y. Succ. I, 52b bot.; Bab. ib. 12b (Ar., Ms. M., Tosef. ib. I, 6 עניצי); a. fr. V. אוּנִין.

אַנִיקָא, v. אַנְיָאקָא.

אֲנִיקָא m. (אנק) *trouble, affliction*. Targ. Y. Gen. XXII, 20; a. e.—*Pl.* אֲנִיקִין, אֲנִיקֵי (often used as a singular). Targ. Lev. XXI, 10 (affliction by death in the family); a. e. Cmp. אֲנַנְקָא.

אֲנִיקוּתָא f. same. Targ. Ps. CII, 21.

אָנַךְ (sec. r. of אך, cmp. חנך) 1) *to rub, polish, finish*, esp. *to glaze vessels, to line* (with onyx). Tosef. Kel. B. Mets. I, 3 כלים .... שֶׁאֲנָכָן באנך וכ׳ (or שאִנְּכָן *Pi.*) clean vessels which one lined with unclean glaze (onyx); v. אֲנָךְ.—2) (cmp. חָכַךְ) *to make sore, to grieve*. Denom. אֲנָךְ II.

***אֲנָךְ** I m. (preced. 2)) *grief, wrong*. B. Mets. 59a all gates are sometimes closed except the gates (of prayer) of those wronged by men (v. אוֹנָאָה), for it says, (Amos VII, 3) "Behold the Lord stands on the wall of *anakh* and in his hand he holds *anakh* (oppression)." Ib. אונאה דכתיב ובידו א׳ the Lord hears the prayer of the wronged, for it says &c.; v. אוֹנָיָתָא.

אֲנָךְ II (b. h., prob. fr. a demonstr. אן, cmp. הן, הוּךְ &c., a. אֲנִי, אָנֹכִי) *plummet, plumb-line*.. Lev. R. s. 33, beg. a. e. א׳ זה סנהדרין וכ׳ by the *plummet* (Amos VII, 7) the Great Sanedrin are meant whose number (71) corresponds with the numerical value of אנך.

אֵינָךְ, אָנָךְ m. (אָנַךְ 1)) *Onyx Agate*, a semipellucid stone of a fine flinty texture. Ab. Zar. 8b Ar. אנך (ed. אינך).—2) *a variety of gypseous alabaster, onyx; a glaze*. Ib. 11b ומחפין .... בא׳ Ar. (ed. באי׳) the streets are paved with &c. (for the procession). Tosef. Kel. B. Mets. I, 3, v. אָנַךְ. Lev. R. s. 33 nothing makes the kettle durable אלא אֲנָכָהּ וכ׳ but its glaze lining; so says the Lord אֲנָכְכֶם וכ׳ I am your lining (stay) in trials (incorr. in some ed. a. Ar. s. v. נך).

אָנֹכִי (b. h.; v. אֲנָךְ II; cmp. אֵינָךְ) *I*. Pesik. R. s. 21, v. אָנוֹךְ. Sabb. 105a א׳ נוטריקון *anokhi* may be interpreted as an acrostichon אנא נפשי כתבית יהבית I myself have written, have given (the Law). Pesik. Baḥod. p. 109b; v. אָנוֹךְ.—*Pl.* אֲנַחְנוּ, נַחְנוּ. Ber. 14b; a. fr. V. אֲנִי, אֲנוּ.

אנלגין, v. next w.

אַנְלוֹגִין m. (ἀναλογεῖον) *reading desk, pulpit*. Kel. XVI, 7 Ar. אנלגין (Var. in R. S. אנליגין, ed. אנגלין; corr. acc.). Y. Meg. III, 73d bot. אנג׳, אירג׳ (corr. acc.). Tosef. Kel. B. Kam. II, 3 או לולגין פרוס׳ וכ׳ ed. Zuck. (Var. אלו לגין, ed. אולו לוגין read אנאלוגין; used as fem.) a reading desk spread out is clean, folded together is unclean (susceptible of levitical uncleanness).

אנלונטית, v. אֲלוּנְטִית I.

אָנַן (b. h.; sec. r. of און, אן, v. אָנַךְ) *to press, oppress, wrong*, v. אָנָה.—אוֹנֵן *one who feels grieved, mourner*, esp. *Onan*, mourner before the burial of a kinsman, contrad. to אָבֵל; v. אֲנִינָה. M. Kat. 14b א׳ מקריב may officiate at sacrifices though being an Onan.—*Pl.* אוֹנְנִין. Snh. 47b לא היו מתאבלין אלא א׳ they observed no mourning ceremonies but lived in silent and retired mourning.—Fem. אוֹנֶנֶת. Keth. 53a.—Denom. אָנִין *complaining, fastidious, feeble*. *Pl.* אֲנִינֵי הדעת *fastidious of taste, easily taking an aversion, delicate*. Pes. 113b. Cmp. אִיסְתְּנִיס.

Nithpa. נִתְאוֹנֵן *to feel wronged, complain of being overreached*, v. אָנָה.

אֲנַן, אֲנַן ch. *to be grieved, to mourn.* Targ. Koh. VII, 4.—Denom. אָנִין; f. אֲנִינָא, with דעתא=h. אָנִין, v. preced. Ḥull. 112ª א׳ דעתיה he was fastidious, delicate. Ber. 24ᵇ; B. Bath. 23ª א׳ דעתאי I am &c.

אֲנַן pl. of אֲנָא.

אֲנָנָא=אֲנָא אֲנָא, v. אֲנָא.

אֲנַנְקָא m. (=אֲנְקָא, נ inserted; אנק)=אֲנִיקָא. Targ. Y. Gen. XXXVIII, 25 אננקי *my distress.—Pl.* אֲנַנְקֵי *troubles.* Targ. II, Esth. V, 1. Targ. Y. II Gen. XXII, 14 (Y. I אֲנִיקֵי). Cant. R. beg. none tells א׳ דידיה (some ed. אונ׳) his troubles except after his release; Koh. R. to I, 12 אנוקי, read אֲנִיקֵי.—Targ. Y. II Gen. XXXVIII, 25 אֲנִינְקֵי Ar. *the distressed* (ed. עיריקא). Cmp. עוק a. deriv.

*__אֲנַנְקֵי__ adv. (ἀνάγκῃ) *perforce, of necessity* (corresp. to בנוהג שבעולם). Gen. R. s. 12 if a human being spreads a tent א׳ ע״י שהות וכ׳ it must in course of time become loose. Cmp. Y. Ber. I, 2ᵈ top.

*__אנקקתא (אֲנַקְקְתָא) אֲנַנְקְתָא__ f. (=h. אֲנָקָה II, נָאקָה) *a full grown camel.* Midr. Till. to CIV, 24 and the lion took pity on him (the dog), for she (the camel), (read דהיא) is a friend of the lion, וכלבא סעדא דא׳ and the dog is a friend of the camel; Yalk. ib. 862 אקנקיתא, אקניקתא, Zay. Raan. a. l. אֲנַקִיתָא.

אָנַס (b. h.; sec. r. of אוס, √אי; cmp. חוס, אנץ, אוץ; as to meaning cmp. כּוּף, אנך &c.) *to bend, force; to do violence; to outrage* &c. Ḥull. 45ª א׳ בסימנים if one in cutting presses the windpipe and gullet out of their natural position. Ib. אָנְסָה עצמה if the animal strained its neck so as to dislocate the organs. Gitt. 44ᵇ; Ḥull. 131ª הרי שאֲנָסוּ וכ׳ if royal officers took forcible possession of (seized,) his barn. Keth. III, 4 האוֹנֵס he who violates a woman. Part. pass. f. אֲנוּסָה *an outraged woman.* Y. Yeb. VI, 7ᶜ; a. fr.—Masc. אָנוּס *the victim of an accident, unavoidably prevented.* Ned. 27ª א׳ רחמנא וכ׳ the Merciful (the Law) acquits from responsibility him who is the victim of an unavoidable accident; a. fr.

Pi. אִנֵּס *to violate.* Num. R. s. 14 לאַנְּסָהּ to violate her.

Nif. נֶאֱנַס *to be forced, overcome, to meet with an accident.* Ber. 13ᵇ נ׳ בשינה overcome by sleep. Ḥull. 31ª נֶאֶנְסָה וטבלה if she dipped in the water by an accident Ib. 45ª ובלבד שלא תֵּאָנֵס provided the animal is not forced so that its organs be dislocated. Keth. I, 10 נאנסה she was outraged; a. v. fr.

אֲנַס, fut. יֵינַס ch. same; 1) *to take by force, snatch, rob.* Targ. II Sam. XXIII, 21; a. fr.—2) *to oppress, rob* (h. עשק). Targ. I Sam. XII, 3; 4; a. fr.—Arakh. 16ª ואזלין ואנסין ליה and they (violent men) go and rob him (or force him to feed them, v. Rashi a. l.). Lev. R. s. 34 אַנְסִינָן (אַנְסִינוּן) אקימנן וכ׳ he forced them, made them managers of public charities.—3) (cmp. ענש) *to distrain, fine.* Targ. Amos. IV, 2; a. fr.; v. אֲנוֹסָא.—4) *to urge, press; restrain.* B. Bath. 57ᵇ one must לְמֵינַס נפשיה restrain himself (turn his eyes away forcibly). Ḥull. 133ª א׳ ליה עידניה time pressed him.—Part. pass. אָנִיס 1) *wronged* &c. Targ. Hos. V, 11; a. e.—2) *unavoidably prevented, forced,* v. preced. Naz. 23ª מינס א׳ he had no will of his own (being drunk). Ned. 27ᵇ; a. fr.

Af. אוֹנֵיס *to oppress.* Targ. Jer. VII, 6 (h. text תונה).

Ithpe. אִתְאֲנִיס, אִתְאֲנַס, contr. אִיתְּנִיס. 1) *to be robbed; to be fined,* (of official extortion); &c. Targ. Is. XXI, 2. Lev. R. s. 34 דאנון מארסוון (read דאתון מִתְאַנְסוּן or דארנון מאנסכון; Yalk. Lev. 665 דאתון מזדמיין, v. זמי) that you will lose through extortion &c.—2) *to meet with an accident, be unavoidably prevented.* Ned. 27ª איתניס ולא אתא he met with an accident and did not come in time. Ib. והא מֵינַס איתניס was he not unavoidably prevented (since he died during the appointed time)? Keth. 16ᵇ אִתְּנוּסֵי הוא דאתנסי they were prevented from forming the bridal procession [prob. alluding to government interference; Rashi: through excessive drinking]. [איתניס *to grow ill,* v. אִיתְּנִיס a. נְסַס.]

אַנָּס m. (preced. ws.) *one who acts violently, a violent man.* B. Bath. 45ª סתם נכרי א׳ הוא as a rule the gentile is violent (lawless). Y. Kidd. I, 60ᶜ top.—*Pl.* אַנָּסִים, אַנָּסִין. Ḥull. 94ᵇ מפני הא׳ on account of the lawless (among the gentiles).—Esp. (law) *Annas, one who is in possession of property bought from one who obtained it by force or consfiscation, owner of reclaimable property.* Kil. VII, 6 (5) הא׳ שזרע וכ׳ if an Annas put seeds into a vineyard (creating Kilayim), and it is reclaimed. Ib. from what time and onward נקרא א׳ is one called an Annas (who may consider himself in undisturbed possession)? Answ. משישקע (v. Y. ib. 31ª) from the time the name of the original owner is sunk (when the property is no longer named after him).—*Pl.* as above. Y. Succ. IV, beg. 54ᵇ, v. הֶפְקֵר.

אֲנַסְיָא, אֲנַסִיא Targ. Y. II Gen. X, 2, v. אוסיא.

אנסיגרון read אַכְסִיגָרוֹן.

אנסיומא read אַכְסְיוֹמָא.

*__אָנַף__ (b. h.; sec. r. of אוּף; v. אפף) *to swell, blow,* whence, *to be angry.—Pi.* אִנֵּף *to quarrel.* Ḥull. 63ª why is it called Anafah? שמְּאַנֶּפֶת עם וכ׳ (not שמנאפת, v. Rashi a. l.) because it quarrels with its kindred.

אַנְפָּא m. (more freq. אַפָּא q. v.) 1) *face, front;* freq. in pl. אַנְפֵּי. Targ. Ps. LXXXIV, 10; a. fr.—2) with prep. ב, *in sight of, before.* B. Mets. 86ª לבבא באנפיה ..... he locked the door before him.—*Pl.* בְּאַנְפֵּי (Targ. also על א׳). Targ. Y. Gen. XXIII, 10; a. e.—Ḥull. 121ª בא׳ נפשיה (=h. בפני עצמו) *for itself, singly.* Targ. Y. Deut. I, 6; a. e. —B. Mets. 22ᵇ.—Keth. 7ᵇ באנפייהו in their presence; a. fr.

*__אַנְפּוֹ__ f. (נפי)=h. תְּנוּפָה *waving.* Targ. Y. II Lev. VII, 30 (20) (some ed. אַנְפּוֹי).

אנפוליא Tosef. Kel. B. Mets. VI, 5 ed. Zuck., read אנפילייא.

אנפוקנין read אנפקינון.

אַנְפּוֹרָא f. (ἀναφορά) *official return. Pl.* אַנְפּוֹרָאוֹת. Pesik. Shek. p. 18^b עשה שתי א׳ made out two military returns (census); Num. R. s. 2 אנפריאות; Pesik. R. s. 11 אפונראות (corr. acc.). [Not to be confounded with אַנְפָּרְיוֹת, pl. of אַנְפָּרוּת.]

אַנְפּוֹרְיָא f. (ἐμπορία) *journey for business, traffic, trade;* also *merchandise.* כלי א׳ merchant's implements (straps, poles &c. for carrying goods). B. Mets. II, 2 כלי א׳ אינו וכ׳ merchant's implements (if found) need not be publicly announced (for return to the owner). Ib. 23^b sq.; Y. B. Mets. II, beg. 8^b; Tosef. ib. 1 (definit. of our w.). Midr. Till. to Ps. CXVIII, 20 התקין א׳ שלו arranged his journey with the caravan. [Also אַנְפּוֹרְיָה.]

אנפטר read אַפְּטֵר.

אנפיא Tosef. Ḥull. III (IV), 27, Var. נפיא, v. אפירן.

***אַנְפִּילוֹגוֹס** m. (ἐπίλογος, epilogus) *concluding speech, argument, inference; peroration.* Koh. R. to X, 16 התחיל א׳ וכ׳ (Solomon) in his wisdom began a concluding argument; (Midr. Till. to Ps. LXXII פרו נובע!)

אנפילוגיס, corr. as preced.

אנפילון, v. אַפִּלְיוֹן II.

אַנְפִּילְיָא, v. אַמְפִּילְיָא.

אַנְפֵּיקְנוֹן, אַנְפֵּיקְנִין, v. אַנְפַּקְנוֹן.

אַנְפַּק, אַנְפְּקָא, אנפק, v. אַנְבַּג.

אַנְפְּקוּת, v. נַפְקוּת.

אנפקיטן, corr. as next w.

אַנְפַּקְנוֹן m. (ὀμφάκινον, sub. ἔλαιον) *oil made of unripe olives.* Targ. Esth. II, 12 אַנְפַּ׳.—Pes. 43^a אנפיקנין (Ms. M. אנפיקנון). Men. VIII, 3; a. e.—Gen. R. s. 98 טן .... (corr. acc.). Cant. R. to IV, 8 איפק׳ (corr. acc.).

***אַנְפָּרוּת** f. (פרר or נפר √פר׳) *a break, division,* whence 1) *the purchase of an odd object, of one of a pair.* Sabb. 80^b (ref. to אַנְדִּיפָא q. v.) וכי אדם עושה מיתיו א׳ will a man buy a half of a thing (as a cosmetic for one temple)?—2) *partial payments, an agreement* (invalid according to Jewish law) *of term payments with the condition of forfeiture on missing one term* (v. אַסְמַכְתָּא), esp. *such an agreement forced upon a Jew by a gentile (Roman) individual or authority.* Gitt. 44^a (v. אָנַס) אם בא׳ if his crop was seized in consequence of an *anparuth,* he is exempt from paying the tithes (of his produces, since he is the loser, whereas if distrained for a real debt, he enjoys the legal benefit of being released of a debt, and therefore must pay the tithes, as if he had sold the crop). Y. Keth. X, end, 34^a בארנונה וכ׳ with reference to annona, capitation tax and forfeiture. Gitt. 58^b הבא מחמת חוב ומחמת א׳ וכ׳ if a gentile (Roman) obtained possession of a Jew's property in consequence of seizure for a debt or of forfeiture and subsequently sold it to a Jew, the Sicarion law finds no application (and the property must, without any indemnity, be restored to its original owner; v. סִיקְרִיקוֹן); וא׳ עצמה וכ׳ and the property seized for forfeiture must have been in the possession of the gentile for twelve months (during which the Jew might have had a chance to reclaim it as illegally seized; v., however, the objection, and subsequent emendation of סיקריקון for א׳, ibid.). Ib. אין א׳ בבבל in Babylon (under the Persian government) there is no *anparuth,* (which is interpreted) אין דין א׳ וכ׳ the laws concerning the purchase by a Jew of property which a gentile had seized for forfeiture find no application in the well regulated Persian state because the owner might have gone to court, if he felt himself aggrieved. Tosef. Gitt. V (III), 2.—*Pl.* אַנְפָּרְיוֹת. Y'lamd. Sh'laḥ. (quot. in Ar.) אני נוטל מהן א׳ וכ׳ I (the Lord) take from them promises to pay in instalments (promises of amending their ways, repentance) and give them extension. Tanḥ. ib., end, a citizen was paying *annonæ* וכותב א׳ and signing agreements of forfeiture; (Num. R. s. 17 אפכרות, v. אַפּוּכֵי). [Ibid. s. 2 אנפריאות, v. אַנְפּוֹרָא pl.]

***אָנַץ** (sec. r. of אוץ, v. אָנַיץ) *to squeeze in, fasten.* Targ. Koh. XII, 11 דאנצין, read דְאַנְיצִין which are fastened (h. text נטועים; gloss דאציתרן, clerical error for דאניצין or דנציבין, embodied in the text of some ed.). Targ. I Sam. XIII, 21, Ar., v. נְצַב.

אנק Y. Bicc. I, 63^d bot. מאונקות, v. אָבַק.

אָנַק (sec. r. of איק, v. חנק), *Pa.* אַנֵּק *to press, choke.* Part. pass. מְאַנַּק *choked, grieved.* Targ. Ezek. IX, 4. Cmp. דְּנַק. V. אֲנִיקָא, אֲנָקְתָא &c.

אנקא B. Mets. 46^b, v. אַנְיָאקָא.

אֲנָקָה I (b. h.; אנק) a species of *lizzard.* Tanḥ. Balak. 9; Num. R. s. 20.

אֲנָקָה II f. *camel,* v. נְאָקָא.

אַנְקוֹרָא, v. אִינְק׳.

***אַנְקְטְמִין, לוּקְטְמִין** m. pl. (a contr. of אנק קטמין, or לולי קטמין, v. אונקלי a. its bibl. equivalent לוּלָי) *loop* or *hook for stumped limbs, a sort of artificial arm* (or *leg;* v. infra). Sabb. VI, 8 א׳ מהורין Mishn. a. Y. (Bab. ed. 66^a ליק׳) an artificial arm (for carrying burdens) is not susceptible to levitical uncleanness, but you must not wear it in walking in the street on the Sabbath (because it is intended for carrying burdens). Y. ib. 8^c bot. (R. Abbahu explains our w.) אונוס קְטְמִין, חמרא די ידיא Ar. (read two words; ed. חונים, corr. acc.) the ὄνος (ass, i. e. pulley) of the stump-handed,—a hand-pulley (ass); Bab. a. l. R. Abbahu (leaving out the etymology) חמרא דאכפא a pulley for loads, v. אַכְפָּא. Oth. opin. ibid. קשירי stilts (artificial legs); פרמא (פדאמי) q. v.—V. Kel. XV, 6

נִירָקְבְּמ. [The definitions by Ar. a. Rashi, referring to nplements of public entertainments, are not in keeping vith the preceding proposition of the Mishnah.]

אנקיינוס, v. אוֹקְ׳.

אנקילין, v. אוּנְקְלִי.

אַנְקִיתָא, v. אֲנַנְקָתָא.

***אנקלווסים, אנקלווסיס**, read אִנְקְווִילִינָטוּס m. (inquilinatus, v. Makeld. Roman Law, ed. Dropsie, § 408) *the lessee's right of dwelling, lease.* Y. B. Mets. VIII, end, 11[d], let him stay עד ימלא א׳ דידיה until his lease expires.

***אֶנְקְלוּמָא (אנקלומה)** (ἐκκαλοῦμαι) *I appeal.* Deut. R. s. 9; Koh. R. to VIII, 8 לומר... א׳ to say before the Lord, 'I appeal against thy decision.' V. next w.

אֶנְקְלִימוֹן (ארנק׳) m. (ἡ ἔκκλητος, v. Sm. Ant. s. v. Appellatio) *appeal* from the decision of a court. Gen. R. s. 49 תולין לו א׳ one is permitted to hang up against him i. e. to announce, an appeal—from the dux &c. Deut. R. s. 9 ליתן לפניו אנקליטין (read ליתלות a. טון...); Koh. R. to VIII, 8 שיתלה א׳ to appeal from his decision. Tanh. Thazr. 7 שלא ירננו עליו אונק׳ וכ׳ (ed. Bub. 9 יתנו, read יתלו). V. next w.

***אנקלימון**, Mus. אנקלימון, read אֶנְקְלֵימָטִין m. pl. (ἔγκλημα, .. ατα) *written complaints, charges.* Deut. R. s. 2; Yalk. Gen. 77; Ex. 167 נתפס בא׳ has been arrested on charges.

אנקלמוס, v. אִרְקוֹנוֹמוֹס.

***אֶנְקְלְסְיָא (אונ׳)** f. (a corruption of ἐνεχυρασία) *taking property in pledge, writ of seizure*=אַדְרַכְתָּא. Tosef. B. Mets. I, 7 אונקליטיא וכ׳ ed. Zuck. (Var. אונקילוסיא, corr. acc.) when a writ of seizure is found, if the debtor admits its correctness, it must be returned to the creditor; if not, it must be returned to neither. Ib. B. Bath. XI, 5 אנקלסיא וכ׳ (אונ׳, אינ׳) a writ of seizure may be written out without notifying the creditor, but not without notifying the debtor and giving him time to protest; v. B. Kam. 112[b]).

אַנְקְקְתָא, אַנְקָתָא, v. אֲנַנְקָתָא.

אֱנָשׁ, v. אִינָשׁ.

אַנְשָׁתָא *her walls*, v. אוּשָׁא

אַנְשׁוֹן. Y. Ter. II, 41[d]; a. e., v. נְשֵׁי *to forget.*

אֲנָשִׁים, v. אֱנוֹשׁ a. אִישׁ.

אַנְתְּ, אַנְתָּה com. (=h. אַתָּה, אַתְּ) *thou.* Dan. II, 29; a. e.—Targ. freq.—Sabb. 30[a] א׳ שלמה thou, O Solomon! Ned. 91[b] אי א׳ לא if it was not thou. B. Mets. 26[b]; a. fr.

***אַנְתָּא** m. (אית, אינת, cmp. אִינְתּוּ for אִיתּוּ) *essence, substance.* Men. 78[a] אימא א׳ דמשחא perhaps by 'loaf of oil', the oil itself is meant?, i. e. a loaf made of congealed oil.

אַנְתּוּ f., v. אִיתּוּ.

אנתונים, read אַנְתּוּנוֹס m. *tunny-fish.* Tosef. Hull III (IV) 27; v. אַטוּנָס.

אַנְתּוּסָאֵי m. pl. *Orthusians*, v. אַרְתּוּסְיָרה. Targ. Gen. X, 17 (Y. ׳אנט).

אַנְתִּימְרוֹס corrupt. of אַנְטִיפַּטְרוֹס, pr. n. m. *Antipater.* Targ. II, Esth. III, 1.

אנתינוס, אנתיניס, v. אנתונים.

***אַנְתִּיקֵי** f. (ἐνθήκη) *store, capital* of the business. B. Bath. V, 1 if one sold a ship, he has not sold with it... את הא׳ the funds and stores belonging to the business. Cmp. ib. 77[b] (definition) עיסקא דאית בה Ms. M. (ed. דבגווה) the business connected with it.

אַנְתְּרוֹפִי m. *anthropeus* (man), an assumed form for ἄνθρωπος, for the purpose of deriving another assumed form (אַנְתְּרוֹפְיָא) *anthropeia* (woman). Gen. R. s. 18; s. 31 did you ever hear people say *gynios* and *gyneia* (from γύνη, woman), or *anthropeus, anthropeia, gabra* (man) *gabratha* (woman)? but you do say (in Hebrew) *ish* and *ish-sha*, both of the same root (as an evidence of the primitiveness of the Hebrew language).

אַנְתְּרוֹפְיָא, v. preced.

אַנְתְּתָא f. (אִתְּתָא) *woman, wife.* Targ. Job XXV, 4; a. fr.—Lev. R. s. 37, beg.; a. fr.—Yeb. 45[b] ... made a gentile woman perform the immersion לשם א׳ as a woman (after menstruation, not as a proselyte).

-אס a formative syllable, v. -אִיס. Words not found under -אס should be looked for under -אִיס.

אס Ex. R. s. 15, v. אִיס.

אסא *to heal*, v. אָסֵי.

אָסָא, אַסָּא I f. (?) (infin. of אסי, as noun) *healing, remedy.* Targ. Jer. XIV, 19 (Regia אַסּוּ). Targ. II Chr. XXI, 18 דְּלֵית א׳ *incurable.*

אָסָא, אַסָּא II m. (preced.) *physician.* Targ. O. Ex. XV, 26 אַסָּךְ (אָסָךְ); Y. אַסְיָאךְ thy &c. V. אַסְיָא, אָסֵי.

אָסָא III m. (contr. of אדסא, v. הדס) *myrtle.* Targ. II, Esth. II, 7; a. e. R. Hash. 23[a] הדס א׳ *hadas* (Is. XLI, 19) is *asa.* Pes. 56[a] א׳ רדא Ar., Ms. O. (ed. דרא) fresh (moist) myrtle. Ber. 9[b] דאמטיית א׳ וכ׳ you had to carry a myrtle-tree to the palace (when forced into public labor, v. אַנְגַּרְיָא). Snh. 44[a] (prov.) א׳ דקאי בינוי וכ׳ a myrtle between willows still is a myrtle by name, and people call it a myrtle.—*Pl.* אָסַיָּא. Targ. Esth. VIII, 15.—Nidd. 37[a] (Rashi, sing.)

*אָסָא, אָשָׁא m. (v. אסר, cmp. אשונא, יָשָׁן, יָשִׁישׁ &c.) *old.* Gitt. 69ᵃ א׳ כלבא (Ar. אשא) old dog (in a charm formula); v. אכסא. Cmp. Assyr. āsi Kalbi, V, R. 8, 12.

*אֲסַב, only in אֲסוּבֵי ינוקא (prob. fr. סב, סבא) *to cause a new-born child to vomit* by putting one's finger into its mouth, to relieve it of phlegm; cmp. חָנַךְ.— Sabb. 123ᵃ, v. Ar. s. v. (Ms. O., Alf., Ash. אסוכי, v. Rabb. D. S. a. l.) [Rashi: *to set an infant's limbs aright,* v. צָבַב Pi.—incongruous with the following אפיקטוריזן . . . .]. [Keth. 10ᵃ אסבוהו, מסבינן, v. סָבָא.]

*אסגנטירין, אסגינטרין, איס׳ &c., a corrupt. of אֶרְגְּוִיסְטְרִין m. (equestris, equester) *one belonging to the equestrian order, knight, nobleman* (v. Sm. Ant. s. v. Eque). Esth. R. to III, 4 אני א׳ של הק״בה וכ׳ (Yalk. a. l. 1054 . . . . אסגנטרינו של) I am the Lord's knight, for . . . . my ancestor (Benjamin) was born in the Land of Israel. Yalk. l. c. וכי א׳ וכ׳ does a knight bow before a commoner?

סְדָה (סְדָה) אַסְדָּה, אַסְדָּא f. (v. סד) *logs joined together, raft.* Ber. IV, 6 באסדא (Ar. סדה, Ms. F. אסכדרא, read אסכדיא; v. infra). Y. ib. 8ᶜ היא א׳ היא אסכדיא וכ׳ *asda, iskhadia* (σχεδία) and *rafsodoth* are the same. Zab. III, 1 אסדה. Neg. XII, 1 אסדה Ar. (ed. אסקריה, Var. אסכדיא; v. אִכְסַנְדְּרָיָא).

אַסְהָדוּתָא, אַסְהָדוּתָא f. (סהד) *attestation, statement of an eye-witness.* Tem. 18ᵇ מאי אסהדותיה what is the object of his statement? Ber. 14ᵇ. Yeb. 64ᵇ.

אָסוֹ, v. אָסוּתָא.—*Pl.* אָסְוָון.

אַסְוָא, v. אַצְוָוא.

אסונן, v. אוּסְיָא.

אַסְוִירוֹס pr. n. m. *Severus,* prob. *Alexander Severus,* Roman emperor. Ab. Zar. 10ᵃ. Nidd. 45ᵃ. V. אַנְטוֹנִינוֹס.

אָסוֹן m. (b. h.; אוס, v. אנס) *accident.* Mekh. Mishp., N'zik. s. 8 אין א׳ אלא מיתה under accident is meant *death* (ref. to Gen. XLII, 38).

אֲסוּפוֹת f. pl. (b. h. אֲסֻפּוֹת, Koh. XII, 11 אסף) *gatherings of scholars, councils.* Y. Snh. X, 28ᵃ bot. Num. R. s. 14. Snh. 12ᵃ בעלי א׳ Sanedrin.

אֲסוּפִי m., אֲסוּפִית f. (אסף) *foundling.* Kidd. IV, 1 (69ᵃ) א׳ כל שנאסף וכ׳ *ăsufi* is a child taken up from the street, whose father and mother are unknown, contrad. to שְׁתוּקִי q. v.—Ib. 73ᵃ if this be so א׳ אסופית לא ישא a male foundling ought not to marry a female foundling. B. Mets. 87ᵃ.

אָסוּר m. (b. h., part. pass. of אָסַר) 1) *prisoner. Pl.* אֲסוּרִים, אֲסוּרִין.—בית הא׳ (b. h.) *prison.* Gen. R. s. 91; a. fr.—2) [Part. of אָסַר, q. v., *forbidden.*]

אָסוּר, v. אִיסּוּר.

אֱסוּר m. ch. (b. h. אֵסוּר) *tie, chain.* Dan. IV, 12. *Pl.* אֱסוּרִין Ezra VII, 26; v. אִיסַר.

אָסוּרָא, אֲסוּרָא m., אֲסָרוּתָא f. same. Targ. Prov. VII, 22 (ed. Walt. אס׳). Targ. Ps. II, 3; v. אִיסַר.

אָסוּרָא, v. אִיסּוּרָא.

אִיסּוּרְיָיתָא, אֲסוּרְיָיתָא f. pl. (אסר; cmp. אֱסָרוּתָא) *bundles, bunches.* Hull. 51ᵇ א׳ bundles of reeds. Bets. 12ᵇ א׳ דחרדלא bundles of mustard stalks. Ib. 13ᵃ א׳ טבלא when in bundles, they are Tebel (v. טֶבֶל).

*אֲסוּרִין m. pl. (v. אָסוּר) prop. *bands,* esp. *certain implements belonging to the wine press.* Y. B. Bath. IV, beg. 14ᶜ, for which Bab. ib. 67ᵇ נסרים, Var. יצרים; Tosef. ib. III, 2 יצירדין, Var. יצירין.

אסורינן Pesik. R. s. 22, v. סור, a. סִיאוּף.

אָסוּתָא, אָסוּ f. (אסי) *cure, remedy.* Targ. Is. LVIII, 8. Targ. Gen. III, 6 (some ed. O. אִיסוּ); a. fr. B. Mets. 86ᵃ top ואסו דרבי וכ׳ and Rabbi's cure shall be effected through him. B. Kam. 85ᵃ, a. fr. מאי אָסוּתֵיה what is the remedy for it? Sabb. 110ᵃ perhaps the Rabbis' snake (excommunication) has bitten him דלית ליה א׳ for which there is no remedy.—*Pl.* אָסְוָון. B. Bath. 58ᵇ בריש כל א׳ אנא חמר I, the wine, stand at the head of all medicines.—אָסְיָתָא. B. Mets. 113ᵇ אָסְוָתַיְיהוּ remedies for them. Lev. R. s. 37 אסייתך (read אָסְוָתָךְ).

אַסְחָרוּתָא f. (סחר) *sitting around the table, banqueting.* Targ. I Kings X, 5. Targ. I Sam. IX, 12 בית א׳ the place of feasting (h. text במה); a. e.

אִסְטְ־ interchanging with אִצְטְ־. [For words not found here below, v. s. אִיסְט׳, or אִצְטְ־.]

אִסְטַטִּיבָה, אִסְטָאטִיבָא f. (stativa, sub. castra) *resting station.* Gen. R. s. 10 end עשה א׳ to take a rest. Pesik R. s. 31 אסטטיא, read אִסְטַטִּיוָא.

אִסְטְבָא, v. אִיסְט׳.

*אִסְטַבְלָא, אִיצ׳, אִיס׳, אִצ׳ II f. (diminut. of אִיסְטְבָא) *colonnade-like walk. Pl.* אִסְטַבְלָאוֹת, אִצ׳ &c. Erub. 24ᵃ עשויין א׳ א׳ Mss. (ed. one א׳, v. Rabb. D. S. a. l.) planted so as to form colonnades.

*אִסְטַבְלָאמָא m. (stabulata, D. C.=stabularius, σταβλίτης) *equerry. Pl.* אִסְטַבְלָאטֵי. Esth. R. to I, 12 קומוס א׳ (read קוֹמֵיס) chief of equerries (comes stabuli) [prob. to be read אִסְטָאבּוּלֵי].

אִסְטַגְיוֹת, אִיס׳ f. pl. (סגי, סוג) *rims, mouldings* around a stove. Kel. VIII, 9; cmp. שְׂפַת, שָׂפָה, לְזִבֵּז.— Y. Ab. Zar. II, 42ᵃ bot. הן ספיות הן א׳ ed. Zyt. (oth. ed. אסטיות) *s'fiyoth* and *istagioth* are the same; cmp. R. S. to Kel. l. c. [Tosef. Kel. B. Kam. VI, 17 .. סטאנאות ... לזיבז ספיות ed. Zuck. (Var. ספונאות, R. S. l. c. סטיראות), prob. corrupt. of סְטַגְיָאוֹת.]

אִסְטַגְנִין, אִצְטַ׳, אִי׳ m. (Ispe. noun of סִגְנוֹן) *observer of constellations, astrologer. Pl.* אִסְטַגְנִינִין, constr. אִסְטַגְנִינֵי &c. Sot. 12ᵇ; 36ᵇ; Ber. 4ᵃ; a. fr. Snh. 49ᵃ, v. אִסְטַגְנִינוּת.

*אִסְטַגְנִינָא, אִצ׳, אִי׳ ch. same.—*Pl.* אִסְטַגְנִינַן (?), אִסְטַגְנִינַיָּא &c. Targ. Y. Ex. VIII, 3; 14; 15. Targ. Job V. 13; a. e.

אִי׳, אִצְ׳, אִסְטַגְנִינוּת f. (v. preced.) *astrological speculation, planetary constellation.* Sabb. 156ª נסתכלתי באיצ׳ וכ׳ ed. (Ms. M. באס׳) I looked at my constellation. Ib. צא מא׳ וכ׳ give up thy astrological speculations, for Israel stands not under planetary influences. Yoma 28ᵇ; a. fr.—Snh. 49ª עדיין א׳ של דוד עומדת Ar. ed. pr., Ms. Oxf. (ed. קיימין ...... אצטגנינו) David's star stands as yet (has not yet gone down).

אִסְטַדִינִין, אִסְטַדְיָה, v. אִיס׳.

אסטו Y. Sabb. VII, 8ᵇ bot., v. אסטומוכריאה.

אִסְטְוָוא I, II, v. אִירְטְוָוא I, II.

אִסְטְוָונָא, אִסְטְוָונִית, v. אִיס׳.

אִסְטְוָורָא, v. אִיסְתּ׳.

אִסְטוֹלָא, v. אִסְטְלָא.

אִסְטוֹלִי, v. אִסְטְלִי I, II.

***אסטומוכריאה**, Y. Sabb. VI, 8ᵇ bot., also in two words אסטו מ׳, quoted from Aquila as a rendition of בתי הנפש (Is. III, 20), read: אֶנְסְטוֹמַכְרִיָא (ἐνστομάχια pl. of ἐνστομάχιον=ἐμπλόκιον; v. explan. ibid. דברים וכ׳) *an ornament of the bosom* (stomach).

אִי׳, אִסְטוֹמְכָא I m. (στόμαχος) prop. *orifice*, esp. *stomach.* Lev. R. s. 4 the food goes מיישטא לא׳ from the gullet into the stomach. Koh. R. to VII, 19 (incorr. order).

אִסְטוֹמְכָא II *muscle, cartilage* &c., v. אִסְחוֹמְכָא.

אסטטיא, Pesik. R. s. 31, read אִסְטָאטִיבָא=אִסְטַטִירָא.

אִסְטְטִיבָא=אִסְטָאטִיבָא.

אִסְטַטְיוֹן, v. אִיס׳.

אִסְטַטְיוֹנַר, v. סְטַטְיוֹנַר.

אִסְטֵיב, אִסְטֵיו, אִסְטֵיב, v. אִיס׳.

אסטיוט, v. סוט׳.

אִסְטְמִיס, אִסְטְמִיס, אסטים, v. אִיסְטְמִיס.

אִסְטְנִיסִית, v. אִסְטְנִית.

אסטית Ex. R. s. 15, read אִסְטֵיב.

אִי׳, אִסְטַכְטוֹן, אִסְטַכְטוֹן m. (στακτόν, sub. ἔλαιον) *oil that runs off without pressing, virgin oil.* Lev. R. s. 5 שמן אסטכ׳ Mus., ed. אסטק׳ (Ar. אסתק׳); Num. R. s. 10 אנטכנון; Cant. R. to IV, 8 אפוקסנין, אפי׳ (corr. acc.).

***אִסְטְכְרָא** com., pl. אִסְטְכְרִינְיָא (אִסְטְכְרִין Ar.) (Ispe. noun of סכר, שכר; cmp. b. h. מַשְׂכִּית, שְׂכִיָּה) prop. *embroidered figures*; hence *embroidered girdle.* Gen. R. s. 19 (ref. to Gen. III, 7) various girdles א׳ גלרין, סדינים (Var. גלרונים, Ar. ed. Koh. גולרין) embroidered girdles (or girdle), wrapping belts, and white linen belts; v. גְּלְרוֹן 3). [*Pl.* in sing. sense, v. גִּלְגְּלִין.]

אִסְטֵל, pl. אִסְטְלִים m., v. אִסְטְלִי.

אִי׳, אִסְטוֹלָא, אִצְטְלָא, אִסְטְלָא f. (Ispe. noun of טלל, טלל; cmp. שְׂלָית) *robe, garment.* Targ. Y. Gen. IX, 23; a. fr.—Sabb. 128ª א׳ הראוויה לו a robe becoming his position. M. Kat. 28ᵇ (prov.) שיול א׳ וכ׳ the grave is a fine robe for the freeman whose outfit is complete (well becoming old and virtuous age). B. Mets. 17ª; a. e.—*Pl.* א׳ דלבושין *a suit of clothes.* Targ. Gen. XLV, 22; (ed. Berl. אוּסְטְלְוָון; ib. Y. אסטלוי ולבוש, read אסטלי דלבוש).—Y. Ber. III, 6ᵈ bot. (v. margin. note ed. Krot.). M. Kat. 24ª. Y. Snh. X, 29ᵇ. Koh. R. to XI, 1 א׳ דלבושן v. supra.—Cmp. אִסְטְלִית.—[Y. Shek. III, 47ᶜ bot. אסטלי של זהב, read אִיסְטְרֵי; v. אִיסְתִּירָא.] [Although our w. coincides, in meaning and sound, with στολή in its poëtic and older sense as 'an outfit', yet the form of its Hebrew equivalent (אסטלית) and the laws regulating the borrowing of words, as well as its appearance in so remote a dialect as the Mandaic (as עצטלא) forbid the derivation from the Greek.]

אִסְטְלָה, אִצְטְלָה, v. אִסְטְלִית.

אִיס׳, אִסְטוֹלִי, אִסְטְלִי f. (טלל, v. preced., =אִטְלִים q. v.) *resting place, road-station.* Y'lamd. to Deut. IV, 30 (quot. in Ar.) עשה אסטולי וכתוב וכ׳ he put up a station for travellers, over which was written, "When this people shall go up &c." (I Kings XII, 27).—*Pl.* אִסְטְלִיּוֹת (fr. אִסְטְלִית). Num. R. s. 23 העמד להם א׳ put up for them (the unintentional murderers fleeing to the place of refuge) resting stations ובכל א .... יות וכ׳ (read אסטלית or אסטל) and let there be an inscription over each of them &c. Tanh. Masé 11; ed. Bub. 8; אִיטְלִיסִיּוֹת, אִיטְלִיס.—Y'lamd. to Deut. III, 9 עמון ומואב עשו אִיסְטְלִים Am. a. Moab erected resting stations for the passing Israelites (quot. in Ar. s. v. ארך 5).

אִיס׳, אִסְטוֹלִי, אִסְטְלִי II f. (a corruption of אֶפִּיסְטוֹלִי q. v.) *letter, dying injunction. Pl.* אִסְטְלִיּוֹת. Y. Sot. VII, 21ᵈ bot. ואי׳ שנתן להם משה ... ליאות and (the stones containing) the dying injunctions of Moses (Deut. XXVII, 8); (cmp. Bab. ib. 35ᵇ). Gen. R. s. 74 end Ar. (ed. a. Var. in Ar. אפיסטולי). *Midr. Sam. ch. XI (ref. to the five verses I Sam. IV, 13—17) הכן לא הוה ליה ממחנון חמשה (?סופרין או חמשה אירסטולין (read טופרין אלא וכ׳ indeed so, not five pencils (writers?) or five messages could kill him, but over the news of the captured ark his neck was broken. [Others read אִיסְטִילִין (*stili*) *styles* used for writing on waxen tablets].

אסטליסטקין, v. אִירְסְטוֹלְסְטִיקָא.

אִי׳, אִצְ׳, אִסְטְלִית f. (טלל, v. אִסְטְלָא, טְלִית) 1) *wardrobe*, esp. *festive suit.* Yoma VII, 1 א׳ לבן a suite of white color. Gitt. VII, 5 אִצְטְלִיתִי Mish. (Bab. 74ª אִירְצְטַלְּחִי, fr. אִירְצְטְלָה) my suit. Ib. 74ᵇ אירצטלתא דוקא (read תִי ..... or תוּ ....). Y. ib. 49ª top כאירצטלות (read לית ....).—2) *station*, v. אִסְטְלִי.

אִסְטְמָא m. 1) (Ispe. noun of אסם=חסם, v. חִיסּוּם, the h. equiv. of our w.) *forging steel, steel-edge.* Ber. 62ᵇ כא׳

לפרולא (Ms. M. אסטימא read אִסְטוּמָא, Ms. O. סטומא, Var. אִיצְ׳, אַצְ׳) what the steel edge is to the iron.—2) *frontlet*, v. אִיסְטְמָא.—3) a word in a charm formula. Sabb. 67ᵃ, v. איסטמאה.

אסטמכרא, v. אסטומיכרייאה.

אסטמותיה, v. איסטמאה.

***אסמן** S'mahoth XIII, end חן בא׳, read או בארזן..., v. אַרְזִין.

אִסְטַנְדְּרָא, אִסְתַּ׳, אִיְ׳ m. (Pers. *ustâd-dâr*, *ustadâr*, Perl. Et. St. p. 104) *major domus*, *vice-roy*. Gitt. 80ᵇ לשום אסט׳ וכ׳ ed. (Ar. אסת׳) in the name of the governor of &c. Kidd. 72ᵇ איסת׳ דמישן the governor of Meshan.

אסטנינותיא, v. אִיסְטְפְנִינֵי.

אִסְטְנִיס, v. אִיסְתְּנִיס.

***אִיסְטַמְּסִית, אִיסְטַמְּסִית, אִסְטָנִית** f. (שׂטן=סטן; cmp. אִיסְטְטְנִית) *a system of information, sycophancy*. Macc. I, 5 (5ᵃ) אסטנית היא זו Ms. M. (ed. איסטטית, Mish. אסטס׳, Y. ed. 1, 7 איסטיסית) this endless prosecution of witnesses on the information by other witnesses testifying to an alibi would be regular sycophancy. [Maim. reads אסטיסית.] Tosef. Macc. I, 10 איסטיטית, ed. Zuck. (Var. ארצטניסית).

אִסְטַסְיָאנִית, v. אִיסְטְטְנִית.

אִסְטַסִּית, v. אִסְטָנִית.

אִסְטַפְנִינֵי, v. אִיסְ׳.

אִסְטַקְטוֹן, v. אִסְטַכְטוֹן.

אִסְטְרָא, pl. אִסְטָרִין 1) *streets*, v. אִסְטְרָטָא.—2) *theatre*, v. אִסְטְרָיָא.

אִסְטְרָא *a coin*, v. אִיסְתִּירָא.

אִסְטְרָאוֹת f. pl. *theatres*, v. אִסְטְרָיָא.

אִסְטְרָאמֵיגָא=אִסְטְרָטֵי׳, v. אִסְטְרַטֵ׳.

אִסְטְרַדְיוֹט=אִסְטְרַטְיוֹט.

אִסְטְרוֹבִיל, אִסְטְרוֹבְלָא, v. אִיסְ׳.

אסטרוגי, איס׳ B. Bath. 143ᵃ, read with Ms. אִסְטְרַטְגֵי.

אסטרוגול, אסטרוגילא, v. next ws.

אִסְטְרוֹלוֹגוֹס (אִיצְ׳, אִיסְ׳; אַצְ׳) m. (ἀστρολόγος) *astronomer*; *astrologer*. Y. Sabb. VI, 8ᵈ top חדא אִסְטְרוֹלוֹגִין (read חד, אר׳) a certain astrol.; a. fr.—*Pl.* אִסְטְרוֹלוֹגִין (אַצְ׳ &c.). Targ. I Chron. XII, 32 ed. Rahm. אירצטרולוגין (Var. אירצטרו׳). Ex. R. 1; a. v. fr.—Cant. R. to VII, 9 אִסְטְרוֹלוֹגוֹסֵי. [Yalk. Ex. 164 איסטרוגילין, a. other corruptions, corr. acc.]—V. also next w.—[As regards צט for סט, v. Recens. Don. b. Librat ed. Filipp. p. 9.]

אִסְטְרוֹלוֹגְיָא (אִיצְ׳) אַצְ׳, (אִיסְ׳, אִסְתּ׳) f. (ἀστρολογία) *astronomy*, mostly *astrology*, *sooth-saying*, *astrological prediction*. Y. Ab. Zar. II, 41ᵃ top הוה חמי בא׳ דידיה he foresaw by dint of astrol. speculation (prob. to be read גרן . . ., v. infra). Pesik. R. s. 14 אסטרוגילא (corr. acc.; cmp. טְרֵיר).—*Pl.* אִסְטְרוֹלוֹגִין prop. *astrologers*, trnsf. *astrological books*, *implements*, *horoscope* &c. Gen. R. s. 85 רואה היתה בא׳ וכ׳ she saw in her astrological books (or horoscope). Deut. R. s. 8 מביט באסטרולוגים; Lev. R. s. 36 אצטרוגלים, לוגים . . . &c. (corr. acc.).

אִסְטְרוֹלוֹגְיָא same. Y. Sabb. VI, 8ᵈ אסת׳ דידיה שקרין his astrological books (or computations) lie.

אסטרון Yalk. Koh. 969, read אִסְטְרַטֵיגִין.

אִסְטְרוֹנְגִילוֹן adv. (στρογγύλον, or στρογγυλοῦν, S.) *in a rounded way*, *circularly* (opp. τετράγωνον, or τετραγώνιον). Pesik. R. s. 10, read: שלא היו יושבין טטרגונין או שורה ארוכה אלא א׳ כחצי גורן עגולה וכ׳ they sat not forming a square or a long line, but in a semi-circle, like the shape of a half of the rounded court-room (v. גּוֹרֶן), so that they could conveniently see each other. V. בוטרגנין.

אִסְטְרוֹפוֹמָטָא, אִיס׳ (variously corrupted, v. infra) m. pl. (στροφώματα) *pivots*, *pins at top and bottom of a door turning in sockets*. Gen. R. s. 66 כמין א׳ הדלתות וכ׳ Ar. (ed. איסטריפומיטא; Yalk. Gen. 115 איסטדומוטא) pivot-like, the doors could be doubled backward. [Yalk. l. c. may be read אסטרופוטא στρόφωτος, v. LXX, Ezek. XLI, 24.] Midd. IV, 1 אירצטרבאמוטא Ar., ed. אירצטרמיטה (corr. as above). Pesik. B'shall. p. 86ᵇ; Yalk. Sam. 152 כאילין אמפומטא &c. (corr. acc.) like doors turning in sockets.

אִסְטְרָטָא, אִיסְטְ׳, אִסְטְרָטָה c. 1) (interchanging with אִסְרָטָא, סְרָטָא, trnsp. אִסְטָרָא; *strata*, sub. via, στρᾶτα S.) *paved way*, *public road*. Targ. Y. II Num. XX, 17 . . . טה; a. fr.—Y. Gitt. IV, beg. 45ᶜ. Y. Snh. II, 20ᵃ top גו א׳ וכ׳ on the road he heard &c. Tosef. Sabb. X (XI) 1 sq. (אסרטא, סרטא, Var. אסתרטא with ת). Ab. d'R. N. XXVIII life is like לאיסטרטא וכ׳ (read טא ....) a public road running between two paths &c. Koh. R. to VII, 7 הוינא עקים אִסְטְרָטִי I was bending my road, went out of my way.—*Pl.* אִסְטְרָטַיָּא, (אִסְטְרָטַיָּא, incorr. אִסְטְרַטְיָא). Targ. Y. Num. XX, 19.—אִסְטְרָטִין usu. *the city walks*, *promenades* (between the colonnades &c.). Y. Sabb. VI, 8ᵃ bot. הוו מטיילין בא׳ were promenading &c. Y. Kil. IX, 32ᵈ top; Cant. R. to V, 13; Y. Keth. XII, 35ᵇ bot. אסטרין. [Deut. R. s. 3 אסטרין, read אסטרטיגין.] [In Targ. mostly אִסְרָטִין, אסטרין.]—2) *theatre*. *Pl.* אִסְטְרָטָאוֹת, v. אִסְטְרָיָא.

אסטרטאות M. Kat. 5ᵃ, read with Ms. M. אִסְטְרַטְיָאוֹת, v. אִסְטְרַטְיָא. V. preced.

אִסְטְרָטָה, v. אִסְטְרָטָא.

אסטרטטי׳ Cant. R. to VII, 9 read אִסְטְרַטְלַטְיָא, v. אִסְטְרַטִילָטָא.

אִסְטְרַטְיָא, אִיסְ׳ I f. (στρατεία, in the sense of στρατόπεδον) *camp*, *encampment*, esp. *an open space in* *front of the royal palace, court;* also *station on the road* for Temple pilgrims. Erub. 26[a] א׳ של מלכים Ms. M. (ed. מלך) camp or court round the royal palace. [Men. 103[b] אירסטריא של מלך, for אירסטרטיא(?), v. however אִסְטְרָיָא.] [Lam. R. to III, 7 באידנא א׳; Ab. d'R. Nath. XXVIII לאר׳, read אִסְטְרָטָא. Targ. Y. Num. XX, 19 רַטְיָא . . . some ed., v. אִסְטְרָטָא.]—*Pl.* אִסְטְרַטְיָאוֹת. M. Kat. 5[a] Ms. M. (ed. טאות . . .); Mekh. B'shall. Vayissa ch. III א׳ *stations* (=רחובות). [Erub. l. c. שהיו . . . טיא . . . , read שהיא, or יאות . . .; v. Rabb. D. S. a. l. note.]

אִסְטְרַטְיָא II (**אִסְרַטְיָא**), **אִיס׳** f. (στρατία) prop. *army;* hence 1) *host* (of heavens, cmp. LXX Neh. IX, 6). Num. R. s. 12 א׳ של מעלה; Midr. Till. to Ps. XCII, end אסר׳ . . . divine army (angels, prophets &c.)—2) *royal suite, court-officers.* Kidd. IV, 5 מוכתב בא׳ של מלך recorded in the king's list of officers (during Agrippa's reign, serving as evidence of legitimate birth; cmp. אַרְכֵי I). Lam. R. to II, 2 אסט׳; Y. Taan. IV, 68[d] bot. אסר׳ the list of Barkokhba's suite. [Y. Ned. XI, 42[d] bot. אסטרטיות read אִסְטְרַטְיוֹטוֹת; ib. אסטרטיות חבק׳ read אִסְטְרַטְיוֹט. Y. Gitt. III, 45[a] top. אסרטיות, v. אִפַּרְטוּסוֹת. Tanh. B'resh. 2 אסטרטיאות, Var. אסטראות, v. אִסְטְרָיָא.]

אִסְטְרַטֵּיג, אִסְטְרַטֵּיגָא m. (στρατήγιον) *camp, regular garrison* (=h. מַצָּב), contrad. to stragglers &c. Targ. I Sam. XIII, 23; XIV, 1; 4; 6; 16; a. e.—*Pl.* אִסְטְרַטֵּיגִין. Targ. II Sam. VIII, 6 (h. text נצִיבים). Targ. I Sam. X, 5 . . . אִסְטְרַטֵּיגֵי (constr.).—גַּיָא . . . . . Targ. I Kings IV, 5 על א׳ chief of camps.

אִסְטְרַטֵּיגוֹס (**אסטרטיג**) m. (στρατηγός) *military commander, general;* (in later Greek) *prefect, city-magistrate;* also *chief of body guards* (στρατηγὸς τῶν πραισενταλίων, D. C.). Ex. R. s. 31 (cmp. Gen. R. s. 58). Ib. s. 37, beg.; a. fr.—Deut. R. s. 10 לאסטרטיגין וכ׳ (read גוס . . . .); a. fr.—*Pl.* אִסְטְרַטֵּיגִין, אִסְטְרַטֵּיגֵי.—Targ. II, Esth. I, 3 איסתרח׳ (corr. acc.) *generals.* Y. Ber. VIII, 12[c] top שני א׳ two chiefs of guards; Gen. R. s. 3; a. fr.—B. Bath. 143[a] בולי ואסטרטיגי Ms. M. (ed. אבולי ואסטרוגי); Y. Yoma I, 39[a] top כולי ואסרטיגי (read בולי ואסטרטיגי, v. בּוּלֵי II). Yalk. Koh. 969 אמר לאסטרון שלו (read לאסטרטיגין) he ordered his guard.

אִסְטְרַטְיוֹט, אִסְטְרַטְיוֹטָא, אִסְטְרַטְיוֹטֵיס m. (στρατιώτης) prop. *soldier,* later *Roman officer* (D. C. Gr. s. v.); *attendant.* Y. Shek. V, 49[a]; Cant. R. to III, 6, end אסטרטיג (corr. acc.). Y. Keth. I, 25[c] top טיוס . . . (corr. acc.).—*Pl.* אִסְטְרַטְיוֹטִין. Targ. I Chr. XVIII, 6 (v. however Targ. II Sam. VIII, 6). Tanh. Haäz. 2, read: באו א׳ the officers came to meet the king.—אִסְטְרַטְיוֹטוֹת. Y. B. Kam. IV, 4[b] top שלח המלכות שני א׳ (read ששלחה) the Roman governm. sent two commissioners. Y. Ned. XI, 42[d] bot. אסטרטיות; v. אִסְטְרַטְיָא II.

אסטרטיוס, אִסְטְרַטְיוֹטֵיס, אִסְטְרַטְיוֹטִין, v. preced.

אסטרטילוס, v. next w.

אִסְטְרַטִילָטָא, אִסְטְרַטִילָטֵיס m. (στρατηλάτης=magister militum, v. Sm. Ant. s. v.) *commander in chief, military governor.* Lev. R. s. 16; a. fr. (everywhere corrupt, corr. acc.). Y. Snh. X, 28[b] top אסרטילטירה (corr. acc.) *his stratelates.*—*Pl.* אִסְטְרַטִילָטִין. Targ. Esth. III, 12; VIII, 9 אסטרטילוסי (corr. acc.). Gen. R. s. 44; a. fr. (corr. acc.). Ib. s. 78 אסטרטלי, read אסטרטילטַי *my stratelatæ.*

אסטרטינוס, read גוס . . . . .

אסטרטלירוס, אסטרטלימוס, v. אִסְטְרַטִילָטָא.

אִסְטַרְיָא, אִסְטַרְיָה, אִסְטַרְיָא, אִיס׳, אִצ׳, אִיצ׳ f. (also אִסְטָרָא m.) cacophemistic appellations of all kinds of gentile sports; cmp. the use of θέατρον and θεατρίζειν in Ad Corinth. I, IV, 9, a. Hebr. X, 33; אסטריא &c., as if a denomin. of סרר, cmp. Syr. אצטרניא, אסטרניא, P. Sm. 304 a. cit. ibid.; אצטריבא, as if fr. צרב; אצטרדיון (v. next w.) as if fr. צרד, v. אִיצְטַדִּין; cmp. אֲבִידָן *theatre, arena, gladiatorial shows,* &c. Ab. Zar. I, 7 (16[a]) גרדום וכ׳ אצטדריא (Ms. M. אצטריבא, but in Gem. 18[b] repeatedly אצטריא; Y. ed. איסטדריא; Mish. Nap. אצטדיא, comment. אצטרדיא) place of execution, of shows &c.; v. Gem. 18[b].—[Men. 103[b] איסטריא של מלך the king's amphitheatre, v. אסטרטיא]. *Pl.* אִסְטַרְיוֹת. Sifra Aharé Par. IX ch. 13. Tanh. B'resh. 2 אִסְטְרָאוֹת Var. (ed. אִסְטְרָטָאוֹת). Ab. Zar. 18[b] אשר לא הלך לאריסטרטאות Ms. M. (ed. לטרטיאות, v. Rabb. D. S. a. l.).—אִסְטָרִין, v. next w.

אִסְטָרִין, אִצְטָרִין, אִיס׳, אִיצ׳ (אִצְטַרְטִיוֹן, אִצְטַרְדִּיוֹן, אִרִיצְטַרְיוֹן, also with rejection of א׳ after prefixes) m. (pl. of אסטרא, v. preced.; used as sing., sub. בית הד׳ &c.) *arena, theatre.* B. Kam. IV, 4 (39[a]) שור האיצטרין Ms. M. (ed. איצטדין, Ms. H. a. R., a. Mish. Nap., a. Y. ed. איסטדין) an ox of the arena (that killed a person). Tosef. Ab. Zar. II, 7 היושב באסטרין וכ׳ Var. (ed. Zuck. איסטרטון, ed. איסטרין) he who visits the amphitheatre is considered a murderer (countenancing bloodshed); Y. ib. I, 40[a] אירצטדין (interchanging with תיאטרון).—*Pl.* אִסְטְרִינִין &c. Ab. Zar. 18[b] אין הולכין לא׳ מפני ש״ד Ms. M. (ed. לאצטדינין מפני מושב לצים . . . ., v. Rab. D. S. a. l. note) you must not attend theatres on account of bloodshed. Ib. (repeatedly) אצטרינָן Ms. M.; Tosef. l. c. 6 לאריצטרטיונין (Var. לצטרדיונין, לצטריונין); 7 לאיצטריונין (Var. לטרזיונין, לצטריונין); Ab. Zar. 18[b] לאצטרינין Ms. M. (ed. טרטיאות, En Yakob I אירצטריאות, v. preced.). [Y. Erub. II, 22[b] bot. איצטדין, אצטדין f. *ruins,* near Tiberias, v. איצטדין.] [אסטרין sometimes for אִסְרָטִין.]

אסטרלימוס, v. אִסְטְרַטִילָטָא.

אִסְטַרְקְלִילָא, v. טְרַקְלִילָא.

אַסִּי (=יוֹסֵי, Frank. Meb. Y. s. v.) pr. n. m. *Assi;* 1) an Amora, mate of R. Immi, disciple of Rab and of Samuel. Sabb. 22[a]; a. fr.—Y. Ab. Zar. V, 45[a] bot. רבסי= רב א׳.—2) a copyist. Y. Keth. II, 26[b] bot. כגון אילין ספריו דא׳ וכ׳ as for instance, if witnesses say, these are the books written by Assi, and like these (in handwriting) must the documents be.

אָסָא, אֲסִי (sec. r. of אוס, v. אנס; cmp. איש, יש, אנש &c.; v. Ges. H. Dict. s. vv. אשה, עשה) *to be strong, well.* [Act. v. *to make well,* v. infra a. אָסֵי.]

Af. אַסֵּי *to cure.* Targ. O. Gen. XX, 17 (Targ. Y. אָסֵי); a. fr.—*Part.* מַסֵּי, מְאַסֵּי.—Ned. 49ª לְאַסָּאָה יתיה, לְאַסָּיֵיה to cure him. Sabb. 111ª איכא מכה מסי where there is a wound, it (the vinegar) heals it. Lev. R. s. 16, end, read: מְאַסֵּינָא ליה לגרמי I shall cure him all alone. Gitt. 56ᵇ מאסיין=מסיין, v. next w.

Ithpa. אִיתַּסֵּי, *Ithpe.* אִיתְּסֵי, אִתְּ׳ *to be cured, to recover.* Targ. Josh. V, 8; a. fr.—Sabb. 33ª. Gitt. 12ᵇ דבעי אִתְּסוּיֵי ביה for he wants to get cured with the money he receives as damages. Yoma 84ª אִיתְּסַאי I got cured. Keth. 62ᵇ איתסיאת she grew well. Koh. R. to I, 8 he went &c. מִיתְאַסְּיָא in order to be cured. Cmp. וֶסֶת.

אָסֵי, אָסְיָא, אָסְיָא, אָסְיָא m. (preced.) *physician, surgeon;* also *thaumaturg,* [*Essene, Therapeut?*] Targ. Ex. XXI, 19; a. e. Y. Yoma III, 40ᵈ bot. חד א׳ וכ׳ a certain thaumaturg in Sepphoris. Y. Taan. III, 66ᵈ אוקיר לאסייך וכ׳ honor thy physician (with presents) ere thou be in need of him. B. Kam. 85ª א׳ רחיקא וכ׳ if the surgeon is far off, the eye will be blind (before he arrives). Num. R. s. 9 תרעא . . . . לא׳ a door which opens not for charity, will be opened for the physician; a. fr. *Pl.* אָסְיָא. Y. Naz. IX, end, 58ª.—אָסַוָותָא, אָסָוָתָא. Targ. Gen. L, 2; a. e. Gitt. 56ᵇ א׳ דמַסְיִין ליה וכ׳ physicians to cure R. Zadok.

אסיא or **אוסיא** a word in a charm formula. Pes. 111ª (Var. lect. v. Rabb. D. S. a. l.)

אַסְיָא, אַסְיָא, עַסְיָא pr. n. *Asia.* 1) *Asia Minor,* or rather the Roman province embracing the Western part of the peninsula of Asia Minor, bequeathed by King Attalus to the Roman republic. Targ. Y. II Gen. X, 3; I Chr. I, 6 (h. text אשכנז). Y. Kidd. I, 61ᵈ top (twice for קני); Gen. R. s. 44 (once for קני, once for קנירי, some ed. אפריה corr. acc.). Y. Meg. I, 71ᵇ bot. (for אשכנז). Sifré Balak 131 (p. 47ᵇ ed. Friedm.) אבריא (corr. acc.); v. Yalk. Num. 771.—B. Mets. 84ª; a. e.—2) name of a town supposed to be *Essa,* east of the lake of Tiberias (v. Neub. Géogr. p. 38; cmp. Rap. Er. Millin s. v.). Y. Kil. IX, 32ᶜ bot. Sabb. 109ª ע׳ (with hot springs). Yeb. XVI, 4 ע׳; Y. ib. 15ᵈ top א׳; a. fr.

אסיאן, v. אוּסְיָא.

אָסְיוּתָא f. (אסי) *cure, recovery.* Targ. Prov. III, 8; a. e.

***אָסֵיט** (v. סיט; cmp. זלל I a. זָלַל) *to be extravagant, squander.* Targ. Prov. XXIII, 20 דְאָסִיטִין וכ׳ (Ms. דְאָסְיטִין, v. infra) who are extravagant in eating meat, v. זלל I.—*Part.* אָסֵיט *extravagant.* Ib. 21.—*Pl.* אָסִיטִין, v. supra.

אסימון Deut. R. s. 7, read אַמְיְינְטוֹן.

***אָסְיָנָא** m. (אסי) *physician.* Y. Sabb. VI, 8ᶜ top אסייניה דר׳ וכ׳ the physician of &c.

אָסִיל, v. אָסֵל.

אָסִימוֹן m. (ἄσημος, -ον) *uncoined metal, bulion.* B. Mets. IV, 1 א׳ קונה וכ׳ the uncoined metal buys the coined, i. e. by delivering the uncoined, which is considered as goods, the purchase is concluded. Ib. 47ᵇ; a. fr.

אָסִינֵי, v. אֲסָנָא.

אַסִּינְתָא, v. אַסְנִיתָא.

***אֲסִינְתָּא** f. (v. אַסְנָא a. חֲסִינָה) *a receptacle for grain.* Keth. 8ª; Ab. Zar. 8ᵇ מכי רמו שערי בא׳ from the time they put barley into the ăsinta (as the first preliminaries of a wedding feast). [Ab. Zar. l. c. read באסינתיה.—Other opin. א׳=אסיתא *mortar,* for pounding barley,—*trough* for brewing beer—*pot* for planting barley for the wedding ceremony, v. Ar. s. v. a. Rashi a. l.]

***אֲסִיסְנָא** m. (redupl. of אסן) *granary, storehouse. Pl.* אֲסִיסְנֵי. Pes. 4ª אכיף ימא א׳ בירואתא on the sea-shore granaries are palaces. [Oth. opin., taking אסיסנא fr. אסס, cmp. אשש, *I would establish* (build) palaces. Oth. opin., reading אסנא or taking our w. to be=אַסְנָא, at the seashore *thorn-bushes* (a thorn-bush) pass(es) for cypresses (a cypress); v. ברותא.] [Gitt. 69ª, v. סִיסְנָא.]

אָסִיף m. (b. h.; אסף) *harvest, crop.*—*Pl.* אֲסִיפִין. Y. Shebi. II, 34ª top, six sowing seasons ושתה א׳ and six crops in one Septennial.

***אֲסִיפָא** m. (=סִיפָּא) *threshold.* B. Kam. 104ᵇ he consummated the transfer of the money (which he authorized him to collect) אגב א׳ דביתיה (Sh'ilt. Ms. סיפא, v. Rashi a. l., v. Rabb. D. S. a. l. note 60) by transferring along with it the threshold of his house (as immovable property); v. אַגַּב. [Oth. vers. סֵיפָא, *end,* extreme wing of the house, v. Rashi a. l.]

אֲסִיפָה f. (b. h. אֲסֵפָה; אסף) 1) *gathering, assembly.* Y. Taan. I, 64ᶜ top אֲסִיפַת עם public meeting for fasting ceremonies. Gen. R. s. 98 ye shall be א׳ אחת one (unanimous) assembly.—2)=אָסִיף. Hag. 18ª חג הבא בזמן א׳ the festival that falls in the harvest season. Ib. א׳ ביו״ט מי שרי Ms. M. (ed. less correct מלאכה) is harvesting permitted &c.?, a. e.—3) (ref. to Num. XI, 22) *the mere taking into the house for consumption,* without the ritual slaughtering (שחיטה). Hull. 27ᵇ. Num. R. s. 19.—4) *being gathered in, death, use of the verb* אסף *with reference to death.* Ib. אֲסִיפַת אהרן the death of Aaron (Num. XX, 24). B. Bath. 16ᵇ גויעה וא׳ the use of גוע a. אסף.

אָסִיר m. (b. h.; אסר) *prisoner.*—*Pl.* אֲסִירִין. Kel. XII, 1 קורות . . . . . של א׳ prisoners' stocks (a metal frame in which the prisoner's feet were shut up).

אָסִיר, אָסִירָא, אֲסִיר m. (אסר) 1) as preced., *imprisoned, prisoner.* Targ. Gen. XL, 3; a. fr.—2) (part. pass. of אֲסַר) *tied, connected.* Fem. אֲסִירָא. Targ. Y. II, Gen. XXV, 1.—3) *forbidden.* Targ. Y. Num. XXV, 6.—*Pl.* אֲסִירִין, אֲסִירֵי, אֲסִירַיָּא; fem. אֲסִירָן. Targ. Gen. XL, 3; 5; a. fr.—Targ. II Sam. III, 34.

אֲסִירָה f. (preced.) *imprisonment.* Gen. R. s. 92 אין כולן בא׳ must not all of them go to prison?

אֲסִיתָא f. (עסי=אסי, עסס; cmp. מְדֹכָה a. דוך) 1) *mortar.* Sabb. 77ᵇ (playful etym.) א׳ חסירתא ed. a. Var. Ar., it is called ásitha because it is caved out (Ms. M. a. Ar. חסידתא pious, submitting to blows). Hull. 105[b] א׳ ובוכנא דתבלי mortar and pestle for spices. Nidd. 36[b] (Issi playing on his name) I am א׳ דנחשא a brazen mortar.— Keth. 49[b] כפו ליה א׳ וכ׳ invert for him a mortar in public (improvise a stand) and let him stand up &c. M. Kat. 22[b] כפי א׳ invert thou a mortar &c.—2) (from its shape) **hip-bone, pelvic bone.** Hull. 52[a] בוכנא וא׳ the pestle and the mortar, i. e. the rib sitting in the hip-bone and the hip-bone.—*3) (cmp. Nidd. l. c.) trnsf. **hard-hearted woman.** Gen. R. s. 17; Lev. R. s. 34 שבוק הדא א׳ Ar. (ed. אנתתא, איתתא בישא; Yalk. Lev. 665; Is. 352 איתתא) divorce that mean woman.

*אַסְכַּדְיָא f. (σχεδία) *raft, float;* cmp. אַסְדָּא. Y. Ber. IV, 8[c] top אסכריא (corr. acc.). Neg. XII, 1 Var.; Naz. 55[a] אסקדיא Mus. (ed. אסקר׳; Tosef. Ohol. XVIII, 5 אכסרא). V. אַכְסַנְדְּרָיָא a. אִסְקָרְיָא.

אִיס׳, אַסְכּוֹלִי f. 1) (σχολή) *school.* Pesik. Bahod. p. 101[b]; Cant. R. to II, 5; Koh. R. to III, 11; Yalk. Ex. 272 (all of which compare to arrive at a corr. text). Ex. R. s. 9. Ib. s. 20, beg.—*Pl.* אַסְכּוֹלִיּוֹת, אִיס׳. Cant. R. to II, 15.—2) (scholæ, sub. palatinæ=scholares, D. C.) *imperial body guard, royal officers.* Deut. R. s. 2 אסכילי פרעה (corr. acc.) Pharaoh's attendants; Cant. R. to VII, 4 אסקולין (corr. acc., or read אַסְכּוֹלָרִין); Midr. Till. to Ps. IV, beg.; Y. Ber. IX, 13[a] אוכלוסין, אוכלסין; Yalk. Ex. 167 איכלוס (corr. acc.).

אַסְכּוֹלַסְטִיקָא, v. אִיס׳.

אַסְכּוּפְּתָא f., pl. אַסְכּוּפָּתָא, v. אִסְקוּפְּתָא. Y. Meg. IV, end, 75[c] א׳ ארעייתא (=אא׳) on the lowest door-sills; Y. Yoma I, 38[c] אסק׳; [the entire passage is obscure].

אסכילי, v. אַסְכּוֹלִי.

אַסְכָּלָה, אַסְכָּלָא f. (סכל, √סך, cmp. Gen. XLVIII, 14) *lattice-work of a fire place, grating, grille.* Pes. VII, 2. Ib. 75[a] א׳ מנוקבת (Ms. M. אי׳) perforated grille (with holes in the upright bars for the spit to turn in, v. Rashi a. l.). Y. Pes. VII, 34[a] bot. צלי אסכלה roasted over the grate.—*Pl.* אַסְכָּלוֹת. Sifré Num. s. 158.—אַסְכָּלָאוֹת. Ab. Zar. 75[b]; Tanh. Hukk. 2.—*Chald. pl.* אַסְכָּלָתָא. Targ. Y. Num. XXXI, 23. Cmp. טַרְטְקַל. [Ἔσχαρα does not correspond in meaning.]

*אִיס׳, אַסְכָּלָא m. pl. (ξύλα,=σκεύη ξύλινα, v. Sm. Ant. s. v. Ships, a var. lect. quoted below) *the wooden implements* of a ship, *oars, ladders, poles* &c. Tosef. B. Bath. IV, 1 he who sells a ship מכר את האיסכ׳ (some ed. איסק׳) sells implicitly the oars &c., (Mish. B. Bath. V, 1 מנהיגין); B. Bath. 73[a] (Rashi אַסְכָּלִין, Ms. M. אסכליא, Ms. R. אסקלה, Ms. O. איסכלניא, read אִיסְכְּלִינָא). [Comm. *ladders*=scalæ.—As to transpos. of כס, cmp. דוכסוסטוס.]

*אַסְכָּמָא (אסכמה) f. (סכם, v. P. Sm. 307 sq. אסכם a. denomin.; an adoption of σχῆμα, -ατος would read אסכימטא) *planning, simulation.* Targ. Prov. VII, 10 (h. text שית); cmp. next w.

אַסְכָּמוּתָא f. (סכם) *consent, agreement.* Targ. Y. Gen. XXXI, 14. Ib. Num. XXXII, 25 בא׳ חדא in one thought; cmp. preced.

אַסְכָּרָה, אַסְכָּרָא f. (סכר; cmp. Ps. LXIII, 12) *choking, croup.* Ber. 8[a]. Taan. 27[b]; a. fr.

אסכריא, v. אַסְכַּדְיָא a. אִסְקָרְיָא.

אֲסֵל, אָסִיל m. (סלל; cmp. Gr. ἄσιλλα) *a pole* or *yoke* carried on two or, more commonly, on one shoulder. Par. VII, 5 וקושרו בא׳ and fastens the bucket to the pole. Kel. XVII, 16 הא׳ שיש בו וכ׳ a carrying yoke in which there is a (hidden) receptacle for money; Koh. R. to IX, 13 אסיל.

אַסְלָא I ch. same. Targ. Y. Num. XIII, 23. Ib. Ex. XXIX, 3.

אַסְלָא II, אַסְלָה, עַסְלָא f. (אסל, עסל, dial. for אצל, נצל, cmp. נִיסֵל) 1) *foot-stool, folding stool.* Sabb. 138[a] מטה וכסא טרסקל וא׳ (Ms. M. ועסלא, Alf. איסקלא, v. Rabb. D. S. a. l. note, v. טְרַסְקַל) couch, folding chair, and foot-stool.—2) *privy, iron frame of a privy-stool* covered with leather. Kel. XXII, 10 הא׳ (Var. in R. S. חסלא); Erub. 10[b] ע׳ ed. (Ar. א׳); Tosef. Kel. B. Bath. I, 4.

אַסְלָא=אַסְלֵי, v. סלי.

אסלמין Y. Ber. V, 9[a] מטיילין בא׳, read אַסְרָטִין or אִגְלֵיסִין; Pesik. R. s. 23—24, p. 122[b] ed. Fr. באנטרי corr. acc.

אַסְלֵי, v. סלי.

אַסְמַכְתָּא f. (סְמַךְ) 1) *support, reliance.* Keth. 67[a] אסמכתייהו אארעא הוא their reliance rests on the landed property.—2) *Scriptural text used as a support for a rabbinical enactment, intimation* (אסמכוה אקרא 'they leaned their enactment against a Bible text'). Hull. 64[b] מדרבנן וקרא א׳ בעלמא it is actually a rabbinical law, and the Bible text (quoted) is a mere support or mnemotechnical aid. Ib. 77[a]; a. fr.—3) (law) *Asmakhta (surety), a promise to submit to a forfeiture of pledged property (or equivalent) without having received a sufficient consideration; collateral security with the condition of forfeiture beyond the amount to be secured;* e. g. A pays a portion of his indebtedness to B, leaving the bill of debt as a security in the hands of a third party, and agreeing to pay *the full amount* on the bill, if, at a stipulated time, he should fail to pay the due balance. B. Bath. 168[a] א׳ לא קניא *asmakhta* does not purchase, gives no title, i. e. gives the claimant no rights (because the law presumes that he who made such a promise, could not have meant it seriously but had in view only to give his transaction the character of good faith and solemnity); ibid. א׳ קניא *asm.* is a valid legal transfer of property. B. Mets. 66[a]; 73[b]. Ned. 27[b]; a. e.—Snh. 24[b] applied to *forfeiture of stake in gambling* (inasmuch as it makes the gambler an immoral person disqualified for witness or judge in court).

אִסְמַרַגְדִין=אִזְמַרַגְדִין.

אוּסְנָא, אִסְנָא m. (אסן=h. חֹסֶן, אָסָם) *store-house, granary.—Pl.* אִסְנַיָּיא. Targ. Joel I, 17 (Var. אוּסְ׳, ח׳).

אַסְּנָא or **אַסְנָא** m. (=h. סְנֶה, v. Ges. H. Dict. s. v.) 1) *thorn-bush, bramble.* Targ. Ex. III, 2; a. e.—Sabb. 67ª א׳ א׳ Ms. M. (ed. הסנה, הסנה) Oh thornbush! Ab. Zar. 28ª גירדא דא׳ parings of the bramble wood.—2) *shrubbery fruit, bramble nut.* Ib.ᵇ קשייתא דא׳ the stones of &c.—*Pl.* אַסְנֵי *a drink* made of shrubbery fruit(?). Pes. 107ª (Ms. M. אַסִינֵי, Ms. M. 2 אַהִינֵי; v. Rabb. D. S. a. l.).

אסנגרין, v. אַכְסִינְרוֹן.

אַסְנִיתָא f.=אַסְּנָא. Sabb. 109ᵇ גורדא דא׳ Ms. M. (ed. אַסְּיַנְתָּא).

אָסְנַפַּר pr. n. m. (prob. identical with Assurbanipal, Schr. K. A. T. p. 376) *Osnappar.* Ezra IV, 10. Snh. 94ª (referred to Sennacherib).

***אָסַס** *to found,* Pes. 4ª, v. אָסִיסְנָא.

אַסְעַר, v. סְעַר.

אָסַף (b. h.; √סף, v. Ges. H. Dict. s. v.; cmp. גרר, a. אגר I) [*to scrape together*], *to gather, harvest.* Snh. III, 3 אוֹסְפֵי שביעית those who harvest the fruits of the Sabbath year (for storage); ib. 26ª אוֹסְפִין (opp. to סוחרין traders in fruits of the Sabbath year).

Nif. נֶאֱסַף 1) *to be gathered; to be taken away* (by death). Num. R. s. 14 (p. 257ᵈ ed. Amst.) והם נֶאֱסָפִים לְשָׁמְעוֹ and they (the people) gather themselves to hear him. Ib. (p. 258ª) בזמן שבעליהם נאספים מהם after their teachers have been taken away from them (when they are dead); Pesik. R. s. 3; Yalk. Koh. to XII, 11; Tanh. B'haăl., 15; a. e.—2) *to be picked up.* Kidd. IV, 1; v. אֲסוּפִי.

Hif. הֶאֱסִיף, mostly הוֹסִיף, v. יָסַף.

אֲסַף ch. same. Y. Keth. V, 30ᵇ top לא מסתברא דלא כאספין וכ׳ (read כאספין) it would be unreasonable not to consider students like harvesters, for they work (even) harder.

אִסְפְּגִין f., v. אִסְפּוּגִית.

***אִסְפְּדִיכָא** m. (Pers. *ispid-ab*; Arab *ispidağ*, Perl. Et. St. p. 48) *white-lead.* Gitt. 69ª אלוא וא׳ Ar. (ed. אספירכא) aloes and white lead.

אִסְפּוּג, אִי׳ m. (ספג, v. סְפוֹג) *sponge-cake, spungy bread.* Targ. O. Ex. XXIX, 23; a. e.—*Pl.* אִסְפּוּגִין. Ib. 2; a. e. (Editions also אֶסְפּוֹג׳).

אִסְפּוּגִית f. h. same. Sabb. 78ᵇ Ms. M. (ed. אִסְפְּגִין, pl., sub. עוּגוֹת).

אספוטמיא, v. אִסְפַּמְיָא 2).

אספון, v. אָסַף.

אספוסין, v. אַפּוֹפְסִין.

אֶסְפּוֹר m. (=h. סַפִּיר) [the glistening] *sapphire.* Targ. Cant. V, 14.

***אִסְפּוּרַק** pr. n. pl. *Isporak.* B. Kam. 94ª top רמן א׳ Ms. M. (ed. דמא׳, Ms. R. דמאיס׳) who came from I.

אִסְפַּטִּי, v. אִסְפַּתִּי.

אספטיא, אספטיה, v. אִיסְפּוֹלִיטַיָּיא.

אַסְפִּי *to feed,* Af. of ספי q. v. B. Bath. 21ª.

אספינדמון, v. אִיסְפֶּנְדְּמָנוֹס.

***אִי׳, אִסְפַּנְקִי, אִסְפְּנִיקִי, אִסְפִּינְקִי** f. (Ispe. noun of פנק) *the free-man's* armor (for h. חֲגוֹר, חֲגוֹרָה q. v.). Targ. II Sam. XVIII, 11; a. e. [Syr. אספניקא, אספנקא *rubro colore tinctus,* P. Sm. 313.]

אִסְפִּיקוּלָא, v. סְפִיקוּלָא.

אספיר, v. אספר.

אספירכא, v. אִסְפְּדִיכָא.

***אִסְפִּירַס** m. (Ispe. noun of פרס, cmp. פַּרְסָה) *the front part of the foot* (where it is split). Num. R. s. 4 הופך א׳ וכ׳ he turned the front of his foot (put his foot on tip-toe) and danced.

***אִסְפְּלִיאָה** f. (Isp. noun of פלא) *solemn declaration.—Pl.* אִסְפְּלִיאוֹת. Deut. R. s. 7, beg. אמן יש בו ג׳ א׳ וכ׳ *Amen* contains three kinds of solemn declarations, oath (vow), consent, and confirmation; v. Shebu. 36ª. V. הַפְלָאָה.

אִיסְ׳, אִסְפְּלִידָא m. (Ispe. noun of פלד; Arab. פלד, *to cut,* v. Ges. H. Dict. s. v.; cmp. פרד); *a cut-off place, recess,* whence 1) *cave, cleft.* Targ. Y. Ex. XXXIII, 22 (h. text נקרה). Targ. Ps. LVII, 1 (ed. אוס׳).—2)=*exedra* (v. אַכְסַדְרָא), *recess in the house, sitting room in the shape of an open hall,* generally supported by columns. B. Bath. 7ª חד מטייה א׳ one of the heirs received a hall as his share. Ib. קא בני...... דא׳ the other built a wall in front of the hall (debarring light and air). Esth. R. to I, 9 בית א׳ *reception rooms.—Pl.* אִסְפְּלִידֵי. Men. 33ᵇ א׳ דאית להו וכ׳ halls supported by columns.

אספלימון, v. אִסְפְּרִיטִין.

אִסְפְּלָנִי=אִסְפְּלָנִיתָא.

אספלניס, v. next w.

***אִי׳, אִסְפְּלָנִית** f. (=אִסְבְּלָנִית or אִסְפַּלְעָנִית, Ispe. noun of בלע or בלי; cmp. בְּלִיתָא, a. סִיפְלְנִי; פ dialect. for ב, induced by preceding sibilant) *rag, plaster, compress* (for softening or healing). Sabb. IX, 2 (expl. ib. 133ᵇ seven portions of fat and one portion of wax). Y. Orl. III, beg. 62ᵈ העושה א׳ וכ׳ he who makes a plaster of the [illegible] Y. Sabb. VII, 10ᵈ top הממרח את הא׳ he who spreads a plaster. Tosef. ib. I, 23; a. fr.—Pesik. R. s. 44 איספלנים (corr. acc.). [Σπληνίον, in Hippocr., seems to be a Greek adaptation of our w.]

אִסְפַּלְנִיתָא, אִיס׳ ch. same. Targ. Job XXX, 24 Ms. (ed. אִסְפְּלְעִיתָא, v. preced.); Var. אַסְכָא.—Sabb. 133ᵇ א׳ דכולהון כיבי וכ׳ a salve for all pains is seven portions of &c., v. preced.—

אִסְפַּמְיָא, אִיס׳ pr. n. (=סְפַּמְיָא, or סִיםְ־מִיא) 1) (prob. of Phœn. origin) *Hispania, Spain.* Nidd. 30ᵇ B. Bath. III, 2 כדי שיהיה בא׳ וכ׳ long enough for the owner to be in Spain, while the present occupant may occupy his property for one year, and for people to travel a year and notify him, and for him to come back the next year (and raise his claim). Ber. 62ᵃ. Yeb. 63ᵃ.—2) (=אַפַּמְיָא q. v.) Apamæa, several towns, esp. one each in Bithynia, Mesopotamia and Syria. Y. Shebi. VI, beg. 36ᵃ (h. קְנוּד); Gen.R.s. 44, end; a. fr.—Gen. R. s. 60, beg. מא׳ ומחבירותיה from Ap. and her sisters (country towns) (in Babylon or Mesopotamia); ib. s. 30 מאספוטמיא; s. 44 ממספ׳ (corr. acc.)—[Targ. Ob. v. 20 Ar. (ed. ספמיא)]. [B. Bath. 74ᵇ פמייס=ימה של א׳ as Ms. M.] V. אִסְפַּנְיָא.

אִסְפָּנִי m. (v. next w.) *Spaniard.—Pl* אִסְפָּנִין. Makhsh. VI, 3 קוליס הא׳ the colias of the Spaniards, a species of thuny-fish (prob. to be read ק׳ הִיסְפָּנִי).

אִסְפַּנְיָא, אִיס׳ pr. n. pl. *Hispania, Spain.* Tanh. Vayetsé, 2 מגליא ומא׳ from Gaul, Spain &s.; cmp. Lev. R. s. 29; Yalk. Jer. 312, a. e. אספמיא.—Pesik. R. s. 32 (p. 56ᵃ ed. Pr.) באספנים (corr. acc.; ed. Fr. s. 31, p. 147ᵃ אספמ׳).—V. אִסְפַּמְיָא.

אספניא, אספנייא Snh. 21ᵇ, v. אַפְּסַנְיָא.

אִסְפַּנְקִי, אִסְפַּנִיקִי, v. אִסְפִּירְנְקִי.

אִסְפַּסְיָנוּס, אִסְפַּסְיָאנוּס pr. n. m. *Vespasian*, the Roman Emperor who, when general, conducted the war against the Jews which ended in the destruction of the Temple. Targ. Lam. I, 19.—Sot. IX, 14 פולמוס של א׳ the Vespasian war. Y. Meg. III, 73ᵈ; Lam. R. introd. (R. Han. 1); a. fr. [Meg. 11ᵃ ושמואל אמר ... נבוכדנצר, read with Ms. M. a. old prints א׳ קיסר.]

אִסְפַּסְיָאנִי (genit. of Vespasianus) *Vespasian's* (followers). Lam. R. to I, 17.

אִסְפַּסְיָנוּס, אִסְפַּסְיָינוּס, v. אִסְפַּסְיָאנוּס.

***אַסְפַּסְתָּא** f. (reduplic. of סְפַס, v. סְפַי; cmp. b. h. מִסְפּוֹא) 1) *fodder for cattle.* Targ. Y. Gen. XXIV, 25; a. fr.—2) (in Talm. Bab.) *any plant especially adapted for fodder, grass* (Pers. *ifsist, clover*, prob. an adaptation of our w.; v. Snh. 93ᵃ: 'to import בזרא דא׳ *aspasta*-seed'; Yalk. Dan. 1060 מא׳, corr. acc.). Yeb. 121ᵇ קטול א׳ cut grass. B. Kam. 20ᵃ; Ab. Zar. 28ᵇ פתילה דא׳ long stalks of asp.— Ib. משחא דא׳ (Ms. a. old ed. דאפרסמא). B. Bath. 28ᵇ.

אספסתורין, v. אִסְפִּתְרִי.

אספקטי, v. אִסְפָּתִי.

אִסְפַּקְלַטוּרָא, אִסְפַּקְלַטוֹר, v. אִיס׳.

אִסְפַּקְלַרְיָא, אִיס׳ f. (specularia) 1) *window-pane made of lapis specularis, window-glass.* Targ. Y. Ex. XIX, 17; a. e.—Kel. XXX, 2 תמחוי שעשאו א׳ a (glass) plate which is used as window-glass.—2) Metaph. *prophetic vision.* Succ. 45ᵇ דמסתכלי בא׳ וכ׳ who contemplate (Deity) through a lucid speculum. Gen. R. s. 91 שראה בא׳ שסברו וכ׳ (play on *sheber, grain*, and *seber, hope*) he saw in the glass of prophecy that his hope (Joseph) was in Egypt. Lev. R. s. 1 א׳ מלוכלכת a dim glass (vision); opp. א׳ מצוחצחת polished glass (clear vision).—*Pl.* אִסְפַּקְלַרְיָאוֹת. Ib.; Yalk. Lev. 432 אִיסְפַּקְלַרְיוֹת.

אספקרפסמי, read אִסְקִיפַּסְטֵי, v. אִסְקְפַּסְטֵי.

***אספר (ספיר)**, Snh. 106ᵃ (וצים מיד כתים) אמר רב ליבון א׳ ed. [missing in Ms. M. and added on margin; Ar. ed. pr. a. ed. Koh. לבין א׳; Yalk. Num. 771 לא לגיון א׳] pr. n. m. (Λέων Ἴσαυρος, Leo Isaurus) *Leo the Isaurian*, Byzantine emperor, leader of the iconoclastic movement which caused a long-continued war between the East and the West of the empire. [The words above quoted are an interpolation of the eighth or ninth century, and refer to "the war between the lion and the lioness"—words immediately preceding our quotation. The interrupted context in Rashi a. l. shows that the commentary to our ws. is also a later addition and that in Rashi's Talmud text there was no such interpolation. As to the impression on the Jews of the iconoclastic agitation, v. Sachs Beitr. I, p. 78. For Var. Lect. v. Rabb. D. S. a. l. and Koh. Ar. s. v.]

אִסְפָּר m. (ספר, cmp. אִסְפּוֹר) *Espar*, a Hebrew name for *Sestertius* (cmp. אִיסָר &c.). *Pl.* const. אִסְפְּרֵי. Maas. Sh. II, 9 (Ms. M. אצטרי, v. אִיסְתְּרָא, Asheri אצפרי); Eduy. I, 10 (he must exchange the fourth Denar) ארבעה א׳ כסף Ms. M. (ed. ארבע) for four sestertii. [Oth. opinions (v. comment.), ἄσπροι, supposed to be worth one fifth of a Denar. There is, however, no evidence of ἄσπροι being used in this sense in the days of the Mishnah.]

אִסְפַּרְגַּל, v. אִיס׳.

***אִסְפַּרְוָוא, אִסְפַּרְוָוה, אִיס׳** collect. n. (prob. a contraction of *explorator viæ*) *forerunner, the commander's van-guard.* Keth. 3ᵇ (Tossaf. take it as singular). V., however, אַפְרְוָורִין.

***אַסְפְּרוֹן** m. (ἄσπρος, ον) *white*, opp. מוורין (μαυρός) *black.* Gen. R. s. 7 מו׳ וחד א׳ Ar. (ed. מיירין) a white fish and a black fish; (Yalk. Gen. 12 חיוור a. אוכם; Y. Kil. I, 27ᵃ bot. לכיסא a. ירוקא).

***אִסְפְּלִימִין, אִסְפְּרִימִין** m. pl. (Ispe. noun of פרט or פלט, v. H. Dict. s. vv.) *separate threads, hangings, fine fringes.* Lev. R. s. 17. Yalk. Ps. 808 איספרטין.

***אִסְפְּרִיסָא** m. (פרס; cmp. אִסְפְּרָס) *that which is to be split, log* (h. בקעת). Lam. R. to III, 12 כבורמא לא׳ (referr. to חץ *arrow*, taken in the sense of חצץ *to split*) as a wedge for the log, i. e. the wedge (Israel) is struck but the log (the hostile nations) is split.

אספרלג, v. אִיסְפַּרְגַּל.

אִסְפַּרְמְקֵי, אִי׳ (אספרקמי) m. pl. (v. Löw Aram. Pfl. p. 152) *smelling herbs, scent-box.* Bets. 36ᵇ בא׳ וכ׳ (ed. בי א׳) in the scent-box of R. A.; Sabb. 121ᵇ בא׳ (Var. באר׳). Men. 43ᵇ אספרקמי ed.

***אָסְפַּרְנָא** (√ פר to *run*, cmp. אַדְרַזְדָּא) *quickly, diligently.* Ezra V, 8; a. e.

אספרקמי, v. אִסְפַּרְמְקֵי.

אַסְפִּתֵּי=אֶצְבְּתֵי q. v. Ohol. XIII, 4.

אִסְפָּטֵי, אִסְפָּתֵי f. (σπάθη, spatha, spata D. C.) *broad sword,* esp. *the executioner's sword.* Pesik. B'shall. p. 81ᵇ באספטר וכ׳ Ar. (ed. איספטר; Yalk. Is. 302 beg. אספקטר; corr. acc.) with the sword with which the Egyptians struck, were they struck.—*Pl.* אִסְפָּתִין. Ex. R. s. 15 עשו א׳ prepare ye the swords; v. ספיקולא.

אִסְפַּתְרֵי m. (σπαθάριος, v. preced.) *carrier of broad sword, one of the imperial body-guard* for which tall men would be selected. Cant. R. to II, 15 אספסהורין (corr. acc.).—*Pl.* אִסְפַּתְרִין. Ib. a province (or city) מגדלת א׳ למלך was rearing spatharii for the king. [Gen. R. s. 65 ענקמון.]

אסקדיא, v. אִסְכַּדְיָא.

אִסְקוּטְלָא I, אִיתְקוּטְלָא m. (Isp. or Ithpe. of קוטל=גודל *thumb*) *snapping with thumb and middle finger, flipping.* Taan. 25ᵃ מחיין לי בא׳ אאפותי Ar. (ed. . . . נרך אפו׳; Ms. M. אאפותאי) he stirred me up by snapping on my forehead.—*Pl.* אִסְקוּטְלֵי. Ab. Zar. 28ᵃ מחויה שתין אס׳ Ar. (ed. אית׳) snap thereon (on the swelling) sixty times.

אִסְקוּטְלָא II f. (scutella, σκοῦτλον) *a salver* or *waiter of nearly square form.* Kel. XXX, 1. M. Kat. III, 7.

אסקולין, v. אִסְכּוּלֵי.

אסקולסטיקא read אִיסְכּוֹ׳.

אִסְקוּנְדְּרֵי, v. אִיס׳.

אִסְקוּפָא, v. אִסְקוּפְתָּא.

אִסְקוּפָּה, אִי׳ f. (סקף, cmp. b. h. מַשְׁקוֹף a. זקף) *cross-piece;* 1) *yard* of a ship. Tosef. B. Bath. IV, 1 ed. Zuck. (Var. אִיזְקָפָה); Y. ib. V, beg. 15ᵃ in selling a vessel one has not implicitly sold את הא׳ the yard (because it is taken down when on land; v. Sm. Ant. s. v. Antenna). Midr. Till. to Ps. CIII (the embryo in the womb) כאדם שנתון באסקופת וכ׳ (some ed. בספינה, read בְּאִסְקוּפַּת הספינה) like a person seated on the yard on open Sea.—2) *lintel, threshold,* gen. *lower door-sill.* Sabb. 6ᵃ; a. fr.; cmp. Y. Ber. V, 37ᵃ, expl. סַף. Y. Snh. VI, 23ᵇ bot. עשה אותי (כא׳) make me the threshold for the Law to pass over me; i. e. let the law have its course at the expense of my life; Yalk. Ps. 688 עשה אסקיפא (corr. acc.).

אסקופת, v. preced.

אִסְקוּפְתָּא, אִסְקוּפָּא, אִיס׳ ch. 1) as preced. 2. Targ. Y. Ex. XII, 22; a. e. (O. שקפא).—*Pl.* אִסְקוּפְתָּא. Targ. Prov. VIII, 34.—Y. Yoma I, 38ᶜ, v. אִסְכּוּפְתָּא. Yoma 53ᵃ מיתווסן א׳ וכ׳ the thresholds . . . . were stained with blood.—אסקופין (better אִסְקוּפָּן). Y. Ab. Zar. III, 42ᶜ top שובעין א׳ . . . seventy door frames were upset.—2) *meat hanging on a crosspiece.* Y. Shek. VII. 50ᶜ bot., ed. Bab. to VII, 4 משוגא (not משיגא) . . . תַּיִרָה to wash his meat in the river; Y. Ab. Zar. II, 41ᵈ bot. תח . . ., read תירה . . .

אַסְקוּתָא f. (נסק) 1) *burning.* Targ. Y. Gen. I, 29.—2) *offering.* Targ. II Chr. XXX, 14; a. e.

אסקלה, v. אִסְכָּלָא.

אִסְקָפָא or **אִסְקָפִי** f. (σκάφη, scapha) *light boat, skiff.* *Pl.* אִסְקָפָאוֹת. Tosef. Succ. III, 12 איספק׳, ed. Zuck. (ed. אספק׳, corr. acc.).

אסקפטי, אסקפי, v. next w.

אִסְקַפַּסְטִי, סְקִיפַּסְטִי f. (σκεπαστή, sub. ἅμαξα, σκεπαστόν=καμάρα; v. Poll. X, 52, Sachs Beitr. I, 171) *tilted wagon, litter with canopy.* Midr. Till. to Ps. 3 אוסקופי, אסקפי (corr. acc.; read מהלכת). Pesik. Bahod. p. 103ᵃ סקיפס׳ Ar. (ed. סקופוטי, corr. acc.). Koh. R. beg. איסקרפסטי (corr. acc.).—*Pl.* סְקִיפַּסְטִיּוֹת, אִסְקַפַּסְטֵיאוֹת &c. Ruth R. to I, 19; Lam. R. to I, 3 אסקפטיות ed. (Ar. סקיפטיות, corr. acc.). Num. R. s. 12 כמנסקי פסקאות, read כמין סקיפסט׳; Yalk. Num. 713 (corr. acc.). [Lev. R. s. 14 בתוך מעיה כמין סקיפסטי Ar., ed. only בתוך מעיה, v. Midr. Till. to Ps. CIII, s. v. אִסְקוּפָּה.]

אִסְקְרָא m., pl. אִסְקְרִין (זקר=סקר) [*the hopper,*] *iskra,* name of a species of locusts born without legs. Hull. 65ᵃ Ar. a. Rashi sing., ed. pl.; Yalk. Lev. 537 (corr. acc.). V. זָחַל.

אִסְקַרְיָא, אִיס׳ f. (סקר *to espy*=b. h. הֵרֶן fr. תור) prop. *espying place,* hence *mast* or rather *yard* (where the captain sits for looking out; cmp. תּוּרְנָא). B. Bath. 73ᵃ, explain. *toren;* v. supra. Taan. 21ᵃ נפילנא מא׳ I would throw myself (into the water) from the sail yard. B. Mets. 69ᵇ. Keth. 69ᵇ א׳ דמכותא mast-yard; Taan. 21ᵃ (v. Rabb. D. S. a. l. note 300).—Neg. XII, 1; Naz. 55ᵃ, v. אִסְכַּדְיָא.

אִסְקְרִיטְוָן f. pl. ch. 1)=next w. Targ. O. Ex. XVI, 31.—*2) read מִקְסוֹטֵירִין (μυξωτῆρες; as LXX Zach. IV, 12) *tubes, lamp-nozzles.* Targ. Zach. l. c.

אסקריטי, v. next w.

אִסְקְרִיטִין, אִי׳ m. pl. (Ispe. noun of קרט; cmp. חֲלַטI a. denom.) *balls; a kind of paste.* Mekh. B'shall Vayas. 5 כעין אסקריטי (read . . . . טין). Hall. I, 4; Pes. 37ᵃ Y. Hall. III, 57ᵈ bot. אי׳ חליטין דשוק isk'ritin are &c., v. חֲלִיטָא III.

אָסַר (b. h.; sec. r. of סור) *to surround, enclose* (v. Schr. KAT Gloss. II, s. v.)—whence 1) *to chain, imprison; to sentence to prison.* Ber. 28ᵇ, v. אֵיסוּר.—2) *to harness, put the horses to.* Mekh. B'shall. 1. Gen. R. s. 55, v. אֲסָרָה.—3) *to bind, obligate.* Lev. R. s. 23 אילולי שא׳ וכ׳ had not the Lord bound himself by an oath; a. e.—4) *to interdict, to declare a thing forbidden according to ritual law,* opp. הִתִּיר to loosen the tie, to allow. Ḥag. 3ᵇ הללו אוֹסְרִין והללו מתירין the ones declare forbidden what the others allow. Lev. R. s. 22 מה שֶׁאָסַרְתִּי לך התרתי לך of whatever I have forbidden thee (as a class) I have allowed thee (a specimen). Erub. VIII, 4 אוֹסֵר עליו he (by residing there) restricts the other (debarring him from carrying things around on the Sabbath).—Part. pass. אָסוּר, f. אֲסוּרָה (*it is*) *forbidden.* Ber. 35ᵃ א׳ לו לאדם ש׳ וכ׳ one must not &c.; a. v. fr.—*Pl.* אֲסוּרִים, אֲסוּרִין; f. אֲסוּרוֹת. Ter. X, 12; a. v. fr. V. אָסוּר.

Nif. נֶאֱסַר *to be forbidden, to become subject to ritual prohibition.* Ib. 11 אוֹסֶרֶת ואינה נֶאֱסֶרֶת affects other things which come in contact with it, but is not affected; a. fr.

אֲסַר, אָסַר ch. same; 1) *to chain, imprison.* Targ. II Kings XVII, 4; a. fr.—2) *to bind by spell, charm.* Targ. Ps. LVIII, 6; a. e.—3) *to tie up, put on* &c. Targ. Y. Gen. XLIX, 11; a. e.—B. Mets. 86ᵇ דקא א׳ ושרי that he tied up (his wound) and untied it. Sabb. 81ᵇ אֲסַרְתָּהּ לארבא she tied (stopped) the ship (by magic spell).—4) *to bind the bowels, check diarrhœa.* Gitt. 69ᵇ לְמֵיסַר.—5) *to forbid.* Ḥull. 109ᵇ כל דא׳ לן וכ׳, v. preced.; a. v. fr. Ib. 111ᵇ; 112ᵃ, a. fr. אָסִיר, אֲסִירֵי *it is, they are, forbidden.*—Ab. Zar. 37ᵇ יוסף אָסְרָא מיבעי ליה he ought to be called, 'Joseph the forbidder.'—Y. Meg. I, 70ᶜ bot. לְוּסַר לפניו to forbid fasting on the day preceding.—6) **to bind one's self by vowing a fast* (cmp. Num. XXX, 3), or *to be bound.* Meg. Taan. XII, end, quoted and discussed Taan. 12ᵃ (v. Var. lect. in Rabb. D. S. a. l. a. notes).

Pa. אַסַּר *to tie* (sheaves). Targ. O. Gen. XXXVII, 7.

Ithpa. אִתְאַסַּר 1) *to be imprisoned.* Targ. Gen. XLII, 19; a. e.—2) (in Talm.) *Ithpe.* אִיתְּסַר *to be forbidden.* Targ. Y. Num. XI, 10.—Ḥull. 101ᵇ ליתסר let it be forbidden. Ib. 115ᵃ מעשה שבת ליתסרו what has been prepared on the Sabbath ought to be forbidden. Yeb. 33ᵃ קא מיתסר במלאכה he is forbidden from doing labor; a. fr.

אֵסָר, v. אִיסָר.

אֱסָר, אִסְרָא, v. אִיסְרָא, אֵיסַר I.

אָסְרָא m. *one who forbids,* v. אֲסַר.

אַסְרַדְיוֹט, א׳ m.=אִסְטְרַטְיוֹט (cmp. stradiot, D. C. s. v. στρατιώτης) *Roman officer.* Koh. R. to XI, 1, V. סְרַדְיוֹט.

אֲסָרָה f. (אסר) *the act of tying* (the horses), *harnessing* (the chariot). Gen. R. s. 55 תבא א׳ שאסר וכ׳ the harnessing which Joseph did himself (in honor of his father, Gen. XLVI, 29) will stand against the harnessing by Pharaoh (to pursue the Israelites, Ex. XIV, 6); i. e. the merits of Joseph's filial love will protect Israel from the hostility of Pharaoh.

אִסְרוּתָא, v. אִיסְרָא I, 2.

אִסְרַטָא, א׳ m.=אִסְטְרָטָא, *road.* Targ., v. אִסְטְ׳.—Y. Shek. VII, 50ᶜ bot. א׳ דגופתא (in Bab. ed. אירסקא דגדפתה corr. acc.). Y. M. Kat. I, 64ᵇ bot.; a. e. (interchanging with אסט׳).—*Pl.* אִסְרָטִין *promenade,* v. אִסְטְ׳. Y. Taan. IV, 68ᵃ bot. Y. Yeb. XII, 12ᵈ top אִסְרָטָן (?). [אִסְרָטִין *troops,* v. אִיסְ׳.]

אִסְרָטָה, same, v. אִיסְ׳.

אִסְרַטְיָא, אִיסְ׳ I f.=אִסְטְרַטְיָא I, *camp, station.* Y. Shek. VII, 50ᶜ bot.

אִסְרַטְיָא, אִיסְ׳ II f. *army, list of officers,* v. אִסְטְרַטְיָא II.

אסרטיגי, v. אִסְטְרָטִיגוֹס.

אִסְרַטְיוֹט, אִיסְ׳ m.=אִסְטְרַטְיוֹט.—*Pl.* אִסְרַטְיוֹטוֹת. Y. Pes. VIII, end, 36ᵇ א׳ היו שומרין וכ׳ (Roman) soldiers were guarding the doors of the Temple in Jerus., and they bathed (as the ceremony of admission into Judaism), and on the same evening partook of the Passover meal. [Tosef. ib. VII, 13, אירצטרדיות ed. Zuck., Var. אצטדריוטות, שתרדיו׳.]

אסרטיון, v. אִיסְרָטִין.

אסרטילוס, אסרטילטא, v. אִסְטְרָטִילָבָא.

אִסְרָטִין, v. אִסְרָטָא a. אִיסְרָטִין.

אִסְרְתָּא, v. אִיסְרָא I, 2.

***אִסְתַּגַּר** (Ithpa. of סגר) *to be locked up, engrossed with,* [Rashi: *to be bewildered, silenced, not knowing what to say*]. B. Kam. 40ᵃ שבקן אסתגרי בקמייתא Ms. F., leave us alone, I am yet engaged in the first question (Rashi: I am not yet ready to answer &c.). [Editions a. Mss. אסתגר, prob. אִסְתַּגִּיר. Ar. אסתניד *I am sick* (?).]

אִסְתְּדִירָא, v. אִיסְטְרִידָא.

אִסְתַּהַר m. (Ithpe. noun of סהר) [*the bright,*] *Venus.* Targ. Job XXXI, 26 (h. text אור, cmp. ibid. ירח=סהרא).—Meg. 13ᵃ why was Hădassa called Esther? או״ה קורין אותה א׳ Ms. M. (ed. על שום א׳) the Gentiles called her *Ist'har* (Esther), (ed. ... after Ist'har); Yalk. Esth. 1053 .... קורין אותה כוכב הנוגה על שם אסתהר called her Venus corresponding to Ist'har. [Cmp. ištar=עַשְׁתֹּרֶת, Schrader KAT 176 sq.] V. אִיסְתְּהִירָא.

אִסְתְּוָרָא, אִסְתְּוִירָא, אִסְתְּוּוּרָא, v. אִיסְ׳.

אִסְתּוֹמְכָא, אִי׳ (אסטומכא) m. (Ithpe. noun of סמך; cmp. סוּבְּכָא) *the thick part,* or *the protection of an organ of the body, muscle, cartilage* &c. Ḥull. 50ᵇ (explaining 'the inner stomach') א׳ דכרסא (Ar. אסט׳) the thick portion of the rumen (?). Ab. Zar. 29ᵃ א׳ דליבא the protector of the heart (or of the stomach), *the cartilago ensiformis, xiphoides,* v. אוּנְקְלִי I, 3; (other opinion rejected in Rashi: *fleshy walls of the heart*).

*אִסְתּוּנְיָא pr. n. pl. *Istunia*, a place near Pumb'ditha, perh. identic with וסתניא q. v. Keth. 111ᵃ.

אסתיוט, v. סוּט.

אִסְתִּירָא, v. אִיס׳.

אסתלגנית, אסתלגיגית, v. אִיסְטַגְלִילִית.

*אִסְתְּלִיתָא=אִסְטְלִית, אִסְטְלָא. Targ. Y. II Deut. XXIV, 13.

אִסְתָּן h., **אִסְתָּנָא, אִיס׳** ch. m. (Ithp. of סן, v. סנן a. שנן) *the clear* or *cold wind*, hence *north-wind, North.* Keth. 23ᵃ; Kidd. 12ᵇ עדים בצד אסתן the witnesses are in the North (Babylon; v. Tosaf. ib. a. v. אורייא).—Targ. Job XXXVII, 22 Ms. (ed. אִסְתְּנָיָא; h. text זהב).—Ber. 59ᵃ אתא אסתנא וכ׳ (Ms. אי׳) the northwind comes and clears the sky. Erub. 65ᵃ a Talmudic decision must be as clear כיומא דא׳ as a northwind day; Meg. 28ᵇ. Sabb. 116ᵇ. Cmp. טִיהֲרָא.

אִסְתַּנְדְּרָא, v. אִסְטַ׳.

אִסְתַּנְיָא, v. אִסְתָּן.

אסתניד, v. אִסְתַּגַּר.

אִסְתְּנִיס, v. אִיסְתְּ׳.

אִסְתַּפְּנִינֵי, v. אִיסְטַ׳.

אסתקמון Ar. for אִסְטַבְּמוֹן.

*אִסְתַּקַּר (Ithpa. of סקר) *to look around.* Keth. 62ᵇ חזיתיה א׳ Ar. (ed. סיי לבה) she saw him looking around in her room (not knowing that a stranger had entered).

אֶסְתֵּר (b. h.) pr. n. f. *Esther*, wife of king Ahasverus. Ex. R. s. 15 ובאה א׳ והאירה and Esther (*bright star*, v. אִסְתְּהַר) came and brought light. Meg. 13ᵃ; a. fr.—מגילת א׳, or only א׳, *the Book of Esther.* Snh. 100ᵃ. Meg. 7ᵃ, a. e. (controversy as to its canonic character).

אסתרולוגיאה, v. אַסְטְרוֹ׳.

אִסְתְּרוֹקָנִית, אִיס׳ f. (Ithp. of סרק) מלח א׳ *desert-salt, fossil salt*, contrad. to מלח סדומית sea-salt. B. Bath. 20ᵇ (Ms. Oxf. אסט׳). Bets. 39ᵃ (Ms. M. אסקלידנית prob. from confounding with סלקונדרית). Men 21ᵃ.

אסתרטיגא, v. אִסְטְרַטֵּיגוֹס.

אָע, אָעָא m. ch. (h. עֵץ) *wood, woods;* also *wooden handle.* Ezra V, 8; a. e.—Targ. O. Lev. XIV, 4; a. e. Y. Sabb. VII, 10ᶜ top, v. אֲלִיקָה.—*Pl.* אָעִין. Targ. Josh. IX, 21; a. e.—Y. Pes. IV, 30ᵈ top.—*Hebr. pl.* אָעִים, *beams.* Y. Erub. I, 19ᶜ; Y. Succ. I, 52ᵃ.

אַעְיָתָא f. pl. (v. preced.) *laths* of a latticed window. Targ. Jud. V, 28 (h. אשנב).

אעל, Y. Sabb. VII, 10ᶜ top, v. אליקה.

אָעֵן, אָעָן=צָאן. Targ. I Sam. XXV, 18.

אַעְרָעָא m. (ערע) *occurrence, adversity.*—*Pl.* אַעְרָעָן. Targ. Ps. XXXIV, 20 Ms.; v. אַרְעָא.

אַף I (b. h.; אפה, cmp. גַּם) *also, too.* Keth. 6ᵇ; a. fr. אַף הוא *the same.* Aboth II, 6.—אַף על פי (abbr. אע״פ) prop. *even following the dictation of;* אַף על גב (abbr. אע״ג) prop. *even on the top of,=notwithstanding, although* (the former mostly in Mishnah, the latter in Gemara). Keth. V, 1 אע״פ שאמרו וכ׳ although the Rabbis have said; a. fr.—Meg. 3ᵃ אע״ג דאיהו לא חזא although he does not see it; a. v. fr.—אַף על פי כן *nevertheless.* Snh. 98ᵃ; a. fr.—*Chald.* same. Targ. O. Num. XVI, 13; a. e. V. אוּף.

אַף II m. (b. h.; v. אָנַף) prop. *breath*, hence 1) *nose.* Midr. Till. to Ps. XVIII, 5 (interpret. *ăfafuni*, ib.) הגיעו הצרות עד א׳ the troubles have risen up to the nose. —2) *panting, anger.*—Du. אַפַּיִם. Y. Taan. II, 65ᵇ bot. ארך אַף ..... ארך אפים וכ׳, it does not read (Jonah IV, 2), Slow of *anger* but of *angers*, which means that He is long suffering both to the righteous and the wicked; a. fr.—3) pr. n. m. *Af*, allegorical name of the angel administering justice. Ex. R. s. 41 end; s. 44; Deut. R. s. 3. —*4) *overheated condition, wearines.* Maksh. III, 8 בשעת האַף when the animal is overheated, Var. יַחַף q. v.

אַף III m. (b. h.; אפף), only in du. אַפַּיִם *face* (*cheeks*).

אַפָּא I ch. c. same; 1) *face, presence.* Targ. Ez. I, 6; a. e.; v. אַנְפָּא.—Gen. R. s. 35, beg. למיחזי סבר אַפַּאי to see my countenance. Ib. s. 87 it is right הדין אַפָּה כסי that the face of this (idol) is covered.—M. Kat. 20ᵇ באַפָּה in her presence, בלא א׳ in her absence.—Transf. *front.* Hull. 47ᵃ אפה וכ׳ the front (of the lungs) facing the examiner.—With -לְ, *towards, opposite.* Snh. 72ᵃ קאי לאפאי he places himself opposite me (for defence). Pes. 111ᵇ לאפיה דשמאליה (Ms. M. לחדיה ש׳) towards, by his left side.— *Pl.* אַפִּין, אַפַּיָא, *face* (b. h. אפים, פנים). Targ. Ez. I, 6; a. fr.— Pesik. R. s. 21 א׳ בא׳ face to face. Cant. R. to III, 11 the angel has חמש א׳ five faces. Lam. R. to V, 5 בשחור א׳ in darkness of countenance, in sadness. Y. B. Mets. IV, 9ᶜ bot ולא אמרין לה לכל א׳ but one must not say so in the presence of all (publicly).—2) (only in pl.) *modes, ways.* Targ. Cant. I, 11.—Ned. 41ᵃ אַפֵּי הלכתא methods of talmudical disquisitions. Lam. R. to II, 2 שיתין א׳ sixty ways of interpretation. Ber. 4ᵇ בתמניא א׳ (Var. אלפין, Ms. M. אלף בית) in eight ways, eightfold acrosticon.— באפי נפשיה *for itself, separately.* Snh. 56ᵇ; a. fr.; v. נַפְשָׁא.—3) esp. in the pl. אַפַּיָא, אַפִּירָא *character, nature* Esth. R. introd. א׳ חציפתא impudent people (h. עזי פנים). Y. Snh. X, 28ᶜ bot. and if the Lord will not hear me כל א׳ שוין all natures (divinities) are alike (proverbial expression of distrust in God); Lam. R. introd. (R. Yitsh. 2) Ar. (ed. אַפִּירִין); Pesik. Shubah p. 162ᵇ; Ruth R. to II, 14. Cmp. אוּפֵי.

אַפָּא II ch.=h. אַף II, *nose.* Targ. Lam. IV, 20; a. e.

אָפָּא m. (contr. of אַפְּעָא q. v.) *a striped wild animal* (of the genus *felis*) of which the male (stronger) and the female species are distinguished, corresp. to h. צבוע q. v.;

leopard, and *hyæna striata (striped hyena)*. B. Kam. 16a (expl. נפרזא leopard); ib. (expl. צבוע); v. discussion ib. Yoma 84a א׳ דיכרא Ms. M. (ed. דדיכרא, corr. acc.) a male *afa*. [Not to be confounded with b. h. אֶפְעֶה, v. Nöld. M. Gr. p. 58 sq. note.]

אפדייני, v. אַפּוּזְיָנֵי.

***אפדכסיס, אפרדכסיס, אפור׳**, read אֶפִּידֶכְסִיוֹס m. (ἐπιδέξιος) *dexterous, clever, refined*. Num. R. s. 10 (alluding to Laban, v. לָבָן) he was surnamed (to his praise) א׳ 'the refined.' R. B. says מלובן ברשע refined in wicked acts. [In parallels Gen. R. s. 60; Ruth R. to I, 22; Yalk. Gen. 109 פרדוכסוס read פְּרִידֶכְסִיוֹס (περιδέξιος).]

אַפַּדְנָא m. (h. אַפֶּדֶן, Pers.; v. Fried.. Del. Proleg. p. 149, note) *country-seat, mansion, palace*. Targ. Jer. XLIII, 10 (h. text שפריר).—M. Kat. 12a. Ber. 56a. Keth. 62a גני בטולא דא׳ sleeps in the shade of his palace (at home, in safety).—*Pl.* אַפַּדְנֵי. Kerith. 6a (read אא׳ or with Rashi על א׳). Keth. 97a.

אָפָה *to bake*, v. אפי.

אַפָּה, v. אַפָּא.

אפו Lev. R. s. 30, read אוֹפִי.

אפודרים, v. אַפִּידְרָא.

אפופלסמון, אָפּוּבַּלְסְמוֹן m. (ὀποβάλσαμον) *juice of the balsam-tree, balsam*. Gen. R. s. 27 היו מביאין א׳ ושף וכ׳ (read ושפין) they would take balsam and smear it on the stones (of the houses of the wealthy); Y. Shebi. V, 55d bot. רושמין בא׳ marked out with balsam. Y. Hor. III, 47c באפי בלסמון (corr. acc.). Gen. R. s. 39, beg. אפופל׳, אפופלסימון (corr. acc.). V. אֲפַרְסְמוֹן.

אפוזיינו, v. next w.

***אַפּוּזְיָנֵי, אֲפוּזִיָּנֵי** m. pl. (ὀψιανός, sub λίθος, obsianus) *obsidian beads* [Rashi: *of gold*, thinking of פז]. Sabb. 57b Ms. M. אפוז׳ (ed. אפוזיינו, Ar. s. v. אב אֲבַז׳; Var. in Mss. אפד׳, אפיד׳, v. Rabb. D. S. a. l.), expl. טוטפת, of Mish., contrad. to חומרתא דקטיפתא balsam beads, v. חוּמַרְתָּא. V. אַפְסְיָן.

אפודרים, v. אַפִּידְרָא.

אֲפוּחָא or **אֲפוּחְיָא** m. (נפח or פוח) *swelling*, whence *bulk, volume*. Pes. 50b נפיש אפוחייהו Ms. Oxf. (ed. אפחזיידהו, v. Rabb. D. S. a. l. note) their bulk is large.

אפוטיין, read אוֹפְסְיָן, v. אַפְסְיָן; cmp. אפוזיינו.

***אפוטיקון** Ex. R. s. 24, in a corrupt passage; cmp. אֵיפּוּס a. Num. R. s. 23, by combination of which the original version may be restored; perhaps; מה הצאן אין מתקינין לה אֵיפּוּסִין אלא רועה בכל יום כך ישראל לא התקינו להם אַפּוֹתִיקָאוֹת במדבר.

אפוטמות, אפוטמים, read מְפוּט׳, v. פָּטָם.

***אַפּוּמְנֵי) אַפִּמ׳, אֲפּוּמְנִיּוֹת)** f. pl. (putealia, or puteana) *enclosures surrounding a well, protected cisterns* (in Noah's ark). Pirké d'R. El. ch. 23, expl. ib. המכסים את אמות חמים וכ׳ (not והמכנריסים) which cover the wells and can be opened and closed. Targ. Y. Gen. VI, 14 אֲפוּמְנְיוּתָא (נְיְרָתָא....?). Tosef. Erub. XI (VIII), 7 כלי אפוכני (ed. Zuck. אב׳ כלים, in oth. ed. omitted) tools for unlocking the puteal.

אפוטרופוס, v. אֶפִּיטְרוֹ׳.

***אפוטריקא** ed., אפוטרכא Ar., read פַּטְרִיאַרְכָא m. (πατριάρχης) *patriarch, religious chief of the Samaritans*. Gen. R. s. 94.

אַפּוּכִי (אוּפְכִי, אִיפּוּכִי) f. (חפך, הפך, cmp. חליפין) *return, exchange, equivalent, settlement* (cmp. esp. Targ. Prov. XXIV, 29, a. P. Sm. s. v. הפך). Lev. R. s. 34, end א׳ דידה הן היא (Yalk. Lev. 665 אִיפּוּכִין, pl.) where is the equivalent for the money spent? Ib. and of all those (praised for their deeds with *ashré*) לא נטל א׳ אלא זה (Yal. l. c. איפוכין) none received the promise of an equivalent except this (Ps. XLI, 2). Gen. R. s. 42 on the day of the destruction of Jerusalem נטלו ישראל׳ אפכי Ar. (ed. אופכי) Israel received full payment for all their sins (ref. to Lam. IV, 22). Ib. א׳ גדולה ample, general settlement; Lam. R. l. c. א׳ שלימה settlement in full. [Tanh. Sh'moth 13, אפופסים, corr. acc.] Num. R. s. 13; Esth. R. introd. Ruth R. introd. אופכין (corr. acc.). [Lam. R. to III, 13 בני אפוכי Mus., *hostages*; v. אוּפְכָא]—*Pl.* אַפּוּכִיּוֹת, אַפְכִיּוֹת. Y'lamd. Sh'laḥ, quot. in Ar.; Num. R. s. 17 a citizen was paying *annonae* וכותב א׳ and writing agreements of converting (security for the case of forfeiture); v., however, אַנְפָּרוּת.

***אַפּוּלְיָא (אפיליא)** pr. n. pl. *Apulia*, the country in the S. E. of Italy. Targ. Ezek. XXVII, 6 some ed., oth. ed. a. Ar. אִיטַלְיָא (h. text כתיים).

אפולירן, Yalk. Ex. 365, read פַּפִּילְיוֹן.

אִיפּוּלִין, אִיפּוּלִים, אֲפוּלִים m. pl. (b. h. פול) *beans*. Tosef. Ter. X, 15 אִיפּוּלִין, אירפולין ed. Zuck. (Var. אפולים, איפולים). Ib. II, 4 איפולין (Var. אופילין). V. אָפוּן.

אפולמוטוס, v. אֶפִּימְלִיטִיס.

אפומטא, v. אמפומטא.

אפומליטיס, read אֶפִּימְלִיטִיס.

***אפומלייא** Y. Ned. II, beg. 40b, read אִיטַלְיָא, v. הֶמְטַלְיָא.

אָפוּן m. *bean* (cmp. אפול s. v. אֲפוּלִים). Y. Yoma IV, 43c bot. עד כא׳ only the size of a bean; v. חָאפוּן. Y. Ab. Zar. III, 43a bot. וכא׳ היה had the shape of a bean. —*Pl.* אִיפּוּנִין, אֲפוּנִים. Kel. III, 2 א׳ הגמלונין Ar., Ms. M. (ed. הגמלנים) large beans; v. גַּמְלוֹן. Sabb. XXI, 3 (143a) שער של א׳ (Ms. L. עפ׳; ed. Sonc. פולין) the silique of the bean. Teb. Yom I, 5; a. fr.

אֲפוּנְדָּה f. (=פונדה q. v., funda) *money bag, purse*, suspended from the neck or from a belt. Y. Sabb. X, 12c. Sabb. X, 3 (92ab) Ar. (ed. פו׳); a. fr.—Trnsf. *womb*. Tanh. Thazr. 3 האפונדיה, אפונדיה; ed. Bub. 5 פונדיה (corr. acc.); [Lev. R. s. 14 ארנקי].

אפונדיה, v. preced.

***אפונס** Hull. 66[b] top; Ab. Zar. 39[a], a. corrupt. of פֵּילָמוּס (πήλαμυς) *pelamys*, a species of *thunny* or *scomber*; Tosef. Hull. III (IV), 27 פולמוס (read 'פי).

אפונראות, v. אַנְפּוֹרָא.

***אַפּוֹסְטְמוֹס, אַפּוֹסְטוֹמוֹס** (Var. פוסטמוס, 'פס) pr. n. m. *Apostomos* (Postomos), one who is mentioned as having burned the Law [and put up an idol in the Temple]. Taan. IV, 6; Y. ib. 68[cd]; Yalk. II Kings 250. [Prob. an officer of king Antioch Epiphanes of Syria; perh. a popul. corrupt. of ἀπόστολος, cmp. II Macc. VI, 1.]

אפוספים, v. אַפּוֹפְסִין.

אַפּוֹפוֹדִין, אי' (frequ. miscopied 'אפיפ, and with ר for ד) c. (ὑποπόδιον) *footstool to the throne or to a high chair of distinction.* Targ. Y. Ex. XXIV, 10 (corr. acc.).— Y. Hag. II, 77[c] bot. after building the throne, he makes 'אפי שלו his foot-stool; Gen. R. s. 1; Lev. R. s. 36 (corr. acc.). Kel. XVI, 1 א' של בעלי הבית (in Talm. ed. בעל) the people's footstool of the household (a folding stool, cmp. אַסְלָא II). Ib. XXIV, 7 ג' פנקסין יש הא' וכ' (corr. acc.) there are three boards or tablets in use (v. פנקס), that which is used as a footsool is susceptible of uncleanness by being trod upon, that with a receptacle for wax (writing tablet) gets unclean by &c. [Gen. R. s. 17; Koh. R. to III, 19, v. אֶפִּיפְּיוֹן.]

אפופירות, v. 'אפי.

אפופלסמון, v. אפובַּלְסְמוֹן.

אפופסים, read

אַפּוֹפְסִין, אַפּוֹפְסִים f. (ἀπόφασις, ἀπόφανσις) *verdict, dispensation.* [Variously corrupted: 'אפופס, 'אירפופסין, אירפפס &c.] Y'lamd. to Gen. III, 1 quot. in Ar. (ref. to Prov. XVIII, 7) the fools give out האפופסין שלהן their own verdict. Pesik. R. s. 44 אפיספים, א־ספיסין (corr. acc.). Ib. s. 46 (ed. Fr. p. 187[b]) נטל א' read ניהן פאופרר he received his verdict (of expulsion from Eden). Y. Sot. VII, 21[d] bot.; Y. R. Hash. I, 57[a] bot. 'איפ; a. fr. [Tanh. Sh'moth 13 שנטלו אפיפסים, read אַפּוֹבֵי.]—Midr. Till to Ps. XVII; Yalk. Ps. 670 two curiosi (v. הנדיוסין) רצין בהפרכוס (באין באירפפוס) (read באפופסים) run (come) each with a verdict; v. בָּאַיִן.—Lev. R. s. 21, beg. אפופסיות Ar., read with ed. אפופסים.

אפופרין Koh. R. to III, 19, v. אֶפִּיפְּיוֹן.

אֲפּוּקֵי, פּוּקֵי m. pl. (פוק, נפק) *exit, end* (=h. מוֹצָאֵי). Y. Pes. IV, 30[d] top בא' שובת' on Sabbath night. Pes. 105[b] א' יומא dismissal of the festive day with benediction; a. fr.—Y. Peah VII, 20[b], top אפיקר (corr. acc.) a. פוקי.— [לאפוקי, v. אֲפֵק.]

אַפּוֹקֵי m. pl. (Af. of נפק) *carrying out.* Targ. O. Lev. XXVI, 5 לא' בר זרעא until seed-time.

אפוקלוס, אפוקליס, v. אֶפִּיקְוֹרִין.

אפוקסנין, read אִסְטְקְטוֹן.

אפורדכים, v. 'אפרכס.

אפורמין Lev. R. s. 25, beg. מפני א', Yalk. Lev. 615 אפרטין, read מפני הַפִּירְקָטִין, v. פִּירְקַיִים.

***אוֹפוֹרְיָיא, אָפוֹרְיָיא** f. (ὀπωρίαι, τὰ) *fruit.* Gen. R. s. 72 בשעת בִּכּוּר כל מיני א' Ar. (ed. א־פ־ריא, read 'או) in the season when all kinds of fruit ripen.

אַפּוּתָא f. (=אַפָּא) 1) *nose.* Targ. Job XLI, 12 (9).— 2) *front of the face, forehead.* Pes. 112[a] יְדָא אא' וכ' the hand on the forehead is one step to sleep. Ber. 44[a], v. הִידְבָא.—Taan. 25[a] מאפותיה out of his forehead. Ib. אאפותיה ed. (read 'אאפ), v. אִסְקוּבְּלָא I.—Ab. Zar. 26[a] אאפותאי Ar. (ed. אפותא, Ms. M. אפותיה, corr.) on its (the child's) forehead. Sabb. 80[b], v. אַנְדִּיפָא.

אפותיק, v. הַפְתֵּק.

אַפּוֹתְיקִי f. (ἀποθήκη) *store-house, store.* Targ. Y. I, Gen. XXIV, 2. Ib. v. 10 שפר א' וכ' the best things of his store (Y. II אפּוֹתִיקֵי . . . ., Ar. only דִיתִיקֵי, v. Gen. R. s. 59).—Y. Sabb. IV, beg. 6[d] bot., opp. to אצל בעה"ב in dwelling rooms, cmp. הַפְתֵּק.—*Pl.* h. אַפּוֹתִיקָאוֹת. Ex. R. s. 30 יש לך א' וכ' hast thou store-houses where to put them?—Ch. אַפּוֹתִיקֵי, אַפּוֹתִיקַיָּא. Targ. Y. I Deut XXXII, 34; a. e.—Y. Ned. IX, 41[c] bot.

אַפּוֹתִיקִי f. (ὑποθήκη) 1) *pledge, mortgage*; an object made a security without being placed in the possession of the pledgee, opp. to מַשְׁכּוֹן.—B. Kam. 96[a] שוויה ניהליה א' וכ' he made it a mortgage by saying, 'You can pay yourself only out of this thing'. Ib. 11[b] עשה עבדו א' if he mortgaged his slave; a. fr.—2) *mortgage-document, deed.* Tosef. Shebi. VIII, 6 שטר שיש בו א' (ed. Zuck. הַפּוֹתִיקֵי) a note (contract) containing a mortgage obligation. Ex. R. s. 31 כתוב לי א' על וכ' give me a mortgage on thy field.—*Pl.* אַפּוֹתִיקָאוֹת. B. Mets. 19[a] דייתיקאות א' וכ' (Ms. M. 'הפותיקי, v. Rabb. D. S. a. l. note) wills, mortgage deeds &c. Tosef. Sabb. VIII (IX), 13 שטרי דייתיקי וא' ed. Zuck. (ed. 'הפות, read 'והפ).

אָפַז (=b. h. פָּזַז) *to dance, leap, sport.* Gen. R. s. 68 (emphasizing *bo*, Gen. XXVIII, 12 as referring to Jacob) אֲפֵזִים בו וכ' sporting with him.

אַפְזִינֵי, v. אֶפּוֹזִינֵי.

***אַפְחָא** f., const. אַפְחַת (נפח), with רוּחָא *grief, cause of grief.* Targ. Y. II Gen. XXVI, 35 ed. (Ar. רְפְּחַן).

אַפְחָזָא m. (פחז) *levity, wantonness.* Snh. 57[a] אפחזוירהו דקא מגלי Ar. (ed. אירחיירהו; Var. lect. v. Rabb. D. S. a. l. note 7) the Bible text describes their wantonness, lewdness.—Pes. 50[b], v. אַפּוּתָא.

אַפְטָא, v. אִירְפְּטָא.

***אפטוניות** Koh. R. to I, 8 עבד בן א', prob. to be read אָפְסוֹנְיוּתָא f. (denom. of אָפְסוֹנִין) *catering, cooking* (for the Jew-Christians living in community of goods). [The entire passage seems to be corrupt or defective. V. Zunz Gott. Vortr. p. 275.]

אפומריקא, v. אפטוריקא.

אַפְטוֹרִיקִי pr. n. m. *Aftoriki.* B. Mets. 5ª אבוה דר׳ א׳; Ḥull. 64ᵇ ... דוסתאי (Dostai) the father of R. A. (Y. Yoma IV, 41ᵈ top פטרוקי אחוה וכ׳ Patruki, brother of R. Darosa).

אֶפְטֵים, אֶפְטֵט m. (=פִּיטְפּוּט; v. בטט) *puppets of clay, a set of clay (or metal) pins to put pots on for cooking, pot-stand.* Tosef. Kel. B. Mets. I, 12 א׳ שיש בו וכ׳ a pot-stand containing metal. Tosef. Nidd. VII, 3 אפטר (corr. acc.).

אפטר Yalk. Deut. 810, read אִיפַּטְרָא.—Tosef. Nidd. VII, 3; v. preced.

אִפְטְיָא, v. אִיפ׳.

אַפְּטְנִיּוֹת, v. אַפּוֹט׳.

אַפְטָרָה f. (פטר, Nif. נִפְטַר *to part;* v. הַפְטָרָה) 1) *farewell-address, homiletic observations made on parting with the host that entertained scholars, toast* (in praise of hospitality, charity, support of students &c.). Gen. R. s. 60 R. Y. עבד לה א׳ used the (preceding) text for a toast; a. fr.—2) v. אַפְטַרְתָּא.

אפטרופולין Yalk. Gen. 9; אפטרפוס, אפטרפא, אפטרפין, v. אֶפִּיטְרוֹפּוֹס a. follow.

אַפְטַרְתָּא f. (v. אַפְטָרָה) prop. *conclusion,* esp. *Aftarah,* or *Haftarah,* i. e. the prophetic lesson read in Synagogue after the reading from the Pentateuch. Pes. 117ᵇ דא׳ (the benediction) belonging to the Aft.—*Gitt. 60ª ספר א׳ (or pl. אַפְטָרְתָא) prob. *a book containing homiletic notes* for toasts &c., v. אַפְטָרָה. [V. Rapap. Er. Mill. p. 167.]—Cmp. הַפְטָרָה.

א׳ בלסמון, אפי Y. Hor. III, 47ᶜ bot., v. אֲפּוֹבַּלְסְמוֹן.

אָפָה, אפי (b. h.; √אף, v. אפף) [*to heat, darken,* cmp. חמץ,] *to bake.* Keth. V, 5 ואוֹפָה and must bake. Pes. 116ª. Y. Ab. Zar. V, 45ª bot. א׳ ג׳ תנורים baked three ovenfulls of bread; a. fr.—Part. pass. אָפוּי baked, (as a noun) *pastry.* Pesik. R. s. 16 א׳ אחד וכ׳ (some ed. עפוי; Pesik. Eth Korb. p. 58ᵇ, Yalk. Num. 777 שבור corr. acc.) I charged thee with the furnishing of one kind of pastry (to supply the governor's household).—*Pl.* אֲפוּיִים. Mekh. Bs'hall. Vay. 4.—Fem. אֲפוּיָה. Gen. R. s. 67 (play on *epho,* Gen. XXVII, 37) פתך א׳ thy bread is baked, thou shalt have to eat without labor. Ib. פורניתא א׳ (read פורניתך), v. פּוּרְנִית a. פּוּרְנִי.

Nif. נֶאֱפָה *to be baked.* Cant. R. to IV, 11 (play on *epho,* v. supra) מי נ׳ בתנור זה who is to be baked in this oven (hell)?—Men. XI, 1; a. e.

Hithpa. הִתְאַפָּה same. Mekh. l. c. היה מִתְאַפֶּה became baked of itself. Sifré Num. 89 המִתְאַפִּים בתנור things baked in the oven.

אֲפָא, אֲפָא (אֲפָה) ,אֲפִי ch. same. Targ. Gen. XIX, 3; a. fr.—Men. 94ª כיון דא׳ לה after he baked it. Sabb. 63ᵇ לְמֵיפָא to bake.—אָפָן, אָפְיָיתָא *baking women, bakers.* Targ. I Sam. VIII, 13.—Ber. 58ᵇ שתין א׳ sixty bakers.—Ib. ואפיין and they used to bake. Y. Bets. IV, 62ᶜ bot. אתת מופה (read מֵיפָה) she came in order to bake; a. fr.

Ithpe. אִתְאֲפֵי *to be baked.* Targ. Lev. VI, 10; a. e.

אַפְיָא, v. אֲפָא.

אַפְיָאן, v. אַפְיָין.

***אַפִּידְרָא** m. (פדר) *stable-floor,* or *cement formed on the stable-floor by moistening and stamping the dung.* Nidd. 28ª he burned the corpse ע״ג פידרא בא׳ Ar. (ed. ע״ג אפודרים) over the dung on the cemented stable-floor. [Oth. opin. *marble-plate,* meaning *a hard cemented substance,* cmp. כלי גָלָל.]

***אִפְיוֹמוֹת** m. pl. (פוט) prop. *able to talk* (sensibly), hence *children* of about six or seven years. Y. Gitt. V, 47ᵇ bot. א׳ פרייא *ifyotoh* (Mish. ib. 8 referred to reads פָּעוּטוֹת q. v.) means *little ones* (v. פרא). Y. Maas. Sh. IV, 55ª פתר לה ...... א׳ וכ׳ expounds the subject by analogy with the law concerning minors, for we read in the Mishnah &c., v. supra.

אפיטריסות, read אֶפִּיטְרוֹפְּסוּת.

אֶפִּיטְרוֹפָּא 1) m. (ch. form=next w.) 1) *guardian, administrator; procurator* (of a Roman district). B. Mets. 39ª א׳ לדיקנני וכ׳ we appoint no guardian for the bearded (adults). Y. ib. III, beg. 9ª לעשות בה א׳ to appoint another person as an administrator of the hired or loaned object. Lam. R. to V, 12 א׳ עליל לקרתא a governor (proconsul) entered a town.—*Pl.* אֶפִּיטְרוֹפַּיָא. Pesik. Asser p. 95ᵇ אילין א׳ וכ׳ those Roman proconsuls that go out visiting the country places (cmp. Ex. R. s. 31, end).—2) fem. *administratrix;* v. אֶפִּיטְרוֹפְּיָא.

אֶפִּיטְרוֹפּוֹס (אַפְט׳, אַפּ׳, אַפִּ׳) 1) m. (ἐπίτροπος) same. Targ. Y. Gen. XXXIX, 4; a. e.—B. Mets. 39ª מעמידין א׳ the court appoints an administrator. Y. Ter. I, 40ᵇ bot. א׳ לעולם a permanent administrator (guardian), א׳ לשעה a temporary administrator (substitute). Ex. R. s. 46 מתגדלת אצל א׳ reared in the house of a guardian; a. fr.—Sabb. 121ª א׳ של מלך royal administrator (of the fiscus).—Tosf. Keth. 13ᵇ, a. e. אין א׳ לעריות there is no guardian (no means of guarding) against inchastity; Y. ib. I, 25ᵈ top א׳ על עריות.—*Pl.* אֶפִּיטְרוֹפְּסִים, אֶפִּיטְרוֹפְּסִין, אַפְטְרְפִין אֶפִּיטְרוֹפִּין. Targ. Y. Gen. XLI, 34. Pes. VIII, 1. Esth. R. to I, 2; a. fr.—Tosef. Ter. V, 7 תרומת א׳ T'rumah set apart by administrators in behalf of minors. Y. ib. l. c.—Gen. R. s. 6; Yalk. Gen. 9 אפיטרופולין (corr. acc.); a. fr. [Yalk. Ps. 771 אפיקורוס twice, read our w.]—2) fem. v. next w.

אֶפִּיטְרוֹפָּא, אֶפִּיטְרוֹפְּיָא (אַפּ׳) f. *administratrix, guardian.* Keth. IX, 6 (86ᵇ) (Mish. ed. פא ..., Talm. ed. פיא ...). B. Bath. 144ª פא .... Y. Keth. IX, 33ª top אפטרפא a. אפטרפוס, אפיטרופא. Tosef. ib. IX, 3.

אֶפִּיטְרוֹפְּסוּת f. (denom. of אפיטרופוס) *guardianship, administration.* Tosef. B. Bath II, 5 (אפיטרוסות ed. Zuck., corr. acc.); Tosef. Keth. IX, 3 יוצא מאפיטרופסותו when he has ceased to be an administrator.

אֲפִיָּה I f. (אפי) *baking.* Y. Sabb. VII, 10[b] bot. א׳ הולדה לבישול baking is a labor forbidden on the Sabbath as a species of cooking; v. אָבII. Men. 94[a]; a. fr.—*Pl.* אֲפִיּוֹת. Y. Pes. III, 30[b] top כדי שתי א׳ twice the time required for baking. [Y. Ned. VII, 40[b] bot. הנודר מן הא׳, read חֲפִירָה as Tosef. Ned. IV, 3.]

אִפִּיַּטְרוֹס m. (ἱππίατρος) *veterinary surgeon.* Num. R. s. 9.

אַפְיָין, אַפְיָאן (עֲפִיָּאן, עַפְיָין) m. (אפי) *bake-fish* (cmp. סולתנית), a small fish believed to grow scales when reaching a certain age. Hull. 66[a] bot. Ar. אפיין (ed. עפיאן); Ab. Zar. 39[a] עפיין ed. (Ms. M. עפאין, read עפיאן, עפיין); Tosef. Hull. III (IV), 27 אנפיא ed. Zuck. (Var. נפיא).

אֲפִיק, v. אָפֵק.

אָפִיל m. (b. h.; אפל) *slow to ripen, late in the season.* M. Kat. 6[a] א׳ late produces, opp. בַּכִּיר. Gen. R. s. 61, beg. זרע בא׳ sow at the advanced season. Fem. אֲפִילָה *advanced autumn, rainy season.* Y. Taan. I, 64[a] bot.—*Pl.* אֲפִילוֹת. Y. R. Hash. III, beg. 47[b] *sheeps which conceive late in the season.*—קרן אפיל, v. אָפֵל II.

אֲפִילָא, אַפְלָא ch. same. M. Kat. 6[b] אפלא וקא משוי לה וכ׳ Ms. M. (ed. א׳ קא, diff. vers. in Rashi) it is a slowly growing garden and by watering he makes it fast growing.—*Pl.* m. אַפְלֵי, אֲפִילֵי. Targ. Koh. XI, 2 *late seeds.* Taan. 3[b] אפילי late clouds (after the rain), v. חַרְפָא. Nidd. 65[b] חרפי ואפלי earlier and later crops (in two succeeding years, so that the interval of time varies). *Pl.* f. אֲפִילָתָא, אַפְלָתָא. Targ. O. Ex. IX, 32. R. Hash. 8[a] late *conceiving,* sluggish sheep, opp. חַרְפָיָתָא.

אֲפִילָה, v. אָפִיל.

אֲפֵילָה adj., v. אָפֵל.

אֲפֵילָה f. (b. h. אֲפֵלָה) *darkness.* Gen. R. s. 89 beg. (mental darkness; trials &c.); v. אוֹפֶל.

אֲפִילוּ (abbrev. אפי׳) (=אַף אִילּוּ) *even if, although, even.* Targ. Ps. XIV, 3 (h. text גם); a. e.—R. Hash. 25[a] (reading אתם Lev. XXIII, 2; 4; 37 as if אַתֶּם) 'which *ye* will proclaim', אתם אפי׳ וכ׳ *ye* even if erring in the appointment of the festive calendar &c., i. e. the appointment of the Supreme Court is definite and binding. Ber. 9[a], a. fr. א׳ לרבנן even if following the opinion of &c.; a. v. fr. [Cant. R. end א׳ להחריבו, v. next w.]

אַפִּילְיוֹן, אַפִּילוֹן I m. (ἀπειλῶν, ἀπειλέων, part. pres. of ἀπειλέω, prob. borrowed fr. Aquila to Ps. CIV, 32) *threatening.* Y. Ber. IX, 13[c] bot. הוא א׳ לעולמו להחריבו He looks upon his world threatening to destroy it. Cant. R. end, that time חושב הקב״ה אפילו לחחריבו וכ׳ (read אפילון לעולמו להח׳) the Lord plans threatening &c. Y'lamd. beg. (quot. in Ar. with ref. to Ps. l. c.) מסתכל אפילון של עולם (read על עולמו) He looks threatening upon His world; cmp. Midr. Till. to Ps. XVIII, 8; Yalk. II Sam. 158.

אַפִּילְיוֹן, אַפִּילוֹן II m. (πυλών, πυλεών) *gate-way.* Ber. 16[b] נכנס לאפילוין Ar. (ed. אנפילון, Ms. F. לבית המרחץ, read לבית החצר, Treat. S'maḥ. I, 10 לחצר).

***אַפִּילְיוֹן** III m. (pilleum, πιλίον) *felt-cap, hat* &c. Kel. XXIX, 1 א׳ של ראש some ed. (others פִּילְיוֹן).—[Sabb. 120[a] פילון, אפילון Ms., ed. אפילות, read אַפִּלְיוֹן, פִּלְיוֹן q. v.]

אפיליות, v. preced.

אפימיות, Pirke d'R. El. ch. X, read אוֹסְפִּרְנִיּוֹת; v. אמפומיות.

אֶפִּימְלִיטֵיס m. (ἐπιμελήτης) *manager, commissioner.* Tosef. B. Bath. X, 5 אפומ׳ ed. Zuck. (ed. אפולמוטוס, corr. acc.). B. Bath. 144[b] פולמוסטוס ed. (Ms. פומלירטוס, oth. var. v. Rabb. D. S. a. l. note 2; corr. acc.). Men. 85[b] פולמוסטוס ed. (Ar. פלמיטוס); corr. acc.

***אָפִּיס, סַר א׳** pr. n. m. (*Sarapis,* Σάραπις) *Serapis,* the Nile-god. Ab. Zar. 43[a] the figure of מיניקה וסר א׳ ed. (Ms. סַרָפִיס; v. Rabb. D. S. a. l.) a nursing woman (Isis) and of Serapis. [Cmp. Sachs Beitr. II, 99 and illustr. in Sm. Ant. s. v. Coma.] [Tosef. Par. V (IV), 2 האפיס ed., read with ed. Zuck. חפאים, v. חַפַּאי.]

אֶפִּיסְטוֹלֵי m. pl. (ἐπιστολαί) *message, injunction, last will.* Gen. R. s. 74 end, ed.; v. אִסְטְלֵי II. Y'lamd. to Deut. II, 2 (quot. in Ar. ed. pr.; oth. ed. פיסטולי).

***אֶפִּיסְטִילְיוֹת** f. pl. (ἐπιστύλιον) *architraves,* lower members of an entablature. Y. Succ. I, 52[a] bot. Mus.; cmp. פִּיסְקְלִיוֹת.

אפיסניות, v. אַפְסַנְיָא.

אפיסתיקתיה, אפיסתקיתיה, v. אִפְסְתְקִי.

אפיפורין, אפיפודין, corruptions of אַפּוֹדִין, אַפּוֹפְסִין or of next w.

***אֶפִּיפִּיּוֹן** m. (ἐφίππιον, ephippium) *saddle cloth,* a figurative expression for the protuberances of the human buttock; v. אַיִן I. Koh. R. to III, 19 (ref. to 'the advantage of man over beast' Koh. l. c.) ואפופרין כפוי עליו וכ׳ (corr. acc.) and an ephippium is pressed over it (the lock of the buttock) in order that he may not look as hideous as a beast; Gen. R. s. 17 אפיפירין (and otherwise, to be corrected after Koh. R. l. c.); Yalk. Koh. 969 אפיפורי פרוסה על רגליו (corr. acc.).

***אַפִּיפוֹרָא** m. (אפיפורא, על פיפורא, v. פִּיפוֹרָא a. next w.) *litter-carrier, chief lecticarius.* Ab. Zar. 11[a] (v. פיפורא for correct versions).

אַפִּפְיָרוֹת, אַפִּיפְיָרוֹת, פִּיפְיָרוֹת f. pl. (פִּיפְרִיּוֹת, —רִיָּה—f. sing.) (√פר, cmp. b. h. פרפר=בקע to *split;* cmp. פַּרְפֶּרֶת, a. פִּרְפְּרָאוֹת פְּרִיפְרִיּוֹת) *split pieces of wood, laths,* slabs used for *espaliers,* also *as frames for decorative* *hangings.* Y. Sot. IX, end, 24ᶜ; Tosef. ib. XV, 9 אבל עושה הוא אפיפרי׳ וכ׳ but one may make lath frames and hang thereon whatever decorations he may desire. [Bab. ib. 49ᵇ פְּפָרְיוֹת; Rashi פְּרִיפְרִית sing.] Kil. VI, 3 על מקצת א׳ on a portion of the espaliers. Ib. VII, 3 מותר א׳ the balance of the espaliers (on which no vine is trained). Kel. XVII, 3 אפי׳ וכ׳ (Ar. פי׳; Mish. אפי׳) frames for hangings to which reeds were fastened from the bottom upward (crosswise) for support. Tosef Kel. B. Mets. VI, 6 (a. freq. in comment.) פִּיפְּאָרוֹת. Ib. פִּיפְּאָרוֹת שאינה וכ׳ a frame (baldachin) which cannot be taken up by its handles and carried through the door (outside).—Ch. פִּיפְּיוֹרָא, פְּיפוּרָא. V. also פוּרְיָא a. אַפִּרְיוֹן. [ר softened into י, cmp. חצוצרה.]

***אפיפסדוס** or **אפיפסרוס** Y. Ter. VIII, 46ᵇ לא מטון א׳ וכ׳, prob. to be read לא מטון לפלמירא וכ׳ they (the would-be captors of R. Isi) had not arrived at Palmyra before all of them (the royal court &c.) were gone (carried into captivity). V. זנביא.

אפיצמלין, v. אִיפְּסְטְלִין.

אָפִיק (b. h.; אפק, √פק, v. פוק, פקק, נפק, פנק; a) *to break through, go forth;* b) *to be a free man, ruler*) 1) *spring, rivulet* (ch. פצידא).—*Pl.* אֲפִיקִים. Ab. Zar. 54ᵇ bot.—2) *ruler. Pl.* as above. Cant. R. to V, 12 (allud. to *ăfîkê mayim*, Cant. ib.) שהם א׳ על זכ׳ they (the scholars) are appointed officers over the waters of the Law.

***אֲפִיקְדוֹנָא**=פִּיקָדוֹנָא. Y. Shebu. VII, 37ᵈ מריה דא׳ (Y. B. Kam. VI, end, 5ᶜ דפ׳).

אֲפִיקוֹלוֹס(?) pr. n. m. *Aphikolos.* Tosef. Hull. VIII, 3; cmp. אבקולס. V. אַפִּיקוֹרִין.

אֲפִיקוֹמִין, אֲפִיקוֹמוֹן, v. next w.

***אֲפִיקוֹמָן** m. (ἐπὶ κῶμον=comessatum ire; cmp. Sm. Ant. s. v. *Comissatio;* Plut. II, 726 Fragm. ed. Wytt.) *'to the aftermeal entertainment!'*=our, *'Remove the cloth'*. Pes. X, 8 אין מפטירין אחר הפסח א׳ after the Paschal meal one must not wind up by saying, 'Now to the after-meal entertainment'; (cmp. אַפְּטָרָה). Y. ib. 37ᵈ top אֲפִיקוֹמָן שלא יהא וכ׳ in order that one should not break loose from his company and join another.—אֲפִיקוֹמִין m. pl. (ἐπίκωμοι) *things belonging to the after-meal, dessert.* Ib. bot. מאי א׳ what are *epicomoi? Fruits, sweet-meats* &c., v. זֶמֶר II. Tosef. ib. 11 אין מפטירין.... אפיקומון וכ׳ ed. Zuck. (read קומין..) we must not offer *epikomoi*, as nuts, dates &c. [Pes. 119ᵇ מאי א׳ אמר רב שלא וכ׳ seems to be a corrupt text; prob. to be read: מאי כגמא אמר רב שלא וכ׳ מאי א׳ אמר שמואל כגון וכ׳; cmp. Y. l. c. top א׳ שלא וכ׳ . . . ; bot. מאי א׳ שמואל אמר וכ׳ . . . .]

אַפִּיקוֹרָא m. (פקר, v. next w.) *an irreverent person, scorner. Pl.* אַפִּיקוֹרֵי. Ned. 23ᵃ דשכיחי א׳ וכ׳ for it occurs frequently that disrespectful persons attack the scholars.

אַפִּיקוֹרוֹס m. (פקרס, enlarg. of פקר, cmp. פרכס &c.; cmp. אפקרסין) *one irreverent of authority* or *religion, sceptic, heretic.* [The peculiar form and also the meaning assigned to our w. found a ready support in its phonetic coincidence with *Epicurus*, the philosopher; cmp. N. T. Acta XVII, 18. The derivatives of our w. and those of the plain root פקר interchange frequently.] Snh. X (XI), 1, the following have no share in the world to come ...'וא and the Ep.; Y. ib. XI, 27ᵈ bot. כהן דאמר אהן ספרא וכ׳ as the one who (speaking of the Law) says (sneeringly) 'That book', or 'Those Rabbis'. Bab. ib. 99ᵇ (similar definition). Ab. II, 14 ודע מה שתשיב לא׳ that you may know what to reply to the sceptic; cmp. Snh. 38ᵇ; a. fr.—*Pl.* אַפִּיקוֹרְסִין, ...סים, ...,אַפִּיקוֹרִ׳. R. Hash. 17ᵃ Yalk. Num. 764. Hag. 5ᵇ מאי תיהדר עלן מא׳ how shall we henceforth cope with the heretics?, i. e. opponents of tradition (Jew-Christians; cmp. מִין a. Snh. 38ᵇ).—Cmp. אַפְקָרוּתָא.—Denom. אַפִּיקוֹרְסִית, v. אַפִּיקוֹרְסוּת.

***אַפִּיקוֹרְן, אַפִּיקוֹרִין**, only in בא׳ as adv. (v. preced. ws.) *without restraint.* Hull. 104ᵇ עוף וגבינה נאכלין בא׳ (Ar. ...רין, ed. ...רן, some ed. אפיק׳, without prefix ב) poultry and cheese may be eaten without restraint, expl. ibid. בלא נטיל׳ וכ׳ without intermission by washing hands &c. *[A marginal note referring to the opinion of אפיקולוס, Tosef. Hull. VIII, 3, has been mistaken for a var. lect. of our w., as אפיקולוס, אפיקלוס, אפקרליס, אפיקולים, and another glossator, prob. thinking of *facialis*, φακιόλης, added פר׳ מטלית— all of which was interpolated in Alfasi a. l., a. in Ar. s. v. אפיקורין.]

אַפִּיקוֹרְסוּת f. (denom. of אפיקורוס) *licentiousness, scepticism.* Kidd. 66ᵇ נזרקה בו א׳ (some ed. רוסית .....) scepticism (Sadduceism) came over him.

אַפִּיקְמְפִיזִין, אַפִּיקְטְוִיזִין (corr. אפו׳) f. (ἀποκοτταβίζειν) orig. *playing at cottabus*, or *squirting wine into a bowl;* trnsf. (S.) *the gourmand's practice of taking an emetic before meal; to vomit.* Sabb. 12ᵃ; 123ᵃᵇ. Ib. XXII, 6. Tosef. ib. XVI (XVII), 22, Var. ed. Zuck. אפקטויזין. Succ. 40ᵇ; B. Kam. 102ᵃ; Sifra B'har ch. I, end אפיקטפיזים (corr. acc.). [A noun ἀποκοττάβισις to which our w. would correspond, is not in the vocabulary.]

פִּיקִילְמִין, אַפִּיקִלְמִין, אַפִּיקִלְמָא m. pl. (ἐμποικιλτά, ποικιλτά, τά) *embroidered garments* (quoted as Aquila's translation of רקמה Ez. XVI, 10; LXX ποικίλα). Pesik. B'shall. p. 84ᵇ. Cant. R. to IV, 11; 12 אפליקטא, איפליקתא (corr. acc.). Lam. R. beg. תרגם אונק׳ אפלקטורין פליקטא (read עקילס, and corr. acc. by striking out one of the two words as var. lect. that came into the text; cmp. Pesik. l. c. note).

אַפִּקִירוֹס, אַפִּיקְרָס, אַפִּיקִירוֹס pr. n. pl. *Epicarus*, a town East of the Jordan (Ptol. V, 16, 9), in Targ. corresp. to h. מַעֲכָה. Targ. Deut. III, 14, O. אפקר׳; Y. II קריית אפיק׳ (Y. I corrupt קירוי ואנטיקירוס). Targ. Josh. XII, 5; XIII, 11; 13.

אפיקלין, v. אוֹפִיקְלִין.

אַפִּקְרוּתָא, v. אַפְקָרוּתָא.

אפיקריתין, אפיקריסון, v. אַפְקַרְסִין.

אֲפִיקְרֶס, v. אֲפִיקִירוֹס.

אַפִּיקַרְסוּת, v. אַפְקַרְסוּת.

אֲפִיקַרְסִי; v. אַפְקַרְסִי.—אֲפִיקַרְסִין, v. אַפְקַר׳.

אפירמין, v. אפורמן.

אַפִּרְיוֹן, v. אַפִּרְיוֹן.

אפירסמן Y. Shek. V, 49ᶜ bot., read אֲפַרְסְמוֹן.

אפיסקיתה, אפיסקיתי, v. אפסתקי.

אָפַךְ (b. h. הָפַךְ q. v.) *to turn, change, reverse, overthrow.* Kil. II, 3 say not I will plant ואח״כ אוֹפֵךְ and then turn the soil over (destroy the previous seed) אלא אוֹפֵךְ Ar. (ed. הוֹפֵךְ) but one must first uproot &c. (cmp. אכל fr. אָכַל). Ter. IX, 1; Tosef. Kil. I, 16 יוֹפֵךְ he shall &c. Ib. end לייפך ed. Zuck. (Var. לוֹפֵךְ) to uproot.

אֲפַךְ, Af. אַפִּיךְ, Pa. אַפֵּךְ ch. 1) *to turn* (act. a. neut.) also *to turn around, to flee; to make turn around, to beat.* Targ. Ps. LXXVIII, 9. Targ. I Chron. VIII, 13; a. fr.— Y. Kil. IX, 32ᶜ top אפיך אפיך turn around, turn around. Men. 25ᵇ, a. fr. איפוך reverse it, or, I reverse it. Ib. ומי מצית אפכת לה how can you reverse it? Gitt. 69ᵇ ונַפְכִיה let him reverse it; a. fr.—(With שבועה) *to reverse the oath, shift the oath over to the opponent.* Shebu. 41ᵃ in a case where the Biblical law prescribes an oath לא מַפְכִינַן we allow it not to be shifted over to the claimant; a. fr. —Sabb. 31ᵃ אפיך ליה he reversed it, i. e. recited the alphabet to him in inverted order. Yeb. 63ᵃ א׳ לה he said to her just the reverse. Gitt. 67ᵇ מֵיפַךְ אפכי they will do the reverse; a. fr.—2) *to overturn, destroy.* Taan. 25ᵃ דאפכיה לעלמא מרישא (Ms. M. דאחרב) that I should destroy the world.—3) (cmp. אִיכְפַּת) *to have to do with, care for, mind.* Y. Bets. I, 60ᵃ bot.; Y. Shebi. IX, 38ᶜ top; Y. Erub. III, 21ᵇ bot. (read:) מה אפך לן פתילה גבי וכ׳ what does the law about wicks concern us when speaking of the egg, i. e. what relation is there between the two? Y. Ter. VIII, 46ᵃ top מה אפך לן מִצְוֹת וכ׳ what relation is there between religious laws and sanitary precautions concerning snake-bitten fruit? Ib. מה אפכייר וכ׳ (corr. acc.).—4) *to move about, travel, traffic.* Ab. Zar. 31ᵇ כ״ע אפכי all the people are about, on the road.—5) *to pay in return, to retaliate*, v. הֲפַךְ a. אַפּוּכֵי.

Ithpe. אִתְּפַךְ, אִתְהַפֵּךְ, אִי׳ *to change off.* Bets. 10ᵇ איתפוכי אתחפך (old ed. correctly אִתְּפוּךְ, mod. ed. אתחפוכי אתחפוך, Ms. M. והפוכי) they changed places. Deriv. אַפּוּכֵי, אִיפְּכָא.

אפכן, אפכייר, v. preced.

אַפְכִיוּת, v. אַפּוּכֵי.

אָפַל, only in Hif. הֶאֱפִיל (denom. of אֹפֶל q. v.) *to make dark, obscure.* Sabb. 86ᵃ bot. מַאֲפִיל בטליתו he makes dark by spreading his cloak (cover) over himself. Y. B. Bath. III, 13ᶜ top עומד ומא׳ the tree stands there and takes the light away.—2) *to be late in ripening, giving birth*, &c.; *to have late crops.* Y. Shebi. V, beg. 35ᵈ שנים מַאֲפִילוֹת years slow in ripening, when the crop is delayed. Gen. R. s. 99 שהיא מַאֲפֶלֶת which has late crops.

אֲפַל ch. same. *Pa.* אַפֵּיל as foreg. Hif. 1). B. Bath. 7ᵃ קא מאפלת עלי thou makest my building dark, obstructest my light.

אָפֵל I m. (√אף, v. אפה; cmp. אבל, הבל) [thick vapory,] 1) *dark.* Sabb. 86ᵃ, a. fr. בית א׳ a dark (windowless) house.—אֲפֵילָה f. *dark place.* Y. Naz. IX, 57ᵈ top; Pes. 81ᵇ במים בא׳, in water or in a dark place (cave).— *Pl.* fem. אֲפֵילוֹת. Lev. R. s. 9 מבואות א׳ dark alleys; a. fr.—2) *heavy, sluggish, slow, late.* Denom. האפיל, v. אָפַל.

אָפֵל II (אָפִיל), קרן א׳ pr. n. pl. *Keren Afel* (Dark-Horn), name of a height. Taan. 22ᵇ עד שישב וכ׳ Ms. M. (ed. שיעמוד) until one sits on *Ker. Afel* and can bathe his feet in water. Ib. חזיוא לי קרן א׳ .... ed. (Ms. חזיא דוכתא) I have seen (that place) K. A.

אַפְלָא, v. אַפֵּלָא.

אפלון, v. אַפִּלְיוֹן.

אַפְלָמוֹר Syr.=אִמְפֶּרְטוֹר q. v.

פַּלְיוֹן, פַּלְיוּם, אַפַּלְיוֹן m. (pallium, παλλίον) *pallium, a sheet worn as a cloak and used for bed-cover.* Sabb. 120ᵃ Ar. a. Rashi (ed. אפילויה, Ms. M. פילין, corr. acc.). Y. ib. XVI, 15ᵈ top פילוין (corr. acc.). Nidd. VIII, 1 וכן בפליום Mish. (Bab. ed. פליוס, corr. acc., Var. פליון). Treat. S'mahoth XII מאפלונר, read כְּאַפַּלְיוֹנֵי.

אפליקטא, אפליקתא, v. אַפִּיקְלָבָא.

אַפַּלְסְמוֹן, v. אַפַּרְסְמוֹן.

אַפַּמְיָא pr. n. pl. 1) (=פַּמְיָיס q. v.) *Paneas* in Northern Galilee (Cæsarea). Y. Kil. IX, 32ᶜ bot. ימא דא׳ the lake of P.—Y. Hall. IV, end; 60ᵇ (?).—2) *Apamœa* in Babylon; v. אַסְפַּמְיָא 2).

אַפַּנְטוֹר, אַפַּנְמוֹרִין=פַּנְתֵּירִין.

אַפַּנְטֵי f. (ἀπαντή=ἀπάντησις) *encountering.*—לא׳ (=εἰς ἀπαντήν, h. לקראת) *to meet, to receive.* Tanh. Emor 22 לא׳ של מלך to salute the king. Pesik. R. Ten Command. 1 לא׳ של מלך וכ׳ (some ed. לאנפני, corr. acc.) to salute his father the king. Cant. R. to I, 12 לאפנתר (corr. acc.). Y. Ab. Zar. II, 41ᵇ bot. לפנטי; Midr. Sam. ch. VII לאפרכי דידיה (corr. acc., or Var. לאפי). [Yalk. Esth. 1058 לאנפטר some ed., read: לְאַנְטְטֵי.]

אַפַּנְטִיסוֹן* (ἀπάντησον) *go to meet* (to join battle). Pesik. R. s. 31 translating *kadd'ma panav* (Ps. XVII, 13). [Correct: אין לנו זוג להזדווג לה אלא אתה קומה ד׳ קדמה פניו א׳ לה; v. Midr. Till. to Ps. l. c.]

פַּנְקְרִיסִין, אַפַּנְקְרִיסִין m. pl. (transposition of קַפְרִיסִין, with נ inserted) *caper-fruit.* Y. Sabb. III, 5ᵈ top א׳ Ar. (ed. פ׳). Ib. I, 3ᶜ bot. פנקריסים (read ין...); Y. Ab. Zar. II, 41ᵈ פ׳. [In parallel places קַפְרִיסִין q. v.]

אַפַּנְתָּא, פַּנְתָּא f. (פנה, v. פנים; cmp. אַפּוּתָא fr. אַף) *upper, (front)*, a kind of *legging* connected with a shoe or sole over which straps are drawn for fastening; corresp. to h. מִנְעָל. Taan. 12ᵇ מסיימי א׳ (Ms. M. פַּנְתָּאֵר pl.) having put on *appantas* (on a public fast-day). Yeb. 102ᵃ הוה ליה א׳ מֵעַל וכ׳ (ed. פ׳; v. Ar. ed. Koh. s. v.) the panta is one 'from on' (referring to Deut. XXV, 9 'and she shall strip his shoe from on his foot'), and the thong a 'from on' of a 'from on', i. e. panta and thong are two coverings. Ber. 43ᵇ ולא אמרו אלא בא׳ (ed. בפ׳) this applies only to the panta (upper).

אפנתי, v. אַפַּנְתֵּר.

אֶפֶס m. (b. h., v. next w.) [*extremity*,] *ankle*.—Dual אַפְסַיִם. Yoma 77ᵇ. Cmp. אוּפְסַיִם.

אָפֵס (אֶפֶס) (b. h., √פס, v. פסס to cut off) 1) *to be gone*.—[As a noun: *there is an end of* . . .] B. Bath. 111ᵃ אפס (דברי) זכריה (v. Rabb. D. S. a. l.) (the words of) Zachariah (to whom you refer as an authority) are (is) gone, i. e. they are no authority.—2) homiletically used as though a Greek word (ἄφες) *let go, leave alone*. Pesik. Vattomer p. 130ᵃ (ref. to *heäfes*, Ps. LXXVII, 9) לשון יוני הוא כמד״א אָפִיס it is a Greek word, as if you were to say, *afes* (let alone); Lam. R. to I, 2 וכמד״א אמר אפס (strike out ואמר, a. read אפיס); Ex. R. s. 45 לשון יוני אפס הניח in Greek *aphes* means, (he) *let go*; Yalk. Ps. 816.—[Gen. R. s. 40 (ref. to *efes* Jud. IV, 9); omitted in Yalk. Gen. 67,—an interpolation from passages quoted above.]

אָפֵס pr. n. m. *Afes*, an Amora. Sabb. 59ᵇ; a. fr.

אָפַס dialect. for אָפַץ q. v.

אפסוגין, read:

אוּפְסוֹנִין, אַפְסוֹנִין m. (ὀψώνιον) *provision, marketing*. Tanh. Tsav 1 כבר שלחתי אפסונין וכ׳ (some ed. ....גין) I have already sent the marketing to thy house (bribing the market commissioner); Yalk. Lev. 479 איפסונין; Mic. 555 אופסינן (corr. acc.).

***אפסחתיה**, Treat. Der. Er. VIII, beg. הוו הולכין את א׳ וכ׳ (v. Var. lect. ibid.) a corrupt and defective passage, to be restored from Lam. R. to IV, 2 a. Tosef. Ber. IV, 8, our w. being a remnant of מִטְפַחַת. V. Koh. Ar. Compl. s. v. I, 224.

***אפסטיא** Erub. 100ᵇ, supposed to be pr. n. pl. (Var. in Rabb. D. S. a. l. note 60 אשפיא, ארשפטא, אשפיפיא). V. Neub. Géogr. p. 348.

***אַפְסְטִיתָה** f. (redupl. of פס, v. פסס) *rake* or *pitchfork*. Y. Sabb. VII, 10ᵃ bot. if one works on flax stalks (on a Sabbath) בא׳ חייב וכ׳ with a rake (spreading them apart), he is guilty of an act resembling winnowing.

אַפְסְטְקִין f. pl. (πιστάκια, τά) *the fruits of the pistachio-tree*. Y. Dem. II, beg. 22ᵇ; Y. Maasr. I, 48ᵈ bot. אִיפ׳; cmp. אַלְצְרִין.

***אַפְסִיּוֹת** f. pl., prob. denomin. of אֶפֶס (אפס דמים I Sam. XVII, 1) of *Ephes*. Y. Dem. II, 22ᶜ bot. תמרין א׳ Ephes dates.

***אַפְסִיִּין** m. (obsianus, ὀψιανός) *obsidian*, a stone used as glass. Tanh. Naso 23. Yalk. Ps. 842 אפוטיין (read אוֹפְסִיִּין). [Midr. Till. to Ps. XCI; Num. R. s. 12 קלְיפין.] Cmp. אַפְזְרִין. V. אמפומיות.

אַפְסִינְתִּין m. (ἀψίνθιον) *absynth, worm-wood*. Ab. Zar. 30ᵃ מַר א׳ the bitter wine is that of absynth (absinthites); v. פסינטון.

אפסיקמא, אפסיקימא, v. אַפְסְקְיָמָא.

אַפְסִירָא, v. אַפְסָרָא.

אַפְסַנְיָא f. (ὀψώνιον, cmp. אַפְסוֹנִין) *provision*, esp. *supply and pay for an army*. Snh. 18ᵇ מלך משום א׳ the king (is excluded from the court deciding on the intercalation of a thirteenth month) on account of the soldiers' pay (it being to his interest to create an embolistic year). Ib. II, 4 (21ᵇ) (Mish. a. Gem. ed. אפס׳ throughout the whole page, Ms. M. אפס׳) כדי ליתן א׳ as much as is required for the stipends he has to pay. Y. Snh. II, 20ᶜ top אפסניא. —*Pl*. אַפְסַנְיוֹת (doubtful, prob. אַבְסַנְיוֹת). Cant. R. to I, 2 שהדה מהלך א׳ (read מחלק, ed. אפסנוות, אפיסנוות). Sifré Deut. 328; Yalk. ib. 946 אַפְסַנְיָאוֹת.

***אַפְסְקְיָמָא, אפסיקמא, אפסיקימא** m. (a corruption of σχίφινος) (*rope*) *twisted of palm-leaves*, (v. Löw Pfl. p. 118). Erub. 58ᵃ ed. a. Ms. (Ar. אפקימא).

אַפְסָר, אִיפְסָר m. (Pers. afsâr, Fl. to Levy Targ. Dict. I, 418ᵇ; ψάλλιον) *bit*. Sabb. V, 1; a. e.

אַפְסָרָא (אַפְסִירָא) ch. same. Targ. Y. Num. XIX, 2.—Trnsf. *the means of taking possession*, as possession is taken of the horse by seizing it by the bit. Kidd. 27ᵃ שטר דא׳ דארעא וכ׳ the deed is valueless in itself as it is merely the bit of landed property. B. Bath. 53ᵇ מיצר א׳ דארעא the balk is &c. (taking possession of which is equal to taking possession of the fields to which it belongs).

***אפסתקי, אפסתיק** f. (supposed to be an adapt. of ὀψοθήκη) *wallet*. Gen. R. s. 70 when Laban could not see (יתיר .... אפי׳ אפסתקיתיה, Yalk. Gen. 124 אפסתיק׳ without אפי׳, Ar. omits אפי׳, Lonz. אפיסטוקתיא, Rashi אפסט׳ without אפי׳) even his (Jacob's) wallet. [Prob. to be read ... חמי אפותיקי דידיה or אַפּוֹתִיקָתֵיהּ, cmp. Targ. Y. Gen. XXIV, 10.]

אַפְעָא m. (contr. אַפְּא; corresp. to h. צָבוּעַ; אפע *to color*, cmp. אפה) [the checkered,] *hyena* or *leopard*. *Pl*. אַפְעַיָּא. Targ. I Sam. XIII, 18 (h. text צְבֹעִים).

אֶפְעֶה m. (b. h.; prob. fr. אפע, v. אוּפְיָא; cmp., however foreg. w.) [the foaming,] *viper, adder*. Bekh. 8ᵃ. Gen. R. s. 20.

אָפַף (b. h.; √אף; cmp. אבב, חפף, כפף &c.) *to swell, to bend; to press, to surround, to heat, to darken*, (v.

אפף, אנה, אפל, אפי׳ן &c.). Midr. Till. to Ps. XVIII, 5, v. next w.—Denomin.

*אֲפָפוֹן m. (or אֲפָפִין m. pl.) *thick web.* Midr. Till. to Ps. XVIII, 5 (explain. *ăfafuni* ib.) when a woman weaves with two double threads חן נקראין א׳ they are called ăfafon (ăfafin); so did David say אפפוני וכ׳ troubles wove around me and came over me doubled.

אָפַס, אֲפַץ (√אף, v. אפה; cmp. חפ׳ן) *to press, squeeze, contract.*—Part. pass. אָפוּץ. Ohol. IX, 3 a gap which was filled with straw או אֲפוּצָה or was made narrower by squeezing the parts together (e. g. pressing the lid down). Tosef. ib. X, 6 אֲפוּסָה a narrowing of the gap by pressing. Y. Sabb. III, 6[c] באפוצה when the wick is compressed in the candlestick. Ib. V, beg. 7[b] בְאֲפוּצִים when the vessels are closely packed. Y. Pes. I, 27[c] top אֲפוּצוֹת.

עֲפַץ, אֲפַץ ch. same, esp. *to use* אַפְצָא q. v., *to dress* or *prepare with gall-nut juice.*—Part. pass. עֲפִיץ, אֲפִיץ. Meg. 19[a] top ולא א׳ Ms. M. (ed. ע׳) a skin not moistened with gall-nut. Gitt. 19[a] הא דאֲפִיצָן Rashi (ed. אפיין) in the one case it means when the parchment has been dressed &c. Ib. 11[a]; 19[b].—Ib. 22[a]; Sabb. 79[a] ע׳.

עַפְצָא, אַפְצָא m. (preced.) [contracting,] *gall-nut.* Gitt. 19[a]; Sabb. 104[b] א׳ (מי) gall-nut juice.—*Pl.* אַפְצֵי, עַפְצֵי. Shebu. 41[b] sq. Ms Fl. א׳, ed. ע׳.—V. עֲפַץ.

אַפֵּק (Af. of נפק q. v.) *to bring out, take away.*—לְאַפּוּקֵי *to the exclusion of.* Ned. 41[a]; a. fr.=למעוטי, להוציא, v. מעט, יצא.

אפקוליס, v. אַפִּיקוֹרִין.

אַפְקוּתָא f. (אפק, v. אֲפִיק) *that which branches off the trunk,* 1) *neck.* Targ. Y. Lev. VII, 30(20). Targ. I Sam. IV, 18 Ar. (Var. אפרק׳, פרק׳, פקותא).—2) א׳ דדיקלא *that portion of the palm-tree where the ramification starts* (Oth. opin. *the ramification, upper portion*). Succ. 13[a]. Nidd. 24[a] אַפְקְתָא וכ׳.

אפקימא, v. אַפְסְקִימָא.

אפקלטורין, v. אַפִּיקִילְטָא.

אֲפִקְלִין, v. אוֹפִיקְוְלִין.

אפקסינן, אפקסוון, read אִסְטַקְטוֹן.

אַפְקַעְתָּא f. (פקע) *cancellation of obligations, exceptional legislation.* א׳ דמלכא *a special royal dispensation* (with reference to the suspensions of rights connected with the Sabbath and Yobel years). B. Mets. 106[a]; 109[a].—Ib. 39[a].

אַפְקְרוּתָא (אַפִּיקְרוּתָא) f. (פקר; v. אַפִּיקוֹרוֹס) *making free, irreverence, contempt of the Law and its teachers.* M. Kat. 16[a] לאפיק׳ לאלתר for contempt of the Law excommunication is pronounced forthwith (without warning). Snh. 100[a] מי מיחזי כי אפק׳ Ms. M. (ed. incorr. נמי מיחזור כו׳) does that look like showing irreverence (to one's teacher)? Erub. 63[a] same (with מתחזי for מיחזי). [Snh. l. c. second time כה״ג מיחזור א׳, corr. as above.]

אפקרייתם, v. אַפִּקְרָסִין.

אפקרסו, Treat. Der. Er. X, Ar., read סוּתוֹ . . .; v. אַפִּקְרָסִין.

אַפִּיקַרְסוּת, אַפְקַרְסוּת f. denom. of אַפִּקְרָסִין q. v.

אַפְקַרְסוּתָא f. (v. אפיקורוס)=אַפְקָרוּתָא. Targ. Y. Deut. I, 12.

אַפִּיקְרָסִי׳, אַפְקַרְסִי m. (v. preced.) *of an irreverent, rebellious disposition.* Y. Snh. X, 27[d] bot.

אִיפ׳, אַפִּיקְרִיסִין, אַפִּיקְרָסִין, אַפְקַרְסִין f. pl. (also used as sing. a. m.) (פקר, with format. ס; v. אפיקורוס; cmp. אַבְרָקִין, פַּקְרָסִין, סַבְרִיקִין, סִפְרָקִין, a. אוּנְקְלִי II) *undress, (negligee),* whence *underwear, the garment next to the skin, shirt, bathing* or *night gown, sheet.* Y. Ber. II, 4[c] top אפיק׳ היה וכ׳ he had an undergarment on beneath; cmp. Pesik. R. s. 22.—Pesik. Shek. p. 15[b] sq. אפיקריסין (sing. a. pl.); Lev. R. s. 24; (Ib. s. 2 פרקסין, פקרסין). Y. Pes. VIII, 36[b] top המעביר בא׳ he who carries a skeleton wrapped in sheets; Y. M. Kat. I, 80[d] top.—Ib. III, end, 83[d] אין א׳ מעכבת (Bab. ib. 22[b] אַפִּיקַרְסוּתוֹ) his underwear (shirt) forms no check (but must likewise be rent; diff. in Rashi a. l.). Treat. S'mahoth XII אפיקריסין (Tur Yor. Deah 203 אפרסקא). [Pesik. R. l. c. אפיקריתים, אפיקרייתם corr. acc.]—Deriv. אַפְקַרְסוּת, אַפִּי׳ &c., *underwear.* Ber. 23[b] one may wrap up &c. &c. באפקרסותו Ar. (Ms. M. באפקרי׳, ed. אפרק׳) in his sheet. Nidd. 48[b] נישוף בא׳ is rubbed against their underwear (corset &c.). Hag. 26[a] ואפי׳ נפל א—ו לתוכו Ms. M. (read נפלה, ed. נפל omitted) even if his underwear fell into it, (the vessel remains clean). Mikv. X, 4 הקשר של אפרקסותו שבכתפו Ar. ed. Koh. (ed. שבפרקסים) the knot of one's bathing sheet which is on the shoulder.

*אַפְקַשְׁיָאן, אַפְקַשְׁיוֹן (Ms. M.) pr. n. m. *Afkashion, Afkashian.* Yoma 28[b] (Var. אפקישן).

אַפְקְתָא, v. אַפְקוּתָא.

*אפר, Y. Bicc. II, beg. 64[c] bot. שתין, א׳ חמשים, א׳—. The entire passage is corrupt, and allows no inference that אפר means (=עבר) *to pass, be past.* The text possibly read: אפי׳ (בן) חמשים ועשה דבר שהוא בחיכרת, אפי׳ (בן) ששים ועשה דבר שהוא בְּעון מיתה מת בחיכרת כהא דתני׳ ר׳ חניני׳ וכ׳. [אבל חדי a. אבל רב חדי ibid. (read: אבל רבותי) is a gloss referr. to S'mahoth ch. III.]

אֵפֶר m. (b. h.; √אף, cmp. אבק, אפה) *ashes.* Ohol. II, 2 א׳ שרופים ashes of persons burnt to death (by accident). B. Bath. 60[b]; Taan. II, 1 א׳ מקלה calcined ashes (symbol of mourning, supplication &c.). Y. ib. II, 65[a] אפרו של יצחק the ashes of (the ram substituted for) Isaac. Gen. R. s. 49. Lev. R. s. 36; a. fr.

אֲפַר m. (√פר, cmp. Ges. H. Dict. s. v. פרא) *pasture-ground* (outside of the town), in gen. *meadow.* Bets. V, 7. Pes. 8[b]; a. fr.

אֲפַר, אֶפְרָא I (אֶפְרָה) ch. same. Targ. Y. II Ex. II, 3; 5 (Var. אפרה; Targ. O. יערא). [Y. Sabb. I, 3ᵇ חד אפר, v. חוּתָא.]

אֶפְרָא II, אֶפְרָה (אִיפְרָא) ch.=h. אֵפֶר. Targ. I Chr. XXI, 15 א׳ דעקדת׳ וכ׳ the ashes of Isaac's offering, v. אֵפֶר.—Y. Taan. II, 67ᵃ a foolish son א׳ בעיני וכ׳ is ashes in the eyes of his mother (תוגת by permutation אפרא; v. א״ת).

אַפְרַגְיָא, אַפְרַגְזְיָא, אַפְרַגְסְיָא f. (ἀπραγία, ἀπραξία) *inactivity, cessation of labor, holiday.* Pesik. Sh'mini, p. 195ᵃ (v. Buber note 66 to p. 193ᵃ) if both of us open (sales) at the same time הרי אנו עושין אפרגיא במדינה (Ar. Var. אפרגיגה, אפרגיזא, read אפרגזיא) we shall create a cessation of labor in the district (as all the laboring people will run to the market town on one and the same day; Yalk. Num. 782 זול from misunderstanding); Cant. R. to VII, 2 אפרגיים (read אפרגייא or אפרגסייא). Pesik. R. s. 41 R. Yonathan . . . . . had goods with him והייתה אפרגים (corr. acc.) and there was inactivity and dull business in consequence thereof [for which Yalk. Ps. 758 ולא היה יכול למוכרה—prob. to be read אַפְּרָטוֹס ἄπρατος; *unsaleable*].

אפרגיזא, אפרגיים, אפרגינא, אפרגים, v. preced.

אפרגל Mekh. Yithro 6 מא׳, read, as Yalk. a. l., מאה פ׳, v. פַּרְגּוֹל.

אפרדוכסוס, v. אפרכסוס.

אֶפְרָה 1) *meadow*, v. אֶפֶר; 2) *ashes*, v. אֶפְרָא II.

אפרהנג, v. פרהנג, פַּרְהַנְגְּרָיָא.

אַפְרוֹדִיטֵי f. (Ἀφροδίτη) *Aphrodite*, a Greek goddess (Venus). Ab. Zar. III, 4 מרחץ של א׳ a bath where A. has a statue. Ib. we do not say, the bath has been built נוי לא׳ וכ׳ as an ornament of A., but we say, A. is an ornamental attachment to the bath. Y. Shebi. VIII, end 38ᵇ מזלפין להדא א׳ squirting water (as a libation) to A.

אפרוודין, read:

אַפְרְוָדִין m. pl., אִפְרוֹדָןָ (אִיפְרָוָן) f. pl. (v. פַּרְוָר, פַּרְבַּר, פַּרְוָרָא, פַּרְוִרְלָא) *those appointed over the outworks of a fortress, runners.* Targ. Ezek. IV, 2; XXI, 27 (h. כָּרִים).

אֶפְרוֹחַ m. (b. h. אֶפְרֹחַ; פרח) *brood, young bird.* Bets. 6ᵇ; Tosef. ib. I, 1; a. fr.—Gen. R. s. 37 אתמול א׳ וכ׳ yesterday a chicken, to-day an egg (lost prestige).

אֶפְרוֹחָא ch. same.—*Pl.* אֶפְרוֹחִין Targ. Deut. XXII, 6 (Var. אֶפְרָחִין); a. e.—אֶפְרוֹחַיָּא. Y. Ber. II, 5ᵃ.

אפרומוס, v. אִפְרוּ׳.

אפרוכוס, read אִיפַּרְכוֹס, v. אִיפַּרְכָא.

אַפְרוֹמְבִּיָא f. (φορβεία) *halter.* Tosef. Kel. B. Mets. IV, 6 sq. V. פְּרוֹמְבְּיָא.

אפרופוס, read אפופסים.

אַפְרַזְתָּא, v. אֲרַזְפְּתָא.

אפרחי Y. Sot. III, 18ᶜ bot., v. פֶּרַח.

אַפְרָחִין, v. אֶפְרוֹחָא.

אפרטומות, read with Mus.:

***אַפְּרַטּוֹסוֹת** f. pl. (apparatus) *military engines.* Y. Keth. II, 26ᵈ; (Y. Gitt. III, 45ᵃ top איסטרטיות *camps*).

אַפִּרְיוֹן, אַפִּרְיוֹן m. (b. h.; אַפְּ׳=פריון, על פריון, פֵּר, פוּר; cmp. פְּרִיָּא, פִּיפּוּרָא, אפיפיירות &c.) [*on a frame,*] *frame and hangings of a palanquin, litter of parade,* esp. for a bride in the wedding procession. Sot. IX, 14 (49ᵃ); Tosef. ib. XV, 9.—Sot. 12ᵃ הושיבה בא׳ (Pesik. R. s. 43 בפוריא), a. e. he placed her in the litter, arranged a wedding procession for her. Num. R. s. 20, end, לישב בא׳ to take her seat in the litter (for the wedding procession); a. e.

***אַפְרִיזָא** m. (פרז) [*the leader*], (archit.) *the king-beam, principal.* B. Bath. 6ᵃ.

אַפְרַיְיָא, v. next w.

אַפְרְיָין m. ch.=h. אַפִּרְיוֹן. B. Mets. end א׳ נמטייה לר׳ שמעון ed. (Ar. הבו ליה אפרייא לר״ל, Var. אִיפּוּרְיָיא, איפריייא; Ms. M. אפרין. Ms. H. אפריון, v. Rabb. D. S. a. l. note) let a palanquin be put up for R. Sh., i. e. he deserves a triumphal procession. Cmp. פִּיפּוּרָא.

אֶפְרַיִם (b. h.) pr. n. m. *Ephraim.* 1) son of Joseph, progenitor of the *tribe of Ephraim.* Gen. R. s. 98; a. fr.—2) name of the expected Messiah, also called *the Messiah, son of Joseph,* in contradist. to the Messiah of the tribe of Judah. Pesik. R. s. 36; 37.—3) a disciple of R. Meïr. B. Mets. 87ᵃ; Gen. R. s. 85 א׳ מקשאה E. the disputant.—4) *E. the Scribe, a disciple of Resh Lakish. B. Mets. end (Ms. M. א׳ מקשאה, v. Rabb. D. S. a. l. note).

אַפְרִין, v. אַפְרְיָין.

אַפְרִיקִי I (אַפְרִיקָא) pr. n. pl. (Africa, Ἀφρική) *Africa,* esp. Northern A., the *Africa Propria* or *Vera* of the Romans. Y. Shebi. VI, 36ᶜ bot. the Girgashite הלך לו לא׳ emigrated to Africa (Carthage). Ib. 'a land like your own' (II Kings XVIII, 32) זו א׳ that means A.; Lev. R. s. 17; Deut. R. s. 5.—Snh. 91ᵃ אפריקיא (corr. acc.). Tam. 32ᵃ sq. מדינת א׳; (Lev. R. s. 27; Pesik. Shor p. 74ᵃ קרטיגנא, v. חֹשֶׁךְ). Lam. R. to I, 5. דוכוס דאפריקא Duke (military governor) of A. (Egypt &c.).—Denom. אַפְרִקִיִּים, ch. אַפְרִיקָאֵי *Africans* (Negroes). Sabb. 31ᵃ.—Targ. II Chr. XXI, 16.

אַפְרִיקִי II, אַפְרִיקָא pr. n. pl. (supposed to be) *Phrygia,* in Asia Minor. Targ. Y. Gen. X, 2 (h. text גֹּמֶר);

Gen. R. s. 37, beg.; (Y. Meg. I, 71[b] bot.; Yoma 10[a] גרממיא). [Y. Ber. IX, 13[c] top; R. Hash. 26[a] (of R. Akiba's journeys)—perh. belonging to preced.]

אַפְרְכוֹס, אַפַּרְכָא, v. אִיפְ׳.

***אפרכוריס** pr. n. pl., prob. אֶפִּיקוֹרוֹס=אֶפַּרְכוּרוֹס q. v. Y. Gitt. IV, 46[a] א׳ צריכא if a slave fled to Ep., it is undecided whether he may be extradited; cmp. אנמריס.

אֶפַּרְכְיָא, אֲפַרְכִי, v. אִיפְ׳.

אפרכלי, Sabb. 45[a] ed., v. פַּרְכָּל, פַּרְכִּיל.

אַרְכָּס transpos. of אַרְפְּכָס.

אֲפַרְכֶּסֶת (אֲפַרְכָּס) f. (פרכס q. v.) [the grinder, moving to and back,] *the hopper, grain-receiver* on top of the millstone. Hag. 3[a]; Hull. 89[a] עשה אזנך כאפ׳ (ed. כארפ׳) make thy ear like the hopper to receive the teachings &c.; Y. Kidd. I, end, 61[d] נקב אזנך כאפרכס הזו perforate (make open) thy ear &c.; Pesik. R. s. 10 הירעשה אזנך וכ׳ shake thy ear, like a hopper, to receive &c.

אֲפַרְסְמָא f.=next w. Targ. Y. Ex. XXXV, 28.—Kerith. 5[b]. R. Hash. 23[a]. Ber. 43[a]. Ab. Zar. 28[b] Ms. M. (ed. אספסתא).

אֲפַרְסְמוֹן, אֲפַרְסְמוֹן (אפלסמון) m. (v. פְּרַסֵּם, פְּרַצֵּם; cmp. also בלסם, בַּלְסְמוֹן) 1) *balsamum.* Yoma 38[b] sq. Y. Ab. Zar. III, 42[c] top; a. fr.—Lam. R. to IV, 15 אפל׳.—2) *balsam-tree, balsam-wood.* Ber. 43[a].

פַּרְסְקִין, אֲפַרְסְקִין (אֲפַרְסְקִים) m. pl. (πέρσικα, τά) *peaches.* Maasr. I, 2; a. fr. V. פַּרְסֵק.

אַפַּרְקִיד adv. (v. פרקד) *on the back.* Ber. 13[b]; Nidd. 14[a] גני א׳ lies on his back. B. Bath. 79[a] top.

אַפְרְקָיָא, v. אַפְרִי׳.

אַפַּרְקְסוּת=אַפִּקְרְסוּת. Ber. 23[b]; 24[b] ed.

אַפְרַשׁ, adv., with לְ־ (v. פְּרַשׁ) *for a time to be defined* (in the future), *indefinitely, forever* (h. לָנֶצַח). Targ. Is. LVII, 16; a. fr.

הַפְרָשָׁה, אַפְרָשָׁה f. (פָּרַשׁ) 1) *separation, setting apart for a sacred purpose,* as the heave-offering (T'rumah, for the priest), or a sacrifice (Korban); also *isolation on account of levitical uncleanness,* or *on acc. of sacredness.* Trnsf. *the thing set apart, offering, gift.* Y. Yoma I, beg. 38[a]; Tosef. Parah III (II), 1 זה (ה)אַפְרָשָׁתוֹ בטהרה וכ׳ (Babli Yoma 8[b] פרישתו) the one is isolated for the purpose of purification (because of uncleanness), the other for sanctification (for the services of the Day of Atonement). Y. Dem. VII, 26[b] bot. תלוי בה׳ depends on the act of setting apart. B. Kam. V, 7 הַפְרָשַׁת הר סיני the isolation of Mount Sinai prescribed as preparation for the giving of the Law (Ex. XIX, 13); a. fr.—*Pl.* אַפְרָשׁוֹת, הַפְרָשׁוֹת. Y. Shek. II, 46[d] top שלש א׳ three kinds of sacred gifts.—2) *crossing the Ocean;* cmp. פְּרַשׁ. Gen. R. s. 6 הפרשת וכ׳; Lev. R. s. 25 פָּרָשַׁת.

אַפְרָשׁוּתָא, אַפְרָשׁוּ ch. as foreg. 1). Targ. Ezek. XLV, 1; a. fr.—*Pl.* אַפְרָשְׁוָתָא, constr. אַפְרָשְׁוַת. Targ. O. Num. XVIII, 8; 19 (some ed. אַפְרָשׁוּת sing.).

אֶפְרָתִי m. (perh.=b. h.) *of Ephratha, Ephrathi.* Y. Keth. XII, 35[a] top יוסף א׳; Y. Kil. IX, 32[b] top יוסי א׳; (Gen. R. s. 100 הַפְרָתִי).—*Pl.* אֶפְרָתִים. Ruth R. to I, 2 expl. פלטריאני *courtiers, noblemen.*—Ch. אֶפְרָתִין. Targ. Ruth l. c. א׳ רבנין (in Ms. our w. omitted).

אִיפְשׁ, אֶפֶשׁ, m. (אפש, √אף, cmp. חפץ; corresp. to b. h. נֶפֶשׁ, v. Jer. XV, 1) *desire, pleasure;* [only with personal pron. as suffix]. Naz. IV, 5 אי אֶפְשִׁי וכ׳ I will not live with an offensive woman. Keth. XII, 3 אי א׳ לזוז וכ׳ I cannot leave my husband's house. Y. Yoma VII, 45[b] bot. אי א׳ שיכפר וכ׳ I do not want the Day of Atonement to bring me forgiveness. Y. Yeb. XIII, beg. 13[b] א׳ בנישואיך I am willing to marry thee. Num. R. s. 13 (alluding to Gen. III, 22) אמר אדם אי א׳ said Adam, I cannot (do penitence). Said the Lord, 'And now',—said Adam 'pen', 'by no means', 'I will not'. Y. Keth. VII, 31[b] bot. אי א׳ אשה (read באשה). Y. Pes. VIII, 35[d] bot. א׳ שתמנה (read אי א׳). Y. Gitt. VI, 1; a. fr. Gen. R. s. 38 אי אֶפְשֵׁנוּ וכ׳ we desire neither him nor his divine protection.

אַפְשָׁה, v. פַּשָּׁה.

אפשלתה, v. אַשְׁפָּלָה.

אֶפְשַׁר, אִיפְשַׁר (אֶוְשַׁר) m. (פשר) *division, space between, alternative,* whence *possibility; it is possible.* Targ. Job XIV, 14; a. fr.—Hull. 11[b] היכא דא׳ א׳ where it is possible (to ascertain facts), it is possible (we must do), but where it is impossible &c. Yeb. 61[b] sq. אין דנין א׳ משאי א׳ we cannot form an analogy between a case where there is an alternative and one where there is none. Sabb. 129[a] לא א׳ ליה he has no means. Y. Sot. VII, 21[c] bot. אי א׳ לומר you cannot say. Taan. 3[b] אי א׳ לעולם וכ׳ the world cannot exist without &c; a. fr.

***אַפְתָּא I** m. *bread.* Ber. 40[b] quot. in Ar., prob. from misreading ריפתא; v. Rabb. D. S. a. l. Ms. M.

אַפְתָּא II f. (פתי) *extension, width,* whence 1) (archit.) *a chamber* or *wing projecting from a building* (with stairs from outside), *balcony-chamber.* B. Bath. 61[a] (explain. יציע). Hull. 92[a] ב״כ דתותי א׳ a synagogue named 'under the balcony'.—2) (bot.) *stole, tuber.* Lam. R. to I, 16, end כהדא א׳ דקרא וכ׳ like that tuber of cabbage, the larger the latter grows, the smaller gets the former.—3) pl. אַפְתֵּי, only with רַמְשָׁא, *spreading of night, nightfall.* Y. Ab. Zar. I, beg. 39[a]. Y. Bath. II, end, 13[c]. Lev. R. s. 25; Koh. R. to II, 20.—באׄ ר׳=בפתי רמשא. Y. Ab. Zar. l. c.; Gen. R. s. 78.

אפתיסיס, v. אִיפּוּתוֹרוֹס.

אַפְתַּנְמִין, v. אֶוּתְּנְמָר.

***הַפְתְּקָא, אַפְתְּקָא** m. (פתק, cmp. הֶפְתֵּק) *ladle with which provision is dealt out.* Snh. 39[a] מחא ביה בא׳

(Rashi באפתקיה, Ms. M. מחייה בחפתקיה) he (the servant) warned him (Ms. M. struck him) with his ladle; (Rashi: struck him on his *neck* (!), v. אַפְקוּתָא).

אַפְּתְּרִין Targ. Y. I Num. XIII, 21 Ar., v. פְּתְרָן.

אִצָּא, v. אִירְצָא I.

אֶצְבַּע f. (b. h.;=עצבע; עצב, צבע, √צב, cmp. Job X, 8; cmp. טבע a. טבעת) 1) *finger, esp. index-finger.* Men. 11ª זו א׳ with this (the fourth from the little finger) the measure of 'a finger' is taken; Keth. 5ᵇ. Y. Taan. IV, 68ᵈ bot.; Lam. R. to II, 2 מקוטעי א׳ (מטיפי) who had their finger cut off (in evidence of devotion to the cause). Yoma I, 7 א׳ צרדה; Tosef. ib. 9 explained א׳ גדולה *middle finger;* cmp. Tanh. Bo, end, expl. אמצעית.—Keth. 71ª הוא נותן א׳ וכ׳ he (the husband) puts his finger between her teeth (and must expect to be bitten), i. e. has to take the consequences of not interfering with her vow in due time.—2) *any projecting limb resembling the shape of a finger.* Hull. 61ª א׳ יתירה *the projecting toe* on a bird's claw. Tam. IV, 3 (31ª) א׳ הכבד the *lobe* of the liver.—Fig. (like יד) *share, part.* Y. Pes. IV, 31ª top; Y. Ab. Zar. I, 40ª top, v. אֶמְצַע.—*Pl.* אֶצְבָּעוֹת. Hag. 15ª; a. fr. (mostly in the sense of *finger's length*).—Pes. 112ᵇ; Nidd. 66ª euphem. for *membra virilia.*—*Dual* אֶצְבְּעַיִים, אֶצְבָּעַיִם. Cant. R. to VIII, 11 גידם א׳ one whose (index) fingers were lopped (stump-like). Ib. that whole trade of mine אינה נקנית אלא בא׳ cannot be acquired except by learning how to use the index-fingers.—Pes. 109ª, a. e. *two finger lengths.*

אֶצְבְּעָא, אֶצְבַּע ch. same. Targ. Ex. XXXI, 18; a. e. —*Pl.* אֶצְבְּעָתָא. Targ. Y. Gen. I, 7; a. fr. Targ. Ps. VIII, 4 אצבעותך. Ned. 49ᵇ באצבעתיה with his fingers. Erub. 53ª we are כי א׳ בקירא לסברא (Ar. אוצבתא) as to reasoning like fingers on wax (hard to be impressed upon), ולשכחה וכ׳ but as to forgetfulness like fingers put in seed (leaving no trace), v. בִּזְרָא; a. fr.

אֶצְבְּעִי m. *of a finger's length, dwarf of the smallest size.* Bekh. 45ᵇ.

אצבעתא, v. אֶצְבְּעָא.

***אִצְבָּתִי** f. (v. צבת, cmp. אצבע) *tongs, snuffers.* Ohol. XIII, 4 (Var. אַסְפָּתִי); Tosef. ib. XIV, 4 לְאִירְצַבְּתוֹ, ed. Zuck. (Var. ולא לצבתו) and for the snuffers belonging to it (the candlestick).

אֲצוֹי Ar., v. אֲצַוְותָא.

אִצְוָא, v. next w.

אִצְוָא f., pl. אִצְוָתָא, אֲצַוְותָא (צור, cmp. צבר a. סבב) *creeper, vine.* Pes. 39ª (expl. חרחבינה) אצווא דדיקלא Ar. (ed. אִצְוָתָא, Ms. M. אסיתא, read אַסְוָתָא, R. Han. אַסָּא, v. Rabb. D. S. a. l. note); Keth. 50ª אִצְוָתָא. Erub. 26ᵇ אצוותא חרוזייתא דדיקלא Ar. (ed. דדיקלא omitted, also in Ms. M., cmp. Rabb. D. S. a. l. note) *arkablin* are the prickling creepers of the palm-tree; v. חִרְזָא. V. אִצְוָותָא.

אֲצָוְחוּתָא, אֲצַוְחָתָא f. (צוח) *cry, noise.* Targ. Ezek. VII, 14.

אֲצוּתָא, אֲצְוָתָא, אֲצַוְותָא f. (אצר, √אץ, cmp. חצב a. denom., a. אֲסִיתָא) *trough, kneading trough;* also *a trough-full, the quantity of bread baked at a time, batch.* Targ. Deut. XXVIII, 5; a. e. (also as plur.) Targ. Ex. VII, 28; a. e.— Pesik. B'shall. p. 91ª כל א׳ וכ׳ the entire batch of bread. Ib.ᵇ (correct acc. to Buber note 198; Var. Ar. אַצְוֵי, אַסְוָתָא, v. Koh. Ar. Compl. s. v.). Cmp. אַצִּיצָא. V. אַצְוָוא.

אֲצְוְחוּתָא, אֲצַוְחָתָא, v. אֲצָוְחָ׳.

אֲצַוְתָא, v. אַצְוָא a. אֲצְוָתָא.

אִצְט־, for words not found here, v. sub אִסְט׳, אִסְט׳ or אִיצְט׳.

אִצְטְדִיָא m. (צדי) 1) *destruction.* Targ. Prov. XVII, 14 (h. text התגלע; for אבטר ib. read אֶטְרֵשׁ, v. נטש).—2) (cacophem.) *theatre, arena;* prevailing vers. אִצְטַדְיָא q. v.

אִצְטְדִינִין, אִצְטְדִין as preced. 2); v. אִצְטְרִין.

אצמלוס, v. next w.

***אִצְטְלוּת** f. (טלל, v. אִסְטְלִית) *covering, lining of a shoe.* Tosef. Kel. B. Bath. IV, 6 שניטל האונטלית שבו ed. Zuck. (R. S. to Kel. XXVI, 4 שניטלו האונטלים; Var. ed. Zuck. האצטלו׳; ed. האצטלים) read שניטלה א׳ the lining of which is off.; v. זרב.

אצמרא, v. אִצְטְרָיָא.

אצטרבאמוטא, v. אִסְטְרוֹפּוֹמְטָא.

אִיס׳, אִיצ׳, אִצְטַרְיָא, אִצְטַרְיָה, אִצְטְרִיָא f. (סרר, cmp. אסטרניא, אצטרניא P. Sm. 304 a. quot. ibid.; cmp. אֲבֵידָן) *place of debauchery,* an opprobrious name for the *theatres, arenas* &c. of the Romans, and a phonetic perversion of *theatrum,* θέατρον. Ab. Zar. I, 7 (16ª) you must not build .... גרדום אצטדריא וכ׳ (Ms. M. אצטריבא, prob. אצטרינא, v. supra; in Gem. 18ᵇ repeatedly אצטר׳, Mishn. Nap. אצטדריא, in comment. ib. אצטרדיא), expl. ib. 16ᵇ בסילקי של גרדום וכ׳ a building for public execution (court) or for public entertainment (amphitheatre &c.)—*Pl.* אִסְטְרִיּוֹת. Sifra Ahare IX, 13. [Men. 103ᵇ אסטריא של מלך royal amphitheatre(?), v. אסטריא.] [Tanh. B'resh. 2 אִסְטְרָטָאוֹת, Var. אִסְטְרָאוֹת *theatres.*] Ab. Zar. 18ᵇ לא הלך לאיסטרטאות Ms. M. (ed. טַרְטְיָאוֹת q. v; En Yak. תרט׳). [For the vers. אִצְטַדְיָא v. s. v.]

אִיס׳, אִיצ׳, אִסְטְרִין, אִצְטְרִין [אִיצְטַדִּין, v. preced. end] f. (prop. pl. of אצטרא, אסטרא, v. preced., used as sing.) same. B. Kam. IV, 4 (39ª) שור האיצטרין Ms. M. (ed. אצטדין, Ms. H. a. R. a. Mish. Nap. אסטדין, Y. ed. איסטדין) an ox of the arena (that killed a person). Tosef. Ab. Zar. II, 7 היושב באסטרין וכ׳ Var. (ed. Zuck. איסטרטון, ed. איסטרין) he who attends the arena as a spectator is like a murderer (countenancing bloodshed); Y. ib. I, 40ª היושב באיצטדין (interchanging with תיאטרון theatrum). *Pl.*

אִצְטְרְדִינִין &c. Ab. Zar. 18[b] אין הולכין לא׳ מפני ש״ד Ms. M. (ed. לאצטדינין מפני מושב לצים . ., v. Rabb. D. S. a. l. note) you must not go to the arenas on account of bloodshed (ed. to theatres on account of 'scorners' seat', Ps. I, 1). Ib. Ms. M. repeat. אִצְטְרְדִין, cmp. אֲבִידָן. Tosef. l. c. 6 לאיצטרטירנין (Var. לצטרדיונין, לצטרריונין); 7 לאיצטרריונין (Var. לטרריונין, לצטרריונין), cmp. טַרְטְיָאוֹת.

אִצְטְרְכַיָּא m. pl. (צרך) *travelling necessaries, provision.* Gen. R. s. 60. Koh. R. to XI, 1.

אצטרמיטה, v. אִסְטְרוֹפוֹמְטָא.

אִצְוָא, אִיצְוָא, אִיצְ׳, אוּצְ׳ f. (אצר, v. אַצְוְתָא) *cut, depression,* (agric.) *bed* as a measure, *row.*—*Pl.* אִצְיָיתָא, אִצְיָאתָא, אוּצְ׳, אִיצְ׳. B. Bath. 12[a] תלת א׳ וכ׳ (Ms. M. אִיצְ׳, Ms. F. איתירתא(?)) three rows containing twelve vine-trees each; (v. Rabb. D. S. a. l. note). Ib. 41[b] he encroached on his neighbor's ground תרתי או׳ ed. (Mss. א׳) two *bed-widths.*

אַצִּיל m. (b. h.; אצל or נצל, cmp. צלע) *the joint which touches the rib, elbow* (with or without יד). Arakh. 19[b] עד הא׳ up to the elbow.—*Pl* אַצִּילִים, constr. אַצִּילֵי. Zeb. 19[a] top כנגד א׳ וכ׳ corresponding to the elbows (where the elbow in natural position touches the body). Y. Yoma V, 42[b] bot.; a. fr.—(Chald.) Lev. R. s. 8, beg. ודין אצילים פריך some ed. (read אַצִּילֵיה) and the other has his elbow (arm) broken.

***אֲצִיפָא, אַצְפָא** m. (v. צִיפָא) *matting* used for bailing dates, cmp. זוּהֲלָא. [Oth. opin: *the flesh sticking to the stone* of half-ripe dates.] Gitt. 89[a] a woman was betrothed בא׳ דהוהלא (Ar. אצפא) with &c. (an object of no value).

אִצִּיצָא, אֲצִיצָא, עֲצִיצָא m. (אצץ, cmp. אַצְוְוֹתָא) *a common bellied vessel.* B. Bath. 144[a] אפי׳ א׳ דהרסנא Ms. (ed. ע׳) even a pot in which fish-hash is kept. Meg. 16[a] א׳ דבית הכסא Ar. (ed. ע׳, Ms. O. עכסים) night-chamber. [Targ. Esth. V, 1 דיעא עֲצִיצָא, read דְּעַ׳ . . . of the night-chamber.] Hebr. עָצִיץ.

***אציתין,** Targ. Koh. XII, 11 a gloss of אנצין, missing in ed. Buxt. a. oth.; v. אֲנָץ.

אֲצַל ($\sqrt{}$צל, v. נצל) *to protect, spare, exempt from taxes.* B. Bath. 55[a], v. אַנְדִּיסְקֵי.—[Bets. 14[a] אצלי, v. צלי.]

אָצֵל or **אָצַל** (b. h.) pr. n. m. *Atsel, Atsal,* mentioned I Chron. VIII, 37 sq.; IX, 43 sq. Pes. 62[b] בין א׳ לא׳ וכ׳ (Ms. . . . מן א׳, v. Rabb. D. S. a. l. note, for var. lect.) the explanation of the repetition of I Chr. VIII, 29 to 38, and IX, 35 to 44 and the verbal discrepancies between the two records would load four hundred camels with discussion; cmp. Rashi to I Chr. l. c.

אֵצֶל (b. h.; $\sqrt{}$צל, v. צלל, צלע) *by the side of, near, with.* B. Mets. V, 1 הרי אֶצְלִי בהן יין thou hast wine with me instead, i. e. I owe thee &c. Ib. 85[b] א׳ מי אתה תקוע by whose side art thou lodged (in the world to come)?; Koh. R. to IX, 10; a. fr.

אַצְלָחוּתָא f. (צלח) *success, prosperity.* Targ. Is. XXXIII, 20; a. e.

אַצְלִי, v. צְלֵי.

אֶצְעָדָה f. (b. h.; צעד) *clasp* or *brooch* for fastening dresses on going out, in Talm. *knee-band*; v. בִּירִית. Sabb. 63[b] בירית זו א׳ what the Mishnah calls *birith* is the Biblical *etsadah*; modified ibid. בירית תחת א׳ וכ׳ *birith* has the function of the *etsadah* (Rashi: *birith* around the knee serves the same purpose as *etsadah* on the shoulder, to save inconvenience in walking).

***אֲצָפָא** or **אַצְפָּא** m. (אצא, v. יָצָא) *trouble, labor.* Targ. Prov. XIV, 23 בכל מן דא׳ לך (h. text עצב) in whatever is a trouble to thee.

אַצְפָּא, v. אֲצִיפָא.

אָצַר (b. h.; sec. r. of צור, cmp. אסר) *to lock up, hoard, gather*; cmp. גָּנַז. B. Bath. 90[b] אוֹצְרֵי פירות those who store up fruit (for speculation). Ib. אין אוֹצְרִין וכ׳; Tosef. Ab. Zar. IV (V), 1 (אצר a. עצר used promiscuously) you must not hoard up (for speculation) such things as are necessaries of life; [correct אין א׳ דברים שיש . . . . כגון יינות שמנים וסלתות ופירות]. Ib. לֶאֱצוֹר (Tosef. לאצר *Pi.*). Ib. לא יְאַצֵּר *Pi.* (Tosef. ולא יַעֲצוֹר, read לא; Var. לא יאציר). Gen. R. s. 45 end (play on נבוכד־אצר) שֶׁאֲצָרָן וכ׳ he locked them up in the desert &c.—Y. Dem. VI, end, 26[a]; Tosef. ib. VI, 4; Ab. Zar. 71[a] אוצר (מוֹצֵר) *government's store-collector, commissary* (apothecarius), or read אוֹצָר q. v.

Pi. אִיצֵּר, *Hif.* הֶאֱצִיר, v. supra.

אֲצַר I, אָצַר ch. same. *Targ. O. Gen. XLI, 35 ויצרון, Var. ויוצרון, ויצרון). B. Bath. 90[b] פוק אצר לי וכ׳ (prob. אַצַּר *Pa.*) go out and buy up for me for storage &c.

Ithpa. אִתְאַצַּר, *Ithpe.* אִתְאֲצַר *to be stored up.* Targ. Is. XXIII, 18.

אַצָּר w. (preced.) אצר פירי *speculator in provision.* Yoma 83[a]; B. Bath. 90[b].

אֲצַר II m. (preced.) *contraction* (h. עֹצֶר). Bekh. 21[b] א׳ חיותא contraction of the womb (and consequent destruction of the fœtus).

אצרות, א׳ רוח, read אוֹצְרוֹת רוּחַ (v. אוֹצָר) *stores of wind,* name of the cavities in the *pearl-shell* in which the pearls are seated, and which contain a kali; v. אַשְׁלָגָא. Y. Sabb. IX, end, 12[b] top.

אַקְהָא, v. אַקְוָוא.

אַקְהָיוּתָא f. (קהי) *bluntness* or *looseness* of teeth. Targ. Amos IV, 6 (h. text נקיון וכ׳) אקהיות שנין=*perplexity.* Cmp. אַקְוָוא.

***אַקְקוּבִּטוֹן, אַקּוּבִּיטוֹן,** m. (accubitum, ἀκκούβιτον) *dining couch* of the Roman nobility of the imperial period in place of the older triclinium. Lev. R.

s. 7 מיסב על א׳ וכ׳ (Pesik. Eth. Korb. p. 61ª הקוביטין; Yalk. Num. 777 איק׳; ib. Lev. 479 קוב׳, קנב׳; ib. Ps. 791 הנני׳ &c., corr. acc.; Pesik. R. s. 16, p. 83ᵇ ed. Fr. הקובטין) reclining on his accubitum.—לחם א׳, or ריפתא (ד)א׳ *bread used at the meals of the nobility, fine bread.* Targ. Y. II Gen. XL, 16 ריפתא קקבטון (read ריפתא דאקקובטון) bread of the nobles (h. text חרי). Pesik. R. l. c. p. 82ª (ref. to לחם הפחה Neh. V, 18) חקקבטין sub. לחם; Pesik. l. c. p. 59ª קקבטון (corr. acc.).

אקובנאה, B. Bath. 73ª bot. Ar., v. קוּפָא a. קוּבְּנָאָה; cmp. אֲקוּנְבֵּי.

אַקְהָא, אֲקָוָא f. (קהי) *what blunts or loosens the teeth, weakening;* fig. (v. Mekh. Bo 18, end) *refutation, arguments. Pl.* אַקְוָיָתָא. Yeb. 110ᵇ יתבי וקמקוו א׳ (Rashi Var. מקהו אַקְהָתָא) they were sitting and raising arguments. Cmp. אַקְהָיוּתָא.

אקומוניס, v. אִיקוֹנוֹמוֹס.

אָקוֹן m. (deriv. of קנה, v. אקן) 1) *reed-basket,* used as a *fisher's cauf.* Kel. XII, 2; XXIII, 5.—2) v. אֲקַן.

אִקוֹנָא, v. איק׳.

אֲקוּנְבֵּי f. (קבב, with נ inserted; Mand. קומבא, Nöld. Mand. Gr. p. 105) *cupola, arched vessel. Pl.* אֲקוּנְבְיָאוֹת. Tosef. Kel. B. Mets. II, 8 א׳ שבמגדלים ed. Zuck. (Var. אקובנ׳, cmp. קובנאה) cupolas on turrets (a piece of house furniture), ornamental vases.

***אָקוּנָס**, a corruption of קוֹלְיָיס m. (κολίας) *colias,* name of a small fish. Ab. Zar. 39ª; Ḥull. 66ᵇ top; Tosef. Ḥull. III (IV), 27 קוליים.

אַקוּפֵּי m. pl. (קָה, נקה) *curlings of the web, anything sticking out of the web* (threads, knots &c.). Sabb. 75ᵇ האי מאן דשקיל א׳ וכ׳ whoever takes threads out of clothes on the Sabbath, is guilty of an act of finishing; v. פַּטְּרֵשׁ. Cmp. אַקְפּוּתָא.

אקופיא, v. קופיא.

אקורפיטא, v. אַקְרַפְטָא.

אֲקוּרְקַרְתָא, v. אַקְרוֹקְתָא.

אֲקוּשָׁא m. (קשי) *hard, hard-baked.* Targ. Y. Lev. XX, 10.—Keth. 39ᵇ. Sot. 4ᵇ, opp. רכיכא. Sabb. 65ª כל חרובין א׳ מידי א׳ anything hard.—*Pl.* אֲקוּשֵׁי. Sabb. 155ª ed. (Ms. M. דאשוני, Ar. דאשרנא).—Targ. Ps. LVIII, 10 אֲקוֹשָׁן (some ed. אַקְשׁוּן).

אַקְטוֹר (אוקטור) m. (actor) *actor publicus,* an officer who had the supervision of slaves and state property.—*Pl.* אַקְטוֹרִין. Mekh. B'shall. Par. 1; Yalk. Ex. 230 אוּ׳.—Targ. Y. Ex. XIV, 5 אוֹקְטְרַיָּא.

קְטִיסְפוֹן, אַקְטִיסְפוֹן pr. n. pl. *Ctesiphon,* a town on the Eastern bank of the Tigris. Targ. Y. Gen. X, 10 ק׳ (for Bibl. *Kalneh*). Yoma 10ª (for Bibl. *Resen*) זו א׳ (Ms. זו אקטספון; Var. קטרספון; טיספוס). Gitt. 6ª. Erub. 57ᵇ אקיסט׳ (corr. acc.; Ms. M. קטר׳; v. Rabb. D. S. a. l. note).

אַקְטַרְתָא f. (קטר) *whatever raises dense smoke when ignited,* hence *roots, twigs* &c. Taan. 24ᵇ bot. ושדייא א׳ (Ms. M. adds בתנורא; v. Rabb. D. S. a. l.) she used to throw twigs into the stove (to make people believe she was baking).

אקי, read: אִיקֵי (εἶκε) *make room!* Y'lamd. to Deut. XI, 22 quot. in Ar. (v. Tanḥ. Ekeb, 4); cmp. Midr. Till. to Ps. XVII.

אקיוס, v. אַקְסִיוֹס.

אֲקִילוֹס (Var. עֲקִילוֹס), pr. n. m. *Akilos* (prob. identic with עקילס q. v.). Gen. R. s. 1 R. Yudan relates בשם א׳.

אקיסטפון, v. אַקְטִיסְפוֹן.

אקיקא, v. אַקְקָיָא.

אַקְלֵד, v. אַקְלִידָא a. קְלֵד.

אַקְלִיבוּסְתָא, v. קְלִיבוֹסֶת.

אַקְלִידָא f. (κλεῖς-δός) *key, lock, fastening.* Sabb. 89ᵇ כבא דא׳ (Ar. s. v. קלד: בבא, Var., v. Rabb. D. S. a. l. note 400) the tooth of the key, *key-bit* (Ar. *'the key-gate'*); Men. 57ª; a. e.—Fig. א׳ דמטרא the key (to the store) of rain; א׳ דת״המ the key (to the gate) of resurrection. Snh. 113ª (Var. קלידא, מפתחא; v. Rabb. D. S. a. l. note 30).—*Pl.* אַקְלִידַיָּא, אַקְלִידֵי. Targ. I Chr. IX, 27.—Gitt. 56ª; a. fr.—Denom. אַקְלֵד, v. קְלֵד.

אקלנדס, read קאלנדס, v. קַלֶּנְדָּא.

אִקְלַס Ithpe. of קְלַס.

אַקְלְפְרִין m. pl. (aquilIferi) *eagle-bearers, bearers of the imperial standard.* Midr. Till. to Ps. XLV (some ed. אלק׳ corr. acc.).

אקמינון, אקמנין Lev. R. s. 34 א׳ פרנסין, read אוקמינון, v. קום.

***אַקְמְתָא** f. (עקם=אקם, cmp. עכביש, עכביתא; Syr. אמקתא?, v. P. Sm. 243) *spider.* Targ. Prov. XXX, 28.

אֲקַן (deriv. of קני) *to grow in stalks, produce stalks* Gitt. 30ª לא צריכא דאקון (Var. דהדר ואקון) in the case before us it means that the seeds which had been despaired off produced stalks (blades) again מהו דתימא אֲקָנְתָא מילתא וכ׳ when you might think this shooting up is *something* (enough to awaken new hopes of recovery), therefore &c.; Taan. 19ª.—Denom. אֲקָנְתָא *growth of stalks;* v. supra.

אקנוס, v. אִיקְנוֹס a. אַקְסִיוֹס.

אַקְנָאתָא, v. אַקְנָיְתָא.

***אַקְנָיוּתָא** f. (קני II) *being provoked.* Targ. I Sam. I, 16 (v. ib. v. 6).

אַקְנָיְיתָא, אַקְנָיָאתָא ch. pl., הַקְנָאָה h. f. (קני I) *giving possession*, whence שְׁטָרֵי אַ׳ or שְׁטַר ה׳ *an agreement by which one's landed estate is mortgaged in the form of a sale from date*, independent of the loan to be consummated afterwards, so that at a certain date the creditor can claim the property, even if sold in the meantime, by referring to the priority of his purchase; *deed of transfer* (v. Bloch Civil-Process, p. 54, notes 5 a. 6 a. quot. ib.). B. Mets. 13[a]; 14[a]; 16[b]. B. Bath. 172[a] שטרא אקניאתא (שטרי, Ms. M. *ib.* a. B. Mets. 16[b] אקנייתא without שטר׳).—אַקְנָיְיתָא בְּמָנֵי *transfers*, or *sales by symbolic delivery*, v. מָנָא; whence *Aknayatha B'manê*, adaptation of the name of *a Babylonian festive time and fair* (cmp. יְרִיד). Ab. Zar. 11[b] Ms. M. a. oth. (ed. אקניתא בחנוני, Var. אקניתיה); [cmp. Y. ib. I, 39[c] where our w. seems to be rendered כנוני].

אקניתא, v. preced.

אקנקיתא, אקניקתא, v. אֲנַנְקָתָא.

אַקְסִיגָרוֹן, v. אַכְסִיגָ׳.

אכסיוס, אַקְסִיוֹס m. (ἄξιος) *worthy, adequate.* Gen. R. s. 46 '*I am God Shadday*' (Gen. XVII, 1) is translated by Aquila אקווס ואקנוס Ar. (ed. אכסיוס, אכסיוט, corr. acc.) ἄξιος and (καὶ) ἵκανος, adequate and sufficient (competent); cmp. ibid. דיידך וכ׳ it is sufficient for thee that I am thy protector.

אַקְסִיל, v. next w.

***אַקְסִילַאלִיאָיין** f. pl. (ξυλαλόη=ἀγάλλοχον) *pieces of bitter aloë-wood.* Targ. Ps. XLV, 9 Ar. (ed. אַקְסִיל אַלוֹאוֹן combine) (h. text אֲהָלוֹת).

הַקְפָּדָה, אַקְפָּדָה f. (קפד, Hif.) *getting excited, ebullition of temper, rashness.* Num. R. s. 10; Y. Ned. I, 36[d] bot. they make the vow of a nazir (ה׳) מיתוך א׳ inconsiderately. Y. Ab. Zar. IV, 44[a]. Tosef. Gitt. VII (V), 6 (opp. ברצון). Y. Naz. I, end, 51[c] הקפדן, read: דָּהָן . . .

אַקְפּוּתָא f. (קה, נקה) *curling the hair.* Targ. Is. III, 24. Cmp. אַקּוּפֵי.

אקקבטון, אקקוביטון, v. אַקּוּבִּיטוֹן.

***אַקַקְיָא** f. (ἀκακία) *the thorny acacia.* Gitt. 69[b] Ar. (ed. אקיקא, corr. acc.).

אַקְרָא f. (dialect. for חַקְרָא in Yer. dial. q. v.; cmp. var. lect. bel.) *fort*, designation of various, mostly Babyl. places. Meg. 6[a] א׳ דתולבקני (Ms. Oxf., L., F. עקרא; v. Rabb. D. S. a. l. note); Kidd. 71[b], v. תולבקני. [Rashi: *fortified ford.*] B. Bath. 127[a], Kidd. 72[a], v. אַגְמָא. B. Mets. 86[a] מא׳ לאגמא from Fort (Agma) to Agma (Var. lect. v. Rabb. D. S. a. l.). B. Bath. 73[b], v. הגרוניא. Macc. 10[a], v. סְלִיקוֹס; a. fr. [The Gr. ἄκρα, orig. *summit*, is a phonetic coincidence.]

אֶקְרַאי m. (קרא, קרה; h. מִקְרֶה) *accidental, chance.* R. Hash. 29[b] בית דינא דא׳ improvized court. Snh. 25[b], a. fr. בעלמא א׳ a mere chance.

אקרופיטא, v. אַקְרַפְטָא.

אַקְרוּקְתָּא f. (קרקר) [*croaker,*] *frog.* B. Bath. 73[b] א׳ (Var. אקורקרתא, &c., v. Rabb. D. S. a. l. note 3) דהויא כי וכ׳ a frog as big as Fort Hag. (others read בי, a frog which was in Fort H.). Ned. 41[a] עקרבא דיתיבא על א׳ ועברה נהרא (corr. ed. acc.) a scorpion sitting on a frog and crossing the river.

אקרפיטא, קְרַפִּיטָא, אַקְרַפְטָא, קְרַפְטָא m. (κράβατος, grabatus) *couch, raised upholstered seat.* M. Kat. 10[b] למבני א׳ Ar. (ed. אקרפיטא, Ms. M. אקרפיטרא) to build up a raised seat (on a frame). [Rashi: אקרופיטא *crib.*] Kidd. 70[a] ליתיב מר אקר׳ sit down, Sir, on the couch; (cmp. אִיצְטְבָא, the Chald. equivalent of our w.).

אָרָא *to treat, argue*, v. ארי.

ארא *fowler*, v. אָרָא IV.

***ארא, ארא׳** (Ms. M. נירי׳; Ar. s. v. פלמודא: פרא or פרא) name of a *fish* or *fish-brine*; perh. אֲרָאיָא (*Raia*) *ray* or *skate.* Ab. Zar. 40[a].

אֶרְאֵל m. (b. h., Is. XXXIII, 7,=אלאל, v. אלל, cmp. אמרכל) *messenger*, esp. (in poetry) *angel.* *Pl.* אֶרְאֵלִים. Keth. 104[a] א׳ ומצוקים וכ׳ the Erelim (angels) and the mortals seized the holy ark (strove for the soul of R. Judah); Y. Kil. IX, 32[b] top וא׳ יצוקים; Y. Keth. XII, 35[a]; Koh. R. to VII, 11; IX, 10; v. יָצַק, מָצַק.

אראני, v. אֲרוֹנִי.

אָרַב (b. h.; √אר, v. ארר, cmp. ארג) 1) *to press into holes, to make holes; to weave; join.* 2) *to look through a hole, to espy, lurk, lie in wait.* B. Kam. 44[b], a. e. (ref. to Deut. XIX, 11) וא׳ לו וכ׳ it says 'And he lurks for *him*' &c., that means the intention to kill *that* man.—Denom. ארבתא, ארבא, ארבא, ארבל׳, אורבא, ארובה.

***אֲרַב** ch. same, part. אָרְבָּא *lurking.* B. Mets. 101[b]; B. Kam. 85[a]; B. Bath. 168[a] thou appearest to me כאריא א׳ like a lurking lion, i. e. I have no confidence in thee.

אַרְבָּא I f. (ארב *to join*, cmp. ארגז, תיבה) *boat.* B. Mets. 101[b] א׳ דחמרא a boat-load of wine; a. fr.—Gitt. 6[a]; Kidd. 72[a] א׳ תניתא וכ׳ Ar. ed. Koh. (ed. תניינא) to the second boat of the (floating) bridge; cmp. Kidd. l. c. והאידנא וכ׳ 'and now the Persians placed the bridge higher up'. [Oth. opin., v. אַרְבְּתָא.]—*Pl.* אַרְבֵּי. B. Mets. 72[b] וא׳.... חיטי the wheat in granaries and ships.

***אַרְבָּא II** f. *a small silver vessel in the shape of a trough* (=עֲרֵיבָה Ar.) B. Bath. 34[b] (Comm.: *ship*).

אַרְבָּא *layer, mesh*, v. אוּרְבָּא.

אָרְבָּא *lurking*, v. אֲרַב.

אַרְבָּאֵי m. pl. *Arabs.* Targ. II Chr. XVII, 11 (ed. Beck; oth. עַרְבָּאֵי).

אַרְבֶּה I m. (b. h.; רבי) *locust* (also collect.). Ex. R. s. 13; a. fr. V. כּוֹבֵשׁ.

אַרְבֶּה II, v. חַרְבָּה.

***אַרְבּוּנָא** m. (ארב, cmp. ערב) *confounding of colors, thickness,* whence *feeble sight.* Pes. 111^b the following three things יהדבי א׳ וכ׳ (Ms. Oxf. עוורונא; Ms. M. v. Rabb. D. S. a. l.) cause defective eye-sight.

אַרְבֵּילָא, v. אַרְבְּלָא.

אַרְבֵּיסַר, v. אַרְבָּעָה end.

אַרְבֵּל I pr. n. pl. *Arbel, Arbela,* in Galilee, near Zepphoris. Y. Ber. I, 2^c בקעת א׳ the Valley of Ar.; Y. Taan. IV, 69^b ארכל (corr. acc.). Y. Shebi. VI, 36^d bot. Koh. R. to I, 18 coarse linen הבאין מא׳ coming from A.; a. e.

אַרְבֵּל II (רְבַל) (denomin. of next w., v. עַרְבֵּל) *to sift, shake.* B. Mets. 26^b דאייתי ארבלא וּמְאַרְבֵּל Ar. (Ms. R. 2 מארביל, ed. מְרַבֵּל וקא מארבל=) that he brought a sieve and sifted the sand. Snh. 39^a וקמרבלינהו Ms. M. (ed. Sonc. וקא מא׳ להו, oth. ed. מהדר להו) and shook them.

Ithpe. אִירְבֵּל (=איתארבל) *to be shaken.* Hull. 49^a מירבל חוא דרביל it was shaken down (by the movements of the animal). [Targ. עַרְבֵּל.]

אַרְבְּלָא, אַרְבֵּילָא, עַרְבְּלָא m. (ארב, cmp. אֲרוּבָּה) *net work, sieve.* B. Mets. 26^b; Snh. 39^a, v. preced.—Macc. 20^b בארבילא (Ms. M. בארבי); Snh. 89^b אכ״ל תמרא בא׳ ate dates out of the sieve, i. e. did a harmless thing.—Targ. Amos IX, 9 ערבלא.—V. עַרְבְּלָאִין.

אַרְבְּלִי m. (אַרְבֵּל I) *a native or resident of Arbel, Arbelite.* Ab. I, 6.—*Pl.* אַרְבֵּלִיִּין. Gen. R. s. 19, beg.; cmp. Koh. R. to I, 18.—[Tosef. Par. XII (XI), 16 כוש הא׳, v. next w.]—Fem. אַרְבֵּלִית. Y. Peah VII, 20^a bot.; Y. Sot. I, 17^b; IX, 24^b bot. סאה א׳ one S'ah of Arbelite wheat. [Ib. IV, end, 19^d top רבי מר עוקבא הורה בארבלי *Arbeli,* supposed to be a place in Babylon. The entire sentence is spurious both from Mar Ukba's title of Rabbi as well as from comparison with Keth. 60^b.]

אַרְבָּן m. (ארב I) *coarse weft,* opp. to פשתין fine flax woof. Parah XII, 8 כוש של א׳ (Var. רוֹבָן) the spindle used for spinning coarse material; [Tosef. ib. XII (XI) 16 כוש הארבלי the spindle used at Arbel; cmp. Koh. R. to I, 18 s. v. אַרְבֵּל I].

אַרְבָּנָא v. אוּרְבָּנָא.

אַרְבְּסְרָאָה, v. אַרְבָּעָה.

אַרְבַּע *four,* v. אַרְבְּעָא I a. אַרְבָּעָה.

אַרְבְּעָא *couching,* v. אַרְבָּעָה II.

אַרְבָּעָה I m., אַרְבַּע f. (b. h.) *four* (frequently represented by ד׳). Hag. 14^b א׳ נכנסו וכ׳ four men entered into theosophical speculation; a. fr.—Constr. אַרְבַּעַת followed by singul. Y. Ber. I, 2^c אַרְבָּעָה מילין=אַרְבַּעַת מיל; Y. Yoma III, beg. 40^b (cmp. Gen. R. s. 50).—*Pl.* אַרְבָּעִים (מ׳) *forty.* Sabb. VII, 2 א׳ חסר אחת thirty nine.—Macc. I, 1, a. fr. לוקה א׳ receives forty (thirty nine) lashes; v. ib. III, 10.

אַרְבְּעָה m., **אַרְבַּע** f. ch. same. Targ. O. Gen. XIV, 9; a. fr.— Constr. a) אַרְבְּעַת Targ. Y. ibid.—b) אַרְבַּעְתֵּי, אַרְבְּעֵי Sabb. 73^a (omitting the object numbered); a. fr.—Targ. Y. Num. II, 3; a. fr.—Y. Gitt. V, 46^d top ארבעתי דינרייא four denars—אַרְבְּעִיתָא, אַרְבְּעַתָּא m. *the fourth* (day of the week). Gen. R. s. 11; Pesik. R. s. 23, beg. Ibid. p. 120^a ed. Fr. ארבעיא, ed. Prag ארבעיתא. Ibid. p. 115^b בְּאַרְבַּעְתָּה on Wednesday.—*Pl.* אַרְבְּעִין *forty.* Targ. Gen. V, 13; a. fr.—Snh. 26^b א׳ בכתפיה forty (lashes) rest on his shoulders, i. e. he is punishable (v. preced.); a. fr.—אַרְבֵּיסַר, אַרְבַּע סְרֵי, אַרְבְּעַסְרֵי *fourteen, fourteenth.* Targ. Y. Gen. XIV, 5 בירבֵיסְרֵי; a. fr. Meg. 2^b בא׳ on the fourteenth of Adar. Sabb. 98^b.—אַרְבֵּסְרָאָה *the fourteenth.* Targ. I Chr. XXIV, 13.

***אַרְבָּעָה** II f. (רבע) *couching.* Targ. Is. VII, 25; LXV, 10 בית א׳ (Var. אַרְבְּעָא, רְבוּעָא) couching place (for animals).

אַרְבַּעְתָּה, אַרְבְּעַתָּא, אַרְבְּעִיתָא, v. אַרְבָּעָה.

אַרְבָּא, אַרְבְּתָא f. (ארב, h. עֲרָבָה, b. h. עֲרָבִים pl.) *[the thickly interwoven,] willow.* Pes. 111^b טולא דא׳ Ms. M., Ar. (v. Rabb. D. S. a. l.; ed. ע׳) the shade of a willow-tree.—*Pl.* אַרְבָּתָא. Sabb. 20^b (Ar. אַרְבָּאתָא; Mss. ע׳). [Gitt. 6^a; Kidd. 72^a ארבא וכ׳ the second willow after crossing the bridge; v., however, אַרְבָּא I.] V. עַרְבָא I, II a. עַרְבְּתָא.

אָרַג, constr. אֲרַג m. (v. רגג, h. ערג) *something desirable.* . . . שפר א׳ the choicest of . . . Targ. Ps. XLV, 14. Targ. Y. Gen. XLV, 18.

אָרַג (b. h.; √אר, v. ארב; cmp. חרג) *to plait, braid, weave.* Sabb. VII, 2 האורג he who weaves on the Sabbath; a. fr.—Metaph. (cmp. גרר) *to argue, conclude, spin out, deduct* &c. Ruth R., Par. 2, beg. (play on *or'gim* II Sam. XXI, 19) they brought a subject up והוא אוֹרְגָהּ and he carried it to a conclusive decision. Ib. שהיו אורגין עמו they argued with him.—Num. R. s. 4 (play on *argaman,* purple) שהוא היה אורג . . . . מִן וכ׳ for it (the purple-covered altar) argued Israel free from sin (pleaded in his behalf). Ib. s. 12 (same play on the word) והוא אורג וכ׳ and He wove (planned) the world so that all creatures should come forth each according to its kind. Ib. א׳ כָּן the Sun weaves (ripens) food.

Nif. נֶאֱרַג *to be woven.* Y. Ter. XI, end, 48^b. Ex. R. s. 50; a. fr.

**Pi.* אִירֵג, part. מְאָרֵג (cmp. עֲרוּגָה) *to follow the grooves of* the garden bed, *to range,* esp. *to select the green and tender onions* (v. חָלַק Hif.). Tosef. Peah I, 9 המארג, quoted in Y. ib. III, 17^c top המירוג (corr. acc.; v. מירוג) a. explained ibid. המחליק וכ׳ he who takes out the green onions for sale and leaves the others to ripen for storage.

אֲרַג ch. same. Snh. 48ᵇ וא׳ בגד וכ׳ and where they weave a garment (directly) for a corpse.

אַרְגְּוָנָא, v. אַרְגְּוָן.

אַרְגּוֹב 1) pr. n. m. (b. h. ארגב) *Argob.* Targ. II Kings XV, 25.—2) v. טַרְכּוֹנָא.

אַרְגּוּבְלָא m. (=b. h. גִּבְלִים) *Giblean* (v. גְּבַל); *master-mason. Pl.* אַרְגּוּבְלַיָּא. Targ. I Kings V, 32 (h. text גבלים); II Kings XII, 13 (h. text גֹּדְרִים). Cmp. אַרְדִּיכָל.

אַרְגְּוָן m.; **אַרְגְּוָנָה** f., **אַרְגְּוָנָא, אַרְגְּוָן** ch. (also ...גְּוָן׳)=b. h. אַרְגָּמָן *purple (garment).* Dan. V, 7; a. e.—Targ. Ex. XXV, 4; a. e.—Tam. 32ᵃ לבישין דא׳ purple garments.—*Pl.* אַרְגְּוָנִים. Pesik. R. s. 33.—אַרְגְּוָנוֹת. Lam. R. to III, 19 א׳ טובות fine purple dresses (for females).

ארגוטרייא, v. אַרְגְּנְטָרְיָא.

אַרְגְּוָנָא, אַרְגְּוָן, v. אַרְגְּוָ׳.

אַרְגָּז m. (b. h.; r. ארג with format. ז; cmp. אַרְבָּא) *box, chest* (joined with tenons &c.). Num. R. s. 4; Hor. 12ᵃ; a. e.—Snh. 46ᵇ *kabor* (to bury, cover) might mean only דעבד א׳ וכ׳ Ms. F. a. Ar. (Var. ארוג, ed. ארון) one makes a chest and puts the corpse in. [Pr. n. pl. v. אַרְגִּיזָא.]

***אַרְגָּזָא** f. (רגז) *provocation, evil deed.* Targ. Ezek. XX, 28 א׳ קורבניהון (prob. to be corr. אַרְגָּזוּת, v. next w.).

אַרְגְּזָוּתָא, אַרְגָּזוּתָא f. same. Targ. I Kings XXI, 22; XV, 30.

אַרְגָּטִיס m. (ἐργάτης) *working man, common laborer.* Y'lamd. Koraḥ (quot. in Ar.) ועשה אותו א׳ (read אותי) and made me (Koraḥ) a working man (Num. VII, 9); Tanḥ. ed. Bub. Koraḥ, p. 96 אור׳.

אַרְגִּיז, אַרְגִּיזָא, אַרְגִּיזָה (ארגז) pr. n. pl. *Argiz, Argiza* (ארזק Schr. KGF 228; *Eragiza*, Ptol. V, 15, 14; modern *Razek*, Koh. Ar. s. v.). Sabb. 19ᵇ; Erub. 63ᵃ חרתא דא׳ Ms. M. a. oth. (v. Rabb. D. S. a. l. notes, ed. חרתא) Ḥadta (Newtown) [Ḥarta] near Ar. [Rashi: *Argiz*, pr. n. m. the builder of the town.] Gitt. 7ᵃ בי א׳, ארגיזה. Zeb. 18ᵇ ארגיזא (Ms. M. אגוזיא, Ms. R. ארגיסא, א־גזיא, Ms. K. ארגידא; v. Rabb. D. S. a. l.).

ארגינימון, ארגינמין, read אֲרוֹנְנוּטִיס, אֲרוֹנְנוּטִין q. v.

אַרְגִּירָא, v. כְּרִיסוֹ.

אַרְגַּלְיָא, אַרְגַּלְיָיא, אַרְגַּלְיָה m. pl. (ἐργαλεῖα, τὰ) *tools, implements.* Ex. R. s. 40, beg. Lev. R. s. 23; Y. Succ. IV, 54ᶜ top; Cant. R. to IV, 8 היא וכל א׳ וכ׳ itself (the brick) and all the implements for making it. [Y'lamd. B'haaloth., quot. in Ar. כלי א׳ implements of a ship.]

אַרְגָּמָן m. (b. h.); *purple-dye, purple garment.* Sabb. 90ᵃ. Kel. XXVII, 12; a. fr.; cmp. אַרְגְּוָן.

ארגנאטרייא, ארגנטורין, v. אַרְגְּנְטָרְיָא.

ארגנטין, v. next w., a. אֲרוֹנְנוּטִיס.

אַרְגְּנְטָרְיָא, אַרְגְּנְטָארִיָּא, אַרְגְּנְטְרִין f. (ἀργεντάρία, argentarium) *silver-case, plate, table service* (of silver or gold). Pesik. Baḥod. p. 106ᵇ ארגנטין Ar. Var. ארגניטין (ארגנטרין ed. Koh.; ed. אנגיטרין); Yalk. Ex. 271 (cmp. versions ibid. a. Ar. s. v., in order to arrive at a correct reading of the whole passage). Y. Peah VIII, 21ᵇ ארגנטורין, אגנטין (corr. acc.). Esth. R. to I, 4 ארגוטדיא, ארגנאטרייא (corr. acc.).

אַרְגֶּסְטִיס (אגריסטיס, ארגסטס) m. (ἀργέστης) *the brightening,* epithet of various winds (cmp. אַסְתָּן); *West-North-West, West-South-West.* Num. R. s. 13 אני מביא רוח א׳ וכ׳ I shall cause to pass over the world an argestes in which both winds (the Northern and the Southern) shall do service; Cant. R. to IV, 16 ארג׳; Lev. R. s. 9 ארגסטס; Ar. Var. אגרסטיס.

***ארגסטירין** Koh. R. to XI, 9, v. אַכְּסִיגְרוֹן.

***אַרְגְּרוֹן** (read אַרְגּוּרוֹן) m. (ἄργυρον) *a small silver coin,* also called *milliarium.* Y. Peah VIII, 21ᵃ top ובלבד וכ׳ provided you do not refuse him his customary *argyron* (the beggar's penny); v. B. Bath. 9ᵃ.

ארד Y. Sot. II, 18ᵃ top, read אָרַר q. v.

אַרְדָּא I m. (Syr. ערדא, v. Löw Pfl. p. 303) *mushroom, morel.* Keth. 61ᵃ Ar. (ed. אַרְדֵּי pl.)—*Pl.* אַרְדֵּי, אַרְדָּיָא. Pes. 119ᵇ ארדיא לה Ar. (ed. אַרְדִּילָא, אַרְדִּילַיָא, אוּרְדִּילַאי, Ms. אַרְדִּילֵי, v. Rabb. D. S. a. l. note); Y. ib. X, end, 37ᵈ ערדילי (read עַרְדִּילֵי or עֲרָדֵי לֵי). Ber. 47ᵃ ארדיא Ar. (ed. a. Ms. אַרְדִּילַיָא). Ab. Zar. 38ᵃ ארדי.

***אַרְדָּא** II prefix of Persian proper nouns, *Arda.*—Gitt. 14ᵇ their names are bewildering בריש ... א׳ וארטא beginning with Arda-, and Arta-, and Phile-.

אַרְדְּבָא, אַרְדַּב f. (ἀρτάβη, Syr. ארדבא, ארטבא) *Artaba*, a Persian and Egyptian dry measure (v. Zuckerm. Jüd. Masse p. 47; Sm. Ant. s. v.). B. Mets 80ᵇ א׳ לעריבה Ar. (ed. אדריב) an Artaba is an unreasonable additional load for a small boat called Arebah. Erub. 102ᵃ Ar. (ed. אדריבא, v. Rabb. D. S. a. l. note 20).

אַרְדַּבְלִיס, v. אדר׳.

אַרְדִּיכָל, אַרְדְּכָל; ch. form אַרְדִּיכְלָא (אדר׳) m. (prob. from a place or country, cmp. אַרְגּוּבְלָא) *artist, artisan* (v. P. Sm. 370 s. v., a. derivat.) esp. *architect, key-stone-setter.* B. Mets. 118ᵇ בנאי ... לא׳ (ed. אדרי׳) when the builder has handed the key-stone over to the architect (to set it). Y. ib. X, end, 12ᶜ ארדכל. Gen. R. s. 8 אר׳; ib. s. 27 אד׳.—*Pl.* אַרְדִּיכְלִין. Targ. II Sam. V, 11 (h. text חרשי אבן קיר); a. e.—Erub. 26ᵃ אַרְדִּ׳ Ar. (Ms. M. דאַרְדִּכְלֵי; ed אדר׳).—אַרְדִּיכְלַיָּא Targ. Ps. CXVIII, 22; a. e.

אַרְדִּילָא m. (dimin. of אַרְדָּא I q. v.).—*Pl.* אַרְדִּילֵי, אַרְדִּלַּיָּא ,אַרְדִּלָּיָא.

אַרְדִּכָל, v. אַרְדִּיכָל.

אַרְדְּלַיָּא, v. אַרְדִּילָא.

***ארדפוי** Targ. Y. Gen. XXX, 37 דלוז וא׳, a corruption; prob. דלוז וּדְאַרְמוֹן, v. אַרְמוֹן III.

אַרְדְּפָנֵי, אַרְדִּפְנֵי m. ch.=h. הַרְדּוּפְנִין; v. הַרְדַּפְנֵי. Targ. Y. I, II Ex. XV, 25.

ארדקסם, read אַרְדִּקְסַט or

אַרְדַּקְסָס pr. n. pl. *Artaxata*, or *Artaxiata*, capital of Great Armenia. Y. Erub. III, beg. 20[c]. Bab. ib. 29[a] עַרְדִּיסְקָא ed. (Ms. M. עֲרְדַּסְקִיס, Var. ערדסקוס, ערדיקס, v. Rabb. D. S. a. l. note). Tosef. ib. IX (VI), 4 ערדסקס, (Var. ערדסקין, ערדסקוס).

אַרְדְּשִׁיר pr. n. pl. *Ardjir*, formerly *Seleucia*, near Ctesiphon. Gitt. 6[a] בי א׳. Erub. 57[b]. B. Bath. 52[a], v. הוֹרְמִיז. Yeb. 37[b] דְּאַרְ=הַרְדְּשִׁיר, sub. הוֹרְמִיז; Yoma 18[b] דרשיש (corr. acc.).

אָרָה, v. ארי.

אֲרוּ (ארי; v. אֲלוּ, cmp. הֲרֵי) *lo!, behold.* Dan. VII, 6; 7; 13.

אֲרוּבָּה f. (b. h. אֲרֻבָּה, ארב) *opening*, whence 1) *an aperture in the roof looking to the ground floor* (answering to the Greek *hypaithron*, Roman *compluvium*), contrad. fr. חַלּוֹן a garret window in the wall projecting above the flat roof. Bets. V, 1 (35[b]); cmp. Rashi a. l. Nidd. 20[b] הסומא בא׳ like a blind man finding his way down from the *ărubbah*, i. e. hitting the truth by chance. Ohol. X, 1; a. fr.—*Pl.* אֲרוּבּוֹת. Ib. 4 sq.; a. e.—2) *the opening panel of folding doors.*—*Pl.* as supra. Yoma 76[a]. [Sabb. 43[a]; 153[b]; Kel. XV, 2 read with Ar. אֲרוּכוֹת.]

אֲרוּגָּה f. (ארג) *web, matting.* Y. Succ. I, end, 52[c] א׳ טמאה a mat (of twigs &c. for covering the festive booth) that became unclean.

***אַרוֹגְנוּטִיס, אַרוֹגְנוֹטִין, אַרוֹגְנוּטֵיס** m. (ἀρωγοναύτης sub. δαίμων) *helper of sailors, Arogonautes*, a demon. Gen. R. s. 63; Y. Ter. VIII, 46[c] top; Yalk. Gen. 110, variously corrupted ארגנטין, ארגינטון, ארגנטרין, אנגיטריס.

אַרְוָא, pl. אַרְוָתָא, אַרְוָת, v. אוּרְיָא Ch.

אָרוֹד, אָרוֹדָא m. *mule*, v. עָרוֹד.

אֻרְוָה f. (b. h.; v. אוּרְיָא II) *manger, crib.*—*Pl.* אֻרְווֹת. Snh. 21[b].

אַרְוָד pr. n. pl. *Aradus* on the Phœnician coast. Gen. R. s. 37 (to *Arvadi*, Gen. X, 18).

אַרְוָדָאֵי m. pl. (preced.) *Aradeans.* Targ. O. Gen. X, 18 (Targ. Y. II אַנְטִירִידְנָאֵי; I לוֹטְסָאֵי, Var. in Targ. I Chr. I, 16 לְטוּסָאֵי).

אַרְוָסָא, v. אַרְוִיסָא.

אָרוּזָא m. *rice*, v. אוּרְזָא.

***אַרְוָסָא, אַרְוִיסָא** m. (a transpos. of אַסְפִּירָא, אַסְפְּרָא) *halter* (Rashi). [Ar. *chain*, Perl. Et. St. p. 21= Pers. arvîs *rope*.] Yeb. 46[a] רמו ליה ארוו׳ וכ׳ Ar. ed. Koh. (ed. ארוי׳, Ar. ed. ארוסיה) they put a halter around his neck (to prevent him from claiming his liberty).

אָרוֹךְ m. (ארך) 1) *long, tall, lasting*; v. infra.—2) (=עָרוֹךְ; cmp. אָרִיךְ) *well-arranged, well-balanced, thinker*, a title of prominent scholars; cmp. אַרְיוֹךְ a. אֲרִיכָא. [In legend intellectual eminence was identified with physical tallness.] Nidd. 24[b] א׳ בדורו *arukh* (the tallest) in his generation. Kidd. 39[b] עולם שכולו א׳ the world in which all is well-balanced (also called שכולו טוב) i. e. *the hereafter*.—*Pl.* אֲרוּכִים. Yoma 71[a] חיים א׳ long life; a. fr.—Fem. אֲרוּכָה. Ber. I, 4 אחת א׳ one lengthy (benediction); a. fr.—Y. Hor. II, 46[d] בא׳ by the long road, slowly; Shebu. 18[ab].—*Pl.* אֲרוּכוֹת. Y. Ber. II, 5[c] top, a. e. א׳ וקצרות long and short roads, i. e. *in all directions.* V. next art.

אֲרוּכָא, v. אַרְכָא III.

אֲרוּכָה I f. 1) fem. of אָרוֹךְ.—2) (noun) *long board, longside of bedstead, bedside.* Succ. 15[b] א׳ ושתי כרעים the long bedside with its two knees (supporters); 16[a].—*Pl.* אֲרוּכוֹת. Ib. I, 8 (Var. ארובות, v. Rabb. D. S. ib. ad 15[a], note 1); Sabb. 43[a]; ib. XXIII, 5 (151[b]) א׳ חמטה (some ed. ארובות, corr. acc.).—[Kel. XV, 2 א׳ של נחתומים Ar. Var. *the long ranging boards* used by the bakers: Maim.; the prevailing versions are אֲרוּבּוֹת or אֲרֵיבוֹת; Tosef. B. Mets. V, 4 ארובות, (Var. ארונות) *basins* or *moulds* in which loaves or cakes are shaped.—Var. Ar. עֲרֵיכוֹת.]

אֲרוּכָה II f. (b. h. ארכה, ארוכה; ארך, v. Ges. H. Dict. s. v.) *the web of new flesh or skin on a healing wound, healing.* העלה א׳ *to produce a new cover, be restored.* Hull. 77[a]; 125[a]; B. Kam. 91[b].

אָרוּם 1) v. אֲרֵי.—2) v אֲרִים.

אֲרוּמָא pr. n. pl. *Aruma.* Erub. 51[b] ed., Ms. M. רוּמָא q. v.

אֲרוּמָאָה m. ch. *Roman.* *Pl.* אֲרוּמָאֵי. Gitt. 17[a]; cmp. אֲרַמָּאָה.

אֲרוּמִי m. h. same. *Pl.* אֲרוּמִיִּים. Gitt. 17[a]; v. אֱדֹם, אֲרַמִּי.

אָרוֹן c. (b. h.; ארן or ארי, √אר, cmp. ארגז, ארבא, עריבה &c.) [joined together,] *chest, box, coffin*, freq. (=אֲרוֹן הַקּוֹדֶשׁ) *the Holy Ark*, in the tabernacle and the Temple, or in Synagogues. Yoma V, 1 הגיע לא׳ reached the place where the Ark stood during the First Temple. Y. Ber. IV, 8[c] top; Gen. R. s. 55 (allegorical etymologies).—Keth. 104[a] א׳ הקודש (figuratively) *a good and learned man's soul*; v. אֲרָאֵל.—Kel. XII, 5 א׳ של גרוסות the grits-dealer's chest. Y. Kil. IX, 32[b] top; Gen. R. s. 100 וחזא

אֲרוֹנִי נקובה (נקופה) וכ׳ let my coffin be perforated at the bottom. Snh. 98^b^ אין לך כל א׳ וא׳ וכ׳ there is no coffin in Palestine in which the Median horses do not eat straw (being used as cribs); a. fr.—*Pl.* אֲרוֹנוֹת. Sot. 13^a^; a. fr. [Y. Keth. VI, 30^d^ bot. וארון, v. אֲרִי I.]

אֲרוֹנָא (אֲרוֹנָה) ch. same. Targ. Ex. XXV, 10; a. fr. Targ. Gen. L, 26 (coffin).—Y. Meg. III, 73^d^ bot. the curtain על א׳ כא׳ over the ark containing the scrolls is as sacred as the ark itself. Y. Ber. II, 5^c^ bot. אֲרוֹנֵיה נַפְקָא his coffin was carried out for burial.

ארונטס, v. אַרְנָטוּס.

***אֲרָאנֵי, אֲרוֹנֵי** m. pl. (prob. pl. of ארונא, so called from closing and opening like chests) name of certain *plants* growing in marshes and closing their leaves at nightfall. Sabb. 35^b^ בדברא עירבי באגמא חזו אדני Ms. M. (ed. עורבי א״נ אדאני . . . .; v. Rabb. D. S. a. l., Ar. הרני, Var. ארוני, Rashi ed. Sonc., Asheri a. R. Niss. early ed. אראני) in the desert you recognize the entrance of the Sabbath (on a cloudy day) by the ravens, in marsh-land you look out for *aroné*.

אֲרוֹנִים, v. אֹרֶן.

אֲרוֹנִית, v. אֵירוֹנִית.

ארונקי, v. אדנדקי.

אֲרוּס, v. אֵירוּס I, II.

ארוסיה, v. אֲרִיוִיסָא.

אֵירוּסִין, אֵרוּסִין m. pl. (אָרַס) *betrothal, preliminary act of marriage*, answering to the Roman *sponsalia; promise in marriage*, disting. fr. נישואין, or כניסה, marriage proper, the latter consisting in conducting the bride to the groom's permanent (or improvised) home. [The betrothal carries with it almost all the legal consequences of marriage, excepting some modifications mostly of a civil (pecuniary) character, and is, according to Talmudic usage, preceded by a benediction (בִּרְכַּת א׳), while the act itself is performed by the bride-groom (or his mandatary) delivering into the hands of the bride (or her mandatary, or her father, if she be a minor) an object representing any value not below the smallest coin (P'rutah), whereby the purpose of the delivery is stated and assented to by acceptance.] Keth. I, 2 אלמנה מן הא׳ a widow whose betrothed died before marriage proper. Ib. V, 1; a. fr. Yeb. 43^a^, a. fr. סעודת א׳ the repast following the betrothal.—Metaph. of the relation between Israel and God, *covenant*. Ex. R. s. 15, end; a. e.

אֲרוּקְתָּא, v. אַרְקְתָא I.

ארורא, Y. Shek. II, end, 47^a^ דארורא צילמא, v. אֲדוּרֵי.

ארורייא, אֲרוּרֵי, v. אֲרַר.

***ארז** (√ אר, v. ארר; cmp. חרז) 1) *to penetrate deeply, to take deep root.*—2) *to be prickly, dry, hard.* Sabb. 155^a^ זירין דאַרְזֵי Zirin are called bundles of twigs which are hard. Ib. כיפין דא׳; [oth. opin., v. אַרְזָא]. Denom. אוּרְזָא, אֲרוּזָא, a. next ws.

אֶרֶז m. (b. h.) *cedar*. Tam. III, 5 של א׳ of cedar wood.—*Pl.* אֲרָזִים. R. Hash. 23^a^; Taan. 25^b^; a. e.—Metaph. *prominent men, scholars*. Sabb. 118^b^ I planted חמשה א׳ five cedars (begot five sons who acquired renown). M. Kat. 25^b^, v. אֵזוֹב.

אַרְזָא ch. 1) same. Targ. Lev. XIV, 4; a. e.—Ab. Zar. 14^a^. R. Hash. 23^a^; a. e.—*Pl.* אַרְזִין, אַרְזַיָּא, אַרְזֵי. Targ. Num. XXIV, 6; a. e.—Y. Ab. Zar. III, 42^c^ top. Sabb. 157^a^. —Ib. 155^a^ זירין דא׳ (Ms. זירין סובי דא׳) *Zirin* means twigs of cedars (Rashi דארזא); [oth. opin. v. ארז].—2) pr. n. pl. תֵּל א׳ *Tel Arza* (Cedar-Hill), in Palestine, scene of massacres during the Bar Kokhba war. Yeb. XVI, 7.— 3) pr. n. m. *Arza*. Tam. VII, 3 בן א׳: Shek. V, 1 ארוזה; Tosef. ib. II, 14.

אַרְזְבוֹנִית f. (cmp. אַרְזוּבָא) *arz'bonith*, a species of *locusts*; cmp. עַרְצוּבְיָא a. פַּרְזוּבָא. Sifra Sh'mini Par. III, ch. 5; Ḥull. 65^a^ חרזובנית.

אַרְזַג, v. אַרְגָּז.

אַרְזָה, v. אַרְזָא.

אַרְזוּבָא m. (=אַרְזַפְתָּא) *hammer*.—*Pl.* אַרְזוּבִין. Targ. I Kings VI, 7.

ארזון, v. אֲרָזִין.

אַרְזִילָא, v. אַרְזָלָא.—אַרְזִילֵי, v. אוּרְזִילָא.

***אֲרָזִין** m. (prob. plur. of אֶרֶז) *box, chest* (for collecting bones). Tosef. Snh. IX, 8 (ed. Zuck. בארון, Var. בארזון). Treat. S'maḥ. ch. XII בגלוסקמא בא׳ (one word inserted by a glossator to explain the other). Ib. בידין (corr. acc.). [Tur Y. D. Abeluth 403: ארזים.]

עַרְסְלָא, עֲרַסֵל, אַרְזִילָא (אוּרְזִילָא), אַרְזָלָא m. (dimin. of עֶרֶס, עַרְסָא) *cradle, hammock* for watchmen in gardens. Targ. Is. I, 8; XXIV, 20 (h. מלונה).—Erub. 25^b^ דעבידא כי אר׳ Ar. (ed. אור׳; Rashi ארזי׳; Tosaf. ערס׳) the roof of the shed has the shape of a cradle, i. e both sides slanting towards the centre.

אַרְזָנָאֵי m. pl. (v. ארזונדא P. Sm. 374, cmp. פרשנדא Neub. Géogr. p. 396) *of Arzania*. Taan. 24^b^ ארבי דא׳ Ar. (ed. דחיטין דפרזינא; Ms. M. דפרזינאי) ships of the Arzanians. Fem. *אַרְזָנְיָיתָא. Git. 70^a^ חיטין א׳ Arzanian wheat (of a large size).

אַרְזַפְתָּא I f. (רזף) *hammer*. Targ. Judg. IV, 26.—Gitt. 56^b^. Meg. 25^a^ (Ms. מַרְזַפְתָּא).

אַרְזַפְתָּא II (אַפְרַזְתָּא) f. (v. זִיףְ, a. הַרְדְּ׳=אַרְזִפְנֵי; cmp. Löw, Pfl. p. 320) *hypericum (barbatum), St. John's wort*, a plant said to be fatal to cattle. B. Kam. 47^b^ באר׳ Ar. a. Ms. H. (Var. חרזיפא, v. Koh. Ar.; ed. אפר׳)

under 'poison' is meant *arzafta* which may also be called *peré* (*fruit*, produces of the earth). B. Bath. 20ª 'אר' Ar. (Ms. 'אר', changed into 'אפ as ed.). Cmp. הֲרִיזִיפוּ.

אָרַח (b. h.; √אר־, v. ארר) 1) *to go through*; v. אָרִיחַ. —2) *to go outside, to travel.* Part. אוֹרֵחַ q. v.—Denom. אוֹרַח *path.*

Pi. אֵרַח (Denom. of אוֹרֵחַ) *to receive a guest, to lodge.* Ber. 63ᵇ הַמְאָרֵחַ. Y. Ab. Zar. I, 39ᶜ bot. לְאָרְחוֹ.

Hithpa., a. *Nithpa.* הִתְאָרֵחַ, נִתְאָרֵחַ *to be received, be the guest of.* Sabb. 13ᵇ a. fr. Y. Hall. IV, 60ª 'מִתְאָ.

אָרַח, אֲרַח ch. same, esp. *to take lodging.* Targ. Jud. XIX, 17. [ארחא ,ארח Yoma 82ᵇ, a. e., Af. of רִיחַ.]

Ithpe. אִתְאֲרַח, contr. אִתְּרַח *to dwell as a stranger, sojourn.* Targ. Y. Deut. I, 6; v. אֲחַר.

אוֹרְחָא, אַרְחָא m. (preced.) *traveler, guest.* Targ. II Sam. XII, 4.—[Y. Ber. I, 2ᵈ top 'לא הוה ארחא אתיא וכ, oth. ed. אתחא, read שַׁחְרָא with oth. ed.].—*Pl.* אַרְחִין, אוֹרְחִין. Y. Peah VIII, end, 21ᵇ, (read as) Y. Shek. V, end, 49ᵇ 'הוה ליה א he had guests. [אוֹרְחָא *path*, v. אוֹרְחָא.]

אַרְחָא *lath*, v. אֲרִיחָא.—ארחין, v. אָרִיחַ.

אַרְטָא prefix of Pers. proper nouns, *Arta-*. Gitt. 14ᵇ, v. אַרְדְּבָא II.

ארטבון, ארטבין Yoma 11ª; Yalk. Deut. 844; Sam. 124—perh. a corruption of טְרִיבּוּן (a Jewish) *tribunus*; cmp. ארטיגוס. [Or pr. n.?]

אַרְטְבִינָא, v. אַרְטְבַנְיָא.

ארטבלאי Targ. Esth. VIII, 10 Levita, v. טְרִיבְלִי.

אַרְטְבָאן, אַרְטְבַן pr. n. m. *Artaban* (IV), the last Parthian king, friend of R. Judah han-Nasi. Y. Peah I, 15ᵈ bot.; Gen. R. s. 35; Yalk. Deut. 844; Prov. 934.—V. אדרבן.

ארטיבנא, אַרְטִינְיָא, אַרְטְבִינָא, אַרְטְבַנְיָא pr. n. pl. *Artabania* (named after Artaban, v. preced.), near Pumbeditha. Erub. 51ᵇ (Var. lect., v. Rabb. D. S. a. l.).

ארטיגוס Yalk. Esth. 1053, read סטרטיגוס or אִסְטְרַ' (Esth. R. to III, 1 טריבונוס, read 'טריב; v. ארטבון).

ארטיקנס, v. אַרְסְקִינָס.

ארטל (א' ליפין), v. ארבי ליפורין.

אַרְטְלַאי, v. טְרִיבְלִי.

***ארסיסיס, ארסמוס, ארטסיס**, Ex. R. s. 13 'יא' נכנס, read: ואין רוטב נכנס בתוכה but no juice enters into it, 'כך נעשה לבו של פרעה ולא היה מקבל וכ so was Pharaoh's heart made and it received not &c.; v. Ter. X, 11.

אַרְטְקְפָא m. (ἀρτόκοπος) *baker*, 'בית א *bakery.* Midr. Sam. ch. XIX 'בית א' שלי (Var. ארתוקופיון q. v.) a rendition of *beth hallaḥmi*, I Sam. XVI, 1) to his (Jesse's) bakery, 'שהוא בא וכ (read with Yalk. Sam. 124 'והוא יבוא וכ) and he (Jesse) shall come out (to the bakery) from Bethlehem (to meet Samuel there). Yalk. l. c. 'ארנקפאן, ארכ (corr. acc.).

אֲרוּם, אֲרֵי (v. next w.; cmp. אֲרוּ) prop. *behold*, in most cases corresponding to b. h. כִּי, *that, so that, because, if; but.* Targ. O. ארי; Targ. Y. ארום; v. fr.

אֲרִי I, אֲרָא (√אר, cmp. ירי) prop. *to point, throw*, hence (in a logical sense) *to argue, question, discuss, treat.* B. Kam. 30ᵇ מדקא ארינן גלל Ar. (ed. איירינן, v. infra) since we pointed out the law about the dung placed in the street as an argument against Rab. Keth. 16ª, a. fr. ודקארי לה מאי קארי לה and he who raised the question, how could he raise it at all, i. e. the answer being so obvious, what must have been the impression he labored under, that he could ask such a question, or raise such an argument?—Y. Keth. VI, 30ᵈ bot. ואין קמו יתמי וארון if the heirs should rise and raise objections (go to law).

Af. אַיְירֵי same. Ned. 2ᵇ איירי בהון he does treat thereof.—Pes. 6ᵇ, a. fr. איידי דאיירי בי incidentally of treating the question of... Kerith. 14ª, a. fr. (באבר אחד) קא מַיְירֵי the argument is up (about one limb). B. Kam. 30ᵇ כי איירינן when we raised the objection (taking our argument from 'the dung', v. supra), it was before R. N. had given his opinion; a. fr.—Deriv. אַרְיָא.

אָרָה, ארי (b. h.; √אר, v. ארר) [*to create a gap,*] *to pluck*, esp. figs. Shebi. I, 2 'הָאוֹרֶה וכ the gatherer and his basket. B. Mets. 89ᵇ day laborers שהיו אורין בתאנים Ar. (ed. 'עודר; v. Rabb. D. S. a. l. note 300) engaged in picking figs. Y. B. Bath. V, 15ª bot.; a. fr.—Num. R. s. 20 Tanḥ. Bal. 4 (homiletic etymology of *araḥ*, Num. XXII, 6).

אֲרִי II, אַרְיֵה m. (b. h.; ארר, v. preced.) [*the light-colored*] 1) *lion.* B. Kam. 16ᵇ 'א תרבות a tamed lion; a. fr.—Transf. *brave man; distinguished scholar* (opp. שועל). Yeb. 122ᵇ. Kidd. 48ᵇ; Snh. 8ᵇ. Gitt. 83ᵇ; Y. ib. IX, 50ª 'אין משיבין את הא' וכ you must not argue against a lion (scholar) after he is dead. B. Kam. 117ª; a. fr.—*Pl.* אֲרָיוֹת.—'זנב לא a tail to lions, i. e. the least among the great (opp. head to foxes). Ab. IV, 15; Y. Snh. IV, 22ᵇ bot.—Hull. 3ᵇ, a. fr. 'גורי א, v. גּוּר.—[Gen. R. s. 28 'א גסטרייה, v. גַּסְטְרָא.]—2) *Leo, Lion* the fifth sign of the Zodiac (corresp. to the month of Ab). Yalk. Ex. 418. Pesik. Dibré p. 116ª; Pesik. R. s. 27 (28, p. 133ᵇ, ed. Fr.); v. אֲרִיאֵל.—3) homiletic surname of *the Lord, Israel* &c. Pesik. l. c.; Pesik. R. l. c.; Yalk. Jer. 259, v. אֲרִיאֵל.

אֲרִי, אַרְיָא (אַרְיֵא) ch. same. Targ. Num. XXIV, 9; a. fr.—B. Mets. 101ᵇ, a. e., v. אֲרַב. Ned. 62ᵇ לאברוחי 'א to drive the lion off, i. e. to get rid of the tax-collector.—Shebu. 22ᵇ, a. fr. 'א' היא דרביע עלה a lion lies on it, i. e. it is unavailable because it is forbidden.—Ab. Zar. 31ᵇ, a. e. 'בר א son of a lion (of a great man).—Hull. 59ᵇ the tiger is 'א' דבי עילאי the lion of the forest of Ilai (v. Schorr He-Haluts VII, 32; cmp. Koh. Angelol. p. 103).—*Pl.* אַרְיָוָתָא, אַרְיָן. Targ. I Chron. XI, 22; a. fr.—

Lam. R. to I, 9) א׳ דאורייתא the lions of the Law (scholars). Y. Shebi. IX, 39ª top. Y. Sabb. I, 4ª top מעלר רישא בין א׳ to put one's head between lions, i. e. to argue against the opinions of great men. [Yalk. Num. 771 גבתא דא׳, v. אֲרִיחַ.]

אַרְיָא, אַרְיְיא, אַרְיָא, אַרְיָא f. (אֲרָא, אֲרִי) *pointing at, argument, topic, subject.* Kerith. 3ᵇ גבי כריתות דאר׳ וכ׳ in speaking of K'rithoth, where this (the punishment of extinction) is the subject proper, I may say, the general term of Sabbath &c. is introduced (relying on those places in the Mishnah where the respective laws are treated in detail). Yoma 74ª, a. fr. אי משום הא לא א׳ were it only for this, there would be no argument (no difficulty). Kerith. 18ª, a. fr. מאי א׳ כי וכ׳ why is the argument brought up only on the presumption (that he has eaten? Supposed, he had not eaten, would not the same argument hold good?). Sabb. 101ª, a. fr. מידי א׳ is this an argument (i.e. how can you compare two cases so unlike each other)?

אֲרִיאֵל (b. h.) *Ariël, Divine Light* (cmp. Ps. CXVIII, 27, v. אֲרִי II); poetic surname of the Temple and Jerusalem. Pesik. Dibré p. 116ª. Pesik. R. s. 27 (28, p. 133ᵇ, ed. Fr.) הבית שנקרא אריה (read אריאל) the Temple which is called Ariël (Is. XXIX, 1). Ib. ישראל שנקרא אריאל (read אריה); בחדש שנקרא אריאל (read אריה); דבריו של אריאל (read אריה; Num. XXIII, 24; Amos III, 8); v. אַרְיֵה.

אָרִיג m. (ארג) *something woven, web.* Sabb. XIII, 1; a. fr. Y. M. Kat. III, end, 83ᵈ, what is meant by ארחוי? Ans. כאריג when it looks as if woven. Meg. 26ᵇ, a. e. טווי לא׳ spinning the flax so as to prepare it for weaving (indirect preparation or designation); Snh. 48ª טווי לַאֲרִיגָה, (Rashi לאריג).

אֲרִיגָה f. (v. preced.) *weaving.* Y. Yoma III, 40ᶜ bot. אֲרִיגָתָן בקודש their weaving must take place within the sanctuary. Snh. 48ª, v. preced.

אַרְיֵה, v. אֲרִי.—אריה Y. Snh. X, 28ᵈ, v. אֲרִיחַ.

***אריהון** (prob. corruption of אֲרִיחַ) pr. n. pl. Cant. R. to II, 17 (ref. to הרי בתר ibid. 'mountains of cutting') כדי שיטלו המלכיות בֶּתֶר א׳ (not שיתלו, v. Matt. Keh. a. l.) that the (Roman) governments may receive (their pay for) the massacre of Ar. (cmp. Joseph. B. J. III, 10, 9 sq. or perh. ref. to the Bar Kokhba war; cmp. טור, גופנית, שמעון a. oth. Y. Taan. IV, 69ª sq.).

אַרְיְוָא, v. אַרְיָא.

אַרְיוֹךְ pr. n. m. (Gen. XIV, 1) *Aryokh,* 1) homiletic surname of Nebuzraddan. Lam. R. to V, 5 (allusion to ארי).—2) (cmp. Dan. II, 14) *Aryokh,* a title of Samuel, the contemporary of Rab. Sabb. 53ª. Kidd. 39ª. Men. 38ᵇ. Hull. 76ᵇ (prob. a Persian adaptation for *judge*).

***אַרְיוֹס** pr. n. m. *Arios.* Sifré Deut. 13; Yalk. Deut. 802.

אריוסטו, v. אוריסטו.

אֲרִיחַ m. (ארח) 1) *bond-timber,* also *small bricks,* which are placed at intervals between the rows of bricks (v. Sm. Ant. s. v. Paries II); *lath* (of half the width of a brick). Erub. I, 3; B. Bath. 3ᵇ; a. e.—*Pl.* אֲרִיחִין. Y. Erub. I, 19ª top ארחין (corr. acc.).—2) *ariaḥ,* a term used in rules for writing certain passages of Holy Scriptures metrically arranged, *the short space filled out with writing,* opp. לבנה (brick, the larger space); v. R. Niss. to Meg. 16ᵇ; [Rashi: א׳ *the writing.* לבנה *the blank*). Y. Meg. III, 74ᵇ bot.; Bab. ib. l. c.; Treat. Sof'rim XII, 10 א׳ ע״ג ל׳ וכ׳ small brick (lath) above brick, and brick above small brick (lath); e. g. (Ex. ch. XV)

ויאמרו לאמר　　אשירה לה׳ כי גאה גאה　　סוס
ורכבו רמה בים　　עזי וזמרת יה ויהי לי

Ib. א׳ ע״ג א׳ וכ׳ small brick (lath) above small brick and brick above brick; e. g. (Esth. IX, 7 sq.)

פרשנדתא　　ואת
דלפון.　　ואת

אֲרִיחַ (אריא, אריה) pr. n. pl. *Ăriaḥ;* [Tarichæa, South of Tiberias, Neub. Géogr. p. 21ᵇ]. Y. Snh. X, 28ᵈ גופתה א׳; Sifré Num. 131 גיבתא דא׳; Yalk. Num. 771 דאריא (Y. l. c. ed. Zyt. אריה) Gufta in the district of Ariaḥ. Tosef. Kil. I, 3; Y. ib. I, 27ª bot. תחום א׳ district of A.

אֲרִיחָא, אַרְחָא ch. (=h. אֲרִיחַ) *lath, bar, pole.* Targ. Num. XIII, 23; a. e. (h. מוֹט). Bets. 32ᵇ נפל לה ארי׳ בתנורא ed. (Ar. ארחא) a binder of the brick wall fell into the stove. Sabb. 129ª a house דשב לבינא וא׳ the width of whose walls was seven bricks and a half; a. e.—*Pl.* אֲרִחִין, אַרְחֵי, אֲרִיחִין, אֲרִיחַיָּא. Targ. Ex. XXV, 27; a. e. (h. בַּדִּים). B. Bath. 3ª כפיסין ארחי K'fissin are bondlaths. Y. Erub. I, 19ª top (also אורחין).

אֲרִיךְ I (b. h. אָרַךְ) *to be long, to project.* Targ. I Kings VIII, 8; II Chr. V, 9.—Y. Ab. Zar. I, 39ᶜ top, v. אִירְכָּא.

Af. אוֹרִיךְ, *Pa.* אָרֵךְ 1) *to be prolonged; to lengthen.* Targ. Ex. XX, 12. Targ. Y. Deut. XXVIII, 67 מְאָרְכָן make appear long; a. fr.—Y. Taan. IV, 68ª מְאָרְכָה יומין to live long; Koh. R. to VII, 7.—2) *to be tall.* Snh. 109ᵇ כי מאריך when one was tall.—3) *to tarry, wait, hope.* Targ. Num. IX, 22. Targ. Job VI, 11.—Y. Yoma VI, 43ᵈ אורכין צבחר wait a while. Y. R. Hash. I, 57ª bot. הוות מוֹרְכָה וכ׳ she waited a whole year. Ib. הוו מורכין. Y. M. Kat. II, 81ᵇ top ארלפא מורכא לך the ship will wait for thee.

אֲרִיךְ II m., **אֲרִיכָא** f. (preced.) 1) *long.* Targ. Ezek. XVII, 3.—Targ. Prov. XIV, 17 דא׳ תרעיתיה whose intrigue is long prepared (h. איש מזמות). V. אֲרִיכָא.—2) (part. pass. of אֲרַךְ *to arrange*) *right, befitting.* Ezra IV, 14.—Succ. 4ᵇ א׳ או לא א׳ is it right or not? B. Mets. 75ª וא׳ and it is proper to do so. Midr. Till. to Ps. I, 2 וא׳ כדין is such a thing right?

אָרִיךְ m. (preced.) *prolonging, retarding.* Targ. Y. I Num. XIV, 18 (II א׳ רתחין, read רותחיה).

אָרִיךְ m. (denom. of אֲרִיךְ II, 2) *preparing, dressing.* Sabb. 33ᵇ הוא קא א׳ ליה לבישריה was dressing (cleansing) his body. Keth. 103[b] וְאָרֵיכְנָא וכ׳ I would dress parchment rolls of deer skins.

אָרִיכָא m. (preced.) [one who arranges arguments,] *Arekha*, title of a lecturer. Sabb. 59[b] גברא רבה א׳ a great man, a lecturer. Esp. known *R. Aḥa Arekha*. Ib. 111[a]; a.e. Ber. 33[a] ed. (Ms. M. Ḥiya); *Abba Arekha* (Rab, v. רַב). [In legend: *tall*, v. אָרוֹךְ.]

***אֲרִיכָא** f. (preced.) *theme of a lecture*. Midr. Till., beg. עבד לה א׳ used that idea of R. Yudan as a theme.

אֲרִיכָא m. (v. אֲרִיךְ II) *long, prolonged*. Bets. 30[b] יומא א׳ Ms. M. (ed. אריכתא); Succ. 45[b] יומא א׳ an adjourned day.—Fem. אֲרִיכְתָא. Ber. 4[b] תפלה א׳ a continued prayer; גאולה א׳ a continued benediction on redemption, v. גְּאוּלָּה. —*Pl.* אֲרִיכָתָא. Keth. 8[a] שית א׳ the six lengthy benedictions.

אֲרִיכָה, אֲרִיכוּת f. (ארך) *prolongation, length; (sub.* אַף, or פנים*) forbearance.* Koh. R. to VII, 8 א׳ שהאריך וכ׳ the forbearance which Samuel showed. Gen. R. s. 70 א׳ פנים. Y. Ḥag. II, 77[b] bot.; a. e. א׳ ימים length of days, long life.—Gen. R. s. 64 א׳ ימים lapse of time.

אֲרִיכוּתָא ch. same. Targ. Is. XXXVIII, 11.

אֲרִיכוּתָא f. (v. אֲרִיךְ II, 2) *preparation, future* (v. ירך, Schr. KAT p. 549). Targ. Jer. XXXI, 5.

אֲרִים (ארום), pr. n. *Arim* (Arum). Y. Ḥag. I, 76[c] bot.; Y. Pes. III, end, 30[b] עליית בית א׳, v. עֲלִיָּה; (Sifré Deut. 41 ערוד; Yalk. ib. 681 שערים; Kidd. 40[b] נתזה).

אֲרִימִין m. (ἔρημα, τὰ) *desert, wilderness*. מקום א׳ a settlement in a desert. Lev. R. s. 35 (ed. אדרימון, Ar. ארימון, corr. acc.). Cant. R. to VII, 11.—Yalk. Jer. 257 אירימון, cmp. אֲרֵימִיאָה.

***אֲרִיס** I m. (ארס) *something tied to the body* (περίαμμα), whence *an emblem set in a ring or chain* (cmp. Deut. VI, 8; Prov. VI, 21, also Sm. Ant. s. v. Amuletum). *Pl.* אֲרִיסִין. Deut. R. s. 3 הכניסה לו שנים א׳ (read שני) brought into his house two emblems (of faith); the king, too, זקק לה כנגדן שני א׳ had two corresponding emblems set for her. Ib. Abraham delivered to his children שני א׳ two emblems (which they should guard, Gen. XVIII, 19).

אָרִיס II m. (ארס) prop. *bound, engaged*, esp. *tenant* who tills the owner's ground for a certain share in the produces, contrad. fr. חכיר tenant who pays the landlord a certain rent in kind, irrespective of the yield of the crops. Y. Bicc. I, end, 64[b]. Y. B. Bath. III, 14[a] bot. א׳ שהוריד א׳ a farmer letting to a sub-farmer. Ex. R. s. 43. Lev. R. s. 1 אֲרִיסוֹ his (the king's) tenant, i. e. Adam (in paradise); a. fr.—*Pl.* אֲרִיסִים, אֲרִיסִין. Y. B. Bath. l. c. Y. M. Kat. III, 82[b] bot. Deut. R. s. 7; a. fr.—Cmp. עָרִיס.

אָרִיס, אֲרִיסָא, אֲרִישָׁא ch. 1) same, also *field laborer*. Targ. Y. Deut. XXIII, 25; 26 Levita (ed. פועל). Targ. Cant. VIII, 11.—Ab. Zar. 21[b] א׳ אריסותיה קעביד the gentile tenant working during the Jewish festive week, works for his tenancy (not as the Jew's employee). Ḥag. 25[b] דינא הוא . . . א׳ וכ׳ it is the tenant's business to procure kegs &c.—*B. Bath. 55[a] דאריסא דפרסאי עד וכ׳ Rashb. a. l. (ed. אריסיתא, Var. דַּאֲרִישָׁן, שָׁאֲרִין . . . , דַּאֲרִישָׁאָן, v. Rabb. D. S. a. l. note, Ms. M. דאריש׳) that the tenant of the Persians is such only up to forty years (after which time he is considered a legitimate owner); v. Nim. Jos. to Alf. a. l. [It seems that the Pers. Jews pronounced אֲרִישָׁא a. אֲרִישׁוּתָא, cmp. דִּישְׁתְּנָא a. דִּיסְתְּנָא.]—*Pl.* אֲרִיסַיָּא. Targ. Job XXIX, 23. אֲרִישָׁאִין, v. supra. [Lev. R. s. 28, v. אֲרִיסְטָא.]—2) *betrothed*, v. אָרַס.

אֲרִיס, אֲרִיסָא *poison*, v. אֶרֶס ch.

אֲרִיסָה Tosef. Kel. B. Bath. IV, 8; v. עֲרִיסָה.

אֲרִיסוּת f. (אָרִיס II) *tenancy, condition of the Aris.* Peah V, 5 בא׳ as a tenancy; a. fr.—*Pl.* אֲרִיסִיּוֹת. Y. Bicc. I, end, 64[b] בעלי א׳ owners of tenanted properties, v. חֲכִירָה.

אֲרִיסוּתָא ch. same. Lev. R. s. 5. Ab. Zar. 21[b]; a. e. B. Bath. 55[a], v. אֲרִיסָא. [M. Kat. 22[b], v. אֲרִישְׁתָּא.]

אֲרִיסְטָא m. (corrupt. of אריסטוטא, ἀριστητής) *breakfasting*, in gen. *invited guest*. *Pl.* אֲרִיסְטִין, אֲרִיסְטַיָּא. Koh. R. to I, 3 שביק א׳ וכ׳ let the guests eat (some ed. אריסטין, *our guests?*). Lev. R. s. 28 אריסיא (corr. acc.). Lam. R. to IV, 2 ביני א׳ among the seated guests.

אֲרִיסְטוֹבְלוֹס, אֲרִיסְטוֹבּוּלוֹס pr. n. m. (Ἀριστόβουλος) *Aristobule*, brother of Hyrcan, son of Alexander Jannai. Men. 64[b]; B. Kam. 82[b]; a. e.

אריסטון, read:

אֲרִיסְטוֹן I m. (ἄριστον) orig. *morning meal*, later *principal meal, dinner, repast*. Y. Ber. IV, 7[b] אין הוויה לכון א׳ כ׳ if ye are invited to a dinner, and the day is advanced, &c. Y. Snh. III, 21[c] top גו א׳ during dinner. Ib. VI, 23[c]; a. fr.

אֲרִיסְטוֹן II pr. n. m. *Ariston*. Hall. IV, 11; Y. Shebi. VI, end, 37[a] (a Syrian land-owner).—Y. Yeb. XVI, end, 16[a] חד א׳ one Ariston. [*'One of the* βουλὴ ἀριστῶν mentioned Cod. Theod. Lib. XII, Tit. 888, Frankel M'bo p. 65[a].]

אֲרִירָה f. (ארר) *cursing, imprecation*. Y. Ber. IV, 8[c] (play on *Aron*, the ark) from there א׳ יוצאה לעולם curse goes forth into the world (for transgressors); a. e.

אֲרִירָן, v. אֲרָרָן.

אֲרִישָׁא or **אֲרִישָׁא, ארישאן, ארישאן, ארישן**, v. אֲרִיסָא.

אֲרִישְׁתָּא or **אֲרִישְׁתָּא (אֲרִיסוּתָא, אֲרִישׁוּתָא)** f. (ארשׁ, v. ארס) prop. *obligation*, hence (sub. סעודה) *a meal which creates an obligation, a meal which is given in the expectation of receiving invitations from the* *reciprocating members of a social club*, opp. פירענא the entertainment in reciprocation for invitations received. M. Kat. 22ᵇ ארדש׳ Ar. (ed. אריסותא, Ms. M. ארשיותא, read ארישו׳).

אֲרִיתָא (אֲרִיתָּא) m. (ארת, √אר, cmp. יְאוֹר) *cut, channel, dyke* Targ. Ps. CVII, 35 (h. text אגם); a. e.—Hull. 107ᵃ א׳ דדלאי dyke for irrigation. B. Kam. 50ᵇ sq.—*Pl.* אֲרִיתָתָא (אֲרִיתֵּי). Targ. O. Ex. VIII, 11. Targ. Ps. LXXVIII, 44. (h. text יְאֹר); a. e. Cmp. חריין.

ארך (√אר, cmp. ארג) *to join, weave;* whence *to arrange, plan;* v. ערך.—V. אֲרִיךְ II, אֲרוּכָה &c.

אָרַךְ or **אָרֵךְ** (b. h.; √אר, cmp. Schr. KAT p. 497 ארג; cmp. also גדל to *plait,* to *be tall*) *to be [pointed, stretched,] long, tall.*

Hif. הֶאֱרִיךְ 1) *to prolong, be long in doing.* Ber. I, 4 אמרו לְהַאֲרִיךְ they commended a lengthy benediction. Ib. 34ᵃ; cmp. אַרְכָן. Yoma 35ᵇ הֶאֱ׳ בתפלתו staid long in prayer.—הא׳ ימים *to live long.* Meg. 27ᵇ; a. fr.—Ber. 8ᵇ, a. fr. מַאֲרִיכִין ימיו his life will be prolonged.—הא׳ רוח, פנים *to be long-suffering, forbearing.* Y. Shebu. IV, beg. 35ᵇ; a. fr.—Y. Taan. II, 65ᵇ bot. when collecting debts (punishing) מאריך וגובה he is slow in collecting (punishes in long intervals, gives extension).—2) *to be long, last long.* Num. R. s. 20, end הא׳ חברזל the point of the spear grew longer, v. infra; a. fr.—3) *[to lengthen the carrying pole,] to make heavy.* Nidd. 16ᵇ כמה הֶאֱרַכְתָּ עלינו how heavy thou hast made our burden (through restrictive laws)!

Nif. נֶאֱרַךְ *to be prolonged, grow longer.* Sifré Num. 131; Yalk. ib. 771; (Num. R. l. c. האריך).

אָרֵךְ, v. אֲרִיךְ I.

אֶרֶךְ m. (b. h.) only with אַף, אַפַּיִם *long-suffering, forbearing.* Y. Taan. II, 65ᵇ; a. fr.; v. אַף.

אַרְכָא I m. (ארך; cmp. אוּרְבָּא); pl. אַרְכֵי *meshes, ranges, intervals.* Sabb. 50ᵇ. Gitt. 69ᵇ. B. Bath. 3ᵃ, v. אוּרְבָּא.—Targ. Esth. VIII, 15 בארכוהי in its (the girdle's) meshes.

אַרְכָא II, אַרְכָּא, אַרְכָה f. (ארך) *duration, term, limit; extension of time.* Dan. IV, 24 (prolongation). Ib. VII, 12 (set term).—Targ. Gen. VI, 3; a. e.

אַרְכָא III f. (=h. אֲרוּכָה) *healing, restoration.* Targ. II Chr. XXIV, 13.—*Pl.* אַרְכָן, (אֲרוּכָן). Targ. Ps. CXLVII, 3 (ed. Vien. ארכא).

***אַרְכַּבְתָּא** f. (רכב) (a rider,) *the uppermost layer of a clay dam around a field.* B. Mets. 103ᵇ בוכרא the first, נפתא the additional (middle), א׳ the uppermost. [Targ. Y. Lev. IX, 17 read אַדְפַּרְתָּה.]

אַרְכָּה f. h. (v. אַרְכָא II) *extension, a certain time.* Num. R. s. 14 (p. 259ᵃ ed. Amst.) נתן להם א׳ וכ׳ allowed them a certain time but finally punished them.

אַרְכּוּבָא=אַרְכּוּבְתָּא.

אַרְכּוּבָה f. (רכב) 1) *the leg from under the hip-bone to the ankle, the knee and its surrounding parts* (containing three sections each of which is called א׳ and defined by a different surname). Hull. IV, 6; v. ib. 76ᵃ (also רְכוּבָה); a. fr.—2) *anything joined, joint.* Kil. VII, 1 הא׳ שבגפן (Tosef. ib. IV, 11, Var. הבריכה שבסלע) that part of the vine which is bent down and laid in the ground to rise at another place. Y. Meg. I, 71ᶜ bot. א׳ של למ״ד the lower joint of the Lammed. Kel. XIV, 8 מפתח של א׳ וכ׳ (Tosef. ib. B. Mets. IV, 15 רוּכְבָה . . . . רכובתו) a key with a joint, broken at the joint.—*Pl.* אַרְכּוּבוֹת. Nid. 30ᵇ. B. Mets. 105ᵃ.

אַרְכּוּבְתָא ch. same. Targ. Esth. V, 9. [Y. Maasr. V, end, 52ᵃ אביבא דפילא, read ארכובא or עניבה; Y. Ned. III, 37ᵈ bot.; Y. Shebu. III, 34ᵈ.]—*Pl.* אַרְכּוּבָתָא. Targ. Koh. XII, 3. Targ. II, Esth. VI, 11.—אַרְכּוּבַיָּא Targ. Job. IV, 4.—V. רְכוּבְתָא.

ארכוליפורין, v. ארכי׳.

אַרְכּוֹנָא, אַרְכּוֹן m. ch. (=h. אַרְכָן q. v.) *ruler, elder* Targ. I Chr. XI, 2 (h. text נגיד). Targ. Job. XXI, 28 (h. text נדיב); a. fr.—Y. Ber. V, 9ᵃ עבר א׳ an elder passed by.—*Pl.* אַרְכּוֹנִין. Targ. II Chr. XI, 11; a. e.—Y. Peah VIII, 21ᵃ (defective sentence); [h. pl. אַרְכּוֹנוֹת, v. אַרְכָן].

אַרְכּוֹנְטֵס, ארכונטוס m. (ἄρχων, -οντος) *archont, city-magistrate, prefect.* Y. Taan. IV, 69ᵃ top. Lam. R. to II, 2; IV, 18. Gen. R. s. 76 ארכונגוס (corr. acc.). [The office of a city mayor or senator in the Roman days was often ruinous to its occupants; v. Sm. Ant. s. v. Senatus.]

***אַרְכּוֹף** m. (רכף, cmp. מַרְכּוֹף) prob. *a screwing contrivance for bending wood; engine of torture, stocks.* Esth. R. to I, 1ᵇ; v. אוּפְּרִיפָא.

אַרְכֵי I f. (ארך, v. עַרְכֵּי; an adaptation of ἀρχή, cmp. אַרְכָן) *term of office, office, court of elders.* Num. R. s. 9 whoever was signed as a witness בא׳ ישנה וכ׳ (Kidd. IV, 5 ערכי q. v.) in the old court of Zepphoris.—Y. M. Kat. II, end, 81ᵇ מעלה לְאַרְכֵיהֶם he (the gentile) takes the deed to their (gentile) office for recording. Y. Gitt. I, 43ᵈ top.—Ruth R. to I, 3 א׳ של בנך דוחקת the time of thy son's accession to office presses. Deut. R. s. 2 הגיע א׳ וכ׳ surrender thy office to Joshua. Ib. a prefect שהיה בא׳ שלו who was in his office; a. fr.—*Pl.* אַרְכִיּוֹת. Ruth. R. l. c. א׳ א׳ הן the terms of office are predestined (cmp. Sabb. 30ᵃ bot. ואין מלכות וכ׳). [עַרְכָּאוֹת, v. עַרְכֵּי.]

אַרְכֵי II, pr. n. pl. קִרְיַת א׳ *Kiryath Arkhi* (=קרית ספר); v. preced. Targ. Josh. XV, 15; a. e.

אַרְכֵי III (Greek pref. ἀρχι—) *chief of* (gen. followed by a pl.) as א׳ בִּרְיוֹנִים *chief of the castle guard.* Pesik. Ekha p. 122ᵇ Ar. (ed. אדני מריונים, corr. acc.); v. respective determinants.

ארכידיקי, Gen. R. s. 50 beg., Mus., v. יודקו.

אַרְכִּיוֹן m. (ἀρχεῖον, archivum) *prefecture, public building, archive.* Tanh. Ki Thetsé ט he went לא׳ של וכ׳

into the Egyptian archive; Pesik. Zakh. p. 27ª לבית א׳ Ar. (ed. ארמון, corr. acc.); Yalk. a. l. ארכוון (some ed. ארמון, corr. acc.). Esth. R. to I, 3 להדא א׳ דגדר as in the state-house of Gadara. [Ex. R. s. 5 בית ארמון corr. acc.]

אַרְכִיטֵיקְטוּס, אַרְכִיטִיקְטוֹן m. (ἀρχιτέκτων, architectus) *architect, engineer.* Gen. R. s. 24, beg. לא׳ שבנה וכ׳ to be compared to an engineer that built the fortifications of a principality; Num. R. s. 9, beg. לארכי קיטון קטאר׳ (corr. acc., and insert שנעשה) to an architect that was appointed &c.; a. fr.—*Pl.* אַרְכִיטֶקְטוֹנִין, אַרְכִיטֶקְטִין. Y. Ber. IX, 13ª top טקטנן .... (corr. acc.).

ארכילוסטקיא, v. אִיסְפּוֹלְסְטִיקָא.

אַרְכִילִיסְטִים, ...לִיסטוּסִין, ארכיליסטוטין, v. next w.

אַרְכִילִיסְטִים m. (ἀρχιλῄστης) *chief robber, leader of a gang.* Gen. R. s. 48; a. fr. [Frequ. ארכיליסטים, divide in two words, v. אַרְכִי III, a. לִיסְטִים.] [Yalk. Ex. 255 ארכיליסטוסין, טוטין . . ., read אִיסְפּוֹלְסְטִיקִין.—Midr. Sam. s. XXV, end ארכיליסטים some ed., v. אַרְכִיסְטִים.]

***אַרְכִילִיפוּרִין** m. (read in two words, v. אַרְכִי III, a. לופר) *chief of the body-guard, executioner;* cmp. ספיקולטור. Pesik. B'shall. p. 91ᵇ ארכוליפורין Ar. (ed. ארטל ליפרן, Var. ארכן ליפרן, ארבו, לפילון ארכופילון, v. Buber a. l. note; corr. acc.).

אַרְכִיסְטִים m. (ὀρχήστης) *dancer.* Y. Succ. V, 55ᶜ top; Y. Snh. II, 20ᵇ bot. ארכסטס; Num. R. s. 4.—*Pl.* אַרְכִיסְטִין or אַרְכִיסְטֵיסִין. Midr. Sam. s. XXV, end ארכיסטריס, Var. ארכיליסטים (corr. acc.).

***אַרְכִיסְטְרָטֵיגוּס, אַרְכִיסְטְרָאטִיגוּס** m. (ἀρχιστρατηγός) *commander in chief;* also *chief magistrate* (v. אִסְטְרָטֵיגוּס). Gen. R. s. 58; (Ex. R. s. 31 אסטרט׳).

ארכיסטריגוס, Gen. R. s. 58, corr. as preced. w.

ארכיסטריס, v. אַרְכִיסְטִים.

ארכיקימון, read אַרְכִיטֶקְטוֹן.

ארכל, v. אַרְבַּל I.

אַרְכָן I m. (ארך, an adaptation of ἄρχων) *elder, magistrate.* B. Bath. 164ᵇ a letter of divorce dated בשנת פלוני א׳ (Var. עַרְכָאן, עַרְכָן v. Rabb. D. S. a. l. note 3 sq.; cmp. עַרְכִי) in the year when—was magistrate; v. הוּגְרָן.—*Pl.* אַרְכוֹנוֹת. Cant. R. to VII, 9. Ch. אַרְכוֹנָא, אַרְכוֹן.

אַרְכָן II m. (אָרַךְ) *one giving long prayers,* opp. קַצְרָן. Ber. 34ª; Mekh. B'shall., Vayassa 1 מארכן (read מה א׳).

אַרְכָנוּתָא f. (אַרְכָן I) *office.* B. Bath. 164ᵇ (Var. עַרְכָנ׳, v. אַרְכָן I).

***אַרְכָסָא** m. (רכס) *thick, well-kneaded.* Men. 43ª חמירא א׳ thick leaven of barley flour.

ארכסטס, ארכסימס, read אַרְכִיסְטִים.

ארכקפאן, v. אַרְטְקַפָּא.

***אַרְכַת** pr. n. pl. *Arkhath, Warka,* S. E. of Babylon (v. Schr. KAT p. 94). Yoma 10ª (expl. *Erekh,* Gen. X, 10) א׳ זו Ms. M. (ed. אוריכות, v. Rabb. D. S. a. l.; Targ. Y. Gen. l. c. חדס; Gen. R. s. 37 חרן; Yalk. 62 ארם).

***אַרְלָא**=עַרְלָא.—*Pl.* אַרְלִין, אַרְלָאִין. Targ. Y. II, Gen. XXXIV, 31 some ed.

אֲרָם pr. n. (b. h.) 1) *Aram,* son of Shem. Targ. Gen. X, 22; a. e.—2) *Aramaea, Syria.* Targ. I Kings XX, 1; a. fr.—3) (a disguise for רוֹמָא) *Rome, Roman empire* (cmp. אֱדוֹם). Pes. 87ᵇ לקבל גזרות אכזריות א׳ ed. (read לסבול... של א׳; in Ms. M. 1 only לסבול גזיר׳, Ms. 2 של... רומיים; oth. var., v. Rabb. D. S. a. l. note; Gitt. 17ª אֲרוֹמָיִים) to endure the severe decrees of Rome.

אַרְמָא, אַרְמָאָה m. (=h. אֲרַמִּי) *Syrian.* Targ. Gen. XXV, 20; a. e.—B. Kam. 59ª דיקלא א׳ Ms. (ed. דא׳ corr. acc.) Syrian palm-tree.—*Fem.* אַרְמֵיתָא. Targ. I Chr. VII, 14 (ed. Rahm. ארמותא).—*Pl.* m. אַרְמָאֵי. Targ. II Chr. XXII, 5; f. אַרְמְיָאתָא. Sabb. 29ª Syrian (dates).—Cmp. אַרְמַאי.

אַרְמָא, אַרָמָא f.=אֲרָמוּתָא 2). Targ. Ex. XXIX, 24; a. e.

אַרְמָאָה, v. אַרְמָא.

אַרְמָאָה, v. next w.

אֲרוֹמָאָה, אַרְמָאָה, אַרְמַיָּא, אֲרַמִּי h., **אַרְמָאִי** ch. m. (=b. h. אֲרַמִּי) *Syrian,* in gen. *gentile, Roman;* cmp. אֲרַמִּי 2). Targ. O. Lev. XXV, 47.—Y. Shebi. IV, 35ᵃᵇ חד א׳ ברומי (Y. Snh. III, 21ᵇ חד בר נש) a gentile in Rome. Ib. או יהודיי וכ׳ (prob. plur.) either be Jewish Jews (living as Jews ought to) or gentile gentiles (Roman Romans). Y. Ab. Zar. III, 41ᶜ top ארמייא וכ׳ the leather bottle of an Aramæan (or gentile) burst open. Yeb. 45ᵇ בר ארמאה son of a gentile. Ḥull. 97ª; a. fr.—*Pl.* אַרְמָאֵי. Targ. Y. Deut. XXXII, 24 (*Romans*); a. e.—Ab. Zar. 31ᵇ.—Gitt. 17ª אֲרוֹמָאֵי (*Romans*). Gen. R. s. 63 אַרְמָאִין. Koh. R. to VII, 11 אַרְמָיִין.—Num. R. s. 7 אַרְמָאִיב (Kel. I, 8 עכ״ום); a. fr. [Lev. R. s. 34 אותן מארמאין, read מיזדמאין, v. זְמַי.] —*Fem.* אַרְמַיְיתָא. Yeb. l. c. V. אַרְמָא.

אַרְמוֹן I m. (b. h., prob. fr. חרם=ארם) *enclosure, palace* (poëtic). Ab. Zar. 24ᵇ praised בדביר א׳ in the innermost of the Palace (Temple). [Ex. R. s. 5 בית א׳; Pesik. Zakh. p 27ª, v. אַרְכִיוֹן.] Cmp. ארם Schr. KAT p. 536.

***אַרְמוֹן II** pr. n. pl. *Armon.* Yeb. 45ª captives coming from A. (v. Neub. Géogr. p. 371; prob. ident. with רִמּוֹן, q. v.).

אַרְמוֹן III m. (v. עַרְמוֹן) *platanus, the oriental plane.* אַרְמוֹנִים. Gen. R. s. 15, beg.; (R. Hash. 23ª; B. Bath. 81ª עַר׳).

אַרְמוּתָא, אֲרָ׳ f. (רום) 1) *raising, rising.* Targ. Is. XIX, 16; a. e.—2) *waving, heave-offering.* Targ. O. Ex.

XXIX, 27; a. e.—*Pl.* אַרְמָוָתָא, const. אַרְמָוַת. Targ. O. Num. XVIII, 11 (Var. אַרְמוּת sing.).

אֲרַמַּי m., אֲרַמִּית f. 1) (b. h.) *Aramaean, Aramaic, Chaldaic.* [Targ. II Kings XVIII, 26.]—לשון א׳ *Chaldaic.* Sabb. 12[b]; a. fr.—2) (=אֲרוֹמִי; v. אֱדֹם 3) *Romish, Roman, heathen.* [Owing to Christian censors as well as timid Jewish copyists, many of the passages originally referring to Romans, Christians, &c., have been altered by substituting *Arammi, Kuthi, Goy* &c., so that only by keen criticism their real application can be ascertained.]—Fem. *gentile woman.* Ber. 8[b] (Ms. M. ארמאית). Snh. IX, 6; a. fr.—Y. Meg. I, 71[c] top ארמית *Latin;* v. בָּדָא.—*Pl.* אֲרַמִּיִּים Meg. 11[a] (some ed. פרסיים; Ms. M. רוֹמִיִּים; Sifra B'hukk. Par. II, ch. 8 אספסיינוס). V. אֲרוֹמִי.

אֲרַמִּיוּתָא f. (preced.) *gentile ways, Romedom, idolatry,* &c. Meg. III (IV), 9 (25[a]) whoever translates (Lev. XVIII, 21), 'Of thy seed thou shalt give none לאעברא בא׳ (Ms. Lond. לאעבורי אומיתא, v. Var. in Rabb. D. S. a. l. note) to become with child in Romedom (identifying Molokh with Rome and misinterpreting *l'haăbir* for the purpose of making it applicable to sexual connection with Romans) must be silenced with a sharp rebuke (v. נְזִיפָה); cmp. Targ. Y. Lev. l. c.—Ab. Zar. 70[a] כד הוינן בארמיותן (Ms. M. הואי בגיותא) when we were yet in our heathendom (prior to our conversion).

אַרְמִי, אַרְמָיָא, v. אַרְמַאי.

***אַרְמִילוּס** pr. n. m. (a disguise of Romulus, Ῥώμυλος=Rome) *Armilus,* a mythical personage, representative of wickedness, answering to the Christian Antichrist. Targ. Is. XI, 4 א׳ רשיעא A. the wicked. Targ. Y. Deut. XXXIV, 3 ארמלגוס (corr. acc.); cmp. אַרְמַנְיָאה. [V. Book of Zerub.; Saadia Emunoth VIII, 2; Graetz Gesch. d. Jud. V, p. 496.]

אַרְמִינְיָא pr. n. *Armenia,* the plateau of Western Asia. Lam. R. to I, 14.—Targ. Y. Gen. VIII, 4 name of a mountain and of a city.

אַרְמֵל (denomin. of next w.) *Nithpa.* נִתְאַרְמְלָה *to become a widow* (a Chaldaism). Keth. II, 1; V, 1; v. אַלְמֵן. Yeb. 42[b]; a. e.

אַרְמְלָא, אַרְמַלְתָּא, אַרְמְלָה f. (=אלמל׳ fr. עלם; v. אַלְמוֹן; v. P. S. s. v. 391) *widow.* Targ. Gen. XXXVIII, 11; a. fr.—Y. Sabb. I, 3[d] top; a. fr.—*Pl.* אַרְמְלָן. Targ. Ex. XXII, 23, a. e.—Y. Keth. I, beg. 24[d].—אַרְמְלָתָא, אַרְמְלָאתָא. Targ. Job XXII, 9; a. e.—Y. Meg. III, 74[a] top; a. e.

ארמלגוס, v. אַרְמִילוּס.

אַרְמְלוּ, אַרְמְלוּת, אַרְמְלוּתָא f. (v. אַרְמְלָא) *(in) widowhood.* Targ. Is. XLVII, 8 sq.; a. e.—Keth. 75[a], v. טַנְדּוּ.—Y. Ned. V, 39[b] top; B. Bath. 98[b] Ms.; ed. אַלְמְנוּת.

אַרְמַלְתָּא, v. אַרְמְלָא.

אַרְמֹן, v. אַרְמוֹן.

אַרְמַנְיָא, 1) v. אַרְמִינְיָא.—[2) Targ. Job I, 1 Nahmanid. in comment., Ms. קושטנטינא, ed. עוץ, v. next w.]

אַרְמַנְיָאה pr. n. pl. *Armannia* (Romania, New-Rome, Constantinople). Targ. Lam. IV, 21 Var. (h. text עוץ).—Deriv. pl. אַרְמַנְיָאֵי. Targ. I Chr. I, 17 ed. Beck. (ed. Rahm. ארמצ׳ corr. acc.).

אַרְמַנְיוּס pr. n. m. (represent. a tribe; v. preced.) *Armanius.* Targ. I Chr. I, 42 (h. text עוץ).

אַרְמַנְיָיא m. *Armenian* (?). Y. Gitt. VI, 48[d] bot. ר׳ יעקב א׳; Y. M. Kat. III, 82[c] top ר׳ א׳ (insert יעקב).

אַרְמַצְיָאֵי, ארמצייאי, v. אַרְמַנְיָאה.

אָרֹן, v. אָרוֹן.

אֹרֶן m. (b. h.; √אר, cmp. אֶרֶז) *pine* (Assyr. ארן *cedar,* Schr. KAT p. 411).—*Pl.* אֳרָנִים. Par. III, 8 (R. Hai Gaon ארנן). R. Hash. 23[a] אֲרוֹנִים (Var. עֲרוֹנִים). B. Bath. 81[a] ע׳.

אַרְנָא m. ch. (=h. אָרוֹן) *chest.* Sabb. 32[a] שקורין לא״הק א׳ who call the holy ark, 'the chest'.

אַרְנָב m.=אַרְנֶבֶת q. v.

אַרְנְבָא, v. אַרְנַבְתָּא.

אַרְנֶבֶת f. (b. h.) *hare;* [pr. n. f., v. next w.]. Meg. 9[b]. Lev. s. 13 הא׳ זו יון *Arnebeth* (Lev. XI, 6) is an allusion to Yavan (Greece); cmp. next w.—*Pl.* אַרְנָבִים. Sabb. 27[a]; Men. 39[b]. [Assyr. Annabu, Schr. KAT p. 498.]

אַרְנְבָא, אַרְנַבְתָּא ch. same. Targ. Lev. XI, 6; a. e.—Lam. R. to II, 10; Ned. 65[a] ארנבא.—Y. Meg. I, 71[d] bot. אמו של תלמי.... ארנתא וכ׳ (corr. acc.) King Ptolemee's mother was named *Hare* (λαγώς); cmp. Meg. 9[b] where the King's wife is named *arnebeth.*

ארנון, Tanh. B'midb. 18, read אָקְטוֹ, v. אֶכְטָא.

***אַרְנוֹן** I m. (deriv. of אָרוֹן) *chest with many cases, trader's chest.* Tanh. B'midb. 20 לאדם פרגמטיוטים שהיה לו א׳ של זכוכית Ar. (ed. incorr.) like a trader that had a chest containing (common) glass beads; cmp. Tanh. ed. Bub. 23a. note; Yalk. Num. 692 (where אבנים must be read ארנון).

אַרְנוֹן II m., **אַרְנוֹנָא, אַרְנוֹנָה** f. (an adaptation of *annona,* cmp. אַנּוֹנָא a. עַסְקָא) [*chest, treasury,* v. preced.] *tax from crops and other farmer's produces delivered in kind.* Y. Keth. XIII, 35[d] א׳ וגלגולת annona and poll-tax.—Pes. 6[a] בהמת א׳ cattle subject to the annona (v. D. C. ed. Hensch, s. v. Annona: 'capitur etiam in pecudibus'); עיסת א׳ dough made of flour subject to annona.—*Pl.* אַרְנוֹנוֹת, אַרְנוֹנִין, אַרְנוֹנִיּוֹת. Targ. Y. Deut. XXVIII, 36. Lev. R. s. 29. Y. Shebi. IV, 35[b]; a. fr.—Y. Snh. III, 21[b] top מיגבי ארנונין to collect taxes Pesik. Shek. 11[b] (description of Roman extortions) אייתי ארנוניך bring thy *annonae.*

אַרְנָטוּס m. (ornatus, ὀρνᾶτος) *decoration.* Lam. R. to IV, 1 שהיה דומה לא׳ של זהב (ed. ארנטס, ארונטס) who was (to the nation) like a gold decoration.

ארנטס, v. preced.

ארנני Yalk. Gen. 47 ארנני קטון, read אַרְכִּיטְקְטוֹן.

אַרְנְסִי, v. אוּרְנוּס.

אַרְנְקָא ch.=next w. B. Bath. 8ª; a. fr.—Trnsf. א׳ דמוחא bag, i. e. *membrane of the brains.* Ber. 19ª.—*Pl.* אַרְנְקֵי. B. Mets. 84ᵇ. Keth. 67ª.

אַרְנָקִי f. (אנק, ר inserted for Dagesh) *merchant's bag suspended from the neck,* cmp. אַבְפְּלִי; in gen. *money-bag, purse.* Y. Kidd. I, 61ª bot. Lev. R. s. 14; a. fr. [Ib. א׳ של כסף, read אוּנְקְיָא.]

ארנקפאן, v. אַרְטְקָפָא.

ארנתא Y. Meg. I, 71ᵈ bot., v. אַרְנַבְתָּא.

אֶרֶס, אִירָס m. (√רס; v. רְסַס; as to modification of meaning cmp. Lat. *virus*) prop. *drop, fluid.* esp. *poison.* Y. Ter. III, beg. 42ª the serpent הטיל בו א׳ threw a drop (of poison) into it. Sabb. 62ᵇ (play on *t'akkasnah,* Is. III, 16) כארס בכעוס (read כא׳ עכיס; v. Var. Rabb. D. S. a. l. note) like the serpent's poison; a. fr.—Y. Maasr. V, end, 52ª an onion שאין לו אירס (read אירס) which has no penetrating moisture.—*Pl.* אֵירְסִין, אֶרְסִין. Y. Ter. VIII, 45ᶜᵈ. Cmp. רִיס.

אֶרֶס, אוּרְסָא ch. same. Targ. Y. Deut. I, 31; Gen. III, 14, some ed. אַרְיְסָא; a. fr.—*Pl.* אֵירְסִין. Targ. Y. Deut. XXXII, 24 (ed. Vien. אֶרְסִין).

אָרַס (b. h. אֵרֵשׂ Pi.; √אר, v. ארר) *to bind, join; to betroth.* Part. pass. אָרוּס, f. אֲרוּסָה *betrothed, engaged.* Keth. 13ᵇ אָרוּס וַאֲרוּסָתוֹ a betrothed couple. Y. Hag. II, 77ᵈ אֲרוּסִי my betrothed, i. e. my beloved citizen.

Pi. אֵרַס, אֵירָס 1) *to betroth to one's self, engage in marriage.* Y. Bets. V, 63ª bot. לְאָרֵס. Ib. הא לאירס יְאָרֵס but betroth he may; a. fr.—Yeb. VI, 4 אירס וכ׳ he betrothed a widow. Keth. I, 6 אֵרַסְתַּנִי, אֵרַסְתִּיךְ; a. fr. [As to the legal status of betrothal, v. אֵירוּסִין.]—2) *to give away in betrothal* (of the bride's father). Ib. IV, 2.—Part. pass. מְאוֹרָסָה. Snh. VII, 9; a. fr.—Ex. R. s. 33 (play on *morashah,* Deut. XXXIII, 4).—

Hithpa. a. *Nithpa.* הִתְאָרְסָה, נִתְאָרְסָה *to be betrothed* (only of the woman). Keth. III, 3; a. e.—Yeb. IV, 10 הנשואות יִתְאָרְסוּ וכ׳ those who have been married before, may get betrothed (before the expiration of three months after separation from their husbands by death or divorce), and those who have been betrothed (and not yet married), may get married (during the above term).

אָרַס, *Pa.* **אָרֵס**, fut. יְאָרֵס, ch. same. Targ. O. Deut. XXVIII, 30; a. fr.—מְאָרְסָא (אֲרְסָא) *betrothed woman.* Targ. Y. Lev. XX, 10. Targ. Ex. XXII, 15 (16).—*Cant. R. to IV, 12 אֲרוּסְתֵּיהּ or אֲרוּסְתֵּיה (Chald. suffix) his betrothed.—[Lev. R. s. 34 דאינון מארסוון, read באנסיבין, v. אֲנַס, or דאתון ביזודמיין, v. זְמַן.]

Ithpe. אִתְאָרֵיס, contr. אִתְּרֵיס (cmp. אֲנַס Ithpe.) *to be betrothed.* בר אִיתְּרוּסֵי *marriageable.* Gitt. 43ª; a. fr.

אַרְסְטֵר, v. אַרִיסְט׳.

***ארסקינון** Koh. R. to I, 7, end, perh. a. corrupt. of אֵירְיוֹקְסִילוֹן m. (ἐριόξυλον) *cotton.* [The entire sentence, however, seems to be misplaced, and a repetition of a preceding one.]

אַרְסְקִינָס pr. n. m. *Ursicinus,* a Roman general delegated against Judea by Gallus who, as Constantine's nephew and associate emperor, resided at Antiochia. Y. Yeb. XVI, beg. 15ᶜ; Y. Sot. IV, 23ᶜ bot. א׳ מלכא U. the king (royal governor?). Y. Shebi. IV, 35ª לא׳....חורון מְפֵּר; Y. Bets. I, 60ᶜ bot. הורי פיתא לא׳ וכ׳ (insert מְפֵּר) the sages allowed to have bread baked on the Sabbath for (the army of) U. because his intercession might be needed. [Diff. explan. of latter sentence, v. Frankel *M'bo,* p. 56ª.] Y. Ber. V, 9ª. Y. Meg. III, 74ª top א׳ אוקיד וכ׳ U. burnt the scrolls of the Law of the congregation of Zennabris.

אָרַע (√רע, v. רעע) *to strike against. Nif.* נֶאֱרַע *to come in contact with* (cmp. זווג), *to happen, befall* (gen. of evil occurrences). Ber. IV, 2 שלא תֶּאֱרַע וכ׳ (Bab. ed. 28ᵇ שלא יֶאֱרַע דבר וכ׳) that no (religious) offence may happen through me (by an erroneous decision &c.). Yoma I, 1 שמא יארע בו פסול lest something may occur to him to unfit him for services. Esth. R. to II, 7 שיארע על ישראל (read שיארע לישר׳) will happen to Israel; a. fr.

Pi. אֵרַע, אֵירַע *to strike, befall;* (neut. v.) *to occur.* Y. Kidd. I, 58ᵈ top ולא א׳ מעשה no accident (illegal act) *occurred.* Gen. R. s. 84 כל מה שאירע לזה וכ׳ whatever befell the one, befell also the other; a. fr.—M. Kat. II, 1 אֵירְעוֹ אבל (Ms. M. אירע בו) mourning in the family befell him; a. e.—Y. Shek. V, 48ᵈ bot. כך וכך אירע; Y. Dem. I, 22ª אירעין....(read אירעו) so and so it happened to him. *Part. Pu.* מְאוֹרָע q. v.

Hithpa. הִתְאָרַע *to be added to, to join.* Y. Sot. I, 17ª אחת מִתְאָרַעַת לאחת וכ׳ one (sin) is added to the other, until the account is full; Num. R. s. 9.

אֲרַע I ch. (in Targ. Y.; in O. usu. עֲרַע q. v.) same; *to join, meet, find; to attack, visit.* Targ. Y. Gen. XIX, 19 תִירְעִינַנִי may befall me Targ. Y. Deut. XXXII, 10 (h. text מצא). Targ. Y. Ex. V, 3 (h. פגע). Ib. IV, 2 (h. פגש; ed. Vien. יַעְרַע read יַאֲרַע). Targ. Y. Lev. V, 7 לא תֶאֱרַע ידיה he will not be able, cannot afford (h. text תגיע וכ׳, cmp. תמצא ידו); a. fr. [Targ. Y. II, Ex. XV, 9 ואֵרַע יתהון (I ונְעַרַע, וגרע) read ואירע and I shall meet them.]

Ithpa. אִתְאָרַע, *Ithpe.* contr. אִיתְרַע, אִירַע or *Pa.* אֲרַע *to be met; to meet.* Targ. Y. I, Num. XXIII, 15 אֶתְעֲרַע (h. text אִקָּרֶה). M. Kat. 18ª, a. e. איתרע ביה מילתא an accident befell him (death in the family).—Lev. R. s. 37 אַרְעַת שעתא it so happened. Koh. R. to XI, 1 ארעת ענת׳ וכ׳ it happened to be the season when the Israelites travelled to Jerusalem. Y. Dem. I, 22ª אירעין, v. preced. Targ. Esth. VIII, 8 התארעין=תִּתְרַן; Targ. Y. Gen. XLIV, 34 תברוז (corr. acc.). [אתרע *to be shaken, weakened,* v. רעע.]

Af. אוֹרַע=Pe. Targ. Ruth II, 3; a. e.—Targ. Ps. LXXXV, 11 אוֹרְעוּן (some ed. אָרְעִין Pe.) meet each other.

***אָרַע** II (√רע, cmp. רוּעַ, *Hif.* הֵרִיעַ, cmp. קְרָא a. קָרָה) *to proclaim a festival.* Sifré Num. 147 אֵירְעוּ במאבל

וכ׳ proclaim it (as מקרא קדש) with special meal and dress; v. Mekh. Bo 9, beg.

Pu. אוֹרַע *to be proclaimed.* B. Bath. 113[b] with והיתה אוֹרְעָה כל וכ׳ (Num. XXVII, 11) . . . משפט the whole section has been proclaimed as of a judicial nature; (Ms. M. הודעה, v. יְדַע).

אֲרַע II (Targ. Y., O. usu. עֲרַע q. v.), *Pa.* אַרַּע, אֲרַע same. Targ. Y. Lev. XXIII, 2; a. fr. Targ. O. Num. X, 2 לְעָרָעָה ed. Berl. (oth. ed. לְאַרְעָא); (Targ. Y. לְעָרְעָא, לְעָרָעָא!). [Targ. Y. Lev. XXIII, 4 דִּי תְעָרְעוּן, corr. דִּי תְאַרְעוּן. Ib. 21, a gloss חיין וקיימין חד בזמן ref. to the festive benediction שהחיינו וקימנו וכ׳.]—Denom. מְעָרְעָא, מְאַרְעָא.

אֲרַע *land,* v. אַרְעָא.—אֲרַע- *nether-, beneath,* v. אַרְעָאָה.

אַרְעָא m. (אֲרַעI) *accident, occurrence.* Targ. Ruth II, 3.—[**Pl.* אַרְעַיָּא *evils, diseases.* Targ. Y. Deut. XXVIII, 60 (prob. to be read מַרְעַיָּא).]

אַרְעָא f. (√רע, h. אֶרֶץ q. v.) [the brittle] *land, earth, ground, field.* Targ. Gen. I, 1. Targ. Y. Gen. XVI, 5; a. fr.—B. Bath. 29[a] חדא א׳ one field; v. בָּאגָא.—Bekh. 25[b] א׳ דחשוכא a land of darkness (Babylon); a. fr.—Sabb. 65[a] בת א׳ (a Chaldaic adaptation of ποδάγρα, podagra) *gout, sore on the toes.*—עם דא׳=עם הארץ, v. אֶרֶץ.—*Pl.* אַרְעָן, אַרְעָתָא, אַרְעָאן. Targ. Jer. XXVIII, 8 Levita, Targ. II Esth. IV, 1. Usu. אַרְעָתָא. Targ. Gen. XXVI, 3; a. fr.—B. Bath. 12[b]; 61[b] *fields.*—B. Kam. 7[a] זול א׳, הוקר א׳ (Ms. M. זיל, sub. דמי) land fell, rose in price. V. לְאַרַע.

אַרְעָאָה, אַרְעָיָה m. (preced.) *earth-ward, that which, he who, is below, nethermost.* Targ. Josh. XVI, 3; a. fr.—Y. Kil. IX, end, 32[d] שלח א׳ to put off the under-garment. Y. B. Mets. X, beg. 12[c] ארעייא who lives in the story below.—*Pl.* אַרְעָאֵי, אַרְעָאִין. Targ. Gen. VI, 16; a. e.—Lam. R. to I, 16 עביד בא׳ וכ׳ deal with the inferiors (females) as thou didst with the superiors (men); ib. to IV, 19; Y. Succ. V, 55[b] (incorr. vers.).—Fem. אַרְעַיְתָא. Targ. Ez. XLI, 7; a. fr.—Y. Maas. Sh. V, 56[c] top.—*Pl.* אַרְעַיָּתָא, אַרְעַיָּיתָא. Targ. Ez. XLII, 5; 6. Y. Yoma I, 38[c]; Y. Meg. V, 75[c] bot., v. אִסְכּוּפְתָא. [Targ. Esth. אֲרַע מדינה, v. לְאַרַע.]

אַרְעַי m. (אֲרַעI) *chance-, occasional, temporary,* v. עֲרַאי.

אַרְעָיָא, אַרְעָיָה, v. אַרְעָאָה.

אַרְעִית f. (v. preced.) *lower portion, bottom.* Y. Kil. VII, beg. 30[d]. Y. Shebi. I, 33[b] top; a. e.

אַרְעִיתָא ch. same. Men. 11[a]; Yoma 48[a] ארעיתיה (read אַרְעִיתֵיה) the bottom of the reversed vessel. Keth. 77[b] א׳ דמוחא the skull(!).—V. אַרְעָאָה.

ארפכוסיא, read אִיפַּרְכוּסְיָא.

אַרְפַּס (אֲפַרְכָּס) ארפכס m. (ἅρπαξ=ὑδράρπαξ, ἁρπάγιον) *clepsydra, water-clock.* Kel. XIV, 8; XXX, 4 אר׳ Ar. (ed. אפ׳). Gen. R. s. 4 הבא אר׳ get me a clepsydra.

ארפכסת, read אֲפַרְכֶּסֶת.

אֶרֶץ f. (b. h.; רצץ; Ch. a. oth. dial. ארע fr. רעע *to press together, stamp*—from the rugged appearance of the surface after the subsidence of the waters) *earth, dry land; country, land, field* (opp. to town). Ex. R. s. 13.... threw dust upon the waters ונעשה א׳ and earth (crust) was formed.—א׳ ישראל (abbr. א״י) *Palestine,* opp. חוצה לָאָ׳, or מדינת הים foreign countries, or distant countries. Gitt. I, 2. Ib. 6[a]; a. fr.—הָאָרֶץ *Palestine,* Hull. 16[b] משנכנסו לא׳ since entering Palestine (under Joshua); a. fr.—עם הָאָ׳ (abbr. ע״ה) *country people,* hence *illiterate, coarse, unrefined* (often applied to an individual); *pl.* עַמֵּי הא׳, opp. תלמיד חכם. Sabb. 63[a]. Hull. 92[a]; a. v. fr.—Esp. ע״ה *those not observing certain religious customs regarding tithes, levitical cleanness* &c., opp. חָבֵר q. v. Dem. I, 2; a. fr.—*Pl.* אֲרָצוֹת. Shebi. IX, 2 שלש א׳ וכ׳ Palestine is divided into three countries with reference to the laws of the Sabbath year. Keth. 111[a]; a. e., v. עִיסָּה; a. fr.

***אַרְצוּת** f. (=אַרְצָאוּת, רצי, cmp. הַרְצָאָה) *persuasion, surrender.* Sot. 4[a] כדי טומאתה וארצותה time required for her pollution (by improper contact) and her surrender to the seducer.

אֲרַק, אֲדַק, עֲדַק m. (ארק, cmp. חרק; אדק, עדק, cmp. חדק) *a perforated vessel,* a sort of clepsydra used in sick rooms. Erub. 104[a] ומטיפין מארק Mus. a. oth. (ed. מיארק read מי א׳, Ms. M. ארוך, indistinct, Ms. Oxf. ארג, Ar. אדק a. ארק, v. Ar. ed. Koh.) you may, on the Sabbath, let water drip from the Arak for a sick person; Y. Erub. X, 26[d] top מטיפין (מוסיפין) בעדק; Tosef. Sabb. II, 8 מן אדק ed. Zuck. (Var. האדק).

אַרְקָא I f. (=אַרְעָא, cmp. רקק, v. אֶרֶץ) *earth.* Jer. X, 11.—Pesik. Bahod. p. 155[a]; Gen. R. s. 13; a. e.

אַרְקָא II pr. n. pl. (Ἄρκη, Ἄρκαι) *Arca,* also called *A. Cæsarea, Cæs. Libani,* at the North-Western foot of Mount Lebanon. Gen. R. s. 37 (interpreting הערקי Gen. X, 17) א׳ דליבנן (some ed. ארקס). [Cmp. ערקת לבנה Bekh. 57[b], v. Neub. Géogr. p. 33; 299.]

אַרְקַבְטָא, v. אַלְקַפְטָא.

ארקבסא, read preced.

ארקולאון, v. אדק׳.

אַרְקוּרְיָאנֵי, אַרְקוּלְיָאנֵי m. pl. *Herculiani,* body of guards instituted by Diocletian, together with the *Joviani,* to supersede the prætorians (Gibb. I, 434; v. Sachs Beitr. I, 113 sq.). Esth. R. to I, 3 יבולנר ובר ק׳ (corr. יוביאני ואר׳).

***ארקלין, ארקילין,** read אַסְקַוְלִין m. (ἀσκαύλης) *performer on the bag-pipe.* Targ. II, Esth. I, 3 א׳ אזיל וכ׳ a bag-piper walks at (over) the head of all (ref. to the wind passing over the flax stalks on the field; in a riddle on linen).

***אַרְקָן** m. pl. *crocus plants.* Mass. Kallah, quot. in Hebr. Dict. fr. Gitt. 70[a], v. מוֹרִיקָא.

ארקלין, v. ארקילין.

ארקליס, read אַרְקְלִיּוֹס pr. n. m. *Heraclius,* the surname of Maximianus, the associate emperor of Diocletian. Y. Ab. Zar. I, 39[d] top אנא דיקל׳ וכ׳ I, Diocletian the king, have instituted the annual fair of Tyre in honor of the genius of my brother Heraclius (Heracles).

אַרְקַפְטָא, v. אַלְקַפְטָא.

אַרְקָתָא I f. (רקק) *beaten, wrought metal*, opp. אַנְדִסְפָּא q. v. Sabb. 59[b] Ar. (ed. אֲרוּקְתָא, Var. רוּקְתָא, v. Rabb. D. S. a. l. note).

אַרְקָתָא II f. *shoe-thong*, v. עַרְקָא, עַרְקָתָא. Yeb. 102[a], v. אַפַּנְתָא.

*__אַרְקָתָא__ III f. (cmp. preced.) name of a parasite worm in the bowels, perh. *fluke-worm.* Sabb. 109[b] ed. (Ms. M. אַרְקָאתָא pl., Ms. O. אורקתא, Ar. ׳עַר). Cmp. עַלְקָא. [Mus.=h. יֵרָקוֹן *jaundice;* cmp. אַרְקָן.]

אָרַר (b. h.; √אר, sec. r. of אור, cmp. חָרַר, *to break through, to make holes, meshes* &c.; v. ארב, ארג, ארה, ארז, ארח, ארך &c.) 1) *to dig, stab;* v. אֲרָרָן.—2) *to point out for execration,* [or *to set outside*]; (cmp. חרם a. נקב, a. also ברך); *to curse.*—Part. pass. אָרוּר, f. אֲרוּרָה, pl. אֲרוּרִים &c. Shebu 36[a]; a. fr.—*Y. Sot. II, 18[a] top מֵי יכול מראה מים ת״ל ארר (read אָרַר) you might infer from the word *mé* (Num. V, 18) that it must have the color of water, therefore the root *arar* is used in connection therewith (i. e. water in which the curse written with ink has been washed off and is recognizable in the mixture); אי ארר וכ׳ (read ארר) from *arar* again you might infer that the drink must have the color of ink, therefore we read *mé*, which means the color of water *and* the color of ink (a colored thin fluid); cmp. Bab. Sot. 16[b] (where the same argument is used with reference to blood).—Part. pass. f. אֲרוּרָה cacophem. for *idol.* Ab. Zar. 51[a] לא׳ זו מיבעיא Ms. M. (ed. לע״ז) so much the more for that cursed (idol).

Pi. אֵרַר, אֵירַר *to curse.* Gen. R. s. 36, end מְאָרֵר. Cant. R. to IV, 11 שאֵרְרָה וכ׳ which Joshuah had cursed. Pesik. R. s. 26 שאֵירְרוּ; a. fr.

Nif. a. *Nithpa.* נֶאֱרַר, נִתְאָרֵר *to be cursed.* Num. R. s. 14 לא נֶאֶרְרוּ וכ׳ they were not cursed before seventy verses were completed (Gen. I, 1 to III, 14; Esth. III, 1 to VII, 10). Y. Sot. IX, 24[b] bot.; Tosef. ib. XV, 2 נִתְאָרְרוּ.

אֲרַר ch. same. Targ. II Kings IX, 34 אֲרוּרְתָא the cursed.—אֲרוּרַיָּא, אֲרוּרֵי m. pl. *Arurs*, the Bible chapters containing the word *arur* (Lev. XXVI, 14—46; Deut. XXVIII, 15—69); [Hebr. תוכחות or קללות]. Y. Meg. III, 74[b] bot.—Meg. 31[b] קא מגמגם .... בא׳ read the *arurs* in an undertone. Koh. R. to VIII, 3.

אֲרִירָן, אֲרָרָן m. (v. אָרַר) *dagger.* Snh. 30[b]; 41[a] אָרָ׳ Ar. (ed. a. Ms. אָרָ׳). [Oth. opin. *club.* Var. ארידן.]

*__אָרַשׁ__ (b. h.; Ps. XXI, 3; √אר, cmp. ארס a. חרש) *to weave, arrange,* trnsf. *to plan.* Gen. R. s. 9 קודם עד שלא יֶאֱרַשׁ וכ׳ before yet my tongue prepares a word. [In later liturgic poëtry ארש is used in the sense of *meditation, devotion.*]

אַרְתּוּסִיָּיה pr. n. pl. (Ὀρθωσίας 1 Macc. XV, 37) *Orthosia,* a Phœnician seaport, South of the river Eleutheros. Gen. R. s. 37 (translat. of *has-sini* Gen. X. 17; Targ. O. ib. אַנְתּוּסָאֵי, Y. I אַנְטוֹסָאֵי, II כַּפְרוּסָאֵי).

ארתוקופיון, read אַרְטוֹקוֹפִּיוֹן m. (ἀρτοκόπιον) *bakery,* v. ארטקפא.

אַרְתִּכָּא, אַרְתִּיכָא m. (רתך) *chariot, vehicle.* Targ. II Chr. X, 18; a. e.—*Pl.* אַרְתְּכִין, אַרְתִּיכִין. Targ. Y. I, Ex. XV, 4 (Y. II רתיכ׳).

אֵשׁ c. (b. h.; אשש 1) 1) *fire.* Sabb. 11[a]; a. e. כא׳ לנעורת as destructive as fire to the flax. Sot. 48[b] כא׳ בנעורת like fire among flax, i. e. inflaming the senses. Gen. R. s. 39 מבול של א׳ (v. מַבּוּל) destruction by fire.—Num. R. s. 2 end א׳ הדיוטית fire from outside of the sanctuary; a. fr. —*Pl.* אִשּׁוֹת. Yoma 21[b]; a. fr.—2) *fever.* א׳ של צמות. Gitt. 70[a].

אִשָּׁא, אִישָׁא, אֶשָּׁתָא, אִישְׁתָּא, א׳ f. ch. same. 1) *fire.* Targ. Gen. XV, 17; a. fr.—B. Mets. 85[b] בעורין דאשא *torches.* Men. 53[a] אישא וכ׳ may fire consume him. —2) *fever.* Targ. Y. Gen. XXI, 15.—Yoma 29[a] אישתא וכ׳ the fever in winter time. Sabb. 66[b] sq. א׳ תלתא *tertian;* א׳ צמירתא *inflammatory fever,* א׳ בת יומא *quotidian.* Yeb. 71[b] דזנתיה אי׳ fever fed its vital energies. Snh. 108[b].

אָשָׁא, v. אוּשָׁא.

אָשָׁא *old,* v. אָסָא.

*__אַשַּׁב__=חֲשַׁב. Part. Ithp. מְאַשַּׁב *respected,* v. חֲשַׁב Ithpa.

אִישְׁבּוֹרֶן, אֶשְׁבּוֹרֶן m. (שבר; cmp. מִקְוֶה) *collection of water, pond; cavity for reception of water,* opp. מִדְרוֹן slope. Pes. 42[a] מקום א׳ place where water poured out would remain stagnant. Ab. Zar. 72[a]; Ohol. III, 3, opp. קטפרס. Toh. VIII, 9; a. e.

אשברוע, read אֶשְׁפְּרוּעַ.

הַשְׁגָּרָה, אַשְׁגָּרָה f. (שגר) *current phraseology* (v. שָׁגוּר part. pass. of שָׁגַר)—אַשְׁגָּרַת לשון (הַ׳) current phrase not meant exactly (arising from one's being accustomed to use a certain word in association with others). Y. Meg. II, 73[b] bot.; Y. Ber. II, 4[d].

אֲשַׁד, אֲשֵׁד, אֲשֵׁיד (√שד, v. שדי; v. H. Dict. s. v. אֶשֶׁד) *to pour out, to shed* (blood), *to deposit* (ashes). Targ. Lev. XVII, 4; a. fr.—Sabb. 156[a] אָשֵׁיד דמא a shedder of blood.—Part. pass. אָשִׁיד *shed, spilt.* Targ. Mic. I, 4; III, 10; a. e.

אִשְׁדְּוָותָא, v. אִשְׁתְּדָיוּתָא.

אֲשִׁדָּתָא f. pl. (שדר=h. יָדוֹת) *lateral supports, arms.* Targ. I Kings X, 19.

אִשָּׁה f. (b. h.; v. איש, אנש), const. אֵשֶׁת, *woman, wife.* Pes. VIII, 1. Ab. Zar. 25[b] א׳ כלי זיינה עליה woman carries her weapon with her, is protected against murder by gentiles (who would rather assault her innocence). Ib. א׳ חשובה a woman of high rank (influential). Ib. אִשְׁתּוֹ כשמירתו his wife's presence guards him from wrong-doing; a. fr.—*Pl.* נָשִׁים (נְשׁוֹת) q. v.

אִשֶּׁה *burnt-offering*, v. אִישָּׁה.

אֲשׁוּהָ, אֲשׁוּוָה, (אֲשׁוּרָא, אֲשׁוּוְ׳) f. (שׁוּי, cmp. אֲשִׁיוְתָא a. אֲשׁוּוְתָא) *skein, reel, clue,* esp. *staff around which the wool is put, spool.* Kel. XXI, 1 the wool which is on the distaff 'ובא Ar. (ed. 'בא corr. acc.) or on the spool. Tosef. Kel. B. Bath. I, 6 צמר שעל גבי האֲשָׁוָוה ed. Zuck. (Var. אשה, cler. err.).

אשוון, v. אֲשָׁזוּן.

אֲשׁוּחֵי m. pl. (Syr. *ashuha* P. Sm. 406, שוח) prop. *the bending, a genus of weak (female) cedar,* disting. fr. ארז male cedar. Sabb. 157[a] (Ms. M. שִׁיחֵי). [Opin. in Ar. *cypresses.*]

אֲשׁוּוָא, v. אַשְׁוָה.

אֲשׁוּן *essence*, v. אִישׁוּן.

אֲשׁוּן, אֲשׁוּנָא *hard*, v. אָשֵׁן.

אֲשׁוּנָא m. (b. h. אָשׁוּן; v. אשן, עשן) *dense vapor, steam; vapor-room in the bath* (sudatio). Y. Ned. IV, 38[d] top he who bathes in the small caldarium (v. Sm. Ant. s. v. Baths) נסב א׳ takes away vapor (and does not benefit his fellow-bather by his presence). Y. Shebi. VIII, 38[a] top אעלליה לי לא׳ take it up for me to the vapor-room. Gen. R. s. 33.

אֲשׁוּר, interj., with הייא (שור) *go on, make haste, quick!* Gitt. 34[a] א׳ חבו לה הייא make haste, give her the letter of divorce; quick! Sabb. 119[a] א׳ הייא א׳ הייא. Ber. 57[b] א׳ צדיקי Ar. (ed. רהוטו) run, ye pious ones.

אַשּׁוּר pr. n. (b. h.) *Ashur, Assyria, Assyrian nation.* Gen. R. s. 37; a. fr.—Yoma 10[a]; Keth. 10[b] א׳ זה סילק (סליקא) Ashur means (the later) Seleucia (ad Tigrim). Snh. 106[a] (referring to the Parthian kingdom). [Yalk. Ezek. 376, v. אֶשֶׁל 3).]

אַשּׁוּרִי m., **אַשּׁוּרִית** f. *Assyrian,* esp. *the modern form of Hebrew type* (square), supposed to have been brought along by the returning Babylonian captives, and made to supersede the older Hebrew (Syriac or Samaritan, עברי) characters. Y. Meg. I, 71[b] א׳ יש לו כתב וכ׳ the Assyrian (trans-Euphratic, Chaldaic) language had a (developed) type of writing, but no tongue (cultivated grammar) &c. [See the whole discussion, ibid.] Cmp. Snh. 21[b]. Meg. 8[b]. Esth. R. to I, 22; a. e.—Meg. I, 8; Y. Sot. VII, beg. 21[b] אשורית *the Hebrew language* in its modern type.

אַשּׁוּת Ar., אִישּׁוּת ed. f. (b. h. אֵשֶׁת Ps. LVIII, 9; אוש or אשש, v. אשש 2) [*groping*, cmp. גשש, גוש,] *mole.* Gen. R. s. 51 (alluding to *esheth* Ps. l. c.) כא׳ זו וכ׳ like that mole which sees not the light. Kel. XXI, 3 מצודת הא׳ the bow for shooting moles (v. Maim. a. l.). M. Kat. I, 4; cmp. ib. 6[b].—Y. ib. 80[c], explained חולדה.

אַשּׁוּתָא ch. same. Targ. O. Lev. XI, 30. Targ. Ps. LVIII, 9.

אֲשִׁיוָתָא, const. אֲשִׁיוַת f. pl. (שור) 1) *meshes*, trnsf. *tricks.* Targ. Is. XXV, 11 (h. text אָרְבּוֹת).—2) v. אֲשִׁיוְתָא.

*__אֲשָׁזוּן__ m. (שזא, cmp. שדא a. אשד) *winnowing.* Targ. Y. I, Gen. XXXV, 16 there was yet סוגעי א׳ עללתא וכ׳ (comment. to Targ. Y. a. l. reads אשזון) much winnowing of the produces of the land &c. (h. text כברת, cmp. Gen. R. s. 82, a. Pesik. R. s. 3, explaining Gen. l. c.). [Targ. Y. II כרוב וכ׳; Targ. Y. Gen. XLVIII, 7 בעיד סוגעי ארעא וכ׳.]

אַשְׁחוּר pr. n. m. (b. h.) *Ashhur.* Sot. 12[a] (I Chr. IV, 5).

אשטמיון, v. אִיסְטַמְיוֹן.

אַשֵּׁי pr. n. m. *Ashshê*, 1) R. A. bar Sinai, president of the academy of Sura (beginning of the fifth century), generally accepted as the redactor of the Gemara (v. גְּמָרָא). Gitt. 59[a]. B. Mets. 86[a]; a. fr.—2) Other Amoraim by that name. Sabb. 75[b]; a. fr. [Y. Ber. I, 3[a] top אשיא.]

אַשְׁיָין, אַשְׁיָיאן, אַשְׁיָאן pr. n. m. *Ashyan*, name of several Amoraim. Y. Ter. I, 41[a]. Ber. 14[a].—Y. Ab. Zar. III, beg., 42[b] A. Nagra (the carpenter).—Y. Yeb. XI, 12[a] bot. Y. Meg. I, 71[c] bot.—V. יַאסְיָן.

אֲשִׁיבְתָּא a word made up as a disguise of שְׁבוּעֲתָא, *oath* (cmp. שְׁבָב=שֵׁיב). Ned. 10[b]; cmp. אֲשִׁיקוּקָא.

אָשִׁיד, אֲשֵׁיד, v. אֶשֶׁד.

אֲשִׁיוֹת f. pl. Snh. 108[b] Ar., v. עֲשָׁשִׁית.

אֲשִׁימָה, אֲשִׁימָא (b. h.) pr. n. m. *Ashima*, idol of the *Hamathcans.* Y. Ab. Zar. III, 42[d] top (ref. to II Kings XVII, 30) אימרא וכ׳ A. is represented as a lamb, as you read *el hāasham* (Lev. V, 16); Snh. 63[b] called 'bald buck' (goat).

אָשִׁין, v. אָשֵׁן.

אשינא, Snh. 96[b], דבורא א׳, v. שִׁינָא.

אֲשֵׁירָא, pl. אֲשֵׁירָיָא, אֲשֵׁירָן, v. אֲשֵׁירְתָא.

אֲשֵׁרָה, אֲשֵׁירָה f. (b. h.) *Asherah, tree* (grove) *devoted to idolatry* (v. Mov. Phœn. p. 567; Sm. Bibl. Dict. s. v.). Ab. Zar. III, 5; 7. Succ. 31[b] א׳ דמשה an Asherah to which the Mosaic law refers (remnant of anti-Mosaic idolatry). Pes. 27[a]; a. fr. *Pl.* אֲשֵׁירוֹת, אֲשֵׁירוּת. Ab. Zar. III, 7; a. fr.—אֲשֵׁירִים. Pirke d'R. El. ch. XXVI.

אֲשֵׁרְתָא, אֲשֵׁירְתָא ch. same. Targ. O. Deut. XVI, 21; a. fr.—*Pl.* אֲשֵׁירָתָא, אֲשֵׁירִין, אֲשֵׁירַיָּא, אֲשֵׁי׳. Targ. II Kings XXIII, 14; XVII, 10. Targ. Is. XVII, 8; a. e.

אֲשִׁישָׁא m. (cmp. next w.) *jug.* Sabb. 141[a] לא ... דא׳ ליהדק Ms. M. a. Ar. (ed. שִׁישָׁא) you must not squeeze a cotton stopper into the mouth of a jug (on the Sabbath). B. Bath. 144[a] א׳ דמשחא ed. (Ms. M. אֲשִׁשָׁא, Ms. H. שישא) a jug of oil. [Pes. 36[b] אֲשִׁישָׁה (q. v.). according to Samuel, identic with our w.=גרבא דחמרא.]

אֲשִׁישָׁה f. (b. h., אשש) *anything made compact and substantial by pressing*, whence 1) *cake, pan-cake* (in Bible *pressed raisin-cake*). Pes. 36[b] excluding from 'bread of misery', חלוט וא' pudding and pan-cake. [Talmudic etymology, ibid., '*one sixth of an epha* of flour made into a cake'.] Y. ib. II, 29[b] bot.—Bab. ib. l. c. Samuel says א' גרבא וכ' *ăshishah* (II Sam. VI, 19) means a jug of wine (v. preced.).—*Pl.* אֲשִׁישׁוֹת (b. h.). Hull. 124[b] אני היום סמכוני בא' to me to-day the Bibl. words apply, 'Support me with cakes' (Cant. II, 5); Bets. 21[a].—2) pl. אֲשִׁישִׁים, אֲשִׁישִׁין *cakes made of boiled lentils impregnated with honey*. Ned. VI, 10; cmp. Y. ib. 40[a] bot.

אֲשִׁישְׁיָין ch. pl. as preced. 1). Targ. Y. Ex. XVI, 31 (h. צַפִּיחִית).

אֲשִׁישִׁים, אֲשִׁישִׁין, v. אֲשִׁישָׁה 2).

אָשִׁית or **אָשׁוּת,** pl. אָשִׁיּוֹת, v. עֲשָׁשִׁית.

אשית, v. אֲשִׁיתָא.

אֲשִׁיתָא or **אֲשִׁיתָא, אוּשִׁיתָא** f. (=h. אָשְׁיָה Jer. L, 15, K'thib אשויה; שׁוּר, cmp. שִׁית) [*meshes, layers*, v. אֲשְׁוָתָא a. אוּרְבָא,] *frame-wall*. B. Bath. 7[a]. Ib. 59[a] תיתרע אשיתאי my framework will be shaken (by the hammering). Ber. 56[a] א' דנפל (read דנפלא; Ms. M. דשא ברייתא) that my wall fell in.—*Pl.* אוּשְׁיָיתָא, אוּשְׁיָתָא, אֲשִׁיָּיתָא, also אוּשְׁוָותָא, אֲשְׁוָתָא. Targ. Ps. XI, 3 (h. text שתות); a. fr.—Ber. 28[a] אשייתא וכ' the walls of his house. B. Kam. 20[b].—[Not to be confounded with אוּשָּׁא *foundation*.] V. אַשְׁוָתָא, אַשְׁוָה.

אֲשִׁיתָא=אִישְׁתָּא *six*.—*Pl.* אֲשִׁיתִּין *sixty*. Y. Taan. IV, 68[d] bot. אֲשִׁיתֵּיסַר, אֲשִׁיתֵּסַר sixteen. Y. Sot. V, 20[b] bot. אשית תיסר corr. acc.

אֶשֶׁךְ m. (b. h.; denom. of אִישׁ) *testicle*. *Pl.* אֲשָׁכִים. Bekh. VII, 5 (44[b]). Tosef. ib. V, 4.—Denom. מְאוּשְׁכָּן *one having large testicles*. Bekh. l. c. (Gem. ed. מאושבן, v. שעבז).

אַשְׁכַּבְתָּא I f. (שכב) *lying down, death*. Keth. 103[b].

אַשְׁכַּבְתָּא II f. (preced.) *butcher's shop*. סכינא דא' *butcher's dissecting knife* [Tosaf. *slaughtering knife*]. B. Mets. 116[a]; Sabb. 123[b].

אֶשְׁכֹּל, אֶשְׁכּוֹל m. (b. h. cmp. סגל) *bunch, cluster* (of grapes). Y. Naz. II, beg. 51[d] תורה קראת לא' וכ' the Bible calls the (berry in the) cluster *must* (*tirosh*, ref. to Is. LXV, 8) while people (at present) call the dried berry must (i. e. in common parlance abstinence from 'berry' means from grape-juice, must &c.).—אשכול של בצים *the ovary* (of birds). Tosef. Zab. V, 9; Bets. 7[a].—Midd. III, 8 א' של זהב a gold imitation of a cluster of grapes.—2) Trnsf. *a distinguished scholar* (opp. עָלִין *leaves=the ignorant*); v. infra. Cant. R. to I, 14, a. e. (play on the word) אִישׁ שהכֹּל בו a man in whom all is contained, i. e. universality of knowledge.—*Pl.* אֶשְׁכּוֹלוֹת, אֶשְׁכָּלוֹת. Hull. 92[a] א' שבח וכ' the grapes thereon (on the nation), that means the scholars; cmp. Lev. R. s. 36.—Esp. *the scholars of the early Maccabean period*. Sot. IX, 9 (47[a]); Tem. 15[b]. Y. Sot. IX, 24[a] top, v. זוגות; Tosef. B. Kam. VIII, 13 אישכלות. Ch. אִתְכָּלָא.

אֶשְׁכִּי, v. אוּשְׁכָּף.

אֶשְׁכֹּל, v. אֶשְׁכּוֹל.

אַשְׁכָּף Ar., אוּשְׁכָּף ed., m. (v. אושכפא) [the saddler,] *a genus of edible locusts*. Hull. 65[b] לחביא הא' to imply the *ashkaf* (among the סלעם).

אשכפא, Keth. 77[b] גירדי דא' Ar. ed., read אַשְׁפָּא as in Ar. ed. Koh. s. v. גרד, v. note ibid.

אֶשְׁכָּרָא m. (prob. a denom. of כַּר) *a wagon, wagon-load*; [b. h. אֶשְׁכָּר *gift, tribute*; cmp. Is. XVI, 1]. *Pl.* אֶשְׁכְּרִין. Targ. Is. V, 10 (h. text צמד). Targ. II Esth. I, 3 א' ומרגלוין (read דמ') loads (gifts) of &c. (after Ps. LXXII, 10).

אֶשְׁכְּרוֹעַ m. (v. P. Sm. 408) *box-tree* or *ebony tree* [prob. a denom. of חשך=אשך, cmp. גּוּשְׁקְרָא]. Neg. II, 1 כא' לא שחורים וכ' like the *eshk'roa*, neither black nor white but of an intermediate color. B. Bath 89[b] אשב' ed. (corr. acc., v. Rabb. D. S. a. l. note 30). Yoma III, 9 (8) גורלות של א' ballot tablets of box-wood (cmp. Sm. Ant. s. v. Buxum); expl. Y. ib. 41[a] top פיקס=פסקינין (πύξινον).

אֶשְׁכְּרוֹעָא ch. same. *Pl.* אֶשְׁכְּרָעִין, אֶשְׁכְּרוֹעִין. Targ. Is. XLI, 19 (h. text תאשור); LX, 13. Targ. Ezek. XXVII, 6 (h. text בת־אשורים!).

אֶשְׁכַּרְתִּי f. (prob. fr. its color, v. preced.) *mole* (?). Hull. 63[a] Ar. Var. s. v. קרפדאי; v. בָּאנַת.

אֶשֶׁל m. (b. h.; אשל *to be firmly rooted*, √אש, v. אשש; v. Ges. H. Dict. s. v.) 1) *tamarisk*, symbol of strength and eminence.—*Pl.* אֶשָׁלִים, const. אֶשְׁלֵי. Y. B. Mets. I, end, 8[a] א' דידנין וכ' the eminent (old) among the Babylonian scholars are but like the pidgeons (the young) among the Palestinean; cmp. Y. Ned. VI, 40[a] bot.—2) *plantation, pleasure-garden, tent*. Sot. 10[a]; Gen. R. s. 54 end (ref. to Gen. XXI, 33, v. Targ. a. l.).—*3) pr. n. *Eshel*, a river in Assyria. Snh. 92[b]. Yalk. Ezek. 376 (אשור).

אֶשְׁלָא, אַשְׁלָא ch. as preced. 1). Targ. I Sam. XXII, 6.—*Pl.* אֶשְׁלֵי.—א' רברבי *great men* (v. preced.). Ab. Zar. 7[b] תלוא בא' ר' it hangs on high tamarisks, i. e. originates from great men. Bets. 27[a]; B. Bath. 31[b].

אַשְׁלָא m. (שלי *to draw up*) *rope, tow; net*. Targ. Job XVIII, 10; a. e. Gitt. 69[a] א' דפוריא עתיקא a rope of an old litter. Keth. 85[a] ממחח לה בא' he pulled it with a rope. B. Kam. 116[b] חד א' one rope's length away from the shore.—*Pl.* אַשְׁלֵי, אַשְׁלַיָּא, אַשְׁלְוָן. Targ. Job XXXVIII, 31. Targ. Y. Gen. X, 26; a. e. [Targ. I Chr. I, 20 אוּשְׁלַיָּא.]—B. Kam. l. c.—Succ. 16[a] משדא א' to twist ropes for a couch. B. Mets. 107[b]; v. מְתַח.—Bekh. 8[b] אייתו א' וכ' bring ye ropes and measure. Keth. 67[a], v. קמחוניא.

אַשְׁלַג m. (שלג) *a kind of alkali*, or *mineral used as a soap*. Nidd. IX, 6; Sabb. IX, 5; Snh. 49[b] קמוניא וא׳ Ms. M. a. oth. (ed. אשלך).

שַׁלְגָא, אַשְׁלְגָא ch. same. Nidd. 62[a] (explaining the *ashleg* of the Mishnah) א׳ שמיה וכ׳ (Ar. שלגא) its name is *ashl'ga*, and it is found in the holes in which pearls sit, and is scraped out with an iron nail; Sabb. 90[a] שלגא Ar. (Ms. M. שולגא, ed. שונאנא). V. אַצְרוֹת רוּחַ.

אַשְׁלִימוּ=אַשְׁלָמוּ.

אשלך, v. אַשְׁלַג.

אַשְׁלָמוּ, אַשְׁלָמוּתָא (אַשְׁלְמְוָותָא, pl. אַשְׁלְמְוָותָא) f. (שלם=h. מִלֻּאִים) (*finishing*) 1) *fitting, setting*. Targ. Ex. XXV, 7; XXVIII, 17; a. e.—2) *initiation*. Targ. Y. Lev. VIII, 28. Ib. 33; 34; a. e. Cmp. חִינּוּךְ.

אָשַׁם (b. h.; שמם) 1) *to be waste* (cmp. Ezek. VI, 6; Hos. XIV, 1). Snh. 97[a] יֶאְשַׁם (in parall. passages יִשּׁוֹם); v. בָּלַק.—2) *to neglect, be guilty*.—Denom.:

אָשָׁם m. (b. h.) *guilt; guilt-offering, asham*, a special kind of offering.—א׳ תלוי (Lev. V, 18) an *asham* to be offered when you are in doubt as to the commission of a sinful act. Kerith. III, 1; a. fr.; (ib. 17[b] differ. opin. as to the nature of the doubt). Ib. VI, 3 אֲשַׁם חסידים the *asham* offered by the over-scrupulous because they *may* have transgressed.—א׳ ודאי the *asham* for the undoubted commission of certain offenses, which are: a) אֲ׳ גזילות for illegal appropriation of private property (after pecuniary reparation; Lev. V, 25); b) אֲ׳ מעילות for misappropriation of sacred property (Lev. V, 16); c) אֲ׳ שפחה חרופה for carnal connection with a slave betrothed to another man (Lev. XIX, 21);—d) אֲ׳ נזיר the offering of a nazarite when interrupting the days of vowed nazaritism by levitical impurity (Num. VI, 12).—Deut. R. s. 1, beg. (alluding to וַאֲשִׁמֵם Deut. I, 13) וַאֲשִׁמְם כתיב it is so written that you may read *v'ashmam* (and their guilt); if you listen not to them אשמה תלוי וכ׳ (read אשמם) their guilt shall fall upon your heads (you will be answerable for what offenses they may commit); differ. in Sifré Deut. 13. [Our Bible editions, however, read ואשימם, *plene*.]—*Pl.* אֲשָׁמוֹת. Kerith. VI, 4. Sifré l. c.; a. fr.

אַשְׁמָא f. (=h. אַשְׁמָה) *guilt*. Targ. Y. Lev. XXII, 16 אַשְׁמַתְהוֹן.

אֲשָׁמָא, אֲשָׁמָא (אֲשָׁמָא) m. (=h. אָשָׁם) *guilt, guilt-offering*. Targ. O. Lev. V, 15; a. fr—*Pl.* אֲשָׁמִין. Targ. II Chron. XXVIII, 10.

אַשְׁמַאי, אַשְׁמַיי m. (v. אָשַׁם 1) *waste* (in mind); *ignorant, neglected*; cmp. בּוּר. Kidd. 32[b] זקן א׳ an uncultured, rough old man. Sifra to Par. III, ch. VII אשמיי (as noun). Cmp. אַשְׁמָה.

אַשְׁמְדַאי, אַשְׁמְדַיי pr. n. m. (Pers. Aêshma, Aêshmadaô, Kohut Jüd. Angel. p. 72; Rapap. Er. Mill. s. v.) *Ashm'day*, chief of demons. Targ. Koh. I, 12.—Pes. 110[a]. Gitt. 68[a]. Num. R. s. 11; a. e.

אַשְׁמָה f. (b. h.; אשם) *negligence, guilt*. Shek. VI, 6. —Gen. R. s. 49 זקני א׳ וכ׳ elders in coarseness (cmp. אַשְׁמַאי) which is (in Chaldaic) elders of shame.—*Pl.* אַשְׁמוֹת, v. אָשָׁם.

אַשְׁמוּרָה, אַשְׁמֹרֶת f. (b. h. אַשְׁמֹרֶת, אַשְׁמֻרָה; שמר) *night-watch, watch, a certain portion* (three or four hours) *of the day, called a watch* (v. Sm. Ant. s. v. *Castra*). Ber. I, 1 סוף הא׳ וכ׳ the end of the first watch of the night; a. fr.—*Pl.* אַשְׁמוּרוֹת. Y. Ber. I, 2[d] top ארבע(ה) א׳ וכ׳ the day is divided into four watches, and so is the night; cmp. Bab. ib. 3[a].

אַשְׁמַיָא pr. n. pl. *Ashmaya*, in the district of Tyre. Y. Dem. II, 22[d] top (corrupt.; for ראש מיא read: דא׳); Tosef. Shebi. IV, 9 דשמיא ed. Zuck. (Var. א׳).

אַשְׁמַיי, v. אַשְׁמַאי.

אָשֵׁן ($\sqrt{}$ אש, v. אשש; cmp. אִישׁ, יֵשׁ, אִית, אֵיתָן) *to be substantial, dense, strong, hard*.—Part. (as adj.) אָשִׁין, אֲשִׁינָא Ar. (ed., Ms. M. אָשׁוּן, אֲשׁוּנָא). Hull. 136[b], opp. רכיך. Ib. 76[a]. Sabb. 155[a] חרובין דאשיני וכ׳ Ar. (Ms. M. אשונא, ed. אקושי) carob fruits which are hard .... aftermath which is hard (dry). Cmp. יָשָׁן.

אַשְׁנָא pr. n. pl. *Ashna*, supposed to be near Tyre. Esth. R. to I, 4 (Var. אַשְׁנָה).

אַשָּׁף m. (b. h.; נשף, v. Fl. to Levy Talm. Dict. I, 283[b]) *enchanter*, (*astrologer*).—*Pl.* אַשָּׁפִים. Tanh. Mikketz 2 (ref. to Dan. II, 2) לא׳ אלו שדוחק׳ במזל the *Ashshafim*, these are those who press (lay stress) upon the planetary constellation, שכן א׳ לשון דחק for the root *ashaf* means *to press* (ref. to שאף, Amos VIII, 4).

אָשַׁף ch. same. Dan. II, 10.—*Pl.* אָשְׁפַיָּא, אָשְׁפִין. Ib. II, 27; V, 11; IV, 4.

***אַשְׁפָא** m. (שפא, שפה) *dressed skin*. Keth. 77[b] גירדא דא׳ the shavings of a hide when it is smoothed. [Ar. s. v. גרד l ed. אשכפא, ed. Koh. אשפא.]

אַשְׁפָּה, אִישְׁפָּה f. (b. h. אַשְׁפֹּת; שפה, שפא. *to heap up*, cmp. Is. XIII, 2, Ps. XXII, 16) *pile, dunghill*. Y. Keth. I, 25[d] bot. הא׳. Hull. 12[a]; a. fr.—שער הא׳ (b. h. ש׳ האשפת, ש׳ השפת) *Hill Gate*, name of a Jerusalem gate. Sabb. 15[a]; a. fr.—*Pl.* אַשְׁפּוֹת. Ex. R. s. 10 ארבע א׳ four heaps (of dead frogs,=b. h. חמרים); a. fr.—Euphem. מגרה לא׳ *using means to prevent conception* (applied to both man a. woman). Keth. VII, 5. (Ib. 72[a], acc. to Boraitha, literally, 'to draw water and pour it out on the dunghill'—as a foolish act). Gen. R. s. 85, ref. to Gen. XXXVIII, 7.—[Homiletic interpretation of בני אשפתו, Lam. III, 13, 'the sons of those laid low' (conquered); Lam. R. a. l., Esth. R. to I, 1[b], v. אוּפְרַכְּא, אוּפִּיְיפָא.]

אַשְׁפּוּרֵי Ab. Zar. 20[b], אַשְׁפָּרָא.

אַשְׁפְּלָה f. (=h. מַשְׁפֶּלֶת q. v.) *basket*, as a measure, cmp. טְעוּנָא. Y. Dem. II, 22[d] top.—*Pl.* אַשְׁפְּלָתָה. Ibid. (ed. אפשלתה, corr. acc.).

אֶשְׁפָּר m. (b. h.; שפר, cmp. שׁוּפְרָא) *a goodly piece* (cmp. דִּשְׁנָא), *a certain quantity of meat, eshpar*. Pes. 36[b] א׳ אחד וכ׳ an eshpar is one sixth of a bullock (as if composed of שש and פר; cmp. אֶסְפָּר).

אַשְׁפָּרָא m. (שפר) *the scourer of dresses*. *Pl.* אַשְׁפָּרֵי. Ab. Zar. 20[b] (Ms. M. אשפירי, ed. אַשְׁפּוֹרֵי).

אִישְׁפּוֹת, אַשְׁפּוֹת f. (b. h. אַשְׁ׳, v. אַשְׁפָּה) *heap, pile, dunghill*. *Pl.* אַשְׁפּוֹתוֹת, אִישְׁ׳. Shebi. III, 2.—Sot. 42[b] אר׳ של וכ׳ piles of slain.

אַשְׁקוּקָה (אשקיקה) *ashkukah*, a fictitious word as a disguise of שְׁבוּעָה, *oath, I swear* (cmp. אֱלֹקִי, אֵיפוֹפִי). Ned. 10[b] א׳ לא אמר כלום if one says *ashkukah*, he has said nothing (his vow is not binding); v. שְׁקוּקָה.

אַשְׁקְלוֹן pr. n. pl. (b. h.) *Ashkelon*, a Philistian town. Y. Shebi. VI, 36[c]; Sifré Deut. 51, v. גְּרִירָא; a. e.—Deriv. אַשְׁקְלוֹנִי m. *Ashkelonian*. Y. Peah I, 15[c] top.—*Pl.* נִיר . . . . אַשְׁקְלוֹנִים Kel. XIII, 7 Ashk. levers; a. e.

אַשְׁקַלְתָּא f. (שקל) *transaction, sale*. B. Bath. 48[b] signed as one of the witnesses אמודעא ואא׳ both on the owner's protest against the forced sale and on the deed of sale.

אִשְׁקָק, אִשְׁקָקָא, אוּשְׁ׳, אִישְׁ׳ m. (v. שְׁקָקָא) *open place, street*. Targ. II Esth. VI, 9; a. e.—Y. Taan. III, 66[c] bot.—*Pl.* אִשְׁקָקֵי &c. Targ. Esth. IX, 14 א׳ מלכא the royal markets. Targ. Y. I Deut. XXIX, 16; a. e.

אֲשֶׁר (b. h. $\sqrt{}$אש, cmp. next w.; v. Ges. H. Dict. s. v., as to opinions on etymol.) *[being,] who, which*. Ber. 11[b] א׳ בחר וכ׳ who hast chosen us; a. v. fr. (in prayer formulas).—In Talm. mostly prefix-שֶׁ.

אָשַׁר (b. h., $\sqrt{}$אש, v. אשש) *to exist, be strong, happy*; v. יָשַׁר.

Pi. אִישֵּׁר, אִשֵּׁר (b. h.) 1) *to exalt, praise, declare happy*. Pesik. R. s. 45 התחיל מְאַשְּׁרָם he commenced by declaring them happy; v. אַשְׁרֵי.—2) *to substantiate*; *to verify, attest to*. Num. R. s. 14 לְאַשֵּׁר את הדין to give strength to the legal decision Y. Gitt. IX, 50[c] bot. אִישַּׁרְנוּהוּ (אישרניהו) we have verified it in the presence of &c.—Part. pass. מְאוּשָּׁר 1) *firm, strong*. Gen. R. s. 15, beg. the bux-tree is called תְּאַשּׁוּר because it is מא׳ וכ׳ the strongest of all (cmp. אָצִיל). Y. Succ. III, 54[a] top; Y. Meg. I, 72[a] top המא׳ שבכלן וכ׳ the strongest (expression) of all, is Hallelujah.—2) *substantial, good, rich*. Gen. R. s. 90, end (ref. to את כל אֲשֶׁר Gen. XLI, 56) המאוּשָּׁרִין שבהם the best stores of all. Ib. s. 28.—Snh. 22[a] is called Ashurith שמאוּשֶּׁרֶת בכתב because its characters are substantial (Ar. שמאושר); Y. Meg. I, 71[b] bot.; Y. Sot. VII, 21[c] top.

Hithpa. הִתְאַשֵּׁר *to be set up, be erected*. Sifra K'dosh. beg. (play on אֲשֵׁרִים) על שם שהם מִתְאַשְּׁרִים מאחרים because they are put up by others.

אֲשַׁר ch. same. [*Ithpe.* אִיתְּשַׁר *to be strengthened*. Targ. Y. Deut. X, 2 יִתְּשַׁר, prob. to be read יִתְיַשַׁר, v. ישר.]

Pa. אַשַּׁר 1) *to make strong*. Keth. 10[b]; Gitt. 70[a] (dates) מְאַשְּׁרָן give strength.—2) *to confirm, verify*; also *to credit, (consider true)*. Keth. 21[a] אַשַּׁרְנוּהִי וכ׳ we verified it &c., v. preced.—Gitt. 30[b] (prov.) חברך מית א׳ וכ׳ if you are told, 'your friend is dead', believe it; 'your friend has grown rich' לא תְּאַשַּׁר don't trust.

אֶשֶׁר m. (b. h.), only in plur. constr. אַשְׁרֵי the *happiness of!, happy is he, are they* &c. Pes. 117[a]; a. fr.—Midr. Till. to Ps. LXXXIV אַשְׁרַאי happy am I.—Yoma VIII, 9 אַשְׁרֵיכֶם happy are ye. Ib. 87[a] אַשְׁרֵיהֶם לצדיקים happy are the righteous; a. fr.

אַשְׁרָא, v. אַשְׁרְתָּא.

אַשְׁרָאִי m. pl. (v. אֲשַׁר Pa.) *sale on trust, debts for goods sold*. Pes. 113[a] כל א׳ וכ׳ in all sales on trust it is doubtful, whether it (the money) will be forthcoming or not, and if it is, it is bad money, (partial payment, bad coins &c).—B. Mets. 63[b] אית ליה א׳ וכ׳ he has debts to collect. B. Bath. 22[a] אית לן א׳ וכ׳ we have outstanding debts to collect (and we must stay until we have collected them).

אַשְׁרַאי, v. אֶשֶׁר.

אַשָּׁרָה, f. *legal attestation*. Y. Gitt. IX, 50[c] bot. אַשָּׁרַת הדיינין; v. אַשַּׁרְתָּא.

אֲשֵׁרָה, v. אֲשֵׁירָה.

אַשְׁרֵי, v. אֶשֶׁר.

אַשְׁרָיוּתָא f. (שרי) *causing to dwell, dwelling*. Targ. Is. LXVI, 1; a. e.

אֻשַּׁרְנָא m. (אשר; cmp. אָשְׁא) *wall*. Ezra V, 3.

אַשַּׁרְתָּא f. (אֲשַׁר) *strength! health!*, a greeting extended to laboring men; cmp. יַשַּׁר. Gitt. 62[a].

אַשָּׁרָא, אַשַּׁרְתָּא f. (אשר) 1) *legal attestation*. Keth. 21[b], a. e. א׳ דדייני the attestation by judges (h. אַשָּׁרַת הדיינין, v. אַשָּׁרָה). B. Bath. 163[a] בין עדים לא׳ (Ar. a. Ms. אשרא) the space between the signature of the witnesses and the legal attestation.—2) (cmp. אַשְׁרָאֵי) *outstanding debts for goods sold*. Gitt. 14[a] R. S. had א׳ דסרבלי וכ׳ money outstanding in Mahuza for garments sold.

אָשַׁשׁ (b. h. r.) 1) ($\sqrt{}$אש) *to glitter, be polished*; v. אֵשׁ a. next ws.—2) (sec. r. of אוש) *to be thick, substantial; to be pressed, dark*, v. אשן, אשונא, אשות, אשל, אשר &c.

Pi. אִישֵּׁשׁ *to make firm, found*. Part. pass. מְאוּשָּׁשׁ. Pesik. Bahod. p. 101[b]; Cant. R. to II, 5 (play on ăshishoth, Cant. l. c.) הלכות המְאוּשָּׁשׁוֹת well-founded decisions. V. אוּשׁ, אוּשָּׁא.

אָשֵׁשׁ m. (preced. 1) *a crystal* or *ball reflecting the light, reflector* (v. next w.). Y. R. Hash. II, 58[a] bot. if the reflection of the moon has been seen באי׳ ובמים in a reflecting glass or in water.

אֶשְׁשִׁיתָא ch. same; v. עֲשָׁשִׁיתָא. Num. R. s. 12 שאשיתא דקנדילא (read אש׳). Yalk. Ex. 186 אשתא; (Tanḥ. Vaëra 14; Ex. R. s. 12 עשש׳).

אשת Y. Ab. Zar. II, 41[d] bot. א׳ קנים, v. חִישָׁה.

אֶשָּׁתָא f. *fire*, v. אֶשָּׁא.—[Yalk. Ex. 186, v. אֶשְׁשִׁיתָא.]

אֶשְׁתָּא *six*, v. אִישְׁתָּא.

אֶשְׁתָּאָה m. *the sixth*. Targ. I Chr. XII, 11.

אֶשְׁתָּדָא, אִישְׁ׳ (contr. of שַׁתָּא דָא, with א׳ pref.) *this year*. Y. Maas. Sh. IV, 55[b].

אֶשְׁתַּדּוּר, אֶשְׁתַּדּוּר m. (שְׁדַר II) *resistance, rebellion*. Ezra IV, 15; 19.—Targ. Lam. I, 1 חובאה א׳ (read חובא דא׳).

*__אֶשְׁתַּדְיוּתָא__ f. (שדי) *being cast about, shaking*. Targ. Is. VII, 2 (Ar. אשדוות).

אשתווא Ithpe. of שוי.

*__אשתומא__ m. (שמם, v. next w.) *confusion, nonsense*. Hull. 84[b] א׳ קאמר וכ׳ he talks nonsense, let his interpreter (אֲמוֹרָא) be taken away from him (v. Rashi a. l. for diff. version, a. conception of אמורא).

אֶשְׁתּוֹמֵם, אִישְׁ׳ (Ithpe. of שמם; cmp. Dan. IV, 16) *he was confounded, stood aghast*. Hull. 21[a]; Sabb. 47[a].

אשתונית Yalk. Lev. 568 זחו הא׳, read זָרֵי האשקלונית.

אַשְׁתּוֹר, עַשְׁתּוֹר pr. n. m. *Ashtor*. Y. Bicc. I, 64[a] top; a. e.

אֶשְׁתַּטִּית, v. אִישְׁ׳.

*__אֶשְׁתַּיָּימָא__ m. (שום) *mark, distinction*. Ab. Zar. 41[a] מעיקרא סבור א׳ וכ׳ Ar. (ed. אִישְׁתַּיָּימָא) at first it was thought the ring in the hand of a statue was a mere distinction (not typical of any religious idea), but afterwards it was found out that (it represents the idea that) he (the bearer of it) seals himself for death as a vicarious sacrifice for the whole world.

אשתי, v. שתי.

אשתין, v. שִׁתִּין.

אֶשְׁתִּיתָא pr. n. m. *Ishtitha*. Erub. 52[a] Ar. (ed. אישתתא, Var. אִישְׁתּוֹ׳, Ms. אישתי׳; v. Rabb. D. S. a. l.)

אֶשְׁתַּלְהָיוּתָא f., constr. אֶשְׁתַּלְהָיוּת (שלהי) *fainting*. Targ. Ps. CXLII, 4.

אֶשְׁתְּמוֹדַע I (v. next w.) 1) *to satisfy one's self from the evidence of friends, to have one identified*. Yeb. 39[b] אשתמודעיניה דאחוה וכ׳ Ar. (ed. אישתמודעינהו) we satisfied ourselves about him that he is the brother &c.—2) *to recognise*. Targ. Gen. XLII, 7; 8; a. fr.—3) *to be recognized, known*. Targ. Y. Ex. XXI, 36; a. fr.—4) *to introduce one's self, to befriend*. Targ. Ruth II, 19; a. e.

אֶשְׁתְּמוֹדַע II m. (Ishtaf. of the form מוֹדַע) *one who proved himself a friend, acquaintance*. Targ. Ruth II, 1; III, 2.

אֶשְׁתְּמוֹדְעוּתָא f. (v. preced.) 1) *partiality, preferment*. Targ. Is. III, 9 (h. text חכרת פנים).—2) *that by which one is recognized, distinctive feature*. Targ. Y. Gen. XLIX, 5 (h. text מְכֵרוֹת=מְכֻרוֹת׳).

אֶשְׁתְּמָמוּתָא, אֶשְׁתְּמָמוּ f. (שמם) *desolation*. Targ. Zeph. II, 13; a. e.

אֶשְׁתַּסַר (contr. of אשתא עסר, cmp. ארביסר) *sixteen*. Targ. I Chr. IV, 27; a. e.

אֶשְׁתָּעוּתָא f. (שעי) *narration, tale, speech*. Targ. Y. Gen. IX, 24. Targ. Y. Lev. XVI, 6; a. e.

אֶשְׁתַּעֲמְמוּ f. (שעמם) *devastation*. Targ. II Chron. XXIX, 8.

אֶשְׁתָּקַד 1) (contr. of שַׁתָּא קַדְמָאָה) *last year*; cmp. אֶשְׁתָּדָא. Y. Gitt. III, end, 45[b] ישן משל א׳ 'old produces' means last year's crop. Bets. 5[b]; a. fr.—2) (contr. of שַׁעְתָּא קַדְ׳) *previously, ere this*. Targ. Y. Lev. XVI, 21.

אֶשְׁתְּרִיוּתָא, corr. אִשְׁתַּדְיוּתָא. Targ. Is. VII, 2, ed. Ven.

א״ת ב״ש, א״ת *Athbash*, a method of interchanging the first letter of the Alphabet (א) with the last (ת), the second (ב) with the last but one (ש), the third from the beginning (ג) with the third from the end (ר), &c. Num. R. s. 13.—Ib. s. 18 ששך באת״בש בבל Sheshach (Jer. XXV, 26) represents Babel by the rule of *athbash*.

אִתְ־ formative prefix of the Ithpa., Ithpe. and Ithpo., and corresponding nouns; in Talmud mostly אִית־; cmp. אִס־ a. אִיס־. [For words not to be found here v. sub אִית־, a. vice versa.]

אַתְּ c. (b. h. אַתְּ f.; contr. of אנת) *thou*. Targ. Gen. III, 11; a. fr.—Y. Snh. I, 19[a] top ואת מר הכן and thou sayest so?—[In Talmudic argumentation את אומר (אתה); Chald. את מר, את אמר *thou sayest*, את צווח ליה *thou callest it*, frequently applied to Scripture texts as though addressing an opponent.] Lev. R. s. 10, end ואת אומר אל פתח וכ׳ and yet the Scripture says, 'To the entrance of the Tabernacle'! i. e. how is this possible?—Y. Pes. V, 32[c] את מר והיה לאבק Scripture says 'And it shall turn into dust'.—Y. Kil. VIII, 31[b] top הן דאת אמר לא אמירה למה את אמר, [add the respective bibl. verses after each אמר a. read אמירה for אמירה] there where it reads, 'thou shalt not' &c. (Lev. XIX, 19), the text gives no reason why; therefore it is repeated (Deut. XXII, 9 adding the reason); a. fr.—[דאת אמר contr. דְּהָ מַר q. v.]—*Pl.* אַתּוּן (תּוּן), (אַתּוּ) m. אַתֵּין f. *ye*. Targ. Ps. CXIV, 6 דאתון Ms. (omitted in ed., and third person). Targ. Is. III, 14. Targ. Ezek.

XIII, 20; a. fr.—Y. Snh. VI, 23[d] top ומה תון בטון (read בעתון) and what is it ye want? Y. Keth. XII, 35[a] אתון אמרתון *ye* said so; a. fr.—Snh. 109[a] דאַתּוּ גנבי (v. Rashi a. l., Ms. דגנבי איח בכו, v. Rabb. D. S. a. l. note) that ye are thieves. V. אַתְּ, אַנְתְּ.

אָת, אַת, אָתָא I, אַתְוָא c. (=b. h. אות; fr. תאה, or תאר, sec. r. of אה or אר; as to reject. of radical ו or ה, cmp. אב, אח &c.) *sign, type; letter* (v. אות II). Targ. Ex. XIII, 16; a. fr.—Targ. Is. VII, 11; a. fr.—*Pl.* אָתִין, אָתַיָּא. Targ. Gen. I, 14. Targ. Ps. LXXIV, 4; a. e.—אַתְוָון, אַתְוָן, אַתְוָותָא, אַתְוָאן, אַתְוָתָא (אָתְן). Targ. Ps. l. c. Targ. O. Num. II, 2 ed. Berl. אַתְוָן, Var. אָתְוָן, אַתְוָון; Y. אתוון (v. Berl. Targ. O. II, p. 39); a. fr.—Koh. R. to I, 13 ה׳ אתואן five letters of acrostics.—אַתְוֵי, (אַתְוֵי, אַתְוַיָּי). Num. R. s. 13, end א׳ דדין וכ׳ the letters composing the one word (קערת) are the same as those composing the other (קרעת).

אֶת, אֵת (b. h.; cmp. יַת, איח; v. Ges. H. Dict. s. v.; cmp. אות III) [*essence*], a particle of the objective case, but also used as a noun, *the thing* (*which*) (cmp. Koh. IV, 3, v. אות III). Ohol. II, 4 את ש.... עליו that upon which ..... Zeb. 72[b]; Bets. 3[b] את שדרכו למנות שנינו we read (Orl. III, 7) that which it is customary to count singly, opp. כל שדרכו וכ׳ whatever is sometimes counted singly; a. fr.—Ber. I, 1 קורין את שמע we read the *Sh'ma'*, a. v. fr.—[The fact that את as a particle of the objective case may be dispensed with, and that את (fr. אתת *to join*) may have the meaning of *with*, gave rise to a method of Biblical interpretation by which, wherever את occurs in the Bible, esp. in laws, an amplification by implication is looked for.] Pes. 22[b] את לרבות וכ׳ the word *eth* (Deut. X, 20 [with] the Lord thy God thou shalt fear [some one else] intimates that we must pay reverence to the scholars next to God. Ib. ואידך את לא דריש and as to the other authority (that differs)? He does not interpret *eth* (as having a particular meaning); a. fr.—*Pl.* אֶתִים, אֶתִין the word *eth* occurring in Scripture, as a substratum for interpretation. Ib. היה דורש כל א׳ וכ׳ used to interpret every *eth* in the Law; a. fr. Num. R. s. 10 זו אחת מג׳ א׳ וכ׳ this is one of the three *eths* &c.

אָתָא I *letter, sign*, v. אָת.

אֲתָא, אָתָא II ch. (b. h. אתה, אתא; sec. r. of אות I q. v.) [*to join*,] *to come, to arrive; to occur to*. Targ. Gen. XIX, 9; a. fr.—Y. Peah III, 17[d] bot. אתאר עובדא וכ׳ the case came before ..... Gen. R. s. 68 (ref. to Gen. XXVIII, 11) א׳ שמשא the Sun (Jacob) has arrived. Snh. 98[b] ייתי ולא איחמיניה he (the Messiah) will come, but I do not desire to live to see him (to pass through the trials preceding his arrival).—תֵּיתֵי לי ד׳ may it come home to me that I did—, i. e. I believe to have merited divine reward. Meg. 28[a]; a. fr.—תיתי לי דלא may it come home to me that I did not—; a formula of assurance, *surely, indeed*. Y. Ber. II, 5[c] bot.; a. fr.; (v. יבוא עלי, s. v. בּוֹא).—Y. Shebi. VI, 36[c] top ייתי די (sub. עלי).—*Imperat.* תָּא (Y. אִיתָא). Gitt. 57[a], a. fr. תא חזי; Y. Dem. VI, 25[b] top איתא חמי; in Bab. usu. תא שמע (abbr. ת״ש) come and see, come and hear, i. e. I will prove it.—אַתְיָא כ׳ it comes like, i. e. it is in accordance with the opinion of. —Y. Naz. VI, 54[d] bot.; a. v. fr.—ואתיא=ואַתְיָא. Ibid.[c] bot. ואתיא כהדא דתני חוקיה (ed. Krot. incorr. ותניא) תֵּיתֵי.—Y. Keth. IV, 28[d] top ואתיין וכ׳ (read ואתיין) and those differences of opinion correspond to .....—אתיא פקידה פקידה the expression *pakad* occurs in two Biblical passages, אתיא זכירה זכירה and the expression *zakhar* occurs in two passages, i. e. draw an analogy between the respective Bible laws in which the same expressions are used, so as to cast a light upon each other. R. Hash. 11[a]; a. fr. [אתא נסיא Y. Meg. II, 73[b], a. e., read אַתְאַנַסְיָא q. v.] [Targ. Y. II Deut. XXXIII, 16 תֵּיתֵין, 3rd pers. fem. fut.]

Af. אַיְתֵי, אַיְתִי, אֵיתִי, אַיְתֵי *to bring, carry, cause to come*. Targ. Gen. IV, 3; a. fr.—מנא תיתי (מנן מחיכא) whence wilt thou bring (evidence), *how will you prove it?* Y. B. Mets. III, beg. 9[a]; a. v. fr.—מֵיתֵי, מַיְתֵי, מַיְיתָה *bringing, to bring*. Y. Peah I, 15[c] top בעי מ׳ וכ׳ he desired to bring it to them. Ib. לא יכילית מייתותי׳ I cannot bring it.—לֵיתֵי, לַיְתֵי let him bring. Sabb. 109[b]; a. fr.—לְאַתּוּיֵי, לְאֵיתּוּיֵי (cmp. אֶת) *to bring in, to include*, opp. לאפוקי; v. אֲפַק. לא׳ מאי what is to be implied (in addition to what is explicitly stated)? Tem. 2[a] הכל לא׳ מאי what does *hakkol* (all) come to imply? a. fr.—*Haf.* הַיְתֵי same. Dan. V, 13; a. e.

Ittaf. אִתְּתֵי (אִתּוּתֵי, אִתְּתֵי) אִתְיְתֵי *to be brought, offered*. Targ. Gen. XXXIII, 11. Targ. Lev. XIII, 2; a. e.

***אָתָא III** f. (b. h. עַיִשׁ, עָשׁ) the constellation called the *Great Bear, Ursa Major*. Ber. 58[b] Ms. M. (ed. יוּתָא, v. Rabb. D. S. a. l., a. Ges. H. Dict. s. v. עָשׁ).

אַתְנָסִיאָה, אֲתַנַסְיָא, אַתְאַנַסְיָא f. (ἀθανασία) *immortality*. Cant. R. to I, 3 (referr. to על־מות, Ps. XLVIII, 15) תרגם עק׳ א׳ וכ׳ Aquila translates it *athanasia* (אל־מות), a world in which there is no death; Y. Meg. II, 73[b] אתא נסיא (combine into one w.); Y. M. Kat. III, 83[b] bot. Ar. (ed. אתנא סירא corr. acc.); Lev. R. s. 11, end (ed. incorr. transp.).

אַתְדְּשָׁא f. (דוש) *stamping upon, trampling*. Targ. Is. XXII, 5.

אַתָּה m., אַתְּ f. (b. h.;=אנתה, v. אָנֹכִי) *thou*. Ber. 11[a]; a. fr.—אתה אומר, v. אַתְּ.—*Pl.* אַתֶּם, אַתֶּן *ye*. Ber. I, 1; a. fr. —R. Hash. 25[a] א׳ א׳ א׳ ג׳ פעמים וכ׳ three times *attem* is written (אַתֶּם, without ו); v. אֶפְרוֹחַ. Sifra Emor IX, 9; a. fr.

אַתּוּ, v. אִיתּוּ.

אַתּוּ *ye*, v. אַתְּ.

אַתְוָא *sign*, pl. אַתְוָון, אַתְוָאן, v. אָת.

אַתּוֹדָאָה, v. איח.

אַתּוּן, v. אַתּוּנָא II. Dan. III, 6; a. e.

אַתּוּנָא I *Athens*, v. אַתִּינַס.

אַתּוּנָא II m. (אתן, sec. r. of אות, v. איח) 1) (cmp. אתן, עַשַׁן, אשונא) *fire-place, stove*. Targ. Ex. XIX, 18;

a. e.—Keth. 67[b] התוא א׳ וכ׳ a fire-place of which the fire has been scraped out. Esth. R. to I, 12 זרוק גופר׳ באתונית cast sulphur into his stove i. e. inflame his passion.—2) v. next w.

אֲתוּנָא (**אַתּוּנָא, אִתּוּנָא**, Ms. **אַתּוּנָא**) m. (v. preced.,=h. אִישׁוֹן) *density, intensiveness, essence.* Targ. Prov. XX, 20 איך א׳ דחשוכא as darkness itself (h. text באישון with ב). Cmp. אֵיתָן.

אַתּוּר, אָתוּר ch.=h. אַשּׁוּר. Targ. Gen. II, 14; a. e.—Deriv. אַתּוּרָאָה, אַתּוּרָיָיה *Assyrian.* Ib. X, 11; a. e.

***אַתּוּרִין** m. pl. (=h. אשורים; שְׁוַר=תְּוַר, v. אִיסְתְּוָורָא) *ankles, footsteps.* Targ. Ps. XL, 3 some ed. (oth. אִיסְתְּוָורֵי).

אִתְחוֹלֵי, v. חָזַל.

אַתְחַלְתָּא f. (חלל) *beginning.* Sot. 41[b] top; a. fr. V. הַתְחָלָה.

אִתְחֲנוּנְתָא or **אִתְחַנָּנוּתָא** f. (חנן) *praying.* Targ. Ps. XXXI, 23.

***אַתִּיךְ** m. (נתך) *cast, hardened, fastened.* Targ. Job XLI, 16 (Ms. נְתִיךְ, h. text יצוק).

אַתִּינָה, v. next w.

אַתִּינַס, אַתּוּנָא (corr. אַתִּינָא), **אַתִּינָה** pr. n. pl. (Ἀθῆναι, acc.—ας) *Athens*, the capital of Attica; in Talm. liter. freq. mentioned for wisdom and wit. Bekh. 8[b] סבי דבי אתו׳ the elders (sages) of the Athenian school. Lam. R. to I, 1, s. v. *Rabbathi*, freq. אתינה a. אתינס.

אַתְּכוּתָא f. (נתך) *smelting, casting.* Targ. Job XXXVII, 10 (some ed. אִתְּ׳). Targ. Y. Lev. XX, 14. Targ. I Kings VII, 24.

אִתְכַּלָא, v. אִיתְכַּלָא.

אִתְכַּנְּעוּתָא, אִתְכַּנְּעוּ f. (כנע) *humiliation.* Targ. Jer. III, 25; a. e.

אִתְכַּפְיָיתָא f. (כפי) *bending.* Midr. Prov. to XXII, 6 אית לה א׳ can be bent.

אַתְלִיטִיס m. (ἀθλήτης) *athlete, prize-fighter.* Gen. R. s. 77 לא׳ (Ar. Var. לה׳).—*Pl.* אַתְלִיטִין. Ib. s. 22.—אַתְלִיטִים Ex. R. s. 21, end. Y'lamd. Emor (quot. in Ar.) תוקעין החלה ואח״כ האתליטין נכנסין first the trumpet is blown (signal), and then the fighters enter (metaphor of the sounding of the Shofar on the New Year, conquest of sin on the Day of Atonement, and carrying the palm on Succoth; v. בָּאֲרִין).

אִתְמְהָא m. (תמה) *strangeness; strange! it sounds curious;* sometimes used as a mere exclamation mark. Gen. R. s. 4 ויעש א׳ וכ׳ and God *made?!* Is it not by his *word* that things were created? Ib. s. 5. Pesik. R. s. 31; a. fr.

אֶתְמוֹל (b. h.=את יום חל, v. חָלָה) *yesterday, on a previous occasion.* Y. Bets. II, 61[b] bot.; a. fr.

אִתְמוֹל ch., v. אִיתְמַל.

אִתְמַכְּכוּתָא f. (מכך) *humiliation, lowliness.* Targ. Ps. CXXXVI, 23.

אִתְמְלוּכָא m. (מלך) *counsel, plan, plot. Pl.* אִתְמְלוּכִין. Targ. Jer. XVIII, 23.

אִתְמְנָיוּתָא f. (מני) *counting, being counted.* Targ. Nah. I, 12.

אִתָּן, v. אֵיתָן.

אתנא, Y. M. Kat. III, 83[b] bot. סירא א׳, v. אַתְאַנְסְיָא.

אַתְנָא, אַתָּנָא, אַתְּנָא f. (h. אָתוֹן) *she-ass.* Targ. Num. XXII, 21; a. fr.—*Pl.* אַתְנָן, אַתְנֵי (אתניי) אַתְנַיָּא (אַתְּ׳). Targ. Gen. XXXII, 15. Targ. I Sam. IX, 3; a. e.

אַתְּ=**אַתְּ אִינְהוּ** *thou art it.* Y. Yeb. XV, 15[a].

אַתְנִיס, v. אִיתְ׳.

אתניסאה, read אתנסיאה, v. אַתְאַנְסְיָא.

אֶתְנַן m. (b. h.; תנה *to hire*) *harlot's hire.* Tem. VI, 2 (29[a]) (as an offering); a. fr.

אַתְנַסְיָא, אַתְנַסְיָאה, v. אַתְאַנְסְיָא.

אִתְנַשְׁיָאת f. (נשי) *oblivion, forgetfulness.* Targ. Is. XLIX, 15.

אִתְעָרוּתָא f. (ערר) *inciting, exciting the funeral escort to weeping.* Targ. Job III, 7.

אתפלגות, Num. R. s. 13, beg. א׳ ר׳ וכ׳ read אתפלגון, v. פְּלַג.

אִתְקוּמְלָא, v. אִסְקוּמְלָא.

אִתְקַטְלָא f. (קטל) *killing.* Targ. Jud. VII, 18 Ar., ed. Buxt. a. oth. מִקְטְלָא.

אִתְקַפְּדַת f. (קפד) *cutting off, destruction.* Targ. Ezek. VII, 25.

אִתְקַפְתָּא, אִית׳ f. (תקף) *seizing;* whence *refutation, objection.* B. Bath. 129[a]; Hag. 9[b] א׳ דר׳ objection raised by. . . . .

אֲתַר, אֲתַר, אַתְרָא, אֲתַר c. (=אתאר, denom. of אָתָא, corresp. to h. מָקוֹם, fr. קום) *place, town.* Targ. Gen. XXII, 3; a. fr.—Ber. 63[a]. Gen. R. s. 39 (prov.) מבית לבית זכ׳ removal from house to house (costs) a shirt;—from town to town, a life. Ex. R. s. 45, end אַתְרִי טפלה לי וכ׳ my (the Lord's) place is an accidental attribute to me, but I am not accidental to my place; cmp. מָקוֹם.—Ned. 49[a], a. fr. מר כי אַתְרֵיה וכ׳ the one follows the custom of his place and the other that of his. B. Bath. 124[b] לאתרין to *our* place.—*Pl.* אַתְרִין, אַתְרַיָּא. Targ. Jud. XIX, 13; a. fr.—Y. Ber. II, 4[c] מן א׳ סגין from many places (passages, authorities); Pesik. R. s. 22 היגים אתריו (corr. acc.)—Denom. אַתְרוּתָא *local custom. Pl.* אַתְרָוָתָא. Gitt. 89[a] א׳

נידוהו the customs of the places are divided.—בְּאַתְרֵי, בְּאַתַר *in place of, instead; in consequence of, because of, for* (corresp to h. תַּחַת). Targ. II Chr. VI, 10; a. fr.—Targ. Job VIII, 4; a. fr.—V. בָּתַר.—על אתר (contr. אַלְּתַר q. v.) *on the spot, presently.* Y. Ber. I, 3[c]. Ib. II, 4[b], a. fr.

אִתְרַבְרְבוּתָא f. (רבּב, Palp. of רב) *boast, pride.* Targ. Zech. XII, 7; a. e.

אִתְרְגוּשָׁא m., **אִתְרְגוּשְׁתָּא** f. (רגש) *noise, noisy crowd, riot.* Targ. Jer. XXV, 31. Targ. Is. XVII, 12; a. fr.—*Pl.* אִתְרְגוּשַׁיָּא, אִתְרְגוּשִׁין, f. אִתְרְגוּשָׁתָא. Targ. Job XVIII, 11. Targ. Ezek. XXXIX, 16; a. e.

אֶתְרוֹג m. (תרג=שרג q. v.) [*the shining,*] *Ethrog,* a kind of orange or citron used with the festive wreath on the Feast of Booths (=פרי עץ הדר Lev. XXIII, 40; v. Targ.). Succ. III, 5; a. fr. Gen. R. s. 15. Lev. R. s. 30, end.—*Pl.* אֶתְרוֹגִין. Maasr. I, 4. Succ. IV, 9 באֶתְרוֹגֵיהֶן with their ethrogim (which they had brought into the Temple); a. e.

אֶתְרוֹגָא, אַתְרוֹגָא ch. same. Targ. II Esth. VII, 10 (tree; fem.).—*Pl.* אֶתְ׳, אַתְרוֹגִין. Targ. O. Lev. XXIII, 40. —Targ. II Esth. III, 8 אֶתְרוֹגִנָּנָא our own citrons.—V. תְּרוֹג.

אֶתְרוּנְגָא m. (an affected pronunciation of אֶתְרוֹגָא; v. תְּרוּנְגָא; Pers. turundj)=אֶתְרוֹגָא. Kidd. 70[a] כל האומר א׳ וכ׳ whoever says *Ethrunga* betrays a third (goodly) portion of haughtiness; either say Ethrog (hebr.) as the Rabbis do, or Ethroga (ch.) as the people do. Cmp. פּוּנְדְּרִיתָא.

אַתְרוּתָא, pl. אַתְרְוָתָא, v. אֲתַר.

אִתְרְחָצָא m. (רחץ) *reliance, trust.* Targ. Is. XXX, 2; 3 (ed. Vien. אִתְרַחֲצָנָא).

אִתְרִיס=אִתְאֲרִיס, v. אָרַס.

אתריסת, v. תְּרֵיס.

אִתְרַן=אִתְאַרְעַן; אִתְרַע=אִתְאֲרַע; v. אָרַע I.

אִתְרַשְׁלוּתָא f. (רשל) *slacking, faintness.* Targ. Jer. XLVII, 3.

אִתְתָא, v. אִיתְּתָא.

ב

ב *Beth,* the second letter of the Alphabet. Its sound lies betwen p (פ) and v (ו), whence its interchange with either, e. g. הפקר and הבקר; בָּא (אֲבָא) and ־וָא.—ב also interchanges with מ, as בולטיתא a. מלטיתא; cmp. b. h. מָלַט a. פָּלַט.

ב often rejected as a last radical letter, e. g. תוב=תו, נסב=נסי.

ב׳ as a numeral letter, *two;* v. א׳.

בְּ־ I prefix (b. h.) *in, within, on* &c. בו ביום on that day; באותו מקום in that very place; מינה וביה from it and in it, i. e. *out of the very thing.* B. Mets. 101[b] אגרא ... מינה וביה she hired carriers, paying them from the very wine which the man had placed in her storeroom.— בְּחוֹן=בּוֹן. Y. Ber. II, 4[c] bot.; a. fr.

בְּ־ II (contr. of בר) *son of.* בר׳ חייא son of R. Ḥiya. Cmp. בְּרַבִּי.

בָּא I m. (=אַבָּא) *1) *father.* Targ. O. Num. III, 24; 30 רב בית בא (and through the entire chapter ed. Berl.; oth. ed. אבא).—2) pr. n. m. *Ba=Abba.* Y. Ber. I, 2[c] top (interchanging with אבא); a. v. fr. in Y., v. אַבָּא II.

***בָּא** II m.=בֵּיתָא, *house.* Targ. Is. V, 8 ed. Ven., oth. ed. בֵּיתָא.

בָּא III m. (part. of בּוֹא) *coming, future.* עולם הַבָּא (abbr. ע״הב) *the world to come, futurity.* Snh. X, 1; a. fr.—לְהַבָּא (Bab.), לְבָא (Y.) *in future.* (מיכן) מכאן ולה׳ from this date and further, opp. למפרע retrospectively, or מעיקרא in the past. Pes. 7[b] לה׳ משמע it refers to an act to be performed. Snh. 27[a] מיכן ולה׳ וכ׳ he becomes disqualified as a witness from now and in future (previous testimonies not being effected). Y. Ter. I, 40[b] bot.; a. fr. —V. בּוֹא.

בָּאב, v. בָּב.

בָּאגָא, בָּגָא m. (בוג dial. for בוק, cmp. בקע) *valley, plain;* (=h. בִּקְעָה) *a group of fields belonging to several owners, rural community.* B. Bath. 29[a] one single field בכולה בא׳ (Ms. H. a. O. בכולה׳) in the whole plain. B. Mets. 22[b] ב׳ בארעא וכ׳ we need not presume an entire plain to be the property of minors; a. e.—*Pl.* בָּגֵי, בָּאגֵי. Pes. 8[b] those students דדיירי בב׳ that are lodged in the rural districts (and come to town for their studies). B. Kam. 113[b] (v. Rabb. D. S. a. l. for diff. vers.). B. Mets. 73[a]; a. e.

באגדתא, Succ. 52[b], v. בַּגְדְּתָאָה.

באגין, באגון, v. בָּאיִן.

***בָּאגָנָא** m. (v. בָּאגָא) 1) *cavity in the field, pool. Pl.* בָּאגְנֵי. B. Kam. 61[b] top, Ms. M. נָאגְנֵי q. v.—2) (cmp. בִּקְיעַ I, a. בקע Josh. IX, 4) *broken* or *burst water-vessel.* —*Pl.* as above. Ber. 58[a] באגני גלויא Ms. M. (read לְיָא, v. אֲיָא I; ed. בגני, read בָּגְנֵי; Ms. F. כאגני דשויג׳ ניגני, read: נָאגְנֵי, v. ב׳ ויש ג(ורסין) נ׳) whither do the broken vessels go? (i. e. what has the blind man to do here?).

בָּדָן, בָּדָאן, בָּאדָן pr. n. pl. *Badan*, a Samaritan place noted for its pomegranats. Tosef. Kel. B. Mets. VI, 10 'בא; Kel. XVII, 5 בדאן. Orl. III, 7; Bets. 3[b].

באחי, Targ. Prov. XXIV, 12 read באקי, v. בְּקָא.

בְּאוּשָׁה f. (b. h. בְּאֻשִׁים) [*sour,*] *an inferior kind of grapes, unripe grapes.* Y. Maasr. I, 48[d] משיקראו' באי' (corr. acc.) when they are called *b'ushah;* v. בְּאַשׁ 4).—*Pl.* באושין. Maasr. I, 2 Y. ed., v. אוּבְשִׁין.

בָּאוֹת f. (בית; cmp. Lat. noctua) 1) *night-bird, owl* (for תִּנְשֶׁמֶת Lev. XI, 18). Ḥull. 63[a] 'בא' שבעופות (Ar. ביאת) the *bavath* among the birds.—2) *groper in the dark, mole* or *salamander* (for תנשמת Lev. XI, 30). Ib. 'ב שבשרצים the *bavath* among the reptiles. [Targ. O. for 1): בֵּיתָא; for 2): אָשׁוּתָא q. v.; v. also סַלְמַנְדְרָא.—Var. in Targ. O. to Lev. XI, 18 בבתא, בּוּתָא, בֵּוְתָא, פּוּסָא, v. Berl. Targ. O. II, p. 34.]

באזי, באזוזי, v. בְּזָא II.

באזיאדן, v. next w.

בָּאזְיָארָן m. pl. (Pers. bâzyâran, Fl., R. Hai Gaon) *falconers.* Sabb. 94[a] 'דב (סוסא) Ar. (some ed. ד for ר; ed. בי ויירדן, Ms. בי זוררין, בי זוריארין, corr. acc.) the falconers' horse (used for carrying falcons, hawks &c. on his back).

בַּטָא, בָּאטָא m. (βάτος) *prickly roach*, a forbidden fish.—*Pl.* בָּטֵי, בָּאטֵי. Ab. Zar. 39[a] דהוה קרי ליה בא'. ed. (Ar. בטי) that he (the Gentile) called the brine *baté.*

בָּטִי, בָּאטִי pr. n. m. *Bati.* Gitt. 11[a] as an un-Jewish name, v. בְּהַק. Ab. Zar. 76[b]; Kidd. 70[b] (בטי) B. bar Tobi, name of a freedman.

באטיון, Yalk. Ps. 662 'פת קלא ב, read אַקוּבִּיטוֹן.

*__בַּיִין, בָּאיִין__ m. (βάϊον-βάϊς, a Coptic word; denomin. βάϊνος; cmp. I Macc. XIII, 51) *palm-leaf, palm-branch.* Lev. R. s. 30; Pesik. Ul'kaḥ. p. 180[a] באגין (read באינין βάϊνον); Tanḥ. Emor 18 אגין (corr. acc.; ed. Bub. 27 אגיז [!]); Yalk. Lev. 651.—Midr. Till. to Ps. XVII יבא; Yalk. Ps. 670 ברמין (corr. acc.); v. אַפּוּפְסִין.

בְּאִימָה (=בי אימה) pr. n. pl. *B'Imah* or *Imah.* Y. Orl. end, 63[b]; Tosef. Kil. II, 16 אומה ed. Zuck. (oth. ed. אימא); v. next w.

בְּאִינָה (=בי אינה) pr. n. pl. *B'Inah* a. B'Imah (v. preced.), two gentile conclaves in Northern Palestine. Y. Orl. end, 63[b]. Tosef. Kil. II, 16 בַּת עֵנָה (Var. בית); cmp. בית ענת, בית ענות Josh. XV, 59; XIX, 38.

בְּאִיר, v. בְּאַר.

בְּאֵשׁ, בְּאִישׁ, בְּאִישׁ ch. (h. בָּאַשׁ) 1) *to be bad, displeasing.* Targ. Gen. XXI, 11; a. fr.—Y. Sabb. VIII, 11[a] bot. 'ובאש לר' וכ it displeased R.... Y. Ber. III, 6[a] bot.; VII, 11[c] top; a. fr.—2) *to be ill, grow sick.* Ned. 40[a] top.—3) (with לבא, עינא, or נפשא) *to be displeased, angry, troubled.* Targ. Deut. XV, 9; 10 (some ed. יַבְאֵשׁ Af.). Targ. I. Sam. I, 8; a. e.—Lam. R., introd., end נפשך בְּאִישָׁא עלך thou art discontented.

Af. אַבְאִישׁ, אַבְאֵשׁ *to make bad; to do evil; to harm one* (with ל or ב of the person). Targ. I Sam. XII, 25. Targ. Is. XIV, 20; a. fr.—Targ. Gen. XIX, 9. Ib. Y. XVI, 12; a. fr.

בְּאִישָׁא c. (preced.) *sick, a patient.* Ber. 22[a b] 'ב' הוה בקילעא וכ Ar. (vers. quot. in marg. note to Ber. l. c. 'ב' הות f.) (ed. באושא הוה עובדא, v. Rabb. D. S. a. l.) there was a patient in the anteroom of &c. Sabb. 30[a] 'מקמי ב for the sake of a patient. Cmp. בִּישׁ.

באישה, v. בְּאוּשָׁה.

בְּאִישׁוּת f., v. בִּישׁוּ.

בָּאִית part. of בית.

בָּלָא, בָּאלָא m. ch. (=h. בול, cmp. יְבוּל) *growth* (of grass); whence *prairie, pasture ground* (in mountains &c.; cmp. Job. XL, 20 expl. in Lev. R. s 22).—Ḥull. 80[a] 'עזי דב *wild goats.* V. תּוּרְבָּלָא.

בָּאלוֹשָׁא, v. בַּלְשָׁא.

בָּאלֵי m. (part. of בלי, contr. of בהל, cmp. b. h. בַּבְּהָלוּת) 1) *hurrying:* Nidd. 26[b] 'ב' ואתי he came in a hurry.—2) *chasing* Ib. 17[a] 'ב' דידבי (Tosaf. בָּלֵי) chased the flies off. [Var. כאלי, v. כלי.]

בָּאלִי pr. n. m. *Bali* (Οὐάλης, Βάλης, *Valens*). Ber. 25[b]; Taan. 18[a]. Sabb. 17[b]; Ab. Zar. 36[b]. Cmp. וָלִיס.

*__כאמי, באמי__ (Mus. a. Maar.), Cant. R. to III, 4, read: פורני פלייאה קקוסכימי πόρνη παλαιὰ κακόσχημε, thou ungainly old harlot, 'מחו את וכ (not מחי) what thinkest thou of thyself? Cmp. פּוֹרְנִי.

*__באנטרין__, read בַּארְגְּטוֹן m. (farctum) *the stuffing of sausage.* Y. Sabb. VII, 10[a] bot. 'כד משקע ב when he puts the stuffing in (on the Sabbath); v. בגומא.

בְּאִנִּי, v. בְּנִי.

בְּאַנְיָא, v. בְּנָאָה.

בָּאצֵי part. of בְּצָא.

בְּאַר (בא√, v. בּוֹא) 1) *to break forth, come to light.* Denom. בְּאֵר; cmp. ביק.—2) *to be open, clear.*—*Pi.* בֵּאֵר (b. h.) *to proclaim* (cmp. Deut. I, 5), *to explain; to make clear (to one's self), to understand clearly.* Y. M. Kat. III, 83[b] top לְבָאֵר משנתו to explain (argue on) what he has learned. Koh. R. to VI, 9 better is he שהוא מְבָאֵר 'משנתו וכ who dwells on his studies to make them clear to himself, than he who learns to recite fluently.—Part. pass. מְבֹאָר *proven, clear.* Yed. III, 1 'מ' הדבר (Talm. ed. 'מ' את הד) from this fact it is proven.

בָּאַר ch., *Pa.* בָּאַר same. Y. M. Kat. III, 83[b] top לא חכמין מְבָאֲרָה know not how to make clear (argue).

בְּאֵר, בְּאֵיר f. (b. h., preced.) *well, spring.* Gen. R. s. 93; a. fr.—Erub. X, 14 (104[ab]), v. חֵקֶר. Taan. 9[a] ב׳ בזכות מרים the well in the desert was given to the Israelites for Miriam's sake; a. fr.— Transf. *origin.* Y. Sot. II, 18[a] (play on בוראיך, Koh. XII, 1) remember בְּאֵירְךָ וכ׳ thy well (whence thou camest), thy pit (grave), thy Creator; Lev. R. s. 18, beg.—*Pl.* בְּאֵרוֹת. Y. Erub. II, beg. 20[a] ב׳ חקר, v. חֵקֶר. V. בּוֹר II.

בְּאֵרָא ch. same. Targ. Cant. I, 1; v. בֵּירָא.

בָּאֲרָג m. (dial. for בִּרְקָא, v. ברק a. deriv.; cmp. בָּאגָא a. בִּקְעָא) *sparkling, effervescent; white-shining.* Ab. Zar. 30[a] מתוק חמר ב׳ Ar. (ed. מי ב׳) by 'sweet wine' we understand effervescent wine (liquid) (*mulsum vinum* or *mulsa aqua*, v. Sm. Ant. s. v. Vinum). —Snh. 98[a] סוסיא ב׳ quot. in Rashi to Ab. Zar. l. c., Ar. s. v. ברקא (ed. ברקא) a white-shining horse. [Deriv. fr. Pers. bârah is refuted by ברקא being used as an equivalent of our w.; v. also Fl. to Levy Talm. Dict. I, 284[a].]

בְּאֶרֶי pr. n. pl. *B'erai,* 1) ident. with בֵּירַי in Galilee. Pesik. R. s. 28; Midr. Till. to Ps. CXXXVII; Yalk. a. l. —2) בֵּי ב׳ in Babylon, v. בֵּירַאי.

בָּאַשׁ (b. h.; √בא, v. בּוֹא) *to be disordered, bad* (cmp. רַע).

Hif. הִבְאִישׁ 1) *to cause decay, to make smell badly.* Ex. R. s. 26; a. e.—2) (with דברים, or sub. דברים) *to use insulting language.* Koh. R. to X, 1.—3) (neut. v.) *to deteriorate, ferment, decay.* Ter. X, 2 אע״פ שה׳ מימיו מותריו Ms. M. (ed. מימיו מימיו corr. acc.) though the barley has begun to ferment &c. Cant. R. to I, 2[b] חמים מַבְאִישִׁים liquids grow stale. Pesik. B'shall. p. 81[b] דג מב׳ ill-smelling fish.—4) (v. בְּאוּשָׁה) [*to begin to ferment, to boil,*] *to be in the early stage of ripening, to be b'ushah.* Maasr. I, 2 grapes are subject to the law of tithes משיב׳ from the time they would be called *b'ushah*, cmp. Y. ib. 48[d]. Shebi. IV, 8. Tosef. Maasr. I, 1.

בָּאתַר, v. בָּתַר.

בָּב, בָּאב, בָּבָא I m. (reduplic. of בא, v. בּוֹא; cmp. b. h. בִּאָה a. מָבוֹא) *entrance, door, gate.* Targ. Esth. V, 14. —Sabb. 32[a], v. חוּטְרָא a. בְּזִיוּנָא I. Ib. 156[b] קרי אב׳ called at the door (begging). Erub. 11[b]; a. fr.—*Pl.* בָּבֵי. Ber. 58[b]; a. fr. Men. 34[a] בָּאבֵי.—Trnsf. (of writings) *section, clause.* ב׳ דרישא the clause of the first proposition. Sabb. 3[a] top; a. fr.—Hence ב׳ קמא (abbr. ב״ק), ב׳ מציעא (ב״מ), ב׳ בתרא (ב״ב) *Baba Kamma, Baba Metsia, Baba Bathra* (first, middle, last section), names of three Talmudic treatises of the order of *N'zikin* (civil law); v. נְזִק. [Tosefta Kelim is likewise divided into three Babas with the same names.].—*Pl.* as above. R. Hash. 33[b] תקיעה דכולי ב׳ the tune T'kiah in all the three sections.

בָּב II, בַּב נַהֲרָא pr. n. *Bab Nahăra* (Gate of the River) name of a tributary or a canal of the Euphrates. Ab. Zar. 39[a] דב׳ נ׳ (Ms. M. דנהרא); Succ. 18[a] (Ms. M. 1 דבנהרא, 2 דפום נהרא), cmp. Yeb. 16[b] sq.).

בָּבָא I, v. בָּב I a. בָּבִיתָא.

בָּבָא II pr. n. m. 1) *Baba* (ben Buta), a disciple of Shammai, blinded by Herod. B. Bath. 3[b]. Kerith. VI, 3. (Cmp. Jos. Ant. XV, 7, 10.)—2) B. father of R. Judah. Eduy. VI, 1; a. fr.

בָּבָה f. (b. h.), only in בָּבַת עַיִן the pupil of the eye. Ex. R. s. 30 ב׳ ע׳ העליונה (some ed. בת; corr. acc.) the Lord's &c. V. בָּבִיתָא I.

בָּבוּ (בבוי) f. *hatred* (only in Targ. Y., =דְּבָבוּ; ד rejected through false analogy, v. דְּבָבָא). Targ. Y. Gen. XXV, 11; a. e.

בָּבוּאָה (in Babli), בּוּבְיָה, בּוּבְיָא (in Y.) f. (onomatop., v. Fl. to Levy Chald. Dict. I, 419 a. Fried. Del. Assyr. Stud. I, 142; v., however, בָּבִיתָא) *reflected image* in metal, water &c.; *image, shadow.* Ned. 9[b] ונסתכלתי בבב׳ שלי (Ar. with two ב, corr. acc.) and I was looking at my image (in the water); Tosef. Naz. IV, 7 (Var. בוביא); Y. Ned. I, 36[d] bot. בובייה; Num. R. s. 10 בוביא. Yeb. 122[a] ב׳ דב׳ a shadow of a shadow. Ab. Zar. 47[a] לב׳ קא סגיד he worships the image (in the water). Gen. R. s. 4 ב׳ גדולה magnified image. Treat. Sof'rim. III, 8 ב׳ שלו the outlines of an effaced letter.

בָּבוּיָא f. (v. preced.) prop. *mirror,* hence (from its shape) a musical instrument, *a little drum, tympanum* (used at orgies, v. Sm. Ant. s. v. Tympanum). Y. Taan. I, 64[b] bot.

בָּבֵי, v. בֵּיבַי.

בָּבִיתָא I בָּבְתָא (בְּבֵייתָא) f. (cmp. בָּב a. בֵּית;=h. בָּבָה, [*the innermost,*] with עֵינָא, *pupil of the eye.* Targ. O. Deut. XXXII, 10 בָּבַת ע׳ (plur.) the pupils of *their* (the Israelites') eyes; [Targ. Y. בבא דעיוניה Ar. (ed. בָּבֵי) the innermost or the gates of His thought, v. בָּב I]. Targ. Prov. VII, 2 בבתא (Ms. בבייתא). Targ. Koh. XII, 2 בבי עינך (some ed. בני, גבי, corr. acc.). Gitt. 69[a] בביתא.

***בָּבִיתָא II** or **בּוּבִיתָא** f. (v. בִּיב a. preced.) *gutter, outlet.* Hull. 85[b] על ב׳ דמיא Ar. (ed. בי׳) over the outlet (wherein the flax is put); v. יְנִיבָא.

***בָּבִיתִין** m. pl. (fr. בָּבָא or fr. בית) *gate* (or *lodging*) *money, contribution for the support of traveling poor.* Y. Dem. III, beg. 23[b].

בָּבֶל (b. h.) pr. n. *Babel, the city of Babylon; Babylonia,* a country of varying limits, chiefly comprising Mesopotamia, a portion of Great Armenia and some neighbouring countries east of the Tigris (v. Neub. Géogr. p. 320). [Owing to the continued political disturbances in Palestine, Babylonia gradually became the centre of Jewish scholarship; hence both the frequent comparisons and jealousies between the East and the West (Babyl. a. Palest.); cmp. אֶרֶץ, חֲנַנְיָה, תַּלְמוּד. Kidd. 69[b]; 71[b]. Sot. 49[b]. Y. Snh. I, 19[a]; Y. Ned. VI, 40[a] bot. כי מב׳ תצא וכ׳ (sarcastic imitation of Is. II, 3). Snh. 24[a] תלמודה של ב׳

Babylonian method (Talmud). עולי ב׳ those coming from Bab. to visit the Temple, pilgrims. Ned. V, 4 דבר של ע׳ ב׳ that in which pilgrims from Bab. (i. e. Jews living abroad) have a share, as the Temple Mount &c. [Macc. 24ᵃ, a. e. המונח של ב׳, read רומי as Ms. M.; cmp. אֲרָמִי.]

בִּבְלָאָה, בִּבְלָאֵי, בַּבְלָיָא, בַּבְלָיְיא m. ch.=h. בַּבְלִי, *Babylonian.* Targ. Josh. VII, 21 (some ed. בַּבְלִי). —Sabb. 105ᵇ ב׳ O, thou Babylonian! B. Mets. 85ᵃ גמרא (Ms. M. תלמודיה דבבל) ב׳ the method he had learned in Babylonia; cmp. preced.—Y. Sabb. VI, 8ᵃ bot.; a. fr.—*Pl.* בַּבְלָאֵי. Targ. Ps. CXXXVII, 3. Hull. 45ᵃ חברין ב׳ our Babyl. colleagues. Keth. 75ᵃ, a. fr. ב׳ טפשאי foolish Babylonians.—Fem. בַּבְלֵיתָא. Targ. l. c. v. 8.—*Pl.* בַּבְלְיָתָא, בַּבְלְיָיתָא. Targ. II Esth. I, 10.—Sabb. 81ᵃ.

בָּבְלוֹן, pr. n. (Βαβυλών) *Babylon.* Cant. R. to I, 6 (a legend about the origin of Rome) and they called it רומי ב׳ Rome-Babylon.

בַּבְלִי m. (preced. ws.) *Babylonian.* Pes. 66ᵃ הלל הב׳ Hillel the Babylonian; a. fr.—*Pl.* בַּבְלִיִּים, בַּבְלִיִּין. Yoma 66ᵇ; Men. 100ᵃ. Cant. R. to VIII, 9; Lam. R. to I, 13 ספסלין מלאין ב׳ וכ׳ students' seats in Palestine occupied by Babylonians; [for מונחי Lam. R. l. c. prob. to be read מומחין].

בַּבְלָיְיא, v. בִּבְלָאָה.

בבליקון, read בַּבִּילֹנִיקוֹן m. (Babylonicum) *Babylonian tapestry.* Yalk. Josh. 18 פורפירא ב׳; (Gen. R. s. 85 בבליא).

בַּבְלִיתָא, v. בִּבְלָאָה.

בָּבְעוּ, v. בָּעוּ.

בָּבְתָא, v. בְּבִיתָא I.

בָּבְתָא, v. בָּאוּת.

בַּג, בַּג בַּג, בֶּן בַּג pr. n. m. *Ben Bag Bag.* B. Kam. 27ᵇ; a. fr. Kidd. 10ᵇ Joh. son of B. B.

בַּגָּא, v. בָּאגָא.

בָּגַד (b. h.; v. infra) *to act violently, to rebel, be faithless.* Snh. 37ᵃ (allud. to Gen. XXVII, 27) א״ת בְּגָדָיו אלא בּוֹגְדָיו do not read *b'gadav* (his garments), but *bog'dav* (his faithless ones). Y. Peah I, 16ᵇ top; Num. R. s. 10, beg.; Cant. R. to V, 16, v. בְּגִידָה.—Mekh. Mishp., N'zikin 3 מאחר שב׳ בה וכ׳ (b'bigdo bah, Ex. XXI, 8) since he &c., treated her contemptuously (opp. to the interpretation of בבגדו as *his garment,* שפירש בגדו עליה he spread his bedcloth over her). [From Targ. renderings as well as from Agadic interpretations it appears that the primitive meaning of בגד ($\sqrt{}$בג) is, *to tear; also to despise,* corresp. to the meanings of $\sqrt{}$בז; v. Targ. Job VI, 5; Is. XXXIII, 1; Prov. XXI, 18; Snh. 94ᵃ, cit. s. v. בזוזא; Esth. R. to I, 10, cit. s. v. בזז; Mekh. l. c.; cmp. also K'thib בג for K'ri בַּז Ezek. XXV, 7.—בֶּגֶד seems to be *a piece, web,* corresp. in meaning and use to φᾶρος.]

בֶּגֶד m. (b. h.; preced.) *web, garment.* Men. 40ᵇ היא ב׳ של וכ׳ if (the garment) itself is a web, but its borders are of leather. Ib. the principal element ב׳ בעינן must be a web (in order to require Tsitsith). Mekh. Mishp., N'zikin 3, v. preced. Sabb. 26ᵇ; a. fr.—*Pl.* בְּגָדִים, constr. בִּגְדֵי. Gen. R. s. 20 ב׳ א״הר Adam's garments, v. אוֹר II, 3. Yoma 60ᵇ ב׳ לבן the Highpriest's white garments (for the Day of Atone, Lev. XVI, 4), contrad. to ב׳ זהב gold-embroidered &c. Ib. 68ᵇ; a. fr.

בַּגְדָא, v. אֲוָנָא II.

***בגדל**, Gen. R. s. 98 ב׳ דין, read מִגְדַּל יוֹן pr. n. pl. *Migdal Yon,* near Sidon; v. Neub. Géogr. p. 295.

בַּגְדַת pr. n. pl. *Bagdath* (prob. Eski Bagdad, Neub. Géogr. p. 360), birth place of R. Hanna. [Kidd. 71ᵇ, v. אֲוָנָא II.]—Hence:

בַּגְדַתָּאָה m. *of Bagdath.* Yeb. 67ᵃ; a. e.—Succ. 52ᵇ Ms. M. (ed. באגדתא, corr. acc.).

***בגומין, בגומא**, read בַּרְגְּמִינִין or בַּרְגְּמִינָא m. pl. (farcimen,—ina) *stuffings of sausage, sausages.* Y. Sabb. VII, 10ᵃ bot. כד מקטע ב׳ when cutting the sausages through (dividing them off), v. באנטרין. Y. Bets. IV, 62ᶜ bot. the sausage-maker is forbidden to work on a Holy Day משום מקטע ב׳ because he cuts the sausage-bags apart; v. סיקורא.

בְּגִידָה f. (בָּגַד) *faithlessness, rebellion.—Pl.* בְּגִידוֹת. Y. Peah I, 16ᵇ top (play on *bigdothekha,* Ps. XLV, 9) כל בגידות שבגדת וכ׳ all sinful acts thou hast committed, shall (after repentance) be like myrrh &c.; Num. R. s. 10, beg.; Cant. R. to V, 16.

בְּגִין, v. גִּין.

***בַּגִּיר, בַּגָּר** m. (בגר) *rough.* Targ. Y. Gen. XXVII, 11 quot. in Tosef. Yom Tob to Keth. III, 8, a. e. (ed. סערן).

בַּגְלָאר, v. גְּלָאר.

***בגלמוררי**, Ms. Oxf. בגלאטורי, Sabb. 103ᵇ, a corrupt. of בּוֹגָלִים לְיטֵירָא (or בּוֹגָאלִים) (vocalis litera) *open sound, vowel.* כיון דאיתיה ב׳ וכ׳ since it has merely the value of a vowel letter, one is guilty for writing two Alephs on the Sabbath (v. R. S.'s opinion ib. מלאכה שכיוצא בה מתקיימת). [Differ. in commentaries.]

בָּגַן, v. פָּגַן.

בָּגַר ($\sqrt{}$בג, v. בָּאגָא; cmp. חֲזָזִית) [*to be rough* (of surface, voice &c.);] *to be wrinkled* (of a female's nipples), whence; *to become of age* (at twelve years and a half). Keth. III, 8 הבּוֹגֶרֶת a girl of beginning maturity (v. Tosef. Yom Tob a. l.). Nidd. V, 7 כיון שֶׁבָּגְרָה as soon as she is mature, v. צָמֵל. Pes. 113ᵃ (prov.) בתך ב׳ וכ׳ has thy daughter become of age? Set thy slave free and give him to her (as husband); a. fr.—Tosef. Keth. III, 8 תִּיבָּגֵר (Nif.); Y. ib. 27ᶜ bot. תִּבָּגוֹר.

בְּגַר ch. same. 1) *to be of age.* Targ. Y. Num. XXX, 11, sq.—2) *to be rough, harsh, husky.* B. Bath. 167ᵇ בגר לה קלא her voice has become rough (from old age).—Denom. בַּגִּיר.

Af. אַבְגַּר *to produce a rough surface, to heat and*

bruise by friction. Nidd. 66ᵃ שפופרת אֲבָגּוּרֵי מבגר לה Ar. Var. אגג׳ מגג׳, ed. אפג׳ מפג׳) will not a tube bruise her?—Keth. 65ᵃ מבגר לה (the ropes of the bedstead) hurt her.

בֶּגֶר m. (preced. ws.) *age of majority* (of females). Y. Kidd. I, 59ᵇ ימות הב׳ the period of majority. Y. B. Bath. IX, beg. 16ᵈ. Kidd. 4ᵃ ב׳ דאיילונית majority of a barren (or wombless) woman (who has no signs of maturity and becomes of age at twenty years). Keth. 38ᵇ יש ב׳ בקבר can the legal consequences of becoming of age enter after the woman's death? [Other form: בּוֹגֶר. Y. Keth. V, 29ᵈ לאחר בּוֹגְרָהּ after her becoming of age.] V. בַּגְרוּת.

בַּגֶּר f. (preced.) *a woman of age.* Tosef. Keth. V, 1 הב׳ כתביעה (read בת׳, Var. ed. Zuck. הבּוֹגֶרֶת בתביעה) she who is of age when asked (by her betrothed) to be married; Y. ib. 29ᵈ הב׳ בשעה (corr. acc.). Ib. נותנין לב׳ וכ׳ a girl of age is allowed twelve months for preparation for her wedding.—Ch. v. בַּגִּיר.

בגרון, Lev. R. s. 28, end, קומוס ב׳, read קוֹמִיס פְּרִיבַטוֹן (κόμης πριουάτων)=*comes privatarum*, v. דומין.

בגרונדרי, v. גּוּנְדְּרָא.

בַּגְרוּת f. (v. בֶּגֶר) *womanhood*, (after twelve years and a half), opp. to נערות, maidenhood (between twelve and twelve and a half) and ילדות childhood (from three to twelve years). Y. Yeb. I, 3ᵃ top אין בין.... לימות הב׳ וכ׳ between the period of maidenhood and that of womanhood there is no more than a six months' interval; Keth. 39ᵃ; a. fr.

בִּיד־, בְּד־ prefix (comp. of בְּ a. דְּ=h. בְּשֶׁל, בְּשֶׁ־) 1) *concerning that (those) of; at the time of; treating of what refers to.* Sabb. 112ᵃ בדטייעי in the case of those (sandals) of the travelling merchants (Arabs). Yoma 78ᵇ, v. הוּצָא. Ḥull. 20ᵃ ומתני׳ בדלא אהדר our Mishnah treats of a case when he did not turn. Gitt. 49ᵃ בדניזק וכ׳ we go in our assessment by (the property) of the injured; a. v. fr.—2) *if, when.* Targ. Y. Gen. XLIII, 5 בִּדְלֵית *unless.* Targ. O. Deut. IX, 4 בְּדִיתַבַּר; a. e.

*__בַּד I__=אֲבַד. Targ. Y. II, Num. XXI, 29 וּבָדְתוּן (Var. וְאַ׳=וּבַדְתוּן). Ithpe. אִתְבִּיד, v. אֲבַד.

בַּד II m. (בדד) *olive press* (cmp. גַּת), *tank.* Shebi. VIII, 6 אין...... בַּבַּד you must not press olives in the tank (in the Sabbath year).—בית הַבַּד *the building containing the tank* and all implements for pressing olives. Sabb. I, 9 קורת ב׳ הב׳ the beam of the press; a. fr.—Bets. 19ᵃ; Tosef. ib. II, 7, v. גַּב.—*Pl.* בַּדִּים, בַּדִּין. B. Bath. IV, 7 בית הב׳. Toh. IX, 7 בד אחד או שני ב׳ a quantity of olives for one tank or for two; a. fr.

בַּד III m. (b. h.; בדד) 1) *single, separate.* Ber. 63ᵇ (play on *baddim*, Jer. L, 36) שיושבין ב׳ ב׳ who study separately (without interchange of ideas). Kerith 5ᵃ expl. Ex. XXX, 34 ב׳ בב׳.—2) with pref. לְ, לְבַד (b. h.) *alone, only.* Sot. 8ᵃ אותה לְבַדָּהּ *her* (Num. V, 19) indicates her alone (each separately); a. fr.—בִּלְבַד (adv.) *only.* Ber. I, 1 ולא זו ב׳ (usu. with אמרו) and not only in this case did they make such a rule. Meg. I, 5 אין בין ... אלא .... ב׳ there is no difference between Festivals and the Sabbath (as to forbidden labors) except only as to the preparation of the necessaries of life; a. fr.—וּבִלְבַד *but only, provided.* Zeb. V, 8; a. fr.

בַּד IV m. (b. h.; בדד) *chosen, fine linen.* Zeb. 18ᵇ ב׳ שיהו של בוץ וכ׳ wherever the Law speaks of garments of *bad*, it means that they must be of byssus, new &c. Ib. how do we know דהאי ב׳ כיתנא הוא that *bad* (as material for garments) means linen (and no other fine stuff)? Answ. Something which grows בד בבד in single stalks (v. preced. a. next w.); Yoma 71ᵇ. Ib. 35ᵃ *bad* is used four times, intimating מובחר בב׳ the choicest of &c (for diff. vers. v. Rabb. D. S. a. l. note); [cmp. Targ. Jer. XLVIII, 30].

בַּד V m. (בדד) *single stalk, twig;* also (b. h.) *pole, bar.* Zeb. 18ᵇ; Yoma 71ᵇ; v. preced. Keth. 17ᵃ ב׳ של הדס myrtle twig. Succ. 44ᵇ even one leaf וב׳ אחד and (on) one twig. B. Mets. 24ᵃ anything on which something is suspended ב׳ קרו ליה is called *bad.*—*Pl.* בַּדִּים. Y. Yoma V, 42ᵇ bot., a. e. בין הב׳ between the bars projecting from the Ark (i. e. their corresponding place in the Second Temple). B. Mets. l. c. בַּדֵּי מחטין וכ׳ poles of peddlars for needles &c. Ib. מאי בדי what does *baddê* mean? Answ. *Twigs.*—And why do they call them *baddê*? Answ., v. supra. V. אַנְפּוֹרְיָא.

בַּדָּא I ch.=h. בַּד II.—*Pl.* בַּדַּיָּא. Targ. Joël II, 24 Ar. (ed. בֵּירַיָּא). Snh. 95ᵃ תותי בי ב׳ under the wine press (Var. בי סריא).

בַּדָּא II m.=h. בַּד IV, *fine linen woof.* Y. Sabb. XIII, beg. 14ᵃ.

בְּדָא, בַּדָּא, v. בדי.

בְּדָא *in this case*, v. דָּא.

בַּדְיָיא, בַּדָּאָה m. ch.=h. בַּדַּאי. Ḥull. 63ᵃ ההוא בריא הוה (corr. acc.; Yalk. Zech. 578 בדאה) that man was a liar.

בַּדָּאוּת, v. בַּדָּיוּת.

בַּדַּאי m. (בדי I) 1) *liar, misrepresenting.* Snh. 89ᵇ (prov.) כך עונשו של ב׳ וכ׳ such is the punishment of the liar &c.; Ab. d'R. Nath. ch. XXX; Gen. R. s. 94 מה טיבו של ב׳ הזה; v. טִיב. Kidd. 49ᵃ he who translates a Bible verse literally (v. צורה), הרי זה ב׳ is a liar (misrepresenting the sense).—2) *invention, fiction.* Deut. R. s. 5, a. fr. דברים של ב׳ fictitious words (mitigating the original report); ib.—דברי ב׳.—*Pl.* בַּדָּאִים, בַּדָּאִין. Y. Gitt. IV, 46ᵃ bot. נמצאו הדברים ב׳ things turned out to be false. B. Bath. 74ᵃ; Snh. 110ᵃᵇ Moses and his laws are true והן ב׳ and they (euphem. for *we*) are liars. Tosef. Keth. II, 1 ב׳ אנו (ed. Zuck. מבוידין) we have been telling a falsehood.

בְּדָאן, בַּדָּאן, v. בָּאדָן.

בָּדַד (b. h.; $\sqrt{}$בד; cmp. בז, *to enter into, split, separate*; v. בדל, בדק, בדר &c.) 1) *to scatter.* Y. Yoma V, 42[c] top בּוֹדְדָהּ ברגלו he scatters it (the frank-incense) with his foot (shoves it apart).—2) *to dig out, create, choose, invent.* Denom. בַּד II, בַּדִּים.—3) *to be lonely. Part.* בּוֹדֵד *lonely.* Pesik. R. s. 29 (30), expl. בדד (Lam. I, 1)= בּוֹדֵד lonely, forsaken. *Part. pass.* בָּדוּד *exiled.* Lam. R. to I, 1 בגדים בדודים Ar. (read בגדי) garments of the exiled (כלי גולה, Jer. XLVI, 19); [ed. בגדי בָדָד, a. בְּדָדִין, v. next w.].

Hithpol. הִתְבּוֹדֵד *to be exiled, homeless.* Lam. R. introd. (R. Alexandri 1) (ref. to Ps. CII, 8) as the bird מִתְבּוֹדֵד וכ׳ is driven (separated from the rest) from roof to roof.

בָּדָד m. (b. h.; preced.) *loneliness,* (adv.) *in a lonely state, in exile.* Snh. 104[a] יהיה ב׳ מושבם the exile shall be their dwelling. Lam. R. to I, 1 בגדי ב׳ garments (outfit) of exile, v. preced.—*Pl.* בְּדָדִים, בְּדָדִין. Ib. בגדי ב׳ (plur. abstr. as חיים &c.).

בַּדָּד m. (denom. of בַּד II) *olive-treader, workingman in the olive press.* Gitt. 62[a].—*Pl.* בַּדָּדִין. Toh. X, 1 sq. Sabb. 19[b] שֶׁמֶן של ב׳ וכ׳ the oil (remnants in corners) belonging to the pressers, and the mats which they use. B. Kam. 119[a] והב׳ לוקחין מהן וכ׳ (read בנשותיהן, v. Rabb. D. S. a. l. note 40) you may buy from the oil pressers' (Rashi: oil producers') wives &c. Tosef. Maasr. I, 10 הב׳ (ה)מדליקין וכ׳ the oil pressers who take their lighting oil (alternately) from one press and another.

בדדיות, v. בְּדִידָה.

***בְּדָדִין** m. pl. (preced. ws.) *stocks* of prisoners. Tosef. Kel. B. Mets. X, end (ed. Zuck. גרדין, v. גַּרְדוֹן).

בָּדָה, v. בדי.

בְּדָה, v. בְּדִי II.

בדו, v. next w.

בְּדוּבַר (Arab. *dubr, back*) *with one's back to.*—Ber. 6[b] (speech of an Arab) ב׳ קיימת וכ׳ Ar. (Ms. M. בדו בר, ed. כדו בר, corr. acc.) with thy back (to the Synagogue) standest thou before the Lord?

בדודיות, v. בְּהוֹרִיה.

בַּדּוּחָא m. (בדח) *merry-maker.*—*Pl.* בַּדּוּחֵי. Taan. 22[a] אינשי ב׳ וכ׳ we are merry-makers and cheer up the sad.

בּוּדְחָא, בְּדוּחָא m. (v. preced.) *cheerfulness.* Targ. Ps. CL, 5 דמשמעין לבדוחא Ms. (ed. incorr. דשמעין בלחודיהון) which are sounded for rejoicing. Ib. LXVIII, 32 בבודחא Ms. (ed. בנוי דחם).

בְּדוּי, v. בדי.

בְּדוֹלַח m. (b. h.) *b'dolah,* name of a jewel, also of a gum, *bdellium.* Gen. R. s. 16, beg. את סבור כב׳ וכ׳ you might think, b'dolah (Gen. II, 12) means the druggists' bdellium—let its neighbor (next word אבן השוהם) explain it (correct. acc. to Yalk. Gen. 21).

בְּדוּלְחָא ch. same. Targ. Gen. II, 12; a. e.

בדולקי, read בְּרוּקְלֵי.

בָּדוֹקָא m. (בדק) *searching, penetrating.*—*Pl.* בָּדוּקַיָּא, בָּדוֹ׳. Targ. Y. Num. V, 19; a. e.

בְּדוּקִי m. (בדק) *one requiring examination,* i. e. *one whose father is unknown,* usually שְׁתוּקִי. Kidd. IV, 2 Abba Saul called the *sh'thuki* ב׳ *b'duki.* Y. ib. II, 65[d] bot.; Bab. ib. 74[a].

בְּדוּר, בְּדוּרָא, בָּ׳ m. (בדר) 1) *dispersion, scattering.* Targ. Is. VIII, 22 (ed. Vien. בְּדוּר), a. e.—2) *one exiled.* Targ. II Sam. XIV, 13 sq.

בדורלהון, בדורוילו, v. פְּרִוִילָא.

בְּדוּתָא f. (בדי I) *fiction, mistake.* B. Bath. 145[a], a. fr. הא דר׳ . . . ב׳ היא R. . . .'s account (or opinion) is a mistake. [Ar. reads בְּרוּתָא q. v.]

בְּדַח, בְּדִיחַ (denom. of $\sqrt{}$דח, v. דָּחָה; cmp. בְּזָרָא) *to be cheerful.* Targ. Y. Ex. XVIII, 9; a. fr.—Ber. 30[b], a. fr. ב׳ טובא was very cheerful. M. Kat. 17[a] בְּדִיחָא דעתאי I feel happy. Sabb. 77[b].—*Hull. 32[a] לא הוה בדיחנא ביה וכ׳ I could not make light of my uncle so as to ask him (Ar. ed. pr. בדיקנא).

Pa. בַּדַּח *to cheer up, make laugh.* Taan 22[a], v. בַּדּוּחָא. Ned. 51[a] have I not cautioned thee דלא תבדחן not to make us laugh? Ib. 50[b] bot. תבדיחן (En Yaak. תבדחן).

בָּדָה, בְּדָא, בדי (b. h., $\sqrt{}$בד, v. בדד) *to dig out,* whence 1) (cmp. ברא) *to take out* (a piece of dough) and *shape, to form.* Men. V, 1; Sifra Emor Par. 10, ch. XIII השאור בּוֹדֶה וכ׳ he gets the leaven required for the loaves out of themselves (taking a piece of dough out of that intended for the loaves).—2) *to create, invent.* Ned. 10[a] לשון שֶׁבָּדוּ וכ׳ terms (for vows) which the Scholars have (arbitrarily) invented (as disguises). Lev. R. s. 9 לשון בָּדוּי an invented expression. Gen. R. s. 100 דברים בְּדוּיִים fictitious words. Ib. s. 48 בדויים (sub. דברים, some ed. בדאות).

Pi. בִּידָּה, בִּידָּא 1) same. Y. Meg. I, 71[c] top בי׳ להן וכ׳ made up for them a false Latin translation (of the Bible) from the Greek; v. בָּרַר.—Y. Keth. II, 26[b] bot. מְבַדִּין הויינן we have been inventing, i. e. speaking in fun; Tosef. ib. II, 1 מבודין אנו (corr. acc.; Var. בדאים). [Y. Kidd. III, 64[d] מבדין אתם וכ׳, prob. to be read בין הדין וכ׳.] [Y. Shebi. IV, 35[b] bot. מבדין בחדשים, v. בָּהָה.]—2) *to disprove, refute.* Tanh. Balak, 14; ed. Bub. 23 (ref. to *baddim,* Is. XLIV, 25) מְבַדִּין וכ׳ they frustrate their predictions.

Hithpa. הִתְבַּדָּה *to be tempted to a falsehood, turn a liar.* Ber. 4[a]; Der. Er. Zut. ch. III train thy tongue to say, I do not know, שמא תִּתְבַּדֶּה וכ׳ lest thou be induced to tell a falsehood and be caught.

בְּדָא, בְּדִי I ch. same, *to invent.* Targ. Y. II. Num. XVI, 28 בַּדְיֵית (Var. בְּדִית).

Ithpa. אִתְבַּדִּי *to be declared wrong, to be mistaken.* Y. Yeb. VIII, 9[c] עברת בִּידָךְ תלתא נהרין ואִיתְבַּדַּת thy story crossed three rivers (coming from Babylonia) and is found to be a mistake; Y. Sabb. II, 9[a] top ואיתבר׳ (corr. acc.).

בְּדִי II, Pa. בַּדִּי, בַּדֵּה (dialect.=בזי) *to despise.* Cant. R. to VIII, 1 (ref. to לא יבוזו לי ibid.; read:) לית דו מבדה לי there is none can despise me (for kissing my brother); [Ex. R. s. 5 beg. corrupt].

בדי, Yalk. Deut. 913 ב׳ פלסטין, v. דִּיפְּלֵי.

בְּדִיאֵי m. pl. (בדי) *fictions.* Bekh. 8[b] מילי דב׳ ed. (Ar. כדי, En Yaak. כדיבי) some stories.

בְּדִיד m. (בדד) *digging instrument, spade, mattock.* Kel. XXIX, 7 יד חב׳ the handle of a spade.—*Pl.* בְּדִידִין. Y'lamd. Sh'laḥ quot. in Ar. ב׳ בברזל (?).—2) *rut, cavity* (cmp. next w.).—*Pl.* as above. M. Kat. 4[b]; Tosef. ib. I, 2; ib. Shebi. I, 7 ב׳ שבעיקרי וכ׳ the cuts around the roots of trees; v. אוּגָיָה.

בּוֹדִידָה, בְּדִידָה f. (בדד, v. בַּד II) *small olive press.* Sifra B'har ch. I one may grind the olives in the large tank ומכניס לבד׳ and then put them into the small press; Shebi. VIII, 6 לבוד׳.—*Pl.* בְּדִידוֹת. Gen. R. s. 31 Ar. (ed. בדריות, בדדיות, corr. acc.).

בַּדָּאוּת, בַּדָּיוּת f. (בדי) *fiction, falsehood.* Lev. R. s. 9. Gen. R. s. 48, v. בַּדָּא.

בְּדִיחַ, v. בְּדַח.

בְּדִיחָא f. (בדח) *joy.* Constr. בְּדִיחַת. Targ. Esth. VIII, 17.

בְּדִיחוּתָא f. (v. preced.) *cheer.* Sabb. 30[b] מלתא דב׳ something humorous. Ber. 55[a] בדיחותיה מפכחא ליה its very cheerfulness frustrates it (the good dream).

***בְּדִינָיֵי** m. (contr. of בי דיינֵי) prop. *court-house,* in gen. *government's building, public building, treasury.* Ber. 56[a] ב׳ דמלכא וכ׳ ed. (Mss. בְּזִיוּנָא, בֵּי זְיוּנָא q. v.) the king's treasury shall be broken into. [Perl. Et. St. p. 25 refers to Pers. *divân* which, however, seems of too late an origin for the Talmudic date, v. Cycl. Brit. 9th ed. s. v. Divan.]

בְּדִיל (comp. of בְּ, דִּי, a. לְ=h. בִּשְׁבִיל) *as to what refers to*— whence; *on account of, for the sake of, in order that.* Targ. O. Gen. VI, 3; a. e.—Lev. R. s. 28, end אזל ב׳ בלנאר he went for (the sake of getting) a bather. Y. Kidd. III, 64[a] ב׳ דלא יכפור וכ׳ in order that he may not deny his owing a cup. Yoma 75[b] ב׳ רבא וכ׳ (v. Rabb. D. S. a. l.) through the merit of the teacher is the scholar supported.—בְּדִילִי, בְּדִילָךְ &c. on my, thy account &c. Targ. O. Deut. III, 26; a. e. (Y. בגלל; b. h. למען).

בְּדִילָה f. (בדל) *separation.* Tanḥ. Mishp. 17 לשון ב׳ an expression meaning 'creating a partition'.

בְּדִין *by right,* v. דִּין.

בִּידִין, בְּדִין m. pl. (h. בַּדִּים; v. בדד, בדי) *fictions,* whence *lying oracles;* trnsf. *conjurers.* Targ. Is. XLIV, 25. Targ. Lev. XX, 27; a. fr.

בְּדִיק, v. בְּדַק.

בְּדִיקָה f. (בָּדַק) *search, examination, test.* Pes. I, 1. Y. ib. I, beg. 27[a] בְּדִיקַת היום ב׳ search (after leavened bread) made in day-time is a (valid) search. Kil. IX, 7; a. fr.—Num. R. s. 9 לב׳ דידיה referring to his search; i. e. intimating that the test by the 'bitter waters' (v. סוטה) will also affect him (the adulterer) (Sot. 28[a] לידיעה).—*Pl.* בְּדִיקוֹת; esp. *cross-examinations of witnesses as to minor circumstances;* v. חֲקִירָה. Snh. V, 2 (40[a]); a. fr.

בְּדִיקוּתָא f. ch. same, esp. *examination of slaughtered animals* as to the condition of the lungs &c., v. בְּדַק. Ḥull. 48[a] לית להו ב׳ וכ׳ no examination will avail them to make them permitted; (ib. 46[a] לית להו בדיקה). Ib. 10[b] מצריך ב׳ וכ׳ declares an examination (of the slaughtering knife) necessary &c.; a. e.

***בְּדִיקְנָאָה** m. (v. בְּדַק Pa., end) *detective, police officer.* Taan. 22[a] ב׳ אנא Ms. M. (ed. זנדוקנא, v. זַנְדּוּקָא). [The description of that officer's doings proves the correctness of the version of Ms. M.]

***בְּדִיתָא** pr. n. *B'ditha,* name of a canal of the Euphrates, v. פּוּמְבְּדִיתָא. M. Kat. 11[a] ב׳ לבאר כוורי (read בב׳, Alf. בפומבדיתא) in the B'ditha the fish were laid dry. [Var. בריתא, ברייתא, v. Rabb. D. S. a. l. note 300.]

בָּדַל (√בד, v. בדד) *to separate, divide, distinguish;* (neut. v.) בָּדֵל *to keep aloof.* Pes. 87[b] בְּדוֹל עצמך וכ׳ withdraw thyself from (touching) her. Y. Ḥag. II, 78[b] top כדי שיהא בָּדֵל מן התרומה in order that he may be careful in handling T'rummah. B. Mets. 59[b] it seems to me שחברים בְּדֵלִים וכ׳ that the colleagues hold themselves aloof from thee (i. e. thou art excommunicated). Ib. 89[a] ב׳ בתמרים to separate (with a tool) dates which stick together (cmp. Rashi a. l.); Y. Maasr. II, 50[a] top הבדיל בתמרים (read הבודל). Ber. 5[a] יסורין בְּדֵלִין וכ׳ pains will stay away from him; a. fr.

Hif. (b. h.) הִבְדִּיל 1) *to sever, set apart, distinguish.* Ḥull. 21[b] מולק ואינו בַּבְדִּיל he nips the bird's neck but must not sever a limb or cut with his nail deeper than required (Lev. I, 17). Ib. I, 7 המבדיל בין וכ׳ He who established distinctions between (the) sanctity (of the Sabbath) and (the) sanctity (of the Festivals); a. fr.—2) (denom. of הַבְדָּלָה or אַבְדָּלָה) *to recite the benediction Hammabdil* on the exit of the Sabbath or Festival, *to say Habdalah.* Ibid. כיצד מבדילין what formula must you use (at the exit of the Sabbath and the simultaneous beginning of a Festival)? a. fr.—Part. Hof. מוּבְדָּל *separated, distinguished.* Num. R. s. 10 beg. מוּבְדָּלִים וכ׳ are different from the doings of other nations. Naz. 7[a] מוּבְדָּלוֹת זו מזו are separated one from another. Tosef. Peah III, 5; a. fr.

בְּדַל, בְּדֵיל ch. 1) as h. Kal (neut.) Ḥull. 116[b] בדילנן

וכ׳ we abstain from them. Ib. לא בדילר וכ׳ do not abstain; a. e.—2) (as foreg. Hif. 2) *to say Habdalah.* Erub. 40^b מי בדלת hast thou said Habd.? . . . אין בדילנא yes, I have &c.

בָּדָן, v. בָּאדָן.

בדסין, v. בִּרְסִין.

בָּדַק (b. h. $\sqrt{}$בד, v. בדר) *to split, break into, penetrate.* Keth. XIII, 9 הנוה היפה בּוֹדֵק the removal to a better residence (and style of living) penetrates (the body and creates disease); v. ib. 110^b מאי ב׳ כדשמואל וכ׳ what does *bodek* mean? Answ. As it is expressed by Samuel . . . ., a change of the mode of living (v. וֶסֶת) is the beginning of abdominal disease.—Esp. 1) *to search, examine, investigate, try.* Sot. V, 1 as well as the water בּוֹדְקִין אותה וכ׳ tries her (eventually makes her sick), so does it try him (the adulterer). Pes. I, 1 ב׳ את החמץ leavened bread is searched after (for the sake of removing it). Ib. 9^b (בית) בָּדוּק a house which has been searched. Snh. III, 6 ב׳ את העדים the witnesses are cross-examined. Ib. IV, 5; v. הֲרִישָׁה. Sabb. 139^a בְּדוֹק בדיינו וכ׳ investigate the doings of the Israelitish judges. Keth. VII, 8 הוא בּוֹדְקָהּ וכ׳ he has her examined (as to bodily soundness) by his female relatives. Ib. 75^b חזקה אין . . . אא״כ בּוֹדְקוֹ the presumption is that nobody will drink out of a cup, unless he has examined it (will not marry a woman before ascertaining her physical condition). Kidd. IV, 4 צריך לִבְדּוֹק אחריה וכ׳ must investigate her family records up to four mothers &c. Ib. 5 אין בודקין מן וכ׳ no family records are searched beyond the altar, i. e. the ascertained fact of a person's admission to priestly services is sufficient evidence of unblemished descent for marriage purposes. Nidd. 30^b ובדקן ומצאן (read ובדקו ומצאו) they (the scholars) examined (made a post mortem examination); Tosef. ib. IV, 17; Bekh. 45^a; a. fr.—2) *to tend, cure* (plants), esp. *to cover with earth or manure.* Tosef. Shebi. I, 12; Y. ib. IV, 35^b bot.

Nif. נִבְדַּק *to be examined* &c. Y. Gitt. I, 43^b; IX, end, 50^d נ׳ השם the report was traced. Nidd. V, 6 נדריה נִבְדָּקִין her vows are subject to examination (to find out whether she knows the import of a vow); a. fr.

בְּדַק, בְּדִיק ch. same; 1) *to split, burst, break into.* Ḥull. 105^a חזא צינורא דבדקא וכ׳ (Ar. דבירדקא) he saw that a sewer had burst into his field (inundating it); v. בִּרְקָא.—2) *to examine, espy; to test.* Targ. Judg. XVIII, 2; a. fr.—Yeb. 65^a אִיבְדוֹק נפשאי I will test myself (as to my virility). Y. Ned. II, 37^b bot. בעי חיפה מִיבְדְּקוּנֵיה Ḥefa wanted to sound his knowledge. Taan. 21^b; a. fr.—3) *to cure the body by means of a purgative.* Ned. 50^b הוה בָּדִיק נפשיה וכ׳ purged himself with &c.; a. e.—Part. pass. בְּדִיק *tested, sure, known.* Y. Sot. V, 20^c bot. לא הוות בדיקה לי was unknown to me (I had not experienced). Taan. 23^b לא בדיקתו לי (not בדקיתו) ye are unknown to me (as to your honesty).—בְּדִיקְנָא *I am sure, I know.* Pes. 111^b בדיקנא ביה במר דלא וכ׳ I am sure you do not know (Ms. M. ב׳ ליה וכ׳, Ms. 2 Oxf. בקינא, v. Rabb. D. S. a. l. note). *Ḥull. 32^a לא הוה בדיקנא ביה וכ׳ Ar. Var. (ed. בדיחנא) I was not so familiar with my uncle that I should have asked him.

Pa. בַּדֵּק *to discover* (by sorcery), *to find out secrets.* Targ. O. Gen. XLIV, 5; 15 . Cmp. בְּדִיקְנָאָה.

בֶּדֶק (b. h., preced.) 1) *breach, defect.*—2) *attendance, repair.* ב׳ הבית (II Kings XII, 8) keeping the Temple in repair. Y. Pes. VIII, 36^a top. Tem. I, 6 קדשי ב׳ הב׳ (Mish. קרבנות) offerings for the Temple repair, opp. to קדשי מזבח objects dedicated for sacrifices. Ibid. VII, 1; a. fr.—*Pl.* בְּדָקִים, constr. בִּדְקֵי. Sabb. 32^a ב׳ מיתה breaches through which death enters, i. e. sins for which one is visited with death; v. דֶּבֶק.

***בֶּדֶק** ch. same, *defect, sin.* Targ. Y. II Num. V, 19 these waters searching לב׳ האילין the defect. [Probably a corrupt reading.]

בִּידְקָא, בִּדְקָא m. ch.=h. בֶּדֶק 1) *breaking into, freshet, bursting dam.* B. Mets. 66^b אתא ב׳ וכ׳ a freshet came and overflooded &c. B. Bath. 41^a שקל בי׳ וכ׳ a freshet swept his field (taking away the fence). Ḥull. 105^a צינורא דב׳ Ar. a channel caused by a freshet, v. בְּדַק. Snh. 7^a strife is likened לצינורא דבי׳ (דמיא) וכ׳ to an inroad made by a burst (of water), once entering it widens more and more; a. fr.—*Pl.* בִּידְקֵי, בִּדְקֵי. Erub. 21^a דשכיחי בי׳ where freshets are of frequent occurrence.—2) *breach, defect.* Targ. O. Gen. XLII, 9 (h. ערוה). Targ. II Kings XII, 6 sq.—*Pl.* Targ. Lam. I, 8 בִּדְקָהָא her shortcomings (h. עֶרְוָתָהּ). [B. Bath. 61^a בדקא, v. בִּרְקָא III.]

***בָּדַר**, Pi. בִּיהֵר as following. Ruth R. to II, 15 חיה מְבַהֵר וכ׳ scattered coins. [Prob. to be read מבקר or מבקיר.]

בְּדַר ($\sqrt{}$בד; cmp. בזר, פזר) 1) *to scatter, strew.*—*Pa.* בַּדֵּר same, also, *to distribute freely.* Targ. Ps. LXVIII, 31; a. fr.—Ḥull. 54^a אי בַּדְּרֵי לה סמא וכ׳ if a powder is strewn upon its wound, it may recover; [Rashb. to B. Bath. 74^b quotes דעבד ליה סמתרי]. Gitt. 56^b ובַדְּרוּ לקיטמיה וכ׳ and scatter ye his (my) ashes over seven waters. Y. Ber. IX, end, 14^d בשעה דמכנשין בַּדֵּר וכ׳ when people gather (are willing to listen to instruction), distribute (teach); when people scatter (throw religion away in neglect), gather in (live in retired study). Cant. R. to VIII, 9 בדרו גרמיכון disperse ye (do not stand in crowds).—Part. pass. מְבַדַּר *scattered.* Y. M. Kat. III, 81^d top אית סגין מנהון מְבַדְּרַן וכ׳ there are more than those (twenty four cases) scattered in Mishnah and Boraitha. Sabb. 20^a, v. infra.—2) *to shake* (in a sieve). Targ. Amos IX, 9. [Ibid. מחזרין, prob. מבדרין.] Cmp. בַּזֵּיל.—3) *to tread olives.* Targ. Mic. VI, 15 (perh. בדר?).

Ithpa. אִיבַּדַּר, אִתְבַּדַּר; *Ithpe.* אִתְבְּדַר, אִיבְּדַר *to be scattered, to disperse.* Targ. Is. XXXIII, 3; a. fr.—Sabb. 20^a קנים מִיבַּדְּרִין (v. Rabb. D. S. a. l. note 300, ed. מבדרן) loose staves in the stove will fall apart (and may require stirring). Lev. R. s. 6 and the denars began מִתְבַּדְּרִין to be scattered. Gitt. 33^b ליבַּדְּרוּ אִיבַּדּוּרֵי (not איבדורי) let them disperse (so as not to be found together). Snh. 8^a bot. ואיבדור and they (the judges) dispersed.—Denom. בִּדּוּר, בִּדּוּרָא.

בדרסין, v. בִּרְדְּסִין.

בָּהָה, בָּהָא, v. בהי.

בְּהָדֵי, v. הַדֵּי.

בֹּהוּ, בּוֹהוּ f. (b. h.; בהי) *chaotic condition;* always with תהו. Gen. R. s. 2; a. fr.

בְּהוּ=אֶבְּהוּ. Ber. 45ª; a. fr. (Ms. M.).

בְּהוֹ ch.=בְּהוֹן *with, in them.* Pes. 72ᵇ; a. fr.; v. הוּ.

בַּהוּלְתָּא, v. בֵּיהוּלְתָּא.

בָּהוֹר, v. בָּהִיר.

בְּהוּתָא f. (בהי) *confusion.* Targ. Prov. XXVI, 21 ed. Wil. (Ms. בְּהַיְתָא; oth. ed. כהותא).

בָּהָה, בָּהָא, בהי (b. h.; √בה, cmp. בוא, *to be broken into; to gasp; to burst forth,* v. בהק, בהר; v. Ges. Hebr. Dict. s. v.) *to be stirred up, confounded, in disorder.* —Gen. R. s. 2, beg. תוהא ובוהא; ib. fem. תוהא ובוֹהָא bewildered and confounded.

**Hif.* הִבְהָה *to clear* (the field), cmp. בָּצָה. Y. Sabb. VII, 10ª top המברה בחרשים (read הַמַּבְהֶה). Y. Shebi. IV, 35ᵇ ומבדין (read וּמַבְהִין or וּמַבְהֶה) you may clear thickets (in the Sabbath year); v. בָּרַךְ Pi.

בְּהֵי ch. same. Part. בָּהֵי, fem. בַּהְיָא *chaotic.* Targ. Y. II, Ex. XII, 42. Targ. Y. Gen. I, 2.

***בהיר**, Targ. Prov. II, 7, read סברא (as in Pesh.) or סַבְהוֹר=ed. Wil. שבהור.

בְּהִילוּ f. (בהל) *haste.* Ezra IV, 23. Targ. Ex. XII, 11; a. e.

בְּהִיקָא, בָּהִיק (בהק) *bright, distinguished.* Targ. Cant. VII, 3; a. e.

בָּהִיר, בָּהוֹר m. (בהר; b. h בהיר) *white, white spot* (cloud).—*Pl.* בְּהִירִין, בְּהוֹ׳. Taan. 7ᵇ (ref. to Job XXXVII, 21) אפי׳ בשעה שהעננים עומדין בהי׳ וכ׳ Ms. M., even when the clouds stand in white spots, there comes a wind &c.; edit. שרקיע נעשה בהו׳ בהו׳ the sky is made (to appear) full of white clouds.

בְּהִירָא, pl. **בְּהִירֵי** same. Targ. Job XXXVII, 21 ב׳ מן וכ׳ white clouds without giving rain &c.

בְּהִית, v. בְּהַת.

בָּהַל (b. h.; √בה, v. בהי) *to hurry, be excited, anxious.* Part. pass. בָּהוּל *excited, pressed.* Pes. 11ª sq. אדם ב׳ הוא וכ׳ man is excited when his property is at stake. Ib. 72ᵇ זמנו ב׳ his time (for doing the thing) is pressed (it cannot be postponed). Yoma 85ª, a. e. ב׳ על מתו anxious to save his dead relative from the fire.

Pi. בִּיהֵל *to agitate, frighten.* Y. Yoma VI, 43ᶜ bot. למה אתה מְבַהֲלֵינוּ why dost thou agitate us.

Hithpa. a. *Nithpa.* הִתְבַּהֵל, נִתְבָּהֵל *to be excited, confounded.* Num. R. s. 14 (ref. to *tibbahel,* Koh. VIII, 3) אל תִּתְבָּהֵל וכ׳ be not intimidated by his wrath. Ib. לא נ׳ מן מעשיה he was not carried away by her (tempting) actions. Ib. לא נ׳ מפנאי וכ׳ he was not confounded on account of his being alone in the house. Pesik. R. s. 36 מתרעשים וּמִתְבַּהֲלִים were in commotion and alarm.—

Part. Hof. מוּבְהָל, or Pual מְבוֹהָל *confounded, hard to pronounce* or *remember.* Gitt. 14ᵇ שמותיהן מוב׳ וכ׳ Ar. (ed. מבו׳) their names are bewildering, beginning with Arda, Arta, Phile.—[Deut. R. s. 9 דעתו מובלגת, read מוּבְהֶלֶת his mind is confused, he cannot collect himself for prayer.]

בְּהִיל, בְּהַל ch. same.—*Pa.* בהיל 1) *to be precocious, inconsiderate, hasty.* Targ. Koh. V, 1; a. e.—2) as h. Piël. Targ. Job XXIII, 16; a. fr.

Ithpa. אִתְבַּהַל, *Ithpe.* אִתְבְּהִיל, אִיתְבְּהַל 1) *to be hurried, to hurry.* Targ. Esth. II, 9.—2) *to be agitated.* Targ. I Sam. XXVIII, 21; a. fr.—Y. Keth. I, 25ª is it possible that the whole town מִתְבַּהֲלָה וכ׳ was excited on account of Naomi?

בֶּהָלָה f. (b. h.; בהל) *suddenness, sudden calamity, shock.* Y. Bicc. II, 64ᵈ top; S'mah. III, 9 לשנים מיתה של ב׳ death after two days' sickness is a shocking death. —Y. B. Mets. II, end, 8ᵈ a rending of garments שאינו של ב׳ וכ׳ which is not done under the influence of the first shock (after the sad news) is considered as if not performed at all.—*Pl.* בֶּהָלוֹת. Num. R. s. 11; Tanh. Naso, 10 באנגריא ובב׳ as a forced duty and in a hurried manner; a. fr.

בַּהָם (בְּהֵמִי?) m. (denom. of next w.) *cattle-driver, cattle-raiser, driver.* Deut. R. s. 3 והבהם עמו and the driver (leader of the ass) was with him. *[Y. Ned. XI, end, 42ᵈ הבּיאם (=בַּהָם) שלי פיתני my stable-man (a gentile) has seduced me. Ib. אין הביאם אוסר (not אסור) (do you believe) the stable-man's connection with thee has no restrictive consequences? [V. Noda Bihudah, 2ⁿᵈ ed., Eb. Haëz. Nr. 12.] Gen. R. s. 86 בהמי (Yalk. Gen. 145 אדם, prob. בהם).—*Pl.* בַּהָמִים, בַּהָמִין. Y. Pes. I, 27ᵇ (in gen. *servants*). Cant. R. to IV, 4 (play on ובבהמתך Deut. VII, 14) there shall be none barren (of knowledge) among thee, אפי׳ בב׳ שבכם even among your cattle drivers; Deut. R. s. 3; a. e.; Gen. R. s. 32 בבהמות (corr. acc.)—Y. Maasr. II, 50ª bot. התריגו לבהמין (not התריגר) give the drivers (field laborers) oranges to eat; [Erub. 53ᵇ אתריגו לפחמין in diff. connection].

בְּהֵמָה f. (b. h.; בהם, Æthiop. *to be dumb;* √בה, v. בהי) *cattle, quadruped domestic animal* (mostly of the horned race); in gen. *dumb beast,* opp. to man. Gen. R. s. 20 ב׳ חיה ועופות domestic animals, wild beasts, and birds; a. fr.—ב׳ גסה *large cattle* (of the bovine race); ב׳ דקה *small cattle* (sheep, goats &c.). Bekh. 8ª; a. fr.— ב׳ ארנינא &c., v. אַרְנוֹנָא, בֶּהֱמַת מְלוֹג, מְלוֹג &c.—*Pl.* בְּהֵמוֹת Gen. R. s. 86; a. fr.

בְּהֵמוֹת m. (b. h.; Coptic p-ehe-mau, *water-ox,* Ges.) in Rabbin. lit. *B'hemoth, a legendary animal* reserved for the righteous in the hereafter; cmp. לִוְיָתָן. Lev. R.

s. 22 in place of the forbidden animals from which you here abstain, ב׳ בהררי אלף (I shall give you in the hereafter) 'the b'hemoth on the thousand mountains' (Ps. L, 10). Ib. s. 13 ב׳ ולויתן וכ׳ b'hemoth a. leviathan are the game of the righteous &c. Ib. ב׳ נותץ וכ׳ b'hemoth shall attack the leviathan with his horns &c.

בַּהַק (b.h.in בֹּהַק; √בה, v. בחי) *to shine with a pale light, be white, glisten.* Bekh. 45[b] בּוֹהַק one glistening (with unsteady eyes, *albino*), diff. fr. לבן white-complected. *Hif.* הִבְהִיק 1) *to shine, be bright.* Y. Pes. I, beg. 27[b] top בשעה שהיו מבהיקים when the candles burned brightly. Ib. מַבְהִיקוֹת; Gen. R. s. 31 מַבְהֶקֶת (of glistening jewels). Ib. s. 40 הבהיקה כל וכ׳ the whole land of Egypt was brightened by her (Sarah's) beauty; a. fr.—2) *to brighten, make bright.* Snh. 100[a].—Part. Hof. מוּבְהָק *distinguished, prominent.* Kidd. 33[a] ברבו המ׳ when his teacher is a distinguished scholar. Gitt. 11[a] שמות מוּבְהָקִין names of a distinctly gentile character (which Jews do not assume). [Sifra Thazr. ch. I שאת מובחקת, read with R. S. to Neg. I, 1 מוגבהת, v. גָּבַהּ.]

בְּהַק ch. same. *Af.* אַבְהִיק *to shine.* Targ. II Sam. XXII, 13.

בֹּהַק, v. בּוֹהַק.

בַּהֲקָא (pl. בַּהֲקֵי), בַּהֲקִי, בַּהֲקִיתָא f.=h. בַּהֶרֶת. Targ. Y. I, II Lev. XIII, 2; XIV, 56; a. e.

בַּהֲקָן m. (בהק) *one afflicted with bohak* (Lev. XIII, 39), *one having an eruption* resembling leprosy, v. בֹּהַק. Gen. R. s. 98 מי שהוא ב׳ וכ׳ one who is a bahakan is hot-tempered. *Pl.* בַּהֲקָנִין. Ib. (ed. פּוֹחֲ׳) ריבה בהן ב׳ (ref. to Gen. XLIX, 7) he let rise among them a large number of bohakanin (hot-tempered men). V. next w.

בוֹהֲקָנִי, בַּהֲקָנִי m. same, *one full of whitish pustules.* Ber. 58[b] Ms. M. (ed. בהקנים plur.). Fem. בַּהֲקָנִית, בּוֹהֲ׳, fem. בַּהֲקָנִיּוֹת, בּוֹ׳. Meg. 24[b] ידיו ב׳ one whose hands are &c.

בָּהַר (b. h.; √בה, v. בחי; cmp. preced. ws.); *Pi.* בִּיהֵר or *Hif.* הִבְהִיר *to shine brightly, be glossy;* trnsf. *to make one's self conspicuous, to boast.* Lev. R. s. 15; Tanh. Thazr. 11 *bahereth* (Lev. XIII, 2) that is Yavan (Græco-Syria) שהיתה מְבַהֶרֶת על וכ׳ (or מַבְהֶרֶת) that lorded it over Israel by her decrees; v. קֶרֶן.—[*Pi.* בִּיהֵר *to make clear.* Pesik. R. s. 33, v. בָּהַר.]

בְּהַר ch., Shaf. שַׁבְהַר q. v.

בְּהָרָא, בַּהֲרָא, v. בַּהַרְתָּא.

בהריקאי, v. חֲרִיקָא.

בַּהֶרֶת f. (b. h., בָּהַר) *bright white spot on the skin,* eventually one of the symptoms of leprosy. Neg. I, 1 ב׳ עזה כשלג *bahereth* means an intensively bright spot (sparkling) like snow. Ib. II, 1 ב׳ עזה וכ׳ an intensely bright spot appears faint on the skin of a Germanus (Teuton), and the faint spot appears bright on a Cushite; (Sifra Thazr., Neg. ch. I, ed. Weiss כב׳, כב׳; Yalk. Lev. 551 גרדמ׳, corr. בכושי, בגרמ׳); a. fr.—*Pl.* בֶּהָרוֹת. Neg. VII, 1. Ib. VIII, 6; Tosef. ib. III, 12.

בַּהֲרָא, בְּהָרָא, בַּהַרְתָּא ch. same. Targ. O. Lev. XIII, 2; a. e.—*Pl.* בַּהֲרָן. Ib. 38; 39. V. בַּהֲקָא.

בְּהֵית, בְּהַת (√בה, v. בחי) 1) (=h. בּוּשׁ, cmp. רוּץ a. רָהַט) 1) *to be confounded, abashed, ashamed.* Targ. O. Gen. XLIX, 8; a. fr.—Y. Shek. I, beg. 45[d] (in Hebr. phraseol.) חן נקרא ולא נבהית (Bab. ed. חנקרא . . . נבעית) can we read this and not feel ashamed? Y. Keth. XII, 35[a] top; Y. Kil. IX, 32[b] top, if I rise among the righteous, לא נבהת I may not feel ashamed. Ib. ומה אנא בהית בעבדאי (read בעובדיי) why should I be ashamed of my doings? Y. Kidd. IV, 65[c] top בָּהֲתִין וכ׳ they are ashamed of one another. Y. Orl. I, 61[b] top בהית מסתכל ביה is ashamed to look at him. Lev. R. s. 31 לא בהתין yet are not ashamed (to worship them).—2) (=בְּעֵית) *to be bewildered.* Keth. 62[a] (prov.) a woman used to abortion (or loss of children through death) לא בהתה is no longer besides herself (when it reoccurs; Ar.: is not ashamed).

Pa. בַּהֵית, *Af.* אַבְהֵית 1) *to put to shame.* Targ. Ps. XIV, 6. Ib. CXIX, 116; a. e.—Y. Shebi. IV, 35[b] bot.; Y. Maas. Sh. V, beg. 55[d] ומבהתין ליה דיעבד and bend the tree down as if in shame, in order that it may bear fruits (cmp. Sabb. 67[a] 'that people may pray for it'). Y. Kil.; Y. Keth. l. c. if I rise among the wicked לא נְבַהֵית (or נְבַהֵת) I may not put (them) to shame.—2) *to frighten, confound.*—Y. R. Hash. II, 58[a] bot. לא תבהית וכ׳ confound not thy Master's children (the Israelites).

Ithpa. אִתְבַּהֵית, *Ithpe.* אִתְבְּהֵית, contr. אִבְּהֵית *to be put to shame.* Cant. R. to II, 5 והוא מתב׳ וכ׳ and he felt ashamed and went away. Y. Sabb. VI, 8[c] top מִבַּהֲתָא she is ashamed.

בֵּיהוּתָא, בְּהִיתְתָא, בַּהֲתָא f. (h. בֹּשֶׁת; בחת, בחי) *shame, disgrace; nakedness* (=h. עֶרְוָה). Targ. Job VIII, 22; a. fr.—Snh. 102[b]; Gen. R. s. 49 סבי דב׳ elders of disgrace, v. אַשְׁמָה. Hull. 56[b] איגלאי בהתייהו their shame (diseased condition) has been revealed. Targ. II Chr. XXXII, 21 בֵּיהוּת.

בּוֹ, v. בְּ-.

בּוֹא (b. h.; √בא, בה, v. בחי, *to enter into, split, insert;* v. בבא, בון; *to be vacant, clear,* v. באר, בור; *to be disordered,* v. בוש, באש) 1) *to enter, come.* R. Hash. I, 2 בָּאֵי העולם those come into the world, i. e mortals. Hull. 54[b] בּוֹאֲכֶם בשלום be welcome!—Tanh. Vaëra 14; Midr. Till. to Ps. LXXVIII, 47, a. e. (play on בחנמל ibid.) בא חן מל [בא נח מל] it (the locust) comes, encamps [rests], and plucks. Y. Shebu. VIII, 38[c] top, a. e. במקום שבאת, v. גְּזֵרָה.—Y. Peah I, 15[c] top, a. fr. יָבֹא עלי אם וכ׳ may (evil) befall me, if—; cmp. אֲתָא; Koh. R. to X, 8 אם לא יבא וכ׳ (corr. acc.).—2) with על (b. h. with אל) *to have sexual connection.* Kerith. I, 1; a. fr.—3) with לְיַד or לִידֵי *to fall into the power of.*—Aboth II, 1 ואין אתה בא לידי עבירה and sin will have no power over thee. Yoma 86[b] בא לידו דבר וכ׳ (not באת) he had the power (the chance) to commit a sin &c.; Kidd. 39[b]; a. fr.—בּוֹא וראה come and see (I will prove). Yoma l. c.; a. fr.

Hif. הֵבִיא 1) *to bring, carry.* Gitt. I, 1 הַמֵּבִיא וכ׳ he who brings (as a messenger) a letter of divorce from abroad; a. fr.—2) *to offer.* Bicc. I, 1; a. fr.—3) *to draw an object toward's one's self,* opp. הוֹלִיךְ, v. הָלַךְ. Hull. II, 3 הוליך ולא ה׳ he put the knife out (in slaughtering) but did not draw it backward; ה׳ ולא וכ׳ or drew it toward himself but did not then move forward; a. fr. —4) *to bring about, produce, cause.* Aboth I, 17 מביא חטא begets sin; a. fr.—5) *to lead, procure admittance.* Ab. Zar. 20[b] Torah מביאה לידי וכ׳ (v. supra) leads to careful conduct &c. Ib. 18[a] אתה מְבִיאֵנִי וכ׳ wilt thou procure me (promise me) admittance into the world to come?; a. fr.

בואנא, v. בְּוָאנָא.

בואת, v. בָּאוּת.

בּוּבְיָא I m. (Syr. *bubia* sartago, P. Sm.; prob.=בי אפיא, פ softened through assimilation, cmp. בי תפייא a. תפי) *a frying pan,* sometimes used as a *coal pan* containing the coal over which things are roasted. Pes. 30[b] האי בוב׳ (Ms. M. 2, Ms. Oxf. Ar. and old ed., v. Rabb. D. S. a. l. note 10); Zeb. 95[b] (Ms. R. 1 מביא, corr. בו׳; Ms. K. בוכיא). Sabb. 29[a] he threw the date stones לבוביא Ms. M. a. Ar. (Y. Bets. IV, 62[c] להפירה, v. Rashi to Sabb. l. c.) into the pan. [Editions vary betw. כוביא a. בוכיא.]

בּוּבְיָא II, **בּוּבְיָה** f. *image,* v. בָּבוּאָה.

בוביא, בוב״ה, Lam. R. to II, 2, v. בִּיבָא.

בוביאר, v. בּוּכְיָאר.

בּוּבְיָה, v. בּוּבְיָא.

בּוּבִיתָא, v. בָּבִיתָא.

בובן *the word* נָבוּב *reversed.* Sabb. 104[a].

***בּוּגְנֵי**, Targ. II Esth. IV, 1 ב׳ נוגמי ארנון, Var. פוגני פוגני נעימי א׳, read (אֶ)פִּיטַגְמָטִין or דִּיטַגְמָטִין (ἐπιτάγματα, διατάγματα) *commands, ordinances;* v. דִּיטַגְמָא.

בּוֹגֵר, v. בָּגַר.—בּוֹגֶרֶת, pl. בּוֹגְרוֹת, v. בָּגַר.

***בּוּדְיָא** c. (denom. of בַּד V) *a mat of reeds.* [The best versions, however, read בּוּרְיָא q. v.]

בּוּדִידָה, v. בְּדִידָה.

בּוּדְחָא, v. בְּדוּחָא.

בּוֹהוּ, v. בֹּהוּ.

בּוֹהֲיוֹן pr. n. m. *Bohăyon.* Pes. 57[a] (Ms. M. בוהין); Tosef. ib. II (III), 20 (Var. בן נבו הירן, נבו חיו).

בֹּהַק, בּוֹהַק m. (b. h.; בהק) *white scurf.* Neg. I, 5. Sifra Thazr., Neg., ch. X.

בּוֹהֲקָא ch. same. Targ. O. Lev. XIII, 38 (ed. Berl. בּוּהֲקָא).

בּוֹהַקְנִי, בּוֹהַקְנִית, v. בֹּהַק.

בּוּוְתָא, v. בַּתְוָא.

בּוּז (b. h., √בז, v. בזז) 1) *to tread upon,* whence *despise.* Aboth IV, 3 אל תהי בָז despise not &c.—2) *to divide;* v. בְּזַבֵּז.

בּוּז ch. same; 1) *to plunder, ransack.* Targ. Gen. XXXIV, 27; a. fr.—Esth. R. to I, 10 (play on בזתא ibid. בוז ביתיה plunder his house.—2) *to tread.* Ib. (play on בגתא ואבגתא ibid. as if from בג, cmp. בגר) בוז ובוזו tread and shatter (v. Targ. Esth. a. l.; cmp. בְּזוֹזָא). [Most of the forms may be derived fr. בזז.]

בּוּזָאָה m. *the Buzite.* Targ. Job XXXII, 2; 6.

***בּוֹזְזָא** m. (בזז, בוז) *plunderer. Pl.* בּוֹזְזַיָּא. Yalk. Jer. 281 (Lam. R. introd. R. Yits. 1 בָּזוֹזַיָּא).

בּוֹזְתָא (בִּיזְתָא) f. (v. בוז) *contempt, contumely.* Targ. Ps. CXIX, 22.—V. בִּיזָא II.

בּוֹחַל m. (בחל I) prop. *aversion, sickness,* hence (cmp. באש) *a certain stage in the growth of the fig* (intermediate between פגה and צמל), *when its head becomes white;* trnsf. *the stage of female puberty* intermediate between childhood (ילדות) and full womanhood (בגרות). Nidd. V, 7 the Scholars have introduced figurative terms for the stages of womanhood: paggah, boḥal &c.; ב׳ אלו ימי נעוריה boḥal means the days of maidenhood. V. בָּחַל.

בּוּטָא pr. n. m. *Buta,* father of Baba, v. בָּבָא II.

***בּוֹטֵט** m. (בְּטַט) *bright spot* (cloud, v. בָּהִיר). Targ. Job XXXVII, 21 (Ms. בּוֹטֵשׁ).

בּוֹטִיטָא, בּוֹטְטָא m. (v. preced.), ב׳ דנורא *spark* (blossom of light, cmp. h. נִיצוֹץ).—*Pl.* בּוֹטִיטֵי, בּוֹטְטֵי. B. Mets. 85[b] בוטטי דנ׳ מחיוה וכ׳ . . . . Ms. M. (ed. . . . בוטי׳ ומחייה, corr. acc.) two sparks came forth and struck the eyes of &c. Ber. 58[a] מילתא אמר ר׳ ששת ונפקו ב׳ דנ׳ וכבינהו (Ms. M. חב ביה מילתא ונפק בוטיתא לעיניה Ar. ed. Koh. דנ׳, omitted in ed., v. Rabb. D. S. a. l. note) R. Sh. spoke a word, and there came forth sparks and blinded him.

בּוֹטֵי m. pl. (בטט) *the poor (broken ones).* Gitt. 37[a]; v. בּוּלְבּוּטִים.

בּוֹטִיטָא, v. בּוֹטְטָא.

בּוֹטִיטָה, v. בְּטִיטָא.

בּוֹטִיתָא, בִּיטִיתָא f. (בטט; cmp. בּוֹטְטָא) *flower-bud of the caper tree, capers.* Ber. 36[b] ושקליה לנִיצא דפרחא והדיא בו׳ Ar. (ed. לפרחא דבי׳ ואיקיים . . . Ms. M. לניצא . . . דפרחא והויא בי׳) the blossom of the caper was cut off, but the bud survived. [Ib. 58[a] בו׳ דנורא Ms. M. read בּוֹטִיתָא, v. בּוֹטְטָא.]—*Pl.* בִּיטְיָתָא, בּוֹטְיָיתָא. Hull. 59[a] שב ב׳ וכ׳ seven blossoming capers (Rashi: stones of the caper fruit). Y. Maasr. IV, end, 51[c] מרמיין . . . בר׳ to remove the buds. [Y. Pes. I, beg. 27[a] באילין בוטיתא, v. בְּטִיטָא.]

בּוּטְלָנָא, בּוּטְלָן m. (בטל) 1) *idleness.* Targ. O. Ex. XXI, 18 (being incapacitated).—2) *indemnity for loss of time.* Ib. v. 19. V. בְּטֵילָא.

בּוּטְמָא m. (בטם, √בט, v. next w.) 1) *terebinth (fruit and tree), pistacia terebinthus* (v. Sm. Ant. s. v. Tereb.). Targ. O. Gen. XXXV, 4; a. e.—*Pl.* (Hebr., fr. בּוּטְמָה) בּוּטְמִין. Y. Kil. I, 27[a] bot. חלוזין והב׳ וכ׳ nuts and terebinths combined produce pistachio.—Chald. בּוּטְמֵי. R. Hash. 23[a] אלונים ב׳ ed. (Ar. אלמונים ב׳; Gen. R. s. 15 אלונים בְּלוּטֵי, B. Bath. 80[b] בּוּטְנֵי, Ms. M. בוטמי), v. אַלּוֹן, אַלְמוֹן I.—2) *pistachio (tree or nut).* Shebi. VII, 5 Ar. s. v. אלה (ed. בָּטְנָה); v. next w.—*Pl.* בּוּטְמִין. Targ. O. Gen. XLIII, 11 ed. Berl. (oth. ed. a. Y. בוטנין).

בּוּטְנָא I m. (b. h. בָּטְנָה; בטן, √בט to be hollow, *swell,* v. Ges. H. Dict. s. v. בטן) *pistachio (nut or tree).* Shebi. VII, 5 Ms. M. a. Y. ed. (Bab. ed. בטנה), v. preced.; Tosef. ib. V, 11 בּוּטְנָה;—*Pl.* בּוּטְנִין, בּוּטְנֵי. Targ. Y. (a. O. some ed.) Gen. XLIII, 11; v. preced. B. Bath. 80[b]; v. preced.

בּוּטְנָא II m. (בטן) *swollen belly, swelling.* Lev. R. s. 18, end; Num. R. s. 7.

בּוּטְנָה, v. בּוּטְנָא I.

בּוּטְנָה pr. n. *Batanæa,* town and district east of the Jordan, reputed for large commercial fairs (יְרִיד). Y. Ab. Zar. I, 39[d]; Gen. R. s. 47 בָּטְנָן. Cmp. בָּשָׁן (b. h.) a. בּוּתְנָן.

בומרגונין Pesik. R. s. 10, read טֶטְרָגוֹנִין; v. אִסְטְרוֹנְגִּילוֹן.

בּוּטְשָׁא, v. בִּיטְשָׁא.

בּוּיְשָׁן, v. בַּיְשָׁן.

בּוּךְ ch. (b. h.; √בו or בח, v. בחר, בהל) *to run to and fro, be agitated.* Part. בָּיֵיךְ, f. בָּיְכָא. Gen. R. s. 87, beg. (expl. חומיה וכ׳ Prov. VII, 11) ביכא חרא וטעיא Ar. (ed. שגשיא; Yalk. Prov. 940 בוכה, corr. acc.) she runs about (revelling) &c. Y. Taan. II, 65[b] (ref. to Mic. VII, 4) (read:) כן גר רא אנן בָּיְיכִין ובבון וכ׳ therefore we are now in trouble. And they wept &c. Ruth. R. s. 3 (before I, 18) קל ברייתא בייבין (read בייכין) the sound of people running in excitement (on business).

בּוּכָאנָא, v. בּוּכְנָא.

בּוּכְיָא* m. (ביך; v. P. Sm. I 526 sq.) 1) *the weaver's shuttle;* 2) *the spider.* Succ. 52[a]; Snh. 99[b] חוט של ב׳ the thread of the shuttle [or spider-web]. [Snh. l. c. כוביא, Mss. vary betw. כוביא a. כוכיא q. v.]—[3) *coal-pan,* v. בּוּבְיָא.]—Cmp. בִּיכֵי.

בּוּכְיאר m. (v. preced.; ר formative, cmp. חליטר) *the weaver's clue.* Sabb. 96[b] ed. a. Ar. (Ms. M. בוב׳, Ms. Oxf. בּוּכְיָיאר, Ar. Var. בּוּכְיָאן).

בוכלין, Y. Shek. VII, beg. 50[c], v. בּוּכְלָיִים.

בּוּכָאנָא, בּוּכְנָא m. (Syr. ܒܘܩܠܐ; בוקלא; בכן, בקל √בך, בק *to split;* cmp. Ges. H. Dict. s. v. בכא) 1) *a club, a stripped smooth pole, bar.* Erub. 102[a] ב׳ קאמרת (Ar. ed. Koh. בכנא) you speak of a club (with a handle used as a door-bar).—*Pl.* בּוּכָאנֵי. B. Kam. 93[b] it says (in the Mish.), 'If one robbed pieces of wood and made utensils out of them' בב׳ דחריינו וכ׳ Ar. (ed. ב׳ with one ב, Ms. H. בביכאני) it means that he made them into clubs, that is 'he polished them'.—2) esp. *a club* (with handles) *used as a pestle* for crushing olives &c. Sabb. 77[b] (playful etymology) בוכנא בּוֹא ואַכְּנה (Ar. ed. Koh. בוכאנא) it is called *bukhana,* 'come and I shall strike'. Y. Bets. I, 60[c] bot. ובוכנה דו כתת ביה and concerning a club, for he pounds with it; Y. Sabb. XVII, 16[b] top במכונה (read בבוכנה). Nidd. 36[b] I am ב׳ דפרזלא וכ׳ an iron pestle which breaks the copper mortar. Bets. 14[a] בו׳ (Ar. ed. Koh. בכ׳).—Trnsf. *the rib resting in the pelvis, hip-joint.* Hull. 52[a], v. אֲסִיתָא.

בּוּכְנָה f. h. (preced.) *the peduncle* (or *upper stem*) deeply seated in the Ethrog (like the rib in the pelvis). Succ. 35[b] בּוּכְנָתוֹ, expl. פִּיטָם.

בּוּכְרָא I m. (בכר) 1)=h. בְּכוֹר, *first-born.* Targ. Ex. XII, 29; a. fr.—Hull. 44[b]; a. fr.—B. Bath. 126[b] ב׳ סכלא (h. בכור שוטה) foolish (wild) first-born, i. e. a first-born by his mother but not by his father (having no privileges).—*Pl.* בּוּכְרִין, בּוּכְרַיָּא. Targ. Ps. CXXXV, 8; a. e.—Fem. בּוּכְרְתָא. Ber. 6[a] ב׳ בת ב׳ a first-born cat whose mother is a first-born.—[2)=h. בִּכּוּרָה. *Pl.* בּוּכְרֵי *first fruits.* Targ. Y. I Deut. XXXIII, 14. (Targ. Y. II בִּכְרָא).]

בּוּכְרָא II f. (v. preced.) *the first,* i. e. *lowest layer* in the clay dam; v. אַרְבַּבְתָּא. B. Mets. 103[b].

בּוּכְרִיָּא, בּוּכְרִיָּה (בַּכַּרְיָא Ar.)* (m. pl.?) f. (baccar, baccaris; βάκχαρις=ἄσαρον; v. Sm. Ant. s. v. Asaron, Löw Pfl. p. 370) *baccar,* an aromatic plant supposed to be *hazelwort* or *spike-nard.* Shebi. VII, 2 (Ms. M. כובריא). Tosef. Kil. III, 12 בורכייר ed. Zuck. (oth. ed. ברכוייד, ברכוייר).

בּוּל I *to mix,* v. בִּיל. [Y. Snh. X, 27[d] קום ב׳ read בּוּל.]

בּוּל II (v. preced. a. בָּלַל) 1) *something kneaded together, a handful, ball, lump.* Sabb. 67[b]; 128[b] ב׳ של מלח a lump of salt. B. Mets. 90[a] ב׳ מאותו המין a handful (fodder) of the same species; v. infra.—*Pl.* בּוּלִים, בּוּלוֹת, בּוּלִין *clods,* v. next w.—Gen. R. s. 13 ב׳ של אדמה clods of moist ground. Num. R. s. 2 sand is thrown into the fire ומוציאו בולים and he brings it out as lumps (of glass); v. בּוּלָס.—2) *fodder.* Lev. R. s. 22 (expl. בול הרים Job XL, 20); Tanh. Pinh. 12.

בּוּל III (prob. fr. נבל) *Bul,* the biblical name for the eighth month (Marheshvan); v. מַרְחֶשְׁוָן. R. Hash. I, 56[d] bot. (etym. of בול) שהעלה נובלת וכ׳ the leaves decay and the ground is cloddy; v. preced.—Tanh. Noah 11, the month is named *bul,* ירח שבוללין לבהמות וכ׳ the month when cattle is given mixed fodder from what is in the house; Pesik. R. s. 7.

בּוּלָאוֹת, v. בּוּלֵי.

בּוּלְבּוּטֵיס, בּוּלְבּוּטֵס m. (corrupt. of βουλευτής) *senator*. Y. Taan. IV, 69[a] ארכינטס ובו׳ (corr. acc.) archont or senator; v. בּוּלֶבְטֵס.—*Pl.* בּוּלְבּוּטֵי. Gitt. 36[b] sq. (explain. פרוסבול) פרוס בולי ובוטי (prob. a Babyl. corruption of πρὸς βουλῇ βουλευτῶν בולי בולבוטי) before the council of senators. Ib. 37[a] (as if two words) בולי ובו׳ וכ׳ bulé are the rich, bute (as if fr. בטט, play on עבט) the poor (broken ones).

בּוּלְבּוּס m. (βολβός, bulbus) in gen. *bulbous root*, esp. *bulbus*, a delicious kind of *onion*, or *musk-hyacinth*. —*Pl.* בּוּלְבְּסִין (בולפ׳). Y. Dem. II, 22[c] bot. (ed. כולכסין, corr. acc.). Ukts. III, 2 בולבסין Var. in Ar. s. v. בלפסין (ed. בלוסין, כלוסין; Maim: ענב אלדיב=*Solanum nigrum*, v. Löw Pfl. p. 296 a. 393). [Gen. R. s. 41 בולבוס some ed., read: בילמוס.]

בּוּלֶבְטֵס, בּוּלֶוְטֵס, corr. **בּוּלֶיוְטֵיס** (incorr. טוס . . .) m. (βουλευτής, v. בולבוטס) *senator, councilman*. Gen. R. s. 76 this one is rich נעבדיניה בל׳ (Yalk. Dan. 1064 בולטוס, corr. acc.) let us make him a senator (to ruin him, v. ארכונטוס). Koh. R. beg. בלווטוס (corr. acc.); Cant. R. beg. בוליוטוס.—Sifré Deut. 309 בלריוסטוס, בלאיוסטוס; Yalk. ib. 942 בלריוסטוס, corr. acc.—*Pl.* בּוּלֶווֹטִין, בּוּלֶבְטֵי, טַיָּיא . . ., טַיָּיה . . . Y. Hag. II, 77[d] bot. Lam. R. to II, 2. Ibid. לאיבדא (לע׳) בולריוטין, read לְאַיעבדא בולריוטיס; v. אַרְכוֹנְטוֹס. Y. Peah I, 16[a] בולווטיה דציפורין the council of Sepphoris. Lev. R. s. 11 אלו הבולריותוס (read טין....). Y. Sabb. XII, 13[c] bot.; Y. Hor. III, end, 48[c] בולווטריא family heads entitled to seats in the Bulé of Sepphoris.

בּוּלְבְּסִין, v. בּוּלְבּוּס.

בּוּלְדָר, בּוּלְדָאר, v. בַּלְדָר.

בּוּלֶוְטֵס, v. בּוּלֶבְטֵס.

בּוּלוֹס, v. בּוּלָס.

בּוּלְבִיתָא f. (בלט, v. בלל; P. Sm. 533) *crumbling, corrosion, being worm-eaten*. Targ. Job XLI, 19 קיסא ב׳ (read דב׳) worm-eaten wood. Targ. Prov. XXV, 20; XII, 4 Ms. (ed. מַלְבִיתָא, Pesh. בל׳).

*__בּוּלֵי__ I pr. n. pl. *Buli* (prob. the assembly building of the Senate in Sepphoris, cmp. בּוּלֶבְטֵס end). Y. Shek. VII, 50[c] bot. (Bab. ed. כילי, oth. כולית׳, קוליתא, ed. Just. ב׳; v. Rabb. D. S. a. l. p. 62, note 30); Y. Taan. I, 64[a] bot. כנישתא דב׳ assembly (or synagogue) of B.—Y. Ab. Zar. III, 43[b] bot. צלמא דב׳ (ed. Krot. דכ׳) a statue (idol) in front of the Bulé(?).

בּוּלֵי II f. (βουλή) *council, assembly*, esp. *senate, city council*. Y. Peah I, 15[c] top בפני כל ב׳ שלו in the presence of the whole council over which he presided; Y. Kidd. I, 61[b] top. Ib. פטר ב׳, v. פַּטְרוֹבּוּלוֹס. Y. Yoma I, 39[a] top כולי (corr. acc.). Y. M. Kat. II, 81[b] אם הזכירוך לב׳ וכ׳ if they have mentioned (nominated) thee for the *bulé*, let the Jordan be thy neighbor, i. e. hide thyself in the bushes near the Jordan. Ib. להפטר מב׳ to be exempt from serving in the *bulé*; Y. Snh. VIII, 26[b] top. Gen. R. s. 6 ב׳ ודימוס senate and people (senatus populusque). Ex. R. s. 15 וכן דימוס וכן כולם (read בולי) and so did the people and so the senate. Gitt. 37[a], v. בּוּלְבּוּטֵס.—*Pl.* בּוּלָאוֹת, בּוּלְיוֹת. Y. Ned. III, 38[a] top; Y. Shebu. III, 34[d] bot. כ״ד ב׳ twenty four city councils, i. e. cities or districts having their own councilmen; [Tanh. Vayikra 7; Matt. 1 ב׳ אלפים עיירות]; Pesik. R. s. 22 אלות (read בולאות). Gitt. 37[a].

בּוּלֶיוְטֵיס, בוליוטוס, v. בּוּלֶבְטֵיס.

בוליטין, v. בּוּרְגִּין.

בוליס, בולים, v. בּוּלָס.

בּוּלְמוֹס m. (βούλιμος, bulimus) *ravenous hunger, bulimy*, esp. *faintness from fasting*. Yoma VIII, 6 (83[a]). Koh. R. to VII, 11 (some ed. incorr. ות . . .); a. fr.—Trnsf. ב׳ של עריות *morbid carnal appetite, sexual passion*. Gen. R. s. 51; s. 41; a. e.

בּוּלָס (בּוּלוֹס) m. (בלס; cmp. ὕαλος, ὕελος) *a shapeless mass, a glass-ball*. Num. R. s. 2 ומוציאו בולים (v. בּוּל II, some ed. בוליס). Y. Ber. I, 2[d] top נוסך כלים (corr. acc.); Gen. R. s. 12 מוצק כלים (read: נוסך ב׳, v. Ar.) casts a lense; v. אֲנַנְקֵי.—Pesik. Par. p. 39[b] גלוריים לכם צפים כהדין ב׳; Pesik. R. s. 14; Yalk. Num. 759 כהדין ב׳ perspicuous (clear) as crystal; cmp. Num. R. s. 19 כהדין סמיא a. Mat. Keh. a. l.

בּוּלָסָא ch. same, esp. *glass-lump*, unshaped and prepared for casting into vessels. Sabb. 154[b] בבלוסא Ar. (ed. בכולסא, read as Rashi a. Ms. בבולסא, v. Rabb. D. S. a. l. note 1) what is meant here are glass lumps (which may be broken without loss).—*Pl.* בּוּלְסִין, בּוּלְסַיָּיא *crystals* or *glass vessels*. Y. Kidd. I, 60[c] top אילין ב׳ those glass vessels (what is the law concerning their division among heirs)? Ib. חכים . . . . בילסיין סגין (corr. acc.) thou art known to have plenty of glass vessels.

בּוּלְסִיף, v. בּוּרְסִיף.

בולפסין, Tosef. Kil. III, 12, v. בּוּלְבּוּס.

בולקס, Y. Taan. II, 66[a], v. בַּלְקִיס.

בּוּלְרָא m. (follis, follera; v. next w. a. Sm. Ant. s. v. Senatus) *follera*, name of a Roman land-tax, adopted by the Persians. B. Kam. 113[b] בב׳ וכרגא וכ׳ Ar. (ed. דברלא ארעא וכרגא, read בב׳ ארנונא וכ׳, Ms. M. בכולארא וכ׳, Ms. R. בכלודא וארנונא ואכרגא, corr. acc.) with reference to follera, annona and charga of the ensuing year.

בּוּלְרִין m. (φολλερόν, S.) *obol*, a small coin. Cant. R. to I, 1 if one drops סלע או ב׳ (Ar. ed. Koh. בלורין, ed. כילרין) a Sela or (even) a folleron. V. פּוּלָר.

בולרין Gen. R. s. 8, v. בלורין.

בולשפטי, v. בֶּלְשָׁפָּט.

בּוּלֶשֶׁת, v. בַּלֶּשֶׁת.

בּוּן I pr. n. m. *Bun*, abbrev. of אָבוּן; name of several Amoraim. Y. Shek. IV, end, 48[c] ר׳ אבון ור׳ ב׳. Y. Ber. III, 6[c] בין some ed. (corr. acc.); a. fr.—Y. R. Hash. I, 56[c] top, a. fr. R. B. bar Ḥiya.—Y. Ter. VIII, 45[c], a. fr. R. B. bar Kahana; v. Fr. M'bo p. 67[b] sq.

בּוּן II *to understand*, v. בִּין.

***בּוּנָא** pl. בּוּנֵי *a handful*, v. בּוּנָא.—Sabb. 67[a] ב׳ כבוניא, v. also בִּינְתָא I.

בּוּנָה pr. n. m. *Bunah*, abbr. of אַבּוּנָה. Y. Gitt. II, 44[b] ב׳ בר שילא (ed. Krot. בינה שילוח, v. marginal note a. l.).

בּוּנִּי or **בּוּנַי** pr. n. m. *Buni* or *Bunai*; 1) name of one of the alleged disciples of Jesus of Nazareth. Snh. 43[a] Ms. M. a. ed. Ven. (omitted in later ed., v. Graetz Gesch. d. Jud. III (2[d] ed.) p. 243; Rœsch Jesusmythen p. 99).—2) name of a pious and liberal man, otherwise named Nakdimon. Taan. 20[a].

***בּוּנְיָא** *Bunia*, a bird. Ḥull. 62[b] ed. (Ar. בְּנָיָא).

בּוּס, v. בָּסַס.

בּוּסְיָא, v. בַּסְיָא.

בּוֹסֶם m. (b. h. בֹּשֶׂם; בסם) *flavor, perfume, spices.* Snh. 108[a] מקום חב׳ (Var. מבושם) place for spices, opp. מקום המנופת.—[Tosef. Kidd. II, 4 נעשה בוסם, ed. Zuck., read בַּסָּם.]

בּוּסַם, בּוּסְמָא, בְּסָמָא, בּוּשָׂם, בּוּשְׂמָא, בְּשָׂ׳ ch. same. Targ. Ex. XXX, 25; a. fr.—*Pl.* בּוּסְמִין, בּוּסְמַיָּא, בְּשָׂ׳, בְּסָ׳, בּוּבָ׳. Ib. 27; 34; a. fr.

בּוּסְמָן m. (preced.) *aromatic fluid* for sprinkling.—*Pl.* בּוּסְמָנִין, constr. בּוּסְמָנֵי. Num. R. s. 13 ב׳ ג״ע (some ed. בּוּ׳) the aromas of paradise (carried by winds).

בּוּסְמָנָא ch. same. *Pl.* בּוּסְמָנָן. Targ. II, Esth. I, 2. V. בּוּסְמָנַיָּא.

בּוּסְמָנוּ, בְּסָ׳ f. (preced.) *art of making perfumes*, Targ. O. Ex. XXX, 25; a. e.

בּוּשׂ׳, בּוּסְמָנִין, בּוּסְמָנַיָּא m. pl. (preced. ws.) *aromas, ointments* &c. Targ. I Kings X, 10. Targ. Ruth. III, 3; a. e.

בּוֹסֶר m. (b. h. בֹּסֶר, בֶּסֶר; בסר II) *half-ripe fruit*, esp. *grapes*. Shebi IV, 8 הב׳ משהביא וכ׳ the *boser* from the time it contains liquid. Gitt. III, 8 (31[a]) בשעת כניסה המים בב׳ when the liquid is beginning to gather in the *boser*; (oth. opin. when it can be put in water for making vinegar; v. Rashi a. l.). Pes. 53[a] הוא ב׳ וכ׳ boser indicates the same stage of ripening as gerua, v. גָּרַע Hif. Y. Maasr. I, 49[a] top; Succ. 36[a] אתרוג הב׳ a half-ripe Ethrog. Y. B. Kam. VI, 5[b] bot.; a. fr.

בּוּסְרָא ch. same. Targ. Ps. LVIII, 10 (h. text נָזִיר); a. e.

בּוּסְרָן m. (בסר I) *contempt*; v. בְּסָרְנוּתָא. Targ. Ezek. VII, 19.

בּוּסְתָּנָא m. (Pers. bûstân) *garden, orchard.* Sabb. 30[b]. Erub. 25[b].—*Pl.* בּוּסְתְּנֵי. B. Bath. 61[b].—Targ. II Esth. III, 8 בּוּסְתָּנָנָא our *orchards* (collect.).

בּוּסְתְּקָא, v. בַּסְתְּקָא.

בּוּעַ, בְּעִי (√בע, cmp. נבע, בְּץ, בט) *to swell, burst forth*, whence (of sound) *to shout, rejoice.* Targ. Is. XIV, 7 (h. text פצח). Ib. LXV, 19; a. fr.—Part. f. בָּיְעָא. Ib. 18 (Var. בָּיְעָא).

בּוּעָא f. (v. preced.) *swelling, abscess*, mostly applied to *tubercles* of the lungs. *Pl.* בּוּעֵי Ḥull. 46[b] sq.; a. fr. V. בּוּעָתָא I.

בּוּעְדָא, v. next w.

***בּוּעֲרָא** m. (בער) *torch, fire-signal.* Targ. Is. XXX, 17 (Var. בּוּעְדָא, v. also בּוּעָתָא III). Targ. Job XII, 5 (Var. בער׳). V. בְּעוּר.

***בּוּעְתָא I, (בּוּתָא)** f. (v. בּוּעָא) *abscess.* Snh. 84[b] למיפתח בוע׳ Ar. (Var. Ar. בותא, ed. כוותא) to cut open an abscess. [Targ. Prov. XXIII, 29 (Var. פודעתא).—*Pl.* בּוּעָתָתָא. Ib. XX, 30 (Var. פודעתא).]

בּוּעֲתָא II f. (בוע) *bursting forth, rejoicing.* Targ. Job XX, 5. Targ. Ps. XLIII, 4 בָּעוּתִי (prob. בּוּעָ׳).

***בּוּעֲתָא III** f. (ביע) *alarm-post, signal-pole.* Targ. Is. XXX, 17 Ar. ed. pr. (h. text תֹּרֶן, taken fr. רנן; oth. ed. Ar. בורעדא, Targ. ed. בּוּעֲרָא q. v.).

בּוּץ I (cmp. בּוּעַ) *to swell, bubble, burst forth, shine.* Pilp. בַּצְבֵּץ.

בּוּץ II m. (b. h.; v. preced.) *linen, byssus.* Yoma VII, 1 (68[b] sq.), v. בַּד IV; a. e.

בּוּץ, בּוּצָא ch. 1) same. Targ. Esth. VIII, 15. Targ. Gen. XLI, 42; a. e.—*Pl.* בּוּצִין. Targ. Job XVIII, 13 Ms. Var. (ed. בּוּצְנִין) *linen garments* (h. text בַּדֵּי).—2) (v. בּוּצִין) *wick.* Targ. Is. XLII, 3; XLIII, 17 (Var. בוצין; h. text פשתה).—3) *swamp*, v. בִּצָּא.

בּוּצִיא, Tosef. Sabb. VII (VIII), 1 a word in a charm formula; v. ימכיא.

בּוּצִינָתָא, v. בּוּצִינְתָא.

בּוּצִין (בּוֹצִין) בּוּצִינָא, בּוּצִין m. (fr. בוץ to shine; orig. a plur. of בּוּצָא) 1) *wicks*; v. בּוּצָא.—In gen. *candle, lamp, light.* Targ. I Sam. III, 3; a. e.—Cant. R. to III, 4 (expl. Is. XXI, 5) אקימת מנרתא אדליקת ב׳ thou hast put up the lamp, lighted the wicks. Sabb. 30[a] לכבות ב׳ דנורא to put out a lamp (Ms. M. omits דנורא).—Snh. 14[a] ב׳ דנהורא bright light (wise man). Gen. R. s. 85 (play on שׁוּעַ, Gen. XXXVIII, 2, v. שְׁעָה) ב׳ דאתרא the light of the town (leader); a. fr.—*Pl.* בּוּצִינַיָּא. Targ. Ex. XXX, 7 sq.; a. e.—2) (in Bab. dialect; cmp. בטר) *a young pumpkin*, contrad. to קרא the full-grown one. Ber. 48[a] (prov.) ב׳ ב׳ מקיניה ידיע Ar. a. Rashi (ed. כקטפיה; Ms. M. בוצינא מקינפיה ידיע, v. Rabb. D. S. a. l. note) the young pumpkin is known by its shaft [by what oozes out of it, מקיטפירה], i. e. the future scholar is recognized by his utterings in childhood. Succ. 56[b] a young pumpkin (now) is better than a large one (later); (differ. in Tosaf. a. l.); a. e.—*Pl.* בּוּצִינַיָּא, בּוּצִינֵי. Targ. O. Num. XI, 5.—Ned. 66[b] (a misunderstanding of בוצינ׳ betw. a Babylonian husband and a Palestinean wife). Yoma 78[a] מצטנן בב׳ Ms. M. (ed. ברנוקא) cooled his hands with young pumpkins.—Meg. 12[a] sq. (prov.) איהו בקרי וכ׳ (Var. בר וכר׳; Sot. 10[a] בר קארי וכ׳) the husband between the old pumpkins, his wife between the young ones, i.e. a faithless husband makes a faithless wife.—*3) (from its shape) ב׳ דריחייא *the pivot* (Rashi); *the hole* (socket) in the lower millstone (Ar.). Pes. 94[b] (Var. סרנא).

בּוּצִית, בּוּצִיתָא, v. בִּרְצ׳.

בּוּצְלָא, בְּצַלָא m. ch. (h. בָּצָל, v. בצל) *onion.—Pl.* בְּצָ׳, בּוּצְלֵי, בּוּצְלַיָּא. Targ. Num. XI, 5.—Kidd. 62[a]; a.e.—Y. Shebi. II, 34[a] bot. ב׳ כופריא וכ׳ country onions which mature no seeds; Gen. R. s. 82, v. בָּצָל. *Ib. s. 95, end וקלף ב׳ peel the onions (i. e. take all we have); [the passage seems to be corrupt; the explanation beginning with פי׳ is a glossator's note].—Kidd. 62[b]; v. next w.

בּוּצְלָנָא m. (v. preced.) *onion-like plants, leeks.* Kidd. 62[b]; v. אֲגַם II.

בּוּצָנָא m. *linen garment;* pl. בּוּצְנִין, v. בּוּצָא.

בוצציא, v. זממיא.

בּוּצְרָאָה, v. next ws.

בּוּצְרָה pr. n. pl. (b. h. בָּצְרָה, v. בצר) *Bozrah* (Fortress), an Idumean town, the home of several scholars. Y. Naz. VII, 56[a] bot.—Denomin.

בּוּצְרָאָה, בּוּצְרִיָּה, בּוּצְרִייָה m. *of Bozrah.* Y. Ned. VI, beg. 39[c]. Cant. R. to VII, 1. Lam. R. to IV, 20 בָּצְרָאָה.—Fem. h. בּוּצְרִית. Y. Bicc. III, beg. 65[c] a Bozrah fig.

בּוּצְרְתָא, v. בְּצוּרְתָא.

בּוּקָא m. (cmp. אָבִיק, b. h. בַּקְבּוּק for which LXX, βῦκος, βίκος; cmp. בוצין, בוּצָא) 1) *an earthen vessel, pitcher.—Pl.* בּוּקֵי. Ab. Zar. 37[b], a. e. לא תתלו ביה ב׳ וכ׳ hang not empty pitchers on R. N., i. e. do not pronounce him the author of such an absurdity; a. fr.—2) (fr. its shape) *hind leg, thigh.* Hull. 42[b]; 54[ab]; v. אַטְמָא. [Ar. s. v. פטם quotes בוכנא.]

בֵּית ב׳, בּוּקְיָא pr. n. pl. *Beth Bukya.* Yeb. 84[a].

בּוּקְיוֹן m. (βουκκίων, bucco; v. Sachs Beitr. II, 121; Sm, Ant. s. v. Atellanæ Fabulæ) *bucco,* the clown in the Atellanæ Fabulæ of the Romans. Ab. Zar. 18[b]; Tosef. ib. II, 6 ב׳ ומוקיון; Y. ib. I, 40[a] בוקיון מופיון (corr. acc.) Bucco and Macchus.

בוקינוס, corr. **בּוּקִינוֹת** (or **בּוּקִינָס**) f. pl. (bucina, βυκάνη) *bucinæ,* horns used in the Roman camps to proclaim the watches of the day and the night. Cant. R. to I, 12 he appointed over them (read:) קלאנין בב׳ ושופר (v. Yalk. Cant. 983) criers with bucinæ and Shofar. Lev. R. s. 29; Pesik. Baḥod. p. 152[a]; Yalk. Lev. 645; Num. 782; Ps. 840 (corr. acc.). [Midr. Till. to Ps. LXXXI, 4 ספק ידרים, read קרנות ב׳ וסלפינגין.]

בוקלסא, בוקלסה, v. בַּקְלָסָא.

בּוֹקֶר, v. בַּקֵּר.

בּוּקְתָא, v. בִּקְתָא end.

בּוּר I ($\sqrt{}$בה, v. בחה) *to be empty, waste, uncultivated.* Y. Dem. VI, 25[b] top שלא תָבוּר א״י in order that Palestine should not lie waste. Ib. יוּבִירוּ ואל וכ׳; (read as) Y. Ab. Zar. I, end, 40[b] יָבוּרוּ let them rather lie waste than rent them to a gentile.—Part. בָּר, בָּרָה a. בּוּרָה. B. Mets. 101[a] שתהא ברה בידו in order that the field may rather lie waste in his own possession; cmp. Y. l. c. [Rashi fr. ברר to be *clear and firm* in his possession, by buying it back from the gentile. R. Ḥan., in Tosaf. a. l., בּוּרָה, *lying* waste in the gentile's possession; v. Rabb. D. S. a. l. note 90.] B. Bath. 168[a] לא צריכא [דאפר׳] בבורה (v. Rabb. D. S. a. l. note) it means to say that even in the case of an unbroken field being rented, the tenant has to pay the scribe's fees; Rashi: even if the field will have to lie fallow for some time to come yet. [Cmp. part. fem. חוּלָה fr. חוּל.]

Hif. הֵבִיר a. הוֹבִיר (fr. יבר, or אבר) *to let lie waste; to neglect.* Arakh. IX, 1 (29[b]) הֱבִירָהּ (הו׳) if he let it untilled. Ex. R. s. 27, end הוֹבִירָהּ. B. Mets. IX, 3 הו׳ (Y. ed. הב׳). Gen. R. s. 82 מַבִירָן (מוֹבִירָן); Koh. R. to IV, 6 מְבַיְּרָן Pi.).

Pi. בַּיֵּיר 1) same. Koh. R. l. c., v. supra. Ex. R. s. 32 (play on שית in אשיתך Jer. III, 19) בִּיַּירְתֶּם עצמיכם ye neglected yourselves (mentally).—*2) (denom. of בּוֹר II or בִּיר) *to prepare a pitfall, to entrap.* Lev. R. s. 19; v. בִּירָנִית 2).

בִּיר, בּוּר ch. as preced. Kal. Targ. O. Gen. XLVII, 19.—Part. בָּיִיר. Taan. 6[b] לא בָּיְירֵי וכ׳ the halls (academies) are not empty (oth. expl.: the gardens do not lie waste). Lev. R. s. 1, beg. he sees חקליה בָּיְירָה וכ׳ (Var. ביירא) his field waste (in the Sabbath year) &c.

Af. אוֹבֵיר as preced. Hif.—B. Mets. IX, 3; Ib. 104[b] אי מוֹבַרְנָא לה if I should let it lie waste.

**Ithpe.* אִתְּבַר *to become empty (stupid).* Targ. Jer. X, 14 (h. text נבער).

בּוּר II m. ch. (cmp. בּוּר I) 1) *something waste, wild-growing,* whence *weed, brier.* Targ. Is. VII, 23; a. e. (always with הוֹבַאר q. v.; h. text שמיר ושית).—2) (adj.) *coarse, indigestible. Pl.* בּוּרִין. Koh. R. to I, 18 the one ate מלין ב׳ coarse food.

בּוּר *to choose,* v. בָּרַר.

בּוּר I m. (v. בּוּר I) *uncultivated, an uncultured person, mannerless, ruffian.* Aboth. II, 5; a. fr.—Mikv. IX, 6 של בּוּר, v. בַּנָּאִים.—*Pl.* בּוּרִים. Num. R. s. 3, beg.

בּוֹר II m. (rarely fem.) (b. h.; v. בּוּר I a. בְּאֵר) 1) *pit, cistern*, often=בְּאֵר. Erub. II, 4 contrad. to בְּאֵר, v. ib. 18ª ב׳ בחפירה . . . באר מים חיים ב׳ מכונסין.—B. Bath. 64ª *bor* means a pit or well gained by mere digging (without masonry), v. הוּה. B. Kam. V, 5 (50ᵇ), a. fr. ב׳ שיח ומערה a narrow pit (about ten hand-breadths deep), a lengthy ditch, and a spacious cavity. Y. Sot. II, 18ª, v. בְּאֵר. B. Kam. 6ª ב׳ תוכיח the word *bor* proves. Taan. 8ª, v. חוּלְדָּה.—Trnsf. *obstacle, danger* (v. Ex. XXI, 33 sq.). B. Kam. 6ª ב׳ המתגלגל a moving danger (e. g. a rolling stone).—ב׳ וסירה v. סִירָה.—ב׳ הגדול the Large Well, ב׳ הגולה the Pilgrims' Well, names of cisterns in the Temple premises. Erub. X, 14; Midd. V, 4.—ב׳ ספינה אלכסנדריה *the tank* of sweet water in Alexandrian merchantmen. Ohol. VIII, 1; Sabb. 35ª; a. e.—[Ib. 77ᵇ ב׳ זונקא, v. בּוּרְזִינְקָא.]—2) *a receptacle for oil or wine in the press.* Maasr. IV, 1 כב׳ קטן like an oil tank on a small scale. Ab. Zar. IV, 8 עד שירד לב׳ until the wine comes into the tank.—*Pl.* בּוֹרוֹת. B. Bath. 17ᵇ; a. fr.—Erub. 104ᵇ ב׳ הקרות, v. הֶקֵּר.—[Y. Snh. I, 19ª bot. אני ובוראך=ובורך I and thy Creator.]

בּוֹרֵא m. (b. h. בָּרָא; ברא) *Creator.* Ab. IV, 22; a. fr. Y. Snh. I, 19ª bot., v. preced.

בּוּרָא I m. ch.=h. בּוּר I. Targ. Prov. XII, 1; XXX, 2 (h. text בַּעַר).—*Pl.* [בּוּרֵי. Ib. XXII, 3 Ms. a. ed. Ven. prob. a gloss for ושברי.] בּוּרַיָּא. Lev. R. s. 18, beg. (opp. חברייא).

בּוֹרָא II m. (doubtful) 1) *little cavity, hole.* Sabb. 103ª לב׳ דקרא Ar. (ed. Koh. לְבֵירָא, ed. בִּיזְרָא q. v.).—2) *female's pudenda.* Ib. 140ᵇ Rashi, Var. (prob. cler. error; ed. כורא), v. בִּזְרָא.

בּוּרבלין. v. פּוּרְבְּלִין.

בּוּרְגָּס, (בּוּרְגָּן) בּוּרְגִּין m. (πυργίον, πύργος burgus) *little turret, isolated place of residence*, often used as a *station* for travellers (*castellum*; v. Sm. Ant. s. v. Mansio). Lev. R. s. 7 הגיע לב׳ וב׳ he arrived at the first station &c.; Pesik. Eth. Korb. p. 61ª Ar. (ed. בורגנין, Yalk. Lev. 479, end בור דגן, corr. acc.). Midr. Till. to Ps. X, 1.—*Pl.* בּוּרְגְּנִין, בּוּרְגָּנִים. Y. Meg. IV, 75ᶜ bot. הדר בב׳ he who takes lodging in &c. (contrad. to פונדקי).—Y. Erub. V, 22ᵇ bot. ע״י מערות וב׳ on account of a connected Sabbath line by means of underground walks and of turrets; (Tosef. ib. VI (V), 8 מגדלות). Erub. 21ª אין ב׳ בבבל the law as to stations in the neighborhood of towns eventually counted as outskirts for measuring Sabbath limits, cannot be applied to Babylon &c. Ib. 55ᵇ והב׳ שבתוכן Ms. M. (ed. שבתוכה) and the station houses in the fields (containing provision and lodging rooms). Maasr. III, 7, v. אַלְקְטִית. Mekh. Yith. Bahod. 1 הרי . . . . את הבּוּרְגָּסִין ואת הבורגמין וכ׳ read ואת הבּוּרְגְּנִין) ye are now forced to keep in repair the large and small stations for those going to the royal vineyards (prob. to be read כרכים fortresses).—Lev. R. s. 37; Erub. 64ᵇ; Y. Ab. Zar. I, 40ª bot. (בורנין, corr. acc.); Tosef. Pes. I (II), 27 אני ב׳ של (הללו) מעיירות I am one of those station guards. Lam. R. to I, 4 it does not read (the roads are in mourning) מבלי ב׳ מבלי בולֵיטִין (Ar. בלויטין, read בַּלִּיסְטְּין) because they are not guarded with turrets and catapults. [Midr. Till. l. c. הבורגן, v. בּוּרְגָּנִי.]

בורגמין, v. preced.

בּוּרְגָּן, v. בּוּרְגִּין a. next art.

בּוּרְגָּנָה, v. next w.

בּוּרְגָּנִי m. (denom. of בורגין) *keeper* or *resident of a station house.* Midr. Till. to Ps. X, 1 when it grew dark, בא לו הכורגן (read . . . . נִי) the *burgani* came to him. Ib. חזר . . . . אצל הב׳ he turned back and came to the *burgani*. Y. Ab. Zar. IV, 43ᵈ אתא גביה בורגנה ed. Krot. (oth. ed. בורגנרה, read בורגני or בורגרי) a station guardsman (burgarius) came to him.

בורגנרה, v. preced.

בּוּרְגָּר m. (burgarius) *castle-guard, station soldier.* Gen. R. s. 36; v. next w.—V. preced.

בּוּרְגָּרוּת f. (denom. of preced.) *station.* Gen. R. s. 36 Noah is called 'a man of the ground' (Gen. IX, 20) בורגר לשם ב׳ as the burgarius is called by the name of the castle; (Yalk. Gen. 61 בורגרתיה, Ar. תֵּה . . . . his station).

בַּרְקָתָא, בּוּרְגָּתָה pr. n. pl. *Burgatha, Barkatha*, a Galilean place north of Samaria; v. Neub. Géogr. p. 173. Y. Ab. Zar. V, 44ᵈ; Bab. ib. 31ª ברק׳.

*__בּוּרְדִּיקָא__ m. (Parthicus, Πάρθικος) *scarlet-colored* (sub. pellis, δέρμα) *leather, scarlet-dyed dress.* Y. Keth. XII, 35ª top אלבישוני ב׳ וכ׳ dress me in scarlet (which is) neither white nor dark; Y. Kil. IX, 32ᵇ top בירדיקא; Gen. R. s. 96 צבועים דבריקא; ib. s. 100 מאנין דבריקה. Yalk. Job 924 בורקיא (for which Sabb. 114ª בגדי האילרין). Cmp. אוֹלָרִין a. חִימוּצָתָא.

בורדיקי, בורדיקאי Pes. 40ᵇ, v. אַבְנְנָּר.

בּוּרְדִּלָא, בַּרְדִּילָא m. (a corrupt. of flagellum, cmp. פְּרַגֵּל; late Lat. burdillus; cmp. late Greek βουρδουλίζειν, Sachs Beitr. II, 88 note) *club, whip.*—*Pl.* בּוּרְדְּלִין *blows, lashes.* Pesik. B'shall. p. 81ᵇ; Yalk. Ex. 225 בורלודין (corr. acc.; Mekh. B'shall. 1 מכות).—בַּרְדִּילַיָּא. Num. R. s. 13 חמית שוטיא וב׳ she beheld the rods and whips.

*__בּוּרְדָּם__ m. (comp. of בּוֹר a. דָּם) [*well of blood*,] *dysentery, bloody flux.* Ned. 41ᵇ ב׳ אין מבקרין ואין מזכירין שמו (Ar. אותו . . . . ברדס) we must not visit (one afflicted with) *burdam*, nor mention its (real) name. [Rashi quotes a vers. בורדס.]

בורדס, v. preced.

בּוּרְדְּסִין, v. בִּרְדְּסִין.

בורדקאי Pes. 40ᵇ, v. אַבְנְנָּר.

בּוֹרָה f. *fallow ground*, v. בּוּר I.

בּוּרוּת f. (בּוּר 1) *emptiness, senselessness*.—דברי ב׳ unmeaning things, nonsense. Nidd. 69[b]; 70[b].

בּוּרְזִינְקָא m. (a comp. of בור a. זינקא, v. זנק) *a leaping well*, i. e. *a well which springs forth periodically to disappear again* (v. Is. LVIII, 11). Sabb. 77[b] ed. in two words (corr. acc.; cmp. בּוּרְקָם; Ms. M. בור זיקנא, corr. acc.), phonetic etymol. בור זה נקי this well is empty. [Syr. בר זנקא *ocrea*, בור זינקא *tiara*, P. Sm. 586 sq., Nöld. Mand. Gr. p. 20 (cmp. בֵּרִית, בּוּרְפַּיִיר) have nothing to do with our w.]

*בּוּרְטְיָא m. (a corrupt. of verutum, βηρύττα, S.) *spit*. Sabb. 146[a] למיברז . . . בב׳ to break open a barrel (of dates) by jamming a spit between the splices (Ms. M. קורבור׳, Alf. ed. Cost. בְּרְזִיתָא). Snh. 27[b] top קתא דב׳ the handle of a burtya.

בּוֹרִי f., pl. בּוֹרְיוֹת, בּוֹרָאוֹת (בּוּר I) *trees which fail to thrive after transplantation*. B. Bath. 95[a] מקבל עליו עשר ב׳ למאה Ms. H. a. Ar. (ed. בורייות, בוריות, Ms. M. טראות לסאה corr. acc.) the owner must be prepared for ten failures out of one hundred trees planted (and has no claim on the contractor).

בֻּרְיִ, בּוּרִי m. (v. בָּרִי) 1) *strength, health, normal condition*. Y. Gitt. VII, 48[c] bot. נשתתק מתוך בּוּרְיוֹ lost his speech while in his normal health (suddenly), opp. מתוך חוליו. Y. Nidd. I, 49[b]; Y. Keth. V, 30[a] bot. פירש מתוך (בָּרְיוֹ) בוריו the child ceased to suck while in normal health. Mekh. Mishp. N'zikin. 6; Y. Keth. IV, 28[c] top (expl. על משענתו Ex. XXI, 19 'on his own support') על בוריו restored to his former health. Mekh. l. c. 13 על בריו.—2) cmp. אָשֵׁר) *certainty, evidence, assertion*. Y. Sot. I, 16[d] עמדי על בורייך stand by thy assertion (be not intimidated). Gen. R. s. 70 מעמידין אותו על בוריו they establish it (the law) on its strength, i. e. arrive at a final decision.

בּוּרְיָא I ch. same. Targ. O. Ex. XXI, 19 על בּוּרְיֵיהּ, v. preced.

*בּוּרְיָא II f. (v. בַּר I;=h. מַחֲצֶלֶת, חוּצֶלֶת) *reed-matting used for partitions, coverings* &c. [Var. בּוּדְיָא, against Syr. בוריא a. best Mss., v. בַּר III.] Succ. 20[b] מסככין בב׳ Ms. M. 2 (ed. a. Ar. with ד, Ms. M. 1 (בכ׳) you may cover the festive booth with matting. Bekh. 8[b]. B. Mets. 67[b] תמרי דאבודיא ed. (Ms. M. דעל בורי׳, v. Rabb. D. S. a. l. note) dates spread on mattings. Erub. 8[a] an alley בריך ב׳ (with ד, ed., Ms. M. with ר) surrounded by a partition of matting.—Ib. 102[a] זיל כרוך ב׳ וכ׳ go and fold the matting up (for the night), but leave a handbreadth of it spread.—*Pl.* בּוּרְיָיתָא. Succ. l. c. Ms. M. בוריתא a. ביריתא (Ms. M. 2 בריתא).

בּוֹרֵיא, בּוֹרְיָא *Creator*, v. בָּרָא.

בּוֹרֵיק, v. בָּרַק.

בּוֹרִית f. (b. h. בֹּרִית, contr. of בהרית, בחר; v. ברר) *a sort of soap, lixivium*, Nidd. IX, 6. Sabb. IX, 5. Ib. 90[a]; Nidd. 62[a], v. אָהָל, אַהֲלָא, זֵירְתָא II a. כַּבְרִיתָא. Kerith. 6[a] ב׳ כרשינה a borith won out of a leek.

בּוֹרִית, v. בֵּרִית.

בּוֹרֶךְ, v. בֶּרֶךְ.

בּוּרְכְּתָא, בּוּרְכָּא f. (v. ברך) *something hollow, absurdity*; cmp. בּוּר I. Keth. 63[b]; Ḥull. 88[b]; Shebu. 12[b] הא ב׳ this is entirely unfounded (or absurd). מאי בורכתיה (הא....) wherein does its absurdity (or hollowness) consist?—[בּוּרְכָּא *knee, shoot*, v. בִּרְכָּא.].

בורכייר, Tosef. Kil. III, 12 ed. Zuck., v. בּוּפְּרְיָא.

בּוּרְכַּיִיר, v. בִּרְכַּיִיר.

בּוּרְכְּתָא, v. בּוּרְכָּא.

בּוּרְלָא, v. בִּירְלָא.

בורלא B. Kam. 113[b] Var., v. בּוּלְרָא.

בורלודין, v. בּוּרְדְּלָא.

בּוּרְמָא m. (פרם=ברם, cmp. P. Sm. I, 616) *a wedge*. Lam. R. to III, 12, v. אִסְפַּרִיסָא.

בּוֹרֶן, v. בְּרִין.

בּוּרְנִי I (ברני) f. (Λιβυρνίς, sub. ναῦς) *Liburnian (ship)*, a light fast-sailing vessel. Targ. Is. XXXIII, 21; Yoma 77[b] (citation of Targ. l. c.). R. Hash. 23[a]. B. Mets. 80[b] ג׳ כורין לב׳ וכ׳ an addition of three *khor* is a culpable overload for a large liburna. [Y. Kidd. I, 61[a] bot. בורניות, v. בְּרִיוֹן.] [Targ. Y. Gen. XXXVI, 2 בורנייתא some ed., v. בּוּרְנָא.]

בּוּרְנִי II pr. n. pl. *Burni*, a place near Lydda. Snh. 32[b].

בּוּרְנִין, v. בִּירַנְתָּא. [Y. Ab. Zar. I, 40[a] bot., v. בּוּרְנִין.]

*נְהַר ב׳, בּוּרְנִיץ pr. n. *N'har* (canal of) *Burnits*, in Babylon. M. Kat. 4[b] ed. (Ms. M. בורנינין or בורנניץ; oth. var., v. Rabb. D. S. a. l. note).

בורסגניות, Cant. R. to II, 2, read פְּרוּסַרְגוּרִיּוֹת, v. פְּרִיסוֹאַרְגִּירָא.

בורסטייתא, Lam. R. to I, 5 Var., v. פְּרִיסְטְיוֹנָא.

בּוּרְסִי II (ברסי) m. (βυρσεύς) *tanner*. Kidd. 82[a] (Ar. ברסי, ed. בורסקי q. v.) read: הגרע והבלן והב׳ אין וכ׳ (v. Tosef. ib. V, 14; Kes. Mish. to Maim. M'lachim I, 6). Keth. 77[a] ב׳ גדול a tanner on a large scale, ב׳ קטון on a small scale (who collects the excrements himself). Tosef. Kidd. II, 2; 4 בורסקי ed. Zuck. (Var. בורסי). Pes. 65[a]; Kidd. 82[b]; a. fr.—*Pl.* בּוּרְסִיִּים. Succ. 51[b] Ms. M. (ed. טַרְסִיִּים).

בּוּרְסִי II pr. pl. *Bursi*, prob. identical with בּוּרְסִיף q. v. Kidd. 72[a].

*בּוּרְסִיוֹן m. (βυρσεῖον) *tannery.* Y. Sabb. V, 7[b] bot. עור מבורסינין (corr. acc.) hide from the tannery.

בּוּרְסִים, בּוּרְסִין, v. בִּרְסִין.

בּוּרְסִיף (בּוּלְסִיף) pr. n. pl. (Βόρσιππα) *Borsif,* a city near the site of Babylon, frequently identified with *Babel.* Snh. 109[a] (phonetic etymol.) בור שפת Ar. (ed. שאפי, Var. שפיא; Yalk. Gen. 62 שפיר, Var. ספר, v. Rabb. D. S. a. l. note 5, a. Schr. KAT. p. 124; p. 278 sq.) an empty pit. Sabb. 36[a]. Gen. R. s. 38 (calling it Bolsif, by play on בָּלַל שְׂפַת, Gen. XI, 9). Ab. Zar. 11[b] בית נבו בכורסי ed. (Ms. M. בית נבו שבבורסין, corr. acc.) the temple of Nebo in Bors. (v. Rabb. D. S. a. l. note). Kidd. 72[a] פרת דבורסי the Euphrates land near B.—Yoma 10[a] כלח זו פרת דבורסיף.

בּוּרְסְקִי f. (βυρσική sub. τέχνη) 1) *the tanning process, tannery,* [fr. (=ב׳ בעל) *the tanner;* v. בּוּרְסִי]. Sabb. I, 2 ולא לב׳ nor must one enter the tannery (to look after the process, shortly before Sabbath). Ib. 9[b] התחלת כ׳ the beginning of the tanner's work. Ib. ב׳ גדולה a tannery on a large scale; v. בּוּרְסִי. B. Bath. 21[b] ולא ב׳ nor to put up a tanner's workshop; a. fr.—2) *Bursiké,* a suburb of Tiberias. Cant. R. to I, 4.

בּוּרְצָא, v. בִּירְצָא.

בּוּרְקִי I *morning star,* v. בְּרַק. Y. Yoma III, 1 Mish.; 40[b]; Y. R. Hash. II, beg. 57[a]. V. בַּרְקַאי.

בּוּרְקִי II, בּוּרְקַיי pr. n. m. *Bor'kay,* an Amora. Y. Kidd. III, 63[d] bot.; a. e. Koh. R. to IX, 9; Yalk. ib. 979 בַּרְקַאי.

בורקיא, Yalk. Job 924, v. בורדיקא.

בורתידה, read קְתִידְרָא.

בורתיה, Targ. Job XV, 33 some ed., read בוסריה, v. בּוּסְרָא.

בּוּשׁ (b. h.; √בה, v. בָּהַת); (as adj.) m. *confounded, abashed, ashamed.* Zeb. 101[a] הודה ולא בוש וכ׳ he confessed and was not ashamed so as to say, 'I have not learned it', but he said &c.; ib.[b] (v. Rabb. D. S. a. l.).—Hag. 22[b] ביש אני=בּוֹשְׁנִי; Tosef. Ohol. V, 11 בּוֹשְׁתִּי. Kidd. 81[b] בּוֹשָׁה she is too bashful to &c. Keth. VIII, 1 אנו בּוֹשִׁין we are confounded (to find a reason); a. fr.—בוש פנים (not בישת) *bashful, chaste.* Aboth V, 20.

Pi. בִּיֵּישׁ *to put to shame, insult, disgrace.* B. Kam. VIII, 1 הַמְבַיֵּישׁ את הישן he who exposes a sleeping person to shame. Ib. הזיק וב׳ he injured and exposed (a person at the same time). Ib. הכל לפי המְבַ׳ והמתבייש all (the fine) according to the social position of the insulter and of the insulted. Succ. 53[a] happy our youth שלא בִּיְּישָׁה וכ׳ which casts no reflection on our old age; a. fr.

**Hif.* הוֹבִישׁ (cmp. הוֹבִיר fr. בור) *to trouble, spoil.* Tosef. B. Kam. V, 12 ed. Zuck. (Var. הבאיש, v. בָּאַשׁ, as Mish. V, 3).

Hithpa. a. *Nithpa.* הִתְבַּיֵּישׁ, נִתְבַּיֵּישׁ *to be put to shame, be exposed, insulted; to be bashful.* B. Kam. l. c. Ned. 20[a]. Num. R. s. 15 התב׳ והטמין he felt ashamed (to offer the king common accommodations) and hid &c. Ib. נִתְבַּיַּישְׁתִּי; a. fr.

בּוּשָׁה f. (b. h.; preced.) *shame.* B. Bath. 75[a] אוי לה לאותה ב׳ Oh, for that shame! Zeb. 113[a]. Y. Shebu. VII, 38[a] top מפני הב׳ in order that they should be ashamed of each other (to swear falsely). Y. Ned. V, 39[b] מפני הב׳ in order to make reparation for putting his neighbor to shame; a. fr.

*בּוּשְׁפִי a word in a charm formula, supposed to mean *night;* v. אוּשְׁפִי. Sabb. 67[b] (Ms. M. בושקי).

בּוּשְׁלָא f. (בשל) 1) *warm and moist* (of a fresh stripped hide). Sabb. 79[a] התם בבו׳ Ar. (ed. בבישולה, early ed. בבושלה, v. Rabb. D. S. a. l. note) there a fresh hide is meant (not dry enough for the first process of tanning).—2) *Pl.* בּוּשְׁלֵי *ripened fruits.* Ber. 40[b] ב׳ כומרא Ar. (ed. כמרא) figs ripened by shrinking (placed in the ground, Ar., overripe through exposure to the sun; Rashi).

בּוּשׂר׳, v. sub. בוסר׳.

בּוֹשֶׁת, בֹּשֶׁת f. (b. h.; בּוּשׁ) (freq. with פנים) *shame, insult; bashfulness, chastity.* Ber. 32[a]; a. fr.—Keth. 67[b] בּוֹשְׁתָּהּ של וכ׳ the shame of a woman (in remaining single).—Trnsf. (sub. דמי) *indemnity for exposure.* B. Kam. VIII, 1 sq. Ib. 85[b] ב׳ דרק ליה וכ׳ an indictable insult (without physical injury) is (e. g.) spitting in one's face. Y. Yeb. VI, 7[b], a. fr. בית הב׳ *pudenda.* Lev. R. s. 14 במקום בָּשְׁתָּהּ near her pudenda.

בּוּת, v. בֵּית.

בּוּתָא, v. בּוּצִינָא I.

בּוּתָא, בְּוֹתָא, v. בְּאוּת.

*בּוּתְנִיאַס, בּוּתְנִיס (?) pr. n. m. a. pl. *Bothneas,* founder of Sidon. Targ. I Chr. I, 13 (Var. כותניאס). Targ. Y. Gen. X, 19 (כותניים, h. text צידן).

בָּתְנַיָּא, בּוּתְנַן, בּוּתְנָיִין, בּוּתְנִיִּים, בּוּתְנַיי pr. n.=h. בָּשָׁן *Bashan,* country East of the Jordan; cmp. ר׳ בְּנָה. Targ. Y. II Deut. XXXII, 14. Ib. I a. II, XXXIII, 22. Targ. Ps. LXVIII, 23 (some ed. כ׳).—Y. Maasr. IV, 51[b] bot. ביתניין. Y. Maas. Sh. IV, beg. 54[d] כות׳ (corr. acc.). Y. Peah I, 16[a] (read:) בּוּתְנַאי, v. חֲנוּתָא.—V. מְתַנַן.

בותרא, Targ. Job XV, 33 בותריה Ms. a. Regia, read בוסריה, v. בּוּסְרָא.

בַּז, v. בְּזַז, בַּזַז.

בְּזָא I, II, v. בזי I, II ch.

בְּזָא, v. בִּיזָא.

*בְּזָאֵר m. pl. (v. בִּיזְעָא, בִּיזָא) *clefts, breaches.* Snh. 95[a] נפק לְשַׁכּוּר ב׳ (Var. לִטְבַר, v. Rabb. D. S. a. l. note) he went out to fill up breaches, v. סְכַר. [Oth. opin. שכר ב׳ name of a place; Yalk. Sam. 155 כפר ב׳, ed. Salon. שכר ב׳, v. Rabb. l. c.]

בַּזְבּוּזָא m. (בזז) *plunder, spoil, ill-gotten goods.—Pl.* בַּזְבּוּזַיָּא. Cant. R. to VII, 7 (expl. נבזביתך Dan. V, 17) בַּזְבּוּזַיִךְ וכ׳ thy ill-gotten goods; you are plunderers, sons of &c.

בִּזְבֵּז (Pilp. of בז, v. בִּזָּא II, a. b. h. בִּזָּה in H. Dict.) 1) *to divide, distribute.* Tosef. Meg. IV (III), 21 אין אדם מְבַזְבֵּז בידיו לעצמו (v. ed. Zuck. Var.) one who distributes (honors) must take none to himself. B. Bath. 142ª a convert died ובזבזו וכ׳ and Israelites divided his property among themselves (he having left no legitimate heirs).—2) *to give away liberally, to give charity on a large scale.* Keth. 50ª הַמְבַזְבֵּז אל יְבַזְבֵּז וכ׳ he who wants to be liberal, must not give away more than &c. Ib. קטנים כתבו ובזבזו 'minors' 'wrote' and 'gave away' (ref. to the order of three traditions concerning minors, transfer of property and charity, related ib. 49ᵇ sq.). B. Bath. 11ª שבזבז וכ׳ who gave away to charities his own and his father's treasures; a. fr.—3) *to spend unnecessarily, squander.* Gen. R. s. 80. [4) *to divide spoils, to plunder,* v. בָּזַז, בַּזְבּוּזָא &c.]

בַּזְבֵּז ch. same; 1) *to shatter.* Esth. R. to I, 10; v. בזז ch.—2) *to give away, to squander.* Targ. Koh. III, 22 למא אנא מְבַ׳ וכ׳ why should I waste money in doing charity? —Keth. 67ᵇ בַּזְבֵּיזָה וכ׳ he gave away (on charity) half of &c. Y. Sot. III, 19ª, a. e. הוות מְבַזְבְּזָה וכ׳ was squandering the estate.—3) (v. בזז) *to treat lightly.* Y. Ter. XI, 48ᵇ; Y. Sabb. II, 4ᵈ top (read:) וכולא מן הדין שמשא [בביתיה] מְבַזְבְּזָא בהקדישא and all this discussion arose from that servant [in R. Ammi's house] dealing lightly with sacred property.

בזבוזא, Y. Sabb. II, 4ᵈ top, v. preced.

בַּזְבְּזֵי, v. בְּזִירֵי.

בַּזְבְּזִיָּה, בַּזְבְּזִיָּה m. pl. [*breakers*], name of messengers from Sodom [or Edom]; a word in a charm formula. Sabb. 67ª (ed. בז בזיה, v. Rabb. D. S. a. l.).

בזבזיך Sabb. 67ª, a word in a formula of incantation; v. preced.

בזבינא, v. next w.

***בַּזְבָּנָא** m. (Pers. bâzwân, bâzbân, Perl. Et. St. p. 117) *collector of bridge toll.* B. Bath. 167ª Ar. (ed. בזבי׳; Ms. M. בזוינא; for oth. var. v. Rabb. D. S. a. l. note).

בַּזְגָּא m. (בזג, cmp. פִּתְקָא) *that which is divided off,* whence *sheaf, bundle.* Hull. 52ª straw ועביד ב׳ (Ar. ed. Koh. בִּיזְ׳) made into bunches.

בזגיתא Y. Kidd. I, 60ᵇ top (ed. Krot. בזגיתא), v. זְגִיתָא.

בָּזָה, v. בזי.

בַּזּוֹז m. (בזז) *robber, plunderer.* *Pl.* בַּזּוֹזִים. Gen. R. s. 1 אומה של ב׳ a nation of robbers.

בַּזּוֹזָא ch. same. Targ. Prov. XXVII, 19.—*Pl.* בַּזּוֹזִין, בַּזּוֹזַיָּא, בַּזּוֹזֵי. Targ. Ps. XXV, 3. Ib. CXIX, 158; a. e.—Snh. 94ª (ref. to ובגד וכ׳ Is. XXIV, 16) עד דאתו ב׳ וכ׳ until the robbers (of the Holy Land) shall have come and those that shall rob it from its robbers. Keth. 112ᵇ.—Lam. R. introd. (R. Yits. 1) איך הוות לנא מב׳ (some ed. מבזוזים, corr. acc.) what an affliction has come to us from the plunderers; v. בּוּזָנָא.

בִּיזָּא, בִּיז׳ m. (בזז) *robbery, plunder.* Targ. Is. XXIV, 16.

***בַּזּוֹזִיתָא (בַּזּוֹנִיתָא)** f. (v. בַּזּוֹזָא) *plunderer.* Targ. Ps. CXXXVII, 8 (Ms. בזוי׳; h. text הַשְּׁדוּדָה!). [Targ. Job XV, 21 בזוזיתיה, בזוזת׳, בזיזות׳, read בַּזּוֹזָא.]

בזותא, v. preced.

בְּזוּל, v. בְּזִיל.

בְּזוּעַ, v. בִּיזוּעַ.

בָּזַז (b. h.; √בז *to divide,* cmp. בִּזָּא II, בָּזַע, בִּזְבֵּז, בָּצַע) *to distribute, to make spoil.* Y. Macc. II, 31ᵈ bot. היה בוזז made booty.—Part. pass. בָּזוּז, f. בְּזוּזָה *robbed, illegitimately conquered.* Gen. R. s. 1 ב׳ היא בידכם it is robbery what ye possess (ye have no title).

בְּזַז I ch. (בַּז) same. Targ. Hos. VII, 9; X, 2; a. fr.—Esth. R. to I, 10, v. בזז. Cant. R. to VII, 7 (prov.) take presents from an heir ולא מן דבָזְזִין ליה but not from one for whom they make spoil (king).

Pa. בַּזֵּיז same. *Num. R. s. 12 דהוא בזיז וכ׳ he robs (the youths of) the noon-day lessons (transl. ישוד Ps. XCI, 6); v. גְּזַז.

Af. אַבִּיז *to cause to be plundered.* Targ. Is. XXIV, 1 מַבִּיז (Var. מְבִיז).

Ithpe. אִתְבְּזִיז *to be robbed.* Ib. 3; a. e.—Ib. 16 מִתְבַּזְזִין = מתבזזין.

***בְּזַז** II *to be shy,* v. בְּזַז.

בזותא, Targ. Job XV, 21, v. בַּזּוֹזִיתָא.

בִּזְזְנָא, Targ. Ps. CXXXVII, 3, v. בְּזִירָא 2).

בְּזָה, בזי (b. h.; √בז *to tread,* v. בוז) *to tread upon,* whence *to despise, spurn, degrade.* Ab. d'R. Nath. ch. XXIX הבוזה את חבירו וכ׳ he who spurns his neighbor (rebuking him) for a sacred cause. Ib. הן בוזין בעצמן they make themselves contemptible (neglecting their appearance). Part. pass. בָּזוּי, f. בְּזוּיָה. Y. Sot. V, end, 20ᵈ שהיתה נבואתו ב׳ his prophetic gift was degraded (by him). Ruth. R. to I, 1 מי שהוא ב׳ בדבריו he who becomes contemptible through his own words (in not practicing what he teaches). Cant. R. to VI, 5 מה עז זו ב׳ as the goat is despised כך בְּזוּיִין וכ׳ so were the Israelites made despicable at Shittim (through debauchery); a. fr.

Pi. בִּזָּה, בִּיזָּה same. Ab. d'R. Nath. l. c. Y. Sot. l. c. he (Isaac) is called Buzi, שבי׳ את וכ׳ because he made all idolatrous temples appear contemptible (by his willingness to be sacrificed to the Lord). Gen. R. s. 30 (play on בוז Job XII, 5) שהיו מְבַזִּים עליו they sneered at him. Snh. 65ᵇ

בְּיַזִּיתוֹ thou hast insulted him. Aboth III, 11 הַמְבַזֶּה את וכ׳ he who disregards the festive weeks (treating them as week days); a. fr.—*Part. Pu.* מְבוּזֶּה, pl. מְבוּזִּין. Ab. Zar. III, 3 המב׳ common vessels, opp. מכובדין ornamental; Tosef. ib. V (VI), 1 בוזיין ed. Zuck. (Var. מב׳); Y. ib. III, 42[d]; a. e.

Hithpa. הִתְבַּזָּה *to be despised, humbled, exposed.* Y. Taan. II, beg. 65[a] you cannot compare המִתְבַּזֶּה מעצמו וכ׳ one who humbles himself to one who is humbled by others. Keth. 97[b]. Ruth. R. to I, 1 אימתי ד״ת מִתְבַּזִּין וכ׳ when are the words of the Law despised by the people? When the scholars make them contemptible (through their conduct); a. fr.

בְּזָא, בְּזֵר I ch. same. Targ. Prov. XIII, 13; a. fr.—Targ. Y. Lev. XVIII, 8 sq. (interchanging with Pa.) לא תבזי not expose. Y. Hag. II, 77[d] bot. לא תִיבְזֵי וכ׳ despise not the children of thy Master (thy fellow-creatures).—Part. pass. בָּזֵי, f. בְּזִית. Targ. Y. II Gen. XVI, 5.

Pa. בַּזֵּי same. Targ. Cant. VIII, 1; a. fr.—Gen. R. s. 63 לא תְבַזּוּן וכ׳ never despise, v. גּוּלְיָיר. Meg. 25[b] if one is ill-reputed שרי ליה לְבַזּוּייה בגי׳מל וש״ין you are permitted to show him your contempt with Gimmel and Shin (v. comment.).

Ithpa. אִתְבַּזֵּי, *Ithpe.* אִיתְבְּזִי, contr. אִיבְּזִי *to be despised.* Targ. Y. I, Gen. XVII, 5 ויתבז איקרי (read ואיתבזי).—Keth. 97[b] דְּתִיתְבַּזֵּי that she (his wife) should be exposed to publicity in court. Ib. דליבְּזוּ that they (his heirs) should &c.

בְּזָא, בְּזֵי II (=בְּזַע q. v.) *to break, divide.* Part. pass. Pes. 110[a] דיקולא בְּזִיָּא ed. (Ms. M. 2 דיקולי בזיין pl., v. Rashi a. l. a. Rabb. D. S. a. l. note) a broken basket.—*Num. R. s. 12 דהוה בזא וכ׳ for he breaks into (compels to interrupt) the lessons of the day (as a ref. to קטב, v. בְּזָז).

Pa. בַּזֵּי *to divide, change off.* B. Bath. 37[a] דבזי בַּזּוּיֵי Ms. M. (ed. דבאזר באזוזי, read with Rashi דבזי בזויי or בּוּזָאֵי; v. Rabb. D. S. a. l. note) he divided the usufruct of each year betw. the trees of each division of the orchard (so as to have actually been in undisturbed possession of the entire orchard for three consecutive years.

Ithpe. אִתְבְּזֵי *to be divided, cut apart.* Targ. Job X, 1 אתבזוירת Ms. Var. (ed. Vien. אתגזרת, Ms. אתכזורית; h. text נקטה).

בִּזָּא, v. בִּיזָא.

בִּזָּה, v. בִּיזָה.

בִּזְיָא, v. בִּיזְיָא.

בִּזָּיוֹן, בִּיזְ׳ m. (b. h.; בָּזָה) *contempt, disgrace.* Y. Ab. Zar. III, 42[d] דבר של ב׳ a common vessel (v. בָּזָה Part. Pu.). Y. Sabb. XI, 13[a] top, a. fr. נהג ב׳ בי׳ to treat disrespectfully. Y. Hag. II, 78[a] top נהג עצמו בב׳ conducted himself disgracefully. Snh. 47[a]; a. fr.

בִּזְיוֹנָא, בִּיזְיוֹנָא ch. same. Snh. 46[b] קבורה משום ב׳ is burial required in order to prevent disgrace (to the dead and his relatives)? Ib. א״א משום ב׳ הוא לא כל וכ׳ (Ms. M. כל . . . . ני דחיי) if you say, burial is required in order to prevent disgrace, he has no such power (as to prohibit it by his last will). Ib. 45[a] [read:] בזיונה דאינש עדיף וכ׳ (the prevention of) disgrace stands to man higher than bodily ease (absence of pain), i. e. one would rather suffer protracted agony than exposure; (Var. lect. v. Rabb. D. S. a. l. note 8); Sot. 8[b].

בֵּי זִירָנָא, בֵּי זִוּוֹנָא, בִּיזְיוֹנָא, בִּזְיוֹנָא I m. (בֵּי a. זִירוֹנָא; v. זוּן II a. זִירָנָא II) *place or means of detention,* whence 1) *prison.* Ber. 56[a] Ms., v. בְּדִירְנֵי. Erub. 11[b] קם אבבא דבי זירנא Ar. (in ed. last two words omitted) placed himself at the prison gate.—*Pl.* בְּזִיוֹנֵי. Sabb. 32[a] (prov.) at the gate of shops (you have) many friends ..., אבב ב׳ וכ׳ (Ms. Oxf. אבי ב׳) at the prison gate—no friends &c.—2) (pl. as a sing. noun) *lock, clasp, buckle.* Sabb. 57[b] what is *ist'ma?* Answ. בזיוני. What is *bizyuné?* Answ. כלוא פרוחי what imprisons the flying (curls), v. אִיסְטְמָא.

בִּזְיוֹנָא, II m. (בְּזֵי II, v. Nöld. Mand. Gr. § 119) *slit.*—*Pl.* בִּיזְיוֹנֵי, בִּזְיוֹנֵי. Ned. 56[b]; Snh. 20[b] a couch is called *mittah,* אעולי ואפוקי בב׳ when the straps go in and out through slits (incisions in the boards), contrad. to אֲבַקְתָּא; (Ms. M. emendation בי זיני, Ms. M. ביזייני; Ned. l. c. בזוני; v. Rashi to Snh. l. c.).

בְּזִין* m. *shy,* v. בְּזַז.

בְּזִיזָא m. 1) (part. pass. of בְּזַז I) *despoiled.* Targ. Is. XVIII, 3; 7 (h. text מְבוּסָה).—2) *sneerer.*—*Pl.* Targ. Ps. CXXXVII, 3 בְּזִיזָנָא (Ms. בְּזוּ׳, ed. Vien. בְּזָזָנָא).

בִּזְבְּזֵי, בְּזִיזֵי* m. pl. (v. בזבז) prob. *distributors,* hence=בְּזִיכָא (cmp. אַפְתִּקָא) *vessels, dishes* with handles. Targ. Y. Ex. XXV, 29 בְּזִיזוֹי Ar., בִּזְבְּזוֹי Mus. (ed. בְּזִיכוֹי).

בזיז a word in an incantation. Sabb. 67[a], v. בזוזיך.

בְּזִיָּא, v. בְּזֵי.

בִּזַּיְיהּ, v. בִּיזְלֵי.

בִּזְיָנֵי, v. בִּזְיוֹנָא II.

בָּזָךְ, בָּזִיךְ m. (בזז, with format. ךְ; v. בְּזִיזֵי) *vessel, dish, censer* (b. h. כַּף). Tam. IV, 3 entrails חנתונים בב׳ which had been put in a vessel. Ib. V, 4. והב׳ היה וכ׳ in the larger vessel was the baz., filled to the brim with incense. Y. Yoma II, 39[c]; a. fr.—*Pl.* בְּזִיכִין, בְּזִיכִים. Men. XI, 5; a. fr.—Num. R. s. 4 (expl. b. h. כַּפּוֹת) בְּזִיכֵי לבונה censers.

בָּזִיךְ, בְּזִיכָא (בַּזִּיכָא, בַּזְכָּא) ch. f. same. Targ. Num. VII, 14; a. fr.—*Pl.* בְּזִיכַיָּא, בַּזִּיכַיָּא, בַּזְכַיָּא. Ib. IV, 7. Targ. Ex. XXV, 29; a. fr.

בזיני, v. בִּזְיוֹנָא II.

בְּזִיעָא f. (בזע) *rent, part.* Targ. Koh. III, 7.—*Pl.* בְּזִיעָן. Targ. Y. Ex. XIV, 21. [Hebr. בְּזִיעִים, expl. בְּזִיוֹנֵי in Rashi to Snh. 20[b].]

בְּזִיקְיָא, v. בּוּקָא.—בזיקים, Tosef. Ned. I, 3, read בְּזִיכִים.

בָּזְבָּא, בָּזָךְ, v. בָּזִיךְ h. a. ch.

בַּזֵּל, בַּרְזֵל (Pa. of בזל, √בז, v. בְּזָא II) *to scatter, to distribute by shaking* (cmp. בְּדַר Pa. 2). Sabb. 66ᵇ ולִיבַזּוּלֵיה וכ׳ Ms. M. a. oth. (ed. לברזוליה, לברזוליה) let him shake it (the ant in the tube) to pieces and carry it off.

בְּזְלֵי, v. בִּיזְלֵי.

בְּזַע (√בז, v. בְּזֵי II; cmp. בצע, פצע &c.) *to split, perforate, rend.* Targ. Gen. XXXVII, 29 (ed. Berl. Pa.). Targ. Ps. LXXVIII, 13; a. fr.—Y. M. Kat. III, 83ᵈ top וּבְזָעוֹן and rent them (his garments); Y. Snh. II, 20ᵃ top ובזעיה (corr. acc.). Lev. R. s. 6; Lam. R. to II, 17 (expl. בצע אמרתו ib.) פורפירויה ב׳ He rent His purple (allowed the Temple curtain to be cut through by Titus).

Pa. בַּזַּע same. Targ. Ps. LXXVIII, 15; a. e. (Var. Pe., v. supra).—Part. pass. מְבַזַּע. Targ. Josh. IX, 4.—Y. Kil. IX, 32ᵇ top; Y. Keth. XII, 35ᵃ top מאנוי מבזעין his garments torn. Y. Kidd. I, 60ᵃ top והיא מְבַזְּעָא בידיה and it (the wine botte) bursts in his hand; v. infra.

Ithpa. אִתְבַּזַּע, *Ithpe.* אִתְבְּזַע, contr. אִיבְּזַע *to be split, rent.* Targ. Num. XVI, 31; a. fr. Y. Ab. Zar. III, 42ᶜ top א׳ ימא וכ׳ the lake of Tib. was split. Ib. מִתְבַּזַּע. Ib. II, 41ᶜ top אתבזעת זיקיה his wine bottle burst. Ib. V, 45ᵃ top והיא מִיבַּזְּעָא בידיה, v. supra. Bekh. 36ᵃ איבזע׳ שיפתיה his lip was slit; a. e.

בָּזָק m. (b. h.; v. next w.) [*shattering, splitting,*] *lightning.* Y. B. Mets. V, 11ᵃ top (citing the Mishnah) וְהִבְרִיקָהּ הַבּ׳ [not דב׳] and lightning struck her (affecting her feet, v. אַבְזָקַת).

בָּזַק (√בז, v. בזר II; cmp. בדק) *to break, crush.* Erub. X, 14 (104ᵃ) בּוֹזְקִין מלח וכ׳ you may crush salt (lumps) on the steps (that the priests should not slip). Gen. R. s. 50, beg. (expl. כמראה הבזק, Ezek. I, 14) כזה שהוא בוזק וכ׳ as one who crushes pieces of peat in the stove (when the flames break forth).

**Nif.* נִבְזַק (cmp. בָּזָק) *to be split in flashes, to flash* (used of the divine spirit). Gen. R. s. 26 הרוח היא נִבְזֶקֶת וכ׳ the spirit flashes in (seizes) one of man's limbs, ... בכל הגוף the entire body.

בְּזַק ch. same.—*Pa.* בַּזֵּק *to cast* (or *shoot*) *a mass of fragments* (as from a catapult). Snh. 108ᵇ ב׳ בהון עפרא וכ׳ Ar. (ed. והויה שדינן) he shot at them with dust and it turned into swords &c. *B. Bath. 73ᵃ והוה כי מבזק ארבעין גירוי דברזלא and there was a flash as if one shot forty arrows of iron (v. Koh. Ar. Compl. s. v. בזק, note 5). —Ed. כי מבזר ארב׳ גריוי דחרדלא like one scattering forty measures of mustard [from a confusion of which two versions the variants in Mss. a. in Ar. arose, v. Rabb. D. S. a. l. note.—Ar. כמיבזק Ithpe.].

Ithpe., contr. אִיבְּזִיק *to be broken.* Yoma 22ᵇ how do you know that *Bazek* (I Sam. XI, 8, v. next w.) is here used לישנא דמיבזיק in the sense of being broken (a fragment of pottery); perhaps it is the name of a place? **B. Bath. 73ᵃ Ar., v. supra.**

בֶּזֶק m. (preced.) *fragment, piece of pottery, pebble* (testa). Yoma 22ᵇ, v. preced. Tanḥ. Ki Thissa 9 ומהו ב׳ וכ׳ what is *bezek?* Answ. he took a pebble &c.

בִּיזְקָא, בִּזְקָא ch. same. Targ. Prov. XXVI, 8. Ar. (ed. ניקצא, Ms. ניסקא).—*Pl.* בִּזְקַיָּא. Pesik. Shek. p. 18ᵃ when they were poor, באילין ב׳ Ar. (ed. בזיקיא) they were counted with broken pieces of pottery, when rich with lambs (ed. reverse order); Num. R. s. 2 בִּזְקָיָּה.

בוזקה, Y. Kidd. I, 60ᵇ top, v. זִיקָא III.

בָּזַר (b. h., √בז, v. בזע) *to strew, scatter.* Kerith. 6ᵇ בּוֹזְרָהּ Ar. (ed. incorr. בזורה, v. Rashi a. l.) he scatters it, lest it may decay.

Pi. בִּזֵּר same. Part. pass. מְבוּזָּר. Sifra B'har ch. I אבל אתה בוצר מן המב׳ ed. Ven. a. oth. (Var. המופקר) but you may gather (in the Sabbath year) the grapes from (broken) branches lying scattered on the ground, opp. השמור בארץ the vine seated in the ground (Y. Shebi. VII, 38ᵇ top המובקר).

בְּזַר ch. same. *Pa.* בַּזֵּר. B. Bath. 73ᵃ, v. בְּזַק.

בִּיזְרָא, בִּזְרָא m. (=בר זרעא, v. Nöld. Mand. Gr. p. 55) *seed.* Targ. Y. Gen. I, 11 sq. (O. בר זרעא). Ib. v. 29.— Snh. 93ᵃ, v. אַסְפַּסְתָּא. B. Mets. 74ᵇ אריסא יהיב בי׳ the tenant furnishes the seed; a. fr. Erub. 53ᵃ ביזרא Ar. (Mss. a. ed. בירא, v. also Rabb. D. S. a. l. note 1); v. אַצְבְּעָא. B. Bath. 73ᵃ; v. בִּזְקָא.—Sabb. 140ᵇ נקיט ב׳ וכ׳ Ar. (ed. reversed order a. כורא, Var. ברזא, סורא, a. בורא דחספא, v. בּוּרָא II) he (R. Ḥisda) took a (valueless) seed grain in one hand and a pearl in the other; the pearl he showed to them (his daughters), but he would not show them the seed grain until they were excited, and then he showed it (as an illustration of the folly of curiosity). [Ar., with a Var. ברזא, translates, *a valueless pebble*=בִּזְקָא q. v., which seems to be confirmed by the vers. בורא דחספא (read בז׳ for בו׳) a fragment of an earthen vessel.] [Rashi's interpretation is grammatically forced and out of harmony with the natural reserve of a father towards his daughters.] [Ib. 103ᵃ לביז׳ דקרא for (putting in) the seed of a pumpkin (Ar. לבורא, ed. Koh. לבירא, Ms. M. לבירא דקירא as a cavity for planting &c.).]—*Pl.* בִּזְרֵי, בִּיזְ׳. Ḥull. 51ᵇ דעביד ב׳ when the flax stalks have seminal vessels. Ib. 60ᵇ שדא ביה ב׳ Ar. (ed. ביזרני) he put seed into it.

בִּיזְרָנָא, בִּזְרָנָא m. (collect. noun, v. preced.); *pl.* בִּזְרָנֵי, בִּי׳ *various seeds.* Kidd. 39ᵃ. Ḥull. 60ᵇ; v. preced. Bets. 15ᵃ דב׳ (צררי) the folds (pockets) wherein the seeds are carried. Gitt. 68ᵇ.

בִּזְתָא f. (בוז) *disgrace.* Targ. Job XII, 19.

בּוּזְתָא f., v. בִּיזָא.

בָּחוּר m. (b. h. בחר) 1) *chosen.* Sabb. 105ᵃ (ref. to אב, Gen. XVII, 5) I have made thee אב a father of the nations, ב׳ נתתיך וכ׳ I have made thee a chosen one among the nations. Gen. R. s. 76, beg.; a. fr.—2) *young* *man, youth, unmarried.* Keth. 7[b], opp. אַלְמוֹן.—Gen. R. s. 39 ב׳ ובתולה מיכן a young man and a virgin on the one side (of the coin). Hag. 14[a]; a. fr.—Fem. בַּחוּרָה. Gen. R. s. 71; a. e.—*Pl.* בַּחוּרִים, f. בַּחוּרוֹת. Num. R. s. 10, beg. לב׳ קול וכ׳ to the young (the strong) 'the voice of the Lord (at revelation) sounded with might', opp. תשים; a. e.

בחורא, בחורין, v. בְּחִירָא.

בחורתא Targ. Y. I, Num. XXI, 27 (28), some ed., read בחודתא, v. חִידָתָא.

***בְּהֵי** (cmp. בחן) *to look out, be cautious.* Lam. R. to I, 16 beg. אילין דבַהְיין וכ׳ (expl. in a. gloss איתבוננו) the cautious did not go out.

בְּחִיר, בְּחִירָא m., **בְּחִירָא** f. (בחר) 1)=h. בָּחוּר, בָּחִיר, *chosen, select.* Targ. II Sam. XXI, 6; a. e.—*Pl.* בְּחִירִין. Targ. Ps. CV, 6; a. e.—Y. Snh. VI, 23[c] bot. תמנין גוברין ב׳ eighty select (young) men; Y. Hag. II, 78[a] top בחו׳ (corr. acc.).—Fem. בְּחִירָן. Targ. O. Ex. XIV, 7.—2) (cmp. בְּחַן) *tried, purified.* Targ. Ps. XVIII, 31; II Sam. XXIII, 31.

בְּחִירָה f. (בחר) *selection, being chosen.* Y. Meg. I, 72[d] top מה ב׳ שנ׳ וכ׳ as the selection (expression בחר) used there &c.—בֵּית הַבְּ׳ (also with omission of בית) *the Temple of Jerusalem.* Snh. 20[b]; a. fr.—Y. Yoma I, 38[c] bot. עידיכם הב׳ וכ׳ your witness, the Temple, shall prove it (Bab. ib. 9[b] בִּירָה).

בְּחִירְתָּא f. ch. (v. preced.) *B'hirta* (selection), surname of the Talmudic treatise named Eduyoth or Ediyoth (עדיות). Kidd. 54[b] bot.; Bekh. 26[a].

בָּחַל I (b. h.; √בח, cmp. √בה s. v. בחי) [1) *to be disordered, sick;* whence בּוֹחַל q. v.].—2) (denomin. of בּוֹחַל) *to be in that stage of ripening when the fig is called bohal;* cmp. בָּאַשׁ. Nidd. 47[a] (quot. fr. Maasr. I, 2) התאנים משיבְחֲלוּ .... משילבינו וכ׳ figs are subject to tithes from the time they are called bohal, which R. . . defines, from the time their heads grow white.

Pi. בֵּיחֵל (בִּיחֵל), *Hif.* הִבְחִיל same. Shebi. IV, 7 בִּיחֲלוּ וכ׳ (Y. ed. בִּיחִילוּ). Y. ib. 35[b] bot.; Y. Maasr. I, 48[d] (חֲיָתָה) מאי ביחילו חֲיִיתָה וכ׳ what is bih.? It (the fig) creates aversion (v. חוּת), as we read (Zech. XI, 8) &c. Maasr. I, 2 משיַבְחִילוּ (Y. ed. שביחילו), v. supra. [Cmp. בָּכַר as to spelling in Talm. Y.]

בָּחַל II (=בהל, v. Prov. XX, 21, cmp. preced.) *to hasten. Pi.* בִּיחֵל *to come early.* Mekh. Bo, Pisha, 2 בי׳ אביב ובא ed. Livorno (oth. ed. בי חל corr. acc.) when the ripening of grains came very early.

Hif. הִבְחִיל *to advance growth.* Y. Sabb. VII, 10[a] top כל דבר שהוא מַבְחִיל (not שהיה מכחיל) whatever is done for advancing the fruits. Ib. לְהַבְחִיל (ed. Krot. להבחיל, corr. acc.).

בָּחַן (b. h.; √בח, v. Ges. H. Dict. s. v.; cmp. בה s. v. בחר) prop. *to distinguish, examine* (cmp. בין, חזר), hence *to try, probe* (of metals); *to find out.* Snh. 107[a] בְּחָנֵנִי try me.—Part. pass. בָּחוּן. Pes. 87[a] בְּחוּנֶיךָ Ms. M. (ed. חנוניך, v. Rabb. D. S. a. l.) thy tried servants. Ib.[b] בְּחוּנַי my tried servants. Yalk. Hos. 515; a. e.

Pi. בִּיחֵן *to inquire.* Yoma 73[b]; Shebu. 35[b] לא ביחנו they did not ask distinctly. Y. B. Kam. IV, 4[b] bot. שב״ד מְבַחֲנִין וכ׳ for the court (appointing him guardian) inquires after his character.

Hif. הִבְחִין *to distinguish.* Snh. 8[b] a. e. לְהַבְחִין בין וכ׳ in order to be able to distinguish between the ignorant and the willful transgressor. Yeb. 42[a]; a. fr.

בְּחַן ch. same. Targ. Koh. II, 6; a. fr.—Y. Maas. Sh. V, beg. 55[d] (read:) דבְחִינַת ליה וכ׳ by whom every Mishnah has been critically examined.

Ithpe. אִתְבְּחַן *to be tried, tested.* Targ. O. Gen. XLII, 15 sq. (Var. אתבחר, v. Berl. Targ. O. II, p. 15).

בָּחַר (b. h.; √בח, v. preced.) 1) *to try, examine;* v. infra.—2) (with ב) *to choose, select, prefer.* Tanh. Mishp. 11 בָּחַרְתָּ ביסורים יותר וכ׳ thou didst prefer sufferings to poverty. Mass. Sof'rim XIII, 9; a. e.—Part. *Hof.* מוּבְחָר *chosen.* מן המ׳ *of the best, the best way.* Bicc. I, 3; a. fr. —מצוה מן המ׳ the most preferable way of performing a religious act. B. Kam. 78[b]; a. fr.—מ׳ מן המ׳ *the very best.* Y. Pes. VI, 33[b] top מ׳ דוחה וכ׳ for doing a thing (in the Temple) in the preferable way, you may set aside (the Sabbath law); for doing it in the best way, you dare not &c.; a. fr.

Pi. בִּיחֵר *to examine.* Pesik. R. s. 33 (ref. to אבחר Job XXIX, 25) הייתי שואלו וּמְבַחֲרוֹ I was in the habit of investigating and examining it; [ed. Fr. emends וּמְבַהֲרוֹ, v. בָּהַר].

בְּחַר ch. same; 1) *to try, test.* Targ. Jer. XVII, 10 (h. text בחן); a. fr.—2) *to choose, select.* Targ. Ps. XXXIII, 12.—Part. בָּחֵר. Targ. Job XV, 5 (not בְּחִיר).—V. בְּחִיר.

**Af.* אַבְחַר *to pick out.* Y. Sabb. VII, 10[a] bot. כד מַבְחַר בקלופייתא when one picks out (the pieces of garlick) in the husks. Ib. כד מכחר (corr. acc.).

בַּחֲרוּת f. (v. בָּחוּר) *youth.* Tana d'be El. ch. XVIII.

בָּחַשׁ (√בח, v. בחן) 1) *to search, examine;* v. next w.—2) *to stir, to go to the bottom of a thing* (v. P. Sm. 508). Ber. 38[a]; Sabb. 156[a], v. שְׁתִית.

בְּחַשׁ ch. same; 1) *to search, examine.* Targ. Y. Gen. XXXIX, 11 לְמִיבְחוּשׁ וכ׳ to examine .... the accounts.—Sabb. 152[a] ארלא אבידנא בָּחִישְׁנָא I am searching for what I have not lost (of the aged man's unsteady walk and bent figure). B. Mets. 5[b] עד דב׳ וכ׳ until I may search and find it. Ib. 86[a] בחוש אבתריה וכ׳ (not בחיש, v. Rabb. D. S. a. l. note 90) search for him and find him. B. Kam. 97[b]. —2) *to stir.* Targ. Esth. I, 14.—Sabb. 30[b] קא בחיש באילני Ms. M. (v. Rabb. D. S. a. l. note) he shook the trees. Ib. 140[a]. Gitt. 45[a] בחשן וכ׳ stirred a (hot) pot with their hands. Ib. 69[b] top.

בַּחֲשָׁא m. (preced.) 1) *stirring ladle, pot-ladle.* Pes. 111[b] [read:] ומיהדר בי ב׳ והדר בי כדא דכמכא (v. comment.)

and he (the shadow-demon) looks like a ladle turning in a vessel &c.—*2) *rakings, hot ashes.* Snh. 39ª [read:] אותיבתה תותי ב׳ she placed it (the roast) under the grate (in the ashes); (Ar. אותיבתיה קמיה בביחוּשָׁיה she placed it before him with the raked ashes clinging to it; Yalk. Gen. 23 אותבי׳ תותי רגליה ב׳, v. Rabb. D. S. a. l. note).—[בחשי, quot. in Ar. fr. Ab. Zar. (60ᵇ), תותי ב׳, read בֵּי שַׁחְיָא, *arm-pit;* v. Y. ib. II, 41ª bot.]

בְּטָא, v. בטי.

בטאריקי, Ex. R. s. 11, read קַטָּאדִיקִי.

בְּטְבּוּט, בְּצִבּוּץ m. (v. next w.; cmp. b. h. בּוּץ) *hemp.* Y. Ab. Zar. V, end, 45ᵇ בט׳; Bab. ib. 75ª בצ׳; Nidd. 65ᵇ.—Tosef. Tohar. XI, 16 בצבץ.

בִּטְבֵּט (Pilp. of בוט or בטט, v. בטי) *to swell.—Hithpa.* הִתְבַּטְבֵּט; *Nithpa.* נִתְבַּטְבֵּט *to swell, grow.* Tanh. Mishp. 9 as the bite of a snake is not felt עד שנ׳ עליו until a swelling sets in, so is usury not felt עד שמִּתְבַּטְבֶּטֶת עליו until it has grown upon him (the debtor). Ex. R. s. 31 שמתבעט, corr. acc.).

בִּטְדָא, v. בִּטְרָא.

בִּטּוּל, בִּטּוּלָא, בִּטּוּי, v. בִּיט׳.

***בִּטְוָיָא** m. pl. (בטי) = h. בָּטַח II, אַבְטַי, *column-like receptacles* (of water). Lev. R. s. 25 (ref. to בטחות, Job XXXVIII, 36, taking ב as a radical letter, 'receptacles of wisdom') מהו בטוחות ב׳ what is battuhoth? Answ. *Bitvaya.* [Ar. reads בטיוטא, taking ב as propos., v. Koh. Ar. Compl. s. v. טיטויא, IV, p. 27. Mat. K. guesses at טויא as a name of *a bird,* as parallel to שכוי.]

בִּטּוּנָא m. (בטן, cmp. Cant. VII, 3) *rounded sheaf, bunch.—Pl.* בִּטּוּנֵי. Hull. 51ᵇ.

בטונין, v. בִּטְנוֹן.

בָּטַח (b. h.; √בט, v. בטי; cmp. רָוַח) *to be at ease, without trouble,* whence *to trust.* Ber. 6ᵇ הו״ל לִבְטוֹחַ וכ׳ he ought to have trusted in the name of the Lord, but did not trust.—Part. pass. בָּטוּחַ *assured.* Y. Naz. IV, end, 53ᶜ.—Lev. R. s. 31 ב׳ שגוזר he may rest assured that &c.; a. fr.

Hif. הִבְטִיחַ *to assure, promise.* Ber. 17ª הבטחה שה׳ the assurance which the Lord has given. Pesik. R. s. 1, beg. אע״פ שמתו המַּבְטִיחִין וכ׳ though those who gave the assurances, the prophets, are dead, but the Lord who promised (through them) is ever-living; a. fr.—*Part. Hof.* מוּבְטָח (=בָּטוּחַ) *confident, sure.* Ber. 4ª מ׳ אני בך וכ׳ I am sure that thou rewardest &c. Ib.ᵇ מ׳ לו may rest assured. Gitt. 58ª מ׳ אני=מוּבְטְחַנִי; a. fr.

בְּטַח I ch. same. Taan. 22ᵇ הואיל וקא ב׳ בע״א since he trusts in idols.

Af. אַבְטַח=preced. *Hif.* Targ. Ruth II, 13.

Ithpe. אִתְבְּטַח *to feel safe.* Targ. Jer. XII, 5.

בָּטַח II, **אַבְטַח (אַבְטַי)** m. (בטח, בטי, v. Ges. H. Dict. s. v. בטח; cmp. מִקְוֶה) *a hollow column-like receptacle of rain water near the house.* [Maim., *a projection in front of the window* to stand upon in climbing.] Ohol. XII, 3 חבטח (Ar. Var. אבטח). Tosef. ib. XIII, 3 אבטי (ed. Zuck. אבטו, corr. acc.). [Cmp. פותי for פותח; טְפֵי IV for טפח.] V. בִּטְוָיָא.

בִּיטָּ׳, בִּטָּחוֹן m. (b. h.; בָּטַח) *trust, faith, hope.* Y. Ber. IX, 13ᵇ bot. יש להם ב׳ there is hope for them (that they will not be punished, if they repent before dying). Sabb. 139ª תלו בִּטְחוֹנָם ב־ they put their trust in &c. Men. 29ᵇ; a. e.

בְּטַט (√בט) 1) (v. בטי) *to swell, burst forth; to shine.* Denom. בּוֹטֵט, בּוֹטְטָא.—2) (=√פט, cmp. בדר) *to tread, to dash to pieces.* Denom. בִּטִּירְטָא.—Cmp. בְּטַשׁ.

בְּטִי, v. בָּאטִי.

בָּטָה, בָּטָא, בטי (b. h.; √בט *to be hollow, to swell;* v. בטן, בטט 1), בטל &c.; v. Ges. H. Dict. s. v.) *to talk inconsiderately, make hasty vows.* Erub. 64ᵇ (ref. to Prov. XII, 18) כל חבּוֹטֶה whoever vows or swears inconsiderately.—Denom. בִּיטּוּי.

בְּטִי f. (v. preced.) 1) *bottom, bathing basin;* v. אַמְבְּטִי.—2) *bottom, depth.* Gen. R. s. 68 Ar. (ed. אמבטי); s. 50; s. 86 (ed. ביטי); v. דְּיוּטָא.

בֶּן ב׳, בַּטִּיחַ pr. n. m. *Ben Battiah,* nephew of R. Johanan b. Zaccai, one of the leaders of the terrorists during the siege of Jerusalem by the Romans. Koh. R. to VII, 11; Lam. R. to I, 5; (Gitt. 56ª אבא סקרא). Kel. XVII, 12.

בְּטִיטָא (בוטיטה) f. (בְּטַט) *cleft, grotto; ruins.* Gen. R. s. 31 בהדא ב׳ דטבריה Ar. (ed. בו׳) in the grotto (or ruins) of Tiberias; cmp. אַלְסִים.—**Pl.* בּוֹטִיטָתָא. Y. Pes. I, beg. 27ª בוטיתא דסדרא רבא (corr. acc.) the ruins of the large colonnade (of Tiberias); cmp. Midr. Till. to Ps. XCIII, s. v. דִּיפְלֵי.

בְּטִיטַיי pr. n. m. *B'titay.* Y. Ber. V, 9ᶜ bot.

בְּטִיל, v. בְּטֵל; בָּטֵיל, v, בְּטֵל.

בְּטִיל m. (בטל) 1) *loose, demoralized* (=בטל מן המצוות). Targ. O. Ex. XXXII, 25 (h. text פרע, v. Rashb. a. l.).—2) *idle, vain. Pl.* בְּטֵלִין, בְּטִילִין. Ib. V, 9. Targ. Koh. V, 2.—3) *idle, resting.* Targ. II Esth. III, 3.—4) *invalid, void,* v. בְּטֵל.

בְּטִילָא f. (בטל; h. בִּיטּוּל) *idleness, loss of time.* Keth. 105ª אגר ב׳ indemnity for loss of time. Ib. קרנא ב׳ דמוכחא (in the case of) Karna, the loss of time was ostensible (i. e. all knew that the fee he took for judging was needed to indemnify him for his loss of time). Y. Ned. IV, 38ᶜ bot. שכר בְּטִילָךְ (in h. phraseol.) indemnity for their loss of time.

בְּטֵין, v. בְּטַן.

בטינין, v. בָּטְנוֹן.

בטינתא, Targ. Jud. XV, 15, v. טִינָתָא.

בָּטֵל I (b. h.; v. בטי) [*to be hollow*]; 1) *to be void, abolished, suspended; to cease to exist.* Keth. 103ᵇ בָּטְלָה קדושה sanctity of life ceased; [oth. opin.: the levitical law concerning the contact with a corpse was suspended in favor of Rabbi; v. Tosaf. a. l.]. Ab. V, 16 ב׳ דבר בָּטְלָה וכ׳ as soon as the (sensual) attraction disappears, love will disappear. Ib. 21 as if dead ועבר וב׳ מן העולם and passed away and disappeared from this world. Y. Meg. I, 70ᵈ top, a. e. בטלה מגלת תענית the *Scroll of Fasts* has been abolished (the festive commemorations enumerated therein are no more observed). Sot. IX, 9 (47ᵃ); a. fr.—2) *to rest from labor, be at ease, be idle.* Ab. IV, 10 אם בָּטַלְתָּ מן וכ׳ if thou choosest not to study the law, there will be many disturbances (excuses) to assist thee. Ib. I, 5 בּוֹטֵל מד״ת he neglects the study of the Law; a. fr.

Nif. נִבְטַל 1) *to be abolished, suspended.* Y. Meg. I, 70ᵈ bot. עתידין לִיבָּטֵל (=לְהִיבָּטֵל) shall in future be abolished (neglected). Gitt. 32ᵃ, v. infra.—2) *to be excused, be exempt.* Ib. II, 16 thou art not a free man לְהִבָּטֵל ממנה so as to be exempt from life's duties.—3) *to remain single.* Gitt. IV, 5 (41ᵇ) יִבָּטֵל shall he never marry?

Pi. בִּטֵּל, בִּיטֵּל 1) *to abolish, suspend, cancel, undo, neglect.* Ab. II, 4 בַּטֵּל רצונך וכ׳ set aside thy will for the sake of the Lord's will, in order that He may set aside the will of others (euphem. for *His will*) for the sake of thy will (withdraw evil decrees at thy prayer). Ib. IV, 9 הַמְבַטֵּל וכ׳ he who neglects the study of the Law on account of his wealth. Sot. IX, 10 (47ᵃ) אַף הוא בִּטֵּל את המעוררין he also abolished (the custom of) the wakers, v. עָרַר. Sabb. 63ᵃ מְבַטְּלָהּ he (the observer of the Law) will cancel it (avert God's evil decree). Mekh. B'shall., Amalek, 2, v. אִיפְּטִירְקוֹס. Macc. 24ᵃ. Ab. Zar. IV, 7 לָמָּה אינו מְבַטְּלָהּ why does He not destroy it (the objects of idol worship)?—Gitt. IV, 1 שוב אינו יכול לְבַטְּלוֹ he can no longer annul it (his letter of divorce). Ib. 2 in former times a man could summon a court in a strange place וּמְבַטְּלוֹ and declare it (the letter of divorce which he had sent off) void. Ib. 32ᵇ אתי דיבור ומבטל דיבור a word (declaration) comes and cancels a word.—Ab. Zar. IV, 4 (42ᵇ) an idolator (gentile) מבטל אליל שלו וכ׳ may (by mutilation &c.) cancel his own or his neigbor's idol (so that it is no longer subject to the law forbidding Jews to derive any benefits from idolatrous paraphernalia), but an Israelite cannot &c. Ib. המב׳ אליל ב׳ וכ׳ in cancelling an idol, one has at the same time cancelled its attachments; a. fr.—ב׳ רשות *to resign possession,* a legal fiction by which the carrying of objects on the Sabbath from one's own place to one common to several persons, may be permitted. Erub. VI, 7 מְבַטֵּל את רשותו he (the brother who forgot to lay the Erub, v. עֵירוּב) must resign his share in the common property. Ib. 68ᵇ מְבַטְּלִין וחוזרין ומב׳ you may resign your share to your neighbor, and then he may resign to you; a. fr.—ב׳ חמץ to renounce (by declaration) the possession of anything leavened that may have remained undiscovered in one's possession. Pes. 6ᵇ הבודק צריך שיְּבַטֵּל after one has searched the house for leavened things, he must renounce (whatever he may have failed to find); a. fr.—*Part. pass.* מְבוּטָּל, f. מְבוּטֶּלֶת. Erub. 69ᵇ רשותי מב׳ לך my possession be resigned to thee (for Sabbath purposes). Gitt. 32ᵃ if a recipient says, מתנה זו מב׳ 'this donation be void', תְּהֵא בְּטֵלָה 'shall be void', opp. to בְּטֵלָה היא 'is a void one', i. e. has been annulled.—Eduy. I, 5; Gitt. 36ᵇ, a. fr. אין ב״ד יכול לב׳ וכ׳ no court can repeal (overrule) the decisions of another court, unless &c.—2) *to neutralize* an admixture of forbidden food &c. in a certain quantity. Hull. 108ᵃ ושאינו מינו ... ומבטלו and the portion of the mixture which is not its kind is prevailing and neutralizes the forbidden portion (as if did not exist at all); a. fr.—3) *to disturb, cause suspense, interfere with.* Erub. 63ᵇ; Meg. 3ᵃ בִּיטַּלְתֶּם וכ׳ ye interfered with the daily offering; a. fr.—Ber. II, 5 לבטל ממני וכ׳ to suspend (shake off) the yoke of heavenly government even one minute.

Hif. הִבְטִיל *to cause interruption, to order suspension.* Succ. V, 5 לְהַבְטִיל את העם וכ׳ to cause the people to cease working.

Hithpa. a. *Nithpa.* נִתְבַּטֵּל, הִתְבַּטֵּל *to be interrupted* &c., v. Nif.—Tan. d'be El. I, 5; II, 3.

בְּטֵיל, בְּטֵל ch. same; 1) as h. Kal 1). Targ. Lam. V, 15; a. e.—Sot. 33ᵃ בטילת עבידתא וכ׳ the decree enforcing idol worship in the Temple has been repealed. Meg. Taan. XI on the twenty second (of Shebat) ב׳ עבידתא was the decree &c. revoked. Sabb. 139ᵃ, Snh. 98ᵃ אי בטלי וכ׳; v. אַמְגּוּשָׁא. R. Hash. 18ᵇ בטילת אדכרתא (Meg. Taan. VII אתנטילת, read אתב׳), v. אַדְכָּרְתָּא; a. fr.—2) as h. Kal 2). Targ. Y. Ex. XVII, 1 [read:] דִּבְטִילוּ אידיהון when their hands were lazy &c.—Part. pass. בְּטִיל *annulled; neutralized* (in a larger quantity, v. preced. Pi.). Hull. 100ᵃ, a. fr. (in Hebr. phraseol.) מין במינו לא ב׳ in a mixture of homogeneous things (of which one is forbidden) the rule of neutralization by quantity takes no effect. Ib. 99ᵃ ברובא ב׳ it is neutralized in any larger quantity (than the forbidden ingredient); a. fr.—Ib. 100ᵃ top ותבטיל, v. Ithpe.

Pa. בַּטֵּיל as h. Pi. Targ. Ps. XXXIII, 10 (some ed. incorr. בְּטִיל); a. e.—Erub. 66ᵇ למאן נִיבַטֵּיל to whom should he resign his right of usage (for Sabbath purposes)? בַּטּוּלֵי . . מְבַטֵּיל לִיבַטֵּיל וכ׳ shall he resign &c.? Ib. 67ᵃ. Pes. 6ᵇ לְבַטְּלֵיהּ let him renounce it (the leavened thing). Ib. ולִיבַטְּלֵיה בארבע let him renounce it at four hours of the day. Gitt. 36ᵇ אֲבַטְּלִינֵּיהּ I would repeal it (that law). Ib. 32ᵃ דבטולי בטליה that he revoked it (the letter of divorce); a. fr.

Af. אַבְטֵיל 1)=Pa. Targ. Y. Gen. VI, 7 אַבְטֵיל I will undo (h. text אמחה); a. e.—2)=h. Hif. Targ. Is. XXX, 11 אַבְטִלוּנָא מ־ make ye us free from tradition.

Ithpe. אִתְבְּטִיל, contr. אִיבְּטִיל. 1) *to be abolished, removed, undone.* Targ. Job XVII, 11; a. fr.—Gitt. 32ᵃᵇ בָּטֵל has two meanings משמע דבטל ומשמע דליבְּטִיל it may mean 'it is void', and may mean 'be it declared void'. Hull. 100ᵃ ותִבְּטִיל ברובא (or ותִבְטִיל) let it be neutralized in the larger mixture; (why is it not &c.?)—2) *to be disturbed, to be forced to be idle.* Targ. Koh. XII, 3; a. e.

בָּטֵל II, בָּטֵיל m. (preced. ws.) 1) *null, void; vain.* Gitt. IV, 1 הוא ב׳ is void (revoked); v. בְּטֵל Ithpe.; a. fr. —*Pl.* בְּטֵלִים, בַּטְלִין, בְּטֵ׳—דברים ב׳ *vanities, absurdities.* Ab. Zar. 16ᵇ; a. fr.—2) *idle, unemployed, not needed.* Snh. 21ᵃ one horse והוא ב׳ when not needed (for war). Koh. R. to VI, 8.—*Pl.* as supra. Y. Meg. I, 70ᵇ bot. עשרה בטילן... לביה״כ (where there are) ten men at leisure for attending Synagogue, v. בַּטְלָן. Ber. 16ᵃ והוא שב׳ ממלאכתן provided they stop working. Ib. 17ᵇ ת״ח ב׳ scholars have to abstain from work; a. fr.—Fem. בְּטֵלָה, בְּטֵילָה. Ab. V, 16, v. בָּטֵל I. Gitt. 32ᵃ, v. בָּטֵל I, Pi.; a. fr.

בַּטָּלָה f. (preced.) *vanity, idleness.* Keth. V, 5 הב׳ מביאה וכ׳ idleness leads to immorality. Ab. III, 4 המפנה לבו לב׳ who turns his mind to vanities. Y. Ber. VI, 10ᵃ bot. להזכיר ש״ש לב׳ to pronounce the name of the Lord for no purpose.—Y. Keth. VII, 31ᵇ bot. דברים של ב׳ useless labors (as carrying water and pouring it out again). Gen. R. s. 91 דבר של ב׳ irrelevant argument. Y. Naz. IV, 53ᵇ על הב׳ for no use. Kidd. 16ᵇ שכר ב׳ compensation for interrupted labor; a. fr.

בַּטָּלוֹן, v. בַּטְלָנוּת.

בַּטְלָן m. (בטל) *unemployed.*—*Pl.* בַּטְלָנִים, בַּטְלָנִין. Snh. 21ᵇ סוסים הב׳ horses not needed for the army. Y. ib. II, 20ᶜ. Meg. I, 3 עשרה ב׳ ten persons having leisure; v. Y. ib. 70ᵇ bot.

בַּטְלָנָא ch. same; *idler, lazy; unemployed.* *Pl.* בַּטְלָנִין. Targ. Ex. V, 8; 17.—בַּטְלָנֵי. Pes. 51ᵇ; 55ᵃ; Ber. 17ᵇ.

בַּטְלָנוּת f., **בַּטָּלוֹן** m. (בטל) *idleness, loss of time.* Treat. Abad. ch. II בַּטְלוֹנוֹ; Sifré Deut. 118 בַּטְלָנוּתוֹ his idleness (during sickness),

בְּטַן, בְּטֵין (v. בטר) *to be pregnant.* Targ. Prov. XXV, 23.—Gen. R. s. 98 (play on *triyah*, Jud. XV, 15, as if τρία, three) בְּטְנָה תרין she was going with two (making together three). Lam. R. to I, 1 רבתי (חד מאת׳ 7). [Targ. Jud. XV, 15 בטינתא, v. בִּינְתָא.]

בֶּטֶן m. (b. h.; v. בטר) *belly.* Nidd. 31ᵇ. Sot. 28ᵃ בִּטְנוֹ וכ׳ the belly of the adulterer; a. fr.

בִּטְנָא ch. f. same. Targ. Jud. XIII, 5; a. e.

בָּטְנַאי *Botnai,* name of a bird. Hull. 63ᵃ.

בִּטְנָה, v. בּוּטְנָא I.—*Pl.* בָּטְנִים, v. also next w.

בִּטְנוֹן m. (בטן) a musical instrument, a sort of *bagpipe;* (oth. opin.) *cittern fastened around the body;* (oth. opin.) *workingman's pinafore.* Kel. XV, 6 (Ar. בטנים, oth. vers. בטינין, בטנינן, v. Ar. Compl. ed. Koh. s. v.).

בָּטְנִי *Botni,* name of a bird. Hull. 63ᵃ (diff. fr. בטנאי).

בָּטְנִית pr. n. *Botnith.* Pes. 57ᵃ Abba Saul ben B.

***בֵּי ב׳ בָּטְנִיתָא** (prob. a geogr. term) (a hen) *of Be Botni.* B. Mets. 86ᵇ זגתא . . . בי ב׳ a black hen &c. [Rashi פטניתא *fattened;* Ar. s. v. זגתא: בדפטמתא, Var. בר פנטיתא, בר פנטיתא; Ms. M. בי פטניתא, Ms. R. 2 בדפטניתא; v. Rabb. D. S. a. l., Koh. in Ar. Compl. l. c.]

בִּטְנָן, v. בּוּטְנָה.

בִּטְרָא (בִּטְדָא) m. (=בֵּי טְרָא, v. עִיטְרָא) *space for spanning one's hand around an object*=h. תְּפִיסָה or אֲחִיזָה. Hull. 50ᵇ.—*Pl.* בִּטְרֵי. Ib. 76ᵃ (ed. ד for ר, as B. Mets. 39ᵇ עיטדא for עיטרא). [Differ. of opin. as to measure: *one finger* or *four fingers.*]

בְּטַשׁ (v. בטט 2) *to tread; to kick, knock down* (with one's foot), *crush.* Targ. Y. I, Ex. XXIV, 10.—Sabb. 116ᵇ אתא חמרא וב׳ לשרגא the ass (offered to the judge as a bribe) came and knocked the (gold) lamp over. B. Kam. 62ᵃ דב׳ בכספתא וכ׳ who kicked the money box aside so that he threw it into the river.

Pa. בַּטֵּשׁ *to stamp.* Targ. II, Esth. III, 8.—B. Kam. 99ᵃ he hired him לְבַטּוּשֵׁי (Rashi a. Ms. R.) for stamping; v. בִּיטְשָׁא.—Transf. *to treat with contempt, sneer at.* Targ. Y. Num. XIV, 9.—Erub. 54ᵃ top. *Shebu. 30ᵇ בטש ביה ואוקמיה לע״ה (Ms. F. only . . אוקמיה) he insulted the ignorant man and made him stand up; v., however, בְּתַשׁ.

Ithpa. אִתְבַּטַּשׁ *to be stamped in, mixed up.* Targ. Y. I, Ex. XXIV, 10.

בִּטְשָׁא, v. בִּיטְשָׁא.

בֵּי 1) (=בְּ־ I) *in, with, at.* Targ. Y. Num. XXII, 28 בי ההיא שעתא at that time. Targ. Cant. I, 9; 13, 14 (ed. Vien. בההיא).—2) (=בין) *between, among.* Sot. 10ᵃ; Meg. 12ᵃ; v. בּוּצִינָא.—Sabb. 109ᵇ בי כיללי (Ms. בכ׳) between the embers; a. fr.—בי שמשי (=h. בין השמשות) during sunset. Ber. 43ᵇ קדושא דבי ש׳ the Kiddush said on Friday night. Keth. 103ᵃ כל בי ש׳ every Friday night.—3) (=בַּר II) *son of;* v. בַּרְבֵּי. Y. Ber. IV, 7ᶜ bot.; a. fr.—4) (=בֵּית) *house of, school of; home, place of* &c. Targ. Job VII, 9; a. e.— . . . תנא דבי ר׳ (sub. תני) a student of the school of R. . . . . taught. Hull. 42ᵃ; a. fr.—Ab. Zar. 6ᵇ בדבי ר׳ או׳ (Ms. M. ב״ר) in (the Boraitha) of the school of R. O. —Yeb. 21ᵇ דבי אימא רבתי one of the family of the grandmother (whether mother's or father's mother). Ib. דבי אבא רבה of the grandfather's family; דבי דודי one of the uncle's relation.—דבי רב the Boraitha of Be Rab (Sifra). Hull. 66ᵃ (v. Rashi a. l.); a. fr.—בי רבנן *college.* Ber. 17ᵃ; a. fr. [For other compounds with בי, v. respective determinants.]

בֵּיָא, בִּיָּא, בִּיָּה, בִּיָּה (בִּיאָה) f. (via, late Gr. βία) *highway, road.* [As regards the import, in the Roman government, of the office of commissioner on highways, v. Sm. Ant. s. v. Via.] Y. Hag. II, 77ᶜ bot.; Midr. Till. to Ps. CXIV, beg.; Yalk. ib. 794; Gen. R. s. 12 (corr. vers. by comparison) אין לך (ניקום ומקום) מדינה ומדינה שאין (לי) לה (איש) אדם ממונה על ב׳ שלו there is not a district (place) which has not an officer appointed over its highways; v. אנגיטוס a. אגדיקוס. Ib. do not read בִּרְיָה

שמו but בִּירָה שמו (Y. l. c. כי יה corr. acc.) (the overseer of) *via* (the maintenance of the world's roads) in His name; cmp. מָקוֹם. [For βία *force*, v. בִּירָא II.]

בִּיאָה II f. (b. h. בִּאָה; בּוֹא) 1) *coming in, entrance.* Men. 4[a]; Sifra Metsor. Neg. ch. IV, Par. 7 (ref. to ושב, Lev. XIV, 39 a. ובא, ib. 44) זו היא שיבה זו היא ב׳ the same rule applies to his coming the second time and to his entering (after a week). Cant. R. to II, 6 (ref. to ביתך . . ., Deut. VI, 10) (on the door post to the right) of thy coming from the street to thy house. Yoma 86[b] ולואי . . . כב׳ oh, that the going out (of office) be (as pure) as the coming into! Ib. sq. ב׳ . . . כיציאה oh, that the coming home (from court) be (as sinless) as the going out (for holding court)! B. Mets. 107[a] ב׳ לעולם birth. Y. Naz. VII, 56[d] top, a. fr. בִּיאַת המקדש entering the Temple. Yoma 53[b] ב׳ ריקנית entering (the Holy of Holies) without incense, i. e. needlessly.—ביאת שמש *sunset.* Ber. 2[a] ב׳ שמשו וכ׳ the sunset of his last day of levitical uncleanness prevents him from &c., i. e. is indispensable for his permission to eat T'rumah, v. מְחַר: a. fr.—*Pl.* בִּיאוֹת. Kidd. 37[b] נאמרו ב׳וכ׳ bibl. passages mentionning entrance into the promised land; a. fr.—2) (v. בּוֹא;=בְּעִילָה) *coition, connection.* Kidd. I, 1; a. fr.—ביאת ערוה incestuous connection. Y. Yeb. II, 3[c] bot.; a. fr.—ב׳ מצוה, v. מִצְוָה.—*Pl.* as supra. Kerith. II, 3; a. fr.—Cant. R. to IV, 12 שתי ב׳ two ways of &c.

***בַּיָּאם**, v. בהם.

ביארי, v. פליא.

בִּיב m. (ביב, v. בָּב) *pipe, gutter, canal.* Erub. VIII, 10 (88[a]). Ab. Zar. III, 4. Gen. R. s. 12 בִּיבָהּ על פתחה its water-spout over its entrance. Ib. בִּיבוֹ man's spout (nose). Ex. R. s. 36 מצא ב׳ he strikes against a gutter; a. e.—*Pl.* בִּיבִים, בִּיבִין. Y. Hag. II, 77[d] bot. במקום ב׳ on a place where there were sewers; Gen. R. s. 1.—Ex. R. s. 6 גורף ב׳ cleaning sewers. Koh. R. to I, 2 בכיבין (corr. acc.)—בִּיבוֹת. B. Kam. 6[a]; 30[a].

בִּיבָא ch. same; *duct, underground walk.* Y. Taan. IV, 68[d] עאל ליה מן ב׳ דמדינתא; (Lam. R. to II, 2 עליל ביה בבובי־ corr. acc.) he came up to him from the duct of the besieged fortress.—[Lam. R. to I, 5 וביבא, v. בִּיבֵי.]

בֵּיבַאי, v. בִּיבַי.

ביבון pr. n. m. Y. Gitt. VII, 48[d] ר׳ ב׳, read as Y. B. Bath. VIII, 16[c] top, בּוּן.

בִּיבֵי (vive) *long live!* Lam. R. to I, 5 ב׳ דומינו וכ׳ Ar. (read דומיני, vive domine imperator) long live my lord the Emperor. [Ed. וביבא מארי אפלטור, Syriac, corr. ביבי.]

בֵּבַי, בִּיבַאי, בֵּיבַי pr. n. m. (b. h., v. Ezra II, 11; Neh. VII, 16) *Bebai.* Shek. V, 1 בן בבי; Yoma 23[a] בי׳. Ib. 34[b] רב ב׳ R. B., an Amora. B. Bath. 36[b]; a. e.—[Y. Maasr. V, 52[a] בעל ביבי, read בֵּבַי q. v.]

***בֵּיבְנֵי** m. (=בי בני, v. בָּנִי) *bath-house.* Y. Ter. VIII, end, 46[c]; (Gen. R. s. 63 בי בני). Y. Sabb. VIII, end, 11[c] גו ב׳ in (the water of) the bath house.

בִּיבָר m. (vivarium, βιβάριον) *vivarium,* an enclosure in which live game, fish &c. (also wild beasts) are kept. Snh. 39[a] לשדיוה לב׳ must be thrown into the vivarium. Ib. שדיוה וכ׳ they threw him &c. but they (the beasts) did not eat him. Bets. 24[a]; a. fr.—*Pl.* בִּיבָרִים, בִּיבָרִין. Ib. III, 1; a. fr. V. בִּיבָרָיָא.

ביברי, Hull. 127[a], read בי ברי, v. בִּירָאִי.

בִּיבְרַיָּא, בִּיבָרַיָּא m. pl. (pl. of vivarium, v. בִּיבָר) *animals kept in the vivarium, game.* Pesik. R. s. 16; Pesik. Eth Korb. p. 58[b]; Yalk. Num. 777; Kings 176; Koh. R. to II, 7 (corrupted צִיב׳, ברב׳ &c.; expl. בַּרְבֻּרִים אֲבֻסִים I Kings V, 3 *chosen, fattened*) מיני ב׳ various kinds of game (deer &c.) from the vivarium. V. בַּרְבְּרַיָּא, end.

בִּידֵר, v. בְּדַר.

בִּידָּא, Pi. of בְּדָא.

בִּידָא m., **בִּידוּ** f. (בְּדֵי I; cmp. בִּדְיָן) *fiction, false report, information.* Y. Sot. IX, 23[c] bot.; Y. Yeb. XVI, 15[c] ואתצידו כולהון מן ב׳ and they were all taken prisoners owing to the information against them. [Rabad Seder hak-Kabb. a. other chroniclers have erroneously ונתלה ר׳ שרירא מידו אחת, read . . . מן בידה or בידו.]

בִּידוּרָא, בִּידוּר, v. בִּדּוּר.

בִּידְיָן, v. בִּדְיָן.

בִּיחוּלְתָּא f. ch.=h. בֶּהָלָה. Targ. O. Lev. XXVI, 16; a. e. (ed. also בַּהוּלְתָּא).

בִּיהוּתָא f. (בהת) *shame.* Targ. II Chr. XXXII, 21, constr. בִּיהוּת; v. בַּהֲתָא.

ביוכא, v. בִּיכָא.

בִּינָא, בִּינוּנְתָּא, בִּינְתָא, בִּינ׳ f. (בין)=בִּינָה *understanding.* Targ. Prov. II, 3; a. fr.

בִּיזָא I, **בִּזָא** m., **בִּיזְתָא** f. (בזי II) 1) *rent, cleft.* Lev. R. s. 19 Ar. [לא] דמי הדין ריסא להדין ב׳ (ed., v. אֲלִיס a. בִּיזְעָא).—*Pl.* בִּיזֵי. B. Bath. 74[a]; Snh. 110[a] אחוי ליה תרי ב׳ Ar. he showed him two clefts in the ground (ed. חזאי תרי ביזעי); Ar. ed. pr. Var. . . . חזאי ביזתא דסליק תננא מינה (Ms. R. בוזתא, v. Rabb. D. S. a. l. note) I saw a cleft out of which smoke rose.—2) *ruin, destruction.* Targ. Is. LX, 18 (h. text שֹׁד); v. next w.

בִּיזָא, בִּזָא II m., **בִּיזְתָא, בִּזְתָא** f.=h. בִּזָּה *dividing; plunder, spoil.* Nah. III, 1. Targ. O. Ex. XV, 9; a. fr.—Lam. R. to II, 13 בערביא וכ׳ in Arabia they call spoil (ביזתא) ăditha (with ref. to אעירך ib.). Cmp. עֲדוּדָה. [Targ. Is. LX, 16 (h. text שֹׁד); v. preced. w.]—Trnsf. בִּיזְתָא *robbed* woman. Midr. Till. to Ps. I, 2 הא ב׳ עלובתא this poor robbed woman; Yalk. Num. 750 (incorr. vers.).

בִּיזָא III m. (בִּיזְתָא f.) (בזז, cmp. בְּזִיזֵי; cmp. שַׁד, שֹׁד) *feeder,* whence *pap, breast.* Targ. Y. Num. XI, 8 (*brisket,* v. בזיזאה; h. text לְשַׁד, cmp. שַׁד).—Y. Kil. I, 27[b] top ליט

'ב' וכ cursed be the breast which nursed such a man.—*Pl.* בִּיזְיָא. Targ. Job XXI, 24 בִּיזוֹי (Var. תדיוהי).—Gen. R. s. 5 'לִיזִיהִין ב' וכ, v. supra; Pesik. Zakh. p. 23[b] (Ar. sing.). Y. Ḥag. II, 77[d] bot.

בִּיזְנָא, v. בִּזְנָא.

בִּיזָה f. (b. h. בִּזָּה; בזז) *spoil.* Num. R. s. 13, end בִּיזַּת הים spoil made at the Red Sea, ב' מצרים made in Egypt; a. e.—*Pl.* בִּיזּוֹת. Lam. R. to II, 13 (ref. to אעידך ib.; cmp. בִּיזְתָא s. v. בִּיזָא II) 'כמה ב' וכ how often did I give you the spoils of your enemies.

בִּיזּוּעַ, בִּזּ' m. (בזע) *rending, rent.* Targ. Joel II, 13. —[ביזועתא, v. בִּיזְעָא.]

***בִּיזְיָא, בִּזְיָא** m. (בזיII) *rag, wreck.* Gen. R. s. 30 ב' סבא old rag (contemptuous designation of an old man).

***בִּיזְיָאה** f. (v. ביזא III) *brisket.* Gen. R. s. 34 Ar. וכבדו ב' דיסקוס נאה (ed. דורון נאה, which is the interpret. of our w. in Ar.).—[The orig. vers. prob. read בביזא נאה על דיסקוס נאה with a fine brisket on a fine plate; v. Yalk. Gen. 60; Ps. 697.]

בִּיזָיוֹן, v. בִּזָּ'.

ביזיונא, v. 'בזיו.

בִּיזְלֵי, בִּזְיָיה m. pl. (בזי II, ל format.) *cuts, rents,* whence *disconnected outskirts* of a community. B. Bath. 68[b] (expl. שרירה) ביזלי. What is bizlé? פיסקי בגי, v. בָּאגָא; Y. ib. IV, 14[c] bot. שורית בזירה (read שְׁרָרָה).

בִּיזְעָא (בִּיזְעָה) בִּיזָעָא m. (בזע) *rent, split, cleft.* Ab. Zar. 70[a] הוה ב' בדשא there was a crack in the door. Cant. R. to IV, 14 (Koh. R. to X, 18 בקיעה), v. אֱלִיס; Lev. R. s. 19, v. בִּיזָא I.—*Pl.* בִּיזְעֵי. Taan. 21[b] דאית ביה ב' ב' Ar. s. v. כסילתא (ed. קרנא דהוה בזיע, Ms. M. v. Rabb. D. S. a. l.), v. פּוּסְלְתָא. Num. R. s. 18 'אזלי וחזאר תרי ב; Snh. 110[a], v. בִּיזָא I.

בִּיזְרָא, בִּיזְרָנָא, בִּיזְרָא, v. 'בִּזְר.

בִּיזְתָא, v. בִּיזָא.

***בִּיזְתָא** pr. n. pl. *Bez'tha* (contr. of בי זיתא Olive-town), near Pumbeditha. Erub. 52[a] 'תהא שביתתי [ב]ב Ar. (ed. בצינתא; Ms. M. בני זיתא read בבי; Ms. O. בוזיתא; v. Rabb. D. S. a. l.) my central point for Sabbath distances be in B.

***בִּיחוּשָׁא**, v. בַּחְשָׁא.

בִּיחֵיל, v. בָּחַל.

ביטא, ביט, Y. Shebu. III, 34[d] bot., read בִּיעָא.

בִּיטָא I (βῆτα) *Beta,* second letter of the Greek Alphabet. Shek. III, 2. Y. ed. (Bab. ב''תא corr. acc.).

בִּיטּוּי, בִּטּוּי m. (בטי) *vain, useless talk,* ref. to vows and oaths which neither benefit nor injure anybody; שבועת ב' a useless oath, contrad. to ש' שוא a false oath or one asserting something impossible. Shebu. III, 9 sq. Ib. 49[b]; B. Mets. 36[a] an oath imposed in court אין בה משום שבועת ב' does not come under the law of vain oaths (as to sacrifices). Ib. ב' שפתים erroneous statement without legal consequences, oppos. to כפירת ממון whereby somebody lost money. [Y. Naz. I, beg. 51[a] שביטוי שבועה, read שְׁבִּיטּוּי.]

בִּיטּוּל, בִּטּ' m. (בטל) *interruption, loss of time; abrogation; relinquishment, renunciation.* Kidd. 33[a] קימה שאין בה ב' rising (in honor of an elder &c.) which causes no interruption of labor.— ב' תורה neglect of the study of the Law. Sabb. 32[b]; a. fr.—Men. 99[a] sq. פעמים שבִּיטּוּלָהּ 'וכ sometimes the neglect of the Law is its establishing. Sabb. XVI, 1 ב' בה''מ neglect of lectures (through reading at home). Y. Peah IV, 18[b], a. e. ב' עניים loss of time to the poor (when compelled to wait for their share in the crop).—Erub. 66[b] ב' רשות, v. בָּטֵל Pi.—Y. Gitt. IV, 46[c] top, a. fr. ב' פריה ורביה neglect of marital life.—Y. Ab. Zar. III, 43[d] bot. יש לה ב' can be cancelled, v. ib. IV, 4 s. v. בָּטֵל Pi.—Pes. 4[b] 'בב' בעלמא וכ a mere relinquishment of possession would be sufficient.; a. v. fr.

בִּיטּוּלָא, בִּטּ' ch. same. Targ. Prov. XV, 22.—Ab. Zar. 53[b].

בִּיטָּחוֹן, v. בִּטָּחוֹן.

בִּיטְּי, v. בְּטֵי.

בִּיטִיתָא, v. בּוּטִיתָא.

בִּיטְנָתָא f. (בטן) *pregnancy, growth of the embryo.* Lam. R. to I, 1 אילין ירחי דב' דילדתא (חד מאת') רבתי 6 (strike out one of the two terms).

בוטשא, בִּיטְשָׁא m. (בטש) *stamping, fulling.* B. Kam. 99[a] (בִּט') 'ב' ב' וכ for every stamping manipulation one M'ah.—*Pl.* בִּיטְשֵׁי Ib. (Var. לבטושי), v. בְּטַשׁ.

בֵּי=בֵּית, v. בַּרְבֵּי.

בִּיָּא I (via), v. בִּיָא.

בִּיָּא II, **בִּיָּה** f. (βία) 1) *force, act of violence, extortion, wrong.* Gen. R. s. 93 (play on *bi,* Gen. XLIV, 18) ב' אתה מעביר עלינו thou passest violence over us (thou treatest us unjustly). Ex. R. s. 20 '. . . ב' וכ שמא do I ever wrong any creature? Deut. R. s. 2 (play on בבאה Ez. VIII, 5) 'הא ב' רבא לעלמא וכ. Oh, this great wrong in this world, v. infra. *Y. Ned. III, 38[a] כן ... כורוסתי ביה that is the way one says to his neighbor (read כריזסתי χαρίζεσθαι βίᾳ) to do a favor perforce (ref. to an invitation accompanied with a vow in case of refusal).—2) interj. (=h. ווי) *woe! help!* Yoma 69[b] 'ב' ב' וכ woe, woe, it is this (the tempter) that destroyed the Temple &c. Yeb. 97[b] 'ב' ב' מאה וכ woe, woe over the brother who is &c. Lev. R. s. 17, end (play on בבאה, v. supra) ב' ב' 'תותבא וכ woe, woe, that the stranger dislodges the owner (idolatry in the Temple).

בייבא, v. בַּיְיכָא.

בייבין, read בייכין, v. בּוּךְ.

בַּיְידָא, v. בַּדָּאָה.

בָּיְיה 1) *road*, v. בִּיָא; 2) *wrong*, v. בִּיָיא.

בַּיְיךְ, v. בּוּךְ.

בַּיְיכָא m. (בוך; cmp. סְבָכָה, סְבָכְתָּא) *net, head-dress.* B. Bath. 146ª 'small presents', תרגמה רבא בייכא וסבכתא Ar. s. v. וייכא (ed. בייבא, Ms. M. ביוב׳, Ms. H. ביוכא, cmp. comment. כגון ב׳; v. Koh. Ar. Compl. s. v.) said R., This means e. g. a net or a cap.

בָּיִיל, v. בִּיל.

ביילין, Tosef. B. Mets. IX, 14, v. בַּיָּרִל.

בַּיִין, v. בִּין ch.

בַּיִיר, בַּיֵּיר, בָּיֵיר, v. בּוּר I h. a. ch.

בַּיָּיר m. (denom. of בֵּיר or בּוֹר, cmp. בּוּר Pi. 2) *superintendent of the well* in rural communities. Shebi. VIII, 5 אין נותנין לא לב׳ וכ׳ (out of the money realized from the fruits of the Sabbath year) you must not pay the well-master &c.; אבל נותן הוא לב׳ לשתות but you may pay the well-master a fee for giving you water to drink. Tosef. B. Mets. IX, 14 הב׳ והבלן וכ׳ (Y. ib. beg. 12ª ed. Krot. הכ׳, corr. acc.) the well-master, the bather &c. when collecting their fees from the owner (individually), may attach only the owner's share in the produces. Ib. VIII, 11ᵈ top שאלה מן הב׳; [Bab. ib. 97ᵇ למישאל מידי מחבריה, read מבַּיָּירָא ch.].

בַּיָּר, בַּיִּיר m. (בּוּר) *untilled, waste ground.* Targ. Deut. XXI, 4 (virgin land, h. text אֵיתָן).—Targ. Is. XXVIII, 25. Targ. Jer. XII, 13 בַּיַּר (!).—Lev. R. s. 1, beg., v. בּוּר ch.

בַּיְישׁוֹנִי, v. בִּישָׁנִי.

ביישא, Y. Bets. I, 60ᶜ bot., read בִּישַׁיָּיא.

בַּיְישָׁן m. 1) (בּוּשׁ) *bashful, chaste; chaste person, bashful man.* Ned. 20ª סימן יפה באדם שהוא ב׳ it is a favorable indication in a man that he is bashful. Ab. II, 5. הב׳ he who is ashamed (to ask questions at school); a. e.—*Pl.* בַּיְישָׁנִין, בַּיְישָׁנִים. Yeb. 79ª. Y. Snh. VI, 23ᵈ בווירשנין (?); Num. R. s. 8; Midr. Sam. ch. XXVIII; Midr. Till. to Ps. I.—2) v. בִּישָׁן.

בַּיְישָׁנִי, בַּיְישָׁנָאָה, v. בישני.

בַּיְיתָא, v. בֵּיתָא I.

בַּיְיתוֹס, v. בֵּיתוֹס.

בַּיָּיתוֹת f. pl. (denom. of בַּיִת) *animals lodged* (at certain seasons) *in sheds within town-limits.* Bets. V, 7 (40ª, Ms. M. ביאתות); Sabb. 45ᵇ; a. e.

*__בִּיכַאי__ m. (v. בּוּכְיָא) name of *a spider.* Tosef. Par. IX (VIII), 6 ed. Zuck. (Var. מובאי corrupt, R. S. to Toh. IX, 2 כובאי).

בִּיכּוּרָה, v. בְּכוּרָה.

*__ביל__ h., Hif. הוֹבִיל *to mix*, v. next w.

בִּיל, בּוּל ch. (cmp. b. h. בָּלַל) *to mix, knead;* trnsf. (cmp. דרש גרס) *to study thoroughly.* Men. 65ª (play on בלשן, Neh. VII, 7; cmp. בלש) הוה בָּיֵיל....ודריש he studied languages and explained them.

*__Pa.__ בַּיֵּיל same; trnsf. *to discuss.* Y. Ab. Zar. III, 43ª מאן דתני אוֹבִיל נייבל (read נְבַיֵּיל) he who reads in the Mish. (III, 5; v. בִּין Hif.) *obil*, means, Let us discuss the subject.

בִּלְגָּה, בִּילְגָּה (b. h.) pr. n. m. *Bilgah*, chief of a priests' division; whence, fem. (sub. משפחת) name of a priests' division, v. מִשְׁמָר. Succ. V, 8 ב׳ לעולם וכ׳ the Bilgah division at all times distributes its shares of the show-bread in the Southern part of the Temple courts. Ib. 56ᵇ; Tosef. ib. IV, 28 בִּילְגָּא ed. Zuck.

בילדין, Targ. Y. II Num. XII, 7, v. לַבְלָר.

בִּילָה f. (=בְּלִילָה, fr. בלל, cmp. נִידָה Lam. I, 8; עִילָה a. עֲלִילָה) *thorough mixture, even distribution of mixed objects.* Zeb. 80ª יש ב׳ a mixture is considered evenly distributed in all its parts. R. Hash. 13ᵇ לכל אין ב׳ none of the mixtures named is a real mixture (of even distribution), except wine and oil (being liquid). Ḥull. 83ᵇ, a. fr. כל הראוי לב׳ וכ׳ wherever from the proportions and properties of the mixture a perfect fusion is possible, the real act of mixing thoroughly is not indispensable.

בילוות, Targ. Job XXXVIII, 37, v. כילוות.

בִּילוֹן, Bekh. VII, 1, v. כִּילוֹן.

בילוניא, v. בְּלִיוֹנָא.

*__בִּילוֹס__ or __כִּילוֹס__, Y. Sabb. VII, 10ᵇ bot. משיח ב׳ (Var. כ׳), read חייב משום לש. [Read the passage as follows: ההן דאגין גידקרין שרי זיפות שרי משריך חייב משום לש —all of which belongs to line 26 fr. bottom.]

בילמי, Pesik. R. s. 21, read צַלְמִי, v. צֶלֶם. [Read: הא ברייה לך חברותך את וחברך בדמותי וצלמי behold, I created for thee thy company; thou and thy neighbor (were made) in my image &c.]

בילן, Bekh. 43ᵇ Ar., v. כִּילוֹן; Kel. XX, 6 Ar., v. וִילוֹן; Targ. Y. Gen. XXV, 25 Ms., Lev. a. oth., v. כִּילָן.

בילני, v. בַּלְנִי.

בילפט, v. בַּלְשְׁפַט.

*__בִּילָּק__ (בָּלָק Ar.) pr. n. m. *Billak*, in conjunction with חִלָּק, חִילָּק, fictitious names for *any men* (similar to our 'Tom, Dick & Harry'). Ḥull. 19ª אנא לא ח׳ וכ׳ I know no Ḥillak and no Billak (I know of no authorities or individual opinions), I only know a tradition. Snh. 98ᵇ ח׳ וב׳ אכלי להו (margin in Ms. M. חלק בלק) shall Ḥ. a. B. (any persons indiscriminately) enjoy it?

בילקאות, Sifré Deut. 36, read בסילקאות, v. בְּסִילְקִי.

בִּילְרִין, v. בּוּלְרִין.

בִּילְתִּין, v. בַּלְתִּין.

בִּימָא, Ab. Zar. 16[b],=next w.

בִּימָה f. (cmp. בָּמָה) *elevated stand for public meetings* (for speakers, readers, holding court &c.). Sot. VII, 8. Succ. 51[b]. Ab. Zar. I, 7 (ib. 16[b] בימא). Gen. R. s. 76 as if seated על ב׳ ודן upon the platform and holding court. Lev. R. s. 13 ונראית כאילו מצעת ב׳ and gives itself the appearance as if holding court (giving the form of legality to robberies). Gen. R. s. 37 ב׳ של רשע the court of injustice (Rome).—Koh. R. to I, 8 (Ab. Zar. 16[b] גרדום; Tosef. Ḥull. II, 24 בָּמָה); a. fr.—*Pl.* (of בימא) בִּימָאוֹת. Pesik. B'shall. p. 84[a] (Ms. O. כסאות; Tanḥ. ed. Bub. B'shall. 5 מגדלים) (wooden) platforms.—בִּימוֹת. Meg. 32[a] הלוחות והב׳ (Ms. M. והבמות; Y. ib. III, 73[d] bot. בימה ולווחין) the tablets (in Synagogues, prob. used for announcements) and the raised seats (for readers or distinguished persons to speak from). [Ar. s. v. במות, ref. to Meg. l. c., explains, לוחות *the board-covers of books*, במות *wooden stands* (עמוד) for exhibiting the Torah scrolls during the services; another opinion quot. in Ar.: לוחות the blank margins between the columns of the scroll, במות the upper and lower as well as the front and back margins; cmp. אריח a. לבנה.] [A derivation of our w. fr. βῆμα is excluded, because the sing., in that case, would be בימא or בימטא a. the pl. בימטין or בימטאות.]

בִּימוֹס, בִּימָס, בִּימָס m. (an adaptation of βωμός, treated in inflection as a cacophemism=בי מיאוס, v. Tosef. Ab. Zar. V, 6, quot. bel., cmp. איצטריא; Syr. בומסא, Ch. בָּמְסָא, בָּמוֹסָא, בִּימְסָא) *pedestal of idolatrous statuary.* Ab. Zar. III, 7 a stone originally hewn לב׳ for an idol's pedestal. Tosef. ib. V (VI), 8 ב׳ שנפגם a broken bomos, (contrad. to מזבח); Bab. ib. 53[b] bot. ב׳ אבן וכ׳ a bomos is made of one stone, an altar of several. Tosef. ib. VI, 10; a. fr.—[Y. B. Mets. X, end, 12[c] העלה על גבי ב׳, read דימוס.]—*Pl.* בִּימָסִ׳, בִּימוֹסִיּוֹת, בִּימוֹסְיָאוֹת, בִּימוּסָאוֹת. Ab. Zar. IV, 6 (53[b]) ב׳ של מלכים (v. Rabb. D. S. a. l., Mish. N. בומסיות) pedestals temporarily put up for the reception of princes (governors). Ib. 54[a] בימסיאות בשעת השמד Ms. M. (v. Rabb. D. S. a. l. note) idolatrous pedestals (or altars) erected during (the Hadrianic) persecution, אע״פ שהשמד בטל איתן הב׳ לא ביטלו although the persecution has been repealed, they (the Romans) have not cancelled these altars; v. בָּטֵל Pi.—Gen. R. s. 53, a. e. (some ed. בִּימָסוֹת) altars. Tosef. Ab. Zar. V (VI), 6 בֵּי מוּסְיָאוֹת ed. Zuck. (Var. בימסיות). [Ab. Zar. I, 7 (16[a]) בימסיות, בימוסיאות, read with Ms. M. a. Ar. דִּימוֹסְיָאוֹת.]

בִּימִי pr. n. m. *Bimi*=אֲבִימִי. Y. Ber. IX, 14[a] top אדא ור׳ ב׳ read: אדא בר ב׳; Y. Taan. I, 64[b] top בר איבומי (איבומ׳); v. Frank. M'bo p. 62[a].

בִּימִין, Yalk. Ps. 670, v. בָּאיִן.

בִּימָס, בִּימָסוֹת, בִּימָסְיָאוֹת, בִּימְסִיוֹת, v. בִּימוֹס.

בִּימְסָא ch.=h. בִּימוֹס. Ab. Zar. 53[b].

בִּין, בּוּן (b. h.; √בה, v. ביא) *to pierce, split, penetrate; whence, to discern, understand;* v. Hif.

**Polel* בּוֹנֵן (cmp. בַּיִן) *to cause to penetrate, to saturate.* Sifra Vayikra, N'dab., Par. 12, ch. XIV (ref. to Lev. II, 13) יכול תְּבוֹנְנֶהוּ from *bammelaḥ* I might judge, 'thou must thoroughly saturate it, ת״ל תמלח therefore it says, 'timlaḥ' (thou shalt strew). Men. 21[a] (quoting Sifra l. c.) מאי תבונהו what does the word *t'bonnehu* mean? Said R. b. U. ה״ק יכול יִתְבּוֹנְנוּ כתבן (taking ת as radical, as if imperat. of a verb תבן, denom. of תֶּבֶן) it means, I might suppose, he must mix it up like straw in clay (v. infra). Said A. to him א״ה יתבוננו מיבעי ליה if so, then it ought to read (in the Sifra) *yithbonennu* (third person). But said A. (taking it fr. בנה) יכול יעשנו כבנין I might suppose, he shall heap the salt upon it like a building (a pile). Said R. to him, א״ה יבננו מיבעי ליה then it ought to read *yibnennu*. But said R. (you must correct the Sifra so as to read) יכול תבינהו (corr. תְּבִינֵהוּ) thou shalt make it savory . . . . . . יתן בו טעם כבינה he shall put a taste into it as does understanding into a man, v. טַעַם. [Yalk. Lev. 454: מאי יתבנהו . . . . יכול יתבלנו כתבן וטיט . . . . תבלנו מ״ל . . . . יכול יעשני כבנין . . . א״ה יבנהו׳ מ״ל . . . יכול תבינהו יכול תבניהו׳ . . . . יכול יתן בו טעם בבינה.—Ar. ed. Koh.: . . . . מאי תבניהו׳ . . . . יכול יתבלנו (הרבה במלח) כתבן בטיט . . . יכול תבינהו יתן וכ׳, correct: יכול יתן בו טעם.]

Hif. *1) הוֹבִין (cmp. הוֹבִיר, s. v. בּוּר) (denomin. of בַּיִן) *to mediate, to be interpreter.* Ab. Zar. III, 5 (45[a]) אני אוֹבִין לְפָנֶיךָ (v. Rabb. D. S. a. l. note 8) let me be thy interpreter (let me explain what you mean) כל מקום וכ׳ (the words על ההרים וכ׳, Deut. XII, 2, are explanatory) wherever thou findest a high mountain &c., know there must be an idol. [In the version אני אחיה אובין וכ׳, אוֹבִין is used as a part. of a verb אָבֵין, denomin. of בַּיִן, to act as a mediator or interpreter.] 2) הֵבִין (b. h.) *to perceive, make intelligible,* esp. *to find analogies* (between two cases). ה׳ דבר מתוך דבר prop. to bring out one thing from between another, i. e. *to form a conclusion by analogy.* Sabb. 31[a] הֲבֵנְתָּה וכ׳ hast thou cultivated thy mind to conclude &c. (ref. to דעת Is. XXXIII, 6). Snh. 93[b] a. fr. Ḥag. II, 1 (11[b]) חכם מֵבִין מדעתו (not יבין, v. Rabb. D. S. a. l. note) a student able to speculate by himself, a thinker.—Ib. 13[a] bot. היה מֵבִין בחשמל speculated over the ḥashmal (Ezek. I, 27); a. fr.

Hithpo. a. *Nithpo.* הִתְבּוֹנֵן, נִתְבּוֹנֵן *to understand one's self, to be careful, to reflect.* B. Kam. 27[b] להתבונן בדרכים to look around on roads (to be prepared for something in their way against which they might strike). Gen. R. s. 34 ויבן כתי׳ נתבונן the word ויבן (he built, Gen. VIII, 20) may be read *vayaben*, i. e. he reflected, argued.

בִּין, בּוּן ch. same; v. infra.—*Pa.* בַּיֵּין, בַּיִּן *to teach, make wise.* Targ. Ps. CXIX, 27. Targ. Job XXXII, 8. Ib. v. 9 יְבִינוּן דינא explain the law (ed. Vienn. יְבִינוּן, Pe., *understand*).

Ithpe. אִתְבַּיַּן *to reflect upon, to understand.* Targ. Job XXXII, 12. Ib. XXVIII, 23; a. fr.

Ithpol. אִתְבּוֹנֵן *to be considerate, cautious.* Lam. R. to ., 16, beg., v. בְּחַי.

בַּיִן m., only in constr. בֵּין, בינת־ (b. h.; preced.; cmp. באירן, בירן) *something split,* or *placed between;* prep. *between, among.*—אין בין...ל־ there is no difference betw. . . . and . . . Meg. I, 5; a. fr.—בין השמשות (abbr. בה״ש) *at twilight, dusk;* v. בֵּי. Ab. V, 6; a. fr.—ב׳ . . . ב׳ . . . *both . . . as well as . . . .* B. Kam. IV, 3; a. fr.—Yeb. 23[a] ב׳ אומרים לו וכ׳ whether the law says to thy father . . ., or &c. Koh. R. to VII, 11 בין ווי לוח וכ׳ owing to the difference between *vay* (woe) and *vah* (ah), R. J. escaped. —דברים שֶׁבֵּינוֹ לְבֵינָהּ private affairs concerning him (the husband) and her (the wife). Ned. 79[b]; a. fr.—*Du.* בֵּינַיִים, בֵּינְתַיִים, בֵּינְתַּיִים (for בֵּינוֹתַיִם) *between two, among, amid.* Gen. R. s. 4 בינייים ובינתיים in the very centre. Y. Ber. II, 5[b] top. Y. Maasr. I, beg. 48[c] טול מבנת׳ take from what is between the two, i. e. qualifications common to both; a. fr.—Constr. בֵּינֵי־. Nidd. 67[b] מפסקת בֵּינֵיהֶן intervening between; a. fr.

בֵּין ch., usu. pl. בֵּינֵי ch. same. Targ. Gen. I, 6; a. fr. —Hull. 114[a]; Sabb. 132[b] אתיא מִבֵּינַיְיהוּ from between the two (from both cases combined) it may be concluded.— מאי בֵּינַיְיהוּ (abbr. מ״ב) wherein do they differ? איכא בינייהו (abbr. א״ב) they differ as to . . . B. Mets. 15[b]; a. v. fr.—ביני וביני a) *in the meantime.* Yeb. 71[b]; a. fr.— b) *the difference between* (these and other goods). Bets. 7[a]; a. fr.—Hull. 47[a] ההוא ב׳ וב׳ a case (of an abnormal lobe) between the normal lungs. [Targ. Am. IX, 9 מִבֵּינָהּ, Var. מבינא, read מִבֵּינֶיהָ from between its meshes.]

בֵּינָא I, בֵּינְתָא f. ch.=h. בִּינָה. Targ. Ps. XLIX, 4. Targ. Job XII, 12; 13; v. בִּיוּנָא.

***בִּינָא II** m. (v. P. Sm. 519) *tamarisk,* (comment.: *willow*). Gitt. 68[b] שורבינא וב׳ (perh. a tautography of שורבינא?).

בִּינָא III m. (בַּיִן, cmp. בֵּין) *a thin thing, hair;* ב׳ דמיא (cmp. נִימָא) *leech. Pl.* בִּינֵי. Gitt. 69[b]. [Sabb. 67[a], v. בִּינִיתָא I a. II.] Cmp. בִּינִיתָא.

בִּינָה f. (b. h.; בין) *intelligence, wisdom.* Nidd. 45[b] (play on ויבן, v. בִּין Hithpa.) the Lord has given to woman ב׳ יתירה greater (earlier maturity of) judgment. Ber. 10[a] במקום ב׳ at the place of understanding (near the heart); a. fr.

בֵּינוֹנִי m. (בין) *central, mean* (between extremes), *average.* Y. Sabb. I, 2[d] bot. לא לח וכ׳ neither wet, nor dry, but between the two (moist). אדם ב׳ a man of average strength. Y. Ber. I, 2[c] bot.; a. fr.—Sot 42[b] ב׳ שבאחיו the middle betw. his brothers (the third of five). —*Pl.* בֵּינוֹנִים, בֵּינוֹנִיִּים. Lev. R. s. 30 בֵּינוֹנֵי המדינה people of the middle class, opp. גדולי; Koh. R. to IX, 7 הבינונים; Tanḥ. Emor 22 ברווני (corr. acc.). R. Hash. 16[b] ב׳ those between the very good and the very bad; a. fr.—Fem. בֵּינוֹנִית. Gitt. V, 1, a. fr. (sub. שדה) *a field of average fertility;* betw. עידית a. זיבורית.—Y. Taan. I, 64[a] bot. הב׳ the intermediate rainy season.—Y. Ber. V, 9[c] bot. there are three things of which too much or too little is obnoxious וּבֵינוֹנִיתָן יפה but a reasonable quantity good. Kel. XVII, 7; a. fr.—*Pl.* בֵּינוֹנִיּוֹת. Ib. 10 היו ב׳ were mean cubits; Y. Shek. VI, 49[d] top הוא כבניינות; Y. Sot. VIII, 22[c] bot. בבינויות (corr. acc.).

בֵּינוּתָא' f.=בִּינָא I. Targ. II Esth. I, 2, beg. בינות ליבא.

בִּינְזָא pr. n. m. *Binza.* Bets. 28[b] (Ms. M. בּיסנא; v. Rabb. D. S. a. l. note).

בֵּינֵי, v. בֵּין ch.

בִּינֵי pl. of בִּינָא III, a. of בִּינְתָא.

בֵּינִים, בֵּינַיִן, בֵּינַיִין m. pl. (בין) *intervals,* empty spaces between the rows of vine. Y. Kil. IV, 29[c] top (R. S. to Kil. IV, 5 בינים). Ib. beg. 29[a], v. בַּרְמוֹן. Cmp. בְּתְוָותָא.

בִּינְיָן, בִּינְיָין, v. בִּנְיָן.

בִּינִיתָא f. (cmp. בִּינָא III; P. Sm. 520) *binitha;* 1) *a small fish* (collect.). B. Kam. 19[b] חמרא דאכל ב׳ an ass that swallowed fish (something unusual). B. Mets. 79[b] bot. ב׳ אכרסה תקלא according to the size of its belly is the weight of fish (if you buy by weight, have the belly first removed; diff. in Ar.). Ib. 59[b] bot. (prov.) if one has a hanged one in his family, say not in his presence זְקוֹף בי׳ hang the fish up; Yalk. Ex. 349 בינתא (corr. acc.); ib. Lev. 617 בְּנִיתָא. Gitt. 69[b] (masc.!) ניתי ב׳ וכ׳ let him take fish and roast it in the smithy.—Bets. 28[a] שב בְּנִיתָא (Var. בִּינְיָיתָא pl., נוניתא, v. Rabb. D. S. a. l. note 9). —2) name of a worm. Macc. 16[b] ב׳ דבי כרבא (Ms. M. מניתא) a worm found between cabbage. [Sabb. 139[b] ב׳ some ed., v. צינריתא.]—3) *hair;* v. בִּינְתָא II.

***בִּינְכָא** transp. of בֵּי כְנָא=בִּיכְנָא, v. כַּנָּא a. כַּנְתָא. Cmp. Syr. בונכא=בוכנא P. Sm. 465; 471.

***בינכי,** Y. Taan. III, 66[c] bot., read בִּינְנָא (?).

בֵּינַת, בֵּינֹת, v. בַּיִן.

בִּינְתָא *understanding,* v. בִּינָא I.

בִּינְתָא I f. collect. noun, or בִּינָתָא pl. (v. בֵּינַת) *the inside part,* whence *the kernel* of seeds. B. Bath. 18[b] bot. אי בב׳ as to the grains (of mustard). Gitt. 69[b] ניזדהר מב׳ let him guard against swallowing the seeds. Sabb. 67[a] בִּינֵי כמונא Ms. M. (ed. בוני) cumin seeds.

בִּינְתָא II (בִּינִיתָא Ar. s. v. בין 2) f. (v. בִּינָא III) *thread, a single hair,* (collect.) *hair.* Targ. Jud. XX, 16 בִּינַת שערא.—Sabb. 140[a] מב׳ דראשי from the hair of my head. Naz. 39[a] עיקבא דב׳ the root of the hair, רישי דב׳ the top of &c.—Yoma 69[b] אשתמיט ב׳ וכ׳ (Ms. M. בניתה) a hair of his beard fell out. Ber. 8[a] כמשחל ב׳ וכ׳ (ed. בניתא) as easy as taking a hair out of the milk.—*Pl.* בִּינֵי. Sabb. 67[a] seven cumin seeds (v. preced.) and ז׳ ב׳ מדיקנא seven hairs from the beard.—בִּינָתָא. Targ. Job IX, 17 חוטר ב׳ (h. text שְׂעָרָה!).

בֵּינָתַיִם, v. בַּיִן.

בִּיסָא c. (=בֵּי עִיסָא) *basin for kneading* the meat-offering. Men. 7a; 24ab. Ib. 57b ב׳ למילש ביה a basin in which to knead.

ביסא pr. n. m. Y. Gitt. IV, 46a top, read נִיסָא.

ביסי *thorns* (Ar.), v. בִּיסָא.

***בִּיסִי** f. (בוס, v. בְּסִיסִי) *tray for wine cups.* Lam. R. to III, 17 מן כל ב׳ וב׳ וכ׳ Ar. (ed. פטים) from each tray (which was handed around) one cup.

בִּיסֵּם *Pi.* of בָּסַם. [Freq. incorr. for בִּיסֵּס, v. בָּסַס.]

בִּיסְמָן, v. בוּסְמָן.

בִּיסְנָא pr. n. m. *Bisna.* Keth. 100a; a. e. V. ברנזא.

בִּיסְתַּרְקָא, בִּסְ׳ c. (=בֵּי אִסְתַּרְקָא, Ithpe. noun of סרק) *receptacle of hackled or hatcheled wool,* whence *mattress, cushion.* B. Kam. 117a חד ב׳ Ms. R. (ed. חדא fem.).—*Pl.* בִּיסְתַּרְקֵי, בִּסְ׳. Targ. Y. Deut. XXXIV, 6 בב׳ מילת (not כב׳) with fine woolen mattresses.—B. Kam. l. c. Bekh. 8b. Taan. 21b bot. מאיך להו ב׳ Ar. (ed. מך) laid down before them mattresses (to sleep on). Yeb. 63a. Snh. 95a. B. Bath. 58a (=חביתא דאודרא in an enigma).

בִּיעַ m. *rejoicing;* v. בּוּעֲתָא II. Targ. Is. XVI, 10; a. e. (Var. בְּיַע incorr.).

בִּיעָא (בִּיעָא), part. f. of בּוּעַ.

בֵּעֲתָא, בֵּיעֲתָא, בֵּיעָה, בִּיעָא f. ch. (=h. בֵּיצָה; בוע) *egg.* Targ. Job VI, 6; a. fr.—Y. Ned. III, 38a top (Y. Shebu. III, 34d bot. סגין, corr. acc.) כגון ב׳ ומרגליתא as e. g. one swearing of an egg that it was a pearl (as an instance of שבועת שקר). Yoma 69b ב׳ בת יומא a fresh egg of the same day; a. fr.—*Pl.* בֵּיעִין, בֵּיעַיָא, בֵּיעֵי, בֵּע׳. Targ. O. Deut. XXII, 6 (Y. ביעיין); a. fr.—Keth. 61a top. Bets. 6b sq. ב׳ דפחיא the eggs of a cackling hen, opp. those found in the killed hen. Ib. ב׳ דדיכרא eggs from a hen impregnated by a cock, opp. ב׳ דספנא מארעא by friction on the ground. Hull. 93a ב׳ חשילתא, v. חֲשִׁילָא. Sabb. 109a ב׳ פיעפועי beaten eggs.—Lev. R. s. 16; a. fr.—זבן בכל בֵּיעֲתָא to buy (the hen) with all the eggs, i. e. to do a thing thoroughly. Lev. R. s. 11; Ruth R. (introd.) to I, 2; Esth. R. beg. ביתא (corr. acc.); v. בֵּיצָה.

בִּיעוּט m. (בעט) *stamping, kick.* B.Kam. 19a. [Targ. Is. LXIII, 3, v. בְּעוֹט.]

בִּיעוּר m. (בער) *removal.* Maas. Sh. V, 3; Shebi. VII, 1, a. fr. (removal of the fruits of the third and sixth years of the Sabbath period).—ב׳ חמץ, v. בָּעַר Pi.—*Pl.* בִּיעוּרִין. Y. Hall. IV, 60a bot. לב׳ as to laws of removal of fruits.

בִּיעוּרָא ch. 1) same. Pes. 6b.—2) *clearing, taking off the last olives.* Targ. Is. XVII, 6; XXIV, 13 (h. לֶקֶט).

בִּיעוּתָא m. (v. בִּיעֲתוּתָא) *fright.* Targ. Job VI, 4; a. e.—*Pl.* בִּיעוּתִין. Targ. Is. XXI, 4; a. e.

בִּיעֲתָא, בֵּיעֲתָא, בִּיעֲתָא *egg,* v. בֵּיעָא.

בִּיעֲתָא *rejoicing,* v. בּוּעֲתָא II. Targ. Ps. XXXII, 7.

בִּיעֲתוּתָא f. (בעת;=b. h. בְּעָתָה) *fright,* v. בִּיעוּתָא. Pes. 3ab ב׳ דגמלים fear of falling down from the camel's back; ב׳ דלילא fear of the night. Sabb. 41a ב׳ דנהרא fear of being drowned. Gitt. 68b הוה ליה ב׳ מיניה he was afraid of him. Sot. 20b fear (פחדא) detains the blood (menstruation), ב׳ וכ׳ sudden fright loosens (produces menstruation). Nidd. 71a.

***בִּיץ**, pl. בִּיצִים Mus., v. הֵינֵץ. Y. Kidd. I, 58d.

בִּיצָא, pl. בִּיצִין, v. בִּצָּא.

בִּיצָה *swamp,* v. בִּצָּה.

בֵּיצָה f. (b. h.; בוץ, בִּצְבֵּץ) 1) [*the bubbling,*] *egg.* Bets. I, 1; a. fr.—Sabb. VIII, 5 (80b) ב׳ קלה a light (easily boiling) egg.—2) *an egg-shaped object, ball, lump.* Ib. בֵּיצַת הגיר Ar. (ed. הסיד) cement (lime) in a lump; Tosef. ib. VIII (IX), 20 בזמן שביצה, Var. שהיא כביצה, when it is as compact as a ball, opp. חבוט.—Par. V, 6; Lev. R. s. 23, end ביצת היוצרים the potter's lump of clay. —3) trnsf. *germ, root,* esp. קעקע ב׳ to stamp out, *to exterminate* (the last germ). Y. Ab. Zar. IV, 44a top. Lev. R. s. 26. Ib. s. 11; Ruth R. (introd.) to I, 2; Esth. R. beg.; v. בֵּיעָא pl.—4) *Betsah,* name of a Talmudic treatise, beginning with that word (in Tosefta יום טוב).—*Pl.* בֵּיצִים, בֵּצִים, constr. בֵּיצֵי. Sabb. VIII, 5; a. fr.—Ab. Zar. 3b; a. e. ביצי כנים, v. כִּינָה.—Y. Snh. XI, 30b bot., [read as] Cant. R. to II, 5 פתפותי בצים הם כאן scrambled eggs are here, i. e. confusion of persons. Y. Shebi. V, 35d bot. עשה ביצים a. עשה ביצה if the leek has formed bulbs. Ib. VII, 37b bot. ביצי נץ חלב, v. חַלְבְּצִין.

בִּיצּוּעַ m. (בָּצַע) *adjustment, compromise* (usually פְּשָׁרָה). Snh. 6a. Y. ib. I, 18b; a. e.—[*Pl.* בִּיצּוּעִין, v. בְּצָעָה.]

בִּיצוּעָא, בִּיצָעָא m. (בְּצַע) *piece, morsel, crumb.*—*Pl.* בִּיצְעֵי, בִּיצּוּעֵי, בִּיצּוּעִין. Targ. O. Lev. II, 6; a. e.—Sabb. 140b לא ליבצע ב׳ he must not eat it by morsels (but enough at a time). Succ. 26a תרתי או תלת ביצעי Ms. M. (ed. ביעי, v. Rashi a. l.) two or three morsels.

בִּיצּוּר (בָּצַר Pi.) *besieging,* trnsf. (by play on בָּצַר Ps. XVIII, 7) *beseeching, entreaty.* Deut. R. s. 2, beg. (in Yalk. Sam. 157 our w. omitted; Yalk. Deut. 811 בצר).

בִּיצּוּרְתָּא, v. בְּצוּרְתָּא a. בְּצוֹרְתָּא.

בִּיצְיָאתָא pl. of בִּיצִיתָא.

***בִּיצִירְתָּא** f. of בְּצִיר, *the lowest.* ~~Targ. Y. Ex. XI, 5.~~

בּוּצִית, בִּיצִית f. (v. בִּצָּה) *dyke-boat, lighting boat,* Babylonian name for Palestinean הוּגִית. B. Bath. 73a; Tosef. ib. IV, 1 בוּ׳; Y. ib. V, beg. 15a בי׳ (v. Rabb. D. S. to B. Bath. l. c., note 5).

בּוּצִיתָא, בִּיצִיתָא ch. same. *Pl.* בִּיצִירָתָא, בִּיצְיָאתָא, בוּ׳. B. Bath. 73a ed. בו׳ (Ms. M. בי׳, Ar. בוציריתא); Sabb. 101a בי׳ דמישן the canal boats of Meshan.

בִּיצְעָא, pl. בִּיצְעֵי *morsels*, v. בִּיצּוּעָא.

בִּיצְעֵי, בִּיצְעִין *ditches*, v. בִּצְעָה.

בִּיצַּרְתָּא, v. בַּצּוֹרְתָא.

***בִּיקָא** m. (בקק) *incisions in muddy ground.* Sabb. 147ᵃ bot. Ar. s. v. פלם (Ms. O. בוקא, ed. פיקא), v. פילומא.

בִּקּוּעַ, בִּיקוּעַ m. (בקע) 1) *splitting, chopping.* Kel. XIII, 3 בית ב׳ that part of the spade (or shovel) which is used for chopping. Ib. XXIX, 7; Y. Meg. I, 71ᵇ top קרדום של ב׳ an axe for chopping, opp. של ניכוש (a hoe) for weeding; Y. Ned. IV, beg. 38ᶜ קורדום של בקער (corr. acc.).—2) (v. בָּקַע) *trimming the* (olive) *tree.* Sifra B'har, beg.

בִּיקּוּר m. (בָּקַר) 1) *examination, investigation.* Pes. 96ᵃ; Arakh. 13ᵇ; Men. 49ᵇ צריך ב׳ requires examination (as to physical defects). Hull. II, 3 (32ᵃ) כדי ב׳ as much time as the examination (of the slaughtering knife) requires; ib. 9ᵃ; [ib. 32ᵃ ביקרו של חכם, read ביקור חכם or בִּיקּוּרוֹ של]. Kerith. 11ᵃ (ref. to בִּקֹּרֶת Lev. XIX, 20) בב׳ תהיה she must first be examined (whether she can endure the punishment required by law).—2) *visiting* (the sick), *visit.* Ned. 39ᵇ ב׳ חולים אין וכ׳ the duty of visiting the sick knows no limits (of time or rank). B. Mets. 30ᵇ; a. fr.

בִּק׳, בִּיקּוֹרֶת f. (b. h. בִּקֹּרֶת, v. preced.) 1) *examination, assessment.* אגרת ב׳ a public announcement inviting buyers to examine the property assessed, i. e. *an announcement of public sale*=אַכְרָזָה. Keth. XI, 5 (99ᵇ); a. fr.—V. אִגֶּרֶת. —2) (b. h. *punishment*). Kerith. 11ᵃ (ref. to Lev. XIX, 20) ב׳ תהיה מלמד שהיא לוקה there shall be *bikkoreth*, this teaches that she shall be lashed. ומינייןְ דהדין ב׳ לישנא וכ׳ how do we know that this bikkoreth has the sense of chastisement? Answ. תהא בקריאה... Rashi (ed. בקראי) she shall have the Bible verses read to her (as customary when chastising in court, v. Macc. III, 14); oth. homilet. interpret. בביקור תהא, v. preced. [Tosef. M. Kat. II, 11 ביקורת ed. Zuck., v. בִּקְרוּת.]

בִּיקְיָא f. (vicia, βίκιον) *vetch.* Y. Maasr. V, end, 52ᵃ. Tosef. ib. III, end בִּקְיָא. Y. Hall. IV, 60ᵇ בִּקְיָיה.

ביקעי, Y. Ned. IV, beg. 38ᶜ, v. בִּיקּוּעַ.

ביקרא, Ab. Zar. 28ᵇ, v. בַּרְקָא II.

בִּיקְתָא, v. בִּקְתָא.

בִּיר m. (=בַּר) *son.* Targ. Y. Ex. I, 15; a. e.—Ber. 5ᵇ; B. Bath. 116ᵃ this is the bone (tooth) דעשיראה ב׳ of the tenth son (that died).—*Pl.* constr. בִּירֵי. Targ. Y. Num. XXXIII, 31 sq. ב׳ עקתא (h. text. בני יעקן!).

בֵּירָא, בֵּיר c. ch. 1)=h. בְּאֵר. Targ. Gen. XVI, 14; a. e. Ber. 56ᵃ. מיבעי עסקך כי הני מידי דנפל לב׳ Ms. M., thy goods will be sought for like something fallen into a well (i. e. thy business will thrive; diff. vers. in ed. a. Mss., v. Rabb. D. S. a. l. note). Sabb. 66ᵇ נפל פותא לב׳ Dyer's Madder, as a remedy, has fallen into the pit (is not practiced). B. Kam. 92ᵇ (prov.) ב׳ דשתית וכ׳ cast no stone into a well out of which thou once didst drink (never despise what once benefitted you).—Hull. 106ᵃ בַּת בֵּירְתָא a little gutter fed by a well.—*Pl.* בֵּירֵי, בֵּירִין. Targ. Gen. XXVI, 15; a. e.—2) (=h. בּוֹר) *pit, hole.* B. Mets. 85ᵃ ב׳ מליא וכ׳ . . . the cavity (created by the taking out of a radish) stood full of water; [Ms. M. כי ב׳ דמיא like a well; v. Rabb. D. S. a. l. note].—*Pl.* as above. Targ. Gen. XIV, 10 (h. text בֶּאֱרוֹת); Gen. R. s. 42.—Snh. 7ᵃ (prov.) שב ב׳ וכ׳ seven pits are open for the righteous man (and he escapes), and one for the evil-doer (into which he falls). Sabb. 110ᵇ. —3) בֵּירָא pr. n. pl. *Bera* (prob. ident. with בֵּירַאי 2, a), native place of R. Simlai. Y. Taan. II, 65ᵈ bot. ר׳ ש׳ דב׳; Y. Meg. I, 72ᶜ bot. דב׳; Koh. R. to III, 14 דבורויירא דיב׳ (corr. acc.).

בֵּירָאָה, בֵּירָיָיה m. (v. next w.) *of Berai*, surname of Ulla. M. Kat. 26ᵃ; a. fr.—Y. Meg. II, 73ᵇ; Y. M. Kat. III, 83ᵇ bot. בֵּירָיָא.

בֵּירִי, בֵּירְיוּי, בֵּירַאי f. (denom. of בְּאֵר, בֵּיר) 1) *watering station*, esp. in Palestine for Temple pilgrims.—*Pl.* בֵּירָיוֹת, בֵּירָיִיוֹת, בֵּירָאוֹת. Erub. II, 1; a. fr. Y. ib. 20ᵇ top לבירייות ולא לבירות (read לבירויי׳ ולא לבירות) for watering stations but not for cisterns; v. Bab. ib. 18ᵃ.—2) pr. n. pl. *Berai* or *Beri*; a) in Galilee. Yeb. 83ᵇ. B. Mets. 84ᵇ בני בירי the inhabitants of B. (Ms. M. בני בר מריון). Y. Pes. IV, 30ᵈ top. Y. Shebi. VI, 36ᶜ top ביריי רבתא (a border-town); (v., however, Hildesh. Beitr. z. Geogr. p. 21).—b) *B.* or *Be-B.* in Babylon, native place of Ulla, R. Dostai, a. oth. Ab. Zar. 40ᵃ. Erub. 56ᵃ מולייתא דבי בי׳ וכ׳ the ascents between Berai a. Narash. Sot. 10ᵃ בי באדר. Erub. 45ᵃ בירי. [Hull. 127ᵃ ביבירי דנרש, read בי בירי ונרש.]

בירבלין, read כּוּרְבְּלִין.

בִּירָה f. (b. h.; ברר, as בִּילָה fr. בלל; cmp. בִּירִית) *cut off, surrounded*, whence 1) *castle, fort.* Gen. R. s. 39; a. fr.—2) *a group of buildings forming one residence.* B. Bath. 61ᵇ בית בב׳ גדולה a house in a large residence (court). Bets. 25ᵃ במפיחין ובב׳; (ib. 24ᵃ בכ׳ בבירות); v. מפיח I, 2.—3) (=בית הבחירה, I Chr. XXIX, 1; 19) *the chosen Divine residence, Temple.* Zeb. 119ᵃ והא בעי ב׳ does it not require a chosen residence (Deut. XII, 18)? Y. Pes. II, 35ᵃ top כל הר וכ׳ the whole Temple mount is named Birah; Pesik. R. s. 14. Zeb. XII, 5 (104ᵇ) בבית הב׳; v. Gem. a. l.—Yoma 9ᵇ עידיכם הב׳ your witness is the Second Temple (which has not been rebuilt; Y. ib. I, 38ᶜ bot. הבחירה). Ed. VII, 3 בִּירַת הפליא (Ms. M. הפליי׳) Fort Haflaya (?).—*Pl.* בִּירוֹת. Bets. 24ᵃ, v. supra. Zeb. 119ᵃ שלש ב׳ וכ׳ there are three Divine residences, Shiloh &c. Ch. בִּירְתָא.—Denom. בִּירוֹן.

בירן, Y. Pes. IV, 30ᵈ top, read בֵּירַי, v. בֵּירַאי.

בִּרְוָן, בִּירְוָון f. pl. *cypress trees*; sing. בְּרוֹתָא, v. בְּרָתָא.

בֵּירוּלִין m. (βηρύλλιον) *beryll*, a precious stone. Targ. Job XXVIII, 16. Ib. 18 (some ed. בֵּירוּצִין q. v., Ms. Var. פֵּירוּצִין). Targ. Y. II Ex. XXVIII, 19 בירזלין (corr. acc.). V. בֵּירְלָא.

בִּירוּס m. (birrus, βίρρος) *birrus*, a travelling cloak, v. בִּרְסִין. Tosef. Meg. IV (III), 30 כירוס, כידוס (corr. acc.).

בֵּירוּץ, בִּירוּץ, בֵּרוּץ m. (ברץ) *heaping, crowding. Pl.* בֵּירוּצִים, בֵּירוּצִין, בֵּר׳. Men. 88ª ב׳ or בֵּירוּצֵי המדות the quantities which remain, when filling from a brimful measure into smaller ones. Y. Shek. IV, 48ª bot. לב׳ goes to the collection of &c. Ib. בירוצי לח the remnants of the overflow of liquids, ב׳ יבש those of dry things emptied over.

***בֵּירוּצִין** m. ch. (Æthiop. אבן ברד, v. Ges. H. Dict. s. v. גָּבִישׁ) *chrystal*. Targ. Job XXVIII, 18; v. בֵּירוּלִין.

בֵּירוּר, בִּירוּר, בֵּרוּר m. (ברר) 1) *clearness, correct sense.* Yalk. Ps. 658 ב׳ של הלכה (cmp. בּוֹרִי) the true sense of the law.—2) *Pl.* בֵּירוּרִין, בֵּר׳ *arbitration.* B. Mets. I, 8, a. e. שטרי ב׳ documents referring to the choice of arbiters, v. קוֹמְפְּרוֹמִיסִין; [anoth. opin. ib. 20ª שטרי טענתא records of evidences, minutes of court proceedings].—3) בֵּרוּרֵי המדות *exact account of wine measures*, whence, *the surplus in the shopkeeper's wine account* arising from measuring quickly and not allowing the wine to settle in the measures. Bets. III, 8 (29ª) ed. (properly omitted in Ms. M., v. Rashi a. l.; Var. in Rashi Ms. בֵּרוּצֵי). Ib. 29ª three hundred *gereb* (v. גרב) of wine מב׳ המ׳ from the surplus found in his account.

בֵּירְזְלִין, v. בֵּירוּלִין.

בִּירַי, v. בִּירָאִי.—[בִּירִי, Hull. 139ᵇ, v. בִּירִי I.]

בִּירְיָא I, v. בִּירִיתָא a. בִּירְיָה.

בִּירְיָא II m. pl. (βίῤῥια, pl. of βίῤῥιον) *birrus*, a kind of cloak, v. בִּרְסִין. Y. Kil. IX, 32ᵈ top quoted in R. S. to Kil. IX, 7 (ed. בריה, corr. acc.).

בֵּירִיאתָא, v. בֵּירוּתָא.

בִּרְיָה, בִּירְיָא f. *creature*, v. בְּרִיָּה.

בֵּירְיוֹן, בֵּירְיוֹנָא m. *palace-guard*, v. בֵּר׳.

בִּירַיִי, v. בִּירָאִי.

בִּירְיִי pr. n. m. *Biryi*, an Amora. Y. Ter. X, 47ᵇ bot. (Hull. 98ª ביריים). Y. Pes. II, end, 29ᶜ (Asheri to Pes. II, s. 13, quotes פראי).

בִּירְיָיה, v. בִּירְאָה.

בִּירְיִים, v. בִּירְיִי.

בירייתכון, Y. Snh. II, 20ᵃ top, read בּוֹרְיֵיכוֹן, v. בִּרְיָיא.

בֵּירֵישָׁא pr. n. pl. *Beresha* (prob. Baris), in the territory of Ruben. Targ. Y. Num. XXXII, 37 (h. text קריתים).

בֵּירִית or **בּוּרִית** f. (בָּרָה, cmp. בְּרִית) *something cut out; ring, hoop.* Tosef. Kel. B. Mets. V, 7 כל הבורית טהורה בְּרִית מחרישה טמאה ed. Zuck. (Var. בורות, בירית) every thing cut in circular form is clean (not susceptible of levitical uncleanness), except the hoop of the plough (cmp. חתיכה ibid.).—Esp. *knee-band, garter.* Sabb. VI, 4. Ib. 63ᵇ ב׳ of the Mishnah is the Biblical אצעדה. Y. ib. VI, 8ᵇ בר׳ כל שהיא וכ׳ it is called *birith* when single, *k'balim*, when the two bands are coupled with a chain. [Ar. ed. Koh. ב׳, oth. ed. בְּרִית. Cmp. Assyr. *birîtu* chain, Schr. KAT 542.]

בִּירְכָא, בִּירְכְּתָא, v. בִּרְכָא, בִּרְכְּתָא.

בִּירְכָּא *knee, shoot*, v. בְּרֵךְ.

בֵּירְלָא, בּוּרְלָא m. (βήρυλλος) *beryll*, a precious stone, prob. the *Chrysoberyll* or *yellow emerald* (h. שֹׁהַם). Targ. O. Ex. XXVIII, 9; 20; a. e.—Targ. Cant. V, 14 (some ed. בְּרְלָא).—*Pl.* בּוּרְלִין. Targ. Esth. I, 4.—V. בֵּירוּלִין.—Targ. Y. Ex. XXXIX, 13 בּוּרְלַת חַלָּא sand-colored beryll. Ib. (I) XXVIII, 20 ובירלוות חלא, prob. to be read בירולין דחלא; Ib. (II) בדולחא (corr. acc.). [Ex. R. s. 38, end פראלוקין, prob. a corrupt. of our w., cmp. LXX].

בִּירָם pr. n. pl. *Biram*, also called *Beth Baltin*. R. Hash. 23ᵃᵇ, a signal station for announcing the New Moon (betw. Syria and Mesopotamia, Neub. Géogr. p. 354). Kidd. 72ª.—Snh. 108ª ועינא רבתי דב׳ Ms. M. (ed. ועינה, corr. acc.) the Great (hot) Spring of B.; v. Hildesh. Beitr. z. Geogr. p. 29, note 206.

בִּירָנִין, v. בִּירָנְתָא.

בִּירָנִית f. (b. h.; denom. of בִּירָה) 1) *castle, palace.* Pes. 118ᵇ (Ms. M. 2 בירה).—*Pl.* בִּירָנִיּוֹת Ibid. (description of Rome; v. Rabb. D. S. a. l. for Var. Lect.).—2) (cmp. בִּירְיוֹן) *a palace-woman, court-lady.*—*Pl.* as supra. Lev. R. s. 19 הושיב ב׳ וכ׳ (Yalk. Kings 249 נשים ב׳) he placed court ladies in Jerusalem (forced them to leave home and serve at the palace); מהו ב׳ what is meant by (why are they named) biraniyoth? בירנן צירדן וכ׳ (not צירדן), he laid a trap for them, he caught them (ensnared them).

בִּירָנְתָא ch.=preced. 1). Targ. Esth. I, 2 (h. text הבירה); a. fr.—*Pl.* בִּירָנְיָתָא, בִּירָנְוָתָא, בִּר׳; constr. בִּירָנְיַת. Targ. Ps. XLVIII, 4 (h. text ארמון). Targ. Am. III, 9 בִּרְנְיַת באשדוד (!).—Targ. Y. Lev. XXV, 29 בִּירָנִין masc. (some ed. בּוּרְנִין) *fortified places.*

בִּירְצָא m. (ברץ) *brim. Pl.* בִּירְצַיָּא. Ab. Zar. 74ᵇ וחתים להו אבִּירְצַיְיהוּ (some ed. אבור׳) and sealed the kegs on their brims. [Gitt. 69ᵇ בירצא, some ed., v. בְּרָצָא.]

בִּירְקָא pr. n. pl. *Birka*, in Babylon. Kidd. 72ª, v. בִּירְתָא.

בירקא, Ab. Zar. 28ᵇ פתילתא ב׳, v. בַּרְקָא II, 2.

בֵּירְתָא f. *well*, v. בֵּיר.

בִּירְתָא f. ch.=h. בִּירָה. Ezra VI, 2. Targ. II Esth. IX, 6, v. בִּירָנְתָא; a. e.—Freq. as pr. n. pl. *Fort.* Y. Ber. II, 5ᵃ top בִּירַת מלכא וכ׳ the royal fort of Bethlehem; (Lam. R. to I, 16, end בירת ערבא). Pesik. Shim. p. 117ᵃ; Yalk. Jer. 263 כד תימוט בירה ב׳ שמה (read בירתא) when a capital declines, it is still called the Capital.—Sot. 38ᵇ ב׳ דשחורי (דשיחורי) the Fort of Shihori. Y. Ab. Zar. V, 44ᵈ בירת סירייקה (Bab. ib. 31ᵃ בירת סריקא (not בירא; Ms. M. ב׳ סירקי) Fort Sirikah in Samaria. Kidd. 72ᵃ ב׳ דסטיא; ib. ב׳ דנדה Ms. Oxf. (ed. only בִּירְקָא) opprobrious by-names of Babylonian places (v. Graetz *Messene*, in Progr. of Bresl. Jew. Semin. 1879); a. fr. [Y. Peah VII, 20ᵃ bot. ב׳ דחרובתא, v. כְּבוּרְתָא.]—[*Pl.* בִּירָתָא (?). Targ. Prov. I, 21, prob. to be read בִּירְיָתָא *streets*, v. Nöld. Mand. Gr. p. 17.]

בִּירְתִין m. pl., v. בִּרְתָא.

בִּירְתִית f. (v. preced. art.) *of Birtha.*—*Pl.* בִּירְתִיּוֹת. Y. Pes. III, 30ᵃ, v. קוּבְטְרוֹת.

בִּישׁ I, **בִּישָׁא** m. (v. באיש) *bad, wrong* (of persons and deeds); also *ill, sick.* Targ. Gen. VI, 5; a. v. fr.—Lev. R. s. 22 (prov.) טב לב׳ וכ׳ when thou hast done good to a bad man, thou hast done evil (to thyself). B. Kam. 115ᵃ חנן בישא Ḥanan, the bad man.—B. Mets. 75ᵇ bot. דב׳ ליה וכ׳ he who fares badly in one place; a. fr.—*Pl.* בִּישִׁין, בִּישַׁיָּא, בִּישַׁיָּא. Targ. Gen. XIII, 13; a. v. fr.—בִּישַׁיָּיא freq. *the sick.* Koh. R. to IV, 6 ומפלגא לב׳ and distributes (the apples) among the sick.—Y. Bets. I, 60ᶜ bot. מבקרא ביש׳ (not בייש׳) to visit the sick.—Fem. בִּישְׁתָא, בִּישָׁא 1) (adj.) *bad;* 2) (noun) *evil, wickedness, illness.* Targ. Gen. XXXVII, 20; a. fr. —Ib. VI, 5, a. fr. בִּישַׁת constr. —Sabb. 129ᵃ ב׳ מי וכ׳ can bad be good? Y. ib. XIV, 14ᶜ bot. טב לבישתא וכ׳ (vinegar is) good for a sore, but bad for a sound tooth. Lev. R. s. 33, beg., from it (the tongue) comes the good ומינה ב׳ and from it the evil; a. fr.—*Pl.* בִּישָׁתָא, בִּישָׁאתָא, בִּישָׁן.—Targ. Gen. XXVIII, 8 (ed. Vien. O. בישא, corr. acc.); a. fr.—Snh. 7ᵃ happy is he who hears (himself insulted) and keeps silence חלפוה בישתיה מאה (corr. חלפוהו בישתא, v. Rabb. D. S. a. l. note 7) a hundred evils pass by him (he escapes &c.); a. fr.

בִּישׁ II, **כְּפַר ב׳** pr. n. pl. *K'far Bish*, prob. *Capharabis* in upper Idumæa. Lam. R. to II, 2; Gitt. 57ᵃ.

בְּאִישׁ, בִּישׁוּתָא, בִּישׁוּת, בִּישׁוּ f. (בִּישׁ I) 1) *bad quality.* Targ. Jer. XXIV, 2; a. e.—2) *wickedness, evil.* Targ. O. Gen. XXXI, 52; a. fr.—Sabb. 156ᵃ חדא לב׳ one quality on the bad side; כולי לב׳ all bad. Lam. R. to I, 1 (רבתי) בישו עבדית וכ׳ (not בישי) have I done wrong that I &c.? Pesik. Zakh. p. 24ᵇ [read twice:] למיגזר לבישא בִּישׁוּתֵיהּ; (Tanh. Ki Thetse 6 בִּישְׁתֵּיהּ, ed. Bub. ib. בישותיה) to repay the bad man his badness. B. Kam. 115ᵃ מפורסם לב׳ notorious for vice.—Men. 52ᵃ מבישותין וכ׳ of our shortcomings they speak to them. Ab. Zar. 65ᵃ ... ב׳ עינא the eye which desires to see your misfortune. Keth. 25ᵇ; Macc. 5ᵇ הדר חזייה לר׳ א׳ בישות he turned around and looked at R. E. with displeasure; Pes. 53ᵇ ... ב׳ חזא ביה Ms. M. 2 a. Oxf. בבישות, v. Rabb. D. S. a. l. note 400).—Y. Taan. III, 66ᶜ bot. ומדינתא אזלא בבאישות and the city perishes in wickedness (by pestilence).

בִּישׁוּלָא, בִּישׁוּל, v. בְּשׁוּ.

בִּישׁוּתָא, בִּישׁוּת, v. בִּישׁוּ.

בִּישֵׁם, v. בְּשַׂם,.—Pesik. R. s. 21, read בִּיסֵּם, v. בְּסַם.

(ביישן) בֵּישָׁן pr. n. pl. (contr. of בית שאן, v. שְׁאָן) *Beshan* (Scythopolis), in Galilee. Y. B. Mets. X, 12ᶜ top בני ביישן דרייא דב׳ the dwelling houses of B.—Pes. 50ᵇ (Ms. Oxf. בישן, Ms. M. מישן).

(ביישני) בֵּישָׁנִי m. (v. preced.) 1) *inhabitant* or *native of Beshan.* Meg. 24ᵇ (ed. בשיני, Ms. M. בשני, corr. acc.).—*Pl.* בֵּישָׁנִין. Y. Ber. II, 4ᵈ bot.; (Meg. l. c. אנשי בית שאן).—Ch. בֵּישְׁנָאֵי. Y. Meg. III, beg. 73ᵈ.—2) *beshani*, name of a species of olives. Peah VII, 1 an olive called ב׳ .... (Ms. M. ביי׳) beshani. Y. ib. 20ᵃ top אית דבעי מימר ב׳ ממש וכ׳ some would say, it means really a beshani (named after Beshan), others would derive its name from the fact (v. בּוֹשׁ) that it shames its neighbor (trees by its richness). [Oth. opin. *a dry olive*, not used for manufacturing oil.]

בִּישְׂרָא, v. בִּשְׂרָא.

בִּישְׂרָנָא m. (v. preced.) *fleshy, stout.*—*Pl.* בִּישְׂרָנֵי. Keth. 61ᵃ.

בִּישְׁתָא, v. בִּישׁ I fem., a. בִּישׁוּ.

בי״ת *Beth*, the second letter of the Alphabeth. Y. Sabb. XVI, 15ᶜ top; a. fr.; v. אל״ף.—Y. Ned. III, 38ᵃ bot. בי״ת תרי וכ׳ the Beth (in ביצחק Gen. XXI, 12) intimates two, a son that is destined to inherit two worlds. Lev. R. s. 19 אם אתה עושה ב׳ כ״ף if thou changest the Beth into a Kaf; a. fr.—*Pl.* בֵּיתִין. Sabb. 103ᵇ one must not write .. בי׳ כפין (Ms. M. בָּתִין) the Beths so as to be taken for Kafs.—Chald. בי״תא. Cant. R. beg.; a. fr. [Shek. III, 2 Mish. ed. ביתא, read בֵּיתָא.]

בַּת, בִּית, inf. בּוּת (sec. r. of בוא) *to go in, lodge, pass the night.* Dan. VI, 19. Targ. Gen. XXXII, 22; a. fr.—Pes. 107ᵃ בת טוות (Dan. l. c.) he went to bed without tasting food. Snh. 95ᵃ (prov.) בת דינא וכ׳ if punishment is procrastinated, punishment is gone. Taan. 24ᵇ ביתו כולי וכ׳ go ye all to bed fasting. Pes. 42ᵃ מיא דביתו (Chald. transl. of the ambiguous מים שֶׁלָּנוּ) water kept in vessels over night. Ber. 60ᵇ בת בדברא he slept in the open field. Snh. 63ᵇ.—Ib. 109ᵃ top בעי לְמֵיבַת he wanted to stay over night; a. e.—Part. בָּאֵית. Targ. Is. LVIII, 5.

Pa. בַּיֵּית same. Erub. 73ᵃ (opp. to taking meals).

Af. אֲבִית *to keep over night, postpone burial.* Snh. 47ᵃ מְבִית ליה למת dare one postpone the burial of the dead?

בַּיִת m. (b. h.; cmp. preced.; v. Ges. H. Dict. s. v. as to various etymological attempts), constr. בֵּית, *pl.* בָּתִּים. 1) *house, household, home.* Yoma 11ᵇ ב׳ מיוחד לדירה

bayith means a building intended for a dwelling. Ib. מי שמייחד ביתו לו (Var. v. Rabb. D. S. a. l. note) he who devotes his house (its contents) to himself exclusively (unaccommodating); Arakh. 16ª מי שמיוחד וכ׳.—בעל הב׳ (abbrev. בע״ה) *owner, landlord; host; private man*, opp. to trader, artisan &c. Ber. 46ª בע״ה בוצע וכ׳ the host breaks the bread, and the guest says the blessing. Tosef. ib. IV, 14 של בע״ה home-made (bread), opp. גלוסקין; Y. ib. VI, 10ᵇ bot.—Sabb. I, 1 בע״ה the donor, opp. עני the recipient. Gen. R. s. 22; a. v. fr.—בן ב׳ *inmate, attendant.* Ab. I, 5; a. fr.—פסול הב׳ the degraded (slave) of the house. Gen. R. s. 70.—2) Esp. (ה)ב׳ *the Temple.* בפני הב׳ in days when the Temple exists, שלא בפני הב׳ when it does not exist. Hull. V, 1; a. fr.—ב׳ שני or ב׳ אחרון *the Second Temple.* Cant. R. to VIII, 9; a. fr.—הר הב׳ Temple Mount, v. הַר.—3) *school, college,* (collect.) *disciples;* בֵּית הלל Hillelites &c. Bets. I, 1; a. fr. Treat. Sof'rim IV, 1 של ב׳ וכ׳ those of the house of &c. [Y. Shebi. II, 33ᵈ bot., a. e. דבית..ר׳, usu. דבי, v. בֵּי].—4) *body.* Ber. 44ᵇ אוי לו לב׳ וכ׳ that human body (Rashi: stomach) is to be pitied where vegetables are a constant guest (being the only food).—5) *wife.* Yoma I, 1 ביתו זו וכ׳ 'his house'—that means his wife. Ib. 13ª והך לאו ביתו היא but this one (designated for him in case of his wife's death) cannot be called 'his house'. Sabb. 118ᵇ; a. fr.—6) Euphem. *pudenda; marital intercourse.* Y. Sabb. IX, 12ª top; Mikv. VIII, 4 שמשה את בֵּיתָהּ she had intercourse. Ib. כבדה את הב׳ she washed &c. Y. Sot. I, 16ᶜ bot. אסורה לביתה is forbidden to her husband. Nidd. 5ª מהומת לביתה she hastens to perform her marital duty. Y. ib. I, beg. 48ᵈ. Cmp. חֶדֶר.—7) *store-house, store-room.* בֵּית העצים wood-room; ב׳ התבן straw-magazine; ב׳ הבקר stable; &c. Yoma 11ª; a. fr.—8) (geogr.) *place, town,* in compounds (for which see the respective determinants), e. g. ב׳ בוקיא Beth-Bukya &c.—9) (anat.) *limb, organ,* in compounds (v. supra 8)), e.g. ב׳ הבליעה œsophagus, &c. —10) *shed* for plants, *covering.* Shebi. II, 4 (pl.). Y. ib. 33ᵈ. —Y. Sabb. VII, 10ª.—11) in compounds, denoting *receptacle, cover* &c., e. g. ב׳ הדיו *inkstand.* Tosef. Kel. B. Mets. IV, 11; ב׳ יד *sleeve,* v. אוּנְקְלִי II, &c.—Men. 34ᵇ, a. e. *cases of the T'fillin.*

Chief compounds: בֵּית אָב, pl. בָּתֵּי אָבוֹת 1) *paternal home, family.* Snh. 38ª שני ב׳ א׳ two families (dynasties); a. fr.—Tosef. Ter. II, 11 אריסי ב׳ א׳=בית אבי׳ *hereditary land-tenants;* B. Bath. 46ᵇ.—2) *priest's division.* Taan. II, 6; a. fr.; v. אֱנוֹשׁ pl.—3) *origin of a law, rule* &c.; cmp. אָב II. Cant. R. to II, 4 ב׳ א׳ של הלכה the origin (principle) of a legal rule. Midr. Till. to Ps. CIV, 29 wherever the root רעש is used, it means cessation of government, ואיזהו ב׳ א׳ שלהם וכ׳ and where is the origin (determining the meaning) of all of them? (Answ. Jer. LI, 29). Lev. R. s. 1, beg. מב׳ א׳ שלהן וכ׳ from the chief passage (Hagg. I, 13 'Haggai, the messenger' &c.) we learn that prophets are called messengers (or angels).—בֵּית דִּין (abbr. ב״ד) *court.* —ב״ד הגדול or ב״ד של שבעים ואחד the Great Sanedrin of seventy one members. Snh. I, 5. Y. ib. 19ª bot.; a. fr.—ב״ד נוטה court of an odd number of judges. ב״ד שקול of an even number of judges. Snh 3ᵇ.—ב״ד שריא a permitting court, opprobrious name of a court too lax in religious affairs. Y. Gitt. VII, 48ᵈ top; Y. Nidd. III, 50ᵈ bot.—[For all other compounds not self-evident, v. respective determinants.] [בית תר, v. בִּיתֵּר.—Gen. R. s. 12 בית שלו, בית של עולם, v. בָּיָא.]

בֵּיתָא, בֵּית, בַּיְתָא I ch. 1) same. Targ. Ex. XII, 3; a. v. fr.—Meg. 16ª ווי מב׳ וכ׳ woe inside, woe outside! Gen. R. s. 32 ההוא ב׳ קלקלתא that house which is a ruin (a Samaritan's designation of the Jerusalem Temple). Y. Snh. I, 18ᶜ ההן ב׳ דלרע that house down there (Rabbi's college); Y. R. Hash. II, 58ª bot. והן ביתא.—Yeb. 109ᵇ דבייתיה כי בייתיה דמי for his (the trustee's) house is like his (the neighbor's) own house (he is familiar with the interior); a. fr.—*Pl.* בָּתֵּי, בָּתַּיָּא, בָּתִּין. Targ. Ex. I, 21; a. v. fr.—B. Bath. 61ᵇ sq. Ib. 67ª, v. בִּירְתָא.—Ber. 6ª *the case of T'fillin,* v. preced. [Playful etymol. בוא אה״ביב בה. Sabb. 77ᵇ.]—2) *night-lodging.* Gitt. 57ª לא יהבי ב׳ לאושפיזא they would not designate a house as a lodging for strangers (Lam. R. to II, 2 דלא הוות מקבלא אכסניא).

בַּיְתָא II f. (=h. בַּת) *bath,* a measure. Targ. Is. V, 10. Targ. Ezek. XLV, 11; a. e.—*Pl.* בַּתִּין, בַּיְתִין. Ib. 14. Targ. I Kings VII, 26.

בִּיתָא *night-bird,* v. בָּאוֹת.

בי״תא, v. בי״ת.

בַּיְתוֹס, בַּיְתוֹס pr. n. m. (Βοηθός) *Boëthus;* 1) the founder of a sect similar to that of the Sadducees, named בַּיְתוֹסִין *Boëthusians.* Ab. d'R. Nath. ch. V.—2) father of one Martha or Miriam, a rich woman in the days of the siege of Jerusalem by Titus. Gitt. 56ª. Lam. R. to I, 16 מרים; Y. Keth. V, 30ᵇ bot. מרתא.—3) B. ben Zonin. Y. B. Mets. V, 10ᵇ top; a. fr.—4) R. B.—Y. Erub. VI, 23ᶜ bot.

בַּיְתוֹסִי, בַּיְ׳ m. *Boëthusian,* v. preced. Sabb. 108ª שאל ב׳ אחד (Mass. Sof. I, 2 שאל אחד, corr. acc.) a Boëthusian asked. Tosef. Yoma I, 8 (Yoma 19ᵇ צדוקי).—*Pl.* בַּיְתוֹסִים, בַּיְתוֹסִין, בַּיְ׳. Men. X, 3. Y. Yoma I, 39ª bot. מפני הב׳ (for which ib. a. Bab. Yoma l. c. הצדוקים); Tosef. l. c. [Ar. ed. pr. בית סי, בית סין, read as one w., like Tosef. l. c. Var.]

ביתור, v. בִּיתֵּר.

בית־יוני, v. הִינִי 3).

בִּיתוּתָא f. (בית) *dwelling.* Targ. Job XXX, 23 Ms. (Var. a. ed. בית קבורתא).

בַּיְתָסִי, ביתיס, Tosef. Yoma I, 18, Var. for בַּיְתוֹסִי.

בִּיתֵּר pr. n. pl. (prob. a contr. of בית תרעא) *Bithter* (Βιθθηρά), known as *Bettar,* a town in Southern Palestine, renowned as the centre of the Bar-Kokhba revolution against Hadrian. [As to its situation, v. Neub. Géogr. p. 130; Graetz Gesch. der Jud. IV, 168). Gitt. 57ª כרך ב׳ the Fortress of B.—Y. Taan. IV, 69ª top. Lam. R. to II, 2; IV, 18; a. fr.—Y. Ber. I, 3ᵈ, a. fr. הרוגי ב׳ those killed in the Bar-Kokhba revolution (whom Hadrian would not allow to be buried). Ḥall. IV, 10 (11) (Y. ed. ביתור; ed. Nap. בייתר, Ven. ביתיר) mentioned as a place not belonging to Palestine proper. Cant. R. to II, 17 בית תר.

*בִּיתְרֵי pr. n. pl. *Bethre.* Snh. 95[a] כי מטו בי תרי (Ms. M. ביטרי) when they came to B.

*ביתרתה, Y. Succ. I, 52[a] bot., read, with Y. Erub. I, 19[c] top; Y. Kil. IV, 29[b], בית חבירתא or תה . . . ., name of a field or an estate.

בָּכָה, בְּכָא, v. בכי.

בכוליאר, Yoma 25[a], v. בּוּכְלְיָים.

בְּכוֹר m. (b. h.; בכר) *first-born* (opp. פשוט, a plain, unprivileged son); also of animals. B. Bath. 126[a] ב׳ ופשוט; a. fr.—Y. Pes. X, beg. 37[b] הוה ב׳ והוה אכיל was a first-born and yet did not fast (on the eve of Passover).—Yeb. 16[a]; Y. ib. I, 3[a] bot. ב׳ שטן (play on קטן) the first in obstinate dispute.—Gen. R. s. 91 (ref. to Gen. XLII, 37) הרי זה ב׳ שוטה וכ׳ is this a foolish first-born son! are thy children not my children? [ב׳ שוטה a first-born son by his mother, v. בּוּכְרָא I.]—Bekh. VIII, 1, a. fr. ב׳ לנחלה a first-born with the privileges of a double share of inheritance (Deut. XXI, 15 sq.), ב׳ לכהן one who must be redeemed from the priest (Ex. XIII, 2). Ib. IV, 4 ראה את הב׳ examined the first-born animal (and declared it defective); a. fr.—*Pl.* בְּכוֹרִים, בְּכוֹרוֹת. Ex. R. s. 18 בְּכוֹרֵי מצרים the first-born of Egyptian cattle; ib. מכת בכורות the plague of the first-born in Egypt; Num. R. s. 4; a. fr.—Bekh. IV, 5 he who receives payment להיות רואה ב׳ for examining first-born animals (as to bodily defects, v. supra); a. fr.—[Y. Shek. III, beg. 47[b] הבכו׳, read הַבְּכִּירוֹת.] Ch. בּוּכְרָא.

בִּכּוּרָא f. ch. (=next w.) *early fig.* Targ. Hos. IX, 10. Targ. Is. XXVIII, 4.—*Pl.* בִּכּוּרַיָּא, בִּכּוּרִין m. *first fruits.* Targ. Lev. II, 14; a. e.

בִּיכּ׳, בִּכּוּרָה f. (b. h.; בכר) *early fruit, esp. fig.*—1) *Pl.* בִּכּוּרוֹת. Gen. R. s. 22 היה אוכל הב׳ וכ׳ ate the early fruits himself and offered the late to the king. Snh. 91[b]; Lev. R. s. 4 ב׳ נאות fine early figs. Ter. IV, 6 בב׳ at the time of early ripening.—2) *Pl.* בִּכּוּרִים m. (b. h.) *first fruits* (to be offered), (sub. מנחת) *offering of first fruits.* Bicc. I, 1; a. fr.—*Biccurim,* name of a treatise of the Mishnah, belonging to the order of Seeds (זרעים).

בְּכוֹרָה f. (b. h.; בכר) 1) *first-born. Pl.* בְּכוֹרוֹת. Ex. R. s. 18 הנקבות הב׳ the first-born females (in Egypt).—2) *first birth, birth-right.* B. Bath. 123[a] נטל ב׳ מראובן וכ׳ took the birth-right from Reuben and gave it to Joseph. Ib. ראויה היתה ב׳ וכ׳ the first birth (of Jacob's children) was destined to issue from Rachel. Ib. 124[a] חלק ב׳ the share of the first-born; a. fr.—3) *the law appertaining to first-born animals,* v. בְּכוֹר.—Bekh. I, 1 חייב בב׳ is subject to the law &c., פטור מן הב׳ is exempt from &c.; a. v. fr.—*Pl.* בְּכוֹרוֹת, v. supra a. בְּכוֹר.—*B'khoroth* (Bekh.), name of a Talmudic treatise, belonging to the order of Kodashim (קדשים).

בְּכוֹרוּתָא ch. same, *birth-right.* Targ. O. Gen. XXV, 31 sq.; v. בְּכֵירוּתָא.

*בַּכּוּשָׁא m. (=בר כושא, v. כשכש; for Syr. בר=בכשא כשא, cmp. הוֹפֵק) *knocker* for giving signals for worship. Y. Meg. III, 73[d] bot. (Var. מַכּוּשָׁא).

בָּכוּתָא, v. בְּכִיתָא.

בָּכָה, בכי (b. h.; √בך *to break through, split,* v. Ges. H. Dict. s. v.; v. בכר) *to weep.* Ḥull. 7[b]; a. fr. Ohol. XVIII, 4 שדה בּוֹכִין weepers' field, a place where the funeral cortege disperses; v. M. Kat. 5[b] שדה שמפטירין בה מתים (Ms. M. שמפסידין) where the funeral addresses are held.

Pi. בִּכָּה 1) *to cause to weep, make cry.* Lam. R. to I, 2 (ref. to בכה תבכה) בוכה וּמְבַכָּה מה״ש עמה she cries and makes the angels cry with her. Ex. R. s. 1 היו מְבַכִּין אותו they made it (the Egyptian child) cry.—2) *to mourn, lament* (Ezek. VIII, 14). Tosef. Kel. B. Bath. II, 8 מְבַכּוֹת מיתיהן lament their dead.

בְּכָא, בכי ch. same, also (act. v.) *to lament.* Targ. Gen. XXIII, 2; a. fr.—Part. בָּכֵי. Ber. 5[b] להחוא שופרא ...קא בכינא I cry over that beauty that it should rot in the ground. Ib. אמאי קבכית why criest thou? Ib. דהוה קא בכי (v. Rabb. D. S. a. l.) that he was crying. Lam. R. to I, 17 בָּכְיָה סלקא בָּכְיָה נחתא weeping she (Israel) goes up (to the ruins of Jerusalem), weeping she goes down. Y. Yoma II, 39[d] top שרון.....בָּכְיִין all the people began to cry.—Y. Ḥag. I, 76[c] bot. בכי בעיינוי blear-eyed.—Taan. 5[b] וכי בכדי בכו בַּכַּיָּיא Ms. M. (ed. ספדו) is it for naught the weepers wept? Gen. R. s. 68, v. next w.; a. fr.

בְּכִי I m. (b. h.; preced.) *weeping.* Gen. R. s. 68; Lev. R. s. 8, a. e. (playing on בכושרות, Ps. LXVIII, 7) ב׳ ושירות weeping and songs, מאן דבעי אומר וכ׳ he who loves (his wife) sings, he who does not, weeps; Snh. 22[a].

בְּכִי f. ch. same. Targ. II, Sam. XIII, 36; v. בְּכִיתָא.

בְּכִי II, בַּעַל ב׳ (עין ב׳) pr. n. pl. *Baalbek* (*En-Bekhi,* later *Heliopolis*), an ancient city of Syria, renowned for its temples and bazaars (יריד). Ab. Zar. 11[b] יריד שבעין ב׳ the bazaar at En B. (with its idolatrous rites). Maasr. V, 8 שום ב׳ ב׳ Baalbek garlic.

בָּכִי m. (b. h. בָּכָא?) a species of *pears,* prob. the pyrum Syrium of the Romans (cmp. LXX a. Vulg. I Chr. XIV, 15). *Pl.* בְּכָיִים. Y. Kil. I, 27[a].

בִּכְיָא f.=בְּכִי. Targ. Is. XXXVIII, 3; a. e.

בַּכְיָא m. (בכי) *weeper, wailer. Pl.* בַּכַּיָּיא. Taan. 5[b], v. בכי ch.

בְּכִיָּה, בכייה f.=בְּכִי I. Y. Taan. IV, 68[d] top בכיי׳ של תפלות; Bab. ib. 29[a] בכי של חנם weeping for no cause. Gitt. 58[a], a. fr. געו בב׳ they sobbed loudly.

בְּכִיוּתָא ch. same. Targ. Y. I Gen. XXXV, 8; (II ib. בְּכוּתָא), v. בְּכִיתָא.

בְּכִיָּה, v. בְּכִיָּה.

*__בַּכְיָן, בַּכְיָין__ m. (preced. ws.) *weeper.* Targ. Esth. II, 21 (Esth. R. ib. בַּרְבָּרֵי).

בְּכֵין *then*, v. כֵּן.

בַּכִּיר m. h. a ch. (b. h. בַּכֻּרָה; בכר) *early, first-ripening*, opp. לקיש or אפיל. Snh. 18[b] אם ב׳ ולקיש וכ׳ when the early and the late seeds blossom simultaneously &c.; Y. ib. I, 18[c] bot.; Y. R. Hash. I, 58[b] bot. (corr. acc.). Gen. R. s. 61; Koh. R. to XI, 6 (ref. to Koh. ib.) אם זרעת בב׳ if thou hast sown in the early season. Ib. הב׳ the early seed. Ib. to VII, 26 לקיש לסטים ב׳ וכ׳ (read ללס׳) the latest of the robbers is the first to be hanged.—Fem. h. בַּכִּירָה. Y. Taan. I, 64[a] bot. הב׳ וכ׳ the early rain sets in on the third (of Marḥeshvan), v. בֵּינוֹנִי. [Y. Sot. III, 19[a] top תאינה ב׳, v. בִּכּוּרָה.]—*Pl.* בַּכִּירוֹת. Y. Dem. I, beg. 21[c] (Tosef. ib. I, 3 בְּכוּרוֹת). Y. R. Hash. I, 56[d] top אלו הב׳ those are the early-bearing sheep; (Y. Shek. III, beg. 47[b] הבכורות, corr. acc.).

בְּכֵרוּתָא, בְּכֵירוּתָא **בְּכֵרוּתָא** f. ch.=h. בְּכוֹרָה 2). Targ. Gen. XXV, 31 (ed. Berl. בְּכוֹ׳); a. fr.—Ber. 7[b] זבנה לבכירותיה (not זבניה) he (Esaw) sold his birthright; ib. שקלו בכירותיה מיניה ויהביה ליוסף Ms. M. (read ויהבוה; ed. incorr.) his (Reuben's) birthright was taken from him and given to Joseph (v. Rabb. D. S. a. l. note). Sot. 13[a] נהר דזבינר לבכירותי וכ׳ though I sold my birthright, have I ever sold my plain heir's right?

בְּכִיתָא (בְּכוּתָא) f. ch. (=h. בְּכִית, בָּכוּת) *weeping, mourning.* Targ. Gen. L, 4. Targ. Deut. XXXIV, 8 (Y. בכותא); a. e.—Gen. R. s. 15, end, Ar. (missing in ed.); Pesik. Ronni p. 142[b]; v. אֲלִיְיתָא.

בכלופסין, בכלוסיפין, v. כְּלוּפְסִין.

בכנא, v. בּוּכְנָא.

בָּכַר (b. h.; √בך, v. בכי, cmp. בָּקַר) [*to break forth,*] *to be early.* [Kal prob. not used.]

Pi. בִּיכֵּר 1) *to be early, produce first fruits.* Tanḥ. Vayḥi 14; Gen. R. s. 99 (פירותיה) מְבַכֶּרֶת has early crops, opp. מלקשת, מאפלת. [Ib. end מבכרין מפירותיהם read מכבדין, v. כָּבַד.]—2) *to bear for the first time* (of animals). Bekh. I, 3 sq. שלא בִיכְּרָה that never before had given birth; a. fr.—3) (neut. v.) *to be first in ripening.* Bicc. III, 1 and sees תאנה שבִּכְּרָה a fig which is first ripe, אשכול שביכר a cluster of grapes which &c. Y. Maasr. I, 49[a] top משיבכר צמריא וכ׳, v. צמריא. Ib. משיבכירו בנות שבע, v. בַּת. Ib. משיבכרו, בִּיכֵּרוּ (v. בָּחַל as to spelling). —4) (b. h.) *to recognize as first-born* (בכור). B. Bath. 130[a] sq.

Hif. הִבְכִּיר same. Bekh. III, 2 המַבְכִּירוֹת those animals which have given birth for the first time.

Hithpa. הִתְבַּכֵּר *to hasten.* Yalk. Gen. 161 עדרא מִתְבַּכֶּרֶת בפירותיה, v. supra.

בְּכַר ch. same.—*Pa.* בַּכַּר 1) *to produce, mature.* Targ. Y. Deut. XXXIII, 14 דִמְבַכְּרָא וכ׳ which his land produces.—2) *to recognize as first-born.* Targ. O. Deut. XXI, 16.

Ithpa. אִתְבַּכַּר *to be dedicated as the first-born.* Targ. O. Lev. XXVII, 26.

בִּכְרָא, v. בּוּכְרָא I, 2.

בִּכְרָא, v. בּוּכ׳.

בְּכֵרוּתָא, v. בְּכֵיר׳.

בַּכַּרְיָא, v. בּוּכַּרְיָא.

בַּל (b. h.; cmp. בלי, v. Ges. H. Dict. s. v.) *not*, frequ. used, in connection with a verb, in the sense of *a prohibitive law.* Erub. 100[a] עובר על בל תגרע he transgresses the law which says 'thou shalt not diminish therefrom' (Deut. XIII, 1). Pes. III, 3 שמוזהרים עליו בבל יראה וכ׳ concerning which we are cautioned by the law prohibiting leavened things to be seen or to be found (Ex. XIII, 7; XII, 19); a. v. fr. [Our w. is also applied to Bible texts in which לא appears.]

בֵּל pr. n. *Bel*, the Babylonian deity. Ab. Zar. 11[b] בית ב׳ בבבל the temple of Bel in Babylon.

*__בָּל__ m. (contr. of בחל, cmp. בָּאלֵי) *care, anxiety.* Dan. VI, 15.

בָּלָא, v. בָּאלָא.

בַּלָּא m. *destroyer*, v. בִּלְעָם.

בְּלָא *to be worn out*, v. בְּלֵי.

בְּלָא, בְּלָא, בְּלָא *without*, v. לָא, לא.

בְּלָיוֹת, בְּלָאוֹת f. pl. (of בְּלָי; בלי) *outworn garments.* Keth. V, 8 מתכסה בבְלָאוֹתֶיהָ וכ׳ she wears her winter clothes in their outworn condition in the summer. Ib. 65[b] מותר ב׳ the entirely outworn clothes (=שחקים Mish. l. c.); a. fr.—2) *the woman's right to claim compensation for the wear or ruin of the things which she brought along as her property* (v. מלוג, a. צאן ברזל). Yeb. X, 1 ...ולא ב׳ nor can she claim compensation for used or spent property (but may take the things in what condition they are, v. comment.). Keth. XI, 6.—[Y. ib. V, 30[b] bot.; XI, 34[a] bot., as in Mish. ib. 7 בליות.]

בלאי, Ned. 91[b] Ar., read with ed. כְּלָאֵי.

בַּלָּאֵי m. pl. *those of* (the family or town of) *Bela*, in Babylon, (prob. a nickname). Kidd. 70[b]; v. טְלָאֵי.

בְּלוֹיִים, בְּלָאִים m. pl. (b. h. בְּלוֹאִים, בְּלוֹיֵי׳, v. בְּלָאוֹת) *fragments, rags.* Succ. 15[b] sq. בְּלָאֵי כלים torn pieces of garments. Ib. V, 3; a. e.—Hull. 107[b] בלאי חמתות fragments of wine bags.—Kel. XXVII, 5 בְּלוֹיֵי נפה וכ׳ (leather) pieces from a winnow or sieve.

בְּלָאִין ch. same. Targ. Jer. XXXVIII, 11; a. e.

בלארי, v. בַּלְנְרִין.

בלבוטס, read בּוּלְבְּטֵס.

בִּילְבֵּל, בִּלְבֵּל (Pilp. of בלל or בול; cmp. בחל) *to mix up; to disarrange, upset, disturb.* Bekh. 38[b] (expl. תבלל, Lev. XXI, 20) דבר המבלבל וכ׳ something which disturbs the arrangement (of the white and the black) of the eye. Snh. 108[a] עמד ובלבל את וכ׳ (Var. ופזר) he upset the bridal canopy. Sot. 46[b] לא בִילְבְּלָהּ did not disturb the town (by pillaging, removing the inhabitants &c.). Y. B. Kam. IV, end, 4[c] one struck him fatally ובא השני ובִילְבְּלוֹ and the other came and made him senseless (accelerating his death).—Part. pass. מְבוּלְבָּל, f. מְבוּלְבֶּלֶת. Succ. 22[a] סוכה מב׳ a festive booth the covering of which is disarranged, v. הָבַל. [Pesik. R. s. 4 נתבלבל, v. בַּלְבֵּל.]

בַּלְבֵּל ch. same. Targ. O. Gen. XI, 9. Targ. Is. XXVIII, 28 וּמְבַלְבֵּל and mixes up (the grain with the chaff, h. text חמם); a. e.—Part. pass. מְבַלְבַּל. Bekh. 44[a] משום דמְבַלְבְּלָן because they (the white and the black of the eye) are mixed up, v. preced.—Denom. מְבַלְבְּלִיתָא *mixture of white and black* (h. תְּבַלֻּל, v. preced.). Ibid. (Ar. ed. pr. מברב׳).

Ithpalp. contr. אִיבַּלְבֵּל *to be disturbed, mixed up.* Hull. 26[b] מִיבַּלְבְּלִי they (water and wine) mix well. M. Kat. 9[b] לִבַּלְבֵּל פתורם thy table (meals) be disturbed (by the noise of children).

בלבסים, בלבסין, v. לִבְסִים a. פְּלוּפְסִין.

בלבקיא, בלבקי, v. גְּלַבְקְיָא.

***בלג,** Deut. R. s. 9 דעתו מובלגת, read מוּבְהֶלֶת, v. בָּהַל, end.

בִּלְגָּה, v. בִּילְגָּה.

***בלגי,** Yoma 83[b] אהדרוהו ב׳ וצער ed. (Ms. M. 1 פלאגר; 2 a. Ar. פלוגר; Ms. Oxf., Yalk. Deut. 959 Ms. לגי, v. Rabb. D. S. a. l. note), take ב as servile letter, v. לוּגָא.

בּוּלְדָּר, בַּלְדָר m. (veredarius, βερεδάριος, with change of liquida) *courier.* Y. Taan. IV, 68[c] bot. ביום ולילה נפק בלדרה וכ׳ could the courier go in one day and night from Jerusalem to Tyre? Gen. R. s. 10. Ib. s. 78; a. e.—*Pl.* בּוּלְדָארִין, בּוּלְדָּרִין. Esth. R. to I, 8 הכתבים והב׳ (strike out either of the two, v. Pesik. Shek. p. 14[a], Cant. R. to III, 4). Ib. ושלח בולדארין והחזיר וכ׳ and sent couriers (after them) and had the letters brought back.

בַּלְדְּרְסִין pr. n. pl. (a corrupt. of Brundisii, Βρεντέσιον) *Brundisium,* a port in Calabria, Italy. Erub. IV, 1 (41[a]); 43[a] Ms. M. (ed. פלנדרסין, Var. פלנדסין, פרנדסין, פלנדריסין, פרדיסין; v. Rabb. D. S. a. l. notes). Cmp. בַּרְדְּסִין.

בָּלָה, v. בלי.

בְּלוֹ f. *a tax* (cmp. Assyr. *biltu,* v. Schr. KAT Gloss. II, s. v. יבל). Ezra IV, 13; a. e.—B. Bath. 8[a] expl. *capitation tax;* Ned. 62[b]. Gen. R. s. 64; Esth. R. introd., v. פרובגירון.

***בַּלְוָתִי** (?) pr. n. m. *Balvati.* Arakh. 11[a].

***בְּלוּזְמָא** f. (בסם, בלסס=בלזם) *drinking of spiced wines,* whence (cmp. בָּסַם) *frolic, carousal.*—*Pl.* בְּלוּזְמָאוֹת. Lev. R. s. 12 והיו שם שתי ב׳ (Yalk. Jer. 320 בלזמיות) two excessive rejoicings took place at the same time. [Num. R. s. 10 a. Midr. Prov. to ch. XI have צהלה.]

בָּלוּט m. (בלט) 1) *acorn, nut.*—*Pl.* בְּלוּטִים, בְּלוּטִין. Men. 63[a] בְּלוּטֵי היונים Grecian nuts (nut-ben; v. Sm. Ant. s. v. Balanus).—2) *oak. Pl.* as above. Y. Keth. VII, end, 31[d]; Gen. R. s. 15, expl. אַלּוֹנִים (v. next w.)—3) (v. Sm. Ant. s. v. Porta) *peg placed in the door-bars* when quite home in the socket. Pesik. R. s. 6 if the gate-bars were wanting ב׳ אחד only one peg.—*Pl.* as above. Ibid.—4) *key-bit.* Y. Sabb. VIII, 11[b] bot. כלוט (corr. acc.); v. חַת.

בְּלוּטָא, בְּלוּט ch. same, *oak.* Targ. Y. II, Gen. XXXV, 8 (h. text אַלּוֹן); a. e.—*Pl.* בְּלוּטֵי, בְּלוּטִין.—Targ. Ezek. XXVII, 6.—R. Hash. 23[a] Ar. (ed. בוטמי a. בלוטי transposed; v. בּוּטְמָא); B. Bath. 80[b].

בְּלוּיִים, v. בְּלָאִים.

בָּלוּל m. (בלל) 1) *mixed up,* v. בָּלַל.—2) *cloudy.* B. Bath. 147[a], v. בָּרוּר.

בלולין, v. לוּל.

בְּלוֹנְיָא, v. בְּלֵיוֹנָא.

בלוניא, Cant. R. to I, 10; Yalk. Cant. 983 בלוניא, בלונדים, read פְּלֵירְנָא, v. לִירְנָא a. חָרֵז.

***בְּלוֹנְקֵי** m. (=בי אלונקי, v. אֲלַנְקֵי) *poles for carrying burdens to market;* cmp. אוּנְקְלֵי I, 2.—Y. Dem. II, 22[c] bot. בלוקח מן חב׳ when buying from the retailer's stand, opp. מן הגינה directly from the garden.

בלוסא, v. בּוּלְסָא.

בלוספין, v. פְּלוּפְסִין.

בְּלוּעָה f. (בלע, v. בְּלִיעָה) *vortex, gulf.* Snh. 108[a] ב׳ דגדר (Ms. O. בְּלִיעָה דגדור, v. Rabb. D. S. a. l. note 300) the gulf of G.

בלופסין, v. פְּלוּפְסִין.

בלורי, v. בַּלְנְרִין.

בְּלוּרְיָא pr. n. f. *B'luria* (Valeria). R. Hash. 17[b], a proselyte. Cmp. בְּרוּרְיָא.

בְּלֵרְיוֹת, בְּלוּרִיוֹת, Gen. R. s. 28; Yalk. Zeph. 566, v. בְּלוּרִית.

***בולרין, בלורין,** read בַּלְנְרִין f. (balnearia) *bath-house.* Gen. R. s. 8; Yalk. Gen. 13 וראה ב׳ אחת מושלכ׳ saw a bath-house cast down.—[Ab. Zar. 18[b], v. בלרין.]

בְּלוּרִית f. (בלר, √בל, v. בלל) *something twisted,* whence 1) *chain, rope* or *wreath* (v. P. Sm. I, 532 בלורא=h. מעשה

מקשה, a. בלוריא vincula jugi).—*Pl.* בְּלוֹרִיּוֹת. Gen. R. s. 28; Yalk. Zeph. 566 ב׳ של זהב (Gen. R. l. c. some ed. בְּלָרִיּוֹת) thick gold chains (as translation of יתר, Job XXII, 20).—2) *plait* or *locks*, esp. the long hair worn by the Roman and Greek youths of the upper classes and offered to the gods on arriving at puberty (v. Sm. Ant. s. v. κόμη). Ab. Zar. I, 3 יום תגלחת זקנו ובלוריתו the day of shaving his (the gentile's) beard and cutting his locks (v. Maim. a. l.). Ib. 29ᵃ. Tosef. Sabb. VI (VII), 1. Deut. R. s. 2 העושה ב׳ וכ׳ he who grows a wig does so for none but an idolatrous purpose. Lev. R. s. 23; a. fr.—Snh. 82ᵃ תפשה בבלוריתה he seized her by her plait.

בְּלוֹרִיתָא ch. same, *woman's plait*. Targ. I. . Num. XXV, 6 (ref. to Snh. 82ᵃ, v. preced.).

בְּלוּשָׁא m. (בלש) *search, examination*. Targ. Ps. LXIV, 7.

בְּלוּשְׁתָּא, בְּלוּשָׁא, v. בִּלֶּשֶׁת, בַּלְּשָׁא.

בלזמיות, v. בְּלוּזְמָא.

***בָּלַח** (cmp. b. h. בלה in בְּבָּהָה, a. בָּחַל), *Hif.* הִבְלִיחַ *to be unsteady, dazzle*. Y. Pes. I, beg. 27ᵃ.

בִּלְחוֹד, v. לְחוֹד.

בָּלַט (√בל, v. בָּלַל; cmp. פלט, מלט, ולד; cmp. Assyr. בלט *to live*, Schr. KAT gloss. I, II) 1) (neut. v.) *to stand forth, project; to be cut in relief*, opp. שָׁקַע to sink, be engraven. R. Hash. 24ᵇ טבעת שחותמה בולט Ms. M. (ed. incorr.) a ring whose seal is cut in relief; Y. Ab. Zar. III, 42ᶜ bot. Gitt. 20ᵃ sq. Sot. III, 4 עיניה בולטות her eyes protruded; Num. R. s. 9.—Yoma 54ᵃ דוחקין ובולטין pressing forth and protruding (from behind the curtain); a. fr.—2) (act. v.) *to drive forth, beat*. Y. Sabb. XII, 13ᵈ בבולט מקום הכתב וכ׳ when he beats out the place of writing, opp. חוקק.

בְּלַט ch. same. Part. pass. בְּלִיט. Targ. II Chr. V, 9. Hull. 45ᵇ בְּלִיטָן, ib. 76ᵃ בְּלִיטֵי protruding sinews, opp. בלועי sunk in the flesh, indistinguishable.

בלטוורא, read בְּבוֹשְׁרוֹת. Cant. R. to II, 15 קיניגין מכללה ודיארטיה עתידים מן ב׳ דא דיחתו וייטורד זה שטיחם אחריהם, read, acc. to intimation in comment. Mat. K., as follows: קיניגין ותייטרן הח״ד מוציא אסירים בכשרות ואח״כ התייטרון זה שנ׳ הבאים אחריהם בים (the passage through the Red Sea and the coming of the noble Egyptians afterwards was) like the order of the kynegion (the actors in the fights of the arena) and the theatron (the spectators), as it says (Ps. LXVIII, 7), 'He leadeth forth the captives with their outfits', and then come the spectators, as we read (Ex. XIV, 28), 'who came after them into the Sea.'

בלי, Y. Ned. III, 38ᵃ top, v. ברייכסין.—Pesik. Bahod. p. 107ᵇ, v. בִּילִי.

בָּלָה, בלי (b. h.; √בל, v. בלל; cmp. נבל) *to be crumbled; to be worn out, to fail, decay, perish*. Koh. R. to I, 4 היא בוֹלָה it (the generation of man) decays (dies out), אינה בוֹלָה it (the earth) does not grow old. Taan. 9ᵃ (play on עד בלי די Mal. III, 10) עד שיִּבְלוּ שפתותיכם מלומר די until your lips grow tired from saying, It is enough; (Y. ib. III, 66ᵈ bot. שיבללו, v. בָּלַל); a. fr.—Part. pass. בָּלוּי *outworn*. *Pl.* בלויים. Midr. Till. to Ps. XXV, 1.

Pi. בִּלָּה *to wear out, outlive, survive*. Lev. R. s. 4 הנפש מְבַלָּה וכ׳ the soul survives the body. Ib. s. 19 (play on אין בלתך, I Sam. II, 2) אין לְבַלּוֹתֶךָ there is none to outlive thee. Koh. R. l. c.; Cant. R. to V, 15 one erects a building ואחר מְבַלֶּה אותו (not מכלה) and another man ruins it. Snh. 105ᵃ, v. בִּלְעָם.

Nif. נִבְלָה, *Nithpa.* נִתְבַּלָּה *to become outworn, fade away*. Esth. R. introd. עתידין לְהִבָּלוֹת (Gen. R. s. 42 לִבְלוֹת) are destined to decay. Deut. R. s. 7, end נִתְבַּלּוּ (the garments) were worn out. B. Mets. 87ᵃ נ׳ הבשר her body was withered. B. Bath. 146ᵃ עשויין לִיבָּלוֹת made to be used up.

בְּלֵי I, בְּלָא, בְּלָה ch. same. Targ. Deut. VIII, 4; ib. Y. XXIX, 4 בלמו, Var. כלמו, read בלת; a. fr.—Lev. R. s. 19 כולו בלה all goes to ruin. Ber. 5ᵇ, v. בְּבָא. Ib. 6ᵃ. Bekh. 9ᵃ ובלו להו ואזול they failed and went to destruction. Ab. V, 22 סיב ובְלֵה בה grow old and frail in it (the study of the Law).—[Targ. Ps. LXII, 11; XCI, 2 Ms., v. בְּלֵי I.]

Pa. בַּלֵּי as preced. *Pi.*—Targ. Is. III, 15; a. e.—Ab. Zar. 20ᵃ that this beauty ב׳ עפרא dust will destroy.—Part. pass. f. מְבַלְּיָא. Lev. R. s. 33 (interpret. בלה נאפים Ezek. XXIII, 43) Aquila translates παλαιὰ πόρνη (old harlot), דהוא מבליא גיירארא ed. (Ar. דהיא מב׳ גיירדייא, Yalk. Dan. 1061 only דהיא מבליא) which means, a wasted harlot (wasted through fornication).

***בְּלֵי II** m. pl. constr. (preced., cmp. בְּלָאוֹת, בְּלוּיִים) *rotten pieces of* (wood). Targ. Is. XLIV, 19 (h. text בול, v. Rashi a. l.; Var. יִבְלֵי).

בְּלִי (b. h., v. preced. ws.) prop. *destruction, naught; not;* v. בְּלִימָה. Ber. 44ᵇ מב׳ בשר if without meat.

בליומוס, v. בּוּלְבְּטֵס.

***בִּילְיוֹנָא, בְּלְיוֹנָא** m. (בלי, formed like בזיונא) [*destruction*,] a cacophem. for idolatrous *phylactery, amulet* (v. Sm. Ant. s. v. Amuletum). ב׳ דגושפנקא (Ar. בילוניא) *an amulet (stone) set in a ring*. Gitt. 57ᵃ עד דמתחזר ב׳ וכ׳ so that the stone of a ring could be distinguished (as to shape, legend &c.) at a distance of a mile (from the illuminated town). Ib. 58ᵃ נקטי ב׳ וכ׳ (Yalk. Lam. 1242 כול׳, כילדינא) they took an amulet (believed to effect the begetting of healthy and handsome children).

בְּלָיוֹת, v. בְּלָאוֹת.

בְּלִיָּתָא, v. בְּלִיתָא.

בְּלִילָה f. (בלל, v. בִּילָה) *mixing, mixture*. Y. Maas. Sh. II, 53ᶜ; Y. Dem. V, 24ᵈ top אין ב׳ אלא וכ׳ b'lilah (an even distribution) applies only to wine or oil. Men. III, 2 זו בְּלִילָתָהּ עבה וכ׳ the one forms a thick mixture (one *Log* of oil to one *Issaron* of flour), the other forms a loose mixture (three Log to one *Issaron*).—*Pl.* בְּלִילוֹת. Tosef.

Dem. II, 7; Men. 18ᵇ; Ḥull. 132ᵇ חב׳ the priest's mixing the offerings (Lev. II, 5; a. fr.).

בְּלִים part. pass. of בָּלַם.

בְּלִימָה (בְּלִי מָה) f. (b. h., v. בְּלִי) [*nothing,*] *air* (fr. Job XXVI, 7). Num. R. s. 14 עשר ספירות ב׳ (some ed. בלי מה) the ten heavenly spheres (cmp. Sepher Yetsir. beg.). Ex. R. s. 15 על אויר העולם על ב׳ ... he rested it (the upper story, the sky) on the atmosphere, on b'limah (Tanḥ. Ḥaye 3 על מה על האויר).

בלינוס, Pesik. R. s. 42, read פְּלִינוֹס.

בְּלִינֵי, v. בְּלְנֵי.

בלינירין, Y. Snh. X, 29ᵃ top, read פְּלִינִידִין.

בליסמורי, v. בַּלִּסְטָרִי.

בליסמין, Cant. R. to II, 14, read כְּלִיסְמִין; cmp. Ex. R. s. 21.

בַּלִּיסְטְרָא (בליצטרא) f. (ballistra, βάλιστρα) *catapult, a war engine for throwing stones,* or (b. manualis) *for arrows.* Lam. R. to II, 2 אבני ב׳ stones thrown from the catapult. Y. Sot. VIII, 22ᵇ bot. ברד כנגד בליצטורא שלהן; (Mekh. Bshall. ş. 2 בלסטראות, pl.; Yalk. Ex. 232 בלסיטראות, read בליסט׳) the hail stones correspond to the catapults in the warfare of men. Pesik. R. s. 17; Pesik. Vayhi p. 67ᵃ אבני בלסתרא (corr. acc.). Pesik. R. s. 29—30 (p. 139ᵇ ed. Fr.) את האבן בליסטרה (read אבן הבל׳). Lam. R. introd. (R. Josh. 2) אבני בליסטרוס (read רא . . .); a. fr.—*Pl.* בַּלִּיסְטְרָאוֹת. Yalk. l. c., v. supra. Tanḥ. Bo 4; Shof'tim 14. Mekh. l. c. Midr. Till. to Ps. XVIII.

בַּלִּיסְטָרִי (בליסטורי) m. (ballistarius, βαλιστάριος) *attendant of the catapult,* also *archer.* Ḥull. 60ᵇ או ב׳ היה .... was Moses a hunter or an archer (to have known the nature of animals so well)?

בליספימיא, v. בְּלַסְפֵּ׳.

בְּלִיעָה f. (בלע) 1) *swallowing, gluttony.* Num. R. s. 14 (play on בֶּלַע Gen. XXXVI, 32) he sold his birthright בשביל בְּלִיעָתוֹ to satisfy his gluttony.—בית הב׳ *œsophagus.* Toh. I, 1; a. fr.—2) *vortex,* v. בְּלוּעָה.

בֵּי בְּ׳, בְּלִיעַ m. (=h. בית הבליעה, v. preced.) *gullet,* whence (cmp. וֶשֶׁט) *straits* (prob. *Scylla and Charybdis*). Bekh. 9ᵃ.—Snh. 110ᶜ בלועי דקרח (corr. acc.) the chasm created for Korah.

בְּלִיַּעַל m. (b. h.) *availing nothing, wickedness.* Snh. 111ᵇ (playing on עוֹל) בנר ב׳ means בנים . . . עול וכ׳ sons who shook off the yoke &c.

בְּלִיעֲתָא f. ch. (=h. בְּלִיעָה) *swallowing,* Targ. Y. I Num. XXVI, 11, constr. בְּלִיעַת.

בליצטורא, בליצטרא. v. בַּלִּיסְטְרָא.

בליקוס, v. בְּלָקִים.

בְּלִיתָא f. (בלי) *rag, shred.* Sabb. 134ᵃ. Ḥull. 8ᵇ ב׳ דפרסא a shred of a curtain (soft rag). Kidd. 48ᵇ צייר בב׳ tied up in a rag.—*Pl.* בְּלָיָיתָא. Yeb. 120ᵃ (some ed. בליתא).

בָּלַל (b. h.; √בל; a) sec. r. of ביל, בול; √בה, בו, cmp. בִּין, *to penetrate, break through,* v. בלט; b) √בל *to crumble, soften,* cmp. √מל; v. בלי, נבל, בלט in בילניתא) *to mix* (with oil), *knead, stir; to mix fodder.* Zeb. XIV, 3 (112ᵇ) הבולל the priest who kneads the meat-offering with oil, v. בְּלִילָה. Dem. V, 5 בולל ונוטל (strike out ואוכל in Bab. ed., Ar. Var. בורר) he mixes the fruits and takes the tithe. Y. B. Kam. IV, beg. 4ᵃ לָבֹול to mix up (coins in a bag.) Y. R. Hash. I, 56ᵈ bot.; Tanḥ. Noah 11, v. בול III; a. fr. —Part. pass. בָּלוּל, f. בְּלוּלָה. Snh. 24ᵃ (play on בבל) ב׳ במקרא וכ׳ mixed up (confused) in Bible study &c. [Y. Yeb. VIII, end, 9ᵈ קריבה בבלל, read בְּכָלִיל.] V. בָּלוּל.

Nif. נִבְלַל, *Hof.* הוּבְלַל *to be mixed.* Y. Maas. Sh. II, 53ᶜ, v. חָפַן. Men. XII, 4 (103ᵇ; 18ᵇ) ששים נבללין sixty measures of flour can be thoroughly mixed; v. בִּילָה. Ib. יכולים לְהִבָּלֵל.—Y. Shek. VI, 49ᵈ bot. אש מוּבְלֶלֶת באש fire mixed with fire.—[Y. Taan. III, 66ᵈ bot. עד שיִּבָּלְלוּ וכ׳ until your speech shall become confounded from repeatedly saying, Enough; v. בלי.] Y. Ber. VI, 10ᵃ top (play on בַּל) יִבָּלְלוּ וכ׳ all blessings shall be kneaded thogether—*Pilp.* בִּלְבֵּל.

בָּלַם I (b. h.; denom. of בְּלוֹם, √בלל, בל, *fodder-bag, nose-bag, muzzle*) *to muzzle, restrain.* Yalk. Num. 743 (read in place of כדו בלום לעמו וכ׳:) פיו בָּלוּם לעמו של משה יכול הוא לִבְלוֹם צפורנו של אחד מהם the mouth of the people of Moses is tied up (we dare not talk), but can he tie up (disable) the nail of any of them (the Canaanites)? Ḥull. 89ᵃ (play on בלימה, Job XXVI, 7) שבּוֹלֵם וכ׳ who restrains himself in strife (refrains from violence, keeps silence &c.).—2) part. pass. בָּלוּם (cmp. אִלֵּם) *unfit for use, lame, sore, swollen, closed by a tumor.* Bekh. 40ᵇ פיו ב׳ one whose mouth is swollen (one opin. in Rashi: *shrunk*); רגליו מְבוּלָּמוֹת (Pu.) one whose feet are swollen (shrunk). Ib. 43ᵇ חוטמו ב׳ Ar. (ed. בולם, corr. acc.) whose nose is obstructed.—Gitt. 67ᵃ אוצר ב׳ a packed treasury of knowledge; v. בָּלַם.—*Part. Pu.* מְבוּלָּם, v. supra.

**Hif.* הִבְלִים *to restrict.*. Y. Ḥag. II, 78ᵃ bot. ובלבד שיַּבְלִים לעיסתו provided that (when cutting &c.) he does only as much as is needed for his dough for the offering; [Tosaf. to Ḥag. 17ᵇ, s. v. אלא, cites שיכלה עיסתו, v. בָּלָה.]

בָּלַם II (v. preced.; cmp. Syr. בלמא *halter*) *to attempt to get rid of the halter; to kick, strike* (of an unruly horse). Pesik. Zakh. p. 24ᵇ (ref. to Ps. XXXII, 9) thou puttest a bit on him והוא בּוֹלֵם and he strikes. Ib. קריב לגביה והוא ב׳ (strike out לא, as Tanḥ. ed. Bub. Ki Thetse, 6 a. Yalk. Ps. 719) you come near him and he strikes; Tanḥ. Ki Thetse, 6; Yalk. Deut. 938, Ps. l. c. (with var. vers.).

בְּלַם ch.=h. בָּלַם I.—1) Part. pass. בְּלִים *tied, mute.* Targ. Is. XXXII, 4; a. e. [Targ. Y. Deut. XXIX, 4; v. בְּלֵי I.]—2) (cmp. כרך) *to put meat between bread, wrap up.* Ḥull. 107ᵇ ב׳ ליה אומצא wrapped up a piece of meat for him (v. Tosaf. a. l.).

בַּלְמָא* m. (preced.; v. בָּלַם) *halter*, trnsf. *guard, protection of the borders of a field*, as fences &c.; cmp. אַפְסָרָא. B. Mets. 103^b^ כל עיקר ב׳ וכ׳ whatever is essential for guarding the limits, the landlord must provide. [Ms. M. כלומ׳, Ar. כלמי, v. בְּלָמָא.]

בַּלָּנִי, בַּלָּן m. (βαλανεύς) *bathing master, bathing attendant* (who receives a small coin as fee, cmp. אוֹלְיָיר). Shebi. VIII, 5; v. בַּיָּיר. Y. B. Bath. IV, 14^c^ bot. מקום חב׳ the bathing master's station (the income therefrom); a. fr.—*Pl.* בַּלָּנִין. Sabb. IV, 2 קורות חב׳ the beams whereon the bathing masters are stationed.

בַּלָּנִי, בַּלָּנָא, בַּלָּנַאי, בַּלָּן ch. same. Lev. R. s. 28 אזל בדיל ב׳ he went after a bather. Ib. אתעביד ב׳ וספר has become a bather and hair cutter; Esth. R. to VI, 10 (בלן); Pesik. R. s. 18.

בלנטיא, Sifra B'har Par. 5, ch. VII (Yalk. Lev. 666 בגלטקא), v. לֶקְטִיקָא a. גְּלוּגְדְקָא.

בַּלְנִי, בַּלָּנִי, v. בַּלָּן, בַּלָּן.

בַּלִּינֵי, בַּלָּנֵי m. pl. (balnea, balineæ) *bath, bathing*. Y. Ber. VI, 10^c^ bot. כהדין דשתי חמרא בתר בלני (read בלינֵי) as if one drinks wine after bathing (for medicinal purposes, when the wine which he drinks after meal cannot be considered as a continuation of the draught taken before meal; v. אֲלוּנְטִית II). Y. Maas. Sh. IV, 54^d^ bot. as much as one will ask (for the fruits left over) on a hot summer day בתר ב׳ after bathing time (when he is anxious to sell).—*Denom. בַּלָּנְיוֹת f. pl. (=balnearia) *bathing apparel*. B. Bath. IV, 5 (67^b^, Bab. ed.) ואת חב׳ (Var. וִילָאוֹת q. v.).

בלנדיא, Y. Sabb. VI, 8^b^ bot., transl. of רעלות Is. III, 19, read בְּלָנִידְיָא.

בַּלְנְרִין (בַּלְרִין) 1) constr. בַּלְנְרֵי (בַּלְרֵי) m. pl. (balnearia) *bathing apparel, bathing utensils*. Y. Kil. IX, 32^a^ bot.; Y. M. Kat. III, 82^a^ ב׳ נשים women's bathing clothes; Sabb. 147^b^ בלרי (some ed. בלורי, corr. בלנ׳); Tosef. Kil. V, 16 בלארי (corr. acc.).—2) *bath-house*, v. בלורין.—V. בַּפְרִיּוֹת.

בָּלַס (√בל, v. בָּלַל) 1) *to mix with all sorts of things, to mix indiscriminately. Part. pass.* בָּלוּס, f. בְּלוּסָה. Sabb. 76^b^ עיסה ב׳ a dough of unsifted flour (with bran &c.). B. Bath. 58^a^ אוצר ב׳ a store room of mixed things (lumber room).—Gitt. 67^a^ אוצר ב׳ a mind full of all kind of knowledge (oth. vers. בלום, v. בָּלַם).—*Pl.* בְּלוּסִין. Mikv. IX, 5 חב׳ utensils soaked with a mixture of colors (stains from use), opp. נקיים shining, polished.—2) (cmp. בלי) *to rot*. Gen. R. s. 28 אוצרות בְּלוּסִים store of spoiled fruits.

בלסימיה, v. בְּלַסְפִימְיָא.

בַּלְסָם, בַּלְסְמוֹן m. (בסם, with inserted ל=ר; hence βάλσαμον which was readopted as בלסמון; cmp. בְּלוּזְמָא) *balsam, aromatic gum*. Gen. R. s. 91 (interpr. צרי) בלסם קטף the gum of the balsam tree.—Targ. Cant. VII, 14. Lev. R. s. 31; Cant. R. to I, 15; a. e. Cmp. פַּלְסְמוֹן a. אַפַּרְסְמוֹן.

בְּלַסְפִימְיָא f. (βλασφημία) *blasphemy*. Y'lamd. to Num. XXVIII, quot. (בלוסס׳) in Ar.—Tanh. ed. Bub. Tol'doth 21 בלסימיה (corr. acc.).

בְּלַסְפִימִיסִין, read בְּלַסְפֵּימֵיסִין (ἐβλασφήμησεν) *he blasphemed*. Y'lamd., ref. to I Kings XXI, 13 quot. in Ar. (interpret. בֵּרַךְ).

בלסתרא, v. בַּלִּיסְטְרָא.

בָּלַע (b. h.; √בל, v. בלל) *to absorb*, opp. פלט; *to swallow, consume*. Y. Shek. VI, 49^c^ bot. . . . שהאור בּוֹלֵעַ בּוֹלַעַת. . . בּוֹלְעִין the flame absorbs a portion of the oil, and so do the wood and the kettle. Hull. 110^b^ the liver when boiled with other meat פולטת ואינה ב׳ gives out (blood) but absorbs nothing from the other pieces. Y. Sabb. XIV, 14^d^ top; Tosef. ib. XII (XIII), 9 but he may sip vinegar וּבוֹלֵעַ and swallow it (opp. פלט to spit it out). Y. Ter. VIII, 45^b^ bot. הלעוס כבלוע what is chewed is to be considered as swallowed. Hull. 71^a^ טומאה בְלוּעָה an unclean object (food) that has been swallowed.—Snh. 110^a^ הַבְּלוּעִין those (of the band of Korah) that were swallowed up. Kel. IX, 6, v. הֶרְבֵּן; a. fr.

Nif. נִבְלַע *to be swallowed;* with בין, *to be absorbed, disappear*. Sot. 36^b^; Tanh. Vayigg. 4; Yalk. Gen. 150 (interpret. the name Bela, Gen. XLVI, 21) שנ׳ בין האומות for he (Joseph) has disappeared among gentiles. Gen. R. s. 94; Yalk. l. c. שנבלע ממני he disappeared to me.

Hif. הִבְלִיעַ *to cause swallowing, to make absorb*. Ex. R. s. 33 הִבְלַעְתָּ לקרח thou mad'st (the earth) swallow Korah. Ber. 24^b^ מַבְלִיעוֹ בטליתו he hides the spittle in his cloak; Y. Sabb. VII, 10^b^ top. Hull. 113^a^ מַבְ׳ דם באברים causes the blood to remain in the meat (prevents it from flowing out).—Trnsf. *to sell something in connection with other things, in a lump, in the bargain*. Bekh. 31^b^ מבליעו וכ׳ he sells it (the meat) in the bargain with the hide &c. B. Mets. 64^a^; B. Kam. 118^b^ one who robs his neighbor וה׳ לו בחשבון and makes up for it implicitly on settling his accounts. V. הַבְלָעָה.

Hof. הוּבְלַע *to be swallowed up; to mingle with*, v. supra Nif.—Part. מוּבְלָע. Ber. 31^b^ מ׳ בין אנשים mixing with people, expl. לא ארוך וכ׳ neither very tall &c. (of average qualities). Erub. IV, 6 מ׳ ביניהן his property is enclosed between theirs (reaches into the limits of each). Y. ib. IV, 21^d^ bot. עיירות המובלעות *inland-towns*, opp. border-towns. Y. B. Bath. VII, 15^cd^ מוּבְלָעִין בה fields which are enclosed by others belonging to the same estate.

Hithpa. הִתְבַּלַּע *to be swallowed up, to disappear*. Midr. Till. to Ps. XIX, beg. מִתְבַּלֵּעַ מן וכ׳ he disappears from the world (forfeits his life).

בְּלַע ch. same. Targ. Ex. VII, 12; a. fr.—Hull. 111^a^ כי היכי דפליט הדר ב׳ as it gives out, so does it again absorb; a. fr.—Part. pass. בְּלִיעַ, בְּלִיעָא. Ib. בליעא דמא filled with blood.—Snh. 110^a^ בלועי דקרח, v. בְּלִיעַ.—

Trnsf. *to receive blows* (cmp. סָפַג). Men. 7ª קולפי טאבי בְּלַעִי וכ׳ I received many blows at the hands of Ab. over &c. Arakh. 22ª. Ber. 56ª.—Targ. II, Esth. III, 7 בְּלִיעָן אינון בידי they are swallowed up (bound to be destroyed) by my hand.

Af. אַבְלַע, as h. Hif. Hull. 67ᵇ אַבְלַע לי let me swallow them (put them in my mouth). Men. 17ª, v. infra. B. Mets. 64ª וא׳ ליה בחשבון, v. preced. Hif.

Ithpe. אִיבְּלַע, אִיתְבְּלַע=as h. Nif. 1) *to be swallowed up, to disappear.* Targ. Y. Gen. XLVI, 21 אתב׳ מניה he was swallowed up (disappeared) from his side; v. preced. Targ. Josh. VI, 5 יתבלע וכ׳ shall sink into the ground beneath it; a. e.—Y. R. Hash. II, 58ª bot. איתב׳ מן קומוי (the moon) disappeared from his sight.—2) *to be given to eat; trnsf. to be taught.* Ber. 24ᵇ הא מילתא אִבְּלְעָא לי בי וכ׳ v. Rabb. D. S. a. l. note) this I have been taught in the school of R. &c.; (Men. 17ª הא מילתא אבלע לי וכ׳ this has R. H. taught me).

בֶּלַע m. (preced.) 1) *absorption, natural loss, leakage.* B. Mets. III, 8 (40ª) לוג ומחצה ב׳ a *Log* and a half is a reasonable leakage (absorbed by new vessels); a. e.—2) pr. n. m. (b. h.) *Bela;* v. בָּלַע a. בְּלִיעָה.—3) בֶּלַע or בְּלַע (cmp. בְּלִי) *a nothing, a mote.* Tanh. Vayak. 7 (ref. to כְּבַלַּע Num. IV, 20) כב׳ הזה שהוא נופל בעין; (Num. R. s. 5 מן העין) as much as a mote which enters one's eye.

בַּלָּע m. *swallower, glutton.* Num. R. s. 14; v. בְּלִיעָה. Snh. 105ª, v. בִּלְעָם.

בְּלַע, בִּלְעָא, בְּלִעָה ch. m. (cmp. בֶּלַע) *the thing swallowed, choking fit.* Y. Ab. Zar. II, 40ᵈ אחן בלעה שרי in a choking attack it is allowed (to apply remedies on the Sabbath) Ib. הוה ליה בלע had a choking fit; Koh. R. to X, 5 הוה ליה חד בלעא. Ib. לאפקא בְּלִעֵיה to get out what he had swallowed.

בלעין, Y. Dem. III, 23ᵇ מחוסר לב׳, read בְּעָלִים=בָּעְלִין, v. בַּעַל.

בִּלְעָם (b. h.) pr. n. m. *Balaam*, the gentile prophet of the Pentateuch. Snh. 105ª ב׳ בַּלָּע עם Ar. (Var. in Ar., a. ed. בִּלָּא) devourer (destroyer) of the people; other homilet. etymology ibid. שבִּלָּה עם he ruined the people (through debauchery; Rashi:=בִּלְבֵּל). Gen. R. s. 65. Ab. V, 19 (as type of false teachers); a. fr.

בלעס (בלע with ס intens.; cmp. בלס, לעס); *Ithpe.* אִתְבְּלַעֵס *to be choked, to choke.* Y. Ter. VIII, 46ª ואיתב׳, ואיתבלעסון (corr. acc.).

***בַּלְצָא** pr. n. m. *Baltsa.* Ex. R. s. 29 שאל ב׳ את ר׳ עקיבא [prob. to be read אלוהי ז״ל=אל׳ ז״ל, cmp. Y. Ber. IX, 13ᶜ; Midr. Till. to Ps. XVIII; CIV end].

בָּלָק, v. בִּיזָּק.

בָּלָק (b. h.) pr. n. m. *Balak*, King of Moab. Ber. 7ª. Num. R. s. 20; a. fr.

בלקטורים, בלקטירין, ...רין, v. בּוּלְקְטַר (collectarius), and בְּלַקְטֵירִין (χαρακτῆρες).

בלקיא, v. גַּלְבְּקָיָא.

בלרא, v. בּוּלָרָא.

בַּלְרֵי, v. בַּלְנָרִין.

בלריון, v. בלרין.

בַּלְרִיּוֹת, v. בְּלוּרִית.

***בלרין**, Ab. Zar. 18ᵇ ב׳ ובלריון Ms. M. (ed. only בלורין; Y. ib. I, 40ª מילרין מילריה, added in Ms. M. l. c. as מלרין ומלריון; Yalk. Ps. 613 בלרין ובלריין) corruption of לִיבְּרָלִין (liberales, sub. ludi, or liberalia) *Bacchanalian games* (v. Sm. Ant. s. v. Dionysia). [The preceding לולין or לולון must prob. be read לודין *ludi.*] V. סגולרין.

בָּלַשׁ (√בל, v. בלל) 1) **to hack and break the clods of earth* (v. בולII; v. Sm. Ant. s. v. Raster). Lev. R. s. 36 on setting a vine בּוֹלְשִׁין אותה וכ׳ (read אותן) you first break them (the large stony clods) under it and then you plant it. Cmp. אַבְלוּשָׁא.—2) (law) *to search* (for concealed goods &c.) *to hold a visitation.* Denom. בַּלָּשֵׁי &c. —3) (milit.) *to patrol.* Midd. I, 7 לִבְלוֹשׁ וכ׳ to patrol the Temple.

בְּלַשׁ ch. same; *to search, examine.* Targ. O. Gen. XXXI, 35; a. fr.

Pa. בַּלֵּשׁ same. Targ. Is. XXII, 5 מְבַלְּשִׁין (ed. Vien. מַבְלְשִׁין Af.); a. e.

Ithpa. אִתְבַּלַּשׁ, *Ithpe.* אִתְבְּלֵישׁ *to be searched, ransacked.* Targ. Ob. v. 6, quot. B. Kam. 3ᵇ; a. e.

בַּלְשָׁא, בָּלוֹשָׁא m. ch. (v. next w.) *searcher; constable.* Nidd. 52ª שדר ב׳ וכ׳ he sent a constable and forced her to leave her (second) husband.—*Pl.* בָּלוֹשִׁין, בָּלוֹשַׁיָּא. Targ. Zeph. I, 12; a. e.—Ber. 44ª בָּלוֹשֵׁי Ar. a. Ms. F. (ed. בָּאלוֹשֵׁי).

בַּלָּשׁ, בַּלָּשַׁאי m. (בלש) *detective, investigator, searching tax-commissioner, constable.* Y. Dem. VII, 26ª מקל ב׳ (not מיקל) the commissioner's pointed staff (with which he searches). Y'lamd. to Gen. XXXVIII, 1 quot. in Ar. בלשיי מסר וכ׳ the constable delivers the prisoner over to the executioner.—*Pl.* בַּלָּשִׁין. Kel. XV, 4 מקל הב׳, v. supra.—בַּלָּשַׁיִין. Y'lamd. to Num. XXIII, 7. [Var. in Hai Gaon בַּלָּסִיי.]

בֵּלְשַׁפַּט pr. n. pl. *Belshafat* (contr. of בי אלישפט), a staple town in Susiana (Khazistan), Syriac name *Beth-Lapetha=Ahwaz* (Neub. Géogr. p. 380). Taan. 22ª בי לפט ed. (Var. בולשפטי, בילפט, v. Rabb. D. S. a. l. note 8). B. Mets. 73ᵇ וולשפט ed. (Ar. לולשפט, Ms. H. בלשפט); B. Bath. 98ª ווֹל שפט ed. (Ar. לולש׳; Ms. M. ולשפט; Var. בי לישפט, לרשפט, וילש׳, ויל שפט, v. Rabb. D. S. a. l. note). [Yoḥăsin s. v. בי אלישפט: ברוקא.]

בַּלֶּשֶׁת, בּוֹלֶשֶׁת f. (בלש) *reconnoitring troop, quartermaster's division, marauders.* Bets. 21ª; Tosef. ib. II, 6. Ab. Zar. V, 6 (Y. ed. בר׳). Y. ib. 45ª top בשלום בו׳ ובמלחמת בו׳ the Mishnah means when the troop comes in peace, or when it comes with hostility. Sabb. 145^b ed. 'בר, Ar. 'בל.

בֵּית ב׳, בַּלְתָּן, בַּלְתִּין, בַּלְתִּי pr. n. pl. *Beth-Baltin* &c., v. בִּירָם. R. Hash. II, 4 (22^b; Ms. M. בילתי, בלתי; v. Rabb. D. S. c. l. note). Ib. 23^a bot. 'מאי בית ב (Ms. M. 1 בילתי, 2 בלתי, Ms. L. בילתין) what is B. B.? Answ. בירם.

במגנימין, Y. R. Hash. I, 57^b, 'כחדא ב, prob. to be read: כחדין אִיפּוֹמְנִימָטִין (ὑπομνήματα) like *the minutes* of the court proceedings, opp. to preced. דירין, read דִּיקִין (δίκη, pl.).

סֵפֶר ב׳, בְּמִדְבַּר m. *the fourth book of Moses* (*Numeri*). Gen. R. s. 3; a. e.—ב׳ רבה the fourth book of Midrash Rabbah (Num. R.).

בָּמָה f. (b.h.; prob. fr. בוא) *entrance, gathering place, ascent* (cmp. b. h. מָבוֹא a. מַעֲלֶה); esp. *Bamah*, name of the legitimate altars prior to, and of the illegitimate after, the establishment of a central sanctuary (at Shiloh) and of the Temple at Jerusalem; *temporary* or *improvised altar*; v. Zeb. XIV, 4—8.—Meg. I, 10 ב׳ גדולה national altar; ב׳ קטנה local altar (during their period of legitimacy); Tosef. Zeb. XIII, 17 sq.; a. fr.—*Pl.* בָּמוֹת Zeb. l. c. Ib. 114^b 'בשעת היתר חב at the period when bamoth were permitted. v. supra; a. fr. [Meg. 32^a 'הלוחות וחב, v. בִּימָה.] Cmp. בִּימָה.

בָּמוֹסָא, v. בָּמְסָא.

בָּמוֹתָא, v. בָּמְתָא.

במיסטאות, Midr. Thron. Salom., Beth-Hammidr. ed. Jellinek V, 2, read בִּימוֹסָאוֹת, v. בִּימוֹס.

בָּמְסָא* m. ch.=h. בִּימוֹס *altar, high-place.* [Targ. Y. II, Deut. XXXII, 13 בָּמְסָא, read בָּמְתָא.]—*Pl.* בָּמְסַיָּא, בָּמוֹסַיָּא (בָּמְסַיָּא) בָּמוֹסִין *idolatrous places of worship.* Targ. II Chr. XIV, 4; a. e.

במרזח, Cant. R. to VII, 10 some ed., read כִּמוֹמֶר חזה.

בָּמְתָא f. ch.=h. בָּמָה. Targ. I Kings III, 4; a. e.—*Pl.* בָּמְתָא (בָּמוֹתָא). Targ. ib. 2; a. e.—[Targ. II Chr. XI, 15 בָּמְתַיָּא.]

בֵּן m., constr. בֶּן (b. h.; בנה) *offspring, son, child.* 'שבוע חב the male child's week, a disguise for *circumcision day*, adopted during the Hadrianic persecutions. Snh. 32^b; Y. Keth. I, 25^c; a. e.—'ישוע חב a disguise for פִּדְיוֹן חבן. B. Kam. 80^a.— . . בְּנוֹ של the son of, v. שֶׁל. בֵּן של קדושים descendant of holy men. Ab. Zar. 50^a; a. e.—*Pl.* בָּנִים, constr. בְּנֵי. Ab. III, 14 ב׳ למקום chosen children of God. Gen. R. s. 82 בָּנֶיהָ של תורה children (followers) of the Law.—Trnsf. *belonging to, fit for* &c.; e. g. בני גולה those belonging to the colony of exiles, Babylonians &c.; בני גליל Galileans; בני אכילה things fit to be eaten &c [For such compounds as are not self-evident, see the respective determinants.] [בני פיקרין, v. בְּנִיפִיקְרִין.]

בַּנָּא, v. בני.

בַּנָּאָה m. (contr. of בַּלָּנָא) 1) *bather.* Targ. II, Esth. VI, 12 Ms. (ed. בַּאנְיָא).—2) pr. n. m., v. בַּנַּאי II.

בַּנַּאי m. h. a. ch. (בני) *builder, mason.* B. Mets. 118^b; a. fr.—Y. Ḥag. II, 77^b top 'אומנתיה דהן ב this boy's trade should be that of a builder. Sabb. 156^b 'ב׳ וסתיר וכ (shall grow to be one) who builds and destroys, destroys and builds (restless). Ib. 115^a; a. fr. V. אַרְדִּיכָל.—[V. בַּנָּאִים, בַּנָּאִין.]

בַּנַּאי II, בַּנָּאָה, a. **רַבַּנַּאי** (=רב ב׳) pr. n. m. *Bannai, Bannaah, Rabbannai*, name of an Amora. Keth. 50^b. Ber. 38^b. [Ib. 55b Ms. M. נהוראי. B. Mets. 2^a, a. e. 'רב, Ms. M. רבינא, v. Rabb. D. S. a. l. note.]

בַּנָּאִין, בַּנָּאִים m. sing. a. pl. (contr. of בן נאים, v. נָאָה) *one of becoming conduct, refined, a cultured person;* opp. בּוּר; (cmp. Sabb. 114^a top, as to a scholar's duty to pay attention to dress). [For oth. opin., v. Sachs Beitr. II, 199; Frankel Monatsschr. 1846, p. 855.] Mikv. IX, 6; Sabb. l. c. 'של ב׳ וכ the garments of a Bannaïm, if stained with pitch on one side cannot be immersed for levitical purposes before the stain is removed (because their owner is more fastidious). Tosef. Mikv. VI (VII), 14 (where גדולה a. קטנה refer to the stain; as to correct vers. v. R. S. to Mikv. l. c.). Sabb. l. c. מאי ב׳ what does B. mean? Answer: 'אלו וכ it means the scholars who are engaged in building up the world (of civilization) all their lives (as if fr. בָּנָה). Ib. (dresses of the B.) אלו 'כלים וכ are the court-garments imported &c., v. אוֹלָרִין.

בנאיתא, v. בְּנְיָיתָא.

בְּנָאתָן, pl. of בְּרַתָּא.

בַּנּוֹיָא m. (בני) *builder.* *Pl.* בַּנּוֹיֵי. Yoma 10^a 'ב׳ ביר וכ shall the builders (of the Temple, the Persians) be delivered into the hands of the destroyers (the Romans)?

בָּנוֹת pl. of בַּת.

בָּנָה, בני (b. h.; sec. r. of בין) [*to combine,*] *to build.* Sabb. XII, 1 הַבּוֹנֶה he who builds (on the Sabbath). Ib. 102^b משום בונה (is guilty) because it is one of the labors classified under 'building'; a. fr.—Metaph. *to educate, train.* Ber. 64^a (ref. to Is. LIV, 93) א״ת בָּנַיִךְ אלא בּוֹנַיִךְ read not *banayikh* (thy children), but *bonayikh* (thy builders, trainers); v. בַּנָּאִים.—Ex. R. s. 23 (play on b'noth, Cant. I, 5) 'בונות וכ the authorities directing the building of Jerusalem; v. Pi.—Ḥull. 78^b זה בונה אב, v. אָב, a. בִּנְיָן. [Tosef. Par. VII (VI), 4 'בְּנָאִ ed. Zuck., v. בָּנָה.]

Nif. נִבְנָה 1) *to be built up.* Y. B. Bath. III, 14^b, a. fr. לִיבָּנוֹת, לְהִיבָּנוֹת.—2) (denom. of בֵּן) *to get children.* Gen. R. s. 71.

Nithpa. נִתְבַּנָּה (denom. of בֵּן) *to be adopted, naturalized.* Pesik. R. s. 43 נִתְבַּנּוּ בישראל they became full Israelitish citizens.

Pi. בִּינָּה *to lay out, plan a city, determine its limits.* Ex. R. l. c. the Great Sanedrin held sessions וּמְבַנִּים אותה (not אותם) and determined the limits of Jerusalem; v. Snh. I, 5.—Part. Pu. מְבוּנָּה *cultivated; built* (of human stature), *well-proportioned.* Keth. 112[a]; Sot. 34[b] חיתה מְבוּנָּה על וכ׳ it (Hebron, in spite of the rocky nature of its soil) was seven times better cultivated than Zoan (one measure of its land yielding as much as did seven measures of the soil of Zoan). Ib. 42[b] (play on *benayim,* I Sam. XVII, 4) מב׳ מכל מום his build was without blemish.

בְּנוֹנִי, v. בֵּינוֹנִי.

בְּנָא, בְּנֵי ch.=h. בָּנָה. Targ. Deut. XXV, 9 (Y. יִבְנֵה); a. fr.—Part. בָּנֵי. Targ. Gen. IV, 17.—M. Kat. 10[b] מִיבְנֵי to erect; a. e.

Ithpe. אִתְבְּנֵי as h. Nif. 1) a. 2). Targ. I Kings III, 2; a. fr.—Targ. Gen. XVI, 2; a. e.—Y. Ber. II, 5[a] מִתְבַּנְיָא will be rebuilt; a. e.

בִּנְיָאתָא, v. בִּנְיָיתָא.

***בִּנִיגְנֵי** pl. (benignae, sub. interpretationes, opp. durae, v. Harper's Lat. Dict. 1882) *favorable side, mitigating circumstances.* Ab. Zar. 4[a] אבקש ב׳ שלהם ed. (Ms. בנו׳; Ar. בניגני, taking ב for a servile letter as do the commentaries) I shall search for what can be found in their favor.

בַּנָּיָה, בַּנָּיָיה I m. ch.=h. בַּנַּאי, *builder.* Y. Yoma III, 40[c]; Y. Gitt. VII, 48[d] bot.; Y. B. Bath. VIII, 16[c] top ב׳ דאורייתא a builder of the law (forming ingenious conclusions).—*Pl.* בַּנָּיִין. Y. Ber. IX, 13[a] top; v. אוּמָּן.

בַּנָּיָיה II pr. n. m. *Bannayah,* an Amora. Y. Peah I, 15[b] bot.; a. fr. (Bab. B. Bath. 57[b] בְּנָאָה, v. בַּנַּאי II).

בְּנַיִים, v. בֵּין.

בִּנְיָינָא, v. בִּנְיָנָא.

בניינות, Y. Shek. VI, 49[d] top, v. בֵּינוֹנִי.

בִּנְיָתָא, בִּנְיָיתָא f. pl. (בני; cmp. ארב, ארג a. denom.) *net-work, veils, curtains* &c. Ber. 61[a]; Sabb. 95[a]; Erub. 18[a]; Nidd. 45[b] שכן בכרכי הים קורין לקלעייתא ב׳ (v. Rabb. D. S. a. l. for vers.) at the sea-towns they call all net-works *binyatha*; Koh. R. to VII, 2 בִּנְיָאתָא (Var. בנאיתא).

בִּנְיָן, בִּינְיָן m. (b. h.; בָּנָה) 1) *building, structure; erection.* Succ. 51[b] מי שלא ראה בח״מ בבִנְיָנוֹ whoever has not seen the Temple in its finished state, expl. ibid. בִּנְיָן הורדוס the Herodian Temple (Ms. M. ראה בנין בח״מ.....; v. Rabb. D. S. a. l. note).—אַמַּת הב׳, v. אַמָּה.—Sabb. 102[b] דרך ב׳ בכך such kind of labor belongs to builders' work. Ib. דמי לב׳ it looks like builders' work; a. fr.—בִּנְיַן אב *standard rule,* v. אָב; v. Hull. 78[b], B. Kam. 77[b] זה בנה אב this (Ex. XII, 5) forms the rule, wherever שה is used &c. (v. Tosaf. a. l.).—Sabb. 114[a] בִּנְיָנוֹ של עולם the preservation of the (mental and moral) world.—2) *human frame, skeleton.* Ohol. II, 1 רוב בניינו the greater portion of a corpse as to size of limbs, contrad. to רוב מניינו the larger as to the number of joints and limbs.

בִּנְיָנָא ch. same. Targ. Koh. III, 3; a. e.

בְּנִיסָא m., **בְּנִיסְתָא** f. (בנס) *sour; angry, sad. Pl.* בְּנִיסִין; f. בְּנִיסָתָא. Targ. Y. Gen. XL, 6 (O. נסיסין). Targ. Prov. XXV, 23. [Y. Shek. IV, 48[b] bot. בנרסין, read: בֵּירְהוֹן, v. בֵּין ch.]

בניסן, Y. Keth. XII, 35[a] ב׳ . . . . חמני, v. בְּנִישָׁא.

בְּנִיפִיקִין (בנפיקין) m. (beneficium, βενεφίκιον) *favor, grant,* esp. *the rights of a privileged person concerning the protection of his character.* Tanh. Korah (ed. Bub.) addit. 2 (cmp. Tanh. ib. 8) משל לשושבינה של בת המלך שביקש בני פיקון מן המלך (corr. acc.) this is to be compared to a sponsor of the King's daughter who claimed satisfaction of the King on the ground of his privileges. He said to the King אם אינך תובע ב׳ שלי if thou wilt not stand up for my privileges &c.; Num. R. s. 18 בנפקין שלך (corr. acc.).

בְּנִיפִיקָרִין m. pl. (beneficiarii, βενεφικιάλιοι) *the commander's attendants, orderlies.* Sifrè Deut. 317 (בני פיקרין, בני פוקרים corr. acc.); Yalk. Deut. 944 אלו ב׳ שלהם those are their (the Roman) beneficiarii.

בְּנִיתָא, v. בִּנְיָיתָא.

***בְּנְכֵּי** m. pl. (√בך, v. בכי) *cavities* dug around the vine to receive the water,=h. בְּדִיד 2). M. Kat. 4[b].

בְּנָן pl., v. בְּרַתָּא.—[V. also בֵּן.]

בְּנַס (sec. r. of בס, v. בסס) *to ferment, get sour;* trnsf. *to be angry, agitated.* Dan. II, 12. Targ. Y. Gen. XL, 2. Targ. Esth. II, 21 בנסו וקצפו (ed. Vien. בְּנִשׁוּ, corr. acc.). Ib. IV, 17 ונסס וב׳ (ed. Vien. וכ׳, corr. acc., h. text ויעבר!); v. נְסַס.—Part. pass. בְּנִיס, v. בְּנִיסָא. Denom. בְּסִין.

בִּנְסָא m. (preced.) *anger, ill-humor.* Targ. Job XVI, 10 (Ms. בנסא, some ed. בְּנָסָא).

בנפיקין, בנפקין, v. בְּנִיפִיקִין.

בַּנְרִיּוֹת f. pl. (=בלנרין; cmp. βανίαριν for βαλνιαρία, S.) *bathing apparel.* Gen. R. s. 45 דליים וב׳ וכ׳ (Ar. בנריות, some ed. סנדיות) buckets and bathing apparel did she make her carry &c.; Yalk. Gen. 79 סנדלריאות (corr. acc.).

בַּנְרְיָיתָא f. pl. ch. same. Y. B. Kam. VII, end 6[a] אנא נסיב בַּנְרְיָיתֵיה I will carry his bathing clothes (i. e. I will be his servant; cmp. B. Mets. 41[a]; Erub. 27[b]; Snh. 62[b]).

בנרסיי, Y. Kil. IX, 32[b] top, v. בִּירְדִּסִין.

בְּנָתָא, בְּנָתָן, pl. of בְּרַתָּא.

בְּנָתַיִים, v. בֵּין, בֵּין.

בנתיקה, Y. Snh. VII, 25[d], v. נְתִיקָה ch.

בְּסָא, v. בסי.

***בסאמה**, Pesik. R. suppl. (p. 197[a] ed. Fr.), v. חַסְטָא.

בסבסטי, Num. R. s. 10, v. סַבַּסְטֵי.

בס״גר a mnemotechnical device, representing בְּהֵמָה, חַסְרוֹן, גְּלוּדָה and חֲרוּתָא. Hull. 42^ab.

בסגר, Lam. R. to III, 7 ב׳ של ערבייא (Yalk. a. l. גנד (גונדא) של ערביים) prob. to be read: הֶסְגֵּר *the locking up* of Jerusalem by the Arabs, v. ib. to I, 5.—[For קסטרא של פרסיים ibid., read רוֹמִיִּים.]

בְּסוּמָא m. (בסם) *sweet-meat, delicacy.—Pl.* בְּסוּמֵי. Erub. 82^b; Meg. 7^b רווחא לב׳ וכ׳ Ms. M. (ed. sing., Var. in ed. בסימא, בסימה) for delicacies there is always room (appetite). V. בָּשׂוּם.

בסוס, read בָּסִיס.

בְּסוּרָא, בְּסוּרְתָּא, v. בְּשׂוֹ׳.

בְּסוּרָה f., pl. בְּסוּרוֹת (בסר) *first-ripe fruits, first priestly gifts.* Keth. 16^b כוס של ב׳ Ar. (ed. בשורה), expl. כוס יין של תרומה. Y. ib. II, 26^b top חבית של בסורות (ed. Krot. בשורות).

***בֶּסְטִיָּא** m. pl. (βέστια, pl.=vestes) *garments.* Num. R. s. 7 כלים וב׳. [Prob. our w. was a gloss to כלים.]

בְּסָא, בסי (v. בסס) *to trample upon;* hence (with ב־) *to despise;* v. בְּזֵי I; cmp. בְּטַשׁ.

Pa. בַּסֵּי 1) same. Y. Ter. VIII, end, 46^c לא מבסי לא ברומי וכ׳ (read תְּבַסֵּי) despise neither a Roman of low standing &c.; (Gen. R. s. 63 לא תבזון).—*2) (Arab. בּס) *to drive, instigate.* Gen. R. s. 79, end, heard an Arab say to his neighbor מה את מְבַסֵּה בי וכ׳ (some ed. מכ׳, corr. acc.) why art thou driving me? and he meant to say מה את מְעַשֵּׂה בי (Var. מְעַסֵּה) why wilt thou force me?—from which they learned the meaning of ועסותם, Mal. III, 21.

בְּסִיָּא (Ar.), **בּוּסְיָא** m. (v. preced.;=h. פְּשִׁיעָה) *indifference, willful negligence.* Targ. Y. Ex. XXII, 8 בבו׳ (corr. acc.). Y. B. Mets. V, 10^b bot. מחה בב׳ if the animal died through negligence; Tosef. ib. V, 10 בבוסיא ed. Zuck. (Var. בב׳). B. Kam. 116^b בבו׳ וכ׳ (Var. בב׳; Ms. M. בבו׳, בְּבִסְיָא).

בסיג׳, v. פסיג׳.

בסילוגוס, בסילגוס, read בָּסִילְיוֹס.

בָּסִילֵיאוֹס (βασιλέως, Genit. of βασιλεύς); v. בָּסִילְיוֹס. Y. R. Hash. I, 57^a bot., v. אַגְרָפּוֹס.

בָּסִילְיוֹן 1) m. (βασίλειον, τὸ) *royal seat, palace.* Y. Snh. II, 20^c מלכא יתיב על ב׳ דידיה וכ׳ (read בר ב׳) the King sits in his palace, and thou sayest thou art the King?—2) (genit. of βασίλεια, τὰ) *of the palace,* or *of the royal affairs.* Gen. R. s. 93 פטרון ב׳ (πάτρων τῶν βασιλείων) *superintendent of* &c.

בָּסִילְיוֹס, בָּסִילֵיוֹס m. (βασιλεύς) *king.* Y. Ber. IX, 12^d bot.; Gen. R. s. 8 (corr. acc.).

בָּסִילְקֵי (בסלקי) f. (βασιλική, sub. στοά) *basilica, a building with colonnades* for holding courts, also *meeting place for merchants, exchange, forum.* Yoma 25^a כמין ב׳ גדולה was built in the style of a large basilica (semicircular). Tosef. Succ. IV, 6 (describing the Alexandrian Synagogue); Succ. 51^b. Gen. R. s. 68 עולים לב׳ וכ׳ one goes up to the basil. and finds the King holding court. Ex. R. s. 15; Tanh. Haye 3 שמא אצל ב׳ וכ׳ perhaps he wanted me to wait for him near the basilica (on the forum). Esth. R. to I, 3. Toh. VI, 8; Tosef. ib. VII, 12; a. fr. [Y. B. Bath. IV, 14^c bot. בסלקי, v. בַּלְפּוֹס.]—*Pl.* בָּסִילְקָאוֹת. Ab. Zar. 16^b שלש ב׳ הן וכ׳ there are three kinds of basilicas, for Kings (holding court), for baths, and royal treasuries (τὸ βασιλικόν, sub. ταμεῖον, S.). Tosef. Ohol. XVIII, 18 selling wheat בב׳ שלהן in their (the gentiles') exchanges. [Lev. R. s. 34 בסלקי, read בפילקי.]

בְּסִים, v. בְּסַם.

בָּסִים, בְּסִימָא m., **בְּסִימָא, בְּסִימְתָּא** f. (בסם) *boiled, ripe,* whence 1) (Var. בְּסִים, בַּסִּים, בַּסִּימָא) *sweet, pleasant, well-seasoned* &c. (=h. ערב). Targ. Ps. CXLI, 2 (h. text ערב, translated in both senses); a. fr.—Keth. 104^a top דמדליא וב׳ אווירא which lies high and whose air is pleasant (temperate). R. Hash. 21^a ב׳ תבשילא וכ׳ (Ms. M. 2 margin כמה ב׳; v. Rabb. D. S. a. l. note 80) how well tastes the food of the Babylonians on the day when in Palestine they observe the Day of Atonement! B. Mets. 60^a לא הוה ב׳ (the wine) was not good. Ib. 69^b דאיכא דב׳ וכ׳ that there is good and bad wine. Ber. 56^a ב׳ חמרך thy wine will be good.—*Pl.* בְּסִימִין, fem. בְּסִימָן, בְּסִימָתָא (also as nouns, as h. נעימים, נעימות). Targ. Y. Num. XXXIII, 28 sq.; a. e.—V. בְּסִימָא.—2) (cmp. חֲלָא) *fermenting, sour.* Y. Maas. Sh. IV, 55^c top חמרא .... מיפוק בסים this man's (thy) wine shall turn sour (ferment); v. בַּסִּין. Lam. R. to I, 1 (7 חד מאתינס) וחד דבסים and one bag with sour wine. Ib. דבסימא חסים the dripping of the sour wine bubbles. Ib. (חד כותאר) ונפיק כוליה בסים and it will all turn sour.

בְּסִמָא, בְּסִימָא m. (v. preced. 2) *fermenting wine, wine turned into vinegar.* Lam. R. to III, 40 אין דעולית׳ מרירן בסימא חמיע Ar. (ed. אית כרנבי ב׳ דסימא חמיע; read אין דכר׳, strike out דסימא) when the endive (the cabbage) is bitter, the fermenting wine turns sour (sin begets sin). Cant. R. end, if the vineyard is cut before its time, אפי׳ בְּסִמֵיה וכ׳ even its vinegar is not good.

בְּסִימָה f. same. Y. Pes. III, beg. 29^d formerly..... the wine (in Judæa) never turned sour, and they put in barley to make it sour, whence it was called ב׳ דרומיא Southern vinegar (fermentation,=h. חומץ האדומי).

בְּסִימוּתָא f. (בסם) *sweetness.* Targ. Ps. XXVII, 4; a. e.

בַּסְּמַיָּא m. pl. (בסם;=h. חֲנֻטִים) *embalming process.* Targ. Y. Gen. L, 3.

***בַּסִּין** m. pl. (בוס) *vinegar.* את מינסב חסין וצבע בב׳ thou wilt take lettuce and dip in vinegar. [Prob. בסים.]

בָּסִיס, v. בְּסַס.

בָּסִיס m. (בסס, בוס; formed like צְצִיץ) *anything to tread upon; footstool, stand, base* (=b. h. מְכֹנָה, כֵּן). Kel.

XI, 7 הפרח והב׳ the bud (receptacle of the candlestick) and the stand. Lev. R. s. 25; Cant. R. to V, 15 like a column which has ב׳ מלמטן וכ׳ a base beneath &c.; Tanh. B'har 1. Y. Ab. Zar. III, 42[d] top בשאין עליהן ב׳ when there is upon them (the idolatrous emblems) no stand (indicating that they were intended for practical use). Ib. כוס בסוס לדרקון וכ׳ (corr. acc.) if the cup serves as a stand for the dragon (idolatrous emblem), it (the cup) is forbidden; a. fr.—Trnsf. (in Sabbath law) *whatever is subservient to another object*, e. g. the case in which a book is kept, the table upon which a lamp is placed. Sabb. 117[a] ב׳ לדבר האסיר subservient to an object which must not be handled on the Sabbath; a. fr.—V. בְּסִיסִית, בְּסִיסִי.

בְּסִיסָא, בְּסִיס f. ch. same. Targ. I Kings VII, 30; a. fr.—Y. Sabb. XVII, 16[b] top ב׳ דידיה its (the delphica's) pedestal. Y. Succ. V, 55[b] bot. whatever (structure) stands isolated being one hundred feet high בעי ב׳ וכ׳ requires a buttress (in the shape of an ascent) of thirty three cubits on each side.—*Pl.* בְּסִיסַיָּא. Targ. I Kings VII, 27; a. e.

בִּסְסִית, בְּסִיסִית, בְּסִיסִי f. (=בְּסִיס; בסס) *footstool, base, stand, step.*—*Pl.* בְּסִיסָאוֹת Ar., בְּסִיסִיּוֹת, בְּסְסִיּוֹת. Kel. XXIV, 6 שלש בְּסְ׳ הן (Ar. בסי׳) there are three stands, one before the bed (step) &c. Num. R. s. 10, beg. בסיסיות, v. בְּסִיס.

בְּסִיר m., **בְּסִירָא** f. 1) (בְּסִ׳) (בסר) *contemned, contemptible.* Targ. Ps. XV, 4; a. fr.—*Pl.* בְּסִירִין, fem. בְּסִירָן. Targ. Mal. II, 9; I, 12. Targ. Jud. IX, 4, v. בַּקָּרָא II.—2) *ripening*, v. בְּסַר II.

בְּסִירוּתָא f. (preced.) *contempt.* Targ. Ps. CXXIII, 3.

בסלקי, v. בְּסִילְקֵי.

בָּשַׂם, בָּסַם (√בס, בש, cmp. בָּשַׁל, *to boil, ripen, be warm, ferment*) *to be sweet, pleasant, pleasing.* Lam. R. to I, 9 יערב לך ויִבְסַם לך may (the sacrifice) be sweet unto thee (Moloch), may it be pleasing unto thee. Gen. R. s. 85 יערב לכם יבושם וכ׳ (Yalk. Gen. 144, Josh. 35 יבסם) may (the wine you drank) be sweet to you, may it well agree with you.—Denom. בּוֹסֶם.

Pi. בִּסֵּם, בִּסֵם, בִּיסֵּם, בִּישֵּׂם *to make a person look well*, esp. (denom. of בּוֹסֶם) *to perfume with oil* &c. Ex. R. s. 23 a bride מקשטין אותה ומְבַסְּמִין אותה is adorned and made handsome (her toilet is attended to).—Part. pass. מְבוּסָּם, f. מְבוּסֶּמֶת, מְבוּשׂ׳ *perfumed, sweet* &c. Num. R. s. 20 מקושטת ומב׳ in full toilet. Tosef. Ber. VI (V), 5 it is not becoming for a scholar שיצא מבוסם to go out with perfumed oil on his head; Ber. 43[b] מבוש׳. B. Bath. VI, 3 יין מב׳ sweet wine (guaranteed as not sour). [Pesik. R. s. 21 בישם העולם; Ruth. R. beg. בִּיסם, read בִּיסֵּס, v. בָּסַס.]

Hithpa. הִתְבַּסֵּם, הִתְבַּשׂ׳; *Nithpa.* נִתְבַּסֵּם, נִתְבַּשׂ׳ 1) *to perfume one's self with oil* &c. Gen. R. s. 17.—2) *to become exhilarated, to feel the wine.* Koh. R. to XI, 9 אכל ושתה ונת׳ he ate and drank and felt well.—3) trnsf. *to grow better, improve.* Gen. R. s. 67, end נִתְבַּסְּמָה דעתו עליו his character grew better (play on בשמת Gen. XXVI, 34).—[Ib. s. 66 נתבשם העולם, v. בָּסַס.]

בְּסַם ch. same. Targ. Ex. XV, 25; a. fr.—*Part. pass.* בְּסִים, v. בְּסִים.

Pa. בַּסֵּים 1) *to sweeten, season*; trnsf. *to make happy, to delight.* Targ. Y. Num. XVIII, 19. Targ. Ps. CXIX, 122; a. e.—Succ. 51[a]; Arakh. 11[a] לְבַסּוּמֵי קלא to sweeten the sound (by means of instrumental accompaniment).—2) *to embalm.* Targ. Y. Gen. L, 2; 26.—Part. pass. מְבַסַּם. Targ. O. XXX, 25.

Ithpa. אִיתְבַּסַּם, *Ithpe.* אִיתְבְּסֵם, contr. אִיבְּסִים 1) *to be sweet, well-seasoned, prepared.* Targ. Job XXIV, 20. Targ. Y. Ex. XXX, 25 מִתְבַּשְּׂם; a. e.—2) *to be embalmed.* Targ. Y. Gen. L, 3.—3) *to be cheerful, feel the wine*; cmp. בְּלוּזְמָא. Snh. 38[a] כיון דאִיבְּסוּם when they were feeling the wine. Sabb. 66[b]. B. Bath. 73[b] bot.—Meg. 7[b] מיחייב אינש לְבַסּוּמֵי וכ׳ (=לאיבסומי, v. Rashi a. l.) one must cheer himself up with wine &c. Ib. איבסום they were feeling the wine (v. Rabb. D. S. a. l. note). [Targ. Cant. II, 5 אתבסם, v. בְּסַס.]

בַּשָּׂם, בַּסָּם m. (preced.) *dealer in*, or *manufacturer of, spices, perfumes* &c.; *druggist.* Kidd. 82[b]. Tosef. ib. II, 2; 4. Y. Ber. IX, 13[c] bot. B. Mets. 56[b] if one sells his (cancelled) notes לב׳ to a druggist (for wrapping paper); a. fr.—[Tosef. Ber. VI (V), 8 ed. Zuck. בושם.]—*Pl.* בַּסָּמִים, בַּשָּׂ׳, בַּסָּמִין. Sabb. 81[a].

בְּסָמָא, v. בְּסִימָא.

בָּסַס (sec. r. of b. h. בּוּס) *to tread, stamp, pile up.* Ukts. I, 5 stalks of eatable plants (straw &c.) שבְּסָסָן בגרן which the owner packed in the barn; Succ. 14[a] מאי בססן what does this *b'sasan* mean? R. . . . says ב׳ ממש he really stamped them (threshed); R. . . says התיר אגדן he untied them (for the purpose of piling the stalks closer by treading upon them). [Pesik. Hahod. p. 45[a]; Pesik. R. s. 15 היו בוססות, read with Num. R. s. 11 כּוֹסְסוֹת, v. כָּסַס.]

Pi. בִּיסֵּס (denom. of בְּסִיס) *to establish firmly, to found, to put on a secure basis.* Cant. R. to I, 9 ומי ב׳ העולם and who gave the world a firm basis?; (ibid. VII, 1; Ruth. R. beg.; Pesik. R. s. 21 בישם, בִּיסם corr. acc.).—Part. pass. מְבוּסָּס *firmly established.* Num. R. s. 15; Tanh. B'haal. 11 כסאו מב׳ למעלן (not מבוסם) His throne is firmly established above, when Israel &c.

Nithpa. נִתְבַּסֵּס *to be firmly established, to rest safely.* Num. R. s. 12 after the Sanctuary was erected נתב׳ העולם the world became firm. Ib. as soon as they made a third leg for the table (v. טרסקל), נתב׳ it stood firm; Tanh. T'rum. 9. Gen. R. s. 66 נתבשם העולם (corr. acc.); Yalk. Ps. 811.

בְּסַס ch. same. Part. pass. בְּסִיס *based, firm.* Targ. Cant. V, 15.

Pa. בַּסֵּיס as preced. Pi. Targ. II Chr. III, 3.

Ithpa. אִתְבַּסַּס as preced. Nithpa. Targ. Cant. II, 5 (not אתבסם).

בְּסְסִית, v. בְּסִיסִית.

בָּסַר I (√בס, v. בסס) *to tread upon*; trnsf. (v. בעט) *to contemn* (with על); *to be overbearing* (with ב). Ex.

R. s. 42, end כך היתה בוֹסֶרֶת עלי so did she slight me. Ib. s. 3 beg.; s. 45 בוֹסֵר הוא על וכ׳ he will treat his prophetic mission lightly. Tanḥ. Ekeb 1 בָּסַרְתִּי בהן have I become overbearing because I observed thy commands? (Tanḥ. ed. Bub. 2 כפרתי, v. note a. l.). Ib. Mikkets 10 לא תהא בוסר בשעת וכ׳ be not haughty in happiness, so as to refuse to pray. Ib. (ed. Bub.) Emor 29 בוסר עליהן; Tanḥ. ib. 20 (some ed. בוחר, corr. acc.) thinks lightly of them.—Part. pass. בָּסוּר, fem. בְּסוּרָה *contemptible.* Tanḥ. Sh'moth 11.

Pi. בִּיסֵּר same. Ex. R. s. 1 וב׳ עליה (some ed. וכיפר) and he despised it (idolatry). Tanḥ. Ekeb 1 some ed. בירסתי, v. supra.

בְּסַר ch. same. Targ. Ps. LXIX, 34; a. fr.

Pa. בַּסֵּר, בְּסַר same. Targ. O. Num. XV, 31 ed. Berl.; a. fr.; [in ed. sometimes בשר].—Targ. I Sam. XI, 12 מבסר למימר spoke sneeringly.—Y. Ber. II, 5ᶜ bot. בר נש דאימיה מְבַסְּרָא ליה one whom his mother (Palestine) despises and his stepmother (Babylon) honors; v. אֵם. Y. Snh. I, 19ª top; Y. Ned. VI, 40ª בעא מבסרתחון (מבסרתחון; read מבסר בחון) he wanted to despise them (reject their authority).

בָּסַר II (√בס, v. בסם) *to begin to boil, to be in the first stage of ripening;* v. next w.—Denom. בּוֹסֶר, בְּסוּרָה. —Trnsf. (v. בָּשַׂר) *to be glad.* Gen. R. s. 34 end (play on לב בשר, Ezek. XXXVI, 26), [read as] Yalk. Gen. 61 לב בוסר בחלקו של חבירו a heart rejoicing in the good fortune of his neighbor.—V. בָּשַׂר.

בְּסַר ch. same. 1) Part. בְּסִיר m., בְּסִירָא f., pl. בְּסִירָן *in the early stage of ripening.* Targ. Y. Ex. IX, 34 בסירן . . . סרווא Ar. (ed. כסידא . . . . סרתא, כסירא, read בסירא; h. text אביב).—2) *to be cheerful;* v. בְּשַׂר.

בְּסַר III, בִּסְרָא *flesh,* v. בְּשַׂר, בִּשְׂרָא.

בסרויא, Pesik. Baḥod. p. 154ᵇ, read קיסרייא.

בַּסְרָנוּתָא f. (בסר I) *contempt.* Targ. Job XII, 21; a. e.

***בַּסְתִּיר** (read בַּסְטִ׳) m. (vestiarius, βεστιάριος S.) *the keeper of the (royal) wardrobe.* Pesik. R. s. 10.

***בִּסְתְּקָא (בּוּס׳)** m. (reduplic. of בסק=בזק; cmp. Mand. עסקא=עזקא, Nöld. Mand. Gr. p. 62; Syr. בירסתא= בירזתא, P. Sm. 520) *jug, pitcher;* cmp. בָּזָךְ. Hull. 49ᵇ.

בִּסְתַּרְקָא, v. בִּיסְ׳.

בְּעָא, v. בעי.

בְּעָאתָא, v. בַּעֲתָא.

בִּעְבּוּעַ m. (v. next w.) *casting bubbles, bulging, bulge.* Mikv. X, 4 (of garments dipped in water until they are soaked through) וינוחו מִבִּעְבּוּעָן and cease from bulging. T'bul Yom II, 8 ב׳ שבחבית (an imperfection in an earthen jug) *a protuberance.*

בִּעְבֵּעַ (Pilp. of בּוּעַ; cmp. בִּצְבֵּץ) 1) *to cast bubbles, to form protuberances, to bulge.* Mikv. X, 4 עד שיְּבַעְבְּעוּ until they (the garments dipped in water) form bulges; v. preced. Yalk. Sam. 157; Midr. Till. to Ps. XVIII, 3 (read:) שהיה שמן המשחה מְבַעְבֵּעַ ויורד עליו the oil of anointment came bubbling down upon him.—2) *to struggle in the water, swim.* Y. Sabb. XIII, 14ᵇ top.; Y. Sot. III, 19ª top. תינוק מב׳ וכ׳ a child struggling in the river. Y. Yoma III, 41ª התחיל מב׳ וכ׳ commenced casting up bubbles from under the ship (Bab. ib. 38ª מבצבצת).

***בַּעְבַּע** ch. (v. בעי) *to ask entrance, knock at the door.* Lev. R. s. 21; Pesik. Aḥare, p. 177ª הוה מבעבע used to knock. [Ar. reads כבכע, quoting Lev. R. l. c. also for a Hebrew verb לכבכע; Rashb. to Pes. 112ª quotes נענע.]

בעד (Arab.) *to keep off.* Imper. IV אַבְעַד. Cant. R. to IV, 1 (ref. to מבעד ib.) ל׳ ערבי וכ׳ it is Arabic; if one desires to say to one, Make room for me (or, Let me alone), he says אבעד לי (some ed. מבעד).

בְּעָה, v. בעי.

בָּעוּ, בָּעוּתָא f. (בעי) *prayer.* Targ. Jer. VII, 16. Targ. II Sam. VII, 20; a. fr.—בְּבָעוּ (in prayer) *I pray* (h. בִּי, נָא). Targ. Gen. XIX, 7. Ib. XLIV, 18; a. v. fr. [Targ. Ps. XLIII, 4, v. בּוּעֲתָא II.]

בְּעוֹד, v. עוֹד.

בְּעוּט m. (בְּעַט) 1) *treading grapes,* or *trodden grapes.* Targ. Is. X, 33; Targ. Joel IV, 13 (ed. בְּעוּט); Targ. Is. LXIII, 3 בִּיעוּט.—2) *a kick with the foot.* Y. Taan. IV, 68ᵈ bot. יהב ליה חד ב׳ וכ׳ he gave him one kick and killed him; Lam. R. to II, 2 חד בעיטא ברגליה.

בָּעוֹר, בְּעוֹרָא (בְּעִיר) m. (בער) *torch, fire* (h. לַפִּיד). Targ. O. Gen. XV, 17 (Y. מבעיר); a. e.—*Pl.* בְּעוֹרִין, בְּעוּרַיָּא. Targ. Nah. II, 5 בְּעוּ׳ (ed. Vien.). Targ. Job XLI, 11; a. e. —B. Mets. 85ᵇ ב׳ דאשא (Ms. M. דנור).

בָּעוּתָא, v. בָּעוּ.

בָּעַט I (√בע, v. בוע) *to swell, bulge.* Midd. III, 8 שלא יִבְעֲטוּ marg. vers. (or יִבָּעֲטוּ Nif.; text יבעט sing.) that the walls should not bulge.

בָּעַט II (b. h.; √בע, akin to בץ, בט) *to trample, strike, kick.* Y. Yoma VIII, 45ᵇ top פרדה בְּעָטָתוֹ a mule kicked him. Ex. R. s. 30 ב׳ בפילקי knocked against the prison door (burst it open). Ab. Zar. IV, 8 גת בְּעוּטָה a wine press packed with stamped grapes.—Trnsf. (with ב) *to resist, reject.* Sabb. 104ª, v. אח״ס.

Pi. בִּיעֵט same. B. Kam. II, 1. היתה מְבַעֶטֶת if the animal kicked. Ber. 32ª; a. e.—Trnsf. *to kick against, rebel, be contumacious.* Sot. 22ª. Y. Ber. IX, 14ᵇ bot., a. e. מְבַעֵט בייסורין bearing suffering with contumacy (instead of showing repentance). Pesik. R. s. 47; Yalk. Job 908 התחיל מב׳ (sub. בייסורין) began to be contumacious (challenging the Lord).

בְּעַט, בְּעֵים ch. same. Targ. Hos. IV, 16; a. e.— Y. Sabb. VII, 11ª bot.; Y. Shek. III, 47ᶜ ב׳ ביה rejected his authority.

Pa. בַּעֵט, בַּעֵיט *to tread (grapes).* Targ. Lam. I, 15.

Ithpe. אִתְבְּעֵיט *to be trodden.* Targ. Joel IV, 13; Targ. Is. LXIII, 3; a. e.

בַּעְטָן m., **בַּעֲטָנִית** f. (preced.) *habitual kicker, butting.* B. Mets. 80ª; Tosef. B. Bath. IV, 6.

בָּעָה, בעי (b. h.; √בע, akin to בח, בו, v. בוא, a) *to enter into, split;* b) *to be empty, bare).* Part. בּוֹעֶה, v. infra.

Hif. הִבְעָה *to lay bare, destroy the crop.* B. Kam. I, 1 הַמַּבְעֶה damaging the crop (ref. to Ex. XXII, 4). Ib. 3ᵇ Rab says מבעה זה אדם the damaging force in the Mishnah means that of a human being (ransacking, searching); for we read (Is. XXI, 12) אם תבעיון בעיו if ye desire to enter &c. (where בעה refers to human action); Samuel says, מבעה זה השן the *mabeh* of the Mishnah refers to the tooth, i. e. to an animal's eating up the crop, for it says (Obad. 6) נבעו מצפניו its hidden treasures were laid bare (made empty,—which refers to eating up). Ib. (argument against Samuel) מי קתני נִבְעָה the Mishnah does not use the Nifal (which may mean *eaten up*); (argument against Rab) מי קתני בּוֹעֶה the Mishnah does not use the Kal (which may refer to human action) but the Hifil "to cause damage"—through the animal.—Tosef. ib. IX, 1.

בְּעֵי I, **בְּעָא** ch. (v. preced.; cmp. בין) 1) *to search, inquire, ask, examine.* Targ. Jud. VI, 29 (h. text בקש); a. fr. —Ber. 2ᵇ ובעי לה מבעיא האי וכ׳ and put it as a question (not as an argument), Does this *uba hash-shemesh* mean &c.? (opposed to preceding ומנא׳ דהאי וכ׳ how can it be proven that &c.). Y. Ḥall. I, 57ᵇ רבנן ... בעיין the Rabbis of ... asked. B. Kam. 33ª בעא ... מרב וכ׳ R. asked R. N.; a. v. fr.—2) *to ask, pray,* frequ. ב׳ רחמין *to ask for mercy, pray.* Targ. Y. Num. XII, 13; a. fr.—Ber. 8ª לבעי איניש רחמי man should pray &c., v. זיבולא. Ib. 10ª בְּעֵי רחמי עלוייהו וכ׳ pray thou for them that they may repent; a. fr.— 3) *to ask, want, desire; to require.* Targ. Ex. II, 15; a. fr.—Pes. 9ª ובָעֵי בדיקה and it (the house) requires searching over again. Keth. 39ᵇ לא בעינא לך I do not want thee. B. Kam. 102ᵇ לא יקרייכו בעינא וכ׳ I want neither your honor nor your disrespect; a. fr.—Pes. 2ª בעו שבוחי *must* give praise.—איבְּעִית, v. אי בעית אימא, usu. איבעית אימא, v. [Y. Yeb. XII, 13ª top בְּעָא תתן לנו, please, give us.]— 4) (ellipt.) *to beg leave to say; to remark, assert.* Y. Ber. I, 2ᵇ top. Y. Peah II, beg. 16ᵈ; a. fr.

Ithpe. אִתְבְּעֵי 1) *to be searched for, to be wanted.* Targ. Jer. L, 20; a. fr.—2) *to be urged, hurried.* Targ. I Sam. XXIII, 26. Targ. II Sam. IV, 4 בְּאִתְבַּעֲיוּתָהּ when she was hurried; v. בְּעַע.

Ithpa. contr. אִיבַּעֵי 1) *to be asked.* Pes. 4ᵇ, a. v. fr. אִיבַּעְיָא להו it was asked by them (the scholars), i. e. the argument came up.—2) *to be required; it ought to.* Ib. 7ᵇ יצא בו מיבעי ליה it ought to read *yatsa bo* (he *has* done his duty). Ib. 15ª מדבריו מ׳ ליה it ought to be *midd'barav* (not *middibrehem*); a. fr.—B. Kam. 21ᵇ א׳ ליה לאסוקי דעתא he ought to have borne in mind; a. fr.—לא מיבעיא *there is no question.* לא מ׳ .... אלא אפילו there is no question as to ...., but even ....; *not only .... but.* Pes. 4ᵇ לא מ׳ באתרא...אלא וכ׳ not only in a place where they pay no wages for searching, but do it themselves, (is there no cause for withdrawing from the agreement,) because a man likes to perform a religious duty: but even in a place where they pay wages, (there is no cause &c.,) for a man likes &c. B. Kam. 54ᵇ לא מ׳ קאמר לא מ׳ שור וכ׳ the Mishnah states a case of 'not only'; not only for an ox ... is he responsible, but even &c.; a. v. fr.— מִיבַּעְיָא *is there any question?*; v. הַשְׁתָּא.

Af. אַבְעֵי *to let burst forth,* v. יְעָא a. נְבַע.

בְּעֵי II (v. בְּעָה, בעי) *to open wide* (the mouth), *to yawn* (of leopards). Targ. II Esth. I, 2 נמרין בעיין.

בְּעָיָא m. 1) (preced.) *yawn, gap.* Constr. בְּעֵי. ב׳ לבא *greed.* Targ. Prov. XXI, 4 (h. text רחב לב).—2) (בעי I) *question.* *Pl.* בְּעָיֵי. Snh. 106ᵇ ד׳ מאות ב׳ four hundred questions. Ib. רבותא למבעי ב׳ is there any greatness in asking questions?

***בְּעָיָא** (מעין) pr. n. m. *Baya* (Mayan), name of a publican. Snh. 44ᵇ ב׳ מוכסא (not מיכ׳); Y. Ḥag. II, 77ᵈ מ׳ מוכס.

בְּעָיָיא f. (part. of בעי) *desirous.* Y. Taan. I, 64ᵇ bot. אנא ב׳ וכ׳ I want to see what I can do to relieve him.— *Pl.* m. בָּעְיֵי. Ib.ª top אימת דאתון בעיי הוא בָּעֵי whenever ye are desirous (that he should come), he is willing to.

בְּעָיָא, v. בֵּיעָא.

בְּעִיט, v. בְּעַט.

בְּעִיטָא, v. בְּעוֹט.

בְּעִיטָה f. (בעט) 1) *kicking.* Y. B. Kam. I, beg. 2ª (of animals). Bab. ib. 27ᵇ לב׳ חמש for kicking with one's foot &c. 2) *beating* (with one's fist). Men. VI, 5 (76ª) שיפה וב׳ בחטין rubbing and beating refer to the preparation of the wheat of the meat-offering (prior to grinding); R. Y. says בבצק (Mish. אף incorr.) beating refers to the dough. Ib. Gem. Var. שיפה בחיטים וב׳ בבצק; Tosef. ib. VIII, 14.

בְּעִיל, v. בְּעַל a. בַּעֲלָא.

בְּעִילָה f. (בָּעַל) *sexual intercourse.* Keth. 3ª שויוה רבנן לִבְעִילָתוֹ בְּעִילַת זנות the Rabbis (in this case) have declared his coition (by which he wanted to establish marriage), a mere act of prostitution (annulled his marriage). Ib. 73ª, a. e. אין אדם עושה בעילתו בעילת זנות the presumption is that nobody wants to make his intercourse with a woman one of prostitution (but wants to make her his wife thereby).—Ib. 4ª בעילת מצוה the marital duty, i. e. first coition; frequ. ב׳ ראשונה. Y. Macc. II, 31ᵈ; a. fr.—*Pl.* בְּעִילוֹת. Sabb. 72ª; a. fr.

בְּעִיץ I m., v. בַּעֲצָא.

***בְּעִיץ** II m. (part. pass. of a verb בעץ, denom. of בעצא) *tinned, wrapt in tin-foil.* Targ. Jer. XXXII, 11 (a. 14, in some ed.) כתיב ב׳ וחתים written, wrapt in tin-foil and tied up (v. חתם) with a seal, opp. to שכרא פתיחא.

בְּעִיר, v. בְּעַר.

בְּעִירָא, בְּעִיר ch. c. (b. h. בְּעִיר; בער; cmp. also בְּעָה) *grazing animal, cattle.* Targ. Gen. I, 24 sq.; a. fr.—Y. B. Mets. II, 8ᶜ bot.; Lev. R. s. 27, a. e. ב׳ דקיקא *small cattle;* v. בְּהֵמָה.—Pesik. B shall. p. 93ᵃ אתקן לי ב׳ get an animal ready for me (for travel). Snh. 105ᵃ (in Hebr. dict., play on בְּעוֹר).

בְּעִית, v. בְּעַת.

בָּעַל (b. h.; √בע, v. בָּעָה, *to enter into, take possession*) [in b. h. *to be master, protect;*] *to have sexual intercourse* (both legal or illicit), *to embrace a woman.* Kidd. 9ᵇ וּבְעָלָהּ מלמד וכ׳ 'and he embraced her' (Deut. XXIV, 1), this intimates that woman can be acquired as wife by intercourse, v. בִּיאָה.—בּוֹעֵל *lover, adulterer,* contrad. to בַּעַל *husband.* Sot. V, 1, a. fr. כשם שאסורה לַבַּעַל לַבּוֹעֵל . . . . as well as the woman suspected of adultery is forbidden to her husband (who must separate himself from her), so is she forbidden to the lover (who cannot marry her after leaving her husband). Yeb. 103ᵃ שבע בעילות ב׳ וכ׳ that wicked man had seven sexual connections &c.; a. fr.—Part. pass. f. בְּעוּלָה *one no longer a virgin,* opp. to בתולה; *married woman,* opp. to ארוסה, v. אָרַס. Keth. 10ᵇ; a. fr.—*Pl.* בְּעוּלוֹת. Y. Kidd. I, 58ᵇ bot.; a. fr.

Nif. נִבְעֲלָה *she had intercourse.* Keth. 5ᵃ . . . נישאת וְנִבְעֶלֶת וכ׳ is married on the fourth day and embraced in the night of the fifth day of the week. Ib. 3ᵇ תִּיבָּעֵל לטפסר וכ׳ must first be surrendered to the (Roman) officer (jus primæ noctis); a. fr.—Masc. נִבְעַל (of the hermaphrodite). Tosef. Bicc. II, 5; Y. Yeb. VIII, 9ᵈ bot.

בְּעֵיל, בְּעַל ch. same. Targ. O. Deut. XXI, 13; a. fr.—Keth. 6ᵇ דבעי לְמִיבְעַל because he is anxious to perform his marital duty. Ib. דטריד דלא בעיל he is excited because he has not &c.; a. fr.

Pa. בַּעֵל, part. pass. f. מְבַעֲלָא *married, having had intercourse.* Targ. Ruth I, 12; a. e.

Ithpe. אִיתְבְּעֵלָא as preced. Nif. Yoma 19ᵇ ואִבְּעוּל כמה, וכ׳ (Ms. M. ואיבעיל) and how many virgins have been seduced (to-day) in Nahardea!

בַּעַל m. (b. h.; preced.) 1) *husband.* Kidd. I, 1 and she becomes her own master בגט ובמיתת הב׳ through a letter of divorce or on the husband's death; a. v. fr.—2) *the idol Baal.* Y. Ab. Zar. III, 43ᵃ bot. ב׳ ראש גוויה הוה וכ׳ the Baal was the phallus and had the shape of a bean [read וכאפון].—3) [*the fructifier,*] *rain* (v. Taan. 6ᵇ; cmp. Is. LV, 10). בֵּית בַּ׳ *a field sufficiently watered by rain* and requiring no artificial irrigation. Tosef. M. Kat. I, 1 שדה (בית) הב׳. B. Bath. III, 1. Tosef. Succ. II, 7 ערבה של ב׳ (sub. בית) a willow in a naturally watered field. Ib. Shebi. II, 4 בשל ב׳ (=בשדה של ב׳), opp. של שוקי. Num. R. s. 16 the Egyptian gods של שקר הם (read שקי) are gods of artificial drainage, but those of Canaan של ב׳ הם are gods of rain; (Tanh. Sh'lah 13, through misunderstanding, שקר... בעלי כח).—4) (mostly in compounds) *owner of, master of, possessed of, given to* &c.; e. g. ב׳ אבידה owner of a lost object; ב׳ אגדה master of Agadah, lecturer; ב׳ דין opponent in court; v. infra. Pes. 86ᵇ ב׳ השם אני I am so named.—*Pl.* בְּעָלִים, בְּעָלִין *owners;* mostly as sing. *owner.* B. Mets. VIII, 1; a. fr. [Y. Dem. III, 23ᵇ bot. לבלערן, read לבעלין.]

Compounds: ב׳ מחשבות *He who knows man's thoughts.* Snh. 19ᵇ.—Ib. בעלי מ׳ *those entertaining considerations* (of fear), *hesitating to do justice.*—ב׳ שיבה *gray-haired.* Ned. III, 8.—ב׳ תשובה *repentant sinner.* Succ. 53ᵃ; a. fr.—ב׳ תשובות *a man of many objections or excuses.* Gen. R. s. 20 beg.—[For other compounds, not self-evident, see the respective determinants.]

בַּעְלָא, constr. בְּעֵיל, בַּעַל ch. same. 1) *husband.* Targ. O. Ex. XXI, 3; a. fr.—Taan. 6ᵇ מטרא ב׳ וכ׳ the rain is the husband (fructifier) of the field; v. preced. 3).—2) *Baal.* Targ. Jud. VI, 25; a. e.—*Pl.* בַּעֲלַיָּא. Ib. II, 11; a. fr.

בַּעֲלָה f. (preced.) *mistress, owner* &c. Gen. R. s. 52 (rendering בְּעֻלַת, Gen. XX, 3, as though בַּעֲלַת) מרתא דבעלה her husband's mistress.—Compounds are mostly self-evident, e. g. בעלת הגט the woman receiving the letter of divorce;—ב׳ איברים an animal of large build. Ber. 32ᵃ; v. בַּעַל.

בְּעָא (v. בָּעָה; cmp. בהל) *to be excited.*—*Af.* אַבְעַ *to hurry.* Targ. I Kings XXII, 9 א׳ מיכיה Ar. (ed. חבע, h. text מהרה) bring . . . . quickly. Targ. Ezek. XXIV, 5.—Part. pass. מַבְעַ, מַבְעָא (מְבַ׳) *quick.* Targ. Deut. XXXII, 35.—*Pl.* מַבְעִין. Targ. Num. XXXII, 17.

Ittaf. אִתַּבַּע *to be in a hurry, be anxious.* Targ. Ps. XXXI, 23 באִתַּבְּעוּתִי Ms. (ed. באִתְּבְעוּתִי). Targ. II Kings VII, 15; Targ. II Sam. IV, 4, v. בְּעַר I.

***בְּעַץ** 1) (dialectic for בְּעַט) *to tread.* Targ. Ps. XCI, 13 תבעוץ some ed. (oth. תבעוט).—2) *to wrap in tin,* v. בְּעִיץ.

בַּעַץ m. (cmp. בּוּץ, v. עבץ a. אבצא) *tin, plumbum album.* Kel. XXX, 3 עשאו בין בב׳ if he mended it either with &c. B. Bath. 89ᵇ (diff. fr. אבר, a. גיסטרא, cassiterum, v. Sm. Ant. s. v. Plumbum). Men. 28ᵇ; a. fr.

בְּעֵיץ, בַּעֲצָא ch. same. Targ. Ezek. XXII, 18. Targ. Y. Num. XXXI, 22 Ar. a. Levita (ed. קסיטרא, O. אבצא).

בָּעַר (b. h.; √בע, v. בָּעָה; cmp. בָּאַר) [*to clear,*] 1) *to burn* (act. a. neut.). Ex. R. s. 2 אש בּוֹעֶרֶת burning fire. Ib. כשם שהסנה בּוֹעֵר וכ׳ as the bush is burning &c. [Num. R. s. 9, end לבוערים בע״ז, read לבוסרים, v. בָּסַר I, Var. לכופרים.]—2) *to be empty.* Denom. בַּעַר.—3) *to eat up.* Denom. בְּעִיר.

Pi. בִּיעֵר 1) *to clear, remove* (out of existence or out of possession). Pes. 6ᵃ זקוק לְבַעֵר is bound to remove (the leaven by burning or otherwise); a. fr.—Shebi. VII, 7 חייב לב׳ is bound to remove (dispose of the fruits of the Sabbath year in due time). [Num. R. s. 9 (p. 230ᵇ ed. Amst.) מבערים את העון, read with Yalk. Num. 708, Sifré Num. 11 מערערין; oth. vers. מבררין, v. בָּרַר.] 2) *to clear, eat up.* B. Kam. 2ᵇ וּבִעֵר זו השן 'and it clears' (Ex. XXII, 4) this refers to injury by the tooth (animal's eating). [3) (b. h.) *to start a fire, enkindle.* V. בְּעֵרָה.]

Hif. הִבְעִיר *to start* or *entertain a fire, to clear a field.* Sabb. 20ª (ref. to לא תבערו וכ׳ Ex. XXXV, 3) בכל.... אי אתה מַבְעִיר 'in all your dwellings' thou art not permitted to start a fire; v. הַבְעָרָה. B. Kam. 60ᵇ הַבְּעֵרָה שֶׁהִבְעַרְתִּי the fire which I set (to Zion). Ib. 55ᵇ (ref. to Ex. l. c. 5) עד דעביד כעין מבעיר only when he acts like the one setting fire (to clear the field, i. e. criminal negligence); a. e.

Hof. הוּבְעַר *to be rekindled, to burn again.* Sabb. 37ªᵇ.

בְּעַר I, בְּעֵיר ch. same. 1) *to burn.* Targ. O. Ex. III, 2 בָּעַר ed. Berl. (oth. ed. בָּעַר, Part.). Targ. Is. LXII, 1. Targ. Ps. XVIII, 9; a. fr.—2) *to remove; to dispose of.* Pes. 5ᵇ בָּעִירוּ חמירא וכ׳ dispose ye of the leavened bread of the (gentile) soldiers (deposited with you).

Pa. בַּעֵר *to enkindle, ignite.* Targ. Ex. XXXV, 3. Targ. O. Lev. VI, 5 (Mss. a. some ed. יַבְעַר Af.).

Af. אַבְעַר same. Targ. O. Lev. VI, 5 (v. supra). *Targ. Y. I Gen. XV, 17 מַבְעִיר שביבין.

***בְּעַר II** (cmp. בְּעֵי II) *to open the mouth wide, to low* (of oxen; cmp. פער). Targ. II Esth. I, 2 בוערין (some edit. גערין).

בְּעֵרָה f. (b. h.; בָּעַר) *fire, conflagration.* B. Kam. VI, 4 השולח את הב׳ ביד וכ׳ he who sends out a deaf and dumb, an idiot or a minor with burning materials (live coal &c.) thus causing or ordering a conflagration. Ib. השולח את הב׳ he who starts a fire (himself). Ib. 60ᵇ, v. בָּעַר.

בְּעַשׁ=בְּאַשׁ *to displease* (in Targ. Y. II). Targ. Y. II Deut. XV, 10 (ed. Vien. באש). Ib. XXVIII, 54 תַּבְעַשׁ (read תִּבְעַשׁ); 56.

בָּעַת (b. h. √בע, v. בָּעָה; interch. with בָּהַת q. v.) *to startle.* [Not used in Kal.]

Nif. נִבְעַת *to be startled, frightened, confounded.* Num. R. s. 18; Tanḥ. Korah 6 נזדעזע אהרן וכ׳ Aaron trembled and was alarmed. Y. Shek. I, beg. Bab. ed. נִבְעִית, v. בָּהַת.

Hif. הִבְעִית *to frighten, bewilder.* Yoma V, 1 (52ᵇ) שלא לְהַבְעִית וכ׳ in order not to alarm the people (by a long delay). Ib. 39ᵇ למה אתה מבעית עצמך why wilt thou be the alarmer thyself (predicting thine own destruction; Ms. M. a. Yalk. Zech. 578 את עצמך, incorr.; Ms. Oxf. בעצמך; Y. ib. VI, 43ᶜ bot. מבהלינו, v. Rabb. D. S. a. l. note).

Hithpa. הִתְבַּעֵת *to be agitated, excited.* Y. Sabb. VI, 8ᵇ top שהוא מִתְבַּעֵת for he is excited.

בְּעַת, בְּעֵית ch. (v. preced.) *to be excited.* Nidd. 66ᵇ משום דבעיתא because she is excited (afraid of falling down).

Pa. בַּעֵת, בַּעִית *to frighten.* Targ. Ps. XVIII, 5 (Ms. בְּעִיתַת Pe.).—Keth. 77ᵇ דילמא מְבַעֲתַת לי lest thou frighten me. Hull. 53ª sq. בַּעוּתֵי קא מְבַעֲתֵי אהדדי they frighten each other. Nidd. 66ª זיל בַּעֲתָהּ go and frighten her (by a sudden noise).

Ithpe. אִתְבְּעִית, אִיבְּעִית *to be afraid; to be agitated, anxious, in haste* (cmp. b. h. חָרַד). Targ. I Sam. XXI, 2. Targ. Is. XXII, 4. Targ. II Kings VII, 15 בְּאִתְבְּהִילוּתְהוֹן Regia (ed. באתבעותהון); v. בְּעָא a. בְּעַר I. Y. Ab. Zar. V, 44ᵈ bot. והוא מתבעת and he is afraid (to touch the wine).—Meg. 3ª האי מאן דמִיבְּעִית when one is suddenly seized with fright. Ib. איבעיתו. Keth. 106ª הוה מיבעית ליה בעותי he ran anxiously to meet him; cmp. Targ. I Sam. l. c.; a. fr.

בַּעְתָא I m. (preced.) *terror.*—*Pl.* בַּעְתַיָּא. Targ. Ps. LXXXVIII, 17, v. בְּרִיעוּתָא.

בַּעְתָא II f. (בעי) *urging, stimulation.* Targ. Prov. XIII, 1; a. e. (h. text גערה).—Ib. XVII, 10 some ed. בָּעָאתָא.

בפה, Y. Meg. I, 72ª top, v. בִּיפָה.

בְּצָא, בְּצַר (√בק=בץ, בע; cmp. בצע) [*to split, break through;*] (cmp. בְּעֵי I) *to search, ransack.* Targ. Prov. II, 4 (ed. Wil. תצביה, read תבציה). Ib. XXV, 27. Ib. XX, 27 (Var. בעיא).—*Part.* בָּצֵי בָּאצֵי. Ib. XXV, 2.

Ithpe. אִתְבְּצִי, contr. אִיבְּצִי *to be searched, found out.* Ib. 3. Ib. XXVIII, 12 מִבְּצֵי.

בְּצָא, בִּיצָא (בוצא) m. (=h. בִּיצָה) *swamp, pond.* Targ. Job VIII, 11 (Var. כיסנא). Targ. Ps. LXIX, 3 בוצא דמצולתא Ms. (ed. מיא).—*Pl.* בִּיצִין, בִּצַּיָּא, בִּי׳. Targ. Is. XIV, 23. Targ. Y. II Ex. VIII, 1 (ed. Vien. בִּיצַיָּא). Targ. Ezek. XLVII, 11.

בִּצְבּוּץ m. *hemp,* v. בִּטְבּוּט.

בִּצְבֵּץ (Pilp. of בוץ or בצץ; v. בְּצָא) *to break through, bubble forth, burst forth.* Sot. 11ᵇ; Ex. R. s. 1 היו מְבַצְבְּצִין וכ׳ they burst forth and came out of the ground. Keth. 111ᵇ the righteous (dead) שמבצבצין וכ׳ will break through (the ground) and rise in Jerusalem.—Pes. 13ª היה חמץ מב׳ the leavened bread crumbled through the bag. Num. R. s. 18, end; Gitt. 56ᵇ דם מב׳ ויוצא blood bubbled forth. Hull. 56ª אם מב׳ if the brains bubble through the hole in the scull.

בַּצְבֵּץ ch. same. Hull. 46ᵇ אי מבצבצא if the lungs (on being put in water, or water being put on the diseased spot) cast bubbles when blown up.

בַּצָּה, בִּצִּים, v. בִּיצָה.

בִּיצָה, בִּצָּה f. (b. h., בצץ; v. בְּצָא; cmp. בִּצְעָה, a. בצאת Ezek. XLVII, 11) *channel, marsh, pond.*—*Pl.* בִּצִּים, בִּי׳. Par. VIII, 10. Tosef. Mikv. I, 14. Snh. 5ᵇ a teacher spoke of מי בֵּיצִים the liquid of eggs, and the students understood בִּצִּים Ar. (Ms. F. ביצים, ed. בצעים, v. בִּצְעָה). V. בִּיצִית.

בְּצוֹצְטְרָא f., pl. בְּצוֹצְטְרָאוֹת (reduplic. of בצר=גִּיזְרָה) a. גְּזוּזְטְרָא; cmp. בְּצוֹרְתָא. Y. B. Bath. III, end, 14ᵇ (for which Tosef. ib. II, 17 גזוזטראות). V. next w.

בְּצוֹצְרָה f. (reduplic. of בצר; cmp. חצוצרה) *a compartment surrounded with bars, balustrade, balcony.* Midd. II, 5 והקיפוה ב׳ וכ׳ and they surrounded the cell (לִשְׁכָּה) with a balcony so that the women could sit above, while the men were seated beneath it; [Succ. 51[b] גזווטרא, Ms. M. גזוזטראות; Tosef. ib. IV, 1 שלש גז׳]. [The variations בצוצטרא, כצוצרא &c., v. Rabb. D. S. to Sabb. 96[a], Erub. 78[b] notes, a. Ar. s. v. גזוזטרא, are clerical errors induced by assonance with the synonymous גזוזטרא. Ἐξώστρα as *balcony*, for h. עלית, Symm. II Kings I, 2, is itself an adaptation of גזוזטרא.]

בְּצַרְצְרִיּוֹת, בְּצוֹצְרִיּוֹת f. pl. (בצר, v. preced.) *engines of siege* or *defence* (v. אֲחָלִית). Pesik. Haḥod. p. 47[a]; Shub. p. 163[b] (for Var. Lect., v. Bub. notes a. l.); Pesik. R. s. 15. Midr. Till. to Ps. II, end שמא אחליות וב׳ אני צריך do I need camps and engines (for demolishing the world)?; Yalk. Ps. 623 צוצריות (corr. acc.). V. קַסְטְרִיּוֹת.

בַּצּוֹרֶת f. (b. h. בַּצֹּרֶת, בַּצָּרָה; בצר) *scarcity of provision, dearth.* Ab. V, 8 רעב של ב׳ וכ׳ a famine in consequence of high prices, when some are hungry, others are satisfied, רעב של מהומה ושל ב׳ a famine through political disturbances and through dearth. Gen. R. s. 33 שנת ב׳ a year of dearth. Taan. III, 1 מכת ב׳, expl. ib. 19[b] מכה המביאה לידי ב׳ a calamity which will produce dearth (want of rain in season).

בַּצּוֹרְתָא (בַּצָּרְתָא, בִּיצּוּרְתָא, בּוּ׳) ch. same. Targ. Jer. XVII, 8 (ed. Wil. בְּצוּרְתָא); a. fr.—Taan. 19[a] נהרא אנהרא ב׳ וכ׳ when provision has to be imported on rivers (canals), it is called ב׳, when from one country to another it is called כפנא. Keth. 97[a].—*Pl.* בַּצּוֹרָתָא. Targ. Jer. XIV, 1 (some ed. בּוּצְרָתָא).

בְּצוּרְתָא (ביצורתא, בצירתא) f.=h. זִוְזָה, *balcony* (v. בְּצוֹצְרָה). Targ. Ezek. XLI, 13 sq.; a. fr.—

בֵּצִים, v. בֵּיצָה.

בִּצִּים, v. בִּצָּה.

בָּצִיר I m. (b. h.; בצר) *vintage, harvesting.* Peah VII, 7; a. fr.—Y. B. Bath. III, 14[a] top ג׳ שנים ..... ב׳ וכ׳ three undisturbed grain crops, three grape harvests &c.; v. Bab. ib. 36[b]. V. בְּצִירָה.

בְּצִיר II, בָּצִיר ch. m. (בצר) *diminished, small;* (adv.) *less, least.* Targ. Y. Gen. I, 16; a. e.—Snh. 108[b]. B. Mets. 21[b] ב׳ מהכי less than this; a. fr.—V. בְּצִירְתָא.

בְּצִיר *to be less*, v. בְּצַר.

בַּצִּירָא, v. בְּצַר, end.

בְּצִירָה f.=בָּצִיר I. Sabb. 17[a] בשעת חב׳ when they are cut; a. fr.—*Pl.* בְּצִירוֹת. B. Bath. 36[b] עד שיבצור ג׳ ב׳, v. בָּצִיר.

בְּצִירְתָא, v. בְּצוּרְתָא.

בְּצַל ($\sqrt{}$בץ, cmp. פצל) *to peel; to split, branch off.* Lam. R. introd.; Koh. R. to XII, 7 (interpret. אם הדרך Ezek. XXI, 26) אמה דבצלית (אם) an arm which branches off (direction post on the cross-road).

Ithpe. איבְּצֵיל (denom. of בְּצַלְא) *to grow bulbous.* Erub. 29[b] top אר׳ זירתא (ed. Pesaro a. Ar. אפציל, Var. אבציל) the bulb has grown to the length of a span.

בָּצָל m. (b. h.; v. preced.) *onion.* Nidd. 17[a]; a. fr.—Maasr. V, 7 (8) ב׳ של רכפה, expl. in Y. ib. 52[a] 'the stalk of which is pressed inward'; oth. opin. 'which has no acerbity', v. אֶרֶס.—*Pl.* בְּצָלִים. Shebi. II, 9 חב׳ הסריסים which produce no seeds. Ib. V, 4 ב׳ הקיצונים summer onions; a. fr.—Ukts. II, 8 עלי ב׳ ובני ב׳ the leek-like sprouts, and the central sprouts of onions. Gen. R. s. 82 (ref. to Obad. 6) קליפת ב׳ (not בצליא) like peeling onions (laying bare Esau's shame).

בְּצַלָא, v. בּוּצְלָא.

בְּצַלְאֵל pr. n. m. (b. h.) *Bezalel*; 1) the artificer of the Tabernacle. Ber. 55[a]. Ex. R. s. 48; a. fr.—2) R. B., an Amora. Cant. R. to III, 11 ר׳ ברכיה בשם ר׳ ב׳ (Num. R. s. 12 בצלה; Pesik. Vayhi, p. 4[b] לוי; Yalk. Ex. 369 only בשם ר׳).

בצלה, v. preced.

עֲלֵי ב׳, בְּצָלִים pr. n. m. *Ăle B'tsalim* (Onion Leaves). Y. Snh. VI, 23[c] bot.; Y. Ḥag. II, 77[d] bot. Miriam, the daughter of A. B. (prob. a nickname).

בְּצַלְצוּל m. (dimin. of בָּצָל) *dwarf-onion, (pallacana).* Kil. I, 3; v. Y. ib. 27[a]. [Maim.: *desert onion.*]

בָּצַע (b. h.; $\sqrt{}$בץ; cmp. בוע, בקע, פצע) 1) *to cut, break,* esp. *to break bread and say the blessing.* Hull. 7[b] מימיו לא ב׳ על וכ׳ never said grace over a piece of bread which was not his own (never accepted an invitation). Ber. 46[a] בע״הב בוצע וכ׳ the host breaks the bread and the guest says grace after meal. Ib. 47[a] אין חבוצע רשאי לִבְצוֹעַ וכ׳ he who is chosen to break the bread, must not begin to break until the Amen of those that respond (to the blessing) is finished; a. fr.—2) *to split the difference, to adjust, compromise.* Snh. 6[b] top נגמר ..... לבצוע after the legal proceedings are closed, thou must not act as an arbiter in a compromise. Ib. אסור לב׳ the court is forbidden to attempt a settlement (you must let the law take its course). Ib. מצוה לב׳ it is a meritorious act to bring about a settlement. Ib. (before having formed an opinion the judge may say) צאו ובִצְעוּ go out and settle; a. fr.

Pi. בִּצַּע *to adjust.* Y. Snh. I, 18[b] top המְבַצֵּעַ חוטא the judge who settles a case is a sinner. Ib. לְבַצֵּעַ (interch. with לבצוע). V. בִּיצּוּעַ.

בְּצַע ch. same. 1) *to break.* B. Bath. 91[b] כד הוה ב׳ ינוקא וכ׳ when a child broke apart a piece of St. John's bread. Sabb. 140[b], v. בִּיצּוּעָא.—*2) *to tear away, rescue* (cmp. פצר). Targ. Job XXXIII, 18 יבצע Ms. (ed. ימנע).

Pa. בַּצַּע *to break.* Targ. O. Lev. II, 6 (Var. בְּצַע Pe.). [Y. Taan. IV, 69[b]; Y. Meg. I, 70[a] bot. מבצע (Cant. R. to I, 16 מצנעה) read: מנצבה, מנצב, v. נְצַב.]

בִּצְעָה f. (בצע, cmp. בִּצָּה) *ditch, dike, pond.*—*Pl.* בִּצְעִין, בִּצְעִים, בִּי׳. Tosef. Snh. III, 4 שתי בצעין ed. Zuck. (Var. ביצועין); Shebu. 16[a] שני בצעים וכ׳ Ar. (read שתי, ed. ביציעין, Ms. M. בצעי׳) there were two ponds (reservoirs) in Jerusalem, the upper &c. Sabb. 31[a] בין בִּצְעֵי המים between the dykes (of the Nile). Snh. 96[a] בִּיצְעֵי וכ׳. Ib. 5[b], v. בִּצָּה.

בָּצַץ (v. בצבץ) *to break through, divide; to ooze, trickle, drip.* Y. Pes. VII, beg. 34[a] כל העצים בּוֹצְצִין משקין all other sorts of wood (used for roasting spits) will drip moisture. Y. M. Kat. I, beg. 80[a]; Tosef. Mikv. I, 13 ההרים בוצצין (ed. Zuck. ביצין) the mountains are trickling (sending the rain water into the rivers; cmp. preced.).

בָּצֵק m. (b. h.; בָּצַק, √בץ, *to break open, split,* v. Deut. VIII, 4; cmp. סדק a. denom.) *dough.* Pes. III, 2 (46[a]) ב׳ הַחֵרֵשׁ deaf dough, i. e. having no indications of rising (which makes it doubtful whether or not fermentation has set in); [oth. reading ב׳ הַחֶרֶשׂ hard and smooth as a potsherd]. Ib. 4; a. fr.—*Pl.* בְּצֵקוֹת. Ib. 40[a].

בָּצַר (b. h.; √בץ, cmp. בצע) *to cut* grapes. Pes. 3[b] בּוֹצְרִין בטהרה one must cut grapes under the rules of levitical cleanness. Gitt. 57[a] בָּצְרוּ .. את כרמיהן וכ׳ the gentiles held vintage in vineyards soaked with Israel's blood; a. fr.

Nif. נִבְצַר 1) *to be cut.* Ex. R. s. 30, beg. עד שתגיע עונתן לִיבָּצֵר until their (the nations') time has arrived to be cut (ripe for punishment). 2) *to be cut off, diminished.* Tanḥ. Noah 18 נִבְצָרִים מן וכ׳ cut off from the world (destroyed). Gen. R. s. 38 יִבָּצֵר מהם shall be denied them.

Pi. בִּיצֵּר, בִּצֵּר *to cut off,* whence (cmp. גדר) 1) *to surround, fortify.* Part. pass. מְבוּצָּר. Y. Pes. VII, 35[b] bot.; Y. Shebu. VIII, beg., 38[b] גג מב׳ a roof surrounded with railings, v. בְּצוֹצְרָה.—Neg. I, 5 מְבוּצֶּרֶת an eruption surrounded with sound flesh; ib. X, 2 sq. מבוצר (of the hair in the flesh affected by the eruption). Deut. R. s. 1 (ref. to עיר מצור Ps. LX, 11, a. מבצר ib. CVIII, 11) עיר שמבוצרת וכ׳ the city (of Rome) which is well fortified &c.—2) *to diminish.* Ib. שמצירה ומבצרה לישראל (Mat. K. וּמְבַצֶּרֶת, Yalk. Ps. 779 מבצרא ch.) the city which troubles and diminishes Israel.

Nithpa. נִתְבַּצֵּר *to be railed around, be set apart.* Meg. 14[a]; Snh. 110[a]; Num. R. s. 18 מקום נ׳ להם וכ׳ a place was set apart for them in Gehenna; Koh. R. to VII, 2.

בָּצַר (v. preced. a. next w.) *to be diminished.* Keth. 7[b] דִבְצָרָה מיום אחד who has less than one day's (celebration of marriage with benedictions at meals).

בְּצַר, בְּצִיר ch. 1) (neut. v.) *to be cut, lessened; to be small; to want.* Ab. Zar. 9[a] כמה בצרן (Rashi בצירן) how much is wanting yet? Targ. Prov. XIV, 28 בציר עמא the population is diminishing.—Ḥull. 42[b] בצר להו חדא there is, according to him, one less (than the number stated); a. fr.—2) (act. v.) *to diminish, lessen.* Targ. Y. Deut. XIII, 1; IV, 2 (Var. תבצרון Pa.). Targ. Job XV, 4.—Nidd. 65[a] לְמִבְצַר לה חדא to allow her one night less; a. fr.

Pa. בַּצֵּר *to cut off; to diminish, deduct.* Men. 37[b] האי מאן דבַצְּרֵיה לגלימיה he who cuts one corner of his cloak off.—Targ. Koh. III, 5. Targ. Deut. IV, 2, a. e., v. supra. —Ab. Zar. 9[b] וּנְבַצֵּר וכ׳ we let him deduct therefrom forty eight. B. Mets. 103[b] בַּצְּרִי לך I let thee have it for less.— Denom. בַּצִּירָא *one who uses the vowel letters sparingly.* Ab. Zar. 9[a b] and as a mnemonical sign (for remembering when to add and when to deduct) ספרא ב׳ וכ׳ the writer of Bible copies writes many words without the vowel letters (defective) which the Mishnah teacher writes *plene.*

בֶּצֶר m. (b. h.) 1)=בָּצִיר *crop,* trnsf. *means of support, (family-) trade.* Ex. R. s. 40, end לעולם . . . . מניח בִּצְרוֹ one should never give up his trade; Pesik. R. s. 6, end מחליף בִּצִירוֹ (Arakh. 16 אומנותו ואומנות אבותיו). Ex. R. l. c. (insert Job XXII, 24—25 as text) the Lord says, אני הוא בִּצְרְכֶן . . . . בִּצְרְכֶן וכ׳ I am your support, give ye never up your support (faith); but also the support of your fathers ye must not give up (labor) &c. Pesik. R. l. c. thou art our God וּבִצְרֵנוּ and our support (ref. to Ps. XCV, 6).—2) pl. בְּצָרִים *fort.* Ex. R. l. c. (ref. to Job l. c.; cmp. Targ.) שנעשה חומותיך He will be thy fortification. [Yalk. Deut. 811, v. בִּיצּוּר.]

בִּצָּרָה, בִּצְּרָאָה &c., v. בּוֹצ׳.

***בֶּצֶת** pr. n. pl. *Betseth,* a Phœnician border-town (perh. identical with Bassa, Neub. Géogr. p. 22). Y. Dem. II, 22[d] top; Tosef. Shebi. IV, 9 (Var. כצת; Hildesh. p. 34 בצץ).

בָּקָא m., **בַּקְתָא** f. (בקק *to enter into, search,* v. P. Sm. 573; cmp. בִּירְנָא III, בִּירִיתָא a. פִּשְׁפֵּשׁ) *gnat.* Ḥull. 58[b] לית ב׳ בר יומא no gnat lives an entire day. Ib. תלו ליה לב׳ וכ׳ they suspended on the gnat's proboscis sixty &c. Ib. אמראי בקת׳ לבקא Ar. (ed. אמרא ב׳ מבקא) the she-gnat quarrelled with the he-gnat, v. מרר.—*Pl.* בַּקֵּי. Succ. 26[a] משום ב׳ on account of the gnats. Sabb. 77[b], v. פִּשְׁפֵּשׁ.

בְּקָא, בְּקִי (√בק, v. preced.; cmp. בצא, a. בין; v. בקר, בקש &c.) *to search, investigate, examine, find out.* Part. בָּקֵי. Targ. Prov. XVII, 3 צרפא בקי Bxt. (ed. נקר). Ib. XXIV, 12 בָּאקֵי Ms. (Bxt. a. oth. בצר; corrupt. באחר; h. text יבין).—B. Mets. 84[b] בְּקִי באבוך וכ׳ (Yalk. Prov. 964 בַּקְרִי) find out what thy father is doing now. Pes. 3[b] בקי מאי דיניה Ms. M. (ed. בדוק) find out his ways and manners. Gitt. 69[b] לִיבְקֵי וכ׳ let one search for the body of one who died on a Sabbath. Koh. R. to XI, 2 (read:) עד דאינון בקיין תרין חיואן וכ׳ (אזלין בעיין.... ונפקין strike out) while they were searching (for the grave), two serpents of fire &c.

בקוותא, Y. Snh. VII, end, 25[d], read בַּקְרוּתָא.

בְּקוֹלְסָא, v. בִּקְלָסָא.

בְּקוּרוֹת, בְּקוֹרֶת, v. בַּקְרוּת.

בְּקוֹרֶת, v. בִּיקוֹרֶת.

בָּקִי, v. בָּקָא.

בָּקִי, בְּקִיא m. h. a. ch. (בקא) *expert, versed, familiar.* Targ. I Chr. XI, 11.—Kidd. 10[b] ב׳ בחדרי תורה well acquainted with the chambers (intricacies) of the Law; Y. Keth. V, 29[d] bot. ב׳ בסתרי וכ׳. Snh. VII, 2 שלא היה

ב״ד ב׳ the court was not versed in the law. Yoma 49a כלום אתה ב׳ ברפואות an expert in medicine. Yeb. 102a ב׳ בר׳ וכ׳ art thou acquainted with R. &c.?; Tosef. ib. XII, 11 ב׳ היה לך בר׳ וכ׳ ed. Zuck. (read ב׳ הו׳ לך ר׳ as oth. ed.) was R. . . . well known to thee? Keth. 6b; a. fr.—*Pl.* בְּקִיאֵי, בְּקִיאִין. Targ. I Chr. XII, 32 (Var. בקיעין). Ḥull. 4a אין ב׳ וכ׳ (the Samaritans) are not so well versed in the details of the Law as &c. Gitt. 86b. Kidd. 30a אינהו ב׳ . . . . אנן לא בְקִיאִינַן they (the ancients) were versed in Biblical orthography (in *defective* and *plene*), we are not.—*Fem.* בְּקִיאָה. Ḥag. 5a. [Targ. Y. II Gen. XLIX, 12 בְּקִיַין בהלכה Ar., ed. כה׳, incorr., Levita in Tishbi בְּקִיאִין; Y. I נקיין מן חלבא!]

בְּקִיָא, בְּקִייא *vetch*, v. בִּיקְיָא.

בְּקִיעַ I m. (בקע; cmp. בְּצִצָה) *fissure, ditch*, esp. *small pond* for washing clothes. M. Kat. 8b נברכת וב׳, expl. as גיהא ובר גיהא a large pond and a small pond. Tosef. B. Bath. I, 2. Ib. M. Kat. I, 9 זו היא נ׳ . . . ב׳ Nibrekheth a. B'kia are the same; Y. ib. I, 80d כל שהוא תושב וכ׳ any permanent cut in the ground is called בקיע (*fissure*, a grave, wash-pond &c.). [Another opin. in Ar. אבן ב׳=ב׳ *a flat stone* whereon washers beat their clothes; Y. l. c. כל שהוא וכ׳ any stone fixed in the ground is called a *b'kia*.—Ms. M. a. ed. Ven. נְקִיעַ, v. נְקַע.]

בְּקִיעַ II m. ch. (בקע=בקא)=בְּקִיא. Snh. 5b ב׳ במומי (Ms. M. פקיע) an expert in judging bodily defects. B. Bath. 164b בקיע some ed. (Ms. M. בקי, F. פקיע).—*Pl.* בְּקִיעֵי, בְּקִיעִין. Targ. I Chr. XII, 32 Var., v. בְּקִי. Shebu. 42a דכמה דנפישי בקיעי טפי (some ed. בקיאי, Ms. F. פ׳) the majority of the experts are supposed to be better versed (than the minority).

בְּקִיעָא m. (בקע) *that which is demolished by chopping*. Lev. R. s. 19, v. אָלִים.

בְּקִיעָה f. (בקע) 1) *cleaving, cleft; that which is cloven, a log*. *Pl.* בְּקִיעוֹת. Koh. R. to II, 23 בקע לי שתי ב׳ chop for me two logs; (Gen. R. s. 27 בקיעות, v. בְּקַעַת). Koh. R. to X, 9; Gen. R. s. 55, end בשכר שתי ב׳ שבקע וכ׳ as a reward for the two pieces of wood which Abraham chopped (Gen. XXII, 3).—2) *crossing, passing over*. Sabb. 101a בְּקִיעַת דגים the crossing of fish under the ship.

בְּקִיעִין, פְּקִיעִין (כפר) pr. n. pl. *B'kiin, (K'far) P'kiin*, modern *Fukin*, a place in Southern Palestine between Lydda and Jabneh, residence of R. Joshua. Y. Ḥag. I, beg. 75d. Snh. 32b; a. fr.

בְּקִיקָא m. (בקק; cmp. בקע, בקיעא) *a broken piece, potsherd*. *Pl.* בְּקִיקִין. Targ. Y. Ex. XII, 12; Num. XXXIII, 4.

בקלאנין, Cant. R. to I, 12 ב׳ בוקינוס וכ׳, read קְלָאנִין בבוק׳ וכ׳, v. קְנָן; v. Yalk. ib. 983.

***בְּקָלְסָא, בּוּקְלְסָא** m. (בקלס, בקל with ס intens., as בלעס a. בלע; cmp. Syr. בוקלא P. Sm. 474; √בק, cmp. בקעת) *club, shepherd's crook*. Gen. R. s. 38 קם נסב בקלסיה (or בקלסא) he stood up, took (his) crook and broke the idols, ויהב בוקלסא וכ׳ and placed the crook into the hand of the largest of them (Rashi בולקסא, corr acc.).—*Pl.* בְּקָלְסֵי, בּוּקְלָסֵי (בְּקוּלְסֵי). Zeb. 105a קיטר לה בבו׳ Rashi (ed. בבקולסי; Ms. M. בקלסי, Ar. s. v. קלס, בקולסי Ms. R. 1 בקינסי, Ms. K. בקונסי) they seize it (the sacrifice to be burnt) with crooks (while standing outside).

בָּקַע (b. h.; √בק, v. בְּקָא) 1) *to split, chop; to break through*. B. Mets. 99a בָּ׳ בו; (Kidd. 47b בִּיקַּע) if he chopped wood with it. Gen. R. s. 55, end; Koh. R. to X, 9; II, 23, v. בְּקִיעָה. Ex. R. s. 21 אני בוֹקֵעַ להם וכ׳ I am going to split the sea for them; a. fr.—Lam. R. to II, 2 בקעו בחיילותיו וכ׳ broke through the lines of N.'s armies; Y. Taan. IV, 69b top ברחו לתוך.—2) *to cross, make a short cut, pass over*. Y. Pes. I, 27b bot. חצר שהרבים בוֹקְעִין וכ׳ a court which people use for crossing. Erub. 16b; Sabb. 101b (a low wall) שהגדיים וכ׳ ב׳ over which the kids pass; v. בְּקַעָה.—3) (cmp. בִּצְבֵּץ) *to break through the ground*, esp. as a legal fiction for a levitical impurity the cause of which is underground, but which affects the things above and beneath. Ohol. VI, 6 טומאה בוֹקַעַת וכ׳ the impurity breaks through the ground and rises, and breaks through and goes down; a. fr.—Koh. R. III, 16 היה הדם בו׳ ועולה the blood broke through and rose. Midr. Till. to Ps. LXXVIII, 45 ב׳ בצור, ב׳ את הצור break through (take root in) the rock; a. fr.

Nif. נִבְקַע *to be split, to burst open*. Ib. הסיפין נבקעין וכ׳ the door sells were burst before them. Ib. נ׳ הספל מאליו the vessel went to pieces of itself. Gen. R. s. 55, end זכה לְהִבָּקַע הים וכ׳ he was rewarded by the sea being divided before the children of Israel. Ḥull. 14b שמא יִבָּקַע הנוד the wine bottle may burst; a. fr.

Pi. בִּיקַּע, בִּקַּע 1) *to split, chop, tear*. Kidd. 47b, v. supra. Y. Bets. I, 60a bot.; Y. Ab. Zar. II, 41c bot. שביקעו (שבקעו) להם וכ׳ of whose flocks the wolves had torn more than &c. Bets. IV, 3 אין מְבַקְּעִין וכ׳ one must not split woods (on Holy Days) etc. Sifré Deut. 183 (ref. to Deut. XIX, 5) מן העץ הַמְבֻקָּע from the *splitting* wood (the handle), opp. העץ המִתְבַּקֵּעַ the *split* wood (the tree). Tanh. Vayetse 9 בַּקֵּעַ וכ׳ chop thou &c.—Part. pass. מְבוּקָּע. Ab. Zar. 65b מְבוּקָּעוֹת grapes burst open.—2) *to jam in, wedge*. Sabb. 67b הַמְבַקַּעַת ביצים (Rashi Var. המקבעת, Ms. M. עצים) one who squeezes egg-shells &c. (a superstitious practice; Tosef. ib. VI (VII), 18 הנותנת בצים . . . . . בכותל).

Hif. הִבְקִיעַ 1) *to cut, clear*. Shebi. IV, 5 הַמַּבְקִיעַ בזתים וכ׳ he who cuts olive-trees down (in the Sabbath year) must not cover the stump with ground.—2) *to lead a line crosswise*. Y. Kil. III, 28d top לְהַבְקִיעַ וכ׳ to plant four rows across a valley from end to end.

Hithpa. הִתְבַּקֵּעַ *to be split; to burst, break*. Sifré Deut. 183, v. supra.—Sabb. XVI, 5. Cant. R. to VI, 4.

בֶּקַע m. (b. h.; בקע) [*a split*,] *beka*, a *weight* and a *coin*, equal to half a Shekel. Gen. R. s. 84; a. e.

בִּקְעָא, v. בִּקְעֲתָא.

בִּקְעָה f. (b. h.; בקע) *cut, notch*, whence *valley, plane; a group of fields*; v. בְּאגָא; esp. *a short cut* for farm-laborers &c. Toh. VI, 7, a. e. חב׳ בימות החמה וכ׳ the path through the fields in summer-time (when used by field laborers) is considered as private ground with regard to Sabbath laws, as public with regard to levitical purity. B. Bath. 61[b] when one sells ... a field בב׳ גדולה within a large group of fields (all belonging to the seller). Ib. (in a place) where they call לשדה ש׳ ולב׳ ב׳ a field *sadeh* and an estate *bikah;* a. fr.—Trnsf. *an unguarded field, moral danger.* Erub. 6[a]; 100[b]; Ḥull. 110[a] רב ב׳ מצא וכ׳ Rab found an unguarded field and fenced it in, i. e. found people transgressing the law in ignorance and instituted preventive regulations.—*Pl.* בְּקָעוֹת. Gen. R. s. 98.—2) (constr.) בִּקְעַת pr. n. pl. *Valley of*—, as ב׳ ידים, ב׳ יזרעאל &c., for all of which see the respective determinants.

בקער, Y. Ned. IV, beg. 38[c], v. בִּיקוּעַ.

בִּקְעָה f. (בקע) 1) *chip, piece of wood; log to be chopped.* B. Kam. 32[b] ניתזה ב׳ וכ׳ a chip slipped out (of the carpenter's hand) and struck his face; Y. ib. III, end, 3[d]. Y. Macc. II, 31[c] bot. Y. Bets. IV, 62[c] bot. אין מכבין את הב׳ you must not extinguish the log; v. כָּסַס. Sabb. 29[a] top; a. fr.—*Pl.* (cmp. pl. of בִּקְעִיּוֹת (בִּיסָה. Ḥull. 37[b] אפי׳ אוכלת ב׳ even if strong enough to bite wood. Koh. R. to III, 17 (a gloss expl. גזירין). Gen. R. s. 27, v. בִּקְעָה.—2) dial. for פִּקְעַת q. v.

בִּקְעָא, בִּקְעִתָא ch. same. Targ. Y. Num. XIX, 6.

בִּקְעָא, בִּקְעָ׳, בִּקְעֲתָא f. ch. = h. בִּקְעָה. Targ. Gen. XI, 2; a. fr.—*Pl.* בִּקְעָתָא.—Y. Shebi. III, 34[c] top, v. פְּקוּעָה.—Constr. בִּקְעַת, pr. n. *Valley of*.... Gen. R. s. 10; a. fr.

בָּקַר (b. h.; √בק, בקע v.) *to enter into, to clear, split;* whence 1) (=בער) *to eat up.* Denom. בָּקָר (=בְּעִיר).—2) (=בער) *to break forth, shine.* Denom. בֹּקֶר.

Pi. בִּיקֵּר, בִּקֵּר (b. h.) 1) *to enter into, examine, search, distinguish* (cmp. בִּין). Keth. 106[a] מְבַקְּרֵי מומין those entrusted with the examination of sacrificial animals. Y. Bets. II, 61[c] top וּבִיקְּרָן מִמּוּמִין and had them examined (and declared free) from bodily defects. Ḥag. 9[b] אין אומרים בַּקְּרוּ וכ׳ we do not say, Examine ye a camel, a swine &c. (i. e. only the deeds of distinguished persons are scrutinized); a. fr.—*Part. pass.* מְבוּקָּר *examined and found fit.* Y. Ber. IV, 7[b] top טלאים מְבוּקָּרִים lambs which passed examination.—2) *to inquire after one's health, to visit the sick.* Ned. IV, 4 (38[b]). ונכנס לְבַקְּרוֹ and comes to see him. Snh. 68[a]; a. v. fr. [Ruth. R. to II, 15, v. infra.]

Hithpa. הִתְבַּקֵּר, *Nithpa.* נִתְבַּקֵּר 1) *to be examined.* Gen. R. s. 81 פנקסו נִתְבַּקְּרָה his account is examined (his sins visited); Tanḥ. Vayishlaḥ 8 מִתְבַּקֶּרֶת. Gen. R. s. 84, read with Yalk. Gen. 141 נתב׳ פנקסי my account &c. 2) *to be visited, attended to.* Num. R. s. 18 as all sick persons מִתְבַּקְּרִין are tended (by physicians).

Hif. הִבְקִיר (Y. Dial. for הִפְקִיר, v. פָּקַר; v. next w.) *to give free, to resign ownership, to declare a property ownerless.* Y. Ned. IV, 38[d]; Y. Peah V, beg. 19[b] [read:] כיון שאדם מַבְקִיר דבר יצא מרשותו as soon as one declares a thing to be free, it has gone out of his control; Y. Dem. III, 23[b] bot. כיון שאדם מ׳ ... ויצא ... הבקירו הבקר as soon as one gives a thing free and it has left his possession, his act is valid; a. fr. [Ruth. R. to II, 15 מבדר, מִבקר, prob. מבקיר; v. בָּדַר.]

Hof. הוּבְקַר *to be declared free, to be free.* Y. Peah VI, 19[c] top.—Part. מוּבְקָר Ib. 19[b] bot. שדי מוּבְקֶרֶת וכ׳ (Tosef. Maasr. III, 11. הרי .. מופ׳) my field shall be free for one day &c.; a. e.

בְּקַר ch. same.—*Pa.* בַּקַּר 1) *to search, examine.* Targ. O. Lev. XIII, 36; a. fr.—2) *to clear, glean.* Targ. Y. I Deut. XXIV, 20 (II תתב׳, read תבקרון, h. text תפאר).—3) *to let the herd graze* (cmp. בער), *to drive unmuzzled animals.* Targ. Y. Gen. XIII, 7.—4) *to visit the sick.* Targ. Y. Ex. XVIII, 20; a. e.—Y. Sabb. VI, 8[c] bot.; a. fr.—5) (=preced. Hif.) *to abandon, leave unclaimed, declare free.* Targ. Y. Ex. XXIII, 11 Ar. (some ed. ותפקר, read ותפקר). Y. Shebi. IX, 39[a] top יַאֲבַקְּרָה קומיהון and I will declare it free goods in their presence. Ib. וּמְבַקְּרִין ליה and declare ye it free property.

בֹּקֶר, בּוֹקֶר m. (b. h.; v. בָּקַר) *morning, early day;* metaph. *light, salvation.* Y. Taan. I, 64[a] top ב׳ לצדיקים וכ׳ a morning for the righteous, a night for the wicked. Ruth. R. to III, 13 בּב׳ בעולם וכ׳ 'in the morning'—that means in the world which is all-good. Esth. R., introd. (ref. to Deut. XXVIII, 67) בבקרה של בבל וכ׳ in the morning (ascendancy) of Babel thou shalt say, Oh that her evening (downfall) would come! Gen. R. s. 21 (ref. to Dan. VIII, 14) לִכְשֶׁיַּעֲשֶׂה בֹּקֶר וכ׳ when the morning of the (persecuting) nations shall become evening, and the evening of Israel morning; Tanḥ. ed. Bub. B'resh. 23. Mekh. Bo, s. 6 in order to define it: לְבָקְרוֹ של ב׳ at the very break of morning; Y. Ber. I, 2[c] top.—*Pl.* בְּקָרִים. Yoma 33[b] חלקהו לשני ב׳ divide the acts prescribed into two mornings, i. e. let another act be inserted between. Ber. 27[a] חלקהו לשני ב׳ take only one half of the morning hours. Y. Pes. V, 31[d] top אית לך מימר תמן בין הַבְּקָרִים then it ought to have read there *ben hab-b'karaim* (as you read בין הערבים, Du.).

בָּקָר m. (b. h.; v. בָּקַר) *a beef;* (collect.) *oxen, cattle.* Sifra Vayikra ch. II, Par. 2 אין לך בבהמה אלא ב׳ וכ׳ under *b'hemah* for offerings (Lev. I, 2) are meant only beeves and sheep; a. fr. בן ב׳ *young cattle, calf.* Ib.; a. fr.—רועי ב׳ *herders* (suspected of feeding upon other people's fields). Snh. III, 2 נאמנין עלי שלשה ר׳ ב׳ (if one says) I have faith in (the arbitration of) three herders.

בַּקָּר m. (preced.) *neat-herd, cow-herd; cattle-driver.* Y. Bets. V, 63[b], v. רָגַל.

בַּקָּרָא I ch. same. B. Mets. 42[b].—*Pl.* בַּקָּרֵי. Sot. 48[a] זמרא דב׳ the song of the drivers (at ploughing).

***בַּקְּרָא** II m., pl. בַּקְּרִין (v. בָּקַר, cmp. b. h. בַּעַר a. בּוּר 1) [*empty,*] *light-minded, thoughtless.* Targ. Jud. IX, 4 Ar. a. Kimḥi (ed. הסירין).

בַּקְרָא c. (בקר) *herd.* Targ. Y. Deut. VII, 13 בַּקְרַת תוריך (h. text שגר אלפיך). B. Mets. 84[a] ב׳ דתורי a herd of oxen, (Var. פדנא, v. Rashia. l. a. Rabb. D.S.a. l. note 2). —*Pl.* m. בַּקְרִין, constr. בַּקְרֵי. Targ. O. Deut. l. c.; Targ. ib. XXVIII, 4.—Fem. בַּקְרָן. Targ. Joel I, 18; Is. VII, 25.

בַּקְרוּת f. (בָּקָר) *cattle-yard, cattle-farm, stock of cattle.* M.Kat. 12ª; Tosef.ib.II, 11 ביקורת (Var. בקרות, בקירות); Y. Pes. IV, 31ᵇ top בקורת. Y. Yeb. IV, 6ª bot.; Y. Nidd. I, 49ᵇ top; Gen. R. s. 20 [read:] בקרות של בית אנטונינוס היתה עוֹבֶרֶת והרביעו (שוורים) ממנה בַקְרוּת של בית רבי the herd of the estate of A. passed by and (some oxen) thereof covered the herd of Rabbi's estate; [perhaps the second בקרות is to be read בְּקָרוֹת fem. pl. of בְּקָרָה; v. Var. lect. in l. c.]

בַּקְרוּתָא I ch. same. Lam. R. to I, 9 חד בענא וחד בב׳ one is employed in the fold and one in the cattle-farm. Y. Snh. VII, 25ᵈ bot. גנב עגל מן בקוותא וכ׳ (corr. מן . . בקר׳ ואייתיה ליה) he stole a calf from the yard and brought it to him.

בַּקְרוּתָא II, **בַּקְרָנוּתָא** f. (v. בַּקְרָא II) *levity, thoughtlessness.* Targ. Jer. XXIII, 32. Targ. I Sam. XVII, 28.

בַּקְרַת, v. בַּקְרָא.

בָּקַשׁ (b. h.; √בק, v. בקא; corresp. to ch. בער); *Pi.* בִּיקֵּשׁ, בִּקֵּשׁ *to seek, desire, beg, ask.* Kidd. 65ª מְבַקְּשִׁין וכ׳ the court begs him to give her a letter of divorce, opp. to כופין. Ber. 12ᵇ בִּקְּשׁוּ לקבוע וכ׳ they (the Rabbis) intended to insert the chapter about Balak &c. Gen. R. s. 84 ב׳ לישב וכ׳ he intended to live in peace; a. fr.—ב׳ רחמים *to pray* (for mercy), v. בער. Ber. l. c. B. Bath. 91ᵇ; a. fr.

Hithpa. הִתְבַּקֵּשׁ, *Nithpa.* נִתְבַּקֵּשׁ *to be sought, to be hunted for* (by detectives); *to be summoned.* Taan. 29ª (a disguised warning given to R. Gamliel) בעל החוטם מִתְבַּקֵּשׁ the well-known man is wanted; v. חוֹטֶם. B. Mets. 86ª, v. רְשַׁבְּח.

בַּקָּשָׁה f. (b. h.; preced.) *desire, prayer.* Ned. XI, 12 דרך ב׳ in the way of a request (to give a divorce, v. preced.). Ber. 9ª, a. fr. אין נא אלא לשון ב׳ the word נָא in the Bible means prayer (I pray &c.). Ib. 57ª תלויה בַּקָּשָׁתוֹ his prayer is held in suspense (its fulfillment is doubtful).—בב׳ ממך *I pray thee*, v. בָּעוּ. Ib. 9ª. Gen. R. s. 75 end; a. fr.—*Pl.* בַּקָּשׁוֹת.

בַּקְתָא, **בִּיקְתָא**, **בִּקְתָא** f. (=בקעא, v. בָּאגָא a. בִּקְעָה) *valley, short cut; group of fields.* Ber. 34ᵇ bot. I consider him arrogant מאן דמצלי בב׳ (Ms. M. a. Ar. בפקתא q. v.) who prays in a valley (where people pass by). Keth. 54ª; 103ª בביתי ולא בביקתי 'in my house' ('as long as you will spend your widowhood in my house'—the marriage contract reads) but not in my estate, i. e. she must be content to live in her late husband's house with his heirs, but she cannot claim a separate residence. [Comment. בי עקתי=בקתי house of my distress, narrow house, i. e. when there is no room for her and the heirs, she loses her claims, v. Sabb. 77ᵇ, etymol. of בי עקתא=ב׳ narrow place.]—בר בי׳ (בת) one of the same rural community; trnsf. *of the same class* or *category*; *neighbor.* Men. 24ᵇ כולהו בנו ב׳ they all belong together. Meïl. 17ᵇ בנו חדא ב׳ of the same category.—Yeb. 84ª בת בי׳ (ed. בוּקְתָא) a parallel case stated immediately after.

בַּקְתָא, v. בַּקָא.

בַּר I m. (b. h.; ברר) [*empty, open*] 1) *uncultivated ground, forest, prairie;* opp. יישוב. Kil. VIII, 6. Hull. 80ª שור הבר the ox of the prairie, *buffalo.* Ib. איל הב׳ forest ram. Y. Sabb. XIV, 14ᵇ bot. חזיר של ב׳ wild swine.—2) *clear, visible,* whence *the outside, surface,* opp. תוך. Yoma 72ᵇ a scholar שאין תוכו כברו whose inside is not as his outside (who is insincere); Ber. 28ª. Y. Pes. VII, 34ª bot. תוך בר the inner parts of the Passover lamb must hang outside (not be put inside, v. R. Akiba in Mish. VII, 1); Mekh. Bo, 6 תוך ובר (read תוכו בר); Pes. 74ª R. Ish. called it תוך בר Ar. s. v. תך 2 (ed. תוך תוך, Var. in Rashi a. Ar. תוכברא q. v.).

בָּרָא, **בַּר**, **בָּר** ch. same 1) (=h. יַעַר, שָׂדֶה) *forest, prairie* &c. Targ. Ps. L, 10sq. Targ O. Gen. III, 1; a. e.—2) (adj.) *living in the forest* &c., *wild.* Targ. Ps. l. c. Var. תרנגול ברא; Sabb. 78ª תרנגולא ב׳ Ms. M. (ed. לת....) woodcock (hen of the prairie).—*3) *peel.* Ib. 139ᵇ ב׳ דתומא the peel of garlic; [Rashi, expl. צלע, must have read אברא].—4) (=h. חוּץ) *outside, outdoors, street.* Targ. Gen. XXXIV, 31 נפקת ב׳ a prostitute, v. חוּץ II; a. fr.—Y. Kil. IX, 32ᵇ מאן בעי לך לבר who wants thee outside? (an intimation to leave the room). Snh. 62ªᵇ; Sabb. 106ª, a. e. פוק תני לברא go out and teach it in the street (i. e. your tradition is rejected).—תנא ברא a Tannai not recorded in the Mishnah, v. בָּרַיְיתָא. M. Kat. 17ᵇ (Rashi: חאי תנא דברייתא); B. Bath. 93ᵇ Ar. (ed. בתרא); cmp. בָּרָאָה.—4) (prep. a. adv.) *outside;* בר מן *outside of, except, without.* Targ. O. Gen. XIV, 24; a. fr.—Ber. 38ᵇ ב׳ מן דין וב׳ וכ׳ without this and without that, i. e. apart from these two arguments. Y. Erub. VII, end 24ᵈ ב׳ מדעתיה without his knowledge; a. fr.—Hull. 62ᵇ וסימניך בר בירה and thy mnemonical sign (as to צרדא a. ברדא, the one being forbidden, the other permitted) be: keep aloof from it (ברדא).—*Trnsf. restriction* (everywhere except . . .), *proviso.* Succ. 45ᵇ; Snh. 97ᵇ who enter the heavenly courts בב׳ with certain qualifications (by special grant), בלא ב׳ without any restrictions.—לְבַר, מִלְּבַר *apart from, outside, exclusively.* Cant. R. to VII, 8 לב׳ מישראל except the Israelites. Hull. 98ª sixtyone, בהדי דידה או... לב׳ מינה the one (egg) included or excluded? B. Bath. 90ᵇ שתותא מלב׳ the sixth part (as an addition) is outside, i. e. to each five portions one is added, an addition of twenty percent, opp. מִלְּגָו. B. Mets. 53ᵇ, v. חוּמְשָׁא.

בַּר II, **בְּרָא** m. ch. (b. h. בַּר poetic; ברי) *son, offspring.* Targ. Gen. IV, 25; a. v. fr.—ב׳ שמואל son of Sam.; בְּרֵיה דר׳ . . . son of . . . . Ber. 3ª, Hull. 11ª; a. v. fr.—B. Mets. 110ª . . בְּרַה דבת the son of the daughter of . . . . Sabb. 116ᵇ במקום ברא ברתא וכ׳ where there is a son, the daughter cannot inherit. Y. Shebi. IX, 39ª bot. אמה דהן ילדת ב׳ this man's mother has born a son, i. e. she may be proud of him; Y. Ab. Zar. IV, 43ᵈ אית לאימיה ב׳ (not ואית); a. v. fr.—*Pl.* [בְּנִין, בְּרִין, בְּנֵי, בְּרֵי. Targ. Y. Ex. X, 9 (some ed.). Targ. Ps. CXXVII, 3 Ms.] בְּנַיָּא, בְּנֵי, בְּנִין.

Targ. Gen. V, 4 בְּנִין וּבְנָן sons and daughters; a. fr.—Keth. IV, 10 (in a marriage contract) בנין דכרין male issue, opp. בְּנָן נוקבין, ib. 11.—Ber. 10ª ב׳ דמעלו good children. Y. B. Bath. VIII, 16ᵇ bot. אין חוון בנוי דהנייה (read בָּנַיי) if my children turn out well; a. v. fr.—בר בת, בר בר, grandson. Esth. R. introd. (expl. נין ונכד) בר ובר בר (not ובר בר) son and grandson; a. fr.

Fem. v. בְּרַת. [The meaning of בר in compounds is generally the same as of בן a. בעל, e. g. ב׳ אולפן *a scholar*, ב׳ אמודאי *a diver*, ב׳ שטיא *a maniac*, ב׳ דעת *a rational being*. בר בי רב, v. בֵּי. For compounds which are not self-evident, see the respective determinants.]

בַּר III m. (b. h.; ברר; v. בַּר I) *clear, bright, clean, pure*. Tosef. Kil. III, 6 (missing in ed. Zuckerm., v. Var. a. l.) שהוא בר ובקי וכ׳ who is clear and well-versed in &c. Num. R. s. 10 (ref. to ברי Prov. XXXI, 2, a. בר Ps. II, 12) the Law שהיא נקראת בר which is called *bar* (clear, pure, Ps. XIX, 9).—*Pl.* בָּרִים. Ib.

בַּר IV, **בָּר** m. (b. h.; v. בָּרַר) [*sifted*] *grain*. Ber. 55ª כשם שא״א לבר בלא וכ׳ as there can be no grain without straw, so there is no dream without idle things; Ned. 8ª.

בָּרָא I *outside, forest* &c., v. בַּר I ch.

בְּרָא II, בְּרָא I *to create*, v. ברי.

בְּרָא II *son*, v. בַּר II.

בָּרָאָה, בָּרְיָיא, בָּרְיָה, בָּרִית m. (v. בַּר I ch.) 1) *external, foreign, not belonging to*, opp. גַּוָּאָה. Targ. II Kings XVI, 18; a. e.—Y. Pes. VII, beg. 34ª תנא ב׳, v. בַּר I ch.—Gen. R. s. 49; Yalk. Gen. 83 (interpret. חָלִלָה Gen. XIII, 25) בריה (בריית) חוא לך it is foreign to thy nature; v. חִיצָה I.—*Pl.* בָּרָאֵי. Kidd. 33ª בתי ב׳ the outer chambers of the bath-house. Ḥag. 5ᵇ בתי ב׳ the outer chambers of the heavens. B. Bath. 30ª בשוקי ב׳ in the market places abroad.—Fem. בָּרְיְתָא, בָּרְיְיתָא. Targ. Ezek. XLII, 1; a. e.—Y. M. Kat. III, beg. 81ᶜ; Y. Ned. X, 42ᵇ top ארעא ב׳ (= h. חוץ לארץ) abroad; v. אֲרַע.—*Pl.* בָּרְיָיתָא, בָּרְיָתָא. Targ. Prov. XXX, 4 ב׳ דארעא the extreme ends of &c.—2) (as noun) *street, open place, field*. B. Bath. 40ᵇ sit down בשוקי ובב׳ Rashi (ed. בשוקא) in markets and open places (i. e. in public). Ḥull. 43; 47ª; 58ᵇ חיוי ב׳ the animals of the prairies, v. בַּר I ch.—Esp. בָּרַיְתָא, בָּרַיְיתָא (sub. מתניתא = h. משנה חחיצונה) *Baraitha* (or *Boraitha*), traditions and opinions of Tannaim not embodied in the Mishnah as compiled by R. Judah han-Nasi. [A collection of such Baraithas is found in the Tosefta (תוספתא) which bears the nearest resemblance to the Mishnah and is called by that name in Talm. Y.—The B. in frequently called מתניתא (Ch.) in contrad. to משנה (Hebr.), v. Num. R. s. 18 (ref. to Cant. VI, 8); Lev. R. s. 30.]—Sabb. 19ᵇ; Erub. 19ᵇ; a. e. ב׳ לא שמיע׳ ליה (cmp. Sabb. 61ª; Pes. 101ᵇ מתנית׳ לא וכ׳) he did not know that Boraitha. Ber. 19ª; a. fr.

בָּרָאִי m. (v. preced.) = אַבְרָאִי *outside*. Ab. Zar. 28ª מכה דב׳ an external wound.—(Adv.) Zeb. 15ª דקאי זר ב׳ the layman stands outside. Ib. לב׳ נפיק וכ׳ does (the blood) run only outside (away from the altar) and not also inside (in all directions)?

בְּרֵאשִׁית (b. h.) *in the beginning*, as a cosmological term (ref. to Gen. I, 1) *creation, primeval period, Nature, Universe*. Targ. Is. XXVIII, 29; a. e.—מִבְּ׳ *from the beginning*. Ib. XLI, 4.—מעשה ב׳ a) *creation*. Gen. R. s. 3; a. fr.—b) *cosmogony*, contrad. to מעשה מרכבה theosophy. Ḥag. II, 1; a. fr.—Y. Shebi. I, beg. 33ª שבת ב׳ the Sabbath commemorative of creation, i. e. the regular weekly Sabbath, contrad. to Holy Days. [In later Hebr. שבת ב׳ the Sabbath on which the first section of the Pentateuch is read.]—Ber. IX, 2 ברוך עושה (מעשה) ב׳ praised be the Author of creation—a formula of benediction for awe-inspiring natural phenomena; v. ib. a. Y. ib. 13ᶜ bot.—ששת ימי ב׳ from the six days of creation. Keth. 8ᵇ נתיב חוא מש׳ וכ׳ this is the way (the lot of humanity) since the world existed.—Tosef. Maasr. III, 14: a. fr.—Y. Taan. II, 65ª bot. מי ב׳; Lam. R. to III, 40 מימי ב׳ primeval waters, *Ocean* &c. (v. Gen. I, 9 sq.).—ספר ב׳ *The Book of Genesis*. Gen. R. s. 3; a. e.—ב׳ רבה *B'reshith Rabbah* (Gen. R.), name of the first book of the Midrash Rabbah.

ברבוי, v. בַּרְבְּרִי.

בַּרְבּוּרִים, v. בַּרְבְּרָא.

בְּרַבִּי, בְּרִיבִּי m. (contr. of בי רבי, *belonging to a school of an eminent teacher*, v. בֵּי 4) *B'rabbi, B'ribbi*, title of scholars, most frequently applied to disciples of R. Judah han-Nasi and his contemporaries, but also to some of his predecessors, and sometimes to the first Amoraim, v. אֲמוֹרָא. B. Mets. 85ª אסמכיה ב׳ he gave him the title of B'rabbi (a scholar of Rabbi Judah). Ḥull. 137ª דברי ברי׳ (ref. to R. Yosé). Ib. 11ᵇ ברבי; Macc. 5ᵇ בריבי (v. Rabb. D. S. a. l. note 100). Sabb. 115ª רבן גמליאל ברי׳ (Tosef. ib. XIII (XIV), 2; Mass. Sofrim V, 15 only ר׳ גמ׳) R. Gaml. son of R. Judah han-Nasi. Erub. 58ª רבי אושעיא ברי׳ (Ms. M. ברב׳, v. Rabb. D. S. a. l. notes 70; 80) R. O. scholar of Rabbi Jud. han-N.—Sifré Deut. 1, end יהודה ברב׳ (Yalk. ib. 792 only יהודה). Y. M. Kat. III, 82ᶜ bot.; Gen. R. s. 100 חד בר׳ אמר a student (Amora) recited &c. Y. Sot. VIII, end, 23ª לית רבי ב׳ [insert או] not even a teacher or a student was exempt. [Snh. 17ᵇ רמי בר ברבי, read ברוכי.]

***בַּרְבֵּיי** m. (abbr. of בַּר בֵּית) *intimate, familiar*. Cant. R. to V, 15; Lev. R. s. 25 אזיל ומתעביד ב׳ (Cant. R. ברבוי, some ed.) he grows to be like an inmate of the house.

ברבר, v. בַּר *son*, a. בַּרְבְּרִי.

בַּרְבְּרָאָה = בַּרְבְּרִי. *Pl.* בַּרְבְּרָאֵי. Targ. Ps. CXIV, 1.

בַּרְבְּרוֹן (βαρβάρων, gen. pl. of βάρβαρος) *of the barbarians*. Lam. R. introd. (R. Josh. 2) נקיטא ב׳ (read ניקיטא, νικῆτα βαρβάρων) O conqueror of the Barbarians (Jews). Y. B. Mets. II, 8ᶜ, v. בַּרְבְּרִי.

בַּרְבַּר, בַּרְבְּרִי m. (βάρβαρος, babbler, Curt. Griech. Etym. p. 290) 1) *foreigner* (in a contemptuous sense), *barbarian*. Esth. R. to II, 21 חב׳ חוה this barbarian (Mordecai, contrad. to Cœlesyrians as Greeks); Targ. Esth. ib. בכרין.—*Pl.* בַּרְבְּרִים, בַּרְבְּרִיִּים. Ex. R. s. 20. Lev. R. s. 11; a. fr.—2) *an inhabitant of Barbaria* (v. בַּרְבַּרְיָא). Gen.

R. s. 60 beg. כושי אחד או ב׳ אחד a Cushite or a Barbar; Cant. R. to II, 8 (for כותי read: כושי). Y. Succ. V, 55[b] top, v. next w.

בַּרְבְּרֵי ch. same. *Pl.* בַּרְבְּרַיָּיא, בַּרְבְּרִיין. Lam. R. to I, 16; IV, 19; Esth. R. introd. עד דאת מכבש ב׳ וכ׳ instead of subjecting the Barbarians (Germans, Britains &c.); Y. Succ. V, 55[b] top (Hebr. diction).—Lev. R. s. 22 נקיטה ב׳, v. בַּרְבְּרוֹן.

בַּרְבַּרְיָא, בַּרְבַּרְיָה, בַּרְבַּרְיָיא, בַּרְבָּרִיאָה f. (barbaria) *foreign* (not Roman) *country*, esp. 1) *Germania Barbara; also Britannia* (as hostile to Rome); 2) *East African coast, Azania*, v. בַּרְבְּרִי. Targ. Y. II Gen. X, 3; Targ. I Chr. I, 6 (for תוגרמה), v. גרמניקיא.—Yeb. 63[b] אנשי ב׳ . . . מרטניא Ar. (ed. מרטנאי, corr. acc.); Sifré Deut. 320 מב׳ ומטונס וממורטניא . . .; Yalk. ib. 945 מב׳ ומבריטניא those from Barbaria [,Tunes] and Mauretania [Britannia] who go naked &c. (v. Brüll, Trachten d. Jud. p. 4 sq.). Cant. R. to II, 8 אחד מכם גולה לב׳ . . . לסמרטיה (Yalk. ib. 586 . . . . לבריטניא) one of you is exiled to B., another to Sarmatia [Britannia]. Midr. Till. to Ps. CIX.—Y. Shek. VI, 50[a] top; Gen. R. s. 23, end כיפי ב׳ the rocks of B. (Azania).—Ib. s. 75 בני ב׳ ובני גרמניא.—Ex. R. s. 18 a king שהלך בנו לב׳ whose son went to a foreign land (conquered province). Koh. R. to II, 7 (ref. to *barburim* I Kings V, 3) a bird &c. היה בא מב׳ וכ׳ came from B. every day. [Ib.; Pesik. R. s. 16; Pesik. Eth. Korb. p. 58[b], מיני ב׳, read with Ar. s. v. ברבר: בַּרְבָּרְיָא.]

ברברית, Y. M. Kat. III, 81[d] bot. תונן בב׳, prob. to be read בְּפַרְדֵּיסָא; cmp. Bab. ib. 17[a].

בַּרְגַּזָא, בַּרְגַּוָא, v. גַּזָא.

בָּרָד m. (b. h.; √בר, v. ברר) [*bright, white,*] *hail* (v. Ges. H. Dict. s. v.). Mikv. VII, 1; a. fr.—אבן הב׳ block of *ice* (or hail stone). Ib.; v. next w.

בַּרְדָּא I ch. same. Targ. Ex. IX, 18; a. fr.—M. Kat. 25[b] כיפי דב׳ hail stones. Ber. 18[b]; v. גְּזִיזָא.

בַּרְדָּא II (cmp. preced. a. אֲשְׁלַג) *barda*, a cosmetic lotion used as a detergent, a mixture of aloes, myrtle and violet. Sabb. 50[b] (Ms. M., once, a. Ar. בר אדא, Alf. Ms. a. oth. בדרא; v. Rabb. D. S. a. l. note)

בַּרְדָּא III m. (v. preced.) *barda*, name of an unclean bird. Hull. 62[b] (Ar. בר אדא).

בַּרְדִּילָא, v. בּוּרְדְּלָא.

ברדין, Tosef. Kel. B. Mets. X, end (ed. Zuck. גרדין), read פַּרְדּוֹן.

ברדנין, ברדינין, Ex. R. s. 38, end, read פַּרְפְּדוֹן.

בַּרְדִּיסִין, v. בַּרְדְּסִין.

בַּרְדְּלָא m. (cmp. b. h. דְּלָיָהוּ, דְּלָיָה) *Bard'la*, surname of several persons. B. Mets. 10[b] אבא כהן ב׳ (Var. כהנא; Ms. M. בר דלא); Gen. R. s. 76, end; Y. Gitt. VIII, 49[c] top; (Y. Peah IV, 18[a] bot. בר דליא).—Succ. 26[a] (Ms. M. 2 בר דלא, v. Rabb. D. S. a. l. note); Gitt. 14[a] רב אחא ב׳. V. בַּרְדְּלָיָא.

ברדלה, v. בַּרְדְּלִיס.

בַּרְדְּלַיָא, בַּרְדְּלַיְיה, בַּרְדְּלָיָה (cmp. ברדלא) pr. n. pl. *Bard'laya*, near Lydda (v. infra). Y. Erub. VI, 24[a] top אנשי בר דליה the inhabitants of B. Y. Shebi. II, 33[d] bot. דברדלייה of B. Y. Peah III, 17[d] bot. R. Jud. b. Pazi דבר דליא (for which Y. Meg. I, 71[a] דברזילה); cmp. Y. Snh. I, 18[c] bot. where R. Jud. b. P. is mentioned as of Lydda. [Num. R. s. 13 ברדליא, some ed., v. בּוּרְדְּלָא.]

בַּרְדְּלִיס, בַּרְדְּלָס m. (πάρδαλις, pardalis; πάρδος, pardus; prob. of Semit. orig.; cmp. b. h. בְּרֻדִּים) *a spotted beast*, whence 1) (v. Sm. Ant. s. vv.) *leopard* or *hyena*, usu. in connection with נָמֵר. Snh. I, 4. B. Kam. I, 4 (expl. ib. 16[a] אַפָּא q. v.). Bekh. 8[a]. B. Mets. VII, 9.—2) (prob.) *marten*, or *mariput* (Rashi: *putois*); usu. in connection with חוּלְדָּה. Pes. 9[b]; Nidd. 15[b]; Ab. Zar. 42[a]; Tosef. Ohol. XVI, 13 ed. Zuck. ברדלה.

ברדניקוס, v. הדרניקוס.

ברדס, v. בּוּרְדָּס.

בַּרְדְּסִין, בּוּרְדְּסִין (. . . סים) m. pl. (a corrupt. of Brundusina, v. בלדרסין) *Brundisian cloaks*, thicker than בִּרְסִין q. v. Kil. IX, 7. Y. ib. 32[d] top בַּרְדִּיסִין. Tosef. Kel. B. Bath. V, 11 ברתסין ed. Zuck. (Var. ברתצין, ברתתצ׳). V. פַּלְדִּיסִין, פַּלְדִּיס.

***בַּרְדֵּק** (Parel of בדק, cmp. הרזק) *to penetrate, go from end to end; to bolt.* Targ. Y. II Ex. XXXVI, 33 לְבַרְדּוּק (h. text לִבְרֹחַ).

בָּרָה 1) fem. of בַּר.—2) v. ברי.

בְּרָוֹן, v. בִּירְוֹן.

ברובה, Y. Hall. I, 57[c], read כְּרוּבָא.

***ברוזא**, read בְּרְזוּזָא m. (בּרז) *perforation.* Targ. Y. Num. XXV, 8 באתר ב׳ in the place of perforation (hole).

ברויירא, Koh. R. to III, 14 שמלאי דב׳., v. בִּיר, בִּירָא 3).

***בֵּי ב׳ בָּרוּךְ** m. (בֵּי, ברך, v. בֵּי) *the neck* of an animal, so named from the benediction (בָּרוּךְ) which precedes the ritual slaughtering.

בְּרוֹכִי pr. n. m. *B'rokhi.* Snh. 17[b] רמי בר ב׳ Ms. M., Ar. a. oth. (ed. ברבי, corr. acc.).

ברולקי, v. בורוקלי.

בְּרָן, v. בִּירְוֹן.

בְּרוּנָא I m. (dimin. of בְּרָא; cmp. אֲבוּנָא) *dear little son, darling.* Pesik. B'shall. p. 83[a] (allud. to termination ני in Rubeni &c.) כאינש דאמר בְּרוּנִי סברוני סביוני as if one says, My own dear son, my features, my looks; Yalk. Num 773; Cant. R. to IV, 12 (corr. acc.); [Ar. s. v. ברן, adds מאבוי from his father (has he this).]

בְּרוּנָא I pr. n. m. *B'runa*, a Babyl. Amora. Ber. 9[b]; a. fr.

בְּרוֹקָא I f. *smaragd*, v. בַּרְקָן.

בְּרוֹקָא II, **בְּרוֹקָה** pr. n. m. *Baroka*, father of R. Johanan. Ab. IV, 4. Erub. VIII, 2; a. v. fr.

בְּרוֹקָא III, **בְּרוֹקָה** m. *morning star*, v. בְּרַק a. בְּרַק. Y. Yoma III, beg. 40b; Y. R. Hash. I, beg. 57d.

***בְּרוּקְלֵי** m. pl. (v. אַמְבּוּרְקְלוֹן) *wrapper, cover*. Midr. Sam. XXII; Yalk. ib. 129 (expl. תרפים as if טרפים, v. טְרַף) ניקורים של ב׳ shreds of (horse) covers (corrupt. בדולקי, Mus. ברולקי).

בְּרוּקְתִּי, v. בַּרְקְתִּי.

בָּרוּר m. (ברר) 1) *clear, bright; certain, firm*. B. Bath. 147a יו״ט ... ב׳ וכ׳ when the day of Pentecosts is bright, sow wheat; opp. בָּלוּל; Tosef. Arakh. I, 9.—Snh. 7b אם ב׳ וכ׳ if the case is as clear to thee as the morning, speak out (thy opinion). Gitt. 89a דבר הב׳ an ascertained fact.—Pes. 50a עולם ב׳ a rightly-conducted world, opp. הפוך.—Y. Ber. II, 5a יחזור ..... הב׳ לו he must begin to re-read from the place which he is certain of having read correctly. Y. Maasr. I, 49b תבשיל חלוט ב׳, v. חָלַט I; ב׳ real boiling (about which there is no legal doubt). Y. Yeb. IV, 5c bot. חלב ב׳ ascertained existence of forbidden fat. Y. Gitt. IX, 50c bot. קיים שריר וב׳ (the formula) valid, firm and established. Y. Kidd. IV, 66a top כהן ב׳ a priest of undoubted genealogy; a. fr.—2) (b. h. בָּרָר, Neh. V, 18) *chosen, best*. Gen. R. s. 23 הב׳ שבהם the best one among them.—*Pl.* בְּרוּרִים, בְּרוּרִין. Y. Kidd. IV, 66a bot. הב׳ שבאחיך the chosen among thy brethren (whose genealogy has been established; v. supra); Num. R. s. 9.

בֵּרוּר, pl. בֵּרוּרִין, constr. בֵּרוּרֵי, v. בֵּירוּר.

בְּרוֹר חַיִל, **ב׳ חַיִל** or **ב׳ חַיִל** pr. n. pl. *B'ror Ḥayil* (*Hail*), seat of R. Johanan b. Zaccai's college, near Jabneh. Snh. 32b (Var. גדור ח׳). Y. Keth. I, 25c; a. fr.

בְּרוּרְיָה, **בְּרוּרְיָא** pr. n. f. *B'ruryah*, daughter of R. Hanania b. T'radjon and wife of R. Meïr, reputed as a learned woman. Ab. Zar. 18a. Ib.b משום מעשה ב׳ Ms. M. (ed. מ׳ דב׳) (R. Meïr left for Babylon) in consequence of what occurred to B. (who defied her husband's opinion regarding woman's weakness and came very near being ensnared by a plot laid against her chastity; v. Rashi a. l.). Tosef. Kel. B. Mets. I, 6.

בְּרוֹשׁ f. (b. h.) *cypress*. R. Hash. 23a; Taan. 25b, a. e. (as a species of cedar); v. בְּרוֹת a. בְּרָתָא.

ברושיתא, Gitt. 69b ב׳ דשיערי, v. פְּרוּשְׁיָיתָא.

בְּרוֹת f.=בְּרוֹשׁ. Sifra Metsora, beg. שהוא של ב׳ that it (עץ ארז, Lev. XIV, 49) means a branch of a cypress; Y. Sot. II, 18a top שלברות (corr. acc.); Tosef. Neg. VIII, 2 של אברית ed. Zuck. (Var. שלא ברית; R. S. to Neg. XIV, 1 אַבְרוֹת).

בְּרוֹתָא ch. same, v. בְּרָתָא.

בְּרוּתָא f. (v. בַּר I ch.) *outside, rejected*; cmp. בָּרַיְיתָא. B. Mets. 9a; a. fr. Ar. (ed. sometimes בְּרוּתָא q. v.).

בְּרַז, **בְּרֵיז**, **בְּרַז** (√בר, v. ברר) [*to get through*,] *to bore, perforate, transfix*. Targ. Y. Num. XXV, 8; a. e. [Targ. Y. Gen. XLIV, 34 דתברז, read דתירון or דתתרן as Targ. Esth. VIII, 6, v. ארע a. ערע.]—Snh. 52b דבריז ליה מיברז that one may put a culprit to death by piercing. Sabb. 146a, v. בּוּרְטְיָא. Snh. 56a; a. fr.

**Af.* אַבְרֵיז *to sting*. Gitt. 84a אי בעי מבריז וכ׳ if he chooses, he may sting himself with thorns and he will not fall asleep (Ar. מחריז, v. חֲרַז).

בְּרָזָא I m. (preced.) *bung-hole, bung*. Ab. Zar. 59b דארישתקיל ברזיה Ms. M. (ed. דארישתקיל לברזא) whose bung was taken out. Ib. כל דלהדי ב׳ all the wine facing the bung-hole (the first gush of wine). Ib. 60a עד דב׳ Ms. M. (ed. הב׳, Rashi ב׳) to a level with &c., i. e. the wine above the bung-hole. Sabb. 139b. B. Bath. 98a שני בב׳ (Ms. H. בברזה) changed the bung-hole (or the bung).

בְּרָזָא II or **בִּרְזָא** m. (בזא II; v. אַבְרְזִין) *cut* (*leather*), *strap; horse-line*. Hag. 9b כי ב׳ סומקא וכ׳ as a red line for a white horse (Ms. M. כוּרְדָא). [Ber. 59a דברזא, read דברדא, v. גְּזִיזָא.]—*Pl.* בְּרָזֵי. Sabb. 117a שקיל ליה בב׳ he stripped the hide strap-wise. Cmp. בִּיזְלֵי.

בְּרַזַג (denom. of בר זוג) *to couple, join* (cmp. איתברנש Syr., P. Sm. 582). Targ. Y. I Deut. XXXII, 4 מכרוג, read מְבַרְזַג (Y. II זְוּוּג). Ib. XXXIV, 6 (Var. למזווגא). Targ. Ps. LXVIII, 7 לבר זוגא (read לְבַרְזוּגָן).

ברזות, v. בִּרְזַיִת.

בַּרְזִיל, v. בַּזֵּל.

ברזולא, v. פַּרְזְלָא.

***בַּרְזִילָה** pr. n. pl. *Barzilah*, v. בַּרְזְלָיָה.

בַּרְזִינָא m. (v. בְּרַז a. בְּרָזָא I) *a tap, sample of wine*, whence *barzina*, a liquid measure, one thirty-second of a Log (Ar.). Sabb. 109b ב׳ לזיבורא a barzina (of urin) is a remedy for a hornet's sting.

בִּרְזַיִת (ברזות b. h.) pr. n. m. *Birzayith* (I Chr. VII, 31). Gen. R. s. 71 end (expl.=בּיר זַיִת).

בַּרְזִיתָא f. (ברז) *spit*, v. בּוּרְטְיָא.

בַּרְזֶל m. (b. h.; ברז) *iron, iron tool*. Gen. R. s. 75 לובשי ב׳ clad in iron armor; a. fr.—צאן ב׳ *flock sold on payment in terms* under the condition that the young be divided until the payment in full has taken place. Bekh. II, 4; v. וָלָד.—ב׳ (נכסי) עבדי צאן *mort-main*, wife's estate held by her husband, which, in case of her death or divorce, he must restore *in specie*, being responsible whith all his landed property for loss or deterioration. Yeb. VII, 1; a. fr.; v. נְכָסִים.

בַּרְזְלָא, **בַּרְזֶל** ch. same. Targ. I Kings XXII, 12; a. e.—Sabb. 66b קול ב׳ (Ms. M. קל פ׳). V. פַּרְזְלָא.

בַּרְזָנִיתָא f. (ברז) *boring, tapping.* B. Mets. 40ᵇ טרחיה ודמי בַּרְזָנִיתֵיה Ar. (ed. בַּרְזַנְיְיתָא pl.; v. Rabb. D. S. a. l. note 30) his (the seller's) trouble and the value of his tapping (the sample; v. בַּרְזִינָא). [Var. in Rashi כרוז׳ his calling out, offering for sale, v. כְּרַז.]

בְּרַח (b. h.; √בר, v. ברר) 1) *to break through, pass through* (Ex. XXXVI, 33). Denom. בְּרִיחַ.—2) *to flee.* Erub. 13ᵇ הבּוֹרֵחַ מן הגדולה he who flees office. Y. Yeb. XIII, 13ᶜ, a. e. בְּרַח מן ג׳ וכ׳ shun three things. Y. Taan. IV, 69ᵇ top, v. בָּקַע; a. fr.

Hif. הִבְרִיחַ 1) *to cause to flee, drive out, exclude.* Y. Yeb. XV, 15ᵃ top לְהַבְרִיחוֹ מנכסיו to force him to flee and abandon his property. Y. Gitt. V, 47ᵃ אדם מַבְרִיחַ עצמו מן חשבועה one will try to shirk the responsibilities of a guardian on account of the oath (which the court asks of him) but one will not do so on account of payment (to which he may eventually be subjected, v. Tosaf. to B. Kam. 39ᵇ).—2) *to abstract, steal, defraud.* B. Kam. 113ᵃ ה׳ את המכס to smuggle. Y. Keth. VI, beg. 30ᶜ שלא תהא מַבְרַחַת משל וכ׳ that she should not take stealthily something which belongs to her husband.

Hof. הוּבְרַח *to be chased, scattered.* Lam. R. to I, 21 הוּבְרְחוּ ענני וכ׳ the clouds of glory were withdrawn (R. Hash. 3ᵃ נסתלקו).

בְּרַח ch. same. *Af.* אַבְרַח as preced. Hif., *to withhold.* B. Kam. 88ᵇ לאברוחינהו לנכסיה מניה in order to withhold his property from &c., i. e. to disinherit.

Ithpe. אִתְבְּרַח *to be driven off, withheld.* Targ. Job VI, 13 (h. text נדחה).

בַּרְחָא m. (ברח, v. בְּרַח 1)) [*one that breaks through,* cmp. Mic. II, 13;] *leader of the flock* (h. עַתּוּד), *bell-wether, buck.* Y. B. Kam. X, end, 7ᶜ if the restored sheep is as distinguishable כגון אחן ב׳ as the barḥa. Ib. what does כגון אחן ב׳ mean? Some say חוטרא &c., v. קַנְהוּרָא a. מַשְׁפּוֹכִית. Bab. ib. 20ᵃ top. Ib. 48ᵃ. Sabb. 18ᵇ. Ib. 152ᵃ ב׳ קרחא a bald buck (sneer at R. Joshua b. Karḥa; v. גַּוְזְנָא).

ברטיא*, Pesik. R. s. 33 חב׳, read חַבְרְבַרְיָא; Alexandria שחיתה אוֹמַנְתּוֹ של כל העולם חב׳ חזה which became the educator of all this world of Barbaria (northern Africa).

בְּרַטְנְיָא, v. בְּרִיטַנְיָא.

בֵּי בִ׳, בֵּרִי, v. בֵּירָאר 2).

ברי I, בָּרָא (b. h.; √בר, v. ברר) 1) *to hollow out, perforate,* v. Hif. a. בָּרַח.—2) *to think out, plan* (cmp. חָקַק, בָּרָא); *to create.* Snh. 38ᵇ when the Lord wanted לִבְראות את וכ׳ ... ואח״כ שב׳ to create man. Gen. R. s. 8 בְּרָאוֹ for He first created all the means of his support and then created him (Adam); a. v. fr.—Part. act. בּוֹרֵא q. v.—Part. pass. בָּרוּא, f. בְּרוּאָה. Gen. R. s. 44 (ref. to Is. IV, 5 וּבָרָא) ככר היא ב׳ וכ׳ it (the futurity) is already created and prepared.

Nif. נִבְרָא *to be created.* Ib. s. 8 אל יִבָּרֵא let him not be created. Snh. 38ᵃ; a. v. fr.

Hif. הִבְרִיא 1) (denom. of בַּר) *to come outside, bore, perforate.* Ḥull. 43ᵇ שמא ה׳ lest it (the thorn found in the throat) may have perforated (the gullet); v. infra.—2) (denom. of בָּרִיא) *to get well, recover; to be strong* or *stout* (fat). Meïl. 17ᵃ יכחיש או יַבְרִיא does he wish him to be lean (feeble) or to be strong?—Y. Peah III, 17ᵈ bot. שמא יבריא for he may get well again. Ḥull. 33ᵃ הרוצה שיַבְ׳ he who wants to be strong. Sabb. XIX, 5; a. fr. [Ḥull. 43ᵇ שמא ה׳ lest the wound created by perforation be healed, Rashi; v. supra.]

בְּרָא, ברי ch. same; 1) *to create.* Targ. Gen. I, 1; a. fr. [Targ. Prov. XX, 12 אלהא אברי, prob. to be read אלהא ברא as ib. XXII, 2.]—Snh. 65ᵇ ברו עלמא they might create a world. Ib. 67 לא מצי ברי he (the demon) cannot create. [Ib. ומיברו, ומיברי, v. Ithpe.]—2) (v. preced. Hif.) *to get well, strong* &c. Ḥull. 93ᵇ מדלא קא בָּרְיִין since they do not grow (develop). Ib. 46ᵇ הדרא בָּרְיָא gets well again. [Taan. 21ᵇ זיל בריא, v. Af.]—3) *to cut, shape.* Targ. Is. XL, 20.—*4) (v. בַּר I ch., a. בָּרָאָה; cmp. זָהַם Pi. 2) *to expel, exile.* Targ. Prov. XXIV, 24 (h. text זעם).

Af. אַבְרִי 1) *to strengthen, make well, make grow.* Targ. II Sam. III, 35 (Var. לְאוֹכָלָא, v. חַבְרָאָה). Succ. 44ᵇ; M. Kat. 3ᵃ אַבְרוּיֵי אילני to make the trees stronger (facilitate their growth); Ab. Zar. 50ᵇ אברויי וכ׳, opp. איקומי to preserve the trees. Nidd. 47ᵇ; Yeb. 97ᵃ אַבְרְיוּהוּ make him grow fat (feed him well). Taan. 21ᵇ זיל אַבְרִי נפשך (ed. בריא, v. Rabb. D. S. a. l.) go and strengthen thyself.—2) *to permeate, perforate.* Ḥull. 112ᵃ דאבריה (the blood) soaked through the bread. Ib. 93ᵇ דין ביה מידי דמברי ליה Ar. (ed. only דין ביה מידי) if he stuck something into it which perforated it (making a passage for the blood).

Ithpe. אִתְבְּרִיא, אִיתְבְּרֵי, contr. אִיבְּרֵי. 1) *to be created.* Targ. Gen. II, 4; a. fr.—Gen. R. s. 78 מן חן דאתברייה (to) where they were created from. Cant. R. to VIII, 5 וכדון אִתְבְּרֵיית וכ׳ now thou hast been created again a new creature (having escaped a great danger).—Ber. 54ᵇ איברי ליה וכ׳ a well was created (arose) before him. Snh. 65ᵇ; 67ᵇ וּמִיבְּרֵי לחו וכ׳ (not ומיברו, Yalk. Ms. איברי, v. Rabb. D. S. a. l. note 4) and a three years' calf was created (arose) before them (Yalk. Ex. 182 וּמִבְרֵי they created).—2) *to become strong.* Y. Snh. VIII, 26ᶜ מכיון דאִבְּרֵי ליביה עלוי וכ׳ since his heart (passion) became so strong over him as to do this (or דאַבְרֵי Af. he allowed his passion to become so strong &c.).—3) (v. בַּר I, בָּרָא) *to grow wild.* Nidd. 50ᵇ (explain. the expression תרנגול ברא used by a scholar) דאיבראי ממרה (=שמרדה) that became too wild (uncontrollable) to her owner.

ברי II, בָּרָה (b. h.) *to cut out* (v. בָּרָא). Part. pass. בָּרוּי, fem. בְּרוּיָה *hollowed out.* Tosef. Kel. B. Kam. III, 3, v. חִידּוּק a. בָּרָה.

Hif. הִבְרָה (b. h.; denom. of בְּרִי, v. ברי I Hif.) *to strengthen, to offer refreshment,* esp. to mourners on coming from the funeral. M. Kat. III, 7 ואין מַבְרִין and no mourner's meal is offered (during the festive week). Snh. II, 3. Ib. 20ᵃ, v. בָּרָה; a. fr. V. הַבְרָאָה. [Y. Sabb. VII, 10ᵃ top חמברה בחרשים read חַמְבְחֵה, v. בחר h.]

בָּרִיא, בְּרִי m. (b. h.; v. בָּרָא) 1) *in natural condition,* whence 1) (cmp. אֵיתָן) *healthy, strong, stout, fat.* B. Bath.

147[b] sq. (opp. sick). Y. Naz. VI, 55[b] top (opp. חש, of tender build); a. fr.—2) *sound, sure, evident.* Y. Succ. I, 52[b] top; Y. Pes. II, 29[b] bot. דבר ב׳ שלא וכ׳ it is sure that he did not &c.—ב׳ לי I am sure. Ḥull. 10[a]; a. fr.—ב׳ ושמא 'sure' and 'perhaps', the plea of two litigants, one asserting a certainty, the other pleading ignorance or offering a possible alternative. Keth. 12[b]; B. Mets. 37[b]; a. fr.—3) *sound, firm.* Cant. R. to III, 4 honey ב׳ כאבן as solid as a stone; a. fr.—*Pl.* בְּרִיאִים. Lev. R. s. 17 ב׳ כמשפחה כאולם as sound as the Temple hall.—Ḥull. 84[a] ב׳ of a healthy, stout family; a. fr.—Fem. בְּרִיאָה. Kidd. 71[b] בבל ב׳ Babylon is sound (as to purity of descent). Erub. 62[a] שכירות ב׳ a sound (legitimate) lease, opp. רעועה rickety; a. fr.—Y. Erub. I, 19[a] בְּרִיָּה a strong, solid rafter.—*Pl.* בְּרִיאוֹת, בְּרִיּוֹת. Ib. top ברויות ed. Krot. (corr. acc.).

בְּרִי, בְּרִיא ch. same. Targ. Koh. X, 6.—Taan. 29[b] דב׳ מזליה when his (the Israelite's) luck is good, opp. ריע מ׳ bad luck.—Yoma 57[a] top השתא ברי וכ׳ now it is sure ye are unclean (rejected by the Lord).—*Pl.* בְּרִיֵּי. Keth. 60[b] sq. בני ב׳ strong children.—Fem. בְּרִיָּא, בְּרִיָּא. Targ. Y. Ex. IV, 7.

בָּרְיָא *Creator*, v. בָּרְיָיא.

בְּרִיָּה, בְּרִיאָה (b. h.) f. (ברא) *creation, formation.* Gen. R. s. 1; Lev. R. s. 36 לב׳ שמים וכ׳ as to creation (plan), the heavens were the first; as to finishing (execution) &c. Gen. R. s. 7, end בְּרִיָּיתוֹ של עולם the creation of the world. Ib. s. 17 man looks למקום ברייתו to where he was created from (the earth), woman … למקום בְּרִיָּיתָהּ to where she was made from (the rib); a. fr.—Mikv. VI, 7 כל שהוא מִבְּרִיַּית חמיים whatever originates in the water (aquatic plants or animals).—Macc. 17[a], a. fr. חיטה אחת כברייתה one wheat grain in its natural condition, נמלה כברייתה an ant in its natural condition (though small). Ib. בריית נשמה the natural condition of an animated being.—Nidd. III, 7 בריית חזכר the formation of a male embryo. B. Kam. 94[b] חוזר לברייתו is changed into its original condition.

בְּרִיּוּת, בְּרִיאוּת f. (בְּרִי) *health, strength, fleshiness.* Esth. R. to I, 3.

בְּרִיּוּתָא, בְּרִיוּתָא, בְּרִיאוּתָא ch. same. Nidd. 47[b] מחמת בריאותָהּ (or read תא . . .) on account of (his) obesity. Bekh. 45[b] ב׳ אתחלא וכ׳ it is (unusual) strength which happened to rest in the left hand (and left-handedness is therefore no defect), opp. כחישותא weakness.

בְּרִיבֵּי, v. בְּרַבֵּי.

בְּרִיָּה, בִּירְיָא, בִּירְיָה, בִּרְיָה f. (ברא) *creature; human being;* (freq. masc.) *man.* Tosef. Kil. I, 9 ברריא. Ber. 17[a]; a. fr.—*Pl.* בְּרִיּוֹת. Ḥull. 127[a] ב׳ גְּדֹלוֹת בים creatures living in the Sea.—חַב׳ (often m.) *people, mankind.* Yoma 86[a]; a. fr.

בְּרָיָה, v. בָּרָאָה.

***בריה**, Y. Kil. IX, 32[d] top, v. בִּירְיָא II.

בִּירְיוֹן, בִּרְיוֹן m. (denom. of בִּירָה) *palace-soldier, castle-guard, keeper.* Ex. R. s. 30 משל לב׳ וכ׳ this is to be compared to a palace-soldier who was drunk &c.; Yalk. Esth. 1056 ללבריון (read לב׳).—*Pl.* בִּרְיוֹנִים, בִּיר׳. Ex. R. l. c. ב׳ שלו וכ׳ his palace-guard sneered at his purple cloak.—בִּרְיוֹנוֹת. Mekh. B'shall., Amalek 1, העמידו עליו ב׳ קשים they appointed over him cruel guards; Tanḥ. ib. 25 עמדו עליו ברוונים וכ׳ (read העמידו); Y. Kidd. I, 61[a] bot. בורניות (corr. acc.). Cmp. בִּירָנִית.

בִּרְיוֹנָא, בִּירְיוֹנָא m. (v. בְּרָא Ithpe. 3, cmp. בְּרִיוּתָא) *rebel, outlaw, highway-man.*—*Pl.* בִּרְיוֹנֵי, בִּר׳. Gitt. 56[a] הנהו ב׳ those rebels (the war party during the last siege of Jerusalem by the Romans). Ib. Abba Sikra ריש ב׳ chief of the rebels.—Ber. 10[a] הנהו ב׳ דהוו וכ׳ there were some highway-men living in the neighborhood of &c. Taan. 23[b] א״נ הנהו בר׳ וכ׳ ed. (omitted in Ms. M. a. oth.). Ib. 24[a] חנך ב׳ Ms. M. (ed. בני מאתיה, v. Rabb. D. S. l. note 2). Snh. 37[a] בְּרִיוֹ׳; a. fr.

בְּרִיּוּת *health*, v. בְּרִיאוּת; בְּרִיוּתָא, v. בְּרִיאוּתָא.

בְּרִיוּתָא f. (v. בִּרְיוֹנָא) *rebellion, defiance of the law.* Sot. 19[b]; 20[a] מחמת ב׳ (refusal to drink the searching water) in defiance, opp. בִרעתותא, רתתא. *[Targ. Prov. XXV, 20, prob. to be read בְּרִיחוּתָא; ed. Lag. בְּרִיוּתָא. The entire verse is a corrupt combination of two versions.]

בְּרִיז, v. בְּרֵז.

בְּרֵיז m. (ברז) *channel, stream.* Targ. I Sam. XIV, 26 (h. text חלך).

בְּרִיחַ m. (b. h.; ברח) *bolt.*—*Pl.* בְּרִיחִים, בְּרִיחִין. Ex. R. s. 52; Yalk. ib. 417.

בְּרִיחָה f. (ברח) *flight.* Gen. R. s. 74; a. e.

בריחי, Sabb. 21[a]; 145[b] *sick persons*, v. בְּרִיחָא.

בְּרִיטַנְיָא pr. n. *Britannia, Great Britain.* Yalk. Deut. 945. Ib. Cant. 586, v. בַּרְבָּרְיָא.

בּוֹרְיָא, בָּרְיָיא m. ch.=h. בּוֹרֵא, *Creator, God.* Targ. Prov. XVII, 5 בָּרְיֵהּ his Maker; a. e.—Y. Ber. I, 2[d] איקריה דבָרְיי the honor of my Maker. Gen. R. s. 68 מה אנא מובר סברי מן בריי why should I give up my hope in my Creator? Y. Hor. III, beg. 47[a] דמי לְבָרְיִיכוֹן is like that of your Maker, v. הוּגְבָא; Y. Snh. II, 20[c] top לבריידתכון (corr. acc.). Lev. R. s. 15 ובוֹרְיָךְ קאים לך and thy Maker will assist thee; a. fr.

בְּרָיָיא *external*, v. בָּרָאָה.

בְּרִיַּית *creation*, v. בְּרִיאָה.

בְּרִיַּית *creature*, v. בְּרִיָּה.

בְּרָיִית *foreign, strange*, v. בָּרָאָה.

בְּרָיְיתָא, v. בָּרָאָה.

בְּרִיּוֹתָא, pl. בְּרִיּוֹתָה, v. בְּרִיתָא.

בְּרִיכָא *shoot*, v. בִּרְכָּא.

בְּרִיכָה f. (ברך) 1) *bending the knee.* Gen. R. s. 39; Y. Ber. I, 3ᶜ bot. (diff. fr. כריעה). Ib. 3ᵈ top לך ב׳ unto thee bending is due; a. e.—2) (denomin. of בֶּרֶךְ) *knee, young shoot.* Orlah I, 5 if a tree has been dying ובו ב׳ וכ׳ but there is a shoot on it . . . . . : the old stem is again like a young shoot (with ref. to the fruits of the first years, v. עָרְלָה). R. Hash. 15ᵇ; Tosef. Shebi. IV, 20 ed. Zuck. אילן העושה ב׳ אחת (ed. ברך) a tree which shoots only once a year (its fruits growing all at once), opp. שתי בריכות (expl. R. Hash. l. c. כעין שתי ב׳) two crops, i. e. early and late fruits.—3) (from the position of the hatching bird) *brood,* esp. of doves. B. Bath. V, 3; Bets. 10ᵃ ב׳ ראשונה the first brood of the year.—*Pl.* בְּרִיכוֹת. R. Hash. l. c.; Tosef. Shebi. l. c. Yeb. 63ᵃ בְּרִכּוֹת, v. בָּרַךְ Hif.

בְּרֵכָה, בְּרֵיכָה f. (b.h.; ברך) *pond, lake.* Mikv. VI, 11 אחד משלש . . . לב׳ one three hundred and twentieth part of the bathing pond. Gen. R. s. 39 (ref. to בְּרָכָה Gen. XII, 12) קרי ביה ב׳ וכ׳ read *b'rekhah,* a pond, as the pond cleanses the unclean (by immersion) &c.; Num. R. s. 11; a. fr.—*Pl.* בְּרֵיכוֹת, בְּרֵכ׳. Makhsh. II, 3.—Cmp. נִבְרֶכֶת.

***בריכסון**, read בְּרִיכְּסִין (=ἔβρεξεν fr. βρέχω; ἐ rejected) *it rained.* Y. Shebu. III, 34ᵈ bot. if seeing that it has rained, one says קורי פלי ב׳, (κύριε πολὺ ἔβρεξεν) 'By God, it has rained much'—this is a vain oath; Y. Ned. III, 38ᵃ top בלי קורי בריקשון (corr. acc.); Pesik. R. s. 22 כלי קרי אברוכסים (corr. acc., read איברייכסין ἔβρεξεν).

בְּרֵיכְתָא f. ch.=h. בְּרֵיכָה. Targ. Is. XXII, 9; a. e.

***רם ב׳, בָּרִין** pr. n. pl. *Ram Barin,* a border town of Northern Palestine (district of Tyre; perh. *Kefr Bureim,* Neub. Géogr. p. 23). Y. Dem. II, 22ᵈ top; Tosef. Shebi. IV, 10 רמכוך, Var. רומברך. Y. l. c. עד כדון for which R. S. to Dem. II, 1 בּוּרָן (prob. the same).

בָּרִיק, v. בְּרַק.

בריקא, בריקה, v. בורדיקא׳.

בריקשון, v. בריכסון.

בְּרִיר, בָּרִיר, בְּרִירָא m., **בְּרִירָא, בְּרִירָה** f. ch.=h. בָּרוּר 1) *clear, pure, certain; polished, bright.* Targ. Ps. XVIII, 27 (h. text נָבָר). Targ. Y. Ex. XXII, 2 (Var. ברור); a. fr.—*Pl.* בְּרִירִין, בְּרִירָן. Targ. Y. I, II Deut. VIII, 9; a. fr. —2) *chosen, peculiar.* Ibid. XXIX, 12.

בְּרִירָה f. (ברר) *sifting, assorting.* Y. Sabb. VII, 10ᵇ top [read:] כל מה שהותר מכלל ב׳ וכ׳ what is allowed on Holy Days as coming under the category of sifting, is not always allowed . . . on the Sabbath; Y. Bets. I, 60ᵈ (usually משום בורר).

בְּרֵירָה f. (ברר) *choosing, choice,* esp. as a dialectic term, *B'rerah, subsequent selection, retrospective designation,* i. e. the legal effect resulting from an actual selection or disposal of things previously undefined as to their purpose, e. g. a letter of divorce must be written with special intention, for the persons concerned; now, "if one says to a scribe, 'Write for me a letter of divorce for one of my wives whom I may choose to divorce', none of them can be divorced with it" (Gitt. III, 1), upon which the remark is made (ib. 24ᵇ) הא קא משמע לן דאין ב׳ this rule of the Mishnah implies the adoption of the principle that subsequent disposal does not react on the original status of the letter of divorce, so as to say that this subsequent selection is equal to a defined intention at the time when the deed was to be written. [The question of B'rerah, i. e. whether a subsequent disposal has or has not a retrospective legal effect, is widely spread in the Talmud, referring both to judicial as well as to ritual cases.] Yoma 55ᵇ ר׳ . . לית ליה ב׳ R. Judah rejects the principle of B'rerah; Y. Shek. VI, 50ᵇ אי אמרינן ב׳ וכ׳ if we adopt the principle of B., let four Zuz (the value of one offering) be taken out of the bag and thrown into the water, and the balance of the money be permitted for use. Hull. 14ᵇ; a. fr.

בְּרִירוּ, v. בְּרִירוּתָא.

בְּרִירוּת f. (ברר) *clearness, pureness, innocence.* Y. Taan. III, 67ᵃ ב׳ כפיך innocence of thy hands (expl. *bor,* Job XXII, 30).

בְּרִירוּ, בְּרִירוּתָא ch. same. Targ. O. Ex. XXIV, 10 (*brightness,* h. text טהר); a. e.—Targ. Prov. XVI, 15 ed. Lag. (Var. ביריאתא).

***פילי ב׳, בריש**, v. אַרְדָּא II. Gitt. 14ᵇ.

בְּרִית f. (b.h.; בָּרָה; v. בִּירִית) prop. *circle, ring, chain,* hence *oath* (of fidelity), *solemn injunction; covenant treatise.* [כרת ב׳ to cut a ring out; to make a covenant; בא בב׳ to enter into the ring, to promise fidelity; הפר ב׳ to break the ring, to break one's oath &c.] Sabb. 137ᵇ; בריתו של אברהם אבינו (sign of) the covenant of Abraham, *circumcision.* Ab. III, 11; a. fr. Y. Peah VIII, 21ᵃ מפני ב׳ של א״א on account of the covenant of Abraham (for the sake of human dignity). Num. R. s. 18, a. fr. ב׳ כרותה לשפתים a law is made for the lips, i. e. words are ominous (ref. to לא נעלה, Num. XVI, 12). Gen. R. s. 34, v. אָוִיר; a. fr.—חַבְ׳ וכ׳ *by the covenant* (an oath), *indeed.* Tosef. Hall. I, 6 ב׳ וכ׳ (Var. חב׳); Pes. 38ᵇ indeed, those are the very words &c.; (some explain) indeed?, are those the very &c. (is it a tradition for which no reason needs to be given)?; Y. Peah V, 19ᵇ bot. חב׳.—*Pl.* בְּרִיתוֹת. Ber. 48ᵇ sq. שלש ב׳ three covenants (three times the word *b'rith,* Deut. XXVIII, 69; XXIX, 8). Tosef. Sot. VIII, 10; 11 ב׳ Var. (ed. Zuck. כְּרִיתוֹת); Sot. 37ᵇ; a. fr.

בְּרִית *a ring, band,* v. בִּירִית. [Y. M. Kat. I, 80ᵇ top, v. כְּרִית.]

בִּרְיָתָא, בִּרְיָא, בִּי׳ f. ch. 1)=h. בְּרִיָּה *creature.* Targ. Is. XXIX, 16; a. fr. Targ. Ezek. I, 9; 11 בִּרְיָא *each* (h. text איש).—*Pl.* בִּרְיָיתָא, בִּרְיָיאתָא, בִּרְיָ׳. Ib. 13 sq. (h. text חַיּוֹת); a. fr. Gen. R. s. 60 הדא דב׳ אמרין that is what people say. Lam. R. to I, 1 מפליא בב׳ (1 חד כותאי) רבתי makes sport of men (interpreting dreams to suit himself). —2) *natural state,* v. בְּרִיָּיה. B. Kam. 93ᵇ.

בְּרִיָּתָא, v. בְּרָאָה.

בריתא, Targ. Y. II Num. XXIV, 6 כב׳ Ar., v. בְּרָתָא end.

בָּרַךְ (b. h.; √בר, v. ברר, ברי) 1) *to cave out.* Denom. בֶּרֶךְ, בְּרֵכָה; cmp. בּוּרְכָּא, בּוּרְכְּתָא.—2) (cmp. ברר) *to select, point out* (cmp. esp. Gen. II, 3) whence *to bless* (Pi.).—Part. pass. בָּרוּךְ *chosen, blessed, praised.* הקדוש ב׳ הוא (abbr. הקב״ה) the Holy One, blessed be He. Pes. 118ᵃ; a. v. fr. Ib. 104ᵇ, a. fr. פותח בב׳ וכ׳ he (who prays) opens the benediction with *barukh* and closes with *barukh* (i. e. ברוך אתה ה׳). Tosef. Sot. I, 10 ב׳ בכלל, v. כְּלָל; a. fr.

Pi. בֵּרֵךְ, בֵּרַךְ, בָּרֵךְ (b. h.) 1) *to praise, bless,* esp. *to recite the due benediction.* Ber. VI, 1. Ib. 5 בר׳ על היין having recited the blessing over wine &c. Pes. X, 9 ב׳ ברכת הפסח having recited the blessing over the Paschal lamb. Ib. 5 אנחנו חייבים... לְבָרֵךְ we are bound to .... praise &c.; a. v. fr.—2) (cmp. נקב) *to blaspheme.* Snh. 56ᵃ עד שֶׁיְּבָרֵךְ שם בשם until he blasphemes the Lord by His name. Ib. שבר׳ את השם בכינוי who blasphemed the Lord by an attribute.—Part. Pu. מְבוֹרָךְ *blessed, praiseworthy.* Ber. VII, 3; a. fr.—3) **to cut through, to clear virgin ground* or *forest.* Tosef. Shebi. III, 20 ed. Zuck. (Var. מגדר); Y. ib. IV, 35ᵇ bot. מבדין; Y. Sabb. VII, 10ᵃ top חמברה, v. בחר h. [Tosef. Shebi. I, 6 מבורכות, v. infra.]

Hithpa. הִתְבָּרֵךְ, *Nithpa.* נִתְבָּרֵךְ *to be blessed* (*praised*); *to be increased* (v. בְּרָכָה). Y. Ber. IX, 14ᵃ top וְיִתְבָּרֵךְ and be blessed. Y. M. Kat. I, beg. 80ᵃ if the waters were scanty וְנִתְבָּרְכוּ and grew plentiful. Yeb. 63ᵃ; a. fr.

Hif. הִבְרִיךְ (denom. of בֶּרֶךְ or בְּרֵכָה) *to form a knee, to engraft;* esp. *to bend a vine by drawing it into the ground and making it grow forth as an independent plant, to sink.* Shebi. II, 6; R. Hash. 10ᵇ; a. fr.—Tosef. Shebi. I, 6 אם היו מוּבְרָכוֹת (incorr. מבורכ׳) if they have been sunk before New Year &c.—Yeb. 63ᵃ (allud. to Gen. XII, 3) שתי ברכות טובות יש לי לְהַבְרִיךְ בך two good shoots (proselytes) have I to engraft on thee, Ruth and &c. (B. Kam. 38ᵇ פרידות וכ׳ . . .).

בְּרֵיךְ, בָּרֵךְ, בְּרַךְ ch. same. Part. Peil בְּרִיךְ *blessed.* Targ. Gen. IX, 26; a. fr.—Sabb. 67ᵃ, a. fr. קודשא ב׳ הוא the Holiness (Holy One), blessed be He. Cant. R. to. IV, 4; Gen. R. s. 32 הדין טורא בְּרִיכָא this blessed mount (Gerizim, revered by the Samaritans; Deut. R. s. 3 קדיש).

Pa. בָּרֵיךְ, בָּרֵיךְ, בָּרֵיךְ as preced. Pi. 1) *to bless* &c. Targ. Deut. VIII, 10; a. fr.—Esp. *to say grace after meal.* Ber. 46ᵃ כי מטי לְבָרוּכֵי וכ׳ when it was time to say grace, he said, Will you please, say grace for us. Y. ib. VI, 10ᵇ מהו למְבָרְכָה בסופה what benediction must be said after it? Ib. bot. לא אנא חכים מברכא I do not know how to say grace after it.—Part. pass. מְבָרַךְ. Targ. Y. II Gen. XLIX, 2.—2) *to blaspheme.* Targ. Job II, 9.—Snh. 56ᵃ לישנא דבורכי in the sense of blaspheming.

Ithpe. אִתְבָּרֵיךְ as preced. Hithpa. Targ. Gen. XII, 3; a. fr.

בֶּרֶךְ (בּוֹרֶךְ) f. (b. h.; preced.) 1) *knee.* Y. Ber. I, 3ᵈ top.—2) *a knee-shaped pole.* Taan. 25ᵇ כמלא ב׳ המחרישה (Var. כוך, v. Rabb. D. S. a. l.) (until the rain penetrates) as far as the knee of the plough enters the soil; Ohol. XVII, 1 בר׳. Kel. XXI, 2 בר׳. [Tosef. Shebi. IV, 20 ברך, v. בְּרִיכָה.]—*Du.* בִּרְכַּיִם. Ber. 34ᵇ; Meg. 22ᵇ; Shebu. 16ᵇ כריעה על ב׳ the word כרע means falling on one's knees. [בִּרְכּוֹת, v. בְּרִיכָה.]

בִּירְכָּא, בִּרְכָּא, בְּרַךְ ch. same, 1) *knee.* Targ. Is. XLV, 23.—*Pl.* בִּרְכַיָּא, בִּרְכֵי, בִּרְכֵּי, בִּר׳. Targ. Jud. VII, 6; a. e.—Ber. 6ᵃ הנהו ב׳ וכ׳ those fatigued knees (of scholars) must be ascribed to them (the demons). Pes. 108ᵃ, v. זָגָא.—2)=h. בְּרִיכָה. *Pl.* בִּירְכֵי *shoots, branches.* Taan. 30ᵃ top (Var. in Rashi בְּרִיכֵי, Ar. בורכי).

בִּירְכָא, בִּרְכָא, f. ch.=h. בְּרָכָה, *blessing, plenty.* Targ. Is. XIX, 24.—בִּרְכָאן plenty for us, *we have enough with.* Gen. R. s. 78 אית במאתן ב׳ we have enough with two hundred fables; Yalk. ib. 133 בִּרְכָן.—*Pl.* בִּרְכָן, בִּר׳; Targ. O. Gen. XXVII, 12 (Y. בִּרְכָאן; ib. 13 בִּירְכָן). [בִּרְכַיָּא Targ. O. Deut. XXVIII, 2, some ed.] V. בִּרְכְּתָא.

בְּרָכָה f. (b. h.; ברך) 1) *blessing, bestowal of prosperity, good wishes, choice, plenty.* Keth. 5ᵃ . . . הואיל ב׳ לדגים because on it the blessing was given to the fish (Gen. I, 22, to be fruitful). Y. ib. I, beg. 24ᵈ אין כתיב ב׳ וכ׳ the blessing (Gen. II, 3) refers not to man but to the day.—Erub. 63ᵇ, a. fr. תבא עליו ב׳ blessing rest upon him (he acts rightly). Keth. 103ᵃ; B. Bath. 144ᵇ בִּרְכַּת הבית ברובה the blessing of a house consists in the number of inmates (every member of a household contributes to its comfort); Tosef. Keth. XII, 3 ב׳ הבית מרובה. B. Mets. 42ᵃ אין הב׳ מצויה וכ׳ blessing (unexpected supply, miraculous increase) will not take place in things which are weighed &c.; Taan. 8ᵇ; a. fr.—Pes. 50ᵇ, a. fr. אינו רואה סימן ב׳ לעולם will never see a sign of prosperity; a. fr.—2) *benediction, prayer to be recited on certain occasions.* Ber. 35ᵃ man must not taste anything בלא ב׳ without a blessing. Ib. 40ᵇ כל ב׳ שאין וכ׳ a benediction in which the Name of the Lord is not invoked, is no benediction; a. fr.—*Pl.* בְּרָכוֹת. 1) *blessings, benedictions.* Ib. 45ᵇ; a. v. fr.—Sabb. 115ᵇ כותבי ב׳ those who write out the formulas of prayer.—2) *B'rakhoth,* the first treatise of the Mishnah, Talmud, a. Tosefta.—Compounds: בִּרְכַּת אבלים the prayer for consolation inserted in the mourners' grace after meal. Keth. 8ᵇ; a. fr.—ב׳ ארוסין benediction preceding betrothal, v. אֵרוּסִין Ib. 7ᵇ.—ב׳ הארץ that portion of the grace after meal which refers to Palestine. Ib. 8ᵇ.—ב׳ הזבח the benediction before partaking of the festive offering (חֲגִיגָה) which accompanies the Paschal lamb. Pes. X, 9 (120ᵃ).—ב׳ הזימון the appeal to the partakers of a meal to say grace, *common prayer.* Ber. 45ᵇ.—ב׳ חתנים benediction on performing the marriage ceremony, also inserted in the grace after wedding meals during seven days. Keth. 8ᵇ.—ב׳ כהנים the priestly benediction (Num. VI, 24—26). Sot. VII, 6.—ב׳ המזון grace after meal. Keth. l. c.—ב׳ המצוות benediction on performing a divine command (of a symbolic nature). Ib. 7ᵇ.—ב׳ רחבה benediction of consolation pronounced in open air on the mourners' return from burial (v. הַבְרָאָה). Ib. 8ᵇ.—ב׳ התורה benediction before and after reading the Law. Y. Ber. I, 3ᶜ.—[For other compounds see the respective determinants.]—3) *blasphemy.* בִּרְכַּת השם. Snh. 56ᵃ sq.; (Tosef. Ab. Zar. VIII (IX), 4 קללת).

בורכייד, ברכוייר, ברכוייד, Tosef. Kil. III, 12, read בּוּפְרָיָא or בּוּפְרִיָּא.

בּוּרְפַּיִיר, בִּרְפַּיִיר m. (=בֵּיר פַּיִיר, v. בֵּירִית a. כּוּר) *the stove-setter's knee-band, the brick-layer's cushion* (on which he kneels at work). Kel. XXVI, 3 (Talm. ed. בּוּר׳).

ברכר, ברכרה, Y. Peah VII, 20ᵃ, v. פַּרְפָּר.

בְּרֵכַת=בְּרֵכָה. Tosef. Mikv. IV, 8.

בִּירְכְתָא, בִּרְכְתָא f. ch.=h. בְּרָכָה. Targ. Gen. XXVII, 36; a. fr.—Ber. 51ᵇ כסא דב׳ (=h. כוס של ברכה) the cup for the grace after meal. Ḥag. 5ᵇ איכו השתא מנעתן מהאי ב׳ how near thou camest depriving us of this blessing; a. fr.—*Pl.* בִּרְכָתָא, בִּר׳. Targ. Deut. XXVIII, 2; a. fr.

בְּרַכְתָּא pr. n. pl. *B'rakhta*. Y. Ber. VI, 10ᵇ bot.; cmp., however, מַבְרַכְתָּא.

בְּרַם h. a. ch. conj. (ברם *to split*, √בר, cmp. פרם, v. בּוּרְמָא) 1) *besides*. Targ. Y. Ex. XXXVI, 7.—2) *however*. Dan. IV, 12; V, 17.—Targ. Ps. LVIII, 3; a. fr.—3) *only, but*. Targ. Gen. VII, 23. Targ. Lam. III, 3 (h. text אַךְ). Targ. Ps. LVIII, 2 חב׳ בקושטא is it only in truth (indeed)?—Sabb. 63ᵇ; Erub. 16ᵇ, a. fr. ב׳ כך אמרו but in fact they said this. B. Mets. 114ᵃ.—3) interj. *truly!, surely!* Sabb. 13ᵇ; Ḥag. 13ᵃ; Men. 45ᵇ ב׳ זכור וכ׳ truly! this man be remembered for blessing!—[Ḥull. 112ᵃ דאברים some ed., read: דאבריה, v. בְּרָא.]

***ברמור**, El. Wil. in Tosef. Kil. III, 12, for ברכויר.

***ברנמין**, Yalk. Ezek. 356, v. לברטין.

בַּרְנֵיש, v. בַּרְנֵשׁ.

ברנקיא, Targ. Is. III, 22 Ar., ed. לבורניקיא q. v.

בַּרְנֵיש, בַּרְנֵשׁ pr. n. pl. *Barnesh*, in Babylon, prob. the modern *Khar-Birnus*, near Helle (Neub. Géogr. p. 345), having in its vicinity a Synagogue named after Daniel. Erub. 21ᵃ. B. Mets. 73ᵇ.

***ברס**, Af. אַבְרִיס *to bray* (used of the wild ass when hungry). Targ. Job VI, 5 (Ms. מַבְרִיס, perh. a denom. of כְּרֵס *stomach, appetite*).

בִּרְסִין (בִּרְסִים) m. pl. (birrus, βίῤῥος, v. בִּירוּס; formed with a geographical termination, cmp. בִּרְדְּסִין) *birrus*, a cloak of thick woolen material. Kil. IX, 7 (Ms. M. a. Ar. בר׳); Y. ib. 32ᵈ top בּוּרְסִין; expl. בריח, v. בִּירְיָא II. Sifré Deut. 234 סרסים read as Yalk. ib. 933 בורס׳.

***בִּרְסָם** m. (Parel of בסם, cmp. בִּלְסָם) *a dripping like balsam*, whence *catarrh of the head*. Ḥull. 105ᵇ קשי לב׳ Ar. (ed. לכ׳, Mus. כרסום) is liable to produce catarrh; לב׳ דחמרא וכ׳ a remedy for a catarrh contracted from drinking the foam of wine, is beer; for thet from beer &c.—Gitt. 69ᵃ לב׳ a remedy for &c. [Ar.: *pleurisy*. Pers. ברסאם, v. Fl. to Levy Talm. Dict. I, p. 228ᵇ.]

ברסנה, v. פַּרְסְנָא.

בָּרַץ (√בר; cmp. בּרז, v. P. Sm. 618) *to break through*. *Pi.* בֵּרֵץ *to cut through* from end to end. Part. Pu. מְבוֹרָץ. Tosef. Kil. III, 10 חריץ המב׳ a ditch which is cut through, going from end to end of the vineyard (Mish. ib. V, 3 מפולש). Men. I, 2 קמצו מב׳ the priest's grasp of the meal offering must be coming forth on both sides.

בְּרַץ ch. same; *Pa.* בָּרֵץ *to bore*. Ab. Zar. 59ᵇ וּבִירְצוּהָ עד דשייפא Ar. (ed. וּבָרְצוּה) and bore into the keg, until it is emptied (Rashi: bend it towards the bung-hole).

בִּרְצוּץ m. (preced., cmp. P. Sm. 618 s. v. ברץ, a. Ges. H. Dict. s. v. פאר) *the crown of the turban*. Targ. Y. Ex. XXXIX, 28 (h. text פארי).

בֵּי ב׳, בַּרְצִיתָא pr. n. pl. *Be-Bartsitha*. M. Kat. 4ᵇ לבי ב׳ early ed. (late ed. לבני בר ציתאי, Ms. M. בר צרתא, v. Rabb. D. S. a. l.).

בָּרַק (b. h.; √בר, v. ברר) *to be bright, shine, flash*. B. Bath. 97ᵇ (יין) בּוֹרֵק white effervescent wine (not fully fermented; Var. בּוֹדֵק searching in the bowels, i. e. causing diarrhœa, v. בָּדַק); Tosef. Men. IX, 9 הַבּוֹרֵיק (sub. יין) the effervescent (wine), v. בָּארַג; Yoma 28ᵇ top, v. next w. Tosef. Ter. VII, 16 [read:] ב׳ והניחו if it was effervescent when he left it.

Hif. הִבְרִיק 1) (cmp. ברץ ברח) *to cut through from end to end*. Y. Kil. V, 29ᵈ bot. עד שיהא מַבְרִיק כדי וכ׳ until it (the ditch in the vineyard) passes through from end to end, wide enough for man and his tilling cattle.—2) (denom. of בָּרָק) *to be affected by lightning, get blind* (or *get vermin*). B. Mets. VI, 3, expl. ib. 78ᵃ אבוזקת a. חוּורִיתא.

בְּרַק I, בְּרֵיק ch. same, *to shine, rise*. Y. Yoma III, beg. 40ᵇ; Y. R. Hash. II, beg. 57ᵈ what is בורקי (Mish. Yoma III, 1)? It means בְּרָקַת, the rising light, as people say in Babylonia בְּרַק ברוקא) בְּרוּק ברוקה) the sparkling (star) shines, meaning אנהר מנהורא the light-giver (morning star) gives light. [Bab. Yoma 28ᵇ (hebr.) בְּרַק ברקאי.] Ber. 59ᵃ (expl. רעמים) ברקא תקיפא דבריק בעננא וכ׳ an intense lightning which flashes through the cloud and breaks pieces of hailstone, (Var. v. Rabb. D. S. a. l.).

Af. אַבְרֵיק *to send forth lightning* (fulminare). Targ. Ps. CXLIV, 6.—Targ. II Esth. III, 8 מבריקן עיניהון their eyes sparkling (in defiance). [Ḥull. 112ᵃ דאבריק some ed., read דאבריה, v. בְּרָא.]

בָּרָק m. (b. h.; preced.) *lightning*. Lev. R. s. 31.—*Pl.* בְּרָקִים. Ber. IX, 2; a. fr.

בְּנֵי ב׳, בְּרַק II (b. h.) pr. n. pl. *B'ne B'rak* (Josh. XIX, 45, modern *Ibn Ibrak*) near Japho, seat of R. Akiba's college. Snh. 32ᵇ. Lev. R. s. 21. Tosef. Sabb. III (IV), 3.

בְּרַקָא I, בְּרַק III m. ch. 1)=h. בָּרָק. Targ. Deut. XXXII, 41 (Y. II בַּרְקָא); a. fr.—Ber. 59ᵃ ב׳ יחידאה a single flash (for vers. v. Rabb. D. S. a. l.); a. fr.—*Pl.* בַּרְקִין, בְּרָקִין, בַּרְקַיָּא, בַּרְקֵי. Targ. Ps. XVIII, 15; a. fr. [Y. R. Hash. II, beg. ברק ברקא, read בַּרְקַאי.] Ber. l. c. וברקיא ירוקתא some ed. (read ירוקרקי as Ms. M.). Ib. דבריק ברקי׳ ומנהמי וכ׳ (read דברוק, v. also Rabb. D. S. a. l.) the lightnings break through and make the clouds rumble &c.—2) *white cataract* (v. בָּרַק Hif.), cmp. בַּרְקִית. Bekh. 38ᵇ וסימנך ברקא

and thy sign (by which to remember which of the two affections of the eye is considered a blemish) take *barka* (meaning *white* and *cataract*, and like the cataract is the floating white spot in the eye a disqualifying blemish). V. next w.

בַּרְקָא II m. (ברק) 1) (adj.) *shining, white.* Snh. 98ª סוסיא ב׳ a white horse, v. בָּאַרְגַּ.—*Pl.* בַּרְקֵי. Y. B. Bath. VIII, 16ᵇ top; Y. Kidd. I, 60ᶜ bot. he let him ride אתרי ריכשי ב׳ on two white steeds (i. e. the donator gave him a doubly fortified document; another opin.: he made him ride on two . ., which run in different directions, i. e. the document is invalid; v. explan. ibid., cmp. B. Bath. 152ª, Keth. 55ª. Gitt. 69ª שודרא ב׳ a string of white hair. Sabb. 67ª; Ab. Zar. 28ᵇ נירא ב׳ a white thread (of hair).—2) (as a noun) *something white, white thread.* Ib. ולירמי ב׳ וכ׳ and let him put a white thread around one end. Ib. פתילי ב׳ Ms. M. (ed. פתילתא ביקרא, corr. acc.) strings of white stuff.

***בַּרְקָא III** m. (v. בָּרַק Hif.) *a compartment near the house with windows on all sides, a kind of piazza.* Erub. 15ª (Rashi Ms. M. בדקא). B. Bath. 61ª ב׳ חלילא Ms. M. a. oth. (ed. בדקא; expl. יציע) a piazza open all around.

בַּרְקַאי I m. *morning star.* Yoma III, 1; 28ᵇ; v. בְּרַק. [Y. ed. בּוֹרְקַי q. v.]

בַּרְקַאי II pr. n. m., v. בּוֹרְקַי II.—2) כְּפַר ב׳ *K'far Barkai*, in Palestine; cmp. בורגתא. Pes. 57ª, ᵇ.

ברקום, Gen. R. s. 98, read לִיבְדְּקוֹס.—Targ. Cant. II, 1, read נַרְקִיס.

בַּרְקוּרְיָאנֵי m. pl. (disguise of Herculiani, cmp. הוּרְמוֹס) *Herculiani*, a cohort of pretorians named after Diocletian (Heraclius). Esth. R. to I, 3 יכולני וכ׳ (read יוֹבְיָינֵי); some ed. בר קוריאני (in two words) Joviani and Herculiani. V. Sachs Beitr. I, 113 sq., ref. to Amm. Marc. XXII, 3, 2.

בַּרְקוּת, v. בַּרְקִית.

בַּרְקִין, v. אַבְרְקִין.

בַּרְקִירְיָא p. n. m. *Barkirya*, an Amora. Y. Kil. IX, 32ᵈ top; Y. Keth. XII, 35ᵇ bot. בר קריא.

בַּרְקִית f. (ברק, v. בַּרְקָא I) *cataract of the eye.* Sabb. 78ª שכן כוחלין לב׳ for they paint the eye with blood as a remedy for a cataract. Tosef. ib. VI (VII), 7 ברקות (Var. ברקי׳). V. בַּרְקְתִּי.

בַּרְקָן m., v. בַּרְקְתָא.

בַּרְקָנַיָּא ch.=next w. Targ. Jud. VIII, 7; 16.

בַּרְקָנִים m. pl. (b. h.) *thistles.* Yoma 69ª (quot. fr. Meg. Taan. ch. IX) they dragged them על הקוצים ועל הב׳ over thorns and thistles.

בָּרֶקֶת f. (ברק) *morning star* (in b. h. *a jewel*, v. next w.). Y. Yoma III, beg. 40ª; Y. R. Hash. II, beg. 57ᵈ, expl. בּוֹרְקַי; v. בְּרַק I.

בַּרְקְתָא f., **בַּרְקָן**, **בְּרוֹקָא** m.=b. h. בָּרֶקֶת, *a jewel*, prob. *smaragd.* Targ. Ex. XXVIII, 17; a. e. Targ. Ezek. XXVIII, 13. Targ. Cant. V, 14 (ed. Vien. בַּרְקָן, corr. acc.); a. e.—Targ. Y. Num. II, 3 ברוקא.

בַּרְקְתָא, v. בּוּרְקְתָה.

בַּרְקְתִּי f. ch.=h. בַּרְקִית. Pes. 111ᵇ קשה לב׳ Ar. (ed. לִבְרוּקְתִּי) is liable to produce a cataract. Gitt. 69ª top לברוק׳ a remedy for &c.

בָּרַר (b. h.; √בר, contr. of באר, בור) [*to clear, clean; to place outside*, whence] 1) *to make clear, prove, ascertain.* Keth. 46ª (interpret. Deut. XXII, 17) ובוֹרְרִין את הדבר וכ׳ and they make the fact as clear (bright) as a new garment.—Part. pass. בָּרוּר q. v.—2) *to single out, select, sift, assort.* Maasr. II, 6 שֶׁאָבוֹר לי which I may select for me. Ib. בּוֹרֵר ואוכל he has a right to pick out and eat (one after the other). Kil. II, 1 יָבוֹר he must take it out entirely. Sabb. VII, 2 הבּוֹרֵר he who sifts (a labor forbidden on the Sabbath). Y. ib. VII, 10ª, a. fr. משום בורר (is guilty) because it comes under the class of sifting. Bab. ib. 74ª בורר ואוכל וכ׳ he may take out singly and eat, take out singly and put it down (rejecting it) ולא יִבְרוֹר but he must not assort (v. discussion ibid.). Gitt. V, 9 לא תָבוֹר she must not help her to sift the grain. Snh. 45ª בְּרוֹר לו וכ׳ choose for the convict the most gentle method of execution; Sot. 8ᵇ, a. fr.—Snh. III, 1 זה בורר וכ׳ each party chooses one judge, and the two judges בּוֹרְרִין וכ׳ elect a third.

Pi. בֵּרֵר, בֵּירֵר 1) *to prove, ascertain.* Snh. 23ᵇ צריך לְבָרֵר the claimant must offer clear evidence. Kerith. 24ª לב׳ עוון to ascertain whether or not the woman was guilty; Num. R. s. 9, v. בָּעַר. Y. Kidd. III, 63ᵈ, v. סִימְפוֹן. Lev. R. s. 11; v. *Nithpa.*—2) *to sift, select.* Y. Ber. IX, 13ᶜ top דש וזרה ובר׳ he threshed, winnowed and sifted. Y. Ned. I, beg. 51ª לשונות שבֵירְרוּ לחן וכ׳ the terms (for oaths, vows &c.) which the Mishnahs have selected (as substitutes for the real expressions of oaths &c.); Bab. ib. 10ᵇ. שבדו, v. בָּדָא. [Esth. R. to I, 22 [read:] בירר להם בלשון רומי מלשון יוני . . . . . interpreted for them (the Bible) in Latin &c., v. בָּדָא. The passage is defective; cmp. Y. Meg. I, 71ᶜ top.] [Y. Snh. X, 28ª בחרו להם ביררי הברזל וכ׳, read בְּרִיּוּת, they selected (as similes for the Law) the soundness of the iron and the fixedness of the tree; cmp. Num. R. s. 14; Koh. R. to XII, 11.]

Hof. הוּבְרַר *to be cleared up, to be decided* (between two alternatives); v. בְּרֵירָה. Bets. 4ª (a hen is bought either for consumption or for breeding) נשחטה הוּבְרְרָה וכ׳ by its being killed, it appears that it was originally intended for slaughtering; Hull. 14ª.

Nif. נִבְרַר *to be selected.* Tanh. Sh'lah. 4 נִבְרְרוּ צדיקים they were righteous at the time they were selected.

Nithpa. נִתְבָּרֵר 1) *to desire clearness, to seek evidence, search for truth.* Lev. R. s. 11 (ref. to II Sam. XXII, 26 sq.) בשעה שנ׳ על עסקיו הק״בה בירר לו וכ׳ when he desired to be enlightened about his affairs (asking, 'Whereby shall I know, Gen. XV, 8), the Lord enlightened him &c. (ib. 13). Ib. בשעה שנ׳ וכ׳ (with ref. to Moses); Midr. Till. to Ps. XVIII, 26 sq.—2) *to be confirmed, established.* Tanh.

T'tsavveh 9, end [read:] נִתְבָּרְרָה כהונה בידם through them the priesthood became established. Pesik. Dibré p. 115[b] [read as:] Yalk. Jer. 258 לא נ׳ . . . . עד שעמד וכ׳ their prophecies were not fulfilled until Jer. arose.

בְּרַר ch.; *Pa.* בָּרֵיר same. Targ. I Chr. XXI, 13. Targ. Is. I, 25; a. e.—Bekh. 57[a] לִיבְרוֹר חד וכ׳ let him take out (for destruction) one lamb as an equivalent of the dog; v. בְּרֵירָה; Y. Shek. VI, 50[b] נברור וכ׳ let him &c.

Ithpe. אִתְבְּרִיר *to be clear, pure.* Targ. Job XXV, 5.

בְּרָרָא m. (ברר) 1) *pureness, unalloyed metal.* Y. Shek. VI, 50[b]; Y. Yoma IV, 41[d] top עד דלא יקום על בְּרָרֵיה וכ׳ as long as the gold ore is not reduced to its pure state, it looses much in the smelting process; but when once brought to its pure state, nothing is lost.—2) *clearness, truth.* Y. Yeb. VIII, 9[b] top; XV, 15[a] דו משים (מקים) . . . על ב׳ because he based the matter on truth (gave a clear decision).

*__בְּרְשָׁן, ברשאן__, Ar. (s. v. בר) בר שאן, *in ecstacy* (?); *naked* (?). Targ. I Sam. XIX, 25 (v. Rashi a. l.; h. text ערום; Var. lect. ביישן).

בְּרַתָּא, בְּרַת I f. (v. בַּר II) *daughter, child, issue; young tree.* Targ. Gen. XXX, 21; a. fr.—B. Bath. 141[a] ב׳ נמי וכ׳ the Lord did not suffer Abraham to be even without a daughter. M. Kat. 9[b] ב׳ אוכמתא Ms. M., v. אוּכָּם. Y. B. Mets. III, 8[c] bot. ב׳ נוקבה female issue. Lev. R. s. 25 ב׳ פחין a mean woman.—ב׳ שבע—בַּת קוֹל=ב׳ קלא, a species of *figs.* Gen. R. s. 15, end (h. בנות שבע). Y. B. Bath. II, end, 13[c] ב׳ שובעין חיוורין white figs; a. fr. [For other compounds, v. respective determinants.]—*Pl.* בְּנָן, בְּנָתָן, בְּנָאתָךְ. [Targ. Y. Ex. X, 9 בְּרָתָנָא our daughters.] Targ. Gen. V, 4; a. fr.—Keth. IV, 11 ב׳ נוקבין, v. בַּר II. Kidd. 71[b] בְּנָתִין our daughters. B. Bath. 141[a] לדידי בנתן וכ׳ I prefer daughters &c.; a. fr.—[Y. Peah VII, 20[a] bot. ב׳ דתרובתא; Y. Sot. I, 17[b] top אורתא, v. בְּרַתָּא.]

בְּרַת II, ב׳ חוורן pr. n. pl. *B'rath Ḥavran* (or *Horan*) prob. ident. with Beth-Horon, v. חוֹרוֹן. Y. M. Kat. I, 80[b] bot.; Y. Shek. I, 46[a]; Y. Ab. Zar. III, 42[c] top; Y. Sot. IX, 23[c] top.

בְּרַתָּא, v. בְּרַת I.

בְּרָתָא, בְּרוֹתָא, בְּרָאתָא c. (=h. בְּרוֹשׁ; ברית or ברר, v. pl. בְּרָוָן; √ בר; v. ברר) [*the chosen* or *strong,*] *cypress,* or *pine-tree.* Targ. II Esth. II, 7 (transl. of Is. LV, 13). Y. Keth. VII, end, 31[d]; Gen. R. s. 15; B. Bath. 80[b] בראתא Ms. M. (ed. בְּרָתֵי pl.; for oth. var. v. Rabb. D. S. a. l.); R. Hash. 23[a] (transl. ברוש). [Y. Peah VIII, 20[d] bot. ב׳ לְהָן אֲהָן צררא סמך הדא what has this pebble to do near this cypress?—an evasive answer or a rebuke; prob. to be read בִּירְתָא.]—*Pl.* בְּרָא׳, בְּרָתֵי, בְּרָתִין. Targ. Cant. I, 17. Targ. Ps. CIV, 17; a. e.—(Fem.) בִּירָנִן, בְּרָנָן, בְּרָוָן. Targ. Is. XLI, 19; a. fr. [Ar. ed. Koh: בִּירָתִין, Targ. II Sam. VI, 5.—Targ. Y. II Num. XXIV, 6 בכרוותיה ed., כבריתא Ar., read בִּבְרָתָא.]

בַּרְתּוֹתָא pr. n. pl. *Bartotha,* in Upper Galilee. Ab. III, 7; Orl. I, 4; a. fr.

בְּרָתֵי, v. בְּרָתָא.—בְּרָתִים, בְּרָתִיִּים, v. פְּרָתֵי.

ברתצין, v. פִּרְקְסִין.

*__בשא__, Ithp. אתבשו, Targ. Lam. I, 14 Var.=אשתבשו, v. שבש (ed. Lag. אִתְרַבְּשׁוּ, corr. acc.).

בִּישׁוּל, בִּשּׁוּל m. (בשל) *ripening, cooking; dish.* Snh. 95[b] זמן בי׳ פירות the season of the ripening of fruits.—Hull. 115[b] sq. איסור ב׳, v. אִיסּוּר. Y. Sabb. VII, 10[a]; Y. Bets. I, 60[b] top הותר מכלל בי׳ permitted as coming under the category of cooking (on Holy Days); a. fr.—*Pl.* בִּשּׁוּלִים, בִּי׳. Ab. Zar. 38[a] בִּישׁוּלֵי נכרים dishes prepared by gentiles. Ib. בישולי של עכ״ום (strike out של, v. Ms. M.); a. fr. [Gen. R. s. 49 אמר בישולה, v. בָּשֵׁל.]

בִּישׁ׳, בְּשׁוּלָא ch. same. Pes. 27[a] דהא קא מקבלא ב׳ מקמיה דניתו וכ׳ Ms. M. (ed. דהא קבלה . . . דניתן) for it receives the dish (to be prepared), before yet they put the wood &c. Ab. Zar. 38[a] קירובי ב׳ וכ׳ to accelerate boiling (make it quicker done) is something essential. Hull. 111[b].

בְּשׂוּם m. (בשם) *delicate food, dainty.* *Pl.* בְּשׂוּמִין, constr. בְּשׂוּמֵי. Cant. R. to I, 12 ריח טוב מב׳ ג״ע the smell of the dainties of Paradise (stimulating their appetites), v. קְהָא.

בשומין, Y. Sabb. VII, 10[a] טריקסימון. ב׳, read שׁוּמִין.

בְּשׂוֹרָא, v. בְּשׂוֹרְתָא.

בְּשׂוֹרָה f. (b. h. בְּשׂרָה; בָּשַׂר) *joy, glad tiding;* in gen. *tidings.* Keth. 16[b] כוס של ב׳ cup of joy (wine carried in the bridal procession of a virgin), v. explan. ib.—Mekh. Bo. s. 12 ב׳ רעה evil prediction. Tanh. Ki. Thetse 4; Pesik. Zakh. p. 24[a] בְּשׂוֹרַת אמו the news of his mother's death; a. e.—*Pl.* בְּשׂוֹרוֹת. Y. Keth. II, 26[b] top חבית של ב׳ the keg of wine carried in the bridal procession, v. supra. Num. R. s. 14 (play on בשר Koh. XII, 12; Ezek. XXXVI, 26) the Lord sends thee ב׳ טובות good tidings. Ber. IX, 2 ב׳ טובות . . . . שמועות רעות Mish. ed. (Talm. ed. 54[a] ב׳ רעות, v. Rabb. D. S. a. l. note 4) good tidings . . . bad news. Sabb. 63[a] אין . . . . ב׳ רעות no bad tidings will reach him.

בְּסוֹרָא, בְּשׂוֹרָא, בְּסוֹרְתָא, בְּשׂוֹרְתָא ch. same. Targ. Job III, 26 (in an evil sense). Targ. II Sam. XVIII, 22; a. e.—R. Hash. 19[a]; Taan. 18[a] (quot. fr. Meg. Taan. ch. XII) אתת ב׳ טבתא good news came. Lam. R. to I, 5 ב׳ ט׳ איתבשרת thou hast received good tidings. Gen. R. s. 81 (in Hebr. phraseol.) ב׳ שמתה אמו the news that his mother died; v. preced.—*Pl.* בְּשׂוֹרָן, בְּסוֹ׳. Targ. Y. II Gen. XLIX, 21.

*__בְּשַׁט__ (cmp. ושט, רשט a. Arab. *basaṭa*) *to send forth in all directions, to shoot wildly.* Targ. Prov. XXVI, 18 ed. Vien.; oth. ed. פשט).

*__בְּשְׁטוּתָא__ f. (v. preced.) *running around in sexual lust.* Targ. Jer. XIII, 27 some ed. (oth. שְׁטוּתָא; ed. Lag. שיט׳).

בְּשִׁיל, v. בְּשֵׁל.

בְּשִׁירוּתָה, בְּשִׁירוּתָא, v. בְּשֵׁרוּתָא.

*בַּשְׁכַּר, v. כַּשְׁכַּר.

בָּשַׁל (b. h.; √בש, sec. r. of באש, cmp. בשם, בשש) *to ripen, boil, be done* (through natural or artificial heat). Y. Snh. VIII, beg. 26ª ב׳ הזרע וכ׳ when the seed boils inside (maturity of genital organs), the pot outside becomes dark (genitals are covered with hair).

Pi. בִּשֵּׁל, בִּישֵּׁל *to mature, cook, roast.* Snh. 95ᵇ לְבַשֵּׁל פירות to make the fruits ripen. Ḥull. 98ᵇ; a. fr.—Pes. 112ª לא תְבַשֵּׁל וכ׳ cook not in a pot which thy neighbor has used before thee (i. e. marry not a divorced woman).—Part. Pu. מְבוּשָּׁל. Ned. VI, 1 הנודר מן המב׳ וכ׳ he who vows abstinence from anything boiled, is permitted to partake of roasts &c. Ib. 49ª באתרא . . . . קרו מב׳ in R. J.'s place they call roast likewise *m'bushshal* (cmp. II Chr. XXXV, 13); a. fr.

Hithpa. הִתְבַּשֵּׁל, *Nithpa.* נִתְבַּשֵּׁל *to be boiled, done, ripe.* Ter. X, 11. Ḥull. VII, 4; a. fr.—Ib. 98ᵇ top, v. בָּשֵׁל.—Sot. 11ª; Ex. R. s. 1 בקדרה שבשלו וכ׳ in the pot they boiled in, they were boiled, (they were done by as they did by others).

בְּשֵׁל, בְּשִׁיל ch. same; as preced. Kal. Targ. O. Gen. XL, 10 ed. Berl. בַּשִׁילוּ (ed. בַּשִּׁילוּ, Pa.); Y. בְּשְׁלוּ; ib. IX, 20.—Part. pass. בְּשִׁיל, בְּשִׁילָא. Targ. O. Num. VI, 19; a. e.—Ab. Zar. 38ª אי לא הוה הפיך בה הוה ב׳ וכ׳ Ms. M. (ed. less corr.) if he (the gentile) had not turned it, it would have been done in two hours.

Pa. בַּשֵּׁיל, בַּשֵּׁל as preced. Pi. Targ. I Kings XIX, 21; a. fr.; v. supra.—Ab. Zar. 38ª לְבַשּׁוּלֵי מנא to bake (in the furnace) the earthen vessel, contrad. to לשרורי to glaze, finish. Ḥull. 110ª ריבעא . . . בער לב׳ how much milk is required to boil a quarter of a litra of meat?

Ithpa. אִיבְּשֵׁל, אִיתְבַּשַּׁל as preced. *Hithpa.* Targ. Y. Deut. XXVI, 2; a. e.—Targ. I Sam. II, 13 כְּמִיבְּשַׁל (Var. כִּמְבַשֵּׁל).—Ab. Zar. 29ᵇ אִיבְּשִׁיל.

בָּשֵׁל m., **בְּשֵׁלָה, בְּשֵׁלָה** f. (b. h.; preced.) *ripe, boiled, done.* זרוע בשלה the boiled shoulder due to the priest (Num. VI, 19). Ḥull. 98ª bot. both derive it מז׳ ב׳ from the process prescribed for the priest's gift &c. Ib.ᵇ top אין ב׳ אלא שלמה when it says, 'the shoulder boiled' it means entire (not carved). Ib. אין ב׳ אלא שנתבשל וכ׳ when it says, 'He shall take &c. from the ram' it means that it must be boiled joined to (or jointly with) the body of the ram. Tanh. Vayera 5 Abraham בלעה בשילה swallowed the fig ripe, i. e. spoke deliberately, opp. פגה; Gen. R. s. 49 אמר בישולה (corr. acc.).

בְּשֵׁלָא ch. same. Targ. Y. Ex. XII, 9.

בַּשָּׁלָא m. (preced.) *cook.*—*Pl.* בַּשָּׁלַיָּא. Targ. Ezek. XLVI, 24 (some ed. בַּשְׁלַיָּא).

בִּשְׁלָמָא (v. שְׁלָמָא) *in peace, well,* whence (as a dialectic term) *granted, it is right, it would be right.* Pes. 7ª ב׳ שבת . . . . אלא וכ׳ it is right as far as 'a Sabbath' is concerned, for it may happen on an eve of Passover concurring with a Sabbath, but (when it says) 'on a Holy Day', how can &c.? Ib. 24ᵇ ב׳ אי . . . שפיר וכ׳ I grant, if . . . ., it would be right (to infer that &c.), but now &c. Ib. 50ª ב׳ למאן דאמר . . . . היינו it is right according to him who says . . . . ., but according to &c.; a. v. fr. ב׳ אי אמרת=אי אמרת ב׳, v. אִי II.

בְּשָׂם, בָּשָׂם &c., v. בֹּסֶם &c.

בֹּשֶׂם m., pl. בְּשָׂמִים (b. h., preced.) *spices, perfumes,* esp. those used for blessings at the exit of the Sabbath. Ber. VIII, 5 sq.; a. fr.

*בַּשְׁקַר (Pashel of בקר) *to search, discover.* Targ. Ps. XLIV, 22 (h. text חקר). Ib. XXVII, 4 ולבשקרה ed. Lag. *to find the truth, speculate* (ed. ולבקרא, h. text ולבַקֵּר).—Yeb. 120ª he passed before them with a plaster on his face ולא בשקרוה and they (the officers) did not discover it (the disguise; for Var. v. Ar. ed. Koh. s. vv. בלוחא a. בשקר). Erub. 19ª ולא מְבַשְׁקַר ליה and he (Abraham) does not discover the disguise; Ar. (taking מב׳ as part. pass.) and he (in his disguise) is not discovered (as a Jew). *Bekh. 36ᵇ חזייה בשקריה he saw him, and discovered his fraud, v. Tosaf.; (ed. a. Rashi חזייה בְּשִׁיקְרֵיה looked at his fraud). [Targ. Y. II Deut. IV, 34 לְמִבְשַׂר, Var. למבשור, read: לְמִבַשְׁקַר.] V. מְבַשְׁקְרָנָא.

בָּשַׂר (v. בָּסַר II a. בָּסַם) *to be sweet, pleasant.*

Pi. בִּישֵּׂר, בִּשֵּׂר *to gladden, to bring good tidings to;* in gen. *to announce.* Ḥull. 87ª מְבַשֵּׂר טובות וכ׳ I am bringing good news. Sabb. 63ª, v. בְּשׂוֹרָה; a. fr.—Part. pass. מְבוּשָּׂר *informed of good news, assured.* Y. Kil. IX, 32ᵇ top יהא מב׳ מחיי העו״הב he shall receive a message from the life in the world to come, i. e. he may be assured of salvation; Y. Keth. XII, 35ª מכושר לחיי וכ׳ . . . (corr. acc.); Y. Shek. III, end, 47ᶜ יהא מב׳ שבן עו״הב הוא. Ex. R. s. 46 אתה מב׳ שמחלתי וכ׳ thou art informed that I have forgiven thee &c. Y. Ber. V, end, 9ᵈ; a. e.

Nithpa. נִתְבַּשֵּׂר *to be gladdened, to receive good tidings.* Pesik. R. s. 42 נ׳ בבנים he was assured that he would have children. Gen. R. s. 47; s. 53 נתבשרה בחלב she was assured that she would nurse her child. [V. בָּסַר II.]

בְּשַׂר, בְּסַר I ch. same, 1) *to be glad;*—*2)=*Pa.* Targ. Y. Gen. XXI, 7. Targ. Y. II ib. XLIX, 21 לְמִיבְשַׂר.

Pa. בַּשַּׂר, בַּסַּר as preced. *Pi.* Targ. Y. I Gen. XLIX, 21. Targ. Jer. XX, 15; a. fr. [Targ. Y. II Deut. IV, 34, v. בַּשְׁקַר.]

Ithpa. אִתְבַּשַּׂר as preced. *Nithpa.* Targ. Ruth I, 6; a. e.

בְּשַׂר, בְּסַר II, v. בִּשְׂרָא.

בָּשָׂר m. (b. h.; v. preced.) [*ripe, warm, sweet, well-looking;* v. Freitag Arab. Dict. s. v. bšr, a. cmp. לֶחֶם] *body* (b. h.); *flesh, meat.* Ḥull. VIII, 1 כל הב׳ any kind of meat. Ib. 16ᵇ בְּשַׂר תאוה meat eaten for satisfying the appetite, i. e. secular meal of meat, opp. to sacrificial meals (v. Deut. XII, 20). Ib. 17ª, v. נְחִירָה; a. fr.—ב׳ ודם (abbr. ב״ו) flesh and blood, i. e. *mortal man.* Ber. 33ª; a. v. fr.

בְּסַר, בְּשַׂר, בִּסְרָא, בִּישְׂרָא I, בִּשְׂרָא ch. same; 1) *body, flesh, meat.* Targ. Gen. II, 21. Targ. Lev. XIII, 2; a. v. fr.—Ḥull. 109ᵇ בעינא . . . בי׳ וכ׳ I desire to eat something tasting like meat with milk. Sabb. 140ᵇ; a. v. fr.—2) *mortal.* Targ. Y. Gen. XL, 23. Targ. Jer. XVII, 5; a. e.

בְּשָׂרָא, בִּישְׂרָא II f. (בשר)=בְּשׂוֹרְתָא. Targ. Y. II Gen. XXI, 7.

***בְּשׂוֹרְתָה** same. Y. Maas. Sh. V, 56[c] top ב׳ וכ׳ (=כסא דב׳) a cup for good news must be full; Y. Ḥag. II, 78[a] bot. בְּשִׂירוּתָה; Y. Bets. II, 61[c] top בשירותא.

בְּשַׁשׁ m. (√בש, v. preced. ws.) *seasoning, relishes.* Targ. Job VI, 6 (h. text טָפֵל.—Ber. 40[a] לית דין צריך ב׳ this (bread, being well seasoned) requires no seasoning relishes to go with it; v. לִיפְתָּן.

בֹּשֶׁת, v. בּוֹשֶׁת.

בַּת I f. (b. h., contr. of בנת) *daughter; maiden, girl; servant-girl* (opp. שפחה slave). Gitt. 89[a] בת לא״א a daughter of Abraham our father, a Jewess. B. Bath. 109[a] בן וב׳ כי הדדי נינהו son and daughter are legally the same. Kidd. II, 3 בת או שפחה גדלת (Bab. ed. מגודל׳) a maid or a slave as hair-dresser; a. fr.—*Pl.* בָּנוֹת, constr. בְּנוֹת. Sabb. VI, 6 חב׳ *girls.* Kidd. 64[a] ב׳ ישראל מקוה וכ׳ Israelitish daughters (married to a degraded priest, v. חָלָל) are a well of purification (means of restoration to priestly ranks); a. fr.—Also Ch. בַּת (v. בְּרַת). Targ. Deut. XV, 12.—Mostly in compounds. Targ. I Sam. I, 16 ב׳ רשעא (h. text בת בליעל); v. infra.—[Y. Keth. II, 26[d] bot., read: בתר איתתיה. Y. Gitt. IX, 50[d] top כבת יוני, read: כתב.]

Compounds of בַּת a. בְּנוֹת (v. בַּר, בֵּן): ב׳ אור *fuel, fit for fuel.* Sabb. 25[b]. בת ארעא.—בנות אזנים, v. אֹזֶן.—בת ארעא a sore on the foot, v. אַרְעָא. Sabb. 65[a] (Mish. צנים).—ב׳ מזגא חמרא Little Wine-Mixer, name of a clean bird. Ḥull. 63[a] top.—ב׳ מינא of the same class or size. Ab. Zar. 28[a].—ב׳ חורין, ב׳ מלך King's, Noblemen's Daughter, name of a demon. Sabb. 109[a]. [ב׳ עין, Ex. R. s. 30, some ed., v. בָּבָה.]—בת ערנא *the hole in the millstone through which the grain passes.* M. Kat. 10[a] (Ms. M. בית טינא).—בת קבריא a species of raven. Esth. R. to I, 4, v. גַּלְגַּל.—ב׳ קול 1) *echo, reverberating sound.* Ex. R. s. 29, end. Cant. R. to I, 3 as the oil (when poured out) אין לו ב׳ קול gives forth no reverberating sound, so does Israel (suffer silently).—2) *Bath-Kol, divine voice,* a sort of substitute for prophecy. Yoma 9[b]; a. fr.—בְּנוֹת שֶׁבַע a species of figs, v. בְּרַת. Maasr. II, 8; a. fr.—ב׳ שוח a species of white figs. Dem. I, 1; a. e.—ב׳ שקמה young sycamore-figs. Ib.; Ber. 40[b], v. דּוּבְלָא.—בת תיהא the small bung-hole in the spicket, to be opened for examining the flavor of the wine. Ab. Zar. 66[b].—[For other compounds, v. respective determinants.]—Chald. pl., v. בְּרַת.

בַּת II f., adv. בְּבַת [*daughter, product of*], בב׳ ראש (=בב׳ זקירת ראש) *headlong;* בב׳ אחת (=בב׳ עשייה אחת, בב׳ כתיבה &c.), *at once, simultaneously, suddenly.* Yoma 38[b] נזקרים בב׳ ר׳ לאחוריהם (Ms. M. בב׳ אחת) staggered backward with a sudden movement (enchanted with the beauty of the music); Cant. R. to III, 6 נסקרין וכ׳; Y. Shek. V, 48[d] bot. נזקרין לו בת ראש (read בב׳) rushed forward to him headlong (to congratulate him). Yoma 67[b] זוקרו בב׳ ר׳ Ar. a. Ms. Oxf. (ed. זורקו) he pushes the scapegoat down the precipice headlong. Succ. 14[b] כדי שיזדקר בה גדי בב׳ ר׳ (Ms. M. גדי ראשו בב׳ אחת . . ., read בב׳ ראשו) wide enough for a goat to leap through with one headlong rush. Erub. 16[a] כדי שלא יזד׳ הגדי בב׳ ר׳ (Ms. M. שלא . . . ירקד הגדי בב׳ א׳; Tosef. Kil. IV, 6 שלא יכנס הגדי . . .; Erub. l. c. bot. (בב׳ א׳) less space than a goat would require &c.—Yoma 38[b] היה כותבה בב׳ א׳ would write a word of four letters (with four pens between his fingers) at a time. Pes. 86[b] who empties his goblet בב׳ א׳ in one draught. Num. R. s. 4 they did not drop the curtain בב׳ א׳ at once, opp. קימעא קימעא; a. fr.

בַּת III c. (b. h.) *bath,* a measure; v. בֵּיתָא II.

***בָּתָה** f. (b. h.; =בחח, v. בתר) *desolation.* Gen. R. s. 31; Yalk. ib. 51 (ref. to קץ . . . בא וכ׳ Gen. VI, 13) their term has come לעשות ב׳ to make (the earth) a waste.

***בַּתְוָא**, pl. **בַּתְוָותָא** f. same, esp. *the untillable cuts* in the valley or field (cmp. בַּתּוֹת Is. VII, 19). Sabb. 110[b] let him cut porret מב׳ דמישרא Ar. (Var. גובתא ed. Koh.; oth. ed. בוותא; Ms. M. ממכתוותא, ed. מכבתותא דמישרי) from the waste parts of the valley; v. בָּתָא.

בְּתוּלָא, v. בְּתוּלְתָא.

בְּתוּלָה f. (b. h.; בתל, √בת, to separate; cmp. בתר; v. Ges. H. Dict. s. v.) [*retired, untouched,*] 1) *virgin.*—*Pl.* בְּתוּלוֹת. Tosef. Shebi. III, 14 sq. שלש ב׳ הן b'thulah is used in three ways, בְּתוּלַת אדם וכ׳ of a human being (virgin), of soil (unbroken), and of sycamores (untrimmed); Nidd. 8[b]; Y. ib. I, 49[a]. Yeb. 61[b] אין ב׳ אלא נערה under b'thulah (in a legal sense) a girl between twelve and twelve and a half years is meant, v. בַּגְרוּת. Ohol. XVI, 4 עד שמגיע . . . לב׳ until he reaches a rock or unbroken ground. Sabb. 90[a] בתולת הוורד a closed rose (Var. quot. in Ar., a. Ms. O. פְּתִילַת). Y. Sot. III, 19[a] ב׳ צריימנית an ascetic maid (retired from social pleasures); Sot. 22[a] ב׳ צליינית (צלויינית) a prayerful (bigoted) maid; a. fr.—2) (only in pl.) *the two posts supporting the beam in the wine-press* (Lat. gemelli, sorores). B. Bath. IV, 5 (67[b]), expl. בלונסות.—3) *Virgo,* sign of the Zodiac. Yalk. Ex. 418. Ib. I Kings 185. Pesik. R. s. 20.

בְּתוּלִין, בְּתוּלִים m. pl. (b. h.; preced.) *virginity, token* or *symptom of virginity.* טענת ב׳ suit of a husband against his young married wife concerning her virginity (Deut. XXII, 13 sq.). Keth. I, 1; a. fr.—Y. Yeb. VI, 7[c] top, a. e. כלו בְּתוּלֶיהָ the symptoms of virginity may have disappeared by absorption. Y. Nidd. 49[a] bot. בתולה לב׳ a b'thulah (virgin) as to virginity, opp. לדמים as to menstruation.

בְּתוּלִין ch. same. Targ. O. Deut. XXII, 14; a. e.—Y. Keth. I, 25[b] bot.; a. e.

בְּתוּלְתָא I, **בְּתוּלָא** ch.=h. בְּתוּלָה. Targ. Gen. XXIV, 16; a. fr.—*Pl.* בְּתוּלָן, בְּתוּלָתָן, בְּתוּלָתָא. Targ. Ps. CXLVIII, 12. Targ. Esth. II, 2. Targ. Lam. I, 15 (read:) וסאיב בְּתוּלָתָא.

בְּתוּלְתָא II f.=h. בְּתוּלִין. Targ. Lam. I, 15.

בִּתְיָה (b.h., I Chr. IV, 18) pr. n. f. *Bithiah*, daughter of Pharaoh; in legend, name of Moses' foster-mother. Lev. R. s. 1, a. e (as if בַּת יָהּ daughter of the Lord, pious). Snh. 31[b] לדודי ליה כבר ב׳ שלם salutation to him whose splendor is like that of the son of B. (Moses).

בְּתֵירָא, בְּתֵירָה, בְּתֵרָה pr. n. m. *B'therah;* 1) father of R. Judah of Netsibin. Yeb. 102[a]; Pes. 3[b]; a. fr.—2) בני ב׳ B'ne B., a scholarly family of Babylonian descent, much favored by Herod. Pes. 66[a]. B. Mets. 85[a] top.

בִּתְנַיָּא, v. בּוּתְנַיָּא.

בֶּתֶר m. h., or בִּתְרָ ch. (b. h.; בתר, √בת to cut, v. בְּתוּלָה) *piece, decree, allotment* (=גְּזֵירָה). Cant. R. to II, 17, v. אריהון a. סולא.—*Pl.* v. בְּתָרִים a. בִּתְרַיָּיא.

בָּתַר, בָּאתַר (= בָּאֲתַר, v. אֲתַר) *after, behind.* Dan. VII, 6; 7.—Targ. Gen. X, 32; a. fr.—With suff. (pl.) בַּתְרַי, בַּתְרָךְ, בַּתְרַאי &c. Targ. O. Ex. XXXIII, 23; a. fr.—Ber. 19[a] spoke (evil) ב׳ ערסי׳ דשמואל Ms. M. (ed. בַּתְרֵיה דמר שמואל, v. Rabb. D. S. a. l. note) of Mar Samuel's private life. Kidd. 71[b] זיל ב׳ שתיקותא follow the rule of silence; i. e. those of a peaceful nature are of pure descent. Pes. 84[a] ב׳ השתא אזלינן we are guided by the present status. Ab. Zar. 10[b] ליהוו למאן דבתרך וכ׳ let them (the presents) pass on to thy successors to be given to my successors that may come after thy death (as bribes to protect them). Y. Dem. II, 23[a] which (opinion of) R. Meïr? ההיא דתנינן לבתרה that opinion of R. M. which is taught below; a. fr.

בַּתְרָא, בַּתְרָאָה, בַּתְרַאי m. (preced.) *the last, latest.* Targ. Ex. IV, 8; a. fr.—Targ. Ps. LXXVIII, 4 בַּתְרַאי Ms. (ed. Vien. בתרי, oth. ed. בַּתְרָאֵי).—Gitt. 47[a] יומא ב׳ the gladiator's last day; a. fr.—בבא ב׳, v. בָּבָא.—*Pl.* בַּתְרָאֵי, בַּתְרָאִין. Targ. Gen. XXXIII, 2; a. e.—Naz. 56[b] קמאי וב׳ the first and the last of the quoted authorities, opp. מרצער.—Hull. 105[b] מיא ב׳=h. מים אחרונים, v. אַחֲרוֹן.—Fem. בַּתְרַיְיתָא, בַּתְרֵיתָא, בַּתְרַיְתָּא, בַּתְרִיתָא. Ab. Zar. 51[a]; a. fr.—בְּבַתְרֵיתָא *in the last place, last.* Targ. O. Deut. XIII, 10; a. e.

בְּתֵרָה, v. בְּתֵירָא.

בְּתָרְיָיא m. pl. ch.=next w. Targ. Y. II Lev. XXVI, 42.

בְּתָרִים m. pl. (v. בֶּתֶר) *pieces of the covenant-offerings.*—ברית בין הב׳ the covenant with Abraham (Gen. XV, 17—18). Cant. R. to II, 17; a. fr.

***בְּתַשׁ** (בת, v. בֶּתֶר) *to make incisions. Pa.* בַּתֵּשׁ with ב *to urge, beg persistently.* Hull. 7[b] הוה מְבַתֵּשׁ ביה טובא he begged him very persistently (to accept the invitation). Shebu. 30[b] בצורבא מרבנן מבתשינן בע״ה לא מבתשינן (Ms. M. מכ׳, with כ, Rashi with ב, v. to Hull. l. c.; ed. diff. vers.) a scholar is urged to sit down (in court), an ignorant man is not urged. [Ib. בטש ביה ואוקמיה לע״ה (read בת׳) he urged him (the scholar, to sit down) and made the ignorant man stand up; v. בְּטַשׁ as to vers.]

***בתת**, Targ. Job XXX, 7 בַּתְתִין Ms. Var. (ed. מִתְחַבְּרִין), read פַּתְתִין, v. פְּתַת.

ג

ג *Gimmel*, the third letter of the Alphabet. It interchanges with כ and ק; cmp. גשרא a. כשורא; גזז a. קצץ &c.; is related to ח, as גבב, חבב; v. letter ח.

ג prosthetic in foreign words before l, v. גלגטיקא, גלוסקא.

ג׳, as a numeral letter, *three*, v. א׳.

גָּאָא, v. גְּאֵי.

גָּאָה, v. גאי.

גֵּאֶה, גֵּיאֶה m. (b. h.; preced.) *lofty; ruler, lord; proud, haughty.* Pes. 113[b] דל ג׳ a proud pauper.—*Pl.* גֵּאִים, גֵּיאִים. Gen. R. s. 63 (ref. to גיים, Gen. XXV, 23) שני גֵיאֵי גוים וכ׳ two rulers of nations (Rome and Israel); Ber. 57[b]; Ab. Zar. 11[a] אל תקרי גוים אלא גֵּיִים read the word גיים not *goyim* (as the Masorah intimates) but *geyim* (lords); (Ms. M. a. Yalk. Gen. 110 גֵּאִים). Sifra B'hụck. Par. 2, ch. V (ref. to Lev. XXVI, 19) אלו הג׳ וכ׳ the 'pride of your power', those are the lordly (patrons) of whom Israel is proud. Cant. R. to III, 10 ארבע ג׳ הם גאה וכ׳ there are four majestic rulers (in the animal kingdom) the ruler among birds &c.; Ex. R. s. 23. Hag. 13[b] שמתגאה על הג׳ who is exalted (rules) over the rulers.—Y. Kidd. IV, end, 66[c]. רובן של עבדים ג׳ most slaves (when raised to power) are overbearing; Treat. Sof'rim XV, 10 נאים (corr. acc.); a. fr.—V. גֵּאִים.

גְּאַר, v. גֵּו ch.

גַּאֲוָה, גַּאֲווּה f. (b. h.; גאי) 1) *haughtiness, pride.* Y. Yoma VII, 44[b] מִפְּנֵי הג׳ to avoid the appearance of pride (on the Day of Atonement).—2) *glory.* Hag. 5[b] (ref. to גוה, Jer. XIII, 17) מפני גַּאֲוָותָן של וכ׳ over the glory of Israel that has been taken from him &c. Ib. מפני גַּאֲוָתָהּ של מלכות שמים over the (lost) glory of the heavenly kingdom (the destruction of the Temple).

גַּאֲוָזָא, v. גַּוְזָא I.

גְּאוּלָּה f. (b. h. גְּאֻלָּה; גאל) 1) *redemption, delivery.* Meg. 15[a], a. fr. מביא ג׳ לעולם causes redemption to come (through his good deeds). Cant. R. to II, 2 בגְאוּלַּת מחר of to-morrow's redemption, i. e. Messianic days.—Kidd. 15[b] גאולת עצמו redemption from service by himself, ג׳ קרובים by relatives, ג׳ אחרים by strangers (Lev. XXV, 47 sq.). Pes. 118[a] מן הג׳ than delivery (from evil); a. fr. [Lev. R. s. 32, end; Koh. R. to IV, 1, read גּוֹאֲלָה, v. גּוֹאֵל.]—*Pl.* גְּאוּלּוֹת. Y. Peah VII, 20[b] bot. שתי ג׳ two redemptions (of fruits).—2) *G'ullah*, a) that section of the prayers between the Sh'ma (שְׁמַע) and the T'fillah (תְּפִלָּה), so called from its contents. Ber. 9[b] סמך ג׳ לתפלה he recited the T'fillah immediately after closing the G'ullah (with the benediction גאל ישראל). Ib. 4[b]; a. fr.—b) *the seventh benediction of the T'fillah, prayer for redemption.* Meg. 17[b].

גְּאוּלְתָּא ch. same, *redemption.* Targ. Y. Num. XXV, 12.

גָּאוֹן m. (b. h.; גאי) *majesty, pride.* Sifra B'ḥuck. Par. 2, ch. V; v. גָּאָה. [In the post-Talmudic period *Gaon* (excellency) was the title of the chiefs of the Babylonian academies.—*Pl.* גְּאוֹנִים.—גְּאוֹנוּת *Gaonate.*]

גאוסטיני, Gen. R. s. 94, v. אָגוּסְטְיָאנִי.

גֵּיאוּתָא, גְּאוּתָא f. (גאי) 1) *haughtiness.* Targ. Prov. VIII, 13 (Ms. גֵּיאוּתָא).—2) *loftiness.* Targ. O. Ex. XV, 1; 21 Var., v. גֵּיוּתָא.

גְּאוּתְנָא, גְּאוּתָן, v. גֵּיוּת׳.

גָּאָה, גאי (b. h.; √גא, גג, גה *to rise; to be arched, caved*) *to rise, swell;* trnsf. *to be elated, proud; to be exalted, majestic.* Mekh. B'shall., Shirah 2, v. infra. [Tosef. M. Kat. I, 7 גּוֹאֶה, v. גָּהָה.]

Pi. גֵּאָה, גֵּיאָה *to exalt.* Mekh. l. c. גֵּאַנִי וגאתיו He (the Lord) exalted me, and I exalt him; Tanḥ. ib. 12 גֵּאֲנִי וגֵאִיתִיו; Yalk. Ex. 242 וגואותיו (corr. acc.). Y. Taan. III, 67[a] top (ref. to Job XXIII, 29) .... אני אמרתי להשפילן לגָאוֹתָן I (the Lord) decreed to humble them (by dearth), and thou--to raise them (Bab. ib. 23[a] הגבהתו).

Hithpa. הִתְגָּאָה, *Nithpa.* נִתְגָּאָה *to show one's self glorious, exalt one's self, be exalted;* (in an evil sense) *to be proud, boast, to lord it.* Mekh. l. c. (ref. to Ex. XV, 1) גָּאָה ועתיד לְהִתְגָּאוֹת He was glorious and will be &c. Ib. מִתְגָּאֶה הוא על כל המִתְגָּאִים He exalts himself above all those who are boastful, שֶׁבַּמֶּה שאו״ה מתג׳ לפניו וכ׳ for that with which the nations boast themselves, becomes the means of their punishment; Tanḥ. l. c.—Ḥag. 13[b], v. גָּאָה. Ib. 5[b] פרנס המתג׳ וכ׳ an officer who lords it over the community. B. Bath. 98[a] המתג׳ בטלית וכ׳ who parades the scholar's cloak. Tosef. Sot. III, 10 sq. לא נִתְגָּאוּ אלא וכ׳ became haughty only in consequence of the bounties &c.; Snh. 109[a]. Ber. 10[b] לאחר שאכל ושתה ונתג׳ זה Ms. M. (ed. לאחר שנתג׳; Yalk. Kings זה ונתג׳ . . . . . .; Lev. 616 לאחר שגאה) after this man has eaten and drunk and become haughty, v. גֵּאִים. Lev. R. s. 10 נתג׳ לבו עליו (Ex. R. s. 37 וזהה דעתו) became overbearing.

גְּאָא, גְּאַר ch. same; *to rise, grow* &c. Targ. I Sam. II, 5 גְּאַן (some ed. גְּגַן).

Ithpa. אִיתְגָּאַר, אִיתְגָּאֵי 1) *to grow high.* Targ. Job VIII, 11 (h. text יִגְאֶה).—2) *to be exalted; to be proud.* Targ. Ex. XV, 1; 21. Targ. Y. II Gen. XXXIV, 31 (I מִלַּגְלֵג); a. e.

גֵּאָיוֹת pl. of. גַּיְא.

גָּאָז, v. גּוּז.

גָּאִים, v. גּוּם a. גַּמַּם.

גֵּאִים m. pl. (abstract noun, v. גְּאָה; cmp. חַיִּים) *loftiness, excellence;* (in a bad sense) *haughtiness.* Hull. 92[a] (play on שָׂרִיגִים, Gen. XL, 10) שלשה שרי ג׳ בכל וכ׳ the three princes of excellence (influential patrons of Israel) in every generation (in Palestine under the Roman, in Babylon under the Parthian government).—Ber. 10[b]; Yalk. Lev. 616 (ref. to I Kings XIV, 9) א״ת גֵּוֶךָ אלא גֵּאֶיךָ read not *gavvekha* (thy body), but *geekha*, thy swelling or pride (applied to taking a meal before prayer), v. גָּאָה.

גָּאַל (b. h.) [*to cover,* cmp. Job III, 4;] *to ransom, redeem, protect.* Pes. X, 6 גְּאָלָנוּ וג׳ וכ׳ has protected us and redeemed our ancestors. Gen. R. s. 78, beg.; Midr. Till. to Ps. XXV, beg.; Lam. R. to III, 23 אמונתך רבה לְגָאֳלֵנוּ thy faith is great enough to redeem us. Gen. R. s. 44.—Kidd. 20[b] לוה וגואל וגוֹאֵל לחצאין he may borrow money and redeem his property (from the sanctuary), and may redeem in instalments. Midr. Till. to Ps. XXXI, beg. גְּאַל אותנו redeem us; a. fr.—V. גּוֹאֵל.

Nif. נִגְאַל *to be redeemed.* Ber. 9[a] כְּשֶׁנִּגְאֲלוּ ישראל וכ׳ when the Israelites were redeemed from Epypt. Kidd. 15[b] (ref. to Lev. XXV, 54) באלה הוא נ׳ וכ׳ through those (his relations) he may be redeemed, but he is not freed after six years of service (Ex. XXI, 2). Ib. 20[b] when the jubilee year arrives ולא נִגְאֲלָה and it (the field) has not been redeemed. Ib. יפה כחו לִיגָּאֵל מיד it has the privilege of immediate redemption. Sabb. 118[b] מיד נִגְאָלִין they would be released (from captivity) at once. Y. Taan. II, 65[d] top וסופן לְהִיגָּאֵל וכ׳ and they will be released &c.; Gen. R. s. 56 לִיגָּאֵל; a. fr.—[In b. h. ג׳ also: *to cover* (with blood), *stain, make repulsive.*]. V. געל.

גְּאַל ch. same.—Part. גָּאֵל, גָּאִיל. Targ. O. Num. XXXV, 12; 19; 21, a. e. ג׳ דמא, v. גּוֹאֵל.

גאלה, Y. Hall. I, 57[d] מלו ג׳, v. מְלִיגָאלָה.

גָּאלֵי, v. גַּלֵּי.

גאלקי, v. גּוּאלְקָא.

גָּאַם, v. גַּם II.

***גְּאַם** = גְּמָא *to swallow.* *Pa.* גַּאֵם *to make swallow.* Hull. 111[a] גַּאֲמוֹ לשבא make (the son of) Sh'ba swallow it (Rashi). [Ar. reads גַּמּוֹ (contr. Pa. of געם or גאם, cmp. Syriac געם P. Sm. 761 sq.) it made (the son of) Sh. feel nauseous (which was his reason for not eating it.]

גָּאנֵי, v. גְּנֵי.

גַּב, v. גַּבָּא.

גַּב, v. גּוּבָא.

גַּב m. (b. h.; גבב) *convex, arched,* whence 1) *the exterior* or *upper part* of a thing, a) *body,* esp. *back* (of an animal's body, usu. אָחוֹר). Gen. R. s. 8, beg. he split the double-faced body (v. פרצוף) ועשאו גַּבַּיִים ג׳ לכאן וכ׳ and gave it two backs, one back on this side &c. —גַּב יָד, גַּב רֶגֶל *a swelling* on the hand, on the foot. Ab. Zar. 28ᵃ; Sabb. 109ᵃ.—b) *eye-brow* (b. h.), *the elevation around genitals* &c. Nidd. 52ᵇ א׳ בגַבָּהּ one hair on the lower surrounding of her genitals, opp. בכריסה, v. כֶּרֶס; B. Bath. 56ᵇ; Snh. 30ᵇ; B. Kam. 70ᵇ, [Rashi: on her finger joints].—c) (also גַּבָּה) גַּבַּת הַזָּקָן, pl. גַּבּוֹת, *chin.* Nidd. 23ᵇ; Y. ib. III, 50ᶜ bot. גומות הזקן (dimples).—*d) *a low fence.* Tosef. B. Mets. XI, 22 (ed. Zuck. גַּג).—*Du.* גַּבַּיִים, גַּבַּיִין. Kel. XXV, 5 outsides of vessels (usu. אֲחוֹרַיִים). Gen. R. s. 8, v. supra.—*Pl.* גַּבִּים, גַּבִּין, גַּבּוֹת. Bekh. VII, 2 שני ג׳ וכ׳ double back and double spine (explain. גִּבֵּן, Lev. XXI, 20); Nidd. 24ᵃ sq.; Ḥull. 60ᵇ.—Nidd. 23ᵇ ג׳ הזקן, v. supra.—עַל גַּבֵּי, עַל גַּב (abbr. ע״ג) *on, upon, by the side of* (cmp. עַל in b. h.). Ḥull. 3ᵃ, a. fr. עומד על גַּבָּיו standing by him, superintending. Nidd. 66ᵃ על גב הנהר by the river-side; Makhsh. I, 4 (v. גִּיף). Succ. IV, 4 על גב ארצטבא (Talm. ed. 42ᵇ גבי), v. אִיסְטְבָא.—Trnsf. *on the basis, on the principle.* אַף עַל גַּב, v. אַף I.—Y. Ḥag. II, 78ᵇ bot. חולין שנעשו על גב הקדש (usu. על טהרת הקדש) layman's food prepared on the principles of sacred food (as though it were sacred food). Bets. II, 3 (17ᵇ); Tosef. ib. II, 7 מטבילין מגב לגב you may (on a Holy Day) immerse vessels for the purpose of changing their use (literally: from principle to principle, from one על גב to another); expl. ibid. רצה לעשות גיתו ע״ג בדו ובדו ע״ג עיסתו הרי זה וכ׳ if one desires to work his wine press on the basis of his olive press, i. e. with vessels originally immersed for the use of the olive press, or his olive press on the basis of his dough, i. e. with vessels originally immersed to be used for kneading, he may immerse his vessels on the same day; Bets. 19ᵃ ע״ג בדו ובדו ע״ג גיתו עושה .... Ms. M. a. Ar. (ed. incorr. כדו) if one wishes to change &c., he might have done so (even without another immersion and, therefore, may re-immerse his vessels on the Holy Day because he does not thereby create a new status).—Cmp. אַגַּב.—Tosef. Sabb. XII (XIII), 1; Y. ib. XIII, 14ᵃ top ע״ג הגס וכ׳ around, or adding to the border of a web &c.; Bab. ib. 105ᵃ על הגס. Hor. III, 3 אין על גַּבָּיו אלא וכ׳ none over him save the Lord his God.—בְּגַב *in the back, behind.* Y. Keth. XII, 35ᵇ top דברים בגב (Bab. 111ᵃ בגו) there is something behind, i. e. there is a reason for it.—Cmp. גַּף.

גַּבָּא, גַּב ch. same; 1) *back, body* &c. Targ. Y. II Ex. II, 3 ג׳ נהרא river-side (Y. I גִּיף). Targ. Job XIII, 12 גב טינא a body (lump) of clay.—Ḥull. 47ᵇ אגבא on top, opp. מגואי inside, below. Sabb. 109ᵃ אג׳ דכרעיה on his foot. Yoma 78ᵃ ג׳ דכרעא הוה it was the back (dórsum) of the foot, cmp. preced. גב רגל; a. fr.—*Pl.* גַּבִּין, גַּבֵּי. Targ. Y. Gen. XXXI, 10; a. e.—[גבירה. Gen. R. s. 8, some ed., read גברים, v. preced.].—עַל גַּבֵּי, עַל גַּב as preced. Targ. II Chr. XXI, 3 ע״ג קרקע, v. אַגַּב. Targ. Y. II Lev. I, 17; a. e.—ע״ג ידא upon one's hand; כע״ג ר׳ (כִּיד ,כד) as upon one's hand, i. e. exposed to danger. Targ. Job. XIII, 14; a. fr.—Also ellipt. כעל גב. Targ. Jud. IX, 17; a. e.—2) (prep.) גַּבֵּי, גַּב *towards, with* &c. Targ. Y. II Num. XXI, 9.—With suffix of pers. pron. Targ. Job XIX, 4; a. fr.—Gen. R. s. 33 יתיב גַּבֵּיה he sat with him. Ib. גַּבְכוֹן in your country. Y. Ned. VI, 40ᵃ sent letters גבי ר׳ יצחק through R. &c. Ib. גַּבָּן (thus we read) in our country. Ber. 10ᵃ ליתי...גַּבָּאֵר let Ezekiel come to me. Gen. R. s. 35 מן גַּבֵּיה ועד גַּבֵּי from those with him &c., from his generation to mine.—Bets. 25ᵇ זיל לגבי דר׳ וכ׳ go to see R. &c.; a. v. fr.

גֶּבָא, גֵּב (גֶּבִי) m. (b. h.; גבי, גבב) *cavity for collecting water, pond, cistern.* Tosef. Mikv. I, 1 המים שבגבא R. S. to Mikv. I, 1 (ed. Zuck. שבגבו, read שבגֶּבִי) the water in the pond. Ib. 3 גבי.—*Pl.* גֶּבָאִים, גֶּבִין, גֶּבִים, גֶּבָאִין, גֶּבָיִים. Cant. R. to I, 2 (ref. to ישקני ib.) יטהרני כאדם שהוא מישק שני ג׳ וכ׳ may He make me pure, as a man levels the surface of two ponds (by which the unclean one is purified). Snh. 94ᵇ. M. Kat. 25ᵇ מי ג׳ stagnant waters, opp. נחל שוטף. Mikv. I, 1. Y. M. Kat. I, 80ᵃ bot.; Tosef. Mikv. I, 13 כמין גבאין ed. Zuck. (read כְּמֵי).

גַּבָּא, v. גּוּבָא.

גְּבָא *to collect,* v. גְּבִי.

גַּבָּאָה, v. גַּבָּיָה.

גַּבָּאוֹת, v. גַּבָּיוֹת.

גַּבַּאי, v. גַּבָּי.

גָּבַב (√גב *to arch, cave, curve;* cmp. √גף, כף &c.) *to curve.* *Pes. 42ᵃ bot. three things ... גּוֹבְבִין את הקומה Ar. (ed. כופפין; Erub. 55ᵇ bot. ed. Sonc. גופפין) curve the erect stature (make man's back high).

Pi. גִּיבֵּב *to heap up, pile,* esp. *to gather twigs, straw* &c.; *to rake.* Shebi. IX, 6 הַמְגַבֵּב ביבש he who gathers dry plants, leaves &c., (opp. מלקט, of green plants). Bets. IV, 6. B. Kam. 101ᵇ; Succ. 40ᵃ גִּיבְּבָן, v. חוֹבָה II. Y. Yeb. VIII, 8ᵈ bot.; a. fr.—Trnsf. (with or sub. דברים) *to pick up frivolous arguments.* Yoma 76ᵃ עד מתי אתה מְגַבֵּב דברים ומביא עלינו (Ms. a. Ar. omit דברים) how long wilt thou rake words together and bring them up against us (i. e. what authority have you for your assertion)?; Sifra Vayikra, N'dab. ch. IV, Par. 4 מגבב ומביא ... (Mekh. B'shall., Vayas. 3 מתמה).

גְּבַב ch., *Pa.* גַּבֵּב same, *to rake, collect.* Targ. Ex. V, 7 וִיגַבְּבוּן ed. Berl. (ed. וִיגַבְּבוּן, Regia וִיגַבְּבוּן; h. text קשש); ib. 12 לְגַבָּבָא ed. Berl. Targ. Ps. CIX, 11 (h. text ינקש); a. fr.—Targ. Prov. VIII, 10 גַּבּוּ לכון וכ׳ hoard ye unto yourselves knowledge. Ib. XXV, 4 גַּבּוּ rake ye out (remove; h. text הגו). Targ. Is. XLVI, 6 גָּבַן וכ׳ they rake together gold (h. text זלים).—Lam. R. to I, 1 רבתי (1 חד כות׳) ההוא גברא מְגַבֵּב כובין וכ׳ this man (thou) will be a gatherer of thorns and when he brings them, all people will run away from him; [Y. Maas. Sh. IV, 55ᵇ bot., v. אִיזָא].

גְּבָבָא m. (preced.) *rakings*, v. next w. ג׳ דעמרא *a ball of clipped wool.* B. Bath. 74ᵃ; Snh. 110ᵃ; Num. R. s. 18. Ber. 9ᵇ בין ג׳ דע׳ חיורא between a lump of white wool &c. Ib. 8ᵃ, v. חִיזְרָא I —*Pl.* גְּבָבֵי. Gitt. 68ᵃ.

גְּבָבָא, v. גִּיבְבָא.

גְּבָבַאי, v. גּוֹבַיָא.

גְּבָבָה f. (גבב) *rakings, small stubble, straw* &c., used as fuel. Sabb. III, 1 sq., Y. ed. (Mish. a. Bab. ed. גְּבָבָא Chald.). Y. ib. III, 5ᶜ bot., Bab. ib. 36ᵇ. Kel. XVII, 1 של בלנין בג׳ the vessels of the bathers cease to be susceptible of levitical uncleanness, when they are so defective as to let small fuel drop out. Par. IV, 3; a. fr.

גְּבָבַיָא, גְּבָבָאֵי, גְּבָבַיֵּי, גְּבָבָיָא, v. גּוֹבַיָא.

גַּבָּה f., v. גַּב.

גָּבָה, v. גבי.

גָּבַהּ, גְּבַהּ, גָּבֵהַּ, גְּבַהּ, v. גּוֹבַה, גְּבוֹהַּ.

גָּבַהּ (b.h.; v. גבב; cmp. גאה) *to be high; to be elated.* Meg. 15ᵃ ג׳ חמן וכ׳ (Var. ג׳ לבו של חמן) Haman is haughtier than Ahasver (he dared what Ah. did not venture); Yalk. Esth. 1056.—Sot. 5ᵃ ולא ג׳ הר סיני למעלה and Mount Sinai did not rise higher (grow proud).

Hif. הִגְבִּיהַּ 1) *to raise, elevate; to make elated.* Taan. 23ᵃ a generation which was to be humbled הִגְבַּהְתּוֹ בתפלתך hast thou lifted up through thy prayer, v. גְּאָה.—Erub. 55ᵃ מי שמַגְבִּיהַּ דעתו עליו כשמים Ms. M. (ed. עליה, ed. Sonc. מגב׳ עצמו כשמ׳; v. Rabb. D. S. a. l.; Yalk. Deut. 940 שמגיס דעתו) who exalts his mind in himself as high as the heavens (who considers himself very wise, ed. who considers himself on account of his knowledge of it as high &c.). Ib. 13ᵇ him who lowers himself חק״בה מַגְבִּיהוֹ the Lord will raise, וכל המגביה עצמו וכ׳ and whomsoever exalts himself, the Lord will lower; ib. 54ᵃ; Ned. 55ᵃ. Tanh. Ki Thissa 14 מַגְבִּיהִים פניהם lifted their faces up; a. fr.—Hall. III, 1 מַגְבַּהַת חלתה she lifts up (dedicates) the priest's share; v., however, גָּבַהּ.—2) *to take up* a lost object in order to take possession of it. B. Mets. 8ᵃ המגביה מציאה לחבירו וכ׳ if one takes up an object in behalf of his neighbor; ib. 10ᵃ; Bets. 39ᵇ; a. fr.

Hof. הוּגְבַּהּ *to be raised.* Sot. 47ᵇ שפלים הוּגְבְּהוּ the low have been raised. Tanh. Ki Thissa 5; Lev. R. s. 8 בלשון זה ה׳ with the word *zeh* (Lev. VI, 13) has he (Aaron) been raised.—*Part.* מוּגְבָּה, f. מוּגְבַּהַת. Y. Shebu. I, 32ᵈ bot. what means שְׂאֵת (Lev. XIII, 2) מוגבחת a raised spot (Sifra Thazr., Neg. ch. 1 מובחקת, corr. acc.).

Hithpa. הִתְגַּבֵּהַּ, *Nithpa.* נִתְגַּבֵּהַּ *to be elated, boastful.* Tanh. Huck. 1 התחיל מִתְגַּבֵּהַּ והולך he beame more and more overbearing (Tanh. ed. Bub. ib.; Num. R. s. 18 מתגבר). Num. R. s. 6, beg. נִתְגַּבְּהוּ בעצמם they were proud of their own selves.

גְּבַהּ, גְּבִיהַּ ch. same, *to be high, elated.* Targ. Ps. CXXXI, 1.—Sabb. 67ᵃ גְּבִיהַּת מכל וכ׳ thou art higher than all other trees. Meg. 15ᵃ ג׳ מלכא וכ׳ Ms. M. (ed. גבר) the King on high is higher than the king below. Hull. 7ᵇ ג׳ טורא וכ׳ a mountain rose between them (separating them). [Y. Ter. X, 47ᵇ bot. גביה מן דאבחתיה, Tosaf. to Hull. 64ᵇ גמיר.]

Af. אַגְבַּהּ 1) *to raise.* Targ. II Chr. XXXIII. 14.—2) *to take up.* Succ. 44ᵇ אַגְבְּהֵיה וכ׳ he took it (the festive wreath) up once as such and a second time for the willow branches thereon. B. Mets. 2ᵇ בהדי הדדי אַגְבְּהוּהָ they took the lost object up at the same time. Ib. 8ᵃ; a. fr.

Ithpa. אִתְגַּבַּהּ, *Ithpe.* אִתְגְּבַהּ 1) *to be high; to grow proud.* Targ. Job XXXV, 5. Targ. Koh. I, 12.—2) *to rise.* Targ. Job XXXIX, 27; a. e.—Hull. 141ᵇ sq. דלִיתְגַּבְּהוּ that the young birds may rise (when frightened).

גַּבְהוּת f. (b. h.; preced.) *height, excellence; pride, haughtiness.* Ber. 10ᵇ (ref. to Ps. CXXX, 1) אין ג׳ לפני וכ׳ there must be no hight (elevated stand during prayer) before the Lord. Esth. R. to IV, 15 מִגַּ׳ לב from haughtiness.—Tanh. Ki Thissa 27 גַּבְהוּתוֹ של עולם the hight of the world, i. e. the Most High.

גַּבְהוּתָא ch. same. Targ. II Chr. XXXII, 26.

גָּבוֹהַּ m. (b. h.; preced. ws.), constr. גְּבַהּ 1) *high, exalted, elevated* &c. Sot. 5ᵃ among men ג׳ רואה את הַגָּ׳ וכ׳ a high person looks up to a higher one, but ignores the lower one. Gen. R. s. 22 (ref. to Ps. XXXII, 1) happy is he שהוא ג׳ מפשעו וכ׳ who is higher than (who controls) his sin, and whose sin is not higher than himself; a. fr.—Snh. 5ᵇ (in Chald. diction) אבוה ... גְּבַהּ עינים הוה this man's (my) father was ambitious.—*Fem.* גְּבוֹהָה. Ab. V, 19 רוח ג׳ *haughtiness*, opp. נמוכה.—*Pl.* גְּבוֹהִים, f. גְּבוֹהוֹת. Esth. R. to IV, 7 הג׳ חושפלו the high were lowered.—Y. Shebi. VI, 36ᶜ top עיניו ... הוו ג׳ my father was ambitious, v. supra.—Esp. הַגָּבוֹהַּ *the Most High.* Y. Snh. VII, 25ᵇ top; ib.ᶜ top ג׳(ה) בעבודתה בעבודת with a service peculiar to it (that idol), or with a service prescribed for the worship of the Lord; Y. Naz. VI, beg. 54ᶜ למלאכת הג׳ referring to a service prescribed for the worship of the Lord (but applied to an idol).—Y. Ned. I, 37ᵃ top; Y. Naz. I, beg. 51ᵃ לשון ג׳ הוא it is an expression alluding to Divinity, v. חֵרֶס.—לַגָּ׳ *for the Lord, on the altar.* Pes. 3ᵇ אליה לג׳ סלקא the fat-tail is offered on the altar; a. fr.—2) *an abnormally tall and slim person with shaking gait.* Bekh. 45ᵇ (explain. כיפח קפח, Mish.) גבוה ed. (Ar. גְּבַהּ).—Fem. גְּבוֹהִית. Ib. (Ar. גְּבַהַת).

גְּבוֹוִין, v. גְּבִיר.

גְּבוּל I (b. h.; גבל) [*heap, mound,*] 1) *landmark, boundary; limit; qualification.* B. Bath. 69ᵇ (ref. to Gen. XXIII, 17) מי שצריך לג׳ סביב such trees as require boundaries (small trees, are included in the sale). Ab. Zar. 24ᵇ ג׳ יש לה this assertion (לוקחין מהן בהמה לקרבן, ib. 23ᵇ) must be qualified. Y. Hall. I, 57ᵇ top (ref. to Is. XXVIII, 25) ע״כ גְּבוּלוֹ של לחם so far goes the definition of bread, i. e. only these species can be called *lehem.*—

2) (in gen.) *country*, contrad. to the sanctuary (מִקְדָּשׁ) and Jerusalem. Keth. 24ᵇ, a. fr. קדשי הג׳ the sacred gifts (T'rumah &c.) set apart and consumed outside of the Temple and Jerusalem.—*Pl.* גְּבוּלִין, גְּבוּלִים. B. Bath. 56ᵃ עיירות העומדות על הג׳ border-towns.—Shek. VII, 3 נמצא בג׳ if found outside of Jerusalem. R. Hash. 30ᵃ; a. fr.—V. גּוֹבַל.

*גְּבוּל II pr. n. *G'bul* (High-land), cmp. גַּבְלָא. Sot. IX, 15; Snh. 97ᵃ אנשי (ה)ג׳ (Ms. M. Snh., a. Cant. R. to II, 13 גָּלִיל).

גְּבוּלָאָה, גְּבוּלָיָיא m. (v. preced.) *of G'bul.* Koh. R. to I, 4 ר׳ יעקב ג׳ (ed. Wil. גְּבוּלָאָה h. form); Y. Hall. III, 59ᵃ ר׳ ר׳ גבולייא; Y. Kidd. IV, 66ᵃ top; Y. Yeb. VIII, 9ᵇ גַּבְלָיָא of Gabla.

גבונתא, Y. Ter. X, 47ᵇ, read זְבִינְתָא.

גִּבּוֹר m. (b. h.; גבר) *strong, brave, mighty; hero.* Ned. 38ᵃ על ג׳ on a strong man; Sabb. 92ᵃ. Ab. IV, 1 איזהו ג׳ who is a hero?; Tam. 32ᵃ; a. fr.—*Pl.* גִּבּוֹרִים. Gen. R. s. 37 פלשתים ג׳ *Philisteans* which means giants, opp. ננסים. Sot. 42ᵇ ד׳ ג׳ four (Philistean) heroes; a. e.

כפר ג׳ חיל, גבור, Meg. 18ᵃ, v. גְּבוּר.

גְּבוּרָא, v. גְּבוּרְתָא.

גְּבוּרָה f. (b. h.; גבר) 1) *superiority, strength, might.* Yoma 69ᵇ זו היא גְבוּרָתוֹ Ms. M. (ed. גְּבוּרַת גבורתו) in this His strength consists (in His long-suffering). Kidd. 49ᵇ י׳ קבים ג׳ וכ׳ ten measures of bravery have come down into the world, nine of which the Persians have taken; Esth. R. to I, 3. Num. R. s. 10 (allud. to Koh. X, 17 a. Is. V, 22) ג׳ של תורה וכ׳ the strength (acquired by the study) of the Law consists in 'happy', the strength of wine in 'woe'; a. fr.—2) הַג׳ *Divine Majesty, the Lord.* Sabb. 87ᵃ. Ib. 88ᵇ, a. fr. מפי הג׳ from the mouth of the Lord.—3) *high age*, v. infra.—*Pl.* גְּבוּרוֹת 1) *manifestations of Divine power, wonders.* Yoma l. c. איה גְבוּרוֹתָיו where are the evidences of His power (that we should call Him גבור)?—2) *G'buroth*, the second section of the T'fillah (v. אָבוֹת), praising the powers of the Lord, also called תְּחִיַּית הַמֵּתִים. Y. Ber. IV, end, 8ᶜ this is the order &c. אבות וג׳ וכ׳ Aboth, G'buroth, and Kiddush hash-Shem (K'dushah).—ג׳ גְּשָׁמִים *the power of rain*, a clause praising the Lord for giving rains, inserted in *G'buroth.* Ber. V, 2 מזכירין ג׳ גש׳ we mention 'the power of rain', i. e. insert the clause, in '*the Resurrection*', contrad. to the prayer for rain (שְׁאֵלָה). Taan. 2ᵃ מאי ג׳ גש׳ וכ׳ why is it named *G'buroth G'shamim?* Ans. מפני שיורדין בגבורה because the rains come down through (God's) wonderful power (ref. to Job. V, 9—10).—3) (allusion to Ps. XC, 10) *the age of eighty.* M. Kat. 28ᵃ שמונים ג׳ (Ms. M. גבורה) 'eighty years' is called g'buroth (g'burah). Treat. S'mahoth III, 8 מיתה של גבורה (Y. Bicc. II, 64ᶜ bot. של זקנה) a death of g'burah (at a high age); Ab. V, 21 בן שמנים לגבורה. M. Kat l. c. הגיע לג׳ if one has reached the age of eighty.

כפר ג׳, גבוריא, Meg. 18ᵃ, v. גְּבוּרְיָא.

גְּבוּרְתָא, גְּבוּרָא, גְּבָרוּתָא, גִּיבָ׳ ch.=h. גְּבוּרָה. Targ. II Chron. X, 10. Targ. Jud. XI, 29 גבורא (ed. Vien. ה....). Targ. Jer. X, 6; a. fr.—*Pl.* גְּבוּרָן, גְּבוּרָתָא, גְּבָרְוָתָא, גִּיבָ׳. Targ. Ps. XX, 7.—Targ. I Chr. XI, 19 (Var. גְּבוּרָאתָא). Targ. Deut. III, 24 (Var. O. גְּבוּרְוָתָךְ, v. Berl. Targ. O. II, 50; ed. Amst. גְּבַרְתָּךְ); a. fr.—Targ. O. ib. XXXIII, 29 גִּיבָּרְוָתָךְ thy mighty deeds (h. text גאותך).

גָּבוּשׁ m. (גבש) *pile of stones. Pl.* גְּבוּשִׁים. Tosef. Ohol. XVII, 9, v. גָּבַשׁ.

גְּבוֹת pr. n. pl., v. גַּבַּת.

גִּבֵּחַ, גִּיבֵּחַ m., **גַּבַּחַת, גִּיבָ׳** f. (גבח=גבה) *high, tall and slim.* Bekh. 45ᵇ Ar., v. גָּבוֹהַּ 2. [In b. h.: *with high forehead, bald in front.*]

גָּבַח; *Pi.* גִּבֵּחַ (v. preced. end) *to shave a bald-pate.* Tosef. Sabb. VI (VII), 1 הַמְגַבֵּחַ, v. גּוּדְגְּדִין.

גְּבַחַת, v. גִּבֵּחַ.

גַּבַּחַת f. (b. h. גבח) 1) *high forehead; baldness in front.* Hull. 65ᵇ חָגָב ואין לו ג׳ a species of locusts which occasionally appear, having no long-stretched heads (=ראשו ארוך ib.); [Ar.: *a protuberance on the back, hump*]. Neg. X, 10 הג׳ a leprous affection on the front of the head (making it bald). Ib. איזו היא ג׳ מן הקדקד וכ׳ which portion of the head is called *gabbahath?* From the crown sliding down forward to where the hair begins on the forehead; Sifra Thazr. Par. 5. ch. X. Tosef. Neg. IV, 11; a. fr.—2) *the front* or *outside of cloth; the nap of new cloth*, opp. קרחת. Sifra l. c. ch. XV בְּגַבַּחְתּוֹ אלו חדשים b'gabbahto (Lev. XIII, 55) means new cloths (v. Targ. O. a. l.).

גבטלא, v. אַנְגְּבִילָא.

גְּבִי, v. גַּבָּא.

גָּבָה, גבי (√גב, v. גבב) *to collect* a bill, taxes &c.; *to make one's self paid, to seize.* Keth. 90ᵃ, a. fr. if a later creditor (second mortgagee) שקדם וג׳ מה שג׳ וכ׳ collected first, what he has collected is his own. B. Mets. 13ᵇ גּוֹבֶה מנכסים ב״ח he may make himself paid of unmortgaged property. Keth. V, 1 גּוֹבָה את הכל she is entitled to the whole amount; a. v. fr.—Lev. R. s. 11 the king sent a treasury officer לִגְבּוֹת to collect (the delinquent taxes); Gen. R. s. 42 לִגְבוֹתָהּ; Tanh. Sh'mini 9. [Lev. R. l. c. וחכו גבור אותו, read וחכו, cmp. Gen. R. l. c.] Ex. R. s. 30 מי ג׳ חירמני חדם וכ׳ who collected from him (punished him for) the blood on his hand? לא ישראל גָּבוּ אותו וכ׳ not the Israelites collected it, but the Gibeonites did.—Gen. R. s. 85; s. 92 end מצא ב״ח מקום לגבות וכ׳ the creditor met with a chance to collect his bill, i. e. the Lord takes this occasion to visit our sins; a. fr.—Part. pass. גָּבוּי *collected, seized.* B. Mets. 58ᵃ על הַגָּ׳ counting on the Shekel contributions collected (though not yet delivered in the Temple treasury); Keth. 108ᵃ; Y. Shek. II, beg. 46ᶜ. Shebu. 48ᵇ, a. fr. כג׳ דמי is considered as if collected (in the possession of the creditor); a. fr.

Nif. נִגְבָּה 1) *to be collected, to be collectible.* B. Mets. l. c. על העתיד לִגָּבוֹת; Y. Shek. l. c. לְחִיגָּבוֹת on what is yet to be collected. Peah VIII, 7 חקופה נִגְבֵּית בשנים the charity fund must be collected by two persons; B. Bath. 8ᵇ; Snh. 17ᵇ; a. fr.—2) *to be collected from, be taxed.* Pesik. R. s. 10 לא היו נִיגְּבִים וכ׳ they were not highly taxed; a. fr.

Hif. הִגְבָּה *to cause to be collected.* Hall. III, 1 מַגְבַּהַת חלתה she orders the priest's gift to be collected; v., however, גָּבַהּ. Gitt. 35ᵇ הַגְבּוּהָ את השאר help her to collect the balance. [Tosef. Sabb. VI (VII), 1 מגבה, v. גָּבַת.]—*Part. pass. fem.* מוּגְבָּה *collected fund.* Tanh. Emor 18.

גְּבָא, גְּבִי ch. same; [1) *to rake,* v. גְּבַב.]—2) *to collect, tax.* Targ. O. Deut. XXII, 19 (h. text ענש). Targ. Koh. VIII, 14; a. e.—Part. act. a. pass. גָּבֵי. Targ. Hos. VIII, 6 (some ed. incorr. גַּבֵּי, v. Rashi a. l.).—B. Mets. 12ᵇ נירחו דלא גָבֵי ... מִגְבָא גָבֵי though it cannot be collected from mortgaged, it may be collected from unencumbered property. Y. Gitt. I, end, 43ᵈ נחתון מִיגְבֵי וכ׳ they went down (to Babylonia) to collect debts there for friends; Y. Kidd. III, 64ᵃ לגביה (read לְמִיגְבֵי); cmp. Gitt. 14ᵇ.—B. Mets. 17ᵇ גָּבְיָא she has a right to collect (seize); a. fr.

Af. אַגְבֵּי as preced. Hif., *to confiscate, fine.* Targ. Am. IV, 5. Targ. Hos. VIII, 13 (some ed. מְגַבַּן Part. pass. Pa.).—Targ. Koh. XI, 4 לא מגבי אגר makes not (people) derive any gain.—B. Kam. 98ᵇ; Keth. 86ᵃ מַגְבֵּי ביה makes him pay. Ib. א׳ ביה כי וכ׳ made him pay the full amount, v. כַּשּׁוּרָא. Shebu. 48ᵇ אַגְבּוּיֵי מַגְבִּינָן ביה we do not order collection on such a bill. [Nidd. 65ᵇ מגבר בה, v. גִּיב a. גִּיתָ.]

Ithpe. אִתְגְּבֵי *to be taxed, fined.* Targ. O. Ex. XXI, 22.

גבי, Y. Succ. V, 55ᵇ bot., v. גְּבִינִי II.

גַּבְיָא I m. (גבי) *collected, hoarded.* Targ. Prov. VIII, 19 סימא סגיא ג׳ ed. Lag., (h. text כסף נבחר) hoarded treasure; XVI, 16.—V. גְּבִי.

***גַּבְיָא II** m. (v. גְּבוֹהַּ a. גִּבֵּחַ) *tall and slim.* Targ. Y. Lev. XXII, 22 דג׳ או דנסיס Ar. (ed. differ. vers., h. text חרוץ או יבלת) extremely tall or of stinted growth; v. גְּבִיחַ. [The vers. of Ar. obviously belonged to Lev. XXI, 20.]

גַּבְיָא III, ג׳ גילא, v. מַגַּבְיָא.

גְּבִיהַּ m. ch.=h. גָּבוֹהַּ (v. גָּבַהּ). Targ. Ps. CXIII, 5 (Var. גְּבִיהַּ).—*Pl.* גְּבִיהִין. Ib. CIII, 11. [Y. Ter. X, 47ᵇ bot., v. גָּבַהּ.]

גְּבִיהָה, גְּבִיהָא pr. n. m. *G'biha.* Snh. 91ᵃ ed. (Ar. גְּבִיפָא).—Ab. Zar. 22ᵃ.

גַּבָּאוּת, גַּבָּיוּת f. (גבי) *collectorship, office of* גַּבַּאי. Y. Dem. II, 23ᵃ top יצא מִגַּבָּיוּתוֹ (not מגביתו); Tosef. ib. III, 4 פירש מגביותו (ed. Zuck. ...ייתו, some ed. מִגַּבָּאוּתוֹ) as soon as he has resigned his office as (Roman) tax-collector.

גַּבָּיוּתָא ch. same. Snh. 25ᵇ עבד ג׳ occupied the collector's office.

גִּבִּיחַ m. ch.=h. גִּבֵּחַ, *extremely tall.* Targ. Y. II Lev. XXI, 20 (second vers. for h. text גִּבֵּן; Var. in Ar. גְּבִיע (not גביני), v. Koh. Ar. Compl. s. v. גבן II, p. 227ᵃ); v. גַּבְיָא II.

גַּבַּאי, גַּבָּיי m. (גבי) *collector* of taxes or charities, *treasurer, manager.* Ned. 65ᵇ when one is reduced to poverty, אינו נופל לידי ג׳ תחלה he does not at once fall into the hands of the public almoner (but is taken care of by his friends). Y. Dem. II, 23ᵃ top; Tosef. ib. III, 4 חבר שנעשה ג׳ if a *ḥaber* (socius, v. חָבֵר 3) becomes a collector (publican), he is expelled from the order; a. fr.—Y. Sabb. XVI, end, 15ᵈ; Y. Yoma VIII, 45ᵇ; Y. Ned. IV, 38ᶜ הניחו לַגַּ׳ שיגבה וכ׳ let the collector collect his debt, i. e. let the divine agency do its mission.—*Pl.* גַּבָּאִים, גַּבָּאִין. Tosef. B. Mets. VIII, 26 הג׳ והמוכסים וכ׳ for tax and custom collectors it is difficult to make reparation; B. Kam. 94ᵇ. Tosef. Dem. III, 17 גַּבָּאֵי צדקה collectors or managers of charity.—Ab. III, 16 הג׳ מחזירים וכ׳ the collectors (divine agencies of justice) go around every day; a. fr.—Chald. גַּבּוֹרָיָא, pl. גַּבּוֹרִין. Targ. Esth. IV, 7 (Bxt. a. oth. גַּבָּאִין). [גַּבְרַיָּא, v. גַּבְרָא I.]

***גַּבְיָין, גְּבָיָין** m. (גבי, cmp. גבב) *saving, thrifty.* Targ. Prov. XXI, 5 (h. text חרוץ).—[גַּבְרַיָּא, v. גַּבְרָא I.]

גבייתי־, read גַּבָּיוּתֵי־.

גְּבִיל m. (גבל) *a mush of flour and water.* Ber. 37ᵇ (defin. טְרִיתָא) ג׳ מרתח a scalded mush (Ms. M. מרתח ג׳), a sort of puff-pastry or trifle.

גְּבִילִית, v. גְּבָלִית.

גְּבִין, v. גְּבִינִין.

גִּבִּין I, גִּבִּינָא m. ch.=(b. h. גִּבֵּן) *hump-backed.* Targ. O. Lev. XXI, 20. Targ. Koh. VII, 13.

גְּבִין II m. h. (v. גַּב) *eye-brow.* Nidd. 23ᵇ הגבין Ar. (ed. הגבן corr. acc.). Bekh. VII, 2 (43ᵇ) ... אין לו גבינין אלא ג׳ אחד וכ׳ if one has no eye-brows or only one eye-brow,—this is the *gibben* of the Bible (Lev. XXI, 20); expl. Gem. ib. זהו מדרש או גבן this is what is deducted by interpretation from *ô gibben* (ib.).—*Pl.* גְּבִינִין, גְּבִינִים. Nidd. l. c.; Y. ib. III, 50ᶜ bot.—Bekh. l. c., v. supra. Ib. (explain. גִּבֵּן, Lev. l. c.) שֶׁגְּבִינָיו שוכבין (not שגבינין) whose eye-brows are lying (overshadowing the eyes).

גְּבִינָא I ch. same; also *eye-lash.* *Pl.* גְּבִינִין, גְּבִינֵי; גְּבִינָתָא. Targ. Lev. XIV, 9. Targ. Y. I, II Lev. XXI, 20 דִגְבִינוֹי שכבן וכ׳, v. preced. (h. text גִּבֵּן).—Targ. Prov. VI, 4; ib. 25 גְּבִינָהָא Ar. (ed. גְּבִינָתָהָא); ib. XXX, 13 (h. text עפעפ׳).—B. Kam. 117ᵃ ומסרחי גבינוה and his eye-lashes were over-hanging (he could not move his eye-lids). Ib. דלו לי גְּבִינַי Mss. (v. Rabb. D. S. a. l. note 3, ed. עיני) lift my eye-lashes for me.

גִּבִּינָא II *hump-backed,* v. גִּבִּין I.

גְּבִינָה f. (b. h.; גבן) *curdled milk, cheese.* Ab. Zar. 34ᵇ גְּבִינַת בית אונייקי Bithynian cheese (prepared by gentiles), v. אוּנְיָיקִי; a. fr.—*Pl.* גְּבִינוֹת. Ib. II, 4; a. fr.—Tosef. Zab. II, 5 הַגְּבִינִין. Treat. Kuthim ch. II הַגְּבִינִים.—Ch. גְּבִינְתָּא.

גְּבִינִי pr. n. m. *G'bini*, name of a Temple crier. Tam. III, 8; Yoma 20b; Y. Succ. V, 55b bot. גבי (corr. acc.).—2) G. ben Ḥarson. Koh. R. to IV, 8.

***גְּבִינְתָּה, גְּבִינְתָּא** f. (גבן, v. גִּבְּנִין I) (the camel's) *hump*. *Pl.* גְּבִינָתָה. Y. Sabb. V, 7b bot. (expl. מטולטלת) כהדא כִּיפָה דהיא משויא ג׳ like a ball (a cushion) to level the humps; cmp. גְּבִיעָה II.

גְּבִינָתָא, pl. of גִּבְנָא I.

גָּבִיעַ m. (b. h.; גבע) *cup*. Gen. R. s. 91; Tanḥ. Mikkets 8; a. e.

גְּבִיעָה, גְּבִיעָא I pr. n. m. *G'biah* (*hump-backed*). Gen. R. s. 61 ג׳ בן קוסם; Snh. 91a ג׳ בן פסיסא Ar. (ed. גְּבִיהָא).

גְּבִיעָה II f. (גבע) *hump*. Gen. R. s. 61 (Alexander the Great to G'biah, v. preced.) אני משוה לך גְּבִיעָתָךְ Var. (ed. פדחתך) I will level thy hump.

גְּבִירָה f. (b. h.; גבר) *mistress*, *lady*. Sot. 12b; Ex. R. s. 1 גְּבִירְתֵּנוּ O our mistress! Taan. 21b (of Palestine, opp. שפחה Babylonia). Y. Ber. III, 6c; a. e.—*Pl.* גְּבִירוֹת. Ex. R. l. c.; Tanḥ. Sh'moth 3 בני ג׳ the sons of the ladies (Leah and Rachel). V. גְּבֶרֶת.

גְּבִישָׁתָא f. pl. (גבש) *hills*. Targ. Zeph. I, 10, v. גִּבְעֲתָא.

גָּבַל (b. h. r.; v. גבב) [*to give a rounded shape*,] *to to knead*, *stamp*. Sabb. XXIV, 3 you may put water into the bran (on the Sabbath) אבל לא גוֹבְלִין but must not mix it to a mass. Tosef. Maasr. III, 13 גובל עיסתו he kneads his dough. Lev. R. s. 29 בד׳ גְּבָלוֹ (Pesik. Bahod. p. 150b גִּיבְּלוֹ) on the fourth day He formed the dust into a mass.

Pi. גִּיבֵּל same. Y. Ter. V, 43c bot. הפריש ואח״כ גי׳ he set apart (the T'rumah) and then made the dough. Ib. מיגבול חמש (read מְגַבֵּל). Taan. 10a שמְגַ׳ את הגבינה that forms a cheese. Ib. 19b שמג׳ את הטיט that stamps clay; a. fr.—Part. pass. מְגוּבָּל. Ib. מ׳ יפה a thoroughly kneaded mass.

Hithpa. הִתְגַּבֵּל *to be kneaded*. Ib. ארנו מִתְגַּבֵּל יפה is not thoroughly kneaded.

גְּבַל ch. 1) same. Y. Sabb. VII, 10b bot. החן דְּגָבֵל כ׳ (or דְּגַבֵּל) he who kneads lime dust. Gitt. 69a ונִיגְבּוֹל .... ונירגדול בדובשא let him knead it with honey. Ib. בחדין קיטמא Ar. (Var. v. גַּרְבֵּל; ed. וניגדבל) let him twist .... and mix (the wick) thoroughly with ashes. Gen. R. s. 34, end גָּבְלִין ליה וכ׳, v. אֲרַמְדְּמָנֵי.—2) (of parasite worms) *to grow*. Ḥull. 67b מיניה קא גָּבְלֵי they grow out of it (originate in the body). Ib. bot. כי קא גָּבְלָן וכ׳ when they grew, they grew as permitted food.

Pa. גַּבֵּל as Pe. 1).—Y. Maas. Sh. V, 56d top וּמְגַבְּלָא אדמיה וכ׳ and to mix its blood with flax-seed. B. Mets. 69a (prov.) גַּבֵּיל לתורא גביל לתורי mix (fodder) for an ox, mix for oxen, i. e. it is the same trouble. Ber. 40a גביל לתורי (if he interrupted himself by saying,) 'Mix fodder for the oxen'. Sabb. 156a.

Ithpa. אִיתְגַּבֵּל, אִיגַּבֵּל *to be kneaded*. Lev. R. s. 6 אִיגַּבְּלוּן בלישה the coins were kneaded with the dough.

גְּבַל, גֵּבַל pr. n., v. גַּבְלָא.

גַּבָּל m. (גבל) *kneader*, *baker*. Pes. 34a ג׳ של בית וכ׳ was the baker for the house of Rabbi. Ib. 46a לג׳ ולתפלה וכ׳ in order to get a kneader (that observes levitical purity), for prayer (in a synagogue) and for washing hands (for a meal) one is bound to walk four *mils* (no more). Keth. 72a פלוני ג׳ תקן וכ׳ a certain kneader prepared for me the dough according to the law of Ḥallah.

גַּבָּלָא ch. same, esp. *one that mixes fodder*. Sabb. 156a ג׳ דבי וכ׳ the *gabbal* of the house of the Nasi, v. preced.

גַּבְלָא, גְּבַל, גֵּבַל (cmp. b. h. גְּבָל) [*Highland*,] *Gabla*, *Gabalena*, a district (and town) South or South West of Jerusalem, occupied by Edomites (v. Graetz Monatsschrift 1875, p. 61 sq.; 1880, p. 481 sq.). Targ. Y. Gen. XXXVI, 20; I Chr. I, 38 (h. text שֵׂעִיר). Targ. Y. I Deut. XXXIII, 2.—Ab. Zar. 59a; Keth. 112a איקלע לג׳ came to Gabla. Cmp. גַּבְלָן.

גַּבְלוּל m. (גבל) *a lump of dough* taken out for forming cakes &c., *a roll of dough*. Y. Ḥall. II, beg. 59a חלה כמין ג׳ the priest's gift must be, in shape and substance, like a roll.—*Pl.* גַּבְלוּלִין. Ib. משתיעשה ג׳ ג׳ from the time that the dough is divided into lumps.

גבלות, v. גִּבְלִית.

גַּבְלָיָא m. *of Gabla*. v. גְּבוּלָאָה a. גַּבְלָא.

גִּבְלִית f. (a geogr. term) *Giblean*, sub. גִּיזְרָה, *a Giblean balcony*. Ohol. XIV, 1 הגיזרה והג׳; Y. Shebi. III, 34c bot. גזורה הגּוּבְלִית. Tosef. Oh. XIV, 9 איזה ג׳ what balcony is called Giblith? כל שמניקה מכאן ומכאן ומשוייר מן האמצע (ed. Zuck. a. oth.) a balcony which sucks from (is girded to the wall on) both sides and left alone (without support) in the middle. [Ar. reads כל שמעוקם מכאן וכ׳ curved on both sides and straight-lined in the middle, and explains our w. to mean אוצר *storeroom*.] [Var. lect. גבלת, גבלות, גבלית.]

חַג׳, גַּבְלָן pr. n. [*Highland*,] *District of Gablan*, *Gabalena* (cmp. גַּבְלָא a. גְּבוּל II). Sot. IX, 15 (49b); Cant. R. to II, 13 והג׳ ישום; Snh. 97a והג׳ יאשם (Ms. F. והגבל) the Gablan will lie desolate; (cmp. Keth. 112a איקלע לגבלא as to the envied fertility of Gabalena). V. גּוּבְלָנָא.

גַּבָּן, v. גְּבְעוֹנִי. [גַּבָּן *with us*, v. גַּב ch.]

גִּבֵּן m. (b. h., denom. of גַּב) *hump-backed*, or one *having defective eye-brows*. Bekh. VII, 2 R. Ḥanina .... says, the *gibben* of the Bible (Lev. XXI, 20) is מי שיש לו שני גבים וכ׳, v. גַּב h.; oth. opin., v. s. v. גְּבִין. [Targ. Y. II *extremely tall*, v. גְּבִיהַ.]

גַּבֵּן, *Pi.* גִּבֵּן (v. גְּבִינָה) *to form cheese*. Sabb. 95a; Tosef. ib. IX (X), 13 המגבין, ed. Zuck. (Var. המגבן); Y. ib. VII, 10c bot. והמְגַבֵּן, v. חבץ.

גִּבְנָא, v. גִּיבְנָא.

גַּבְנוּן m. (b. h. גִּבֵּן; גבן) *humpy, humpbacked. Pl.* גַּבְנוּנִים. Mekh. Yithro, Baḥod. 4 (ref. to Ps. LXVIII, 17) כלכם ג׳ אתם וכ׳ ye are all humpbacked (blemished) as we read (Lev. XXI, 20) &c., v. גִּבֵּן; (Meg. 29ª בעלי מומין); Yalk. Ex. 284; v. Tanḥ. B'midbar 7; Yalk. Ps. 796.

גִּבְנוּנִי, v. גִּבְעוֹנִי.

גִּבְסִים, v. גִּיפְסוֹס a. גִּפְסִים.

גָּבַע (cmp. גבח) *to be arched.*—Part. גָּבִיעַ, v. גִּבֵּחַ.

**Af.* אַגְבַּע *to waddle.* Y. Dem. I, 22ª top saw one mouse (which had swallowed a jewel) ואתי מַגְבַּע come in waddling.

גֶּבַע (b. h.) pr. n. pl. *Geba*, a Samaritan town. Kel. XVII, 5 חֲצִירֵי ג׳ leeks of G.; Y. Orl. III, 63ª bot. חריצר ג׳ (corr. acc.); Tosef. Kel. B. Mets. VI, 10 חצר ג׳ של בית חכותים.—[Tosef. Sot. XI, 14 (ref. to Zech. XIV, 10) גבע רמון, Yalk. Zech. 585 ג׳ ורמון.]

גִּבְעָה f. (b. h.; גבע) 1) *hill.* Lev. R. s. 10 כמין ג׳ like a hill (the bullock between the two rams). Cant. R. to IV, 6 עשה ערלותיהן ג׳ he piled up their preputia; Gen. R. s. 47 העמידן גִּבְעַת ערלות; a. e.—*Pl.* גְּבָעוֹת. Ḥag. 15ª ברא הרים ברא ג׳ He created mountains, and (corresponding to them) hills. Taan. 8ᵇ (ref. to Job XXXVII, 13) אם לשבט בהרים וג׳ if He sends rain as a scourge, He sends it on mountains and hills. Ab. Zar. 17ª הרים וג׳ ye mountains and hills! Sot. 5ª; a. fr.—2) pr. n. pl. *Gibeah.* Gitt. 6ᵇ עסיק בפלגש ג׳ studying the case of the woman murdered in Gibeah (Jud. XIX sq.). Pesik. R. s. 11 בפלגש בג׳ in the war about the woman of G.; a. e.—Shebu. 35ᵇ שמות האמורין בג׳ Rashi (ed. בגִבְעַת בִּנְיָמִין) the names (*Adonai, El* &c.) used in the chapter about Gibeah (Jud. XX).

גִּבְעוֹל m. (b. h.; גבע, ל dimin.; cmp. גָּבִיעַ) *calyx* or *capsule* of plants. Par. XII, 2 (of hyssop).—*Pl.* גִּבְעוֹלִין. Ib. 2; 5; Yoma 14ᵇ.—Ib. 75ª זרע פשתן בגבעולין (Ms. M. 2 בגִבְעוֹלָיו) the seed of flax in (its) capsules; v. גַּד II. Num. R. s. 7 נעשה ג׳ the flax had formed capsules; Lev. R. s. 18 ומצאה ג׳ (when no longer good for linen). Par. XI, 7, v. גָּמַל; a. fr.

גִּבְעוֹנָאֵי, v. next w.

גִּבְעוֹנִי m. (b. h.) *Gibeonite, one not admissible as a member of the congregation of Israel*, v. נָתִין. Pesik. R. s. 26 (ref. to Jer. XXVIII, 1). Yeb. 71ª ג׳ מהול (Ar. ed. Koh. גבנוני, oth. ed. גבן) a circumcised G.; Ab. Zar. 27ª גִּבְנוֹנִי; Yalk. Gen. 81 Ms. גבעוני (v. Rabb. D. S. to Ab. Zar. l. c. note 40).—*Pl.* גִּבְעוֹנִים. Num. R. s. 8; Ex. R. s. 30; Yeb. 78ᵇ; a. fr.—Ch. גִּבְעוֹנָאֵי. Targ. II Sam. XXI, 1; a. e.—Kidd. 70ᵇ, v. גּוֹבַיָּא; a. e.

גִּבְעֲתָא f. ch. = h. גִּבְעָה. Targ. Jud. VII, 1; a. e.—*Pl.* גִּבְעָתָא. Targ. Zeph. I, 10 (ed. Lag. גברשתא).

גָּבַר (b. h.; v. גבב) *to be uppermost, prevail; to be strong.* Num. R. s. 7 לשון גָּבַר, v. אָנוּשׁ. Sot. IX, 15 גָּבְרוּ בעלי זרוע the violent prevailed. Y. Bets. II, 61ᶜ top; Tosef. Ḥag. II, 11; Bets. 20ª גָּבְרָה יָדָן וכ׳ the Shammaites prevailed over (outnumbered) the Hillelites; a. fr.

Pi. גִּבֵּר, גִּיבֵּר *to make strong, strengthen, sustain.* Lam. R. to III, 1 גִּבְּרַנִי לעמוד בכולן he made me strong enough to survive all these calamities; ib. 12. Cant. R. to II, 14 מְגַבְּרָן לישראל (ed. Wil. מַגְבִּירָן Hif.) sustains Israel. Ib. III, 7 שהן מְגַבְּרִין את וכ׳ they (the sixty words of the priestly benediction) strengthen Israel. Mekh. B'shall., Amalek, s. 1 וכי . . . מְגַבְּרוֹת ישראל can Moses' (uplifted) hands make Israel victorious?; a. fr.—Part. pass. מְגוּבָּר, v. infra.

Hif. הִגְבִּיר 1) same; v. supra.—2) *to grow strong.* Ib. עתידין . . לְהַגְבִּיר בד״ת וכ׳ (Moses' uplifted hands indicated that the Lord remembered that) Israel would in the future be strong in the Law which was to be given through his (Moses') hands, opp. לחמיך; Yalk. Ex. 264.

Hithpa. הִתְגַּבֵּר, *Nithpa.* נִתְגַּבֵּר *to rise, swell; to grow strong, gather courage; to make one's self master.* Tanḥ. B'resh. 7 המים מִתְגַּבְּרִין the waters of the Nile rose. Num. R. s. 19 ומִתְגַּבֶּרֶת שם and rose there. Ib. מלא מים מִתְגַּבְּרִין full of high waters. Snh. 96ª לא נ׳ עד וכ׳ had no courage until he came to Dan. R. Hash. III, 8 היו מִתְגַּבְּרִין they were victorious. Ḥag. 16ª, a. e. if one feels שיצרו מתג׳ עליו that his passion threatens to make itself master over him; Kidd. 80ᵇ. Ned. 81ª מפני שהן מתגברין על הצבור because they lord it over the people (Ar. מתגדרין, v. גָּדַר). Num. R. s. 18, v. גָּבַהּ. Yalk. Is. 287 (ref. to Is. XVII, 11) מכה מִתְגַּבֶּרֶת (Lev. R. s. 18 מגרת, corr. acc. or מגברת) an affliction which makes itself the master, v. אָנוּשׁ. Gen. R. s. 76; a. fr.

גְּבַר I ch. same. Targ. Ps. CIII, 11.—Gitt. 60ᵇ, v. אֵילִים. Pes. 76ª, a. fr. עילאה ג׳ in the case of a contact between warm and cold substances, the upper one prevails (heating or cooling the substance into which it is poured); תתאה ג׳ the lower prevails.

Pa. גַּבַּר as preced. *Pi.* Targ. Am. V, 9. Targ. Zech. X, 6; a. e.—Part. pass. מְגַבַּר *growing, swelling.* Targ. Is. VIII, 8.

Af. אַגְבַּר *to make strong, to cause to overpower.* Targ. Is. XLI, 25.—Snh. 38ª אַגְבְּרוּ חמרא וכ׳ let the wine get the better of the young men, i. e. give them plenty to drink, that they may become mirthful.

גֶּבֶר m. (b. h.; גבר) 1) *man, master.* Lam. R. to III, 1. Kidd. 80ᵇ (ref. to Lam. III, 39) וכי ג׳ על חטאיו הוא (Rashi) is man master over his sins (sinless)?—2) *cock.* Yoma I, 8 בקריאת הג׳ at the time of the crowing of the cock; ib. 20ᵇ; Y. Shek. V, 48ᵈ bot.; Y. Succ. V, 55ᶜ disputed meaning: *man's (the cryer's) crying*, or *the cock's crowing*, v. פְּרוֹזָא.—3) (euphem.) *membrum virile.* Bekh. VII, 5 (44ᵇ) בעל ג׳ a man with an abnormally large membrum.

גְּבַר II, **גַּבְרָא** ch. same; *man.* Targ. Gen. II, 24; a. v. fr.—Ber. 63ª באתר דלית ג׳ כ׳ where there is no man, (leader). B. Mets. 97ª (prov.) ג׳ דנשי וכ׳ for a man whom women killed there is no law or judge. Erub. 53ᵇ, v. אִיסְפְּרִיזָא.—Men. 42ᵇ, a. e. חובת ג׳ personal duty, opp. ח׳

טלית the duty resting on the garment (whether or not you wear it).—חהוא גברא a certain man. B. Mets. l. c.; a. v. fr. [Frequ. חאי גברא, חהוא, or גברא, euphem. for *I*, or *thou;* v. החוא.]—Bekh. 36ᵃ בלא גברא (Rashi גברי) without naming an authority.—*Pl.* גַּבְרִין, גַּבְרַיָּיא, גַּבְרֵי. Targ. O. Deut. I, 13; a. v. fr.—Lev. R. s. 23 יחוון גַּבְ׳ בכל מילייא (Cant. R. to II, 2 גּוּבְרִין) they shall be strong (trained) in all things. B. Kam. 92ᵇ (prov.) כד חוינן זוטרי לג׳ וכ׳ when we were young, we were esteemed as men, now that we are old &c.; a. v. fr.—Keth. 6ᵃ בלא ג׳, v. supra. Ib. 53ᵇ סימן דגברי שַׁק זוֹרַק the mnemonical sign for the authorities quoted is &c. (פפא, רבא, אלעזר, לקיש, ששת).—Fem. גַּבְרְתָא, only assumed for argument, v. אַנְתְּרוֹפֵי. V. also גּוּבְרָא.

גַּבְרָא, v. גִּיבְרָא.

גַּבְרְוָתָא, v. גִּיבַּר.

גַּבְרוּתָא, v. גְּבוּרְתָא.

גַּבְרִיאֵל pr. n. (b. h.) *Gabriel*, name of an angel (*Divine Strength*). Dan. VIII, 16; a. e. Gen. R. s. 1, beg. Ex. R. s. 1. Y. Ber. I, 13ᵃ bot. לא יצווח לא לג׳ וכ׳ man in distress must not invoke Gabriel &c.; a. v. fr.

גַּבְרִית f. (denom. of גֶּבֶר) *cock-like.* Sabb. 67ᵇ kill this hen שקרתה ג׳ for she crowed like a cock (a superstitious practice); (Tosef. ib. VI (VII), 5 שקראה כזכר).

גְּבֶרֶת f. (b. h.)=גְּבִירָה. Gen. R. s. 51 בן גְּבִרְתָּהּ her mistress' son. Ib. s. 45 גְּבִרְתִּי (גְּבִיר׳) my mistress; a. e.

גַּבְרְתָא, v. גְּבַר II.

גַּבְרְתָן m. (denom. of גְּבִירָה) *brave, hero.* Sifré Deut. 305; Yalk. ib. 941 ג׳ (ש)כמותך a hero (who is) like thyself.

גַּבְרְתָנִית f. (v. preced.) *powerful, overwhelming.* Num. R. s. 7 (ref. to אָנוּשׁ Is. XVII, 11, v. גָּבַר) leprosy is called a strong disease מפני שהיא מכה ג׳ (not חג׳) because it is an overpowering affliction; Lev. R. s. 18 מכה ג׳ ומתשת an overpowering and weakening &c.

גָּבַשׁ *to be high, piled up;* denom. גָּבוּשׁ.

Pi. גִּבֵּשׁ *to fill with piles of stones.* Tosef. Oh. XVII, 9 שֶׁגִּבְּשׁוֹ בגבושים which he filled up &c.; (Oh. XVIII, 5 רְצָפוֹ באבנים).

גְּבַשׁ ch. same; *to heap up.* Targ. Prov. VI, 8 ed. (Ms. גדש׳).

גַּבְשׁוּשִׁין, v. גַּבְשׁוּשִׁיתָא.

גַּבְשׁוּשִׁית f. (גבש) *heap of stones, pile, mound.* Sabb. 73ᵇ. Ib. 152ᵃ (ref. to Koh. XII, 5 מגבוה ייראו) שאפי׳ ג׳ קטנה וכ׳ even a small mound appears to him (the aged man) like the highest mountains. Y. Erub. II, 20ᵃ, opp. חָרִיץ.—*Pl.* גַּבְשׁוּשִׁיּוֹת. Y. Sot. VII, 21ᶜ שתי ג׳ וכ׳ (not שית . . . .) they put up two mounds and named them Mount Gerizim &c.

גַּבְשׁוּשִׁיתָא ch. same. Targ. Koh. XII, 5.—Targ. Cant. IV, 1, v. גַּלְשׁוּשִׁיתָא.—*Pl.* גַּבְשׁוּשִׁין m. (fr. גַּבְשׁוּשָׁא). Y. Snh. VII, 25ᵈ מינוקיא עבדין ג׳ (Jewish) children (in Rome) made little piles &c.

גַּבַּת pr. n. pl. *Gabbath*, later name for Biblical *Gibbethon*, in the territory of Dan. [Cmp. as to change of Biblical names Y. Meg. I, 70ᵃ bot.] Y. Taan. IV, 69ᵇ; Ruth R. introd.; Cant. R. to I, 16 מג׳ ועד אנטיפרס וכ׳ between G. and Antipatris there were sixty myriads of townships; Y. Meg. l. c. מגבות; Lam. R. to II, 2 מגיבתון.

גַּבְתָּא, v. גּוּבְתָא I.

גַּג m. (b. h.) 1) *roof.* Midd. V, 3. Pes. 13ᵇ, v. אִיסְטְבָא; a. v. fr.—Yoma 47ᵃ עלה לגג excelled all, v. זֶרֶד.—2) in gen. *upper portion, top, apex.* Y. Yeb. VIII, 9ᵃ רוב גַּגָּהּ של עטרה the largest portion of the top of the membral corona, contrad. to רוב גּוּבְהָהּ, v. גּוּבָה; Y. Sabb. XIX, end, 17ᵇ רוב גוב׳ עטרה (corr. acc.).—Hull. 67ᵇ ג׳ תמרה the outer covering of a date.—*Pl.* גַּגּוֹת. Erub. IX, 1; a. fr.—Men. X, 2 (64ᵇ), v. צְרִיפִין.

גַּגִּית, v. גִּיגִית.

***גַּגְמֵי** or **גּוּגְמֵי** m. pl. (=גמגמי, r. גמא?) *stone-like peas.* Hor. 13ᵃ Ar. (Var. Ar. a. ed. פְּלִימֵי).

גד, v. גדד a. נגי׳.

גָּד pr. n. m. *Gad* 1) son of Jacob. Gen. R. s. 71; a. fr.—תנאי בני גד, v. תְּנַאי.—2) the prophet in the days of David. B. Bath. 15ᵃ דאסקיה ג׳ החוזה וכ׳ Gad, the seer, and Nathan, the prophet, continued the Book of Samuel (from XXVIII, 3; Ms. O. דאתא ג׳ . . . . וסיימוה).

גַּד I, גָּדָד m. (גדד, cmp. חד) [*cutting,*] *bitter, acrid.* Ex. R. s. 5 (ref. to Num. XI, 7) מר וגד bitter and acrid. Targ. B'shall., ed. Bub. 21 גד ולענה (read כלענה; Yalk. Ex. 258 מר כלע׳).—*Pl.* גַּדִּים, גַּדִּין, גְּדָדִין. Gen. R. s. 71 (play on *Gaddi*, Num. XIII, 11) [read:] גְּדָדִין ומררין acrid and bitter (people); Yalk. Gen. 126 כגידרין מררין, v. גִּידָא II; Yalk. Ezra 1067 בר גדי׳ (corr. acc.). [גדרין, Targ. Y. Num. XXII, 7 Ar. s. v. גדרין, read אַגְרִין.]

גַּד II m. (b. h.; cmp. כַּד II) *a rounded-off seed grain, coriander,* (in Talm. a. Midr.) *linseed.* Yoma 75ᵃ (ref. to Ex. XVI, 7) עגול כגִידָא וכ׳ the manna resembled a grain by its rounded shape, and a pearl by its white color; even so it has been taught גד שדומה לזרע וכ׳ the word *gad* (grain) is used, because the manna resembled linseed; Yalk. Ex. 261; Num. 734. Mekh. B'shall., Vayassa, 5 (ref. to Ex. l. c.) איני יודע של מי דומה I do not know to which the comparison refers (to shape or to color); דומה לזרע וכ׳... it resembles (in form) linseed: but you might think &c., ת״ל לבן therefore 'white' is added.

גַּד, גָּד III m. (b. h.; גדד, cmp. גזר) 1) *decree, fate,* esp. *Gad* (*Fortune*), a god worshipped by the Babylonians and the Jewish exiles. Snh. 63ᵇ ג׳ נמי מיכתב כתיב Gad is also one of the names of idols mentioned in the Bible.

Sabb. 67[b] ג׳ אינו אלא לשון ע״א Gad is nothing else than a designation of an idol, v. next w.—2) גַּד יָוָן pr. n. *Gad Yavan* (*Greek Fortune*) near Jerusalem. Zab. I, 5 כְּמִן ג׳ י׳ לשילוח as long as it takes from G. Y. to Siloah; Tosef. ib. I, 10 כְּמִגַּדְיָוָן לשילה; Snh. 63[b] כְּמִיגַּדְיָוָן לשילה (corr. acc.)—[*Gad Yavan* is prob. the name of a pool connected with the Siloah, perh. *Fount of the Virgin*, v. Sm. Bible Dict. s. v. Siloam.] [Toh. VI, 6; Erub. 22[b] בית גד גד, v. גַּלְגּוּל.]

גַּד, גַּדָּא ch. same, *luck; genius, godhead.* Targ. O. Gen. XXX, 11 גַּד; Y. II גַּדָּא (not גְּדָא). Targ. Esth. VIII, 15 גַּדָּא (not גְּדָא).—Gen. R. s. 71 ג׳ דביתא the good genius of the house. Sabb. 67[b] גד גַּדִּי וסינוק לא (Ms. M. צינוק), a charm formula supposed to mean, *Be lucky, my luck, and tire not* (prob. *Grow, my luck* &c., v. נְגַד). Ḥull. 40[a] לג׳ דהר to the godhead of the mountain. Ned. 56[a] (explain. ערסא דג׳ (דרגש) the bed reserved for the domestic genius (bed of state). Y. Ab. Zar. I, 39[d] top לְגַדֵּיה וכ׳, v. ארקליס. Gen. R. s. 65 [ביה] ג׳ דע״ז דאת קאים by the idolatrous godhead by whom thou standest, i. e. to whom thou referrest in saying, 'Let my father rise' (Gen. XXVII, 31). Y. Sabb. XVI, end, 15[d]; Y. Yoma VIII, 45[b]; Y. Ned. IV, 38[d] בְגַדָּךְ מדלר (not בגרך) doest thou rely upon thy good luck? Koh. R. to VII, 26 מה ביש ג׳ וכ׳ how bad is this woman's (my) luck!; a. fr.—*Pl.* גַּדַּיָּיא, גַּדַּיָּא. Y. Ab. Zar. III, 43[a] bot. ג׳ קורין אותה גליא a place called *Gaddaya* is cacophemistically named *Gallaya* (dung-hills); Tosef. ib. VI (VII), 4 גדגיא ed. Zuck. (ed. גריא, corr. acc.).

גַּדַּאי pr. n. m. *Gaddai* (b. h. גַּדִּי). Keth. 105[a].

גדבל, v. גַּרְבֵּל.

גְּדָבְרָא m.=גִּזְבָּר. *Pl.* גְּדָבְרִין, גְּדָבְרַיָּא. Dan. III, 2; 3.—Targ. Koh. II, 7.

גדגד, v. גַּלְגּוּל.

גדגדות, Y. Shek. to IV, 4 in Bab. ed. (Var. גדגניות), v. גְּרוֹגְרוֹת.

גְּדִגְדְּנִיּוֹת, גּוּדְגְּ׳ f. pl. (cmp. גַּד II) *melilot*, a kind of clover, v. הִנְדְּקוֹקָא. Y. Erub. III, 20[d] top; Y. Peah VIII, 21[a] top; Erub. 28[a]. Ber. 57[b].—[In later ritualistic literature our w. designates *cherries*, v. Löw Pfl. p. 94.]

גדגיא, Tosef. Ab. Zar. VI (VII), 4 ed. Zuck., v. גַּדָּא.

גדגלידא, v. גַּרְגְּלִידָא.

גדגניות, v. גדגדות.

גָּדַד I (b. h.; cmp. גזז, קצץ) *to cut, cut off.* Par. II, 2; Bekh. 44[a] יָגוֹד let him lop off (the black tops of the horns or hoofs).—[V. גָּדַר.]—Trnsf. (cmp. קצץ) *to fix the price.* B. Bath. 13[a] גּוֹד או אָגוֹד either fix you a price for my share, or I shall do so (and buy your share); דינא דגוד או אגוד the right of settling by *god o agod.* Ib. אגוד איכא גוד ליכא the offer to buy is applicable in this case (the half-freed slave can offer to buy his other half), but the offer to sell cannot be made (since there is no price for a free man).—*Part. pass.* גָּדוּד *stripped* (of branches); trnsf. *empty-handed.* Gen. R. s. 68, beg. ג׳ שלחו (Yalk. ib. 117 גדודי) Isaac sent Jacob away without anything valuable.

Pi. גִּדֵּד *to cut off, level.* Gen. R. s. 71 (play on בא גד, Gen. XXX, 11) בא מי שעתיד לְגַדֵּד וכ׳ he has come who is destined to level the fastnesses of the nations (idolatry). Tanḥ. Ki Thissa 13 (play on מגדל גד, Josh. XV, 37) from there the Lord יוצא וּמְגַדֵּד וכ׳ will proceed and level &c.; Ex. R. s. 40 ומגידד (corr. acc.).

Nif. נִגְדַּד *to be cut off.* Keth. 51[a] כל העומד לִיגָּדֵד כְּנִגְדּוּד דמי Ar. (ed. ליגזז, v. גָּזַז).

Hithpol. הִתְגּוֹדֵד *to make incisions in one's own body.* Yeb. 13[b], v. גּוּד. Tanḥ. Sh'laḥ. 15; Num. R. s. 17 קבר מת לא תִתְגּוֹדְדוּ when one buried a dead, the law says, Ye shall not &c. (Deut. XIV, 1). V. גְּדִידָה.

**Polel* גּוֹדֵד same. Yeb. l. c. א״כ לימא קרא לא תְגוֹדְדוּ if it were so (that Deut. XIV, 1 meant only to forbid incisions in the body) it ought to read *lo t'god'du,* ye shall make no incisions.

גְּדַד ch. same. [Dan. IV, 11; 20.] Targ. Deut. XIV, 1 תִגוֹדְדוּן, v. preced. Hithpol.—Bets. 6[a] אפי׳ לְמִיגַּד ליה וכ׳ Ar. a. Ms. M. (ed. לְמִיגַּז) even to cut a shroud for him (the dead, on the second Holy Day); Sabb. 150[b], v. גָּזַז.

גָּדַד II, v. גּוּד.

גָּדָד m. *acrid,* v. גַּד I.

גְּדוּד I m. (b. h.; v. גּוּד) *troop, band.* Pesik. R. s. 20, end ג׳ מלאכים a troop of angels. Ber. 3[b]; Snh. 16[a] לכו ופשטו ידיכם בג׳ go ye and stretch your hands out (for booty) as a band (of marauders). Pesik. R. l. c. ג׳ של מלאכי חבלה a troop of angels of destruction.—*Pl.* גְּדוּדִים, גְּדוּדִין. Ib. Deut. R. s. 11, end. Ber. 29[b] במקום גְּדוּדֵי חיה וכ׳ in a place where there are hords of wild beasts or robbers; Tosef. ib. III, 11 Var. ed. Zuck.

גְּדוּד II pr. n. pl. *G'dud.* Arakh. IX, 6 (32[ab]); Y. Meg. I, 70[a] bot. גְּדוֹר q. v.

גְּדוּד, v. גְּירוּד.

גְּדוּדָא, גְּדוּרָא, v. גִּירוּדָא.

גְּדוּדָא f. (גדד, v. גָּדַד part. pass.) *a tree stripped of all branches.* Erub. 100[b] (Ar. גרדא, Var. גרודא; Ms. M. גרידא, ed. Sonc. גדור, גרויא; v. Rabb. D. S. a. l. note). [גדודאן, Targ. Is. XXXVIII, 12, v. גִּירוּדָא.]

גְּדוּדִי m. *stripped, empty-handed,* v. גָּדַד.

גְּדוּדִית f. (dimin. of גְּדוּד) *small troop.* *Pl.* גְּדוּדִיּוֹת. Sifra B'ḥuck. beg. (ref. to Lev. XXVI, 31) I shall lay waste your sanctuaries מן הג׳ even of the troops (of travellers; Rashi: of pilgrims).

גְּדוּדִית II f. (גָּדַד I; cmp. Ps. LXV, 11) *ruins.* *Pl.* גְּדוּדִיּוֹת. Erub. V, I (52[b]) ג׳ גבוהות וכ׳ (Ms. M. omits גבוה׳) debris ten palms high. Cmp. גַּדָּא I.

גדודקי, v. גורזקי.

גדודתה, Y. Dem. I, 21[d] במקום שהיתה ג׳ R. S. to Dem. I, 2 (ed. גררתה), prob. במקום גדודי חיה, v. גְּדוּד.

גָּדוֹל m., **גְּדוֹלָה** f. (b. h.; גדל) 1) *great, distinguished;* (noun) *a great man, leader.* Sabb. 94[b], a. fr. ג׳ כבוד הבריות וכ׳ human dignity is something great, for it overrules a prohibitive law &c. Ned. 49[b] ג׳ מלאכה וכ׳ labor is something great, for it honors him who pursues it.—Sot. I, 9 ג׳ ממנו his superior. Gen. R. s. 100 גְּדוֹל העולמים the Great One of the worlds, the Lord.—Snh. 21[b] גְּ׳ העולם a world-renowned man (Solomon). M. Kat. 22[a] גְּ׳ הדור a prominent man of his days. Y. ib. III, 82[c] top גְּ׳ המשפחה the chief of the family; a. v. fr.—2) *adult, of age, older.* Yeb. II, 8 בג׳ on the eldest brother. Ib. XIII, 11 ג׳ וקטנה if one of the brother's widows is of age, and the other a minor; a. fr.—כהן גדול (abbr. כ״ג) *Highpriest.* Ib. IX, 1; a. fr.—*Pl.* גְּדוֹלִים, גְּדוֹלִין; גְּדוֹלוֹת. Koh. R. to VII, 8 גְּדוֹלֵי הדור scholars, v. supra; ג׳ ירושלים prominent citizens of Jerusalem.—Ab. Zar. 18[a] ג׳ רומי Roman dignitaries; a. fr.—Ber. 23[b], a. e. גדולים (sub. נקבים) the larger functions of the body, movement of the bowels; v. דַּק.

גְּדוֹל, v. גְּדִידוֹל.

גְּדוּלָּה f. (b. h.; גדל) *greatness, distinction, dignity, wealth, high position, office.* Gitt. 59[a] תורה וג׳ במקום א׳ learning and high office combined in one person. Ber. 61[a] בג׳ מתחילין מִן הגדול וכ׳ for distinction the superior is first mentioned, for degradation the inferior. Erub. 13[b] מחזר על הג׳ hunting for office. Ib. 54[a] עולה לג׳ will rise to distinction. Y. Ter. V, 43[c] top למשחה לג׳ וכ׳ '*for ointment*' (Num. XVIII, 11) means for installation in office, for unguent, and for lighting. Meg. 31[a] גְּדוּלָּתוֹ של הקב״ה Ms. M. (ed. גבורתו) a description of the greatness of the Lord. Ex. R. s. 3 end הלב ששמח בגדולַּת אחיו וכ׳ the heart (of Aaron) which rejoiced over a brother's distinction shall wear the Urim &c.; a. fr.

גְּדוּף, גִּדּוּפָא, v. גִּדּף.

גִּדּוּפִי f. (גדף) *blasphemy.* Sabb. 75[a], v. אַמְגּוּשְׁתָּא.

גְּדוֹר, v. גְּדִידוֹר.

גְּדוֹר pr. n. pl. *G'dor,* in Peraea. Y. Meg. I, 70[a] bot.; Arakh. 32[ab] (repeatedly גדוד). Ib. גמלא בגליל וג׳ בעבר הירדן Gamla in Galilee, G. in Peraea. Y. R. Hash. II, 58[a] top הרי מכוור וג׳ (as stations for signalizing the New Moon) the mountains of Mikhvar and G'dor (Bab. ib. 23[b] חרים וכייר וגֶדֶר, corr. acc., v. גֶּדֶר); Y. Shebi. IX, 38[d] bot.

גָּדוּר, גְּדוּרָא *a stripped tree,* v. גְּדוּדָא.

גְּדוּרָה, גְּדוּרָא pr. n. pl. *G'durah* (Gadara) near Tiberias, giving the name to a species of carob. Y. Maasr. I, beg. 48[c] חרובי ג׳; Y. Orl. I, 61[a] top גידודה; Gen. R. s. 79 חרובין של גרודא; Yalk. ib. 133 גידורא.

גדורקרי, v. גורזקי.

גָּדוּשׁ (גְּדִישׁ, גָּרִישׁ) pr. n. m. *Gadush.* Tosef. Maas. Sh. I, 14; Erub. 27[a] (v. Rabb. D. s. a. l.).

גְּדֵי* (v. גדד I) *to cut, divide, assign.*

Pa. גַּדֵּי *to cut off, excommunicate.* Nidd. 36[b] ואי לא צאית גְּרַיֵּיה הוא סבר גַּדְּיֵיה א״ל and if he does not obey, drag him over (v. גרי, i. e. force him with arguments), but he (R. Assé) understood that he told him *gadd'yeh* (excommunicate him). Ib. לָא צייח גדייה he (Shila bar Abina) did not obey, and he (R. Assé) excommunicated him (Rashi). [Tosaf. read for גרייה: גַּדְּיֵיה, fr. גדי, a sec. form of נגד, *draw him over.*—Ar. s. v. צנע 2 reads גַּדְּיֵיה *lash him* (ref. to Deut. XIV, 1), without referring to any misapprehension, while s. v. גר 10 הוא סבר גרייה א״ל is quoted—obviously a later insertion of a copyist.]

גְּדִי m. (b. h.) 1) *kid,* in gen. *young animal.* Ḥull. 113[ab] (ref. to Gen. XXXVIII, 17) כאן ג׳ עזים וכ׳ here it reads *g'di izzim* from which we learn that wherever *g'di* without any qualification is used, it includes cow and sheep. Men. XIII, 7; a. fr.—*Pl.* גְּדָיִים, גְּדָיִם, גְּדָיִים. Snh. 11[a]; Tosef. ib. II, 4 מפני הג׳ וכ׳ on account of the kids or lambs (being too young for offerings on Passover).—Y. ib. X, 28[b] bot.; Gen. R. s. 42, a. e. אם אין ג׳ אין תישים when there will be no kids (young students), there will be no wethers (leaders, scholars). Y. ib. I, 19[a] top ג׳ שהנחת וכ׳ the kids (young scholars) thou hast left behind (in Palestine) have grown to be wethers; a. e.—Trnsf. *the tender grain in its husks.* Pesik. Asser p. 99[b]; Tanḥ. R'eh 17; Yalk. Deut. 892 (homiletic interpret. of Deut. XV, 21) אל תגרמו לי לבשל ג׳ וכ׳ do not cause me to ripen the grains in their mothers' womb (husks, so as to be blown out by the East wind).—2) *the Capricorn,* a sign in the Zodiac. Pesik. R. s. 20. Yalk. Ex. 418; Kings 185. [Yalk. Num. 785 הרי נכנס הזאב לגדי, v. גדיגוד.]

גַּדְיָא, גַּדְי I ch. same. Targ. O. Gen. XXXVIII, 17; 20 (Y. גדיי, גדיר, גדיר (?)); 23 O. a. Y. גַּדְיָא.—Pes. 3[b] גדי מסנקן, v. סַנְק. Sabb. 18[b] דג׳ (השרא) meat of a kid. Ib. 20[a]. Ḥull. 51[a].—*Pl.* גַּדְיָן, גַּדְאַן, גַּדְיָין, constr. גַּדְיֵי, גַּדְיֵי. Targ. Deut. XIV, 4. Targ. Gen. XXVII, 16 ed. Berl. גַּדְיֵי; 9 גַּדְיֵי; a. e. Midr. Sam. ch. XX (expl. הר׳ צי החלב I Sam. XVII, 18) גדיין מניעין וכ׳ kids taken away from their mothers.—גַּדְיְתָא. Targ. Y. Num. XV, 27 (h. text עֵז).

גַּדְיָא II pr. n. m. *Gadya.* Y. Sot. IX, 24[b] אצל בית ג׳ (Snh. 11[a] בעלייה בית גּוּרְיָא). Tanḥ. Ki Thetsé 9; Pesik. Zakhor p. 25[ab] יודן בן ג׳; Lam. R. to III, 64 גדייא; Yalk. Ps. 827 (Yalk. Sam. 123 Ms. O. גּוּרְיָא, v. Bub. Pesik. l. c. note 76).

גַּדְיָא, v. גַּבָּא.

גדיאן, Ḥull. 65[a] ed., read נַדְיָאן v. נַדְיָין a. גְּדוֹנָא.

גדיגוד, גדיגור, גדיגוד, Y'lamd. Mattoth quot. in Ar., הרי נכנס הזאב לג׳ . . . . . read with Yalk. Num. 785: הרי לגְּדִי

(or לִגְדִיו) the wolf is coming to get his kid; cmp. Tanh. Matt. 4 עד שהזאב בא לצאן פרשו לו הַמְצודה while the wolf goes for the sheep, spread ye the snare for him.

גְּדִידָה f. (גָּדַד I Hithpa.) 1) *incision in the flesh, wounding.* Kidd. 35b או אינו אלא (אף) לג׳ perhaps the exemption of females (intimated by בנים Deut. XIV, 1) refers (also) to the law forbidding incisions? Ib. שריטה וג׳ אחת היא *s'ritah* and *g'didah* are legally the same. Macc. 21a שריטה ביד וג׳ בכלי *s'ritah* is done with the hand (nails), *g'didah* with an instrument.—2) *cutting dates,* v. גְּדִירָה.

גְּדִידִים pr. n. m. *G'didim.* Kidd. 66a Judah b. G.

גְּדִיָּה, גַּדְיָה f. *she-kid* (v. גְּדִי). Men. XIII, 7 (107b).—Trnsf. *the tender grain in the husks. Pl.* גְּדִיּוֹת. Pesik. R. s. 25 הריני מבשל את הג׳ וכ׳ I shall make ripe &c., v. גְּדִי.

גַּדְיָא, v. גַּדְיָא II.

גַּדְיְתָא, v. גַּדְיָא I.

גָּדִיל m. (גדל) *growing,* esp. *one entering on puberty.* Tosef. Mikv. VI, 10, v. כְּשׁוּת.—*Pl.* גְּדֵילִים, v. גָּדַל I.

גְּדִיל m. (b. h.; גדל II) 1) pl. גְּדִילִין, גְּדִילִים *twisted threads, fringes,* v. צִיצִית. Men. 39b; Yeb. 5b גדיל שנים ג׳ ארבעה *gadil* (a twist) means at least two threads, *g'dilim* means four threads (which doubled make eight). Sifré Num. 115; a. e.—2) *twist, table-cloth.* B. Bath. 57b שני שלישי ג׳ . . גלוי וכ׳ Ar. a. Ms. O. (ed. גלאר) two thirds of the width of the table covered and one third uncovered for putting on dishes and vegetables.

***גְּדִיל** m. ch. (גדל) *liberal, heaped measure,* opp. מחיק. Y. Pes. IV, end, 31c (Esth. R. to I, 4 גדיש).

גְּדִילָא ch.=h. גְּדִיל. Men. 39b top וג׳ מיגדיל and the fringe is twisted (without leaving loose threads). *Pl.* fem. גְּדִילָתָא, v. גְּדִילְתָּא.

גְּדִילָה I f. (גָּדַל I) *growth.* דרך ג׳ *the way a thing grows, in natural position.* Nidd. 67a דרך גְּדִילָתָהּ in her natural position (not pressing limbs together). Succ. 45b דרך גְּדִילָתָן as the plants grow (not upside down); a. e.

גְּדִילָה II f.=גְּדִיל 1). Sifré Num. 115 שתהא ג׳ יוצא וכ׳ the twisted fringe must start from the border, and the loose fringes out of the twist; Yalk. ib. 750.

גְּדִילוּ f. (גדל) *plaiting, wreathing.* Targ. O. Ex. XXVIII, 14; a. e. (h. text עבת).

גְּדִילְתָּא f. (preced.) *rope, chain, plat of hair, fringe.* Targ. Is. V, 18.—*Pl.* גְּדִילָן, גְּדִילָתָא. Targ. Jud. XV, 13 sq. Targ. Y. II Deut. XXII, 12. Targ. O. Ex. XXVIII, 4; 24; a. e.

גַּדִּין, v. גְּדִי ch.—[Targ. Y. Num. XXII, 7 Ar., read אַגְרִין.]

גַּדִּיפִין, v. גִּדְהוּפָא.

גָּדִיר m. (b. h. גָּדֵר; גדר) *fence, guard, precaution against trespassing the law.* Y. Dem. I, 21d מפני גְדִירָהּ, מפני גְדִירוֹ in order to guard it against transgressing. Gen. R. s. 79 (גְּדֵרָן) פרצת גְּדִירָן של וכ׳ thou hast broken down the guard (enactment) which the scholars have erected; a. fr.

גְּדִירָא, גַּדִּירָא c. ch. same, *fence, partition.* Targ. O. Num. XXII, 24; a. e.—ג׳ מיצעא דאודנא the central fence of the ear, *anti-helix.* Targ. Y. Lev. VIII, 23, a. e. (h. text תְּנוּךְ).—B. Kam. 23b לגדור מר ג׳ וכ׳ erect you a fence in your field.

גְּדִירָה f. (preced.) *fence, fortification;* trnsf. *guard, self-restraint.* Cant. R. to IV, 12 גְּדֵירַת ערוה moral restraint, v. גָּדֵר.—*Pl.* גְּדִירוֹת. Pesik. R. s. 26 saw the Temple (which the angels had set on fire) עשור לו ג׳ של אבנים (Yalk. Jer. 300 גזורות של אבנים) surrounded with stone fences (fortified).

גְּדִירָה f. (גדר) *cutting dates, date harvest.*—*Pl.* גְּדִירוֹת. B. Bath. 36b (Ar. a. ed. Pes. גדיד׳), v. גָּדַר.

גָּדִישׁ m. (גדש) *heaped, liberal measure.* Esth. R. to I, 4; v. גְּדִיל.

גָּדִישׁ I m. (b. h.; גדש) *a heap,* esp. of sheaves, *shock* or *stack of grain;* [in b. h. also *mound*]. B. Mets. V, 7 פוסק עמו על הג׳ he may conclude a bargain with him (the early harvester) for the grain in the stack (though no price has been published as yet). Peah VI, 2. Yad. IV, 7.—*Pl.* גְּדִישִׁין, גְּדִישִׁים. Gen. R. s. 51 end. B. Kam. 60b. Pesik. Shubah p. 164a ג׳ ג׳ של עבירות heaps of sins; a. e. [V. גָּדוּשׁ.]

גְּדִישׁ, גְּדִישָׁא ch. same, *pile; mound,* Targ. Y. Ex. XXII, 5. Targ. Job V, 26.—Y. Sabb. XVI, 15d, end, spread his cloak על ג׳ over a burning stalk.—*Pl.* גְּדִישִׁין. Targ. O. Ex. XXII, 5. Targ. Job XXI, 32.

גַּדִּישׁ m. ch. (גְּדַשׁ II) *staff, leader of a blind man.* Lev. R. s. 22; Yalk. Koh. 972 והוה חחיא . . ג׳ ליה וכ׳ and the seeing man was a leader to the blind man.

גְּדִישׁוּתָא f. (גְּדַשׁ I) *heaped measure.* Targ. Y. Lev. XIX, 35.

גַּדְיְתָא, v. גַּדְיָא I.

גָּדַל, גָּדֵל I (b. h.; v. גדל II) *to be high, to grow, be large, tall.* Ex. R. s. 1 שהיה גָּדֵל שלא וכ׳ he was extraordinarily tall for his age. Ib. וכי אין הכל גְּדֵילִים do not all children grow?—Y. Maasr. I, 49a, v. טָפוּס; a. fr. Fem. גְּדֵלָה, pl. גְּדֵלוֹת. Succ. 34a; a. fr.

Pi. גִּדֵּל, גַּדֵּל 1) *to raise* (of live stock and of plants); *to rear, train.* Kil. VIII, 1 מותרים לְגַדֵּל you are permitted to raise. Snh. 19b מיכל גִּדְּלָה Michal reared (Mirab's children). Ib.; Meg. 13a המְגַדֵּל יתום וכ׳ he who educates an orphan in his house. Gen. R. s. 98 הדר . . מְגַדְּלִים שער

they let their hair grow (in mourning). Erub. 100[b] מְגַדֶּלֶת שֵׂעָר she lets her hair grow (does not cut it); a. fr.—2) *to raise to dignity, make famous; to praise.* Hor. 9[a] (ref. to Lev. XXI, 10) whence do we know אם אין לו שחייבין לְגַדְּלוֹ when he (the Highpriest) is poor, that they (the brethren) are bound to raise him (make him independent)? Ib. גַּדְּלֵהוּ משל אחיו raise him by a collection from his brethren (v. Rabb. D. S. a. l.). Esth. R. to III, 1 למה גִּדְּלוֹ for what purpose did (the Lord) raise him? Yalk. Esth. 1053 עד היכן גִּידְּלוֹ וכ׳ how high did he raise him? Fifty cubits (to the gallows); a. fr.—Y. Meg. III, end, 74[c] (ref. to הגדול, Neh. VIII, 6) במה גִידְּלוֹ wherewith did he magnify the Lord (describe His greatness)?; Yoma 69[b] ג׳ בשם וכ׳ he praised the Lord by pronouncing the tetragrammaton; Y. Ber. VII, 11[c] גודלו (corr. acc.)—Part. pass. מְגוּדָּל *well grown.* Ber. 11[a]; a. fr.—Kidd. 49[a], [b], v. גַּדֶּלֶת.

Hif. הִגְדִּיל *to grow up, to become of age.* Yeb. X, 9 וּמִשֶּׁהִ׳ and after he is of age. Ib. XIII, 1 עד שֶׁתַּגְדִּיל until she becomes of age; a. fr.

Hithpa. הִתְגַּדֵּל, *Nithpa.* נִתְגַּדֵּל 1) *to be raised* to dignity. Esth. R. to III, 1 יִתְגַּדֵּל ואח״כ יתלה let him first become great and then be hanged. Gen. R. s. 99, end (play on פֹּרָת, Gen. XLIX, 22) ע״י פָּרוֹת נ׳ by means of cows (Pharaoh's dream) was he raised to power; a. fr.—2) *to be magnified.* Y. Ber. IX, 14[a] top; Y. Taan. I, 64[b] top יִתְגַּדֵּל וכ׳ may Thy Name be glorified, sanctified &c.; a. e.—3) *to glorify one's self, to boast, parade.* Ned. 62[a]; Ab. IV, 5 אל תעשם עטרה לְהִתְגַּדֵּל בהם make them (the words of the Law) not a crown to parade therewith.—4) *to grow, prosper, be nursed.* Tanh. V'zoth 1; Pesik. ib. p. 199[a] הרי .... מִתְגַּדֵּל עמו the poison-bearing tree will be nursed along with it (the health-giving tree). Tanh. B'resh. 7 נִתְגַּדַּלְתָּ וחטאת thou didst grow older and didst sin, opp. תינוק הייח; a. fr.

גְּדַל I ch. same. Kidd. 71[b] ג׳ ולא נסיב was grown up and not yet married.

Pa. גַּדֵּל *to raise, rear.* Hag. 4[b] מרים מְגַדְּלָא דרדקי Miryam, the childrens' nurse.

Ithpa. אִתְגַּדַּל *to be exalted.* Targ. Ps. CIV, 1.

גָּדַל II (v. preced.; cmp. גדש) [*to heap up, round;*] *to plait, dress the hair.* Kel. XVI, 7 גּוֹדְלֵי מצנפות cap-weavers (on a model head, v. אמוּם). Ib. XV, 3 וגוֹדְלוֹת and dress their hair. Sabb. X, 6 הַגּוֹדֶלֶת she who plaits her hair (on the Sabbath). Ib. 94[b] bot. גודלת משום אורגת plaiting the hair (is forbidden on the Sabbath) as an act of weaving; ib. 95[a] (another opin.) ג׳ . . . משום בונה as an act of building. Y. ib. VII, 10[d] הגודל כלי צורה he who forms raised figures on a vessel. M. Kat. 11[a] ג׳ תנור *to build* a stove.

גְּדַל II ch. same. Gitt. 69[a] ניגדול תרתי וכ׳ let him twine two threads. M. Kat. 11[a] לְמִיגְדַּל אהורי to weave nets; למי׳ תנורא to build a stove, v. preced.

Pa. גַּדֵּל same. Hag. 4[b] מרים מְגַדְּלָא נשיא Ms. M. (ed. מג׳ שיער נ׳) Miriam the women's hair-dresser (v. Rabb. D. S. a. l. note); Snh. 67[a]; Sabb. 104[b] (missing in later editions). Succ. 37[a] הנהו מְגַדְּלֵי הושענא those twining the willow twigs (v. הוֹשַׁעְנָא).

גַּדָּל, v. גִּידּוֹל.

גַּדְלוּן m. (גדל) *elevation to dignity, rise.* Yalk. Ps. 777, v. גִּידּוֹל.

***גַּדְלָיי** (גדל II) *weaver.* Y. Keth. XII, 35[a] bot. (Y. Kil. IX, 32[b] bot. גרדיי).

גּוֹדֶלֶת, גַּדֶּלֶת f. (גדל II) *hair-dresser.* Kel. XV, 3 the sieve-like receptacle של גד׳ (Mish. ed. גּוֹדְלוֹת pl.) of the hair-dresser. Kidd. II, 3 ע״מ שיש לי בת או שפחה גד׳ וכ׳ (Y. a. Talm. ed. 49[b] מגודלת, Ar. מגדלת) under the condition that I shall have a (free) girl or a hand-maid as a hair-dresser, and she has none, or 'that I shall have none', and she has. Ib. 49[a] מי סברת מאי מגודלת גדולה ממש מאי מגודלת גדלת וכ׳ do you think *m'guddeleth* of the Mishnah means really *a well-trained* (girl or hand-maid)? It means *a hair-dresser*, when she may see, I want none to take up my words and carry them to my neighbors. Y. ib. II, 62[c] bot. כיני מתניתן בת לגוֹדַלְתֵּיךְ ושפחה לשמשותיך the Mishnah means this: a girl for thy hair-dresser (or thy governess), and a hand-maid for thy attendant. Lev. R. s. 19 נפרים לַגַּ׳ וְהַגַּ׳ וכ׳ let us win the favor of the (queen's) hair-dresser (or *governess*), and the hair-dresser will win the queen and the queen the king; Gen. R. s. 100.

גָּדַם (v. גדד I) *to lop off, stump.*—Part. pass. גָּדוּם, f. גְּדוּמָה. Zeb. 62[b] אמה ג׳ (Y. Yoma IV, 41[c] bot. גְּמוּדָה) a reduced cubit, v. אַמָּה. [Gen. R. s. 12 אמה ג׳, read גְּרוּמָה, v. גָּרַם.] Tosef. Bekh. V, 4 אצבעותיו גְּדוּמוֹת ed. Zuck. (Var. גרומות) with stump-like fingers.

Hithpa. הִתְגַּדֵּם *to be cut off, lopped.* Taan. 21[a] . . . ידי יִתְגַּדְּמוּ may my hands .... be stumped (through sickness).

גְּדַם ch. same. *Parel* גִּרְדֵּם.

גִּדֵּם, v. גִּדֵּם.

גַּדְפָּנָא (גַּדְנְפָּא) גִּדְנְפָא m. (גדף, with inserted נ) *rim, enclosure.* Targ. O. Ex. XXV, 25, a. e. (ed. Berl. גַּדְ׳, Y. גפוף, h. text מסגרת). Targ. Ezek. XLIII, 13; 17 (h. text גבול).—Succ. 20[b] דאית ליה ג׳ (Ms. M. גדפנא, Ar. גדפא) when the matting has a rim (so as to be used as a receptacle for fruits). Ab. Zar. 76[ab] אהדר ליה ג׳ דלישא made a rim of dough around the kettle.—*Pl.* גַּדְנְפַיָּא, גַּדְנְפִין. Targ. I Kings VII, 28 sq. Targ. II Kings XVI, 17. V. גַּדְפָּא.

גָּדַע (b. h.; v. גדד I) *to cut, chop, lop off.*—Y. Sabb. IV, end, 7[a] חריות שֶׁגְּדָעָן וכ׳ twigs which one cut off (trimming the date tree) with the intention of using them for &c. (Bab. ib. 50[a] גדר).—Part. pass. גָּדוּעַ, f. גְּדוּעָה; pl. גְּדוּעִים, גְּדוּעוֹת. Midr. Till. to Ps. LXXV, end קרני ישראל ג׳ the horns (power) of Israel are lopped off (checked).

Pi. גִּדַּע, גִּידַּע. Ib.; Midr. Sam. ch. V, end קרנות שגי׳ צדיקו וכ׳ the horns which the Righteous One of the world (the Lord) has lopped.

Nif. נִגְדַּע *to be lopped, diminished.* Cant. R. to III, 7 נ׳ גובה וכ׳ (Var. נגרע, v. גרע) Adam's high stature was reduced. [V. גָּרַע.]

גְּדַע ch. same. *Targ. II Sam. X, 4 (ed. Lag. גרע).

Ithpa. אִתְגַּדַּע *to be cut, mutilated.* Targ. Y. Ex. XII, 12; Num. XXXIII, 4.

גָּדַף (b. h.; cmp. preced.) *to cut, scrape.* Part. pass. גָּדוּף, pl. גְּדוּפִין. Pes. 42ª מים חג׳ Ar., v. גָּרַף.—מיתה גְדוּפָה, v. infra.

Pi. גִּדֵּף, גִּידֵּף 1) *to hollow out, scrape* or *chisel so as to form an enclosure* or *rim* (cmp. גדנפא, גדפא).—2) *to scrape, to empty to the dregs.* Kerith. 7ᵇ (explain. מגדף, Num. XV, 30, as a metaphor) as one says to his neighbor גִּדַּפְתָּ את הקערה וחיסרת Ar. (ed. גֵּירַ׳; Sifré Num. 112 גֵרַרְתָּ מן וכ׳) thou hast scraped out the dish and lessened the thickness of the vessel (i. e. besides worshipping the forces of Nature to impair, so to speak, the supremacy of the Creator); he who thus explains, is of the opinion that מגדף means blaspheming the Divine Name; ג׳ הקערה ולא וכ׳ thou hast scraped the dish clean but not impaired it (i. e. to worship natural forces without denying the Divine supremacy); he who thus explains, is of the opinion that מגדף is a worshipper of idols; [Y. Snh. VII, 25ᵇ top גיר׳ את כל וכ׳ thou hast emptied the whole dish and left nothing in it, i. e. thou hast erased the entire Law; Sifré l. c. גררתה וכ׳].—Trnsf. (cmp. ארר, נקב, קלל) *to blaspheme* (God); *to revile, reproach.* Kerith. I, 2 אַף הַמְגַדֵּף the blasphemer is also excluded from the rule (and has not to offer a sacrifice in the case of sinning through ignorance); expl. ib. 7ᵇ, v. supra. Snh. VII, 5; a. fr.—Num. R. s. 10 לפי שהיה מחרפם וּמְגַדְּפָם בנחיצה לכך מת מיתה גְדוּפָה וכ׳ because be (Sisera) disgraced and reviled them (the Israelites) with oppressive measures, therefore he died an ignominious death, for (the Lord) delivered him into the hands of a woman; a. fr.

גְּדַף ch., *Pa.* גַּדֵּיף 1) same, *to blaspheme.* Targ. I Kings XXI, 13; a. e.—Y. M. Kat. III, 83ᵇ; Y. Snh. VII, 25ᵇ top.—2) (with ב) *to sneer at.* Snh. 40ᵇ; Ab. Zar. 35ª מְגַדֵּף בה ר׳ R. . . . sneered at the opinion.

גַּדְפָּא m. (v. גָּדַף Pi. 1) *hollowed out,* whence 1) *rim, border.* Succ. 20ᵇ; Ab. Zar. 76ªᵇ Ar., v. גַּדְנְפָא.—2) (cmp. כָּנָף) *wing.* Targ. Job XXXIX, 13. Targ. O. Deut. IV, 17 (ed. Berl. גַּפָּא, v. Berl. Targ. O. II, p. 50); a. e.—B. Bath. 73ᵇ דלי ג׳ (Rashbam דליא לי גדנפא, Ms. O. גפא, v. Rabb. D. S. a. l. note 40) lifted (towards me) a wing.—Trnsf. *bird; feather, plumage.* Keth. 105ᵇ פרח ג׳ וכ׳ a bird flew on his head. Gitt. 86ª בג׳ דאווזא with a goose feather; Ab. Zar. 28ª. Hull. 46ᵇ we put on it ג׳ או רוקא a feather or some spittle.—*Pl.* גַּדְפִין, גַּדְפֵי (גַּר׳). Targ. Job XXXVIII, 13 borders of the earth. Targ. Ex. XXXVII, 9. Targ. Y. Gen. I, 21; a. e.—B. Bath. l. c. דשמטי גַדְפֵּירְהוּ וכ׳ whose feathers fell out on account of their fatness. Hull. 31ª we see גידפי דמ׳ צר אי that the rims of the cut throat stand apart (Rashi: that the plumage of the throat is cut through).

***גדפה,** Y. B. Mets. IV, beg. 9ᵈ לג׳, read מבקרא, as Y. Gitt. IV, 48ᵇ top; cmp. Y. Peah III, 17ᵈ bot.

גַּדְפֵי, v. כַּתְפֵי.

גַּדְפָן, גּוֹדְפָן m. (גדף) *blasphemer.*—*Pl.* גַּדְפָנִין, גּוֹד׳. Y. M. Kat. III, 83ᵇ משרבו הגד׳ וכ׳ since the (gentile) blasphemers (of the Lord) became too numerous, they (the Israelites) ceased to rend their garments (on hearing blasphemy); Y. Snh. VII, 25ᵇ top הגר׳ (corr. acc.).—Y. Yoma VII, 44ᶜ top; Cant. R. to IV, 4 על הגד׳ (Lev. R. s. 10 על הַמְגַדְּפִים) atones for the blasphemers.

גָּדַר *to roll,* v. גַּנְדַּר I.

גָּדַר (b. h.; v. גדד I) 1) *to cut,* esp. *to harvest dates.* B. Mets. 89ᵇ (Ar. גדד, v. Rabb. D. S. a. l. note 300). B. Bath. 36ᵇ עד שיגדור ג׳ גדירות until he has reaped three date harvests.—Y. Sabb. VII, 9ᶜ top; Bab. ib. 73ᵇ (terms equivalent to קוצר); Y. ib. 10ª ed. Krot. הגורד (corr. acc.).—Sabb. 50ª; 125ᵇ חריות . . . . שֶׁגְּדָרָן לעצים twigs of a date tree which one cut with the intention of using them for fuel; v. גָּדַע.—Tosef. Ber. IV, 21; a. fr.—*Part. pass. גָּדוּר *cut down.* Tosef. Shebi. IV, 13 כרם ג׳ בציפורי (Var. גדול; R. S. to Shebi. VI, 4 גריד) a ruined vineyard in Zepphoris.—2) *to surround with a* גָּדֵר, *fence in; to limit, control, ward off.* B. Kam. 23ª שהיה לו לְגוֹדְרָהּ ולא גְדָרָהּ he ought to have fenced it in and did not do so. Tosef. M. Kat. I, 7 חומה . . . גּוֹדְרִין אותה if a city wall is broken into, we may fence it in (repair it, during the festive week).—Gen. R. s. 49 (play on *haaf*, Gen. XVIII, 23) אתה גודר את האף והאף לא יִגְדְּרָךְ Thou controllest the anger, but the anger does not control Thee.—Y. Ber. IX, end, 14ᶜ וגוֹדְרָהּ, v. זָקַן I.—Mikv. V, 6 גודר כלים one may form a dam with garments (Tosef. ib. IV, 10 גרר, corr. acc.). Y. Ber. III, 6ᶜ דבר שהוא גוֹדֵר את ישראל מן וכ׳ a custom which guards Israel from sin. Lev. R. s. 24 מי שהוא גודר עצמו וכ׳ (Y. Yeb. II, 3ᵈ top פורש) he who guards himself against sin (restraining himself from anything unchaste) is called holy. Gen. R. s. 70 גָּדְרוּ עצמן וכ׳ trained themselves to chastity; a. fr.—*Part. pass.* גָּדוּר *abstinent, chaste.* Lev. R. s. 22 ומעצמו הוא ג׳ and he will become abstinent of his own accord. Gen. R. l. c. אנשי מזרח גְּדוּרִים וכ׳ the people of the East are chaste; a. fr.—ג׳ פרצה (or sub. פרצה) to fence in a breach, *to remedy calamities,* also *to check lawlessness* by preventive measures (v. גְּזֵרָה). Ber. 19ª שתִּגְדּוֹר וכ׳ that Thou repair our breaches (relieve us); B. Bath. 91ᵇ.—Lev. R. s. 1 (play on *Abigdor* I Chr. IV, 4) הרבה גוֹדְרִין וכ׳ Israel had many fencemakers (guardians against sin). Ruth. R. s. 2, a. fr.—Erub. 6ª, a. e. ג׳ בה גדר, v. בִּקְעָה.—[Y. Erub. X, 26ᵇ bot. דלת גודרת וכ׳; Tosef. ib. XI (VII), 18 גוררת ed. Zuck., Var. גוד׳, v. גָּרַר.]—[Y. Sabb. XV, 15ᵇ top וגדרתא, read וּגְדַרְתָּהּ.]

Nif. נִגְדַּר *to be guarded; to guard one's self.* Y. Sabb. XVII, beg. 16ª כיון שנִגְדְּרוּ (ib. III, 6ª top שנִתְגַּדְּרוּ) when they had been trained (to guard against desecrating the Sabbath). Lev. R. s. 32 נ׳ כל הנשים וכ׳ all women were made chaste through her meritorious example; a. e.

Pi. גִּידֵּר *to cut into.* Gitt. 56ᵇ; Lev. R. s. 20; 22; Num. R. s. 18 וגיד׳ את הפרוכת and cut into the curtain (Koh.

R. to V, 8; Tanh. Huck. 1 'יגד'). [Tosef. Shebi. III, 20 מְגַדֵּר בחורשין Var. (ed. Zuck. מברך) to cut into, to clear thickets, v. בחה.]

Hithpa. הִתְגַּדֵּר 1) [*to cut one'sself off from others,*] *to distinguish one's self, to excel; to raise one's self above others, to arrogate power, be presumptuous.* Ber. 17ª כשם שהוא אינו מִתְגַּדֵּר וכ׳ as he cannot excel in my work (study), so can I not in his (field labor). Hull. 7ª my predecessors have left room for me לְהִתְגַּדֵּר בו to distinguish myself; Yoma 78ª; (Y. Dem. II, 22ᶜ bot. עטרה להתעטר, Ar. להתגדר).—Ned. 81ª כדי שלא יִתְגַּדְּרוּ על וכ׳ in order that they may not be presumptuous towards the people; v. גָּבַר Hithpa. [Mekh. B'shall., Vayassa 1 כבן שמתגדר וכ׳, v. גָּדַר II.]—2) *to be trained,* v. supra Nif.

גְּדַר ch. same; 1) *to fence in; to check.* B. Kam. 23ᵇ, v. גְּדִירָא. Yeb. 90ᵇ מִיגְדַּר מילתא שאני a measure to check something (an extraordinary measure for checking lawlessnes) is something different, allows of no analogies.—*2) *to cut off, deduct.* Esth. R. to I, 4 גַּדְרָאנֵיה מן פורני I will deduct it from my dowry. [Ib. to I, 9 אנא מגדיר, v. גְּדַר.]

גָּדֵר I m. (v. גְּדִיר) *fence, partition.* Peah II, 3. Y. ib. 16ᵈ ג׳ מחובר a hedge, v. חָבַר. B. Kam. 23ª [read:] ונפל הג׳ (v. Rabb. D. S. a. l.) and the partition wall fell in; a. v. fr.—Trnsf. *guard against trespassing the law, restraint, preventive measure* (v. גְּזֵרָה). Tosef. Shebi III, 13 לא גזרו אלא ג׳ שיכול לעמוד they (the scholars) erect only such a fence as can stand, i. e. enact only practicable measures (v. גָּזַר). Snh. 21ª ג׳ גדול גָּדְרָה וכ׳ Tamar erected a great guard at the time (became a warning to girls). Lev. R. s. 26 the serpent פרץ גְּדֵרוֹ של עולם made a breach in the fence of the world (opened the way to lawlessness). Ib. s. 24, a. fr. ג׳ ערוה guard against immorality, *chastity,* v. גָּדַר; a. fr.—Y. Pes. I, 27ᶜ bot. ויש ג׳ לג׳ can a preventive rabbinical law (גְּזֵרָה) be enacted as a guard for another preventive law?—*Pl.* גְּדֵרוֹת. Lev. R. s. 24; a. e., v. גָּדִיר.

גֶּדֶר II, הַגֶּדֶר pr. n. pl. *Geder (Gadara),* capital of Peraea, v. גָּדוֹר. Pesik. R. s. 21 (p. 107ª ed. Fr.) מן הגודר (read גדור or גדר), v. פֵּיוּס; ib. (p. 108ª) מן הג׳.—R. Hash. 23ᵇ, v. גָּדוֹר. Esth. R. to I, 3, v. אַרְכִּיוֹן.—Y. Kidd. III, 64ᵈ top מי ג׳ חמתא דג׳ Hamtha (Hot Springs) near G.—Sabb. 109ª springs of G.—Erub. 61ª; Tosef ib. VI (V), 13 שיהו בני ג׳ יורדין וכ׳ that the inhabitants of G. were permitted to go down to Hamtha (on the Sabbath), but &c., v. טַטְרַג.

גַּדְרָאנֵיה=גַּדְרָנֵיה=אנא גַּדְרָא ליה, v. גְּדַר.

גדרסן, Targ. Jud. XVI, 14 some ed., read גַּרְדְּאָין, v. גַּרְדִּי.

גדרפוס, v. גנדרופוס.

גָּדֵשׁ pr. n. pl. *Gadesh,* in Gilead. Midr. Sam. ch. XXX; XXXII (expl. חגלעדה II Sam. XXIV, 6).

גָּדַשׁ *to heap up, to put up stacks of grain.* Pes. 56ª; Men. 71ª גּוֹדְשִׁין לפני העומר they put the stacks of grain up before offering the Omer (v. עוֹמֶר); Tosef. Pes. II (III), 19 (corr. acc.). Tosef. B. Kam. VI, 24 השאילו לִגְדּוֹשׁ . . . וגָ׳ וכ׳ if he lent him a spot to pile wheat on it, and he piled barley; a. fr.—2) *to give heaped measure,* opp. מחק to strike. B. Bath. V, 11 where the usage is למחוק לא יִגְדּוֹשׁ וכ׳ to strike grain, one must not heap (even for special remuneration) &c.; a. fr.—Part. pass. גָּדוּשׁ, f. גְּדוּשָׁה, *brimful, overflowing, heaped.* Tam. V, 4. Yoma 48ª גְּדוּשׁוֹת, v. כַּפָּה I. Gen. R. s. 22 חטאו ג׳ . . . . ומגודש the measure of thy sin is heaped to excess.—Sabb. 153ᵇ; Tosef. ib. I, 17; Y. ib. I, 3ᶜ בו ביום גָּדְשׁוּ (את ה)סאה on that day (of rabbinical enactments) they overfilled the measure (of laws).

Nif. נִגְדַּשׁ *to be heaped up, to tower up.* Men. IX, 5 היו נִגְדָּשׁוֹת were heaped, v. גּוֹדֶשׁ. Sot. 34ª the waters נִגְדָּשִׁין ועולין rose more and more.

Pi. גִּידֵּשׁ same. Part. pass. מְגוּדָּשׁ, v. supra.

Hif. הִגְדִּישׁ *to pile up stacks.* B. Kam. VI, 3.

גְּדַשׁ I ch. same. Targ. Prov. VI, 8 Ms. (ed. גבש׳).

גַּדַּשׁ II, *Pa.* גַּדֵּשׁ (cmp. נְגַד III a. נגיד) *to lead a blind man.* Lev. R. s. 22; Koh. R. to V, 8; Yalk. ib. 972; v. גַּדִּישׁ.

גָּהָה, גָּחָה (for dialect. change of ה a. ח, cmp. גבח a. גבה) *to swell, bulge; to hang over* (cmp. בָּעַט I). M. Kat. 7ª כותל הגּוֹהֶה וכ׳ Ar. (ed. ח) a wall inclining towards the public road; Tosef. ib. I, 7 גּוֹאֶה ed. Zuck. (Var. גוחה); Y. ib. I, 80ᶜ bot.; a. e.—Succ. 45ª כדי שיהו גוהות על וכ׳ (ed. גוחות, Ms. M. גבוהות) that the willows might overtop the altar one cubit. [Cmp. Ps. XXII, 7 גֹּחִי *bending over me, protecting.*]

גָּהַט, גָּחַט (cmp. גחין) *to polish over, erase.* Part. Peïl גָּהוּט, גָּחוּט, *erased.* Ber. 56ª ו״ו דפטר חמור ג׳ וכ׳ (for right vers. v. Rabb. D. S. a. l.) the Vav in *Peter Ḥămor* (Ex. XIII, 13) of thy T'fillin is erased (had by mistake been written and its erasure could be noticed).

גְּהִינָּם, v. גֵּיהִינָּם.

גהיקן, גהיקין, v. גַּמִּיקִין.

גָּהַץ (cmp. גהט) *to be bright, glad, willing.* Gen. R. s. 39 [combine text of ed. with vers. of Ar. and read:] וא״ת שלא ג׳ אברהם ושמח על דבור המקום שאילו ג׳ ושמח למה לא יצא and if you will say, Abraham was not glad and joyful over the command of the Lord (to leave his home), for if he were so, why did he not emigrate (until he was commanded)?

Pi. גִּיהֵץ, *Hif.* הִגְהִיץ *to polish* (clothes), *iron, gloss.* Cant. R. to IV, 11 the cloud rubbed their clothes ומְגַהֵיצָן and polished them; Midr. Till. to Ps. XXIII ומְגַהֲצָן; Yalk. Deut. 850; Ps. 691 ענני כבוד היו מְגַהֲצִין וכ׳; Pesik. B'shall. p. 92ª מְגַהֲצִים וכ׳; (Deut. R. s. 7 ומלבנן). Ib. אין מג׳ אלא באור (v. אַמְיַינְטוֹן) is cleansed only by fire.—*Part. Pu.* מְגוּהָץ, pl. מְגוּהָצִין. Pes. 109ª. Y. M. Kat. III, 82ª bot.

Hithpa. הִתְגַּהֵץ *to be polished.* Cant. R. l. c., a. parallel, passages, v. supra.

גַּהַק, *Pi.* גִּיהֵק (onomatop.) *to belch.* Ber. 24[a]. Ib.[b] מְגַהֵק.

גַּהַר, v. גָּחַר.

גֵּו, גַּו m. (b. h.; cmp. גב) *belly, body;* prep. *within, among.* Keth. 15[a]; B. Kam. 44[b], a. e. זורק אבן לגו one who throws a stone into (a crowd); Yalk. Deut. 921 לגוּר (corr. acc.). Keth. 111[a]; Kidd. 44[b] דברים בגו there is something in it, v. גַּב end.

גַּו, גֵּיו, גַּו, גַּוָּא, גּוֹ, constr. **גּוֹ, גּוֹא** ch. same; 1) (=h. קֶרֶב) *belly; innermost.* Targ. Ex. XXIX, 13; a. e. Targ. Prov. XXVI, 24. Targ. O. Deut. III, 16 (h. text תּוֹךְ); a. fr.—Sabb. 152[b] לגַוֵּיה דביתא (insert ולידזול) and go home. Cant. R. to IV, 8 like the hen דמנערא גפה מגווא קטמא (read מִגּוֹא) that shakes her wings off (rising) from between the ashes (Gen. R. s. 75 beg. מן קיטמא). Cant. R. to I, 7 יומא דהוה קאים בגַוֵּיה the day on which he stood, i. e. that every day; a. fr.—*Pl.* גַּוַּיָּא. Targ. Prov. XX, 27 (ed. Lag. גַּוַּיֵּיה).—2) (with or without ב) *among, amid; in, into.* Targ. Ex. XIV, 22; a. fr.—Y. Peah VIII, 20[d] bot. מן גוא לפסא out of the pot. Hull. 41[a] אית ליה שותפות בגַוָּהּ he owns a share in it. Ib. 48[b] קופא לגַיו if the head of the pin is towards the inside. Lev. R. s. 12 את מפני מלגאו מלבר . . . pour thou out from inside (the hole), and I shall drink from outside. B. Mets. 53[b] sq., v. בַּר I ch. a. חוּמְשָׁא.—Pes. 110[b] אתית לגאו, אתית לגו I have come among (you). Y. Keth. XII, 35[b]; Y. Kil. IX, 32[c] bot. גוא ארעא וכ׳ in a unclean land. Y. Keth. l. c.[a] bot.; Y. Kil. l. c.[b] bot. גו בני (גובני) in the bath-house. Y. Ned. IX, 41[b] bot. גו שמשא in the sun (in sunlight); a. v. fr.—מן גו, מִיגּוֹ, מִגּוֹ *because, in consequence of.* Y. Taan. II, 65[b], v. בּוֹךְ. Y. Ber. I, 3[b] top מן גו דאינון ציבחר because they are brief.—B. Mets. 39[b] מיגו דמוקמינן וכ׳ since we have to appoint a guardian for &c. Ib. 5[b], a. fr. מ׳ דחשיד אממונא וכ׳ since he is suspected of wrong-doing in money matters, he is also suspected of swearing falsely; a. fr.—Hence מִגּוֹ, מִיגּוֹ *Miggo*, 1) (=h. מִתּוֹךְ, Shebu. 45[b], and מֵאַחַר, v. אַחַר) *a legal rule according to which a deponent's statement is accepted as true on the ground that, if he had intended to tell a lie, he might have invented one more advantageous to his case* (cmp. B. Bath. 31[a] מה לו לשקר אי בעי וכ׳ why should he lie? If he wanted to lie, he might have said &c.). Keth. 16[a] התם מאי מ׳ איכא what *miggo* is there in that case, i. e. what choice did she have in inventing a statement, if she intended to tell a lie? Ib. מכדי האי מ׳ והאי מ׳ וכ׳ since in this case there is the legal presumption of a *miggo*, and so is in the other, what is the difference between the one *miggo* and the other?; a. fr.—2) (cmp. אַגַּב) *an action declared valid because one part of it was indisputably legitimate,* or *because the legal status required for its legitimacy might easily have been obtained.* B. Mets. 9[b] מ׳ דאי בעי מפקר וכ׳ since, if he wanted, he might have declared his possession public property, in which case he would have obtained the legal status of poverty entitling him to the corner of the field (פֵּאָה), and since (if he had resigned his property) he would have been entitled to take possession of the corner for himself, he has a right also to take possession of it in behalf of his neighbor. Ib. תרי מ׳ לא אמרינן two *miggos* cannot be accepted, i. e. two conditions required to make an action legitimate cannot be dispensed with. Ib. 8[a]. Ned. 88[b]; a. e.

גּוָּאָה, גַּוָּאִי, גַּוַּר׳, (גַּוָּיָא) m. (preced.) *inner, inside* (adj. a. adv.) Targ. I Kings VI, 27; a. e.—Zeb. 15[a] דקאי ג׳ stands inside. Ib. לג׳, v. בְּרָאֵי. Y. Sabb. VIII, 11[a] top בחהן גויוא of the inside (reed), opp. בראה.—*Pl.* גַּוָּאֵין, גַּוָּאֵי. Targ. Y. Num. VI, 4.—Hull. 47[a] bot. מג׳ from the inner lungs (lower part), opp. אַגַּבָּא. B. Bath. 29[b] שכוני ג׳ the interior compartments. Hag. 5[b] בתי ג׳ the inner chambers of the heavens; a. fr.—Fem. גַּוַּיְתָא. Targ. Ezek. XL, 27; a. e.—*Pl.* גַּוַּיאָתָא. Erub. 25[b] גודא ג׳ (read גודרי, Ms. M. גודרי גואר) inner partitions.

גַּוָּאזָא, v. גַּוְזָא.

גּוֹאֵל m. (b. h.; גָּאַל) *vindicator, redeemer, relative entitled to redemption* (Lev. XXV, 25 sq.); in general *relation.*—ג׳ הדם *avenger of blood, nearest relation* (Num. XXXV, 19 sq.). Macc. II, 7. Ib. 12[a] [read:] אב שהרג בנו בנו נעש׳ לו ג׳ הדם when a father killed a son of his, his (surviving) son becomes the avenger of blood. Tanh. Masé 11 וימצא אותו הג׳ and the avenger may meet him; Num. R. s. 23 ג׳ הדם. Macc. 10[a] (ref. to Deut. XIX, 6) בג׳ הדם הכתוב וכ׳ the text means the avenger (is not punished); a. fr.—*Pl.* גּוֹאֲלִין, גּוֹאֲלִים. B. Kam. 109[a]; Kidd. 21[a] (ref. to Num. V, 8) וכי יש אדם שאין לו ג׳ is there a person ... without relations (heirs)?; Snh. 68[b] גואל. B. Kam. l. c.[b]; Snh. 69[a] בידוע שאין לו ג׳ it is known that the minor has no heirs (offspring); a. fr.—Esp. *the redeemer from captivity,* also *the Lord.* Lev. R. s. 32 end; Cant. R. to IV, 7; Koh. R. to IV, 1 (ref. to וְגֻלָּהּ, Zech. IV, 2) one reads גּוֹלָה (He emigrates), and one reads גּוֹאֲלָהּ (not גאולה) her Redeemer (goes at the head of Israel). Ib. מאן דאמר גואלה פרוקא (not גאולה) he who reads גואלה means 'the Redeemer' as it says (Is. XLVII, 4), Our redeemer &c.—Pesik. S'lih. p. 166[b] אין . . . אלא בג׳ מלא they will be redeemed only through a *complete* redeemer (ref. to גואל Is. LIX, 20 written *plene*). Ex. R. s. 26 beg.; a. fr.—*Pl.* as above. Gen. R. s. 85; Yalk. ib. 145 מהיכן ג׳ עומדים (not גדולים) whence will the redeemers rise (if not from Judah)? Ib. ג׳ אני מעוברת I am going pregnant with redeemers (of Israel).

גּוּאַלְקָא, גּוּלְקָא, גּוּוָלְקָא m. (Arab. guwâlik, Pers. gawâlakh=hippopera, Freytag s. v.) *long pouch as a receptacle for grain,* thrown over the shoulders or across an animal's back, *haversack.* Taan. 23[b] הבו לי גואלקי וכ׳ (Ar. קא . . .; Ms. M. 2 שקיל גולקא, v. Rabb. D. S. a. l. note 200) get me my haversack, and I shall go and buy &c.—*Pl.* גּוּאַלְקֵי, גּוּאַלְקָאן. Targ. Lam. V, 5.—Sabb. 154[b], v. חֲבַר (where Var. lect. are quoted). Succ. 20[b] חזו לגואלקי Ms. M. (ed. לגולקי) are fit for haversacks.

גַּוָּאן, v. גַּוּון.

גּוֹב, *Pa.* גַּיֵּיב, v. גִּיב I. [Targ. Prov. IX, 3 Ms., v. גִּיב II.]

גּוֹב m. (גבב, גבב, cmp. גֻּבָּא) *pit;* ג׳ אריות *lions' den.* Ex. R. s. 18, end הצרל לדניאל מג׳ א׳ He rescued Daniel from the lions' den. Deut. R. s. 2; a. e.

גּוֹב, גּוּב, גּוּבָּא, גֹּב, גַּבָּא, גּוּבָּה ch. 1) same. Dan. VI, 8; 13; 17 sq.—Targ. Ex. XXI, 33 sq. (some ed. גּוּבָא); Targ. Ps. XLIV, 26 (ed. Vien. גּוּבָא); a. e.—Y. Ab. Zar. IV, 44ª bot. נפל לג׳ fell into a wine pit, v. זָחַל.—*Pl.* גּוּבִּין, גּוּבַּיָּא, גּוּבֵּי, גּוּב׳. Targ. Jer. II, 13. Targ. Gen. XXXVII, 20 ed. Berl. גּוּבַּ׳ (Y. גּוֹב׳).—2) (cmp. גַּב, גַּבָּא) *body, trunk, untrimmed log.*—*Pl.* גּוּבֵּי or גּוֹבֵי. B. Kam. 96ª ג׳ דדיקלא logs of a date-tree. Ib. ג׳ ועבדינהו וכ׳, v. כְּשׁוּרָא. Sabb. 109ᵇ the swallowed serpent came out of his body ג׳ ג׳ in single trunks (sections of the body). M. Kat. 24ª ג׳ דדיקנא chin, v. גַּב (Rashi: *the dimples* of the chin).—3) *back, top.* Targ. Prov. IX, 3 Ms. על ג׳ (cmp. על גַּב; ed. גִּיב, h. text גַּפֵּי).—4) *prep. (cmp. גַּבֵּי s. v. גַּב) מן גובי *out of.* Y. Keth. II, 35ª ומן גובידן עבד וכ׳ and out of these (seventeen years) he spent thirteen years suffering with tooth-ache; Y. Kil. IX, 32ᵇ ומן גובעין (corr. acc.).

גּוֹבָא m. *locust,* v. גּוּבַאי. Targ. Ex. X, 4; a. fr.—**Pl.* גּוֹבַיָּיא. Targ. Y. II Gen. XXIII, 2 ed. pr. a. ed. Ven. (later ed. גובריא *giants,* Anak and his three sons, v. Gen. R. s. 58; h. text ארבע).

גּוֹבָאה, v. גּוֹבְהָא.

גּוֹבַאי, גּוֹבַיי m. (b. h. גּוֹב, גּוֹבַי; גבה, cmp. גִּבֵּחַ) [*the hump-backed,*] *gobay,* a species of edible locusts. Ber. VI, 3. Sabb. 32ᵇ. Y. Taan. I, end, 64ᵈ שני דברים...וג׳ two calamities, drought and locusts. Ib. III, 66ᵈ (homiletic etymology) why is it called גוביי? דו גבי דינא וכ׳ because it collects the (fines of) judgment of the Lord.

גּוֹבָאי, גּוֹבֵי ch. same. Targ. Y. I Deut. XXVIII, 38. Targ. Ps. CV, 34. Am. VII, 1; a. e. (mostly גּוֹבָא; Var. גּוֹבַאי, גּוֹבֵי).

גּוֹבָאֵי m. pl. *inhabitants of Gobaya,* v. גּוֹבַיָּא.

גּוּבַבְתָּא, גּוּפַפְתָּא f. pl. (גבב) *hills,* esp. *Gob'batha,* near Sepphoris. Gen. R. s. 98 (ref. to גת החפר, 1 Kings XIV, 25) אילין ג׳ דציפורין that is G. near Sepph. Koh. R. to IX, 10 the lamentations over the death of Rabbi at Sepph. were heard עד גובבתה וכ׳ (some ed. גובתתה, גובת׳, corr. acc.) as far as Gob., a distance of three *mil;* ib. to VII, 11 גופתתא; Y. Kil. V, 32ᵇ top לגו פפתה (combine in one w.); Y. Keth. XII, 35ª top לגו פתתה (corr. acc.). [Y. Snh. VII, end, 25ᵈ גופתא דציפורין; Y. Ber. III, 6ª bot.; Y. Naz. VII, 56ª top גופנא דציפ׳ (corr. acc.). Y. Shek. VII, 50ᶜ bot.; Y. Succ. II, 53ª top גופתא—prob. the same as גובב׳.] V. גּוּבְתָא.

גּוֹבַהּ m. (b. h. גֹּבַהּ; גָּבַהּ) *height, elevation; thick, fleshy part* (cmp. גַּב). Midd. IV, 1 גָּבְהוֹ Ib. 6. גּוֹבְהוֹ; a. fr.—Men. 37ᵇ ג׳ שביד the thickest part of the upper arm (קיבורת); ג׳ שבראש the highest point of the forehead. Y. Yeb. VIII, 9ª; Y. Sabb. XIX, end, 17ᵇ; Bab. ib. 137ᵇ גּוֹבְהָהּ של עטרה the thickest part of the apex.

גּוֹבְהָא ch. same. Targ. Y. Ex. XIII, 9 (corresp. to Men. 37ᵇ, v. preced.). Targ. Job V, 7 (some ed. גובאה, corr. acc.).

גּוֹבַיָּא pr. n. *Gobaya,* a Babylonian place or district, (v. Graetz, *Koenigr. Messene,* in programme of the Rabbin. Semin., Breslau 1879). Kidd. 72ª; Y. Yeb. I, 3ᵇ top; גווכריא (corr. acc.); Y. Kidd. IV, 65ᵈ top גַּבְבַיָּא.—Denom. pl. גּוֹבָאֵי. Kidd. 70ᵇ (phonetic play) ג׳ גבעונאי Gobeans are legally considered like Gibeonites (v. גִּבְעוֹנִי); Y. Yeb. l. c. גווכאי (corr. acc.); Y. Kidd. l. c. גַּבְבָאֵי, גַּבְבָיֵי. Ber. 17ᵇ ג׳ טפשאי foolish Gobeans.

גּוּבַיְינָא m.=h. גִּיבּוּי, *collection.* Yeb. 66ᵇ, a. e. מחוסר ג׳ wanting collection (not yet collected). B. Mets. 110ᵇ landed property כיון דלג׳ קיימא וכ׳ because it is ready to be collected from, (is seizable for debts and cannot be hidden), is considered as if collected.

***גּוּבִיתָא** f. (v. h. גַּב d) *a low fence.* Y. Orl. III, end, 63ᵇ עבר חנן ג׳ וכ׳ Hanan passed over the fence and tore the mixed seeds out.

גּוֹבַל m. (גבל, v. גְּבוּל) *border of the field, balk, ridge.* Kil. III, 1 sq. Ms. M. (ed. גבול). Y. ib. 28ᶜ (R. S. to Kil. III, 1, reads: גבול).—*Pl.* גּוֹבְלִין. Ib.

גּוּבְלָא m. (גבל; v. גְּבִיל) *a thick dough-like mass.* Ber. 38ª ג׳ בעלמא הוא it is a mere thick mass (no bread).

גּוֹבְלָאֵי m. pl. (v. גַּבְלָא) *of Gabla, Idumeans.* Targ. Ps. LXXXIII, 8 ed. (Var. גּוֹבְנָאֵי, Ms. גִּיבְלַי).

גּוֹבְלִית, v. גִּבְלִית.

גּוּבְלְנָא, גּוּלְדָנָה ch.=h. גַּבְלָן. Y. Ab. Zar. II, 41ᶜ top לגובלנ׳; Y. Meg. III, 73ᵈ bot. לגוולנה.

גּוּבְנָא ch. m.=h. גְּבִינָה, *cheese.* Y. Shek. VII, 50ᶜ bot. עיגול דג׳ a loaf of cheese. Y. M. Kat. III, 83ᵇ bot.—*Pl.* גּוּבְנִין. Targ. I Sam. XVII, 18. Targ. Jud. V, 25 (*cream,* h. text חמאה). Targ. Ps. LV, 22 (h. text מ(חֲמָאוֹת)). Targ. Job XX, 17; XXIX, 6 Ms. (v. לְוָוֵאר).

גּוּבְנַי=גּוּ בְנֵי, v. גַּו.

***גּוֹבְנָאֵי**, v. גּוֹבְלָאֵי.

גּוֹבְעִין, Y. Kil. IX, 32ᵇ, v. גּוֹב ch., end.

גּוּבְרָא m. 1)=גַּבְרָא, *man, husband.* Targ. Koh. V, 11.—Y. Taan. I, 64ᵇ bot.; a. fr.—*Pl.* גּוּבְרִין, גּוּבְרַיָּא. Targ. Y. Deut. I, 13; a. e.—Snh. 65ᵇ מה גבר מגו׳ what is the difference between man and men (you and common people). Ber. 31ᵇ גברא בגו׳ a man among men (a distinguished man). Gitt. 45ª עדיי ג׳ וכ׳ these (our captors) are men and those (our husbands) in Nehardea are men (Rashi: *our masters, husbands*), a. fr.—2) *strength, skill.* Nidd. 25ᵇ; 64ᵇ דרב גּוּבְרֵיה because his skill (physiological knowledge) was great.

גּוּבְשָׁא f. (גבש) *hill, mound.*—*Pl.* גּוּבְשָׁתָא. Targ. Zeph. I, 10 Kimhi (ed. גִּבְעָתָא).

גּוּפְתָּא, גַּבְתָּא, גּוּבְתָּא f. (v. גּוּבַבְתָּא) *hill* (or *pit*), esp. *Gubta, Gabta,* name of several places, as ג׳ דאריח, v. אֲרִיחַ; גּוּבַת שמאי, v. סִימַאי &c.

גּוּבְתָּא f. (cmp. גֵּב) *little reservoir*, whence *tube, channel.* Targ. II Esth. I, 3 ג׳ דכוחלא the tube containing the eye-paint; Ber. 18ᵇ גּוּבְתָּאִר דכ׳ my tube &c.—Sabb. 90ᵇ רמי ליה בג׳ דנחשא one puts it into a bronze tube. Ib. 146ᵇ ג׳ to insert a tube into the barrel. Hull. 58ᵇ ההיא ג׳ וכ׳ a channel was discovered forming the passage from the second stomach &c. Yeb. 75ᵇ ג׳ דשכבת זרע the channel for the effusion of semen.

גוּגְיֵיתִית, v. גִּיגִּיתָא.

גּוּגַלְתָּא=גּוּלְגַּלְתָּא.

גּוּגְמֵי, v. גַּגְמֵי.

גּוּד 1) (sec. r. of אָגַד I) *to bind;* denom. גִּיד.—[Polel גּוֹדֵד, fr. which גְּדוּד.]—2) (denom. of גדוד) *to form a faction;* (b. h. *to attack in small bands*). Yeb. 13ᵇ (ref. to Deut. XIV, 1, v. גָּדַד I) if *lo tithgod'du* were meant only in the one sense of 'ye shall form no factions', it would have read לֹא תָגוּדוּ.

Hithpol. הִתְגּוֹדֵד *to form bands, factions.* Ib. 14ᵃ כי אמרינן לא תתגודדו the law against factions applies only to &c.—Sifré Deut. 96; [Pesik. Zutr. R'eh (p. 43) מלשון גדוד].

גּוּד or **גּוֹד**, forms of גדד a. נגד.

***גּוּד** m. (נגד) [*stretched,*] *leather bag* for wine, milk &c.; which travellers at night stretch like a tent in order to let the cool air strike it, *large leather bottle.* Sabb. 138ᵃ הג׳ . . . לא יעשה (Ms. M. הניד a. O., v. Rabb. D. S. a. l. note) one must not stretch the bag &c. on the Sabbath. Ib.ᵇ, v. כֶּסֶךְ.

***גּוּדָא** ch. same. Succ. 48ᵇ out of this man's (thy) skin משוינן ליה ג׳ (Ms. M. 2 נודא) we shall make a bottle.

גּוּדָא I f. (גְּדַר) 1) *partition, wall.* Targ. Ps. LXII, 4 (ed. Vien. גּוּדָא; Ms. גודרא, h. text גדר). Targ. Koh. X, 8 ג׳ דעלמא the world's fence (morality).—B. Bath. 2ᵃ (explain. מחיצה, Mish. ib. I, 1) it means ג׳ *wall* (not פלוגתא division). Ib. 36ᵃ מג׳ דערודי ולבר the land outside the fence which is erected to protect the fields from beasts. Sabb. 110ᵇ בין תנורא לג׳ between the stove and the wall. Taan. 21ᵃ ג׳ רעיעא (Ms. M.; Yalk. Deut. 897 אשיתא) a ruinous wall. Koh. R. to X, 7 טריף רישיה אג׳ he knocked his head against the wall. B. Kam. 92ᵇ (prov.) קרית חברך . . . רמי ג׳ רבה שדי ביה (Ms. M. דחי גידא רבא וכ׳, Ms. R. a. Yalk. Ez. 364 דחי ג׳ רמי שדי עילויה) when thou hast called thy neighbor (cautioning him), and he would not answer, push down a big wall and throw it at him (he deserves to suffer).—*Pl.* with suff. גּוּדַּיָּא. Targ. Ps. LXXX, 13 (ed. Vien. גּוּדְרָהָא, Ms. גדירהא, h. text גְּדֵרֶיהָ).—2) (cmp. גִּידּוּד) *banks.* Taan. 24ᵇ; Yoma 77ᵇ ג׳ דנהר וכ׳ the banks of &c. *Gitt. 73ᵃ אַגּוּדָא דנהר וכ׳ Ar. (ed. אגידא, v. next w.) on the banks of &c.

גּוּדָא, גִּידָא m. (גּוּד) *junction, joined boards.* Hag. 15ᵃ כי גו׳ דגמלא (Ms. M. 2 כגידא) as the boards of a landing bridge are placed side by side (leaving small slits). Snh. 7ᵃ דמי לגו׳ דגמלא וכ׳ (Ms. M. לגי׳, v. Rabb. D. S. a. l.) like the junction of a landing bridge (which is at first shaky, but,) once put up, grows firmer.—*Gitt. 73ᵃ bought poppy seed, אגידא דנהר וכ׳ deliverable at the landing of &c.; v. preced.—Y. Meg. I, 71ᵈ top גו׳ דרצועתא the seam of the straps (of the phylacteries). V. גִּידָא.

גּוּדָא II pr. n. m. *Gudda.* Ab. Zar. 32ᵃ (Ms. M. גּוּרָא, v. Rabb. D. S. a. l. note).

גודאות, Yalk. Gen. 55, read גור׳, v. גּוּרְיָה.

גּוּדְגְּדָא, גּוּדְגְּדָה pr. n. m. *Gudgada,* father of R. Johanan. Hag. II, 7; Gitt. V, 5; Yeb. XIV, 2; Eduy. VII, 9. ר׳ נחוניה בן ג׳ ed. (Ms. M. יוחנן).

***גּוּדְגְּדִין** m. pl. (v. גַּד h. a. ch.) *good luck, Fortune.* Tosef. Sabb. VI (VII), 1 המגבח לג׳ ed. Zuck. (Var. גורגדין; oth. ed. המגבה לגרגרן) he who shaves his head (makes a bald-pate) for good luck (a superstitious practice).

גּוּדְגַּדְנִיּוֹת, v. גַּדְגַּ׳.

גּוּדְיוֹן, v. גּוּזְיוֹן.

גּוֹדֶל m. (b. h. גֹּדֶל; v. גדל) 1) *greatness.* Erub. 21ᵇ כבודי וגוֹדְלִי, my glory and my greatness.—Ex. R. s. 29; Cant. R. to I, 2 גָּדְלוֹ His greatness.—Ib. to II, 4; Num. R. s. 2 (play on ודגלו, Cant. l. c.) וגודלו עלי אהבה even his (the child's) elevating himself over Me (by putting his finger on the Divine Name) is (a token of) love; (Tanh. B'midb. 10 ודגלו; ed. Bub. ib. note וגידודלו Ms. R.).—2) *pile.—Pl.* גּוֹדָלִין. Y. B. Mets. II, beg. 8ᵇ עשוירן ג׳ (coins found) piled up (assorted according to their sizes, pyramid-like; Bab. ib. 25ᵃ כמגדלין).

גּוּדָל m. (גדל, v. אֲגוּדָל) *thumb, great toe.* [Cant. R. to II, 4 גּוּדָלוֹ עלי וכ׳ the child's pointing with his finger (comment.); v., however, preced. w.] Y. Ber. I, 2ᶜ top עקב בצד ג׳ heel touching toe (in walking); Sabb. 62ᵇ (expl. הלוך וטפוף, Is. III, 16).—*Pl.* גּוּדָלִין, גּוּדָלִים, constr. גּוּדְלֵי. Sabb. 151ᵇ ג׳ רגליו his great toes.

גּוּדְלָנָא m. (גדל, v. גְּדִיל) *the heap, the difference between stricken and heaped measure.* Y. Pes. IV, end, 31ᶜ [read:] אנא מחשכנא ג׳ וכ׳ I will deduct the difference from my dowry, v. חֲשַׁךְ.

גּוֹדֶלֶת f. *governess* or *hair-dresser,* v. גַּדֶּלֶת.

גּוּדְמָא, v. גִּידְמָא.

גּוּדַע pr. n. m. *Gudda.* Ab. Zar. 32ᵇ (Ms. M. גּוּרַע, v. גּוּדָא II).

גּוּדְפָן, v. גַּדְּפָן.

גּוֹדְרוֹת f. pl. (denom. of גדרה *fold,* Num. XXXII, 16) *animals living in folds* (which they leave in day-time), in gen. *moving live stock.* B. Bath. 36ᵃ; Gitt. 20ᵇ; Keth 84ᵇ הג׳ אין להם חזקה the possession of fold-animals is no evidence of ownership (as they may have come over by accident). B. Mets. 69ᵃ בג׳ כ״ד חדש fold-animals (small cattle given out for raising on half-profit) must be attended to twenty four months (before a division of profits can be demanded by the keeper).

גּוּדְרִיתָא f. (גדר) *partition;* ג׳ דקני (=h. חיצת קנים) a hedge of reeds spreading from a common stem. Erub. 19ᵇ (Ms. M. גּוּדְרִיְיתָא, pl.; Ar. גורדדיתא). Sabb. 50ᵇ בגורד׳ דקני ed. (corr. בגודר׳, Ms. M. בגרירתא, corr. בגדיר׳; Ar. בי גזרתא) (to put a knife) between the branches of a hedge of reeds. [The vers. of Ar. proves גודר׳ to be the proper version and גורד׳ or גריר׳, corruptions.]

גּוּדֶשׁ m. (גדש) *the heap, the top over the level of a dry measure.* Zeb. 62ᵇ כמחק ג׳ סאה as thick as the instrument for striking off the top of a S'ah. Men. IX, 5 (90ᵃ) היה גּוּדְשָׁהּ לתוכה (Var. גְּדָשָׁהּ) its heap was added to the measure, i. e. the additional quantity forming the top of other measures, was contained in the Highpriest's measure which was so much larger.

גּוּדְשָׁא ch. same. Erub. 14ᵇ ההוא לג׳ this refers to heaped measure (dry quantities). Ib. ההוא ג׳ תילתא הוי that top in dry measures amounts to one third of the entire quantity; Sabb. 35ᵃ.

גּוּהָא (Ms. M. גִּיהָא) m. (גנח=גנה, or גוח=גוה, v. Nöld. Mand. Gr. p. 52) *an abrupt sound, a subterranean thunder, earthquake, rumbling.* Ber. 59ᵃ defining זְוָעוֹת (Mish. IX, 2). Ib. גנח ג׳ (Ms. M. גנא גי׳) a thunder roared (a rumbling was heard). Ib. ג׳ ג׳ עביד it really comes in one rumbling sound after the other.

גּוּהַר, v. גִּיהַר.

גּוּהַרְקָא I f. (a corrupt. of גרהוקא, carruca, καροῦχα, καῤῥοῦχα) *a carriage used by persons of distinction* (v. Sm. Ant. s. v.). Taan. 20ᵇ ג׳ דדהבא a gilt carruca (aurea carruca, v. Sm. Ant. l. c.); Gitt. 31ᵇ. B. Mets. 73ᵇ מעייל להו בג׳ דרבא made them draw Raba's carriage. Ib. 85ᵇ ג׳ דר׳ חייא the carriage in which R. Ḥiya will rise to heaven.—*Pl.* גּוּהַרְקֵי. Ib. בכולהו ג׳ Ms. H. (v. Rabb. D. S. a. l. note 90).

גּוּהַרְקָא II m. (=גֵּוּ הַרְקָא; cmp. Syr. חרוק acerbus P. Sm. 1384, a. h. חַרְצָן) *sour and hard berry.*—*Pl.* גּוּהַרְקֵי. Naz. 34ᵇ גוה׳ ed. (Ar. גורקי) undeveloped grapes.—Pes. 25ᵇ גוהרקי Ms. M. (ed. גוהרקיה, Ar. גרקי) undeveloped olives (used for rubbing the skin in fever).

גַּוַּר, v. גֵּו.

גַּוָּא, גַּוָּאָה, v. גַּוָּא, גַּוָּאָה.

גַּוָּזָא I m. (גוז)=h. גֶּזַע, 1) *trunk, stem.* Ber. 40ᵃᵇ איתיה לג׳ וכ׳ (Ms. F. גִּזְעָא, Ar. גְּזָא) there remains a stem which produces fruits again. Ab. Zar. 35ᵇ קטפא דגַוָּזָא ed. (Ms. M. גוווזא, Ar. גזא, גנזא, v. Koh. Ar. Compl. s. v. גז II, p. 262); Nidd. 8ᵇ קטפא דגווזא the gum which oozes out of the stem, opp. דפירי.—Ned. 50ᵃ (became rich) מן גַּוָּזָא through a (hollowed out) trunk. Ib. לא אשכחו אלא גווזא וכ׳ they found on the sea shore nothing (of the wrecked ship) except a trunk. Ib. וכולי עיסקא מחית בההוא גוזא (Ar. גיאזא, read גו׳) and the entire treasure of the ship was hidden in that trunk; [Rashi: chest, v. גּוּזָא].—2) [*that which is cut off,*] *branches;* [*that which is chopped,*] *wood.* Ḥull. 8ᵇ פסק ביה ג׳ לע״ז (Ar. גואזא) he cut wood with it for idolatrous purposes. B. Kam. 22ᵇ ג׳ סילתא וכ׳ (Ms. O. a. Ar. גואזא) chopped wood, kindling chips and light. Sabb. 154ᵇ גואזא פרסכנא ed. (Ms. M. גווזא ופ׳, v. Rabb. D. S. a. l. note) low and spreading ramifications (forming the fourth wall of a *Succah*). Gitt. 69ᵇ, v. מרמהין.—גַּוָּזֵי. Sabb. 155ᵃ let him rest the ladder אגוזי וכ׳ Ms. M. (ed. אַגַּוָּאזֵי, Ms. O. גואזא) on the branches spreading beyond the circumference of the tree (Rashi: *on pegs* reaching beyond &c.).—3) pl. גַּאוְּזִין (cmp. אִיסקוּזוֹת) *lots, division by lots.* Lam. R. to I, 1 רבתי (חד מאת׳ 1) נעביד ג׳ let us divide by lots (comment.: *pieces of wood* on which names are written for raffling).

גַּוָּזָא, II m. (v. preced.) *castrate, eunuch;* in gen. *servant, guardsman.* Targ. I Kings XXII, 9; a. fr. (var. גַּוְּזָא, גַּוְאָזָא, גַּוָּזָאָה &c.—Sabb. 152ᵃ ההוא גַּוְזָאָה ed. (ed. Sonc. גַּוָּזָא, v. Rabb. D. S. a. l. note 40; Ar. גאזא, v. Koh. Ar. Compl. s. v. גוז, p. 256 notes).—*Pl.* גַּוָּזֵי &c., גַּוְּזָאִין. Targ. II Kings IX, 32.—Meg. 28ᵃ (Ms. M. גוזאי, Ar. גואזי). Kidd. 33ᵃ משדר גוזאי used to send guardsmen.

גְּוִיָּה, v. גְּוִיָּה.

גְּוִיתָא, גְּוִויְתָא, v. גְּוִייְתָא.

גוּכִיא, v. גּוּבָא.

גוּלְנָה, v. גּוּבְלָנָא.

גּוּלְקָא, v. גּוּאלְקָא.

גַּוָּן, גָּוֶן (גּוּן, constr. גּוֹן) m. (גון) *surface, color; resemblance.* Erub. 53ᵇ (as specimen of elegant language) מאי גַּוָּן טליתך of what color is thy cloak?—Midr. Till. to Ps. XC, end מפני מה [בחר] תכלת מכל ג׳ why has the blue been preferred to any other color?—*Pl.* גַּוָּנִים, נִין.... Ber. 6ᵇ. Nidd. 24ᵇ ג׳ תנן the Mishnah (III, 2 גנינים) speaks of variegated colors. Num. R. s. 12 מינין הרבה וג׳ הרבה many qualities and many colors; a. fr.—Trnsf. כְּגוֹן (cmp. כְּעֵין s. v. עַיִן) *like, similar to; for example.* כגון שׁ־ (Chald. כגון ד׳) *for instance if, when.* Ps. 119ᵇ כג׳ תמרים וכ׳ such things as dates, roasted ears &c. Ib. כג׳ אורדילאי לי e. g. mushrooms for me. B. Mets. 101ᵃ כג׳ דא צריכא רבה something like this was very necessary to be said. Ḥull. 84ᵃ כג׳ אנו people like ourselves (in our condition). Y. Ber. I, 3ᵇ top כג׳ אנו שעוסקין וכ׳ people like ourselves who are engaged &c. Shebi. VIII, 1; 3. Tosef. ib. IV, 8. Orl. II, 7. B. Kam. 108ᵃ כ׳ שטען וכ׳ e. g. if he claims &c. B. Mets. 69ᵃ כ׳ דאית וכ׳ if he has &c.; a. v. fr.—Denom. גִּוֵּן *to color.* Sabb. 140ᵃ top the egg is put in לְגַוֵּן (Ar. לְגַוָּאן, Ms. M. לגיאן, O. לירגון) only for coloring.

גַּוְנָא, גַּוָּנָא, גָּוֶן, גַּוָּן ch. same. Targ. Esth. I, 6. Targ. Y. Lev. XV, 3 גּוּנֵיהּ. Ib. 19 גַּוֵּן ed. Amst.—Targ. Koh. I, 13 ג׳ ביש a sort of evil (h. text ענין); a. e.—Nidd. 24ᵇ בחד ג׳ הוה קאי it would constantly have only one color.—Trnsf. *way, manner.* Targ. Y. Lev. V, 4 לכל גּוֹנָן די in what way soever. Targ. Is. L, 11 ובהדא גַּוְנָא (some ed. גוונא) and in this manner; a. e.—כי האי ג׳ (abbr. כה״ג) *like this, in this way, in a case like this.* Targ. Ruth IV, 6.—B. Mets. 30[b] ומי הוי הפקר כי האי ג׳ is there a renunciation of property like this, i. e. is such a conditional renunciation valid? Ib. 69[b] top כה״ג צריך וכ׳ in such a case he must give notice; a. v. fr.—*Pl.* גַּוְונֵי, גַּוְונִין. Targ. Y. Num. II, 3; 10; a. e.—Targ. Y. Ex. XIV, 2.—B. Mets. 8[b] תרי גוני מנהיג there are two ways of driving. B. Kam. 108[a] תרי ג׳ ממונא two sorts of indemnities or fines; a. fr.—Ib. 86[a] (ארדישיה) בעי מחוי גוני wants to show faces (pantomimes, by moving his head).—גְּוָון, v. preced. [Snh. 98[a], v. חָוָר.]

גַּוְתָן, גַּוְתָּנָא=גֵּוְתַ׳.

גוז (b. h., v. גזז) *to cut* (the way, air), *pass, fly.*—*Hif.* הֵגִיז *to carry across, drive up.* Mekh. Yithro, Baḥod. s. 5; Tanḥ. Vayikra 3; Yalk. Lev. 427.

גוז ch. same, 1) *to cut, cut off.*—Part. גָּאֵיז, גָּיֵיז. Gitt. 67[b] זימנין דג׳ ליה לדיבוריה sometimes one cuts his speech short (does not finish his sentence).—Ned. 68[a] בעל מֵיגַז גָּיֵיז does the husband (betrothed) cut the vow apart, i. e. annul half the vow of his betrothed, leaving it to her father to annul the other half?, opp. מיקלש קליש he weakens the stringency of the entire vow.—2) *to cross, pass.* Targ. Is. LI, 10.—Koh. R. to VII, 8 גי״ז וכ׳ passed the street riding on horse-back (Yalk. ib. 974 עבר). Lev. R. s. 37 [read:] מן דגיידין בחד נהר when they were crossing a river.

Af. אָגֵיז *to carry across.* Gen. R. s. 10 מְגִיזָה יתיה וכ׳ carried it across the river; Koh. R. to V, 8; Yalk. ib. 972 מְגִיזָא; Lev. R. s. 22 ומגזותיה (corr. וּמְגִיזְתֵּיה). Koh. R. l. c. אֲגִיזְתֵּיה she carried it over; Lev. R. l. c. אגיזותא (corr. acc.).

גּוּזָא, v. גּוּזְזָא.

***גּוּזָא** m. (גנז, cmp. גַּזָּא) *chest, money chest.* Nidd. 50[a] Rashi, v. גּוּזְזָא I.

***גּוֹזָא** pr. n. *Goza*, a river or channel in Babylon. Ab. Zar. 39[a] נהר ג׳ (Ms. M. נתן; Succ. 18[a] איתן, Ms. M. נתן, v. Rabb. D. S. a. l. note).

גּוּזָאָה *castrate*, v. גּוּזְזָא II.

גּוּזְזִין m. pl. (גזז) 1) *cut wool.* Targ. Ezek. XXVII, 24 (Ar. גודרזין, h. text גלומי).—2) v. גְּזָזִין.

גּוֹזֵל *robber*, v. גַּזְלָן.

גּוֹזָל m. (b. h., cmp. Syr. זוגלא, a. זַגְתָּא) *brood, chick,* esp. *pigeon.* Kinnim II, 1. Gen. R. s. 44 (expl. תור וג׳, Gen. XV, 9) תור ובן יונה.—*Pl.* גּוֹזָלִים, גּוֹזָלוֹת. Y. Ned. I, beg. 40[b] לים . . .; Tosef. ib. IV, 1 לות . . . . Snh. 94[b]; a. fr.—Trnsf. *young children.* Pes. 49[a] ומייתם גּוֹזָלָיו ed. (Ms. M. a. Yalk. Am. 545 בניו) and causes his children to become orphans. Y. B. Mets. I, end, 8[a] גזלי הדיינין (read גּוֹזְלֵי), v. אֶשֶׁל.

גּוֹזָלָא I ch. same.—*Pl.* גּוֹזָלִין, גּוֹזָלַיָּא. Targ. Cant. IV, 1. Targ. Y. II Deut. XXXII, 11. Targ. Ps. LXXXIV, 4; a. e.—Y. B. Mets. I, 8[a] top. Pes. 119[b]; a. e.

גּוֹזְלָא II m. (גזל) *robber. Pl.* גּוֹזְלִין. Targ. Y. II Gen. VI, 11.

גּוֹזְלָן, v. גַּזְלָן.

גּוּזְמָא m. (גזם) *a figure of speech, hyperbole.* B. Mets. 104[b] ג׳ בעלמא הוא דקגזים he used only a hyperbolical expression ('a thousand Zuz'). Arakh. 11[a] וסימנך מתניתא ג׳ and thy mnemotechnical sign (to remember who said a hundred and who a thousand) be: the Boraitha (or Mishnah) frequently uses hyperboles. Bets. 4[a]; a. fr. —V. חֲבַאי.

גַּוְזַנְיָא pr. n. pl. (a fictitious denom. of גּוּזְזָא II) *Gavzania* (*Eunuchia*), a fictitious place. Sabb. 152[a] a eunuch (*gavvaza*) asked R. Joshuah ben Karḥah (Baldhead) מהכא לקרחינא כמא how far is from here to Karḥina (Baldburgh), upon which R. Josh. replied כמהכא לג׳ (Ms. M. לגוווזאה) as far as from here to Eunuchia (v. Sachs Beitr. II, p. 132).

גּוֹזֵר m. (גזר) *circumciser, surgeon.* Y. Sab. XIX, beg., 16[d]; Bab. ib. 130[b] ר׳ יהודה הג׳ R. J. the surgeon. [Cmp. גְּזוֹרִי.]

גּוֹזְרָיָא, v. גְּזוֹרִי.

גּוּזַרְתָּא, v. גְּזוּרְתָּא.

גּוּחָא, גּוּחַ, v. גִּיחַ, גִּיחָא.

גּוּחְכָא m. (גחך) *laughter, sneer.* Targ. Prov. XIV, 13 (h. text שְׂחֹק). Targ. Ps. LXXIX, 4 (ed. Vien. גוּ׳, Ms. גְּחֹ׳; h. text קלס).

גּוּמָא, גּוּמְּה, גּוּמֵי, גּוּמֵס, read גּוּסָה, v. גָּסָה.

גּוֹי m. (b. h.; cmp. גֵּו) *crowd, people, nation;* pl. גּוֹיִם *gentiles*, fr. which גּוֹי = נָכְרִי or עכו״ם, *gentile, idolator.* Tosef. Ab. Zar. III, 4 sq.; Y. ib. IV, 41[a] top contrad. to כותי (Bab. ib. 29[a] נכרי); a. v. fr.—*Pl.* גּוֹיִים, גּוֹיִם. Ab. Zar. I, 1 sq. in Y. ed. ג׳ (Bab. ed. עכו״ם, נכרים, Mish. עכומ״ז, נכרים indiscriminately); a. v. fr.—Fem. גּוֹיָה *gentile woman.* Y. Yeb. II, 4[a] top ואין בנך מן הג׳ וכ׳ thy son from a gentile is not called thy son but her son (Bab. ib. 23[a] נכרית); a. fr.—*Pl.* גּוֹיוֹת. Y. ib. IV, 6[a] bot. [Y. Gitt. I, 43[b] top, a. e. גוים לוקין, v. גַּוּוּס.]

גְּוִיָּא, גְּוִיָּתָא, v. גְּוָאָה.

גְּוִיָּא, v. גְּוִירְתָּא.

גְּוִיד, Targ. Prov. XVI, 30 some ed., read גְּזַם, v. גְּזַם.

גְּוִיָּה, גְּוִיָּה, גְּוִיָּה f. (b. h.; cmp. גֵּו) 1) *inner body, creature.* Y. Ber. IV, 8[b] top לכל ג׳ וג׳ וכ׳ to each creature its needs. Mikv. X, 7 לפסול את הג׳ to make the inner body unfit (for receiving T'rumah); Toh. I, 3 הַגְּוִיָּה; a. fr.—*Pl.* גְּוִיּוֹת, גְּוִיוֹת. Yoma 80[b] טומאת ג׳ some ed. (oth. sing.)

the uncleanness of the inner body.—2) *membrum.* Nidd. 25ª; Y. ib. III, 50ᵈ. Kidd. 25ª; a. fr.—*Pl.* גְּוִיּוֹת. Midr. Sam. ch. XX גוויה some ed. (corr. acc.).

גְּוִויתָא, גְּוִיר׳ ch. same, *body.* Targ. Y. Gen. VII, 23; a. fr.—*Pl.* גְּוִיָּיתָא. Targ. Is. VI, 2 גוויתהון Kimhi in ed. Ven. I, read גְּוִיָּיתְהוֹן (ed. תֵּיה . . ., corr. acc.). Targ. Ezek. I, 11.

גְּוִיל m. (גלל) 1) *a rolling stone, rough untrimmed stone, cobble.* B. Bath. I, 1; expl. ib. 3ª ג׳ אבני דלא וכ׳ untrimmed stones. B. Mets. 117ᵇ.—2) *a roll of parchment.* Y. M. Kat. III, 83ᵇ bot. must rend his garments חג׳ בפני עצמו וכ׳ once for the burnt parchment and a second times for the writing; Bab. ib. 26ª אחת על הג׳ Ms. M.—Ib. (ref. to Jer. XXXVI, 27) המגילה זה הג׳ Ms. M. (v. Rabb. D. S. a. l.) *m'gillah* refers to the writing paper, *hadd'barim* to the writing.—*Pl.* גְּוִילִין. Ab. Zar. 18ª I see ג׳ נשרפין וכ׳ En Yakob (v. Rabb. D. S. a. l. note 50, ed. incorr. גליון) the parchment burned but the letters soar upward. —Esp. *g'vil*, a certain kind of parchment, v. דוּכְסוּסְטוּס. Tosef. B. Bath. IV, 7 (if one sold) ספר של צבאים . . . של ג׳ a book for deer-skin and it is found to be *g'vil.* Mass. Sof'rim I, 4. Sabb. 79ᵇ; a. e.

גְּוִילָא ch. same, *parchment, roll.* Targ. Y. Deut. XXXI, 24 (h. text ספר). [Y. Meg. IV, 75ᵇ bot., v. גּוּל.]

גְּוִיעָה f. (גָּוַע) *exspiration, use of the verb* גָּוַע *with reference to death.* B. Bath. 16ᵇ, v. אֲסִיפָה.

***גּוּל** (b. h.; √גו, cmp. גבל) *to form a ball, circle; to roll up* a scroll of the Law. Y. Yoma VII, 44ᵇ top שארן גָּלִין וכ׳; Y. Meg. IV, 75ᵇ bot. שארן גולים (read גָּלִים or גּוֹלְל׳, v. גָּלַל) the Book of the Law must not be rolled up (to prepare the place to be read from) in the presence of the congregation. Denom. גִּיל, גְּוִיל, גּוֹל. [In b. h. גּוּל or גִּיל *to dance, rejoice.*]

גּוּל ch. same. Part. גָּיֵיל (גָּאֵיל). Y. Yoma VII, 44ᵇ top [read:] תהא גייל לה לאחורי פרוכתא thou must roll it (the scroll, v. preced.) behind the curtain; Y. Meg. IV, 75ᵇ bot. (corr. acc.).

Hitpol. אִתְגּוֹלֵל, v. גָּלַל Ithpalp.

גּוֹל *clapper,* v. גִּיל.

***גּוּלָא** m., constr. גּוּל (גול) *ball, roll.* Targ. Is. XXXVIII, 12 some ed. כג׳ גרדאין like the weavers' roll (v., however, נְוּלָא *web;* oth. ed. כנחל גרדאין, מנחל גידודין).

גּוּלָא *cloak,* v. גּוּלְתָא.

גולאי, Zeb. 116ᵈ, v. גִּילְאֵי.

גּוּלְבָּא m. (גלב) *spelt.* Pes. 35ª, explain. כּוּסְמִין (ib. Mish.) ג׳ (Ms. M. גּוּלְבֵּי pl.); Men. 70ªᵇ.

גּוּלְבּוּנָה, גּוּלְבִּינָא m. *a species of peas,* (Vicia sativa, Lathuros cicera, v. Fl. to Levy Talm. Dict. I, 433ᵇ). Y. Kil. I, 27ª top, explain. פורקדן of Mish. I, 1 (v. quot. in R. S. a. l.).

גּוּלְגָא, v. גַּלְגָּא.

גּוּלְגּוּלְתָא, גּוּלְגּוֹלֶת, v. גֻּלְגֹּלֶת, גּוּלְגַּלְתָּא.

גולגודקין, read גַּלְגִּילוֹקִין m. pl. (calceoli) (*Roman*) *shoes* which leave the toes uncovered (v. Sm. Ant. s. v.). Y. Bets. V, 63ª bot. we saw his toes מן ג׳ דידיה reaching out of his *calceoli.*

גולגית, v. גַּלְגִּית.

גולגל, v. גַּלְגַּל.

גּוּלְגְּלָא ch.=next w. Y. Snh. VII, end, 25ᵈ נסב חדא ג׳ וכ׳ took a skull and threw it upward.—*Pl.* גּוּלְגְּלַיָּא *capitation taxes.* Lev. R. s. 33 (Yalk. Dan. 1061 גֻּלְגְּלִיּוֹת).

גֻּלְ׳, גּוּלְגּוֹלֶת, גּוּלְגֹּלֶת f. (b. h.; גלל) 1) *head, skull.* Ab. II, 6. Snh. 65ᵇ הנשאל בג׳ he who consults a skull (as a conjurer). Koh. R. to XII, 6 'the golden bowl' (גולה ib.) is the head (bowed down in old age); a. e.— *Pl.* גּוּלְגְּלִיּוֹת. Num. R. s. 19; Tanh. Huck. 20 ג׳ וזרועות וכ׳ innumerable skulls, arms &c.—2) *capitation tax.* Y. Keth. X, end, 34ᵇ; ib. XIII, 35ᵈ, v. אַרְנוֹנָא. Tanh. Ki Thissa 1; a. fr.—*Pl.* as above. Y. Peah I, 15ᵇ bot.—Yalk. Dan. 1061, v. preced.; a. fr.

גּוּלְגּוּל׳, גּוּלְגַּלְתָּא ch. same, 1) *skull, head.* Targ. Ex. XVI, 16; a. fr. Targ. II Esth. III, 9 גּוּלְגַּלְתָּא.—Tam. 32ᵇ והבו ליה ג׳ חדא they gave him (Alexander the Great) a skull. Ib. ג׳ דעינא, v. גּוּלְגְּלָא.—2) *capitation tax.* B. Bath. 8ª; Ned. 62ᵇ כסף ג׳, v. בְּלוֹ. Pesik. Shek. p. 11ª גּוּלְגַּלְתֵּיךְ thy capitation tax (for the Roman government); a. e.

גולגסיים, v. גַּלְגָּאס.

גּוּלְדְּנָא, v. גַּלְדְּנָא.

גּוֹלָה, גּוֹלֶה, part. of גָּלָה.

גּוֹלָה f. (b. h.; גלי) *exile,* esp. (with or without בני) *the diaspora, Jews living abroad,* esp. *Babylonians.* Ab. Zar. 30ᵇ. R. Hash. 18ᵇ באת שמועה לג׳ the report came to the captivity (in Babylonia); a. fr.—ראש ג׳ (ch. ריש גלותא) chief of the Babylonian Jews, *Resh G'lutha.* Snh. 38ª; Hull. 92ª ר׳ ג׳ שבבבל; a. e.—עולי ג׳ those returning from Babylonian captivity. B. Bath. 15ª bot.—V. גָּלוּת.

גֻּלָּה f. (b. h. גֻּלָּה; גלל) *cup, bowl.* Lev. R. s. 32, a. e. (used for play on גּוֹלָה, a. גּוֹאֲלָה), v. גּוֹאֵל.

גולהי, גולהא, v. גּוּלְהֵי.

גולור, v. גּוּלְיֵיר.

גּוּלְיָא *cloak,* v. גּוּלְתָא.

גַּלְיֵיר, גּוּלְיֵיר m. (galearius) *soldier's boy, common soldier.* Gen. R. s. 63 never despise a low Roman ולא בג׳ זעיר (Y. Ter. VIII, end, 46ᶜ בחבר) not even a low galearius. Num. R. s. 9; Tosef. Sot. III, 14, v. סַפָּן. Esth. R. to III, 1. Ib. to VI, 12 practiced in four trades a bather, a barber

גלויר וכ׳ (read גלייר) a soldier's servant and a crier; a.e.—*Pl.* גּוּלְיָרִין. Pesik. R. s. 15; Pesik. Haḥod. p. 45[b] גולרירין (corr. acc.); Num. R. s. 11; a. e. the subordinate divine messengers.—Naz. 66[b] גּוּלְיָרִים מתגרין וכ׳ the common soldiers begin the battle and the heroes (veteran soldiers) wind up with victory; Ber. 53[b] גולרירין (Var. גלוורין, corr. acc.).

***גּוּלִילָא** m. (גלל) *threshing roller.* Targ. I Kings XIV, 10 ed. Lag. (ed. גּוּלְלִין, Var. גְּלִילָא); v. גַּנְדַּר I.

גוליקוס, v. גְּיוּס.

גּוּלִית, v. גְּלִית.

גּוּלִיתָא, v. גּוּלְתָא.

גּוֹלֵל m. (גלל, cmp. גַּל) *the stone placed on top of a burial cave, top-stone,* contrad. to דּוֹפֵק. Ohol. II, 4; a. fr.—סתימת הג׳ the closing of the tomb with the *golel.* Snh. 47[b]; Sabb. 152[b] עד שיסתם הג׳.—Erub. 15[b]; Succ. 23[a] cannot be used ג׳ לקבר for closing up a grave, i. e. if put on top, it is not considered a *golel* in levitical law, v. Ḥull. 72[a].

גּוֹלְלָא ch. same. Targ. Job. XIV, 22; a. e.

גּוֹלֶם m. (b. h. גֹּלֶם, גלם) *a rolled up, shapeless mass,* whence 1) *lump, a shapeless or lifeless substance.* Y. Nidd. III, 50[d] and the other limbs of the embryo look כמין ג׳ מצומתים like a lump, squeezed together. Gen. R. s. 14 העמידו ג׳ He made him stand, a large, lifeless mass. Ib. s. 24 ג׳ בראו וכ׳ He formed him into a huge body, which extended from one end &c. Ib. (ref. to Ps. CXXXIX, 16) ג׳ שראו עיניך (read גּוֹלָמִים) the embryos which Thy eyes have seen, have all been recorded (preordained) &c.; Pesik. R. s. 23; a. fr.—Ib. s. 33 גלומי׳ הוו (read גְּלוּמִין or גולמין) they were (hard) lumps (blocks).—2) *unfinished matter, a vessel wanting finishing,* opp. פשוט plain surface, forming no receptacle. Snh. 22[b] אשה ג׳ היא ואינה וכ׳ woman (unmarried) is an unfinished vessel, and she makes a covenant with (cares for) none but him who made her a vessel.—*Pl.* גּוֹלָמִים, גְּלָ׳, constr. גּוֹלְמֵי. Kel. XII, 6 ג׳ כלי מתכות unfinished metal vessels, v. defin. Ḥull. 25[a]; Tosef. Kel. B. Mets. II, 10.—Ib. VII, 12 גְּלָמִין (ed. Zuck. גלמי) pumpkins in their natural shape, opp. to חתוכין ומנוקבין.—Sifré Num. 158 כלים ולא גלומים (Yalk. ib. 786 גּוֹלְמִין) 'vessels' which means finished vessels but not half-finished.—Trnsf. *uneducated, unrefined.* Ab. V, 7.—3) *body. Pl.* as above. Sifré Num. 131; Yalk. ib. 771 the spear entered בשני ג׳ both bodies.

גּוֹלְמָא ch. same; 1) *unfinished vessel.*—2) *Pl.* גּוֹלְמַיָּא, גּוֹלְמֵי. Targ. Y. Num. XXXI, 22 (after Sifré Num. 158, v. preced.).—Sabb. 52[b] בִגְלָמֵי; 123[a] בגולמי׳ it treats of unfinished (needles).—2) (cmp. גְּוִיל) *stone. Pl.* גּוֹלְמִין. Targ. Esth. IX, 5 קטילת ג׳ (for b. h. הֶרֶג) death by stoning.—Snh. 95[a] [read:] אייתו לי ... גולמא (דטינא) ונירגמינה bring ye unto me, each of you a stone (lump of clay), and we shall stone it (overthrow the city with mere stones); cmp. Yalk. Is. 284; Ar. s. v. גולמהרג.—3) *hill,* v. גְּלִימָא II.

גולמהרג, גולמר, Snh. 95[a], v. preced.

גּוֹלְמִי m., **גּוֹלָמִית** f.=*like a* גּוֹלֶם, *roughly shaped. Pl.* גּוֹלָמִיּוֹת. Ex. R. s. 30, v. גָּלַם.

גּוֹלְמִישׁ m. (גלם, with formative ־ִישׁ; cmp. עַכְבִּישׁ) [*hard, stone-like,* v. גולמא,] *golamish,* a species of *cedar.* R. Hash. 23[a], (explain. אדרא); Snh. 108[b] (v. Rabb. D. S. a. l. note 1).

גְּלַמְשָׁא, גּוֹלְמִישׁ ch. same. Targ. Y. Num. XIX, 6 (h. text ארז).—*Pl.* גְּלַמְשִׁין. Targ. Cant. V, 15 (h. text ארזים).

גּוֹלָן (b. h.) pr. n. pl. *Golan,* in Bashan (Gaulanitis). Targ. O. Deut. IV, 43 (Y. דברא). Targ. Jos. XX, 8; a. e.—Macc. 9[b].

***גּוֹלָנִית** f. (preced.) *a coin* named after *Golan.* Tosef. Maas. Sh. IV, 13 Var. (ed. Zuck. נולגית).

גּוּלְפָא m. (גלף) *stone pitcher, jug.* Yoma 12[a] it is usage to leave in the inn ג׳ ומשכא the (empty) wine pitcher and the hide (of the slaughtered animal). Ned. 49[b] שקיל ג׳ וכ׳ would carry a pitcher (on which to sit during the lectures) on his shoulder.—*Pl.* גּוּלְפֵי, גּוּלְפַיָּא. B. Bath. 71[a] the house דמחזיק מאה ג׳ which has room for one hundred jugs (placed in rows). Ab. Zar. 32[a] בג׳ חיורי in unglazed jugs. Ḥag. 25[b] למיטרח אג׳ to provide jugs (for the harvest). [גולפין, Targ. Esth. IX, 5, a clerical tautography of גולמין, v. גּוֹלְמָא.]

גּוּלְקָא, v. גּוּאַלְקָא.

גּוּלְתָא f. (גול, גלל; cmp. גְּלִימָא) [*wrapper,*] *a long woolen cloak of state used at prayers.* Sabb. 77[b] (playful etymology) ג׳ גלי ותיב Ar. a. Rashi, roll it up and sit down (Ms. O. גלי ואייתי travel abroad and import it, ed. גלי ואתיב uncover thyself and put it down). Y. Kil. IX, end, 32[d] to wrap up money גו גּוּלְתֵה וכ׳ in one's cloak and tie it up with linen cords. Y. Taan. III, 66[d] top עצור גּוּלְתָךְ וכ׳ save thy cloak from the rain (a sneer at an unefficacious prayer for rain). Ib. IV, 67[c] את יהב לי גולתי׳ וכ׳ give me my cloak that we may pray at the time of closing the gates (sunset). B. Mets. 85[a] ג׳ דדהבא וכ׳ they spread over thee a gold-trimmed cloak (at graduation ceremonies); a. fr.—*Pl.* גּוּלְתָא, גּוּלְיָתָא, גּוּלִין. Targ. Y. II Num. XV, 38 גּוּלְתְהוֹן, I גּוּלְיָתְהוֹן a. גּוּלֵיהוֹן. Targ. Y. ib. XVI, 1 גּוּלְיָתֵיה his cloaks. Ib. 2 גּוּלֵיהוֹן. Targ. Y. I Deut. XXII, 12 גּוּלְיָיתֵ־, II גּוּלְתֵי־. Ib. XXXIII, 19.—Gen. R. s. 36 (expl. סרבלי־ Dan. III, 21) בגולֵיהוֹן (fr. גּוּלָא) in their fine cloaks; Cant. R. to VII, 9; Esth. R. to I, 12. Bets. 38[b] גּוּלְתָיכוּ שקלי have I taken your cloaks (that you laugh at me)?—[Gen. R. s. 19 גולין Ar. ed. Koh., v. גְּלָיוֹן end.]

גּוּם I m. *bent, joint,* v. גַּם II.

גּוּם II *to cut off,* v. גְּמַם.

גּוֹמָא m. h. a. ch. (b. h. גֹּמֶא, cmp. אגם, אגמא) *bulrush, papyrus.* Targ. Is. XIX, 6. Targ. O. Ex. II, 3. Targ.

Job VIII, 11 (some ed. גומרא). [Y. Sabb. VII, 10ª bot.; Y. Bets. IV, 62ᶜ bot., v. בגומא.]—*Pl.* גּוּמַיָּא, גּוּמֵי. Targ. Y. Gen. XLI, 2. Targ. Y. Ex. II, 3.—Y. Sabb. VII, 10ª גומי.

גּוּמָא f. (גמא to scrape, v. Targ. Job XXXIX, 24) *hole, indentation*, Ḥull. II, 9 (41ª). B. Bath. 16ª for each hair עצמה בפני ג׳ a separate follicle. Y. Keth. I, 25ᵇ לעושה ג׳ וכ׳ like one making a depression in flesh which fills up again; a. e.—*Pl.* גּוּמוֹת. Ab. Zar. 76ᵇ a knife שאין בה ג׳ which is not battered. Tosef. Maasr. III, 18 ג׳ הלוק (ed. Zuck. גּוּמַת, sing.), v. לוּק.—Y. Nidd. III, 50ᶜ bot. ג׳ הזקן dimples, v. גַּב.—גומיות, v. גּוּמָמִית.

גּוּמָאצָא, v. גּוּמָצָא.

גּוֹמֶד m. (b. h. גֹּמֶד, v. גָּמַד) 1) *gomed, a length-measure, supposed to be the cubit less the hand's length; arm.* [Arakh. 11ª וגַמְדָּהּ אמה Ar. and the arm of the scraper was one cubit, contrad. to היא itself, i. e. the perpendicular part; ed. וגובהּ.]—*Pl.* גּוֹמְדִים, גּוֹמְדִין. B. Bath. 100ª שני גמ׳ ed. (Ms. M. a. Ar. גו׳).—2) *a veil of a square gomed*, used by Arabs in cold weather for covering the face.—*Pl.* גּוֹמְדִין. Kel. XXIX, 1 הג׳ של ערביין.—Denom. גָּמַד *to measure by the gomed.* Tana d'be El. I, ch. XXXI (v. Lattes Saggio p. 84).

גומיא, v. גּוּמָא.

גומים, v. גָּמַם.

גּוּמָל pr. n. m., v. גַּמְלָא III.

גּוּמְלָא, v. גַּמְלָא.

גּוּמָמִית f. (גמם, v. גּוּמָא) *hole, excavation.* *Pl.* גּוּמָמִיּוֹת. Y. Kil. III, 28ᶜ ג׳ שיש בהן וכ׳ depressions in a field of the width of &c.—Y. Ab. Zar. IV, 44ª bot. מותר ג׳ what is left in the depressions in the vat.; Tosef. ib. VII (VIII), 5 גומיות ed. Zuck. (Var. גממיות).—Tosef. Mikv. III, 4; Hag. 19ª גּוּמָמִיּוֹת.

גומנני, v. גַּמְזוּדְנַיָּיה.

גּוּמָסִית, v. גַּמּוּסְסִית.

גּוּמָצָא, גּוּמְצָא f. (b. h. גּוּמָץ) *pit.* Targ. Prov. XXII, 14 Ms. (ed. גומאצא). Ib. XXIII, 27. Ib. XXVI, 27 masc.

גּוּמְרָה, גּוּמְרָא f. (גמר to consume) *burning, glowing coal.* Targ. Y. Ex. XXVII, 5.—Y. Bets. II, 61ᶜ top; Y. Maas. Sh. V, 56ᶜ top; Y. Ḥag. II, 78ª bot. (prov.) כל ג׳ דלא כויה וכ׳ a coal which does not burn you in its time, will never burn you.—*Pl.* גּוּמְרִין, גּוּמְרַיָּא, גּוּמְרֵי. Targ. Y. Gen. III, 24. Targ. Job V, 7; a. e.—Targ. Y. Ex. XXXVIII, 4 גורמיא (corr. acc.), v. גַּרְמָא. Ḥull. 93ᵇ. Gen. R. s. 51 (ref. to פחים, Ps. XI, 6) ג׳ ומצדין burning coals (=פחמים) or snares; Yalk. Ps. 655, cmp. Midr. Till. to Ps. XI. Sabb. 110ª; a. e.

גּוּמַרְתָּא f. 1) same. Ḥull. 11ª דמנח ג׳ וכ׳ he may put a burning coal on it.—2) *a local skin-disease*, prob. *a burn.* Y. Ab. Zar. II, 40ᵈ top; Y. Sabb. XIV, 14ᵈ top.

גּוּמְתָא f. ch.=h. גּוּמָא. Targ. Job XXXIX, 24 יעביד ג׳ (prob. גּוּמָתָא pl., h. text יְגַמֵּא).

גּוּן (cmp. גָּנַן *to surround*; with על, *to cover.* Denom. גָּנַן. *Hif.* הֵגֵין same, *to protect.* Midr. Till. to Ps. I מה המגן הזה מֵגֵין את . . מֵגֵין על וכ׳ as the shield surrounds the body, so does the Lord protect man. Sot. 10ª [read:] מה הקב״ה מגין על . . . אף שמשון ה׳ וכ׳ as the Lord protects the whole world, so did Samson in his generation protect Israel; Yalk. Jud. 69. Sot. 21ª; a. fr.

גּוּן ch., v. גִּין.

גּוּן, גּוּנָא, גַּוָּן, v. גּוּו׳.

גּוּנְבָא *tail*, v. גּוּנְבְּתָא.

גּוּנְבָא *bed-cloth*, v. גּוּנְכָא.

גּוּנְבְרָא, v. גִּינְבְּרָא.

גּוֹנֶבֶת f. (גנב) *inclined to steal.* Deut. R. s. 6; Tanḥ. Vayesheb 6; v. מַשְׁמְשָׁנִית a. גַּנְּבִית.

גּוּנְדָּא I c. (=גּוּדָא; גוד or גדד, v. גְּדוּד I) *a band, troop.* B. Mets. 86ª ג׳ דפרשי a troop of horsemen. Ab. Zar. 11ª ג׳ דרומאי a troop of Roman (soldiers). [Ib. הדר שדר גונדאי דרומאי וכ׳, read with Ms. M. גונדא אחרינא, v. Rabb. D. S. a. l.). Ber. 58ª; a. e.—Ned. 32ª ג׳ דחימה the troop commanded by Ḥemah (angel of wrath).—*Pl.* גּוּנְדֵּי. Ḥull. 60ª ג׳ דנפישי Ar. (ed. חילותיה) His armies are too numerous.

גּוּנְדָּא II f. (=גּוּדָא) 1) *wall.* *Pl.* גּוּנְדֵּי. Sot. 22ᵇ דחריפי ג׳ (Ar. s. v. חך 5, v. infra) who scratch themselves against the walls (in saintly self-chastisement).—2) *gunda*, name of a domestic overall used at work for the protection of one's clothes, *duster.* *Gitt. 68ᵇ (in Hebr. diction) גּוּנְדּוֹ his duster (was all that was left to Solomon) (Snh. 20ᵇ (Ms. M.) Yalk. Kings 177, Tanḥ. Aḥăre 1 קודו; Koh. R. to II, 10 קודיה; Y. Snh. II, 20ᶜ bot. קניא). Sabb. 119ª R. Anan (while preparing for the Sabbath) לבוש ג׳ (Ms. O. גורנא, Alf. Ms. גודנא, Asheri ed. Ven. גונרא, v. Rabb. D. S. a. l. note 2) put a *gunda* on.—*Pl.* גּוּנְדֵּי. Sot. 22ᵇ מהני דחפו ג׳ .... בי דינא let the great Court call to account those who are wrapt up in overalls (hypocrites whom you cannot see through; Rashi: those who wrap themselves in cloaks as though they were true Pharisees; oth. vers., v. supra).

***גּוּנְדְּלִית** f. (גדל II; נ inserted, cmp. next ws.) *spiral form*, (sub. כתב) *writing in spiral form* (cmp. Greek *bustrophedon*), esp. signatures of witnesses alternately in Hebrew handwriting (from the right to the left) and in Greek (from the left to the right). Gitt. 87ᵇ (ref. to two documents side by side on the same sheet with two Hebrew and two Greek signatures going through from under one document to the other), דילמא ג׳ חתים וכולהו וכ׳ perhaps it was signed *gund'lith*, and all the signatures belong to

Hebrew
Hebrew
Greek
Greek

one document (to the one on the right in the case of Hebrew commencing the spire, to that on the left, if Greek begins the spire). Ib. (ref. to a case when Hebrew and Greek signatures alternate with each other) דילמא ג׳ חתים ותלתא וכ׳ perhaps it was signed *gund'lith*, so that three of the signatures belong to one document, and only one to the other. [For oth. interpret. v. comment. a. Ar. Compl. s. v. גנדל.]

Greek
Greek
Hebrew
Hebrew
Hebrew
Hebrew
Greek
Greek

גונדרי, v. גְּרוּנְדֵּי.

גּוּנְדְּרִיתָא f. (גדר, נ inserted; cmp. preced. art.) *balustrade, ledge.* Kidd. 70ᵃ פורתא דג׳ וכ׳ (Ar. by cler. error זנא . . . .) I am only making a little bit of a balustrade (a word considered too affected in place of b.h. מעקה, Talmudic מחיצה).

גּוּנִי, גִּינִי f. (γυνή) *woman.* Gen. R. s. 18; s. 31; v. next w.

גּוּנְיָא, גִּינְיָא m. (an assumed form corresp. to γυνεος) *man*, v. אַנְתְּרוֹפִי. Gen. R. s. 18; s. 31.

גונירות, v. גְּרִינָּאר.

גונין, v. גְּרִינִין.

גוניסר, גוניסריות, v. גְּרִינֵּיסַר.

גּוּנְבָא m. *bed-cloth, blanket.* Targ. Jud. IV, 18 (h. text שמיכה). Targ. II Kings VIII, 15 (h. text מכבר). [Var. גּוּנְבָא.]

***גּוּנְתָּאִי** m. (v. גּוּתְיָא) *a Goth.* Lam. R. to II, 2 (Y. Taan. IV, 69ᵃ top כותריא, Yalk. Deut. 946 גינאר).

גוּס I (cmp. גאה.) *to swell, be bold* (gen. with לב). Keth. 12ᵃ כדי שיהא לבו גַּס בה in order that he may become bold towards her (become intimate). Ib. 28ᵃ שאין לבו גס בה for he is not intimate enough with her (not having been married to her). Sot. I, 6 לבו גס בהן she is too proud towards them (their appearance may only harden her heart). Gitt. VII, 4 לבה גס בשפחתה she is too proud towards her handmaid (so that her presence has no restraining influence). Ab. IV, 7 הגס לבו בהוראה he who gives decisions in haughtiness. [Ib. גס רוח, v. גַּס.] Tosef. Maasr. III, 7 לא גס לבי וכ׳ I did not venture to say &c.

Hif. הֵגִיס (with לב or דעת) *to embolden one's heart;* (reflexive) *to become bold.* Ex. R. s. 6 מי ה׳ את לבך who made thee so bold i. e. who has encouraged thee to take such liberties? Y. Maasr. II, beg. 49ᶜ לְהָגֵס את לבו שיאכל to encourage him to eat. Y. Snh. I, 18ᵃ bot. ה׳ דעתו לדון he dared to judge singly. Num. R. s. 2 הֵגִיסוּ את לבם they became presumptuous; Lev. R. s. 20 גיסו לבם (corr. acc.)—Num. R. s. 19 היה מֵגִיס בינו וכ׳ (sub. לבו) was arrogant (towards the king) in privacy; ה׳ במעמד וכ׳ was arrogant in the presence of his legions; a. fr.

גוּס ch. same. Ber. 47ᵃ גַּס דעתיה Ms. M. he has become proud. Snh. 8ᵃ קא גָּאֵיס (ביה) (Ms. O. גַּיֵּיס, v. Rabb. D. S. a. l. note) he was arrogant.

Af. אַגֵּיס as h. Hif.—Targ. Y. Deut. XVII, 20. Ib. Lev. IX, 7 א׳ מנדעך take courage. Ib. Ex. XXVIII, 39 מַגְיְסֵי רעיוניהון the haughty (cmp. גסי רוח, s. v. גַּס).

Ithpa. אִתְגַּס *to become bold, haughty.* Targ. II Chr. XXVI, 16 (h. text גבה). Targ. Koh. I, 12 (Var. אתגבה).

גוּס II *to come in contact, touch, be connected.* Denom. גִּיס; גַּיִּיס. [Ukts. II, 6 שׁיגוס, v. נָגַס.]

Hif. הֵגִיס *to stir* (with a ladle &c.). Makhsh. V, 11 מְגִיסָה בקדרה she stirs the pot. Ab. Zar. 38ᵇ top וּמְגִיסָה and may stir it.—Sabb. 67ᵇ המגיס בפני אפרוחים (missing in Ms.) who stirs a dish before chickens (a superstitious practice). Meil. 17ᵃ, a. e.

Pi. גַּיֵּיס, v. s. v. גַּיִּיס.

גוּס ch. same 1) *to come in contact, meet.* Pes. 110ᵇ גַּס ביה וכ׳ an Arab met him. Gitt. 65ᵇ מִיגַס גָּאֵיס בה (Ar. גַּיִּיס) he may meet him.—Adj. גַּיִּיס, גִּיס *familiar*, v. גִּיס. —2) *to recline, dine*, v. גְּסַס.

***גּוּסִי** m. (גָּסָה) *nauseousness, indigestion.* Sifra B'har Par. 3, ch. IV (ref. to Lev. XXV, 19) אוֹכֵל ולא ג׳ eating (with gratification), but not to produce indigestion. [Prob. to be read אוכל ולא גוּסָה, v. גָּסָה.]

גוסין, Ex. R. s. 9 some ed., v. גִּיס.

גּוֹסֵס m., **גּוֹסֶסֶת** f. (Pol. of גוס=גוז, Syr. גוס P. Sm. 686) *rapidly passing away, sinking, dying.* Ohol. I, 6; a. fr.—Kidd. 71ᵇ עילם ג׳ Elam is to be despaired of (with reference to purity of descent, v. בָּרִי).—*Pl.* גּוֹסְסִים, גּוֹסְסִין; f. גּוֹסְסוֹת. Gitt. 28ᵃ, a. fr. רוב ג׳ למיתה the majority of those believed to be in a dying condition, really die. Shebu. 37ᵇ.—Y. Yeb. I, 3ᵇ top (of genealogical descent, v. supra). V. גְּרִיסָה, גְּרִזָה.

***גּוֹסְפְּנִין** m. *chariots* (?). Targ. Is. X, 32 (missing in ed. Lag. I, p. XXVIII⁷; Snh. 95ᵇ has קרנות).

גוסרדליא, v. גָּסָה.

גָּוַע (b. h.; cmp. קָוִיץ, קְוִיץ) 1) [*to shrink,*] *fail, fall away.* Gen. R. s. 31 (explain. יגוע, Gen. VI, 17) רצמוק (Yalk. Gen. 55 רנמוק), v. צָמַק. Ib. s. 12 גזעה; s. 19 גרעה, read: גָּוְעָה וכ׳ his stature was reduced.—2) (act. v.) *to diminish.* Tanh. Noah 7; ed. Bub. 10 והן גָּוְעוּ אותן וכ׳ and they (the wild beasts) diminished their numbers, as it says (Gen. VII, 21) and there were diminished &c.

גוּף I, perf. a. part. גָּף (=גָּפַף) [*to join* body to body,] *to squeeze, cork, bung.* Nidd. 6ᵇ היתה גָּפָה וכ׳ was corking (pitching) wine jugs. M. Kat. 11ᵇ כדו לָגוּף we take for the mourner his wine jug for corking. [Ib. Mish. II, 1 וגף, omitted in Ms. M., v. Rabb. D. S. a. l. note.] Maas. Sh. III, 12 אע״פ שֶׁגְּפָן; Tosef. ib. II, 18 שֶׁגְּפָם (Var. גּוֹפָם fr. גָּפָה) though he corked them; a. e.

Pi. גַּיֵּיף *to embrace, hug.* Y. Yoma III, 41a גַּיְּיפוֹ he put his arms around it.

Hif. הֵגִיף (Neh. VII, 3) *to fill up* (a hole), *close* (a door), *fasten.* Par. VI, 1. Ohol. XIII, 3 הֱגִיפָהּ ולא וכ׳ he filled the hole out but not entirely. Zab. III, 2 מְגִיפִין או פותחין if both close or open a door simultaneously. Tosef. Ohol. XIV, 1; a. e.—Part. pass. מוּגָף fastened. Y. Keth. VII, 31c מ׳ צריכה if the door (behind the suspected couple) was closed (but not locked), it is doubtful (whether the woman is to be considered a *Sotah*, v. סוֹטָה).

גּוּף ch. same 1) *to close.* Targ. Mal. I, 10; a. e.—2) [*to embrace,*] *to have illegitimate intercourse, to commit adultery with.* Targ. O. Lev. XX, 10 (Y. גּוּר); a. e.—Part. גָּיְיפָא, גָּיֵיף. Targ. Hos. IV, 2; 13; a. e.—Lev. R. s. 3; Koh. R. to IV, 6 (prov.) ג׳ בחזורין וכ׳ (Ar. גָּיְרָא) she prostitutes herself for apples and distributes them among the sick (sinning and doing charity).

Af. אֲגִיף, אַגֵּיף, אָגֵף *to close.* Targ. II Sam. XIII, 17 אִיגוֹף ed. Lag. (ed. אֲגֵיף) close thou &c. Ib. 18 אגף (ed. Lagarde (ed. אגיף); a. e.—B. Kam. 105a אגף חציירה he closed half of the opening.

Pa. גַּיֵּיף as Pe. 2. Targ. Hos. IV, 14 מְגַיְּ׳ (ed. Lag. גייפן). —V. גּוּפָה a. גּוּר II.

גּוּף II m. (b. h. גּוּפָה, גַּף, cmp. גְּוִיָּה, גֵּו) 1) *body, person, self.* Kidd. 20a (expl. *b'gappo* Ex. XXI, 3) בגופו נכנס וכ׳ of himself he entered, of himself he shall go out (free, in the seventh year) but not, like a gentile slave, on losing a limb. Snh. 91a ג׳ ונשמה וכ׳ the body and the soul may try to escape judgment (shifting the responsibility one on the other). Kidd. 37a, a. fr. חובת הג׳ *personal duty*, contrad. to ח׳ קרקע laws connected with the (Palestinean) soil. Y. Taan. I, 64d top, a. e. אותו הג׳ הקדוש that holy body (saint). R. Hash. 17a בגופן by defiling their bodies. Ab. IV, 6 גופו מכובד וכ׳ will himself be honored by men.—Trnsf. *Guf*, the fictitious storehouse of souls in heaven. Yeb. 62a, a. e. the son of David shall not come עד שיכלו .... שֶׁבַּג׳ before all souls in the *Guf* are exhausted (i. e. sent to live on earth).—2) *essence, substance.* Y Ber. I, 3c גּוּפָהּ של שמ״ע an integral portion of the Sh'ma (confession of faith). Y. Sabb. II, 5a top גופה של פתילה the wick itself. Gitt. IX, 3 גּוּפוֹ של גט וכ׳ the essential formula of a letter of divorce is &c. Yoma 74b גופו של מעשה the deed (of sexual gratification) itself; a. fr.—Pes. 112b מצוה וגוף גדול עושה פירות ולו שכר (Ar. a. Ms. M. 2 a. O., ed. ולא) a charity and at the same time a good investment is the act of him who helps to produce fruits, while he has the reward (e.g. one who loans money to a husbandman on security, allowing payment in small instalments); מצוה וג׳ טהור וכ׳ a religious act by which one preserves his body pure does he perform who marries a wife &c.—*Pl.* גּוּפִין, constr. גּוּפֵי. Gen. R. s. 31.—Y. Sabb. II, 5b bot. ג׳ הלכות; Tosef. ib. II, 10 ג׳ תורה essential parts of the Law; Ab. III, 18; Hag. I, 8 (10a); 11b. —3) *membrum.* Lev. R. s. 25, end.—4) *surface, color* (cmp. גַּוָּון). Men. 44a top גופו דומה וכ׳ its color resembles that of the Sea, contrad. to ברייה shape; Mass. Tsitsith ed. Kirchheim p. 23.

גּוּפָא ch. same, 1) *body.* Targ. I Sam. XXXI, 10; 12 (h. text גויה). Targ. Prov. XVII, 22 (h. text גהה); a. e.—Lam. R. to I, 1 (רבתי) ג׳ כולא the entire body (of the chicken). Sabb. 65b דלא לילפן ג׳ נכראה that they might not become used to bodily contact.—2) *self, substance* &c. Bets. 3a, a. fr. היא ג׳ גזרה this law is itself only a precautionary measure. Nidd. 46a, a. fr. הא ג׳ קשיא this contains a contradiction in itself.—3) *Gufa (text)*, a talmudical term used for taking up a text or subject after an interruption by a discussion or digression; *our text says; returning to our subject,* &c. Hull. 54b; a. v. fr.—Lev. R. s. 5; s. 6; s. 8. [Y. Keth. XII, 35b bot. גוף רמא, read גּוּפָה.]—*Pl.* גּוּפַיָּא, גּוּפֵי. Targ. I Sam. XXXI, 12.—Zeb. 82b תרי ג׳ two subjects.

***גּוּפָן** m. (גפן, v. H. Dict. s. v.) *curve,* trnsf. *character of letters.* Meg. 9a בג׳ שלנו in our (Hebrew) characters, בג׳ שלהן in their (foreign) characters. [Ar. reads גיפן.]—Y. ib. II, beg. 73a שתיתה כתובה גיגנטון, read: שתהיה כתובה בגופנן it must be written in our characters (though in a foreign language).

***גּוּפָן, pl. גּוּפְנִין** m. a species of *dill.* Tosef. Kil. I, 1 [read:] השבת והג׳ anise and *gof'nin.*—2) *late grapes.* Dem. I, 1 (Y. ed. גופנן), expl. Ber. 40b שלהי גופני the late fruits of the grape-vine. [Y. ib. 21d top explains גופנן with שמירה (read שׁוּמָרָה) *dill;* Maim. a. l.: a species of vegetables similar to שבת, v. supra.]

גּוּפְנָא, גּוּפַן c. ch. 1)=h. גֶּפֶן, *vine,* esp. *grape-vine.* Targ. O. Gen. XLIX, 22 ed. Berl. (some ed. גּוֹפֶן, Y. גופנן). Targ. Ezek. XVII, 7 גופנא fem. (ib. 6; 8 גֶּפֶן m.). Targ. Hos. IX, 10; a. fr.—Lev. R. s. 12 הדא ג׳ מסתמכ׳ וכ׳ the grape-vine is supported with so many reeds and props &c. Ib. ג׳ מתקרייא וכ׳ the vine (with its product) goes by three names.—2) *the cotton-tree,* עמרא דג׳ *cotton.* Sabb. 110b. Gitt. 69b ודעמר ג׳ and (rags) of cotton cloth. Y. Kidd. III, 64c bot. a proselyte is like לעמרא (ד)ג׳ וכ׳ cotton, if you desire to combine it with wool, you may do so (without violating the law of כִּלְאַיִם) &c.—*Pl.* גּוּפְנִין, גּוּפְנַיָּא, גּוּפְנֵי. Targ. Joel I, 12. Ib. 7 (ed. Lag. גפ׳). Targ. Ps. CV, 33; a. e.—Ber. 40b, v. preced. B. Kam. 92a. Keth. 79a. B. Bath. 69b; a. fr. [Targ. Y. Num. VI, 4 מגופנין מִקְלִיפִין, read בִּק׳ מג׳ being a misplaced gloss to מגופנא.]

גּוּפְנָא pr. n. pl. *Gofna, Gophna,* fifteen miles northwest of Jerusalem (v. Neub. Géogr. p. 157). Y. Taan. IV, 69a bot.; Lam. R. to II, 2 גּוּפְנָא. Ib. to I, 5 Vespasian went מסחי בהדא גפנא to take a bath at G.—Ber. 44a בית גופנין (Ms. M. גּוּפְנִין).—Tosef. Ohol. XVIII, 16 גּוּפְנִית. [Y. Ber. III, 6a bot.; Y. Naz. VII, 56a top, v. גּוּבְבָתָא.]

גּוּפְפְתָא, v. גּוּבְבָתָא.

גּוֹפֶר m. (b. h. גֹּפֶר, v. גפר) *gofer,* a resinous tree. Snh. 108b, v. זַבְלִיגָא. [Tanh. Noah 5 (ref. to Gen. VI, 14) identifies our w. with ארזים.]

גּוּפְרִיתָא f. ch.=h. גָּפְרִית *sulphur.* Targ. O. Gen. XIX, 24; a. e. [Some ed. גָּפְ׳.] V. כִּבְרִיתָא.

גּוּפְתָא, v. גּוּבְתָא a. גּוּבְבְתָא, also גּוּפְפְתָא.

גּוּפְתָּיָיה m. (v. preced.) *of Gufta.* Y. Sabb. V, 7[b] חנין מג׳, read ח׳ ג׳ Ḥanin of G.

גופתתא, v. גּוּבְבְתָא.

גּוּץ I ch. (cmp. קָצַע) *to gnaw* (of mice). Part. גָּיֵיץ, pl. גָּיְיצֵי. Hor. 13[a].

גּוּץ II m. (v. preced.; cmp. קָנַץ) *short, dwarfish.* Ber. 31[b], v. בָּלַע.—*Pl.* גּוּצִים. Pesik. V'zoth p. 200[a] ג׳ ממנו of a lower stature; (ib. Baḥod. p. 108[a] קוצים כיוצא בו; Sifré Deut. 343 only קוצים; Yalk. Ps. 776; Ex. 286).—*Fem.* גּוּצָה. Yeb. 106[b] הוא ארוך והיא ג׳ if he is very tall and she dwarfish.

גּוּצָא, גּוּץ ch. same. Targ. Job XIV, 1 (Ms. גוזז; h. text קצר).—B. Mets. 27[b] גופו דאריך או ג׳ Ms. M. a. H. (ed. דארוך) insufficient signs of the body for identification—e. g. 'very tall', 'dwarfish'. Snh. 109[b] כי ג׳ וכ׳ when he was short, they stretched him. Meg. 27[b] איניש ג׳ הוה was a very short man. Ned. 50[b] ג׳ ורבה כריסיה short and very stout.—*Pl.* גּוּצֵי. Ḥull. 63[a]. Sot. 38[b] אריכי באפי ג׳ the tall in front of the small.—*Fem.* גּוּצָא. B. Mets. 59[a] (prov.) אתתך ג׳ וכ׳ if thy wife is dwarf, bend down and listen to her (advice), v. לְחַשׁ.

גּוּצְּין *sparks,* v. גֵּיץ.

גּוּר I (b. h.) [*to move around* (cmp. סחר),] *to be a stranger, sojourn, dwell.* Sot. 36[b] גֵּרָא שֶׁגָּר וכ׳ he is named Gera (Gen. XLVI, 21), because he (Joseph) dwells in exile; Gen. R. s. 94. Yeb. 96[b] is it possible לָגוּר וכ׳ בשני to dwell (simultaneously) in two worlds? Sabb. 104[a], v. ג״ר. Sifré Deut. 301 (ref. to Deut. XXVI, 5) מלמד ... להשתקע אלא לָגוּר שם it proves that he (Jacob) did not go down to be permanently settled, but only to sojourn there; a. fr. —Denom. גֵּר.

Pi. גִּיֵּיר (denom. of גֵּר) *to make a proselyte, to initiate into the Jewish faith.* Gen. R. s. 39 (ref. to Gen. XII, 5 'the souls which they had made') אלו הגרים שֶׁגִּיְּירוּ that means the proselytes they had made. Ib. כל מי שמקרב . . . וּמְגַיְּירוֹ וכ׳ whoever befriends a gentile and effects his conversion, is considered as though he had created him. Sabb. 31[a] גַּיְּירֵנִי וכ׳ make me a Jew with the condition &c.; a. fr. [For גִּיֵּיר *to dress with lime,* v. גִּיר.]

Hithpa. הִתְגַּיֵּיר, *Nithpa.* נִתְגַּיֵּיר *to become a proselyte.* Ber. 57[b] עתידים לְהִתְגַּיֵּיר they will adopt the Jewish faith. Yeb. 47[b] גר שבא לחתג׳ if a stranger comes (appears before Jewish authorities) desirous to become a Jew. Ab. Zar. 3[b] מִתְגַּיְּירִין shall ask to be admitted &c.; a. fr.

גּוּר ch. same. Taan. 25[a] גָּרֵי (גָּיְרוּ) בך גיירי Ar., ed. Ven. a. oth. (v. Rabb. D. S. a. l. note 1, ed. גָּיְרֵי) proselytes shall dwell with thee (in heaven); (for oth. vers. v. גִּיר III).

Pa. גַּיֵּיר *to convert.* Targ. Y. Gen. XII, 5, v. preced. Targ. Y. Ex. XVIII, 7; 27; a. e.—Sabb. 31[a] גַּיְּירֵיהּ he accepted him for initiation. Yeb. 76[a] גִּיּוּרֵי גַּיְּירָהּ he made her an Israelite. Gen. R. s. 76, end לאו גַּיְּירְתֵּיהּ would she not have converted him?; a. e.

Ithpa. אִיתְגַּיֵּיר, אִתְגַּיֵּיר 1) *to reside as a stranger.* Targ. Lev. XVI, 29; a. fr.—2) *to become a Jew, to embrace the Israelitish faith, to be converted.* Targ. Y. Ex. XVIII, 6. Targ. Ps. LXVIII, 19; 32; a. e.

גּוּר II (euphem., cmp. גּוּהַּ ch.) *to have illegitimate intercourse;* (also as act. v.) *to seduce.* Targ. Job XXXVI, 20 תגור Ms. (ed. תְּגַיֵּיר). Targ. Y. Lev. XX, 10 (O. גּוּהַּ); a. e.—Part. גָּיֵיר, גָּיְרָא. Lev. R. s. 3; Koh. R. to IV, 6 ג׳ בחזורין Ar. (ed. גָּיְפָא), v. גּוּהַּ ch.—Ab. Zar. 10[b] הוה ליה ברתא דשמה גירא וכ׳ he (the emperor) had a daughter whose name was Gira (Ar. גילא), and who did wrong (was seduced); he sent to him (Rabbi) גרגירא (Ar. גרגילא) a *gargira* (rocket, play on גירא).

Pa. גַּיֵּיר *to seduce.* Targ. Job XXVI, 20, v. supra. Targ. Prov. VI, 32 דגַיֵּיר איתתא Ar. (ed. דְּגַיֵּיר בא׳).

גּוּר III m. (b. h.; גרר, cmp. בני כרוך אחריו Ḥull. 78[b]) *young animal, whelp, cub.* Yalk. Job 926 עלה ג׳ אחד וכ׳ a young (R'êm) appeared in Palestine; Gen. R. s. 31 גורא א׳ (corr. acc.).—*Pl.* גּוּרִים. Ib. גּוּרָיו וכ׳ his (the R'êm's) whelps went into the ark. Ib. s. 98 גבורה של ..... של גוריו the strength of the lion and the daring of his whelps.—גּוּר אַרְיֵה pr. n. m., v. גּוּרְיָא II.

גּוּרָא, גּוּר ch. same. Lev. R. s. 19 (prov.) ג׳ טב מכלב בישׁ וכ׳ raise not a gentle cub of a vicious dog, much less a vicious cub &c.—[*Pl.* גּוּרֵי. Y. B. Bath. II, 13[b] bot. מן קל ג׳, prob. גַּיְרֵי, v. גִּיר III.]

גּוּרָא, pl. **גּוּרָאוֹת**, v. גּוּרְיָה II.

גּוּרְגָּא m. (גרג) *wicker-net* used in vine and oil presses.—*Pl.* גּוּרְגֵּי. Ab. Zar. 75[a] (Ms. M. indistinct: גמגדי, גוזגדי, or גודגדי).

גורגדנא, v. גּוּרְגְּנָא.

גּוֹרְגּוֹס pr. n. m. (Γόργος) *Gorgos.* Treat. S'maḥ. II, 4 (Asheri to M. Kat. 141 גורגנוס).

גּוּרְגּוּתְנִי, v. גַּרְגּוּ׳.

גּוּרְגְּלִידָא, v. גַּרְגְּ׳.

***גּוּרְגְּנָא** m. (v. גַּרְגְּתָא) *connected with a wheel work.* Arakh. 10[b] (expl. הרדולים hydraulis) ג׳ טבלא Ar. (ed. גורגדנא, read גּוּרְגְּנָא) a musical instrument (of pipes) worked by the pressure of water, v. טַבְלָא I (Rashi: *bell,*—which, however, does not correspond to the context in which הרדולים is used; v. esp. Tosef. Arakh. I, 13).

גּוּרְגְּרָן, v. גַּרְגְּרָן.

גורדיון, v. next w.

גּוֹרְדְּיָינִי, גּוֹרְדְּיָינוֹן, גּוֹרְדְּיָ׳ m. (Gordianus) *Gordian,* name of a *gold denar* coined by one of the Roman emperors of that name. Y. Yoma IV, 41[d] top; Num. R. s. 12;

Cant. R. to III, 10 Diocletian possessed (of that sort of gold) משקל דינר ג׳ only the weight of a Gordian denar. Lev. R. s. 7 כעובי דינר גרדיון היה בו (corr. acc.) the bronze plate on the altar was as thick as a G. denar; Y. Ḥag. III, end, 79d.—Cant. R. l. c. משקל גורדינון; Num. R. l. c. משקל דינר גורדייני; Men. 29a דינר זהב קורדיקיני (corr. קורדייני).—Y. Gitt. IV, 47b [read:] קרקע דינרא גרדיינא רביע מעות טרימיסא (ed. דינר אגרמא . . . . סרימיסין) for a piece of land bought for a Gordian denar,—if he chooses to pay to the original owner the due indemnity of the fourth portion in money (instead of land), he must pay him a *tremis;* cmp. Bab. ib. 58b רביע בקרקע שחן שליש במעות. Y. Kidd. II, 62d דינר קורדיינא; Y. Keth. VII, 31d top דינרא ק׳. Ḥull. 54b קורדינאה a. קורדנאה (corr. acc.).

גורדייתא, v. גּוּדְרַיְיתָא.

גּוּרְדִינוֹן, v. גּוּרְדְּיָינִי.

גּוּרְדְּלִי m. (גרד) *scraper, scratcher, gurd'li,* a nickname for an inferior white wine, adopted as a play on חרדלי a dark red wine (mustard-colored). Gen. R. s. 98 יין חרדלי . . . יין ג׳ וכ׳ if thou drankest *ḥard'li,* thou drankest wine; if *gurd'li,* thou drankest bad wine. Sabb. 62b sq. (an obscene disguise for a fair-complected woman).

***גורזקי** *a trap* or *cage.* Sabb. 106b עד שיכניסנו לג׳ שלו until he forces him (the lion) into his &c. [Ms. M. גדורקרי (or גדוד׳); O. גרודרקי; Ar. גרדלקי; s. v. גדיגוד גדורקי; ed. Sonc. גודקי; ed. Ven. גרזקי.—Prob. our w., combined with the suspicious שלו, is an old clerical corrupt. of גיקרופלוס κεκρύφαλος *the pouch of a hunting net,* v. Sm. Ant. s. v. Retis. For a similar Babylonian corruption of an imported Palestinean term, cmp. אנדכתרר.]

גּוּרְיָא I m. (v. גּוּר III) *cub, young lion.* Snh. 64a כג׳ דנורא fire in the form of a young lion.—*Pl.* גּוּרְיָין. Ib. 95a (play on בֵּיתְרֵי q. v.) when they came to Bethré, they said בין תרי ג׳ קטלין א׳ (read קטלן) Ms. M. (ed. בתרי ג׳ קטלו לאריא, read בי תרי a. קטלן) between (us) two cubs (David and Abishai)—can we kill the lion (Goliath)?

גּוּרְיָא II, **גּוּרְיָה** I (v. preced.) pr. n. m. (*Abba*) *Gurya.* Kidd. IV, 13.—Mekh. Mishpat. 20 (ed. Friedm. p. 104a; 109a) איסי בן גוריה; Yalk. Ex. 351; ib. 359 איסי בן יהודה a. בן גור אריה.

גּוּרְיָה II m.=ch. גּוּרְיָא *cub. Pl.* גּוּרָאוֹת, גּוּרְיוֹת. Zeb. 113b; Yalk. Gen. 55 *young R'êms.*

גּוּרְיוֹן, גּוּרְיָין, גּוּרְיָן pr. n. m. *Guryon, Guryan.* 1) a Tannai (Abba) G. Kidd. IV, 13.—2) an Amora. Y. M. Kat. III, 82d bot.; a. fr.—3) G. of Isporak. Tem. 30b; B. Kam. 93b sq.

גּוּרְיְיתָא, גּוּרְיְתָא f. (v. גּוּרְיָא) *a young female cub* (dog or lion). Erub. 86a (prov.) נבח בך כלבא עול נבחא בך גוריתא וכ׳ Ar. (ed. נבח בך גורייתא, corr. acc., v. Rabb. D. S. a. l. note 400) if the dog barks at thee, go in; if the bitch barks at thee, go away, i. e. you can endure a quarrelsome son-in-law, but not a quarrelsome daughter-in-law. Sabb. 67a (in a charm formula) אאוסי דגורייתא (Rashi דגוריית׳) on the nostrils of a lioness.—*Pl.* גּוּרְיָתָא, גּוּרְיָאתָא. Ib. 155b בג׳ זוטרי it means young dogs (which eat flesh with difficulty). Keth. 61b she plays בג׳ קיטנייתא with little cubs (Ar. קיסנייתא), v. נדשיר. [Ar. גוריתא, name of a bird, v. גּוּרְיְתָא.]

גּוֹרָל m. (b. h.; גרל, cmp. גלל) [*a little ball* or *stone,*] *lot.* Yoma 39a; a. fr.—*Pl.* גּוֹרָלוֹת. Ib. IV, 1; a. fr.—Denom. הִגְרִיל *to cast lots.* Ib. 39b; a. fr. V. הַגְרָלָה.

גּוֹרֶן c. (b. h. גֹּרֶן; גרר) [*collection,*] 1) (cmp. מְגוּרָה Hag. II, 19) *granary, threshing floor; harvesting season.* Pesik. R. s. 10 הרי הג׳ בא when harvesting comes. Ib. ומשיירים את החטים באתה הג׳ when harvest time came. Ib. לג׳ and they reserved the wheat for storage; Midr. Till. to Ps. II; Gen. R. s. 83, end; Cant. R. to VII, 3 עד שתבוא הג׳; (נכנסו אל הג׳) באו לג׳. Tosef. B. Mets. VIII, 27; Y. ib. 11d גּוֹרְנוֹ his store of pottery. Maasr. I, 5 איזהו גָּרְנָן למעשרות (comment. גּוֹרְנָן) what is their harvesting time for making them liable to tithes?—*Pl.* גְּרָנוֹת. Y. Peah I, 16c bot.; a. fr.—2) (cmp. כְּרִי a. כְּירָה) *circle, meeting, court-room, court* (v. I Kings XXII, 10). Pesik. R. l. c.; v. אִסְמְרוֹנְגְּרִילוֹן; Snh. IV, 3. Koh. R. to I, 11 the Lord will be seated כבג׳ as in a court; Lev. R. s. 11 end כג׳ (corr. acc.); Ex. R. s. 5 the Lord will seat the elders of Israel כג׳ as the Sanedrin used to be seated. Ib. it is the habit of kings (councils) לישב כג׳ עגולה (read בג׳) to sit in a round court-room; Ḥull. 5a (ref. to II Kings l. c.) אלא כי ג׳ ממש וכ׳ a real court,—ג׳ but it means like the court (of the Sanedrin, ref. to Snh. l. c.). Cant. R. to V, 11 גָּרְנָהּ של תורה the gathering for studying the Law (Lev. R. s. 19; Yalk. Prov. 964 רְנָּה). Cmp. אִדְּרָא.

גּוּרְנָא ch. same, esp. *gathering of rain water, reservoir* (Syr. labrum lapideum in quo homines se abluant, P. Sm. 692). Y. Meg. II, 74a bot. washed his hands and feet מן גּוּרְנָה (with water) out of its (the Synagogue's) reservoir. [Var. גודנה incorr.]

גּוּרְסִינָא, v. גִּירְסָנָא.

גּוּרְסַק pr. n. m. *Gursak.* Erub. 29a (Var. גורסאק, גורסקי, גירסיק, v. Rabb. D. S. a. l. note 40).

גּוּשׁ I (v. גשש) *to be hard, thick.* V. גִּישׁ.

Af. אָגִישׁ, or אַגֵּשׁ (fr. גשש) *to harden,* (with אפא) *to be bold.* Lam. R. to I, 21 אַגְּשִׁתּוּן אפיכון (or אַגְּשָׁתּוּן) Ar. (ed. a. Var. Ar. אקשיתון) have ye the hardihood (to come back to me)?; Pesik. Anokhi p. 138b הא אגשתון אפיכון Ms. O. a. Parma (ed. ארגישתון). Ib. אַגְּשַׁת אפך Ar. a. Ms. O. a. Parma (ed. ארגשת, Lam. R. l. c. אקשית) hast thou &c.?

גּוּשׁ II m. (b. h.; גשש, v. preced.) *something substantial, lump, clod, ball.* Nidd. 23a ההיא ג׳ איקרי such a shapeless fetus is called *gush* (a ball, stone). Y. ib.

II, 50[b] ג׳ של אדמה a clod of earth. Y. Kil. IX, 32[d] top; Y. Keth. XII, 35[b] bot. ג׳ עפר a handfull of Palestine earth. Toh. V, 1 ג׳ מארץ העמים a lump of imported clay, v. Sabb. 14[b].—Y. Hall. III, 59[a] when the dough is formed into ג׳ אחד one cohesive mass; a. fr.—*Pl.* גּוּשִׁין. Lam. R. to I, 20 (explain. חמרמרו ib.) עשאן ג׳ ג׳ their bowels were pressed to lumps (v. חמרים Ex. VIII, 10). B. Mets. 101[a] נעקרו בגוּשֵׁיהֶן they were uprooted with their clods of earth (attached to the roots). Y. ib. VIII, end 11[d] [read:] בששטפן בגושיהן when the river swept them away with their clods.—גּוּשׁ חָלָב pr. n. pl. (*Fat Ground*) *Gush-Heleb*, *Giscala* (Neub. Géogr. p. 230) in Galilee. Arakh. IX, 6. Tosef. Men. IX, 5; a. e.—גּוּשׁ חַלְבָאֵי m. pl. *inhabitants of Giscala*. Pesik. B'shall. p. 94[a]; Koh. R. to XI, 2.

גּוּשָׁא ch. same, esp. *ground, soil*, contrad. to air, atmosphere. Naz. 54[b]; 55[a] (ib. 19[b] גושה). Sabb. 15[b].—*Pl.* גּוּשַׁיָּיא. Nidd. 20[a] בגושייהו with their clods of ground. V. גּרְגְּשְׁתָּא.

גּוּשְׁמָא, m. (גשם, cmp. גֶּשֶׁם) *matter, substance, body.* Targ. Ps. XXII, 21; a. fr.—Targ. Job XX, 20 (h. text חמודו).—*Pl.* גּוּשְׁמִין, גּוּשְׁמַיָּא. Targ. II Chr. XX, 24. Targ. Ps. LXXXVIII, 11; a. e. V. גַּשְׁתָּא.

גושפנא Ar. in some ed. s. v. בלן, read גושפנקא, v. Koh. Ar. Compl. s. vv.

גּוּשְׁפַּנְקָא m. (prob.=גוש פנקא *the freeman's lump* or *cylinder*) *signet; seal; signet-ring.* Targ. Koh. I, 12. Targ. Esth. III, 10; a. fr.—Ber. 6[a] בג׳ דפרזלא with an iron signet. Gitt. 57[a]; 58[a], v. בְּלוֹרָא.—*Pl.* גּוּשְׁפַּנְקֵי. Sabb. 66[b] בשתין ג׳ with sixty seals.

***גּוּשְׁפְּקֵי** m. pl. (prob. of the same origin as Latin *gausapa*) *rough shaggy cloth, bed-cover* for the winter. Gitt. 70[b], Var. for גלופקרי.

גּוּשְׁקְרָא (גָּשְׁקְרָא) f. 1) *wheat flour of the second course, dark flour*, opp. חִיוַּרְיָתָא. Gitt. 56[a]. [Fl. to Levy Targ. Dict. II, 570[b] refers to Arab. *hushkâr*, derived fr. the Persian, *bran-bread.*]—2) *a cotton-like plant.* Sabb. 20[b] (Var. קוש׳); v. אַגְבִּין.

גּוּתָאֵי, גּוּתָיָא m. (cmp. גּוּנְתָאֵי) *a Goth; servant, body-guard.* *Pl.* גּוּתָיִין. Y. Hor. III, beg. 47[a]; Y. Snh. II, beg. 19[d] גנתין (corr. acc.). Y. Bets. I, 60[c] bot. was leaning on תרין ג׳ two servants (Goths).

גּוּתְיָא pr. n. *Gothia*, the land of the Goths. Y. Meg. I, 71[b] bot. (explain. Magog); Targ. I Chr. I, 5 (Vers. in ed. Rahmer) גיתייא. V. Neub. Géogr. p. 422.

גְּוִתְנָא, v. גִּירְתְנָא.

גֵּז m. (b. h.; גזז) *shorn wool, fleece,*—רֵאשִׁית הַגֵּז the first shorn wool (the priest's gift), Deut. XVIII, 4). Hull. XI, 1; a. e.—*Pl.* גִּיזִין. B. Kam. 118[b]. V. גִּיזָה.

גַּז (גַּס) m. (dialect.=עַז, cmp. b. h. equivalent עזניה) *gaz*, name of a bird of prey, supposed to be *the falcon.* Hull. III, 1 הגז Ar. (ed. הגס). Tosef. ib. III, 3 הגס. [Alleged name of a species of bees, v. הָגְזִין or הָגְזִין.]

בַּר גַּ׳, גַּזָּא ch. same. Targ. Y. Lev. XI, 13 (O. עָזְיָא). Targ. Y. II Deut. XIV, 12 (also in one w. בַּרְגְּזָא; Y. I בר גִּיזָא). [גזר, Nidd. 17[a] Ar., v. זַגָּא.]

גַּזָּא or **גַּזָא** m. (=גנזא; גנז; fr. which γάζα) *treasure, collection.* בי ג׳— *treasury.* Sabb. 63[a] ומשתכחא בי ג׳ וכ׳ Ms. M. a. Ar. (ed. בְּגַנְזָא) it is found in the treasury (among the collections) of queen &c. Yoma 51[a] בי ג׳ דאהרן Aaron's (the Highpriest's) fund. Hor. 9[a] דדילך או דג׳ (Ms. M. דידיך דג׳, insert או, v. Rabb. D. S. a. l. note) from thy (the Highpriest's) private money or from the fund?—Meïl. 17[b] עולו לבי ג׳ Ar. (ed. עיילינהו לגנזיה) go ye into the treasury (he took them to &c.). Hull. 139[a] wherever the vowed sacrifice stands, בבי ג׳ דרחמנא וכ׳ it is in the Lord's treasury (it is to be considered as if its delivery had taken place). —[גַּזָּא Ber. 40[ab] Ar., v. גַּזְוָזָא I.]

גזא דפטר, v. גזירפטר.

גַּזָּא pr. n. m. *Gaza.* Sabb. 145[b] (Ms. M. גדא, Rashi Ms. גדיל).

גַּזָא, v. גזר.

גִּיזְ׳, גִּזְבָּר m. (late b. h.; גזב, cmp. קַצָּב, with format. ר) *manager, treasurer.* Ex. R. s. 21 עשיתיך ג׳ עליו I have appointed thee its (the Sea's) commander. Ib. s. 51 ג׳ לעצמו sole treasurer. Sabb. 31[b]. Tosef. Hor. II, 10 אמרכל קודם לגז׳ the *Amarkhal* in the Temple is of a higher rank than the *Gizbar*; Y. ib. III, 48[b] לגיבר (corr. acc.); a. fr.—*Pl.* גִּזְבָּרִין, גִּזְבָּרִים, גִּיזְ׳. Meïl. III, 8. Shek. V, 2; a. fr.—Fem. גִּזְבָּרִית. Sabb. 62[a] אשה ג׳ a woman engaged as treasurer (wearing a signet ring).

גִּיזְ׳, גִּזְבְּרָא ch. same. Targ. Esth. X, 3 ג׳ וסבא commander and elder (h. text גדול).

גִּזָּה, v. גִּיזָה.

גָּזָה, v. גָּזַר.

גְּזוּזְטְרָא, גְּזוּזְטְרָה f. h. a. ch. (=גְּזוּזְרָה, reduplic. of גזר; b. h. equival. גִּזְרָה q. v.; cmp. בְּצוֹצְרָה) *enclosure, balcony.* Ohol. XIV, 1 הזיז וכ׳ the *ziz* is a projection the finished side of which faces the ground, והגז׳ וכ׳ Ar. s. v. זיז (ed. והגזוזרה) while *g'zuztra* is one facing upward. Zab. IV, 1 על גז׳ Ar. (ed. כצוצרא).—Targ. Ezek. XLI, 13 גז׳ Ar. (ed. Koh. כזוזטרא; Targ. ed. בצורתא). Midd. II, 5 ג׳ Ar. (ed. כצוצרא).—*Pl.* גְּזוּזְטְרָאוֹת (טְרוֹת . . . .). Tosef. Succ. IV, 1; Succ. 51[b] Ms. M. (ed. sing.). [Ar. גְּזוּזְרִיוֹת, כצוצטראות, כצוצריות, כסוסטראית, כסוסראות, גְּזוּזְטְרִיוֹת.] [Tosef. Erub. IX (VI), 27 גזוסטרא ed. Zuck., Var. גזוז׳.]

גְּזוּזְטְרִית, v. preced.

גְּזוֹזִין, v. גָּזִין.

גְּזוּזְרִית, v. גְּזוּזְטְרָא.

גזולא, v. גְּזִילָא.

גּוֹזֵם, v. גִּרְזוּם.

***גּוּזְמָא** m. (גזם, v. P. Sm. s. v. גזמא 699) *violent man.* Targ. Ps. VIII, 3 Ms. (ed. גְּזָו׳, גיזומא; Levita גוזם; h. text מתנקם).

גּוּזְסְטְרָא, v. גּוּזְוְטְרָא.

גּוֹזְרָא m. (גזר) *circumciser, surgeon.—Pl.* גּוֹזְרַיָּא. Y. Keth. V, 30[a] אנא חכים לגוזרה וכ׳ (corr. לְגוֹזְרַיָּה) I (as an infant) could distinguish the surgeons that attended me at circumcision.

***גְּזוֹרָאָה** m., pl. גְּזוֹרָאֵי *inhabitants of Gezer (?),* prob.=גְּדוֹרָאֵי, v. גְּדוֹרָא. Y. Erub. V, 22[d] bot.

גְּזוֹרָה *circumcision,* v. גְּזוּרְתָא.

***גּוֹזְרִי, גְּזוֹרָיָא** m. *of Gezer (?),* v. גְּזוֹרָאָה. Y. Meg. I, 71[a] top ר׳ יודן גזר׳. Y. R. Hash. III, end, 59[a] ר׳ יודה גוז׳. [Cmp. גּוֹזֵר.]

גְּזוֹרָה, גְּזוּרְתָא, גְּזוֹרְתָא, גְּזוֹרְתָא f. (גזר) *circumcision, feast of circumcision; the circumcised membrum.* Targ. Y. Ex. IV, 25 sq. Targ. Y. Gen. XXIV, 25 גּוּזַ׳; v. גְּזֵירְתָא.—Y. Succ. III. 53[a] גזורה דר׳ וכ׳ the feast of circumcision at R. &c. Y. Ab. Zar. III, 42[c] top יהב נפשיה כל ג׳ he staked his life for the ceremony of circumcision. Y. Meg. I, 72[b] bot. חמי גְּזוֹרְתִי see that I am circumcised; ib. III, 74[a]; Y. Snh. X, 29[c] גזור׳; Koh. R. to IX, 10 גזורתי.

גָּזַז (b. h.) *to cut, shear.* Pesik. R. s. 11 (play on גינת אגוז, Cant. V, 11) הגינה שאני גוזז אותה וכ׳ the garden which I trim at all times. Ib. when they sin מיד אני גוֹזְזָם I cut (punish) them at once; Yalk. Cant. 992.—Ḥull. 138[a] הא צאנו לָגוֹז but when he hires his (the gentile's) sheep for shearing (Rashi לִגְזוֹז). Ib. לגוזז; a. e.—Part. pass. גָּזוּז (v. גִּזָּה) *covered with fleece.* Koh. R. to I, 9 a time will come when the wolf להיות ג׳ וכ׳ shall have a fleece of fine wool.

Nif. נִגְזַז *to be cut, trimmed, shorn.* Ukts. I, 4 את שדרכם לִיגָּזֵז וכ׳ those plants which usually are cut but which have been taken out with their roots. Pesik. R. l. c.; Yalk. l. c. כל דבר שהוא נ׳ מיד וכ׳ whatever (plant) is cut (trimmed) soon drives new shoots and grows better. Cant. R. to VI, 11 מה האגוזה נִגְזֶזֶת וכ׳ as the nut-tree is trimmed and shoots anew. Ib. כצפרנים הללו כך כל שֶׁנִּגְזָזִין וכ׳ as the nails are cut and grow again, מה שישראל נגוזין מעמלן וכ׳ so the more Israel is shorn of his worldly toil and given up to the toils of the study of the Law.

גְּזַז, גְּזֵיז, גְּזַז ch. 1) same. Targ. Gen. XXXVIII, 13 לְמִיגַּז ed. Berl. (Y. לְמֶיגְזַז). Targ. Deut. XV, 19 תִיגּוֹז ed. Berl. (Y. תֵּיגוֹז); a. e.—Y. Sabb. VII, 10[a]. Succ. 30[a] bot. לא תְגוֹזוּ אתון לִגְזוּזְהָ אינהו וכ׳ (v. Rabb. D. S. a. l. note) do ye not cut (the myrtle) yourselves, but let them cut it. Ḥull. 138[a] מעידנא דאתחיל למיגז from the time he commenced shearing; a. e.—Bets. 6[a], v. גְּזַר. Nidd. 17[a] גז מידי וכ׳ if he cut something else afterwards.—Part. pass. גְּזִיז *cut, broken, shortened.* Targ. Ps. LXXII, 6 עסבא דג׳ (Ms. M. גריז) grass eaten up &c. (h. text גֵּז). Targ. Cant. IV, 2. Targ. Job XIV, 1, v. גּוּצָא.—*Yoma 78[b] מאני גְּזִיזֵי דפחרא *defective* earthen vessels (Ms. M. 1 פזירי, 2 a. Ar. גזירי, Ms. L. מאני דפחרא בזוזא, v. Rabb. D. S. a. l.).—2) *to cross, pass* (v. גוז). Targ. Is. LI, 10; a. fr., v. גּוּז.—Ruth R. to III, 13 גָּזֵיז בשוקא וכ׳ passing the street on horse-back; (Koh. R. to VII, 8 גריז). Pes. 111[b] לִגְזוֹזֵי לה (v. Rabb. D. S. a. l. note) to go out of its way, v. גזר. Lev. R. s. 12 גזוז נטוריא Ar. ed. Koh. (oth. ed. גזון, differ. vers. in ed.) the watchmen are past.—3) *to castrate.* B. Mets. 90[b] top Ms. M., v. גְּבַח II.

Pa. גַּזֵּיז *to cut into, interrupt.* Lam. R. to I, 3 ג׳ סיגיא וכ׳ interrupts the study of the midday, v. בַּזַּז I.

Ithpe. אִתְגְּזִיז *to be cut.* Targ. Am. VII, 1.

גַּזָּז m. (preced.) *wool-cutter.—Pl.* גַּזָּזִין. Gen. R. s. 86, end, will you import ג׳ בדמשק wool-cutters to Damascus? (Mat. K. גְּזָזִין *wool*).

גְּזָזִין, גּוֹזְזִין m. pl. (=b. h. גֹּזְזִים; גזז) *(feast of) wool-shearing.* Targ. Gen. XXXVIII, 12 גָּזְזֵי (Y. גוֹ׳). Targ. I Sam. XXV, 7 גוזזין ed. Lag. (ed. גוז׳); 11 גָּזְזַי. Targ. II Sam. XIII, 23 sq. גוזזין ed. Lag. (ed. גְּזָ׳).

גְּזַר, גְּזָא (v. גזז) 1) *to cut.* Sabb. 150[b] למיגזא ליה אסא (Ms. M. למיגז, v. גְּזַז) to cut a myrtle branch for one (attending a wedding, Rashi לה for the bride); ib. למיגזא ליה גלימא (Ms. M. למיגז, Ar. s. v. גד: למיגד 'to cut', v. גדד, or 'to sew', v. אֲגַד I) to cut a shroud for the dead; Bets. 6[a] למיגז (Ms. M. למיגד, v. Rabb. D. S. a. l. note). Snh. 106[a] (prov.) when the camel asked for horns, אודניך דהוו ליה גָּזְרִין מיניה they cut off the ears he had. Ib. 96[a] אתי אִיגְזַיְרִיךְ אנא I myself will cut thy hair. Succ. 37[b] למיכל לְמִגְזְרֵיה he may be induced to cut it (Ms. M. . . . למיתלש). Gitt. 3[a] אתי למיגזריה he may cut it short, i. e. say only a portion of a lengthy legal formula, v. גזז. Y. ib. V, 47[b] top ומה דאת גְּזַר גְּזַר and what crop thou mayest cut, cut, i. e. enjoy the crop as my tenant; a. e. —2) *to pass, go out of one's way.* Pes. 111[b] לגזורי לה Rashi, v. גְּזַז. Ib. וגזר לה (Ms. M. גריז ליה, v. גוז) he went out of the demon's way.—Targ. Jer. VIII, 6 דְּגָזְיָא Ar. s. v. גז 4 (ed. גזר, corr. גזר) which passes swiftly (h. text שׁוֹטֵף).—3) *to deal out, dispense, repay.* Pesik. Zakhor p. 24[b] [read:] לְמִיגְזֵי לטבא טיבותיה ולמ׳ לבישא בישותיה (v. Bub. note 68 sq.) to repay the good man his goodness &c.; Tanḥ. Ki Thetsé 6 לגזירה (corr. acc.); ed. Bub. ib.; Treat. Sof'rim XIV, 7 למזגא, למגזא (corr. acc.); Yalk. Ps. 719.—Y. Taan. IV, 69[c] top וגזי ליה and he (R. Ba bar Zabda) retaliated to him (R. Elazar) his refutation; Y. Meg. I, 70[c] top וגזה ליה.

Pa. גַּזֵּי *to cut, design.* Targ. Is. XLIV, 13.

גְּזָיָא, v. preced.

גְּזִיב pr. n. pl. *G'zib,* v. כְּזִיב a. אַכְזִיב.

גְּזִירָא m. (גזז) *cut off,* whence 1) *branch, club.* Snh. 7[a] אדריה לִגְזִירֵיה וכ׳ lifted up his club and stood (against me;

Rashi: his *fist*). B. Kam. 5ª תבריה ר״ע לגזיזיה R. Akiba has broken the force of his club (Rashi: *fist*), i. e. modified his opinion; ib. 42ᵇ.—2) *piece.* ג׳ דברדא *a piece of ice.* Targ. I Chr. XI, 22 חבר ג׳ דב׳ וכ׳ he cut a hole in the ice and bathed; Ber. 18ᵇ גְּזִיזֵי.—*Pl.* גְּזִיזֵי. Ib. 59ª גְּזִיזַיָּה דברדא Ar. (ed. גזיזי דברזא) hail-stones (Ms. M. בְּזִיזַיָּה דנורא or בְּזָאָה, Ms. F. גְּזִיזֵי, v. Rabb. D. S. a. l. note).

גְּזִיזָה f. (גזז) 1) *shearing wool.* Yalk. Num. 750 (Korah, beg.) זמן הג׳ (Midr. Till. to Ps. I זמן גיזה) the season of shearing. Hull. 135ª מחוסר ג׳ וכ׳ wants shearing, redemption &c. Gen. R. s. 74; s. 85; Midr. Sam. ch. XXIII כל מקום שנ׳ ג׳ וכ׳ wherever shearing is mentioned in biblical accounts, it marks (an important epoch).—2) (=חתיכה, v. preced.) *piece, shred.*—*Pl.* גְּזִיזוֹת. Y. Orl. III, 63ª top (in Chald. diction) what profit is it to him גזים גזיזית (read זות ...) to cut it into shreds?

גְּזִיזְתָא f. pl. (גזז) *cuts* (of the road), *paths, narrow passages.* Pes. 19ᵇ (Ms. M. גזירי׳, clerical error). Ib. 113ª top.

גְּזִיל־, v. גְּזַל.

גְּזֵילָא, גְּזִילָא m. ch.=h. גְּזֵלָה. Targ. Lev. V, 21 (Y. גְּזוּלָא); a. e.—*Pl.* גְּזִילַיָּא. Y. B. Kam. X, beg. 7ᵇ אזל תנייה לג׳ the Tannai (Tosef. B. Mets. V, 26) goes over (from usurers' gains) to robbed objects.—*Pl. f.* גְּזֵילָתָא, גְּזֵלָ׳. Targ. Koh. V, 7.

גְּזֵלָה, גְּזֵילָה f. (b. h. גָּזֵל, גְּזֵלָה; גזל) *robbery, robbed object, illegitimate gain.* B. Kam. 98ᵇ משלם כשעת הג׳ he must make retribution according to the value of the object at the time it was robbed. Y. ib. X, 7ᵇ bot. ג׳ מפורסמת a well-known robbery or robbed object. Treat. S'maḥ. ch. IX מרובה גְּזֵלַת המת וכ׳ severer is the crime of robbery (or wrong) committed against a dead person &c. —*Pl.* גְּזֵלוֹת, גְּזֵילוֹת. Snh. I, 1 ג׳ וחבלות law-suits of larceny and mayhem. Gitt. 55ᵇ that it may not be said מזבח אוכל ג׳ the altar receives illegitimately acquired goods; Y. ib. V, 47ᵇ top.—Keth. 105ª; ib. XIII, 1 דייני ג׳ Y. ed. (Bab. גזירות) judges in suits of robbery; Bab. ib. 105ª (harmonizing the two versions) גוזרי גזירות על ג׳ decreeing fines in cases of robbery. [Targ. Cant. VI, 6 גְּזֵלָה a. גְּזֵילוֹת h. forms.]

גְּזִים, v. גְּזַם.

גְּזִיר, pl. גְּזִירִין, v. גְּזַר.

גְּזֵירָא f. ch.=h. גְּזֵרָה, *decree, law.* Targ. Gen. XLVII, 26 (ed. Berl. גְּזֵירָה, h. text חֹק). *Pl.* גְּזֵירָן. Targ. Esth. I, 19 archive of decrees.—גְּזֵירָן. Targ. Ezek. XX, 25. V. גְּזֵירְתָא.

גְּזֵירָה, v. preced. a. גְּזֵרָה.

גזירה, Lam. R. to IV, 7, v. גְּזִיזָה.—Y. Keth. V, 30ª חכים לג׳, v. גְּזוֹרָא.

גְּזִירְפַּטֵּי, גְּזִירְפַּטֵּר, גְּזוֹרְפַּטֵּי m. pl. (ἀζαραπατεῖς, Pers. hazâr paiti; v. Perl. Et. St. p. 118, a. authorities quot. ib.) name of a class of oppressive *Persian officers* (chiliarchi). Taan. 20ª. Snh. 98ª; Sabb. 139ª. [Ar. גזיר דפ׳, גאזר דפטר; Var. גזיר פ׳, גזיר דפ׳, גרז דיפטר, גירזפטי, גוזרפ׳ &c., v. Rabb. D. S. a. l. c.]

גְּזֵרְתָא, גְּזֵירְתָא f. ch. (גזר) 1) *circumcision, foreskin,* v. גְּזוּרְתָא. Targ. Y. II Ex. IV, 25 sq. (some ed. גְּזִיר׳).—2) (=h. גְּזֵרָה) *decree, edict, ordinance.* Targ. Ex. V, 14 גְּזֵירַתְכוֹן your decreed task. Targ. I Kings X, 25 גְּזֵירַת וכ׳ the decreed (tax) of every year. Targ. O. Ex. I, 8; a. fr.—Gitt. 55ᵇ ג׳ קמייתא the first (Roman) decree (after the capture of Jerusalem). Ab. Zar. 35ª כי גזרי ג׳ וכ׳ when they published a (religious) enactment in Palestine.—*Pl.* גְּזֵירָתָא. Targ. Job XIV, 5.

גָּזִית f. (b. h.; גזז) *hewn stone; wall of squared stones.* B. Bath. I, 1, contrad. to גְּוִיל. B. Mets. 117ᵇ; a. fr.—לשכת הג׳ *the cell of Gazith,* name of a Temple compartment, the seat of the Great Sanedrin. Midd. V, 4; a. fr.—Trnsf. אבן ג׳ (*squared stone*), *a plain interpreter of Bible texts* (*Midrash*). Ab. d'R. N. ch. XXVIII; 2ᵈ vers. ch. XLVI.

גָּזַל (b. h.) *to tear away, rob* (with accus. of person or of object); *to take illegitimately.* B. Kam. X, 5 הגוזל שדה מ־ he who robs a field from his neighbor (takes forcible possession). Ib. 6 הגוזל את וכ׳ he who robs his neighbor (takes illegitimately what belongs to his neighbor). Ib. 7 גְּזַלְתִּיךָ I have wronged thee (and owe thee retribution). Ber. 35ᵇ כאילו גוזל להקב״ה as though he robbed the Lord. Taan. 16ª ג׳ מריש ובנאו בבירה if one robbed a beam and placed it in a large building; a. v. fr.—*Part.* גּוֹזֵל *robber,* pl. גּוֹזְלִין. Y. B. Bath. III, 14ª bot. האומנין והג׳ וכ׳ mechanics (who take working material to their homes) and robbers cannot claim the right of possession, v. חֲזָקָה.—*Part. pass.* גָּזוּל *robbed, illegitimately acquired.* Succ. III, 1; a. fr.

Nif. נִגְזַל *to be robbed* (of object taken, or of person deprived). B. Kam. 95ª, a. e. קרקע אינה נִגְזֶלֶת landed property cannot be robbed, i. e. can never become legitimate property by the law of limitation, v. יֵאוּשׁ.—Part. נִגְזָל *the person robbed* of his property, *claimant.* Shebu. VII, 1; a. fr.

גְּזַל I, גְּזֵיל ch. same. Targ. Lev. V, 23; a. e.—B. Kam. 103ª מִיגְזַל גְּזִלוּהָ they acquired it illegitimately. Ib. 96ª; a. fr.—[גזל *to spin,* Targ. Y. Ex. XXXV, 26, quoted in Ar. s. v. כש 3, read כזל.]

גָּזֵל, גֶּזֶל m. (b. h. גָּזֵל; גזל) *robbery, wrong, oppression.* Sabb. 32ᵇ בעון ג׳ וכ׳ as a punishment for the crime of oppression, the locust rises &c. (ref. to Am. IV, 1 a. 9). Gen. R. s. 31, beg. שטופים בזימה ובג׳ steeped in lust and violence. Pes. 113ᵇ Canaan bequeathed to his sons .... אהבו את הג׳ love ye violence. B. Kam. 80ᵇ אין בו משום ג׳ the law of robbery does not apply to it (it is not private property). Erub. 100ᵇ we should have learned ג׳ מנמלה the regard of property from the ant. B. Kam. 109ª עד שיוציא גְּזֵלוֹ וכ׳ until he dispossesses himself of his robbery. Ib. שיוציא גזילה (corr. acc.). Ib.ᵇ גזלו יוצא וכ׳ his robbery must go out of his possession. Y. B. Mets. II, 8[c] גזילו של גוי וכ׳ what has been illegitimately taken from a gentile, is forbidden (must be restored). Y. Gitt. IV, 45[c] מפני ג׳ השבט in order to protect the (priestly) tribe from loss; Y. Orl. II, 61[d] bot. מפני גזל השבט (corr. acc.); a. fr.

גַּזְלָא, גְּזֵלָא, גְּזֵילָה, v. גזיל׳.

גזלי, Y. B. Mets. I, 8[a] bot. ג׳ הדריינן, v. גּוֹזָל.

גַּזְלָן, גּוֹזְלָן m. (גזל) *robber*. B. Kam. 62[a] (defin.) חמסן ... ג׳ לא יהיב וכ׳ *ḥamsan* (violent man) is one who (takes by force and) pays; *gazlan*—who takes without paying. Snh. 26[b] ג׳ דאורייתא a robber in the strict (Biblical) sense; ג׳ דרבנן a robber in a wider (Rabbinical) sense, e. g. a gambler &c.; ib. 25[b].—Y. Snh. VIII, 26[b] he who takes an object in the presence of witnesses is called thief (גַּנָּב), he who takes in the owner's presence—ג׳ a robber; v. B. Kam. 79[b]. Y. Kidd. II, 62[b] bot. כל המשנה וכ׳ he who changes the use of a loaned object without the owner's consent נקרא גז׳ is called a robber. Ib. I, 60[c] top גז׳; a. fr.—*Pl.* גַּזְלָנִים, גַּזְלָנִין, גּוֹזְלָ׳. Snh. l. c. Ib. 38[a]; a. fr.

גַּזְלָנָא ch. same. B. Bath. 30[b]; a. e.—*Pl.* גַּזְלָנִין, גַּזְלָנֵי. Snh. 26[b]. B. Kam. 79[b].

גַּזְלָנוּת f. (preced.) *robbery*. B. Bath. 47[a] הוחזק על שדה זו בג׳ (not החזיק, v. Rabb. D. S. a. l. note) he is known as possessing this field through illegitimate means.

גַּזְלָנוּתָא ch. same. Snh. 23[b] ערער דג׳ an objection raised against the fitness of witnesses on account of their illegitimate trade. Ib. 27[a] פסלינהו בג׳ they disqualified them by denouncing them for robbery.

גְּזַלְתָּא, v. גְּזֵילָא.

גָּזַם (v. גזז) *to cut, trim.*

Pi. גִּזֵּם 1) *to cut branches off* (for letting the sap drip), *to tap.* Ab. Zar. 50[b] אין מְגַזְּמִין you must not tap (in the festive week or in the Sabbath year).—2) Trnsf. (cmp. b. h. קרץ a. Targ. Prov. XVI, 30) *to threaten mischief.* Num. R. s. 14 שהיא מְגַזֶּמֶת לעשות לו which she was threatening to do unto him.

גְּזַם, גְּזֵים ch. same, 1) *to cut.* Y. Orl. III, 63[a] top גְּזִים וכ׳, v. גְּזִירָה.—2) *to threaten.* Targ. Prov. XVI, 30 (h. text קרץ). Shebu. 46[a] עביד איניש דגזים וכ׳ a man frequently threatens mischief and does not do it. Ib. הכי נמי ג׳ וכ׳ (not דג׳, v. Rabb. D. S. a. l.) in this case, too, he may have threatened and not done it.—3) *to speak hyperbolically.* B. Mets. 104[b], v. גּוּזְמָא.

***גָּזַע** (cmp. גָּדַע) *to cut off, lop off.* [Gen. R. s. 12 גזעה קומתו, read גְּרָעָה, v. גָּרַע.]

גֶּזַע m. (b. h.; preced.) *trunk, stem, stump; that which grows out of the trunk, shoot.* B. Bath. V, 4 העולה מן הג׳ whatever shoots out of the trunk, opp. שרשים; defined ib. 82[a] כל שרואה ... מן הג׳ whatever sees (when shooting) the light of day is 'from the *geza*' (and belongs to the owner of the tree). Ib. דקל אין לו ג׳ a date tree has no *geza*, i. e. the purchaser of a date tree has no claim on shoots growing out of the trunk; ib. אין לו ג׳ לבעל הדקל לפי שאין לו ג׳ Ms. M. (ed. שאין מוציא ג׳, v. Rabb. D. S. a. l. note) the owner .... has no claim &c., because the stump of a date-tree has no shoots. Ib. 80[b] אין גִּזְעָן מחליף their stump grows no new shoots. Nidd. 55[a] שער .... גִּזְעוֹ מחליף hair, if cut, grows again. Ib. בשר ג׳ מחליף flesh, if cut, regenerates; a. fr.—Trnsf. (of persons) ג׳ ישישים *a shoot, offspring of worthy men* M. Kat. 25[b].

***גְּזַף** (cmp. קצף) *to be wrath.—Ithpe.* אִיגְּזַף *wrath is enkindled.* Ab. Zar. 55[a] דכי מִגְּזַף בעלמא ולא אתי מטרא וכ׳ Ar. where, when the world is cursed, and no rain comes, he (the idol) appears to them in a dream &c.; [Ms. M. מנדיף, Ag. Hatt. מינזף עלמא, v. נְזַף; En Yakob מנגיב עלמא, v. נְגַב; ed. דכי מצטריך עלמ׳ למיטרא].

גָּזַר (b. h.; v. גזז; cmp. גדר) 1) *to cut*; v. גּוֹזֵר.—2) *to cut off, to guard*; v. גְּזִירָה a. גְּזֵרָה;—trnsf. *to institute a precautionary measure* (גְּזֵרָה); *to enact a prohibition, to decree* (mostly in a restrictive sense). Sabb. I, 4 .. ושמנה גָּזְרוּ בו ביום they issued eighteen enactments on that day. Ib. 14[b] ג׳ טומאה על וכ׳ declared metal vessels (of gentiles) unclean (even when broken and remolten, v. ib. 16[b]). Ib. 17[b] גזרו על פתן מִשּׁוּם וכ׳ they prohibited their (the gentiles') bread in order to prevent the use of their oil &c. Ib. 30[a] מלך בו״ד גּוֹזֵר גזירה a mortal king issues a decree. Ber. 61[b] גָּזְרָה מלכות הרשעה שמד על ישראל שלא וכ׳ Ms. M. (v. Rabb. D. S. a. l. note) the wicked (Roman) government decreed religious persecution over Israel, that they should not study the Law &c. R. Hash. 18[b] גזרו תענית they ordered a public fast. Ib. II, 9 גּוֹזְרַנִי עליך וכ׳ I order thee to come to me &c. Yoma 67[b] (ref. to גזרה, Lev. XVI, 22) אני ה׳ גְּזַרְתִּיו וכ׳ I, the Lord, have ordained it; a. v. fr.

Nif. נִגְזַר *to be decreed, ordained.* R. Hash. 17[b] נִגְזְרָה גזרה it has been decreed. Ber. 58[b]; a. fr.

Hithpa. הִתְגַּזֵּר 1) *to be cut to pieces.* Yoma l. c. (ref. to גזרה, Lev. l. c.) דבר הַמִּתְגַּזֵּר where an object thrown down is shattered to pieces. [2) *to be cut off, be steep.* Ib. Ms. 2 מקום המתג׳ a steep place.]

גְּזַר ch. same, 1) *to cut, split.* Targ. Ps. LXXIV, 13 (h. text פרר). Targ. Y. Lev. XXV, 3 sq. (h. text זמר); a. e.—B. Kam. 81[b] גזרתינהו לשקך וכ׳ ed. (Ar. גְּזִירִית, Ms. R. גְּזַרִי, Ms. F. אַגְזַרְתִּינְהוּ Af.) I should have split thy shoulder with the iron weapon (i. e. should have excommunicated thee).—ג׳ קיימא *to make a covenant* (h. כָּרַת בְּרִית). Targ. Gen. XV, 18; a. fr.—2) *to circumcise, have one's self circumcised.* Targ. Gen. XVII, 10; 11; a. fr.—Targ. Y. Lev. XIX, 23 ג׳ גזרא (h. text ערל ערלה, v. עָרְלָה).—Part. pass. גְּזִיר, pl. גְּזִירִין. Targ. Y. Gen. XVII, 13. Targ. Josh. V, 5; a. e.—Macc. 11[a] (prov.) שְׁכֶם נסרב ומבגאי גזיר (Gen. R. s. 80 ומגבאי קטע) Shechem wants to marry (Dinah), and Mabgai (his subject) must submit to circumcision. Gen. R. l. c. גְּזוֹר be thou circumcised. Y. Kidd. III, 64[d] bot. מהו מִיגְזוֹר וכ׳ how about circumcising .... on the Sabbath? Y. Sabb. XIX, 16[d] bot. הוה ליה עובדא

למיגזור וכ׳ had a case, when he was to have his son... circumcised (on a Sabbath). Y. Meg. I, 72[b] bot. אזל וג׳ he (Antoninus) went and had himself circumcised; (Y. Snh. X, 29[c] וגייר גרמיה); Koh. R. to IX, 10 הוה גזיר was circumcised; a. fr.—3) *to decree; to enact a prohibition as a precautionary measure, to prohibit, guard.* Targ. Job XXII, 28; a. e. Targ. Is. XXI, 17 גְּזִיר כן it is so decreed.—Ab. Zar. 36[a] ואתי ארנהו וגְזוּר וכ׳ and they came and forbade (gentile bread &c.) even in the field. Sabb. 14[a] טומאה . . . גְּזַרֵי ביה declared him unclean.—Ib. 53[b] ולא גְּזַרִינַן דילמא וכ׳ and we do not prohibit it (from fear) lest he may &c. Ab. Zar. 38[b] גזרינן הא אטו הא we may forbid one thing in order to ward off from another thing; a. v. fr. V. גְּזֵרָה.

Ithpe. אִתְגְּזֵיר, אִתְגְּזַר 1) *to be cut off.* Targ. Job XVIII, 14; a. e.—Ms. מתגזירר׳; h. text יתמלל׳. Targ. Ps. LVIII, 8 (Var. מתגורר׳).—2) *to be decreed.* Targ. Koh. VIII, 4; a. e.

גְּזָר m., constr. גְּזַר (גזר) *decree,* גְּזַר דִּין *sentence, legal decision, divine dispensation.* Keth. 8[b] אפי׳ נחתם לו ג׳ ד׳ של וכ׳ even if a divine decree granting seventy years of happiness were sealed to him; Sabb. 33[a]. Lev. R. s. 26 בלי שטר ובלי ג׳ ד׳ without a note of indebtedness and without a judicial verdict. Ib. כמה גזר דין, corr. גְּזֵרֵי דִינִין.—Y. Snh. III, 21[d] top עבדון ליה ג׳ ד׳ the court passes sentence over him; a. fr.—*Pl.* גְּזֵרֵי דִינִין, גְּזֵרִין. Lev. R. l. c. Y. M. Kat. III, 82[a] bot. (expl. גזירות ב״ד, Mish. III, 3) אילו גז׳ ד׳ that means judicial verdicts.

גְּזִיר, (גְּיזָר), גְּזָר m. (גזר) *piece* (of wood), *log, club.* Y. Shebi. IX, 39[a] top; Y. Shek. VI, end; 50[b] מביא גז׳ אחד he may offer one log; (Bab. ed. Var. גזיר).—*Pl.* גְּזָרִין, גְּזִירִין, גִּיזְרִין. Tam. II, 3. Yoma II, 5 גְּזִרֵי עצים; Y. Shebi. l. c.; Y. Shek. l. c. גזירירי (corr. acc.); Bab. ed. גזרי. Tosef. Kel. B. Kam. I, 6 פצעין את מוחו בגז׳ they split his scull with clubs; Snh. IX, 6 בגזר׳ Mish.; ib. 82[b] בגיזר; Taan. 18[b] בגיזר; (Sifra Emor Par. 8, ch. IX בבקעיות, v. בִּקְעַת); Koh. R. to III, 17 בגזר׳; a. e.

גִּיזְרָא, גְּזָרָא I ch. 1) same, *piece; club.* B. Kam. 81[b] ג׳ דפרזלי (Ms. H. a. F. גְּזָרֵי, R. גִּיזְרֵי), v. גְּזַר.—*Pl.* גְּזָר׳, גְּזָרֵי, גִּיזְ׳, גְּזָרִין (v. preced.). Targ. I Kings III, 25 להרין ג׳ (ed. Lag. only לתרין) into two pieces (h. text לשנים).—2) *what is to be cut* (h. עָרְלָה). Targ. Y. Lev. XIX, 23, v. גְּזַר.—3) (cmp. גְּזֵרָה) *a guard.* Sabb. 54[b] דעבדו ליה לגז׳ (a strap on the foot of the ass) which is put on him as a guard (against knocking the feet against one another).

גִּיזְרָא, גְּזָרָא II m. (cmp. h. גִּדְרוֹת) *sheep in folds, fold, flock.* Targ. Prov. XXX, 31 בית גיז׳ Ms. (ed. גיזורא) between the flock.—*Pl.* constr. גְּזָרֵי. Targ. I Kings XX, 27 (h. text חשיפי).

***גְּזָרָאֵי** m. pl. (גזר) *persecutors* (v. גְּזֵרָה). Targ. Y. II Deut. XXXII, 33.

גְּזוּרָה, גְּזֻזְרָה f. (b. h.; גזר) *enclosure; balcony.* Ohol. XIV, 1, v. גְּזוּזְטְרָא; Y. Shebi. III, 34[c] bot., v. גַּבְלִיָּה.—*Pl.* (from גְּזֻרִית) גְּזֻרִיּוֹת. Ohol. VIII, 2 Mish. (Talm. ed. גְּזֻזְרִיּוֹת, Ar. גזוזטראות, R. Hai Gaon גְּיזְרָאוֹת, v. Koh. Ar. Compl. II, p. 264, note 3).—2) (cmp. גָּזִית a. גְּזִיר) *hewn stone block.* Pesik. Aniya p. 135[b] (ref. to ספיר גזרתם, Lam. IV, 7, v. Bub. note 24) כל ג׳ וג׳ וכ׳ every block which will be placed in the future Jerusalem, will be as handsome as sapphire; Yalk. Is. 339 גְּזִירָה; Lam. R. to l. c. כל גזירה וגזר׳ שהיתה וכ׳ every stone block in Jerusalem was as hard as sapphire.

גְּזֵרָה, גְּזִירָה, גֵּזָרָה f. (b. h.; גזר) 1) *a secluded and narrow place, dale, precipice.* Yoma 67[b] ומנין שבצוק ת״ל ג׳ and how do we know that the place (Azazel) must be precipitous? We read *g'zerah* (Lev. XVI, 22); Sifra Aharé Par. 2, ch. II. Gen. R. s. 98, beg. איזה לשם ואיזה לג׳ which (goat) for the Lord and which for the precipice.—2) *decree, edict, divine dispensation;* (in an evil sense) *persecution* by foreign governments. Sifra l. c. ch. VI, Par. 5 יכול יהא גְּזֵרַת מלך lest you may think it is a royal ordinance (the reason of which is not known); v. vers. in Yalk. Lev. 576. Num. R. s. 19 ג׳ גזרתי . . . על גְּזֵרָתִי I have decreed it, thou art not permitted to transgress my decree (though knowing no reason).—R. Hash. 18[b] גְּזֵרַת המלכות (Ms. M. שמד) political persecution. Sabb. 145[b] to reflect איזו ג׳ קשה אביא וכ׳ what hard dispensation to send them; a. fr.—3) *a rabbinical enactment issued as a guard* (v. גְּדֵר), *preventive measure;* in gen. *prohibition, restriction.* B. Bath. 60[b], a. e. אין גוזרין ג׳ על וכ׳ we must not impose a restriction on the public which the majority can not endure. Bets. 2[b], a. fr. ג׳ משום וכ׳ it is prohibited in order to prevent &c. Ib. 3[a] ג׳ לג׳ a guard to a guard, i. e. a preventive measure enacted in order to prevent the violation of another preventive measure; a. fr.—*Pl.* גְּזֵרוֹת, גְּזֵירוֹת. B. Bath. l. c. ג׳ רעות וקשות Ms. M. (v. Rabb. D. S. a. l. note) bad and severe enactments (persecutions). Sabb. 30[a] Moses, our teacher גזר כמה ג׳ issued so many restrictions. Macc. 24[a] ארבע ג׳ גזר וכ׳ four hardships did Moses pronounce over Israel. Erub. 21[b] הרבה ג׳ גזרתי על עצמי וכ׳ many restrictions did I (Israel) impose upon myself beyond those which thou (the Lord, in the Torah) &c. Pes. 87[b], v. אָרַם; a. fr.—M. Kat. III, 3, v. גְּזַר.—4) (logics) *category,* esp. ג׳ שָׁוָה *G'zerah shavah, an equal or identic category,* i. e. an analogy between two laws established on the basis of verbal congruities in the texts, e. g. Pes. 66[a], נאמר מועדו בפסח וכ׳ the Passover law contains the word *moădo* (due season, Num. IX, 2) and the law concerning the daily sacrifices uses the same word (ib. XXVIII, 2): as the word *moădo* in the latter indicates that it applies also to the Sabbath day (superseding the ordinary Sabbath law concerning labor), so does it in the former intimate that it supersedes the Sabbath law (if the eve of Passover occurs on a Sabbath). Ib. אין אדם דן ג״ש מעצמו you cannot establish an analogy from congruent expressions of your own accord, i. e. it must be authorized by tradition that the verbal congruity is applied to a certain analogy and no other.—Y. Yeb. XI, 11[d] top ג״ש במקום שבאת an analogy can be drawn wherever it occurs, i. e. a textual analogy once established must be carried through all details; ib. VIII, 9[c] bot. ג״ש במקום

שכתוב (corr. acc.); Y. Kidd. IV, 65[d] top; Y. Snh. IX, 26[d] bot.; a. e.—Sabb. 97[a] ג״ש לא גמיר he had no tradition concerning that analogy; a. fr.—In gen. ג״ש *analogy.* Bets. I, 6; a. e.—*Pl.* גְּזֵירוֹת שָׁווֹת. Gen. R. s. 46; Lev. R. s. 25. [Y. Ber. VIII, 12[b] top גזירה דהוא רבע, read גזירת or גזירנא I command that &c.; Y. Keth. V, 30[a] גזירה דגזרין, v. גְּזוֹרָא.]

גְּזֵרְתָּא, v. גְּזֵירְתָא.

גַּזְתָא, v. גִּיזְתָא.

גָּחָה, v. גְּחָה.

גָּחוֹן m. (b. h.; preced.) *belly.* Gen. R. s. 20.

גְּחִיךְ, v. גְּחַךְ.

גְּחִילְנָא, v. כּוֹחִילְנָא.

גְּחִין, v. גְּחַן.

גְּחִירָא, v. גִּיחוּרָא.

גְּחַךְ, גְּחִיךְ, (corresp. to b. h. צחק) 1) *to laugh, jest.* Targ. Y. Gen. XVIII, 13; 15 (O. חייך, h. text צחק). Y. Naz. VII, 56[c] top אתחמי ג׳ he appeared to be laughing. Y. Kidd. III, 64[a] bot. גְּחָכִין they laughed. Y. Ber. VI, 10[c] top [read:] גחיך ליה חבריה his colleague laughed at him (Bab. ib. 39[a] לגלג . . . חבירו). Y. Kil. IX, 32[c] bot. ג׳ לקבליה he received him with a smile; Y. Keth. XII, 35[b]. Gen. R. s. 30 גְּחוּךְ צבורא לקליה the audience laughed at what he said; a. fr.—2) *to sport, to be obscene* (of obscene idolatrous practices). Targ. II Chr. XV, 16; a. e.

Pa. גַּחֵךְ same, 1) *to jest.* Targ. Y. Gen. XIX, 14.—2) *to be obscene.* Targ. Y. ib. XXI, 9. Targ. Y. Ex. XXXII, 6; a. e.

Ithpe. אִיגְּחַךְ *to be made sport of.* Y. B. Mets. IV, 9[d] it is no honor to me that people should say (of me) פלוני א׳ that man was fooled (allowed himself to be taken advantage of).

גַּחְכָן m. (preced.) *jester.* Snh. 39[a] אלהיכון ג׳ וכ׳ your God is a jester (making sport of the prophet).

גַּחַל, v. next w. pl.

גַּחֶלֶת f. (b. h.; גחל) *burning coal.* Bets. V, 5; Tosef. ib. IV, 7 הג׳ כרגלי וכ׳ if one takes burning coals from his neighbor on the Holy day, they may be carried only as far as the owner is permitted to go; contrad. to שלהבת. Y. Ber. VIII, 12[b] bot.; a. e.—Yeb. 63[b] כניצוץ מבעיר ג׳ (as dangerous) as a spark kindling coals. Ab. II, 10 והוי זהיר בגַחַלְתָּן וכ׳ take care of their (the scholars') burning coals (do not treat them lightly) that thou mayest not be burnt. Gen. R. s. 78 end שלא נִכְוֶה בגַחַלְתּוֹ וכ׳ (we are afraid) that we may be burnt by the coal of Jacob, i. e. come to grief through contact with a godly man.—*Pl.* גֶּחָלִים. Yoma IV, 3. Gen. R. s. 51 רדת ג׳ she took coals out of the oven; a. fr.

***גַּחֲמוּן** m. (imper. of a verb גחם *to burn,* Arab. *gaḥama,* adopted for homiletical play on גחם, Gen. XXII, 24) *burn them.* Yalk. Gen. 102, end (from Gen. R. s. 57, end) גחם גחמון Yalk. a.l. [Midr. ed. גמחון.—The entire passage seems to be a late gloss.]

גָּחַן (v. גחה) *to bend.* Pesik. R. s. 26 היה גוֹחֵן לארץ וכ׳ he bent down to the ground and kissed the foot-prints. Num. R. s. 4, beg. אמו גוֹחֶנֶת עליו וכ׳ his mother bends over him and lets him suck; (Tosef. Sabb. XV (XVI), 5 שידהו מהלכין שוחה).—*Part. pass.* גָּחוּן *bent.* Gen. R. s. 20 גְּחוּנִין וכ׳ (v. Yalk. ib. 31) that they walk bent (with grief) over their dead.

גְּחַן, גְּחִין ch. same. Targ. Y. Gen. XXIII, 7 (O. סגיד). Targ. Ps. XCV, 6. Targ. I Kings XVIII, 42 (h. text גהר); a. fr.—Gitt. 57[b] גחין ושקליה bend down and take it up. B. Mets. 59[a], v. גּוּצָא.—Sot. 40[a] ג׳ וזקיף עליה bends down (to listen to him) and stands up by his side (as an Amora).—Part. pass. גְּחִין, pl. גְּחִינֵי. Sabb. 43[a] בתי ג׳ houses *with low ceilings.*

גָּחָר, גַּחַר m. (גחר or גהר; cmp. I Kings XVIII, 42) *projection, jetty.* *Pl.* גְּחָרִים, גְּהָרִים. Ohol. VIII, 2 גה׳ ed.; Ar. גח׳, R. S. גְּחִירִים. [Ar.: *an opening* in a wall for admitting *light;* oth. opin.: *cave.* Cmp. גִּיהָה a. גִּיחוּר.]

גֵּט (גִּיט־) m. (חטט, גטט, cmp. חטט) [*engraving,*] *a legal document.*—ג׳ אשה (often without אשה) letter of divorce. *Pl.* גִּיטֵּי נשים. Gitt. I, 5; 4; a. fr.—ג׳ חוב (usu. שטר) note of indebtedness. B. Kam. 95[a]; Keth. 51[b].—ג׳ חֲלִיצָה a certificate stating compliance with the law of *ḥălitsah* (Deut. XXV, 5—10). Yeb. 106[a]. Ib.[b] דמקרי גט חליצה who pronounces the words to be said at the act of *ḥălitsah* (Deut. XXV, 7 a. 8).—ג׳ מִיאוּן a certificate stating a woman's protest against her marriage. Ib.—ג׳ אשה=ג׳ כריתות. Snh. 11[a].—ג׳ מעושה a document (of divorce) made out under compulsion. Gitt. IX, 8; a. fr.—[For other compounds see respective determinants].—Ib. II, 5 a woman may write את גִּיטָּהּ her own letter of divorce. Ib. 7 להביא את גִּטָּהּ to carry her letter of divorce. Ib. VI, 1, a. fr. גִּיטְּךָ, גִּטָּהּ, גִּיטִּי, גִּטִּי &c. Ib., a. fr. הרי זה ג׳ the letter of divorce is valid. Ib. אינו ג׳ it is not valid. Ib. ג׳ ואינו ג׳ it is of doubtful validity.—*Pl.* גִּטִּין, גִּיטִּין; constr. גִּטֵּי, גִּיטֵּי. Ib. III, 2; II, 2; a. fr.—Hence *Gittin,* name of a Talmudic treatise.

גִּיטָא, גִּטָּא, גֵּט ch. same. Targ. O. Deut. XXIV, 1 (ed. Berl. גֵּט). Targ. Y. Gen. XXI, 14; a. fr.—Gitt. IX, 3 ג׳ פטורין=h. גט כריתות, v. preced.—Yeb. 106[b] ג׳ דחליצתא=h. גט חליצה, v. preced.; a. fr.—*Pl.* גִּיטִּין, גִּיטֵּי. Gitt. 84[b].

גמורין, v. הוּגְמַטְרִין.

גמישא, גמשא, Targ. Y. II Lev. I, 16 Ar., v. נִטְשָׁא.

גַּיְא f. (b.h.; גאר) *glen, wady.* Constr. גֵּיא. Erub. 19[a]; Succ. 32[b], v. גֵּיהִינֹּם.—*Pl.* גֵּאָיוֹת. Shebi. III, 8 מדרגות על פי הג׳ steps leading to the ravines (for carrying up the water for irrigation); Tosef. ib. III, 4. Ab. Zar. 54[b].

גֵּיאָה, v. גֵּאָה.

גֵּיאוּתָא, v. גֵּאוּתָא.

גֵּיאוּתָנָא, v. גֵּיוְתָנָא.

גֵּיאוּתָא, v. גֵּאוּתָא.

גִּיאָרָא, v. גִּיּוֹרָא.

גיאתר, גיאתן, v. גִּיתְּוֹן.

גִּיב I. or גּוּב (denom. of גַּב; cmp. דברים בגב s. v. גַּב), *Pa.* גַּיֵּיב *to reply.* Gen. R. s. 80 מְגַיֵּיב will he be able to reply (argue)?

Af. אָגִיב same. Y. Ber. I, 3[b] top מְגִיב ליה חבריה upon which his colleague remarked. Ib. IV, 8[b] top. Y. Kidd. I, 61[b] [read:] אמרה לון . . . אמרה לכון אכין ואגיבונתה אכין; . . . אימיה אכין ואגיבונה אכין R. Tarfon's mother spoke to you thus (as reported), and ye answered her accordingly; R. Yishmael's mother spoke to us thus, and we &c. [Nidd. 65[b] דמגבי, read דְּמְגִיבֵי; v. גִּיחַ.]

גִּיב II m. (=גַּב) *back, top.* Targ. Prov. IX, 3 ed. (Ms. גּוּב).

גִּיבְבָא m. (גבב, v. preced.) *hump* of a mountain, *summit.* Targ. Ps. LXVIII, 16 Var., v. גִּיבְנָא.—*Pl.* f. גִּיבְבָתָא. Gen. R. s. 98 some ed., v. גּוּבְבָתָא.

גיבביי, Y. Kidd. IV, 65[d] top, some ed., v. גּוּבַיָּא.

גִּיבּוּי m. (גבי) *collection* of debts, dues &c. Bekh. 5[a] בג׳ כסף in the Bibl. account concerning the collection of silver (Ex. XXXVIII, 25 sq.). Keth. 68[a] קודם שיבוא לידי ג׳ before it becomes due for collection through the court.

גִּיבּוּל m. (גבל) *kneading.*—בר ג׳ fit, designed to be kneaded. Sabb. 18[a]; 155[b].

גִּיבּוֹר, v. גִּבּ׳.

גִּיבְלֵי, v. גּוּבְלָאֵי.

גִּבְנָא, גִּיבְנָא m. (גבן) *hump.* Targ. Ps. LXVIII, 16 אתעביד להון ג׳ (Var. גיבבא) became hump-backed (unfit for sacred purposes, v. גִּבֵּנַן). **Pl.* גִּיבְנַיָּא. Sifré Deut. 51 ed. Fr. גִּבְנֵ׳ דאשקלון the heights of A., v. גַּפָּא.

גיבס׳, v. גִּיפְסוֹס a. גֶּפֶס.

גִּבָּר, גִּיבָּרָא, גִּבְ׳ I, m. ch.=h. גִּבּוֹר, *strong; hero; giant.* Targ. Gen. X, 8; a. e.—*Pl.* גִּיבָּרִין, גִּיבָּרַיָּא, גִּבְ׳. Targ. O. a. Y. II Gen. XLIX, 5; a. e.—Targ. O. Gen. XXXVI, 24 (Y. כודנייתא, h. text ימם). Targ. O. Gen. XV, 20 גִּיבָּרַיָּא ed. Berl. (ed. גִּבָּרָאֵי, Y. גִּבָּרָאֵי, h. text רפאים); Deut. II, 10; 11 (Y. גִּבָּרַיָּא, h. text ענקים). Ib. 20; 21.—Snh. 100[b] גברי גיברין קטל דויא grief kills the strongest man.—Fem. pl. גִּיבָּרְוָותָא, גִּבְ׳. Ber. 31[a] כמה הלכתא ג׳ וכ׳ (Ms. M. גִּבָּרָתָא) how many *important* rules can we learn &c.!

גִּיבְרָא, גִּבְ׳ II m. (v. אֵיבְרָא a. גְּבַר) *membrum virile.* Targ. Job XL, 17 Ms. a. Ar. s. v. שעבו (ed. וְיִתְנַיָּא; h. text גידיו). Targ. Y. Num. XXV, 8 בית גִּיבְרֵיה his parts.—*Pl.* גִּיבָּרַיָּא. Targ. Y. Ex. XVII, 13; Deut. XXV, 18 (v. Tanḥ. Ki Thetse 10).

גִּיבָּרוּתָא, v. גְּבוּרְתָא.

גִּיגִית f. (cmp. גַּג) *something arched, roofing, a huge vessel, tub, tank* (for brewing beer); *reservoir.* Sabb. 18[b] ג׳ . . . מ״ט שרו וכ׳ why do the Hillelites permit the preparation of beer in the tank (where the process is continued on the Sabbath)? Ib. XXIV, 5 אם יש בג׳ whether there is in the roofing (which connected two buildings) &c. Ib. 157[b] ג׳ סרוקה וכ׳ a defective roofing rested over them. Ib. 108[b] sq. יד לג׳ כ׳ the hand which is put in the beer tank (in the morning, before being washed); [Ar.: a hand used for taking beer to tap out of the tank]. Snh. 77[a] כפה עליו ג׳ if one inverts a tank over a man (causing his death indirectly). Sabb. 88[a] כפה . . . כג׳ the Lord arched the mount over them like a tank; Ab. Zar. 2[b]; a. e.—*Pl.* גִּיגִּיּוֹת. Y. Snh. VII, 25[b] bot. מה שבג׳ וכ׳ what lives in reservoirs or in *vivaria.* Succ. IV, 6 ג׳ של זהב gilt tanks.

גִּיגִּיתָא ch. same. Y. Ter. VIII, 45[c] bot.; Y. Ab. Zar. II, 41[a] bot. [read:] איתגליא ליה גִּיגִּיתֵיה his water (or beer) tank was left uncovered.—*Pl.* גִּיגִּיָּיתָא. Y. Sabb. I, 3[d] top; Y. Ter. VII, 45[d] bot. גוגייתיה (corr. acc.).

גִּיגַּל, v. גַּלְגְּלָא.

***גיגנמון**, Y. Meg. II, beg. 73[a], read בְּגוּפְנַן, v. גּוּפֶן.

גִּיד m. (b. h.; גוד) *thread, chord, sinew, artery, tendon.*—ג׳ הַנָּשֶׁה (b. h.) *nervus ischiadicus.* Ḥull. VII, 1 גיד הנ׳ נוהג וכ׳ the law concerning the nervus ischiadicus (Gen. XXXII, 33) applies &c. Ib. 89[b], a. fr. איסור ג׳ (sub. הנשה) the prohibitory law concerning &c.—Euphem. *membrum virile.* Kidd. 25[a].—*Pl.* גִּידִים, גִּידִין, constr. גִּידֵי. Ḥull. VII, 5. Ib. 100[b], a. fr. אין בג׳ בנ״ט the rule for mixtures of forbidden and permitted things to be decided by taste-giving quantities applies not to tendons. Ib. 90[b] ג׳ צואר the blood vessels of the throat, contrad. to ג׳ בשר soft tendons.—Y. Meg. I, 17[d] top תופרין בג׳ the T'fillin are sewed with threads of dried tendons.—Gen. R. s. 20 ג׳ של אדמה fibres of dried roots in the ground. Maasr. I, 2 [משירטילו ג׳ [אדומים (v. comment.) when they (the peaches) get [red] veins; Y. ib. I, 48[d] bot.—Denom. גַּיֵּיד q. v. [גִּיד, pl. גִּידִין *wormwood,* v. גִּידָא II.]

גִּידָא ch. same. Targ. Gen. XXXII, 33.—Targ. Y. Deut. XXIII, 2 *membrum.*—Ḥull. 97[b] גיד הנשה=ג׳ נשיא, v. preced.—Y. Meg. I, 71[d] top גודא דרצועתא the thread with which a thong of the T'fillin was pieced together.—*Pl.* גִּידִין, גִּידַיָּא. Targ. Ez. XXXVII, 6. Targ. Job X, 11.

גִּידָא I m. ch.=h. גַּד II, *grain, coriander* &c. Targ. O. Ex. XVI, 31; Num. XI, 7 (Y. כּוּסְבַּר).—Yoma 75[a], v. גַּד II.—*Pl.* גִּידֵי. Sabb. 109[b] ג׳ דרוביא Ms. O. (ed. גירדי) grains of fenugreek, v. גִּיר III, 2.

גִּידָא II, (**גִּידְדָא**) m. (גדד, v. גַּד I) *worm-wood, bitter herb.* Targ. Am. V, 7. Targ. Prov. V, 4 גידדא ed. Lag. (ed. גידרא, גירא, corr. acc.; Ar. גִּידֵּי pl.).—*Pl.* גִּידִּין. Targ. Jer. IX, 14 Ar. (ed. גידרין, corr. acc.). Ib. XXIII, 15; a. e.—(In h. diction) Yalk. Gen. 126, v. גַּד I. Tanḥ. B'shall., ed. Bub. 22 (play on גד) שהיה בפיהם כג׳ מרין the manna was in their (the gentiles') mouths like bitter worm-wood. Sabb. 87^a (play on וַיַּגֵּד, Ex. XIX, 9) דברים שקשין לאדם כַּגִּידִּין words (of warning against punishment) which are as hard (distasteful) to man as worm-wood. [Targ. Y. I, II Gen. XLIX, 23 גידרין, גידריא some ed., read גיר׳, v. גִּיר III.]

גִּידָא, v. preced.

*__גִּידּוּד__ m. (גדד) *full of incisions, wrinkled,* [or *acrid*(?), v. גַּד I]. Y. Dem. II, beg. 22^b ג׳ הוא; v., however, גְּדוּדָא.

גִּידּוּד, גִּדּוּד m. (גדד) *a steep* or *straight embankment.* Erub. 93^b (Ms. M. גִּדּוּד, v. Rabb. D. S. a. l. note 10); Gitt. 15^b ג׳ חמשה ומחיצה וכ׳ an earth embankment of five cubits and on it a partition wall of five.

גִּידּוּדָא, גִּדּוּדָא ch. same. *Pl.* גִּידּוּדִין, גִּידּוּדֵי. *Targ. Is. XXXVIII, 12 נחל גי׳ ed. Lag. (Rashi גְּדוּדָאָן) a wady between steep embankments (Var. נְגַל גְּדָדָאָן, h. text אֹרֶג).—Sabb. 41^a לית ליה גי׳ (Ms. M. גד׳) has no steep banks. Erub. 6^a דאיכא גי׳ where there are yet embankments (remnants of ruined buildings).—בית ג׳ *soil full of cuts, rough places.* Targ. Is. XL, 4 (h. text רכסים).—Trnsf. *snares.* Targ. Ps. XXXI, 21 גידודי גיבריא (h. text רכסי) snares of mighty (violent) men (Ms. גברי גדודי).

גידודה, v. גִּדּוּדָא.

גִּידּוּל, גִּדּוּל I m. (גדל) 1) *rearing* of children. Snh. 19^b צער ג׳ בנים the trouble of rearing children; Gen. R. s. 20; Erub. 100^b.—2) *growth.* Ber. VI, 3 דבר שאין גִּדּוּלוֹ וכ׳ (Y. ed. גִּידּוּלָיו pl.) whatever does not grow out of the soil (animal food &c.); a. fr.—*Pl.* גִּידּוּלִין, constr. גִּידּוּלֵי. Y. ib. V, 9^c top דרך גִּידּוּלֵיהֶן the way they grow, v. גְּדִילָה.—Ned. VII, 6 אסור בחלופיהן (ובגיד׳) ובגִידּוּלֵיהֶן it is forbidden to eat or enjoy what has been exchanged for the fruits or what has grown of their seeds. Ib. גידולי ג׳ growths of the second degree. Y. Ter. VII, end, 45^a ג׳ איסור products of forbidden seeds. Ber. 40^b ג׳ קרקע products of the ground; a. fr.—3) *raising to dignity, elevation.*—*Pl.* as above. Gen. R. s. 55 beg. ג׳ אחר ג׳ (Yalk. ib. 95 גְּדוּלָּה, Yalk. Ps. 777 גְּדָלוֹן).

גִּידּוּל II, **גִּידֵּל, גִּדֵּל** pr. n. m. *Giddol,* name of several Amoraim. Y. Meg. III, end 74^c ר׳ גי׳; Yoma 69^b ר׳ גדל. Y. Bets. I, 60^a (without title). Kidd. 59^a ר׳ גידל; a. fr.—G. b. Binyamin, b. Minyamin (Minyomi). Y. Pes. VIII, end, 36^b.—Y. B. Bath. III, 14^a; Bab. ib. 39^b; a. fr.—G. b. R'ulai. Gitt. 34^a.

גידומי, v. גְּדוּמֵי.

*__גִּידּוּדִין__ m. pl. (v. גִּידּוּדָא) *valleys, ravines.* Targ. Is. XXI, 14 ג׳ פוקו למיא ed. Lag. (v. notes p. XXIX, 21) come forth, ye ravines, to receive the waters (ed. Buxt. a. oth. נְגָדִין). [Our w. prob. a corrupt. of גִּידּוּדִין.]

גִּידּוּעַ m. (גדע) 1) *felling.* Y. Ab. Zar. IV, 44^a (ref. to Deut. VII, 5).—*Pl.* גִּידּוּעִין, constr. גִּידּוּעֵי. Bab. ib. 45^b ג׳ ע״א the execution of the laws concerning the destruction of objects used for idolatry.—2) *that which grows out of a stump;* cmp. גֶּזַע. Ib. שגִּידּוּעָיו אסור וכ׳ the fresh growth of which is forbidden while the root is permitted; 48^a.

גִּידּוּף, גִּדּוּף m. (b. h. pl.; גדף) *blasphemy, reviling.* Gitt. 56^b; a. e.—*Pl.* גִּידּוּפִין, גִּד׳. Y. Ter. I, 40^d תפלתו ג׳ his prayer is blasphemy. Ex. R. s. 41, beg.; a. e.

גִּידּוּפָא ch. same. B. Kam. 38^a דגד׳ הוא for (their way of consoling) is blasphemy.—*Pl.* גִּידּוּפִין, גִּידּוּפַיָּא, גִּד׳. Targ. I Sam. II, 3. Targ. Y. I Deut. XXXII, 3 (II גִּדִּיפִין, גִּדִּ׳).—Cant. R. to I, 6 מדינתא דתירופיא וג׳ a city full of scorn and blasphemy (Cæsarea).

גִּידּוּר, גִּדּוּר m. (גדר) *fencing in, self-restraint.*—ג׳ ערוה *chastity.* Lev. R. s. 32; v. גָּדֵר a. גְּדִירָה.—Y. Dem. III, 23^c top מפני גידורו, read גְּדִירוֹ, v. גְּדִיר.—Erub. 93^b, v. גִּידּוּד.

גִּידֵּל pr. n. m., v. גִּידּוּל.

*__גִּידֵּל__ m. (גדל, Pi.) *pupil.* Yalk. Gen. 84 ג׳ בית אברהם וכ׳ (Gen. R. s. 50 בביתו של א״א, corr. acc.) he (Lot) was a pupil of the house of Abraham; v. Tanḥ. ed. Bub., Vayera 15.

גִּידֵּם, גִּדֵּם m. (גדם) *one whose hand or fingers are cut off* or *stumped.* Men. 37^a; Taan. 21^a; a. fr.—*Pl.* גִּידְּמִים, גִּידְּמִין, גִּד׳. Snh. VIII, 4; Y. ib. VIII, 26^b top; a. e.—Fem. גִּידֶּמֶת, גִּד׳. Y. Yeb. XII, 13^a top; Gen. R. s. 81, beg. Sabb. 53^b אשה ג׳ a woman with a stumped finger.—Hull. 79^a גידמת an animal whose tail and ears are lopped off. Cmp. קִיטֵּם.

גִּידְמָא (גּוּדְמָא) ch. m. (v. preced.) *trunk; twig, branch* (cmp. גֶּזַע). Gitt. 37^a ג׳ דדיקלא ed. (Ar. גו׳ בדיקליה) trunk of a palm tree (Ar. a branch on his &c.). Macc. 8^a ומחייה לג׳ Ar. (ed. גרמא, Ms. M. גירמא) and struck a branch.—*Pl.* גִּידְמֵי, גּוּד׳ Sabb. 110^a אסא וגי׳ ed. (Ar. וגו׳, Ms. O. גירד׳, v. Rabb. D. S. a. l.) myrtle and palm branches.

גידונא, v. גִּירְדּוֹנָא.

גִּיהַ m. (נגה; cmp. גִּיחַ) *flame, light.* Targ. Job XVIII, 5 (Ms. Var. גִּיין).

גִּיהָא I m. (גיה=גִּיחַ, cmp. בְּקִיעַ) *cavity, pond.* M. Kat. 8^b (explain. נברכת בקיע a. ג׳ ובר ג׳) (Ms. M. גִּיהֲאָה) a pond and a pool derived from a pond.

גִּיהָא II *rumbling,* v. גְּהָא.

גִּיהוּץ m. (גהץ) *calendering clothes, fine laundry work.* Y. M. Kat. III, 82^a bot. איזהו ג׳ כלי וכ׳ the process called *gihuts* applies to woolen garments when they are new, and to white linen garments when laundried. Taan. 29[b] ג׳ שלנו כביבוס שלהם (Ms. M. always גִּיהוּיִן) our (Babylonian) laundry work is like their (Palestinean) plain wash. Ib. אין בהן משום ג׳ are not included in the prohibition of laundry work (in the festive week &c.). Keth. 10[b] top.

גִּיהָיָא, גִּיהְיָא, גִּיהָ m. (v. גִּיהָ) *flame-colored.* Bekh. 45[b] (expl. גיחור) as people say סומקא גיה׳ Ar. (ed. גיה׳) flame-red.

גִּיהִיאָה, v. גִּיהָא I.

גֵּיהִינֹּם, גֵּיהִנָּם, גֵּיהִינָּם, גְּהִינָּם c. (b. h. גֵּיא, גֵּיא חִנֹּם בֶּן חִנֹּם) pr. n. *Gehinnom, Gehenna,* a glen to the south of Jerusalem where Molokh was worshipped; whence *place of punishment of the wicked in the hereafter, hell,* opp. גן עדן paradise. Erub. 19[a]; Succ. 32[b] שתי תמרות ..... וזו היא פתחה של ג׳ two palm-trees are in the Valley of Ben Hinnom .... and this is the entrance to Gehenna. Sot. 4[b], a. fr. דינה של ג׳ future punishment. Yoma 72[b] לא תירתו תרתי ג׳ be not the heirs of two G. (here and hereafter, by laborious study of the Law without living up to its requirements). R. Hash. 17[a]; a. fr.

גִּיהַר, גִּיהֲר, גּוֹהַר m. (cmp. גִּיהְרָא, גִּיהוֹר) *gihar,* name of a precious stone, *ruby.* Targ. Cant. V, 14 (ed. Lag. גו׳).—*Pl.* גּוֹהֲרִין, v. יוֹהֲרָא.

גיובריא, v. גִּינְבְּרָא.

גִּיוֹר, v. גֵּר.

גֵּיוָה f. ch.=h. גַּאֲוָה *pride.* Targ. Is. III, 24 מחלבן בג׳ (h. text פתיגיל!).

***גִּיוְטָאֵי** m. pl. *inhabitants of Coptos* (Κόπτος) in Upper Egypt. Targ. Y. I Gen. X, 13 (some ed. גי׳); Targ. I Chr. I, 11 גיוטאי ed. Rahmer (Var. ניוט׳, ed. Lag. כאטאי, h. text לודים). Cmp. גִּיפְטַר.

גִּיוְתָנָא, v. גֵּיוְתָ׳.

גִּיוְרָא, v. גַּאֲוָה.

גיונברי, v. גִּזְבְּרָא.

גָּיוֹס, גַּיְּיוֹס (גייס) pr. n. m. *Caius, Gaius,* 1) (mostly corrupt) used, in connection with לוקיוס (Lucius), to represent gentile names in general. Pesik. R. s. 21 (ed. Fr. p. 107[ab]) ג׳ מן הגודר ולוקיוס מן וכ׳ e. g. Gaius of Gadara and Lucius of Susitha (Hippos). Ib. 108[a] (corr. acc.).—Y. Gitt. I, 43[b] top גוים לוקין וכ׳ (corr. acc.) G. a. L. are the signers and ye ask yet (whether the signers must be personally known as Jews to the witnesses)? [Bab. ib. 11[b] לוקוס ולוס, prob. ל׳ וגיוס.]—Y. Ter. X, 47[b]; Y. Ab. Zar. III, 42[a] [ref. to letters accompanying a ship load(?)]. —2) *Emperor Caius Caligula.* Y. Sot. IX, 24[b] top גייס גוליקס (גוליקס); Bab. ib. 33[a] גסקלגס; Cant. R. to VIII, 9 גיוסלוקין (corr. גיוס קליגולס=Καλιγούλας).

גִּיוּפָא, v. גִּירְפָא.

גִּיּוֹר, גִּיּוֹרָא m. ch.=h. גֵּר 1) *stranger.* Targ. O. Ex. XXIII, 9; a. fr.—Erub. 9[a]; B. Kam. 42[a]; Yoma 47[a] יציבא וג׳ בשמי שמיא . . the native below and the stranger on top! i. e. what a paradox is this!—2) *proselyte.* Targ. Y. Ex. II, 12; a. e.—Y. Sabb. VI, 8[d] top. Y. Kidd. VII, 64[c] bot. חתן ג׳ וכ׳, v. גּוּפְנָא. Snh. 94[a]; a. fr.—*Pl.* גִּיּוֹרִין, גִּיּוֹרַיָּא. Targ. I Chr. XXVIII, 2; a. e.—Fem. גִּיּוֹרְתָא *proselyte.* Ber. 8[b]; Pes. 112[b].

גִּיּוֹרָא (גִּיּוֹרָא) גַּיּוֹרָא m. (גיר II) *adulterer, wencher, lewd man.* Targ. Job XXIV, 15 Ms. (ed. גיופא). Targ. Y. Lev. XX, 10 גִּיּ׳.—*Pl.* גִּיּוֹרִין, גִּיּוֹרַיָּא, גִּיּוֹרֵי (גִּי׳). Targ. Y. Ex. XX, 13. Targ. Ps. L, 18 Ms. (ed. גיורפי); a. e.—[Targ. Prov. XXX, 31, read with Ms. גִּזְרָא II.]—Fem. גִּיּוֹרְתָא. Targ. Y. Lev. XX, 10 גִּיּוֹ׳. Targ. Prov. XXX, 20 גַּיַּרְתָּא.

בר ג׳, גִּיּוֹרֵי pr. n. m. *Bar-Giyore* (son of proselytes). M. Kat. 18[a] בר ג׳ (Ms. M. גיורא); Erub. 62[a].—Gen. R. s. 35 יודן בר ג׳; Yalk. Josh. 31 (some ed. גירי); M. Kat. 9[a]; Tanh. B'resh. 13 יהודה בן גרים.

גִּיּוֹרֶת, fem. of גֵּר.

גִּיּוֹרְתָּא, fem. of גִּיּוֹרָא.

גַּיּוֹרְתָּא (גִּיּוֹ׳), fem. of גַּיּוֹרָא.

גֵּיוּת, גֵּיוּתָא, גֵּיוּת f. (denom. of גּוֹי) *gentile status.* Keth. 11[a] בגיותה while she may live as a gentile (as she may protest against her conversion in childhood).

גֵּיוְתָא f. (גאר, v. גֵּאוּתָא) 1) *grandeur.* Targ. Ezek. XXVIII, 13. Targ. O. Ex. XV, 1 ed. Berl.—2) *pride, haughtiness,* v. גֵּיהוּ.

גֵּיוְתָן, גֵּאוֹתָן, גֵּיוָתָ׳, גֵּיוְתָ m. (v. preced.) *haughty, proud man.* Gen. R. s. 85 גיו׳; Yalk. Dan. 1063 גאו׳.—*Pl.* גֵּיוְתָנִין &c. Ex. R. s. 8; Tanh. Vaëra 9 הג׳ שעושין וכ׳ the haughty who declare themselves as gods. Treat. Der. Er. II, beg. גֵּפְ׳ גִּיפְתָּנִין.

גֵּיוְתָנָא, גֵּאוֹ׳, גַּוְ׳ (גִּיפְ׳) ch. 1) same. Targ. Ps. XXXVI, 12. Targ. Is. XLIX, 25 (Vers.); a. e.—*Pl.* גֵּיוְתָנִין &c. Targ. Ez. XVI, 49.—2) (in a good sense) *exalted.* Targ. Job XXII, 29.

גֵּיוְתָנוּתָא, גִּיפְ׳ f. (preced.) 1) *exaltedness, glory.* Targ. Ps. XLVI, 4. Targ. Y. Ex. XV, 7; a. e.—2) *pride, haughtiness.* Targ. Ps. XXXI, 19; a. e.

גִּיזָא I f., v. גִּיזְתָא.

גִּיזָא II m., v. גִּזָּא.

גִּיזְבָּר, גִּיזְבְּרָא, v. גִּזְ׳.

גִּיזָה, גִּזָּה f. (גזז) *shearing; wool cut* or *to be cut.* Bekh. 14[a]; 25[a]; Hull. 135[a] אסורים בג׳ must not be shorn. Ib. בני ג׳ permitted to be cut. Y. Sabb. XIX, 17[a] top; Y. Pes. VI, 33[a] בגיזתו (בגיזתה) between its wool (Bab.

ib. 66a בצמרו); a. fr.—Midr. Till. to Ps. I זמן ג׳, v. גְּזִיזָה.—*Pl.* גִּיזוֹת, גִּיזּוֹת. Ḥull. l. c. חוץ מִגִּיזּוֹתֶיהָ with the exception of its wool. Midr. Till. l. c. ללבוש מִגִּזּוֹתֵיהֶן to have garments from their wool.

גִּיזָה f. *agony*, v. גִּיסָה.

גִּיזוּזָא m. (גזז) 1) *cutting off, shearing.* Constr. גִּיזּוּז. Targ. Is. III, 24; XXII, 12 (h. text קרחה).—2) *trimming.* B. Bath. 4a.

גִּיזּוּם, גִּזּוּם m. (גָּזַם) *cutting, tapping.* Ab. Zar. 50b ג׳ אברויי וכ׳ tapping is an act of strengthening the tree. Ib. סכין שמן לג׳ you may put oil on the cut (to stop the flow of sap).

גִּיזִין, v. גֵּז.

***גִּיזִית**, pl. גִּיזִיּוֹת (גזז, v. גְּזִירָא, cmp. גֶּזַע) *twigs.* Y. Sabb. IV, 7a top, tie ye ראשי ג׳ the tops of twigs (as bundles to sit on). [The passage is defective.]

גִּיזֶר, v. גֶּזֶר.

גִּיזְרָה, גִּיזְרָא, v. גִּזְרָא, גזרה.

גיזריפטי, v. גִּזְרִיפַּטֵי.

גִּיזָא, גִּיזְתָא f. ch.=h. גִּיזָה *fleece.* Targ. Jud. VI, 37. Targ. Deut. XVIII, 4; a. e.

גִּיזְתְּיָא, v. גֵּיתֵי.

גִּיחַ, גוּחַ (cmp. גִּיחַ) 1) *to break forth, stir up.* Dan. VII, 2. Targ. Job XXXVIII, 8 בְּמִגְחֵיה (h. text בגיחו) when he breaks forth. [Targ. Ps. XLII, 5 למגח Ms., read למחג, v. חגג].—ג׳ קרבא, v. infra.—2) (cmp. meanings of בּוּעַ) *to low* (of oxen). Targ. Job VI, 5 (some ed. יגעי, h. text יגעה).

Af. אַגִּיחַ, אָגַח (אַגַּח), esp. with קרבא (Af. a. Pe.) *to attack, fight.* Targ. O. Ex. I, 10; XIV, 14. Targ. Y. Gen. XXI, 10.—Targ. Ps. LX, 2 אֲגִיחַ עם (sub. קרבא). Targ. O. Deut. XX, 4; a. fr.—Tosef. Sot. XIII, 5; Sot. 33a לְאַגָּחָא קרבא to wage war. Nidd. 65b כתובה דמַגְחֵי וכ׳ Ar. (ed. מגבי, v. גְּבַב, Var. דמגחי) a marriage deed over which they fight much before signing.

Ithpa. אִתְּגַח (with קרבא) *to be fought.* Targ. O. Ex. XVII, 16; a. e.

גִּיחוּךְ m. (גחך) *laughter, sport; obscenity.* Nidd. 23a לידי ג׳ וכ׳ . . הביאו tried to make R. laugh, but the latter did not laugh.—Sabb. 64a כומז (Num. XXXI, 50) is translated מחוך, דבר המביא לידי ג׳ ed. (Ms. M., Yalk. Num. 786 מחוך) something which leads to obscenity.

גִּיחוּכָא ch. same. Targ. II Chron. XV, 16 (h. text מִפלצת).

גִּיחוֹן pr. n. (b. h.) the river *Giḥon.* Gen. R. s. 16 (play on גָּחוֹן).

גִּיחוּץ, v. גִּיהוּץ.

גִּיחוֹר m. (v. גִּיחַ a. גִּיחְוָרָא) *red-spotted* in the face. Bekh. VII, 6, expl. ib. 45b סומקא. Ber. 58b; a. e.

גִּיחוֹרָא ch. same. *Pl.* גִּיחוֹרֵי. Ber. 59b והאי דג׳ משום דמשמשי וכ׳ (Ms. M. שפירי, inserting גיחורי in place of דנהידי עינייהו ed.) that they are red-spotted arises from sexual intercourse in day-time; (Ar. והאי דגִחִירֵי משום דדיירי בבתי אפלי because they live in dark rooms).

גִּיחְיָא, v. גִּיחְוָרָא.

גִּיחֲכָא, v. גּוּחֲכָא.

גִּיטָא, גֵּיט, v. גֵּט, גִּטָּא.

***גַּיֵּר**, *Pa.* גַּיֵּר (cmp. גאר) *to manifest power, treat with rigor.* Gen. R. s. 33 חן דמחיית גַּיֵּרת where Thou strikest, Thou showest Thy power (crushest; Rashi a. l. גַּזֵּית thou cuttest; Lev. R. s. 27; Pesik. Shor 74a; Tanḥ. Emor 6 את מדקדק). V. גֵּיתֵי.

גַּיֵּיד *Pi.* (denom. of גִּיד) *to cut an artery through, to bleed to death* (a gentile mode of execution). *Lev. R. s. 6 מְגַיֵּיד את הגנבים והורג וכ׳ Ar. s. v. גד 12 (Var. מנגיד, Ar. Compl. ed. Koh. 239²) had the thieves bled to death and the receivers of stolen goods decapitated (ed. הורג את הקבלנין ומתיר את הגנבים).—Part. pass. מְגוּיָּד *he who had his arteries opened, bled to death.* Ohol. I, 6 אפי׳ מג׳ even if his arteries are cut open (and he is dying). Yeb. XVI, 3 (120a). Ib.b למימרא דמג׳ חי does this intimate that one whose arteries have been severed, may survive?—Y. ib. XVI, 15c bot. אפי׳ ראוהו מ׳ וכ׳ (Tosef. ib. XIV, 4 נִתְגַּיֵּיד) even if witnesses have seen him bleeding from severed arteries, I say, the operation may have been performed with a glowing knife and he may have recovered. Tosef. Gitt. VII (V), 1; Bab. ib. 70b מְגוּיָּד; Y. ib. VII, 48c bot.

Nithpa. נִתְגַּיֵּיד, v. supra.

גַּיֵּיד ch. same. Snh. 67b וגַיְּדֵיה לגמלא (read לגמליה, v. Rabb. D. S. a. l. note 8) and severed his camel's arteries; Yeb. 120b.

***גַּיְדוֹר** m. (γαῦδαρος, Sachs Beitr. I, 155; mod. Greek γάδαρος; prob. an adaptation of עָרוֹד, v. S. s. v. γαράσδοειδής) *a small ass.* Y. B. Mets. VI, 11a. Cmp. גִּירְדוֹנָא.

גַּיּוּס, v. גַּיִּס.

גַּיּוֹרָא, גַּיּוֹפָא, v. גַּיּוֹ׳.

גֵּיִם, v. גֵּאֶה.

גֵּיֵס, v. גּוּס II.

גַּיִּס m. (גּוּס II) *troop,* esp. *ravaging troop, invaders, robbers* (=b. h. גְּדוּד). Pes. III, 7 (49a) (if one left his home) להציל מן הג׳ Y. ed. a. Ms. M. (ed. גויים, עכום, v. Rabb. D. S. a. l. note) to rescue (Israelites &c.) from an invading troop. Yeb. 122b רדף אחרינו ג׳ a band pursued us; a. fr.—*Pl.* גַּיָּיסוֹת. Ib. XVI, 7 (122a) the country is משובשת בג׳ in confusion on account of invaders. Ruth R. to I, 5; a. fr.—Denom. גַּיֵּיס *to arrange battle, to order* *out troops; to array.* Ib. כמה גייסות... לַגַּיֵּיס how many troops can I send out. Ib.; Lev. R. s. 17 התחיל מְגַיֵּיס חיילותיו וכ׳ he began to arrange his armies for battle; a. fr. [גייס pr. n. m., v. גַּיּוּס.]

גַּיְיסָא ch. same. Targ. II Chr. XXXII, 7 (h. text המון).—Y. Sot. VIII, end, 23ᵃ (translation of Gen. XLIX, 19) ג׳ אתי מְגַיֵּיסְתֵּיה וכ׳ an army comes to ravage him, but he &c.; Gen. R. s. 98.—Ber. 60ᵇ bot.; a. e. *Pl.* גַּיְיסִין. Targ. Ps. LXV, 11 גַּיְסָתָא ed. Vien. (ed. גרי׳, Ms. גַּיְיָ׳).—Denom. גַּיֵּיס = h. גַּיֵּיס, v. preced.—Gen. R. l. c.; a. e.

גַּיְיסָא, v. גַּיְסָא II a. גיס II.

גַּיֵּיף, גַּיֵּיף, v. גּוּף I h. a. ch.

גַּיְפָא, גַּיּוֹפָא, גַּיָּפָא m. (preced.) *adulterer, wencher, lewd man.* Targ. Job XXIV, 15 (v. גַּיּוֹרָא). Targ. O. Lev. XX, 10.—*Pl.* גַּיְּיפִין, גַּיְּיפַיָּא, גַּיּוּפֵי. Targ. Jer. VII, 9. Targ. Ps. L, 18 (v. גַּיּוֹרָא); a. e.—Fem. גַּיַּיפְתָּא, גַּיְּפ׳. Targ. O. Lev. l. c.—*Pl.* גַּיָּיפָן. Targ. Ezek. XVI, 38; a. e.

גַּיֵּיר, גַּיֵּיר, v. גּוּר h. a. ch.; also גִּיר II.

גַּיָּארָא, גַּיּוֹרָא m. (גּוּר II) *adultery, whoredom.—Pl.* גַּיּוּרַיָּא. Lev. R. s. 33, v. גְּלַד.

גִּיל I (b. h., v. גול) *to form a circle, to gather; to rejoice.* Y. Ber. V, 8ᵈ bot. (ref. to Ps. II, 11) לכשיבוא יום רעדה תָּגִילוּ when the time of trembling comes (in a disposition of reverence) shall ye assemble (for prayer); cmp. גִּילָה.

גִּיל II m. (b. h.; preced.) *circle, association of coevals.* B. Mets. 27ᵇ; Yeb. 120ᵃ the same mark מצויה בבן גילו is frequently found with those born at the same hour (under the same planetary influences, cmp. מַזָּל). Meg. 11ᵃ בן גילו וכ׳ of the same character. Ned. 39ᵇ בן גילו (Ar. בני) of the same age; B. Bets. 30ᵇ. Ruth R. to I, 3 מת אחד מן הג׳ ידאג כל הג׳ if one of the circle (of the coevals) died, the whole circle must take it to heart.—*Pl.* גִּילִין. Ib.—v. גִּילָאֵי. [Y. Orl. II, 61ᵈ bot. גיל השבט, v. גֶּזֶל.]

גִּיל III m. (גול) *ball, clapper of a bell.* Lev. R. s. 27, beg.; Tanh. Emor 5 גול; ed. Bub. ib. 7 גיל.

גִּילָא I pr. n. f. *Gela (Coelia?).* Ab. Zar. 10ᵇ Ar., v. גּוּר II.

גִּילָא II, **גִּילָּא, גְּלָא** m. (גלל) 1) *something rounded.* Succ. 34ᵃ חילפא ג׳ a willow with rounded leaves. Sabb. 110ᵃ; Men. 42ᵇ (מ)גבריא ג׳ (v. מַגַּבְרָא) liquid alum in rounded form (στυπτηρία στρογγύλη, v. Sm. Ant. s. v. Stypteria).—2) (cmp. גַּלְגַּל Ps. LXXXIII, 14) *[rolled about,] stubble, straw.* Targ. Job XIII, 25.—Hull. 46ᵇ a feather, spittle, או ג׳ or a piece of straw. Ib. 56ᵇ top ג׳ דחיטתא a piece of wheat straw. Nidd. 26ᵇ דרמינן ליה בג׳ דחטתא on whom we may throw wheat chaff, i. e. embarrass with petty questions.—*Pl.* גִּילֵי, גִּילַּיָּא, גִּילֵּי. Targ. Ex. V, 12. Targ. Job XLI, 20 sq.—Snh. 108ᵇ, v. גִּיר III.—Succ. 14ᵃ בְּגִילֵּיהוֹן (grains) in their haulms.—בֵּי גִּילֵי *dumping ground, marsh.* גילדנא דבי ג׳ the small fish living among the reeds in the swamps. Ber. 44ᵇ; Keth. 105ᵇ.

גִּילָאֵי m. pl. (גִּיל II) *persons of the same age and circle.* Zeb. 116ᵇ תרי עולמי ג׳ (some ed. גו׳, v. Rabb. D. S. a. l. note 3) two youths of the same &c.

גִּילְבוֹנָה, v. גּוּלְבְּרִינָא.

גִּילְגְּלִין, גִּילְגְּלָא, גִּילְגַל, גִּילְגָל, גִּילְגּוּל, v. גלג׳.

גִּילְדָנָא, גִּילְדְּאָה, גִּילְדָא, גֶּלֶד, v. גְּלַד, גִּלְדָ׳.

גִּילָה f. (b. h.; גִּיל I) *gathering; rejoicing.* Ber. 30ᵇ (ref. to Ps. II, 11) במקום ג׳ שם תהא רעדה where there is a gathering (for prayer and the like) there shall be trembling, v. גִּיל I.

גִּילָּה, v. גִּלָּה.

גִּילְהֵי, גּוּלְהֵי m. pl. (גלי; cmp. שִׁילְהֵי fr. שלה) *[uncoverings,] flashes, the glowing horizon.* Taan. 3ᵇ ג׳ דליליא (Ms. M. גו׳) the glow after sunset. Pes. 13ᵃ top בגי׳ וכ׳ Ms. M. (ed. בגילוליא) he was standing in the glow before sunrise (mistaking it for the flashing of sunrise, v. הָנֵץ); Snh. 42ᵃ (ed. בגילוריא).

גִּילּוּחַ m. (גלח) *shaving, hair-cutting.* Macc. 21ᵃ ג׳ שרש בו וכ׳ a cutting with which a destruction is connected (which attacks the roots); a. fr.

גִּילּוּחַ, גְּלוּחַ ch. (preced.) *shaved beard* (in mourning). Targ. Is. XV, 2; Jer. XLVIII, 37, v. גְּלִבָא.

גִּילּוּי, גִּלּוּי m. (גלי) 1) *uncovering.*—ג׳ עריות uncovering of nakedness, *incest* (Lev. XVIII, 6; a. fr.). Yoma 9ᵃ; a. fr.—ג׳ ראש *bareheadedness.* Sabb. 118ᵇ.—ג׳ פנים *barefacedness, defiance.* Sot. 42ᵇ, v. גָּלְיָת. Erub. 69ᵃ מומר וג׳ פנים an apostate and a defiant person, expl. מומר בג׳ פ׳ a defiant apostate; a. e.—2) *the law forbidding the use of liquids that were left uncovered* (as possibly poisoned by serpents). Ter. VIII, 4 אסורים משום ג׳ are forbidden on account of *gilluy;* a. fr.—*Pl.* גִּילּוּיִים, גִּילּוּיִין. Y. Ab. Zar. II, 41ᵃ bot.; Y. Ter. VIII, 45ᶜ bot. [read:] שהיה מלגלג בג׳ (not מגלגל, not בגילוי יין) who sneered at the law of *gilluy.*

גִּילּוּיָא, גִּילּוּיָיא, גְּלִ׳ ch. 1) same. Targ. Y. Gen. VI, 2 גִּילּוּי בשרא nakedness. Ib. XIII, 13; Num. XXXV, 25 ג׳ עריותא = h. גִּילּוּי עריות.—Esp. *liquids left uncovered, law concerning them.* Hull. 49ᵇ כי הוה להו ג׳ when they had a case of uncovered liquids. Gitt. 69ᵇ לג׳ וכ׳ against the danger from drinking uncovered liquids apply &c. Ab. Zar. 30ᵃ אג׳ לא קפדי they care not for the law concerning uncovered liquids; a. fr.—גִּילּוּי דעתא intimation of meaning. Gitt. 34ᵃ בג׳ ד׳ בגיטא וכ׳ they differ with regard to one intimating the annulment of a letter of divorce.—2) *bright, polished surface.* Zeb. 38ᵇ אַגִּילּוּיֵיהּ on its (the altar's) top surface cleared of ashes.—Snh. 42ᵃ; Pes. 13ᵃ, v. גִּילְהֵי.—Targ. Nah. II, 8 בְּגִילְיָא ed. Lag. (oth. ed. בִּגְלָיָא) *openly* (not in a covered carriage), v. גְּלֵי.

גִּילּוּל, pl. גִּילּוּלִים, v. גִּלּוּל.

גִּירְלוּלַיָא, v. גִּירְלָא.

גִּירְלוּעַ m. (גָּלַע) *exposure, attack.* Y. Yeb. VIII, end, 9[d], v. גָּלַע.

גִּירְלַיָא, v. גִּירְלוּרָא.

גִּירְלְיוֹן, v. גִּלָּיוֹן.

גִּירְלָלִין, v. גִּלָּה.

גִּירְלשְׁלֵי, v. גלשלי.

גִּימוֹל m. (גמל to wean, train) *a pointed pole tied to the neck of a calf to prevent it from sucking* (v. שִׁירְחוּעַ), or *a little yoke* put on the calf for breaking it in. Y. Sabb. V, 7[c] top אית תניין תני ג׳ some teachers read (Mish. V, 4) *gimol* (in place of *gimon*) in the sense of גמל in I Sam. I, 24; v. next w.

גִּימוֹן m. (גמם to couple, tie) *a little yoke* (בר נִירָא), or *a board tied* to the head of a calf (פִּרִנְקְסָה), or *a pointed pole* (שִׁירְחוּעַ, v. preced. w.). Sabb. V, 4; expl. Y. ib. V, 7[c]; Bab. ib. 54[b].—Y. l. c. מאן דמר ג׳ וכ׳ he who reads *gimon* supports the opinion of R. Ḥisda (פרנקסה); he who reads *gimol* supports the opinions &c. (שררתוע or בר נירא).—*Pl.* גִּימוֹנוֹת, v. next w.

גִּימוֹנִית f. (v. preced.) *chord, band. Pl.* גִּימוֹנִיּוֹת. Succ. III, 8 ג׳ של זהב gold bands; Tosef. ib. II, 10 גִּימוֹנוֹת.

גִּמַטְרִיָּא, גִּימַטְרִיָא, גִּימְטְרִיא f. (a transpos. of γραμματεῖον, . . . ἄτια, pl.) 1) *accounts.* Y. Ter. V, 43[c] bot. חשבון ג׳ arithmetical calculation.—2) *the use of letters for their numerical value; homiletic interpretation based on the numerical value of letters.* Ber. 8[a] תוֹצָאוֹת בגי׳ וכ׳ the word *totsaoth* (Ps. LXVIII, 21) intimates 903 (causes of death). Lev. R. s. 21 חשטן גי׳ וכ׳; Midr. Till. to Ps. XXVII השט״ן בגי׳ וכ׳ *hassatan* (the accuser) counts 364; a. fr.—3) *learned writing, cifer.* Snh. 22[a] בגי׳ איכתיב (Ms. M. איתחזר) the inscription of the wall was in cifers (א״ת ב״ש).—*Pl.* גִּימַטְרִיָּאוֹת *arithmetic.* Ab. III, 18.

גִּימַטְרִיקוֹן, גִּימַטְרִיּוֹן m. (γραμματεῖον, γραμματικόν) same, *cifer-writing.* Y. Taan. III, 67[a] לישן ג׳, גימטריון וכ׳, v. אֶפְרָא. Pesik. R. s. 43 לשון גרמטריקון הוא תהו הוא אסף it is cipher speech, *Tohu* (I Sam. I, 1) is (in א״ת ב״ש) *Asaf.*

גִּימ״ל m. *Gimmel,* third letter of the Alphabet; numerical value, *three.* Shek. III, 2; a. fr.—Sabb. 104[a] (childrens' mnemonical play) גי׳ דל״ת גמול דלים (Ms. M. גמל) Gimmel-Daleth intimates, Do good to the poor. Ib. כרעיה דג׳ the foot of the Gimmel; a. fr.—*Pl.* גִּמְלִין. Ib. 103[b] one must not write ... ג׳ צדין וכ׳ Ms. M. (ed. גַּמִּין) Gimmels so as to be possibly taken for Tsaddes.

גִּימֵל pr. n. m., v. גִּמְלָא.

גִּימְלָא, v. גִּמְלָא a. גַּמְלָא I, 2.

גִּין I (v. גנן), Af. אַגִּין (with על) *to cover, surround with; to protect.* Targ. Y. I Deut. XXXII, 10 (II אקיף). Targ. II Kings XX, 6. Targ. Is. XXVII, 3 מְגִין (ed. Lag. מגן, v. גְּנַן); a. e.

Ithpe. אִתְגִּין *to be protected.* Targ. Zeph. II, 3 (ed. Lag. יתגן). V. גְּנַן.

גִּין II m. (preced.) *protection.* Targ. Is. XXVIII, 15.—בְּגִין *for the sake of, on account of; in order that.* Targ. Y. Gen. XII, 13 (O. בדיל). Ib. XVIII, 24; a. fr.—[In Talm. h. a. ch.] Yeb. 89[b] אוכלת בְּגִינוֹ וכ׳ on his account (as his wife) she is permitted to eat T'rumah. Y. B. Kam. X, 7[c] top בג׳ כן therefore; a. fr.—בגין ד׳ *because, since.* Y. Gitt. IX, 50[b] ב׳ דרב וכ׳ because Rab and Samuel, both of them, said. Y. Bicc. II, 64[d] top ב׳ דכתיב because it is so written; a. fr.

גִּינָא, v. גִּינְּתָא a. גַּנָּא.

גִּינָּאָה m. (denom. of גִּינָּא) *gardener, dealer in vegetables.* Ḥull. 105[b]. Sabb. 110[b].—*Pl.* גִּינָּאֵי. Gitt. 14[a]. Taan. 20[b] פריש להו לג׳ (Ms. M. יתיר לגַנָּאֵי) was left over with the gardeners (was not sold).

גִּינַּאי, גִּינַּיִר, גִּינַּאר I f. (denom. of גַּן, גִּינָּה) *a group of gardens, country residences.*—*Pl.* גִּינָּאוֹת. Midr. Till. to Ps. XLVIII, end; Yalk. ib. 756.—B. Bath. 75[b] Ms. M. (ed. גינואות, v. Rabb. D. S. a. l. note); Yalk. Zach. 568; v. טֶפֶה. [Ar. גינואות, גונרות, v. ed. Koh. s. v. גרננא p. 320.]—[Yalk. Deut. 946, v. גִּינְתָאר.]

גִּינַּאי, גִּינַּיִר, גִּינַּאר II m. (denom. of גִּינָּא; cmp. preced.) *dyke for irrigating gardens;* also pr. n. *Ginnai.* Ḥull. 7[a] ג׳ נהרא the rivulet Ginnai; Y. Dem. I, 22[a] top. Y. Shek. VI, 50[c] bot. ג׳ שטף זיקין an overflowing dyke carried off wine bottles.

גִּינְבְּרָא m. (cmp. ζιγγίβερις a. זַנְגְּבִיל) *ginger.* Gitt. 86[a].

גִּינְבְּרָא, v. גִּנְבְּרָא.

גִּינְגְּלוֹן, v. גִּלְגְּלִין.

גִּינדרונא, v. גִּירְדוֹנָא.

גִּינַּת, v. גַּן. [Chald. = גִּינָּא.]

גִּינּוּן, v. גִּנּוּן.

גִּינּוּנִיתָא, v. גִּנּוּנִיתָא.

גִּינוּסִין, גִּינוּסִים, גִּינוּסְיָא, גִּינוּסְיָא, v. גִּינִיסְיָא.

גִּינּוֹסַר, v. גִּינֵּסַר.

גִּינְזַק, v. גִּנְזַק.

גִּינְיָא, גִּינְיָא, גִּינַּר, v. גּוּנַר a. גּוּנְיָא.

גִּינִיאָךְ, גִּ׳ טַעֲוָתָא read גִּינָּיָא דט׳. Targ. Is. LXV, 3; LXVI, 17 (Buxt. a. oth. ed. גִּינָן), v. גִּינְּתָא.

גִּינַּיִר, v. גִּינְאַר.

***גִּינַּיִן (גּוּכִין)** m. pl. (גנן) *protective armor, cuirass* (?). Tosef. Kel. B. Mets. III, 1. [V. גַּנָּא.]

גִּינִיסְיָא, גִּינִיסִין (גִּנוּ׳, גִּינוּ׳, גְּנוּ׳) m. pl. (γενέσια, τά) 1) (with יום) *bithday festival, anniversary of death*; in gen. *commemorative festival*. Targ. Esth. III, 8. Targ. Y. Gen. XL, 20 גְּנוּסָא (v. גִּנִיסָא a. גְּנוּסַיָּא).—Ab. Zar. I, 3 (8ª) יום ג׳ של מלכים royal anniversaries, expl. Y. ib. 39ᶜ birthday festival (with ref. to Gen. XL, 20, v. supra); Bab. ib. 10ª (after discussion) יום שמעמידין בו המלך installation of a king (Roman emperor). Y. R. Hash. III, 59ª top; Yalk. Hab. 564. Ex. R. s. 15 יום ג׳ an anniversary (commemorative of his delivery); a. e.—2) (=γενέθλια) *descent, nobility of birth*. Pesik. Naḥămu p. 126ᵃᵇ; Yalk. Gen. 162 הודעתם ג׳ שלי (Gen. R. s. 100 הודעתי הוגנסים corr. acc.), ye have made known my noble descent. Pesik. Haḥod. p. 53ª בת גִּינוּסִים; Pesik. R. s. 15 בת גינסין (read גִּנִיסִין, Yalk. Ex. 190 only בת טובים) a woman of noble birth. Cant. R. to I, 2; a. fr. [Sot. 36ᵇ גִּנִיסֵי מלכות וכ׳ Ar. (ed. גְּנוּנֵי) I recognize in him royal nobility.]

גִּינֵיסַר (גְּנוּ׳, גְּנֵי׳, גִּינוּ׳) pr. n. pl. (Γεννησάρ, Γεννησαρέτ, a hellenization of כִּנֶּרֶת) *Gennesar, Gennesaret*, lake, town and district of G. Pes. 8ᵇ פירות גינו׳ Gennes. fruits. Gen. R. s. 98 (etymology) גנוסר=גני שרים princely gardens; Meg. 6ª, v. כִּנֶּרֶת; a. e.—*Pl.* גִּינֵיסַרְיוֹת. Y. Meg. I, 70ª bot. שני גנ׳ היו (corr. acc.) were there two places of the name of G.?

גינירות, Tosef. Men. IX, 3, Var. ניטרות, read נירורות, v. נִיר.

גִּינְבַיָא, v. גִּבָּא.

גינסין, v. גִּינִיסְיָא.

גִּינְתָא, גִּינָּא, גִּנ׳ f. (גנן, v. גַּן) *garden*. Targ. O. Gen. II, 8. Targ. Y. I Gen. XLXI, 4 גינא (Y. II גִּנָּא). Targ. Ps. LVI, 14 (second vers.). Constr. גִּינַּת. Targ. Deut. XI, 10; a. fr.—Gen. R. s. 80 (prov.) לפום ג׳ גננא as the garden so the gardener (as the people so the leader); Y. Snh. II, 20ᵈ top כגִּנְּתָה כן גננה. B. Bath. 54ª; a. fr.—*Pl.* גִּינָּתָא, constr. גִּינַּת. Targ. Koh. II, 5.—גִּנָּן, גִּינָּן. Targ. Is. LXV, 3; LXVI, 17 (some ed. גִּנָּן; v. גינואך). V. גִּבָּא.

גִּיס m. (גנס; cmp. גנז a. כנס; Syr. גסא divitiae P. Sm. 757) *spoils, heaped up treasures*. *Pl.* גִּיסִין. Ex. R. s. 9 (ref. to Esth. I, 4) ששה ג׳ וכ׳ he showed them six collections every day, and not two of them alike; Esth. R. to l. c. ששה ג׳ היה פותח וכ׳ (ed. נוסין, נרסין, corr. acc.) six treasuries he opened to them &c.; (Yalk. Esth. 1046 תסבורייות; Targ. II Esth. I, 4 בי גנזר).

גִּיס II, גָּיִיס m. (גוס II) *intimate, familiar*. Keth. 85ᵇ ואי . . דג׳ ביה הא ג׳ ביה (Ar. גס ביה . . . דגייס . . .) but if it is one who is familiar with him (so as to use his name without a title), then, we may say, he spoke of him in a familiar way.—Fem. גָּיִיסָא. Kidd. 81ª ג׳ ביה she was on familiar terms with him.—*Pl.* גִּיסֵי, גָּיִיסֵי. Ib. 33ª דגי׳ בה רבנן where scholars are a familiar sight (and no attention is paid them). Keth. 28ª גיי׳ בהדדי they are intimate with each other.

גִּיס II m. (v. preced., cmp. גִּיסָא III) *the wife's sister's husband, brother-in-law*. Snh. III, 4 (27ᵇ) גִּיסוֹ (Y. ib. III, 7 אֲגִיסוֹ); a. fr.—*Pl.* גִּיסִין. Y. Shek. I, end, 46ᵇ; a. e.

גִּיסָא I, אֲגִיסָא ch. same. Y. Snh. III, 21ᵇ bot. אֲגִיסֵיה דר׳ וכ׳ R. H.'s brother-in-law.—*Pl.* גִּיסֵי. Snh. 28ᵇ אחי וג׳ brothers and brothers-in-law (two brothers having married two sisters). Ib. תרי ג׳.

גִּיסָא II, גָּיִיסָא m. (גוס I) *bold man*. Hull. 18ᵇ he called out over him ג׳ ג׳ (Ar. ed. Koh. גיי׳ וגיי׳) bold man that thou art!

גִּיסָא III m. (גוס II) *neighborhood, side*. Kidd. 33ª באידך ג׳ on the other side (of the river); Erub. 16ᵇ. Sabb. 110ª בההוא ג׳ וכ׳ in a certain neighborhood of &c. —Yoma 77ᵇ. Bekh. 44ᵇ אַגִּ׳ sideways. Koh. R. to VII, 9 when the kettle boils over, על גיסיה שפיך it pours over its own sides (wrath will hurt none but the man himself); a. fr.—Trnsf. *way, manner*. Gitt. 67ᵇ some argue להאי ג׳ וכ׳ one way and some the other way; a. fr.— Nidd. 66ª [read:] לא תגלי . . . דכי היכי דתהוו עליך להן ג׳ וכ׳ (v. Ar. ed. Koh. s. v. דם IV, 752) do not tell thy friends, for as they wondered over thee on the one side (over thy bad luck), they may wonder on the other side (over thy good fortune, and bewitch it). [Hull. 17ᵇ אתרי גִּיסָנֵי, Sh'eltoth d'R. Ahai 92, ed. אתלת רוחתא.]

גִּיסָה, גִּיזָה f. (v. גּוֹסֵס) *agony of death, dying stage*. Y. Sot. IX, 23ᵈ bot. מקום גִּיסָתָהּ the place where the expiatory heifer died; Tosef. ib. IX, 1 גִּיזָתָהּ.

גִּיסְטְרָא, גִּסְטְרָא, גִּצְטְרָא f. (=גורזרא, a reduplic. of גזר; for assimilation of sibilants cmp. Nöld. Mand. Gr. p. 45 sq.) *something defective, mutilated*; 1) *a large vessel which turned out defective or unwieldy*, by having its handles broken off or being cracked, and is therefore used as a *receptacle for refuse*, as *a pickling pot*, as *a receiver of drippings* from a leaking vessel &c. Kel. II, 6 גס׳ שנמצאת וכ׳ (Ar. גצרא) a defective vessel found in the furnace (in which vessels are put for baking); Tosef. ib. B. Kam. III, 10 ואם היתה גסטרה but if the jug turned out a *gistra*, contrad. to נפחתה. Ib. אי זו היא גסטרא כל שנסדקין אזניה וכ׳ (Kel. IV, 3 גיס׳ . . . . כל שניטלו וכ׳) when is a vessel called *gistra*? When its handles are split (broken off) &c. Ib. 2 גי׳ שנתרועעה וכ׳ if a *gistra* is broken so as to be no longer a receptacle for liquids, though it may yet receive eatables, it is not susceptible of uncleanness, for there is no fragment of a fragment, i. e. a fragment of a *gistra* is no longer considered a vessel. Sabb. 96ª (a leaking *gistra* is not considered a vessel) because nobody says הָבֵא ג׳ לג׳ bring a *g.* to be put under a *gistra*; a. fr.— 2) *an animal body maimed to disfigurement*. Hull. 21ª; 32ᵇ עשאה ג׳ נבלה if one made an animal a *gistra* by lacerating some of its limbs, it is considered a carcass. Ib. 52ª ג׳ קאמריתו ye speak of a maimed body (a rib on each side disjointed)! Ib. 27ª דלא לישוייה ג׳ that in cutting the animal's throat one must not make it a *gistra* (by cutting the head off). Snh. 52^b^ דעביד ליה ג׳ that the culprit be cut in two.—Hull. 124^a^ דעבדיה ג׳ he split the stove lengthwise.—*Pl.* גִּיסְטְרָאוֹת, גִּיסְטְרָיוֹת. Tosef. Kel. B. Kam. III, 8 שרובן מן הג׳ for most of the fragments of pottery found in the potter's place come from misshaped vessels. Makhsh. II, 3 ג׳ שישראל וכ׳ pots into which Israelites and gentiles cast their refuse.—Y. Sabb. III, beg. 5^c^ ממלא גִּצְרָא וכ׳ one may fill a large pot with hot ashes &c.—3) (castra) *camp*, v. גִּסְטְרָא.

גיסטרון, v. גַּסְטְרוֹן.

גִּיסְסָא I m. (גּוּס II, v. גִּיסָא III a. גֶּסֶס) 1) *side, arm.* —*Pl.* גִּיסְסִין. Targ. Is. LX, 4; LXVI, 13 (h. text צד).— 2) *Pl.* גִּיסְסַיָּא, גִּס׳ *loins.* Targ. O. Lev. III, 4; 15 (h. text כסלים, Y. כפליא).

גִּיסְסָא II m. (cmp. גִּשּׁוּשׁ) *long pole.*—*Pl.* גִּיסְסִין, גִּס׳. Targ. II Sam. XVIII, 14 (Ar. גִּסְסִין, h. text שבטים).

גיסתרא, v. גִּסְטְרָא.

גִּיעֲגוּעַ, v. גַּע׳.

גִּיעוּל I m. (גָּעַל) *the cleaning of an impure vessel* by means of boiling water (Num. XXXI, 23), v. הַגְעָלָה. Zeb. 97^a^; Ab. Zar. 76^a^ כל יום ...... ג׳ לחבירו every day the boiling done in the sacred vessel is the means of absorbing the soakings of the previous day.—*Pl.* גִּיעוּלִים, constr. גִּיעוּלֵי; (עכו״ם, גוים) ג׳ גכרים vessels of gentiles which require cleaning with boiling water before they may be used by Jews. Ib. 67^b^; 75^b^; a. fr.

גִּיעוּל II m. (גָּעַל, v. Job XXI, 10), pl. constr. גִּיעוּלֵי, ג׳ בצים *abortive eggs* driven off by striking the hen. Tosef. Ter. IX, 5; Y. ib. X, 47^b^ bot.; Hull. 64^b^ (Rashi: *eggs scalded in hot water* together with forbidden eggs, v. preced.).

גִּיף m. (b. h. גַּף) *side, shore.* Makhsh. I, 4 על ג׳ הנהר Ar. (ed. גַּב, R. Hai Gaon גַּף, v. Koh. Ar. Compl. s. v. note 9).

גִּיפָא, גִּיף ch. same. Targ. Y. Ex. XIV, 9. Ib. XV, 9 (Y. II some ed. גַּף). Ib. II, 5 (Y. II גַּב, O. כֵּיף); a. e.— Y. Kidd. I, 58^d^; Y. Keth. VI, end 31^a^ אייתיבוני על ג׳ נהרא וכ׳ place me at the shore of a river, and if I do not ...., cast me into the river. Ib. XIII, 35^b^ bot. (גוף, corr. acc.); Y. Kil. IX, 32^c^ bot.; a. fr.

***גִּיף** m. (גּוּף I) *adultery, sensuality.* Sabb. 104^a^, v. אח״ס.

גִּיָּפָא, v. גִּירָפָא.

גִּיפּוּף m. (גפף) 1) *embracing, hugging.* Snh. 56^b^ ג׳ ונישוק embracing and kissing idols.—2) *closing up.* Y. Sabb. III, 5^d^ bot. אחר גִּיפּוּפוֹ according as the stove is closed up.

גִּיפּוּף, גִּיפּוּפָא, גִּפ׳, גֵּפ׳ ch. (cmp. preced.) *railing, rim.* Targ. Y. Ex. XXV, 25; 27 (h. text מסגרת; O. גדנפא).—*Pl.* גִּיפּוּפִין, גִּיפּוּפֵי. Targ. Y. I Deut. XXII, 8 (II גופה). Erub. 89^b^.

גִּיפְטִי m. (Αἰγύπτιος) *Egyptian, Coptic.*—*Pl.* גִּיפְטִים. Meg. 18^a^ גיפטית לג׳ (Ar. גפתית לגפתים) to Egyptian Jews &c.—Fem. גִּיפְטִית *in Egyptian or Coptic language.* Ib.—Sabb. 115^a^. Ib.^b^ תנא דג׳ the author of the rule concerning sacred writings in Egyptian &c. (ib.^a^). Cmp. גִּירְוּטָאֵר.

גִּיפֶן, v. גּוֹפֶן.

גִּיפְסוֹס m. (γύψος) *gypsum.* Y. Sabb. II, 5^a^ top; v. גִּפְסִים.

גִּיפְסִים, גִּיפְסִיס, גיפסים, v. גִּפְסִים.

גִּיפֵף, v. גַּפַּף.

גִּיפֵר, v. גַּפַּר.

גִּיפְתָּא (גּוּפ׳) ch.=h. גֶּפֶת a sort of *peat* or *turf.* Y. Sabb. IV, 6^d^ [read:] כמראר גו ג׳ I kept it warm in *gifta.* Ib. על ג׳ on top of *g.*

גיפתי, Erub. 64^a^ (missing in Ms. M.), marginal version דיפתי q. v.

גִּיפְתָּן, גִּיפְתָּנָא, גִּיפְתָּנוּתָא, v. גִּיוּת׳.

גִּיצָא m. ch.=h. גֵּץ *spark.* Targ. Job XVIII, 5 Ms. Var. for גִּיהָה.—*Pl.* גִּיצִין, גִּירְצִין. Targ. Job V, 7 (Ms. גִּי׳ (ed. גִּי׳, ed. Vien. כצין). Ib. XLI, 11 Ms. (ed. גּוּצִין). Targ. Ps. CXL, 11 (ed. Vien. כיצין).

***גִּיר** I (Syriac גיר, P. Sm. 709 sq., prob. fr. גרר, cmp. גְּרָרָא) *as a consequence, for* &c. Targ. Prov. XXIX, 19 (agreeing with Peshito) ידע ג׳ דלא בליע ed. Lag. (Var. ולא, ed. דידע ג׳ ולא וכ׳, Peshito .... בלע) for he understands (from being spoken to) only that he will receive no blows. [Ib. XXIII, 14 אנת ביר וכ׳ Ms. (missing in ed.), read: גיר (as in Peshito) thou, therefore, &c.]

גִּיר II m. (b. h. גִּר; גרר or גור *to boil, effervesce,* v. H. Dict. s. v.) 1) *lime.* Sabb. 80^b^ ביצת הג׳ Ar. (ed. הסיד), v. בֵּיצָה.—Denom. גִּייֵּר *to plaster.* Lam. R. to IV, 11 Ar. (ed. סייד).—Hull. 88^b^ bot. הג׳ והזרניך quot. in Rashi to Ex. XVI, 14 (ed. only חו׳) powdered lime and orpiment.— 2) *ink-stone, or sulphate of iron (sory).* Bets. 15^a^ ביצת הג׳ a lump of inkstone (for blackening leather).—In gen. *powder*, in compounds גִּירְגִּבְסִין *powder of gypsum;* גִּירְקִרְקִין *wax dust,* v. אֲגִּין. Y. Sabb. VII, 10^b^ bot. (perh. to be read in two words: lime, gypsum &c.).—3) *froth.* Men. VIII, 7 (87^a^) זרק הג׳ (Mish. ז׳ את הגיד, corr. acc.) if the froth (of the fermenting wine) burst forth; Tosef. ib. IX, 11 ג׳ של שמרים.

גִּירָא, גִּיר I ch. same, *lime, plaster.* Dan. V, 5.— Targ. O. Ex. XVI, 14 דעדק כג׳ thin and brittle like a coat of lime (h. text מחספס). Targ. Y. Deut. XXVII, 2 (h. text סיד); a. e.—2) *froth, foam. Pl.* גִּירִין Targ. Y. Ex. XV, 10 ג׳ דימא the foaming billows. [Targ. Jer. IX, 14, read כגירדין, v. גִּירְדָא II.]—3) name of *a disease, a sort of fever (?).* Gitt. 69^b^, v. next w.

גִּיר III, גִּירָא II, גִּירְרָא m. (גרר, גרי; cmp. b. h. שֶׁלַח) 1) *projectile, arrow.* Targ. Is. XXXVII, 33. Targ. Job XLI, 20; a. fr.—Gitt. 56ª שדא ג׳ וכ׳ he shot an arrow eastward. B. Kam. 26ᵇ בעידנא דשדייה פסוקי מפסקי גִּירֵיה (v. Rabb. D. S. a. l. note) at the time he let his arrow off, its force was broken, i. e. when he threw the vessel down, polsters were there to prevent its breaking. Succ. 38ª דין ג׳ בעיניה וכ׳ this is an arrow in the tempter's eyes, i. e. this enables us to defy him. Kidd. 30ª I should say to Satan ג׳ בעיניך I defy thee; ib. 81ª.—Taan. 25ª אגרי בך גִּירַי I shall let my arrow loose against thee (v. Rabb. D. S. a. l. note; oth. vers. v. גּוּר I ch.). Pes. 28ª, v. גִּירָאָה; a. fr.—ג׳ דלילתא (Ar. דלוליתא) the arrow of Lilith, supposed to be a wedge-shaped meteoric stone. Gitt. 69ᵇ לגירא ליתי ג׳ דל׳ as a remedy for *gira* (v. preced.) let one get a *gira* of &c.—*Pl.* גִּירְרִין, גִּירֵי, גִּירַיָּא, גִּירְרִין; גִּירְרַיָּא. Targ. II Sam. I, 22. Targ. Y. I, II Gen. XLIX, 23 (not גיד׳). Targ. Ps. CXX, 4; a. fr.—Snh. 108ᵇ גרלי והוו ג׳ he threw chaff and it turned into arrows. B. Bath. 73ª; v. בִּזְק. Y. ib. II, 13ᵇ bot. מן קל גורי וכ׳ (corr. acc.) from the hissing sound of the arrows; a. fr.—2) *shoot* of a plant. *Pl.* גִּירֵי. Sabb. 109ᵇ ג׳ דרוביא shoots of fenugreek; (oth. opin. in Ar. *flax-seeds,* Ms. O. גידא, v. גִּרְדָּא I).

גִּירָא III m. (גרר; cmp. גִּרָרָא) *direct consequence* of an act. *Pl.* גִּירֵי. B. Bath. 22ᵇ בגירי דידיה (Rashi דיליה); ib. 25ᵇ sq. בגִּירֵיה דיליה (Ms. M. only בגירריה, v. Rabb. D. S. a. l. note); B. Mets. 117ª בגירי דיליה when the damage is a direct result of his act. Ib. 44ª גירי דידיה וכ׳ it is his act that helped it (to get sour). [Rashi: *his arrows* in a metaphorical sense, v. preced.]

גִּירָא IV pr. n. f., v. גִּילָא.

גִּירָא ch.=h. גֵּר. *Pl.* גִּירֵי. Taan. 25ª, v. גּוּר I ch.

גִּירָאָה m. (denom. of גִּירָא II) *shooter,* (Rashi:) *arrow-maker.* Pes. 28ª (prov.) ג׳ בגִּירֵיה מקטיל וכ׳ (ed. גירא, corr. acc., v. Rabb. D. S. a. l. note) when the shooter (arrow-maker) is killed by his own arrow, he is paid from the spinnings of his own hand.

גִּירְגְּבְסִין, v. גִּיר II, 2).

גִּירְגֵּר, v. גַּרְגַּר.

גִּירְדָא I m. (גְּרַד) *scraping, rind.* Sabb. 109ᵇ גר׳ דאסניתא (ed. גר׳ דאסינתא) the paring of &c., v. אַסְנִיתָא. Keth. 77ᵇ, v. אַשְׁפָּא. Ab. Zar. 28ª גִּירְדָא דיבלא וגר׳ דאסנא (Ms. M. וגוררא . . . גרדא, early ed. וגורדא) scraped root of cynodon and the paring of the bramble. Sot. 10ᵇ; Num. R. s. 9 (prov.) קמי דשתי חמרא חמרא קמי רפיקא גר׳ דיבלא before wine drinkers, place wine; before a ploughman—a dish of scraped roots &c. V. גִּרְדָּא.

גִּירְדָא II m. (גדד, with ר inserted) *stump, stem.* Pes. 111ᵇ top גר׳ דדיקלא (Var. גידא, גידא, v. Rabb. D. S. a. l. note 30) the stem of a palm tree (Ar.: *rind,* v. preced.). B. Mets. 86ª (Ms. M. גידרא, Ms. R. 2 גיררא, v. Rabb. D. S. a. l. note).

גִּירְדָא, גִּירְדַאי, v. גִּרְד׳.

גִּירְדוֹנָא (גִּידְרוֹנָא) m. (cmp. גַּדְּדוֹר) *a young ass.* Ned. 41ª.

גִּירְדָנָא, גִּירְדַי, v. גִּרְד׳.

גִּירָה, v. גֵּרָה.

גִּירָה, Pi. of גרי.

גִּירוּי m. (גרי) *instigation, provocation, stirring up.* Sifré Deut. 87, v. הַסָּתָה; Yalk. ib. 886. Tanh. Balak. 2 (ref. to Deut. II, 19) כל מיני ג׳ any sort of provocation (is forbidden); Num. R. s. 20, beg. גירור (corr. acc.); Yalk. ib. 765.

גִּירוּמִין, גִּירוּמִים m. pl. (גרם) *that which goes along, customary addition to weight* or *measure* at sales. B. Bath. VI, 11 נותן לו גִּירוּמִיו (Bab. ed. 88ᵇ מין . . ., Y. ed. מים . . . .) he must give him the due surplus. Sifra K'doshim Par. 9, ch. VIII.

גירומסין, v. גרמסין.

גירונין, Targ. II Chr. XX, 25, some ed., read רירגונין.

גִּירוּעַ I m. (גָּרַע) I) *deduction* from the price of redemption according to the years of possession (Lev. XXVII, 18). Arakh. 24ª ליגאל בג׳ to be redeemed with due deduction. B. Mets. 106ª the Sabbath year לא תעלה לו בג׳ Ar. (ed. מן הג׳, v. Rabb. D. S. s. l. note 90) ought not to be counted in for deduction.—*Pl.* גֵּירוּעִין. Y. Shebu. VI, beg. 36ᵈ סוף גֵּירוּעֶיהָ the final redemption of the Hebrew hand-maid.

גִּירוּעַ II, גֵּרוּעַ m. (גָּרַע II) *the formation of globules* or *kernels* in the grape. Ber. 36ᵇ; Pes. 53ª חוא בוסר חוא ג׳, v. בּוֹסֶר.

גירור, v. גֵּירוּר.

גִּירוּשִׁין, v. גֵּרוּשִׁין.

גִּירוּת, v. גֵּרוּת.

גִּירוּתָא f. *girutha,* name of an unclean bird, supposed to be *moor-hen.* Hull. 62ᵇ; Nidd. 50ᵇ expl. *the hen of the marshes.* Hull. 109ᵇ we are forbidden ג׳ to eat *girutha.* [Ar. גּוּרִיתָא, v. Koh. Ar. Compl. II, 378ª.]

גִּירִי m. (denom. of גֵּר) *belonging to a convert family, descendant of proselytes.* Kidd. IV, 1 (collectively); v. Tos'foth Yom Tob a. l. s. v. כהני.

גִּירְמָא, v. גַּרְמָא.

גִּירְמַנִיקִי, גִּירְמַנְיָא, v. גַּרְמ׳.

גִּירְסָא I, גִּרְסָא m. (גְּרַס II) *acquired learning, tradition, study by heart.* Targ. Cant. I, 2 בג׳ for study by heart (oral tradition).—Meg. 6ᵇ לאוקומי ג׳ וכ׳ to preserve (remember) what one has learned, requires divine assistance. Sabb. 21ᵇ ג׳ דינקותא acquired in early youth (which is better remembered). Ib. 30ᵇ לא ... פומיה מג׳ did not cease studying by heart; B. Mets. 86ᵃ מִגִּירְסֵיהּ.—*Pl.* גִּירְסַיָּא. B. Bath. 22ᵃ they may be disturbed. מִגִּירְסַיְיהוּ in their studies. [In later literature גִּירְסָא *version*.]

גִּירְסָא II, v. גִּירְצָא.

גִּירְסָנָא (גּוּרְסִינָא) m. (גְּרַס II; b. h. גְּרֻשָׁה, גֶּרֶשׁ, Ezek. XLV, 9) *acquisition, saving*. Yeb. 117ᵃ. Ib. גִּירְסָנִי (Rashi גִּירְסָנָאִי) what is accumulated for me.

גִּרְ׳, גֵּירָעוֹן m. (=גֵּירוּעַ I) *deduction*. Arakh. 25ᵇ בת ג׳ subject to the law of deduction. Ib. IX, 7 (33ᵃ) .. יוצאים ובג׳ כסף go back to their owners in the year of Jubilee or with a deduction from the purchasing price (Lev. XXV, 27). Kidd. I, 2 (of the Hebrew slave); a. e.

גִּירָצָא m. (גרין, v. גְּרִיצָה) *putting layers of dough on each other*. Pes. 37ᵃ נפישא בג׳ Ar. (ed. Koh. בלישא, ed. בגירסא, בלִישָׁה) because it grows thick by combination.

גִּירְקְרְדִין, v. גִּיר II, 2).

גִּירָרָא *arrow*, v. גִּיר III.

גיררתו, Koh. R. to IV, 14 מבית ג׳ של פרעה, read: גְּדֵירָתוֹ (v. גְּדֵירָה) from Pharaoh's *fortress* (where he was in prison).

***גִּישׁ** m. (v. גְּרַס I) *familiar*. Yeb. 117ᵇ דג׳ לה וכ׳ Ar. (ed. דרגיש) annoyance of family quarrels is familiar to her.

גִּישָׁה f. (נגש) *drawing near* the altar (Ex. XXX, 20). Yoma 32ᵇ. Zeb. 19ᵇ; a. fr.

גִּישְׁרָא, v. גִּשְׁרָא.

גִּישְׁתָּא, v. גִּשְׁתָּא.

גִּישְׁתְּמָא m. (reduplic. of גשם) *door-sill, door-stop*; v. גַּשְׁמָה.

גִּיתָא m. (גאה, cmp. גֵּו, גּוּי) [*growth, accrued property*,] *herd, flock* (corresp. to h. מִקְנֶה). Targ. I Chr. XXVIII, 1.—*Pl.* גִּיתֵי, גִּיתִין. Targ. Am. I, 1. Targ. Gen. XLVI, 34; a. fr.—Ned. 38ᵃ (quot. fr. Targ. Am. l. c.).

גִּיתֵי m. pl. (v. preced., cmp. גֵּאִים) *haughtiness, tyranny*. B. Kam. 114ᵃ דדייני בג׳ (Rashi בגִיזְתָא, Ms. H. בגִיזְתָה, Ms. R. בגִיתֵי, v. Rabb. D. S. a. l. note 2 for Var. lect.) whom they (the gentile judges) convict tyrannically (not listening to arguments), opp. to Jewish judges who go by argument, points of law &c. [Rashi a. v. מגרזתא, B. Mets. 30ᵇ, quotes our w. גִּיזְתָא; Ms. F. has גִּיזְתֵי, fr. גזז with anomalous pl. *arbitrary decisions*, v. מִגְזָתָא.]

גַּל m. (b. h.; גלל) 1) *heap of stones, bones* &c., esp. *rubbish, ruins*. Sot. IX, 2 if the body of a murdered person was found טמון בג׳ buried in a heap. Keth. 15ᵇ לפקח עליו את הג׳ as to removing debris for saving one's life (on the Sabbath). Sabb. 34ᵃ עשהו ג׳ של עצמות changed him into a heap of bones; a. fr.—*Pl.* גַּלִּים, גַּלִּין. Nidd. IX, 5. Kil. I, 2, v. חֲזֶרֶת. Cmp. גִּילָא.—2) *wave, billow*. Mikv. V, 6 ג׳ שנתלש a wave thrown on shore. Yeb. 121ᵃ; a. fr.—*Pl.* as above. Ex. R. s. 19 הגיעוה ג׳ waves overcame her, i. e. she encountered storms; a. e.—3) *revolving door, turning on hinges or pivots*. Sabb. 81ᵃ של ג׳ the pivot of a revolving door. V. גַּלָּה.—4) (v. LXX Hos. XII, 12) *turtoise*. *Pl.* as above. Sifra Sh'mini, ch. IV, Par. 3.

גַּלָּא ch. same, 1) *heap*. *Pl.* גַּלִּין. Targ. Is. XXV, 2.—2) also גַּלְלָא *wave*. Koh. R. to XI, 1.—*Pl.* גַּלִּין, גַּלַּיָּא, גַּלֵּי, גַּלְלַיָּא, גַּלְלֵי. Targ. Zech. X, 11. Targ. Ps. XLII, 8 (some ed. גִּלּוּלֵי); a. e. Targ. Y. I Ex. XV, 18 [read:] בֵּינֵי גַּלְלַיָּא between the waves.—Yeb. 121ᵃ גלי אשפלו the waves may have cast him out (alive).—3) *revolving door*. B. Kam. 112ᵃ. Snh. 113ᵃ bot. דטרקיה לגַלֵּיה וכ׳ who locked his door and lost the key.—*Pl.* גַּלֵּי. Ber. 28ᵃ טרוקו ג׳ close ye the (college doors); Ab. Zar. 58ᵃ. B. Mets. 108ᵃ, v. אַגְלָא.—4) pl. גַּלֵּי, גַּלַּיָּא *excrements, ordure*. Targ. Ezek. IV, 12; 15 (incorr. גְּלֵי).—5) (v. גִּלּוּל) *Gallaya*, cacophemism for similarly sounding idolatrous names. Y. Ab. Zar. III, 43ᵃ bot.; Tosef. ib. VI (VII), 4, v. גַּדָּא (Ab. Zar. 46ᵃ; Tem. 28ᵇ; v. גַּלְיָא II). Meg. 6ᵃ בית גליא שלהן their house of idolatry. [גלין, Sabb. 138ᵃ, v. גַּלָּה.] [Targ. II Kings XXIII, 6; Jer. XXVI, 23, v. גְּלֵי.]

גְּלָא, v. גְּלֵי.

גלא, ג׳ קסינון, v. גַּלַאקְסִינוֹן.

גְּלָאִי, v. גְּלֵי.

גְּלָאלָא, Yalk. Zech. 578, v. גַּלְלָא.

גַּלַאקְסִינוֹן m. Ar. (ed. גלא ק׳) (γαλῆ Ἀξεινῶν) [*fur of*] *the weasel imported by the Axeinoi* (living around the Pontus Axenus or Euxenus); *ermine* (v. Sm. Ant. s. v. Pellis). Gen. R. s. 20, end גלי ק׳ (גלא). Y. Sabb. II, 4ᵈ bot. (rendition of תַּחַשׁ) גלקטינון; Koh. R. to I, 9 גלטינן (corr. acc.). Ib. והכלב גלבטינון (read גלכסינון) and the dog shall wear ermine fur.

גַּלַּב (cmp. גלח, גלש) *to scrape, shave*. Targ. Y. Lev. XIX, 27.—V. גְּלִירְבָא.

גְּלָב m. (preced.) *razor, knife*. Targ. Y. Num. VI, 5; VIII, 7 (גְּלַב).—*Pl.* גִּלְבִין. Gen. R. s. 31 (transl. חרבות צרים Josh. V, 2) ג׳ דטינרי flint knives.—[Targ. Ezek. XXVII, 24, v. גְּלָה.]

גַּלָּבָא, גַּלָּב ch. (preced.) *barber*.—*Pl.* גַּלָּבַיָּא. Targ. Ezek. V, 1.

גלבטא, v. אַנְטְבִילָא.

***גִּלְבִין** m. pl. (גלב)=קַלְפִין, *scales*. Targ. I Sam. XVII, 5 שריין ג׳ (Var. גלבין; h. text קשקשים). V., however, גִּלְדָא.

***גְּלַבְקְיָא** f. (γλαύκιον, glaucion) *juice of glaucion*, a plant like the horned poppy. Sifra Vayikra, Hoba, Par. 12, ch. XXII המערב ... ג׳ בשמן Ar. (ed. גלוביא, Var. בלבקיא &c., v. ed. Weiss p. 28ᵈ note) he who adulterates oil with the juice of glaucium (selling it for poppy-oil); Koh. R. to

IX, 13 בלבקי; ib. to VI, 1 בלקיא; Tosef. B. Bath. V, 6 מי כגלקיא ed. Zuck. (Var. בלקיא); Yalk. Lev. 479 בלנקי (corruptions of פְּלַוְקְיָא or כְּלַבְקְיָא; cmp. Löw Pfl. p. 205 a. 257). [Ar. a. Mus. seem to think of *Lycium*.]

גְּלַג, *Pa.* גַּלֵּיג (reduplic. of גל, v. גלח) *to reveal* (v. P. Sm. 723), *to announce*. Gen. R. s. 36 זיל גַּלֵּיג וכ׳ Ar. (ed. זיל גְּלוֹג, not זילא) go, tell thy mother the good news; Lev. R. s. 5.—Ib. s. 25; Koh. R. to II, 20 איזילי גליג לאימיך (not גליגי) I will go and tell thy mother. Pesik. Aniya, p. 137[a] [read:] כל מה דאת יכיל למיגלג גלג למישבח שבח as much as thou canst tell, tell; as much as thou canst praise, praise; Yalk. Is. 339 (corr. acc.); (Pesik. R. s. 32 דרוש וכ׳).

Ithpe. אִיגַּלֵּיג *to boast*. Lev. R. s. 10 is it these דאת מְגַלֵּיג עליהון of whom thou art so boastful?

גְּלָגָא, pl. גְּלָגִין m. (preced.) *revelation, preaching*. Y. Sot. I, 17[b]; Lev. R. s. 26 [read:] מאר את בעי מן גַּלְגוי דהדין do not mind this man's boastful talk.

גלגוטיקא, v. גלוגדקא.

גִּלְגּוּל, **גִּ׳ל׳** m. (גלגל) 1) *rolling, turning*. Y. Sot. I, 16[c] bot. כדי ג׳ ביצה as much time as is required for roasting an egg in the ashes; Num. R. s. 9.—Y. Pes. III, 30[a] לאחר גִּילְגּוּלָהּ after the dough has been rolled (formed).—Keth. 111[a] ע״י ג׳ by rolling under the ground (for resurrection in the Holy Land).—2) (with or without שבועה) *the rule permitting the court to insert in an oath an affirmation to which the person concerned could not have been compelled directly; an oath by implication*. Kidd. 27[b]. Y. ib. I, 60[d]. Yeb. 58[b]; Kidd. l. c. ע״י ג׳ by implication (the woman including in her oath the time of her betrothal); a. fr.—4) (cmp. גַּל) בית ג׳ *a field full of hills and depressions*. Toh. VI, 6; Erub. 22[b] (Var. in Ar. גדגד, ref. to גְּדוּדוּד). [Tosef. B. Bath. II, 16 בית גרלגל, v. גִּלְגֵּל.]

גִּלְגּוּל, **גִּ׳ל׳** ch., v. גִּלְגְּלָא.

גִּלְגֵּיל, v. גִּלְגֵּל.

גִּלְגִּילָא, v. גַּרְגִּירָא.

גלגילון, v. גִּלְגְּלִין.

גִּלְגֵּל (b. h., Pilp. of גלל) 1) *to roll, turn*. Pirké d'R. El. ch. XXXVI לְגַלְגֵּל וכ׳ to roll (move) the stone.—Y. Sabb. III, 6[a] top מְגַלְגְּלִין ביצה וכ׳ you may roll an egg (for roasting) on &c. Hall. III, 1 (בחטים) גִּלְגְּלָה when she has formed the dough (of wheat) by rolling; a. fr.—*Part. pass.* מְגוּלְגָּל, f. מְגוּלְגֶּלֶת; pl. מְגוּלְגָּלִים, מְגוּלְגָּלִין; מְגוּלְגָּלוֹת. 1) *rolled*. Pes. 7[a] עיסה מג׳ a formed dough. Y. Sot. I, 16[c] bot. ביצים מג׳ roasted eggs; a. fr.—2) *rounded*. B. Bath. 16[b] מה עדשה זו מְגוּלְגֶּלֶת אף אבילות מְגַלְגֶּלֶת וכ׳ as the lentil is rounded, so does mourning roll and go around (different version in Ms., v. Rabb. D. S. a. l. note, a. in Yalk. Gen. 110, v. גִּלְגַּל). [Men. 86[a], v. גַּרְגֵּר.]—2) (with על) *to roll upon, to put on one's shoulders, to burden, tax, assess*. Keth. VIII, 1 (78[a]) אתם מגלגלים עלינו וכ׳ you burden us with old restrictive laws. Y. Shebi. IV, 35[b] אתם מג׳ וכ׳ ye impose upon us taxes &c. Y. B. Bath. I, beg. 12[d] מג׳ עליו וכ׳ you make him bear the expenses for &c.—3) *to bring about, cause*. Sabb. 32[a]; Tosef. Yoma V (IV), 12 מגלגלין זכות ע״י וכ׳ good things are brought about through the agency of good men &c.; a. fr.—4) (v. גָּלַל Nif.) *to overcome* (one's own feelings), *to put up with, bear with*. Keth. 67[b] רצונך שתְּגַלְגֵּל עמי בעדשים will you bear with me when I offer you only lentils? ג׳ עמו וכ׳ he tried to live with him on lentils, and died. Ib. 111[a] ג׳ בעצמו he conquered his love and remained single. Y. ib. VII, beg. 31[b] מגלגלת עמו וכ׳ she has to bear with him thirty days longer. Y. Yeb. VIII, 8[d] top גַּלְגֵּל עמהן וכ׳ bear with them twelve months (give them time for reconsideration).

Hithpalp. הִתְגַּלְגֵּל, הִתְגַּ׳, *Nithpalp.* נִתְגַּלְגֵּל 1) *to be rolled*. Erub. X, 3 נ׳ חספר מידו the scroll rolled out of his hands (down the roof). Hall. III, 1 עד שתִּתְגַּלְגֵּל בחטים in the case of wheat flour, until it (the dough) is rolled, v. supra. Y. Kil. IX, 32[c] top; Y. Keth. XII, 35[b] top מִתְגַּלְגְּלִין their bodies are rolled underground, v. גִּלְגּוּל. B. Kam. 17[b] ונתג׳ למקום אחר but the barrel rolled to another place. Pesik. R. s. 6 מא״י נִתְגַּלְגְּלָה וכ׳ from Palestine it (the stone) rolled and arrived just for this momentary use; a. fr.—2) *to be turned, changed, transferred, caused*. Pirké d'R. El. ch. XLIX נתגלגלה המלכות על וכ׳ the royal dignity was transferred on Esther. Shebu. VII, 8 נ׳ לו שבועה וכ׳ if by chance an oath is imposed upon him in another law-suit (with the same persons), the court makes him swear by implication &c.; v. גִּלְגּוּל.—3) (of waters) *to tower, gather*. Pirké d'R. El. ch. V; ch. XXIII.—4) (with רחמים) *to prevail* (over hatred &c.), *be moved*. Pesik. R. s. 20 נִתְגַּלְגְּלוּ רחמיו וכ׳ the Lord's compassion was moved. Tanh. Vayigg. 4; a. e.—5) *to throw one's self upon, to attack*. Yalk. Is. 350 (ib. 288 נתגאה).

גַּלְגֵּיל, **גַּלְגֵּל** ch. same, *to roll*. Targ. Y. I Gen. XXVIII, 10 (II גלל). Ib. XXIX, 8 (O. גנדר); a. e.—Y. Shebu. VI, 37[a] wait עד דִּיגַלְגֵּל עלך וכ׳ until he heaps upon thee all his claims, and then swear concerning all of them. Ib. VII, end, 38[a] או אישתבע ליה כל דמְגַלְגֵּל עלך or thou must swear to him concerning all that he asks thee to swear to by implication.—*Part. pass.* Ber. 44[b] ביעתא מְגוּלְגַּלְתָּא an egg roasted in ashes, v. preced.

Ithpalp. אִתְגַּלְגַּל, אִיתְגַּלְגַּל, אִיגַּלְגַּל; אִתְגּוֹלַל (fr. גְּלַל), אִתְגּוֹלַל (Ithpolel of גּוּל) 1) as preced. Hithpalp. 3. Targ. Job XXX, 14.—2) (with רחמין) as preced. Hithpalp. 4. Targ. I Kings III, 26 איתגלגלו ed. Lag. (ed. אִיתְגַּלְגְּלוּ). Targ. O. Gen. XLIII, 30 אִתְגּוֹלְלוּ). Targ. Hos. XI, 8 מתגללא ed. Lag. ed. אִתְגּוֹלְלוּ). Targ. Jer. XXXI, 20 אִתְגּוֹ׳. Targ. II Chr. XXXIII, 13. Targ. Y. Num. XXVI, 1; a. e.—3) *to come about, to happen*. B. Mets. 40[a], a. e. ארגלגל מילתא it so happened in the course of time.—4) (denom. of גולגלתא) *to crown, adorn one's self*. Esth. R. to I, 4 whether with its own or with strange (feathers) מִתְגַּלְגֶּלֶת בת קבריא the raven will adorn itself; ib. 9.

גַּלְגַּל m. (b.h.; preced.) 1) *wheel*, esp. *the wheel-work at wells, crane* &c. Midd. V, 4. Tosef. B. Bath. II, 16

בית גולגל לרבים ed. Zuck. (Var. גילגל) a public well. B. Bath. IV, 5 את הג׳ the crane of the wine or oil press, v. חוּמְרְתָּא. Erub. X, 14; a. fr.—2) *globe, celestial sphere, esp. the sphere of the zodiac.* Yoma 20[b], a. e. ג׳ חמה the revolution of the Sun. Pes. 94[b] ג׳ קבוע ומזלות וכ׳ the sphere of the zodiac is stationary, and the planets make the circuit; ג׳ חוזר וכ׳ the sphere (wheel) turns around and the planets are stationary; a. fr.—B. Bath. 16[b] Ms. M. מה עדש זה דומה לג׳ וכ׳ as the lentil resembles a sphere, so is mourning a sphere making a circuit in the world; (diff. in ed., v. גַּלְגַּל); Yalk. Gen. 110 מה עדשים האלו ג׳ וכ׳.—3) *the eye-ball.* Gen. R. s. 42; Lev. R. s. 11; Ruth R. introd. 6 (ref. to עין משפט Gen. XIV, 7) ג׳ עינו של עולם the eye-ball of the world (Abraham). Snh. 108[a] בשביל ג׳ העין וכ׳ on account of (the covetousness of) the eye-ball (v. next w.); a. e.—*Pl.* גַּלְגַּלִּים. Makhsh. III, 8 wheel works. B. Bath. 58[a] שני גַּלְגַּלֵּי חמה two Sun-globes.—Y. Nidd. III, 50[c] bot. ג׳ אדם וכ׳ the apples of man's eyes are round.—Trnsf. *the rotation of fortune, changes* (v. B. Bath. 16[b] quot. above). Sabb. 151[b] (ref. to בִּגְלַל Deut. XV, 10) ג׳ הוא וכ׳ a wheel rotates in this world, i. e. changes of fortune take place constantly; Ex. R. s. 31, a. e.—3) (=גַּרְגַּר) *globule, grain.* Sabb. 64[b]; 65[a], v. גַּרְגַּר.—*Pl.* as above. Y. Maasr. V, end, 52[a]; Tosef. ib. III, 14 Egyptian beans are those שגַּלְגַּלֵּיהֶן חדין (ed. Zuck. גלוגל׳, Var. גלגל הן, corr. acc.) whose globules are pointed.

גִּלְגְּלָא, גַּלְגַּל ,גִּיל׳ ch. same; 1) *wheel.* Targ. Ezek. I, 15 sq. גִּיל׳ ed. Lag. Targ. Ps. LXXXIII, 14; a. e.—Erub. 104[a] למימלא בגי׳ to fill (draw water) with the wheel. Lev. R. s. 34, v. אַנְטַלְיָא.—2) *globe, celestial sphere.* Targ. Ps. LXXVII, 19. Targ. Job XXXVIII, 33.—B. Bath. 74[a] ג׳ דרקיע וכ׳ the sphere of the zodiac which turns around. —3) *eye-ball.* Targ. Ps. XVII, 8 גִּילְגּוּל ed. Lag. (oth. ed. גַּלְגּוּל; Ms. גִּיגַל).—Tam. 32[b] they handed him ג׳ דעינא Ar. (ed. גולגלתא incorr.) an eye-ball. Ib. גולגלתא דעינא וכ׳ (read גילגלא) the eye-ball of a mortal which is never satisfied. B. Bath. 73[b].—4) *stubble.* Targ. Is. XVII, 13.—*Pl.* גִּיל׳, גַּלְגְּלַיָּא. Targ. Ezek. I, 16 sq.—Targ. Ex. XIV, 25 גַּלְגְּלֵי ed. Berl. (ed. a. Y. גַּלְגַּלֵּי). Targ. Y. II ib. גַּלְגְּלַיָּא; a. e.—Koh. R. to XII, 6; Lev. R. s. 18; a. e.—4) (v. next w.) *a sort of girdle.* *Pl.* גַּלְגַּלַּיָּיה. Y. Sabb. VI, 8[b] bot. (transl. of גליונים, Is. III, 22), v. גִּלְיוֹן 3.

גַּלְגְּלוֹן m., v. next w.

גִּילְגְּלִין ,גַּלְגְּלִין m. pl. (used as sing.; גלל) *girdle of net-work, bandage, wrap.* Eduy. III, 4 (Ms. M. גנגלון, v. infra). Neg. XI, 11 גלגלון.—Y. Naz. VII, 56[b] bot. נקבר אפי׳ ג׳ קטן וכ׳ if there is buried with the corpse even a small wrap (or belt), the law concerning decayed corpses (v. רָקָב) finds no application. Ib. if two corpses are buried beside each other נעשה ג׳ לזה וכ׳ each acts as *gilg'lin* to the other (suspending the law of *rakab*); Bab. ib. 51[a]; Nidd. 27[b] גנגרלון. Tosef. Kel. B. Bath. V, 9 גנגלין. Sifra Sh'mini ch. XI, Par. 10 גנגלים וגנגרליון (a fusion of two versions); ib. Aḥăré Par. 8, ch. XII גרנגלרון; a. e. [Var. lect.: גנגלים, גנגלון, גנגילון, influenced by the Latin *cingulum* to which our w. nearly corresponds.]

גַּלְגֹּלֶת, v. גּוּלְגּוֹלֶת.

גַּלְגַּלְתָּא f. (גלל) *ball, round stone.* Gitt. 47[a] חריתא וג׳ a bag and a stone (in it).

גָּלַד *to form a coating; to congeal, become solid.* Y. Ber. I, 2[c] bot. יִגְלֹד הרקיע let the (liquid mass of the) firmament solidify; Gen. R. s. 4, beg. גָּלְדָה טיפה וכ׳ the intermediate layer of water solidified.—*Part. pass.* גָּלוּד, f. גְּלוּדָה (denom. of גֶּלֶד) *skinned, flayed* in consequence of bruises, scabs &c. Hull. III, 2; Tosef. ib. III, 7; a. e.

Hif. הִגְלִיד 1) same. Tosef. Par. IX (VIII), 8 הִגְלִידוּ froze. Nidd. 56[b]; Tosef. ib. VI, 13 מַגְלִיד forms a clodded surface, opp. מקדיר penetrates.—2) *to form a rind, scab;* v. infra.

Hof. הוּגְלַד *to be covered with a scab* (of a wound). Hull. 51[a] הו׳ פי המכה Rashi a. Ar. (ed. הִגְלִיד) if the top of the wound is covered with a crust; Keth. 76[b]; Tosef. Hull. III, 11 הגליד.

גְּלַד ch. same.—*Part. pass.* גְּלִיד *hoar-covered.* Sabb. 152[a] טור תלג סחרנוהי גְּלִידִין (v. Rabb. D. S. a. l. note) the mountain (my head) is snow-covered, its sides (beard) hoary. [Lev. R. s. 7, v. next w.]

Ithpe. אִיגְּלִיד *to be flayed.* Hull. 46[b], v. אַהֲרִינָא; Succ. 35[b].

גֶּלֶד m. (b. h.; גלד) 1) *coating, skin; thickness.* Y. B. Bath. III, 13[c] top עד מקום שעושה ג׳ the fifty cubits of legal distance from the inhabited place are counted from the end of the town to the place where he flays the carcass. Yoma 44[b] [read:] בכל יום היה גִּלְדָּהּ עב והיום דק (v. Rabb. D. S. a. l.) all the year around the pan was of a thick size, and this day (Day of Atonem.) it was thin. Num. R. s. 13 קערה גִּלְדָּהּ .... גִּלְדּוֹ דק the charger was of a heavy size, the bowl &c. R. Hash. 27[b] if he scraped the Shofar והעמידו על גִּלְדּוֹ and reduced it to its due size. Lev. R. s. 7 וא״ת דהוה ג׳ (Ar. גְּלִיד) but you may think the bronze on top of the altar was a solid mass, v. גּוּרְדְּוָנָא.—2) *scab* of a wound, *crust.* Mikv. IX, 2 ג׳ שחוץ למכה (Maim. גֶּלֶד שעל גבי וכ׳) the scab surrounding the wound (Maim.: on the wound).—*Pl.* גְּלָדִים, constr. גִּלְדֵי, גִּילְדֵי. Ib. ג׳ צואה וכ׳ the scabby, dirty spots on one's body.

גִּלְדָּא ,גִּיל׳ ch. same; 1) *plate, covering.* Targ. Y. I Num. VII, 13 גי׳ סמיך (=גֶּלֶד עב, v. preced.).—*Pl.* גִּלְדִין. גי׳ Targ. Ezek. XXVII, 24 חפן ג׳ (gold, or silver) plated.—2) *scab, scurf.* *Pl.* גִּלְדֵי, גי׳. Hull. 46[b] lungs full ג׳ of scabs. —3) *skin, leather.* Targ. I Sam. XVII, 5 (v. Lag. I, p. XVI) שריין גלבין (ed. שריין דגלד נוני ימא) a coat of mail made of the skin of sea-fishes (h. text קשקשים).—Snh. 110[a]; Pes. 119[a] אקלידי וקלפי דג׳ (Ms. M. קיפלי, v. Rabb. D. S. a. l. note) the keys and the locks (the stiff rims of the bags usually of metal) were of leather (so as to be of light weight). Ber. 43[b] בגי׳ on the leather of the shoe, opp. פנתא, v. אַפַּנְתָּא (Rashi: *heel*).

גַּלְדָּאָה ,גִּיל׳ m. (preced.) *worker* or *dealer in leather, harness-maker* &c.—*Pl.* גִּיל׳, גַּלְדָּאֵי. B. Mets. 24[b]; Hull. 48[a] sq. שוקא דג׳ harness-makers' place.

גִּלְדְּנָא, גִּיל׳ m. (גלד) *gildana*, name of a certain fish with a *thick fatty skin*. Snh. 100ᵇ לא תנטוש גיל׳ וכ׳ (Ms. M. תפשוט) do not begin to strip the *gildana* from its gill, lest its skin go to ruin (a citation from Ben Sira). B. Bath. 73ᵇ ההוא ג׳ וכ׳ that was a sea *gildana* (a small fish among the sea monsters). Hor. 12ᵃ; Ker. 6ᵃ. —*Pl.* גִּלְדְּנֵי, גִּיל׳. Tam. 32ᵇ ג׳ דמלחא Rashi (ed. גולדנא) salted g. Ber. 44ᵇ; Keth. 105ᵇ, v. גִּילָא II.

גְּלָלָה, גִּילָה f. (גלל, cmp. גַּל 3) *a valve, folding*. Y. Sabb. XII, beg. 13ᶜ מטה של ג׳ folding couch.—*Pl.* גְּלָלִין. Bab. ib. 138ᵃ כסא ג׳ camp chair.

גְּלָה, v. גּוּלָּה.

גָּלָה, v. גלי.

גְּלוֹ, v. גְּלוּתָא.

גלובדק, v. גְּלוּגְדְקָא.

גלוביא, v. גְּלַבְקְיָא.

גְּלוּגְדְקָא (גלוגדק), גְּלֶקְטִיקָא f. (popular corruption of *lectica*; for the prefixed guttural cmp. laena and χλαῖνα, lectum and κλίνη; v. Liddell & Scott's Greek Dict. s. lit. Γ) 1) *litter, sedan-chair*. Bets. 25ᵇ Ar. (ed. גלודקי, Ms. M. גלודקי). Cant. R. to V, 5; Koh. R. to IX, 11 אפי׳ בגלק׳ לא וכ׳ could not even be carried in a *lectica*. Cant. R. to IV, 8 בכל קדיקה; Yalk. Ps. 838 כל קרקיא (read בִּגְלֶקְדִיקָא). Ib. Lev. 666 שלא יטייל אחריך בגלטק׳; Sifra B'har Par. 5, ch. VII ... יטול .... בלנביא) he (the Hebrew servant) shall not walk behind thee when thou art carried in the lectica, v. לֶקְטִיקָא. Sifré Deut. 37 גלגוטיקא; Yalk. Kings 238 גלוגיקא.—*2) (=lecticula) *bier*. Targ. Job XV, 24 איטימוס לגלוגדיקא Ar. ed. Koh. (ed. לגלוגדק) ready for the bier (for death, cmp. LXX).—3) **foot-stool* to the throne. Targ. Y. Ex. XXIV, 10 אתקניה גְּלוּגְדָק וכ׳ (גיל׳ some ed.) made the sapphire brick a footstool in place of the *hypopodion* &c.—Targ. Lam. II, 1 גלוגדקא דרגלוהי (h. text הדום רגליו).

גלוגות, v. חֲלַגְלוֹג׳.

גלוגיקא, v. preced. art.

גלוגלין, Tosef. Maasr. III, 14, v. גַּלְגַּל.

גלודקי, v. גְּלוּגְדְקָא.

גלודי, v. גִּילְהֵי.

גלואי, Lam. R. introd., beg., v. גָּלוֹיָא.

גלוקי, v. גּוּאַלְקָא.

גָּלוּי m. (part. pass. of גָּלָה) *appearance, outside*. Gen. R. s. 45 אין סיתרה כגלויה her private conduct is not like her public appearance (she is insincere); ib. s. 71.—בַּגָּ׳ *in public, visible to all*, opp. בסתר. Ab. IV, 4 he will be punished בג׳ in an ostensible way. Sot. 3ᵃ; a. fr.

גָּלוּר, v. גִּירְבּוּרָא, גִּירְבּוּר.

גָּלוֹיָא m. (גלי) *exile, stranger*. *Pl.* גָּלוֹיֵי. Lev. R. s. 5 גלויא בר גלויי Ar. (ed. גלויי בר ג׳, corr. acc.) thou stranger, son of strangers. Lam. R. introd. beg. גלוואי, read גָּלוֹיָאֵי (Ar. גְּלוֹלָאֵי).

גָּלוּיֵי, v. גלי ch.

גִּילּוּל, גִּלּוּל m., pl. גִּלּוּלִים, גִּי׳ (b. h.; גלל) *filth* (v. גָּלָל), *idols*. Meg. 13ᵃ to clean herself מִגִּלּוּלֵי בית אביה from the contamination of her paternal idolatry. Ib. מרדה בגילולי וכ׳ she rejected &c.—עבודת ג׳, עובד ג׳ (abbr. ע״ג) *idolator, idolatry*. In some ed. for עכ״ום, ע״ז &c.; v. זָר a. כּוֹכָב.

גָּלוֹלָא m. (גלל) *cast about, homeless*. *Pl.* גְּלוֹלָאֵי, גְּלוֹלַיָּא. Lam. R. introd., beg. Ar., v. גָּלוֹיָא; Pesik. Dibré, p. 110ᵇ גליליא (Var. גְּלוֹ׳, v. Bub. note a. l.). V. גְּלִילָה.

גָּלוֹם, v. גּוֹלֶם.

גלוסא, v. גְּרִיסָא.

קְלוֹסְטְרָא, גְּלוֹסְטְרָא (claustra, clostra, pl.) *fastening, lock, bar*. Erub. X, 10 נגר שיש בראשו ג׳ a door bolt which has on its top a (movable) fastening contrivance (which may occasionally be used as a pestle). Sabb. 123ᵇ ג׳ (Ar. ק׳, Ms. M. repeatedly גלוסקי) the law about claustra, ref. to Kel. XI, 4 ק׳. Sabb. 124ᵃ ג׳.

גְּלוֹסְטְרָאָה m. (preced.) *locksmith* (claustrarius). Ber. 22ᵃ R. Yehudah גלוסטרא (corr. acc., Ms. M. קלסתראה, Yoḥăsin Completum p. 148ᵇ קְלוֹסְטְרָאָה).

גְּלוּסְקָא, קְלוּסְקָא, קין ... c. (a contraction of גלופסיקא or גלוסביקא, Lesbiacus, Lesbiaca, v. בְּלוּפְסִין, בְּלוּפ׳, קְלוּפ׳, לְבָסִים; as to guttural before ל, v. גְּלוּגְדְקָא) *relating to Lesbos* (an island of the Aegean Sea, noted for its fertility and luxuries), *Lesbian*, whence 1) [in Syriac] name of *a brand of white flour* (P. Sm. 726), *a white and delicate bread* (cmp. Athenæus Deipnosophistæ III, 111). Tosef. Ber. IV, 15 שלמה של גלוסקין an unbroken loaf of *g'luskin*, opp. של בע״הב home-made. Dem. VI, 12 buy for me גְּלוּסְקָן אחד ed. (accus.; Ms. M. גלוסקא אחת, Ar. קין אחת ....., R. S. קלוסקין) one loaf &c. Y. Ab. Zar. I, 40ᵃ bot. קלוסקין אחת; Erub. 64ᵇ גלוסקין pl.—Pes. 6ᵇ he may find ג׳ יפה ודעתו עליה Rashi (ed. ודעתיה עילויה, Ms. M. יפיפיה) a fine *gl.* which he may have the intention of eating (in place of burning). Lam. R. to I, 16 גלוסקאן; a. e.—*Pl.* גְּלוּסְקָאוֹת, גְּלוּסְקִין, קְלוּ׳. Sabb. 30ᵇ. Gen. R. s. 88, beg. Lam. R. to II, 12 גלו׳ (Ar. ed. Koh. קלסקין); a. e.—2) *a superior sort of olives already pressed when appearing in the market* (θλασταί, σταφυλίδες, v. Athenæus l. c. II, 56; cmp. בְּלוּפְסִין). Ab. Zar. II, 7 זיתי קלוסקא המגולגלין Y. ed. II, 10 (Mish. זתים גלוסקאות, Bab. ed. 39ᵇ זיתי ג׳, Mish. Nap. קלוסטא, Ar. ed. Koh. s. v. גלגל: קלוסטרא, קלוסטא). Bab. ib. 40ᵇ (ed. Pes. a. oth. קלוסקא, Alf. early ed. גלוסטא, v. Rabb. D. S. a. l. note 4). Y. ib. II, 42ᵃ bot. הן זיתי ק׳ וכ׳ *zethé k'luska* is the same as *rolled olives*. [Ex. R. s. 30 גלוסקאות, v. גְּלוּסְקְמָא.]

גְּלוּסְקָאן, v. preced.

גְּלוּסְקוֹם, גלוסקוים, v. next art.

גְּלוּסְקִין, v. גְּלוּסְקָא.

דְּלוּסְקְמָא, גְּלוּסְקוֹם, גְּלוּסְקְמָא m. (γλωσσόκομον, v. LXX, II Chr. XXIV, 8; as to ד for ג׳, v. Liddell & Scott s. lit. Δ) *case, chest, coffin.* Y. Sot. VII, 22[d] כמין גלוסקום a kind of casing; Y. Shek. VI, 49[d] bot. גלוסקוים (corr. acc.).—Gitt. III, 3 if he found the document בג׳.. Ar. (ed. בד׳) in a case; expl. ib. 28[a] טליקא דסבי a box for elders (for keeping documents &c.); B. Mets. I, 8 Y. ed. ג׳ (Bab. 20[a], [b] a. Mish. ד׳). Meïl. VI, 1 ג׳ (Bab. ed. 21[a] ד׳). M. Kat. 24[b] (ד׳) ג׳ הניטלת באגפיים a coffin carried by its handles.—*Pl.* גְּלוּסְקְמִין, גְּלוּסְקְמָאוֹת, ד׳. Meg. 26[b] דְּלוּסְקְמֵי ספרים (Alf. Ms. קְמָאוֹת..., ed. סקאות...) cases for books &c.—Ex. R. s. 30, end פותח הגלוסקאות (corr. acc.) he opens the cases (containing his goods).

גְּלוּף, v. גְּלַף.

גְּלוּפְסִין, v. כְּלוּפְסִין.

גְּלוּפְקְרָא, v. next w.

קְלוּבְקְרִין, גְּלוּפְקְרִין, גְּלוּפְקְרֵי m. pl. (cubicularia, sub. gausapina &c.) *woolly bed-covers, blankets.* Targ. Y. I Deut. XXIV, 13 (h. text שַׂלְמָה).—Sabb. 51[a]; Tosef. ib. III (IV), 20, opp. סדין linen sheets. Gitt. 70[b] ג׳ וסדיני (Var. גושפקר) shall we ascertain his sanity of mind, according to the season, by asking him whether he desires heavy or light covers? Ib. 35[a] גלופקרין אחד Ar. (ed. גלופקרא) one set of bed-clothes.—Kel. XXIX, 2 קלובקרין אחד (Bart. גלופקרין, Bab. ed. אחת). Tosef. Sabb. VI (VII), 4; Yalk. Lev. 587.

גלורין, Num. R. s. 11, read גַּלְיָרִין, v. גּוּלְיָיר.

גְּלוֹשׁ m. (גלש) *bald-headed.* Targ. O. Lev. XIII, 41.

גְּלוֹשׁוּתָא f. (preced.) *bald forehead.* Targ. O. Lev. XIII, 42 sq. (some ed. גְּלוֹשְׁתָא).

גָּלוּת f. (b. h.; גלי) *exile;* also (sub. בני) *the exiled community, diaspora.* Ab. I, 11 שמא התחובו חובת ג׳ ye may be condemned to exile. Ber. 56[a], a. e. ג׳ מכפרת עון exile (leaving home) is an expiation. ג׳ בבל Babylonian captivity; ג׳ יון Greek (Syrian) dominion; ג׳ אדום Roman dominion. Ex. R. s. 15.—Esp. *banishment to the city of refuge* (Num. XXXV, 11 sq.). Macc. II, 6; a. fr.—*Pl.* גָּלֻיּוֹת. Arakh. 12[a] שלש ג׳ three divisions of exiles; Num. R. s. 23, end סנחריב הגלה . . . . ג׳ Sennacherib carried them off in three divisions.—Pes. 88[a] קבוץ ג׳ the reunion of the exiled. Men. 110[a] ג׳ של שאר וכ׳ the exiled of other countries (besides Babylonia). Bets. 4[b] שני ימים טובים של ג׳ the two Holy Days (in the place of the one Biblical) observed by those living abroad (whom the communications of the Palestinean authorities could not reach); a. fr.

גְּלוּתָא, גָּלוּ ch. same. Targ. Y. Ex. XX, 14. Targ. Am. I, 6; a. e.—ריש ג׳ *Resh-Galutha*, chief of the Babylonian Jews. Succ. 31[a]; a. fr.—*Pl.* גַּלְוָותָא. Targ. Ps. LXIX, 1 גַּלְוָות ed. Lag. (oth. ed. גָּלוּת sing.). Targ. Y. Ex. XL, 10. Targ. O. Deut. XXX, 4 יהוין גָּלְוָ׳ ed. Berl. (ed. יהי גָּלוּ׳, corr. acc.) thy exiles; a. e.—Snh. 11[b] בני ג׳ דבבל וכ׳ the diasporas of Babylonia and all other diasporas (v. Rabb. D. S. a. l. note). Hull. 60[b] that the Egyptians might not call his brothers ג׳ *exiles.*

גָּלַח (b. h.; cmp. גלב), *Pi.* גִּלַּח, גִּלֵּחַ *to cut the hair, shave.* Naz. VI, 3. Ib. IV, 6 ג׳ או גִּילְּחוּהוּ וכ׳ if he himself or his friends cut his hair. M. Kat. III, 1 ואלו מְגַלְּחִין וכ׳ the following are permitted to cut their hair during the festive week. Ib. 14[a] מותר לְגַלֵּחַ; a. fr.—Part. pass. מְגוּלָּח, f. מְגוּלַּחַת. Naz. IV, 5 אשה מְגֻלַּ׳ a woman with her hair cut; Y. ib. IV, end, 53[c].

גְּלַח ch. Pa. גַּלַּח same. Targ. O. Lev. XIII, 33; a. fr.—M. Kat. 17[b] איבעי ליה לְגַלּוּחֵי וכ׳ he ought to have his hair cut &c.

Ithpa. אִתְגַּלַּח, אִיגַּלַּח *to have one's hair cut.* Targ. Jud. XVI, 17; 22.—Sabb. 110[b] לִיגַּלַּח וכ׳ let him have the middle part of his head shaved.

גַּלְחִי pr. n. pl. *Galḥi*, a legendary place in the district of Sodom. Nidd. 69[a] האי דינא .... דדיני בג׳ such justice which is injustice is dealt out in G.

גלטורי, v. בגלטורי.

גלמינון, v. גְּלַאקְסִינוֹן.

גְּלָה, גלי (b. h.) 1) *to be uncovered.* Tosef. Mikv. III, 1 a pit שֶׁגָּלָה ed. Zuck. which was left open.—*Part. pass.* גָּלוּי *open, revealed.* Sabb. 55[a] ג׳ וידוע וכ׳ it is open and known to me. Ber. 60[b]; a. fr. V. גָּלוּי.—2) (of a place) *to become bare of inhabitants* (v. Jud. XVIII, 30; Jer. I, 3); (of the inhabitants) *to leave home, go into exile.* Y. Taan. I, 64[a] top בכ״מ שגָּלוּ ... גָּלַת וכ׳ whithersoever Israel went as exiles, the Divine Majesty went with them (ref. to נגלה, I Sam. II, 27); Meg. 29[a]; a. e.—Pesik. Haḥod. p. 48[a] אם ג׳ אחד מכם ... כאילו גְּלִיתֶם כולכם if one of you is banished (by the Roman Government) to &c.: . . . as though ye all had been banished; Pesik. R. s. 15; Cant. R. to II, 8. Arakh. 12[a]; Meg. 11[b] גָּלוּ בשבע they were transported to Babylonia in the seventh year (after the subjection of Jojakim). Macc. II, 1 אלו הן הַגּוֹלִין the following (involuntary homicides) have to leave for the city of refuge. Ib. אינו גּוֹלֶה is not bound to flee to &c. Ib. 3 האב גולה ע״י הבן a father is banished for killing his son; a. fr.

Hif. הִגְלָה *to banish; carry into captivity.* Macc. 12[b] היו ... מַגְלִין וכ׳ the Israelites executed the law of banishment in the desert. Num. R. s. 23, end. Ruth R. to I, 1 ומַגְלָם מארצם and is the cause of their exile &c.; a. fr.—Koh. R. to XII, 6 (play on גלת ib.) 'the golden bowl' is the gullet, שהיא מַגְלָה את הזהב ומריצה וכ׳ (not שהיה; Lev. R. s. 18 שמכלה, corr. acc.) which banishes the gold and makes the silver run, i. e. which impoverishes the glutton.

Nif. נִגְלָה *to be discovered, exposed to view; to reveal one's self, appear.* Tanḥ. Sh'moth 19 נ׳ עליו בקולו וכ׳ He revealed Himself to Moses with the voice of Amram &c.; Ex. R. s. 3. Ib. s. 2, end בכ״מ שהשכינה נִגְלֵית wherever the Divine Glory appears. Snh. II, 1, v. פָּסָה II; a. fr.

Pi. גִּלָּה, גַּלֵּה to *uncover, remove; to discover, reveal, publish.* Ex. R. s. 15, beg. גִּלּוּ הצדיקים וכ׳ the righteous uncovered their heads. Sot. V, 2; Gen. R. s. 21 מִי יְגַלֶּה עפר וכ׳ Oh that one would remove the dust from over thy eyes, i. e. Oh, that thou wouldst resurrect!; Y. Ber. IX, 13ᵈ bot.—Sabb. 88ᵃ מי גי׳ וכ׳ who revealed this secret to my children? Meg. 3ᵃ; a. fr.—ג׳ משפחות *to expose to suspicion* the legitimacy of families. Tosef. Naz. I, 3; Kidd. 71ᵃ.—(ג׳ פנים בתורה (שלא כהלכה a) to interpret the Law in opposition to the adopted sense, *to misinterpret, pervert.* Ab. III, 11; a. e. b) *to put the Law to shame* by treating its teachers irreverently. Snh. 99ᵃ; a. e.—ג׳ פנים (in gen.) *to expose, put to shame.* Pirkê d'R. El. ch. XLIV, v. לָבַן II.—*Part. pass.* מְגוּלֶּה, f. מְגוּלָּה *uncovered.* Par. XI, 1; Ḥull. 9ᵇ; a. fr. *Pl.* מְגוּלִּין. Ib.; a. fr.

Nithpa. נִתְגַּלָּה, נִתְגַּל *to be revealed; to be exposed.* Pirkê d'R. El. ch. XXIII ונתגל בתוך האהל his nakedness was exposed &c. Yoma 9ᵇ נתג׳ עונם their sins were public (they did not hide them); נתג׳ קיצם the end of their captivity was revealed (through prophecy). Naz. 23ᵇ נ׳ קלונו his disgrace is published.—Pes. 119ᵃ; a. fr.—Tanḥ. Mishp. 6; Yalk. Prov. 956, v. גָּלַע.

גְּלָא, גְּלָא, גְּלֵי ch. same; 1) *to reveal, uncover.* Targ. Num. XXII, 31. Targ. Am. III, 7; a. fr.—Part. גָּלֵי. Targ. Prov. XX, 19.—2) *to go into exile, go away, disappear.* Targ. Hos. X, 5.—Ib. XI, 11 דִּיגְלוֹ those who were exiled. Targ. Am. V, 5 מִיגְלָא יִגְלוֹן (some ed. ילפון, corr. acc.); a. fr.—Ber. 56ᵃ אִגְלֵי I will leave home; גלא לבי רומאי he emigrated into Roman territory. Pes. 49ᵃ לא גְלָאִי I should not have emigrated; לא גלאי כדגלי ארנשי I did not emigrate (voluntarily) as others do. Koh. R. to IX, 10 את הוית גָלֵי וכ׳, v. אֲלַה II.—Part. גָּלֵי, pl. גָּלַיָּא, f. גָּלָן *exiles.* Targ. Nah. II, 8 בגָלַיָּא ed. among the exiles (on foot; ed. Lag. בגִילַיָּא, v. גִּילוֹיָא, h. text גֻּלְּתָה). Targ. Am. VI, 7 גָּלָן the exiled communities.—Targ. II Kings XXIII, 6 קברי ג׳ (some ed. גָּלֵ׳) the graves of the homeless (h. text בני העם).—*Part. pass.* גְּלֵי, גְּלֵי, גָּ׳, גְּלִיא *known, revealed; uncovered.* Dan. II, 19; 30. Targ. Job XXIII, 10. Targ. I Sam. III, 1; a. fr.—Targ. O. Ex. XIV, 8 ברויש ג׳ openly (h. text ביד רמה).

Pa. גַּלֵּי as preced. Pi.—Targ. Lev. XVIII, 6 sq.; a. fr. Gitt. 31ᵇ ג׳ לדרעיה he uncovered his arm. Ab. Zar. 28ᵃ; Yoma 84ᵃ דלא מְגַלֵּית that thou wilt not divulge it. Ib. מְגַלֵּינָא I shall divulge. Ḥull. 113ᵃ תנא סיפא לגַלּוּיֵי רישא the second clause is stated in order to throw light on the first. Gitt. 34ᵃ גַּלּוּיֵי דיתא, v. גִּילוּיָא. Y. Maasr. V, end, 52ᵃ מן דגַלֵּית לך חספא אשכחת מרגניתא (not דגלויית) after I removed the potsherd, thou foundest the pearl, i. e. but for my teaching, you would not have found the truth which you now claim as your own discovery; Y. Keth. IX, 33ᵇ bot. (corr. acc.); [in Babli דלאית, v. דלי].

Af. אַגְלֵי *to banish.* Targ. II Kings XV, 29; a. fr.—Snh. 94ᵃ. [הַגְלִי Ezra IV, 10; a. e.]

Ithpe. אִיתְגְּלִי, אִיגְּלִי 1) *to be uncovered, revealed* &c. Targ. Is. LXII, 1. Ib. LI, 9 אִיתְגְּלָא reveal thyself (h. text עורי). Targ. II Sam. VI, 20 דא׳ who exposed himself; a. fr.—Snh. 109ᵇ אִיגְּלַאי מלתא the fact became known. R. Hash. 22ᵇ; a. fr. כל מילתא דעבידא לאִיגַּלּוּיֵי וכ׳ people are not presumed to tell a lie which is likely to be found out. Sot. 22ᵇ מאי דמִגַּלְּיָא מגליא what is visible is visible, i. e. man judges only by what he can ascertain, opp. מטמרא.—R. Hash. 21ᵇ whence do we know that *alil* has the meaning of being clearly visible? לישנא דמִיגַּלֵּי הוא Ab. Zar. 30ᵃ איגלי ליה חמרא his wine was found uncovered. Bets. 3ᵃ מִגַּלּוּ וקיימי remain visible; a. fr.—2) *to be led into captivity.* Targ. Jer. XL, 1.

גְּלָאי, גְּלֵי m. (גלי, cmp. גִּילְהֵי) *flash.* בְּגְ׳ *as a flash, suddenly, rapidly.* Targ. Is. XLI, 2; 25; Targ. Hos. XI, 11.

***גָּלִי** f. (cmp. γάλιον) *galium, bed-straw,* an odoriferous plant. Targ. Y. Num. XXI, 12 [read:] דמרבי חילפי וג׳.

גְּלָיָא, גְּלֵי, גְּלִי, גְּלֵי, part. pass. of גְּלָא.—*Pl.* fem. גְּלְיָין. Targ. Prov. XXXI, 27 (ed. Lag. גלין).

גַּלְיָא I pr. n. (Gallia) 1) *Gaul, country of the Gauls* in Europe. Yeb. 63ᵃ ships going מג׳ לאספמיא from Gaul to Spain.—2) *Gallia* or *Galatia* in Asia Minor. R. Hash. 26ᵃ. Keth. 60ᵃ Naḥum איש ג׳ the Galatian.

***גַּלְיָא** II f. (גלי) *revelation.* בית ג׳ *a place or temple for oracles.* Ab. Zar. 46ᵃ היו קורין אותה בית ג׳ קורין אותה בית כריא when they (the idolators) call a place *Beth-Galia,* Israelites should call it *Beth-Kharia,* v. כַּרְיָא; Tem. 28ᵇ.—Meg. 6ᵃ (ref. to Zech. IX, 7) זה בית ג׳ שלהן that means their temple. V., however, גַּלָּא a. גַּדָּא.

גַּלַּיָא, v. גַּלָּא a. preced.

גָּלַיָּא *exiles,* v. גְּלֵי.

גליאס, גליאסין, read גַּלִּיגָאס, גַּלִּיגָאסִין.

***גְּלִיבָא** m. (גלב) *shaved face.* Targ. Is. XV, 2 Kimḥi (ed. גרלות).

***גְּלִיבְמוֹן** m. (γλυπτόν) *carved.* Y'lamd. to Deut. IV, 4 quot. in Ar., expl. פטורי ציצים (I Kings VI, 18).

***גַּלִּיגָאס, גַּלִּיגָס** m. (caliga, adopted fr. acc. pl. caligas) *nail-studded shoe of the Roman soldier.*—*Pl.* גַּלִּיגָאסִין. Lam. R. to II, 7 [read:] ועשו מסמרות של גליאסין שלהן רושם בארץ and the nails of their shoes left marks in the Temple floor. [Vers. in Ar.: ועושין רושם במסמרות הגלגוסרים בקרקע בירהמ״ק.]

גְּלִיד m. (גלד) 1) *ice-coating* on the water. Ohol. VIII, 5. Mikv. VII, 1.—2) v. גֶּלֶד.

גְּלִידָא, גְּלִיד ch. same; *ice, hoar-frost* (h. כפור, קרח). Targ. Ps. CXLVII, 16. Targ. O. Gen. XXXI, 40 (Y. קרושא).

גִּלָּיוֹן, גִּלְ׳, גִּילְ׳ m. (b. h. גִּלָּיוֹן; גלי) 1) *blank parchment, margin of scrolls.* Yad. III, 4 ג׳ . . . שמלמעלן וכ׳ the blank portions of a sacred book, the upper, the lower margins and those at the beginning and the end; Sabb 116ª Ms. M. (ed. pl.). Men. 30ª.—*Pl.* גִּלְיוֹנִין, גִּלְ׳. Sabb. l. c., v. supra. Ib. הג׳ של ס״ת (Ms.M.sing.) blank parchments of, or intended for, a sacred book.—2) (a satirical adaptation of εὐαγγέλιον, v. אָוֶן) *gospel.* Tosef. Sabb. XIII (XIV), 5 הג׳ וספרי מינין; Sabb. l. c. הג׳ וספרי הצדוקים (Ms. M. הגליון . . . מינין) the gospels and books of heretics; [disputants, Sabb. l. c., take our w. in the sense of *blanks*]. Ib. sq., v. אָוֶן.—3) (v. Is. III, 23; cmp. גְּלַגְּלִין) *a girdle* of fine material. Gen. R. s. 19 (Ar. גלוונים; ed. Koh. גולין, corr. acc.).

גליוה, Lev. R. s. 20 יודן ג׳, read גְּלִילָאָה; cmp. Tanḥ. Aḥaré 3 יודן דמן גלילא.

גְּלַיְיר, v. גּוּלְיָיר.

גָּלִיל pr.n. (b. h.) [*District,*] esp. *Galilee* in Northern Palestine. Shebi. IX, 2 ג׳ העליון Upper Galilee, ג׳ התחתון Lower Galilee. Sot. IX, 15 (49ᵇ) הַגָּ׳. Keth. 9ᵇ; a. fr. [ג׳ בגוים, Snh. 94ᵇ, v. גְּלִילָה.]

גְּלִילָא ch. same; 1) *district, circuit.* Targ. Ezek. XLVII, 8.—*Pl.* גְּלִילֵי, גְּלִילִין. Targ. Josh. XXII, 10; a. e.—2) *Galilee.* Ib. XX, 7; a. e.—Sabb. 47ª; 78ª בג׳ שנו it refers only to Galilee.—Tosef. Snh. II, 5; Y. Maas. Sh. V, 56ᶜ top, a. e. ג׳ עילאה Upper Galilee, (ארעיתא) ג׳ תיתאה Lower G.; Snh. 11ᵇ גלילאה (corr. acc.).—Erub. 53ᵇ בר ג׳ a Galilean.

גְּלִילָא, pl. **גְּלִילַיָּא**, v. גְּלוֹלָא.

גְּלִילָאָה m. ch.=h. גְּלִילִי, *Galilean.* Erub. 53ᵇ ג׳ שוטה (Ms. M. גלילא) foolish Galilean, v. אִימַר.—Snh. 113ª ההוא ג׳ a certain Galilean; Sabb. 88ª. Ḥull. 27ᵇ; a. e.—*Pl.* גְּלִילָאֵי. Y. B. Bath. VI, 15ᶜ top.

גְּלִילָה f. (גלל) *casting about, contempt.* Snh. 94ᵇ (play on גְּלִיל הַגּוֹיִם, Is. VIII, 23) אנ׳ עוש׳ אותו ג׳ בגוים Ms. M. (ed. אעשה לו גליל) I will make him (Sennaherib) contemptible among the nations; Yalk. II Kings 237.

גְּלִילִי m. (גָּלִיל) *Galilean.* Yad. IV, 8 צדוקי ג׳ Mish. ed. (Talm. ed. only צדוקי) a Galilean Sadducee (heretic).—ר׳ יוסי הג׳ R. José the Galilean. Pes. 28ª; a. v. fr., v. יוֹסֵי.—**Pl.* גְּלִילִין, גְּלִילִים. Kel. II, 2 הפכים הג׳ Galilean flasks; Tosef. ib. B. Kam. II, 2 הפכין והג׳ (read הפכין הג׳); ib. 9. [Cmp., however, גָּלָל.]

גְּלַלְנִיתָא, גְּלִילְתָא f. (v. גְּלָה) *folding.* Sabb. 47ᵇ מטה גליל׳ Ms. M. (ed. גללני׳, Ar. גרליתא) *folding couch, cot.*

גְּלִימָא, גְּלִים I m. (גָּלַם 1) *wrapper, cloak.* Targ. O. Gen. XXV, 25 ed. כִּגְלִים (ed Berl. כִּכְלָן, v. כְּלָן, Var. כִּגְלָם). Targ. II Esth. VIII, 15.—Sabb. 77ᵇ it is called *g'lima,* שנעשה בו כגולם ed. (Ms. M. שנעשית כגו׳) because one looks in it like a shapeless (armless) body (Ms. M. it is rolled up like a lump). Snh. 102ᵇ שיפולי ג׳ trail of the cloak; a. fr.—*Pl.* גְּלִימֵי. Ib. 110ª.

גְּלִימָא II, **גַּלְמָא** f. (גלם 2) 1) *height, hill*—*Pl.* גַּלְמָתָא, גְּלִימָתָא. Targ. Y. I, II Num. XXIII, 9; Targ. Y. II Gen. XLIX, 26 גּוּלְמָתָא (read גּוּלְמָ׳). Targ. Y. II ib. 11 sq. גּוּלְמָתֵיה his hills. Targ. Ps. LXXII, 3 גַּלְמָ׳.—2) *valley.* Targ. Job XXXIX, 21. Targ. Josh. XVIII, 28 Var. (ed. Lag. I, p. VIII³⁰ גְּלִימַת).—*Pl.* גַּלְמָתָא, גְּלִימָתָא. Targ. Job XXXIX, 10. Targ. Y. Num. XXI, 19.—גְּלִימִין. Pesik. B'shall. p. 93ª ומחית ליה ג׳ (Ar. גַּלְמָן) and carried him down the valleys.

גָּלִינֵי f. (γαλήνη) *calm, stillness of wind and wave.* Y. Yeb. XV, 15ᵈ top אם (הירה) הים ג׳ וכ׳ if there was a calm sea, and you looked around and there was none &c.; Y. Erub. IV, 21ᵈ bot. גלנו ed. Krot. (corr. acc.).

גְּלִיפָא m. (v. next w.) *shaping* (of writing), *impress, poetry.* Targ. Ps. XVI, 1 ג׳ תריצא a well-arranged poetry (h. text מכתם). Ib. CXIX, 130 גְּלִיף דבריך the impress of thy words (h. text פֵּתַח).

גְּלִיפָה f. (גְּלַף) *shaping, formation* (of speech, cmp. גוּזְמָא, גזם). Pesik. R. s. 33 גְּלִיפַת שפתים eloquence (ref. to Is. LVII, 19).

גַּלִּיצוּר pr. n. *Gallitsur,* name of an angel. Pesik. R. s. 20 (defined מְגַלֶּה טעמי צור revealing the reasons of the Creator); Yalk. R'ubeni, Mishpatim end ג׳ המכונה רזיאל G. surnamed Raziël.

גָּלְיָת, גּוֹלְיָת pr. n. m. (b. h.) *Goliath,* the Philistine. Sot. VIII, 1 בנצחונו של ג׳ relying on the strength of G. Ib. 42ᵇ גלית . . . בגילוי פנים וכ׳ he is named G., because he stood before the Lord with barefacedness (defiance). Lev. R. s. 5; a. fr.

גלכין, v. גְּלָבִין.

גָּלַל (b. h.) 1) *to roll, unfold, fold.* Meg 32ª he opens (the scroll), sees the place (to read from), גולל ומברך rolls it up again and says the benediction. Ib. הגולל ס״ת וכ׳ he who rolls the scrolls up (preparing the place to read from). B. Mets. II, 8 (29ᵇ) גּוֹלְלָן he must roll the scrolls over (for the purpose of airing); a. fr.—2) (v. Gen. XXIX, 3) *to roll off* (one's shoulders), *disregard.* Gen. R. s. 21 (play on גללו, Job XX, 7) על שג׳ מצוה וכ׳ because he disregarded a light command.

Nif. נִגְלַל *to be rolled, folded.* Cant. R. to V, 14 והיו נִגְלָלִין they could be folded up. Snh. 68ª my two arms which are like two scrolls of the Law שנגללין rolled up (not unfolded, i. e. with me learning is buried which I was prevented from teaching).—Trnsf., with על, *to be rolled on top of, to prevail.* Ber. 7ª יִגּוֹלּוּ רחמי על וכ׳ may my mercy prevail over my attributes (of justice &c). Ib. יגולו רחמיך; v. גַּלְגֵּל.

Hof. הוּגְלַל *to be rolled up, folded.* Taan. 21ᵇ; Men. 95ª הוּגְלְלוּ הפרוכות when the curtains (of the Tabernacle) were folded up (for removing).

גְּלַל ch. same, *to roll, unfold.*—Part. pass. גְּלִיל *unfolded, visible.* Targ. Cant. V, 14.

Pa. גַּלֵּל *to roll off.* Targ. Y. II Gen. XXVIII, 10 (some ed. לְגַלְלָא Pe.).

Ithpe. אִתְגְּלַל, v. גַּלְגֵּל, Ithpalp.

גַּלָּל, constr. **גְּלַל** m. (b. h.; preced.) 1) *rolling along with, appendage.* Men. 15^a; Pes. 13^b לחם ג׳ תודה the bread is an appendage of the thank-offering; Men. 80^a לִגְלַל תודה.—בִּגְלַל *in consequence of, on account of,* v. next w.—2) *something rolled, rounded, ball, ordure, excrement, dung.* B. Kam. III, 3 ההופך את הג׳ he who upturns (throws up) ordure into the street.—*Pl.* גְּלָלִין, גְּלָלִים. Sabb. 153^b להטיל ג׳ to cast excrements (of animals). Lev. R. s. 16; Esth. R. to III, 1 מה הג׳ הללו וכ׳ as the dung is repulsive.—3) (with כְּלֵי) *a material used for vessels,* supposed to be *baked ordure.* Kel. X, 1. Par. V, 5. Mikv. IV, 1; Sabb. 16^b. Men. 69^{ab}; a. fr. [Rashi to Sabb. l. c. expl. ג׳=שייש, *marble,* to Men. l. c.=צפיעי בקר.]

גְּלָלָא, גְּלָל ch. same; 1) *untrimmed stone, cobble* (v. גְּוִיל). [Ezra V, 8.]—Ḥull. 63^a אתא ג׳ a stone fell (from on high); Yalk. Zech. 578 גלאלא. Gitt. 47^a Ar. (ed. גַּלְגַּלְתָּא). Ab. Zar. 22^b, v. דַּבָּלָא.—2) *lump.*—*Pl.* גְּלָלֵי. Ḥull. 112^a bot. תרי ג׳ דמלחא Rashi (ed. ג׳ מלחא) two lumps of salt.—3) *ordure,* v. גְּלָא.—*Pl.* as supra. B. Kam. 92^b (prov.) a dog in his hunger ג׳ מבלע (Ms. H. sing.) will swallow excrements (Rashi: stones).—4) *wave,* v. גַּלָּא.—5) *consequence;* בג׳ *on account of, in order to.* Targ. Ps. XL, 12 (Ms. ג׳ הרכנא). Targ. II Chr. XXIV, 25; a. e.

גְּלָלִיתָא f. (preced.) 1) *ball-shaped lump.* מילח׳ ג׳ *salt in lumps, rock-salt.* Ḥull. 114^a; Kidd. 62^a.—2) *folding,* v. גְּלִילְתָּא.

גָּלַם (b. h.; cmp. גלל) 1) *to roll up, to unshape.* Denom. גּוֹלֶם.—2) (denom. of גּוֹלֶם) *to calculate in a lump, fix an arbitrary price,* opp. דקדק to calculate exactly. Sifra B'har, Par. 6, ch. IX; B. Kam. 113^b יכול יִגְלוֹם עליו you might think, he (the redeemer of the Jewish slave in possession of a gentile) was permitted to force an arbitrary price upon him (the gentile); [Rashi: (גלם *to double*) he (the gentile owner) might be permitted to ask an exorbitant price].—Part. pass. גָּלוּם, f. גְּלוּמָה 1) *wrapt up.* Sot. 42^a, v. גַּלְמוּד.—2) *roughly shaped, unfinished.* *Pl.* גְּלוּמִים, גְּלוּמוֹת. Sifré Num. 158, v. גּוֹלֶם. Ex. R. s. 30 מצות גלומות rough laws (containing no details, assigning no reasons; Var. lect. גוֹלְמִיּוֹת, גולמות, fr. גּוֹלְמִי).

גְּלַם ch. same; 1) *to roll, wrap up.* Denom. גְּלִים, גּוֹלְמָא I, גְּלִימָא.—2) *to arch, cave.* Denom. גְּלִימָא II.

גְּלַם, v. גְּלִים.

גַּלְמָא, גְּלַם, v. גּוֹל׳.

גַּלְמָא, v. גְּלִימָא II.

גַּלְמוּד m., **גַּלְמוּדָה** f. (b. h.; גלם; ד format., v. Fürst H. Dict. s. v.) *like a shapeless, lifeless lump,* whence (cmp. דמם) *lonely, melancholy.* Sot. 42^a in the sea-towns קורין לנדה ג׳ they call the menstruous woman *galmudah;* R. Hash. 26^a. Ib. (phonetic etymol.) גמולה (דא) מבעלה she is weaned (separated) from her husband; [Ar. ed. Pes. a. Ven. גלומה, which version, however, disagrees with the reference to Gen. XXI, 8 in Ar. s. v.]. Gen. R. s. 31; s. 34 (ref. to Job XXX, 3) when there is want in the world &c. ג׳ הוי רואה . . . כאילו ג׳ be lonely; look upon thy wife, as if she were menstruous; Y. Taan. I, end, 64^d עשה אשתך ג׳ make thy wife lonely. [Cmp. Snh. 22^b, quot. s. v. גּוֹלֶם.]

גַּלְמוּדָא f. (preced.) (euphem.) *a menstruous woman.* Gen. R. s. 79, end they heard a woman say to her friend ג׳ אנא I am *galmuda* (for נדה), from which they learned the meaning of *galmudah* in Is. XLIX, 21 (v. corr. vers. in 'Rashi' a. l.).

גַּלְמוּדָה, v. גַּלְמוּד.

גַּלְמָתָא, גַּלְמָן, v. גְּלִימָא II.

גלנר, v. גַּלִּינֵר.

גָּלַע (b. h.; cmp. גלח a. גרע) *to scratch off, rub; lay open.* *Nif.* נִגְלַע *to be opened through rubbing or scratching, to bleed.* Nidd. VIII, 2 (58^b) והיא יכולה לְהִגָּלַע וכ׳ (Bart. להתגלע) and it (the wound) may have been bruised so as to bleed.

Pi. גִּלַּע, גִּלֵּעַ (with ב of person) *to detract from, lay bare the ignorance of, attack.* Y. Yeb. VIII, end, 9^d משום שלא לְגַלֵּעַ בו וכ׳ (did they send him off) in order not to see him exposed, or because he was not fit (to argue)? What is the difference? היה דרכו לְגַלֵּעַ א״ת משום שלא לגלע בו וכ׳ It was his (Rabbi's) habit to begin with vehement argument; now, if you were to say, 'in order not to see him exposed', his exposure was in his own hand (he being the attacking part) &c. Ib. מה היה לו לְגַ׳ בו what could he have attacked (on that subject of *androgynos*)?

Hithpa. הִתְגַּלֵּעַ, *Nithpa.* נִתְגַּלֵּעַ 1) *to be scratched open,* v. supra. 2) *to be laid bare, be argued.* Snh. 6^b; Y. ib. I, 18^b (ref. to Prov. XVII, 14) (עד שלא נתג׳) קודם שנתג׳ הריב נטוש before the case of litigation has been laid open (fully argued), you (the judge) may compromise it &c.; Tanḥ. Mishp. 6; Yalk. Prov. 956 נִתְגַּלֶּה, יִתְגַּלֶּה).

גַּלְעֵד, גִּלְעָד, v. גַּלַּשׁ.

גַּלְעִינָה, גַּלְעִין, v. פַּרְעִינָה, פַּרְעִין.

גָּלַף (cmp. גלב) *to dig out, engrave; to shape, form.* Gen. R. s. 47; s. 53; s. 63 ג׳ לה הקב״ה וכ׳ the Lord shaped a womb for her.—Part. pass. גָּלוּף *engraven.* Tanḥ. Balak 14.—*Pi.* גִּלֵּף same. Pesik. Ăniya, p. 137^a מְגַלְּפִין בו shaping it; Pesik. R. s. 32 מפליגים (corr. acc.).

גְּלַף I ch. same. Targ. I Kings VII, 36. Targ. Ex. XXVIII, 9; a. e.—Part. pass. גְּלִיף. Targ. Y. ib. 11; a. e.—*Pl.* גְּלִיפָן, גְּלִיפִין. Targ. Ex. XXXIX, 6; a. e.

גְּלַף II, **גְּלוֹף** m. (preced.) *engraving, setting.* Targ. Ex. XXVIII, 11. Targ. Hag. II, 23; a. e.

גַּלְפִיתָא f.=אִגַּלְפּוּתָא. Targ. Y. II Ex. XXXV, 33.

גַּלְפַּטְרָה pr. n. f. *Cleopatra,* queen of Egypt. Tosef. Nidd. IV, 17 ed. Zuck., v. קְלֵיאוֹפַּטְרָא.

גלקטינון, v. גַּלַאקְסִינוֹן.

גַּלְקְטִיקָא, v. גְּלוּגְדְּקָא.

גָּלַשׁ (b. h.; cmp. גלה) 1) *to come in sight, to come forth.* Cant. R. to IV, 1 (ref. to שגלשו מהר וכ׳ ib.) הר שגלשתן מתוכה עשיתיו גלעד לאו״ה (not תי . . . .) the mountain (of trouble) out of which ye came in sight again (ye escaped), I (the Lord) made it a hill of witness (a warning) to the nations; אי זה זה ים סוף what is this? It is the Red Sea [which R. Joshua . . . translated into Chaldean: טורא דאתנהרתון מן גווה]; ib. to IV, 4 הר שג׳ . . . . הר סיני I made your escape memorable to the nations, it is Mount Sinai (by the giving of the Law); ib. repeatedly (referring to various escapes from dangers).

Hif. הִגְלִישׁ *to bring to light, to publish.* Ib. to IV, 1 ומה הגלשה הִגְלַשְׁתִּי וכ׳ (Ar. ed. Koh. גלשה) and what publication (institution or law) have I (the Lord) brought to light out of that event?

**Hof.* הוּגְלַשׁ (denom. of גֶּלֶשׁ *baldness*) *to be made hot enough for scalding the hair or feathers of an animal's skin.* Part. מוּגְלָשׁ, pl. מוּגְלָשִׁין *seething water.* Pes. 37[b] (Rabad to Eduy. V, 2 quotes a version מַגְלוּשִׁין *scalding water,* Ar. מֵי גְלָשִׁים, fr. גֶּלֶשׁ; Y. Ḥall. I, 58[a] top חַמִּין).

גְּלַשׁ ch. same; *to shine, be bald;* v. גְּלוֹשׁ, גְּלוֹשׁוּתָא &c. —Part. pass. גְּלִישׁ=h. מוּגְלָשׁ (v. preced.) *brought to scalding heat, boiling over.* Koh. R. to VIII, 9, v. גִּירְסָא III.

***גֶּלֶשׁ** m. (preced.) *baldness. Pl.* גְּלָשִׁים. מֵי ג׳ *scalding water,* v. גָּלַשׁ Hof.

***גַּלְשָׁא**, m., pl. **גַּלְשִׁין** *bright* or *bald lines.* Cant. R. to IV, 1 (a gloss to גלש) a woman whose hair is thick הדא מוצינא עבדא לה ג׳ ג׳ parts it so as to show white lines; כההוא לפי טבאות הוא עבד ג׳ ג׳ (prob. to be read . . . בוצינא . . כד הוא) a young pumpkin, when it sprouts nicely, produces bright stripes.

גִּלְשָׁה, v. הַגְלָשָׁה.

גַּלְשׁוּשִׁיתָא f. (גלש) *public monument.* Targ. Cant. to IV, 1 (v. Cant. R. to ib. s. v. גָּלַשׁ). [Ar. reads גבשושיתא, but the phonetic interpretation refers to שגלשו of the Hebrew text.]

גִּלְשְׁלָשׁוּתָא, גַּלְשְׁלָשְׁתָא, גַּלְשׁוּלְשְׁתָא, גַּלְשְׁלוּשְׁתָא, גִּיל׳= גְּלוֹשׁוּתָא. Targ. Y. Lev. XIII, 42 sq.

גְּלַשְׁלְשַׁן=גְּלוֹשׁ. Targ. Y. Lev. XIII, 41.

גַּלְתָא, v. גּוּלְתָא.

גַּם I (b. h.; גמם) [*junction,*] 1) *too, also.* Snh. 108[b]; Taan. 21[a] ג׳ זו לטובה this, too, is for the best. איש גם זו, v. גַּמְזוֹ.—2) *the particle gam* in the Bible text. B. Kam. 94[a] ג׳ לב״ה קשיא *the gam* (Deut. XXIII, 19) is unaccounted for according to Beth Hillel's opinion; Tem. 30[b]. Esth. R. to I, 9 (ref. to גם ib.) אין ג׳ אלא ריבוי *gam* intimates an amplification, a. e.—*Pl.* גַּמִּים, גַּמִּין. Gen. R. s. 1; Y. Ber. IX, 14[b] bot. אתין וג׳ ריבויין the *eths* and the *gams* intimate an extended qualification (by implication), v. אֵת.

גַּם II, **גַּאם (גמא)** m. (preced.) *joint, angle,* esp. *two sides of a rectangle.* Erub. 55[a] כמין גם Ar. (ed. גאם) in the shape of a right angle. Zeb. 53[b] גמא (Yalk. Lev. 441 גאם). Pes. 8[b] שורה אחת כמין ג׳ one row of wine vessels, in the shape of &c., i. e. the front and the whole upper layer. Y. ib. I, 27[b] bot. קולפו כמין גם.—Kel. XIV, 8 (מפתח) של גם שנשבר מתוך גומו a key whose bit is joined (opp. to של ארכובה of one piece) broken at its junction. [Sabb. 105[a] על הגם Ar., ed. על הַגַּס, q. v.]—*Pl.* גַּמִּים, גַּמִּין. Y. Pes. l. c. קולפו כמין שני ג׳ he takes off for examination two front and two upper layers, v. supra. Ib. if the vessels are arranged like steps קולפו ג׳ ג׳ he must examine by front and upper layers on each landing. B. Mets. 28[a] מדת גַּמָּיו the combined measure of both dimensions of a piece of goods, square measure, opp. מדת ארכו ומדת רחבו the measure of each dimension specified.—Sabb. 103[b] גַּמִּין, v. גר״מל.—[Commentators explain our w.=*Greek Gamma,* Γ, whence the Var. גַּמָּא.]

גַּמָּא m. (Γάμμα) 1) *Gamma,* the third letter of the Greek alphabet. Shek. III, 2 אלפא ביתא ג׳ Ms. O. (ed. גמלא).—2) *the shape of a Gamma,* Γ, v. preced.

גָּמָא (b. h.), גָּמַע, גָּמָה *to take a draught, quaff; to sip, suck up.* Y. Maas. Sh. II, beg. 53[b] he melted fat וגְמָיְיו וּגְמָעוֹ and sipped it; Y. Yoma VIII, 45[a] top וגמייו. Sabb. XIV, 4 (111[a]) לא יִגְמָא בחֹמץ וכ׳ Ar. (ed. יִגְמַע, or יגמ׳ *Pi.,* v. infra) he must not quaff vinegar through his teeth. Y. Maasr. III, 50[d] bot. כמה . . . . לִגְמוֹת בכוס how large a portion of the cup one must quaff at a time. Y. Shebi. II, end, 34[b]; Y. Ned. VII, beg. 40[b] the leaves of the colocasia must not be used (in case of a vow of abstinence from vegetables, or in the Sabbath year) לגמות וכ׳ to sip water out of them (v. Sm. Ant. s.v. Colocasia); a. fr.

Pi. גִּמֵּא, גִּמֵּעַ same. Sabb. 111[a] מְגַמֵּעַ ופולט תנן (Ms. M. לא יְגַמֵּעַ ויפלוט) the Mishnah means, he must not quaff and spit out; Bets. 18[b]; Y. Shebi. VIII, 38[a] top מְגַמֵּא; a. fr.

גְּמָאִין m. pl. (preced.) *sweetmeats, delicacies.* Esth. R. to I, 9 (play on גם ib.) מיני ג׳ various delicacies.

גִּמְגֵּם (Pilp. of גמם) [*to peel, scrape;* trnsf., cmp. חָסַם II, חָכַךְ] *to hesitate, stammer, to speak with an expression of uncertainty* or *of scruple.* Kidd. 30[a] אל תְּגַמְגֵּם ותאמר לו that thou need not hesitate in answering him; Sifré Deut. 34. Ber. 22[a] היה מְגַמְגֵּם למעלה וכ׳ (Ms. M. a. Rashi מג׳ וקורא) was speaking hesitatingly over (as the Amora of) R. Judah &c. Ib.[b] מג׳ וקורא he should read in a hesitating manner (rapidly murmuring); Y. ib. III, 6[c] bot. התחיל מג׳ בה he commenced stammering over it (hesitating to pronounce the Divine Name). [Cant. R. to VII, 1 מתגמגם, transpos. of מתמגמג, v. מְגַג.]

גַּמְגֵּם ch. same. Hag. 15[b] מְגַמְגֵּם בלישניה a stotterer (Ar. מלגם). Meg. 31[b] קא מג׳ וכ׳ (v. Rabb. D. S. a. l. Var. Lect.) read the curses (v. אֲרַר) rapidly murmuring; Koh. R. to VIII, 3.

גֹּמֶד, v. גּוֹמֶד.

גָּמַד (v. next w.) *to contract.* אמה גְמוּדָה a reduced cubit, v. גְּדַם.—*Pi.* גִּמֵּד, v. גּוֹמֶד.

גָּמַד (cmp. קמט, קמץ) *to contract, shrink, be tight.* Pes. 111[a] גְּמוּד מסאניה (Ms. M. גמד) his shoes shrank (became too tight). Ḥull. 43[a] גמדא ליה (the gullet) contracts. Gitt. 57[a] גמדא the land shrinks, opp. רווחא. Yoma 69[a]; Bets. 15[a] חאר נמטא גמדא דנרש וכ׳ the shrunk (hard) mattress of Narash (which does not warm) is permitted (does not come under the law of כִּלְאַיִם).—Part. pass. גְּמִיד *contracted, atrophied.* Targ. Jud. III, 15; XX, 16 (h. text אִטֵּר q. v.).

גַּמְדָּא I, v. preced.

גַּמְדָּא II *Gamda;* 1) pr.n.m. B. Kam. 72[a] Rab. G.— Pes. 64[a]; 73[b]; Ḥull. 30[a] R. Ḥiya bar G.—2) G., name of a river or canal in Babylonia. Ab. Zar. 39[a]; Succ. 18[a] נהר ג׳.

גָּמָדָה, v. גָּמָא.

גמד, Ḥull. 111[a], v. גְּאַם.

גָּמוּד m., **גְּמוּדָה** f. (גמד) *contracted, reduced.* Y. Yoma IV, 41[c] bot., v. גָּרַם a. אַמָּה.

גְּמוּל m. (b. h.; גָּמַל) *deed, reward, recompense.* Keth. 8[b] בעל הג׳ . . . גְּמוּלְכֶם may He who rewards, pay you for your good deed.—*Pl.* גְּמוּלִים, גְּמוּלִין. Gen. R. s. 13 ג׳ טובים וכ׳ goodness bestowed on the guilty. Tosef. Shebi. VII, 9 ואין משלמין מהן ג׳ and favors received must not be repaid with them (the fruits of the Sabbath year); ib. Peah IV, 16.—גְּמוּלוֹת. Deut. R. s. 1 ג׳ אני פורע (some ed. גמי׳ incorr.) I repay according to deeds.

גְּמוּלָא f. ch. same.—*Pl.* גְּמוּלָן. Targ. Ps. CXVI, 12.

***גּוּמָּסִית, גְּמוּמְסִית** f. (גמס, *to couple;* cmp. גמז) *coupling song,* a sarcastic adaptation of γάμος, to deride the *hymenean songs* in their licentious application to sodomy and to copulation of animals (cmp. אֶרְפּוֹתוֹרוֹס).—*Pl.* גּוּמָּסִיּוֹת, גְּמוּמְסִיּוֹת (Ar. ed. Koh. גַּמְסִיּוֹת). Gen. R. s. 26 the generation of the flood were not doomed to destruction עד שכתבו ג׳ לזכר ולבהמה until they composed hymenean songs for sodomy &c.; Tanḥ., ed. Bub., B'resh. 22 גמיקריסום; 33 קמיסמסין, Var. קמיסקסין, Y'lamd. quot. in Ar. גמיסרקין—(perversions arisen from confounding our w. with גַּמִּיקִין q. v.); Yalk. Gen. 43 גממטיות (corr. acc.); Lev. R. s. 23 גומסיות לזכר ולנקבה (corr. acc.).

***גמורקין** or נמ׳, Koh. R. to III, 9, a corruption of אַמְבּוּרְקְלוֹן, v. אַנְבּוּרְקְרָאוֹת=אַנְבּוּרְקָרִין.

גָּמַז (cmp. גמומסית), *Pi.* גִּמֵּז *to couple,* esp. *to suspend branches of the wild fig on the cultivated* (the process called caprification, v. Sm. Ant. s. v. Caprificatio). Tosef. Shebi. I, 11 ומצדדין ומְגַמְּזִין ed. (missing in ed. Zuck.).

***בַּר ג׳, גַּמְזָא** pr. n. pl. *Bar Gamza.* Lam. R. to I, 15 (Ar. s. v. סח 3: בורגרא).

גִּמְזוֹ (b. h.) pr. n. pl. *Gimzo,* in Judea. Taan. 21[a], a. fr. נחום איש גם זו; Tosef. Shebu. I, 7 מנחם וכ׳ (always in two words).

גַּמְזוּז m. (v. גמז) *a fig or carob ripened through caprification.* Lam. R. to I, 5 (Ar. גמזזן).

גַּמְזוּזִיבַיָּיה m. pl. (preced.) *a dish of gamzuz* (prepared with wine), v. אוּרְזָנַיָּא. Y. Maas. Sh. II, beg. 53[b]; Y. Yoma VIII, 45[a] top גומננר; Y. Shebu. III, 34[b] bot. גמרירה (corr. acc. or גַּמְזוּזִירָה).

גַּמְזִית f., pl. **גַּמְזִיוֹת** (גמז) 1) *branches used for caprification.* Pes. IV, 8 (55[b]) ומתירין ג׳ של הקדש (ed. Y. בג׳, Var. מתזירין) they considered as permitted the use of branches of (carob or sycamore) trees belonging to the Temple treasury; Tosef. ib. III, 19 (Var. גזוזיות, גיזות); Men. 71[a] ג׳ . . . . של חרוב וכ׳; Pes. 56[a]; Y. ib. IV, 31[b]; Y. Peah VII, end, 20[c]. [R. Hai Gaon reads גַּזְאזִיוֹת *twigs,* cmp. גוזזיות Var. Tosef., v. supra.]—2) *fruits ripened through caprification,* v. גַּמְזוּז. Tosef. Ter. V, 7.

גַּמְחוֹן, v. גַּחְמוֹן.

גַּמְטְרִיָּא, v. גִּימ׳.

גְּמַע, גְּמַר I, *Pa.* גַּמַּע, גַּמֵּר ch.=h. גָּמָא, גָּמַע, to *swallow, quaff.* Targ. Job XXXIX, 30 גָּמְעָן (Ms. גַּמְצָאן).—Y. Ab. Zar. II, 41[c] bot. (expl. שורפה, Mish. II, 7) גמר לה (ed. גמילה, corr. acc.) he quaffs it, sucks it out. Succ. 49[b] לִיגְמַע גַּמּוּעֵי let him quaff (take full draughts); ib. אגמע גמועי (read: מְגַמַּע with Rashi, or גַּמַּע, v. Rabb. D. S. a. l. note 300). Sabb. 109[b] ולגמע.

גְּמִי II m.=גּוֹמֶא *bulrushes, reed-grass* (used for ropes). Kil. VI, 9. Sabb. VIII, 2. Y. Erub. I, 18[d] וגמי על גביהן and a reed-rope over them; a. fr.—Chald. form גְּמִירָא. Ib.

גְּמִיאָה, גְּמִירָה, גְּמִיעָה f. (גָּמָא, גָּמָה, גָּמַע) *quaffing, full draught.* Sabb. VIII, 1 (76[b]) כדי גמיא׳ Ms. O. a. Ar. (ed. גמיע׳) as much as is quaffed at a time. Ib. 77[a] (discussion about spelling with א or ע); Tosef. ib. VIII (IX), 8 (with ע); Y. ib. VIII, beg. 11[a] גמירה. Gen. R. s. 60 גמיר׳ אחת (some ed. גְּמִיָּה) only one quaff; Tanḥ. Pinḥ. 13 כדי גמיא׳; Num. R. s. 21 גמיריא (corr. acc.); Midr. Prov. ch. XIII גמיאה.—Num. R. l. c. הוא עושה גמיע׳ אחת the Leviathan swallows with one quaff; Pesik. R. s. 16 (with א); a. fr.

גְּמִיד, v. גָּמַד.

גְּמִירָא, v. גְּמִי II.—[Num. R. s. 21 כדי גמירא, v. גְּמִיאָה.]

גְּמִיָּה, גְּמִיָּיה, v. גְּמִיאָה.

גָּמִיל, v. גְּמַל.

גמילה, Y. Ab. Zar. II, 41[c] bot., v. גְּמַר I.

גְּמִילָה, constr. **גְּמִילַת**, v. גְּמִילוּת.

גְּמִילוּת f. (גמל), ג׳ חֲסָדִים (also גְּמִילַת, v. גְּמִילָה) *deeds of love, charity* (abbr. ג״ח). Peah I, 1. Ber. 5[a]. Sot. 14[a] the Torah תחילתה ג״ח וכ׳ begins with charity (clothing the naked, Gen. III, 21) and ends with charity (burying the dead, Deut. XXXIV, 6); a. v. fr.—[Deut. R. s. 1, v. גְּמוּל.]

גמיסיקין, גמיסקוס, גמיסקין, v. גַּמִּיקִין a. גְּמוּמָסִית.

גְּמִיעָה, v. גְּמִיאָה.

גמיקון, v. next w.

גַּמִּיקִין m. pl. (γαμικά, τά) *marriage, nuptial feast* (the guests of which are the witnesses of the marriage; v. Sm. Ant. s. v. *Marriage*); *wedding contract.* Pesik. Haḥod. p. 52[b]; Yalk. Ex. 190 a king married many wives ולא כתב להם לא ג׳ ולא איפטיא but did not order in their behalf a record of the nuptial act or of the date of marriage וכיון שנשא . . וכתב לה ג׳ וכ׳ but when he married a woman of noble descent, he had her marriage recorded as we read (Esth. II, 16) &c., v. אִיפַּטְיָא; Pesik. R. s. 15 כתובת גחיקן (read גמ׳). Ex. R. s. 32 שאין ביניהם גמיסקין for there is between them no wedding feast to testify to their alliance. Ib. s. 47 כתב לה גמיסקוס משלו he had a marriage contract written at his own expense; עֲשֵׂה לה ג׳ ולואי וכ׳ prepare thou the certificate, and would I could prevail upon myself to lend my signature to it! [Var. in ed. a. Ar. גמיסקוס, גמיסקין, גמיקון, גמיקן, v. Ar. ed. Koh. s. v. גמס, note.—The nouns γαμισκος, γαμισκα, as if from γαμίσκω, are not otherwise recorded in the Greek vocabulary, and seem to be cacophemistic perversions; cmp. גמומסית.]

גמיקיסום, v. גְּמוּמָסִית.

גְּמִירָא, גְּמִיר m. (Part. pass. of גְּמַר) 1) (=h. כָּלִיל) *finished, perfect.* Targ. Ez. XVI, 14.—2) *holocaust, entirely burnt.* Targ. Lev. VI, 16; a. fr.—3) (=h. כָּלָה) גְּמִירָא f. (with or without כלייה) *entire destruction, extermination.* Targ. Gen. XVIII, 21 (Targ. Y. II, v. כְּלָיְיה). Targ. Jer. V, 18; a. fr.—4) *concluded, decision.* Targ. I Sam. XX, 33; a. e.—V. also גְּמַר II, III.

גמ״ל, v. גרמ״ל.

גָּמַל (b. h.) [*to tie, couple, load,*] 1) *to load (good or evil) on, to deal with,* esp. *to do good to.* Gen. R. s. 38 שהוא ג׳ עליך תחלה for he was the first to do thee good; Yalk. Prov. 956.—Sabb. 104[a] גְּמוֹל דלים, v. גרמ״ל.—ג׳ חסד *to be kind, charitable.* Ib. שכן דרכו של גּוֹמֵל חסדים וכ׳ (Ms. M. דרכן של גּוֹמְלֵי) for such is the habit of the charitable to run after the poor. Yeb. 79[a]; a. v. fr.—2) *to make even, repay.* Dem. IV, 6 אע״פ שהן כגוֹמְלִין זה את זה although it has the appearance as if they were repaying each other (by mutual recommendations). Ab. Zar. 61[b] חיישינן לגומלין we reject witnesses suspected of favoring each other; Keth. 24[a].— 3) (cmp. גָּמַר a. חָסַל) [*to finish,*] *to wean.* B. Mets. 87[a] on that day שג׳ אברהם וכ׳ when Abraham celebrated the weaning of Isaac &c.; Yalk. Gen. 93; Deut. R. s. 1 שמל (corr. acc.). Pesik. R. s. 25 תינוק הַגָּמוּל וכ׳ a Jewish infant just weaned; a. fr.—4) *to ripen, be fully developed.* Par. XI, 7 *yon'koth* are גבעולין שלא גָּמְלוּ capsules of hyssop which are not yet developed; (Tosef. ib. XI (X), 7 גָּמְרוּ).

Nif. נִגְמַל *to be weaned.* Gen. R. s. 53 נ׳ מחלבו weaned from his mother's milk; נ׳ מיה״ר weaned from the evil inclination (able to resist temptation); a. fr.

Pi. גִּמֵּל *to take turns.*—Y. M. Kat. III, 82[b] bot. פרה מְגַמֶּלֶת a cow engaged for working in a team in turns; v. גַּמְלָא I, 2.

גְּמַל ch. same, *to do one good* or *evil.* Targ. I Sam. XXIV, 18; a. fr.—Y. Ḥag. II, 77[d] bot. the whole town stopped work מִיגְמוֹל ליה חסד in order to show kindness to him (to give him an honorable funeral).—Y. Ab. Zar. III, 42[c] top גָּמֵיל חיסדא the charitable.

Ithpe. אִתְגְּמַל *to be laden with; to be bestowed.* Targ. II Esth. V, 2 (Targ. I אטעינת, h. text וַתִּשָּׂא).—Y. Ḥag. l. c. לא איתג׳ ליה חסד nobody cared to attend his funeral, v. supra.

גָּמָל m. (b. h.; גמל) [*carrier of loads,*] *camel.* Bekh. 8[a]. Ber. 56[b]; a. fr.—*Pl.* גְּמַלִּים. Keth. 67[a] ג׳ של ערביא וכ׳ camels in Arabia can be levied for a wife's portion (כְּתוּבָּה); a. fr.

גַּמָּל m. (preced.) *camel-driver.* Kidd. IV, 13 one must not rear his son to be חמר ג׳ וכ׳ an ass-driver, or a camel-driver &c.; Y. ib. IV, end, 66[c]; a. e.—*Pl.* גַּמָּלִין. Ib.—Y. M. Kat. III, 62[a] bot. גַּמָּלָיו his drivers.—חַמָּר (ו)גַמָּל ass-driver and camel-driver in one person (the camel-driver walking by the head of his beast, the ass-driver behind), *one walking forward and backward,* i. e. one who, owing to the loss of the object with which he appointed the central point for the movements of the day (v. עֵירוּב), may walk only from his home to that spot and back. Erub. III, 4 (35[a]); Tosef. ib. V (IV), 2; Y. ib. III, 21[b] top.

גַּמְלָא, גִּימ׳, גּוּמ׳ (גְּמ׳) m. ch.=h. גְּמוּל. Targ. Is. III, 11. Targ. Ps. XCIV, 2. Ib. CXXXVII, 8 גְּמ׳ Ms.; a. e.—*Pl.* גַּמְלַיָּא. Targ. Is. XXXV, 4.—Lev. R. s. 4 גַּמְלַיי טבוייה דגמלית עימיך my benefits which I bestowed on thee.

גַּמְלָא I c., ch. 1) =h. גָּמָל *camel.* Targ. Lev. XI, 4; a. e.—Snh. 106[a] (prov.) ג׳ אזלא וכ׳ the camel went to ask for horns, and had her ears cut off.—Macc. 5[a] ג׳ פרחא a flying (swift) camel, *dromedary;* Yeb. 116[a].— Ib. 45[a] (prov.) ג׳ במדי וכ׳ in Media a camel can dance on a *kab* (bushel), i. e. in Media everything is possible. Sot. 13[b]; Keth. 67[a], a. e. (prov.) לפום ג׳ שיחנא according to the camel is his load, i. e. the greater the man, the greater his responsibility.—*Pl.* גַּמְלֵי, גַּמְלַיָּא, גַּמְלִין. Targ. Gen. XXIV, 10 sq.; a. fr.—Gen. R. s. 38.—Y. Hor. III, 48[a] bot. אבא יודן דגַמְלוֹי Abba Yudan who is busy among his camels; Lev. R. s. 5 דגמלי; a. fr.—2) *couple, teaming arrangement.* M. Kat. 11[b] הוה להו ג׳ דתורא בהדי הדדי (Asheri 33 . . . . עבוד גִּימְלָא) had an arrangement between them to team their oxen for mutual work. Ib. פסקיה לְגַמְלֵיה he broke the arrangement (Ms. M.; as corrected, לגמלא ולא שדריה . . ., v. Rabb. D. S. a. l. note); v. גָּמַל Pi.—3) *a small bridge, crossboard* (cmp. גֶּשֶׁר). M. Kat. 6[b] והוא דליכא גשרא . . . ג׳ provided there is neither bridge nor crossboard. Snh. 67[b], v. אִיסְקָנִיתָא. B. Bath. 21[a] ג׳

contrad. fr. תיתורא. Snh. 7ᵃ, v. גּוּדְרָא.—4) *large-sized*, v. גַּמְלָנָא.

גַּמְלָא II pr. n. pl. *Gamala*, in Galilee. Arakh. IX, 6. Tosef. Macc. III (II), 2; Y. ib. II, 31ᵈ גַּמְלָה.

גַּמְלָא III pr. n. m. *Gamla* (abbrev. of Gamliel). Yoma 18ᵃ; Yeb. VI, 4; B. Bath. 21ᵃ Joshua ben G., a highpriest.—Gitt. 30ᵇ Abba Elazar b. Gamla; Bets. 13ᵇ גרמל; Bekh. 58ᵇ, Men. 54ᵇ גומל (Ms. M. גמל).—Snh. 111ᵃ R. Ḥănina b. Gamla (v. Rabb. D. S. a. l. note), usu. b. Gamliel.

גמלא, Shek. III, 2, v. גַּמָּא.

גַּמְלָה, v. גַּמְלָא II.

גַּמְלוֹן m. (deriv. of גָּמָל) *large-sized* (bean).—*Pl.* גַּמְלוֹנִין, גַּמְלוֹנִים. Shebi. II, 8; Kil. III, 2. גמלנים ed., v. אָפוּן.—Tosef. Kil. II, 8 פולין הג׳ (v. ed. Zuck. note). Tosef. T'bul Yom I, 1.

גַּמְלִיאֵל pr. n. m. (b. h.) *Gamaliel, Gamliel*; 1) Tannaim, a) Rabban G. senior (הזקן), grandson of Hillel. R. Hash. II, 5. Gitt. IV, 2; a. fr.—b) Rabban G. (of Jabneh), grandson of the former. Ber. I, 1. Peah VI, 6.—Ber. 27ᵇ sq. Tosef. Nidd. IX, 17; a. fr. (v. Frank. Darkhé Mish. p. 69).—2) Amoraim, a) R. G. B'ribbi (Bar Rabbi) I, son of R. Judah han-Nasi I. Y. Ḥall. IV, 60ᵃ top ר׳ ג׳ ב״ר. Keth. 103ᵇ. Ib. 10ᵇ. Men. 84ᵇ; a. e. [Ab. II, 2.]—b) R. G. B'ribbi II, son of R. Judah han-Nasi II. Y. Ab. Zar. I, 39ᵇ.—c) (also גַּמְלִיֵּיל) G. Zuga. Y. Ḥall. IV, 60ᵃ top; a. fr.; a. others (v. Frank. M'bo p. 72ᵃ sq.).

גַּמְלִין, pl. of גרמ״ל.

גַּמְלָן, v. גַּמְלוֹן.

גַּמְלָנָא m., **גַּמְלָנִיתָא** f. ch.=h. גַּמְלוֹן, *large-sized*. Sabb. 66ᵇ שומשמנא ג׳ Ar. (ed. גמלא) a large ant.—Ab. Zar. 28ᵇ, v. חִיפּוּשִׁיתָא.

גַּמֶּלֶת f. (גַּמָּל) *a caravan of camel-drivers*. Snh. X, 5 (111ᵇ); ib. 112ᵃ; B. Bath. 8ᵃ.

גַּמְלְתָא f. (גַּמְלָא) *stock of camels*. Gen. R. s. 75 (ref. to generic sing. שור חמור, Gen. XXXII, 6) it is a popular expression חמורתא ג׳ (as we say in Chald.) the stock of asses, of camels.

גָּמַם 1) *to join, connect*. Denom. גַּם I, II.—2) *to make even, level, smoothen, peel, raze*. Shebi. IV, 5 גּוֹמֵם מִן הארץ Ms. M. (ed. מֵעַל, Y. מֵעַם) he razes (the tree) even with the ground; B. Bath. 80ᵇ ג׳ מעם. Tosef. Maas. Sh. V, 18 גּוֹמְמִין אותו you may raze it (the vineyard with the fourth year's fruits). Ter. IX, 7 עד שיגוֹם את האוכל (Y. ib. end, 46ᵈ האוכלין) until he has entirely cut off what is eatable. Y. l. c. כיני מתניתן עד שי׳ בעלים the Mishnah means, until he has razed the plant while it was yet bearing leaves. Y. Kil. V, 30ᵇ bot.; Y. Shebi. I, end, 33ᶜ הגוֹמֵם את כרמו וכ׳ he who razes his vineyard lower than a hand-breadth (above the surface); עד שיגום מעם הארץ until he razes it even with the ground.—Ḥull. 92ᵇ גּוֹמְמוֹ עם וכ׳ he peels the fat off even with &c., opp. to חָטַט. Tosef. Kel. B. Mets. VII, 3 עד שֶׁיְּפַּח ויָגֹם (R. S. to Kel. XVII, 12 שיְּנַפֵּחַ ויגֹם Nif.) until one has blown it up and scraped it (polished the leather surface).—*Part. pass.* גָּמוּם *levelled, smoothened*. Ḥull. 59ᵃ פיה ג׳ her mouth is smooth i. e. toothless (Rashi: *cut off*); v. infra. Tosef. Bekh. IV, 16 איזהו גמום וכ׳ (ed. Zuck. גמום, corr. acc.) what animal is called *gamum?* That which lacks horns, i. e. whose horns are not projecting, v. next w. Ib. 15 הגומים (ed. Zuck. הנימום) read: הַגְּמוּמִים.

Nif. נִגְמַם *to be levelled, smoothened, razed*. Shebi. I, 8 אילן שנ׳ (Ms. M. שנפגם) a tree which has been cut off (near the ground). Bekh. VI, 4 (39ᵃ) the incisors שנפגמו ושנִגְמְמוּ which are broken off or levelled (with the gum; cmp. Ḥull. 59ᵃ quoted above). Ḥull. 70ᵃ נגממו כותלי וכ׳ if the sides of the womb are peeled (diminished in size). Tosef. Kel. B. Mets. l. c. נגממו after the leather bottles have grown too thin for holding liquids. Kel. XVII, 4 נגממו if they are worn off (the sides of a vessel having become too thin), opp. נפרצו broken into (Maim.: the sides have been cut off, so that nothing but the bottom remained); Tosef. ib. B. Mets. VI, 9 נפגמו ed. Zuck. (R. S. to Kel. l. c. נגממו).—Trnsf. *to be degraded, disgraced*. Esth. R. to I, 9 (play on *gam* ib.) Vashti's time has come לִיגָּמֵם to be disgraced (explained ליבצר).

Pi. גִּמֵּם as Kel. Gen. R. s. 38 when a vineyard yields no fruits, מְגַמְּמִין אותו the owner cuts it down.

גְּמַם (גּוּם) ch. same. Y. Kil. II, 27ᵈ גַּם כרמיא razed his vineyards. Ḥull. 50ᵃ גּוּם שדי peel it off and throw it away. Ib. 92ᵇ גָּאִים ליה ed. (Ar. גיים) peeled it off (on the surface, opp. מרטט). Ib. 96ᵃ.

Ithpe. אִיגּוּם as preced. Nif. Ib. 44ᵃ אִיגּוּם אִיגּוּמֵי וכ׳ the chin was razed, detached without laceration from the neck, opp. איעקור forcibly torn off. Bekh. 44ᵃ אִיגּוּם אִיגּוּמֵי the horns are levelled (not projecting), opp. איעקור uprooted.

גַּמְמִיּוֹת, v. גּוּמְמִית.

גַּמְסִית, v. גְּמוּמְסִית.

גמניא, v. גַּרְמַנְיָא.

גַּמַע, גָּמַע, v. גַּמָּא a. גָּמַר I.

גְּמַץ (v. גמם) *to finish a pit*. Targ. Ps. VII, 16.—Denom. גּוּמְצָא.

גָּמַר I, *Pi.* גִּמֵּר (denom. of מוּגְמָר, v. גּוּמְרָא) *to perfume (clothes) with burned spices*. Bets. 22ᵇ לְגַמֵּר for the purpose of perfuming clothes. Ber. 53ᵃ.

Hithpa. הִתְגַּמֵּר *to be perfumed, soaked with perfume*. Sabb. 18ᵃ you may put *mugmar* under the clothes on the eve of Sabbath, וּמִתְגַּמְּרִין והולכין וכ׳ and the process of soaking is continued during the entire Sabbath day. Bets. l. c. הבית מִתְגַּמֵּר מאליו the room is perfumed of itself.

גְּמַר I ch., *Ithpe.* אִתְגַּמַּר as preced. *Hithpa.* Targ. Cant. III, 6. Targ. Ps. XLV, 9.

גָּמַר II (b. h.; cmp. v. גמם) 1) *to polish, touch up, finish.* Y. Sabb. VII, 10ᵃ bot. ג׳ מלאכתו when he gives to his work the finishing touch; a. fr.—2) (in gen.) *to complete, end.* Pes. X, 7 גּוֹמֵר עליו את החלל he reads over it (the fourth cup) the Hallel to the end, v. הַלֵּל.—Tosef. Succ. III, 2 גּוֹמְרִין בהן וכ׳ on those occasions the *entire* Hallel is read; Ber. 14ᵃ; Arakh. 10ᵃ; Taan. 28ᵇ. Ber. 13ᵇ חוזר וגוֹמְרָהּ (after the disciples left) did he take it up again and read the whole of the Sh'ma?—Y. Yeb. II, beg. 3ᶜ הביאה גּוֹמֶרֶת בה coition consummates the levir's marriage (Bab. ib. 18ᵃ קונה קניין גמור), v. מַאֲמָר.—Y. Ber. VI, 10ᵈ top ג׳ מלאכול after he has finished eating; a. fr.—Euphem. *to gratify the sexual appetite.* Kerith. II, 4. Pes. 87ᵃ (play on *Gomer*, Hos. I, 3) שהכל גּוֹמְרִים בה all people could gratify their lust on her.—וְגוֹמֵר (abbr. וגו׳, וג׳) *and one finishes* (the sentence quoted)=*and so forth, &c.*, a clerical term used in Bible citations to save the writing out of the entire quotation. Ḥull. 98ᵃ. Gen. R. s. 51, beg.; a. fr.—**Part. pass.* גָּמוּר, f. גְּמוּרָה *finished, complete, real, valid.* Kidd. 40ᵇ, a. fr. צדיק ג׳ a perfectly righteous man (without faults); רשע ג׳ a wicked man throughout (without any good quality). Yeb. 18ᵇ, a. fr. קניין ג׳ real (legal) possession.—*Pl.* גְּמוּרִים, גְּמוּרוֹת. Ḥull. 89ᵃ; a. fr.—Bets. 2ᵇ, a. e. בצים ג׳ perfectly developed eggs (with shells), v. infra.—3) *to destroy.* Pes. 87ᵇ (play on *Gomer*, v. supra) בזוז וְגָמְרוּ (Ms. M. גמרו וגמרו) they plundered and destroyed (they destroyed thoroughly).—4) *to conclude, determine, decide.* Kel. XVI, 1. Ber. 17ᵃ גְּמוֹר בכל לבבך וכ׳ be determined with all thy heart &c. Shebu. 26ᵇ ג׳ בלבו he resolved (vowed) in his heart, opp. הוציא בשפתיו; Ḥag. 10ᵃ.—Erub. 13ᵇ, a. fr. נמנו וגמרו they were counted (their votes were taken) and they decided.—Snh. III, 7 (42ᵃ) גמרו את הדבר when they had closed the case (being ready for publishing the sentence); a. fr.—5) *to draw a conclusion by analogy.* Sabb. 96ᵇ ג׳ העברה העברה מיוה״כ one forms an analogy between the expressions *heĕbir* &c.; a. fr.—6) *to be fully developed.* Tosef. Par. XI, 7, v. גָּמַל.—בצים גמורות, v. supra.

Pi. גִּמֵּר 1) *to destroy.* Pes. 87ᵇ בקשו לְגַמֵּר וכ׳ they intented to destroy the possessions of Israel in her (Gomer's) days, v. supra.—2) *to develop, mature, ripen.* Y. Shebi. V, beg. 35ᵈ אין פירותיה׳ מְגַמְּרִין וכ׳ their fruits ripen only every three years.

Nif. נִגְמַר *to be finished, completed.* Snh. VI, 1 נ׳ הדין when proceedings are finished (sentence pronounced). Gen. R. s. 12 נִגְמְרָה מלאכתן they were finished; a. fr.

גְּמַר II ch. same; 1) *to finish.* Targ. Ps. LVII, 3 דִּיגְמַר (ed. Lag. די גמר, corr. acc.); a. fr.—Pes. 55ᵃ גַּמְרִינַן we dare finish a work commenced. Ib. מִיגְמַר אין אתחולי לא to finish is permitted, but not to begin; a. fr.—2) *to consume, destroy.* Targ. Job I, 16. Ib. XXII, 20; a. fr. (also *Pa.*).—3) *to end, cease.* Targ. Ps. XII, 2 גְּמִירוּ they are gone. Targ. Prov. V, 11. Ib. XXII, 8; a. e.—4) *to conclude, derive.* Ḥull. 98ᵇ וְלִיגְמַר מינה now let one draw a conclusion from this (by analogy)! Ib. מחדוש לא גָמְרִינַן from an exception we draw no conclusions; a. fr.—5) *to be perfect, ready to answer, to know well.* [Targ. Y. Deut. VI, 7 וְתִגְמְרִינוּן וכ׳, read וְתַגְ׳, v. infra.]—*Part.* גְּמִיר. Sabb. 63ᵃ והוה גְּמִירְנָא וכ׳ and I knew well the whole Talmud (v. Rabh. D. S. a. l.). Taan. 7ᵃ bot. דִגְמִירֵי who are learned; ib.ᵇ top טפי הוו ג׳ they would be more learned; a. fr.—Whence: *to learn by heart*, esp. *to learn traditional law* (cmp. גְּרַס II). Targ. Job XXII, 22 (h. text קח, cmp. לֶקַח).—Sabb. l. c. לִיגְמַר איניש והדר ליסבר one must first learn traditions, and then he may reason; Ab. Zar. 19ᵃ, v. גְּרַס II.—Ber. 43ᵃ וברכת ... גְּמִירִינַן and we are not sufficiently familiar with the laws concerning grace at meals. Yoma 29ᵃ מִיגְמַר בעתיקא וכ׳ to remember well something old (to refresh the memory) is more difficult than to commit to memory a fresh thing. Sabb. l. c. למיגמר מינה from whom to receive traditions. Sot. 36ᵇ לא הוה קגמר he could not remember; a. fr.—Sabb. 96ᵇ גמרא גְּמִירֵי לה they (the scholars) know it by tradition; ib. 97ᵃ גְּמִירֵי.—הילכתא ג׳ לה they have a tradition, *it is a well-known maxim.* Snh. 37ᵇ bot. Sot. 34ᵃ. Gitt. 47ᵃ; a. fr.

Pa. גַּמֵּר *to finish; to consume.* Targ. Job XXI, 13 ed. (Ms. גָּמְרִין Part. Pe.). Ib. XIII, 28; a. fr.

Af. אַגְמֵיר *to teach verbally.* Targ. Y. Deut. VI, 7 [read:] ותַגְמְרִינוּן and thou shalt teach them (v. Ber. 13ᵇ).—Sot. 36ᵇ אַגְמְרֵיה ולא גמר he taught him (the Hebrew language), but he (Pharaoh) could not remember it. Ḥull. 45ᵇ אַגְמְרָךְ גמרא I will teach thee a tradition. B. Kam. 17ᵃ לְאַגְמוּרֵי as to teaching. Ber. 13ᵇ, v. גְּרַס II.

Ithpe. אִתְגְּמַר, אִגְּמַר *to be finished; to be destroyed.* Targ. Job XXIII, 17. Targ. Ps. CIX, 23.—Targ. Y. Num. XVIII, 14 דִמְגַּמַּר (h. text חֵרֶם). Targ. Y. Ex. XXII, 19 יִתְגַּמְּרוּן (h. text יָחֳרָם).

גְּמַר, constr. **גְּמַר** m. (preced.) *finishing, last touch; consummation.* Sabb. 103ᵃ, a. fr. ג׳ מלאכה the finishing work.—Snh. 6ᵇ; a. fr. ג׳ דין close of legal proceedings.

גְּמַר III ch. 1) same, *finish, perfection, beauty.* Snh. 8ᵇ, a. e. ג׳ דינא, v. preced. Targ. Ez. XXVII, 24 ג׳ מינר וכ׳ the perfection of all valuable things (h. text מכללים). Ib. XXIII, 6 ed. Lag. (ed. גמיר, h. text תכלת). Ib. 12 (h. text מכלול).—2) (cmp. גּוּמְרָא) *carbuncle*, a precious stone. Targ. Is. LIV, 12 (h. text אקדח).

גְּמָרָא f. (v. גְּמַר II, 5) *memorizing of verbal teachings, tradition.* Ab. Zar. 19ᵃ bot. הנ״מ סברא אבל ג׳ מחד רבא וכ׳ (v. Rabb. D. S. a. l. note) this refers to reasoning (dialectics), but as to traditional laws (rules &c.), it is better to study only with one teacher, in order not to be confused by varying wording; Yalk. Ps. 614.—Gitt. 6ᵇ הא ג׳ היא וג׳ לא שמיע ליה this is merely a tradition (not to be arrived at by way of reasoning) and one may not have heard that tradition (and yet be an able man). B. Mets. 33ᵃᵇ ג׳ verbal study (opp. to משנה which had been put to writing). Arakh. 29ᵃ רב גְּמָרֵיהּ גמיר (not גמור) Rab had his own tradition about it (had it from his teacher that the Mishnah was corrupt). Erub. 60ᵃ ג׳ גמור וזמורתא תהא if it is a tradition, learn it by heart, let it be like a song (the wording of which you dare not change); Sabb. 106ᵇ; Ab. Zar. 32ᵇ; Bets. 24ᵃ (variously interpreted in comment.).—Yoma 14ᵇ, a. fr. משמיה דג׳ as a tradition (without knowing the reasoning process, cmp. ib. 33ᵃ bot. ג׳ גמירנא

וכ׳); a. fr.—*G'mara*, that part of the Talmud containing those discussions, decisions &c. which, after the reduction to writing of the Mishnah, were the materials of verbal studies until they, too, were put to writing.—Abbrev. גמ׳, a clerical mark in the Talmud Babli editions, to indicate where the Mishnah ends, and the G'mara begins.

גַּמְרֵי (infin. Pa. of גמר) לְגַ׳ *entirely.* *Targ. Job XXX, 24 Ms. (ed. לגרמיה).—Pes. 55^b^. B. Kam. 35^b^; a. fr.

גמריוה, Y. Shebu. III, 34^b^ bot., v. גַּמְזוּזִרְכָּיָה.

גַּמְרָנָא m. (Denom. of גְּמָרָא) *a teacher of traditions.* Pes. 105^b^.

גְּמַשׁ (cmp. כמש) *to contract, bend.* Yoma 67^a^ Ms. M. 2 (v. Rabb. D. S. a. l. note 20) זימנין דגְמִישׁ רישיה ולא חזי ליה sometimes the animal's head (in falling) is bent, and he (the man) cannot see the chord.

Pa. גַּמֵּישׁ same. Ib. ed. זימנין דג׳ ליה לרישיה ולאו אדעתיה the animal may bend its head, and the man may not think of looking after the chord.

גַּן, c., **גַּנָּה**, **גִּינָּה** f. (b. h.; גנן) *a fenced-in place, garden.*—גַּן עֵדֶן *paradise, place of future reward*, opp. גֵּיהִינָּם. Pes. 54^a^; Ned. 39^b^; a. fr.—Gen. R. s. 15 beg. גן גדול מעדן the garden was larger than Eden (Eden was a portion of the garden, ref. to Ez. XXXI, 9). Taan. 10^a^ וגן אחד וכ׳ and the garden was one sixtieth portion of Eden.—Gen. R. l. c. כפיגר שהיא נתונה בגנ׳ like a spring in a garden. Kil. II, 2 זרעוני גנה garden plants. Ex. R. s. 31 גלגל שבגנ׳ the wheel works of the well in the garden; a. fr.—Trnsf. (cmp. hortulus a. κῆπος) *woman.* Pirké d'R. El. ch. XXI אין גן אלא האשה וכ׳ *gan* (Gen. III, 3) means woman who is compared to a garden (ref. to Cant. IV, 12), מה הגנה זו וכ׳ as a garden &c. Cant. R. to IV, 12 גַּפְתִּי נעולה והיא מתגנייא my consort (Israel) is closed (chaste), and yet defamed.—*Pl.* גַּנּוֹת. Lev. R. s. 3, beg. better off is he who owns גינה one garden and &c. ממי שנוטל ג׳ של וכ׳ than he who takes other people's gardens on half-shares; a. fr.—Gen. R. s. 85 חורש בגנות (euphem. for sexual intercourse).

גִּינָּא, **גַּנָּא** ch. same. Targ. Job XXXVIII, 18 גַּן עדן Ms. (ed. גינתא דע׳); a. fr.; v. גִּינְּתָא.—*Pl.* גִּינִּין, גִּינַּיָּא, גַּנַּיָּ׳. Targ. II Kings IX, 27.—Lev. R. s. 3, v. אֲגַר II.—ג׳ דאשקלון *the gardens* (or *the forts?*) *of Ascalon*, name of a Palestinean border place (v. Hildesh. Beitr. p. 72). Y. Shebi. VI, 36^c^; ib. מן מה דתני גנויה וכ׳ (corr. גנייה) from the expression 'the gardens of A.', we derive that A. itself is considered as foreign land; Tosef. ib. IV, 11 גינייא דא׳; Sifré Deut. 51 גבנייא דא׳ (prob. גַּנַּיָּ׳); Yalk. ib. 874 גִּינַּיָּא.

גְּנָא, v. גְּנַח I a. גנר.

גְּנָאָה, v. גִּינָּאָה.

גְּנַאי m. (גנר) *disgrace, shame, blame; obscenity.* Ab. Zar. 46^a^ a byname לג׳ of reproach, (cacophemistic, opp. לשבח). Kidd. 33^b^; Y. Shek. V, 49^a^ bot. חד אמר לג׳ one says 'they looked after Moses' (Ex. XXXIII, 8) with the purpose of fault-finding; Tanh. Ki Thissa 27. Meg. 25^b^ כל המקראות . . לג׳ וכ׳ words in the Torah which, as they are written (v. כתיב), have become obscene, are in reading changed &c. (שגל changed into שכב &c.). Ber. 33^b^ ג׳ הוא לו it would be offering an insult to him; a. fr.

גְּנַאי, **גְּנַיי** ch. same. Targ. II Esth. I, 2. Targ. Y. Lev. XX, 17; a. e.

גָּנַב (b. h.) [*to put behind, aside,*] *to steal.* Y. Snh. VIII, 26^b^ top לא תִגְנוֹב את . . . . גּוֹנֵב do not carry off steathily thine own property from the thief, lest thou appear to be stealing.—Snh. 86^a^ גונב נפש one who kidnaps a person. B. Kam. VII, 2 ג׳ על פי שנים if he is convicted of stealing through two witnesses; a. fr.—ג׳ דעת *to deceive, to create a false impression.* Ḥull. 94^a^ אסור לִגְנוֹב דעת וכ׳ it is forbidden to create &c. (e.g. to make believe as if you opened a fresh barrel of wine as a special attention to your guest, while you would have had to do it at any rate). Shebu. 39^a^; a. fr.—ג׳ עין *to deceive by a false impression on the eye, to delude.* B. Mets. IV, 12.—Part. pass. גָּנוּב, f. גְּנוּבָה. Ab. Zar. 44^b^; Meil. 7^b^ תשובה ג׳ a fallacious reply; v. גְּנוּבְתָא II.

Pi. גִּנֵּב *to keep behind.* Ex. R. s. 5 היו מְגַנְּבִין את עצמן וכ׳ they kept themselves at a distance from Moses and then withdrew.

Nif. נִגְנַב 1) *to be stolen, kidnapped.* B. Mets. III, 1. Gen. R. s. 84; a. fr.—2) *to be deceived* (sub. דעת). Tosef. B. Kam. VII, 8 sq.; Mekh. Mishp. N'zikin, s. 13.

Hithpa. הִתְגַּנֵּב *to sneak in.* Pesik. R. s. 21, היו מִתְגַּנְּבִים וכ׳ they used to have stealthy intercourse &c. Mekh. l. c. המִתְגַּנֵּב אחר וכ׳ who steals himself (into the college room) behind a neighbor.

גְּנֵיב, **גְּנַב** ch. same. Targ. Y. Gen. XXXI, 30. Ib. 20. Targ. O. Deut. XXIV, 7 גָּנֵיב (Y. גְּנִיב, corr. acc.); a. fr.—Part. pass. גְּנִיב. Targ. O. Gen. XL, 15 גְּנֵיבְנָא ed. Berl. I have been stolen.—Ruth R. introd. 3 (a trial before a Roman court) גְּנַבְתּוּן לא גְנַבְנוּן "Ye have stolen".—'We have not' . . . .; לא גְנַבְתְּ מאן ג׳ עמך "thou hast not stolen? Who has been stealing with thee?"; Gen. R. s. 37; s. 63. B. Kam. 65^b^ תורא גַּנְבִי מינך was it an ox I stole from thee?—Ib. 67^b^ עד דגְנֵיב תרי (he is not bound to pay) unless he stole two animals; a. fr.

Pa. גַּנֵּיב 1) same. Targ. Jer. XXIII, 30.—2) *to go round about.* Keth. 19^a^ גַּנּוֹבָא גַּנּוּבֵי למה לך וכ׳ O thou cunning man, what is the use of thy going round about?; Yeb. 91^a^; B. Bath. 133^a^ גַּנָּבָא גנובי Ms. R. (ed. גנבא גנבי, corr. acc.).—Part. pass. מְגַנַּב *crooked.* Targ. Jud. V, 6 אורחן מְגַנְּבָן (h. text עקלקל׳).

Ithpa. אִיתְגַּנַּב, *Ithpe.* אִיתְגְּנֵב, אִיגְּנַב 1) *to be stolen.* Targ. Ex. XXII, 11. Targ. Y. Gen. XL, 15; a. e.—B. Mets. 34^a^ top מי יימר דמִיגַּנְּבָא who can say that it will be stolen? Ib. 24^a^ אִגְּנִיב כסא וכ׳ a silver goblet was stolen from the inn; a. e.—2) *to sneak away.* Targ. II Sam. XIX, 4.

גַּנָּב m. (b. h.) *thief.* Y. Snh. VIII, 26^b^ top גנב בפני עדים גַּ׳ וכ׳ if one carries an object off in the sight of witnesses, he is a thief (amenable to the law Ex. XXI, 37), if in the owner's presence, he is a robber. B. Kam. 57^a^

since he keeps himself hidden ג׳ הוא he is a thief (not a robber). Ib., a. fr. טוען טענת ג׳ he pleads that a thief had stolen the object in his charge. Snh. 26^b ג׳ ניסן וכ׳ a thief (a laborer or tenant who takes fruits) in Nisan or in Tishri is not a thief (to be considered unfit to testify in court); a. fr.—*Pl.* גַּנָּבִים, גַּנָּבִין. Tosef. B. Kam. VII, 8; Mekh. Mishp., N'zikin, s. 13; a. fr.

גַּנָּב, גַּנָּבָא ch. 1) same. Targ. Ex. XXII, 1; a. e.—Ber. 5^b (prov.) בתר ג׳ גנוב וכ׳ steal after the thief (take thine own stealthily from him), and thou hast a taste (of theft), v. גְּנַב. Snh. 22^a (prov.) חסריה לג׳ נפשיה וכ׳ when strength fails the thief, he pretends to be honest.—*Pl.* גַּנָּבִין, גַּנָּבַיָּא, גַּנָּבֵי. Targ. Y. Ex. XX, 13; a. fr.—Ab. Zar. 70^a. Snh. 109^a, v. אַתְ; a. fr.—2) *cunning.* B. Bath. 133^a, v. גְּנַב *Pa.*

גֶּנֶב m.=גְּנֵיבָה q. v.

גְּנֵבָא, v. גְּנַב ch.

גְּנֵבָה, v. גְּנֵיבָה.

גַּנֶּבֶת f. (denom. of גַּנָּב) *inclined to steal. Pl.* גַּנָּבִיּוֹת. Gen. R. s. 45, v. גּוֹנֶבֶת.

גִּינְבְּרָא, גַּנְבְּרָא m. (=גִּיבַּר) *strong man, giant.*—*Pl.* גַּנְבְּרַיָּא, גַּנְבְּרֵי. Targ. Prov. IX, 18 גנברי ed. Lag. (ed. Vien. גוברי, some ed. גנסרי, corr. acc.). Targ. Y. Gen. XIV, 1 גיובריא (read גִּינְבְּ׳). Targ. Y. Deut. II, 10 sq. [Ib. 11 מישר גיונברי, corr. acc.]

גִּנְבְּרָא *ginger,* v. גִּינְ׳.

גַּנְבְּתָא f. (גנב) *thief.* Gen. R. s. 92 גנבא בר ג׳ thief (Benjamin), son of a thief (Rachel); Tanh. Mikk. 10 (ref. to Gen. XXXI, 19).

גְּנְגִּידִין m. (γιγγίδιον) *gingidium,* a kind of chervil (bitter herb; v. Sm. Ant. s. v.). Y. Pes. II, 29^c top (expl. תמכה).

גִּינְגִּילוֹן, גִּנְגְּלוֹן, גִּינְ׳ m. (cingulum) *girdle,* v. גִּלְגְּלִין.

גנגלים, v. גִּלְגְּלִין.

גַּנְדֵּר I (גדר *to be rounded,* v. גַּד II; cmp. כדר; v. Nöld. Neusyrische Gramm. p. 39) *to roll.* Targ. O. Gen. XXIX, 3; 8; 10 (ed. Berl. נדר, v. Berl. Targ. O. II, p. 10; Targ. Y. ib. 13 נדר, some ed. גדר). Targ. I Kings XIV, 10 כמא דמְגַנְדְּרִין בגולגלא (Var. דמנדרין) as they roll with a (threshing) roller (h. text יבער הגלל..).—Gitt. 69^b ונִיגַנְדְּרֵיה וכ׳ (Rashi ולג׳) and let him roll it sixty times. Ab. Zar. 28^a ונִיגנדר (some ed. וניגדר).

Ithpa. אִיגַּנְדַּר *to be rolled; to roll one's self.* B. Kam. 35^a למקלייה ואִיגַּנְדּוּרֵי בקיטמא Ms. M. (ed. ואיגנדר, v. Rabb. D. S. a. l. note) to burn the stack in order to roll himself in the ashes. Ib. קמִגַּנְדַּר בקיטמיה Ms. M. he did roll himself in its ashes. Gitt. 77^b איג׳ גיטא Ar. (ed. אזל, Rashi to Sabb. 80^a quotes איג׳) the letter of divorce (thrown over to the woman) rolled and fell &c. Yeb. 17^a (prov.) קבא רבא .... מִיגַּנְדַּר וכ׳ the large and the small measure (both instruments of fraud) roll together and arrive at hell, and from hell &c., i. e. all the low elements meet in those Babylonian places.

גַּנְדֵּר II (גדר, cmp. גָּדַר *Hithpa.*), *Ithpa.* אִיגַּנְדַּר *to lord it.* Taan. 23^b מִגַּנְדְּרָא עלי she lords it over me (being proud of her beauty; (Ms. M. אתא ומרדא ליה).

קֻנְטְרוֹפוּס, גַּנְדְּרוֹפוּס m. (corrupt. of κυνάνθρωπος or of λυκάνθρωπος, sub. νόσος; for rejection of ל, v. בּוּרְיָר) *lycanthropy,* a form of melancholy, the patient so afflicted believing himself to be a wolf (or a dog) and spending his nights among tombstones; also (ὁ λυκάνθρωπος) *the person so afflicted.* Hag 3^b אימר גנדריפס אחדיה ed. (Ms. M. גדרפוס, Var. גנדרופס, גנס׳, גרדפוס, v. Rabb. D. S. a. l. note) say, lycanthropy has seized him.—Y. Gitt. VII, beg. 48^c חיוצא בלילה קניטרופיס; Y. Ter. I, 40^b קנוטרוכוס (corr. acc.) he who goes out at nights is merely a lycanthrope (but not insane).

גנדריפס, v. preced.

גַּנֵּה, v. גְּנַה I.

גַּנָּה, גִּנָּה, v. גַּן.

גְּנָה, v. גנר.

גְּנוֹבָא (=גַּנָּבָא) *cunning.* Keth. 19^a, v. גְּנַב *Pa.*

גְּנוֹבָא m. (גנב) *stolen, secret. Pl.* גְּנוֹבַיָּא. Targ. Prov. IX, 17 (Ms. גְּנִיבֵי).

גְּנוּבְתָּא I f., **גּוֹנְבָא** m. (גנב) *tail.* Targ. Job XL, 17 Ms. (ed. דונביה). Targ. Y. Deut. XIV, 9 גּוֹנְבֵיה. Sabb. 77^b. M. Kat. 17^a; a. e.

גְּנוּבְתָּא II f. (גנב) 1) *theft, stolen object,* v. גְּנֵיבוּתָא.—2) *fallacy, fallacious reply* (v. גְּנַב). Ab. Zar. 44^b מאי גְּנוּבְתֵּיה wherein lies the fallacy of his answer? Ib. גְּנוּבְתָּה מהכא its fallacy comes in from here (consists in this).

גְּנוּגֶנֶת, גְּנוּגְנִית* f. (גנן, cmp. גַּנּוּן) a sort of *parasol made of osier* and used by field laborers. Kel. XVI, 7 גנוגנת העני Ar. (Mish. גְּנוּגְנוֹת pl., Talm. ed. גנוגנית, Maim. comment. ed. Derenbourg גְּנוּנֶת). [Ar. a. R. S.: *the poor man's bag.*]

גִּנּוּי* m. (גנר, cmp. גְּנַאי) *shame.* Y. Yoma VI, 43^c the order of confession is עוו פשעו חטאו in order not to mention גִּנּוּיָין של ישראל the shame of Israel (by bringing the name of Israel in direct connection with פשעו as the harshest of the three expressions).

גנויה, Y. Shebi. VI, 36^c. v. גִּנָּא.

גַּנּוּן, גִּינּוּן m. (גנן) *baldachin* (the Greek θάλαμος), *bride-chamber, state room.* Cant. R. to I, 4 (play on *ganno,* ib. IV, 16) לגַנּוּנו to his state room (the Tabernacle). Ib. to V, 1; Num. R. s. 13. Pesik. R. s. 5.—Num. R. l. c.

מהו גַּנִּי גִּנּוּנִי מה חכילה וכ׳ *ganni* (Cant. IV, 16) means "my state room"; as the bridal curtain is embroidered in variegated colors, so was the Tabernacle &c.; a. e.

גְּנָנָא, גְּנוּנָא, גִּינּוּ׳, גִּנּוּן ch. same; 1) *cover, shade, baldachin;* esp. *bridal chamber, state-room.* Targ. Y. Gen. XIV, 13 גננא cover. Targ. Is. IV, 5 בגנון (read כג׳, ed. Lag. כגנון, h. text חפה). Targ. Job XV, 32 Var. his enclosure (v. כְּילְתָא) shall not be גנונא ed. Lag. (ed. גננא) a (wreathed) state-room (h. text רענגה; cmp. Cant. I, 16). Targ. Y. Ex. II, 1 גי׳ דהדלולא. Targ. Ps. XIX, 6; a. e.—Y. Yeb. XIII, 13ᶜ bot. עבד לה גנון if a bridal room is prepared for her. Y. Ber. II, 5ᵃ they went מיעבד גְּנוּנֵיה דר׳ וכ׳ to prepare the bridal chamber of &c.; Bab. ib. 16ᵃ קטרין ליה גננא wreathed the bridal chamber of &c. Ruth R. to I, 17 (sect. 3) [read:] דיהא גְנוּנָךְ חסר וכ׳ that thy state-room in the hereafter have one jewel less than &c., i. e. that the jewel given thee in this world be deducted from thy future reward.—2) (v. גנר) *couch, breeding place.* Targ. Job XL, 22. Ib. 31.

גְּנוּנִים, v. גְּנִירִים.

גְּנוּנִית f. (v. גִּנּוּן) *couch.*—*Pl.* גְּנוּנִיּוֹת. Y'lamd. to Deut. X, 12 quot. in Ar. (ref. to בַּגַּנִּים, Cant. VIII, 13) when the students at college sit ג׳ ג׳ arranged by couches (school forms).

גְּנוּנִיתָא, גִּינּוּ׳, גְּנוּנִיתָא f. (v. גַּן) (*hortulus,*) *garden at the house, pleasure-garden.* Targ. Y. Ex. II, 21.—Ber. 43ᵇ. Y. Kidd. IV, end, 66ᵈ ג׳ של ירק vegetable garden; a. fr.—*Pl.* גְּנוּנְיָיתָא, גְּנוּנְיָאתָא. B. Bath. 68ᵃ ᵇ.—Esp. (=גַּן עֵדֶן) *paradise.* Targ. Y. Gen. XLVI, 17; a. e.

גְּנוּנִיתָא pr. n. f. *G'nunitha,* (*gardener*) legendary name of Esther's attendant for the third day of the week (with ref. to Gen. I, 11). Targ. Esth. II, 9.

גְּנוּנֶת, v. גְּנוּגְנִית.

גְּנוּס, pl. גְּנוּסִים, גְּנוּסִין, v. גִּירְנִיסְיָא.

גְּנוּסָא, v. גְּנִיסָא.

גְּנוּסְיָא, v. גִּירְנִיסְיָא a. גְּנִיסַיָּא.

גְּנוּסַיָּא, v. גְּנִיסַיָּא.

גְּנוּסֵר, v. גִּינּוּסַר.

גְּנוּת f. (גנר; v. גִּנּוּי) *blame, disgrace.* Pes. X, 4. Arakh. 16ᵃ בא לידי גְנוּתוֹ may be induced to speak of his shortcomings; a. fr.

גְּנוּתָא ch. same. Targ. Y. Gen. XXXIV, 14. Targ. Koh. V, 5.

גָּנַז [*to cut off, set aside,*] 1) *to save, hoard up, reserve.* B. Bath. 11ᵃ; Tosef. Peah IV, 18 אבותיך גָּנְזוּ וכ׳ thy ancestors saved (treasures) and increased the savings of their fathers. Ḥag. 12ᵃ למי גְּנָזוֹ for whom has He reserved it?; a. fr.—*Part. pass.* גָּנוּז, f. גְּנוּזָה *reserved.* Pes. 119ᵃ; Snh. 110ᵃ.—2) *to remove from sight, hide* (in order to prevent desecration). Tosef. Sabb. XIII (XIV), 5; Sabb. 116ᵃ. Meg. 26ᵇ a book of the Law in a state of decay גּוֹנְזִין אותו וכ׳ is buried by the side of a scholar; a. fr.—3) *to declare a book apocryhal, to suppress, prohibit the reading of.* Pes. 56ᵃ ג׳ ספר רפואות suppressed the Book of Remedies. Sabb. 115ᵃ אף הוא צוה עליו וּגְנָזוֹ he (R. Gamliel junior), too, gave orders about it and suppressed it; Tosef. ib. XIII (XIV), 3; a. fr.—Sabb. 30ᵇ בקשו חכמים לִגְנוֹז וכ׳ the scholars wanted to suppress (declare uncanonical) the Book of Koheleth; a. fr.

Nif. נִגְנַז 1) *to disappear, be hidden.* Yoma 52ᵇ משנ׳ הארון נִגְנְזָה וכ׳ when the Holy Ark was removed, there disappeared with it &c.; Tosef. ib. III (II), 7. Tosef. Sot. II, 2 מגילתה נִגְנֶזֶת וכ׳ the scroll used for the suspected wife (סוטה) was hidden away under the door pivot of the Temple; a. fr.—2) (of books) *to be prohibited, suppressed.* Sabb. 13ᵇ אלמלא הוא נ׳ וכ׳ but for him, the Book of Ezekiel would have been suppressed; Ḥag. 13ᵃ; Men. 45ᵃ; a. e.

גְּנַז ch. same, *to save.*—Targ. II Kings XX, 17.—Part. pass. גְּנִיז, f. גְּנִיזָא 1) *hidden, stored up, reserved.* Targ. II Chr. XXXIV, 15. Targ. I Sam. XXV, 29.—*Pl.* גְּנִיזִין, גְּנִיזָן. Targ. O. Deut. XXXII, 34. Targ. Hos. XIII, 12.—Targ. Prov. XXX, 18.

Ithpe. אִתְגְּנִיז *to disappear.* Targ. Y. Num. XX, 2; 13.

גֶּנֶז m. (b. h.; preced.) *store, treasure.*—*Pl.* גְּנָזִים, constr. גִּנְזֵי. Ḥag. 12ᵇ. Pes. 119ᵃ בית גְּנָזָיו של וכ׳ Korah's storehouse. Ib. 118ᵇ bot. בית גְּנָזֵיהֶם Ms. M. 2 (Ms. M. 1 גְּנָזָיו; ed. גנוזה, corr. acc.).

גִּנְזָא, constr. גְּנַז, גְּנִיז ch. 1) same. Targ. I Sam. XXV, 29 גְּנָז; Targ. Y. Deut. XXXI, 16 גְּנִיז.—*Pl.* גִּנְזִין, גִּנְזַיָּא, גִּנְזֵי. Targ. Ps. CIV, 13. Targ. Hos. XIII, 15. Targ. Y. Deut. XXXIII, 19 the hidden treasures.—Koh. R. to XI, 1 [read:] ועול לבי גנזי הירדי וכ׳ and go into my treasury and take from there seven suits of clothes.—2) *garments kept in the royal treasury* (cmp. Koh. R. l. c., a. טַרְזִיָּא). Targ. Esth. I, 3 גנזי מילתא fine woolen garments. [Ab. Zar. 35ᵇ, v. גַּפְוָזָא I.]

גנזבייה, v. גִּנְזַכָּיָה.

***גִּנְזַכָּה** f. (b. h. pl. גִּנְזַכִּים; גנז, with format. ך, cmp. בזך) *treasury, store.* Gen. R. s. 61 (homiletic interpret. of קטורה, cmp. קוֹרְטוֹר׳) כזה שהוא חותם ג׳ ומוצאה וכ׳ (not ומוציאה) like one who seals up a store and finds it sealed and knotted; Yalk. ib. 109 גניזבא some ed. (corr. acc.); ib. Chron. 1074.

***גִּנְזַכָּיָה** (v. next w.) *of Ginzak.* Y. Ber. II, 5ᵇ top Benjamin of G. (Nidd. 65ᵃ מנימין סקסנאה).

גִּינְזָק, גִּנְזָק pr. n. pl. *Ginzak, Gazaka,* a city in the North of Media Atropatene (v. Neub. Géogr. p. 375). Kidd. 72ᵃ; Yeb. 17ᵃ, expl. נהר גוזן (II Kings XVIII, 11). Ab. Zar. 34ᵃ; 39ᵃ; Gen. R. s. 33 (mentioned in connection with R. Akiba); Taan. 11ᵇ (v. Rabb. D. S. a. l. note 7). Treat. S'maḥ. ch. XII.

גְּנַח (v. גּוּהָא) *to groan*, esp. 1) (with or without מלבו) *to sigh heavily under an attack of angina pectoris.* Tem. 15^b; B. Kam. 80^a; Tosef. ib. VIII, 6; Keth. 60^a.—2) *to cough and spit blood.* Gen. R. s. 32, end ג׳ דם; Tanh. Noah 9 ג׳ וכוהה דם, v. כָּהַח.

גְּנַח I ch. same, *to groan, rumble* (of the underground thunder at earthquakes). Ber. 59^a ג׳ גוהא (Ms. M. גְּנָא, Ms. O. גְּנַה), v. גּוּהָא.

Pa. גַּנַּח same, esp. *to utter disconnected sounds* (staccato), opp. to ילל to utter a trembling plaintive sound (tremolo). R. Hash. 34^a.

***גְּנַח** II *to cut, pass swiftly.* Targ. Ps. VIII, 9 Ar. (ed. חָלִיק, h. text עובר).

Pa. גַּנַּח *to castrate.* B. Mets. 90^b top they take them stealthily וּמְגַנְּחִין יתהון (Ms. M. וגוזין, v. גְּזַז; v. Rabb. D. S. a. l. note). [גנח prob. misread for גוזו, a. מגנחין for מְגַוְּזִין, denom. of גַּוָּזָא II. Cmp. form of letters, Sabb. XII, 5; 103^b; 104^b.]

גְּנָה, גני (cmp. גָּנַן) *to cover, be covered.*

Pi. גִּנָּה, גִּינָּה *to overshadow, to obscure, to put to shame; to censure.* Snh. 92^b היו מְגַנִּין את החמה וכ׳ obscured the sun with their beauty. Gitt. 58^a היו מג׳ את הפז וכ׳ they outshone the finest gold with their beauty. Snh. l. c. בקש לְגַנּוֹת וכ׳ he would have attempted to excel all the praises &c.—Sabb. 33^b שגי׳ who criticised (the Roman government); a. fr.—Part. pass. מְגוּנֶּה *deserving to be covered up, reprehensible, indecent; ugly.* Pes. 3^a דבר מג׳ an ugly expression e.g. טמא in place of לא טהור. Ber. 33^b הרי זה מג׳ he is to be reprehended; ib. 45^b, opp. משובח; a. fr.

Hithpa. הִתְגַּנָּה *to make one's self reprehensible, to become repulsive.* Hag. 15^b ומה לִמְתְגַּנִּין בה וכ׳ if such regard is paid to those who abuse the knowledge of the Law &c., opp. משתבוחין. Kidd. 41^a he may see in her דבר מגונה וְתִתְגַּנֶּה עליו something objectionable, and she may become repulsive to him. Yoma 78^b, v. אִיבָה. Keth. 65^b; a. fr.

גְּנָא, גְּנֵי ch. same, *to be shaded, to lie down, sleep.* Targ. Job XL, 21. Targ. Y. Deut. XXIV, 13. Targ. II Esth. I, 4 מיגנֵי to recline for meals, *to dine;* a. fr.—Gitt. 68^a וּגְנָא and fell asleep. Sabb. 65^a did not allow his daughters גַּנְיָאן גבי הדדי (Ms. M. דגַנְיָין) to sleep together. Ib. 129^a וניגְנֵי וכ׳ let him lie in the sun. Yoma 78^b ולִיגְנֵי and let him sleep (in his sandals). Snh. 109^b גְּנֵי אפוריא lie down on the bed. Y. Taan. I, end, 64^b כותלא דגָנְאֵי ביה a wall of a room in which people sleep; ib. IV, 64^d bot. דגַנְיֵי.—B. Bath. 58^a גָּנֵי Ar. (ed. גָּאנֵי) is lying. [Ber. 59^a Ms. M., v. גְּנַח I.]

Pa. גַּנֵּי (with על) *to cover, protect.* Targ. Is. IV, 5. Targ. Y. Deut. XXVIII, 15.

Af. אַגְנֵי *to cause to lie down.* Targ. II Esth. I, 3 (2) ואַ׳ וכ׳ and made them lie down (for meals),—Snh. l. c. they had a bed דהוו מַגְנֵי עלה וכ׳ upon which they made strangers lie. Num. R. s. 18; Tanh. Korah 10 ואַגְנִיתֵיה וכ׳ and made him lie down on his bed; Snh. l. c.—B. Mets. 84^b [read:] אַגְנְיַין בעליתאי hide me, I pray, in my room (v. Rashi a. Rabb. D. S. a. l. note 7). Ib. [read:] אגניתיה בעליתיה I kept his body in his room.

Ithpe. אִיתְגְּנֵי, אִיגַּנֵּי (v. preced. Hithpa.) *to be disgraced, become repulsive.* Targ. II Chr. XV, 16.—Y. Ab. Zar. III, 42^c bot. [read:] דלא יהוון מִיתְגַּנְּיִין בי that they may not be disgraced through me (be ashamed of me). Sabb. 140^b ואתי לְמִתְגַּנְיָא and he may be disgraced. Ib. 65^a מידי דמִיתְגַּנְיָא ביה something by which she is exposed. Keth. 65^b תִּתְגַּנֵּי ותִתְגּ׳ let her look repulsive (her husband being dead).

גְּנֵיב־, v. גְּנַב.

גְּנִיבָה, גְּנִיבָא pr. n. m. *G'niba.* Gitt. 31^b; 62^a. Y. ib. VI, 48^a bot. כהדא ג׳ אתאפק וכ׳ as in the case of one G'niba who was carried out to be put to death.

גְּנֵבָה, גְּנֵיבָה f. (b. h.; גנב) *theft, the stolen object; deception.* B. Kam. X, 3 ויצא לו שם ג׳ בעיר and the report of his being robbed had spread in town. Ib. 8 did not know בִּגְנֵיבָתוֹ that it had been stolen. Y. Sot. III, end, 19^b ג׳ אחת one theft; Kidd. 18^a. Ib. גְּנֵיבוֹ אלף if what he has stolen is worth one thousand (Shekel &c.); a. fr.—*Pl.* גְּנֵבוֹת, גְּנֵיבוֹת. Ib.—Mekh. Mishp., N'zikin, s. 13 גנב שלש ג׳ וכ׳ he committed three frauds &c., v. גָּנַב. Num. R. s. 7; a. fr.

גְּנֵיבוּת f. same; ג׳ דעת *deception.* Y. Snh. VI, 23^d bot., sq.

גְּנֵיבְתָא, גְּנֵיבוּתָא, גְּנֵב׳ ch.=h. גְּנֵיבָה. Targ. Y. Ex. XXII, 2 sq. (O. גְּנוּבְתָא); a. fr.—*Pl.* גְּנֵיבָתָא. Ab. Zar. 26^a עבוד ג׳ committed thefts.

גְּנִיגְרִי *hunter*, v. קְנִיגְרִי.

גְּנִיזָא, גְּנִיז 1) Part. pass. of גְּנַז.—2)=גִּנְזָא.

גְּנִיזָה f. (גנז) *removal of sacred objects.* Sabb. XVI, 1 טעונים ג׳ must be removed (in case of their being unfit for use). Meg. 26^b זו היא גְּנִיזָתָן this (their use for shrouds) is their removal.—[Pes. 118^b בית גניזה, v. גְּנַז].

גְּנֵירִי, v. גְּנַאר.

גנירין, v. גְּנִינִים.

גנין, v. גִּפּוּן ch.

גְּנִינִים, גְּנוּנִים m. pl. (contr. of גְּוָונוּנִ׳, v. גִּוּוּן) *of many colors.* Nidd. III, 3 (24^b) שפיר מלא גנו׳ (an abortion consisting of) a bag full of a many-colored substance; (Ar. גנו׳—for which in Gem. ib. גוונים; incorr. opin.= גבנונים *lumps of a fleshy substance*, v. Ar. s. v.); Bekh. VIII, 1 גנו׳ (Talm. ed. 47^b גנו׳); Kerith. I, 5 גנו׳ (Talm. ed. 7^b גנו׳).—Esp. *a sort of flour containing all shades of colors.* Tanh. T'savveh 13 סאה גנו׳ (ed. Bub. 10 גבונים, Ms. R. גנרינך, oth. corrupt. v. ib. note 63) one measure full of all sorts of flour; Y. Peah VII, 20^a bot. גנירין (corr. גנינין; omitted in Yalk. Hab. 565).—Sot. 36^b גְּנוּנֵי מלכות royal *manners* (v. גִּוּוּן a. גִּוְּנָא; Ar. גְּנוּסֵי, גְּנִיסֵי, v. גְּנִיסְיָא).

גְּנִיסָא, גְּנִיסְתָּא (גְּנוּ׳) f. (adopted fr. γένος) *gens, family, gentry.* Targ. Y. Ex. XII, 47. Targ. Y. Deut. XXIX, 17.—Targ. Y. Gen. VI, 9 גְּנִיסַת נח (גְּנִסַּת) of the family of Noah; a. fr.—*Pl.* גְּנִיסָתָא, גְּנִיסָאתָא, גְּנִיסָן. Targ. Y. Deut. X, 6. Targ. Y. Num. XXVI, 7 (some ed. גניסתא read סְתָא . . .). Targ. Job XXXI, 34; a. e.—Masc. pl. גְּנִיסַיָּא. Targ. Ps. CVII, 41, v. next w.

גְּנִיסַיָּא, גְּנוּ׳ m. pl. (v. preced. a. גְּרִנִיסְיָא) *nobles, gentry.* Targ. Y. Gen. XXXVI, 29 sq.; Deut. II, 12 (some ed. סְרַיָּא . . ., corr. acc.; h. text חֹרִי).

גְּנִיסִין, v. גְּרִנִיסְיָא.

גְּנִיסַר, v. גְּרִנֵיסַר.

גְּנִיסְתָּא, v. גְּנִיסָא.

גָּנַן (b. h.) *to protect, surround.* Denom. גַּן.

גְּנַן ch. same. Targ. Zech. VIII, 4.

Af. אַגֵּין same. Targ. O. Gen. VII, 16 (some ed. אֲגֵין, fr. גִּין, Y. I אַגֵּין, h. text סגר). Targ. Ex. XXXIII, 22. Targ. Is. I, 6; a. fr. (interchanging with אֲגֵין).—Sot. 21[a] אגוני מַגְּנָא does protect, contrad. fr. אצולי to rescue. Keth. 77[b] אגוני לא מגנא will it (the Law) not protect (me)? Ab. Zar. 15[b] bot. מגנו עלוייהו they (the bucklers) protect them. Ib. 16[a] מגנו עלוון they (the Persian soldiers) protect us.

גַּנָּן m. (denom. of גַּן) *gardener.* Lev. R. s. 5.—*Pl.* גַּנָּנִין, גַּנָּנִים. Kel. XVII, 1. Yoma V, 6; a. e.

גַּנָּנָה, גַּנָּנָא ch. same. Y. Snh. II, end, 20[d]; Gen. R. s. 80, v. גִּינְתָא.

גְּנָנָא, v. גְּנוּן.

גְּנֶסֶת, v. גְּנִיסָא.

גנסרי, v. גִּנְבְרָא.

***גַּנְפָא**=גַּפָּא.—*Pl.* גַּנְפֵי. Targ. Mic. I, 16 (ed. Lag. a. oth. גרפ׳), v. גַּדְפָא a. גַּדְנְפָא.

גַּנְתָּא, v. גִּינ׳.

גַּס I m. *falcon,* v. גַּז.

גַּס II m. (v. next w.) *the thick part of the web, border, hem.* Tosef. Sabb. XII (XIII), 1 כ״ג הגס (Var. הנס; Y. ib. XIII, beg. 14[a] הגב, corr. acc.), v. גַּב; Bab. ib. 105[a] על הגס (some ed. הנס).

גַּס III m., **גַּסָּה** f. (גסס, cmp. גּשׁשׁ) *bulky, huge, large.* Hull. III, 1 עוף הגס large fowl (goose, hen &c.), opp. דק.—(בהמה)גסה *large cattle* (beeves &c.), opp. דקה sheep, goats &c. Ib. Y. Pes. IV, 30[d] bot.; a. fr.—Dem. II, 4 sq. בגסה, במדה ג׳ in large quantities, *wholesale.*—Ber. 6[b] פסיעה ג׳ large, hasty step. Pes. 107[b] אכילה ג׳ a large, full meal.—Shebi. IV, 1 (to gather wood or stones) את הגס הגס the larger the better, i. e. picking out the largest for using them in buildings &c., clearly indicating that it is not done for the purpose of improving the field; expl. Y. ib. beg. 35[a] כדרך שהוא מלקט .... בין דקים לגסים as one gathers in his neighbor's field distinguishing between the small and large pieces.—Nidd. 2[b] הַגַּס הַגַּס she noticed the menstruation only when coming in large quantities (in clods, while the blood had previously been imperceptibly gathering).—*Pl.* גַּסִּים, גַּסִּין, f. גַּסּוֹת. Y. Shebi. l. c. Hag. 26[a]; a. fr.—גַּס רוּחַ *presumptuous, haughty.* Ab. IV, 7. [Ib. גס·לבו, v. גוּס.]—*Pl.* גַּסֵּי רוח. Y. Pes. V, 32[a] bot.; a. fr.—גַּסִּים (sub. נקבים) *movement of the bowels,* v. גָּדוֹל end. Y. Ber. II, 4[d] top; a. e.

גַּסָּא ch. f. (sub. מִידָּה) *large quantity.*—בג׳ *intemperately.* Esth. R. to I, 8 לפום דהמן שאתן ג׳ because there (at the Persian court) they used to drink immoderately.

גָּסָא, v. גַּסָּה.

גִּסְבַּר, Tosef. Shebi. II, 7 השבת והג׳ some ed., v. כּוּסְבַּר.

גָּסָה (denom. of גַּס; cmp. אכילה גסה, s. v. גַּס) 1) *to swallow large quantities at a time, to glut.* Der. Er. Zutta ch. V ולא יִגְסֶה בפני וכ׳ must not eat or drink like a glutton in the presence of &c.—Pesik. Vattomer, p. 131[a] (ref. to לחם הקלקל, Num. XXI, 5) I (the Lord) selected for them light food . . . . ., שלא יהא אחד מהם גּוֹסֶה ודלריא אוחזהו lest one of them should eat too much and be seized with diarrhœa; Sifré Deut. 1 Ms. (v. ed. Fr. note 26); Yalk. Num. 764 גוער (corr. acc.); ib. Deut. 790 גוסרודלריא (read גוס׳ ודולריא); ib. Is. 332 גוטס (corr. acc.); Lam. R. to III, 37 גּוֹסָא.—2) *to feel inflated, nauseous; to belch.* Nidd. 63[b] (among the symptoms of approaching menstruation) וגוֹסָה.—V. גּוּסֵר.

גַּסּוּת f. (גַּס III) (with or without רוח) *presumptuousness.* Succ. 29[b]. Kidd. 49[b]; a. fr.

גַּסּוּתָא ch. same. Targ. Ps. X, 2. Ib. CI, 5 גסות עיינין haughty look; a. fr.

גִּסְטְרָא, v. גִּיס׳.

גַּסְטְרָא f. (castra, v. קַסְטְרָא) *military camp, fort.* Sabb. 121[a] אנשי ג׳ של וכ׳ Ar. (ed. גיסט׳, גיסת׳, גרזט׳, v. Rabb. D. S. a. l. note 1) the Roman garrison of Sepphoris. Ber. 32[b] (Ms. M. גרסט׳, Yalk. Is. 332 גסתרא) ועל כל לגיון ולגיון בראתי בו שלשים ג׳ וכ׳ Ms. M. (v. Rabb. D. S. a. l.) for each legion (of minor planets in the constellations) I created thirty camps, and for each camp thirty squares, v. קרטון.—Sot. 13[b] sq. שלחה מלכות הרשעה אצל ג׳ בית וכ׳ the Roman government sent to the camp of Beth Peor; (Yalk. Deut. end גיס׳; Pesik. Zutr. Deut. p. 134 בלכות של חצרה ושל בית וכ׳).—Hence: pr. n. pl. *Castra.* Lev. R. s. 23 כגון ג׳ לחיפא as Castra is hostile to Haifa; Lam. R. to I, 17 קסטרא.—*Pl.* גַּסְטְרִיּוֹת. Gen. R. s. 28 אריות ג׳; Yalk. ib. 47 חיילות גי׳, read אהלויות וג׳, v. אֲהָלִית.—*2) (cmp. castellum) *reservoir.* Lev. R. s. 15 Ar., Var. קִנְצִיבְרָא (cisterna, κινστέρνα) *cistern* (not extant in ed; B. Bath. 16[a] דְּפוּס).

גַּסְטְרוֹן, v. גַּסְּיטְרוֹן.

גַּסְטְרְיוֹת, v. גַּסְטְרָא.

גַּסִיוּטָאֵי* m. pl. n. gent. (Κασιώτις, Κάσιος) *inhabitants of Casiotis*, a district surrounding Mount Casius, East of Pelusium in Egypt. Targ. Y. I Gen. X, 14 נסיוט׳ (corr. ג׳, Y. II פְּילוּסָאֵי; h. text פתרסים); Targ. I Chr. I, 12 נסיוט׳, נסאט׳ (corr. acc.).

גַּסִּיטְרוֹן m. (κασσίτερος) *tin*. B. Mets. 23[b] [read:] של ג׳. Men. 28[b] ושל גיסט׳ (corr. acc.); cmp. קַסִּיטְרָא.

גסיסין, v. גִּיסְסָא II.

גָּסַס (v. גּוּס II; cmp. גִּיסְסָא III) *to recline, to dine*. Y. Snh. III, 21[c] top אשגח למִיגוס גו וכ׳ cared to remain undisturbed at a banquet among the guests. Esth. R. to I, 8 דבעי מֵיגַס וכ׳ where one wants first to dine and then to drink. Lev. R. s. 28 why dost thou not allow the guests דיִגְסוּן to eat? Koh. R. to II, 17; a. fr.—Denom. מְגַס, מְגִיסְתָּא &c.

גֶּסֶס m., pl. גְּסָסִים (v. preced. a. גִּיסְסָא) *side, arm*. Nidd. 48[b] על גְּסָסֵיהֶן upon their (left) arms.

גִּסְסָא, v. גִּיס׳.

גסתרא, v. גַּסְטְרָא.

גְּעָא, v. גְּעַר.

געא, Koh. R. to XI, 1 לבי געא וגנזר, read לבר גִּנְזִר or לבר גַּזָּא.

גְּעָגוּעַ, גִּיעֲגוּעַ, m., pl. גְּעָגוּעִים, גְּעָגוּעִין, גִּי׳ (reduplic. of געו) *lowing, roaring* trnsf. 1) *homesickness, longing* (as the cow lows after her calf). Sabb. 66[b] בן שיש לו גיע׳ וכ׳ Ms. M. (ed. omit לו) a son who is homesick for his father. Snh. 39[a]. Ib. 63[b].—2) *sulky, rebellious conduct, howling* (of children). Tanh. Shmoth 1; Ex. R. s. 1, beg. שהיו לו ג׳ על אברהם וכ׳ who behaved rebelliously against his father.

גְּעַגַע (=פגעג, cmp. קעקע) *to roll*. *Hithpa*. הִתְגַּעְגַּע, חִגַּ׳ *to roll one's self*. Cant. R. to IV, 11 מִתְגַּעְגְּעִין היו וכ׳ they would roll themselves in the plants around the well (to make their garments flagrant); (Pesik. B'hall. p. 92[b]; Yalk. Deut. 850 מתלכלכין); Midr. Till. to Ps. XXIII מִגַּעְגְּעִין; Yalk. Ps. 691; (Deut. R. s. 7, end מתעגגין).—Lev. R. s. 20, v. next w.

גְּעַגַע, *Ithpa*. אִתְגַּעְגַּע, אִיגַּעְגַּע ch. same, *to roll one's self, wallow*. Lam. R. to II, 2 as long as that hen מִתְגַּעְגְּעָא בקיטמא wallows in the ashes (as Israel lives in its religious element). Koh. R. to XI, 1 מנין מְגַעְגְּעִין בדמא clothes rolled in blood (suspicious of murder).—Tanh. Aharé 3 (ref. to Job XXXIX, 30) חמי אפרוחיו מגעגעין בדם וכ׳ he sees his brood wallowing in blood (Aaron sees his sons dead), and is silent; Lev. R. s. 20 ראה . . . . בְּאַדְמָא Ar. (ed. באדמה); Pesik. Aharé p. 171[b] מְעַגְעֲגִין באדמה (Ms. Carmoli מגעגעין באדמא). [Targ. I, II Gen. XLIX, 11 מעגעגין באדמא.]—Trnsf. *to enjoy one's self, play*. Targ. Ps. CXIX, 117 ואֶתְגַּעְגַּע Ms. (ed. וַאֲגַעְגַּע, h. text שעשע).

גִּעְגְּעָא m. (preced.; cmp. חוגג) *rolling*; (ג׳ דמיא) *cataract*. Lam. R. to I, 17, v. אָגוּגָא.

גָּעָה, גער (b. h.; cmp. גוח) *to burst forth, to roar, low*. Midr. Till. to Ps. CXXXVII, beg., a. e. גָּעוּ וכ׳, v. בְּכִיָּה.—Gen. R. s. 31, end וגָעֲתָה אמו and the whelp's mother roared. Yalk. Gen. 101 ג׳ געירה וכ׳ cried loudly. Hull. 38[a] top גּוֹעָה if the animal lows (when taken to slaughter). Tosef. Bekh. VII, 10 גּוֹעוֹת. Y. Taan. II, beg. 65[a] חָשְׁבֵנוּ כאלו גּוֹעִים וכ׳ regard us as if we were lowing before thee (in agony) like cattle; a. fr.

גְּעָא, גְּעַר ch. same. Targ. I Sam. VI, 12. [Ib. II, 5 וגען some ed., corr. וְגָאַן, v. גאר]. Targ. Job VI, 5, v. פְּרַח.—Y. Taan. II, 65[b] והוו אילין גָּעֲיִין וכ׳ and they lowed from this side &c.; Pesik. Shubah, p. 161[a] מְגַעֲיִין. Y. Ber. II, 5[a] top גָּעַת תורתיה his cow lowed; Lam. R. to I, 16, end.

Pa. גַּעַר same, v. supra.

גְּעִיָּה, גְּעִירָה f. (preced.) *roaring, crying in agony*. Yalk. Gen. 101, v. גָּעַר. Tana d'be El. I, ch. III בכו וגעו ג׳ אחת they wept and burst forth in one loud cry of agony.

גְּעִיּוּתָא ch. same. Lam. R. to I, 16.

גְּעִילָה f. (next w.) *loathing, rejection*. Lam. R. to V, 20; Pesik. R. s. 31; Yalk. Is. 332.

גָּעַל (h. h.; cmp. גאל) *to be covered with impurity, be loathsome; to loathe*. V. preced.

Hif. הִגְעִיל *to remove impurity by means of hot water, to cleanse*. Ab. Zar. V, 12 את שדרכו לְהַגְעִיל יַגְעִיל a vessel which ordinarily is cleansed with hot water, must be purified for ritual purposes by means of hot water. Ib. 76[a] כיצד מַגְעִילָן וכ׳ how must one disinfect them? You put a smaller vessel into a larger one &c.; a. fr.—Y. Ter. XI, 48[a] מַגְעִילָהּ בחמין removes the soakings of T'rumah &c. [Y. Maasr. I, end, 49[b] שיגעיל, read משיעגל, v. עָגַל.] V. הַגְעָלָה.

Nif. נִגְעַל *to be removed through boiling*. Y. Ter. l. c.

Nithpa. נִתְגַּעַל *to be soiled*. Zeb. 88[a].

גְּעַל ch. same. *Ithpa*. אִתְגַּעַל, *Ithpe*. אִתְגְּעֵל, אִיגְּעַל *to be polluted, soiled*. Targ. Is. I, 6.—*Part. pass. Af*. מְגַעַל. Ib. VI, 5; XXVIII, 8.

גְּעַר (b. h. גָּעַר) *to shout, to rebuke*. Targ. Zech. III, 2 ed. Lag. (ed. יְזִיף).—Kidd. 81[b] רחמנא נִגְעַר ביה וכ׳ the Lord rebuke Satan. Gen. R. s. 56 ההוא גברא דִיגְעַר ביה that man of whom it is said, Rebuke him (Satan; with ref. to Zech. l. c.).

גָּעַשׁ (b. h.) 1) *to rush forth, to quake, be agitated*. Yalk. Josh. 35 (cit. fr. Sabb. 105[b], ref. to הר געש Josh. XXIV, 30) מלמד שג׳ עליהם החר להרגם it intimates that the mountain over them quaked (threatening) to slay them; Sabb. l. c. שרגש. Cant. R. to III, 10 ג׳ הים וכ׳

the sea rushed forth and flooded the cave.—2) *to cough* or *sneeze*. Lev. R. s. 3 ג׳ השור וכ׳.

Hif. הִגְעִישׁ *to shake, cause to reel.* Koh. R. to VII, 1 להרעיש וגם לְהַגְעִישׁ וכ׳ to shake and even make reel the mountain &c., v. supra.

Hithpa. הִתְגָּעֵשׁ, *Nithpa.* נִתְגָּעֵשׁ *to be agitated, very busy, anxious.* Ruth R., introd. 2 נִתְגָּעֲשׁוּ ... מעשות ג״ח וכ׳ the Israelites were too much engrossed (in settling) to attend the funeral of Joshua; Koh. R. l. c.—Pesik. R. addit. s. 2 (ref. to יגעשו, Job XXXIV, 20) מִתְגָּעֲשִׁים וכ׳ marched hurriedly to get out &c.

גַּעְתּוֹן pr. n. pl. *Gaton* (*Gatan;* v. Hildesh. Beitr. p. 13 sq.). Y. Shebi. VII, 36[c] ראש מי ג׳ וג׳ עצמה the head of the brook of G. and G. itself; Tosef. ib. IV, 11 ריש מיא דג׳ וג׳ גרמא Var. (ed. ריש מעון רגעתן וכ׳, corr. acc.); Sifré Deut. 51 מגיאתו וגיא׳ עצמה (read מי ג׳ וג׳); Yalk. ib. 874.

גַּף I m. (b. h.; גַּפָּה, v. גּוּף) *body.* בְּגַפּוֹ *alone*; explained Kidd. 20[a] בגופו נכנס בגופו יצא he came with his body, and so he shall go out, i. e. he has no claim for injuries received during servitude; oth. expl. יחידי נכנס וכ׳ if he entered a single man, he must leave a single man, i. e. his master has no right to give him a Canaanite slave for propagating purposes.

גַּף II c. (גנף, cmp. כָּנָף a. כַּף; v. אֲגַף) [*bent, joint,*] 1) *the long portion of the wing.* Zeb. VII, 5 שיבש גַּפָּהּ (Talm. ed. 68[b] שיבשה, v. Rabb. D. S. a. l.) whose wing is withered. Hull. 57[a] שמוטת גַּף a bird whose wing is dislocated.—*Du.* גַּפַּיִם, גַּפַּיִם. Ib III, 4 נשתברו גַּפֶּיהָ whose wings are broken, contrad. to כנפ wing feathers.—2) *arms, shoulders* of a human being. Ohol. VII, 4 נִיטֶּלֶת בג׳ carried by her arms (put around the necks of her supporters); v. אֲגַף.—3) *handles* of a vessel, *sides* &c. Kel. VIII, 3. Tosef. ib. B. Mets. X, 5; a. e.—V. גֵּיף.

גַּפָּא I ch. same; 1) *wing,* also *winged animal* (interch. with גַּדְפָא). Targ. Prov. I, 17; a. fr.—Cant. R. to IV, 8 דמנערא גפא (Gen. R. s. 75 גרמה, Var. אגפה), v. גַּו.—*Pl.* גַּפֵּי, גַּפַּיָּא, גַּפִּין. Targ. Koh. X, 20. Targ. Ez. I, 6; a. fr.—Lam. R. to I, 1 רבתי beg.—*2) *a pole with a hook* for cutting off fruits on high trees; [oth. opin. *a ladder hooked* into the tree.] Ned. 89[b] (a proverbial phrase) רהיט בג׳ ותובלריא he ran with hook and ropes (or baskets); i. e. he tried his utmost.

גַּפָּא II m. (גַּפָּה, cmp. אֲגַף) *city-gate.* B. Bath. 8[a]; B. Mets. 108[a], v. אִגְלָא.—V. next w.

גַּפָּה f. (גַּפָּא m. ch.) (v. preced.) 1) *stone fence with gate.* Peah VI, 2 סמוך לג׳ ולגדיש (Ms. M. לגפא ולגדר, Ar. לגפא) near the stone fence (ready for being carried out) or the stack; Eduy. IV, 4. Kil. II, 8 (Ms. M. א . . .). B. Mets. II, 3.—2) ג׳ של רומי (Ch. גפא דרומאי) *the Capitol of Rome.* Sifré Num. 115 ג׳ של ר׳ (Var. גפר) by the Capitol of Rome (an invocation used by a gentile woman). Men. 44[a] ג׳ של פרס (read רומי, Ar. גפא דרומי). Pes. 87[b] ג׳ דרומאי ed. (Ms. M. דרומי, omitted in some ed.).

גַּפָּה, part. גּוֹפֶה, v. גּוּף I.

גֵּפוּף, גִּפּוּף, v. גִּיפוּף.

גַּפִּי, v. גַּפָּה.

גפל, Y. Sabb. XIII, 14[a] bot. מגפל, v. גָּפַף.

גֶּפֶן c. (b. h. גפן, v. גַּפָּה) *vine,* esp. *grape-vine.* Kil. VII, 2; a. fr.—פרי הג׳ *wine.* Ber. VI, 1; a. fr.—צֶמֶר ג׳ *cotton, cotton tree,* v. גּוּפְנָא. Kil. l. c.—*Pl.* גְּפָנִים. Ib.; a. fr.

גּוּפְנָא, גַּפְנָה, גַּפְנָא, v. גּוּפְנָא.

גָּפַס (גָּפַת) (v. גּפף) *to make air-tight, to paste with gypsum, clay* &c. Kel. X, 5 שֶׁגְּפָסָן עם וכ׳ Ar. a. R. H. G. (ed. שֶׁגְּפָתָן); Tosef. ib. B. Kam. VII, 7 שגפסן (Var. שגפת׳, R. S. to Kel. l. c. שֶׁגְּפָפָן) which one closed up by connecting the paste with the rim (leaving an empty space between the cover and the body of the vessel).

Nif. נִגְפַּס *to harden and be closely consolidated with the ground.* Mikv. IV, 3 Ar., Maim. a. Rabad (v. Tos'f. Yom Tob a. l.; ed. נכבש).

גִּיפְסִים, גְּפָסִים m. pl. (preced.; cmp. גַּפָּה) *paste, plaster,* esp. *gypsum.* Kel. X, 2 we must use בסיד בג׳ וכ׳ lime or gypsum &c. Y. M. Kat. I, 80[b] bot. גירבסם; Y. Shebi. III, 34[c] bot. גִּיפְסוֹס, v. infra. Tosef. Kel. B. Kam. III, 4 גְּפָסִית ed. Zuck. (oth. ed. גְּפָסִים). Hull. 8[a] גפסית רותח; Pes. 75[b] גפסים רותח, Ar. גפסים רותחין. Tosef. Mikv. IV, 7 גפסים; a. fr. [Greek adoption: γύψος, readopted גִּיפְסוֹס, גִּירְבְסוֹס.]

גְּפָסוֹס, v. גִּיפְ׳.

גְּפָסִיס m. (denom. of גפס) *plastering material, gypsum,* v. גְּפָסִים.

גְּפָסִית f. same, v. גְּפָסִים.

גָּפַף (v. גּוּף) *to bend, to join; to press, close;* v. גָּפַס.

Pi. גִּיפֵּף 1) *to attach a rim, to surround.* Kel. XV, 2.—2) *to throw arms around, embrace* (v. גַּף). Yoma 66[b] גי׳ ונשק Ar. (ed. גפף ונישק) whosoever embraces or kisses an idol; Snh. VII, 6 (60[b]) הַמְגַפֵּף.—Pesik. R. s. 26 גִּיפְּפָן וכ׳ he hugged and kissed them. Ib. מְגַפְּפוֹת את וכ׳ threw their arms around the columns.—Y. Keth. VII, 31[c] מְגַפְּפִין סוטה if they have been seen embracing one another, she is amenable to the law of Sotah (v. סוֹטָה); a. fr.—*Part. pass.* מְגוּפָּף *closed, enclosed, surrounded from all sides.* Y. Kil. IV, 29[b] bot.; Y. Erub. I, 19[c] מְגוּפֶּפֶת וכ׳ enclosed on four sides; a. fr.—Tosef. Bekh. IV, 16 שאזניה מְגוּפָּפוֹת וכ׳ whose ears are closed.

Hif. הֵגֵף *to lock up, shut.* Y. Sabb. XIII, 14[a] bot. [read:] ולא כְּמֵגֵף לתוכה וכ׳ we are not treating the case of one shutting (the animal) up in the vivarium; (Y. Bets. III, beg. 61[d] בְּנָגֵל).

גְּפַף ch. same, *to embrace.* Y. Erub. III, 20[d] bot.; VII, 24[d] top נסתיה גַּפְּפֵיה she took him and hugged and kissed him &c.—Snh. 82[b] גַּפְּתָה לאמה (Yalk. Num. 372 גפתא) did she hug her mother there? [Rashi: she made her mother a prostitute.]

Pa. גַּפֵּיף, גַּפֵּיף 1) *to embrace.* Targ. O. Gen. XXIX, 13 ׳גַ (Ms. a. Y. some ed. ׳גַּפְּ). Ib. XXXIII, 4; a. fr.—2) *to fold hands* (in idleness). Targ. Koh. IV, 5.

גָּפַר (v. נפק) *to make thick, tighten.* Denom. גָּפְרִית; fr. which

Pi. גִּיפֵּר *to make water-tight.* Part. pass. מְגוּפָּר, f. מְגוּפֶּרֶת *water-tight.* B. Bath. 97[b]; Tosef. ib. VI, 3 מְגוּפָּרוֹת (defective clay vessels) made tight by a lining of sulphur or pitch.

Hithpa. הִתְגַּפֵּר *to be darkened through sulphur fumes.* Sabb. 18[a]; Y. ib. I, 4[a] top; Tosef. ib. I, 23 מִתְגַּפְּרִין they (the silver vessels) go through the process of sulphuring.

גְּפַר, *Pa.* גַּפֵּר as preced. *Pi.* Y. Sabb. VII, 10[c] top מְגַפֵּר, v. אֱלִיקָה.

גָּפְרִית f. (b. h.; גפר, cmp. כַּבְרִיתָא) *sulphur* [or *bitumen, pitch*]. Sabb. 18[a], a. e., v. גָּפַר Hithpa.

גֶּפֶת, v. גֶּפֶס.

גֶּפֶת f. (גפף) *a pressed hard mass, peat, turf.* Sabb. IV, 1. Ib. 47[b] ג׳ של זתים peat made of olive peels, דשומשמין of poppy seed (after the oil is pressed out). Kel. IX, 5; a. fr.—Ch. גּוּפְתָּא.

גפתא, גפתה, v. גַּפָּה.

גִּפְתִּי, v. גִּיפְטִי.

גֵּץ m. (גהץ, v. Targ. Job. XVIII, 5 s. v. גִּיצָא) [*shining,*] 1) *spark* from the forger's hammer. B. Kam. VI, 6 (62[b]); B. Bath. 26[a]; Sabb. 21[b]. Gen. R. s. 84; Tanh. Vayesheb 1.—2) (cmp. Arab. ג̈ץ *gypsum*) ג׳ יוני *a white earth, chalk; a cross-path laid out with whitened pegs of baked mud or clay* (=יתדות הדרכים). Mikv. IX, 2 ג׳ ד׳ the lime of the crossings sticking to the feet or clothes; cmp. Tosef. ib. VI (VII), 14.

***גַּצָּא** m. (preced.) *lime, pypsum.* בג׳ ואגורא quot. in Ar. fr. Erub. beg.—not to be found.—גצא, M. Kat. 10[b] Var., v. גַּצָּא, נוּצְיָא.

גִּצְמְרָא, גצרא, v. גִּיסְטְרָא.

גקרמונין, Pesik. Shor p. 74[b], read גַּרְזְמִין.

ג״ר ד״ק, ג״ר, a transmutation of letters, v. א״ת. Sabb. 104[a] גופו טימא ארחם עליו though he defiled his body, I shall have mercy &c. Ib. אם... גּוּר בדוק: ג״ר ד״ק (Ar. גּוּר בדוק תהיה) if thou doest so (be chaste), dwell thou in heaven (a dweller . . . shalt thou be).

גֵּר m. (b. h.; גּוּר) 1) *a dweller.* Sabb. 104[a], v. preced.—2) *a stranger.* Tanh. Vayigg. 4 ג׳ גרא שנעשה he is named Gera, because he (Joseph) became a stranger, v. גּוּר.—Esp. *a proselyte, convert to Judaism.* Yeb. 46[b]; Ber. 47[b] לעולם אינו ג׳ וכ׳ one is not a proselyte until he has been &c. Yeb. l. c.; Kidd. 62[b] ג׳ צריך שלשה a proselyte requires a court of three for making declaration and immersion. Kerith. II, 1 ג׳ מחוסר כפרה a proselyte who has not yet offered a sacrifice in the Temple; a. v. fr.—ג׳ צֶדֶק a full, true proselyte, ג׳ תּוֹשָׁב one who, for the sake of acquiring limited citizenship in Palestine, renounces idolatry. Snh. 96[b]; Gitt. 57[b]; a. fr.—ג׳ שקר an insincere proselyte (from impure motives). Y. B. Mets. V, 10[c].—*Pl.* גֵּרִים, constr. גֵּרֵי, גֵּירֵי.—ג׳ גרורים self-made converts, not formally admitted. Ab. Zar. 3[b]; 24[a]; a. e. —גרי אריות *lion-proselytes,* i. e. proselytes from mere fear (with ref. to II Kings XVII, 25 sq.). Hull. 3[b], opp. גרי אמת. Kidd. 75[b]; Snh. 85[b]; a. fr.—גרי חלומות proselytes converted by the advice of a dreamer or an interpreter of dreams; גרי מרדכי ואסתר such as joined the Jewish ranks from motives like those prevalent in the days of Mordecai and Esther (Esth. VIII, 17). Yeb. 24[b]. —Nidd. VII, 3 (56[b]) גרים טועין Ar. (ed. וטועין) proselytes not living in accordance with the Jewish usages.—בן גרים a descendant of proselytes. B. Mets. IV, 10 (58[b]).—Sabb. 33[b] יהודה בן ג׳. [Mode of admission, v. Yeb. 47[a].—Views about converts, v. Num. R. s. 8; Nidd. 13[b]; Pes. 87[b]; a. fr.]. Fem. גִּיֹּרֶת. Gen. R. s. 88, end.—Usu. גִּיּוֹרֶת. Keth. IV, 3; a. fr.

גְּרָא, v. גְּרֵי.

גָּרָא, Targ. Y. Gen. XXX, 11, v. גַּדָּא.

גַּרְאִין, v. גַּרְעִין.

גְּרָאפָּא f. (גרף) *a dish prepared on the hot oven plate after the removal of the coal.* Esth. R. to I, 4 ג׳ דטלופחין lentil cakes baked in the clean oven, contrad. to דטמאשא baked in the ashes.

גָּרֵב pr. n. pl. *Gareb,* near Shiloh, supposed to have been the seat of the Image of Micah (Jud. XVII, 7 sq.). Snh. 103[b].

גְּרַב (cmp. גרף) 1) *to scrape,* v. next ws.—2) *to rob, seize, levy.* Sabb. 148[a] זיל גְּרַבֵיה go and seize him (take his coat until he appears). Ib. לא בדינא גְרַבְתִּיךְ was I not right in summoning thee? Hag. 5[b] גַּרְבוּהוּ they (the royal officers) seized his property. Gitt. 45[a] משום דלא לִיגַרְבוּ וכ׳ in order that robbers should not be tempted to kidnap persons and then offer them for ransom. Ib. 46[b] גרבי להו seized them (for debts).

Ithpe. אִיגְּרַב *to be robbed.* Y. B. Mets. IV, 9[d] אִיגְּרַבְת thou hast been robbed of one Denar.

גָּרָב I m. (preced.) *the quantity collected on emptying the wine or oil press* (v. next w.); in gen. *bottle, keg* as a measure. Ter. X, 8 וכל ג׳ וכ׳ Ms. (ed. כל) and one measured the keg and it contained (as usual) two S'ah.—*Pl.* גְּרָבִים, constr. גַּרְבֵי. Sabb. 13[b]; a. e. three hundred ג׳ שמן *garab* of oil. Bets. 29[a].

גַּרְבָּא, גְּרַב I ch. same, *bottle.* Targ. Jer. XIII, 12; Targ. I Sam. I, 24 (h. text נֶבֶל). Ib. XVI, 20 (h. text נֹאד);

a. e.—[B. Mets. 15^b, v. גְּרִירָא.]—*Pl.* גַּרְבִּין. Targ. I Sam. XXV, 18. Targ. Hag. II, 16 (h. text פּוּרָה, quantity pressed at a time). Targ. Joel I, 17 (h. text פרדות!).

גָּרָב II m. (b. h.; גרב) *itch, scurf.* Bekh. VI, 12; classified ib. 41^a.

גְּרַב, גַּרְבָּא II ch. same. Targ. Y. II Lev. XXI, 20 (Y. I חרסין יבשין, v. Bekh. 41^a). Targ. Deut. XXVIII, 27.—Denom. גַּרְבָּן *one affected with itch.* Targ. O. Lev. l. c.

גַּרְבָּא m. (גרב) *plundering troop.* Ber. 60^b bot. אתא ג׳ וגרביה למתא Ar. (ed. גייסא שבייה) a troop came by night and carried the inhabitants off.

גַּרְבִיתָא f. (גרב) *the scouring* or *sweeping* (wind); ג׳ רוחא North-wind. Targ. Prov. XXV, 23 (h. text צפון). Ib. XXVII, 16 גַּרְבִּיתָא, גַּרְבִּיר׳ (h. text צְפֻנֶיהָ צָפַן!).

גַּרְבֵּל (Parel of גבל) *to knead, roll.* Gitt. 69^a וּנְגַרְבֵּל קיטמא Ar. (ed. ונגד׳, corr. acc.) let him roll (the wicks) in the ashes.

גַּרְבָּן, v. גָּרָב II ch.

גַּרְבְתָא f. (euphem. transpos. of גברתא, v. גֶּבֶר 3) *abnormal length of the membrum virile.* Bekh. 44^b, v. next w.

גִּרְבְּתָן m. (v. preced.) *one having an abnormally long membrum* (one of the blemishes unfitting for priestly service). Bekh. 44^b הג׳ זה בעל קיק (for Mish. בעל גבר). Ib. בעל קיק בביצים ג׳ בגיד Ar. *baal kik* refers to the testicles, *g'rabtan* to the membrum (ed. קרין ... גרבתא וכ׳, v. preced.).

גַּרְגַּ, *Pa.* גַּרְגֵּג (=גרגר) *to be rough, to roughen,* whence 1) *to incite, stir up.* Targ. Prov. X, 12; XXIX, 22 (h. text ערר, גרה). Ib. VI, 3 גַּרֵג הביל חברך ed. Lag. (Var. הביל, חביל) stir up, now, thy friend (for whom thou hast vouched), v. Peshittô a. Syr. Hexapla.—2) *to be excited, impatient.* Targ. Ps. XXXVII, 1; 7; 8 (Ms. תִּגְרַג Pe., h. text תתחר).—3) (v. P. Sm. 773, s. v. גרג 2, cmp. גַּרְגּוּתְנִי, אֲרוּכָה II) *to cover with scurf, heal up.* Targ. Job XXX, 24 יְגָרֵג מחתיה he will heal up the wound he has inflicted.

גַּרְגּוּשְׁתָּא, v. גַּרְגְּשְׁתָּא.

גַּרְגּוּתָא, גַּרְגִּיתָא, גַּרְגְּרִיתָא f. (=גלגליתא, v. גַּלְגְּלָא, cmp. גַּרְגֵּר) *wheel-work, well for irrigating fields.* Ber. 58^a; B. Bath. 91^b (prov.) אפי׳ ריש ג׳ וכ׳ (Ber. ed. גרגר׳, Ms. M. גדגיד׳, corr. acc., v. Rabb. D. S. a. l.) even a superintendent of the well (cmp. בִּירָא) is appointed in heaven. B. Kam. 27^b. B. Mets. 103^a if one says, 'Lend me ג׳ ההוא the use of *this* well', he may restore &c.; בי ג׳ 'a place (in the field) for a well',—he may go on digging wells until he strikes one that suits him. B. Bath. 56^a.—*Pl.* גַּרְגּוּתֵי. B. Mets. l. c.

גַּרְגּוּתְנִי (גַּרְגְּתְנִי Ar.) f. (v. גּוּרְגָּא) 1) *a wicker* or *net work* in the *wine or oil press.* Ab. Zar. 56^b החזיר ג׳ לגת if he placed the net (once used) back into the vat. Hag. 22^b גורג׳ some ed.; Tosef. ib. III, 4. Lev. R. s. 22 he gathered the vessels of the Temple ונתנן לתוך ג׳ and placed them in a net; Gitt. 56^b he took the curtain ועשאו כמין ג׳ and shaped it like &c. Tosef. Kel. B. Mets. VI, 5.—2) (from its shrivelled surface) *the scarry and lifeless surface of a healed up wound, eschar.* B. Kam. 85^a העלתה מכתו ג׳ if, through neglect of medical advice, the wound became scabby; Y. ib. 6^b bot. [read:] עלתה בו ג׳.

גַּרְגִּילָא, v. גַּרְגִּירָא.

גְּרָגִים m. pl. (v. preced. art. a. גּוּרְגָּא) *nets, filters.* Tosef. Kil. V, 25 ed. Zuck., v. אכסלית.

***גַּרְגִּינָא** m. (v. preced.) *wicker-work.* Gen. R. s. 79; Yalk. ib. 133 שוקא דג׳ wicker market (differ. in Koh. R. to X, 8).

גַּרְגִּיר m. (גרר) 1) [*the stimulating plant,*] *garden-rocket, Eruca* (v. Sm. Ant. s.v.). Yoma 18^b; Yalk. Kings 228. Tosef. Shebi. II, 9; Erub. 28^a sq. (Ar. ed. Koh. גרגל).—Shebi. IX, 1 גרגר של אפר (comment. גרגיר) *field-rocket, Eruca agrestis.*—[2) *grain, berry,* v. גַּרְגֵּר.]

גַּרְגִּירָא ch. same; 1) *rocket.* Yoma 18^b ג׳ מצרנאה rocket growing on the balk (Ms. M. מצראה). Sabb. 109^a (Ar. ed. Koh. גַּרְגִּילָא; Yalk. Kings 228 גַּרְגִּירָא).—Gitt. 69^b גַּלְגְּלָא ed. (Ar. s. v. בזר: גַּרְגִּילָא). Ab. Zar. 10^b, v. גזר II.—[2) *berry, grain,* v. גַּרְגְּרָא.]

גַּרְגִּישְׁתָּא, v. גַּרְגְּשְׁתָּא.

גַּרְגִּיתָא, v. גַּרְגּוּתָא.

גַּרְגְּלִידָא m. (=גלגליד׳; גלד) *slice;* ג׳ דליפתא *a slice of turnip,* esp. the upper slice. Bekh. 43^b one whose head resembles לגרגלידה דל׳ Ar. (ed. לגדגלידא, corr. acc.) the upper portion &c. (expl. לפתם ib. VII, 1).—*Pl.* גַּרְגְּלִידֵי. Ber. 39^a (Ar. גורג׳). Ib. 56^a (Var. in Ar. ראשי לפתות). Keth. 61^a.

גַּרְגַּף, v. גְּרַף.

גַּרְגֵּר, גִּירְגֵּר 1) (denom. of גָּרוֹן, גַּרְגֶּרֶת) *to pour down the throat,* opp. שתה to set the lips to the vessel. Par. IX, 4; Tosef. ib. IX (VIII), 6.—*Gitt. 89^a גִּירְגְּרָה בשוק if she quaffs outdoors; [Rashi: walks with outstretched neck (גָּרוֹן)].—2) denom. of גַּרְגַּר) *to pick single berries.* Maasr. II, 6 מְגַרְגֵּר ואוכל he may pick grapes (from the hanging cluster) and eat; ib. III, 9; Y. ib. II, 50^a top.—3) (denom. of גְּרוֹגֶרֶת) *to let the olive shrivel* (on the tree or in the sun on the roof), *to mark out for shrivelling.* Ex. R. s. 36 that olive—while it is yet on its tree, מְגַרְגְּרִין אותו they mark it out for shrivelling (in order to use it for the press). Men. VIII, 4 מְגַרְגְּרוֹ בראש הזית he lets it shrivel on the top of the olive tree; מג׳ בראש הגג in the sun on the roof; [for oth. opin. v. Rashi a. l.].—Ib. 86^a מְגַרְגְּרוֹ תנן או מְגַלְגְּלוֹ תנן does it read *m'garg'ro* (he lets it shrivel) or *m'galg'lo* (he lets it hang until it is fully rounded)?

גַּרְגַּר ch. (v. preced.) *to grow berries, to ripen into full berries.*—Part. pass. מְגַרְגַּר. Targ. Ps. I, 3 ed. Lag. (some ed. סגרגר).

גַּרְגַּר m. 1) (b. h.; גרר=גלל) *berry, grain, heap* (*of pebbles*). Peah VII, 4 ג׳ יחידי single berries (not growing in bunches). Shebi. III, 7 (Bart. גרגיר) a heap of pebbles. —Tosef. Sabb. II, 8 גרגיר של מלח a globule of salt. Sabb. VI, 5 בפלפל בגרגיר מלח (Y. ed. גרגר, Bab. ed. 64[b], 65[a] גלגל, Ms. O. גרגר).—*Pl.* גַּרְגְּרִים, גַּרְגְּרִין. Peah VI, 5; a. e.—2) (=גְּרוֹגֶרֶת) *the shrivelled olive. Pl.* as above. Men. VIII, 3 (85[b]), v. גַּרְגֵּר.—[3) *rocket*, v. גַּרְגִּיר.]

גַּרְגְּרָא ch. same, 1) *berry.*—*Pl.* גַּרְגְּרִין. Targ. Is. XVII, 6.—Targ. Y. I Deut. XXXII, 14 גַּרְגְּרֵי חיטיהון their wheat grains.—[2) *rocket*, v. גַּרְגִּירָא.]

גַּרְגְּרַיִין f. pl. (גרר, v. next w.) *wheel-works* of a well. Targ. II Esth. I, 2 (3) ג׳ דאע wooden wheel-works.

גַּרְגְּרִיתָא, v. גַּרְגּוּתָא.

גַּרְגְּרָן, גַּרְגְּרָן, גּוּרְגְּרָן m. (v. גַּרְגֶּרֶת) *glutton, bibber.* Y. Ber. VI, 10[c] top, v. גַּרְגְּרָנוּת. Pes. 86[b]; a. fr.—Nidd. X, 8 (of one unable to control his sexual appetite).—*Pl.* גַּרְגְּרָנִין. Yoma 39[a] bot., opp. צנועין.—Fem. גַּרְגְּרָנִית. *Pl.* גַּרְגְּרָנִיּוֹת (unable to resist tasting temptation). Gen. R. s. 45; Deut. R. s. 6 (ref. to Gen. III, 6).

גַּרְגְּרָן, גַּרְגְּרָנָא ch. same. Targ. Y. Deut. XXI, 20.—*Pl.* גַּרְגְּרָנֵי. Keth. 60[b] Ar. Var. (ed. גירדני, v. גַּרְדָּנָא).—Fem. גַּרְגְּרָנִיתָא. Targ. Lam. I, 11 (h. text זוללה).

גַּרְגְּרָנוּת f. (preced.) *greed.* Y. Ber. VI, 10[c] top לא לזה גורגרן . . . . בגַרְגְּרָנוּתוֹ וכ׳ not this greedy man must be laughed at, but thou, the sneerer; he acted hastily in his greed &c.

גַּרְגְּרָנִית, גַּרְגְּרָנִיתָא, v. גַּרְגְּרָן h. a. ch.

גַּרְגֶּרֶת (b. h. pl. גַּרְגְּרוֹת *neck*; גרגר; v. גָּרַר, a. גָּרָה) *throat, gullet*; (in ritual law) *wind-pipe, trachea.* Koh. R. to XII, 6; Lev. R. s. 18, v. גָּלָה Hif.—Ex. R. s. 24 the Lord created for man מעין בתוך גַּרְגַּרְתּוֹ a well (mucous membranes) in the trachea. Hull. II, 4 פסק את הג׳ he tore open (instead of cutting) the trachea. Ib. III, 3 פסוקת הג׳ an animal with a split between the rings of the wind-pipe.

גַּרְגִּישׁ׳, גַּרְגּוּשׁ׳, גַּרְגִּישׁ׳, גַּרְגְּשְׁתָּא f. (=גּוּשׁ׳; גשש) =h. גּוּשׁ, 1) *clod, lump of earth.* Targ. Ps. XVIII, 43. Targ. Job VII, 5 (h. text גוש). Targ. Y. Gen. I, 24; a. fr.—*Pl.* גַּרְגִּישׁ׳, גַּרְגְּשָׁתָא. Targ. Job XXI, 33; XXXVIII, 38 (h. text רגבים).—2) *a certain reddish clay*, used also as medicine. B. Mets. 40[a] משום ג׳ the difference of opinion as regards leakage (v. בָּלַע) arises from the different qualities of the clay used for the vessels. Nidd. 20[a] bot. broke apart קורטא דג׳ a piece of potter's clay. Keth. 60[b] דאכלה גרגוש׳ a woman who eats *gargushta* (as an astringent or in place of a cosmetic; v. Sm. Ant. s. v. Creta). Ab. Zar. 38[b].

גַּרְגְּתָנֵי, v. גַּרְגּוּתָנֵי.

גָּרַד (b. h.; v. גרר) 1) *to scratch, scrape, comb.* Sabb. VIII, 6 (81[a]) לִגְרוֹד Ar. a. ed. Y.; a. fr. [Editions a. Mss. mostly גָּרַר q. v.]—*Part. pass.* גָּרוּד *stripped*, v. גַּרְדּוּם.—2) (denom. of גֶּרֶד 2) *to cut the web with its fringes off the loom.* Yoma 72[b] (expl. בגדי השרד Ex. XXXV, 19) בגדים שגּוֹרְדִין אותן כברייתן מכליהן וכ׳ webs which they cut off the looms in their needed shape (so as to require no tailoring), leaving a small portion of the unwoven threads.

גְּרַד ch. same; 1) *to scrape, comb, strip*; trnsf. *to chastise.* Targ. Jud. VIII, 16 וגרד Regia (ed. Lag. גרר, oth. ed. תַבַר; h. text וַיֹּדַע).—Naz. 4[b], v. גְּרֵי.—Part. pass. גְּרִיד. Sabb. 109[b] דגְרִידָא מעילאר וכ׳ which has been stripped of its rind from the top downward.—2) *to rub, create friction* (of sexual connection).—Part. גָּרֵיד. Yeb. 75[b].—[3) *to stimulate the appetite.* Ber. 35[b], a. fr. Ar. (ed. a. Ms. mostly גְּרַר).] [*Ithpa.*, v. גְּרַר.] V. גרר, גרע.

גֶּרֶד m. (גרד) 1) *erasure.* Men. 30[b] Ar. (ed. גֶּרֶר).—2) *that which is combed, fringe.*—*Pl.* גְּרָדִין. Ib. 42[b]; Succ. 9[a].

גַּרְדָּא ch. same, 1) *combing*; ג׳ דסרבלא *the removal of the woolly surface of a thick cloth.* B. Kam. 99[a]; B. Mets. 112[a].—M. Kat. 23[a] went out בג׳ דס׳ (Ms. M. 2 בגרדא) in a fresh scraped and smoothed cloak.—2) *fringe, thread.* Sabb. 134[a] דילמא מידביק ג׳ מיניה (Var. מדביקא גרדתא, v. Rashi a. l.) lest a thread of it stick to the membrum.—*Pl.* גַּרְדִּין, גַּרְדֵּי, גַּרְדַּיָּא. Targ. Y. Num. XV, 38 (ref. to Men. 42[b]). —Bekh. 8[b] כרוכו לי ג׳ מיניה וכ׳ twist for me threads pulled out of it, and I will sew it. Men. 31[b]. [גַּרְדָּא or גְּרָדָא *scraping*, v. גְּרִירָא.—גְּרָדָא *cud*, v. גְּרָרָא I.]

גַּרְדַּאי, v. גַּרְדֵּי.

גַּרְדּוּם m. (גרדם) *a stump.* Ruth R. s. 1 end וילך איש ג׳ 'and a man went' (Ruth I, 1)—a stump, i. e. without any description as to what he took with him (opp. to the description of the return to Palestine, Ezra II, 66); [Yalk. Ezra 1067 גָּרוּד, v. גָּרַד; ib. Ruth 598 גָּרוּד *stripped, alone*, cmp. גְּרִידָא.]—*Pl.* גַּרְדּוּמִין, constr. גַּרְדּוּמֵי. Tosef. Par. XII (XI), 2 ג׳ אזוב stumped stalks of hyssop; ג׳ ציצית (not ציצה); Men. 38[b] ג׳ תכלת remnant of the *tsitsith.* Sifré Num. 115 שיריה וגַרְדּוּמֶיהָ what is left of it or the stump of it; Men. 39[a] שיריו וגַרְדּוּמָיו, expl. ibid. דבעינן שירא לגרדומיו a small remnant of the threads must remain on the stumps; a. e.

גַּרְדּוֹן, גַּרְדּוֹם m. (גרד, cmp. Targ. Jud. VIII, 6 s. v. גְּרַד; cmp. סָרַק) *place of torture and execution,* (*Roman*) *executioner's scaffold, gallows.* Sabb. 32[a] העולה לג׳ לידון he who ascends the scaffold to be punished. Ab. Zar. I, 7 בסילקי ג׳ וכ׳ a basilica, a scaffold &c., interpreted ib. 16[b] בס׳ של ג׳ a basilica for tortures, executions &c., i. e. a basilica for holding court. Pesik. Shimu, p. 118[b] תלאו בגרדון ordered him to be suspended on the gallows (for torture); Y. Taan. IV, 69[b] top תְּלָיָין בג׳ (cmp. Gitt. 57[b], a. e. מסריקנא וכ׳). Tosef. Kel. B. Mets. X, end והגרדין טהור ed. Zuck. (ed. ברדין; corr. acc.) the torturer's block is not affected by levitical impurity.

גַּרְדּוּמָא ch.=h. גַּרְדּוּם.—*Pl.* גַּרְדּוּמֵי. Bekh. 44[a] אשתיור ג׳ roots of the eyebrows remained visible.—Gen. R. s. 33, v. גַּרְזִימֵי.

גַּרְדּוֹן, גרדין, v. גַּרְדּוּם.

גַּרְדִּי, גַּרְ׳, גִּירְ׳ m. 1) (גרד) *wool-dresser*, in gen. *common weaver*, diff. fr. טַרְסִי. [Our w. adopted in Greek a. Latin γέρδιος, gerdius.] B. Bath. 21ª one of the inmates of a court הרוצה לעשות ג׳ . . . that wants to open a business as . . . . weaver. Kel. XII, 4 מסמר הג׳ the weaver's pin (of the shuttle). Sabb. 93ᵇ קנה של ג׳ the weaver's cane (quill); Y. ib. X, 12ᶜ bot. גיר׳; a. fr.—*Pl.* גַּרְדִּיִּים, גַּרְדִּין. Kidd. 82ª; Tosef. ib. V, 14. Eduy. I, 3; Sab. 15ª.—Kil. IX, 10 גרדין, v. אוּת II.—[2) (=גַּדְרִי) *of Gadara*, v. אַבְנִימוֹס.]

גַּרְדִּי, גַּרְדַּאי, גִּירְ׳ ch. same. Targ. Y. Ex. XXXIX, 22; a. e.—Koh. R. to IX, 10 חד גַּרְדַּיי (some ed. גרדייא, corr. acc.); Y. Kil. IX, 32ᵇ bot.; Y. Keth. XII, 35ª bot. גדליי (corr. acc.)—*Pl.* גַּרְדָּאִין, גַּרְדָּאֵי, גִּירְ׳. Targ. Jud. XVI, 14 (some ed. גדרסן, corr. acc.). Targ. Is. XXXVIII, 12 (v. גִּרְדּוּדָא); a. e.—Y. Ab. Zar. I, 39ᶜ bot. גירדאי.—Yoma 20ᵇ, v. אֲבוּב. Sabb. 151ᵇ, v. אַכְסָן.

גרדיון, v. גּוּרְדְּיָרִי.—גרדין, v. גַּרְדּוֹן.

גרדיקי, v. גְּרָרִיקִי.

גַּרְדִּיתָא f. (גרד) *web* or *thread*. Targ. Job VII, 6 גרדית מחי (Ms. גַּרְדָּיַית pl.; h. text ארג) the weaver's thread.

גַּרְדֵּם (Parel of גדם) *to cut off, to lop*.—Ithpa. אִיגַּרְדֵּם 1) *to be lopped*. Men. 38ᵇ איג׳ תכלת וכ׳ if the blue fringe has been lopped off, but the white remains &c. Ib. 39ª גרדומיו דאִיגַּרְדּוּם אִיגַּרְדּוּמֵי does not *gardumav* intimate that they (the fringes) are entirely cut off (leaving no remnant)?—2) אִיגַּרְדַּם, אִיתְגַּרְדַּם (=גרזם, v. גַּרְזִימֵי) *to be nibbled at*. Targ. Ps. XXXIX, 12 היך עמר דאית׳ (Ms. דאיג׳) like wool nibbled at (by moths; h. text כָּעָשׁ).

גרדמני, Sifré Thazr., Neg. ch. I some ed., read גְּרָמָנִי.

גַּרְדָּנָא, גַּרְ׳, גִּירְ׳* m. (גרד) 1)=גַּרְדַּי, *weaver*. Ab. Zar. 26ª there was among them חד גר׳ Ms. M. (ed. גיר׳) one weaver. Ib. ג׳ דלא טריון, v. טַרְיָן. [Var. גרדן, גרדנאר in Rashi a. l., v. Rabb. D. S. a. l. note 90.]—2) *scabby, afflicted with an itch*.—*Pl.* גַּרְדָּנֵי, גִּירְ׳. Keth. 60ᵇ, v. גַּרְגְּרָנָא.

גרדקי, v. גְּרָרִיקִי.

גָּרָה, v. גרי.

גֵּרָה I f. (b. h.; cmp. גַּרְגַּר) 1) *gerah* (a grain), name of a coin. Bekh. 50ª.—2) *the seed of St. John's bread*, v. next w.

גֵּרָה II f. (גרר, v. גִּירָא II) *a shoot, stalk* (of flax or asparagus). Mekh. Mshp., N'zikin, s. 13 המערב את הג׳ בחלתן (Var. גִּירָה, גררה) he who mixes (other) stalks among stalks of fenugrec; Yalk. Ex. 343; Tosef. B. Kam. VII, 8 גידה ed. Zuck. (Var. גירה, גורה). [Löw Pfl. p. 317: *seed of St. John's bread* among seeds of fenugrec.]

גֵּרָה III f. (גרר, cmp. גָּרוֹן, גַּרְגֶּרֶת) 1) [*the rough*, cmp. τραχεῖα,] *throat, larynx with wind-pipe, lungs and heart*. Tam. III, 1. Ib. IV, 3. Yoma II, 7.—2) (b. h.; cmp. גרס) *ground food, cud*. מַעֲלֵה ג׳ *ruminant*. Bekh. 6ª; Sifra Sh'mini Par. 2, ch. III; a. e.

גֵּרָה IV f., v. גֵּר.

גְּרוֹגְרוֹת, בַּר ג׳ pr. n. m. *G'rog'roth, Bar G'rog'roth*, surname of one Judah. Y. Shek. IV, 48ª ר׳ יהודה ג׳ (Bab. ed. גדגדניות, גדגדות, Ms. M. גרוגרות, v. Rabb. D. S. a. l., p. 34, note 20). Yoma 78ª בר ג׳ (Ms. M. בר גרוגרת).

גְּרוֹגֶרֶת f. (גרר, v. גֵּרָה III) [*the rugged, shrivelled*,] *the dry fig*. Sabb. 80ª; B. Bath. 55ᵇ; Kerith. 17ª גרוגרות (corr. acc.). Lam. R. to I, 11 כג׳ of the size of &c. Y. Naz. II, beg. 51ᵈ people call לג׳ תירוש dry figs, too, *tirosh* (Tosaf. to Men. 103ª לגרוגרות); a. e.—*Pl.* גְּרוֹגְרוֹת. Naz. II, 1 if one says, I will be a Nazir abstaining from *g'rog'roth*, he is a Nazir; Tosef. ib. II, 1; v. פְּרִיגּוּר. Maasr. I, 8; a. fr.

גָּרוּד (גָּרוּר) m. (part. pass. of גָּרַד or גָּרַר) *stripped, bare*. Yalk. Ruth 598, v. גַּרְדּוּם.—*Pl.* גְּרוּדִים. Ab. Zar. 33ª גרוד׳ wine jars not lined with pitch; Tosef. ib. IV (V), 10 גְּרוּדִין.—Fem. pl. גְּרוּדוֹת. Y. ib. II, 41ᵇ bot.

גְּרוּדָא* pr. n. pl. *G'ruda*, near Tiberias. Gen. R. s. 79, v. גְּדוּרָא.

גרוזמי, גרוזמין, גרוזמיתא, v. גַּרְזִימִי.

גְּרוּטִי f. (γρύτη) *trash, frippery, broken ware*. Kel. XI, 3 a vessel made משברי כלים מן הג׳ Ar. (ed. גרוטים, Bart. גרוטאות) out of fragments of vessels, or out of small ware &c.—*Pl.* גְּרוּטָאוֹת. Sabb. 123ª זורקה לבין הג׳ (Ms. O. גְּרוּטָאוֹתָיו; R. S. to Kel. l. c. גְּרוּטוֹתָיו) he cast it among the rubbish (considering it no longer a vessel); B. Mets. 52ᵇ בין גרוטותיו (Ms. M. לתוך גריטות׳). Bekh. 13ᵇ; Ab. Zar. 53ª; 71ᵇ; Tosef. ib. V (VI), 3. Tosef. Ḥull. I, 18.

גרויא, v. גְּרִייָא.

גְּרוּם, גְּרוּמָה, v. גְּרַם.

גְּרוּמֵי, גְּרוּמְנֵי m. pl. (γρυμέα, crumena, v. Lidd. a. Scott s. v.;=γρύτη) *trumpery, broken pieces of iron, glassware* &c. B. Bath. 89ᵇ top דיגרומי ed. (Ms. M. דגרומני, Ar. בגרמני) scales used for weighing &c.

גְּרוּמִין, v. גִּירוּמִין.

גְּרוּמְתָא, גְּרוּמִיתָא, v. גַּרְמִיתָא.

גָּרוֹן m. (b. h.; v. גֵּרָה III) *throat, palate*. Gen. R. s. 94 להוט אחר גְּרוֹנוֹ anxious to gratify his appetite, to receive sustenance, v. לָהַט. Ber. 36ª, a. e. חשש בגרונו to have a sore throat; a. e.

גְּרוֹנָא ch. same. Targ. Is. LVIII, 1; a. e.—Succ. 49ᵇ שבע מִגְּרוֹנֵיה he finds satisfaction from his palate, i. e. by taking draughts large enough to gratify his taste.

גְּרוּנְדָּא m. (גרד, cmp. גָּרִיד) *hard, stony clod*.—*Pl.* גְּרוּנְדֵּי. B. Mets. 80ª ואי דמחזקא בג׳ Ms. M. (v. Rabb. D.

S. a. l. note; ed. דמחזקא גונדרי, corr. acc.) if the field is known for its stony clods.

גְּרוֹסָה h. a. ch. m. (v. גָּרִיס) *grist-maker* or *dealer*. Y. Ber. I, 2[d] bot. R. Jacob ג׳. Y. Maas. Sh. IV, 54[d] bot. חזוי פירין לג׳ showed the produces to a grist-dealer (to value them).—*Pl.* גְּרוֹסִים, גְּרוֹסוֹת. Men. X, 4; Lev. R. s. 18 רחיים של ג׳; Pesik. R. s. 28 גרוסת (corr. acc.) the grist-grinders' mills; Pesik. Haomer, p. 69[a] גריסות (corr. acc.); a. e.—Y. Pes. IV, 30[d] top; Y. M. Kat. II, end, 81[b] גְּרוֹסֵי צפורין the grist-makers of Sepphoris.

גְּרוֹסְיָא f. (גרס) *a dish of beans* (a remedy for melancholy). Targ. II Esth. III, 8 (cmp. Gen. R. s. 94, beg.).

גרוסת, v. גְּרוֹסָה.

גְּרוֹעִין, גְּרוֹעַ, v. גֵּירוּעַ.

גְּרוֹעַ, v. גָּרַע.

גְּרוֹף m.=גְּרוֹפִית *block* or *shoot*. Gen. R. s. 53 lest people say ג׳ מביתו וכ׳ (Isaac is) a shoot taken from the house of Abimelekh. Tanḥ. B'huck. 5, v. גְּרוֹפִית.

גרופי, גרופות, גרופי, v. גְּרוֹפִית.

גְּרוֹפִינָא, v. אַגְרוֹפִינָא.

גְּרוֹפִית f. (גרף, cmp. אֶגְרוֹף) [*as large as a fist*,] *little stump* or *shoot*. Kel. XII, 8 ג׳ של זית a vessel made out of a piece of an olive tree; Tosef. ib. B. Mets. II, 19 he who makes vessels מג׳ של זית R. S. to Kel. l. c. (ed. Zuck. גפי, גרפות, corr. acc.).—Metaph. ג׳ של שקמה block of a sycamore tree, i. e. *a man barren of thought, ignorant; barren of merits, worthless*. Tanḥ. B'huck. 5 Jephtah was as poor in the Law כגְרוֹפִי׳ של שקמה (ed. Bub. 7 גרופות של ש׳ היה, note: גרופית) as a block &c.—Y. Ab. Zar. II, 40[c]; Gen. R. s. 25, end; Ruth R. s. 1, opp. ג׳ של זית one rich in merits; a. e.—*Pl.* גְּרוֹפִיּוֹת. B. Bath. V, 3 if one buys olive trees for felling, מניח שתי ג׳ he must leave a stump of two fists' size (out of which new shoots may rise); Tosef. ib. IV, 7 (v. Tos'f. Y. Tob a. l., a. B. Bath. 80[b]).—Gen. R. s. 31, end ג׳ לזתים Ar. (ed. sing.) shoots for future olive plantation.

גָּרוּר, v. גָּרַר a. גָּרוּד.

גָּרוּשׁ m., **גְּרוּשָׁה** f. (part. pass. of גָּרַשׁ) *a divorced spouse*. Pes. 112[a] ג׳ שנשא ג׳ a divorced husband who married a divorced wife. Ib. ג׳ בחיי בעלה marrying a divorced wife while her husband is yet alive. Ned. 20[b] גְּרוּשַׁת הלב divorced at heart, one whom her husband is determined to divorce; a. fr.—*Pl.* גְּרוּשִׁים, f. גְּרוּשׁוֹת. Yalk. Jer. 268 וכי ג׳ אתם לי are ye divorced from me (the Lord)?

גֵּירוּשִׁין, גֵּרוּשִׁין m. pl. (גרש) *sending off, divorce*. Gen. R. s. 19; Lam. R. introd. 4 (ref. to Gen. III, 23 sq.) דנתי אותו בשלוחין ובג׳ I punished him with expulsion and banishment.—Gitt. 64[a] שליש אומר לגי׳ the trustee says (the letter has been given me not as a deposit but) as a letter of divorce which I was authorized by thy wife to receive in her behalf.—Y. Kidd. I, 58[c] top גוים אין להן ג׳ the law of divorce (according to Deut. XXIV, 3) does not apply to gentiles. Ib. או שאין להם ג׳ וכ׳ either they have not the institution of divorce, or either may divorce the other; Gen. R. s. 18; a. fr.

גֵּירוּת, גֵּרוּת f. (denom. of גֵּר) 1) *the stranger's civic condition*. Gen. R. s. 44; Pesik. R. s. 15, a. e., v. אִיסוֹפּוֹלִיטְיָא. —2) *conversion to Judaism*. Gitt. 85[a].

גְּרְזֵימֵי, גְּרְזֵימִיתָא, גְּרְזְמִיתָא f. (גְּרְזִימִין m. pl.) (גרזם, Parel of גזם, cmp. b. h. כַּרְסֵם) *nibblings, dessert* (mostly of fruits, v. infra). Lam. R. introd. 10 I wished they had made me (the Lord) כגרזימי חזו וכ׳ ed. (Var. גרזמי, Ar. גרוז׳) like dessert which (at least) is served up at the end; Esth. R. to I, 9 כִּכְרְזִימִין חזה (!); Yalk. Is. 318 כגרומזי וכ׳ (corr. acc.). Y. Ber. VI, 10[c] bot. גרזמתה, גרזימי ed. Krot. (Ar. גרוזמתא)=פַּרְפֶּרֶת a. פַּיסָנִין. Gen. R. s. 33 גרוזמי דדהב וכ׳ Ar. Var. (ed. גַּרְדּוּמֵי, גַּרְדּוּמֵי, v. גדם) golden fruits on a golden tray; Lev. R. s. 27 גרוזמין דדהב Ar. (ed. רמונין . . . חזורין); [Pesik. Shor, p. 74[b] . . . בחורין ורימונין . . וגקרמונין (corr. בחזורין . . . וגרוזמין); Tanh. Emor 6 ובלחמא].

גרזקי, v. גורזקי.

גָּרָה, גרי (b. h.) 1) *to be rough, grating, scraping*; v. גָּרוֹן, גֵּרָה &c.—2) *to be hot, burn, singe* (cmp. חָרָה).

Pi. גֵּרָה, גִּירָה *to incite, stir up, let loose*. Snh. 107[b] שגר׳ דובים וכ׳ because he let the bears loose against the children. Ex. R. s. 21 ג׳ לפרעה He incited Pharaoh &c. Gen. R. s. 19, end (interpret. *hishshiani*, Gen. III, 13) גֵּירַנִי. Cant. R. to I, 4 (play on משכני ib.) ממה שגֵּרִיתָ בי שכני הרעים from my hostile neighbors whom thou hast incited against me.—Trnsf. ג׳ את הדוב ב־ *to let temptation loose against*. Gen. R. s. 87 אני מְגָרֶה בך וכ׳ I shall lay temptation in thy way; a. fr.—Lev. R. s. 17 ביום שיְגָרֶה וכ׳ on the day when the Lord shall stir up his anger &c.

Hithpa. הִתְגָּרָה, *Nithpa.* נִתְגָּרָה 1) *to be inflamed, jealous; to rival*. Snh. 19[a] מִתְגָּרוֹת זו בזו jealous of one another.—2) *to engage in battle, to fight*. Ber. 7[b]; Meg. 6[b] מותר לְהִתְגָּרוֹת וכ׳ it is permitted to enter into combat with the wicked (with reference to b. h. התחרה).—Num. R. s. 19 נתג׳ בהם he attacked them.—3) *to be let loose*. Esth. R. introd. נִתְגָּרְתָה אותה הדוב that temptation was aroused (against Joseph), v. supra; Num. R. s. 13 מִתְגָּרַת.—4) *to have a passion for, to indulge freely in*. Yoma 76[b] wine is called תִּירוֹשׁ, because he המִתְגָּרֶה בו נעשה רש who indulges in it becomes poor. Ab. Zar. 18[b]; 19[b] אֶתְגָּרֶה בשינה I will freely indulge in sleep (idleness).—5) (denom. of תִּגְרָה) *to incite*. Num. R. s. 18; Tanḥ. Korah 3 לְהִתְגָּרוֹת בו את וכ׳ to incite Israel against him.

גְּרָא, גְּרֵי ch. same.—Pa. גָּרֵי 1) *to incite, let loose*. Targ. Num. XXI, 6; a. fr.—2) *to let off, drive, thrust*. Naz. 4[b] דילמא גָּרוּיֵי ג׳ בהו perhaps he thrust (the jaw bone) at them (without touching them; Ar. a. Rashi: גרדויי גרד וכ׳, obviously for גרדויי גרד, cmp. גירדא, v. Koh. Ar. Compl. s. v.). Taan. 25[a] אֲגָרֵי בך וכ׳, v. גִּירָא II. [3) *to drag* (cmp. גרר). Nidd. 36[b], v. גְּדֵי.]

Ithpa. אִתְגְּרֵי, *Ithpe.* אִיגְּרֵי 1) *to attack.* Targ. Deut. II, 5; a. fr. Targ. I Sam. XIII, 4 (h. text נבאש!). [Targ. Ps. XXII, 8 ed. Lag., v. גְּרַר.]—Lam. R. to I, 5 מלכיותא מִתְגָּרְיָן בכון kingdoms will attack you; a. e.—2) *to be let loose, hurled.* Targ. Y. Deut. XXVIII, 60; a. e.—Y. Peah I, 16ᵃ top הא דובא מִתְגַּרְיָא לך that same temptation will be let loose &c., v. preced. Hithpa.—3) *to become impassionate, be hot with sexual passion.* Snh. 64ᵃ דלא מִיגְּרֵי איניש בקרובתיה Ms. M. (ed. איגרו) that one does not fall in love with his nearest kindred. Ab. Zar. 22ᵇ כיון דמיגרי בה because the animal will show his sexual desire by running after her (and thus betray her sin).—Denom. תִּגְרָא.

גְּרִיבָא m., pl. גְּרִיבֵי, v. גְּרִיוָא.

***גְּרִיבָה** pr. n. *G'ribah,* name of a street or open place in Tiberias. Koh. R. to X, 8, v. גַּרְגְּנָא.

גָּרֵיד, v. גָּרַד.

גְּרִיד m. (גרד) [*rind, crust,* cmp. גָּרָב.] *the parched surface of the field, arid land, unbroken* or *untilled ground.*—ימי הג׳ *dry season, summer.* B. Mets. V, 10.—Ib. חרוש עמי בג׳ plough thou with me in dry ground (in summer), opp. רְבִיעָה.—מקום הג׳ *dry ground,* opp. מקום (הטינא) הטיט muddy ground. Pes. 55ᵃ; Y. Kil. II, 27ᵈ top; Y. Ḥall. I, 57ᶜ.—M. Kat. 6ᵇ שדה ג׳, opp. מטוננת.—Y. Kil. II, 28ᵃ bot. ג׳ unbroken ground between tilled fields. Gen. R. s. 33, end נעשה כג׳ וכ׳ (the earth, after the flood had subsided) became like hard unbroken ground; they planted but nothing would grow.

גְּרִידָא ch. same, *rind,* v. גְּרִידְתָא.

גְּרִידָא m. (גרד) [*stripped,*] *alone, mere, unqualified* (v. גַּרְדּוּם). Ab. Zar. 37ᵃ אם מתי ג׳ the mere formula 'If I die' (without qualification). Yeb. 20ᵃ לא תנשה ג׳ הוא it is merely a prohibitory law; a. fr.—*Pl.* גְּרִידֵי. Ib. 79ᵇ חייבי לאוין ג׳ trespassers of a mere prohibitory law, opp. לאוין דשאר referring to incest. Ḥull. 2ᵇ; a. fr.—Fem. גְּרִידְתָא. Sot. 32ᵇ אמירה ג׳ the expression אמר not qualified by ענה. Keth. 73ᵇ טעות אשה אחת ג׳ a plain error concerning one woman (where you cannot say that the case may be considered as though concerning two different persons); a. fr.—[Targ. Y. II Ex. XIV, 25, v. גְּרַר.]

גְּרִידָה f. *scraping,* v. גְּרִירָה.

גְּרִידוּתָא f. (גְּרַד 2) *friction* (at sexual intercourse). Yeb. 75ᵇ (Ar. גרידתא).

גְּרֵידְתָא, v. גְּרִידָא. [Yeb. 75ᵇ Ar., v. preced.]

גְּרִיוָא, גְּרִיוָה, (גְּרִיבָא) f. (גרב, גרף, labial softened) [*a quantity carried at a time to and from the handmill* (cmp. גָּרָב I),] 1) *griva,* a dry measure (=סְאָה). Ab. Zar. 43ᵃ והוא דנקיט ג׳ וכ׳ provided the statue (of Serapis) has a *grivah* (modius) as a symbol of measuring (v. Sm. Ant. s. v. Coma). Erub. 29ᵇ גרויא (corr. acc., v. Rabb. D. S. a. l. note 1). Pes. 32ᵃ. Ned. 51ᵃ כל ג׳ וכ׳ whatever measure I may want.—2) בר ג׳ or ג׳ *the size of a field needed for a griva of seed* (cmp. סְאָה). B. Kam. 96ᵃ ג׳ דארעא a *griva* of land; B. Mets. 110ᵇ; ib. 15ᵇ גרבא ed. (Ms. M. גרויא, Ms. F. גריבא, Ms. R. גרויא, v. Rabb. D. S. a. l. note).—*Pl.* גְּרִיוֵי. Erub. 14ᵇ. B. Bath. 73ᵃ, v. בָּזֵק. Ned. 50ᵇ sq.

גריוזמי, גריוזמתה, v. גַּרְזִימִי.

גְּרִימוֹת, v. גְּרוּמִי.

גרימני, v. גַּרְמָנִי.

גְּרִיס, v. גְּרַס.

גְּרִיס m., pl. גְּרִיסִין (b. h. גֶּרֶשׂ; v. גָּרַס I) [*split, broken,*] *grits* 1) esp. *pounded beans; beans used for pounding.* Gen. R. s. 94, beg.; Nidd. IX, 6 sq.; Tosef. ib. VIII, 9, v. חֲלוּקָה a. שְׁעוּעִית.—Maasr. V, 8 ג׳ הקלקין Cilician beans. Tosef. ib. III, 14 [read:] אילו הן ג׳ הקלקין (אילו) הַגַּסִּין המרובעין (v. Maim. a. R. S. to Maasr. l. c.) Cilician beans are the large and quadrangular; a. fr. [גריסות, v. גְּרוֹסָה.]—כג׳ *the size of a bean.* Sifra Thazr. Neg. ch. I. Kel. XVII, 12 ג׳ נגעים כג׳ וכ׳ the *garis* as a standard for eruptions is the Cilician bean.—2) (pl.) *a dish of pounded grains.* Koh. R. to II, 2; Tanḥ. Aḥaré 1, a. e. קערה של ג׳ a dish of boiled grit; Ruth R. to II, 14 גְּרִישִׁין. [Ib. to 15 היה מבקר גרישין, read with Yalk. ib. 604 גְּרִישִׁין, v. גְּרִישׁ.]

גְּרִיסָא ch. same. Y. Sabb. III, 6ᵇ top פינכא דג׳ a dish of beans; Y. Maasr. I, 49ᵃ top דגלוסא (corr. acc.).—*Pl.* גְּרִיסִין. Targ. Y. Lev. XIV, 37. [Ex. R. s. 43 קאקי גריסין, v. קָאקִיגוֹרוֹס.]

גְּרִיעַ, גְּרִיעָא, v. גְּרַע.

גְּרִיעוּתָא f. (גרע) *diminution; lesser degree; disadvantage.* Ber. 56ᵃ מפשר ליה לג׳ he interpreted his dream unfavourably, opp. למעליותא. B. Kam. 99ᵇ . . . עביד בך תרתי לג׳ he has doubly injured thee (through his verdict). Yeb. 122ᵇ top מאי ג׳ וכ׳ whereon is the inn-keeper's lower status (lesser trustworthiness) based? Ḥull. 5ᵇ wherever the Bible uses *b'hemah* (beast), ג׳ היא does it necessarily imply contempt?

גְּרִיפָה f. (גרף) *removal of coal and ashes, scraping.* Bets. 28ᵇ גְּרִיפַת וכ׳ the cleaning of stoves &c.

גריפס, גריפוס, v. אַגְרָפּוֹס.

גְּרִיץ, pl. גְּרִיצִין, גְּרִיצִים, v. גְּרִיצָה.

גְּרִיץ, גְּרִיצָא, pl. גְּרִיצִן, v. גְּרִיצְתָא.

גְּרִיצָה f. (גריץ to cut, cmp. גרס) *slice. Pl.* גְּרִיצוֹת *bread or cake formed of slices twisted together* or *layers above one another, twists.* Bets. II, 6 (21ᵇ) אין אופין פָּתָן ג׳ Ms. M. a. ed. Y. (ed. פִּתִּין גְּרִיצִין, Ar. פתן גריצין) they must not (on Holy Days) bake their bread in the form of twists; Y. ib. 61ᶜ bot.—Tosef. Ab. Zar. VII (VIII), 2 מוליכין עמו ג׳ לתנור you may carry your cakes, to be baked with his, to the confectioner's oven.—Snh. 100ᵇ, v. next w.

גְּרִיצְתָּא f., גְּרִיץ m. ch. same. Targ. Ex. XXIX, 23 (O. צִתָּא . . . ., Y. גריץ, h. text חַלָּה). Targ. Prov. VI, 26 (h. text כִּכַּר); a. e.—*Pl.* גְּרִיצָן, גְּרִיצָתָא. Targ. Gen. XVIII, 6 (h. text עגות). Targ. Lev. VII, 12 sq.—Snh. 100[b] תרתין גריצים, read גְּרִיצָן.

גְּרִירָה f. (גרר) 1) *scraping off.* Hull. 84[a] וג׳ .... מחוסר requires the acts of pouring out the blood, scraping off the blood stains &c. Ib. 93[a] בעי ג׳ . . . ריש מעיא the top of the small bowels up to a cubit's length must be scraped (in order to remove the fat).—2) *dragging, pulling, moving an object without lifting.* Sabb. 22[a]; Pes. 101[a]; Men. 41[b] בג׳ ... הלכה the law decides in favor of ... with reference to dragging an object on the Sabbath, v. גָּרַר. Y. Kidd. I, 60[d] top מהו שיקנו בג׳ can they be taken possession of by moving without lifting?—3) *carrying with, involving.* Y. Pes. VII, 34[c] top ג׳ . . . מאי נפקא what is the difference between them? They differ as to the majority of one tribe carrying with it (determining the legal status of) the whole nation, v. גָּרַר 3.—Sabb. 71[a] ומי אית ליה ג׳ . . . does R. adopt the opinion that one action can be involved with another so as to be considered one continuous act (e. g. cutting grain and immediately grinding it)? Ib. ג׳ דג׳ an application of this principle in the second degree, that the action involved should involve a third action.

גְּרִישׁ m., pl. גְּרִישִׁין, v. גְּרִיס.

גְּרַל, Hif. הִגְרִיל, v. גּוֹרָל.

גְּרַם (v. גרר) *to drag along, carry with it.*—Part. pass. גָּרוּם *added in boot, additional measure,* v. אַמָּה.—גְּרוּמִין אַמָּה גְּרוּמָה *a large cubit.* Gen. R. s. 12 [read:] כאמה ג׳ the size of a liberal cubit (equal to a cubit and a half of strict measure; some ed. גד׳; vers. in 'Rashi' a. l. גרמידא ומחצה).—Y. Shek. VI, end, 50[b] אמה גרו׳, read גְּדוּמָה, v. גָּדַם. [Tosef. Bekh. V, 4 אצבעותיו גרומות Var., ed. Zuck. גדומות.]—Trnsf. *to carry with it, to be the cause of, to engender.* דבר הגורם לממון something which may be the cause of pecuniary profit or loss. B. Kam. 71[b] if one steals objects dedicated to the sanctuary for which the original owner is responsible in case of loss &c., he is bound to pay the thief's fine (כֶּפֶל) to the owner; אלמא דבר הג׳ למ׳ כממון דמי which proves that that which may cause a pecuniary loss, is to be considered as the property of him to whom it may cause it. Ib. 98[b] according to the opinion of R. Shimeon who says מיחייב ... דבר הגורם that what is the cause of monetary gain is considered as money, he who burns a note of indebtedness is bound to pay the full amount of the note; a. fr.—Snh. 104[a] גורם גלות לבניו causes his children to be exiled. Ber. 5[b] bot. ג׳ לשכינה וכ׳ is the cause of the Divine Presence departing from Israel. M. Kat. 25[a] בבל גָּרְמָה לו Babylonia was the cause (that the Shekhinah did not rest upon him). Ab. Zar. 8[b] bot. המקום גורם the place makes the act legal, i. e. only in the Temple hall can the Sanhedrin judge capital cases; Snh. 14[b] המקום ג׳ only in the Temple hall can a rebellious elder be judged; ib. 87[a].—Y. Yeb. I, 2[c] top דבר שהוא בא מחמת הגורם וכ׳ if a prohibition arises from a cause (a person that causes it, e. g. the prohibition against C.'s marrying B. because B.'s sister A. is his wife)—when the cause is removed (through A.'s death), the prohibition ceases; but a prohibition which has not its cause in the action of a person (but in natural kinship, e. g. C.'s daughter married to C.'s brother whereby she becomes forbidden to him also as his brother's wife), is not removed with the removal of the cause of the (additional) prohibition, i. e. C. cannot perform the levir's marriage with his brother's wife since she has not ceased to be his daughter; ib. III, beg., 4[c]; IV, 6[a] top.—זה וזה גורם *a product of combined causes.* Tem. 30[b] זה וזה ג׳ אסור a product of combined causes is forbidden, e. g. the offspring of a dam unfitted for the altar, and of a sire fit; Pes. 27[a]; a. fr.—Ib. 26[b] זה וזה ג׳ מי שמעת ליה can you prove that Rabbi adopts the rule forbidding the product of combined causes?—Nidd. 31[a] (homiletical play on Gen. XLIX, 14) חמור ג׳ לישׂשכר the braying of an ass was the cause of Isachar being begotten; Gen. R. s. 99; v. next w.

Pi. גֵּירֵם same. Gen. R. s. 39 הדרך מְגָרֶמֶת וכ׳ traveling is the cause of three evils.

Nif. נִגְרַם *to be indirectly engendered.* Ab. Zar. 55[b] אסור לִיגָּרֵם וכ׳ no assistance must be given to making unclean &c.

Hif. הִגְרִים *to leave a comb* (גָּרוּם) *in striking a measure off,* whence (in ritual slaughtering) *to cut in a slanting direction, to let the knife slide beyond the space prescribed for cutting.* Hull. 19[a]; 20[a]; a. fr.—Part. pass. f. מוּגְרֶמֶת an animal slaughtered by a slanting cut. Ib. 18[b]; a. fr.—Denom. הַגְרָמָה.

גְּרַם I ch. same. Targ. Is. III, 9; a. fr.—Meg. 12[b] אנא גְּרָמִי וכ׳ Ms. M. (ed. גרים) I am the cause that M. was born. Ber. 7[b] שמא גָרֵים a person's name has an influence on his fate or character. Ab. Zar. 19[b] ע״א מאן קא גרים לה what action caused the work to be called an idol?—Gen. R. s. 98 [read:] ישׂשכר חמור גְּרֵמֵיה (play on גרם, v. preced. w.) the braying of an ass caused him to be begotten (by announcing Jacob's arrival upon which Leah went forth to meet him; v. ib. s. 99, Nidd. 31[a]).

גְּרַם II, גְּרֵים (denom. of גַּרְמָא, cmp. עצם) *to be substantial, strong.* *Targ. Prov. XVIII, 10 ויגריס ביה Ms. a. Var. in ed. Lag. (read וְיִגְרְים; ed. ונתרים). Ib. V, 19 תִּגְרַם (some ed. תִּגְרֵם, Ms. תגרס) thou shalt grow strong.

Pa. גָּרֵים 1) *to strengthen, comfort.* Targ. Y. II Gen. XXXV, 9 וגָרֵימַת וכ׳ (some ed. וגרי׳ Pe.) and Thou didst strengthen him (in his trouble).—2) *to eat up to the bone, to pick off.* Targ. Ps. XXVII, 2 לְגַרְמָא (Ms. a. Regia לְגַמְרָא, v. גְּמַר).—B. Bath. 22[a] אדמְגַרְמֵיתוּ גרמי וכ׳ (Ms. M. מגרדיתו fr. גְּרַד; Ar. דמגרמיסתו fr. גְּרַם; v. Rabb. D. S. a. l. note) in place of picking off bones (receiving scanty instruction) in the school of A., go ye and eat flesh &c.

Af. אַגְרֵים *to make substantial, harden.* Targ. Prov. VIII, 28 (Var. אוגריס, h. text אמץ).

גְּרָם m. (גָּרַם) *cause, indirect production of an effect.* Sabb. 120ᵇ גְּרַם כיבוי indirect extinction of a fire (by placing vessels filled with water in its way), v. גְּרָמָא.

גֶּרֶם m. (b. h.; גרם *to strip;* cmp. גרד, גְּרִידָא) [*stripped, bare,* cmp. II Kings IX, 13,] *skeleton, bone;* (cmp. עֶצֶם) *self, strength.—Pl.* גְּרָמִים. Gen. R. s. 98 מה חמור זה גְּרָמָיו ברורים as the bony frame of the ass is clearly discernible.

גַּרְמָא ch., constr. גְּרַם, גֶּרֶם same, 1) *a bare twig,* opp. כִּבְבָא. Macc. 8ᵃ (Ms. M. גִּירְמָא).—2) *bone.* Targ. Gen. II, 23; a. fr. [Targ. Y. Ex. XXVII, 5 גומא read גַּר׳ or גּוּרְמָא.]—Gen. R. s. 70 [read as Yalk. ib. 124, cmp. Dan. VI, 25) כחדין ג׳ אנא מהדק לך like a bone I shall crush thee. Ber. 5ᵇ; B. Bath. 116ᵃ, v. בִּיר.—*Pl.* גַּרְמַיָּא, גַּרְמֵי. Targ. Gen. l. c. גַּרְמַי (Y. גַּרְמֵי). Targ. Ezek. XXXVII, 4; a. fr.—Targ. Y. Ex. XXXVIII, 4 [read:] גּוּמְרַיָּא וְגַרְמַיָּא or גורמיא וגומריא, v. supra.—B. Bath. 58ᵃ חביתא דג׳ a vessel of bones (an enigmatical phrase for *an animal*). Ib. 22ᵃ, v. גְּרַם II.—Bets. 11ᵃ תברא ג׳ a block on which bones are chopped; a. fr.—3) *body, self.* ג׳ ג׳ *each for itself, one after the other.* Ib. 11ᵇ. Hull. 113ᵃ.—With suffixes of personal pronouns: גַּרְמִי *myself* &c. Targ. Job I, 3 לְגַרְמֵיהּ as his own, לְגֶרֶם אתתיה (Ms. לגרם) as his wife's sole property. Targ. Y. Lev. VII, 29 בְּגַרְמֵיהּ himself; a. fr.—Gen. R. s. 75, beg., v. גַּפָּא I. Y. Ber. III, 6ᶜ bot. קטר גרמיה tied himself; a. fr.—Ber. 48ᵃ, a. fr. לג׳ הוא דעבד he did so for himself, i. e. this is no authoritative precedent.—Y. Orl. I, 61ᵃ top ג׳ אמר he gave his own opinion. Y. Erub. III, 21ᵃ bot. בשם גרמיה in his own name; Y. Kidd. II, 63ᵃ top.—Y. Keth. III, end, 28ᵃ כל גַּרְמָהּ אמרה this very fact (thing) proves; Y. Shebu. V, end, 36ᶜ; Y. Keth. IX, beg. 32ᵈ; Y. Pes. IX, end, 37ᵃ כל גרמא (corr. acc.).

גְּרָמָא ch.=h. גְּרָם, 1) *cause.*—מ״ע שהזמן ג׳ (in Hebr. diction) a positive command the observance of which depends on a certain time of the day or season of the year. Kidd. I, 7 (29ᵃ); a. fr.—2) *indirect effect.* Sabb. 120ᵇ ג׳ שרי indirect effect (e. g. effacing the Divine Name in consequence of bathing) is permitted, opp. עשייה the direct act. B. Kam. 60ᵃ ג׳ בניזקין פטור damage by indirect action is not actionable. B. Bath. 22ᵇ ג׳ בניזקין אסור to cause indirect damage is forbidden.—*Pl.* גְּרָמֵי. B. Kam. 98ᵇ מאן דדאין דינא דג׳ he who holds the opinion that one who is the cause of damage to another person is responsible; ib. 100ᵃ; 117ᵇ; a. e.

גרמומיא, v. גַּרְמַמְיָא.

***גְּרַמַּטְיוֹן** m. (γραμματεῖον) *bond, document.* Ex. R. s. 15 גרמסיון (corr. acc.).

דינא דג׳, גַּרְמֵי, v. גְּרָמָא.

גַּרְמִידָא m. (=גַּמִּידָא, v. גּוֹמֶד) *arm, elbow, cubit.* Targ. Y. Ex. II, 5. Targ. Jud. III, 16 (h. text גמד).—B. Mets. 64ᵃ בני ג׳ of an arm's length.—*Pl.* גַּרְמִידֵי. Targ. Y. Ex. XVI, 29; a. e.—Snh. 7ᵃ. Erub. 14ᵇ.

גרמיני, v. גַּרְמָנִי.

גַּרְמִיתָא f. (dimin. of גַּרְמָא) *a small bone* or *sinew.* Hull. 103ᵇ Ar. (ed. גְּרוּמִיתָא, גְּרוּמִיתָא).

גַּרְמַמְיָא, גַּרְמַנְיָא, גִּיר׳ pr. n. *Germamia, Germania,* 1) *the land of the Cimmerii* (v. Schr. KAT p. 428). Targ. I Chr. I, 5; Targ. Y. Gen. X, 2 (for *Magog*); Y. Meg. I, 71ᵇ bot.; Yoma 10ᵃ (for *Gomer*); Gen. R. s. 37, beg. (for *Magog*). Ib. (also for *Togarmah,* v. גַּרְמַנִיקְיָא).—2) (של רומי or ג׳ של אדום) *Germania, the Roman province of Germania.* Meg. 6ᵃᵇ; Yalk. Ps. 888. Gen. R. s. 75, v. בַּרְבַּרְיָא. [Y. Sabb. VI, 8ᶜ bot. read גַּרְמָנִי.]

גרמנא, v. next w.

גַּרְמָנִי m. (Germanus, v. preced. art.) *German, one of the Caucasian race, white man,* opp. כּוּשִׁי. Gen. R. s. 86 everywhere you find ג׳ מוכר כושי one of the white race sells a dark man. Neg. II, 1, v. בַּהֶרֶת.—Y. Yoma VIII, 45ᵇ top ג׳ עבדיה וכ׳ a German, a slave of &c.; Y. Sabb. VI, 8ᶜ bot. גרמניא (corr. acc.); Y. Ab. Zar. II, end, 42ᵃ גרמנא.

גרמני, B. Bath. 89ᵇ Ar., v. גְּרוּמֵי.

גַּרְמַנְיָא, v. גַּרְמַמְיָא.

גַּרְמָנִיקְיָא, גִּיר׳ pr. n. pl. *Germanicia,* town (and district) in the province of Commagene, near the borders of Cappadocia. Y. Meg. I, 71ᵇ bot.; Yoma 10ᵃ; Gen. R. s. 37 (for *Togarmah,* v. Schr. KAT p. 428); [Targ. Y. II Gen. X, 3; Targ. I Chr. I, 6 בַּרְבַּרְיָאה.]

גרמסיון, v. גְּרַמַּטְיוֹן.

***גרמסין**, prob. to be read גְּרַמְּטִין m. pl. (γράμμα, -ατος,=scrupulum, v. Sm. Ant. s. v.) *gramma,* 1/24 of an ounce. Y. Shek. II, 46ᵈ top, half a Shekel which makes שיתא ג׳ (Bab. ed. to II 3 also גירומסין, Ms. M. גירמוסין, Yalk. Ex. 386 גרמיסין) six *grammata.*

גָּרֶן, v. גּוֹרֶן.

גָּרַן, denom. of גּוֹרֶן q. v.

גרנן, v. גּוֹרֶן.

גָּרַס (b. h.; v. גרר), *Pi.* גֵּירֵס *to crush, split, grind.* Tosef. T'bul Yom II, 12 fat figs שלא גֵירְסָהּ which he has not yet crushed (into a cake). V. גְּרִיס.

גְּרַס I ch.; *Pa.* גָּרֵיס, *Af.* אַגְרֵיס same. B. Bath. 22ᵃ, v. גְּרַם II *Af.* [Targ. Prov. VIII, 28, v. גְּרַם II Af.]

גְּרַס II, גְּרֵיס (cmp. גרר, גּוֹרֶן) *to scrape together; to collect, accumulate.* Denom. גּוּרְסִינָא. [Targ. Prov. XVIII, 10; V, 19, v. גְּרַם II.]—Trnsf. *to acquire knowledge, to commit traditions to memory,* as a preliminary stage to speculation and analysis compared to grinding, v. טְחַן. Ab. Zar. 19ᵃ לעולם ליגמר ואע״ג דמשכח וליגרס ואע״ג דלא ידע וכ׳ Ms. M. one must at all events acquire readiness (v. גְּמַר II), though one may afterwards forget, and one must study by heart though one does not understand, for Holy Writ says (Ps. CXIX, 20) *gar'sah* &c.; it says גָּרְסָה and not טָחֲנָה (my soul *heaps up*, but not it *grinds*, learns but not analyzes); (ed. לִיגְרִיס, and other Variants); Yalk. Ps. 876.—Ber. 8ª חוה גָּרֵיסְנָא בגו ביתאי Ms. M. (v. Rabb. D. S. a. l.) I used to study in my house; Meg. 29ª. Ber. l. c. bot. turned his face וגריס and reviewed (what he had learned). Taan. 10ᵇ לְמִיגְרַס to recite traditions, opp. לעיוני to speculate. Ber. 13ᵇ (ref. to Deut. XI, 18, v. Targ. Y. a. l.) teach your children..., כ׳ היכי דלִיגְרְסוּ בהו (Ms. M. ונִגְרְסוּ בהו) so that they be able to review them (by themselves); a. fr.—*Part. act.* גָּרֵיס *well-versed, knowing by heart.* B. Bath. 21ª ג׳ ולא דייק knowing Bible verses by heart, but being inexact.—*Part. pass.* גְּרִיס, f. גְּרִיסָא *known by heart.* Men. 32ᵇ מיגרס גְּרִיסָן; Meg. 18ᵇ מיגרס גְּרִיסָן they are known by heart.

גִּירְסָא, גִּרְסָא I f. (preced.) 1) *acquired learning, study of tradition.* Targ. Cant. I, 2 בג׳ for verbal study.—Meg. 6ᵇ לאוקומי ג׳ וכ׳ to preserve (in memory) what one has learned requires divine assistance. Sabb. 21ᵇ ג׳ דינקותא what has been learned in youth (which is better remembered). Ib. 30ᵇ לא הוה פסיק פומיה מג׳ did not cease reciting. Erub. 68ª אנא .... בגִרְסָאִי I am busy studying; a. fr.—*Pl.* גִּרְסַיָּיא, גִּיר׳. B. Bath. 22ª דלא ליטרדו מגִּרְסַיְיהוּ Ms. M. (ed. אתו ליטרדו מג׳) that they may not be disturbed in their studies.—2) (editorial note) *version.* Yalk. Gen. 84 ג׳ אחרינא זה וכ׳ another version (for זה איוב, Gen. R. s. 50) is, 'This alludes to the tribe of Levi'. [Frequently in commentaries.—Denom. גרס *to read.* הכי גרסינן (abbr. ה״ג) such is the proper reading.]

גִּרְסָא, גִּיר׳ II, v. גִּירְצָא.

גַּרְסִי m. (v. גְּרִיס) *grits-dealer* or *maker*, v. גְּרוֹסָה. Midr. Prov. ch. IX; Erub. 21ᵇ יהושוע הג׳ (not רבי, v. Rabb. D. S. a. l. note).

גָּרַע I (b. h.; v. גרר) *to scrape off, to diminish, deduct.* Snh. 29ª כל המוסיף גּוֹרֵעַ he who adds (to the truth) diminishes (whoever does too much does too little). R. Hash. 28ᵇ, a. fr. עובר על בל תִּגְרַע transgresses the law which prohibits diminishing from what the Law prescribes (Deut. XIII, 1, v. בַּל). Yoma 48ª גּוֹרְעִין ומוסיפין ודורשין we may take away (one servile letter from one word of the text) and add it to another and thus interpret the law (e. g. מדם הפר explained as: דם מהפר); B. Bath. 111ᵇ; a. fr.—Y. Yeb. VIII, end, 9ᵈ, v. פָּלַע.—[Gen. R. s. 19, a. e. גרעה קומתו, v. גָּרַע.]—*Part. pass.* גָּרוּעַ *inferior. Pl.* גְּרוּעִים. Gen. R. s. 28. [Ber. 36ª ומי גרע, read with Ms. M. גריער.]

Hif. הִגְרִיעַ *to deduct from, to calculate the price of redemption in proportion to the years served and those to be served*, v. גֵּרָעוֹן. Kidd. 11ᵇ מַגְרַעַת מפדיונה she makes a deduction from her redemption money; ib. 14ᵇ מגרעת פדיונה she lessens &c.; ib. 16ª מגרע פד׳ (corr. acc.). Y. Kidd. I, 58ᶜ bot.; Y. Shebu. VI, beg. 36ᵈ מגרעת (ב)מעה וכ׳ she redeems herself by deducting a M'ah for each year.

Nif. נִגְרַע *to be deducted, to be redeemed by deducting the compensation for the time served.* Y. Kidd. l. c. אם בקשה לִיגָּרֵעַ if the desires a redemption by deduction &c.; Y. Shebu. l. c. למיגרע (read: לְהִיגָּ׳ or לִיגָּ׳). Kidd. 11ᵇ תִּיגָּרֵעַ עד פרוטה she can redeem herself by deductions until she comes down to a P'rutah.

גְּרַע ch. same, esp. *to shave, cut the hair* (dialectically interchanging with גרד). Targ. Jud. XVI, 19; II Sam. X. 4 Ar. (ed. גדע, ed. Lag. II Sam. l. c. גרע; cmp. Is. XV, 2, Jer. XLVIII, 37).—Lam. R. to I, 1 רבתי (8 חד מאת׳) ג׳ רישיה he shaved his head. Snh. 96ª (prov.) גְּרַעְתֵּיה לארמאה וכ׳ Ar. (ed. גרידתיה, Ms. M. גרידתיה) if you shave a gentile, he likes it; hang fire on his beard, and you will get no end of his fun (i. e. if he finds it convenient, he will submit to indignities).—Part. pass. גְּרִיעַ, f. גְּרִיעָא 1) *shaved.* Lam. R. l. c.—2) *inferior, less.* Yeb. 51ª ג׳ ממאמר is inferior (as to legal power) to &c., v. מַאֲמָר. Gitt. 70ª ג׳ דכולהו the worst of all.

Af. אַגְרַע as preced. *Hif.* [Targ. Y. II Gen. XXX, 11, read מגדעא.] Kidd. 11ᵇ מַגְרְעָה ואזלה she deducts more and more every year. Ib. [read:] מאי מגרעה what is there for her to deduct from?—Arakh. 25ª, v. infra.

Ithpe. אִיגְּרַע as preced. *Nif.* Arakh. 30ᵇ מִיגְּרְעָא ואזלא his obligation grows less (every year, if he chooses to redeem her). Ib. 25ª לא מִגְּרַע ליה (Rashi מיג׳) no deduction is allowed him (for fractions of a year).

גָּרַע II (b. h.; cmp. גַּרְגַּר) *to form globules, to drop.* Denom. גַּרְעִין.

Pi. גֵּרַע, *Hif.* הִגְרִיעַ (denom. of גרעין) *to form globules* (one of the early stages of development of the grape). Shebi. IV, 10 גפנים מִשֶּׁיְּגָרְעוּ grape vines (must not be cut down in the Sabbath year) from the moment they form stones, Maim.; oth. opin. ovules containing moisture; Y. ib. IV, end 35ᶜ משיגריעו (Hif.), defined משיזחלו מים, with ref. to Job XXXVI, 27; Ber. 63ᵇ; Pes. 52ᵇ sq. משיגרייעו (Ms. M. 2 משיגרעו).

גָּרָע m. (גרע I) *scraper, barber,* in gen. *low class surgeon, blood-letter* &c. Kidd. 82ª. Kel. XII, 4; Tosef. ib. B. Mets. II, 11 גָּרוֹעַ, v. מַסְמֵר.

גַּרְעוֹן, v. גֵּרָ׳.

גַּרְעִין, גַּלְעִין, גַּרְאִין c. (v. גָּרַע II) *globule,* esp. *the stone* or *kernel* of a stone fruit, *nut* &c.—*Pl.* גַּרְעִינִין, גַּלְעִינִין, גַּרְאִ׳. Sabb. VII, 4 (76ᵇ) גרעינין Ms. M. (ed. גַּרְעִינֵיהֶן); Y. ed. גַּלְעִינֵיהֶן. Bab. ib. 77ᵇ top, question as to spelling with א or ע (decided by ref. to ונגרע Lev. XXVII, 18). Shebi. VII, 3 גל׳. Ter. XI, 5 גַּרְעִינֵי תרומה (Ms. M. גל׳) stones of fruits which are the priest's share. Tosef. ib. X, 1; a. fr. V. גַּרְעִינָה.

גַּרְעִינָא, v. גַּרְעִינוּתָא.

גַּרְעִינָה, גַּלְעִינָה f.=גַּרְעִין (collect. noun, used promiscuously with גַּרְעִינִין). Ukts. II, 2 גל׳ של רוטב the stones of moist olives; Y. Ter. XI, 47ᵈ bot. גלעיני הרוטב. Y. Maasr. I, 48ᵈ bot.; a. fr.

גַּרְעִינוּתָא f. ch. same. Ber. 39ª גַּרְעִינוּתֵיה (Ms. M. גַּרְעִינֵיה) the stones (of an olive).

גָּרַף (b. h.; v. גרר) *to scrape, sweep, esp. to remove ashes and coal from the stove; to scrape together, collect.* Kel. VIII, 11 היתה גוֹרַפְתּוֹ if while she was sweeping it (the stove) &c. Sabb. III, 1 עד שֶׁיִּגְרוֹף not before he has swept it.—Y. Peah VII, 20^b top (ref. to Joel I, 17) תחת שהיינו גוֹרְפִים וכ׳ in place of collecting honey (from bee-hives or trees), we collected foul matter. Sabb. XVII, 2 לִגְרוֹף בה וכ׳ to grab with it the figs out of the barrel; a. fr.—Gen. R. s. 67 גּוֹרֶפֶת מחוטמה blowing her nose (v. גָּרַר).—*Part. pass.* גָּרוּף, f. גְּרוּפָה *cleared* of ashes &c., *swept.* Sabb. III, 4, v. אַנְטִיכִי; a. fr.—[Gen. R. s. 53 ג׳ מביתו של וכ׳ (Isaac is) the refuse of &c., comment.; v., however, גְּרוֹף.]

Pi. גֵּירֵף same. Kerith. 7^b; Y. Snh. VII, 25^b top, v. גָּרַף.

גְּרַף ch. same. Targ. II Esth. III, 8 גרפין חמיעא they remove leavened things.—Y. Pes. II, end, 29^c גְּרוֹף מן תוחתיהון scrape them at the bottom. Y. Bets. IV, 62^c bot. [read:] איזלי גְּרַפִין go thou and sweep them (the stones) out. Y. M. Kat. I, 80^b bot.; a. fr.

Ithpe. אִתְגְּרִיף *to be scraped out, removed.* Targ. II Esth. l. c.

Ithpalp. אִיתְגַּרְגֵּיף same. Targ. Job VII, 12 like the Ocean דמִתְגַּרְגֵּף וכ׳ Ms. which, at certain times, is swept (pours itself out over the shores; ed. דמתרגיף, v. רְגַף).

גרפות, גרפות, v. גְּרוּפִית.

גרקי, v. גּוּתַרְקָא II.

גָּרַר I (b. h.; v. גָּרָה) [*to produce a grating, scraping sound,*] 1) *to scratch, scrape, shave* (v. גָּרַע, גָּרַד I). Sabb. VIII, 6 (81^a) כדי לִגְרוֹר וכ׳ (Ar. a. Y. ed. לגרוד) large enough to scrape with it the top &c. R. Hash. 27^b גְּרָרוֹ Ms. M. (ed. גרדו), v. גָּלַד. Keth. 60^a; Kerith. 21^b גּוֹרְרוֹ וכ׳ he must scrape the blood off before eating the bread; a. fr.—Part. pass. גָּרוּר, v. גָּרוּד.—2) *to drag, to move without lifting;* (also neut. verb) *to follow.* Sabb. 29^b, a. fr. גורר אדם וכ׳ one may, on the Sabbath, pull or push a couch &c. (on the floor). Y. Kil. I, 27^b bot. לא יָגוֹר אדם וכ׳ one must not pull &c. Tanh. Thazr. 8 גְּרָרוּהוּ מקברו they dragged him out of his grave. Tosef. Erub. XI (VIII), 13; Tosef. Bets. II, 19 דלת הגּוֹרֶרֶת ... הגּוֹרְרִים (Y. Erub. X, 26^b bot. גוררת, corr. acc., v. גָּדַר) a door which drags along the ground (on opening), a matting which is moved by dragging, or large kegs which &c.; Erub. 101^a דלת הַנִּגְרֶרֶת ... הנגרר. Cant R. to II, 15 אני גוֹרְרוֹ למבולו I will drag him to the flood in which to perish; a. fr.—Tanh. Thazr. 9 (ref. to Ps. V, 5 יגרך) אין אתה נגרר .... ואין הרעה גוֹרֶרֶת אותך וכ׳ neither art thou dragged behind (attracted by) evil, nor does evil drag (have power over) thee, nor does it dwell with thee; Yalk. Kings 231 אין אתה גורר אחר .... גוררת אחריך.—Part. pass. גָּרוּר *dragged along, hanging on.—Pl.* גְּרוּרִין, גְּרוּרִים. Num. R. s. 18 ח׳ ג׳ eight threads dragged along (as fringes; Tanh. Korah 12 ח׳ חוטין). Ab. Zar. 3^b, a. e. גרים ג׳ proselytes who have attached themselves but have not been admitted, v. גֵּר.—3) *to carry with it, to cause; to affect* (v. גָּרַם). Y. Hor. I, 46^a bot.; Y. Pes. VII, 34^c שבט אחד גּוֹרֵר וכ׳ (a majority of) one tribe affects the legal status of the entire nation, i. e. the majority of tribes (seven) decides, though it may be a minority of the people as a whole. Lev. R. s. 13, end (play on *gerah*, Lev. XI, 4 sq.) גָּרְרָה מלכות וכ׳ carried another government after it, i. e. was followed by another oppressive government. Ab. IV, 2 מצוה גּוֹרֶרֶת וכ׳ a good deed begets a good deed &c. Tosef. Sabb. XV (XVI), 6 [read:] אין גּוֹרֵר וכ׳ it is not considered a corpse so as to cause uncleanness to man or vessels.—4) *to saw, split.* Sabb. XVII, 2 (122^b) a saw (may be used on the Sabbath) לָגוֹר בה וכ׳ (Ms. M. לִגְרוֹר, Mish. ed. Pes. לִגְרַר, v. Rabb. D. S. a. l. note) to saw cheese with it. Ohol. XV, 8 עתיד לָגוֹר Ar. intended to be sawed apart (ed. לגוד, fr. גדד, v. Tosef. ib. XV, 8). Tosef. Kel. B. Mets. II, 18 לָגוֹר וכ׳ to saw off a part &c.

Nif. נִגְרַר 1) *to be dragged, pulled.* Erub. X, 11 נגר הנג׳ a bolt which is dragged along (with the door, i. e. attached and hanging down). Ib. 101^a, v. supra. Tanh. Thazr. 9, v. supra. Bets. II, 10 (23^b) אינה נִגְרֶרֶת; ib. אין נִגְרָרִין must not be dragged or pulled, a. fr.—2) *to be scraped, planed.* B. Kam. 119^b הנ׳ במגירה shavings, opp. נפסק במגירה chips.—Nidd. 55^b נִגְרָרִין דרך הפה (secretions of the nose) scraped (discharged) through the mouth (v. גָּרַף).

Pi. גֵּרֵר, גֵּירֵר 1) *to drag.* Pes. IV, 9 (56^a) ג׳ עצמות וכ׳ he had the bones of his father carried out on a bed of ropes. Ib. I, 2 (9^a); a. fr.—Tosef. Sabb. VI (VII), 1 (a superstitious custom) הַמְגָרֶרֶת בנה וכ׳ Var. (ed. Zuck. המגוררת) one who drags her son among the dead (to the cemetery).—2) *to scrape, plane.* Ib. XVI (XVII), 19 מְגָרְרָן he may scrape them (clean his feet of mud). Tosef. Kel. B. Mets. II, 17; Hull. 25^a עתיד . . . לְגָרֵר requiring planing for finish; a. fr.—Part. pass. מְגוֹרָר a) *scratched, full of scabs.* Gen. R. s. 64 (play on מגרר, Gen. XXVI, 26) ד״א מג׳ וכ׳ another explanation is *m'gorar*, for eruptions grew on him (with ref. to Job II, 8); Yalk. ib. 111; v. גָּרַר II. b) *planed.* Tosef. Sot. XV, 1 היו מְגוֹרָרוֹת במגר׳ Var. (ed. Zuck. היה מְגָרֵר) the stones were planed with a plane.

Hithpa. הִתְגָּרֵר *to be scraped.* Tosef. Sabb. XVI (XVII), 19 אין מִתְגָּרְרִין במגוררת ed. Zuck. (Var. מגרדין במגרדת, Sabb. 147^b גודרין במגרדת, Ms. M. במגירדה, corr. acc.) one must not be scraped with a strigil. Ib. XXII, 6 (147^a) מתגררין, Talm. ed. (Mish. מִתְגָּרְדִין, v. Rabb. D. S. to 147^b, note 70).

גְּרַר ch. same; 1) *to drag, pull, push.*—Part. pass. גְּרִיר *dragged, following, guided by.* Targ. Y. II Ex. XIV, 25 גְּרִירָן וכ׳ (some ed. גריד) pushed from behind.—B. Kam. 18^b בתר גופיה גְּרִירָן they are clinging to his body. Taan. 24^a אנן בתרייהו גרירינן Rashi (ed. גררינן, read גְּרִירִינָן, Ms. M. קאזלינן) we must be guided by their order. Ab. Zar. 72^b all the wine in the barrel ג׳ .... אגישתא moves towards the siphon. B. Mets. 85^a דג׳ עלמא וכ׳ that all the world followed David.—2) *to scratch, scrape.* Targ. Jud. VIII, 16, v. גְּרַד.—Hull. 83^b וְלִיגְרְרֵיה ונכסי (Ar. גרד) let him scrape off the blood and cover it. Ib. וּנְגְרוֹר.—*Part.* גָּרֵיר Ib.—3) *to rub, to whet the appetite.* Ber. 35^b כי היכי דִנְגְרְרֵיה לליביה (Ar. everywhere גרד) in order to stimulate his appetite. Ib. טובא גָּרֵיר a large quantity has an appetizing effect. Pes. 107^b מִגְרַר גָּרֵיר. Sabb. 140^b משום דג׳ because it stimulates the appetite.

Pa. גָּרֵיר *to make appetizing.* Esth. R. to I, 9 [read:] אנא מְגָרֵיר וכ׳ I will make their drinks appetizing (induce them to get intoxicated, interpreting Jer. LI, 39; differ. in comment.).—2) *to saw off*. Targ. Y. Deut. XXXIII, 20 דמְגָרֵר וכ׳ (or דמַגְרַר Af., ed. דמְגָרַר, corr. acc.) for he cuts off the arm &c. (II מְפָרֵק).

Ithpa. אִתְגָּרַר 1) *to be dragged*. Y. Kidd. I, 60[d] large bags דארחידהון מִתְגָּרְרָה which are commonly dragged (not lifted).—2) *to stimulate, instigate one another*. Targ. Ps. XXII, 8 מִתְגָּרְרִין (some ed. מִתְגָּרְדִין, ed. Lag. מִתְגָּרֵין, fr. גרי; h. text יפטירו).

*גָּרַר II (fr. a Polel of גּוּר; cmp. גָּלַל) *to roll*; cmp. גַּרְגַּר.—Part. pass. מְגוֹרָר *whirled, reeling*. Gen. R. s. 64 (play on מגרר, Gen. XXVI, 26) מג׳ ... שנכנסו וכ׳ reeling (after a night revel) &c.; v. גָּרַר I.

Hithpa. הִתְגָּרֵר, *Hithpol.* הִתְגּוֹרֵר (v. Jer. XXX, 23, cmp. XXIII, 19) *to roll one's self*, esp. (cmp. חָבַט II, חָנַן, נָפַל Hithpa.) *to lie in contrition, asking forgiveness*. Mekh. B'shall., Vayassa 1, [read as in] Yalk. Ex. 256 (ref. to וישלך אל המים, Ex. XV, 25, as if meaning, 'and he caused them to throw themselves down in contrition over their sin by the sea-side'). היו ישראל מתחננים ומִתְגָּרְרִים ..... כבן שהוא מתחנן לפני אביו וכתלמיד שמִתְגּוֹרֵר לפני רבו כך היו ישראל מתחננין ומִתְגּוֹרְרִין וכ׳ the Israelites prayed beseechingly and rolled themselves in contrition before &c.

גֵּרַר, v. גֵּרָד.

גְּרָרָא I f. (=h. גֵּרָה III, 2) *cud*. Targ. Y. II Deut. XIV, 6 sq. (some ed. גְּרָדָא).

גְּרָרָא II f. (גרר) 1) *that which is carried along*; אגב ג׳ *incidentally, occasionally*. B. Mets. 4[b]; Shebu. 40[b]. [2) *scraping*, v. גִּירָדָא I.]

*__גְּרָרָה__ *stalk*, v. גֵּרָה II.

גררין, Bets. 24[b] top, Ar., v. גֶּנֶר.

גרריקו, v. next w.

גְּרָרִיקִי f. (a Greek formation fr. גְּרָר, LXX Γέραροι) *Gerarikê, the district of G'rar* in Philistea. Targ. Y. Gen. XX, 1 (Ar. a. Lev. גרדקי, corr. acc., ed. גְּרָר); ib. XXVI, 1.—Gen. R. s. 64 גרדיקי (corr. acc.); Y. Shebi. VI, 36[c] bot. גרריקו (corr. acc.).

גררתה, Y. Dem. I, 21[d], v. גדודתה.

גָּרַשׁ (b. h.) 1) *to stir up, to set in commotion*. Sifré Deut. 39; Yalk. ib. 859 יכול יהו מים גּוֹרְשִׁין את העפר ממקום בקעה וכ׳ you might suppose the (rain) water will stir up the (fat) ground of the valley, and thus the valley will lack (drinking) water.—2) (cmp. טָרַד) *to banish; to send off, divorce* (a wife).—Part. pass. גָּרוּשׁ, f. גְּרוּשָׁה q. v.

Pi. גֵּירֵשׁ, גֵּרֵשׁ *to send off, banish*. Gen. R. s. 21.—Esp. *to give a letter of divorce*. Gitt. IX, 1 הַמְגָרֵשׁ וכ׳ if one divorces his wife and says, on handing her the letter, &c.; a. v. fr.—Ib. VI, 5 if one says (to his delegates)... גָּרְשׁוּהָ *ga'rshuha*, they are authorized to write and deliver to her a letter of divorce (*geresh* being the colloquial term for divorcing).

Pa. גּוּרַשׁ *to be banished*, &c. Pirkê d'R. El. ch. XIX; ג׳ ויצא וכ׳ XX he was banished and he left paradise.—*Part.* מְגוּרָשׁ, f. מְגוּרֶשֶׁת. Gitt. VII, 4 מג׳ ואינה מג׳ she is and is not divorced, i. e. her divorce is doubtful, and she has to suffer the disqualifications of a married and of a divorced woman. Ib. 5; a. v. fr.

Hithpa. הִתְגָּרֵשׁ, *Nithpa.* נִתְגָּרֵשׁ 1) *to be banished; to be divorced*. Midr. Till. to Ps. XCII. Gitt. 65[a] מִתְגָּרֶשֶׁת בקידושי וכ׳ she is entitled to receive a letter of divorce for herself even though her father had contracted the marriage in her behalf; a. v. fr. [2) *to be stirred up, become muddy, thick*. Midr. d'R. Akiba, Alef (Jellinek Beth Hammidrash III, 13).]

גְּרַשׁ I ch. same. *Pa.* גָּרֵישׁ. Pes. 110[b] דגָרְשָׁהּ לאיתתיה Ms. M. (ed. דגרשא, corr. acc.) who had divorced his wife. Ber. 56[a] תרי נשי מְגָרֵשְׁת it will be thy destiny to divorce two wives. Arakh. 23[a] דלִיגָרֵשׁ לדביתהו that he should divorce &c. Ib. אטו כל דמְגָרֵשׁ וכ׳ does every one who divorces his wife, give divorce in court?; a. fr.

Ithpe. אִיגְּרֵשׁ, infin. אִיגְּרוּשֵׁי *to be divorced*. Gitt. 78[a] בת אי׳ in a fit condition to receive a letter of divorce.

*__גְּרַשׁ II__ (cmp. גרר *to drag*) *to hoist up*. Y. Kil. IX, 32[c] top. Y. Keth. XII, 35[b] top [read:] ואין ענייה אתון גרשין לי and if I call, ye will hoist me up; (Koh. R. to IX, 10 שרר; Mat. K. quotes גדש, v. גְּרַשׁ II).

גֶּרֶשׂ m. (b. h.; v. גָּרִיס) *grits*. Sifra Vayikra, N'dabah, ch. XIV, Par. 13 אפשר יקלנו ג׳ I might think he must roast it after being pounded; Men. 66[b].

גַּרְשָׂא ch. same. Targ. Y. Lev. II, 14; 16 Levita (ed. פירוכ׳).

*__קְרֵטִיקוֹן, גְּרֵתִיקוֹן__ m. (γῆ κρητική, creta) *chalk, white earth* used for cleansing silver ware. Sabb. 50[a] גרתי׳ Ar. (ed. גרתקין, גרתקון); Y. Bets. IV, 62[c] bot. קרטי׳; Tosef. ib. IV, 10 קירטון ed. Zuck. (Var. קריתין, קרקתין). [Rashi to Sabb. l. c. expl. אלום, describing *tartar* deposited in wine vessels; Ar.: pulverised *resin*.]

גַּשׁ, v. נְגַשׁ.

גְּשַׁגַּשׁ, v. גָּשַׁשׁ.

גְּשׁוֹרָא, pl. גְּשׁוֹרֵי, v. גִּשְׁרָא.

גָּשׁוֹשׁ m. (גשש), ג׳ של ספינה prob. *framework* of a ship (v. גְּשִׁישׁ); comment.: *sounding pole*. Sabb. 125[b] (Ms. M. אגושש, Ms. O. גשיש; v. Sm. Ant. s. v. Contus).

גַּשּׁוֹשָׁא, גַּשּׁוֹשָׁאָה m. (v. preced.) 1) *one carrying the sounding pole in advance of the ship, sounder*. *Pl.* גַּשּׁוֹשֵׁי Sabb. 100[b] (Ms. O. גַּשּׁוֹשָׁאֵי).—2) *one tracing treasures buried in the ground*.—*Pl.* גַּשּׁוֹשָׁאֵי. B. Mets. 42[a].

גְּשִׁישׁ m. (גּוּשׁ, גָּשַׁשׁ; formed like עָצִיץ) [1) *sounding apparatus*, v. גָּשׁוֹשׁ.]—2) *a frame on which the couch is spread* (sponda). Zab. III, 1; 3 ג׳ של מטה; Tosef. ib. IV, 4. Ib. Mikv. VI (VII), 17 הג׳ החיצון the outer frame (of a double bed, sponda exterior, v. Sm. Ant. s. v. Lectus).

Esth. R. to I, 6.—*Pl.* גַּשְׁרְשָׁרִים, גַּשְׁרְשִׁין. Tosef. Kel. B. Mets. VIII, 8 חג׳ של קיטליזקי (ed. Zuck. קיטליאקי, read ס for א) the bed-frames of the little bed-chambers (κοιτωνίσκοι—which are taken apart or placed against the wall in day time).—*Tosef. Mikv. VI, 8 ג׳ ע״ג חשבר Ar. (ed. קשקשים, Sabb. 53ª קשישין) *splints.*

גָּשַׁם (b. h., v. גוש) *to make the earth cloddy* (v. Ges. H. Dict.[10] s. v.).—*Part. pass.* גָּשׁוּם *cloddy* in consequence of ample rains. Y. Yoma V, 42ᶜ top שנת גְּשׁוּמָה שחונה וכ׳ (sub. ארץ) a year in which the earth forms clods, then is parched so as to form scabs, and then moistened with dew; Bab. ib. 53ᵇ שנת שחונה שנת ג׳ Ms. M. (ed. שנה ג׳ ושח׳, v. Rabb. D. S. a. l. note), expl. אם שח׳ (היא) תהא ג׳ if it is to be parched, let it first be soaked with heavy rains; Lev. R. s. 20; Tanh. Aḥăré 3 (corr. acc.); ed. Bub. ib. 4.

Hof. הוּגְשַׁם (denom. of גֶּשֶׁם) *to be frought with rain, rain-bringing.* B. Bath. 25ᵇ since the destruction of the Temple לא הוּגְשְׁמָה וכ׳ the south wind has not been rain-bringing.

גֶּשֶׁם I m. (b. h.; preced.) *heavy, continuous rain.* Taan. 3ᵇ לא אמר מוריד הַגֶּ׳ if he failed to insert in the second benediction (v. גְּבוּרָה) 'Who sendeth rain'.—*Pl.* גְּשָׁמִים. Taan. I, 1, a. fr. גבורות ג׳, v. גְּבוּרָה. Ib. 2 שואלין את הג׳ we insert the petition for rain in the ninth benediction, v. שְׁאֵלָה.—ימות הג׳ *rainy season, autumn and winter.* Ib. 3ᵇ. Toh. VI, 7, v. בִּקְעָה; a. v. fr.—שְׂדֵה ג׳ (or sub. שדה) *a field naturally watered by rain,* opp. שלחין. Bekh. VI, 3 של ג׳ from fields with natural irrigation; cmp. בַּעַל. [In later Hebr. literature גֶּשֶׁם *substance,* v. next w.].

גֶּשֶׁם II, **גִּשְׁמָא** m. ch. (גשם, v. גּוּשְׁמָא) *body, self.* Dan. IV, 30.—*Pl.* גִּשְׁמַיָּא. Lam. R. to I, 5 לא יהבין גִּשְׁמֵיהוֹן (Koh. R. to VII, 11 גרמיהון) they will not devote themselves to warfare.

גִּשְׁמָה (גִּשְׁמָא) f. (v. preced., cmp. גָּשִׁישׁ) *frame, door-stop* against which the door shuts. Erub. 101ª (explain. 'a widowed door') דלית לה ג׳ (Ms. M. בשמא, a clerical error for כשמא, oth. Var. גְּשָׁאמָא, קְשָׁאמָא, v. Rabb. D. S. a. l. note; גִּישְׁתְּמָא, reduplic. of גשם, cmp. גוזטרא, v. Ar. ed. Koh. s. v. גשם) which does not shut against a frame.

גשף, Men. 50ᵇ איגשף Ar., v. נְשַׁב, נְשַׁף.

גִּשְׁקְרָא, v. גִּשְׁקְרָא.

גָּשַׁר (v. גשש) *to join,* esp. *to make a bridge.* Ab. Zar. 2ᵇ הרבה גשרים גָּשַׁרְנוּ we have built numerous bridges.

גְּשַׁר ch. same. B. Kam. 113ᵇ קטלי .. וגַשְׁרֵי גִּשְׁרֵי they (the government officials) fell trees (belonging to private persons) and build bridges.

גֶּשֶׁר m. (preced.) *bridge, ferry.* Erub. 55ᵇ; Tosef. ib. VI (V), 4 הקבר והג׳ וכ׳ graves and bridges (in the outskirts of towns) which have a place of shelter.—Gen. R. s. 76, end עשה עצמו כג׳ וכ׳ Jacob constituted himself a ferry, taking persons from one shore and setting them down on the other (Mat. K. כגַּשָּׁר like a *ferry-man*).—*Pl.* גְּשָׁרִים, גְּשָׁרִין. Erub. V, 1. Ib. IX, 4 ג׳ המפולשים bridges under which there is an open passage. Ab. Zar. 2ᵇ; a. fr.

גִּישְׁרָא, גִּשְׁרָא ch. same, 1) *board, joist* (cmp. כָּשׁוּרָא).—*Pl.* גִּשְׁרִין. Targ. Ezek. XXVII, 5 Levita (ed. גִּשְׁרִיךְ, גַּשְׁרָךְ).—2) *bridge.* Ber. 59ᵇ he who sees the Euphrates אג׳ דבבל from the bridge (or ferry) of Babylon; a. fr.—*Pl.* גִּשְׁרַיָּא, גִּשְׁרֵי, גִּישְׁ׳. Targ. Y. I Ex. XX, 26. Targ. Nah. II, 7 (h. text שערי).—B. Kam. 113ᵇ, v. גְּשַׁר. B. Bath. 73ᵇ.—[Sabb. 67ª top וז׳ סרכי מז׳ גָּשׁוּרֵי (Ms. M. גשרי)—prob. a Var. of preceding וז׳ צרבי מז׳ כשורי, v. כָּשׁוּרָא.]

גָּשַׁשׁ (b. h.; v. גוש) *to touch a substance, to strike against.* Hall. II, 2; Y. ib. 58ᶜ top הספינה גוֹשֶׁשֶׁת the ship touches the ground (in harbor).

Pi. גִּישֵׁשׁ *to feel, grope.* Y. Yoma V, 42ᶜ היה מְגַשֵּׁשׁ וכ׳ entered groping &c.

Pilp. גִּשְׁגֵּשׁ (cmp. קשקש, כשכש) *to beat, ring.* Lev. R. s. 8 (ref. to Jud. XIII, 25, cmp. פַּעַמֹן) התחיל רוה״ק לְגַשְׁגֵּשׁ וכ׳ the holy spirit began to ring in Samson.

Hithpa. הִתְגַּשֵּׁשׁ, *Hithpol.* הִתְגּוֹשֵׁשׁ, *Hithpalp.* הִתְגַּשְׁגֵּשׁ, *Nithpa.* נִתְגַּשֵּׁשׁ 1) *to wrestle, fight.* Gen. R. s. 22; s. 77; Cant. R. to III, 6. Ex. R. s. 28, beg.—2) *to exercise one's strength, practice.* Pesik. S'liḥoth, p. 166ª גבור שהוא מִתְגּוֹשֵׁשׁ וכ׳ a warrior practicing on a stone-cutter's stone.

גְּשַׁשׁ ch., *Pa.* גַּשֵּׁשׁ same, *to feel, touch.* Targ. Y. Gen. XXVII, 12; 22 (h. text מוש). Gitt. 67ᵇ bot. גַּשְּׁשֵׁיה he (being blind) touched it (and felt the bone).

גִּשְׁתָּא, גִּישְׁ׳ I f. (preced.) *feeling, touch.* Hull. 47ᵇ resembling wood בג׳ in touch. Ib. 122ᵇ; Sabb. 107ᵇ.

גִּשְׁתָּא, גִּישְׁ׳ II f. (preced.; cmp. גּוּשְׁשָׁא) *sounding tube;* ג׳ ובת ג׳ *a large and small tube,* i. e. *a siphon.* Ab. Zar. 72ᵇ אסיק חמרא בג׳ brought up wine through the siphon. Ib. a gentile came and put his hand אג׳ on the large tube. Ib. גרירר . . . אג׳, v. גְּרַר.

גַּת I pr. n. pl. *Gath* in Philistea. Snh. 102ª; a. e.

גַּת II f., with suffix גִּיתּ־, גִּתּ־ (contr. of גִּנַּת) *a marked-off space.* Tosef. Ohol. XV, 7 'the court of a burying place' זו הגת . . . לתוכה (R. S. to Ohol. XV, 8, ed. Zuck. גל, Var. לתוכו) is the marked space into which the caverns open.—Par. IV, 2 שרפה חוץ מִגִּתָּהּ if he burnt the cow outside of the place selected for the purpose; Zeb. XIV, 4; Tosef. Par. III, 9 sq.—*Pl.* גִּתּוֹת, גִּית׳. Par. l. c.

גַּת III f., with suffix גִּיתּ־, גִּתּ־ (b. h.; contr. of גנת, cmp. גִּיגִּית) *vat for wine pressing;* (שעת)הג׳ *the season of wine pressing.* Ab. Zar. V, 11 ג׳ של אבן a stone vat, של חרס an earthen. Ib. IV, 8, v. בָּעַט. Hag. III, 4 (24ᵇ) מניחה לג׳ הבאה he may reserve it for the next season (and give it to the priest). Ib. 25ᵇ דבר שאין לו ג׳ something which has no special manufacturing season (e. g. date wine); a. fr.—Lam. R. introd. 32 (play on מבלגִּיתִי, Jer.

VIII, 18) עשיתי לביתי גּוּתִּי I made my house my vat (cmp. Lam. I, 15).—Pl. גִּיתּוֹת, גִּתּ׳, גִּתּ׳.—בית חגר׳ the press room. Tosef. Ter. III, 7; Y. ib. II, 41[b] bot. בית חגיתי׳ (corr. acc.)—Tosef. l. c. שתי ג׳ לבור וכ׳ two vats for one pit; a. fr.

*גִּתִּית, גִּיתִּ׳ f. (denom. of preced.) *woman engaged in the wine press, wine treader.*—Pl. גִּיתִּיּוֹת, גִּתִּ׳. Gen. R. s. 71 [read:] אף חג׳ מאחורי הקוריים וכ׳ even the wine-treaders behind the beam handlers (of loose character) maligned her. Esth. R. to I, 10 (play on אבגתא) אביא ג׳ מא׳ ק׳ I shall bring the wine treaders &c. (to deride her).

ד

ד *Daleth*, the fourth letter of the Alphabet; it interchanges dialectically with ז, e. g. דב, זב; with צ, e. g. אֶצְבַּע, אֶדְבַּע.—ד eliminated in קַדְמָא=קַמָּא, אוּדְנָא=אוּנָּא.

ד׳ as a numeral, *four*, v. א׳.

דְּ־ (דִּי) a prefix, corresp. to h. שֶׁ־, *of, who, which, that* (quod). Targ. Gen. XXXI, 42. Ib. IX, 5; a. v. fr.—Ber. 2[a] זמן ק״ש דעַרבית the time of reading the Sh'ma of bed-time (Deut. VI, 7). Ib. ליתני׳ דערבית וכ׳ let him first state *that of* (the law concerning) the evening prayer. Ib. הא קמ״ל דכפרה וכ׳ we are given to understand (by implication) that &c. Ib. ממאי דהאי וכ׳ whence is it proved that this *uba* &c.? Ib.[b] ואינהו דמחשכי וכ׳ and it was *they* who (as an exception) worked late and early; a. v. fr.—[This prefix is used for the formation of what may be named *Difel nouns*, as דִּבְרָא, דִּכְבָא &c., a. *Dispeel nouns* as דִּיסְקַרְתָּא &c.]

דָּא I, דָּה f. (=h. זאת, זו) *this*; with prefix ה, הָדָא (הָדָא), cmp. אָדָא I. Targ. Gen. II, 23; a. fr.—Ned. 41[a] (prov.) דְּדָא ביה וכ׳ in whom there is this (wisdom), in him there is everything.—דא ודא this and that, both. Sabb. 52[b] ד׳ וד׳ (אחת) חדא היא all sorts of rings come under the same law; a. fr.—Y. Succ. I, 52[c] top הדא אמרה היא הדא this proves &c., v. אָדָא I.—הדא היא דכתיב (abbr. הה״ד) וכ׳ it is this which Scripture says, thus we read. Y. Sot. I, 17[b] bot.; Gen. R. s. 2; a. v. fr.—Y. Gitt. IV, 45[d] bot. introduced his lecture בדה with this.—לא בְדָא *not in this case*, i. e. the law does not apply to this. Y. Ber. I, 2[b] bot.; a. fr.—Y. Taan. II, 66[a] bot. לא בדא הלכה וכ׳ not in this case is the practice in agreement with the anonymous opinion.

דָּא II, דא דא *da da*, the camel-drivers' call. Pes. 112[b]. [דא, Cant. R. to II, 15, v. בלטוורא.]

דָּאַב (b. h.; cmp. זוב, דוב) *to melt, pine away, languish.*—*Hif.* הַדְאִיב *to melt, to cause to languish.* B. Bath. 79[a] (play on מידבא, Num. XXI, 30) עד שתַּדְאִיב נשמתן (Var. תדיב, תדוב, v. Rabb. D. S. a. l. note 2) until it (the fire of Gehenna) shall melt their soul. Ned. 22[a] (ref. to Deut. XXVIII, 65) שמכלה .... ומַדְאִיב וכ׳ which ruins the eyesight and makes life languid. Ch. דְּאֵיב.

דְּאָב, דָּאִיב m. (preced.) *languor, weariness.* Targ. Y. II Deut. XXVIII, 65.

דָּוָונָא, דָּבוֹנָא, דָּאבוֹנָא same. Targ. Job XLI, 14 (דאב fem., h. text דאבה).—Targ. Ps. XIII, 3 דב׳ Ms. (ed. דוו׳; h. text יגון). Targ. Y. Num. XXI, 30 בְּדָבוֹ׳ (some ed. כְּדָ׳, h. text דיבון, cmp. B. Bath. 79[a], s. v. דָּאַב); a. e.

*דַּאֲבֵן (denom. of preced.) *to make languid.* Targ. Prov. XVIII, 8 מְדַאַבְנָן ed. Lag. (oth. ed. מרכנן, h. text כמתלהמים).

דֹּאֵג, v. דּוֹאֵג.

דָּאַג (b. h.) [*to melt,*] cmp. דאב a. רצף, *to be low-spirited, to sorrow, fear.* Snh. 106[b] (play on דאג, I Sam. XXI, 8, a. דוֹיג, ib. XXII, 18) at first יושב הקב״ה ודואג וכ׳ the Lord sat in anxiety, that he (Doeg) might degenerate; after . . . ., He said ווי שיצא זה woe that he did &c. Ber. 40[a] יִדְאַג מריח וכ׳ must be in fear of contracting &c. Succ. 29[a]. Ḥag. 13[a] שלבו דואג בקרבו whose heart within him is in fear of sin (reverential). Sabb. 105[b] sq. יִדְאֲגוּ כל האחין all the brothers should feel troubled (examine their ways). Midr. Till. to Ps. XLVIII a man committed a sin והיה דואג בלבו and was troubled in his heart; a. fr.

דָּאָה I (b. h.) *to float, fly.* Pirké d'R. El. ch. IV הוֹאֶה על וכ׳ (ref. to Ps. XVIII, 11).

דָּאָה II f. (b. h.; v. דַּיָּה) *Daah*, name of an unclean bird. Ḥull. 63[b] ד׳ וראה וכ׳ Daah and Raah and Ayyah and Dayyah are the same genus; Sifré Deut. 103.

דָּאוֵי=דָּוִי, v. דוי, דְּוָא II.

דאומטיקוס, read: רֶאוּבְטִיקוֹס.

דאוסיניסי, Y. Ab. Zar. V, end, 45[b], v. דְּנִיסְטֵיס.

דַּאי m. (v. די) *sufficiency.*—יותר מִדַּאי more than enough, *too much.* Keth. 111[a]; a. fr.—כְּדַאי, v. כְּדַי.

דְּאֵיב (v. דאב) *to flow.* Targ. Ps. CV, 41 (h. text זוב).—Part. דָּאֵיב, v. דּוּב.

דָּאִיב *languor*, v. דְּאָב.

דָּאִיק, דָּאֵיג, v. דּוּק, דּוּג.

דָּאִיסְקַרְתָּא, v. דִּיסְקַרְתָּא.

דאיסרטוס, Y. B. Mets. II, 8[c], v. דְּנִיסְטֵיס.

דָּאִיר, דָּאִיץ, v. דּוּר, דּוּץ.

דאית, Targ. Prov. XII, 12 some ed., read רָאִיג.

דָּאִיתָאָה, pl. דָּאִיתָאִין, v. דִּיתָאָה.

דָּאלוּ, v. דָּלוּ.

דאפלא, v. דיופלא.

דָּאצִיפֵי, דִּיוּצִיפֵי m. pl. name of a species of *doves*. Hull. 62ª ed. (Ar. דוי׳).

***דָּאַר** (v. דּוּר) *to turn, circle.* Targ. Ps. CXXIX, 3 דַּארוּ דַּאֲרָיָא ed. Ven. (cmp. Pesh.) the turners turned (planned my destruction, h. text חרשו חרשים; ed. Lag. ראדו ראדריא, oth. ed. רדו רדייא, v. רְדֵי).

***דַּאֲרָא** m. *turner*, pl. דַּאֲרַיָּא, v. preced.

דָּארוּ pr. n. m. *Daru*, name of R. Naḥman's slave. B. Mets. 64ᵇ; a. e.

דארזי, v. ארז a. אַרְזָא.

***דְּאַת** (h. דשא) *to sprout.* *Af.* אַדְאִית *to bring forth.* Targ. C. Gen. I, 11, v. דִּיתְאָה.

דֹּב, v. דּוֹב.

דֵּב (v. דֵּיבָא) *wolf.* Gen. R. s. 99 לדב כתיב דב הוה שמה it reads (Dan. VII, 5) לדב (instead of לדוב)—*deb* (wolf) was her (Media's) name (with ref. to Jer. V, 6); Lev. R. s. 13; Esth. R. introd.

דְּבָא, v. דבר.

דִּבָּא, v. דִּיבָּא.

דָּבָא *to drip, overflow.* Sifré Deut. 42 (ref. to Deut. XXXIII, 25) כל הארצות דּוֹבְאוֹת כסף וכ׳ all countries will send their overflow of silver to the land of Israel (to buy fruits); Yalk. Deut. 963; Lev. R. s. 35 ד׳ כסף ומביאין לא״י. [Sifré l. c. הארצות דובאות למלאות וכ׳, read באות; cmp. Lev. R. l. c.]

דָּבַב I (b. h.) *to drip, flow; to murmur, speak lowly, whisper.* Yeb. 97ª (ref. to Cant. VII, 10) מ׳ה כומר ... כ׳ה כומר דּוֹבֵב as the heated mass of grapes drips as soon as you apply your finger, כך . . . דּוֹבְבוֹת וכ׳ so do the lips of scholars in the grave murmur when their names are cited; Snh. 90ᵇ; Bekh. 31ᵇ (Y. Ber. II, 4ᵇ bot. רוחשות, Ar. דובבות); a. e.—2) **to drop pitch.* Y. Ab. Zar. II, 41ᵇ bot. נכרי עובדן ודוֹבְבָן a gentile may tan them (the leather bottles) and pitch them; [Tosef. ib. IV (V), 10 זופתן ed. Zuck. (Var. רובבן; Bab. ib. 33ª ריבבן; Tosaf. a. l. quotes fr. Tosef. רובד׳, v. רָבַב a. רָבַד.]

דָּבַב II (deriv. of דִּבָּה or דְּבַב) *to speak evil, be hostile*, only in part. pass. דָּבוּב, f. דְּבוּבָה. Y. Erub. VII, 24ᶜ bot. a woman שהיתה ד׳ לחבירתה who was on bad terms with her neighbor (ib. III, 20ᵈ bot. דבר׳, corr. acc.).—*Pl.* דְּבוּבִין, דְּבוּבוֹת. Cant. R. to III, 11 two legions ד׳ זה עם זה hostile to each other. Ib. fire and hail ד׳ זה וכ׳ are hostile elements; Pesik. Vayhi, p. 4ª רכו׳ (corr. acc.).

דְּבַב I ch. same, *to murmur.* דַּבְבָן Ar. (prob. quot. of B. Kam. 117ª bot. חזינהו לשיפוותיה דקא חזא דפריט׳ שיפוותיה Ms. M.).

דְּבַב m. (=דִּבָּה, v. דָּבַב) *whisper, evil speech;* only in בַּעַל ד׳, pl. בַּעֲלֵי ד׳ *man of evil speech*, i. e. *opponent, informer*. Cant. R. to VII, 10 (play on *dobeb*, ib.) הייתי נעשה בעל ד׳ וכ׳ I should have become an opponent of those (patriarchs) sleeping &c. Sifra B'ḥuck. Par. 2, ch. IV בעלי ד׳ וכ׳ informers shall surround you from without; Yalk. Lev. 673 בעל דבבא. Sifra Emor, Par. 14, ch. XIX the whole congregation shall act כבעלי ד׳ לו as if they were his accusers.

דְּבַב II, **דְּבָבָא** ch. same, with בְּעֵיל, בְּעַל. Targ. Ps. VIII, 3 (h. text אוֹיֵב); a. fr.—Gitt. 55ᵇ וב׳ דְּבָבֵיה בר וכ׳ and his enemy was Bar K., opp. רחמיה.—*Pl.* בעלי ד׳, also דְּבָבַיָּא, ב׳ דְּבָבִין. Targ. Ps. LXVIII, 24. Ib. XXXVII, 20.—Targ. Lam. I, 2; a. fr. [Sifré Num. 42, v. next w. Yalk. Lev. 637, v. preced.]

דְּבָבָה f. same. Sifré Num. 42 במקום ... ושנאה ובעלי ד׳ (not דבבא) there (in heavens) where there are neither hatred . . . . nor slanderers; Yalk. ib. 711.

דְּבָבוּ, דְּבָבוּתָא ch. same, *hatred.* Targ. Gen. III, 5; a. e.—Targ. Is. XIV, 21 ed. Lag. (ed. דבב).

דַּבְדְּבָנִיּוֹת f. pl. (reduplic. of דבב) *lumps of dripping grapes* (exposed to heat; v. דָּבַב). Ab. Zar. II, 7 (39ᵇ) והדבר׳ (Mish. ed. דברניות, Ms. M. דברבנ׳; Y. ed. דכדב׳, corr. acc.; Mish. Nap. הַמְּדְמָנִיּוֹת). Y. Sabb. I, 4ª bot.; Y. Bets. II, 62ª top דמדמ׳. Cmp. אֲדַמְדְּמָנֵי.

דִּבָּה, דִּיבָּה f. (b. h.; רבב) *evil report, calumny.*—Trnsf. *an ill-reputed* woman. Pes. 87ᵇ (play on *Diblayim*, Hos. I, 3) ד׳ רעה בת ד׳ וכ׳ an ill-reputed woman daughter of &c.; cmp. דּוּמָה I.

דִּבּוּ f. (דֵּב) *she-wolf.* Cant. R. to III, 4 כבין ד׳ לכלב about that stage of the morning when you begin to distinguish between a wolf and a dog (v. Ber. 9ᵇ).

דְּבוֹנָא, v. דְּאבוֹנָא.

דִּבּוּק, דִּבּוּר, דְּבוּרָא, v. דִּיב׳.

דְּבוֹר, דְּבוֹרָא, v. דְּבוֹרְיָא.

דְּבוֹרָה f. (b. h. דְּבֹרָה; דבר *to lead, join*) 1) [*swarm,*] *bee.* Yalk. Deut. 795 (play on הדברים, Deut. I, 1) מה הד׳ הזו בניה מתנהגין וכ׳ as the bee is followed by the young, so are the Israelites led by the righteous &c.; (Deut. R. s. 1 כִּדְּבוֹרִים היו וכ׳ like bees my children were guided &c.). Ib. מה הד׳ הזו וכ׳ as the bee whose honey &c.; a. fr.—*Pl.* דְּבוֹרִים. Kel. XVI, 7 מדף של ד׳ the vessel used for smoking the bees out. Bekh. 7ᵇ דבש ד׳ bee-honey. Deut. R. l. c., v. supra.—2) pr. n. f. *Deborah*, the heroine and prophetess. Meg. 14a; a. fr.—שִׁירַת ד׳ *the song of Deborah* (Jud. V). Y. Meg. III, 74b bot.; Treat. Sof'rim XII, 10; a. e.

דְּבוֹרְיָא (דְּבוֹר, דְּבוֹרָא) f. *bee-swarm, bee-hive.* B. Bath. 108a (in Hebr. Diction). הרחק חרדלך מִדְּבוֹרַיי Rashi (ed. מִן דְּבוֹרָאֵי, Ms. F. a. R. דבורי) remove thy mustard plants from my bee-hive. Ib. דְּבוֹרְיָיךְ Rashi (ed. דבורך).—*Pl.* דְּבוֹרְיָין. Y. Peah VII, 20b top דבש דד׳ bee-honey.

דְּבוֹרִיתָא, v. דַּבָּרְתָּא.

דְּבַח I ch.=h. זָבַח, *to slaughter, to sacrifice, feast.* Targ. Ps. LIV, 8; a. fr.

Pa. דַּבַּח same. Targ. Ex. V, 8; a. fr.

דְּבַח II, **דִּיבְחָא, דִּבְחָא** ch.=h. זֶבַח, *slaughtering, sacrifice, feast.* Targ. II Kings V, 17. Targ. Prov. XXI, 3; a. e.—*Pl.* דִּבְחִין, דִּבְחַיָּא, דִּיבְ׳. Targ. Num. XXV, 2 דִּבְחֵי (some ed. O. דַּבְ׳). Targ. II Sam. XV, 12; a. fr.—Esp. *the feast of Passover.* Sabb. 110a בין ד׳ לעצרתא between Passover and Pentecost.

***דְּבָא, דְּבִי** (=דְּוָא) *to look out, lie in wait.*—*Pa.* דַּבֵּי *to lurk for, hunt.* Sabb. 106b הני לא בעי דַּבּוּיֵי Ms. M. (ed. לא עבידי לדבויי ד׳) the ones need no hunting; Bets. 24a בעיין לְדַ׳ Ms. M. (v. Rabb. D. S. a. l.; ed. עבידי לד׳), v. דְּבֵי.

דביבה, v. דָּבַב II.

דִּבְיוֹנִים m. pl. (b. h.; דבב=דבח) *excrements*, a softer expression in the *K'ri* instead of the *Kethib* חריונים (II Kings VI, 25). Meg. 25b.

דְּבֵילָה f. (b. h.; דבל, cmp. דבב) *a thick viscid mass, cake of pressed figs; fig used for pressing.* Pes. 87b (play on *Diblayim*, Hos. I, 3) she was sweet in the mouth of all כד׳ like figs; כד׳ . . . הכל all trod upon her as figs are trodden upon. Gen. R. s. 31 הכניס עמו ד׳ he took the provision with him in a pressed state; רוב מִכְנָסוֹ ד׳ most of his storage was &c. Yoma 76a; Tosef. Ker. I, 20, a. e. ד׳ קעילית preserved figs from Keilah (which are intoxicating). Y. Bicc. III, beg. 65c ד׳, opp. גרוגרות; a. fr.—*Pl.* דְּבֵילוֹת. Naz. 9a (alternating with sing.).

דִּיבְלָא, דְּבֶלְתָּא, דְּבֵילְתָא ch. same. Targ. Jud. IX, 11 (h. text התנובה); a. e.—*Pl.* דִּיבְלִין. Targ. 1 Chr. XII, 40.—דְּבֵילָתָא, דִּבְלָ׳. Targ. I Sam. XXX, 12 (some ed. sing.). Targ. Y. Num. XXXIII, 46.

דְּבֵילְתָּה same. Y. Dem. II, 22c.

דְּבִיק, דָּבִיק, v. דָּבֵק.

דְּבִיקָה f. (דבק) 1) *embrace.* Ex. R. s. 33 דרך דְּבִיקָתָן in the position of their embrace.—2) *attachment.* Gen. R. s. 80; Midr. Till. to Ps. XXII בד׳ with the expression דבק (ref. to Deut. IV, 4).

דְּבִיר m. (b. h.) 1) *the Holy of Holies* in the Temple. Y. Ber. IV, 8c top.—2) *the Book*, a word in use among the Persian Jews. Ab. Zar. 24b (ref. to Jud. I, 11).

דְּבִירָא, v. דִּירְבָּא.

דְּבִיתָא f. (Difel noun of בֵּיתָא, v. letter ד) [*of the house,*] *wife*, only with suff. of person. pron. דְּבִיתְהוּ ד׳ *the wife of.* Ber. 27b. Taan. 23b ד׳ דמר your wife; a. v. fr.—דְּבִיתְהַי *thy wife.* Ned. 51a.

דבלא, Targ. Is. XXXIV, 4, some ed., read נִבְלָא.

דְּבֵלָה, v. דְּבֵילָה.

דַּבְלוּל m., pl. דַּבְלוּלִין (denom. of דְּבֵלָה, cmp. σῦκον, συκῆ, ficus) *piles, excrescences; trnsf. lumps.* Tosef. Kel. B. Mets. IX, 2 היו ד׳ יוצאין וכ׳ (cmp. מֵעִירִין ib.) if lumps of upholstery protrude from the couch. Ib. VII, 11 היו ד׳ . . . חימנה if lumps or irregular pieces of reeds hang down from the matting.—Denom. מְדוּבְלָל a) *lumpy.* Bekh. III, 4 הצמר המ׳ (Talm. ed. 25b המדולדל) the clumps in the wool.—b) (cmp. Arab. *dubal*) *melancholy, miserable-looking.* Succ. II, 2 סוכה הַמְדוּבְלֶלֶת a miserable looking Succah, expl. ib. 22a (by Rab) as עגיה or מדולדלת (Y. ib. 52b bot. מדוללת, v. דַּלַל a. דִּלְדֵּל) beggarly, thinned; (by Samuel) as קנה עולה וקנה יורד or מבולבלת disarranged.

דַּבְלֵל, part. pass. מְדוּבְלָל, v. preced.

דְּבֶלְתָּא, v. דְּבִילְתָא.

דָּבֵק, דָּבַק (b. h.) *to cleave, adhere, stick.* B. Bath. 91b, v. infra.—Yalk. Gen. 133 דבקו כל החיל וכ׳ the whole army was close to the fortress.—Ib. Deut. 824 ד׳ לסדומיים he joined the Sodomites.—2) *to join, glue, affix.* Y. Meg. I, 71d top הוּבְקִין בְּדֶבֶק the parchment is joined with glue.—*Part. pass.* דָּבוּק, f. דְּבוּקָה *attached, close, cleaving.* Sot. 42b (ref. to Ruth I, 14) בני הדבוקה the descendants of her who was attached (to Naomi). Gen. R. s. 20 דְּבוּקִין לעור close to the skin. Snh. 64a (ref. to Deut. IV, 4) like two dates הַדְּבוּקִים וכ׳ which stick to one another (easily separated); ib. דבוקים ממש really glued (inseparable); Yalk. Deut. 824 כשתי . . . הַדְּבוּקוֹת; a. fr.

Nif. נִדְבַּק *to be joined, attached, affixed.* Keth. 111b; Yalk. l. c. is it possible for man לִידָּבֵק וכ׳ to be joined to the Divine Majesty? Ib. כאילו נ׳ בשכינה (Keth. l. c. מִדַּבֵּק) as though he were joined. B. Bath. 91b ששבה ונִדְבְּקָה וכ׳ (Ms. H. ודָבְקָה) (Ruth) who came back and remained attached to Bethlehem (v. supra); a. fr.

Pi. דִּיבֵּק, דִּבֵּק 1) *to glue.* R. Hash. III, 6 (27a, b).—2) *to invite one to join in travel.* Gen. R. s. 29 ראה אחד ודִיבְּקוֹ he saw a person and made him go with him.—Part. pass. מְדוּבָּק Yalk. Deut. l. c. שמְדוּבָּקִים לחיין וכ׳ who cling to the Life of the World (the Lord).

Hif. הִדְבִּיק *to paste, fasten.* Pes. 37a הרתיח ולבסוף ה׳ he heated the pot and then pasted the dough to its wall. Ib.b.

Hithpa. הִתְדַּבֵּק, הִדַּבֵּק *to be joined.* Gen. R. s. 59 אין ארור מִתְדַּבֵּק בברוך (Yalk. Hos. 528 מִדַּבֵּק) the cursed (Eliezer) shall not be joined (through marriage) to the blessed (Isaac). Keth. l. c., v. Nif.—Yalk. Deut. l. c. מִדַּבֶּקֶת; a. fr. [Sabb. 113b [read:] לִידַּבֵּק עם הנשים or לדבר, v. Rabb. D. S. a. l. note.]

דְּבַק, דְּבֵק ch. same, *to adhere* &c. Targ. Ps. XLIV, 26. Targ. Prov. XVIII, 24 דָּבֵיק ed. Lag.; a. e.— Keth. 111ᵇ וכי אפשר לִדְבוּקֵי, v. preced. Nif.

Pa. דַּבֵּק *to paste, glue.* Men. 11ᵃ הַדְבְּקִיה לקומ׳ץ וכ׳ if he pasted the handfull of dough to the wall of the vessel.

Ithpa. אִתְדַּבַּק, *Ithpe.* אִיתְדְּבֵיק, אִידְּבַק *to be attached, join.* Targ. Ruth I, 14; a. fr.—Gitt. 56ᵇ מחו לְאִידְּבוּקֵי בהו how about joining their ranks?—Pes. 49ᵃ לְאִידְּבַק אנא בזרעיה Ms. M. (ed. דאדבק בזרעיה) that I should be connected with his descendants. Sabb. 113ᵇ. Gen. R. s. 14 אית חספין מִתְדַּבְּקִין can broken earthen vessels be joined together?

Af. אַדְבֵּק, אַדְבֵּיק 1) *to reach, overtake, attain to, obtain* (corresp. to h. הִשִּׂיג). Targ. Gen. XXXI, 23. Targ. O. Lev. XIV, 21 sq.; a. fr.—Part. pass. מְדַבַּק *joined work.* Targ. I Kings VII, 29 (h. text לִיוֹת; v. 30 עובד דיבוק).— 2) *to join* (plans), *to contrive fraud* (nectere dolos; h. text הצמיד). Targ. Ps. L, 19 (Ms. *Pa.*).

דֶּבֶק m. (b. h.; preced.) 1) *glue, paste.* Y. Meg. I, 71ᵈ top, v. דֶּבֶק. Sabb. VIII, 4, v. שַׁבְשֶׁבֶת.—2) *junction.* Hull. 50ᵃ מקום הד׳ the place where the entrails adhere to the hip.— *Pl.* דְּבָקִים *followers.* Yalk. Deut. 824 אתם ודִבְקֵיכֶם ye and your followers.—3) *nexus, cause.* *Pl.* as above; constr. דִּבְקֵי, דִּיבְ׳.—ד׳ מיתה duties the neglect of which is the cause of premature death. Sabb. 32ᵃ (a Variant of בדקי, v. בֶּדֶק); Y. ib. II, 5ᵇ bot.; Tosef. ib. II, 10 דיבק ed. Zuck. (corr. acc.); Ber. 31ᵇ.

דָּבַר (b. h.) *to join, arrange, lead* (the flock); v. next w.

Pi. דִּבֵּר, דִּיבֵּר (b. h.) *to converse, speak.* Ber. 31ᵇ, a. fr. דִּבְּרָה תורה כלשון ב״א the Torah speaks according to the language of men, i. e. uses metaphors and phrases adapted to human understanding. Sot. 12ᵇ שעתיד לְדַבֵּר וכ׳ destined to speak to Divinity. Ter. I, 2 חרש שדִּבְּרוּ .... מְדַבֵּר wherever the scholars use the word *ḥērēsh,* they mean one who neither hears nor talks. Mekh. Bo 7, end, a. fr. או אינו מְדַבֵּר אלא ב־ or does perhaps the text speak only of—? [מְדַבֵּר as a noun, v. s. v.].

Nif. נִדְבַּר *to hold communion, converse.* Mekh. Bo, introd. לא נ׳ עמו וכ׳ the Lord did not hold communion with him outside the capital of Egypt. Ib. fr.

Hithpa. הִדַּבֵּר, same, esp. part. f. מִדַּבֶּרֶת *being on terms of intimacy with a man.* Keth. I, 8 ראוה מד׳ עם אחד (omit בשוק); expl. ib. 13ᵃ. Ib. VII, 6 מד׳ עם כל אדם she is intimate with everybody. Ib. לכשהיא מד׳ בתוך ביתה וכ׳ when her neighbors can hear her voice in moments of intimacy with her husband.

Hif. הִדְבִּיר *to make submissive, persuade,* v. דִּיבּוּר. Macc. 11ᵃ דִּבֵּר לחוד יַדְבֵּר לחוד the Piel *dibber* has one meaning (speaking harshly), and the Hif. *yadber* another.

דְּבַר ch. same, 1) *to seize, take, lead, drive.* Targ. Gen. XIX, 15; a. fr. (h. לקח).—Ib. XXXI, 18; a. fr. (h. נהג).— 2) *to conduct one's self* (cmp. נָהַג). Erub. 14ᵇ, a. e. פוק חזי מאי עמא ד׳ go out and see how the people conduct themselves (what the religious usage is). Koh. R. to IX, 10, v. כְּלוּם.

Pa. דַּבַּר 1) *to lead, drive.* Targ. O. Ex. III, 1 ed. Berl. (ed. דְּבַר). Ib. XIV, 21 (ed. דְּבַר, h. text ויולך). Targ. Ez. XVI, 12; a. e.—Keth. 62ᵇ sq. עד כמה קא מְדַבְּרַת אלמנות חיים how long yet wilt thou lead a life of living widowhood (separation from a living husband)?—2) *to carry off.* Targ. Ezek. XXXIII, 6; a. e.

Af. אַדְבִּיר *to take, lead.* Targ. Is. XIV, 2; a. fr.—Bets. 21ᵇ אַדְבְּרֵיה וכ׳ took him out on a walk; ib. 29ᵃ. Y. Yeb. XIII, 13ᶜ bot. מַדְבְּרִין לה גבר they introduce to her a suitor.

Ithpa. אִתְדַּבַּר, אִיתְדַּבַּר, *Ithpe.* אִידְּבַר 1) *to be seized, taken away.* Targ. Prov. XXIV, 11. Targ. Ez. XXXIII, 6. Targ. II Kings II, 9 sq.; a. e.—2) *to conduct one's self.* Targ. Gen. XXXIII, 14 אִידַּבַּר ed. Berl. (h. text אתנהלה).

דָּבָר m. (b. h.; preced.) 1) *word, utterance, command* (cmp. דִּיבּוּר). B. Bath. 56ᵇ (ref. to Deut. XIX, 15) ד׳ ולא חצי ד׳ a statement (testimony) but not a partial statement. Mekh. Bo, introd. היה דְּבַר ה׳ לאהרן (Tanḥ. ib. 5 דבור) the word of the Lord came to &c.; a. fr—דְּבַר תורה according to the Biblical law. Erub. 81; a. fr.—*Pl.* דְּבָרִים, constr. דִּבְרֵי. ד׳ תורה Biblical laws; ד׳ סופרים Rabbinical laws. Ib. Yeb. IX, 3; a. fr.—ד׳ קבלה prophetic exhortations or incidental utterances in other Biblical books than the Pentateuch. Hag. 10ᵇ; Nidd. 23ᵃ; a. e.—B. Mets. 49ᵃ; Bekh. 13ᵇ ד׳ יש בהם משום מחוסרי אמנה to word of mouth the rules concerning the faithless are applied, i. e. a verbal agreement is morally binding. B. Mets. 48ᵃ הנושא ונותן בד׳ וכ׳ he who contracts verbally has no legal claim. Ib. ד׳ וארכא ... קאי באבל he who retracts a verbal transaction with which a payment of money was connected, comes under the category of those against whom the words 'but the scholars declared' (ib. IV, 2) has been pronounced.—דִּבְרֵי הַיָּמִים *the Book of Chronicles.* Lev. R. s. 1. B. Bath. 14ᵇ.—דָּבָר אַחֵר (abbrev. ד״א) another interpretation (is this). Gen. R. s. 1, beg.; a. fr.—2) *thing, affair, object, occurrence* &c. Sot. 28ᵇ ד׳ שיש בו דעת לישאל an object which has sense to ask, i. e. a rational being, opp. ד׳ שאין וכ׳ dumb creatures &c.—Num. R. s. 11 ד׳ שבינך לבינו that which concerns only thy relation to God; v. בֵּין.—ד׳ שבממון a monetary affair. B. Mets. 94ᵃ; a. fr.—ד׳ הלמד מענינו a thing (law) derived from the context on the very subject. Sifra, introd.; a. fr.—ד׳ אחר (abbr. ד״א) something not to be named, a) *idolatry.* Men. XIII, 10 ואין צריך לומר לד״א much less priests who have been offering to idols; a. fr.—b) *swine.* Ber. 43ᵇ (prov.) תלה ליה קורא לד״א וכ׳ hang a palm shoot around the swine and it will follow its habits (of wallowing in the mud). Sabb. 129ᵃ sq.; a. e.—c) *leprosy* Ib. אי פגע בד״א קשה לד״א if he meets a swine (after blood letting), he is in danger of becoming a leper.—d) *unchaste conduct, sexual intercourse, sodomy* &c. Ib. 17ᵇ על בנותיהן משום ד״א ועל ד״א משום ד״א they forbade connection with their daughters on account of idolatry, and decreed something else (that a gentile child should be unclean as though afflicted with gonorrhœa) on account of sodomy. Ber. 8ᵇ צנועין בד״א chaste in marital life; a. fr.—*Pl.* as above. —בעל ד׳ *the person to deal with, opponent, party.* B. Mets. 14ᵃ לאו ב״ד דידי את I have nothing to do with thee; a. fr.—לא היו ד׳ מעולם there were no such things,

I deny it outright. Shebu. 41[b]; a. fr.—ד׳ בגו, ד׳ בגב, v. גַּו, גַּב.

דֶּבֶר m. (b. h.; cmp. דְּבַר Pa. a. Ithpe., esp. Targ. Ez. XXXIII, 6) *death, pestilence.* Ab. V, 8. Sabb. 33[a]; a. fr.—Esp. *the plague of pestilence in Egypt.* Ex. R. s. 12. Tanh. Vaëra 14; a. fr.

דַּבָּר m. (דבר) *leader.*—*Pl.* דַּבָּרִין. Snh. 8[a] ד׳ אחד וכ׳ a generation must have one leader, but not two.

דַּבָּרָא I, דְּבָרָא m. (דבר, cmp. נָהַג) *drive, way of moving.* Targ. II Kings IX, 20.—*Pl.* דַּבָּרִין. Targ. Jud. V, 20 כבשי ד׳ (h. text מְסִלּוֹת).

דַּבָּרָא II, pl. דַּבָּרֵי *bees,* v. הַבַּרְתָּא.

דַּבְרָא m. (דבר) 1) *pasture, field.* Taan. 4[b]. Ab. Zar. 68[b] בדר׳ concerning a field mouse; a. e.—2) pr. n. pl. *Dabra.* Targ. Y. Deut. IV, 43 (h. text גּוֹלָן).

דִּבְרָה, pl. דִּבְּרוֹת, v. דִּיבֵּר.

דַּבְרוֹנָא (דברונה) m. (דבר) *drift, flow, current* (cmp. דַּבָּרָא I). Ab. Zar. 47[a] לד׳ דנהרא וכ׳ Ms. M. a. Rashi (ed. לדברונה דמיא) he worships the current of the river (the whole connection from its source to its mouth).

דברותא, Yalk. Gen. 22 ד׳ דמיא, v. זַבְרוּתָא.

דַּבָּרִיתָא (דַּבָּרְיוּתָא) דַּבָּרִית, f. (v. דַּבָּר) *leader.* Midr. Till. to Ps. XXII, 6; Yalk. Jud. 42; Ps. 686 (play on דבורה) חשיך דרא דאתתא ד׳ poor is the generation whose leader is a woman.

דַּבְּרָן m. (דבר) *spokesman.* Yalk. Gen. 151 למה אתה ד׳ why art thou the spokesman?

דַּבְּרָן m. (preced.) *eloquent.* Targ. Y. Ex. IV, 10.

דַּבְּרָנִית f. (cmp. preced.) *talkative, loquacious.* Gen. R. s. 18, beg.—*Pl.* דַּבְּרָנִיּוֹת. Ber. 48[b]. Gen. R. s. 45; Deut. R. s. 6; a. e. [Ab. Zar. II, 7, v. הַדְבְּבָנִיּוֹת].

דִּבַּרְתָּא I f. (דְּבַר)=h. מַלְקוֹחַ, *booty.* Targ. Num. XXXI, 11; a. e.

דִּבַּרְתָּא II f. (דְּבַר)=h. דֶּבֶר, *pestilence.* Taan. 21[b].

דְּבוֹרְתָא, דַּבַּרְתָּא f. ch.=h. דְּבוֹרָה, *bee.* *Pl.* דַּבַּרְיָתָא, דְּבוֹרְיָתָא. Targ. O. a. Y. II Deut. I, 44. Targ. Jud. XIV, 8.—דַּבָּרֵי. Y. Sabb. I, 3[b].

דָּבַשׁ, *Hif.* הִדְבִּישׁ *to become liquid, to ferment* (of honey). B. Mets. 38[a]. Snh. 101[a]. Sabb. 154[b].

דְּבַשׁ m. (b. h.; preced.) *glutinous substance, honey* (of bees, dates &c.). Bekh. 7[b]. Ter. XI, 2 ד׳ תמרים; a. fr.

דִּבְשָׁא, v. הוּבְשָׁא.

מַדְבַּשְׁתָּא, דְּבֶשְׁתָּא pr. n. pl. *D'beshta, Madbashta* (Honey-Town) in Gad. Targ. Y. I, II Num. XXXII, 34. Targ. Y. ib. 3 מד׳ (O. מלבשתא ed. Amst., ed. Berl. דיבון).

דָּג m. (b. h.) *fish.* ד׳ טמא unclean fish, forbidden in dietary laws, ד׳ טהור clean, permitted. Bekh. I, 2; a. fr.—*Pl.* דָּגִים. Hull. VIII, 1; a. fr.—M. Kat. 25[b] דְּגֵי רקק, v. קְ—. מַזַּל דָּגִים (or without מזל) *The Fishes, Pisces,* twelfth sign of the Zodiac. Pesik. R. s. 20; a. e; v. גְּדִי.

דָּגָה f. (b. h.) same, mostly collect. *all kind of fish, pieces of fish.* Ned. 51[b] if one says, 'I will taste no דג, he is forbidden to eat large fish &c.; if he says דגה he is forbidden small fish &c. Ib. ד׳ משמע גדולים וכ׳ *dagah* implies both large and small (in Biblical language), but in vows the popular usage is followed. Y. Bets. II, 61[b] top; a. fr.

דְּגוּגָא m. (preced., v. דוּגִית) *fisher boat, light shallow-going boat.* *Pl.* דְּגוּגִין. Targ. Is. XVIII, 2 (Var. דּוּגְגִין).

דְּגוּגִית f. same.—*Pl.* דְּגוּגְיָתָא. Targ. Am. IV, 2 דְּגוּגִית (Var. דוּגִית, דגוגית sing.).

דָּגוּל, v. דִּיגּוּל.

דָּגוּל, v. דָּגַל.

דָּגוֹן (b. h.) pr. n. *Dagon,* name of the Philistean god. Tosef. Sabb. VII (VIII), 2 דגן על שם ע״ז וכ׳ Dagan (in the charm *Dagan v'Kidron*) reminds of idolatry, as it is said &c. (Jud. XVI, 23). Y. ib. VI, 8[c] bot. [read:] ד׳ משום ע״ז.

דְּגוֹרָא m. (דְּגַר I) *heap, pile, mound.* Targ. O. Gen. XXXI, 46. Targ. Hab. III, 15 (piled up waves, h. text חֹמֶר).—*Pl.* דְּגוֹרִין. Targ. O. Ex. VIII, 10; a. e.—[Y. Kil. I, 27[a] top חסדיגרגון, read חס דגורין, R. S. to Kil. I, 2 חסא דארגרין, cler. error, for דדגורין; v. חֲסָא.]

דְּגִירָה f. (דָּגַר b. h.) *brooding,* the expression דגר. Hull. 140[b] אתיא ד׳ ד׳ there is an analogy betwen *dagar* (Jer. XVII, 11) and *dagar* (Is. XXXIV, 15).

דָּגַל I, *Pi.* דִּגֵּל, דִּיגֵּל (denom. of דֶּגֶל) *to outgeneral, play tricks* (cmp. στρατηγέω a. καταστρατηγέω). Cant. R. to II, 4 (play on ודגלו ib.) אפי׳ אותן הַדִּיגּוּלִין שדִּיגֵּל.. באביו even those devices with which Jacob deceived his father.

Hif. הִדְגִּיל same. Sabb. 63[a] (play on ודגלו, v. supra) two students הַמַּדְגִּילִים זה לזה וכ׳ who outwit each other with sophistries (Tosaf. to Ab. Zar. 22[b]). [Rashi: *who form an assembly* (דֶּגֶל) for studies, in the absence of a teacher.]

דַּגַּל ch., *Pa.* דַּגֵּיל same. Targ. Prov. XVI, 10 לא נְדַגֵּיל פומיה Ar. (ed. נדגול) his mouth is not tricky (h. text מעל).

דָּגַל II, part. pass. דָּגוּל, v. דֶּגֶל.—*Nif.* נִדְגַּל (denom. of דֶּגֶל) *to be divided in troops, arranged.* Part. pl. f. נִדְגָּלוֹת *those arranged in troops, the hosts of heaven.* Num. R. s. 2 (ref. to Cant. VI, 4) ובמה אתם כנ׳ and wherein do ye (Israelites) resemble the angels?; Yalk. Cant. 992.

Hif. הִדְגִּיל 1) *to put up a flag, to signalize.* Tanh., ed. Bub., B'midb. 15 (ref. to Cant. II, 4) ולוי הוא מַדְגִּיל עלי אהבה (Tanh. ib. 14; Num. R. l. c. מגדיל) Oh, that He would let the flag of love wave over me!—2) *to arrange an assembly.* Sabb. 63ᵃ, v. דָּגַל I.

דֶּגֶל m. (b. h.) *troop, division, cohort* (cmp. *caterva*); *standard.* Cant. R. to II, 4 וְדִגְלוֹ Michael and his band (of angels); a. e.—*Pl.* דְּגָלִים. Num. R. s. 2 והיו כולם עשויים ד׳ ד׳ וכ׳ and all of them (the angels) were arranged in divisions, as it is said (Cant. V, 10) *dagul* (surrounded by divisions) of a myriad each (with ref. to Ps. LXVIII, 18). Ib. עֲשֵׂה אותם ד׳ וְכ׳ divide them into cohorts as they desired (with ref. to Num. II, 2); v. Cant. R. to II, 4; Tanḥ. B'midb. 10.—Ex. R. s. 15 אין ד׳ אלא צבאות *d'galim* means hosts. Ib. דִּגְלֵי השמים ... וד׳ הארץ וכ׳ the heavenly hosts are the angels, the earthly hosts (of the Lord) are Israel. Ib. s. 24, end; a. fr.—Sabb. 5ᵃ; 98ᵃ דומה לְדִגְלֵי מדבר resembling the marches of the Israelites in the desert.

***דִּיגְלָא, דִּגְלָא** m. (v. preced.) *a carrying pole in the shape of a standard,* Ar. (ed. a. Mss. mostly רִגְלָא, רִיגְ׳ q. v.) Bets. 30ᵃ. B. Mets. 83ᵃ (v. Rabb. D. S. a. l. note, a. to Sabb. 148ᵃ).

דַּגָּלָא (דִּיגָּאלָא) m. (דְּגַל) *cunning; false.* Targ. Prov. XIX, 28 דיגא׳ ed. Lag. (oth. ed. דגל׳, ר׳). Ib. XXIV, 28 (h. text חנם). Ib. XX, 17 (h. text שקר).—Ab. Zar. 22ᵇ (prov.) מכתבא ... ד׳ בחבריה ידע Ar. (ed. a. Ms. M. רגלא) the pencil splits the stone (marble), a schemer finds out his like.

דגלוס, דגלום, Koh. R. to V, 12 ד׳ פטרגוס, a corrupt. arising fr. two Var. to ערטיל ibid., פודלגוס a. פודגרוס (ποδαγρός, ποδαλγός); cmp. Y. Kidd. I, 61ᵃ; Sot. 10ᵃ; Tanḥ. Masé 12.

דַּגָּלוּתָא f. (דְּגַל) *cunning, scheme.* Targ. Prov. XVII, 4 ed. Lag. (Var. ר׳). Ib. XXX, 8 דיגלתא ed. Lag. (Var. דיג׳); v. דַּגָּלָא.

דִּגְלַת, v. דִּיגְלַת.

דָּגֶם, v. דּוּגְמָא.

דגמטרין, דגמטורין, v. דוגמטרין.

דָּגָן m. (b. h.; v. next w.) *pile; grain, bread, breadstuff.* Pesik. R. s. 10 דְּגָנוֹ של עולם are the store of the world. Tosef. Ber. IV, 15; Y. ib. VI, 10ᵇ שהוא הד׳ וכ׳ the more preferable kind of bread. Tosef. l. c. כל שהוא מין שבע ואינו מין ד׳ whatever belongs to the seven produces (Deut. VIII, 8) but not to breadstuffs; Bab. ib. 37ᵇ. Pes. III, 1; a. fr.—Ned. VII, 2 הנודר מן הד׳ וכ׳ he who vows abstinence from *dagan,* is forbidden dry Egyptian beans, v. next w.—*Pl.* דְּגָנִים. Pesik. R. s. 41 מנפח את הד׳ swells the grains; (Yalk. Ps. 755 מנפנק את רגליה, read דְּגָנֶיהָ). Tosef. Ber. VII (VI), 8 Var.—בֵּית דָּ׳ pr. n. pl. *Beth-Dagan* in Judea. Tosef. Ohol. III, 9. [Tosef. Sabb. VII (VIII), 2, v. דָּגוֹן.]

דְּגַן, *Ithpe.* אִידְּגַן *to be piled up, stored.* Ned. 55ᵃ shall we judge (fr. R. Meir's opinion VII, 2, v. preced.) כל דמידגן משמע *dagan* implies everything which is piled up?—Ber. 47ᵇ; Bets. 13ᵇ האי (אִךְ׳) אר׳ וכ׳ the one (the piled up) has become *dagan,* the other (standing in the ears) is not yet *dagan* (with ref. to Num. XVIII, 27).

דִּגְנָא ch.=h. דָּגָן. Targ. Y. Ex. XXIII, 19 (cmp. Tanḥ. R'eh 17 s. v. גְּדִי).—Y. Ned. VII, 40ᶜ top (ref. to R. Meir's opinion ib. VII, 2, v. preced.) דִּגְנָהּ דארעא dry Egyptian beans are the bread of the land (Palestine, therefore implied in *dagan*); (ref. to the Rabbis' opinion, ib.) דגנה מעבורה 'its bread' means its home growth.

דְּגַר I (h. דָּגַר) 1) *to heap,* v. דְּגוֹרָא.—2) *to brood.* Targ. Job XXXIX, 14.

Ithpe. אִידְּגַר *to be piled up* (of bowels in pain). Targ. Lam. I, 20. Ib. II, 11 אידגארן ed. Lag. (h. text חמרמר, cmp. חֹמֶר=דְּגוֹרָא).

***דְּגַר II** (cmp. זקר) *to leap.* Hull. 51ᵃ ד׳ נפל מאיגרא (our w. omitted in Ar. s. v. אירפומא) it leaped [and] fell from the roof (Rashi).

דֹּד, v. דּוֹד.

דַּד m. (b. h.;=דודו, v. דוה; cmp. דְּהִין) *breast, nipple, teat.* Sabb. 144ᵇ. Sifré Num. 89; Tosef. Sot. IV, 3 (ed. Zuck. שד); a. e.—Trnsf. *spigot.* Yoma III, 10.—*Pl.* דַּדִּים. Ber. 10ᵃ. Y. Yeb. II, 3ᵈ; a. fr.

דַּד, דַּדָּא ch. same. Ab. Zar. 26ᵃ she may smear poison לד׳ מאבראי on her breast outside.—*Pl.* דַּדַּיָּא, דַּדִּין. Targ. Is. XXXII, 12 (ed. Lag. תדין).—Lam. R. to I, 1 (6 חד מאת׳) יתרין מזגין אדלין תרין דדיא (not דדא) רבתי the two bottlers (in the riddle) are the two breasts. Gen. R. s. 98 יתברכון ד׳ וכ׳ blessed are the breasts which nursed such a son.

דִּדְבָא, v. דִּידְבָא.

דֹּדָה, v. דּוֹד.

דָּדָה, v. דדי.

דדהובא, v. דְּהוּבָא.

דְּדֵהִין, v. דְּהַן II.

דַּדְוָתָא, v. הוּדָא.

דָּדָה, דדי (b. h.; cmp. זוז) *to move nimbly, hop, trip.* —*Pi.* דִּדָּה 1) *to walk, pull* (a young child or beast unable to walk by itself). Sabb. XVIII, 2 מְדַדִּין עגלין וכ׳ you may lead or pull calves &c. (on the Sabbath). Ib. אשה מְדַדָּה וכ׳ a mother may walk her child. Ib. 128ᵇ דוחין אין מדדין לא push you may, but make them hop, no. Pes. IV, 7 (55ᵇ) מְדַדִּין ומחזורין וכ׳ Ar. (ed. only מחזירין). Sabb. 88ᵇ and the angels מְדַדִּין אותן led them (the frightened Israelites) back; א״ת ידודון אלא יְדַדּוּן read not (Ps. LXVIII, 13) *yiddodun* but *y'daddun* (they led them). Cant. R. to VIII, 11 the angels מְדַדִּין להם וכ׳ led the Israelites away, והיו מְדַדִּין לפני וכ׳ and they themselves tripped timidly before the Lord, v. infra. Y. Sabb. XVII, end, 16ᵇ; Y. Erub. X, 26ᶜ top מְדַדֵּהוּ וכ׳ he makes the bolt slide with his finger tips. Cant. R. to IV, 8 [read:] אדרין, מְדַדִּם ואינם וכ׳ He had just been leading them (through the Red Sea), and they should not trust?—ד׳ פיתקין to shake stones (ballots), i. e. to protest against. Esth. R. to I, 2 מה״ש מְדַדִּין פיתקין וכ׳ the angels protested against the Lord's decision; Cant. R. to VIII, 11 יְהוּדוּן בהם ממדדין פיטקין (read מדדין) they (the angels) were excited against them, they protested (ref. to Joel IV, 3).

Hithpa. (b. h.) הִדַּדָּה to hop, trip (of young or tied birds). B. Mets. 25ᵇ אי מִידַּדִּין Ms. M. (ed. אי בְּמַדַּ׳) if the tied birds (deposited in a certain place) hop from spot to spot. B. Bath. 23ᵇ; Bets. 11ᵃ.

דדי, *Pa.* דַּדֵּי ch. same. Sabb. 128ᵇ דַּדּוּיֵי מְדַדִּינָן pull them we may, opp. עקר.

Ithpa. אִידַּדֵּי 1) as preced. Hithpa. B. Bath. 24ᵃ כל דמִידַּדֵּי וכ׳ any young bird which hops, will hop only within sight of its nest. Bets. 11ᵃ אִידַּדּוּיֵי אִידַּדּוּ they came hopping (from the nest). Sabb. 99ᵇ דלא לִדַּדּוּ וכ׳ that the boards should not shake.—2) to move about. Y. Kidd. III, 64ᵃ top כינר אורחא דזובנה מִדַּדְיָיה it is the habit of traders to travel from place to place.

דדינין, דדינון, Y. Sabb. II, beg. 4ᶜ, v. דְּרִינוֹן.

דדכאות, v. דִּירְכֵי.

דדנייא, Lam. R. to II, 2, v. הוּדָא.

דְּדָנִים m. pl. (b. h.) *Dedanites*, a nomadic tribe on the borders of Idumaea. Tanh. Yithro 5.—V. הוּדָנִים.

דדנין, Y. R. Hash. II, 58ᵃ top, expl. עצי שמן (Mish. ib. II, 2), prob. דַּדִּינִין (δᾴδινος, pl.) *pine-wood*, (used for torches; Bab. ib. 23ᵃ אפרסמא; v. Sm. Ant. s. v. Taeda).

דדרא, v. דִּרְדָּא I.

דַּדֶּקֶרֶת, v. דּוֹקֶרֶת.

דָּה, v. דָּא.

דָּהַב (cmp. זהב, צהב) to be red (or yellow).—*Hif.* הִדְהִיב to redden, make red (with anger). Lev. R. s. 15, end (play on *madhebah*, Is. XIV, 4) שהיא מַדְהֶבֶת וכ׳ that reddens with indignation the face of every one coming near her.

דְּהַב, דַּהֲבָא m. ch.=h. זָהָב, *gold*. Targ. Gen. II, 11; a. e.—Y. B. Mets. II, 8ᶜ bot. קופר דד׳ a golden piece resembling meat; Tam. 32ᵃ; a. fr.—B. Mets. 70ᵃ; B. Bath. 166ᵃ ד׳ פריכא broken pieces of gold (for the melting pot). Ib. 165ᵇ ד׳ אין פחות וכ׳ if a note has the word 'gold' (without any further definition), it means no less than a Denar in gold (v. Rabb. D. S. a. l. note).

דַּהֲבַאי pr. n. m. (preced.) *Dahăbai* (Goldsmith). Hag. 2ᵃ.

דַּהֲבוּנָא m. (preced. ws.) *price in gold, cash*. Targ. II Esth. III, 11 (ed. Lag. ר׳, corr. acc.).

דַּהֲבִי m.=h. זַהֲבִי, *goldsmith*.—*Pl.* דַּהֲבִין. Cant. R. to V, 5 דהבים (corr. acc.).

דַּהֲבָן ch. same. Y. Gitt. IV, 46ᵃ.

דַּהֲבַת (דִּיהָ׳) pr. n. pl. *Dahăbath*. Taan. 7ᵇ Ms. M. (ed. דִּה׳).

דָּהָה *to be faint*, v. דִּירְחָה.

דְּהוֹן (דְּרְהוֹן, רְהוֹן) m. (v. דְּהִין) *fattening substance, urin-soaked dung; a concrete of dung used for vessels*, cmp. גָּלָל. Y. Ab. Zar. II, 41ᵇ bot. אהן ד׳ של מימי וכ׳ a vessel made of dung prepared with urin absorbs no liquids.—Gen. R. s. 39, end (ref. to *Bethel*, changed into *Beth-aven*, Josh. VII, 2) [read:] לא זכתה . . . . בית העמל חרי . . . . בית העמד תמן קריין לפועלא טבא עמלא עמידה . . . (ולְדְרְהוֹן) ולדהון she did not deserve even to be named *Beth Heamal* (house of toil, cmp. עמל ואון Ps. XC, 10), now she is named *Beth-Heamad* (dung-house); there (in Samaria, Galilee &c.) they call the good laborer *amela* (the industrious, v. עמל), and the dung prepared with urin *amidah* (concrete, cmp. עָמַד Hif.); Y. Sabb. IX, 11ᵈ; Y. Ab. Zar. III, 43ᵃ bot.; Yalk. Josh. 17 (v. Koh. Ar. Compl. s. v. הרהון).

דְּהִיק, דְּהַק=דְּחַק. Targ. Job XI, 3. Targ. Ps. II, 4 ed. Lag.

דְּהַן, דְּהִין (cmp. דוה; interch. dialectically with רחן, cmp. רוה) *to drip, to be fat* (corresp. to h. רָוָה a. דָּשֵׁן). Targ. Prov. XI, 25 תדהן ed. Lag. (Var. תורכן, תורכן, corr. acc.); a. fr.

Pa. דַּהֵין 1) *to fatten*. Targ. Ps. XXIII, 5. Targ. Prov. XV, 30; a. e.—2) *to grow fat*. Targ. Y. Deut. XXXI, 20.—[Targ. Ps. XX, 4, v. דַּהֲנַאן.]

Ithpa. אִידַּהַין *to drip, be fat*. Targ. Is. XXXIV, 6.—Shebu. 47ᵇ, v. next w.

דְּהִין, דְּהִינָא m. (preced.) *fat, sappy*. Shebu. 47ᵇ קרב לגבי ד׳ ואִידַּהַין go near a fat man, and be fat.—*Pl.* דְּהִינִין. Targ. Ps. XCII, 15. Ib. XXII, 30 (Var. רח׳).

דְּהִינוּנִיתָא, v. דַּהֲנוּנִיתָא.

דְּהַק, v. דְּחִיק.

דַּהֲכָא, v. הוּכָא.

דְּהַן I *to be fat*, v. דְּהִין.

דְּהַן II, דַּהֲנָא m. (preced.) *fat*. Targ. Ps. XXXVI, 9 (Var רחן). Targ. Is. LV, 2 ed. Bxt. בד׳ (ed. Lag. a. oth. בדִדְהֵין; cmp. דִּירְבָא).

***דַּהֲנַאן** (denom. of preced.; cmp. דַּאֲבַן) *to consider fat, to accept*. Targ. Ps. XX, 4 (ed. Wil. יְדַהֵן; h. text יְדַשְּׁנֶה).

דַּהֲנִיתָא f. (רחן, cmp. דְּהוֹן) *manure*. Targ. Ez. XXXII, 6 (ed. Lag. דוה׳).

דְּהִינוּ׳, דַּהֲנוּנִיתָא f. (preced. ws.) *of a fat land*. תמרתא ד׳ (a fat-land date) *a species of dates of strong* *perfume*. Keth. 61ª דחני׳; Sot. 49ª דחיני׳ (corr. דחיני׳). Ib. ריחא דחיני׳ (read דרחיני׳) the flavor of a *d'hinunitha*.

דחק, v. דחק.

דו I (=דהוא, cmp. דִּי) *who, which is, since he, it*, &c. Y. Sabb. XIX, beg. 16ᵈ דו אמר ... היא דאמר the same that says ..., says also &c. Y. Peah I, 15ᶜ top בגין דו בעי וכ׳ because he wants to teach &c. Y. Maasr. I, 49ª bot. מן דו from the time that. Y. Gitt. IX, 50ᶜ top nobody says 'even' אלא דו מודה וכ׳ except he admits the preceding; a. fr.

דו II c. (=הֵן) *this, that*. Y. Naz. IV, end, 53ᶜ. Y. Erub. V, 22ᶜ top דו ואַלְפַּיִם itself (the whole area of the town) and two thousand cubits beside.

דו III (δύο, only in certain compounds) *two, double*. Lev. R. s. 14, beg. דו פרצופין נברא Adam was created with two faces (male and female persons combined); Gen. R. s. 8, beg. דיו; Ber. 68ª; a. e.—Ex. R. s. 5 דו פרצ׳ היה יוצא the word of the Lord went forth in two characters (killing and reviving). V. דְּיוֹ II.

דְּוָא, v. דְּוִי.

דּוֹאֵג (b. h. דֹּאֵג) pr. n. m. *Doeg*, 1) the servant of Saul. Snh. 106ᵇ; a. e.—2) one D. ben Joseph. Lam. R. to I, 16; Sifra B'huck. ch. VI.

דַּוֵּאר, Pa. of דור I ch.

דַּוָּאר I, **דַּוָּואר**, **דַּוָּור** m. (דור I, cmp. preced.) 1) (transl. of cursor) *mail-carrier, despatch-bearer*. Tanh. Ekeb 11 ד׳ שהיה מהלך וכ׳ a *cursor* who travelled with an ordinance in his hand. Sabb. 19ª קביע ד׳ במתא Ms. M. (ed. בי ד׳) the mail-carrier (ed. the post office) is permanently located in town.—2) (Pers. dâvar, judge, ruler, Fl.) בֵּי ד׳ *the (Persian) circuit court* consisting of regular law scholars, opp. דייני דמגיסתא squires in country places ignorant of the law. B. Kam. 114ª (Ms. R. אַבֵּי ד׳ in the &c., Ms. M. בודאור, corr. acc.). Gitt. 58ᵇ כיון דאיכא בי ד׳ וכ׳ since there exists (in Persia) a lawful court, and he did not sue (the tax officer). Ab. Zar. 26ª נקיטנא לי זימנא לבי ד׳ I am summoned to court (and have no time). [In later Hebr. literature בי דואר is used in the sense of *post-office*.]

***דַּוָּאר** II m. (cmp. preced.) *davvar*, a species of lizard. Ex. R. s. 15 end [prob. to be read עָרוֹד, v. Hull. 127ª, or חֲוַרְבָּר, v. Sifra Sh'mini ch. VI, Par. 5].

דּוּב, **דִּיב** ch.=h. זוב, *to flow, drip*. Targ. Ps. LXXVIII, 20 (Var. וְדַיְיבָן). Targ. Lev. XV, 25 יְדוּב.— Part. דָּאִיב, דָּיֵיב. Ib. 33.—Hull. 8ᵇ bot.—Pes. 74ᵇ מֵדַב דָּיֵיב it drips. Nidd. 22ª עד דמידב ד׳ it must be fluid. Hull. 133ª.

דּוֹב, **דֹּב** c. (b. h.; דבב) [*murmurer*,] *bear*. Kidd. 72ª; Ab. Zar. 2ᵇ; Meg. 11ª (used of Persians, ref. to Dan. VII, 5). —Allegorically: *temptation*. Num. R. s. 13; a. e., v. גֵּרָה.— *Pl*. דּוּבִּים. Snh. 107ᵇ

דּוּבָּא, **דֹּב**, **דּוֹב** ch. same. Targ. II Sam. XVII, 8. Targ. Is. XI, 7 (some ed. דיבא, corr. acc.).—Kidd. 72ª. Taan. 25ª.—Gen. R. s. 87, beg. הא ד׳ קמך here is the temptation before thee.—*Pl*. דּוּבַּיָּא, דּוּבִּין. Targ. II Kings II, 24.—Taan. l. c.; B. Mets. 106ª.—[דּוּבָא, דּוּבָא wolf, v. דֵּיבָא.] [Targ. I Kings XIV, 28, v. דּוּבָא.]

דִּיבָא, **דְּוָיָא**, **דּוּוָא**, **דּוּבָא** m. ch.=h. זוֹב, *flux, gonorrhœa, abnormal menstruation*. Targ. Lev. XV, 2 sq. [Targ. Y. ib. 3 דְּיֵיתָה, read דְּוָיְתָה]; a. e.

דּוּבִּיאֵל pr. n. m. *Dubbiël* (bear-god), the genius of the Persians (v. דוב). Yoma 77ª, v. אִיסְרָא II.

דּוּבְלָא m. (v. דְּבֵלָה) *a species of figs* or *sycamore*. *Pl*. דּוּבְלֵי. Ber. 40ᵇ (defin. בנות שקמה). [דובלא, Sot. 10ª, v. רַבְלָא.]

דּוּבְנָא m. (v. דּוּבָא)=h. זָב, *one afflicted with gonorrhœa*. Targ. Lev. XV, 4; 7; a. e.

דּוּבְקָא, v. דִּיבְקָא.

דּוּבָר *back*, v. בְּדוּבָר.

***דּוּבֶשׁ** m. (v. דְּבַשׁ) *honey-crop*. Deut. R. s. 1 דּוּבְשָׁהּ לבעלה what honey the bee produces, belongs to its owner; Yalk. ib. 795. [Hall. I, 4 דובשין, Mish. ed., v. דּוּבְשָׁן.]

דּוּבְשָׁא m. ch.=h. דְּבַשׁ. Targ. Jud. XIV, 8; a. fr.— Ber. 37ᵇ. Ib. 38ª ד׳ דתמרי date honey; a. e.—Yoma 83ᵇ some ed. דיבשא.

דּוּבְשָׁן m. (preced. wds.) 1) *honey-crop, honey-store*. B. Kam. 114ᵇ. Snh. 101ª. B. Bath. 80ª דּוּבְשָׁנָן their own stock of honey.—2) *honey-cake*.—*Pl*. דּוּבְשָׁנִין. Hall. I, 4 (3), expl. Y. ib. 57ᵈ מלי גאלה meligala, honey and milk cake (Mish. ed. דובשין, corr. acc.).

דּוּבְשָׁנִיתָא f. (preced. wds.) *honey-like*. Gitt. 69ª חלבניתא ד׳ sweet galbanum.

דובשקא, v. דִּפְשְׁקָא.

דּוּג ch.=h. דָּאַג, *to be anxious, troubled*. Part. דָּאִיג, דָּיֵיג. Sabb. 156ᵇ הוה דָּאִיגָא וכ׳ she was very much troubled over it. M. Kat. 28ª הוו קא דָיְיגֵי רבנן the rabbis were troubled (over R. Huna's sudden death).

דוגזר, v. רוּגְזָר.

דּוּגֵי m. pl. (דוג, v. דָּאַג) *drippings* from melting fat.— בֵּי ד׳ a receptacle for the drippings of a roast. Hull. 111ᵇ.

דוגיאות, Yalk. Deut. 923, v. כדכיאות.

דוגין, Y. Keth. II, 26ᵈ, v. זוֹג.

דּוּגִית f. (=דגוגית, denom. of דָּג) *fisher-boat, light-going boat for shallows*, Palestinean word for Babylonian בְּצִיָּרִית. B. Bath. 73ª; 78ᵇ; Y. ib. V, beg. 15ª.

דּוּגְמָא, **דִּיגְמָא**, **דּוּגְמַת** f. (δεῖγμα, cmp. παράδειγμα) 1) *simile, illustration* (cmp. מָשָׁל לְ-, משל למה חרבר דומה). Cant. R., introd. עד.. היתה ד׳ up to Solomon's days the method of argument by illustration was unknown (in Hebrew literature).—2) *show, exhibition, public appearance.* Y. Hor. III, beg. 47[a] ד׳ דידכו דמי וכ׳ (prob. to be read דמ״א) your appearance resembles that of your Maker. Eduy. V, 6; Ber. 19[a] ד׳ השקוה it was for show that they made her drink, i. e. they merely pretended to give her the real 'bitter waters'; [oth. opin. they performed the act on one who was, *like themselves*, a descendant of gentiles; Y. M. Kat. III, 81[d] דִּכְמָה השקוה, (a popular adaptation of our w.; v. דִּכְמָא), expl. דִּכְוָותָהּ something like it]. Midr. Sam. ch. XX (expl. תפקד לשלום, I Sam. XVII, 18) ד׳ דידהון how they look.—3) *sample, example, token* (corresp. to h. אות). Ḥag. 16[a] (play on דגול מרבבה, Cant. V, 10) דוּגְמָא הוא ברבבה שלו He is exemplified by His myriad (of angels), i. e. the Divine nature is recognized indirectly from the nature of His ministering messengers, v. Cant. R. to V, 9.—Keth. 28[b] קחו לכם ד׳ וכ׳ take a warning example &c. Taan. 23[a] ד׳ לדורות a sample (of great fertility) as a lesson for future generations. Sabb. 30[b] I will show thee דוּגְמָתָן וכ׳ (Ms. M. דוּגְמָתוֹ) the like thereof in this world.—Ib. 11[b] the dyer must not go out on the Sabbath בדו׳ שבצוארו (Ar. בדו׳ שבאזנו; Tosef. ib. I, 8 בדו׳ שבאזנו) with the sample of colors around his neck, v. אות II.—Num. R. s. 6 (expl. Job XXXVI, 7 עינו) ד׳ דידהו that which is like his own doing, i. e. some realization of his ideal, v. עֵדְנָא; Midr. Sam. ch. XXVIII דוגמה דידהון; Gen. R. s. 71 דוגמת דידיה (corr. acc.), v. next w.; a. fr.—*Pl.* דוּגְמוֹת. B. Kam. 119[b], v. אות II (Var. Ms. דוּגְמָאוֹת). [Our w., owing to its phonetic resemblance to דִּכְמָא, is inflected as though it were a native, whence the forms: דוּגְמָה, דוּגְמַת, דוּגְמַת־, דוּגְמוֹת, and even a Var. to Tosef. Sabb. I, 8 דָּגְמוֹ, as though fr. דָּגֵם.]

דוּגְמַטְרִין, דוּגְמַטְרִין (דוגמטורין,) **דִּגְמַטְרִין,** (דיגמטורי) m. pl. (a transpos. of διαγράμματα; cmp. דִּימַטְרִיָּא) *plans, designs.* Gen. R. s. 11 מראה לאלו מעין ד׳ שלהן וכ׳ Ar. (ed. דוגמא גטורין, some ed. in one w., corr. acc.; Tanḥ. Ki Thissa 33 מעין דוגמא שלהם) He shows to these (the righteous) something corresponding to their designs (reward) and to those &c. Tanḥ. P'kudé 11 (ref. to Job XXXVI, 7) the Lord refuses not to the righteous man ד׳ שלו a realization of his designs (ideals), v. preced.

דוגמניות, Midr. Till. to Ps. CXVIII, read הֶגְמוֹנִיּוֹת, v. הֶגְמוֹנְיָה.

דָּוִד, דָּוִיד (b. h.) pr. n. m. *David*, King of Israel. Ber. 4[a]; a. v. fr.—בן ד׳ or ד׳ (=משיח) the son of David (the David of the future), the redeemer of Israel from captivity. Snh. 98[b] ד׳ אחר a second David. R. Hash. 25[a] (a secret watchword) ד׳ מלך וכ׳ David, the King of Israel, is alive &c. Y. Ber. II, 5[a] top. Yeb. 62[a]; a. fr.

דֹּד, דּוֹד, דּוּד (b. h.) 1) *friend, lover, beloved;* (allegor.) *the Lord*, as the beloved of Israel. Cant. R. to I, 4, v. גִּנּוּן; a. e.—2) *uncle, father's brother.* Sifra K'dosh. Par. 10, ch. XI; Yeb. 54[b].—Fem. דּוֹדָה, דֹּדָה *aunt.* Ib.—*Pl.* דּוֹדִים 1) **friends**, *related.* Y. Snh. XI, 30[a] bot.; Y. Ber. I, 3[b] bot. (ref. to Cant. I, 2) ד׳ דברי וכ׳ the words of the scholars are related to the words of the Law; Cant. R. to l. c. Ab. Zar. 35[a] דברי דודים Ms. M. (ed. דודיך) the words of the friends (the scholars); Num. R. s. 14. Gen. R. s. 37 בני דוֹדֵיהֶן וכ׳ cousins (related nation).—2) (abstr. noun) *friendship, love.* Ab. Zar. II, 5 (29[b]) do you read כי טובים דודיך מיין .... דּוֹדֶיךָ מיין Ms. M. (v. Rabb. D. S. a. l. a. Cant. R. l. c.) better is thy (God's) love, or thy (Israel's) love?

דּוֹדָא ch. same. Gen. R. s. 37, beg. בני דוֹדֵיכֶן אנן we are your cousins (Yalk. Chr. 1073 דוֹדֵיכוֹן, pl.).—*Pl.* דּוֹדַיָּא. Y. Taan. IV, 69[a] top כן ארחתון דבני ד׳ עבדין is this the way cousins act?; Lam. R. to II, 2 דדנייא (corr. acc.).

דּוּדָא m. (b. h. דּוּד) *boiler, caldron, pot.* Targ. II Kings IV, 38; a. e.—Snh. 64[a], v. אֲבָרָא; a. fr.—*Pl.* דּוּדֵי, דּוּדַיָּא. Targ. Zach. XIV, 20; a. e.—Nidd. 68[a] ד׳ חסרת thou wantest boilers (for hot water). B. Kam. 101[a] top, v. כַּפְרָא. Sabb. 41[a], v. אַנְטִיכִי.—Fem. דּוּדָה, דּוּדְוָותָא. Targ. Y. Ex. XVI, 3; XXXVIII, 3; a. e. Targ. Y. Lev. VIII, 31 דּוּדְוָותַיָּא (!).

דודאי, v. דּוּדָאִי.

דּוּדְבָא, v. דִּידְבָא.

דּוּדָה, v. דּוּד.

דּוּדְוָותָא, v. דּוּדָא.

דודורין, v. דַּרְדּוּר.

דּוּדְנִיָּא, v. דַּרְדְּנָיָא.

דּוֹדָנִים m. pl. (b. h. דֹּדָנִים) *Dodanites*, a Javanic tribe, v. דַּרְדְּנָיָא. Gen. R. s. 37, beg.; Yalk. Chr. 1073 (ref. to דֹּדָ׳, Gen. X, 4, a. רוֹדָ׳, I Chr. I, 7).

דָּוָה, v. דוי.

***דּוּוִי** f. (דוי) *menstruation.* Y. Ab. Zar. II, 40[d] bot.; v., however, זַכְרוּתָא.

דּוּחֲנָא m.=דֹּחַן II. Targ. Prov. III, 8 ed. Lag. (ed. רוח׳, Ms. רֵוָּח׳, h. text שקוי).

דּוּחֲנִיתָא, v. דַּחֲנִיתָא.

דּוּרָא, v. דּוּבָא.

דַּוָּאר, v. דַּיָּאר.

דַּוְודָא, v. דִּיוְודָא.

דָּוֶה, pl. דָּוִים, v. דוי.

דְּוִי, v. דְּוַי.

דְּוָל, דַּוְלָא, דְּוַל, דַּו׳ m. (דול) *bucket;* (collect.) *irrigation* by means of buckets. Targ. Is. XL, 15 (ed. Vien. דוּל׳).—Erub. 20[b] דלי ליה לד׳ בהדיה he might carry the bucket with him.—B. Mets. 104[a] top בד׳ ... איבעי לך you ought to have brought the water over from the large well by irrigating works. Ib. 77[a] מאן .. לד׳ if one hired working men for irrigating work. M. Kat. 4[a] הוה דלי ד׳

was doing irrigating work. Yeb. 97ᵇ דלאי דדלו ד׳ ye water drawers engaged in irrigation.—*Pl.* דַּוּלְּין. Targ. II Esth. I, 2.

דַּוְלָלָא, v. דַּוְלָלָא.

דָּוֹן m.=דַּאֲבוֹן. Ab. II, 7 Ar. (ed. דְּאָנָה).

דְּוָנָא, דָּוֹנָא, דְּוָון, v. דְּאבוֹנָא.

דַּוְקְנָא, דִּיוְקָא, v. דְּוֹק.

דַּוּר, v. דּוּר.

דָּוָר, v. דָּאַר.

דָּוְשָׁא m. (דּוּשׁ) 1) *treading, passage.* Sabb. 81ᵇ משום ד׳ because of treading down (injuring a neighbor's field). B. Bath. 22ᵇ ד׳ דחכא וכ׳ the passage between the walls (stamping the ground) is beneficial to both buildings.—2) *ordinary course, habit.* B. Kam. 116ᵇ דַּוְשֵׁיה נקיט ואזיל he (the boatman) took his wonted course. Ber. 16ᵃ דוושיה נקיט Ar. (ed. סרכיה) he followed his habit (in recitation).

דְּוּתָא* f. (דוי) *the sick man's draught, medicine for the appetite.* Targ. Job VI, 7 (Ms. זוותא; h. text כדוי).

דְּוָתָא, דְּוָתָא f. ch. (=h. דָּוָה; v. דּוּבָא) *a menstruating woman.* Targ. Y. Num. XXXI, 23 (some ed. דְּוָתָא).

דוזגר, v. רוּזְגַר.

דוּחַ, *Hif.* הֵדִיחַ (b. h.; v. הֵחַ) [*to brighten,*] *to wash off, cleanse, rinse.* Mikv. VII, 3. Ḥull. 8ᵇ מֵדִיחַ he must wash the meat (at the place where the knife passed); a. fr.—Tam. IV, 2 בית המְדִיחִין the washers' hall where the offering meat was washed.—Y. Ab. Zar. III, 42ᵈ bot. לְהָדִיחַ=לְדִיחַ.

Hof. הוּדַח *to be washed, cleansed.* Makhsh. IV, 3 בשביל שתוּדַח in order that the dish may be washed by the rain; Ḥull. 16ᵃ; Sabb. 11ᵇ; a. fr.

Nif. נָדוֹחַ, נִידּוֹחַ *to be washed away.* Koh. R. to VII, 1; Midr. Sam. ch. XXIII.

דוּחַ ch., *Af.* אֲדִיחַ same. Targ. II Chr. IV, 6.

דוּחָה, Yeb. 80ᵇ; Gitt. 57ᵃ, v. הֵידָחָה.

דוּחִינָא ch.=h. דוֹחַן. Targ. Y. Num. XV, 19.

דּוּחָכָא m. (חֲחַךְ) *laughter, scorn.* Targ. Job XXXIV, 7 (Lev. חֲחָכָא).

דּוֹחַן m. (b. h. דֹּחַן) *a species of millet.* Pes. 35ᵃ. Ber. 37ᵃ; a. fr.

דֹּחַק, דּוֹחַק m. (דחק) [*pressure;*] 1) *need, distress.* Ḥag. 5ᵃ בשעת דּוֹחְקוֹ just when he needs it (no sooner); Yeb. 63ᵃ (v. Tosaf. a. l.). Ab. II, 3 בשעת דָּחְקוֹ when he is in need (of official protection). Y. Ber. V, 9ᵇ בד׳, v. אַזְפָּה.—2) *crowd,* v. דּירחוּק.—3) *emergency,* v. דְּחַק.

[In later Hebr. הוּחַק *a forced opinion* or *reply,* v. next w.]

דּוּחְקָא, דּוּחֲקָא ch. same; 1) *squeezing, forcing.* Targ. Y. Num. XXII, 24 בד׳ in a narrow place.—Pes. 14ᵇ, a. e. מאי דּוּחֲקֵיה דר׳ וכ׳ what forces R. . . . (logically) to put it &c.—Ḥull. 8ᵇ ד׳ דסכינא the force of the knife (the blade forcing its way).—2) *crowded state, pushing.* Ber. 6ᵃ ד׳ דכלה Ms. M. (ed. ד׳ דחוה בכלה) the pushing at public lectures, v. כַּלָּה. Ib.ᵇ, v. אַגְרָא I.—3) *oppression, extortion, distress.* Targ. Ex. III, 9; a. e.—Gitt. 45ᵃ משום ד׳ דְצִיבּוּרָא because the exorbitant price is an extortion of the community.—4) *difficulty.* Bets. 30ᵃ דדרו בד׳ (Ms. M. רחקא) a load carried (on ordinary days) with a great effort.

דְּוָה, דוי (b. h.; cmp. דָּאַב) [*to drip, melt away,*] *to mourn, repine.* Nidd. 23ᵇ (ref. to Deut. XXI, 17 אֹנוֹ, cmp. דְּוַי) מי שלבו דָּוֶה עליו a child over whose death his (the father's) heart is grieved. Ber. 16ᵇ אל יִדְוֶה לבנו may our heart not sink. Kidd. 81ᵇ יִדְווּ כל הַדְּווּים let all those mourn who feel the affliction; Naz. 23ᵃ. Yeb. 47ᵃ the Israelites ... are דווים (some ed. דְּווּיִים, Part. pass.) broken down (under persecution). Gen. R. s. 60; s. 74; a. fr.

Nif. נִדְוֶוה *to be afflicted.* Pesik. Asser, p. 96ᵃ כל אותו שנ׳ האיש over this man (me) in his affliction; Tanḥ. R'eeh ed. Bub. 7 (Tanḥ. ib. 10 שנידוהו, Yalk. Deut. 892; Prov. 962 שנדוהו, corr. acc.).

Hif. הִדְוָה *to afflict.* Y. R. Hash. I, 57ᵇ bot. מַדְוָה לה וכ׳ afflicts it (the year, causes prayers and fasting from fear of failure of the crop) in its beginning.

דְּוָא, דוי I ch. same. Targ. Jer. XLVIII, 17; a. e.

Ithpe. אִדְּוִי *to feel pain, groan.* Ḥull. 51ᵃ מִדְוּוּ וקריבי they groan constantly.

דְּוָא, דוי II (v. preced; cmp. b. h. כָּלָה, כָּסָה) *to look out for, espy.* Sabb. 35ᵃ דָּוֵי למזרח Ar. (ed. דָּאֵוֵי) he looked eastward (for the reflection of the setting sun). Ib. 53ᵇ they raise their nostrils [read:] ומסגי כי דָּוֵי (Ms. O. כדובי) and march like looking out (for the wolf). Ker. 6ᵃ דְּוִי לפומיה וכ׳ Ar. (ed. חזו) watch the lips of &c. Tam. 26ᵇ דוי לחכא וכ׳ he (the watchman) looks out in both directions.

דְּוֵי, דְּוֵי m. (דְּוָא I) *sad, depressed.* Targ. I Kings XX, 43; XXI, 4 (ed. Vien. דְּוַי).—*Pl.* דְּוָון, דְּוָן. Targ. Is. XVI, 7 (ed. Lag. חו׳, corr. acc.); 11.

דְּוַי, דְּווּי, דְּוָיָא m. ch. (=h. דְּוַי, v. preced.) *grief, affliction.* Targ. Gen. XXXV, 18 (h. text אוֹנִי, v. דְּוָה). Targ. Y. ib. XLII, 38 דְּווֹי (O. דוונא).

דְּוָיָא m. same. Snh. 100ᵇ (cit. fr. the Book of Ben Sira) לא תעיל ד׳ וכ׳ suffer not grief to enter thy heart &c.; v. גִּיבַר.

דְּוָיָא, v. דּוּבָא.

דִּיוֹן m. (דוי) *grief.* Yalk. Jer. 279 דִּיוֹנוֹ של בית the grief over the (destroyed) Temple (differ. in Lam. R. introd. 32).

דּוּרִיל m. (דּוּל Af.) *winding; clue,* only in דוריל ידיה the clue which one's own hand wound up, i. e. *one's own doing.* Pes. 28^{a}, v. גְּרִירָאָה. Cmp. דַּלִּיל.

דּוּךְ I (b. h.) 1) *to pound, break.* Y. Bets. I, 60^{d} top וידוך וכ׳ but why should he not pound a day before?—Part. pass. דַּךְ, v. דַּךְ.—2) *to designate, mark off,* v. דּוּךְ II. [Gen. R. s. 5, v. דּוּךְ III.]

Nif. נָדוֹךְ, נִידוֹךְ, *to be pounded, crushed.* Bets. I, 7 נְדוֹכִין כדרכן are pounded (on Holy Days) in their usual way. Ib. 14^{a} לְדוֹכָהּ וכ׳ as to pounding it (salt) alone. Yoma 75^{a} דבר שנ׳ וכ׳ something which is pounded in the mortar (spices); a. fr.

Pol. דּוֹכֵךְ, part. pass. מְדוֹכָךְ *crushed.* Yalk. Ps. 848 מְדוֹכָכִים אנו we are crushed (Gen. R. s. 5 מדוכנין, v. דָּכָן).

דּוּךְ ch. same. Part. דָּאֵיךְ, דָּאִיךְ. Targ. O. Num. XI, 8. Bets. 14^{a} דוּךְ, v. infra.

Pa. דַּיֵּיךְ same. Bets. 14^{a} כי דַיְיכַתְּ וכ׳ ed. (Ms. M. דייכת) . . . . דוק when thou poundest (on a Holy Day), bend the mortar sideways and pound.

Af. אֲדִיךְ (cmp. דעך) *to extinguish.* Kidd. 81^{a} אתו כ״ע לְאַדּוֹכֵיהּ Ar. s. v. אדך (missing in ed.) people came to put the fire out.

דּוּךְ II, דּוּכָא m. (cmp. דַּךְ; Assyr. דכי *to muster,* Schr. KAT p. 209^{9}) [*marked off, pointed out,*] *place, stand, hall.* Targ. I Kings XIV, 28 (ed. Lag. דובא, some ed. רובא, corr. acc.); Targ. II Chr. XII, 11 (h. text תָּא).—Ber. 18^{b}. Ib. 42^{b}. V. דּוּכְתָּא.

דּוּךְ III m. (v. preced.) *leader, chief commander,* only in דּוּךְ דּוּכְנִין (an adaptation of dux ducum, δοὺξ δουκῶν, v. Du Cange s. v.) the leader of the services of the Levites, v. דּוּכָן. Y. Sabb. X, 12^{c}; Num. R. s. 7 (rendering of נשיא נשיאי Num. III, 32). Ib. s. 4, end [read:] אלעזר הוה דוך דוכנין וכ׳ Eleazar was chief commander, prince over princes; cmp. דּוּכּוּס.—**Pl.* דּוּכִים. Gen. R. s. 5 (play on דָּכְיָם, Ps. XCIII, 3) ('the rivers lift up their voices', saying to the waves of the Sea) דּוּכִים קבלונו ye leaders, receive us; [Yalk. Ps. 848 דַּכִּים אנו we are crushed].

דּוּכָא, v. דּוּךְ II.

דּוּכּוּס, דּוּכָּס m. (dux) *dux, commander.* Ex. R. s. 15; a. fr.—[Gen. R. s. 5 לדוכוס ים Rashi, v. דכסס.]—*Pl.* דּוּכָּסִים, דּוּכּוֹסִין. Cant. R. to II, 15 עשו ודוּכָּסֶיהָ (read ורומי) Rome and her *duces.* Gen. R. s. 78 דּוּכָּסַי my (Rome's) *duces;* a. fr. [Lev. R. s. 16 דוכוסיא ודאני, read as ed. Wil. דוכוס אחד ד׳.] V. דּוּכָּסָא.

דוכוסיא, v. preced.

דּוּכִיתָא f. (דּוּךְ) *mortar* (h. מְדֹכָה). Targ. Y. I Num. XI, 8.

דּוּכָן m. (cmp. דּוּךְ II) *place to stand on, stand, stage,* esp. *Dukhan,* the priests' stage from which they pronounce the benediction. Midd. II, 6; a. fr.—סלק לד׳ to go up the stage, *to officiate as priest.* Sabb. 118^{b}; a. e.—2) *religious service from the stand, the Levite's singing, teaching.* Meg. 3^{a}; Arakh. 4^{a} the Levites מְדוּכָנָן Ms. M. (ed. בד׳) must interrupt their services.—*Pl.* דּוּכָנִין, דּוּכָנִים, v. דּוּךְ III. Cmp. דָּכוֹן.

דּוּכָן, דּוּכָנָא ch. same. Targ. Y. Num. VI, 23. Targ. Ezek. XLII, 12 (h. גדרת); a. e.—In gen. *teacher's platform, pulpit.* B. Bath. 21^{a} ריש ד׳ *superintendent of the platform,* title of a tutor who assists the teacher of a primary class numbering more than twenty five pupils.—Cmp. דִּכְוָון.

דּוּכְנָה f. (דוך, v. דכן) *pounding, pounded dish.* Y. M. Kat. I, 80^{d} bot. buy for us שיתורין לד׳ peas for pounding.

דּוּכָּס, דּוּכָּסָא ch. = דּוּכּוּס. Lam. R. to I, 5. Ab. Zar. 11^{a}; a. e.—*Pl.* דּוּכְּסִין, דּוּכְּסַיָּא. Targ. Cant. VI, 8; a. e.—Gen. R. s. 67; a. fr.—Koh. R. to X, 18; Lam. R. introd. (R. Alex. 2) (ref to Is. XXII, 8 מסך) [read:] גלי דִּכְסַיָּיה He uncovered (disgraced) its (the Temple's) commanders (cmp. דּוּךְ III).

דוכסוסטון, v. next w.

דּוּכְסוּסְטוֹס m. (transpos. of δύσχιστος) *hard to split,* an inferior kind of *parchment,* opp. to קלף, a split parchment of superior quality. Men. 31^{b}. Ib. 32^{a} sq.; Sabb. 79^{b}; a. fr.—*Pl.* דּוּכְסוּסְטִין. Y. Sabb. VIII, 11^{b} (not טון . . . . .).

דּוּכְסוֹסְיָא m. (v. דּוּךְ III, a. סוּסְיָא; a popular adaptation of טַכְסִיוֹטָא, ταξεώτης) *the magistrate's officer, sergeant.* Meg. 27^{a} דוכסו׳ ed. (Ms. M. דוכסס׳, Ar. דכסס׳), expl. by R. Shesheth פרשא דמתא the riding messenger of the town. [Cmp. דורקטי.]

דּוּכְסוּתָא f. (denom. of דּוּכָּסָא) *dukedom, (ducatus), governorship.* Cant. R. to VI, 12 [read:] הב לי ד׳ דגובבתא give me the governorship of G. (v. גּוֹבַבְתָּא). Ib. כד נסב ד׳ וכ׳ having entered the office he came down from there (to Sepphoris).

דוכסן, Y. B. Mets. II, 8^{c} bot. בד׳, some ed., v. פַּרְבַּסִין.

דוכסס, v. דִּכְסַס.

דוכססיא, v. דּוּכְסוֹסְיָא.

דּוּכְרָא, v. דְּכַר II.

דּוּכְרָן, דּוּכְרָנָא, v. דָּכְרָן.

דּוּכְרָנִית f. (denom. of דּוּכְרָא) *ram-like,* or *man-like.* Keth. 11^{a}, v. אַיְלוֹנִית.

דּוּכְתָּא f. (v. דּוּךְ II) *place.* Ber. 42^{b} (interch. with דּוּךְ). Ib. 4^{b} בכל ד׳ everywhere else (in Rabbinical writings). Yeb. 62^{a} בד׳ אחריתי in another place (of the Scriptures). B. Mets. 93^{b} bot.; a. v. fr.

דּוּל (v. דְּלָא) *to wind, draw water.* Denom. דַּוְולָא, דַּוָל.

**Af.* אַדְיל *to wind up, make skeins, prepare for spinning.* Yeb. 63^{a} זבון ולא תדויל Ar. s. v. דל 5 buy (ready-made) and do not wind skeins (ed. זבין ולא תיזול, v. זול I a. II).

Ithpe. אִידִּיל, אִידְּוִיל, *to be drawn from, to give water enough for irrigation.* B. Bath. 8^{a} ודילמא לא מִידְּוִיל but perhaps the well (to be dug) will prove unfit for irrigation? Ib. 12[b].

דּוּלָא, דְּוַל, v. דְּוּל.

דּוּלְבָּא, v. דְּלוּב.

דּוּלְבְּקִי, v. דְּלַפְקִי.

דַּוְולָא, דַּוְלָא m. (דּוּל, v. דְּוִיל) *clue, skein.—Pl.* דַּוְלֵי. Ḥull. 60[a] they give the leper a reel וסתר דַּוְלֵי ed. (Ar. דוולא) and he must wind up the clues or skeins.

דּוּלְפִינִין m. pl. (δελφίν) *dolphins* (a fish about which many fables were circulated among the ancients, cmp. Sm. Ant. s. v.). Bekh. 8[a] דולפנ׳ (Var. דּוּלְפִּרְנָא, corr. acc.; Ar. ed. pr. דִּילְ׳); Tosef. ib. I, 11.

דּוּלְפָנָא m. (דלף) *blear-eyed.—Pl.* דּוּלְפָנֵי. Keth. 60[b]. [דולפנין, Bekh. 8[a]; v. preced.] [דולפני, Tosef. Kel. B. Bath. I, 9, read דולפקי.]

דּוּלְפְּקִי, v. דְּלַפְקִי.

דולפקס, דולפקוס, Sifré Deut. 231, v. לִיבְדְּקוֹס.

דולריא, v. דַּרְדְּיָא.

דוֹם, imper. of דָּמַם.

דּוּם, דִּים (cmp. דבב, דמם) *to speak in a low voice, to suspect.* Part. pass. דָּיִים *suspected.* Yeb. 52[a] מִידָם הוה ד׳ מחמתיה he was suspected of illicit relations with his mother-in-law; Kidd. 12[b] דַּיְימָא חמתיה מיניה .... (v. Rashi to Yeb. l. c.) his mother-in-law was suspected &c.; Yeb. 69[b] sq.

דּוּמָא pr. n. *Duma.* Tosef. Par. II (I), 1 וד׳ היתה נקראת the cow was named Duma (Var. וד׳ שמו the owner's name was D., v. דָּמָא); Yalk. Num. 759 דמה.—V. דּוּמָה II.

דּוּמָה I f. (v. דּוּם) 1) *evil report, rumor.* Nidd. 66[a], v. דִּימָה.—2) *a woman of ill repute.* Sot. 27[a]. Gitt. 69[b] ד׳ בת ד׳ דשדתיה which an ill reputed daughter of an ill-reputed mother has spun.

דּוּמָה II f. (b.h.; preced.) *silence, land of death.* Masc. *Dumah,* the guardian angel of the deceased. Ber. 18[b] (Ms. M. דּוּמָא). Ḥag. 5[a] משלימנא ליה לד׳ I (the angel of death) hand him over to Dumah. Sabb. 152[b].

דּוּמוֹס, v. דִּימוֹס.

דומסיריא, v. דִּימוֹסִין.

דּוּמִי f. (דּוּם) *evil report, gossip.* M. Kat. 18[b]; Yeb. 25[a] ד׳ דמתא וכ׳ the gossip of a place must remain undenied for a day and a half (in order to be acted upon legally).

דּוּמְיָא m. (דָּמָא) *resemblance, (there is) an analogy; (under) analogous conditions.* Kidd. 19[a] בנו ד׳ דידיה וכ׳ 'his son' (Ex. XXI, 9) means a son like himself (the father), as he (the father) is of age, so must his son (to whom he designates her) be of age. Shebu. 40[b]; B. Mets. 4[b] ד׳ דכלים וכ׳ under similar conditions as the just stated claim of chattel and landed property. Meg. 2[a] זמניהם ד׳ דזמנם מה וכ׳ *z'mannehem* (their respective seasons, Esth. IX, 31) is analogous to *z'mannam* (ib. 27); as *z'mannam* means two days &c.—M. Kat. 4[a]; a. fr.

דּוּמִיטְיָנוּס pr. n. m. *Domitian,* the Roman Emperor. Y. Sabb. XIV, 14[d] ברתיה דדמיטי׳; Y. Ab. Zar. II, 40[d] דתימטינים (corr. acc.).

דומין, Esth. R. to VI, 10 ד׳ פנטון, read קוֹמִים פְּרִיבָטוֹן, v. בגרון. V. קוֹמִים.

דומינו, read דּוֹמִינֵי (vocat. of dominus) *O Lord.* Lam. R. to I, 5 Ar., v. פִּיבֵּר. [דומינון, דומינין, דומינו, Gen. R. s. 8; Koh. R. to VI, 10, read הֵימְנוֹן.]

דּוּמְנִיקִי, דּוּמִינְקִי f. pl. (dominicae, sub aedes, v. Revue des Etudes Juives, 1884, p. 277) *churches.* Snh. 74[b] חני קוּקֵי וד׳ היכי יהבינן להו נורא Ms. M. (ed. omit. נורא; Var. lect., v. Rabb. D. S. a. l.) how dare we give fire to those churches (on Sundays)? [קוּקי, קוואקי &c., misnomer of κυριακή, the name used by the Greek teachers of Christianity, corresp. to the Latin dominica.—For another explan. v. Revue des Etudes Juives 1885, p. 195 sq.]

דּוּמְכָא, v. דִּמְכָא.

דּוּמָם, v. דָּמַם.

דּוּמְנִיקִי, v. דּוּמִינְקֵי.

דומסיא, v. דִּימוֹסְיָא.

דומקיא, Yeb. 17[a], v. רומקי.

דּוּן, v. דִּין.

***דּוֹן** m. (v. דַּנָּא) *keg, measure.* B. Bath. 90[b] they called it ד׳ פפא (quot. Tosaf. to Yeb. 79[a] ed. רוז, Ms. M. רז, Ms. H. כוז) and they named it (the measure introduced by Papa) ד׳ פפא *Papa's keg.*

דּוֹנָךְ, v. דָּוִין.

דּוֹנָטִיבָא, דּוֹנָאטִיבָא m. pl. (donativa, pl.) *imperial donations.* Gen. R. s. 10, end (בח..., corr. acc.); Yalk. ib. 16 דונאט׳. Ex. R. s. 41 דונה טיבה some ed. (corr. acc.). Num. R. s. 7; a. fr.

דּוּנְבָא, v. דִּנְבָא.

דּוֹנַג, v. דִּינַג.

דּוֹנַג m. (b. h.) *wax.* Lam. R. to I, 4 נעשו כד׳ they became (yellow-complected) like wax.

דונגר, v. רוּנְגָר.

דונה, דונה טיבה, דונהטיבה, v. דּוֹנָאטִיבָא.

דּוּס (=דּוּשׁ) *to stamp;* denom. דַּיְיסָא.

דּוֹסָא pr. n. m. (prob. an abbrev. of Dositheus, v. דּוֹסְתַּאי) *Dosa,* a Tannai, usu. named *R. D. ben Harkhinas,* or *Hork'nos.* Eduy. III, 1.—Tosef. Kel. B. Bath. IV, 14; a. fr.—Erub. 83[a] [read:] ר׳ נתן אומר ר׳ ד׳ אומר (v. Rabb.

D. S. a. l.). [Y. Shek. VII, 50^d ר׳ די, Men. 50^b ר׳ יוסי.] V. חֲנִידָא, a. חַרְפִּינָס.

דוסאי, v. דּוֹסְתַּאי.

דוסיקאות, Tosef. Kel. B. Mets. II, 3, v. דִּיסְקָא.

דוסקמא, דוסמקא, Tanh. Noah 1, v. דּוּרְמַסְקִית.

דּוֹסְתַּאי pr. n. m. (Δοσίθεος) *Dostai*, 1) a disciple of Shammai. Orlah II, 5.—2) D. father of Abba José. Tosef. Peah IV, 2 ed. Zuck. (Var. דוסאי); Yoma 22^b; a. fr.—3) R. D. son of R. Judah. Tosef. Shebi. II, 18; a. e.—4) R. D. son of R. Jannai. Tosef. Ber. VII (VI), 8. Nidd. 31^b; a. fr.

דופורון, דופורין, read: רִיפּוּדִין m. (repudium) *divorce*. Gen. R. s. 18 (among gentiles) the wife may divorce him והיא נותנת לו ד׳ and she gives him the *repudium* (v. Sm. Ant. s. v.).

דּוֹפִי f. (b. h. דֳּפִי, דְּפִי; r. דָּפָה *to strike against, damage*; cmp. דפן) *damage to reputation* (cmp. meanig of גָּדַף), *taint, reproach*. Yoma 22^b לא היה בו שום ד׳ no reproach rested on Saul's descent. Tem. 15^b; Tosef. B. Kam. VIII, 13; a. fr.—Snh. 99^b הגדות של ד׳; v. דָּרַשׁ.—Pes. 30^b earthen ware אינו יוצא מידי דופיו לעולם (Ms. O. מדפני, v. Rabb. D. S. a. l. note 50; Ab. Zar. 34^a דופני, Ms. M. דָּפְיוֹ) can never get rid of its defect (once made unclean, it cannot be cleansed by any process, v. תַּקָּנָה).

דּוֹפְיָא ch. same. Targ. Ps. L, 20 (Var. דָּפְיָא, דופי, Regia דָּפְיוֹ fem.).

דופלומטר, v. דיפלומט׳.

דופלין, v. דיפלון.

***דּוֹפֶן, דֶּפֶן** m. *damage, defect*. Ab. Zar. 34^a, v. דופי.

דּוֹפֶן, דֹּפֶן c. (דפן, v. דָּה) 1) *board-partition*, esp. a wall of the festive booth (סוּכָּה). Succ. 4^a ד׳ האמצעי the middle of the three walls. Ib. ד׳ עקומה *the curved wall*, a legal fiction by which a part of the ceiling may be considered as part of a curved wall.—Ib. 6^b; a. fr.—2) (trnsf.) *side* of a vessel, oppos. to bottom, rim &c. Ohol. IX, 16 תחת דָּפְנָהּ under the belly of its side; Tosef. ib. X, 9 הוֹפְנָהּ. Ib. VII, 10 side of a cave, opp. to שקוף &c.; a. fr.—3) *the chest surrounding the lungs, ribs*, also *a single rib*. Hull. 48^a, a. fr. ריאה הסמוכה לד׳ lungs adhering to the chest. Snh. 49^a ד׳ חמישית the fifth rib (counting from the lowest).—4) *the paries of the abdomen*. יוצא ד׳ a fetus extracted by means of *the cesarean section*. Nidd. V, 1; a. fr.—Metaph. תלה בד׳ to suspend from the wall, i. e. *to leave a decision in suspense*. Y. Kidd. IV, 65^b bot.; Y. Snh. VI, 23^c bot. בריפן (corr. acc.).—*Pl.* דוֹפָנִים, constr. דוֹפְנֵי; mostly דְּפָנוֹת. Hull. 45^b דופני ריאה *the grooves between the lungs*, דפנות *ribs*. Ib.^a שתי ד׳ two sides of the chest.—Succ. I, 1; a. fr.—Tosef. Ohol. VI, 2 בצד דופני וכ׳ ed. Zuck. on the *wall-like* side of the tent. Ib. עם דופני של אוהל, ed. Zuck., read (with R. S. to Ohol. V, 7) דפנות or (with ed.) דוֹפְנוֹ.

דּוֹפְנָא, דִּפְנָא ch. same. B. Mets. 23^b אי דדפני Ar. (ed. דדפקא) whether the piece is from the ribs.—*Pl.* דוֹפְנַיָּיתָא. Targ. Y. Lev. XXIII, 42 (דוֹפְנַיָּיתָא).—דַּפְנָתָא. Y. Succ. I, 51^d.

דּוֹפְנִי, v. דוֹפֶן.

דּוֹפֶק m. (דפק; cmp. אַגָּף) *that against which a turning body knocks, frame*, esp. *dofek, the frame supporting the movable stone of a tomb*, v. גּוֹלֵל. Ohol. II, 4; a. e.—*Pl.* דּוֹפְקִין. Ib. דופק ד׳ the frame supporting the frame stones or sills.

דּוֹפְקָא ch. same. Targ. Y. Num. XIX, 16; 18.

דּוֹפְקָנִין m. pl. (דפק) *knockers*, name of a parasite plant growing on thorns, cmp. כְּשׁוּת. Tosef. Erub. XI (VIII), 11 קרנין וד׳ (Var. קוצין) 'horns' and 'knockers'.

דופרה, v. דִּיפְרָא.

דּוּפְשְׁקָא, v. דִּפְשְׁקָא.

דּוּץ I, דִּיץ (b. h.) *to skip, dance; to rejoice*. Denom. דִּיצָה.

דּוּץ, דִּיץ ch. same. Targ. Job XLI, 14 תדיץ ed. Lag. (Ms. תדוץ, some ed. תדיח, corr. acc.).—Targ. II Sam. I, 20. Targ. Ps. XXI, 14 (ed. Lag. נְדוּצְצָא *Pol.*); a. fr.—*Part.* דָּאִיץ, דָּיְצִין. Targ. Hab. I, 15. Targ. Prov. XXIX, 6; a. e.

דּוּץ II (contr. of דָּצַץ) *to prick, stick, squeeze*. Sabb. 50^b דָּצָהּ שלפה וכ׳ if he stuck it in, pulled it out &c.—Ib. 156^b דָּצַתָּה בגודא (Ms. O. דעיצתא בביזעא, v. Rabb. D. S. a. l. note 30) she stuck it (the brooch) into the wall. Hull. 93^b אי דָּץ ביה מידי if he stuck something into the nostrils (so as to keep them open). Succ. 37^b לא לְדוּץ וכ׳ one must not squeeze the palm branch between the myrtle and willow (after they have been tied together). [B. Bath. 74^a דציצה Ar., v. דְּצִיץ.]

דּוּק m. *a withered spot in the eye*, v. דַּק II.

דּוּק (cmp. דוּךְ) 1) *to pound, beat; to powder*. Bets. 14^a, v. הוּךְ.—Part. Peil דָּיִיק *powdered*. Ib.^b ד׳ נפי fine-powdered. Hull. 51^b, v. פִּיתְנָא. V. דָּקַק.—2) (cmp. בִּין, בָּקַר a. oth.) *to examine carefully, to be particular, exact in expression; to pay special attention, to mind*. Ib. 6^a, a. fr. דָּק ואשכח he examined and found. Succ. 8^a לא דק he did not express himself exactly; a. fr.—*Part.* דָּיֵיק *careful*. Keth. 18^b מֵידַק ד׳ he is very careful (as to what witnesses he uses). Yoma 83^b הוה ד׳ בשמא minded a man's name (considering it an indication of his character). Ib. לא הוו דַּיְיקִי בשמא did not mind &c. Ib. דַּיְיקִיתוּ ye mind.—Part. Peil דָּיִיק (v. *Pa.*) *proved, conclusive*. B. Kam. 3^b those verses לא כמר דַּיְיקֵי וכ׳ are no evidence either for the one or the other.—Denom. דִּיּוּקָא, דַּיְקָא, דַּוְקָא.

Pa. דַּיֵּיק 1) *to grind, to chew carefully*. Sabb. 155^a bot. דדַיְּיקָה ואכלה Ms. M. (ed. דדיקה באוכלא) she grinds her food carefully.—2) *to argue by pressing a word, to analyze, prove*. Keth. 31^b ד׳ מרישא takes his argument from the first clause; a. fr.—3) *to calculate exactly*. Targ. Y. Lev. XXVII, 18. Ib. XXV, 50, v. דְּקְדֵק; a. e.

Af. אַדִּיק, אודיק *to be punctilious, get impatient*. Koh. R. to III, 9 א׳ מלכא the king was irritated. Pesik. B'shall.

p. 86[b]; Yalk. Sam. 152 אודיקַת סרח וכ׳ Serah . . . grew *angry;* cmp. דִּקְדֵּק.—2) *to examine, look with anxiety, wait attentively.* Targ. Prov. VII, 6. Targ. Ps. XIV, 2; a. fr.—Gen. R. s. 17 אודיק . . . לקלהון R. . . . . examined into the noise they made; Lev. R. s. 34; Yalk. Lev. 665; Yalk. Is. 352. Y. Keth. XII, 35[a] top; Y. Kil. IX, 32[b] top א׳ לון חכ׳ Bar K. looked out for them (waiting for them to ask him).

דְּוּקָא, דּוּקָא, דִּוּקָא m. (preced.) 1) *exactness, minuteness.* Nez. 7[b] נחית לד׳ enters into minuteness (saying 'one and a half').—2) (as an adv.) *exactly, exclusively, only.* Yeb. 76[a] ד׳ שערתא a real barley corn it must be (nothing else). Men. 30[a] באמצע שיטה ד׳ only in the middle of a line.—Gitt. 44[a] ד׳ או לאו ד׳ is this meant exactly (one hundred), or not exactly? Men. 27[b] אל ד׳ *el* (towards) is meant in its exact sense; a. fr.

דּוּקָא I m. (דוק)=h. דַּק, *chaff.* Targ. Is. XL, 15. Ib. XXVIII, 28.

דּוּקָא II m.=h. דַּק, *a withered spot in the eye* (or *withered in growth, dwarf*). Targ. O. Lev. XXI, 20 (Y. II ib. ננס).

דּוּקְיָא m. (דוק) *evidence by conclusion, exact meaning.* Keth. 31[b] בד׳ דהא וכ׳ they differ as to the conclusion to be drawn from this Mishnah. Zeb. 31[b] (Rashi: דִּיוּקָא).

דּוֹקְיָא m. pl. (δόκια, pl. of δόκιον) *beams of the ceiling.* Lam. R. to I, 1 חד בר נש) רבתי, an oneirocritical interpret. of Kappadokia) *Kappa* in Greek is *twenty,* ד׳ בל״י קורות (not דיקיא) *dokia* in Greek is *beams;* v. דִּיקָא.

דוקלינוס, v. דִּיקְלִיטְיָנוּס.

דּוּקִים (v. דּוּק) pr. n. pl. *Dukim* (cmp. צוּפִים), *Dokos,* a stronghold near Jericho. Y. Ab. Zar. I, 39[c] טקסיס דד׳ the garrison of D.

דּוּקִינָר m. (ducenarius, δουκηνάριος S.) *commander, procurator.* Y. Ab. Zar. I, 39[b] (Bab. ib. 6[b] מינאה).

דּוּקְלִיטְיָאנוּס, v. דִּיקְלִיט׳.

דְּוּקְנָא, דּוּקְנָא, דִּוּקְנָא m. (דּוּק) *calculating, accurate scholar.* Ab. Zar. 10[a] ספרא ד׳ an accurate scribe (paying attention to exact historical dates).—*Pl.* דּוּקָנֵי, דִּוּ׳. Men. 29[b] ספרי ד׳ careful copyists of the Bible. Yeb. 43[a] משום דמסיימי בה ד׳ זו וכ׳ because exact scholars report a traditional addition (to the Halachah in question), 'These are the words of R. S.'

דִּיקְנִי, דּוּקְנִי f. (denom. of דָּקָן; adopted in Hebr.) *trimming shears* on a pole. Y. Maasr. III, end, 51[a] היתה ניטלת בד׳ if the fruit is taken off with trimming shears (by a person standing outside the garden). Ib. צור צור דּוּקְנִיתָךְ וכ׳ wrap well up (keep well thy question about) the pruner (sophistical as it is), it is better than anything (the Agadists have to say).—Tosef. Kel. B. Mets. III, 9 האיזמל של דד׳ one knife of the shears.

דּוּקְנִיתָא, v. preced.

דּוּקְרָא m. ch. (דקר) *fork-like reed,* opp. to קני plain stems; prop. *Pl.* דּוּקְרִין, דּוּקְרֵי. Succ. 13[a] ד׳ דקני the pronged reeds (corresp. to אַפְקוּתָא of the palm-tree, Rashi). Lev. R. s. 12.

דֻּקְרָן, דּוּקְרָן m. h. same, *fork, fork-like reed, pronged pole.* Y. Erub. I, 18[c] קנה וד׳ reed-stem and prongs. Ib. 19[c] כמין דק׳; Y. Kil. IV, 29[b] כמין דוק׳; Y. Succ. I, 52[a] bot. כמין דְּקָרִים (v. דֶּקֶר). Y. Shebi. II, 33[d] top עושה לה דיק׳ (corr. acc.) he puts under it a pronged prop. Tosef. Kel. B. Mets. III, 14 הדוק׳ ed. Zuck. (Var. דורקין).—*Pl.* דֻּק׳, דּוּקְרָנִין, דּוּקְרָנִים. Y. Kil. l. c. he took דוק׳ וסותם forked reeds with which he closed the breach; Y. Erub. I, 19[c] top; Y. Succ. l. c.—Tosef. ib. I, 4 if one made a ceiling of the Succah בקנים ובד׳ with (plain) reeds and with forked reeds; Bab. ib. 13[a] קנים וד׳ (Ms. M. 2 קנים הד׳, v. Ar. s. v. דקר), expl. קנים של ד׳ pronged reeds. Tosef. Men. XI, 6 דומין לדק׳ shaped like forks; Men. XI, 6 (96[a]) מפרצלין . . . . כמין ד׳ Ar. (ed. omit. כמין ד׳).—*Denom. מְדוּקְרָן *fork-shaped.* Tosef. Kil. IV, 5 קנים מְדוּקְרָנִים; Erub. 16[a]; 11[b] קנים הדוקרניך (Ms. M. הדוקרים).

דֻּקְ׳, דּוּקְרָנָא ch. same.—*Pl.* דֻּקְ׳, דּוּקְרָנִין. Y. Yoma III, beg. 40[b] כמין תרין דק׳ וכ׳ like two prongs of light; Y. Ber. I, 2[c] דקור׳ (corr. דוקר׳); Gen. R. s. 50 Ar. (ed. תרתין קרנין).

דּוּר I (b. h.) [1) *to form a circle or enclosure* (v. Fl. to Levy Talm. Dict. I, p. 440[a] sq.).—Denom. דּוּר II, דּוֹר, דִּירָה &c.].—2) (denom. of דִּירָה) *to reside, dwell.* Ber. 8[a] לעולם יָדוּר וכ׳ one must try to live in the same place with his teacher. Keth. 72[a]; a. fr. אין אדם דָּר וכ׳, v. כְּפִיפָה. Ib. 110[b] בל הַדָּר בא״י whoever lives in Palestine.—Succ. 35[a] (ref. to *hadar,* Lev. XXIII, 40) א״ת הָדָר אלא הַדָּר דבר שֶׁדָּר וכ׳ ed. (Ms. M. הָדָר דבר הַדָּר וכ׳) read not *hadar* but *haddar,* something which remains on its tree from year to year (without withering); a. fr.—3) *to lodge,* v. infra.

Pi. דַּיֵּיר 1) *to cause a circuit;* ד׳ שדה *to let cattle change folds within a field, to collect manure in a field, by letting cattle live on it.* Shebi. III, 4. Y. ib. 34[c] bot. מְדַיְּירִין בטובה you may let your cattle live on one's field as a favor; a. e.—2) *to lodge,* v. infra.

Hif. הֵדִיר *to lodge.* Pesik. R. s. 3, beg. (play on דָּרְבָן) שמֵדִיר בינה בפרה it (the goad) causes understanding to dwell in the cow; Pesik Baḥod. p. 153[a] שמורה (ed. O. שמדיר); Koh. R. to XII, 11 [read:] שהוא מְדַיֵּיר; Num. R. s. 14 שדּר; Y. Snh. Tanḥ. B'haăl 15 הָדַר אצל הפרה וכ׳.—[Num. R. l. c. the words of the wise הָדָּרִים בינה וכ׳ lodge understanding with men.]

Nithpa. נִדַּיֵּיר *to be manured* by cattle living in folds, v. Piel. Shebi. IV, 2; M. Kat. 13[a]; a. e.

דִּיר, דּוּר ch. same, *to dwell.* Targ. Ps. CV, 23; a. fr.—Pes. 113[a] top (v. Rabb. D. S. a. l. note 6).—Part. דָּיֵיר, דָּאִיר. Targ. Ps. LVII, 5 דָּיְירָא Ms. (ed. חיירא).—Yeb. 52[a] דאיר בבי חמוה he resides with his father-in-law. B. Mets. 117[a] דהוו דָּיְירֵי who occupied. Taan. 24[a] דָּיְירְנָא וכ׳ I live in a poor village.

Pa. דַּיֵּיר, דַּיָּאר, דַּיּוּר 1) *to go around, to peddle* (cmp. h. סָחַר). R. Hash. 9[b] (expl. דְּרוֹר, Lev. XXV, 10) כְּמְדַיֵּיר כי דיירא ומוביל וכ׳ Ms. M. (ed. בי דיירא, Ar. s. v. דר 3: מְדַיָּאר דריא) as a traveller is licensed to go around and carry his goods through the whole district.—2) *to deposit manure*, v. preced. *Pi.*—B. Kam. 113[b] חני דְּדַיְּירֵי דיירי Rashi (ed. דרר, Ms. R. דִּמְדַיְּירֵי דיירי, v. Rabb. D. S. a. l. note) those (gentiles) who manure fields for pay by letting cattle live on them in folds.—3) *to place around (in a row*, Rashi). Kidd. 81[a] ד׳ גולפי placed jugs around (as a partition).—*4) *to round a person, to overtake.* B. Kam. 92[b]; B. Mets. 107[b] (prov.) רהוט . . . ולא דַּיּוּרוּהוּ וכ׳ Ar. (ed. אמטו, מטו) runners run but overtake not one who has taken a morning meal.

דּוּר II m. (preced., cmp. זֵר) *rim, wreath.* Kel. XVI, 3.—*Pl.* דּוּרִים. Ib.

***דּוּר** III m. *a stuffed bag.* Lam. R. to I, 1 רבתי (חד כות׳2), v. אֲדַר I. [Y. Snh. X, 28[a] top; Num. R. s. 14; 15; Tanh. B'haal. 15, v. כַּדּוּר.]

דּוֹר m. (b. h., דּוּר I) [*circle, period*, cmp. גּוֹרָל] *generation, contemporaries.* Arakh. 17[a] ד׳ לפי פרנס as the leader so the generation; a. v. fr.—ד׳ הפלגה the generation which witnessed the separation of races; ד׳ המבול which perished in the flood; ד׳ המדבר which perished in the desert, &c. Snh. X, 3 (107[b], sq.); a. fr.—*Pl.* דּוֹרוֹת. Ib. 99[a]; a. fr.—לְדוֹרוֹת *for all time to come; permanent*, opp. הוראת שעה, לשעה a temporary ordinance. Ib. 16[b] (ref. to Num. VII, 1) אותם במשיחה ולא לד׳ וכ׳ only they were installed with ointment, but not as a precedent for future installations; a. fr.—Men. 19[b], a. e. ד׳ משעה לא ילפינן a permanent law cannot be derived from a special temporary legislation.—פסח ד׳ annual Passover celebration, opp. to פסח מצרים the one observed in Epypt. Pes. IX, 5; a. fr.

דּוּר imperat. of נָדַר. Kidd. 41[a]; a. fr.

דּוּרָא I m. (v. דּוּר 1) *district, settlement, village* (corresp. to h. חָצֵר). B. Bath. 54[b] ד׳ דרעותא Ms. M. (ed. דרעיאתא); Erub. 12[a] דּוּרָה דרעותא *Shephardville* (v., however, Berl. Beitr. z. Geogr. Babyl. p. 30).—Pes. 40[a] ד׳ דבי וכ׳ the settlement of Be-Hashu.—*Pl.* דּוּרָתָא. Targ. Ps. X, 8 ed. Lag. (Var. דרתיא, v. דַּרְתָּא; Ms. דּוּרַאתָיָיא).

דּוּרָא II m. (b. h. דַּר, v. Ges. H. Dict. s. v.) *dura*, name of *a jewel, mother of pearl*(?). Targ. Esth. I, 6 ד׳ דכרכי וכ׳ the dura of the Sea places.—Esth. R. to l. c. אית אתר . . למרגליתא דּוּרָה there is a place where a pearl (or jewel) is called *durah;* Meg. 12[a] there is a precious stone in the Sea places ודִירָה שמה Ms. M. (ed. דָּרָה) whose name is *dirah (darah)*; Y. Snh. X, 28[a] top תמן קריין . . דירה there (at a certain place) they call &c.

דּוּרָא III or **דִּירָא** m. (דּוּר I) *a parasite worm* in the bowels. Num. R. s. 7 [read:] שאחיה נותן ד׳ במעיהן; v. דִּרְיָא.

דּוּרָא IV m. (דור II) *burden, load.* B. Kam. 92[b] (prov.) אי דלית ד׳ וכ׳ (our w. missing in Ar. s. v. דלא) if thou wilt lift the burden, I shall lift (if you will share the responsibility, I shall take the lead).

***דּוּרָא** IV, or **בֵּי ד׳, דַּוָּרָא** (cmp. דַּוָּאר I) *Be-Dura (Davvara)*, a station near Hagronia. Ber. 31[a] ed. (Ms. M. דיירא, without בי; Ms. F. בי דירא; oth. var. דראר, דרא, בי דודא, v. Rabb. D. S. a. l. note).

***דּוֹרָאטָא** m. pl. (δώρατα, irreg. pl. of δῶρον, v. LXX, II Chr. XXXII, 23 ed. R.) *gifts.* Y'lamd. to Num. XV, 1 quot. in Ar. s. v. דרדה.

***דּוּרַאי** m. (v. דּוּרָא) *county governor*,—מרי ד׳ (Mylord, the governor), title of an officer. Yoma 82[b]; Snh. 74[a]; Pes. 25[b] (Ms. M. דוראי; Rashi: the lord of *my village*, v. דּוּרָא I).

דּוּרְבָן, v. דָּרְבָן.

דּוּרְבָנָא m. (contract. of דברברנא, reduplic. of דבר, v. דַּבָּר; cmp. דּוּרְבָנָא a. דָּרְבָן) *a haughty leader.* Targ. Job XXXIV, 20 ed. Lag. (ed. Vien. דּוּרְבָּנֵי).—*Pl.* דּוּרְבָּנַיָּא, דּוּרְבָּנֵי. Ib. XXXV, 9 (Var. רַבְרְבָנ׳). Targ. Prov. VIII, 16 Var. ed. Lag. דוכרני (corr. acc.). Targ. Ps. XXXI, 24.

דּוּרְגּוֹן, דַּרְגּוֹן m. (דרג) *a suite of graded officers.* Y. Hor. III, beg. 47[a] הוא וכל דו׳ דידיה Himself and His entire staff (of angels); Y. Snh. II, 20[a] top דר׳. Ex. R. s. 1 הניח מניח דר׳ שלו he (Moses) left his escort.—Y'lamd. to Num. XII, 1, quot. in Ar. דרוגין. Num. R. s. 4 שיהיו עושין דר׳ לפניו that they should form a hierarchy of officers before him. Y. Keth. XII, 35[a] bot. חמא דורגין דידיה וכ׳; Koh. R. to IX, 10 דרגין (corr. acc.) he saw his (R. Hiya's) suite in the future world, and his eyes became dim.

דּוּרְדָּא m. (Pers. *durd*, cmp., however, דרד) *sediment, lees, dregs.* Ab. Zar. 32[a].—*Pl.* דּוּרְדֵּי, דּוּרְדַּיָּא (used as sing.). Targ. Ps. LXXV, 9.—Meg. 12[b] like wine resting על דּוּרְדְּיֵהּ upon its lees (Jer. XLVIII, 11). Ab. Zar. 34[a]; a. e.

דּוּרְדְּנְיָא, v. דַּרְדְּנָיָא.

דּוּרְדֵּס, v. דַּרְדֵּס.

דּוּרְדָּיָא pr. n. m. *Durdaya.* Ab. Zar. 17[a] El. ben D. (Var. דרודיא).

דּוּרָה, v. דּוּרָא I, II.

דּוּרוֹן I pr. n. pl., כרם ד׳ *the vineyard of Doron.* Y. Kil. VII, 20[a] bot.

דּוּרוֹן II, ch. form דּוּרוֹנָא m. (δῶρον) *present, honorary gift.* Targ. Ps. CXLI, 2. Ib. XL, 7; a. e.—Zeb. 7[b] עולה ד׳ הוא the burnt offering is a votive gift (not a means of atonement). Pes. 118[b]; a. fr.—*Pl.* דּוּרוֹנִין. Targ. Y. Ex. XII, 46; a. e.—דּוּרוֹנוֹת. Gen. R. s. 79. (Yalk. ib. 133 דּוֹרְנִית); a. fr.—Chald. form. דּוּרוֹנְיָתָא. Targ. Ps. XX, 4 ed. Lag. (Ms. a. some ed. דוכר׳ incorr.). Cant. R. to VIII, 11 דורוניות, v. next w.

דּוֹרְיָא f. (δωρεά) same. *Pl.* הוֹרְיוֹת, הוֹרָאוֹת. Gen. R. s. 85, end, the one sent (to Babylon) dates, and the other (to Palestine) דורייות gifts of honor (purple cloak, ref. to Josh. VII, 21); Cant. R. to VIII, 11 דורוניות (corr. acc. or הוֹרוֹנוֹת).—Ex. R. s. 5 דוראות של עטרות gifts consisting of crowns.

דְּרוֹרִיָּה, דּוֹרִיָּיה, דּוֹרִיָּה f. (דרר, דור, v. דְּרוֹר) *freedom, remission of tribute* or *fine, pardon.* Gen. R. s. 53 (play on יִצְחָק) [read:] יצא חוק לעולם ליתן דו׳ לעולם a law was issued to give a grant (remission of sin) &c.; Yalk. ib. 92 יצא חוק דרור׳ וכ׳. Gen. R. l. c. [read:] מה עשייה . . . ליתן ד׳ לעולם אף עשייה . . . . ליתן ד׳ לעולם as the verb עשה used there (Esth. II, 18) means to grant a remission to the world, so does the verb עשה (Gen. XXI, 8) etc.; Pesik. Sos, p. 146[a] דורניא (corr. acc.); Yalk. Gen. 93 דרור׳.—Y'lamd. to Lev. XXI, 10, quot. in Ar. ד׳ שלימה full pardon.

דּוֹרְיוֹת, v. הוֹרְיָא.

דּוֹרִיָּיה, v. הוֹרִיָּה.

דּוֹרְכָא m. (דרך) *threshing.* Targ. Y. II Deut. XXV, 4 הוֹרְכֵיה (Y. I דָּרְכֵיה, h. text דיש).

דּוֹרְכָאוֹת f. pl. (v. preced.) *pomace.* Tosef. Maas. Sh. I, 10 ד׳ של תְּמרה ed. Zuck. (Var. דירכאות).

דּוֹרְכָאוֹת, דּוֹרְכִיאוֹת, דּוֹרְכִיּוֹת *reliefs,* v. דִּידְכֵי.

דּוּרְמוֹס m. (a disguise of Ἕρμης, or Mercurius, the divinity of commerce to whom a great annual fair, prob. of Tyre, was dedicated, v. Y. Ab. Zar. I, 39[d] top, quot. s. v. ארקליס) *Durmos,* name of *a great annual fair.* B. Mets. 72[b] (Ms. M. אסרטיון, v. Rabb. D. S. a. l. note).

דורמוסקית, v. הוּרְמַסְקִית.

דורמילוס, דורמלוס, דורמליס, v. דרומילוס.

דורמסיאות, דורמסיות, דורמייס׳, v. אנדרולומוסיא.

דורמסקין, v. הַרְמַסְקִינָא.

דּוּרְמַסְקִית pr. n. f. *Durmaskith* (*of Damascus*). Sifré Deut. 1 R. José ben D.; Ḥag. 3[b]; Tosef. Yad. II, 16 דורמוס׳; Tosef. Sot. III, 9; a. fr.—Mekh. Yithro, Baḥod. 1 Abba José b. D.—[Tanḥ. Noah 1 דוסקמא, דוסמקא (corr. acc.), Var. קצרתא, v. Tanḥ. ed. Bub. ib.] [*Pl.* הוּרְמַסְקִיּוֹת, v. הַרְמַסְקִינָא.]

דורמסקנא, דורמסקניות, דורמסקנין, v. הַרְמַסְקִינָא.

דורניא, Pesik. Sos p. 146[a], v. הוֹרִיָּה.

דורניאות, Esth. R. to I, 1, read הוֹרוֹנִיּוֹת, v. הִידְכֵי.

דורסות, Tosef. Maas. Sh. I, 10 Var., v. הִרוּסוֹת.

דורסים, Y. Kidd. I, 58[d], v. הְרוֹסָה.

דּוֹרְסָן m. (דרס) *place where hides are trodden or fulled* before tanning. Bets. I, 5 (11[a]) you must not place the hide לפני הד׳ in front of the *dor'san* (Mish. Nap. a. oth. בית הדריסה, Y. ed. לפני הדריסה).

דּוֹרְצִינֵי, v. הַרְצִינֵי.

דּוֹרְקְטֵי f. (a perversion of τρωκτή, sub. σταφυλή, v. infra) *grape used for dessert,* fit for eating but yielding no wine, fig. *a woman who has no menstruation.* Nidd. IX, 11. Ib. 64[b]; Keth. 10[b] (phonetic etymology) דור קטיע [hence the perversion] a cut-off race (bound to die out). Ib. משפחת ד׳ a family the women of which have neither menstruation nor symptoms of injured virginity. Y. ib. I, 25[a] bot. quoting Mish. Nidd. l. c. טְרוֹקְטֵי.

דורקין, דורקן, Tosef. Kel. B. Mets. III, 14 Var., v. הוּקְרָן.

דּוֹרֵשׁ m. *lecturer,* v. דָּרַשׁ.

דּוֹרְשִׁינֵי m. (comp. of הוּר a. שִׁינֵי, pl. of שִׁינָּא) [*row of teeth,*] *gum.* Sabb. 65[a] לד׳ (some ed. לדורשו׳, incorr.; Ms. M. דורשני, Var. a. Ar. in two words, v. Rabb. D. S. a. l. note) a remedy for the gum. Cmp. הַדְרָא I.

דּוֹרְתָא, v. הַרְתָא.

דּוּשׁ (b. h.), part. a. perf. דָּשׁ 1) *to tread, trample, thresh.* Sabb. VII, 2 הַדָּשׁ he who threshes (on the Sabbath); a. fr.—Euphem. for sexual contact. Nidd. 41[b]. Gen. R. s. 85. Pes. 87[b]; a. e.—דוש בעקב to trample with one's heel, *to treat lightly, not to heed.* Ab. Zar. 18[a]. Lev. R. s. 27.—2) *to walk about, be familiar, well-known.* Meg. 24[b] אם היה דש בעירו if he has been a familiar figure in his town (so that people do not mind his bodily disfigurement); Y. Taan. IV, beg. 67[b]; a. fr.

Pi. דַּיֵּישׁ *to trample.* Ex. R. s. 15 חייתם מְדַיְּישִׁין את העץ וכ׳ you used to tread upon this piece of wood. Midr. Till. to Ps. VIII, 3 מְדַיֵּישׁ עליך כעפר even one who treads upon thee as upon dust. Gen. R. s. 44 הַיְּישֵׁם tread upon them.

Polel הוֹשֵׁשׁ, v. דָּשַׁשׁ.

דּוּשׁ ch. same, 1) *to thresh.* Targ. Ruth II, 17.—Zeb. 116[b]; Men. 22[a], v. הַשְׁתָּאָה.—2) *to tread upon, trample* (to death). Targ. II Kings VII, 17; a. fr.—B. Kam. 9[a] דָּיֵישׁ אמצרי he sets his foot upon the landmark (symbol of possession).—3) *to be used to, not to mind.* Sabb. 129[b] כיון דדשו ביה רבים since the people are in the habit of doing it. Gitt. 56[b] כיון דדש דש being used (to the hammering) the gnat did not heed it. Keth. 62[a] דָּשְׁנָן בה we are used to it.—Targ. Prov. VIII, 33 תְּדִישׁוּן, v. Af.

Af. אַדִּישׁ, אָדֵישׁ *to pass over, to leave unheeded, to be listless.* Targ. Prov. IV, 15; XIII, 18; XV, 32 Ar. a. Mss. (ed. Lag. אר׳, מר׳ with ר, h. text פרע); ib. VIII, 33 (v. supra, ed. Lag. תירשון).—Snh. 7[a] (prov.) טוביה לדשמע ואדיש (Ms. M. ואריש) happy he who hears (himself abused) and minds it not; he will escape a hundred evils.—Y. Peah I, 15[c] bot.; Y. Kidd. I, 61[b] אכול ואַדִּישׁ . . . . ומַדְשִׁין eat and care not (do not share in our conversation), for so do dogs eat and mind not. [Targ. Y. II Num. XI, 8 אדשין, v. דְּקַשׁ.]

Ithpe. אִידַּשׁ, אִתְדַּשׁ *to be trampled upon, threshed.* Targ. Is. XXIV, 3. Ib. XXV, 10.—[Targ. Jer. XLVIII, 26, v. דְּשַׁשׁ.] *Polel* דּוֹשֵׁשׁ. *Palp.* דַּשְׁדֵּשׁ, v. דְּשַׁשׁ.

דּוּשָׁא, v. דּוּשָׁא.

דּוֹשֶׁן m. (דשן) *fat pasture ground.* Sifré Num. 81; Deut. 62 דּוֹשְׁנָהּ של יריחו (cmp. הַדֶּשֶׁן Jer. XXXI, 39).

דּוּת, דִּוּת, חֲדוּת f. (sub. בית) m. *a subterranean masoned store-room, cistern, cellar.* [Syr. חדותא *grex, horreum,* P. Sm. 1200.] [In Mishnah Seder Tohăroth חדות, v. R. S. to Ohol. XI, 8.] B. Bath. IV, 2 he who sells a house, has not sold with it לא את הבור ולא את הד׳ either the pit or the *duth.* Ib. 64ª אחד הבור ואחד הד׳ וכ׳ *bor* and *duth* are subterranean, בור בהפירה ד׳ בבנין a *bor* is made by digging, a *duth* by masonry. Tosef. Erub. XI (VIII), 18; Tosef. Pes. I, 3 הריצע והד׳; Y. ib. I, 27ᵇ top והחד׳. Ib. בח׳ שיש לה וכ׳ treating of a *ḥadduth* which has a lid. R. Hash. III, 7.—Y. Ab. Zar. II, 40ᶜ bot. עולה ... לחרות (corr. acc.) when going up with him to the upper story or down to the cellar &c. Kel. V, 6 ed. Derenb. הח׳. Ohol. XI, 8 הח׳; Tosef. ib. XII, 4 הד׳; a. fr.—*Pl.* הּוּתִיּוֹת. Tosef. B. Bath. III, 1 (Var. הּוּתוֹת, Mish. ib. IV, 2 sing.).—חֲדוּתִין. Y. ib. IV, 14ᶜ bot. חרותין ed. Krot. (corr. acc.). [Our w. seems to be originally חדות, fr. יחד. As to rejection of ח cmp. חֲלַבְּצִין.]

דְּוָתָא, דְּוִתָא, v. דְּוִיתָא.

דְּחָא, דְּחָא, v. דחי.

***דָּחַד**, *Pa.* דַּחֵד (=חדחד) *to set apart of each kind.* Targ. Y. I Deut. XV, 14 (O. פרש, h. text ענק Hif.) מְדַחֲדָא תְּדַחֲדוּן ליה (ed. Amst. מדחר׳ תדחר׳, corr. acc.).

דְּחָה, v. דחי.

דָּחַח, דַּחַח (cmp. זָהָה) *to be merry, wanton.*—Denom.:

***דַּחֲוָא** f. *jester, dancer.*—*Pl.* דַּחֲוָן. Dan. VI, 19 (cmp. דַּחֲוָיָא; oth. opin.=next w.).

***דַּחֲוָוֹנוֹת** f. pl. (v. preced.) *boards used at weddings as tables.* Tosef. Kel. B. Mets. V, 3 Kimḥi (ed. Zuck. רחויני ר, Var. רחזוינות).

דְּחוּתָא m., pl. דְּחוּתֵי (דחח, v. דָּהָה) *wantonness.* Targ. Ps. LXII, 9 ed. Lag., v. וְחוּתָא.

דְּחוּי, v. דחי.

דְּחוּי, v. דִּיחוּי.

דְּחוּכָא m. (דְּחֵיךְ) *feast, wedding entertainment.* Koh. R. to II, 2 [read:] דדחוּכֵיה מערבבא וכ׳ he whose feast is disturbed,—what has rejoicing to do with him?; Pesik. Aḥaré p. 169ᵇ הן דרחבה מעורבב (read הָןְ דִּדְחוּכֵיה); Lev. R. s. 20.

דְּחוּק m. (דחק) 1) *oppression.* Targ. Ex. VI, 6. Targ. Ps. XLIII, 2.—2) *need, stint.* Targ. II Chr. XVIII, 26; I Kings XXII, 27.

דְּחָה, דְּחָא, דְּחָא, דחי (b. h. דָּחָה) 1) *to push away, thrust.* Tosef. Yoma IV (III), 14 דְּחָאוֹ ולא מת; Y. ib. VI, 43ᶜ bot. דְּחָייוֹ if the man thrust the goat down the precipice, and it did not die. Snh. 107ᵇ, a. e. תהא שמאל דוחה וכ׳ let the left hand repel them and the right invite; a. fr.—Transf. ד׳ בקש, or בקנה *to dismiss with a vague or paltry reply.* Ḥull. 27ᵇ. Tanḥ. Ḥuck. 8; Num. R. s. 19; a. fr.—2) *to expel.* Tosef. Dem. III, 4; Bekh. 31ª; Y. Dem. II, 23ª top, v. חֲבֵירוּת.—3) *to suspend, make inoperative, supersede.* Ohol. VII, 6 אין דוחין נפש מפני וכ׳ we dare not set aside the regard due to one human life for the sake of saving another human life; Gen R. s. 94 כך עושין דוחים וכ׳ is it thus one must act? dare you sacrifice one life &c.?—Y. Snh. VIII, 26ᶜ top ד׳ את הספק to disregard the doubt the benefit of which is to be given to the criminal.—Y. Shek. IV, 47ᵈ bot. דְּחִינוּ אותו וכ׳ we postponed it (the fast) to the first day of the week; Meg. 5ᵇ דְּחִינוּהוּ; Erub. 41ª דְּחִינֻהוּ.—Pes. VI, 1 . . אלו דברים דוחין וכ׳ the following performances needed for the Passover offering take precedence of the Sabbath (cause a suspension of the Sabbath laws); a. v. fr.—*Part. pass.* דָּחוּי a) *pushed, hurried.* M. Kat. 28ª מיתה דחויה a hurried death.—b) *suspended, superseded.* Yoma 7ᵇ, a. fr. טומאה דְּחוּיָה היא וכ׳ the law about levitical purity is only suspended for the sake of an entire community (and its suspension requires atonement), opp. טומאה הותרה the law &c. is inoperative. Zeb. 12ª ד׳ מעיקרו unfit from the start, opp. נראה ונדחה, v. infra.—[Yeb. 80ᵇ; Gitt. 57ª דוחה, v. דִּיהָה.]

Nif. נִדְחָה *to be pushed aside, suspended; to give way.* Meg. 5ᵇ הואיל ונ׳ יִדָּחֶה the fast being once suspended (on account of the Sabbath), let it remain so (and not be taken up on Sunday). Pes. 66ᵇ איש נ׳ . . . ואין צבור נִידְחִין an individual (if unclean on Passover) is suspended (postpones the celebration) until the second Passover (Num. IX, 10 sq.), but not a community. Yoma 64ª בעלי חיים אינן נידחין animals (dedicated for sacrifices) cannot be removed forever from sacred use (as long as the obstacle lies not in their physical unfitness). Ib. נראה ונ׳ once fit and then discarded (on account of a temporary unfitness).—Ber. 64ª כל הנ׳ . . שעה נִדְחֵת מפניו to him who gives way to time (yielding patiently to circumstances), time will give way, v. דָּחַק.

Hif. הִדְחָה 1) *to remove hurriedly.* M. Kat. 22ª מַדְחֶה מיטתו he who is anxious to remove the bier of a relative (hurries the burial).—2) *to thrust.* Arakh. 30ᵇ אַדְחֶה אבן אחר וכ׳ Rashi (ed. אידחה, corrupt. of אֲדַדֶּה; Ar. דְּחֵה imperat. Kal) I will throw a stone after the fallen man (not give the sinner a chance to return). [Naz. 16ᵇ מדחיך בה Ar., read with ed. כדהוינן בה.] [Tosef. Toh. VIII, 8 המדחה, v. כָּחַס.]

דְּחָא, דְּחֵי ch. same, 1) *to thrust, push, knock down.* Targ. O. Num. XXXV, 20 דְּחָהִי he knocked him down (h. text הדף; Y. דַּחְיֵיה). Targ. Ps. CXVIII, 13; a. e.—2) *to suspend, supersede* &c., v. preced. 3). Zeb. 12ᵇ הוא ד׳ נפשיה בידים he debarred himself from offering (on account of his apostasy). Pes. 69ᵇ אימא לִידְחֵי I might think they take precedence of the Sabbath. Ber. 23ª גברא דְּחוּיָא הוא the person was for the time in an unfit condition to pray (and his prayer does not count at all).

Af. אַדְחֵי, *Pa.* דַּחֵי *to push aside, drive off.* Pes. 57ᵃ דַּחוּיֵי קא מַדְחֵי לן he sends us off (with a vain promise). *Ithpa.* אִידְּחֵי, *Ithpe.* אִידְחִי 1) *to be thrust down.* Targ. Ps. XXXVI, 13 אִידְּחִיַּין Ms. (ed. יִדַּחֲיַן); a. e.—2) *to be superseded, postponed* &c. (v. preced. Nif.). Targ. Y. Num. IX, 10.—Zeb. 12ᵇ ממילא אי׳ he was debarred from offering through no fault of his. Ib. גברא אי׳ the person was unfit; a. fr.

דְּחִיָּה, דְּחִיָּיה f. (preced.) 1) *thrusting, knocking down.* Snh. 45ᵃ (ref. to דוחפו, Mish. ib. VI, 4) מנין שבד׳ whence do we derive the law that he must be knocked down?; Y. ib. VI, 23ᶜ top מניין שטעון ד׳.—*Pl.* דְּחִיּוֹת, דְּחִיּוֹת. Ib.—2) *postponement, suspension.* Y. Sabb. XIX, beg. 16ᵈ עיקר דְּחִיָּיתָן וכ׳ what they chiefly supersede is the Sabbath and that which is required for their execution is labor (otherwise forbidden).—[דְּחִיּוֹת in later Hebr. literature: *the reasons for shifting the first day of Tishri* in the Jewish calendar.]

דַּחֲיָיא m. (v. דַּחֲוָא) *feaster, reveller.*—*Pl.* דַּחֲיִין. Lev. R. s. 33, v. דִּיאוֹנִיסִין.—Fem. דַּחֲיְיתָא. Lam. R. introd. (R. Johan. I) קרתא ד׳ (translation of קריה עליזה Is. XXII, 2; Targ. חדאה).

דְּחַךְ, דְּחֵךְ, דְּחִיךְ (cmp. דחה) *to laugh; to deride.* Targ. Job XI, 3; Targ. Ps. II, 4, v. דְּחִיךְ. Targ. Ps. XXII, 8 (ed. Lag. רחב). Targ. Prov. I, 26 (Var. דחק, incorr.).—Pesik. B'shall. p. 93ᵇ דַּחֲכָא וכ׳ laughing and weeping (Koh. R. to XI, 2 חריכת).

Pa. דַּחֵךְ *to make sport of, to play.* Gen. R. s. 79 לית אנא מְדַחֵךְ בהדין וכ׳ (Koh. R. to X, 8 מגהך) will I not make sport of that elder of the Jews?! Koh. R. to III, 2 children מְדַחֲכִין וכ׳ (ed. Wil. מדה׳) playing in front of a dwelling.

דְּחַל, דְּחֵיל (cmp. זחל a. Arab. *dahala*) [*to be depressed, bent,*] *to fear, be afraid of, shun; to worship, revere.* Targ. Gen. XVIII, 15. Targ. Ps. XXXIII, 8; a. fr.—*Part.* דָּחֵיל, דָּחֵיל; constr. דְּחֵיל. Targ. Ex. IX, 20. Targ. Gen. XIX, 30; a. fr.—Sabb. 23ᵇ דד׳ מרבנן he who reveres the scholars. Y. Naz. IX, end 58ᵃ (play on מורה a. מורא, v. Mishn. ib. IX, 5) מה ביזרא ד׳ וכ׳ as the grain is afraid of the iron (scythe), so is the hair &c.; a. fr.—Sabb. 31ᵇ, a. fr. דְּחֵיל חטאין shunning sin.

Pa. דַּחֵל *to frighten, to cause fear.* Targ. II Sam. XIV, 15 דַּחֲלוּנִי ed. Lag. (ed. דחלונני).

Af. אַדְחֵיל *to frighten, scare.* Cant. R. to III, 6 מן הדא את מדחיל לי with this (fire) wilt thou frighten me?—Koh. R. to VII, 1 (prov.) whom a snake once has bitten, חבלא מדחיל ליה a rope will frighten.

Ithpe. אִידְּחִיל *to be afraid.* Lev. R. s. 9 אִידְּחִילַת מיניה she was afraid of him.

דְּחִילָא, דְּחִיל m. (preced.) 1) *fearing,* v. preced.—2) *fearful, terrible, awe-inspiring.* Targ. Y. Gen. XXVIII, 17. Targ. Ps. LXXVI, 5 דְּחִיל Ms. (ed. נהיר דחיל, combin. of two versions). Targ. Deut. X, 17. Ib. VIII, 15; a. fr.—Lev. R. s. 9 מה ד׳ הדין שליטא how severe is this ruler!—*Pl.* דְּחִילִין, f. דְּחִילָן. Targ. Hab. I, 7. Targ. Ps. XLV, 5 (noun).

דְּחִילָא m. (preced.) *fear, reverence.* Targ. Jon. I, 16 (ed. Lag. דַּחֲלָא).

דְּחִילוּ f. same, *fear, worship.* Targ. O. Gen. XXVIII, 17 מא ד׳ אתרא וכ׳ Oh, the fearfulness of this place!—**Pl.* דְּחִילָוָון *manifestations of worship.* Targ. Is. LXVI, 20 ed. Ven. I a. Levita (ed. Lag. רחילוון, oth. ed. רחילין; h. text צַבִּים (!); cmp. חושבהן for כרכרות ibid.).

דחינוניתא, v. דַּהֲנוּנִיתָא.

דְּחִיס, v. דָּחַס.

דְּחִיף, v. דְּחַף.

דְּחִיפָה f. (דחף) *pushing, knocking down.* Y. Sabb. VII, 9ᵈ bot. נגיחה וד׳ אב goring and knocking down are chief actionable damages, v. אָב (Y. B. Kam. I, beg. 2ᵃ נגיפה).

דְּחִיק, דְּחֵיק, v. דְּחַק.

דָּחִיק m., **דְּחִיקָא** c. (דחק) 1) *narrow, pressed.* Targ. Y. Num. XXII, 26. Targ. I Kings VIII, 64 (not ר׳); a. e.—Taan. 21ᵃ ד׳ להו מילתא טובא they were hard pressed (in great distress); B. Mets. 114ᵇ.—*Pl.* דְּחִיקִין, f. דְּחִיקָן. Targ. Ez. XLII, 5 sq.—2) *forced.* B. Kam. 43ᵃ, a. e. שינויא ד׳ a forced answer (argument).

דְּחַל, v. דְּחֵיל.

דַּחֲלָא I m. (preced.) *fearer, worshipper.*—דד׳ ד׳ *God-fearing.* Targ. Gen. XXII, 12; a. e.—*Pl.* דַּחֲלַיָּא. Targ. Ps. CXXXV, 20; a. e.—Targ. Is. LV, 13 דחלי חטאה shunning evil.—Fem. דַּחֲלְתָא. Targ. Prov. XXXI, 30 דד׳ ד׳ Ms. (ed. דחלתיה דאלהא). Targ. II Kings IV, 8.

דַּחֲלָא II, דַּחֲלְתָא f. (preced.) *fear.* Targ. Ps. II, 11. Targ. Prov. I, 7; a. fr.—Y. B. Mets. II, 8ᶜ bot. בגין דַּחֲלְתֵיךְ from fear of thee; a. e.—Trnsf. (cmp. יִרְאָה) m. *deity.* Targ. Is. II, 22. Targ. Y. II Deut. XXXII, 15. Targ. Y. I ib. 18 דַּחֲלַת (Ms. דחלא); a. fr. *Pl.* דַּחֲלָן. Ib. 17; a. fr.—דַּחֲלָתָא. Targ. Ps. LV, 5.

דחלא, Pesik. Zakhor, p. 26ᵇ, read: זַחֲלָא.

דַּחֲלוּלָא m., pl. **דַּחֲלוּלֵי** *scarecrows.* B. Bath. 27ᵇ ובד׳ בעלמא סגי ליה Ms. (v. Rabb. D. S. a. l.) and the putting up of scarecrows (to keep the birds off) would be sufficient (Rashi: cutting *gaps* between the branches).

דַּחֲלוּנָא m. (v. דַּחֲלָא) *God-fearing, conscientious.*—*Pl.* דַּחֲלוּנַיָּא. Y. Maas. Sh. V, 56ᵇ bot., v. חָבֵר.

דַּחֲלְתָא, דַּחַלְתָּא, v. דַּחֲלָא.

דחם, v. next w.

דָּחַס (דָּחַשׁ) (cmp. דחי) *to press, crowd.*—*Part. pass.* דָּחוּס, f. דְּחוּסָה *crowded, thick, full.* Lev. R. s. 30 ד׳ בעלין Ar. (ed. רחוש) thick with leaves; ד׳ בבנים richly blessed with children; Pesik. Ul'kah. p. 184ᵃ דָּחוּשׁ Ms. O. (ed. ר׳, v. Ar. Compl. ed. Koh. s. v. חש 3, a. Koh. Ar. Compl. s. v. דחס).

Pi. דִּחֵס same. Tosef. Toh. VIII, 8 המְדַחֵס כליו וכ׳ (ed. Zuck. המדחם, ed. המדחה; R. S. to Toh. VII, 7 חרש, corr. acc.) if one stuffs his bathing apparel into the bather's window closet (opp. to המניח).

דְּחַס (v. preced.) *to press, stamp.* Targ. Lam. II, 2 ed. Lag.—Yeb. 103ª צריך למְדַחְסֵיה לכרעיה must press his foot (rest it firmly on the ground). Y. B. Mets. IX, beg. 12 הוו דחשין (read: דַּחִישִׁין or דְּחִיסִין) they were crowded, opp. דְּלִיל.

Pa. דַּחֵיס same. Ib. [Targ. Y. Deut. XXV, 9 ויחדס ed. pr., oth. ויחכס, prob. וִידַחֵס.]

דְּחָסָה f. (דָּחַס) *squeezing, pressure* (on the abdomen). Yeb. 42ª bot.

דָּחַף (b. h.; cmp. דחי) *to push, thrust, knock down* (interchanging with דָּחָה). Yoma VI, 6 דְּחָפוֹ וכ׳ knocked him down backward. Ib. 66ᵇ דחפו (Tosef. ib. IV (III), 14 דחאו), v. דחי. Snh. VI, 4; a. e.—Part. pass. דָּחוּף, f. דְּחוּפָה *impelled, hastened.* M. Kat. 28ª מיתה ד׳ (stronger than דְּחוּיָה, v. דחי; Var. סחופה, v. Rabb. D. S. a. l. note).

דְּחַף ch. same. Targ. Y. Lev. XXIV, 23 (v. Snh. 45ª quot. s. v. דְּחִיָּה). Targ. Y. Deut. VI, 19 (some ed. דחי; h. text הדף). Targ. Job XVIII, 18 Ms. Var. (ed. הדף).—*Part. pass.* דְּחִיף, pl. דְּחִיפִין *hastened, hurried.* Targ. II Esth. III, 15; VIII, 14 (Targ. I Esth. סחיפין, cmp. preced.). [Targ. Prov. I, 26, v. דְּחִיק.]

Ithpe. אִידְּחַף, אִתְדְּחַף *to be pressed against, to hold firm.* Targ. Y. I Deut. XIX, 5 Levita תתד׳ (ed. תִּדְּחַף, Pe., Var. תִּדְ׳; Y. II תִּתְקַף, h. text נדחה).

דָּחַק (b. h.; cmp. preced.) *to press, squeeze, crowd, stamp.* Pes. 95ᵇ, a. e. דָּחֲקוּ זבין וכ׳ if persons afflicted with .... forced their way &c.—Men. 98ᵇ top הוּחֲקִין ובולטין וכ׳ pressed against and protruded &c. Ab. II, 15 בעה״ב דוחק the employer (the Lord) presses (urges to work). Ber. 64ª ד׳ את השעה to force time, be importunate, v. דָּחָה. Lev. R. s. 28; Pesik. Haom. p. 70ᵇ; Pesik. R. s. 18; Yalk. Job 998 (ref. to וּשְׁאָף, Job V, 5) מי ד׳ (ל)(ב)ממונו וכ׳ who trampled upon the wealth of &c.?—Sifra Vayikra Par. 1, ch. II ד׳ להיות מדבר וכ׳ (Yalk. Lev. 430 נדחק) He pressed himself (confined His Presence) between the Cherubim &c.—*Part. pass.* דָּחוּק *pressed, scarce.* Ab. Zar. 35ᵇ.

Nif. נִדְחַק *to be pressed, confined,* v. supra.

דְּחַק I, דְּחֵיק ch. same, 1) *to push, squeeze* &c. Targ. Jud. I, 34; a. fr.—2) *to impel, hurry, press.* Targ. Josh. X, 13 (h. text אוץ). Targ. Y. Deut. XV, 3; a. fr.—M. Kat. 28ª דָּחֲקָא רגליה וכ׳ the foot of Bar Nathan is pressing (his predestined term of office has begun).

Pa. דַּחֵק *to press* (a debtor). Targ. Y. Deut. XV, 2 לְמִדְחֲקָא (ed. Vien. למדח׳).

Ithpe. אִדְּחֵק, אִידּ׳ 1) *to be pressed, squeeze one's self.* Targ. O. Num. XXII, 25 (Y. אִדְּחָקַת, read אִדּ׳).—2) *to be distressed.* Targ. I Sam. XIII, 6; XIV, 24.

דְּחָק m. (preced.) 1) *emergency.* Nidd. 9ᵇ, a. fr. בשעת הד׳ in a case of emergency.—2) *pressure, need,* v. דּוֹחַק.

דְּחַק II, דַּחֲקָא ch. same, *oppression, distress.* Targ. Y. Deut. XXVI, 7 דְּחָקָן (O. דּוּחְקָנָא).

דַּחֲקָא m. (preced.) *oppressor. Pl.* דַּחֲקַיָּא. Targ. Jud. II, 18.

דַּחֲקוּתָא f.=דַּחֲקָא. Targ. Y. Gen. XXX, 8.

דחש, v. דחס h. a. ch.

***דמסים**, Y. Bets. III, beg. 62ª top; Y. Sabb. III, 14ª bot., read: רֵיטֵיס (retis) כהח״א ר׳ a stoppage in the river as one made with a net (v. Sm. Ant. s. v. Retis).

דִּי (h. זֶה, cmp. דֵּין; corresp. to h. שֶׁ־, שֶׁל, אֲשֶׁר) 1) *who, which, where, whom* &c. Dan. IV, 5; a. fr.—Targ. Gen. XXIV, 27. Targ. Ps. LXXIII, 27; a. fr.—Mostly as prefix: דְּ־, דִּ־, דַּ־, v. ד־.—With personal pronouns דִּידִי, דִּילִי; דִּידָךְ, דִּילָךְ; דִּידִיךְ, דִּילִיךְ; דִּידֵיהּ, דִּילֵיהּ; דִּידָהּ, דִּילָהּ; דִּידַהוֹן, דִּידְהוֹן; דִּידְכוֹן, דִּלְכוֹן; דִּידְכֵן, דִּידְכוֹן; דִּלָן *mine, thine* &c. Targ. O. Gen. XXXI, 16 דילנא (Y. די לנא). Targ. O. ib. XXXIII, 9; a. fr.—B. Bath. 4ᵇ דידי ודידיה הוא it is mine and his. Ib. עבד דידיה he made the *ḥazith* on his side, v. חָזִית. Ber. 2ᵇ בין השמשות דידך thy definition of *ben hash-sh'mashoth.* Tam. 32ª דידי טבא מדידכו my advice is better than yours. Gitt. 84ᵇ דילכון your countryman (Rab Kahăna). B. Kam. 117ᵇ דילכון אמרי דילהון היא I believed (learning) was yours (the Palestineans'); but it is theirs (the Babylonians'); Succ. 44ª דִּלְכוֹן, דִּלְהוֹן.—Ḥull. 42ᵇ תנא דידן the author or compiler of our Mishnah. Deut. R. s. 2 ר״י דידיה אמר R. J. said in his own name. Ab. Zar. 17ª פלוגא דידיה אדידיה there is a discrepancy between two opinions of his. Y. Ḥag. II, 78ª top מן דידכן; Y. Snh. VI, 23ᶜ bot. מן דידכון one of yours.—2) *that (quod).* Dan. IV, 3; a. fr.—Y. Taan. IV, 67ᶜ bot. די תעניתא that it is a fast-day.

דִּי II=דְּאִי, *for if.* Y. R. Hash. I, 56ᵇ די לא כן. Also דִּלָא, דִּילָא *for if not.* Y. Ter. V, 43ᶜ; a. fr.—דִּילָכֵן, דִּלָכֵן *for if not so.* Y. Shebi. IV, 35ª bot.; a. fr. V. דל.

דַּי m. (b h.; דָּיָה, cmp. דַּאי) *sufficiency, plenty;* constr. דֵּי *enough for;* דַּיִּי *enough for me,* דַּיֶּיךָ *enough for thee* &c. Nidd. I, 1 דַּיָּין שעתן they have enough for the time being, i. e. the unclean condition, now discovered, has no retrospective effect, opp. מִפְּקִידָה לפקידה. Pes. 8ᵇ דַּיֵּינוּ we should have been contented. Taan. 24ᵇ דַּיּוֹ בקב וכ׳ (Ms. M. דַּיי לו קב) he is contented with a Kab of &c. B. Kam. II, 5 (25ª) דיו לבא מן הדין וכ׳ it is sufficient for the law which is derived by conclusion *ad majus* to be as strict as the law from which it is derived, i. e. you cannot go beyond the latter. Ib. ור״ט לית ליה דיו does R. T. not follow the principle of *dayyo* (that the derived law cannot go beyond the original)? והא דיו דאורייתא הוא is not the principle of *dayyo* biblical?—Gen. R. s. 21 דייך פפוס it is enough for thee, Papus, i. e. say no more; a. fr.—With prefix כְּדַי (v. כְּדֵיי), constr. כְּדֵי *as much as is required for, corresponding to,* as conj. *in order to.* Maasr. V, 6 ומצא כ׳ מדתו and found a quantity corresponding to what he had measured into it (reasonably increased); יותר על כ׳ מדתו more than the reasonable quantity.—כ׳ דיבור or תוך כ׳ ד׳ as much, within as much, time as is needed for an utterance (e. g. a greeting, v. Y. Ber. I, 4ᵇ). B.

Kam. 73ª, a. fr. תוך כ׳ דיבור כדיבור דמי two statements following each other immediately are considered one. Ib.ᵇ תרי ת׳ כ׳ ד׳ there are two different intervals comprised under the expression *tokh k'd'e dibbur*. Snh. 31ᵇ bot. כ׳ לחלוק וכ׳ in order to give honor to &c. Ib. 32ª bot. כ׳ שלא תנעול דלת וכ׳ in order not to make loans too difficult, v. דֶּלֶת; a. fr.

דִּי־ (representing δις-, δύο) *two, twice,* cmp. דּוּ III.

***דִּיאו** m. (דאב=דאו formed like עִוֵּר, v. דְּוִי) *longing, faint, love-sick.* Cant. R. to II, 9, v. דְּוִי.

***דִּיאו**, Y. Ab. Zar. I, 39ᶜ top, קָלוֹן ד׳, read דִּיאָן (calo diem) *I proclaim (welcome) the day,* an etymology of *calenda* (v. Sm. Ant. s. v. Calendar). V. קָלֶנְדָּס.

***דִּיאוֹנִיסִין** m. pl. (διονύσια, τά) *the Dionysian feast, bacchantic revels.* Lev. R. s. 33 (ref. to Ezek. XXIII, 42) מובאים קאניסין וכ׳ (corr. acc.) *'carried along'* (in procession) refers to the Dionysia, 'drunken', means the revellers, v. דִּהְיָרָא.

דִּיאֶטְמָא, v. דִּייטְמָא.

(דְּיוֹטְ׳) דִּיטַגְמָא, דִּיאֲטַגְמָא f. (διάταγμα) *edict, ordinance.* Targ. II Esth. III, 15; a. e.—Sifré Deut. s. 33 כדיוט׳ ישנה like an antiquated ordinance. Lev. R. s. 1; a. fr.—*Pl.* דִּיאֲטַגְמָאוֹת, דִּיטַ׳, דְּיוֹטְ׳. Ex. R. s. 30; a. e.—דִּיאֲטַגְמָטִין. Y. Shebu. VII, 38ª bot. דיאטיגמתין; Y. Keth. IX, 33ᵇ bot. דין מוגמרין (corr. acc.).

דִּיאֶטְמָה, pl. **דִּיאֶטְמוֹת**, v. דִּייטְמָא.

דיאטיגמתין, v. דִּיאֲטַגְמָא.

(דְּיוֹ׳) דְּיַי׳, דִּיאַטְרִיטִין, דִּיאַטְרִיטָא m. pl. (diatreta, v. Sm. Ant. s. v. Vitrum) *cut or engraved glass vessels.* Ex. R. s. 27, end [read:] ב׳ כוסות הללו ד׳ these two cups of cut glass. Esth. R. to I, 7 כוסות דיוטירי׳ (corr. acc.). Gen. R. s. 19 דיוטרי׳ (corr. acc.). Ruth R. to I, 1 כוסות דיוטריטון (corr. acc.); a. fr.

***דִּיאוֹקִיטֵיס, דִּיאוֹקִיטָא** m. (διοικήτης, dioecetes) *overseer of the treasury, treasurer.* Lev. R. s. 5 (prov.) unfortunate the district where the physician has the gout, ודאיקוטטא בחד עינא ed. (Mus. ודייקטסא, corr. acc.) and the treasurer only one eye (is unable to examine the coins).

דִּיאָלָא, v. דִּיילָא.

דיאלקמו, v. אֲלַקְמוּ.

דיאנה, דיאנא, Men. 77ª ed., v. זִיָּנָא II.

***דיאתימון**, read דִּיאֲתֵימִין (διεθέμην, sec. aor. med. of διατίθημι) *I disposed by will.* Y. B. Bath. VIII, 16ᶜ top אף הכותב ד׳ בלעז וכ׳ even if one writes in Greek διεθέμην (*I willed*, instead of *I will*), it is to be considered as if it were a gift (cmp. ib. יחזק עשיתי &c.); ib. חיזרתי וכ׳ I went around to all linguists to find out what ד׳ was &c.; Tosef. ib. IX, 14 דיותימין (ed. Zuck. דייתיקי, corr. acc.).

(דְּיוֹ׳) דְּיָיתִיקִי, דִּיאַתִיקִי f. (διαθήκη) *a disposition of property,* esp. *by will and testament; covenant, contract,* v. Y. Peah III, 17ᵈ bot. for difference between ד׳ a. מתנה.—Targ. Y. Gen. XXIV, 10 ד׳ דריבונא Ar. (ed. שפר אפותיקי); Gen. R. s. 59, end (ref. to Gen. l. c.) זו ד׳ this means (his master's) will (in favor of Isaac).—Y. Ber. V, 9ᵇ top בד׳ נתתיו לו וכ׳ have I given it to him as a bequest (which may be cancelled)? I have given it to him as a donation. Y. B. Bath. VIII, 16ᵇ bot. ויחזור בִּדְיָיתִיקָתוֹ he may change his will. Ib.; Bab. ib. 152ᵇ ד׳ מבטלת ד׳ the later will cancels the prior. Y. B. Mets. I, end, 8ª אין . . . לפנים דייתיקין וכ׳ nobody is likely to make a defective will (by anticipating in it the receipt of a debt before it has been collected).—*Pl.* דְּיָיתִיקָאוֹת. B. Mets. 19ª. Tosef. B. Bath. XI, 6; a. e.

דִּיב, v. דִּוּב.

דִּיבָא m. (=h. זְאֵב), *wolf.* Targ. Y. I Gen. XLIX, 27 (II דּוֹב). Targ. Is. XI, 6 (Regia דּוּבָא); LXV, 25.—*Pl.* דִּיבִין. Targ. Zeph. III, 3.—[Targ. Is. XI, 7 דיבא *bear,* v. דּוּבָא.]

דִּיבָא m. 1) *flux, gonorrhoea,* v. דּוּבָא.—2) סני דיבא or סניא דיבי *a certain part of the maw,* v. סַנֵּי.

דִּיבָא f. ch.=h. דִּבָּה. Targ. O. Gen. XXXVII, 2 דִּיבְּהוֹן, דִּבְּהוֹן, ed. Berl. טִיבְהוֹן.

דִּיבָבָא m. (cmp. זְבוּב) *fly.* Targ. Koh. X, 1 (h. text זבובי מות, ed. Buxt. דבובא).—*Pl.* דִּיבָבֵי, דִּיבָבַיָּא. Targ. Is. VII, 18 (ed. Lag. דבב׳, ed. Buxt. דְּבוּבַיָּא). Targ. Y. Lev. XI, 20 דִּיבָבֵי (read דִּי׳); Targ. Y. Deut. XIV, 19. V. דִּידְבָא.

דִּיבָה, v. דִּבָּה.

דיבוון, דיבון, Targ. Y. II Num. XXXII, 24 some ed., v. דִּבְוָן.

דיבונא, Targ. Prov. XXIV, 2, v. דִּיפּוּנָא.

דִּבּוּק, דִּיבּוּק m. (דבק) 1) *attachment, junction, intimacy.* Cant. R. to II, 6 (ref. to Deut. XI, 22) איזהו ד׳ what is the form of intimacy? [Ab. ch. VI (Boraitha) ד׳ חברים (some ed. דקדוק) the friendship of students (the care in selection of friends).—2) *glue, paste, solder.* Y. Sabb. III, 6ª bot. שמא נתאכל דִּיבּוּקוֹ (read: שלא יתא׳ וכ׳) lest its solder may be consumed (if the vessel be left without water). [Hull. 52ª, read דִּבּוּק if the bird is caught by means of glue, v. דֶּבֶק.]

דִּבּוּק, דִּיבּוּק ch. same, *joining.* Targ. I Kings VII, 30 עובד ד׳ joiner's work.

דִּבּוּר, דִּיבּוּר m. (דבר) *utterance, speech, dictate.* Cant. R. to III, 4 ד׳ קשה of the various expressions for prophecy *dibbur* is the severest; Gen. R. s. 44; Macc. 11ª; (Sifre Num. 99 דִּבֵּר). Lev. R. s. 1 (play on ויקר, Num. XXIII, 4, a. ויקרא Lev. I, 1) the Lord reveals Himself to the gentile prophets בחצי ד׳ only with half a word (defective revelation), opp. ד׳ שלם. Ex. R. s. 28 ד׳ זכור וכ׳ the commandment, 'Remember the Sabbath'. Y. Ned. III, 37[d] bot.; a. fr.—תוך כדי ד׳, v. הַדִּ׳.—Esp. הַדִּ׳ *revelation, Divine Speech*, (hypostasized) *the Word, the Dibbur.* Lev. R. s. 1, beg. קול הד׳ עצמו the direct voice of the Dibbur. Yeb. 5[b], a. fr. לפני הד׳ prior to the revelation. Cant. R. to I, 2; a. fr.— על פי הד׳ following the Divine order. Y. Sabb. VII, 10[c]; a. fr.—*Pl.* דִּיבּוּרִים, דִּיבּוּרִין, דִּבּ׳. Gen. R. s. 38 ד׳ אחדים mysterious words (accounts), v. אֶחָד. Cant. R. l. c.; a. fr. V. דָּבָר.—2) (homilet., v. Ps. XLVII, 4) *being led, submission.* Sabb. 63[a] אין ד׳ אלא נחת the root דבר (in Mal. III, 16 נדברו) means submission; Macc. 11[a] (corr. acc.).

דִּבּוּרָא, דִּבּ׳, דִּבְּרָא, דִּיבּוּרָא ch. same, esp. *revelation.* Targ. Ez. I, 24; 25 ed. Lag. דבר׳ (oth. דבו׳, some ed. די בירא, read דִּיבְּרָא). Targ. Y. Num. VII, 89; a. fr.—R. Hash. 6[a] אימא ד׳ לא כלום הוא I might have thought a mere word (without action) was of no effect. Ib. לא קיימיה לדיבוריה he did not substantiate his word (by an action). Ned. 41[a] ד׳ קשר וכ׳ talking is injurious to the eyes; a. fr.—*Pl.* דִּבּ׳, דִּיבְּרַיָּא, דִּבְּרַיָּא, דִּיבּוּרַיָּא, esp. *the Ten Commandments.* Targ. Y. Ex. XX, 1 (II דִּיבְּרַיָּא); a. fr.—Y. Meg. IV, 75[b] bot. קטע בדיבר׳ וכ׳ cut the Ten Commandments apart, so that our children may be able to study them.

דִּיבְחָא, v. דִּבְחָא.

דִּיבִי, v. דִּיבָא.

דִּיבֵירָא, *of Bera, Bire,* v. בִּירָא.

דִּיבֵּירָא, v. דִּיבּוּרָא.

דִּיבְלָא, v. דְּבֵילְתָּא.—[דיבלא Yoma 78[b], v. בְּלָא.]

דִּיבְקָא, דּוּבְקָא m. (דבק) *joining, combination.* Meïl. 16[b] האי ד׳ דידך היא Ar. (ed. דּוּבְקָא) this is merely thy own combination (that Rab's opinion was delivered in connection with the Mishnah), but Rab himself recited merely a tradition (without reference to that special clause of the Mishnah).

דִּבֵּר, דִּיבֵּר (b. h.) m.=דִּיבּוּר, esp. *revelation.* Sifra Thazr., Neg., ch. I. Mekh. Bo, beg. (Tanh. ib. 5 דבור); a. fr.—*Pl.* דִּיבְּרוֹת (fem.). Mekh. l. c., v. כְּלוֹל. Y. Ber. IV, 8[c] top; a. fr.—Esp. *the Ten Commandments.* B. Kam. 54[b] ד׳ הראשונות the text of the Decalogue in Exodus, ד׳ האחרונות the one in Deuteronomy. Snh. 67[a], מִדִּבְּרוֹתֶיךָ, v. כָּלָה.

דִּיבְרָא, דִּבְרָא, v. דִּיבּוּרָא.

דִּיבְשָׁא, v. דּוּבְשָׁא.

דִּיגְאלָא, v. דַּגָּלָא.

דִּיגּוּל m. (דָּגַל I) *stratagem, deception.* Cant. R. to II, 4 דִּיגּוּלוֹ his (Jacob's) stratagem (Gen. XXVII, 16).—*Pl.* דִּגּוּ׳, דִּיגּוּלִין. Ib.; v. דָּגַל.

דִּיגּוּן m. (v. דגן) *storing of grain, piling up.* Gitt. 47[a] דִּיגּוּנְךָ ולא ד׳ נכרי (the word דגנך, Deut. XIV, 23 means) what thou (the Israelite) storest up (is subject to tithes), but not what the gentile stores up, opp. to דְּגָנְךָ וכ׳ the grain growing on thy ground (Palestine). B. Mets. 88[b] ד׳ בני Ms. F. (ed. גורן, v. Rabb. D. S. a. l. note 100) adapted for storage.

דִּיגוֹן m. 1) (δίγονος) prop. *born a second time,* in gen. *for a second term, twice* (Lat. *bis*). B. Bath. 164[b] such is the custom of that nation ארכן שניה קורין לו ד׳ (Ms. M. דוגין) an archont in his second term is called *digonos* (bis, iterum consul). Ib.; Naz. 8[b] if one says, I vow to be a Nazir .... די׳ שתים *digon,* he has to be a Nazir twice in succession; Tosef. ib. I, 2 טריגון ed. Zuck. (Var. דריגון, corr. acc.).—2) (by analogy with τριγώνιον, τετραγώνιον) *having two corners.* Tosef. Neg. VI, 3 (בית) דיגון וכ׳ ed. Zuck. (corr. acc.) a house which has only two corners (semicircularly built); B. Bath. l. c.; Naz. l. c.

דיגמסיס, v. דִּיגְנוֹסִיס.

דִּיגְלָא, v. דִּגְלָא.

דִּיגְלַת, דִּיג׳ pr. n. (h. חִדֶּקֶל) *the river Tigris.* Targ. Gen. II, 14.—M. Kat. 25[b] bot. נשוק כיפי ד״ וכ׳ the shores of the Tigris touched each other (the water forming a level with the banks). Kidd. 71[b]. Yeb. 121[a]. Ber. 59[b]. Taan. 24[b] שפוך מרזבי דמחוזא לד׳ (not דציפורי, v. Rabb. D. S. a. l. note) the gutters of Maḥuza emptied themselves into the Tigris.

דִּיגְמָא, v. דּוּגְמָא.

דִּיגְנוֹסִיס f. (διάγνωσις) *decree.* Targ. II Esth. II, 8 ed. Lag. (ed. דיגט׳, corr. acc.).

דִּידִי, v. דִּי.

דִּידְבָא, דּוּדְבָא (דִּדְבָא) m. (=דבדבא, v. דִּיבְבָא) *fly.* Hull. 58[b] לית די׳ בת שתא (Ar. דד׳) no fly lives a whole year. Ber. 44[a] עד דהוה שריק ליה דו׳ וכ׳ (Ms. M. דשריא .. דור׳; v. Rabb. D. S. a. l. note) so that a fly would glide down his (fat and smooth) face.—Gitt. 86[b] דִּידְבְתָא דבינֵי כיפי a large fly found among sheaves.

***דִּידְיוֹנִי** f. (reduplic. of דוי or דוע; cmp. אוּדְיָיתָא) *the vapor room.* Nidd. 67[a] אימר בד׳ נפל Ar. s. v. ארדוותא (ed. רדיוני) I say, it (the mud) fell off in the vapor room (where she entered after the bath).

דִּידְכֵי f., pl. **דִּידְכָאוֹת** (διαδοχή, v. דייתיכוס) *relays, guards at stations.* [Popular adaptation דרכ׳, as if fr. דֶּרֶךְ.] Yoma VI, 8 (68[b]) דיד׳ Y. ed. (Mish. דִּרְכָאוֹת; Bab. ed. דִּיהְכָ׳, Ms. M. דִּיהֲבָ׳, Ms. L. דיד׳, דוד׳; Mish. Nap. דִּירְכָּוֹת, v. Rabb. D. S. a. l. note). Mekh. B'shall. s. 1 דורכיות היו לו Pharaoh had guards at stations (communicating with one another).—Gen. R. s. 10; Yalk. ib. 16 [read:] הרבה להן בריצה והרבה להן בְדִידוֹכִין he increased for them the speed (of the mail bearers), and the number of mail stations. Esth. R. to I, 1 דורכ׳ עם דורנאות וכ׳ postmen carrying gifts will be numerous &c.

דַּיָּה f. (b. h.; v. דָּאָה) *Dayyah* name of several unclean birds. Hull. 63[a] *ḥăsidah* (Lev. XI, 19) זו ד׳ לבנה is the white *dayyah* (stork), *anaphah* (ib.) זו ד׳ רגזנית the irascible *dayyah*; v. הַיְיתָא.

דִּיהַּ (cmp. דוי) *to be faint.—Af.* אַדִּיהַּ *to make fainter, paler.* Nidd. 20ª אַדִּיהוּ לֵיה וכ׳ they showed him a fainter color, and he declared it clean.

דִּיהֶה, דִּיהָא m. (preced.; cmp. form and meaning of כֵּהֶה) *faint, feeble, dim; light* in substance, *thin.* Neg. I, 2 של סיד דֵּיהָה הימנה the red within the lime-colored leprosy is fainter than the latter, opp. עז; Tosef. ib. I, 3 דוֹהָא. Tosef. Nidd. III, 11 ד׳ מכאן if fainter than this (shoe-black), opp. עמוק; Nidd. II, 7; 20ª ד׳ מכן. Ib. ד׳ דד׳ extremely faint. Gitt. 57ª דיהה מן האור Ar. (ed. דוחה, read דוֹהָה, fr. דָּהָה) gets faint from the effect of the heat. Yeb. 80ᵇ; Tosef. ib. X, 6 שכבת זרעו דוחה his semen is watery, opp. מקושר cohesive; Tosef. Zabim II, 4 דוהה; Nidd. 35ᵇ.—Y. B. Bath. VIII, 16ª bot. wherever the word מורשה (heirloom) is used, לשון דיהא it is a faint (vague) expression (not meant in its true sense as a real inheritance). Ib. (ref. to Deut. XXXIII, 4) לית ד׳ סיגין וכ׳ there is none vaguer than this (*morashah*), for whosoever labors (studies), obtains the whole of it.—*Pl. f.* דֵּיהוֹת. Y. Ter. III, 42ᵇ top ענבים ד׳ the juice of grapes is light in substance (incohesive).

דִּיהְדֵי (=דִּי הָדֵי) *of this* (certain event). Targ. Y. Gen. XXV, 33 כיום ד׳ as if it were the day of a certain event (of Isaac's death and Esau's succession, cmp. Targ. Y. ib. 31); Targ. O. ib. 31, 33 הִלְהֵר ed. Berl. (ed. הִלְהֵין, הִילְהֵין, cmp. הֵילֵי, הִלֵּיה, s. v. הֵי).

דִּיהֲנָא=דַּהֲנָא. Targ. Ps. LXV, 12.

דַּיּוּ, v. הַיְיתָא.

דְּיוֹ I f. (b. h.; דוי) *fluid, writing ink.* Ab. IV, 20. Sabb. 133ᵇ. Y. Sot. II, 18ª top, v. אֶרֶר; a. fr.—*Pl.* דְּיוֹאוֹת, דְּיוֹת. Midr. Sam. ch. XXVII, end (דיוא׳); Gen. R. s. 58; Yalk. ib. 102; Yalk. Kings 170 כמה ד׳ וכ׳ how many ink drops have been spilt . . . . to write 'the sons of Heth' ten times!

דְּיוֹ II (δι-) *two, double,* a Greek prefix, sometimes used as a separate word (δύο) for etymological purposes, and sometimes separated from its junction. Erub. 18ª (explain. דיומדין, v. דְּיוֹמַד) דיו עמודין two columns; ib. (expl. דיופרא, v. דִּיפְרָא) העושה ד׳ פירות bearing fruits twice a year.—ד׳ זוגר, ד׳ פרצוף, דיוס׳ &c., v. דיוז׳, דיוי׳ &c.

דיו־ a Greek prefix.—1)=δι-, v. preced.—2)=δια-.

***דְּיוּ** m. (v. דְּוַי) 1) *faintness, trouble, sickness.* Y. Ber. IX, 13ª bot. ד׳ ליה וכ׳ he was in trouble; (so) we let him pass.—2) interj. expressive of love-longing (cmp. אוי &c.) *Oh! Ah!* Cant. R. to II, 9 (play on דודי) את אומר לנו ד׳ ד׳ וכ׳ thou (O Lord) sayest to us, Oh! Oh! [strike out the gloss פי׳ דיאו דיאו]. *Thou* art sighing for *us* first (instead of our aspiring for thee)! Ib. (twice more; correct slight inaccuracies). Pesik. R. s. 15 [read:] את אמרת לנו דיו, דיאו את לגבן, את אתת לגבן קדמאה; Num. R. s. 11 [read:] את אמרת לנו דיו אה אתת וכ׳.

דְּיוָא m. (v. preced. a. דְּוַי) *grief.* Targ. Prov. XXIII, 29 ed., Ms. דְּיוָדָא.

דְּיוֹבִיט m. (διαβήτης, diabetes) *siphon.* Y. Erub. X, 26ᵈ top מעלין בד׳ you may draw liquids by means of a siphon on the Sabbath; Tosef. Sabb. II, 8; Erub. 104ª בדיופי׳ (popular perversion, as though=דְּיוֹ פִּי *double mouth,* v. דְּיוֹ II).

***דְּוָדָא, דְּיוָדָא** m. (reduplic. of דוו, v. דוי) *grief.* Targ. Prov. XXIII, 29 Ms. דד׳, ed. Lag. דוד׳; ed. דְּיוָא (Var. in ed. Lag. p. XII רדוא, corr. acc.). [Prob. a corrupt. fr. דְּיוּוּיָא, v. next w.]

דִּיוּוּי m. (דָּוָה) *grief.* Gen. R. s. 74 חזר לדיוּוּיוּ Ar. s. v. קרקר 2; Yalk. Gen. 130 (ed. Gen. R. לסורו) he (Laban) went back to his grief.

דיוזגי, דיוזגר, v. next w.

דְּיוֹזוּגֵי (a popular perversion of διαδοχή, as though= דְּיוֹ זוּגֵי *two sets,* v. דְּיוֹ II) *succession in government, surrender of office.* Sot. 13ᵇ אותה שבת של ד׳ היתה וכ׳ (Ar. דיוזגי; Yalk. Deut. 941 דיוזגי) it was the week of transmission of office when the office was taken from the one (Moses) and given to the other (Joshua, hence 'Moses and Joshua went' &c., Deut. XXXI, 14); v. דייתיכוס.

דְּיוֹמָא, v. דְּיֵיטָר.

דְּיוֹמַטְגָּמָא, v. דְּיאַטַגְמָא.

דיומס, read דְּיוֹמָא.

דְּיוֹמְרִימוֹן, v. דִּיאַטְרִיטָא.

דיומרין, Gen. R. s. 62, a corrupt. of דיומי, v. דְּיֵיטָר.

דְּיוֹמַד m. (perh. a perversion of δίδυμος, *forked,* cmp. LXX, Josh. VIII, 29; popular etymol.=דְּיוֹ עַמּוּדִין, v. דְּיוֹ II; Erub. 18ª) *a corner-piece* made of two boards rectangularly joined or of a block dug out in the shape of a trough, four of which corner-pieces form, in legal fiction, an enclosure of wells &c. (v. פַּס), making the ground so enclosed a private place for Sabbath use. Erub. 15ª, a. fr. נידון משום ד׳ is considered as a *diomad* (two fictitious walls). Y. ib. II, 20ª top, opp. פשוט a plain bar; a. fr.—*Pl.* דְּיוֹמְדִין. Ib. II, 1 ארבע ד׳ נראין כשמונה four corner pieces having the appearance of eight bars; a. fr. [דיומדין, Y. Shebi. VII, beg. 37ᵇ, v. דִּימוֹרוֹן.]

דיומסית, דיומסת, v. דִּימְסִית.

דִּיוּנָא m., pl. דִּיוּנִין (דין) *quarrels.* Lev. R. s. 12 (ref. to מדנים, Prov. XXIII, 29) למאן ד׳ Ar. s. v. פט (ed. דינין).

דְּיוֹסוֹס or **דְּיוֹסִים** pr. n. m. (prob. intended for Dionysos) name of one of Haman's ancestors. Targ. Esth. V, 1; Targ. II Esth. III, 1 (strike out בר דיוס, Var. דיוסף).

דיוסטוס, Ex. R. s. 31, beg., read דְּיִסְקֻיס.

דִּיוֹסְטַר m. (an adaptation of διωστήρ, treated as a compound of ־דִּיוֹ and סְטַר) *a pole reaching from end to end* (LXX Ex. XXXVIII, 4; Aquila Ex. XXX, 4) 1) *the transverse staff of the upright loom* (v.Sm. Ant. s.v. Tela). Kel. XX, 3; Tosef. ib. B. Mets. XI, 5 דיסטר.—2) (adj.) *double-edged.* Targ. Ps. CXLIX, 6 סייפא דיוסטרא ed. (Ms. דיו סטר).—3) ד׳ ביפסלת *the engraving on both sides of the tablets* (Ex. XXXII, 15). Targ. Ps. LXXIV, 6 (corresp. to גליפיהא ib.; Ms. דִּיוֹ סְטְרָא).

דִּיוֹסְפְּרָא pr. n. pl. *Diosp'ra* (prob. Diospolis=Lydda). Sabb. 46ª.

דיוסק, v. דִּיסְקָא.

דיוסקום, דיוסקוס, v. דִּיסְקוֹס.

דיופוטא, Var. of טַפִּיטָא.

דִּיוֹפְּמִין, דִּיוֹפִיטִין m. pl. (διαβήτης=circinus, cmp. דִּיוֹבִיט) *compasses.* Sifré Deut. 7 ye need no arms, אלא קובע ד׳ ומחלק but one has only to put up compasses and divide (the land in shares); Yalk. ib. 801 לא קובע ד׳ (some ed. רופיטון, corr. acc.); Targ. Y. Deut. I, 8 קבעו דִּיפְּטַיָּא וכ׳ (דִּפ׳) put up the compasses &c.

דִּיוֹפִי, v. דִּיוֹבִיט.

דִּיוֹפִיטִין, v. דִּיוֹפְּטִין.

דִּיוֹפְלָא f., pl. **דִּיוֹפְלֵי** (a corrupt. for tabula or tabella,—ae) *letter, despatch.* Ab. d'R. Nath. ch. IV [read:] עד שבאה אליו ד׳ וכ׳ when he received a letter from Rome announcing the death of the Emperor &c.; (Ed. Schechter 2nd vers. ch. VI: באו לו אגרות). Meg. Taan. ch. XII עד שבאת עליו דיופלה של רומי ופצעו וכ׳ when a despatch arrived against him, and his head was split with clubs (v. Sm. Ant. s. v. Fustuarium); Koh. R. to III, 17; Taan. 18ᵇ דאפלי מרומי Ms. M. (ed. דיופלר מהעיר); Sifra Emor Par. 8, ch. IX.

דיופלוסמון, v. דִּיפְלֵי.

דיופלין, Gen. R. s. 59, v. דיפלון.

דִּיוֹפְרָא, v. דִּיפְרָא.

דִּיוֹפְרוֹסוֹף, דִּיוֹפַרְצוּף, v. דִּיפְרוֹסוֹף.

דִּיוּקָא m. (דוק) *deduction, argument, implied opinion.* B. Mets. 8ª מהיכא . . . . דִּיוּקֵיהּ דרמי whence does Rami . . . . draw his deduction? Keth. 17ᵇ ד׳ דמתניתן וכ׳ he reports what is to be derived from the Mishnah by implication; a. fr.—Meil. 16ª, v. דִּיבְקָא.

דיוקולגין, v. דִּיקוֹלוֹגוֹס.

דיוקמניאות, v. דִּיקוֹמָנִי.

דְּיוֹקָן f. (a reverential transformation of אִיקוֹן q. v.) *image, likeness.* M. Kat. 15ᵇ דמות דְּיוֹקָנִי a likeness of My image (a human life; Y. Ber. III, 6ª top; Y. M. Kat. III, 83ª top אִיקונין); v. פָּפָּה. B. Bath. 58ª בדמות דיוקני דְּיוֹקָנִי עצמה וכ׳ . . . thou hast been permitted to see the likeness of My image (Abraham), but My image itself (Adam) &c. Hull. 91ᵇ דְּיוֹקְנוֹ של מעלה his (Jacob's) image in heaven (Gen. R. s. 68 איקונין). Sot. 36ᵇ באת דמות דיוקנו וכ׳ Ar. ed. Koh. (ed. באתה דיוקנו) a vision resembling his father's countenance appeared; Tanḥ. Vayesh. 9; a. fr.—Sabb. 149ª דְּיוֹקָנָהּ עצמה the statue itself.—*Pl.* דְּיוֹקְנָאוֹת (fr. דיוקני). Sabb. l. c.; Tosef. ib. XVII (XVIII), 1 ed. Zuck. (Var. פַּיְיקְנָאוֹת, הַיְקְנָאוֹת) *statues, busts,* differ. fr. צורה painting (Y. Ab. Zar. III, 42ᵇ bot. אִיקוֹנִיּוֹת). B. Mets. 115ª שכר ד׳ remuneration for pictures(?)

דְּיוֹקְנָא ch. same. Targ. Y. Gen. I, 26. Targ. Y. Deut. XXI, 23. Targ. Ps. XXXIX, 7; a. e.—*Pl.* דְּיוֹקְנִין. Targ. Y. Lev. XXVI, 1.

דְּיוֹקְנָה, v. דְּיוֹקָן.

דְּיוֹקְנִי f. (v. preced.) *figure,* esp. *a figure in place of a signature* (v. Gitt. 36ª, quot. s. v. פְּוּרָא). B. Kam. 104ᵇ you must not deliver trust money to a mandatary בד׳ ואפי׳ וכ׳ if the power of attorney is signed with a mere figure, even if witnesses are signed on it identifying the signature.—*Pl.* דְּיוֹקְנָאוֹת, v. דְּיוֹקָן.

***דִּיוּקְתָא** f. (דוק) *the examination of family records required for pure marriages* (v. בָּדַק); in gen. *family record.* B. Mets. 59ᵇ (prov.) בדיוּקְתֵּיה...דזקיף וכ׳, quot. Yalk. Ex. 349 (ed. בדיותקיה, Ms. M. בריסתקי, Ms. H. בדוּקְתֵּיה, Ms. F. בדותקיה, &c., v. Rabb. D. S. a. l. note) if there is a case of hanging in one's family record, say not to him, Hang this fish up for me. [Sh'ilt. d'R. Aḥai s. 41 has three times דוקתא, s. 153 דותקא. For the etymol. of דיותקא, דות׳, v. Perl. Et. St. p. 80.]

דִּיוּר, דִּיִּיר m. (דור) *dwelling,* esp. *temporary residence, lodging.* Y. Erub. V, 23ª top לשם דייר as a lodging place; a. e.—*Pl.* דִּיוּרִין, דִּיוּרִים. Ib. ד׳ ממש real lodging places, ראוי׳ לד׳ fit for shelter. Tosef. ib. X (VII), 12; a. fr. V. דִּיר.

דַּיָּיר, דַּיּוֹר m. (דור) *inhabitant, lodger, tenant.* Y. Maasr. II, 50ᵈ top, opp. to בעה״ב landlord; a. e.—*Pl.* דַּיּוֹרִים, מאי ד׳... ד׳ ממש אטו ד׳ וכ׳ Ib. 10ª .Succ. I, 2 .הַיָּירִין, דַּיּוֹרִין what is meant by *dayyorin?* Do you mean that no dwellers occupy the upper story?—Does the fitness of a residence depend on the existence of real dwellers?—Gen. R. s. 28; a. fr.

דַּיָּיר, דַּיָּר, דַּיּוֹרָא, דַּיּוֹר (not דִּי׳) ch. 1) same. Targ. Y. II Gen. XLIV, 18. Targ. Y. Ex. XII, 45. Targ. O. Deut. XXIII, 8 (h. text גֵּר).—Gen. R. s. 58 (expl. גר, Gen. XXIII, 4).—*Pl.* דַּיּוֹרִין, דַּיָּרֵי &c. Targ. Y. Deut. l. c.; a. e.—2) *traveller, pedlar.* R. Hash. 9ᵇ, v. דּוּר *Pa.*—3) *proselyte.* Gitt. 54ª; Bekh. 30ª ד׳ בר דַּיַּירְתָּא proselyte son of a proselyte.—4) *pl.* דַּיּוֹרֵי, דַּיּוֹרָאֵי *innkeeper.* Taan. 21ª; Snh. 109ª.—*Fem.* דַּיַּירְתָּא *proselyte,* v. supra. [Y. Snh. VIII, 26ᵇ top נסבה דיורין, read דינרין, cmp. Bab. ib. 71ª.]

דְּיוֹרָא, דְּיָירָא ch.=h. דִּיוּר, esp. *inn.* Taan. 21ª בחהוא דיר׳ Ms. M. (ed. דִּיָּר׳, Var. דורא) in a certain inn.

Ib. 'אמטו לחווא דיו Ms. M. (ed. . . . כי אתו ביתו) they reached the same inn; Snh. 109ᵃ 'דיו Ms. M. (ed. 'דייר).—B. Kam. 113ᵇ, v. דִּירָא.

דִּיוּתָא f. ch.=h. דְּיוֹ, *ink.* Targ. Jer. XXXVI, 18.—Ḥull. 47ᵇ 'כד like dried ink. Nidd. 20ᵃ 'פכחותא דד the watery part of the ink, 'חרותא דד the sediment. Ib. 'קורטא דד a piece of dry ink (a sort of Indian ink, v. Sm. Ant. s. v. Atramentum).—Denom. דַּיֵּית *to dot with ink-marks.* B. Bath. 163ᵃ מְדַיֵּית ליה Ar. (ed. מְטַיֵּיט).

דיותקא, v. דְּיוּקְתָא.

דִּיחוּי, דִּחוּי m. (דחי) *suspension, removal of a consecrated object from its purpose; disability.* Kidd. 7ᵇ; Zeb. 12ᵃ, a. e. 'ד' מעיקרא הוי ד a primary disability (existing at the time of the vow) is considered like a removal (through a cause of a later date), (opp. to נראה ונדחה, v. דָּחָה Nif.). Ib. יש ד' בדמים the law concerning suspension or removal applies also to such objects as are consecrated only for the value they represent; a. e.—*Pl.* 'דִּיחוּיִין, דח. Yoma 63b 'דלית ליה ד who rejects the opinion concerning unfitness (of the scape-goat on account of an accident to the sacrificial goat). Zeb. 12ᵇ; a. e.

דִּיחוּק m. (דחק) *crowd.* Tosef. Yoma IV (III), 17 ed. Zuck. (Var. דּוֹחַק).

דיחתו, Cant. R. to II, 15, v. בלטוורא.

דִּיטַגְמָא, v. דִּיאֲטַגְמָא.

דיטי, v. דִּייָטָא.

דַּיִו, v. דַּי.

דְּיֵיאוֹן=דִּי יְהוֹן, *that they be.* Y. Ḥall. I, 58ᵃ top.

דַּיֵּיג, v. דּוּג.

דְּיֵיה, Targ. Y. Lev. XV, 3, v. דּוֹבָא.

דִּיאַטִי, דִּיוֹטָא, דְּיֵיטִי, דְּיֵיטָא f. (δίαιτα, diaeta) 1) *chamber, sitting-room* (generally up-stairs); *compartment, story.* Sabb. XI, 2 (96ᵃ) בדיוטי אחת Y. ed. a. Ar. (Bab. דיוטא, v. Rabb. D. S. a. l. note 1) in the same story (of separate buildings). B. Bath. 63ᵃ 'דיוי' העליונה Ar. (ed. 'דיו) upper story. Y. Yeb. I, 3ᵃ bot. 'לד' התחתונה וכ to the nethermost room of the nether world (utmost degree of damnation; Gen. R. s. 68, a. e. אמבטה, אֲמְבְּטֵי; בֵּטֵר, ביטר). Tosef. Erub. IX (VI), 21 דיוטא ed. Zuck. (Var. דיאטה, ed. דיאטס, corr. acc.); a. fr.—Gen. R. s. 62 they buried him בדיוטרין שלו (corr. acc.) in the compartment designated for him.—*Pl.* דְּיוֹטָאוֹת, דְּיוֹטוֹת, דְּיֵיטוֹת. Erub. VIII, 11 (88ᵃ) 'שתי ד' וכ two upper compartments opposite each other (with a common yard between them). Tosef. ib. VIII (V), 11, v. אַלְקְטֵר. Ib. XI (VIII), 4; a. fr.—2) *arbitrator's office,* whence *diaeta,* name of a prison in Cæsarea in the Roman days. Esth. R. introd., beg. (some ed. דְּיָטֵר).

דְּיֵיטוֹנָא f. (διάτονος, diatonus) *band-stone* running through the thickness of the wall. Lam. R. to I, 1 רבתי (חדא אתתא), 'ד' דבייתי וכ Ar. (Var. עֲדִיתָא) the bandstone of my house was broken.

דַּיָּאלָא, דַּיּוֹלָא m. (דול) 1) prop. *one who pours water over another person's hands* (cmp. II Kings III, 11) hence (=שַׁמָּשׁ) *attendant, waiter,* esp. *attendant of a dining club,* serving at the table and collecting assessments, fees &c. Sabb. 148ᵃ; B. Kam. 119ᵃ 'אדא ד (Y. Sabb. II, 4ᵈ top אדא שמשא) Ada, the waiter. Pes. 86ᵇ 'והוא דרגש בהו ד provided the club-keeper has taken notice of them (Ms. M. 1 'דגַשׁ וכ the club-keeper knows them well; Ms. M. 2 'דהדר בהו ד that he went around for them to see whether they are all in).—2) in gen. *beadle, constable.* Yoma 18ᵃ (prov.) 'אי בר אחתיך ד' הוי חזי בשוקא קמיה וכ if thy sister's son has been appointed a constable, look out that thou pass not before him in the street (for he knows thy affairs well and may blackmail thee).

***דִּיוּלָא** f. (דול) *pouring, sprinkling.* Y. Pes. V, 32ᶜ bot. (ref. to Num. XIX, 13) הא ד' קיים גבה זריקה of this sprinkling act the expression זרק is used, and yet (in Num. XIX, 18 sq.) you call it הַזָּיָה.

דַּיָּן, דַּיָּין m. (b. h.; דון) *judge,* generally at the same time *lecturer, spiritual leader.* Snh. 7ᵇ. Sabb. 10ᵃ; a. fr.—*Pl.* דַּיָּינִין, דַּיָּינִים. Snh. l. c. 'כלי הד the judges' implements (stick, strap &c.). B. Bath. 51ᵃ דַּיָּינֵי גולה the judges of the Diaspora (Karna a. Samuel; v. Snh. 17ᵇ). Keth. XIII, 1, v. גְּזֵירָה; a. fr.—*Fem. pl.* דַּיָּינוֹת. Koh. R. to II, 8 דיינים 'זכרים וד' נקבות male judges and female judges (leaders; Yalk. ib. 968 דַּיָּינִין . . וְדַיָּינָן נקבות).

דַּיָּין, דַּיָּינָא, דַּיּ' m. ch. same. Targ. Ps. VII, 12; a. fr.—Keth. 94ᵇ 'אנא ד' וכ I am an authorized judge &c. Snh. 7ᵇ 'אוקמו ד' דלא וכ appointed a judge (lecturer) who had not studied; a. fr.—*Pl.* 'דַּיָּינִין, דַּיָּינַיָּא, דַּיָּ. Targ. Deut. XVI, 18; a. fr.—B. Bath. 29ᵃ ד' דשפלי דַיָּינֵי הכי Ms. M. (ed. ד' דשיפלי הכי דָאָרְנֵי) ignorant judges will so decide; ib. 133ᵇ 'ד' דחצצתא וכ compromising judges (who know not the law) &c.; a. fr.

דַּיְסָא, דַּיְסָא f. (דוש=דוס) *a dish of pounded grain* (wheat or barley), *grit.* Taan. 24ᵇ 'פינכא דד a plate of grit. Ber. 36ᵇ ד' גרידא a plain dish of &c. (without admixture of honey). Bets. 16ᵃ. Ned. 49ᵇ.

דייספק, v. דִּיסְפַּק.

דייסיקיא, v. דִּיסְקָיָא.

דייסקי, v. דִּיסְקָיָא a. דִּיסְקָא.

דַּיְיצִיפֵי, v. דָּאצִיפֵי.

דַּיְיקָא m. (דוק) *evidence by implication.* Pes. 99ᵃ 'מתניתין נמי ד our Mishnah, too, is evidence thereof; a. fr. V. דַּיְקָא.

דייקולגין, v. דִּיקוּלוּגוּס.

דייקוסין, v. דְּקַרְנְתִּין.

דייקי, v. דִּיקִי.

דייקינתון, דייקינטין, v. דְּקִינְתִּין.

דייקלירא, דייקלר׳, Y. Ber. III, 6[d] bot., perh. a corrupt fragment of *perpendiculum* (פרפנדיקלון), *plumb-line* (hanging with its weight downward).

דייקניתא, v. דְּקִינְתִּין.

דַּיָּרָא, דַּיָּיר, v. דַּיּוֹר, דַּיּוֹרָא.

דָּיָרָא, דָּיָיר, v. דִּיוֹרָא.

דַּיֵּיר, דָּיֵיר, v. דּוּר.

דיירומין, v. דִּיאטְרִיטָא.

דַּיִּישׁ, v. דַּיִשׁ.

דַּיֵּית 1) (*Pa.* of דית, cmp. Syr. דעת P. Sm. 933, a. דור) *to drip, sweat.* Pes. 30[b] מְדַיְּיתִי Ms. M. (ed. מִידַּיְּיתֵי Ithpa.) (the glazed vessels) exude (are porous).—2*) *to languish, faint.* Targ. Job IX, 13 דייתין, Ar. (ed. Lag. דיתין, Var. דייתן, ed. שָׁיְתִין).—3) denom. of דִּיתָא q. v.

דַּיּוּ דִּיתָא, דַּיְיתָא f. ch.=h. דַּיָּה. Targ. Lev. XI, 14. Targ. Y. ib. 19 (v. דַּיָּה). Targ. Deut. XIV, 13 (Targ. Y. V ib., v. אִרְפּוּ). Targ. Y. ib. 18.—Keth. 50[a] דיו חיוורתא Ar. (ed. דַּיָּה). B. Mets. 24[b] דיו (masc.).—Y. Shek. VII, 50[c] bot.; Y. Ab. Zar. II, 41[d] bot.

דְּיֵיתִיכוֹס m. (corrupt. of διάδοχος) *successor.* Sifré Deut. 334 בא ד׳ שלו (sub. זמן) the time of his successor (surrender of office) had arrived (cmp. דיווגי); Yalk. Deut. 947 דיתיקוס. Sifré ib. s. 27 דייתיכוס (corr. acc.); Yalk. Deut. 814 דוכוס (read דיידוכוס).

דייתיקי, v. דִּיאַתִיקִי.

דִּיכָה f. (דּוּךְ) *pounding.* Sabb. 19[b], contrad. to שחיקה pulverizing.

דִּיכְוָון, v. דִּכְוָן.

דִּיכְוָות־, v. דִּכְוָת־.

דִּיכּוּן m. (דָּכַן) *the crushing* of the bulb or tuber in the ground. Y. Shebi. V, 35[d] bot. ד׳ כעיקור crushing is equivalent to tearing the plant out with the root.

דִּיכּוּנָא, דִּכּוּנָא m. (preced.) *crushing, oppression.* Targ. Prov. XXIV, 2 (ed. Lag. ריכונ׳, Var. ריבונא, ed. Vien. רִבּוּ׳; h. text שֹׁד). Ib. XXI, 7 ed. Vien. דכ׳ (ed. Lag. ריכ׳, Var. ריב׳).

דִּיכְוָת־, v. דִּכְוָת.

דַּיְכִי, v. דִּךְ.

*__דַּיְכֵי__ m. pl. (דּוּךְ II) *marks, points.* B. Bath. 4[b] סניפי ד׳ מלבר Ms. M. a. Ar. (ed. סינופי דרכי) the points (stinging boughs of the thorn hedge) must be directed outside (towards the neighbor). [Oth. opin. in Ar. *the staves supporting the hedge.*]

דִּיכְמָה, דִּיכְמָא, v. דִּכְמָא.

דיכסאים, Gen. R. s. 5, v. דִּכְסָס.

דיכפת, v. דִּיכְפַּת.

דִּיכְרָא, v. דְּכַר II.

דִּיל־ (דִּילָךְ, דִּילִי &c.), v. דִּי I.

דִּילָא, דִּיל־=דְּאִי לָא, v. דִּי II a. דִּל.

דִּילְבִּין, דִּילְבָּא, v. דְּלוּב.

דִּילְדּוּל, v. דִּלְדּוּל.

דִּילְדֵּל, v. דִּלְדֵּל.

דִּילּוּג m. (דָּלַג) *leap, skipping.* Num. R. s. 5 בד׳ in a leap (hurriedly).—Ib. s. 2 (play on ודגלו, Cant. II, 4) ודילוגו עלי וכ׳ even his skipping from subject to subject is to me a token of love. Cant. R. to l. c. (ref. to a child's skipping over the Name of the Lord in reading exercises and to an ignorant person's misreading); Yalk. ib. 986.

דִּילוּעִין, v. דְּלַעַת.

דִּלָּטוֹר, דִּילָטוֹר m. (delator) *informer, sycophant.* Snh. 43[b]; a. e.—*Pl.* דִּילָטוֹרִין, דִּלָ׳. Y. Peah I, 16[a]; Lev. R. s. 26; a. fr.

דִּילָטוֹרָא, דִּלָ׳ ch. same. [Targ. Y. Gen. III, 4 דְּלָטוּר, v. next w.]—*Pl.* דִּילָטוֹרַיָּא. Esth. R. introd. מן דסגין ד׳ וכ׳ when the informers increased, the plundering (confiscation) of people's property increased; Yalk. Esth. 1044; Yalk. Job 920.

דִּילָטוּרָא, דִּלָ׳ f. (delatura) *information, sycophancy.* Targ. Y. Gen. III, 4 (corr. acc., v. preced.).—Pesik. R. s. 33 אמר ד׳ על בניי spoke evil of My children.

דִּילָטוֹרְיָא, דִּלָ׳ f. (delatoria, sub. verba) same. Gen. R. s. 19; a. fr. [Y. Peah I, 16[a] bot. חיה לחן דר׳, read: חוו בחן דִּילָטוֹרִין, v. דִּילָטוֹר.]

דִּילְכֵן, v. דִּי II.

דִּילְמָא, דִּלְמָא I (=דִּי לְמָא, v. Ezra VII, 23;=h. שֶׁלָּמָּה=שֶׁמָּא) *for why,* whence 1) *lest, perhaps.* Targ. Deut. VII, 22; a. v. fr.—Ab. Zar. 35[a] ד׳ איכא וכ׳ lest there may be one who &c. Ber. 29[b] מסתפינא ד׳ וכ׳ I am afraid, lest I may become confused; a. fr.—2) (without the meaning of apprehension) *perhaps, it may be.* R. Hash. 3[a]; a. e. כִּי has four meanings: אי ד׳ אלא הא *if, perhaps* (*lest*), *but, because.* Ber. 2[b] top ד׳ ביאת וכ׳ is it not possible that the word *uba* indicates the arrival of *his* sun (the morning of the eighth day)? Ib. או ד׳ or may it not be; a. v. fr.—[Pesik. Shek. p. 13[a] דד׳, corr. דילמא, as Tanh. Ki Thissa 5.]

דִּילְמָא, דִּלְמָא II (=הָא (הִיא) אַלְמָא=, v. אַלְמָא) *here is a confirmation*, a heading used in the Palest. dialect for introducing a story as *an illustration* (corresp. to h. מעשה; v. Ruth R. to I, 17 a. Ex. R. s. 52). Koh. R. to V, 11. Pesik. Baḥod. p. 155[a]. Y. Ber. I, 2[c]. Y. Peah III, 17[d] bot.; a. fr. (in Talm. Y.).

דולמא, דילמא, Y. Kil. IX, 32[d] top, a fragment of a Variant of the following דלמטיקרין; read: חבררסין והדלמטיקין קולבין ומעפורין.

דילניה, Y. B. Mets. II, 8[c], a corrupt., perh. of כְּלִידוֹנָהּ, v. כְּלִידוֹן, *her bracelet*.

דִּילְפָא, דִּילְפָה, v. דִּלְפָּה, דִּלְפָא.

דִּילְפִינִין, v. דּוֹלְפִינִין.

דִּים, v. דּוּם.

דִּימְדּוּם, v. דִּמְדּוּם.

דִּימָה f. (דמם or דום) *evil talk, gossip, envy* (cmp. דבב a. derivatives). Nidd. 66[a] שמא דִּימַת עיריך וכ׳ ed. (Ar. דמות) perhaps the envy of thy towns-women has risen against thee (bewitched thee).

דימוניקי, v. דּוּמְנִיקִי.

דִּימוֹס I, דּוּמוֹס m. (δόμος, v. LXX, I Ezra VI, 24) *a row* or *layer* of stones, bricks &c. in a wall. Y. Erub. I, 19[a] top דו׳ של ארחין a row of bond timber, v. אָרִיחַ. Sabb. 102[b] ד׳ של אבנים a row of stones in a wall; Tosef. ib. XI (XII), 1. B. Mets. 118[b] על הד׳ .. הניח placed a stone in its position. Sot. 44[a] if in rebuilding his house הוסיף בו ד׳ אחד he made it one layer higher; a. fr.—*Pl.* דִּימוֹסִים, דִּימוֹסִין. [Ex. R. s. 50, read with Gen. R. s. 3 הַדִּימַלְיוֹסִים.] Num. R. s. 7, beg. דמוסין (corr. acc.). [דִּימוֹסִין *baths*, v. דִּימוֹסְיָא.] Chald. form דִּימוֹסָא, *pl.* דִּימוֹסַיָּא. Y. Ber. II, 5[a] bot. מנית ד׳ I counted the layers (during prayer).

דִּימוֹס II m. (δῆμος) 1) *people* (populus). Gen. R. s. 6; Ex. R. s. 15, v. בּוּלֵי II.—2) *popular gathering, public festival with games* (δημοτικὸς ἀγών) given by Emperors or high officials and connected with amnesty; in gen. *amnesty, pardon*. Y. Ber. IX, 14[b] when the king נותן ד׳ grants a general pardon, opp. ספיקולה.—Kidd. 63[a] עשה בד׳ הזה act as was done in that public game (Ar. הדומוס). —Lev. R. s. 29, a. fr. יצא בד׳ he was pardoned. Gen. R. s. 79 when he heard a divine voice say ד׳ ד׳ *demos, demos* (pardon), the bird escaped, opp. ספיקולא; Y. Shebi. IX, 38[d] top; Pesik. B'shall. p. 88[b] דיניס (corr. acc.); a. fr.—[Ex. R. s. 2, beg. ינתן בד׳, v. דִּימוֹסִין.—Gen. R. s. 8 דִּימוֹסָה, v. דִּימוֹסְיָא.]—*Pl.* דִּימוֹסִין *public games*. Cant. R. to VII, 12 נטייל בד׳ וכ׳ let us take a walk among (observe) the amusements of the world.

דִּימוֹסָא, pl. **דִּימוֹסַיָּא**, v. דִּימוֹס I, end.

דִּימוֹסְיָא (דמוסיא) f. (δημόσια, τά) 1) *public affairs*. Gen. R. s. 8 בד׳ של מדינה Ar. (ed. בדימוֹסָה; Yalk. Job 907 בדימוסים) with the public affairs of the country.—2) (δημόσιος=fiscus) *state property*. Y. Snh. X, 28[b] top ואחד ד׳ לכולן and one golden calf was the common property of all the tribes. Gen. R. s. 84, end; Yalk. ib. 143 they sold him לדמ׳ של וכ׳ to the public treasury (as a state slave).—3) (also as pl.) *state-tax, confiscation*. Lev. R. s. 30 למגבי דמ׳ וכ׳ to collect the taxes &c. Ib. ... התיר מדמוסא שלהן (corr. acc.) he remitted one third of their due taxes; Pesik. Ul'kaḥ. p. 182[b]. Ib. Shek. p. 11[a] sq. אייתי דימוסיך bring thy *demosia*; Yalk. Ex. 386 דִּימוֹסַיִיךְ; Yalk. Prov. 953.—*Pl.* (Hebr.) דִּימוֹסִיּוֹת, דִּימוֹסְיָאוֹת. Lam. R. to III, 7.—4) *public bath*, v. דִּימוֹסִין.

דִּימוֹסִיִין, v. next w. a. preced.

דִּימוֹסִין m. (δημόσιον) 1) (sub. βαλανεῖον) *public bath*. Y. Snh. VII, 25[d] top, a. fr. ד׳ דטיבריא the baths of Tiberias. Koh. R. to V, 11 דִּימוֹסִין; a. fr.—*Pl.* דִּימוֹסְיָאוֹת, דִּימוֹסִיּוֹת (דמוס׳). Ab. Zar. I, 7 (16[a]) דימוסיא׳ Ar. (Ms. M. דומסיא׳, ed. בימ׳, corr. acc.). Gen. R. s. 1 דמוסיות. Ib. s. 8; a. fr.—Y. Shebi. VIII, 38[b] bot. דומסייא read דִּימוֹסַיָּא public baths, opp. פריבטה private baths.—2) *prison*. Ex. R. s. 2, beg. בדימוס (corr. acc.).

דימוסיס, v. דִּימוֹסְיָא.

דִּימוֹסִית, v. דִּימְסִית.

דִּימוֹסִיּוֹת, v. preced. a. דִּימוֹסְיָא.

דימסנאי) דִּימְסוֹנָאֵי, דִּימוֹסְנָאֵי*) m. pl. (a corrupt. of δημοσιῶναι=publicani) *farmers of public revenues* under the Roman government. Meg. Taan. ch. III, quot. in Snh. 91[a] [read:] איתבטילו ד׳ וכ׳ (v. Rabb. D. S. a. l. note) the *demosionai* were removed.

דִּמּוּעַ, דִּימּוּעַ m. (דָּמַע) *mixture of T'rumah and Ḥullin*. Tosef. Dem. V, 2; Y. ib. IV, 24[a] אימת הד׳ conscientiousness in observing &c. Ib. V, end, 25[a]; a. e.—Nidd. 47[a] דמ׳ דרבנן the law concerning mixture &c., which is merely of rabbinical origin.

דִּיימוֹרוֹן, דִּימוֹרוֹן m. (diamoron) *a medicament composed of the juice of black mulberries and honey*. Y. Shebi. VII, beg. 37[b] Mus. (ed. דיומדין, corr. acc.).

דִּימַחְמְרָא, v. דִּמַחְמְרָא.

דִּמְסִית, דִּימְסִית pr. n. pl. (cmp. דִּימוֹסִין) *Dimsith* (*Bath*), identical with Emmaus, v. אֶמָּאוּס. Sabb. 147[b] קרקעיתה של ד׳ Ar. (ed. דיומסת, דיומסית, corr. acc.) the mud of D.—Ib. מיא דיומס׳ (read מיא דדימסית, v. Rabb. D. S. a. l. note 20). Ab. d'R. N. ch. XIV, end (cmp. Sabb. l. c., a. Koh. R. to VII, 7).

דִּימְעָתָא, v. דִּמְ׳.

דִּינוּ, דִּין, v. דֵּן.

דִּין I, דּוּן (b. h., v. Ges. H. Dict. s. v.) [*to rule*,] 1) *to hold court, pass sentence, punish*. Snh. II, 2 המלך לא דָן ולא דָנִין וכ׳ the king must not act as judge, nor be summoned before court. B. Kam. 82[a] ודנין בשני וכ׳ court is held on Mondays and Thursdays. Snh. VII, 5 דנין את

ידרן העדים וכ׳ witnesses are examined &c., v. בִּירּוּר. Ib. 5[a] ידרן dare he hold court? He dare; a. fr.—2) *to argue, conclude.* Pes. 27[b] דָּנוּ דין אחר they argued differently. Maas. Sh. II, 9; Eduy. I, 10 הַדָּנִין לפני חכמים those who argued before the scholars; Snh. 17[b] by 'those who argued &c.' are meant R. Shimeon &c. Ab. Zar. III, 5 (45[a]) אני אובין וְאָדוּן (v. Rabb. D. S. a. l. note 8), v. בִּין. R. Hash. 7[a] דנין שנה . . . משנה וכ׳ we compare the word *shanah* (year), used in connection with *months*, with *shanah* used &c. (Num. XXVIII, 14 with Ex. XII, 2); a. fr.—3) *to judge, form an opinion of.* Ab. I, 6, v. זְכוּת; a. fr.

Nif. נִדּוֹן, נִידּוֹן (b. h. נָדוֹן) *to be judged, be called to account, summoned, punished, sentenced.* R. Hash. I, 2 העולם נ׳ sentence is passed upon the world (prosperity or failure decreed). Ib. 16[a] נִידּוֹנֶת לשעבר sentence has been passed upon it in the previous year (on the Passover, *before* the seed was sown), נ׳ להבא on the Passover of this same year (after the seed has been planted). Ib. אדם נ׳ בכל יום judgment is passed on man every day. Ib. 12[a] ברותחין נִידּוֹנוּ they were punished with (found their death in) hot water. Ab. III, 15 בטוב העולם נ׳ the world is ruled with divine mercy. Hull. 45[a] נ׳ כמוח is subject to the same law as the brain. B. Kam. II, 5 להיות כנ׳, v. דַּי; a. fr.

Pi. דַּיֵּין *to argue, discuss, dispute.* Koh. R. to II, 8 היתה מְדַיֶּינֶת וכ׳ she argued (contended) with him. Ib. שמְּדַיְּינִין בהלכה who argue legal questions.—Gen. R. s. 3 היו מְדַיְּינִין זה עם זה contended with one another; a. fr.

דּוּן, דִּין ch. same. Targ. I Kings XX, 40; a. e.—*Part.* דָּאֵין, דָּיֵין, דָּאֵן. Targ. Is. XVI, 5. Targ. O. Ex. XVIII, 16 דְּאֵרְנָא ed. Berl. (Var. דָּאֵינְנָא, דָּאֵרְנָא, v. Berl. Targ. O. II, p. 25; Y. דָּיְינָא).—Ib. מֵידוּן, מֵידַן. Targ. O. ib. 13 לְמֵידַן (ed. Berl. לְמֵדַן, Y. לְמֵידוּן); a. e.—Y. Snh. I, 18[a] bot. יתיב הוי דָּיְינִין דַּיָּין וכ׳ sat holding court single-handed. Ib. קומי וכ׳ had a law-suit before &c. Keth. 27[b] דָּאֵינְנָא I decide (v. supra). B. Bath. 29[a], v. דַּיְּינָא; a. fr. [Sabb. 67[b], v. דנר.]—דּוּן מִינָּהּ ומינה judge from it and (all) from it, i. e. an analogy (v. גְּזֵירָה) must be carried through all points so that the case deduced agrees throughout with the case from which the deduction has started, opp. דון מינה ואוקי באתרה judge from it and place the deduction back on its own basis, i. e. let the deduction won by analogy be regulated by the rules of the original case, e. g. Shebu. 31[a] an analogy between testimony and trust with reference to false oaths (Lev. V, 1 sq., a. 21 sq.). Yeb. 78[b]; B. Kam. 25[b]; a. fr.

Pa. דַּיֵּין 1) *to dispute, quarrel.* Targ. Y. Ex. XV, 12; a. e.—2) *to decide.* Shebu. 32[b] היכי לְדַיְּינֵי דַּיָּינֵי וכ׳ how shall the judges decide this case?; ib. 47[a] לִידַיְּינוּ; a. e.

Ithpe. אִתְדָּן, אִתְּדָן, אִד׳ *to be judged, decreed upon, punished.* Targ. Y. Ex. XVIII, 11. Targ. Is. LIX, 4; a. fr.—R. Hash. 16[a] אימת אִיתְּדוּן when were these sentences passed?—Ib. חד דינא מִתְּדָנָא sentence is passed upon it (the grain) once only; תרי דינֵי מתדנא sentence is . . . . twice.

Ithpa. אִידַּיַּין, אִיתְדַּיַּין 1) same. Targ. Ps. XXXVII, 33; a. e.—2) *to argue, dispute, have a law-suit with.* Targ. II Chr. XXII, 8; a. e.—Y. Snh. III, end, 21[d] [read:] והוון מִיתְדַּיְּינִין וכ׳ and contested before &c.; a. e.

דִּין II m. (b. h.; preced.) 1) *law-suit, claim; judgment, justice, law.* Yeb. 92[a]; Snh. 6[b] יקוב הד׳ את ההר let the law cut through the mountain (justice under all circumstances). Ib. 2[b] אין דִּינֵיהֶם ד׳ their decision is not binding. Keth. IX, 2 אין מרחמין בד׳ compassion must have no influence on the decision of the law. Ib. IX, 1 ד׳ ודברים אין לי וכ׳ I have no claim whatever &c. Snh. l. c. שנים שבאו לד׳ two persons who come before court. Ib. VI, 1, v. גָּמַר.—B. Mets. 30[b], a. fr. ד׳ תורה strict law, opp. לפנים משורת הד׳ inside the line of the law, *equity.*—Sabb. 33[a] עינוי הד׳ vexations of the law, unnecessary delay of sentence, עיוות הד׳ perversion of the law, partiality and sophistry; קילקול הד׳ disregard of the law, wrong sentence through carelessness.—Ab. Zar. 18[a], a. fr. יום הד׳ the day of judgment (in the world to come). Ib., a. fr. הצדיק את הד׳ to declare God's judgment right, to submit to God's decree with resignation, צידוק הד׳ resignation.—Ab. IV, 22, a. fr. נתן ד׳ to give an account, to be made responsible.—Gen. R. s. 28 נטלו דִּינָם suffered punishment. Ib. s. 22 לתבוע דינו של וכ׳ (Ar. דקיון) to make responsible for &c., cmp. דִּיקְיוֹן; a. fr.—Ib. s. 12 end, a. fr. מידת הד׳ the attribute of justice, Divine Justice, opp. מידת הרחמים Divine Mercy; v. מִדָּה.—בֵּית דִּין (abbr. ב״ד) court, v. בַּיִת.—גְּזַר ד׳ decree, v. גְּזַר.—Kidd. 65[b], a. fr. בעל ד׳ litigant, opponent in court.—Snh. 32[b] ד׳ מרומה proceedings in court which bear evidences of fraudulent claims or statements.—Ber. 55[a] מוסר ד׳ על חבירו וכ׳ one who appeals to the Lord for judgment on his neighbor.—2) *argument, analogy.* Snh. 4[b]; Zeb. 38[a] מפני הד׳ by analogy from equal expressions, v. גְּזֵרָה. Ib. וחלא ד׳ הוא is not this an analogy?—Esp. *conclusion from minor to major* (קַל וָחוֹמֶר). Y. Kidd. I, beg. 58[b]; Bab. ib. 4[b], a. fr. ד׳ הוא it is a proper conclusion; מה . . . . אינו ד׳ if a Hebrew hand-maid . . . . . . is acquired by means of money, אינו ד׳ וכ׳ is it not so much the more proper that a wife &c.—Snh. 54[a], a. fr. אין עונשין מן הד׳ the tresspass of a law derived by conclusion *ad majus* is not punishable.—לבא מן הד׳ וכ׳, v. דַּי.—Snh. 2[b], a. fr. ובד׳ הוא די and by right &c. Ib. הוא הד׳ דאפי׳ the same applies also to &c.—*Pl.* דִּינִין, דִּינִים, constr. דִּינֵי. Hag. I, 8 הד׳ the interpretations of laws, v. ib. 11[a].—Snh. IV, 1, a. fr. דיני ממונות civil cases, ד׳ נפשות capital cases. R. Hash. 21[b] ד׳ שבלב שלא וכ׳ sentences from a mere inner conviction, without witnesses &c.; a. fr.

דִּינָא, דִּין ch. same, 1) *law, decision; cause* &c. Targ. Is. LVIII, 6, v. מַסְטֵי. Targ. Prov. XX, 8; a. fr.—Gen. R. s. 45 יבעי דִּינִי גבך may my cause be required at thy hands, i. e. you wronged me, cmp. דִּיקְיוֹן.—Snh. 8[a] יומא דד׳ court day. B. Kam. 39[a]; B. Mets. 117[b] נחית לעומקיה דד׳ he enters into the depth of the case before him. B. Bath. 173[b] ד׳ דפרסאי Persian law (arbitrary). B. Kam. 113[a], a. fr. ד׳ דמלכותא ד׳ the law of the (secular) government is law (must supersede the Jewish law in civil affairs). B. Mets. 83[a] ד׳ הכי is this the law? Ber. 5[b] דעביד ד׳ בלא ד׳ that He will pass sentence without justice (punish without cause). Nidd. 69[a], v. פַּלְחִי. Gitt. 56[b] bot. ד׳ דההוא גברא במאי what is this man's (thy) punishment (in the nether world)? Lev. R. s. 27 אילו הוה הדין ד׳ וכ׳ if such a case would come up in your country. Ib. דִּינְכוֹן אתיתי למחמי (Tanh. Emor 6 דיצבון, read: דִּינֵיכוֹן pl.) I came to see your administration of the law; a. fr.—2) *contest, quarrel.* Targ. Prov. XVII, 1; a. fr.—*Pl.* דִּינִין. Targ. Y. Gen. XIII, 7 [read:] והוו דינין. Targ. Y. Ex. I, 10 בהלין ד׳ by what laws; a. fr.—[Y. Keth. IX, 33[b] bot. דין מוגמרין, v. דִּיאָטֵגְמָא.]

דִּינָא, דַּיָּן, v. דַּיָּין.

דִּינָאטוֹס m. (δυνατός) *able, capable.* Y'lamd. to Deut. IV, 30 אני ד׳ וכ׳ Ar. ed. R. (Var. דינסטוס &c., v. Koh. Ar. Compl. III, p. 97[b]).

דִּינַג, דּוּנַג pr. n. f. *Dinag (Dunag)*, daughter of R. Naḥman. Kidd. 70[a] דר׳ Ar. (ed. דו׳).

דִּינָה pr. n. f. (b. h.) *Dinah*, daughter of Jacob. B. Bath. 15[b]; a. fr.

דִּינוּ, v. דַּיִן.

דִּינוּן=דְּאִינוּן (v. אִיהוּ). Y. Bicc. II, end, 65[b] ד׳ מרין who say (v. הוּ I). Y. B. Bath. X, 17[c] bot. (a note which contains the words) זוזין ד׳ וכ׳ '—*zuz* which are', and the number is effaced (Mish. ib. 2 דאינון). Y. B. Mets. V, 10[b] top ומה ד׳ וכ׳ and what profit they may bring; a. e.

דִּינוּן, v. הֵן.

דִּינוּר, נהר ד׳ pr. n. *N'har Dinur* [*Fire-River*] a fictitious river (v. Dan. VII, 10). Yalk. Is. 373 the Sun bathes in a river of fire which is called נ׳ ד׳. Gen. R. s. 78; Hag. 13[b] (Ex. R. s. 15 נהר של אש).

דיניס, Pesik. B'shall. p. 88[b], v. דִּימוֹס II.

דִּינָמִיס f. (δύναμις) *power, ability.* Cant. R. to IV, 8 (not דינמוס, interpret. אֵל, Is. XLV, 14).

דינסטיס, v. דְּנִיסְטֵיס.

דינקאי, Koh. R. to X, 8, v. נִקַּאי.

דִּינָר m. (denarius) *denar* (silver denar=1/24 of a gold denar, v. Zuckerm. Talm. Münz. p. 19 sq.; Sm. Ant. s. v. Denarius). Y. Kidd. I, 58[d] top; cmp. B. Mets. 44[b]; a. fr.—*Pl.* דִּינָרִין, constr. דִּינְרֵי. Y. Ber. IX, 13[d] bot.; a. fr.—V. גּוֹרְדִּינוֹן a. אִיסָר.—B. Bath. 166[a] דִּינְרֵי (sub. זהב) *gold denars*, דינרין *silver denars.*

דִּינָרָא, דִּינָרָא, דִּינָר ch. same. Targ. Y. Ex. XXX, 13.—Y. Keth. VII, 31[d] top; Y. Kidd. II, 62[d], v. גּוֹרְדִּינוֹן. Ab. Zar. 52[b] ד׳ טריינא והדריינא שיפא Ms. (ed. חדר׳ טורו׳) a Trojanic, Hadrianic denar which is rubbed off (i. e. Jewish coins restamped by Trojanus &c.). Ib. 6[b] ד׳ קיסראנא (some ed. קיסרנאה, Rashi קס׳) a Cæsarean denar (Ms. M. ד׳ דקיסר a denar coined in commemoration of coronation; cmp., however, דִּיסְקוֹס); a. fr.—*Pl.* דִּינָרִין, דִּינְרֵי. B. Bath. 166[a]; a. fr.

דִּיסָא, v. דַּיְיסָא.

דיסגנים, v. דִּיסְקָנֹס.

דִּיסְטוּרִין, v. דִּיסְתּוֹרָא.

דִּיסִיקְיָא, v. דִּיסַקְיָא.

*__דִּיסְפָּק__ (דייסס׳ Ar., ed. דִּיסְפָּק) m. a *litter carried by mules* (Lat. Basterna). Ḥull. 79[a] אר מעיילת לי . . . בד׳ when you hitch for me the mules to the litter. Gitt. 55[b]; 57[a] שקא דד׳ the shaft of a litter. [Prob. named after the city of Thapsacus.]

דִּיסְקָא (דִּסְקָא) m. (δίσκος) *disc* (always used in the sense of *tabula, tabella*), 1) *tablet.*—*Pl.* דִּיסְקֵי. Men. 40[a] לִיכתביה אד׳ (Rashi אדיסקי׳, Ms. R. 2 a. K. אר׳) let it be published on public tablets (inscriptions; comment.: in official letters from Palestine to Babylon, v. infra).—2) *official document, letter.* B. Kam. 112[b] נקיט ד׳ מב״ד וכ׳ (M. M. דיסקא, v. Rabb. D. S. a. l. note) he held a letter from the Supreme Court (authorizing him to take depositions of witnesses). Kidd 70[a] ד׳ דזמינותא Ar. (ed. פיתקא דהזמנא, פיסקא) summons to appear before court. Ib.[b], v. דַּסְקָא.—*Pl.* דִּיסְקֵי. Men. 40[a], v. supra. Gitt. 36[a] their signatures in the shape of figures (as a fish, bough &c.) were known to the public בדסקי (Rashi בדיס׳, Ar. בדייס׳) by the official letters which they issued. Ib. 88[a] רב בדי׳ וכ׳ (Ar. בדייי׳) Rab put his signature sideways only in official letters.—[דיסקאות, v. דִּיסַקְיָא.]

דִּסְקוֹס I, דִּיסְקוֹס m. (δίσκος) *disk, plate, trencher.* Ex. R. s. 15 ד׳ של לבנה the disc of the Moon. Ib. דס׳ שלה her (the Moon's) disc. Y. Ab. Zar. I, 39[b] ד׳ מלא דינרין (Bab. ib. 6[b] דינרא קיסרנאה, v. דִּינָרָא) a plate full of (gold) denars. Gen. R. s. 33 דס׳ דדהב a golden plate. Ib. s. 11 דייסקוס אחד טעון וכ׳ (corr. acc.; Var. Ar. טרפזין; Sabb. 119[a] שלחן; Pesik. R. s. 23 תמחוי) a large trencher carried on sixteen poles. Esth. R. to I, 19; a. e.—*Pl.* דִּיסְקוֹסִים, דִּיסְקוֹסִין. Gen. R. s. 10 a bath-tub in which were שני די׳ נאים Ar. (ed. דיו׳; Yalk. Gen. 16 דיסקסי׳, דסקוס׳; Yalk. Prov. 961 רסיקוסין, corr. acc.) two fine disks.—Ib. דיסקים, v. דִּיסְקָרִין.

דִּיסְקוֹס II pr. n. m. (or place). Tosef. Mikv. I, 17; Y. Ter. VIII, 45[b]; Kidd. 66[b] דסקים, v. מְגוּרָה I.

דִּיסַקְיָא f. (δισάκκιον=bisaccium S.) *bag with two pouches, saddle.* Tosef. B. Bath. IV, 2; B. Bath. 78[a].—Ber. 18[a] לא יתנם בדי׳ ויניחם וכ׳ Ms. M. (once דיסיקיא, ed. דסקיא) one must not put them in the saddle bag and place them across the back of an ass. Sabb. 142[b] די׳ Ms. M. (ed. דס׳); a. fr.—Y. Ber. III, 6[d] bot. דייסקי; Y. Erub. VI, 23[c] top דייסקיא (corr. acc.). Y. Sabb. VII, 10[c] אזנים של דיסיקיא (corr. acc.) locks of &c.—*Pl.* דִּיסַקְיָאוֹת. Tosef. Kel. B. Mets. II, 3 דוסיקאות ed. Zuck. (R. S. to Kel. XII, 1 סיטונות; Kel. l. c. דיסקאות).

דִּיסְקִיפְּלִינָא f. (disciplina) *instruction, habit.* Y'lamd. Vayikra, end, quot. Ar.

דִּיסְקָנֹס (דיסקניס, דיסגניס, דיסגנים) m. (a popular corrupt. of דִּיקְסְטַנֹס, דיג׳, dextans) *dextans*, a copper coin, 5/6 of an As. Y. Maas. Sh. I, 52[d] top מעות

ד׳ של money consisting of small coins (Tosef. ib. I, 4 (פרוטות קטנות וכ׳), v. תורמסר.

דיסקרא, דיסקרי, v. next w.

דִּיסְקָרִין, דִּס׳ m. (δισκάριον, v. דִּיסְקוֹס) *salver, saucer.* Gen. R. s. 78 דיסקרא, דסיקרין (corr. acc.).—*Pl.* דִּיסְקָרִין. Ib. s. 93 (translat. משכיות, Prov. XXV, 11; Yalk. Prov. 961 דִּיסְקִים, v. דִּיסְקוֹס). Pesik. Bahod. p. 101ª; Pesik. R. s. 14; Lev. R. s. 20 דיסקרי (read: שני דיסקרין); Pesik. Par., p. 36ᵇ קיטונין (corr. acc.); Koh. R. to VIII, 1; a. e.

דִּיסְקַרְתָּא, דְּאִיסְקַרְתָּא, דִּס׳ c. (a Dispael of קַרְתָּא, v. דְּ־) *part of a town, settlement, private town* (עיר של יחיד). Erub. 59ª 'a private town which became public ground' כגון דאיס׳ וכ׳ ed. (Ms. M. דיס׳) e. g. the *diskarta* of the Resh Galutha. Ib. דיס׳ דנשואר Ms. M. (ed. דנתזואי). Gitt. 40ª דס׳ דעבדי a settlement of slaves. Meg. 16ª סגי ליה בחדא ד׳ Ms. M. (ed. בחד) he is sufficiently rewarded with a township (as a royal grant, v. דִּיסְתָּקָא).—Sot. 6ᵇ רב יהודה מד׳ Rab Judah of *Diskarta.* [Fl. to Levy Targ. Dict. II, 577ª identifies our w. with Pers. *dastcharah, dascharah.*]

דִּיסְתּוּדָר, דִּס׳ m. (Dithpe. or Dispe. of סודר; v. preced.) *shreds of a turban.* Sabb. 48ª ed. (Ms. M. סוּדְרָא).

דִּיסְתּוֹרָא, דִּיסְתּוֹרָן sing., **דִּיסְטוּרִין, דִּס׳** pl. m. (Dithpe. or Dispe. of אסר; v. preced.) *a binding relation, the relation of a serf* or *peasant, a sort of tenancy.* Arakh. 28ª סגיא ליה בדיסתורין ed. (Ar. a. Yalk. Lev. 678 דיסטורין) (when consecrating all of his fields) he may still make a living by working as a serf. Kidd. 60ᵇ דנקיט בדיסתורא ed. (Ar. דסטורין) when he holds the land shown to her as a peasant (but owns it not).

דִּיסְתְּנָא, דִּס׳ I c. (dial. for דשתנא, reduplic. of הֶשְׁנָא) *gift, portion.* Sabb. 156ᵇ אנא שקלת דד׳ דיהבו לי וכ׳ Ms. M. (v. Rabb. D. S. a. l. note, ed. שקלתי דיסתנאי דיהבת) I took the portion which was given to me (the bride) and gave it &c. Ber. 42ª שדא . . . . ד׳ Ms. M. (read שדר; ed. שדרו לחו ד׳ מבי וכ׳) the Resh Galutha sent them an honorary portion. Gitt. 67ᵇ ד׳ דחנקא חמותא Ar. (ed. ר׳ . . . . חמתא) a gift which chokes a mother-in-law (a colloquial expression for a treacherous gift, as from a diseased animal &c.; differ. in Rashi). Ber. 50ᵇ שקל . . . . פתק . . . ד׳ Mar Z. took (some of the fruits) and threw them to R... as his portion of honor (Ms. M. זרק . . . רומנא).

דִּיסְתָּנָא, דִּס׳ II (dial. דִּשְׁתָּנָא) f. (Difel, v. דְּ־, denom. of וֶסְתָּא) *a menstruous woman.* Taan. 22ª דיס׳ ed. (Ms. M. דיש׳). Sabb. 110ª דיס׳ Ms. O. (ed. דיש׳, Ms. M. דש׳). Ab. Zar. 18ª דש׳. Ib. 24ᵇ כמאן קרו פרסאי לנדה דש׳ (Ms. M. אמרי for קרי) on what authority do the Persians call a menstruous woman *dishtana* (for the usual *distana*)? Answ. (ref. to Gen. XXXI, 35 as if fr. דוש, cmp. דַּיְשָׁא, having the *course* of women). [פרסאי does not necessarily refer to the Persian language, as evidenced by the preceding חֲבִיר. Persian *dashtân* may be borrowed from Aram.—Syr. דשתנא, P. Sm. 958.]

דִּיסְתְּקָא, דִּס׳ m. (dial. for דשתקא, v. preced.; Dithpe. denom. of שָׁקָא; cmp. Syr. אסתקא, דסתקא, P. Sm. 325; 931) *handle* of an axe, sword &c. Targ. Jud. III, 22.—Y. Erub. V, 22ᵈ bot. דשקתא דגזוראי (read: דִּשְׁתְּקָא) the handle of a wood-cutters' axe (wedged in between two buildings of a court). [Correct s. v. גְּזוֹרָאָה: (גזר) *wood-cutter.*]

***דִּיסְתְּקָא, דִּס׳** f. (dial. for דשתקא, v. preced.; Dithpe. denom. of שׁוּקָא, שְׁקָקָא) *market-town, settlement.* Targ. II Esth. VI, 10 ed. Frf. (ed. Lag. רוסתקא, oth. ed. ריס׳; Meg. 16ª דִּיסְקַרְתָּא).—Ber. 54ª דס׳ דמחוזא; B. Mets. 83ª; B. Bath. 12ᵇ; Yalk. Ex. 346 ריס׳ the market-town (outside) of M'hoza; v. רִיסְתָּקָא.

דִּיעֲבַד m. (=דְּאִיעֲבַד, Dithpe. of עֲבַד) *having been done, diabad,* a dialectical term to indicate that the case before you is dealt with as a fact, and not with reference to its direct permissibility in the premises, לכתחילה; *as a fact, decision ex post facto.* Hull. 2ª הכל שוחטין לכתחילה ושחיטתן כשרה ד׳ the words of the Mishnah (I, 1), 'All slaughter' mean a direct permission (all *may* &c.), whereas the immediately following clause, 'And their slaughtering is ritually legitimate' indicates a decision after the fact (which implies that deaf-mute persons &c. must not be admitted to the slaughtering act)!—Ib.ᵇ איכא הכל לכ׳ איכא הכל ד׳ sometimes 'All...' means a direct permission (all *may*), and sometimes a sanction after the fact. Ib. תרתי ד׳ למה לי why should there be in the Mishnah two *diabads?* Men. 105ᵇ ד׳ אין לכ׳ לא if it has been done, it is legitimate, but directly permissible it is not. Ber. 15ª; a. v. fr.—בְּד׳ *as a diabad.* Hull. 15ᵇ לא קא מכשיר . . . אלא בד׳ R. H. declares the action legitimate after it has been done, but he does not directly authorize it; a. fr. [Zeb. 75ᵇ דאיערב, read: דאיעבד.]

דֵּיעָה, v. דעה.

דִּיעֲתָא f. (=h. זֵעָה) *sweat.* Targ. O. Gen. III, 19 (ed. זֵיעֲתָא, v. Berl. Targ. O. II, p. 2).

דִּיף, Targ. Job XLI, 14 חדיף, some ed., read: חדיץ, v. חוץ I, ch.

דיפל, v. next w.

דִּיפְלָא f. (dupla, sub. pecunia) *a double price,* in gen. (=mulcta, v. Du Cange s. v.) *fine.* Y. Ab. Zar. I, 39ᵈ bot.—Y. Sabb. VI, end, 8ᵈ מאי גרם ליה ד׳ (not דיפל) what was the cause of his being fined?; v. מוּכְסָא.

דיפלומטר, Ex. R. s. 20, beg., v. פלומטר.

***דיפלין**, read: דִּיפְלִין m. pl. (pl. of διπλός) *double (years), double age,* i. e. 140 years (Ps. XC, 10). Gen. R. s. 59 (expl. בא בימים, Gen. XXIV, 1) בא בדי׳ (some ed. בדיופ׳, Yalk. ib. 103 בדוּפְלִין) he was entering into his double age (approaching his one hundred and fortieth year; cmp. Gen. XXI, 5; XXV, 20); comment.: *double world* (this life and the hereafter).

דִּיפְלֵי f. (διπλῆ, sub. στοά, v. Lübker Reallex. s. v. Stoa) *a double colonnade.*—ד׳ איסטבא an *ist'ba* (v. אִיסְטְבָא)

with a double row of seats, v. אִיסְטְוָונִית. Y. Succ. V, 55ª bot. (describing the basilica-synagogue of Alexandria). Yalk. Ps. 848 ד׳ אירטוון של וכ׳ the basilica-synagogue of Tiberias; Midr. Till. to Ps. XCIII, end דפליסט׳ (corr. acc.).—Contracted: דִּיּוּפְלוֹסְט׳, דִּיפְלִיסְטוֹן (v. סְטָיו). Succ. 51ᵇ (v. Rabb. D. S. a. l. note 40); Tosef. ib. IV, 5; Yalk. Deut. 913 די פלסטין (corr. acc.).—[Y. Pes. X, 37ᶜ top דיפלי פוטירין, read: פירלי דפוטירין, v. פְּרָלִי a. פּוֹטֵירִין.]

דִּיפְלִס׳, דִּיפְלִיסְטוֹן, v. preced.

דִּפְ׳, דוּפְ׳) דִּיפְרָא) m. (δίφορος) *bearing twice a year*, a species of *figs*. Dem. I, 1 דופרה ed. (Ms. M. דיפרא, read רא . . .; Ar. דיופרא). Shebi. IX, 4 דו׳; Tosef. ib. VII, 15 דר׳.—Erub. 18ª דיופרא, v. דּוּ II.—*Pl.* דִּיפְרִין. Y. Shebi. IX, 39ª top דפרין, דפרים (corr. acc.).—[Gen. R. s. 65 דיפרא סופא, v. פְּרָאסוֹפָא.]—V. דִּיפְרַיאוֹת.

דִּיפְּרוֹסוֹף, דִּיפַרְצוּף m., pl. **דִּיפְּרוֹסוֹפִין, דִּיפַרְצוּפִין** (διπρόσωπος) *double-faced*. Erub. 18ª דיו פרצוף פנים וכ׳ ed. (Ms. M. דו פרצוף, Ar. דיו פרצוף) Adam had two faces. Ber. 61ª דו פרצופין ברא וכ׳ (Ms. M. שני) the Lord created Adam with two faces; Gen. R. s. 8 beg. דיו פרצופים וכ׳; Yalk. ib. 20 דיו פרצופין (Ar. דיו פרוסיפון, corr. פרוסופין); Tanḥ. Thazr. 1; a. fr.—Trnsf. *double-natured*. Ex. R. s. 5; Lev. R. s. 1 דו פ׳ היה וכ׳ the Word (v. דִּיבּוּר) went forth with a double nature, bringing life and death; Cant. R. to II, 3 דִּיפְרוֹסְפִין.

***דִּיפְרַיאוֹת** f. pl. (v. דִּיפְרָא) prop. *bearing twice a year*, in gen. *several crops in one year*. Tanḥ. T'tsavveh, ed. Bub., 10 והיא עושה לי שלש ד׳ כל שנה (Ms. R. דופריות, Tanḥ. ib. 13 רפיאות, ed. Amst. רפאיות; Yalk. Hab. 565 צופריאות) and it brings me three crops every year.

דִּיפַרְצוּף, v. דִּיפְּרוֹסוֹף.

דִּפְתִּי, דִּיפְתִּי pr. n. pl. *Difti*, in Babylonia (v. Neub. Géogr. p. 390). Ḥull. 87ᵇ. [Erub. 64ª גיפתי, marginal correct. ד׳; missing in Ms. M.; ed. Sonc. גובתא; Ms. O. זיפתי &c., v. Rabb. D. S. a. l. note.]

דִּפְ׳, דִּיפְתְּרָא m. (διφθέρα) 1) *hide prepared for writing* (contrad. to מצה a. חיפה, v. also דוכסוסטוס). Meg. II, 2 (opp. to ספר). Ib. 19ª defined דר׳ דמלוח וכ׳ *diphtera* is a skin prepared with salt and flour, but not with gall-nut, v. עֲפָץ; Sabb. 79ª; Gitt. 22ª.—2) *record, document, list*. Tanḥ. Vaëra 5 ד׳ של אלוהות a list of the deities; Yalk. Ex. 175.—*Pl.* דִּפְ׳, דִּיפְתְּרִין, דִּיפְתְּרָאוֹת. Y. Peah II, 17ª bot. דִּפְתְּרֵיהֶן their (national) records. Pesik. R. s. 8 ד׳ כתובות וכ records are written before the Lord &c.

דִּיץ I, *to dance*, v. הוּץ I.

דִּיץ II, **דִּיץ, דִּיצָא** I m. (preced.) *dance, rejoicing*. Targ. Is. XXXII, 13. Targ. Job III, 22 (h. text גִּיל); a. e.

דִּיצָא II f. (הוּץ II) *pricking pain* in the eye. Bets. 22ª; Ab. Zar. 28ᵇ.

דִּיצָא m. (הוּץ I)=b. h. זֶמֶר, an animal of the *deer* or *gazelle* species. Targ. O. Deut. XIV, 5.—*Pl.* דִּיצִין. Targ. Y. ib.—Fem. דִּיצְתָא. Targ. Prov. V, 19 (h. text יעלת).

דִּיצָה f. (הוּץ I) 1) *dancing, rejoicing*. Keth. 8ª. Pesik. Ronni, p. 141ᵇ ומעיילין ד׳ and insert *ditsah* (in place of הריצה); Cant. R. to I, 4; Ab. d'R. N. ch. XXXIV.—2) דִּיצַת הערבִיין (sub. תריס) *a shield* used at Arabian sports. Kel. XXIV, 1. [Gen. R. s. 10, beg., read רִיצָה, v. דִּידְכֵי.]

דִּיצוּתָא f. (preced.) *rejoicing*. Targ. I Chr. XVI, 27 (h. text חדוה).

דִּיצִיבוֹן, Tanḥ. Emor 6, read: דִּינֵיכוֹן, v. דִּינָא.

דִּיצְתָא, v. דִּיצָא.

דִּיק, v. הוּק.

דִּיקָא m. (preced.) *evidence by conclusion*. Sabb. 154ᵇ, a. fr. ד׳ נמי there is also an evidence, i. e. I can also prove it. V. דַּיְקָא.

***דִּיקָא** (δέκα) *ten*. Ber. 56ᵇ (oneirocritical analysis of *Kappadokia*) קפא כשורא ד׳ עשרה *Kappa* (v. כִּיפָּה) means *beam*, *deka* means *ten*; [v., however, דּוּקְרְיָא, a. Gen. R. s. 68].

דִּיקְדֵּק, דִּיקְדוּקָא, דִּיקְדוּק, v. דִּקְד׳.

דִּיקוֹ, Num. R. s. 22 ד׳ שלכם, read: דִּיקִי.

דִּיקוּלָא m. (דקל; v. דְּקַל) *anything made of thin twigs* or *reeds* (cmp. דִּיקוּרָא); 1) *basket* of twisted osiers or reeds. Snh. 7ª (prov.) היא נימא וד׳ שפיל when she slumbers, the basket (upon her head) drops (laziness begets ruin). Meg. 7ᵇ (prov.) if a peasant become a king, ד׳ מצואריה וכ׳ the basket will never come down from his neck (he will always betray his low birth). Pes. 112ᵇ ריש תורא בד׳ וכ׳ even when the ox has his head in the fodder basket, &c. Ned. 51ª.—Ḥull. 98ª, v. next w.—*Pl.* דִּיקוּלֵי. B. Mets. 83ᵇ ד׳ ד׳ וכ׳ basketfuls of fat. Ab. Zar. 75ª דקולי ed., v. חַלְתָּא.—*2) *a shoe made of twisted reeds* &c.—*Pl.* דִּיקוּלֵי. Yoma 78ᵇ בדיקו׳ Ar. (Ms. M. בדקולי, ed. בדי־בְלֵי, Var. in Mss. דיקורי, רכולי, v. Rabb. D. S. a. l.).

דִּיקוּלָא m. (דקל; cmp. תִּימוּר, תָּמַר) 1) ד׳ דמיא (=h. קִילוּחַ) the *column* or *jet* of boiling water poured upon wheat &c. for scalding. Pes. 40ª (Ar. דיקלא).—2) (=h. קְלוּחַ) *seething kettle*. Ḥull. 98ª דר׳ דבישרא a kettle of boiling meat; [Ar.: a kettle containing *a basketful* &c.; v. preced.]. [Keth. 10ᵇ לד׳, v. דִּקְלָא׳.]

דִּיקוּלָאָה m. (v. דִּיקוּלָא) *basket maker*.—*Pl.* דִּיקוּלָאֵי. B. Bath. 22ª ד׳ דאייתי דיקולי Ms. M. (ed. . . . דיקלאי) basket-makers who brought wickerwork for sale; [Rashi: 'one opinion': *kettle-makers*, v. preced.].

דִּיקוֹלוֹגוֹס m. (δικολόγος) *pleader, advocate*. Lev. R. s. 29 מנה לך דקליקוס Ar. (corr. acc., ed. נִיקוֹלוֹגוֹס q. v.).—*Pl.* דִּיקוֹלוֹגִין. Yalk. Num. 738 שני ד׳ וכ׳ two pleaders stood before Hadrian; Yalk. Prov. 946 דיוקולגין (corr. acc.).

דיקולר, v. דייקלירא.

דיקומייני, דיקומוני, read:

דִּיקוּמָנֵי m. pl. *Decumani*, soldiers of the tenth Roman cohort. Esth. R. to I, 3, end, v. אָגוּסְטְנָאנֵי. Gen. R. s. 94 דיוקמניאות, דיקומנירית (corr. acc.).

דיקונת־ה, v. קוּנְתִּירָה, קָנַת.

דִּיקוּקָא m. (דקק) *crushing, fragments*. Targ. Is. XXX, 14.

דִּיקוּרְיוֹן m. (decurio) *decurio*, commander of ten horsemen. Sifré Deut. 322 דיקריון (corr. acc.); Yalk. ib. 946.

דִּיקֵי f. (δίκη) *right, justice, punishment, satisfaction*. Ex. R. s. 19 עשיתי ד׳ שלהם בבני (not דייקי) I gave them (the Gibeonites) satisfaction (for their wrongs) on My children (II Sam. XXI, 1 sq.).—Cant. R. to II, 7 (ref. to Is. XXXII, 1) [read:] עד שנובה ד׳ שלו until He collects His debt of justice (punishes Israel for his sins). Gen. R. s. 45 חבע ד׳ דידי Ar. (ed. דקיון) plead my cause; a. e.—Num. R. s. 22; Tanḥ. Matt. 3 [read:] אינו אלא ד׳ שלכם מתבקשים it is your cause which is taken up.—*Pl.* דִּיקִין. Y. R. Hash. I, 57[b] כהדין דירין (corr. acc.) like court proceedings, v. במגנרמיק.

דִּיקִיוֹן, v. דִּקְיוֹן.

דיקיוס, Yalk. Gen. 15. v. דִּקְיוֹן.

דיקייא, Lam. R. to I, 1 (חד בר נש) רבתי, v. הוּקְיָיא.

דַּיְיקְ׳, דִּיקִינְתִּין m. pl. (ὑάκινθος; די for חי or יי to avoid the use of letters of the Tetragrammaton; Ar. reads וייקינטין) *hyacinth*, a precious stone. Ex. R. s. 38, end לוי ד׳ (not דייקני) Levi was represented on the Highpriests' breast-plate by a hyacinth (h. ברקת). Y'lamd. to Deut. X, 1, quot. in Ar. המרגליות ודי׳ (Yalk. ib. 854 דייקינטין, דייקיסנין, corr. acc.) the pearls and hyacinths. Gen. R. s. 79, end (after interpreting קְשָׂט in קְשִׂיטָה, Gen. XXXIII, 19) what function have *Yod Hê* here? [read:] אלו חליות ד׳ וזמרגדין שדרכן וכ׳ (v. 'Rashi' a. l. a. Yalk. ib. 134) these are the links of hyacinths and smaragds with which jewelry is decorated, i. e. the vowel letters connecting the consonants, but which also have an allegorical meaning (v. the sentence following: מי כותב וכ׳).

דִּיקִינְתִּינוֹן m. (ὑακίνθινον, v. preced.) *hyacinth-colored*. Esth. R. to I, 6 (quoted as Greek translation of כרפס ib.) יקינטינון Mus. (ed. טרינון, corr. acc.); v. אלטינון.

דִּיקְלָא, v. דִּקְלָא a. דִּיקוּלָא.

דיקלאי, v. דִּיקוּלָאָה.

דִּיקְלוּט pr. n. m. (Diocles, etis) *Diocles*, the name of the emperor Diocletian before his accession to the throne. Y. Ter. VIII, end, 46[b] ד׳ חזירא D. the swineherd; ib.[c], v. דִּיקְלֵיטְיָנוּס.

דיקלון, Y. Sabb. II, 5[a] top וקוקה ד׳, read: ז׳ דדיקלין *a strainer made of reeds*, v. דִּיקוּלָא.

דִּיקְלֵיטְיָנוּס, דִּיקְלֵיטְיָינוּס, דִּיקְלֵטְיָאנוּס (abbrev. דִּיקְלוּט) pr. n. m. *Diocletian*, Roman emperor. Y. Ter. VIII, end 46[c] (v. דִּיקְלוּט) we despised Dioclet the swineherd, ד׳ מלכא וכ׳ D. the King we do not despise; Gen. R. s. 63. Y. Ab. Zar. I, 39[d] top דיקלטיא׳. Y. Naz. VII, 56[a] דוקלינוס (corr. acc.); a. fr.

דִּיקְנָא, v. דִּקְנָא.

דִּיקְנֵי, v. הוּקְנֵי.

דִּיקְנָנָא, v. דִּקְנָנָא.

דיקריון, v. דִּיקוּרְיוֹן.

דֵּיר I m. (=זֵיר) *crown, rim*. Targ. Ex. XXV, 11; (Targ. O. ed. Berl. זֵיר, v. ib. II, p. 27); a. fr.

דֵּיר II m. *tent*, v. דִּירָא.

דיר, *Pi.* דִּיֵּיר, *Pa.* דַּיֵּיר, v. הוּר.

דִּיר m. (דּוּר) *shed*, esp. for cattle, wood &c.; *stable, store-house*. B. Kam. VI, 1; a. fr.—Yalk. Ex. 191 מִדִּירוֹ (Pesik. Haḥod. p. 55[a] מדירן, Var. מדורות, Pesik. R. s. 15 מִדִּירוֹת) when taken directly from its stable.—*Pl.* דִּירִים. Ned. I, 3 כד׳ (Y. a. Bab. ed., 10[b], דִּירָיִים *Du.*) as forbidden as the Temple sheds for cattle or wood. Ib. 13[a] דירים; Y. ib. 37[a]; Tosef. ib. I, 3 דירריים.

דִּירָא (דִּיירָא), דֵּיר, דִּיר ch. same, *shed*, also *tent* for human residence. Targ. Mic. II, 12. Targ. Prov. XXI, 20 דִּירֵיה וכ׳ (ed. Vien. דִּירֵיה) the dwelling of the wise man; a. fr.—*Pl.* דִּירִין. Targ. Y. Num. XXXII, 16; 24 (Targ. Y. II ib., v. דִּבְרָן). Targ. Is. XXXII, 19.—B. Kam. 113[b] דירי דיירי Rashi (ed. דרי), v. הוּר Pa.—[דירין, Y. R. Hash. I. 57[b] כהדין ד׳, v. דִּיקֵי.]

דִּירָא, v. דְּיוֹרָא.

דִּירָה I f. (preced.) *human dwelling*. Yoma 10[a] בית ד׳ a compartment in the Temple designated for a dwelling. Ib.[b] דִּירַת קבע permanent residence, opp. ד׳ עראי. Ib. ד׳ בעל כרחה וכ׳ a dwelling not freely chosen (as the Highpriests' in the Temple) is not called a dwelling (to require *M'zuzah*). Ib. 11[b] מיוחד לד׳, v. יָחַד; a. fr.—*Pl.* דִּירוֹת. Pesik. R. s. 15; v., however, דִּיר.

דִּירָה II f. name of *a grain worm*. Par. IX, 2; cmp. הוּרָא III.

דִּירָה III f. name of *a jewel*, v. הוּרָא II.

דִּירְכָא, v. דִּרְכָא.

דִּירְכָאוֹת, דִּירְכִיוֹת f. pl. *guards at stations*, v. דִּירְכֵּי.

דִּירְתָּא f. ch.=h. דִּירָה I.—*Pl.* דִּירְוָותָא, constr. דִּירְוָות. Targ. Jer. IX, 9. Targ. Ps. LXXXIII, 13 Ms. (ed. עדירת; h. text נאות).—דִּירְתָא, דִּירָאתָא. B. Bath. 67[a]. Lam. R. to I, 1 העיר; v. דַּרְתָּא.

דִּישׁ, דַּיִשׁ, דִּיִשׁ m. (b.h.; דוש) *treading, threshing.* Meil. 13[a] (ref. to בדישו, Deut. XXV, 4) דִּישׁוֹ שלך וכ׳ what the ox threshes of thine own, but not of sacred property; Y. Ter. IX, 46[c] bot. בד׳ שהוא מותר לך. Tosef. Kel. B. Mets. IV, 3 מקום הדיי׳ the threshing place. Gen. R. s. 69, a. e. מה עפר עשוי ד׳ לכל as the dust is trodden upon by all.—B. Mets. 90[b] לאו בדִישׁוֹ הוא he did not muzzle it in the threshing place.

דִּישׁ, דִּישָׁא, דַּיִשׁ, דִּיִשׁ ch. same. Targ. O. Deut. XXV, 4. Targ. Is. XXVIII, 18; a. e.—Hull. 6[b] (prov.) תורא מִדִּישֵׁיה וכ׳ the ox has a right to eat of what he threshes.

דִּישָׁאָה m. (preced.) *thresher.*—*Pl.* דִּישָׁאֵי. Zeb. 116[b] [read:] דדיישין ביה ד׳ (Ms. M. דדישי דִּישָׁתָאֵי) with which the threshers thresh; Men. 22[a] דדשו בה דִּישְׁתָּאֵי; Ab. Zar. 24[b] דדיישן (קורקסא) ed. (Ms. M. דדייש׳ ביה הַשִּׁירָתָא); Yalk. Sam. 122 דְּדָיְשָׁא-(קורקשא), v. preced.

דִּישָׁה f. (דוש) *threshing.* Sabb. 75[a]. Pesik. Haḥod. p. 46[a], a. e. בדִישָׁתָן in their law about threshing (Deut. XXV, 4). B. Mets. 90[b].—Euphem. *coitus, friction.* Nidd. 41[b].

דִּשּׁוּן, דִּישׁוּן m. (דשן) *removal of ashes, cleaning.* Yoma 21[a] ד׳ מזבח הפנימי the ashes removed from the inner altar, ד׳ המנורה the snuffs of the candlesticks. Ib. 33[a] ד׳ מזבח וכ׳ the cleaning of &c. Tam. III, 9.

דִּישָׁן pr. n. gent. *Dishan.* Targ. Gen. XXXVI, 21; Targ. I Chr. I, 38 דִּיתָן.

דִּישְׁנָא, v. דִּשְׁנָא.

דִּישְׁרָא m. *rye.* Pes. 35[a] (expl. שִׁיפוֹן, cmp. דוש a. שׁוּת).

דִּישְׁתָּאָה, pl. **דִּישְׁתָּאֵי** m. *threshers*, v. דִּישָׁאָה.

דִּישְׁתָּנָא, v. דִּיסְתְּנָא II.

דית, v. דַּיִית.

דַּיְתָא, v. דַּיי׳.

דִּיתָא, v. next w.

דִּית׳, דִּיתְאָה m. ch. (v. דאת)=h. דֶּשֶׁא, *sprouting, plants.* Targ. O. Gen. I, 11; a. fr.—Meg. 27[b] Rab. H. Ar. a. Ms. M. 2 (ed. ריתא, Ag. Hatt. דיתא) אסר דיי׳ had grass tied around (in place of a belt).—*Pl.* דִּיתְאֵי, דִּיתְאִין. Targ. Jer. XIV, 5. Targ. Ps. XXIII, 2 (some ed. הָאִיתְאִין). Targ. Y. Gen. l. c.

דִּיתִיכוֹס, v. דְּיַיִת׳.

דיתכאות, v. דִּידְכֵי.

דִּיתָן, v. דִּישָׁן.

דֵּךְ, דֵּיכִי, דָּךְ m., **דָּךְ** f. (דא with format. ך; cmp. דּוּךְ II) *this, that.* Ezra V, 16; a. fr. Ib. IV, 13; a. fr.—Targ. Gen. XXXVII, 19 דֵּיכִי ed. Berl. (ed. דֵּיכִי). Targ. Jud. VI, 20; a. fr.—Gen. R. s. 5; Yalk. Ps. 848; (play on דָּכְיָם, Ps. XCIII, 3) לְהָהֵךְ ימא unto this sea there; Midr. Till. to Ps. l. c. להדך פלן, expl. לדוכתא פלן. B. Mets. 86[a] מרי דדכי the lord of this (breeze) here.

דַּךְ m. (b. h.; דכך) *crushed, broken; afflicted, contrite.* Lev. R. s. 34; Midr. Prov. ch. XXII דך (שהוא) מדוכדך the poor man is called *dakh* because he is crushed.—*Pl.* דַּכִּים. Sabb. 104[a], v. דכ״ץ. Ib. 105[a], v. נצטר״ק. Yalk. Ps. 848, v. דּוּךְ III.

דְּכָא, *Pi.* דִּכֵּא (b. h.; v. preced.) *to crush, humble.* Midr. Till. to Ps. XCIII, 3 (play on דכים ib.) אני מְדַכְּאָן וכ׳ I will crush them (the Philistines) by means of severe afflictions. Ib. וִידַכְּאוּ ישראל וכ׳ and crush Israel by means of persecutions; a. e.—*Part. pass.* מְדוּכָּא, pl. מְדוּכָּאִין. Keth. 8[b].

דְּכָא, v. דְּכַר.

דכדבניות, v. דִּבְדְּבָנִיּוֹת.

דִּיכ׳, דִּכְדּוּךְ m. (next w.) *being crushed.* Y. Hag. II, 77[c] top; Ruth R. to III, 13 (ref. to דכא, Ps. XC, 3) עד דִּכְדּוּכָהּ של נפש מקבלין up to the time when life is crushed, are repentant sinners received.

דִּכְדֵּךְ (Pilp. of דוך) *to crush.*—Part. pass. מְדוּכְדָּךְ. Lev. R. s. 34, v. דַּךְ.

דַּכְדֵּךְ ch. 1) same. Targ. Ps. CXLIII, 3.—2) *to act humbly, to dissemble humility.* Ib. X, 10 יְדַכְדֵּךְ ed. Wil. (Ms. יִדַּכְּךְ, h. text דכה).

דְּכוּ, v. דְּכוּתָא.

דִּי׳, דִּכְוָון f. pl. (v. דּוּךְ; cmp. דִּכּוֹן) *marked off places, folds.* Targ. Y. II Num. XXXII, 16; 24 (Targ. Y. I דִּירִין, h. text גדרות).

דִּכְוָתַ־, v. דִּכְוָתַ־.

דִּכּוֹן m. (דכן, cmp. דִּבְוֹן, דוּכָן) *an elevated spot* in the kitchen or in the bath-house for vessels &c., *stand* (fixed to the stove or portable). Kel. VII, 2. Tosef. ib. B. Kam. V, 7 דָּכִין. Ib. 8 ד׳ של אולירין the bathers' stand.

דִּכּוֹנָא, דִּכּוֹן, v. דִּיכ׳.

דְּכוּרָא m. (דְּכַר II) *male person, male population.* Targ. O. Gen. XVII, 14 (Y. דְּכוּרָאָה). Ib. 10; a. fr.

דְּכוּרוּ f. *necromantic apparitions,* v. זְכוּרוּ. Targ. II Chr. XXXIII, 6.

דִּכְוָתַ־, דִּיכְוָתַ־ (only with suffix of personal pronoun; v. כְּוָת) *the like of, resemblance, appearance.* דִּכְוָתִי the like of me, &c. Targ. Ex. XI, 6. Targ. Y. ib. דדִּכְוָתֵיה לרליא וכ׳ that there was never a plague like that of this night &c.; a. fr.—Y. M. Kat. III, 81[d] (expl. דכמת, v. דּוּגְמָא) דִּכְוָותָהּ a resemblance of it. Yalk. Sam. 134 (prov.) מולידין ולא דִּכְוָתְהוֹן וכ׳ (Cant. R. introd. דלית כְּוָותְהוֹן)

parents of incomparable virtue often rear children not like them at all; a. fr.—Cmp. דִּכְמָא.

דְּכוּ, דְּכוּתָא f. (דכי) *purity, levitical cleanness.* Targ. Lev. XII, 4; a. e. [Targ. Y. ib. 6 דְּכִיתָא.]—*Pl.* דַּכְוָוְתָא, דַּכְיָ׳ *affairs concernig levitical cleanness.* Targ. I Chr. XXIII, 28.

דָּכָה, דכי, *Pi.* דִּכָּה (Aramaism, v. next w.) *to declare clean.* Nidd. 25ª לא דִּכּוּ וכ׳ the scholars never declared clean &c.

דְּכָא, דְּכִי (=h. זָכָה) [*to be clear* (cmp. דָּכַךְ),] 1) *to be clean, pure; to be cleared, acquitted, cleansed from sin.* Targ. Lev. XII, 7 וְיִתְדְּכֵי O. ed. Berl. (ed. ות׳ incorr., Y. וְיִתְדְּכֵי). Ib. XVI, 30 תִּדְכּוֹן O. (Y. תֵּידְכוּן). Targ. Ezek. XXIV, 13 תִּדְכִּין (Nun emphat.; ed. Lag. תדכן); a. fr.—2) *to be deserving, privileged, admitted* (cmp. זכי). Targ. O. Deut. XXIII, 2 sq —Targ. Ruth II, 10. Ib. 13 מִדְּכֵי (sub. למיעל).—Lev. R. s. 34 [read:] זכי בי או דכי בי, v. זְכֵי.—*Part.* דָּכֵי, f. דַּכְיָא. Targ. Is. LXV, 5 דַּכִּינָא וכ׳ I am purer than &c., v. דְּכֵי. [Targ. Prov. VI, 11, v. דְּרַךְ.]

Pa. דַּכֵּי *to clear, purify; to restore to levitical cleanness, to cleanse.* Targ. Ezek. XXIV, 13. Targ. Lev. XVI, 30; a. fr.—Gen. R. s. 79 לית אנן מְדַכָּן יתה וכ׳ should we not restore it (Tiberias) to levitical cleanness from the slain (buried there)?; Yalk. ib. 133 מְדַכְּיִין. Gen. R. l. c. [read:] צרוכין אנו מְדַכְּיָהּ לטבריא we must cleanse Tiberias (Pesik. B'shall. p. 89ᵇ למזכייה); Koh. R. to X, 8.—Ib. דדַכְּיֵיה which he had declared clean. Y. Shebi. IX, 38ᵈ מְדַכֵּי טיבריא.—Nidd. 8ᵇ מְדַכָּן וכ׳ observe the same levitical cleanness as required for Temple offerings, v. חֲבֵרָא.

Ithpa. אִידַּכֵּי, אִתְדַּכֵּי 1) *to became clean, be cleansed* (from sin), *be purified.* Targ. II Sam. XI, 4. Targ. Lev. XIV, 4 לְדְמִדַּכֵּי ed. Berl. (Var. לַמִּידַּכֵּי; Y. לְדְמִדְכֵּי); ib. 7; a. fr.—2) *to be cleared away, be removed, be gone.* Ber. 2ᵇ אִדַּכֵּי יומא the day is past; v. טְהַר.

Af. אַדְכָא *to polish;* trnsf. *to train.* Targ. Prov. XXII, 6 ארכא ed. Lag. (Ms. אדכיה, read אַדְכֵּיה; some ed. אַדְרְכָא; h. text חנך).

דְּכֵי m., **דַּכְיָא** c., **דַּכִיתָא** f. (preced.) *clear, pure, clean, guiltless.* Targ. Ex. XXV, 11. Ib. XXVII, 20.—Ib. XXXI, 8; a. fr.—*Pl.* דַּכְיָין, דַּכָּן; f. דַּכְיָתָא. Targ. Lev. XIV, 4. Targ. O. Gen. XXVII, 15; a. e.—Eduy. VIII, 4 דַּכָּן they are clean (permitted), v. אַיִל; ib. דאינון דַּכְיָין ed. (Ms. M. דכן) that they are clean (not susceptible of levitical uncleanness); Pes. 16ª; Ned. 19ª; Ab. Zar. 37ª.—Yoma 76ᵇ חיטי דכייתא fine wheat flour.

דכיח, v. דְּכִי *Af.*

דְּכִיךְ m., **דְּכִיכְתָא** f., v. דְּכַךְ.

דָּכַיִן, v. דְּכוֹן.

דְּכִיר m. (v. דְּכַר)=h. זָכוּר, *remembered, reminded, mindful.* Targ. Ps. CIII, 14 ד׳ קדמוי it is remembered before Him.—Targ. Gen. IX, 15 דְּכִירְנָא I shall remember; a. fr.—Taan. 20ᵇ בינקותיה לא דכירנא I do not remember his young days. Hull. 137ᵇ.—*Pl.* דְּכִירִין, דְּכִירֵי. Targ. Y. Deut. V, 15; a. e.—Snh. 29ᵇ.—Fem. דְּכִירָא. Targ. Lam. I, 7.

דְּכִירָא f. 1) v. preced.—2)=דִּכּוּרוּ. Targ. Y. II Num. XXIV, 1.

דָּכַךְ (v. דכא), *Pi.* דִּכֵּךְ *to crush.* Part. pass. מְדוּכָּךְ, pl. מְדוּכָּכִים. Midr. Till. to Ps. XCIII מד׳ אנו we are crushed, worn out (Gen. R. s. 5 מדוכנין, v. דָּכַן).

דְּכַךְ ch. same. Part. Peil. דְּכִיךְ, f. דְּכִיכְתָא *crushed, melancholy.* Targ. Prov. XVII, 22 (h. text נכאה). [Ib. VI, 11 ויתדכוך some ed., v. דְּרַךְ.]

Pa. דַּכֵּךְ *to crush.* Targ. Job IV, 19.

Ithpa. אִדַּכַּךְ, אִתְדַּכַּךְ *to be crushed.* Targ. Job XXXIV, 25.

דִּכְמָא, דִּכְמַת, דִּיכ׳ f. (compound of דִּי, כְּ a. מָא, v. כְּמָא a. דִּי) *appearance, resemblance, the like of.* Y. M. Kat. III, 81ᵈ, v. דְּכְוָות. With suffix of pers. pronoun: דִּכְמִי, דִּכְמֵיהּ, דִּכְמוֹתִי &c. Targ. Job I, 8; II, 3; a. e.—Constr. דִּכְמַת, with suffix דִּכְמָתִי &c. Targ. II Chr. XVIII, 3 ed. Lag. Targ. Job XII, 3; a. fr.—*Targ. Ps. LXXIII, 15 דִּכְמָתְהוֹן (ed. Lag. דמכמתחון), v. כְּמַת.

דָּכַן, pl. of דְּכֵי.

דָּכַן, *Pi.* דִּיכֵּן (cmp. דכך) *to pound* bulbous plants in the ground in order to stop the growth of the tuber (differ. fr. ריכן, v. רָכַן). Y. Shebi. V, 35ᵈ bot. דִּיכְּנוֹ וכ׳ he crushed the tuber in the Sabbatical year and took it out after &c. [Tosef. ib. II, 10 לדכן Var., read with ed. Zuck. לרכן; cmp. Y. ib. 36ª top.]—Part. pass. מְדוּכָּן, pl. מְדוּכָּנִין. Ned. 58ª במד׳ it treats of onions which had been pounded in the preceding agricultural year; Y. Shebi. VI, end, 37ª במורכנין (corr. acc.).—Gen. R. s. 5, v. דָּכַךְ.

דְּכַן ch. same, *to crush.* Targ. Prov. XI, 3.

***דָּכַס** (cmp. preced. a. Arab. دكس in Wahrmund Arab. Handwörterbuch) *to crush, weaken.* Y'lamd. to Gen. XXIV, 1 quot. in Ar. חלי דוכסן (חולי דוכסן) read דָּכְסוֹ or דִּיכְּסוֹ disease broke his energies (I Kings XI, 4). Gen. R. s. 5, v. דְּכָסָס.

דְּכַסוּמֵנִי, דְּכְסוּמֵינִי, דּוּכ׳ f. (δεξαμενή) *reservoir, tank.* Pesik. R. s. 4.—Y'lamd. to Num. XX, 8 quot. in Ar.

דכסוסיא, v. דּוּכְסוּסְיָא.

דכסיא, דכסייא, v. דּוּכְסָא.

דכסן, v. דָּכַס.

דְּכָסָס, דּוּכְסָס, דּוּכ׳ m. (דָּכַס, cmp. Arab. *dakasan*) *masses stamped upon each other, mounds, piles.* Gen. R. s. 5 (play on דָּכְיָם, Ps. XCIII, 3) לד׳ ים Yalk. Ps. 848 (ed. Gen. R. לדוכסאים, לדוכ׳) unto the piled up waters of the Sea.

דכ״ץ, v. אח״ס. Sabb. 104ª דכים הם כנים הם צדיקים הם they are humble, sincere, righteous.

דְּכַר I=h. זָכַר [*to mark,*] *to remember.* Targ. Lam. III, 19 sq. Targ. Ps. LXXXVIII, 6; a. fr.—Sabb. 12ᵇ רחמנא

וכ׳ יִדְכְּרִינָךְ the Lord remember thee for health.—Part. דְּכִיר, pass. דְּכִירָא, דְּכִיר remembering, reminded. Targ. Ps. CXXXVII, 1 הוינא דְכִירִין (ed. Lag. דְּכִירִין). Targ. Gen. VIII, 1; a. fr.; v. דְּכִיר.—2) to mention, remind. Targ. Gen. XL, 14 (with על).—[Targ. Y. I Num. XXIV, 1, v. Af.].—Sabb. 57ª, a. fr. מאן ד׳ שמיה who mentioned his (its) name, i. e. what has this to do here?

Af. אַדְכַּר to remind, call to remembrance. Targ. Gen. XLI, 9. Targ. Y. II Num. XXIV, 1 (Y. I מַד׳, corr. acc.); a. e.—Ber. 31ª, a. e. אַדְכַּרְתָּן מילתא וכ׳ thou recallest to my mind what R. . . . said; Succ. 53ª bot.—Snh. 82ª אַדְכְּרֵיה רב לגמריה (by reciting the verse) he recalled to Rabs' mind a tradition, v. גְּמָרָא. Nidd. 24ᵇ דכי מַדְכְּרוּ ליה מַדְכַּר that when they mention it (the reason), one should be reminded (that he has heard the law before). Keth. 20ª מַדְכַּר חד לחבריה one (witness) may recall (the circumstances) to the other's mind. Ber. 18ᵇ לְאַדְכּוּרֵיה to recall it.

Ithpe. אִיתְדְּכַר, אִדְּ׳. 1) to be remembered. Targ. Jer. XI, 19 יִדְּכַר (not יִדְּכַּר).—2) to be reminded, recollect. Targ. Ps. XXV, 6; a. e.—Keth. 20ᵇ. Nidd. 24ᵇ, v. supra; a. e.

דְּכַר II, דִּכְרָא, דִּוּכ׳, דִּיכ׳ m.=h. זָכָר [marked,] 1) male, man. Targ. Gen. I, 27; a. fr.—Gen. R. s. 33 בר ד׳ male offspring, opp. ברתא נוקבא. Bets. 7ª ביעי דרכ׳ eggs originating from fructification by a cock, opp. דספנא וכ׳ from self-friction. Pes. 56ª כופרא דד׳, v. כּוּפְרָא III.—Pl. דִּכְרִין, דִּכְרַיָּא, דִּכְרֵי, דְּר׳, דּוּ׳. Targ. Ex. XIII, 15; a. fr.—Keth. IV, 10 (52ᵇ) בנין דיכרין male issue, opp. בנן נוקבן. Gen. R. l. c. הוא מן ד׳ וכ׳ he is a descendant of Judah by the male side.—2) (sub. דענא) the male of the flock, ram. Targ. Num. XXVIII, 11; a. fr.—Pl. as above. Targ. Ex. XXIX, 1; a. fr.—Hull. 51ª הנהו ד׳ וכ׳ wethers which thieves carried off (by throwing them over the fence)—Gen. R. s. 70, end, v. דִּכְרָנֵי. [עדנבי דיכרין, v. כְּרוּמָא a. כְּרֵה.]

דִּכְרוֹן, דִּכְרוֹנָה=next w. Ezra VI, 2.

דָּכְרָן, דָּכְרָנָא, דוּכ׳ m.=h. זִכָּרוֹן, memorial, record. Targ. O. Gen. IX, 16; a. fr.—Snh. 29ᵇ bot. דו׳ פתגמי a memorial of judicial proceedings (but not the verbatim reproduction of the words of the witnesses).—Pl. דָּכְרָנַיָּא. Targ. Job XIV, 17; a. e.

דִּכְרָנִי, דִּיכ׳ m. (דְּכַרII, 2) ram-like, lewd, unchaste. Pl. דִּכְרָנִין. Gen. R. s. 70, end 'Rashi' (ed. דכרון, דכרין).

דֵּל, דִּיל (contract. of הָאִי לָא) for if not. דֵּל כֵּן (joined דֵּלְכֵן, דֵּילְכֵן, v. דִּי II) for were it not so. Y. Yoma VIII, 44ᵈ bot. Y. Gitt. VII, beg. 48ᶜ; a. e.—Y. Ber. II, 5ª bot.—Y. Shebi. IV, 35ª bot. אכול דילכן וכ׳ eat, for if thou (doest) not so, I shall kill thee.

דַּל I (imperat. of דְּלַל) lessen, deduct; (adv.) less. Sabb. 89ᵇ ד׳ עשרין deduct twenty years. R. Hash. 7ᵇ ד׳ רגלים leave out festivals. Succ. 2ª ד׳ עשתרות וכ׳ imagine the Succah outside of the hollow, and there remains the shade of the roof; ד׳ דופנין imagine the walls removed. Ib. 56ᵇ נימא ליה דל בדל let the retiring division of priests say to the coming in, 'less for less', i. e. take ye one loaf less and those relieving you will also take one less. Midr. Prov. ch. XXII דל עוד מחייו deduct also from the years of his life; a. e.

דַּל II m. (b. h.; דָּלַל) thin, sparse; poor, needy. Kil. V, 1 כרם ד׳ a sparsely planted vineyard; Y. ib. 29ᵈ bot. ד׳ בגפנים וכ׳ poor concerning vines, and rich as regards labor (requiring as much labor as a thickly planted vineyard). Lev. R. s. 34, v. דִּלְדֵּל; a. fr.—Pl. דַּלִּים. Sabb. 104ª, v. גימ״ל. Tanh. B'har 3 ד׳ כמיצ״ט they were void of good deeds. Num. R. s. 5 ד׳ במנירן small in numbers; a. fr.—דַּלּוּת, v. דַּלֵּי דַלּוּת.

דָּלָא, v. דַּל.

דְּלָא that not, which not, v. דִּי.

דְּלָא to draw, v. דלי.

דַּלָּאָה m. (preced.) drawer of water, worker on an irrigating apparatus.—Pl. דַּלָּאֵי. B. Kam. 50ᵇ; Hull. 107ª, v. אֲרִיתָא. Yeb. 97ᵇ, v. דְּוֵל.

דָּלַג (b. h.) to contract, go back; to leap (cmp. קָפַץ). Taan. 27ᵇ; Meg. 22ª הדּוֹלֵג the second reader goes back, i. e. takes up the last verse read by his predecessor. Ib. נִדְלוֹג let us take up the last verse.

Pi. דִּילֵּג to leap, skip. Cant. R. to II, 9 מְדַלֵּג וכ׳ skips from mount &c. Meg. IV, 4 מְדַלְּגִין בנביא in reading from the Prophets you may skip (read two portions separated in the text). Num. R. s. 2 מד׳ מהלכה וכ׳ skips (digresses) from subject to subject. Tosef. Dem. III, 17 charity collectors מד׳ על פיתחיהן וכ׳ must skip the doors of (take no contributions from) those eating the fruits of the Sabbatical year; a. fr.

דְּלַג ch. same; Pa. דַּלֵּג to reduce. Gitt. 82ª top מְדַלֵּג ותני חד חד (the author of the Boraitha, Tosef. ib. VIII (VI), 9) drops only one by one (seven foldings with six signatures, six with five &c.). [Targ. Y. Gen. XLI, 14 דלגיה, some ed., דלגיה Buxt., read דלוניה, v. דְּלֵי.]

דִּלְדּוּל, דִּיל׳ m. (v. next w.) 1) a limb torn in shreds, strips &c. Hull. 46ª דד׳ זה וכ׳ as to this case of (נדלדלה) the liver found to be torn &c.—2) wart with a thin neck, v. יַבֶּלֶת. Pl. דִּלְדּוּלִין, דִּיל׳. Neg. VI, 7 (Tosef. ib. II, 2 תלתלין); Sifra Thazr., Neg., Par. 1, ch. II. Bekh. VII, 6 (45ᵇ, Rashi בעלי הד׳ (תלתולין) persons or animals afflicted with large warts. Neg. VI, 8 הד׳ שבראש וכ׳ (hairless) warts on the head or chin (Tos'f. Yom Tob: isolated hair-grown spots).

דִּלְדֵּל, דִּיל׳ (Pilp. of דְּלַל) to reduce, weaken. Sot. 9ᵇ (play on דלילה) דִּילְדְּלָה את כחו וכ׳ she weakened his strength, his understanding, his merits; Num. R. s. 9. Tanh. B'har 3 מְדַלְדְּלוֹ וכ׳ the Lord reduces his income, and he must sell his property.—2) to loosen, detach. Kidd. 24ᵇ דד׳ בו עצם he loosened a tooth in the slave's jaw.—Part. pass. מְדוּלְדָּל a) loosely connected, hanging down, detached. Lev. R. s. 34 he is called dal מד׳ מן הנכסים which means detached from his property (homeless); Midr. Prov. ch. XXII דל מנכסיו (insert מדולדל). Ker. III, 8 אבר המ׳ (Talm. ed. 15ª sq. הַמְדוּלְדֶּלֶת) a limb hanging down from the body (not yet entirely detached). Hull. IX, 7

חִמְדּוּלְדָּלִין . . האבר limb or a part of flesh hanging down in tangles. Bekh. III, 4; v. דַּבְלוּל.—b) *poverty-stricken, beggarly.* Succ. 22[b], v. דַּבְלוּל. Tanh. Vayakhel 7 עניים וּמְדוּלְדָּלִים poor and miserable.

Hithpalp. הִידַּ׳, הִתְדַּלְדֵּל; *Nithpa.* נִתְדַּלְדֵּל, נִידַּ׳ 1) *to become thin, sparse; to be reduced.* Num. R. s. 5 (play on דל, Prov. XXII, 22) והם מִתְדַּלְדְּלִים וכ׳ they (the Levites) expose themselves to diminution for your sake.—2) *to be detached, loosely connected, disarranged, parted into shreds.* Y. Ab. Zar. V, 44[d] top ני׳ חותמן the berries are forcibly detached from the stalk, v. חוֹתָם. Hull. 46[a] נִידַּלְדְּלָה כבד וכ׳ the liver is parted into shreds and mixed up with the fat layers. Ib. 44[a] סימנים שֶׁנִּדַּלְדְּלוּ וכ׳ gullet and windpipe which are torn loose from their connection so that the larger portion of their circumference is detached.—3) *to be disregarded.* Sot. IX, 15 (49[a]) נִדַּלְדְּלוּ וכ׳ miracle workers are not appreciated.

דַּלְדֵּל ch. (preced.) *to become poor, neglected.* Sot. IX, 15 אזלא וְדַלְדְּלָה become more and more abandonned.

Ithpalp. אִידַּלְדַּל *to be torn loose.* Hull. 44[a] אִידַּלְדַּל אִידַּלְדּוּלֵי Ar. (ed. אִיפְּרוּק וכ׳; v. Tosaf. a. l.).

דַּלְדָּלוּת, v. דַּלּוּת.

דל״ח, Y. Naz. II, 51[d] bot. לשון חסר הוא דל״ח מל״ח קבר״ת בר״ה (Var. מל״ח דל״ח), read as ib. V, end, 54[b]: לשון הפוך הוא דלא קברת בריה the language (Mish. ib. V, 6, 'I will be a Nazir that this is &c.') has a negative meaning, as in the phrase 'that she will not bury her son' (where the opposite is meant).

דָּלָה, v. דלי.

דִּלְהֵי, דִּלְהֵין, v. דִּיהִי.

דְּלוֹ f. (דלי) *irrigation.* B. Bath. 12[a] דוולא . . . . בי ד׳ יומא Rashi (ed. דָּאלוֹ, Ar. בדלי) a well can be divided between heirs only when there is for each enough for one day's irrigating work.—*Pl.* דַּלְוָותָא. Gitt. 74[b] דלו תלת ד׳ irrigate three times a year.

דּוּלְבָּא, דְּלוּב m.=h. עַרְמוֹן, *plane-tree.* Targ. O. Gen. XXX, 37.—Gen. R. s. 73, end דְּלוּף (דליף); Yalk. ib. 130 דלוב.—*Pl.* דּוּלְבֵּי. R. Hash. 23[a]; B. Bath. 81[a]; Y. Keth. VII, end, 31[d]; Gen. R. s. 15, beg. דִּילְבִּין (not ון . . .). [Ber. 40[b] דולבי Ms. M., v. דּוּבְלָא.]

דלובקס, דלובקוס, read: לִיבְּדְקוֹס.

דְּלוּבְקֵי, v. דַּלְפְּקֵי.

דַּלְוָתָא, v. דְּלוֹ.

דְּלוֹ׳, דְּלוּחָא m. (דְּלַח) *fear; object of fright.* Targ. Job III, 25. Targ. Ps XXXI, 12; a. fr.—*Pl.* דְּלוֹחַיָּא, דְּלוֹ׳. Targ. Y. Deut. XXV, 18. Targ. Job XV, 21; a. e.

דְּלוּס, v. דֶּלֶס.

דְּלוּסְקְמָא, v. גְּלוּסְקְמָא.

דְּלוּעִין, v. דְּלַעַת.

דְּלוּף, v. דְּלוּב.

דלופקי, v. דַּלְפְּקֵי.

דַּלּוּת f. (דלל) 1) *poverty.* Midr. Prov. ch. XXII; a. fr.—בד׳ in poverty, i. e. sacrifice of poverty (birds), opp. בעשירות lambs, goats &c.; בְּדַלֵּי ד׳ the sacrifice of extreme poverty (flour). Kerith. 10[b]. Hor. 9[a] (v. Ms. M. a. l.). Kerith. l. c. עָלֶיהָ דְּדַלּוּת upon the person coming under the category of *dalluth;* עליה דדלי דלות upon the person coming under the category of extreme *dalluth.* Y. Hor. II, 46[d] (ref. to Lev. XIV, 21) מי שהוא ראוי לבוא לידי ד׳ only he who may possibly come under the category &c. (Bab. ib. l. c. בא לידי עניות).—*2) *vacillation.* Yoma 9[b] (ref. to דלת, Cant. VIII, 9) שעליתם בד׳ (Ms. M. 2) that ye left the Babylonian captivity with vacillation, opp. to כחומה, 'as a wall', i. e. all combined and firm; (Ms. Ms. 1 שעשיתם עצמיכם כדלת, ed. שעליתם כדלתות; Ar. ed. pr. s. v. סמגור quotes בדלדלות, Ms. Koh. בדלי דלות; Yalk. Cant. 994 Ms. בדלי דלות).

דְּלַח 1) (as in Hebr. a. Syr.) *to stir up, make turbid.* Targ. Is. XXX, 14 ed. (ed. Lag. זלח, h. text חשׂף) a sherd with which למִדְלַח מיא וכ׳ to stir up some water out of a (dried up) pool.—2) *to be troubled, to fear.* Targ. Job III, 25. Targ. Ps. XXVII, 1; a. e.—[Targ. Job XXXVIII, 25 דלח Ms., ed. דְּלָא.]

Pa. דַּלַּח, *Af.* אַדְלַח *to frighten.* Targ. Job IV, 14 דַּלַּח Buxt. (some ed. a. Ms. דְּלִיחַ).—Targ. Prov. XXVIII, 14.

דְּלַטְ׳, v. דִּילְט׳.

דָּלָה, דלי (b. h.; דָּלַל) [*to be suspended, swing;* denom. דְּלִי; whence] 1) *to draw water.* Gen. R. s. 93; Cant. R. to I, 1. Ex. R. s. 1 אנשים דּוֹלִים וכ׳ men draw the water and women water the flock; a. fr.—Yoma 28[b] (play on דמשק, Gen. XV, 2) שדולה ומשקה וכ׳ he (Eliezer) drew and gave to drink of his master's teachings.—2) *to lift up, relieve.* Midr. Till. to Ps. I, 3 וכשידְלֵנִי וכ׳ and when the Lord shall lift me up out of the depths of suffering. Cant. R. to II, 1.

Hif. הִדְלָה 1) *to draw water, to irrigate.* B. Kam. 51[b] הַמַּדְלֶה מים וכ׳ he who draws water (to irrigate his field &c.); ואני אַדְלֶה and I will &c.; a. fr.—2) (denom. of דָּלִית) *to suspend, to train a plant to an espalier* &c. Succ. I, 4 ה׳ עליה וכ׳ if he trained a vine over the festive wreath. Kil. VI, 4; a. fr.—*Part. pass.* מוּדְלֶה, f. מוּדְלָה. Ib. Midd. III, 8. Y. B. Mets. X, 12[c], v. דָּלִית.—Bab. ib. 91[b] במודלות Ms. F. (ed. במודלית) when figs and grapes overhang one another. [Y. Shebi. II, 33[c] bot. מודלה, v. מִדְלַעַת.]

Pi. דִּלָּה *to sprinkle.* Part. מְדַלֶּה, pl. מְדַלִּין. M. Kat. 4[a] sq., v. דָּלַל.

דְּלָא, דְּלֵי ch. same, 1) *to be suspended.* Part. pl. דַּלְיָין suspended. Targ. Esth. I, 6.—2) *to draw, raise.* Targ. Ex. II, 19. Targ. II Esth. I, 2 buckets דדלו אבנא which draw stone; a. fr. [Targ. Y. Num. XIV, 14 read מַדְלֵי Af.] [Pes. 40[a] מדלייהו, v. מְדַלָּא.]—3) *to lift up.* B. Kam. 92[b] דְּלִינָא, דְּלֵית, v. דּוּרָא IV.—Ber. 18[a] דַּלְיֵיה (Yalk. Koh. 979; Yalk. Sam. 152 סלקיה) lift it (the cloak) up. Kidd. 81[a] דַּלְיֵיה וכ׳ he carried it by himself.—Yeb. 92[b]; B. Mets. 17[b] אי לאו דדְלַאי לך וכ׳ had I not taken up (removed) the sherd for thee, thou wouldst never have found the pearl under it, i. e. but for my intimation you would not have reached the conclusion &c.; Macc. 21[b].— M. Kat. 28[b], v. דְּלַל.

Pa. דַּלֵּי (v. דלל) 1) *to relieve, lighten.* Targ. Y. Deut. XXXII, 51 ולא דַּלּוּ מיניה (Var. דְּלוֹ, fr. דְּלַל) and they would not relieve him (give him a respite). Ib. דַּלֵּי מיני (Var. דְּלֵי) respite me.—Meg. 13[a] דַּלֵּי כרגא he lightened the taxes (Esth. II, 18).—2) *to lift up.* Ber. 6[b] דַּלּוּיֵי lifting up the voice at funerals, v. דְּלַל.

Af. אַדְלֵי *to lift, suspend.* Sot. 34[a] טעונא דמַדְלֵי וכ׳ a load which one can lift up and put on his shoulders, is the third portion of the weight he can carry.

Ithpe. אִידְּלֵי 1) *to be suspended.* Y. Sabb. XVI, end, 15[d], a. e. בגדך מִדְּלֵי (sub. אַתְּ) doest thou depend on thy good luck?, v. גַּדָּא.—2) *to be elevated, high.* Pes. 8[a] דמִידַּלְיָא (a bed) which stands on high legs (leaving space under it).—3) *to be relieved.* B. Bath. 16[b]; Yalk. Gen. 106 (prov.) (מִידְּלֵי) א׳ יומא א׳ קצירא when the day (sun) is high, the sick man is relieved.

דְּלִי, דֶּלִי m. (b. h.; דָּלָה) 1) *bucket,* also used as *cover* of the well. B. Kam. 51[b] משימסור לו דָּלְיוֹ from the moment he delivers his bucket (Rashi: cover) to him; Y. Kidd. I, 60[b] top; Y. B. Bath. III, beg. 13[d] דָּלְיוֹ. Tosef. Ber. IV, 16 ד׳ של צונן a bucket of cold water; a. fr.—*Pl.* דְּלָיִים. Gen. R. s. 45, v. בַּנְרִיּוֹת. [Y. B. Bath. l. c. (perhaps) דְּלָיָיו].—2) *Aquarius,* a sign of the zodiac. Yalk. Ex. 418.—3) בֵּית ד׳ pr. n. pl. *Beth Doli.* Yeb. XVI, 7; Eduy. VIII, 5 (Ms. M. מדלי).—4) *tangle,* v. דָּלִיל.

דליא, דליה, בר ד׳, v. בַּרְדְּלַיָּא.

דְּלִיָּה f. (דָּלָה) *drawing water.* Ex. R. s. 1 ד׳ אחת דלה one draft (bucketful) he drew.

דָּלִיל m. (דלל, cmp. דִּלְדֵּל) *anything irregularly wound, tangle; tow, oakum* &c. B. Kam. II, 1 היה ד׳ קשור וכ׳ (Ms. M. a. Var. noticed in comment. דְּלִי) if the cock's feet were entangled &c. Ib. 19[b] בעל הד׳ the owner of the tangled material.

דָּלִיל m. (part. pass. of דָּלַל) *thin, sparsely planted.*— *Pl.* דְּלִילִין. Y. B. Mets. IX, beg. 12[a], opp. רחשין, v. רָחַס.

דְּלִיפָה, v. דֶּלֶף.

דְּלִיק, דָּלֵיק, v. דְּלַק, דְּלֵק.

דְּלֵקָה, דְּלֵיקָה f. (דלק) *fire, conflagration.* Sabb. XVI, 1 sq.; a. fr.

דְּלֵק, דְּלֵיקְתָּא ch. 1) same. Targ. Ex. XXII, 5. Targ. Num. XI, 3.—Nidd. 36[b] are you not afraid מד׳ of the fire (punishment for disobeying a rabbi, cmp. גַּחֶלֶת)? Y. Yoma VIII, 45[b]; a. fr.—2) (=h. דַּלֶּקֶת) *fever.* Targ. O. Deut. XXVIII, 22 ed. Berl. (ed. דַּלְקְתָא, דְּלֶקְתָּא).

דָּלִית f. (b. h.; דלי) [*suspended,*] *branches of the vine trained to an espalier* &c.; also *grapes of the espalier.* Peah IV, 1 במחובר לקרקע ובד׳ וכ׳ of that which is directly connected with the ground as well as of the hanging fruits (grapes) and of the palm tree; Tosef. ib. III, 16. Y. B. Mets. X, 12[c] ד׳ אחת וכ׳ a grape vine which was overhanging a neighbor's peach tree; a. fr.— *Pl.* דָּלִיּוֹת. Men. VIII, 6 (86[b]) wine for libation must not be offered מן הד׳ (Tosef. ib. IX, 10 sing.) from grapes of the espalier, opp. רגלויות. Pes. 53[a] ד׳ של וכ׳; Tosef. Shebi. VII, 15 ד׳ שבאשכול וכ׳ the hanging grapes of Abel.

דִּלְכּוֹן, v. דּ׳.

דִּלְכֵן, v. דּ׳ל.

דָּלַל (b. h.) [*to be thin, swing, hang,*] *to be poor.* Lev. R. s. 34 דַּלּוּ מן המצות they became poor in good deeds.

Hif. הֵדַל, הֵידֵל 1) *to thin, to take off grapes,* or *take out plants* in order to give the remainder more room. Peah III, 3 המֵדַל (Y. ed. המֵידַל) he who thins the vineyard; Tosef. ib. I, 10. Peah VII, 5; a. fr.—M. Kat. 4[a] sq. (a Boraitha quoted by Rabina) והתניא מְדַלִּין לירקות וכ׳ (v. דָּלָה) are we not told, you may irrigate the vegetable garden during the festive week, if you intend to use the vegetables during the festive days? Said Rabbah to him [read:] מי סברת מדלין מיא מאי מדלין שלופי you think this *m'dallin* means you may draw water, it means: *to pluck* (ref. to Peah VII, 5).—Said Rabina to him: והתניא מדלין מים לירקות וכ׳ But it reads, *M'dallin mayim* you may sprinkle *water* &c.—*Part. Pual* מְדוּלָּל, f. מְדוּלֶּלֶת *beggarly.* Y. Succ. II, 52[d] bot.; v. דַּבְלוּל.

דְּלַל ch. 1) *to lift up* (v. דְּלֵי). Keth. 72[a] דִּידַל יְדַלּוּנֵיה him who lifts up (his voice in funereal lamentations), they will lift up (praise him at his funeral); M. Kat. 28[b].— 2) *to thin,* v. דָּלִיל.

Ithpa. אִידַּל *to lift one's self up, be proud.* Ib. [read:] דלא אִידַּל ידלוניה him who did not praise himself, they will &c. (Ms. M. 2 לא לִידַּל דדידלוניה, read: דְּיִדַלּוּנֵיה, let one not praise himself, in order that they may &c.).

דְּלוּם, דֶּלֶם m. (דלל, with format. מ) *diminution, defect* (cmp. דּוֹפִי). Pes. 57[a] that the workmanship was good ואין בהם ד׳ Ms. M. 1 a. ed. (Ms. M. 2 דליס, Ar. דלוס, דליס, v. Koh. Ar. Compl.) and there was no defect in them; Tosef. Men. XIII, 19 שלא נטה בו דלום ed. Zuck. (ed. כלום).—Tosef. B. Kam. VII, 8 אין השמן מקבל דליס (Var. כלום; Mekh. Mishp. N'zikin. s. 13 מַבָּל; Yalk. Ex. 343 מַעַל) oil admits of no dilution through admixture (cmp. Cant. R. to I, 3).

דִּלְמָא I, II, v. דִּילְמָא I, II.

דלמטיקון, דלמטיקון, read:

דַּלְמָטִיקִין m. pl. (δαλματική, dalmatica) *dalmatics,* long undergarments of Dalmatian wool. Kil. IX, 7; expl. Y. ib. 32[d] top קובלין (read קולובין κολόβιον, v. Sm. Ant. s. v. δαλματική).

דֶּלֶס, דְּלוּס, דָּלִיס m. (דלל; cmp. Samaritan דלס

דלס Gen. XXI, 23, Arab. *dallasa*) *adulteration, fraud.* V., however, הֶלֶם. [V. Fränkel Aram. Fremdw. p. 188.]

דלסתי, v. דַּלְתָא.

דְּלַעַת f. (דלע, cmp. הֲלִי a. זְלוּעַ) [*bottle-shaped,*] *gourd*, a general name for *cucumbers, pumpkins* &c. (v. Sm. Ant. s. vv. Colocynthe a. Colocynthis). Kil. I, 2 ד׳ מצרית וכ׳ Ms. M. (ed. חמצרי, corr. acc.) Egyptian gourd and the Bitter-gourd may be planted together (v. כִּלְאַיִם). Ned. VI, 1 דלעת הרמוצה, variously explained ib. 51ª; Y. Kil. I, 27ª top; a. fr.—Sot. 16ª מגלחו כד׳ he shaves his body as smooth as a gourd; Y. Kidd. I, 59ᵈ top כדלת (corr. acc.). *Pl.* דִּלּוּעִים, דִּלּוּעִין, דיל׳. Sabb. XXIV, 4. Ned. VII, 1; a. fr.—Tosef. Maasr. III, 14 הַדִּלּוּעוֹת.—Erub. 104ª הַדָּלָיו, v. מִדְלַעַת.

דָּלַף (b. h.; cmp. זלף) *to drip.* Bekh. 44ª his eyes are דומעות הוֹלְפוֹת וכ׳ tearing, dripping or running.

דְּלַף ch. same. Targ. Prov. XIX, 13 דָּלֵף (Var. דָּלֵיף).—Sabb. 43ª דשכיחי דְּדַלְפֵי which are liable to have leaky roofs.

דֶּלֶף m. (preced.) *drippings* from the roof; *leak* in the roof. Bets. V, 1; Sabb. 43ª. Pes. 39ᵇ שנפל לתוכו ד׳ on which the drippings from the roof have fallen. Makhsh. IV, 4 sq.; a. e.

דִּלְפָא, דִּיל׳, דְּל׳ ch. same. Targ. Prov. XIX, 13; XXVII, 15.—Y. Maas. Sh. IV, 55ᶜ top; Lam. R. to I, 1 חד כות׳ (1) רבתי.

דִּלְפָה, דִּיל׳ f. (preced.) בֵּית ד׳ *receptacle of drippings*, name of the second roof of the Temple made for protection against an eventual leak in the upper roof. Midd. IV, 6 (Maim. הַדְּלִיפָה).

דְּלוּפְקִי, דְּלְפְּקִי f. (δελφική=δέλφιξ, delphica, sub. mensa) *delphica*, a three-legged table used as a toilet table or a waiter, contrad. fr. שלחן eating table (v. Becker Gallus, ed. Göll II, p. 354). Kel. XXV, 1. Ib. XXII, 1; Tosef. ib. B. Bath. I, 9 דולפני (corr. acc.). Ab. Zar. V, 5 (69ª) דלפ׳ Ar. (Ms. M. דלוב׳, ed. דולב׳, v. Rabb. D. S. a. l. note). Y. Dem. VI, 25ᵈ statuary made כמין ד׳ like a kind of delphica (for practical use and not for idol worship, cmp. בְּסִיס). *Ex. R. s. 43 מגפפת לד׳ hugging the statuary figure supporting a delphica (Num. R. s. 2 סריס).—*Pl.* דְּלְפְּקִיּוֹת. Y. Ab. Zar. III, 42ᶜ bot.

דָּלַק, דְּלֵיק (b. h.) 1) *to burn; to be illumined.* Gen. R. s. 39 saw a castle הוֹלֶקֶת lighted. B. Kam. VI, 5 וְדָלְקוּ and they caught fire. Y. Sabb. II, beg. 4ᶜ והיא דְּלֵיקָה והולכת that it may continue to burn. Ib.ᵈ דְּלֵיקִין are burning.—Part. pass. דָּלוּק *enkindled, burning.* Gen. R. s. 11 מצאתי אותו דָ׳ (Yalk. ib. 16 הוֹלֵק) I found it still burning. Midr. Till. to Ps. VII, 14 (ref. to לדלקים ib.) שלבם דָ׳ עליהם (Yalk. a. l. דולק) whose hearts within them are burning (with lust).—Lam. R. to IV, 19 [read:] שהיו שמשליכין דולקין אחריהם מֵעֲבִיּוֹת (Koh. R. to V, 2 דֶּלֶק אחריהם) they (the Romans) sent fire after them from their engines (tormenta), v. עֲבִית.—2) *to pursue eagerly.* Lam. R. l. c. הוֹלְקֵיהֶם של ישראל (Koh. R. l. c. רודפ׳; Midr. Till. l. c. שונאין) Israel's persecutors.

Nif. נִדְלַק *to be burnt, destroyed by fire.* Orl. III, 1 יִדָּלֵק; יִדָּלְקוּ must be burnt. Ib. 2 sq.; a. fr.—Y. B. Kam. IV, 5ᶜ top דרכן לִידָּלֵק liable to take fire.

Hif. הִדְלִיק *to kindle, light.* Sabb. II, 1 במה מַדְלִיקִין what material may be used for the Sabbath lights? Ib. 7 הַדְלִיקוּ וכ׳ light the lamps. Y. ib. II, 4ᶜ bot.; Y. Ter. XI, 48ᵇ top באת לְהַדְלִיק וכ׳ she came to get a light from a priest's wife; a. fr.—V. הַדְלָקָה.

דְּלֵיק, דְּלַק ch. same; 1) *to burn.* Targ. Am. V, 6; a. e.—Meg. 12ᵇ דָּלְקָה ביה חמתיה Ms. M. (v. Rabb. D. S. a. l.)=חמתו בערה בו (Esth. I, 12).—2) *to pursue*, v. infra.

Af. אַדְלֵיק 1) *to kindle a light, start a fire.* Targ. Num. VIII, 2. Targ. Ex. XXII, 5; a. e.—Sabb. 22ᵇ וְאַדְלוּקֵי and kindle (the chip). Ib. bot. לצורכו הוא דְאַדְלְקָהּ he lighted it for his use. Ib. 23ª מַדְלְיקֵי עלי וכ׳ they light the Hanuckah lamps in my behalf at home; a. e.—2) *to pursue.* Targ. Lam. IV, 19. [Ib. III, 66 תַּדְלוּק׳, read תִּדְלוּק׳ or תַּדְלִיק׳.]

דֶּלֶק m. (preced.) *light, burning material, wick, wood* &c. Y. Sabb. II, beg., 4ᶜ לא הוצת האור ברוב הד׳ the larger portion of the burning material was not enkindled (on the entrance of the Sabbath). Midd. I, 4 שער הד׳ the Temple gate by which the burning material was brought in. Koh. R. to V, 2, v. דָּלַק.

דלקמירין, v. פּוּלְקְמָרִין.

דַּלֶּקֶת f. (b. h.; דלק) *fever.* Y. Ab. Zar. II, 41ª bot.

דִּלְקָא, דֶּלֶק׳, דַּלֶּקְתָּא, v. דְּלֵיקְתָא.

דלריא, v. הִדְרָיָא.

דל״ת *Daleth*, the fourth letter of the Alphabeth. Sabb. 104ª, v. גימ״ל. Y. ib. VII, 10ᵈ top היה ד׳ וכ׳ if one changed a *Daleth* into a *Resh.* Maas. Sh. IV, 11 ד׳ דמאי the mark *Daleth* intimates that the contents are *D'mai* (v. דְּמַאי); Tosef. ib. V, 1; Y. ib. IV, 55ᵇ top. Y. Snh. X, 28ᵇ top; a. fr.—*Pl.* דַּל״תִין, דַּל״תִים. Sifré Deut. 36; Sabb. 103ᵇ.

דֶּלֶת f. (b. h.; דלל) *door, lid* on hinges, *shutter.* Erub. 101ª, v. אַלְמָנָה.—נעל ד׳ בפני לוין to shut the door to borrowers, *to render credit difficult.* Snh. 32ª; a. fr.—B. Kam. 80ᵇ ד׳ הננעלת וכ׳ a door once shut is not easily opened, i. e. it requires ardent prayer to regain divine grace after a calamity has set in; a. fr.—Tosef. Kel. B. Mets VI, 7 של ד׳ *on hinges*, v. מַסְחֵיט.—*Pl.* דְּלָתוֹת, constr. דַּלְתוֹת. Sabb. XVII, 1. Lev. R. s. 14 יש ד׳ וכ׳ a woman's womb has doors (muscles, ref. to Job III, 10); a. fr.—Par. III, 2; Tosef. ib. III (II), 2 על גביהן ד׳ a seat of boards on hinges upon the backs of the oxen; Succ. 21ª.—Yoma 9ᵇ כד׳ vacillating like doors, v. הַלּוּת. [Y. Kidd. I, 59ᵈ top, v. דְּלַעַת.]

***דַּלְתָא** ch. same. *Pl.* constr. דַּלְתֵי. Targ. Job III, 9 (10) דלתתי דהנון דשי, a gloss to פאתי or פרתי. [Ed. Lag. דלסתי; Ms. ולסתייר.]

***דלתותא**, Targ. Prov. XIX, 14 Var. (v. ed. Lag. II, p. XII⁴), a corruption of ירותתא.

דָּם m., constr. דַּם (b. h.; דום or דמם, cmp. דבב) *liquid; blood; life.* Men. 44ª בְּדָמוֹ (not בדמה, v. Rabb. D. S. a. l. note) with the juice of the purple shell.—Sabb. 31ᵇ רביעית ד׳ וכ׳ one fourth of a Log of blood did I (the Lord) put in your body (the smallest quantity required to sustain life, v. Sot. 5ª). Snh. 72ᵇ (ref. to Gen. IX, 6) הצל דָּמוֹ וכ׳ save the life of the one (who is pursued) at the expense of the life of the other (the pursuer).—דַּם ברית= ד׳ של מילה the blood lost at circumcision. Tosef. Sabb. XV (XVI), 9 צריך לְהַטִּיף . . . ד׳ ב׳ he must cause the blood of the covenant to flow from him (even if born without preputium). Ib. 8; a. fr.—Pes. 16ᵇ ד׳ שהנפש וכ׳ the blood with which life escapes when cutting the animal's throat is called a *fluid* (with regard to levitical purity, v. כָּשֵׁר); a. v. fr.—*Pl.* דָּמִים. Keth. 9ᵇ טענת ד׳ complaint of absence of the token of virginity.—שְׁפִיכוּת ד׳ (abbr. ש״ד) *murder.* Yoma 67ᵇ; a. fr.—Midd. III, 1, a. e. ד׳ העליונים blood sprinkled against the upper part of the altar, opp. ד׳ התחתונים.—Snh. VIII, 6, a. fr. (with ref. to Ex. XXII, 1) יש לו ד׳ his blood is revenged, אין לו ד׳ may be killed with impunity. Ib. 72ª בד׳ קנגהו he acquired possession of them by risking his life.—[דָּמִים *equivalent,* v. דָּמִים.)

דָּם, דְּמָא ch. same 1) *blood; life.* Targ. O. Gen. IV, 10. Targ. ib. IX, 6; a. fr.—B. Bath. 58ᵇ בריש כל מַרְעִין אנא ד׳ וכ׳ at the head of all diseases (chief cause of physical disorders) am I, the blood. Yoma 82ᵇ, a. e. מאי חזית דד׳ דידך וכ׳ what right hast thou to assume that thy blood is redder than thy neighbor's (you have no right to commit murder even under compulsion). Kidd. 81ª נשויתיה (שויתה) לִדְמָךְ וכ׳ I should have valued thy life two *M'ah,* i. e. I should not have spared thee; Pes. 112ᵇ Ms. M. (ed. סכנתיך, v. Rabb. D. S. a. l. note 200, a. note 3). Keth. 60ᵇ bot. על דמא דחמרא Ar. s. v. גרדן (ed. רמא) on the blood of an ass.—*Pl.* דְּמֵי. Targ. Gen. IV, 11; a. fr.—Gitt. 57ᵇ, v. דְּמֵי I.—2) *congestion.* Ab. Zar. 28ᵇ; Bets. 22ª ד׳ דמעתא וכ׳ congestion of the eye, tears &c. Gitt. 68ᵇ לד׳ דרישא for congestion of the head (head-ache). [דְּמֵי *equivalent,* v. דָּמִין.] V. אַרְדָּמָא.

דְּמָא *to resemble,* v. דְּמֵי.

דָּמָא pr. n. m. *Dama,* name of a gentile of Ascalon, praised for his filial reverence. Ab. Zar. 23ᵇ (Var. רמא, רמה, v. Rabb. D. S. a. l. note 90); Kidd. 31ª; Y. Peah I, 15ᶜ top דָּמָה; Yalk. Ex. 364. Cmp. דּוּמָא.

דְּמַי, דְּמַאי m. (דמי) *suspicion, talk,* whence (cmp. דּוּמָה, שְׁתוּקִי) *D'mai,* fruits about which there is a suspicion as to the tithes therefrom being properly taken, opp. וַדַּאי. Y. Maas. Sh. V, end, 56ᵈ [read:] דמאי דְּמַי תיקן דְּמַי לא תיקן *D'mai* means, There is a talk that he has given the tithes, there is a talk that he has not; Y. Sot. IX, 24ᵇ top ומי לא תיקן (read דְּמַי). Y. Dem. II, 22ª top; Y. Shek. V, 48ᵈ top אפרישתון דְּמַיָּין have you set apart what is due of them (the barley) according to the law of D'mai?—Dem. I, 1. Ib. 3 פטור מן הד׳ is exempt from the law of D'mai (no tithes required of them on account of doubt); a. fr.—*D'mai,* name of a treatise of *Mishnah, Tosefta* a. *Y'rushalmi* of the Order of *Z'raïm.* [Not to be confounded with ד־מאי=דְּמַאי *of what.*]

דְּמָאִין m. pl. (דמי, v. P. Sm. 913 sq.) *figures.* Targ. Jud. XVII, 5; XVIII, 14; a. e.

דִּימ׳, דְּמָדוּם m., pl. דִּי׳ דְּמָדוּמִין, (דָּמַם) *stand-still, stillness;* דִּמְדּוּמֵי חמה the time in the morning and the evening when the sun appears to stand still or be silent (cmp. Yoma 20ᵇ), *dawn and sunset.* Sabb. 118ᵇ; Ber. 29ᵇ; a. fr. Y. Pes. V, beg. 31ᶜ ד׳ החמה sunset.

דִּמְדֵּם (Pilp. of דמם) *to silence.* Part. pass. מְדוּמְדָּם *unable to speak, overcome by wine.* Y. Ter. I, 40ᵈ bot.

דַּמְדֵּם ch. same. Part. pass. מְדַמְדַּם *overwhelmed.* Cant. R. to III, 4 הוה מ׳ וכ׳ he lay in a stupor the whole night, opp. פרפר to be restless.

Ithpalp. אִידַּמְדַּם *to be dumb.* Targ. Y. II Ex. XV, 16 [read:] יִדַּ׳.

דַּמְדְמָנִיּוֹת, v. הַדְּבָנִיּוֹת (cmp. דָּם).

דָּמָה pr. n. m., v. דָּמָא.

דָּמָה, v. דמי.

דַּמְהַרְיָא pr. n. pl. *Damharia,* in Babylonia. R. Hash. 21ª. Erub. 6ª דמה׳ Ms. M. (ed. דמח׳). Men. 81ª Ms. M. (ed. דַּמְהוּרְיָא). V. Berl. Beitr. z. Geogr. p. 30.

דְּמוּ f.=דְּמוּתָא. Targ. Y. Deut. V, 8. Targ. O. Ex. XX, 4 ed. Berl.; a. fr.

דְּמוּי, דְּמוּ m. same. Targ. Y. Ex. XX, 4; a. e.

דְּמוּךְ, v. דְּמַךְ.

דְּמוּכָא m. (preced.) *sleep.* Targ. Esth. II, 21 בית ד׳ bed-room.

דמולא, Targ. Prov. VI, 31 Ms. (ed. מולא), read מוֹדְלָא.

דמוסא, דמוסיא, v. דימ׳.

דְּמוּעַ, v. דִּימ׳.

דָּמוֹת *gossip,* v. דִּימָה.

דְּמוּת f. (b. h.; דמי) *resemblance, image,* esp. *man's divine image* (Gen. I, 26). Yeb. 63ᵇ כאילו ממעט הד׳ as though he diminished the divine image (by neglecting the propagation of man). Num. R. s. 19 מדמין ד׳ גבורה של מעלה וכ׳ they compare the appearance of Divinity to the shape of man; a. fr.—*Pl.* דְּמוּיוֹת. Pesik. R. s. 33 כמה ד׳ נדמיתי וכ׳ in how many images (visions) did I appear to you!—Yalk. Ex. 422 שני ד׳ אחד וכ׳ (!) two embroidered *designs,* one on each side.

דְּמוּתָא, דְּמוּת ch. same. Targ. O. Ex. XX, 4 (v. דְּמוּ). Targ. O. Deut. IV, 15 sq.; a. e.—Pesik. Parah, p. 41ª כִּדְמוּתֵיהּ אנא וכ׳ whenever I see a vision resembling him &c.; Pesik. R. s. 14 בדמותיה (corr. acc.).

דִּימ׳, דְּמַחֲמְרָא m. (Difel of מְחַמַּר, v. חֲמַר I, a. דְּ־) *that which is ruined; ruins, debris.* Targ. Is. XXIII, 13; XXV, 2 (h. text מפלה).

דָּמָה, דמי (b. h.; v. דום, דמם) 1) *to mumble, think* (cmp. דבב); *to be silent.* Denom. (דִּימָה, דְּמוּת.—2) *to imagine, compare.* Denom. דְּמוּת.—3) (denom. of דְּמוּת) *to resemble, be like, to imitate.* Sabb. 133b הוי דומה לו imitate Him. Ber. 29b שתפלתו דוֹמָה עליו וכ׳ to whom his prayer appears like a burden. Taan. 22b אין דורו דומה יפה (v. Rabb. D. S. a. l. note 20) his generation was not considered worthy. B. Kam. 92b; Yalk. Jud. 67 ובן אדם לדו׳ לו (not ובני)and man associates with his equal. Sifra Sh'mini Par. 10, ch. XII; Hull. 76b הַדּוֹמֶה that which resembles the animal specified in the Bible (species); הד׳ לַדּוֹמֶה what resembles the animal classified with the animal specified in the Bible (genus); a. fr.—אֵינוֹ דּוֹמֶה there is no resemblance, *you cannot compare.* Yeb. 64a א׳ ד׳ תפלת.... לתפלת וכ׳ you cannot compare the prayer of .... to the prayer of &c. Sabb. 119b; a. fr.—Hull. 48b זו דּוֹמָה לזו these are analogous cases, v. Pi.—(משל) למה הדבר דומה (abbrev. לה״ד, מלה״ד) (a simile:) to what can this be compared?, a phrase introducing a simile. Taan. 25b. Yoma 86b; a. v. fr.

Nif. נִדְמָה [1) (b. h.) *to be silenced, undone*].—2) *to be compared, to be imagined; to appear in the disguise of; to seem.* Kidd. 32b כמה״ש נִדְמוּ לו that they appeared to him as ministering angels; נדמו לו לערביים they appeared to him as if they were Arabs. Succ. 52a צדיקים נ׳ להם כהר וכ׳ to the righteous sin will appear like a high mount; a. fr.—נִדְמֶה an animal *suspected* to be a hybrid or looking like one (cmp. הַכַּאי), esp. *a lamb looking like a kid,* and vice versa. Bekh. 12a 'a ewe which gave birth to what looked like a kid'. Hull. 38b; a. fr.

Pi. הִדִּימָה 1) *to compare, judge from analogy.* Lev. R. s. 32 דִּמִּיתִיךָ להם I made thee like them (beasts). B. Bath. 130b ובלבד שלא יְדַמֶּה וכ׳ but one must not decide ritual cases by analogy; v. Hull. 48b.—2) *to have an opinion* without authority to refer to. Gitt. 19a; 37a מפני שאנו מְדַמִּין because we have such an opinion.—*Part. pass.* מְדוּמֶּה, pl. מְדוּמִּין; כמ׳ אני *it seems to me,* כמ׳ אנו *it seems to us* &c. Men. 18a. Taan. 23a; a. fr.—Y. Ber. II, 5b bot. כמ׳ הייתי I thought.

דְּמָא I, דְּמֵי ch. same, 1) *to be dumb.* Targ. Hab. II, 19 דַּמְיָא (some ed. incorr. ר׳).—2) *to imagine, suspect, consider,* Targ. I Kings VIII, 27 דָּמֵי (incorr. חמי).—Part. act. a. pass. דָּמֵי *suspected, considered; resembling, like.*—Yeb. 114b אמרה בדְדָמֵי she speaks of what was to be suspected (under the circumstances, though she has not seen it).—שפיר דמי it is considered as right, *it is right.* Ab. Zar. 38b ש׳ ד׳ it is all right (is permitted). Ber. 13b הא מיגנא ש׳ ד׳ but to lie (on the back) is permitted; a. v. fr.—Ber. 25b כוליה ביתא .... ד׳ the entire house is to be considered (for legal purposes) as four cubits. Ib. 4b כתפלה אריכתא דַּמְיָא is to be considered as one continued prayer, v. אֲרִיכָא; a. fr.—היכי דמי (abbrev. ה״ד) what is it like? *in what case?* Yeb. 63b ה״ד אשה רעה what do you call 'a bad wife'? Sabb. 4a ה״ד אילימא וכ׳ what case do you mean? Do you mean the case of an involuntary transgressor &c.?; a. v. fr.—Targ. Y. I Deut. XXXII, 32, v. *Pa.*—Erub. 54a כהלולא ד׳ is like a wedding feast (soon passing away). B. Kam. 85a דָּמְיָת עלי כאריא וכ׳, v. אֲרַב. Taan. 21b דָּמְיָן מעייהו ל- their entrails look like those of human beings; a. fr.—Pes. 14b, a. fr. מי דָּמֵי is this like (the other)?, i. e. there is no analogy between them.

Pa. דַּמֵּי 1) *to compare.* Targ. Is. XL, 25; a. fr.—Hull. 55b, a. e. טרפות קא מְדַמֵּית להדדי you compare cases of *T'refoth* to one another (form an analogy)? (v. preced. *Pi.*). Snh. 47a מי קא מדמית וכ׳ can you compare &c.?—Part. pass. מְדַמֵּי, f. מְדַמְיָא, pl. מְדַמְיָין. Targ. Y. II Deut. XXXII, 32 sq. (Y. I דמי׳).—2) *to imagine, speculate.* Targ. Jud. XI, 23. Targ. Is. XLV, 9; a. e.

Ithpe. אִתְדְּמֵי, אִידְּמֵי, אִדּ׳ 1) *to be like, to take an example.* Targ. Prov. VI, 6 אִתְדְּמָא וכ׳ imitate the ant (ed. Vien. אִתְרְמֵי, read אתד׳). Targ. Ps. CII, 7; a. e.—Y. Shek. IV, 48d top; Y. Dem. I, 21d bot. לא אִידְּמִינָן we cannot compare ourselves. Gitt. 57b איתו דמי ולא אִידְּמוּ they brought blood of animals but it did not look like (the blood of the prophet); a. fr.—2) *to appear* in the disguise of. Kidd. 81a ... א״ ליה שטן כ Satan appeared to him as a woman &c. Ib. 29b א״ ליה וכ׳ (a demon) appeared to him as a monster &c. Snh. 95a א״; a. fr.

דְּמֵי II, 1) pl. of דְּמָא.—2) *value,* v. דָּמִין.

דְּמֵי, v. דְּמַאי.

דְּמִיטְיָנוּס׳, v. דּוֹמִיט׳.

דְּמִיכְתָּא, constr. דְּמִיכַת f. (דמך) *sleep.* Targ. Koh. V, 11.

דָּמִין, דָּמִים m. pl., constr. דְּמֵי (דמה) *equivalent, compensation;* (cmp. שָׁוֶה) *price, value; payment.* Pes. 112b בשעה שאין לך ד׳ do not bargain when thou hast no money to pay with. Kerith. 13b ד׳ וערכין the assessment of an object to be redeemed or of an object the value of which was dedicated, v. עֵרֶךְ.—Pes. 32a ... לפי מידה או לפי ד׳ וכ׳ must he pay the fine according to quantity or according to value?—Kidd. I, 6 כל הנעשה ד׳ באחר whatever is used as payment for another object; expl. ib. 28a כל הנישום ד׳ וכ׳ whatever is assessed as an equivalent, i. e. an exchange is meant and not a sale for cash. Ib.b החליף דמי שור בפרה if he gives a cow in payment of money which he owes for an ox; a. fr.—Keth. 103b נהוג נשיאותך בד׳ Ar. conduct thy office of Nasi as something valuable (Var. in Ar., a. ed. בִּרְמִים).

דְּמֵי, דָּמִין, דְּמֵי constr. **דְּמֵי** ch. same. Targ. Lam. V, 4 (h. text מְחִיר); a. fr.—B. Mets. 5b he thinks (as a mental reservation) דמי קא יהבנא ליה I am willing to compensate him. Ib. לא תחמוד לאינשי בלא ד׳ משמע להו common people understand the law, 'thou shalt not covet' (Ex. XX, 16) to mean coveting to get our neighbor's property without compensation. B. Kam. 46a אי דְּמֵי רדיא וכ׳ if he paid the market price of a ploughing ox, he surely bought him for ploughing; a. fr.

דָּמִין (or דַּמִּין) pr. n. pl. *Damin* (D'min), later name of *Ădami* (Josh. XIX, 33). Y. Meg. I, 70a bot.

דְּמַךְ, דְּמִיךְ, דְּמוּךְ *to sleep; to die, to lie in the grave.* Targ. Ps. III, 6. Ib. IV, 9; a. fr.—Gen. R. s. 72, beg. עמך הוא דמיך he (Jacob) will lie with thee in the grave.

Ib. s. 91, a. fr. כד ד׳ וכ׳ when R... was dead; a. v. fr.—Ruth R. to III, 13; Koh. R. to VII, 8 ודָמְכַת לה and the fire over the grave died out.

Pa. דַּמֵּךְ same. Targ. Koh. V, 11. Targ. Job III, 13, some ed.—Y. Maas. Sh. IV, 55[c] top והוא גברא יתיב מְדַמֵּךְ (not מדרך) and this man (I, thou) dreamt that he was sitting and sleeping.

Ithpe. אִידְּמִיךְ to feel the approach of death. Y. Kil. IX, 32[c] bot.; Y. Keth. XII, 35[b].

דַּמְכָא, דְּמָכָא, דּוּמ׳ m. (preced.) *sleep; couch.* Targ. Ps. CXXXII, 4. Targ. Y. Deut. XXVIII, 16; a. e.—*Pl.* דַּמְכִין. Targ. Ps. CXLIX, 5 דַּמכירהון Ms. (ed. דּמ׳) their resting places.

דַּמְכוּתָא f. (preced.) *death.* Y. Ab. Zar. III, 42[c] top.

דָּמַם (b. h.; v. דָּמָה, הוּם) 1) *to be silent, dumb, at rest; to be stricken dumb.* Pesik. R. s. 33 (ref. to Is. VI, 5) היאך היה לי שֶׁדָּמַמְתִּי how did it happen to me that I was silent (did not join in the praises of the angels)? Taan. 20[a] דָּמְמוּ הרוחות when the winds subside. Snh. 91[a] כאבן הדּוֹמֵם like a dumb stone. Ber. 19[a] יושב ודוֹמֵם sits in silence; a. fr.—*Part. pass.* דָּמוּם, f. דְּמוּמָה. Lam. R. to I, 17 (ref. to אֶדַּדֵּם, Ps. XLII, 5) ועכשיו ד׳ סלקא וכ׳ and now in silence does she (Israel) go up (to the ruins of Jerusalem), and in silence &c.—V. דִּמְדֵּם.—2) *to leave off.* Midr. Till. to Ps. IV, 5 (ref. to ודמו ib.) [read:] ובלבד שתָּדוֹם וכ׳ provided that thou leavest off from the sin &c.; Yalk. ib. 627.

Hif. הִדְמִים *to silence, bring to a stand-still.* Ex. R. s. 29 end ה׳ כל העולם He made the world stand still. Gen. R. s. 97 שהוא מַדְמִים וכ׳ who will bring to a stand-still sun and moon.

דַּמַּסְקָאָה, v. דַּמֶּשֶׂק.

דַּמַּסְקוֹס pr. n. pl. (Damascus) *Damascus* in Syria. Y. Bicc. III, 65[d] כד מסקום read בד׳ in D.

דָּמַע (b. h.) *to flow, shed tears.* Tosef. Bekh. IV, 4 אם..... דּוֹמַעַת if his eye is tearing. Bekh. 44[a], v. דָּלַף. [Sifré Deut. 157 שזולגו עיניו ... עד שיהו דומעות, read: דְּמָעוֹת; v. Sot. VII, 8.]

Pi. דִּמַּע (denom. of דֶּמַע II) *to make a thing, otherwise exempt, subject to the law of T'rumah, to mix secular grain, wine, oil &c. with T'rumah in proportions sufficient to make the whole prohibited to non-priests;* in gen. *to mix secular with sacred things.* Orl. II, 4; 6 הַמְדַמֵּעַ; a. fr.—Ter. III, 1 אינה מְדַמַּעַת וכ׳ does not make *Dema* by itself (if mixed with secular fruits). Ib. 2 אינה מְדַמַּעְתָּן does not make them *dema;* מְדַמְּעוֹת בקטנה וכ׳ make *dema,* the smallest of the two being considered as an admixture; a. fr.—Part. pass. מְדוּמָּע. Ib. V, 6 אין המדומע מדמע וכ׳ that which became subject to the law of T'rumah through an admixture, can affect a second mixture only in proportion, i. e. according to the quantity of real T'rumah contained therein. Ḥag. III, 4 wine jars or oil jars הַמְדוּמָּעוֹת which have been mixed up; expl. ib. 25[b] מד׳ דקדש containing liquids, a portion of which was designated for libations.

Nif. נִדְמַע *to become Dema through mixture.* Ter. l. c. Nidd. 46[b] עיסה שנִדְמְעָה if a sufficient quantity of T'rumah has been put in a dough to make it forbidden to non-priests; a. e.

דְּמַע ch. *to tear, drip.* Targ. Jer. XIII, 17 (some ed. דַּמַּע .. *Pa.*). Targ. Lam. II, 18.

דֶּמַע I m. (b. h.; preced.) 1) *tear, weeping.* Men. 30[a]; B. Bath. 15[a] Moses wrote בד׳ (Ms. M. בִּדְמָעוֹת) with tears (so that he could not speak).—*Pl.*, v. דִּמְעָה.

דֶּמַע II m. (b. h.; cmp. נִיב, תְּנוּבָה) *fruits,* whence (sub. רֵאשִׁית, מַתְּנַת, v. Ex. XXII, 28) *the priest's share of the produces, T'rumah.* Mekh. Mishp. s. 19; Yalk. Ex. 351 T'rumah has three names, *Reshith, T'rumah* וד׳ and *Dema;* Tem. 4[a]. Ohol. XVI, 4 אוכל בדְמָעוֹ he may partake of his priestly share. Tosef. Ter. X, 16 בית הד׳ place in the barn designated for T'rumah.

דִּמְעָא f. 1) *tear.* v. דִּמְעֲתָא.—2) as preced. Targ. O. Ex. XXII, 28.

דִּמְעָה f. (b. h.; preced. wds.) *tear,* collect. *tears, weeping.* Lam. R. to II, 11 דִּמְעַת חסם וכ׳ (Ar. החסית, Var. חשום, v. Ar. Compl. ed. Koh. s. v. חסית) tears caused by pungent matter, mustard &c. Ib. ד׳ הקרר Ar. l. c. (ed. Amst. הקבר, ed. Lam. R. בית הכסא, v. Sabb. 152[a] top); Ab. d'R. N. II, ch. XLVIII (ed. Schechter, p. 132 הדקר) tears caused by severe cold; a. e.—*Pl.* דְּמָעוֹת. Ib.; Sabb. 151[b]; Ab. d'R. N. ch. XLI (XLVIII, v. supra); a. fr.—B. Bath. 15[a], v. דֶּמַע.

דִּמְעֲתָא ch. same. Targ. Is. XXXVIII, 5; a. fr.—*Pl.* דִּמְעָן, דִּמְעָתָא. Targ. Ps. CXVI, 8. Targ. Lam. II, 11 (ed. Lag. דִּמְעִין m., fr. דִּמְעָא). Targ. Jer. XIII, 17 דמען ed. Lag. (oth. ed. עין ..); a. fr.—Bets. 22[a]; Ab. Zar. 28[b] דִּמְעֲתָא (or עֲתָא .. sing.) constant tearing of the eyes.—Sabb. 33[b] דִּמְעָה עיניה (some ed. דִּמְעַת, Ms. M. דִּמְעִיה) tears dropped from his eyes.

דְּמַר*, *Ithpa.* אִתְדַּמַּר (v. P. Sm. p. 921) *to be stupefied, astonished.* Targ. Prov. VI, 30 לא לְמִיתְדַּמְּרוּ (Ms. a. some ed. למתר׳, corr. acc.) let them not be astonished (h. text יבוזו, v. LXX).

דַּמֶּשֶׂק (b. h.) pr. n. pl. *Damascus.* Targ. O. Gen. XIV, 15 (Y. I דַּרְמָשֶׂק). Targ. Is. XVII, 1; a. fr.—Sifré Deut. 1 שאני מד׳ I (R. José b. Durmaskith) am from D., v. דּוּרְמַסְקִית; a. fr.

דַּמַּשְׂקָאָה m. *of Damascus.* Targ. O. Gen. XV, 2 (ed. Berl. דַּמַּס׳).

דְּמֵת, v. דּוּמָא.

דָּן (b. h.) 1) pr. n. m. *Dan,* son of Jacob. Pes. 4[a] מדן קאתי he is a descendant of Dan; a. e.—2) pr. n. pl. *Dan* in northern Palestine. Pesik. Shek. p. 15[a] מזבח שבדן the altar (erected by Jeroboam) in Dan.—Targ. Y. II Num. XXXIV, 15. Targ. Cant. V, 4; Pirké d'R. El. ch. XXVII expl.=פמיאס, *Paneas;* Midr. Sam. ch. XXX; XXXII פנירס (יען) דנה.—Y. Dem. II, 22[c] bot. כְּפַר דָּן.—3) name of an idol *Dan.* Sabb. 67[b]; Tosef. ib. VII (VIII), 3; Y. ib. VI, 8[c] bot. (ref. to Am. VIII, 14).

דֵּן, דֵּין, emph. **דְּנָא, דְּנָה** c. (cmp. דָּא, הָדֵן) *this, that.* Targ. Is. VI, 3. Targ. Deut. II, 3 הָדֵן (ed. Berl. הָא ד׳=הָדֵין); a. v. fr.—Lev. R. s. 7 מן הד׳ קריא from this verse (it is proven). Ib. s. 8 ד׳ אמר לינא בעיא לד׳ וכ׳ the one said, I do not want this (woman) &c. Sabb. 112[b] לית ד׳ ב״א this is not (an ordinary) human being; ib. כגון ד׳ וכ׳ a man like this is worth the name of a human being; a. fr.—Y. Ab. Zar. II, 41[d] bot.; a. e. אסיר לך דנא this (piece) is forbidden to thee.—מן קדמת דנא ere this, formerly. Y. Sot. II, 17[d]; a. e.—כְּדֵי a)=h. פֹּה, *here* (cmp. כָּא, הָכָא). Targ. Jud. XVIII, 3. Targ. Is. XXII, 16 (some ed. כְּדֵין); b) *like this, thus.* Targ. Gen. XXXII, 4. Targ. Jud. XVIII, 4; a. fr. [Targ. Ps. II, 10 read; כְּדוּן.]—B. Bath. 75[a] (play on כדכד, Is. LIV, 12) לִיהוֹי כד׳ וכד׳ let it be as this one says, and as that one; Pesik. Aniy. p. 135[b]; Pesik. R. s. 32.—בְּכְדֵין in this manner. Targ. 1 Kings XXII, 20.—מְדֵין=h. מַה־זֶּה, *why.* Targ. Jer. XXVI, 9; a. e.—אֵי מְהֵדֵין *from what, which.* Targ. Jon. I, 8.—הֵינוּ (=הֵין הוּ) *this.* Y. Erub. VII, 24[c] top, a. e. חֵי ד׳ צד וכ׳ (=h. אֵיזֶהוּ) which is 'side', and which &c.?, v. הֵיידֵינוּ.—*Pl.* הֵינוּן, הֵינֵי. Y. Snh. IV, 22[b] bot. חי ד׳ וכ׳ which are the two additional ones?—[הָדֵין *then,* v. הֵיידֵין.]

דְּנָא 1) v. preced.—2) v. דְּנָה. [Targ. Prov. VIII, 7 דנא, Var. ed. Lag., v. רְנָא.]

דַּנָּא m. (v. אוּדְנָא II) *a cylindrical vessel, jar* (dolium). Yoma 28[b] ד׳ דחלא a jar of vinegar (which emits a stronger smell through a slight opening than when open). Ab. Zar. 60[a], v. כּוּבָא II. Sabb. 157[b], v. אוּדְנָא II.

דָּנָב* pr. n. pl. *Danab.* Tosef. Dem. I, 13 אוצרה של ד׳ Var. (ed. Zuck. ר׳). Tosef. Shebi. IV, 8 (Var. ed. Zuck. דנב, דגב, text ר׳); Y. Dem. II, 22[d] top דבב.

דּוּנְבָא, דַּנְבָא m. (=h. זָנָב) *tail.* Targ. Jud. XV, 4. Targ. Job XL, 17, v. גְּנוּבְתָּא I. Targ. O. Ex. IV, 4 ed. Berl. (ed. זַנ׳); a. e.—*Pl.* דַּנְבֵי, דַּנְבַיָּא. Targ. Jud. l. c. Targ. Y. Gen. XXXVII, 2; a. e.—Snh. 37[a] בדנבי (Ms. M. בד׳) among the last (in the front row).

דַּנְגָּאֵר, v. זִינְגָּאֵר.

דַּנְדְּנָה, דַּנְדְּנָא f. *mint* (Maim.). Shebi. VII, 1 עלה ד׳ חור the leaves of *dandana;* 2 עקר ד׳ חור the root of &c. (Y. ed. חור׳, corr. acc.); Nidd. 51[b] (v., however, Löw Pfl. p. 108 sq.).

דְּנָא, דְּנָה 1) v. דֵּן.—2)=הָאֲנָא *which I.* Y. Pes. V, 32[c] bot. (Y. Taan. III, 67[a] bot. דאנא).

דְּנַח *to shine, be bright* (corresp. to h. זרח). Targ. Gen. XXXII, 32; a. fr.—Lev. R. s. 27 ושמשא דַּנְחָא וכ׳ does the sun shine in your country?; Gen. R. s. 33 אית גבכון שמשא דנח; Tanḥ. Emor 6; Y. B. Mets. II, 8[c] bot.

דני a word in a charm formula. Sabb. 67[b] הוּנוּ דָּנֵי *be strong, my vessels* (Rashi, v. דָּנָא); Y. ib. VI, 8[c] bot.; Tosef. ib. VII (VIII), 3 דני דני.

דָּנִיאֵל (b. h.) pr. n. m. *Daniel,* 1) the Babylonian exile. Snh. 93[a]; a. fr.—Erub. 21[a] בי כנישתא דד׳ a synagogue named from D., v. בְּרְנִשׁ.—B. Bath. 14[b]; 15[a] *the Book of Daniel.*—2) name of an Amora. Y. Succ. IV, 54[b] bot. Hull. 62[a]; a. fr.—3) one Daniel, 'the tailor', a scholar. Lev. R. s. 32, end; Koh. R. to IV, 1.

דָּנִיסְטֵיס, v. דָּנִס׳.

דַּנְכוֹ pr. n. m. *Dankho,* name of an expert money changer. B. Kam. 99[b] (Ms. M. בנכו, דנכו).

דְּנָן, דֵּינָן c. (=דֵּן) *this one; there.* Targ. Ps. XXIV, 6; a. e.—Targ. Gen. XXV, 32; Targ. Num. XI, 20 למא ד׳= h. למה זה.—B. Mets. 15[a]. Ib. 18[a]; Keth. 89[b].—כְּדְנָן *thus.* Targ. Gen. XXXII, 5; a. e.

דָּאנ׳, דָּנִיס׳, דָּנִסְטֵיס m. (δανειστής, danista) *money-lender, usurer, creditor.* Ex. R. s. 29 טוס .... (corr. acc.). Ib. s. 31, beg. דיוסטוס (corr. acc.). Num. R. s. 9, beg. הד׳ משבר שיניו the lender breaks the debtor's teeth (enforces his claim). Y. Sabb. II, 5[b] top (ref. to יַשִּׁי, Ps. LV, 16) he makes the angel of death ד׳ שלו (some ed. דיני) his creditor (to collect his debts, visit his sins). Y'lamd. Thazr. end (quot. in Ar.) דנסטס, (Var. דינסטיס, corr. acc.). [Ib. to Deut. IV, 30 אני דינאסטוס וכ׳ ed. Koh. (v. Var. ib.), v. דִּינַאסְטוֹס.]—*Pl.* דָּנִסְטִין. Ib. to Deut. XXIV, 10.—Y. B. Mets. II, 8[c] ארלין דאירסטוס; Y. Ab. Zar. V, 42[b] bot. אילין דאוסיניסי, read: דָּאנִסְטִיסֵי.

דְּנַק (Difel of אנק, v. דּ־) *to feel narrow, to choke.* *Ithpe.* אִידְּנַק 1) *to sigh, sob* (corresp. to h. אנק). Targ. Ezek. XXIV, 17. Targ. Mal. II, 13. Targ. Ezek. IX, 4 מידני ed. Lag. (ed. מאנ׳).—2) (cmp. חֲנַק) *to regret, despair.* Ib. VI, 9; XX, 43; XXXVI, 31.

דָּנְקָא m. (Pers. dânkh; δανάκη) *Danka,* a small Persian coin, *the sixth of a Denar,* in gen. *one sixth.* B. Mets. 60[b] מאה בד׳ one hundred *P'rutah* for a *d.*—Ib. 39[b] ואידך תילתא יהבינן ד׳ וכ׳ and of the remaining one third we give one sixth to the sister, and for the other one sixth we appoint &c.—Zeb. 48[a]; Kerith. 22[b] בר ד׳, בת ד׳ worth a *d.*—Sabb. 35[a] [read with Rashi:] א״ב פלגא דד׳ the difference between two thirds and three fourths (of a mile) is half a sixth.—*Pl.* דַּנְקֵי. R. Hash. 26[a] (identified with מָעָה a. קְשִׁיטָה).

דנקאי, Gen. R. s. 79, v. נַקָּאי.

דנרסי, v. הַדְּהֵסִין.

דְּסִ־, for words under דְּס׳, v. under דִּיס׳.

דסיקרין, v. דִּיסְקְרִין.

דַּסְקָא* m., an assumed word for טַסְקָא q. v. Kidd. 70[b] (criticising the spelling דסקא for דיסקא, in a summons issued by R. Naḥman) הא גברא והא ד׳ this word (ג, ב, ר, a. א) is read *gabra* and so this word (ד, ס, ק a. א) must be read *daska* (which you must have meant for *taska*).

דעד, Targ. Nah. III, 12 some ed., v. רְעַד.

דַּעֲדֵּק (=רקדק, v. דקק) *to crush, break into small fragments; to humiliate.* Targ. II Chr. XXXIV, 7. Targ. Job XVI, 12 (Ms. Var. רצדק׳, corr. acc.). Ib. XL, 12.

דַּעֲדֵּק m. (preced.) *powdered; minute, tender, young.* Targ. O. Ex. XVI, 14 (Y. הְקִיק) *something powdered.*—Targ. Am. VII, 1; a. e.—*Pl.* דַּעְדְּקִין, דַּעְדְּקַיָּא; f. דַּעְדְּקָן. Targ. Jer. XVI, 6. Targ. O. Num. XXIII, 10; a. e.—Targ. Ez. XVI, 61.—Tosef. Snh. II, 5 וכאימריא ד׳ and that the spring lambs are yet tender; Snh. 11[b] Ms. M. (ed. ערקין, Var. עדקין, v. Rabb. D. S. a. l. note). V. הַקִּיק a. הְרַקְּ.

דֵּיעָה, דֵּעָה f. (b.h.; ידע) *knowledge, understanding, reason; view; taste.* Snh. 92[a] אדם שיש בו ד׳ a man that has obtained knowledge. Lev. R. s. 1 (prov.) ד׳ קנית וכ׳ if thou hast acquired knowledge, what doest thou lack? &c. —Cant. R. to IV, 3 ד׳ סרוחה של וכ׳ the corrupt mind of, i. e. the fool, Ahasver; a. v. fr.—*Pl.* דֵּיעוֹת, דֵּעוֹת (used also in Chald. phrases). Shebu. 42[a] אזלינן בתר רוב ד׳ we are guided by the majority of opinions; Yoma 83[a]; Tem. 27[b] בתר ד׳ אזלינן. Shebu. l. c. כיון דנחית לד׳ since he cared to mention a certain number of minds (as witnesses). Y. Sot. I, 17[a]; Tosef. ib. V, 9; a. e. כשם שיש ד׳ וכ׳ as men differ in tastes (sensibilities) as regards food and drink, so do husbands differ &c. Pes. 112[a] ארבע ד׳ וכ׳ there are four thoughts &c. (the husband thinking of his first wife and the wife of her first husband); a. fr. V. דַּעַת.

דֵּעָוֹן, דֵּעְוֹן f. pl. ch. (preced.) *opinions.* Y. Yeb. I, 2[c] bot.; Y. Keth. VI, beg. 30[c] ד׳ ד׳ אית וכ׳ there are different opinions related in behalf of &c.; ib. V, 30[a] top רעיון העיון (corr. acc.).

דָּעַךְ (b. h.; cmp. דּוּךְ) *to crush, stamp upon.* Sifré Num. 160.

Nif. נִדְעַךְ *to be stamped upon, crushed, annihilated.* Pesik. R. s. 35 נִדְעֲכוּ והלכו להם they were annihilated (their resistance broken) and gone.

דְּעַךְ ch. same, esp. *to extinguish, quench.* Targ. Prov. XVI, 14 נִדְעֲכִנֵּיה ed. Lag. (some ed. נדעיר׳, corr. acc.).—דְּעֵיךְ *to be quenched.* Targ. Is. XLIII, 17 דְּעִיכוּ (ed. Lag. דער׳). Targ. Prov. X, 7; XIII, 9, a. e. נִדְעַךְ shall be quenched.

Af. אַדְעֵיךְ *to quench.* Ib. XV, 18.

דְּעַץ (v. הוּץ II) *to prick, squeeze, fix, stick.*—Part. pass. דְּעִיץ *fixed.* Targ. Y. Ex. II, 21.

Pa. דְּעֵיץ same. Targ. O. Gen. XXX, 38 ed. Berl. (some ed. וד׳; Bxt. וְדְעִיץ *Pe.*).—B. Bath. 74[a] דַּעֲצִיתֵהּ וכ׳ (Ms. M. אנחיתיה, Ar. דַּצְיֵיה, v. Rabb. D. S. a. l. note). I stuck it on the point of the lance.

דַּעַץ, Snh. 22[a] Var. in Ar. s. v. רעץ, v. רַעַץ.

דעקין, Y. B. Kam. X, 7[c] top בר נש ד׳, v. עָקָא.

דַּעַת f. (b.h.; v. דֵּעָה) *knowledge, mind; temperament, physical disposition, constitution.* עלתה על ד׳ *to occur to one's mind, to strike.* Sot. IX, 6 (45[b]); a. fr.—שיקול הד׳ weighing of opinions, i. e. decision between opposite views. Snh. 6[a] טעה בש׳ הד׳ made a mistake in deciding, against the common practice, a case concerning which there are opposite authorities, opp. to a decision against an established law; ib. 33[a]; Y. Keth. IX, 33[a]; Y. Snh. I, 18[a] bot.—Y. Ḥag. II, 77[b] top אין דַּעְתָּן נקיה their mind is not pure (unfit to study esoterics).—B. Mets. 11[b], a. e. ד׳ אחרת מקנה a deputized person (or fictitious person, e. g. one's ground) can take possession. Snh. 25[a] sq. תולה בד׳ עצמו one who makes the chance of a game dependent on his own action, e. g. throwing dice, תולה בד׳ יונו who makes it dependent on his dove's flight.—Tosef. Ḥull. VII, 1 וד׳ מכרעת reason decides in favor &c.; Ḥull. 90[b] מאי ד׳ ד׳ תורה by saying 'reason decides' does he mean a reasonable interpretation of the Biblical law, or is he in doubt and 'reason decides' means ד׳ נוטה his opinion inclines in favor of &c.?—מִדַּ׳, לְדַ׳ *with the consent of, with the knowledge of,* opp. בעל ברח־, v. בּוֹרֵחַ. Kidd. 44[a] מד׳ אביה with her father's consent; מִדַּעְתָּהּ with her consent. Ib. שלא לד׳ אביה without her father's consent; a. fr.—ד׳ יפה good physical constitution, מי שדעתו ד׳ *not fastidious* in taste, opp. אִיסְטְנִיס q. v.—ד׳ קצרה *impatience, greed,* ד׳ רחבה *contentedness.* B. Bath. 145[b] bot.; Snh. 101[a] top.—Ber. 29[b] דַּעְתָּם קצרה they are impatient (Rashi: they do not understand how to express their wishes).—Pes. 113[b] אין הד׳ סובלתן whom the mind cannot endure; a. fr.—*Pl.* דֵּעוֹת, v. דֵּעָה.

דַּעְתָּא ch. same. Targ. Job XV, 2; a. fr.—Ber. 18[b] אחלישתיה לְדַעְתֵּיה thou madest him feel badly; Ḥull. 94[b]. —Ber. 33[b] bot. לא כיון דעתיה he had not his mind directed on it, recited without devotion. Ib. 36[a] צנון .... אַדַּ׳ וכ׳ people plant radishes with the intention of eating them when they are young. Ib. מאי דַּעְתָּךְ כר״ע (in doing so) what was thy opinion? Is it that thou holdest to R. A.?—Kidd. 81[b]; Ber. 26[a], a. fr. לאו אַדַּעְתָּאִי I did not think of it. Keth. 3[a], a. fr. כל דמקדש אַדַּ׳ וכ׳ whosoever betroths a wife to himself does so with the implicit understanding that his act is in agreement with the rabbinical enactments.—M. Kat. 17[a], v. בְּדַה. Gitt. 70[b] ד׳ צילותא a clear mind, full consciousness; ד׳ שגישתא a confused mind, delirium. M. Kat. 26[b] bot. כמה לית ביה ד׳ וכ׳ how little sense (manners) has this scholar!—סלקא דעתך (abbr. ס״ד) it enters thy mind, i. e. you may think. Ber. 41[b] כל שיעוריה ס״ד 'all its measures',—you cannot mean that?—Pes. 2[a], a. fr. קא ס״ד וכ׳ (abbr. קס״ד) thy first impression naturally was that he who said 'light' meant really &c. (an editorial remark for the sake of introducing a discussion on premises finally to be upset). Ib. 14[b] דאי ס״ד וכ׳ for if we were to think that it was a rabbinical law; ib. 18[a]; a. fr.—Ib. top ואי ס״ד מכלים וכ׳ if we were to assume that he withdrew his opinion only as to vessels &c.; ib. 19[a]; a. fr.—Sot. 46[a] ס״ד אמינא .... צריכא you may possibly think we say, i. e. you may be misled to interpret &c.; therefore (to obviate such a misinterpretation) a Biblical intimation is required; a. fr.

דַּף m. (דפף, *to hammer, join;* cmp. דפן) *board, plank;* trnsf. *a column* in the scroll (later Hebr. *a leaf* of a book).

Kel. XV, 2 ד׳ של נחתומות וכ׳ the (metal) plank of the bakers joined to the wall; B. Bath. 66a, b. Yad. IV, 8 בד׳ on the same column. Tosef. Gitt. IX (VII), 10; a. fr.—*Pl.* דַּפִּין, דַּפִּים. Ab. Zar. 75a; Nidd. 65a הד׳ the planks used as frame in the wine press. Num. R. s. 14 (ed. Amst. p. 258c) מקיים הד׳ keeps the joined boards (of the door) together. Men. 30a בת שלש ד׳ (יריעה) a sheet of parchment wide enough for three columns. Ib.b לבין הד׳ in the space between the columns. Neg. XI, 9 דַּפֵּי חלוק the strips (widths) of a shirt; a. fr.

דַּפָּא ch. same. Targ. O. Ex. XXVI, 16 (Y. לוחא, h. text קֶרֶשׁ); a. fr.—Y. Meg. III, 74b bot. the word *ish* (Esth. IX, 6) בריש ד׳ must be written on the top of the column.—*Pl.* דַּפֵּי, דַּפַּיָּא, דַּפִּין. Targ. O. l. c. 18; a. fr. [Some ed. דַּפִּין, דַּפַּיָּא, דַּפָּא.]—B. Mets. 74a בי דפי the frame of the oil press, v. preced.—Succ. 36b ד׳ ד׳ דעבידא when the Ethrog was artificially moulded so as to look like planks joined together (angular); [Rashi: as the wheel of a water mill].

דפאטא, v. גְּזִירְדַּפְטֵּר.

דְּפוּס m. (interch. with טְפוּס; דַּף, cmp. form דְּלוּס) [*joined boards forming a frame*, v. דַּף pl.,] *frame, mould* for cakes &c. Men. XI, 1 (94a) ד׳ (Mish. ט׳). Dem. V, 4 מכל ד׳ וד׳ Ar. (ed. ט׳; Y. טִיפּוּס) from each cake-form. Succ. 36b גדלו בד׳ if one trained it (the Ethrog) in a frame.—B. Bath. 16a (ref. to Job XXXVIII, 25) to each rain drop in the clouds I created ד׳ בפני עצמה a special mould (that no two of them commingle).—Sabb. 64a ד׳ של דדין a cast of female breasts; a. e.—*Pl.* דְּפוּסִים, דְּפוּסִין. Men. 94a. Ib. 97a by קערותיו (Ex. XXV, 29) אלו הד׳ the cake-moulds are meant; Num. R. s. 13 (ed. Amst. p. 254a) דפוסי׳ (some ed.) read דְּפוּסָיו. V. טְפוּס, cmp. טוֹפֶס. [In modern Hebr. ד׳ *print*, בית הד׳ *printing office*; מַדְפִּיס *printer*, נִדְפַּס *printed*.]

דפוס, Targ. Y. II Gen. XLIX, 11 ד׳ ערגבין, read with Bxt. רְפוּס.

דפוסיו׳, דפוסות, דפוסי׳, v. דְּפוּס.

דפוקא, Num. R. s. 9 some ed., read רְפוּקָא.

דפטא, v. גְּזִירְדַּפְטֵּר.

דִּפְטִיָּא, v. דִּיוֹפְטְרִין.

דִּפִי, דָּפִיא, דְּפִיו, דְּפִי, v. דּוֹפִי, דּוֹפְיָא.

דְּפִיחַ, דְּפִיעַ, Var. of רְפִיעַ, רְפִיחַ q. v.

דפליסט׳, v. דִּיפְלָר.

דָּפַן (cmp. דַּף) *to hammer, force into a groove* &c.—Part. pass. דָּפוּן, f. דְּפוּנָה. Kel. II, 3 חבית ד׳ וכ׳ an attachment in the shape of a jar fitted into the projecting rims of a vessel (to serve as a handle).

Pi. דִּפֵּן *to force, enforce the law against.* Sifra Emor ch. I מנין אם לא רצה דַּפְּנוּ whence do we prove the rule, 'If he refuses (to dismiss her), force him'; Yeb. 88b מנין שאם וכ׳ (read אם). Ib. צריכא למימר דפנו (not דד׳, v. Yalk. Lev. 629). Ib. דפנו בעדים proceed against him by procuring counter-evidence.

דְּפַן, *Pa.* דַּפֵּן ch. same. B. Mets. 107b דַּפְּנוּהוּ they prosecuted him.

דַּפְּנָא m. (preced.) *beadle.*—*Pl.* דַּפְּנִין. Gitt. 34a משום דַּפְּנוֹי on account of his (R. Shesheth's) beadles (who forced him).

דַּפְנָא *partition*, v. דּוֹפְנָא.

דַּפְנָא m. (cmp. δάφνη which is prob. of Semitic origin, v. preced.) *Bay-tree* used for hedges. M. Kat. 7a; B. Bath. 4a; v. הוּצָא. Pes. 56a שירכא דד׳ the juice of the bay-fruit.

דפנא, דפנו, v. דַּפְנֵי.

דִּפְנוֹת pl. of דּוֹפֶן.

דַּפְנֵי (דָּפְנִי) pr. n. pl. *Daphne*, a suburb of Antiochia in Syria. Targ. Y. Num. XXXIV, 11 (h. text רבלה).—Lev. R. s. 19 ד׳ של וכ׳ (not דפנו) Daphne Antiochena; Y. Shek. VI, 50a bot. דופני; Y. Snh. X, 29c bot. (not דפנא).

דָּפַק (b. h.) *to knock, strike against.* Denom. דּוֹפֶק. [Gen. R. s. 44 שירהו מתדפקות, read מִתְרַפְּקוֹת, v. רָפַק.]

דְּפַק, *Pa.* דַּפֵּק ch. same, *to knock.* Lev. R. s. 5 [read:] מְדַפְּקָא לה she knocks at the door.

דִּפְרָא, v. דִּיפְרָא.

דִּפְשְׁקָא m. (Dif. of פשק, dial. for פסק, פתק, v. דְּ־; v. Koh. Ar. Compl. s. v. דבשקא; corresp. to בִּצְּעָה) *dyke, ditch.* *Pl.* דִּפְשְׁקֵי. Sabb. 21a ומד׳ רבי ed. (Ar. ובדוב׳, Mus. s. v. פשק quotes ומִפְשְׁקֵי in Rashi, דופש׳ in Talm.) and they grow in dykes.

דִּפְתְּרָא, דִּפְתִּי, v. דִּיפְתִּי.

דַּץ, v. דּוּץ.

דצדק, v. הַצְדֵּק.

דַּצּוֹצָא m. (דצץ, reduplic. of דּוּץ II) *a pullet in the egg-shell.* Bekh. 8b (some ed. ר׳, Ar. רציצא; Rashi הַצִּירָצָא).

דְּצִי (sec. r. of דּוּץ II) *to stick.* *Pa.* דַּצֵּי. B. Bath. 74a דַּצְּיֵיה, v. דַּעַץ.

***דְּצִיָּא** f. (רצי, sec. r. of דּוּץ I) *cheering up.* Targ. Prov. VI, 22 דַּצְיָיךְ Ms. (ed. רציך; h. text תשיחך).

***דְּצִיצָא** m. (דצץ, redupl. of דּוּץ I, cmp. preced.) *rejoicing.* Targ. Is. LXVI, 10 Ar. (ed. דִּיץ).

ד׳ עד״ש באח״ב, דצ״ך, *the initials* of the names *of the twelve Egyptian plagues.* דם, צפרדע, כנים; ערוב, דבר, שחין, ברד; ארבה, חשך, מכת בכורות. Ex. R. s. 5; s. 8 end; Tanh. Vaëra 9.

דַּק I m. (b. h.; דקק) *thin, fine, tender*, opp. גַּס. Hull. III, 1 עוף הד׳ small fowl (doves, birds &c.). Ib. VI, 7

זבל הד׳ powdered ordure, חול הד׳ fine sand; a. fr.—*Pl.* דַּקִּין, דַּקִּים. Ib. III, 1; a. fr. הד׳ the *small bowels.*—Y. Ber. II, 4[d] top בדקים (sub. נקבים) concerning the smaller functions of the body (urinizing, usu. קטנים), opp. גסים (usu. גדולים), v. גָּדוֹל.—Kel. II, 2 הד׳ שבכלי חרס the fine and small earthen vessels; a. fr.—Fem. דַּקָּה. ד׳ (בהמה), small cattle, v. גַּס. Ḥull. l. c. B. Kam. VII, 7. Ib. 80[a] חיה ד׳ small forest animals (deer, fox &c.). בד׳ (sub. מדה) in small quantities, *retail.* Dem. II, 5; Y. ib. 23[a] bot.; Tosef. ib. III, 12, v. לוּמָא.—Yoma IV, 4 ד׳ powdered frank incense, ד׳ מן הד׳ the very finest; a. fr.—*Pl.* דַּקּוֹת. Ḥull. 56[a]; a. fr.

דַּק, דַּקָּא ch. same.—*Pl.* דַּקִּיק. Naz. 59[b] לד׳ with the small bowels (of the sacrifice).

דַּק II, דֹּק, דּוּק m. (b. h.) *a veiled* or *withered spot* in the eye, *cataract.* Sifra Emor ch. II, Par. 3 דק זה חדוק the Biblical *dak* is what is now called *doḳ.* Bekh. 38[b] דוק שחור a black spot, ד׳ לבן a white spot.—*Pl.* דּוּקִין. Gitt. 56[a]; Ab. Zar. 51[a] ד׳ שכעין; a. e.—V. דּוּקָא II.

דִּקְדּוּק, דִּיק׳ m. (דִּקְדֵּק) 1) *crushing, humiliation, suffering.*—*Pl.* דִּקְדּוּקִים. Erub. 41[b] דִּקְדּוּקֵי עניות the sufferings of poverty.—2) *nicety, fine point, subtility, detail, minuteness;* [in later Hebr.: *grammar*]. Ab. ch. VI ד׳ חברים the fine points discussed among scholars. Snh. 99[a] חוץ מד׳ זה except this single point (in the adopted interpretation of the Law). Bekh. 30[b].—Y. Ber. II, 4[d] אלו צריכין ד׳ (not צריך) the following pairs of words require special care in pronouncing; Deut. R. s. 2 ד׳ אותיות.—*Pl.* as above, constr. דִּקְדּוּקֵי, דִּיק׳. Ḥull. 4[a] ד׳ מצות the details of ritual laws. Succ. 28[a] ד׳ תורה the subtile points in the interpretation of Biblical laws, ד׳ סופרים the special points in rabbinical enactments. Lev. R. s. 22 שני ד׳ שחיטה וכ׳ there are two defined rules concerning the cutting of animals. Y. Yoma III, 41[a]; Y. Sot. II, 18[a] כל ד׳ הפרשה all the particulars of the section; Tosef. ib. II, 1; a. fr.

דִּקְדּוּקָא, דִּיק׳ ch. same.—*Pl.* דִּקְדּוּקִין. Targ. Cant. V, 13.

דִּקְדֵּק (Pilp. of דוק or דקק) 1) *to crush, grind;* v. *Nithpa.*—*Part. pass.* מְדוּקְדָּק *broken, humiliated, afflicted.* Ex. R. s. 31 מדו׳ בענוות afflicted with poverty. Gen. R. s. 100 עני מדו׳ a very poor man.—2) *to even a woof by beating.* Tosef. Sabb. VIII (IX), 2; Sabb. 75[b]; 97[b] (v. Rashi a. l.).—3) *to examine minutely, search, investigate* (charity cases); *to trace genealogical records* (corresp. to בָּדַק); in gen. *to be very strict* in religious observances; (with עם) *to deal strictly with* (esp. used of divine retribution). Y. Peah VIII, 21[a] מְדַקְדְּקִין בכסות וכ׳ you must make inquiries if one asks for clothes, but you must not &c., if food is asked for; Lev. R. s. 34 (B. Bath. 9[a] בודקין).—Y. Kidd. IV, 65[d] אין מד׳ אחריה you must not trace its past records. Y. B. Bath. IV, end, 14[d] it is the custom in sales להיות מְדַקְדְּקִין to be strict, opp. בעין יפה liberal. Ex. R. s. 31 מד׳ עמהם he is stinting (illiberal) towards the poor. Y. Succ. I, 52[b] top לא ד׳ בה he paid no particular attention to its preparation. Ḥull. 4[a] חרבה מד׳ בה יותר וכ׳ they are very strict in the observance, even more so than &c.; Tosef. Pes. I (II), 15.—Yeb. 121[b] (ref. to Ps. L, 3) הקב״ה מד׳ עם וכ׳ the Lord deals with those around Him (the good) strictly, to a hair's breadth; Y. Shek. V, 48[d]. Lev. R. s. 27; a. fr.—Tanḥ. Mishp. 11 למה אתה מְדַקְדֵּק בהכאתה why art thou so severe in punishing her?

Nithpa. נִדַּקְדֵּק (=נִתְדַּ׳) *to be crushed, powdered.* Ohol. II, 7.

דַּקְדֵּק ch. same, 1) *to crush, humiliate,* v. דַּקֵּק. Lev. R. s. 27, v. גִּיר.—2) *to investigate; to be strict.* Targ. Job IX, 17 (cmp. Yeb. 121[b] in preced. w.)—Lam. R. to I, 22 (ref. to עולל, ib.) דַּקְדֵּק עליהון מה דדַקְדַּקְתָּא עלי be as strict in punishing them as thou hast been in punishing me.

Ithpa. אִיתְדַּקְדֵּק *to be crushed, powdered, broken.* Targ. Mic. I, 7 ידקדקון Var. (ed. Lag. ידקקון; Vien. ידקרון, corr. acc.). Targ. Is. XXI, 9 יִדַּ׳ (not יְדַ׳). [Targ. Nah. III, 10= יזדקוק they will be chained, v. זְקַק.]

דַּקְדְּקָא m. (preced.) *powder.* Targ. II Chr. XXXIV, 7 (ed. Lag. ארדקא, h. text הֵדֵק).

דַּקְדְּקִירָא c. (דקדק, with format. ר; cmp. סמוקרי &c.) *very thin, light.* Y. M. Kat. II, 81[b] top [read:] דזיפתה ד׳ for its pitch coating is very light, opp. גלידא.

דַּקְדַּקְתָּא, v. דַּקְתָּא.

דַּקָּה, v. דַּק I.

דָּקָה m. (v. דוק Af.) [*a look-out,*] *a small door* or *bar* at the foot of a stairway, leading to a court or river bank. Erub. 60[a]. Ib. 61[a].—*Pl.* (Chald.) דָּקֵי. Ib.

דִּקוּלָא, v. דִּיקוּלָא.

דקונתיה, v. קֵנָה, קוּנְתֵּיהּ.

דִּקוּקָא, v. דִּיקוּקָא.

דקוקיא, read דקי׳, v. דַּקִּיק.

דָּקוֹר m. (דקר) *chisel* or *borer.* Kel. XIV, 3 ד׳ של חרש the carpenter's &c.

דְּקוּרָא m. (דקר; cmp. דּוּקְרָא) *wickerwork, basket; jug inclosed in wickerwork.*—*Pl.* דְּקוּרֵי, דְּקוּרַיָּא. B. Mets. 84[a] כי ד׳ דהרפניא (Ms. M. כדקוראי) of the size of the baskets of H.; Sabb. 127[a] כד׳ וכ׳ of the size of the jugs of H.—Ḥull. 4[a] דקוריא דציפורי baskets with slaughtered birds (v. Tosaf. a. l.; Rashi: *strings of birds,* fr. דקר *to perforate*).

דקוריא, Y. Maas. Sh. IV, 55[b] bot. ד׳ עָסָא, read: דּוּקְרַיָּא *twenty beams.*

דִּקְיוֹן, דִּיק׳ m. (דְּקָה=b. h. דָּכָה; cmp. דקק ,דוק) *crushing; oppression, wrong.* תבע ד׳ של־ *to ask satisfaction for one's wrongs, to take one's part;* Gen. R. s. 9, end תובעת ד׳ של וכ׳ protects the wronged; Yalk. Gen. 15 דיקיוס (corr. acc.). Num. R. s. 20 וכי ד׳ של וכ׳ did the angel take up the cause of the ass?; a. e. Cmp. עִלְבּוֹן.

***דִּקִלָן, דִּקִילִין**, Targ. II Sam. XVII, 19, prob. to be read דִּקִיקָן or דְּקִיקָן (Pesh. דוישא) *pounded grits;* v. next w.

דַּקִּיק m., **דַּקִּיקָא** c. (דַּק, v. דקק) 1) *broken, powdered, pounded.* Targ. O. Ex. XXXII, 20 (some ed. a. Y. דְּקָק׳). Targ. Y. Ex. IX, 8 דְּקִ׳ a pounded mass (v. דַּעְדַּק; h. text פִּיחַ); a. e.—*Pl.* דַּקִּיקִין, דְּקִי׳, f. דַּקִּיקָן. Targ. O. Lev. XVI, 12.—2) *minute, tender, little, young.* Lev. R. s. 27, a. e. בעיר ד׳, v. בְּעִיר.—*Pl.* בעירא דקיקא, דַּקִּיקַיָּא, דַּקִּיקִין &c. Targ. II Chr. XXXIII, 11.—Y. Snh. I, 18[d] top; Y. Maas. Sh. V, 56[c] top גוזליא ד׳ the pigeons are yet very small. Y. Bets. I, end, 61[a] טליין ד׳ young children. Y. B. Mets. VI, end, 5[c] בנין ד׳ *minors.* Ib. מהו דיימרון דקיקייא וכ׳ can the minors say to the adults &c.? Ib. דקוקיא (corr. acc.).—[Targ. Y. Gen. XIX, 11 מְדַקִּיקִיתוֹן Ar., ed. מטליא.]—Y. Ber. I, 2[a] כופרניא ד׳ (the inhabitants of) small villages (living in scattered dwellings).—Fem. דַּקִּיקָא, דַּקִּיקְתָא. Targ. II Esth. IX, 19 קירוי ד׳ (h. text ערי הפרזות).—Y. Gitt. V, 47[c] top ארלין ד׳ the traps for small animals. Y. Dem. V, 24[c] bot.—V. דְּקָקָה.

דִּקִירָא, v. אִיתִּי II.

דְּקִירָה f. (דקר) *act of digging, quantity of ground broken with one stroke.* Bets. 8[b].—*Pl.* דְּקִירוֹת. Ib.

דַּקִּיתָא f. collect. noun (דקק) *young shoots.* Targ. Y. Gen. XXII, 3 [read:] ד׳ דתאנ׳ (=מרבדות של תאנה, v. Tam. 29[b]).

דְּקִיתָא f. (v. preced.) *the lowest joint of the vertebra* (=h. עָצֶה). Targ. Y. Lev. III, 9. [Targ. Y. Deut. XVIII, 3 ד׳ Ar., v. רְקִיתָא.]

דֶּקֶל m. (cmp. דקר) 1) *palm-tree.* Peah IV, 1. Tam. 29[b]; a. fr.—B. Bath. 36[b] ד׳ נערה (Ms. H. a. O. נעורה, v. Rabb. D. S. a. l. note 3) a young palm bearing more than once a year (oth. opin.: one dropping its fruits prematurely). Ab. Zar. I, 5 ד׳ טב a variety called *dekel tab* (Chald.: *good palm*). Sifra Thazr., Neg., Par. 5, ch. XIII ד׳ הרים אתה thou art a mountain-palm (too rash, v. Men. 84[b] top; Var. in R. S. to Neg. XI, 7 דוקר וכ׳ cutting through mountains, sophistical; Yalk. Lev. 552 עוקר).—*Pl.* דְּקָלִים, דְּקָלִין. Gen. R. s. 88.—Tosef. M. Kat. II, 10; Sabb. XIV, 3 מי דקלים (Var. דקרים, Tosef. ib. XII (XIII), 13 דקר׳, Var. ed. Zuck. דקלין) a potion used as *a purgative* (said to be the water of a well springing forth between two date-trees); Y. ib. XIV, 14[c]; Bab. ib. 110[a]; Y. Ber. VI, end, 10[d].—2)=דֶּקֶר. Y. Sot. II, 18[a].

דִּקְלָא, דִּיקְ׳ ch. same, *palm-tree.* Targ. Ps. XCII, 13. Targ. Y. Gen. XXII, 3; a. e.—B. Kam. 59[a] ד׳ ארמאה Ms. M. (ed. דארמ׳, incorr.) an Aramean palm, ד׳ פרסאה a Persian palm. Ib. 92[b] (prov.) מטייל ואזיל ד׳ וכ׳ the bad palm will travel to meet a barren cane (like meets like). Ber. 55[b] bot. none see in a dream ד׳ דדהבא a golden palm-tree (a thing not experienced in reality). Erub. 51[a] ד׳ דסביל וכ׳ a palm-tree which supports its neighbor. Ib. ד׳ דפריק וכ׳ a palm which pays its owner's taxes. Keth. 10[b] כי נרגא לדיקלא (not לדיקולא) as injurious as the axe to the palm-tree.—*Pl.* דִּקְלִין, דִּקְלַיָּא, דִּקְלֵי, דִּי׳. Targ. Ex. XV, 27. Targ. Deut. XXXIV, 3.—Y. R. Hash. II, 58[a] top, a. e. ד׳ דבבל the Babylonian palms. B. Bath. 26[a]; a. fr. [Sabb. 110[a] שני דקלי, read: דקלים as Ms. M.]—Fem. form דִּיקְלְתָא. Sabb. l. c. תרתי ד׳ Ms. O. (ed. תלאר, Ms. M. תילתא, corr. acc.), v. Y. ib. XIV, 14[c].

דַּקְלַי m. (preced.) *a palm-gardener.* Gen. R. s. 41, beg.; Num. R. s. 3; Midr. Till. to Ps. XCII (Yalk. Ps. 845 אדם).

דִּקְנָא, דִּיקְ׳, דְּקַן m. ch.=h. זָקָן, *beard, bearded chin, hair-growth.* Targ. Lev. XIII, 29 sq.; a. fr.—B. Bath. 58[a] תפשיה בדיקניה seized him by his beard. Gen. R. s. 72 (prov.) הניאת לסבי מן דיקני thou pleasest my grandfather (with hair) from my beard, i. e. you wish to be liberal at other people's expense; (Yalk. Gen. 129 חבאת לפני מן דאקני, corr. acc.). Naz. 39[a] bot. [read:] כד צבער סביא דיקניהון when old men dye their beards. B. Mets. 60[b] צבעיה לרישיה ולדיקניה he dyed the hair of his head and beard; ib. ולד׳ . . . חווריה he washed it white again; a. fr.—*Pl.* דִּקְנִין, דִּי׳. Targ. Y. Lev. XIX, 27; a. e.—B. Mets. 39[a], v. next w.

דִּקְנָנָא, דִּיקְ׳ m. (preced.) *bearded,* i. e. *adult, major.*—*Pl.* דִּקְנָנֵי, דִּי׳. B. Mets. 39[a] לדיקנני (Ar. לדיקני *for beards,* i. e. adults), v. אפיטרופא. Ib. 70[a] אפי׳ בד׳ וכ׳ is permitted even for the benefit of adult orphans.

דָּקַק (b. h.; cmp. הוּק, דּוּק) *to crush, pound, powder.*—Denom. דַּק.—*Pilp.* דִּקְדֵּק q. v.

Hif. הֵדֵק, הֵידֵק 1) same. Kerith. 6[b] היטב הידק הידק היטב pounding well &c.; Y. Yoma IV, 41[d] bot. כשהיה מידק חיה אומר הָדֵק וכ׳ when the attendant pounded, the superintendent called, Pound well &c. [Sifré Deut. 207 לחרוק פשתן, read לְהָדִיק or לִפְרוֹק.]—2) *to be fine, small.* Part. מֵדַק, מֵידַק. Succ. IV, 9 (48[b]) one was wide (מעובה), ואחד מדק Ms. M. (ed. דק; Y. ed., Ms. M. 2, a. Mish. ed. Pes. מי׳; Mish. Nap. מודק Hof.) and the other tube was narrow; Y. ib. 54[d] top (they thought) חמ׳ של יין the narrow was for wine. Y. Yoma III, 41[a]; Y. Sot. II, 18[a] top מידק small and thin type of letters. Arakh. 25[a] מי׳ a sparsely sown field.

Nif. נָדַק, נִדּוֹק *to be crushed.* Mekh. Bo. s. 13 נִידָּקוֹת; Pesik. R. s. 17 נִידֶּקֶת; Pesik. Vayhi, p. 64[b] נָדֶקֶת. [Zeb. 22[a] טיט הנדוק, read הנרוק, v. רָקַק.]

דְּקַק ch. same, v. דקיק.—Imperat. דוק (v. הוּק). Sabb. 152[a] ד׳ בככי וכ׳ grind with thy jaws (eat well), and thou wilt find (its effect) in marching.

Pa. דַּקֵּק same. B. Kam. 101[a] ודקינהו and pounded them.—*Part. pass.* מְדַקַּק (מְדַקְדַק). Targ. Is. XXX, 14 (h. text כָּתוּת).—*Palp.* דַּקְדֵּק q. v.

Af. אַדֵּק, אַדִּיק (הַדֵּק) same. Targ. II Kings XXIII, 15; Targ. II Chr. XXXIV, 4 אודיק.—Gen. R. s. 70 מְהַדֵּק, v. גַּרְמָא. Lam. R. introd. (R. Ḥănina 2) אכלה ומַדְּקָה (fr. Dan. VII, 7). [Targ. Y. II Num. V, 19 הִזְקִי=הֵדַקִי, v. זְקַק.]

דַּקְקָה f. (דקק, v. דקיק) *a tender child.* Y. R. Hash. II, 58[b] top כחדא ד׳ as the nails of a young child; Y. Snh. I, 18[c] bot. ed. Krot. ד׳ (corr. acc.).

דָּקַר (b. h.) 1) *to dig, bore, pierce.* Sabb. 110ª, a. e. (explain. מי דקרין, v. דָּקֶל) שהם הוקְרִין וכ׳ because they make an opening in the bile. Y. Ned. IX, 41ᵇ bot. ודוקרה בלבו and sticks it (the sword) into his own heart. Gitt. 56ª, v. next w.—Kidd. 22ᵇ; a. fr.—2) (cmp. דָּקֶל) *to spread, branch off.* Succ. 13ª Ar.; Erub. 11ᵇ; 16ª קנים ההוקְרִים (ההוקְרִין) reeds which spread, i. e. the top reeds, v. הוּקְרָן.—*Part. Pu.* מְדוּקָּר *ramified,* formed like a הוּקְרָן. Erub. 11ᵇ Ar.

Nif. נִדְקַר *to be pierced, stabbed.* Tanḥ. Pinḥ. 1; Num. R. s. 21, beg.

דְּקַר ch. same, *to stab.* Gitt. 56ª בעו למִדְקְרֵיה (the guardsmen) wanted to stab his body (to see whether R. Joḥ. was really dead). Ib. (Hebr.) יאמרו רבן דָּקְרוּ they (the Romans) will say, they stabbed their teacher. [Ex. R. s. 47 ודקרין, v. קְרֵי.]

דֶּקֶר m. (preced.) *a pronged tool, mattock* (v. Sm. Ant. s. v. Raster). Bets. I, 2; 7ᵇ. Ib. ד׳ נעוץ וכ׳ the mattock was stuck into the ground on the eve of the Festival. Shebi. V, 6.—Y. Sot. II, 18ª יחפור בדֶקֶל (twice).—*Pl.* דְּקָרִים, דְּקָרִין. מֵי ד׳ *a purgative water,* v. דָּקַר a. דֶּקֶל. Sabb. 110ª (differences about spelling דקר׳ or דקל׳); Y. ib. XIV, 14ᶜ; a. e.—Y. Succ. I, 52ª bot. כמין ד׳ like prongs, v. הוּקְרָן.

דַּקְרוּנָא, pl. **דַּקְרוּנִין,** v. הוּקְרָנָא.

דַּקְרָנָא, דַּקְרָן, v. הוּקְרָ׳.

דַּקְתָּא f. (דוק) *stalks of flax beaten once* (still hard and knotty), contrad. to דַּקְדַּקְתָּא *thoroughly beaten, tow.* Ḥull. 51ᵇ ד׳ חיישינן וכ׳ if a bird falls upon *dakta,* we must apprehend internal injury, if on *daktakta,* we need not. B. Bath. 26ª top הוה אזלא ד׳ וכ׳ Ms. M. a. oth. (ed. ד׳, v. Rabb. D. S. a. l. note 2) pieces of stalks flew off and injured people.

דָּר, v. דּוּר.

דָּר part. of דּוּר.

דָּר m. (דּוּר) *row.*—*Pl.* דָּרִין. Gen. R. s. 20 (explain. דַּרְדַּר) שהיא עשוייה ד׳ ד׳ because it consists of rows above rows (of the imbricated form of the artichoke).

דָּר, דָּרָא I ch. 1) same, *row, range, order.* Keth. 60ª בד׳ דנשי in a row of women. B. Kam. 117ª בד׳ קמא in the first row of scholars. Ḥull. 11ª top ד׳ דגברי a row of men. Ib. 47ª בד׳ דאוני within the ranges of the lobes of the lungs. Ib. 53ª בד׳ דסיחופיה in the order in which the claws of the lion's paw appear when he assaults an animal. Snh. 97ᵇ ד׳ קמא דקמי וכ׳ Ms. M. (ed. ד׳ דקמי; Ms. K. a. Ar. דָּרֵי, pl.) the first row (of righteous men) before the Lord; Succ. 45ᵇ (v. Rabb. D. S. a. l. note 9).—Kidd. 36ᵇ ר״י דדריה R. J. his class-mate; a. fr.—*Pl.* דָּרִין, דָּרֵי. Meg. 12ª (expl. דַּר, Esth. I, 6) ד׳ ד׳ ranges of mosaics. Nidd. 20ª תלתא ד׳ וכ׳ there are three ranges of leaves, and three leaves in each. Ber. 28ª ד׳ חוורתא rows of white hair. Ib. 62ᵇ (phonetic etymol. of אדמקיפנא (קפנדריא אַף׳ וכ׳ in place of going around the rows of houses &c. Ab. Zar. 28ª ומייתי דמא מבי דרי ed. (Ms. M. מבי ככי); Yoma 84ª ואתי דמא מבי ד׳ (Ms. M. ומייתי ליה דמא מבי ככי ושיני) and he makes blood come (and blood will come) out from between the rows of teeth. [Ib. בככי דריה, v. דַּרְדָּא.] [Taan. 3ᵇ; B. Mets. 73ª; B. Kam. 113ᵇ בי ד׳, v. דָּרֵי.]—2) *a range of wood, pyre.* Cant. R. to III, 4 ד׳ יקידא יקדת a burning pyre hast thou set on fire, v. יְקַד.—*Pl.* as above. Targ. Ps. LXXXII, 15 Ms. (ed. זרזי).—3) (v. דּוּר) *period, generation.* Targ. Deut. XXXIII, 7. Targ. Job. VI, 17; a. fr.—Ḥag. 5ª עד דמלי להו לד׳ until they have completed the period (lived the years allotted to them). Snh. 97ᵇ בכל ד׳ וד׳ (Ms. M.) in each generation; a. fr.—*Pl.* דָּרִין, דָּרַיָּא, דָּרֵי. Targ. Is. LI, 8 sq.—Targ. Ps. XLIX, 12 (Ms. דָּרָתָא); a. fr.—Ḥull. 93ᵇ; Yeb. 39ᵇ אכשור ד׳ have the generations (the present) grown better?

דָּרָא II f. *court,* v. דַּרְתָּא.—דירא *shed,* v. דִּירָא.

דְּרָא 1) *to winnow;* 2) *to carry,* v. דרי I, II.

דרא, Pes. 56ª, אסא ד׳, v. דְּדָא.

דרבאני, v. דַּרְבְּנָאָה.

דרבון, Deut. R. s. 6, read דַּרְקוֹן.

דַּרְבוֹנֵי, v. דַּרְבְּנָאָה.

דָּרְבָן m. (b. h.; a contr. of דברבין, v. דָּבַר) [*leader,*] *goad, the iron point on the staff* (מַלְמֵד); also *the spud at the end of the handle of the ploughshare* (v. Sm. Ant. s. vv. Aratrum a Catrinos). Ḥag. 3ᵇ מה ד׳ זה וכ׳ as the goad directs the cow &c. Kel. IX, 6 מלמד שבלע הד׳ a goad (handle) in which the iron point was driven in so that nothing could be seen of it. Ib. XXV, 2, v. מַהֲצֶע. Tosef. ib. B. Mets. IV, 4. Pesik. Baḥod. p. 153ª; Y. Snh. X, 28ª, a. e., v. הדור I. Ib. אדם עושה ד׳ לפרתו וכ׳ man makes a goad to direct his cow, and to his (evil) inclination should he not &c.?—*Pl.* דָּרְבוֹנוֹת, דָּרְבָנוֹת. Koh. R. to XII, 11; Num. R. s. 15 (quoted fr. Koh. l. c.); a. fr. [Num. R. s. 14 א״ת כד׳ אלא כדרבנות, v. כַּד I.]

***דַּרְבְּנָאָה** m., pl. **דַּרְבְּנָאֵי** (v. preced.) *goad-bearers* (an adaptation of δορυφόροι in speaking of Athens), *guardsmen.* Bekh. 8ᵇ (Ar. דַּרְבוֹנֵי).

דָּרַג *to leap, step.*—*Hif.* הִדְרִיג *to make a step* (מַדְרֵגָה), i. e. *to fell trees at uneven heights from the ground,* so as to make the stumps appear like steps, opp. החליק to cut at even heights. Y. Shebi. IV, 35ᵇ bot. [read:] לא יהא מחליק ומַדְרִיג מדריג ומחליק וכ׳ he must not cut one portion even and another step-like, but must make the stumps equally high; מקום . . יַדְרִיג לַדְרִיג יחליק where it is the custom to cut even, he must (in the Sabbatical year) cut uneven &c.; Tosef. ib. III, 14 [read:] ה״ז לא יחליק ויַדְרִיג וכ׳. Y. Erub. VII, beg. 24ᵇ, v. כּוּפְתָּ.

דַּרְגָּא, דַּרְג c. (v. preced.) *step, stairs, ladder.* Targ. II Esth. I, 2. Targ. II Kings IX, 13 ד׳ שַׁעֲרָא (h. text גרם המעלות, v. גֶּרֶם).—Sabb. 77ᵇ; Keth. 10ᵇ (phonet. etymol.)

דרך גג a way to the roof. Sabb. 155ᵃ, v. אַמְּדְלָא. Yeb. 63ᵃ נחות ד׳ ... סק ד׳ וכ׳ go down a step when taking a wife, go up a step in choosing a groomsman; Y. Kidd. IV, 66ᵃ. Pes. 112ᵃ ד׳ לפחדא, לשינתא inviting fear, sleep; v. אוּסֵי.—*Pl.* דַּרְגִּין. Targ. O. a. Y. II Ex. XX, 23; a. e.—Targ. II Sam. VI, 13 דרג׳ Regia a. Kimḥi (ed. זוג׳).

דּוּרְגּוֹן, דַּרְגּוֹן m. (דרג) *a suite of graded officers, staff.* Y. Hor. III, beg. 47ᵃ הוא וכל דו׳ דידיה He and His entire staff (of angels); Y. Snh. II, 20ᵃ top. Ex. R. s. 1 שהיה מניח ד׳ שלו Moses left his suite. Num. R. s. 4 עושין ד׳ וכ׳ (not דרגין) to form his staff (on bringing up the Ark, II Sam. VI, 1 sq.).—Y'lamd. to Num. XII, 1, quot. in Ar.; ib. to Deut. XI, 22 דרו׳, a. דור׳ (v. Koh. Ar. Compl. s. v. אקר).—[Tosef. Naz. I, 2 דרגון, v. טְרִיגוֹן, דִּיגוֹן.]

דַּרְגּוּשָׁה, v. דַּרְגָּשָׁא.

דרגיבת, דרגי, Y. Sabb. VI, 8ᶜ bot., read with Tosef. ib. VII (VIII), 2 דגן וקדרון, a charm formula.

דַּרְגִּישִׁין, v. דַּרְגָּשָׁא.

דַּרְגֵּשׁ c. (דרג, with formative ש) 1) *the footstool in front of a high bed (Scamnum)*; 2) *state bed with its footstool;* (v. Ned. 56ᵃ sq. the discussions about the meaning of our w., a. Maim. comment. to Mish. a. l.). Ned. VII, 5 הנודר ... . מותר בד׳ if one vows abstinence from 'bed', he is allowed the use of the footstool. Snh. II, 3 (20ᵃ). M. Kat. 27ᵃ, v. פְּגָא; Y. Ber. II, 5ᵈ bot.; Y. Ned. VII, end, 40ᵉ; a. e.

דַּרְגָּשָׁא ch. same, in gen. *couch.* Targ. Y. Gen. XLVII, 31 (Y. II דַּרְגּוּשָׁה). Ib. XLVIII, 2. Targ. Ps. VI, 7; a. e.—*Pl.* דַּרְגָּשִׁין. Targ. Esth. I, 6 (ed. Lag. דַּרְגִּישִׁין). Targ. Ez. XXIII, 41; a. e.

דרד, *Pa.* דַּרֵּד (=רדרד, cmp. רדה, ירד) *to take down, remove ashes.* Targ. Y. Ex. XXVII, 3 (למ׳) לְמִדַרְדָא וכ׳ to cleanse it (the altar, h. text דשן); Targ. Y. Num. IV, 13 וִידַרְדוּן.

Ithpe. אִידְּרִיד *to glide down.* Sot. 44ᵃ מִדְּרִיד ונפל (the uncleanness coming out sideways) glides down and falls to the ground. Cmp. מְדְרוֹן.

דַּרְדּוּגֵי, v. דַּרְדֵּיג.

דַּרְדּוּר m. (דרר) *a large barrel carried on wheels*, or *rolled.* Kel. XV, 1 ד׳ עגלה a water tank on wheels. Sifra Sh'mini ch. VII, Par. 6 מוציא דרור עגלה (corr. acc.). Ib. ארבה ד׳ עגלה; Yalk. Lev. 538 דַּרְדַּר. Pirké d'R. El. ch. XXX (ref. to חמת Gen. XXI, 14) לקח את הד׳ וכ׳ Abraham took the water barrel and tied it to her loins that it might drag behind her &c. [Sifré Num. 115, read דְּרִיד, as Yalk. ib. 750.]—*Pl.* דַּרְדּוּרִין. Tosef. Ab. Zar. IV (V), 5 (Var. הדרורין); Ab. Zar. 32ᵃ. Tosef. ib. VII (VIII), 9; Ab. Zar. 59ᵇ top Ms. M. (ed. דור׳, corr. acc.). [Yalk. Cant. 992 דרדורי׳, v. דַּרְדַּר.]

דַּרְדֵּיג (Paʿpel of דרג, cmp. זרק; v. Fl. in Levy Talm. Dict. I, 444ᵃ) *to drip.* Keth. 17ᵇ ד׳ משחא וכ׳ he dripped oil on the head of scholars at his son's wedding. Ib. הַדַּרְדּוּגֵי משחא וכ׳ the act of dripping oil &c. (indicating that the bride is a virgin).

דַּרְדַּנְיָא pr. n. *Dardania,* a district and city of Upper Mysia. Targ. Y. I Gen. X, 4 (some ed. הוֹרְדַּנְיָא; Y. II הוֹד׳); Targ. I Chr. I, 7 (h. text דדנים, רד׳); Gen. R. s. 37, beg.; Y. Meg. I, 71ᵇ bot. דַּרְדַּנְיָה.

דַּרְדְּסָא m., pl. **דּוּר׳, דַּרְדְּסִין** (Paʿpel of דרס) *cloth-shoes* or *slippers, socks.* Y. Kil. IX, 32ᵈ top (explain. מנעלות הפינון Mish.). Ib. דילבש ד׳ דעמר ע״ג ד׳ וכ׳ who puts woolen socks over linen &c. Ib. bot. ד׳ דע׳ בחדא וכ׳ a woolen shoe on one foot &c.—Gen. R. s. 100 ואלבשוני דַּרְדְּסַאי וכ׳ dress me in my slippers .... and place my sandals by my feet (v. Sm. Ant. s. v. Solea); Y. Kil. IX, 32ᵇ top בנרסיי; Y. Keth. XII, 35ᵃ top דנרסיי, read דַּרְדְּסַיי. Y. Orl. III, 63ᵃ top מעבדיניה דורדסין (ed. Krot. דודר׳, corr. acc.) to make socks of them.

דַּרְדְּקָא, דַּרְדַּק m. (Parpel noun of דקק; cmp. הַקִּיק a. הַדְּקַק) *tender, young, small*; esp. *pupil of a primary class.* Targ. Job III, 19.—B. Mets. 66ᵃ ד׳ קריעה גברא רבא וכ׳ was it a child that destroyed the note? A great man &c. Ib. ד׳ קריעה דכולי עלמא וכ׳ it was a beginner in learning that tore it, for, in civil law, all people are beginners &c.—*Pl.* דַּרְדְּקֵי, דַּרְדְּקִין. Targ. Job XXX, 1 ד׳ מיני my juniors; a. e.—B. Mets. l. c.—B. Bath. 21ᵃ מקרי ד׳ teacher of primaries (Bible teacher); Bekh. 46ᵃ. Sabb. 104ᵃ. B. Kam. 92ᵇ, v. גַּבְרָא. Keth. 111ᵇ מקרי ד׳ דר״ל the teacher of Resh Lakish's children.

דַּרְדֵּר (Pilp. of דרר, v. Fl. to Levy Talm. Dict. I, p. 444ᵃ); *Hithpalp.* הִדַּרְדֵּר *to roll.* Cant. R. to VI, 11 כולן מְדַּרְדְּרִין ומתגלגלין all of them get in commotion and roll (Pesik. R. s. 11 מתרעמין ומרגשין). V. דַּרְדּוּר.

דַּרְדַּר m. (b. h.; v. דַּר) *thistle, artichoke* (v. Löw Pfl. p. 100; 427). Gen. R. s. 20.—*Pl.* דַּרְדָּרִים, דַּרְדָּרִין. Shebi. VII, 1. Lev. R. s. 23; Cant. R. to II, 2 חוחים וד׳ thorns and thistles.—Pesik. R. s. 10 בקוצין ובד׳ וכ׳ with hedges of thorns &c.; Yalk. Cant. 992 דרדורי׳. [Yalk. Lev. 538, v. דַּרְדּוּר.]—V. עַכָּבִית.

דַּרְדָּרָא ch. same.—Gitt. 70ᵃ מאי ד׳ what kind of *Dardara?* Ans. מוריקא דחוחי 'the crocus of thorns', i. e. Carthamus tinctorius (Löw Pfl. p. 199).—*Pl.* דַּרְדָּרִין. Targ. Y. II Gen. III, 18.—Pesik. B'shall. p. 93ᵃ [read:] ומעבר ליה חקלוון דד׳ (v. Bub. note 225) and he carried him over fields full of thistles.

דָּרוֹכוֹת m. pl. (דרך) *grape or olive treaders.* Ter. III, 4. Y. ib. 42ᵃ bot.; Y. Ab. Zar. IV, 44ᵇ top דרוכית (corr. acc.).

דרולמוסיא, v. אנדרולומוסיא.

דָּרוֹם m. (b. h.) *South, southern region.* Yoma 21ᵇ כלפי ד׳ towards the South. Gen. R. s. I, beg. דְּרוֹמוֹ של רקיע the southern section of the sky; a. fr.—Esp. הַדָּ׳ (b. h. הַנֶּגֶב) *the South of Palestine,* south of Lydda (with a town of the same name: *Darom*, v. Neub. Géogr. p. 63). Pes. 70[b]. Yeb. 45[a]; Zeb. 22[b] זקני ד׳; Y. Erub. VI, 23[c] bot. זקני הד׳ the scholars of D.

דְּרוֹמָא, דְּרוֹמָה ch. same. Targ. Gen. XXVIII, 14; a. fr.—Targ. Deut. XXXIV, 3; a. fr.—Lev. R. s. 20 [read:] רבנן דד׳ (or דְּרוֹמָאֵי)=זקני דרום, v. preced.—Y. Hor. III, end, 48[c] מטבריה אִמְּדָּרוֹמָה from Tiberias or from Daromah?—Y. Ber. VIII, 12[a] top; a. fr. [Y. Erub. VI, 23[c] bot. ר׳ נתן דרומה, v. next w.]—בַּר דְּ׳ *Bar-Daroma*, name of a leader during the Bar-Kokhba rebellion. Gitt. 57[a].

דְּרוֹמָאָה m. (preced.) *inhabitant of Darom* or *Daroma, Daromean.* Y. Erub. VI, 23[c] bot. ר׳ נתן ד׳ (not דרומה).—*Pl.* דְּרוֹמָאֵי. Zeb. 22[b]. Y. Taan. III, 66[c] bot. דְּרוֹמָאֵיֵ (?). Ib. IV, 69[b] bot. ד׳ נהגין הגה the Daromeans, in their custom of observing mourning for the destruction of the Temple, refer to חַגָּהּ (Hos. II, 13) (and mourn from the 'festive day', i. e. the first day of Ab, to the ninth; v. Bab. ib. 29[b] sq.). V. דְּרוֹמָיָא.

***דְּרוֹמוֹס** m. (δρόμος) *the runner's race in the stadium; course;* in gen. *contest* at public games. Kidd. 63[a] act before me כד׳ הזה Ar. (ed. הִימוֹס) as is done in that certain *dromos.*

דרומוסקוס, v. הוּרְמַסְקוֹס.

דְּרוֹמִי m., **דְּרוֹמִית** f. (דָּרוֹם) *southern; Daromean.* Y. Peah III, 17[d] חציירה ד׳ its southern half; Y. Kidd. I, 60[d] top.—Gen. R. s. 91, v. אָבָל. Y. Sabb. I, 3[d] top, a. e. ר׳ שמלאי הד׳ R. Simlai the Daromean.—B. Bath. 25[b], a. fr. רוח ד׳ southern wind.—Zeb. V, 3, a. fr. ד׳ מזרחית South-East. Y. Pes. V, 32[a] bot. לד׳ a Daromean (Bab. ib. 62[b] לוודים); a. fr.—*Pl.* דְּרוֹמִיִּים. Shek. VI, 3 Y. a. Bab. ed. (Mish. הָרוֹמִים).

דְּרוֹמַיָּא, דְּרוֹמָיָה ch. same. Y. Ber. III, 6[b] bot. ר׳ יעקב ד׳; a. fr.—Ib. I, 2[b] bot. דרומנה (corr. acc.).—*Pl.* דְּרוֹמָיֵי. Y. Pes. V, 32[a] bot. Y. Ber. II, 5[b] דְּרוֹמָיֵיא, דְּרוֹמָיֵא. V. דְּרוֹמָאָה.

דרומילוס, Gen. R. s. 48; Yalk. ib. 82 דרומלות, prob. a corrupt. of דִּיפִּילוֹס m. (δίπυλος) *double-gated (passage).*

דרומיסקוס, v. הוּרְמַסְקוֹס.

דרומנה, v. דְּרוֹמָיָא.

***דְּרוּמָתָא** pr. n. pl. *Darumatha.* M. Kat. 27[b] ed. (Ms. M. 1 דארו מ׳ 2, דראו מ׳, v. Rabb. D. S. a. l. note).

דְּרוֹסָא, דְּרוֹסָה pr. n. m. *D'rosa, D'rosah.* Y. Yoma IV, 41[d] top ר׳ ד׳; Num. R. s. 12 דְּרוֹסָאִי; Cant. R. to III, 10 דרוסה.—בן ד׳, v. אֲבִילָה.

דְּרוֹסָה m. *Darosah (Wine-Treader)*, name of a coin, = $1^3/_4$ As. Y. Kidd. I, 58[d]; Bab. ib. 12[a] חַדְרִיס; Tosef. B. Bath. V, 12 חַדְרֵס.—*Pl.* הוֹרְסִים. Y. l. c. ג׳ ד׳ למעה (Bab. l. c. חַדְרִיסִין; Tosef. l. c. הַדְרֵסִין) three *d.* make one *M'ah.* [V. legends of Jewish coins in Conder Handbook to the Bible, 3rd ed., p. 177, sq.]

דְּרוֹסָה, v. דָּרַס.

דְּרוּסוֹת f. pl. (דרס) *pomace* of dates in an advanced stage, contrad. to הוּרְקָאוֹת. Tosef. Maas. Sh. I, 10 (Var. דורסות).

דְּרוֹעָא, v. דְּרַע III.

***דְּרוֹפְתְקִי** m. sing. a. pl. (a comp. of דרי *to carry*, a. pl. of פִּתְקָא; cmp. מקבלי פתקין Sabb. X, 4) *bag for official documents, mail bag.* Snh. 99[b] [read with Ms. M.] כולהו גופי ד׳ ניניהו טוביה לדזכו והוו ד׳ דאורייתא שנ׳ כו׳ . . בבטנך (Ar. דרפתקי) all human bodies are mail bags (carrying the decrees of the Lord); happy they who are found worthy to be receptacles of the Law, as it says &c. (Prov. XXII, 18).

***דְּרוּקָא** m (cmp. Lat. drungus, v. Sachs Beitr. I, p. 96) *a troop of soldiers.* Keth. 62[a] ד׳ דמלכא Ar. (ed. פריסתקא).

דרוקרא, v. next w.

דְּרוּקֶרֶת (דְּדְקֶ׳, דַּרְקֶרֶת) pr. n. pl. *Drukereth* (*Darkereth, Dadk.*) a Babylonian town (cmp. דְּרוּמָתָא, v. Berl. Beitr. Geogr., p. 31). Taan. 21[b] (Ms. M. דרו׳). Nidd. 58[b]. Sabb. 94[b] דרוקרא (corr. acc.).

דְּרוֹר m. (b. h.; דרר, v. דור) [*moving about,*] 1) *freedom, privilege, amnesty.* Midr. Till. to Ps. XC ליטול ד׳ to ask a privilege. Ib. שתתן לי ד׳, v. מֶרֶד I.—Esp. *merchant's license.* Meg. 12[a] (cmp. דוּר ch. *Pa.*).—2) צפור ד׳ *a free bird*, living in the house as well as in the field. Sabb. 106[b]. Neg. XIV, 1 שתי ציפרי ד׳ (corresp. to חיות, Lev. XIV, 4); Tosef. Naz. VI, 1 שני צפרים ד׳; Y. ib. VIII, 57[a] bot. Tosef. Neg. VIII, 3 שתי ציפרין ד׳ ואלו וכ׳ two free birds which means such as are around in the city. Neg. XIV, 5 נמצאת שלא ד׳ it is discovered that it is not a free bird; Tosef. ib. VIII, 7 [read:] ונמצאת שנייה שלא ד׳ (v. R. S. to Neg. l. c.).—[Y. Snh. X, 28[a] top כד׳ נאות, read: כהור בנות like the *jewel* of girls, v. הִירָא II.]

דְּרוֹרִיָּה f. (preced., formed like שערוריה) *freedom*, v. הוֹרִיָּה.

דְּרוֹשָׁא, דְּרוֹשָׁה m. ch.=h. דַּרְשָׁן *lecturer.* Y. Sot. I, 16[d] bot.; Lev. R. s. 9; Num. R. s. 9.—*Pl.* דְּרוֹשַׁיָּא. Succ. 38[b] in Alf. (ed. דָּרְשַׁיָּא). [Y. Yeb. VIII, 8[d] top דְּרוֹשָׁה, v. דְּרַשׁ.]

דְּרֵי I, דְּרָא (=h. זָרָה) *to scatter, strew; to winnow.* Targ. O. Ex. XXXII, 20 דרא ed. Berl. (some ed. זרא); Y. דרה. Targ. Is. XLI, 16. Ib. XXX, 24; a. fr.—B. Mets. 74[a] מִידְרָא winnowing. Ab. Zar. 44[a] what proof is there that *vayissaëm* (II Sam. V, 21) לישנא דְּדְרוּיֵי הוא Ar. a. ed. Pes. (v. Rabb. D. S. a. l. note 7; ed. זרויי) has the meaning of scattering (to the winds)? Ans. (ref. to Is. XLI, 16) ומתרגמינן תדרינון (Ms. M. תבדר׳, ed. תזרי׳, v. supra) and we translate (*tissaëm*) 'shall scatter them'.

דְּרֵי II, דְּרָא (cmp. דלי, a. b. h. נָשָׂא quoted in preced. art.) *to carry away, to lift, bear, sustain.* Sabb. 66[b] a big ant דדָרֵי מידי which is carrying something. Meg. 28[a] ד׳ מרא וכ׳ was carrying a rake over his shoulder. Ib.

אתא ..... וקא ד׳ מיניה ed. (Ms. M. a. Ar. שקיל) R. H. came and took it from him (to carry it himself). Ib. אי רגילת דדָרֵית במתך דְּרִי if thou, in thy own place, art accustomed to carry (such things), carry it. Ab. Zar. 44ª it was a magnetic stone דהות דָּרְיָא ליה Rashi (ed. דרא, Yalk. Ms. II Sam. to XII, 30 דליא, v. Rabb. D. S. a. l. note 9) which sustained it (held the crown suspended).—Ab. Zar. 32ª ודרו בהדייהו and they carry (the fragments of soaked clay vessels) with them (Ms. M. ודרו ליה במיא, v. תְּרִי); a. fr.—Sabb. 77ª כל חמרא דלא דרי וכ׳ a wine which bears not an admixture of three (measures of water) to one, is no wine; B. Bath. 96ᵇ דָּארֵי; Erub. 29ᵇ. V. דּוּרָא IV.

Ithpe. אִידְּרִי *to be carried off; to get up involuntarily* to save something. Ab. Zar. 59ᵇ; 60ᵇ. Y. Sabb. III, 5ᵈ top ואִידְּרוּן חברייא וכ׳ the colleagues jumped up trying to bring him back.

דָּרֵי, בֵּי ד׳ m. (=בֵּי אִדְּרֵי, v. אִדַּר; v. Fl. to Levy Targ. Dict. I, p. 417ᵇ) *barn.* Taan. 3ᵇ מיבעי לבי ד׳ (v. Rabb. D. S. a. l. note 4) (the strong wind) is needed in the barn (for winnowing). B. Mets. 73ª הפוכו בבי ד׳ turn around (busy yourselves) in the barn. B. Kam. 113ᵇ מאן ... בבי ד׳ he whose grain is found in the barn.—[Ab. Zar. 28ª, v. דָּרָא I.]

דריא, R. Hash. 9ᵇ Ar., v. דור ch. *Pa.*

דריאבון, Tosef. B. Bath. XI, 2, v. דַּרְפּוֹן.

דריגון, Tosef. Naz. I, 2, v. דִּינוֹן a טְרִיגוֹן.

דָּרְיָוֶשׁ (b. h.) pr. n. m. *Darius*, King of Persia. Lev. R. s. 13; Esth. R. to IV, 4 ד׳ האחרון וכ׳ Darius the Second was the son of Esther.

דְּרֵיךְ, v. דְּרַךְ.

דְּרִיכָה f. (דרך) *treading* grapes &c. Sabb. 145ª bot. דְּרִיכַת זיתים Ms. M. (ed. דריסת).

דְּרִיכוֹן, v. דַּרְפּוֹן.

דריכות, Ter. III, 4 some ed., v. דְּרוֹכוֹת.

דְּרִינוֹן* m. (corrupt. of κέδρινον) *cedar-wood*, the wool-like substance of which is used for wicks. Y. Sabb. II, beg. 4ᶜ (explain. לֶבֶשׁ; Bab. ib. 20ᵇ שוכא דארזא). V. קֶדְרִינוֹן.

דְּרִיס, v. דְּרַס.

דְּרִיסָה f. (דרס) *treading; walking, crossing.* Sabb. 145ª דְּרִיסַת זיתים וכ׳ (Ms. M. דְּרִיכַת) treading olives &c. Meg. I, 6 דריסת הרגל entering one's ground, the benefit of crossing; Y. Erub. VI, 23ᵈ bot.—Y. Bicc. I, 63ᵈ top מקום ד׳ a place for crossing, (right of way but not ownership of the interior of the soil). Lev. R. s. 3, beg. ד׳ אחת וכ׳ one passing which the Lord passed.—Y. Sabb. I, 2ᵈ bot. כל המעכב דרסה (corr. acc.) whatever prevents from crossing; a. fr.—Bets. I, 5, v. דּוֹרְסָן.

דָּרִישׁ m. *lecturer*, v. דְּרַשׁ.

דְּרִישָׁה f. (דרש) 1) *inquiry.* Snh. 11ᵇ כל ד׳ שאתה דורש וכ׳ whatever inquiry about common affairs you have to make.—2) *examination of witnesses, cross-examination*, v. חֲקִירָה. Snh. IV, 1; a. fr.—3) *interpretation* of the Biblical text. Pes. 22ᵇ; a. e., v. פְּרִישָׁה.—*Pl.* דְּרִישׁוֹת. Lev. R. s. 13, beg. שתי ד׳ two queries.

דָּרַךְ (b. h.) *to tread, stamp, walk.* Ter. I, 9 ונמלך לְדוֹרְכָן and after consideration decided to use them for pressing. Ex. R. s. 15 עתיד לִדְרוֹךְ וכ׳ He will tread with His shoe upon &c.; a. fr.

Nif. נִדְרַךְ *to be trodden, pressed.* Ter. I, 8 ענבים הַנִּדְרָכוֹת (Mish. ed. הַנִּדְרָכִים) grapes in the press or intended for the press.

Hif. הִדְרִיךְ *to lead, rear, train.* Snh. 76ᵇ; Yeb. 62ᵇ הַמַּדְרִיךְ בניו וכ׳ he who leads his sons ... on the right path.

דְּרַךְ, דְּרֵיךְ ch. 1) same. Targ. O. Deut. I, 36. Targ. Is. LIX, 8; a. fr.—Keth. 60ᵇ bot. דְּדָרְכָא על וכ׳ who stepped upon &c. Sabb. 109ª דדרכא ליה וכ׳ Ms. M. (ed. דדריכא) that an ass had stepped on his foot. [Y. Maas. Sh. IV, 55ᶜ top יתיב מידרך, read: מְדַמֵּךְ, v. דְּמַךְ.—Lev. R. s. 27 דרכת עד, read: אוֹרְכַת, v. אֲרִיךְ I.]—2) *to overtake*, v. infra.

Af. אַדְרַךְ 1) *to thresh.* Targ. Is. XXVIII, 27 sq.; a. e.—2) *to lead.* Targ. Prov. XXII, 6, v. דְּכֵי *Af.*—Targ. Ps. XXV, 9; a. e.—3) *to trace, overtake.* Targ. Prov. VI, 11; XXIV, 34 וְתַדְרְכִיךְ (ed. Lag. וְתִירִךְ, Var. ותדרוך, ותדכיך, ותרכיך, h. text כמהלך).—Keth. 60ᵇ; Ab. Zar. 15ᵇ ולא אַדְרְכֵיה and did not find him.

דֶּרֶךְ c. (b. h.; preced.) *way, road; method, manner.* Kidd. 2ᵇ ד׳ לשון וכ׳ *derekh* is feminine gender &c. Ib. דַּרְכּוֹ של איש וכ׳ it is man's way to carry war, and not woman's.—Y. Ned. I, beg. 36ᶜ, a. e. התורה דיברה כִּדְרָכָהּ, v. לָשׁוֹן. Succ. II, 1 לפי דַּרְכֵּינוּ by our way (incidentally). Ab. Zar. 15ᵇ כד׳ שאסור ... כך וכ׳ Ms. M. (ed. כד׳ שאמרו אסור) on the same principle that &c.; a. v. fr.—ד׳ אֶרֶץ (abbrev. ד״א) the way of the land, a) *good manners;* b) *secular occupation, trade;* c) (euphem.) *sexual connection.* Ab. II, 2 study עם ד״א combined with a trade. Tosef. Sot. VII, 20 לימדה.. ד״א וכ׳ the Torah teaches incidentally the proper conduct that one must first build a house &c.—Gitt. 70ª bot. ד׳ וד״א וכ׳ travelling, marital connection &c. Gen. R. s. 18, end. Ib. s. 22, beg.—Ib. s. 80 כְּדַרְכָּהּ natural gratification of sexual appetite, שלא כד׳ unnatural. Ib. s. 18, end; a. fr.—Snh. 31ᵇ העביר עלי את הד׳ mutilated me (oth. interpret.: wronged me in business).—*Pl.* דְּרָכִים. Kidd. I, 1. R. Hash. 17ª פירשו מִדַּרְכֵי ציבור they deviated from the ways of the community, became heretics.—דרכי אמורי, v. אֱמוֹרִי.—דרכי שלום ways of peace (ref. to Prov. III, 17); מפני ד׳ ש׳ because the ways of the Law are ways of peace (differ. fr. משום איבה, v. אֵיבָה), i. e. it is a demand of equity, good manners &c., though no special law can be quoted for it. Gitt. V, 8 sq.; a. fr.—דרך ארץ (ד״א) *Derekh Erets (Manners)*, name of a treatise attached to Talmud editions, divided into *Rabba* (Large), and *Zuta* (Small).

דַּרְכָא, דִּירְכָא ch. same. Kidd. 2ᵇ ד׳ דמיכלא וכ׳ it is usual for excessive eating to produce &c.—Ab. Zar. 48ᵇ ד׳ אחרינא another road.

דּוֹרְכָא, דָּרְכָא m. (דרך) *threshing, threshing time.* Targ. Y. I, II Deut. XXV, 4. Targ. Y. Lev. XXVI, 5 (הַרְכָא).

דרכון, Y. Kil. I, 27ª bot., v. יַרְבּוּז.

דַּרְכּוֹן m. (late b. h. אֲדַרְכֹּן, hellenized Δαρεικός) *Daric,* a Persian gold (and silver) coin, v. infra.—*Tosef. B. Bath. XI, 2 דָּרִיכוֹן ed. Zuck. (Var. דריאבון).—*Pl.* דַּרְכּוֹנוֹת.— Shek. II, 1 (in carrying the half-Shekel contributions to Jerusalem) מצרפין שקלים לד׳ (old ed. לדרב׳) you may exchange them for Darics. B. Bath. X, 2 (165ᵇ) if in a note is found ד׳ דאינון וכ׳ (Var. דַּרְכְּמוֹנוֹת) 'Darics which are'—and the rest is blurred. Shek. II, 4 after the Jews came from Babylonia היו שוקלין ד׳ they offered their half-Shekels in (half-)Darics of silver (this being the standard coin); Y. ib. 46ᵈ top ד׳ דינרין *Darics,* which is *denars* (of silver, v. דִּינָר). Tosef. ib. II, 4; Y. ib. III, 47ᶜ bot. דרכונות של זהב (Bab. ed. Var. דַּרְכְּמוֹנֵי זהב; Ms. M. דַּרְכּוֹנֵי).

דרכל, v. זַרְכֵּל.

דַּרְכְּמוֹן m. (late b. h.)=דַּרְכּוֹן.—*Pl.* דַּרְכְּמוֹנוֹת, v. דַּרְכּוֹן.

דרכמונין, Lam. R. to I, 6, a corrupt. for מָנִין (v. מָנֶה) with a numeral before it, perh. ארבע or ד׳.

דָּרַם, *Hif.* הִדְרִים (denom. of דָּרוֹם) *to turn southward.* B. Bath. 25ᵇ יַדְרִים shall face South(-East) in prayer.— *Part. Hof.* מוּדְרָם *exposed to the southern sun;* pl. f. מוּדְרָמוֹת. Men. 85ª.

דְּרַם ch., *Af.* אַדְרֵים same. B. Bath. 25ᵇ אַדְרִימוּ אַדְרוּמֵי face ye South-East.

דַּרְמוּסְקוֹס, v. דַּרְמַסְקוֹס.

דרמינון, Y. Shebi. II, beg. 37ᵇ, read: רוֹדוֹמֵילוֹן m. (ῥοδόμηλον) *a marmelade of quinces and roses.*

דַּרְמַסְקוֹס, דַּרְמוּס׳ (דרומיס׳) pr. n. pl. (*district of*) *Damascus.* Gen. R. s. 44, end דרמו׳; Yalk. ib. 78 דרמס׳ (expl. הקיני, Gen. XV, 19); B. Bath. 56ª ערדיסקוס.

דַּרְמַסְקִינָא, דַּרְמַסְקִינִין m. pl. (pl. of δαμασκηνόν) *Damascene plums.* Y. Sabb. I, 4ª bot.; Y. Bets. III, 62ª top דורמסקנא, נה ..... Ber. 39ª דורמסקין (Ms. M. margin דורמסקנין; Y. ib. VI, 10ᵇ bot. אַחְוָנַיָּיא).—B. Kam. 116ᵇ top דורמסקנין. Tosef. Ter. VII, 13 דרמסקנין. Tosef. Dem I, 9 דורמסקיות ed. Zuck. (Var. הַדּוּרְמַסְקְנִיּוֹת).

דֶּרֶן m. (cmp. b. h. הֵרָאוֹן) *deren,* name of a parasite worm.—*Pl.* דְּרָנִים, constr. דַּרְנֵי. Ḥull. 67ᵇ. Sabb. 54ᵇ ד׳ ראשה the worms in the sheep's head.

דַּרְנָא ch. same, also *moth* in clothes; *wood worm.* Sabb. 75ª top (in Hebr. diction) יריעה שנפל בה ד׳ a curtain of the Tabernacle which was attacked by moths. Ib. קרש שנפל בו ד׳ Ms. M. (ed. שנפלה).—*Pl.* דַּרְנֵי. Ḥull. 67ᵇ. V. זַרְנָא.

דרניקוס, v. חדרניקוס.

דָּרַס 1) *to tread, stamp.* B. Kam. II, 1 דָּרְסָה על וכ׳ if she trod upon a vessel. Y. Maasr. II, 49ᵈ bot. והוא עתיד לדוֹרְסָן dates which he intends to stamp; a. fr.— בית הדּוֹרְסִין, v. מַעְגִּיל.—Part. pass. דָּרוּס, f. דְּרוּסָה.—דְּרוּסַת איש (calcata a viro) *defloured.* Keth. I, 7.—2) (ritual) *to press,* i. e. *to cut the throat of an animal by pressing the knife* (adding muscular force to the cutting capacity of the knife, instead of passing the latter to and back). Ḥull. 20ᵇ. Ib. 30ᵇ שמא יִדְרוֹס זה על זה lest they press the knife by one adding to the strength of the other.— Denom. דְּרָסָה.—3) (of animals of prey) *to attack with paws or claws.* Ib. 53ª. Pes. 49ᵇ; Snh. 90ᵇ; a. fr.—Ḥull. III, 6 עוֹף הַדּוֹרֵס a bird of prey (that seizes food with its claws or eats animals before they are dead).—דְּרוּסָה f. *an animal known to have been attacked by a beast or bird of prey* (which are suspected of leaving a poisonous substance in the body). Ib. III, 1 (42ª) דְּרוּסַת הזאב an animal saved from the attack of a wolf.—יש דרוסה ל- the case of a *d'rusah* applies to one attacked by &c. Ib. 52ᵇ; a. fr.—4) *to stuff food into the camel's mouth,* contrad. to אָבַס a. הִלְעִיט.—Sabb. XXIV, 3; Gen. R. s. 63; Num. R. s. 21.

Nif. נִדְרַס *to be trodden down, to be effaced* (by treading or otherwise). B. Mets. 22ª עשוי לִידָּרֵס liable to be effaced; ib.ᵇ.

דְּרַס, דְּרֵיס ch. same, 1) *to tread.* Targ. Y. I Deut. XXVIII, 56; a. e.—Lev. R. s. 28, end דְּרוֹס עלי step on me.—Part. pass. דְּרִיס. Targ. Y. Deut. XXVIII, 33 *oppressed.*—2) *to press, use as a rest* (v. מִדְרָס). Nidd. 32ᵇ הא קא דָּרֵיס לכולהו Ar. (ed. הא דרס להו).—3) as preced. 2). Ḥull. 9ª זמנין דשהי ודָרֵיס וכ׳ he may sometimes pause or press unawares.—4) as preced. 3). Part. act. דָּרֵיס, pass. דְּרִיס, f. דְּרִיסָא. Targ. Y. Lev. XX, 25; a. e.—Ḥull. 53ª דדָרֵיס ופסקוהו לידיה when people cut its forefeet off, while it was attacking; a. e.

Ithpe. אִידְּרַס as preced. *Nif.* B. Mets. 22ᵇ sq. משום דמִדַּרְסָא because the mark is likely to be effaced.

דְּרָסָה f. (דָּרַס 2) *pressing the knife* (which makes the animal so cut ritually forbidden). Ḥull. 9ª; a. e. [Y. Sabb. I, 2ᵈ bot., v. דְּרִיסָה.]

דְּרַע I=זְרַע *to sow.* Targ. Koh. II, 5. Targ. Job XXXI, 8 Ms. (ed. זרע). [דרעינא, Ḥag. 5ª, v. רְעָא I.]

דְּרַע II, דַּרְעָא m. (preced.) *seed, produce; offspring.* Targ. Y. Gen. IV, 3 (ed. Amst. מזרע). Targ. Cant. I, 14; a. e.—Targ. Ps. XXXVII, 26 (ed. Lag. ז׳, Var. ד׳).

דְּרַע III, דְּרָעָא (דְּרוֹעָא) c. ch.=h. זְרוֹעַ, *arm,* (of animals) *shoulder.* Targ. Ex. VI, 6. Targ. O. Num. VI, 19 (Y. אֶדְרוֹעָא); a. fr.—Gitt. 31ᵇ; Ber. 5ᵇ לִדְרָעֵיה, v. גְּלֵי. Keth. 65ª [read:] איגלי דְּרָעָהּ her arm was uncovered; a. fr.—[Gen. R. s. 80 שגלה בה דרועה, a corrupt., prob. to be read: שגלתה את זרועה.]—Yoma 33ᵇ עבורי ד׳ וכ׳ it is forbidden to forego the arm in favor of the forehead, i. e. to reverse the order of putting on T'fillin (Deut. VI, 8; oth. interpret. v. Tosaf. a. l.). Ib. מד׳ (Ms. M. מאדרדעא).—*Pl.* דְּרָעַיָּא, דְּרוֹעַ׳. Targ. Ps. XXXVII, 17 דְּרוֹעֵי.—

Targ. O. Gen. XLIX, 24.—דְּרָעָתָא. Targ. Job XXII, 9 וּדְרָעַת Ms. (ed. אדרעת).

דרפתקי, v. דְּרוּפְתְקֵי.

דרצונא, v. next w.

דּוּרְצִינִי, דָּרְצִינִי f. (Pers. *dâr sini*, Lag. Ges. Abh. 35, Löw Pfl. p. 346) [*Chinese wood,*] *cinnamon.* Sabb. 65ª דורצניי Ms. M. (ed. דרצונא, Ar. דרצין; v. Rabb. D. S. a. l. note).

דְּרַק=זְרַק *to sprinkle, strew, thrust.* Targ. Job II, 12. Targ. Y. Ex. XIX, 13; a. e.

Pa. דָּרֵיק same. Targ. II Chr. XXIX, 22.

דְּרָקוֹן m. (δράκων) *dragon, Boa Constrictor* (v. Sm. Ant. s. v.). [Its figure was used as a military ensign of the Roman cohorts. In Talm. it is considered an emblem of idolatry.] Ab. Zar. III, 3 if one finds vessels ... ועליהם צורת ד׳ upon which is the figure of the sun .... or of a dragon. Tosef. ib. V (VI), 2 איזהו מין ד׳ שאסור (v. ed. Zuck. note) what kind of serpent is forbidden (as an emblem of idolatry)?; Y. ib. III, 42ᵈ top.—Lev. R. s. 16, beg. (ref. to תעכסנה, Is. III, 16; cmp. עֲכָסִים) שהיתה צורת ד׳ וכ׳ the figure of a serpent was on her shoes; Lam. R. to IV, 15 דרקין (corr. acc.). B. Bath. 16ᵇ. Gitt. 56ᵇ וד׳ כרוך עליה and a serpent wound around the barrel (allusion to the city of Jerusalem under the terrorism of the extremists). [Deut. R. s. 6 בא הדרבון, corr. acc.] [Y. Kil. I, 27ª bot. Ar., v. תַּרְבּוּז.]

דְּרָקוֹנָא, דְּרָקוֹן ch. same. Gitt. 56ᵇ. Ber. 62ᵇ אתא ד׳ וכ׳, v. כַּרְכַּשְׁתָּא II; Gitt. 57ª דרקנא (corr. acc.).

דרקונים, דרקונוס, v. הדרניקוס.

דְּרָרָא I m. (דְּרָא I) [*row of teeth,*] *the gum* (cmp. דּוּרְשׁוּרֵי). Ab. Zar. 28ª; Yoma 84ª רמי מידי בי כביה ואתי (רמי . . . (ואתא) ומיתי דמא מבי דררי) דמי מִדְּרָרֵיה Ar. (ed. if he puts anything between his teeth, his gums will bleed. Ib. ודַבֵּיק בי דרריך Ar. ed. Koh. (read: דְּרָרָיךְ; ed. Ab. Zar. ביה דררי; Yoma בבכי דרריה, Rashi דרריה; v. Rabb. D. S. a. l.) and stick it into the inside of thy gums.

דְּרָרָא II m. (דור, v. דרר) [*the object around which the question revolves,*] *stake, risk.* ד׳ דממון *fixed sum.* Targ. Esth. IV, 7.—In Talm. ד׳ דממונא *money at stake, eventual loss.* B. Mets. 2ᵇ. Keth. 23ᵇ; a. fr.—Hag. 21ᵇ ד׳ דטומאה מדאורייתא an eventual violation of the Biblical law of purity; Nidd. 6ª.

דְּרַרְיָא f. (an adaptation of διάῤῥοια, as if fr. דְּרִי I; as to dialectic variations, v. infra) *diarrhœa.* Lev. R. s. 18 (explain. זָרָא, Num. XI, 20) R. Ebiathar says, *l'zara* means לד׳ Ar.; Num. R. s. 7 לד׳ שאהיה נותן דורא וכ׳ (not אותן) Ar. (ed. לקרדא or לקדרא) it will cause diarhœa, for I will put a worm in their entrails. Sifré Deut. 1 דולריא; Pesik. Vattom., p. 131ª דרר׳ Ar. (Var. in Ar. a. ed. דלר׳, Ms. O. דרד׳, Ms. Parma דר אריא), v. גֶּסָה. Gitt. 70ª (כילכמה) אוחזתו דל׳ will be seized with diarrhœa. [Ib. (מיושב) אוחזתו דל׳ ed., Ar. אלריא q. v.] Ib. מאי דל׳ (insert סם) what is the remedy for *d.*? Ans. כַּרְדָּרָא q. v.

דָּרַשׁ (b. h.) 1) *to examine, question.* Denom. דְּרִישָׁה.—2) *to expound, interpret.* Ber. I, 5 עד שדְּרָשָׁהּ בן זומא until Ben Zoma found an intimation of it in the Biblical wording. Taan. 5ᵇ מקרא אני דוֹרֵשׁ I find it intimated in a Bible verse. B. Mets. 104ª היה ד׳ לשון הדיוט interpreted the popular (Chaldaic) wording used in documents. Pes. 22ᵇ, v. אֵת; a. v. fr.—Part. pass. דָּרוּשׁ, f. דְּרוּשָׁה. Y. Yeb. VIII, 8ᵈ top והלא ד׳ הוא has not the word ממזר been employed for interpretation?, opp. מופנה.—Denom. מִדְרָשׁ, דְּרִישָׁה.—3) (in gen.) *to teach, lecture.* Hag. II, 1 אין דּוֹרְשִׁין בב׳ you must not lecture on &c. Snh. 99ᵇ ודורש בהגדות וכ׳ lectured on topics with the object of fault-finding; a. v. fr.—דּוֹרֵשׁ *lecturer.* Ex. R. s. 42, beg. אבא הַד׳ Abba, the lecturer. Ib. s. 8, end, v. אֲמֵירָא.—*Pl.* דּוֹרְשִׁים. Snh. 38ᵇ; Ab. Zar. 5ª דור דור ודוֹרְשָׁיו every generation with its preachers. חוֹמֵר, דּוֹרְשֵׁי חמורות, v. חוֹמֶר; ד׳ רשומות, v. רְשׁוּמָה. [M. Kat. II, 5 (13ᵇ) הדרשין Ms. M. (ed. עושין), read הוֹשְׁשִׁין.]

Nif. נִדְרַשׁ *to be interpreted, expounded.* Sifra, introd. rules שהתורה נִדְרֶשֶׁת בהן by which the Law is interpreted. Y. Peah II, 17ª דברים הַנִּדְרָשִׁין מן הכתב things which are derived by interpretation from the written code (Torah); הנדרשין מן הפה derived from the oral code (Mishnah). Y. Meg. I, 70ª top נתנה לְהִידָּרֵשׁ is a legitimate object of interpretation.

Hithpa. הִתְדָּרֵשׁ same. Y. Keth. III, 27ᵈ top מִתְדָּרֵשׁ (מִתְדָּרְשָׁה) ולו וכ׳ the words *v'lo* &c. are open for interpretation, v. גְּזֵרָה.

דְּרַשׁ ch. same. [Targ. Jer. XLVIII, 26, some ed., וידרשון, v. דְּשַׁשׁ.] Targ. Jud. V, 9.—Succ. 51ᵇ bot. קרא אשכחו ודְרוּשׁ they found a Bible verse and interpreted it. Arakh. 30ᵇ איכא לְמִידְרְשִׁינְהוּ וכ׳ it may be interpreted in favor of a lenient practice &c.—Sot. 21ª לְהאי קרא ... דְּרַשִׁיה R. .... interpreted this verse. Ib. מאי דְרוּשׁ what verse did they interpret (to guide them in their action)?—Bets. 28ª דְּרַשִׁינַן הוה ליה . . . משמך we taught in thy name. Yeb. 94ª לְמִידְרַשׁ וכ׳ R. El. might have given a valuable interpretation &c., v. מַרְגָּנִיתָא. Lev. R. s. 9 עד דיחסל מִמִּדְרַשׁ until he ended his lecture. Ber. 28ª נִדְרוֹשׁ מר וכ׳ shall this teacher lecture one Sabbath, and the other &c.? Ib. לְדָרוֹשׁ ר׳ (v. Rabb. D. S. a. l. note); a. v. fr.—דָּרֵישׁ *lecturer.* Y. Yeb. XII, 13ª top ד׳ ודיין וכ׳ to serve as lecturer, judge &c.

Ithpe. אִידְּרִישׁ *to be interpreted.* Ber. 63ª . . . האי קרא מִידְּרִישׁ וכ׳ this verse (Ps. CXIX, 126) can be interpreted in its regular order (it is time to work &c., because people neglect the law) or in inverted order (the teachers ignore the letter of the law, because it is time to work for the Lord by guarding its spirit); ib. 60ª; Snh. 70ª.

דְּרָשָׁא, pl. **דְּרָשַׁיָּא**, v. דְּרוֹשָׁא.

דְּרָשָׁא, (h. form) **דְּרָשָׁה** f. (preced.) *interpretation, argument, attempt to harmonize.* Pes. 62ᵇ ת׳ גמלי דדרשה (Ms. M. דְּרָשֵׁי pl., v. Rabb. D. S. a. l. note), v. אֲצִיל.—Yeb. 54ᵇ לד׳ אתי is required for an argument to be based upon it. Ib. ומאי ד׳ and what is the argument based upon it?

Ib. 70[b] בו לדרשה וכ׳ the word *bo* (Ex. XXII, 44, a. e.) is inserted for interpretation (emphasis); a. fr.

דַּרְשָׁן m. (preced. wds.) *interpreter of the law, lawyer, lecturer.* Lev. R. s. 30, beg.—*Pi.* דַּרְשָׁנִין, דַּרְשָׁנִים. Sot. 49[b]; Tosef. ib. XV, 5 דּוֹרְשָׁנִים. Gen. R. s. 5. Koh. R. to VII, 5; a. fr.—Fem. דַּרְשָׁנִית, pl. דַּרְשָׁנִיּוֹת. B. Bath. 119[b] ד׳ היו (not חן, v. Rabb. D. S. a. l.) were good lawyers (arguers).

דָּרָא, דָּרְתָא, דַּרְתָּא f. (דור) 1) *court-yard.* Targ. Ex. XXVII, 12; a. fr.—[Targ. II Esth. V, 1; VI, 5 דרא; I Esth. דרתא.]—Y. Snh. X, 28[a] bot. עד דַּרְתֵּיה דר׳ וכ׳ (ed. Krot. דַּרְתֵּה) to the court of R. H.'s residence. Yoma 72[b]; Sabb. 31[b] דלית ליה ד׳ וכ׳ he who has no court, but makes a gate-way for his court (who possesses erudition but no fear of the Lord).—*Pl.* דָּרָתָא (דַּרְתַּיָּא), דָּרְאָתָא. Targ. II Kings XXI, 5 (ed. Lag. דָּרַת constr.). Targ. Ps. X, 8 דורתיא ed. Lag. (Var. דדרתיא, Ms. דּוּרְאָתָיָא). Targ. I Chr. XXIII, 28 דרתיא ed. Lag. (ed. Rahmer דראתא).—2) *buildings, dwellings* in a court.—*Pl.* דָּרְתָא. B. Bath. 67[a] if he said דִּירָתָא, all agree, it meant *houses;* they differ only when he said דַּרְתָּא (Ms. O. דָּרָאתָא), the one says, the court is meant &c. Ib. if he said דָּרָאתָא (Ms. M. דרתא).

דרתא, Targ. O. Lev. II, 7, v. רְדָתָא.

דרתנא, Targ. Prov. XVI, 28, v. חַרְתָּנָא.

דַּשׁ, v. דּוּשׁ.

דֶּשֶׁא m. (b. h.) *tender grass, herbage.*—*Pl.* דְּשָׁאִים, דְּשָׁאִין *herbs.* Ber. VI, 1. Ex. R. s. 17, beg. Hull. 60[a]. Y. Kil. I, 27[b] top. R. Hash. 11[a] what month is it שהארץ מוציאה ד׳ וכ׳ in which the earth produces fresh green while the trees are full of fruits?—Ib. הארץ מליאה ד׳ the ground is covered with herbs.

דַּשָּׁא (דָּשָׁא, ד׳) m. (=דרשא, Sam. דרשה; דרש, cmp. also דּוּשׁ) *entrance, door-way* (v. דְּרִיסָה); *door.* Targ. O. Gen. XIX, 6 דַּשָּׁא ed. Berl. (oth. ed. a. Y. דָּשָׁא). Targ. O. Ex. XXI, 6 דַּשָּׁא ed. Berl. (Y. דָּ׳); a. fr.—Hull. 52[b], v. אֲחַד. Sabb. 77[b]; Keth. 10[b] (phonetic etymol.) דשא דרך שָׁם. Ib. כי עברא לד׳ (as strengthening) as the bolt to a door. Ber. 56[a] ד׳ דבריתא דנפל (read דביתאי, v. Rabb. D. S. a. l. note) (I dreamt) that the door of my house fell down; a. fr.—*Pl.* דַּשֵּׁי, דַּשַּׁיָּא, דַּשִּׁין, ד׳. Targ. Job XXXVIII, 8. Targ. O. Deut. III, 5; a. e. [Targ. Esth. I, 6 ודשרין וכ׳, read וַדַּשִּׁין וכ׳ (or וַדְרָשִׁין, v. supra) and there were turning doors of silver.]—Men. 33[a] תלי דשי וכ׳ (some ed. דשא) hang the door frames in first.

דַּשְׁדֵּשׁ, v. דְּשַׁשׁ.

דִּשּׁוּן, v. דִּישׁ׳.

דשונא, v. רְשׁוּנָא.

דשונה, Tanh. Aharé 3, read שְׁתוּנָה, v. גְּשֵׁם.

דָּשׁוֹשׁ m., pl. **דָּשׁוֹשׁוֹת** (cmp. דָּרוֹכוֹת) *wheat-stampers, groats-makers.* M. Kat. II, 5 (13[b]; Ms. רשתות, רששות, v. Rabb. D. S. a. l.).—Constr. דָּשׁוֹשֵׁי. Ib. 13[b] ed. (Ms. ר׳). V. דְּשַׁשׁ.

דַּשִּׁישׁ, דְּשִׁישׁ, v. דְּשַׁשׁ.

דְּשִׁיתָא pl. (דוש, cmp. דָּשׁוֹשׁוֹת a. פְּתִיּוֹת) *threshing* (women) or *gritsmakers.* Ab. Zar. 24[b] דדיישן ביה ד׳ Ms. M. (ed. only דדיישן); Zeb. 116[b] דדיישן דישאי ed. (Ms. M. דדיישי דִּישְׁתָּאֵי); Men. 22[a] דדשו בה דִּשְׁתָּאֵי (fr. דשש) wherewith the threshers (or gritsmakers) crush the grain.

דָּשֵׁן (b. h.; cmp. דֶּשֶׁא) *to be moist, sappy, fat.*

Pi. דִּשֵּׁן 1) *to bless with rich pastures.* Ber. 29[a] דַּשְּׁנֵנוּ בנאות וכ׳ (cmp. Ps. XXIII, 2) give us pasture on the meadows of thy land.—2) (b. h.; denom. of דֶּשֶׁן) *to remove the ashes, to clean* (the lamps). Tam. III, 9 מְדַשְּׁנָן trims them. Yoma II, 3 מי מְדַשֵּׁן וכ׳ who shall do the cleaning of the inner altar. Tam. III, 1; a. e.

Nithpa. נִתְדַּשֵּׁן 1) *to become sappy, vigorous.* Pirké d'R. El. ch. XXXII, end.—2) *to be treated like the charred wick, to become unfit for sacred use.* Men. 88[b] נר׳ השמן נִידַּשְּׁנָה וכ׳ the oil as well as the wick has become unfit.

דֶּשֶׁן m. (b. h.; v. preced.) 1) *fat, honorary gift,* v. next w.—2) *ashes* (of burnt flesh &c.). Zeb. V, 2, a. fr. בֵּית הד׳ the place where the ashes of sacrifices were deposited.—*Pl.* דְּשָׁנִין. Ib. 104[b] שלש בֵּית הַדְּשָׁנִין (!)

דִּישְׁנָא, דִּשְׁנָא ch. same, *fat piece, honorary gift, present.* Snh. 94[b] (ref. to II Chr. XXXII, 1 in connection with the preceding account) האי ד׳ להאי פרדשנא Ar. (ed. דיש׳; Ms. M. רש׳, corrected into דש׳, oth. Mss. דיש׳, v. Rabb. D. S. a. l. note; Yalk. Kings 235 דיש׳) such a treat for such a gift, i. e. is this an adequate reward? V. דִּיסְקָנָא I.

***דשקתא**, Y. Erub. V, 22[d] bot., v. דִּיסְקְתָא.

דשרין, Targ. Esth. I, 6, v. דַּשָּׁא.

דָּשַׁשׁ (v. דּוּשׁ) *to crush grain, make groats.* M. Kat. 13[b] (Ms. M. ר׳), v. דָּשׁוֹשׁ.

דְּשַׁשׁ ch. same, *Pa.* דַּשִּׁישׁ, *Polel* (of דּוּשׁ) דּוֹשֵׁשׁ *to stamp upon.* Targ. Esth. VI, 1.—Targ. Jer. XLVIII, 26, v. infra.—Targ. Jud. V, 21. Targ. Ps. XVIII, 43 דושי׳ Ms. (ed. Lag. ר׳); Targ. II Sam. XXII, 43. Targ. II Chr. XXXII, 1; a. e.

Af. אַדֵּשׁ *to crush, pound.* Targ. Y. Num. XI, 8.

Palp. דַּשְׁדֵּשׁ *to tramp, reel* (of a drunken person). Targ. Is. XIX, 14; Targ. Jer. XLVIII, 26 וִידַשְׁדְּשׁוּן Ar. (Kimhi וידדשון, ed. Lag. וִידַדְשׁוּן=וידשד׳).—Part. pass. מְדַשְׁדַּשׁ *stamped upon.* Targ. Is. XIX, 14 (h. text מובס).

דִּישׁ׳, דִּשְׁתָּאָה m. (=דשאה; דשש) *thresher* or *gritsmaker.* *Pl.* דִּשְׁתָּאֵי, דִּישׁ׳. Men. 22[a], v. דְּשִׁיתָא.

***דִּשְׁתַּיְיהִי** pr. n. f. *Dishtayhi.* Pes. 110[a] א״ל אם ד׳ מְכַשְּׁפָנִיּוֹת Ms. M. (Ms. O. דיש׳, v. Rabb. D. S. a. l. note; ed. רישתינהו דנשים כשפניות) Mother D. of the sorceresses told me.

דשתן, Y. Shek. V, 49[b] top, v. רַשְׁוָתָא.

דִּשְׁתָּנָא, v. דִּיסְקְנָא II.

דִּשְׁתְּקָא, v. דִּיסְתְּקָא.

דַּת=דְּאַתְּ. Y. Snh. X, 27[d] bot., a. fr. כמה דת מר (=כמה דתימר) as thou sayest, i. e. as we read in Scriptures &c.—Y. Ab. Zar. II, 42[a] top הדא דת מר וכ׳ (interch. with הדא דתימא=הדא דאת אמר) that which thou sayest (hast recited), applies only &c.—Y. Snh. X, 29[d] top על דעתך דת מר according to thy opinion who sayest; a. fr.

דָּת f. (b. h.; =דנת, fem. form of דִּין, Arab. *dîn* corresp. to our w.) 1) *custom, law; judgment, punishment.* Esth. R. to I, 8 כְּדָת כל מקום וכ׳ in accordance with the usages of &c.—Keth. VII, 6 דַּת משה Mosaic (ritual) law, ד׳ יהודית Jewish custom (chastity, decency); Tosef. ib. VII, 6 ד׳ משה וישראל. Ib. 7 שעברו על הדת who disregard the Jewish custom. Esth. R. to I, 15 כדת just dealing, v. אַכְזְרִיּוּת. Meg. 12[a] ד׳ של תורה the Biblical dues (sacrifices); a. fr.—2) *religion.* Succ. 56[b] המירה דָתָהּ (Tosef. ib. IV, 28 נשתמדה) she changed her faith, became an apostate. Yeb. 70[b]; Pes. 96[a] (ref. to Ex. XII, 43, v. דְּרָשָׁא) בו המרת דת וכ׳ to eat of *it* (the passover lamb) apostasy does unfit, but &c.—*Pl.* דָּתִין. Koh. R. to VII, 19 (play on ידותון, I Chr. XXV, 3) הנבא על הד׳ ועל הדינין וכ׳ (Asaph) who prophesied over the judgments and dispensations that passed over him; Cant. R. to IV, 4 (corr. acc.). [As to derivation of our w. from the Persian, v. Ges. H. Dict.[10] s. v.]

דָּתָא, דָּת ch. same. Dan VI, 16. Ib. II, 15; a. fr.—*Pl. constr.* דָּתֵי. Ezra VII, 25.

דְּתָאָה, v. דִּיתָאָה.

דְּתָבְרַיָּא m. pl. (v. Fl. to Levy Talm. Dict. I, 440[b]; 444[b]) *judges.* Dan. III, 2.—Cant. R. to VII, 9, expl. איסכולסטיקי, v. אִיסְכּוֹלַסְטִיקָא.

ה

ה *He,* the fifth letter of the Alphabet.—It interchanges dialectically with א as הֲדָא a. דָא, הִידַיִין a. אִידַיִין, הַגָּדָה a. אַגָּדָה &c.; with ח as דְּהַךְ a. דְּחַךְ, גָּחָה a. גָּהָה &c.; with ו as בְּהִית a. בּוּשׁ, רְהַט a. רוּץ &c.—ה a formative prefix of verbal nouns, e. g. הֶסְפֵּד, הוֹלָכָה &c.

ה׳ as a numeral, *five,* v. א׳.

הֲ־, הַ־, הֶ־ (b. h.) an interrogative prefix. Targ. O. Gen. IV, 9; a. e.—With לא, הֲלָא ch. (=b. h. הֲלֹא) *is it not?, behold, indeed.* Targ. Gen. IV, 7; a. fr.

הַ־, הָ־, הֶ־ (followed by Dagesh forte) 1) the definite article, *the.* Ber. I, 1 הָאַשְׁמוֹרָה הָרִאשׁוֹנָה the first night watch. Ib. הַשַּׁחַר the dawn; a. v. fr.—2) an interjection, *ly.* Sabb. 145[a], v. אֱלוֹהַּ; a. fr.—3) (ch.)=הָא q. v.

הֵא, הֵ״א, הֵ״י *He,* name of the fifth letter of the Alphabet. Y. Maas. Sh. V, 56[a] לא מתמנעין רבנין דרשי (not דרב׳) בין ה״א לח״ת the rabbis do not hesitate to draw analogies between words written with *He* and those with *Ḥeth* (as *hillulim* and *ḥillulim*); Y. Peah VII, 20[b] bot. Y. Meg. I, 71[c] bot. צריך לכתוב ה״א וכ׳ you must write the *He* of *laădonay* (Deut. XXXII, 6) so that it extend below the foot of the *Lammed.* Y. Sabb. VII, 9[b] bot. ה״א תמניא וכ׳ *He* may count for eight, as the rabbis do not hesitate &c., v. supra.—Men. 37[a] מידכה (כתיב בה״י) כהה (v. Rabb. D. S. a. l. note) it is derived from *yad'khah* (Ex. XIII, 16) with a *He,* which intimates (יד כהה) the weak (left) hand; a. fr.—*Pl.* הֵ״הִין. Y. Ber. II, 4[d] bot. עושין ה׳ חיתין they pronounce *He* like Ḥeth. Sabb. 103[b].

הָא I f. (demonstr. pronoun) *this.* Yoma 26[a] הא שכיחא והא וכ׳ the one is a frequent (daily) performance, but the other is rare. Ber. 2[a] והא קמ״ל and this he intimates. Ib. 4[b] והא דקאמרי וכ׳ and as to this (the fact) that they say, 'Until midnight', it is said in order to prevent &c. Ib. 9[a] הא דר׳ אחא as to this (opinion) of R. Aḥa. Ib. 15[b] הא דידיה והא דרביה the one represents his own opinion, the other that of his teacher; a. v. fr.—הא והא *both.* Taan. 25[a] bot.; a. fr.—Contractions: הָנִיחָא=הא ניחא this would be right. Yoma 3[a]; a. fr.—וְהָדְתַנְיָא=והא דת׳ and as to it being taught in the Boraitha. B. Kam. 12[a]; a. fr.—With prefixes: דְּהָא *of this.* Yoma 13[b] דגיטא דהא וכ׳ that the letter of divorce for this wife is invalid; a. fr.—אַהָא=על הא *referring to this.* Keth. 40[b] אַתּוּן אהא וכ׳ ye cited it (Resh Lakish's opinion) with reference to that, we used to cite it with reference to this; a. fr.—2) *here, here is.* Targ. Gen. XXII, 7; a. fr.—B. Kam. 12[a] הא עולא וכ׳ here is (the opinion of) Ulla, here &c.; a. fr.—3) (as conjunction) [*there is this,*] a) introducing a self-evident consequent, *then of course.* Yoma 13[a] מיתה חד הא קיימא הא if that one dies, there is the other one living; a. fr.—דְּהָא *for, of course.* Ber. 3[b] דהא אשה וכ׳ for, of course, a woman is not liable to be found in the open field; a. fr.—b) introducing a counter-argument, [*here is a case speaking against you,*] *but, is'nt it?* &c. Ib. 4[b] ואי אמרת . . . הא לא קא סמך . . . דהא וכ׳ and if you be right in saying that one must &c.; then he failed to do so, since he had to say *hashkibenu* between. Ib. 9[b] הא בלילא נמי וכ׳ are they not by night, too, distinguishable?—Ib. 13[a] לקרות והא קא קרי you say, 'if he directed his heart' (Mish. II, 1) means the intention to read in the Law? well, was he not reading?—Ib. ולרבי נמי הא כתיב שמע but according to Rabbi's opinion, too, does not the text say *sh'ma* (you must understand)?—Contractions: הָכְתִיב=הא כתיב, הָאָמַר=הא אמר, הָתַנְיָא=הא תניא do we not read?, did he not say?, has it not been taught? &c. Yoma 26[a]. R. Hash. 34[b]. Ber. 14[b]; a. fr.—c) introducing an inference of limitation, *this means to say but.*— Ib. 13[b] מקרא ... הא מיגנא ש״ד *read* he dare not (while lying on his back), but sleeping in that position is permitted?, והא ר׳ וכ׳ but did'nt R..... say &c.?—Y. Succ. V, beg. 55[a] (ref. to Mishnah: 'playing the flute &c.) הא של קרבן דוחה this allows the inference that at offerings the playing does supersede the Sabbath.—[Targ. Y. Ex. VII, 23 הא some ed., read דָא.]

הָא II, **הָא** I (v. preced.) an interjection, 1) (cmp. הָה) *Oh!* Targ. Jer. IV, 30 (not והא).—Ned. II, 2 (15[b]) הא קרבן שאוכל לך (Mish. a. Y. ed. קרבן) Oh, the sacrifice, that I will (not) eat this which belongs to thee!. Ib. 16[a] לא שנו ליה קרבן...הקרבן draws no distinction between *korban* and *ha-korban* (v. marginal note to Rashi a. l.). Ib. II, 2 הא שבועה שאוכל לך (Mish. a. Y. ed. שבועה) Oh, an oath that &c. Ib. 16[a] מכלל דהא שבועה שאוכל וכ׳ we infer from this that 'Oh, an oath that I will eat' means that I will not eat.—2) *behold* (h. הֵן, הִנֵּה). Dan. III, 25.—Targ. Gen. III, 22. Ib. XX, 15; a. fr.—Dan. II, 43 הָא־כְדִי *as if.*— Targ. Ps. CXXIII, 2 הָא כמא *as,* .... הא כדין Ms. (ed. הָכְדֵין) *so.*—3) introducing a question, *is it that?* Targ. Job XV, 7; a. e.—Ib. XXXVIII, 19 הא דין Ms. (ed. אֵידֵין) *where?*

הָא II, **הֵא הֵא** pr. n. m. *He-He.* Ab. V, 23 בן הא הא. Ḥag. 9[b] בר הֵי הֵי (Ms. M. 2 הֵיהֵי); Yalk. Is. 328; Yalk. Mal. 591 בר הא הא (v. Rabb. D. S. to Ḥag. l. c. note 19).

הָא III name of *a worm,* v. הֵה.

הַאֲזָנָה f. (אָזַן) *giving ear, close attention,* contrad. to שְׁמִיעָה. Sifré Deut. 306.

הַאי c. (=הָ־אִי) *this, that.* Targ. Ruth IV, 6, v. גְּוָונָא. Ber. 2[a] ה׳ וטהר this *v'taher* (Lev. XXII, 7). Ib. 4[b] ה׳ אחד this 'one' (Is. VI, 6). Ib. 6[a] ה׳ מאן דְּבָעֵי וכ׳ he who wants &c. Ib. 7[b] bot. מאי כולי ה׳ (Ms. M. למה לך כולי ה׳) what is all this for?—Ib. 8[b] בה׳ שעתא at that hour. Erub. 10[a]; a. fr. ה׳ מאי what is that, i. e. what has this to do here?, this is no argument.—Ber. 43[a] ה׳ משחא וכ׳ as to balsam oil &c. Ḥag. 4[b] כולי ה׳ ואולי all that (suffering) and yet only 'perhaps'!—Ib. ה׳ קרא this (following) verse; a. v. fr.—With suffix ך (*locale*) הַאיְךְ *the one there, the former.* R. Hash. 2[b] בשלמא ה׳ ... אלא האי וכ׳ I grant it as to the former (verse), for it says distinctly . . ., but as to the latter &c. Snh. 4[b] ירשיעון דהאיך והאי (Ms. M. האיך והאי) *the Elohim* which is the subject to *yarshiun* (Ex. XXII, 8) is the same in the preceding clause as in this, i. e. it means the same number of judges, and the repetition of *Elohim* does not intimate a differently construed court. B. Bath. 167[b] איתתיה דה׳ the other one's wife; a. fr.

הָאיְדְּנָא, v. אִידְּנָא.

הַאיְךְ, v. האי.

הָאֵיק, Targ. Job. XXIV, 16, v. חוּק ch.

הַאיתָא f. *cream,* v. הַאיְתָא.

הַאיתָא=הָא אִיתָא, v. הָא I a. אִית.

הָאֵל, הָאל (cmp. הָלְאָה) 1) *farther off, far* (of space). Targ. Y. Gen. XXXII, 25 מן ה׳ on the other side of. Targ. Y. Num. XVII, 2 לה׳ far away.—2) לה׳ *onward* (of time). Targ. Y. Ex. XVI, 21.

הַאֲמָנָה f. (אמן) 1) *confirmation, fulfillment.* Shebu. 36[a] הַאֲמָנַת דברים prayer for fulfillment, v. אָמֵן II.—2) *faith.* Yalk. Is. 296; Yalk. Hos. 519 (interchanging with אֱמוּנָה a. אֲמָנָה). Tosef. B. Bath. V, 8 some ed.; a. fr.

הָאן (=הא אן) *where? whither?* Targ. Y. Gen. XXII, 7. Targ. Job XXIV, 25 Ms. (ed. הָן). Targ. Ps. CXXXIX, 7 Ms. (ed. Lag. והאן . . אן; ed. ואן . . אן); a. e.—V. הָן.

הָאֲנָא (=הא אנא) *behold I.* Targ. Jer. XXIII, 32 (ed. Wil. הָאֲנָא). Targ. Y. Gen. XXII, 7 (ed. Amst. הָא נָא, two words); a. e.

*__הָאַסְטוּ__ f. (a Samaritan word, cmp. הָ־ a. סטר) *Oh, the perversion* (of the law)! Y. Shebi. IV, 35[a]; Y. Snh. III, 21[b] top [read:] חד משמרייא הוה עבר בשמיטתא .... אמר לון ה׳ שרי לכון מירדא וכ׳ a Samaritan passed (by Jewish fields) in the Sabbatical year and saw them throw up the ploughed clods, when he said to them, Oh, that perversion of the law! You have been given permission to plough (in the Sabbatical year, because of the government's' edict), but have you been permitted to &c.?

הָאֵק, Targ. Job XXIV, 16, v. חוק ch.

הַאֲרָה f. (אור) 1) *kindling.* Sifra Tsav, Par. 11, ch. XVI, end הַאֲרַת הנרות kindling the lights in the Temple (quoted by Hai Gaon to Zeb. ch. III; differ. vers. in ed.).— 2) הַאֲרַת פנים *shining of divine countenance, grace.* Midr. Till. to Ps. LXXX, end; Yalk. ib. 830.

הַב 1) abbrev. of יְהַב. Ab. Zar. 76[b] והב ליה לבאטר and gave it to B.—Ib. והב ליה למר וכ׳ Ms. M. (ed. הב). Y. Ber. I, 2[d] bot. there are people הָבִין וכ׳ who pay money for the permission to visit the palace.—2) Imperat. of יְהַב. [הב הב, Targ. Prov. XXX, 15 ed. Wil., v. הַבְהֵב.]

הֲבָאָה f. (בּוֹא) 1) *carrying, bringing.* Bicc. II, 2 require הֲבָאַת מקום to be brought to the Temple place (Deut. XII, 5 sq.). Ḥag. 4[b] ישנו בה׳ is subject to the law of offering festive sacrifices. Y. Sabb. III, 6[a] הבאת לונטיות carrying home the bathing sheets; Y. Erub. VIII, 25[b] top; a. fr.—*Pl.* הֲבָאוֹת. Yoma 47[a] (ref. to Lev. XVI, 12) הבאה ה׳ . . ולא שתי ה׳ the Law speaks of *one* carrying in but not of offering in two instalments.—2) *bringing about, making.* Peah I, 1 הבאת שלום וכ׳ making peace between &c; Yeb. 109[a]; a. e.—[3) *drawing home* of the slaughtering knife &c., opp. to הוֹלָכָה moving forward; (used in commentaries and digests).]

הֲוַאי, הֲבַאי m. (הבי, הוי, cmp. הבל) [*breath,*] *vanity, vain talk; impossibility, exaggeration, rhetorical phrase.* Ned. III, 1 נדרי הב׳ vows made dependent on an impossibility, expl. ib. 2 קונם וכ׳ I may be forbidden...., if I have not seen &c. (a mere exaggeration not meant literally). Ib. 24b שבועות ה׳ oaths affirming &c. (Shebu. III, 8 שבועת שוא). Ḥull. 90b לשון הב׳ Ar. (ed. חו׳) exaggeration in rhetorical speech; Tam. 29a; a. e. V. גּוּזְמָא.

חַבְאָשָׁה f. (באש) *disfigurement through disease.* Yalk. Deut. 942 (Tana d'be El. Zut. ch. III בּוּשָׁה).

חָבַב, חֲבַב, v. חַבְחֵב, חַבְחֵב.

חַבְדָּלָה f. (בָּדַל) 1) *cutting apart.* Hull. 20b מצות ה׳ the law ordering the separation of the head from the body (Lev. I, 15). Ib. ישנו בה׳ must be cut apart; a. fr.—2) *separation.* Gen. R. s. 3 ויבדל ה׳ ממש *vayyabdel* (Gen. I, 4) means real separation (in space, not logical differentiation). Ḥag. 15a דהואי . . . . . . ה׳ the separation (of the waters) took place on the second day.—3) *Habdalah,* a formula of prayer for the exit of the Sabbath or Festivals, v. אַבְדָּלָה. Ber. VIII, 5; a. fr.—*Pl.* הַבְדָּלוֹת *the distinctions referred to in the Habdalah.* Ḥull. 26b bot.; Pes. 104a סדר ה׳ the order of the subjects of distinction. Ib. מעין ה׳ האמורות וכ׳ corresponding to the distinctions mentioned in the Bible (Lev. X, 10 &c.).

חִבְהֵב I (Pilp. of חבב *to glow;* cmp. חבל) 1) *to singe, parch.* Y. Maasr. IV, beg., 51a הַמְהַבְהֵב שיבולין באור if one parches ears over the fire; Tosef. ib. III, 1 המה׳ בשדה וכ׳ (sub. שיבולין). Men. X, 4 (66a). Bets. 34a. Sabb. II, 3 ולא הִבְהֲבָהּ and did not singe it (to prepare it for a wick).—Snh. 37a is it possible for fire to be in contact with flax ואינה מְהַבְהֶבֶת and not to singe?—*Part. pass.* מְהוּבְהָב *lightly roasted.* Y. ib. VIII, beg., 26a.—2) *to be like coals giving heat without flame; to nod consent without showing anxiety.* Ber. 34a שנים מחבחב (Y. ib. V, 9c bot. מעמעם) if asked a second time, he must not consent &c.

Nithpa. נִתְהַבְהֵב *to be affected by flames.* Yoma 41b נ׳ הלשון if the band caught fire.

חַבְהֵב ch. same; part. pass. מְהַבְהַב 1) *glowing with passion, greedy. Pl. fem.* מְהַבְהֲבָן. Targ. Prov. XXX, 15 ed. Lag. (ed. Wil. הב הב).—2) *lightly roasted; rare.* Targ. Y. Lev. II, 14 (h. text קלוי). Targ. Y. II Ex. XII, 9 (Y. I a. O. כד חי, h. text נא).—Yalk. Ex. 191 (symbolizing Ex. XII, 9) לא תַבְעוּנָה מְהַבְהֲבָה desire not to consume her (Rome) half-done (but well ripe for destruction); Pesik. R. s. 15; Pesik. Haḥod. p. 56b (corr. acc.).

חַבְהֲבָא m. (preced.) *glow, heat.* Targ. Y. II Gen. XLIV, 19.

חָבוּ, בַּר חָבוּ pr. n. m. *Bar Habu (Ḥabu),* a writer of T'fillin and M'zuzoth. Ber. 53b אדבי בר ה׳ Ms. M. (Ar. ה׳, ed. אבהו) over the lights in the house of Bar H.—Meg. 18b (v. Rabb. D. S. a. l. note 60). B. Mets. 29b.

חַבָּטָה f. (נבט) 1) *looking at, keeping in sight.* Gen. R. s. 44 (ref. to Gen. XV, 5) אין ה׳ אלא מלמעלה וכ׳ the use of *hibbit* indicates a looking down from above. Lam. R. to V, 1 ה׳ מקרוב *hibbit* is used for looking at a near object, contrad. to ראייה.—2) *superintendence, watching owner-less objects,* as fruits of the Sabbatical year, v. הֶפְקֵר. B. Mets. 118a כאן בהגבהה כאן בה׳ in the one case the laborer was hired for taking up abandoned objects, in the other for watching. Ib. ה׳ בהפקר קני watching gives the right of possession of *hefker.* [Ms. M. has חֲבָטָה; Ar., s. v. בט 2, hesitates betw. ה׳ a. ח׳.]

חבטח, v. בָּטַח II.

חַבְטָחָה f. (בָּטַח) *assurance, divine promise, faith.* Ex. R. s. 38 באתה הה׳ the promise came true. Ber. 17a גדולה ה׳ וכ׳ the divine promise (of reward) to women is greater &c. Ib. V, 4; Sot. 38b ואם הַבְטָחָתוֹ וכ׳ but if he is confident that &c. Gen. R. s. 76 אין ה׳ לצדיקים וכ׳ the rigtheous do not rely on the divine promise in this world (they are afraid, lest their sin may have caused its withdrawal, v. Ber. 4b). Mekh. Yithro s. 2 אנשי אמת אלו בעלי ה׳ (Var. אֲבְטָחָה) 'men of truth' (Ex. XVIII, 21) that means men having faith in God; a. e.—*Pl.* הַבְטָחוֹת. Ex. R. s. 19 הרי כל ה׳ וכ׳ are these all the promises held out to the proselyte &c.?; a. fr.

חֲבִיל, Targ. Prov. VI, 3 some ed., v. חֵיכִיל.

חֲבִיר *dark, sad,* v. חֲפִיר.

חֲבִירָא m. (חבר, cmp. חבל) *vapor, mist, darkness.* Targ. Prov. IV, 19 Ar. (ed. Lag. חֲבִירָא, oth. ed. חכירא, חכירה). Ib. VII, 9 (ed. Lag. חֲבִירְתָּא, oth. ed. חכירה).—*Pl.* חֲבִירַיָּא. Targ. Ps. XXXV, 6 Lev. (ed. Lag. חכירייא, ed. Wil. חסירא, corr. acc.; Ms. חֲבִירְיָאתָא; h. text חלקלקות). V. חֶבְרָא.

חֲבְכִין (=חא בכין) *Oh then, yea then.* Targ. Ps. LI, 21; a. e.

חָבַל, *Hif.* הֶחֱבִיל (cmp. חבב) *to be affected by hot air, begin to steam.* Sabb. I, 6 (17b) long enough before the Sabbath כדי שיַּחֲבִילוּ for the flax stalks to begin &c.

חֲבַל ch. (=b. h. הָבַל, denom. of הֶבְלָא) 1) *to do vain things.* Targ. Job XXVII, 12.—2) *to be wanton, to sport.* Targ. Ps. LXII, 11 תְּהַבְלוּן ed. Wil. (Bxt. תִּתְהַבְּלוּן *Ithpa.*; ed. Lag. תקבלון, Ms. תתחבלון).

הֶבֶל m., constr. הֶבֶל or הֲבַל (b. h.) 1) *breath, vapor, air, heat.* Sabb. 88b בה׳ שבפיהם with the (fiery) breath of their mouths. Ib. 119b ה׳ תינוקות וכ׳ the breath of school children. Ib. ה׳ שאין בו חטא a sinless breath (of children). Y. Ab. Zar. III, 42d bot. ה׳ המרחץ וכ׳ the vapor of the bath room is injurious to the teeth. Yeb. 80b אין בשרו מעלה ה׳ his body (after bathing) does not steam. Pesik. Bahod. p. 154a; Lev. R. s. 29 (ref. to Ps. LXII, 10) עד שהן עשויין ה׳ בתוך וכ׳ while they are yet a gas (in the first embryonic stage) . . . ., they are predestined for marital union. Y. Ter. X, 47a bot. הה׳ כובש the heat (of the fresh bread placed on top of an open wine casket) keeps the evaporations of the wine down. B. Kam. 50b לְהַבְלוֹ for injuries suffered through the bad air of the pit (into which the animal fell), opp. to לחבטו injuries arising from knocking against the ground. Koh. R. to I, 2 ה׳ של תנור the hot air of the stove; ה׳ של עליונה the vapor of the topmost pot; Yalk. ib. 966 ה׳ שביציה; a. e.—

2) (b.h.) *vanity*. B. Bath. 16[b] תנחומין של ה׳ vain consolations. Koh. R. l. c.; Yalk. l. c. (ref. to Ps. CXLIV, 4) לאיזו ה׳ to what kind of *hebel* (breath) man is like; a. fr.—*Pl.* הֲבָלִים. Ib. שבעה ה׳ וכ׳ the seven times that Solomon used the word *hebel*. Pesik. Bahod. l. c.; Lev. R. l. c. כל ה׳ וכזבים וכ׳ all the vain things and falsehoods which the Israelites commit.

הֲבָלָא, הַבְלָא, constr. הֲבַל, הֲבֵל ch. same, 1) *breath* &c. Targ. Ps. XC, 9.—B. Mets. 36[b] ה׳ דאגמא the vapors of the marsh. Sabb. 95[a] מצטער מה׳ suffering from the close air of the room. Hull. 8[a] ואתי ה׳ וכ׳ and the effect of the hot iron comes and removes the traces of the stroke; ה׳ קדים וכ׳ the burn takes effect first &c. Bekh. 7[a] bot. ה׳ דבישרא וכ׳ it is the exudations of the body (which make the urin thick). B. Kam. 50[b] דאית ביה ה׳ in which the air is injurious (v. preced.). Ib. אין ה׳ למיתה ויש ה׳ וכ׳ the air is not bad enough to cause death, but enough to cause injury; a. fr.—2) *vanity*. Targ. Job XXVII, 12 ה׳. Targ. Koh. I, 2.—*Pl.* הַבְלִין, הַבְלַיָּא. Ib.—Ib. XII, 8.

הֲבָלוּתָא, הֲבָלוּ f. (preced.) *vanity*. Targ. Koh. I, 2; XI, 8; a. e.

הַבְלִילָא m. (בלל) *stomach* (first or second). Succ. 34[a]; Sabb. 36[a] ה׳ בי כסי וכ׳ Ar. (ed. הוּבְלִילָא) formerly they called the second stomach *hablila*, and now the first, v. הֲמְסֵס, a. כּוֹס, כַּפָּא.

הַבְלָעָה f. (בלע) [*absorption*,] *payment for a thing included in the bargain* (and not mentioned); *indirect sale* or *purchase*. Erub. 27[b] שנתן דמי .... בה׳ he paid the full value of the salt and water indirectly (by paying so much more for the oil for which he bargained). Bekh. 31[b] מוכרין אותו בה׳ it is sold in connection with other things. Ned. 37[a] ה׳ היא the teacher's fee for the Sabbath lessons is included in the general engagement (by the week, the month &c.).

הֶבְעֵר m. (בער) *damage through carelessness in handling fire*. B. Kam. I, 1; cmp. Y. ib. beg. 2[a]; Tosef. ib. IX, 1.

הַבְעָרָה f. (preced.) 1) *the law* (Ex. XXXV, 3) *forbidding the kindling of fire on the Sabbath*. Sabb. 70[a] ה׳ ללאו יצאת the law, 'ye shall kindle no fire &c.' is singled out in order to indicate that its transgression is a plain offence (לָאו). Ib. ה׳ לחלק יצאת that law is specified in order to intimate that each transgression of a Sabbath law is to be atoned for separately (if several of them have been committed in one act); Pes. 5[b]. Y. Sabb. II, 5[a] bot.; a. fr.—2) *removal, destruction*. Y. Snh. VII, 24[b] bot. we read here (Deut. XIX, 19) ובערת, and there (ib. XXI, 9) תבער, ה׳ ה׳ וכ׳ compare the analogous expressions for analogous modes of execution &c.—3) *heating, fire*. Pesik. R. s. 16, end כדי ה׳ אחת sufficient for one altar fire: Tanh. Ki Thissa 10.

הֶבְקֵר, Palest. dialect for הֶפְקֵר q. v.

הַבְרָא (הַבְרָה) הַבְרָא m. (v. הֲבִירָא; Syr. חברא, P. Sm. 1186) *mist, darkness*. Tam. 32[a] דפרשי בה׳ which travel in the dark (fog). Ker. 5[b] bot. בביתא דה׳ Ar. (ed. דבהתא) in a half-dark house; Hor. 12[a] דה׳ Ar. a. En Yakob (v. Rabb. D. S. a. l. note 1, ed. דח׳). Pes. 112[b] לא ליזיל בה׳ בלא מסאני Ms. M. (ed. הברא a. oth. differ., v. Rabb. D. S. a. l.) one must not walk without shoes in the dark (twilight).

הַבְרָאָה f. (בָּרָה) 1) *recovery to health*. Sabb. 137[a] יום הַבְרָאָתוֹ the day on which the child recovers.—[2) *refreshment*, esp. סעודת ה׳ *the meal of comfort given the mourner after funeral*, v. ברי II Hif. In commentaries and digests.]

הַבְרָה, v. הַבְרָא.

הֲבָרָה f. (חבר, cmp. הֲבִירָא; Neo-Syr. חברא P. Sm. 1185 bot.) 1) *confused sound* (contrad. to tune), *noise*. Yoma 19[b] כדי שישמע ... קול ה׳ that the Highpriest might hear the reverberating noise (of people awake at night). R. Hash. III, 7 ואם קול ה׳ וכ׳ but if he heard only an indistinct sound (echo, opp. קול שופר).—2) *report, rumor*. Y. Dem. I, 22[a] נפלה ה׳ בעיר the report spread in town. Y. R. Hash. IV, 59[b] bot. נפלה ה׳ וכ׳ an alarm spread. Gitt. 89[a] שמעו קול ה׳ they heard only an indistinct rumor (gossip). Gen. R. s. 10; a. fr. [In modern Hebrew ה׳ *syllable*.]

הָגָא, v. הגי.

הֶגָא m. ch. (h. הֶגֶה; הגי) *thought, utterance*. Targ. Job XXXVII, 2.

הַגְבָּהָה f. (גבה) 1) *lifting, taking up a found object*. B. Mets. 118[a], v. הַבָּטָה. B. Bath. 76[b] ה׳ קונה בכל מקום lifting gives possession everywhere (on private or public ground); Kidd. 22[b]; a. fr.—2) *elevation*. Ex. R. s. 45 השפלתי זו הַגְבָּהָתִי my humiliation is my elevation; Lev. R. s. 1.

הַגְבָּלָה f. (גבל) *setting bounds, marking off*. Sabb. 87[a] מצות ה׳ the command concerning the setting of bounds at Mount Sinai (Ex. XIX, 12).

הַגָּדָה, הַגָּדָה f. (נגד) 1) *telling, communication, evidence*. Snh. 30[b] (ref. to Lev. V, 1) מקשינן ה׳ לראייה the laws regulating the witnessing of the act must also apply to the evidence before court (that the two witnesses must be together).—2) (v. אַגָּדָה) *homiletics, popular lecture*, opp. to הֲלָכָה legal interpretation. Hag. 14[a] מה לך אצל ה׳ what hast thou to do with homiletics? Ib. בעלי ה׳ Ms. M. (ed. א׳) lecturers. Ib. 3[a] במה היתה ה׳ וכ׳ what was the subject of to-day's lecture?; a. fr.—3) *Haggadah*, the recitations at the home service on Passover nights, v. אַגַּדְתָּא. Pes. 115[b]; 116[b].—*Pl.* הַגָּדוֹת, הַגָּ׳. Y. Peah II, 17[a] bot. אין למדין מן הה׳ we must not derive laws from homiletical interpretations.

הגדום, הגדיס, v. הוגדס.

הֶגְדֵּר m. (גדר) [*restriction*,] *hegder*, a word made up as a substitute for (הֶקְדֵּשׁ) *hekdesh*, v. כִּינּוּי. Y. Ned. I, beg. 36[c].

הָגָה, v. הגי.

הֶגֶה m. (b. h.; preced.) *thought, study.* Gen. R. s. 49 (ref. to Job XXXVII, 2) אין ה׳ אלא תורה *hegeh* (thought, speculation) means study of the Law.

הָגָה, v. הֵיגָה.

הָגִין, v. הַגְזִין.

הֶגְזֵר m. (גזר) [*restriction,*] *hegzer,* a word made up as a substitute for הֶקְדֵּשׁ. Y. Ned. I, beg. 36^{c}, v. הֶגְהֵר.

הָגָה, הגי (b. h.; v. אָגָא) [*to point, pierce,*] 1) *to reason, argue, deduct.* Koh. R. to I, 16 חלב הוֹגֶה the heart reasons (ref. to Ps. XLIX, 4 הָגוּת). Deut. R. s. 11 הוֹגִים those who study the Law, contrad. to עוֹשִׂים.—Y. Meg. I, 72^{b} ה׳ נח תורה וכ׳ Noah deducted a new law from a given law. Gen. R. s. 49 שהוא הוגה בתורה וכ׳ who shall discuss the Law in seventy languages; a. fr.—2) *to pronounce, recite, spell.* Midr. Till. to Ps. XC, 9 (ref. to הֶגֶה, ib.) זה נער שהוא הוגה like a boy that spells (with difficulty). Snh. X (IX), 1 ההוגה וכ׳ he who pronounces the Divine Name as it is written, v. אָגָא. Koh. R. to XII, 12 (ref. to לַהַג ib.) לְהָגוֹת ניתנו וכ׳ they are good for reading exercises but not for painful study; v. הִגָּיוֹן. Y. Meg. IV, 74^{d} bot. לא יהא הוגה מפיו וקורא he must not spell (the letters of a Biblical book) from memory and dictate for writing a scroll.—3) *to murmur a charm,* v. *Hif.*

Nif. נֶהֱגָה *to be spelled, read.* Sabb. XII, 4; 5, נֶהֱגִין זה עם זה letters which can be read together (give sense).

Pi. הִגָּה (also from יָגָה) *to pierce, sting;* ה׳ מכה *to prickle, open a wound;* trnsf. *to lay bare a person's disgrace.* Lam. R. to I, 4 (interpret. נוגות, ib.) they assaulted her . . ., עד שהִגּוּ את מכתה and then laughed at her disgrace. Ib. to III, 33 (ref. to וַיַּגֶּה); Cant. R. to VII, 8.

Hif. הֶהֱגָה *to murmur charms.*—*Part.* מַהְגֶּה, pl. מַהְגִּים, מַהְגִּין. Sot. 12^{b} (ref. to Is. VIII, 19) מ׳ ואינן וכ׳ they murmur but know not what &c.; Ex. R. s. 1 הוֹגִין. Lev. R. s. 6 המ׳ אלו המנהמין *hammahgin* (Is. l. c.) that means the humming (sorcerers).

הָגָא, הגי ch. same; *to reason, speak, study.* Part. הָגֵי. Targ. Josh. I, 8.—*Pl.* הָגְיָין. Targ. Y. Deut. VI, 7. [Targ. Y. Num. XI, 1, v. next w.]

Af. אַהְגֵּי same; Y. Ber. V, 9^{a} הוא מַהְגֵּי באורייתא סגין ed. Lehm. (ed. מנהגור, מנהגירה) meditated much in the Law.

Pa. הַגֵּי (v. preced. *Pi.*) *to sting, to point at with scorn.* Targ. Is. XXVII, 8 מַגֵּי עליהון וכ׳ (ed. Lag. מיגר, Bxt. הָגֵר, ed. Wil. הגר, corr. acc.) he pointed at them with words (of scorn).

הַגְיָא, הָגֵי m. (preced.) *speech, meditation.* Targ. Y. Num. XI, 1 הַגְיָאן their speech. Y. Ber. V, 9 מִנְהֲגִיה וכ׳, מִן ה׳=) מִנְהֲגוֹ) because of his meditating in &c., v. preced.

הִגָּיוֹן m. (b. h.; preced. wds.) *recitation, reading lesson.* Y. Snh. X, 28^{a} top (ref. to לַהַג, Koh. XII, 12) לה׳ ניתנו וכ׳ they are good for recitation, not for painful study, v. הָגָה. Ber. 28^{b} מנעו בניכם מן הה׳ restrain your children from recitation (parading a superficial knowledge of the Bible by verbal memorizing).

הִגְיוֹנָא ch. (הגי, v. *Pa.*) *derision, boastful talk.* Targ. Lam. III, 62 (Var. לְהֶגְיוֹנ׳).

הֲגָיָה f. (הָגָה) *speaking, recitation, study.* Y. Ber. I, 3^{c} top (ref. to Josh. I, 8) שתהא הֲגָיַית יום וכ׳ that the recitation of the day and the night be alike; Midr. Till. to Ps. I, 2.

הָגִים, הָגִין, v. הֵיגָה.

הַגְלָשָׁה f. (גָּלַשׁ) *publication, revelation.* Cant. R. to IV, 1, v. גָּלַשׁ (Ar. גְּלָשָׁה).

הֶגְמוֹן (אֶגְמוֹן) m. (ἡγεμών) *general.* Targ. Is. IX, 13; XIX, 15 (ed. Lag. הֵיג׳; h. text זנב).—Sabb. 145^{b} ה׳ א׳ וקמטון ed. (Ms. O. ה׳; Ms. M. א׳ וקמוטרי, Ar. ה׳ וקומיון, read וקמיטרין) a general with his suite (comites). Taan. 29^{a} Ms. M. (ed. אָדוֹן). Y. Snh. I, 19^{b} top; a. fr.—*Pl.* הֶגְמוֹנִים, הֶגְמוֹנִין. Targ. II Esth. VIII, 7.—Ex. R. s. 31, end. [Tanh. Yithro 5 הגמונות, v הֶגְמוֹנְיָא.]—Ch. form הֶגְמוֹנָא. Ab. Zar. 11^{a}.

הֶגְמוֹנְיָה, הֶגְמוֹנְיָא f. (ἡγεμονία) 1) *commandership, consulship.* Gen. R. s. 50, beg.; Lev. R. s. 26 נטל ה׳ וכ׳ got an appointment as a consul from the King. Cant. R. to I, 6; Lam. R., introd. (R. Yitsh. 3) וכולן עשו ישראל ה׳ (אחת) וכ׳ and Israel declared all these gods one government and worshipped all of them; Esth. R. to I, 9 אומוניאה (read: אֶגְמוֹנְיָאָה, cmp. אֶגְמוֹן).—*Pl.* הֶגְמוֹנְיוֹת *staff of commanding officers.* Tanh. Yithro 5 לה׳ שעליהם (not להגמונות) to the staff appointed over them (to take them to the exile). Midr. Till. to Ps. CXVIII, 6 he will send forth דוגמניות על וכ׳ (corr. acc.) staffs to all countries &c.—2) (v. Sm. Ant. s. v. Eisagogeis) *court, administration, jurisdiction, district.* Gitt. I, 1 מה׳ לה׳ from one jurisdiction to another.—*Pl.* as above. Ib. 4^{b} there were in one town שתי ה׳ וכ׳ two jurisdictions jealous of each other.

הָגַן (v. Ez. XLII, 12) *to balance, make corresponding.*—*Part. pass.* הָגוּן (cmp. הָגוּי רָאוּי) *fit, worthy.* Hull. 133^{a} תלמיד שאינו ה׳ an unworthy student. Esth. R. to II, 4 מי ה׳ לדבר זה who was well-fitted for this mission?; Midr. Sam. ch. XIII.—B. Kam. 80^{a} לא נתכוונה אלא לה׳ לה she had in her mind only such a one as would be worthy of her; a. fr.—*Pl.* הֲגוּנִין. Gen. R. s. 48 Ar.

Pi. הִגֵּן, part. pass. מְהוּגָּן=הָגוּן; pl. מְהוּגָּנִים, מְהוּגָּנִין. B. Kam. l. c. ב״א שאינן מ׳ unworthy people (not her equals). Ib. 16^{b} ב״א שאינן מ׳ unworthy recipients of charity. Keth. 22^{a} אנשים מ׳ worthy men (proposing to me). Kidd. 70^{a} בנים שאינן מ׳ degenerate children; a. fr.—V. הוּגָּן.

**Hif.* הֶהֱגִין *to be of the same weight.* Y. Keth. I, 25^{b} top טבריינייות מַהֲגִינוֹת וכ׳ (not סב׳) the Tiberian Selaim are of the same weight as &c.

הָגַן same, only in *part. pass. Pa.* מְהַגַּן, f. מְהַגְּנָא= מְהוּגָּן, v. preced. Targ. Y. Gen. XXIV, 12; 26. Targ. Y. Num. XXII, 32 לא מְהוּגְּנָא displeasing.—Taan. 22^{b} מילתא דלא מה׳ an unbecoming word.—*Pl.* m. מְהַגְּנִין. Targ. Y. I Num. XII, 1.

הַגַּס, v. גַּס.

הַגָּעָה f. (נָגַע) *striking.* Mekh. Bo, Pisha, s. 11, v. טְבִילָה.

הַגְעָלָה f.=גִּיעוּל, *the cleaning of an impure vessel by means of boiling water.* Ab. Zar. 76^{a} ה׳ בחמין *hagalah* is always done with hot water. Ib. מאי ה׳ דקתני התם מריקה וכ׳ Ms. M. (ed. differ.) the *hagalah* there (in the Mishnah) means in general scouring and rinsing (also with cold water).

הֲגָפָה f. (גוף) *shutting up, closing.* Yoma 18ᵃ הֲגָפַת דלתות (some ed. הֲגָפוֹת pl.) locking the Temple doors; Arakh. 11ᵇ; a. fr.—Sot. VIII, 1 (קול) הגפת תריסין noise made by fastening the cuirasses (to frighten the enemy); Sifré Deut. 192; a. e.—Mekh. B'shall. 2 אֲגָפַת תריסין (not תריסטין).

הָגַר, Ned. 49ᵇ והוגרני Ar., v. חָגַר.

הָגָר (b. h.) pr. n. f. *Hagar*, hand-maid of Sarah. Gen. R. s. 45, beg.; a. fr.

הַגְרָאָה, v. next w.

הַגְרָה pr. n. *Hagrah*, an Arabian district; cmp. חַגְרָא. Num. R. s. 13, beg. גלות ה׳ the diaspora of H.—Denom. ch. הַגְרָאָה m. *Hagrean.* Targ. I Chr. XXVII, 31.

הגרול, v. הֶגְרֵיל.

הגרום, v. הוגדס.

הַגְרוֹנְיָא pr. n. pl. *Hagronia* (Agranum), a Babylonian town, seat of several scholars (v. Neub. Géogr. p. 347). Ber. 31ᵃ. Sabb. 11ᵃ סבי דה׳ the elders (scholars) of H.; a. fr.

הֶגְרֵיל m.=next w. Y. Yoma VI, 43ᶜ הֶגְרֵילוֹ של וכ׳ (ed. Krot. הגרולו, incorr.) the designation by lot of the first animal.

הַגְרָלָה f. (גרל) *casting lots*, esp. for the sacrifices of the Day of Atonement (Lev. XVI, 8). Y. Yoma IV, 41ᶜ ה׳ מעכבת casting lots is indispensable for the legality of the entire act. Bab. ib. 62ᵇ. Kerith. 28ᵃ; a. e.

הֶגְרֵם m. (v. next w.) *hegrem*, a word formed as a substitute of הֶקְדֵּשׁ [prob. to be read הֶגְדֵּם, v. גַּדַּם]. Y. Ned. I, beg. 36ᶜ, v. חֶגְהֵר.

הַגְרָמָה f. (גָּרַם Hif.) *cutting the animal's throat in a slanting direction*, letting the knife slide beyond the space ritually designated for cutting. Hull. 9ᵃ. Ib. 27ᵃ; a. fr.

הַגָּשָׁה f. (נָגַשׁ) 1) *drawing near, coming forward.* Gen. R. s. 49; s. 93 ה׳ למלחמה the verb נגש is used for drawing near for battle; ה׳ לפיוס for persuasion, &c.—2) *bringing near, offering.* Sifra Vayikra, N'dabah, ch. XII, Par. 11. Men. V, 5, sq.; a. fr.—*Pl.* הַגָּשׁוֹת. Ib.; a. fr.

הַגְתָא, v. הֵיגְ׳.

הֲדֵי a prefix (a compound of הָא a. דִּ־), pl. הֲדֵיֵ, 1) with prefix ב and suffix of personal pronoun: בַּהֲדִי, בַּהֲדַאי ;בַּהֲדָךְ ;בַּהֲדֵיה ;בַּהֲדָן ;בַּהֲדָנָא ,בַּהֲדַיְיכוּ ;בַּהֲדַיְיהוּ *with myself, in my presence; with thyself* &c. Targ. Job VI, 4. Ib. XV, 10; a. e.—B. Bath. 41ᵃ בהדאי in connection with myself. Sabb. 118ᵃ הא דאיכא בהדך אוכליה eat what thou hast with thee; מלוינן ליה .... בהדיה we give him a meal along. B. Bath. 73ᵇ אחלוי בהדן וכ׳ a certain Arab joined us. Hull. 57ᵇ מלכא הוה בהדייהו the king was among them; a. fr.—2) בַּהֲדֵי *in the presence of, with.* Targ. Y. Deut. XXII, 15.—Pes. 112ᵇ a law-suit ב׳ תלתא with three opponents. Sabb. 33ᵇ ב׳ פניא near twilight. Keth. 103ᵇ ב׳ דידי מינצת with me wilt thou dispute?—B. Kam. 92ᵃ, v. הוּצָא; a. fr.—לַהֲדֵי ,ב׳ הדדי, v. הֲדָדֵי.—לַהֲדֵי *towards, near.* Sabb. 134ᵃ ל׳ יומא towards the light. Ib. ל׳ פומיה (not פומי, Ms. M. בהדי פומי) close to his mouth. Ab. Zar. 30ᵇ טיף ל׳ טיף טיף (Ms. M. .. טיף טיף בהדי) drop immediately after drop. Pes. l. c. לַהֲדֵיה כרעיה (Ms. על גבי) at his feet; a. fr.—3) (conj.) בהדי די *during the time that, while.* Gitt. 68ᵃ top ב׳ דקא מעיינו ואתו while they were going on searching. Hull. 53ᵃ ב׳ דדריס while he inserts his nails, ב׳ דשליף in the moment he takes them off; a. fr.

הָדָא, v. דָּא.

הֲדָדֵי (=הדי־הדי, v. הדי) *each other, mutually.* Targ II Esth. I, 7 הדא להדא=להדדי (ed. Lag. לחדדי, Var. לה׳; cmp. Syr. חדדא P. Sm. 1196). Gitt. 68ᵃ כבשינהו אה׳ (=הדא אהדא) squeeze them against each other. Ib. 69ᵃ בהדי ה׳ with one another (in immediate contact). Hull. 43ᵃ, v. הֲנֵיזָ; a. fr.—כי ה׳ (=הדא כי הדא) *like each other.* Snh. 4ᵇ (*heleb* a. *ḥăleb*) דכי ה׳ נינהו which are written alike. Erub. 69ᵇ כי ה׳ וכ׳ are in the same legal category. Yeb. 14ᵃ כי ה׳ of equal rank in scholarship; a. e.

הָדָה I, v. דָּא.

הָדָה II (interj., v. preced.) *hoa! look out!* Tosef. Sabb. VI (VII), 10 [read:] החוסס אוד בכותל ואומר ה׳ (Var. חדה, v. ed. Zuck. note) if one strikes a brand against a wall and says *hada* (a superstitious practice to frighten away evil spirits). Ib. 11 (Var. חדא). Ib. 12 (v. ed. Zuck. note).

הדורין, Tosef. Toh. VIII, 6 Var., v. חֲדוּרִין.

הֲדוֹם m. (b. h.) *stool.* Macc. 24ᵇ בית ה׳ רגלי וכ׳ the house which was the foot-stool of our God; Sifré Deut. 43.

***הדוסטא**, Y. Sabb. VI, 8ᵃ top, a corrupt., prob. for היפודימטא m. pl. (ὑποδήματα) *half-shoes*, contrad. to sandals or soles which may accidentally be fastened with the front backward.

הָדוּק, v. חִדּוּק.

הָדוּר, v. הָדַר.

הֲדוּר ch. (=h. הָדוּר) *splendid, handsome.* Targ. Y. Gen. XXIV, 65.

הִדּוּר, v. הידור.

הָדוֹר, v. הידור.

הֲדוּרָא ,הֲדָרָא m. (הָדַר) *coil, convolution.* ה׳ דכנתא *the coils of the ileum.* Hull. 48ᵇ. Ib. 113ᵃ (ed. הדרא).—*Pl.* הֲדוּרֵי (cmp. Is. XLV, 2) *spiral road, a field which* *can be tilled only by spiral movements, steep hill.* B. Bath. 12ᵃ בה׳ in the case of a steep ascent (which requires more time).—בית ה׳ *Beth-Hădurê*, name of a summit from which the scape-goat was thrown down (Lev. XVI, 21 sq.). Targ. Y. Lev. XVI, 22.—Yoma VI, 8 (68ᵇ) Ms. M. in Gemara (Mish. הרורי, indistinctly corrected, v. Rabb. D. S. a. l. note 3 a. 6, ed. חדודו, Y. ed. חורון).

הֲדוֹרָה f. (הדר) *circuit, round-trip.* Y. Hor. III, 48ᵃ bot., v. חֲזִירָה.

הדות, v. הוּת.

הֲדָחָה f. (הוּחַ) *washing off, rinsing.* Ḥull. 107ᵇ. Ab. Zar. 60ᵇ; a. fr.

הֲדֵי, v. הַדּ־.

הֶדְיָא (v. preced.) *presence, directness;* בה׳ *openly, explicitly.* Snh. 39ᵃ לשקליה בה׳ (Yalk. Gen. 24 בַּהֲדֵיה, v. הַדּ־) He ought to have taken it (Adam's rib) openly (while he was awake). Sabb. 133ᵇ גדול בה׳ כתיב ביה וכ׳ as to an adult, is it not said distinctly concerning him, 'And any male' &c.?—Pes. 27ᵃ הא תניא בה׳ is it not explicitly taught?; a. fr.

הַדְיָא II, הַדָּיָה, בַּר ה׳, בֶּן ה׳ m. (corresp. to h. דָּאָה or דַּיָּה, v. discussion Ḥull. 63ᵇ) 1) a bird of the *hawk* species. Sifra Sh'mini Par. 3, ch. V (ref. to למינהו, Lev. XI, 16) 'after its kind' לחביא בן ההדייה חנץ refers to *ben hădaya;* Ḥull. 63ᵃ בר חיריא ed., Ar. בר הוּדְיָא. Lev. R. s. 5, beg. הדין בר הדיה וכ׳ ed. (Ar. חוריא, v. ed. Koh. s. v.) this hawk sees its food at a distance of &c. (v. Ḥull. 63ᵇ, ref. to רָאָה a. דָּאָה).—2) pr. n. m. *Bar Hădaya.* Ber. 56ᵃ (an interpreter of dreams). Ab. Zar. 30ᵃ.

הַדְיֵב, v. הַדְיֵיב.

הַדָּיָה, v. הֶדְיָא.—[Targ. Prov. XXXI, 25 הדיה, some ed., read הֶדְרָא.]

הֶדְיוֹט m. (an adaptation of ἰδιώτης) *private man* (opp. to priest, officer &c.), *commoner; ignoble, ignorant.* Targ. I Sam. XVIII, 23; a. fr.—Meg. 12ᵇ, a. e. (prov.) הח׳ קופץ בראש the lowest man rushes ahead (is the first to give an opinion).—Yeb. 59ᵃ, a. fr. כהן ה׳ a common priest, opp. כהן גדול. M. Kat. I, 8 הח׳ the untrained tailor, opp. אומן the professional. Ib. 10ᵃ היכי דמי ה׳ when do you call one a *hedyot?*—B. Mets. 104ᵃ לשון ה׳ the popular terms, v. הֶדְיֵשׁ. Gen. R. s. 96 משל ה׳ a popular adage; a. fr.—*Pl.* (Ch.) הֶדְיוֹטִין. Targ. Job XXX, 8; a. e.—(Hebrew) הֶדְיוֹטוֹת. Snh. X, 2 (90ᵃ) three kings וארבעה ה׳ and four private persons. Ib. 21ᵇ bot. לה׳ for the common people (Samaritans). Tosef. Sabb. XIII (XIV), 1; Y. ib. XVI, 15ᶜ top שטרי ה׳ private (not Hebrew) writings; Bab. ib. 116ᵇ; a. fr. Num. R. s. 8 הֶדְיוֹטִים (some ed.).—Fem. הֶדְיוֹטִית. Ruth R. to I, 19 פרה ה׳ a cow of common stock (not trained for work).

הדיוכין, Gen. R. s 10, read: הֶדְיוֹכִין, v. הֵידְכַר.

הַדְיֵיב, הַדְיֵב (ח׳) pr. n. *Adiabena,* a district of Assyria between the rivers Lycus and Caprus. Targ. Jer. LI, 27 (ed. Lag. ח׳; h. text אשכנז). Targ. Ez. XXVII, 23 (h. text עדן).—Gen. R. s. 37 Ar. (for ריפת, Gen. X, 3; ed. הַדְיֵיב); Y. Meg. I, 71ᵇ bot. חדיית (corr. acc.). Y. Sabb. XIV, beg. 14ᵇ חדיית (corr. acc.); Bab. ib. 121ᵇ ח׳ (Ms. M. חריב, corr. acc.; v. Rabb. D. S. a. l. note). M. Kat. 28ᵃ זווא דמה׳ Ar. (ed. זוג׳); Nidd. 21ᵇ זוגא דמן ה׳ Z. of Ad.—Yeb. 16ᵇ sq. חבור זו ה׳ Ḥabor (II Kings XVIII, 11) is *Ḥadyab.*

הַדְיְבָא m. (preced.) *of Adiabena.* B. Bath. 26ᵇ (Ms. H. חריייבא, Var. in ed. חדריבא, חדייבא, בר אבא, v. Rabb. D. S. a. l. note 300).

הַדָּיֵיה, v. הֶדְיָא.

הדיין, v. הֵידֵיין.

הַדְיֵיף, הדיית, v. הַדְיֵיב.

הַדִּימָא *dissected,* v. הֲדַם.

הדימה, v. ארקולאון.

הַדֵּין, הָדֵין, v. הֵין a. הֵידֵין.

הַדֵּיף, v. הַדְיֵיב.

הֲדָךְ, v. הָךְ.

הַדְלֵיקָא f. (דלק) *fire.* Targ. II Esth. III, 8 (ed. Lag. ה . . .).—[Num. R. s. 15, beg. הדליקתן some ed., read הַדְלָקָתָן, v. next w.).

הַדְלָקָה f. (דלק) *lighting, kindling.* Sabb. 23ᵃ ה׳ עושה מצוה the kindling (of the Ḥanukhah lights) is the ceremony prescribed, contrad. to הנחה the placing it. Ib. II, 6 (31ᵇ) הַדְלָקַת הנר kindling the Sabbath lights. Y. Ter. V, 43ᶜ top למשחה לה׳ *l'moshḥah* (Num. XVIII, 8) means (also) for lighting purposes (cmp. מְשִׁחָא). Num. R. s. 15, beg. על הַדְלָקָתָן וכ׳ concerning feeding them with olive oil.

הֲדַם, *Pa.* הַדֵּם (אַדֵּם) 1) *to dissect, dismember, tear to pieces.* Targ. Jud. XIV, 6. Ib. XIX, 29; XX, 6 (v. Ar. ed. Koh. s. v.); a. e.—Ab. Zar. 38ᵇ דילמא הַדּוֹמֵי הַדְמוּהָ וכ׳ Ms. M. a. Ar. (ed. אדמורי אַדְמוּהָ, read אַדּוֹמֵי) perhaps they carved the bird and then put it into the pot. Erub. 30ᵃ דאַדִּימֵי הַדּוֹמֵי נְהַדְּמִיה shall we cut him apart?—Bets. 24ᵇ (ed. Sonc. a. Ven. דהַדִּימֵי, v. Rabb. D. S. a. l. note) fish that were dissected (Rashi: *red,* v. אֲדִימָא).—2) אַהֲדֵם (denom. of next w.) *to arrange the parts of an animal.* Gitt. 67ᵇ אַהֲדִמוּ לִי הַדָּמֵי דחיותא arrange before me the limbs of the (dissected) animal.

הַדָּמָא, הַדָּם m. (v. preced.) *part, member.*—*Pl.* הַדָּמִין, הַדָּמֵי. Dan. II, 5; III, 29.—Gitt. 67ᵇ, v. preced.

הֲדָן, v. הֵן.

הַדְנָא (=האידנא) *then.* Targ. II Esth. II, 13; cmp. הֵידֵין.

הדס (חדס) הָדַס, *Pi.* הִידֵּס (ח׳) (cmp. דחס) *to make incisions, mark* (cmp. הנדז) esp. (of chickens) *to leave marks of the feet, to scratch.* B. Kam. II, 2 היה מְהַדֵּס וכ׳ it was scratching and broke vessels; expl. ib. 17[b] bot. הד׳ והתיז it scratched and caused the smashing of the vessel by rolling it against a hard object. Ib. הוו מְהַדְּסִין על וכ׳ left marks on dough or fruits, or soiled &c.; Y. ib. II, beg. 2[d] שהידסו את וכ׳. Ib. הידסו עפר על וכ׳ (Bab. ib. l. c. העלו עפר) they threw dust by scratching; a. e. [Ar. reads חדס; Syr. הדס *to study.*]

הֲדֵס* (ch. v. preced.; cmp. אִסְפִּירֵס) *to dance on tiptoe.* Y. Peah I, 15[d] הוה מְהַדֵּס קומי כליא (ed. Krot. מקלס) used to dance before the bridal couples; (Keth. 17[a] מרקד).

הדס, הֲדַס pr. n. pl. *Hadas,* (prob.) *Edessa* in Mesopotamia. Targ. Y. Gen. X, 10 (h. text אֶרֶךְ, v. אַרְכַּת).

הֲדַס m. (b. h.) *myrtle branch* (with three leaves on top), used for the festive wreath on the Feast of Booths (Lev. XXIII, 40). Succ. III, 2. Ib. 32[b] ה׳ שוטה wild myrtle (with one or two leaves on top); a. fr.—*Pl.* הֲדַסִּים. Ib. III, 4 שלשה ה׳ three myrtle branches are required for the festive wreath. Meg. 13[a] the righteous שנקראו ה׳ who are named myrtles (Zech. I, 8); a. e.

הֲדַסָּא, הֲדַס ch. same. Targ. II Esth. II, 7.—*Pl.* הֲדַסַּיָּא, הֲדַסִּין. Targ. Lev. XXIII, 40. Targ. Zech. I, 8; a. e.

הֲדַסָּה f. (b. h.) same; also pr. n. f. *Hădassah,* name of Esther. Esth. R. to II, 7. Meg. 10[b]; 13[a]; [Targ. II Esth. II, 7].

הדסמ״ב, mnemonical abbrev. for חבאת וידוי אסור טומאה ביעור. Yeb. 74[b] שכן ה׳ for they (the tithes of the third year) require bringing to the Temple and confession, are forbidden to the mourner (אונן), must not be removed in levitical uncleanness, and must be removed (Deut. XXVI, 12—14).

הדף (חדף) הָדַף (b. h.) *to thrust down, hurry.—Part. pass.* הָדוּף, f. הֲדוּפָה *hurried.* Y. Bicc. II, 64[d] top מיתה ה׳ (Var. ח׳; cmp. M. Kat. 28[a] s. v. חָטַף). [Pesik. R. s. 21 פנים חרופות, v. חָרַף.]

הֲדַף ch. same, *to thrust.* Targ. Y. Num. XXXV, 20 הדוף (read: חדפיה); ib. 22. Targ. Job XVIII, 18.

הדק, הֲדַק, v. דָּקַק.

הָדַק, *Pi.* הִידֵּק, *to squeeze,* v. חָדַק.

הֲדַק ch., *Pa.* הַדֵּיק same. Sabb. 141[a] לא לִיהְדּוֹק וכ׳ one must not squeeze cotton into the mouth of a bottle (as a stopper). Ib. 125[b] דהַדְקָה, v. חֲדַק; a. fr.—B. Kam. 85[b] דהַדְקִיה, v. הַרְיָק.—*Part. pass.* מְהַדַּק, v. infra.

Ithpe. אִיהְדַק *to be squeezed in, rabbeted.* Sabb. 65[a] הא דמִיהְדַק ed. (Ar. מְהַדַּק, v. supra) in the one case it means that it is squeezed into the ear. Pes. 109[b] הֲדוּקֵי הוה מיהדק the parts of the table were rabbeted. Ab. Zar. 31[a] דיקולא ומי׳ a basket squeezed over the wine casket.

הָדַר (b. h.; cmp. חדר, דור, חזר) *to enclose, go around. Part. pass.* הָדוּר 1) *rounded.* Hull. 59[b] הֲדוּרוֹת בעינן Ar. (ed. חֲדוּרוֹת, v. חָדַר) the horns must de rounded (not flat; Ar.: showing circular layers).—2) (b. h.) *distinguished, adorned, beautiful.* Gen. R. s. 60 (ref. to הלזה, Gen. XXIV, 25) ראתה אותו ה׳ she saw his commanding appearance; Midr. Till. to Ps. XC, end.

Pi. הִדֵּר, הִי׳ 1) *to crown, adorn, distinguish.* Lev. R. s. 30 שהִדְּרוֹ הקב״ה וכ׳ whom the Lord crowned with old age. Kidd. 32[b] יְהַדְּרֶנּוּ בממון that he must show him honor even at a material sacrifice; a. e.—*Part. pass.* מְהוּדָּר. Lev. R. s. 3 שיהא המזבח מה׳ וכ׳ that the altar may appear adorned by the poor man's offering; a. e.—2) *to go around searching,* whence *to be zealous in religious observances, to look out for the best method of doing good.* Sabb. 21[b] המְהַדְּרִין the zealous, המה׳ מן המה׳ the most zealous. V. הידור.

Hithpa. הִתְהַדֵּר *to be crowned, glorified.* Gen. R. s. 1 הוא לבדו מִתְהַדֵּר וכ׳ He alone is glorified through His world.

הֲדַר ch. (preced.) *to go around, come back, return.* Targ. Y. Gen. III, 19; a. fr.—B. Mets. 14[a] what thou takest from him, עלי דידי ה׳ comes back on my property (I am responsible for it). Ib. 69[b] הַדְרָא בעינא is returned bodily. Pes. 29[b], a. fr. ה׳ ביה went back on himself, changed his opinion. B. Mets. 65[a] הָדְרִי בי I take it back. B. Bath. 84[a] לא מצית הָדְרַת בך וכ׳ thou wouldst not have been at liberty to retract (the transaction), and now thou shouldst &c.?; a. fr. [Frequ. used adverbially.] B. Mets. 6[a] שתיק מעיקרא וה׳ צוח first he kept silence and then (reconsidering) he protested. Gitt. 8[b] ה׳ אמר אביי another time A. said. Hull. 76[b] הָדוּר שלחו (חדר) another time they sent word; a. fr.

Pa. הַדַּר (v. preced. *Pi.*) 1) *to honor, distinguish.* Dan. IV, 31.—Targ. O. Lev. XIX, 15 (ed. Berl. תַהְדַּר *Af.*).—B. Bath. 8[b] הַדְּרֵי, v. הוּדְרָא.—2) *to go around searching, be zealous, anxious.* Hull. 76[b]; Nidd. 65[b] הַהוּרֵי אפירכא what need is there to go around searching for an argument (why do you resort to unknown authorities)? Sabb. 23[a] הוה מְהַדַּר מר וכ׳ my teacher used to be anxious for puppy-oil. Ib. מהדרא אמשחא (read: מהדר אמ׳); a. fr.—3) *to restore; 4) to review;* v. *Af.*

Af. אַהְדַּר 1) *to return, restore; to lead back; to turn around.* Targ. Y. Deut. XXII, 3 (some ed. *Pa.*). Targ. Cant. VII, 5; a. fr.—B. Mets. 26[a] אי ... לאַהְדּוּרָהּ אַהְדְּרוּהָ ניהלי if they had had the intention of returning it, they would have returned it to me. Ib. אמרי קמייהו .... לִיהַדְּרוּ לי ולא הַדְּרוּ לי וכ׳ (differ. in Mss., v. Rabb. D. S. a. l. note) I spoke in their presence several times (of my loss); they might have returned it to me, but did not; will they now return it?—Hull. 20[a] בדלא א׳ when he did not turn round (the windpipe &c.). Hag. 5[b] ... עמא דאַהְדַּרִינְהוּ מיניה a people from which its master has turned away his face; a. fr.—2) *to repeat, review.* M. Kat. 28[a] אַהְדְּרֵי לתלמודאי that I may review my studies. Ber. 38[b] מַהְדַּר תלמודיה (or מְהַדַּר); a. fr.—3) *to reply.* Hull. 34[a] מאי אהדרי

וכ׳ what did . . . . reply to one another?; a. e. — 4) *to carry around in procession.* Yeb. 110[a] Ar., v. פּוּרְסְיָא; v. אֲדוּרֵי.

Ithpa. אִיתְהַדַּר, *Ithpe.* אִיתְהֲדַר 1) *to go around begging.* Sabb. 151[b] אֲהְדוּרֵי אפיתחא לא מִיהֲדַר he will not be forced to go around begging. — 2) *to go back.* Ned. 50[a] איהדר לאחורי I will go back again.

הָדָר m. (b. h.; preced.) 1) *adornment, crown, beauty, glory.* Ab. Zar. 24[b] ברוב הֲדָרֶךָ in the abundance of thy glory. Gen. R. s. 39 (ref. to Ps. CX, 3) מֵהֲדָרוֹ של עולם וכ׳ from the glory of the world (the East) have I consecrated thee; (Yalk. Ps. 869 בהררי קדש בהררי של עולם וכ׳ 'in the mountains of holiness', among the mountains, i. e. the distinguished, of the world &c.).—Y. Succ. III, 53[d] a tree שפריו ה׳ וכ׳ whose fruit is beautiful &c.—Lev. R. s. 30; a. fr.—[Ib. תרגם עקילס הגר הדר Aquila in his translation read our w. *haddar*, v. הדּוּר I.]—2) עֵץ הָדָר (b. h.) the tree *Hadar.* Ib.; a. fr.

הֲדָרָא, הֶדְרָא ch. 1) same. Targ. Prov. XXXI, 25 (Ms. הֲדָרָה). Ib. XIV, 28.—Targ. Y. II Deut. XXXIII, 17, v. הֲדָרְתָא. Y. Maas. Sh. IV, end, 55[c] (ref. to a dream about אֲדָר) בה׳ דאורייתא וכ׳ through the glory of the Law thou shalt be raised, cmp. אַדְרוּתָא.—2) הֶדְרָא=הִדּוּרָא q. v.

הַדְרָאָה f. (הדר) *flour of the second course.* פת ה׳ bread made of seconds (opp. פת נקייה). Pes. 37[a] (Ar. הַרְדָאָה trnsp.). Tosef. Sabb. XIII (XIV), 7. Y. Pes. II, 29[b] bot.; Bab. ib. 36[b], opp. מצה של שְׁלֹמֹה.

הַדְרַאוּלִיס, v. הִדְרַוְלִיס.

הֲדָרָה, constr. הַדְרַת (b. h.; v. הָדָר) *beauty, dignity.* Sabb. 152[a] ה׳ פנים זקן the beauty of the face is the beard. B. Mets. 84[a] ה׳ פנים לא הויא ליה he had no beard.

הֲדִירָה, v. הֲדָרָא.

הדרונא, v. הִדְרוֹנָא.

הִדְרוֹקָן m. (ὑδρωπικόν or ὑδερικόν, sub. πάθος) *dropsy;* ה׳ (חולה) *one afflicted with dropsy.* Erub. 41[b] חיה וחולי מעיים וה׳ Ms. M. (ed. חיה misplaced, v. Rabb. D. S. a. l. note) a lying-in woman, and sufferers from bowel diseases or dropsy. Ber. 25[a]; 62[b]; Bekh. 44[b]; Tam. 27[b]. Sabb. 33[a] (Ms. M. הִדְרָקוֹן); a. e. [Ar. reads everywhere הדרקון.]

הדרוס, v. הַדְּרֵס.

הַדְרִיָינָא m. *Hadrianic.* Ab. Zar. 52[b] דינרא טריינא וה׳ Ms. M. (ed. differ. order, v. Rabb. D. S. a. l. note) the Trajanic and the Hadrianic Denarius; Bekh. 50[b].

הַדְרִיָינוּס pr. n. m. *Hadrian,* v. אַדְרִיָינוּס.

הַדְרִייָנֵי, v. אַדְרִיָינֵי.

הדרינתא, v. הַדְרָנִיתָא.

הֲדִירֵיס, v. הַדְּרֵס.

הַדְרָנָא m. (הֲדַר) 1) *one who goes back on his word, shuffler, rogue;* cmp. הַדְרָנִיתָא. Keth. 53[a] שוידה נפשך ה׳ וכ׳ I do not advise thee to make a rogue of thyself.— 2) v. הוּדְרָנָא.

הַדַרְנִיאֵל pr. n. *Hădarniel (surrounding God),* name of an angel. Pesik. R. s. 20.

***הַדְרָנִיקוֹס** m. (a corrupt. of ὑδερικός or ὑδρωπικός, cmp. הִדְרוֹקָן; for Var. lect. v. infra) *one afflicted with dropsy.* Ber. 58[b] ואת הננס ואת ה׳ (Ms. M. ואת הרדינקס, Ms. F. והננס ה׳); Tosef. ib. VII (VI), 3 (absent in ed. Zuck., added in note); Tanh. Pinh. 10 . . . הבהקנין ואת דרניקוס; ed. Bub. ib. 1 ואת הדרקונוס . . . הננס (Mss. הדריקינוס, הדרקונים); Y. Ber. IX, 13[b] bot. (absent); [absent in Bekh. VII, 6, among bodily blemishes disqualifying for priestly service]. [Our w. is obviously a gloss to one of the anomalies enumerated in the text, prob. to קִפֵּחַ.—Ar. reads והברדניקוס, in the place of קפח in our text, giving it the meaning of כִּפֵּחַ q. v., but records also הדר׳ in letter *He;* Alf. reads בדרקינוס, בדריקנוס, leaving out קפח.—For other definitions of our w., v. commentaries.]

הַדְרָנִיתָא f. (הדר; v. הַדְרָנָא) *swindler, a woman who sells property and afterwards reclaims it on a mortgage held by herself.* Keth. 97[a] דלא ליקרו לה ה׳ (some ed. הדרינתא) that they may not call her a swindler.

הַדְּרֵס, הֲדִירֵיס m. a popular contraction of הַהוּרֵס, *pl.* (by false analogy) הַדְּרֵסִין, הֲדִירֵיסִין, v. דְּרוֹסָה.

הַדְרְסִיּוֹת, v. הַרְדְּסִיּוֹת.

הִדְרָקוֹן, v. הִדְרוֹקָן.

הַדְרְתָא f., constr. הֲדָרָא=הַדְרַת. Targ. Y. I Deut. XXXIII, 17.

הֲדָתְנַיָּא, v. הָא I.

הָהּ (b. h.; interj.) *ah, alas!* Esth. R. to I, 2 (play on *hahem*) הה לאותן הימים alas, for those days (of feasting)!

הֵה m. *heh,* name of *a worm* in the pomegranate. Sabb. 90[a] (Var. הָא, הָה, v. Rabb. D. S. a. l. notes 200 a. 300; Alf. ed. הח).

הַהוּא, הַהִיא, v. הוּא, הִיא.

הָהֵן, הַהִין m. (=הא חין) *this, that.* Y. Yeb. III, 5[a] bot. ח׳ תרתיי ה׳ וכ׳ this one is guilty of two sins, and that one is &c.—Y. Gitt. IX, 50[b] כל ה׳ פירקא (ib. VIII, 49[c] bot. כל הדא) all of this chapter is the teaching of R. M. Y. Snh. VII, 25[d]. Y. Erub. V, 22[c] bot., v. next w.; a. fr.

הָהֵנוּ (=ההן הוא, v. preced.) *this is.* Y. Erub. V, 22[c] bot. אין חמשה כן ההן ה׳ אמצעי וכ׳ (not חמשה) if you commence measuring from this (village), that one will be the central village, &c. Y. Pes. II, beg. 28[c] ה׳ איסור וכ׳ (ed. Krot. הָהֵנֵי) this is implied in the prohibition of benefit. V. דִּינוּ.

הו, v. הוּא ch.

הוּא m., **הִיא** f. (b. h.) *he, it; she; it is* &c. Snh.

III, 3 (24[b]) if he has no trade אלא חוא (Y. ed., Erub. 82[a] חיא) except this (gambling &c.); יש לו אומנות שלא חוא (חיא) if he has a trade besides this (v. Rabb. D. S. a. l. note 80).—חיא—חיא, חוא—חוא it is the same, i. e. there is no difference between the two. Y. Ber. I, 3[b] היא היא both are equally precious. Gen. R. s. 9, end הוא מאד הוא אדם the word מאד has the same letters as אדם. Ber. 2[b] דילמא ביאת אורו הוא perhaps it is (means) the arrival of his day, v. אור II; a. v. fr.—[Shebi. III, 8 עושה הוא; IV, 5 מכסה הוא, Y. ed. מְכַסֶּהוּ, עוֹשֵׂהוּ; ib. X, 6 מזכה הוא; Ms. M., Gitt. 37[a] מְזַכֵּהוּ.]—ולא היא but it is not so (it has a different reason &c.). Ber. 57[a]; a. fr.—כל שהוא (כל שהיא) a) *whosoever, whatsoever (is)*. Peah II, 4 כל ש׳ אוכל whatever is eatable &c.; a. fr.—b) *whatever it may be, a minimum*, v. כָּל. Shebi. X, 6 כל שהוא; Gitt. l. c. כל שֶׁהוּ; a. fr.—ספר היא *the Book Hi*, name of a Pentateuch scroll in the Temple in which היא occurs nine times (for the archaic הוא), whereas in others it appears eleven times (v. Ab. d'R. N. ch. XXXIV, ed. Schechter). Sifré Deut. 356; Y. Taan. IV, 68[a] bot.—הַהִיא, הַהוּא, mostly in Chald. diction, v. next w.—*Pl.* הֵם m., הֵן c. Ber. 2[b] והלא כהנים . . . הם טובלים but do not priests bathe &c.?—Meg. 14[b] רחמניות הן are compassionate. Hull. 127[b] הרי הן וכ׳ they are to be treated as if &c.; a. v. fr.—הן . . הן are the same. Y. Ab. Zar. II, end, 42[a], v. אִסְטַגְּרוֹת.—With prep. לָהֶם, מֵהֶן, בָּהֶם &c.

הוּא, הוּ m., **הִיא, הִי** f., ch. same. Targ. Ex. I, 16; a. v. fr.—היא הדא, v. הָא.—Y. Shebi. VII, 37[c] top בהוא אתר (R. S. to Shebi. VII, 3 בההוא אתרא) in the same place.—כל דהוי whatsoever, v. preced. Arakh. 2[a] נפשות כל דהו human beings of any nature, v. כָּל.—Y. Kil. VI, 31[b] top כהיא דאמר וכ׳ (in Babli כי הא) as (that which) R... said.—*Pl.* הֵן (perhaps only in Hebr. phrases); הִינּוּן, הִינִּין. Targ. Y. Ex. I, 10; Ib. 19 (O. אִינ׳); a. fr.—With prefix ה: הַהוּא, הַהִיא. Targ. Y. Ex. XXI, 20; a. fr.—In Talmud frequ. used to introduce a case. Pes. 3[b] ה׳ ארמאה דר׳ it occurred that a gentile &c. Keth. 78[b] ה׳ איתתא דר׳ the case came up of a woman that &c.; a. v. fr.—ה׳ גברא, ה׳ איתתא frequ. euphemistically for *myself, thyself* (to avoid ominous speech or curse). Y. Maas. Sh. IV, 55[b] bot. אבוי דה׳ ג׳ thy father. Ib.[c] top חמית ה׳ א׳ I saw; בעלה דה׳ א׳ thy husband; a. v. fr.—With prefix ד: דהוא, דהיא, contr. דְּהוּ, דִּי, דְּהִי, v. דִּי a. הוּ.—With prefixed prep. בְּהוֹן, בְּהוֹן, לְהוֹן, לְהוֹן.

הֲוָא, v. הוי.

הֲוָאר, v. חֲבַאר.

הוֹאִיל conj. (=הוֹיִיל, v. יָאַל) [*it helps, or help,*] followed by ד, *because, since*. Ab. Zar. III, 7 ה׳ ולצורה וכ׳ since they worship the figure (but not the tree). Y. Shek. III, beg. 47[b] ה׳ ואילו וכ׳ since they say so and the others &c.; a. v. fr.—Also in Chald. phrases. Targ. Y. II Gen. XVIII, 17; a. e.—Yeb. 22[a] ה׳ ואתי לידן since we are at these subjects. Bets. 18[b] ה׳ ובשבת שרי וכ׳ since it is allowed on the Sabbath, it is also allowed on Yom Kippur. Ib. ומי אית ליה לרבא ה׳ does Raba adopt the principle of *hoïl* (because something is permitted in one case, the permission must be extended to all analogous cases)?; a. fr.—Yeb. 117[a] ה׳ דלא ידעה וכ׳ it helps (we believe her that her husband is dead), for she did not know &c. (marginal correction משום).

הוּבָאר m. (בחר) *desolation, waste; desert plants, thorn*. Targ. Is. VII, 23; a. e. (with בּוּר II q. v.).—*Pl.* (of הוּבָאֵי (הוּבְאֵי. Targ. Job XXX, 4 Ms. (ed. הובאר, ed. Wil. הוּבִי, h. text מלוח). Targ. Y. Num. XXXIII, 41 (some ed. הובאר וכור, corr. acc.).

הוֹבָדָא, constr. הובד m. (אבד) *destruction*. Targ. Esth. IX, 5.

הוּבְדָנָא m. (v. preced.) *ruin*. Targ. Ps. XCII, 12 (ed. Wil. טוּב׳, corr. acc. or אוֹ׳).

הוֹבִיר, *Hif.* of בּוּר I.

הוּבְלִילָא, v. הַבְלִילָא.

הוּבְעִיּוֹת=אוּבְעִיוֹת, v. אַבְעָיָה. Peah IV, 5 Ms. M.

הוֹבְרָא, הוֹבְרָיָא, אוֹ׳ f. ch. (=h. הַבְרָאָה; ברי) *mourners' meal on returning from burial*. Gen. R. s. 49 זו ה׳ this (צדקה Gen. XVIII, 19) means the custom of offering mourners the meal &c. Y. M. Kat. III, end, 83[d] עבדון ליה איב׳ (read אוֹ׳) they prepared for him &c.

הוֹבְרִים m. pl. (v. b. h. הָבַר) *astrological specula, horoscopes*. Num. R. s. 20 היה רואה בהוֹבְרָיו וכ׳ he saw in his horoscopes that &c.

***הוּגְדָס** (Var. v. infra) pr. n. m. *Hugdes*. Yoma III, 11 Y. ed. (Mish. a. Bab. ed. (38[a]) הגרים, Ms. M. הגר׳, v. Rabb. D. S. a. l. note); ib. 38[b] הוגרס (Ms. M. אגרס, v. Rabb. D. S. a. l. note); Tosef. ib. II, 8 אוגדס (Var. אגדיס, some ed. הגדיס); Shek. V, 1 הוגרס (הוגדס, v. Rabb. D. S. a. l. p. 40, note 6).

הוֹגִין m., pl. הוֹגְנִים, הוגנין (הגן) [*balance-holder,*] *anchor, ballast*. B. Bath. V, 1 ההוגין Y. ed. (Mish. a. Bab. ed. עוגין q. v.).—Gen. R. s. 12; Yalk. Is. 314 נין, הוגנים.....—Gen. R. s. 83 הוגין Ar. (ed. pl.). Sifré Deut. 346 וקשרים בהוגנים וכ׳ and tied the two ships to anchors and iron weights, and made them rest upon them; Yalk. ib. 953; Yalk. Am. 548.—Y. Sabb. XVII, beg. 16[a] אף ההוגין; Tosef. ib. XIV (XV), 1 אף אגוז שבספינה ed. Zuck. (Var. ארגן, עוגין) also a ballast stone in the ship (may be handled on the Sabbath).

הוֹגֶן m. (preced.) *balance*; only in כְּה׳ (adv.) *appropriately, reasonably, correspondingly*. Gen. R. s. 93 כה׳ וכשורה עשה he acted (according to balance and line) exactly right. Taan. 4[a] שאלו שלא כה׳ made an unreasonable demand (making their actions dependent on chance); לשנים השיבו כה׳ two of them were answered properly (Providence favoring their ways); Gen. R. s. 60; Lev. R. s. 37. Yeb. 110[a] הוא עשה שלא כה׳ וכ׳ he acted improperly, therefore the court deals with him improperly (more strictly than the law would justify) and declares his marriage invalid; B. Bath. 48[b]; a. fr.

הוֹגֶן m. *border, rim,* v. אוֹגֶן.

הוֹגָן, only in fem. הוֹגֶנֶת (=מְהוּגֶּנֶת, v. הָגַן; cmp. הוֹגֶן) *befitting, corresponding to; well-regulated.* Yeb. XII, 6 (106[b]) עֵצָה הה׳ לו an advice befitting his case. Gitt. VIII, 5 (79[b]) לשום מלכות שאינה ה׳ (Mish. אחרת) in the name of a government not corresponding (to the country in which the document was written, or not recognized in the country). Kidd. 70[a] אשה שאינה ה׳ לו a wife beneath the social standing of her husband (eventually degrading the priestly status of the issue); Y. Gitt. I, 43[c] bot.; a. fr.—*Pl.* (from הָגוּן, הָגַן, v. הָגַן) הֲגוּנוֹת. Snh. 93[a] ה׳ לכהונה fit to be married by priests.

הוֹגְנָא, הוֹגְנָא m. (הגן, v. preced. wds.; v. meanings of Arab. stem hagan in Fl. to Levy Targ. Dict. I, 423[a]) *young camel,* or *dromedary.* *Pl.* הוֹגְנִין, הוֹגְנֵי. Targ. Is. LX, 6 (ed. Lag. הגרי, h. text בכרי). Targ. II Chr. IX, 1.—Y. Ḥag. II, beg. 77[a]. Snh. 52[a] (prov.) . . . נפישין משכי דה׳ many old camels are laden with the hides of the young ones (many old men survive the young).

הוגנוס׳, v. הוגניס׳.

הוֹגְנִין, הוֹגְנִים, v. הוגין.

הוגניסים, הוגניסים, Gen. R. s. 100, v. פְּרִיסְקָא.

הוּגְנַס m., pl. הוּגְנְסִין (εὐγενής, v. אבגרנוס) *of noble birth.* Gen. R. s. 48 . הוגנסין . הגונין Ar. (ed. ב״א גדולים . . . מהוגנין).

הוגרס, הוגרם, v. הוּגְנַס.

הוֹד m. (b. h.) *distinction, pride, majesty.* Ex. R. s. 47 קרני ה׳ the rays of majesty (from Moses' face). Y. Yeb. II, 3[d] (play on לְהָדְפָהּ, II Kings IV, 27) he placed his hand בהוד שביופיה וכ׳ on the most distinctive of her charms, &c.

הוֹדָאָה, הוֹדָיָה f. (ודי) 1) *confession, admission.* Shebu. VI, 1 הה׳ בשוה וכ׳ the amount admitted to be due must be at least one P'rutah. B. Mets. 3[b], a. fr. הוֹדָאַת בעל דין וכ׳ the admission of indebtedness by the defendant is worth as much as a hundred witnesses; a. fr.—2) *confession before the Lord, thanksgiving.* Sot. IX, 10 (47[a]) הוֹדָיַית המעשר (Mish. הוֹדָיוֹת, pl.) the confession to be recited on having given away the third year's tithes (Deut. XXVI, 12 sq.); ib. 47[b] הוֹדָאַת; Maas. Sh. V, 15 (Mish. ed. הודיות). Gen. R. s. 71 Leah seized פלך ה׳ the shuttle of confession (made gratitude her duty, Gen. XXIX, 35); בעלי ה׳ men of confession (ready to admit their wrong or to thank the Lord): Midr. Sam. ch. XXVIII.—Ber. IV, 2 (28[b]) אני נותן ה׳ וכ׳ I offer thanks for my lot (being permitted to teach). Y. ib. I, 3[d] top ה׳ ושבח וכ׳ thanks and praise are due to &c.; a. fr.—3) *Hodaah, the first of the last three sections of the Prayer of Benedictions* (תפלה), so named from the words *Modim* &c. Ber. 34[a] בה׳ התחלה וכ׳ in reciting the Hodaah one must bend at the beginning &c. Ib.[b] בה׳ ובה׳ של הלל on reading the Hodaah or the thanksgiving in *Hallel* (הודו). Ib. ה׳ דבה״מ the thanksgiving in the grace after meal (נוֹדֶה לְּךָ וכ׳). Y. Taan. II, 65[c] bot. הודייה.—*Pl.* הוֹדָאוֹת, הוֹדָיוֹת. Taan. 6[b] ברוך רוב הה׳ blessed be He to whom a multitude of thanks is due; אל הה׳ the Power to whom (all) thanksgivings are due; Y. Ber. I, 3[d] top; a. fr.—Y. Taan. III, 66[d] bot. פר של ה׳ the bullock over which the confessions are uttered.—Esp. *Hodâaoth, proceedings resting on evidences of the defendant's admission of his indebtedness.* Snh. 2[b]; B. Kam. 84[b]; a. e.; cmp. אוֹדָיְתָא.

הוֹדָאָה ch. (preced.) *confession of guilt.* Targ. Josh. VII, 19 (ed. Lag. אוֹדָאָה).

הודאה, Sifra Sh'mini Par. 3, ch. V, a corrupt Var. lect. for הֲדָרְיָא, which came into the text; v. הֲדָרְיָא.

הוֹדּוּ I pr. n. (b. h. הֹדּוּ) *India.* Targ. Zeph. III, 10 (h. text כוש); v. הִנְדְּיָא.—Esth. R. to I, 1; Meg. 11[a]; a. e.

הוֹדוּ II (ודי) *hodu* (*thank ye* the Lord), a section of Hallel. Succ. III, 9; a. e.

הוֹדְיָא, v. הֲדָיָא.

הוֹדָיָה, הוֹדָיָיה, v. הוֹדָאָה.

הוֹדַע, *Af.* of יְדַע; v. also יָדַע.

הוּדְרָא m. (הדר) *trimmed (and thin) beam for ornament,* opp. כשורא a supporting joist.—*Pl.* הוּדְרֵי. B. Bath. 3[b] שרגי ליבני והדרי ה׳ וכ׳ (v. Rabb. D. S. a. l. note) if the officers of the congregation have had the bricks (for the new Synagogue) piled up, the beams trimmed &c. Ib. 6[a] אחזיק לְהוּדְרֵי וכ׳ if one has acquired, by the law of limitation, the right of laying beams in the neighbor's wall, he has not the right of laying joists. [For transpos. of ד a. ר, cmp. מְדוּרָא.]

הוּדְרָנָא m. (הדר) *circle,* only in הֲדַר ה׳ *all-around.* Pes. 76[a] סולת דה׳ הוּדְרָנֵיה (missing in Ms. M., v. Rabb. D. S. a. l.) the flour around it. Sabb. 77[b] לאפוקי הדר הו׳ (Ms. M. ה׳ הדרנא; in ed. הדר left out, v. marg. note a. Rabb. D. S. a. l.) to exclude what is required for rubbing all around the sore.

הַוָּה f. (b. h.; הוי, v. Pi.) [*change,*] *misfortune.*—*Pl.* הַוּוֹת. Num. R. s. 12 (expl. מִדֶּבֶר הוות, Ps. XCI, 3) מִדָּבָר שמביא ה׳ בעולם from the word which produces misfortunes &c.; Midr. Till. to Ps. l. c. שמביא הַוָּה לעולם (insert מדבר).

הֵוָה* pr. n. pl. *Hevah.* Y. Yeb. III, 5[a] top R. H. דמן ה׳ of H.; (Gitt. 86[b] הונא or הוגא, Var. חֵיפָא).

הָוָה, v. הֲוִי.

הָוָה *ah!*, v. וָהּ.

הוֹהֲרָא, v. אוֹהֲרָא.

הוּוּ only in ה׳ ד־, *he who.* Targ. Prov. XVI, 19, a. fr. (in Targ. Prov.) ed. Lag. (Ms. הוֹן, v. הָן; ed. Wil. הוּא).

הוֹוְיָה, v. הֲוָיָה.

הוֹוְנָא, v. הֲוָנָא.

הוֹוִינָא, הֲוֹוִינַן = הֲוֵי׳, v. הֲוֵי.

הוּכריא, misread by Mus. for הוּבְרְיָא q. v.

הָוְנָא, v. הֶוְנָא.

הוועדה, Y. B. Kam. IV, 4b top בה׳, read בהוַּעֲדָה, v. עוד.

הוותיאוס, v. אֶוְותִיאוֹס.

הוּזְמָא, v. הִיזְמָא.

הוּמְבָא (הִימְבָא) הוּמְבָא, v. חוּטְבָא.

הוּמְלָס, v. הֶטְלֵיס.

הוֹי (b. h.) *woe!, ah!* Ex. R. s. 24, beg. (ref. to Deut. XXXII, 6) כלומר ה׳ (ה)ליר׳ וכ׳ as if saying, Woe unto &c.—Y. Snh. X, 29b bot., v. וָהּ; a. fr.

הֲוָה, הָוָה, הֲוִי (b. h.) *to exist; to be, become; to occur, come to pass.*—With part. ה׳ מביט *he looked;* ה׳ אומר *he said,* freq. *used to say.* Gen. R. s. 1, beg. אני ה׳ הקב״ה מַבִּיט וכ׳ ... הָיִיתִי וכ׳ I was the implement &c. Ib. the Lord looked into the Law (as often as a thing was to be created). Ab. I, 13 הוא ה׳ אומר the same used to say. Gen. R. s. 2 ה׳ ללמה ולא כלום became a nothing; a. v. fr.—Apocopate forms: יְהֵא, יְהִי, תְּהֵא, תְּהִי, אֶהֱא, אֱהִי; יְהוּ (=יִהְיוּ), תְּהוּ (=תִּהְיוּ). Yoma 66b אהא בשלום אני וכ׳ (Tosef. ib. IV (III), 14 נִהְיֶה) may I and you be as well; Y. ib. VI, 43c bot. כן תהוּ וכ׳ so may ye be well. B. Mets. 35a תהא במאמינו let this be (speak of a case) when he accepts his opponent's statement; a. v. fr.—Part. הֹוֶה, הֹוָה 1) *frequent, usual.* Sabb. VI, 6 דברו חכמים בה׳ the scholars (in using the words 'Arabian women') speak of the ordinary custom (not to the exclusion of other people); a. fr.—2) *existing, enduring.* Pesik. R. s. 11, end הם הויים ודומים [להקב״ה] they shall be existing for themselves (not merely as an attachment) and resembling [the Lord]; ib. אַף הם הויים אש וכ׳ they, too, shall endure as a consuming fire.—Cant. R. to II, 13 עניות ירבה ויוקר הווה (read תרבה) poverty shall increase, and prices remain high (different in Snh. 97a a. Sot. 49b, v. אָמַר II). *Imper.* הֱוֵי, הֱוָא; pl. הֱווּ. Ab. I, 4. Ib. II, 3; a. fr.—הֱוֵי אוֹמֵר, also elliptically הֱוֵי *say,* i. e. *you must admit, this proves, that is meant by saying.* Taan. 2a which is the service of the heart? ה׳ אומר זו תפלה you must admit, it is prayer. Tosef. Nidd. I, 6 ה׳ לא אמרום וכ׳ that is to say, the scholars have spoken &c. Cant. R. to I, 6 ה׳ כרמי שלי וכ׳ this is meant by 'my vineyard &c.'—Y. Shebu. VII, 38c top הוי לא צורכה וכ׳ it is evident that it would not have been necessary &c.; a. fr.

Pi. הִוָּה, חִיָּה (v. חֲוָיָה 1) 1) *to change one's legal status, to dispose of.* Keth. 40b (ref. to תהיה Deut. XXII, 19) במְהַוָּה עצמה וכ׳ the text speaks of a woman who can dispose of herself.—2) *to produce, make.* Kidd. 58a (ref. to והיית, Deut. VII, 26) כל שאתה מְהַוֶּה הימנה whatever thou makest out of it; Tem. 30b מְהַוֶּה ממנה; a. e.

הֲוֵי, הֲוָא, הֲוָה, fut. יֶהֱוֵי, יְהֵי, תְּהֵא, תְּהֵי ch. 1) same. Targ. Gen. I, 3; a. v. fr.—Koh. R. to IX, 10 הוא הוה גלי he emigrated, v. גְּלֵי. Ib. לא הֲוֵינָא גלי did I not emigrate?—Ib. ויהוי מה דהוי (read דיהוי) and come what may. Ber. 3a (in Hebr. diction) ג׳ משמרות הוי וכ׳ the night consists of three watches. Ib.b תרי נשפי הוו there are two נשף (twilights); a. v. fr.—Y. Maasr. IV, end, 51c הֲווֹן מפקדין וכ׳ (=הֲהֲווֹן, or read: הֲווֹן) give orders to your wives &c., דיהוון מרימרין וכ׳ that they (the laborers) should &c.—B. Bath. 73b, a. fr. הוה אזלינן it happened that we &c.—Kidd. 31b הֲוָאִית (=הֲוָאת) מרבינתיה הואי she was his foster-mother. Ned. 50a אי הואי לי (Rashi הוי) if I become wealthy. Y. Shek. V, 49b top אית הוה סבין וכ׳ (Bab. ed. איתהוה, איתהוון, corr. acc.) there used to be old men &c.; Y. Peah VIII, 21b אית הוו.—Imper. הֱוֵי, v. preced. Ib. זיל הוי בי רב go and stay at college; a. fr.—In Palest. dialect יָא, יְהָא=יֵיא. Y. Taan. IV, 68c top יֵיא שלמא וכ׳ peace be with the hand &c.; a. fr.—V. יָבָא, יֵיאבָךְ.—2) *to dwell upon, discuss,* v. infra.

Pa. הַוֵּי, הַוִּי, הַוָּא 1) *to produce.* Y. Taan. III, 66d bot. דהַוְּיָה וכ׳ (not דהוית) where the ground used to produce &c.; Midr. Till. to Ps. CXXVI דהַוְיָה; v. זְוִויר.—2) (also Peel) with ב or על *to dwell upon, to discuss, argue, oppose,* cmp. קום. Y. R. Hash. I, 57a top על דב״ה אינון הַוּוּי they were discussing the question on the basis of Beth-Hillel's opinion (differing as to the application of B. H.'s principle). Keth. 72b הוי בה ר׳ פפא R. P. (when that subject was up) raised the question.—Usu. והוינן בה, וה׳ עלה on its being brought up at college we raised the point. Ber. 45b. Gitt. 4b; a. fr.—Naz. 16b וכולה כדה׳ בהאלימא וכ׳ and all this must be understood, in accordance with what we have discussed (ib. 5a sq.), in the sense of &c.—Kidd. 50b, a. fr. מאי הַוֵּי עלה what have they decided upon it?, what is the result?—[Nidd. 66a תהוו... נתהוו, v. תְּהָא.]

הֲוָיָה, הֲוָיַת, הֲוִית, הַוָּיָה f. (preced.) 1) *existence, status, condition, stability.* Ab. Zar. 54b (ref. to תהיה, Lev. XXV, 12) בהֲוָיָתָהּ תהא it shall remain in its status. Y. Ber. II, 4d bot. (ref. to והיו, Deut. VI, 6) כדרך הֲוָיָתָן יהיו they shall remain (be read) in the order in which they stand. Y. Shek. IV, 48b top שתהא ה׳ בקודש that it must retain its sacred character. Cant. R. to VI, 4 (ref. to ויהיו, Num. VII, 5) נתן להם ה׳ he gave them stability; Num. R. s. 12, end ניתן לחם ה׳ (read ניתנה). M. Kat. 15a הויה the use of the word היה in the Biblical text; Men. 28a; a. e.—Esp. (with ref. to והיתה לאיש, Deut. XXIV, 2, v. הָיָה *Pi.*) *legal status of marriage,* Kidd. 5a מקיש ה׳ ליציאה וכ׳ the text puts entrance into marriage on an equality with going out (divorce), as divorce takes place by means of a deed, so may marriage be contracted &c. Yeb. 13b (ref. to לא תהיה, Deut. XXV, 5) לא תהיה בה ה׳ לזר she shall have no legal status with another man; Y. ib. I, 2c bot. לא תהא לה ה׳ וכ׳ (not יהא); a. fr.—*Pl.* הֲוָיוֹת, הֲוָיָ׳. Keth. 46b, a. e. איתקוש ה׳ להדדי the various modes of entrance into marriage correspond to each other.—2) הַוָּיָה, or הַ׳ (v. preced. *Pa.*) *discussion, argument.* Y. Maasr. II, 49d bot. הוי׳ דר׳ מנא the result of a discussion stated by R. M.—*Pl.* הֲוָיוֹת or הַוָּ׳. Succ. 28a ה׳ דאביי וכ׳ (Ms. M. sing.) arguments raised by A. &c.; B. Bath. 134a (Ms. H. sing., Ms. R. הַוָּיֵי; v. Rabb. D. S. a. l. note 40).

הוּנְגְּרָאָה, הוּנְגְּרָאֵי m. (v. הַגְרָה) *inhabitants of Hagra.* Targ. Ps. LXXXIII, 7. Targ. I Chr. V, 10; a. e.

הוּן I *he*, v. הֵן. [לְהוֹן, בְּהוֹן, v. הוּא ch.] [Targ. Y. II Gen. XIV, 5 בְּהוֹן, taking בְּהֶם=בְּהָם; Y. I הֶמְתָּא.]

הוֹן II m. (b. h.; contr. of הָוֹן; הוה; cmp. Gr. οὐσία) 1) *possession, wealth.* Y. Peah I, 15[d] top (ref. to Prov. III, 9) בין שיש לך ה׳ וכ׳ whether or not thou art wealthy; Pesik. R. s. 23—24; a. e.—Ib. s. 25 (interpreting מהונך, Prov. l. c.) ממה שחננך from whatever He has graced thee with; Pesik. Asser, p. 97[a]; a. e—2) *natural condition, nature; faculty; health, sanity.* Pesik. R. l. c. כבד....שאם... נוי וכ׳ honor the Lord with thy nature; if thou art handsome &c. Ib. (another interpretation) מהוֹנֶיךָ וכ׳ (pl.) while thou art in possession of thy powers (health); honor thy physician &c.; Ib. בקולך . . . with thy voice; Pesik. l. c.; a. fr.—Pesik. R. l. c. עד שהונו עליו while his mind was sound. Gen. R. s. 78 (interpret. לאטי, Gen. XXXIII, 14) להוני להוני אני מהלך I shall walk suitably to my condition (at my ease, slowly). Lam. R. to I, 13 לְהוֹנָךְ לה׳ come to thy senses (be not rash)!

הֲוָן, הוֹנָא, הוֹן, הֲוָן ch. same. Targ. Prov. XXXI, 5 (h. text מְחֻקָּק) *proper conduct.* Ib. XXVIII, 16 ed. Lag. (oth. ed. הֲוָיָנָא, h. text תבונות). Ib. V, 19 הוונא ed. Lag. (ed. Wil. תְּרַיְנָא).—Pesik. Asser, p. 97[a] (ref. to מהונך, Prov. III, 9, v. preced.) עבוד בהֶוְנָךְ עד וכ׳ (or בהוֹנָךְ) do (good) while in thy senses, ere thou be unable to do through the loss of thy senses; Tanḥ. R'eh 12; a. e.—Lev. R. s. 34 (play on האביון) אהן מסכינא הב הֲוָנָךְ מיניה here is this poor man, give; thy nature is the same as his; Ruth R. to II, 19 האביון הֲוָנָךְ ביה.

הוּנָא pr. n. m. *Huna* (in Y. also חונא, הונה, חונה) 1) Rab Huna, disciple of Rab. Keth. 106[a] מתיבתא דר׳ ה׳ the college of R. H.—Gitt. 59[b]. Y. B. Kam. X, end, 7[c]; Y. Shebu. VI, end, 37[b]; a. v. fr.—2) R. H., an Amora of the fourth gener. Y. Peah III, 17[d] bot. (ה׳).—3) R. H. Rabbah (Roba) of Sepphoris. Y. Ber. IV, end, 8[c]; Y. R. Hash. IV, end, 59[d]. Gen. R. s. 8; a. e.—Yoma 77[b]; Hull. 51[a] ר׳ ה׳ צפוראה (prob. the same).—4) *Mar Huna, Resh Galutha.* Y. Kil. IX, 32[b] (read מר for רב). [Ib. bot., strike out ריש גל׳, v. M. Kat. 25[a]]; a. others. V. Fr. M'bo, p. 73[a], sq. [חונא, Gitt. 86[b], v. הָוָא.]

הוֹנָאָה, הוֹנָיָה f. (=אוֹנָאָה; ינה) *oppression, wrong.* Sifra B'har ch. III, Par. 3 הניית ממון ... הניית דברים, read הוֹנָיַת.—Esp. (law) *imposition, fraudulent representation; redress in case of overreaching*, v. אוֹנָאָה. B. Mets. IV, 6 Y. ed. (Mish. IV, 7 אי׳) ההוניה וכ׳ the overreaching, to be actionable, must be at least four M'ah &c. Y. Keth. XI, 34[c] top אין לְמִקַּח ה׳ וכ׳ against purchase there is no claim for overreaching, i. e. the purchase itself is not invalidated. Y. B. Mets. IV, 9[d] top ה׳ מצבה the actual amount overcharged. Ib. הוֹנָיָתוֹ the amount with which he was overcharged. Sifra l. c. יש ה׳ legal redress can be claimed; a. v. fr.—*Pl.* הוֹנָיוֹת, v. אוֹנָיָה.

הונגמוס, v. אגניטוס.

הֲוִיָּנָא, v. הֲוָנָא.

הוֹכִיחַ m. (יכח) *evidence, precedent, rule.* Y. Dem. II, 22[c] top; ib. III, 23[c] this one day has become ה׳ לכל הימים a precedent by which to judge all other days. Y. Nidd. II, 50[a] top הוֹכִיחָהּ קיים her evidence (the cloth with which she examined herself) exists; Bab. ib. 16[b] מוֹכִיחָהּ.

הוֹל (cmp. חלל) *to be merry.—Polel* הוֹלֵל *to deride, laugh at* (cmp. שָׂחַק). Pesik. Aḥăré, p. 169[a] (ref. to Koh. II, 2) אמר שלמה שלשה . . . מה״ד הוֹלַלְתִּים Solomon said, Three things which Divine Justice scorned (and prohibited)—I laughed at them; Tanḥ. Aḥăré 1 (read: ששחקה, a. הוללתים); Y. Snh. II, 20[c] top חיללתים (corr. acc.); Koh. R. to II, 2 (read: שלמה for שמואל, a. הוללתים for תם . . .).

הוּלְיָא (interj.) *hulya!*, sailor's cry. Pes. 112[b], v. הַיְרָא.

הוֹלָכָה f. (הָלַךְ *Hif.*) 1) *leading, carrying.* Yoma 27[a] הוֹלָכַת איברים וכ׳ the carrying of the portions of the sacrifice to the altar ascent. Zeb. 14[a] ה׳ שלא ברגל לא שמה ה׳ carrying without moving the feet (handing over without walking from the spot) is not called *holakhah.* Ib. 15[a] ה׳ זוטרתי immediate sprinkling from a slaughtering place near the altar, opp. ה׳ רבתי actual carrying.—שליח לה׳ a delegate sent by the husband to deliver the letter of divorce, opp. שליח לקבלה a delegate authorized by the wife to receive &c. Gitt. 62[b]; a. fr.—[2) *drawing the slaughterer's knife in a forward direction*, v. הֲבָאָה.]

הוֹלֵלָה f. (b. h. הוללות *confusion;* חלל, cmp. חלל, חוּלְחַלְתָּא, חֲלַחוּלִית) [*creating confusion,*] *intrigue, schemes.* Koh. R. to II, 12 ה׳ של מלכות the diplomatic schemes of the (Roman) government (cmp. Targ. a. l., I, 17, a. e.) Ib. ה׳ של מינות the intrigues of the heretics.—*Pl.* הוֹלֵלוֹת. Lev. R. s. 17 (ib. s. 20 חלחליות), v. חַלְחוּלִית; Midr. Till. to Ps. V, 6.

הוּמְהוּם, v. אוּמָּאָה.

הוֹמוֹנְיָא f. (ὁμόνοια) *concord, union*, opp. מחלוקת. Lam. R. introd. (R. Alexandri 1) נעשו כולן ה׳ all of them (formerly divided into factions) became unanimous (Mekh. Yithro, Baḥod., s. 1 הושוו לב אחד; Lev. R. s. 9 חנייה אחת). [Lam. R. l. c. (Zibdi b. Levi 1) ה׳ אחת; Yalk. Ps. 795 הומני׳, read: הֶגְמוֹנְיָא.]

הוּמַם *to become defective*, v. מום.

הוּמַנְיָא, הֲו׳ pr. n. pl. *Humania,* [*Hymenia*, v. Neub. Géogr. p. 367, below Ctesiphon], a town in Babylonia hostile to Jews. Kidd. 72[a]. Ib.[b]; Yeb. 16[b] כגון ה׳ וכ׳ as hostile as H. against Pum Nahăra. [Ar. ed. Koh. הימוניא, Ms. O., quoted in Neub. l. c. הימניא.] [Yalk. Ps. 795 הומני׳, v. הֶגְמוֹנְיָא.]

הומניות, v. הֲמָנִיוֹת.

הוֹמֶר, v. חוֹמֶר.

הונדקס pr. n. m. Y. Sabb. XVI, 15[d] top מהניתא דר׳ ה׳, prob. a corruption for יוסה, v. Mishn. a. l. [The entire passage seems to be corrupt, v. Bab. ib. 117[b], sq.]

הוֹנָיָיה, v. הוֹנָאָה.

הוּנְיָיקִי, v. אוּנְיָיקִי.

הונים, v. אֲנִקְטְמִין.

הוּפָא, v. אוּפָא a. חוּפָא.

הוּפְכָא m. (הפך) *perverseness.* Targ. Prov. II, 14.

הוֹפָעָה f. (יפע) *the appearance* (of Deity). the use of the verb הוֹפִיעַ. Midr. Till. to Ps. XIV.—*Pl.* הוֹפָעוֹת. Sifré Deut. 343; Yalk. Ps. 759. Snh. 92[a] הופעות (corr. acc.); Ber. 33[a] Ms. F. (ed. נקמות, v. Rabb. D. S. a. l. note 40).

הוֹפָעוּתָא ch. same. Targ. Jud. V, 4 (ed. Lag. הוֹפָעַת).

הוֹפַעְתָא, הופעיות, v. preced. wds.

הופקנה, Targ. Prov. XXV, 16, correct (with Bxt.): סוּפְקָנְךְ, v. סוּפְקָנָא.

הוּץ I *fastened,* pl. הוּצִין, v. אוּץ.

הוּץ II m., pl. **הוּצִין** (v. next w.) *palm-leaves.* Y. Sabb. VII, 10[c] top he who beats סיב ה׳ וכ׳ bast, palm leaves or papyrus. Ib. XVIII, 11[b] top; Bab. ib. 78[b]; Tosef. ib. VIII (IX), 10. [Succ. 12[b]; 15[a] סככה בה׳ Ms. M., ed. חֵץ, v. חִיצִין.]

הוּצָא I m. (הוץ; cmp. חוץ, נוץ) 1) (adj.) *prickly.* B. Kam. 80[a] שרצא ה׳ Ms. M. (ed. חרצא) a prickly creeping animal, v. חַרְזָא.—2) *the long and thin foliage of a palm-branch spreading from the stem.* Succ. 32[a] a *Lulab* דסליק בחד ה׳ which spreads its foliage on one side only.—*Pl.* הוּצֵי. B. Kam. 96[a] if one stole a palm-branch ועבדינהו ה׳ and tore it into leaves. Yoma 78[b] בדה׳ in shoes made of &c.—3) *prickly shrubbery used as fence, hedge.* B. Kam. 92[a] (prov.) בהדי ה׳ לקי כרבא with the shrub the cabbage is smitten (the good suffer with the bad). Ned. 49[b] אכיל בה׳ ate with a thorn (as a fork). Ib. 91[b] פרטיה... לה׳ וכ׳ the lover parted the hedge and ran off. B. Bath. 4[a] דנהיגי בה׳ ודפנא where it is customary to make fences with shrubbery or bay-trees.—Ib.[b] ה׳ ליה ליה וכ׳ where they use hedges for fences, the exclusive ownership of one neighbor can only be secured by a deed.—*Pl.* הוּצֵי. Ib.

הוּצָא II pr. n. pl. *Hutsa.* Y. Ned. IX, 42[c] יהודה איש ה׳; v., however, הוּצָל.

הוֹצָאָה f. (יצא, v. יְצִיאָה) 1) *carrying out.* B. Kam. 30[a] שעת הוֹצָאַת זבלים the season for carrying out dung; a. fr.—הוֹצָאַת המת *funeral escort.* Meg. 3[b]; a. e.—Esp. (with ref. to Sabbath law) *carrying out of the house,* in gen. *transferring an object from one territory to another* (from private to public ground a. vice versa, v. רָשׁוּת). Sabb. 2[b] שתים דה׳ two forbidden acts in taking out of the house, opp. הכנסה, carrying in. Ib. תנא הכנסה נמי ה׳ וכ׳ the teacher of the Mishnah calls the carrying in, too, *hotsaah* (Mish. יְצִיאָה), *transfer.* Ib. כל עקירת... ה׳ וכ׳ any removal of an object from its place is implied in the term *hotsaah.* Y. ib. I, 2[b]; a. fr.—2) *bringing forth, sprouting.* Y. Shebi. V, 35[d] bot. מהוצאת עלין from the time that the leaves come forth.—3) ה׳ נפש *the escape of life, last dying movement.* Hull. 38[a].—4) *the time consumed by the laborer to go out to the field.* Gen. R. s. 72 ה׳ כְּשֶׁל בעה״ב the time for going out to the place of labor is included in the working hours belonging to the employer (B. Mets. 83[b], a. e. יציאה).—5) *expenditure, outlay, cost; marketing.* Y. Peah IV, beg. 18[a] ה׳ משל בעה״ב the cost (of cutting the fruits of the tree) must be borne by the owner (and not by the poor). Y. Shek. I, end, 46[b] ה׳ דרכים expense for keeping the roads in repair. Keth. 80[a] אם הי׳ שבח יותר על הה׳ if the income from the improvement exceeds the outlay. Sabb. 117[b] ה׳ שבת the marketing for the Sabbath; a. fr.—*Pl.* הוֹצָאוֹת. Keth. VIII, 5 המוציא ה׳ על וכ׳ if one spends money for improving his wife's estate. Num. R. s. 14, end כמה ה׳ יוצאות וכ׳ how large the expenses are for the royal table; a. fr.

הוּצָל pr. n. pl. *Hutsal,* 1) an old fortress in Palestine. Sabb. 92[a], sq. (?) Meg. 5[b], also called ה׳ דבית בנימין, or דבר בנימין (v. Rabb. D. S. a. l., a. Neub. Géogr. p. 152).—2) H. in Babylonia. Ib. 29[a]. Yoma 52[a], sq. Kerith. 13[b]; a. fr. (v. Berl. Beitr. z. Geogr. p. 32).

הוּצָן m. (cmp. הוץ II a. הוּצָא), only in pl. constr. הוּצְנֵי פשתן (*hard*) *flax-stalks* before they are prepared for spinning, opp. אֲנִיצֵי, v. אָנִיץ. Tosef. Succ. I, 5; Succ. 12[b]; Y. ib. I, 52[b] bot. V. הוּשָׁן.—Tosef. Maasr. III, 8 ה׳ פשתן (Var. אוצני) read: ה׳ תלתן stalks of fenugrec.

הוֹקָעָה f. (יקע *Hif.*) *making an abomination, exposure; hanging.* Snh. 34[b] מנין לה׳ וכ׳ how do we know that *hokaah* (Num. XXV, 4) means hanging?

הוֹר or **הוֹרֶה** m. (b. h. in pl.; ירה) *teacher, father.* Deut. R. s. 1 (play on הַהָר הזה, Deut. II, 3) הוֹרוֹ זה וכ׳ this his *hor,* that is his father.—*Pl.* הוֹרִים. Gen. R. s. 68; Yalk. Ps. 878, v. מְעַבְּדָנָא. Pesik. R. s. 23—24 הוֹרָיו his parents. Pirké d'R. El. ch. XXXII אהבתו הולכת אחר הוריו his love follows (is given to) his parents. Gen. R. s. 76; a. fr.

הוֹרָאָה, v. הוֹרָיָה.

הוּרְדָא, v. הוּדְרָא.

הוֹרָדָה f. (יָרַד) *leading down, letting down; descent.* Y. Sot. IX, 24[a] top משעת ה׳ from the moment the calf is led down (Deut. XXI, 4). Midd. IV, 7 בית הוֹרָדַת המים (Talm. ed. הורדות pl.) an enclosure in the Temple serving as a spout for the rain water.

הוֹרְדוֹס, הוֹרְדוּס pr. n. m. *Herod,* the Idumean, King of Judæa. B. Bath. 3[b]. Ib. 4[a], a. e. בנין ה׳, v. בִּנְיָן. Lev. R. s. 35; Taan. 23[a]; a. fr.

הוֹרָה I f. *conception*, v. הוֹרָת.

הוֹרָה II f. (b. h.; v. הור) [*mother*,] (homiletically) *teaching.* Cant. R. to III, 4 (interpret. חדר הוֹרָתִי, ib.) זה אה"מ .. בהוריה that means the Tabernacle, for from there issued the obligation of Israel to abide by legal decisions; Lev. R. s. 1; Cant. R. to II, 3, v. next w.

הוֹרָאָה, הוֹרָיָיה, הוֹרָיָה f. (ירה, *Hif.*) *decision, instruction; teacher's* or *judge's office.* Y. Ber. IV, 8^c top *Moriah* שמשם ה' וכ' because instruction goes forth &c.; Taan. 16^a יוצאה ... הוראה (not יצא); Gen. R. s. 55; Pesik. R. s. 40.—Cant. R. to III, 4, a. e., v. preced.—Y. Shebi. VI, 36^c top אין הוֹרָאָתוֹ הוריה his decision is not binding. Kerith. 13^b לא סגי ליה בלא ה' he could not help giving a practical decision (cases constantly coming before him). Y. Sot. VIII, 22^d bot. ואסור בה' and (he who drinks it) is forbidden to give a decision. Hor. I, 1 ראוי לה' authorized to teach; a. v. fr.—הוֹרָאַת שעה (הוֹרָיַת) *a decision under an emergency, a special dispensation* (not to be taken as a precedent), opp. ה' לדורות. Yoma 69^b; a. fr.—מוֹרֵה ה' *an authorized teacher, judge.* Pes. 3^b; a. fr.—*Pl.* הוֹרָיוֹת, הוֹרָאוֹת. Y. Naz. IV, end, 53^c עד שתורה ה' בישראל before being appointed a teacher in Israel. Hor. I, 5 (5^a) הוריות ב"ד (Mish. ed. הוֹרָיַית); a. fr.—*Horayoth* (*Horaoth*), name of a treatise of Mishnah, Tosefta, Talmud Babli a. Y'rushalmi, on liability for erroneous decisions.

הורכינוס, הורכיינוס, Tosef. Gitt. VIII (VI), 3, read with ed. Zuck. הִיפַּרְכִיוּת.

הוֹרְקִינוֹס, v. הִרְקִינָס.

הוֹרְמִיז pr. n. 1) *Ormuzd* (Ahuramazda), the good principle in the Zendavesta. Snh. 39^a, v. אֲהוֹרְמִין.—[B. Bath. 73^a bot., v. next w.].—2) a gentile (Persian) proper noun, v. בַּתְק. Gitt. 11^a.—3) איפרא ה', v. אִיפְרָא.—4) ה' ארדשיר pr. n. pl. *Hormiz(Ormuzd)-Ardjir*, prob. identical with Ardjir, v. אַרְדְּשִׁיר. B. Bath. 52^a.

הוֹרְמִין m. *Hormin*, name of a demon, cmp. אֲהוֹרְמִין. B. Bath. 73^a bot. ה' בר לילית (Ar. a. Ms. H. a. Var. in comment. הורמיז).

הוֹרְמִינֵי, v. חַרְמִינֵי.

הוֹרְקְנוֹס pr. n. m. *Hyrcan*, 1) a Maccabean prince and High-priest, brother to Aristobule. B. Kam. 82^b; Sot. 49^b.—2) father of R. Eliezer. Ab. II, 8; a. fr.—3) son of R. Eliezer. Snh. 68^a.

הוֹרָת or **הוֹרָה** f. (denom. of Hofal of הָרָה) *conception, being conceived.* Snh. 58^a, a. fr. הוֹרָתוֹ שלא בקדושה he was conceived in an unhallowed condition (when his mother was a gentile). Ex. R. s. 1 הוֹרָתָהּ בדרך she was conceived on the road. Ib. מה הורתה שלא בצער as she conceived without pain; a. fr.

הוֹשָׁטָה f. (יָשַׁט) *reaching over, handing over*, opp. הוֹלָכָה q. v.—Y. Sabb. VII, 10^d ולמה לא תנינן ה' עמהון why is not reaching an object over (from one territory to another) counted among the labors forbidden on the Sabbath? Zeb. 14^a כדי הוֹשָׁטַת ידו as far as one may reach over with his hand (without moving from his place).

הוֹשֶׁן m., only in pl. constr. הוֹשְׁנֵי פשתן *flax-stalks* in an intermediate station of preparation, contrad. to אַנִּיצֵי a. הוּצְנֵי (v. אָנִיץ a. הוּצָן). Succ. 12^b בה' פ' איני יודע Ms. M. (v. Rabb. D. S. a. l.) if one covered the Succah with *hosh'neh* . . ., I do not know (whether or not the Succah is *kasher*). Ib. וה' פשתן עצמן א"י מהן Ms. M. (v. Rabb. D. S. a. l.) nor do I know what *hosh'ne* . . . are (in which stage they are called so).

הוֹשָׁעָה f. (יָשַׁע) *relief, delivery.* Yalk. Num. 725.

הוֹשַׁעְיָה, הוֹשַׁעְיָא pr. n. m. *Hoshaya* (in Bab. אוֹשַׁעְיָא, q. v.) 1) R. H. the Elder (רַבָּה). Y. Kidd. I, 60^a bot.; Y. Keth. IX, 32^d, sq. אבי המשנה the author of the Mishnah (Tosefta); a. fr.—2) several Amoraim by that name. Y. Ter. VIII, 45^c. Y. Bets. I, 60^c bot.; a. fr. Y. Frank. M'bo p. 74^a, sq.

הוֹשַׁעְנָא f. (=הוֹשִׁיעָה נָא=הוֹשַׁע־נָא) [*help, I pray,*] *Hosanna*, name of parts of, or of the entire, festive wreath (*Lulab*) carried in procession on the Feast of Booths. Succ. 30^b ה' דאוונכרי וכ' the traders' own H. (myrtles). Ib., sq. מעיקרא ... והשתא ה' before its use was designated it was called *asa* and now it is called H.—Ib. 37^a כי גדליתו ה' when ye tie the festive wreath; a. fr.—Targ. II Esth. III, 8.—Esp. *the separate branches of the willow tree carried in procession on the last day of Succoth*, whence יומא דה', יום ה' *the seventh day of the Feast of Booths* (now called ה' רַבָּה); v. עֲרוּבְתָא.

הותא, Targ. Prov. XXVI, 21 בְּחוּתָא Ms., v. בְּחוּתָא.

הַזָּאָה, v. הַזָּיָה.

הֲזָדָה f. (זוד) *wilful act; use of the stem* זיד *in the Bible text.* Snh. 16^a אתיא ה' ה' וכ' an analogy is drawn between the law concerning the false prophet (יזיד Deut. XVIII, 20) and that concerning the rebellious elder (בזדון, ib. XVII, 12). Ib. והא ה' כי כתיבא וכ' but is not the term 'wilfulness' used in connection with death penalty?

הוזמר, v. זֶוֶט.

הַזָּאָה, הַזָּיָיה, הַזָּיָה f. (נזה) *sprinkling* of the blood of sacrifices, of the water of purification upon the unclean. Zeb. V, 1 ודמן טעון ה' וכ' and their blood must be sprinkled on the space between the bars &c.—Y. Ber. V, 9^d top הַזָּיָיתוֹ כשרה the rite of sprinkling which he performed is valid. Pes. VI, 2 הזאה תוכיח (Y. ed. הזייה) let the sprinkling (on the unclean) prove it; a. fr.—*Pl.* הַזָּאוֹת, הַזָּיוֹת. Y. Yoma V, 42^d top. Bab. ib. 55^a. Men. III, 6; a. fr.

הז"ו, ל"ך, ה"ך, mnemotechnical formula for *the six portions into which the song of Hadzinu* (Deut. XXXII, 1—43) *is to be divided in public recitation*: v. 1—6 האזינו; v. 7—12 זכור; v. 13—18 ירכיבהו; v. 19—26 וירא; v. 27—35 לולא; v. 36—43 כי. R. Hash. 31^a (v. Tosaf. a. l. for another division); Treat. Sof'rim XII, 8.

הֲזָוִיה, v. הֲזָיָה.

הֶזֵּיקָא, הֶזֵּיק, v. הֶיזֵּק.

הַזְכָּרָה f. (זכר; v. אַזְכָּרָה) 1) *giving a debtor notice* in order to prevent loss of right by limitation. Keth. 104ª גובה שלא בה׳ has a right to collect (after the lapse of twenty five years) even if he has given no notice.—2) *Hazkarah* (=הַזְכָּרַת גשמים), the insertion of a reference to rain in the second section of the Prayer of Benedictions, v. גְּבוּרָה, contrad. to שְׁאֵלָה. Taan. 2ᵇ; a. e.—3) *the Tetragrammaton.* Y. Ber. III, 6ᶜ bot.—*Pl.* הַזְכָּרוֹת. Ib. IV, 8ª top י״ח ה׳ וכ׳ eighteen invocations in Ps. XXIX. Lev. R. s. 1 י״ח ה׳ שבק״ש eighteen invocations in the recitation of Sh'ma, v. שְׁמַע; a. e.

הַזְמָא, pl. **הַזְמֵי**, v. הֵיזְמָא.

הֲזָמָה f. (זמם) *the refutation of witnesses by proving an alibi,* contrad. to הכחשה counterevidence; *the conviction of false witnesses* (Deut. XIX, 19). B. Mets. 4ª בתורת ה׳ subject to the law of *hăzamah*. Keth. 20ª ה׳ שלא בפניהן evidence of an alibi taken in the absence of the witnesses concerned. Macc. 2ª דין ה׳ the punishment for evidence disproved by an alibi (retaliation); a. e.

הַזְמָנָא m. (זמן) *summons.* Kidd. 70ª פיתקא (פיסקא) דהז׳ (Ar. דיסקא דזמינותא) a document containing a summons (to appear before court).

הַזְמָנָה f. (זמן) *preparation, designation* of an object for a certain purpose. Snh. 47ᵇ, a. e. ה׳ מילתא designation is a reality, i. e. the designation of an object for a certain (sacred) purpose is equal to its having been used. Bets. 26ᵇ ה׳ designation for use on the coming Holy Day; a. e.

הַזְמָנוּתָא f.=הַזְמָנָא. Kidd. 70ᵇ, v. דִּסְקָא.

*__הזמת__ (Arab. *ḥuzmath*) *a bunch.* Snh. 26ᵇ bot., quot. in Ar., a gloss to כפא which came into the text, v. כַּפָּא a. קָפָא.

הֶזֵּק, v. הֶיזֵּק.

*__הַזָר__ (Pers. hazâr, v. Perles Et. St. p. 16) *a thousand.* Snh. 98ª (speaking to the Persian king) אית לך כאר ה׳ גונא Ar. hast thou (Khar hazâr gûnah, Persian) an ass of a thousand colors? [Ed. בר חיור גוני, Ms. M. חמר בר גוני, Ms. F. חיור מאה גוונג, Ms. K. גוונג; Yalk. Zech. 576 Ms. מי אית ליה גווני דאית ליה לחמריה has he (your horse) the colors which his (the Messiah's) ass has?; v. Rabb. D. S. a. l.]

הֶחְלֵט m. (חָלַט II) *final decision,* esp. *ascertained condition of leprosy* after the probationary days of confinement (הֶסְגֵּר, v. Lev. XIII). Y. M. Kat. III, 82ᶜ bot. לה׳ הכא הוא עבד here (in Miriam's case) the confinement was ordered for a definite case of leprosy, opp. להסגר for probation; ib. ימי ה׳ the seven days of Miriam's leprosy (Num. XII, 14 sq.); Gen. R. s. 100.—V. חֲלִיטָה III.

הַחְלָטָה f. *paste,* v. חֲלִיטָה II.

החרפותא, Pesik. Parah, p. 35ª, read חַרְסְפִיתָא.

הֲטָבָה f. (טוב) 1) *doing good,* esp. *a vow to benefit one's self* (or *others*), opp. הרעה self-abnegation (or harm to others). Shebu. III, 5 דברים שיש בהן הרעה או ה׳ vows in which a self-abnegation or an enjoyment is implied. Ib. 27ª מה ה׳ רשות וכ׳ as well as the vow of enjoyment refers to something religiously indifferent, so &c. Ib. הֲטָבַת אחרים a vow comprising a benefit to others; a. fr.—2) (v. Ex. XXX, 7) *preparing, trimming.* Yoma 14ᵇ; ib. 33ª; a. fr.—Lev. R. s. 32; Cant. R. to II, 14, a. e. (ref. to היטיבו, Deut. XVIII, 17) ה׳ כהֲטָבַת הנרות a well considered word (which has its effect) like well-trimmed lights; כה׳ הקטורת like the well-prepared frank-incense.

הַטְבָּלָה f. (טָבַל I) *immersion* of vessels for levitical purification. Bets. 18ª, v. הַשְׁקָה; a. e.

הִטּוּי m. (נָטָה Hif.) *inclination, sliding.* Bets. 9ᵇ ה׳ סולם וכ׳ the question about moving a ladder by sliding from one window to another.

הֲטוּלִים (חֲטוּ׳), עֲטוּלִין m. pl. (*wine of*) *Hătul* or *Ătul,* a place mentioned as producing the most preferable wine for libation. Men. VIII, 6 ה׳ (Talm. ed. 86ᵇ ע׳ (Ms. M. קְלוּטְיִים, v. Rabb. D. S. a l., note; Ar. ה׳).

הֶטֵּחַ m. (טוּחַ I) *plaster.* Tosef. Ohol. VII, 4 אם יכול הֶטֵּחַ וכ׳ if the plaster on them is thick enough to stand by itself.

הַטָּחָה f. (טוּחַ II) 1) *throwing* (a stone &c.), Y. B. Kam. III, 3ᶜ top אם כדרך ה׳ הטיח if one hit (him who was carrying a flask) in the way of throwing a stone (not merely by letting a stone lie in the road).—2) *contusion.* Y. Sabb. VI, 8ᶜ bot. דומה . . . ה׳ זו בלבד it seems that I am not to carry off from this place anything except this contusion (of my finger).

הטיומא, Tanh., ed. Bub., B'reshith 6, read קטיומא.

הֲטָיָיה, הַטָּיָיה f. (נטה) 1) *being inclined,* i. e. *giving a verdict according to the majority of votes* (Ex. XXIII, 2 אחרי רבים לחטות). Snh. I, 6 לא כהַטָּיָיתְךָ וכ׳ thy verdict against the defendant must not be given in the same way as thy verdict of acquittal; for the latter suffices a majority of one, for the former there must be a majority of two.—2) *perversion of justice* (Ex. XXIII, 6). Sot. 47ᵇ הַטָּיַית משפט.—3) (euphem.) *performing coition with a virgin without causing a bleeding.* Keth. 6ᵇ.

חמלים, v. next w.

הוּמְלָס, הַמְלִיס m. (כלל, v. אַטְלֵיז) *bazaar, shop, public place* (cmp. חָנוּת). Gen. R. s. 19; s. 20 I shall die ואתה יושב לך ה׳ (some ed. המלים, corr. acc.), and thou wilt sit in public places (with none to care for)?—*Pl.* הוּמְ׳, הַמְלִיסִין. Ib. s. 37 היו מעמידין ה׳ (some ed. סִין . . ., corr. acc.) they arranged bazaars (with entertainments) where they would exchange their wives. Ib. s. 79 (ref. to ויחן, Gen. XXXIII, 18; cmp. חנות) התחיל מעמיד ה׳ וכ׳ he was the first to put up bazaars and sell cheap.

הֶטְלִיס* (a popular exclamation containing a disguised oath; v. פִּינּוּר) *I swear!* Gen. R. s. 87; Yalk. Gen 145; Yalk. Job 920.

הַטְמָנָה f. (טָמַן) *preserving*, esp. (v. Sabb. IV, 1) *putting a dish in a warm place or under covers to keep it warm for the Sabbath.* Sabb. 39ᵃ. Ib.ᵇ בטלה ה׳ וכ׳ the permission to keep a dish in matter which adds heat was abolished. Ib. 50ᵃ יחדן לה׳ he designated them to be used for keeping dishes warm; a. fr.

הַטָּפָה f. (נָטַף) *flow of words, prophetic speech* (Mic. II, 11). Gen. R. s. 44; Cant. R. to III, 4 (one of the biblical terms for prophecy). [Tosef. Kel. B. Mets. IV, 1 הטפה, v. חֲטִיפָה.]

הֶטְרֵחַ m.=טוֹרַח, *preparation.* Koh. R. to IX, 8.

הַטְּרִית, הַ׳ f. (נטר, v. אַטְרִי, טְרִית) *a preserve of gourd.*—*Pl.* הַטְּרִיוֹת. Ned. 49ᵃ ה׳ רכות וכ׳ soft preserves with which the sick eat their bread; Y. ib. VI, 39ᶜ bot. (for הרופא read החולה); Tosef. ib. III, 1 טריות רכות ed. Zuck. (Var. סיטרות רכות, ארמר וחרכיה, read: .. ארטריות, הוטריות).

הֶטְרְשָׁא, Y. B. Mets. V, 10ᶜ bot., v. טַרְשָׁא.

ה״י, v. ה״א.

הֵי I pr. n. m., v. הֵא II.

הֵי II 1) interj. (b. h. הָא) *behold, here is.* Y. Succ. V, beg. 55ᵃ הי לך מצה here is unleavened bread for thee. Combined הֵילָךְ. Ib.—B. Mets. 4ᵃ I owe thee only fifty Zuz, וה׳ and here they are.—Hence (law) *helakh, the instantaneous delivery of the amount confessed,* while the creditor claims a larger amount. Ib. ה׳ פטור וכ׳ if one delivers one portion of the claim (says, 'here it is'), he is exempt from taking an oath (as one who confesses a part of a claimed debt otherwise must do); a. fr.—2) (interrog.) *which?* Hull. 14ᵃ הי ר׳ יהודה which R. Judah, i. e. to which opinion of R. J. do you allude? Sabb. 9ᵇ הי כסוך וכ׳ which 'near Minhah' is meant in the Mishnah?—Hull. 49ᵇ הי מינייהו which of them (eventually closes up a hole in the entrails); a. fr.—3) *where?* Ber. 31ᵃ הי תורה וכ׳ where is the law, and where the good deeds to protect us?—Targ. Y. Deut. V, 23, v. הֵן.—הי דינו, v. הֵיךְ.—4) *as, like.* Targ. Y. I Deut. XXXII, 41 הֵיא ברק (not חיא) as lightning. Mostly הי כ־; comb. היכ־. Targ. Y. Lev. XXV, 40, v. הֵיךְ.

הִי I she, v. הוּ.

הִי II, m. (b. h. Ez. II, 10;=נְהִי) [*grief,*] *woe! oh!* Snh. 11ᵃ הי חסיד וכ׳ alas, the pious man (is no more)! (Y. Sot. IX, 24ᵇ הוי). Meg. 28ᵇ הי צנא . . . דחסר (Ms. M. אי, omitting דחסר) alas for the lost basket full of books (dead letter learning)! Ib. 11ᵃ, v. יַי.

הִיא she, v. הוּא.

הֵיאָ=הי.

הֵיאַךְ h. (interrog.=הֵיךְ) *how!* Ab. Zar. II, 5 ה׳ אתה קורא (Y. ed. האיך) how do you read?—Y. Ber. IV, 7ᶜ top. Pesik. R. s. 1; a. fr.

הִיגָא m.=הִיגָה, v. הִיגְתָא.

הִיגָא ch., pl. הִיגֵי, v. הִיגְתָא.

הִיגָה m., pl. הִיגִים, הִיגִין (v. הֲגָה, cmp. אֶגֶה) *a prickly shrub* or *tree* (v. Sm. Ant. s. v. Acanthus II, Acantha), prob. *hollow.* Erub. 34ᵇ החי׳ וכ׳ Ms. M. (ed. החג׳); Tosef. Kil. III, 15 ed. Zuck. החגין, oth. ed. חבין, corr. acc.) *hegin* belong to the class of trees. Lam. R. introd. (R. Naḥman) (play on חגים ינקופו, Is. XXIX, 1; v. הִיגְתָא) the deserted roads מעלין הי׳ (Yalk. Is. 302 הי׳ וקוצים) are overgrown with shrubs (and thorns).

היגים or **היגיס**, Pesik. R. s. 22 ה׳ אחריו, v. אַתְרָא.

הִיגְיְתָא, v. הִיגְתָא.

הֶיגְמוֹן, v. הֶגְ׳.

הִיגְתָא f. ch.=h. הִיגָה. Targ. II Esth. II, 7 (translating נעצוץ, Is. LV, 13, some ed. הִיגֵי׳). Sabb. 110ᵇ חרגוגא דהה׳ רומיתא a thistle growing among Roman thorns (prob. Corduelis spinosa, v. Sm. Ant. s. v. Acantha and succeed. wds.)—*Pl.* הִיגֵי. B. Bath. 83ᵇ ה׳ רומייתא (Ms. H. היגא רומיתא). B. Kam. 119ᵇ (in Hebr. dict.) מנקפי ה׳ (Rashi a. Ms. M. הִיגָא) those who trim thorns (collecting the twigs for themselves). Ab. Zar. 47ᵇ דגדיר ליה בהיזמי והיגי Ms. M. a. Ar. (ed. הינגי) he makes a fence by means of thorns and shrubs; a. fr.

הִידִי, הִידָה, הִידָא f. (=הֵי דָא הֵי, הֵי דָא, v. אִידִין a. הִידְּדָא) 1) *what now?, who now?, where now?* Targ. Y. I Deut. IV, 7; 8 (II הִידְּדָא). Targ. II Esth. VIII, 7.—Koh. R. to IX, 18.—2) (ellipt.) ה׳ לי־ ,ה׳ ל־ *what is this here in reference to? what hast thou to do with—?* Gen. R. s. 87 חן אדני הי׳ לדקמך (Yalk. ib. 145 הידה לקומך) 'here is my lord' (thy husband), what hast thou to do with the one before thee (me)?—Y. B. Kam. V, beg. 4ᵈ אידדי ליקומיך what claim hast thou against me?—Lev. R. s. 26 הידא לִיגַבֵּר שנאך וכ׳ (not לי גבי) why dost thou call on thy enemy &c.?—[הִידָא, הִידְּדָא, v. הִידְּדָא.]

הִידוּאָה m. *Indian.* Targ. Jer. XIII, 23 ed. Lag. (oth. ed. הִנְדְּוָאָה, הִינְדְּוָאָה; h. text כּוּשִׁי).

הִידּוּס m. (הָדַס) *damage done by scratching chickens.* B. Kam. 17ᵇ; 18ᵇ; v. מִדְּבַר.

הִידוֹר m. (ὕδωρ) *water.* Succ. 35ᵃ א״ת הָדָר אלא ה׳ וכ׳ Ms. M. 2 (ed. אדור, Ar. הדור) read not *hadar* (Lev. XXIII, 40) but *hydor*, for in Greek water is called h.; Yalk. Lev. 651.

הִידּוּר, הִידוּר m. (הָדַר, Pi.) *paying respect; honoring, adorning.* Kidd. 32ᵇ (ref. to Lev. XIX, 32) קימה במקום שיש ה׳ rising in such a way as to show your respects (being near enough). Ib. ה׳ שאין בו וכ׳, v. חֶסְרוֹן. Lam. R. to I, 1 (ונד מתלבי׳) רבתר בהידורה של תורה וכ׳ thou shalt die in the glory of the Law (as a great scholar), v. הֲדָרָא.— ה׳ מצוה doing a religious act in the handsomest way. B. Kam. 9b ה׳ מצוה עד וכ׳ the expense for adorning a religious act (e. g. buying a fine copy of the Law) must not exceed one third (of the ordinary expense); a. e.

הִידִי, v. הִידָא.

הָדֵין, הִידֵין (contr. of הארדנא, v. הַדְנָא) *then*. Targ. Prov. I, 28 (h. text אז); a. fr.—Targ. Ps. CXIX, 6 ed. Lag. (some ed. הָדֵין). Ib. XIX, 14 (Reg. אֲזֵין, cmp. אֵיזִי).

הִידֵין *which?*, v. הַיידֵן.

הִידְנוּ, הֵידֵינוּ, v. הַיידְנוּ.

הִיוּתִיאוּס, הִיוּתָאוּס, v. אֶוּוּתִיאוּס.

הִיזֵיק, הִיזֵיקָא, v. הֶיזֵּק, הֵיזְקָא.

הִיזְמָא, הִיזְ׳, אִיזְמָא m. (חוס, cmp. חוס) *a prickly shrub*, prob. *Spina Regia* (v. Löw Aram. Pfl. p. 231 a. quot. ib. from Plin. Hist. Nat.). Tosef. Kil. I, 11 you must not plant *cuscuta* על גבי הא׳ ed. Zuck. (Var. אזמאזמא, corr. acc.) on *izma*.—*Pl.* הִיזְמֵי. Targ. Job XXXI, 40 הי׳ (Ms. חו׳).—Keth. 77b שכר של הי׳ beer containing (in place of hops) cuscuta growing on *hizmê*.—Mostly in connection with הִיגֵי, v. הִיגְתָא. Sabb. 107b; a. fr.

הִיזְמְתָא f. (preced.) *shrubbery of hizmê*. Erub. 28b דקטלינן לה לה׳ וכ׳ for the cuscuta dies when the *hizmê* are cut.

הֶיזֵּק m. (נזק) *injury, damage, loss; danger*. Gitt. 53a, a. fr. ה׳ שאינו ניכר a damage not discernible in the object itself (e. g. if an unclean person touches food, whereby its value is reduced, because the scope of its use is limited). B. Kam. 2b שן יש הנאה לְהֶיזֵּקָהּ the damage done by the tooth is connected with a benefit (to the animal). Ib. רגל היזקה מצוי the damage by the foot is an ordinary occurrence (and must be guarded against). Y. Ber. IX, 14b top ה׳ חמין possible injury to health by the hot bath. Gen. R. s. 82 דבר של ה׳ an obnoxious thing (animal); a. fr.

הֵיזְקָא, הִיזְ׳ ch. same. Pes. 8b היכא דשכיח ה׳ where danger is to be expected. B. Kam. 22b ברי ה׳ the damage is sure to occur. Ib. 5a ה׳ דמינכרא=h. היזק ניכר, v. preced.; a. fr.

הִיזְרָא, v. חִיזְרָא.

הִיטְבָא, v. חוּטְבָא.

הִיטְּנֵי m. pl. (v. אִיטָן) *calamus, reeds*. Yoma 78b בהי׳ in shoes made of reeds. [Rashi: מין שעם; Ms. M. a. oth. רהיטני; oth. vers. חיטני; Asheri: shoes made of *wheat-straw*.]

הִיטְּרִית, v. הֵטְ׳.

הַיי c. 1) (=הַאי) *this, that*. Y. Keth. XII, 35a bot. ה׳ שיניך וכ׳ (Y. Kil. IX, 32b bot. האי) how is that tooth of thine?—[Y. Snh. VIII, beg. 26a חיי די ליה אב, v. הַיידָא.]—2) (=הֵי) *which?* (generally with הֵין or דָּא, v. הַיידָא, הַיידֵן).

Y. Shek. V, 48d (read היי) אהיי דין... וה׳ דין וכ׳ which wine was good for the bowels, and which &c.—Y. R. Hash. I, beg. 56a ה׳ דין שני.. וה׳ וכ׳ which *sheni* refers to months, and which to years?—Y. Meg. I, 72a top ה׳ לין אינון וכ׳ (=ה׳ אילין); Y. Succ. III, 54a top הַיילֵין which are the headings of chapters?—Y. Keth. VII, 31c top [read:] כהיי דא מתניתא דר׳ חנין בשם ר׳ שמואל with which of them does the Boraitha cited by R. Ḥ.... agree?—Ib. IX, 32d bot. [read:] היי לין רבנין (Y. B. Bath. VIII, 16b מאן אינון) who are meant by 'the Rabbis'?—With prefixes: כְּיי, לְיי. Y. Ber. I, 3a top כיי דמ׳ר ר׳ וכ׳ (=כהא דאמר) as (that which) R... said. Y. Erub. III, 21a top; a. fr.—Y. Shebu. II, 33d לְהַיידָא) ליי דא מילה) with regard to what?; a. e.—Y. Gitt. IX, end, 50d ואדיין את ליי (usually לזו), v. אֲדַיִין.

הַיְיא (traditional pronunc. חייא) only in אַהַייא (=אַהֵי הָא) *to which* (of the clauses &c.) does *this* refer? Kidd. 74a; Keth. 12a; v. אִילֵימָא; a. fr.

הַיְיא adv. (=חייא, cmp. חָיוֹת, Ex. I, 19) 1) *quickly, rapidly*. B. Kam. 84a; Sabb. 134b סליק בישרא ה׳ (Ms. M. הַיָא, v. Rabb. D. S. a. l. note) the flesh grows fast (the wound heals quickly). Ib. 119a bot. דליקומי ה׳ that they may soon rise.—2) (an exclamation of encouragement) *quick! go on!* Gitt 34a, a. e., v. אַשּׁוּר.—Pes. 112b (sailors' cry) ה׳ ה׳ Ms. M. (ed. היליי ה׳ הילא והילוק הוליא, v. Rabb. D. S. a. l. note; Mus. in Ar. ed. Koh.: הליוני ה׳ הילא הילוק). [Y. Peah I, 15d דהדיין סבא ה׳ ed. Amst., ed. Krot. חייר, Y. Ab. Zar. III, 42c top חייא, read חַיי.]

הַיידָא, הַיידְה f. (=היי דא) 1) *this very thing, even this, it is this*. Y. Dem. I, 22b top ה׳ מחלוקת this very thing is controverted. Y. Sabb. VII, 10c bot. ה׳ משום נטילת וכ׳ this is because it is an act of killing. Y. Taan. V, 67d top וה׳ אמר and this he said.—2) (=הֵי דָא) *which? where?* Y. Maas. Sh. V, 56a top בה׳ אתיתא by which road did you come? Ib. ולא חכים בה׳ and he did not know by which.—Y. Sabb. II, 5a bot. ה׳ היא which (transgression) is it (that he is guilty of)? Ib. VII, 10c, a. fr. וה׳ אמרה דא and what (Mishnah, Boraitha) says this (where is your authority)?; Y. Pes. II, 29b bot. וְהַיידָא.—Contr. הַיְדָא. Ib. VII, 34b bot. ה׳ אמר and it is this he said; i. e. in this connection he said it.—לְהַיידָא, v. חיי.—הויידא ל־ (cmp. h. הִנֵּה) *behold, there is*. Y. Bicc. II, beg. 64c הַהַיידָלוֹן חמשים וכ׳ (=וה׳ לון) and behold, here are fifty two.—Gen. R. s. 84 (ref. to הַלָּזֶה, Gen. XXXVII, 19) הוידא חי׳=) הַיידֵי ליה וכ׳) behold, it is himself, he comes carrying his dreams; (Yalk. ib. 141 דילדה, corr. acc.).—Y. Snh. VIII, beg. 26a חיי די ליה אב וכ׳ behold, he is a father and not a son.

הַיידֵי, v. preced.

הַיידֵין, v. הַיידֵן.

הַיידֵינוּ, v. הַיידְנוּ.

הַיידָלוֹן, v. הַיידָא.

הַיידֵן m. (=היי דן, v. הַיידָא) *which now? who?* Y

Peah VIII, 21[a] top ח׳ וינון (read י״נון or אינון) which are they?; [Y. Erub. III, 20[d] top אילין אינון, read: אִילֵּין].— Y. Dem. II, 23[a] ח׳ ר׳ מאיר, v. חֵי II.—Y. Sabb. XIX, 17[b] (also חיי דין). Y. Gitt. II, 44[a] bot. ח׳ הוא למחר what is meant by 'to-morrow' (the next following or the day after the next)?; a. fr.

חֵידְנוּ, חֵיידְנוּ (also חיי דנו) c. (=חיי דן הו, v. preced.) *which now is?* Y. Erub. V, 22[c] bot. ח׳ אמצעי which do you call 'the central'? (v. הָהֵנוּ). Y. Pes. I, 27[d] top חיי ד׳ שעת הביעור which 'time of removal'? Ib. V, 32[c] top וחַיידֵינוּ לשמו פטור and what case do you mean when saying *lishmo patur?*—Y. Yeb. IV, 6[b] top חֵידֵינוּ רבה which is greater?—Y. Snh. V, 22[d] top חיידינו כולל וח׳ מונה what is meant by *kolel*, and what by *moneh?*; Y. Naz. III, 52[d] bot. חיי די נו (corr. acc.).

חֵיילֵין, v. חֵיי.

חיימים, חיימ״ס, read: חֵמִייפּוּס.

חֵיינוּ c. (=חיי נִיהוּ) *it is this, it is he; it is the same, it corresponds to.* Ber. 25[b] bot. ח׳ דבעא וכ׳ it is this that R. J. asked. Pes. 50[a] ח׳ דכתיב וכ׳ it corresponds to what is written &c., v. בִּשְׁלָמָא. Y. Ter. II, 41[b] bot. וח׳ חמשה וכ׳ this is analogous to the case of 'five sacks' &c. Sabb. 118[b] ח׳ ורדימס ח׳ וכ׳ Vardimas and Menahem are names of the same person; a. v. fr.—Ber. 2[b] חכמים ח׳ ר׳ מאיר what difference is there between what 'the scholars' say and what R. M. says? Ib. ר׳ חנינא ח׳ ר׳ וכ׳; a. fr.— [דְּהַיְינוּ *which means.* Gen. R. s. 87 (in a gloss) דח׳ בעליך viz. thy husband.]

חֵיכ־ prefix, v. next w.

חֵיךְ: ch. (=חֵי כְּ) 1) *how?* (v. הֵיאַךְ). Y. Erub. I, 19[b] bot. ח׳ עבידא how can it happen?, i. e. name a case to which this rule will apply.—2) *as, like;* in Targ. editions mostly with double comparison: חֵיךְ כְּ־.—Targ. Ps. XXII, 15, sq.; a. v. fr.—ח׳—ח׳ *as—so.* Targ. Ps. CXXXIX, 12.— ח׳ מה *as that which, even as.* Targ. Y. II Num. XXIV, 1, v. infra.—ח׳ מה דאת אמר (abbr. חמד״א) even as you read in the Scriptures. Gen. R. s. 1, beg.; a. v. fr.—Y. Succ. III, 54[a] top ח׳ מה דאמרת וכ׳ the same words which you spoke to the one, you spoke to the other!—Combined חֵיכְמָה, חֵיכְמָא. Targ. Y. Gen. XXI, 1; a. fr.—Y. Erub. I, 19[b]; a. fr.—As prefix to nouns חֵיכ־. Targ. I Chr. II, 54 חיכנטופא (ed. Lag. חי כנ׳). Ib. 55 (ed. Lag. חי כ־); v. חֵי II.—*[3) (v. next w.) *where?* Targ. Ps. LXXXIX, 50 Ms. (ed. אָן).]

חֵיכָא (=חֵי כָּא) *where?*, (relat.) *where.* Targ. Jer. III, 2 (ed. Lag. אֵיכָא); a. e.—Targ. Prov. XXVI, 20 Ar. (ed. חֵיכְנָא).—Ber. 2[a] תנא ח׳ קאי וכ׳ where does the Tannai (of the Mishnah) stand, that he starts with, 'From what time'?, i. e. to what law does he refer?—Yeb. 106[a] אבוך ח׳ where is thy father?—Snh. 93[a] לח׳ אזלו where did they go to (what became of them)? Ib. ודניאל לח׳ אזל where was Daniel at the time?; a. v. fr.—Hull. 11[b] ח׳ . . . דלא וכ׳ (not חיכי), v. אֶפְשַׁר. Yoma 2[b] ח׳ דליכא דדמי ליה where there is nothing resembling it. B. Mets. 102[a] כל ח׳ דאיתו וכ׳ in all cases in which he can acquire possession himself; a. v. fr.—Emph. חֵיכָן (in Hebr. diction). Pes. 2[b] וכי ח׳ מצינו do we find anywhere &c.? Succ. 23[a] ח׳ סוכתך where is thy Succah?

חֵיכְדָא (=חֵי כְדָא, v. Dan. II, 43 הא כדי) *even as.* Targ. Y. Deut. XVI, 21 sq. (some ed. חֵיכְמָא).

חֵכ׳, חֵיכְדֵין (v. preced.) 1) *even so.* Targ. Y. Deut. XVI, 21; a. e. [Targ. II Esth. III, 8 ח׳—ח׳ ed. Lag., oth. ed. כח׳—ח׳ even as—so.]—2) (interrog.) *how now?.* Targ. Ps. LXXIII, 11 (not הֵכְ׳).—3) (exclam.) *Oh, how!* Ib. 19.— 4) *one like this.* Pesik. Zakh., p. 23[b]; Yalk. Gen. 135, v. בִּיזָא III.

חֵיכִי (=חי כי) 1) *how?* Ber. 4[b] ח׳ מצי סמיך how can he join?; a. fr.—ח׳ דמי (abbr. ח״ד), v. דְּמֵי I.—Emphat. חֵיכִין *how now?* Ned. 51[b] ח׳ משמע how is it now to be decided?—2) כי ח׳ a) *as well as,* v. כִּי ch.—b) *so that, in order that.* Ber. 8[a] כי ח׳ דתורכו חיי in order that you may prolong your lives. Ib. 6[b] כי ח׳ דלא ליחוק lest he may be injured; a. v. fr.

חֵיכֵיל* (cmp. preced., v. P. Sm. 1006 s. v. חכיל; cmp. b. h. כְּבַל) *therefore, now.* Targ. Prov. VI, 3 Ms. (ed. Lag. הכיל, ed. חביל, חב״ל; Pesh. הכיל).

חֵיכִין, v. חֵיכִי.

חֵיכֵּירָא, v. חֵיכָּרָא.

חֵיכָל m. (b. h.) *palace, the Temple;* esp. *the Holy,* the hall containing the golden altar &c., contrad. to the Holy of Holies, v. דְּבִיר. Midd. IV, 1; a. fr.—Ned. I, 3 כח׳ as forbidden as the offerings of the Temple (a vow formula). Y. Succ. V, 55[c] ומשחיתים לח׳ (not ומשתחוים, v. Rashi to Ez. VIII, 16) and offended the Temple (through indecency); a. fr.—*Pl.* חֵיכָלוֹת. Y. Shek. V, end, 49[b] (quot. fr. Hos. VIII, 14).

חֵיכְלָא, חֵיכָלָא ch. same. Targ. I Kings VI, 3; a. e.—Kidd. 71[a] ח׳ by the Temple!—Y. Taan. III, end, 67[a] קום לך קומי ח׳ stand up facing the Temple (for prayer). Cant. R. to I, 1, end (ref. to Am. VIII, 3) שבחות דח׳ praises of the Temple (religious songs).

חֵיכְמָה, חֵיכְמָא, v. חֵיךְ.

חֵיכָן, v. חֵיכָא.

חֵיכְנָה, חֵיכְנָא (v. חֵיךְ) 1) *thus, in the following manner, even as.* Targ. Prov. VI, 8. Targ. Ps. XLVIII, 9; a. fr.—2) *Oh, how!* Targ. Prov. V, 12.—[Ib. XXVI, 20 ח׳ . . . וח׳ *as—even so* (Ar. חֵיכָא).]

חֵיכֵּר m. (נָכַר) *recognition, sign, indication.* Men. 33[a]; Erub. 11[b] ח׳ ציר a mark in the door posts (holes) for the hinges, v. אַבְקָתָא. V. חַכֵּר a. חַכָּרָה.

חֵיכֵּירָא, חֵיכָּרָא ch. same. Sabb. 16[a] עבדי בהו רבנן ח׳ the Rabbis made a distinction (a somewhat different, law) concerning glass ware. Yoma 2[a] כי היכי דליהוי להו ה׳ in order that they be distinguishable (from other sacrifices). Hor. 13[b] לא בעי . . . ה׳ וכ׳ ought there not to be a distinction (in honors) between myself and them? Pes. 114[b] ה׳ לתינוקות some distinction to attract the attention of the children.—*Pl.* הֵיכֵּרֵי. Zeb. 21[b] בי תרי ה׳ הוו עבדי two signals were given at a time.

הִילָא I pr. n. m.=אִילָא. Y. Yoma VI, 43[c] top; a. e.

הִילָא II *hila*, a sailor's cry, v. הַיְיא.

הִילוּן, v. חָלוּן.

הִילּוּךְ, הִילוּךְ, הִלּוּךְ m. (הָלַךְ) 1) *walk*. Keth. 111[a]. Sabb. 113[b] הִילּוּכָךְ של שבת thy way of walking on the Sabbath. Nidd. 31[a] ה׳ רגלים faculty of walking.—Gen. R. s. 20 ה׳ מעים כדרך וכ׳ (not בדרך) natural movement of the bowels (Ber. 57[b] שלשול).—2) *walking* (lengthwise and breadthwise) *through a field*, as a form of taking possession. B. Bath. 100[a]; Y. Kidd. I, 60[c].—3)=הוֹלָכָה, *carrying to the altar*. Zeb. I, 4. Ib. 15[b] ה׳ שצריך להלך (לילך) a carrying necessary for the purpose.

הִילוּכָא ch. same, 1) *walking*. Sabb. 148[a] הא קא מפשי בה׳ they would have to do so much more walking; ib. 113[b] קא מפיש בה׳; a. e.—2) as preced. 2). B. Bath. 100[a].

הִלּוּל, הִילוּל, הִלּוּל m. (הלל) 1) *recitation of Hallel* (v. הַלֵּל), *singing praises*. Num. R. s. 3, beg. לולבין לה׳ the branches are employed (on Succoth) for reciting Hallel with them. [Ib., a. e. לְהַלֵּל.]—2) *occurrence of the stem* הלל *in Bible texts*. Ber. 35[a] (ref. to the plural הלולים, Lev. XIX, 24) אייתר ליה חד ה׳ לברכה one *hillul* is remained over to be employed as an intimation that you must give praise (when drinking wine).—*Pl.* הִילּוּלִים. R. Hash. 32[a] עשרה ה׳ ten times הלל in Ps. CL; Meg. 21[b] (omitted in Ms. M., v. Rabb. D. S. a. l. note).—Pes. 117[a] *hal'luyah* means חללוהו בהי׳ הרבה praise him with many praises.

הִלּוּלָא, הִילּוּלָא ch. same, esp. *praising the bride in dancing before her* (v. Ps. LXXVIII, 63; Keth. 17[a]), in gen. *wedding*. Targ. Koh. III, 4; a. e.—Ber. 31[a]; a. fr.—Snh. 105[a] (prov.) when mouse and cat עבדי ה׳ מבישרא וכ׳ Ms. M. (ed. מתרבא) make a wedding feast, it is from the flesh (fat) of an unlucky (victim).—בי ה׳ *wedding house, feast*. Ber. 6[b] אגרא דבי ה׳ מילי (Var. הִלּוּלֵי pl.) the meritorious act in attending a wedding consists in words (cheering songs, addresses &c.); a. e.—*Pl.* הִילּוּלֵי, הִלּ׳. M. Kat. 28[a] בי ר׳ חסדא שתין ה׳ sixty weddings were celebrated in the house of R. H. Gitt. 57[a] ובהך גיסא ה׳ ותרנגי׳ and on the other side of the town were weddings and feasts; a. e.

הִילּוּף (or הִילּוּק) *hiluf* (or *hiluk*), a sailor's cry; v. הַיְיא.

הִילְיוֹנִי *hilyoni*, a sailor's cry, v. preced.

הִילְיִסְטוֹן, v. אֲלִיִסְטוֹן.

הִילֵין, v. הָלֵין.

הִילָךְ, v. הֵי II.

הִילָךְ, הֵילָךְ=אֵילָךְ. Y. Yeb. X, end, 11[c].—Zab. III, 2 ה׳ . . . ה׳ this way . . ., the other way; a. fr.

הִילְכָא f., pl. **הִילְכָן**, v. הִלְכְתָא.

הִלְכָךְ, הִילְכָךְ (=הֵי לְכָךְ) *therefore*. Yoma 74[b] הי׳ מאן וכ׳ therefore (since sight aids in satisfying the appetite) &c. Meg. 21[b] הי׳ therefore (since the opinions differ); a. fr. [Ms. M. 2 reads הולכך, v. Rabb. D. S. vol. VI, preface, p. I, note.]

הִילְכְתָא, הִילְכָן, v. הִלְכְתָא.

הִילֵּל pr. n. m. *Hillel*, v. הִלֵּל. [הִילֵּל, Pi. of הָלַל q. v.]

הִילְמֵי (corr. חַלְמֵי) f. (ἅλμη) *brine for pickling*. Sabb. XIV, 2. Ib. 108[b]. Y. ib. XIV, 14[c] top הי׳ צריכה אומן the preparation of *halmé* requires a trained person. Erub. 14[b] בהלמי Ar. (ed. בהי׳) in the law concerning *halmé* (Sabb. l. c.)—*Pl.* הִילְמִין or הַלְמִין. Y. Ter. X, 47[a] bot. מהלימין הוו, read: מהילמין הוה it (the taste) came from the brine.

הִילְמֵי, Pesik. R. s. 23—24, read מִילְקֵי, v. לקי.

הִילְנִי I pr. n. f. (Ἑλένη) *Helen*, 1) mother of king Munbaz, a convert to Judaism. Succ. 2[b] (Ms. M. הלני, Var. הלנית, v. Rabb. D. S. a. l. note); Tosef. ib. I, 1. Yoma III, 10; Tosef. ib. II, 3 (not הרלני). Naz. III, 6.—2) mother of R. Hillel. Lev. R. s. 12, end; Yalk. Jer. 320 ר׳ הילל בר ה׳; (Lam. R. to II, 8 ר׳ אילם).

הִילְנִי II, *hilni*, a sailor's cry; v. הַיְיא.

הֶלְקֵט, הִילְקֵט m. (לקט, v. אֲלָקְטִית; cmp. b. h. יַלְקוּט) [*receptacle, store*,] 1) *the ciborium* (seed vessel) *of the Egyptian colocasia* (v. Sm. Ant. s. v. Colocasia; v. קוּלְקָס).—*Pl.* הִילְקְטִין, הֵלְ׳. Tosef. Maasr. III, 14; Y. ib. V, end, 52[a] whose stalks are few, והֶלְקְטֵיהֶן מרובין and ciboria numerous.—2) *stack of grain, pile of fruits in the field*.—Pl. as ab. Naz. 8[b] כמנין הִילְקְטֵי קיץ (as many days a Nazir) as the number of piles during the fig crop.—[3) *a bird's pouch*; v. next w.]

הִלְקֵט, הִילְקֵט (denom. of preced.) 1) (of circumcision) *to trim the preputium*, by splitting and drawing it upwards so as *to form a sort of pouch* around the denuded cone. Sabb. 133[b]; Tosef. ib. XV (XVI), 4 מְהַלְקְטִין וכ׳ you must denude the cone &c.—2) *to fill a bird's pouch* or *crop, to stuff*. Sabb. XXIV, 3. Ib. 155[b]; Tosef. ib. XVIII, 4 distinction between מהלקטין a. מַלְקִיטִין (Hif. of לָקַט).

הִילְקְטֵי f. (v. אֲלָקְטֵי) *winding staircase*. Tosef. Erub. VIII (V), 11, v. אֲלָקְטֵי. *Sabb. 157[a] bot. הִלְ׳ קטנה וכ׳ (Ms. M. הילקה, Rashi a. Tosaf. הילקט) a small passage (Rashi) was between, covered with a defective roofing; (Tosaf. *pile, shed*, v. אֲלָקְטִית).

חֵימ־ prefix (=b. h. ־מִמ) *from, of.* חֵימֶנִּי from me; חֵימָךְ from thee; חֵימֵּנּוּ, חֵימֶנָּה from him, her (it). Ned. 9ª he said הריני עלי חימנו 'I will be' (a Nazir), 'upon me' (shall the vow of an offering rest), and 'from it' (I will abstain). Keth. 27ᵇ חוץ מחימנה except herself. Y. Shebi. VIII, 38ª bot. אין לוקחין חֵימֶנּוּ וכ׳ (Bekh. IV, 7, sq. ממנו, Talm. 29ᵇ ח׳ interch. with ממנו) you must not buy of him &c. Gen. R s. 87 למעלה חימנה on top of it (the bed). Ib. s. 38 ויצילך חימנו and save thee from it (the fire); a. fr.—לא כל חימנו not all depends on him, i. e. he has no right, it is not in his power. Ib. לא כל חימנו לבור וכ׳ He had no right to choose for Himself the heavens &c. Num. R. s. 4 לא הימך לומר ליתן וכ׳ you had no right to order &c. Ex. R. s. 15 וכל חימך וכ׳ have you a right to say &c.? v. כֹּל.

חֵימַג, v. חֵמַג.

חֵימוּ ch.=h. הֵם; די ח׳ *which are.* B. Bath. X, 2 Y. ed. (Mish. a. Babli אינון).

חִימוּם (חימוס), v. חֲמָם.

חימונא, Y. Keth. I, 25ª top, v. הֵימוּמָא.

חימוניא, v. הוּמָנְיָא.

חימוס, v. חִימּוּם.

חימוסיון, v. חימיסיון.

חימוּצְיָאתָא, v. חִימוּצָּתָא.

חֵימִין *to trust*, v. חֵימַן.

***חֵימִיסוּ, אֵי׳** (ἡμίσυ) *half.* Tanh. ed. Bub., additam. to Sh'laḥ. 19 (ref. to הֵמַסּוּ, Deut. I, 28) 'they divided our hearts' לשון אליונוסטי אֵימִיסוּ (read ארלינוסטי) the Greek *hemisy;* v. Num. R. s. 17; v. מָסַס.

חֵימְיָנָא, v. הֶמְיָנָא.

חימוס׳, חימסיון, חימיסיון, read: חֲמִיתִיסְטִיּוֹן or אֲמִיתִיסְטִיּוֹן m. (ἀμεθύστιον, dim. of ἀμέθυστος) *amethyst*, a jewel in the Highpriests' breast-plate. Ex. R. s. 38, end (v. LXX Ex. XXVIII, 19).

***חֵימְלְטָא, חֲמַלְטָא** m., pl. **חֵימְלָטֵי** (denom. of מֶלֶט, v. מְלָטֵט) *the casings for the beams in wall openings.* B. Bath. 6ª אע״ג דמנח ביה חמלטא Ar. (ed. Koh. חַמְלָטָה, Ms. M. דמתנח ביה חמולט׳, ed. דעביד ליה חימלטי) although he placed sills thereon (intimating that the neighbor may in future rest beams on them). V. מְעַזִּיבָה.

חֵימַלְתָּא, חֲמַלְתָּא, אֲמַלְתָּא f. (חמל=חמל) [*heating spice,*] *preserved ginger.* Ber. 36ᵇ האי חמ׳ דאתיא וכ׳ (Ms. M. חֲמַ׳, marginal correction חימ׳); Yoma 81ᵇ הד׳ (Ms. M. הד׳, Var. חמ׳, אמ׳, v. Rabb. D. S. a. l. notes) that preserved ginger coming from India; cmp. חֲמַם.

חֵימִין, חֵימַן (Af. of אמן;=h. הֶאֱמִין) *to credit, trust, confide; to loan on trust; to admit as evidence.* Targ. O. Gen. XV, 6. Targ. ib. XLV, 26; a. fr.—B. Kam. 115ª חֵימוּנֵי הֵימְנֵיה he loaned him on trust (without a pawn). Keth. 22ᵇ הֵמְנוּהָ רבנן כבי תרי the Rabbis declared his evidence as legal as if there had been two witnesses. Shebu. 41ᵇ לא לדידיה הֵימְנֵיה he did not trust him by himself (without witnesses). Y. Ber. II, 4ᶜ top לאילין דברישך הֵימְנִית I trusted those (T'fillin) on thy head; a. fr.—*Part. pass.* מְהֵימַן (=h. נֶאֱמָן) *faithful, reliable; credited, admitted as evidence.* Targ. Num. XII, 7 (Y. II הֵימַן); a. fr.—Sabb. 10ᵇ דמתרגמינן אלהא מְהֵימְנָא for we translate (Deut. VII, 9) &c. (only the participle being used as a divine attribute, not the abstract noun).—Keth. 27ᵇ מְהֵימְנָא she is admitted &c. Ib. מהימני (corr. acc.). Y. Gitt. V, 47ª [read:] בעי בר נש מ׳ מיתן כמה ומתקרי a man would sacrifice any amount in order to be called trustworthy; Y. B. Kam. IV, 4ᵇ bot. חימן; a. fr.—B. Mets. 86ᵇ לא מהימנא לך (ed. (=מהימן אנא, part. act.) I do not trust thee (Mss. לא הימן ביה he (Abraham) did not rely on him).

חֵימָנוּ, v. חֵימָנוּתָא.

חֵימֶנּוּ, v. חֵימ־.

חִמְ׳, חִימְנוֹן m. (ὕμνος, acc.) *hymn.* Ex. R. s. 45. Gen. R. s. 8; Koh. R. to VI, 10 דומינין, דומינון, דומינו (corr. acc.); Yalk. Gen. 23; Yalk. Is. 261; a. fr.

חֵימָנוּ, חֵימָנוּתָא f. (חימן) *trust, confidence, faith.* Targ. Y. Gen. XV, 6; a. fr.—B. Mets. 15ᵇ, a. fr. דליקום בְּהֵימָנוּתֵיה (דליקום) to keep up his reputation for honesty (his credit). Ib. 86ᵇ לית ח׳ בעבדי no reliance can be placed on servants.—As an affirmation: *faith! on my word!* Ned. 49ᵇ ח׳ בידא וכ׳ my word in the hand of this woman, i. e. I pledge thee my word. Snh. 38ᵇ ח׳ בידך Ms. M. I assure thee (ed. ח׳ בידן we have the evidence in our hands).—Sabb. 10ᵇ שרי למימר ח׳ וכ׳ it is permitted to say 'faith!' in an unclean place, v. חֵימַן.

חימני׳, Erub. 94ª, v. הֶמְיָנָא.

חֵימַנְיָא, v. הוּמָנְיָא.

חֵימְנִיק, v. חַמְנִיק.

***חֵימָנִית** f. (הֵימַן) *reliable, steady;* רוח ח׳ even-tempered disposition, opp. רוח קפדנית rash. Yalk. Num. 776 (quoted fr. Sifré Zuta).

חימנק, v. חִינָק.

חימסיון, v. חימיסיון.

חִימְצָא m. (=h. חֹמֶשׁ, v. Nöld. Mand. Gr. p. 46) *the fat around the large stomach of ruminants;* בַּר ח׳ *the fat covering the less curved side of the large stomach* (opinions undecided). Hull. 49ᵇ Ar. (ed. חִי׳ a. בַּר חִי׳).

חימצותא, v. חִימוּצָּתָא.

חִין 1) *yes*, v. הֵן.—2) (=b. h. הֵן) *behold!, now.* Sifra Vayikra, Ḥobah, ch. XI, Par. 8 חין אם האומר וכ׳ now, if he who speaks (seducing to idolatry) is not punishable, how can he &c.? (Yalk. Lev. 470 only אם האומר).

***חִין** I=אין II. Y. Bicc. I, 63ᵈ top ח׳ תימר (interchanging with אין).

הִין II m. (b. h.) *Hin*, a liquid measure, equal to twelve Log. Eduy. I, 3; Sabb. 15ª Hillel said מלא ה׳ וכ׳ a *hin* of &c., (using *hin* instead of *twelve Log*) because one must use his teacher's words, v. לָשׁוֹן. Men. IX, 2. Ib. 88ª הוה ה׳ דעבד משה וכ׳ there was (in the Temple) the *hin* which Moses made for &c.; a. e.—2) homiletical interpretation of *hin tsedek* (Lev. XIX, 36)=הֵן, *yes*. B. Mets. 49ª שיהא הן שלך וכ׳ that thy *yes* be true and thy *no* be true. Y. Maas. Sh. IV, 55ᵇ top והיגו הין צדק and where is (what becomes of) the *hin tsedek* (that thy *yes* must be true &c.)?; Y. Gitt. VI, 47ᵈ bot. וְהֵן הוא ה׳ צ׳.

הִינָא ch. same. Targ. O. Ex. XXX, 24; a. e.

הֶינָא m. (ἕνα, acc. of εἷς) *one*, v. הֵן.

***הִינָא** f. (cmp. הַיְיָא a. חַי) *quick-baked, half-baked*. Pes. 37ª מצה ה׳ ed. a. Asheri (Ms. M. 2 נָא, v. Rabb. D. S. a. l. note 3); Men. 78ᵇ Ms. (ed. נא; v. Rabb. D. S. a. l. note 4).

הִינַג, v. הֵנַג.

הִינְגֵּר, v. הֵינְתָא.

הִינְדָּא m. *Indian vetch*. Bekh. 37ᵇ מאי כרשינה what kind of *karshinah* is meant? Ans. ה׳ Indian; v. כַּרְשִׁינָה II.

הִינְדְּבִי, v. אַנְטוּבִין.

הִינְדְּוָן, הִינְדְּוָאָה, הִינְדְּוָא m. ch. *Indian*. B. Bath. 74ᵇ ר׳ יהודה ה׳ (v. Rabb. D. S. a. l. note 100) R. J. the Indian. Ab. Zar. 16ª פרזלא ה׳ Indian iron (used for armour).—Targ. Jer. XIII, 23, v. הִידוֹאָה.—*Pl.* הִינְדְּוָאֵי.—בֵּי ה׳ *India*. Ber. 36ᵇ; Yoma 81ᵇ (Ar. הִנְדְּוֵי).

הִנְ׳, הִינְדְּוִי, הִינְדְּוּוִי h. same. *Pl.* הִינְדְּוִין, הִינְדְּוִוין, הִנְ׳. Yoma III, 7 (Y. ed. הינדוון, corr. acc.) Indian linen garments. Y. ib. 40ᵈ top.—בֵּי הִנְדְּוֵי, v. preced.—V. הִינְדִּיקִי.

הִינְדְּוָא, v. הִנְדְּ׳.

הִנְ׳, הִינְדְּיָא pr. n. *India*. Targ. Esth. I, 1 (h. text הֹדּוּ). Targ. II Esth. VIII, 13; a. e.

הִנְ׳, הִינְדִּיקִי f. (Ἰνδική, sub. γῆ) *India*. Targ. Y. Gen. II, 11 ארע ה׳ (Ar. הִנְדִּיקִין; h. text חוילה). Ib. XXV, 18 הנדקי (Y. II הינדיקיא).—Denom. הִנְ׳, הִינְדְּקָאֵי, הִינְדִּיקָאֵי *Indians*. Targ. I Chr. I, 9.

הִינוּ, בית ה׳, B. Mets. 88ª, v. הִינִי.

הִינוּ (=הֵי נִיהוּ, cmp. הַיְינוּ) *where is?* Y. Maas. Sh. IV, 55ᵇ top, v. הִין II, 2.

הִינּוּחַ m. (נוח) *setting down, temporary deposit*. Y. B. Mets. II, beg. 8ᵇ דרך ה׳ in the way an object is laid down (to be taken up again), opp. משוקע hidden away. Ib.; Bab. ib. 21ª דרך ה׳, opp. דרך נפילה accidental dropping. Ib. 25ᵇ ספק ה׳ a case which leaves it doubtful whether an object was laid down to be called for again, or dropped.—Zeb. 27ª מחשבת ה׳ the intention of letting the blood of the sacrifice stand over the due time (v. ib. III, 6).

הִינוּמָה, הִינוּמָא f. (נוּם, formed like preced.) *slumbering couch*, esp. (a popular adaptation of ὑμέναιος) *henuma, a curtained litter on which a virgin bride was carried in procession* (cmp. Sm. Ant. s. v. Lectica, about κλίνη a. φορεῖον). Keth. II, 1 שיצאת בה׳ that she was carried out of her father's home in a *henuma* or with loosened hair; Y. ib. I, 25ª top הימונא (corr. acc.). Bab. ib. 16ᵇ עדי ה׳ witnesses testifying to her having been taken out in a *h*.—Ib. 17ᵇ מאי ה׳ what is *henuma*? Answ. תנורא דאסא an oven-shaped (frame) draped with myrtles; oth. opin. קלתא דמנמנמא בה וכ׳ (not קריתא דמנמנא, v. Rashbam to B. Bath. 92ᵇ) a curtained couch on which the bride reclines as though slumbering. Y. Keth. II, 26ª bot. תמן נמנומא וכ׳ there (in Babylon) they call it *namnuma* (a slumbering couch), the Rabbis here call it פוריומא q. v.

הִינוּן m. pl. (=הָא אִינוּן) *those, exactly those*. Y. R. Hash. II, 58ª bot. בה׳ דהוון קיימין וכ׳ in the case of such witnesses as had been standing (at the time of observation) &c. Gen. R. s. 9, end ה׳ אותיות דדין ה׳ וכ׳ the same letters form both words (מאד a. אדם).

הִינְטִין, v. איפוטנקריק.

הִינִי 1) pr. n. pl. *Hini*, a Babylonian place near Pumbeditha, a twin-town of Shili. Gitt. 80ª. Bets. 25ᵇ. B. Mets. 72ᵇ.—2) pr. n. m. *Hini*. Sabb. 147ª אסי בר ה׳ (Ms. M. ר׳ א׳ בר חני, v. Rabb. D. S. a. l. note).—3) בית ה׳ pr. n. pl. *Beth Hini* [Bethania], a place near Jerusalem (v. Neub. Géogr. p. 149 sq.). B. Mets. 88ª חנויות של בית הינו (Ms. H. חנן; Y. Peah I, 16ᶜ bot. בני חנון; Sifré Deut. 105 בני חנן) the shops of B. Pes. 53ª בית ה׳ (Ms. M. בייתני); Tosef. Shebi. VII, 14 ביתיני, ביתאני; Erub. 28ᵇ ביתיוני (Ms. M. בית ואני); v. אוֹנִי II.

הִינְיָיקִי, v. אוּנְיָיקִי.

הִינָּם I, v. הִנָּם.

הִינָּם II, **הִינָּן** *they are*, v. הֵן.

הִינְצִין, v. בֵּין.

הִינָק (?) pr. n. m. *Hinak*. Pes. 101ᵇ the school of רב ה׳ . . בר ה׳ Rab H., or according to some, Bar H.; (Ms. M. רב הינק a. רב הימנק; v. Rabb. D. S. a. l. note).

הֵיסֵב, *to recline*, v. סָבַב.

הֵיסֵבָה, הֵיסֵב, v. הֶסֵּב, הֲסִבָּה.

הֶיסַּח m. (נסח) *removal*, only in ה׳ הדעת *discarding from the mind, being given up, diverted attention*. Y. Ter. VIII, 46ᵇ top לא נפסלה בה׳ הד׳ it (the T'rumah) has not become degraded by your giving up the hope of using it. Ib. ה׳ הד׳ דבר תורה the law declaring T'rumah degraded by being given up is Biblical. Snh. 97ª three things happen בה׳ הד׳ when least thought of. V. הֶסֵּיעַ.

הֶסֵּט, הִיסֵּט m. (יָסַט or סוּט) *shaking an object so as to move it from its place*, differ. fr. רעדה vibration (v. Tosef. Zab. IV, 6), esp. *hesset*, one of the causes of levitical uncleanness. Toh. X, 1 אינן בקיאין בה׳ are not familiar with the laws of *hesset*. Meg. 8ᵇ מלטמא . . בה׳ so as not to make earthen vessels unclean by shaking them; a. fr.—*Pl.* הֶסֵּטוֹת, הֶיסֵּיטוֹת *laws concerning hesset*. Y. Dem. II, 23ᵃ top. Y. Sot. V, 20ᵃ top.

הֶיסֵּי׳, הֶיסֵּטָא ch. same. Targ. Y. Num. XIX, 22.

הֶיסֵּיטוֹת, v. הֶיסֵּט.

הֶיסֵּק, v. הֶסֵּק.

הֶיסֵּת m. (יסת, v. וֶסֶת) *consuetudinal law, equity;* only שבועת ה׳ *consuetudinal* or *equitable oath*. [שבועת ה׳ is applied, if one who is sued for a debt, denies the latter entirely (כופר הכל), in contradist. to the legal oath which is required when the defendant admits a part of the claim (מודה במקצת). It being presumed that nobody will go to law unless he have a claim, it is a matter of equity to put the opponent to an oath, to which he may in return put the claimant.] Shebu. 40ᵇ; B. Mets. 5ᵃ; 6ᵃ.

הִיפַּטִיקוֹס (variously corrupted) m. (ὑπατικός) *consular, governor*. Sifré Deut. 309 [read:] אם היה ה׳ שגדול משניהם if he were a hypaticos who is higher than either of them; Yalk. ib. 542.—Sifré ib. 330.—*Pl.* הִיפַּטִיקִין. Ib. 327; 317 הפינקים (corr. acc.). Y'lamd. to Gen. XXV, 23 quot. in Ar. חפאטיקון (read הִפַּאטִיקִין). V. אִיפַּטִיקוֹס.

הֶיפֵק, v. הֶפֵק.

הֶיפֵּר, v. הֶפֵּר.

היפרכון, v. הִפַּרְכוֹס.

הִיפַּרְכְיָה, הִיפַּרְכְיָא, v. הִפּ׳.

הֶיקֵּים, Hif. of קוּם.

הֶיקֵּיף, הֶיקֵּיפָא, הֶיקֵּישׁ, הֶיקֵּישָׁא, v. sub הֶיקְשָׁא, היקפא.

הֶיקֵּם, v. הֶקֵּם.

הֶקֵּף, הֶקֵּיף, הִיקֵּיף, הֶיקֵּף m. (נקף II) 1) *circumference, surface*. Y. Erub. VII, beg. 24ᵇ ה׳ תשעים וכ׳ a circumference of ninety &c. Sabb. 20ᵃ רוב הֶיקֵּפוֹ the larger portion of the surface of the wood (burning), opp. רוב עביו. Succ. 7ᵇ אם יש בְּהֶקֵּיפָהּ וכ׳ if there is room enough in the circumference of a round Succah to seat &c. Erub. I, 5, a. e כל שיש בהיקפו וכ׳ whatever (circle) has a circumference of three hand-breadths, has a width (diameter) of one. B. Bath. 13ᵇ כדי לגול ה׳ enough (blank parchment) to be wrapt around the entire rolled-up scroll. Ib. 14ᵃ קשיא הקף this is in contradiction to what has been said above 'enough to be wrapt &c.'; a. fr.—2) *outstanding debt*, v. הַקָּפָה. Tosef. B. Mets. VIII, 27 כדי שיגבה הקיפו sufficient time, to collect his outstandings (to wind up his business).

הֶיקֵּיפָא, הֶיקֵּפָא m. (v. preced.) *enclosure, fence*. B. Kam. 20ᵇ את גרמת לי ה׳ יתירא thou (on account of the situation of thy field) hast put me to the trouble of erecting an additional (or larger) fence.

הֶקֵּשׁ, הֶקֵּישׁ, הִיקֵּישׁ, הֶיקֵּשׁ m. (נָקַשׁ) [*clapping together*,] *comparing, correspondence;* esp. *hekkesh*, the analogy between two laws which rests on a biblical intimation (as Lev. XIV, 13) or on a principle common to both. Y. Pes. VI, beg., 33ᵃ מה׳ הואיל ותמיד וכ׳ he derived the law that the Passover sacrifice supersedes the Sabbath (v. דָּחָה) by drawing an analogy: as the daily offering is &c., (contrad. to גזירה שוה, v. גְּזֵרָה). Zeb. 49ᵇ, a. e. דבר הלמד בה׳ חוזר וכ׳ a law which is derived by analogy may be used for deriving another law by analogy; a. fr.

הֶיקֵּישָׁא, הֶיקְשָׁא ch. same. Snh. 85ᵇ בה׳ פליגי they differ as to the application of the *hekkesh* (between striking and cursing). Kerith. 4ᵇ; a. fr.

(חַרְדּוּף) הִירְדּוּף m. *hirduf, a shrub* or *tree* with bitter and stinging leaves, supposed to be *rhododaphne, oleander* (v. P. Sm. 1050 הרדוף; Löw Pfl. p. 130). Succ. 32ᵇ ואימא הר׳ (Ms. M. 2 ה׳, v. Rabb. D. S. a. l. note 8) but might not *hirduf* be meant (by *ets aboth*, Lev. XXIII, 40)?—Pes. 39ᵃ ואימא הר׳ might not *h.* be meant (by *m'rorim*, Ex. XII, 8)?

הירדופני, v. הִרְדַּפְנֵי.

הִירְהוּן m. (denom. of הִרְהִין, v. רְהַן) *pledge*. Y. Keth. II, 26ᵈ שנייא היא בה׳ it is different in the case of a woman being placed among gentiles as a pledge.

הִירְהֵר, הִירְהוּרָא, הִירְהוּר, v. הִר׳.

הֶישְׁבּוֹן, v. הֶשְׁ׳.

הֶיתֵּירָא, הֶיתֵּיר, v. הֶיתֵּרָא, הֶיתֵּר.

הִיתְלוּת, הִיתְלוּ pr. n. pl. *Hithlu, Hithluth*. Yeb. 59ᵇ; Tosef. Nidd. I, 9 (ed. Zolk. חיתלה).

הֶתֵּר, הֶתֵּיר, הֶיתֵּר m. (נתר, Hif. הִתִּיר) *release, legal permission, permitted object, legitimate action*, opp. אִיסּוּר. Yoma 86ᵇ, a. fr. נעשית לו כה׳ it appears to him like a legitimate act.—Y. Sabb. VII, 9ᵈ top יש לה ה׳ וכ׳ there is a time when the legal restriction concerning her is removed. Gen. R. s. 76, end; s. 80 beg. לחשיאה דרך ה׳ to give her in marriage, in a legitimate way. Num. R. s. 10, beg. אלו שהיו נוהגין ה׳ וכ׳ those who consider the connection with hand-maids permitted. Y. Yeb. I, beg. 2ᵃ לְהֶיתֵּירָהּ הראשון to the original status of free choice; a. fr.—Esp. ה׳ (נדרים) *the release from a vow by the declaration of a scholar after finding due reasons for its annulment*, v. פֶּתַח. Hag. I, 8 ה׳ נ׳ פורחין באויר the rules concerning the release from vows hang in the air (have no biblical foundation). Y. Naz. IX, beg. 57ᶜ ה׳ חכם dispensation by a scholar's decision; a. fr.

הֶתֵּ׳, הֶיתֵּירָא, הֶיתֵּרָא ch. same. Ab. Zar. 39ᵇ, a. e. לא שבק ה׳ ואכל וכ׳ one will not let stand what is permitted and eat what is forbidden. Hull. 111[b] ה׳ בלע it absorbed permitted substances. Ib. ה׳ דאתי לידי איסורא a permitted substance which is bound to become forbidden (when coming in contact with milk). Ber. 60[a], a. fr. כה דה׳, v. כְּהָא; a. fr.

הָךְ, fut. **יְהָךְ**, inf. **מְהָךְ** (contr. of הלך) *to go.* Ezra V, 5; a. e.—Targ. Gen. XX, 13; a. fr.—*Part. Af. pl.* מַהֲכִין. Targ. Ps. CXV, 7 ed. Lag. (oth. ed. מהלכין).

הָךְ, הַךְ f. (=הָא with affixed ךְ locale) *this, that.* B. Bath. 58[a] הך איתתא this woman here (myself). Yoma 13[a] מיתא הא קיימא הך if this one should die, the other will be (his wife). Ib. והך לאו ביתו היא but this one (appointed to become his wife eventually) is not 'his house' (not being his wife).—Yeb. 23[b], a. fr. היינו הך is not this the same case?; a. fr.

הָכָא, הָכָה (=הָא כָא; cmp. preced.) *here, hither; in this case, now.* Targ. Gen. XXII, 5; a. fr.—Y. Hag. II, 78[a] top היך אתית להכה how didst thou come hither?—Y. Snh. VI, 23[c] bot. ומעייל להכא וכ׳ and I shall bring hither &c.—Succ. 4[a], a. fr. התם..ה׳ there (in the case first mentioned) . . ., here (in this case). R. Hash. 4[a], a. fr. מה׳ from the following (Biblical passage &c.). Pes. 114[a], a. fr. ה׳ נמי וכ׳ (abbr. ה״נ) in this case, too, &c.; a. v. fr.—In Babli: ה׳ here, in Babylonia, התם, תמן in Palestine; in Y. the reverse. Snh. 5[a]; a. fr.—Y. Ber. I, 3[d] bot. דבנן דה׳ Palestine scholars. Y. Keth. II, 26[a] bot., v. הֵימוּמָא; Lev. R. s. 30 מן ה׳ from now, v. הָלָא; a. v. fr.

הַכָּאָה, הַכָּיָיה f. (נכה, Hif.) *striking, beating, assault.* Macc. 8[b] sq., a. e. ה׳ שאין בה שוה פרוטה a striking for which no P'rutah can be claimed as damages. Y. B. Kam. IV, 4[c] הַכָּיַית מיתה a fatal blow; a. e.—*Pl.* הַכָּאוֹת. Tanh. Thazr. 9 לסבול ה׳ to suffer blows.

הכאכא, Tosef. B. Kam. IX, 28 ed. (Var. in ed. Zuck. כאי, הכחכא); Tosef. Shebu. VI, 2 הנחכין ed., v. חביבאי.

הִכְדֵּין, v. הֵיכְדֵין.

הכחכא, v. הכאכא.

הֶכְחֵשׁ, הֶכְחֵישׁ m. (כחש) *contradiction, incongruity in details of legal evidence.* Y. Yeb. XV, 15[a] bot. ה׳ עדות בתוך עדות an incongruity in the statements of witnesses concerning the details of the main fact to be ascertained; ה׳ עדות לאחר עדות concerning circumstances subsequent to the main fact.

הַכְחָשָׁה f. (v. preced.) 1) *contradiction,* the denial by one set of witnesses of the deposits of the preceding set; *counterevidence* (contrad. to הֲזָמָה), *rejection of evidence owing to counterevidence.* B. Mets. 3[b] ישנן בה׳ וכ׳ are subject to rejection through counterevidence or proof of alibi. Ib. אינו בה׳ וכ׳ (the debtor's own admission) cannot be upset by counterevidence &c. B. Kam. 73[b], a. e. ה׳ תחלת הזמה וכ׳ counterevidence is a preliminary procedure to be finished by proving an alibi, i. e. both are one continued process of law; a. fr.—2) *failing, waste of flesh,* in gen. *deterioration.* B. Kam. 94[a] ה׳ דהדר (sub. בישרא) a deterioration which can be raplaced (by good food), ה׳ דלא הדר which cannot be replaced (e. g. a fracture).

הָכִי (=הָא כִי) *so, in this manner, thus.* Snh. 109[b] ה׳ אתני בינייהו thus they agreed between themselves. Ber. 2[b], a. fr. ה׳ קאמר ליה he may say so to him, i. e. this is his argument. Succ. 26[b], a. fr. חסורי . . . וה׳ קתני something is left out (in the Mishnah), and it must read thus. Naz. 2[a], a. fr. וה׳ קאמר (abbr. וה״ק) and he means this.—אי ה׳ (abbr. א״ה) *if this be so,* introducing an argument. Gitt. 5[a]; a. v. fr.—בר ה׳ *fit for such a thing, old enough* &c. Sot. 26[b] לאו בר ה׳ הוא he is unable to copulate; a. fr.—אדה׳ וה׳ אַדְּהָ׳ *in the meanwhile.* Ber. 16[a]. Ib. 18[b] אדה׳ וה׳ חזייה וכ׳ Ms. M. (ed. only אדה׳) while this was going on, he saw &c.; a. fr.—כל ה׳ *all this, that much.* Snh. 107[a]; a. fr.—בתר ה׳ *afterwards.* Targ. Prov. XX, 25.—מטול ה׳, משום ה׳, אמטו לה׳ *on account of such* (a thing), *therefore.* Targ. Ps. XLIX, 15.—Pes. 31[a]. Tam. 32[a]; a. fr.; v. אֲמְטוּ, מְטוּל. Zeb. 14[a] לה׳ therefore.—השתא דאתית לה׳ *now after coming so far, at this stage of the argument.* Ber. 15[b]; a. fr.—ה׳ השתא, v. הַשְׁתָּא.—אפילו ה׳ *even so, at any rate.* Targ. Y. Gen. XXVII, 33.—ה׳ נמי, v. נַמִּי.

הַכָּיָיה, v. הַכָּאָה.

הָכֵין I, II, v. הָכֵן I, II.

***הֲכִינָה** f. (denom. of כֵּן; cmp. כנה *Pi.*) *by-name.* Taan. 20[b] בַּהֲכִינָתוֹ (v. Rabb. D. S. a. l. note 8); Meg. 28[a] בח׳ ed. (v. Rabb. D. S. a. l. note 300), v. חֲנִיכָה.

הָכֵינִי (=הָכֵין הִי) *it is thus.* Y. Yoma II, 39[c] bot. ה׳ it is thus (R. H. said).

הֵיכִיצַד=הָא כֵיצַד, v. כֵּיצַד.

הָכֵירָא, v. הֵיכִ׳.

הַכֹּל, v. כֹּל. [B. Kam. 116[a] תשפך הכל, v. חֲבַל.]

הַכְמָנָה f. (כָּמַן) *hiding, the appointment of witnesses to lie in wait* in order to overhear the seducer to idolatry. Snh. 67[a].

הָכֵן, הָכֵין I (=הָא כֵן) *thus.* Targ. Prov. XXIII, 7. Targ. Is. LI, 6; a. e.

הָכֵן, הָכֵין II m. (inf. Hif. of כּוּן, used as a technical term with ref. to הכינו, Ex. XVI, 5) *preparing, designation for use on the Sabbath or Holy Day.* Y. Sabb. III, 6[b] there is nothing that exists in the shape in which it is used, ואינו בְּהָכֵן which may not be considered as designated for use (on the Sabbath &c.). Y. Bets. 62[a] top ספק ה׳ where there is a doubt as to whether a thing has been ready for use when the festive day began. Ib. הגוי צריך ה׳ that which a gentile offers on a Holy Day requires designation in due time. Ib. I, beg. 60[a] בַּהֲכִינָה של אמה because its mother (the hen) was designated for slaughter on the Holy Day; a. fr. [In Babli הֲכָנָה.]

הֲכָנָה f. (preced.) 1) same. Bets. 2[b] משום ה׳ on account of the law requiring readiness for use on the preceding day. Ib. 4a ה' דרבה the law about readiness as interpreted by Rabbah (ib. 2b); a. fr.—2) (ref. to תכין Deut. XIX, 3) *marking out the road* to the city of refuge for the involuntary manslayer. Macc. 10b.

הַכְנָסָה f. (כָּנַס) 1) *carrying in, putting in.* Sabb. 2b, v. הוֹצָאָה; Y. ib. I, beg. 2b. Y. Hor. I, 46a; a. fr.—Yeb. 55b הַכְנָסַת עטרה insertion of the corona of the membrum virile; B. Mets. 91a ה' the coupling.—Y. Yeb. XII, 12c; Y. B. Bath. III, 14a top הַכְנָסַת פירות the bringing home of the crop.—Num. R. s. 17 ה' ישראל לארץ the leading of Israel into the promised land.—ה' כלה the leading of the bride into the chamber, in gen. *wedding ceremonies.* Succ. 49b.—Meg. 3b; Keth. 17a; a. e.—ה' אורחים *hospitality.* Sabb. 127a; a. fr.—2) *entering, coming home.* Y. Yoma V, 42b bot. ה' יתירה an unnecessary entrance into the Holy of Holies.—Gen. R. s. 72 ה' the time required by the laborer for going home from the field, v. הוֹצָאָה 4).

הַכֵּר (imper. Hif. of נכר) *recognize!, the word hakker.* Sot. 10b בה' בישר וכ' with the word *hakker* (Gen. XXXVII, 32) he brought the news to his father, with *hakker* did they &c. (Gen. XXXVIII, 25). Gen. R. s. 85 (the account of Tamar follows that of the sale of Joseph) כדי לסמוך ה' לה' in order to let one *hakker* follow the other *hakker*.—ה' פנים *partiality.* Ex. R. s. 30 (ref. to Prov. XXIII, 23).

הכרא, Pes. 112b, v. הַבְרָא.

הַכָּרָה f. (b. h.; נָכַר *Hif.*) *recognition.*—הַכָּרַת העובר recognition of the embryo, *certainty of pregnancy.* Nidd. 8b; Y. Yeb. IV, 6a; a. e.—הכרת פנים *that by which a face is recognized, means of identification; nose, features.* Y. Sot. IX, 23c bot. from the nose, מקום ה' פ' the place of identification. Y. Yeb. XVI, 15c; Gen. R. s. 65, a. e. העביר ה' פניהם של ישראל he (Abijah) mutilated the features of Israelites (slain in battle). Y. Nidd. III, 50c עד שתצא ה' פניו until that portion of the fetus comes to light by which its nature can be ascertained. Ib. הַכָּרוֹת פניו; a. fr.

הַכְרָזָה f. (כְּרַז) *public announcement.* Snh. 26b ה' בבי"ד announcement in court proclaiming a person disqualified as a witness. Ib. 89a צריכין ה' must be published, as to the nature of the crime for which they are to be executed. Deut. R. s. 11 ממונה על הה' appointed to announce the divine decrees.

הֶכְרֵיעַ, pl. **הֶכְרֵיעִים**, v. next w.

הֶכְרַע m. (כָּרַע *Hif.*) 1) *customary additional weight in retailing, boot,* v. פִּירוּמִים. B. Bath. 89a. Ker. 5a בה' הוא שוקל וכ' must he weigh (the frank incense) with boot or exactly (v. עַיִן)? Snh. 102a אחד מכ"ד בה' לליטרא one twenty fourth of the overweight of a litra (a minute portion).—2) (Gramm.) *decision as to the junction of a word with the preceding or the following word* (v. next w.), *construction, syntax.* Yoma 52a in five verses אין לחם ה' the grammatical construction is undecided; Gen. R. s. 80; Tanh. B'shall. 26; Mekh. B'shall., Amalek 1; a. e.—*Pl.* הֶכְרֵיעִים. Y. Meg. IV, 74d bot. (ref. to Neh. VIII, 8 (ויבינו) אלו הח' that means the grammatical constructions.

הַכְרָעָה f. same, 1) *overweight.*—*Pl.* הַכְרָעוֹת. Kerith. 5a הקב"ה יודע (ב)ה' the Lord takes notice of overweights (liberality) in offerings.—2) *grammatical construction. Pl.* as above. Cant. R. to I, 2 he might have diverted his mind מחמשה ה' וכ' by referring him to one of the five disputed constructions of Bible verses, v. preced.; (Y. Ab. Zar. II, 41c bot. השיאות). Gen. R. s. 36, end (ref. to Neh. VIII, 8, v. preced.) אלו הח' והראיות that means the disputed constructions and the arguments for and against; Yalk. Gen. 61.—3) *casting vote, verdict by a majority of one.* Y. Snh. I, 18b even arbitration in court requires הַכְרָעַת הדעת a majority of one. Hull. 137a אין הכרעת שלישית מכרעת (sub. דעת) a casting vote consisting of a third divergent opinion is not binding; B. Kam. 116a; Pes. 21a; Naz. 53a.

הֶכְשֵׁר, הֶכְשֵׁיר m. (כָּשֵׁר) *preparation; fitness,* esp. 1) *direct cause, responsibility.* B. Kam. I, 2 חבתי . . כה' כל נזקו I am bound to pay such compensation as though I had been the entire cause of the damage. Y. ib. 2a לה' נזקין it refers to responsibility for damage, opp. נזקי גופו infliction of bodily injuries; Y. Gitt. V, beg. 46c.—2) *finishing.* Gen. R. s. 14 הֶכְשֵׁירוֹ באור (an earthen or glass vessel) is finished in fire.—3) *that which makes a thing legal, that which is ritually fit* (v. כָּשֵׁר). Y. Gitt. III, 44d מפסולו את למד הכשירו from what makes a letter of divorce invalid you can learn what makes it valid. Y. Pes. V, 32b top לבור פסולו מתוך הכשירו to distinguish the unfit element of it from the fit element.—4) (levitical law) *fitness to become unclean* (which arises from contact with certain liquids), *cause of fitness* (הוכשר לקבל טומאה, v. כָּשֵׁר). Hull. 36b עשאוהו כה' מים they declared it (slaughtering, pressing grapes) to be equal in its effect to the fitness for uncleanness which arises from contact with liquids. Ib. 121a ה' מים ממקום אחר the liquids which produce the fitness to become unclean must come from without. Ib. ה' למה לי why should contact with liquids be necessary at all? Ib. צריך ה' requires contact with liquids in order to become fit &c. Y. Kil. VII, end, 31a; Sabb. 95b ה' זרעים (v. Rabb. D. S. a. l.) the requirement that the plants (in the pot) must come in contact with liquids in order to be fit for uncleanness; a. fr.

הֶכְשֵׁירָא ch. same, *proper ritual act.* Hull. 19b.

הַכְשָׁרָה f. same, *making fit* for use. Taan. 10a (play on חַשְׁרַת, II Sam. XXII, 12, a. חשכת, Ps. XVIII, 12) [read as Ms. M. 2:] שקול . . . וקרי ביה הַכְשָׁרַת מים take the *Kaf* and add it to the *Resh* and read *hakhsharath mayim,* sweetening of the waters. [Ed. only הכשר', Ms. M. 1 ח', v. Rabb. D. S. a. l. note. As to the interchange for homiletical purposes between ה a. ח, v. ח"א.]

הַכְשָׁרוּת f. (v. preced. wds.) *fitness; virtue, charity.* Mekh. Bo s. 16; Yalk. Ex. 220 (play on בכושרות, Ps. LXVIII, 7) נהג עמהם בה' He dealt with them charitably; Tanh. Bo 11 בְּכַשְׁרוּת; Yalk. Ps. 795.

חַל־, definite art., v. הַלָּז, הַלֵּזוּ.

חל, Y. Sabb. I, 4ª אתקין לחל, a corrupt.; read: מותרין לקבל, v. Bets. 24ᵇ; Y. ib. III, 62ª top.—Y. R. Hash. II, 58ᵇ top, v. next w.

הָלְאָה (b. h. הָלְאָה; cmp. הָאֵל) *further on*, with prefix ל. Lev. R. s. 30 מן הכא ולה' נחל וכ' (ed. Wil. מן הכא נחל) from now and onward we shall begin a new account. Y. R. Hash. II, 58ᵇ top מן ההוא הרעא דלהל (read ולהלא) from this court session and for all future ones.

הָלָא, v. הַלֵּי.

הַלְבּוֹן, dial. for חַלְבּוֹן.

הלבשוש, הלבשיש, v. הַלְפּ'.

הַלָּה (tradit. pronunc. הֲלָה) m. (cmp. הָלְאָה) *that one there, this one;* (mostly in legal proceedings) *the person concerned.* B. Mets. III, 2. Shebu. VI, 6, sq. וה' אומר וכ' and the defendant says &c. B. Mets. 113ᵇ; a. v. fr. [Eduy. IV, 9 ה' תצא fem., v. הַלָּז.]—*Pl.* הַלָּלוּ. Erub. 54ª ה' ניצצין וה' וכ' these blossom and those fade. Hor. 14ª מי הם ה' שמימיהם וכ' who are those whose waters we drink &c.?—Bets. 15ᵇ ה' בעלי וכ' these here (now leaving the assembly) are &c.; a. fr.

הַלְהוּלְתָּא, v. חוּלְחוּלְתָּא.

הַלְוָאָה f. (לוה) *loan.* B. Mets. 81ᵇ בשעת הַלְוָאָתוֹ at the time the loan was transacted. Ib. 14ª, a. fr. שטר ה' note of indebtedness, promissory note; a. fr.

הַלְוַאי, הַלְוָאי, הֲלַוַּאי, v. אַלְוַאי.

הַלְוָיָה, הַלְוָיָה, הֲלָוָיָה f. (לוה) *escort on parting, attendance to a departing friend's needs; following a funeral procession.* Sot. 46ᵇ, v. לְוָיָה.—Y. ib. IX, 23ᵈ bot.

הַלּוּךְ, הִלּוּל, הלולא, v. הִילּ'.

הַלּוּם, v. אֲלוּם.

הֲלֹם (b. h. הֲלֹם; cmp. הָלְאָה) *here, hither; thus far.* Zeb. 102ª (play on הֲלֹם, q. v.) אין ה' אלא מלכות *hălom* alludes to royalty, as we read (II Sam. VII, 18) &c. עד ה' thus far (to be king). Ib. וכל הכא דכתיב ה' וכ' does *hălom* in the Bible always intimate royalty for all time to come?

הַלָּז m. (b. h.; v. הַל־ a. זֶה) *this here, that there.* Snh. 11ᵇ ה' סופר ed. (missing in Ms. M.; Tosef. ib. II, 6 הלה, Var. הלך); Y. ib. I, 18ᵈ top; Y. Maas. Sh. V, 56ᶜ top ה' הסופר the, then, scribe; v. נָזוּק.—Keth. 36ᵇ. Y. Erub. I, 18ᶜ bot. פירצה של ה' the breach on the other side.—*Fem.* הַלֵּזוּ. Yeb. XIII, 7 (109ª) ה' תצא (missing in Mish. ed.) the other sister is free. Ib. וה' תצא. Ib. 51ᵇ; (Eduy. IV, 9 הלה).

הַלָּזָה f. (לוז III) *talk, sneer.* Tosef. Keth. II, 3 נפלה ה' וכ' ed. Zuck. (Var. חלוה, חלוזן, corr. acc.) talk (against the court's action) spread in town, opp. ערער legal protest.

הַלֵּזוּ, v. הַלָּז.

הַלְטָאָה* f.=לְטָאָה, *a species of lizard.* Pes. 88ᵇ גישתא דה' נמצאת ה' a lizard was found. Hull. 122ᵇ the touch of the skin of &c. [In Mishn., Tosefta a. Sifra לטאה, with defin. article ה.]

הַלְטְתָא ch. same. Targ. O. Lev. XI, 30 (ed. Berl. הַלְטְתָא, Var. חולטיתא, v. Berl. Targ. O. II, p. 34).

הֲלָא, הֲלֵי (synon. with לאי, להי) *to be faint, to labor.* Targ. Is. XLII, 4 ed. Lag. (ed. ילהי). Ib. LXV, 23 יהלון (some ed. רח'; ed. Lag. ילהון). Targ. Jer. LI, 58.

Af. אַהְלֵי, *Pa.* הַלֵּי *to fatigue.* Targ. Is. VII, 13 מַהְלֵן (Buxt. מְהַלָּן).

הֲלִיוֹנֵי, v. הִילְ'.

הֲלִיסְמוֹן, v. אֲלִיסְמוֹן.

הֲלִיךְ, v. הֲלַךְ.

הֲלִיכָה f. (b. h.; הָלַךְ) *going, going away; walking; run.* Pes. 8ᵇ בַּהֲלִיכָתָן on their going (opp. חזירה, return). Keth. 111ª אל תרבה בה' do not walk too much. Sot. 12ᵇ אין ה' זו וכ' this 'going' (Ex. II, 5) means death. Hull. I, 2 בדרך הֲלִיכָתָהּ in the direction in which its indentations run (not against them); a. fr.—[Y. B. Kam. X, 7ᵇ bot. שֶׁגְּזָלוֹ מן הה', read: הַהֲלָכָה, v. Y. Keth. II, end, 27ª.]—*Pl.* הֲלִיכוֹת. Meg. 28ᵇ; Nidd. 73ª, v. הֲלָכָה.

הֲלִיכְתָא ch. same. *Pl.* הֲלִיכָתָא, constr. הֲלִיכַת. Targ. Ps. LXVIII, 25. [Ib. הֲלִיכוֹת, corr. acc.]

הֲלִילָא, v. הֲלָא.

הלים, v. וּלִים.

הליסמין, read: הֲלִיסְמוֹן.

הֲלֵךְ, v. הֲלַךְ.

הָלֵין m. pl. (contract. of הָאִילֵּין) *these, those, these things.* Targ. Prov. XXIV, 23. Ib. XXXI, 8.—Ned. 91ᵇ. Ib. 79ᵃ ה' וה' both; a. fr.—Lev. R. s. 25 הָלֵין תאיניא (Koh. R. to II, 20 הלין) these figs here.

הָלֵין (=הָדֵין) *which? what?* Targ. Y. Ex. I, 10 בה' דינין by what laws.

הָלַךְ (b. h.) *to go, go away; to walk.* Yeb. 84ª כשהָלַכְתִּי וכ' when I left home to study with &c. Macc. 10ᵇ, a. e. בדרך שאדם רוצה לֵילֵךְ בה מוֹלִיכִין אותו whatever way one desires to go, one is led; a. v. fr.—הוֹלְכֵי מדברות travellers through the desert. Taan. 27ᵇ; a. e.—Y. Kidd. I, 61ᵈ כהולכים בתורת ד' (not בה') as though they did walk in the law &c.—Imper. לֵךְ, לְכָה, v. כְּלָה *Pi.*, a. כַּלֵּךְ.

Pi. הִלֵּךְ, הִילֵּךְ 1) same, *to walk, tread upon.* Hull. IX, 2 (122ª) אי שהי' בהן (Mish. ed. שהלך) or trod upon them for tanning purposes. Erub. 100ᵇ שֶׁיְּהַלֵּךְ ע"ג וכ' to tread upon plants. Gen. R. s. 39 מְהַלֵּךְ בארם וכ' travelling through Aram &c.—Keth. 60ª; Ker. 22ª מְהַלֵּךְ שתים

walking on two legs (human beings); a. fr.—2) *to cause opening of the bowels.* Y. Kil. I, 27ª top מְהַלֶּכֶת את בני מהלך לפניהן מיעים; cmp. הִילּוּךְ. [Y. Keth. XII, 35 top הַלַּך אל הארץ, v. חָלַד.]

Hif. הוֹלִיךְ 1) *to lead; to carry.* Macc. 10ᵇ, v. supra. Gitt. 4ª המוֹלִיךְ וכ׳ he who carries abroad a letter of divorce, contrad. to המביא he who brings a letter from abroad. Ab. Zar. III, 9 יוֹלִיךְ הנאה וכ׳ let him cast the profit (one loaf's value) into the Sea. Gitt. VI, 1 הוֹלֵךְ גט וכ׳ carry this letter of divorce (as a messenger). Ib. 63ª sq. (distinction between הילך, here is the letter of divorce, i. e. take possession of it in behalf of my wife, and הולך carry it, i. e. be my messenger). Ib. 64ª, a. e. הולך כזכי דמי 'carry' (the letter of divorce) is equal to 'take possession' (in behalf of her who authorized thee); a. fr.

Hithpa. הִתְהַלֵּךְ *to go away, withdraw.* Cant. R. to V, 1; Gen. R. s. 19 (ref. to Gen. III, 8) מְהַלֵּךְ . . . אלא מִתְהַלֵּךְ וכ׳ it does not say *m'hallekh* (walking) but *mithhallekh*, He hastened and went upward. Ib. מתהלך לו (ed. מת הלך, corr. acc., v. Matt. K.) is he (Adam) going away (from God)?, v. אתמהא.

הֲלַךְ, הֲלִיךְ ch. same, *to walk.* Targ. Ps. CXXVI, 6 (Ms. *Pa.*). Targ. Y. II Gen. XXII, 8 הֲלִיכוּ (some ed. הַלְ׳). Contr. מְהָךְ, יְהָךְ, v. הוך.

Pa. הַלֵּיךְ, הַלֵּךְ same. Targ. O. Gen. V, 22. Targ. I Sam. XXX, 31; a. fr.

Ithpa. אִתְהַלַּךְ same. Targ. Ps. CI, 2. Ib. CXVI, 9.

הֲלָךְ m. (Ezra IV, 13) name of *a tax*, prob. *sustenance of marching troops.* B. Bath. 8ª; Ned. 62ᵇ expl. as אַרְנוֹנָא. Gen. R. s. 64, a. e., v. אַנְגַּרְיָא.

הֵלֶךְ m. (b. h.; הלך) *traveller.* Succ. 52ᵇ (ref. to II Sam. XII, 4) מתחלה קראו ה׳ וכ׳ at first he calls him (the tempting sin) a traveller &c.

הַלְכָא, הָלְכָא=h. הֵילָךְ, הִילָךְ, *hither, thither.* Targ. O. Ex. III, 5 (h. text הֲלֹם). Targ. Jud. XIV, 15 (h. text הֲלֹא, v. הֲלָא). Targ. Y. Num. XXI, 35; a. e.

הֲלָכָה f. (הלך) 1) (cmp. מִנְהָג) *practice, adopted opinion, rule.*—ה׳ כ־ in practice, the opinion of . . . . is the rule. Keth. 77ª ה׳ כמותו; a. v. fr.—ה׳ למשה מסיני a usage dating from Moses as delivered from Sinai, i. e. *a traditional law* or *a traditional interpretation of a written law.* Kidd. 38ᵇ; a. fr.—2) in gen. *traditional law, tradition, custom.* Orl. III, 9 הערלה ה׳ the application of the laws of Orlah (v. עָרְלָה) outside of Palestine is traditional or a custom (הילכות מדינה, v. Kidd. 38ᵇ).—Y. Bets. II, 61ᵇ top לה׳ as a traditional opinion (of a teacher), opp. לעובדא as his own decision for practice. Y. Dem. III, 23ᶜ bot., sq. מה׳ according to a custom. Ker. 13ᵇ 'which the Lord has spoken' (Lev. X, 11) זו ה׳ that means traditional interpretations. Ib. III, 9 (15ᵇ) אם ה׳ נקבל אם לדין וכ׳ if it is a tradition, we must accept it, but if it is a logical inference, there may be an objection to it.—3) *law*, contrad. to אַגָּדָה. Ber. 31ª מתוך דבר ה׳ from discussion about a law, opp. ה׳ פסוקה a decision arrived at after discussion. Ib. 47ᵇ ....בה׳ המחדדין who whet each other's wits in legal discussion. Snh. 82ª נתעלמה ממנו ה׳ the law had escaped his memory. Ib. ראה . . ונזכר ה׳ he saw an act and recalled the law; a. v. fr.—*Pl.* הֲלָכוֹת, constr. הִלְכוֹת, הִילְ׳. Kidd. l. c. הי׳ מדינה (v. R. S. to Orl. III, 9; ed. הלכתא מדינה, corr. acc.) the usages of the country (outside of Palestine). Y. Hor. III, end, 48ᶜ אילו ה׳ that means the collections of laws (Mishnah). Tem. 14ᵇ כותבי ה׳ those who reduce traditions (oral law) to writing. Snh. 67ᵇ הי׳ כשפים the laws concerning the punishment of witchcraft. Ib. הלְ׳ יצירה mystic practices. Sabb. 32ª; Tosef. ib. II, 10; a. v. fr.—[הלכה in Talmud Y., heading of ***Mishnah***, in Talm. Bab. מתני׳.]

הִלְכוֹת, הִלְכְוָתָא, pl., v. הִלְכְתָא.

הִלְכָךְ, v. הִיל׳.

***הַלְכְּשׁוּשׁ, הַלְכְּשִׁישׁ** m. (redupl. of לבש, cmp. לֶבֶשׁ) *swelling, bruise, sore.* Targ. Y. Ex. XXI, 25 (ed. Amst. הַלְבְּ׳; h. text חַבּוּרָה).—*Pl.* הַלְכְּשׁוּשִׁין, constr. הַלְכְּשׁוּשֵׁי. Targ. Ps. XXII, 18 (ed. הַלְבְּ׳); ib. XXXVIII, 6 (ed. הלב׳, Ms. הלפ׳, h. text חַבּוּרֹת־). Targ. Job IX, 17 (ed. הלב׳; h. text פְּצָעַ־).

הִלְכְתָא, הִילְ׳ ch. f. (v. הֲלָכָה a. הֲלִיכָה) 1) *step.* Targ. Prov. XVI, 9.—*Pl.* הִלְכָתָא, הִילְכָתָא. Ib. XXVI, 7 (ed. Wil. הִלְכְתָא). Ib. XXIX, 5; a. e.—Targ. Ps. XXIII, 3 הִלְכְוָתָא ד־ Ms. (ed. Lag. הִילְכַת צ׳, ed. Wil. הִלְכַת).—2) *custom, habit.* Targ. II Kings XI, 14. Targ. Y. Gen. XLIII, 33.—3) *law, rule.* Targ. Y. Ex. XII, 6; a. e.—Snh. 51ᵇ ה׳ למשיחא it is a *halakhah* for the Messianic days (without present application). Erub. 65ª הי׳ בעיא וכ׳, v. אַסְתְּנָא; a. fr.—Pes. 64ª, a. fr. למאי ה׳ for what practical issue &c.?—*Pl.* הִלְכָתָא. Ber. 31ª, v. פִּיבָר; a. fr.—Targ. Koh. XII, 11 הִילְכָתִין.—Lev. R. s. 3, beg. בר הִילְכָן (fr. הִילְכָא) a scholar.

הִלֵּל, הִילְ׳ pr. n. m. *Hillel*, 1) H. the Babylonian (הבבלי) or Senior (הזקן). Pes. 66ª. Tosef. Snh. VII, 11. Yoma 35ᵇ ה׳ מחייב וכ׳ the example of Hillel condemns the poor (who plead poverty as an excuse for not studying the Law); a. v. fr.—בֵּית ה׳ *Beth-Hillel, the School of H., the Hillelites.* Bets. I, 1; a. v. fr.—2) H., son of Rabban Gamliel. Pes. 51ª; Tosef. M. Kat. II, 16; a. fr.—3) R. H., son of אָלֵס or וָולָס, an Amora. Y. Kil. IX, 32ª top. Gitt. 59ª; a. fr.—[Y. Bets. V, 63ª bot. ר׳ ליל, prob. a corrupt. or abbrev. of H.]—4) name of several Amoraim. Y. Ber. II, 5ª bot.; a. fr. V. Frank. M'bo p. 76ª.—5) one Rabbi H. Snh. 98ᵇ, sq.

הָלַל (b. h.) *to be bright, shine.*—*Pi.* הִלֵּל *to praise.* Pes. X, 5 לְהַלֵּל. Midr. Till. to Ps. CXIII צריכים אתם לה׳ לו you must give praise to Him. Ib. מנין הַלְלוּ the numerical value of *hal'lu* (71).

Hithpa. הִתְהַלֵּל *to praise one's self, boast.* Yalk. Jer. 284.

הַלֵּל m. (preced.) *Hallel* (Praise), recitations for Holy Days, consisting of Ps. CXIII to CXVIII, called ה׳ המצרי Egyptian H. (with ref. to Ps. CXIV), contrad. to ה׳ הגדול

the Large H. (v. differ. opinions Pes. 118[a]). Pes. X, 7, v. גְּמַר. Taan. 28[b]; a. fr.

חַלָּא, חֲלֵילָא, חֲלֵילָה ch. same. Ber. 56[a] ה׳ מצראה (Ms. M. חלי׳ דמצראי) Egyptian Hallel, v. preced.—Cant. R. to II, 14; Pes. 85[b] bot.; Y. ib. VII, 35[b] bot., v. זֵיתָא I.—Taan. 28[b] ה׳ דבריש ירחא (Ms. M. הלל דר״ח) the recitation of Hallel on the New Moon Day. Meg. 14[a] קרייתא זו ה׳ the reading of the *M'gillah* takes the place of Hallel; a. e.

חָלַם (b. h.; cmp. חָלָם a. Arab. ḥilm *friend;* v. Fl. to Levy Talm. Dict. I, p. 558[a]) 1) *to join, weld.* Gen. R. s. 44 (ref. to הוֹלֵם פעם Is. XLI, 7) וח׳ את כל וכ׳ and welded all mankind to follow one road to the Lord; Yalk. ib. 76; Yalk. Is. 313.—2) *to be attached, fit closely.* Ab. Zar. 44[a] שמתנשא לה׳ (ed. מִתנשא שביקש להולמו ולא הולְמתוֹ Ms. M. corr. acc.) 'he exalted himself' (I Kings I, 5) means that he attempted to fasten (the crown to his head), but it would not fit him; Yalk. Kings 166; Snh. 21[b].—[Tosef. Bekh. IV, 13 מוהלמות, read: מְבוּלָּמוֹת, v. בָּלַם.]

Hif. הֶחֱלִים *to attach closely, paste on.* Y. Ter. X, 47[a] bot. מַחֲלִימִין היו they made the pastry adhere to the mouth of the vessel.

חֶלְמוֹן, חַלָּמָה, v. חל׳.

חַלְמִי, v. הילְמִי.

הַלָּן, הַלָּן or (v. הַלָּא) *there*, opp. כָּאן. Y. Keth. IV, 28[d] bot.; Y. Gitt. V, 46[d] bot. בני בנים של כאן בני בנים של ה׳ the 'grandchildren' here (with reference to maintenance) are legally the same as the 'grandchildren' there (with reference to the duty of propagation, i. e. 'grandchildren are like children'). Lev. R. s. 10 תבא לקיחה של כאן .... של ה׳ (ed. Wilno שֶׁלְּהַלָּן, v. infra) the 'taking' here (Lev. VIII, 2) shall atone for the 'taking' there (Ex. XXXII, 4).—Mostly לְהַלָּן *there.* B. Kam. 84[a] מה לה׳ ממון אף כאן ממון as below (Ex. XXI, 36) *taḥath* means pecuniary compensation, so here (ib. 24) &c. Sot. 38[a] נאמר כאן .. ונאמר לה׳ here (Num. VI, 27) the expression *sum shem* is used, and there (Deut. XII, 5) &c.; a. fr.—Gen. R. s. 50 (expl. גש הלאה, Gen. XIX, 9) קרב לה׳ get nearer there (go away).

חֲלָנָה f. (לוּן I) *leaving over night, undue delay over night.* Meil. 4[b] ה׳ דקעביד בידים the illegal delay of the sprinkling of the blood, an offence which he commits with his hands (omission of an act), opp. to מַחֲשָׁבָה undue thought.—הֲלָנַת דין the reserving of the verdict for the next morning. Snh. 17[a]; 34[a]; 35[a].

חֲלָנָה f. (לוּן II) *murmuring, rebellion.* Ex. R. s. 25 ומה ה׳ וכ׳ what cause was there for rebellion?

הִלְנִי, v. הילְנִי.

הֲלָעֲטָה f. (לָעַט) *stuffing.* Sabb. 155[b] ה׳ למקום שיכולה להחזיר by *halatah* is meant a stuffing to a point of the throat from which the animal can bring it back again to the mouth, opp. הַמְרָאָה pushing far down the gullet.

חלפשיש, v. חַלְפְּשִׁיט.

חֶלְקֵט, חֲלֻקְט, חֲלָקְטֵי, v. sub חיל׳.

חֲלָקִיב, Sabb. 156[a] מהלקיטין, v. לָקַט.

חֲלָקָשָׁה f. (לָקַשׁ) *doing late, procrastination.* Num. R. s. 1, beg. (interpret. מאפליה, Jer. II, 31) לשון ה׳ it means procrastination; ib. s. 23; Tanh. Masê 9; a. e.

הֵם m. pl. of הוּא.

הֲמָא, v. הֲמִי.

הֵימַג, הֵמַג, הֵמַג m., only in בַּר ה׳ *Bar-Hemag*, a subspecies of *abratha* (hyssop). Sabb. 109[b] (defining h. אֵזוֹב), v. אַבְרָתָא.

בֵּית ה׳, הַמְגַּנְיָה, הַמְגַּנְיָא pr. n. pl. *Beth-Hamgania.* Kil. VI, 4 (v. Rabb. D. S. a. l. note).

הַמְדַאי, v. הַמְדָן.

בַּר ה׳, הַמְדוּדֵי pr. n. m. *Bar-Hamdudê* (Var. בר הַמְדוּרֵי *Bar-Hamdurê*). Yoma 87[b] (v. Rabb. D. S. a. l. note 8). Sabb. 107[b]; 125[a] בר המדורי(מר) ed. (Ms. ... דר, ... דא). Yeb. 83[b] רר .... Men. 38[b] (v. Rabb. D. S. a. l. note 40).

בר ה׳, הַמְדוּרֵי, v. preced.

המדך, v. הַרְמֵיךְ.

הַמְדָן pr. n. pl. *Hamdan* (*Hamadân*, v. Schr. KAT[2] p. 378), *Ekbatana*, capital of Media, v. אַחְמְתָא. Kidd. 72[a] (ed. חַמְדָן).—[Targ. I Chr. I, 5 Var. in ed. Rahmer המדן (ed. הַמְדַאי, ח׳, not ..דְּאֵי); Targ. Y. Gen. X, 2 הַמְדַּיי (not ..הדיי).]

הֲמָת, v. חמי.

הָמוֹן m. (b. h.; preced.) *noise, tumult; multitude.* Yoma 20[b] קול הֲמוֹנָהּ של רומי Ms. M. (ed. העיר); Lam. R. to V, 18; Macc. 24[a] קול ה׳ של רומי Ms. Ms. (ed. בבל); Yalk. Is. 278 המוני של כרך גדול (read: הֲמוֹנוֹ), the din of the city of Rome, v. פוֹטִירוֹלִין. Macc. 10[a] (ref. to Koh. V, 9) ללמד בה׳ to teach before large crowds; (Yalk. Koh. 971 ללמוד בה׳ to study among a crowd of students).—*Pl.* הֲמוֹנִים. Ex. R. s. 11 אתם עשיתם ה׳ ה׳ וכ׳ you arranged troops against my children &c.—Cant. R. to VIII, 11 (play on המון, ib. באו עליהן המונות (read: המונים) hordes came against them. Ib. שהמו אחריהם הֲמוֹנֵי מלאכים (not מלכים) troops of angels rushed for them (to prevent them from receiving the Law, v. הֲדָה). Ib. שהמו אחר המוני המוניות, read: שהמו אחריהם המוניות, v. הֲמוֹנוֹת.

הָמוֹן, הֲמוֹנָא ch. same, *multitude.* Targ. Is. XIII, 4. Targ. II Kings XXV, 11; a. e.

הֲמוֹנוֹת, הֲמוֹנִית or **הֲמוֹנִיּוֹת** f., pl. (preced. wds.) *troops, crowds.* Cant. R. to VIII, 11 (v. הָמוֹן, end) שהמו

דמלכוותא ה׳ אחריהם the hosts of kingdoms were greedy for them (to have a foothold in their country). Lam. R. to I, 17 formerly I used to go up to the Temple ה׳ ה׳ של חגיגה in (singing) troops of pilgrimage. Lev. R. s. 33 הייתם נעשים הומניות הו׳ לע״ז (corr. ׳המו) ye used to form troops (noisy processions) for idolatry; v. הִיאוֹנִיסְין.

המונייא, Cant. R. to V, 14, read: הֲמוּנְיָה (v. חמי); v. Pesik. B'shall. p. 90[b].

הֶמְטַלְיָא f. (a popular corrupt. of ἡπατόριον, v. Sm. Ant. s. v. Eupatorium) *liver-wort*, in gen. *herbs used for cooling the blood* (cmp. חוּמְצָן). Y. Ned. VII, beg. 40[b] במיני אפומליא וכ׳ (read: אפוטליא or ׳אימט) the various kinds of *hepatoria*, e. g. Napu, Melissophylon and Colocasia.—Tosef. Maasr. III, 7 ׳אמיטל׳ נהגו בה וכ (Var. ׳המטל) for *hepatoria* the scholars allowed no exemption &c. Tosef. Ab. Zar. IV (V), 11 המיטליא וכ׳ (Var. ׳המוט) *hep.* &c. prepared by gentiles; Y. ib. II, 41[d], Y. Sabb. I, 3[c] bot. הרי מוט׳ (read: ׳הֲהִימ); Ab. Zar. 38[b] החמטליא Ms. M. (ed. ׳המט). Ib. היא ה׳ וכ׳ ed. (Ms. M. ׳ח) *hemtalia* is (legally) the same as &c., v. פְּסִילְיָא. Cmp. חוּמְטַרְיָא.

הָמָה, המי (b. h.; cmp. המם) *to be noisy, excited*, with אחר *to rush after, be greedy, envious* &c.—Cant. R. to VIII, 11 הָמוּ, v. הָמוֹן a. הֲמוֹנוּת. Part. הוֹמֶה, v. infra; fem. הוֹמִיָּה. Y. M. Kat. III, beg. 81[c] (in a riddle) ה׳ בירכתי ביתה she (the soul?) is restless in the corners of her house. Midr. Till. to Ps. LXXVII הוֹמִים are in commotion.

Pi. הִמָּה same, *to covet* (with אחר). Lev. R. s. 22 (ref. to אוהב בהמון, Koh. V, 9) כל מי שהומה וּמְהַמֶּה אחר הממון whosoever is greedy and covetous for money; ib. הומה ומה׳ אחר תורה ambitious to accumulate learning; a. e.—*Part. pass.* f. מְהוּמָּה *anxious*. Nidd. 5[a], v. בַּיִת.—Denom. מָמוֹן.

הֲמָא, המי ch. same, *to be excited, to roar, rumble*. Targ. Jer. IV, 19. Ib. V, 22; a. e.—[Targ. Prov. XXVIII, 27 מהמי Ar., v. חֲמָא.]

הֶמְיָה, הֶמְיָיה f. (b. h.; preced.)=הָמוֹן, *din* of a large city. Sifré Deut. 43 [read:] קול ה׳ של רוכבי מפוטירולין, v. הָמוֹן a. פּוּטִירוֹלִין.

הֶמְיוֹנֵס (corr. הֶמְיוֹנוֹס) m. (ἡμίονος) *mule* whose sire is an ass. Gen. R. s. 82, end; Y. Ber. VIII, 12[b] top (expl. יֵמִם, Gen. XXXVI, 24); v. הֶמְיִיפּוּס.

הֶמְיִיה, v. הֶמְיָה.

הֶמְיָין m. (Pers. *hemyân*, Fl. in Levy Targ. Dict. s. v. הֶמְיָנָא) *belt, girdle*. Erub. X, 15 (104[b]).—*Pl.* הֶמְיָינִין. Succ. V, 3 (51[a]) וּמֵהֶמְיָינֵיהֶן הֵיוּ מפקיעין ed. Y. a. Ms. M. (v. Rabb. D. S. a. l. note) out of their (old) belts they made wicks.

הִימְ׳, הֶמְיָנָא, הֶמְיָינָא ch. same. Targ. O. Ex. XXXIX, 29 (ed. Berl.; oth. ed. ׳הֶמְ); a. fr.—Erub. 94[a] שקילו הֶמְיָינֵיה וכ׳ Ms. M. (ed. ׳הימני, corr. acc.) take his belt and tie &c. Meg. 27[b] משכנתיה לְהֶמְיָינַאי I pawned my belt. Zeb. 19[a] הוה מִדְּלֵי לִי המיינאי וכ׳ (Ms. M. ׳הִימְיָנַאי) my belt had slipped upward and he himself pulled it down.—Sabb. 59[b] הֶמְיָינָא.—*Pl.* הֶמְיָינִין, ׳הִמְיָ, ׳הֶמְיָנֵי, ׳הֶמְ, ׳הִמְ. Targ. O. Ex. XXVIII, 4 (ed. Berl.; oth. ed. ׳הִ).—Sabb. l. c., v. קַמְרָא.

המיינטון, Y. Sabb. VII, 10[c] top, v. אַמְיַינְטוֹן.

***הֶמְיִיפּוּס** or **הֶמִיפּוּס** m. (ἡμίιππος, S.) *half-horse, a mule whose sire is a horse.* Gen. R. s. 82, end (expl. יֵמִם, Gen. XXXVI, 24) חמיסו (corr. acc., in oppos. to המיונס); Y. Ber. VIII, 12[b] top ורבנן אמרין הירימס (corr. acc.).

הָמִים m. (המם) *confused in mind, delirious*. Y. Gitt. VII, beg. 48[c], expl. קורדייקוס.

הֵמִין, v. ׳הִימ.

הֶמְיָנָא, v. הֶמְיָינָא.

הֶמִינָא m. (ἡμίνα, hemina) *hemina*, a liquid measure, half a sextarius (nearly half a pint English).—*Pl.* הֶמִינִין. Targ. II Esth. I, 8 (ed. Lag. המינון, corr. acc.).

המיסו, v. הֶמְיִיפּוּס.

הֲמִיצְתָא, v. חִימוּצְתָא.

המירוס, המירום, v. next. w.

הֲמִירָם (prob.) pr. n. m. *Hămiram*, a person from whom certain secular books are named: ספרי ה׳ (cmp. בן תַּגְלָא, בן לַעֲנָה, בן סירא). Yad. IV, 6 (comment. מִירָם, בִּירָם); Y. Snh. X, 28[a] top ספרי ה׳ (contrad. to ספרים החיצונים). Hull. 60[b] worth to be burnt כספרי בירון Ar. ed. Koh. s. v. מרום (Var. בִּירוֹן, הַמִּירוֹס, missing in ed.). [Conjectures: *Homeros* (Homer); Ἡμερησία (βίβλια) *diaries*; symbolical name='the Lord remove them'. V. Koh. Ar. Compl. s. v. מרום.]

המירס, v. preced.

הֶמְלְכָא, v. הִימְלְכָא.

הֶמְלְתָא, v. הִימְלְתָא.

הָמַם (b. h.; cmp. הוּם) 1) *to confound*. Tanh. Vayera 22 הֲמָמוֹ והלך וכ׳ He confounded him (took him by surprise), and thus he (Abraham) went to sacrifice his son; Gen. R. s. 55.—Mekh. B'shall. s. 5 (ref. to Ex. XIV, 24) הֲמָמָן ערבבן He confounded them, He brought confusion into their ranks; ib. s. 2; a. e.—2) *to stir up, sweep* (v. next w.). Lam. R. introd. (R. Abbahu 2) (expl. הכביד, Is. VIII, 23, and ref. to Targ. Is. XIV, 23) הֲמָמָם במכבבד he swept them as with a broom (Num. R. s. 23, end, a. e. הכבידן, v. כָּבַד); Yalk. Is. 282 .ה׳ במכבר [הוּמָם, denom. of מוּם q. v.]

הֲמַם I ch. same; *Pa.* הַמֵּם, or *Af.* אַהֲמֵם *to sweep*. Targ. Is. XIV, 23 (h. text טאטא).

הֲמַם II, *Ithpa.* אִיהֲמַם (denom. of מוּם) *to mutilate one's self* (h. התגודד). Targ. O. Deut. XIV, 1 (ed. Berl.

תחת', v. Berl. Massor. p. 90). Targ. I Kings XVIII, 28 Kimḥi (some ed. 'אתח'); a. e.—Part. מִתְחַמַּם *mutilated*. Targ. Jer. XLI, 5; XLVIII, 37 (some ed. 'מתח').

הֲמָמָא f., constr. הֲמָמַת (הֲמַם I) *sweepings, refuse*. Targ. Amos VIII, 6 המֵמת ed. Lag. (ed. Wil. 'מַהּ, h. text מַפַּל).

הֲמָמָה f. (המם) *confusion, perplexity*. Mekh. B'shall. s. 5 אין ה' אלא מגפה the word *hamam* (Ex. XIV, 24) means pestilence.

הָמָן pr. n. m. (b. h.) *Haman*. Snh. 61ᵃ נעבד כה' worshipped as H. wanted to be. Ḥull. 139ᵇ ה' מן התורה מנין where is Haman alluded to in the Pentateuch?—Meg. 10ᵇ ה' הרשע; a. fr.

הֲמְנוֹן, v. הִימְנוֹן.

המנוכא, v. הַמְנִיכָא.

הַמְנוּנָא pr. n. m. *Hamnuna*, name of several Amoraim. Y. Taan. IV, 68ᵃ רב ה' דבבל R. H. of Babylonia.—Y. Hor. III, 47ᶜ top. Shebu. 34ᵇ; a. fr.—Y. B. Bath. VI, end, 15ᶜ רב ה' ספרא R. H., the scribe.

הַמְנִיכָא m. (מני, with format. ך, cmp. בְּזִיךְ) [*emblem of appointment to office*,] *necklace*. Dan. V, 7, a. e. (Kethib: המונכא, המנוכא).—Targ. Prov. I, 9 (some ed. המניכה).—*Pl.* הַמְנִיכִין. Targ. Esth. II, 9.—V. מְנִיכָא. [Greek transformation μανιάκης, fr. which מוּנְיָיק.]

***הִימְ', הַמְנִיק** m. *a sort of spoon* or *fork*, with one end pointed and the other broad (similar to the *cochlear*, v. כּוֹכְלְיָאר). B. Mets. 25ᵇ סכיני וה' (Ms. R. המנק) knives and fork (which may have been cast on the dunghill inadvertently). Succ. 32ᵃ דעביד כהימנק (Ms. M. והוא דעביד לה כי חימניק) when the palm-branch is formed like a *himnek* (Rashi: like the top of the stylus).

המסי, *Ithp.* אִתְהַמְסִי, v. מְסִי.

הֶמְסֵיסָא, v. הֶמְסֵסָא.

מַסְמָסָה, הֲמַסְמָסָה f. (מְסַס) *melting, softening* of the brain or spinal column. Ḥull. 45ᵇ איזוהי .. ואיזוהי ה' which (of the defects) is *hamrakhah*, and which *hămasmasah*? Answ. מַסְמָסָה כל שאינו יכול לעמוד וכ' when the column does not remain upright (when held in the hand). Ib. 53ᵇ המ' *decayed flesh*.

הֶמְסֵס or **מֶסֶס** m. (מָסַס) [*the dissolving* (*digesting*) *receptacle*,] *the first stomach of ruminants*, cmp. הַבְלִילָא. Ḥull. III, 1 המסס (=הַהֶ', or הַמֶּסֶס). Lev. R. s. 4; Midr. Till. to Ps. CIII, beg. המ' לטחון the first stomach has the function of grinding (the food). Lev. R. s. 18; Koh. R. to XII, 3 'the grinders' (ib.) זו ה' that is the stomach. [From later usage, e.g. Tur Yoré Deah 49, and from its Chald. equivalent it would seem that our w. is הֶמְסֵס, and the definite article fused with the ה of the noun.]

הֶמְסֵיסָא, הֶמְסֵסָא ch. same. Lev. R. s. 3; Koh. R. to VII, 19 'המסי; Yalk. Koh. 976 'חמסס.

הַמְעָסָה, הַמְעִיסָה, v. מְעִיסָה.

***הֲמַר** m. constr. (מור) *substitute*. Ḥull. 112ᵃ Ar., ed. חמר, v. הֲמָרָא I.

הַמְרָאָה I f. (מרי I) *stuffing food down the throat of an animal*. Sabb. 155ᵇ, v. הַלְעָטָה.

הַמְרָאָה, הַמְרָיָה II f. (מרי II) *rebelliousness, rebellion; contempt of court*, v. מַמְרֵא II. Snh. 16ᵃ מֵהַמְרָאָתוֹ from the Scriptural text treating of his (the elder's) rebellion.. Ib. 14ᵇ ה' המראתו his rebellion is legally punishable; a. fr.—*Pl.* הַמְרָיוֹת. Midr. Till. to Ps. CVI, 7; Yalk. ib. 864 שתי ה' המרו וכ' they rebelled twice.

הֲמָרָה f. (מור) *change*, הֲמָרַת הַדָּת, *change of religion, apostasy*. Pes. 96ᵃ (Ms. M. משומדות); Yeb. 71ᵃ top.

הַמְרָיָה, v. הַמְרָאָה II.

הֲמְרָכָה f. (מָרַךְ) *softening* of the brain or the spinal column into a liquid state, contrad. to הֲמַסְמָסָה, into a cohesive, pulpy substance. Ḥull. 45ᵇ.

הַמְשָׁכָה f. (מָשַׁךְ) *conducting water through a channel*. Tem. 12ᵇ.

הַמְתָּא (הֲמְתָא) pr. n. pl. *Hamtha*. Targ. O. a. Y. I Gen. XIV, 5 (h. text הָם).

המתגרה, Koh. R. to III, 14, read: חֲמַת גֶּדֶר.

הֵן *they*, pl. of הוא, הִיא.

הֵן, הֵין, הֵן h. a. ch. (b. h. הֵן) 1) *here is, behold*. הֵינָם, הֵינָן *behold, they are*. Ned. V, 6 (48ᵃ) והר' לפניך אלא וכ' Bab. ed. (Mish. ואינן; Y. ed. והן בפניך עד) and behold they are before thee (thine), but only in order that my father &c.—2) (introducing a question or exclamation) *how?, indeed!* Y. Shek. I, 45ᵈ bot. הן נקרא ולא וכ' can we, indeed, read this and not feel ashamed? (Bab. ed. הֵיקרא, marginal correct. Ms. M. 'הן נק).—3) *if*. Dan. II, 5, sq.; a. fr.—הֵן—הֵן *whether—or*. Ezra VII, 26.—B. Bath. VII, 2 הן חסר הן יתר whether it be less (than a Beth Kor) or more. Ib. 3; a. e.—4) *yes* (cmp. הֵין I). B. Mets. 49ᵃ, v. הֵין II. Mekh. Yithro s. 4 answer על לאו לאו ועל הן הן *no* to a prohibition and *yes* to a positive command. Ib. s. 5 ה' וה' yes, indeed; a fr.—Ned. 11ᵃ, a. fr. מכלל לאו אתה שומע הן from the negative we derive the affirmative by implication; Y. ib. I, end, 37ᵃ, a. e. ממשמע לאו וכ'. Men. X, 3 (65ᵃ).

הָן (הוֹן) 1) ה' ד־ *he who*. Targ. Prov. XIX, 1, a. fr. in Ms., ed. Lag. הֲוֵן q. v.—Pesik. Aḥaré, p. 169ᵇ, v. הִיהוּכָא; a. e.—2) *this one, that one*. Y. Meg. I, 72ᵃ . . . לְהָן הִיךְ וכ' (Y. Succ. III, 54ᵃ top לדין), v. הֵיךְ. Y. Kil. IX, 32ᶜ top [read:] מה הן שאל להן וכ'; Y. Keth. XII, 35ᵇ top מה הין דשאיל להון (corr. acc.) from all that this one asked that one &c.; a. fr.—3) *what?* Y. B. Mets. II, 8ᶜ לְהָן, v. אָהֵן.—4) *where* (relat.), *where?* Esth. R. to I, 12 [read:] הן דליסטאה מקפח וכ' where the robber waylays, there he is executed. Y. Snh. I, 19ᵃ top; Y. Ned. VI, 40ᵃ bot. הן דמטא מטא where he came to, he came to (and his order was obeyed). Y. Kil. IX, 32[c] bot. [read:] להן דאשתלחית מינסבינן to the place whither I was sent to take them; Y. Keth. XII, 35[b] להון דשלחית (read דאשתלחית). Gen. R. s. 78, v. בְּרָא. Y. Ber. II, 5[c] bot. להן ייזיל whither shall he go? Ib. II, 5[a] top מן הן הוא where is he from?; a. fr.—*Pl.* הָנָךְ, הָנֵי, הָנְהוּ *those, these.* Targ. Esth. I, 10; a. e.—Tam. 32[b]. B. Mets. 117[a], v. הַהוּא.—Gitt. 6[a] . . . הנך דהני והני ברהנך וכ׳ those (the inhabitants of Ctesiphon) know the signatures of these (of Ardshir), but the latter do not know &c. Bets. 10[b]; a. v. fr.—**Fem. pl.* הָיַן. Y. Bets. V, 63[b] top רבנין . . . . . מפרשין לה׳ the Rabbis of Cæsarea report these (controversies) more explicitly (stating the opinion of each by name; Y. Pes. VIII, 36[a] top מפרשין להון).—הני מילי (abbrev. הנ״מ) these words (have been said), i. e. *this is the case only* &c. Ber. 21[a] bot. (הוה אמינא) הנ״מ יחיד ויחיד I might have thought this refers only to &c.—Ib. 15[a] והנ״מ לק״ש but this applies only to &c.; a. v. fr.—מנא הני מילי, v. מְנָא II.—Emphatic. הָנָא, הָנָּה. Gen. R. s. 87 הנה טבא וכ׳ is this (slave) good? Is the omen favorable?; Yalk. ib. 145 הא טב וכ׳ (corr. acc.).

הֲנָא, v. הֲנֵי.

הֲנָאָה I *enjoyment*, v. הֲנָיָיה.

הֲנָאָה II (נוא, Hif. הֵנִיא) *intervention, objection.* Sifré Num. 153 (ref. to הניא, Num. XXX, 6) ה׳ זו מה היא what this 'objection' means; v. הֲפָרָה.

בַּר ה׳, הֵינַג, הֲנַג m. (cmp. הֲמַג) *Bar-Henag,* surname of a species of *abrathah* (אַבְרָתָה). Sabb. 109[b] (defin. h. אזוב יון).—[*Pl.* הֲנִיגִין, הֵינָ׳, v. הֵיגְתָא.]

הֲנְדָאָה, v. הִינְדְוָואָה.

הֲנְדְבֵי, v. אַנְטוּבְּגִין.

הַנְדְוָאָה, הַנְדְוָוי, הַנְדְוִי, v. הִינ׳.

הַנְדֵּס, הַנְדֵּז (v. חָדַס, *Pi.*) *to mark by means of incisions* (cmp. פָּסַס). B. Bath. 89[b] באתרא דמְהַנְדְזֵי Ms. (ed. דמְהַנְדְסֵי) in a place where the authorities mark vessels used for measuring. Ib. (כל) כמה דלא מהנדז לא שקיל Ar. (Ms. H. כל כמה דלא חזי הינדוא; ed. only לית לן בה) what is beyond the mark of the vessel the purchaser will not accept (merely on the faith of the seller as to the quantity).

Ithpe. אִיתְהַנְדֵּז *to be incised.* Hull. 43[a] זימנין דמִיתְהַנְדְזִין וכ׳ at times (when the animal stretches its neck) the perforations in the two skins of the oesophagus may just exactly cover each other.

הִינְדְזָא, הַנְדְזָא m. (preced.) *mark; calculation of proportions.* B. Bath. 89[b], v. preced. Gitt. 60[b] ואשקי בה׳ and use the water in proportion (as much as is due to thy share). [Later Hebr. הַנְדָּסָה *geometry.*]

הנדיוסין, Midr. Till. to Ps. XVII; Yalk. Ps. 670, read: קִירְיוֹסִין; v. אַפּוֹפְסִין.

הנדוקא, v. הִנְדְקָא.

הִנְדִּיקִי, v. הִינְדִיקִי.

הִנְדִית f. (preced.) *Indian.* Midr. Till. to Ps. VI חרב ה׳ an Indian sword.

הִנְדְקָא m. (prob. הִנְדְּקָאֵי pl., v. הִינ׳) *Indian.* נהמא דה׳ *Indian bread,* a dough roasted on the spit and poured over with oil, or eggs and oil. Ber. 37[b] (Asheri דהנדוקא).

הִנְדְקָאֵי, v. הִינ׳.

הִנְדְּקוֹקֵי m. pl. (דקק, with prefixed ה a. נ inserted; corresp. to h. גַּרְגְּרָנִיּוֹת) *melilot,* a kind of clover used as a relish.—Erub. 28[a] ה׳ מדאי Median Melilot. Y. ib. III, 20[d] top; Y. Peah VIII, 21[a] top.

הֵנָּה, v. הֵן.

הִנֵּה (b. h.; v. הֵן) *behold, here is.* Koh. R. to V, 6 ה׳ שׁל בו״ד the 'here is' of a human being (Esth. VIII, 7), ה׳ של הק״בה the 'here is' of the Lord (Zech. XIV, 1).—הִנְנִי here am I. Gen. R. s. 55 ה׳ לכהונה I am ready for priesthood; a. fr.

הִנְדָה, v. הני.

הַנְהָגָה f. (נָהַג) *driving* an animal, a form of taking possession. B. Mets. 9[a], v. מְשִׁיכָה.

הֵנְּהוּ, v. הֵן.

הֲנָחָה f. (b. h.; נוּחַ) *rest, ease, relief.* Gen. R. s. 87, beg. (ref. to Ps. CXXV, 3) אין לו ה׳ וכ׳ finds no ease in the company of &c.—הֲנָחַת רוח *peace of mind, appeasement.* Y. Dem. VII, beg. 26[a] (interch. with נחת רוח). Y. Peah I, 15[c] bot.; Y. Kidd. I, 61[a] bot. בעושה ה׳ רוחו וכ׳ when he gives his father ease of mind (by obeying his wishes).

הַנָּחָה f. (נוּחַ *Hif.*) *putting down, depositing, laying down* (v. הֲנוּחַ). Sabb. 22[b], sq. ה׳ עושה מצוה the real religious ceremony consists in putting the lights in their appropriate place. Ib. 4[a], a. e. עקירה וה׳ the lifting up (of a burden on the Sabbath) and the putting down.—Kel. VIII, 8 מקום הַנָּחַת העצים the place (in the oven) where the wood is placed. Ib. XXII, 1 מקום הנחת וכ׳ enough (left of the side board) to set down the cups; enough . . to set down portions of meat; Y. Ab. Zar. II, end, 42[a] היא מקום ה׳ הכוסות וכ׳ (not תחת) both terms mean the same. Taan. 2[b]; 4[a] משעת הַנָּחָתוֹ from the time it (the Lulab) is stored away (the seventh day of Succoth).

הֵנָּךְ, v. הֵן.

הֲנִי, הֲנָה (denom. of הֲנָאָה), *Nif.* נֶהֱנָה (=נָאוֹת, v. אות I) 1) *to be pleased, to enjoy, to profit.* B. Kam. 20[a], a. fr. זה נה׳ the one is benefitted &c., opp. חָסֵר. Ib. II, 2 משלם מה שֶׁנֶּהֱנֵית he must pay for what the animal has enjoyed (eaten or drunk), contrad. to מה שהזיקה what she has damaged. Ber. 10[b] הרוצה לֵהָנוֹת יֵהָנֶה וכ׳ (Rashi

(ליה׳) he who desires to make use (of people's hospitalities), may do so following the example of Elisha. R. Hash. 28[a], a. fr. מצות לא ליהנות ניתנו religious ceremonies are not considered an enjoyment (as regards the use of sacred property &c.); a. v. fr.—2) *to be enjoyed.* Ber. 35[a] דבר שנ׳ something which is enjoyable (can be eaten &c.).

Pi. הִנָּה *to benefit, to entertain, to cause to share.* Snh. 92[a] אינו מְהַנֶּה ת״ח וכ׳ allows no scholar to share his wealth. Ber. 63[b] bot. ומְהַנֵּהוּ וכ׳ and invites him to partake of his wealth. Yad. IV, 3 הרי אתה כמְהַנָּן וכ׳ you appear to benefit them pecuniarily, but &c. Ab. Zar. 16[b] sq. שמא דבר מינות . . . . והִנָּאךָ (v. Rabb. D. S. a. l. note 20) perhaps a heretical idea was communicated to thee and it pleased thee; Yalk. Prov. 937; a. fr. [Snh. 102[b] הֶהֱנָה *Hif.*, marginal note היה מְהַנֶּה; v. Yalk. Kings 207.]

הֲנָא, הֲנִי ch. (preced.) *to please, to profit.* Targ. Jer. XXXI, 25 הֲנָתְנִי ed. Lag. (oth. ed. הֲנָאתְנִי). Targ. Is. XLIV, 10 לְהָנָאָה (h. text הוֹעִיל); a. e.—*Part.* הָנֵי. Gen. R. s. 8 עביד מה דה׳ לך do what pleases thee.—*Pl.* הַנְיָין. Gen. R. s. 3; s. 9 דין ה׳ לי יתהון לא ה׳ לי these (worlds) please me, those did not &c.; Midr. Till. to Ps. XXXIV; Koh. R. to III, 11, v. הֵן.

Af. אַהֲנִי 1) *to please, do good, benefit.* Targ. Hab. II, 18; a. fr.—Snh. 99[b] bot. מאי אַהֲנוּ לן רבנן (not אהני) what good have the Rabbis done us? Ab. Zar. 14[b] אַהֲנַאי לכון וכ׳ I did you good inasmuch &c. Y. Ber. I, 4[b] bot. ומה מְהַנְיָא ליה (ed. Krot. ומה missing) what good will it do him?; Y. M. Kat. III, 83[c] bot. ומה אנים ליה (corr. acc.); a. fr.—2) *to take effect, be legal.* Tem. 4[b] אי עביד מַהֲנֵי if (what the law forbids) has been done, the act has its legal effect. Ber. 43[a] מְהַנְיָא ליה הסבה the lying down of a company for a meal has an influence (in that one says the benediction in behalf of all); a. fr.

Ithpe. אִתְהֲנֵי, *Ithpa.* אִתְהַנֵּי *to profit, enjoy, be gratified.* Targ. Y. Deut. I, 6 א׳ לכון it benefitted you (v. Sifré Deut. 5). Targ. O. Gen. XXXVII, 26.—Targ. II Sam. XVII, 16 דלמא יִתְהֲנֵי וכ׳ (ed Wil. יִתְהֲנֵי) perhaps it will please the king (h. text יְבֻלַּע). Targ. Ez. XVI, 31; a. e.—Ned. 50[a] דאִיתְהֲנֵי וכ׳ that I should enjoy this world's goods. Hag. 15[a] לִיתְהֲנֵי וכ׳ let him (myself) enjoy the world. Yeb. 103[a] מִתְהַנְיָא מעבירה she derived gratification from a sinful act. Y. Snh. X, 29[b] top ובר נש לא מִתְהֲנֵי כלום (not מיתהנים) and none were benefitted; a. fr.

הֲנָיָא, v. הֲנָיָה ch.

הֲנָאָה, הֲנָיָה f. (denom. of נְאוֹת, v. נאות I; cmp. נָאֶה) *enjoyment, pleasure, benefit.* Taan. 8[a] מאי ה׳ יש לך what does it profit thee (to bite)?—Sifré Deut. 5 (ref. to רב, Deut. I, 6) ה׳ גדולה וכ׳ your dwelling &c. was of great benefit to you; a. v. fr.—Snh. 26[b], a. fr. בעל ה׳ *a worldling.*—נדר ה׳ מן to vow refusal of any benefit or favor from a person. Ned. IV, 1, sq.; a. fr.—Kidd. 41[a] דור ה׳ ממנו vow that you will have no favor at his hands. [Sifra B'har ch. III, Par. 3 הנוית, v. הוֹנָיָה.]

הֲנָאָה, הֲנָיָא, הֲנָיָה ch. same. Targ. Jer. XVI, 19. Targ. Koh. II, 2; 12.—Targ. Y. Lev. V, 16 הֲנָיַית קודשא enjoyment of sacred property. Targ. Y. Gen. XXXVII, 26; a. fr.—Ex. R. s. 6, end; Tanh. Vaëra 2 (prov.) מן שטיא לית הניא וכ׳ of acacias there is no profit except you cut them down, i. e. a wicked man can be converted by suffering only.—Taan. 23[b] מקרבא הֲנָיָיתָהּ Rashi (ed. הנייתא; what good she does is a direct one (by giving bread); ואנא . . . ולא מקרבא הנייתיה (read: הֲנָיָיתִי) but I give money, and what good I do is indirect; Keth. 67[b] ומקרבן אהנייתי (read: ומקרבא הֲנָיָיתִי, or ומקרבן הֲנָיָיתִי, pl.).—Y. B. Bath. V, 16[b] bot. בנוי דה׳ (cmp. מְעַלֵּי) good, worthy children.—2) *loveliness, beauty* (cmp. נָאֶה). Targ. Ps. XXIII, 2 הֲנָיַית דיתאין loveliness of plants (h. text נְאוֹת!).

הֲנָיָיתָא, v. preced.

הֲנִיפָה, v. הֲנָפָה.

הֲנֵיץ, v. הֲנֵץ.

הֲנִית, v. הֲנָיָה ch.

הֲנָךְ, v. הֵן.

הַנְכָּיָה f. (נכי) *deduction, diminution.* Y. Ber. IX, 14[b] bot.; Y. Sot. V, 20[c] bot. [read:] פרוש מִן הנ׳ מן מאי דאית לי אנא מנכי עביד מצוה a Pharisee 'from deduction' (who says), I take from what is mine (I stint myself) in order to do a good deed.

הִנֹּם m. (homiletically=חִנָּם; v. ה״א) *gratuitous, purposeless act, vanity.* Erub. 19[a] (play on גיהנם) ... גיא שהכל יורדין בה על עסקי ה׳ (v. Rabb. D. S. a. l. note 50) the valley which all enter for affairs of vanity (worldly lusts).

הֲנָן, v. הֵן.

הָנֵף m. (Inf. Hif. of נוף) *waving ceremony* in the Temple.—יום ה׳ (Lev. XXIII, 10—12) *the second day of Passover.* R. Hash. IV, 3; Succ. III, 12; Y. Hall. I, 57[c] top; a. e.—Tosef. Arakh. I, 11 ביום ה׳ on the same weekday as the second day of Passover; Arakh. 9[b]; v. עִבּוּר.

הֲנָפָה f. (b. h.) same; *brandishing, swinging.* Pesik. R. s. 41 (ref. to יפה נוף Ps. XLVIII, 3) היפה בהֲנָפַת העומר שלה who is beautiful when she waves the Omer; Yalk. Ps. 755; Yalk. Ex. 417 בהֲנִיפָתָהּ.—Y. Maasr. II, 50[a] top הֲנָפַת מגל the swinging of the sickle.

הֶנְפֵּק m. (נפק) *producing* before court, esp. *the legal endorsement of a note, stating that it has been produced in court and found valid.* B. Mets. 7[b]; 16[b]; a. e.

הֲנֵיץ, הֲנֵץ [*the blossom,*] name of *a coin; pl.* (through false analogy, v. הֲרוּסָה) הִינְצִין, הֲנֵצִין. Tosef. B. Bath. V, 12[a]; Kidd. 12[a], v. נֵץ.

הָנֵץ m. (Inf. Hif. of נָצַץ) *sparkling,* ה׳ החמה *the first sparklings of the rising sun.* Taan. III, 9. Ber. I, 2; a. fr.

הֲנָצָה f. (נוץ, v. preced.) *sprouting forth.* Men. 69[a] שתי . . . . ה׳ שרזין וכ׳ (Rashi) does the offering of the two loaves cause the permission to use plants which had sprouted forth at the time of the offering, or is a distinct formation of fruits required?, v. חֲנָטָה. Ib. ה׳ דפירא the coming forth of the fruit, ה׳ דעלה of the foliage.

הַנְתּוּכִין m. pl. (תוך, חכך, with prefix הנ; cmp. הנדקוקא) *pannelled ceiling.* Targ. I Kings VI, 9 (h. text גֵּבִים).

הֵיסֵב, הֶסֵּב m. (סבב, Hif.) *placing the divans around the table; in. gen. banquet, meal in company* (v. מֵסֵב). Y. Maasr. IV, 51[b] top עשה הד׳ בשדה if one arranges a meal in company in the field. Y. B. Bath. IX, 16[d] bot. ועשה לו ה׳ וכ׳ and he made the wedding meal for him in the *triclinium.* Y. Taan. IV, 68[a] bot. סדר ה׳ the position of couches at a banquet. Ib. the patriarchs lie in the grave דרך ה׳ in the same position to one another as at meals (distinction between seniors and juniors; v. Sm. Ant. s. v. Triclinium).

הֵיס׳, הֵסִיבָּה, הֲסִבָּה I f. same; *lying down for a meal in company.* Ber. 43[a], v. הֵנִי. Ib. היסבה (Ms. M. הֶסֵּב), v. preced. Ib. 52[b] הֲסִבַּת גוים Ms. M. (ed. מְסִבַּת) a banqueting of gentiles. Pes. 108[a] הֲסִיבַּת ימין lying on the right side at the Passover meal; a. fr.

הֲסִבָּה II f. (סבב; v. Num. XXXVI, 7) *the transfer of landed property from one tribe to another.* B. Bath. 111[b] הֲסִבַּת הבעל ed. (Ms. H. a. Rashb. סִיבַּת, סִבַּת) the transfer which would be caused by the husband's succeding to his wife's property. Ib. 112[a] ה׳ הבן Ms. R. (ed. סיבת, סבת) the eventual transfer through the son's succession.

הֶסְגֵּר m. (סָגַר; v. Lev. XIII, 4, a. e.) *locking up* the leper for trial; cmp. הֶחְלֵט. Y. Meg. I, 71[b] מתוך ה׳ after being locked up. Y. M. Kat. III, 82[c] bot.; a. fr.

הַסְגָּרָה f. same. Lev. R. s. 17 אין ה׳ וכ׳ locking up (סגר, I Sam. XVII, 46) alludes to leprosy.

הָסָה (b. h.) *to be silent.* Num. R. s. 23 וְהָסוּ כל וכ׳ and all Israel was silenced before him (to listen to him); Tanh. Masé 5 הסכו; ed. Bub. 4 ותסו.

הסוקים, Y. Snh. VIII, beg. 26[a], read: אכל חסחוסים, v. חַסְחוּס.

הַסְחוּס, v. חַסְחוּס.

הַסֵּט, v. הֵיסֵט.

***הַסְטָא** f. (hasta) *spear.* Pesik. R. suppl. (p. 197[a] ed. Fr.) עושה להם בסאטה בתוך הארץ (read: שולח להם ה׳ וכ׳; corresp. to ירה חצים, Pesik. Vayhi, p. 66[b]) he sends (or throws) a spear into their land (as a declaration of war, v. Sm. Ant. a. Luebker Reallex. s. v. Hasta).

הֲסִיבָּה, v. הֲסִבָּה.

הֶסֵּיחַ, v. הֵיסֵ׳.

הֶסֵּיעַ m. (נָסַע)=preced. w., (with or sub. הַדַּעַת) *discarding, giving up.* Y. Pes. I, 28[b] top ה׳ דבר תורה, v. הֵיסֵחַ. Y. Shek. VII, beg. 50[c] ה׳ דעת טעון וכ׳ sacrificial meat whose existence has been forgotten (is unfit and) requires decomposition before it is burnt. Y. Meg. IV, 75[c] top מפני ה׳ ד׳ because his attention may be diverted (by looking at the priests); Y. Taan. IV, beg. 67[b] מסיע (corr. acc.). Y. Pes. X, 37[d] bot. מפני ה׳ הד׳ because the thought of eating it has been abandonned.

הֲסַם Ar., v. חֲסַם.

הֶסְפֵּד m. (סָפַד) *funeral ceremonies, manifestations of mourning, funeral address, eulogy* &c. M. Kat. III, 8 שלא להרגיל את הה׳ in order not to invite lamentation. Tosef. ib. II, 17 ה׳ על לב *hesped* means beating on the heart. Y. Ber. III, 6[b] top [read:] הסופד וכל העסוקין בה׳ (v. Tosef. ib. II, 11 ed. Zuck., Var.) the leader of the lamentation and all those engaged in it. Y. Succ. V, 55[b] bot. הֶסְפֵּידוֹ של וכ׳ the mourning for &c. Sabb. 153[a] מהספדו של אדם וכ׳ from the way a person is mourned for you can learn whether he deserves future happiness; a. fr.—קשר ה׳ *to compose and arrange a funeral song.* Y. Yeb. XVI, 15[d] top מצא ה׳ קשור וכ׳ found that lamentations were prepared in his house. Y. Yoma I, 38[b]; Y. Sot. I, end, 17[d]. Lam. R. introd. (R. Joh. 1).

הֶסְפֵּי׳, הֶסְפֵּדָא ch. same. Targ. Lam. I, 18; a. e.—Ber. 6[b]. Succ. 52[a]; a. fr.

הֲסָתָה f. (יָסַת or סות) *seduction, enticement.* Yoma 22[b] דאוריה ודה׳ the sin against Uriah and that of counting the people to which he was enticed (II Sam. XXIV, 1). Hull. 4[b] אין ה׳ בדברים *enticing* (the verb הסית) never applies to verbal persuasion (but only to sensual influences). Sifré Deut. 87 אין ה׳ אלא טעות *enticing* means leading astray; אין ה׳ אלא גירוי it means instigation.

הַסְתֵּר m. (Infin. Hif. of סָתַר) ה׳ פנים (from Deut. XXXI, 18) *hiding of face, divine anger, refusal to answer prayer.* Hag. 5[a] כל שאינו בה׳ פ׳ וכ׳ he who is not subject to the hiding of face (who does not suffer under general persecution) is none of them (not of Israelitish descent). Ib.[b].

הַעֲבָרָה f. (עָבַר) 1) *carrying, bearing.* R. Hash. 27[b], a. e. (ref. to והעברת, Lev. XXV, 9) דרך הַעֲבָרָתוֹ (leave the horn) in the way in which it was borne by the living animal (in its natural shape).—2) (=הַעֲבָרַת קול) *causing the sound to pass over a certain space, proclamation.* Ib. 34[a] דיליף ה׳ ה׳ ממשה Ms. M. (ed. דגמר עברה ע׳) we learn the meaning of העביר (Lev. l. c.) from the meaning it has in reference to Moses (Ex. XXXVI, 6). Sabb. 96[b]; Yalk. Ex. 413.—3) *leading across, passing; in gen. use of the stem* עבר. Y. Snh. VII, 25[b] bot. (interch. with עברה); Sifra K'doshim ch. VIII, Par. 4 מה ה׳ וכ׳ as the 'passing' there (Deut. XVIII, 10) means through fire, so does the 'passing' here (Lev. XVIII, 21). Bekh. 32[a] ה׳ ה׳ ממעשר analogy between the first-born and the tithes founded on the use of the stem עבר (Ex. XIII, 12, a. Lev. XXVII, 32); (Zeb. 9ª, a. e. עברה).—4) (from Num. VIII, 7, VI, 5, a. e.) הַעֲבָרַת שיער *passing the razor over the hair, shaving.* Naz. 58ᵇ, sq. ה׳ ש׳ removing the hair of the body. Y. ib. II, end, 52ᵇ לה׳ ש׳ for the purpose of removing the hair, opp. גדול שיער.

הַעֲדָאָה f. 1) (עוּד, *Hif.*) *testimony, deposition.* B. Mets. 3ª, ᵇ הַעֲדָאַת עדים evidence through witnesses; a. e.—2) (יָעַד) *warning given to the owner of a mischievous animal* (Ex. XXI, 29); *law concerning damages payable after warning,* v. מוּעָד. B. Kam. 18ᵇ יש ה׳ וכ׳ the law &c. applies to &c. (and full damages must be paid). Y. ib. II, beg. 2ᵈ; a. fr.

הַעֲדָפָה f. (עָדַף) *surplus; addition, increase.* Keth. 43ª לה׳ concerning the surplus of the value of labor over the cost of sustenance. Ib. 66ª ה׳ ע״י הדחק a surplus gained through an extraordinary exertion. B. Kam. 87ᵇ. Gitt. 12ª; a. e.—Ib.ᵇ לה׳ for additional support (not included in the sustenance furnished by the master).

הַעֲלָיָה, הַעֲלָאָה f. (עָלָה *Hif.*) 1) (fr. Lev. XIX, 19) *throwing over one's shoulders, wrapping,* opp. to לבישה putting on of a dress. Yeb. 4ᵇ. Yoma 69ª.—2) *bringing up, offering on the altar, placing on the table.* Pesik. R. s. 16, end כדי ה׳ אחת sufficient for one offering; Tanh. Ki Thissa 10. Hull. 104ª ואנן נגזר ה׳ and shall we forbid the serving on the table for fear that &c.?—3) (v. Lev. XVI, 9) *taking the lot out of the ballot box.* Y. Yoma IV, 41ᶜ top.

הֶעְלֵם c. (Inf. Nif. of עָלַם) *being unknown,* esp. (with ref. to Lev. IV to V) *unconsciousness, forgetfulness* as the cause of a transgression. Shebu. 26ª ה׳ שבועה forgetting that he had sworn; ה׳ חפץ forgetting the subject of the oath. Sabb. 70ᵇ ה׳ שבת unconsciousness of its being the Sabbath day; ה׳ מלאכות of the sinful nature of those labors. Ib. אם עשאן .. בה׳ אחד if he did all the forbidden labors in one state of unconsciousness (without being reminded between); Y. ib. III, 9ᵇ top בה׳ אחת. Ib. I, 2ᵇ בעלם אחד (interch. with בהעלם); B. Bath. 55ᵇ בה׳ (Ms. H. בעלם); Ker. IV, 2 (17ᵇ) בה׳ אחת; ib. III, 2 בה׳ אחד. Sifra Vayikra, Hobah, Par. 1, ch. I; a. fr.—*Pl.* הֶעְלֵימוֹת. Y. Sabb. l. c. בשני ה׳ in two discontinuous states of forgetfulness. Y. Shebu. I, 32ᵈ top כמה ידיעות וה׳ many moments of consciousness and intervening forgetfulness. Y. Snh. VII, 24ᶜ top; a. e.—Usu. הַעֲלָמוֹת (fr. הַעֲלָמָה, v. next w.), or הֶעְלֵמוֹת. Sabb. 80ª בשתי ה׳; Ker. 17ª; B. Bath. l. c. בשני ה׳. Tosef. Ker. III, 2; 7 בשני ה׳; a. fr.—[Midr. Till. to Ps. IX, 1 הַעֲלָמוֹת, v. עֶלֶם.]

הַעֲלָמָה f. same. Shebu. 4ª ה׳ למלקות מאי עבידתיה how can an act committed through forgetfulness be punished with lashes?—Ib. 14ᵇ ה׳ היא is this to be considered a sin committed through ignorance (not preceded by knowledge)?—*Pl.* הַעֲלָמוֹת, v. preced.

הַעֲמָדָה f. (עָמַד) *placing, being placed, appearance.* B. Kam. 34ª, a. e. בשעת ה׳ בדין according to the condition of the animal at the time of appearance in court. Bekh. 32ᵇ, a. e. בעי ה׳ והערכה must be placed (before the priest) and appraised (Lev. XXVII, 11). Ib. בכלל ה׳ וכ׳ subject to the law requiring placing &c. Yoma 41ᵇ אה׳ קאי does it refer to the placing of the sacrifice (to והעמידו, Mish. ib.)?—Y. Maas. III, 54ᶜ top ה׳ והערכה (interchanging with עמדה).

הַעֲנֵק, הַעֲנָקָה m. (Inf. Hif. of עָנַק, with ref. to Deut. XV, 14) *the outfitting of the emancipated slave.* Kidd. 17ᵇ לה׳ ('and also to thy handmaid shalt thou do likewise', Deut. XV, 17) refers to the outfit (not to the marking of the ear); Y. ib. I, 59ᶜ bot.; Sifré Deut. 122.

הַעֲרָאָה, v. הַעֲרָיָה.

הֶעֱרֵב m. (Inf. Hif. of עָרַב) ה׳ שמש *sunset,* required for the unclean person, after purification, to be entirely clean (Lev. XI, 27; a. fr.). Yoma 6ª והא בעי ה׳ חש׳ does he not require the sunset to pass before he may officiate?; a. fr.

הַעֲרָבָה f. (denom. of עֶרֶב) 1) *going home in the evening from labor* (=הַכְנָסָה), opp. to הַשְׁכָּמָה. Y. B. Mets. VII, beg. 11ᵇ [read:] שתהא השכמה משל בעה״ב וה׳ משל פועלין that the time needed for going out &c., v. הוֹצָאָה 4). Ib. (not ערבית) ובערבי שבתות בין . . . . ה׳ וכ׳ on Sabbath eves both are deducted from the employer's time.—2) *night work.* Lev. R. s. 19; Midr. Sam. ch. V דברי תורה צריכין השחרה וה׳ הפרנסה מנין the words of the Law require early and late study, whence shall sustenance come?

הַעֲרָאָה, הַעֲרָיָה f. (עָרָה, v. Lev. XX, 18) *sexual contact, the first stage of sexual connection.* Tosef. Sot. I, 2; Y. ib. I, 16ᶜ bot. כדי ה׳ time long enough for arriving at the intimacy of the first stage. Yeb. 55ᵇ, a. e. ה׳ זו הכנסת וכ׳, v. הַכְנָסָה; a. fr.

הַעֲרָכָה f. (עָרַךְ) *appraisement.* Bekh. 32ᵇ; a. e., v. הַעֲמָדָה.

הַעֲרָמָה f. (עָרַם) *trickery, legal evasion, improper means to avoid a religious duty.* Y. Peah V, 19ᵇ bot.; Y. Ned. IV, end, 38ᵈ לא חשו לה׳ the Rabbis did not apprehend an evasion. Ib. V, end, 39ᵇ a donation like that of Beth-Horon (v. Mish. ib. 7) שהיתה בה׳ which was made for the sake of circumventing (a vow). Tosef. B. Mets. IV, 3 הַעֲרָמַת רבית an evasion of the law of usury; B. Mets. 62ᵇ; Y. ib. V, 10ᵇ top; a. fr.

הָפוּךְ, הֲפוּךְ, v. הָפַךְ.

הפות, Tosef. Kel. B. Mets. II, 12, v. הָפוּת.

הִפּוֹתִיקָאוֹת, הִפּוֹתִקִי, הִפּוֹתִיקִי, pl., v. אַפּוֹתִיקִי.

הַפְטָרָה f. (פָּטַר, v. אַפְטָרָה) 1) *farewell-address, toast on parting.* Gen. R. s. 69, end.—2) *Haftarah, prophetic lesson* read in Synagogue after the reading from the Pentateuch, v. אַפְטַרְתָּא. Meg. 30ᵇ.—*Pl.* הַפְטָרוֹת. Ib.; a. e.

הַפִּיָא Ar., v. חוּפְיָא.

הפיטקי, v. הִיפָּטִיקוֹס.

הָפִיךְ, v. הָפַךְ.

הָפִיךְ adv., v. הָפַךְ.

הָפִיכָא f. (הָפַךְ) *perverse.* Targ. Prov. X, 31 Ms. (ed. הַפִּיכוּ).—*Pl.* הַפִּיכָתָא *perverse things, perverseness.* Ib. XVI, 30.

הֲפִיכָה f. (הָפַךְ) *upturning, displacing,* as a symbol of possession. Y. B. Kam. III, 3[c] bot., contrad. to הַגְבָּהָה. [הֲפִיכוֹת, v. הֲפֵכָה.]

הֲפִיכוּ f. (הָפַךְ) *perverseness.* Targ. Prov. X, 31, v. הָפִיכָא.

הֲפֵיכְתָּא, v. הֲפֵכְתָּא.

הֲפִינוֹס (הפינס) *of Haipha*(?). Gen. R. s. 100 יוסי ה׳; v. חֵפָנִי.

הָפַךְ (b. h.) 1) (act. verb) *to turn; to change; to reverse; to pervert, subvert, destroy.* Ex. R. s. 18 הָפְכָה המדינה שעבודה וכ׳ a country perverted the rules of forced labor for the captives (treating them inhumanely); ה׳ עליהם את הדין וכ׳ he changed the law against them and put them to death by night (against the Jewish law, v. Snh. IV, 1). Ib. ה׳ סדום He destroyed Sodom. Ber. 55[b] כשם שהָפַכְתָּ וכ׳ as thou didst turn the curse ... into blessing, כן הֲפוֹךְ וכ׳ so do thou turn &c. B. Kam. III, 3 החוֹפֵךְ את הגלל he who upturns (changes the place of) the dung (taking possession); a. v. fr.—*Part. pass.* הָפוּךְ. Pes. 50[a] עולם ה׳ ראיתי וכ׳ I saw a reversed world, the uppermost below &c. Sabb. 108[b] הֲפוּכָה סדום וכ׳ Sodom is subverted and what is said about it is perverted. Sifra Thazr. Par. 3, ch. III הפוכה ,הפוך when its color is changed; a. v. fr.—Y. Naz. V, end, 54[b] לשון הפוך, v. הֵפֶךְ.—2) (neut. verb) *to change.* Sifra ch. IV אי כולו ה׳ לבן if the whole of it has turned white. Neg. IV, 3; a. fr.

Nif. נֶהְפַּךְ 1) *to be upturned, destroyed; to be changed.* Yalk. Esth. 1056 כשנ׳ סדום when Sodom was subverted. Gen. R. s. 50 ומדינה נֶהְפֶּכֶת, v. אַדְרַבְלָא. Tanh. Sh'moth 25 נ׳ לחם מן וכ׳ the voice turned around, as if coming from &c.; a. fr.—2) *to roll about,* v. *Hithpa.*

Pi. הִיפֵּךְ 1) *to reverse, pervert, turn.* Gen. R. s. 20 שהי׳ דברים וכ׳ who spoke perversely of the Creator. Kidd. 59[a] עני מְהַפֵּךְ וכ׳ a poor man turns the cake, and another comes and takes it, i. e. one who buys away what another is negotiating for.—2) *to scheme,* v. infra.

Hithpa. הִתְהַפֵּךְ, *Nithpa.* נִתְהַפֵּךְ 1) *to be changed, disguise one's self.* Gen. R. s. 21 end שהם מִתְהַפְּכִים they (the angels) assume various shapes.—2) *to turn one's self around.* Ib. שהיא מִתְהַפֶּכֶת וכ׳ for it (the fiery sword) turns around man &c. Yeb. 35[a]; Keth. 37[a] מתהפכת she turns herself (makes violent motions). Ib. נִתְהַפְּכָה (Keth. l. c. נֶהֶפְכָה).—Tanh. Vayetsé 11 היה מ׳ עליו prevaricated (changing terms).—3) *to scheme.* Ruth R. introd. 3 שהוא מִתְהַפֵּךְ ובא וכ׳ he (Esaw=Rome) schemes and comes against &c.; Yalk. Prov. 959 בא ומִתְהַפֵּךְ על וכ׳. Ib. שהם מִתְהַפְּכִים וכ׳; Ruth R. l. c. שמְהַפְּכִין וכ׳.

הֲפַךְ, הֲפֵיךְ, יְהַפוֹךְ ch., fut. יְהַפוֹךְ, same (v. אֲפַךְ) 1) *to turn, change.* Targ. Ps. CV, 29; a. fr.—Y. Sabb. XVI, end, 15[d] ה׳ אפוי he turned his face off.—2) *to overturn, destroy.* Targ. Gen. XIX, 25; a. fr.—3) (neut. verb) *to turn around.* Targ. Prov. XXVI, 11; a. e.—Num. R. s. 12 כהדין ברנש . . . . הָפוּךְ לאחוריה like one going down a ladder backwards; Y. R. Hash. II, 58[a] כאילין דסלקין בסולמא הָפִיךְ like those who ascend a ladder backward; Yalk. Job 912 [read:] כהדין דסלקין בסולמא הפוך (v. Lattes Saggio p. 106).—4) (with ב) *to be engaged in, to handle.* Pes. 113[a] (prov.) הֲפוֹךְ בנבילתא ולא תֵיפוֹךְ וכ׳ deal in carcasses, but deal not in words (gossip, sophistry &c.). Y. B. Kam. IV, beg. 4[a] אנא חפך ומיתהפך בדידי וכ׳ I turn around my stock of goods (selling and buying again), so that I reach thee in profits. Ab. V, 22 הֲפוֹךְ בה וכ׳ study it over and again; a. fr.—V. הָפִיכָא.

Pa. הַפֵּיךְ 1) (=h. הֵשִׁיב) *to turn; to bring back, restore; to turn off* (wrath), *to appease; to give in return, reply.* Targ. Prov. XXV, 13.—Ib. XXIX, 8.—Ib. XXIV, 29 Ms. (ed. אַהְפֵּיךְ *Af.*).—Ib. 26.—2) *to handle, be engaged in, barter, study* (v. Pe. 4). Kidd. 59[a] דוה מְהַפֵּךְ בההיא וכ׳ was negotiating about a field. Sabb. 119[a] כמה דלא מְהַפִּיכְנָא בזכותיה before I study what might be said in his favor. Pes. 40[a] דמְהַפְּכֵי כיפי who handle sheaves; כי מְהַפְּכִיתוּ הַפִּיכוּ וכ׳ (Ms. M. חפכיתו) when ye handle (them), handle them with the thought that they will be used for a religious purpose.—*Part. pass.* מְהַפַּךְ. Y. Maasr. III, end, 51[a] היא חפכה והיא מְהַפְּכָה it turns and is turned in all directions (studied over and again), but we can learn nothing from it.

Af. אַהְפֵּךְ, v. supra.

Ithpa. אִתְהַפֵּךְ, *Ithpe.* אִתְהֲפֵיךְ 1) *to be turned, changed; to turn about, deal in* &c. Targ. Lev. XIII, 3. Targ. Job XXX, 21; a. fr.—Y. Maasr. III, end, 51[a], v. supra.—2) *to roll about.* Targ. Jud. VII, 13; a. e.

הֵפֶךְ m. (b. h.; preced. wds.) 1) *reverse, opposite.* לְשׁוֹן ה׳ a phrase which means the reverse (euphemism). Y. Naz. II, 51[d] bot. (ed. Krot. חפר, corr. acc.); ib. V, end, 54[b] לְשׁוֹן הָפוּךְ.—2) *upturning* (a pile), *displacing.* B. Kam. 29[b] כל ה׳ למטה וכ׳ the term 'upturning' means a movement within three cubits (Var. v. Rabb. D. S. a. l. note 80).

הֲפֵכָה, הֲפִיכָה f. (preced. wds.) 1) (b. h.) *destruction.*—2) *change, turn.*—*Pl.* הֲפֵכוֹת, הֲפִי׳. Ber. 55[b] שלש ה׳ three verses in which *change* (the expression חפך) occurs.

הַפַּכְנָא m. (preced. wds.) *fickle-minded.*—*Pl.* הַפַּכְנִין. Targ. Y. I Deut. XXXII, 20.

הֲפַכְפַּךְ m. (b. h.) same. Yalk. Esth. 1056, v. next w.—*Pl.* הֲפַכְפְּכִין. Ruth R. introd., 3; Yalk. Deut. 945 (Sifré Deut. 320 הֲפַכְפְּכָנִים, v. next w.).

הֲפַכְפְּכָן m. same. Meg. 15[b] (Yalk. Esth. 1056, v. preced.).—*Pl.*, v. preced.

הֲפֵכְתָּא, הֲפֵי׳ f. (הֲפַךְ) *destruction.* Targ. Gen.

XIX, 29. Targ. O. Deut. XXIX, 20 (Ms. מֵהֲפֵיכְתָּא); a. e.—*Pl.* הֲפֵיכָתָא.—Targ. Y. II Gen. XVIII, 2.

הַפְלָאָה f. (פָּלָא) 1) *distinction, peculiarity, use of the word* פלא. Sabb. 138ᵇ ה׳ זו וכ׳ this peculiarity of punishment (Deut. XXVIII, 59) &c.; ה׳ זו תורה it means the Law (afflictions causing the Law to be forgotten, ref. to Is. XXIX, 14).—2) *distinct and solemn specification of a vow* (from Lev. XXVII, 2; Num. VI, 2; v. אִיסְפְּלִיאָה). Tosef. Naz. III, 19 לא ניתנה נזירות אלא לה׳ the law of the *nazir's* vow applies only to distinct utterance (where there is no doubt); Naz. 34ᵃ; a. e.—Ib. 62ᵃ of the two *ki yafli* (Lev. l. c., Num. l. c.) אחד ה׳ לאיסור ואחד ה׳ וכ׳ one intimates a distinct binding expression, and one a distinctness which opens the way to absolution (v. הֶתֵּר); Ḥag. 10ᵃ אחת ה׳ וכ׳.

הֶפְלֵג, הֶפְלֵיג m. (פָּלַג) 1) *separation, interruption, interval.* Y. B. Kam. II, end, 3ᵃ בה׳ נגיחות it refers to gorings at intervals (not in three consecutive days). Y. Yoma III, 40ᵇ bot. אם להפליג if the conversation lasted long enough to be considered a discontinuation of the services, opp. לשעה. Ib. עשו אותה כה׳ they declared it (the going out for easing one's self, v. מסיכה) to be like a discontinuation.—2) *digression.* Y. Ab. Zar. III, 42ᵈ bot. תשובת ה׳ השיבו he made a reply only to divert his mind (Bab. ib. 44ᵇ תשובה גנובה, v. גָּנַב).

הַפְלָגָה f. (preced.) *separation,* הדור ה׳, v. דּוֹר. Snh. X, 3; a. fr.

הֶפְלֵיג, v. הֶפְלֵג.

הֶפְסֵד m. (פסד) *decrease, loss; injury; disadvantage; waste.* Pes. 15ᵇ ה׳ חולין an unnecessary destruction of &c.—Ib., a. fr. ה׳ מרובה a considerable loss, opp. ה׳ מועט. Ab. II, 1 ה׳ מצוה the loss (inconvenience, sacrifice) connected with the performance of a good deed. Ib. V, 11, sq. יצא שכרו בהֶפְסֵדוֹ his advantage is set off by his disadvantage. Lev. R. s. 34 הֶפְסֵדָהּ the disadvantage of (punishment for) neglecting it, opp. שכרה reward for observing it. B. Kam. 115ᵇ מפני ה׳ כהן because it is an injury to the priest (entitled to it). Sabb. 147ᵇ ה׳ אוכלין a waste of eatables; a. fr.

הֶפְסֵדָא ch. same. B. Kam. 115ᵇ דאיכא ה׳ (ed. הפסדה, corr. acc., Ms. R. a. F. הפסד). V. פְּסֵידָא.

הֶפְסֵק m. (פסק) *interruption, suspension, end.* Erub. 54ᵃ אין לו ה׳ וכ׳ there is no end to it for all eternity. Y. Ber. XI, 10ᵃ bot. ה׳ ברכה an unlawful interruption between the blessing and the partaking of food. Ib. II, 5ᵇ top ימי ה׳ intervening days during which menstruation ceased. Ib. IX, 13ᶜ bot.; Midr. Till. to Ps. CIV, 32 ה׳ מלכות interregnum, anarchy. Y. Yeb. II, 3ᵈ bot. שניות אין להן ה׳ the secondary degrees of forbidden marriages have no limitation; a. fr.

הַפְסָקָה f. (preced.) *ceasing, interruption, interval.* Gen. R. s. 33 Sivan, the seventh month להַפְסָקַת וכ׳ counting from the time the rains ceased (Yalk. ib. 59 לירידה). Taan. 4ᵇ לה׳ with reference to ceasing to insert the mention of rain in the prayers. Lev. R. s. 1, end אין כאן ה׳ there is nothing intervening (between ויקרא a. וידבר, Lev. I, 1); a. fr.—*Pl.* הַפְסָקוֹת. Num. R. s. 14, end ה׳ the intervals in revelations, i. e. passages in the Pentateuch not introduced by *vayikra* and *vaydabber*.—Esp. *Hafsakah*, the Sabbath intervening between the four Sabbaths on which the sections of the Torah, *Sh'kalim, Zakhor, Parah* and *Haḥodesh* are severally read, v. פָּרָשָׁה. Meg. 30ᵃ שנייה לה׳ 'the second Sabbath' means that following the Hafsakah.

הַפְצָא Ar., v. חַפְצָא.

הַפְקִירָא, v. הֶפְקֵרָא.

הַפְקָעָה f. (פָּקַע; cmp. אַפְקַעְתָּא) *cancellation, release from debt.* B. Kam. 113ᵇ הַפְקָעַת הלואתו the cancellation of his (the gentile's) loan.

הֶפְקֵר (Y. dial. הֶבְקֵר) m. (פָּקַר) *declaring free, renunciation of ownership* in favor of whosoever would take possession of the object renounced; *confiscation; public property.* Eduy. IV, 3 הפ׳ לעניים הפ׳ Ms. M. (ed. הב׳, v. Rabb. D. S. a. l. note) renunciation of ownership (of the standing crop) in favor of the poor is valid (exempting from tithes); (oth. opin.) אינו ה׳ עד שיפקיר וכ׳ Ms. M. (ed. שיובקר) it is not valid unless the owner make it free for the rich, too; Peah VI, 1 (v. Rabb. D. S. a. l.); B. Mets. 30ᵇ הפ׳. Yeb. 89ᵇ; Gitt. 36ᵇ ה׳ ב״ד ה׳ the confiscation by the court (disposing of private property by the process of law) is valid; Y. Shek. I, 46ᵃ bot. הב׳. Peah I, 6 ונותן משום ה׳ or he may set aside a portion of his crop as public property. Y. ib. III, 17ᶜ bot. וה׳ חייב בפיאה is public property ever subject to the laws of *Peah?* Ib. V, 19ᵇ אין הֶבְקֵירוֹ ה׳ his renunciation is ineffectual. Ib. אין ה׳ יוצא..אלא בזכייה renounced property does not go out of the owner's possession, until somebody takes possession of it; Y. Ned. IV, 38ᵈ (corr. acc.). Y. Snh. VI, 23ᵇ, beg. ה׳ טעות הוא it is a confiscation under an erroneous presumption (and invalid); a. fr.—Gen. R. s. 80, end בני אדם של ה׳ *outlaws.* Yeb. 66ᵃ מנהג ה׳ נהגו בה people took liberties with her (because she had neither the legal status of a freed woman nor that of a slave).

הֶפְקֵרָא, הֶפְקִירָא m. (פקר, cmp. אַפְקְרוּתָא) 1) *unbridled lust, lawlessness.* Gitt. 13ᵃ עבדא בה׳ ניחא ליה a slave prefers the dissolute life with a slave (to regular marriage with a free woman); Keth. 11ᵃ.—2) as preced. word. B. Kam. 115ᵇ מה׳ קא זכינא (in securing the honey from a broken vessel on the road) I took possession of renounced goods.—Targ. Y. Deut. XXV, 5 הֶפְקֵרָא (הַפְקְרָא) *an unprotected woman.*

הֵפֵר m. (Inf. Hif. of פּוּר, פָּרַר; fr. Num. XXX, esp verse 13) *the law of 'hafer', the husband's* (or *father's*) *right* of declaring void his wife's (or *daughter's*) *vow invalidation.* Ned. X, 7, a. fr. את שבא לכלל הקם בא לכלל ה׳ whatever comes under the law of *hakem* (confirmation) comes under the law of *hafer* (invalidation), i. e. as yo cannot confirm a vow before it has been made, so you cannot invalidate a vow in advance. Ib. 69ª; 79ª על הח׳ in a case where the right of invalidation might have been exercised. Tosef. ib. VII, 5 חומר בהקם שאינו בה׳ there are restrictions in the law of confirmation which do not apply to the law of invalidation &c. Y. ib. X, 42ª bot. ה׳ נדרים מעת לעת, v. next w.; a. fr. [In comment. our w. is spelled הפר and הֵיפֵר indiscriminately, which would intimate that it is pronounced הֵפֵר, fr. Num. XXX, 9.]

הֲפָרָה f. (preced.) *invalidation, declaring void;* also *absolution for cause* (v. הַתָּרָה). Ned. X, 8 הֲפָרַת נדרים כל היום the right (of the father or the husband) to declare a vow void lasts the whole day on which it came to his notice (to sunset); Y. ib. 42ª bot. הפר נדרים מעת לעת twenty four hours; Tosef. ib. VI, 1; Sabb. 157ª.—Ned. 87ᵇ מה הקמה ממנו אף ה׳ ממנו as the confirmation may be partial, so may the invalidation &c.; a. fr.—Gitt. 36ª אין לו ה׳ cannot be absolved from. Shebu. 29ᵇ top כי היכי ..... ה׳ in order to make absolution impossible.

הִיפַ׳, הַפַּרְכָא (not הַפּ׳) m. (ὕπαρχος) 1) *governor, lieutenant.*—*Pl.* הִי׳, הַפַּרְכֵי, הַפַּרְכִין. Targ. Esth. III, 12.—Ab. Zar. 8ᵇ.—2) *subject (land), colony.* Targ. Esth. X, 1 הַפַּרְכֵי ימא (h. text איי הים); Targ. Y. Gen. XLIX, 13.

הַפַּרְכוֹס, הִי׳ m. same, *lieutenant.* Ex. R. s. 18, beg. Yalk. Ps. 875 (to Ps. CXVI, 15) [read:] משל למלך ששלח ה׳ (v. Midr. Till. to Ps. l. c.); a. e. [Ib. ה׳ אחרת, read בהפרכוס הפרכיא (v. next w.).—Midr. Till. to Ps. XVII, some ed. ה׳ בא, v. אַפּוֹפְסִין.]—*Pl.* הִי׳, הַפַּרְכִין. Tosef. Gitt. VIII (VI), 3 לשום הירפרכון (corr. acc.). V. אִיפַּרְכוֹס.

הִי׳, הַפַּרְכְיָה, הַפַּרְכְיָא f. (ὑπαρχία) *lieutenancy, provincial government, province.* Sifré Deut. 330; Yalk. ib. 946 [read:] היפטיקוס נכנס לתוך ה׳ שלו אם יכול ליפרע מכל הוא נפרע ואם לאו וכ׳ a consul enters his province; if he is able to collect (taxes) from all &c. Yalk. Ps. 875 הפרכוס אחרת (corr. acc.; v. preced.)—*Pl.* הִי׳, הַפַּרְכִיּוֹת. Tosef. Gitt. VIII (VI), 3 ed. Zuck. (v. הורכיינוס).

הפרניא, v. הַרְפַּנְיָא.

הֶפְרֵשׁ m. (פָּרַשׁ) *difference.* Sabb. 155ᵇ ומה ה׳ בין וכ׳ and what is the difference between the two? Pes. 27ᵇ אמר להן ה׳ said he to them, There is a difference; a. fr.

הַפְרָשָׁה, v. אַפְרָשָׁה.

הֶפְשֵׁט m. (פָּשַׁט) *stripping, flaying.* Zeb. V, 4 טעונה ה׳ ונתוח requires flaying and carving (Lev. I, 6). Ib. 50ᵇ שלא בה׳ carving without previous flaying. Y. Pes. VI, 33ª bot. הֶפְשֵׁיטוֹ the flaying of it; a. fr.

הַפְשָׁטָה f. same. Sabb. 116ᵇ קודם הַפְשָׁטַת העור before the hide (up to the chest) is stripped off. Sifra Vayikra, N'dabah, Par. 4, ch. VI (ref. to Lev. I, 6) נתחים שהיו בכלל ה׳ such pieces as are affected by the order of flaying (to the exclusion of the head which is cut off before flaying); a. e.

הֶפְשֵׁיט, v. הֶפְשֵׁט.

הֶפְשֵׁר m. (פָּשַׁר) *making tepid, warming.* Sabb. 40ᵇ הֶפְשֵׁרוֹ זהו בשולו warming is to oil what cooking is to other liquids (a forbidden labor).

הֶפְתֵּיק, הֶפְתֵּיקָא, v. הֶפְתֵּק, הֶפְתֵּקָא.

הפתכי, הפתכו, Yalk. Deut. 942, read: הִיפָּטִיקוֹס.

הֶפְתֵּק m. (פתק *to cut, divide off;* Var. lect. v. infra) *the store-room* in the dwelling house out of which the daily portions of provision and work are distributed; also *the retailer's shelves* &c., contrad. to אוצר ware-house. Ab. Zar. II, 7 (39ᵇ) הבאין מן הה׳ the preserved locusts which the merchant takes from the shelves, contrad. to מן הסלולה, those laid out in baskets in front of the counter. Ib. 40ᵇ מן הה׳ מן האוצר ומן הספינה (not הסלולה, v. Rabb. D. S. a. l. note 5); Tosef. ib. IV (V), 12 מן הפתק וכ׳ ed. Zuck. (Var. הפתיק, cmp. הַמֶּכֶס for fusion of article) from the shelves, the ware-room or the ship.—Sabb. 50ª; Tosef. ib. III (IV), 19 גיזי צמר של ה׳ cut wool stored in the pantry (intended for spinning; Rashi: from the merchant's shelves). [Ar. s. v. אפתק reads: אוּפְתֵּיק, noting a Var. ה׳. One Ms. Ar., a. Mish. ed. Nap. read אפותיק for אוּפְתֵּיק, induced by phonetic resemblance to ἀποθήκη. V. Ar. ed. Koh. s. v. אפתק, a. Rabb. D. S. to Ab. Zar. 39ᵇ note 8.]

הִיפְתֵּי׳, הַפְּתֵי׳, הַפְּתֵקָא ch. (preced.) *treasury.* Targ. Y. Gen. XLVII, 14. Ib. Deut. XXIII, 22 (constr.) בהַפְתֵּיק וכ׳ in the treasury of the Lord (v. Hull. 139ª quot. s. v. גְּזָא).

הַפְתְּקָא *ladle,* v. אַפְתְּקָא.

הפתקאות, read: הַפּוֹתִיקָאוֹת; **הפתקי**, read: הַפּוֹתִיקִי.

הצאתה, v. הַצָּתָה.

הַצָּבָה f. (יצב) *standing, use of the verb* יצב. Num. R. s. 18, beg.; Tanh. Korah 3 (analogy betw. Num. XVI, 27 a. I Sam. XVII, 4, a. 16). Pesik. Zutr. Nitsab. beg. יש ה׳ לטובה וכ׳ the word יצב is sometimes used in a good sense (as firmness) and at times in a bad sense (as provocation); v. יְצִיבָה.

הַצְלְבוֹנִי, v. הַצְלֶפּוֹנִי.

הַצָּלָה f. (b. h.; נצל) *rescue, relief.* Meg. 16ᵇ הַצָּלַת נפשות saving of human lives. Gitt. 56ª (in Chald. diction) אפשר דהוי ה׳ פורתא may be some little relief (by royal favor) can be had; ib.ᵇ וה׳ פורתא נמי וכ׳ and even a little favor will not be shown. Hull. 52ᵇ הצלת עצמה the animal's own effort to save itself; ה׳ אחרים the human efforts to save the animal. Ex. R. s. 1 ה׳ מים saving from drowning; a. fr.

הַצְלֶלְפּוֹנִי (b. h.) pr. n. f. *Hazzelelponi,* alleged name of Samson's mother. Num. R. s. 10; B. Bath. 91ª צְלֶלְפּוֹנִית ed. (Ms. R. הצללפונית, Ms. R. צלולפונית).

הַצְלֶפּוֹנִי pr. n. (cmp. preced.), בני ה׳ prob. name

fo *a family* settled in Babylonia. M. Kat. 22ª (Ms. M. חצלבוני).

הַצְנֵעַ m. (Inf. Hif. of צנע) *chastity*. Pesik. Sos, p. 146ᵇ; Yalk. Job 906; (Yalk. Gen. 93 הַצְנִיעוּת).

הַצָּעָה f. (יָצַע) *making a couch, laying out of mattresses, carpets* &c. Keth. 4ᵇ, a. e. הַצָּעַת המטה making the bed (for her husband). Yoma 69ª בה׳ שרי for spreading under (to sit or lie on), garments of mixed materials (כלאים) are permitted. —V. מַצָּע.—Trnsf. *arrangement, structure, construction*. Ḥull. 49ᵇ כך היא ה׳ של משנה וכ׳ the construction of the Mishnah (Boraitha) is as you stated, but reverse the first clause. Snh. 51ª; a. e.

הַצָּתָה f. (יָצַת) *kindling*. Y. Sabb. II, beg. 4ᶜ צריכה הצאתה ברוב וכ׳ (corr. acc.) must be kindled so that the larger portion be on fire, v. הֶלֶק. Y. Yoma II, 39ᶜ top; Bab. ib. 24ᵇ הַצָּתַת וכ׳ kindling of &c.

הַקְבָּלָה f. (קבל, v. קַבָּלָה), הַקְבָּלַת פָּנִים *reception*. Shebu. 35ᵇ; Sabb. 127 (Ms. M. קַבָּלַת) ה׳ פני שכינה receiving the Divine Presence.

הֶקְדֵּשׁ, הֶקְדֵּישׁ m. (קדש) 1) *that which is dedicated to a sacred purpose*, esp. *sacred* or *Temple property*. Yeb. 66ᵇ bot., a. fr. ה׳ וכ׳ a pledged animal which the debtor dedicates as a sacrifice &c., v. פָּקַע. Gen. R. s. 60 ה׳ דמים; Arakh. VIII, 7 ה׳ עילוי dedication of the value of an object; opp. ה׳ מזבח dedication for the altar (allowing no redemption). Ib. VII, 1 אין מחשבין חדשים לה׳ months are not counted for redeeming dedicated property, i. e. fractions of a year count for a year in favor of the treasury. Kidd. 2ᵇ דאסר לה אכ״ע כה׳ because (by betrothing her to himself) he makes her forbidden to all other men like sacred property (v. קָדַשׁ). Taan. 24ª הרי הן ה׳ עליך וכ׳ they shall be to thee sacred property (like charity funds); a. v. fr.—2) *dedication*. Arakh. 2ª; Tem. 2ª תחלת ה׳ a preliminary act of dedication, סוף ה׳ the final dedication (laying hands on the animal's head prior to sacrificing it). Ib. 9ᵇ; B. Mets. 54ᵇ ה׳ ראשון the original dedication, ה׳ שני the substitution (for an animal which became defective); a. fr.—*Pl.* הֶקְדֵּשׁ׳, הֶקְדֵּישׁוֹת- 1) *sacred objects*. Lev. R. s. 5; a. fr.—2) *laws concerning dedication*. Tosef. Erub. XI (VIII), 24; ib. Ḥag. I, 9 (ed. Zuck. וחקרקעות, corr. acc.); a. e.

הַקָּזָה f. (נקז) *letting blood, opening a vein*. Ker. V, 1 דם ה׳ שהנפש יוצאה בו the blood of arteries with which life goes out, i. e. the splashing blood; ib. 22ª. Nidd. 19ᵇ. —Gitt. 70ª הַקָּזַת דם blood-letting. Sabb. 29ª סעודת ה׳ Ms. M. (ed. ה׳ דם) the meal taken after blood-letting; a. fr.

הֶקְטֵר m. (קטר) *letting rise in smoke, burning on the altar*. Ber. I, 1; a. fr.

הַקְטָרָה f. same. Y. Pes. VII, 34ᶜ top. Y. Yoma II, 39ᶜ; a. e.—*Pl.* הַקְטָרוֹת. Tosef. Dem. II, 7 הה׳; Men. 18ᵇ Ms. M. (ed. הק׳); Ḥull. 132ᵇ הק׳ (v. הֶמְסֵס as to fusion of article).

הֶקֵּיף, הֶקֵּיפָא, v. הֵיקֵ׳.

הֶקֵּישׁ, הֶקֵּישָׁא, v. הֵיקֵ׳.

הָקֵם m. (Inf. Hif. of קום, formed for analogy with הָפֵר q. v.) *confirmation, the privilege of confirming a vow*. Ned. X, 7; a. fr. (comment. write indiscriminately הקם a. הֵיקֵם, analogous to הֵיפֵר).

הֲקָמָה f. (קום) 1) same. Ned. 69ª ה׳ ראשונה the first confirmation (when he said the first קיים ליכי). Ib. ולא תיחול ה׳ but my confirmation shall not take effect; a. e.—2) *erection*. R. Hash. 2ᵇ לַהֲקָמַת המשכן dating from the erection of the Tabernacle. Y. Yoma I, 38ᶜ top; Num. R. s. 12, a. e. ה׳ חלילה the putting up (of the Tabernacle) by night; a. e.—*Pl.* הֲקָמוֹת. Ib. הֲקָמוֹתָיו his repeated acts of putting up.

הַקְנָאָה f., v. אַקְנַיְיתָא.

הֶקֵּף, הֶקֵּפָא, v. הֵיקֵ׳.

הַקְפָּדָה, v. אַקְפָּדָה.

הַקָּפָה f. (נָקַף II) 1) *surrounding, going round*. Yoma 59ª ה׳ ברגל the sprinkling was done in walking around; ה׳ ביד by circular movements of the hand. Pesik. R. s. 41 הַקָּפַת המזבח going around the altar in procession with the Lulab; a. e.—2) (ref. to Lev. XIX, 27) *shaving the hair of the head all around*. Naz. 29ª ועביד ה׳ and he (the Nazir) may shave &c. Ib. הַקָּפַת כל הראש shaving the entire head, opp. to ה׳ פאה shaving the ends, v. פֵּאָה. Y. Sot. II, beg. 17ᵈ ה׳ נזירות the shaving required by Nazir laws (Num. VI, 18); a. e.—3) *growth of hair around a limb*. Y. Yeb. X, end, 11ᶜ; Snh. 68ᵇ.—4) *debts for merchandise* payable at certain seasons (cmp. תְּקוּפָה). Shebi. X, 1; Tosef. ib. VIII, 3 הקפת חנות וכ׳ shop-debts are not subject to the law of limitation in the Sabbatical year.—*Pl.* הַקָּפוֹת. Gen. R. s. 41 he came back לפרוע הַקָּפוֹתָיו to pay his debts; Yalk. ib. 69.

הֲקָצָה I f. (קִיץ) *waking up*. Midr. Till. to Ps. XVII, 15 הֲקָצַת המתים resurrection of the dead.

הַקָּצָה II f. (קוץ, קָצַץ) *cutting*, הַקָּצַת שפתים (cmp. Prov. XVI, 30) cutting the lips, i. e. contracting the mouth for a blasphemous expression. Snh. 65ª Ar. a. Ms. K. (ed. עקימת, v. עֲקִימָה).

הָקֵר m. (Inf. Hif. of קוּר; cmp. Jer. VI, 7) *welling, pouring forth* (cmp. מָקוֹר). בְּאֵר ה׳ (בּוֹר) *well*, opp. to cistern; esp. *B'er Haker* name of a certain well. Erub. X, 14. Ib. 104ᵇ כל הבורות ה׳ Ms. M. (ed. incorr. הקרות); Y. ib. II, beg. 20ª.

הַקְרָבָה f. (קָרַב) 1) *offering*, use of the verb הִקְרִיב. Men. 11ª בת ה׳ היא it is an object which may eventually be offered. B. Kam. 12ᵇ חזי לה׳ fit for offering (if the Temple existed). Erub. 63ᵇ, a. e. גדול ... מֵהַקְרָבַת התמידין study of the Law is more important than the offering of daily sacrifices. Lev. R. s. 2, end נאמר ה׳ וכ׳ the term

חקריב is used &c. Ib. s. 20 they died על חקריבה ועל ה׳ (=הַקְ׳) for coming near (Lev. XVII, 1) and for offering (Lev. X, 1); a. fr.—2) *drawing nigh for attack.* Ex. R. s. 21 הקרבת פרעה (Ex. XIV, 10).

הַקְרָיָה, הַקְרִיָּה f. (קָרָה Hif.) *preparation, arrangement.* Sifra Num. 159; Yalk. ib. 787 (interpret. הקריתם, Num. XXXV, 11).

הֶקֵּשׁ, v. הֵיקֵּ׳.

הַקָּשָׁה f. (נָקַשׁ) *clapping, knocking together.* Snh. 65ᵃ הַקָּשַׁת זרועותיו the clapping of his (the necromancer's) arms; Ker. 3ᵇ.—*Pl.* הַקָּשׁוֹת. Ib. (Snh. l. c. always sing.).

הַר (הֲרָר) הַר m. (b.h.; הרר) *mound, mountain; trnsf. eminent person.* Midd. II, 1, a. fr. הַר הבית the Temple mount. Yeb. 17ᵃ (play on הַרְפַּנְיָא) הַר שהכל פונין בו a hill to which all turn (whose spurious descent prevents them from getting wives elsewhere); a. v. fr.—Hull. 39ᵇ (in Chald. diction) רישיך והר here is thy head and here the mountain (a colloquial phrase for compelling one to give up a bargain).—Ex. R. s. 28 (ref. to Ex. XIX, 3) בזכות הה׳ for the merit of the distinguished one (Abraham), ואין הה׳ אלא אבות *har* means the patriarchs (ref. to Mic. VI, 2). Snh. 107ᵃ ה׳ שבכם the most prominent of you; a. fr.—[For proper nouns composed with הר, v. respective determinants.]—*Pl.* הָרִים, הֲרָרִים. Tam. 32ᵃ, a. e. הָרֵי חושך, v. חוֹשֶׁךְ.—Snh. 24ᵃ עוקר הרי הרים uprooting the highest mountains (a figure for dialectical ingenuity). Y. Yeb. I, 3ᵃ bot. בין שני הָהָ׳ וכ׳ between the two high mountains (great scholars). Ex. R. s. 15 ואין ה׳ אלא אבות, v. supra.—Hag. I, 8 כה׳ תלויין בשערה like mountains suspended on a hair (a slender Bible text for numerous Talmudic laws); a. v. fr.

הֲרָא, *Af.* אַחְרֵי (cmp. חרי, חרר, חרי) *to heat, irritate.* Targ. Prov. XXV, 20 מַחְרָא (Var. מַחְרָה) ed. Lag. (ed. מחרא, ed. Wil. מחדא, corr. acc.); v. בְּרִיוּתָא.—Cmp. חַרְחֵר, חִרְחֵר.

הַרְבָּה (Inf. Hif. of רָבָה) *to increase; the numerical value of the letters* הרבה=212 (days). Gen. R. s. 20 (play on הרבה ארבה, Gen. III, 16) כל שהוא ה׳ ארבה וכ׳ if an embryo is 212 days old, I shall cause it to grow (it is vital); Y. Nidd. I, 49ᵇ top כל שהוא בה׳ הרי הוא בארבה; v. אל״ך.

הַרְבָּעָה f. (רָבַע) *the (forbidden) coupling of heterogeneous animals.* Snh. 56ᵇ הַרְבָּעַת בהמה; Sifra Ahare Par. 9, ch. XIII. Hull. 71ᵃ לה׳ with reference to forbidden coupling; a. e.

הָרַג (b.h.) [*to cut*, v. חֲרַג,] *to kill, put to death.* Num. R. s. 21, beg. בא לְהָרְגְךָ השכם לְהָרְגוֹ if one comes to kill thee, be the first to kill him; Ber. 58ᵃ; Snh. 72ᵃ ..לְהוֹרְגָךְ. Gitt. 56ᵇ כסבור ה׳ את עצמו להורגו he (Titus) thought he had killed himself (euphem. for *the Lord*); a. v. fr.—*Part. pass.* הָרוּג. Tosef. Gitt. V (III), 1 הֲרוּגִין שנהרגו לפני מלחמה ובשעת מלחמה (ed. Zuck. בשעת) those executed (by the Roman government) before and during the Vespasian war; Y. Gitt. V, 47ᵇ top [read:] הֲרוּגֵי המלחמה ולפני וכ׳. Y. Ber. I, 3ᵈ, v. בִּיתֵּר. Pes. 50ᵃ; B. Bath. 10ᵇ, a. e. הרוגי מלכות martyrs under the Roman government (R. Akiba and his fellow-martyrs), v. לוּד; a. fr.

Nif. נֶהֱרַג *to be killed, executed.* Taan. 18ᵇ נֶהֶרְגוּ were put to death (by the Roman government). Gitt. 56ᵃ יֵהָרֵג is to be put to death. Snh. 74ᵃ עבור ואל תֵּהָרֵג transgress or thou wilt be killed; a. fr.

הָרָג m. (preced.) *murderer, highway-man,* contrad. to חָרַם the oppressor who does not threaten to kill. Y. B. Mets. IV, end, 9ᵈ.—*Pl.* הָרָגִין. Ned. III, 4, v. נָדַר.

הֶרֶג m. (b. h.; preced. wds.) *execution by decapitation with a sword.* Snh. VII, 1; a. fr.

הַרְגֵּז, הַרְגִּיז m. (prob.=אַרְגָּז q. v.) euphem. for *buttocks* (or *testicles*). Bekh. VI, 6 הַרְגִּיזוֹ Maim., Ar. Var. הַרְגּוֹזוֹ, ed. אֲכוּז q. v.

הַרְגִּיפִין, v. חַרְגָּ׳.

הֶרְגֵּל m. (רגל, v. רָגִיל) 1) *habit;* לשון ה׳ habit of the tongue, fluency acquired by memorizing. Koh. R. to VI, 9.—2) *leading to, occasion for.* מפני ה׳ עבירה because it offers an occasion for sin. Sabb. I, 3; Pes. 30ᵃ; 36ᵃ; a. e.—Ab. Zar. 17ᵃ ה׳ דבר (euphem.) preliminaries of sexual connection.

הרגנא, v. חַרְגָּנָא.

הַרְגְּפִין, v. חַרְגְּפִין.

הַרְגָּשָׁה f. (רָגַשׁ, Hif.) *sensation, perception, sensuous affection.* Nidd. 43ᵃ נעקרה בה׳ he felt the effusion coming, ויצתה שלא בה׳ but the discharge was not perceived. Ib. 57ᵇ הַרְגָּשַׁת מי וכ׳ the sensation of discharging urin; a. fr. Yalk. Jud. 42 לכל ה׳ וה׳ to every *sense.*—*Pl.* הַרְגָּשׁוֹת *senses.* Num. R. s. 14 כנגד חמש ה׳ וחמש מורגשות corresponding to the five senses and the five perceptions.

הַרְגַּת, v. חַרְגָּא.

הַרְדָּאוּלִיס, v. הַרְדְּוּלִיס.

הַרְדּוּבְלִין f. (ὑδραυλις) *water-organ.* Targ. Ps. CL, 4 Ms. (Regia הרדיב׳, ed. חֲלִילִין).

הַרְדּוּלִיס m. same. Arakh. 10ᵇ (not לים...); Tosef. ib. I, 13 הרדאולים לא היו וכ׳ ed. Zuck. (corr. acc.; ed. הַרְדָאוּלִ׳ לא היה); cmp. אַדְרַבְלִיס.

***הַרְדּוּס** m. (transpos. of דרס, v. מִדְרָא, מִדְרוֹן &c.) *the copulation of birds;* מעשה ה׳ *unnatural gratification on a woman's body.* Snh. 66ᵇ Ar. (ed. חידודין; v. חִרְדּוּרִים). [Ar.: *doing of Herod,* ref. to B. Bath. 3ᵇ; v. הוֹרְדּוֹס.]

הַרְדּוּף, v. הִרְדּוּף.

הַרְדּוּפָה, v. הִרְדְּפָה.

הַרְדּוּפְנֵי, v. הַרְדַּפְנֵי.

הַרְדּוּפְנִין m. (comp. of הר=חר, a. הוֹפֶן; v. חַרְחֲבִינָה) *wall-ivy*, the leaves of which may be used for bitter herbs on the Passover night. Pes. 39ª (Ms. M. הַרְדְּפ׳). V. הַרְדַּפְנֵי.

הַרְדְּסִיּוֹת, הַרְדְּסִיאוֹת (הדרס׳) f. pl., יוני ה׳ *a species of domesticated doves* (prob. so named from the manner of their fructification, v. הַרְדּוּס). Ḥull. XII, 1; Bets. 25ª; Tosef. ib. I, 10; Tosef. Ḥull. X, 9 הרד׳ ed. Zuck. (Var. הדר׳). Ḥull. 139ᵇ חד תני הדר׳ וחד תני הרד׳ וכ׳ one reads *hadr.*, and one reads *hard.*, the one deriving our w. from Herod, the other from the name of a place.

***הַרְדָּפָה** f. (הדף, with ר inserted; cmp. הִירְדּוּף) [*removal, isolation,*] *imprisonment within a narrow enclosure of reeds or poles,* a punishment for contempt of court (v. נִידּוּי). M. Kat. 16ª (explain. לִשְׁרֹשִׁי, Ezra VII, 26). Ib. (a version of the Gaonim quoted by Asheri a. l., Nr. 53) מאי ה׳ א״ר פפא נצבי דקני what is *hardafah?* Said R. P., Poles of reeds (fastened in the ground). [In ed. a. Mss. the answer to מאי ה׳ is absent.] [Ar. ed. Koh. הַרְדּוּפָה.]

הרדפוני, v. next w.

הַרְדּוּפְנֵי, הַרְדַּפְנֵי m. (Chald. form of הַרְדּוּפְנִין) *a creeper* the berries of which were known to be injurious to animals. Ḥull. III, 5 (58ᵇ); Tosef. ib. III, 19.— Mekh. B'shall., Vayassa 1 (ref. to Ex. XV, 25) זה עץ ה׳ it was the trunk of an ivy; Ex. R. s. 50; (ib. s. 23 הירדינון); Yalk. ib. 256 הרדפוני (corr. acc.); Tanh. B'shall. 24 מר ה׳ חיה; Tanh., ed. Bub., ib. 19.—[Var. הירדופני, v. Koh. Ar. s. v.]—Targ. Y. Ex. XV, 25 אַרְדַּפְנֵי.

הַרְדְּפְנִין, v. הַרְדּוּפ׳.

הָרָה (b. h.) *to conceive, be with child.* Yalk. Ex. 168, end. Y. B. Kam. V, 5ª top; Bab. ib. 49ª.

Hof. הוֹרָה *to be conceived;* *(homilet.) *conception*, v. הוֹרָה. Gen. R. s. 64; Yalk. Job 894 that she would have said to him, ה׳ גבר is this a time for conception, man? ('Rashi').

הַרְהוֹן I, v. הִרְ׳.

הַרְהוֹן II m. *urin-soaked dung*, v. הָהוֹן a. הָהִין.

הִרְ׳, הַרְהוּר m. (הִרְהֵר) 1) *thought, meditation*, opp. דִּיבּוּר loud recitation. Ber. 20ᵇ ה׳ כדיבור דמי reviewing in mind (a Biblical passage &c.) is as good as loud recitation. Sabb. 150ª (ref. to Is. LVIII, 13) דיבור אסור ה׳ וכ׳ talking (business on the Sabbath) is forbidden, thinking (planning) is permitted.—2) *heated imagination, esp. impure fancies.* Ber. 12ᵇ ה׳ עבירה unchaste imagination, ה׳ ע״ז idolatrous fancy. Nidd. 13ᵇ המביא עצמו לידי ה׳ who allows sinful fancies to take a hold of him. Zab. II, 2; a. fr.—*Pl.* הַרְהוּרִים. Yoma 29ª top הִרְהוּרֵי עבירה וכ׳ sinful (obscene) imaginations are more injurious to health than the sin itself. Esth. R. to III, 1 (play on ahar) הרהורי דברים היו שם plans (schemes) were there.

הִירְהוּרָא, הַרְהוּרָא ch. same. Targ. O. Deut. XXIX, 18. Targ. Y. ib. XXIII, 11; a. e.—Snh. 45ª חיישי לה׳ take into consideration the possibility of creating impure thoughts (among the spectators); Sot. 8ª.—*Pl.* הִרְ׳, הַרְהוּרִין, הַרְהוֹרִין. Targ. Y. Lev. VI, 2. Targ. Ez. XXXVIII, 10; a. fr.

הִרְ׳, הִרְהֵר (Pilp. of הרר; v. הָרָה, cmp. esp. Is. LIX, 13) 1) *to conceive in mind, to think, meditate, plan.* Ber. III, 4 מְהַרְהֵר בלבו thinks (recites the Sh'ma) in his heart, v. הִרְהוּר. Gitt. 57ᵇ הר׳ תשובה בדעתיה he conceived the idea of repentance.—2) *to be heated, entertain impure thoughts.* Ḥull. 37ᵇ לא הִרְהַרְתִּי ביום I allowed no impure thoughts to rise in me in day-time; a. fr.—3) (followed by אחר) *to disparage, criticise, detract from.* Snh. 110ª הַמְהַרְהֵר אחר רבו who speaks evil of his teacher. Num. R. s. 7 אם הִרְהַרְתָּ וכ׳ if thou criticisest them &c. Ber. 19ª אל תְּהַרְהֵר אחריו ביום do not think evil of him the day after (for he surely repented). Sifré Deut. 307 אין לְהַרְהֵר אחר מִדּוֹתָיו you must not criticise His dealings with man; a. fr.—4) *to heat, make sick with fever.* Lev. R. s. 17 (play on חַרְצֻבּוֹת, Ps. LXXIII, 4; v. ה״א) לא הִרְהַרְתִּים בחלאים (Var. הרהר׳; Ar. s. v. זרצב: ערער׳) I did not make them hot with diseases; Yalk. Ps. 808. [Ukts. III, 11, v. חִרְהֵר.]

הַרְהֵיר, הַרְהֵר ch. same. Targ. Y. Gen. VI, 2.— Targ. Job II, 10 הַרְהַר; a. fr.

הרוגייב׳, Y. Kil. I, 27ª, v. גְּרִירְנָא.

הַרְוָחָא m. (v. next w.) *profit*, opp. פְּסֵידָה. M. Kat. 2ª.

הַרְוָחָה, הַרְוָחַת f. (b. h. הַרְוָחָה; רֶוַח) 1) *relief, release.* Ex. R. s. 10, end; Tanh., ed. Bub., Vaëra 22; Yalk. Ex. 186 (cmp. הַמֶּסֶס as to fusion of article). Tanh. Mikk. 10, v. בָּסַר I; a. e.—2) *plenty, liberal provision; comfort.* Snh. 21ᵇ לא צריכא לה׳ the word לוֹ is to intimate a liberal appropriation (for the army). Sifré Deut. 306 ואין לשון פתיחה אלא לשון ה׳ the word 'opening' has the meaning of comfort, opp. לשון דוחק. Keth. 43ª אלמנתו לא ניחא ליה בה׳ וכ׳ as to his widow he cares not for her living comfortably (from her own earnings besides the legal alimentation) &c.

הרויין, Tosef. Toh. VIII, 1, v. חֲרוּיִין.

***הֲרוּרִים** m. pl. (הרר, v. הִרְהֵר) *heating*, מעשה ה׳ *unnatural gratification on a woman's body.* Snh. 66ᵇ, Resp. Gaon. ed. Cassel, p. 110; v. הַרְהוּס, a. הִידּוּד.

הַרְזְבָנ׳, הַרְזְבוּנִית, v. אַרְזְבוּנִית.

הַרְזִיפָא, v. אַרְזִיפְתָּא II, a. next w.

הַרְזִיפוּ, הַרְזִיפֵי f., m. pl. (Rashi) (v. אַרְזִיפְתָּא II) name of a *bitter herb* (not generally used as food). Pes. 39ª (Ms. M. 2 אַרְזִיפָא, Ms. O. הדרוף, v. הִירְדּוּף; v. Rabb. D. S. a. l. note 9).

הִרְזֵק, הִרְזִיק (=הִזֵּק, v. חזק) *to imprison.* B. Kam. 85[b] הִרְזִקֵיה באנדרונא וכ׳ Ar. (ed. הדק׳) he kept him locked up in a room and forced him to be idle.—*Part. pass.* מְהַרְזֵק. Ned. 91[b] דהוה קא מ׳ בביתא וכ׳ Ar. (ed. מִתְהַרְזִיק *Ithpa.*) who was locked up in a room with a woman.

הִרְזִיקִי m. pl. (preced.) בֵּי ה׳ *guard-house, a gate house* with one door opening to the court and another leading to the entrance to the inner rooms or buildings; cmp. פְּלָאֵר. Men. 33[b].

הִרְזֵק, v. הִרְזִיק.

הַרְחָצָה f. (רָחַץ) *washing, bathing.* Sabb. 134[b] הַרְחָצַת כל גופו bathing the child's entire body; ה׳ מילה bathing the wound of circumcision. Keth. 96[a].

הַרְחֵק or **הַרְחָק** (רָחַק) 1) *distance.*—ה׳ עדות a) *an unlawful space between a deed and the signatures of the witnesses.* Y. Gitt. I, 43[c] bot. עדים פסולין אינן נעשין כה׳ ע׳ the signatures of disqualified witnesses, between qualified ones, are not to be looked upon as if they were a blank creating an unlawful distance; ib. IX, 50[c]; ib. VIII, end, 49[d] (insert: עדים פסולים אינן).—b) *distance of relationship,* i. e. *testimony not objectionable on account of kinship.* Y. Keth. II, 26[d] top [read:] ואם אין את מאמינו שהוא בנו יעשה כה׳ ע׳ וכ׳ and if you do not believe him that he is his son, let his statement (that he is a priest) be considered a stranger's testimony &c.—2) *a precautionary measure, a preventive law.* Y. Maasr. I, 49[b] top.

הַרְחָקַת f. as preced. 2. Pes. 2[b]. Ab. Zar. 31[b] ה׳ יתירתא an extraordinary precaution.

הַרְטָבָה׳, v. רְטִיבָה.

הֲרֵי I, הָרֵי m. (=הראי; ראה) *aspect, characteristic points, case.* B. Kam. I, 1 (ref. to the four cases of damage Ex. XXI, 28; XXI, 33; XXII, 4; XXII, 5) לא ה׳ השור כה׳ וכ׳ (Y. ed. לא השור כה׳ וכ׳) the case of the goring ox is not analogous to that of the eating animal, nor are the cases of both of them which are animated beings, analogous to the case of damage through fire which is inanimate &c. (i. e. the four cases had to be specified in the Biblical text); yet the points common to all are that they are liable to do damage &c. Mekh. Mishp., N'zikin, s. 5 לא ה׳ הדיין כה׳ וכ׳ the case of (cursing) the judge is not analogous to that of (cursing) the prince, yet the point common to both &c. [In G'marah רְאִי, v. B. Kam. 4[a].]

הֲרֵי II (v. preced.,=b. h. הֵן, הִנֵּה) 1) *behold, here is.* Gen. R. s. 91, end ה׳ הכסף וכ׳ here is the silver &c.—Ab. III, 4, a. fr. ה׳ זה וכ׳ such a person is &c. Bets. V, 3, a. fr. ה׳ אלו וכ׳ in this case they are &c. B. Kam. IX, 2 ה׳ שלך לפניך here is thy property before thee (take it in the condition in which it is); a. v. fr.—ה׳ אני=הֲרֵינִי behold, I am, will be &c. Naz. I, 1 ה׳ נזיר I will be a Nazir. Kidd. 31[b] ה׳ כפרת וכ׳ may I be the atonement for his rest (a blessing formula for a deceased father); a. fr.—2) ה׳ ש׳- *here is a case of one, if.* Meg. 3[b] ה׳ שהיה וכ׳ if one is going to slaughter &c.; a. fr.

הֲרִיגָה f. (הָרַג) *killing.* Sabb. 107[b].—Esp. *execution of capital punishment, decapitation.* Y. Keth. II, 26[d] נגמר דינה לה׳ if she has been sentenced to death. Y. Snh. VII, 24[b] ה׳ decapitation, v. הֶרֶג. Ex. R. s. 1; a. fr.

הֵרִידוּס pr. n. m. *Hōredos* (Herod), one of Haman's ancestry. Targ. II Esth. III, 1 (ed. Lag. הדירוס).

הֵרָיוֹן m. (b. h.; הָרָה) *conception, coition.* Nidd. 16[b]. Gen. R. s. 64. Y. B. Kam. V, 5[a] top בעל ה׳ the natural father (not step-father); a. e.—B. Kam. 49[a] בית הה׳ womb, abdomen.

הריוסן, Y. Ter. XI, 48[a], v. הַרְסָן.

הריית, v. חֲדִירִית.

הָרִיס, v. חָרִיץ.

הֲרִיעָה f. (רוּעַ) *shouting* for joy. Pesik. Ronni, p. 141[b] one of the expressions for rejoicing (Cant. R. to I, 4, reads תְּרוּעָה). Cmp. הֲרָעָה II.

הֲרִיפָה f. (רוּף, רפה) *trembling,* only in הֲרִיפַת עין *wink of the eye,* בה׳ ע׳ in a wink. Koh. R. to XI, 1 (ed. Wil. כה׳).

הֲרִיפוֹת or **הֲרִי׳** f. pl. (b. h.; הרף, cmp. חָרַף) *grits, polenta.* Sot. 42[b] (homiletical play on *Harafah,* II Sam. XXI, 16, a. *Orpah,* Ruth I, 4) why was she called Harafah? שהכל דשין אותה כה׳ because all pounded (used) her like grits, v. דּוּשׁ. [Cmp. Y. Kidd. I, 59[a] top a. Kerith. 11[a] where חרף is taken as the equivalent of כתש, with reference to הריפות Prov. XXVII, 22. Cmp. הַלְטָאָה for obliteration of radical ה.—Targ. I Chr. XX, 4; 6; 8 reads ערפה for h. text הרפא, הרפאים.]

הֲרִיקָא, v. חֲרִיקָא.

הרך, v. חֲרָךְ.

הַרְכֵּב m. (רָכַב) *carrying (a lamb) on one's shoulder.* Pes. VI, 1 הַרְכֵּבוֹ Y. ed., Ms. M. a. Mish. Nap. הַרְכִּיבוֹ (ed. הַרְכָּבָתוֹ) the carrying of the Passover lamb to the Temple. Y. ib. 33[b] top.

הַרְכָּבָה f. 1) same, v. preced.—2) *grafting.* Shebi. II, 6; a. fr.

הרכיא, v. חַרְכָּיָא.

הֶרְכֵּיב, v. הַרְכֵּב.

הַרְכִּינַס pr. n. m. (Ἀρχῖνος) *Harkinas,* father of R. Dosa. R. Hash. II, 8 (25[a]) הר׳ Mish. a. Ms. M. (ed. הור׳); Mish. Pes. a. Y. ed. ארכינס, v. Rabb. D. S. a. l. note). Tosef. Neg. I, 6 הרכ׳; (ib. Kel. B. Bath. IV, 14 הורקנס). Yeb. 16[a]; a. fr.

הַרְכָּנָה f. (רָכַן) *inclination,* הַרְכָּנַת הָרֹאשׁ *nodding assent.* Y. Gitt. VII, 48[c] bot.; Y. Ter. I, 40[b] top.

הֲרָמָה f. (רום) 1) *lifting, removal.* Y. Yoma II, beg. 39[b] יצא זה שהוא בה׳ this (service) is excluded, since it consists only of removing (the ashes). Ib. 39c; a. fr.—2) *separating the priest's gift* &c. Bets. I, 6 (12b) אינו זכאי בַּהֲרָמָתָהּ (v. Rabb.D. S. a. l.) nobody obtains a privilege by its being set apart; a. fr.—3) *lifting up, elevation.* Yalk. Ps. 624 (ref. to ומרים, Ps. III, 4) . . . תחת שהייתי תלוי ראש נתת לי הֲרָמַת ראש וכ׳ while I deserved hanging down the head (in the consciousness of guilt), thou hast granted me a lifting up of the head (forgiveness, II Sam. XII, 13); ib. (ref. to תשא Ex. XXX, 12) . . . . תחת שהיינו תלוי ראש . . . ה׳ ראש; Pesik. Shek. 10b, sq. (corr. acc.); Midr. Till. to Ps. l. c.; Yalk. Ex. 365 (corr. acc.). Tanh. Emor 16.

הַרְמוּצָא, v. רְמוּצָה, s. v. רָמַץ.

הַרְמֵךְ, הַרְמֵיךְ pr. n. pl. (*Be*) *Harmekh* in Babylonia. Gitt. 60b בי ה׳ Ar. (ed. בי ח׳). M. Kat. 4b הרמיך Ms. M. (ed. בר חמדך). Zeb. 2b בי ח׳ (v. Rabb. D. S. a. l. note 6).

(הוּרְמִינִי) הַרְמִינֵי pr. n. *Harmine* (*Hurmini*), prob. a province of Armenia. Targ. Jer. LI, 27 הור׳ ed. Lag. a. oth. (h. text מִנִּי). Targ. Am. IV, 3 הר׳ (ed. Lag. הור׳; h. text הרמונה). Targ. Mic. VII, 12 הור׳ רבתא (Var. ed. Lag. הור׳) *Armenia Major* (?).

הַרְמֵךְ, v. הַרְמֵיךְ.

הַרְמָנָא m. (מני, with preform. הר, cmp. הרפתקי) *appointment to office, authority, royal patent.* Targ. Job I, 12; II, 7. Targ. Y. Num. XVII, 11.—Ber. 58a holding court בלא ה׳ דמלכא without royal appointment. B. Mets. 84a ה׳ דמלכא הוא (Ms. R. 2 הור׳) it is a royal appointment (which I cannot decline). Hull. 57b ה׳ דמלכא לא ליבעו would they not have asked for royal authority? Ib. ה׳ דמלכא הוו נקיטי they were in possession &c.; (Ar. ed. Koh. the king was among them ומה׳ דמלכא עבוד and they did it by royal authority). B. Bath. 46b, v. next w.—*Trnsf.* (cmp. רְשׁוּת) *office, bureau*, esp. *Resh Galutha's office.* Erub. 59a משום דשכיחי רבנן גבי ה׳ (v. Rabb. D. S. a. l. note 300) because scholars are accustomed to meet at the Resh Galutha's office (Ar. קהרמנא).

הַרְמָנְיָא f. same. B. Bath. 46b ה׳ בעלמא שויוה they (the owners) considered it (the transmission of the land to subtenants) merely an appointment (agency); (Asheri הרמנא שַׁוְיָה; Ar. הרמנא; v. Rabb. D. S. a. l. note 90).

הרנגול, a clerical slip in Ar. s. v. הַרְנוֹגָא.

הַרְנוֹגָא m. 1) *harnoga*, name of a bird, one of eight about which there is a doubt as to being clean. Hull. 62b.—2) *a thorn*, v. חַרְנוֹגָא.

הרני, v. אֲרוֹנֵי.

הרנירק, v. אנדכתרי.

הָרַס (b. h.) 1) *to break, to destroy, demolish.* Midr. Till. to Ps. IX, 7 הוא הוֹרֵס את וכ׳ He destroys your plans; Yalk. Mal. 587.—*Part. pass.* הָרוּס; f. הֲרוּסָה. Gen. R. s. 45; a. e.—Y. Ber. IV, 8a; a. e.—2) *to break through, rush.* Yalk. Ex. 284 (expl. פן יהרסו, Ex. XIX, 21) שמא ידחקו, v. דָּחַק; Mekh. Yithro, Bahod., s. 4.

הֶרֶס m. (preced.) *destruction.* Men. 110a (interpret. עִיר הַהֶרֶס, Is. XIX, 18) קרתא . . . דעתידא למיחרב (v. Rabb. D. S. a. l.) the town of Beth Shemesh which is doomed to destruction; v. חֶרֶס.

הַרְסָן, v. חַרְסָן.

הַרְסָנָא m. (הרס; cmp. Arab. הריסת, Fl. to Levy Talm. Dict. I, p. 559b; cmp. חֲרוּסֶת) *fish-hash.* B. Bath. 144a, v. אַצְרָצָא.—כַּסָּא דה׳ a pie of fish-hash and flour. Bets. 16a, sq.; Ab. Zar. 38a; a. fr.

הֲרָעָה I f. (רָעַע, Hif. הֵרַע) *doing harm*) to one's self or others); *self-abnegation; vow to injure;* v. הֲטָבָה. Shebu. III, 5; a. fr.

הֲרָעָה II f. (רוּעַ) *sounding the trumpet, a certain note or signal.* Y. R. Hash. IV, 59c bot., v. טרימוטה.—Cmp. תְּרוּעָה, הֲרִיעָה.

הֶרֶף m. (רפה, v. הֲרִיפָה) *trembling;* ה׳ עַיִן *wink, an indefinable portion of time.* Y. Ber. I, 2b bot. בין השמשות כה׳ ע׳ the time called *ben-hash-sh'mashoth* is really like a wink of the eye. Ib.c top. Ib.d top; Lam. R. to II, 19; v. רֶגַע. Cant. R. to III, 6 בה׳ ע׳ (not כה׳) instantaneously; a. fr.

הָרָפָה pr. n. f. *Harafah.* Sot. 42b, v. הֲרִיפוֹת.

הרפותיא, v. חַרְסְפִיתָא.

הרפיא, v. חַרְפַּיָּא.

הַרְפַּנְיָא pr. n. pl. *Harpania* (*Hipparenum*, Neub. Géogr. p. 335; p. 352) in Babylonia, a rich industrial town with a Jewish population of spurious descent. Yeb. 17a what a great man, אי לאו דה׳ מאתיה were not H. his native town! Ib. מאי ה׳, v. הַר. Sabb. 127a (Ms. M. הרפנאי, read הַרְפְּנָאֵי *Harpanians*); B. Mets. 84a דה׳ Ms. M. (ed. דְּהַרְפְּנָאֵי), v. דְּקוּרָא. Ab. Zar. 74b. Snh. 48b (Ms. M. נהר פניא). [Kidd. 72b Ms. O. הפרניא והימניא, ed. only הומניא.]—Denom. הַרְפְּנָאָה m. *of H.* Erub. 59b (v. Rabb. D. S. a. l. note 90).—*Pl.* הַרְפְּנָאֵי, v. supra.

הַרְפַּתְקָא, pl. **הַרְפַּתְקֵי** m. (פתק with preform. הר, cmp. הַרְמָנָא; v. פִּיתְקָא) [*portions, allotments,*] 1) *measure, limitation.* Targ. Job XVIII, 2 (h. text קִנְצֵי).—2) *destinies, reverses, experiences* (cmp. גְּזֵרָה). Ib. XII, 5 ה׳ זמנא the changes of time (h. text מועדי רגל; cmp. רֶגֶל).—R. Hash. 16a כל הנך ה׳ דעדו וכ׳ all those preordained changes that passed over the standing crop (up to Passover).

הַרְצָאָה, הַרְצָיָה f. (רָצָה) 1) (v. Lev. I, 4) *acceptability of a sacrifice, gracious reception, qualification for offering, atonement.* Hull. 81a לילה לקדושה יום לה׳ the eve of the eighth day qualifies it for dedication, the morning for an acceptable offering. Zeb. 28b, a. e. (ref. to Lev. XXII, 27 a. XIX, 7) כְּהַרְצָאַת כשר וכ׳ the same ceremonies which are needed for the atoning efficacy of the legally performed offering, are required for making it an unfit offering (the eating of which is punishable with extinction). Ker. 9[a] (הַרְצָאַת דם (דמים reception into the covenant through the sprinkling of blood (Ex. XXIV, 5 sq.).—Sifra Vayikra, N'dabah, Par. 5, ch. VII לאחר הרציה after the sprinkling of the blood. Zeb. 45[b] בני ה׳ those for whom a sacrifice may effect atonement. Sifra Emor ch. III, Par. 4 מה חילול . . . ה׳ as the desecration *there* refers to a sacrifice which has an atoning effect; a. fr.—2) *making willing, conciliation.* Men. 27[a] וכן ישראל בה׳ .... באגודה אחת (Ms. M. .... וכן ישראל עד בה׳ אחת) and so is it with Israel's conciliation (with God), which can be achieved only when they are all one brotherhood; (Yalk. Lev. 651: וכן ישראל לא ישובו לארצם עד וכ׳). Kidd. 14[b] להרצאת אדון to make the master willing to dismiss his slave (Deut. XV, 18).—3) (v. רָצָה *Hif.*) *discourse* (on theosophy).—*Pl.* הַרְצָאוֹת. Hag. 14[b].

הַרְקָדָה f. (רָקַד) *shaking* (in the sieve), *sifting.* Pes. 11[a] טחינה וה׳ מא״ל in grinding and sifting (the flour) what change from the ordinary process can he make? Ib. ה׳ ע״ג נפה he does the sifting on the back of the sieve. Y. Sabb. VII, 10[b] bot.; a. e.—Tosef. Men. XI, 4 הַרְקֵידָן.

הרקיא, הרקיה, v. חַרְקִיָּא.

הֶרְקֵיד m. *sifting*, v. הַרְקָדָה.

***הֶרַקְלִיאוֹפוֹלִיס** pr. n. pl. *Heracleopolis*, in Middle Egypt. Pesik. Vayhi, p. 63[b] עיר ההרס זה הרקנו. (corr. acc.) *Ir Haheres* (Is. XIX, 18) is Heracleopolis; Pesik. R. s. 17 סרק אני (corr. acc.). [V., however, Men. 100[a].]

הֶרֶר, pl. הֲרָרִים, v. הַר.

הַרְשָׁאָה f. (רָשָׁה, *Hif.*) *authorization, authority, power of attorney.* Keth. 95[a] נכתבו ה׳ להדדי let the two purchasers of the same property write out a power of attorney to one another (to sue the seller). Shebu. 31[a] הבא בה׳ he who comes before court with a power of attorney (not in his own case). Bekh. 47[b]; a. fr.

***הֶרֶת** f. (b. h., v. Jer. XX, 17; הָרָה) *womb* of an animal. Ber. 44[b]; 57[b]; Ab. Zar. 29[a]. [Oth. opin. *sweetbread, pancreas;* v. רֶתֶת.]

הַרְתָּא f., v. חַרְתָּא.

הרתת, v. רֶתֶת.

הָשֵׁב m. (Inf. Hif. of שוּב) *restoring, giving back.* B. Mets. III, 6 (38[a]) מפני ה׳ אבידה Ms. M. a. Y. ed. (ed. מפני שהוא כמשיב) because the taking care of a trust comes under the duty of restoring a neighbor's lost property; Y. Yeb. II, end, 4[b]; a. e.; v. next w.

הֲשָׁבָה f. same, הֲשָׁבַת אבידה the duty of restoring a neighbor's lost property. B. Kam. V, 7 (54[b]) לה׳ א׳ (Ms. M. a. Y. ed. לְהָשִׁיב; Y. ib. V, end, 5[a] לְהָשֵׁב, v. preced.); Yalk. Ex. 281; a. fr.—*Pl.* הֲשָׁבוֹת. B. Kam. 57[a]; B. Mets. 31[a] מפני . . ריבתה ה׳ הרבה because the Biblical text speaks frequently of restoration (but does nos intimate that the owner must be notified of the restoration).

הֶישׁ׳, הֶשְׁבּוֹן m. (preced.) *making amends for robbery, fraud* &c. (according to Lev. V, 20—26). Yeb. 47[b] לא ניתן לה׳ has not the privilege of making amends (and being atoned for); Ab. Zar. 71[b]. B. Bath. 35[b] לא ניתן לה׳ has no opportunity of &c.—B. Mets. 48[a] להי׳ as amenable to the law &c.

הַשְׁבָּתָה f. (שָׁבַת *Hif.*) *removal* (v. Ex. XII, 15). Pes. 5[a] הַשְׁבָּתַת שְׂאוֹר.—*Pl.* הַשְׁבָּתוֹת. Ib. 10[b] שלש ה׳ בתורה the three injunctions in the Torah concerning the removal of leavened things.

הֶשֵּׂג m. (נָשַׂג) *reaching*, ה׳ יד *regard to one's wealth, the law regulating the payment of certain vows according to one's means* (Lev. XXVII, 8). Arakh. 5[a] נידון בה׳ יד does he come under the law of &c.?—Ib. IV, 1 ה׳ יד בנודר the law of *hesseg yad* is regulated by the means of him who makes the vow; a. e.

הַשָּׂגָה f. same, הַשָּׂגַת יד (Lev. XXV, 26) *having* or *obtaining the necessary means.* Y. Kidd. I, 59[b] top ה׳ יד של עצמו his own obtaining the means of redemption; ה׳ ידי אחרים the furnishing the means by others.

הַשְׁגָּרָה, v. אַשְׁגָּרָה.

הַשְׁכָּרָה f. (denom. of שַׁחַר) *getting up early; early work, study.* Lev. R. s. 19, beg., v. הַעֲרָבָה.

הַשְׁחֵת (Inf. Hif. of שָׁחַת) pr. n. *Hashheth* (*Destruction*), allegorical name of an angel of justice. Ex. R. s. 41, end (ref. to Ps. CVI, 23); ib. s. 44; (Deut. R. s. 3, a. e. מַשְׁחִית).

הַשְׁחָתָה f. (שָׁחַת) 1) *destruction.* Y. Shek. I, 45[d] bot. (ref. to Zeph. III, 7) כל ה׳ . . . בהשכמה וכ׳ whatever destructive work the Israelites undertook, they did with early rising (eagerly). Ex. R. 10, end הַשְׁחָתַת הצפרדעים the injury (to their bodies) caused by the frogs (Ps. LXXVIII, 45); a e.—2) (with ref. to Lev. XIX, 27) *shaving with a razor.* Naz. 57[b]; Kidd. 35[b] כל שישנו בה׳ וכ׳ he to whom the law, 'Thou shalt not destroy' (Lev. l. c.) applies, is subject to the law, 'Ye shall not take off all around &c.', v. הַקָּפָה. Ib. גילות שיש בו ה׳, v. גִּילּוּחַ; a. fr.

הַשִּׁיאָה f. (נָשָׂא, Hif.)=הַסִּיעַ, *diverting the mind* from a question which must not be answered, a *Biblical puzzle of interpretation* used for diverting the mind.—*Pl.* הַשִּׁיאוֹת. Y. Ab. Zar. II, 41[c] bot. (ref. to השיאו, Mish. ib. II, 8) he ought to have diverted his mind by means of one מחמש ה׳ בתורה of the five puzzles &c., v. הַכְרָעָה.

הָשִׁיב, v. הֲשָׁבָה.

הַשְׂכֵּל m. (b. h.; שָׂכַל) *reflection, wisdom.* Lev. R. s. 3, end; a. e.—Esp. *haskel*, one of the expressions for hymns (ref. to מַשְׂכִּיל in Psalm inscriptions). Y. Succ. II, 54[a] top; Y. Meg. I, 72[a] top; (Pes. 117[a] מַשְׂכִּיל).

הַשְׂכָּלָה f. (preced.) *wise reflection, thoughtfulness.* Gen. R. s. 60 (ref. to Prov. XVII, 2) ומהו הַשְׂכָּלָתוֹ and what was his (Eliezer's) reflection?; Yalk. Prov. 956.

הַשְׁכָּמָה f. (שכם, *Hif.*) 1) *early rising, early morning hour.* Sabb. 86[a] בה׳ עלה he went up early in the morning. Sifra K'dosh. ch. III, Par. 2 צא בה׳ start early.—Sabb. 127ª הַשְׁכָּמַת בה״מ coming in good time to college; a. fr.—Trnsf. *eagerness*. Y. Shek. I, 45ᵈ bot., v. הַשְׁחָתָה.—2) *going to labor in the morning*. Y. B. Mets. VII, beg. 11ᵇ שתהא חשלמה (corr. acc.), v. הַעֲרָבָה.

הַשְׁלָחָה f. (שָׁלַח), הַשְׁלָחַת יד *stretching forth of hand, Divine punishment*. Lev. R. s. 20; Num. R. s. 2 (ref. to Ex. XXIV, 11) מכאן שהיו ראויין לה׳ יד from here we learn that they would have deserved punishment at that time. V. הִשְׁתַּלְּחַת.

הַשְׁלָכָה f. (שָׁלַךְ, *Hif.*) *casting away* by the side of the altar (Lev. I, 16). Sifra Vayikra, N'dab., Par. 7, ch. IX אותה אותה בה׳ וכ׳ 'it' intimates, only it (the bird sacrifice) is subject to the rule, 'And he shall cast' &c.

הַשְׁלָמָה f. (שָׁלַם) *completion*. Naz. 8ᵇ מי הוי ה׳ כלל how could he ever have finished the days of vowed nazirate?—Esth. R. to III, 7 הַשְׁלָמַת החומה וכ׳ the completion of the wall of Jerusalem.—Y. B. Mets. VII, beg. 11ᵇ, v. הַשְׁכָּמָה.

הַשְׁמֵד (Infin. Hif. of שָׁמַד) [*extermination*,] *Hashmed*, allegorical name of an angel of justice. Ex. R. s. 41, end; s. 44; Midr. Till. to Ps. VII; a. fr.; (Deut. R. s. 3 (מְכַלֶּה).

הַשְׁמָדָה f. (preced.) *extermination, use of the verb* שמד. Lev. R. s. 7; s. 10.

הֲשָׂמָה f. (שׂוּם, Hif.), הֲשָׂמַת עַיִן *putting an eye upon, paying kind attention to* Gen. R. s. 93 [read:] זו היא ה׳ ע׳ שאמרת נהפך הדבר לסמיות עינים is this the kindness thou hast promised (Gen. XLIV, 21)? This is blindness; (Yalk. Gen. 150 בִּימַת).

הַשְׁמֵט m. (Inf. Hif. of שָׁמַט, v. Deut. XV, 3) *cancelling*, esp. ה׳ כספים *cancelling of (cash) debts in the Sabbatical year*. Y. Shebi. X, 39ᶜ bot.; Y. Gitt. IV, 45ᶜ bot., sq. Y. Macc. I, 31ª bot. כה׳ כספים הוא it is, like a cash debt, forfeited by limitation.

הַשְׁמָטָה f. same. Y. R. Hash. III, 58ᵈ bot. הַשְׁמָטַת כספים. Arakh. 4ª ה׳ קרקע the return of landed property to the seller in the year of the jubilee. Kidd. 38ᵇ ה׳ כ׳ חובת הגוף הוא the remission of cash debts is a personal obligation (not dependent on the land of Palestine); a. fr.

***הֲשָׁפָה** f. (שוף) *smoothing, rubbing, finishing by rubbing*. Tosef. Kel. B. Mets. IV, 1 ed. (ed. Zuck. חטפה, v. חֲטִיפָה).

הַשְׁפָּלָה f. (שָׁפֵל) *lowering, removal from office*. Gen. R. s. 96 ואין מות אלא לשון ה׳ death (Koh. VIII, 8) means removal &c. Ex. R. s. 45 הַשְׁפָּלָתִי, v. הַגְבָּהָה; Lev. R. s. 1; a. e.

הַשְׁפֵּעַ m. (Inf. Hif. of שָׁפַע) *plenty, liberality*. Esth. R. to X, end.

הַשְׁקָאָה, v. הַשְׁקָיָה.

הַשָּׁקָה f. (נָשַׁק, *Hif.*) [*causing contact*,] *dipping of a vessel, filled with an unclean liquid, so as to make its surface level with the surface of the water into which it is dipped*, a ceremony of levitical purification, contrad. to הטבלה, immersion. Bets. 18ª נגזור ה׳ אטו הטבלה let us prohibit levelling as a precaution against immersion (on the Holy Days). Ib.ᵇ קשיא ה׳ the Mishnah permitting *hashshakah* is contradictory (to what Rabbi said in the Boraitha). Hull. 26ᵇ לא סלקא להו ה׳ למיא the *hash.* will not affect the liquid (in the vessel).

הַשְׁקָאָה, הַשְׁקָיָיה, הַשְׁקָיָה f. (שָׁקָה, *Hif.*) *giving to drink*, esp. (הַשְׁקָיַית סוֹטָה) *handing the bitter water to the suspected wife* (Num. V, 24). Meg. II, 7 (20ᵇ) ולהשקיית וכ׳ (Ms. M. ולְהַשְׁקוֹת, Ms. L. לְהַשְׁקָאַת, v. Rabb. D. S. a. l. note). Y. Sot. III, 18ᵈ top מוזיקה סמוכה לה׳ the blotting out must be immediately followed by the giving to drink. Snh. 87ª השקאת; a. fr.

הַשְׁקָפָה f. (שָׁקַף, *Hif.*) *the looking down, the use of the verb* הִשְׁקִיף. Y. Maas. Sh. V, 56ᶜ bot. כל ה׳...ארירה וכ׳ (not ארורה) wherever in the Torah *hishkif* is used, it means curse (punishment), but this (Deut. XXVI, 15) means blessing. Tosef. ib. V, 25 'from thy holy dwelling' זו מקום ה׳ וכ׳ ed. (ed. Zuck. ממעון קדשך השקיפה) that is the place of looking down, i. e. *hashkifah* (Deut. l. c.) refers only to 'thy holy dwelling', 'and bless' to 'from (the store of) the heavens'.

הַשְׁרָשָׁה f. (שָׁרַשׁ, *Hif.*) *taking root*. Pes. 55ª ובה׳ and as to counting the third day after planting for taking root. Y. Shebi. II, 34ª top אחר ה׳ we go by the date of taking root. Y. Kil. I, 27ᵇ אינו רוצה בהַשְׁרָשָׁתָן he has no interest in their taking root; Y. Maasr. V, 51ᵈ top. Men. 69ª; a. fr.

הַשְׁתָּא (=הָא שַׁעְתָּא) 1) *now*. Targ. Prov. VII, 24; a. fr.—Sabb. 91ª, a. fr. בתר ה׳ אזלינן we go by the present condition. Pes. 4ª וה׳ דקי״ל and now that it is established that &c. Hull. 97ª ה׳ דאמר וכ׳ now that R. . . says &c.; a. v. fr.—ה׳ הכי *so now!, indeed*, i. e. *how can you compare these two cases?* Snh. 41ᵇ; a. fr.—2) (introducing an argument) *since, when, if*. Hull. 5ᵇ, a. fr. ה׳ בהמתן . . . . לא כל שכן since the Lord does not allow any evil to come through a beast belonging to the righteous, how much less through the righteous themselves? Ib. 6ᵇ ה׳ מיגזל גזלה חלופי מיבעיא if she would take what is not her own, is there any question that she would eventually exchange her own for what belongs to her neighbor?; a. fr.

הִשְׁתַּחֲוָאָה, הִשְׁתַּחֲוָיָה, ...יָיה, הִשְׁתַּחֲו׳ f. (שָׁחָה, *Hithpa.*) *prostration* for prayer. Ber. 34ᵇ; Meg. 22ᵇ ה׳ זו פישוט וכ׳ prostration means spreading out hands and feet. Y. Ber. I, 3ᵈ top לך ה׳ before Thee prostration is due; a. fr.—[Y. Ab. Zar. IV, 43ᵈ top שְׁתַּחֲוָיָה.]—*Pl.* הִשְׁתַּחֲוָיוֹת, הִשְׁתַּחֲוָ׳. Shek. VI, 1. Ber. 31ª מפני כריעות וה׳ in consequence of his repeated kneelings and prostrations.

הִשְׁתַּלַּח m., v. next w.

הִשְׁתַּלְּחוּת f. (שָׁלַח, *Hithpa.*) ה׳ יד *being stricken by divine hand, divine visitation*, v. הַשְׁלָחָה. Num. R. s. 15 Var. (ed. הִשְׁתַּלְּחָה); Tanh. B'haäl. 16 להשתלח; (ib. ed. Bub. 27 לְטִירוּף).

השתק, Koh. R. to I, 5 מערטלו ומהשתקו ומנרתקו, read: מערטלו מְנַרְתְּקוֹ, or מִנַּשְׁתְּקוֹ; v. נַרְתֵּק a. נַשְׁתֵּק.

***הֲתוֹבְתָא** f. (תּוּב *Af.*) *argument, objection.—Pl.* הֲתוֹבָתָה. Y. Peah IV, 18[b] top כל אילין ה׳ וכ׳ all objections which R. Z. brought forth. V. תְּיוּבְתָּא.

הַתָּזָה f. (נָתַז) *knocking off, cutting off.* Y. Snh. VII, 24[b] bot. הַתָּזַת הראש decapitation.

הַתְחָלָה f. (חלל *Hif.*) *beginning, preliminary act.* Sabb. 9[b] הַתְחָלַת התספורת the preparations for hair-cutting.—Ex. R. s. 1 אין ויואל אלא לשון ה׳ *vayoël* (Ex. II, 21) has the meaning of beginning (attempting). Ber. 14[b] היא ה׳ is considered a beginning of the recitation (and you must finish it); a. fr.—*Pl.* הַתְחָלוֹת. Mekh. Yithro, Bahod., s. 2 כל ה׳ קשות all beginnings are difficult. Cmp. אַתְחַלְתָּא.

הֲתֵירָא, הֲתֵיר, v. הֵיתֵ׳.

התך, *Pi.* הִיתֵּךְ (sec. verb of נתך, fr. *Hif.*) *to melt. Part. pass.* מְהוּתָּךְ; חלב מה׳ melted tallow. Y. Sabb. II, 4[d] top; Bab. ib. 21[a].

הַתְלִיטִים m., Ar., Var. for אַתְלִיטִים.

הַתְלָעָה f. (תָּלַע *Hif.*) *being worm-eaten, rottenness.* B. Kam. 52[b] הוי פושע לענין ה׳ he is guilty of criminal carelessness when the cover of the pit became rotten.

הָתָם (=הָא תָּם, v. תָּם II) *there; in that case;* opp. הָכָא q. v. Y. Ber. I, 3[d] bot. רבנן דה׳ the Babylonian teachers. Snh. 5[a] מה׳ לה׳ from Palestine for Palestine. Ib.[b] ה׳ שאני there, in the case just cited, it is different; a. v. fr.

***התם**, Y. Ber. VII, 12[a] אכלין ה׳ אכל בה׳ (some vers. כה׳); בה׳ (some vers. כי ה׳, כה׳), read בְּמַפָּה; v. Hull. 107[a], sq.

הַתְקָנָה f. (תָּקַן, v. תַּקָּנָה) *amendment*, i. e. *a rabbinical measure* to prevent transgression of a law. Y. Succ. III, end, 54[a] ה׳ אחר ה׳ a rabbinical measure to fortify a rabbinical measure; cmp. גְּזֵירָה.

הֶתֵּרָא, הֶתֵּר, v. הֵיתֵ׳.

הַתְרָאָה, v. הַתְרָיָה.

הַתָּרָה f. (נָתַר *Hif.*) 1) *untying, loosening.* Y. Yeb. XII, 12[c], a. e. ה׳, or הַתָּרַת הרצועות the untying of the shoe strings by the brother's wife, v. חֲלִיצָה. Sot. I, 16[c] bot. ה׳ הסינר loosening of the pantaloons; a. e.—2) (=הֵיתֵר) *permission, declaring permitted.* Y. Sabb. XVII, 16[a] bot. קודם לְהַתָּרַת כלים prior to the passage of the law permitting the handling of tools on the Sabbath (Mish. XVII, 1); Bab. ib. 123[b]. Snh. 58[b] מאימת הַתָּרָתָהּ when is she again considered free?

הַתְרָאָה, הַתְרָיָיה, הַתְרָיָה f. (תָּרָה *Hif.*) *making one acquainted with the law on a certain subject,* esp. *the legal warning, by witnesses, given to the offender immediately before committing the offense.* Snh. 8[b], a. e. חבר אינו צריך ה׳ וכ׳ a student requires no warning, for the law requiring warning is intended only to enable the court to decide between the willful and the ignorant offender. Shebu. 3[b], a. fr. הַתְרָאַת כספק a warning under doubt, e. g. one swears that he will do a certain thing during this day, when the actual moment of the offense (of omission) cannot be defined, so as to make the warning precede it immediately. Y. Pes. V, 32[c] top מקבלין התרייה על ספק warning is accepted (considered legal) on a doubtful offense; a. fr.—*Pl.* הַתְרָאוֹת, הַתְרָיוֹת. Y. B. Kam. VII, 5[d] bot.; a. e.

הַתְרָעָה f. (תָּרַע, *Hif.*) *sounding the alarm on public fast-days* (with the Shofar and prayer עֲנֵינוּ). Taan. 14[a].—*Pl.* הַתְרָעוֹת. Ib.

ו

ו *Vav*, the sixth letter of the Alphabet. It interchanges wit ב, as אִיסְטָוָוא a. אִיסְטַבָא, a. fr.; v. letter ב; also with ע as וָתִיק a. b. h. עָתֵק (v. וֶסֶת); v. also letter י. In inflections ו interchanges with, and is the equivalent of י. [To give ו the value of a consonant, וו is frequently used for ו, as ווסת and וֶסֶת.—For lexicographical purposes ignore the second ו in words beginning with וו.—As a vowel sign *u* or *o* (וּ, וֹ). In words of foreign derivation וּ (*u*) is frequently inserted where the originals have *a*, as גּוּלְיָיר for *galearis* &c.]

ו׳, as a numeral, *six*, v. א׳.

וְ, וּ, a prefix, *and, but;* often introducing a question: *but, is it indeed so?* Hull. 2[a] וכל הכל וכ׳ is it so that wherever הַכֹּל is used, it means &c.? Ib. והא כתיב וכ׳ is it not written &c.?; a. fr.

ווא, ווה pr. n. m. *Va, Vah,* abbrev. of אַבָּא. Y. Ber. III, 6[d] bot. Ib. 6[a] top; a. fr. V. אַבָּא II.

וא"ו, וי"ו, ו"ו, *Vav*, name of the sixth letter of the Alphabet. Kidd. 30[a] וא"ו דגחון חציין וכ׳ the Vav in *Gahon* (Lev. XI, 42) marks the (first) half of the number of letters in the Pentateuch. Ib. וא"ו . . מהאר

גיסא וכ׳ does the Vav of *gahon* belong to the first half or to the second?—Gen. R. s. 58 Ephron (Gen. XXIII, 16) is spelt חסר וא״ו without Vav; a. fr.—Y. Shebu. I, 33ª bot. ושעיר וי״ו מוסיף וכ׳ the Vav in Us'ir (Num. XXVIII, 22) adds to the preceding subject, i. e. a goat in addition to &c. Kidd. 66ᵇ וי״ו דשלום וכ׳ the Vav in Shalom (Num. XXV, 12) is curtailed (so that it may be read *Shalem*, unblemished). Ḥull. 16ª, v. אוּפְתָּא. B. Mets. 87ª; Meg. 16ᵇ, v. לִבְרוּת.—Yoma 45ª, a. fr. וא״ו לא דרשי they do not use the Vav for interpretation; a. fr.—*Pl.* וָוִי״ם, וָוִי״ן. Y. Meg. I, 71ᶜ top (deriving from ווי העמודים, Ex. XXVII, 10) שיהא ווים וכ׳ that the shape of the Vav in the Pentateuch is column-like (as in כתב אשורית); Snh. 22ª ....מה אף ווים וכ׳ as the columns have not changed (their shape), so has not the shape of the Vav. Y. Naz. I, 51ᵇ top עד שיזכיר ו׳ he must utter the Vav conjunctive. Ib. IV, beg. 53ª מאן תאנא ו׳ who is it that says the Vav must be uttered?; Y. Kidd. II, 62ᵇ; a. fr.

וָאי=וַי; v. וָה.

וְאֵלֶּה שְׁמוֹת, ו׳ *V'elleh Sh'moth* (*and these are the names of*), name of the second Book of Moses, *Exodus*. Gen. R. s. 3; Yalk. ib. 4.

וָאלִי f. (ואל, cmp. b. h. יָאַל a. הוֹאִיל) *propriety.* לא ו׳ *it is unbecoming.* Ned. 8ᵇ לא ו׳ למישרא וכ׳ Ar. (ed. שרי, Var. יאי; Naḥm. יאלי) it is unbecoming (for a pupil) to absolve from a vow in a place where his teacher lives. Contr. וָלָא.

וָואנַיי, וָאנַי pr. n. *Vânay*, name of a river or canal in Babylonia. Kidd. 71ᵇ נהר ואני Ar. (ed. יואני); Y. ib. IV, 65ᵈ top וואניי; Y. Yeb. I, 3ᵇ top וואניי. Gen. R. s. 16 (א)עברות נהר ו׳ Ar. (ed. only נהרא) at the ford of &c. [Erub. 28ᵇ בית ואני Ms. M., v. הִינִי 3.] ['Nahr-Avan, a canal east of the Tigris', Neub. Géogr. p. 324.—'Nahrvân in Irak Arabi', Koh. Ar. Compl. s. v. ואני.]

וַארְדוּנְיָא, v. וַרְדִּינָא II.

ובא, Midr. Till. to Ps. XVII, v. בְּאִיָּן.

וביבא, Lam. R. to I, 5, v. בִּיבִי.

וגודי, Yalk. Gen. 150, v. זוֹגָא.

וַדָּאָה f., pl. וַדָּאוֹת (v. next w.) *certainties.* B. Mets. 83ᵇ ו׳ שלכם cases in which you act on ascertained facts.

וַדַּאי, וַדִּי, וַוַדִּי m., **וַדָּאִית, וַדָּיִית (וַדָּאָה)** f. (ידע) 1) *well-known, certain; distinct, real.* Ber. 33ᵇ הו׳ (v. Rabb. D. S. a. l. note) Thou, the known one!—Arakh. I, 1 זכר ו׳ a person distinctly male, נקבה ודאית distinctly female (no hermaphrodite &c.). Yoma VIII, 8, a. fr. אשם ו׳, v. אָשָׁם.—Sabb. II, 7 הו׳ that which undoubtedly requires the separation of the tithes, opp. דְּמַאי.—Y. Bets. I, 60ᵇ וַדָּיָיתָהּ, וַדָּיוֹ where there is no doubt about it, opp. ספיקה, ספיקו. Kidd. IV, 3 (74ª) וַדָּאָן the sure cases among them.—Num. R. s. 2, end אכילה וודייה Ar. ed. Koh. (ed. ודאית) the eating (in Ex. XXIV, 11) was a real one (physical refreshment, no metaphor); a. v. fr.—2) (gramm.) *emphatic form* by means of *He* paragogic. Ex. R. s. 3 לכה וודאית וכ׳ (strike out the gloss הה״א בסוף וכ׳) the word *l'khah* (Ex. III, 3) is emphatic (as if=לָךְ *unto thee* it belongs), if not thou &c.; Y. Succ. IV, 54ᶜ top לך יודייה (read: לכה וו׳) the *l'khah* (Ps. LXXX, 3) has the emphatic form (*unto thee* as well as unto us).—3) (noun) *certainty, undisputed fact.*—אין ספק מוציא מידי ו׳ doubt cannot take a case out of the status of certainty. Ab. Zar. 41ᵇ הוי ספק וו׳ ואין וכ׳ here is a doubt (the idolatrous character of an object may have been given up) against a certainty (that it *was* an idol) and the doubt cannot set aside the certainty. Pes. 9ª; a. fr.—בְּו׳, ו׳ (adv.) *surely, indeed; in reality.* Y. Keth. V, 29ᵈ. Gen. R. s. 98 עלית בו׳ 'thou didst ascend' thy father's couch (Gen. XLIX, 4) means in reality (no metaphor). Ib. חללת ו׳ 'thou didst defile' (ib.) is to be taken literally. Pes. l. c. דו׳ מעשרי for it is sure that they separate the tithes. Gen. R. s. 55 נסה אותו בו׳ He tried him in the true sense of the word (gave him time); a. e.

וָדָה, *Pi.* וִידָּה, *Hithpa.* הִתְוַדָּה, v. יָדָה.—Denom. וִידּוּי.

וודי, v. יְדָאִי.

ודי, *Pa.* וַדִּי, *Af.* אוֹדִי, v. ידי.

ודנין, Tosef. Dem. I, 27, Var. ed. Zuck., v. יירדנון.

וְדַע, וָדַע, v. יְדַע, יָדַע.

וודעא, Y. Bicc. III, 65ᶜ bot., v. וַיְעְדָא.

וָוה pr. n. m., v. וָוא.

וָהּ, וָוהּ (הֲוָהּ) (interj.; cmp. b. h. הֶאָח, הָהּ) *vah* (*hăvah*), an exclamation of pleasure; *ah!* &c., contradist. to ווי (woe!). Lam. R. to I, 5 לכה אמרת ווי אמר וה אמרי (Ar. ואי) why didst thou exclaim, *Vay* (woe!)? Said he, I said *Vah.* Ib. בין וי לוה וכ׳ between *Vay* and *Vah* R. Joh. escaped.—Pesik. Asser, p. 97ᵇ בתחלה הם אומרים וה ולבסוף הם אומרים ווי at first (on entering the hot and again the cold place) they say *Vah* (how pleasant!), but finally they say *Vay* (woe!); Tanh. R'eh 13 הוה; Tanh. ed. Bub., ib. 10; Yalk. Deut. 892; (diff. versions: Y. Snh. X, 29ᵇ bot.; Yalk. Ps. 737). Pesik. l. c. (play on הֶאָח, Ps. XL, 3) ממקום שאומרים וה ווי (not שאומר) from the place where they (the wicked) say *Vah* and (then) *Vay*; Tanh. ed. Bub. l. c. וה ווי; Tanh. l. c. (corr. acc.); Yalk. Deut. l. c. הי ווי; (differ. vers. in Yalk. Ps. l. c. a. Y. l. c.).

וָו m. 1) (b. h.) *hook.*—*Pl.* וָוִים. Ex. R. s. 51; a. fr.—2) the letter *Vav.*—*Pl.* וָוִים, וָוִין; v. וא״ו.

וָו ch. same.—*Pl.* וָוִין, וָוַיָּא. Targ. Ex. XXXVIII, 28. Ib. XXVII, 10; a. fr.

וּו=יְהוּ. Y. Snh. X, 29ᵇ top וא״ל and he said to him.

וזרד, Tosef. Kil. III, 15 Var. ed. Zuck., v. יְזַרְד.

וחי, *Af.* אוֹחִי, אַיְוחִי, v. יְחִי.

וחר, *Af.* אוֹחַר, אַיְוחַר; *Pa.* ווחר, v. אחר.

*וָטִיב, וָטוּב m. (ויטב) *sexual gratification.* Shebu. 18ª Ar. (read וְטִיבוֹ) עד שימות וטיבו until his gratification dies out; [Ar.: membrum virile; Hal. G'dol. אבירו, v. Perl. Et. St. p. 65].—Ed. וְטוּבֵיה Chald. form; [Rashi: וְטוּבֵיה *and well is it with him,* in which case it must read עד שימות הגיד ו׳, v. Ar. s. v. מת].

ווס, v. sub וס.

וַי, וַיי, וָוי, וָי m. h. a. ch. 1) *woe;* (interj.) *oh! woe!* Targ. Prov. XXIII, 29 ed. Wil. (ed. Lag. וָיָא or וַיָּא).—Targ. Ps. CXX, 5; a. fr.—Gen. R. s. 26 לא ישלה ווי מפומך the word *woe* shall never cease from thy lips. Ib. ווי דלא וכ׳ woe that my son does not eat &c. Ab. Zar. 11ᵇ ו׳ לדין כד וכ׳ woe to this one (Esau), when that one (Jacob) shall rise. Meg. 16ª ווי מביתא וכ׳ woe from inside, woe from outside! Ib. 11ª (play on *vayhi,* Esth. I, 1) ווי והי הדא וכ׳ (Ms. M. ווי הוה מה וכ׳; v. Rabb. D. S. a. l. note, a. marg. note in ed.) woe and grief, as it is written &c.; a. fr.—2) *the preformative* וַי in the Imperfect with Vav Conversive.—*Pl.* וַוִין. Snh. 70ª י״ג ו׳ נאמרו ביין thirteen times do we read *vay* (woe) in the chapter about wine (Gen. IX, 20 to 24); Gen. R. s. 36 כתיב בה ו׳ י״ד פעמים fourteen times &c. (ib. 20 to 25).

וַיָּא, וָיָא, v. preced.

וַיְדַבֵּר *Vaydabber (and he spoke),* name of the Fourth Book of Moses, *Numbers.* Gen. R. s. 64 ספר ו׳. Ib. עביד ו׳ תלתא וכ׳ divided the Book of Numbers into three books. Yalk. Gen. 4 ספר ו׳ (Gen. R. s. 3 בְּמִדְבַּר).

וִידּוּי m. (יָדָה) *confession of sin, prayer for pardon.* Tosef. Yoma V (IV), 14; Yoma 87ᵇ מצות ו׳ ערב וכ׳ the proper time for confession (on the entrance of the Day of Atonement) is &c. Ib. וחותם בו׳ and closes the benediction with an allusion to confession (forgiveness). Y. ib. VI, 43ᶜ הו׳ מעכב the confession (by the Highpriest, Lev. XVI, 21) is indispensible for the legality of the act. Snh. VI, 2 וידוויו his (Achan's) confession; a. fr.—*Pl.* (Chald.) וִידּוּיִן, וִידּוּיִין. Shebu. 14ª תרי ו׳ (Ms. F. שני; Rashi וידויי) two confessions (Lev. XVI, 6 a. 11).

וויי, v. וַי.

ווייאדן, v. בְּאַזְוָארָן.

ווייִדָא, v. חַיְידָא.

וויירינון, v, ויירינון.

ווייִתְנִיא, v. וְתָנָא.

וִילוֹן, וִילָאוֹת, v. next w.

וִילוֹן m. (velum, βῆλον) *door-curtain, curtain.* Targ. Y. Ex. XXXVI, 37.—Kel. XX, 6 ועשאו ו׳ (Ar. בילן) and made of it a curtain (or sail); Tosef. ib. B. Mets. XI, 8. Bets. 14ᵇ bot. ו׳ טמא וכ׳ a door-curtain is subject to levitical uncleanness, because &c. Sabb. 138ª; Erub. 102ª. Gen. R. s. 52, beg. [read:] ווילון מונח בינרהם with a curtain let down between them; ib. s. 74; Lev. R. s. 1; Yalk. Job 897. Esth. R. to I, 6 נגללין כו׳ זה וכ׳ they were rolled up like the curtain before the ark of the Law; a. fr.—Esp. *Vilon* (Curtain), the lowest of the seven heavens. Hag. 12ᵇ. Ber. 58ᵇ ו׳ הוא דמגלגל Ms. M. (ed. דמקרע דמגלגל, one of which is a gloss) the Curtain is rolled up (torn apart).—*Pl.* וִילָאוֹת. B. Bath. IV, 6 (67ᵇ) את הו׳ Mish. a. Ms. M. (Bab. ed. בלנרות, Y. ed. בולניות) the curtains belonging to the bath-house. Ib. 67ᵇ בית הו׳ the room in which the curtains are kept. Tosef. ib. III, 1 [read:] לא את הו׳ (ולא את הוילסאות ולא את המרחצאות), Var. הוילסאות, being a copyist's corrupt tautography).—Chald. pl.: וִילָוָתָא. Targ. Ps. CV, 39 (not וִילָתָא).—וִילָוָן. Targ. Y. Ex. XXVII, 9 (ed. Amst. וִילָוָן; Y. II וִילָוָון, read: וִילָוָון); ib. XXXVIII, 9 וִילָוֵי (corr. acc.). Ib. 12; 14 וִילָוָן (corr. acc.). Ib. 15 וִלָוָן.—וִילָוָתָא, constr. וִילָוַת. Ib. XXXV, 17 וְוִילָוַת (corr. acc.). Targ. Y. Num. III, 26 וִלָוַות.

ווילסאות, v. preced.

וִינוֹן=וְאִינוּן, v. וִינוּן.

וַיְנָיָא (וַהוּנ׳) וַיְנַיָּיה, m. pl. (denom. of וַי or וָה) *woe-makers,* a word coined in opposition to הוללים (merry-makers), and defined by אללי as a play on הולל-. Pesik. Ahăre, p. 170ª קרי להון ווי נייה אלו שביאין אללי וכ׳ (Ar. וחיינא, corr. acc.) called them (the hol'lim, Ps. LXXV, 5) *vayyanaya,* those who bring *al'lay* (woe) &c.; Lev. R. s. 17 זהוניא (corr. acc.; ib. s. 20 אלליא); Tanh. Ahăre 2 זה והנייא ed. princ. (later ed. פסוק זה הוללים, corr. acc.); Tanh., ed. Bub., ib. 3 דהוניא; Yalk. Lev. 524 וי ויניה (corr. acc.); Yalk. Ps. 811 זוהוניא, זוהונייא (corr. acc.).

וויס, v. ווס sub וס.

וויסט, v. וָשֶׁט.

וויסלאות, v. וִילוֹן.

וִיעוּד m. (יָעַד; cmp. וַועַד) *place of meeting, appointment.*—*Pl.* וִיעוּדִין. Lam. R. to II, 13; Pesik. Nah., p. 125ª כמה ו׳ ויעדתי בכם how many appointments did I arrange with you (Tabernacle, Temple &c.)!

וַיִּקְרָא *Vayyikra (and he called),* name of the Third Book of Moses, *Leviticus.* Gen. R. s. 3 ספר ו׳; ib. s. 64; v. וַיְדַבֵּר.

וִיתּוּר m. (וָתַר) *the retailer's customary addition to exact measure.* Ned. 32ᵇ; B. Bath. 57ᵇ, a. e. אפילו ו׳ אסור וכ׳ if one forswears himself any benefit from his neighbor, he dare not even accept the customary addition &c.

וִיתִּינְיָא, v. וְתִינְיָא.

וויתוקין, v. וִיתֵּק.

וויתירה, Y. Keth. IV, end, 29ᵇ, v. וָתַר.

ווִיתְנִיא, v. וְתָנָא.

וִיתֵּק m. (ותק; cmp. עתק) 1) *frail, weak-nerved.*—*Pl.* וִיתְּקִין. Gitt. 70ª ו׳ הוויין ליה בנים (Ar. וַתִּיקִין, וחוקין) will have sickly children; Nidd. 17ª הוין לו וכ׳; Keth. 77ᵇ ויתיקין (Asheri ויתקין; Alf. נִכְפִּין *epileptic*); Treat. Kallah ויתקין (some ed. וותר׳).—2) (sub. מַכָּה or a similar w.) f. *senility, debility.* Gitt. l. c. אחזתו ו׳ debility will befall him.

ויִתְּרוֹן m. (וָתַר) *rest, remnant.* Gen. R. s. 98 (expl. אל תותר, Gen. XLIX, 4) אל יהר לך וִיתְּרוֹן עון שלך there will be no remnant of thy sin left (but will all be forgiven.)

וְכַח, וָכַח, v. יְכַח, יָכַח.

וִול, ו׳ שְׁפָט, B. Bath. 98ª, v. בַּלְשְׁפָט.

וָלָא m. (v. וְאִלִּי; P. Sm. 1062 ולא) *(it is) becoming.* Targ. Prov. XXIV, 26 ו׳ שיפותיה וכ׳ Ms. (in ed. our w. omitted) it is becoming that the lips be kissed of those &c.

וְלַד, וָלָד, v. יְלַד, יָלַד.

וָולָד, וָלָד, constr. וְלַד m. (b. h.; יָלַד) *child, infant; young of an animal; offspring; embryo.* Y. Yeb. VII, 8ª וְלַד בהמת וכ׳ the young of a domestic animal &c., v. מְלוֹג; ו׳ שפחה וכ׳ the child of a slave &c.—Sabb. 63ᵇ כבר נד ו׳ the embryo is already loosened (abortion must follow). Snh. 22ª; Sot. 2ª קודם יצירת הו׳ before the embryo assumes distinct shape. Lev. R. s. 14 צורות הו׳ the successive shapes of the embryo. Kidd. III, 12 הו׳ הולך אחר הזכר the child has the legal status of the father. Ib וְלָדָהּ כמותה her child has her legal status; a. fr.—*Pl.* וְלָדוֹת, וְוָלָ׳; constr. וְלְדֵי. B. Kam. VIII, 2 דמי ו׳ damages for causing abortion. Bekh. II, 4 ולדי ו׳ the second generation of sheep sold on condition of dividing the young with the (gentile) seller until payment in full, v. בַּרְזֶל; a. fr.—Y. Keth. VII, 31ᵇ bot. המקללת את וְלָדָיו בפני יולדיו who curses his (her husband's) children in the presence of his parents; Bab. ib. 72ᵇ מולידיו . . רולידיו, v. יָלַד.—וְלַד הטומאה, v. אָב.

וַלְדָּא (וָולַד) וְלַד ch. same. Targ. Gen. XI, 30; a. fr.—Sabb. 63ᵇ איתעקר וַלְדָּהּ her foetus was loosened; v. preced.—*Pl.* וַלְדִּין. Targ. Y. II Gen. XXXII, 16; a. e.—בית ולדא *womb.* Targ. Y. Gen. XX, 18; O. פְּתַח ו׳.—Targ. O. Gen. XL, 20 יום בית ו׳ דפ׳ the festival of Pharaoh's *mother.*

וַלְדָנִית f. (preced.) *a handmaid intended for breeding slave children, breeder.* Y. B. Kam. V, 5ª top שפחה ו׳ אני וכ׳ I sell thee a breeder.

וָלֵס, וָלִיס p. n. m. (Οὐάλης, Valens) *Valis,* an Amora, father of R. Hillel. Gitt. 59ª; Snh. 36ª (Ms. M. ולס, Ar. ed. Koh. ווילס); Y. Kil. II, 32ª top; ib. I, 27ª top אלס.—Y. Ḥall. I, 57ᶜ bot. חלים (ed. Krot. ה׳, read: וו׳). V. Frank. M'bo p. 76. Cmp. בָּאלִי.

וְסִי, וִיס, ווּס (Arab. *vasha* colorare) *to color, stain.*—*Ithp.* אִיתְוָוס, אִיתְוִיס, אִיתְוְסָא *to be stained, soiled.* Sabb. 75ᵇ דְּלִיתְוִיס בית השחיטה (Ms. M. דניתויס) that the throat of the slaughtered animal be stained with blood. Ib. 124ᵇ אִתְוִוס מסנאיה טינא Ms. O. (ed. אתוסאר, Ar. ed. Koh. איתווס מאניה; ed. Sonc. אִתְוְוסַר) his shoes were soiled with mud. Pes. 65ᵇ; Zeb. 35ª מִיתְוְוסֵי מאנייהו their garments would be soiled (with blood). Yoma 53ª מִתְוְוסָן אסקופתא וכ׳ (Ms. M. 2 מִתְוְוסָא sing.) the thresholds &c.—B. Kam. 18ª דמתווס בלישא Ar. a. Ms. F. (v. Rabb. D. S. a. l. note 80, ed. דמאוס, corr. acc.) the rope was covered with dough (which attracted the chickens).

וֶסֶת, ו׳ וֶוֹ׳ f. (וָסַת, intensive of עָשָׂה; as to ע a. י (ו), v. Nöld. Mand. Gr. p. 72) [*habitual doing, condition,*] 1) *regular diet.* Snh. 101ª; Keth. 110ᵇ, a. e. שינוי ו׳ וכ׳ a change of diet is the beginning of bowel diseases.—2) *conduct, way, manner.* Y. Yoma I, 38ᶜ bot. כל ו׳ טובה וכ׳ every kind of good manners was found among them. Gen. R. s. 87 כך הו׳ וֶסֶתָן של וכ׳ this was the custom of the gentiles. Ned. IX, 9 כך היא וֶסֶתוֹ של וכ׳ such is that man's way of acting.—3) *regular date,* or *regular premonitory symptoms, of menstruation.* Nidd. I, 1 כל אשה שיש לה ו׳ every woman of regular days &c. Ib. 4ᵇ שלא בשעת וֶסֶתָהּ out of her regular time. Ib. 11ᵇ אשה שאין לה ו׳ a woman who has no regular time. Ib. IX, 8 (63ª) שיש לה ו׳ that has regular symptoms of approaching menstruation, v. infra. [Ib. 12ª; 14ᵇ שיעור ו׳, v. אֱוְותִיאוֹס.] Tosef. ib. I, 11 כיוונה שעת וסתה she had her courses again (after an intermission) exactly at the usual date; Y. ib. I, 49ᶜ top כיוונה מחמ׳ הווסת (corr. acc.). Ib. וו׳ ארוכה a delayed menstruation (which may be expected any time), contrad. to הפסק עונה a skipping over of one course; a. fr.—*Pl.* וֶסֶתוֹת. Ib. IX, 8 ואלו הן הו׳ and these are the symptoms of approaching &c. Ib. 63ª התם בו׳ דיומי there (ib. I, 1) regularity of date is meant, הכא בו׳ דגופא here regularity of symptoms. Ib. 15ª, a. e. ו׳ דאורייתא the rule requiring a woman to examine herself on the regular day is of biblical origin. Yeb. 64ᵇ bot. ו׳ ושור וכ׳ the law concerning the mode of establishing a regularity of menstruation (Nidd. IX, 10) &c.—Gen. R. s. 48 (expl. עדנה, Gen. XVIII, 12), v. וֶוסְתָּנִית; a. fr.

וֶוסְתָּא ch. as preced. 3. Targ. Y. Lev. XV, 31 (v. Nidd. 63ᵇ). [Lev. R. s. 28, end מטי׳ ווסתיה, read מנר מסותיה, v. מְסוּתָא.]

וַוסְתַּנְיָא pr. n. pl. *Vastania,* birth-place of R. Ḥiya. Taan. 9ª bot.; Zeb. 112ª Ms. R. a. K. (Ms. M. חסדא מיוסתניא, ed. חייא מיוסתני׳; perhaps identical with הוסניא, Yeb. 21ᵇ); v. also אִסְתּוּנְיָא. [V. Neub. Géogr. p. 391; Berl. Beitr. Geogr. p. 37.]

***וֶוסְתָּנִית** f. (וֶוסֶת) *a woman with regular menstruation.* Yalk. Gen. 82 (expl. עדנה, Gen. XVIII, 12) עדנה עדנין ו׳ *ednah* is related to *iddanin* (Dan. VII, 25, periods), and means a woman &c. (differ. in Gen. R. s. 48, v. וֶוסֶת).

וָעַד, *Pi.* וִיעֵד, v. יָעַד.

וַעַד, ו׳ וַ׳ m. (preced.) 1) *meeting, appointment.* בֵּית ו׳ *meeting place.* Ab. I, 4 let thy house be בית ו׳ וכ׳ a meeting place for scholars.—Esp. בית ו׳ a) *scholars' meeting place,* *college, Beth-ham-Midrash.* Y. Ber. IV, 7c bot. . . למחר לבית הו׳ to-morrow, when I come to college &c. Y. Macc. II, 31d bot. עושים לו בית ו׳ you must provide a school-house for him. Sot. IX, 15 (49b) בי ו׳ יהיה וכ׳ the school-house will be used for debauchery. Gen. R. s. 1; a. fr.—b) בֵּית הַוַּ׳ *the Temple.* Y. Naz. VIII, 57a bot. . . . שלא תנעול מבית הו׳ so as not to lock out repentance from the Temple.—2) *fair, public games.* Hull. 127a; cmp. אֲבִידָן.

ווַעֲדָא ch. same; בי ו׳ (בית) *college.* Y. Ber. II, 5c bot. Y. Meg. I, 71d נעביד בי ו׳ let us have school; a. fr.

וְעָדָה f. (preced. wds.) *appointment, designation of time; insuspensibility.* Y. Yoma VI, 43d bot. ו׳ שכתוב בה במועדו לית שמע מינה כלום from an appointment (of time or space) in a biblical law where the word בְּמוֹעֲדוֹ is used, we can derive nothing (for other actions). Ib. [read:] ואמר ליה רבי בון בר חייה קיים בפר משיח ו׳ and he said to him, R. B. bar H. applied the designation of time, i. e. the rule of insuspensibility, even to the offering of the anointed priest.

ועדוין, v. וְעוֹדִי.

וְעוֹד m. [*and something besides,*] *addition, increase.* Erub. 83a כמה ו׳ how much is that 'and something'?—*Pl.* וְעוֹדוֹת *additions.* Ib. אייתי ו׳ דרבי וכ׳ bring along the additions which Rabbi speaks of, and add them thereto. Ib. bot. בו׳ דרבי Ms. M. a. Rashi (ed. ועודיות של רבי, corr. acc.).

וְעוֹדִי m. (denom. of preced.) *with addition, large measure.*—*Pl.* וְעוֹדִיִּין. Men. VII, 2 (78a) שש עשרונות ו׳ Talm. ed. (Mish. ועדוין, read: וְעוֹדִיִּין; v. Rabb. D. S. a. l., note 9) six tenths (of an Epha), large measure.—[וְעוֹדִיּוֹת, v. preced.]

ועי, *Af.* אַוְעֵי, v. וְעָא.

ווּעידא, Targ. Prov. VII, 20 Ms. ליומא ו׳, ed. ליומא דעידא, v. עִידָא.

וועצא, Targ. Cant. II, 2 some ed., read נִעְרְצָא.

ווקלמה, Y. Sabb. VII, 10a bot., Or Z'rua Sabb. Nr. 57 בוקלמה, read: וּמִלְקְמָן, v. מסבסלה.

וקתא, Targ. Prov. XIV, 3, v. זַקְתָּא.

***וֶרֶד** I m. (ירד; cmp. מוֹרָד I) *valley.* Lev. R. s. 23; Cant. R. to II, 2 שושנה אחת של ו׳ a lily of the valley (שושנת העמקים, Cant. II, 1).

וֶרֶד II m. (Arab. *vard* flos arboris; rosa) 1) *rose, rose-tree;* (collectively) *roses.* Shebi. VII, 6 הו׳ the rose-tree. Ib. 7 ו׳ חדש roses of the new crop. Y. ib. beg. 37b עיקר הו׳ the rose-tree itself (the wood); Tosef. ib. V, 7 חרוב (corr. acc.). Sabb. XIV, 4 שמן ו׳ rose-oil; a. fr.—Y. Kil. V, end, 30a הקנים והאגין והו׳ וכ׳; Tosef. ib. III, 15 והוורד ed. Zuck. (Var. והוורד); Erub. 34b Ms. M. והאורדין (Rashi והוורדין, ed. omitted; corr. acc. or plur.).—*Pl.* וְרָדִים, וְרָדִין. Maasr. II, 5 גינת ו׳ rose-garden (for the cultivation of fine fruits &c.).—2)* *rose-colored, red wool,* &c. Keth. 72b טווה ו׳ כנגד פניה she spins red material holding it up to her face (to make it look bright; Tosaf.); [Maim.: she spins in the street בו׳ with a rose in her hair; Rashi (who seems to read וְרָד fr. רדד): with the thread in front of her body, i. e. she spins in the street in an indecent position.]

וַרְדָּא, וַרְד ch. same, 1) *rose.* Targ. Cant. II, 1 sq. (h. text שושנה). Targ. Ez. XXVII, 24 Ar., v. כּוּשְׁפָּא.—Y. Shebi. VII, beg. 37b מהו לכבוש מן החן וו׳ is it permitted to use roses for preserving in the Sabbatical year?—Sabb. 152a רנקותא כלילא דו׳ youth is a wreath of roses. Gitt. 68b ו׳ חיורא דקאי וכ׳ a white rose (or blossom) whose leaves are all on one side. B. Bath. 69a, v. וַרְדָּנָא.—*Pl.* וַרְדֵּי, וַרְדִין. Targ. Cant. VI, 2. Ib. VII, 3.—B. Bath. 84a דחלפא אבי וו׳ דג״ע (Ms. H. אַבֵּי. . .) he (the sun) passes the rose-garden of Paradise. Ab. Zar. 65a יתיב . . . . בי וו׳ Ms. M. (ed. בוורדא) seated up to his neck in roses.—2) *rose-color.*—Hull. 46a bot. וסימנך כיתונא דוו׳ וכ׳ and thy sign-word (for remembering which of the two membranes of the lungs is of vital import) is, the rose-colored (precious) shirt, in which the lungs lie (i. e. the interior membrane).—3) עינוניתא דוו׳ *the little rose-lobe,* name of an additional lobe of the lungs found with animals of the steppes (וְהִירְדָּא). Ib. 47a bot.

וַרְדָּאן (preced.) *Vardan,* surname of R. Ḥin'na. Gitt. 64b (Rashi: ורדא׳ *of Vardania,* v. וַרְדִּינָא II).

וַרְדּוּנְיָא, v. וַרְדִּינָא II.

וַרְדִּימוֹס ,וַרְדִּימַס ,וַר׳ pr. n. m. (a corrupt. of Εὐρύδημος) *Vardimos, Vardimas.* Ned. 81a. Sabb. 118b הייגו ו׳ וכ׳ V. is Menahem (etymology fr. וֶרֶד).—Sifra Emor Par. 10, ch. XIII אֲוַרְדִּימַס. Y. Shebi. VIII, 38b top אבירודימוס.

וַרְדִּינָא I m. (v. וַרְדָּא) *(wild) rose-bush, thorn-hedge.* Sabb. 67a.—*Pl.* וַרְדִּינֵי. B. Kam. 80a.

וַרְדִּינָא II (**וַרְדּוּנְיָא, וַרְדַּנְיָא**) pr. n. pl. *Vardina (Vardania, Vardunia),* a town in Babylonia, near Be-Berai. Sot. 10a וַארְדּוּנְיָא ed. (some ed. וַרְדּוּנֵי, Ar. וורדינא). Erub. 49a אנשי ורדינא (Ms. M. incorr. ורדינאה, Ms. O. ורדנא, v. Rabb. D. S. a. l. note; R. Ḥănanel: וורדאן, v. Berl. Beitr. Geogr. p. 34, note 3) the men of V. (known for their stinginess). V. וַרְדָּאן.

וַרְדִּינָאָה m. (preced.) *of Vardina.* Nidd. 19b אמי ו׳ Ammi of V. (oth. opin. 'handsome as a rose'; Gitt. 41a א׳ שפיר נאה).

וַרְדָּנָא m. (וַרְדָּא), בי וו׳ *flower-garden* (v. וֶרֶד II pl.). B. Bath. 69a והוא דקרו ליה בי וו׳ דפ׳ Ms. M. (ed. לה וורדא; oth. Mss. וַרְדֵּי, v. Rabb. D. S. a. l. note) provided it goes by the name of 'the flower garden of that man.'

וַרְדַּנְיָא, v. וַרְדִּינָא.

וְרִיד m. (ירד, cmp. יָרִיד a. וַרְדָּן) *the large blood vessel, jugular vein* (leading from the head to the heart).—*Pl.* וְרִידִין. Hull. II, 1 עד שישחוט את הו׳ he must sever the jugular veins; Tosef. ib. II, 1.—Zeb. 25ª sq. צריך שיתן 'וו' וכ he must let the blood of the jugular veins run into the center of the receiving bowl. Ber. 8ᵇ; Snh. 96ª 'הזהרו בוו be careful in slaughtering that you sever the veins, v. supra; a. e.

וְרִיר m. (אור)=חֲוַרְוָור white spots (λεύκωμα) in the eye. Tosef. Bekh. IV, 2; 3 (ריר, corr. acc.); 4; (Bekh. VI, 3, Talm. ed. 38ᵇ חורוור q. v.).

***וְרְשְׁכָא** f. silk-strain.—Pl. וְרְשְׁכֵי. Kidd. 13ª. B. Mets. 51ª (Ms. R. 1 'ריר). [Koh. Ar. Compl. s. v. refers to Pers. ברשך belt. Oth. interpret. of our w.: beads, frontlet.]

וֶשֶׁט m. (יָשַׁט) [something stretched and narrow,] 1) gullet. Hull. III, 1 'נקובת הו an animal whose gullet is found to have been perforated.—Nidd. 23ᵇ וֶשְׁטוֹ נקוב if the infant's gullet is perforated (there being a hole in the throat); 'ו אטום if its gullet is closed; a. fr.—Yalk. Ps. 687 (translating מַלְקוֹחַי, Ps. XXII, 16) לְוֶושְׁטִי; Midr. Till. to Ps. l. c. לוירסטי (corr. acc.; cmp. Lat. fauces) to my throat.—2) (cmp. בְּלִיעַ, בְּלוּעָה) straits, canal. Ber. 8ª (Rashi: loop-hole for the rope), v. פִּיטוּרִין a. צִיפּוּרִין; M. Kat. end; Lev. R. s. 4; Tanh. Mikk. 10; ed. Bub. 15; Koh. R. to VI, 6.

וֶשְׁטָא, 'וֶ ch. same, gullet. Y. Snh. IX, 27ª top. Lev. R. s. 3; Koh. R. to VII, 19; Yalk. Koh. 976.

וַת, לְוַת &c., v. יַת.

וַת=וְאַתְּ, and thou. Y. Snh. XI, 30ᵇ bot. ות מר הכין and thou (the Biblical text) sayest so (that he died in the same year)? Y. Shebu. I, 33ᵇ top; a. e.—Y. Macc. II, end, 32ª וַתְּמַר אכן (=ואת אמר).

וָוְתָא f. (v. וָו) stork (from the shape of its beak and neck). Targ. Ps. CIV, 17 (ed. Lag. וָוְתָא, Regia ותיא). Targ. Y. II Deut. XIV, 13 (belonging to v. 18, h. text חסידה, v. אִיבּוּ).

וְתוּנְיָא, וְתוּנְיַיקִי, וְתוּבְיָא, וְתוּבְיָיא, v. 'וְתִינְ.

ותוקין, v. וִיתֵּק.

ותיא, v. וָוְתָא.

וְתַיָּא=וְאַתְיָא, v. אֲתָא.

ווֹתִינָא, v. וִיתְנָא.

וְתִינְיָא, 'וְתוּ pr. n. (Βιθυνία) Bithynia, a province in the N. W. of Asia Minor. Targ. Y. Gen. X, 2 'וְוִתִינְ, 'וְיָתִינְ (read: 'ווית; h. text תבל); Targ. I Chr. I, 5 (corr. acc.).—Gen. R. s. 37, beg. (misplaced, v. אוסיא); Y. Meg. I, 71ᵇ bot. (Yoma 10ª בית אונייקי).

וְתִינְיַיקִי, 'וְתוּ f. (preced. Βιθυνιακή) Bithynian. Y. Ab. Zar. II, end, 42ª 'גבינה וו, v. אוּנְיָיקִי. Ab. Zar. II, 5 Y. ed. 'ותיר (corr. acc.).

וָתִיק m. (ותק, cmp. Arab. vatik, a. b. h. עָתֵק) enduring; trusty; strong; distinguished.—'תלמיד ו a faithful student, distinguished scholar. Y. Ber. II, 5ᶜ; Cant. R. to VI, 2; a. fr.—Sabb. 105ª 'ו נתתיך באומות (omitted in Ms. M., a. Yalk. Gen. 81) I made thee distinguished among the nations.—Pl. וְתִיקִים, וְתִיקִין. Sifré Num. 92; ib. Deut. 13, v. פָּסַק.—Tosef. Hor. I, 1. Y. Snh. X, 29ª.—Esp. Vᵉthikin (Ancients), the conscientiously pious men of former days. Ber. 9ᵇ 'ו היו גומרין אותה עם וכ (Tosef. ib. I, 2 'מצותה עם וכ, v. Rabb. D. S. a. l. note 60) the V. used to finish the reading of the Sh'mah &c.; ib. 25ᵇ; 26ª; Y. ib. I, 3ª bot. 'הוו.—R. Hash. 32ᵇ. [וַתִּיקִין, Gitt. 70ª, v. וִיתֵּק.]

וַתִּיקָא m. (v. preced.) name of a certain pastry, tart. Pes. 39ᵇ.

ותירייקי, v. וְתִינְיַיקִי.

וַתְּמַר, v. וַת.

וְוִתְנָא m. (יתן, cmp. אֵיתָן) sinew, vein (h. גִּיד).—Pl. וְוִתְנַיָּא. Targ. Job XL, 17 (ed. Lag. 'וְוִתִינַ, Var. 'וַרִּי, 'וַרִּ).

וְתַנְיָה, v. וִתְנָא.

וְתַק, Pa. וַתֵּק (privative verb, v. וָתִיק; cmp. עתק Targ. Lam. III, 4) to unnerve (v. וִיתֵּק); to break, shatter. Targ. I Kings XIX, 11 מְוַותֵּק Ar. Ms. quoted in Buxt. s. v. (ed. מפרקין).

וָתַר, וְוָתַר (v. יָתַר) to be plentiful. Y. Succ. V, 55ᶜ (ref. to Jer. II, 13) הא וָתְרוּ לְאלף (not וותרה) were they not numerous up to a thousand?; Cant. R. to I, 6 הא ווּתרו למאד (read: לְמֵאָה).

Pi. וִיתֵּר 1) to do more than justice requires, to be liberal; to forego one's rights. Y. Ned. I, beg. 39ª if they had agreed על מנת לְוַתֵּר to yield their rights (to allow each other the use of the entire court). B. Bath. 126ª 'ו . . . . בכור if a first-born accepted an equal share (of a field) with his brothers, he has renounced his privilege; Y. Keth. IV, end, 29ᵇ חזקה ויתר (read: וִויתֵּר). Ib. וִיתְּרָה (=ויתרה). B. Kam. 9ª 'ו he has renounced his rights (cannot resort to his co-heirs for redress). Ruth R. to I, 8 'שויתרו לה וכ they relinquished their claim on her &c.; a. fr.—2) to be indulgent, forgive. Y. Hag. I, 76ᶜ 'ו' הקב"ה על וכ the Lord overlooked Israel's idolatry, but did not &c.; Lam. R. introd. (R. Abba 2). Y. Sot. V, end, 20ᵈ שהיה מְוַותֵּר על קללתו he pardoned those who cursed him. Deut. R. s. 9 'נְוַותֵּר לו עוד יום וכ (not עד) let us give him a respite of one day or two.—Num. R. s. 21 לא יהא אדם מוותר על התורה man must not be more liberal than the Law; a. fr.—Snh. XI, 5 (89ª) המו' על דברי נביא he who disobeys a prophet from mere soft-heartedness (v. I Kings XX, 35, sq.).—3) to give additional space to a plant by removing surrounding plants, to make open space. Y. Shebi. II, 33ᵈ top מְוַותְּרִין בגפנים you may clear (in the Sabbatical year) between the grape vines; ib. 'מקום שנהגו לוותר וכ where it is customary to clear before the festive month; Tosef. ib. I, 7 מְוַתְּרִין; ib. להתיר ed. Zuck. (read: לְוַותֵּר).

Nif. הִוָּותֵר (v. נָתַר) 1) to be let loose, set free. Midr. P'tirath Mosheh אֶוָּותֵר (Jellinek Beth-ham-Midrash I, 125; v. Lattes Saggio 107).—2) to be outlawed, v. infra.

Hithpa. הִתְוַתֵּר, *Nithpa.* נִתְוַתֵּר (v. נָתַר) 1) *to become loose* (of bowels).—2) *to be declared free, be outlawed.* Cant. R. to III, 4 נִתְוַתְּרוּ מעיו וכ׳ (Yalk. Is. 288 נתרזו בני מ׳) his bowels were loose that whole night. B.Kam. 50a bot. יִתְוַתְּרוּ חייו Ms. M. (ed. יִוָּתְרוּ, *Nif.*, v. supra) his life shall be let loose i. e. shall be outlawed; Ar. ed. Koh. יִתְוַתְּרוּן מעיו וחייו (v. Rabb. D. S. a. l. note); Tanh. Ki Thissa 26 יתותרון בני מעיו his bowels &c., v. next w.; Yalk. Ps. 648 יִוָּתְרוּ חייו his life be outlawed.

וָתַר, *Pa.* וַיתֵּר 1) *to give a surplus, to profit, avail.* Targ. Prov. X, 2.—2) *to be indulgent, to overlook.* Lev. R. s. 10, beg. אם אין את מְוַותֵּר צִיבְחַר וכ׳ unless thou overlook something &c.; Gen. R. s. 49; a. e.

Ithpa. אִיוַּותַּר, אִתְוַותַּר 1) *to be loosened.* Y. Bets. II, end, 62b מאן דאמר ... יִתְוַתְּרוּן בני מעור וכ׳ whoever says, the Lord is lax in dealing out justice,—may his bowels become relaxed; He is merely long-suffering &c.; Y. Shek. V, 48d; Y. Taan. II, 65b bot.; Midr. Till. to Ps. X, 2 לִיוַּותְּרוּן מעוהר; Esth. R. to III, 15; IV, 1; Yalk. ib. 1056 יִוַּתְּרוּ מ׳ Yalk. Gen. 115 יִוַּתְּרוּ.—2) *to be declared free, outlawed;* v. preced.

וַתְּרָן m. (preced. wds.; also in Chald. diction) *liberal, benevolent, indulgent.* Snh. 102b ו׳ ... היה was very liberal (supporting scholars). Y. Sot. V, end, 20d (ref. to Job I, 1) ו׳ היה he (Job) was liberal; ומאן דלית הוא ו׳ וכ׳ but if one is not liberal, may he not be virtuous (shunning evil)?; but it means forgiving &c., v. וָתַר.—Num. R. s. 9, beg. תהא ו׳ בתוך וכ׳ be lenient in thy house (be not angry when anything gets broken &c.). Y. Gitt. IV, 45c bot. אילולי דאנא ו׳ if I were not lenient.—Esp. *lax in the practice of justice.* B. Kam. 50a; Y. Bets. II, end, 62b, a. fr., v. preced.—*Pl.* וַתְּרָנִים. Gen. R. s. 53 [read:] .. בביתו ו׳ היו in the house of Abraham they were kind-hearted.—Fem. וַתְּרָנִית. Y. Ab. Zar. I, beg. 39a (they said) ע״ז ו׳ היא the heathen deity is benevolent (entertaining the worshippers).

ז

ז *Zayin*, the seventh letter of the Alphabet; it interchanges with ד, q. v.; with צ, as זהר a. צהר, זוודא a. צדה &c.; with ס a. שׂ, as זור a. סור, עלז a. עלס &c. ז as final formative (*Palez=Pales*), as אטליז, אושפיזא &c.

זְאֵב m. (b. h.) *wolf.* B. Mets. VII, 9 ז׳ אחד וכ׳ the attack by one wolf is not considered an accident relieving from responsibility; a. fr.—*Pl.* זְאֵבִים, זְאֵיבִין. Ib. בשעת משלחת ז׳ at a time when wolves are coming forth in hordes, v. מִשְׁלַחַת; Y. Shebi. IV, 35b top; Y. Ter. XI, end, 48b. Esth. R. to IX, 2, v. כִּבְשָׂה; a. fr.—Fem. זְאֵבָה. Midr. Till. to Ps. X, 13 נזדמנה הז׳ וכ׳ a she-wolf was provided for them who gave them suck; v. רומוס; ib. to XVII, 14 וזמנת להם ז׳ and Thou didst provide &c.; Yalk. Ps. 652.

זָאזָא m. (reduplic. of זע=זא, v. זוּעַ a. זעזע) *foliage, spray; young twigs.* Targ. Job XIV, 9; a. e.—Sabb. 20b (expl. עצים של בבל) ז׳ dry twigs and leaves used as fuel.

זַאֲטוּט, v. זַעֲטוּט.

זְאֵיב, v. זְאֵב.

זְאַר (cmp. זור, דור) *to pass around.* Targ. Job XXVIII, 8 (ed. Wil. זְאוֹר, Lev. זיאר read זָאִיר, part.; Ms. דָּר; h. text עדה).

זֹאת, v. זֶה.

ז״ב, an abbreviation for זְמַן a. בָּמָה. Zeb. 28b דדמיר ליה בז״ב because both subjects have reference to *time* and application to the *improvised altar* (v. בָּמָה) as well as to the Temple.

זָב m., **זָבָה** f. (b. h.; זוב) 1) *faint.* Y. Kidd. I, 61a (expl. זב, II Sam. III, 29) תָּשִׁישׁ q. v.—2) *one afflicted with gonorrhœa.* Zab. I, 5 זב גמור a real *zabh* (subject to all the laws in Lev. XV, 1—15; 19—24). Ib. V, 6; a. v. fr.—*Pl.* זָבִים, זָבִין; f. זָבוֹת. Sifra Metsora, Zabim, Par. 1 מטמאים כז׳ (not בז׳) they make unclean like Israelitish *zabim;* Nidd. 34a שיהו כז׳ וכ׳; a. v. fr. [Sabb. 110b מִזּוֹבִיךְ, v. זוֹב.]—*Zabim*, name of a treatise of the Mishnah a. Tosefta, and of a section of the Sifra to Metsora.

זְבַד (b. h. זָבַד) *to present with, outfit.* Targ. Y. Gen. XXX, 20 (some ed. עבד, corr. acc.).

זַבְדָּא, v. זַבְדַּי.

זְבַדַּאי, v. זַבְדִּין.

זַבְדַּי pr. n. m. *Zabday*, 1) name of an Amora *Z. bar Levi.* Zeb. 28b; (Kerith. 5a זַבְדָּא). Y. Dem. VII, beg. 26a. Y. Ab. Zar. III, 42c זַבְדַּיי בר ליואר; Gen. R. s. 62 זבדי בן לוי; a. fr.—2) Y. Ber. III, 6c bot. אבא בר זבדא. Ib. יעקב בר זבדי.

זְבַדְיָה (b. h.) pr. n. m. *Zebadiah*, name of an Amora. Y. Ber. III, 6c bot.—[Y. Sot. I, 16d, v. זְכַרְיָה.]

בֵּית ז׳, זַבְדִּין pr. n. pl. *Beth-Zabdin*, prob. in Galilee. Y. Meg. I, 70c bot.; Y. Taan. II, 66a; M'gillath Taan. ch. XII בֵּית זַבְדַּאי (v. Graetz Gesch. d. Jud. III^2, p. 423).

זָבָה, v. זָב.

זְבוּב m. (b. h.; זבב) *fly*. Sabb. 121[b] ז׳ שבארץ מצרים the Egyptian fly (whose sting is dangerous). Tosef. Sot. V, 9; Gitt. 90[a]. Pesik. Zakhor, p. 26[b] לז׳ שהוא וכ׳ (Amalek resembles) the fly which is greedy for a sore; a. fr.—*Pl.* זְבוּבִין, זְבוּבִים. Y. Sabb. XIV, beg. 14[b]; Tosef. ib. XII (XIII), 4. Keth. 77[b] ז׳ של בעלי וכ׳ (not זבובי) flies which sucked from those afflicted with gonorrhœa (carrying contagion); a. fr.

זְבוּגָא* m. *lizard.*—*Pl.* זְבוּגֵי. Nidd. 56[a] ז׳ דמחוזא (Ar. זַבְזֵגֵי, Mus.: זבובי, prob. clerical error) (skeletons of) lizards of Maḥuza.

זָבוּד pr. n. pl. *Zabud*, on the northernmost border of Galilee. Gen. R. s. 98 (ref. to Gen. XLIX, 13 על צידון) ז׳ דגלילה (*Safet*, Lit. Centralblatt 1879, p. 1188).

זְבוּדָא m. (זבד) *gift, outfit.*—*Pl.* זְבוּדִין. Targ. Y. Gen. XXX, 20 (h. text זֶבֶד).

זבוזין, Y. Ter. VIII, 45[b] bot. ׳בז, in a corrupt sentence which prob. read: שקץ זיזין והגזין וכל שקצים שהפרישו, v. Sifra Sh'mini Par. 10, ch. XII.

זְבוּל m. (b. h.; זָבַל) [*place of offering* or *entertainment*,] 1) *residence*, esp. *Temple*. R. Hash. 17[a]; Y. Ber. IX, 13[b] bot. פשטו ידיהם בז׳ they laid hand on the Temple; a. e.—2) *Z'bul*, name of the fourth heaven. Ḥag. 12[b] ז׳ שבו . . . ומזבח וכ׳ it is called *Z.*, because there are (the heavenly) Jerusalem and the Sanctuary with the altar erected &c.—3) יום ז׳ *festival* of a heathen divinity. Pesik. R. s. 6 יום ז׳ נילוס היה it was the festival of Nilus; [cacophemistic disguise: נבול, Gen. R. s. 87; Cant. R. beg. ניבול וזבול;—Yalk. Gen. 146 גידול; Sot. 36[b] [חֲגָם]. V. זִיבּוּל.

זְבוּלֻן, זְבֻלוּן, זְבוּלוּן (b. h.) pr. n. m. *Zebulun*, 1) son of Jacob; *tribe of Zebulun; country of Z.* Gen. R. s. 98. Pes. 4[a]; a. fr.—2) one *Z. ben Dan.* Kidd. 30[a].

זְבוּנָא m. (זבן) *purchase*. Targ. Y. II Deut. XVIII, 8 בר זְבוּנֵיה that which he bought. *Pl.* זְבוּנִין. Ruth R. to I, 17 (sect. 3) זבן ז׳ he made his purchases.—V. זְבִינָא.

זְבוּנָא, v. ׳זיב.

זַבּוֹנָה, זַבּוֹנָא m. (preced. wds.) *buyer, merchant.* Targ. II Esth. III, 11.—Y. Kil. II, beg. 27[c].—Y. Kidd. II, 64[a] top קרן ז׳ וכ׳ the merchant packed his goods on his wagon and went off; v. דַּהֵר.

זַבּוּנֵי, v. זְבַן *Pa.*

זְבוּרָא, v. ׳זיב.

זְבוּרִית f. (זבר, cmp. צבר a. also זַרְבּוּבִית) 1) *a receptacle for drippings fastened* (or *belonging*) *to the bottom of a vessel, saucer.* Mikv. X, 71 בלא ז׳ if the vessel to be immersed has no saucer (a rim at the bottom, wider than the belly of the vessel and which forces the water into the latter); (Var. זִירְבָּרִין, זוּבְרִית, זִיבּוּרִית, זְחִבּוּרִית). [Rabad to Maim. Mikv. III, 12 reads זַרְבּוּבִית q. v.].—2) *lowest land*, v. זִיבּוּרִית.

זַבְזְגָא* m., pl. זַבְזְגֵי 1) (reduplication of זגא, v. זָגֵי; for inserted ב, v. זַבְלְגַן) *nest, brood, hatch.* M. Kat. 28[b] (in a funeral song) אחנא תגרא אזבזגיה מיבדקי (or:) תגרי .... דאזבזגי מיבדקו (v. Rabb. D. S. a. l.; Rashi a. l.) our brother, the merchant, will be judged by the brood he left behind, (or) our brethren, the merchants, will be judged by the broods (allusion to Jer. XVII, 11). [En Yakob reads תגרי.. דאזבזגי מיבדקי our (departed) brethren are merchants who (on crossing the frontier of life) are searched for goods.—Ms. M. 2 דאזיקי וכ׳ who are searched for the wine bags they carry, v. זִיקָא II a. זוק.]—2) v. זְבוּגָא.

זָבַח (b. h., cmp. זבל) [*to give a feast*,] *to slaughter, sacrifice.* Ḥull. II, 3 (ref. to Deut. XXVII, 7) מה שאתה זוֹבֵחַ וכ׳ thou mayest eat what *thou* (a human hand) cuttest. Snh. 60[b] בזובח לעכו״ם of one sacrificing to an idol; a. fr.—Part. pass. זָבוּחַ. Lev. R. s. 10 (play on מזבח, Ex. XXXII, 5) מֵהַזָּ׳ לפניו וכ׳ he was afraid on account of him who lay killed before him (Hur); a. fr.

Pi. זִיבַּח same. Snh. 62[a] ז׳ וקיטר וכ׳ if he slaughtered a sacrifice, and burnt &c. (to an idol). Ib. VII, 6 (60[b]) הַמְזַבֵּחַ Talm. ed. (Mish. הזובח) he who offers an animal (to an idol), a. fr.—V. זָבַל.

Nif. נִזְבַּח *to be sacrificed, to be slaughtered; to die as a martyr.* Zeb. I, 1 שנִּזְבְּחוּ שלא לשמן which were offered not for the purpose for which they were dedicated. Y. Snh. X, 29[c] top (play on עלי זבח, Ps. L, 5) שעילו אותי ונזבחו על שמי who raised me and sacrificed themselves for my name's sake; a. fr.

זֶבַח m. (b. h.; preced.) *a slaughtering, sacrifice*, esp. (*festive*) *peace-offering* (חֲגִיגָה). Pes. X, 9. Tosef. ib. X, 14. Tosef. Ber. V, 22; a. fr.—*Pl.* זְבָחִים, constr. זִבְחֵי. Ib. Zeb. I, 1 כל הז׳ all animalic offerings; a. fr.—*Z'baḥim*, name of a treatise of the Mishnah, Tosefta and Talmud Babli (also called שְׁחִיטַת קָדָשִׁים).

זְבִיד pr. n. m. *Z'bid*, name of several Amoraim. Ber. 46[b], a. fr. (Z. bar Levi).—Ib. 38[a].—Ab. Zar. 56[a].—Y. Sabb. I, 3[b], v. next w.

זְבִידָה, זְבִידָא pr. n. m. *Z'bida, Z'bidah*, name of a Palestinean Amora. Y. Orl. I, 61[a] bot.—Y. Sot. VII, 21[d].—Ib. ר׳ יודה בר זביד. Ib. bot. ר׳ סימון בר זביד. Y. Sabb. I, 3[b] רב זביד.

זְבִיחָה f. (זָבַח) *slaughtering ceremony.* Ḥull. 31[b] כוונה לז׳ intention to slaughter according to ritual, contrad. to חתיכה the cutting operation as such. Snh. 60[b] ז׳ יצתה slaughtering for idolatry is especially mentioned (Ex. XXII, 19); a. fr.

זְבִיק or **זַבִּיק**, v. זוּב.

זַבִּילָא m. (v. זָבַל; Syr. זבילא, זנב׳, P. Sm. 1074; 1140) *a basket* (or *book-chest*) *of palm leaves.*—*Pl.* זַבִּילֵי. Meg. 26[b] ז׳ דחומשי receptacles for Pentateuch copies; [Ar.: *leather casing.*]

זְבִילָא m. (v. זָבַל) [*an implement for forming heaps,*] *shovel, mattock.* Taan. 21[b] שיול מרא וז' וכ' he lent mattock and shovel for burial. B. Mets. 103[b]. [Ber. 8[a], v. זִיבוּלָא.]

זְבֵין, v. זְבַן.

זְבִינָא I pr. n. m., v. זְמִינָא.

זְבִינָא II, constr. זְבִין m. (זבן) 1) *object of purchase, goods.* Targ. O. Gen. XVII, 12 (Y. זְבִינֵי pl.). Targ. Ez. VII, 13; a. e.—Y. Kidd. III, beg., 63[c] זבין ז' bargaining for an object. Pesik. R. s. 21 הא ז' והא וכ' here are the goods and here the salesman; a. e.—2) *purchase.* Targ. Y. Lev. XXV, 42 (O. זִיבּוּן).—*Pl.* זְבִינֵי, זְבִינִין. Targ. O. Lev. XXV, 14 (Y. some ed. זַבִּינֵי).—Targ. Gen. XLIX, 32 (Y. some ed. 'זַבִּ); a. e.—Pes. 113[a], v. זְבַן *Pa.*—3) *purchase money.* Targ. Lev. XXV, 16 (Y. some ed. 'זַבִּינ); a. e.

זַבִּינָא m. (preced.) *sale, sold goods, merchandise.* Targ. Y. Gen. XLIX, 32, a. e.; v. preced.—Pes. 113[a] (prov.) while the dust is yet on thy feet, זַבִּינָךְ זבין sell thy goods.—*Pl.* זַבִּינֵי *sale.* B. Bath. 47[b] זַבִּינֵיה ז' his sale is valid; a. fr.

זְבִינְתָּא f. (preced.) *goods; bargain.* Y. Ab. Zar. II, 42[a] אלא ע"י ערלא ז' וכ' but, I say, through some accident the goods (in the ship) were upset; Y. Ter. X, 47[b] גבינתא (corr. acc.).—B. Mets. 51[a] עד דמתרמי ליה ז' כזְבִינְתֵּיה until he strikes upon goods like those he bought. Ib. קים ליה בז' he knew the value of his goods; a. fr.—*Pl.* זְבִינָתָא. Ruth R. to I, 17 (s. 3) ואילין ז' וכ' what do these purchases (marketing) mean?

זְבוּת, Y. Taan. I, 64[b] bot., v. זְבַן.

זָבַל I (b. h.; cmp. זבד) *to entertain liberally.*—Denom. זִבּוּל.

Pi. זִבֵּל (cmp. זבח) *to offer to idols, make merry with idolatrous ceremonies.* Ab. Zar. 18[b] שמְזַבְּלִין שם וכ' because they have there (in their theatres) idolatrous entertainments; Tosef. ib. II, 5 (ed. Zuck. מזבחין). Y. Ber. IX, 13[b] bot. if one sees people מז' לע"ז engaged in idolatrous services; a. fr.

זָבַל II, *Pi.* זִבֵּל (denom. of זֶבֶל) *to deposit foliage in the field* for manure, *to manure.* Shebi. III, 2 עד כמה מְזַבְּלִין how many piles may be deposited? Ib. II, 2 מְזַבְּלִין וכ' you may manure &c. Keth. 10[b] the rain waters ומְזַבֵּל and *softens* (corresp. to מוג, Ps. LXV, 11, cmp. בּוּל II). Cant. R. to I, 1 אנחנו לא נְזַבֵּל וכ' (not נזבלים) should we not improve (our minds) even as those carrying out foliage and straw?; a. fr.—Part. pass. מְזוּבָּל *manured.* Y. M. Kat. I, 80[b].

Nif. נִזְבַּל, *Nithpa.* נִזְדַּבֵּל *to be manured.* Midr. Sam. ch. IV.—Ab. Zar. 49[a] שדה שנִזְדַּבְּלָה וכ' a field which has been manured with material connected with idolatry (foliage from a worshipped tree &c.).

זְבַל ch. same.—*Ithpa.* אִיזְדַּבַּל *to be manured.* Ab. Zar. 49[a] (read אִזְדַּבְּלָא).

זֶבֶל m. (cmp. Assyr. zabâlu, KAT², p. 550; cmp. צָבַר) [*heaped up,*] esp. *foliage piled up for forming manure, manure, deposits.* Sabb. IV, 1 you must not keep dishes warm for the Sabbath בז' וכ' in foliage . . . . whether dry or moist. Ab. Zar. III, 8 (48[b]) והוָה להן לז' and serves for them as manure. Yoma V, 6 נמכרין . . . לז' is sold to the gardeners for forming manure. Tosef. B. Mets. XI, 8 זִיבְלוֹ his heaped-up foliage. B. Mets. V, 7 (72[b]) עד שיהיה לו ז' באשפתו Ms. M. (ed. אלא א"כ היתה וכ') unless he has manure piled up; a. fr.—*Pl.* זְבָלִים. Shebi. III, 1 מאימתי מוציאין ז' וכ' when may deposits of foliage be carried out for piling up in the fields.—Gen. R. s. 31 לז' (Snh. 108[b] sing.) for deposits of excrements &c.—Tosef. B. Mets. l. c. שעת הז' the season for carrying out foliage; a. fr.—בית הז' *a field dependent on manuring.* Men. VIII, 3 (85[a]).

זַבָּל m. (preced.) *one carrying foliage for making dung.*—*Pl.* זַבָּלִים. Cant. R. to I, 1 ז' ותבנים carriers of foliage and of straw.

זַבְלְגָן m. (זָלַג, with inserted ב=זולגן, cmp. זבזגא a. next w.) *blear-eyed.* Meg. 24[b].—*Pl.* זַבְלְגָנִים, זַבְלְגָנִין. Bekh. 43[b]; Tosef. ib. V, 2.

זַבְלִיגָא, זַמְבְּלִיגָא (זַמְלִיגָא) m. (זלג, v. preced.) *a resinous tree,* a species of *cedar.* Snh. 108[b], (expl. גּוֹפֶר) ז' Ar. s. v. אדר (Var. in Ar. 'זמל); ed. זו מבליגא (corr. acc.); R. Hash. 23[a] 'מ ed. (Ms. M. 'זו מ, v. Rabb. D. S. a. l. note; corr. acc.).

זַבֶּלֶת f. (v. זֶבֶל) *the place in the field where foliage is piled up.* Tosef. B. Mets. XI, 8 להוציאו לזַבַּלְתּוֹ ed. Zuck. to carry it out to his field &c.

זְבַן, זְבֵין (cmp. זמן, a. Syr. זבן) [*to plan,*] *to bargain, buy.* Dan. II, 8.—Targ. Gen. XXV, 10; a. fr.—B. Bath. 30[a, b] [read:] מפלניא זְבִנְתָּהּ דזַבְנָהּ מינך I bought it of such a person who has bought it of thee. Ib. אֵיזְבּוּן דינאי I will buy what by law belongs to me (to avoid litigation); a. v. fr.

Pa. זַבֵּין *to sell.* Targ. Gen. XXV, 31; 33; a. fr.—B. Bath. l. c. זַבְנָהּ ניהלי sell it to me. Ib. 90[a], a. e. (prov.) זְבַן וזַבֵּין . . . איקרי buy and sell and be called a merchant, i. e. will a man buy and sell without profit?—Pes. 113[a] מילי דזבינֵי וזבּוּנֵי Ag. hat-Torah (v. Rabb. D. S. a. l. note 50; ed. מילי דעלמא) rules about buying and selling. Ib. כל מילי זבין וכ' as regards all things, sell and regret, except wine דתִזַבֵּין ולא וכ' Ms. M. (ed. דזבין) which you must sell and never regret. Meg. 26[b] זַבּוּנָהּ to sell it. Gitt. 47[a] ז' נפשיה וכ' sold himself to &c.; a. fr.—Y. Taan. I, 64[b] bot. זבית ערסי (read: זַבְּנִית) I sold my bedstead.

Ithpa. אִזְדַּבַּן *to be sold, to be bought; to sell one's self.* Targ. Ps. CV, 17; a. fr.—B. Mets. 40[b] הוה מִזְדַּבַּן לי (Ms. M. הוה זבנתיה) it would have been saleable with me. Kidd. 69[a] ואִיזְדַּבַּן וכ' and get thyself sold as a Hebrew slave.

זְבֹרִין, v. זִבּוּרִית.

זָג m. (b. h.; זוג) 1) *pl.* זַגִּים, זַגִּין (cmp. דכך) *pomace of grapes, husks* or *kernels and flesh.* Naz. VI, 2 (34[b]) חרצנים . . . הז' אלו הפנימים *hartsannim* (Num. VI, 4) means the exterior, *zaggim* the interior; (ib. contrary opinion, v. זוג).—Tosef. Toh. III, 1 הגפן והזוגין וכ' ed.

Zuck. (oth. ed. זַגִּין; some ed. זומין, corr. acc.) the grape vine (clusters) and the pomace which have been treated in cleanness. Sabb. IV, 1.—Naz. l. c. זַג זָגָן Mish. (Y. ed. זגין, Bab. ed. זג; Tosef. ib. IV, 2 זגא ed. Zuck., Var. זג) *the husk* (or *the interior*) of one berry.—2) *bell*, v. זוג.

זַגָּא ch. same, 1) *husk* or *kernel and flesh* of one berry, v. preced.—*Pl.* זַגִּין. Targ. Y. Num. VI, 4 ז׳ גוואין וכ׳ the interior *zaggin*, v. preced.—2) *bell*. Targ. O. Ex. XXVIII, 34; a. e.—*Pl.* זַגִּין, זַגַּיָּא, זַגֵּי. Ib. 33; XXXIX, 25.—Nidd. 17ᵃ מקרקש זגי וכ׳ made the bells of his curtains ring; [Ar. מק׳ פַּגֵּי chased the *flies*, v. חַגְזִין].

זָגָא, v. זְגַר.

זַגָּג m. (זגג *to clear*, cmp. זכך a. דכך, v. Ges. Thes. s. v.) *glass-maker; dealer in glass-ware*. M. Kat. 13ᵇ; Pes. 55ᵇ בית הז׳ the glass-maker's work-shop.—Gen. R. s. 19 חנותו של ז׳ a glass-dealer's shop. Ib. s. 25; a. fr.—*Pl.* זַגָּגִין. Kel. XXIV, 8 מטה של ז׳ the frame used by the glass-makers to put their ware on. B. Kam. 31ᵃ.

זַגָּגָא ch. same. *Pl.* זַגָּגַיָּא. Y. Ab. Zar. II, 40ᶜ bot. לא אלפון ז׳ the glass-makers did not teach their art.

(זוּגְדָּס) זַגְדָּן, זַגְדּוּם m. (contr. of זוג a. גד fr. גדד, cmp. גדודא juvenis cælebs, P. Sm. 652) *unmatched*; esp. *one with an unequal pair of eyes or eye-brows*. Bekh. VII, 3 זוגדם Mish. (v. infra; Talm. ed. 43ᵇ זגדן). Ib. 44ᵃ זגדום אחד שחור וכ׳ Z. is one who has one black and one white eye-brow; כל זוגא .... ז׳ קרי ליה any unequal pair is called Z. Ib. זַגְדְּיָיא מחוי וכ׳ (ch. form of our w.); Tosef. ib. V, 2, sq. סגריס (read: סַגְּדוּם *Safel* of גדד). Sifra Emor ch. II, Par. 3 זגדוס (read ם ....). [Ar. זגדוס, influenced by the etymol.: זוג, and דוס=δίς.]

זַגְדְּיָיא, v. preced.

זוּגִיתָא, זְגוּגִיתָא f. (זגג, v. זַגָּג) *glass, crystal; glass-ware*. Targ. Job XXVIII, 18 (in one version); a. e. Targ. II Esth. I, 2 (3) בית זוג׳ glass-house.—Ber. 31ᵃ כסי דזוגוג׳ Ar. ed. Koh. (ed. כסא דזוג׳ חיורתא, v. Rabb. D. S. a. l. note 10) cups (a cup) of (white) glass; Yalk. Ps. 881. Hull. 84ᵇ בזוגיתא וכ׳ (corr. acc.) it means white glass (crystal). Gitt. 68ᵇ זוג׳. [Pes. 74ᵇ כזוּגָא חיורא Ar. a. Ms. O. like white glass; ed. זווא.]

זִגְזֵג (Pilp. of זגג, v. זַגָּג) *to clarify*. Y. Nidd. III, 50ᵈ top שהוא מתון וּמְזַגְזֵג (Tosef. ib. IV, 11 רך ומזכך; Bab. ib. 25ᵇ מצחצח) oil is cohesive and clarifies.

זַגְזָגְאֵל pr. n. m. (v. preced.) *Zagzagel* (*Divine Clearness*, cmp. אספקלריא), name of an angel. Deut. R. s. 11, end. Targ. Y. Ex. III, 2 זגנוגאל (corr. acc. or זַגְזַגְאֵל).

זְגָא, זְגַר *to lie down, recline*. Meil. 14ᵇ דילמא בעי לְמִיזְגָא וזגא עלוייהו he may desire to lie down and will lie down on them. Gitt. 47ᵃ לְמִזְגָא עליה to recline on (while eating). Pes. 108ᵃ זְגַרְנָן אברכי וכ׳ we reclined (at the Passover meal) against the knees &c.—Sabb. 124ᵇ חזו למזגא עלוייהו they may be used for sitting on them (when seats are improvised). Snh. 85ᵇ דז׳ עליה he leaned on him. [Tanh. Ki Thetsé 6, a. e. למזגר, v. זְגַר.] [Targ. Y. Deut. X, 22 למזגר ed. pr., v. מְסַגֵּר.]

Af. אַזְגַּר *to lay down*. Sabb. 119ᵃ top לא מַזְגַּרְנָא וכ׳ some ed. מַזְרְגְנָא *Pa.*) I do not rest my head upon my pillow before &c.

זָגִיד m. (v. preced., cmp. אפרקד) *in a brooding position*. Hull. 62ᵇ מרדו ז׳ ואכיל (Rashi מרה) *mardu brooding and eating* (name of a bird, prob. an adaptation of a foreign word), contrad. to סגיד ואכיל kneeling down and eating (like a bird of prey). [R. Gerson Ms. to Hull.: מרדו מזרג, leaving out אכיל; Ar. ed. Koh. III, p. 319.]

***זְגִיתָא** f. (=זְגוּגִיתָא) *a crystal vessel*. Y. Kidd. I, 60ᵇ top החן דנסב בז׳ (ed. Krot. כזיתא, corr. acc.) if one takes up a crystal vessel (to take possession).

זָגָן, v. זַג.

זגנוגאל, v. זַגְזָגְאֵל.

זַגְתָּא or **זָגְתָא** f. (זגר) 1) *a clucking hen*. Bekh. 8ᵇ. B. Mets. 86ᵇ, v. בַּרְנִיתָא.—2) ז׳ על אפרחהא (*the clucking hen over her chickens*,) *the Pleiades*. Targ. Job XXXVIII, 32 (Ar. ed. pr. על בנהא).

זֵד m. (b. h.; זוד) *wicked*.—*Pl.* זֵדִים. Tanh. Korah 12 ברכת הז׳ the additional (twelfth) section of the Prayer of Benedictions, also called ב׳ הצדוקים or המינים, v. מִין.

זֵידוֹן m. (preced.) *violent man*.—*Pl.* זֵידוֹנִין. Der. Er. ch. II, beg.

זָדוֹן m. (b. h.; זוד) *premeditated, conscious sin*, opp. שְׁגָגָה. Ab. IV, 13 a scholar's error in teaching עולה ז׳ is accounted for a wilful wrong. Ker. 25ᵇ, a. fr. דבר שזדונו כרת a sin which if wilfully committed, is punished with extinction, Sabb. 69ᵃ דבר שחייבים על ז׳ וכ׳. Ib. בזדון שבת when he is fully conscious that this is a Sabbath day (whereon certain labors are forbidden); a. fr.—*Pl.* זְדוֹנוֹת. B. Mets. 33ᵇ ששגגות ... כז׳ to whom errors are accounted &c.—Yoma 36ᵃ; a. fr.

זְדוֹן ch. same. Targ. O. Deut. XXIX, 17.—*Pl.* זְדוֹנַיָּיא *passions*. Targ. Ps. XIX, 14 Ms. (ed. זֵידְנַיָּא, זֵידוֹנַ׳, v. זֵידְנָא).

זְדוֹנְתָא, זְדוֹנָא f. (preced.) *haughtiness, violence*. Targ. Hab. I, 3. Targ. Prov. XI, 2 Ms. (ed. זֵידוֹנְתָא).

זְדוֹנוּתָא, v. next w.

זְדָנוּתָא, זְדָנוּ f. ch.=h. זָדוֹן *wilfulness, rashness*. Targ. Y. II Lev. XXIV, 12. Targ. O. Deut. XXIX, 18 (ed. Berl. זֵידְנוּתָא; Y. זְדוֹנוּתָא). Targ. Y. ib. XV, 9 (ed. Amst. זְדָנוּתָ׳); a. e.

זדנו, v. זוז I.

זֶה m., **זאֹת, זוֹ** f. (b. h.) *this, that*. Men. 53ᵇ יבא זה ויקבל זה מזה וכ׳ let this one come and receive this &c.; זה משה

'this one' that means Moses; זאת זו התורה 'this'—that means the Law. Gen. R. s. 4 לגיון זה this legion; a. v. fr.—זְהוּ=זה הוא, *this is.* Sabb. 40[b] הפשרו זהו בישולו (also זה הוא) warming it is the cooking of it, v. הֶפְשֵׁר; a. fr.—Gitt. VIII, 4 אי זהו Y. ed. (Mish. אֵיזֶהוּ); a. v. fr.

זָהַב, *Hif.* הִזְהִיב (denom. of זָהָב) *to glitter,* contrad. to הצהיב (v. צָהַב). Hull. 22[b] משיַזְהִיבוּ when their plumage is glittering.—*Part. Hof.* מוּזְהָב, f. מוּזְהֶבֶת *gold-embroidered.* Sabb. 59[b].—*Pl.* f. מוּזְהָבוֹת. Tosef. Sot. XV, 9, v. זְהוֹרִית.

זָהָב m. (b. h.) *gold, gold coin,* v. דִּינָר. Snh. 92[b] יוצק ז׳ רותח וכ׳ molten gold be poured into &c. Ex. R. s. 33 מכל עשרך . . . ושל ז׳ than all thy (Korah's) wealth of silver and gold; a. fr.—B. Mets. IV, 1 הז׳ קונה את הכסף וכ׳ the delivery of gold coin effects the purchase of silver &c., i. e. in an exchange of coined gold for silver &c., the superior metal is the merchandise and the inferior the money; Y. ed. הכסף קונה את הז׳; v. Bab. ib. 44[a]; a. fr.—*Pl.* זְהָבִים, זְהָבִין. Ex. R. s. 35; Cant. R. to III, 10 שבעה (מיני) ז׳ וכ׳ seven kinds of gold were used in the Temple. Yoma 44[b] שבעה ז׳ וכ׳ there are seven &c.—Erub. 53[b] (in allegorical speech) והרקיעו לז׳ וכ׳ Ms. M. (ed. ארקיעו) make the gold (glowing coals) sky-blue (fan them so as to give blue flames) and prepare for me two tellers in the dark (cocks).

זְהָבִי m. (preced.) *goldsmith, jeweller.* Ex. R. s. 5; a. e.—*Pl.* זְהָבִים, זְהָבִין. Succ. 51[b]; Tosef. ib. IV, 6. Sabb. 123[a]. Ex. R. s. 35 (play on זהב סגור, I Kings VI, 20, a. e.) שהיה סוגר כל הז׳ (Cant. R. to III, 10 בעד כל בעלי הז׳) it closed up the shops of all gold dealers.

זָהָה, זָהַח [*to glisten,*] *to be proud, wanton.*—Denom. זָהוּהַ.

Hif. הִזְהִיהַּ, הִזְהִיחַ *to charge one with wantonness.* Hull. 7[a], אין מַזְהִיהִין אותו Ar., (ed. מַזְהִיחִין) you must not reproach him as a haughty person, v. זָנַח a. זוּחַ.

זְהָה, זְהַח ch. same.—**Pa.* זַהֵיהַּ, זַהֵיחַ *to make haughty.* Targ. Ps. XLIV, 19 לא זר פליג וזהוחית לבנא (ed. Lag. זהוחנן, Ms. זהוהן), read: וזהית יה וכ׳ (or וזחיה) no stranger divided and made haughty our heart.

זְהוּ, v. זֶה.

זָהוּב m. (זהב) *a gold coin.* Tosef. Shebu. V, 9 דינר זהב ז׳ a gold denar in coin, contrad. to דינר זהב the value of a gold denar; Shebu. 40[a]. Y. Shebi. X, end, 39[d] מה בין ז׳ וכ׳ what is the difference between a gold coin (as a pledge) and a gold ring?—ז׳ דרכו להשתנות a gold coin may be exchanged (the pledgee being permitted to use it). Ex. R. s. 35; a. v. fr.—*Pl.* זְהוּבִים. Cant. R. to I, 1; a. fr.

זָהוּהַ, זָחוּחַ m. (זָהָה) *proud, boastful, wanton.*—*Pl.* זְחוּחִים, זְהוּהִים; only in זְחוּחֵי הלב (זְחוּחֵי). Sot. 47[b] זה׳ Ar. (ed. זח׳); Tosef. ib. XIV, 9 זְהִיהֵי Var. (ed. Zuck. זהורי, corr. acc.); Hull. 7[a].

זְהוּהָא, זְחוּחָא ch. 1) same.—*Pl.* זְהוּהִין, constr. זְהוּהֵי. Targ. Job XXXVI, 13, a. e.—2) *wantonness, pride.* Targ. Lam. III, 33 ed. Lag. (oth. ed. זְהוּהָה).—*Pl.* as above. Targ. Ps. LXII, 9 (ed. Lag. דהוהי).—[Ib. XLIV, 19, v. זְהָה.]

זְהוּנִיא, v. זַוִּיגָנְיָא.

זָהוֹר, pl. **זְהוֹרִים**, fem. **זְהוֹרוֹת**, v. זְהוֹרִית. [Tosef. Sot. XIV, 9 זהורי הלב, v. זָהוּהַ.]

זְהוֹרָא, v. זֵיהוּרָא.

זָהוֹרָא, v. זִיהוּרָא.

זְהוֹרִי m. (v. next w.) *safran-colored* or *crimson.* Targ. Y. Gen. XXXVIII, 28; 30, v. זְהוֹרִיתָא.

זְהוֹרִית f. (זהר; v. P. Sm. 1115 s. v. זהור׳) *crimson; crocus; crimson* (or *safran*) *colored material,* esp. *silk* (b. h. שָׁנִי). Kel. XXVII, 12 ז׳ טובה fine crimsom *silk.* Y. Succ. III, 53[d] (defining אדמדם) ז׳ עמוקה deep crimson. Pesik. R. s. 26 ומלבשתן ז׳ (some ed. זהורים) and clads them in silk. Nidd. 25[b] כב׳ . . . של זְהוֹרִין like two threads of silk (woof); כב׳ . . . זהורית (prob. to be read זְהוֹרוֹת) like two threads of silk (warp); Y. ib. III, 50[d] של זהורות; Lev. R. s. 14. Yoma VI, 8 לשון של ז׳ a crimson-colored strap. Tosef. Sabb. IV (V), 5 ז׳ שבין עיניו crimson ornament between his (the horse's) eyes; Sabb. 53[a] זְהַרוּרִית (Ar. זהור׳); a. e.—*Pl.* זְהוֹרִיּוֹת. Tosef. Sot. XV, 9 ז׳ מוזהבות (Sot. 49[b] זהורית מוזהבות, corr. acc.) gold-embroidered silks used for brides' canopies.

זְהוֹרִיתָא ch. same. Targ. O. Gen. XXXVIII, 28; 30. Targ. Is. I, 18 (ed. Wil. זְהָרִיתָא; h. text תּוֹלָע); a. e.—Gitt. 69[b] חוטא דז׳ a (crimson) silk thread.

זְהִיגָא m. (זהה) *a wanton jester.* Lev. R. s. 20 Ar.; v., however, זַוִּיגָנְיָא.

זָהִים m. (זהם) *a filthy person, one wearing a laboring suit.* Targ. Job XXXVIII, 14.

זָהִיר m., **זְהִירָה** f. (זהר) *looking out; strictly observant; careful, on one's guard.* Ab. II, 1 הוי ז׳ וכ׳ be as strict in the observance of minor religious duties &c. Ib. IV, 13; B. Mets. 33[b] הוי ז׳ בתלמוד be careful in teaching the Law, v. זָדוֹן. Snh. 76[b] הוי ז׳ במי שיועצך וכ׳ Ms. M. (ed. מן היועצך, v. Rabb. D. S. a. l. note) beware of him who advises thee to his own advantage. Sabb. 23[b] הז׳ במזוזה he who is strict in the observance &c.; a. fr.—*Pl.* זְהִירִין, f. זְהִירוֹת. Ab. II, 3 הוו ז׳ ברשות beware of the officials. Sabb. II, 6 על שאינן ז׳ וכ׳ because they are not careful in the observance of the laws concerning &c.; a. fr.

זְהִיר, זְהִיר ch. same. Targ. Y. Gen. XLIX, 26 וז׳ ביקרא וכ׳ guarding the honor &c.—*Pl.* זְהִירִין. Ezra IV, 22.—Targ. Y. Deut. XII, 16.—V. זְהַר.

זְהִירָא *poison,* v. זִיהֲרָא.

זְהִירוּת f. (v. זהיר) *strictness, care.* Ab. Zar. 20[b] תורה מביאה לידי ז׳ וכ׳ study leads to strictness, strictness to zeal (differ. vers., v. Rabb. D. S. a. l., note, a. Sot. IX, 15).

זָהַל, v. זָחַל.

זָהַם (b. h.; cmp. זהח) [*to be glistening;* cmp. צחן a. צחנה)] *to be filthy, smell offensively, be offensive.*—Part. זוֹהֵם, or part. pass. זָהוּם. Y. Ab. Zar. II, 41[c] bot. ר"ל אמר ככוס ז׳ (not בכוס) R. L. says, It is like drinking out of an offensive cup; השותה בכוס ז׳ וכ׳ he who drinks (sacred wine &c.) out of &c. Y. Nidd. IV, end, 51[b] דם נדה זהום (Tosef. ib. IX, 10 זוהם; Bab. ib. 65[b]) the blood of a menstruant is sticky (or ill-smelling).

Pi. זִיהֵם 1) *to smear plants with rancid oil* for keeping off vermin, [oth. opin.: *to cover a wound in a tree with dung and tie it up.*] Shebi. II, 4. Y. ib. 33[d] (expl. מְזַהֲמִין of Mish.) מתלעין to keep the worms off. Ib. המְזַהֵם אינו וכ׳ oiling a plant is merely like appointing a watchman (it does not advance growth). Y. Sabb. VII, 10[a] top, v. כָּחַל II.—*Part. pass.* מְזוּהָם, f. מְזוּהֶמֶת *ill-smelling, filthy, offensive.* Bekh. VI, 12 ומז׳ and an animal of offensive smell or sight. Ber. 53[b] מז׳ an offensive-looking priest. Y. Gitt. VIII, 49[d] top מז׳ היא מלפניו she is disgusting to him (on account of her conduct); a. e.—*Pl.* מְזוּהָמִים, מְזוּהָמִין; fem. מְזוּהָמוֹת. Ber. l. c. ידים מ׳ smelling hands (after a meal, when not perfumed). Lev. R. s. 16; Esth. R. to III, 1 מה ... מ׳ וכ׳ as ordure is offensive, so is he (the leper); a. e.—2) *to declare unfit for priestly or levitical service (or connection), to reject.* Bekh. 47[a] אין מְזַהֲמִין וכ׳ the child is not rejected (as the child of a gentile).—Y. Yeb. X, 11[a]; XIII, 13[d] bot. ואין ב״ד מזהמין אותה but the court does not declare her unfit to marry a priest.—3) (v. זוֹהֲמָא) part. pass. מְזוּהָם, pl. מְזוּהָמִין *inclined to lasciviousness, unchaste.* Sabb. 145[b] bot.

**Hif.* הִזְהִים *to become unfit for offering through offensiveness.* Pesik. Vayhi, p. 10[a] לא הִזְהִימוּ (perh. to be read הוּזְהֲמוּ Hof.; (Yalk. Num. 713 הוזמו, expl. חוסמו, corr. acc., or הוּסְמוּ as Num. R. s. 12, end, a. e., v. Bub. note to Pesik. l. c.).

זְהַם ch. same. Part. pass. זְהִים q. v.

Pa. זַהֵם *to create aversion, to sicken.* Lev. R. s. 16 (to the leper) לא תְזַהֵם ברייתא (ed. Wil. תזוהום, read תְּזַהִים) do not sicken people with thy sight.

Ithpe. אִזְדְּהֵם, *Ithpa.* אִזְדַּהַם 1) *to be soiled, to empty the bowels.* Targ. Ps. CVI, 20.—2) *to become offensive.* Ab. Zar. 26[a] לא מִיזְדַּהֲמָנָא וכ׳ I do not desire to become offensive to my husband (get ungainly through nursing).

זָהַר (b. h.; cmp. זהח) 1) *to shine;* v. זָהוֹר, זְהוֹרִית.—2) *to look out, beware, be strict* (corresp. to b. h. שָׁמַר); v. זָהִיר.

Pi. זִהֵר *to brighten.* Midr. Till. to Ps. XC, 16 וזִהֲרוּ and brightened his countenance.

Nif. הִזָּהֵר (=b. h. הִשָּׁמֵר) *to be careful, be strict; to beware, take heed.* Ber. 8[b] הִזָּהֲרוּ בוורידין be careful to cut the jugular veins, v. וְרִיד. Ib. ה׳ בזקן וכ׳ beware of disregarding an old man who &c. Ned. 81[a] ה׳ בבני עניים וכ׳ take heed of (do not disregard) the children of the poor; a. fr.

Hif. הִזְהִיר *to caution, forewarn,* esp. *to prohibit by a special law,* v. אַזְהָרָה. Yeb. 22[b], a. e. אין מַזְהִירִין מן הדין a law derived from analogy (v. דִּין) is not considered a specified law on which punishment can be executed after due warning. Zeb. 106[b], a. e. לא ענש אא״כ ה׳ the Bible text did not pronounce punishment without having expressed a warning ('thou shalt not' &c.); a. fr.

Hof. הוּזְהַר *to be forewarned, to be forbidden from doing* (by a special law). Yeb. 84[b] לא הוּזְהֲרוּ וכ׳ there is no specific law prohibiting women of legitimate birth to marry men of illegitimate birth.—Part. מוּזְהָר, f. מוּזְהֶרֶת. Ib. מלמד שהאשה מ׳ (the repeated expression, 'they shall not take', Lev. XXI, 7) intimates that woman is included with man in the prohibition; ib. כל היכא דהוא מ׳ היא מ׳ wherever the man is cautioned not to marry, the woman (in the same social relation) is cautioned; a. fr. [Ib. היא לא מוזהרא, read: מוזהרת.]

זְהַר, זְהִיר ch. same, 1) *to shine, bloom.* Targ. Job XXII, 28 (ed. Wil. יַזְהַר *Af.*). Targ. Hos. XIV, 6; a. e.—2) *to look out, guard.*—Part. pass. זְהִיר. Hag. 23[a] מֵיזְהַר זהיר בהו he guards them (from levitical impurity). Hull. 107[b] דזְהִיר he is careful (not to touch), contrad. to זריז taking precaution. Y. Ber. V, 9[a] bot. זְהִירָא לה watches it (the cloak). Y. Ab. Zar. III, 41[a] bot. לא הוינא ז׳ לך was I not on my guard against thee?; a. fr.

Pa. זַהַר 1) *to emit light, to glisten.* Targ. Zech. IX, 15.—2) *to caution.* Targ. Cant. V, 2.

Af. אַזְהַר 1) *to give light, shine.* Targ. Is. IX, 1; a. e.—2) *to explain.* Targ. Ex. XVIII, 20.—3) *to caution.* Targ. Ez. III, 18; a. e.—Snh. 66[a] bot. דילמא אקודש א׳ וכ׳ perhaps in saying 'thou shalt not curse *Elohim*' (Ex. XXII, 27) the Law gave warning with regard *to holy Elohim* (God), but not with regard to secular *Elohim* (authorities)?

Ithpe. אִזְדְּהַר, *Ithpa.* אִזְדַּהַר 1) *to take heed, beware.* Targ. Y. Ex. X, 28; a. e.—Ab. Zar. 28[a], v. זִיקָא I. Ib. 12[b], v. שַׁבְרִירִי; a. fr.—2) *to watch.* Y. Ber. V, 9[a] bot. מִזְדַּהֲרָא ליה was watching it. B. Bath. 29[a] תרתי . . מִזְדְּהַר the first two or three years man takes care of the deed. Ib. הוה מִזְדַּהֲרְנָא וכ׳ I should have taken care &c.; a. e.

זָהֳרָא, זַהֲרָא I, (זהר) 1) *light.* Y. Yoma III, beg. 40[b], v. אִיבְּרַיְיתָא. Cant. R. to VII, 3 (ref. to הסהר ib., v. אַגָּן) אית . . . לזהרא סהרא (some ed. לזהרה) there are places where they write and pronounce *sahăra* for *zahăra.*—2) *brightness, splendor; moon,* v. זִיהֲרָא a. זִיהֲרָא I.

זַהֲרָא II *poison,* v. זִיהֲרָא II.

זַהֲרָה, v. זַהֲרָא I.

זְהוֹרָא, v. זִיהֲרָרָא.

זְהוֹרָא, זִיהֲ׳ m. (זהר) *red light, glare, reflex.*—*Pl.* זְהוֹרֵי, זִי׳. Pes. 13[a] וז׳ בעלמא וכ׳ (Ms. M. זהרוריה, Ms. M. 2 וזהרורי) and what he saw was merely the glare, v. גִּילְהֵי; Snh. 42[a].—B. Mets. 84[a] והנהו ז׳ דנפקי מיניה מעין וכ׳ Ms. M. (ed. והחוא ז׳ מעין; Rashi: זי׳) and those reflexes issuing from it are a specimen of the beauty of &c.

זְהוֹרִית, v. זְהוֹרִית.

זְהוֹרִיתָא, v. זְהוֹרִיתָא.

זוּ, v. זֶה.

זוּב (b.h.; cmp. דבב, דוה) *to flow, drip.* Bets. 3[a], a. fr. משקין שזָבוּ juice of fruits which flowed out (on a Holy

Day). Hull. 27ª (play on וזבחת, Deut. XII, 21), ממקום שֶׁזָּב יַחְתּוֹ from where (the blood) will flow (the jugular veins), there break (its life), v. חָתַת; a. fr.—V. זָב.

זוֹב m. (b. h.; preced.) *flux, gonorrhea, prolonged menstruation.* Nidd. 35ᵇ ז׳ דומה the flux (of the gonorrhea) resembles &c. Ib. יולדה בז׳ one giving birth while suffering with flux; a. fr.—Men. 64ᵇ שמא בז׳ סיכנה perhaps she was in danger from a severe *hemorrhage*, v. זִיבָה a. זֵיבָה.

זוֹב or **זָבָא** ch. same. Sabb. 110ᵇ (in an incantation) קוּם מזוֹבִיךְ (Ms. M. a. some ed. מִזָּבִיךְ) rise (be cured) from thy flux.

זוֹבָן m. (denom. of זָנָב) *the bag which contains a male animal's membrum.* Bekh. VI, 5; expl. ib. 39ᵇ כיס ולא וכ׳ the bag but not the organ itself; Tosef. ib. IV, 6.

זָוַג, *Pi.* זִוֵּג, זִיוֵּג, זִוּוּג 1) *to join, couple, match; to adjust.* Tosef. Kil. V, 11 הַמְזַוֵּג את הכלאים he who harnesses together two heterogeneous animals; B Mets. 90ᵇ הַמְזַ׳ בכל׳. Y. Gitt. III, 44ᵈ bot. הגע עצמך שזיווג but supposed that one matched it, i. e. found a letter of divorce just containing the names of the persons under consideration (though not written for that special transaction). Ib. כיון שאינו מצוי לְזַוֵּג אפי׳ ז׳ כמי שלא ז׳ since it is so rare to find such a matching combination, even if one did, we consider it as if he had not done it, i. e. such rare chances are not taken into consideration. Y. Shek. V, 49ª bot. הגע.. שז׳ אותו היום supposed somebody produced a ticket with the mark of the same day of the week?—Ib. אפי׳ לזויג וכ׳ (read as above: כיון שאינו וכ׳). Y. M. Kat. I, end, 80ᵈ bot. מְזַוֵּג את האומריות one who knots the fringes two by two (instead of making a regular network).—Y. Shek. V, 48ᵈ bot. מְזַוֵּג את הפתילות (Bab. ed. מְזַוֵּג) he adjusted the length of the wicks (to the length of the time they had to burn); Y. Yoma II, 39ᵈ bot.—Esp. 2) *to join in wedlock, to wed.* Sot. 2ª אין מְזַוְּוגִין לו לאדם וכ׳ a wife is selected (in heaven) for each man according to his deserts. Ib. קשין לְזַוְּוגָן וכ׳ to wed couples is as difficult as the splitting of the Red Sea. Gen. R. s. 68; Lev. R. s. 8, beg. מְזַוֵּג זיווגים וכ׳ He joins couples, decrees who should be married to whom. Ib. אני יכולה זווגן בלילה לְזַוְּגָם וכ׳ I can couple them in one hour. Ib. וכ׳ (read: זִוְּגָתָן); a. fr.—3) *to join* in a hostile sense, *to attack.* Cant. R. to III, 6, v. לָבַב.—4) *to match in misery, to comfort by pointing out a similar case* (cmp. Lam. II, 13). Pesik. R. s. 30 מזדווג בה וכ׳ (read מְזַוֵּג לה) He shows her (the country) a fellow-sufferer to comfort her. Ib. מזדויג לה אלכסנדריה וכ׳ (corr. acc.) he pointed out to her Alexandria. Ib. בא יואל וזי׳ לה Joel came and comforted her (by pointing to the Lord's sympathy).

Hithpa. הִזְדַּוֵּג, *Nithpa.* נִזְדַּוֵּג 1) *to be joined; to join, meet.* Y. Yoma VI, 43ᶜ top שיִזְדַּוֵּג לו חבירו that the other bullock must be joined to him (they must belong to the same couple). Snh. V, 5 (40ª) מִזְדַּוְּוגִין זוגות וכ׳ they met in couples (for consultation). Y. Taan. I, 64ª top (ref. to Is. XXI, 11, play on אֵלַי וכ׳) אֵלִי מארכן נז׳ לי וכ׳ whence did my God join me again? From Seir (Rome); a. fr.—2) (in a hostile sense) *to join in battle, attack.* Ex. R. s. 1; Tanh. Sh'moth 5 בוא ונִזְדַּוֵּג וכ׳ come and let us plan how to get at that nation. Lev. R. s. 11 נִזְדַּוְּוגוּ לו שלשה וכ׳ three enemies attacked it jointly. Ib. באו ברבריים כ׳ לו barbarians attacked him; Esth. R. introd.; a. fr.—3) *to be wedded.* Cant. R. to I, 4 (נגרלה); Pesik. Sos, p. 147ª כשם שנִזְדַּוַּגְתֶּם וכ׳ as you have been married with festivities.

זְוַג ch., *Pa.* זַוֵּג, זַוֵּיג, זַוֵּיג same, *to join, couple* &c. Targ. Y. Deut. XVI, 21. Targ. Ps. LXVIII, 7. Targ. Y. I Deut. XXXIII, 7; a. e.—*Part. pass.* מְזַוַּג *joined.* Targ. Y. Ex. XXVI, 24 (h. text תאמים). Targ. Y. II Num. VII, 3 מְזַוְּגָן with teams and harness (h. text צָב).

Ithpa. אִזְדַּוַּג as preced. *Hithpa.* Targ. Y. Deut. V, 27; a. e.—Targ. Y. Ex. XXI, 13 (h. text צדה); a. e.

זוֹג m. (זגג) *bell, the body of the bell,* contrad. to עינבל, clapper. Naz. VI, 1 כז׳ של בהמה (*zag* means the shell) like the bell of an animal; החיצון ז׳ וכ׳ the outer part is called *zog*, the inner *inbol*. Sabb. V, 4. Tosef. Kel. B. Mets. I, 13 ז׳ של דלת door-bell. Tosef. Sabb. V (VI), 7, sq.; Sabb. 58ª, sq.; a. fr.—*Pl.* זוּגִין, זְוָגִין. Tosef. Kel. l. c. העושה זג׳ וכ׳ he who fastens bells to a mortar. Ib. 14 חזקת ז׳ וכ׳ the rule concerning bells &c. Y. Gitt. III, 45ª top ז׳ bells (among the appurtenances of siege, v. כַּרְכּוֹם II); Y. Keth. II, 26ᵈ דוגין (corr. acc.). Tosef. l. c. [read:] אמר לְאוּמן עשה לי שני ז׳ אחד לדלת וכ׳ if one says to the artisan, Make for me two bells, one for a door &c.; Y. Gitt. III, 44ᵈ top (corr. acc.); a. fr. [זוגין *grape-shells,* v. זַג.]

זוּג m. (זָוַג) 1) *couple, pair, set.* Erub. X, 1 מכניסן ז׳ ז׳ he must bring them in, one set at a time (on his head and arm). Snh. 12ª (in a secret letter) ז׳ בא וכ׳ a couple (of scholars or messengers of Jewish authorities) came from Rakkath (Tiberias), and the eagle (Rome) caught them; a. fr.—בֶּן ז׳ *partner, equal, match, counterpart.* Gitt. 90ᵇ אין זה בן זוגו׳ וכ׳ this (second husband) is not the equal of the first husband (is morally inferior). Gen. R. s. 11 שאין לו בן ז׳ it (the seventh day) has no match (the week having three couples of days and one single day). Ib. כ״י היא בן זוגך the congregation of Israel be thy match. Ib. s. 7 בהמות יש לו בן ז׳ the B'hemoth has a partner (is created male and female).—*Pl.* זוּגוֹת. Ib. אין להם בן ז׳ (for בני זוג, cmp. ברזוג) have no partners (females). Deut. R. s. 2 שמים וארץ ז׳ וכ׳ heaven and earth are couples, sun and moon are couples &c.—Pes. 110ᵇ יש בו משום ז׳ the apprehension of danger from even numbers applies to it, v. זוּגָא; a. fr.—Esp. *Zugoth*, the two chiefs (*Nasi* and *Ab Beth Din*) of the Supreme Court since its reorganization after Simon the Just (v. Ab. I, 2; 4, sq.). Naz. 56ᵇ; Peah II, 6. Y. Sot. IX, 24ª top וכל הז׳ היו וכ׳ were all the *Zugoth* no accomplished scholars? Ib. כל הז׳ שעמדו (Tosef. B. Kam. VIII, 13 האשכולות). Ib. bot.; Y. Maas. Sh. V, end, 56ᵈ העמיד ז׳ he (John Hyrcan) appointed double sets of guards.—2) (*pair of*) *scissors.* Kel. XIII, 1 ז׳ של ספרים barbers' scissors. Neg. IV, 4; Nidd. VI, 12; a. fr.

זִוּוּג, **זִוּג** m. (preced.) *marriage.* Sot. 2ª; Gitt. 90ᵇ בז׳ ראשון in first marriage; Snh. 22ª בזווג. Yalk. Jud. 70, v. זירוג.

זוג *to be clear*, v. זרג.

זוּגָא, זוּג, זוֹג, זוֹגָא I ch.=h. זוג 1) *pair, couple, team, set.* Targ. II Kings IX, 25. Targ. Jud. XVII, 10 זוג לבושין a set of garments; a. e.—בַּר זוּג *match, wife.* Targ. Y. II Gen. II, 18; a. e.—Snh. 43ª מסרינן ליה ז׳ דרבנן we give him two scholars (to escort him); Yoma 85ᵇ (Ms. M. זְוָוא). Y. Ḥag. II, 78ª top כל דמטי יחכום זוגיה whosoever has a chance shall select his partner (as if for a dance); a. fr.—*Pl.* זוּגֵי. Pes. 110ª Ashm'dai . . . . is appointed אכולהו ז׳ overseer of all even numbers (of cups &c., which were believed to invite dangers); a. e.—Keth. 71ª, v. זְוָוא I.—Sot. 13ᵇ דרו ז׳, v. הֵידוֹזוּגֵר.—2) (cmp. above זוג לבושין, a. זְוַד) *an outfit for travelling, travelling cloak.* Targ. Y. Lev. XV, 9 (not זונא) garment for polster.—Erub. 100ᵇ bot. זבינא לך זוגא דמטו וכ׳ ed. (Ms. M. זרנא דמטרא, v. Rabb. D. S. a. l. note) I shall buy thee garments reaching to thy feet.—*Pl.* as above. Gen. R. s. 92 לבש זוגוי put on his travelling equipments; Yalk. Gen. 150 וגוהי read זוּגוֹהִי.—3) *scissors.* B. Mets. 116ª, a. e., v. זְוָוא I.

זוּגָא II, **זוּגָה** pr. n. m. *Zuga*, name of several Amoraim. Y. Maasr. V, end, 52ª; Y. Dem. II, 22ᶜ; a. e.—Gamliel Z. Ib.ᵈ top; a. e. (v. Fr. M'bo p. 77ª; 71ᵇ).—M. Kat. 28ª, a. e., Ar. זְוָוא II.

זוּגָא *glass*, v. זְגוּגִיתָא.

זוגדס, זוגדוס, v. זַגְדוּס.

זוּגָה I pr. n. m., v. זוּגָא II.

זוּגָה II f. (זוג) *intended, beloved.* Keth. 63ª זוּגָתָךְ נזכרת didst thou think of thy girl (that thou camest home before thy time was up)?

זוד, v. זיד.

זְוַד, *Pa.* זַוֵּיד, זַיֵּיד (cmp. זבד; =b. h. צוד) *to endow, outfit*, esp. for travelling. Targ. Y. II Deut. XV, 14 (h. text הַעֲנֵק).—Ab. Zar. 17ª זַוְּידוּ לה זוודתא (editorial insertion; Ms. M. טרחו, v. Rabb. D. S. a. l. note) prepare her shrouds; R. Hash. 17ª זוידו Ms. M. (ed. צביתו).

Ithpe. אִזְדְּוַד, *Ithpa.* אִזְדַּוַּד 1) *to provide one's self for a journey, lay in provision.* Targ. Josh. IX, 12 (h. text הִצְטַיַּדְ).—2) *to tie up bundles.* Ib. 4 (h. text הצטיר, v. צָרַר, צוּר).

זְוָדָא, זְוַודָא, זְוָדְתָא c. (preced.) 1)=h. צידה, *outfit for travelling, provision; dying outfit, shroud;* trnsf. *good deeds.* Targ. Ps. CXXXII, 15.—*Pl.* זְוָ׳, זְוָדִין. Targ. O. Gen. XLII, 25; a. e.—Keth. 67ᵇ זְוָדַאי קלילי my provision (for the journey of death) is scanty. M. Kat. 28ᵇ דשלימו זְוָדֵיהּ whose outfit for death is completed, v. אִסְטְלָא.—זְוָדְתָא. Ib. 27ᵇ צבית ז׳ לאידך prepare the burial outfit for another son. R. Hash. 17ª; Ab. Zar. 17ª, v. preced.; a. fr.—2) *bag, bundle.* Kidd. 12ª ז׳ דאודרי (Ar. ed. Koh. זְוָדֵי, pl.) a bundle of tow cotton (being of small value).

זוּהֲ, Snh. 96ᵇ, part. f. זֵיהָא, v. זוח ch.

זוּהֲמָה, זוּהֲמָא f. (זהם) 1) *froth; filth, decayed matter, evil smell.* Pes. 42ᵇ שואבת את הז׳ absorbs the froth of boiling meat. Ter. X, 1 ליטול את הז׳ to carry off foul matter; Y. Ab. Zar. III, 41ᶜ top את שהוא ליטול את הז׳ a substance which is used for &c.—Ber. 53ª שמן . . . . . את הז׳; Y. ib. VI, 10ᵈ שמן לז׳ oil used for perfuming the hands after the meal, v. זָהַם.—2) *moral impurity, obscenity, voluptuousness.* Yalk. Lev. 525 דבר של ז׳ (ed. Lemb. זומא), v. זִימְּמָא. Yeb. 103ᵇ שדי בה ז׳ he infected her with sensuality. Ib., a. e. הטיל בה ז׳ the serpent infected her (Eve, i.e. the human race) with lasciviousness. Ib. פסקה זוּהֲמָתָן their sensual passions ceased (were checked through the influence of religion); a. fr.—3) ז׳ דשמשא *the sultry air produced by the passage of the sunrays through a cloudy atmosphere.* Yoma 28ᵇ ז׳ דש׳ וכ׳ (Ar. a. Ms. L. זִיהֲרָא, Ms. O. זוֹהֲרָא, v. Rabb. D. S. a. l. note) the sultry heat is more intense than that of direct sunlight. [Sabb. 123ª ז׳ לירסטרון, v. זוֹמְלִיסְטְרוֹן.]

זוּהֲמַאי pr. n. m. *Zohămai*, by-name of a scholar. Ber. 53ᵇ, v. זָהַם.

זוּהֲמָה, v. זוּהֲמָא.

זוּהֲרָא m. (זהר), ז׳ דשמשא *reflected sun-light.* Yoma 28ᵇ, v. זוּהֲמָא.

זָוָא I, זָרָא m. (זְוַד; cmp. זוג, fr. זָג) *pair, set; change of clothes; scissors* (corresp. to, and interchanging with זוּגָא). Meg. 16ª לית לי זווא Ms. M. I have no scissors; אתא אליהו ושדא ליה ז׳ Elijah came and dropped a pair of scissors; (ed. זוזא, a. entirely differ. vers.; Ar. זווא). B. Mets. 116ª bot. זוגא דסרבלי ed. (Ms. M. זוזי, Ms. F. זוזא; Ar. זווי) scissors for shearing shaggy woolen stuff; B. Bath. 52ª; Shebu. 46ᵇ; Ab. Zar. 75ᵇ זוזא (Ar. זוו׳). Taan. 21ᵇ bot. זווא דרבנן ed. Pes. a. oth. (oth. ed. זוזא, oth. זוגא, v. Rabb. D. S. a. l. note 100) a delegation of scholars. Meg. 7ª; Succ. 4ᵇ; Sabb. 54ᵇ (an editorial gloss) בכוליה סדר מועד כל כי האי זווא וכ׳ Ar. (ed. זוגא) in the entire Order of Moëd, wherever this combination of authorities appears, some take out R. Joh. and insert R. Jon.—Ber. 22ᵇ חד מהאי זווא וכ׳ Ar. (ed. זוגא) one of the first combination of scholars, and one of the second combination.—*Pl.* זְוָוֵי (זוזי). Keth. 71ª ז׳ ז׳ קתני Ar. (ed. זוגי) they are arranged in couples (two scholars for the one opinion and two for the other). Pes. 111ª הנהו ז׳ בכשפים עסיקן Ms. M. (ed. ודאי וכ׳) these are of the couples engaged in sorcery. Erub. 97ª צבתים ז׳ ז׳ (v. Rabb. D. S. a. l. note 90) *ts'vathim* (Mish. ib. X, 1) means bundles of one set (of *T'fillin*) each. Ib. 37ª עולא זוזי זוזי קתני ed. (Ms. M. זווי, v. Rabb. D. S. a. l. note) Ula arranges the authorities quoted in couples (two on each side, v. supra). Sabb. 129ᵇ דקדימא מאדים בז׳ (Ms. M. בזוּזֵיהּ, Ms. O. בזוזי, Tosaf. to Erub. 56ª בזוגי) when the planet Mars rules at even-numbered hours of the day. Y. Ab. Zar. I, 39ᶜ bot. רחוץ בז׳ אוחרי bathe in another suit of clothes.—Sabb. 19ᵇ כרכי דזוזי (Ms. O. כריכי דזוגי) *coupled* (hinged) mattings used for roof-like protections for goods; [Var. quoted in Rashi: זִיזֵי meaning *ships;*] ib. 156ᵇ (where Rashi has זווי *ships*).

זְוָרָא II pr. n. m. *Zava*, v. זוּגָא II.

זְוּג, v. זִיווּג.

זְוָרְדָא, זְוַד, זָוַג, זֵוּג, v. זְוָדָא, זְוַד, זְוַג, זֵוּג.

זְוָרֵי m. pl. (v. זְוָיָא) *change of* (cmp. חלף); prep. *instead, in place of*. Y. Taan. III, 66^d bot. ז׳ דהוות וכ׳ (v. חֲוִי) where it (the ground) used to grow vineyards &c.; Midr. Till. to Ps. CXXVI (corr. acc.).

***זְוָתָא** f. (v. זְוָיָא I; cmp. פָּרָךְ) *what is taken with food, relish*. Targ. Job VI, 7 Ms. (ed. דְּוּתָא q. v.).

זְוְתָּכָא, v. זְיוְתְ׳.

זוּז I, perf. a. part. זָז (reduplic. of זא or זע, v. זוּעַ, cmp. זָאזָא) *to move, go away, depart*. Keth. XII, 3 לָזוּז, v. אֶפֶשׁ.—Yeb. 30^a, a. fr. ומשנה לא זָזָה ממקומה but the Mishnah was not removed from its place, i. e. it was left in the collection as it was, though afterwards repealed or modified. Gitt. 58^a איני זז מכאן וכ׳ I shall not leave this spot until &c. Tanh. Matt. 6; Num. R. s. 22, end, a. e. (play on זוזים *coins*) שֶׁזָּזִים וכ׳ they leave the one and are given to the other; a. v. fr.

Hif. הֵזִיז *to move, shake; to remove.* Ab. III, 17 אין מְזִיזִין וכ׳ they cannot move it (the tree) from its place; Taan. 20^a מְזִיזוֹת; Snh. 106^a.—Ex. R. s. 45 אין אתה יכול לְהָזִיז וכ׳ thou canst not remove thy love from them. Koh. R. to I, 13 אינו מֵזִיז ואינו מזיע וכ׳ he will not give up studying &c.; a. fr.

Hithpalp. (with anorganic נ) הִזְדַּנְזֵז, הִזְדַּעְזֵעַ v. זִעְזֵעַ.

זוּז ch. same. Targ. Y. Num. XIV, 44.

Af. אָזִיז *to shake*. Hull. 38^a אֲזוּזֵי אודני the shaking of the ears (as a symptom of vitality).

זוּז II m. (=זוזה, v. זוהה) [*the glittering*, cmp. אִיסָר, אַסְתִּירָא &c.) *Zuz*, 1) *a silver coin*, one fourth of a Shekel, =דִּינָר. Keth. I, 5; a. fr.—*Pl.* זוּזִים, זוּזִין. Num. R. s. 22, end, a. e., v. זוז I; a. fr.—2) *a weight*. Ter. X, 8; Tosef. ib. IX, 1 (Var. זִין); Y. ib. X, 47^b top זִין.—*Pl.* זוזים. Tosef. l. c. ed. Zuck.; Y. l. c. זִינִין.

זוּזָא I ch. same. Targ. I Sam. IX, 8 (h. text רבע שקל).—Kidd. 12^a קום כ״ד בז׳ twenty four Isar went on a Zuz: when the Isar was reduced, קום ל״ב ז׳ thirty two Isar went &c.—Sabb. 66^b ז׳ חדורא a new silver coin; Pes. 74^b, v. זְגוּגִיתָא. Hag. 5^a (prov.) ז׳ לעללא וכ׳ a Zuz for provision is not on hand, but for (saving from) hanging it is, i. e. charity often waits for the extremest distress. B. Kam. 11^a (prov.) כשורא במתא בז׳ וכ׳ a joist in town costs a Zuz, a joist in the woods the same, i. e. the cost of transportation has no influence on the price; a. fr.—*Pl.* זוּזֵי, זוּזִין; also in gen. *money*. Targ. II Esth. I, 8; a. e.—Hag. 9^b. B. Mets. 63^b אי הוו לי ז׳ וכ׳ if I had money. Ib. ז׳ דאינשי וכ׳ people's money does the brokership for them (with cash in hand you need no broker); a. fr.—Ib. 65^b זוּזַאי the money due to me.—Keth. 65^b; 67^a ז׳ פשיטי (=ז׳ מדינה) *country Zuz*, one eighth of the town Zuz (or Tyrian) in value; (v. Zuckerman Münzen, Jahresber. des Jüd. Theol. Seminars, Breslau 1862, p. 6; p. 24).

זוּזָא II *couple* &c., v. זְוָיָא I.

זוֹזִין m. *zozin*, name of a jewel in the Highpriest's breast-plate. Targ. Y. Ex. XXVIII, 19 (h. text לשם).

זוּחַ I (cmp. זָחַח, cmp. זוא P. Sm. 1092) *to be elated, cheerful*; (in an evil sense) *to be proud, overbearing*. Keth. 67^b כדי שֶׁתָּזוּחַ דעתו עליו in order that his mind be elevated (that he may not feel himself humiliated).—Ex. R. s. 37 זָחָה דעתו עליו he became overbearing. Snh. 38^a אם תָּזוּחַ דעתו עליו if he become overbearing; a. e.—[Y. Sabb. VIII, 11^b bot. הזיח, v. next w.]

זוּחַ ch. same. Y. Sabb. VIII, 11^b bot. הא דלא זָיְחָה דעתי עלי (not הזיח) this happened because I am not cheerful (I am too poor to collect my thoughts).—Snh. 96^b קא זָיְחָא דעתיה (Rashi זָחַח) he became overbearing.

זוּחַ II or **זָחַח** (b. h. זחח; cmp. זוּעַ) *to be unsteady, move*.—Part. זָח *faint-hearted, distracted*. Keth. 69^b; M. Kat. 28^b; Yalk. Am. 545, v. כַּר II.

Hif. הֵזִיחַ or הֵזִיחַ *to remove, to cause to move, to force one to yield* to others' opinions. Hull. 7^a אין מְזִיחִין אותו (with ref. to יִזַּח, Ex. XXVIII, 28) we do not make him give up his opinion; v. זָחַח.—Keth. 10^b מזבח מֵזִיחַ (or מְזִיח) the altar removes (evil decrees).

זוּחַ ch. 1) same. Targ. Y. Deut. XX, 3 (O. זוע; h. text יֵרַךְ). Targ. Job VIII, 14.—*2) (act. verb) *to remove, turn away*. Targ. Y. Num. IV, 19 (prob. to be read: וְיַזִּיחוּן Af.).

Af. אָזִיחַ *to cause to tremble*. Targ. Jer. L, 23 (ed. Lag. מזיע, v. זוּעַ).

זוּחֲלָא, זוּחַל m. (זחל) *creeper, worm*. Targ. Y. I Num. XXI, 35.—Tanh. Ki Thetsé 9, v. זַחֲלָא.—*Pl.* זוּחֲלִין. Targ. Mic. VII, 17 (ed. Lag. a. oth. זָחֲלֵי); a. e. V. זַחֲלָא.

זוּט or **זוֹט** m. (זוט, זוּט, cmp. צָבַת, צְבָט) 1) *a catch, a bag-like receptacle for catch in the fisher's net; the solid web of the net-work*. Kel. XXIII, 5 החרם טמא מפני זוטו Ar. (ed. הזוטו, R. Hai G. הזוּבָן, Var. הזובן) the net is fit for levitical uncleanness on account of its bag (being a receptacle of solid web). Ib. XXVIII, 9 ... החרם .. העושה ומזוטו טמא (ed. Dehr., Ar. ed. Koh. ומן הזוטו) a garment made out of a net is clean, but one made out of its solid portion &c.—2) (cmp. שלולית, שָׁלָל) *what the Sea throws out, deposits after the tide; the deposit* or *ore of a mine*. B. Mets. 21^b בזוטו של ים ובשלוליתו וכ׳ things found among the deposits of the Sea or the alluvium of a river. Ib. 24^a; Ab. Zar. 43^a.—Cant. R. to IV, 8 מה החרמון הזה כל טוב נתון בזוטו (not טובו; Yalk. Cant. 988 בתוכו) as in the Hermon all good things are deposited in its mines &c.—Y. Ber. IV, 7^b bot. (ref. to צולה, Is. XLIV, 27) זו בבל שהיא זוטו של עולם that means Babylon which is the deposit of the world (the treasury of booty and commerce); Lam. R. introd. (R. Josh. 2) זוטא (corr. acc.).

זוּטָא c. (contract. of זעטוטא, reduplic. of זע, זא, v. זוּעַ. cmp. forms like גּוּזְמְרָא a. פִּיסְתְּרָא) *slender, young; small*;

Targ. I Chr. XVIII, 17. Ib. XI, 22 יומא ז׳ *short* day.—B. Bath. 36[b] פירא ז׳ small crop (as grass, aftermath &c.), opp. פ׳ רבא grains &c.—Keth. 66[b] שומא ז׳ the taxation on a small scale; a. fr.—Ib. 106[a], v. אֱלָדְּהוּ. [Y. Yeb. IV, 5[d] top, read: זוּטָא.—Lam. R. introd. (R. Josh. 2), v. preced.]—*Pl.* זוּטֵי. Ab. Zar. 8[a] יומי ז׳ the short days of the Winter. Ib. 10[b] [read:] ז׳ . . . מחייה מיתי נינהו (v. En Yak. a. l.) even the least among you can revive the dead.—זוּטָא, זוּטֵר (as surname) *junior*. Keth. 69[a]; B. Bath. 66[b].—Ib. 120[a].

זוֹטוֹס pr. n. m. (Ζῶτος; Jos. Ant. XX, 2, 1 Ἰζάτης) *Zotos, Izates*, a prince of Adiabena. Gen. R. s. 46, v. מוּנְבָּז.

זוּטֵי m. 1) *junior*, v. זוּטָא.—2) pr. n. m. *Zuti*, an Amora. Ned. 77[a]; Sabb. 157[a] רב ז׳ דבר רב פפר; ib. ז׳ דבי רב פפא (Ms. M. רב זוטרי . . פפר).

זוּמַן, v. זְוַן.

זוּטַר I (v. next w.) *to be small, young*. Hag. 5[a] שכיב אֲדָז׳ (Ms. M. 2 אדריניק) died young.

Ithpe. אִיזְּוּטַר, אִתְזוּטַר *to shrink; to appear small.* Ned. 50[b] עד דמִתְזוּטְרָא כי וכ׳ until it is so reduced in size that you can swallow it.—Snh. 95[a] אי׳ בעיניה (En Yak. אִזְדוּטַר) it seemed to him a small enterprise.

זוּטַר, II, זוּטְרָא I m. (a contract. of זעירער; cmp. זוּטָא) *small, young, junior*. Targ. Ps. CXIX, 141; a. e.—Taan. 23[b] ז׳ (ינוקא) the younger child. Keth. 66[b] עסקא זוטא דזוטר רווחא a small investment which brings a small profit, v. זוּזָא III; a. fr.—*Pl.* זוּטְרֵי. B. Kam. 92[b], v. גַּבְרָא; a. e.—Fem. זוּטַרְתִּי, זוּטַרְתָּא. Ber. 33[b] מילתא ז׳ a trifle. Ab. Zar. 29[a], v. מְלוֹא ch.—*Pl.* זוּטְרָתָא. Targ. Ps. CIV, 25 Ms. (ed. זעירי).—Zeb. 63[a] בז׳ Ar. (v. marginal note, ed. בזכרותא) counting the little fingers (of which six go on a *Tefah*).

זוּטְרָא II pr. n. m. *Zutra* (corresp. to זְעֵירָא), 1) *Mar Z.*, name of several Amoraim. Ber. 43[b]; a. fr.—2) *Rab Z.* Ib.; a. v. fr. (v., however, Rabb. D. S. a. l. notes 5, 6, 7).—רב זוּטְרֵי, v. זוּטַר.

זוּטַרְתָּא, זוּטַרְתִּי I, v. זוּטַר II.

זוּטַרְתִּי II pr. n. *Zutarti*. Ber. 12[b] (Var. זוטרא, זוטראי, v. Rabb. D. S. a. l. note 9).

זָוֵי *to join, couple*. Denom. זָוִית, זָוְיָא &c.

זָוֵי m. (זוח, cmp. Syr. זוא *tumuit*, P. Sm. 1092) [*breast*,] 1) *projection, bay-window*. Targ. I Kings VII, 4 (h. text מחזה).—2) *a projection of a wall formed by abruptly reducing its thickness*, so as to give space for *a balcony*.—*Pl.* זָוֵי. Targ. Ez. XLII, 3 (Levita זְוֵי; h. text אתיק).—זְוִיָּא. Ib. 5 (ed. Lag. זְוִיזָא).

זויד, Tosef. Bekh. V, 9, v. זִידּוּר.

זָוְיָא m. = זָוִיתָא, *corner*. Lam. R. to I, 1 (7 חד מאה) רבתי בחד ז׳ in a corner (aside from the road). [זְוִיִּין, v. זָוִיתָא.]

זָוִיר, v. זִידּוּר.

זָוִית f. (b. h.; v. זָוְיָא) *joint, angle, corner*. Ber. 31[a] בז׳ זו in one corner of the room, בז׳ אחרת in another corner; Pes. 10[b].—M. Kat. 18[a] מז׳ לז׳ from one corner of the lips to the other (mustaches); a. fr.—קרן ז׳ (*the horn of juncture*), *corner-piece, shelf*. Gitt. 13[a] צבורין ומונחין בק׳ ז׳ heaped up and ready on the shelf; Kidd. 66[a]; a. e.—*Pl.* זָוִיּוֹת. Neg. XII, 3 בשני כתלים בז׳ Mish. ed. (Talm. ed. sing.) on two adjoining walls; Sifra M'tsora, Neg., Par. 7, ch. V.

זָוִיתָא ch. same. Targ. Ez. XLVI, 23; a. e.—Taan. 23[b].—*Pl.* זָוְיָתָא, constr. זָוְיַת; זָוְיָן, זְוִיָּן, זו׳. Targ. Ex. XXV, 26; a. fr.

זוּל I (b. h., v. זָלַל) *to be of slight value, to be cheap; to be despicable, mean.* Sabb. 55[b] (play on פּחז, Gen. XLIX, 4) פּוחה חבחה זַלְתָּה (not זלתא, v. Rabb. D. S. a. l. note 300) thou wast rash, becamest guilty, degradedst thyself. Snh. 98[a] מלכות הַזָּלָה the despicable (Roman) government (Rashi: 'the slightest trace of tyranny').—2) (cmp. בוז) *to squander, be excessive in sensual enjoyments, be dissolute*. Num. R. s. 10 (ed. Amst. p. 240[a]) חבורה של זַלְלִין a company of dissolute men.—*Polel* זוֹלֵל, only as part. 1) *low, mean*. Midr. Prov. to II, 4 (ref. to Jer. XV, 19) כל . . . להוציא ד"ת מז׳ he who succeeds in making the words of the Law come forth from a low man (who educates an abandoned person).—Pesik. R. s. 21 נעשה העולם זוֹלֵלָה the world became an object reduced in value.—2) *spendthrift, glutton*. Sifré Deut. 219 ז׳ בבשר *zolel* (Deut. XXI, 20) refers to excesses in eating meat (v. Snh. VIII, 2).

Hif. הֵזִיל 1) *to become cheap, fall in price*. Y. Keth. XII, beg. 34[d] היו ביוקר והֵזִילוּ if provisions were dear and fell in price.—2) *to treat with contempt*. Treat. Der. Er. ch. II מְזִילֵי הרבים those who treat the public &c. [B. Bath. 25[a], v. נָזַל.]

Hof. הוּזַל *to fall in price*. B. Mets. V, 8 והוּזְלוּ and (the wheat) fell. Ib. 75[a]; a. fr.

זוּל ch. same; perf. זָל, Part. זוֹל, זִיל 1) *to disregard*. Targ. Y. II Gen. XVI, 5 (perh. fr. זְלַל).—2) *to be worthless, cheap*. Targ. Y. Deut. XXVIII, 68 בדמין זוֹלִין for a low price.—B. Mets. 77[a] זל עבידתא (sub שכר) labor has become cheaper. Ib. זל עביד׳ מעיקרא labor was originally cheap. Ib. זיל עביד׳ Ms. M. (v. Rabb. D. S. a. l. note 40). Ber. 63[a] (prov.) זָלָא קמץ קניה Ms. M. (ed. זַלְתְּ קבוץ קנה מינה, Ar. קפוץ) if a thing is cheap, be quick and buy it. B. Mets. 64[a] bot. אי יקרא אי זילא וכ׳ whether it will rise or fall, it shall be in my possession (gain or loss shall be mine). Ab. Zar. 70[a] זִילָה עלייהו she is contemptible in their sight. B. Bath. 110[a] זִילָא בי מילתא such occupation is beneath my dignity. Yeb. 63[a] זַבִּין ולא תִּיזוּל sell (part of thy clothes to start a business) in order not to be disgraced by poverty; (oth. explan., v. next w.).

Af. אוֹזִיל *to sell cheap, make easy terms*. B. Mets. 77[a] אוזילו אינהו גביה זווא וכ׳ at the start they had agreed to work for one *zuz* less (than the market price of labor), and wages were generally reduced afterwards. Ib.[b] אוֹזְלֵי מוֹזיל וכ׳ he will lower the price and sell (some of his movable goods in order to raise money). Ib. 73[a] top מוֹזְלֵי גבייהו they will be easier in selling them. Ib. bot. אוזילי דקא מוזלי גביכו (better אחולי . . מחלי, v. Rabb. D. S. a. l. note 1) they are liberal towards you (paying more than the ordinary wages). Gen. R. s. 39 חלא מְזִיל חמרא

vinegar cheapens wine, i. e. where bad wine is plentiful in the market, good wine sells cheaper; a. fr.

Ithpe. אִתְּזִיל *to be degraded, disgraced.* Keth. 53[b] לא ניחא ליה דתִתְּזִיל he does not want her to be disgraced (by dependence on public charity).

זוּל II (cmp. אָזַל II) *to spin.* Yeb. 63[a] זָבְנִין ולא תָזוּל buy (ready-made cloth) and do not spin; (oth. opin., v. preced.); v. הזול a. זוֹלָלָא.

זוֹל m. (זוּל I) *low price.* Sub. 70[a] (ref. to זוֹלֵל) עד שיקח בשר בז׳ וכ׳ until he buys meat and wine at the lowest prices (in order to have large quantities). B. Mets. 73[a] מקום הז׳ the place where prices are low. Maas. Sh. IV, 2 בשער הז׳ at the lower (the wholesale) market price. Y. Keth. XII, beg. 34[d] היו בז׳ וכ׳ if provision at the time was cheap and it rose. Ib. נותן בז׳ he pays alimentation according to the lower prices; a. fr.

זוֹלָא ch. same. Y. Kil. IX, 32[c] top תמן ז׳ there everything is cheap. B. Mets. 64[b] מקבל עליה ז׳ he takes the risk of a reduction in prices.

זולמא, v. זַלְתָּא.

זוֹלַל, v. זול I Ib.

זוֹלְלָא or **זְוָלְלָא** m. (זול II) *skein.*—*Pl.* זוֹלָלֵי. Hull. 60[a], quoted in Tosaf. to Yeb. 63[a] for הַזָּלְלָא, q. v.

זוֹלְשָׁפְט, v. בֶּלְשָׁפָט.

*__זוּם__ (cmp. זהם) [*to glisten,*] *to be fat, greasy, filthy.*—*Part. Polel* זוֹמֵם. Sabb. 152[b] (where the souls of the righteous are compared to clean, and those of the wicked to filthy garments) ושל רשעים זוֹמְמוֹת והולכות while the souls of the wicked are getting more and more greasy.

זוֹם m. (preced., cmp. זָמִית) *juice, brine.* Num. R. s. 7 הז׳ של בשר the juice (or brine) of meat.—Pes. III, 1, v. next w.

זוֹמָא I m. (preced.) same, *broth, pulp.* Pes. III, 1 (42[a]) ז׳ של צבעים Ms. M. 2 a. oth (v. Rabb. D. S. a. l. note 1, Koh. Ar. s. v.; ed. זוֹמָן, v. preced.) the dyers' broth (made of bran, to make the dye adhesive). Y. ib. III, beg., 29[d] זומי של וכ׳ (corr. acc.).—[Yalk. Lev. 525 דבר של ז׳, v. זוֹהֲמָא.] [ז׳ ליסטרא, v. זוֹמְלִיסְטְרוֹן.]

זוֹמָא II pr. n. m. *Zoma.*—בן ז׳, or שמעון בן ז׳ (*Simon*) *ben Zoma*, a Tannai. Ab. IV, 1; a. fr.

זוֹמִילִיסְטְרָא, זוֹמָאלִיסְטְרוֹן, v. זוֹמְלִיסְטְרוֹן.

זוֹמוֹת, Y. Shebi. V, end, 36[a], v. זִימְיָא.

זומי, ז׳ ליסטרא, ז׳ לסטרון, v. זוֹמְלִיסְטְרוֹן.

זוֹמִית, v. זָמִית.

זוֹמְלִיסְטְרוֹן (variously corrupted) m. (ζωμάρυστρον=ζωμήρυσις) *soup-ladle*, with a spoon on one side and a fork on the other. Kel. XIII, 2; XXV, 3 זומל׳ Ar. ed. זומא ליסטרא, זומי לס׳, Var. in Ar. זומניסטרה). Tosef. b. B. Bath. III, 6 זומליסטרין. Y. Sabb. XVII, beg. 16[a] זומי ל׳; Tosef. ib. XIV (XV), 1 זומה ל׳ (Var. זומא); Sabb. 123[b] זוהמא ל׳; Hor. 13[b] זוהמא ל׳.

זוּן (cmp. זוד) *to provide, outfit; to sustain*, esp. *to feed.* Gitt. I, 6 שלא לָזוּן את וכ׳ not to sustain his slave. Ib. 12[a] איני זָנְךָ I will not support thee. Y. Keth. V, 29[d] top שתהא זוֹנְתוֹ ומפרנסתו (for זָנְתוֹ) that she should provide for all his wants. Sabb. 104[a] ז״ח זן . . . וחן וכ׳ He supports and graces thee; a. fr.—Ber. 35[b], a. e. כל הזן עלי I vow abstinence from whatever sustains the body.—Trnsf. *to feed the eye, to derive pleasure from a sight* (mostly of an illicit sight). Ohol. XIII, 4 one makes an opening in the wall לזון את עיניו for the sake of enjoying a view; Tosef. ib. XIV, 4. Pes. 26[a] כדי שלא יזונו עיניהם וכ׳ that the laborers might not look at the Holy of Holies. Lev. R. s. 20 לא זן עיניו מן וכ׳ did not look at the Divine Majesty. Ib. s. 23, end ואינו זן וכ׳ and does not allow his eye to rest on an obscenity; a. fr.

Nif. נִזּוֹן, נִיזּוֹן *to be fed, sustained.* Gitt. 12[b] נ׳ מן הצדקה must be supported from the public charity. Ib. (distinction betw. נ׳ a. התפרנס, v. פַּרְנֵס). Taan. 24[b]. Keth. XI, 1 נִיזּוֹנֶת מנכסי וכ׳ must be supported from the estate &c.

Hif. הֵזִין *to bless with plenty.* Keth. 10[b], v. זוּהַ II.

Pi. זַיֵּין *to outfit, decorate; to gird, arm* (cmp. זָיְוָא I, a. P. Sm. 1102 sq.) Lev. R. s. 34 (ref. to יחליץ, Is. LVIII, 11) ישמוט יְזַיֵּין וכ׳ it has the meanings of 'he will loosen', 'he will arm', 'he will rescue', 'he will give rest'.—*Part. pass.* מְזוּיָּן, מְזוּיָּן. B. Kam. 57[a] לסטים מ׳ a robber in arms; טוען בטענת ל׳ מ׳ he pleads that he has been robbed by &c. Ib. 58[a]; a. e.—*Pl.* מְזוּיָּנִין. Ex. R. s. 20 (expl. חמשים, Ex. XXIII, 8) שיצאו מ׳ they went out fully equipped; Mekh. B'shall., beg.; a. e.

Hithpa. הִזְדַּיֵּין *to arm one's self, to fight.* Tanh. Ki Thabo 3 מִזְדַּיֵּין על וכ׳ He goes to war in defense of him &c.

זוּן I ch. same, *to support, nourish.* Targ. Gen. XLVII, 12 (h. text כלכל); a. fr.—Bets. 32[b] ומיזן לא זָנוּ ליה Ms. M. (ed. זַיְנוּהוּ *Pa.*) and they also refused to assist him (from the charities).—Part. זָיֵין. Ber. 35[b] מִשְׁחָא ז׳ oil nourishes, contrad. to סעיד to satisfy. Num. R. s. 9 אחין זָ׳ ומפרנס this one feeds and supports (his wife). Yalk. Lev. 665 והוה ז׳ להון וכ׳ (Lev. R. s. 34 מפרנס) and he supported them as long as they lived; a. fr.

Pa. זַיֵּין 1) same. Bets. 32[b], v. supra. Y. Yeb. IV, 6[b] אנא מְזַיְּינָנָא ירחי I shall supply the wants of the household during my month (one month every year). Bab. ib. 65[a] אית ליה לְמֵיזַיְינִינְהוּ (some ed. למיד׳, read למיז׳) he has the means to support all of them; a. e.—2) *to equip, arm, decorate.* Targ. Y. Gen. XIV, 14 (O. זריז, h. text וירק).—*Part. pass.* מְזַיַּן, מְזַיֵּין. Targ. Gen. XLIX, 19; a. e.

Ithpe. אִתְּזִין, אִתְּזַן *to be supported, managed.* Ib. XLI, 40 (h. text ישק). Targ. Koh. III, 22.—Keth. IV, 11 (in a marriage deed) ומִיתְּזַנְנָא and shall be supported.

Ithpa. אִזְדַּיַּן *to be equipped, armed.* Targ. Joel II, 9 (h. text ישקו). Targ. Y. II Num. XXXI, 3.

זוּן II (cmp. preced.) [*to gird, tie*], (cmp. אסר) *to detain.*—Denom. זְיְנָא, זִירָנָא.

זֵרֶן or **זוֹן** m. (cmp. זָנָא a. זַרְ) *girdle, laborer's apron.* Kel. XXVI, 3. Cmp. זֻנִיתָא.—[זונים, v. זוֹנִי.]

זוֹנָארָא, v. זוֹנָרָא.

זוֹנְבָא=הוּנְבָא. Targ. Job XL, 17 Ms.

זוֹנֶה, v. זוֹנִין.

זוֹנָה f. (b.h.; זָנָה) [*degenerate, degraded,*] 1) (in marriage law) *one unfit to marry a priest* (v. זָהַם). Yeb. VI, 5 שהיא ז׳ האמורה וכ׳ for that (אַיְלוֹנִית) is the *zonah* meant in the Law (Lev. XXI, 7, as one not married for propagation). Ib. אין ז׳ אלא וכ׳ a *zonah* (unfit to marry a priest) is none but a proselyte, a freed-woman and one who has had connection in forbidden grades of relationship. Ib. 61[b], a.e. פנוי . . . עשאה ז׳ if an unmarried man has had connection with an unmarried woman without the intention of marriage, he has made her a *zonah* (for priesthood). Ib. ז׳ כשמה the Biblical *zonah* means what the name indicates (a faithless wife); ib. ז׳ מופקרת *zonah* means a prostitute; a. fr.—2) *harlot.* Ber. 23[a]. Ḥag. 15[a] (in Chald. diction) אשכח ז׳ he met a prostitute. Snh. 82[a]; a. fr.—*Pl.* זוֹנוֹת. Ab. Zar. 17[b], a. e. קובה של ז׳ (Roman) house of prostitution. Snh. 95[b]; a. fr.

זוֹנִי f. (ζώνη) *belt; cuirass, armour* (v. Sm. Ant. s. v.). Num. R. s. 4 end חגור מתניו בזונו (corr. acc.) he had a belt around his loins. Y'lamd. Vaëthh., quot. in Ar. התיר ז׳ שלו untied his belt (removed from office).—*Pl.* זוֹנָס (ζώνας, accus. pl.), זוֹנָאוֹת, זוֹנִין. Lev. R. s. 13, beg. התיר זוניך שלהן (Ar. s. v. זנס: זונס) untied their belts (made them weak). Cant. R. to IV, 4 [read:] ואחד אוסרו זְוָנוֹ מהו זינו ר׳ הונא . . . אמר זונס and one angel girded him with his armour (outfit). What is meant by &c.? . . . . *zonas* (belts of magistracy); Pesik. Naḥ., p. 124[b] (expl. זיינו, Ar. זונו, read: זוינו or זינו) זונו . . . ר׳ הונא; Pesik. R. s. 21 (expl. מוסרו זונא, read: אוסרו זינו) זונס; ib. s. 33 (expl. זוֹנִיוֹת, v. זונית וכ׳) זוֹנָארוֹת; Tanḥ. T'savveh 11 זוֹנָארוֹת; Tanḥ. ed. Bub., Sh'lah, addit. 1 זינם (read זונס); Yalk. Ps. 858 זוֹנָאוֹת; Midr. Till. to Ps. CIII זונראות (corr. acc.).

זוֹנִיחָה, v. זְנוּחָא.

זוֹנִין, זוֹנַיָּיא m. pl. ch.=next w. Gen. R. s. 28, end הוו זרעין . . . . . מפקא ז׳ they sowed seeds and the earth produced rye-grass. Ib. אילין ז׳ וכ׳ that rye-grass is a growth dating from the generation of the flood.

זוֹנִין I m. pl. (of זוֹנֶה; זָנָה) [*degenerate wheat,*] *a weed growing among wheat, darnel* or *rye-grass* (Lolium perenne, v. Löw Pfl. p. 133). Kil. I, 1. Y. ib. 26[d] מין חטין וכ׳ they (zonin) are a kind of wheat, only that fruits degenerate, v. זָנָה. Tosef. Ter. VI, 10 ז׳ שבה (Var. זוגין) the darnel in it; Y. ib. V, end, 43[d] ז׳ טנופת (strike out ט׳ as a gloss).

זוֹנִין II *belt*, v. זוֹנִי.

זוֹנִין III, **זוֹנָן** pr. n. m. *Zonin, Zonan.* Ab. Zar. V, 2 (65[b]) זונין Ms. M. a. Y. ed. (v. Rabb. D. S. a. l.; ed. זונן); Y. B. Mets. V, 10[b] top, v. בִּירְתּוֹס. Sabb. 81[a]; a. fr.

זוֹנִיראוֹת, v. זוֹנִי.

זוֹנִית or **זְוָנִית** f., pl. זוֹנִיּוֹת (v. זֵרֶן) *outfit, armour* Pesik. R. s. 33, v. זוֹנִי.

זוֹנִיתָא I or **זְוָנִיתָא** f. ch. (v. preced.) *laborer' apron.* Pesik. Haomer, p. 72[a] אסר זוֹנִיתֵיה וכ׳ (Ar. זונסתיה Var. זוסתיה, a corrupt. of מני מסותיה) he tied his apro around him and went on &c.; Pesik. R. s. 18 זוניתא. V מְסוּתָא.

זוֹנִיתָא II f. ch.=h. זוֹנָה, *harlot.* Lam. R. to I, 16.

זוֹנָן, v. זוֹנִין III.

זוֹנָס, v. זוֹנִי.

זוֹנסתיה, v. זוֹנִיתָא I.

זוֹנָרָא m. (ζωνάριον) *belt.* Targ. Prov. XXXI, 24 (ed Wil. זוּנָארָא).—Y. Snh. X, 29[a] top hast thou any clai on us אלא הדין ז׳ וכ׳ except this belt and this cloak (in signia of office)?—*Pl.* זוֹנָרִין. Y. Sabb. VI, 8[b] bot. (expl חריטים, Is. III, 22) ז׳ מצויירין girdles embroidered wit figures.

זוסטא, זוסטה, v. זוֹסְמָא.

זוֹסִימִי pr. n. f. (Ζωσίμη) *Zosime.* Y. Shebi. VIII, 38 top, v. אוּדְרִיתָא II.

זוֹסְמָא m. (ζῶσμα=ζῶμα, in the sense of περίζωμα *cook's apron.* Num. R. s. 4, end לובש מקורעים וזוסטא (cor acc.) puts on ragged garments and an apron. Y. Meg I, 71[b] top החק זוסטה וכ׳ (corr. acc.) an apron whos meshes are wide &c.; Y. Ned. IV, beg. 38[c] זוסטה נחק (corr. acc.).

זוסתיה, v. זוֹנִיתָא I.

זוּעַ (b. h.) 1) *to drip,* v. *Hif.*—2) *to move, shak tremble.* Pesik. R. s. 26 איברי זָעוּ עלי (read with Yalk Jer. 262: קרבי) my bowels within me trembled.

Hif. הֵזִיעַ, הֶזִיעַ 1) *to perspire, drip.* Zeb. 18[b] (ref. t ביזע, Ez. XLIV, 18) במקום שמַזִּיעִין on that part of th body where one perspires. Toh. IX, 1; Meil. 21[a] משיַּזִּיעוּ Ar (ed. משיזועו) from the time the olives begin to drip, v מַעֲטָן. Sifra B'huck., Par. 2, ch. V השמים מַזִּיעִים the heaven perspire (vapors, rain); הנחושת מזיע (read: מַזִּיעָה) bronz sweats. Gen. R. s. 20 (ref. to Gen. III, 19) הִזִּיעוּ פניו hi face began to drip (tears, v. Pes. 118[a]); a. e.—2) *to mov* Tosef. Shebi. III, 4 מחרישה מְזִיעָתָן, v. זְעָזַע. Koh. R. t I, 13, v. זוז I.—3) *to be agitated.* Cant. R. to IV, 4 אפשר שלא הז׳ וכ׳ is it possible that the sensual desire was no at all agitated?

זוּעַ ch. same *to move, tremble; hesitate.* Targ. O. a Y. II Ex. XX, 15. Targ. O. ib. XIII, 17 (h. text ינחם); a fr.—Ab. V, 22 מינה לא תָזוּעַ thou shalt not move (deviate from it (the Law).—Part. זָיֵיעַ. Targ. Jer. IV, 24; a. e.– Lev. R. s. 10 מן . . לית את ז׳ thou shalt never leave m palace.

Pa. זַיַּיע 1) *to shake, frighten.* Targ. Y. Num. VI, 2 מְזַיְיעֵי frightening demons.—2) *to sweat, drip.* Targ. Y

Lev. XXVI, 19 (cmp. Sifra a.l., quot. in preced. w.); Targ. Y. Deut. XXVIII, 23 מְזִיעַ (Af.).

Af. אַזִיעַ 1) *to shake, frighten.* Targ. Jud. VIII, 12; a. fr.—Part. pass. מְזָעָא, f. מְזַעֲתָא. Targ. Prov. XXV, 19 Ms. (ed. מוערא).—2) *to sweat;* v. supra.

Ithpe. אִתְזִיעַ *to be frightened.* Part. מִתְזְעַ. Targ. Prov. XVII, 12.

זִיעָא, זוֹעָא f. (preced.) 1) *trembling, fear.* Targ. Y. Deut. II, 25 זִיעָתָךְ the fear of thee (v. זוֹעֲפָא).—2) *tempest* Targ. Job XXXVII, 9 Ms. (ed. זִיעָא).

זְוָעָה f. (b. h.; preced.) *earth-quake.*—*Pl.* זְוָעוֹת. Ber. IX, 1. Ib. 59ª, v. גּוֹהָא. Y. ib. IX, 13ᶜ; Tosef. B. Mets. XI, 7; a. e.

זוֹעֲפָא f. (זעף) *fear.* Targ. O. Deut. II, 25 some ed. (ed. Berl. 1 'זוֹעָ, v. זוֹעָא).

זוֹעַר pr. n. pl. (=b. h. צוֹעַר) *Zoar,* a Sodomitic place. Targ. Y. Gen. XIX, 22, sq.—Y. Yoma III, beg. 40ᵇ (Y. Ber. I, 2ᶜ צוער).

זוּף I (cmp. זוב) *to drip, be viscid.*—V. זיף I a. זֶפֶת.

Pi. זַיֵּיף 1) *to make thick, viscid; to adulterate.* Sot. 48ᵇ (expl. דבש זיפים) דבש שמְזַיְּיפִין בו a honey which is used for mixing with other substances in order to make them appear viscid (differ. in comment.).—2) *to be unctuous, false, treacherous.* Ib. (ref. to זיפים, Ps. LIV, 2) בני אדם הַמְזַיְּיפִין Ar. (Rashi שמזייפין; ed. המ' דבריהם) people who are unctuous (ed. who *make* their words *unctuous,* i. e. insinuate themselves). Sifré Deut. 26 דומה שז' משה בתורה it seems as if Moses was not sincere in writing the Law (smoothing over his own shortcomings).—3) *to falsify, forge; to prove the fallacy of, refute; to denounce as false, deny.* Y. Sot. VII, 21ᶜ 'זִיַּיפְתֶּם תורתכם וכ ye (Samaritans) have falsified your Torah (adding שכם to Deut. XI, 30) but to no purpose; Bab. ib. 33ᵇ.—Ib. בדבר זה זִיַּיפְתִּי ספרי 'וכ with this argument I showed the fallacy of the books of the Samaritans; Snh. 90ᵇ. Ib. 'זִיַּיפְתֶּם ולא וכ Ms. M. (v. Rabb. D. S. a. l. note, ed. ז' תורתכם) ye disputed (our evidence from Deut. XXXI, 16), but it does not avail you (for the idea of resurrection is evident from Num. XV, 31).—*Part. pass.* מְזוּיָּיף, f. מְזוּיֶּיפֶת *false, informal, faulty* (of documents signed by disqualified witnesses). Gitt. 10ᵇ (גט) מז' מתוכו וכ' a document which has its rejection in itself (being signed by disqualified witnesses, although it would have been valid without the signature of witnesses) is illegal; B. Bath. 170ª; a. e.—Ib. ונמצאת עדותן מז' and their evidence (signature) is found out to be informal (because they are disqualified).

Hithpa. הִזְדַּיֵּיף *to be falsified, forged.* Gitt. II, 4 מפני שהוא יכול לה' because (on such writing material) forgery (erasing and writing over) is made easy. Ib. 19ᵇ כתב שאינו יכול לה' a writing which cannot be forged (i. e. written on material dressed with gall-nut, v. אֲפַץ). [*Hif.* הוזיף, v. רָזַה.]

זוּף ch. same.—*Pa.* זַיֵּיף *to falsify, forge.* Targ. Jer. VIII, 8 לִמְזַיְּיפָא ed. Lag. (ed. לְזַיְּפָא).—Keth. 36ᵇ זַיֵּיפוּ לִי forge for me (erase &c.). Ib. זַיֵּיף ז' וכתב he practiced imitation of handwriting and then wrote himself. B. Bath. 163ª דילמא מְזַיֵּיף וכתב וכ' he may imitate and insert (over the signatures) whatever he desires. Ib. כל דמזייף לאו וכ' (not המז', v. Ms. M.) whoever desires to forge will not go to the scribe; a. e.

זוּף II (cmp. זקף) [*to be rough,*] *to be angry, threaten.* Targ. Is. XVII, 13. Targ. Zech. III, 2 יְזִיף (ed. Lag. יגער). Targ. Mal. III, 11; a. e. [*Af.* אוזיף, v. רְזַה.]

זוּפְרִין, v. זִפְרִין.

זוּק, זִיק, *Pa.* זַיֵּיק (denom. of זִיקָא II) *to blow up, fill with air.* Hull. 109ᵇ זַיְּיקוּ לה וכ' blow up for her an udder for roasting; (Rashi: *put . . . on the spud,* i. e. prepare a זוקתא *udder,* v. P. Sm. 1147).

זִיקָאנָא m. (preced.) *blown up, swollen, afflicted with dropsy* (v. Syr. זקיא, P. Sm. 1147).—*Pl.* זִיקָאנֵי. Ab. Zar 31ᵇ (Ms. M. זַיְקִינֵי; early ed. 'זְוִוקָא).

זוּקִינָא, v. preced.

זוּקְפָא m. (זקף) *rising, elevation, pride.* Targ. Job XX, 6 (h. text שִׂיא).

זוּקְתָא, v. זִיקְתָא.

זוּר I (b. h.; cmp. הוּר) *to go around,* with מִ־ or הרמ־ *to turn away, be estranged; to deviate.* Yoma 72ᵇ זָרָה הימנו the Law departs from him (is forgotten); v. זָר. Midr. Till. to Ps. XC, 5 (play on זְרַמְתָּם, ib.) זָרוּ מתו ותמו they deviated (from the Law) &c.; זרו מתורתיך וכ'; Yalk. Ps. 841.

זוּר ch. same; 1) (with מִ־) *to turn away.* Targ. Num. XVI, 26 (h. text סור); a. e.—2) (with לְ־) [*to turn from the road to,*] *to enter as a guest, to lodge.* Targ. Gen. XIX, 2, sq.; a. fr.

Pa. 1) זַוֵּור *to turn, roll.*—*Part. pass.* מְזַוַּור. Bekh. 44ª דמְזַוְורָן עיניה Ar. (ed. דמְזַוֵּר עיניה, Rashi דמזוורן, read: דמזוורן) one whose eyes are rolled about (ed. who rolls his eyes); v. זִיוּר.—2) זַיֵּיר (cmp. צוּר, זרר) *to tie up, keep* (as a pledge); *to press.* B. Mets. 16ᵇ ז' ליה . . . אפשיטי he keeps the document until the writer's fee is paid. V. זוּרְזָא, מְזוֹרָה, זַיָּירָא &c.

זוּר II m. (preced. v. זִיר) *crown, wreath;* (bot.) *capsule.* Tosef. Maasr. III, 14 כל שאין לו אלא ז' אחד המקיף וכ' (ed. Zuck. דִּיר I) (a garlick plant) which has only one capsule of seeds crowning the stem; Y. ib. V, end, 52ª חור (corr. acc.).

זוּרָאן, v. זוּרְיוֹן.

זוּרד, Tosef. Kil. III, 15, v. וֶרֶד II.

זוּרְזַיָא, v. next w.

זוּרְיָא m. pl. (זור; cmp. זִיר) *bunches.* Y. Maas. Sh. IV, 54ᵈ bot. מסיק לזוּרְיֵיה (ed. Zyt. זוּרְזַיֵּיה, v. זִירְזָא) when he takes up his bunches (the remnants of his stock), v. בַּלְּנֵר.

זְרִיוֹן, זוּרְיוֹן m. (זרי, cmp. זרר) *wringing,* מי ז' *water flowing from flax when wrung out, flax-water.*

Pes. 107ª אישתי מי זו׳ (Ms. O. זר׳; Ms. M. זוראן, v. Rabb. D. S. a. l.) I will rather drink flax-water than &c. [Cmp. זורי, P. Sm. 1114.]

זוּתָן, זוֹתַבְנַיִן, v. זִיוְתָן.

זַזֵּר, v. זֵוַר.

זַח m. *distracted*, v. זוּחַ.

זָחוּחַ, זָחוּחָא, v. זְהוֹהָא, זָהוּהַ.

זָחַח, זְחַח, v. זָהַה, זְהַה; also זוּהַ II.

זָחִיל, זְחֵיל m. (זחל) *worm*. Targ. Job XIII, 28; a. e.

זָחַל (b. h.) 1) *to creep*.—2) *to flow, run*. זוֹחֲלִין, זוֹחֲלִים *running waters*, opp. to נוטפין dripping water (collected rain water &c.). Mikv. V, 5 הז׳ כמעין running waters are like a well (for levitical purposes). Ib. נוטפין שעשאן ז׳ collected rain water which was made running (by causing an overflow into a channel). Eduy. VII, 3, sq. Sabb. 65ᵇ; a. e.—Y. Shebi. IV, end, 35ᶜ משיַזְחִילוּ מים when the berries are sufficiently developed to yield running drops when squeezed, v. גָּרַע II. [Num. R. s. 13, beg. ווזחלות; Yalk. Cant. 988 זוחלת, read זולח׳, v. זָלַח.]

Hif. הִזְחִיל *to let collected water run into a channel*. Mikv. V, 5 אין מַזְחִילִין בו you must not use it for &c.

זְחַל I ch. same, 1) *to creep*. Targ. Jer. XLVI, 22; a. e.—2) *to flow*. Targ. Ps. CXLVII, 18 Ms. (ed. זלח׳, h. text יזלו). [Targ. II Esth. I, 2 זחלין בוסמ׳, read זלחין, v. preced.]

Pa. זַחֵל *to let run off, to empty* (by opening the spicket). Y. Ab. Zar IV, 44ª bot. עד דתְזַחֲלוּן גובה until ye shall have emptied the pit.

זְחַל II (cmp. זחח, צהל) *to be bright, brighten up*. Y. Snh. XI, 30ᵇ top; Koh. R. to VIII, 1; Pesik. Par., p. 37ᵇ וחלין (corr. acc.); Yalk. Koh. 977 וחלין (corr. acc.).

זָחַל m. (preced.) *zahal*, name of a species of *locusts* born without legs. Tosef. Ḥull. III (IV), 25. Ḥull. 65ᵇ, v. אַסְקְרָא.

זַחְלָא, זַחֲלָא ch. 1) same. Targ. Am. IV, 9; a. fr.—Yalk. Deut. 938 (play on עמלק) עם ילק פרח כהדין ז׳ a people of locusts, quick like the *zahla*; ib. Ex. 262; Pesik. Zakh., p. 26ᵇ דחלא (corr. acc.); Tanḥ. Ki Thetse 9 פרח כזוחל (corr. acc.).—*Pl.* זַחֲלַיָּא. Targ. Is. XXXIII, 4 Ar. (ed. sing.).—2) (זְחַל I)=זוֹחֲלָא *worm, moth*. Targ. Job IV, 19. Targ. Y. Deut. XXVIII, 39. [Targ. Y. II Deut. XXXII, 24 זחלל עפרא, read: זַחֲלֵי creeping in the dust.

זחלל, v. preced.

זחרתיה, Yalk. Gen. 116, v. נַחְרְתָא.

***זַחְתָן** m. (זחח, formed like גֵּיוְתָן) *haughty*.—*Pl.* זַחְתָנִין. Treat. Der. Er. ch. II, beg.

***זט**, prob. an abbreviation of זְרִירָךְ טָב *may thy sneezing be for good*. Y. Ber. VI, 10ᵈ top אסור למימר ליה זט Ar. (explaining=ζήτω, live!); ed. יי סעדך=ייס the Lord help thee!

זַטּוּט, v. זַעְטוּט.

זמחא, v. זְנוּחָא.

זַטַּר, v. זוּטַר.

***זַטְרִי** pr. n. m. *Zatri* (v. זוּטְרֵי). Pesik. Vatt. 133ᵇ (v., however, Bub. ib. note 70).

זיאטמווס, Yalk. Ps. 631, v. זִיטְרַטוֹס.

זִיאַר, v. זְאַר.

זִיאָרָא, v. זַיְרָא.

זִיבָה I f. (זוב) *gonorrhœa, protracted menstruation, legal condition of one suffering from* &c., v. זָב. Zab. II, 2; Naz. IX, 4 משנזקק לז׳ as soon as he is declared a *zab*. Y. Maas. Sh. II, end, 53ᵈ; a. fr.—Men. 64ᵇ לְזִיבָתִי I offer a sacrifice for my recovery from the condition of a *zabah* (v. זָבָה), or from a severe hemorrhage, v. זוּב; Y. Shek. V, 48ᵈ, v. next w.—*Pl.* זִיבוֹת. Ker. I, 7; a. fr.

זִיבָה II or **זִיבַת** f. (popular diatectical pronunciation for זְאֵבָה) *wolf*. Y. Shek. V, 48ᵈ a woman said לְזִיבָתִי (v. preced.) which was interpreted as possibly meaning זאב בא ליטול את בנה a wolf had come near carrying off her son (and hence the thanks-offering); [differ. in Men. 64ᵇ, v. זוּב].

זְבוּחַ, זִיבּוּחַ m. (זבח) *slaughtering* of a sacrifice, *festival*. Snh. 63ª; 65ª; a. fr.—Tanḥ. Vayesh. 9 זִבּוּחוֹ של נילוס, v. זבול 3).

זְבוּל, זִיבּוּל m. (זבל) (*idolatrous*) *sacrificing and merriment*. Pesik. R. s. 6 יום זְבוּל . . . . . לזי׳ נילוס it was the festival of Nilus, and all went out for the entertainment in honor of N.; v. זְבוּל 3).

זִיבּוּלָא f. (v. זְבִילָא) *a shovelful, clod*. Ber. 8ª (prov.) (Ar. זבילא) עד ז׳ בתרייתא שלמא . . אפי׳ ליבעי man ought to pray for peace even to the last clod of earth thrown on his grave.

זִבּ׳, זִיבּוּנָא m. (זבן) *sale*. Targ. O. Lev. XXV, 42; a. e.

זִיבּוּרָא m. (זבר; cmp. h. דְּבוֹרָה) *bee, wasp*. Targ. Y. Lev. XI, 20.—Gitt. 70ª האי מאן דבלע זי׳ וכ׳ he who swallowed a wasp cannot live.—Midr. Till. to Ps. I, end אמרין לז׳ וכ׳ (not אומרין) people say to the wasp, we want neither thy sting nor thy honey. Ab. Zar. 28ᵇ bot. וקרירי לז׳ and cold water is good for the sting of a wasp. Ḥag. 5ª evils opposing each other כגון ז׳ ועקרבא as a bite of a wasp (requiring cold water) and one by a scorpion (requiring hot water); a. e.—*Pl.* זִיבּוּרֵי. Targ. Y. Lev. l. c.; a. e.—Snh. 109ᵇ; a. e.—*Fem.* זִיבּוֹרְתָא. Ab. Zar. 17ᵇ Ms. M. (ed. זיבוריתא). Meg. 14ᵇ חדא שמה ז׳ one was named wasp (Deborah).—*Pl.* זִיבּוּרְיָתָא. Targ. Ps. CXVIII, 12 (ed. Wil. זִבּ׳).

זִבּ׳, זִיבּוּרִית f. (זבר, v. זִבּוּרִית) 1) *the lowest* (*worst*) *land of an estate* (classified into עידית best, בינונית mean and ׳ז). Gitt. V, 1. Ib. 49ª top כגון . . . כו׳ דמזיק when the claimant's best land was only as good as the defendant's worst. B. Kam. 7ᵇ ז׳ . . אין לו אלא if one has only third class land; a. fr.—2) v. זִבּוּרִית.

זִיבוּת (זָבוּת) f. (זוב) *gonorrhea.* Lev. R. s. 18.

זִיבְחָא m. ch.=h. זֶבַח *sacrifice.* Tem. 31ᵇ עיקר ז׳ sacrifice in its strictest sense, i. e. cattle dedicated for the altar.

זִיג, *Pi.* זַיֵּיג, v. זָוַג.

זִיג (v. זגג) 1) *to be clear, bright, transparent.*—Part. זָיֵג, זַיֵּיג. Pes. 74ᵇ דזיג וכ׳ ed. (Ar. דזייג) it was as clear as &c., v. זְגוּגִיתָא. Sabb. 134ª והיכא דז׳ and where there is a transparent spot in the child's rump. Nidd. 25ª. Hull. 76ᵇ כיון דזִיגֵי וכ׳ (Ar. דזייגי) when they are transparent although not white.—2) (cmp. Lat. vitrea bilis) *to be glass-like.* Keth. 61ᵇ זג לה she got a greenish bilious complexion (was *swollen*, Rashi).

זִיגָא, Erub. 100ᵇ bot., v. זוֹגָא.

זִיגּוֹד, זִיגָּד pr. n. m. *Ziggad, Ziggod* (cmp. אַרְזְגַּד). Pes. 113ᵇ; Macc. 11ª (prov.) טוביה חטא וז׳ מנגד Tobias sinned and Z. was punished (because he was a single witness).

זִיגוּתָא, read זְגוּגִיתָא, v. זְגוּגִיתָא.

זִיד, זוּד (b. h.; cmp. הוּד) *to flow over, boil.* Sot. 11ª; Ex. R. s. 1, expl. זדו (Ex. XVIII, 11), v. בָּשַׁל.

Hif. הֵזִיד 1) *to boil, cook.* Snh. 69ª (ref. to יזיד Ex. XXI, 14) איש מֵזִיד וכ׳ a man (adult) cooks (prepares semen virile) and begets; Y. ib. VIII, beg. 26ª משיָּזִיד from the time he prepares &c.; a. e.—2) *to plan evil, to act with premeditation, in full consciousness of doing wrong.* Sabb. 69ª ה׳ בזה ובזה זו מֵזִיד וכ׳ if he acted in full consciousness of both (of its being a Sabbath day and of such a labor being forbidden on the Sabbath), that is the wilful sinner meant in the Law (punishable). Ib. שגג . . וה׳ במלאכה if he labored under a mistake as to the Sabbath day, but was aware of the sinful nature of the labor (if done on the Sabbath). Ex. R. s. 5, end; a. fr.—Part. מֵזִיד, f. מְזִידָה, v. supra. Y. Sot. V, beg. 20ª; a. fr.—במ׳ if done wilfully, opp. בשוגג. Ker. 18ª; a. fr.—*Pl.* מְזִידִין. Bets. 30ª, a. e. מוטב . . ואל יהיו מ׳ it is better that they be ignorant than that they know and transgress wilfully; a. fr.

זִיד, זוּד ch. same.—*Af.* אָזֵיד *to plan* &c. Targ. Y. Ex. XV, 21. Targ. O. ib. XXI, 14 ed. Berl. (ed. ירשע).

זִידוּ, זְדוּ f. (preced.) *premeditation, malice.* Targ. Ez. XXIV, 7.

זֵידָנָא, זֵידוֹנָא m. (preced.) 1) *wilful, violent; tyrant.* Targ. Prov. XXI, 24. Targ. Job XXXI, 3. Targ. Y. Deut. XVI, 22.—*Pl.* זֵידָנִין, זֵידוֹנִין. Targ. Ps. LXXXVI, 14 (ed. Lag. זְדוֹנִין).—2) *seething, boiling over; trnsf. passion.*—*Pl.* זֵידָנַיָּא, זֵידָנִין, זֵידוֹנַיָּא. Targ. Ps. CXXIV, 5 (Ms. זידונין).—Ib. XIX, 14 זֵידוֹנֵי׳ ed. Lag. (ed. Wil. זֵיד׳), v. זָדוֹן ch.

זִידָל, v. זְרִידָל.

זֵידָנוּתָא, v. זְדָנוּ.

זִיהָא, v. זוּהָ.

זִיהָא m. (זהה, cmp. זיו) *reflected light, reflexion.* Yoma 28ᵇ, v. זוֹהֲמָא. Ber. 58ᵇ זִיהֲיה Ar. (some ed. זיהרא, incorr.; ed. זְיוּיה) its (the comet's) reflexion.

זִיהֲרָא, v. זִיהוֹרָא.

זִיהוּם m. (זָהַם) 1) *the covering of plants with rancid oil,* or *tying up with manure* (v. זָהַם). Ab. Zar. 50ᵇ ז׳ אוקומי וכ׳ *ziham* is a means of preserving the tree, v. ברר I ch.—2) *offensive, turbid substance.* Nidd. 65ᵇ, v. זָהַם.—3) *social disqualification, spot in the family record* (not subject to legal disqualification). Y. Yeb. X, 11ª אין לה אלא משום ז׳ כהונה וכ׳ there is nothing against her except a social disqualification for priesthood, but the court cannot declare her &c., v. זָהַם; ib. XIII, 13ᵈ bot. אין בה וכ׳; Y. Gitt. VIII, 49ᶜ bot. אין בה משום ייחוס כהונה (corr. acc.).

זִיהוּמָא ch. same, as preced. 1).—*Pl.* זיהומי. Ab. Zar. 50ᵇ תרי ז׳ איכא Ms. M. (ed. זִיהֲמוּמֵי) there are two different processes called *zihum.*

זִיהוּמְתָא f. (preced.) *fat, filth, sediment.* Targ. Ez. XXIV, 6 (h. text חֶלְאָה).

זִיהוּרָא m. (זהר) *what is worth guarding, possession, treasure.* Targ. Prov. IV, 23 (Bxt. זהו׳, h. text מִשְׁמָר). V. זִיהֲרָא III.

זִיהוֹרָא m. (זהר) *splendor, brightness.* Targ. Ez. VIII, 2 ed. Lag. (ed. זְהֲרָא).—Targ. Ps. XVIII, 13 זיהור Ms. M. (ed. זְהוֹר; Targ. II Sam. XXII, 13 זיו). Targ. O. Deut. XXXIII, 2. Targ. Ps. XIX, 5 זיהורא Ms. (ed. Lag. זִיהֲרָא, ed. Wil. זיהרא, oth. זיהוא).—*Pl.* זִיהוֹרַיָּא. Targ. Ez. I, 13 (ed. Lag. sing.) [Ib. XXXII, 8 ניהוריא ed. Lag., ed. זְהָרַיָּא).

זִיהִיא, v. זִיהָא.

זִיהֲמוּמֵי, v. זִיהוּמָא.

זִיהֲרָא I, זְהָרָא m. (זהר) *moon, moon-light.* Targ. Y. Deut. IV, 19 (O. סיהרא). Ib. XVII, 3 ז׳ Ar. (ed. ס׳); a. e.—Kidd. 81ª נפל ז׳ באיפומא Ar. (ed. נהורא) moon-light fell through the opening (impluvium). Y. Taan. IV, end, 69ᶜ אשלם ז׳ full-moon arrived.—V. זְהָרָא.

זִיהֲרָא II (זְהָרָא, Ar.) m. (זהר, cmp. זהה a. זהם) [*a glittering substance,*] 1) *gall* (cmp. Syr. זהרא P. Sm. 1091, זהירא *acerbus*, ib. 1090); trnsf. *anger, injured pride.* Gitt. 45ᵇ אימליא ז׳ she was filled with gall (anger). Ber. 51ᵇ.—2) *venom, a fatal substance discharged by animals of prey on attacking.* Ab. Zar. 30ᵇ זִיהֲרֵיה חליש Ms. M. (ed. זיהרא קליש) its (the serpent's) poison grows weaker with old age. Hull. 53ª שדי זיהריה it discharges its venom. Ib. 52ᵇ ז׳ אית ליה . . . . זיהריה it issues a fluid but its discharge does not burn. Nidd. 55ᵇ נהר דז׳ וכ׳ Ar.

(ed. רוזחי׳, corr. acc.) though the poison is removed from the body (through the secretion of the nose), the fluid itself (put in the eye) is not removed.

זִיהֲרָא III m. (זהר) [*that which is guarded*, cmp. בְּלָמָא a. זִיהוּרָא;] *landed estate* (comprising fields, gardens &c., to the exclusion of private dwellings, contrad. to נכסין). B. Bath. 61[b] bot. אי א״ל זִיהֲרִי וכ׳ Ms. M. a. oth. (ed. א...) if he said (in the agreement), I sell thee my landed estate, the sale includes even orchards &c.

זִיהֲרוֹרָא, זִיהֲרָרָא, זה׳ m. (preced.) *owner of large estates, rich landlord.—Pl.* זִיהֲרוֹרֵי &c. B. Bath. 55[a] הנהו ז׳ דזבין ארעא....... דזבינהו זבינהו (Ms. O. הזבינהי ארעייהו, Var. זהורי, זיארי, זיאהררי, v. Rabb. D. S. a. l. note) as to those landlords, whoever sells land to them for the taxes, the sale is valid. [Ar: '*land-tax collectors*—whosoever buys from them' &c.]

זִיהֲרוֹרָא *glare*, v. זְהֲרוּרָא.

זִיהֲרָרָא, v. זִיהֲרוֹרָא.

זִיו m. (b. h.;=זהוי; זחח) 1) *splendor, glory, countenance.* Sot. IX, 15 (49[a]) ז׳ החכמה the glory of learning, ז׳ הכהונה of priesthood. Ber. 64[a] ז׳ השכינה Divine Glory; a. fr.—ז׳ איקונין, v. אִיקוֹנִין.—2) *good looks, bloom* of health. Koh. R. to III, 11 עדיין לא בא זיוו וכ׳ my son's former good look has not come back yet; Cant. R. to II, 5 עדיין לא בא בני בזיוו הנשתנה וכ׳ my son has not yet recovered his bright looks which changed &c. Koh. R. l. c. זִיוָן של בני; Cant. R. l. c. זיותן וכ׳ (corr. acc.); Yalk. Ex. 272.—3) *bloom, forth-coming vegetation.* Y. R. Hash. I, 56[d] bot. 'the month of Ziv' (I Kings VI, 1) שבו זיוו של עולם because in it the world appears in bloom. Cant. R. to VI, 11 זיון של ירק (read זיוו) the beauty of a vegetable garden.—4) (b. h. זו) *Ziv*, name of the *Spring-month.* R. Hash. 11[a], a. e., v. supra. Pesik. Bahod., p. 106[b]; a. e.

זִיו, זִיוָא I ch. same. Targ. Y. Ex. XXXIII, 11; a. fr.—Targ. I Kings VI, 1; 37 ירח ז׳ ניצניא, v. preced.—R. Hash. 11[a] דאית בה ז׳ לאילני for in that month (Ziv) there is the bloom of trees. Y. Yeb. XVI, 15[c] bot.; Lev. R. s. 18 זִיוְוהוֹן דאפוי his features.—Snh. 31[b], v. בְּתִיָה; a. e.

זִיוָא II, v. זִיזָא I.

זִיוַאי pr. n. m. *Zivay*, son-in-law of R. Meïr. Ber. 53[b] (v. Rabb. D. S. a. l. note). Yalk. Koh. 989 ז׳ חתנו של ר׳ מ׳ (ed. Lemb. ז׳ omitted); Sabb. 153[a] זריזאי Ms. M. (Ms. O. ר׳ זיתאי, ed. omitted, v. Rabb. D. S. a. l. note).

זִיוְוד, Tosef. Bekh. V, 9, v. זִיוֵּר.

זִיוָן, זִיוָא, זִיוו, v. זִיוָא, זִיו.

זִוּוּג, זִיוּוּג m. (זָוַג) *coupling, matching, marital destiny.* Gen. R. s. 68, beg. ארץ זִיוּוּגוֹ של וכ׳ man's conjugal destiny is decreed by the Lord; (Yalk. Jud. 70 זוגו׳ or זִוְּגוֹ, v. זָוָג). Ib. יש שהוא הולך אצל זיווגו וכ׳ (Yalk. זוגו) one must travel to meet her who is designated for him, to another she travels to meet him. Midr. Till. to Ps. LIX ייחד הב״ה שמו על הז׳ the Lord has His special name connected with marriage (Gen. XXIV, 50; Jud. XIV, 4; Prov. XIX, 14); a. fr.—Trnsf. *a corresponding case, solace offered by pointing to a similar case* (v. זָוַג). Pesik. R. s. 30 מבקשים ז׳ לירושלים וכ׳ were looking out for a similar bereavement as a solace to Jerusalem and could not find any (ref. to Lam. II, 13). Ib. the Lord said אני אהיה זיווגך I will be thy partner in misery (ref. to Is. XLIII, 14).—*Pl.* זִוּוּגִים, זִיוּוּגִין, זִוּו׳. Gen. R. l. c.; Lev. R. s. 8, beg.; a. e.

זִיוְויין, v. זַיְיתָא.

זִיוּוּעַ m. (זוע) *trembling.* Targ. Nah. II, 11 ed. Lag. (ed. Wil. זִיעָ, oth. ed. זִיוּעַ).

זִיוּוּר, v. זִיוֵּר.

זִיוְתָן, v. זִיוְתָן.

זִיוִיד, Tosef. Bekh. V, 9, v. זִיוֵּר.

זִיוּן m. (זון) 1) *putting on armour, going to war.* Num. R. s. 14 (p. 257[a] ed. Amst.) (ref. to נשק, Ps. CXL, 8) כיום זִיוּנָם של וכ׳ on the day when the thirty and one kings went to war against Joshua.—2) *the decoration of letters with crownlets.—Pl.* זִיוּנִין. Men. 29[b] seven letters (in the Torah-scrolls) require שלשה ז׳ each three crownlets (flourishes).

זִיוּנָא I, **זִיוּן׳** m. (זון I) 1) *food, alimentation.* Targ. O. Ex. XXI, 10.—Ber. 44[a] ז׳ food, contrad. to מזונא satisfactory meal.

זִיוּנָא II m. ch.=h. זִיוּן 2).—*Pl.* זִיוּנֵי. Sabb. 105[a] דבעי ז׳ when the letters (he has written) want crownlets for finishing touches.

זִיוּנָא III m. (זון I) *management, expenses and risks of business.* Keth. 66[b] עיסקא זוטא דזוטר ז׳ a small capital the management of which is easy.

זִיוּנָא m. (זון II) בֵּי ז׳ *prison*, v. בְּזִיוּנָא I.

זִיוּעַ, זִיוַע, v. זִיוּוּעַ.

זִיוּף m. (זוף, *Pi.*) *informality, fault.* Y. Gitt. II, 44[a] bot. זה זִיוּפוֹ מד״א such a document (written in day-time and signed by night) would be defective on account of a condition not perceptible from the document itself, opp. מזויפין מתוכו, v. זוף I.

זִיוֵּר (זִיוִיר) m. (זור) *one whose eyes are unsteady*, v. זוור ch.—Bekh. 44[a] Ar. (ed. זריד, corr. acc.); Tosef. ib. V, 9 זִיוִיד. זרויד (corr. acc.).

זִיוְתָן m. (fr. זִיוָה, fem. form of זִיו, formed like פִּיוְתָן) *bright, distinguished, noble. Pl.* זִיוְתָנִין, ...ִים, constr. זִיוְתָנֵי. R. Hash. 11[a] (play on זו, I Kings VI, 1) שבו נבראו ז׳ עולם for in that month were created the nobles of the world (the patriarchs).

זִיוְתָן, זִיוְתָנָא ch. same. Targ. Job XXXI, 26.—Targ. II Esth. X, 3 דמזהר וז׳ (missing in ed. Lag.). Targ.

Is. XIV, 12. Targ. Zech. X, 3 (ed. Wil. זִוְתָן).—Sabb. 156ᵃ גבר ז׳ a distinguished (or handsome) man.—*Pl.* זִיוְתָנִין, זִיוְתָנַיָּא. Targ. Cant. VI, 10 זִיוְתָ׳ ed. Lag. (ed. Amst. זִוְתָ׳).— Targ. Y. II Gen. XIV, 5 זיות׳ (corr. acc.); Gen. R. s. 42 זיותניא דבהון (ed. Wil. נה . . . ., corr. acc.) the brightest among them (h. text זוזים בהם, v. הוֹן I).—Keth. 61ᵃ בני זִיוְתָנֵי handsome children.—Targ. Ps. CXLIV, 12 זיותנין (read זִיוְתָנָן fem., Ms. זְוִתַּנְיָן!).

זִיז I m. (זוז or זעזע) 1) ז׳ שבעדשים name of *a mite* in lentils.—*Pl.* זִיזִין, זִיזִים. Hull. 67ᵇ; Sifra Sh'mini Par. 10, ch. XII; Y. Ter. VIII, 45ᵇ bot.—2) *spider.*—*Pl.* as above. Y. Sabb. XIV, beg. 14ᵇ (differ. in Bab. ib. 106ᵇ, a. Tosef. ib. XII (XIII), 4).—[Tosef. Bekh. I, 8 דבש הזיזין ed. Zuck. Var. הגודין, v. חַגְזִין.]—3) name of a fabulous *bird* (ref. to Ps. L, 11). Lev. R. s. 22, end. B. Bath. 73ᵇ.

זִיז II m. (=זוז, v. זְוִי, זָוִית) *an attachment, a projection* from the door frame serving as *a shed* over the entrance, or *a moulding* projecting from a window-sill serving as *a bracket.* Ohol. XIV, 1 (difference betw. our w. a. גיזרה, v. גְּזוּזְטְרָא). Ib. 4 ז׳ שהוא סיבב וכ׳ a moulding which runs around the entire building (or room) and forms a part of the door frame. Erub. X, 4 ז׳ שלפני חלון וכ׳ a bracket in front of a window. Yalk. Deut. 898 והז׳ עליו אכילה וכ׳ and on the bracket (in front of the palace) are spread eatables, drinks &c.; a. v. fr.—*Pl.* זִיזִין, זִיזִים. Ohol. VIII, 2. B. Bath. III, 8; a. fr.

זִיזָא I ch. same. Targ. I Kings VI, 5 (ed. Wil. a. oth. זִיזָא). Targ. Ez. XLI, 6 (ed. Lag. *pl.*).—B. Mets. 83ᵃ; Yalk. Ex. 346 ז׳ דמחוזא (not זו׳) a Mahuza balcony or bay-window (cmp. גַּבְלִית). B. Bath. 60ᵃ—*Pl.* זִיזַיָּא, זיזין. Targ. I Kings VI, 6. Targ. Ez. XLII, 5; a. e., v. זְוִי. [B. Bath. l. c. זיזין דהוה נפיק, read with Ms. M. זיזא . . . מפיק.]

זִיזָא II ch.=h. זִיז I, 1. Targ. Y. Deut. XIV, 19.

זִיזָא III, **בַּר ז׳** pr. n. m. *Bar-Ziza.* Y. B. Kam. VI, 5ᶜ bot.; Y. Shebu. VI, 37ᵈ.

זִיזְיוֹן, זִיזְיָן, זִיזְיָן, זִיזְיָין pr. n. pl. *Zizyon, Zizyan.* Tosef. Shebi. IV, 8 זיזין ed. Zuck. (Var. זיזיין, ed. זיזיון); Y. Dem. II, 22ᵈ top חיזיון.

זִיחַ, v. זוּחַ.

זִיטָא (זִיטָה) זִיטָא (ζῆτα) the Greek letter *Zeta* (numerical value ζ' *seven*), used in phonetic play like ζῆτω, *live!* Gen. R. s. 14, beg., a. e., v. אִיטָא; Y. Yeb. IV, 5ᵈ top זיטא (corr. acc.).

זיטוטוס, read:

זִיטִיטוּס or **זִיטֵיטוּס** m. (ζητητός or ζητευτός, sub. θανεῖν, cmp. Tobit I, 19, a. מתבקש Taan. 29ᵃ) *one who is sought for to be put to death, a fugitive from justice, outlaw.* Gen. R. s. 32, beg.; s. 38, beg.; (Yalk. Ps. 631 עשה זיאטטוס; Ar. ed. Koh. זיטיטוס, Var. זיטוט׳, זיטוס׳) אותו ז׳ declare him an outlaw, and he will be like (legally) dead &c.

זִיטְמָא, זִיטִימָא m. (ζήτημα) *judicial inquiry,* דבר

של ז׳ *something subject to investigation, charge, suspicion* (of heresy, cmp. Acta XVIII, 15; XXIII, 29, or of il-loyalty). Num. R. s. 4 זיטים׳ Mus. (ed. זיטמא). Pesik. Aḥaré, p. 173ᵇ זיטר׳ Ar. s. v. זנם Var. (ed. זינומירא; Ar. זינרמון, read זִיטִיסִין=ζήτησις); Lev. R. s. 20 זינרמון Ar. (ed. שְׁמָצָה; Yalk. Lev. 525 זוהמא, זומא).

זִיזָארָא, v. זַיְירָא.

זִיג, v. זַגָּ.

זַיְדָל, זַיְדָל pr. n. m. *Zaydal.* Y. Ab. Zar. II, 41ᵃ top; Y. Ter. VIII, 45ᶜ top.

זיודן, v. בָּאזְרָק.

זִין, זַיִן, v. זוּן.

זַיִן, זַיִן. m. (זון) *armament, armor, weapon* (collect.), *steel*; כלי ז׳ *implements of war.* Tosef. Ab. Zar. II, 4 אין..לא ז׳ ולא כלי ז׳ you must not sell them either armor (steel) or implements &c. Snh. 104ᵃ ז׳ אוכל ז׳ וכ׳ he showed them steel consuming steel, i. e. the manufacture of hardened steel (cmp. ib. 96ᵇ); Cant. R. to III, 4 ז׳ בולע ז׳. Tanh., ed. Bub., Lekh 23 חריני חוגרו זִיינִי I will gird him with my (royal) armor. Cant. R. to IV, 4; Pesik. Nah., p. 124ᵇ, a. e., v. זוֹנִי. Ex. R. s. 45 (ref. to עדי, Ex. XXXIII, 5), cmp. זוֹנִי; a. fr.—Ab. Zar. 25ᵇ; Yeb. 115ᵃ אשה כלי זַיְנָהּ עליה a woman has her armor with her, i. e. her physical weakness is her protection from murderous attacks. [Num. R. s. 4, end בזינו, v. זוֹנִי.]—*Pl.* זַיְינוֹת. Pirké d'R. El. ch. XLVII, beg.

זַיי״ן *the letter Zayin.*—*Pl.* זַיי״נִין. Sabb. XII, 5. Ib. 103ᵇ.

זַיְנָא I, **זֵינָא** m. *weapon, ornament,* v. זַיִן.

זִינָא II m. (זין II) *restriction, loss* (cmp. רְוָוחָא). Targ. Y. Num. XXI, 27 זִינָא, opp. אגרא.—Men. 77ᵃ ז׳ Ar. (Ms. M. זִיאנָא, v. Rabb. D. S. a. l. note; ed. דיאנא; B. Bath. 90ᵃ פסידא), opp. רווחא.

זִינְקִי, v. סִיאַנְקִי.

זִיעָא, v. זִיעַ.

זִיף, זַיִף, v. זוּף h. a. ch.

זִיוּף, v. זִיף.

זַיְפָא m. (זוף) *forgery, a forged document.* B. Bath. 32ᵇ שטרא ז׳ הוא (Ms. H. זויפא) the document is a forgery. Keth. 36ᵇ דז׳ הוא that it is a forged document.

זַיְיפִי or **זַיְפִי** (v. preced.) *Z'yafi* or *Zayafi,* a fictitious name of one of the Sodomite judges. Snh. 109ᵇ (Rashi זויפא).

זַיְיפָנָא m. (preced. wds.) *forger, deceiver.* Ab. Zar. 11ᵇ.

זַיְיפָנוּתָא f. (preced.) *forgery, deceit.* Ab. Zar. 11ᵇ.

זַיְרָא, זִירָה, זִירָא m. (זור Pa) *press, the perforated tub containing the object to be pressed or beaten.*

Y. Sabb. XVII, 16^b top; Y. Bets. I, 60^c bot. בז׳ ובמזורה וכ׳ as regards the handling on the Sabbath of a press-tub &c. Ib. ז׳ דו עצר ביה וכ׳ *zayyara* is that in which an object is squeezed, *m'zorah* is that with which the beating is done. Ab. Zar. 60^a מִעצרא וזירא Ms. M. (ed. מִעצרא דזי׳, Rashi to Sabb. 123^a מִעצרתא זירארא) the vat or the press-tub (used by a gentile for making wine).—*Pl.* זַיְירֵי. Sabb. 123^a סיכי ז׳ ומזורי (Ar. ed. Koh. זַיְאֲרֵי) the dyer's pins, tubs and beams.

זַיְיתָא, זַיְיתַיָּה, זַיְיתִין, pl. v. זֵיתָא I, II.

זִיכַּיָא, זִיכֵּי m. pl. (זכי, Pa.) *clearings*, i. e. *twigs, roots &c. collected for clearing the ground, rubbish.* M. Kat. 10^b; B. Bath. 54^a האי מאן דזכי ז׳ (Ar. זַכָּיָא, Var. in Mss. &c. זִכֵּ׳, דִכֵּ׳, דִיכְּיָא, v. Rabb. D. S. a. l. note) he who clears away rubbish.

זִיל *to be worthless*, part. זִיל, v. זוּל.

זִיל imperat. of אֲזַל.

זִילָא 1) part. f. of זוּל; 2) m.=זִילוּתָא *low valuation.*—*Pl.* זִילֵי. B. Mets. 52^b, v. זְלַל.

זִילַאי pr. n. m. *Zilay.* Ber. 53^b.

זִילּוּף, זִלּ׳ m. (זָלַף) *sprinkling* (with aromatic wine &c.). Pes. 20^b ראוי לז׳ (Ms. O. through entire page זֶלֶף) fit for sprinkling. Ib. תַּעֲשֶׂה ז׳ may be used for &c.—Num. R. s. 13, beg. (ref. to יזלו, Cant. IV, 16) זה ז׳ that means aromatic sprinkling. Succ. 40^b; B. Kam. 102^a לאכלה ולא לז׳ 'to be eaten' (Lev. XXV, 6) but not to be used for perfumes; v. זֶלַח.

זִילוּתָא f. (זול) 1) *cheapness, low price.* Targ. II Chr. IX, 27. Targ. Job XXVIII, 17 Ms. a. Levita (ed. קילותא).—2) *disregard, disgrace.* Targ. Lam. I, 8.—Yeb. 100^a משום ז׳ because it is a disgrace (for a woman to stand waiting). Macc. 24^a דלא שמע בז׳ וכ׳ he does not hear a scholar defamed and keeps silence. B. Kam. 102^b bot. לא יקרייכו ... זִילוּתַיְיכוּ וכ׳ I want neither your honor nor your insults; a. fr.

זִילְזוּלָא m. (זְלַל) *disregard.* Ab. Zar. 35^a לזי׳ בה, read with early eds. לִזְלְזוּלֵי.

זִילְחָא, v. זִלְחָא.

זִימָא m., pl. זִימֵי (v. זמם III) *secretory vessels, nostrils, gils* (Syr. זומא P. Sm. 1101). B. Bath. 74^a זִימֵיה (Var. אוּסְיה, v. Rashb. a. l.; Ms. O. זהוריה, Ms. H. קימיה, a. oth. Var., v. Rabb. D. S. a. l. note).

זִימָּה, זִמָּה I f. (b. h.; זָמַם III) 1) [*filth* (cmp. זוּהֲמָא),] *obscenity, libidiousness, carnality.* Sabb. 152^a שטוף בזי׳ excessive in carnal gratification. Snh. 106^a אלהיהם של אלו שונא ז׳ הוא their (the Israelites') God hates libidiousness. B. Kam. 16^b (play on זנים, II Chr. XVI, 14) כל המריח . . . ז׳ גָּרִידֵי whoever smells them becomes lusty. Ab. II, 7 מרבה זמה increases unchastity; a. fr.—Ab. Zar. 17^b (ref. to מזמה, Prov. II, 11, v. next w.) מדבר זי׳ וכ׳ she (the Torah) will guard thee from improper conduct.—2) (homilet.; cmp. זָמַם I, הַמַּאי הוּמְדוּ &c.) *suspicion, parental uncertainty.* Sifra K'dosh., Par. 3, ch. VII ממלא . . ממזרים שנ׳ ז׳ זה מה הוא he fills the world with bastards, as it says (Lev. XIX, 29) the land will be full of *zimmah*, 'what is this person?'; Yeb. 37^b הכי קאמר זו מה היא R. El. b. Jacob means by *zimmah* doubts as to paternity.

זִימָּה, זִמָּה II f. (b. h.; זָמַם I) *thought, plan, counsel;* (in an evil sense) *cunning, evil plan.* Ab. Zar. 17^b (ref. to מזמה, Prov. II, 11, and reading מְזִ׳) מאי מזי׳ וכ׳ what do you understand by *mizzimmah?* Do you mean the Law in which the word *zimmah* is used in the sense of *counsel* (in Lev. XVIII, 17) since it is translated (in Targ. O.) 'counsel of the wicked' &c.?—Then it ought to read *zimmah* (divine counsel shall guard thee).—(Ans.) ה״ק מדבר ז׳ וכ׳, v. preced. (v. Rabb. D. S. a. l. note 2).—Deut. R. s. 2 (ref. to Ez. XXII, 11) מאי בזי׳ במחשבה what does this *b'zimmah* mean? With reasoning.

זִימּוּן, זִמּוּן m. (זְמַן) 1) *designatian for a purpose*, v. הַזְמָנָה. Ned. 7^a ז׳ מועיל has designation the same effect as virtual use (=הזמנה מילתא)?; Ber. 26^a יש ז׳; a. fr.—2) *summons to appear before court;* 3) *appointment for a common meal, the appeal to partakers ta say grace after a common meal.* Snh. 8^a ז׳ בשלשה *zimmun* requires three persons, מאי ז׳ . . . ברכת ז׳ what is meant by *zimmun?* Shall we say, it means the grace after meal &c.?—But we read ז׳ וברכת ז׳ וכ׳ *z.* and the grace &c. require three persons .... אלא מאי ז׳ אזמוני וכ׳ consequently, *zimmun* (not qualified) means summons before court. Ber. VII, 5 מצטרפים לז׳ can be counted together for common grace. Ib. 45^b אין ברכת הז׳ בינידהם (not המזון) the appeal and answer to common grace must not take place between them. Ib. אין ז׳ למפרע the appointment for a meal and benediction in common cannot be made retroactive (it must be made before the meal commences); a. fr.—*Pl.* זִימּוּנִים *appointments, meeting places.* Pesik. R. s. 33 כמה ז׳ נזדמנתי אִתְּכֶם how many meetings have I not appointed with you!; v. וִיעוּד.

זִימוּנָא pr. n. m., v. זְמִינָא.

זִימּוּם m. (זָמַם I) *intention, planning; conspiracy.* Y. Hag. II, 78^a top עד כדי ז׳ even the planning of a breach of law may be punishable in extraordinary times.

זִימֵי, v. זוּמָא I.—[זִימֵי, B. Bath. 74^a זימיה, v. זִימָא.]

זִימְיָא f. (ζημία) *fine, penalty*, esp. *the oppressive penalties of the Roman government.* Tanh. Naso 10; Num. R. s. 11 שלא תבוא ז׳ למדינה that no *zemia* may be decreed over the district.—*Pl.* זִימְיָין. Y'lamd. Aharé (quot. in Ar.); Yalk. Cant. 985.—זִימְיוֹת. Y. Ab. Zar. IV, 44^b; Y. Shebi. IV, 35^b; ib. V, end, 36^a זומות (corr. acc.). Y. Peah I, 15^b bot.; Yalk. Prov. 935 המזימיות (corr. acc.). Yalk. Jer. 312; Pesik. Bahod. p. 151^a זמיות (corr. acc.).—V. next w.

זִימְיוֹן, זִמְיוֹן m. (זמה=ch. זְמֵי I; adapt. of ζημία,

v. preced.) *penalty, tax.*—*Pl.* זִימְיוֹנִית, זִמְ׳. Gen. R. s. 1; (Y. Peah I, 15[b] bot. זימיות). Y. Gitt. VI, end, 47[c] (Y. Shebi. IV, 35[b] זימיות).

זִימְיוֹנָא, זִמְ׳ m. (זְמַר II) *plan.*—*Pl.* זִימְיוֹנִין, זִמְ׳. Targ. Job XXI, 27; a. e.

זִימִין, v. זִימְרָא.

זִימְנָא pr. n. m., v. זְמִינָא.

זִימְנָא *time*, v. זְמַן II.

***זִימְנָה** f. (זמן) *summons* for public labor. Pesik. R. s. 23—24 אייתון ז׳ וכ׳ they issued a summons for millers; (Y. Peah I, 15[c] bot. אתת צמות; Y. Kidd. I, 61[b] bot. אתא מצוותא).

(זִימְרָא,) זִימְרָה, v. זִמְרָה.

זִין I *to outfit, provide*, v. זוּן.

זִין II m. *Zin*, name of a weight, v. זוּז.

זַיִן m. *armor* &c., v. זַיְין.

זִין I *kind*, v. זַן.

זִין II, זֵינָא, זַי׳, זַיְינָא (זַיִן, זַיְינָא) m. ch.=h. זַיִין. Targ. O. Gen. XLI, 44. Targ. O. Deut. XXII, 5 תִּקּוּן זֵין man's outfit; a. fr.—B. Bath. 4[a] אם זַיְינָךְ עלך וכ׳ though thou art armed (like a free man), thy record is here (showing that thou art a slave).—*Pl.* זַיְינִין, זַיְנִין &c. Targ. Y. II Gen. XLIX, 19. Targ. Cant. IV, 4. Targ. Ps. VII, 14 זֵינֵי Ms. (ed. זַיְ׳); a. e.

זינאות, v. זוּנִי.

זִינְגָּאֵי, זִנְ׳ m. pl. *Zingaë*, name of a Cushite tribe, prob. named from *Zeugis, Zeugitana Regio* in Africa Propria (cmp. τὰ Ζίγγα or Ζίγγα in Numidia, Strabo XVII, 831). Targ. Y. Gen. X, 7; Targ. I Chr. I, 9 (Var. in ed. Rahmer דנ׳; h. text סבתכא).

זינומריא, Pesik. Aḥaré, p. 173[b], v. זִיטְרְמָא.

זינומתא, זנו׳, Targ. Y. Num. V, 21, a corrupt. of מוֹמְתָא or אוֹמָתָא.

זִינּוּק m. (זָנַק) *squirting, splash, water rushing through a spout.* Ḥull. 38[a]. Zeb. 25[b] תחת הז׳ under the spout. Ib. במזרק שא״א לו בלא ז׳ when receiving the blood of the sacrifice in the bowl, which cannot be done without splashing. Yalk. Deut. 962 (ref. to Deut. XXXIII, 22 יזנק) מה ז׳ זה וכ׳ as the jet comes from one place and divides itself in two directions.—*Pl.* זינוּקים. Pesik. R. s. 43.

זינימון, Ar. s. v. זנם, v. זִיטְרְמָא.

זִינְקָא m. (זְנַק) *leap.* Sabb. 77[b], v. בּוּדְזִינְקָא.

זִיעַ m. (זוּעַ) *trembling, agitation.* Lev. R. s. 11; s. 27; Sifra Sh'mini, Milluim, a. e. באימה ברתת ובז׳ in fear, trembling and commotion.

זִיעַ, זִיעָא, זִיעֲא f. ch. (preced.) 1) *earthquake.* Targ. Am. I, 1 (ed. Lag. זִיעְיָא).—2) *tempest.* Targ. Job XXXVII, 9, v. זוֹעָא.—3) *sweat*, v. זִיעֲתָא.—4) *trembling commotion.* Targ. Is. XXI, 3 זיעא ed. Lag. (ed. זִיעְיָא). Targ. Ps. XLVIII, 7 Ms. זִיעָא (ed. זַעֲוָא, זַעְוָא, not זַעְוְיָא). Targ. Jer. XXII, 23 זִיעַ (some ed. זיעתא).

זֵיעָה f. (b. h. זֵעָה; זוּעַ) 1) *moisture, dripping, sweat, vapor.* Makhsh. II, 1 זֵיעַת בתים the drippings of damp walls in houses &c. Toh. IX, 1, v. מַעֲטָן. Ber. 57[b]; Gen. R. s. 20; a. fr.—V. next art.—2) *commotion, agitation.* Cant. R. to IV, 4, v. זִיעַ.

זִיעֲזֵעַ, v. זַעְ׳.

זִיעֲתָא, זִיעָא, זֵי׳ f.=h. זֵיעָה 1) *sweat.* Targ. O. Gen. III, 19, v. דִּיעֲתָא.—Y. Ab. Zar. II, 41[a] bot. כל זיעה וכ׳ (Y. Ter. VIII, 45[d] top זיעא) every perspiration of man is poisonous &c.—Gen. R. s. 78, beg. מן זיעתהון וכ׳ from the sweat of the Ḥayoth (Ez. I, 5).—Ber. 38[a] (זיעה) זיעא בעלמא mere exudation (of the dates). Pes. 24[b] ז׳ בעלמא merely the juice pressed out (not manufactured drink).—2) *trembling, fear.* Targ. Jer. XXII, 23, v. זִיעַ. Targ. O. Deut. II, 25 זִיעֲתָךְ Var., v. זוֹעָא. Targ. II Esth. IV, 2 (fr. Deut. XXVIII, 67).

זִיף I, verb, v. זוּף a. זְיַף, רְיַף.

זִיף II m., pl. זִיפִּין, זִיפִים (זוּף I; b. h. צוּפִים) *thick honey.* Makhsh. V, 9 דבש הז׳ (R. S. דבש וזו׳), expl. Sot. 48[b], v. זוּף I.

זִיף III (b. h.) pr. n. pl. *Zif*, in the territory of Judah.—Denom. זִיפִי, pl. זִיפִים, זִיפִין *inhabitants of Zif.* Sot. 48[b] (expl. דבש זיפים, v. preced.) על שם מקומו the honey of the Ziphites.—Ib. (ref. to Ps. LIV, 2) ע״ש מקומן *Zifim* means men of Zif (Josh. XV, 24).

זַיִף, זִיף m. (v. זוּף II), pl. זַיְפִים, זַיְפִין, זַיְ׳, זַי׳, 1) *bristles.* Y. Sabb. VII, 11[b] זַיְפֵי חזיר bristles of a swine; Tosef. ib. IX (X), 2 שני זיפין (Var. זַפִּין).—2) *eye-brows.* Bekh. 44[a] שתמו זיפיו (ed. זיפין, incorr.) one whose eye-brows are gone.

זִיפָא, זַי׳ ch. 1) same, *eye-brow.* *Pl.* זַיְפִין, זַי׳. Bekh. 44[a] דנפישי זיפיה whose eye-brows are extremely large.—*2) *graving tool, chisel.* Targ. O. Ex. XXXII, 4 זַי׳ ed. Berl. (ed. Amst. זִיפָא); [oth. opin. *shaggy mat, cloth*, v. שׁוּשִׁיפָא] (h. text חרט).

זִיפּוּת m. (זֶפֶת) *coating of pitch.* Y. Sabb. VII, 10[b] bot. שרי ז׳ he who dissolves the pitch-lining, v. בּירלוֹס.

זִיפִירִין, v. זְפִירִין.

זִיפְלַן, v. זִפְלַן.

זִיפְרִין, v. זְפִירִין.

זִיפְתָא, זִיפְתּ׳, v. זִפָא, זֶפֶת.

זִיפְתִּי, v. דִּיפְתִּי.

זִיק m. (זנק), pl. זִיקִין (b. h. זִקִּים, זִיק׳, זִיקוֹת) *sparks, burning arrows* (b. h.); *meteors, shooting stars* [or *comet*]. Ber. IX, 1, expl. ib. 58[b] ככבא דשביט.—2) *a blast of wind,* [also imagined as *a spirit* (cmp. רוּחַ)]. B. Mets. 107ᵇ.—(Mikv. IX, 5 Ar., v. זְקַק.]

זִיקָא I ch. same, 1) *shooting star*, or *comet*. Y. Ber. IX, 13ᶜ.—*Pl.* זִיקֵי, זִיקִין. Targ. Y. Ex. XX, 2, sq.—2) *blast, wind, draught* (*spirit*). Targ. Y. Lev. XVI, 22 רוח ז׳. Targ. Job IV, 15; a. e.—Ab. Zar. 28ᵇ ויזדהר מז׳ and let him beware of exposing his ear to a draught.—Ber. 40ᵇ תמרי ז׳ dates blown down by the wind. Ned. 28ᵇ איכא ז׳ נפישא a strong wind is blowing (threatening to mow down the standing crop). Esth. R. to I, 12 פוז ז׳ וכ׳ blow a blast into his belly (arouse his anger). Taan. 24ᵃ נשב ז׳ (not נשא), a wind arose (gathering clouds); ib. 25ᵇ; B. Mets. 85ᵇ; a. e.—Sabb. 129ᵃ היכא דכריך ז׳ in a room where the air is turned around, i. e. in a draught.—Gen. R. s. 50, beg. (ref. to כמראה הבזק, Ez. I, 14) כרוחא לז׳ as the wind drives the sparks at a conflagration; [comment.: as the wind shakes the suspended leather-hose, v. next w.]; ib. כז׳ לעננא as the wind scatters the clouds. Ber. 59ᵃ כז׳ על פום דני like the rumbling sound produced by blowing into wine vessels; a. fr.

זִיקָא II c. (v. preced.) [*sprinkler*,] *hose, skin* for wine, water &c. (Syr. זוקתא uter). Targ. Ps. XXXIII, 7 (h. text נֵד); a. e.—Gen. R. s. 50, v. preced. Ab. Zar. 60ᵃ ז׳ בין מליא וכ׳ a tied up wine skin whether entirely filled &c. Y. ib. V, 45ᵃ top אהן דנגד בז׳ וכ׳ if one drags a skin (to take possession) and it bursts; Y. Kidd. I, 60ᵇ בזקה; a. fr.—*Pl.* זִיקַיָּא, זִיקִין. Targ. Y. Ex. XV, 8 (h. text נֵד). Targ. Josh. IX, 4 (h. text נֹאדוֹת); a. e.—Lev. R. s. 12 (quot. in Ar., not found in ed.) נפרוק ארלין זיקייא בהדין משכבא let us unload these bottles in this burial ground.

זִיקָא III m., pl. זִיקִין (זקק; cmp. b. h. זִקִּים) *fetters, chains*. Targ. II Sam. III, 34. Targ. Jer. XL, 1 זִיקַיָּא Levita (ed. עִיקַיָּא).—[זִיקָא f. *obligation*, v. next w.]

זִיקָה f. (זָקַק; cmp. חֲבִילָה fr. חבל) [*tie, chain*,] 1) *obligation, duty*. Y. Ter. VI, end, 44ᵇ זיקת תרומה וכ׳ the obligation to pay *T'rumah* and tithes. Y. Maasr. II, 50ᵃ top לא בא לז׳ וכ׳ it has not yet come under the obligation of tithes. Treat. S'maḥ. ch. XIII ז׳ שמירתו עליו the duty of watching the corpse rests upon him. Yalk. Gen. 151 חוץ לזיקא הן עומדין (corr. acc.) they are not pledged.—2) *legal restriction*. Snh. 50ᵇ זיקת הבעל marital ties, betrothal.—Esp. *zikah, the interdependence of a childless widow and her late husband's brothers, the levirate relation*. Yeb. 17ᵇ, a. fr. יש ז׳ the relation between a woman and her eventual *yabam* is a real connection, i.e. carries with it all legal consequences as regards the laws of incest and the right of interference with her vows, אין ז׳ the levirate relation is no marital connection as long as the levirate marriage is not consummated. Ib. III, 9, v. יָבָם. Y. ib. I, 2ᵈ; XIII, beg. 13ᵇ ממאנת ... לעקור זיקת המת she may refuse the *yabam* so as to annul retrospectively the relation between herself and her deceased husband, v. מָאַן; a. fr.

זִיקוּ, Tanḥ. Matt. 3, v. דִּיקֵי.

זִיקוּק m. (v. זִיק) *dart, spark*.—*Pl.* זִיקוּקִין. Deut. R. s. 7 שני ז׳ של אש two darts of fire (Tanḥ. Vayak. 7 ניצוצין).

זִיקוּקָא I, זִקוּקָא ch. same.—*Pl.* זִיקוּקִין, זִק׳. Targ. Hab. III, 4. Targ. Y. Ex. XXIV, 17 זִיקוּקֵי אישא.—Y. Ber. V, 9ᵃ תריך ז׳ דנור, v. preced.

זִיקוּקָא II m. (dimin. of זִיקָא II) *bottle*.—*Pl.* זִיקוּקִין. Y. Ab. Zar. II, 41ᶜ top ז׳ זעירין small bottles.

זִיקְנָה, זִיקְנוּת, v. זָקֵ׳.

זִיקְפָא, v. זִקְפָּא I, II.

זִיקְתָא f. (collect. noun; denom. of זִיקָא I) *sharpshooter*. B. Mets. 94ᵃ כך וכך ז׳ פסיקא לן Ms. M. (ed. זוקתא; Ar. כאן וכאן ז׳ איכא בהדן) so many sharp-shooters are assigned to us for our protection. [זיקתא *goad*, v. זְקַת.]

זִיר, *Pa.* זַיֵּיר, v. זור.

זֵיר, זִיר, זֵר m. (b. h. זֵר; זור) 1) *crown, wreath, rim*. Yoma 72ᵇ מאי (ו)משהו ז׳ what purpose serves the 'something' (over ten handbreadths)? It is the space for the rim. Ib. כתיב זר וקרי זיר וכ׳ it is written (in the Bible) זר (which allows the reading זָר) and is read *zer*; if you are worthy, the Law is to you a crown, &c., v. זוּר; a. fr.—*Pl.* זִירִין. Ib. שלשה ז׳ three crowns (of vessels of the sanctuary).—2) *crest, customary addition to dry measure*; v. גִּרוֹמִין. Sifra K'dosh. Par. 3, ch. VIII 'in *m'surah*' (Lev. XIX, 35) זו ז׳ הגדול that means the large crest.—3) (bot.) *capsule of seeds, seed-pot*.—*Pl.* as above. Maasr. IV, 5; Ab. Zar. 7ᵇ השבת ... זרע וירק וז׳ the dill-plant is subject to tithes when its seeds are collected, or when its leaves are used as vegetable, or when its pods are eaten. Y. Maasr. IV, 51ᵇ bot. זרעה לז׳ if he planted it for the sake of the pods; Tosef. Shebi. II, 7 זרעה ז׳ (read לז׳). B. Kam. 81ᵃ.—4) (v. זור *Pa.*, cmp. זֶרֶת) *small bundle, bunch*, contrad. to חֲבִילָה.—*Pl.* as above.—Y. Ter. X, 47ᵇ top; Y. Orl. III, 63ᵃ bot. ה׳ כ״ה ז׳ a *ḥăbilah* is twenty five bunches. Sabb. XXIV, 2, contrad. to פִּיפִין a. פְּקִיעִין; expl. ib. 155ᵃ ז׳ דארזו, v. אַרְזָא; ib. (anoth. defin.) ז׳ תלתא they are called *zirin* when tied with three bands; [Var. lect. זֵרִין, זירדין, זְרָדִין, זירין, v. Rabb. D. S. a. l. note 80, a. marginal note in Talm. ed.].

זִירָא, זֵרָא, זִיר ch. same, *wreath, crown, rim*. Targ. O. Ex. XXV, 11 ed. Berl., v. זִיר I.

זִירָא, v. זְעֵירָא.

זֵירָא pr. n. m. (=זְעֵירָא) *Zera* (*Little*), name of several Amoraim. Keth. 110ᵇ; a. fr.—Ib. 43ᵇ, a. fr.; v. זְעֵירָא.

זִירָה f. (זור) *circle*, esp. *wrestlers' ring*. Ex. R. s. 27 (play on זר, Prov. VI, 1) אתה הכנסת עצמך לז׳ וכ׳ thou (by assuming an office) hast placed thyself in the arena &c. Ib. אני ואתה עומדים בז׳ we two stand in the arena (combatting each other).

זֵירוּד I m. (זָרַד *Pi.*) *cutting shoots off, trimming, thinning*. Shebi. II, 3; Y. ib. 33ᵈ זֵירוּדָהּ של חמישית the trimming] as it is done in the fifth year of the year-Sabbath.

זֵירוּד II pr. n. m. *Zerud.* Ab. Zar. 30ª ישמעאל בן ז׳ ed. (Ms. M. שמעון בן זכור, or זבור, v. Rabb. D. S. a. l.). Snh. 14ª שמעון בן ז׳ ed. (Ms. M. זירוז, v. Rabb. D. S. a. l. note).

זֵירוּז m. (זָרַז *Pi.*) *quickening, urging on, encouraging.* Sifré Num. 1; Num. R. s. 7 אין צירוי . . אלא ז׳ the verb צוה has everywhere the meaning of encouragement. Gen. R. s. 56, a. e. (the repetition of a call) לשון חיבה לשון ז׳ expresses endearment, encouragement. Kidd. 29ª; a. e.—*Pl.* זֵירוּזִין.—נדרי ז׳ vows intended for urging to buy or sell, vows uttered while bargaining. Ned. III, 1. Ib. 21ª נדרא הוי או ז׳ הוי is it a real vow or merely (a vow for) bargaining?—Y. ib. III, 38ª top שבועות ז׳.—[זירוז pr. n. m., v. preced.]

זֵירוּעַ, v. זֵר׳.

זֵירְזָא m. (זרז, v. זוּרְזָא) *bundle, bunch.* Yeb. 101ᵇ ז׳ דקני a bundle of reeds; Sabb. 8ᵇ.

זֵירְנָא, v. זַרְנָא.

זֵירְפָא, v. זִרְפָא.

זֵירְקְתָא, זְרִיקְתָא.

זֵירְתָא, v. זַרְתָא.

זַיִת m. (b. h.; זות; cmp. הַדְּיוּת) 1) *outflow, run.* Men. 86ª שמן זית מְזִיתוֹ 'olive-oil' (Ex. XXVII, 20) that means of that which flows of itself (before pressing). Ib. (VIII, 4) ז׳ ראשון the first run.—2) *olive;* (sub. עץ) *olive tree.* Ib. בראש הז׳, v. גַּרְגֵּר; a. v. fr.—כַּזַּ׳ the size of an olive; כחצי ז׳ half the size of &c. Bets. I, 1 זה וזה בכז׳ the legal size for both is that of &c. Zeb. III, 3. Kel. XVII, 8, v. אֱגוֹזִי; a. v. fr.—*Pl.* זֵתִים, זֵיתִים. Ber. 57ª הרואה ז׳ וכ׳ one who dreams of olives. B. Mets. VIII, 5 המוכר זֵיתָיו וכ׳ he who sells his olive trees for the use of the wood. T'bul Yom III, 6. Ḥall. III, 9 זֵיתֵי מסיק, v. מָסִיק; a. fr.—Tanḥ. ed. Bub. Ki Thetsé 10 כַּזֵּ׳ כַּזֵּ׳ in pieces of olive-sizes; Pesik. Zakh., p. 25ᵇ ז׳ ז׳; Pesik. R. s. 12.—Ukts. III, 6 פריצי ז׳ the proud among the olives; expl. Tosef. ib. III, 6 היוצאין מתחת וכ׳ such as come out uncrushed from under the press; B. Mets. 105ª רשעי ז׳ (yielding very little oil).

זֵיתָא I ch. same. Targ. Hag. II, 19. Targ. Gen. VIII, 11; a. e.—Ḥull. 98ª ההוא כז׳ וכ׳ fat of the size of an olive. Ib. פלגא דז׳ half the size of &c.; תלתין פלגין דז׳ thirty times the size of half an olive. Y. Pes. VII, 35ᵇ (prov.) כז׳ פסחא וכ׳ with an olive's size of the Passover meat (for each participant), the Hallel (sung on the roof) seems to burst the roof (i. e. joy in simplicity is the purest); Bab. ib. 85ᵇ; Cant. R. to II, 14 פסחא בבריתא (read כז׳).—*Pl.* זֵיתִין, זֵיתַיָּא, זיתי. Targ. Mic. VI, 15.—Targ. II Kings XXIII, 13 טור ז׳ (h. text הר המשחית); Targ. II Sam. XV, 30 (h. text הזתים).—B. Mets. 21ᵇ. Ned. 68ª תרין ז׳ two olives.—Y. Maas. Sh. IV, 56ᶜ top זיתאי (read זיתיא).—Y. Taan. III, 66ᵈ bot. זֵיתָיִן; a. fr.

זֵיתָא II m. (v. זַיִת 1; cmp. Syr. דועתא P. Sm. 933, זתא 1163) *resin,* name of *an alkali* used for cleansing. Nidd. 62ª (expl. בורית) ז׳ Ar. s. v. זתא (ed. כבריתא).—*Pl.* זֵיתַיָּה or זֵיתְהָיָה, v. next w. [R. Hai Gaon to Nidd. IX, 6 read זאתא, ואתא, v. Löw Pfl. p. 42, sq.]

זִיתוּם or **זִיתוֹס** m. (ζῦθος, zythum, an adapt. of an Egyptian w.; cmp. preced. w., a. דועתא דחטי sudor tritici, P. Sm. 933, sq.), ז׳ המצרי *Egyptian beer.* Pes. III, 1 (42ª; readings vary betw. ם a. ס, v. Rabb. D. S. a. l. note 1); described ib. 42ᵇ; Y. ib. III, beg. 29ᵈ זיתים המצרי (corr. acc.), defined: זֵיתְהָיָה (v. preced.) *decocts* (sudores tritici &c., v. supra).

זִיתִים, v. preced.

זַךְ m. (b. h.; זכך, v. זָכָה) *clear, transparent; pure.* Men. VIII, 5 (86ª). Ib. 86ᵇ אין זך אלא נקי *zakh* means pure.

זְכָא, v. זְכֵי.

זַכָּאָה f. h., v. זַכַּאי.

זַכָּאָה m. a. f. ch. (preced., v. זַכַּאי) *clear, innocent.* Targ. Ps. II, 7. Targ. Num. V, 19; a. e.—*Pl.* זַכָּאִין, v. זַכַּאי ch.

זַכָּאוּתָא f. (preced.) 1) *innocence.* Targ. Gen. XX, 5.—2) *justifying.* Targ. Job XXXII, 2 מטול זַכָּאוּתֵיהּ וכ׳ because he justified himself more &c.

זַכַּאי I m. (זָכָה) 1) *clear, guiltless, righteous; deserving, worthy* (corresp. to b. h. צַדִּיק), opp. חַיָּיב. Sabb. 32ª, a. e. מגלגלין זכות ע״י ז׳, v. גִּלְגֵּל.—יום ז׳ a lucky day, anniversary of joyous events. Taan. 29ª; a. e.—Snh. 11ª אין דורו ז׳ לכך his generation is not deserving it (Sot. 48ᵇ זכאין, pl.); a. fr.—2) *acquitted, not guilty.* Snh. III, 6 שנים אומרים ז׳ if two vote, 'Not guilty'; a. fr.—3) *entitled to possession* or *disposal, having authority, a right* &c.; v. זָכָה.—Keth. IV, 4 האב ז׳ בבתו וכ׳ the father has authority over his (minor) daughter to give her away in marriage by receiving a consideration &c.; וז׳ במציאתה וכ׳ and has the right of possession of what she finds . . . . . and of interference with her vows; a. fr.—*Pl.* זַכָּאִין. Ab. I, 8 כז׳ as if both (claimant and defendant) had been right. Sot. 48ᵇ, v. supra; a. fr.—Fem. זַכָּאָה. Snh. 45ª שמא תצא...ז׳ she may be acquitted in court.

זַכַּאי ch. same, *righteous, innocent.* Targ. Gen. VI, 9; a. e.—*Pl.* זַכָּאִין. Targ. Jer. XIX, 4; a. e.—V. זַכִּי.

זַכַּאי II pr. n. m. (b. h. זַכַּי) *Zakkai,* 1) father of R. Johanan. Snh. 41ᵇ כי היה למד בן ז׳ וכ׳ when he was a student, they called him Ben Z. &c. Ab. II, 8; a. fr.—2) בן (בר) ז׳ *Ben (Bar) Z.* Ḥull. 52ª.—3) *R. Z.,* also זַכִּיי name of several Amoraim. Y. Sabb. VII, 9ᶜ top; Snh. 62ª (Ms. M. רב ז׳); Y. Yeb. VIII, 9ᶜ זכירה (corr. acc.); a. e.—Y. Keth. IV, 28ᵈ top ר׳ ז׳ דאלכסנדריה; Y. Yeb. VII, 8ᵇ bot. ז׳

ר׳ ז׳ אלכס׳ (cor. acc); a. e.—Y. Meg. IV, 75[b] bot. ר׳ ז׳ דכבול.—Ib. 74[d] bot. ר׳ ז׳ טבחא Z., the butcher.

זְכָה, v. זכי.

זְכוּ, זְכוּ, v. זְכוּתָא.

זְכוּכִית f. (b. h.; זכך, cmp. זְגוּגִיתָא) *glass, crystal.* Meg. 6[a] (ref. to Deut. XXXIII, 19) חול זו ז׳ לבנה 'sand' alludes to white glass.—Sabb. 14[b] גזרו טומאה על כלי ז׳ declared glass vessels subject to the laws of levitical purity. Ib. 15[b]; a. fr.—*Pl.* זְכוּכִיּוֹת *glass beads.* Num. R. s. 21.—B. Kam. 30[a] זְכוּכִיּוֹתָיו his *broken glass ware.* Ib. זְכוּכִיּוֹתֵיהֶם (ib. III, 2 sing.).

זְכוּכִיתָא ch. same. Targ. Job XXVIII, 17.

זָכוּר I part. pass. of זָכַר.

זָכוּר II m. (b. h.)=זָכָר *male* (mostly used in connection with pederasty). Snh. VII, 4. Ib. 54[b]; a. fr.—Snh. 65[b], v. זְכוּרוּ.—*Pl.* זְכוּרִים *necromantic incantation,* v. זְכוּרוּ. Pesik. R. s. 23.

זְכוּרָא, pl. **זְכוּרִין** (v. preced.) *necromantic apparitions.* Targ. Y. II Deut. XVIII, 11.

זְכוּרוּ f. (זָכָר; cmp. Lat. fascinum=*witchcraft* a. *membrum virile*) *necromantic incantation* (by means of a membrum); *necromantic apparition.* Snh. 65[b] המעלה בז׳ he who conjures up the dead by means of &c.; Gen. R. s. 11; Y. Snh. VII, 25[c]; Lev. R. s. 26.—Snh. l. c.; Yalk. Deut. 918 (interpret. מעונן, Deut. XVIII, 11, fr. עונ) הַמַּעֲבִיר שבעה מיני זָכוּר על העין (Ar. ed. Koh. זמר זכורן, cler. error) he who lets pass before one's eyes seven sorts of apparitions; (Sifra K'dosh. Par. 3, ch. VI; Sifré Deut. 171 מעביר על העין only).

זְכוּרוּ ch. same. Targ. O. Lev. XIX, 31, a. e., v. דְּכוּרוּ. Targ. Y. ib. מסיק ז׳, read: בז׳.

זְכוּת f. (זָכָה) 1) *acquittal, favorable judgment, plea in defence.*—לִמֵּד ז׳ *to plead in favor of the defendant.* Snh. IV, 1 הכל מלמדין ז׳ all are permitted to plead for the defendant. Ib. פותחין לז׳ the opening argument must be for the defence. Ib. מטין על פי אחד לז׳ a majority of one is sufficient for acquittal; a. fr.—Ab. I, 6 הוי דן .... לכף ז׳ judge every man with an inclination in his favor. Sabb. 32[a] הבא ז׳ והפטר bring pleaders in thy favor (good deeds) and be acquitted; a. fr.—2) *doing good, blessing.* Taan. 29[a], a. fr. מגלגלין ז׳, v. גִּלְגֵּל.—Y. Naz. VII, 56[a] bot. נתכוונתי לז׳ I had the intention of doing good; Treat. S'maḥ. IV, end. [Ib. תחלת זכותי, read: תשמישי.]—3) *the protecting influence of good conduct, merit.* Y. Peah I, 16[b] top הז׳ יש לה קרן וכ׳ good deeds have a capital and interests (reward the author and protect his offspring).—R. Hash. 11[a] בז׳ אבות for the sake of the Patriarchs; בז׳ אימהות for the sake of the Mothers (Sarah &c.). Ber. 27[b] לית ליה ז׳ אבות has no distinguished ancestry to rely on. Gen. R. s. 44 זְכוּתְךָ עומדת וכ׳ thy guarding influence shall stand by them. Snh. 12[a] בז׳ הרחמים ובִזְכוּתָם through Divine mercy and their own merits; a. fr.—4) *advantage, privilege, benefit.* B. Mets. 19[a] ז׳ היא לעבד וכ׳ liberty is a benefit to the slave. Tosef. Gitt. I, 5 היאך נמצא ז׳ וכ׳ ed. Zuck. (Var. מפני מה זכין) how dare we obtain a benefit for this slave?; a. fr.—*Pl.* זָכִיּוֹת. Yoma 86[b] זדונות נעשו לו כז׳ wilful wrongs are accounted to him (who repents) as though they were merits. Taan. 20[b] מנכין לו מִזָּכִיּוֹתָיו it is deducted from the rewards for his good deeds. Ex. R. s. 38, end; a. fr.

זְכוּתָא, זְכוּ, זְכוּ ch. same. Targ. Gen. XV, 6. Targ. Y. Deut. VI, 25. Targ. Y. Num. XX, 2; a. fr.—Lev. R. s. 30 מוליה ז׳, v. preced. a. אֱלָה II. Ber. 10[a] ז׳ דידי ודידך my merit and thine. Keth. 10[b] מאי ז׳ where is the benefit (that the word זכה can be used)?; a. fr.—*Pl.* זַכְוָתָא, זַכְוָן, זַכְוָ׳. Targ. Deut. XXXIII, 21.—Sabb. 140[a] מנכו לי מז׳ וכ׳ (Ms. O. מִזַּכְוָתָאִי, v. Rabb. D. S. a. l.) it may be deducted from my reward in the world to come. Ḥag. 15[a] למיכתב ז׳ וכ׳ to record the merits of Israel; למימחק ז׳ וכ׳ to wipe out the record of &c.; a. e.—Esp. (pl.) *verdict in favor, title, claims.* Keth. 85[a] כתבו לי ז׳ וכ׳ give me in writing your decision in my favor, that they must pay &c. Ned. 27[a] דאתפרס ז׳ וכ׳ whose papers were deposited in court; לירלון הני זַכְוָתָאִי these my papers (claims) shall be void.

זְכִין, v. זָכַךְ.

זָכָה, זכי (b. h.; cmp. זַךְ) [*to be pure, clear,*] 1) *to be acquitted, be right.* B. Mets. 107[b] זוכה בדין he will be successful in his plea before court. Ber. 7[b] זוכה בדין (v. Rabb. D. S. a. l. note) he will be found righteous in Divine judgment; a. fr.—2) *to be found worthy of, to be privileged, to succeed.* Ib. I, 5 ולא זָכִיתִי וכ׳ I did not succeed (in proving) that &c. Ib. 5[b] לא .... זוכה לשתי וכ׳ not every one is privileged to enjoy two tables (this world and the hereafter). Ḥag. 5[b] תִּזְכּוּ להקביל וכ׳ you will be privileged to receive &c. Pes. 19[a] זָכִינוּ שאין וכ׳ it was a good thing for us that &c. Erub. 54[a] ז׳ תאוות וכ׳ if one is favored, 'thou givest him the desire of his heart' (without prayer), if less favored &c. Yeb. 63[a], v. נֶגֶד; a. fr.—3) *to take possession, have authority; to own* (cmp. קָנָה); *to gain, obtain a privilege.* B. Mets. I, 3 אני זָכִיתִי בה I took possession of it for myself; ז׳ בה it is his. Ib. 4 זה שהחזיק בה ז׳ בה the one that took a hold of it, is the legitimate owner. Ib. זָכְתָה לי שדי my field (in which the object lies) has taken possession for me. Y. Kidd. I, 60[a] top הראוי לִזְכּוֹת ע״י עצמו וכ׳ he who is legally qualified to acquire ownership through his own act, can obtain ownership through another person.—Erub. VII, 11 (81[b]), a. fr. זָכִין לאדם שלא בפניו you may obtain a privilege in behalf of a person in his absence, but you cannot act in his behalf to his disadvantage; a. fr.—4) (v. *Pi.*) *to benefit another person by one's own merit, to transfer blessing* &c. Eduy. II, 9 האב זוֹכֶה לבן וכ׳ a (good) father transmits to his son the benefits of beauty &c. Tosef. ib. I, 14 עד הפרק זוכה לו up to the age of majority the father's merit stands by him, מכאן ואילך זוכה לעצמו after that he lives on his own merits.—5) *to deserve well of, be of service to.* Lev. R. s. 34 (ref. to Ps. XLI, 2) הוי . . . היאך לִזְכּוֹת עמו reflect well how to be of real service to him. Ib. לזכות בו to deserve divine reward through him. Ib. שיהו זָכִין אלו לאלו that they may deserve well of each other (the poor being the instrumentality of bliss to the giver); a. fr.

Pi. זִכָּה, זִיכָּ׳ 1) *to acquit, to argue* or *vote for acquittal.* Erub. 19ª יפה זִכִּיתָ וכ׳ thou wast right in acquitting, in condemning. Snh. III, 5 שנים מְזַכִּין if two vote for acquittal; a. fr.—2) *to obtain a privilege for, take possession in behalf of; to transfer, make an assignment to.* Y. Kidd. l. c. זה זי׳ לבן דעת the one obtained a privilege for a rational being. B. Bath. VIII, 6 זי׳ בה לאחר if in his will (found on his body) he made an assignment to somebody else (as executor); a. fr.—3) *to transfer divine favor, to exercise a protecting influence on.* Snh. 111ª מְזַכֶּה לא דיין את כל וכ׳ protects the entire town. Yoma 87ª לא דיין שזוכין לעצמן אלא שמְזַכִּין וכ׳ Ms. M. not only do they obtain divine grace for themselves, but they also transfer the same on their children &c.; a. fr.—4) *to lead to righteousness, to convert, make better, purer.* Ib.; Ab. V, 18, a. e. כל המזכה את וכ׳ whoever causes a community to do good. Macc. III, 16 רצה הקב״ה לְזַכּוֹת וכ׳ the Lord desired to make Israel pure; a. fr.

Hithpa. הִזְדַּכָּה, *Nithpa.* נִזְדַּכָּה 1) *to be acquitted, to be found not guilty.* Snh. 30ª מדבריהם נז׳ פלוני the defendant has been acquitted by their (the court's) verdict. Y. ib. V, 22ᵈ top ובאיזו מִזְדַּכֶּה פוטרין אותו and on whichsoever (of the two counts) he is found not guilty, he is acquitted; a. fr.—2) *to have favorable evidence* or *argument offered.* Ib. 23ª נ׳ מפי עצמו if the defendant himself offers &c. Ib. הרי שנ׳ מפי עצמו (read מפי עדו).

זְכָא, זְכִי ch. same, 1) *to be clear, pure.* Targ. Job IX, 15. Ib. X, 15 זְכִיתִי (some ed. זְכִי׳, corr. acc.); a. e.—2) *to go unpunished* (h. נקה). Targ. Jer. XXV, 29; a. e.—3) *to deserve well, do good, to obtain a claim on divine favor.* Lev. R. s. 34 [read:] אדם . . . זְכֵי בי אי זְכֵי בי the beggar says . . . . 'obtain a claim &c. through me', or 'become pure through me', (which means) זְכֵי גרמך בי benefit thyself through me. Ib. אנן זָכְיָין בך we shall give thee something. Ib. ז׳ בהאר אתתא give this woman (me) something. Y. Ḥag. I, 76ᶜ bot. שלח . . מְזַכֵּי וכ׳ sent his son to Tiberias for his improvement (through study); Y. Pes. III, 30ᵇ bot. יזכי (corr. acc.); a. fr.—4) *to become worthy of divine grace, to be privileged to enjoy, to live to see.* Targ. Job XX, 17; a. e.—Ber. 17ª נשים במאי זָכְיָין wherewith do women (who do not study the Law) deserve divine grace?—Sabb. 21ᵇ אי זָכֵאי if I had been worthy (if the Lord had permitted me). Lev. R. s. 25 אי זָכִית אכלית if the Lord permit, I may eat thereof. Ib. אם זָכִית (תיכול) אכול if thou shalt live long enough to eat thereof. Ḥull. 50ª; Bets. 27ª, a. e. אִזְכֵּי ואסיק וכ׳ the Lord permitting I will go &c.; a. fr.—4) *to take possession, acquire a title.* B. Mets. 8ª מיגו דזָכֵי לנפשיה since he has a right to take possession for himself, v. מִיגוֹ, s. v. גוֹ.—B. Kam. 12ᵇ; a. fr.

Pa. זַכֵּי 1) *to clear* (from rubbish). M. Kat. 10ᵇ; B. Bath. 54ª, v. זִיכֵּי.—2) *to clear, acquit, justify; to leave unpunished.* Targ. O. Ex. XX, 7 (Y. מְזַכֵּי, read: מְזַכֵּי). Targ. Cant. VII, 3; a. fr.—3) *to cleanse.* Targ. Ps. LXXIII, 13 זַכָּאִית Ms. (ed. זַכִּית, ed. Wil. זַכְוָת, corr. acc.); a. e.—Lev. R. s. 34, v. supra.—4) *to win, defeat.* Ab. Zar. 10ᵇ; Snh. 39ª כל דז׳ מלכא Ms. M. (ed. למלכא) whosoever defeats the king in argument. Ib. 107ª עבדא ז׳ למריה (old ed. כפריה) the servant conquered his master. Bekh. 8ᵇ אי זַכִּיתוּ לי if you defeat me; ואי זַכִּינָא בכו (read לכו) and if we defeat you. Ḥull. 31ᵇ זַכְּנְהוּ וכ׳ R. N. defeated the Rabbis; a. e.—5) *to entitle, give possession to.* Pes. 78ª שטרא מְזַכֵּי לבר תרי a document giving a title to both contestants, i. e. one agreeing with two opposite opinions.

Ithpa. אִזְדַּכֵּי, *Ithpe.* אִזְדְּכֵי *to be cleared, to go unpunished; to clear one's self, to defend one's self.* Targ. Y. Gen. XXIV, 8. Ib. XLIV, 16; a. e.

זַכִּי m.=זַכַּאי, *innocent, righteous.* Targ. O. Num. XXXV, 33 ed. Berl. (ed. Amst. זכאי). Targ. O. Deut. XIX, 10; a. e.—Fem. זַכְיָא. Targ. Y. I Gen. XXXVIII, 26 (Y. II זכאי).—*Pl.* זַכָּאִין, v. זַכַּאי; זַכְיָין. Targ. Y. II l. c.; Targ. Ez. XVI, 52 (some ed. זַכְוָן).

זַכִּיא, v. זִיכִּי.

זְכִיָּה, v. זְכִייה.

זַכִּיר pr. n. m., v. זַכַּאי II.

זכויה, Y. Yeb. VIII, 9ᶜ, v. זַכַּאי II.

זְכִיָּה f. (זָכָה) *possession, taking possession, claim.* Y. Peah V, beg. 19ᵇ, v. הֶפְקֵר. Y. Pes. II, 29ª top מאן דאמר ז׳ according to the opinion that renounced property does not go out of the owner's possession until somebody took possession of it. B. Kam. 12ᵇ אית להו לכהנים ז׳ בגויה Ms. M. (ed. בגוויהו) the priests have a claim on it. Ib. ולית אית ליה להו זכיה Ms. M. (omitted in ed.). B. Mets. 12ª ז׳ לנפשיה has a right to take possession in his own behalf; a. e.

זַכִּיכָא, זַכִּיךְ m. ch.=h. זַךְ. Targ. Y. Lev. XXIV, 2. Targ. Y. Gen. XLIX, 12 (of wine).

זְכִירָה f. (זָכַר) 1) *remembrance, thinking.* Men. 43ᵇ (ref. to Num. XV, 39) ראייה מביא לידי ז׳ ז׳ וכ׳ seeing leads to thinking, thinking to doing. Gen. R. s. 33 (ref. to Gen. VIII, 1) מה ז׳ נזכר לו what (meritorious deed) remembered He to him. Meg. 15ª אביגיל בזְכִירָתָהּ Abig. suggested licentiousness by alluding to her being remembered (I Sam. XXV, 31); a. e.—2) *recitation.* Ib. 2ᵇ (ref. to Esth. IX, 28) ז׳ recitation of the Book of Esther, contrad. to עשייה celebration of the Festival.

זכירי, Yeb. 31ᵇ, read דְּכִירֵי, v. דְּכִיר.

זָכַךְ (b. h.; v. זָכָה) *to be clear.*

Pilp. זִכְזֵךְ *to make clear.* Tosef. Nidd. IV, 11 שמן רך ומְזַכְזֵךְ oil is softly flowing and clears (the embryonic mass; Nidd. 25ᵇ ומצחצחו).

זָכַר (b. h.; ch. דְּכַר) [*to mark,*] *to remember, mention; to celebrate* (by a ceremony &c.). Pes. 106ª (ref. to Ex. XX, 8 זכור) זָכְרֵהוּ על היין Ms. M. (ed. זוֹכְרֵהוּ) remember the Sabbath (distinguish it) by a benediction over wine; Bets. 15ᵇ זכרהו מֵאַחֵר שבא וכ׳ mark the Sabbath (by a ceremony) from another (Holy Day) which (preceding the Sabbath) may cause the neglect of it (Ms. M. לאחר, Rashi מֵאַחֵר, v. אָחַר; v. R. Nissim a. l.). Men. 43ᵇ ראה . . . וזָכוֹר וכ׳ see this ceremony and be reminded of another

&c.; a. fr.—*Part. pass.* זָכוּר, f. זְכוּרָה a) *reminded, remembering, mindful.*—ז׳ אני, contr. זְכוּרַנִי *I recollect.* Sabb. 115ᵃ ז׳ אני בי׳ I recollect about &c.—Bets. 18ᵃ ז׳ היא she will remember. Snh. 52ᵇ; a. fr.—b) *thought of, remembered.* B. Mets. 11ᵃ ז׳ ולבסוף שכוח if the sheaf had been thought of and was afterwards forgotten.—ז׳ לטוב (abbr. ז״ל) *remembered for blessing.* Gen. R. s. 16 end אליהו ז״ל El. of blessed memory, v. זִכָּרוֹן.—Sabb. 13ᵇ, a. e., v. בְּרַם; a. fr.—*Pl.* זְכוּרִים. Pesik. R. s. 13, end; a. e.

Nif. נִזְכַּר *to be reminded, to remember* (with accus.). Pes. 66ᵃ; Snh. 82ᵃ ראה מעשה ונ׳ הלכה he saw the practice and recalled the tradition. Yoma 38ᵃ כבוד אבותי נִזְכַּרְתִּי I was thinking of the vanished glory of my ancestors. Ex. R. s. 45 הִזָּכֵר remember; a. fr.

Hif. הִזְכִּיר 1) *to cause to be remembered, to recall.* Ber. 55ᵃ, a. e. ג׳ דברים מַזְכִּירִים וכ׳ three occasions cause the sins of man to be remembered; a. fr.—2) *to cite* (as an argument), *to take into account.* Ib. 60ᵃ; a. e. אין מזכירין מ״נ miracles must not be cited as evidence. Kidd. 40ᵇ אין מזכירין לו שוב רשעו his wickedness is not counted; a. fr.—3) *to recite* (in prayer), *quote.* Hor. 14ᵃ ושמותם אין אנו מז׳ whose names we do not quote (as authorities). Ber. I, 5 מזכירין י״מ וכ׳ we must recite the going out from Egypt (Num. XV, 37 to 41) in night prayers; a. fr.

Hof. הוּזְכַּר *to be mentioned.* Kel. XVII, 5. Toh. VI, 6; a. e.—*Part.* מוּזְכָּר, f. מוּזְכֶּרֶת *clearly defined.* Kidd. 77ᵃ.

זָכָר m. (b. h.; preced.) [v. זָכוּר,] 1) *male* (of man and animals), *male child; opp.* נקבה. Nidd. III, 7 תשב לז׳ וכ׳ she shall observe the laws as after the birth of a male child &c. (Lev. XII, 4). Ib. בריית הז׳ the formation of the male embryo. Y. B. Bath. IX, 16ᵈ bot. שמחת ז׳ the rejoicing over the birth of a boy; a. v. fr.—*Pl.* זְכָרִים. Nidd. 31ᵇ. Zeb. V, 3, a. fr. זִכְרֵי כהונה the male members of the priestly tribe.—Gen. R. s. 13, a. e. המים העליונים ז׳ וכ׳ the waters from above are the males (fructifiers), &c.—2) (v. דְּכַר II) (ז׳ (של רחלים *the male of the flock, ram.* Bekh. V, 3; Yeb. 121ᵇ.—Shek. V, 3 ז׳ משמש עם וכ׳ that with the inscription 'male' was used only for libations connected with rams.—*Pl.* as above. R. Hash. III, 4, sq. בשל ז׳ with horns of rams; a. fr.—3) *membrum* (of animals). Tosef. Bekh. IV, 6, v. זוּבָן.—4) (of inanimate objects) *the thinner, pointed side of a double tool,* v. זַכְרוּת. Kel. XIII, 2 הז׳ the pointed side of the cosmetic tube, contrad. to כַּף the broad part.—5) *the marrow of horns, reeds* &c. Tosef. Kel. B. Mets. VII, 12. [Ib. Par. II (I), 2, v. זַכְרוּת.]—6) (gramm.) לשון ז׳ *masculine gender.* Kidd. 2ᵇ אשכחן דרך דאיקרי ל׳ ז׳ we find (in the Bible) *derekh* in the masculine gender. Mekh. B'shall., Shirah 1 בל׳ ז׳ in the masculine form (שִׁיר); Cant. R. to I, 5; a. e.

זֵכֶר, זֶכֶר m. (b. h.; זָכַר) *memorial, remembrance, symbol, mnemonical allusion.* Succ. III, 12 ז׳ למקדש as a reminiscence of the Temple usages; Pes. 115ᵃ. Ib. 116ᵃ ז׳ לתפוח typical of the apple tree (Cant. VIII, 5; v. Sot. 11ᵇ); ז׳ לטיט typical of the clay (which the Israelites had to tread). Ber. 2ᵇ; Tosef. Sabb. VII (VIII), 4, a. e. אע״פ שאין . . . ז׳ לדבר although there is no proof for it (in the Bible), there is a mnemonical allusion to it; a. fr.

זִכָּרוֹן m. (b. h.) same, *memory, memorial.* Kidd. 31ᵇ, a. e. זִכְרוֹנוֹ לברכה (abbr. ז״ל) of blessed memory, v. זָכַר. Y. Shek. II, 47ᵃ top דבריהן הן זִכְרוֹנָן their words are their monument; Gen. R. s. 82 זִכְרוֹנֵיהֶם (pl.). R. Hash. 27ᵃ ז׳ ליום ראשון typical of the first day of creation; a. fr.—Esp. *a Biblical verse in which Divine remembrance is alluded to, citation of verses* &c. R. Hash. IV, 6 ז׳ . . . של פורענות citation of remembrance . . . . for evil. Ib. 32ᵇ ז׳ של יחיד a verse treating of the remembrance by the Lord of an individual; a. fr.—*Pl.* זִכְרוֹנוֹת. Ber. 6ᵃ ספר הז׳ the Divine records; a. fr.—Esp. *Zikhronoth, that portion of the Musaf of the New Year's Day which treats of Divine remembrance.* R. Hash. IV, 5, sq.; a. fr.—Constr. זִכְרוֹנֵי, v. supra.

זַכְרוּת f. (denom. of זָכָר) 1) *male genitals; male sex.* Y. Snh. X, 28ᵈ bot.; Num. R. s. 20, end.—Ab. Zar. 44ᵃ (expl. מִפלצת, II Chr. XV, 16) כמין ז׳ a phallus. Men. 6ᵃ תמות וז׳ בבהמה unblemished condition and male sex of sacrifices are required only of cattle. Y. Yeb. VIII, end, 9ᵈ צד ז׳ the male side of the hermaphrodite; מכח זַכְרוּתוֹ in as much as he is a male; a. fr.—2) *the thin and pointed side of a double tool.* Bets. 31ᵇ ז׳ שלו the sharper side of a hatchet (used for splitting), opp. נקבות שלו the broader side. Cant. R. to I, 3 [read:] כאדם שמטביל זַכְרוּתוֹ של מכחול בים as much as one takes up when dipping the point of the painting staff into the paint bottle.—3) *the fructifying principle, germ, bud, eye* or *strophiole* (in plants); *germinating spot* (in eggs) &c., v. next w.—Y. Sabb. VII, 9ᵈ bot.; XII, 13ᶜ bot. כדי לִיטַע זַכְרוּתָהּ של חיטה deep enough to plant the wheat grain up to its eye (so that it can take root). Y. Ter. X, end, 47ᶜ ז׳ של חלמון that part of the yolk where germination sets in; ib. ז׳ של מוח the germinating point in the white of the egg (the more substantial and cohesive part).—4) *the bony inside of an animal's horn* or *hoofs, the bony projection over which the horny substance grows.* R. Hash. 27ᵇ. Y. Erub. I, 19ᵇ bot. Bekh. 44ᵃ (Tosef. ib. II (I), 2 הַזָּכָר). [Zeb. 63ᵃ בזכרות, v. זוּטְרָא I.]

זַכְרוּתָא ch. same, 1) *male genitals.* Y. Ab. Zar. II, 40ᵈ bot. מן זכרותיה דדוחר; Y. Sabb. XIV, 14ᵈ bot. מן יברותה דדירדי or דדירדי; Tosaf. to Ab. Zar. 27ᵇ זכרות דחזור, read: מן זכרותא דבַּחְזוּר (v. הִתְיָא, הַתְיָא) a medicinal drink prepared of the phallus of Dionysian revellers; [oth. opin. v. infra].—2) (cmp. preced. 3) *source, fountain-head, feeder.* Bekh. 55ᵃ ז׳ דירדנא וכ׳ the chief supply of the Jordan comes from the cave of Paneas. Ib. ז׳ דדמא וכ׳ the liver is the fountain-head of the blood. Ib. ז׳ דמיא וכ׳ (Yalk. Gen. 22 דברותא, read הַכְרוּתָא or זַכ׳) the Euphrates is the supplier of water (for the world), cmp. אֱוְתְּנָטֵר.—[Y. Ab. Zar. l. c. מן ז׳ דדוחר from the source of menstruation, v. supra.] [Zeb. 63ᵃ, v. זוּטְרָא I.]

זְכַרְיָה, זְכַרְיָהוּ (b. h.) pr. n. m. *Zechariah,* 1) the prophet-priest slain in the Temple court (II Chr. XXIV, 20, sq.). Targ. Lam. II, 20.—Gitt. 57ᵇ; Y. Taan. IV, 69ᵃ bot.; Lam. R. to II, 2; a. e.—2) *Zechariah,* the prophet. Erub. 21ᵃ. Macc. 24ᵇ. Snh. 99ᵃ; a. e.—3) Z. ben *K'butal,* a survivor of the Second Temple. Yoma I, 6; ib. 19^b (v. Rabb. D. S. a. l. notes 3, 4).—4) R. Z. son of Eucolus, a Tannai. Tosef. Sabb. XVI (XVII), 6, v. אֶבְקוֹלָס; Gitt. 56^a; a. e.—5) R. Z., the butcher's son, a Tannai. Eduy. VIII, 2. B. Bath. 111^a; a. e.—6) name of several Amoraim. Y. Snh. I, 18^b top. Y. Pes. I, 27^b top; Y. Sot. I, 16^d זבדיה; Num. R. s. 9 זכר׳.—Snh. 67^b; a. e.

זִכְרָן m. (זָכַר) *one having a good memory.* Der. Er. Zuta ch. III כונס וז׳ a receptive and retentive mind.

זָל, זַל, v. זָלַל, זול.

זְלָא, v. זְלֵי.

זָלַג (cmp. זלח, זלף) *to drip, flow.* Sot. VII, 8; Pes. 118^a זָלְגוּ עיניו דמעות his eyes shed tears. Y. Snh IV, 23^b bot. זלגו עיניהם (sub. דמעות). Yalk. Job 897 עינו של ימין זוֹלֶגֶת דם his right eye was dripping blood; Gen. R. s. 93 שני שלטונין זולגות (corr. acc.); a. e.

זְלַג ch. same. Targ. Ps. LXXVII, 3. Targ. Lam. I, 2 זָלְגָן Ar. (ed. זלגן); a. e.

זַלְדְקָן m. (a comp. of זַל, v. זלל, a. דִקְנָא) *thin-bearded, one with a downy beard.* Snh. 100^b (a citation fr. Ben Sira) ז׳ קורטמן (Ms. M. דלדקן, Var. זיל ד׳ ,דל דקן &c., v. Rabb. D. S. a. l. note) a thin-bearded person is sharp-minded. Y. Taan. IV, beg. 67^b; Y. Meg. IV, 75^c top היה מעבר ז׳ removed one with a downy beard (from pronouncing the priestly benediction).

זְלוֹחָאָה m. (זלח) *sprinkler.—Pl.* זְלוֹחָאֵי. Hull. 60^a הנך . . ז׳ וכ׳ these (the winds and rains) are the sweepers and sprinklers that march before the Lord.

זְלוֹעַ m. (זלע Syr. to draw water, P. Sm. 1129; v. דלי) *pitcher.* Targ. Jer. XIX, 1; a. e.

זְלוֹף, v. זִילּוּף.

***זְלוּקְפָא** m. (transpos. of זלפק, Palel of זפק, v. זֶפֶק) *craw* of birds. Targ. Y. Lev. I, 16 Ar. (ed. זְרוּקְפָא; Ar. s. v. לקט: זְלַפְקְקָא).

זַלְזְלָא m. (זלזל, v. זול a. זלל) *spendthrift, debauchee.—Pl.* זַלְזְלֵי. Targ. Prov. XXVIII, 7 (ed. Lag. a. oth. זְלִילֵי).

זַלְזֵל, זִלְזֵל, v. זָלַל, זְלַל.

זַלְזְגָנָא m. (preced.) *intemperate, gluttonous.—Pl.* זַלְזְגָנֵי. Keth. 60^b.

זָלַח (cmp. זלג) 1) *to drip, be wet.* Y. B. Mets. VI, beg. 10^d שדהו זָלְחָה his field was too wet (for work).—2) *to sprinkle* aromatic fluids. Num. R. s. 13, beg. מכבדות וזולחות וכ׳ (not וזוחלות) the winds sweep and sprinkle all the perfumes &c.; Yalk. Cant. 988 זולחת ומכבדת, read: מכ׳ וזוֹלֶחֶת; cmp. זְלוֹחָאָה.—Tosef. Shek. I, 12 יַזְלַח לו זֶלַח וכ׳ (or יְזַלֵּחַ) one may use it for sprinkling before his bier (Y. ib. II, 47^a top יעשה לו זלוח).

Pi. זִילֵּחַ *to sprinkle* the floor for cooling or perfuming the air. Tosef. Sabb. XVI (XVII), 3 אין מְזַלְּחִין את הבית וכ׳ (not החבית) one must not (on the Sabbath) sprinkle the house with any kind of sprinkling fluids.

זְלַח ch. same, *to sprinkle, rain.* Targ. Job XXXVI, 28 (Ms. זחל). Targ. Cant. V, 13; a. e. [Targ. Is. XXX, 14, v. חֲלַף.]

Af. אַזְלַח, אַזְלִיחַ *to cause a flux* or *diarrhœa* by fright. Targ. Ps. XXIX, 9 (h. text יחולל).

Ithpe. אִזְדְּלַח *to be sprinkled, to gurgle forth,* v. זִלְחָא. Targ. Job XXVIII, 4 מִיזְדְּלַח מרזביא (Ms. מזדלף) gurgling (and forming) gutters (h. text נַחַל).

זֶלַח m. (preced. wds.) *sprinkling fluid, perfume.* Tosef. Shek. I, 12, v. זָלַח.—*Pl.* זְלָחִין. Sifra B'har, Par. 1, ch. I ולא לעשות . . ז׳ but not for preparing perfumes, v. זִילּוּף. Tosef. Sabb. XVI (XVII), 3, v. זָלַח.

זִלְחָא, זוּלְחָא ch. same, *sprinkling, gurgling, jet of water.* Sabb. 95^a שרי ז׳ permitted sprinkling the floors on the Sabbath. Meg. 28^b ז׳ דמטרא a shower.—*Pl.* constr. זִלְחֵי (זָלְ׳), ז׳. Targ. Job XXVIII, 11 Regia (ed. קלילי, h. text בכי). Targ. Ps. XLII, 8 ז׳ מרזבין the gurgling of gutters, v. זְלַח *Ithpe.*

***זְלָא, זְלֵי,** *to flow, glide.* Targ. Prov. IV, 21 (v. זְלַל).

זְלִיל m. (v. זלל)=h. זוֹלֵל, *reckless in spending and eating.* Targ. O. Deut. XXI, 20 זְ׳ בסר (ed. Amst. זַלְ׳) wasteful in buying and eating meat; cmp. זול I h. a. זול.

זְלִיל m., **זְלִילָא** I f. (זלל) *light, easy; insignificant, valueless.* Targ. II Chr. IX, 27. Targ. Prov. XIV, 6.—Y. Pes. IV, end, 31^{b, c} כמריש וז׳ shrunk and cheap.

זְלִילָא II m. (preced.) *common man, humble; low.* Targ. Prov. XII, 9.—*Pl.* זְלִילֵי. Ib. XXVIII, 7 (some ed. זְלְזִילֵי).

זְלִילָה m. ch. (preced.) *cheap.* Y. B. Mets. V, 10^c bot. בשער ז׳ . . שתא (not בשעה, בשעת) at the lowest price of the entire year.

זְלִיפָה f. (זָלַף) *emptying* from vessel to vessel. Ab. Zar. 36^a זְלִיפָתָן של . . אוסרתן the fact that they pour (into their oil vessels) residues of unclean (of forbidden) vessels makes their oil forbidden.

זְלִיקָא m. (זלק, cmp. P. Sm. 1125; 1131, a. זרק) *spark.—Pl.* זְלִיקֵי. Targ. Prov. XVI, 27.

זָלַל (b. h; cmp. דלל) *to be light, slender.*—זוֹלֵל, v. זול.

Pilp. זִלְזֵל 1) *to treat lightly, to despise, neglect* (with ב). Ber. 6^b (ref. to Ps. XII, 9) ובני אדם מְזַלְזְלִין בהן and which people treat slightly. Y. Peah I, 15^d, sq. מז׳ בבני וכ׳ they despise the sons of the handmaids; Gen. R. s. 84. Sabb. 62^b המזלזל וכ׳ he who is neglectful in the observance &c. Ab. Zar. 36^a לודאי מזלזלין הן Ms. M. (ed. דמזלזלו) the Lyddeans are neglectful of religious observances; a. e.—2) ז׳ מעות *to disregard money-matters.* Y. Snh. VIII, 26^b top; ib. XI, beg. 30^a (the rebellious son that took what belonged to his father) אינו חייב עד שיְזַלְזֵל מ׳ cannot be made responsible, unless he disregards money, expl. ib. 'he takes an object and sells it for its exact cost price' (thus proving both his rationality and his wastefulness).

זְלַל ch. same, *to be of little value, disregarded.* Targ. Prov. III, 21 לא נְזַל בעינך (h. text ילזו). Ib. IV, 21 לא יְזִלְּן בעיניך Var. ed. Lag. a. oth. ed. (ed. Lag. בעינך, v. זְלֵי; h. text יליזו מ־).

Palp. זַלְזֵל 1) *to disregard, despise.* Targ. Y. Deut. XXVII, 16. Targ. Y. Gen. XVI, 4 זלזלת (ed. pr. זַלְּלַת) she disregarded.—Ḥull. 133ᵃ זַלְזוּלֵי קא מְזַלְזֵל וכ׳ does he show that he treats religious observances with disrespect?, opp. חבב.—Ab. Zar. 35ᵃ ואתי לזַלְזוּלֵי בה Ms. M. (ed. לזילזולא) and he may be induced to disregard it; a. e.—2) *to count the lowest price.* B. Mets. 52ᵇ מְזַלְזְלִינַן במעשר שני in redeeming second tithes we are permitted to count closely. Ib. תרי זילי לא מז׳ two lowerings of value must not be applied to it (to value closely and then to count a defective coin for full).

Ithpalp. אִיזְדַּלְזֵל; contr. אִיזַּלְזֵל *to be despised; to lower one's self.* Targ. Job XL, 4. Targ. Koh. IX, 16.—Targ. Y. Deut. XXVIII, 16.

זָלַף (cmp. דלף, זלח) 1) *to pour, empty over.* M. Kat. II, 1, sq. זוֹלֵף וכ׳ he may empty the contents of the vat into the press and finish the process &c. Y. ib. 81ᵃ bot. זוֹלְפִין את יינו they put his grapes for him into the press. Tohar. X, 7 חזולֵף את חבור if one empties the wine or oil pit.—2) *to sprinkle.* Par. VI, 2 זָלַף וכ׳ (R. S. זִילֵּף) if he used all the water for sprinkling. Ib. 3 יזלף ed. (comm. זוֹלֵף; Yoma 58ᵃ זולף והולך) he may sprinkle &c. (Bart. a. Rashi to Yoma l. c. he may empty the water into bottles &c.). Ib. VII, 8 זולף (Maim.: he empties &c.); a. fr.

Pi. זִילֵּף *to drip, sprinkle.* Par. VI, 2, sq., v. supra.—Y. Sabb. IX, 12ᵃ מְזַלְּפִין וכ׳ you may drip hot water on the wound; Tosef. ib. XV (XVI), 4. Sabb. XIX, 3; a. e.

Hif. הִזְלִיף *to flow, squirt* (neut. verb). Ab. Zar. 59ᵇ מַזְלִיף (Ms. M. מזלף; Tosef. ib. VII (VIII), 5 מנתז).

זְלַף ch. same. Targ. Job XXXVI, 27 יִזְלְפוּן Ms. (ed. יזַלְּ׳ *Pa.*).—Y. Ab. Zar. IV, 44ᵇ bot. Ib.ᵃ bot. וזַלְפוּן וכ׳ and receive the wine at his hands.—Part. זָלִיף. Targ. Hab. II, 15.

Pa. זַלֵּיף *to squirt, drip.* Targ. Job XXIX, 6.—Keth. 67ᵇ מְזַלְּפֵי ליה וכ׳ they sprinkled old wine before him as a perfume, v. זלח.

Ithpe. אִזְדְּלֵף *to flow out, to empty itself.* Targ. Job XX, 28. Ib. XXVIII, 4, v. זְלַח.

זֶלֶף m., v. זִילּוּף.

זְלִתָּא f. (זלל; cmp. זְלוּעַ) *bucket, hod.* Yeb. 46ᵃ ז׳ דטינא Ar. (ed. זולטא, prob. corrupt. of זלועא) a hod with clay. [Sabb. 55ᵇ זלתא, v. זול I h.]

זְמָא, v. זְמַי.

זְמַבְלִיגָא, v. זִבְלִיגָא.

זִמָּה, v. זִימָּה.

זְמוּם m. (זָמַם II) *muzzle, bit.*—*Pl.* זְמוּמִים. Gen. R. s. 60 (interpret. ויפתח, Gen. XXIV, 32) התיר זְמוּמֵיהֶם he took their muzzles off; Yalk. Gen. 109 זְמָמֵיהֶן, v. זָמַם II.

זְמוּן, v. זִימּוּן.

זְמוֹרָא c. (v. P. Sm. 1138; prob. from the color of peeled vine shoots, v. זְמוֹרָה) *bluish-black* or *bluish-gray.*—*Pl.* f. זְמוֹרָן. Gen. R. s. 85 חוין עינוהי ז׳ his eyes were &c.

זְמוֹרֵד, v. אזמורד.

זְמוֹרָה f. (b.h.; זָמַר I) 1) *vine-shoot, vine-rod.* Sabb. XVII, 6 ז׳ שה״א וכ׳ a rod which is tied to a pitcher (to let it down into the well); a. e.—Esp. *the rod as an officer's badge and punishing instrument.* Num. R. s. 18 וליתן לו ז׳ and to give him the rod (appoint him an officer).—בעל הז׳ *carrier of the rod* (among the Romans *Centurio*, v. Sm. Ant. s. v.). Sabb. 145ᵇ ובעלי ז׳ Ms. M. (ed. ובעל) and Centuriones, v. הֶגְמוֹן. Y. Sot. IX, 24ᵇ top (rank of officers) בעל האגמון בעל הז׳ וכ׳ cane-bearer, rod-bearer, strap-bearer; Tosef. ib. XV, 7 (variously corrupted, v. Var. in ed. Zuck.). Midr. Till. to Ps. LXXIII, end; Yalk. ib. 808. Ex. R. s. 21, end; a. fr.—*Pl.* זְמוֹרוֹת. Gen. R. s. 31, end ז׳ לפילים vine-rods as food for elephants; ז׳ לנטיעות shoots for future plantation.—2) *membrum virile, phallus.* Tanḥ. Ki Thetsé 10 the Israelites did not know מה טיבה של ז׳ the idolatrous function of the phallus (with ref. to Ez. VIII, 17). Ib. חיכך . . את הז׳ Esau giggled and produced the phallus; Pesik. Zakhor, p. 27ᵇ. Num. R. s. 13. Pesik. R. s. 7 בחירופיו . . ובז׳ with his (Amalek's) blasphemies and by throwing up the phallus (taken from the mutilated Israelitish bodies). Ib. זְמוֹרָתָם של וכ׳ the membra of Israelites; Num. R. s. 13 (זִכְרוּתָן).

זְמוֹרְתָּא f. (זְמַר II) *song.* Sabb. 106ᵇ, a. e., v. זִמְרָא.

זַמְזוּמֵי m. (infin. of זמזם *tinnire*, P. Sm. 1132, v. זָמַם I) *playing on a tingling instrument.* Erub. 104ᵃ כי קלא דז׳ as the sound of tingling; [Ms. M. דמן מזומה, Ms. Alf. כי זמומי; Asheri: כמו זִרְמְזוּמֵי; Sefer ha-Ittim כַּמְזַמּוּמֵי].

זְמֵי, זְמָא I, (v. זָמַם II) *to bind over, to fine* (cmp. זוב, אסר &c.). Targ. Y. Deut. XXII, 19 (h. text ענש).

Af. אַזְמֵי same. Ruth R. to I, 1 יזמי להון, read מַזְמֵי he (the Roman officer) fines them; Yalk. Prov. 959 מזמי להון (corr. מז׳); Pesik. Shek., p. 11ᵇ ומזמיה ליה, Ms. O. ומזמי ליה; Yalk. Ex. 386 (corr. acc.).

Ithpe. אִזְדְּמֵי *to be fined; to lose.* Lev. R. s. 34 דבני אחתיה מִזְדַּמְיִין ת״ש וכ׳ Ar. (ed. מתבעין מן מלכותא) that his sister's son will be fined (or lose) seven hundred Denars. Ib. או אתון מארמאין (read: מִזְדַּמְאִין, *Ithpa.*; Yalk. Lev. 665 מזדמיין) or you will pay &c. Ib. דלמא . . . דאנן מז׳ (Yalk. l. c. דאינון, corr. acc.) didst thou know that we are destined to lose &c.? Ib. דאינון מארסוון (Yalk. l. c. דאתון מזדמיין), v. אֲנַס.

זְמֵי II (cmp. זמם I a. דמי) *to think.* Denom. זִימְיוֹנָא.

זְמִיוֹנָא, זְמִיוֹן, v. זִימְ׳.

זְמִימָה, v. זָמַם I.

זָמִין, part. pass. of זְמַן.

זְמִינָא I m. (זְמַן) *invited guest.* Ned. 24ᵃ.—*Pl.* זְמִינַיָּא. Targ. I Sam. IX, 22 (ed. Wil. זְמַנ׳, corr. acc.).

זְמִינָא II pr. n. m. *Z'mina* (interch. with זְבִינָא). Y. Bicc. III, 65[d] top ר׳ ז׳.—Y. Kil. IX, 32[d] top אבא בר זבינא; Y. Shek. V, beg. 48[c] זמ׳; Sabb. 112[b] רבא בר זימונא ed. (Ms. M. זימנא); a. fr.

זְמִיר, v. זְמַר I.

זְמִירָא m.=זְמָרָא, *song*. Esth. R. to III, 1 (Yalk. Esth. 1054 זמרי).

זְמִירָה I f. (זָמַר I) *pruning the vine*. Y. Kil. VIII, 31[c] top; Y. Sabb. VII, 10[a]; a. e.

זְמִירָה II f. (b. h.; זָמַר II), pl. זְמִירוֹת *songs*. Cant. R. to II, 12. Sot. 35[a] קרא לד״ת ז׳ he called the words of the Law songs (an entertaining secular study); v. זֶמֶר I.

זְמִית (זוּמִית) f. (זהם=זום; Syr. זמיתא, P. Sm. 1134) [*foam*,] name of *a brine*. Ber. 36[a]; 40[b] (Ms. F. זו׳); Ned. 55[b] זו׳.

זָמַם I (b. h.; cmp. דמם, דבב) *to mumble; to meditate, plan* (mostly in an evil sense, cmp. דִּבָּה).—*Part.* זוֹמֵם *planning evil*, esp. (with ref. to Deut. XIX, 19) a) *giving false testimony, amenable to the law of retaliation;* b) *rebutting witness*. Tosef. Macc. I, 1 עד ז׳ a witness convicted of false testimony; a. fr.—*Fem.* זוֹמֶמֶת (sub. עדות). Macc. I, 9 נמצאת אחת מהן ז׳ if one evidence (of one set of witnesses) has been disproved; a. e.—*Pl.* זוֹמְמִים, זוֹמְמִין. Ib. 4 אין אלו ז׳ they do not come under the law of retaliation. Ib. נעשים ז׳ are declared amenable to the law &c.; a. fr.—Tosef. ib. I, 10 זוֹמְמֵיהֶן those witnesses on whose evidence they had been declared guilty of false testimony. Y. ib. I, beg. 31[a] זוֹמְמָיו those who witnessed falsely against him. Tosef. Snh. VIII, 2 העדים וזוממיהן וזוֹמְמֵי זוממיהן the original witnesses and their refuters, and the refuters of their refuters; a. fr.

Hif. הֵזִים *to make a person a* זוֹמֵם, *to refute witnesses by testifying to an alibi, to rebut*. Macc. I, 5 if other witnesses came again והֵזִימּוּם and rebutted them. Keth. 20[a], v. כָּחַשׁ; a. fr. Macc. I, 4 (5[a]) שיזימו Bab. ed., read שֶׁיּוּזַמּוּ, v. infra.

Hof. הוּזַם, *Nif.* נִיזּוֹם *to be refuted, to be declared liable to the law of retaliation*. Snh. 10[a] פלוני .... והוּזַמּוּ if witnesses declared, This man did &c., and were declared guilty &c. Macc. 3[a] הוּזַמְנוּ וכ׳ we have been convicted &c. before that certain court, and made to pay. Ib. I, 4 עד שֶׁיּוּזַמּוּ את עצמן (Ar. בעצמן, Bab. ed. שיזימו corr. acc.) unless an alibi is established against their own persons (not an alibi of any of the alleged actors in the case). Ib. 5[b] עד שיזומו שניהם unless both of them are refuted; a. fr.

Pi. זִמֵּם *to rebut*. Part. מְזַמֵּם, pl. מְזַמְּמִין, contr. מְזַמְּרִים. Y. ib. I, 31[b] top.—*Part. pass.* מְזוּמָּם *one accused by false witnesses*. Snh. VI, 2 אם היה יודע שהוא מ׳ if he knew that he was innocent.

Nithpa. נִזְדַּמֵּם 1) *to be refuted* &c., v. *Hof.* Y. Macc. I, beg. 31[a] נִזְדַּמְּמוּ=נִיזּוֹמוּ.—2) *to be mumbled*. Gen. R. s. 81, beg. (ref. to זמות, Prov. XXX, 32) אם נִזְדַּמְּמוּ אחריך דברים וכ׳ (Yalk. Prov. 964 נִזְמְמוּ *Nif.*) if thou hast been slandered, put thy hand to thy mouth; v. זָמַם II.—Denom. זְמָם I.

זְמַם I ch. same.

Af. אַזֵּים=preced. *Hif.* Targ. Y. Deut. XIX, 18 דמַזְמִין who rebut.—B. Kam. 73[b] bot. דאפכינהו ואַזְמִינְהוּ they reversed their statement of the case and also testified to an alibi as to time and place.

Ithpa. אִיתַּזַּם, אִיתַּזַּים *to be proven a false witness*. Ib. 73[a] כי מִיתַּזְמֵי אטביחה when they were proven false witnesses with reference to slaughtering; ואִיתַּזְמוּ להו אגניבה and they are considered as false witnesses also with reference to stealing. Ib. אטביחה דקא מִיתַּזְמֵי אִיתַּזּוּם as regards the testimony to slaughtering on which they were refuted, they are refuted; a. e.—*Ithpe.* אִתְּזוּם. Macc. 3[b] א׳ חד מינייהו against one of them an alibi was proven.

זָמַם II (cmp. צמם) *to tie up, to muzzle* (b. h. חָסַם). Ber. 63[b] (ref. to זמות, Prov. XXX, 32, v. preced. w.) אם ז׳ וכ׳ if he muzzles his mouth (is ashamed to ask his teacher), he will have to put his hand to the mouth (when he in turn is asked). Ter. IX, 3 לא זוֹמֵם he does not muzzle his animal (complies with the law, Deut. XXV, 4); a. e.—*Part. pass.* זָמוּם, f. זְמוּמָה; pl. זְמוּמִים, זְמוּמוֹת *muzzled, prevented from grazing*. Gen. R. s. 41. Pesik. R. s. 3. Gen. R. s. 59, end; a. e.—Denom. זְמָם II.

זְמַם ch.=same, *to muzzle*. Targ. Y. II Gen. XIII, 7.

Pa. זַמֵּים same. Targ. Y. Deut. XXV, 4.

זָמַם III *to be filthy*, v. זוּם.

***זְמַם** III, *Ithpe.* אִתְזְמִים (cmp. דמם) *to be confounded*. Targ. Is. XXIX, 9 אִתְזְמִימוּ (ed. Wil. אִדְזְמִימוּ fr. דמם; absent in ed. Lag.; h. text השתעשעו, rendered by אשתגרשו a. our w., of which one is a gloss). [For אדז׳ cmp. חֲתַקֵּר s. v. דְּקַק.]

זְמָם I or **זָמָם** m. (זָמַם I) *false testimony*. Macc. 2[b] בגניבתו ולא בזְמָמוֹ 'one is sold for theft' (Ex. XXII, 2), but not for false testimony (which might eventually have caused the sale of the alleged thief); Y. Sot. III, end, 19[b]; Tosef. Macc. I, 1 בִזְמָמוֹ.

זְמָם II m. (זָמַם II) *muzzle* (v. זְמוּם). Gen. R. s. 81 (play on זמות, Prov. XXX, 32, v. זָמַם I) אם חשבת... נוח לך ליתן ז׳ וכ׳ if thou hast planned to do a good deed ...., it would have been better for thee to put a muzzle on thy mouth. Ib. s. 75 (ref. to זממו, Ps. CXL, 9) עשה לו ז׳ וכ׳ put a bit to Esaw (Rome); .. ומהו ז׳ וכ׳ and what is the bit (to check Rome's power) &c.?; Meg. 6[a] bot. זְמָמוֹ אל תפק וכ׳ 'do not loosen his bit' (Ps. l. c.), that means Germania &c.—*Pl.* זְמָמִים, v. זְמוּם.

זְמָם, זְמָמָא ch. same, also the camel's *ring* or *staff through the nose* and the *basket* fastened thereto. Targ. Is. XXXVII, 29. Targ. Ps. XXXII, 9; a. fr.—Sabb. 107[a], v. אִיפָּה. Ib. 111[b], sq. קיטרא דקטרי בז׳ the loop which is made to fasten the camel's basket to the ring; קיטרא דז׳ גופיה the (permanent) knot in the bit itself; v. אִיסְטְרִידָא.

זָמַן (b. h.; cmp. זבן) *to arrange, designate.*

Pi. זִימֵּן 1) *to invite,* esp. *to a meal.* B. Kam. 79b; a. v. fr.—*Part. pass.* מְזוּמָּן, f. מְזוּמֶּנֶת; pl. מְזוּמָּנִים, מְזוּמָּנוֹת a) *invited.* Pesik. R. s. 41, end מי שהיא מ׳ לסעודה he who is invited to the feast. Ib. (expl. מִקְרָאִי, Is. XLVIII, 12) מְזוּמָּנִי My invited guest (Israel); a. e.—b) *designated, chosen.* Ber. 43a הוא מ׳ לברכה he is the one designated (by the host) to say grace. Ab. Zar. 17a מ׳ לחיי וכ׳ chosen for the bliss of futurity.—Snh. 102a עת היא מ׳ וכ׳ there is a time designated for &c. Ib. יום מזומן (not עת היא, v. Rabb. D. S. a. l. note 8); Yalk. Is. 330; ib. Jer. 287.—c) *ready at hand, in one's possession.* B. Mets. 102a; Sifré Deut. 227, a. e. כי יקרא פרט למ׳ 'if it chance' (Deut. XXII, 6) this excludes that which is at thy disposal (in thy court yard); a. e.—2) *to appoint a meal in common,* so as to say grace together; *to preface the grace after meal by saying, Let us praise* &c.; v. זִימּוּן. Ber. VII, 1 שלשה ... חייבין לְזַמֵּן if three dine together, they are bound to make an appointment for common grace. Ib. מְזַמְּנִין עליו common grace may be appointed by making him one of the party (offering him something to eat). Ib. אין מ׳ עליהן you cannot count them in (to make up the requisite number). Ib. 2 עד כמה מזמנין how much must one eat of the meal in order to be counted one of the company? Ib. 3 כיצד מ׳ how is the appeal for common grace made?; a. fr.

Hif. הִזְמִין 1) *to cause to prepare, to notify.* Dem. VII, 1 המַזְמִין את חבירו וכ׳ if one notifies his friend that he will dine with him (on the Sabbath).—2) *to designate for use;* v. הַזְמָנָה. Ber. 26a הִזְמִינוֹ וכ׳ if he designated a building for &c.—3) *to summon,* v. next w.

Nithpa. נִזְדַּמֵּן 1) *to meet, to come to hand* (providentially); *to join one's self to.* Snh. 96a אותו מלאך שנ׳ לו וכ׳ that angel who was commissioned to accompany Abraham. Ib. נ׳ לו רגלי אחד a footman was joined to him (to meet his challenge). Ab. Zar. 25b ישראל שנ׳ לו וכ׳ (Ḥull. 91a שנטפל) an Israelite whom a gentile joins on the road. Shebi. VII, 4 שנִזְדַּמְּנוּ להם וכ׳ who accidentally caught unclean animals; a. fr.—2) *to make an appointment for meeting one another.* Pesik. R. s. 33, v. זִימּוּן.

זְמַן I ch. same.—*Part. pass.* זְמִין *ready, prepared.* Targ. Ex. XXXIV, 2 (Y. זְמִין, זַמִּין, incorr.).—Ib. XIX, 11; 15 זְמִינִין (Y. II מְזַמְּנִין, v. infra).—V. זְמִינָא.

Pa. זַמֵּין 1) *to invite; to appoint; to summon; to prepare.* Targ. Mic. III, 5. Targ. Ex. XIX, 10; 14 (ed. Berl. זַמֵּין, v. Berl. Targ. O. II, p. 25); a. fr. [Ib. XXV, 22 ואִזְּמֵן, ed. Berl. ואִזְדַּמֵּין, Y. אִיזְּמַן, Ithpe.].—M. Kat. 16a מְזַמְּנִינַן ליה וכ׳ we summon him &c. Cant. R. to V, 13 ביומוי דזַמֵּינַן וכ׳ (not דזמניין) in those my days when we invited two parties of scholars (for discussions).—*Part. pass.* מְזַמַּן (hebraism: מְזוּמָּן). Targ. Ps. LXXII, 17 (h. text ינון).—*Pl.* constr. מְזַמְּנֵי. Targ. Y. Num. I, 16 (h. text קריאי). [Ib. XXVI, 9 מנמנמי Ar., read מזמני; ed. מערעי).—2) *to appoint a meal in common, to say grace in common.* Ber. 45b נִיהְדַּר ונְזַמֵּן let us go back and agree (retrospectively) to make our meal a common one.

Af. אַזְמֵין same. Targ. Y. Gen. XXIV, 7. Targ. I Sam. XVI, 3. Targ. Ex. XIX, 10 וְתַזְ׳ some ed. v. supra; a. fr.—Ber. 50b אַזְמוּן עלייהו they counted them in for common grace, v. preced. *Pi.*—Snh. 48a דאַזְמְנֵיה וכ׳ which one designated for &c.—B. Bath. 58a sq. אי אתי איניש מעלמא ומַזְמֵין ליה לדינא Ms. M. (ed. incorr.) if any unknown man will come and sue him; a. fr.

Ithpa. אִזְדַּמַּן 1) as preced. *Nithpa.* Targ. Job XXXIII, 23.—Targ. Y. II Gen. XIX, 31 לְמִיזְדַּמְּנָא וכ׳ to join us in wedlock (cmp. זָוַג).—Targ. Am. III, 3; a. e.—2) *to prepare one's self.* Targ. Josh. VII, 13; a. e. [Targ. Y. II Gen. XXII, 8 יזדמן, read יְזַמֵּן.]—Contr. אִיזַּמַּן, *Ithpe.* אִיזְּמִין, v. supra.

זְמַן m. (b. h.; preced.) 1) *appointed time, term, time.* Kidd. I, 7, a. fr. הז׳ גרמא, v. גְּרָמָא.—B. Kam. 113a קובעים לו ז׳ וכ׳ we appoint (in the summons to appear before court) a Monday, Thursday and Monday in succession. Gitt. 72a, a. fr. זְמַנּוֹ של שטר the date of the document.—Taan. 14b, a. fr. בז׳ הזה in our days (after the dissolution of the Jewish common-wealth). Ib. הכל לפי הז׳ all depends on the season (whether it is advanced or retarded, v. Rabb. D. S. a. l. note 400). Ib. זְמַנָּהּ של רביעה the rainy season; a. v. fr.—*Pl.* זְמַנִּים. Meg. 2a ז׳ הרבה various dates (for reading the Megillah).—בִּזְמַן שֶׁ־ *in the case of, when, if.* Erub. VI, 7 אימתי בז׳ וכ׳ in what case (is this said)? When they carry &c. Ib. 6 ומודים בז׳ וכ׳ they all agree that, if some of them &c.; a. v. fr.—בִּזְמַנָּהּ, בִּזְמַנּוֹ &c. *in its prescribed, due time;* חוץ לִזְמַנּוֹ &c. *out of time, beyond its due time.* Zeb. I, 1. Ib. II, 3; a. v. fr.—2) *festive season* (cmp. מְאַרְעָא, מִקְרָא); *'Z'man', that section of the benediction on the entrance of a Festival which refers to the return of the festive season* (שהחיינו והגיענו לזמן הזה ....). Pes. 102b מדלא אמר ז׳ since he did not mention the benediction of *Z'man*, v. יקנה״ז. Succ. 48a שמיני ... ז׳ בפני עצמו the eighth day (of Succoth) ... is a festive season for itself, requiring the insertion of *Z'man;* a. fr.—*Pl.* as above. Y. Ab. Zar. I, 39c ג׳ ז׳ בבבל there are three festive seasons (idolatrous fairs) in Babylonia. Tosef. Ber. III, 13 חותם ברוך ... והז׳ you must close with 'Blessed be He .. who sanctifies the Sabbath, Israel, and the Seasons.—[Snh. 101a הקורא ... שלא בזמנו he who cites a Biblical verse at a banquet out of its *context* (perverting its sense for lascivious purposes); Treat. Kallah beg.]

זְמַן II, **זִמְנָא**, **זְמָנָא**, ז׳ ch. same. Targ. O. Gen. XVIII, 14 (Y. ז׳ חגא, h. text מועד). Ib. II, 23 הדא ז׳ this time (h. text הפעם); a. fr.—Targ. Jer. XVIII, 7, 9 ז׳ .... וז׳ at one time ... another time.—Ḥull. 105b ליקבע לי מר ז׳ וכ׳ set me a term, and I shall pay. M. Kat. 16a דקבעינן ז׳ that (in legal summons) a date is fixed for appearing in court. Ib. ז׳ בתר ז׳ one term after the other (in case of failing to appear on the first summons). Ḥag. 4b אזיל בלא זִמְנֵיה dies before his destined time; a. v. fr.—B. Bath. 73b, a. fr. ז׳ חדא once upon a time (introducing a story).—*Pl.* זִמְנִין, זִי׳. Targ. Ex. XXIII, 17; a. e.—Zeb. 94b, a. fr. ז׳ סגיאין many times.—ז׳—ז׳ *at times ... at other times.* Ber. 20b, a. fr.—מַשְׁכַּן זִמְנָא=h. אֹהֶל מוֹעֵד. Targ. Ex. XXVIII, 43; a. fr.—Targ. Ps. LXXIV, 4 משכני ז׳=זְמָנֶךָ.—Targ. Jer. XLVII, 6 לְבֵית ז׳ to thy destined home (the sheath; h. text הַתַּעְרֵךְ!).—[Targ. Ps. CXLI, 4 בזמן

משתיהון Ms. (ed. בזמר בית מ׳) at their *appointed banquets*, v. preced. wds.]

זָמַר I (b. h.) *to nip; to prune; to cut.* Sabb. 73[b] זוֹמֵר וצריך וכ׳ if one trims a tree (on the Sabbath) for making use of the wood. Snh. 26[a] כהן וזומר (not וזוכר) a priest is he, and he prunes the vine (in the Sabbatical year)!; a. fr.

Nif. נִזְמַר *to be pruned*, trnsf. *to be checked, unnerved, defeated.* Cant. R. to II, 12 (ref. to זמיר ib.) הגיע זמנה של ערלה שתִּזָּמֵר the time for pruning the preputium (circumcision) has come (v. Ex. R. s. 19); הגיע . . . שיִזָּמְרוּ the time has come for the Egyptians to be checked; Pesik. Haḥod., p. 50[a]; Pesik. R. s. 15.—Lev. R. s. 9, beg. Akhan is named Zimri (I Chr. II, 6, cmp. with Josh. VII, 24) שנִזְמְרוּ . . על ידו because through him the Israelites were unnerved (Josh. VII, 5); a. e.

זְמַר ch., *Af.* אַזְמִיר same. Y. Shebi. IV, 35[a] חמא חד א׳ וכ׳ (not איז׳) saw one prune &c. (in the Sabbatical year).

זָמַר II (b. h ; cmp. זָמַם I) *to tingle, make music, sing.* V. זֶמֶר.

Pi. זִמֵּר 1) *to sing one's praise.* Cant. R. to II, 16 הוא זִמְּרַנִי . . וזִמַּרְתִּיו (or זִמְרָתִיו, זִמְּרַנִי) He praised me, and I &c.—Gen. R. s. 91, end (expl. מזמרת, Gen. XLIII, 11) דברים שהן מְזַמְּרִין וכ׳ things which men praise all over the world.—2) *to review a lesson in recitative chant* (v. זִמְרָה). Snh. 99[b] top זַמֵּר בכל יום chant every day; Tosef. Ohol. XVI, 8 ז׳ בי הדירה ז׳ (the Law says) review me steadily &c.; ib. Par. IV (III), 7; cmp. גִּמְרָא.

זְמַר ch., *Pa.* זַמֵּיר same, 1) *to sing.* Targ. Ps. XVIII, 50; a. e.—Sot. 48[a] זַמְּרֵי גברי וכ׳ when men sing and women respond.—2) *to sing a satire, deride.* Targ. Lam. III, 14.

***זָמַר** III, *Hif.* הִזְמִיר (cmp. זְמוֹרָא) *to look bluish.* Y'lamd. to Num. XXV, 14, quot. in Ar. (play on זמרי) עד שה׳ בשרו כביצה מוזרת until his flesh (through his lewdness) had the color of a smashed (rotten) egg; (cmp. Tanh. Pinh. 2, Num. R. s. 21, beg., Snh. 82[b]—where our w. is omitted).

זֶמֶר I m. (זָמַר II) *music, song*; כלי ז׳ (or sub. כלי) *musical instrument.* Sot. 48[a] בארבעה מיני ז׳ to the music of four instruments. Y. ib. VII, 21[c] top לעז לז׳ Greek is adapted for song; Y. Meg. I, 71[b] bot.—Snh. 101[a] ועושה אותו כמין ז׳ and treats it (a verse of Song of Songs) like a (secular) song; Yalk. Prov. 953; a. fr.

זֶמֶר II m. (זָמַר I; cmp. זמרה, Gen. XLIII, 11) *fruits*, (grapes &c.), *dessert.* Y. Pes. X, 37[d] bot. (expl. אפיקומין) מיני ז׳ various dessert fruits (Bab. ib. 119[b] תמרים וכ׳; Tosef. ib. X, 11 אגוזים וכ׳).

זַמָּר m. (זָמַר I) *musician, singer.* Kel. XVI, 7 מרכוף של ז׳, v. מַרְכּוֹף. Yalk. Lam. 1001.

זַמָּרָא ch. same.—*Pl.* זַמָּרַיָּא. Targ. Koh. II, 8.—Fem. pl. זַמָּרָתָא. Ib.

זְמָרָא ch.=זֶמֶר I.—ז׳ זְנֵי (זִינֵי)=מִינֵי זֶמֶר (כְּלֵי) *musical instruments.* Dan. III, 5; a. e.—Targ. Koh. II, 8.—Targ. Ez. XXXIII, 32 זְמַר אבובין flute-music.—*Pl.* זְמָרַיָּא. Targ. Lam. V, 14.—Ib. III, 63 זְמָרֵיהוֹן object of their derisive songs, v. זְמַר II.

זְמָרָא, זִימְ׳ I m. same, *song, music.* Gitt. 7[a] ז׳ מנא לן וכ׳ how is it proved that music (at banquets, after the destruction of the Temple) is forbidden? Ib. ז׳ דמנא instrumental music, ז׳ דפומא vocal music. Sot. 48[a] ז׳ בביתא וכ׳ music in the house—destruction at the threshold. Ib. ז׳ בטיל prohibited musical entertainments.—Sabb. 118[b] פסוקי דז׳ verses of praise (Ps. CXLVIII a. CL; v. Rabb. D. S. a. l. note 200).—*Pl.* זְמָרִין, זִמְ׳. Y. Meg. III, 74[a] bot. היה דמיך וקאים בז׳ used to go to bed and rise with music.—V. זִמְרָה.

זְמָרָא, זִמְ׳ II pr. n. m. *Zimra*, father of R. Yosé, v. יוסי. Keth. 96[a]; a. fr.

זְמַרְגַּד, זְמַרְגְּדָא (זמרגדד, זמרגדו) m. (σμάραγδος) *smaragd, emerald, colored crystal* (v. Sm. Ant. s. v.). Targ. Prov. XXV, 12; a. fr. (in the sense of a precious stone [v. next w.], and as crystal or spar of copper mine).—*Pl. h.* זְמַרְגְּדִין. Lev. R. s. 2 (precious stones).

זְמַרְגְּדִין, זְמַרְגְּדִין m. (σμαράγδιον) *emerald*, a precious stone. Targ. Y. II Ex. XXVIII, 19, v. אִזְמַרְגַּד.

זְמֹרָה, v. זְמוֹרָה.

זִמְרָה, זִימְ׳ f. (זָמַר II) *chant on reciting Talmudic lessons.* Meg. 32[a] (some ed. זימרא); Treat. Sof'rim III, 10.

זִמְרִי (b. h.) pr. n. m. *Zimri*, slain by Phinehas (Num. XXV, 14). Snh. 82[b], a. e., v. זָמַר III. Y. Taan. III, 66[c] bot. כמה ז׳ וכ׳ how mani Zimris (lewd men) are in our days!; a. fr.

זְמָרְתָא, pl. **זַמָּרָיָתָא**, v. זַמָּרָא.

זִימְתָנֵי, זִמְתָנֵי nom. gent. pl. (denom. of זִמָּה=זמתא) *Zimthanê* (schemers). Targ. Y. Deut. II, 20 (Targ. O. חשבני; h. text זמזמים).

זַן, זִין, זְנָא I (b. h. זַן; Syr. זן qualitas, modus, P. Sm. 1138, sq.; cmp. זֶה, a. מִין a. מַה) *quality, nature; kind, species.* Targ. Gen. I, 11 לִזְנֵיהּ after its kind. Targ. Lev. XI, 14 לִזְנָהּ; a. v. fr.—Ber. 32[a] (prov.) מלי כריסיה זנא בישא Ar. (ed. זיני בישי) filled stomachs are a bad sort (plenty is tempting).—*Pl.* זְנִין, זְנֵי. Targ. Gen. I, 21; a. fr.—Dan. II, 5, v. זְמָרָא.—B. Kam. 16[b] (expl. זנים, II Chr. XVI, 14) זני זני Ms. M. a. Ar. (ed. זיני) various species.

זְנָא II *to go astray*, v. זְנֵי.

זַנָּאי m. (זני) *adulterer; voluptuous.* Sabb. 156[a].—*Pl.* זַנָּאִין. Targ. Jer. IX, 1; a. e.—Targ. Ez. XXIII, 45 (h. text נֹאֲפֹת).

זָנָב m. (b. h.) *attachment, tail.* Bekh. VI, 9 זְנַב הגדי the tail of a kid; a. fr.—Yoma 41[b] ז׳ לשון the tail-end (fringes) of the band. Erub. 18[a] (ref. to צלע, Gen. II, 22) ז׳ it means the tail (with which Adam was originally created). Kil. IV, 6 ואחת יוצאה ז׳ and one vine projects like a tail. Ukts. I, 3 ז׳ של אשכול the skeleton of the cluster of grapes (the thin branches), opp. to יד, the stem; a. fr.—Trnsf. *the last, least.* Ab. IV, 15, v. אַרִי.—Euphem. *membrum virile.* Tanh. Ki Thetsé 10 (expl. ויזנב, Deut. XXV, 18) הכה אותן מכת ז׳ Amalek mutilated them by cutting off &c.; Pesik. Zakh., p. 27ª; Pesik. R. s. 12; Num. R. s. 13; v. זְמוֹרָה.—Denom.

זִנֵּב *Pi.* (b. h.) 1) (v. Ukts. I, 3 quot. in preced. w.) *to cut off the extreme branches of the vine, to trim.* Shebi. IV, 6 המזנב בגפנים he who trims grape-vines.—Trnsf. ז׳ באשכולות [*to thin the clusters,*] *to diminish the scholars* by persecution (v. אֶשְׁכּוֹל). Gen. R. s. 42; Lev. R. s. 11; a. e.—2) *to attack, force a passage.* Gen. R. s. 74 בקש לְזַנֵּבָן Joab wanted to force his passage through their territory; Yalk. Sam. 147.

זַנְבָא, v. דַּנְבָּא.

זְנוֹבְיָה pr. n. f. *Zenobia*, queen of Palmyra. Y. Ter. VIII, 46ᵇ bot. ז׳ מלכתא (not מלכותא).

זַנְגָאֵי, v. זִיגְ׳.

זנגבילא, Targ. Cant. III, 9, read: זְמִבְּלִינָא=זַנְבְּלִינָא.

זַנְגְּבִילָא f. (ζιγγίβερις, zingiber) an Arabian *spice plant*, prob. *ginger.* Yoma 81ᵇ; Ber. 36ᵇ (v. Ms. M. in Rabb. D. S. a. l.), v. הִימְלְתָא.

זַנְדּוּקָא m. (Syr. זנדיקא, P. Sm. 1141;=זודוקא, reduplic. of זקק, cmp. זִיקָא III; for inserted נ cmp מזדנדזין s. v. זעזע) *jailer.* Taan. 22ª ז׳ אנא Ar. (ed., a. Ar. ed. Koh. זַנְדּוּקָנָא, v. Rabb. D. S. a. l. note 50; Ms. M. בְּדִיקְנָאָה) I am a jailer.

זָנָה, v. זני.

זְנוּ, v. זְנוּתָא.

זָנוֹחָא pr. n. pl. *Z'noḥa* (b. h. זָנוֹחַ, Josh. XV, 34; 56) in Judaea. Men. VIII, 1 (83ᵇ) Ar. a. Rashi (ed. זנחא, Ms. M. זוניחא, Mish. ed. מזוניחה, Mish. Nap. וזוניחא; v. Rabb. D. S. a. l. note); Tosef. ib. IX, 2 זו לחה (corr. acc.).

זְנוּנִים m. pl. (b. h.; זָנָה) 1) *prostitution;* בני ז׳ *children begotten in prostitution.* Pes. 87ª bot. בני ז׳; ib.ᵇ ובניך בני ז׳ Ms. M. (ed. בנים ז׳, ובניך ז׳, v. זָנָן).—2) *sensuality.* Ib. 111ª אחדא ... רוח ז׳ sexual passion will seize him (her).

זְנוּק, v. זינוק.

זְנוּת f. (b. h.; זָנָה) *prostitution, unchastity, voluptuousness.* Sot. IX, 15 (49ᵇ) בית הועד יהיה לז׳ (=לבית ז׳) the scholars' meeting house shall become a place of licentiousness (where low people assemble). Num. R. s. 13 על ז׳ אחותו for seducing his sister. Ab. Zar. 36ᵇ דרך ז׳ a meretricious connection, opp. אישות. Gen. R. s. 26 .. על הכל חוץ מן הז׳ .... the Lord is long-suffering to everything except debauchery. Keth. 3ª, v. בְּעִילָה; a. v. fr.

זְנוּ, זְנוּתָא ch. same. Targ. Y. Gen. XXXIII, 2. Targ. Hos. IV, 11; a. fr.—Targ. Job XXXVI, 14 מרי ז׳ keepers of brothels.—Sot. 3ᵇ ז׳ בביתא וכ׳ faithlessness in the house is like a worm in poppy-plants.

זָנַח (b. h.) *to glisten* (cmp. דנח) *to be fat; to be greasy, foul* (cmp. meanings of זהם, צחן, v. Ges. Thes. s. v. זנח); 1) (act. verb) *to loathe.* Midr. Till. to Ps. LX; Yalk. Ps. 777 אני זְנַחְתִּי אתכם אתם זְנַחְתֶּם אותי did I loathe you? You loathed me.—2) *to be loth.* Pesik. R. s. 41 (ref. to זונה, Ps. LXXIII, 27) שרחקו וזנחו הימך because they removed themselves from and were loth of Thee.

Hif. הִזְנִיחַ 1) *to declare rejectable, unclean;* (cmp. זהם) *to reject;* (cmp. סאב, רחק) *to remove.* Hull. 7ª אין מַזְנִיחִין אותו we must not detest him (remove him from college). Pesik. R. l. c. מַזְנִיחִים עצמם הימך they (through their sins) remove themselves from thee.—2) *to polish, cleanse.* Lev. R. s. 1, beg. (ref. to אבי זנוח) I Chr. IV, 18) that is Moses שהיה אב לַמַּזְנִיחִים שהִזְנִיחָם מע״ז for he was the father of the cleaners, for he cleansed them from idolatry; Yalk. ib. 428.

Pi. זִנַּח *to make glistening, to stroke, dress.* Num. R. s. 20; Tanh. Balak 12 באתר ... זִנַּחְתִּיהָ I had come to kill her, and now I had to polish her up; (Tanh. ed. Bub. ib. 20 זינחתה; Yalk. Num. 768, Matt. K. to Num. R. l. c. quotes in Tanh. l. c. דכיתיה).

זנח, Targ. Ps. XV, 5 יזנח ed. Lag., read יזוּח or יזוּע.

זָנָה, זני (b. h.) 1) [*to run to and fro, wander;*] (with אחר) *to run after,* (with מאחרי) *to run away from;* esp. *to run about as a prostitute, to be faithless, be unchaste* (cmp. ch. נפקת ברא for זוֹנָה, a. מעי for our w.). Sabb. 55ᵇ (play on פחז, Gen. XLIX, 4) פסעת ... חטאת זָנִיתָ thou hast trespassed upon religion, sinned, been unchaste (v. זול).—Snh. 100ᵇ שמא תִּזְנֶה lest she may go astray (be seduced); a. v. fr.—2) *to commit an offense.* Gitt. 6ᵇ explain. ותזנה עליו, Jud. XIX, 2, cmp. Targ. a. l.

Pi. זִינָּה same, also *to invite faithlessness, to excite the senses.* Sabb. 88ᵇ עלובה כלה מְזַנָּה בתוך חופתה (v. Rabb. D. S. a. l.) bold is the bride who thinks of faithlessness while getting married; Gitt. 36ᵇ שזִינְּתָה בקרב וכ׳. Sot. 10ª כל הַמְזַנֶּה ... מְזַנֶּנֶת עליו if a man is lewd, his wife will think of faithlessness against him; Yalk. Job 918 מְזַנָּה תחתיו. Meg. 15ª רחב בשמה זִינְּתָה וכ׳ Rahab suggested impure thoughts by her name (*Rahab hazzonah*), Jael with her call (Jud. IV, 18) &c., v. זְכִירָה; a. fr.—Trnsf. (of plants) *to degenerate.* Gen. R. s. 28, end אף הארץ זינתה the earth, too, became degenerated in her produces; v. זוּנִירָא. Y. Kil. I, beg. 26ᵈ הפירות מְזַנִּין the produces may degenerate (ref. to Lev. XIX, 29).

זְנָא, זְנִי same. Targ. Y. Gen. XXXVIII, 24 זַנְיַית (O. זַנִּיאַת); a. e.

Pa. זַנִּי same. Targ. O. Deut. XXII, 21 לְזַנָּ׳ ed. Berl. (ed. Amst. לְזַנָּאָה); a. e.—Keth. 81ª ספק זַנַּאי וכ׳ there is a doubt, did she or did she not commit adultery?—*Denom. אַזְיָין f. *a runner (after men).* Snh. 106ª bot. (prov.) מסגני ושילטי הואי א׳ לגברי נגרי (נגדי) after (living with) princes and governors she became a runner after ship draggers (or carpenters). [Our w. is absent in Yalk. Num. 785 as well as in Ms. M., the latter having a marginal version אזלא הויא.]

זְנִיוּתָא, Ms. זְנָיוּ׳, Targ. Prov. XXIX, 3, read: זַנְיָתָא, זַנְיָ׳, v. next w.

זַנְיָתָא, זַנִּיתָא (זַנָּיָ׳) f. ch.=h. זוֹנָה. Targ. Joel IV, 3 (ed. Wil. זַנְיְתָא). Targ. Prov. VII, 10. Ib. VI, 26;

a. e.—Pesik. R. s. 21 בר׳ דז׳ the son of the whore (heretic). —*Pl.* זְנִיָּיתָא, זַנְּרֵי׳, זַנְּרֵי׳. Targ. Hos. IV, 14. Targ. Prov. XXIX, 3, v. preced. Y. Taan. I, 64[b] bot. מיגר ז׳ hiring out prostitutes.

זְנָן (sec. r. of זָנָה) *to be faithless, suspected of faithlessness.*—*Part. pass.* זָנוּן, pl. זְנוּנִים *of spurious paternity.* Pes. 87[a] bot. ותוליד לך בנים ז׳ and she will bear thee spurious sons; ib.[b] ובניך ז׳; v. זְנוּנִים.

Pi. זִנֵּן *to think of faithlessness.* Sot. 10[a], v. זָנָה.

זָנַק, *Pi.* זִינֵּק (b. h.) 1) *to squirt, sputter, eject with force.* Nidd. 59[b] בִּמְזַנֶּקֶת it means a woman discharging urin in a gush. Hull. 38[a] זִינְּקָה the animal's blood sputtered (when its jugular arteries were cut). Y. Yoma I, 39[a] bot. חוטמו מְזַנֵּק תולעים his nose discharging worms.—2) [*to make a persons' mouth water,*] *to make a person sick by withholding from him a desired dish.* Ex. R. s. 16, end אתם זִינַּקְתֶּם את בני וכ׳ ye made my children sick by withholding from them meat, when ye ate &c.

Hif. הִזְנִיק *to drop, to pour.* Y. Sabb. VIII, 11[b] bot. בִּמַזְנִיק שנו the Mishnah means when one uses pitch or sulphur in a liquid state.

זָע, v. זוּעַ a. זעזע.

זעאתא, Targ. Prov. XII, 21 some ed., v. עאתא.

זְעוּר, זְעוּרָא, v. זְעֵיר, זְעֵירָא, a. next w.

זְעוּרֵי m. pl. (זְעַר)=h. נְעוּרִים, *youth, youthful days.* Targ. I Sam. XII, 2 (ed. Wil. זְעֵרֵי). Targ. II Sam. XIX, 8 זְעוּרָךְ (sing.); a. e.

זְעָזוּעַ m. (זעזע) *shock, fright.* Targ. Y. Gen. XXVII, 33.

זִיעַ׳, זַעֲזַע (Pilp. of זוּעַ) *to move, shake, agitate, trouble.* Ex. R. s. 15, end ז׳ את הימים וכ׳ He stirred the seas up and showed to him (Moses) &c. Y. Ber. IX, 13[c] bot. אני מְזַעֲזֵעַ עולמי I will make my world quake. Orl. I, 3 זִיעְזַעְתּוֹ המחרישה the ploughshare loosened it (the roots of the tree); זִיעְזָעוֹ ועשאו בעפר he (the husbandman) lifted the tree and placed it in soft earth (v. comment.).

Hithpalp. הִזְדַּעְזֵעַ, *Nithpa.* נִזְדַּעְזֵעַ 1) *to be shaken, frightened.* Shebu. 39[a]. Y. Ber. IV, 7[b] נִזְדַּעְזְעָה החומה the wall was removed from its place; B. Kam. 82[b] נז׳ א״י Palestine quaked. Cant. R. to III, 7 מתיראין ומִזְדַּעְזְעִין וכ׳ were frightened and shaken; a. fr.—2) *to rise in rebellion.* Yalk. Num. 763 שנזדעזעו בני המדינה against whom the inhabitants of the country rebelled; a. fr.—Contracted part. מְזְדַּיְּיִין, or מִזְדַּנְדְזִין (=מזדעזען). Hull. 48[a] התלמידים מזדנז׳ בדבר ed. (Ar. מזדנדז׳) the students oppose it.—3) *to cause to quake.* Midr. Till. to Ps. XVIII, 8 אתה הִזְדַּעְזַעְתָּ . . . אֲזַדְּעְזַע וכ׳ . . . thou hast made thy limbs tremble . . . , so will I make my world quake, v. supra.

זַעֲזַע ch. same. Targ. Ps. LX, 4; a. fr.

Ithpalp. אִזְדַּעְזַע *to be frightened.* Targ. Y. Gen. XXVII, 33; a. fr.

זַעֲטוּט (זַאֲטוּט, זַטּוּט) m. (redupl. of זעט, v. זוּטָא) *young man, youth, student.*—*Pl.* זַעֲטוּטִים, constr. זַעֲטוּטֵי (a Variant of נערי, Ex. XXIV, 5, because נערי admits of the meaning of *servants, slaves,* Greek παιδές). Sifré Deut. 356 (v. מָעוֹן a. חָיָא) and one manuscript existed in the Temple which was named ספר זעטוטים the Book of Za'ăṭûṭim (containing זעטוטי for נערי); Treat. Sof'rim VI, 4 זאטוטי; Y. Taan. IV, 68[a] bot. זעטוטי.—Meg. 9[a] (reported as one of the changes in the Greek translation of the Pentateuch, and ref. to נערי l. c., and to אצילי Ex. XXIV, 11:) זאטוטי ed. (Ms. Par. זט׳, oth. mss. a. Yalk. Gen. 3 זטוטי) 'the youths' (νεανίσκοι, in place of παιδές, v. LXX Ex. l. c.).

זַעֲטוּטָא, pl. **זַעֲטוּטֵי** ch. same. Targ. Y. Ex. XXIV, 11 Lev. (ed. עולימיא). Targ. Cant. VI, 5.

***זְעִי** (v. זְעֵיר I) *to be small, diminished.* Targ. Prov. X, 27 נזעין Ms. a. Var. ed. Lag. (ed. Lag. a. oth. זעה).

זְעֵייָא, זְעֵיָא, v. זְעֵרָא.

***זְעֵיוָתָא** f. pl. (v. זְעַר) *small.* Targ. Prov. VII, 6 Lev. a. Buxt. (ed. Lag. זעירתא, Var. זעירי׳).

זְעִיק, v. זְעַק.

זְעֵיר I, זְעַר, זְעַר, זְעַר, fut. נִזְעַר, יִזְעַר (cmp. זוּעַ; b. h. זְעֵיר) 1) *to be slender, small; to be reduced, diminished.* Targ. Prov. X, 27, v. זְעִי. Targ. Jer. XXIX, 6; a. fr.—Y. Sabb. VIII, 11[a] bot. זְעֵרַת ולא ז׳ וכ׳ it (the measure) was reduced, but was not made as small as it had been before; v. *Ithpe.*—2) (cmp. צער) *to get sick.* Gen. R. s. 33 ותִזְעַר נפשיה and he may get sick.—3) *to restrain.* Targ. II Sam. XVIII, 16 ed. Lag. a. Ar. (ed. מנע; h. text חשך).

Af. אַזְעֵר, אַזְעַר, אַזְעֵיר 1) *to reduce, do little.* Targ. Ex. XVI, 17; 18 (h. text הַמַּמְעִיט). Targ. Lev. XXV, 16; a. fr.—Targ. Y. Num. XXII, 6 לְאַזְעוּרֵיה to reduce (defeat) him (h. text נכה).—2) *to be small.* Targ. O. Ex. XII, 4; a. e.

Ithpe. אִזְּעַר, אִזְדְּעַר *to be made smaller.* Targ. Y. Gen. I, 16.—Y. Shek. III, 47[c] top [read:] אִזְעֵירָא ולא אִזְעֲרַת וכ׳ it was reduced, but not made as small &c., v. supra.

זְעֵיר II, זְעֵירָא, זְעֵירָא m., **זְעֵירְתָּא, זְעֵירְתָּא** f. (preced.) *small, young, tender; lesser; a little.* Targ. Gen. I, 16. Targ. O. ib. XLIV, 25.—Targ. Gen. XIX, 31; a. fr.—Y. Ber. II, 4[b] דרבה . . לא ז׳ the inferior does not greet the superior; Y. Shek. II, 47[a] top דז׳ (not ר׳ ז׳).—Y. Snh. III, 21[a] bot. בשום דזעיר מיניה in behalf of one his junior. Y. Keth. V, beg. 29[c] ז׳ ובר and said something small (insignificant). Ib. והדא היא ז׳ is this something small?; a. fr.—זְעֵירָיָא, זְעֵירִין. Targ. Y. Ex. XII, 4. Targ. Ps. CXV, 13; a. fr.—Y. M. Kat. III, 82[d] top והוא שאיל לז׳ and he asked the inferior (scholars)?—Fem. זְעֵירָתָא, זְעֵירָן. Targ. O. Gen. XXXII, 10.—Targ. Ps. CIV, 25 (Ms. זוטרתא).

זְעֵיר III pr. n. m. *Z'er (Little),* an Amora. Y. Ter. VIII, 46[b] bot. ז׳ בר חיננא. Y. Ber. V, end, 8[d] ר׳ ז׳; a. e.

זְעֵירָא I, v. זְעֵיר II.

זְעֵירָא II pr. n. m. *Z'era,* [also: זְעוּרָא, רָה . . .] name of several Amoraim. Y. Ter. XI, 47[d] bot.; a. fr. (in Bab. זֵירָא).—Y. Ber. VI, 10[d] top; a. e.—Ib. I, 3[a] top תנאי ר׳ ז׳.—Ib. VIII, 12[c] top; Gen. R. s. 3 ר׳ ז׳ בר אבהו.—Y. Sabb. I, 3[d] ר׳ ז׳ בר אבינא. V. Fr. M'bo p. 77[b], sq.

זְעֵירוּתָא f. (זעיר) *smallness, small number.* Targ. Lev. XXV, 16; a. e.

זְעֵירְתָּא, v. זְעֵיר II.

זָעַם (b. h.) *to be excited, angry.—Part. pass.* זָעוּם; f. זְעוּמָה; pl. זְעוּמוֹת. Num. R. s. 11 פנים ז׳ morose countenance, opp. מאירות; cmp. זָעַף.

זַעַם m. (b. h.; preced.) *anger, displeasure.* Num. R. s. 11 פנים של ז׳, v. preced. Kidd. 66ᵃ ויבדלו . . . בז׳ and Israel's scholars parted under (the king's) displeasure.

זעע, v. זעזע, a. זוע.

זָעַף (b. h.; cmp. זָעַם) *to be excited, troubled, serious.—Part. act.* זוֹעֵף; f. זוֹעֶפֶת, pl. זוֹעֲפוֹת, part. pass. זָעוּף; f. זְעוּפָה; pl. זְעוּפוֹת. Pesik. R. s. 21 פנים זוע׳ (a. זער׳) serious (commanding) countenance. Pesik. Baḥod. p. 110ᵃ; Yalk. Ex. 286 פנים זו׳, contrad. to בינוניות indifferent, מסבירות inviting, kind countenance.

זְעַף ch. same, *to rage, threaten, storm.* Targ. Ps. L, 3 (h. text נשערה). Ib. X, 5 (h. text יפיח).—Gen. R. s. 63 בעא רבי דיזעוף ביה Rabbi wanted him (R.S.) to threaten him; Yalk. ib. 110 דיזעף (Y. Ter. VIII, end, 46ᶜ למינזף).

זַעַף m. (b. h.; preced. wds.) *stormwind, vehemence; anger.* Taan. III, 8 התחילו לירד בז׳ the rain began to come down with vehemence. Pesik. R. s. 15, v. אַגְרִיאָן. Treat. S'maḥ. III, 9 מיתה של ז׳ a sudden death (by the anger of the Lord); cmp. M. Kat. 28ᵃ, s. v. דָּחָה.

זַעְפָּא ch. same, *stormwind, hurricane.* Targ. Job I, 19 (ed. Wil. זִיקָא); a. e.—Ber. 59ᵃ (expl. הזוועות Mish. ib. IX, 2).

זְעַפְרָנָא m. (Arab. a. Pers. zafrân) *saffron.* Targ. Y. Lev. XV, 19 (ed. Amst. זְעְפְרָנָא).

זָעַק (b. h.) *to cry.* Ex. R. s. 1 (ref. to Ex II, 23) אין וַיִּזְעֲקוּ אלא וכ׳ 'they cried' has the meaning of lamenting.

Hif. הִזְעִיק *to cause to cry.* Gen. R. s. 67, v. זְעָקָה.

זְעַק, זְעֵיק ch. same. Targ. Ex. II, 23; a. e.

זְעָקָה f. (b. h.; preced. wds.) *cry, prayer.* Yalk. Deut. 811; Yalk. Sam. 157 (as one of the expressions for prayer; Deut. R. s. 2 צְעָקָה). Gen. R. s. 67 ז׳ אחת וכ׳ Jacob caused Esau to utter one cry.

זעקפי, Gen. R. s. 98, v. זְקִיפִין.

זְעֵרְתָּא, v. זְעֵיר II.

זִפְתָּא, זִיפְתָּא, זֶפָא f. ch. 1)=h. זֶפֶת *pitch.* Targ. Is. XXXIV, 9. Targ. Ex. II, 3.—2)=זיפות *pitch-coating.* Y. M. Kat. II, 81ᵇ top [read:] דזיפתה, v. הַקְדְּקִירָא.

זִיפְרִין, זִיפִירִין, (זוּפְרִים, זוּפ׳, זִפְרִין) pr. n. pl. (Ζεφύριον) *Z'firin, Zifirin* &c., prob. *the headland of Cyprus* (v. Sm. Class. Dict. s. v. Zephyrium a. Neub. Géogr. p. 391), a place mentioned in connection with R. Akiba's travels. Y. B. Kam. IX, end, 7ᵃ זופ׳; Sifré Num. s. 4 זופרי, זפרונה; Num. R. s. 8 זיפ׳; B. Kam. 113ᵃ זפר׳ (v. Rabb. D. S. a. l. note); Yalk. Num. 701 כופרי.

זִיפְ׳, זִפְלָן c. pl. (Syr. זפלן, P. Sm. 1146; פלא, v. פְּלָן, with preform. ז׳) *a certain number, so and so many.* Targ. II Esth. I, 8.

זָפַף (v. זוף a. זֶפֶת), *Pi.* זִיפֵּף *to line vessels with pitch.—Part. pass. Kal* זָפוּף, *Part. Pual* מְזוּפָּף. Tosef. Ab. Zar. IV (V), 10 זפופות; Ab. Zar. 33ᵃ מְזוּפָּפִין. B. Mets. 40ᵇ בכז׳ when the oil vessels are lined. V. זֶפֶת.

זֶפֶק m. (זפק, cmp. ספק, כּוֹפֶק; cmp. אִרְכֻּפְּקָא) *bird's crop.* Ḥull. III, 4. Ib. 6 (one of the signs of clean birds). Lam. R. to IV, 15 ז׳ של תרנגולת, v. שַׁלְפּוּחִית.

זֶפֶק, זַפְקָא ch. same. Targ. O. Lev. I, 16.—Targ. Y. Deut. XIV, 11 זפק; ib. Lev. XI, 13 זַפְקְתָא. V. זְלוּקְפָא.

זַפְקְתָא f., v. preced.

זִפְרִין, זִפְרוֹנָה, v. זִפִירִין.

זָקָה, v. זִיקָא II.

זָקוֹף m. (זקף, cmp. אסקופא) *lintel;* trnsf. *upper lip.* Targ. Ps. CXLI, 3 (h. text דַּל, cmp. דֶּלֶת).

זָקוּף, v. זָקַף.

זָקוֹף, pl. **זְקוֹפִין, זְקוֹפִים**, v. זְקִיפִין.

זְקוּפָה, זְקוּפָא f. (a. Hebraism, v. זָקַף) (קומא) קומה ז׳ *erect stature, pride.* Targ. Hos. XI, 7. Targ. Y. Lev. XXVI, 13. [זקיפה *gallows,* v. זְקִיפָא II.]

זְקוּקָה m. ch. (זקק) *strainer.* Y. Sabb. II, 5ᵃ top, v. דִּירְקְלִין.

זְקִינָה, v. זָקֵן II.

זָקַף *to erect,* v. זָקַף.

זְקִיף, זְקִיפָא I m. (preced.) 1) *erect, upright.* Pes. 40ᵃ ז׳ אסיר if it (the pot) stands upright (so that the moisture cannot run out), the grain is forbidden. [Ms. M. זִיקְפָא as a noun, *an upright standing vessel.*]—2) *elevated, projecting.* Targ. Y. Lev. XIII, 2 שומא ז׳ (h. text שְׂאֵת; some ed. זְקִיפָא).—*Pl.* זְקִיפִין. Targ. Y. Ex. XXVII, 2.

זְקִיפָא II (זִיקְפָא) m. (preced.) 1) *pole, scaffolding, gallows.* Targ. II Esth. II, 7; a. e.—Targ. I Chr. X, 10 בז׳.—Meg. 16ᵇ וי״ו . . . למימתחה כז׳ (Asheri כד ז׳; ed. זיק׳ incorr.; v. Rabb. D. S. a. l. note 6) you must extend the *Vav* of ויזתא (Esth. IX, 9) as long as a pole; כולהו בחד ז׳ וכ׳ (ed. זקיפה, Ms. H. 2 בז׳ חדא; Asheri בחדא ז׳) they were all hanged on one pole (at the same execution, v. infra).—B. Mets. 83ᵇ תותי ז׳ under the gallows. Ab. Zar. 18ᵇ אסקוה לז׳ they took him out for execution.—2) (part. pass. of זְקַף) *hanged, culprit.* B. Mets. 59ᵇ, v. דִּיוּקְתָא.—3) (fem.) *execution,* v. supra.

זְקִיפָא m. (preced.) *raising, lifting up.* Targ. Y. Gen. XV, 12. [Targ. Y. Lev. XVIII, 2, v. זְקִיפָא I.]

זְקִיפָה f. (זָקַף) *putting up, erection.* Ab. Zar. 46ᵃ דמינכרא זְקִיפָתָהּ the erection of which is noticeable.

Succ. 43b דלמא בז׳ perhaps the proper ceremony consists in posting it (by the side of the altar).—M.Kat. 24a, a. e. זְקִיפַת המטה the putting up of the couch (on the Sabbath during mourning), opp. כְּפִיָּיה.

זְקוֹפִין, זְקִיפִין m. pl. (זָקַף) *officers for restoring the line of battle, guards against desertions.* Sot. VIII, 6 (44a זקי׳; Y. ed. זְקוֹפִים, Rashi זוֹקְפִין). Gen. R. s. 98 זעקפי מלחמה (read זְקִיפֵי or זוֹקְפֵי).

זְקִיפְתָּא m. (זָקַף) *rising up.* Targ. Lam. III, 63. [Ab. Zar. 46a האי זקיפת׳, read: זְקִיפְתָּה, v. זְקִיפָה.]

זְקִירָא m. (זְקַר) *leap.* B. Kam. 22a top (Rashi: זְקִירָה h. fem.).

זְקִירָה f. (preced.) *leap,* v. preced.—R. Hash. 18a Ar., v. סְקִירָה a. זָקַר.

זְקִיתָא f. (זקק) [*the transparent one,* cmp. זְבוּגָא,] *chamæleon* (v. Sm. Ant. s. v.). Snh. 108b ed. (Ms. M. זקותא, Ms. F. רקיתא); Yalk. Gen. 59 (some ed. רקיתא). [Mus. derives our w. fr. זיקא, cmp. זַיְקָאנָא, the chamæleon being believed to live on air.]

זָקֵן I (b. h.) [*to be thin, shrunk, hard,*] *to be old.* Gen. R. s. 48 (ref. to Gen. XVIII, 13) ואני זָקַנְתִּי מלעשות וכ׳ am I (the Lord) too old to do wonders?

Hif. הִזְקִין 1) *to grow old.* Snh. 100b הִזְקִינָה שמא וכ׳ when she arrives at old age, he is afraid lest &c. Erub. 56a מַזְקִינִים בחצי וכ׳ they age in the middle of their days (prematurely). Sabb. 152a כל זמן שֶׁמַּזְקִינִין the older they grow; a. fr.—2) *to make old, consider old (feeble).* Gen. R. s. 48 אתם . . . ומזקינים חביריכם you consider each himself young, and each his partner old (Yalk. ib. 82 ומז׳ אדוניכם and believe your Lord too old [to do wonders]); v. supra.

Nif. נִזְקַן, *Nithpa.* נִזְדַּקֵּן 1) *to become old, weak, frail.* Y. Ber. IX, end 14c (ref. to prov. XXIII, 22) אם נִזְדַּקְּנָה אומתך וכ׳ if thy nation is decaying (in faith), stand up and fence her in (prevent her being trodden upon); Yalk. Prov. 960.—2) (cmp. דקדק) *to be maturely considered, be clear* (beyond doubt);—3) (cmp. קשיש) *to be hard, difficult.* Tosef. Snh. VII, 7 (the presiding judge declares) נִזְקַן הדין (נִיזְקַן) ed. Zuck. (Var. נזדקן, נזדקק); discussed in Snh. 42a מאי נזד׳ הדין what does *nizdakken* mean? Does it mean קש דינא the case is hard (difficult, so as to demand a reconsideration)? . . . . It means חכם דינא the case is clear; Y. Snh. V, end, 23a.

זְקֵן ch. same.

Af. אַזְקֵן 1) *to make old, weaken.* Erub. 56a הני מולייתא אַזְקְנוּן . . those ascents . . . made us (me) old, v. בִּירָאר.—2) *to grow old.* Nidd. 47a אַזְקְנָא לה (some ed. אזקונא, Asheri אזקנה) this would be a sign that she has entered old age (passed the change of life).

זָקֵן II m. (b. h.; preced.) 1) *old man.* Gen. R. s. 39, opp. בחור. Y. Bicc. III, 65c bot. עמידת ז׳ (Yalk. Lev. 670 מצות ז׳) the duty of standing up before an old man. Hag. 14a; a. fr.—2) *elder, judge, scholar.* Ib. (ref. to Is. III, 2) ז׳ זה שראוי וכ׳ *zaken* means one fit to sit in college sessions. Ber. 8b ז׳ ששכח וכ׳ a scholar who forgot what he had learned, &c., v. אוֹנֶס. Kidd. 32b אין ז׳ אלא חכם under *zaken* (Lev. XIX, 32) a scholar is meant; Sifra K'dosh. Par. 3, ch. VII אין זקן אלא זה שקנה חכמה a *zaken* is he who has acquired wisdom (through study).—ז׳ אשמאי, v. אַשְׁמַאי. Yoma 28b ז׳ ויושב בישיבה a scholar and member of college. Y. M Kat. III, beg. 81c איני מכירך ז׳ I shall not recognize thee as (give thee the diploma of) a *zaken;* a. fr.—*Pl.* זְקֵנִים. Snh. I, 3, v. סְמִיכָה. Num. R. s. 14 מצות הז׳ rabbinical law. Ber. 11a זִקְנֵי ב״ש the graduates of the Shammai school; a. v. fr.—3) *grandfather, ancestor.* Ex. R. s. 1 מעשה זְקֵנָן the conduct of their ancestor (Abraham). Pesik. Zakh., p. 27b; a. fr.—Fem. זְקֵנָה, זְקֵינָה. 1) *old woman.* Gen. R. s. 39.—Nidd. 9a ז׳ *one who is past the change of life.* Ibb; a. fr.—2) *grandmother, ancestress.* Kidd. 31b הוה ליה ההיא אמא זקי׳ had a grandmother. Gen. R. s. 93 זְקֵינָתוֹ של זה this man's (my) ancestress (Sarah); a. e.—3) (sub. נְטִיעָה) *old plantation.* Tosef. Shebi. I, 2; a. e., opp. נטיעה young plantation.—*Pl.* זְקֵינוֹת. Y. ib. I, 33b bot.; a. e.

זָקָן m. (b. h.; cmp. דִּקְן) *beard, hair-covered spot.* Ber. 11a זְקָנְךָ וכ׳ thy beard is &c., v. גָּדַל. Snh. VIII, 1 (68b) עד שיקיף ז׳ התחתון וכ׳ until he grows a beard, by which is meant the hair of the genitals &c.; a. fr.—*Pl.* זְקָנִים. Lev. R. s. 3.

זִקְנָה f. (b. h.; זָקֵן) *old age; frailty.* Ber. 39a ז׳ אין כאן is there not (the claim of) old age here?—Sabb. 152a ז׳ קופצת עליו frailty of old age will overtake him (prematurely). B. Bath. 120a מפלג בז׳ extremely old. Snh. 17a, a. e. בעלי ז׳ men commanding repect for their age. B. Mets. 87a; Snh. 107b עד אברהם לא הואי ז׳ (v. Rabb. D. S. a. l. note 1) up to Abraham's days, there was no distinction in appearance of old age (v. Gen. XXIV, 1); a. fr.

זִקְנוּת f. same. Kidd. 82b זקנותו (interch. with זִקְנָתוֹ). Y. Bets. I, 60c bot. שימרתי כחי לזיקנותי I save my strength for my old age; a. fr.

זִקְנְתָא, זִקְנוּתָא ch. same. Targ. Ps. LXXI, 18 (Ms. זקנו׳).

זָקַף (b. h.) 1) *to join, put together, put up, erect, restore* (to proper position). Bets. II, 6 אין זוֹקְפִין וכ׳ you must not set up (put together the links of) a lamp on a Holy Day (v. ib. 22a). M. Kat. 27a מאימתי זוֹקְפִין וכ׳ from what time on the eve of the Sabbath are the mourners' couches put up again? Ab. Zar. 46a ז׳ לבינה וכ׳ if one put a brick up to worship it, v. זְקִיפָה; a. fr.—Part. pass. זָקוּף, f. זְקוּפָה. M. Kat. III, 7 מטה ז׳ a put-up couch, opp. מ׳ כפויה an upset couch whereon mourners are seated; a. fr.—2) (cmp. לָוָה a. Lat. nexus) *to establish a loan, to obligate, enjoin upon* (with עַל). B. Mets. 72a וְזוֹקְפָן עליו במלוה and the creditor settles the interests on the debtor as a loan (the note stating the combined amount of principle and interest as principle). Gitt. 18a עד שתפגום וְתִזְקוֹף until she accepts partial payment (of her widowhood) and settles the balance as a loan (by

taking a note &c.). **Ib.** זָקְפָה ולא פגמה if she allows her **widowhood** to be entered as a loan without taking a partial payment. Ib. אונס ... שזְקָפָן במלוה indemnity for outrage, fines . . . which were settled in the way of a loan; a. e.—3) (neut. verb) *to stand upright, to be restored again.* B. Mets. 59[b] לא נפלו . . ולא זָקְפוּ the bent walls did not fall, nor did they assume their straight position. Ber. 11[a] וז׳ ר׳ ישמ׳ R. Y. remained upright, opp. הִטָּה. Ib. כשאני . . אתה זָקַפְתָּ when I bowed, thou didst remain upright. Y. ib. IV, beg. 7[a] זוֹקֵף he erects himself (from his bowed position).—Part. pass. זָקוּף, f. זְקוּפָה *upright, erect.* Ber. l. c.—קומה זקופה erect stature, *proud carriage.* Ib. 43[b]; a. fr.

Nif. נִזְקַף 1) *to be put up, to erect one's self.* Tosef. ib. I, 6; Sifré Deut. 34; a. e.—2) *to be converted into a loan.* Gitt. l. c. מאימתי נִזְקָפִים במלוה from what time are fines &c. considered as converted loans (so as to be subject to limitation)?

זְקַף, זְקוֹף ch. same, 1) *to put up, rear, erect, raise* (arms, head &c.). Targ. Gen. XXXI, 45. Targ. Y. Ex. XVII, 11 זְקִיף; a. fr.—Bets. 22[a] ז׳ לה לשרגא he put the lamp up. M. Kat. 25[a] זַקְפֵיה לארוניה he set his coffin upright.—*Part. pass.* זְקִיף q. v.—2) *to stand erect.* Targ. Job XXIX, 8. Ib. XXIV, 24 זקופי Ms. (ed. אוריכו) stand undiscouraged (wait).—3) *to hang up.* Targ. I Chr. X, 10; a. e.—Part. pass. זְקִיף *hanged.* B. Mets. 59[b], v. דִּיזְקְתָא.

Af. אַזְקִיף *to elevate,* Targ. Ps. XXX, 2 (Regia *Pe.*; h. text דלה).

Ithpa. אִזְדַּקַּף, *Ithpe.* אִזְדְּקִיף 1) *to be erect, to rise.* Targ. Gen. XXXVII, 7. Targ. Ps. XXI, 14; a. e.—2) *to be hanged.* Meg. 16[b] אִזְדַּקִּיפוּ, v. זְקִיפָא II.

זְקִפוּתָא f. (preced.) *raising, lifting up.* Targ. Ps. CXLI, 2.

זָקַק (b. h.; cmp. זכך a. דקק) [*to make thin, fine, clear,*] 1) *to distil, smelt,* v. *Pi.*—2) (cmp. צָרַף) *to rivet, forge; to chain, to join; to bind, obligate.*—*Part. pass.* זָקוּק, f. זְקוּקָה; pl. זְקוּקִים, זְקוּקִין, f. זְקוּקוֹת, with ל *chained to, connected with, dependent on.* Men. 27[a] העושין פירות יהיו ז׳ וכ׳ the fruit-bearing species of the festive wreath shall be combined with those which bear no fruits. Y. Ber. VI, 10[a] bot. כשהיו כולן ז׳ וכ׳ when they were, all of them, dependent on one loaf (for saying grace). Pesik. R. s. 43 כנגד שלש . . . זקוקות להן (not זקוקין) corresponding to the three laws for which, our Rabbis taught, women are made responsible (Sabb. II, 6). Y. Ab. Zar. II, 41[a] top ז׳ למלכות in constant intercourse with the government.—Num. R. s. 9 לשנים היא זקוקה she is responsible to two (her husband and the Lord).—Shebu. VI, 3 נכסים ..... זוֹקְקִין וכ׳ movable chattel binds the immovable with reference to the obligation of making oath, i. e. the two claims preferred in one suit are considered as one lawsuit, and the oath must refer to both; Y. Keth. XII, 36[a] bot. [read:] לזוֹקְקָן לשבועה to combine the two (as one lawsuit) with regard to the oath. Yeb. II, 5 זוקק את וכ׳ he holds his brother's wife tied to the leviratical marriage, i. e. she cannot marry otherwise until released from him; a. fr. V. זִיקָה.

Nif. נִזְקַק (cmp. זָוַג *Nithpa.*) 1) *to join, meet; to be engaged in.* Gen. R. s. 20 מעולם לא נ׳ וכ׳ the Lord never engaged in communication with woman. Ib. s. 42; Pesik. R. s. 5; a. e. נ׳ המלך וכ׳ the king was attached to, took an interest in the affairs of the country. Sabb. 12[b] אין מ״ה נִזְקָקִין לו the angels do not attend to his prayers.—[2) (in a hostile sense) *to attack.* Gen. R. l. c. באו ברברים לִיזָּקֵק לו (Pesik. R. l. c.; Ruth R. introd., a. e. לְהִזְדַּוֵּוג) Barbarians came to attack him.]—3) *to live with; to be coupled.* Ruth R. to IV, 3 ע״מ שלא אֶזָּקֵק לה with the condition that I will not live with her. Gen. R. s. 20 איני נִזְקֶקֶת וכ׳ I shall never again live with &c.—Pesik. R. s. 15; Pesik. Haḥod., p. 43[b] שיהא אדם נִזְקָק לביתו in order that man be attached to his house (love his wife); Yalk. Ps. 738; a. e.

Hif. הִזְקִיק *to oblige.* Succ. 28[a] הִזְקַקְתּוּנִי וכ׳ will you force me to say &c.?

Hof. הוּזְקַק *to be made dependent on, to obligate one's self, to be obliged to regard.* B. Bath. 170[a] אם הוּזְקְקוּ וכ׳ Ms. M. (ed. אם כתוב בו הוּזְקַקְנוּ) if they (the parties to the deed) bound themselves to depend on the signatures of witnesses, &c. (ed. if it was written in the document, we obligate ourselves &c.).

Nithpa. נִזְדַּקֵּק 1) *to be engaged in, to care.* Tanḥ. Korah 6 לא נִזְדַּקְּקוּ לחשיבו (Yalk. Num. 750 נִזְקְקוּ) they did not care to answer him.—2) *to attach one's self to, to make love to.* Num. R. s. 9.—3) (in an evil sense) *to get at, to harm.* Ib. s. 5 בקש לְהִזְדַּקֵּק להם wanted to harm them.

Pi. זִיקֵּק (b. h.) *to smelt, refine, distil.* Lev. R. s. 31 עד שמְזַקְּקוֹ until he has refined the gold.—*Part. pass.* מְזוּקָּק, f. מְזוּקֶּקֶת. Pesik. R. s. 14 התורה .... ומז׳ וכ׳ the Torah is clarified and distilled in forty nine ways.—2) *to chain, tie, connect.*—Part. pass. as ab. Y. Ḥag. III, beg. 78[d] במז׳ לקדש it treats of an object which is tied (has been made subject) to the law regulating sacred matter, i. e. treated as if it were sacred matter, v. טָהֳרָה.

זְקַק ch. same, 1) *to refine.*—*Part. pass.* זְקִיק. Targ. Ps. XII, 7. Targ. Cant. I, 11; a. e.—2) *to chain.* Part. pass. as above. Targ. Is. LX, 11 זְקִיקִין led in chains (h. text נהוגים).—3) *to obligate.* Part. pass. as ab. Y. Ber. I, 3[c] bot. זְקִיקִינָן למברכה we are bound to say the blessing. Y. B. Mets. X, beg. 12[c] ז׳ את וכ׳ thou art bound to carry me (the lower story must be kept in repair at the expense of its owner). Ib. דאינון זקוקין (read: זקי׳).

Pa. זַקֵּיק 1) *to refine.*—Part. pass. מְזוּקָּק (Hebraism). Targ. Cant. I, 11.—2) *to obligate, tie.* Yeb. 22[b] top מיזקק נמי זַקִּיקָה Rashi (ed. זקיק) he (the bastard brother) also ties her (prevents her from remarrying).

Ithpa. אִזְדַּקַּק, contr. אִיזַּקַּק *to be cleared.* Targ. Y. II Num. V, 19 הִדַּכַּי (h. text הִנָּקִי).

Ithpe. אִיזְדְּקִיק as preced. *Nif.* Ned. 77[a] איזדקיקו ליה רבנן וכ׳ the Rabbis attended to (the absolution from vows of) the son &c. Ib., sq. א׳ ליה רב וכ׳ Rab attended to Rabbah's vows in a private room of the school-house &c.—Y. Keth. II, 26[c] bot. אִיזְדְּקִיק וכ׳ to sleep with &c.

זַקָּק m. (denom. of זִיקָא II; cmp. זִיקוּקָא II) *maker of and dealer in leather bags.*—*Pl.* זַקָּקִין. Mikv. IX, 5 ז׳ של saddles used by the dealers in hose (Ar.: של זיקקין saddles on which hose is carried).

זָקַר (cmp. Syr. זקר P. Sm. 1151) 1) *to thrust, fling.* Yoma 67[b] זוֹקְרוֹ בת וכ׳ Ar. a. Mss. M. 2 a. O. (ed. זורקו, v. Rabb. D. S. a. l. note), v. בַּת II.—2) *to cast lots; to decide.*

Nif. נִזְקַר, *Nithpa.* נִזְדַּקֵּר 1) *to be thrown; to leap, to stagger.* Ib. 38[b], v. בַּת II.—2) *to be decided upon, to be decreed upon.* Erub. 52[b] למקום שרובו הוא נזקר (Var. נזר׳) he is judged to belong to where the larger portion of his body is.—R. Hash. 18[a] כולן נזקרין בזקירה אחת Ar. (Var. Ar., a. ed. נסקרין . . . בסקירה) the fate of all of them is decided in one decree.—Ber. 46[a] אל יִזְדַּקֵּר וכ׳ (Alf. a. oth. יִזְדַּקֵּק, v. זָקַק, v. Rabb. D. S. a. l. note 40) may there not occur to him (our host) or to us anything that suggests sin &c.

זְקַר ch. same, *Ithpa.* אִזְדַּקַּר *to leap forth, to leap with joy; to stagger, reel.* Gitt. 57[a] אִזְדַּקּוּר וכ׳ they leaped and ate and drank. Nidd. 17[b] אִזְדַּקְּרָה she staggered, jumped backward; ib. 57[b].—Lev. R. s. 5 (ref. to Is. XXII, 17, v. גֶּבֶר) כהדא תרנגולא .... מְזַדַּקֵּר Ar. (in ed. a. Yalk. Is. 291 our w. omitted) like a (slaughtered) cock that rolls from place to place in spasmodic thrusts.

זִיקָ׳, זְקָתָא, זְקַת m. (זקת *to sting*, P. Sm. 1151; cmp. זִיקָא ,זִיק) *goad.* Targ. I Sam. XIII, 21 (h. text הַדָּרְבָן). Targ. Prov. XIV, 3 (some ed. זק׳, corr. acc.).—*Pl.* זְקָתִין, זִיקָ׳. Targ. Koh. XII, 11. [B. Mets. 94[a], v. זִיקְתָא.]

זַר, v. זֵיר.

זָר m. (b. h.; v. זור a. זרר) 1) *stranger;* (in Talm. mostly) *non-priest, layman.* Zeb. II, 1. Ib. 14[a]; Yoma 49[a]; a. fr.—Fem. זָרָה. Yeb. 85[b] ותהא ז׳ וכ׳ granted that she is not of a priestly family;—is not a lay-woman permitted &c.?—2) *oppressor, enemy.* Y. Ned. IX, beg. 41[b] (ref. to אל זר, Ps. LXXXI, 10) זר שבקרבך וכ׳ do not make the enemy within thyself thy king; Sabb. 105[b] איזהו אל זר וכ׳ which is the tyrannical power within thee?—Ex. R. s. 34 (play on זֵר a. זָר, v. זֵיר) if one is worthy נעשים לו זר ואם לאו זר they are to him a crown, if not—an enemy; Tanh. Vayakh. 8.—Fem. זָרָה. Yoma 72[b] נעשית לו ז׳ Ms. O. (Ms. M. נעשית ז׳ ממנו) the Law appears to him a tyrant (Ms. M. she becomes estranged from him, v. זור).—3) *outcast; shunned, loathsome* (v. זָרָא). Num. R. s. 7 (play on זָרָא, Num. XI, 20) והיאך נעשה ז׳ וכ׳ and how does he become an outcast? Leprosy overcomes him.—*Pl.* זָרִים. Ib. ז׳ מן הקהל excluded from the congregation.—Zeb. III, 1; a. fr.

זָר ch. same. Targ. Ps. XLIV, 19, v. זְהֵה.—Sabb. 82[b], v. כְּבַר.

זָרָא m. (b. h.; v. preced. a. next w.) *nausea, loathing.* Num. R. s. 7; Lev. R. s. 18, v. הוֹרָא III, הַדְרָיָא ,זָרָנָא.

זְרָא, v. זרי ch.

זֵרָב m. (v. next w.) *rim, lining, trimming.* Kil. IX, 7 מנעול של ז׳ Ms. M. a. oth. (v. Rabb. D. S. a. l. note; ed. זרד) a cloth-lined shoe; Y. ib. 32[d] top.

זָרַב *to surround, line, trim.* Y. Kil. IX, 32[d] top (ref. to מנעול של זרב, v. preced.) אית אתרין דזַרְבִין עימרא וכ׳ (not עימיה) there are places where they put wool around the shoe from inside.

Ithpe. אִזְדְּרִיב (denom. of preced.) *to be made to flow over the rim, to be upset.* Yoma 78[a] משום דמִזְדְּרִיב ed. (Ar. משום דאתי לא׳, Ms. O. דילמא אתי לאִזְדַּרְבּוּיֵי, v. Rabb. D. S. a. l. note 70) because the silver vessel (being smooth) may be upset and liquid flow over. V. זְרִיזָה.

זַרְבּוּבִית f. (v. זָרַב) *a tray* or *saucer* fastened to the bottom of a drinking vessel for the reception of drippings; in gen. *saucer, dish, disk.* Pesik. R. s. 35 שנדמה כז׳ קטנה וכ׳ (ed. Fr. זרבוכ׳, corr. acc.) whose face appeared (over the camp) like a small disk of fire; Yalk. Dan. 1062 כבבית (corr. acc., or כִּגְרִיגַת).—*Pl.* זַרְבּוּבִיּוֹת. Lev. R. s. 5; Num. R. s. 10 (expl. מזרקי, Am. VI, 6) כוסות שיש להם ז׳ cups with saucers; Yalk. Am. 545 שאין בהם זכיכית (corr. acc.).

זרבונין, v. זַרְבּוּזָה.

***זַרְגּוֹן** m. (v. זרג a. denom. P. Sm. 1154) *zargon*, name of a plant, prob. a species of *beet.* Y. Kil. I, 27[a] bot. ז׳ ולפת *z.* crossed with carrot. [It is evident that our w. cannot mean a vine-shoot, as Fl. to Levy Talm. Dict. I, 564, a. Löw Pfl. p. 87 suggest.—R. S. to Kil. I, 4 reads זגדין or וגדין.]

***זַרְגּוּנָה** m. *zargunah*, name of a *tree* or *shrub* with copious twigs, but bare beneath. Y. Succ. III, beg. 53[c].

זֶרֶד m. (v. זרז) 1) *strength, alertness, valor.* Yoma 47[a] (a metaphor in imitation of Prov. XXXI, 29) כל הנשים . . ז׳ זַרְדוּ וז׳ אמי עלת׳ לגג Ar. (read עלה; ed. הנשים זרדו וז׳ אימא וכ׳; Ms. M. זֶרֶז זָרְזוּ אימא, insert ז׳; Ms. M. 2 זריד זרדו וז׳; v. Rabb. D. S. a. l. note) all women have done valiantly, but the valor of my mother excelled them all (a metaphor of careful maternity).—2) (v. next w.) pl. זְרָדִין, זְרָדִים *shoots, greens.* Tosef. Sabb. IX (X), 16; Sabb. 103[a] הַמְזָרֵד ז׳ וכ׳ he who cuts greens, if for human food &c. Ib. XVIII, 2 (126[b]) חבילי ז׳ bundles of greens (young reeds &c., available for fodder); ib. 128[a]; Tosef. ib. XIV (XV), 10 זרדן ed. Zuck. (read זרדין, Var. דים . .).—Esp. לולבי ז׳ *the young sprouts of the service-tree*, the interior of which is eaten as a relish. Shebi. VII, 5. Tosef. Sabb. VIII (IX), 9 לולברן וז׳ (corr. acc.); Tosef. Maas. Sh. I, 13; Tosef. Ukts. III, 9; Ukts. III, 4.—3) pr. n. (b. h.) *Zered*, name of a brook, נחלא דז׳. Targ. O. Num. XXI, 12; a. e.—Tosef. Shebi. IV, 11; Y. ib. VI, 36[c]; Sifré Deut. 51 דוירד; Yalk. Deut. 874 נחלת דור (corr. acc.); v. Hildesh. Beitr. p. 66.

זַרֵד (denom. of preced.) ז׳ זֶרֶד (=עשה חיל) *to do valiantly.* Yoma 47[a], v. preced.

Pi. זֵירֵד [*to strengthen, accelerate growth*; cmp. בְּרָא *Af.*,] *to trim, nip shoots off.* Sabb. XII, 2 המקרסם והמְזָרֵד he who cuts off dry twigs, or young shoots. Ib. 103[a], v. preced. Ab. Zar. III, 10 (49[b]). Tosef. Sabb. IX (X), 16 וזֵרֵד ed. Zuck. (Var. וזירד).

זַרְדָּא m. (זרד) *coat of mail, armour* (v. P. Sm. 1154, sq. s. vv. זרדא, זרגנא, זרגא). Sabb. 62[a], expl. שריון.

זרדן, Tosef. Sabb. XIV (XV), 10, v. זֶרֶד pl.

זַרְדְּתָא (זַרְתָּא) f. (זרד) *bushes of sorb*, or *service-tree*, growing in unhealthy marshes (v. Löw. Pfl. p. 289) Pes. 111[b] דבי ז׳ שידי (v. Rabb. D. S. a. l. note 400) the spirits of the sorb-bushes are named *shiddé* (demons). Ib. ז׳ סמיכא למתא וכ׳ a sorb-bush near a town has no less than sixty *shiddé*; [Ms. M. זַרְתָּא, זירדְתָא, זַרְדְּתָא; v. Rabb. D. S. a. l. notes).—Kidd. 73[b] ז׳ . . . יש בו וכ׳ a child exposed in a sorb-bush near a town (where it is likely to die) is considered a foundling (אֲסוּפִי). Keth. 79[a] אבא ז׳ וכ׳ a forest (of timber), a sorb plantation and a fish-pond.

זָרָה, fem. of זָר q. v.

זָרָה' I, II, v. זרי I, II.

***מְלַח דְּז׳, זַרְוַאי** pr. n. pl. *Melaḥ d'Zarvai*, a border place on the east side of the Jordan. Tosef. Shebi. IV, 11 מלח דז׳ Var. (ed. Zuck. מלי חורואי); Y. Shebi. VI, 36[c] מלח דזרכאיי (read זַרְ׳=זַרְבָ׳, v. Hildesh. Beitr. p. 61, sq.); Sifré Deut. s. 51 עלית זירוא; Yalk. ib. 874 מילית ווירואר. [Hildesh. l. c. a. Neub. Géogr. p. 20 emend מוּלְיָא or מְלִתָא (מליתא) for מלח.]

זָרוּז, pl. **זָרוּזִין**, v. זֵירוּז.

זְרוֹעַ f. (b. h.) *arm*; (with animals) *fore-leg*, *shoulder*; *strength*, *force*. Ber. 17[b] ניזונין בז׳ receive their sustenance from the Lord by dint of their strength (virtue), opp. בצדקה by divine grace. Y. Taan. IV, 69[a] top זְרוֹעָן של כל ישראל the arm (defence, protection) of all Israel. Sabb. 56[a] נטלו בז׳ they took by force. Lev. R. s. 2 כבא על חבירו בז׳ like one coming against his neighbor with force (confident of victory).—Ḥull. X, 1 הז׳ the law concerning the shoulder as the priest's share (Deut. XVIII, 3). Ib. 98[a] ז׳ בשלה, v. בָּשֵׁל; a. fr.—*Pl.* זְרוֹעוֹת, constr. זְרוֹעֵי. Sot. 49[b]; Tosef. ib. XIV, 3 ז׳ תורה the supports of the Law.—בעלי ז׳ violent men. B. Mets. 118[a]; a. e.

זְרוּעַ, זֵרוּ׳ m. (=b. h. זֵרוּעַ; זרע) *sowing*; *seed*. Targ. O. Lev. XI, 37.—*Pl.* זֵרוּעִין, זֵרּ׳. Targ. Is. LXI, 11 זֵרוּעֲהָא (ed. Lag. זֵירוּעָהּ sing.). [Y. Sabb. IX, 12[a] top; Y. Kil. III, beg. 28[c] (ref. to Is. l. c.) זֵירוּעֶיהָ מלא *zerûēha* is spelt *plene* (with ו); v. ראנא.]

זָרוֹק pr. n., נהר ז׳, v. רֶזֶק.

זְרוּקִינְיָא pr. n. pl. *Z'rukinya*, in Babylonia. Ḥull. 111[a].

זְרוּקְפָא, v. זְלוּקְפָא.

זרורזי, Cant. R. to II, 9, v. זְרַז I.

זָרוּת f. (denom. of זָר) *the legal status of the non-priest*, *the laws concerning non-priests*. Y. Ter. V, 43[c] איסור ז׳ the prohibition as far as it concerns the T'rumah to be eaten by non-priests. Y. Bicc. II, 65[a] היתר ז׳ inasmuch as they are permitted to non-priests. Y. Orl. II, end, 62[c] משום ז׳ for violating the law forbidding non-priests &c.—Yeb. 68[b], a. e. (ref. to וכל זר, Lev. XXII, 10) ז׳ אמרתי לך וכ׳ the Law treats of non-priests, but not of the mourners; a. e.

זָרַז (reduplic. of זר, v. זרר; cmp. אזר) *to be strong*, *vigorous*, *quick*, v. זָרַד.—Part. pass. זָרוּז, v. זָרִיז.

Pi. זֵרֵז 1) *to strengthen*, *to make active and ready*, *to instigate*. Pes. 89[a] קאמר . . כדי לזָרְזָן he said so in order to awaken their emulation in religious acts. Nidd. 31[a]; Yoma 47[a] זֵירְזָתְנִי, v. זָרָה I.—*Part. pass.* מְזוֹרָז a) *strong*, *vigorous*. Nidd. l. c.; Snh. 70[b]; a. e., v. לָבָן II.—b) *active*, *zealous to do good*, *valiant*. Macc. 23[a] אין מְזָרְזִין אלא למְזוֹרָזִין Ar. (ed. מזורז; some ed. מזרז, corr. acc.) only the strong-minded it is worth encouraging; Yalk. Deut. 937; Sifré Num. 1 לִמְזוֹרָזִים; a. e.—2) (with ב) *to admonish*, *be severe*. Tanḥ. Korah 6 התחיל מְזָרֵז בהן (Num. R. s. 18 לדבר להם) he began to speak to them earnestly.

Hithpa. הִזְדָּרֵז, *Nithpa.* נִזְדָּרֵז 1) *to be alert*, *zealous*, *conscientious*. Pesik. R. s. 6 (ref. to מהיר, Prov. XXII, 29) נִזְדָּרַזְתָּ במלאכתך thou hast been zealous (conscientious) in thy own occupation. Tanḥ P'kudé 11; a. fr.—V. זָרִיז.—3) *to be armed*. Yalk. Num. 785, v. next w.

זְרַז I, *Pa.* זָרֵיז same; 1) *to be quick*, *to hurry*. Targ. Y. II Gen. XXIV, 20 (h. text מהר).—Targ. Ps. LXX, 2 זָרֵיז ed. (Ms. זָ׳; h. text חוש); a. e.—*Part. Pe.* זָרִיז, *Pa.* מְזָרֵז; pl. מְזָרְזִין, זָרְזִין, זְרִיזִין. Targ. Y. I, II Num. IX, 8, opp. מתון; v. also זָרִיז.—2) *to quicken*, *strengthen*. Yeb. 102[b] (expl. יחליץ, Is. LVIII, 11) זָרוּזֵי גרמי it means quickening the bones. Cant. R. to II, 10 זָרוּזִי גרמיך (not זרורזי) make thyself ready; Pesik. R. s. 15 זָרֵזִי.—3) (cmp. אֲזַר, זְיַר) *to tie around*, *gird*, *arm*; *to harness*, *saddle*. Targ. O. Gen. XIV, 14. Targ. Job XXXVIII, 3 זָרֵיז Ms. (ed. זְרַז, זָרֵיז). Targ. O. Ex. XXIX, 9; a. fr. —*Part. pass.* מְזָרַז, pl. מְזָרְזִין, מְזָרְזַיָּא *armed*. Ib. XIII, 18. Targ. Is. XV, 4; a. fr.—Yeb. l. c. (ref. to וחלצה, Deut. XXV, 9) ואימא זָרוּזֵי הוא may I not say, it means *tying on?*

Ithpa. אִזְדָּרַז, *Ithpe.* אִזְדְּרִיז 1) *to strengthen one's self* (so as not to give way to emotion). Targ. Y. Gen. XLIII, 31. Targ. Esth. V, 10.—2) *to gird one's self*, *be armed*. Targ. Num. XXXII, 17; 20; a. e.—Targ. Prov. XXX, 31, v. זַרְפַּל.—Sifré Num. s. 157 אין החלצו אלא אִיזְדָּרְזוּ *heḥal'tsu* (Num. XXXI, 3) means, be armed; Yalk. ib. 785 הִזְדָּרְזוּ (Hebr.).

זְרָז (זְרִיז) m. (preced.) 1) *strength*, *valor*, v. זְרַד.—2) *belt*, *belt-saddle*. Kel. XXIII, 2 זָ׳ האשקלוני Ar. a. ed. Dehr. (ed. זריז) the Ashkelonian saddle; Sifra M'tsora, Zabim, Par. 2, ch. III; Yalk. Lev. 568 זהו האשתונית (corr. acc.).—*Pl.* זְרָזִין, constr. זַרְזֵי (זְרִיזֵי). Erub. 18[b] ז׳ תאנים *garments* of fig-leaves (v. next w.).

זְרָז II, זְרָזָא, זְרִיז ch. same. Targ. I Sam. XVIII, 4; a. fr.—Targ. Is. V, 27 זְרִיז (constr., ed. Lag. זרז).—*Pl.* זַרְזִין, זְרָזִין *garments*, *equipment*. Targ. O. Gen. III, 7 (h. text חֲגֹרֹת). Targ. Jud. XIV, 19 זרזיהון ed. Lag. (ed. Wil. זְרָזָהוֹן, h. text חליצות׳).—Targ. Ps. LXXXIII, 15 זַרְזֵי טוריא the *crests* of mountains (cmp. זִיר; Ms. דְּרֵי, v. דְּרָא I).

זַרְזֵף, זַרְזֵיף (redupl. of זרף, v. זרב) *to flow over*. Cant. R. to I, 3 מה השמן . . . מְזָרְזֵף בשאר . . . מְזַרְזְפִים וכ׳ (not כשאר) as oil on top of another liquid, when the cup is full, does not flow over with other liquids, so will the words of the Law not flow over (the lips) in connection with words of frivolity.

זַרְזִיפָא m., pl. **זַרְזִיפֵי** (preced.) *squirtings from a vessel poured out from a height.* Yoma 87ª ז׳ דמיא (Var. זַרְזִיפְתָּא f., pl. זַרְזִיפָתָא, v. Rabb. D. S. a. l. note 6). [Cmp. b. h. זַרְזִיף.]

זַרְזִיר I, זַרְזָר m. (v. זִירָה) *wrestler, antagonist, gladiator.* Y. R. Hash. I, 57ª bot. זה . . לנצח זַרְזִירוֹ וכ׳ each is anxious to defeat his antagonist.—*Pl.* זַרְזָרִין, זַרְזִירִין. Lam. R. to V, 1 אדם . . שני זרזירין . . . כובש וכ׳ (not כבוש) if a man trains two gladiators in his house, he will restrain the stronger one &c. [Bib. Hebr. זַרְזִיר *quick*, or *armed*, v. זרז.]

זַרְזִיר II m. (Syr. זרזירא P. Sm. 1156, Ar. *zurzur;* prob. fr. זור *to circle*) *starling,* also (collect.) *flock of starlings.* Hull. 62ª לחביא את הז׳ (Sifra Sh'mini, Par. 3, ch. V חַזַּרְזִירִים, Ar. . . . רין) to include the starling (in the genus raven). Hull. l. c.; B. Kam. 92ᵇ (prov.) לא לחנם הלך ז׳ וכ׳ not without cause does the starling follow the raven &c.; Gen. R. s. 65, beg. Ib. עלה ז׳ אחד וכ׳ a flock of starlings came to Palestine.—*Pl.* זַרְזִירִים, זַרְזִירִין. Ib. s. 75 אין שני ז׳ וכ׳ two flocks of starlings cannot sleep on one board (two nations cannot rule at the same time). Tosef. Hull. III (IV), 23.

זַרְזִיף, v. זַרְזִיפָא.

זַרְזָר, pl. **זַרְזָרִין**, v. זַרְזִיר I.

זָרַח (b. h.; cmp. next w.) [*to spread,*] *to shine, sparkle, rise* (cmp. הָנֵץ). Hull. 91ᵇ וכי שמש . . . זָרְחָה did the sun rise for him (Jacob) alone? Y. Snh. VIII, end, 26ᶜ . . . וכי החמה זורחת does the sun shine on him (the thief) alone? a. fr.—Tanh. Tsav 13, a. fr. צרעת זרחה וכ׳ leprosy broke out on &c.

Hif. הִזְרִיחַ 1) *to make shine.* Gen. R. s. 22 ה׳ לו הצרעת the Lord made leprosy glisten on his face. Ib. ה׳ . . . חמה he caused the globe of the sun to shine bright for him (a sign of pardon). Lev. R. s. 28, beg. דיין שהקב״ה מַזְרִיחַ וכ׳ it is reward enough for them that the Lord lets the sun rise &c. Macc. 10ª (ref. to מזרחה, Deut. IV, 41) הִזְרַחְתָּ שמש וכ׳ let the sun shine on unwilling manslayers (give them safety). Ib. הִזְרַחְתָּ וכ׳ thou (Moses) hast &c.—2) (neut. verb) *to glisten.* Shebi. IV, 7 משיַזְרִיחוּ (Ms. M. משהַ׳) when the young figs begin to glisten.—3) (denom. of מִזְרָח) *to go east.* Gen. R. s. 61, end (ref. to Gen. XXV, 6) כל מה . . . . לְהַזְרִיחַ תַּזְרִיחוּ go as far east as you can.

זָרָה, זרי I (b. h.) *to scatter, to winnow.* Sabb. VII, 2 הזוֹרֶה he who winnows (on the Sabbath).—Ib. 73ᵇ היינו זורה וכ׳ is not winnowing the same process as sifting &c.?—Ab. Zar. III, 3 שוחק וזורה לרוח he must grind it and cast it to the wind; a. fr.—Euphem. *to emit semen.* Gen. R. s. 85, v. הוּשׁ.

Pi. זֵירָה same, also *to sift, select.* Pesik. R. s. 10 שיחקו וזי׳ וכ׳ he ground and scattered it &c.—Nidd. 31ª; Yoma 47ª (ref. to ותזרני II Sam. XXII, 40, a. ותאזרני Ps. XVIII, 40) זֵירִיתַנִי וזרזתני thou didst sift me (select the best semen for embryonic formation, cmp. זֶרַד) and make me healthy.

זְרָא, זרי ch. same, *to scatter.* Targ. O. Ex. XXXII, 20 (Var. דרא).

זָרָה, זרי II (sec. r. of זור) *to deviate, to do wrong.* Midr. Till. to Ps. LVIII, 4 (ref. to זרו ib.) מרחם זְרִיתֶם while in the womb you were wrong-doers; Yalk. Ps. 776. Midr. Till. to Ps. XC, 5, v. זור I.

זְרִיבָה f. (זָרַב) *flowing over, boiling over, scalding.* Lev. R. s. 7, end (ref. to Job VI, 17, applied to the deluge) זְרִיבָתָם לחלוטין וכ׳ their scalding (destruction by hot water) was final (there is no resurrection for them); Gen. R. s. 28, end; Y. Snh. X, 29ᵇ bot. (cmp. חֲלוּטִין a. צְמִיתוּת).

זָרִיד m. (זרד) 1)=זֶרֶד.—2) (from its strengthening effect) *a broth* or *porridge of broken grain.* Ber. 37ª ז׳ ועיסן וכ׳ Ms. M. (ed. זָרִיז); expl. (in Ms. M. a. Ar., v. Rabb. D. S. a. l. note 30) ז׳ ארבע ארבע the dish is called *zarid,* when the grain is broken into four pieces (v. Sm. Ant. s. v. Alica; v. M. Kat. 13ᵇ). Y. Ned. VI, 39ᶜ bot. [Bekh. 44ª, v. זִיוּר.]

זְרִיָּה, זְרִייָה f. (זָרָה II) *deviation,* (cmp. זְנָה) *lewdness.* Midr. Till. to Ps. XC, 5 (ref. to זרמתם ib., v. זור I) זְרִיָּתָם לשעה היתה their debauchery was only for a while; Yalk. Ps. 841 זְרִיָּתָם.

זְרִיוֹן, v. זוּרְיוֹן.

זָרִיז m. (זָרַז) 1)=זֶרֶז.—2)=זָרִיד.—3) (adj.) *strong, quick; scrupulous; industrious.* Snh. 70ᵇ בן ז׳ a healthy child; Num. R. s. 10 זָרוּז.—Tosef. Bekh. VI, 10 אם היה בנו ז׳ if his son is a bright student; Kidd. 29ᵇ. Pes. 50ᵇ יש ז׳ ונשכר one is industrious and will be rewarded &c.; Tosef. Yeb. IV, 8, opp. שפל lazy.; a. fr.—*Pl.* זְרִיזִין, fem. זְרִיזוֹת. Pes. 4ª, a. e. ז׳ מקדימין למצות the zealous do their religious duty as early as possible. Sabb. 20ª, a. fr. כהנים ז׳ הן priests are presumed to be scrupulous.—Pes. 89ª, a. e. נמצאו בנות ז׳ וכ׳ the daughters proved to be zealous &c.; a. fr.

זָרִיז, זְרִיז ch. same. Targ. Prov. XXIV, 5 (some ed. זרין, corr. acc.). Targ. Y. Lev. XXIV, 12, opp. מְתוּן; a. fr.—Hull. 107ᵇ דז׳ because he is scrupulous, contrad. to זָהִיר.—*Pl.* זְרִיזִין, fem. זְרִיזָן. Targ. Esth. III, 15; a. e.—Targ. Y. Ex. I, 19 (not . . . זרן).

זָרִיז m. *belt,* v. זְרָז II.

זְרִיזוּת f. (זָרִיז) *strength, quickness, zeal, industry.* Ab. Zar. 20ᵇ, v. זְהִירוּת. Sot. 12ᵇ בז׳ כעלמה quick like a girl. Lev. R. s. 11, end (ref. to על-מות, Ps. XLVIII, 15) בעלמות בז׳ with *almuth,* that is with alertness. Sifra Sh'mini, beg. בז׳; a. fr.

זְרִיזוּתָא ch. same. Targ. Y. Lev. IX, 8, v. preced.—Hull. 16ª קמ״ל . . זְרִיזוּתֵיה the Bible verse quoted intimates only Abraham's zeal.

זְרִיחָה f. (זָרַח) *rise, brightness.* Y. Erub. V, 22ᶜ זְרִיחַת החמה sunrise, East. Gen. R. s. 68 בִּזְרִיחָתָהּ in its rise. Pes. 2ª כן ז׳ שמש וכ׳ Ms. M. (ed. כעין) so will be the sunshine for the righteous &c.; a. fr.

זְרִיָּה, v. זְרִיָּה.

זְרִיעַ, v. זְרַע I.

זְרִיעָה f. (זְרַע) *sowing, seed.* Ber. 35[b] בשעת ז׳ at seed-time. Sabb. 91[a] לז׳ to use it for seed; a. fr.

זְרִיקָה f. (זָרַק) 1) *sprinkling* the blood on the altar. Zeb. 25[b]. Y. Pes. VII, 34[b] bot.; a. v. fr.—2) *thrusting.* Sabb. 96[b] ז׳ תולדה וכ׳ thrusting (on the Sabbath from one area, רשות, to another) is forbidden as a subspecies of carrying (v. הוֹצָאָה). Y. Erub. IV, beg. 21[d] ע״י ז׳ by means of thrusting from place to place; a. fr.

זִירְקְתָא, זְרִיקְתָא f. (זרק) *that which is thrown off, pickings in the woods,* used as fuel. Targ. Is. XXXIII, 4 זריק׳ ed. Lag. (oth. ed. זִרְקָ׳, זְרַק׳; h. text גֵּבִים, cmp. גְּבָבָה); v. אֲזִי.

זְרִירָא m., pl. **זְרִירִין** (זרר; cmp. זרי; cmp. Lat. sternuo) *sputtering, sneezing.* Targ. Job XLI, 10 זְרִירוֹי (זְרִירוֹהִי) (Var. מַקְקָא).

זריתיה, v. זִרְתָּא.

זרכאי, v. זַרְוַאר.

זַרְכֵּל, *Ithpa.* אִזְדְּרְכֵּל (orig. Ithpa. of דרכל, fr. דרך, cmp. אתדרכל P. Sm. 952; v. ib. 1157 s. v. זרכל a. sq.) *to walk proudly.* Targ. Prov. XXX, 31 מִיזְדַּרְכֵּיל ed. Lag. (ed. Wil. מְזַדְּרֵז, v. זְרַז), v. אַבָּבָא.

זַרְמִית, זַרְמִית f. ch. (=b. h. זֶרֶם; cmp. זרב, זרי) *shower, storm.* Targ. Is. IV, 6 Ib. XXVIII, 2; a. e.

זַרְנָא m. (זרר, cmp. זְרִירָא) *vomiting, nausea.* Lev. R. s. 18, end (expl. זָרָא, Num. XI, 20); (Num. R. s. 7 לְזָרָא; Ar. s. v. בוטנא: זֵירָנָא).

זַרְנוּקָא m. (*Parel* of זנק, cmp. זִיקָא II) *leather bag, hose.* Targ. Ps. CXIX, 83 (h. text נֹאד).—B. Mets. 103[b] דוולא וז׳ buckets and hose (for irrigation). B. Bath. 58[a] ז׳ אמרה לכו (comment. זרונקא, Ms. O. זרקונא, corr. acc.) she means a hose (which had been made of the hide of the animal stolen from her). Ib. 167[a] קם אז׳ (some ed. אזרונקא, v. Rabb. D. S. a. l. note) he wrote standing on a hose (to imitate a trembling hand-writing).—*Pl.* זַרְנוּקִין. Targ. Job XXXII, 19 Ar. (ed. לגינין, insert חיך).

זַרְנִיךְ m. (v. P. Sm. 1158) *arsenic, orpiment* (v. Sm. Ant. s. v. Arsenicon). Hull. 88[b] bot.

זָרַע (b. h.; cmp. זרי) *to strew, sow.* Kil. I, 9. Ib. II, 3 אֶזְרַע, v. אָפַךְ; a. fr.—Part. pass. זָרוּעַ, f. זְרוּעָה; pl. זְרוּעִים &c. Ib. ז׳ חטים sown with wheat; a. fr.—Y. Sot. I, 17[b] top כשם . . . . בנותיהן זרועות וכ׳ as well as their vineyards are sown with mixed seeds, so are their daughters &c. (faithless wives).

Nif. נִזְרַע *to be sown, to be stocked with seed.* Gen. R. s. 83, end, a. e. בשבילי נִזְרְעָה וכ׳ the field has been sown for my sake. Shebi. IV, 2 תִּזָּרַע may be sown; a. fr.

Hif. הִזְרִיעַ *to emit semen* (also used of women emitting a secretion at coition). Ber. 60[a], a. e. איש מַזְרִיעַ תחלה when the male is the first to emit semen; אשה מַזְרַעַת וכ׳ when the female is the first &c.; a. fr.

זְרַע I ch. same. Targ. Jud. VI, 3; a. fr.—Part. זָרֵעַ, זָרְעָא (זָרֵיעַ). Targ. Prov. XI, 18; a. fr.—Targ. Is. XXVIII, 25 זָרֵעַ. Ib. XXXII, 20 זָרְעִין.—R. Hash. 16[a] לִיזְרַע חרפא let him sow early seed (barley &c.). Y. Peah VII, 20[b] top הוה ז׳ חקלא וכ׳ planted carrots on his field; a. fr.

Ithpa. אִזְדְּרַע, *Ithpe.* אִזְדְּרַע as preced. *Nif.* Targ. O. Deut. XXIX, 22; a. e.—Y. Peah l. c. אִזְדַּרְעוּן they have been planted.

Af. אַזְרַע as preced. *Hif.* Y. Kil. I, 27[a] bot. ומַזְרְעִין and they copulated.

זֶרַע m. (b. h.; preced.) *seed;* animalic *semen* (mostly שִׁכְבַת ז׳). Gen. R. s. 73 נעשו חמים ז׳ וכ׳ the water in their bellies turned into semen. Y. Kil. I, 27[a] bot. נוטל חימנו ז׳ he may take seed thereof. Shebi. II, 8 שזרעו לז׳ which he planted for the sake of obtaining seed, opp. לירק for using it as vegetable; a. fr.—Trnsf. *issue, descent.* Gen. R. s. 23; s. 51 אותו ז׳ שהוא וכ׳ that issue which was to come from a foreign place (Moab). Ber. 31[b] ז׳ שמושח וכ׳ a descendant who will anoint two men; a. fr.—*Pl.* זְרָעִים. Peah II, 3 הכל מפסיק לז׳ all of them form a partition with regard to seeds (making each field separately subject to Peah), opp. to trees. Kil. III, 2 כל מין ז׳ all kinds of seeds (small vegetable), opp. ירקות large beans &c.; a. fr.—Y. Shebi. II, 34[a] top ששה זְרָעִין six *sowing seasons* during a Sabbatical period.—סֵדֶר ז׳ or ז׳ *Order of Seeds, Z'raim,* the first of the six orders of the Mishnah a. Tosefta. Sabb. 31[a]. Esth. R. to I, 2.

זְרַע II, **זַרְעָא** ch. same. Targ. O. Gen. I, 11; a. fr. בר ז׳ that which is fit for propagation, *seed-capsule,* v. בִּירָא. Targ. Prov. XI, 21; a. fr.—Targ. Ps. XXXVII, 26 Ms. (ed. דרעיה, v. דְּרַע II).—Y. Snh. VII, end, 25[d] ז׳ דכיתן flax-seed.

זֵרָעוֹן, pl. **זֵרְעוֹנִים, זֵרְעוֹנִין** m. (b. h.; preced. wds.) *rows of plants in one bed,* also (=זְרָעִים) *seeds.* Kil. II, 2 זֵרְעוֹנֵי גנה וכ׳ garden seeds which are not used for food, i. e. seeds of vegetables; Tosef. Maasr. III, 14; Sabb. IX, 7. Tosef. l. c. ז׳ שדה field seeds (e. g. vetch &c.). Kil. III, 1 חמשה ז׳ five rows of different seeds; a. fr.

זרעות, Snh. 37[a], v. זַרְעִית.

זַרְעִי f., v. זַרְעִיתָא.

זַרְעִית f. (preced. wds.) *descendants, family.*—*Pl.* זַרְעִיּוֹת. Snh. IV, 5 (37[a]) דמו ודם זַרְעִיּוֹתָיו Mish. a. Y. ed. (Bab. ed. זרעותיו, v. Rabb. D. S. a. l. note 10) his own (the murdered man's) blood and that of his eventual descendants; Gen. R. s. 22; Yalk. Gen. 38.

זַרְעִי, זַרְעִיתָא, זַרְעִית ch. same. Targ. O. Deut. XXIX, 17. Targ. Josh. VII, 14; a. e.—Y. Kil. IX, 32[c] top זַרְעִיתֵיה לא פסיקה וכ׳ his race shall never cease; Y. Keth. XII, 35[b] top זרעייתא (corr. acc.). Koh. R. to IV, 9 והא ז׳ ז׳ וכ׳ here is the third generation of that family &c.—*Pl.* זַרְעָיָתָא, זַרְעָיָין; constr. זַרְעֲיַת. Targ. O. Gen. IV, 10 (cmp. Snh. IV, 5 quot. in preced.; ed. Berl. זַרְעָיָן). Targ. Zech. XII, 12 14 (not זרעין). Targ. O. Ex. VI, 14 (ed. Berl. זַרְעֲיַת); a. fr.—Kidd. 70[b] תרתי ז׳ איכא וכ׳ there are two families in N. &c.

זְרַף, Ab. Zar. 18ᵇ נזרפיה Ar. (ed. לייתיה, Var. Ar. נטרפיה, Ms. M. לתפסיה) prob. a corrupt. for נִגְרְבֵיה, v. גְּרַב.

זְרַף, *Pa.* זָרֵיף (cmp. זרב) *to form a rim* or *elevation around a wound* (cmp. סַפַּחַת, פְּתִית), *to cause a swelling and inflammation.* Ab. Zar. 28ᵇ מִיזְרַף זָרֵיף the operation with the hand creates soreness. Hull. 77ᵃ; Yeb. 76ᵃ פרזלא מז׳ ז׳ cutting with an iron tool causes inflammation.

זִיר׳, זַרְפָּא m. (preced.) *inflammation, swelling of a wound.* Sabb. 67ᵃ דעבדי ליה לז׳ Ms. M. (ed. דעבדי לזר׳) it is applied for healing an inflammation &c.

זָרַק (b. h.; cmp. זרי) *to sprinkle; to cast, throw.* Keth. 103ᵇ זָרוּק וכ׳, v. מָרָה I. Sabb. XI, 1 הזורק מרשות וכ׳ he who throws an object from private to public ground; a. fr.—Esp. *to sprinkle blood on the altar* (Lev. I, 5). Yoma III, 4 קבל .. וזרקו he received the blood and did the required sprinkling. Zeb. I, 4; a. fr.—Yoma 67ᵇ, v. זָכַר.

Nif. נִזְרַק *to be sprinkled.* Pes. V, 3; a. fr.

זְרַק ch. same. Targ. O. Ex. XXIV, 6 (Y. דריק); a. fr.—Gen. R. s. 53, end; s. 86, end [read:] זְרוֹק חוטרא . . . נפיל throw a stick in the air and it will fall back to its origin (the ground), i. e. innate disposition will always come forth; (cmp. Tanh. Balak 17; Num. R. s. 20).

Ithpe. אִזְדְּרֵיק *to be sprinkled.* Targ. Num. XIX, 13; a. e.—Pes. 78ᵇ bot. אשתקד כי איז׳ דם last year when the blood of the Passover sacrifice was sprinkled.

זְרַקְתָּא, v. זְרִיקְתָּא.

זָרַר (b. h.; v. זור a. זָרָה) 1) *to press, stamp;* 2) *to scatter.*

Nif. נִזַּר, נִיזַּר *to be scattered.* Pesik. Vayhi, p. 64ᵇ היתה . . . נדקת ונזרת was crushed, ground, and scattered; Pesik. R. s. 17; Yalk. Ex. 186; Mekh. Bo s. 13 . . . ונזָרוֹת (pl.).

Hof. הוּזַר *to be smashed.* Part. מוּזָר, fem. מוּזֶרֶת, pl. מוּזָרוֹת. ביצה מ׳ an egg smashed in the nest, *rotten* (cmp. מָאַס). Snh. 82ᵇ; Tanh. Pinh. 2; a. e., v. זָמַר III.—Nidd. 35ᵇ. Hull. XII, 3.

זֶרֶת f. (b. h.; preced.) *span* (the spread fingers); *distance from the little finger to the thumb of a spread hand.* Keth. 5ᵇ; Men. 11ᵃ זו ז׳ this one (the little finger) is used for measuring the span. Tosef. Kel. B. Mets. VI, 12 ז׳ אמורה וכ׳ *zereth* mentioned therein (in measures), is half a cubit of six handbreadths; a. fr.—*Du.* זַרְתַּיִם, זֵירְ׳. Men. 85ᵃ; Tosef. ib. IX, 3 קנה זרת ושבולת ז׳ the halm one span long, and the ear two; Taan. 5ᵃ זֵרְתַּיִם.

זֵירְתָא, זַרְתָּא ch. same, also *fist, hand.* Targ. Ex. XXVIII, 16 (ed. Amst. זְרְתָא). Targ. Is. XL, 12; a. e.—Gen. R. s. 63 (play on זרו, Ps. LVIII, 4) זר׳ מתיחא וכ׳ Ar. (ed. זֵירְתֵיהּ) his fist was directed against him (Jacob); Yalk. Gen. 110; Yalk. Deut. 938 זירתיה;—Tanh. Ki Thetsé 4; Yalk. Jer. 261; Yalk. Ps. 868 זרתיה; Tanh., ed. Bub. l. c. זירתיה.

זַתָּא, v. זֵיתָא.

זֵתִים, v. זַיִת.

ח

ח *Heth*, eighth letter of the Alphabet. It interchanges with א, ה a. ע, v. letters א, a. ה; also with ג a. ק, as חבב, גבב, a. קבב; חָרָה a. גָּרָה &c.—For dialectical pronunciation, v. א״ה a. ח״ה.

ח׳, as a numeral letter, *eight.*

חָאֵי, part. of חָיֵי.

חָאִיךְ, חָאִיס, חָאִיק, v. חוּךְ, חוּס, חוּק (חָקַק).

***חָאִיתָא** f. (חוי, cmp. חבב, *to be arched*, cmp. גְּבִינָה; Syr. חאותא, P. Sm. 1166) *clotted cream.* Targ. Prov. XXX, 33 Ms. (Var. ed. Lag. ח׳; ed. Lag. a. oth. חֶמְאָתָא).

חאסטו, v. הָאַסְטוּ.

חָאפוּן m. (v. חָפַן) *a handful, a grab.* בן ח׳ *grabber* (a play on פָּאפִּין, v. אָפִּין). Y. Yoma IV, 43ᶜ bot. (Bab. ib. 39ᵃ sq. בן חָמְצָן).

חָאק, v. חוּק ch.

חָב, חַב, v. חוּב.

חַבָּא, חָבָא, v. חבי.

חָבָא, חוּבָּא.

חָבָא, B. Kam. 101ᵇ, v. חֵבָה.

חָבַב I (b. h.) [*to be arched;* denom. חוב II;] *to bosom, love.*

Pi. חִבֵּב, חִיבֵּב 1) same, *to love, cherish;* with לפני or בפני, *to prefer.* Ex. R. s. 27; Tanh. Yithro 4 Yithro is named חוֹבָב, שח׳ את וכ׳ because he loved the Law; Sifré Num. 78. Sabb. 13ᵇ היו מְחַבְּבִין את הצרות they cherished the memory of past troubles (devoting memorial days to the relief from them). Ib. 51ᵃ, a. e. כמה מחבבין זה את זה how they honor each other. Pes. 100ᵃ בכל יום היית מחבב . . . בפני thou didst always prefer my opinions to those of R. J., and now thou embracest his opinion in my presence; Y. ib. X, beg. 37ᵇ; Tosef. Ber. V, 2; a. fr.—2) (denom. of חָבִיב) *to make beloved.* Gen. R. s. 39 כדי לְחַבְּבָהּ בעיניו in order to make him feel the dearness of home; כדי לְחַבְּבוֹ וכ׳ to make him feel how dear was his son to him.

חֲבַב ch., *Pa.* חַבִּיב same, 1) *to love, honor.* Targ. Prov. IV, 8 חַבְּבָהּ honor her. Targ. O. Deut. XXXIII, 3; a. fr.—2) *to make beloved.* Targ. Y. ib.—Sabb. 130ª is it משום חַבּוּבֵי מצוה (Rashi חִיבּוּב) in order to show the high appreciation of the ceremony (of circumcision)?—Ib. אלא לְחַבּוּבֵי (Ms. M. לְחַבֵּב). Ḥull. 133ª חבובי קא מְחַבֵּב וכ׳ does he (by taking hastily) prove his anxiety for the divine command, or &c.?

Ithpa. אִיתְחַבִּיב *to be tied together* (in affection). Targ. I Sam. XVIII, 1 (h. text נקשרה).

חֲבַב* II (v. preced. wds.) *to embrace* (in a fight), *to wrestle.* Tosef. Shebu. VI, 2 כל זמן שהיו חוֹבְבִין זה את זה (Var. חוֹכְבִין) as long as they were fighting each other, i. e. if the case comes up immediately after the fight took place; ib. B. Kam. IX, 28 חוכבין; Y. Shebu. VII, 37ᵈ bot.. חוכבין.—V. חֲבִיבָאֵי.

חֲבָבָאֵי, v. חֲבִיבָאֵי.

חִיבָּה, חִבָּה f. (preced. wds.) *love, esteem, honor.* Koh. R. to V, 14 בא לעולם בח׳ וכ׳ man enters the world with love (caressed by his nearest), and leaves with love. Y. Bicc. II, 64ᵈ top לשבעה מיתה של ח׳ a death after seven days of sickness is a death of (divine) love; (ib.ᶜ bot. לשבעים מיתה של ח׳, read שֵׁיבָה).—Ab. III, 14 ח׳ יתירה וכ׳ the greater divine love consists in its being made known to him &c. Ḥull. 33ª, a. e. חִיבַּת הקדש מכשרתן the honor in which sacred objects are held makes them fit for levitical uncleanness (even without contact with liquids, v. כָּשֵׁר). Ex. R. s. 2, a. fr. לשון ח׳ the repetition of a name intimates endearment. Y. Succ. IV, 54ᵈ top לשון ח׳ (the word שֵׁבֶר, Num. XXVIII, 7) expresses something dear; (Bab. ib. 49ᵇ; Num. R. s. 21 שתייה).—Keth. 56ª חיבת חופה וכ׳ the affection produced by the seclusion in the bridal department is the final act of possession. Gen. R. s. 93; Yalk. ib. 150 [read:] על חיבת העין כך כל בעל אכסניא וכ׳ if this was done for a dear object of sight (our sister), how much more shall we do in defence of the host of the Lord (Benjamin, v. אוּשְׁפִּיזְכָן); a. fr.—Ch. חִיבְּתָא.

חֵיבָה, חֵבָה f. (חבא) *reserve, storage.* B. Kam. 101ᵇ שגיבבן בחיבה Ms. M. (oth. בחבה; ed. בְּחֵבָא, v. Rabb. D. S. a. l. note) which he gathered up for storage; Succ. 40ª לחיבה ed. (Ms. Ms. 2 בחיבה, v. Rabb. D. S. a. l. note 200).

חָבוּ, pr. n. m. בר ח׳, v. חֲבוּ.

חָבוּבָא, v. חִיב׳.

חבוורתא, Ḥull. 57ᵇ, v. חֲבַרְוּתָא.

חָבוּט, חִיב׳.

חָבוּט m. (חָבַט) *pressed down*, esp. *ḥabut*, a legal fiction by which an inclined projection is assumed to be like a horizontal plane. Erub. 9ª או לבוד ... או ח׳ אמרינן וכ׳ either we assume the fiction of a junction (v. לָבוּד) or of *ḥabut*, but both of them we do not assume. [Rashi reads חֲבוֹט or ch. חבוט, as imperative: *press it down.*]

חָבוּטָא, v. חַבְטָא, a. חָבַטָא.

חָבוּל, v. חָבַל I, II. [Y. Kidd. IV, 65ᵈ top ח׳ יומא, v. חֲבִיל.]

חֲבוּלָא, חָבוּל, v. חִיב׳.

חֲבוּלָה f. (b. h. חֲבֹלָה; חָבַל 1) *pledge.* Tanh. B'shall. 19 (ref. to חבל תחבל, Ex. XXII, 25) . . . חָבַלְתָּ ח׳ אחת חֲבוּלוֹת הרבה if thou seizest a pledge once, thou wilt finally be seized many times (cmp. Ex. R. s. 31, quot. s. v. מַשְׁכּוֹן); Yalk. Ex. 257; Mekh. B'shall., Vayassa, s. 1 (corr. acc.). Tosef. Keth. XI, 8 המלוה . . . על חֲבִילָה וכ׳ if one gives a loan on a pawn &c.—*Pl.* חֲבוּלוֹת, v. supra (Yalk. l. c. חֲבֹלוֹת).

חֲבוּלָא m. *injury, loss*, v. חֲבִילָא.

חִיב׳, חִבּ׳, חֲבוּלְיָא f. (חבל; v. Nöld. Mand. Gr. p. 146, sq.) *interest, usury* (h. נֶשֶׁךְ). Targ. O. Ex. XXII, 24 חֲ׳ ed. Berl. (oth. ed. חִ׳). Targ. Ps. XV, 5; a. e.—M. Kat. 28ᵇ (in a funeral dirge) מותא כי מותא ומרעין חי׳ death is death (paying a debt), but sufferings are the interests.

חָבוּר, v. חִיב׳.

חֲבוּרָא c. ch.=h. חֲבוּרָה, *company, party.* Targ. O. Ex. XII, 46 (Y. ed. Amst. חַב׳).—*Pl.* חֲבוּרָן. Targ. Y. Deut. XXXIV, 6; a. e.—Masc. חֲבוּרִין. Targ. Y. II Deut. XIV, 1 (some ed. חַב׳; Ar. חבורן; cmp. אֲגוּדָה).

חַבּוּרָא I, v. preced.

חַבּוּרָא II m. (חבר) *charmer.*—*Pl.* constr. חַבּוּרֵי. Targ. Y. II Deut. XVIII, 11 חַבּוּרֵי חֲבוּרֵי בִישִׁין (not חֲבוּרָא) those who conjure up companies of evil (demons).

חֲבוּרָה I f. (חָבַר) *company, association, party;* esp. *those united for eating the Passover lamb in company* (Ex. XII, 4); *the colleagues at school* (v. חָבֵר); *the college.* Pes. VII, 3, a. fr. בני ח׳ the members of a Passover party. Ib. אם חֲבוּרַת כהנים if it is a party consisting of priests only. Y. ib. X, 37ᵈ top שלא יהא עומד מח׳ זו וכ׳ that one should not rise from one party and join another; Bab. ib. 119ᵇ, v. אֲפִיקוֹמָן; a. fr.—Ber. 9ᵇ במעמד כל הח׳ in the presence of the whole college. Ned. 81ª הזהרו בח׳ beware of disregarding the benefits of collegiate studies. Lev. R. s. 2, end חֲבוּרָתוֹ של משה the disciples of Moses; a. fr.—Y. Dem. II, 23ª top דוחין אותו מחבורתו, v. חֲבֵירוּת.—*Pl.* חֲבוּרוֹת. Pes. IX, 10; a. fr.

חַבּוּרָה (חֲבוּרָה) f. (b. h.; חָבַר 4) *a mark of violence, wound, discoloring.* B. Kam. VIII, 1 מקום שאינו עושה ח׳ a spot on which no wound is made by burning (e. g. on the nail). Snh. XI, 1 (85ᵇ) עד שיעשה בהן ח׳ unless by striking them he creates a wound; Y. ib. XI, beg. 30ª באיזו ח׳ כחבורת שבת כח׳ נזקין what wound is meant here? One the creating of which would be a Sabbath offence (discoloring), or one of the kind required for claiming damages?; Mekh. Mishp., N'zikin, s. 5 מכה שיש בה ח׳ (in order to be punishable with death) it must be a beating which makes a wound (or a sore). Sabb. 107ᵇ ח׳ שאינה חוזרת a permanent discoloring. Ib. מניין לח׳ שאינה וכ׳ whence is it proven that by *ḥabburah* a permanent (not a momentary) discoloring is meant?—

Keth. 3[b] עושה ח׳ he makes a wound (by tearing the hymen). Ib. 5[b] מקלקל בח׳ destroying by making a hole, מתקן בח׳ amending by &c.; a. v. fr.—*Pl.* חבורות. Gen. R. s. 23; a. e.

חֲבוּרְתָּא ch. same. Yalk. Gen. 38, v. חֲוַרְתָּא.

חֲבוּרְתָּא ch.=h. חֲבוּרָה, *company* &c.—Y. Ber. II, 5[c] top וַחֲבוּרְתֵּיה and his disciples. Y. Ter. II, 41[c] כד הוה מורי בחבורתיה when teaching in his college; a. e.—*Pl.* חֲבוּרָתָא. M. Kat. 27[b] ח׳ איכא במתא there are burial societies in the place.

חַבּוּשׁ m. (Syr. חבושא, P. Sm. 1187) name of *a fruit, quince* (v., however, Löw Pfl. p. 143)—*Pl.* חַבּוּשִׁין. Sabb. 45[a]: Bets. 26[b]. Tosef. Ter. VII, 13 חובשין ודרמסקנין ed. Zuck. (Var. עובעין; Y. ib. VIII, 45[d] ענבים ואובשין). [חָבוּשׁ *prisoner*, v. חָבַשׁ.]

חַבּוּשָׁא ch. same. Keth. 60[b].—*Pl.* חַבּוּשֵׁי. Snh. 39[a].

חֲבוּשָׁא m. (חבש) *imprisonment.* Koh. R. to XI, 9 לַחֲבוּשֵׁי לֵית את סקר my being imprisoned thou dost not take into consideration.—Targ. Y. II Gen. XXXIX, 20 בית חֲבוּשָׁה (Ar. חֲבוּשְׁיָא) *prison.*

חָבַט (b. h.; cmp. חבש, חבל) [*to use force,*] 1) *to press down.* Erub. 42[b] תקרת . . . חוֹבֶטֶת the roofing of the house presses upon him (keeps him mindful of the Sabbath limit); v. חָבוּט. B. Mets. 80[b] חֲבָטוֹ לאלתר (Ar. חבסו, v. חָבַס) the load pressed him down immediately (before he could find out that it was too heavy for him). Snh. 19[b] חֲבָטָן בקרקע pressed them into the ground. Succ. IV, 6 (45[a]) חוֹבְטִין אותן ע״ג קרקע בצידי המזבח Ms. M. (v. Rabb. D. S. a. l. note 10) they laid them down closely upon one another on the ground by the altar (opp. to זוקפין, ib. IV, 4). Keth. 39[a] צער שֶׁחֲבָטָהּ ע״ג וכ׳ 'the pain' (Mish. ib. III, 4) refers to his pressing her down on the hard ground.—2) *to force, to knock open,* esp. *to knock upon olives* to make them burst, before putting them under the press, or *upon ears* to thresh the grain out. Ex. R. s. 36, beg. מורידין . . . . ונחבט ומשחוֹבְטִין וכ׳ they take the olive down and it is knocked upon, and after knocking it, they put it into the vat (corresp. to כתש, Men. VIII, 4). Ib. באין או״ה . . . . וחובטין .. ממקום וכ׳ the gentiles come and knock them (the Israelites) from place to place. Men. X, 4; a. e.—*Part. pass.* חָבוּט *mashed.* Sabb. 80[b] בח׳ when the lime is mashed (and mixed with water); Y. ib. VIII, 11[b] bot. בחביט (corr. acc.).—3) *to lay down for receiving lashes,* in gen. *to punish, bind over.* Gitt. IX, 8 ובנכרים חובטין אותו וכ׳ but when the gentile authorities bind him over and say, Do as the Israelites tell thee, (the letter of divorce so enforced) is valid (differ. vers. in Y. ed.); Tosef. Yeb. XII, 13.—Tosef. Sot. XV, 7 מסרוהו לבעל זמורה וַחֲבָטוֹ ed. Zuck. Var. (Y. ib. IX, 24[b] top וחבשו) they gave him in charge of the rod-bearer (v. זְמוֹרָה), and he tried to force him (into submission). Midd. I, 2 חוֹבְטוֹ במקלו he punishes him with his cane.

Nif. נֶחְבַּט *to be knocked upon; to strike against.* Ex. R. s. 36, v. supra.—Keth. 36[b] מפני שֶׁנֶּחְבֶּטֶת וכ׳ because the blind girl may have struck against something (and fallen, so as to have lost her virginity by the shock). Hull. 51[b] עוף שנ׳ על וכ׳ a bird that fell with force upon water.—Koh. R. to VII, 8, v. infra.

Pi. חִיבֵּט *to press down, throw down.* Keth. l. c. חִיבְּטָהּ ע״ג שיראין if he forced her down on (soft) silk garments.

Hithpa. הִתְחַבֵּט, נִתְחַבֵּט *to prostrate one's self* (in prayer, in deep commotion). Gen. R. s. 91 היה מִתְחַבֵּט לפני רגליו וכ׳ he threw himself to the feet of every one &c. (with ref. to Gen. XLII, 21). Ib. s. 70; Num. R. s. 8, end; Yalk. Gen. 123 דבר שנתח׳ וכ׳ a thing for which that patriarch (Jacob) begged in prostration; Koh. R. to VII, 8 שֶׁנֶּחְבַּט. Deut. R. s. 2, beg. עכשיו הוא מתחנן ומתח׳ now he supplicates and prostrates himself; a. fr.

חֲבַט, חֲבֵיט ch. same, 1) *to knock; to strike, punish.* Targ. O. Deut. XXIV, 20. Targ. Jud. VI, 11. Targ. Is. XXVIII, 27 (Regia: מְחַבְּטִין *Pa.*).—Targ. Prov. XXVIII, 3 מטרא חֲבִיטָא (not חֲבִיטָא) a prostrating rain (h. text סחף). Y. Sabb. XVII, 16[b] top דו חֲבֵיט ביה; Y. Bets. I, 60[c] חֲבַט, v. זְזִירָא.—Gen. R. s. 7, a. e. חֲבוֹט חבטך, v. חֲבָטָא. B. Bath. 58[a] חֲבוֹטוּ (not חובטו), v. חֲבִיטָא.—2) *to throw down.* Y. Snh. VI, 23[c] top חַבְטִין תורא בחילא Ash. to Hull. 51[a] (ed. בחייליה) threw an ox down with force (before slaughtering).—*Part. pass.* חֲבִיט, f. חֲבִיטָא *prostrated.* Keth. 10[a] מברכתא ח׳ ליה is Mabrakhta (i. e. all the women of ill repute of M.) prostrated before him (so that he is an expert in such matters)? [Y. Sabb. VIII, 11[b] bot. בחביט, v. preced.]

Pa. חַבֵּיט *to shake, agitate.* Targ. Y. Num. XXV, 8 (ed. Amst. Pe.) he shook (the spear). Targ. Esth. VI, 1.—Succ. 44[b] ח׳ ח׳ ולא וכ׳ he shook it repeatedly but said no benediction.

Ithpa. אִיחַבַּט as preced. *Nif.* Keth. 36[b] כולהו נמי חֲבוּטֵי מִיחַבְּטֵי all girls (even if not blind) may receive a shock by falling.

חֶבֶט I c. (חָבַט 1) *fastening;* ח׳ של סנדל *thongs of a sandal joined in a knot* (v. Sm. Ant. s. v. Sandalium). Mikv. X, 3.—*Pl.* חֲבָטִין (חוֹבְטִין). Y. Yeb. XII, 12[d] top והן שיהו חו׳ של עץ this means that the thongs be of wood (of the vegetable kingdom; oth. vers. תרסיות, מעמידין). Ib. נפסקו חֲבָטָיו (omitted Tosef. Kel. B. Bath. IV, 5, a. Sabb. 112[a]) if its thongs are broken; נפסקה . . . אחת בח׳ if one set of its thongs is broken; Y. Sabb. V, 8[a] חבהיו (corr. acc.; omitted Tosef. ib. XII (XIII), 14).

חֶבֶט II m. (חָבַט, v. *Nif.*) *shock, lesion through a fall.* B. Kam. 50[b] לְחַבְטוֹ, v. הֶבֶל. Ib. חבטו קרקע וכ׳ (not חבטא or חבטה, v. Rabb. D. S. a. l. note 1; Yalk. Ex. 341) as to the shock which the animal suffered, it is the natural ground which injured it, v. קַרְקַע.

חַבְטָא ch. same, also *stroke, blow.* Hull. 8[a] ח׳ קדים וכ׳ does the effect of the blow come first (and create an inflammation, שחין), and the effect of the heat follows (creating a burn, מכוה) &c.?—B. Mets. 116[b] אי בחבסא נפל אי בח׳ נפל whether the building fell through pressure (in which case the lower portion of the materials would be more affected), or through a shock.—Gen. R. s. 7 חבוט

חֲבָטָךְ go on with thy beating; Koh. R. to VII, 23; Tanh. Huck. 6 חֲבִיטָךְ; Y. Kidd. III, 64^c bot. חבוטך.—Esp. *the beating of olives.* Lam. R. to I, 1 רבתי (2 חד כות׳) בשעת ח׳ in the season of beating; ib. חבטה (corr. acc.).—*Pl.* חֲבַטַיָּא *olives ready for beating.* Y. Maas. Sh. IV, 55^b bot. [read:] חחוא חוח בנציא ואת בת׳ that one (dreamt of olives) in the blooming stage, but thou of olives ripe for beating.

*חֲבָטָה f. (חָבַט) *seizing an object violently* in order to take possession of it. B. Mets. 118^a, v. חֲבָטָה. [B. Kam. 50^b, v. חֲבַט II.—Lam. R. to I, 1 רבתי (חד כות׳ 2), v. preced.]

חבטי, Y. Shebu. VII, 37^d, v. חֲבִיבָאֵי.

חָבָה, חָבָא, חבי (b. h.) *to cover, hide.*—*Part. pass.* (fr. חבה) חָבוּי, f. חֲבוּיָה. Cant. R. to II, 1 (play on חֲבַצֶּלֶת, ib.) חבויה בצלן של מצרים hidden (disregarded) in the shade of Egypt; ח׳ בצלו של ים nearly covered up by the darkness of the Sea; ח׳ בצלו של סיני nearly covered up by the shade of Sinai (threatening to fall upon me) &c.—Ib. שה׳ בְּצָלָהּ its (the young lily's) onion is hidden (its leaves not being unfolded).—Ib. כל מתי . . חֲבוּיִים בי all the dead of the world are buried in me (the earth).

Nif. נֶחְבָּא *to be hidden.* Sabb. 60^a היו נֶחְבָּאִין וכ׳ they hid in a cave. Taan. 23^b, v. infra.

Hif. הֶחְבִּיא *to hide.* Taan. l. c. they named him חנן הנחבא מפני שה׳ עצמו Ms. M. (ed. שחיה מַחְבִּיא) because he hid himself (in his modesty). Y. Kil. V, 30^a top (play on בתי כְלָאִים, Is. XLII, 22) בית שמַּחְבִּיאִין . . . כִּלְאַיִם a garden house in which it is permitted to keep plants of a different species (from the surrounding vines). Sot. 34^b (play on נחבי׳ וכ׳) שה׳ he hid (suppressed) the word of God (truth); Tanh. Sh'lah 6 שה׳ את דבריו he suppressed the words he ought to have said; ib. Haäz. 7. [Lam. R. introd. (R. Josh. 2) מחבי חבריים, read: מחבר חבריים, v. חָבַר.]

Hithpa. הִתְחַבֵּא *to hide one's self.* Midr. Prov. ch. IX; Tanh. Ki Thabo 2 מִתְחַבְּאִים trying to hide themselves.

חֲבָא, חֲבִי ch. same. Bekh. 43^b, v. infra.

Ithpa. אִתְחַבָּא, *Ithpe.* אִיתְּחֲבִי *to hide one's self; to be hidden, covered.* Targ. Lam. I, 3. Targ. Y. Gen. VII, 19, sq. (ed. pr.=O. אתחפ׳).—Bekh. 43^b דחַבְיָא מִיתְחַבֵי (Rashi, ed. מִתְ׳) when the head is hidden (between the shoulders). B. Kam. 60^b מִתְחַבֵי חַבּוּרֵי וכ׳ he hides himself and walks (by the way-sides).

חֲבַי pr. n. m *Hăbay.* Yeb. 115^b bot. (a name of frequent occurrence in Mahuza).—B. Kam. 72^a Ms. M. (ed. חֲבִיבֵי); Erub. 57^a Ms. M. (ed. הֲגִילָאֵי).

חָבִיב I m. (חָבַב) *beloved, dear, precious; favored, privileged.* Ab. II, 10 יהי . . . ח׳ עליך וכ׳ let thy neighbor's honor be as dear to thee as thine own. Ib. III, 14 ח׳ אדם וכ׳ man is privileged (favored of God) in that he was created &c.; a. v. fr.—*Pl.* חֲבִיבִים, חֲבִיבִין. Ber. 5^b ח׳ עליך יסורין are sufferings dear to thee (as divine trials)?—Yoma 52^a ח׳ ישראל וכ׳ Israel is favored, for the Lord made them independent of a mediator; a. v. fr.—*Fem.* חֲבִיבָה. Tosef. Ber. VII, 24; Ber. 63^a; Y. ib. IX, end, 14^d כמה ח׳ תורח וכ׳ the Law is appreciated. Pes. 68^b כמה ח׳ מצוה בשעתה how much more preferable is a religious act when done betimes; a. e.—*Pl.* חֲבִיבוֹת. Sot. 13^a כמה ח׳ . . . על וכ׳ how dear were religious acts to Moses.

חֲבִיבָא I, חָבִיב, חַבִּ׳, חָ׳ ch. same. Targ. Jer. XXXI, 19; a. fr.—*Pl.* חֲבִיבִין, חֲבִיבַיָּא. Targ. Is. I, 4. Targ. Y. II Deut. XXVI, 18; a. e.—*Fem.* חֲבִיבָא; חֲבִיבְתָּא (as noun). Targ. Y. Gen. XLIV, 30 (h. text קשורה, cmp. חָבַב *Ithpa.*).—Targ. Cant. VI, 4.

חֲבִיבָא II, חָבִיב m. (preced.) [*connected,*] *uncle, father's brother.* Targ. Y. Lev. X, 4; a. e.—B. Bath. 41^b. Y. B. Kam. X, beg., 7^b; a. fr.—*Fem.* חֲבִיבְתָּא 1) *aunt, father's brother's wife.* Targ. Y. Ex. VI, 20; a. e.—*2) *mother-in-law.* Targ. Y. II Deut. XXVII, 23 (h. text חתנת).

חֲבִיבָא III, חֲבִיבָה pr. n. m. *Hăbiba,* name of several Amoraim. Yoma 10^a; B. Mets. 85^b רב ח׳ בר סורמקי (Ms. M. חֲבִיבֵי, v. Rabb. D. S. a. l. note).—Ib. אמר רב ח׳ (v. Rabb. D. S. l. c.). Sabb. 54^b, a. e., v. זְוָוא I. Y. Meg. I, 70^b top ר׳ חביבה; a. fr.—V. Fr. M'bo p. 79^b.

*חֲבָבָאֵי, חֲבִיבָאֵי m. pl. (v. חָבַב II) *wrestlers, a case of assault and battery without witnesses.* Tosef. Shebu. VI, 2 ר׳ יהודה היה קורא אותה ח׳ (Var. ed. Zuck. הנחבכן) R. Judah called such a case (in Chald.) *hăbibaê;* ib. B. Kam. IX, 28 (our w. a. אותה omitted in ed. Zuck., Var. אותה כאר, אותה הכחבא); Y. Shebu. VII, 37^d bot. קורא חבטי.

חֲבִיבָה, v. חָבִיב I, a. חֲבִיבָא III.

חֲבִיבוּתָא f. (חָבִיב) *love, attachment, divine favor.* Sabb. 88^b ועדיין ח׳ היא גבן (Ms. M. חֲבִיבוּתֵיה הוא) and yet (in spite of our defection) the divine love is with us; Gitt. 36^b; Yalk. Cant. 983. Arakh. 16^b אגב ח׳ וכ׳ on account of the extreme friendship &c.

חֲבִיבַי pr. n. m. *Hăbibay,* v. חֲבַי a. חֲבִיבָא III.

חֲבִיבְתָּא, v. חֲבִיבָא I a. II.

חֶבְיוֹנָא m. (חבי; b. h. חֶבְיוֹן) *secret place, recess.*—*Pl.* constr. חֶבְיוֹנֵי. Targ. Cant. II, 14 ח׳ הַדַּרְגָּתָא (ed. Lag. הַדַּרְגִּיתָא, h. text סתר המדרגה). Targ. Koh. X, 20.

חֲבִיוֹנָה f. (dimin. of חָבִית) *a small vessel, flask* with flat sides.—*Pl.* חֲבִיוֹנוֹת. Kel. II, 2; Tosef. ib. B. Kam. II, 2 אֲבִיוֹנוֹת (ed. Zuck. אובינות).

חֲבִיטָא, חָבִיט m. 1) part. pass. of חָבַט.—2) (חָבַט) *flail, cudgel.* [Tanh. Huck. 6 חביטך, v. חֲבָטָא.]—*Pl.* חֲבִיטֵי. B. Bath. 58^a [read:] שקילו ח׳ חבוטו אקיברא וכ׳ (v. Ms. M. a. Rabb. D. S. a. l. note) take cudgels and beat on the grave of your father, until &c.

חבויים, Lam. R. introd. (R. Josh. 2) מחבר ח׳, read: מחבר חבריים, v. חָבַר.

חֲבִיל (v. חֲבַל I) *to get sick.* B. Mets. 97^a ח׳ ומית got sick (from overeating itself) and died.

חֲבִיל *woe!,* v. חֲבַל II. [Targ. Prov. IV, 13, v. הֲחִיבַל.]

חֲבִיל, ח׳ יַמָּא (v. חֲבַלָּא II) pr. n. *Ḥăbel Yamma* (*district of the sea*), a Babylonian district (v. Berl. Geogr. p. 34, sq.; Neub. Géogr. p. 327). Kidd. 72[a]; Y. ib. IV, 65[d] top (not חבול); Gen. R. s. 37 חֲבַל.

חֲבִילָא I f. (חבל) *injury, loss.* M. Kat. 28[b] ווי לאזלא ווי לח׳ (Ms. M. לְחֲבוּלָא) woe for him that is gone, woe for the loss!—Bekh. 8[b] מנא דלא שוי חֲבִילֵיה (Rashi חבליה) a utensil which is not worth the damage which it causes.

חֲבִילָא II (v. next w.) *bundle.—Pl.* חֲבִילִין. Lev. R. s. 14 (prov.) אשתרי חד חבלא אשתרו תרין ח׳ if one rope is untied, two bundles are loosened. [Ar. ed. Koh., a. ed. Wil. חַבְלִין.]

חֲבִילָה f. (חָבַל 2) 1) *connection, whatever is in a connected state.* Kel. XVIII, 9 המטה מיטמאת ח׳ וכ׳ a couch gets unclean only when combined, and can become clean again &c., opp. איברים; Succ. 16[a].—2) *bundle, load, baggage, luggage.* Y. Ter. X, 47[b] top, v. זֵיר. B. Mets. 72[b] המוליך ח׳ וכ׳ if one carries a load (as a messenger) from one place to another (where prices are higher). Kidd. 65[b] וח׳ עמהם and have luggage with them. B. Mets. 78[a] כשבאת ח׳ לידו when the working man has left a bundle (of tools) with him (as a pledge that he will come to work); a. fr.—*Pl.* חֲבִילוֹת, חֲבִילִין, constr. (mostly) חֲבִילֵי. Sabb. XVIII, 2 ח׳ קש וכ׳ bundles of straw &c.—Y. Ber. VII, beg. 11[a] מג׳ ח׳ from three different bundles (of hyssop). B. Kam. 10[a] bot. מרבה בח׳ Ms. M. (ed. sing.) one adding bundles (of dry twigs) to the fire. — Ber. 49[a], a. e. אין עושין מצות ח׳ ח׳ we must not perform religious duties bundle-wise (but pay attention to each singly). Erub. 54[b] (ref. to Prov. XIII, 11) אם עושה . . ח׳ ח׳ מתמעטת Ms. O. (v. Rabb. D. S. a. l. note) if one studies bundle-wise (too many subjects at a time), his learning will decrease (ed. מתמעט he will become poorer in learning). B. Mets. 84[b] הקפתנו ח׳ תשובות וכ׳ Ms. M. (v. Rabb. D. S. a. l. note) thou hast surrounded us with bundles of arguments which contain no substance; a. fr. — 3) *band, bandage.* Ab. Zar. 10[b], sq. נתפרדה ח׳ the bond (of friendship between the two nations) is severed —*Pl.* חֲבִילִין. Lev. R. s. 14; Yalk. Job 905 עשוייה .. ח׳ ח׳ consists of cells, convolutions and bands (muscles).—4) *pledge,* v. חֲבוֹלָה.

חבין, Tosef. Kil. III, 15, v. הֵיגָה.

חֲבִינָאוּת, v. חֲבִינָנוּת.

חבינגא, v. חֲכִינָּנָא.

חֲבִינָנוּתָא, חֲבִינָנוּת f. (חבן, denom. of חוּבָּא, v. P. Sm. 1181, *to fold hands in the bosom*) *idleness.* Targ. Prov. XXXI, 27 ולחמא דחבנוותא ed. Lag. (Var. חכינאנות, ed. Wil. חכינג׳, corr. acc.). Ib. XXII, 13 בחבננותיה ed. Lag. (Var. a. ed. Wil. בחכינ׳, corr. acc.).

חביץ, Y. Peah I, 16[a] בר ח׳, v. חוּבָּץ I.

חָבִיץ m. (חבץ) *a dish of flour, honey and oil beaten into a pulp;* ח׳ קדרה a *habits* boiled in a pot. Ber. 36[b], v. אַבְרוּשָׁךְ.—Gen. R. s. 48.

חֲבִיצָא ch. 1) same. Ber. 37[b]; Men. 75[b] חֲבִיצָה (fem.; Ms. M. חמיצא, v. Rabb. D. S. a. l. note). Y. Ned. VI, beg. 39[c].—2) ח׳ דתמרי *a cake of pressed dates.* B. Mets. 99[b] (Ar. חִיבּוּצָא, Ms. H. חוצצא).

חֲבִירר, v. חָבַר.

חַבִּ׳, חֲבִירָא, v. חֲבִירָא.

חֲבִירָה, חֲבֵירוּת, חֲבֵירְתָּא, v. חָבֵר, a. חַבְרָא.

חֲבִישָׁה f. (חָבַשׁ) *imprisonment.* Snh. 78[b] ח׳ מנא לן whence do we derive the right of committing to prison (to await the result of wounds afflicted)?—Y. Yeb. XII, 12[d] bot. בית ח׳ דר׳ וכ׳ the prison where R. Akiba was confined.

חָבִית f. (חבב, as גָּזִית fr. גזז, v. Fl. to Levy Talm. Dict. II, 202[1]) *an arched, pouched vessel, (earthen) wine jug.* B. Kam. III, 1 (27[a], identical with כַּד); a. fr.—Kel. II, 3 ח׳ של שייטין the swimmers' bottle (used for practicing).—*Pl.* חָבִיּוֹת. Ib. 2 ח׳ לודיות Lyddean jugs, smaller than לחמיות Bethlehem bottles. Nidd. 6[b], v. גּוּף I h.; a. fr.

חָבִיתָא ch. same. B. Kam. 27[a]. Sabb. 74[b] דעביד ח׳ who makes an earthen jug (on the Sabbath); a. e.—*Pl.* חָבִיָּיתָא. Ib. 110[a] אתרתי ח׳ Ms. M. (ed. חָבְיָתָא) on two jugs.

חֲבִיתִּים, חֲבִיתִּין f. pl. (b. h. חֲבִתִּים; חבת, cmp. חבץ, חָבִיץ) *a sort of cakes* (cmp. מַחֲבַת). Y. Yoma I, beg. 38[a] נאמר תמיד בח׳ the word *tamid* is used in connection with *hăbittin* (Lev. VI, 13). Ib. אין ח׳ מעכבת (sub. הקרבת) the offering of the cakes at the Highpriest's inauguration is no indispensable requirement. Men. XI, 3 חֲבִיתֵּי כ״ג the cakes at the Highpriest's inauguration.

חָבַל (b. h.; cmp. חבב) 1) *to seize, to take a pledge.* Mekh. B'shall., Vayassa, s. 1, a. e., v. חֲבוֹלָה.—B. Mets. IX, 13 (115[a]) החובל את הריחים he who seizes millstones (for his debt); a. fr. — 2) *to twist* (v. חֶבֶל); *to do violence, unshape; to inflict a wound, to hurt* (followed by ב of the object). B. Kam. VIII, 1 החובל בחבירו he who injures his neighbor. Sabb. XIV, 1. Ib. 106[a] חובל בצריך לכלבו one who wounds (an animal on the Sabbath is guilty) when he needs the blood for his dog. Ib. חובל בעלמא one who wounds generally (not for a purpose); a. fr.—3) *to writhe, travail,* v. *Pi.*

Nif. נֶחְבַּל 1) *to be seized.* Yalk. Ex. 351 שניתן לֵיחָבֵל ביום (B. Mets. 114[b] לַחֲבוֹל) which may be seized as a pledge in day time. — 2) *to be injured.* Tosef. B. Kam. IX, 29 אע״פ שלא .... מן הנֶחְבָּל וכ׳ although the injurer does not ask the injured (to pray for him), the injured must pray &c.; a. fr.

Pi. חִיבֵּל 1) *to injure, wound; to unshape, ruin, spoil.* Ber. 51[a] יש לי ... לְחַבֵּל I have permission to injure (kill). B. Kam. 91[b] לחבל בעצמו to mutilate one's self. — Kel. XIV, 2 משיְּחַבֵּל from the moment he batters (the tube, for fitting it into the top of the staff); Tosef. ib. B. Mets. IV, 5 משיחבול, v. חָבַר. Num. R. s. 10 (play on חֲבַל, Prov. XXIII, 34) שחִבְּלַתּוֹ יעל וכ׳ whom Jael mutilated on his head. Yalk. Ex. 301 חִבַּלְתֶּם מעשיכם you have ruined (turned to evil) your deeds. Snh. 24[a] מְחַבְּלִין זה לזה וכ׳ (Ms. K. זה את זה) wound each other's feelings in discussions; a. fr.—2) *to travail.* Taan. 8[a] bot. מְחַבֶּלֶת ואינה יולדת (Rashi: חוֹבֶלֶת) travails but cannot give birth.—*Pass. pass.* מְחוּבָּל *ruined.* Ex. R. s. 30.

Hithpa. הִתְחַבֵּל *to be spoiled, ruined.* Mekh. B'shall., Vayassa, s. 1 נותן דבר המְחַבֵּל לתוך דבר המִתְחַבֵּל he puts a thing which spoils (the taste) into a thing which is spoiled.

חֲבַל I, חֲבִיל, fut. יַחְבּוֹל same, *to wrong, be violent.* Targ. Job XXXIV, 31.

Pa. חַבֵּיל 1) *to injure; to ruin, destroy* &c. (corresp. to b. h. הִשְׁחִית). Targ. O. Lev. XIX, 27. Targ. Gen. VI, 12; a. fr.—*Part. pass.* מְחַבַּל *mutilated, blemished.* Targ. O. Deut. XXIII, 2. Targ. Mal. I, 14.—B. Kam. 87[a] אי בעי מְחַבֵּל בה לא מצי חַבֵּיל Ms. M. (ed. מחח׳, incorr.) if he desired to wound her (his daughter), he dared not.—2) *to travail.* Denom. מְחַבַּלְתָּא.

Ithpa. אִתְחַבַּל *to be corrupted, destroyed.* Targ. Gen. VI, 11, sq. Targ. Job XVII, 1; a. e. [Targ. Ps. LXII, 11, v. חֲבַל.]—*Ithpe.* אִיתְּחַבַל *to get sick.* B. Mets. 97[a] ואי׳ ומיית Ms. H. (ed. חָבִיל).

חֲבַל II m. (preced.) 1) *injury,* v. חַבְלָא I.—2) *woe!, Oh!* (cmp. בְּיָיא II). Targ. Job X, 15 (Var. חֲבוֹל, חֲבֵיל); a. e.—[Also in Hebr. diction] Ned. 74[b] ח׳ עליך וכ׳ woe unto thee! (a pity) that &c. Snh. 111[a]; Ex. R. s. 6, a. e. ח׳ על דאבדין וכ׳ Oh, for those who are gone and cannot be replaced! Ib. s. 26; Mekh. B'shall., Vayassa, s. 6 (prov.) נפל ביתא ח׳ לכוותא (not אבל) when the house falls, woe to the windows!; a. fr.—3) (adv.) *to ruin.* Pes. 20[b] ח׳ תשפך (v. Rabb. D. S. a. l. note 9) it must be poured out (and go) to ruin; B. Kam. 116[a] (ed. חבל, corr. acc., v. Rabb. D. S. a. l. note 30), opp. to תעשה זילוּת, v. זִילוּת.

חֲבֵל, v. חֲבִיל.

חֶבֶל m. (b. h.; חָבַל) 1) *rope, a measure of dimensions, rope's length.* Gen. R. s. 93 קשר ח׳ בח׳ tied rope to rope, v. נִימָא; Cant. R. to I, 1. Erub. V, 4 אין מודדין אלא בח׳ וכ׳ Sabbath distances must be measured with a rope of fifty cubits' length. Ib. 58[a], v. אַפְסַקִימָא. B. Bath. VII, 2 (103[b]) מדה בח׳ measured with the rope (exact dimensions). Peah IV, 5 על חח׳ in a straight line, v. לָמֶט; a. fr.—*Pl.* חֲבָלִים. Erub. l. c. ג׳ ח׳ הם וכ׳ there are three kinds of ropes (used for legal purposes).—Trnsf. *share, possession.* Sifré Deut. 312 אין ח׳ אלא גורל *hebel* means lot; a. e.

חֵבֶל m. (b. h.; חָבַל) 1) *writhing, throes of birth, agony.* Snh. 98[b], a. e. חֶבְלוֹ של משיח the sufferings which are to precede the advent of the Messiah.—*Pl.* חֲבָלִים, constr. חֶבְלֵי. Nidd. 31[a] ח׳ נקבה the pains at giving birth to a female. Ib. חבלי של נקבה (read: חבלים). Ib. וזהו ח׳ אשה and this is the cause of woman's throes.—2) *damage, injury.* Mekh. Mishp., N'zikin, s. 8 ח׳ אשה לבעל the damages for a wife's injury belong to her husband.

חִיב׳, חֶבְלָא ch. same.—*Pl.* חִיב׳, חֶבְלִין, חֲבָלִין. Targ. Is. XIII, 8. Ib. XXI, 3; a. e.

חַבְלָא I, חַבָּלָא m. (preced.) *injury, ruin.* [Dan. III, 25 חֲבָל. Ezra IV, 22 חֲבָלָא.]—Constr. חֲבַל. Targ. Job V, 21. Ib. 22 (ed. Wil. חַבַּל). Targ. Y. II Gen. XXII, 10 גובא דח׳ (=h. בְּאֵר שַׁחַת). Targ. Jon. II, 7; a. e.—B. Kam. 89[b] בחבליה for the injury he sustained. Bekh. 8[b] חַבְלֵיה Rashi, v. חֲבִילָא. Snh. 100[b] לידול לח׳ go to ruin.

חַבָּלָא, חַבְלָא f.=h. חַבָּלָה, *destruction.* Targ. Y. I Ex. IV, 25 מלאך ח׳ (II מְחַבְּלָא). Targ. Y. I Gen. XXII, 10 (II some ed. חַבָּלָה), v. preced.

חַבְלָא II, חֲבָלָא ch.=h. חֶבֶל, 1) *rope, measure.* Targ. II Sam. VIII, 2.—Y. Sot. VIII, end, 23[a] צווח לסיפיה דח׳ וכ׳ called the ending point of a rope measure its head. Lev. R. s. 14, v. חֲבִילָא II.—Koh. R. to IX, 10 אייתון חַבְלָה וכ׳ get a rope and tie it &c. Gen. R. s. 49 את תפיש ח׳ וכ׳ thou seizest the rope by both ends (demanding justice and mercy); Lev. R. s. 10, beg.; a. fr.—*Pl.* חַבְלֵי, חַבְלִין. Targ. II Sam. l. c. Targ. Prov. V, 22; a. e.—Y. Sabb. VII, 10[c] top, v. אֲלִיקָה. Y. Meg. IV, 74[d] bot. עבד ח׳ וכ׳ make ropes and catch deers.—2) *district.* Constr. חֲבַל, v. חֲבִיל.

חַבָּלָה, v. preced.

חֲבָלָה f. (חָבַל) *injury, mayhem; damages for mayhem.* B. Kam. 87[a] ח׳ למי to whom belong the damages? Ib. 91[a] bot. כי לא . . . לח׳ דחסריה ממונא we disallow payment in instalments only for the injury, because he caused a loss of money (to the wounded person); a. fr.—*Pl.* חֲבָלוֹת. Ib. Snh. I, 1, v. גְּזֵילָה; a. fr.

חַבָּלָה f. (preced.) *destruction.* מלאכי ח׳ angels of destruction, *demons.* Kidd. 72[a]; a. fr. [Chald. חַבָּלָה or חַבְּלָה, v. חַבְּלָא.]

חַבְלוּתָא f. (preced.) *act of destroying.* Targ. Y. Ex. XII, 27.

חֲבִלָּן, חַבְלָנִית, v. חוֹבְלָ׳.

חבננא, v. חֲבִינְנָא.

חַבְנָנוּתָא, v. חֲבִינָ׳.

חָבַס (cmp. חָבַט) *to crush, press down.* B. Mets. 80[b] Ar., v. חָבַט.

Nif. נֶחְבַּס *to be crushed.* Hull. 42[b] גולגולת שנֶחְבְּסָה וכ׳ a skull the larger portion of which is crushed.

חַבְסָא m. (preced.) *crush through pressure.* B. Mets. 116[b], v. חֲבָטָא.

חָבַץ, *Pi.* חִיבֵּץ (cmp. חָבַט) *to beat* milk &c. into a pulp, *to make a pulp, to scramble.* Sabb. 95[a]; Tosef. ib. IX (X), 13. המְחַבֵּץ והמגבן he who makes thick milk (on the Sabbath, oth. opin. in Rashi: *who presses thick milk* in a bag to let the fluid run out). Ib. XII (XIII), 14 ובלבד שלא יְחַבֵּץ (Var. יַחְבּוֹץ, v. ed. Zuck. note) provided, he does not beat it into a pulp. T'bul Yom II, 4 אם חי׳ if the unclean person stirred (the jelly with the oil on top).

Y. Maasr. II, 50[a] top; a. e. [Y. Orl. I, 61[b] top המחבץ, read: המחמץ.]

חֲבַצֶּלֶת f. (b. h.; prob. a comp. of חב, v. חוב II, a. בצל; v. Ges. H. Dict.[10] s. v.) *young lily*, before its leaves are unfolded. Cant. R. to II, 1 כ״ז שהיא קטנה קורא אותה ח׳ וכ׳ as long as the lily is small, it is named *ḥ.*, when it is full-grown it is named *shoshannah;* v. חָבָא.

חָבַק (b. h.; cmp. חבב a. אבק) *to embrace, press, fasten. Part. pass.* חָבוּק, pl. חֲבוּקִין *clinging to, creeping* (of vines). Y. Kil. VI, beg., 30[b] ח׳ לכותל creeping up the wall.

Pi. חִיבֵּק *to embrace.* Pesik. R. s. 3 באין ומְחַבְּקִין וכ׳ they shall come and embrace Rachel's grave; a. fr.

Hithpa. הִתְחַבֵּק *to embrace one another, make love.* Y. Bets. II, 61[c] מִתְחַבֵּק עם וכ׳ making love to thy wife; Y. Sabb. II, 6[a] bot. מְחַבֵּק.

חֲבַק, *Pa.* חַבֵּק 1) same. Targ. Prov. IV, 8 חַבִּיקְיָה embrace her (Wisdom). Ib. V, 20; a. e.—Pes. 111[b] חַבְּקֵיה לדיקלא (Ms. M. חנקיה, v. Rabb. D. S. a. l. note, Rashi נפלא אדיקלא, Rashb. נפקא אד׳) he threw his arms around the tree.—2) *to fold hands*, cmp. חֲבִינָנוּתָא. Targ. Prov. VI, 10 (h. text חִבֻּק).

חֶבֶק m. (preced. wds.) *junction;* 1) *loop of ribands on the shoe, ankle loop.* Nidd. 58[a] עד מְקום ח׳ the part of the leg to the place where the loop sits (is called the inside of the leg); וח׳ עצמו and (if blood is found) on the ankle itself. [Oth. opin.: 'the place where the leg meets the thigh in a squatting position', Ar.—'the knee-hole with its sinews', Rashi.]—2) *riband around the neck.—Pl.* חֲבָקִין. Sabb. 57[a].—3) *a band with which the saddle or housing of an animal is fastened around its belly;* [oth. opin.: *the housing itself*]. Kel. XIX, 3. Sifra Sh'mini, Sh'rats., Par. 6, ch. VIII; Sabb. 64[a]. B. Bath. 78[a], v. קִילְקִי.

חָבַר (b. h.) 1) *to join, befriend, assist.* Y. Ab. Zar. I, 39[b] top (ref. to Ps. LVIII, 6) [read:] כל מי שהיה חוֹבְרוֹ הוא חוברו whoever assisted him (in his political ambition), him he befriended.—Esp. חוֹבֵר, pl. חוֹבְרִים, חוֹבְרִין *having a share in the ownership of a sacrifice*, v. חֲבוּרָה. Men. IX, 9 (93[b] bot.) אחד מניף לכל החו׳ Ms. M. (ed. חֲבֵרִים) one of the compauy does the waving in behalf of all of them. Ib. 94[a] נתמעטה בחו׳ is reduced in numbers as regards the participants (only one of them being required to act). Tem. 2[a]; Arakh. 2[a] בעלי ח׳ (sub. קרבן) partners of a sacrifice (also בעלי קרבן).—2) with על (cmp. זָוַג) *to join against, protest.* B. Bath. 11[a] חָבְרוּ עליו וכ׳ his brothers &c. combined to protest against his actions.—3) *to tie, fascinate, charm.* Lam. R. to I, 5 מביאין חובֵר וחוֹבְרִין וכ׳ they procure a charmer and charm the serpent. Sifré Deut. 172 ח׳ מרובה ח׳ he who charms large objects; Ker. 3[b] ח׳ גדול; Snh. 65[a] חַבָּר גדול. Ker. l. c. חובֵר חֶבֶר דבלאו הדין הוא but what kind of charmer (Deut. XVIII, 11) is he that is liable only to lashes (v. לַאו)?; a. fr.—[4) (cmp. חָבַל) *to unshape, wound.* Denom. חַבּוּרָה.]

Pi. חִיבֵּר 1) *to join, fasten.* Yalk. Job 927 (ref. to Job XL, 30) מי שח׳ עצמו במצות whoever befriended himself with good deeds; Tanḥ. Nitsab. 4 (corr. acc.). Kel. XIV, 2 וחִבְּרָהּ לו (or וְחִבְּרָהּ) and he fastened the tube to it (the staff). Ib. משיְּחַבֵּר from the moment he attaches it, opp. משיחבל, v. חָבַל.—Part. pass. מְחוּבָּר. Ib. XII, 2 כל המ׳ וכ׳ whatever is fastened (belonging) to an object fit to become unclean &c.—מ׳ (לקרקע) *fixed, immovable*, opp. תלוש. B. Mets. 89[a] אוכל במ׳ may eat of what is standing in the field (Deut. XXIII, 25, sq.). Peah IV, 1, v. דָּלִית. Y. ib. 18[a] ואינו מ׳ and when the Mishnah says בדלית ובדקל, it does not mean במ׳ בדלית וכ׳ 'of that which is attached to the vine and tree'; אין תימר מ׳ הוא וכ׳ if you say, it means that which is attached, then the Mishnah means to say that the owner must designate the *Peah* while it is up (on the tree) &c.—Ib. II, beg. 16[d] (in a passage misplaced and corrupted) הא גדר מ׳ ואינו מ׳ this 'fence' (Mish. ib. II, 3) is to be considered as something attached to the ground (like a growth) and (in other respects) as not attached.—2) *to charm.* Lam. R., introd. (R. Josh. 2) התחיל מְחַבֵּר חֲבָרִים (not מחבי חביים) he began to consult charmers (with ref. to Ez. XXI, 26). Snh. 65[a] מקטר לְחַבֵּר he burns incense for charming purposes (to exorcise the demons); a. fr.

Nif. נֶחְבַּר *to be joined, gathered.* Gen. R. s. 80 (ref. to Hos. VI, 9) as the priests נֶחְבָּרִים על וכ׳ are grooped around &c.; Macc. 10[a] מִתְחַבְּרִין וכ׳.

Hithpa. הִתְחַבֵּר, *Nithpa.* נִתְחַבֵּר 1) same; v. supra.—2) *to associate, make friends with.* Ab. I, 7.—Num. R. s. 20, beg. נִתְחַבְּרוּ מואב וכ׳ Moab and Midian formed an alliance; Tanḥ. Balak 3.—3) *to be charmed, spellbound.* Ib. B'shall. 18 מיד נתח׳ וכ׳ at once the bird is spellbound (by the snake looking at its shadow) and falls to pieces; Yalk. Ex. 255 מית (read מתחבר); Mekh. B'shall., Vayassa, s. 1 מִתְחַבֵּר על צלו (not ומת׳ אל) it remains spell-bound over its own shadow.

חֲבַר, *Pa.* חַבֵּר ch. same, 1) *to fasten, join.* Targ. Ps. CXIX, 69 (Ms. חָבְרוּ *Pe.*; h. text טפלו).—2) *to combine against.* Targ. Job XVI, 4 (h. text אחבירה).—3) *to charm.* Targ. Y. I Deut. XVIII, 11.—4) *to wound*, v. infra. [Y. Maas. Sh. V, 56[b] bot., v. חֲבַר.]

Ithpa. איתְחַבַּר, אִתְחַבַּר 1) *to associate.* Targ. Hos. IV, 17; a. e.—2) *to be wounded.* Keth. 5[b] דם מיפקד פקיד או חַבּוּרֵי אִיתְחַבַּר is the blood (in the womb) stored up, or is it the result of a wound?; ib. 6[a] דם חבורי מִיתְחַבַּר.

חָבֵר m. (b. h.; preced. wds.) (with suff. חֲבֵיר־) 1) *associate, friend, partner* (in sacrifices); *colleague, fellow-student; fellow-being; of the same kind* (also of things). Ab. II, 9 ח׳ טוב a true friend; ח׳ רע a false friend. Ib. 10 כבוד חֲבֵרְךָ thy neighbor's honor. Sabb. 63[a] top בח׳ טוב with a good friend (an obscene disguise for a fair woman, v. גּוּרְדְּלִי); a. v. fr.—ח׳ ותלמיד, (in Babli) תלמיד ח׳ colleague and pupil, a title of distinction for a student, *fellow.* Y. Shek. III, beg. 47[b]; Y. B. Bath. IX, end, 17[b], a. e. ח׳ ות׳ הוה וכ׳ was a fellow under R. Ak.; Bab. ib. 158[b]. Ber. 27[b] דתלמיד ח׳ הוה who was a fellow (under Rab).—2) *Ḥaber, Fellow*, a scholar's title, less than חַכָּם or זָקֵן. Kidd. 33[b] (in Chald. phras.) אתון חכימי, אנא ח׳ ye are *ḥakkime* (doctors), and I merely a fellow. Snh. 8[b], a. e. ח׳ אינו וכ׳, v. הַתְרָאָה; a. fr.—Gen. R. s. 84 (play on חֶבְרוֹן) חָבֵר הנאה וכ׳ that worthy scholar buried &c.—3) *Ḥaber*, *member of a religious or charitable association*, esp. *member of the order for the observance of levitical laws in daily intercourse*. Dem. II, 3. Tosef. ib. II, 2 מקבלין אותו להיות ח׳ is accepted as a member of the order; a. v. fr.—*Pl.* חֲבֵרִים, חֲבֵר׳. Ber. 28ᵇ ולא יכשלו חֲבֵרַי וכ׳ that my colleagues (in court) may not fail in a decision of the law. Ib. הזהרו בכבוד חֲבֵרֵיכֶם take heed of your fellow-students' honor. Bekh. 30ᵇ בפני שלשה ח׳ in the presence of three members of the order. Pesik. R. s. 11 חֲבֵרֵיהֶם שלהם עוסקים וכ׳ the members of societies among them are engaged in charitable work. Ib. ואין חביריהם מרגישים and their neighbors (the fruits in the same bag) are not affected; a. v. fr.—*Fem.* חֲבֵרָה, חֲבֵרָה, חֲבֶרֶת, חֲבֶירֶת. Snh. 8ᵇ אשה חבירה a scholarly woman (acquainted with the law). Ber. 48ᵇ, a. fr. אין מלכות נוגעת בחֲבֶרְתָּהּ וכ׳ one term of office does not touch upon its successor even at a hair's breadth (duration of power is preordained). Deut. R. s. 7 אין טיפה מתערבת בחברתה one rain-drop does not mix itself with the other; a. fr.—*Pl.* חֲבֵרוֹת. Sabb. 129ᵃ חֲבֵרוֹתֶיהָ וכ׳, v. אֲגַם; a. fr.

חֶבֶר m. (b. h.; preced. wds.) 1) *association*.—חֶבֶר עיר *a town organization, congregation* (for divine services, study, charities). Ber. IV, 7. R. Hash. 34ᵇ. Meg. 27ᵇ top (Rashi: חֲבַר עיר a scholar maintained by the town, v. preced. w.).—2) *charm*. Snh. 65ᵃ; Ker. 3ᵇ, v. חָבַר.—*Pl.* חֲבָרִים. Lam. R. introd. (R. Josh. 2), v. חָבַר, *Pi*.—3) ח׳ גואלקי *a load of sacks tied across* an animal's back, to unload which you must lift them before untying, contrad. to אֶבֶר גואלקי a load kept in balance by equal weight on both sides, to unload which you need only untie the knot on the animal's back. Sabb. 154ᵇ מאי לאו בחבר גוולקי וכ׳ ed. (Ms. M. באבר גזול or גדול) do you not think (when it says, ib. XXIV, 1, 'he unties the ropes and the sacks drop of themselves') a *ḥeber* is meant which must be lifted along the sides of the animal?; לא באבר גואלקי וכ׳ Rashi Ms. a. Ar. (ed. בחבר אגלווקי, Ms. M. בגאלקי מפייהו, read: גופייהו, v. Rabb. D. S. a. l. note 7) no, a balanced load is meant &c.; v. Ar. Compl. ed. Koh s. v. חבר. Cmp. אַבְרְוֹרֵי.

חַבָּר m. (b. h. *associate*; Talm.=חוֹבֵר, v. זַבָּר) 1) *charmer*. Snh. 65ᵃ, v. חָבַר. Deut. R. s. 7; a. e.—2) *magus* (v. אַמְגּוּשָׁא), *Parsee priest, guebre* in gen. *Parsee government*. Sabb. 11ᵃ תחת נכרי ולא תחת ח׳ (v. Rabb. D. S. a. l. note 80) rather under heathen (Roman) government, than under a Parsee.—*Pl.* חַבָּרִים, חַבָּרִין. Kidd. 72ᵃ חראנו ח׳ let me see (give me a description of) the Parsees (as opposed to Persians). Pes. 113ᵇ. Yeb. 63ᵇ (ref. to Deut. XXXII, 21 גוי נבל) אלו ח׳ this means the Parsees.

חַבָּר, חַבָּרָא ch. same, 1) *charmer*, v. חַבּוּרָא II.—Lev. R. s. 22; Yalk. Koh. 972 אתא חד חבר (Gen. R. s. 10; Koh. R. to V, 8 גבר, corr. acc.) a charmer (of snakes) came; Tanh. Ḥuck 1.—*Pl.* חַבָּרַיָּא. Snh. 65ᵇ מן ח׳ את thou art a creation of the charmers.—2) *Parsee*. Gitt. 16ᵇ, sq. אתא החוא ח׳ וכ׳ a Parsee came and took the lamp from them.—*Pl.* חַבָּרֵי. Sabb. 45ᵃ מקמי ח׳ from fear of the Parsees (that they might see the lights). Yeb. 63ᵇ אתו ח׳ לבבל the Parsees have entered the Jewish colonies of Babylonia. Bets. 6ᵃ but nowadays דאיכא ח׳ when there are Parsees (forcing to public labors).

חַבְרָא m.=h. חָבֵר 1) *friend, neighbor, fellow-being* &c. Targ. Prov. X, 24 (h. text רֵעַ!); a. fr. [Targ. Hos. III, 1 בחבריה, v. חַמְרָא I.]—B. Bath. 28ᵇ, a. fr. חַבְרָךְ ח׳ אית ליה וכ׳ thy friend has a friend, and thy friend's friend has a friend (you cannot claim ignorance). Sabb. 31ᵃ דעלך סני לחברך וכ׳ do not unto thy neighbor what would be hateful to thee; a. v. fr.—*Pl.* חַבְרִין, חַבְרֵי. Targ. Jud. XIV, 11; a. fr.—B. Bath. 16ᵇ אי חברא כח׳ דאיוב וכ׳ either a friend like those of Job, or death; a. e.—Esp. *Ḥaber*, a) *scholar* (v. preced.), *fellow-student*; b) *member of an order*. Bets. 25ᵃ חַבְרִין our fellow-student (Rab Ḥisda); בר ח׳ the son of &c. (Rab Huna).—Y. Taan. I, 64ᶜ ר׳ חנניא חַבְרְהוֹן וכ׳ R. H. the 'Fellow of the Rabbis'.—*Pl.* חַבְרַיָּא, חַבְרִין, חַבְרִין. Targ. Job XII, 2. Ib. XL, 30 Ms. (ed. חַכִּימַיָּא). Nidd. 6ᵇ ח׳ מדכן וכ׳ the *Ḥăberim* observe &c., v. דְּכֵי. Ḥull 12ᵇ אושעי׳ זעירא דמן ח׳ O. junior, of the *Ḥaberim* (Tosaf.: of *Ḥabaria*, pr. n. pl.); Taan. 24ᵃ. Gen. R. s. 13, end אבימי מן ח׳ וכ׳ A., one of the *H.*, visited a sick person, v. חַבִּירְתָּא.—Fem. חֲבַרְתָּא, חֲבֵירְ׳, חֲבֵרָ׳. Targ. Ps. CX, 1 (v. Ber. 48ᵇ quot. s. v. חָבֵר fem.). Targ. O. Ex. XI, 2; a. e.—Yeb. 63ᵇ (prov.) בחַבְרְתָהּ ולא בסילתא correcting a bad wife by giving her a rival will be more effective than thorns; a. fr.—*Pl.* חֲבַרְתָּא, חֲבֵרָ׳. Targ. Jud. XI, 37, sq. [ביתרתה, v. בית זבוררתא.]

חֲבַרְבַּר (denom. of זְבִירָא) *to darken*. Targ. Ps. CXXXIX, 11 מְחַבְרַבַּר ,מְחַבְּ׳ (ed. Wil. מַחֲ׳).

חֲבַרְבַּר m. (v. preced.) [*hiding in the dark*,] *ḥabarbar*, a species of *lizard*. Sifra Sh'mini, Sh'rats., ch. VI, Par. 5 (a subspecies of צב; Ḥull. 127ᵃ ערוד). Gen. R. s. 82, end ויצא מהם ח׳ (not ויצאת; Ḥull. l. c. ערוד); Y. Ber. VIII, 12ᵇ, v. זְבִינָה. Ib. V, 9ᵃ bot. (Bab. ib. 33ᵃ, Tosef. ib. III, 20 ערוד).—Y. Yoma VIII, 45ᵇ top חֲוַרְבָּר.

חֲבַרְבָּרָא ch. same. Y. Ber. V, 9ᵃ bot. הדין ח׳ (not בריא . . .).

חֲבַרְבְּרֵי m. pl. (preced. wds.) *groping in the dark, temporary loss of direction*. Targ. Y. II Gen. XIX, 11 Var. (ed. חַרְבָּלִיה, read זברברייה); v. חִירוּרָנַיָּא.

חֲבֵרָה, pl. **חֲבֵרוֹת**, v. חָבֵר.

חֶבְרוֹן (b. h.) pr. n. pl. *Hebron*, in Judea. Macc. 9ᵇ. Gen. R. s. 84 (ref. to Gen. XXXVII, 14) וחלא אין ח׳ וכ׳ is not H. situated on a mountain? Yoma III, 1 עד שבח׳ up to the horizon over H.; a. fr.

חֲבַרוּרָא m. (reduplic. of חבר) *companionship, association*. Keth. 65ᵃ לך ולחברך ולַחֲבְרוּרָךְ for thine own sake, and for the sake of thy friend and thy association (social standing). [Yalk. Is. 292, ed. Salon., fr. Pes. 118ᵇ לַחֲבְרוּרִיךָ, v. Rabb. D. S. a. l. note 300.]

חֲבֵרוּת, חֲבֵי׳ f. (חָבֵר) 1) *the condition of a Ḥaber* with reference to levitical pureness; *the Order of Hăberim*. Bekh. 30ᵇ הבא לקבל דברי ח׳ he who comes before scholars to take upon himself the obligations of a *ḥaber*. Tosef. Dem. III, 4 דוחין אותו מַחֲבֵירוּתוֹ ed. Zuck. (Var.

מחבורתו) is expelled from the order; Y. ib. II, 23ª top מחבור׳ (cor. acc); a. fr.—2) *the position of a scholar, 'fellowship'*. Y. Ber. V, 9ª bot. אפי׳ תואר ח׳ וכ׳ even the appellation of fellowship (if you had called us *ḥăberim*) would not have been unbecoming to us.

חֲבָרוּתָא, חַבְרוּתָא ch. (preced.) 1) *attachment; companionship, friendship*. Targ. Ps. CXXXIX, 2 (h. text רֵעַ).—Taan. 23ª (prov.) או ח׳ או מיתותא (Ms. M. אי חברא אי מותא) either companions or death; B. Bath. 16ᵇ (v. Rabb. D. S. a. l. note 90). Ber. 34ª top ח׳ כלפי שמיא (מי איכא) is there a social equality with reference to Heaven (dare man treat prayer as he would a talk with a friend)?; Meg. 25ª.—2) (collect. noun) *scholars of the college*. Yeb. 96ᵇ ח׳ נמי the fellows (my pupils), too, are quoted against me?—Y. Shebi. VII, 37ᶜ top ר׳ יוחנן וחברותיה (v. חֲבוּרְתָא).—*Pl.* חַבְרְוָותָא. Ḥull. 57ᵇ Rashi (ed. חבוורתא, corr. acc.).

חבריות, Y. M. Kat. I, 80ᵇ top, v. כְּרִית.

חֲבֶרְתָּא, חֲבֶרֶת, v. חֲבָרָא, חָבֵר.

חָבַשׁ (b. h.) *to tie;* 1) *to saddle, harness*. Gen. R. s. 55, end חבשה שח׳ וכ׳ the harnessing which Abraham did.—2) *to imprison, chain*. Y. Sot. IX, 24ᵇ top; Tosef. ib. XV, 7 (Var. lect.) חֲבָשׁוֹ attempted to force him by imprisonment, v. חָבַט. Deut. R. s. 2 היה חוֹבֵשׁ וכ׳ he could imprison (condemn) whom he wanted to, opp. פָּדָה. Y. Pes. VIII, 36ª bot. חֲבָשׁוּהוּ ישראל if Israelites keep him in prison (and promised to let him free for Passover); a. fr.—Part. pass. חָבוּשׁ, חֲבוּשָׁה. Ber. 5ᵇ, a. e. אין ח׳ מתיר וכ׳ a prisoner cannot release himself from prison (one cannot do as much for himself as he can for others). Ib. 54ᵇ. B. Bath. 20ª חֲבוּשֵׁי מלכות imprisoned by royal authority; a. fr.—3) (agric.) *to narrow in, to plant one species too near another species, to produce Kilayim* (כִּלְאַיִם). Y. Kil. III, beg., 28ᶜ; Y. Sabb. IX, 11ᵈ bot. אין מין פוגע בחברו לחוֹבְשׁוֹ one species must not meet with the other (in the soil) so as to prevent its growth. Y. Kil. III, 28ᵈ אורכו בכמה חוֹבֵשׁ at what distance, lengthwise, does one interfere with the other (so as to be forbidden to plant)? Ib. II, 28ª אין אדם חובש וכ׳ one cannot make forbidden as Kilayim that which is not his own (by planting too near); a. fr.—*Part. pass.* חָבוּשׁ, f. חֲבוּשָׁה *too closely planted between different species*. Ib. I, end, 27ᶜ שעורה ח׳ באמצע barley planted between.

Nif. נֶחְבַּשׁ 1) *to be imprisoned, be detained*. Keth II, 9 האשה שֶׁנֶּחְבְּשָׁה וכ׳ a married woman that has been detained in the power of gentiles, if for money &c.; a. e.—2) *to be planted too closely, to become forbidden as Kilayim*. Y. Kil. III, 28ᵈ bot. נ׳ בשמונה becomes forbidden by a neighborhood of eight cubits. Ib. שלא יֵחָבֵשׁ אלא וכ׳ that it is not made forbidden at a distance of more than eight cubits.

Hif. הֶחְבִּישׁ *to be the cause of prohibition as Kilayim*. Ib. שלא יַחְבִּישׁ וכ׳ that it does not cause a prohibition at a distance of more &c.

Hithpa הִתְחַבֵּשׁ *to be kept as prisoner*. Sabb. 152ᵇ והן יִתְחַבְּשׁוּ וכ׳ (Ms. M. יֵחָבְשׁוּ) and they, themselves, shall be kept in prison.

חֲבַשׁ ch. same, *to imprison*. Y. B. Bath. V, end, 15ᵇ חַבְשִׁין ליה ought to be put in prison.—*Part. pass.* חֲבִישׁ *closely packed*. Ḥull. 52ª כל דח׳ חיישינן Ar. (Var. חביט, ed. דלא משריק יש בו וכ׳) whatever is closely packed (e. g. wheat) is liable to cause injury to an animal falling upon it.

Ithpa. אִתְחַבַּשׁ *to be imprisoned*. Lev. R. s. 30 אתח׳ בפילקי he was put in prison; Pesik. Ul'kaḥ., p. 182ª אִתְחַבַּשׁ Ar. (ed. אתייהב).

חֲבָשָׁה f. (preced. wds.) *saddling, harnessing*. Gen. R. s. 55, end (ref. to Gen. XXII, 3, a. Num. XXII, 21) תבוא ח׳ ותעמוד על ח׳ let (Abraham's) act of harnessing (anxiety to obey the Lord's behest) come and stand (protect) against (Balaam's) harnessing (anxiety to curse); Mekh. B'shall. s. 1 חוֹבָשָׁה.

חבת, Y. Sabb. V, 8ª חבתיו, v. חֶבֶט I.

***חַבְתָּא** pr. n. pl. *Habta*, home of a Highpriest Phineas (Josephus B. J. IV, 3, 8 *Aphtha*). Tosef. Yoma I, 6 פנחס איש ח׳ (Lev. R. s. 26, end פנחס הסתת).

חֲבִתָּא, v. חֲבִיתָּ׳.

חֲבִתִּין, v. חֲבִיתִּ׳.

חָג, חַג, v. חגג, חוג.

חַג m. (b. h.; חגג; cmp. מוֹעֵד, אֵיד) 1) *anniversary, festival*. Lev. R. s. 29; Pesik. Baḥod. p. 153ª ויש לו חג וחגו בן יומו a New-Moon of a month in which there is a festival and whose festival coincides with the New-Moon, v. כֶּסֶה I. Y. Taan. IV, 69ᵇ bot., v. דְּרוֹמָאָה. Sot. 36ᵇ יום חַגָּם their (the Egyptians') festive day; a. fr.—Esp. *ḥag* (*festive period*), *the Feast of Booths with its Eighth Day of Convocation* (שמיני עצרת). Succ. IV, 2 י״ט הראשון של חג the first Holy Day of the *ḥag*; ib. 5 י״ט האחרון וכ׳ the last &c. (the eighth day); a. fr.—2) *pilgrim's festive offering*. Ḥag. 10ᵇ, v. next w., a. חֲגִיגָה.—*Pl.* חַגִּים, constr. חַגֵּי. Ber. 33ᵇ ח׳ נדבה periods of free-will offerings.

חַגָּא I ch. same. Targ. Deut. XVI, 16.—Targ. Y. Gen. XVIII, 14 זמן ח׳ (h. text מוֹעֵד); a. fr.—Ḥag. 10ᵇ (ref. to Ex. XII, 14) how can you prove that this *ḥag* means (festive) offering, דילמא חוגו חגא וכ׳ perhaps it means 'celebrate a feast'?—Ib. דילמא . . . אכלו . . וחוגו ח׳ וכ׳ perhaps the text means to say, 'eat and drink and have a feast (rejoice) before me' (without alluding to special pilgrims' offerings)?—Ib. (ref. to Ex. XXIII, 18) ואי ס״ד דחגא הוא וכ׳ Ms. M. (ed. דחוגא) if you would say, חַגִּי means feast (merry-making) &c.—Koh. R. to III, 2 בין ח׳ וכ׳ between the Feast of Booths and Ḥanuckah. Y. Sabb. VIII, beg. 11ª; a. fr.—*Pl.* חַגַּיָּא, חַגִּין. Targ. Ez. XLVI, 11; a. fr.

חַגָּא II pr. n. m. (abbr. of Haggai) *Ḥagga*, an Amora. Ab. Zar. 68ª. B. Kam. 42ª Ms. M. (ed. חַגַּי).

חֲגָה, pl. **חֲגִין**, v. חִיגָה.

חָגָב m. (b. h.) 1) *hopper, locust*. Sabb. IX, 7 ח׳ חי טהור a living clean (eatable) locust.—*Pl.* חֲגָבִים, חַגָבִין.

Ḥull. 63ᵇ מיני ח׳ species of locusts. Pes. III, 5 (spreading apart) כקרני ח׳ like the proboscides of locusts. Sabb. 106ᵇ; Tosef. ib. XII (XIII), 5. Gen. R. s. 38 the palm-trees appeared to them כאלו ח׳ as though they were locusts (v. חֲגָזָא).—2) (metaph.) *pudenda*. Sabb. 152ᵃ, v. עֲגָבָה. V. also קַרְסוֹל.

חֲגָבָא ch. same. Targ. O. Lev. XI, 22 ed. Berl. (oth. ed. חֲגָבָא; Y. כרזובא).

חָגַג (b. h.; cmp. חוג) [*to turn*,] (denom. of חַג) *to celebrate an anniversary, to observe a festival, to make a periodical pilgrimage*. Num. R. s. 20 אומה החוֹגֶגֶת וכ׳ a nation that celebrates three pilgrims' festivals.—Esp. *to offer the pilgrim's festive sacrifice* (חֲגִיגָה). Ḥag. I, 6 מי שלא חַג... חוגג וכ׳ he who failed to offer on the first day . . . ., may do so during the entire festive season. Pes. 70ᵇ חֲגַגְתֶּם חגיגה you have offered &c.; a. fr.

חֲגַג ch. same, 1) *to turn, draw a circle*. Targ. Prov. VIII, 27 (Ms. חֲגַל).—2) *to celebrate a festival; to feast*. Targ. O. Deut. XVI, 15 תֵּיחוֹג (Y. תְּחַגּוּן). Targ. I Sam. XXX, 16.—Ḥag. 10ᵇ חוגו חגא, v. חַגָּא I.

חַגְוָא m., pl. constr. חַגְוֵי (b. h. constr. חַגְוֵי; חגא, cmp. הֵיגָא) *rugged places, clefts*. Targ. Cant. II, 14.

חָגוּר, v. חִגְּרָא.

חֲגוֹר m. (b. h.) *girdle, outfit*, v. next w.

חֲגוֹרָה f. (b. h.; חגר) 1) *girding, wearing apparel for travelling, outfit*.—Pl. חֲגוֹרוֹת, constr. חֲגוֹרֵי. Gen. R. s. 19 (ref. to Gen. III, 7) חגורה אין... אלא חגורות חגורי חגורות it does not say *ḥăgorah* (a girdle) but *ḥăgoroth* which means sets of outfits; [Ar. חגור חגורי וחגורות]; v. אִסְטְכְרָא.—2) *an enclosure, rope-fence*, contrad. to מְחִיצָה a. פַּסִּין. Erub. II, 4 (Ar. חֲגִירָה).

חֲגָז, חָגָז m., pl. **חֲגָזִין** (cmp. חגס, חגב) a species of *wild bees*, or *locusts*. Sabb. 106ᵇ הצד חגבים ח׳ וכ׳ Ms. O. (Alf. ed. Const. חִיגְזִין, Rashi חַגָּ׳, ed. גזין, v. Rabb. D. S. a. l. note 200) if one catches (on the Sabbath) locusts, *ḥăgazin* &c.; Y. ib. XIV, beg. 14ᵇ חגירן וחושין, read חגזין ויחושין.—Bekh. 7ᵇ דבש חגזין והצירעין (=הח׳, cmp. חֶכְסֵס; Makhsh. VI, 4 חגזין omitted) the honey of &c.

חַגְזָא* ch. same.—Pl. חַגְזַיָּא or חַגְ׳. Y. R. Hash. II, 58ᵃ top the palm-trees of Babylon appeared to us כאילין חגייא (corr. acc. or חֲגָבַיָּא); v. Gen. R. s. 38, quot. s. v. חָגָב.

חַגַּי (b. h.) pr. n. m. 1) *Haggai*, the Prophet. Naz. 53ᵃ. Yeb. 16ᵃ; a. fr.—2) also חַגָּיי, name of several Amoraim. Y. Ber. II, 5ᵇ top.—Y. Dem. III, 23ᵇ bot. B. Kam. 42ᵃ, v. חַגָּא II. V. Fr. M'bo, p. 79ᵇ, sq.

חֲגִיגָה f. (חָגַג) 1) *celebration*, esp. *pilgrimage to Jerusalem for the festivals*. Ber. 33ᵇ חֲגִיגַת הרגל the pilgrimage of the festive season. Lam. R. to I, 17, v. חֲמוֹנוּת.—2) *the festive offering of the visitors of the Temple on the festivals* (Ex. XXIII, 14, a. e). Ḥag. I, 2. Y. ib. 76ᵃ bot. חֲגִיגָתוֹ his festal sacrifice; a. fr.—Pl. חֲגִיגוֹת. Ḥag. I, 8 *the laws concerning festive sacrifices*; Tosef. Ib. I, 9.—3) *Ḥăgigah*, a treatise of the Mishnah, Talmud Babli a. Y'rushalmi, a. Tosefta.

חגידה, v. חֲגִירָה.

חַגִּיר, v. חִגֵּר.

חגייא, Y. R. Hash. II, 58ᵃ top, v. חַגְזָא.

חַגִּירָא, חֲגִיר, חַגִּיר m. (=h. חִגֵּר) *lame, halting*. Targ. Lev. XXI, 18. Targ. Job XXIX, 15; a. e.—Pl. חַגִּירִין. Targ. Is. XXXIII, 23.

חֲגִירָה f.; v. חֲגוֹרָה 2).—בֵּית ח׳ pr. n. *Beth-Ḥăgirah*, name of a family. Y. Meg. I, 71ᵈ bot. של ב׳ ח׳ (ed. Krot. חגידה) those of the family of &c.

חֲגַל (cmp. עגל) 1) *to draw a circle*. Targ. Prov. VIII, 27 Ms., v. חֲגַג.—2) *to go around*, v. infra.

Pa. חַגֵּל *to go around* (visiting, peddling, begging; cmp. P. Sm. 1191). Y. Sot. III, 19ᵃ bot. (expl. שובבית) [read:] מְחַגְּלָה ונסבת וכ׳ she goes about visiting and gets a bad reputation. [Gen. R. s. 17 והוות חַגְּלַת נגידה לה Ar. ed. Koh.; Yalk. Is. 352 והוות חגלה נגידא ליה and she (his wife) went around begging, leading him.]

חֲגַס m. (cmp. חגב, חגז) *rabbit*, or *cony*.—Pl. חֲגָסֵי. Targ. Prov. XXX, 26 (Ar. s. v. גס: הגסי; some ed. חנסי, corr. acc.).

חָגַר I (b. h.) *to encircle; to gird*. Sabb. 63ᵃ אם ת״ח... חֲגְרֵיהוּ על מתנך if a scholar be even revengeful . . like a serpent, bind him around thy loins (be not afraid of him). Midd. III, 1 וחוט.. חוֹגְרוֹ וכ׳ and a red line went around it.—Gen. R. s. 71 לא ח׳ מתניו כנגדה did he not gird his loins (in bold prayer) in her presence (Gen. XXV, 21)? Ex. R. s. 43, beg. התחיל חוגר בתפלה (sub. מתניו) he began to pray boldly. Taan. 14ᵇ לַחְגּוֹר שק to put on sackcloth (for prayer); a. fr.

חֲגַר ch. same. Y. Ned. III, beg. 37ᵈ ח׳ עליה מיתנא tied a rope around it, i. e. made the law more stringent. Bab. ib. 49ᵇ וחוֹגְרָנִי צדעי (Rashi: וחוגר אני, Ar. וח׳) and I had my forehead tied up.

חָגַר II (v. חִגֵּר) *to halt, to limp; to hesitate*. Hull. 18ᵃ כדי שֶׁתַּחְגּוֹר וכ׳ a notch deep enough for the nail to halt on passing over the edge; Bekh. 37ᵇ; Tosef. ib. IV, 1 והיא חוֹגֶרֶת and it (the finger nail) is caught.

Hif. הֶחְגִּיר same. Y. Pes. VII, 35ᵇ top כדי שתהא היד מַחְגֶּרֶת enough for the finger to be caught. Zab. III, 1 מַחְגִּירִין they halt (do not stand firm).

Nithpa. נִתְחַגֵּר *to become lame*. Tosef. Eduy. I, 14.

חֲגַר ch. same, *to be lame*. Targ. II Sam. IV, 4.

Af. אַחְגִּיר same. Targ. II Esth. I, 2. Targ. II Sam. XIX, 27 מַחְגִּיר ed. Ven. (ed. Lag. מחוגר, oth. ed. חַגִּיר). [חֲגַר constr. of חִגְּרָא q. v.]

חִגֵּר, חִיגֵּר m. (חָגַר I; cmp. אִלֵּם) [*tied*,] *limping, lame*. Ḥag. I, 1. Snh. 91ᵇ; a. fr.—Pl. חִגְּרִים, חִגְּרִין, חִי׳.

Ib. VIII, 4. Mekh. Yithro, Baḥod., s. 9; a. e.—Fem. חֲגֶּרֶת, 'חָג. B. Kam. 78b; Tosef. ib. VII, 15 'החג a lame animal. [Y. Shebi. VII, 37c top החגר, read: הַתֶּגֶר.]

חָגַר pr. n. *Hagar* (*Petra*), a district, cmp. next w. Gitt. I, 1 'ומן הח and from the district of H., v. next w.

חַגְרָא I, חֲגָרָה ch., pr. n. *Hagra*, 1) a town and province in the desert of Shur. Targ. O. Gen. XVI, 14 (h. text ברד). Ib. 7 (h. text שור). Targ. Gen. XX, 1.—Targ. O. Gen. XXV, 18 (v. חֲלִיצָא).—2) *Petra*. Tosef Shebi. IV, 11 'רקם דח ed. Zuck. (Var. ורכה דדוגרא, corrupt.); Sifré Deut. 51 תחגרא; Yalk. ib. 874 'רגם דח. V. Hildesh. Geogr. p. 51, sq. [Yeb. 116a Anan b. Hiya 'מח, v. מְחַגְּרָא.]

חַגְרָא II pr. n. m. *Hagra*. Y. Meg. I, 71c bot.—Y. Peah IV, end, 18c (Tosef. Kil. I, 12, a. e. אַגְרָא q. v.).

חַגְּרָא m. ch.=h. חִגֵּר 1) *lame*. Targ. Job XXIX, 15 Var.—Sabb. 32a (prov.) 'רעיא וח' וכ the shepherd lame, and the sheep running (i. e. in critical moments man's sins come home to him).—2) constr. חֲגַר *hesitating in speech*. Targ. Y. I Ex. IV, 10 (Y. II חגּוּר). Ib. VI, 12; 30 Ar. (ed. קשר).

חֲגָרָה, v. חַגְרָא I.

***חִיג', חַגְרְתָא** f. (v. חַגְּרָא) *lameness, frailty*. Gen. R. s. 23; Tanḥ. B'resh. 11 אסיא אסי חִיגַּרְתָּךְ (Yalk. ib. 38 חֲבוּרְתָּךְ) physician, cure thy own infirmity.

חַגְּתָא f. (v. חַגָּא) *pilgrims' festive season*. Ab. Zar. 11b 'ח דטייעי the travelling merchants' season (Arabic fair).

חַד I m. (b. h.; חדד) 1) *pointed, sharp*. Hull. 64a ראשה אחד חד if one side of the egg is pointed, the other rounded (כַּד); ib. (Chald.) רישיה חד חד.—*Pl.* חַדִּין. Ib.—Fem. חַדָּה. Snh. 94a. Ber. 10a 'אפי' חרב ח' וכ even if a sharpened sword is laid on one's throat, one must not despair of praying for divine mercy. Gen. R. s. 16 (play on חִדֶּקֶל, Gen. II, 14) 'שהיתה קַלָּה וחדה וכ (Greece) who was rash and sharp in her decrees.—2) *swift*. *Pl.* as ab. Ber. 59b (play on חדקל) its waters 'ח וקלין are swift and light.—V. חַדָּה.

חַד II m., חֲדָא c.=h. אֶחָד, *one, singular, particular*. Targ. Gen. I, 5; a. v. fr.—חד בשבא first day in the week. Targ. II Esth. III, 7.—Targ. Ps. XXVII, 4. Targ. Ez. XVIII, 10 (some ed. חדת); a. fr.—Y. Ab. Zar. I, 39b bot. בחד בשובא, v. supra. Meg. 11a, a. fr. '. . . וחד וכ חד one authority . . . ., another authority &c. Ber. 28a חדא הוא 'לך או חדת וכ is this a unique subject to thee (the only thing learned from R. Joh.) or a novel (strange) thing?—Gitt. 44a; Bekh. 3a טפי חד one time more (eleven times the value of the sold object); a. v. fr.—[Sabb. 67a bot. חד חד, v. חַדְחַד.]—כַּחֲדָא [*like one*,] *together, simultaneously*. Targ. Ps. II, 2; a. fr.—לַחֲדָא *singularly, very much, too much*. Targ. Gen. I, 31. Targ. Ps. CXIX, 8; a. fr.

חֲדָא I, v. preced.

חֲדָא II *to be glad*, v. חֲדֵי.

חדא, Tosef. Sabb. VI (VII), 11, Var., v. הָדָה II.

חֲדָאָה m. (v. חֶדְיָא) *merry*. Targ. Is. XXII, 2.

חדאקנו, Pesik. Vayhi, p. 63b, v. הֶרְקְלִיאוּפוֹלִים.

חָדַד (b. h.) [*to cut, point*,] *to be sharp, pointed*.

Pi. חִידֵּד *to sharpen, whet, point*. Y. Bets. V, 63b top 'לְחַדֵּד ראשו וכ they differ as to pointing the top of the spit (on the Holy Day)—Trnsf. *to whet the mind, to try somebody's acumen, to puzzle*. Taan. 7a (ref. to Prov. XXVII, 17) 'אף . . מְחַדְּדִין וכ so do two scholars whet each other's mind &c. Naz. 59b, a. e. לא אמר . . . לְחַדֵּד 'בה וכ R. J. said it only in order to encourage the students in raising points; a. e.—*Part. pass.* מְחוּדָּד *sharpened, well discussed, clear and ready*. Kidd. 30a (ref. to ושננתם, Deut. VI, 7) שיהו ד"ת מְחוּדָּדִים בפיך that the words of the Law be ever ready in thy mouth (Sifré Deut. 34 מְסוּדָּרִים), v. גַּבְגַּס.

Hithpa. הִתְחַדֵּד *to be whetted*. Gen. R. s. 69 אין סכין 'מִתְחַדֶּדֶת וכ a knife is whetted on the broad side of another, 'כך אין ת"ח מִתְחַדֵּד וכ so is a student's mind whetted by a fellow-student, v. supra.

חֲדַד ch. same. Targ. Job XLI, 22. [Targ. Y. I Deut. I, 44 דִחַרְדָן which *sting*; some ed. דחדרן, v. חֲדַר.]

Pa. חַדֵּד 1) as preced. *Pi.* Sabb. 32a (prov.) נפל תורא חַדְּדֵיה לסכינא Ms. M. (ed. חדד, Ms. O. חַדְּדוּ) when the ox is thrown down, sharpen the knife (in critical moments man's sins are visited, v. חַגְּרָא). Hull. 43b, a. fr. לְחַדּוּדֵי 'וכ to try Abbayis' acumen.—*Part. pass.* מְחַדַּד *ready in answering questions, well-versed, quick* (v. preced.). Erub. 13b האי דִמְחַדַּדְנָא מחבריי Ms. M. (ed. מחבריא) the reason that I am readier than my fellow-students. Yeb. 14a ב"ש מְחַדְּדֵי טפי those of the school of Sh. were more acute. Nidd. 14b מחדדי שמעתתיה (read: מְחַדַּדְןָ), v. infra.—2) *to cheer up, entertain*. Gitt. 68b, v. חֶדְוְתָא.

Ithpa. אִיתְחַדַּד *to be well studied, ready at hand*. Keth. 62b [read:] מְחַדַּדָן שמעתתיה (Rashi: מחדדן) he recited his lessons (traditions) well.

חַדָּה f. 1) fem. of חַד I; 2) *sharp side, edge*. Y. Ber. I, 2b bot. [חדה, Tosef. Sabb. VI (VII), 11 Var., v. הָדָה II.]

חֶדְוָ, חֶדְ' f. (חדי) *joy*. Targ. Is. XXXII, 14.—Cant. R. to I, 4, v. חֶדְיָתָא. Ber. 55a חֶדְוֵיה, v. מִסְתְּיָרָא.

חֶדְוָא, חֶדְוְוא, חַד' f. 1) same. Targ. O. Gen. XXXI, 27 חֶדְוָא ed. Berl. (Y. חדווא; some ed. חֶדְוָן pl.). Targ. Is. XXXII, 14; a. e.—2) (an exclamation of joy) *aha!* (h. הֶאָח). Targ. Ps. XXXV, 21 (Var. חֶדְוָה). Ib. 25 Ms. (ed. 'וחדיאת וכ, v. חֲדֵי).—*Pl.* חֶדְוָן, v. supra; חֶדְוָתָא, v. חִידְיָתָא.—3) *enigma, allegory; Pl.* חֶדְוָן, v. חִידְיָתָא.

חִדּוּד, v. חִידּוּד.

חֲדוּדוֹ, בית ח', v. הֲדוּרָא.

חדודי, Targ. Y. Deut. XVIII, 10; 14 some ed., v. יְדוֹעָא.

חֶדְוָה f. (b. h.; חֶדְוָה) *joy, rejoicing.* Bets. 15[b] (ref. to Neh. VIII, 10) וקיימו מצות ח׳ Ar. (missing in ed.) and fulfill the law of festive rejoicing. Keth. 8[a] (in the wedding benediction).—V. חֶדְוָא 2).

חֶדְוָוא, חֶדְוָותָא, v. חֶדְוָא, חֶדְוָתָא.

***חֲדוּוִין** m. pl. (cmp. חֲדוּת, a. Syr. חדוא P. Sm. 1200) *subterranean stores.* Tosef. Toh. VIII, 1; 6 (Var. חרויין ed. Zuck., R. S. to Toh. VII, 1 חררין; to ib. 6 הדרין).

חִדּוּק, חִדּוּשׁ, v. sub חִיד׳.

חֲדוּת, v. הוּת.

חֶדְוָתָא, חֶדְוְתָא, חֶדְוְותָא ch.=h. חֶדְוָה. Targ. Ps. IV, 8. Targ. Y. Deut. XVI, 10 חֶדְוַת; a. fr.—Cant. R. to I, 4 (האי ח׳ שלימא חדו על חדו (נגילה this is a complete rejoicing, joy upon joy. Lev. R. s. 20; Koh. R. to II, 2, v. הִתּוּכָא. Gen. R. s. 27 בשעת ח׳ ח׳ (Yalk. ib. 47 חדוה חדוה Hebr.), v. אֶבְלָא.—*Pl.* חֶדְוָן׳, חֶדְוָתָא. Targ. Ps. XVI, 11; a. e. [חֶדְוָתָא, חֶדְוָן׳, pl. of חַדְיָא II.]

חֲדוּתָא, חֲדוּוְתָא, חֲדוּוִיתָא f. (preced., cmp. דַּחְיָא) 1) *dancer, reveller.* Kidd. 81[b] אנא ח׳ דהדרי מיומא Ar. (ed. חרותא דהדר, corr. acc.) I am a reveller returning from a day (of carousing).—2) *a wedding party.* Gitt. 68[b] he saw ח׳ דחוו מְחַדְּדָן לה a wedding party whom people entertained with riddles &c. [Y. Ber. VI, 10[a] top לבי חנוותא (ed. Lehm. לְמֵי חַטְתָא) prob. to be read לבי חד׳ to a wedding.]

חֲדָא, חֲדִי (b. h. חָדָה, cmp. חדר) *to be bright, glad; to rejoice.* Targ. O. Deut. XXVIII, 63 ed. Berl. (oth. ed. a. Y. חֲדִי, incorr.). Targ. Ps. CXXII, 1; a. fr.—Pes. 68[b] חֲדַאִי נפשאי (Ms. M. נפש, v. Rabb. D. S. a. l.) be glad, my soul!—Snh. 39[b]; Meg. 10[b] מי ח׳ קודשא וכ׳ (v. Rabb. D. S. a. l.) does the Lord rejoice in the downfall &c.?; a. e. [Y. Snh. VI, 23[c] bot.; Y. Ḥag. II, 78[a] top, v. next w.]

Af. אַחְדִּי *to gladden.* Targ. Ps. XXX, 2; a. fr.—[Targ. O. Ex. XXVIII, 28 וְיַחֲדוּן, fr. אָחַד.]—Y. Snh. l. c., v. infra.

Pa. חַדִּי 1) same. Targ. Ps. XXI, 7; a. e.—Y. Ḥag. l. c. וּמְחַדֵּי לכון who will entertain you (Y. Snh. l. c. וּמַחֲדֵי).—2) *to observe a festival,* v. חֶדְוָה. Y. M. Kat. II, 81[b] top מְחַדֵּי את מועדא וכ׳ wouldst thou enjoy the festival? Drink &c.

חַדְיָא, חֲדִייא, חֲדִי I, חֲדִ׳ ch. 1) *bright, clean, glossy.*—*Pl.* חַדְיָן, חַדְיֵי, חַדְיָן, f. חַדְיָן. Targ. Prov. XVII, 24 (Var. חַדְיָן, incorr.).—Y. Snh. IV, 23[c] bot. לבושי מאנין נקיים חדרי (read: נקיי וחדיי) dressed in clean and glossy garments (in spite of the rain, v. Rashi to Snh. 44[b]); Y. Hag. II, 78[a] top הווי עמכון חדיי (corr. acc.).—2) *merry, noisy.*—*Fem.* חַדְיְתָא. Yalk. Is. 289 (transl. עליזה, Is. XXII, 2), v. חֶדְוָה a. הַחְיָא.—*Pl.* חַדְיֵי (abstr. noun) *joy.* Targ. II Esth. 1, 2 (3), opp. נְסִיס.

חַדְיָא, חֲדִייא, חֲדִי II m.=h. חָזֶה, *breast, chest, bosom.* Targ. Ex. XXIX, 26, sq.; a. e.—Targ. Prov. XXIV, 33.—בֵּי ח׳ *bosom.* Kidd. 70[b] מִבֵּי חַדְיֵהּ out of his bosom. Sabb. 13[a] אבי חַדְיַיהוּ on their bosoms.—*Pl.* (fem.) חַדְוָתָא, חַדְיָוָתָא. Targ. Lev. IX, 20.

חָדִיד (b. h.) pr. n. pl. *Hadid,* near Ono. Arakh. IX, 6 (32[a], sq.); Y. Meg. I, 70[a] bot. (not הדיר).

חֲדְיֵיב, v. חַדְיֵיב.

חֲדְיַית pr. n. pl. *Ḥadiath,* in Assyria. Targ. Y. Gen. X, 11, sq. (Var. חר׳, חד׳, Y. I, verse 11, פריות, h. text כלח). V. Schr. KAT², p. 98.

חֲדִינָא, v. חֲרִינָא.

חֲדֵיסַר, v. חַדְסַר.

חָדַל (b. h.) [*to be cut off,*] *to cease, to omit.* Gen. R. s. 48 (expl. חדל, Gen. XVIII, 1, by ref. to Deut. XXIII, 23 and Num. IX, 13) פסק.

חֲדָלָה f. (preced.) *omission, use of the root* חדל. Ned. 22[a].

חָדַס, v. הָדַס.

חדס, Targ. Y. Deut. XXV, 9, v. הָחַס.

חֲדַסַר m., **חֲדַסְרֵי** f. (=חד עסר) *eleven, eleventh.* Targ. Y. I Deut. I, 2. Ib. 3 ח׳ ירח eleventh month. Targ. Y. Ex. XXVI, 7; a. e.—R. Hash. 21[a] top בח׳ וכ׳ on the eleventh of Tishri. Arakh. 12[a] וחדסרי (some ed. חד ס׳). Taan. 18[b] חֲדֵיסַר (Ms. M. חד סר) the eleventh (of Adar).

חֲדַסְרָאִי, חֲדַסְרָאָה m. (preced.) *the eleventh.* Targ. I Chr. XXIV, 12 (ed. Lag. two words). Targ. Y. Num. XXV, 8 (ed. Amst. חֲדַסְרָאֵי).

חֲדַסְרֵי, v. חַדְסַר.

חָדַק, חֲדַק, חֲדַק *to cut into, prick.*—*Part. pass.* חָדוּק, fem. חֲדוּקָה, pl. חֲדוּקוֹת. Hull. 59[b] ח׳ בעינן Ar. the horns must be prickly (rough); ed. חרוקות, v. חָרַק.

Pi. חִדֵּק *to squeeze into, drive in.* Erub. 101[a] (play on חדק, Mic. VII, 4, a. והדקות, ib. IV, 13) שמְחַדְּקִין אוה״ע וכ׳ Ms. M. (ed. שְׁמָהַ׳ את הרשעים) those who force the nations into Gehenna; Yalk. Mic. 556. Y. Sabb. X, end, 12[d] לְהַדֵּק בה וכ׳ to close with it (to stuff it into) defective bags.

Hithpa. הִתְחַדֵּק *to be driven into, to stick to.* Tanḥ. Ki Thissa 1; Pesik. R. s. 10, beg. (ref. to Prov. XV, 19) as the thorn מִתְחַדֶּקֶת בבגדיו וכ׳ sticks to the garments &c.

חֲדַק ch. same. *Part.* חָדֵיק *pricking, injuring* (by being forced into). Sabb. 78[b] כיון דח׳ במנא Ms. M. because a rope injures a vessel by being forced into a hole (ed. חריק, v. חֲרַק).

Pa. חַדֵּק *to force into, to fill a gap.* Yoma 72[a] חַדְּקִינְהוּ fasten them by forcing the chords through the rings. Sabb. 125[b] כיון דחַדְּקֵיהּ Ms. M. (ed. דה׳) since he squeezed the stone in (made it immovable).

חֵדֶק (b. h.), **חֲדֶק** m. (preced.) 1) *thorn.* Erub. 101[a] it is written about you (Jews) טובם כח׳ (Mic. VII, 4) the best among them is like a thorn.—2) *anything used for filling a gap, stop-gap.*—*Pl.* חֲדָקִים, חֲדָקִין, ח׳. Ib. כשם

שח׳ וכ׳ (Ms. O. שח׳) as the stop-gaps protect the breach &c.—Ib. X, 8 (101ª) וח׳ שבפרצה (Bab. ed. חוּדְקִים, Ms. M. הדקין, Var. חורקין, חרקין, v. Rabb. D. S. a. l. note) and the stop-gaps in a breach.

חִדְקָא, חִידְ׳ I ch. same, 1) *thorn.* Targ. Mic. VII, 4. —*Pl.* חִדְקַיָּא, חִי׳. Y. Taan. II, 65ᵇ top (ref. to Mic. l. c., v. preced.).—2) חִידְקֵי *parts* or *limbs* of a candlestick *fastened in their places*, opp. חוליות movable limbs. Sabb. 46ª ed. a. Ms. M. (Ar. חרקי).

חִדְקָא, חִי׳ II pr. n. m. *Ḥidka*, a Tannaï, disciple of R. Akiba. Sabb. 117ᵇ; Keth. 64ᵇ. B. Bath. 119ª.

חִדְקָאָה m. (derisive denominative of חִדְקָא I) *descendant of a thorny race.* Erub. 101ª; Yalk. Mic. 556 (with ref. to Mic. VII, 4, v. חֵדֶק; our w. absent in Ms. M., v. Rabb. D. S. a. l. note).

חִדֶּקֶל (b. h.) pr. n. *Hiddekel, Tigris.* Gen. R. s. 16; Ber. 59ᵇ, v. חַד I.

חָדַר (b. h.) [*to cut off,*] *to surround, enclose. Part. pass.* חָדוּר *rounded,* v. חָדַר.

חֲדַר ch. same, *to swarm around.* Targ. Y. I Deut. I, 44 היכמא דהַדְרָן וחיישן וכ׳ (some ed. דחדרן, v. חֲדַר) as the wasps swarm around (man) and hie away (cmp. חזר in Targ. Ps. CXVIII, 11, sq.).

חֶדֶר m. (b. h.; preced. wds.) *enclosure, chamber, secret compartment.* B. Bath. IV, 1 חח׳ וכ׳ the special enclosure for storage inside of the building; a. fr.—Trnsf. *the inner part of the female genitals, the upper end of the vagina or uterus.* Nidd. II, 5. Ib. 17ᵇ; Y. ib. II, 50ª top.—*Pl.* חֲדָרִים. בחדרי ח׳ in the remotest recesses, in strict secrecy. Bets. 9ª, a. fr., v. מַרְאִית. Cant. R. to I, 4 (הביאני) ח׳ בהמות וכ׳ the mysteries of Behemoth &c.; ח׳ מרכבה, v. מֶרְכָּבָה; Yalk. Cant. 982.

חֲדְרוֹנָא, v. חֲרְהוֹנָא.

חַדְרָךְ (b. h.) pr. n. pl. *Ḥadrakh.* Sifré Deut. 1; Cant. R. to VII, 5 (ref. to Zech. IX, 1) I am from Damascus ויש שם מקום ושמו ח׳ and there is a place there named Ḥ.; Yalk. Zech. 575. Ib. (play on the word) חד . . ורך וכ׳ severe . . . and mild. Cant. R. l. c. שעתיד להדריך וכ׳ he (the Messiah) will lead the entire world &c.

חָדַשׁ (b. h.) [*to be bright,*] *to be new.*

Pi. חִידֵּשׁ, חִדֵּשׁ 1) *to renew, renovate, polish.* Lev. R. s. 29 (ref. to בחדש, Ps. LXXXI, 4) תְּחַדְּשׁוּ מעשיכם ye shall polish (cleanse) your doings. Gen. R. s. 78, beg. (ref. to Lam. III, 23) אתה מְחַדְּשֵׁנוּ וכ׳ thou renewest our lives every morning; אתה מח׳ לבוקרן וכ׳ thou inspirest us with new life in the morning (rise to power) &c., v. בֹּקֶר; a. fr.—2) *to commence anew, do again.* R. Hash. 7ª, a. e. (ref. to Num. XXVIII, 14) חַדֵּשׁ והבא וכ׳ commence a new account and offer T'rumah of the new produces.—3) *to promulgate a new law, to establish a new interpretation of a Biblical law; to find a new point.* Sabb. 104ª, a. fr. (ref. to Lev. XXVI, 46) אין נביא רשאי לְחַדֵּשׁ וכ׳ (v. Rabb. D. S. a. l.) since the promulgation of *these* laws no prophet has a right to issue a new law. Y. Erub. V, 22ᶜ bot. it is called the New Gate, because there חִידְּשׁוּ וכ׳ (not חו׳) the Sof'rim instituted the interpretation (*Halakhah*); a. fr.

Hithpa. הִתְחַדֵּשׁ, *Nithpa.* נִתְחַדֵּשׁ 1) *to be renewed, to be established as a new interpretation* (cmp. Lat. novellae); *to be offered as a new point* (דבר חדש). Y. Yeb. VIII, 9ᶜ top (ref. to I Chr. VIII, 9) שעל ידיה נִתְחַדְּשָׁה הלכה וכ׳ at her instance the new interpretation (of the law Deut. XXIII, 4) was established; Midr. Sam. ch. XXII; Ruth R. to II, 5 כבר נ׳ הלכה the law has been interpreted long before. Sot. 3ᵇ, a. fr. לא נשנית אלא בשביל דבר שנ׳ בה the section is repeated for the sake of a new point added. —2) *to change turns.* Yoma 26ª משמרות מִתְחַדְּשׁוֹת the Temple attendants are relieved.

חָדָשׁ m. (b. h.; preced.) *new, fresh, additional.* Ber. IX, 3. Sifra introd. לידון בדבר ח׳ in order to be defined by a new point (not included in the general law); a. fr.—Esp. הֶחָ׳ or ח׳ *the new produces of the field* not permitted for use before the Omer day (Lev. XXIII, 10—14). Kidd. I, 9 (37ª) אַף (מן) חח׳ also with the exception of the new produces (the law concerning which applies even to foreign countries). Ib. 39ª תני ח׳ read 'the new fruit' (leaving out 'also'). Dem. IV, 7 שלי ח׳ הוא mine is new fruit (not yet permitted); a. fr.—*Pl.* חֲדָשִׁים. Yoma II, 4 ח׳ לקטורת בֹּאוּ new men for offering incense (such as never before have performed that function), come and &c. Ib. ח׳ גם ישנים new men and also old ones (who have officiated before this). Lev. R. s. 2, end (ref. to Cant. VII, 14) ח׳ the later leaders, opp. to ישנים the patriarchs; a. fr.—Fem. חֲדָשָׁה. Ib. s. 13 תורה ח׳ a new law, expl. חִדּוּשׁ תורה a novel interpretation of the law (concerning slaughtering). Pesik. Baḥod., p. 102ª פרוזדוגמא ח׳ a recent decree; a. fr.

חֹדֶשׁ, חוֹדֶשׁ m. (b. h.; preced.) 1) *new moon,* i. e. *the first appearance of the crescent.* R. Hash. I, 9, a. e. מי שראה את הח׳ he who sees the new moon (when it was his duty to travel to the place of the Supreme Court to testify). Ib. יוצאין לעדות הח׳ they travel for the purpose of testifying to the sight of the new moon; a. fr.—2) *month.* Snh. V, 1 באיזה ח׳ in what month?; בכמה בַּח׳ on what day of the month?; a. v. fr.—ראש ח׳ (abbr. ר״ח) *the first day of the month, the festival of New Moon.* Meg. 21ᵇ פרשת ר״ח the section of the Law read on the New Moon Day (Num. XXVIII, 1—15); a. fr.—*Pl.* חֳדָשִׁים. Ib. III, 4 בראשי ח׳ on New Moon Days. R. Hash. I, 3 על ששה ח׳ וכ׳ for the proclamation of six New Moon Days messengers are sent abroad. Keth. 60ª שלשה ח׳ at an age of three months; a. fr. [Pesik. Baḥod., p. 154ᵇ ניטש מח׳ וכ׳, read חוֹרֶשׁ.—Y. Shebi. IV, 35ᵇ bot. בחדשי׳, read בחרשי׳, v. חוֹרֶשׁ.]

חֲדָשָׁה I f. 1) fem. of חָדָשׁ.—2) *dedication of a new building.* Sifré Deut. 229 (ref. to חדש, Deut. XXII, 8) משעת חֲדָשָׁתוֹ וכ׳ (Yalk. ib. 930 חִדּוּשׁוֹ) you must make a battlement as soon as you dedicate it (not delay).

חֲדָשָׁה II (b. h.), עיר ח׳ pr. n. pl. *Ir Hădashah*, in Judæa. Erub. V, 6 (v., however, Y. ib. 23ª top).

חֲדַת, חַדְתָּא m., **חַדְתָּא, חֲדַתָּא** f. ch.=h. חָדָשׁ. Targ. Num. VI, 3. Targ. Ex. I, 8 (Y. ed. Amst. חֲדַת); a. e.—Targ. Deut. XXIV, 5 (ed. Berl. חֲדַתָּא); a. e.—Targ. Jer. XXXI, 21 חדתא a new event.—Ber. 28ª, v. חַד II.—Yoma 19ᵇ (expl. אחת, ib. I, 7) על חדת for (showing) something novel.—*Pl.* חַדְתִּין; fem. חַדְתָּן, חֲדַתָּן, חַדְתָּתָא. Targ. Is. LXV, 17. Ib. XLVIII, 6; a. e.—Shek. VI, 5 תקלין ח׳ וד׳ new Shekels (of this year's contributions). Y. Gitt. V, 47ª מה ח׳ יימרון (read: יומא דין) what were the novel things to-day (at college)?; Y. Yoma III, 40ᶜ bot. חדתון (corr. acc.); Y. B. Kam. IX, 6ᵈ bot. חידות.—Men. 35ª, sq. חדתתא new *T'fillin*.—Denom.:

חַדֵּת, חַדֵּית=h. חִדֵּשׁ 1) *to renew, restore.* Targ. I Sam. XI, 14; a. fr.—[Targ. O. Deut. XXXII, 12, v. infra.]—2) *to add something new, to change; to make an exception.* Targ. Y. Lev. XXVII, 34 (v. חָדַשׁ, Pi. 3); a. e.—Keth. 45ª ח׳ רחמנא the biblical text states an exceptional law.

Ithpa. אִתְחַדַּת *to be renewed* &c. (v. חָדַשׁ). Targ. O. Deut. XXXII, 12 לְאִתְחַדָּתָא ed. Berl. (oth. ed. לְחַדָּתָא, לְחַדְתָּא which He will renew).—Targ. I Chr. VIII, 9 (v. נְרִשׁוּאָרִין ch.). Targ. Y. Deut. XXXII, 1.

חַדְתָּא, חֲדַתָּא, v. חֲדַת.

חדתון, v. חֲדַת.

חַדְתּוּתָא f. (preced. wds.) *new condition.* Targ. O. Lev. XIII, 55 (h. text גַּבַּחַת q. v.).

חַדְתָּנָא m. (preced. wds.) *a new-fangled (deity).*—*Pl.* חַדְתָּנִין. Targ. Y. II Deut. XXXII, 17.

חו, Y. Sabb. I, 3ᵇ חו רב וכ׳, v. חוֹתָא.

חֵוָא, constr. **חֵוַת**, v. חֵיוָא.

חֲוָא, v. חֲיֵי.

חוּב (b. h.), perf. חָב, part. חַיָּיב, חָב [*to be bound over, seized,*] 1) *to be declared guilty, be sentenced; to be punishable; to be (legally, morally or religiously) bound, to be responsible.* B. Kam. I, 1 חב המזיק he who caused the damage must pay. Ib. 6ᵇ חב . . . חייב . . . מיבעי לה the Mishnah says *ḥab*, ought it not rather to read *ḥayab* (part.)?—[Answ.: they are the words of a Jerusalem Tannai.]—Ib. I, 2 כל שֶׁחַבְתִּי בשמירתו וכ׳ for whatever I am legally bound to guard, I am legally answerable in case of injury. Sabb. I, 1 העני חייב the recipient (the person standing outside) is guilty (of transgressing the Sabbath law).—Y. Ned. I, 36ᵈ top חב על כל וכ׳ he is punishable for each separately.—Ber. IX, 5 חייב אדם וכ׳ man must praise the Lord &c. Ḥag. 4ª, a. e. כל מצוה שהאשה חַיֶּיבֶת בה וכ׳ whatever religious act is obligatory on woman, is also obligatory &c.—Ib. מה להלן נשים חַיָּיבוֹת as there (Deut. XXXI, 12) women are included in the obligation; a. v. fr.—2) *to act in behalf of a person to the latter's disadvantage.* Erub. VII, 11 ואין חָבִין וכ׳, v. זָכָה. Y. B. Kam. IV, 4ᵈ bot. בתחלה . . . צ״מ לָחוּב להן וכ׳ originally guardians are not assigned to minors that they may eventually act to their disadvantage &c.; ואם חָבוּ וְזָכוּ but if they have done so, their action is legal (and they cannot be held responsible); Y. Gitt. V, 47ª top.—Y. Keth. XI, 34ᵇ bot. נמצאתה חב וכ׳ then you would cause a disadvantage to the relics; a. fr.—ח׳ בעצמו *to be alone answerable* for one's loss. Ber. I, 3 כדאי היית לָחוּב בעצמך thou wouldst have deserved to be made answerable &c., i. e. if you had met with an accident you would have had none but yourself to blame.—3) *to owe, be indebted.* Shebu. VII, 5; a. fr.—ח׳ חטאת *to be bound to bring a sin-offering;* ח׳ מיתה *to be subject to death penalty.* Sabb. VII, 1. Ib. XI, 6 כל חַיְּיבֵי חטאת וכ׳ all those eventually bound to bring &c., are not bound, unless &c. Snh. 58ᵇ; a. fr.

Pi. חִיֵּיב *to declare guilty, to convict, sentence* (opp. פָּטַר, זִיכָּה). Snh. 6ª ח׳ את הזכאי if a judge (by an illegal decision) convicted one who ought to have been acquitted. Ib. III, 6 ואחד מְחַיֵּיב and one votes for acquittal. Shebu. IV, 13 ר׳ מאיר מח׳ וכ׳ R. M. says, he is guilty (of blasphemy); a. v. fr.—Ex. R. s. 32, beg. חִיַּיבְתֶּם עצמיכם you have given judgment against yourselves. B. Mets. 3ᵇ פיו אין מְחַיְּיבוֹ ממון וכ׳ the defendant's own statement cannot cause a judgment against him to pay a penalty, but causes the imposition of an oath. Yoma 35ᵇ הלל מח׳ וכ׳, v. הִלֵּל.—*Part. pass.* מְחוּיָּב, מְחוּיָּיב=חַיָּיב, *sentenced, bound.* Y. Keth. III, 27ᵇ מְחוּיְּיבֵי מיתות those sentenced to death, מ׳ מכות sentenced to lashes.—Ber. 20ᵇ, a. fr. כל שאינו מ׳ בדבר וכ׳ whatever is not obligatory upon a person himself, cannot be done by him as a representative of the community, v. חוֹבָה; a. fr.

Hithpa. הִתְחַיֵּיב, *Nithpa.* נִתְחַיֵּיב 1) *to be convicted, amenable to law.* Keth. 30ᵇ מי שנ׳ סקילה he who (under Jewish jurisdiction) would have been sentenced to death through stoning. Ib. כבר נ׳ בגניבה וכ׳ he was amenable to punishment for theft, before he transgressed &c. Ib. מִתְחַיֵּיב בנפשו לא הוה וכ׳ but guilty of a deadly sin he was not until he ate it; a. fr.—2) *to be responsible.* Ab. III, 4, a. fr. הרי זה מתח׳ בנפשו he is responsible for his life, would have himself to blame, if any accident should befall him (v. Ber. 3 quoted above).—3) *to be doomed, to have the misfortune to.* Tosef. Shebu. III, 4 אין אדם מתח׳ לשמוע וכ׳ one has not the misfortune to hear (a curse &c.), unless he sinned himself (ref. to Lev. V, 1). Ib. הרואה . . עבירה נ׳ לראות if one sees people sin, (we say) he had the misfortune to see, opp. זכה.

חוּב ch., perf. a. part. חָב, חַב same, esp. *to incur guilt, to sin.* Targ. Ex. XXXII, 31. Targ. Lev. IV, 22; a. fr.—Targ. O. Num. XV, 28 בְּמֵיחָבֵיה ed. Berl. (oth. ed. בְּמֵיחַ׳, בְּמֶחֱבֵיה).

Pa. חַיֵּיב 1) as preced. *Pi.* Targ. Job XXXIV, 17; a. fr.—Lam. R. to II, 1 (expl. יָעִיב, ib.) איך ח׳ וכ׳ how did the Lord . . condemn &c.; there are places דצווחין לְחַיָּיבָא עייבא where *ḥayaba* (the guilty) is pronounced *ʿayaba*, v. עוּב.—B. Kam. 68ᵇ לא לִיחַיְּיבֵיה (omitted in Ms. F.) do not condemn him (to pay a fine). Ber. 20ᵇ וכל מ״ע נְחַיְּיבִינְהוּ וכ׳ we might just as well by rabbinical ordinance declare them subject to all positive religious duties; a. fr.—*Part. pass.* מְחַיַּיב (interch. with מִיחַיַּיב, v. infra).—2) *to induce to sin.* Targ. II Kings XXI, 16; a. e.

Ithpa. אִיתְחַיַּיב, אִיחַיַּיב 1) *to become guilty, to be induced to sin.* Targ. I Sam. XIX, 5 (ed. Lag. את מחייב). Targ. Y. Lev. V, 19; a. e.—2) *to be convicted, sentenced* &c.; *to be amenable to law, be bound.* Targ. Ps. XXXIV, 23; a. e.—Keth. 85ª דְאִיתְחַיְּיבָא שבועה וכ׳... ההיא a woman was declared bound to make oath in the court of &c. R. Hash. 29ª מִיחַיְּיבֵי are bound (subject to the law about Shofar). Ib. אימא.. לא לִיחַיְּיבוּ I might have thought they ought not to be bound. B. Kam. 72ᵇ כי קא מִיחַיַּיב (v. supra) when does he become responsible; a. v. fr.

חוֹב I m. (b. h.; preced. wds.) *debt, indebtedness.*—בעל ח׳ (abbr. ב״ח) *creditor.* Keth. IX, 2 והניח.. וב״ח וכ׳ and left a widow, a creditor (claiming a debt) and heirs. Ib. 3 וב״ח יותר על חובו and the creditor (seized) more than his debt amounted to. Ib. 69ª בת בעלת ח׳ הויא a daughter (of a deceased father) has the privileges of a creditor, contrad. to יורשת, heiress; a. fr.—שטר ח׳ *note of indebtedness.* Ib. XIII, 8 המוציא ש׳ ח׳ וכ׳ if one produces a note against &c.; a. fr.—*Pl.* חוֹבִין. Ned. 47ᵇ בעלי ח׳ creditors.

חוֹב II m. (b. h. חֹב; חבב) 1) *bosom,* trnsf. *the full ramification of a tree,* opp. חוּד the point, the body of the tree reaching above the main branches. B. Kam. 81ª bot. חובו של אילן Ar., Ms. H. a. F. (Rashi version: וזיבו; ed. איבו, v. אֵב).—2) *seam, rim.*—*Pl.* חוֹבִין. Ib. 119ᵇ top ולא.. שלשה ח׳ he must not use (of the cloth for stretching and hackling) more than three widths of a seam; [Tosef. ib. XI, 13 ed. Zuck. חבין, also some Mss. B. Kam. l. c., Ms. F. a. R. חָפִין, v. Rabb. D. S. a. l., note; v. חָפָה].

חוֹבָא, חוֹבָה ch.=h. חוֹב I 1) *debt.* Targ. Y. Deut. XIX, 15 חוֹב ממון. Targ. Is. III, 12 מרי ח׳ creditors (h. text נֹשִׁים!).—2) *sin, guilt.* Targ. Gen. XX, 9 (O. ed. Amst. חוֹבָאָה); a. fr.—Y. Hag. II, 77ᵈ bot. דין עבד חדא ח׳ this one comitted one sin and died in it; Y. Snh. VI, 23ᶜ חד חובה. Ib. ומה ח׳ וכ׳ and what was the sin he committed?—*Pl.* חוֹבִין, חוֹבַיָּא, חוֹבֵי. Targ. Koh. X, 4. Targ. I Sam. XIII, 1; a. e.—Lam. R. to I, 2 ח׳ בישיא וכ׳ (not בישא) bad debts have you contracted &c.

חוּבָא *storage,* v. חֲבָה.

חוּבָּא I ch.=h. חוֹב II, *lap, bosom.* Targ. Prov. VI, 27; a. e. (ed. Lag. עוב׳, v. עוּבָא; h. text חֵק). Targ. Y. Ex. IV, 6.

חוּבָּא II, **חוּבָּה** I *hubba,* name of a bird. Hull. 62ᵇ.

חוֹבָאָה f., v. חוֹבָא.

חוּבָּה II pr. n. f. *Hubbah,* wife of R. Huna. B. Kam. 80ª (Ms. M. חִיבָּה); Naz. 57ᵇ.

חוּבָה *storage,* v. חֲבָה.

חוֹבָה f. (חוב) *obligation, duty;* (sub. קרבן) *obligatory sacrifice,* opp. נְדָבָה. Naz. II, 8 הרי אני נזיר ח׳ I am a Nazir by obligation (because the condition of my vow was fulfilled), opp. נזיר נדבה a voluntary nazarite without a conditional vow. Ib. הראשון ח׳ in that case my first nazariteship was obligatory. Kinnim I, 1 הח׳ the obligatory sacrifices, opp. נדרים ונדבות. Ber. 27ᵇ.. תפלת רשות או ח׳ is the evening prayer elective or obligatory? Zeb. I, 1 לא עלו... לשם ח׳ they are not accounted to those who offered them as a compliance with the obligation under which they are. Ber. 8ᵇ, a. fr. יוצא.. ידי חוֹבָתוֹ has paid his obligation (of reading the Sh'ma). Ib. 20ᵇ, a. fr. אינו מוציא.. ידי חוֹבָתָן cannot be the medium through which others pay their obligation (v. חוּב); a. fr. חובת הגוף, חובת גברא, &c., v. גַּבְ׳א, גּוּף &c.—Y. Ber. IX, 14ᵇ bot. פרוש אדע חוֹבָתִי וכ׳ a Pharisee of the class (of those who say), 'I want to know my obligation, and I will pay it', expl. חי דא חובתא וכ׳ what wrong have I done that I may do a good act to make up for it.—*Pl.* חוֹבוֹת. Succ. 56ª, v. רֶגֶל; a. e.—2) *condemnation, doom.*—*Pl.* as ab. Midr. Till. to Ps. IV, 8 פותחין בח׳ begin with predictions of doom, opp. נחמות. [חוֹבָה Ch., v. חוֹבָא.]

חוֹבְטִין, חוֹבְטִ, pl. **חוֹבְטִין**, v. חָבַט.

***חוּבְטָא, חֲבוּטָא** m. (חבט) [*hash,*] *giblets.* Lam. R. to I, 1 נסב ח׳ ומע׳א (רבתי) Ar. (ed. Koh. חבו׳, Var. קרביא; ed. בני מעיא) he took the giblets with the entrails.

חוֹבְלָן m. (חָבַל) *a wasteful, reckless person.* Treat. S'mah. IX, end שלא יהא ח׳ (Var. חבלן) not to be reckless by throwing garments upon the dead to be buried with them.

חוֹבְלָנִית f. (v. preced.) *a court which does not spare human lives, tyrannical.* Macc. I, 10 (Y. ed. a. Bab. 7ª חַבְלָנִית).

חוּבָּץ I, **בַּר ח׳** pr. n. m. *Bar-Hubbats.* Y. Peah I, 16ª, v. next w. Ib. בר חביץ (corr. acc.).

חוּבָּץ II, **חוּבְּצָא** m. (חבץ) 1) *soft cheese.* Y. Pes. I, 33ᶜ.—Lam. R. to I, 1 ח׳ דעיזא וכ׳ (4 חד מאת׳) רבתי cheese from a white goat.—*Pl.* חוּבְּצִין. Ib. Y. Peah I, 16ª אמר חד ח׳ said one, Let us have cheese (indirectly denouncing one Bar-Hubbats who had absented himself from a meeting, v. preced.).—2) ח׳ דתמרי *a mash of pressed dates.* Keth. 80ª (differ. fr. חֲבִיצָא; Ar. חִיבּוּצָא), v. שִׁיגְרָא.

חוֹבֵר m. (חָבַר) 1) (b. h.) *charmer,* v. חָבַר 3).—2) *assistant, partner,* v. חָבַר 1).

חוּבְשָׁה, v. חֲבָשָׁה.

חוּבְשִׁין m. pl. *quinces,* v. חָבוּשׁ.

חוֹבְתָא, חוֹבְתָּה f. ch.=h. חוֹבָה, 1) *debt.* Targ. Ez. XVIII, 7 (ed. Wil. חוֹבָתָא, pl.). Targ. II Kings IV, 7.—2) *obligation, duty.* Targ. Koh. VII, 18 נפק ית ידי חובת וכ׳, v. חוֹבָה.—3) *guilt, sin, sin-offering.* Targ. Lev. V, 6, sq.—Targ. Ps. CIX, 7; a. e.—Y. Sot. V, 20ᶜ bot. אירדד ח׳ וכ׳; Y. Ber. IX, 14ᵇ bot. חי דא חובתה, v. חוֹבָה.—4) *disadvantage; condemning evidence.* B. Mets. 28ᵇ לא מייתי אינש ח׳ וכ׳ one is not supposed to offer evidence against himself.—*Pl.* חוֹבָתָא, v. supra.—Targ. Lam. IV, 22 חוֹבוֹתַיִךְ (h. form).

חוּג v. חָגַג, חָנַג.

חוֹגֵג (חוֹג) חוּג m., pl. **חוֹגְגִים (חוּגִים)** (=b. h. חַגְוֵי, v. חָגַג a. חַגְוָא) *clefts, precipices*. Midr. Till. to Ps. XLII, 5 (ref. to חוג, ib.) לשון יוני הוא ח׳ של מים (ed. חוגים, Yalk. Ps. 742 חוגגים) it is a Greek phrase 'precipices of water' (καταρράκτης); cmp. אֲגוֹגָא.

חוּגְתָא f. (חָגַג) *circle, limit*. Targ. Prov. VIII, 27.

חוּד (v. אָחַד) 1) *to connect, finish an arch* by inserting the keystone. Y. Ab. Zar. I, 40ª bot. דהוא חָיֵיד כל וכ׳ for he finishes the entire arch (cmp. Bab. ib. 19ᵇ מכוש אחרון, v. מַכּוֹשׁ II).—2) (cmp. Syr. אחד claudere enigma, P. Sm. 116) *to bring to a point, to compose an enigma, allegory &c.* Targ. Jud. XIV, 12, sq. Targ. Ez. XVII, 2. [*Af.* אָחִיד *to connect*. Targ. Is. XLIV, 13 מְאָחֵיד (מְאַחֵיד), fr. אָחַד.]

חוּד m. (חוד) *point, thin part*. Cant. R. to V, 2 כחוּדָהּ של מחט as the point of a needle. B. Kam. 81ª bot., v. חוֹב II. Zeb. 53ª חוּדוֹ (חוּדָהּ) של קרן the point of the horn of the altar. [Tosef. Kel. B. Mets. III, 9, v. חוֹר I.] V. חַדָּה.

חוּד ch. v. לְחוּד.

חוּדָא=h. חוּד. Hull. 18ᵇ ח׳ דכובעא the projecting point of the Adam's apple.

חוּדַאי, חוּ׳ m. (חוד) *enigma*.—*Pl.* חוּדָאִין, חוּ׳. Targ. I Kings X, 1 (ed. Lag. מתלין).

חִידְתָּא, חוּדְתָּא, חוּדִיתָא same, also *allegory*. Targ. Jud. XIV, 12; 13; 16.—Targ. Y. Num. XXI, 27 (some ed. חורתא, corr. acc.).—*Pl.* חוּדָן, חֻדָּן, חוּדְּיָן, חִידָן. Targ. O. Num. XII, 8 חוּדִּין ed. Berl. (ed. Amst. חִידְיָן). Targ. Ps. LXXVIII, 2. Targ. II Chr. IX, 1 מותלוון וחידְיָן ed. Lag., v. preced. w.

חוֹדֶק, pl. חוֹדְקִים, v. חֵדֶק.

חוֹדְקִי, v. חִידְקִי.

חוֹדֶשׁ, v. חֹדֶשׁ.

חוּדְתָא, v. חוּדִיתָא.

חַוָּה (b. h.) pr. n. f. *Havvah, Eve*, Adam's wife. Gen. R. s. 22 ח׳ הראשונה the original Eve. Sabb. 95ª; a. fr.

חוודרוריא, v. חִירוּרָיָא.

חֶוְיָא, v. חִיוְיָא.

חַוְיָא f. (חֲוֵי) *instruction, law*. Targ. Y. II Lev. VII, 7 (h. text תורה).

חֲוִילָא, v. חוּלָא II.

חֲוּוּק or **חֲוֹוק** m. (חוק) *rundle of a ladder*.—*Pl.* חֲוָיקִין or חֲוִוּקִין. B. Bath. 59ª. Lev. R. s. 29 חֲוָוקים Ar. (ed. צְוִיקִים).

חֲוָור, חִוָּור, חַוּוֹרָא, v. חֲוַר, חִיוַּר.

חֲוַרְבָּרָא, v. חֲבַרְבָּרָא.

חֲוַרְוָור, v. חֲוַרְוָור a. next w.

***חֲוַרוּלִין** m. pl. (cmp. חַרוּל) *thistles*, used for bitter herb (מָרוֹר); cmp. חַרְחָבִין. Pes. 39ª Ar. (ed. חזרת יולין, Ms. M. חזרת אלין, Ms. M. 2 היובלין, Ms. O. חארולין, v. Rabb. D. S. a. l. note); Tosef. ib. I (II), 33 חוורוור ed. Zuck. (Var. חרדל, prob. corrupt., for חָרוּל).

חֲוַרְוָר, v. חִירְוָור.

חֲוּוּרְוָרָיָא, v. חִירוּרָיָא.

חַוְרָן pr. n. pl. (b. h. חַוְרָן, v. Wetzst. to Delitzsch Job p. 597, cmp. חָרֵר) *Havran, Auran*, a signal station, for proclaiming the New-Moon, in the country east of the Jordan named Auranitis. R. Hash. II, 4 (22ᵇ) (Mish. Pes. חורון, Mish. Nap. חברון; Ms. O. חורון); Tosef. ib. II (I), 2 (Var. חַוְרָן).—בֵּית ח׳ (בְּרַת) *Beth-(Brath-)Havran*, prob. the same place. Y. Shek. I, 46ª; Y. M. Kat. I, 80ᵇ bot., a. e. ר׳ חוניה דב׳ ח׳; Bab. ib. 3ᵇ ר׳ נחוניא איש בקעת בית חַוְרְתָן (Ms. M. בקעת חור׳); Succ. 34ª Ms. M. (missing in ed.). Erub. 11ª בקעת בית חורתן Ms. M. (ed. חרויתן).

חוורנס, Y. Ab. Zar. II, 42ª top, read: הַרְסָנָא; cmp. Bets. 16ª; Ab. Zar. 38ª.

חֲוּוּרְתָּא, v. חִיוַּר׳.

חֲוּרְתָן, v. חַוְרָן.

חוּז, v. חָזָה.

חוֹזָאָה I m. (חזי) *a visionary, fiction-teller*. Pes. 105ᵇ לא ח׳ אנא ולא חכימא אנא Ms. M. (ed. ח׳ .... חכימאה וכ׳, v. Rabb. D. S. a. l.) I am neither a poet (inventing a story) nor a speculator. [Rashi explains: מַגִּיד.]

חוֹזָאָה II, v. next w.

בֵּי ח׳, חוֹזָאֵי pr. n. *Be-Hozaë*, a district, on the caravan road, along the Tigris and its canals. M. Kat. 20ª (Ms. M. 2 בי חוזאה). Sabb. 51ᵇ sent money לבי ח׳ וכ׳ to (the merchants in) Be-H. to buy him a Lybian ass (v. Neub. Géogr. p. 380). Taan. 21ᵇ ארבא מותנא בי ח׳ there is an epidemic in B. H.—Keth. 85ª ... . בי ח׳ הוו מסקי men of B. H. had a claim against him.—Denom. חוֹזָאָה. Ab. Zar. 41ᵇ רב חנינא ח׳; Sabb. 130ᵇ; a. fr.

חוֹזֶה m. (b. h. חֹזֶה; חָזָה) *seer*. Gen. R. s. 90; Yalk. ib. 148 (interpret. ח of צָפְנַת פַּעְנֵחַ, Gen. XLI, 45).—*Pl.* חוֹזִים. Lam. R. introd. (R. Joh. 1).

חוֹזִי m. (חָזָה; formed like חוֹלִי) *aspect, nature*. Tosef. Ohol. XV, 12 איני יודע חוזיו . . . מהו וכ׳ I do not know the nature of the case, but (I do know) that &c.

חוֹזְרָנָא m., pl. **חוֹזְרָנִין (חֲזַר)** *surroundings*. Targ. Y. Gen. XXXV, 5. Ib. XLI, 48.

חוֹזְרָנוּתָא f. (collect. noun) same. Targ. Y. Deut. XIII, 8. V. חֲזִרְנוּתָא.

חוֹזֵרֶר, v. חִזְרֵר.

חוֹחַ m. (b. h.; =חוחו, v. חָיָה) *thorn*. B. Kam. 16ª, v. next w.

חוּחָא ch. same. Targ. II Kings XIV, 9.—Y. Sabb. I, 3[b] (read:] קמושא מתעביד ח׳ דאפר ח׳ דאפר מתעביד שד (not קִמְקְמָה ... חורב וכ׳) the *kimmosh* (v. קִימּוֹשׁ) changes into a thorn of the meadow (to distinguish fr. ח׳ *plum-tree*), the thorn .. changes into a demon; v. B. Kam. 16[a].—*Pl.* חוּחִין, חוּחֵי. Targ. Is. XXXIV, 13. Gitt. 70[a], v. הִדְרָרָא. [Syr. חוחא, *plum-tree*, v. אַחְוָנַיְרָא.]

חוּט, pl. **חוּטִּין** f. (חטט) *incisors*. Bekh. VI, 4 (39[a]) ח׳ החיצונות (Mish. ed. חִיטְּרֵי, read חוּ׳) the central two incisors, הפנימיות (Bab. ed. הפנימים) the one each to the right and left of the central incisors. Ib. 35[a]; 37[a].

חוּט I (v. חָטַט) *to dig, perforate.—Pol.* חוֹטֵט, *Hithpol.* הִתְחוֹטֵט, v. חָטַט.

חוּט ch., *Pa.* חַיֵּיט same. Targ. Y. Ex. XXI, 6.—B. Bath. 58[a], v. חֲטִיטָא.

חוּט II *to fasten*, esp. (denom. of חֲוָט) *to provide a shoe with straps*. Y. Kil. IX, 32[d] top לא יָחוּט ליה מסאניה that he should not make for his (woolen) shoes straps of flax but leather thongs. Ib. מהו מֵיחוּט מסאניה בכיתן (not דכ׳) is it permitted to put flax straps on &c.?

Pa. חַיֵּיט, חַיֵּט 1) same, *to fasten, strap*. Targ. Y. Deut. XXV, 9.—2) *to sew*. Targ. Job XVI, 15; a. e.—Men. 37[b] האי מאן דחַיְיטֵיה לגלימיה he who sewed the trail of his cloak up. Y. Shebi. IV, 35[a] bot. הוה מְחַיֵּיט וכ׳ was doing tailor's work at &c.; a. fr.—3) *to mend, patch*. Lam. R. to I, 1 ח׳ ליה מן וכ׳ (1 חד כות׳) רבתי he patched it in one place &c.; a. e.—4) *to form a net of straps, plait*. Ab. Zar. 75[a] דחַיְיטֵי בחבלי וכ׳ Ms. M. (ed. דחַבְטֵי) which they plait with chords &c.

חֲוָט m. ch.=h. חֶבֶט I, *shoe-thong*. Y. Kil. IX, 32[d] top, v. חוּט II.

חוּט III m. (b. h.; preced. wds.) 1) *thread, chord, strap; sinew*. Kel. XXIX, 3 ח׳ משקולת chord of the plumb-line; ib. 4 ח׳ מאזנים of the balances.—Yeb. 121[b], a. fr. ח׳ השערה a single hair, v. הַקָּדָק.—Hull. III, 1, a fr. ח׳ השדרה the spinal chord.—Hag. 12[b] הקב״ה . . . . ח׳ של חסד the Lord strings around him a chord of grace (protection). Meg. 13[a] ח׳ של חסד וכ׳ a chord of (divine) grace was strung &c. Men. 39[a] נפסק החו׳ מעיקרו the twining thread of the show-fringes is broken at the top. Ib. ח׳ של כרך the thread used for twining; a. fr.—Y. Sabb. VI, 8[b] bot. חוטמה וכ׳, read: חוט דומה לשערה a band (of hair) resembling her own hair.—*Pl.* חוּטִין, חוּטִים. Snh. 52[a], a. e. שני ח׳ של אש two threads (lines) of fire. Lev. R. s. 14, v. זָהוֹרִית.—Men. 39[b] חוּטֵי צמר woolen threads (as show-fringes). Sabb. VI, 5 חוטי שיער bands made of hair. Ib. 6 בח׳ וכ׳ with threads .... in their ears (in place of earrings). Hull 93[a] ח׳ שביד the veins of the fore-foot; a. fr.—2) (Geogr.) *air-line*. Tosef. Ter. II, 12. Ib. 13 מן הח׳ ולפנים וכ׳ what is inside (East) of the line is considered as belonging to the land of Israel.—[Tosef. Kel. B. Bath. V, 14 יוצאת החוט, v. חוּץ II.]

חוּטָא ch. same, 1) *thread* &c. Targ. Gen. XIV, 23 (cmp. חֲוָט); a. fr.—B. Bath. 91[b] ח׳ דדובשא a continuous flow of honey; a. fr.—2) *border-line* (v. preced. 2). Y. Shebi. VI, 36[c] bot. ח׳ דנוה the border-line of Naveh (separating the territory occupied by Jews from the neighboring heathen colony for levitical purposes).—*Pl.* חוּטִין, חוּטַיָּא, חוּטֵי. Targ. O. Ex. XXXIX, 3; a. fr.—Hull. 93[a] חמשא ח׳ הוו there are five veins or sinews which must be removed; a. fr.—Esp. *the show-fringes* (צִיצִית). Ib. 110[a] לא רמי ח׳ had no show-fringes put on his garment; a. fr.

חוּטְבָא m. (חֲטַב) 1) *embroidery, design.—Pl.* חוּטְבֵי. Ned. 49[b] גלימא דח׳ (Rashi a. Tosaf. דחו׳, Ar. דחיט׳) an embroidered cloak.—2) (v. חֲטַב I) *chiselling; trnsf. design, plot*. Targ. Ps. LXXIII, 7 חוּטְבֵיהוֹן (Lev. חָט׳).

חוֹטֶם m. (חטם, v. חתם) [*seal, mark*,] 1) *the distinctive feature of the face, nose, nostril*. Yeb. XVI, 3 (120[a]) identification of a corpse can be established only בפרצוף פנים עם הח׳ on seeing the face with the nose on. Y. Sot. IX, 23[c] bot., v. הַכָּרָה. Lev. R. s. 18, beg. והירח זה הח׳ 'the moon' (Koh. XII, 2) is a metaphorical expression for the nose; Sabb. 151[b]; a. fr.—Taan. 29[a] בעל הח׳ a disguise for *the well-known man*, v. בָּקַשׁ. [Y. Sabb. VI, 8[b] bot. חוטמה, v. חוּט III.]—2) *the oblate part of a spheric body*. Nidd. 47[a]; Tosef. ib. VI, 4 ראש הח׳ the top (central circle) of the oblate part of a female breast. Succ. 35[b] bot. חוֹטְמוֹ the oblate top of the Ethrog; Y. ib. III, 53[d]; a. fr.—*Pl.* חוֹטְמִין. Tosef. Nidd. IV, 10 שני חוֹטְמֵי the indications of the two nostrils of the embryo; Nidd. 25[a] חוטמין (read חוטמיו); Lev. R. s. 14 (Y. Nidd. III, 50[d] נקובי חוטמו). Bekh. 39[a] ניקבו ח׳ וכ׳ if the partitions of the nostrils are perforated into one another.—Trnsf. 3) *snout*. *Pl.* as ab. Midd. III, 2 (Mish. some ed. חוטין, incorr.). Succ. IV, 9 (48[b]) ומנוקבין כמין שני ח׳ the two bowls had cavities (outlets) like two slender snouts, v. דָּקַק (v. Rashi a. l.).—4) *the knotted strappings of a shoe*. Tosef. Sabb. XII (XIII), 14 (cmp. חַרְטוּמָא).

חוּטְמָא ch. same, *nose*. Targ. Y. Lev. XXI, 18.

חוּטְרָא, חוּטֵר I c. (=b. h. חֹטֶר, v. חֲטַר; cmp. גִּזְרָא I) *staff, scepter*. Targ. Num. XVII, 17. Targ. Ps. XLV, 7; a. fr. [Also חֹטֶר, חֻטְרָא, constr. חֻטַר.]—Gen. R. s. 53, v. זְרַק. Yeb. 65[b]; Keth. 64[a]; v. מְרָא II.—Lev. R. s. 18 ח׳ ותרתין וכ׳ the (old man's) staff and two feet. Sabb. 109[b] ח׳ דרעיא Ms. M. (ed. יחידאה) the Shepherd's Staff (the Lonely Staff), name of a plant, v. חוּטְרָרָא.—Y. Kidd. I, 60[b] top, a. e., v. מַשְׁכּוֹנִית; a. fr.—*Pl.* חוּטְרִין, חוּטְרַיָּא. Targ. Gen. XXX, 37; a. fr.

חוּטְרָא II, חֻטְרָא m. (v. חֲטַר, cmp. גִּזְרָא II) *fold, enclosure*. Targ. Mic. II, 12.—Sabb. 32[a] (prov.) אבב ח׳ מילי וכ׳ at the gate of the fold, there are words (bargaining), but in the stalls (where the sheep are delivered), strict account (in critical moments a woman's sins are visited, v. תִּגְרָא).—*Pl.* חוּטְרִין, חֻט׳. Targ. O. Num. XXXII, 16 זִט׳ ed. Berl. (ed. Lisb. חֻט׳). Targ. I Sam. XXIV, 4 חו׳ ed. Lag. (oth. ed. חֻט׳).

חוּטְרָא III, חוּטְרָה, חוּטְרַיָּה pr. n. pl. *Ḥutra, Ḥutraya*, near Nehardea. Y. Sabb. I, 4[a] bot. Ib. V, end, 7[c] R. Idi דחוטריה; Y. Bets. II, end, 61[d] דחוטר׳.

חוּמְרָנָא m. (חוּטְרָא I) *striped like a staff* (v. Ge. XXX, 37). Sabb. 110ᵇ דבר אחר ח׳ a striped (checkered) swine. [Oth. opin. in Ar.: *hump-backed*, v. next w., a. P. Sm. 1250.]

חוּמֶרֶת f.=חֲטוֹטֶרֶת, *camel's hunch.* Sabb. 54ᵃ ובחוּטַרְתּוֹ (Alf. בחֲטוֹטַרְתּוֹ) and tied to is hunch.

חָוָה, חוי, *Pi.* חִוָּה (b. h.) 1) *to point.* Meg. 16ᵃ הויתה מְחַוָּה וכ׳ she was pointing at Ahasver.—2) *to show, teach, tell.* Gen. R. s. 20 (play on חַוָּה) ח׳ לה אדם וכ׳ Adam told her &c.

חֲוָא, חוי ch., *Pa.* חַוִּי same, *to show; to tell.* Targ. Y. II Deut. XXXIV, 1. Targ. Jud. IV, 12; a. fr.—Y. Kil. VII, 31ᵃ top ח׳ סלעא וכ׳ (not סלעיה) showed a Sela to R. E. (for examination).

Af. אַחֲוִי same. Targ. Y. Deut. l. c.; a. e.—B. Kam. 100ᵃ א׳ ליה דינרא וכ׳ showed a Denar to R. E. (v. supra). Ib. 116ᵇ דאחוי אַחְוִיָּה (not אחזוי) he pointed the field out (to the officials for confiscation). Ib. ואמרי ליה אַחְוִי ארעתיה (not אחויי, v. Rabb. D. S. a. l. note 70) and the officials said to him show (us) his field. Snh. 107ᵇ Mss. a. old eds. (omitted in later ed.) א׳ ליה בידיה he made a sign to him with his hand; a. fr.—Y. Yeb. XII, 12ᶜ top .. ר׳ מַחְוֵי וכ׳ R. Z. told R. Ba that &c. [Targ. II Esth. II, 21 מחוי חיויא, read with ed. Lag. וּמְחַוִּיָּה, v. מְחָא II.]

Ithpa. אִתְחַוִּי *to be announced; to be told.* Targ. Gen. XXVII, 42. Targ. Ps. LXXXVIII, 12 (not דיִ תחוי).

חֵוַי, חֵוֵי, חִוְיָא, חִוֵי, v. חִוְיָא.

חווילאות, v. חוּלָא II.

חוך *to rub, scratch*, v. חָכַךְ.

חוּךְ I ch. same. Sabb. 54ᵇ דלא הדר חָיֵיךְ ביה that the animal might not turn to scratch (and make the wound sore again).

חוּךְ II (onomatop., v. preced.) [*to hawk,*] *to laugh,* (=צְחַק) *to jest with, caress; to laugh at.* Part. חָאֵיךְ, חָיֵיךְ. Targ. Y. Gen. XXVI, 8. Targ. Prov. XXIX, 9 חָאֵךְ, ed. Lag. חאיך (Lev. אֲחֵיךְ *Af.*).—Gitt. 55ᵇ לא תחוכו, v. infra. M. Kat. 17ᵃ לא בדידך קא חָיְיכְנָא Ms. M. (ed. מְחַיְּכְנָא) I do not laugh at thee; a. fr.

Pa. חַיֵּיךְ, חָאֵיךְ same, 1) *to hawk.* Gen. R. s. 67, v. חָכַךְ.—2) *to laugh.* Targ. Jud. XVI, 25. Targ. O. Gen. XXI, 9 מְחָאִיךְ (Ms. מְאַחֵיךְ). Ib. XVIII, 12; a. fr.—Pesik. B'shall. p. 90ᵃ אנא .. וּמְחַיֵּיךְ בהדין וכ׳ (Ms. O. מדחיך, Ms. Carm. מגחך) I will go and make sport of &c. (v. חַיֵּיךְ). Snh. 26ᵇ אַחוּכֵי קא מְחַיְּיכַת בן does thou make sport of us?—M. Kat. 17ᵃ חייך ed. (Ms. M. אַחֵיךְ). Ib. קא מחייכנא, v. supra.

Af. אַחֵיךְ same. Targ. O. Gen. XXI, 9; a. e., v. supra.—Ber. 18ᵇ מ״ט אַחִיכַת (Ms. M. חייכת) why didst thou laugh (with joy)? Ib. 19ᵃ לא תַחִיכוּ עלה do not laugh at it (v. supra).—Ned. 51ᵃ א׳ רבי (not אחוך); a. fr.—V. מִיךְ.

חוּךְ I m. *scab*, v. חִיכּוּךְ.

חוּךְ II; חֵיךְ, חוּכָא m. (חוּךְ II) *laughter, gladness, object of derision.* Targ. O. Gen. XXXVIII, 23. Targ. Jud. XVI, 27; a. fr.—Targ. Job XII, 4 חיך (ed. Lag. חַיִיךְ).—Ber. 9ᵇ לא פסק ח׳ וכ׳ laughter did not vanish from his lips (he felt happy) &c. Shebu. 34ᵇ מאי ח׳ what is the cause of the laughter?—Erub. 68ᵇ, v. אַבְלוּלָא; a. e.

חָכְ׳, חוּכְמְתָא, חוּכְמָא f. (חכם) 1) *wisdom, learning.* Targ. Ex. XXVIII, 3; a. fr.—Sabb. 90ᵇ לח׳ for acquiring wisdom. Ib. 30ᵃ אן חָכְמְתָךְ where is thy wisdom? M. Kat. 28ᵃ חוּכְמְתִיה וכ׳; a. e.—2) *subtlety.* Targ. Gen. XXVII, 35.

חוּכֵר m. *farmer*, v. חָכִיר.

חוּל (b. h.; cmp. חלל) [*to turn around, circle,*] 1) *to dance.* Part. חָל, חוֹל; perf. חָל. Taan. IV, 8 יוצאות וחולות וכ׳ used to go out and dance in the vineyards; Lam. R. introd. (ר׳ זעירא) וְחָלוֹת (ed. Wil. וחוֹלוֹת). Koh. R. to I, 11 חָלִין לפניו dance before Him, v. חוֹלָה. Gen. R. s. 74 חָלִים; Cant. R. to VII, 1; a. e.—2) (cmp. חַג) *to come in turn, to occur.* Meg. I, 1 חל להיות וכ׳ if the fourteenth fell on a Monday. R. Hash. IV, 1; a. v. fr.—3) (with על) *to hover around one's head, to rest upon one as a duty; to take effect* (as a law). Shebu. 25ᵃ הנדרים חָלִים על וכ׳ vows are binding even if referring to a religious obligation. Ib. שבועות חָלוֹת וכ׳ oaths are binding &c.; Ned. 15ᵃ. Ib. 17ᵃ אין חָלָה וכ׳ one vow of nazaritism does not take effect &c.; Hull. 101ᵃ אִיסוּר חל וכ׳, v. אִיסּוּר. Y. Sabb. VII, 9ᵃ top; a. v. fr.

Hof. הוּחַל [*to be made to circle,*] *to be commenced, established.* Ber. 31ᵃ הוּחֲלָה it (prayer at fixed times) was instituted.

חוּל ch. same, 1) *to dance.* *Part.* חָיֵיל. Targ. Y. Ex. XV, 20 סיילן (read חָיְלָן).—2) *to take effect.* Yoma 14ᵃ חָיְילָא עליה וכ׳ the observation of mourning rests upon him. Ned. 17ᵃ ח׳ נזירות וכ׳, v. preced. Shebu. 24ᵇ ח׳ אתאנים takes effect with reference to figs. Hull. 103ᵃ אתי ... ח׳ comes and takes effect in addition to &c. Ib. .. ובמיתי מֵיחַל (מֵיחוּל) וכ׳ and they differ as to whether or not the prohibition of . . . . comes to take effect &c.; a. fr.—3) *to hover over one's head, be impending.* Targ. Jer. VII, 20; a. e.

Ithpa. אִתְחַיֵּיל *to turn in a circle, dance.* Targ. Ps. XLII, 5 (h. text אדדם).

חוּל II (v. חָלָה) *to be smooth, quiet*, v. infra.

Hithpol. הִתְחוֹלֵל *to be quieted.* Ber. 30ᵇ כדי שֶׁתִּתְחוֹלֵל דעתו עליו (Ms. M., Yalk. Ex. 392, Deut. 813 שֶׁתָּחוּל) until his mind is quieted (collected for prayer).

חוּל ch. same, *to be smooth, lax; to be forgiving, renounce; to be sweet.* Targ. O. Gen. IV, 26 חָלוּ וכ׳ men became lax in worshipping.—Keth. 86ᵃ top תיזיל וְתֵיחוּל וכ׳ Alf. (ed. ותיחלה, Asheri ותימחל) let her go and renounce her mother's widowhood in favor of her father.—Gitt. 47ᵃ דְּלֵיחוּל אַדְמֵיה that he (the gladiator) may be in a forgiving mood for his life (which he is forced to risk); [oth. opin. דְּלֵיחוּל אַדְמֵיה that his blood may be *sweet*, Ar. s. v. ארכא].

Pa. חַיֵּיל *to sweeten* (by adding good wine), *to improve.* B. Mets. 60[a] דילמא טפי ומְחַיֵּילֵיה וכ׳ lest he may add unmixed wine and improve it, and then sell it (for pure wine).

Af. אַחִיל (אַחֲלֵי, fr. חלי) *to be liberal, to forgive.* Ber. 12[b] אַחִילוּ ליה מן וכ׳ they in heaven forgave him. Sabb. 30[a] דא׳ להו עון וכ׳ He pardoned them for the violation of the Day of Atonement; M. Kat. 9[a]. Keth. l. c. אַחִילְתֵּה she renounced it, v. supra.—B. Mets. 73[a] מַחֲלֵי . . . אֲחוּלֵי Ms. R. (ed. אוזולי . . מוזלי, v. זול I ch.) they were liberal towards you. B. Bath. 144[a] אחולי אַחֲלָה she resigned her claim. [M. Kat. 17[a] מִתְחֲלִיל=מיתחיל, v. חֲלַל.] V. מְחַל.

חוֹל I (b. h.; חול I or חלל; cmp. גלל, גל) *sand, sand-region, esp. the sand used for glass-making.* Sabb. VIII, 5 ח׳ הדק fine sand (marl used for manure); ח׳ הגס coarse sand (for cementing). Meg. 6[a], v. זְכוּכִית. [Sabb. 90[a] בורית זה ח׳, v. אֲהָל.]—*Pl.* חוֹלוֹת *sandy region, sea-shore, desert.* Sabb. 31[a] בין הח׳ on an oasis surrounded with sand-land. Meg. 6[a] Cæsarea שהיא יושבת בין הח׳ which was situated between the sea-places, v. חוֹלָה.—Lev. R. s. 5 ח׳ אנטוכיא, v. חוֹלָה.—Y. B. Kam. I, 2[c] top בחופר בח׳ if one digs a pit in sandy ground. Sifré Deut. 39 בית הח׳, v. חוֹלְסִית.

חוֹל II m. *Ḥol*, name of a fabulous bird (Phoenix). Gen. R. s. 19 (ref. to Job XXIX, 18); Midr. Sam. ch. XII; Yalk. Job 917. Cmp. אֲזִירַשְׁנָא.

חוֹל III (b. h.; חלל) [*outside of the sanctuary, foreign,*] *profane, common*, opp. קוֹדֶשׁ; *week-day*, opp. שַׁבָּת, מוֹעֵד. Pes. 104[a]; Hull. 26[b] בין קודש לח׳ between what is sacred and what is secular. Shebu. 35[b] כל שמות . . . חוץ מזה שהוא ח׳ all names of lordship (*Adonay*) . . . are sacred, except the following which is secular (referring to persons).—חוֹלוֹ של מועד, or חול המועד the half-festive days intervening between the first and the last days of Passover or of Succoth. Meg. 22[b]; a. fr.—Maas. Sh. III, 8 פתוחות לח׳ having an entrance on secular ground; ib. תוכן ח׳ their inside is secular ground. B. Mets. 84[b] כלי .... ישתמש בו ח׳ shall the vessel once used for sacred things, be used for secular purposes (shall R. Eleazar's widow marry Rabbi)?; a. v. fr.—*Pl.* חוּלִּין *profane things, animals &c. not consecrated, ordinary objects.* Hull. 2[b], a. e. ח׳ שנעשו על וכ׳ ordinary food (not T'rumah) prepared with the precautions required for the levitical cleanness of consecrated food.—Pes. 22[a], a. fr. ח׳ שנשחטו בעזרה animals not consecrated for sacrifices which were slaughtered in the Temple court. Ib., a. fr. ח׳ . . . דאורייתא the law forbidding the use of ordinary animals slaughtered &c., is not Biblical. Gitt. 62[a] עיסת חוּלָּיו his ordinary dough; זיתי חוליו (not ...ים), v. טָהֳרָה. Hag. I, 3 באות מן הח׳ are procured from secular funds, opp. to proceeds from second tithes; a. fr.—Ber. 32[a] (play on ויחל, Ex. XXXII, 11) ח׳ הוא לך וכ׳ it is too foreign to thy nature to do such a thing; Yalk. Gen. 83, v. חָלִילָה.—*Hullin* (=שְׁחִיטַת ח׳), name of a treatise of the Mishnah, Tosefta and Talmud Babli, of the Order of Kodashim, containing the laws concerning ordinary meat.

חוּלָא (חוֹלָא) ch. same. Targ. Lev. X, 10; a. fr.—*Pl.* חוּלִּין, חוּלֵּי (חוֹלֵי). Targ. Y. Ex. XXII, 30 ח׳ בדכותא (=חולין שנעשו על טהרת הקדש, v. preced.). Targ. Y. Lev. VI, 21.—Targ. Y. Gen. XVIII, 25 ח׳ הוא לך, v. preced.

חוּלָא I *vinegar*, v. חַלָּא III.

חוּלָא II f. (cmp. חֵיל) *a fortified place, castle.* Yalk. Num. 743 שלא קנה חוּלָאוֹ וכ׳ who does not own his castle (named after him; Sifré Deut. s. 37 חוּלָאוֹת).—*Pl.* חוּלָאוֹת. Ib. (Sifré l. c. Var. חֲוִילָאוֹת, v. ed. Fr. note; ib. חוּוילאות, corr. acc.).

חוּלְדָא ch. = next w. Targ. O. Lev. XI, 29 (h. text חֹלֶד; Y. כרכשתא).

חוּלְדָּה I f. (חֹלֶד; cmp. b. h. חלד) 1) *mole.* Y. Hag. I, 80[c], v. אֲשׁוּת.—Kel. XV, 6.—2) *weasel.* Pes. I, 2. Ib. 118[b]. Taan. 8[a] מח׳ ובור from the story about weasel and well (v. comment.). Y. Sabb. XIV, 14[c] top; a. fr.—חוּלְדַּת הַסְּנָאִים (סְנָאִין, סְנָיִי׳) *the porcupine*, v. חַרְזָא. Kil. VIII, 5. Tosef. B. Kam. VIII, 17.—*Pl.* חוּלְדוֹת. Lev. R. s. 6, beg.—B. Kam. 80[a] ח׳ הסנאין Ms. H. (ed. סנאים).

חוּלְדָּה II f. (v. preced.; cmp. חַלּוֹן) *a back-gate.* חוּלְדַּת הַמּוֹלִים *the mule-drivers' gate*, entrance for loads. Y. Yoma I, 38[c]; Y. Meg. IV, end, 75[c].—Midd. I, 3 שני שערי ח׳ two Temple-Mount gates formed like a *huldah;* Cant. R. to II, 9 שער ח׳.

חוּלְדָּה III (b. h. חֻלְדָּה) pr. n. f. *Huldah*, the prophetess. Meg. 14[b] (transl. בַּרְקוּשְׁתָּא). Y. Naz. IX, 57[d] bot. קברי בני ח׳ the graves of the sons of H.; Treat. S'mah. ch. XIV קבר ח׳; a. e.

חוֹלֶה m. (b. h. חֹלֶה; חָלָה) *sick; a patient.* Ber. 10[a] לך ובקר את החו׳ go and visit the sick (King). Ib. 54[b] מי שהיה ח׳ וכ׳ he who has been sick and recovered. Ib. bot. ח׳ חתן וכ׳ a sick person, a bridegroom &c.; a. v. fr.—*Pl.* חוֹלִין, חוֹלִים. Cant. R. to II, 5 ח׳ מן השעבוד suffering from oppression. Gitt. 28[a], a. fr. רוב ח׳ לחיים the majority of the sick recover again. Ib. 61[a] מבקרין חולי נכרים וכ׳ you are bound to visit the sick of the gentile community alike with &c.; a. fr.—בִּיקוּר ח׳, v. בִּיקּוּר.—*Fem.* חולה. Sot. 36[b] ח׳ היא that she was sick.—Midr. Till. to Ps. XLVIII, 14 (play on לחילה, ib.) לאותה הח׳ שהיא עתידה להיות ח׳ (pay attention) to that sick (nation), for she is destined to be sick (suffering). Cant. R. l. c.; a. fr.

חוֹלָה I f. (v. preced.) *evil, bad.* Koh. R. to V, 12 וכי יש רעה ח׳ וכ׳ is there a bad evil and a good evil?

חוֹלָה II f. (חול;=b. h. מָחוֹל) *chorus of singers and dancers.* Y. Meg. II, 73[b] (ref. to חילה, Ps. XLVIII, 14) עתיד . . . להרעשות ראש ח׳ וכ׳ the Lord will be chosen the leader of the chorus (choragus) &c.; Cant. R. to I, 3; VII, 1 [read:] לֵירָעְשׁוֹת וכ׳; Lev. R. s. 11, end להיות ראש ח׳; (Yalk. Is. 294 מחול; Koh. R. to I, 11 מחולה); ib. לחולה כח׳ שנעשה וכ׳ לחו׳ כתיב read *l'holah.* Cant. R. l. c. like the chorus which was arranged for us &c.

חולונאי, v. חִילּוֹנָאָה.

חולות, v. חול I, a. חוֹלַת. [V. also חול I h.]

חוּלְזָא m. (חלז), pl. חוּלְזִין *loins.* Targ. II Esth. VI, 11 חַלּוּז, חוּלְזוּר, v. חֲלַז.

חולחול, read חִילְחוּל.

חוּלְחוּלִית, pl. **חוּלְחוּלִיּוֹת**, v. חַלְחוֹלִית.

חוּלְחוּלְתָּא, חוּלְחַלְתָּא, חַלְחוּל׳ f. ch.=h. חַלְחוֹלִית, *intrigues, trickery.* Targ. Koh. II, 12 חל׳ ed. Lag. (Var. חַלְחוּל׳, v. חוֹלְלָה); VII, 25; X, 13.

חוּלְחָלִית, pl. **חוּלְחָלִיּוֹת**, v. חַלְחָלִית.

חוּלְמֵיתָא, v. חִלְטְתָא.

חוּלְטָנִית, v. חַלְטָנִית.

חוּלֵי, חו׳ *sweet*, v. חֲלֵי.

חוּלִי *disease*, v. חֳלִי.

חוּלְיָא I, חוּלְיָה, חוּלְיִי׳ f. (b. h. חֶלְיָה; חלי, cmp. חָלַל III; cmp. גְּלָה) [*loose part, something movable,*] *limb, link; vertebra of the spinal column.* Bekh. VI, 5 בין ח׳ לח׳ (Talm. ed. 39[b] מח׳ לח׳) between two vertebrae.—Hull. 52[a] if a rib is displaced וח׳ עמה and a vertebra with it. Ib. 42[b]; a. fr.—Y. Succ. I, 51[d] ח׳ של עמוד *a segment* of a column. Men. 38[b] ח׳ *a joint* of the plaited show-threads.—*Pl.* חֲלָיוֹת, חוּלְיוֹת. Kel. XI, 8 a chain שח׳ שלה וכ׳ the links of which are of metal stringed on &c. Ib. ח׳ של אבנים וכ׳ links consisting of jewels, pearls &c. Gen. R. s. 79, v. דִּיקְנִיתִין. Ohol. I, 8 שמונה עשרה ח׳ eighteen vertebrae.—Bets. 22[a] מנורה של חליות a candlestick which can be taken apart. Sabb. 46[a], v. חֻדְקָא. Kel. V, 8; 10 חתכו ח׳ if he cut the burned clay of an oven into tiles; a. fr.—Esp. *a segment of earth* cut out in digging a pit and piled up on its borders; (collect.) *the entrenchment around a well* (increasing its capacity). Ber. 3[b]; 59[a] (prov.) אין הבור מתמלא מחוּלְיָתוֹ a pit cannot be filled up with its own earth, i. e. a community cannot live on its own resources. Sabb. XI, 2 (99[a]) חוּלְיַת הבור (חוּלְיַיִת, Mish. חוּלְיוֹת, pl.) the entrenchment of a well. Erub. 78[a]; Sabb. 99[a] בור וחוּלְיָתָהּ (וחוליי׳) וכ׳ the depth of the well and its entrenchment are counted together to make up ten handbreadths. Ib.[b] בור תשעה . . . ח׳ if the pit was nine handbreadths deep, and he took out of the bottom one segment (which had been cut before this). Ib. ונתן לתוכה ח׳ and threw a segment in. B. Kam. 51[a] עקרו שניהם ח׳ וכ׳ both of them took the last segment out together, so as to complete the legal depth &c. Yoma 84[b] עוקר ח׳ break loose one segment of the entrenchment; a. fr.

חוּלְיָא II, חוּלְיָיא m. ch. (v. חֲלֵי) *something sweet, sweetness.* Targ. Jud. XIV, 14. Ib. IX, 11.—Meg. 7[b] אנא שדרי ליה ח׳ I sent him something sweet. Pes. 115[b] אגב חוּלְיָיהּ Rashb. (ed. חליוה דתבלין, read: חוּלְיָא, v. Rabb. D. S. a. l. note 60) on account of the sweetness in it &c.

חוּלְיָה, חוּלְיָיא, חוּלְיָה, v. preced. wds.

חוּלִילָא m. (חָלַל) *chisel* (h. גרזן). Targ. Is. X, 15.—*Pl.* חוּלִילִין. Targ. I Kings VI, 7 (Var. חוּלֳלָא, חַלְּלָא).

חוּלִין, v. חול III.

חוֹלֵץ, חוֹלֵיץ m. (חָלַץ) *tongs.* Tosef. Kel. B. Mets. IV, 5 [read:] ח׳ של נגר . . המסמרים the carpenter's tongs with which he pulls nails.

חולית, v. חוֹלַת.

***חולית**, Targ. Esth. VIII, 15 חולת ח׳, a corruption, prob. to be read: חוּלְחוּלִית f. (חלל) (the hollow) *sheath* of a sword.

חוֹלֵל m. (b. h.; חול I) *dancer.* *Pl.* חוֹלְלִים. Yalk. Ps. 729, v. חֵירָה.

חוּלְלָא, v. חוּלִילָא.

חוּלָסִית f. (denom. of חול I) *sand-field, ground from which sand for glass-making is dug.* [Cmp. Gr. ὕαλος, ὕελος.] B. Bath. 67[a] (Ms. M. חול׳, Var. חֵל׳, v. Rabb. D. S. a. l. note); Arakh. 32[a]; Meg. 6[b] (missing in censured editions) ח׳ ומצולה (Ms. M. חרסית, v. Rabb. D. S. a. l.), v. מְצוּלָה.—Sifré Deut. 39 Var. בית הח׳ glass-sand soil, v. חול I.—*Pl.* חוּלְסָאוֹת.—בית הח׳ glass-shop on sandy soil. B. Bath. l. c. (Ms. F. חחוּלְסוֹת, Ms. H. ובתי החילסאות, v. Rabb. D. S. a l. note 60).

חוֹלֵף m. (חָלַף) *slaughtering knife.* Tosef. Kel. B. Bath. VII, 3 ושל ח׳ and the handle of &c. Ib. בן ח׳ (not בין, v. R. S. to Kel. XXIX, 8) a small slaughtering knife.

חוּלַף, constr. of חוּלְפָא, v. חֲלַף II.

חוֹלְפָה or **חוֹלֶפֶת**, pl. **חוֹלְפוֹת** *shoots*, v. חֵלֶף a. חֲלִיפָה.

חוּלְפָנָא m., constr. חוּלְפַן (חלף) *value received in exchange* (h. מְחִיר). Targ. O. Deut. XXIII, 19.

חולפניתא, Vers. in Ar. for חַסְפְּנִיתָא.

חוֹלֵץ, v. חוֹלֵיץ.

חוּלַק, חוּלְקָא m. ch.=h. חֵלֶק, *portion, share.* Targ. Deut. XIV, 27. Targ. Gen. XLVIII, 22; a. fr.—Y. Yeb. VII, 8[b] top נסבה ח׳ וכ׳ she is entitled to a share with her sisters. B. Bath. 142[b] אית ח׳ לטליא או וכ׳ is the young man (to whom a share equal to that of the eventual future issue from a second wife was promised as a donation) entitled to that share besides the inheritance with the other children, or not?—*Pl.* חוּלְקִין, חוּלְקַיָּא. Targ. Gen. XLVII, 24 (Y. חוּלְקִין). Targ. Ez. XLVIII, 21 (ed. Lag. חָלְקַיָּא); a. e. V. חֻלְקָא.

חוּלְשָׁא (חוּלְשָׁא) m. (חלש) *faintness, weariness.* Targ. Is. XL, 23.—B. Mets. 80[b]. Yoma 56[b] משום ח׳ דכה״ג וכ׳ on account of the faintness of the Highpriest (under the excitement of the services of the Day of Atonement) he may not take notice of it. Sabb. 87[a] ח׳ דאורחא weariness from travelling. Ber. 40[a] ח׳ דלבא indigestion.

חוֹלַת, חוֹלִית f. (חול I) 1) *sand-plain, sterile shore-land.* Arakh. III, 2 (14ª) חולת המחוז the sand-plain of the Maḥoz (district of Samaria), opp. to pleasure gardens of Sebaste; Tosef. ib. II, 8 חולית של מחוזא. Ib. חולית של יבנה, opp. to pleasure gardens of Jericho. [Comment. take our w. fr. חול III: *the surroundings of a town, promenade.*]—2) ח׳ אנטוכיא pr.n.pl. *the Harbor [Suburb] of Antiochia.* Y. Hor. III, 48ª bot.; Deut. R. s. 4 חוּלְתָא של א׳ (ed. Wil. חִילְּתָה); Yalk. Prov. 956; Lev. R. s. 5 חולות א׳.

חוּלְתָא (חִי׳, חַ...תָה) (preced.) pr. n. pl. 1) ח׳ של אַנְטוֹכְיָא, v. preced.—2) ימא דח׳ *Sea or Lake of Ḥulta,* prob. the navigable portion of the Orontes up to Antiochia. Y. Kil. IX, end, 32ᶜ; B. Bath. 74ᵇ ימה של חולתא Ms. M. (ed. חילת׳; Yalk. Ps. 697 עכו).

חוּלְתָא pr. n. f. *Ḥultha* (the Week-Day-Servant). Targ. Esth. II, 9 (attendant on the first day of the week, v. גְּנוּנִיתָא).

חוּם (v. חמם) *to be warm.* Part. חָאֵים, חָיֵים. Hull. 8ᵇ לכי חָיֵימָא when it (the knife) gets warm; v. infra.

Af. אַחִים *to warm; to affect* (hearers). M. Kat. 12ᵇ מיא דא׳ וכ׳ water which a gentile cook had warmed.—Sabb. 153ª א׳ באספידא דהתם וכ׳ ed. (Ms. דאנא . . . א׳ מר, Ms. O. א׳ לי) arouse the feelings of the people when delivering my funeral address, for I (my soul) shall be present. Ib. הא דמַחֲמוּ . ליה וחאים Ms. M. (Rashi Ms. וְחַיֵּים; ed. ואחים, v. Rabb. D. S. a. l. note) in the one case (that of the righteous man) they speak warmly of him, and one becomes warm &c.—Ib. מאן א׳ הספ׳ (Ms. M. חאים, corr. acc.) who will arouse mourning for thee?

חוּם m. (b. h. חֹם; חמם) *summer, heat.* B. Mets. 106ᵇ; Gen. R. s. 34. Ib. s. 48 בארבע... אין ח׳ אלא וכ׳ four hours after sunrise there is heat only where the sun shines; a. e.

חוּמָא, חוּמָּא I m. same. Targ. Gen. VIII, 22; a. e., v. חוּמְתָא.—Gen. R. s. 87 (in Hebr. dict.) בכל חוּמָאו in his full heat (of youth).

חוּמָא II pr. n. f. *Homa,* wife of Abbayi. Keth. 65ª; Yeb. 64ᵇ חוּמָה.

חוֹמָה f. (b. h.; חָמָה *to surround, protect,* v. Ges. H. Dict. s. v. חמה) *wall,* esp. *fortification* Yeb. 62ᵇ (ref. to Jer. XXXI, 21) בלא ח׳ lives without (moral) protection. Meg. 5ᵇ שימה חוֹמָתָהּ whose lake is her fortification. Ib. I, 1 מוקפין ח׳ fortified all around; a. fr.—*Pl.* חוֹמוֹת. Cant. R. to V, 7 חוֹמוֹתֶיהָ של וכ׳ the walls of; a. e.

חוּמְטָא I f. (חמט) *darkness.* Targ. Y. Gen. XV, 17; cmp. אֲמִיטְתָא.

חוּמְטָא II m. (v. preced.; prob. from its gray-blackish color) *a lizard (chamæleon).* Targ. O. Lev. XI, 30 (h. text חֹמֶט).

חוּמְטוֹן m. (חמט, cmp. חמץ, *to be salty, bitter,* v. Fl. to Levy Talm. Dict. II, p. 205ᵇ) *ḥumton,* a sandy soil containing salty substances and used for the preservation of wheat. Sabb. 31ª קב ח׳ (Ms. M. חוּמְטִין) a Kab of ḥ powder.—ארץ ח׳ pr. n. *Land of Ḥ.*, a district of northern Palestine. Ib. 54ª א׳ ח׳ וכ׳ the district presented to Hiram was the Land of H.

חוּמְטִין m. pl. *ḥumton powder,* v. preced

חוּמַטְרְיָא f. (a popular corrupt. of εὐπατώριον, ἠπατόριον, v. Sm. Ant. s. v.; v. P. Sm. 80; 83, 995) *Eupatorium, a drink made of liver-wort.* Sabb. 109ᵇ, v. אַבּוּב.—V. חֲמַטְלְיָא.

חוּמָס, ח׳ סוּבְנִי m. (a corruption of ἡμισάβανον) *a half-size sabanum, linen cloth.* Gitt. 59ª (sent to Rabbi) סובני וח׳ סובני וכ׳ Ar. (ed. סיבני וח׳ only) a full-size sabanum and a half-size, which were compressed to the respective sizes of a nut and half a nut.

חוֹמֶס, חוּמסא, v. חָמָס.

חוּמְסָא m. (חמס) *a violent man. Pl.* חוּמְסִין. Targ. Y. II Gen. VI, 12.

חוּמְסָן, v. חַמְסָן.

חוּמְעָא m. (חמע) *vinegar.* Targ. Prov. X, 26 Ms. (ed. חוּמְצָא).

חוֹמֶץ m. (b. h. חֹמֶץ; חָמֵץ) *vinegar.* Pes. III, 1 ח׳ האדומי Edomite (Roman) vinegar (wine fermented with barley). Ib. 42ᵇ (when the wine of Judæa could only be soured by an admixture of barley) הוו קורין אותו ח׳ סתם וכ׳ they called it plain *vinegar,* and now ... they call it *Edomite* (Roman, Cæsarean) *vinegar* (to distinguish it from pure vine vinegar). Dem. I, 1 הח׳ שביהודה the vinegar made in Judæa, v. supra. Y. Sabb. XIV, 14ᶜ bot. חוֹמֶץ של פירות fruit-vinegar; a. fr.—B. Mets. 83ᵇ ח׳ בן יין vinegar son of wine (bad son of a good father).

חוֹמֵץ m. (b. h.) *violent man,* v. חַמְצָן.

חוּמְצָא I. v. חוּמְעָא.

חוּמְצָא II, v. חִימְצָא.

חוּמְצָאֵי m. pl., v. חָמֵץ end.

חוּמְצָן m., pl. **חוּמְצָנִין** *dishes prepared with vinegar* (חוֹמֶץ), *salads* (for cooling). Ruth R. to II, 14 מיני ח׳; Yalk. ib. 603 חימוצין; Lev. R. s. 34 חֲמִצִים.

חוֹמֶר I m. (חָמַר II) *[weight, load,] ritual restriction; great importance.* Ḥag. III, 1, sq. ח׳ בקודש מבתרומה there are restrictions in the law regarding Temple sanctuaries which do not apply to T'rumah. Ib. 4 ח׳ בתרומה (sub. מבקודש); a. fr.—*Pl.* חוֹמָרִין, חוֹמָרִים. Tosef. Kil. V, 4 מטילין אותו לשני ח׳ we subject it to both restrictions (by classifying it with domestic animals and with beasts of the field). Y. Erub. IX, end, 25ᵈ לח׳ (ח׳) double restrictions are imposed. Y. Snh. XI, 30ª bot.; a. fr.—חוֹמְרֵי בית הלל restrictions adopted by the Hillelites. Hull. 44ª. Ib. אי כב״ש כקוליהן וכחוֹמְרֵיהֶן וכ׳ either you follow the Shammaites in their easier and their stricter practices, or &c. Ib. 18ᵇ ח׳ המקום וכ׳ the restrictive usages of the place &c.; a. fr. — קַל וָחוֹמֶר *Kal Vaḥomer, a conclusion a minori ad majus.* Sifra introd. (ref. to Num. XII, 14, sq., a. Gen. XLIV, 8). Pes. 66[a] קו״ח הוא מה תמיד וכ׳ we conclude (that the Passover sacrifice must be offered on a Sabbath day) by the syllogism &c.: if the daily sacrifice &c., v. דִּין; a. fr. — Gen. R. s. 23 קו״ח של חושך an absurd syllogism. — *Pl.* קַלִּים וַחֲמוּרִים (fr. חָמוּר). Ib. s. 92, end אחד מעשרה ק׳ וח׳ וכ׳ one of the ten conclusions a minori in the Bible; Yalk. Sam. 132.

חוֹמֶר II (הוֹמֶר Ar.) m. (חָמַר I; v. P. Sm. 1310 s. v. חומרא) [*whatever joins or is joined,*] *bead, little ball* (bulla) hung around the neck; *jewel, clasp, seal;* trnsf. כמין ח׳ like a jewel, i. e. *a precious ethical principle* (cmp. Prov. I, 9, a. מַרְגָּלִיתָא), *a symbol.* Kidd. 22[b] הירה דורש ... כמין ח׳ interpreted this in a symbolical way (giving the practical Biblical law about perforating the slave's ear an ethical signification); Mekh. Mishp, N'zik., s. 2 כמו חומר (Var. אומר, corr. acc.). Sot. 15[a] אדרשנה כמין ח׳ I shall interpret it symbolically. — *Pl.* חֲמוּרוֹת (fr. חמור, cmp. חֲמוּרְתָּא). Ḥull. 134[b] דורשי ח׳ (Ar. הוֹמְרוֹת) symbolizing interpreters.

חוּמְרָא I m. = חוֹמֶר I. Snh. 49[b] ח׳ בעלמא a mere restrictive measure (which does not allow a conclusion as to the rank of the successive functions of the High-priest). Ib. bot. ומאי ח׳ wh·ein consists the greater import (the greater gravity of the crime)? Pes. 11[a] משום ח׳ דשבת וכ׳ on account of the great import of the Sabbath (the grave penalty for its desecration) people are careful &c. — Ḥull. 9[b] ספק סכנתא לח׳ where there is a doubt about a prohibition based on danger to health the stricter practice is preferred; ib. ספק איסורא נמי לח׳ the same is the case with a doubt about a ritual prohibition. Bets. 3[b]; a. fr. — [Targ. II Esth. III, 3, v. חֵימָרָא.]

חוּמְרָא II m. (v. חוֹמֶר II) *joint, knot, bead, amulet.* Kidd. 73[b] תלי ח׳ וכ׳ Ar. (ed. רמי חוּמְרֵי) if the child is found with an amulet (beads, by which the mother intimated the hope of future identification) ... it is not considered a foundling (v. אֲסוּפִי). — *Pl.* חוּמְרֵי. Ib. 9[a] top ח׳ פתכריתא glass-beads. Sabb. 147[b] bot. ח׳ שדרא the vertebrae (v. חוּלְיָא I). Gitt. 69[a] top עקרבא דשב ח׳ a scorpion with seven joints (Rashi: seven shades of *color, stripes*); v. חוּמַרְתָּא.

חוּמְרָא III m. (v. preced.) *accumulated sum, result of calculation.* Ab. Zar. 9[a] ומשכח ליה לחוּמְרֵיה (Ar. אחמריה, אחמריה) and he will find the sum he wants.

חוּמְרָא m. (חמר) *weight* for holding the tent, *socket.* Targ. Y. Ex. XXXVIII, 27 (h. text אדן). — *Pl.* חוּמְרִין, חוּמְרַיָּא, constr. חוּמְרֵי. Ib.; a. fr.

חוּמַרְתָּא f. (v. preced. wds.) 1) *a ball* (bulla), *bead, charm.* Sabb. 57[b] (expl. טוטפת) ח׳ דקטיפתא a charm containing balsam. Ib. 62[a] (expl. כובלת); Gitt. 69[b] ח׳ דפילון a charm containing phyllon. M. Kat. 12[b]; Erub. 69[a] ח׳ דמדושא (Ms. O. מר׳) a *bulla* containing a jewel for sealing (differ. opin. v. Rashi to Erub. l. c.). — 2) *bud, (ball).* Gitt. 69[a] bot. ח׳ דכשותא the bud of cuscuta. — 3) *weight-stone, lever.* B. Bath. 67[b] (expl. גלגל) ח׳ the weight used for hoisting the beams of the press. Zeb. 21[b] בחוּמַרְתֵּיה with its wheel work. — 4) *smoothing weight* in the laundry. Keth. 10[b] top. — 5) *stone* or *sand in the bladder.* Gitt. 69[b] bot. ח׳ דנפקא מיניה the stony substance which he passes.

חוֹמֶשׁ m. (b. h. חֹמֶשׁ; חמש) 1) *one fifth,* esp. one fifth of the value to be added as *fine* on restoring misappropriated property or redeeming dedicated property (Lev. V, 16; 24; XXVII, 27). B. Kam. IX, 6. B. Mets. 54[a] חוֹמְשׁוֹ של קרן the fifth part of the principal (assessed value), i. e. one plus one fifth, v. next w.; a. fr. — 2) *Ḥomesh, one of the five books of Moses,* also *one of the five books of Psalms.* Sot. 36[b] ח׳ הפיקודים the Book of Numbers; ח׳ שני the Book of Exodus; a. fr. — *Pl.* חוּמָשִׁין, חוּמָשִׁים. B. Mets. IV, 8 חמשה ח׳ הן there are five things to which the law ordaining the addition of one fifth applies. — Ḥag. 14[a] חמשה חוּמְשֵׁי תורה the five books of the Law. Y. Meg. III, 74[a] top ח׳ single parts of the Pentateuch. Kidd. 33[a] שני ח׳ two books of the Psalms.

חוּמְשָׁא, constr. **חוּמַשׁ** ch. same. Targ. Lev. V, 24. Targ. Y. Gen. XLVII, 26; a. e. — B. Mets. 53[b] ח׳ מלגיו the one fifth is included in the amount, i. e. the addition is one fifth of the principal (v. preced. w.); ח׳ מלבר the one fifth is excluded, i. e. the addition must form one fifth of the principal plus the addition (25 percent), v. בַּר I ch. — Ib. 54[b] ח׳ דח׳ a fine of one fifth for misappropriating the addition of one fifth; a. fr. — *Pl.* חוּמְשֵׁי. B. Kam. 108[a].

חוּמְתָא f. = חוּמָא, *heat.* Targ. Y. Ex. XII, 39 (ed. Amst. חוּמְתָא). Targ. Cant. I, 7 (ed. Amst. חוּמָתָא, pl.). — [Targ. Prov. XXIX, 11, v. חֵימְתָא.]

חוּמְתָא ch. = h. חוֹמָה; constr. חוּמַת. Lam. R. to II, 2.

חוּמְתֵי f. (חמם; corresp. to Gr. πύρεθρον) name of *a plant, pellitory* (Parietaria). Gitt. 69[a] bot. ח׳ כי ממרו וכ׳ (Ar. incorr. ח׳ ומ׳) pellitory leaves are in such a case as good as Mamru, but the root of p. &c.

חוּן, v. חָנַן.

חוּנָה, חוּנָא pr. n. m., v. חוּנָא.

חוֹנִי pr. n. m. (abbrev. of נְחוּנְיָא) *Ḥoni, Onias,* 1) *Ḥ.* surnamed *M'aggel* (circle-drawer). Taan. III, 8; Ber. 19[a]. — 2) his grandson. Y. Taan. III, 66[d] bot.; Midr. Till. to Ps. CXXVI. — Tosef. R. Hash. IV (II), 11 ח׳ הקטן.

חוּנְיָא, חוּנְיָה, חוּנְיִי׳ pr. n. m. (preced.) *Ḥonia,* name of several Amoraim. Y. Sabb. XIV, 14[c] bot. R. Ḥ. Jacob of Ephrataim. Y. Shek. I, 46[a]; Y. M. Kat. I, 80[b] bot.; a. e. v. חֲוּרָן. — V. נְחוּנְיָא.

חוֹנְיו (חוֹנְיִי) pr. n. m. (preced.) *Onias,* the founder of the Onias Temple, בֵּית ח׳, in Egypt. Men. XIII, 10. Ib. 109[b]; a. e. — V. נְחוּנְיוֹן.

חוּנְיָא, חוּנְיָה, חוּנְיָיא, v. חוּנְיָא.

חוּס (b. h.) 1) [*to bend over, have affection for* (v. Jon. IV, 10),] *to protect, spare, have consideration for* (with על). Neg. XII, 5 אם כך חָסָה התורה וכ׳ if the Law has such consideration for man's property of small value &c. Sot. 14ª אם כבה ח׳ וכ׳ if the Law made such considerate provision for those transgressing &c. Y. Keth. IV, end, 29ᵇ חָסוּ על כבודן וכ׳ cared more for their honour than &c.; a. v. fr.—[2) *to be connected, related.*—Denom. חִיּוּס.]

חוס ch. same. Targ. Ex. XII, 27 (h. text פסח). Targ. II Chr. XXXVI, 15 חָאִיס ed. Lag. (oth. ed. חָס); a. fr.— Taan. 24ª גברא ... חָס עלי דידי היכי חָיֵיס will a man that has no consideration for his son . . ., care for my concerns? Pes. 39ª מאי חסא דחס וכ׳ what typical meaning has *ḥasa* (חַסָּא)? The Lord spared us (in Egypt, v. Targ. Ex. l. c.); a. e.

Pa. חַיֵּיס *to commiserate, grace, favor* (h. חָנַן). Targ. Ps. XXXVII, 21; a. fr.

Af. אַחִיס, אֲחִיס *to have affection for.* Targ. Mal. III, 17 (ed. Lag. חייס; h. text חמל).—[Targ. Is. XXX, 14 נחוס some ed., read בְּחָיָס.]

חוּסְכָּא m. (חָסַךְ) *rubbing off, reduction by wear and tear.* B. Mets. 70ª; cmp. חָסוֹךְ II.

חוּסָם, v. חָסוּם.

חוּסְמָנָא, pl. **חוּסְמָנַיָּא**, v. אוּסְמָנָא.

חוֹסֶן m. (חסן I; cmp. b. h. חָסוֹן) 1) *strength.* Ex. R. s. 30 (ref. to Dan. IV, 27) הח׳ שלי the strength is Mine.— 2) *tow, oakum.* Sabb. II, 1, expl. ib. 20ᵇ 'flax pounded but not carded'; Y. ib. II, beg. 4ᶜ.

חוּסְנָא m. (v. preced.) 1) *fort, castle.* Targ. Ps. XXXI, 3 (h. text צור).—2) *strength, dominion.* Targ. Cant. V, 16.—3) *store-house*, v. חִסְנָא.

חוּסְקִי, v. חִידְקִי.

חוֹסֶר m. (b. h. חֹסֶר; חָסַר) *want, scarcity of provision.* Gen. R. s. 34, v. חֶסְרוֹן.

חוּסְרָנָא, חוּסְרָן ch. same, *need, want; loss.* Targ. Deut. XV, 8 (Var. חֶסְרוֹנָא). Targ. Jud. XVIII, 10 (ed. Wil. חָס׳). Targ. Prov. XXI, 5; a. e.

חוּף I h. *to rub, cleanse*, v. חָפַף II.

חוּף ch. same. Gitt. 68ª bot. חָף ביה he scratched himself against it. Snh. 95ª הוה קא חָיֵיף רישיה he cleansed his head. Ib. 107ª וְזִיְיפָא (וְחִיְיפָה) she &c. Nidd. 66ᵇ לְמֵיחַף (fr. חפף) to wash her hair.

חוּף II *to bend over*, v. חָפַף I.

חוּפָא m. (חפף I) *rim, felloe.*—*Pl.* חוּפִּין, constr. חוּפֵּי. Targ. I Kings VII, 33 (h. text חשק׳).

חוּפָאָה m. (חפא) 1) *cover, roofing.* Targ. Ex. XXVI, 14; a. fr.—Targ. Ez. XXVII, 6 בית ח׳ a house (theatre) with awnings.—2) *coating, plate.* Targ. O. Num. XVII, 3, sq. (ed. Berl. חוּפ׳), v. חִפְיָא.

חוּפָּה f. (b. h. חֻפָּה; חפף I) 1) *covering, canopy*, esp. *bridal chamber*; also (=כניסה לח׳) *the entrance of the bride into the bridal chamber; wedding.* Kidd. 5ª, a. fr. ח׳ קונה the introduction into the bridal chamber constitutes possession (legitimate marriage). Ib. 3ª למעוטי ח׳ to exclude, as a form of marriage, the delivery by her father to take her into the bridal chamber. Gen. R. s. 94 לא ראה בחופתי was not present at my wedding. Snh. 108ª עשה ח׳ לבנו arranged a bridal room for his son. Ab. V, 21 בן י״ח לח׳ at eighteen years one is fit for marriage. Y. Succ. II, 53ª top; Bab. ib. 25ᵇ בני ח׳ wedding party; a. fr.— *Pl.* חוּפּוֹת. Lam. R. to III, 19 כך וכך ח׳ וכ׳ so many state rooms will I arrange &c. Y. Sot. IX, end, 24ᶜ; Tosef. ib. XV, 9 אלו הן ח׳ חתנים these are the bridal canopies (which were interdicted after the destruction of the Temple); (Bab. ib. 49ᵇ חופת sing.). Lev. R. s. 25, beg.; a. fr.— 2) *seat of the Divine Majesty, sanctuary.*—*Pl.* as ab. Y. Meg. I, 72ᵈ top כל ח׳ שהיו וכ׳ all sanctuaries (Shiloh, Gilgal &c.) which existed &c.

חוּפוֹרוֹת, Tosef. B. Mets. IX, 14, v. חָפוּר.

חוּפְיָא m. (חוף I) 1) *rubbing.* Ber. 6ª מח׳ דידהו from their (the demons') rubbing against their clothing.— 2) *broom.* Succ. 32ª דעביד כי ח׳ it has the shape of a broom. B. Kam. 96ª if one stole palm-leaves ועבדינהו ח׳ and made a broom of them. [Ar. הָפְיָא, Var. חוּפְיָא, v. Rabb. D. S. to Succ. l. c. note 2.]

חוּפְנָא, חוֹפֶן, v. חָפְנָא, חֹפֶן.

חוֹפֶר, v. חָפוּר.

חוּץ I (cmp. אוּץ), perf. a. part. חָץ [*to squeeze in; to be wedged in,*] 1) *to be tight, immovable.* Makhsh. III, 8 בשביל שיָּחוּצוּ that they may become tight (by swelling). Mikv. X, 3 בזמן שהיא חוצה (cmp. part. fem. חוֹלָה, fr. חול) if it is tight (immovable).—2) *to tighten, tie closely.* Y. Ḥag. III, 79ª top חָצִים אותה (חָצִין) they tie it watertight.— 3) חוּץ or חָצַץ *to wedge in, form a partition; to intervene*, esp. (at bathing) *to prevent the water from touching the body.* Erub. III, 1 (27ª) יכול לָחוּץ (לָחוֹץ) ולאכול Ms. M. (Bab. ed. לח׳ ולילך וכ׳, Mish. לילך לח׳ ולאכ׳, Y. ed. לח׳ ולוכל, v. Rabb. D. S. a. l. note) he may form a partition (between himself and the uncleanness, by sitting in a vehicle &c.) and eat. Zeb. 19ª מהו שיָּחוּץ (שתָּחוּץ) does it form a partition between the body and the water (so as to make the immersion ineffective)?—Y. Sabb. VII, beg. 7ᵈ שהן חָצִין וכ׳ for they form an interposition at bathing after menstruation. V. חָצַץ.

חוּץ ch. 1) same. Part. חָיֵיץ, f. חָיְיצָא same. Zeb. 19ª, v. preced. Ib. חָיְיצֵי (Rashi: וְזָיְיצָן)—2) (v. נְזִירִין) *to form a partition, to build a wall by piling up material without cementing;* (of persons) *to form a lane.* Y. Shebi. III, end, 34ᵈ דחָיְיצֵי, v. חָיֵיץ ליה.—Keth. 17ª; Meg. 29ª וכ׳, v. אבוּלָא.

חוּץ II m. (b. h.; preced.) 1) *that which is divided off, outside, street.* Kel. XXVIII, 9 חלוק של יוצאת חח׳ the shirt of the runabout (prostitute; v. Sm. Ant. s. v. Coa Vestis a. Diaphane Heimata; Tosef. ib. B. Bath. V, 14 יוצאות חחוט going out of the *line* of custom). Zeb. 57ᵇ; Yoma 57ª ח׳ ופנים Ar. (v. Rabb. D. S. a. l note 2, a. Tosaf.

to Zeb. l. c.) what is done outside the Temple and what inside. Hull. VI, 2 השוחט ... בח׳ he who slaughters unconsecrated animals within the Temple court, or consecrated animals without. Ib. 85[a] שחוטי ח׳ consecrated animals slaughtered outside the Temple court. Ib. 68[a] יצתה ח׳ למחיצתו was carried outside of its legal limits; a. fr.—בַּח׳, מִבַּח׳ *outside, from outside,* לַח׳ *out* (through the window &c.). Sabb. I, 1. Ab. Zar. 11[a]; a. v. fr.—2) (followed by מ־) *except, without.* Hull. I, 1 ח׳ מחרש וכ׳ except a deaf and dumb &c. Gen. R. s. 49 ח׳ מדעתו without consulting him; a. v. fr.

חוּצָב *stone-cutter,* v. חַצָּב.

חוּצָה f. (b. h.) 1)=חוּץ II; (followed by ל־) *outside of, out of.* Ab. Zar. I, 4 ח׳ לה outside the town limits.—ח׳ לארץ outside of Palestine, *foreign territory.* Hull. V, 1 בח׳ לא׳ abroad; a. v. fr.—2) *an outskirt,* not included in the Sabbath community (ערוב). Erub. V, 6.

חוּצָה II f. (preced.) 1)=חִיצוֹנָה, *outsider, stranger* (not related). Yeb. 13[b] (interpret. Deut. XXV, 5) אשת המת הח׳ the deceased's wife who is a stranger (to the brother); Y. ib. I, 3[a]. Ib. דאינון דרשין הח׳ החיצונה (the Samaritans) who interpret *haḥutsah* like *haḥitsonah.*—2) *a strange, unnatural act.* Yalk. Is. 303, v. חִיצָה I.

חוּצַל m., v. next w.

חוּצֶלֶת f. (חצל, v. חצץ; cmp. מַחֲצֶלֶת, בּוּרְיָא II) *matting used for partitions, coverings &c.*—*Pl.* חוּצָלוֹת. Eduy. III, 4; Succ. 20[a] כל הח׳ וכ׳ all kinds of mattings are liable to uncleanness by contact with corpses; v. מַרְזוּבְלֵי. Tosef. Kel. B. Bath. IV, 14 החוּצְלִים ed. Zuck. (Var. חולצות; ed. חוצלות).

חוּצְנָא m., pl. **חוּצְנַיָּא** (denom. of חוּץ) *outworks, outposts.* Targ. Jer. LI, 12 (h. text אֹרְבִים).

חוּצְפָּא, חוּצֵף m. (חצף) *barefacedness, boldness, impudence.* Targ. Jer. III, 3. Targ. Y. Num. XVI, 2; a. e.—Sot. 49[b] (IX, 15) in the Messianic period ח׳ יסגא impudence will prevail (Snh. 97[a] העזות תרבה). Snh. 105[a] ח׳ אפי׳ וכ׳ boldness will carry its point even against heaven. Ib. ח׳ מלכותא וכ׳ insolence is a royal power without a crown. B. Bath. 155[b], a. e.

חוּצְפִּית pr. n. m. *Hutspith,* surnamed the Interpreter, a Tannai, one of the martyrs of the Hadrianic persecution. Shebi. X, 6; Tosef. ib. VIII, 10. Hull. 142[a]. Ber. 27[b]. Y. ib. IV, 7[d] top (some ed. חצפית).

חוק (cmp. חוג) *to round, arch, hollow.* Denom. חָוִיק, חֵיק.

חוק ch. same.—*Part.* חָאִיק. Targ. Job XXIV, 16 ed. Lag. (Var. חָאֵיק, ed. Wil. חָאֵק, oth. ed. דאיק, corr. acc.; h. text חתר).

Pa. חַיֵּיק *to dig out.* Sabb. 109[b] וּלְיחַיְּיקִיה לגוּיה Rashi a. Ms. O. (v. Rabb. D. S. a. l. note 200) let him dig out its interior. Snh. 56[a] (ref. to נקב. Lev. XXIV, 16) ואימא דח׳ שם וכ׳ may it not mean that he cut out the Divine Name in the edge of the knife?, v. נָקַב.

חוֹק m. (b. h. חֹק; חקק, v. preced.) [*circle, drawing, engraving,*] *law, rule, custom; assigned share, mark.* Erub. 54[a] אניח לבני ח׳ I will leave to my sons a due share (a fixed living). Sabb. 137[b] ח׳ בשארו שם He ordered a mark to be put on his (Abraham's) flesh. Snh. 111[a] שמשייר אפי׳ ח׳ אחד (some ed. חֹק) who leaves even one law unobserved. Ib. למי שלא עשה אפי׳ ח׳ וכ׳ Ms. M. (ed. differ., v. Rabb. D. S. a. l. note) who observed not even one law; a. fr.—*Pl.* חֻקִּים, חוקים. Kidd. 39[a] (ref. to Lev. XIX, 19) ח׳ שחקקתי וכ׳ the lines which I have drawn long ago (by creating separate species); Y. Kil. I, 27[b] top (it is forbidden) משום ח׳ ... בעולמי as coming under the interpretation of (Lev. l. c.) "the lines which I have drawn &c." Tam. 31[b] חוּקֵּי העמים customs of gentiles. Sifra Aḥărê ch. XII, Par. 9 ח׳ החקוקים וכ׳ (idolatrous) usages practiced by them and their fathers &c, v. next w.; a. fr.

חֻקָּה, חוּקָּה f. (b. h.) same, esp. *firmly established distinctive usage, religious observance.* Ab. Zar. 11[a] שריפה לאו ח׳ הוא the burning of costly materials at funerals is not a specific (gentile) religious custom. Num. R. s. 19, beg. חקה חקקתי I have ordained a ceremony (without giving a reason). Ib. four (laws) דכתיב בהן ח׳ in reference to which the word *ḥukkah* (rule without reason) is used. Ib. לך אני מגלה ... אבל לאחר ח׳ unto thee I reveal the reason . . ., but to anybody else it is a rule; a. fr.—*Pl.* חֻקּוֹת, חוקות. Tanh. B'huck. 4 מצותי וְחֻקּוֹתַי; a. fr.

חָוַר (b. h.; cmp. אור) *to perforate; to be transparent, white, clear.*

Pi. חִוֵּור, חִיֵּ׳ *to make clear, evident.* Mekh. Mishp., N'zikin, s. 13 (ref. to Deut. XXII, 17) מְחַוְּורִין .. כשמלה they must make the fact as clear as a (white) sheet. Gen. R. s. 98 (ref. to כבס, ib. XLIX, 11) שהוא מְחַוֵּור וכ׳ he will make clear to them the words of the Law; שהוא מח׳ להם טעיותיהם he will prove to them their errors; a. e.—*Part. pass.* מְחוּוָּר *clear, proved, evident.* Y. Shek. III, end, 47[c] מ׳ שבכולן the clearest of all the quoted Biblical evidences. Gen. R. s. 47, end; Y. Ab. Zar. I, 39[d] top מ׳ שבכולן the least doubtful of all. Y. Succ. V, beg. 55[a] משם שאינו מח׳ because the use of the flute is not clearly stated in the Law. Y. Ter. II, 41[c] bot. זה אחד . . . שהן מְחוּוָּרִין וכ׳ this is one of the three interpretations (of the Rabbis) which are clearly indicated in the Bible text. Y. Erub. III, 21[a] bot. הגיעוך סוף ... שאינן מח׳ thou must finally admit that the law of Sabbath limits finds no proof in the Biblical words. Y. Ber. II, 5[a] bot. הגיעוך סוֹף מלאכות תפלה שאינן מח׳ מד״ת ed. Lehm. (oth. ed. corr. acc.) thou must admit that for labors permitted or forbidden during prayer no support is to be found in &c.; a. fr.

Hithpa. הִתְחַוֵּור *to be made clear.* Y. Keth. IV, 28[c] top (ref. to Deut. XXII, 17) עד שיִתְחַוְּורוּ וכ׳ the facts must be as clear &c., v. supra.

חֲוַר, חֲוַור ch. same, 1) *to be white, to shine.* Targ. Joel I, 7. Targ. O. Gen. XLIX, 12 יִחְוְּרָן ed. Berl. (ed.

Lsh. יֶחֱוַרְן, oth. ed. 'יְחַוְ). Targ. Is. I, 18 (some ed. *Pa.*); a. e.—Keth. 61^b top דְּחָוַור אפיה that he looked pale. B. Kam. 69^a כי היכי דניחְוַור טפי that it may appear still more white (glistening from a distance). Naz. 39^a, sq. חֲוֹרִין עיקבי נימהון the lower ends of dyed hair are white (which proves that the growth comes from beneath); a. fr.—2) (of eyes) *to be bright, to look with gratification.* Targ. Prov. XXIII, 33. Ib. XVII, 24 חֲיָירָן Ms. (ed. חדיין, v. חדי). [Ib. IV, 25, emend. by Luzzatto Oheb Ger p. 108, v., however, אור I ch.]—Kidd. 39^a לא חֲוַורִיתוּ you do not see clearly (the law is not clear to you).

Pa. חַוַּור 1) *to whiten, wash, cleanse.* Targ. II Sam. XIX, 25; a. fr.—B. Mets. 60^b 'חַוְורֵיה וכ, v. דְּקַן. Hull. 95^b top מְחַוֵּור, v. חֲלַל II. [Y. Taan. IV, 69^b bot. מרוח, read מְחַוֵּר or מְחוֹר to wash.]—*Part. pass.* מְחַוַּור, f. מְחַוְּורָא *blanched.* Targ. Y. Ex. IV, 6.—2) *to make evident, to prove.* Gen. R. s. 27 'דִּמְחַוֵּור וכ which will prove it better; Yalk. Koh. 968.—מְחַוַּורְתָּא *it is proven, obvious.* Hull. 117^a. Pes. 55^b; a. fr.

Af. אַחְוַור *to make white.* B. Kam. 85^b ואַחְוְורֵיה לבשריה and it (the corrodent) made his skin look white (like a leper's; Var. v. Rabb. D. S. a. l.). B. Mets. 58^b באַחְוְורֵי אפי (they guard against) whitening faces (putting persons to shame); Yalk. Ex. 349.

חָוֵר, חִוְרָא, חִוַּרְתָּא, חָוֵר, v. חִיוַּר.

חוּר I, or חָרַר (cmp. preced. wds.) *to bore.* Sabb. 103^a חָר חורתא he bored a hole.

חוּר I, חוֹר II m. (b. h.; preced. wds.) 1) *hole, cavity.* Pes. 8^a 'ח שבין אדם לחבירו a cave between two residences of neighbors.—Sabb. 52^b מחט שניטל חוּרָהּ (Ms. M. חוּרְדָהּ, Ms. O. חֲרָרָהּ, some ed. חוּדָהּ) a needle whose eye is broken off; ib. 123^a חֲרָרָהּ (Ms. M. חוּדָהּ); Kel. XIII, 5 חֲרִירָהּ; Tosef. ib. B. Mets. III, 9 חודה.—*Pl.* חוֹרִין. Pes. l. c. Ib. 'חוֹרֵי בית וכ the upper and the lower holes in the wall; a. fr.—2) *ant's store,* v. חוֹרָר. [Pesik. Shor p. 74^b חורין דדהב, v. חֲוַּור.] [Y. Maasr. V, end, 52^a חור אחר, v. זוּר II.]

חוֹר II m. (b. h.), *pl.* חוֹרִין [*white garments,*] *freedom;* 'בַּת ח, 'בֶּן ח *free, freed,* opp. to slave. Gitt. IV, 4 ויעושה 'בן ח . . . and he must declare him free. Ib. 5 חציו עבד 'וחציו בן ח half a slave and half a freedman; a. fr.—*Pl.* 'בְּנֵי ח. B. Kam. I, 3 'עדים ב' ח' וכ witnesses who are freemen and of the Jewish faith. Esth. R. to I, 6 (expl. חור ib.) 'בגדים שב' ח' וכ garments which freemen wear; a. fr.—'נכסים) בני ח) *free* (not mortgaged) *property,* opp. משועבדים. B. Kam. 8^b; a. fr. [Bibl. Hebr. חוֹרִים, חֹרִים *noblemen.*

חוּר III (b. h.) pr. n. m. *Hur,* the husband of Miriam. Mekh. B'shall., Amalek 1. Pesik. R. s. 12. Ex. R. s. 48 (grandfather of Bezaleel); a. fr.

חוֹרָא I ch. = h. חוֹר I, *hole.* Targ. II Kings XII, 10 (ed. Wil. 'חוּ); a. fr.—Arakh. 30^a, a. e. (prov.) לאו עכברא 'גנב אלא ח' גנב not the mouse is the thief but the hole (which hides the theft, i. e. fine the purchaser of the slave but not the seller). Ib. . . . אי לאו, 'ח מנא ליה but for the mouse (which steals), whence would the hole have something to hide?—*Pl.* חוֹרַאי. Targ. I Sam. XIV, 11.—Meg. 12^a (expl. חור Esth. I, 6) Ms. חוֹרֵי חוֹרֵי F. (ed. חֹרֵי חֹרֵי) webs full of holes, *net-work.*

חוֹרָא II ch. = h. חוֹר II, pl. חוֹרִין, חוֹרֵי, חֹרֵי; 'בַּר ח *free man.* Targ. Ex. XXI, 2; 5. Targ. Deut. XV, 13; a. fr.—Gen. R. s. 92 בר חֹרַיָּא thou freedman.—B. Mets. 13^a, sq. 'בני ח unencumbered property; Y. B. Kam. X, beg. 7^b; a. fr.

חוֹרָאֵי (v. preced.) pr. n. gent. *Horaë* (Freemen). Targ. O. Deut. II, 12 (Y. גִּנּוּסַיָּיא, h. text חֹרִים); cmp. אֱלֵיוְתֵּרוּסוֹלִים.

חוֹרֵב m. (b. h. חֹרֶב; חָרַב) *waste.* Pesik. R. s. 35, end; (Yalk. Is. 337 ארץ).

חוֹרְבָּא I m. (v. preced.) 1) *heat, dryness.* Targ. Ps. XC, 6.—2) *desolation, waste.* Targ. Ez. XXIX, 10 חוֹרַב (constr.).—3) *injurious confusion of ideas.* Arakh. 12^a (ed. חורבה). V. next w.

חוֹרְבָּא II, חָרְבָא f., constr. חָרְבַת = next w. Targ. Ez. XXIX, 9; a. fr.—Keth. 13^b ח' דדברא (חורבה) a ruined building standing in the field. Sot. 48^a, v. זְמָרָא I; a. e.—*Pl.* חוֹרְבָתָא, חָרְבָתָא; constr. חָרְבַת. Targ. Mal. I, 4. Targ. Is. LXI, 4; a. fr.—Snh. 71^a ח' סגירתא (Tosef. Neg. VI, 1 חוֹרְבָתָה סגירתה) a place named Leprous Debris (deposit of debris of leprous houses).

חָרְבָה, חוֹרְבָה f. (b. h.; חָרַב) *ruin, ruins, deserted building.* Ber. 3^a. Y. Dem. VI, 25^c top אויר חוֹרְבָתוֹ (if one sells) the space filled with debris belonging to him. Ib. 'תלוש מן הח' וכ break some stones from this ruin by which thou mayest take possession of the space; a. fr. [Arakh. 12^a, v. חוֹרְבָּא I.]—*Pl.* חוֹרָבוֹת, חֲרָבוֹת. Ber. l. c. 'חורבה אחת מחוֹרְבוֹת וכ one of the ruins of Jerusalem.

חֻרְבָּן, חוּרְבָּן m. (v. preced.) *destruction, desolate condition.* Hag. 5^b חֻרְבַּן בה"מ the destruction of the Temple. M. Kat. 26^a בחוּרְבָּנָן in their ruined state. Y. Kil. IV, end, 29^c בחוּרְבָּנוֹ in its (the vineyard's) waste state, opp. מַטָּעָה. Ab. Zar. 9^b 'לח' הבית ח from the destruction of the Second Temple. Yoma 39^b; a. fr.—*Pl.* חוּרְבָּנוֹת, 'חֳרָ. Gen. R. s. 56; Yalk. Gen. 102 'שהיתה . . בשני ח for she (Palmyra) took a part in both destructions of the Temple; Lam. R. to II, 2 'בשתי ח (fem.).

חוּרְבָּנָא ch. same. Targ. Is. XXXIV, 11. Targ. Lam. I, 2 חוּרְבַּן (constr.).—Snh. 96^b. B. Bath. 14^b 'סופיה ח the end of the book speaks of destruction. Ib. 'סמכינן ח' לח in arranging the order of the Biblical books, we join the record of destruction (at the end of one book) to that of destruction (at the beginning of the other).

חֹרֶג, חוֹרֵג m. (חרג) [*filling a gap,* v. חֲרִיקָא,] *step-son.* Snh. III, 4 (27^b) (חֹרְגוֹ) חוֹרְגוֹ לבדו his step-son alone (not his relations). Yeb. 21^a; a. e.—*Pl.* חוֹרְגִין. Y. ib. II, 3^d bot. 'שני ח' וכ two step-children (of different parents) brought up in the same house.

חוֹרְגָּה f. (preced.) *step-daughter.* Y. Yeb. II, 3^d bot. חוֹרְגָתוֹ one's step-daughter; Bab. ib. 21^b; a. e.

חוּרְגְּתָא ch. same. Sot. 43[b] ח׳ חגדילח וכ׳ a man's wife's daughter brought up among step-brothers.

חוּרוּד, v. next w.

חוּוָרוֹר, חֲוַרְוָר m. (חָוַר, v. Sm. 1231) *white spots on the cornea* (λεύχωμα). Bekh. VI, 3 (38[b]; Mish. ed. חורוד, v. Koh. Ar. Compl. s. v.); v. וָרִיר. Cmp. חִיוַּרְוָרָא.

חוֹרוֹן, בֵּית ח׳ pr. n. pl. *Beth-Horon*, a border town between Benjamin and Ephraim. Nidd. 61[a]; Snh. 32[b] מעלות בית ח׳ the ascent to Beth-H. (narrow); Erub. 22[b] מעלות בית ח׳ ed. Sonc. (ed. מָרוֹן; ed. Sal. בית מ׳ a. בית ח׳, v. R. Hash. 18[a], a. D. S. a. l. note 4). [R. Hash. II, 4, v. חַוְורָן.]

חוּרוֹן, pl. **חוּרוֹנִין**, v. חוֹרָן.

חֲוַרְוָר, v. חִוַּרְוָר.

חוּרֵי m. pl. constr. = אֲחוֹרֵי (v. אֲחוֹרָא) *behind, after.* Y. Shebi. IV, 35[a] bot. פרי ח׳ חמרא וכ׳ running after (driving) an ass on a Sabbath (being forced to public labor). Y. Snh. I, 18[c] bot. [read:] קם ליה מן חורוי מצלי (Y. R. Hash. II, 58[b] top מן אחורויי) stood up from behind him to pray. Y. Sot. VII, end, 22[a] לח׳ פרוכחא, v. גּוּל ch.— Y. Ber. II, 5[a] bot. תרין . . . לחורויי two thirds of the load on his back; a. fr.

חוֹרִי I m. = אָחוֹרִי, *another, second.* Y. Peah VIII, 21[a] אתא חד סיעא ח׳ a second caravan came.—*Pl.* חוֹרֵי. Y. Ber. IX, 14[a] bot. אית לך ח׳ there are other cases for you to quote.—*Fem.* חוֹרִי, חוֹרִיתָא, חוֹרָנִי׳ (noun) *something else.* Lev. R. s. 33 אמר ח׳ gave another explanation. Y. M. Kat. I, 80[c] bot. ח׳ היא it is another sore (not the one seen before). Ib. II, 81[b] top בשתא ח׳ (ed. Krot. חוריתאי) in the year following. Y. Succ. V, beg. 55[a] בשובתא ח׳ the next Sabbath; a. e.

חוֹרִי II f. (b. h.) *cakes*, v. חֲרָרָה.

חוּרְלָא m. ch. = h. חָרוּל.—*Pl.* חוּרְלֵי. Targ. Prov. XXIV, 31.

חוֹרֵם m. *net-maker*, or *fisher*, v. חָרַם.

חוּרְמָה, v. חָרְמָה.

חוּרְמָן, חוּרְמָנָא m. (חרם, v. P. Sm. 1375) 1) (adj.) *burning, venomous.* Targ. Y. Num. II, 25 (ed. Amst. חָרְמָן). Targ. O. Gen. XLIX, 17.—2) *basilisk.* Targ. Y. ib.—*Pl.* חוּרְמָנַיָּא, חוּרְמָנִין. Targ. Y. I Num. XXI, 6. Targ. Job XX, 16; a. e.

חוּרָן, v. חַוְרָן.

חוֹרָן, חוֹרָנָא, חוֹרָנָה, חָרָ׳ (חֲרִינָה) m. = אוֹחֲרָן, *another, next; last.* Targ. Y. Lev. XIX, 6. Targ. Y. Ex. IX, 6. Targ. Job XX, 18; a. e.—Y. Pes. VI, 33[a] bot. דח׳ מקדש וכ׳ that another man will sanctify &c. Y. Peah II, 17[a] bot. וחרנה אמר and the other (scholar) says; Y. Ter. II, 41[c] top וחרנה; a. fr.—*Pl.* חוֹרָנִין, חוֹרוֹנִין. Targ. I Chr. XXIII, 17; a. e.—Y. Peah VIII, 21[b] top לח׳ to other people (not himself).—*Fem.* חוֹרָנִיתָא, חוֹרָנִי׳, חוֹרָנְתָא (...תָּה). Targ. Y. Ex. XXI, 10 (ed. Amst. אוֹחְרָנִיתָא). Targ. II Chr. III, 12; a. e.—Y. Sabb. II, 5[a] sq. למה ח׳ why the other sacrifice?—*Pl.* חוֹרָנְיָיתָא, חוֹרָנְיָין. Targ. I Chr. XXIII, 27.—Y. Sabb. X, end, 12[d]; a. fr.

חוּרְסְפִיתָא, v. חֲרָס.

חוֹרֶף m. (b. h. חֹרֶף; חרף) [*severe season,*] *Midwinter.* B. Mets. 106[b], a. e. (ref. to Gen. VIII, 22) חצי כסלו . . . ח׳ half of Kislev, Tebeth and half of Sh'bat form the midwinter. Yoma 10[a] בית ח׳ וכ׳ they are called Winterhouse or Summerhouse, but not house without qualification. Koh. R. to VI, 3; Esth. R. to I, 2 ימות הח׳ winter-season.

חוּרְפָא m. (חרף) *sharpness, edge; pungent taste.* Snh. 56[a] ח׳ דסכינא the sharp edge of the knife. Ab. Zar. 39[a] חוּרְפָּה דחלתיתא (not פיה . . .) the pungency of *assa foetida*; a. fr.—Trnsf. *acumen, ingenuity.* B. Mets. 96[b] לפום ח׳ וכ׳ as great as a man's ingenuity, is the mistake he makes; Nidd. 33[b]. Erub. 90[a] אגב חוּרְפֵּיה לא וכ׳ relying on his ingenuity he did not study it carefully; B. Bath. 116[b].—*Pl.* חוּרְפֵּי. Targ. Y. Lev. XIX, 16 תרין חוּרְפּוֹי its double edge.

חוּרְפָא f. (v. Ges. H. Dict.[10] s. v. חרף I; cmp., however, R. Hash. 8[a] s. v. אֲפִילָא) *a young lamb* (used as a standard value in exchange). Targ. Job XLII, 11 (h. text קשיטה, Ms. a. Ar. Var. מיצא, מרגליתא; v. Gen. R. s. 79, end).—*Pl.* חוּרְפָן. Targ. O. Gen. XXXIII, 19 (Y. מרגלוין). Ib. XXI, 28; a. fr.

חוּרְפִיתָא pr. n. f. *Hurphitha* (the quick maid), name of one of Esther's servants (for Friday). Targ. Esth. II, 9; v. גְּנוּנִיתָא.

חוֹרָר m. (חרר IV) *pile, esp. ant's store.*—Pl. constr. חוֹרְרֵי, contr. חוֹרֵי; only in ח׳ הנמלים. Peah IV, 11 ed. חורי (Y. ed. חוררי, Mish. Nap. חֲרָרֵי); Maasr. V, 7 (Y. ed. חוררי; Ms. M. חררי); Y. ib. 52[a] top; Y. M. Kat. I, 80[c] חוררי.

חוֹרֶשׁ m. (b. h. חֹרֶשׁ, v. Ges. H. Dict. s. v. חרש II, cmp. חֵרֶשׁ) [*difficult of accession,*] *thicket, wild-growing bushes.* Y. Ab. Zar. I, 39[c] ונעשה ח׳ גדול and it grew to a large thicket of reeds; Cant. R. to I, 6. Lev. R. s. 29 ניתש מח׳ זה וכ׳ tears himself loose from one thicket and is caught in another; Y. Taan. II, 65[d] top; Pesik. Bahod., p. 154[b] חרש (corr. acc.), v. נָטַשׁ; Yalk. Lev. 645.—*Pl.* חֳרָשִׁים, חוֹרָשִׁין, חוֹרָשִׁים. B. Kam. 81[a] top שהיו מרעין בח׳ that people shall have the privilege of pasture on untilled lands. Ib. 79[b], opp. יישוב. Ib. 80[a]. Y. Sabb. VII, 10[a] top, v. בָּהָה; Y. Shebi. IV, 35[b] bot. בחר׳ (corr. acc.).

חוּרְשָׁא ch. 1) same. Targ. Ps. LXXX, 14; a. fr.— Cant. R. to I, 1 ח׳ של קנים, v. חֲרִישָׁה III. Ib. to III, 4 (ref. to Ps. LXXX, 14 יער with suspended ע) אם זכיתם . . . מן ח׳ if you will do good, your invaders shall be (like animals) from the water (יְאוֹר), if not, they shall be (like animals) from the forest; Yalk. Ps. 830.—2*) (P. Sm. 1386 *angina*) *narrow place in the throat, windpipe.* Shebu. 6[b]

בחוּרְשֵׁיה קא אכיל ליה that man eats into his windpipe (asks a dangerous question; Rashi: eats in his *forest*, i. e. knows not what is going on in the world; R. Hai G. in Ar.: *he scratches his eye-sore*).—*Pl.* חוּרְשַׁיָּא, חוּרְשֵׁי. Targ. Jer. IV, 29.—Gen. R. s. 24, beg. (ref. to Is. XXIX, 17, cmp. Targ. a. l.) ח׳ דבני ארנש thickets of people (crowded population).

חוּרְתָא f.=חוּרָא I, *cave*. Ned. 50[b] על לח׳ (ed. לְחַרְתָּא) the monkey went into a cave. [Targ. Y. Num. XXI, 27, v. חוּדִיתָא.]

חוּרְתָן, v. חֲיוּר׳.

חוּשׁ I m. (חָשַׁשׁ, cmp. גּוּשׁ) *thick substance*.—*Pl.* חוּשִׁים. B. Bath. 143[b] (play on חושים, Gen. XLVI, 23) מרובים כח׳ של קנה numerous as the leaves [or the *knots*] of reeds.—V. חִישָׁה.

חוּשׁ II (b. h.; v. preced.) [*to feel, press*,] 1) *to feel pain, be affected*. Erub. 54[a] חָשׁ בראשו if one has a headache; ח׳ בגרונו one whose throat is affected; a. fr.—2) *to apprehend, consider*. Y. Peah V, 18[d] bot. וחש לומר וכ׳ but then he reconsidered saying &c.—Ex. R. s. 3 אל תָּחוּשׁ do not mind it.—3) *to be anxious, quick, to hurry*. Y. Yeb. VIII, 9[c] top (play on בֶּעְרָא .. חוּשִׁים, I Chr. VIII, 8) חָשׁ כנמר וּבִיאֵר וכ׳ he was quick like a panther and made clear &c.—4) *to think, be silent*, v. חָשָׁה.—V. חָשַׁשׁ.

חוּשׁ ch., pret. חָשׁ, part. חָשׁ, חָיֵישׁ, same, 1) *to feel, suffer, be troubled*. Targ. Ps. LXXIII, 21. Targ. Prov. XXVI, 10; a. e.—Sabb. 140[a] חש ביוקרא דלבא suffered with heaviness of the heart.—Ib. וְחָשְׁאִי בנפשאי וכ׳ Ar. (ed. וְחָשַׁר, Ms. P. וחשר בי, fr. חָשְׁאָ, חָשַׁר) and I felt the cooling effect from the hair &c.—2) *to apprehend, care for*. Targ. Y. Num. XII, 3; a. e.—Y. Ber. VI, 10[b] bot. מֵיחוּשׁ.... הואיל וחש לה since R. Z. cared to do it, we must do likewise. Pes. 84[a]; Yoma 46[a], a. e. לא (חייש) חש לקימחיה cares not what flour he grinds (what argument he offers). Keth. 21[a] וחש .. לבי״ד טועין and S. took into consideration that a court might have a mistaken opinion (and was more explicit in his document than the law required); Yeb. 106[a] דחָיְישִׁינָן וכ׳ for we must take into consideration &c.; B. Bath. 164[a]. Ib. (וניחוש) וְלֵיחוּשׁ וכ׳ but should we not apprehend that perhaps &c.; a. fr.—3) *to be anxious, hasten to, flee*. Targ. Cant. II, 9. Targ. Ps. CXLI, 1 חִישׁ לִי hasten to my help. Targ. Y. Deut. I, 44, v. חָדַר.

Af. אָחִישׁ *to provide for with anxiety*. Targ. O. Deut. XXXII, 11 מְחִישׁ (Y. מְחִישׁ). [Targ. Ps. LV, 9 אוֹחִישׁ Ms. (ed. אַרְחִישׁ).]

חוּשְׁבְנָא m.=h. חֶשְׁבּוֹן, *calculation, number, measurement*. Targ. Ex. XXX, 12. Targ. Koh. IX, 10 (Ms. חֶשְׁבּוֹנָא); a. e.—Yoma 17[b] ח׳ בעלמא הוא it is merely an account of measurements (without observing a particular order). Hull. 95[b] השתא ח׳ בעלמא ידע now I see only that he understands astronomical calculations. Y. Ber. II, 5[a] top חוּשְׁבָּנֵיה דהדין וכ׳ the numerical value of the letters of the one (צמח) is the same as of those of the other (מנחם). Lev. R. s. 30 מן חכא נחיל ח׳ from now let us commence a new account; Koh. R. to IX, 7; Pesik. Ul'kaḥ. p. 103[a]. Sabb. 32[a], v. חוּטְרָא II. Lam. R. to I, 5 ח׳ דאצבע (Ar. חוּשְׁבָּנַיָּא דאצבעד) calculation with fingers (Roman notation?); a. fr.—*Pl.* חוּשְׁבְּנַיָּא, constr. חוּשְׁבְּנֵי. Targ. Cant. VII, 5.—Lam. R. l. c., v. supra.

חוֹשֶׁךְ, v. חֹשֶׁךְ.

חוּשְׁכָא, v. חֲשׁוּכָא II.

חוּשְׁלָא m. (חשל; v. P. Sm. 1404) 1) *pounded grain*. Targ. Ez. XXVII, 17 quot. in Rashi (ed. ריחוש).—2) *peeled barley*. Yoma 79[a] without the husk ח׳ קרי לה Ms. M. a. Ar. (ed. אוּשְׁלָא) it is called *hushla* (not שעורה). Snh. 27[a] bot. Hull. 51[a].—*Pl.* חוּשְׁלֵי. B. Kam. 30[b] bot. אפקר ח׳ ed. (Ms. M. אוּשְׁלֵי, Ms. H. חֲשִׁילֵי) declared as free property peeled barley (which one had spread on public ground for drying). M. Kat. 16[b] קא מניפה חוּשְׁלָאֵי (omitted in Ms., v. Rabb. D. S. a. l.) was winnowing peeled barley.

חוֹשֶׁן, חֹשֶׁן m. (b. h.; חשן, cmp. חשל) *breast-plate*. Zeb. 88[b] ח׳ מכפר וכ׳ the Highpriest's breast-plate brings atonement for wrong judgments. Sabb. 139[a] זכה לח׳ המשפט וכ׳ was privileged to wear the breast-plate of judgment upon his heart. Yoma 72[a] המזיח ח׳ מעל וכ׳ he who loosens the breast-plate from the *Ephod*; a. fr.

חוֹשֶׁן, חוּשְׁנָא ch. same. Targ. Ex. XXVIII, 4; a. fr.

חוּת (cmp. חתת) *to shrink from, to loathe*.—*Part.* חָת, f. חָתָה, חָתָה, חוֹתָה (cmp. חָלָה a. חוֹלָה fr. חוּל). Y. Ter. VIII, 45[c] top (ref. to שקץ) כל דבר שנפשו ..... חָתָה ממנו anything loathsome. Pesik. R. s. 11 ונפשו של אדם חתה מהם וכ׳ and one shrinks from eating them. Esth. R. to I, 7 נפשו של אדם ח׳ וכ׳ does not man rather loathe to drink out of golden cu ? [Y. Yoma IV, 41[c] bot. לחות, read לחתות, v. חָתָה I.]

Pi. חִיֵּית, חַיֵּית *to create aversion*. Y. Shebi. IV, 35[b] bot.; Y. Maasr. I, 48[d], v. בָּחַל.

חוֹתָל c. (חתל b. h. *to tie around, swaddle*) *wrapper of reed-matting* in which dates are packed, *bale*. Tosef. Kel. B. Mets. VI, 4 ח׳ של וכ׳ a mat for dates which is intended to be thrown away when the dates are eaten. Kel. XVI, 5 ח׳ שהוא וכ׳ a bale which you can add to or take from (without cutting it open) &c. Y. Sabb. I, end, 4[b] ח׳ שהוא מלא וכ׳ a bale filled with fruit stones. Ukts. II, 2, v. חוֹתָם.—[Y. Keth. VIII, 32[b] top מלא חותלה אסר וכ׳, read חותל . . . ר׳ אסר וכ׳.]—*Pl.* חוֹתָלוֹת. Sabb. 146[a].

חותלה, v. preced.

חוֹתָם m. (b. h.; חָתַם) 1) *seal, stamp, die; enclosure locked up with a mark*. Sabb. VIII, 5 כדי ח׳ המרצופין as much sealing clay as required for a seal on bags. Ib. ח׳ האיגרות seal on letters. Snh. IV, 5 אדם טובע ... בח׳ אחד a human being prints many coins from one die &c., but the Lord טבע .... בחוֹתָמוֹ של וכ׳ stamped every human being with the die of Adam, and yet not one is like the other; Y. ib. IV, 22[b] bot. מח׳ וכ׳. Sabb. 58[a] העבד בח׳ שבצוארו the slave with the mark hanging down from his neck, בח׳

שבכסותו with the mark tied to his garment; a. fr.—Trnsf. *sexual innocence; purity.* Yalk. Num. 766, v. infra. —*Pl.* חוֹתָמִים, חוֹתָמוֹת. Y. Snh. l. c.—Bets. 31[b] ח׳ שבקרקע וכ׳ knots which serve as marks on doors of subterranean stores, may be untied &c.; a. e.—Tan. d'be El. ch. XX, בחוֹתָמֵיהֶן in their innocence.—2) [*lock,*] *the oblate side of a berry to which the stalk is attached.* Y. Ab. Zar. V, 44[d] top. Toh. X, 5 ח׳ . . . . . גרגר a single berry, if its oblate part with the stalk is intact; Tosef. ib. XI, 10. Ib. מקום ח׳ the place where the stalk (now torn out) was seated (and where now juice is oozing out).—3) *the membraneous enclosure separating the stone of a date from its flesh, pericarp* (as far as not eatable). Tosef. Hull. I, 23 חח׳ טמא ביבשה quot. by R. S. to Ukts. II, 2 (ed. Zuck. חח׳ omitted; oth. ed. הזיתים in place of the preceding העמים) the pericarp is counted in with the unclean matter in dry dates; Ukts. l. c. ח׳ של יבשה R. S. (ed. a. Maim. חותל).—4) *concluding formula of prayers.*—*Pl.* as ab. Taan. II, 3 חוֹתָמֵיהֶן. Y. Ber. I, 3[d] bot. חוֹתְמוֹתֵיהֶן, v. חִיתּוּם.

חוֹתָמָא ch. same. Targ. Job XLI, 7. Ib. XXXVIII, 14 (Ms. חוֹתָמִין, *pl.*).

חוֹתֶמֶת f. (b. h.) same, *seal.* Gen. R. s. 61.

חוּתְרָא m., pl. **חוּתְרִין**, v. חַתִירָא.

חֵז, pl. **חֵזִין**, v. חֲזִיז.

חֲזָא, v. חֲזֵי.

חזאיא Ar. ed. Koh. III, p. 356, v. חֵזִיזָא II.

חֲזוּ, constr. of חֶזְוָא.

חֵזוּ, חֵיזוּ f.=next w. Targ. O. Gen. XXIV, 16 (ed. Berl. למיחזי).—Ib. Num. XII, 8; a. e.—*Pl.*, v. חֶזוּתָא.

חֵיזְוָא, חֶזְוָא, חֶזְוָא I m. (חזי) *looks, appearance; vision.* Targ. Gen. XXIX, 17. Targ. Y. I ib. XVI, 13 (ed. Amst. חֶזְוָא).—Targ. Is. LIII, 2 חֲזוּ) חֵיזוּ חולא) the appearance of an ordinary being; a. fr.—Koh. R. to V, 2 ח׳ הוא דין this is a vision (not a mere dream); Yalk. Esth. 1057 [read:] דין בחלמא חזאר או ח׳ הוא (for חיזווא some ed., read חֵיזְוָוא) did I see this in a dream, or was it a vision?—*Pl.* חֶזְוִין, חֵיזְוִין, חֵיזְוָנָא. Targ. O. Num. XII, 6 (some ed. חֵיזְוָן, fr. חֵיזוּ). Targ. Esth. VI, 1; a. e.—2) *look-out, cross-road.*—*Pl.* constr. חֲזוֵי, חֵיזְוֵי (חֵיזוֹרֵי). Targ. Y. Gen. XIII, 18; XIV, 13; Deut. XI, 30, v. next art.

חֲזְוָנָא, v. חֵזוֹנָא.—**חֶזְוָנָא**, v. חֶזְוָנָא.

חֲזוֹזָא m.=**חֶזְוָא**. Targ. Y. II Ex. III, 3 (I חֶזְוָנָא). —Targ. Y. II Gen. XII, 6; XIV, 6; XXXV, 9 (quot. of XVIII, 1).

חֲזוֵיא (חֲזוֵ׳, חַזוֵ׳) m. (חזי) *seer.* Targ. I Sam. IX, 9. Targ. II Sam. XXIV, 11; a. e.

חזוויתיה, Y. Ab. Zar. II, 40[d] top, v. חֲזָזִיתָא.

חָזוֹן m. (b. h.; חָזָה) *vision.* Lev. R. s. 1 בדבור ובח׳ in word and in vision.

חָזוֹנָא m. (חזי) *seer.* Targ. I Chr. XXIX, 29 (ed. Lag. חֶזְוָיָא, oth. ed. חֶזְוָנָא).

חֵזוֹנָא, חֵיזוֹ׳, חֶזוֹ׳, חֵז׳ m. (preced. wds.) *vision, astounding spectacle; wonder.* Targ. O. Ex. III, 3; a. e.—*Pl.* חֶזְוָנִין. Targ. Deut. XXVI, 8 (ed. Berl. sing.). Ib. XXXIV, 12 (ed. Berl. sing.; Y. II חֶזְוָוָתָא, pl. of חֵזוּ). [Targ. I Chr. XXIX, 29, v. preced.]

חִזּוּק, v. חִיזּוּק.

חֲזוֹר (חֲזוֹר) m. (חזר) *surrounding.* ח׳ ח׳ *all around.* Targ. Y. Ex. XIX, 12; a. e.—Targ. Ps. L, 3 (ed. Wil. ח׳). Y. Bicc. I, end, 64[b] חר׳ חר׳ וכ׳ around Zepphoris.

חֵי׳, חֲזוֹרָא, חֵיזוּרָא, חֵיזוּר, חֵיזוֹר, חֲזוּר m. (v. preced.; cmp. הָדָר) *apple; apple-tree; apple-shaped ball, bell* &c. Targ. Joel I, 12 (ed. Lag. *pl.*). Targ. Ex. XXV, 33 (h. text כפתר); a. fr.—Lev. R. s. 12 trees are called by their names (of the fruits) חזורא מתקרי חיזור there is the apple, it (the tree) is also called apple(-tree).—*Pl.* חֵי׳, חֵיזוּרֵי, חֵיזוּרִין. Targ. Prov. XXV, 11; a. e.—Lev. R. s. 27. Gen. R. s. 93 (retransl. from Aquila Prov. l. c.); Yalk. Prov. 961; a. e.—Targ. Y. Ex. XXXIX, 25 חֵיזוּרַיִין.

חָזוּת f. (חָזָה) *polish, lustre, beauty.* Yoma 70[a] כדי להראות חָזוּתוֹ וכ׳ to show the people the beauty of it (his copy of the Law); Tosef. ib. IV (III), 18 חֲזִיָּתָן.—B. Mets. 21[b] הזותו מוכיח עליו (masc.) the looks of the olive proves the owner; [Ar. Var. זֵיתוֹ].

חָזוּתָא ch. same, 1) *vision.* Targ. Job XX, 8.—*Pl.* חֵיוָ׳, חֶזְוָותָא, v. חֶזְוָנָא.—2) *watch-tower.*—*Pl.* as ab. Targ. Is. XXIII, 13. Targ. Y. Num. XXXV, 11 (v. חֵיוּתָא).—3) *appearance, color.* B. Kam. 101[a] ח׳ מילתא היא appearance (improved by dying) is a substantial improvement. Hull. 47[b] בח׳ resembling wood in appearance, v. גּוּשְׁתָּא I. Sabb. 77[a] התם משום ח׳ there it treats about color.—*Pl.* as ab. Targ. Y. Deut. XXVIII, 27 ח׳ דמסמיין which dull *the eye-sight* (h. text עפלים).—Hull. 46[b] ח׳ ח׳ Ar. (ed. חֶזְוָתָא) several spots of abnormal colors.

חֲזַז, Hif. הֶחֱזִיז, v. חָזָה.

חֲזָזָא, v. חֲזָזִיתָא.

חֲזָזִית f. (חזז *to make incisions*) *lichen,* a cutaneous disease connected with desquamation and sometimes ulceration. Bekh. VI, 12 בעל ח׳ an animal afflicted with lichen. Ib. 41[a] (expl. ילפת, Lev. XXII, 22) ח׳ המצרית Egyptian lichen; ח׳ דעלמא ordinary lichen.—Succ. III, 6 (34[b]) עלתה ח׳ if an Ethrog is covered with lichen (scabs). Ruth R. to III, 8 (ref. to וילפת ib., a. ילֶּפֶת) כח׳ (לפתתו) לפפתו she twisted herself around him like lichen.—[Y. Yoma VIII, 45[b] top רוח ח׳, v. חֲזָזִית.]

חֲזָזִיתָא ch. same. Targ. Y. I Lev. XXI, 20 ח׳ מצריתא (h. text ילפת), v. preced.—Gitt. 70[a] top (some ed. חֲזִיתָא). Y. Sabb. XIV, 14[d] top לְחֲזָזִיתָה (putting spittle on) a scab; Y. Ab. Zar. II, 40[d] top לחזויתיה (corr. acc.).—*Pl.* חֲזָזִין (חֲזָזָא m.). Targ. Y. II Lev. l. c.

חֲזָזָן m. (preced.) *one afflicted with lichen.* Targ. O. Lev. XXI, 20; XXII, 22.

חָזָה, חזי (b.h.) [*to divide,*] *to discern, see* (cmp. בּוּן). B. Bath. 91ª חֲזִיתֶם נעמר וכ׳ have you seen what has become of Naomi &c.?

Pi. חִזָּה *to distribute kindled chips between logs of wood.* Sabb. I, 11 (19ᵇ) וּמְחַזְּזִין Mss. (ed. Ven. מחיזין; Y. ed. Krot. ומחוזין, read וּמְחַזְוִזִין, *Hif.* of חזז, or מְחַזְּזִין), v. אָחַז.—V. חָזִית.

חֲזָא, חזי ch. same, *to see, recognize, to decide.* Targ. O. Gen. XXIX, 10; a. fr.—Ber. 45ª; Erub. 14ᵇ, a. e. פוק חֲזִי וכ׳, v. דְּבַר. Ib. 13ᵇ דַּחֲזִיתֵיהּ לר״מ וכ׳ (not דחזיתא) because I have seen R. M. &c. Hull. 59ᵇ בעינא דאֶיחֱזֵי וכ׳ I want to see your God Erub. 63ª ח׳ לנפשיה may examine the knife for his own use; a. fr.—*Part. pass.* חֲזֵי, חֲזֵי, f. חֲזְיָא (cmp. רָאוּי) *pointed out, fit for, prepared;* (*it is*) *proper.* Targ. Job XV, 11. Targ. O. Lev. V, 10; a.e.—Keth. 21ª כִּדְחָ׳, כִּדְחָזֵי as it is proper. B.Bath.19ᵇ ח׳ לבהמתו fit for his cattle as feed; a. fr.—Sabb. 90ª, a. fr. למאי חזיא what is it good for (what use can be made of it)?—*Pl.* חֲזוּ, חָזוּ. Ib. top ח׳ למתק וכ׳ they may be used for seasoning &c. Bets. 26ᵇ; a.fr.—חזי לי it was pointed out to me, *I saw.* Gitt. 57ª. Taan. 25ᵇ; a. fr.

Af. אַחֲזֵי *to show, let see, reveal; to lay before a teacher for examination* or *decision.* Targ. O. Gen. XLI, 28; a. fr.—Hull. 59ᵇ בעינא דמַחֲזִית וכ׳ I want thee to show it to me. Bets. l. c. אַחֲזְיֵיה לחכם וכ׳ as soon as he showed it to an expert (and the latter decided favorably) &c.; a. fr.

Pa. חַזֵּי same. Targ. II Esth. II, 8.—B. Mets. 67ª ואודיק חַזְיָתַן אירלונית and when he looked at me (and noticed that I was going to object by referring to אוֹנָאָה), he pointed out to us the case of אִירְלוֹנִית (v. Rabb. D. S. a. l. note 50; Ms. R. חַזְתַן).

Ithpe. אִתְחֲזֵי, אִיתְחֲזֵי, אִיתְחֲזֵי 1) *to be seen, to appear.* Targ. Jud. XIII, 10; a. fr.—Ber. 17ᵇ מִיתְחֲזֵי כיוהרא it looks like assumption; a. fr.—2) *to look at each other.* Targ. O. Gen. XLII, 1.—3) *to become fit, adapted for use.* Bets. 26ᵇ אי דאִתְחֲזוּ בה״ש א׳ if on the entrance of the Sabbath they became fit for use, they have become so (for the entire Sabbath). Ib. אחזו . . . . אחזו והדר they had been fit (on the entrance of the Sabbath), and were unfitted (through rain), and became fit again; a. fr.—4) *to be shown, to be laid before the scholar for decision.* Ib. אתח׳ לחכם וכ׳ it had been shown to (and decided upon by) the expert on the eve &c.; a. fr.

חֲזְיָא *fit,* v. preced.

חֶזְוָא I m., v. חֶזְוָא.

חֶזְוָא II f., pl. **חֶזְוָן** (preced.) *mirror.* Targ. Y. II Ex. XXXVIII, 8 (ed. Amst. חֶזְוַית constr.).

חֶזְוָי f. same. Targ. Y. Num. XII, 6 (h. text מַרְאָה); cmp. אִסְפַּקְלַרְיָא. [Ib. 8 חיזיו, some ed., read with ed. Amst.: חֵיזוּ, h. text מַרְאָה.]

חִזָּיוֹן I m. (b. h.; preced. wds.) *vision.*—*Pl.* חֶזְיוֹנוֹת (fem.). Snh. 39ᵇ (play on והזונות, I Kings XXII, 38) כדי למרק שתי ח׳ Ms. M. (v. Rabb. D. S. a. l.) in order to polish (make clear) two visions. Ib. (play on לחכו, ib. 34) כדי לתמם שתי ח׳ to fulfill two visions. Gen. R. s. 13; Yalk. ib. 20 (ref. to חֲזִיז, q. v.) שעושה ח׳ ברקיע וכ׳ He creates (awe-inspiring) sights in the sky and causes holy inspiration to rest &c. [Ar. s. v. אד: חֲזִיזִיּוֹת, fr. חֲזוֹרִית, *breaks, splits.*]

חִזָּיוֹן II m. or חֶזְיוֹנָה (v. חֲזָזִית) 1) *lichen, moss.* B. Mets. 105ᵇ ramification (סוכה) is considered weak, שנתבאת בְחֶזְיוֹנָה (or בחזיונה) when it is hidden under (fully covered with) moss. [Ar. ed. בחיזונה, ed. Koh. בחזונה; comment.: *the grip of the hand,* fr. אחז; marg. emend.: בְּאֶחֱזְיוֹנָה, v. Tosaf. a. l.]—Erub. 28ª אבל לא בחזין ולא בחזנות Ms. M. (Rabb. D. S. a. l. note quotes חזיונות) but neither with lichens nor with lichen dishes (Lecanora esculenta).—2) pl. חֶזְיוֹנוֹת *lichen, scab;* trnsf. *irregular lumps* of clouds. Y. Taan. III, 66ᶜ bot. a cloud is called *ḥaziz* (v. next w.) שהוא עושה . . ח׳ ח׳ וכ׳ for He makes the sky full of irregular lumps (cumuli), as we read (Zech. X, 1), the Lord makes *ḥăzizim.*

חֲזִיז, חָזִיז m. (b. h.; v. חֲזָזִית) 1) *cloud with uneven surface* (like scabs or swollen lumps), *cumulus* (which brings rain). Gen. R. s. 13 (allegorical explanation), v. חִזָּיוֹן I. Y. Taan. III, 66ᶜ bot., v. preced.—Bab. ib. 9ᵇ.—*Pl.* חֲזִיזִים. Ib. מאי ח׳ what are *ḥazizim* (Zech. X, 1)? Answ. פורחות eruptions (defined: 'a thin under a thick cloud').—2) [Readings vary between חזיז a. חָזִין, pl. of חָז] *lichen,* used as food (Lecantora esculenta). Erub. 28ª, v. חִזָּיוֹן II.—B. Kam. 119ᵇ כשות וח׳ וכ׳ the law of robbery does not apply to cuscuta and lichen. Keth. 60ᵇ.—3) [Readings vary as ab.] *young blades of grain* used for pasture. Taan. 5ª אוכל ח׳ מן התלמים Ms. M. (some ed. חזיז) eats the young green from the furrows. B. Kam. 58ᵇ bot. [Tosef. Ohol. XIII, 11 שני חזידן, read: חזיזין, v. זיז II.]

חֲזִיז I (or חַזִּזָן f. pl.) same, *young green.* Targ. Ps. CXXVI, 6 ed. Lag. חזיז (Lev. חזין, not found in oth. editions).

חֲזִיז II, **כְּפַר ח׳** pr. n. pl. *K'far Ḥaziz.* Kil. VI, 4 Ms. M. a. Ar. (ed. עֲזִיז).

חֲזִיזָא I ch.=h. חָזִיז 1), *cloud.* Targ. Cant. II, 9.—*Pl.* חֲזִיזֵי. Targ. Job XXVIII, 26.

חֲזִיזָא II m. (v. חָזִיז) *shaggy.* Bekh. 44ª גדיא ח׳ a shaggy goat (called צִימָּה, with long hair lumps and long-dependent ears, Capra Syriaca, v. Encyclop. Brit. s. v. Goat).

חֲזִיזִיּוֹת, v. חִזָּיוֹן I.

חֲזִירָה, v. חָזוּת.

חֲזִיזָא, חֲזִיזְנָא m. ch. (חזי, cmp. חֲזִיז, חֲזִיזָא &c.) *prickly bur, chestnut.* Kel. XIV, 2 a cane with a metal knob כמין ח׳ (ed. Dehr. חזיזנה) of the shape of a chestnut bur (as a weapon).

חֲזִיר m. (b. h.) *swine.* Hull. IX, 2 ח׳ של ישוב domesticated swine; ח׳ חבר wild boar. Num. R. s. 12 מה . . . . אִיסוּר לְחָזִ׳ וכ׳ is the swine more strictly forbidden than other unclean animals?—Lev. R. s. 13 ואת הח׳ זו פרס

(read רומי or אדום). Ib. מה ח׳ וכ׳ as the swine . . . stretches out its cloven feet (sign of cleanness), ... so does the Roman government &c., v. בִּימָה. Gen. R. s. 65, beg.; a. fr.—*Pl.* חֲזִירִים, חֲזִירִין. Kidd. 49ᵇ תשעה נטלו ח׳ nine (measures of plagues) did swines receive. B. Kam. VII, 7; a. e.—Fem. חֲזִירְתָּה, חֲזִירָה *sow.* Esth. R. to III, 1. Ib. to I, 15 לח׳ כדת וכ׳ the swine (Vashti) to be treated according to law, but the holy people &c.!, v. אַכְזְרִיּוּת.

חֲזִירָא, חֲזִיר ch. Targ. Ps. LXXX, 14. Targ. Lev. XI, 7 (some ed. חֲזִי׳).—Y. Ber. II, 4ᶜ bot. אתן ח׳ וכ׳ the swine is a moving privy. Sabb. 155ᵇ לית . . . . מן ח׳ none is poorer than the dog, none richer than the swine (finding its food everywhere); a. e.—*Pl.* חֲזִירִין, חֲזִירֵי. Gen. R. s. 63; Y. Ter. VIII, end, 46ᶜ, v. דִּיקְלֶטְיָאנוּס. Taan. 21ᵇ ארבא מותנא בח׳ there is an epidemic among the swine; a. e.—Fem. חֲזִירְתָּא, Lam. R. to I, 16, end כחדא ח׳ וכ׳ like the (nursing) sow, the more their young fatten &c.

***חַזִּירָא** m. (preced.) *swine-herd.* Y. Ter. VIII, 40ᵇ sq., v. הִיקְלוּט.

חֲזִירָה I *sow,* v. חֲזִיר.

חֲזִירָה II f. (חָזַר) 1) *return, going back,* opp. הֲלִיכָה. Y. B. Mets. VI, beg. 10ᵈ שכר הליכה וח׳ indemnification for loss of time in going to the field and returning. Lev. R. s. 5 בַּחֲזִירַת רבותינו לשם when the teachers came again to that place, v. חֲדוּרָה.—Y. Yoma III, 43ᶜ bot. דרך ח׳ on the way homeward. Koh. R. to XI, 9 . . . . מעט בריצה בח׳ slacken thy speed, that thou mayest not have too far to return (regret and punishment will reach you); a. fr.—2) *reconsideration, reversion of judgment.* Y. Hor. I, beg. 45ᵈ bot. וכן בח׳ the same rule applies when the court reverses &c.—3) *going round.* Y. Sot. I, 16ᶜ bot. כדי חֲזִירַת דקל (Bab. ib. 4ᵃ חֲזָרַת) the time required for going round a palm-tree.—4) *restoration,* v. חֲזָרָה.

חֲזִירְתָּא, חֲזִירְתָּה, v. חֲזִיר.

חָזִית f. (חזז; cmp. גָּזִית fr. גזז) *cutting; rough, unfinished side.* Tam. II, 4 חֲזִיתָהּ מזרחה the uneven side of the pile (where the thinner and pointed ends of the logs leave gaps and make the front uneven) was eastward. Par. III, 8. Y. Meg. IV, end, 75ᶜ bot. נותן בח׳ he puts (the M'zuzah) on the rough door (which is more used by the inmates); חיו שניהן ח׳ if both are of rough work.—Esp. *the rough side of a fence or wall,* indicating that the neighbor had no right to it, *border-mark.* B. Bath. I, 2 (2) כונס . . ועושה ח׳ מבחוץ he moves back on his own ground and builds, and makes the border-mark outside. Ib. 4ᵃ מאי ח׳ וכ׳ wherein consists the border-mark? Answ. He bends the pegs on top outward.—2) *rough sore, contusion.*—*Pl.* חֲזִיּוֹת. Y. Ber. IX, 13ᶜ bot. (emended in ed. Lehm. כתית, as Sabb. 77ᵇ). Cmp. חֲזָזִית.

חָזִיתָא f. (preced.) *contusion.* Gitt. 70ᵃ top some ed., v. חֲזָזִיתָא.

חָזַם, *Hif.* הֶחֱזִים (cmp. גָּזַם) *to cut, trim, thin.* Dem. III, 2 הרוצה לְהַחֲזִים וכ׳ he who desires to trim leaves of vegetables for the sake of lightening the burden; Tosef. ib. IV, 2 לְהַחֲזִים Var. ed. Zuck. (ed. לְהַחזיר, corr. acc.).

חֲזַם ch. same, *to cut off, nip off.* Targ. Y. I Lev. I, 15 (Y. II יַעֲזִים; h. text מלק).

חַזָּן or **חָזָן** m. (חזי) *superintendent, officer;* 1) (school) *governor* superintending children at their studies. Sabb. I, 3 הח׳ רואה וכ׳ on Friday night the governor may look in where the children read, but must not read himself.—2) (in collegiate debates) *one who announces the order of proceedings, crier, janitor* &c. Y. Ber. IV, 7ᵈ top אמרו לר׳ זינון הח׳ וכ׳ they said to R. Zinon the hazan, 'Say, Commence' (the debate)!—3) (in synagogue) *superintendent at prayer-meetings,* giving the signals for responses, assigning seats &c., *sexton.* Succ. 51ᵇ וח׳ הכנסת וכ׳ and the sexton stood upon it with the flag in his hand. Yoma VII, 1; Sot. VII, 8.—4) (in court) *crier, sheriff* (collecting the votes, executing punishment). Macc. III, 12. Y. Sot. VII, 21ᵈ top.—*Pl.* חַזָּנִים, חַזָּנִין (חָזָ׳). Tam. V, 3 (Temple sextons).—Tosef. Snh. IX, 1 הח׳ קורין וכ׳ the criers call out each judge's name (to take his vote); Y. ib. V, end, 23ᵃ חַזָּנֵי כנסיות. Macc. 23ᵃ אין מעמידין ח׳ וכ׳ we must appoint as constables (for punishing) men of lesser physical strength &c. Sabb. 56ᵃ.

חַזָּנָא or **חֲזָ׳** ch. 1) same. Y. Ber. V, 9ᶜ bot. עאל ח׳ וכ׳ the sexton came and urged one to go up (to read the prayers). Y. Meg. IV, 75ᵇ bot.; Y. Sot. VII, end, 22ᵃ.—2) חַזָּן מתא *town-guard* (watching the flocks of the common and guarding the town by night). B. Mets. 93ᵇ.—*Pl.* חַזָּנֵי מתא. Ib.

חָזַק (b. h.; cmp. חדק, הדק, אדק) [*to squeeze together,*] (neut. verb) *to be thick, solid; to be strong.* Y. Ber. I, 2ᶜ bot. (ref. to Gen. I, 6) יֶחֱזַק הרקיע וכ׳ let the expanse become solidified, let it coagulate, congeal; Gen. R. s. 4; (Yalk. ib. 5 ותחזק, *Hithpa.*).

Pi. חִיזֵּק *to join, repair, tighten, strengthen.* Snh. 94ᵃ (expl. חזקיה) שחי׳ את ישראל וכ׳ (Ms. M. שהחזיק, *Hif.*) he joined Israel to their Father &c. Ib. שֶׁחִזְּקוֹ יה the Lord strengthened him. Pes. 45ᵃ שעשור לְחַזֵּק Ms. M. where the dough in the cracks is put in for repairing the trough. Sabb. 146ᵇ לְחַ׳ (העשור) when the hole was filled up for making the vessel sound, opp. לשמר to prevent evaporation; a. fr.—*Part. pass.* מְחוּזָּק, *pl.* מְחוּזָּקִים. Sifré Num. 1 אין מְחַזְּקִים אלא המח׳ (ed. תמוחז׳) only the strong-minded it is worth while to strengthen (encourage).

Hif. הֶחֱזִיק 1) same, v. supra.—ח׳ טובה ל־ *to attach merit to, to account as merit, to be grateful.* Ab. II, 8 אל תַּחֲזִיק ט׳ לעצמך do not claim credit for it (be not proud). Yoma 86ᵇ אלא שמַחֲזִיק לו ט׳ but He even gives him credit (for his sins when he repents). Men. 53ᵃ הַחֲזֵק לי וכ׳ give me credit for making Thee known &c. Keth. 68ᵃ, a. e. בואו ונַחֲזִיק וכ׳ let us be thankful to the fraudulent poor &c.; a. fr.—2) (with יד) *to strengthen, to encourage, abet.* Gitt. V, 9 לפי שאין מַחֲזִיקִין וכ׳ because we must not encourage (by favors) those who do wrong. Ib. ומחזיקין ידי עכו״ם וכ׳ we may encourage (greet with תחזקנה ידיכם, Zech. VIII, 9) gentiles at agricultural work in the Sabbatical year; a. fr.—3) *to hold, contain.* Ib. 57ᵃ אין עורו מחזיק וכ׳ its skin (once flayed) can not again cover its entire body (it shrinks). Ib. (in Chald. dict.)

אפי׳ שתין . . . לא מ׳ it would not have room even for sixty myriads of reeds. Par. VII, 8 בשביל שתַּחֲזִיק וכ׳ in order that it (the reservoir) might hold more water. Ukts. III, 12 לא מצא .. מחזיק וכ׳ the Lord found no vessel so fit to contain all blessings as peace; Deut. R. s. 5 end; a. fr.—4) (with ב) *to take a hold of, seize, take possession.* Hull. 4ª, a. e. כל מצוה שהֶחֱזִיקוּ וכ׳ whatever Jewish law the Samaritans have adopted &c., v. הֶקְדֵּק. B. Mets. I, 4 וה׳ בה and took a hold of it. B. Bath. III, 3 בּמַחֲזִיק when one is in possession (basing his claim on possession). Ib. המַ׳ בנכסי הגר he who takes possession of the estate of a convert (who has no heirs in law). Ib. 2 ויַחֲזִיק שנה that he may be in possession for one year, v. אִסְפְּמְיָא; a. fr.; v. חֲזָקָה.—Y. Hag. I, 76ᶜ, a. e. שלא הֶחֱזִיקוּ בשכר וכ׳ they did not cling to the duty of maintaining teachers &c.—5) (v. חֲזָקָה) *to presume, to be under a certain impression, to be convinced.* Y. Kidd. IV, 66ᵇ היו מַחֲזִיקִין בו שהוא בנו וכ׳ if people were under the impression that a certain person was their neighbor's son, but in his dying hour he declared &c. Ib. היו מ׳ אותו שהוא וכ׳ if people took him to be a relation of his; a. e.—Hag. 19ª, v. infra.

Hof. הוּחְזַק (denom. of חֲזָקָה) *to be presumed, be held for, be known for.* Gitt. 14ª בשה׳ כפרן when the man is known to be a liar. Shebu. 34ᵇ, a. fr. ה׳ כפרן (in such a case) he is considered a confirmed liar.—Y. Kidd. l. c. bot. הוּחְזְקוּ if they were generally assumed (to be husband and wife); a. fr.—Hag. 19ª הטובל לחולין וה׳ לחולין if one takes an immersion for the purpose of being enabled to partake of ordinary food and is considered (by himself) to have immersed for that purpose. Ib. טבל ולא ה׳ if he did immerse but did not have a certain purpose in view. Ib. עודיהו . . . . ה׳ לדבר קל מחזיק עצמו וכ׳ as long as he has one foot yet in the water, when he had had in view a minor purpose for his bath, he may still change it for a higher purpose. Ib. אם לא ה׳ מחזיק if he had had no particular object in view, he may on coming out define the object for which he has bathed.—*Part.* מוּחְזָק 1) *held in possession, adhered to.* Bekh. VIII, 9 ולא בראוי כבמ׳ nor does he take a double share of what is coming due to the estate as he does of what is held in possession; B. Bath. 55ª; a. fr.—Sabb. 130ª עדיין היא מוּחְזֶקֶת בידם it is still strongly adhered to, opp. מְרוּפָּה, v. רָפָה.—2) *being known, approved.* Sifra K'dosh. Par. 3, ch. V במ׳ לך when he is known to thee (to be a proselyte); a. e.—3) *being sure, convinced, knowing from experience.* Keth. 25ᵇ מוּחְזְקַנִי בזה וכ׳ (=מ׳ אני) I know this man to be a priest; a. e.—Sifré Num. 1, v. supra.

Hithpa. הִתְחַזֵּק, *Nithpa.* נִתְחַזֵּק 1) *to become solid, strong.* Yalk. Gen. 5 יִתְחַזֵּק, v. preced.—2) *to feel encouraged, take courage.* Ber. 32ª נ׳ בתפלה became emboldened to pray.

חֲזַק ch. 1) same.—*Part. pass.* חֲזִיק *tied up, bandaged.* Y. Ber. II, 4ᶜ top דהוה ח׳ רישיה when his head was tied up (with a turban); Pesik. R. s. 22 (not רישין, v. notes in ed. Fr.). Y. Pes. X, 37ᶜ וח׳ רישיה וכ׳ and his head was tied up (or he felt like having a bandage around his head) &c.; Y. Shek. III, 47ᶜ top והוה חזוק (read חזיק); וחזק (corr. acc.).—2) *to take possession.* B. Bath. 52ᵇ, sq. חֲזַק וקני take possession and acquire; a. fr.

Pa. חַזֵּיק *to fasten.*—Lev. R. s. 21 [read] חַזֵּק כפתור tighten his muzzle, v. פִּיפְתָא.—*Part. pass.* מְחַזַּק. Targ. Y. Gen. L, 1.

Af. אַחֲזֵיק as preced. *Hif.*; 1) (with טיבו &c.) *to give credit to.* Y. Ber. II, 5ª bot. אנא מַחֲזִיק טיבו לראשי וכ׳ I give credit to my head, which bends of itself &c. Bab. ib. 19ª לאַחֲזוּקֵי ליה וכ׳ that due credit for the preservation of Israel be given to Moses.—2) *to presume.* Shebu. 46ᵇ לאַחֲזוּקֵי אינש בגנבי לא מַחֲזְקִינַן we must not put a person in the category of thieves (on the charge of one individual); a. e.—3) *to adhere to, adopt.* Hull. 4ª כיון דאַחֲזִיקוּ בחו א׳ בחו since they (the Samaritans) have adopted it, they observe it (also for Israelites). Ib. אַחֲזוּק ולא א׳ וכ׳ as to their observance or non-observance of adopted unwritten customs for Israelites there are differences of opinion; a. fr.—4) *to take possession, to claim possession.* B. Bath. 29ᵇ כי היכי דלא תַחֲזְקוּ אהדדי ed. (differ. in Ms. M., v. Rabb. D. S. a. l.) that you might not claim possession against one another. Ib. 36ª האי מאן דא׳ וכ׳ if one claims a field on the ground of possession, if it lies outside &c., v. גּוּדָא I. Ib. לא מַחֲזְקֵי בן ולא מַחֲזְקִינַן בהו they have no claim of possession against us (for one might have been afraid to disturb them), and they have no claim against us (for, being wealthy, they might not have cared to drive one out); a. fr.—5) *to be strong, encouraged.* Gitt. 62ª אַחֲזוּקוּ 'be strong' (a greeting to field laborers, v. preced.).

Ithpa. אִתְחַזַּק, *Ithpe.* אִתְחֲזִיק 1) *to adhere to.* Targ. Prov. IV, 13; a. e.—2) *to be known, be under the presumption.* Targ. Y. Lev. XIX, 33 (v. preced.).—Hull. 10ᵇ היכא דלא א׳ where no presumption (of leprosy) has as yet been formed. Snh. 89ᵇ דמִיתְחֲזַק וכ׳ Ms. M. (ed. מוחזק) where one is approved (as a righteous prophet), it is different.

חֶזְקָא m. = next w., *presumption, ascertained status.* Hull. 10ᵇ אוקי אַחֶזְקֵיה (strike out מילתא) place everything on its once ascertained status as long as you have no evidence of a change. Yeb. 31ª אַחֶזְקָהּ upon her condition as it would be if there were no evidence at all.

חֲזָקָה f. (חָזַק) 1) *taking hold.* Y. M. Kat. III, 83ᶜ top (ref. to II Sam. I, 11) אין ח׳ וכ׳ taking hold (of a garment to rend it in mourning) means no less than a hand-breadth of it.—2) (law) *taking posssession, posession, usucaption; claim based on undisturbed possession* during a legally fixed period. B. Bath. III, 1 חֶזְקַת הבתים וכ׳ the legal period of undisturbed possession (in order to give a title) is for houses .... three years. Ib. 29ᵇ (in Chald. diction) אכלית שני ח׳ I had the undisturbed usufruct for the period prescribed by law. Ib. 36ª עבדים יש להם ח׳ does the law of possession apply to slaves?—Ib. אין להם ח׳ לאלתר וכ׳ present possession gives no title (as is the case with inanimate movable chattel), but a possession of three years does. Ib. III, 2 שלש ארצות לח׳ there are in Palestine three districts with different usages of possession. Ib. 3 כל ח׳ שאין וכ׳ possession without a plea (of purchase or any other mode of legal acquisition) gives no title; a. v. fr.—3) *presumption, presumptive continuance of an actual condition until evidence of a change is produced; legal status.* Hull. 9ª בהמה בחייה בחֶזְקַת איסור וכ׳ the animal when alive, has the status of a forbidden object (v. אֵבֶר),

until you ascertain by what means it has been ritually slaughtered; when it is slaughtered הרי היא בח׳ היתר וכ׳ it has the status of a permitted object, until you find out how it became forbidden. Gitt. III, 3 בחזקת שהוא קיים under the presumption that her husband (though sick or old when the messenger was deputed) is alive. Keth. 75ᵇ ח׳ דגופא a presumption as regards physical condition, ח׳ דממונא the fact of possession against which the claimant has to produce satisfactory evidence. Ib. ח׳ אין אדם שותה וכ׳ the presumption is that no man drinks out of a cup without examining (that none will marry without having ascertained the woman's physical condition). Yeb. 31ᵇ top חזקת בר שטיא the legal status of an insane person's property; a. v. fr.—*Pl.* חֲזָקוֹת. Kidd. 80ᵃ סוקלין .... מלקין על הח׳ we execute punishment on the basis of actual facts (though not provable by legal evidence, e. g. man and wife and children living together and treating each other as such, are legally considered as being one family), v. חָזַק *Hof.*—Y. Ḥall. IV, 60ᵃ bot. לח׳ with reference to the local usages of usucaption (Gitt. III, 2, v. supra); a. e.

חִזְקִי, v. חִידְקִי.

חִזְקִיָּה, חִזְקִיָּהוּ (b. h.) pr. n. m. *Ezekiah, Hizkiah, Hizkiahu;* 1) King of Judæa. Snh. 98ᵇ. B. Bath. 15ᵃ ח׳ וסיעתו וכ׳ Ez. and his assistants edited the books of Isaiah, Proverbs &c.; a. fr.—2) name of several Amoraim. Zeb. 75ᵇ. Y. Shebi. VIII, 38ᵃ top; a. fr.—Y. Snh. III, 21ᵈ ח׳ חוקוק (v. Fr. M'bo, p. 81ᵇ).—Y. Sabb. XIV, 14ᵈ top.—Y. Shebi. III, 34ᵈ top.

חֶזְקְתָא f. ch.=h. חֲזָקָה. Targ. Y. Gen. XIII, 17. [In Talmudic Chald. the Hebrew forms are retained; v. also חֶזְקָא.]

חָזַר 1) *to go around* (searching). Koh. R. to VII, 8 הוא חוזר עליה he searches it again (tries to recover his scholarship); ib. יכול הוא לַחֲזוֹר עליה he may recover it; a. e.; v. infra.—2) *to turn around, return; to retract, repent.* Ib. חֲזוֹר בך come back (repent)! Eduy. V, 6 חזור בך withdraw thy opposition.—Dem. IV, 1 חָזְרָה למקומה came back to its place (was mixed up again). Maas. Sh. I, 5 יַחְזְרוּ דמים וכ׳ the money shall return to its former condition, i. e. the sale is annulled, and the money has again its sacred character. Ker. 8ᵃ נַחֲזוֹר על הראשונות let us go back to what was said first. Sabb. 118ᵇ; Arakh. 15ᵇ מימי . . וְחָזַרְתִּי לאחורי I never said a word (about a fellowman) on which I went back (when confronted with him). Kidd. 59ᵃ וְחָזְרָה בה and she reconsiders (her consent to be married); חוֹזֶרֶת she may do so; Gitt. 32ᵇ. Ib. חוזר ומגרש בו dare he use the same letter of divorce again (after he has revoked it)? Ter. IV, 3 ח׳ והוסיף then again he added. Gitt. VI, 5 חָזְרוּ לומר then again they said (added); a. v. fr.

Pi. חִיזֵּר *to go around from one to the other.* Yeb. 53ᵃ צריכה לְחַזֵּר על וכ׳ she must apply to all the brothers successively; (ib. 26ᵇ; 51ᵇ לַחֲזוֹר). Y. Taan. IV, 68ᵃ bot. חִיזַּרְנוּ על כל וכ׳ we searched the whole Bible; Y. Ab. Zar. I, beg. 39ᵃ חי׳ בכל וכ׳; (Sifré Deut. s. 1 חָזַרְנוּ). Y. B. Bath. VIII, 16ᶜ top, v. דיאתימון. Kidd. 2ᵇ לְחַזֵּר על אשה to go around in search of a wife (to woo). Ib. מי חוזר על מי (Kal) which of them goes around &c.?; Nidd. 31ᵇ מי מְחַזֵּר וכ׳.

Hif. הֶחֱזִיר 1) *to restore, give back.* Ber. 27ᵇ הַמַּחֲזִיר שלום לרבו he who returns the plain salutation (*shalom*) of his teacher (without adding, 'My teacher'). Ib. 32ᵇ לא ח׳ לו שלום did not answer his greeting. B. Mets. 7ᵇ יַחֲזִיר לאשה he must restore (the lost document) to the wife. Keth. 73ᵇ וְהֶחֱזִירָהּ and re-married her; a. fr.—2) *to revoke; to reconsider, to grant a new trial.* Gitt. VI, 3 אם רצה לְהַחֲזִיר לא יַחֲזִיר if the husband wants to revoke the letter of divorce, he cannot do so.—Snh. IV, 1 דיני נפשות מַחֲזִירִין וכ׳ in capital cases verdicts may be reconsidered in favor of the defendant. Ib. VI, 1 מחזירין the convict is brought back for a new trial; a. fr.—[Ib. 33ᵇ אין חוזר, Ms. F. מחזירין (ed. חוזרין).]—Eduy. V, 7 החזרת בך, Mish. ed. חֲזוֹרְתָּ, v. supra.—3) *to make one read over, to cause correction.* Y. Meg. IV, 74ᵈ מחזירין אותו we order him to read it over again correctly. Ber. 29ᵃ; a. fr.

חֲזַר ch. same. Targ. Ps. XLVIII, 13. Ib. CXIV, 3. Targ. Y. II Gen. XLIX, 19; a. fr.—Y. Shek. V, end, 49ᵇ א״ל מֵיחֲזַר he said to him, on coming back (I shall give thee something); ח׳ ואשכחיה מית when he came back, he found him dead. Koh. R. to VII, 8 חֲזוֹר עול לך go home again. Ib. ולית את חוזר בך (h. form) and thou dost not repent? [Usually הֲדַר.]

Af. אַחֲזַר, אַחְזַר 1) *to surround, go around.* Targ. Ps. XXII, 13. Ib. XXVI, 6; a. e.—Targ. Y. Num. XXI, 4 לְאַחֲזָרָא (not לְאַחֲזֵ׳).—2) *to cause to turn back, to cause to flee.* Targ. Ps. XLIV, 11.—3) *to turn* (one's face). Targ. II Chr. VI, 3.—4) *to restore.* Targ. Y. II Deut. XXIV, 13; a. e.—Targ. II Kings II, 8 וא׳ *he rolled up* (his cloak).—*Part. pass.* מַחְזַר, v. infra.

Pa. חַזֵּר 1) *to turn around, twist.* Targ. Hos. X, 2.—2) *to move to and back, to winnow.* Targ. Am. IX, 9 (cmp. חִירָרָא II). [Targ. Job XL, 22 יְחַזְרִי׳ some ed., read יְחַזְ׳.]—*Part. pass.* מְחַזַּר *turned off, going backward.* Targ. O. Gen. IX, 23 (ed. Berl. מְחַזְּרִין; Targ. Y. אפיהון מְאַחְזְרִין, h. text אחרנית).—Y. Meg. IV, 74ᵈ bot. חד מְחַזֵּר מנא וכ׳ one (of the scholars mentioned) ordered the translator using the word *mâna* (vessel, in translating טֶנֶא, Deut. XXVI, 2) to go over it again (and say סַלָּא, basket) &c.; Y. Bicc. III, end, 65ᵈ חד אמר מה׳ (strike out אמר); v. חֵרוֹקְנָא.

חֲזָרָא m. (preced.) [*turner,*] *spit, a pointed twig improvised as a spit.* Bets. 33ᵃ Ms. M. (ed. fem., Ar. חִירָרָא).

חֲזָרָא, v. חִיזָר.

חזורד, v. חֲזָרֵר.

חֲזָרָה f. (חָזַר) 1) *return; retraction, reconsideration.* Keth. 73ᵇ אין חֲזָרָתָהּ ח׳ גמורה her return (as a minor, to her husband after divorce, i. e. her remarriage) is not fully valid. Ḥull. 116ᵇ קודם ח׳ before the editor of the Mishnah had changed his opinion. Yeb. 64ᵇ אבין ישנו בח׳ Abin (being constantly with R. Joh.) is aware of an eventual change of his teacher's opinion; [oth. explan.: is in the habit of *reviewing* his traditions).—2) *restoration, amendment; atonement, repentance.* Y. R. Hash. I, 57ᶜ top ויבדק ויחזור בו ח׳ גמורה and he is examined and gives evidence of true reformation; ib. חֲזִירַת ממון לא חֲזָרַת דברים (by which is meant) restoration of ill-gotten gain, not a mere return in words; Y. Shebu. VII, 37[d] bot.; Snh. 25[b] חֲזָרַת ממון.—3) *turning backward, turning inside*. M. Kat. 24[a] חֲזָרַת קרע לאחוריו turning the rent in the mourner's garment inside (during the Sabbath); Gen. R. s. 100; Y. M. Kat. III, 82[d] bot. חֲזִירַת.—4) *going around*, v. חֲזָרָה.

חֲזָרִין, חֲזָרִים, v. חֲזֶרֶת.

חזרינותא, v. חֲזָרָ׳.

חַזְרָן m. (חָזַר, v. הָדַר) *zealous in the execution of religious duties*. Sabb. 156[a] ח׳ במצות. [Tosef. Kel. B. Mets. IX, 6 ח׳ some ed., read מְזֻרָן.]

חַזְרָן ch. same, *busy*. Sabb. 156[a] גבר ח׳ a busy, active man, expl. חזרן במצות, v. preced.

חַזְרְנוּתָא f. (v. חוּזְרָנוּתָא) *surrounding*. Targ. Ps. XLIV, 14 (ed. Lag. חזרני׳). Targ. Job XLI, 6 (constr.); a. e.

חַזְרָר (חֲזָרָד) חֲזָרָר m. (v. חֲזוּר) [*little apple*,] *crab-apple* (Malus Coronaria), similar yet heterogeneous to apple. Kil. I, 4 Ms. M. (ed. חזרד).—*Pl.* חֲזָרָרִין. Y. Ter. II, 41[c] bot. קטנות כח׳ (not כב׳) as small as crab-apples; (Y. Sabb. III, 5[d] כחזו׳; Bab. ib. 38[a] כעוזרדין, v. חֲזָרָר). Maasr. I, 3 Ms. M. (ed. עוזרדין).

חֲזֶרֶת f. *lettuce*. Kil. I, 2 ח׳ וח׳ גלין (garden) lettuce and hill-lettuce (wild lettuce). Pes. II, 6 (expl. ib. 39[a] חסא). Ib. X, 3; a. e.—*Pl.* חֲזָרִין, חֲזָרִים. Ukts. I, 2. Ib. II, 7. Y. Sabb. I, 3[b] bot. לקנב חיזורין (read: חזורין).

חָח m. (b. h.) *fastening, clasp, chain*. Ex. R. s. 48, end.

חחי, Gitt. 70[a] קורטמי דח׳, v. חָרִיָא.

חַט, v. חֵטָא a. חַטְאָה.

חַט, pl. **חַטִּין**, v. חוּט.

חַט, חַט, v. חָטַט I.

יַחַט Targ. Is. XIV, 19, v. יָחַט.

חַטָא, חֵטָא, v. חטר.

חֵטְא m. (b. h.; preced.) *failure, sin*. Ber. 4[a] שמא יגרום החט׳ perhaps sin is the cause (preventing the fulfillment of divine promise). Ib. אלא שגרם החט׳ but for sin that prevented it. Sabb. 119[b], v. הֶבֶל; a. fr.—יְרֵא ח׳, יִרְאַת ח׳, v. יָרֵא a. יִרְאָה.—In Talm. Y. also חֵט. Y. Sabb. I, 3[c] top; a. fr.—*Pl.* חֲטָאִים. Ber. 10[a] (ref. to חַטָּאִים, Ps. CIV, 35) מי כתיב חוֹטְאִים ח׳ כתיב does the text read *ḥot'im* (sinners), it may be read *ḥăṭaim* (sins). Ib. כיון דִּיתַּמּוּ ח׳ וכ׳ when sins shall cease, the wicked shall be no more. Yoma IV, 2; a. fr.

חֵטָא ch., v. חֶטְאָה.

חַטָּא I m. (חטט), *line drawn with a stylus*.—*Pl.* חַטֵּי. Keth. 69[a] top בינֵי ח׳ between the lines, v. חֲלֵי.

חַטָּא II, pl. **חַטַּיָּא**, *wheat*, v. חִיטְּתָא.

חַטָּא, v. next w.

חַטָּאָה, חַטָּ׳ ,חַטָּ m. (חָטָא) 1) *sinner*. Ber. 60[a] ח׳ את art thou a sinner?—*Pl.* חַטָּאֵי, חַטָּאִין ,חַטָּ׳ ,חַטְּאַיָּא, חַטָּיָיה, חַטָּיָא. Targ. Prov. I, 10. Targ. Ps. CIV, 35.—Gen. R. s. 12; Yalk. ib. 19. Pesik. Naḥ. p. 128[b]; Yalk. Ex. 391; a. e.—2) *searcher of sin, accuser*. Targ. Zech. III, 1 (ed. Lag. יַחְטָא).

חִיטָא, חֵט, חֵטָא, חֶטְהָא, (חֵט׳) חֶטְאָה m. ch.=h. חֵטְא. Targ. Deut. XIX, 15. Targ. I Sam. X, 26. Targ. Gen. IV, 7 (ed. Berl. חֶטְאָה, some ed. חַטָאת). Targ. Prov. XXI, 4 (ed. Lag. חטהא); a. e.—M. Kat. 16[a] פרטינן חטא חֶטְאֵיה וכ׳ we must specify his sin publicly. Snh. 37[b] חֶטְאֵי, חִיטְ׳, חֶטְאִין. *Pl.*—אחריתי the sin of another act. Targ. Jer. XIV, 19 (ed. Lag. חובין). Targ. O. Lev. XVIII, 7 (v. זִימָּה II). Targ. Prov. XIV, 34 (ed. Lag. חֶטְהֵי); a. fr. [Ib. XXVIII, 13 חֵטוּר, v. חֲטַר.]

חַטָּאת f. (b. h.; חָטָא) 1) *mistake, inadvertence, sin*.—*Pl.* חַטָּאוֹת. B. Mets. 33[b] (ref. to Is. LVIII, 1) חַטֹּאתָם אלו וכ׳ 'their mistakes', this refers to the ignorant whose wilful sins are accounted to them as errors.—2) *sacrifice expiating inadvertent sin, sin-offering*. B. Bath. 10[b] (ref. to Prov. XIV, 34) וחסד לישראל ולאמים ח׳ (differ. in Ms. M., v. Rabb. D. S. a. l. note) but benevolence is a sin-offering for Israel as well as for gentiles. Ib. כשם שחט׳ מכפרת וכ׳ (differ. in Ms. M.) as well as the sin-offering brings atonement to Israel &c. Zeb. I, 1; a. fr.—*Pl.* חַטָּאוֹת; constr. חַטֹּאת, חַטְּאוֹת. Ib. V, 3 ח׳ הצבור congregational sin-offerings. Ib. 112[a] הפריש שתי ח׳ וכ׳ if he sets apart two sin-offerings for security's sake; a. v. fr.

חַטָּאתָא, חַטָּתָא (חַטָּאת) ch. same, 1) *sin, stumbling*. Targ. Prov. X, 16 Ms. (ed. חַטּוּתָא). [Ib. XXI, 4 חטהא Ms. (ed. חטהא, חטאה).]—Y. Keth. II, 26[c] bot. חטאת דחנניה (prob. חֶטְאֵיה).—2) *sin-offering*. Targ. Ex. XXIX, 36; a. fr.—*Pl.* חַטְוָתָא, חַטָּוָ׳. Targ. Num. XVIII, 9. Targ. Hos. IV, 8.

חָטַב I (b. h.; cmp. חָטַט) *to split, cut, chop*.—Part. pass. חָטוּב. Macc. 8[a] אם מצא חָטוּב (אינו חוֹטֵב) if he finds cut wood (for the religious purpose), he need not cut it.

Pi. חִיטֵּב *to eraze*. Treat. Sofrim V, 1 מְחַטֵּב (Var. lect. מעבב, מעטב); (Treat. Sefer Torah, ed. Kirchh. V, 1 מַחְטִיב *Hif.*).

חָטַב II (cmp. Arab. *ḥaṭab*, a. חִטָּה) *to fall in love, to woo*. Koh. R. to VII, 26 היתה חוֹטֶבֶת באדם וכ׳ she would propose to a man in the street (some ed. חוֹטֶפֶת). [Lam. R. to I, 1 חטבו ממנה, v. חָטַף.]—V. חֲטִיבָה.

חֲטַב, חֲטִיב ch. 1) same, *to select, betroth one's self to*. Targ. Deut. XXVI, 17, sq.—2) (=חטף) *to seize violently*. Targ. Y. I Gen. XLIX, 5 (h. text חמס).—3) *to embroider, design*, v. חוּטְבָא.

חַטְבָא, v. חוּטְבָא.

חֲטָבָה f. (חָטַב I) *cutting, chopping*. Macc. II, 2 חֲטָבַת עצים; Sifré Deut. 182 חֲטִיבַת. Macc. 8[a] ממאי דמח׳ עצים דרשות וכ׳ how can you prove that we derive the rule from an ordinary cutting of wood, perhaps a cutting of wood for a Succah is meant &c.?

חֻטָּה f. *incisor*, v. חוּט.

חִיטָּה, חִטָּה f. (b. h.; v. חָנַט) [*the clean, bright*, cmp. פת נקיה, s. v. נָקִי,] *wheat-grain*, (collect.) *wheat*. Midr. Till. to Ps. II, 12; Cant. R. to VII, 3 מה ח׳ זו סדוקה as the wheat-grain is slit. Shebu. V, 3 אמר ח׳ if he says *ḥittah* (in the sing.). Ib. 38ª אפי׳ ח׳ בכלל חטין even *ḥittah* means a quantity of wheat. Tosef. Ned. III, 7; Y. ib. VI, end, 40ª חי׳ שאני וכ׳ if one vows, 'I will not taste *ḥittah* (wheat-grains)', contrad. to חִטִּין; a. fr.—*Pl.* חִטִּים, חִטִּין, חִי׳. Ib. Pes. II, 5. Ib. 35ª כוסמין מין ח׳ spelt is a species of wheat; Men. 70ª. Gen. R. s. 15 ח׳ היו 'the tree of knowledge' was wheat. Shebu. l. c.; a. fr.

חִטְדָא, v. חֶטְאָה.

חֲטוֹמָא, v. חֲטִימָא.

חֲטוֹטֶרֶת, חֲטֶרֶת f. (חטר, cmp. חוֹטֶר II) (*camel's*) *hunch, hump*. Ḥull. IX, 2 (Talm. ed. 122ª חטר׳). Sabb. 54ª, v. חוֹטֶרֶת.—*Pl.* חֲטָרוֹת, חֲטוֹטָרוֹת. Bekh. VII, 1 (43ª) בעלי חטוטרות Maim. (Mishn. *sing.*; Talm. ed. חטרות) humpbacked men; Tosef. ib. V, 2.

חֲטוּי, v. חִיטּוּי.

חֲטוּלִים, v. חֲטוּלִים.

חֲמוֹנִיא, Y. Maas. Sh. IV, 54ᵈ bot., v. סִיטוֹנָא.

חֲטוֹפָא, חֲטוֹף m. (חֲטַף) *violence, robbery, robbed goods*. Targ. Jud. IX, 24; a. fr.—*Pl.* חֲטוֹפַיָּא, חֲטוֹפִין. Targ. Ps. LXXII, 14; a. e.

חַטּוֹפָא m. (preced.) *robber, violent man*.—*Pl.* חַטּוֹפִין, חַ׳. Targ. Ob. 5; a. e.

חֲטוּרָא f. ch., *pl.* constr. חֲטוּרַאת=h. חֲטוֹטֶרֶת. Targ. Is. XXX, 6 Ar. ed. Koh. (Ar. Ms. חטוטרה; ed. Lag. חִיטוּרְיַת, oth. ed. חֲטוּרְיַאת).

חֲטוּתָא, v. חֲטָאתָא.

חִטְחֵט, v. next w.

חָטַט 1) *to dig, cut out* (of the sucket), *hollow out*. Mikv. IV, 3 החוטט בצינור וכ׳ if one makes a cavity in a water pipe for the deposit of pebbles. Gen. R. s. 34 היה חוטט את וכ׳ the embryo would cut its way through &c. Kidd. 24ᵇ וחֲטָטָהּ and he (the master) cut it (the eye) out.—2) *to rake, clean a well*. M. Kat. I, 2 וחוֹטְטִין אותן and you may clean the wells. Ib. 5ª ח׳ .. ואין חופרין וכ׳ you may clean..., but not dig (deepen) &c. [Ib. ולא חוטטין לתוכן you must not rake pebbles into them; v., however vers. Ms. M., Rabb. D. S. a. l.]—Y. ib. 80ᵇ bot. חוטטין אותן גרפין לון וכ׳ (not חוטכן) *ḥot'tin* means 'they rake them', as we read (Mikv. l. c.).—3) *to take sheaves out with a rake*. Succ. I, 8 החוטט בגדיש וכ׳ if one takes sheaves out of a stack, so as to form a shed (Succah). Ib. 15ª.

Pi. חִטֵּט 1) *to rake*. Y. Sabb. III, beg. 5ᶜ צריך לְחַטֵּט ביד וכ׳ he must rake (coals and ashes out of the oven) with a handle, which proves that he must clean thoroughly.—2) *to make holes, to pick*. Tosef. Mikv. VII (VIII), 2 אוצין צריך לחטט Var. (ed. Zuck. לְחַטֵּט) if the holes in the baskets are filled up with grapes &c., one must clean them by picking. B. Kam. 18ª תרנגולין שהיו מְחַטְּטִין וכ׳ chickens that picked on the rope of a bucket. Tosef. B. Mets. VIII, 30 שמְחַטְּטִין את וכ׳ (Var. שמְחַטְחֲטִין) for they pick holes in the walls.—3) (with אחר) *to dig after, to trace with the knife*. Ḥull. 74ᵇ; Tosef. ib. VII, 4.—4) *to trim*. Sabb. 90ª; Men. 107ª, v. מָחַט.

Pilp. חִטְחֵט same. Y. Orl. III, 63ª מצוי לְחַטְחֵט אחריו it is likely that they dig after it (to take it out of the ground); a. e. (v. supra).

Nif. נֶחֱטַט *to be dug out, picked out*. Kidd. 24ᵇ נֶחְטְטָה עינה if the bird's eye was picked out; Zeb. VII, 5 (68ᵇ) Ar. (ed. נסמית).

Hithpa. הִתְחַטֵּט *to be exhumed*. Yeb. 63ᵇ מתים מִתְחַטְּטִין the dead are exhumed (by the Guebres).

Polel (of חוט), *part.* מְחוֹטֵט (v. מַחַט) *stinging* (the eye), *dazzling*, v. infra.

Hithpol. הִתְחוֹטֵט *to be cut* (of jewels), *to be polished, glisten*. Meg. 12ª (play on בַּהַט, Esth. I, 6) אבנים שמִּתְחוֹטְטוֹת על בעליהן וי״א אבנים המְחוֹטְטוֹת לעינים במקומן Ms. F. (v. Rabb. D. S. a. l. note 5) stones which glisten on those who wear them, and some say, Stones which dazzle the eyes in the place where they are found.

חֲטַט I ch. same, *to dig, hollow out*. Ḥull. 25ª; Sabb. 103ª דחט קפיזא וכ׳ Ar. (ed. דחק) he hollowed out a K'fiza (smaller measure) whereas the material was large enough for a Kab. Pes. 28ª (prov.) כפא דחט נגרא בגויה נשרי חרדלא ונרשלוף Ms. M. (read: ונירשוף; ed. דחט׳ נגרא בגווה נשרוף וכ׳; Var. דחק) in the ladle which the artisan hollowed out, he shall have mustard soaked and shall swallow it (man is paid with his own coin).

Pa. חַטֵּט *to dig after, exhume*. Yeb. 63ᵇ קא מְחַטְּטֵי שכבי they (the Guebres) exhume the (Jewish) dead. [B. Bath. 58ª, v. חֲטִיָא.]

חֲטַט II, *Pa.* חַטִּיט (sec. r. of חוט II) *to sew*. Targ. Gen. III, 7. Targ. Ez. XIII, 18.

חֲטָט, חֲטָטִים, חֲטָטִין *pl.* (חָטַט, cmp. חֲזָזִית) *scab, scurf, sores*. Yoma 77ᵇ. Lev. R. s. 19.

חֲטָטָא ch. same. Targ. Job XXX, 24 חֲטָטֵיה ed. Lag. (oth. ed. חֲטָטֵי, *pl.*; h. text פיד).

חֲטֶמֶרֶת, v. חֲטוֹטֶ׳.

חָמָה, חָמָא, חָמַי I [*to stroll idly, saunter* (v. Fl. to Levy Targ. Dict. I, 424²),] *to live in luxury, to be like a nobleman, to be well-dressed, clean* &c. (cmp. פנק, פרנק).

Pi. חִטֵּא, חִטָּה *to make look well, polish, dress, cleanse, prepare*. Ḥull. 27ª (play on וְשָׁחַט, Lev. I, 5) ממקום ששח חַטֵּהוּ from the place where the animal bends (its head, the front of the neck), cleanse it (let its blood run out). Ib. ממאי דהאי חטהו לישנא דדכויי הוא how can you prove that this *ḥattehu* has the meaning of cleansing?—Ib. ממקום שסח חטהו from where it utters sound, cleanse it. [Cant. R. to VII, 2, v. infra.]

Hithpa. הִתְחַטֵּא, הִתְחַטָּה, *Nithpa.* נִתְחַ׳ 1) *to enjoy, to be gratified*. Cant. R. to VII, 2 [read:] כל חִיטּוּיִין.. שישראל מִתְחַטְּין וכ׳ all luxuries and enjoyments which Israel indulge in and enjoy. Men. 66[b] (play on נִתְעַלְּסָה, Prov. VII, 18) נשא ונתן ונעלה ונשמח ונתחטא באהבים let us have a conversation, then let us go up and rejoice and delight ourselves with dalliances; Sifra Vayikra, N'dabah, ch. XIV, Par. 13. Men. l. c. (play on נֶעֱלָסָה Job XXXIX, 13) נושא עולה ונתחטא; Sifra l. c. נושא ועולה וּמִתְחַטֵּא he (the bird) raises (his wings) and rises and enjoys himself (differ. interpret. in Rashi).—2) *to show one's self a nobleman, to be generous, proud.* Cant. R. to VII, 7 שהיה מתחטא על וכ׳ he was generous towards &c. (ref. to Gen. XIV, 23, Dan. V, 17).—3) *to be imperious, to lord it, to ask petulantly.* Taan. III, 8 אתה מתח׳ לפני thou comest petulantly before the Lord כבן שהוא מתח׳ על וכ׳ like a son that lords it over his father &c. Cant. R. to V, 6 (explain. חמק, ib.) נתח׳ וכ׳ he became petulant, he got angry with me.

חֲטִי ch. same; *part.* חַטְיָא *used to comfort, tender, delicate.* Targ. Y. Gen. XXXIII, 13 טליא חַטְיָין (h. text רכים).

Pa. חַטֵּא *to cause to be generous, to persuade to leniency.* Koh. R. to IX, 18 אנא אזלא וּמְחַטְּא ליה I will go to appeal to his generosity (Midr. Sam. ch. XXXII ומפייסה).

Ithpe. אִתְחַטִּי *to be raised in luxury. Part. pass.* מִתְחַטַּי, fem. מִתְחַטְּיָא, מִתְחַטַּיְיתָא *delicate.* Targ. Y. I, II Deut. XXVIII, 54; 56.

חָטָא, חֲטִי II (b. h.) [*to miss,*] *to fail, err, sin.* Yoma IV, 2, sq. Ber. 17[a]; a. fr. R. Hash. 26[a] חוטא בל יקריב he that sinned (with gold by making the golden calf) shall not bring nigh (the gold, enter with gold garments); ח׳ בל יתגאה he that sinned (with gold) shall not parade himself (with it).—Keth. 11[a] שלא יהא חוטא נשכר that the sinner may not profit by his sin; Yeb. 92[b]; a. e.

Pi. חִטֵּא *to expiate* (*cleanse from sin,* v. חָטָא I). Yoma V, 5 (58[b]) מְחַטֵּא ויורד he expiates (sprinkles) and goes down (sprinkling downward; Rashi: moves his arm downward). Ib. במקומו היה עומד ומח׳ he remained in his place and sprinkled. Zeb. 53[a].

Hif. הֶחְטִיא *to cause to sin.* Midr. Till. to Ps. IV, 5; Pesik. Shubah, p. 158[a]. Ab. V, 18; a. fr.

חֲטָא, חֲטִי ch. same. Targ. Y. Gen. XLIX, 3. Targ. Josh. VII, 11; a. fr.—Sabb. 56[a] מִחְטָא נמי לא חטאו but at all events they did not sin; ib.[b] ומירחטא וכ׳.—Pes. 113[b]; Macc. 11[a], v. זִיגּוּד; a. fr.

Af. אַחְטִי *to cause to sin.* Targ. Y. Num. XXVII, 3; a. e.

Pa. חַטִּי same. Targ. Y. II Num. XXIV, 14 חַטִּי יתהון (ed. Ven. חַטֵּי) seduce them (to immorality).

Ithpe. אִתְחַטִּי, אִיתְחַטִּי *to be tempted.* Y. Taan. I, 64[b] bot. תִּתְחַטֵּי that thou be not tempted to sin (through thy husband's absence).

חֵטְי m. = חֵטְא, esp. *unexpiated sin, consequence of sin.* Y. Taan. IV, 68[c] top חֶטְיוֹ של וכ׳, v. אוּנְקְיָא. V. חֶטְיָיה.

חֲטִי ch. same. Dan. IV, 24.—*Pl.* with suffix חֲטוֹי. Targ. Prov. XXVIII, 13 (Ms. חֲטוֹי, some ed. חֶטוֹי).

חִטַּיָּא *wheat,* v. חִיטָּא.

חַטַּיָּא, חַטַּיְיא, חֲטָיָא, v. חַטָּאָה.

חַטְיָא, ח׳ m. (חֲטִי II) *sinner.* Targ. Prov. XIV, 21. Ib. XIX, 2 (Var. חַטְיָיא, read חַטָּיָיא; incorr. חֶטְיָא).

חֲטִיאָה, כפר ח׳, Gen. R. s. 65, v. חִישָּׁיָא.

חֲטִיבָא f. ch. = next w. Targ. Y. I Deut. XXVI, 17, sq.

חֲטִיבָה I f. (חָטַב II) 1) *object of love.* Ber. 6[a]; Hag. 3[a] (ref. to Deut. XXVI, 17) אתם עשיתוני ח׳ אחת וכ׳ you made me the only object of your love in the world, and I shall make you &c. (ref. to II Sam. VII, 23); Tanh. Ki Thabo 2.—2) *declaring love.* Ib. עושין ח׳ וכ׳ declare their love to God; Tanh., ed. Bub., ib. 4.

חֲטִיבָה II, v. חֲטָבָה.

חַטִּיטָא (חַטּוּטָא) m. (חֲטַט I) *digger;* חַטִּיט שכבר one who exhumes the dead, grave-robber. B. Bath. 58[a] הוה ח׳ ש׳ (Ms. H. קא מְחַיִּיט מערתא, early eds. חַיִּיט, fr. חוט I).—*Pl.* constr. חַטִּיטֵי. Yeb. 63[b] (some ed. חָטוֹטֵי).

חֲטִיטָה f. (חָטַט I) 1) *cleaning* a well, *raking.* M. Kat. 5[a] ח׳ אין וכ׳ cleaning is permitted, but digging &c. Ib. ח׳ מי שרי is cleaning permitted?; a. e.—2) *hollowing out.* Tosef. Kel. B. Mets. II, 17; Hull. 25[a] מחוסר ח׳ a block requiring hollowing out for becoming a receptacle. Ib. מחוסר ח׳ פשיטא is it not a matter of course that a block requiring hollowing out is not fit for uncleanness?; v. חָטַט.

חַטִּיטוּב* m. (reduplic. of חָטַב I) *battle-axe.* B. Mets. 58[b] Ms. R. a. oth. (v. next w.); Tosef. ib. III, 24 (Var. וחטיטוס, וחטיטום).

חַטִּיטוּם* m. (reduplic. of חטם, v. חוֹטֵם) *buckler.* B. Mets. 58[b] סוס וסייף וח׳ ed. (Ms. R. 1 וסייף ותריס חטיטוב, Ms. R. 2 סייף וסוס וחטיטוב, Ms. F. וסייף ותריס וְחַתִּיתוּם, חטיטוב, v. Rabb. D. S. a. l. note 6, Ar. Compl. ed. Koh.) horse and sword (and battle-axe) and buckler; (Y. ib. IV, end, 9[d] סייף וסוס ותריס).

חַטָּיָא *sinner,* v. חַטְיָא.—**חַטָּיָיא**, v. חַטָּאָה.

חֲטָיָא, חֲטָיָה, חֲטָיָיא f. = חֵטְי, *sin, misconduct, failing.* Ex. R. s. 26 (ref. to Ex. XVII, 5) עבור על ח׳ שלהם pass over (ignore) their misconduct; (Yalk. ib. 262; Mekh. B'shall., Vayassa, s. 6 חֵטְא). Pesik. R. s. 13 והואיל ומפני ח׳ של אבותיהם וכ׳ (not עונותיהם) since Amalek came in consequence of the sin of their fathers (at Rephidim), says He to them, Remember &c. (Deut. XXV, 17)?—Gen. R. s. 18, end מאיזו ח׳ וכ׳ (Yalk. Gen. 25 מאיזה טעם) on account of what impropriety of conduct &c. Num. R. s. 9, end מפני ח׳ אחת וכ׳ on account of one single misconduct (in making the golden calf) &c. Deut. R. s. 2 תכתב ח׳ שלי וכ׳ let my failing be recorded (Yoma 86[b], a. e. סורחני).

חֲטַיָּיה, כפר ח׳, v. חִישָּׁיָא.

חַטִּים, חַטִּין, v. חִיטָּה.

חֲטִיפָה f. (חָטַף) *pinching* off the rough edges. Kel. XIV, 1 מחוסר ח׳ (ed. Dehr. חֲטָפָה, Var. חֲגָפָה) a fragment of a vessel needing &c. in order to be used; Tosef. ib. B. Mets. IV, 1 חטפה, v. חֲשָׁפָה.

חֲטִיפִיתָא, v. חֲטִפִיתָא.

חֲמִיתָא f. (חֲטַר I) *tenderness, delicate health.* Targ. Y. II Deut. XXVIII, 56.

חֲטָם m. (v. חוֹטָם) *the young camel's ring or staff* put through the nose, v. זְמָמָא. Sabb. V, 1 (51[b]); Y. Bets. II, 61[c] bot.

חטן, Y. Shebi. VII, beg. 37[b], v. טָנַן, טִין.

חָטַף (b. h.; cmp. חָטַט, a. גָּזַל with גָּזַז) 1) *to seize, rob.* Y. Ber. I, 3[c] bot. (ref. to I Kings VIII, 54) כפיים הללו שלא חָטְפוּ בבנין וכ׳ ed. Krot. (oth. ed. נטפו, prob. נִטְנְפוּ, v. טָנַף) like those hands which did not rob anything at building the Temple. Lam. R. to I, 1 וחָטְפוֹ ממנה and snatched it (the letter of divorce) out of her hands; a. fr.—Koh. R. to VII, 26, v. חָטַב.—2) (cmp. Lat. carpo) *to do a thing with haste,* esp. (v. Ber. 35[a] sq., Tosef. ib. IV, 1) *to break without benediction.* Tosef. Pes. X, 9 חוֹטְפִין מצה לתינוק *matzah* is distributed among the children before the regular turn in the Passover ceremonies, in order that they may not fall asleep; Pes. 109[a] (v. Rabb. D. S. a. l. note 50; oth. opin. in comment.). *Part. pass.* חָטוּף, f. חֲטוּפָה *snatched, abrupt.* M. Kat. 28[a] מת פתאם מיתה ח׳ if one dies suddenly, it is called an abrupt death (snatched by death); Treat. S'mah. ch. III לארבעה ... מיתה ח׳ after four or five days of sickness, it is called &c.; v. דָּחַף.—אמן ח׳, v. אָמֵן II.

Hithpa. הִתְחַטֵּף *to be snatched, hurried.* Y. Ber. VIII, end, 12[c] he who says 'a hurried Amen'—יִתְחַטְּפוּ שנותיו his years will be hurried (he will die an untimely, sudden death, v. supra); Bab. ib. 47[a].

חֲטַף, חֲטִיף ch. same, 1) *to seize, snatch.* Targ. Jud. XXI, 21. Targ. I Kings XX, 33 וחטפוהא מיניה they snatched the word hastily from him (h. text ויחלטו הממנו); a. e.—B. Bath. 33[b], sq. דמִיחְטַף חַטְפָהּ מיניה that he took it from him forcibly. Hull. 133[a] הוה חָטֵיפְנָא מתנתא I used to take the priest's gifts eagerly (v. חָבַב). Erub. 54[a] חֲטוֹף ואכול וכ׳ make haste and eat &c. (enjoy life, while you live).—2) *to do violence, strain* (the text), *to misinterpret.* Targ. Ez. XXII, 26.—3) (of animals of prey) *to tear.* Targ. II Esth. I, 2 דובין חטפין (read: דֵּיבִין) the wolves (on Solomon's throne) made an attempt to tear (the false witness). Ib. למחטוף לבהון וכ׳, as if to tear the hearts &c.

Pa. חַטֵּף same. Ib. (of hawks).

Ithpe. אִתְחֲטֵף *to be robbed, be snatched.* Targ. Prov. XIII, 2.—Y. Kidd. I, 60[b] top והוא מִתְחַטְפָא and it is taken by force (confiscated).

חִיטְפָא, חַטְפָא m. (preced.) *robbery, violence.* Targ. Ez. XLV, 9. Targ. Is. LX, 18.

חֲטָפָה, חַטְפָא, v. חֲטִיפָה.

חֲטִיפִיתָא, חֲמִיפִי׳ f. (preced. wds.) name of an unclean bird (h. תַּחְמָס), *ostrich* (?). Targ. Y. Lev. XI, 16; Deut. XIV, 15.

חָטַר 1) *to cut off* (denom. חוּטְרָא I, *twig,* cmp. גָּזַז &c.). —2) *to fence in* (cmp. גדר, גזר &c.). Targ. Job XIX, 8.—Denom. חוּטְרָא II.—3) (denom. of חוּטְרָא I) *to whip, strike.* Sabb. 67[a] בלועא דחמרא חֲטַרְתֵּיהּ (Ms. M. חטבתיה) with an ass' jaw I should strike him.

Pa. חַטֵּר *to provide with a vertical stroke* (חוּטְרָא). Men. 29[b] דהוו חַטְרֵי להו לגגיה דחי״ת (Ms. M. חַטְרֵי ליה Pe.) they used to put a vertical stroke on the roof of the Heth.

חֲטַר, חַטְרָא, חֲטַר, חֵט׳, v. חוּטְרָא. [Y. M. Kat. III, 83[d] top נחית מן חטריה, read: חֲמָרֵיה.]

חֲטֹרֶת, v. חֲטוֹטֶרֶת.

חַטָּתָא, v. חַטָּאתָא.

חַי m. (b. h.; חָיָה) 1) *living, alive; living creature; healthy.* Ber. 27[b] אלמלא אני חי והוא מת יכול החי וכ׳ if I were alive and he dead, the living one might give the lie to the dead. Ib. V, 5 זה חי this one is destined to live (recover). Sabb. 94[a], a. e. החי נושא את עצמו a living being carries itself (the carrying of a living being on the Sabbath is not unlawful). Ib. X, 5 את ה׳ זי במטה (he who carries) a living person on a couch; a. v. fr.—אבר מן החי, v. אֵבֶר וכ׳.—*Pl.* חַיִּים, חַיִּין. Ab. IV, 22 והח׳ לידון and the living are destined to be judged. Sabb. 94[a] בין ח׳ ובין שחוטין whether alive or slaughtered; a. fr.—Ab. Zar. 5[b] (ref. to החי, Gen. VI, 19) שחיין ראשי וכ׳ the ends of whose limbs live (exist).—2) *in natural condition, raw* (opp. בשול); *unmixed* (opp. מָזוּג). Snh. 70[a] בשר חי raw meat, יין חי unmixed wine. Ab. Zar. 38[a], a. fr. הנאכל כמות שהוא חי what is eatable in its natural state; a. fr.—*Fem.* חַיָּה. Hull. 42[a] (ref. to Lev. XI, 2) ח׳ אכול וכ׳ what is in a healthy condition (viable), you may eat, v. טְרֵפָה. [V. חַיָּה.]

חַי, חַיָּא, חַיָּיא ch. same. Targ. Gen. IX, 3; a. fr.—Targ. Ex. XII, 9 כד זיר (half-)raw; a. fr.—Sabb. 18[b] קרא חייא raw cabbage.—Midr. Till. to Ps. XXII, 7 [read:] חשיך חי דבעי למיתא luckless in the living one that is dependent on the dead; Yalk. ib. 686; a. fr.—*Pl.* חַיִּין, חַיֵּי, חַיַּיָּא. Targ. Ps. XXXVIII, 20. Targ. Num. XVII, 13; a. fr.—Snh. 98[b] אי מן ח׳ הוא if he is one of the living (the present age); Y. Ber. II, 5[a] top; a. fr.—*Fem.* חַיָּא, חַיָּתָא, חַיְיָ׳, חַיְּא. Targ. Gen. I, 20. Targ. Y. ib. XXXVII, 2; a. e.—Sabb. 18[b] קדרא ח׳ a raw dish.—*Pl.* חַיָּין, חַיָּתָא. Targ. Y. Gen. I, 21; a. fr.—Targ. Y. II Ex. I, 19 (*strong*).—[B. Kam. 38[b] דהוה חַיָּה (h. form.) that she would have lived.

חַיָא, v. חַיִי.

חַיָּב, חַיָּבָא, v. חַיָי׳.

חִיבָּה, v. חִבָּה.

חִיבּוּבָא, חִבּ׳, חִיבּוּב, constr. חִבּ׳ m. (חבב) *love; loved object.* Targ. Mic. VI, 7; a. e.—Sabb. 130[a], v. חָבַב.

חִיבּוּט, חִבּ׳ m. (חָבַט) *laying down, pressing.* Succ. IV, 6 יום ח׳ חריות the day of laying down the twigs. Ib. 43[b].

חִיבּוּל, חִיבּוּלָא, חִיבּ׳ (חֲבַל) 1) *wound, injury.* Targ. Lev. XIX, 28; XXI, 5.—M. Kat. 28ᵇ, v. חֲבִילָא I.—2) *moral defect, corruption.* Targ. Job XI, 15. Ib. XXXI, 7; a. e.

חִיבּוּלְיָא, v. חֲבוּלְיָא.

חִיבּוּצָא, v. חוּבְצָא.

חִבּוּר, חִיבּוּר m. (חָבַר) *junction, connection.* Kel. III, 6 אינה ח׳ is not considered a connection (touching the stopper by an unclean person &c. does not affect the contents of the cask). Ib. XVIII, 2; Sabb. 44ᵇ; 46ᵃ.—Ab. Zar. 56ᵇ, a. e. נצוק ח׳ the jet produced by pouring out is a connection (the liquid at one end, if touched by a gentile &c., affects that in the vessel); Toh. VIII, 9; a. v. fr.—Y. Sot. VIII, 22ᵈ אין ... ח׳ לעיר we do not consider it as connected with the town (as regards Sabbath limits). Y. Kil. IX, end, 32ᵈ ח׳ לבגד considered as connected (woven) with the garment; a. fr.

חִיבּוּרָא, חִב׳ ch. same. Targ. Y. I Lev. XIX, 10 בְּחִיבּוּרְהוֹן on the tree (v. Y. Peah IV, 18ᵃ, s. v. חָבַר).

חִיבְּתָא, חִבְ׳ ch.=h. חִבָּה. Targ Cant. II, 4; a. fr.—*Pl.* חִיבָּתָא. Ib. IV, 10.

חִיגֵּר, חִיגְּרָא, חִיגַּרְתָּא, v. sub חִג׳.

חֵידָא, Targ. Ps. LVII, 5 ed. Wil., v. חֲדֵי.

חֵידוּ, v. חֵדוּ.

חִדּוּד, חִידּוּד m. (חָדַד) 1) *the effect of the sharp edge, cut.* Hull. 8ᵃ חִידּוּדָהּ קודם וכ׳ (in cutting with a heated knife) the effect of its edge precedes the effect of the heat.—2) (b. h. חִדּוּד) *pointed projection, prong.* Kel. II, 5 ויש לו ח׳ and (the lid) has a pointed knob (which prevents the use of it separately as a receptacle). Ib. או שהיה ואין לו ח׳ (ed. Dehr. ואינו חָדוּד, v. חָדַד). Ib. IV, 1 בו ח׳ or (the vessel cannot stand straight) because it has a pointed bottom which makes it incline; a. fr.—*Pl.* חִידּוּדִים, חִדּ׳, חִידּוּדִין. Ib. 3 היו בה ח׳ יוצאין if there are prongs projecting from the bottom of the misshaped vessel.—Snh. 94ᵃ (play on ויחד, Ex. XVIII, 9) נעשה בשרו ח׳ ח׳ Ms. M. (v. Rabb. D. S. a. l.) he felt like cuts in his body; Yalk. Ex. 268 חד׳ חד׳.—3) *sharpening, whetting* (euphem. for *unnatural gratification*). Snh. 66ᵇ, v. הֶרְדּוּס.

חִידּוּק, חִד׳, ח׳ m. (חָדַק, ח׳) *that which is squeezed in to fill a gap, repair, insertion.* Hull. 57ᵇ one who had a hole in the (fractured) scull, ועשו לו ח׳ של קרויה וכ׳ ed. (Ar. ח׳ של קרא . . .) and they inserted a piece of a pumpkin shell, and he recovered. Kel. III, 5 ח׳ ק׳ הכרויה R. S. (ed. only ח׳ס׳) the lining of a pumpkin shell that has been hollowed out (to be used as a drawing vessel, i. e. the earthen vessel or clay which has been fitted in as a protection); Tosef. ib. B. Kam. III, 3 ח׳ הק׳ הברויה (v. בָּרָה a. כָּרָה); Y. Pes. III, 30ᵃ top ח׳ קירויה וכרויה (read הכרויה).

חִידּוּשׁ, חִד׳ m. (חָדַשׁ) 1) *renovation, the first stage of the crescent moon.* Y. Ber. IX, 13ᵈ הרואה ... בְּחִידּוּשָׁהּ he who sees the moon in her first stage. Y. Shek. I, 46ᵃ bot. שמרהו שיבוא בְּחִידּוּשׁוֹ observe it that it (the maturing of the crops) should coincide with the first part of the month of Nisan. R. Hash. 25ᵃ אין חִידּוּשָׁהּ של לבנה וכ׳ (Ms. M. חֲדָשָׁהּ, v. חֹדֶשׁ) the renovation of the moon takes no less than twenty nine days and a half &c.—2) *restoration.* Y. Taan. II, 65ᶜ bot. ח׳ בית וכ׳ the restoration of thy sanctuary.—3) *novel interpretation, novel idea, additional legislation* (novellae). Hag. 3ᵃ א״א לבה״מ בלא ח׳ it is impossible for a college session to pass without a novel remark. Ib. מה ח׳ היה וכ׳ what was the news in college to-day?—Cant. R. to IV, 16 ובואי דבר של ח׳ 'and come' (ib.) intimates a novel rule (adding thanks-offerings); Y. Meg. I, 72ᶜ top, a. e.—Lev. R. s. 13, v. חָדַשׁ; a. fr.—4) *strange law, exception, unique law* (which allows of no conclusion by analogy), *anomaly.* Sub. 27ᵃ עד זומם ח׳ הוא וכ׳ the law concerning the punishment of false witnesses is an anomaly, (for why must we trust the one set more than the other?) אין . . חִידּוּשׁוֹ ואילך therefore you cannot go beyond what it says distinctly, i. e. previous evidences of refuted witnesses cannot be assailed. Pes. 44ᵇ מבשר וחלב ... דח׳ הוא you can draw no analogy from the law concerning the mixture of flesh and milk, for it is an anomaly; ומאי חידושו and wherein is it an anomaly? Y. Ter. VII, beg. 44ᶜ לְחִידּוּשׁוֹ יצא the law (Deut. XXII, 13 sq.) is specified for its anomalous nature; a. fr.

חִידוּת, Y. B. Kam. IX, 6ᵈ bot., read: חִידּוּשׁ or חדתין חוו, v. חֲדַת.

חִידְקָא, v. חֵדֶ׳.

חִידְקִי (חִזְקִי, חוּסְקִי, חִירְקִי, חוּדְ׳) pr. n. pl. *Hidki* in Assyria. Yeb. 17ᵃ; Kidd. 72ᵇ (v. Var. in Neub. Géogr. p. 373).

חִידְתָּא, v. חוּדְ.

חִיָּה, v. חיי.

חַיָּה I f. (b. h.; חַיָּה) 1) (adj.) v. חַי.—2) *animal,* esp. *beast of chase, deer* &c., contrad. to בְּהֵמָה. Hull. VI, 1 ונוהג בח׳ ובעוף and applies to beasts of chase and birds; a. fr.—Ab. V, 9, a. fr. ח׳ רעה the plague of wild beasts. Ex. R. s. 35 (ref. to Ps. LXVIII, 31) ח׳ הדרה וכ׳ the beast that lives between the reeds (Rome).—Sabb. 151ᵇ; Snh. 38ᵇ, a. e. אין ח׳ רעה שולטת וכ׳ no wild beast has power over man, unless he appears to it to resemble a brute creature; a. fr.—*Pl.* חַיּוֹת. Taan. 8ᵃ לע״ל . . . כל הח׳ וכ׳ in the future all the wild beasts shall gather and come to the serpent &c. Bets. 25ᵇ כלב בח׳ the dog (is the most irrepressible) among the wild beasts. Ber. 61ᵇ פקח שבח׳ the shrewdest of all animals; a. v. fr.—Esp. *Hayoth,* legendary celestial creatures (Ez. I, 5). Hag. 13ᵃ; a. fr.

חַיָּה II f. (חָיָה) 1) [*recovering,*] *lying-in woman, woman in confinement.* Yoma VIII, 1 הח׳ תנעול וכ׳ a woman after confinement may wear shoes (on the Day of Atonement). Ber. 54ᵇ וחולה ח׳ וכ׳ a sick person, a lying-in &c.; a. fr.—*Pl.* חַיּוֹת. Y. Kil. IX, 32ᵇ bot.; Gen. R. s. 96, end אי לכם ח׳ וכ׳ woe to you, lying-in women in Palestine; a. fr.—2) [*physician,*] *midwife.* Tosef. B. Bath. VII, 2 נאמנת ח׳ וכ׳ the midwife is an admissible witness as to which (of twins) was the first-born; Y. Kidd. IV, 69ᵈ bot.; Y. B. Bath. III, beg. 13ᵈ הח׳ בשעה וכ׳ the midwife (is an admissible witness) only as long as she is seated by the obstetric chair (not after she left the mother). Y. Yeb. XVI, end, 16ᵃ עשו אותו כח׳ וכ׳ they place him in the same category as a midwife whose testimony is valid on the spot; a. e.—*Pl.* as ab. Cant. R. to IV, 5 מרים .. חַיּוֹתֵיהֶן וכ׳ Miriam .... were the midwives of Israel; a. fr.

חֵיוָא, חֵיוְתָא f. ch. = constr. חֵיוַת, חֵיוּת = h. חַיָּה I, *animal,* mostly collect. *beasts.* Targ. Y. Gen. XXXVII, 2. Targ. Gen. I, 25; a. fr.—Yeb. 121ᵇ ושדי לְחֵיוָאִי and cast it before my cattle; Snh. 74ᵇ לְחֵיוְתָא (ed. Sonc. לְחֵיוְתָאִי); a. fr.—*Pl.* חֵיוָאן, חֵיוָון. Targ. Y. Gen. XXV, 27.—Koh. R. to XI, 2 תרין ח׳ דנור two animals of fire (M. K. חִיוָן serpents). Ib. חֵיוָן.—(Masc. pl.) חֵיוֵי. Hull. 43ᵇ, a. e. ח׳ בריתא, v. בְּרָאָה.—V. חֵיוְתָא.

חִיוָאי pr. n. m. *Hivai.* Yeb. 121ᵇ מאן אִיכָא בי ח׳ וכ׳ who is here belonging to the house of Ḥ.?

חִיּוּב, חִיוּב m. (חוב, v. חָיַיב) *obligation; restriction, disadvantage; conviction.* Sabb. 2ᵇ מהן לח׳ ומהן לפטור some of them are mentioned for conviction (as punishable), and some as not punishable. Ib. 3ᵃ ח׳ חטאת obligation to bring a sin-offering. Y. Keth. IX, beg. 32ᵈ מזכותו אתה למד חִיּוּבוֹ from his privilege you can deduct his restriction (what he has no right to).—Y. Ḥall. III, beg. 59ᵃ מפטור על ח׳ from what is exempt (from Ḥallah) for what is subject (to Ḥallah); a. fr.

חִיּוּב, חִיּוּבָא, חִיּ׳ ch. same, 1) *guilt, wickedness.* Targ. Job XXXV, 8.—2) *obligation, conviction.* R. Hash. 28ᵃ בח׳ as an obligation; זמן ח׳ the time when one is bound to hear the Shofar; מקום ח׳ a place where one is bound. Succ. 56ᵃ ח׳ דיומא the obligation of the day (to dwell in booths). B. Kam. 68ᵃ חִיּוּבֵיהּ לאחר יאוש הוא his obligation begins after the object has been despaired of; a. fr.—*Pl.* חִיּוּבֵי, חִיּוּ׳. Sabb. 2ᵇ; a. e.

חִיּוּבְתָּא f. (preced.) *guilt.* Targ. Y. Ex. V, 16.

חֵיוָא, v. חֵיוָא.

חיומא, read חֲיָיטָא.

חִיוּרָא, חִיוּרְתָּא, חִיוַּור, v. sub חִיוַּר׳.

חֵיוְתָא, v. חֵיוְתָא.

חִוְיָא, חִוְיָא, חִוְיָי, חִוְיֵי m. (חוי, v. Ges. H. Dict.¹⁰ s. v. חוה) *serpent.* Targ. Gen. III, 1. Targ. O. Ex. IV, 2 חִוְיֵי ed. Berl. (Var. חִוְוי, חִוְיֵי); a. fr.—Y. Sabb. I, 3ᵇ ודבר נשא ח׳ and the spine of a human being is turned into a serpent. Sabb. 85ᵃ (play on הַחִוִּי) שהיו מועמין את הארץ כח׳ they tasted the ground (for agricultural purposes) like a serpent. Gen. R. s. 20 (play on חַוָּה) ח׳ חִוְיָךְ ואת ח׳ דאדם the serpent is thy (Eve's) serpent (seducer), and thou art Adam's serpent. Sabb. 110ᵃ ח׳ דרבנן טרקיה the Rabbis' serpent bit him, i. e. he was bitten by a serpent as a punishment for disregarding rabbinical ordinances (with ref. to Koh. X, 8); Ab. Zar. 27ᵇ. Ber. 12ᵇ זקף כח׳ erected himself (in prayer) like a serpent (raising his head first); a. fr.—*Pl.* חִוְיָא; (*fem. pl.*) חִוְיָן, חִוְיָנְ, חִוְיָן. Targ. Num. XXI, 6, sq.; a. fr.—[V. אִוְיָא.]

חיווין, pr. n. pl., v. זִיזְיָן.

חִיוְלָא, v. חַיְלָא.

(חִוָּר, חִוָּר) חִוָּרָא, חִוָּר, חִיוַּר m. (חור) 1) *white.* Targ. Gen. XXX, 35; a. fr.—B. Mets. 58ᵇ דאזיל ואתי ח׳ .. the red color (of the face) disappears, and the white takes its place; a. fr.—*Pl.* חִוָּרִין, חִוָּרִין, חִוָּרֵי. Targ. Zech. VI, 3 (ed. Wil. חִוָּ׳); a. fr.—Ber. 28ᵃ, v. חֲצָבָא; a. fr.—*Fem.* חִוַּרְתָּא, חִוָּרָא, חִוַּר׳. Targ. Lev. XIII, 4 (ed. Berl. חִוָּרָא); a. fr.—(As a noun) *white skin, white spot* &c. Targ. Y. Lev. XXII, 22.—Gitt. 68ᵃ וח׳ באוכמתא a white spot on a dark skin, v. אוּכָּם. Ib. 56ᵃ חיורתא (Ar. חִוַּרְיָתָא) *white flour,* v. גּוּשְׁקְרָא; a. fr.—*Pl.* חִוָּרָתָא, חִוָּרָן, חִוָּ׳, חִוָּרָן, חִוָּרֵי. Targ. Lev. XIII, 38, sq.—Ber. 28ᵃ לית לך ח׳ thou hast no gray hair (art too young for the office); v. דָּרָא I. Sabb. 110ᵃ top תליסר חמרי ח׳ thirteen white she-asses. Hull. 7ᵇ; Yoma 49ᵃ כרעיהו (רישו) דח׳ when their legs are white; a. fr. [Snh. 98ᵃ חיור גונו, v. הָדָר.]—[Pes. 42ᵇ מיא דחיורי, v. חִיזְרָא II.]—2) *leprous, leper, white-spotted* (from disease), *blanched.* Targ. O. Ex. IV, 6 (Y. ed. Amst. מְחַוְּורָא, h. text מצרעת).—Gitt. 68ᵃ טעמא דח׳ the taste of a leprous (white-spotted) animal. Snh. 98ᵇ ח׳ דבי רבי שמו the name of the Messiah is 'the leper of the house of Rabbi'; a. fr. [חמר חיור יין, v. חִיוַּרְיָין.]

חִוַּרְוָרִיָּא m. pl. (v. preced.) [*dazzling appearances,* (cmp. שַׁבְרִירַיָּא a. b. h. סַנְוֵרִים),] *temporary loss of direction, bewilderment.* Targ. Y. I Gen. XIX, 11 Ar. ed. Koh. (ed. R. חַוּוּרְוָרִיָּא; Targ. ed. חוודרוריא, חוורור׳, חוורר׳), v. חֲבַרְבְּרֵי; cmp. חִרוּרָא.

***חִיוַּרְיָין, חִיוַּרְיָן, חִיוַּרְיָין** (also חיור יין) pr. n. pl. *Ḥivvar-yayin, Ḥivv'rayin.*—חֲמַר ח׳ name of a *wine* of inferior quality and color, cmp. פָּרַק. B. Bath. 97ᵇ חמר חיוריין מהו (Ms. H. חיור יין, v. Rabb. D. S. a. l. note 20) how about the use of Ḥ. wine for religious purposes?—Kerith. 6ᵃ חמר חיור יין עתיק old Ḥ. wine (used as a substitute of caper wine for soaking onycha); Y. Yoma IV, 41ᵈ חיוורין.

חִיוַּרְיָתָא, v. חִיוַּר.

חִיּוּת f. (b. h.; חָיָה) *living, support.* Ber. 61ᵇ במקום חִיּוּתֵנוּ (חַיּוּתֵינוּ) in the element in which we live (the water). Gen. R. s. 20 (play on חַוָּה) ניתנה לו לְחַיּוּתוֹ וכ׳ she had been given to him for his strength, but she advised him like a serpent; a. e.—*Pl.* חִיּוּת, v. next w.

חַיּוּתָא ch. 1) same, *life, livelihood.* Yoma 85ᵃ עיקר ח׳ וכ׳ the real life is in the nose (cessation of breath from the nostrils is the main sign of death); Sot. 45ᵇ.—Hull. 19ᵇ כי נפקא ח׳ when life escapes. B. Bath. 21ᵇ פסקת לה לְחַיּוּתָאִי Ar. (ed. חַיּוּתִי, v. Rabb. D. S. a. l. note 20) thou disturbest my livelihood. Macc. 10ᵃ עבד ליה ח׳ וכ׳ Ms. M. (ed. עביד .. מידי דתיהוי ליה ח׳) make life for him so that he may live (give him security of life); ib. עביד ליה מידי דתיהוי ליה ח׳ prepare for him something which secures life (religious study); Yalk. Deut. 829; 921.—Gitt. 12[a] עביד ליה ח׳ טפי you must allow him a more ample living (than under ordinary conditions).—Pes. 89[a] (ref. to מהיות, Ex. XII, 4) מֵחַיּוּתֵיה דשה from the lamb while it is yet alive (you may withdraw). Ib. ור״ש סבר מחַיּוּתָיו דשה Ms. M. 2 (Ar. מחיותיה, ed. מֵחֲיַיּתֵיה) R. S. says, from the life of the lamb in both senses (during life proper and as long as the blood has not yet been sprinkled; v. Rabb. D. S. a. l. note 70).—2) *womb*. Bekh. 21[b], v. אֲצַר II.—3) *animal*, v. next w.

חֵיוְתָא, חֵיוָ׳ f. (preced.) 1)=חֵיוָא. Targ. Y. Gen. IX, 5 חֵיוְתָא. Targ. Is. XXXVIII, 13.—Snh. 74[b], v. חֵיוָא. B. Mets. 5[a]. Ib. 93[a]. B. Bath. 29[b] אוקומי בה ח׳ to place cattle there for grazing. Lev. R. s. 13; Cant. R. to III, 4, v. מְכַר.—*Pl.* חֵיוָתָא, constr. חֵיוַות; חֵיוָון, v. חֵיוָא.—2) (v. preced.) *living, provision*.—*Pl.* חֵיוְוָתָא. Targ. Y. Num. XXXV, 11 בתי ח׳ ed. pr. (ed. חזוותא, corr. acc.) deposits of breadstuff (v. מִחְיָה).

חֵיזוּנָא, חֵיזְוָא, חֵיזְוָא, חֵיזוּ v. sub חז׳.

חֵיזוֹן, v. חִזָּיוֹן II.

חִיזּוּק, חִזּ׳ m. (חָזַק) 1) *repairing, supporting*. Y. Erub. V, 22[d] bot. לח׳ בתים וכ׳ (the handle of an axe wedged in between two buildings) was intended to support the houses, v. דִּיסְתְּקָא.—2) *effort, mental energy*. Ber. 32[b]; Yalk. Josh. 5.—3) *fastening, stringent measures for the protection of the law*. Keth. 83[b], a. e. חכמים עשו ח׳ לדבריהם וכ׳ the scholars protected their own enactments more than the biblical laws. Erub. 3[a] סוכה דאורייתא לא בעי ח׳ וכ׳ the law of Succah being Biblical requires no protection, but that about &c. Keth. 56[b]; a. fr.

חֵיזוּר, חֵיזוּר, v. חָזוּר a. חַזּוּר.

חֵיזוּתָא, v. חֲזוּתָא.

חֵיזָ״ךְ, v. חָזָ׳.

חִיזָּק m. (חָזַק) *fastening, band, ring* &c. Num. R. s. 3, beg. even its bast הולך לח׳ (ed. Wil. לחִיזּוּק) is used for bandage; Midr. Till. to Ps. XCII, 13 (Gen. R. s. 41 לחבלים).

חִיזְקָא ch. same, *clasp, ring*.—*Pl.* חִיזְקַיָּא. Y. Sabb. VI, 8[b] bot. (expl. טבעות, Is. III, 21); cmp. עִיזְקָא.

חִיזְרָא, חִזְ׳ I c. (חזר, cmp. חֲזִיר) 1) *prickly, knotty thorn*. B. Mets. 103[b] קני דח׳ וכ׳ (Ar. Var. חרזא, חזרזא, v. Ar. ed. Koh. s. v. ארכבתא) the poles for the shrub (to be put up as a hedge on top of the earth mound) must be supplied by the landlord, but the shrub itself by the tenant. Ned. 41[b] top כח׳ לדיקלא as its prickles protect the palm-tree (v. Num. R. s. 3, beg.). Ber. 8[a] כח׳ בגבבא דעמרא וכ׳ (Ms. M. לח׳ דשלפא מגבבא וכ׳) as a thorn in a ball of wool which (if one tries to tear loose) lacerates backward (in the opposite direction of its knots), v. נְשַׁר I.—*Pl.* חִיזְרֵי. Sabb. 63[b]; Bets. 29[b], a. e. (proverbial expression) אח׳ שקילא טיבותיך ושדיא (שקילי.. ושדי) thy good-natured advice is taken and thrown over the hedge, i. e. thy advice comes too late.—2) *a flexible and strong reed, bamboo-cane*. Ber. 12[b] כרע כח׳ he bent (in prayer) like a cane (when it is swung).

חִיזְרָא, חִזְ׳ II m. (חָזַר; cmp. הַדְרָאָה) *second course, bran*. B. Mets. 60[b] מיא דח׳ (Ms. F. דחזירא, Ms. R. 1 דחִזְרֵי, Ms. R. 2 דחזורי) bran-broth (which bloats the animal fed on it); Pes. 42[b] מיא דחיז׳ Ms. M., Ar. a. oth. (v. Rabb. D. S. a. l. note; ed. דחירורי, read: דחִיזְרֵי pl.), v. זוּמָא I.

חִיזְרָד, v. חִיזְרָר.

חִיזְרִין, Y. Sabb. I, 3[b] bot., v. חֲזֶרֶת.

חִיזְרָר, (חִיזְרָד) חִזְ׳ m. (cmp. חֲזָרָר) *medlar* (Mespilus Azarolus, v. Löw Pfl., p. 288, a. Sm. Ant. s. v. Mespile), being considered homogeneous to quincy. [In Mish. a. Babyl. dialect עוּזְרָר (עוּזְרָד), but different from חֲזָרָר.] Y. Kil. I, 27[a] תפוח ע״ג חיזרד; (Tosef. ib. I, 3 אוּזְרָד).—*Pl.* חִיזְרָרִין. Y. Sabb. III, 5[d] קטנים כח׳ boiled down to the size of medlars; (Bab. ib. 38[a] עוזרדין; Y. Ter. II, 41[c] bot., v. חֲזָרָר).

חִיטָּא, חִטָּא, חִטֵּ׳, חִיטִּי, חִיטִּין, חִיטַּיָּא m., pl. ch. (=h. חִטָּה) 1) *wheat*. Targ. I Chr. XXI, 20. Targ. Ps. LXXXI, 17; a. e.—Ber. 58[b] חִטֵּי.—Ib. 64[a]; B. Bath. 145[b]; Hor. 14[a] (prov.) הכל צריכין למרי ח׳ all people depend on the owners of wheat, i. e. sound learning is the bread, while dialectics and homiletics are the spices of study; a. fr.—2) *glands, nipples, protuberances*. Hull. 18[b] פגע בח׳ if, in slaughtering, the knife struck the glands near the windpipe. Y. Hag. II, 77[d] bot. ח׳ ביזייא the nipples of the breasts; Y. Snh. VI, 23[c] bot. ח׳ מחייא (corr. acc.). V. חִנְטָא a. חִיטְתָא.

חִיטָּה, v. חִטָּה.

חִיטּוּר, חִטּוּר m. (v. חטר I, II) 1) *cleansing, purification*. Sifré Num. 126 לכלל ח׳ under the law of purification (ref. to Num. XIX, 12, Naz. 61[b] טהרה).—2) *delicacy, luxury, enjoyment*.—*Pl.* חִיטּוּרִין. Cant. R. to VII, 2 חיטטין (corr. acc.), v. חָטָא I.

חִיטּוּרָא m. ch. (v. preced. 2), *being raised in luxury, being delicate*. Targ. Y. I Deut. XXVIII, 56. [Some ed. חִיטּוּיָא.]

חִיטְמִין, v. חִיטּוּר.

חִיטַּיָּא, כְּפַר ח׳ pr. n. pl. *K'far Ḥittaya*, near Tiberias (*Ḥattin*). Y. Hor. III, beg. 47[a]. Y. Meg. I, 70[a] (expl. הצדים, Josh. XIX, 35). Gen. R. s. 65 כ׳ חטיאה. Pesik. R. s. 16 חִטַּיָּה; Pesik. Eth Korb., p. 61[a] חטייא. Hag. 5[b].

חִיטִּין 1) pl. of חִטָּה a. of חִיטָּא.—2) *reed*, v. אִיטָן.

חִיטְנֵי, v. חִיטְנֵי.

חִיטְפָא, v. חֲטָפָא.

חִיטְתָא f. (v. חִיטָּא) *wheat crop of a field*. Y. Snh. IV, end, 22[c] אפי׳ חיטתא או ח׳ וכ׳ (ed. Krot. חיטטא, corr.

acc.) even the crop of figs or of wheat of one field is not like the other. [Y. Ned. VI, end, 40ª הדרין ח׳, read: חִיטָּא.]

חִיָה, חיי (b. h.) 1) *to live.* Tam. 32ª מה ... וִיחְיֶה what must man do in order to live (long)?; a. v. fr.— *Part.* חַי (v. חַי).—Keth. I, 6 לא מפיה אנו חָיִין we do not live on what comes from her lips, i. e. we do not go by her evidence. Y. ib. II, 26ᶜ bot. אנו כחיין מפיה we (the court) are again in the condition of dependence on her own evidence. Y. Shebi. II, 34ª top שהן חָיִין מִמֵּי וכ׳ they live (draw nourishment) from the waters of last year; ib. הוא חָיָה (הוא חָיָה) it draws &c.—Snh. 108ª לא חיין ולא נידונין they have no share in the resurrection nor will they be judged; a. fr.—2) *to heal; to recover, regain health.* Keth. 6ª, a. e. עד שתִּחְיֶה המכה until the wound is healed up. Hull. 7ᵇ וְחָיָה and did recover; וְחָיְתָה and it (the wound) healed up; a. fr. [Y. Maasr. I, 48ᵈ חיותה; Y. Shebi. IV, 35ᵇ bot. חריתה, v. חוּת.]

Nif. נֶחְיָה *to be recalled to life, to resurrect.* Ab. IV, 22 והמתים לְהֵחָיוֹת and the dead are destined to be revived. Snh. 90ᵇ שעתיד להחיות that he (Aaron) will resurrect.

Pi. חִיָּה, חִיָּיה 1) *to keep alive, sustain.* Tam. 32ª יְחַיֶּה את עצמו let him feed himself (his passions, be selfish). Yoma 71ª מְחַיֶּה חיים He who sustains the living; a. fr.—2) *to recall to life, to revive.* Snh. l. c. הקב״ה מְחַיֶּה מתים the Lord revives the dead. Ib. מה שאני ממית אני מְחַיֶּה what I put to death, I revive again; a. fr.

Hif. הֶחְיָה, הֶחֱיָיה same. Ib. 92ᵇ מתים שה׳ יחזקאל the dead whom Ezekiel revived (Ez. XXXVII). Ib. והֶחֱיָיה מתים וכ׳ and revive the dead in the valley of Dura; a. fr.

חִיָא, חִיי ch. same. Targ. Gen. V, 3; a. v. fr.—*Part.* חַיי, חַאי. Targ. Y. Num. XXI, 8. Targ. Deut. VIII, 3; a. fr.—Taan. 25ª דחְיִית ... אי דחָיֵינָא (v. Ms. M. a. Rashi) is what I have lived more or what I have yet to live? Answ. דחְיִית what thou hast lived. Snh. 81ª מאן דעביד לכולהו הוא דח׳ will he only live who practiced all these virtues?; a. fr.—Hull. 7ᵇ הא קחזינא דחָיֵי but do'nt we see that they do recover?—Snh. 91ª דחָיִין מיתי דמיתי חָיִין if those who live must die, can those who died, live again?; a. fr.

Pa. חַיֵּי as preced. *Pi.* Targ. Ps. LXXI, 20 תְּחַיֵּי (some ed. תְּחַי). Targ. Job XXXVI, 6; a. fr.

Af. אַחַי, אַחְיֵי, אַחְיָיא same. Targ. II Kings VIII, 1.—Targ. Y. II Deut. III, 1; a. e.

חַיֵּי 1) *life,* v. חַיִּין.—2) *the living,* v. חַי ch., a. preced.

חַיָּיא *midwife,* v. חַיְּתָא.

חַיָּיא 1) *life,* v. חַיִּין.—2) *the living,* v. חַי ch.

חִיָּיה, חִיָּיא pr. n. m. (abbr. of אֲחִיָּה) *Hiyya,* name of several Amoraim. Esp. R. H. Robah (the elder, רובה, רבה, רבא), the redactor of the Tosefta in conjunction with R. Oshaya. Taan. 21ª. Y. Meg. IV, 74ᵈ bot. Keth. 103ᵇ; a. v. fr.—R. H. of Sepphoris. Y. Orl. III, 63ª.—R. H. bar Abba (Ba). Y. Sabb. I, 3ª; a. fr.—R. H. bar Ada I a. II. Y. Maasr. I, 48ᵈ top; a. fr.—Y. Dem. II, 22ᶜ top; a. fr.; and many more, v. Fr. M'bo, p. 81ᵇ, sq.

חַיָּיב m. (חוּב) 1) *debtor.* B. Mets. 12ᵇ בשה׳ מודה when the debtor admits (that the note has not been paid); a. fr.—2) (*he is*) *bound,* (*he is*) *guilty.* Peah IV, 7 ח׳ he is bound (to leave the poor man's corner). Keth. 30ᵇ ולרבא ח׳ and according to Raba's opinion he must pay; a. v. fr.—Sabb. I, 1 ח׳ is guilty (of Sabbath-breaking, eventually bound to bring a guilt-offering); a. v. fr.— *Pl.* חַיָּיבִין. Ber. III, 1 ח׳ are bound (to read the Sh'ma); a. fr.—*Fem.* חַיֶּיבֶת. Hag. 4ª, a. e. שהאשה ח׳ בה which woman is bound to observe; a. fr.—*Pl.* חַיָּיבוֹת. Ib.; a. fr.—3) *wicked.*—*Fem.* as ab. Mekh. B'shall. s. 1 מלכות ח׳ wicked government (usu. רְשָׁעָה).

חַיָּיב, חָיָב ch. same. Targ. Mal. I, 14.

חַיָּיב, חַיָּבָא, חַיָּבָא m. (preced.) *sinner, wicked man.* Targ. Gen. XVIII, 23; a. fr.—Lam. R. to II, 1, v. חוב Pa.—*Pl.* חַיָּיבַיָּא, חַיָּיבִין. Targ. Job XXXVIII, 13. Targ. II Sam. XXII, 5; a. fr.—Snh. 91ª; a. e.

חַיָּיה, v. חַיָּיא.

חִיוּוּב, חִיוּוּבָא, v. חִיּוּב, חִיּוּבָא.

חַיָּיט m. (denom. of חוט III) *seamster, tailor, clothmender.* Sabb. I, 3; Tosef. ib. I, 8; a. fr.—*Pl.* חַיָּיטִין. Y. Pes. IV, 31ᵇ top.

חַיָּיט, חַיָּיטָא ch. same. Gen. R. s. 11; Koh. R. to IV, 1, v. דָּנִיאֵל. Y. Sabb. XV, beg. 15ª חיוטא (corr. acc.). Cant. R. to VI, 12, v. יוֹסְטָא.

חָיֵיךְ, חַיֵּיךְ, חַיֵּיךְ, v. חוּךְ.

***חַיָּיךְ** m. (חוּךְ I) *stammerer.* Tanh. D'barim 2 אם אתה ח׳ וכ׳ if thou art a stammerer, study the Law repeatedly.

חַיֵּיל, v. חוּל I ch.

חַיֵּיל, v. חַיִל.

חַיִל, חַיֵּיל m. (b. h.; חוּל I) 1) [*surrounding, protection,*] *army.*—*Pl.* חַיָּילוֹת, חַיָּילִים. Mekh. B'shall. s. 1. Ib., Shirah, s. 3. Ib. 4 לספק אכסניות לכל חַיָּילוֹתָיו to provide pay for all his troops. Midr. Till. to Ps. XLVIII, 14 (ref. to לְחֵילָהּ ib.=לְחַיָּילוֹתֶיהָ וכ׳ (לְחֵילָה to her (Jerusalem's) hosts that shall enter it (as pilgrims); a. fr.—2) *strength, health.* Gen. R. s. 54 יישר חֵילְכֶם may your strength be confirmed (I thank you)!; Midr. Sam. ch. XII חֵילְכֶם; Yalk. Sam. 103 חֵילְכֶן. Num. R. s. 10 (ref. to Prov. XXXI, 3) זה חֵילָהּ של תורה that is the strength which the Law gives.—בְּרוֹר ח׳, v. בְּרוֹר.

חַיֵּילָא, v. חֵילָא.

חיילותא, Targ. Cant. VIII, 4, read: חֵילְוָת׳, v. חֵילָא.

חַיִּים m. pl. (b. h.; חָיָה) *life, support; health.* Sabb. 33ᵇ חַיֵּי עולם everlasting life (future world), ח׳ שעה temporary life (physical wants).—חיי נפש *necessaries of life.* Y. Ned.

IX, 42ᶜ כביסה ח׳ נ׳ washing clothes belongs to the necessaries of life (which the poor must be supplied with). Ib. ח׳ העיר הזאת the support of the poor of one's own place. Pes. 113ᵇ חַיֵּיהֶם אינם חיים whose life is no life (deserving the name); a. v. fr.—חַיֶּיךָ, בְּחַ׳ by thy life!, *as thou livest!* Lev. R. s. 15; a. v. fr.—Ber. 3ᵃ, a. e. חַיֶּיךָ וחַיֵּי ראשך by thy life, and by thy head!—(עד) יורד עמו לחַיָּיו persecutes him even as far as to deprive him of his livelihood. Kidd. 28ᵃ. Ex. R. s. 1, beg.; a. fr.—Lev. R. s. 19 בית חַיֵּינוּ our house of life (the Temple). Mekh. Yithro, Amal., s. 2 (ref. to Ex. XVIII, 20) הודע להם בית חַיֵּיהֶם make known to them their house of life (prayer, study; v. Targ. Y. Ex. l. c.); B. Mets. 30ᵇ; B. Kam. 99ᵇ, sq. (v. comment.).—[חַיִּים *the living ones*, v. חַי.]

חַיֵּי, חַיִּין, חַיַּיָּא ch. same. Targ. Y. II Gen. XLV, 28. Targ. Gen. II, 7. Ib. 9 (Y. ed. Amst. חַיָּיא); a. fr.—Y. Ab. Zar. III, 42ᶜ top חייא דאהן וכ׳ Oh, what a (blessed) life that man has led that &c.; Y. Peah I, 15ᵈ חיוי (corr. acc.; Gen. R. s. 59 חמון וכ׳). B. Bath. 58ᵇ בראש כל חיין אנא חמר at the head of all life-giving things, am I, the wine. Sabb. 67ᵇ (drinking toast) חמרא וח׳ וכ׳ wine and health to our teachers!; a. fr.

חַיְנָא, v. חִינָא.

חַיִּיס, חָיֵיס, v. חוס.

חַיִּיס I (חוס 2) *connection, relationship, legally recognized ancestry* or *descent*. Kidd. 69ᵃ עבד אין לו ח׳ a slave has no legal relations (paternity); Yeb. 23ᵃ. B. Kam. 88ᵃ שאין להם ח׳ בנים who have no legitimate sons (i. e. slaves); שאין להם ח׳ אבות who have no legitimate parentage. Ib. גר נהי דאין לו ח׳ למעלה וכ׳ the proselyte, though he has no relationship upwards (with his relations before his conversion), has relations downwards (with his children born in Judaism); a. e.

חַיִּיס II m. (חוס 1) *protection*. Mekh. Bo, Pisḥa, s. 11, v. חֲסִית II.

חַיְיסָא, חַיְסָא, v. חַיָּס. [Targ. Prov. III, 25 וזריסא, חריסא, v. חִיפְּא I.]

חָיֵיץ, v. חוץ ch.

חַיִּיץ m. (b. h. חַיִּץ; v. חוץ 1 h. a. ch.) *a pile of loose and uneven material, a rough extemporised embankment*, opp. to earth-covered and finished. Shebi. III, 8 עושה ח׳ הוא (Y. ed. עוֹשֶׂהוּ) he may make (it) a loose embankment; Y. ib. 34ᵈ מהו ח׳ חָיֵיץ ליה what is *ḥayits?* He partitions it up (ref. to Ez. XIII, 10, v. Targ. a. Rashi a. l.).

חַיְיצָאוֹת, v. חִיצָא.

חָיֵיש, v. חוש ch.

חַיְיתָא, חַיְתָא I, 1) (adj.), v. חַי.—2) (noun) *living creature*. Targ. O. Gen. I, 28. Ib. 30 חֵיַת (constr.); a. e.

חַיְיתָא, חַיְתָא II, f. ch.=h. חַיָּה II, 1) *lying-in woman*. Targ. Y. Deut. XXVIII, 12 (cmp. Taan. 2ᵃ, sq.). Koh. R. to III, 2 ולמה .. לה ח׳ וכ׳ and why do they call her *ḥay'tha?* Because she was dying and is recovering.—3) *midwife*. Targ. Gen. XXXV, 17.—Y. Keth. V, 30ᵃ, v. חָכַם. Gen. R. s. 60 (prov.) בין ח׳ למחבלתא וכ׳ between the midwife and the travailing woman, the child of the poor woman dies.—*Pl.* חַיָּתָא, חַיָּיתָא, חַיָּן. Targ. Ex. I, 15.—Y. Sabb. XIII, end, 16ᶜ שאלון לח׳ ask the midwives (about their usages on the Sabbath); אמרה ליה ליכא חַיָּיא said she to him, there is no midwife (in the place).

חַיְיתָא, חַיְתָא III, f. (b. h. חַיָּה; חָנָה, v. II Sam. XXIII, 13) *encampment, lodge*. Targ. Ps. LXVIII, 11. Targ. II Sam. XXIII, 11.

חַיְתָא, חַיְיתָא IV m. (חות, cmp. נַחַת a. Syr. חתא *pera a. trabs*, P. Sm. 1408) *pouch, bag*. Gitt. 45ᵇ ח׳ דתפילי a bag containing T'fillin. Hull. 45ᵃ (by play on חייתא *life* a. *bag*) וסימניך ח׳ דמתנח ביה וכ׳ and thy sign (to remember which of the two skins is essential for life), the bag in which the cerebrum lies. Keth. 93ᵃ; B. Kam. 9ᵃ, a. e. ח׳ דקטרי וכ׳ thou wast satisfied to buy a pouch sealed with knots, i. e. it is your fault that you did not examine the purchase.—Gitt. 47ᵃ, v. גַּלְגַּלְתָּא. Ib. כל ... אמחיה ח׳ ופלגא I will give each of you one blow with the whole bag, and one blow with half of it.

חֵיךְ m. (b. h. חֵךְ; חָנַךְ) *palate; taste*. Gen. R. s. 99 (play on חכלילי, Gen. XLIX, 12) חִיכִּי ערב לי the taste in my mouth is sweet to me (Matt. K. חִיכּוֹ its taste); חיך לי לי sweet taste is mine, is mine; Yalk. ib. 160; Keth. 111ᵇ כל ח׳ שטועמו וכ׳ every palate which tastes it, says, (Give) me; Tanh. Vayhi 10 ח׳ לי לי מיינה וכ׳ (give) me a taste of the wine of the Law.—Trnsf. (cmp. טַעַם) *good sense, persuasive word*. Cant. R. to V, 16 (ref. to חִכּוֹ, ib.) יש לך ח׳ גדול (מתוק) מזה is there anything more persuasive than this?

חִכָּא, חִיכָּא ch. same. Targ. Prov. V, 3.

חִיכּוּךְ m. (חָכַךְ) *scab, itch* (as an epidemic). B. Kam. 80ᵇ. Taan. 14ᵃ (Ms. M. 2, a. Ar. חִחוּךְ).—Tanh. ed. Bub., R'eh 10, v. חָכַךְ.

חִיכּוּכָא, חִכ׳ ch. same. Targ. Y. I Deut. XXVIII, 27 (h. text חרס), v. חֲכוּכָא.

חַיִל, v. חֵיל.—בְּרוֹר חַ׳, v. בְּרוֹר.

חֵיל, חֵל I, m. (חול, v. חֵירָל) *surrounding*, esp. *Ḥel*, a place within the fortification of the Temple. Midd. I, 5. Snh. 88ᵇ. Par. III, 11; Targ. Y. Num. XIX, 9; a. fr.

חַיֵּל, *Pa*. חַיֵּיל, חַיֵּל (denom. of חֵילָא) 1) *to strengthen*. Targ. Job IV, 4. Ib. XVI, 5 (incorr. ed. אאח׳); a. e.—2) *to serve*. Targ. Num. IV, 23; a. e.

Ithpa. אִתְחַיֵּיל 1) *to be strengthened*. Targ. Job VI, 16; a. fr.—2) *to move into war, to gather together*. Targ. Num. XXXI, 7. Targ. Job X, 17 (some ed. מתיירל׳, corr. acc.).

חֵיל II, חֵילָא I (v. חַיִל) 1) (adj.) *strong*. Targ. Job VIII, 2 Ms. (ed. רַבָּא). Keth. 62ᵃ דחיל מר כולי האי Ar. ed. Koh. (Var. דחֵילָא דמר; ed. דהכי) that you are so strong (that such is your strength).—2) (noun) *strength*. Targ. Job XX, 11 (ed. Lag. חֵיוּל׳; some ed. חֲיַיל׳). Targ. Prov. V, 10; a. fr.—Keth. 62ᵃ, v. supra. Y. B. Mets. IV, beg. 9[c] עד דרוח חֵילָךְ עלך while thou wast yet in thy strength (of manhood). Y. Yeb. IV, 6[b] לית בְּחֵילִי I cannot do it. B. Mets. 84[a] חילך לאורייתא give thy physical strength to the study of the Law; a. fr.—Trnsf. *logical support, evidence, argument.* Y. Pes. V, 32[a] top נסיב חֵילֵיה מן וכ׳ borrowed his argument from &c. Y. Maasr. I, 49[b] top; a. e.—3) *army, host; service.* Targ. Num. I, 3; a. fr.—Targ. Ps. LXVIII, 12 Ms. (ed. חֵילְוַת).—*Pl.* חֵילַיָּא, constr. חֵילֵי; חֵילְוָתָא, constr. חֵילְוַת. Targ. Ex. XII, 41. Targ. I Kings XXII, 19; a. fr.—Targ. Ps. XXXIII, 16; a. fr. Targ. II Esth. I, 4 ed. Amst. חֲלְוָתָא. Targ. Ps. XLIV, 10 ed. Lag. חֵילְוָתָנָא (oth. ed. חֵילָוָנָא, חַלְוָנָא).—Ḥull. 60[a] נפישן חֵילְוָותֵיה (not נפישי) his troops are too numerous.

חֵילָא II m. *valley*, v. חֵילְתָא.

חֵילָא III m. *vinegar*, v. חֲלָא III.

חֵילָה f.=חוֹלָה II, *dance, song; rejoicing.* Midr. Till. to Ps. XLVIII, 14 ד״א לח׳ לשירה another interpretation (v. חֵייל), *l'helah* (Ps. l. c.) means, to song; עתיד הקב״ה לעשות ח׳ וכ׳, v. חוֹלָה II.—Deut. R. s. 1 (ref. to התחולל Ps. XXXVII, 7) when afflictions befall thee, קבל אותן בח׳ receive them with rejoicing; (Yalk. Ps. 729 כחוֹלְלִים like dancers).

חֵילְוָא, v. חֵיל II.

חִילוּזָא, v. חִלּוּז.

חִלּ׳, חִילּוּי m. (חָלָה, *Pi.*) *sweetening, softening;* trnsf. *entreaty, ḥilluy*, one of the expressions for prayer (v. זְעָקָה). Ex. R. s. 43 (ref. to ויחל, Ex. XXXII, 11) לשון ח׳ it means *sweetening.*—Yalk. Deut. 811; Yalk. Sam. 157; (Sifré Deut. s. 26 חילול, corr. acc.).

חִלּ׳, חִילּוּל m. (חָלַל) 1) *desecration, defamation.* Y. Shebu. VI, end, 37[b] ח׳ שבועה the desecration committed by an unnecessary oath. Sabb. 33[a], a. fr. ח׳ שבת desecration of the Sabbath; ח׳ השם defamation of the Name of the Lord, *disgracing the Jewish religion.* Yoma 86[a] ה״ד ח׳ השם what act, for instance, would be a profanation &c.?—Kidd. 40[a] אין מקיפין בח׳ וכ׳, v. נָקַף I, II. Ber. 19[b]; a. fr.—2) *redemption of sacred objects, secularization.* Ib. 35[a] טעון ח׳ requires redemption. Y. Naz. II, beg. 51[d] משמשין לשון ח׳ mean redemption; a. fr.—*Pl.* חִילּוּלִים, חִלּ׳. Y. Peah VII, 20[b] bot. (interpret. הלולים, Lev. XIX, 24), v. ח״א.—3) *the loss of priestly status, becoming a ḥalal* (v. חָלָל II). Y. Ter. VII, 44[d] bot. את שחִילּוּלָהּ וכ׳ whose loss of priesthood was caused by &c.—*Pl.* חִילּוּלִין, חִלּ׳. Keth. 29[b] ח׳ הוא עושה he causes loss of priesthood (to his offspring). Snh. 50[b] בחִילּוּלֵי שבוגות וכ׳ the text speaks of desecration effected through illicit intercourse (not of Sabbath breaking).—[Sifré Deut. s. 26, v. preced. w.]

חִילוֹנַאי, חִילוֹנָאָה, חִילוֹנַי m. (חוֹל; v. חוֹל III) *outsider, stranger, non-priest, non-Israelite.* Targ. Is. XXIV, 2. Targ. Ex. XXIX, 33 (O. ed. Amst. ...נָאָה, incorr.); a. fr.—*Pl.* חִילוֹנָאֵי. Targ. Y. Deut. XXIII, 3 (not חול׳).—*Fem.* חִילוֹנֵיתָא. Targ. Ps. CXXXVII, 4 ארעא ח׳ unholy land.—Targ. Prov. II, 16 (Ms. חִילוֹנֵייְתָא).

חִלּ׳, חִילוֹנִי h. same. Lev. R. s. 24.

חִילוֹנִיתָא, חִילוֹנְיְיתָא, v. חִילוֹנָאָה.

חִלּ׳, חִילּוּף m. (חָלַף) 1) *exchange, relief.*—*Pl.* חִילּוּפִים, חִילּוּפִין *those who relieve.* Ber. III, 1 the carriers וחִילּוּפֵיהֶן וחִילּוּפֵי וכ׳ and those designated to relieve them, and those who are to relieve the relief.—Gen. R. s. 91 יש לחם ח׳ can be replaced; (Y. Ber. II, 5[c] חֲלִיפִין). Num. R. s. 10 (ref. to חלוף, Prov. XXXI, 8) שהן חִלּוּפֵי אביהם for they take the place of their father; a. fr.—2) *the contrary, reverse.* Ab. Zar. 46[b] או ח׳ is it not rather the reverse?; (Y. Taan. III, 67[a] או חֲלֶף); Y. Ab. Zar. V, 45[b] top; a. fr.—ח׳ הדברים the things are just the reverse. Ab. Zar. 51[b]. Y. Ter. II, 41[c] bot.; a. fr.—*Pl.* as ab. Y. Peah I, 16[b] top אבל בגוים ח׳ but as regards gentiles, the opposite takes place.

חִלּ׳, חִילּוּפָא ch. same, 1) *opposite, reverse.* Targ. Y. Deut. XI, 26; a. e.—Ab. Zar. 28[b], sq. וח׳ סכנתא and to do the reverse is dangerous.—*Pl.* חִילּוּפִין. Y. Yoma III, 40[d] top לא מסתברא אלא ח׳ the reverse stands to reason; Y. Shebu. I, 33[b] bot. דאילא ח׳ (corr. acc.).—Y. Gitt. IV, 45[d] bot. לא מסתברא ח׳ does not the reverse stand to reason?—2) *exchange, substitute.* Targ. O. Lev. XXVII, 10.—*Pl.* constr. חִילּוּפֵי. Targ. Y. Num. XVIII, 31 in exchange of; a. e.—3) (pl.) *change* from life to death. Targ. Job XIV, 14.—4) (pl.) *crisis, decision.* Y. Sot. I, 17[b] bot. things were coming לידי ח׳ to a crisis (either David or Absalom must be king); Num. R. s. 9.

חִילּוּץ, v. חִלּוּץ.

חִלּ׳, חִילּוּק m. (חָלַק) 1) *distribution.* Keth. II, 1 ח׳ קליות וכ׳ testifying to the distribution of roasted ears (at the wedding) is an evidence (of the bride having been a virgin). Tosef. ib. III, 1 ח׳ גרנות taking a share at the distribution of priest's gifts of the threshing floor; a. fr.—2) *division, separation, specification.* Y. Sabb. VII, end, 9[c] bot. יצא . . . לח׳ it was specified, after being implicitly intimated, for division of the general law, i. e. that each of the implied acts is punishable for itself. Bab. ib. 70[a] ח׳ מלאכות the separate treatment of each labor as a transgression of the Sabbath law. Macc. 21[b]; a. fr. [חלוקי כפרה, v. חָלַק.]

חֵילְוָתָא, v. חֵיל II.

חִילְזוֹן, חִילְזוֹנָא, v. sub חלז.

חִילְחוּל, v. חַלְחוּל.

חֵילִיא, Y. Ab. Zar. II, 41[a] bot., read: חֵיוְיָא.

חִילִיז, v. חִלִּיז.

חִילְמָא, v. חֶלְמָא.

חִילְמִית, v. חַלְמִית.

חֵילֶף, חֲלַף m. (חלף) *a species of rush* (so named from its sharp edges, v. Fl. to Levy Targ. Dict. I, 425[1], a. Sm. Ant. s. v. Schoenus). Tosef. Succ. I, 10 של קנים ושל ח׳ (a matting) of reeds or rushes; Succ. 20[a] Ar. (ed.

חִילת, Ms. M. חוּלית). Sot. 49[b] Ar. (ed. חילת).—Kel. XVII, 17. —[*Pl.* חִילְפִין, v. חֲלִיפִין a. חֲלֵה.]

חִילְפָא I, חִלְ׳ ch. same. Gitt. 68[b] bot.—*Pl.* חִילְפֵי, חִלְ׳. Hull. 62[b], v. בְּרָזָא. — ח׳ דִּימָא *sea-rush, Schoenanth, Juncus odoratus* (v. Löw Pfl., p. 168; Sm. Ant. s. v. Schoenus), *a spice.* Gitt. l. c. חילפא וח׳ דימא rush and sea-rush. Ber. 43[b].—[Targ. Y. Num. XXI, 12 only חילפי, v. חִלָּף.]

חִילְפָא II m. (חלף) a species of *willow* with serried leaves (v. preced.; Fl. to Levy Targ. Dict. I, 425[1] "so called from its fast growth"). Succ. 34[a] משכחת לה בח׳ גילא Ms. M. a. Rashi (ed. פי תניא האי בח׳ וכ׳) ('a willow the leaves of which are not serried like the teeth of a saw, but like those of a sickle') refers to a willow with rounded leaves.—[Ib. ח׳ ערבתא Rashi, v. חִלְפְתָא.]—*Pl.* חִילְפֵי. Sabb. 152[a] סבותא כלילא דח׳ old age is a crown of willow rods (heavy to wear). Ib. 77[b]. Snh. 44[a], v. אָסָא III.

חִילְפָא III m., pl. **חִילְפֵי**=h. חֲלִיפִין, *shoots rising out of a trunk.* Hull. 110[a] קדחו בהו ח׳ shoots had made their way through them (proving that the peats of grapes deposited there had been abandoned by its owner).

חִילְפוֹת, v. חֲלֵה.

(חִלְפַי) חִילְפַיי, חִילְפַי pr. n. m. *Hilfay* (Graecised Ἀλφαῖος, P. Sm. 1292), 1) an Amora (in Babli אִילְפָא, אִילְפַי). Y. Maasr. II, 49[d] bot. Y. Keth. VI, end, 31[a]; a. e.—2) H., grandson of R. Abbahu. Y. Bicc. II, 64[d] top.

חִילְפִין, v. חֲלִיפִין.

חִילֵק I, חֵלֶק m. *helek*, name of a small fish preserved in brine, *helek-brine.* [Latin: alec, alex, halec, allec, the variations indicating foreign origin; cmp. חִילְקָא II.] Ab. Zar. II, 6 (Mish. Nap. חלק). Ib. 39[a], expl. סוּלְתָּנִית. Ib. 34[b] ח׳ אומן *helek*-brine prepared by a professional man.

חִילֵק II m. (חָלַק) *a tree too smooth for climbing, young or clipped tree. Pl.* constr. חִילְקֵי. Peah IV, 1 ח׳ אגוזים Y. ed. (Bab. ed. a. Mish. חֲלִיקֵי) smooth nut trees.

חִילָּק, חִלָּק *Hillak*, a fictitious name, v. בִּילָּק.

חִילְקָא I *field*, v. חַלְקָא.

חִילְקָא, II, חִילְקָה f. (חָלַק; cmp. Lat. alica, halica, a. חֵילֶק I) *split grain, grist, spelt used for halica* (v. Sm. Ant. s. v. Alica). Makhsh. VI, 2 חילקה Mish. (Talm. ed. חֲלִיקָה). Y. Sabb. I, 3[c] bot. M. Kat. 13[b] ח׳ הדא לתרתי it is called *helka* when each grain is broken in two parts; Ber. 37[a] Ms. ח׳ דמתברי באסיתא תרתי תרתי *hilka* is wheat pounded &c.—M. Kat. l. c. (another opin.) ח׳ כונתא h. is spelt. Ib. it is called *helka* (*smooth*), דשקיל חלקייהו Ar. (ed. דשקל) because its husks have been taken off (cmp. חִילֵק II); v. חִלְקָא.

חִילֵשׁ m. constr. (v. חָלַשׁ) (*something rounded, hollow*, v. P. Sm. 1295 חלשא *specillum*) *reed.* Targ. Zech. XI, 13 ח׳ כתבא (ed. Lag. חלש, ed. Ven. חִילַשׁ) writing reed.

חִילַת I f. (חלל; cmp. preced.) name of a *reed*, v. חִילֵשׁ.

חִילַת II pr. n. pl. *Helath.* Targ. Ez. XXVII, 18 (h. text חֶלְבּוֹן, v. Schr. KAT[2] p. 425, sq.); cmp. חִילְתִּיה a. חֶלְבְּנָה.—B. Bath. 74[b] ימה של ח׳ (Ms. M. שחלר׳); Yalk. Ps. 697; (Y. Kil. IX, end, 32[c] ימא דחילתא).]

חֵילָא, חִילְתָא, חִילְתָא f., **חֵילָא** m. (חלל) *hollow, glen, valley.* Targ. Deut. III, 29. Targ. Is. XXVIII, 1; a. e.— *Pl.* (m.) חִילַיָּא. Ib. XL, 4; a. e.—[B. Bath. 74[b], v. חוּלְתָא.]

חִילְתִּית, חִלְתִּ׳ f. (v. חִילַת II) *assa foetida*, an umbelliferous plant used, as a resin or in leaves, for a spice and for medicinal purposes. Ukts. III, 5. Sabb. XX, 3 (140[a]) אין שורין את הח׳ וכ׳ (Mish. ed. חִילְתִּית) you must not dissolve the resin of asa-foetida in warm water (on the Sabbath). Y. ib. XX, 17[c] bot. מי ח׳ a solution of &c. Ib. ח׳ עצמה וכ׳ *asaf.* itself is used in food for healthy persons. Hull. 58[b] (distinction between the medicinal properties of the gum and those of the leaves). Ab. Zar. II, 6 קורט של ח׳ tears of &c. (Ar. עלה וכ׳ leaves). Sifré Deut. s. 107; a. fr.

חִילְתִּיתָא, חִלְ׳ ch. same. Ab. Zar. 39[a]. Y. Shebi. VII, 37[c] top חלתותא (corr. acc.).

חִימָה, v. חֵמָה.

חִימּוּד m. (חָמַד) *desire, lust.* Nidd. 20[b] דם ח׳ discharge of blood owing to sexual appetite.

חִימּוּם m. (חָמַם) 1) *warming, sitting in the sun.* Gen. R. s. 48 ח׳ יפה וכ׳ basking in the sunshine is good for a wound; Yalk. ib. 82 החמין (corr. acc.).—2) *heated state, excitement.* M. Kat. 24[a] בשעת ח׳ at the moment of excitement (immediately after a death in the family). Yoma 18[a] לידי ח׳ to sexual excitement (pollution).—3) *a spice*, v. חָמָם.

חִימּוּס m. (חָמַס) *violence, oppression.* Gen. R. s. 31, beg. ח׳ ממון oppression in money affairs, ח׳ דברים violence in speech (blasphemous language).

חִימּוּעַ m. ch. (חמ״ע)=next w. Pes. 39[b], sq. Ms. M. (ed. חִימּוּץ).

חִימּוּץ, חִמּ׳ m. (חָמֵץ I) *becoming sour, fermentation, leavening.* Pes. 39[b] שאינן באין לידי ח׳ which will not ferment (so as to become חָמֵץ). Ib., sq. (in Chald. diction) ואתי לידי ח׳ and may ferment. Bets 7[b] שחימוצו קשה which is a strong leavening agent. Y. Hall. I, beg. 57[a] אין חִימּוּצוֹ חמץ ברור the fermentation which it produces is not real leavening. Nidd. 63[a] כמה הִמּוּצָן how long must urin stand to be considered as fermenting?—*Pl.* חִימּוּצִין *salads*, v. חוּמְצָן.

חִימּוּצָא, חִמּ׳ m. (חמץ, v. Ges. H. Dict.[10] s. v. חמץ) *shame.* Targ. Prov. XVII, 21 (h. text תוגה).

חִימּוּצִיתָא, חִימּוּצִיאָתָא, v. next w.

חִימּוּצְתָא f. pl. (חמץ, v. Ges. H. Dict.[10] s. v. חמץ; cmp. Is. LXIII, 1) *scarlet-colored garments*, in gen. ח׳ רוֹמָיָתָא dyed Roman garments, contrad. to white (cmp.

טורְדִיקָא a. אולָרִין). M. Kat. 23ª ח׳ ר׳ סומקתא חדתי ed. Ms. M. חימוציאתא דדומי, Ar. חמיצתא, Mus. חמיצתא) Roman dyed garments, red and new.

חימות, Nidd. 51ᵇ, v. חֲמָם.

חימסא, Gen. R. s. 45 some ed., v. חֲמַס.

חִימְצָא (חוּמְצָא) m. 1) a species of *small peas* (Cicer Arietanus).—*Pl.* חִימְצֵי. Yeb. 63ª (Ar. חוּ׳). Hull. 52ᵇ (some ed. חֻמְצֵי).—2) v. חִימְצָא.

חֵימָרָא, חֵימְ׳, חֵמָ׳ m. ch.=h. חֵמָר, *asphalt* (from its dark color, Ges. H. Dict.[10] s. v.), used as *cement*. Targ. O. Gen. XI, 3. Targ. Ex. II, 3.—Targ. II Esth. III, 3 ורידתא דגלגלוי כחימָרָא ed. Lag. (oth. ed. ורידתא לגלוי בחוי, read: דִגְלָוי כח׳) and the odor of its billows is like that of asphalt.

חֵימְתָא (חוּ׳) f. ch.=h. חֵמָה, *anger, passion*. Targ. Prov. XXVII, 4. Ib. XXIX, 11 (some ed. חוּ׳); a. e.

חימתא *mother-in-law*, v. חֲמָתָא.

חִינָא, חֵין, v. חֵן, חִנָא.

חֵינָא, חִיָינָא, v. חֲנָא.

חִינְגָא, חִנְ׳ m. (חגג, with נ inserted) 1) *circle; dancing, chorus, feast*.—*Pl.* חִינְגֵי, חִינְגִין, חִינְגַיָא, חִנְ׳. Targ. Jud. IX, 27 (vintage feast).—Gitt. 57ª, v. הִילּוּלָא.—2) *dancing place* in the vineyards (v. מָחוֹל). Targ. Lam. I, 4 (cmp. Taan. IV, 8).—*Pl.* as ab. Targ. Jud. XXI, 21; 23. Targ. I Sam. XVIII, 6.—3) *ḥinga*, name of a musical instrument (h. מָחוֹל a. חָלִיל). Pes. 111ᵇ תלו ח׳ בגוריה they had a *ḥ*. suspended in the hollow of the tree.—*Pl.* as ab. Targ. I Kings I, 40. Targ. Ps. V, 1 (h. text נחילות). Ib. CL, 4; a. fr.—4) *fair*, esp. *cattle market*. Sabb. 54ᵇ; Bets. 33ª כמאן דאזיל לח׳ like one going with his beast to market.

חִינְגִיתָא, חִנְ׳ f. (preced.) *a musical instrument*. Targ. Ps. IV, 1 (ed. Lag. נְגִינָתָא, Ms. חִינְגְנָתָא, v. next w.).

חִינְגְנָא m., pl. חִינְגְנַיָּא, חִנְ׳ same. Targ. Ps. LXXXVII, 7 (some ed. חנגריא, h. text חללים).—*Fem. pl.* חִינְגְנָתָא, v. preced.

חִינּוּגָא m. (חָגַג, a denom. of חִינְגָא) *festivity*. Targ. Lam. V, 15.—*Pl.* חִינּוּגִין. Ib. I, 4.

חִינּוּךְ, חִנּ׳ m. (חָנַךְ) 1) *finishing*. Y. M. Kat. I, 80ᵈ top איזהו ח׳ קברים what finishing of tombs (is meant in the Mishn. ib. 6)?—2) *inauguration*. Men 78ª חִינּוּכוֹ his inauguration as a common priest, contrad. to משיחתו his anointment as highpriest. Y. Shek. VI, 50ᵈ top חִינּוּכוֹ his (the highpriest's) inauguration.—3) *gradual introduction of children into religious practice, training*. Yoma 82ª אי זה ח׳ wherein does the child's training (to fast on the Day of Atonement) consist?—Ib. ומי קרי לח׳ השלמה is fasting the entire day called initiation?—Naz. 29ª ח׳ מדרבנן the training of minors for religious practices is a rabbinically ordained duty; a. e.

חִינּוּכָא, חִנּ׳ ch. same.—*Pl.* חִינּוּכֵי, חִנּ׳. Yoma 82ª תרי ח׳ הוו there are two modes of initiation (gradual training to fasting by hours, and making the child fast a whole day before he has reached religious maturity).

חִינּוּן, חִנּ׳ m. (חָנַן) *prayer for grace*, *ḥinnun*, one of the expressions for prayer, v. זְעָקָה. Sifré Deut. s. 26 (ref. to Deut. III, 23); (Deut. R. s. 2 תחנונים; Yalk. Sam. 157; Yalk. Deut. 811 תחנה).

חינוניתא, Sot. 49ª, v. הַהִנּוּנִיתָא. [Ar. s. v. חן: *Hinnunitha*, pr. n. pl.]

חִינְטַיָא, חִינְטִין, חִינְטָא, v. sub חִנְ׳.

חִינְכֵי m. pl. ch.=h. חֲנִיכַיִם, *jaws*. Gitt. 69ª לח׳ for pains of the jaws. B. Kam. 35ª כריבין ליה חינְכֵיה Ms. H. (ed. כריבין) had pains in his jaws.

חִינְנָה, חִינְנָא pr. n. m. *Hin'na*, name of several Amoraim. [Vers. frequ. vary with חנינא, חגא). Pes. 75ª רב ח׳ סבא (Ms. M. חגא).—Ib. Ḥ. bar Idi (Ms. M. חנינא). Y. Maas. Sh. II, beg. 53ᵇ; (Y. Yoma VIII, 45ª top חנניה); a. fr. V. Fr. M'bo, p. 84ª, sq.

חֵינָנָא, v. חֲנָ͏א.

חִיס, חֲיָסָא, חֲיָ׳ m. ch.=h. חַיִּים II, *protection, mercy*. Targ. Ex. XII, 27 (ed. Amst. חַיִּס, חֲיָיסָא). Targ. Jer. IV, 4. Targ. Is. I, 31; a. e. [Targ. Prov. III, 25, v. חֵיפָא I.]

חִיסְדָא, חִיסְדַאי, חִיסְדַיי, v. sub חִסְ׳.

חִיסּוּד m. (חָסַד II) *shame, rebuke; revilement*.—*Pl.* חִיסּוּדִים. Pesik. Shek., p. 12ᵇ (ref. to וחסד וכ׳, Prov. XIV, 34) ח׳ וכ׳ . . . מקבלין the Israelites must bear reproaches from the nations, when they sin.

חִיסּוּדָא, חִסּ׳ ch. same. Targ. O. Gen. XXXIV, 14 (ed. Berl. חִיסּוּדָא). Targ. Prov. XIV, 31; a. fr. (interch. in ed. with חִסְדָּא, חִסְדָּ׳).—*Pl.* חִיסּוּדִין, חִסּ׳. Targ. Is. XXXVII, 3; a. e.

חִיסּוּלָא, חִסּ׳ m. (חָסַל) *finished work, perfection*. —*Pl.* חִיסּוּלִין, חִסּ׳. Targ. Ps. CIII, 2 חִיסּוּלוֹי His perfect deeds (v. Ber. 10ª, h. text גמוליו).

חִיסּוּם I *muzzle*, v. חֲסוּם.

חִיסּוּם, חִסּ׳ II m. (חָסַם II) [*finish, polish*,] 1) *the steel-coating of cutting tools, steel-edge* (cmp. אִסְטָמָא). Kel. XIII, 4 נטל חִיסּוּמָן if their steel-edge is worn off.—2) *varnish, coating, uppermost layer*. Y. Ber. IX, 14ª אין הארץ ... לפי חִיסּוּמָהּ the earth drinks (absorbs the rain) only as far as its upper layer (crust) goes; Y. Taan. I, 64ᵇ; Gen. R. s. 13, end; a. e.—Tosef. Ukts. II, 4 (T'bul Yom) ח׳ העליון (ed. Zuck. סל) the uppermost layer of the bone.

חִיסּוּר, חִסּ׳ m. (חָסֵר) *lack, want*. Cant. R. to IV, 11 אם חסרה ח׳ וכ׳ if she is suffering from the absence of one of them.

חִיסְחוּן m. (חסח, reduplic. of חוס), v. next w.

חִיסָּכוֹן, חִסָּ׳ m. (חָסַךְ) *sparing, regard to expense* in religious laws. Men. 86[b] (expl. התורה חסה וכ׳, v. חוס); ib. 76[b] חיסחון (Ms. Vatic. חיסכ׳); a. e.

חִיסְנָא, v. חִסְנָא.

חִיסָּרוֹן, v. חֶסְרוֹן.

חִיפָּא I m. (חוּף I, cmp. חוּפְיָא) [*sweep,*] *impetuous attack*. Targ. Prov. XXVII, 4 (h. text שֶׁטֶף). Ib. III, 25 ed. Lag. (ed. חיסא, corr. acc.; h. text שֹׁאָת).

חִיפָּא II, pr. n. pl., v. חֵיפָה I.

חִיפָּא m. (חפף I; cmp. b. h. חֹף) *border* in webs. Sabb. 96[b] מטו הדדי בח׳ Ms. M. (Ar. חִיפָּה, חָפָּה, ed. חֶפֶת, v. Rabb. D. S. a. l. note) the weavers, if placed near each other, would have touched one another on making the border.

חִיפָּה f. h., v. preced. a. חֶפֶת.

חֵיפָה I, **חֵיפָא**, **בֵּית ח׳** pr. n. pl. *Haifā, Beth-Ḥaifā,* a harbor of the Mediterranean Sea, south of Ptolemais. Sabb. 26[a]. Y. Erub. II, 20[a] top (חיפא). Koh. R. to XII, 7 חיפס (corr. acc.). Meg. 24[b] בית ח׳ (Ms. M. only ח׳).—Denom. חֵיפָנִי an inhabitant of H (noted for indiscriminate pronunciation of א a. ע). Ib.—*Pl.* חֵיפָנִין. Y. Ber. II, 4[d] bot., .. ח״א.—V. חֶפָנִי.

חִיפָּה II (or חִיפָּה) f. (חוּף, חפף I, חפה) *ḥefa* (or *ḥippa*) *a skin which has been salted*, but has not gone through the consecutive stages of tanning with flour and gall-nut. Sabb. 79[a]; Gitt. 22[a]. Sifra Sh'mini, Sh'ratsim, ch. VII, Par. 6 עור האִיפָּה.

חֵיפָה III pr. n. m. *Ḥefa* (=עֵיפָא). Y. Ned. II, 37[b] bot.; Y. Shebu. III, 34[d] top, (Bab. ib. 28[b] עֵיפָא, Ms. F. איפה). Y. R. Hash. I, 56[b] top.

חִיפּוּי, v. חִפּוּי.

חִיפּוּפֵי m. pl. (חפף I; cmp. חִיפָּא) *border-stones, pegs* or *stakes along the road*, to prevent vehicles from trespassing on private property. [Rashi: from חפף II, pegs against which vehicles *rub*.] Sabb. 6[a].

חִיפּוּפִין m. pl. h., constr. חִיפּוּפֵי same. Keth. 24[b].

חִיפּוּפִיתָא f. (חפף II) *scabs, scurf*, arising from uncleanness. Yalk. Num. 787 (fr. Ned. 81[a], where ed. have עִירְבּוּבִיתָא, Ar. חרפופיתא. v. Koh. Ar. Compl. s. v. חרף). V. חֲפָפִית.

חִיפּוּשׂ m. (חָפַשׂ) *search, use of the root* חפש. Pes. 7[b] we learn מציאה מח׳ the meaning of מצא (Ex. XII, 19) from the expression חפש (connected with מצא, Gen. XLIV, 12), i. e. you must search after leavened bread before Passover, &c.

חִיפּוּשָׁא (אִיפּוּשָׁא) m. [*mud-fish,*] name of an unclean fish. Ab. Zar. 39[a] דהיה דמי לח׳ (Ms. לא׳). V. חֲפִיתָא.

חִפּוּשִׁית, חִיפּוּשִׁית f. (חָפַשׂ) *scarabee, beetle*. Sifra Sh'mini, Sh'ratsim, Par. 10, ch. XII; Hull. 67[b].—Par. IX, 2 (doubtful; perh. *scorpion*, v. next w.).

חִפּ׳, חִיפּוּשִׁיתָא ch. same. Cant. R. to I, 1 (prov.) מה ילדת ח׳ וכ׳ what does the beetle beget? Insects worse than itself; (Yalk. Sam. 134 חפושית, expl. *scorpion*).—Ab. Zar. 28[b] ח׳ גמלניתא a large-sized beetle (Rashi: '*hanneton*', *cockchafer*).

חִיפָּזוֹן, v. חִפָּזוֹן.

חִיפְנִי, חִיפס, v. חֵיפָה I.

חִיפְצָא, v. חִפְצָא.

חֵיפְתָא, v. חֶפְתָא.

חַיִץ, v. חַץ.

חִיצָא or **חִיצִי** f. (חוּץ I) *partition, screen*.—*Pl.* חִיצָאוֹת. Gen. R. s. 28 מפקיע בח׳ breaking into the screens (of the bridal chamber); Yalk. ib. 47 בַּחִיצָאוֹת.

חִיצָה I (or חוּצָה) f. (חוּץ II, cmp. חָלִילָה) *a strange act, unnatural deed*. Pesik. R. s. 40 (play on חצה, Is. XXXIII, 7) חי׳ חיא בידך מכושרני read *ḥitsah*, the angels cried חי׳ כתב (read: מיכוס יתיה) it is unnatural on thy part to have him (Isaac) slaughtered; Gen. R. s. 56 ח׳ היא בְּרִיָּה וכ׳ it is an outrage! A creature to kill his own son!; Yalk. Is. 303 חו׳ היא לך חו׳ היא לאבא למיכס ית בריה; Lam. R. to I, 2 חי׳ היא גביה וכ׳ it is unnatural for him (Abraham) &c., cmp. בְּרִיָּה.

חִיצָה II (חוּץ, cmp. חַיִץ) *partition*, only in חִיצַת קנים *single reeds planted around a well*. Erub. 15[a]; 19[b]; Succ. 24[b] מחיצת; Tosef. Erub. II, 4 (Var. מחיצת); (Y. ib. II, 20[a] ארשות).—Tosef. Shebi. III, 19 חישת ed. Zuck. (Var. חִיצוֹת pl.). V. חִישָׁה.

חִיצּוּי m. (חָצָה) *dividing off*, esp. dividing the altar into two compartments by means of a net (Ex. XXVII, 5). Zeb. 119[b] יש ח׳ division is required.

חִיצוֹן m. (b. h.; חוּץ I) *outer, external*. Zeb. V, 1 מזבח הח׳ the outer altar (in the Temple court); a. fr.—Nidd. V, 1 בית הח׳ *vagina*.—*Fem.* חִיצוֹנָה. Y. Yeb. I, 3[a], v. חוּצָה II.—Num. R. s. 18 משנה הח׳=בְּרַיְיתָא.—*Pl.* חִיצוֹנוֹת. Sabb. 31[b] מפתחות הח׳ the outside keys (of the treasury); Yalk. Deut. 855; Yalk. Is. 302; En Yakob Sabb. l. c. (מפתחות) החיצוניות the keys to the outer room.

חִיצוֹנִי m. (preced.) *strange; separatist; heretical*.—*Pl.* חִיצוֹנִים. Meg. IV, 8 (24[b]) דרך הח׳ the manner of the separatists (who follow their own interpretations of the Law, irrespective of public usages). Snh. X, 1 (90[a]) ספרים הח׳ profane books, expl. Y. ib. 28[a] top; Bab. ib. 100[b].—*Fem.* חִיצוֹנִית, v. preced.

חִיצְרָא, v. חַצְרָא.

חֵיק m. (b. h.; חוק) 1) *lap, bosom, embrace*. M. Kat. 24[a] a child יוצא בח׳ is carried out in one's arms (without a coffin); Kidd. 80[b]; Treat. S'maḥ. III, 2.—Y. M. Kat. III, beg. 81[c] הניח ח׳ אמו וכ׳ left his mother's lap (Palestine). Tosef. Yeb. IX, 4 מח׳ בעלה directly from the embrace of her husband; a. e.—2) *receptacle, cavity, bottom*. Men. 97[b]; Erub. 4[a] (ref. to Ez. XLIII, 17), v. יסוד.

חִיקָא ch. same. Targ. II Sam. XII, 3, v. חֵנָא.

חִיקוֹק pr. n. pl. (v. Josh. XIX, 34; I Chr. VI, 60) *Hikok* (*Ḥukok*), in Northern Palestine. Y. Shebi. IX, beg. 38[c].—Denom.: חִיקוֹקָאָה, חִיקוֹקָיָא (חֲקוֹקָאָה, חֲקוֹקָא, חֲקוֹקָה) m. *of Ḥ.* Y. Pes. I, 27[c] bot. יוחנן חי׳; Bab. ib. 3[b] חק׳ (v. Rabb. D. S. a. l. note); a. e.

חִירָא, Targ. Ps. LVII, 5, some ed., v. חֲרִי.

חִירְגָא, v. חִרְגָא.

חִירָה f., pl. **חִירוֹת** (חור) *cavernous rocks* resembling human figures. Mekh. B'shall. s. 1 (ref. to *Pi-Haḥiroth*, Ex. XIV, 2) מה ח׳ וכ׳ what was the nature of these rocks? —They were not slanting but abrupt &c. Ib. הח׳ מצד וכ׳ the rocks were on one side, and Migdol &c. Ib. אין ח׳ אלא מקום חֵירוּתָן וכ׳ *ḥiroth* means the place of Israel's liberty (licentiousness); Yalk. Ex. 230; Num. R. s. 20.

חֵירוּ, v. חֵירוּתָא.

חֵירוּם m. (חָרַם) *exclusion, disassociation*, esp. *interdiction of travel* between two countries at war with each other. B. Bath. 38[a] בשעת ח׳ at a time when commercial intercourse was cut off. Ib.[b] יהודה . . . ח׳ דמו Judaea and Galilee are generally to be considered as if in a state of interdiction (possession in one country is no valid claim when the owner lived in the other); Y. ib. III, 14[a] top.

חֵירוּף, חירוּף m. (חָרַף) *blasphemy*.—*Pl.* חֵר׳, חֵירוּפִין. Ex. R. s. 41, beg. Lev. R. s. 7; a. fr.

חֵירוּפָא, חֵר׳, ch., pl. **חֵירוּפִין, חֵר׳** same. Targ. Y. Num. XVI, 27.

חֵירוּת, חֵרוּת, חרוּת f. (חור II) *freedom, liberty, libertinism; leisure*. Mekh. B'shall. s. 1, v. חִירָה. Gitt. 42[a] יצא לח׳ becomes free (ib. 8[b], a. fr. בן חורין). Erub. 54[a] (play on חָרוּת, Ex. XXXII, 16) א״ת חרות אלא חר׳ read not *ḥaruth* (engraven) but *ḥeruth* (liberty) on the tablets (you are free, if you observe the law); Ex. R. s. 32, beg. ח׳ מן המלכיות liberation from political oppression, ח׳ ממלאך המות liberation from the angel of death (pestilence); a. fr.

חֵירוּ, חֵירוּתָא, חֵירוּת ch. same. Targ. Lev. XXV, 10. Targ. Is. LXI, 1; a. e.

חִירְזָא, חִרְזָא m. (חָרַז) *a thorny shrub* used for hedges. B. Mets. 103[b] Ar. Var., v. חִיזְרָא I.

חִירְחוּר m., pl. **חִירְחוּרִים** (חִרְחֵר) *heated contest*. Gitt. 57[b] (ref. to Job V, 2) בְּחִירְחוּרֵי לשון תחבא in the contests of the tongue (prayer) thou shalt seek refuge (when persecuted).

חִירְיָא, בַּר ח׳, v. חַדְיָא.

***חִירָיָה** pr. n. pl. *Ḥirayah*, in Zebulun. Y. Meg. I, 70[a] bot. (rendition of Yidălah, Josh. XIX, 15; corresp. to El-Hariṭiye, on Fischer-Guthe's Neue Handkarte v. Palaest.).

חִירְיָנָא, v. חִרְיָנָא.

חִירְמָא, v. חִרְמָא.

חִירָנִית, v. אירונית.

חִירְפָא m. (חרף) *sharp-edged knife, slaughtering knife*.—*Pl.* חִירְפֵי. Targ. Prov. XXX, 14 (ed. Lag. a. oth. חָרִיפֵי; h. text מאכלות).

חִירְקָא, v. חִרְקָא.

חִירָר m. (חרר) *freedom, emancipation*. Targ. Y. Deut. XV, 17 (cmp. שִׁיחְרוּר).

חִירְשָׁא, v. חִרְשָׁא.

חִירְתָא f. ch.=h. חִירָה.—*Pl.* חִירָתָא. Targ. Ex. XIV, 2; Targ. Num. XXXIII, 7 פומי ח׳, פום ח׳ (h. text פי החירות, v. חִירָה).

חִישׁ, v. חוש.

חִישָׁה or **חִישַׁת** f. (v. חוש 1) *thicket, inaccessible place* to be cleared by fire in order to be made arable, v. אֲגַם.—חִישַׁת (חִישַׁת) קנים *reed-thicket*. Y. Sabb. VII, 10[a] top המצית את האור בח׳ ק׳ he who sets fire to a reed-thicket; [Y. Shebi. IV, 35[b] bot. בְּאִישַׁת; Y. Ab. Zar. II, 41[d] bot. באשת, cmp. אוש a. אָשַׁשׁ].—Tosef. Shebi. III, 19, v. חִיצָה II.

חִישּׁוּב m. (חָשַׁב) *(astronomical) calculation*. Sabb. 75[a]. Snh. 10[b].

חִישׁוּתָא f.=b. h. חוּשׁ, *sense, sensation*. Targ. Job XX, 2 Ms a. Regia (ed. רְחִישְׁתָּא, a. רְגִישְׁתָּא).

חִישַׁת *thicket*, v. חִישָׁה.

חִישְׁתָּא I ch., constr. חִישַׁת, same. Targ. Mic. III, 12; Targ. Jer. XXVI, 18 (h. text בָּמוֹת).

***חִישְׁתָּא** II pr. n. *Ḥishta*, a canal in Babylonia. Pes. 40[b] ed. (Ms. M. אישתא, cmp. חִישָׁה).

חי״ת *Ḥeth*, the eighth letter of the Alphabet. Y. Peah VII, 20[b] bot., a. e., v. ה״א. Lev. R. s. 19; a. fr.—*Pl.* חֵי״תִין. Y. Ber. II, 4[d] bot. Sabb. 103[b].

חִיתָא, חַיְתָא, v. חֵירְתָא.

חִיתָה, v. חות.

חִיתּוּךְ, חִתּ׳ m. (חָתַךְ) 1) *cut, incision, articulation*. Nidd. 25[a] ח׳ ידים וכ׳ indications (in the embryo) of hands and feet. Y. Sabb. VII, 10[c] bot.—2) *(cmp. גְּזֵירָה) *sentence, (condemning) verdict*.—*Pl.* חִתּ׳, חִיתּוּכִין. Lam. R. to II, 1 (expl. תָּו, Ezek. IX, 4) ח׳ ופספס sentences and verdicts (Mus. s. v. פספין: כתיטא בפ׳ like the letter θ, for θάνατος, at voting; Yalk. Ez. 349 only פס׳: Ar. s. v. פספס: חתיכה פספסן, ed. pr. הֲתִיבָה).

חִיתּוּכָא ch. same, 1) *cut.* Hull. 47ᵇ ח׳ דאוני the incisions marking the lobes of the lung.—*Pl.* חִיתּוּכֵי. Ib. 48ᵃ ח׳ דאוני ed. (Rashi: מקום חיתוכה דאוני) the place in the neck where the lungs begin to separate.—2) *a portion cut off, segment* (חֲתִיכָה). Ib. 48ᵇ מחטא . . . בח׳ דריאה (Rashi: בחִיתּוּכָה) a needle was found in a segment of the lungs.

חִיתּוּם, חִתּ׳ m. (חָתַם) 1) *signature.* B. Bath. X, 8 לאחר ח׳ שטרות after the deeds were signed. Ib. 176ᵃ; a. fr.—2) (ברכות) ח׳ *the formula with which a prayer closes, concluding benediction* ('Blessed be thou, O Lord. who &c.'). Ber. 12ᵃ הכל הולך אחר ח׳ ב׳ Ms. M. (ed. only חוח׳) the concluding formula decides the appropriateness of a prayer. Ib. או אחר ח׳ ב׳ אזלינן Ms. M. (ed. חתימה) or do we go by the concluding phrase?—*Pl.* חִיתּוּמִין. Y. Ber. I, 3ᵈ bot. אחר חִיתּוּמֵיהֶן according to their conclusions; (ib. חוֹתְמוֹתֵיהֶן, v. חוֹתָם); Y. Taan. II, 65ᶜ bot.

חִיתּוּן m. (חָתַן) *marriage; wedding ceremony,* only in *pl.* חִיתּוּנִין, חִיתּוּנִים. Num. R. s. 12 (ref. to Cant. III, 11) ח׳ הוי וכ׳ the law-giving on Sinai was a wedding (between God and Israel), as we read (Ex. XIX, 10) &c., v. קִידּוּשִׁין; Pesik. Vayhi, p. 5ᵃ; Cant. R. to l. c. כחתנים (corr. acc.).

חִיתּוּנָא ch. same. Targ. Y. Gen. XXXIV, 9.—*Pl.* חִיתּוּנִין. Targ. Y. Deut. VI, 7; XI, 19 חִיתּוּנֵיכוֹן (ed. Amst. חיתּוּנְכוֹן *sing*).

חיתמא, Y. Snh. IV, end, 22ᶜ, read: חִיטְּתָא.

חִיתִּית, חִתִּ׳ f. (b. h.=חתחית; חָתַת) *being broken, subdued;* esp. *dread inspired by superiors, fear.* Gen. R. s. 34 (ref. to Gen. IX, 2, compared with I, 28) מורא וח׳ חזרו (not וחתות) the fear and dread (of man) were restored (after the deluge), but subjection was not. R. Hash. 17ᵃ (applying Ez. XXXII, 24 sq.) שנתנו חִיתִּיתָם וכ׳ those (leaders) who tyrannize the land of the living.—Lev. R. s. 18; Koh. R. to XII, 5 (ref. to חתחתים, ib.) [read:] חִיתִּיתָהּ של דרך וכ׳ the dread of travelling befalls him.

חֵךְ, v. חֵיךְ.

חִכָּא, v. חֵיכָא.

חכאכית, v. אַבְאָבִית a. אַבְאָבִית.

חָכָה, v. חכי.

חַכָּה f. (b. h.; חָכַךְ I; cmp. חָח) *hook, fish-hook.* Y. Pes. IV, 30ᵈ top. M. Kat. 25ᵇ נפלה ח׳ וכ׳ . . בנהל if the fish-hook is thrown into the rapid river (to catch the fish), what can the waters in the pond do (if the great die, what can common humanity expect)?—Erub. 19ᵃ מטילין לו ח׳ וכ׳ they put a hook into the convict's mouth &c.; a. e.—*Pl.* חַכִּין. Tosef. B. Kam. VIII, 17. Sifré Num. s. 44 גררום בחַכֵּי ברזל they dragged them out of the sanctuary with iron hooks (on shafts, v. בַּקְלוּסָא); Yalk. ib. 712 בקנר (corr. acc.); Sifra Sh'mini, introd. חנית של ברזל (read: חַכִּים). Tosef. B. Kam. XI, 13 שלש חכין (Var. כופין, חוטין) three fuller's hooks (for stretching clothes; v. חוב II, 2).

חִכּוּךְ, חִכּוּכָא, v. חִיכּוּ׳.

חֲכוּכָא m., constr. חֲכוּךְ (חָכַךְ) *scratching.*—ח׳ חספא scratching with a potsherd, *eruption.* Targ. Y. II Deut. XXVIII, 27, v. חִיכּוּכָא.

חָכוּר, v. חָכִיר.

חכה, חכי (b. h.), *Pi.* חִכָּה 1) (denom. of חַכָּה) *to insert a hook, to fish with the angle, to fasten.* Y. Sabb. IV, end, 7ᶜ אם לְחַכּוֹת בו if it is a *sûgar* (v. סוגר) with which to fasten a dog (by inserting the hook of a chain), opp. בשביל שלא לאכול one intended to prevent from eating (a muzzle); Y. Bets. II, end, 61ᵈ (not להכות). B. Kam. 81ᵃ וּמְחַכִּין בימה וכ׳ and that people be free to fish with the angle in the lake of Tiberias.—2) (b. h.) *to lie in wait* (v. Hos. VI, 9); *to wait for, hope, be anxious for* (with ל). Snh. 97ᵇ (fr. Hab. II, 3) חַכֵּה לו wait for it (the redemption); ib. אנו מְחַכִּין והוא אינו מְחַכֶּה we are anxious, but He is not (ref. to Is. XXX, 18). Pesik. R. s. 34; Yalk. Zeph. 567; a. e. [Yalk. Lev. 604 כחכה, v. חָקָה.]

חכי, *Pa.* חַכֵּי ch. same. Pesik. V'zoth, p. 196ᵃ (ref. to Is. XXX, 18) כחדין צײדא דמחכי וכ׳ like the hunter that waits for prey; Yalk. Deut. 950.

חָכִים I, חַכִּים, v. חָכָם.

חַכִּים II, חַכִּימָא, חֲכִים m. ch.=h. חָכָם, *wise; sage, scholar.* Targ. I Kings III, 12. Targ. Y. Lev. XIX, 32; a. fr.—Ab. Zar. 76ᵇ מאן ח׳ למיעבד וכ׳ who but R. . . . is wise enough to do that?; Pes. 76ᵃ.—Taan. 32ᵃ אידן מתקרי ח׳ who is to be called a wise man?; a. fr.—Esp. *Ḥakham,* a scholar's title, inferior to Rabbi. B. Mets. 86ᵃ top ח׳ יתקרי וכ׳ shall be called a *Ḥakham,* but not a Rabbi. Y. Taan. IV, 68ᵃ דמנייתך ח׳ that I have appointed thee a *Ḥ.* (intimating that he would never be a Rabbi); a. e.—*Pl.* חַכִּימִין, חַכִּימַיָּא, חַכִּימֵי. Targ. Deut. I, 13. Targ. Job XL, 30 (h. text חַבָּרִים, cmp. חָבֵר); a. fr.—Nidd. 20ᵇ כמה ח׳ יהודאי how wise the Jews are. Sot. IX, 15 (49ᵃ) שרו ח׳ וכ׳ the *Hăkhamim* began to be (in scholarship) like common school teachers. Succ. 38ᵇ; a. fr.—*Fem.* חַכִּימָא, חַכִּימְתָּא. Targ. II Sam. XX, 16; a. e.—*Pl.* חַכִּימָתָא. Targ. Jer. IX, 16. Targ. Jud. V, 29 חַכִּימַת (constr. pl.).

חַכִּימָאָה m. (preced.) *one pretending to be a scholar.* Pes. 105ᵇ ed. (Ms. a. comment. חַכִּימָא).

חַכִּימוּתָא f. ch.=h. חָכְמָה, *wisdom.* Targ. Ex. XXXV, 35; a. e.

חַכִּימְתָּא, v. חַכִּים II.

חֲכִינָא, v. חֲכִינָה.

חֲכִינַאי, חֲכִינַיי pr. n. m. *Ḥăkhinai.* Keth. 62ᵇ, a. fr. R. Ḥanania, son of H.—Y. M. Kat. III, 81ᵈ top.

חכינאנות, v. חָבֵר׳.

חֲכִינָה, חֲכִינָא f. (חכן, cmp. עכן) *hăkhina,* name of a large snake, prob. *annulated snake.* Y. Ber. V, 9ᵃ bot.

(in Chald. dict.), v. זְהַר. Ib. VIII, 12ᵇ; Gen. R. s. 82, end (Hull. 127ᵃ נחש). Y. Snh. X, 28ᵈ top כריסָה של ח׳ (not ככריסה) like the venom of a h.; Ruth R. to III, 13. Y. Taan. IV, 69ᵃ top ח׳ כריכה עליו (read: כרוכה) a snake wound around him; (Lam. R. to II, 2 עכנא כריכא).—*Pl.* חֲכִינִים. Cant. R. to VII, 8 [read:] חבר שהיה לו שתי ח׳ a charmer who had two snakes.

חכינה, Meg. 28ᵃ בחכינתו, v. חֲכִינָה.

חכינותא, v. חֲבַר׳.

חֲכִינָנָא m. (v. חֲכִינָא) *wound, snake-like; insidious.* Targ. Prov. XVIII, 8 Var. ed. Lag. (ed. Lag. a. oth. חבננא, oth. ed. שיגושא; h. text נרגן).

חֲכִינְתָּה f. ch.=h. חֲכִינָה. Y. Sabb. VI, end, 8ᵈ.

חָכִיר, חַכִּיר m. (חכר, cmp. חכינא) *bent, bowed down.* Targ. Ps. XXXV, 14; XXXVIII, 7 (Ar. חֲבִיר; Ms. חָמַר I).

חָכִיר, חָכוּר m. (חָכַר) 1) *tenant* on a fixed rent payable in kind, v. אָרִיס II. Y. Bicc. I, end, 64ᵇ ח׳ לשעה a tenant for a fixed term, ח׳ לעולם a permanent tenant (on ground rent). B. Mets. 104ᵃ חוֹכֵר; a. fr.- *Pl.* חֲכִירִין, חֲכוּרוֹת, חֲכִירוֹת (חוכרין) חֲכוּרוֹת, חֲכַר׳. Y. Bicc. l. c. חֲכוּרֵי בתי אבות hereditary tenants. Tosef. Peah III, 1. Ib. Ter. II, 11 חוכרין ed. Zuck. (Var. חכורות, חכירות). Y. M. Kat. III, 82ᵇ bot. חֲכִירָיו.—2) *the fixed annual rent in kind.* B. Mets. IX, 2 (103ᵇ) מנכה לו מן חֲכִירוֹ Talm. ed. (Mish. חֲכוֹ׳) he deducts from the stipulated rent (in proportion). Ib. 4 (105ᵃ) הואיל ואני נותן לך חֲכִירָךְ (Y. ed. חֲכוּרָךְ, Mish. חֲכוּרָהּ) as long as I give thee thy rent (Mish.: the rent for it).

חֲכִירָא ch. = same. — *Pl.* חֲכִירֵי. B. Mets. 68ᵃ, v. נַרְשָׁאָה.

חכירא, חכיריא, v. חֲבִירָא.

חֲכִירוּת (חֲכוּרוּת) f. (v. חָכִיר) 1) *tenancy, tenure* on rent in kind. Bicc. I, 11 בעלי אריסות וח׳ *landlords* of properties held in tenure, on shares, or on fixed rent; or *tenants* on &c.; expl. Y. ib. 64ᵇ either חכירי בתי אבות (v. חָכִיר), or בעלי אריסיות וחֲכִירִיּוֹת (not וחכורות).—2) *stipulated rent.* Tosef. B. Mets. IX, 24 ח׳ של שתי שנים Var. (ed. Zuck. only חכורי) the rent for two years in advance.— *Pl.* חֲכִירִיּוֹת, v. supra.

חָכַךְ I (v. Fl. to Levy Talm. Dict. II, 204²) 1) *to restrain, fasten, hook.*— Denom. חַכָּה.—2) *to grasp* (one another), *to wrestle*; v. חָבַב II.

חָכַךְ II (onomatop.) 1) *to be rough; to rub, scratch.* Naz. 59ᵃ מהו לָחוֹךְ how about (removing the hair by) rubbing (Tosaf.: לחוך ולהִתְחַכֵּךְ about rubbing or being rubbed)?—2) (cmp. חָרַט, a. חָיַיךְ) *to hesitate.* Ned. I, 1 היה חוֹכֵךְ בזה להחמיר had some hesitation about deciding in favor of greater stringency (for the expression מנודה; oth. opin. in R. N. to Bab. ib. 7ᵃ: denom. of חֵךְ, *had a taste for* &c.).

Hithpa. הִתְחַכֵּךְ, *Nithpa.* נִתְחַכֵּךְ *to rub one's self against a rough object; to be rubbed.* B. Kam. IV, 6 שור שהיה מִתְחַכֵּךְ וכ׳ an ox that scratched himself against a wall; Tosef. ib. IV, 6. B. Kam. 3ᵃ נִתְחַכְּכָה וכ׳ she (the animal) scratched herself against a wall for her gratification (without intention to do injury) &c.—Naz. 59ᵃ, v. supra; a. fr.

Pi. חִיכֵּךְ (v. חוּךְ II) *to hawk; to deride.* Gen. R. s. 67 (play on חכר, Gen. XXVII, 36) התחיל מְחַכֵּךְ בגרונו וכ׳ he began to hawk with his throat (to express contempt), like one that hawks and spits; Tanh. Ki Thetsé 10; Pesik. Zakh., p. 27ᵇ, v. זְמוֹרָה; [Ar. ed. Koh. s. v. זמר: חִיכְחֵךְ, *Pilp.*].—Cmp. כָּחַח.

חֲכַךְ ch., *Ithpa.* אִתְחַכֵּךְ as preced. *Hithpa.* B. Kam. 44ᵃ.

חֲכַךְ m. (preced.) 1) *scab, sore*; trnsf. *tribulation, visitation.* Y. M. Kat. III, 81ᵈ top; (B. Mets. 59ᵇ אַךְ, Var. אַף). — *Pl.* חֲכָכִים *inflammations.* Gen. R. s. 19, beg. (v., however, אֲבַעְבּוּעוֹת).—2) *cough, catarrh.* Y. Snh. X, 29ᵇ bot. בתחלה הוא . . . ח׳ first He causes a cold to enter them; (Tanh., ed. Bub., R'eh 10 חִיכּוּךְ); Pesik. Asser 97ᵇ הקב״ה ח׳ (insert מכניס בהם); v. זָהָ.

חָכַם (b. h.; v. חָכָם) 1) *to be wise, to know.* Nidd. 70ᵇ מה יעשה אדם ויֶחְכַּם what must one do in order to be wise?—2) (denom. of חָכָם) *to meet for deliberation.* Ib. לכשיחיו נֶחְכַּם להן when they resurrect, we shall meet to discuss their case.

Hif. הֶחְכִּים 1) *to grow wise, to become a scholar.* B. Bath. 25ᵇ הרוצה שיַּחְכִּים he who desires to become a scholar; ib. 175ᵇ (Ber. 63ᵇ שיִתְחַכֵּם). Ab. II, 5 . . . לא כל מַחְכִּים not every one that has a large trade, becomes wise (experienced); a. fr.—2) *to make wise, to stimulate a person's mind by ingenious suggestions, questions* &c. Hag. 14ᵃ תלמיד המַחְכִּים וכ׳ a student who enlightens his teachers. B. Mets. 107ᵇ ומַחְכִּימַת פתי and makes the simple wise.—3) *to subtilize, philosophize.* Ex. R. s. 6, beg. ח׳ על גזרתו וכ׳ philosophized on (tried to find out the reasons for) the Lord's law. Ib. מה שהייתי מַחְכִּים וכ׳ when I philosophised . . . . . and made myself believe . . . . ., it was all vain boast &c.

Hithpa. הִתְחַכֵּם, *Nithpa.* נִתְחַכֵּם *to become wise.* Ber. 63ᵇ, v. supra. B. Bath. 25ᵇ מתוך שמִתְחַכֵּם מִתעשר because by becoming wise, he will get rich. Pesik. R. s. 33 beg. מאליו נתח׳ became wise by his own speculation.

חֲכַם, חֲכִים, also **חַכִּים** (adj. with verbal inflection) 1) *to be wise, shrewd; to be learned.* Targ. I Kings V, 11. Targ. O. Ex. XV, 8 חֲכִימוּ (חַכּ׳, h. text נערמו). Targ. Is. XXIX, 16; a. fr.—Gitt. 56ᵇ דחַכִּמִיתוּ וכ׳ that you are so wise. Taan. 23ᵇ דניחַכְּמִים טובא that we may become well-learned; a. fr.—2) *to recognize, to know, remember.* Targ. Y. II Gen. XXXVII, 33 (some ed. חַכֵּם *Pa.*).—Targ. II Esth. II, 18; a. fr.—Lev. R. s. 30 ח׳ את וכ׳ doest thou know anything in favor of this man?—Y. M. Kat. III, 83ᵇ top, v. בְּאַר.—Y. Ber. II, 4ᵈ top וחַכְמִין אינון כלום do they (the dead) know anything?—Y. Shek. VII, 50ᶜ bot. יַחְכְּמוּן שפריא קיטריהון let the wine-dealers identify their knots (marks on the wine bottles). Y. Keth. V, 30ᵃ bot. [read:] חֲכִים אנא לחייתא דמילדא לי (or חַכִּים) I (as an infant) recognized the midwife that assisted at my birth (when she came to nurse my mother). Y. Ter. XI, end, 48[b] לא אנא ח׳ לאבא I never knew my father. Y. Hag. II, 78[a] top יַחְכִּים shall select (Y. Snh. VI, 23[a] bot. יטול), v. זוּגָא.—2) (euphem.=b. h. יָדַע) *to sleep with.* Targ. Y. Gen. IV, 1. Ar. (ed. ידע). Targ. Y. II ib. XX, 16; a. e.—Y. Maas. Sh. IV, 55[b] bot.; Lam. R. to I, 1 חד כותאר) רבתי 1) a. e.—3) *to be clear, evident.* Snh. 42[a], v. זָקֵן I.

Pa. חַכִּים 1) *to make wise, teach.* Targ. Y. Deut. XXXIV, 10. Targ. Job XXXV, 11; a. e.—2) *to outwit.* Targ. O. Gen. XXVII, 36 (Rashi a. l. quotes וכמני, v. כְּמַן, v. Berl. Targ. O. II, p. 10).

Ithpa. אִתְחַכַּם 1) *to become wise.* Targ. Ps. CV, 22; a. e.—2) *to be informed, aware; to learn.* Ib. XXXV, 8. Targ. Y. Ex. II, 4.—3) *to hold counsel.* Targ. O. Ex. I, 10.—4) *to be recognized.* Y. Sot. IX, 23[c] bot.; Y. Yeb. XVI, 15[c] מאן דבעי דלא מִתְחַכְּמָה he who desires to disguise himself; לא מִתְחַכְּמִין they were not recognized, v. נְחִירָא.

Af. אַחְכִּים *to teach, make wise.* Targ. Ez. III, 2; a. e.—B. Bath. 158[b] אוירא דא״י מַחְכִּים the climate of Palestine makes wise.

חָכָם m. (b. h.; v. Fl. to Levy Talm. Dict. II, 204²) [*retentive,*] 1) *one who knows.* חֲכַם הרזים He who knows the secrets (minds of men). Ber. 58[a]; Tosef. ib. VII (VI), 2; Num. R. s. 21, beg.—2) *wise man, scholar; esp. Hakham,* a scholar's title, less than Rabbi. Ab. IV, 1 איזהו ח׳ who is a wise man? Snh. 21[a] (ref. to II Sam. XIII, 3) איש ח׳ לרשעה a man wise for wickedness (artful). Gitt. 67[a] ח׳ וסופר is a scholar and a scribe; ח׳ לכשירצה might be a scholar, if he wanted. Hor. 13[b] ר״מ ח׳ R. M. was the *Hakham* (counselor); a. v. fr.—*Pl.* חֲכָמִים, frequ. in the sense of *a number of scholars,* as opposed to a single authority. Hull. 85[a] ראה רבי . . ושנאו בלשון ח׳ Rabbi approving of R. Meir's opinion . . . ., recorded it in the Mishnah as the opinion of 'scholars'. Ber. I, 1; a. v. fr.—חַכְמֵי אומות העולם gentile scholars (philosophers), חכמי ישראל Jewish scholars. R. Hash. 12[a]. Pes. 94[b]; a. fr.—תַּלְמִיד חָכָם (=ת״ח, תלמיד וח׳, cmp. חָבֵר, abbr. ת״ח) title of a student, *disciple, scholar.* Hag. 15[b] ת״ח אע״פ שסרח וכ׳ a scholar's learning is not to be despised, even if he has gone astray. Hull. 9[a] ת״ח צריך וכ׳ in order to be recognised as a *Talmid Hakham,* one must have learned three things &c.; a. v. fr.—*Pl.* תַּלְמִידֵי חֲכָמִים. Ber. 64[a] ת״ח מרבים וכ׳ scholars increase the peace of the world; a. v. fr.

חכם, Y. Erub. IX, end, 25[d] וחח׳, read והחמים, v. חָמִים.

חַכְמָא, v. חוּכְמָא.

חַכְמַאי pr. n. m. *Hakhmai.* M. Kat. 9[a] bot. ר׳ יונתן בן ח׳ Ms. M. (ed. עסביר, read: עכ׳); Y. Ter. XI, end, 48[b] עַכְּבַאי.

חֲכָמָה f. 1) fem. of חָכָם. Y. Shek. V, 48[d] top הרי זו ח׳ that is a wise court; Snh. 17[b] שלרשית ח׳ a Sanhedrin containing three orators is a wise one.—2) *female physician, midwife.* R. Hash. II, 5; Erub. 45[a] ח׳ הבאה לילד a midwife called for assisting at birth. Sabb. XVIII, 3 וקורין לה ח׳ וכ׳ and we must call for her a midwife from another place (on the Sabbath); a. fr.

חָכְמָה f. (b. h.; חָכַם) *wisdom, learning, art.* Ber. 17[a] תכלית ח׳ וכ׳ the perfection of wisdom is repentance and good deeds. Ib. 33[a] ברכת ח׳ the benediction of wisdom (the fourth of the Prayer of Benedictions). Gen. R. s. 17 חָכְמָתוֹ מרובה וכ׳ his (Adam's) wisdom is greater than yours. R. Hash. 29[b] שהיא ח׳ ואינה מלאכה it is an art and not a labor; a. v. fr.—לשון ח׳ *enigmatical speech.* Erub. 53[b].—חָכְמַת יוונית, v. יְוָנִי.

חַכְמָנִית f. (preced.) *well-educated, smart.*—*Pl.* חַכְמָנִיּוֹת. B. Bath. 119[b].

חָכְמְתָא, v. חוּכ׳.

חכן, Y. Erub. VI, 23[d] bot., read חָכֵן.

חָכַר (cmp. חָבַר) *to contract, farm,* esp. *to give* or *to take in rent on a fixed annual rental payable in kind,* contrad. to אָרִיס, שָׂכַר or קִבֵּל q. v.—B. Mets. IX, 2 חֲכוֹר לי וכ׳ give me in rent &c. Tosef. Dem. VI, 2 החוכר שדה if one takes in rent a field. Ib. מה בין שוכר לחוכר what is the difference between the *sokher* and the *hokher?;* a. fr.—V. חָכִיר.

Hif. הֶחְכִּיר *to give in rent. Part.* מַחְכִּיר *landlord.* B. Mets. 104[a]; a. e.—*Part. pass.* מוּחְכָּר, f. מוּחְכֶּרֶת. B. Bath. 123[b], sq. פרה ב׳ a cow rented out *for half-profit* (Rashi).

חֲכַר ch. same. B. Mets. 68[a] חֲכִרָה, v. מַשְׁכֵּן. Y. Maas. Sh. V, 56[b] bot. [read:] כד . . . חָכְרִין . . . תַּחְכְּרוּן וכ׳ when you rent land, rent only from God-fearing men.

חַכְרָנוּתָא f. (preced.) *tenancy.* B. Mets. 104[a] (Rashi: חֲכִירוּת).

חכשרה, v. הַכְשָׁרָה.

חל, Y. Ned. IV, beg. 39[c] bot כגון החל מן נונירה, read: כגון הדין חַלְמוֹן כ׳ as, for instance, *fish-raw.*—Y. Ab. Zar. II, 40[d] top כחל לה, read: בחללה, v. חַלְלָא.

חַל, perf. a. part. of חוּל.

חַל I, v. חֲלַל.

חַל II m. (חלל, cmp. חָלֵי) *weak, mild* (wine). Targ. Y. Deut. VIII, 8, opp. חֲרִיף.

חַל III *vinegar,* v. חָלָא III.

חָלָא m. (חלל, cmp. גלל) *a globular concretion.*—*Pl.* חָלֵי. Bekh. 7[b] ח׳ דיחמורתא ball-like concretions found in the *yahmur* (fallow-deer), v. יַחְמוּרָא.

חָלָא I m.=h. חוֹל I, *sand.* Targ. Gen. XXXII, 13; a. fr.—Pes. 113[a], v. אַדָּ.—*Pl.* חָלְתָא (fem.). Sabb. 110[a] בי ח׳ between the sand-mounds.

חָלָא II m.=חוֹל II. Targ. Job XXIX, 18.

חָלָא III, **חַלָּא**, **חַל** m. (חוֹל or חלל) [*turned, spoiled,*] *vinegar.* Targ. O. Num. VI, 3 חַל; Y. חַלָּא. Targ. Ps. LXIX, 22 ח׳ ed. (Ms. חָ׳). Targ. Prov. XXV, 20 חלא ed. Lag. (ed. חֵילָא, Ms. חוֹ׳). Targ. Ruth II, 14.—Ab. Zar. 12[b]. Gen. R. s. 39, v. זוּל I ch.—Hull. 120[a] ח׳ דקריש Ar. (ed. חלב) a jellied vinegar sauce of meat; a. fr.—Y. Maasr. III, 50[d] bot. ח׳ בר חמרא a deteriorated son, v. חוֹמֶץ; Hull. 105[a]. [Y. Ter. VII, 45[d] bot. בחלא, read: בַּחַקְלָא.]

חָלָא *to be sick*, v. חָלִי.

חֶלְאָה (b. h.) pr. n. f. *Helah*, an Agadic surname of Miriam. Ex. R. s. 1, v. כָּזַר.

חֲלָאִים, v. חָלִי.

חָלָב m., constr. **חֲלֵב** (b. h) [*secretion*,] *milk*. Ab. Zar. II, 6 ח׳ שחֲלָבוֹ וכ׳ milk (of a cow) milked by a gentile. Makhsh. VI, 5 מי ח׳ serum of milk; a. fr.—בשר בח׳ *the boiling of meat with milk, the prohibitory law concerning* &c. (Ex. XXIV, 19; XXXIV, 26; Deut. XIV, 21). Pes. 54[b], v. חִידּוּשׁ.—Ḥull. 110[a] לא גמירי דב׳ בח׳ אסור they did not know that boiling meat with milk was forbidden; a. fr.—חֲלַב בֵּיצִים *white of eggs*. Y. Ter. X, 47[b] bot., cmp. חֶלְבּוֹן.—(ח׳ (ח) נֵץ *ornithogalum, Star of Bethlehem*, a bulbous plant. Shebi. VII, 1, v. חֶלְבְּצִין; Ukts. III, 2.—Trnsf. חח׳ *white wine*. Gen. R. s. 98, opp. אדום.

חֲלָב, חַלְבָּא, חֲל׳ ch. same. Targ. Gen. XVIII, 8. Targ. Job X, 10; a. fr.—Y. Ter. VIII, 46[a] חַלְבּוּן ח׳ milked. Ḥull. 109[b], v. בִּשְׂרָא I. Ib. 110[a]; a. e.

חָלַב (denom. of חָלָב) *to milk; to yield milk*. Ab. Zar. II, 6, v. חָלָב. Bekh. 20[b] רוב .... חוֹלְבוֹת וכ׳ the majority of animals secrete no milk unless they have given birth; a. fr.

Nif. נֶחְלַב *to be milked*. Sabb. 53[b] לֵיחָלֵב when the bag is tied on for milking purposes (to support the udders), opp. לִיבש for drying up.

חֲלַב ch. same. Y. Ter. VIII, 46[a], v. חָלָב.

חֵלֶב m. (b. h.) *fatty concretion* (cmp. חֶלְאָ), esp. *that abdominal fat of cattle which it is forbidden to eat, ḥeleb* (Lev. III, 17), contrad. to שומן. Kerith. III, 1. Ḥull. 113[b] המבשל ח׳ בֶּחָלָב if one boils fat with milk. Snh. 4[b] חֵלֶב וְחָלָב דכר וכ׳ *ḥeleb* a. *ḥalab* which are written alike, v. אֵם; a. fr.—*Pl.* חֲלָבִים, חֲלָבִין. Ber. I, 1 ח׳ ואברים the pieces of fat and the limbs belonging to the altar; Tam. VII, 3 שלחן חח׳ the (marble) table designated for the fat-pieces (and limbs).—Ker. 12[a], sq. חֲלָבִין laws concerning the eating of *ḥeleb*; Y. Yeb. X, 11[a] top מדמי לח לח׳ (not לחלבון); a. fr.—[Y. Ter. X, 47[b] bot. לובן חלבין, v. חֶלְבּוֹן.]—גוש ח׳, v. גּוּשׁ.

***חֲלַב** ch. m. (preced.) *a viscous substance, glair*. Ḥull. 120[a] ח׳ דקריש ed. (v. Rashi); v. חֶלְאָ III.

חֶלְבּוֹן (חִלְבּוֹן Ar.) m. (v. preced. wds.) *glair, white of an egg*. Ab. Zar. 40[a]; Ḥull. 64[a], v. חֶלְמוֹן; a. fr.—Y. Ter. X, 47[b] bot. בלובן חלבין, read: בחלבון (v. cit. in Tosaf. to Ḥull. 64[b]).

חֶלְבּוֹנָא, constr. **חֶלְבּוֹן** ch. same. Targ. Y. Gen. XXXIX, 14; 20. Targ. Job VI, 6.

חֶלְבֵּיצִין, v. חֶלְבְּצִין.

חֶלְבְּנָא, חֶלְבְּנַיָּא, pl., v. חֶלְבְּנִיתָא.

חֶלְבְּנָה f. (b. h.; cmp. חָלָב, חֵלֶב, v. חִילְתִּית) *galbanum*, a gum-resin used as an ingredient of frank-incense, smelling like asafoetida. Ker. 6[a]. Ib.[b]; Yalk. Ex. 389 ח׳ ריחה רע ומנאה וכ׳ the smell of galb. is evil, and yet the Bible counts it among the spices (so are the wicked with the righteous combined in prayer).

חֶלְבְּנִיתָא (חֶלְבְּנְתָּא, חֶלְבְּנְתָּא) ch. same. Targ. O. Ex. XXX, 34; Targ. Y. וְחֶלְבְּנַיָּא, pl.—Gitt. 69[a], v. הוּבְשָׁנִיתָא.

חֶלְבְּצִין, חֶלְבִּי׳ m. (compound of חָלָב a. בֵּיצָה) *bulb of ornithogalum*. Shebi. VII, 2; expl. Y. ib. 37[b] bot. בֵּיצֵי נֵץ חָלָב eggs (bulbs) of &c., v. חָלָב; Tosef. ib. V, 6; Nidd. 62[a] חַלְבְּרִיצִין (absorbing ח); Sabb. 90[a] חחל׳. Tosef. Kil. III, 12 חלבוצין.

חֲלַגְלוֹג m., pl. **חֲלַגְלוֹגִין, חֲלַגְלוֹגוֹת** (חלג, cmp. חלק) *purslane*. Erub. 28[a] ובחל׳ (Ms. M. ובגלוגות, read: וּבַגְּלַ׳, v. Rabb. D. S. a. l. note, ח absorbed, v. preced.); Y. Peah VIII, 21[a] top; Y. Erub. III, 20[d] top, expl. פרפחיניה. Shebi. IX, 1 (Mish. ed. גיח ...., read: גוח ..; v. Rabb. D. S. a. l. note). Y. ib. 38[c] (Rabbi's maid said) נתפזרו חֲלוֹגְלוֹגוֹתֶיךָ thy purslane plants have been scattered; R. Hash. 26[b] חֲלוֹגְלוֹגְךָ (Ms. M. לגלוגך). Ib. לא ידעי רבנן מאי חלוגל׳ (Mss. לגל׳).

חָלַד (cmp. חלל) *to undermine, cave, dig*. Pes. 118[b] שחוֹלֶדֶת בעיקרי וכ׳ Ms. M. (ed. as in Ḥull. 20[b] חוררה) which undermines the foundations &c. V. חוּלְדָּה.

Hif. הֶחְלִיד 1) same. Y. Kil. IX, 32[c] top מַחְלִיד הקב״ה את וכ׳ .... the Lord caves the ground before them and they roll &c.; Y. Keth. XII, 35[b] top .. אל מחלך (corr. acc.). B. Bath. 19[b] מפני שמַחְלִידִין וכ׳ because their roots undermine the ground.—2) *to pass the slaughtering knife under cover, to squeeze in*. Ḥull. II, 4. Ib. 20[b]; a. fr.—Tosef. Kel. B. Bath. I, 5 מפני שהכובס אומן מַחְלִידוֹ לתוכו (R. S. to Kel. XXI, 1) because so much of it does the professional fuller fold up for inserting a rod into it (v. חוב II, 2).

חֲלַד ch. same; Part. pass. חֲלִיד *covered with earth, mouldering*. Targ. Job XI, 17 Ms. (ed. דחלך, דחלך, corr. acc.).

חֶלֶד m. (b. h.; preced.) *mould*; trnsf. *earthly life*. Midr. Till. to Ps. XVII, 14 אין ח׳ אלא ארץ *ḥeled* means earth (ref. to Ps. XLIX, 2). Tanḥ. Ki Thabo 2 (ref. to Ps. XVII, 14) הן מתים מח׳ they die away from this world, v. חֲלוּדָה.

חֲלָדָה f. (חָלַד Hif.) *passing the knife under cover*. Ḥull. 9[a]; 27[a]; a. e.

חלדאות, v. חֲלוּדָה.

חֲלָדוּתָא f. ch.=h. חֲלוּדָה, *rust*. Targ. Y. Num. XXXI, 22 (v. Rashi a. l.).

***חֲלָדִין** m. pl. (preced. wds.) *cave-dwellers*. Gen. R. s. 37, transl. of חִוִּי (Gen. X, 17); cmp. חִוְיָא.

חֲלָה, v. חלי.

חַלָּה f. (b. h.; חלל) 1) [*rolled, rounded*] *cake*.—*Pl.* חַלּוֹת. Ukts. III, 5 ח׳ חריע (Tosef. Maas. Sh. I, 13 חַלַּת

(collect. noun), a.e., v. חֲרִיעַ.—Men. III, 6 שתי ח׳ the two loaves (offered on the Feast of Weeks, Lev. XXIII, 17).—B. Bath. V, 3; Ukts. III, 11 ח׳ דבש *honey-combs;* a. fr.—2) (with ref. to Num. XV, 20, sq.) *Ḥallah, the priest's share of the dough.* Sabb. II, 6, v. זָהִיר. Ḥall. I, 1 וחייבין בח׳ are subject to the law of *Ḥallah.*—Ib. II, 7 שיעור הח׳ the quantity to be set aside for the priest. Ib. 8 מעיסה שלא הורמה חַלָּתָהּ Ms. M. (v. Rabb. D. S. a. l. note) from a dough from which the priest's share has not yet been taken; a. fr.—*Pl.* as ab. Pesik. Shimu, p. 118[a] שתי ח׳ two portions (one for being burnt, and one for the priest); Y. Erub. III, end, 21[c]; Cant. R. to I 6; a. e.—Trnsf. *ḥallah, the sanctification of creation, man.* Gen. R. s. 14, beg.; Yalk. Prov. 962, a. e. (ref. to Prov. XXIX, 4, ואיש תרומות) שחיה גמר חַלָּתוֹ וכ׳ that is Adam who was the final sanctification of the world; Gen. R. s. 17, end.—*Ḥallah,* name of a treatise of the Mishnah, Tosefta a. Talm. Y., of the Order of Z'raïm.

חֲלוּגְלוּג, v. חֲלַגְלוּג.

חֲלוּדָה f. (חָלַד) [*covering of earth &c., mouldering from being in a cave,*] 1) *rust, mould.* Kel. XIII, 5 העלתה ח׳ became rusty; Tosef. ib. B. Mets. III, 10; a. fr.—Trnsf. *sin.* Tanḥ. Ki Thabo 2 (ref. to חלד Ps. XVII, 14) [read:] אמרו זה לזה ח׳ הם מלאין חטאין יש בידן (v. Tanḥ. ed. Bub. ib. 4) they (the gentiles) say to one another, they (the Israelites) are full of rust, there are sins in their hands.—2) *a skin disease arising from living in caves.* Midr. Till. to Ps. XVII, 14 (v. supra) אלו שהעלה גופן ח׳ they are those (persecuted Jews) whose bodies became afflicted with sores, &c.; Y. Shebi. IX, 38[d]; Gen. R. s. 79.—*Pl.* חֲלוּדוֹת. Pesik. B'shall., p. 88[b]; Esth. R. to I, 9 חֲלוּדָאוֹת (some ed. חלדואות, corr. acc.).

חַלְוָן pr. n. pl. *Halvan* (*Ḥolvân*) in Assyria (b. h. חלח, v. P. Sm. 1277, Neub. Géogr. p. 373). Kidd. 72[a]; Yeb. 16[b] Ms. M. (ed. חלזון, corr. acc.).

חָלוּז, חִילוּזָא (חִי׳) m. (חלז) *knot* or *sling of the upper garment when lifted,* (*sinus*). Targ. II Esth. I, 2 (3) וחליזות חִילוּזָהּ she lifted her garment.—Pes. 113[a] תמרי בחֲלוּזָךְ וכ׳ if thou bringest dates home, with thy *sinus* (before ungirding) run to the brewery; [comment.: with the dates tied up in thy *bag*]. V. חוּלְזָא.

חָלוּט m.=הֶחְלֵט. Tosef. Neg. VIII, 6 בימי חִלּוּטוֹ during his days of declared leprosy.

חָלוּט m., v. חָלַט.

חֲלוּטִין m. pl. h. a. ch. (חָלַט II) *final action, decision.* לַחֲ׳ *finally, permanently, absolutely* (b. h. לִצְמִיתוּת). Targ. Lev. XXV, 23; a. e.—Ex. R. s. 3; Arakh. 15[b]; Snh. 106[b].—Lev. R. s. 7, end, v. יְרִיבָה.—V. חַלְטָנִית.—בח׳ *by final decision* (from which there is no appeal). Gen. R. s. 42; Yalk. ib. 72; Koh. R. to V, 15 היך מה דאתא בחלו׳ וכ׳ Ar. ed. (בחלי׳) as man enters this world by final decision, so does he leave it it (cmp. Ab. IV, 22).—[Gen. R. s. 94, beg. חלוטין, v. חֲלִיטָא III.]

חָלוּל, חַלּוּי, v. sub חִי׳.

חָלוּל m. (חָלַל) *hollowed; pipe, channel.*—*Pl.* חֲלוּלִים, חֲלוּלִין. Sifra K'dosh. Par. 1; Yalk. Lev. 604 the idols are called אֱלִילִים על שם שהם ח׳ because they are hollow.—Ber. 60[b] ח׳ ח׳ Ms. F. a. oth. (ed. חֲלָלִים) full of channels (bowels &c.).

חָלוּם m. *sane,* v. חָלַם I.

חֲלוֹם (b. h.; v. חָלַם II) *dream.* Ber. 55[a]; a. fr.—*Pl.* חֲלוֹמוֹת. Ib.[b]; a. fr.—Ib. 10[b] בעל הח׳ the genius of dream.—[חלומות דהרואה that portion of the chapter Haroëh, in B'rakhoth, treating of dreams: Ber. 55[a] to 57[b]; often quoted in Ar. a. oth.]

חַלּוֹן c. (b. h.; חלל) *perforation, aperture, window.* B. Bath. III, 6 ח׳ המצרית וכ׳ the Egyptian window (a very small aperture in the wall) gives no privilege (v. חֲזָקָה), i. e. the neighbor may build against it, contrad. to הצורית a Tyrian window. Gen. R. s. 31, expl. צהר (Gen. VI, 16); a. v. fr.—*Pl.* חַלּוֹנוֹת. Y. R. Hash. II, 58[a]; Ex. R. s. 15 שס״ה ח׳ וכ׳ 365 apertures did the Lord create in the sky; a. fr.

חִלּוּף, חִלּוּפָא, v. חִי׳.

חִלּוּץ m. (v. חָלַץ *Hif.*) *strength, quickness.* Ber. 16[b] חיים של ח׳ עצמות (missing in Mss., v. Rabb. D. S. a. l. note 5) a life of healthfull energy (v. Is. LVIII, 11).

חֲלוּצָה, חֲלוּצָא I pr. n. pl. or district *Hălutsa.* Targ. Y. II Gen. XVI, 7; Ex. XV, 22 (h. text שׁוּר). Targ. Y. Gen. XVI, 14 (h. text בָּרֶד).—Gen. R. s. 45; Yalk. ib. 79 (expl. בדרך שור, Gen. XVI, 7) באורחא דח׳ on the road of H.—V. חַגְרָא I.

חֲלוּצָה II f., v. חָלַץ.

חָלוּק I m. (חָלַק, v. חָלָק) *plain, smooth garment,* in gen. *undershirt.* Kel. XXVIII, 9, v. חוּץ II.—M. Kat. 14[a], a. e. כל . . . אלא ח׳ אחד he who has only one shirt. Ab. Zar. 34[a] ח׳ לבן a plain white frock, v. אִימְרָה. Y. Taan. II, 65[d] (ref. to I Sam. VII, 6) לבש שמואל חֲלוּקָן וכ׳ Samuel put on the common shirt of all Israelites, i. e. included himself among the sinners; a. fr.—Trnsf. a) *a shirt-shaped bandage.* Sabb. XIX, 2 (drawn over the circumcised membrum).—b) *a row, layer.* Y. Pes. I, 27[b] bot. מפשיטו ח׳ אחד he strips it of one shirt, i. e. removes one row all around the pile of bottles.—*Pl.* חֲלוּקִים, חֲלוּקִין, חֲלוּקוֹת. M. Kat. 22[b]. Y. l. c. שני חלקות (read: חלוק׳) two rows. Tosef. Kil. V, 6 שני ח׳ two shirts of different materials (כִּלְאַיִם). Lam. R. introd. (R. Abbahu 2); ib. to III, 13 והח׳ שלו עליו (the camel) with his covers on; a. fr.

חָלוּק II 1) *divided,* v. חָלַק; 2) *empty, smooth,* v. חָלָק.

חִלּוּק, v. חִילּוּק.

חֲלוּק, חֲלוּקָא ch.=h. חָלוּק I. Targ. Y. Ex. XXII, 26 ח׳ תותביה ed. pr. (later ed. only תות׳).—Lam. R. introd. (R. Abbahu 5); ib. to III, 13 כח׳ דיהודאי וכ׳ as long as a Jewish Sabbath shirt (transmitted from father to son).—Sabb. 134ª ח׳ דינוקא the child's bandage, v. חָלוּק I.

חֲלוּקָּה f. (b. h. חֲלֻקָּה; חָלַק) *division, partition.* B. Bath. 122ª לא כח׳ של עוה״ז וכ׳ the distribution of land in the future will not be like the one of the present. Ib. 126ª יש לו לבכור קודם ח׳ the first-born is the legal owner of his share before the partition has taken place. Keth. 26ª בתורת ח׳ as an heir's share. Ib. 94ᵇ ח׳ עדיפא division among two claimants (where evidence is wanted) is preferable (to discretionary adjudication to one, v. שׁוּדָא); a. e.

***חֲלוּקָה** f., constr. **חֲלוּקַת**, only in (פול) ח׳ נפש [*smoothing the soul,*] name of a species of *bean*=שעועית. Nidd. IX, 7 (expl. מי גריסין) לעיסת גריסין של פול ח׳ נ׳ a chewed mass of grist of beans named *ḥălukath nefesh* (Rashi: *beans split to the core*, v. חִילְקָא II); [Tosef. ib. VIII, 9 עז עיקת נפש ed. Zuck. (Var. (ער עוקת נחש); Gen. R. s. 94, beg. פול שהוא על עיקת נפש; Yalk. ib. 152 שבארן על עָקַת נפש the bean-grist used for (relieving) the pressure of the soul; cmp. Y. Kil. I, 27ᵇ top, etymol. of שְׁעוּעִית, a. B. Bath. 16ª, quot. s. v. עֲדָשָׁה.—Our w. is prob. a popular re-adaptation of *Alica*, v. Sm. Ant. s. v.]

חֲלוּתָא *hosts*, v. חֵילָא I.

חֲלַז, *Pa.* חַלֵּיז (cmp. חלץ) *to gird, to form a sinus; to lift the cloak.* Targ. II Esth. I, 2 (3), v. חֲלוּז.—*Part. pass.* מְחַלַּז. Ib. VI, 11 ומְחַלְּזִין חולזוי his loins girt (his cloak lifted up, ready for labor).

חָלָז, חִילָז, חִלָּזוֹן m. (v. preced.) 1) *conchiferous animal, snail, oyster*, esp. *purple-fish, purple-shell used for dying t'kheleth* (תְּכֵלֶת). Snh. 91ª ח׳ אחד (ed. אחת, v. Rabb. D. S. a. l. note 60 a. Ar. s. v.). Pesik. B'shall. p. 92ª ח׳ הזה וכ׳ as the snail grows, its shell grows with it; Deut. R. s. 7, end —Sabb. 26ª (expl. יגבים, Jer. LII, 16) צידיי ח׳ וכ׳ the shellfishers from &c. Men. 44ª. Meg. 6ª; a. fr. — *Pl.* חִלְזוֹנוֹת. Snh. l. c.—2) name of a *beetle* or *locust*, v. next w.—Y. Sabb. I, 3ᵇ. Yalk. Ex. 185; Tanh. Vaera, ed. Bub. 19.—3) (cmp. Lat. Cochlea) *a snail-shaped piece of a chain, screw.* Kel. XII, 1; Tosef. ib. B. Mets. II, 3.—4) *an eye-disease*, also called נחש. Bekh. VI, 2; ib. 38ᵇ. Sifra Emor ch. II, Par. 3.—[Kidd. 72ª; Yeb. 16ᵇ, v. חַלְוָון.]

חִלְזוֹנָא ch. same, 1) *purple-fish; snail.* Targ. Y. I Deut. XXXIII, 19 (v. Meg. 6ª).—*Pl.* חִלְזוֹנֵי. Ab. Zar. 28ᵇ, v. מַשְׁקְדֵי.—2) *beetle* or *locust.* Targ. Y. Deut. XXVIII, 42 Ar. (ed. חלנונא, h. text צלצל).—3) *an affection of the eye.* Targ. Y. I Lev. XXI, 20 Ar. a. oth. (ed. חִלָּזוֹן; Y. II ריחלזווה, read: דחִלְזוֹנָה; v. חֲלִיז).

חִילְחוּל, חַלְחוּל m. (חַלְחֵל) *penetration of a poisonous substance, poison.* Tanh. Mishp. 18; ed. Bub. 12 (חול׳, corr. acc.) הח׳ היה נכנס וכ׳ the poison (of the flies) entered their bodies; Yalk. Ex. 359.

חַלְחוּלִית f. (v. preced.) *winding;* pl. חַלְחוּלִיּוֹת *intrigues.* Lev. R. s. 20 (expl. להוללים, Ps. LXXV, 5) ח׳ רעות ..... למערבביא אלו שלבם (some ed. חַלְחוּלִיּוֹת) to those creating confusion, those whose hearts are full of evil intrigues; Tanh. Aḥăré 2 חלחל׳; Yalk. Lev. 524 חולחלויות; Yalk. Ps. 811; [Lev. R. s. 17 (ref. to Ps. LXXIII, 3) במערבא אומרים אלו . . חוללות וכ׳ (read: בְּמְעַרְבְּבַיָּא אלו), v. הוֹלֵלָה].

חַלְחוּלֶת f. (next w.; v. preced. wds.) *mesentery*, a membrane keeping the entrails in position. Hull. 50ª.

חִלְחֵל (b. h.; Pilp. of חלל) 1) *to penetrate into cavities; to perforate.* Sot. 7ᵇ; Num. R. s. 9 מְחַלְחֵל ויורד (the powder on a wound) penetrates and goes down (into the body). Gen. R. s. 98 ריסו מח׳ וכ׳ its venom penetrates (the body of the bitten one) after (the serpent's) death.—2) *to shake, roll* (in a vessel &c.); *to rinse.* Makhsh. III, 6 ח׳ לתוכן if he washed olives by rolling them in the rain water.—*Part. pass.* מְחוּלְחָל, f. מְחוּלְחֶלֶת *hollow, blown up; loosely put in.* Oh. IX, 7 כלי מח׳ a hollow vessel (not packed entirely), opp. אֲפוּצָה. Kel. X, 3 מגופת החבית המח׳ וכ׳ (Bart. הַמְּחַלְחֶלֶת) the stopper of a keg which can be moved around, without, however, falling out of itself. Teb. Yom I, 1; a. fr.

Hithpalp. הִתְחַלְחֵל, *Nithpalp.* נִתְחַלְחֵל 1) *to permeate.* Num. R. s. 9 שהם מִתְחַלְחְלִים וכ׳ that they will permeate all her limbs.—2) *to be shaken in a hollow space, to be thrown about.* Mikv. IV, 3 היו צרורות מתח׳ וכ׳ if pebbles rolled about in the spout.—3) *to be permeated* (with poison) *to be affected, injured.* Y. B. Kam. I, beg. 2ᵇ ונתח׳ כולו and the whole of it is damaged (by the heat &c.).—4) (cmp. חָלָה) *to be weakened, be neutralized.* Y. Ter. VIII, 46ª top ע״י מליחה מתח׳ through salting it, the poison is neutralized.

חַלְחֵל ch. same, *to penetrate, to hollow out.* Hull. 119ᵇ חַלְחוּלֵי מְחַלְחֵל the hair perforates the skin.—*Part. pass.* מְחַלְחַל *hollow; loosely filled.* Ber. 59ª ענני חלחולי מְחַלְחֲלֵי (Ms. F. עיבא . . מיחלחל) the clouds are not entirely filled with water. Pes. 74ª אירדי דמח׳ because the wood is hollow (having marrow inside); a. e.

Ithpalp. אִיחַלְחֵל, אִתְחַלְחַל 1) *to be perforated, be open.* Ber. l. c. Ms. F. v. supra.—Esp. *to be permeated by poison, feel the effect of poison.* Y. Ab. Zar. II, 41ª bot.; Y. Ter. VIII, 45ᶜ bot. לא אספיק . . עד דאיתח׳ he had scarcely drank of it when he became affected (collapsed). Y. Ab. Zar. II, 40ᵈ top חמתה מִתְחַלְחֲלָה he saw that the plaster was poisoned.—2) *to tremble.* Targ. Ps. XCVII, 4. Targ. Y. Ex. XXXII, 11 (h. text ויחל); a. e.

חָלַט I (v. חָלַט II, a. Syr. חלט P. Sm. 1277) *bind up, mix*, esp. *to stir flour in hot water*, v. חֲלִיטָה II.—*Part. pass.* חָלוּט a paste prepared by stirring, *dumpling.* Y. Ḥall. I, 58ª top; Y. Maasr. I, 49ᵇ ח׳ ברור a real *ḥalut* (concerning which there is no doubt as to the obligation of *Ḥallah*). Y. Ab. Zar. II, 42ª top ח׳ מחוסר וכ׳ the *ḥalut* (prepared by a gentile) wants finishing through fire (frying or boiling); a. fr.

Nif. נֶחְלַט *to become consistent through stirring.* Y. Ḥall. l. c. נֶחְלְטָה כל צורכה sufficiently stirred to be a consistent paste-ball.

חֲלַט ch. same, 1) *to make a paste.* Targ. II Sam. XIII, 6.—2) (cmp. next wds. a. צמת) *to cause contraction* by scalding or by putting in vinegar. *Part. pass.* חֲלִיט. Hull. 111[a] וה׳ הוי מעיקרא Rashi (ed. מִיחֲלַט הוה ח׳ ליה וכ׳) it (the liver) was first scalded (so as to emit no blood in boiling).

Pa. חַלֵּיט *to cause contraction, to scald, put in vinegar.* Ib. חַלְּטֵיה ליה וכ׳. Pes. 74[b] bot. חלא דח׳ ביה וכ׳ vinegar which one has used once for drawing the blood from meat and contracting the blood vessels, must not be used a second time.

Ithpa. אִתְחַלַּט, *Ithpe.* אִיתְחֲלַט, אִיחֲלֵט 1) *to be mixed up, to mingle.* Targ. Prov. XX, 19; XXIV, 21 (h. text תתערב).—2) *to be confused.* Ib. XIV, 16 (h. text מתעבר!).—3) *to be contracted,* v. supra.

חָלַט II (b. h.; cmp. חָלַץ) [*to surround, tie up* (corresp. to b. h. צמת),] 1) *to make final. Part. pass.* חָלוּט, f. חֲלוּטָה *permanently sold, irredeemable.* Arakh. IX, 4 הגיע ... היה ח׳ וכו׳ (Talm. ed. 31[a] היתה ח׳, read: חלוטה) when the last day .... had passed and it (the house) was not redeemed, it was his forever ..., for we read לצמיתות (Lev. XXV, 30); (Tosef. ib. V, 10 צמת). Arakh. l. c. בראשונה ... שיהא ח׳ לו formerly the purchaser used to hide himself on the last day .... in order that it might become his irredeemably; Sifra B'har ch. V, Par. 4 שתהא חלוטה לו. Arakh. 31[b] לְמִי ח׳ to which (of the two buyers) did it belong finally?; a. fr.—V. חֲלוּטִין.—2) *to pass final judgment on a leper* after probationary enclosure (Lev. XIII). Zeb. 102[a] אני מסגירה ואני חוֹלְטָהּ וכ׳ I will lock her up, declare her a leper and discharge her.

Hif. הֶחֱלִיט 1) *to pass final judgment, to make valid; to adjudicate.* Y. Dem. VII, beg. 26[a] צריך לְהַחֲלִיט וכ׳ he must make the consecrating conditions valid by speech. Y. Keth. X, 33[d] bot. אי זה .. לְהַחֲלִיט מַחֲלִיטִין which of them the court chooses to declare valid, it may &c. Gen. R. s. 61 שלא תַחֲלִיט להם וכ׳ lest thou surrender the country to them (through bad argument); Yalk. ib. 110 (insert להם). Y. Ab. Zar. I, 39[b] top גסות ... היא הֶחֱלִיטַתּוּ his haughtiness made Jerob. a confirmed sinner; a. e.—2) *to declare a person a leper.* Y. M. Kat. I, 80[c] bot. מטמא ומַחֲלִיט declares him unclean and this a decided leper; ורבנן ... ומַחֲלִיטִין and the Rabbis say, he must be examined as if it were a new case, but at all events they declare &c.—*Part. pass.* מוּחְלָט, f. מוּחְלֶטֶת 1) *irrevocable, confirmed.* Yoma 86[b] תשובת המוּחְלָטִין the repentance of the confirmed sinners.—2) *the declared leper,* opp. to מוּסְגָּר. Meg. I, 7. Yeb. 103[b]. Tosef. Naz. VI, 1 מ׳ בספק one declared a leper from doubt; Y. ib. VIII, end, 57[b]; a. fr.

חֲלַט ch. same, 1) *Part. pass.* חֲלִיטָא, חֲלִיט, *irredeemably sold.* Targ. Y. Gen. XLVII, 20.—2) *to sentence a leper.* Targ. Y. Deut. XXI, 5 לְמַחְלוּט, v. *Af.*

Pa. חַלֵּיט *to sell irredeemably, to forfeit.* Y. Pes. IV, 31[b] bot. ולא יְחַלְּטוּן בניהון that they might not forfeit their pledged children. Y. Shebi. VI, 36[c] bot. [read:] בגין דלא תְחַלְּטוּן .. ביד that you might not surrender the government to their (the Samaritans') hands. Y. Keth. IX, 33[b] bot. אנן מְחַלְּטִין וכ׳ we shall declare their property forfeited. Arakh. 31[b] ולחַלְּטֵיה הקדש let the sacred treasury be declared its permanent owner; a. e.

Af. אַחְלֵט *to sentence a leper.* Targ. Y. Lev. XIII, 11.—Part. pass. מַחְלַט, f. מַחְלְטָא. Ib. 51.

Ithpe. אִיתְחֲלַט *to become irredeemable.* Arakh. 32[b] וירושלים מי מִיחְלַט בה are buildings in Jerusalem ever irredeemable?

חֲלָטָא f. (preced.) *final decision, adjudication.*—*Pl.* חֲלָטָתָא. B. Mets. 16[b] שטרי ח׳ legal documents giving the claimant the title for the seized property.

חוּל׳, חֲלָטָנִית f. = חֲלוּטִין, *final action;* לח׳ *irredeemably.* Y. Gitt. IV, end, 46[b] (expl. לִצְמִיתות, Lev. XXV, 23) לחול׳; Y. Dem. IV, 24[d] bot.—Gen. R. s. 28, end, v. זְרִיבָה; a. e.

חֲלַטְרַיָּא, v. חֲלִיטַר.

חַלְטָתָא f. *lizzard,* v. חֲלַטְּתָא.

חָלָה, חָלִי (b. h.; cmp. חלל) 1) *to be lax, to be sick, faint away, grieve.* Ex. R. s. 43 (expl. ויחל, Ex. XXXII, 11 ח׳ משה Moses was sick (grieved). Kidd. 71[b], a. e. מדי חוֹלָה Media is sick, v. פּוּסָס.—Ber. 28[b] כשח׳ וכ׳ when R. ... fell sick; a. fr.—V. חוֹלֶה.—2) *to be smooth* (to the taste), *sweet.*

Pi. חִלָּה 1) *to soften, sweeten; to soothe, assuage* (by prayer, gifts &c.). Ex. R. l. c. מהו וַיְחַל שהכניס וכ׳ what does *vayḥal* (Ex. l. c.) mean? He offered &c. (ref. to Ps. XLV, 13). Ib. מהו ויחל עשה את המר וכ׳ he made sweet what was bitter. Ib. חַלֵּי מרירתן וכ׳ sweeten thou the bitterness (sin) of Israel &c.—Ib. מי שיְּחַלֶּה וכ׳ one to sweeten the bitterness &c. (by prayer). Yalk. Ex. 392 אביי אמר עד שֶׁחִלָּהוּ לחקב״ה בתפילתו (v. infra) Ab. explained *vayḥal,* until he assuaged (the anger of) the Lord &c. Deut. R. s. 3 הרי בניך מרים חַלֵּה אותן thy children are bitter, sweeten them. Ib. היאך יהא א״ל הוי חל אתה היאך אהא אומר א״ל הוי אומר חַלֵּה את המרים, read: רחמים what shall I say? Said He, Say, sweeten &c.; Yalk. Ex. 392. Lam. R. to I, 2 לא חִלִּינוּ פניך we did not assuage thee by repentance; Ex. R. s. 45 חִלִּינוּ מלפני הקב״ה we prayed &c.; a. fr.

Hif. הֶחֱלָה 1) *to assuage, soften.* Ber. 32[a] אביי אמר עד שֶׁהֶחֱלָהוּ לחקב״ה בתפלה Ms. M. (v. D. S. a. l.) until he assuaged &c., v. supra. [Ib. שה׳ עליהם וכ׳, read: שֶׁהֵחֵל, v. חָלַל.]—2) *to make sick, wear out.* Ib. עמד משה ... עד שהחלהו (Ms. M. עד שחלה) Moses stood in prayer ... until He wore Him out (by his persistency, v. Rashi a. l. a. Rabb. D. S. a. l. note 3).—3) (v. חָלַל a. חִלְחֵל) *to permeate, affect.* B. Mets. 107[b] bile is called *maḥlah* (v. מַחֲלָה) שהיא מַחֲלָה וכ׳ (Ms. F. שמְּחַלֶּלֶת) for it goes through the entire body [perh. מְחַלָּה, fr. חָלַל].

Hof. הוּחֲלָה *to be made sick.* Ber. l. c. עמד .... עד שה׳ ed. Sonc. a. oth. (v. supra) until He was worn out.

חֲלָא, חֲלִי ch. same, 1) *to be soft, sweet.* Targ. Prov. XXVII, 7. Targ. Y. II Lev. II, 11 (h. text דבש); a. e.—

2) *to be sick, grieve.* Yoma 22ᵇ; B. Kam. 20ᵇ כמה לא ח׳ וכ׳ how little does he whom the Lord supports need to grieve or trouble himself! — 3) *to remit.* Keth. 86ᵃ top וּתִיחֲלָה, v. חול II ch.

Pa. חַלֵּי 1) *to sweeten.—Part. pass.* f. מְחַלְּיָא. Cant. R. to III, 4 בשעת מְחַלְּיַית שינתא during the sweetest sleep. Ab. Zar. 39ᵃ מח׳ שמנוניתא Ms. M. the fatty substance (absorbed in the knife) becomes sweet again (loses its bad taste); ed. מְחַלְּיָא ליה ש׳ (read: לש׳) it (the strong taste of assa foetida) sweetens &c. [Ber. 6ᵇ קא מחליין ed., Ms. מחללי, v. חָלַל I.]

Ithpe. אִתְחֲלִי (אִתְחַלֵּי) *to become sweet.* Targ. Y. II Ex. XV, 25.

חֲלֵי m. (preced.) *sweet.* Targ. Y. II Gen. XLIX, 21. Targ. Y. II Deut. XXIX, 17 (ed. Amst. חֲלֵי; Y. I חוֹלֵי, חוּלֵי).—Arakh. 10ᵇ (play on חָלִיל) דח׳ קליה because its sound is sweet.—*Fem.* חֲלִיתָא, חֲלֵיאֲתָא, חֲלָיָא. Targ. Prov. XXIV, 13 דחליא ed. Lag. (ed. Wil. דְחֵלְיָא, corr. acc.). —Targ. Ps. XIX, 11 (Ms. חֲלָיָיאתָא, pl.)— Sabb. 109ᵇ אתרוגא חליתא a sweet orange.—*Pl.* חֲלָיִין, חֲלַיִין (חוּלֵיי). Targ. Ps. CXIX, 103. Targ. Prov. IX, 17 (some ed. חלים, corr. acc.) Ib. II, 16.—Ab. Zar. 38ᵇ חוּלֵיי as to sweet ones, v. אֲהִינָא.

חֳלִי, חוֹלִי m. (b. h.; חָלָה) 1) *disease.* Snh. 64ᵃ אם תעמוד . . . מֵחָלְיָהּ if this woman (I) shall rise from her sickness. Ib. מוטב שתחזור . . לְחוֹלְיָהּ I would rather relapse into my disease; a. fr.—B. Mets. 87ᵃ דחָלָה ח׳ אחריתי (missing in Mss., v. Rabb. D. S. a. l. note) that he had been sick once before.—*Pl.* חֳלָיִים, חֳלָיִם, חֳלָאִין, חֳלָאִים. Sot. 47ᵃ. Gen. R. s. 56; a. fr.—2) (sub. בעל) *patient, sufferer.* Ḥull. 110ᵃ; a. fr.

חֲלְיָא m. (חלי) *secretion, serum.* Pes. 74ᵇ חֲלְיֵיהּ אסיר its serum is forbidden. [Ib. 115ᵇ חלייה דחבלין, v. חוּלְיָא II.]

חֲלִיאֲתָא, v. חֲלֵי.

חֲלִין, חִילּ׳ m. (v. חִלָּזוֹן) *one afflicted with an eye-disease called* חִלָּזוֹן. Targ. O. Lev. XXI, 20 (ed. Berl. חִלִּין, v. Berl. Masorah p. 72).

חֲלִין, *Pa.* of חֲלַז.

חֲלִיטָא I f. part. of חָלַט.

חֲלִיטָא II f., pl. **חֲלִיטָתָא** (v. חָלַט II) *strings, necklace.* Targ. Is. III, 20 (h. text לחשים). Targ. Hos. II, 15 חֲלִיטַת וכ׳ (constr.) her pearl-strings (h. text חלית).

חֲלִיטָא III (חֲלִיטָה, חָלוּ׳) c. ch.=h. חֲלִיטָה II or חָלוּט (v. חָלַט I). Y. Ned. VI, beg. 39ᶜ; Y. Naz. V, 55ᶜ top. Y. Ab. Zar. V, 44ᵈ bot. חֲלִיטָן their (the Samaritans') *ḥalut.—Pl.* (fem.) חֲלִיטָתָא; (masc.) חֲלִיטִין. Targ. II Sam. XIII, 6; 8.—Y. Ḥall. I, 57ᵈ ח׳ דשוק *ḥ.* sold in the market (mixed with oil), v. אִסְקְרִיטִין.—Ib. (expl. חלת מסרת) ח׳ דמייר water-*ḥ.* (for which Pes. 37ᵇ חלוט של בעלי בתים). Y. Erub. III, 20ᵈ אכל חלוטן (read: חליטין or חליטא); Gen. R. s. 94, beg. חֲלוּטִין (Ar. אֲלִיטִין, dial. for ח׳).

חֲלִיטָה I f.=ch. חֲלִיטָא II. Y. Meg. I, 71ᶜ bot. היה כתבו עשור כחצי ח׳ if the writing was in the shape of half a necklace (of three or more strings, i. e. in decreasing lines).

חֲלִיטָה II (הַחֲלָטָה) f. (=חָלוּט, v. חָלַט I) *a paste made of flour stirred in boiling water, dumpling.* Ḥall. I, 6; Y. ib. 58ᵃ top ח׳ קמח לתוך חמין *ḥălitah* is flour put into hot water, contrad. to מעיסה which is חמין לתוך קמח (v. Tosef. ib. I, 1); Pes. 37ᵇ (Ms. O. החלטה; v. vers. in Rabb. D. S. a. l. note 6); Y. ib. II, 29ᶜ.— Y. Ber. VI, 10ᵇ.

חֲלִיטָה III f. (חָלַט II, v. הֶחְלֵט) *the priest's final decision on leprosy.* Sifra Thazr. Par. 3, ch. IV לאחר חֲלִיטַת מחיה וכ׳ (R. S. to Neg. VIII, 1 חִלּוּט) immediately after having originally declared it unclean on account of a sound spot in the sore (Lev. XIII, 10, sq.). [Ib. החלט מחיה].

חֲלִיטְרָא, חֲלִיטַר m. (denom. of חֲלִיטָא III) *seller of pastry, confectioner.* Y. B. Bath. II, beg., 13ᵇ, v. אִיסְטִיב. Y. Ḥall. II, 58ᶜ bot.; a. e.—*Pl.* חֲלִיטְרַיָּא. Y. Shebi. VII, 37ᶜ top חלטריא.

חליית, Pes. 115ᵇ, v. חוּלְיָא II.

חָלַל (v. חָלַל) *to turn, bore, chisel.* Targ. Is. X, 15.

חָלִיל m. (b. h.; חָלַל, v. preced.) *fife, flute;* frequ. הֶחָלִיל *the flute-players, the music in the procession.* Arakh. II, 3 הח׳ מכה וכ׳ the fluters play in front of the altar. Ib. 10ᵇ היינו ח׳ היינו אבוב *ḥalil* and *abbub* are the same. Bicc. III, 3 הח׳ מכה לפניהם the fluters precede them playing. Succ. V, 1 הח׳ חמשה וכ׳ for musical performance (on the Succoth festival) there are five and six days respectively; a. fr.—*Pl.* חֲלִילִים, חֲלִילִין. Arakh. II, 3. B. Mets. VI, 1 לחביא ח׳ וכ׳ to bring pipers for a wedding or a funeral. Kinnim III, 6; a. fr.

חֲלִילָא ch. same. Targ. Y. Deut. XVI, 14.—*Pl.* חֲלִילִין. Targ. Ps. CL, 4 (h. text מִנִּים).

חֲלִילָא c. (v. preced.) 1) *hollow.* Constr. חֲלִיל. Targ. Ex. XXVII, 8 (h. text נְבוּב).—2) *rounded, going all around.* B. Bath. 61ᵃ, v. בַּרְקָא III.—Ab. Zar. 10ᵇ, v. קמוניא.—*Pl.* חֲלִילַיָּא, f. חֲלִילָתָא. Targ. II Chr. XXVI, 15.— Sabb. 57ᵃ ח׳ תיכי chains composed of chord rings (v. חוּלְיָא I).

חֲלִילָה adv. (v. preced.) 1) *round about, in turn.* Succ. V, 6 חוזרין ח׳ they take turns all around. Keth. X, 6. Tosef. Zeb. I, 1 חזרנו ח׳ we are moving in a circle, i. e. this way of arguing will lead to no conclusion; Zeb. 10ᵇ חוזרני ח׳ ed. I am moving &c.; a. e.—2) (b. h.; cmp. חוּלִין s. v. חול III) *outside, foreign to.* Gen. R. s. 49; Yalk. ib. 83 (expl. חללה, Gen. XVIII, 25), v. בְּרָאָה, a. חול III; Tanḥ. Vayera 8 חָלָלָה כתיב it may be read *ḥălalah* (desecration), לא חול הוא לך is it not too profane for thee?

חֲלִים m. ch. (cmp. חָלוּם s. v. חָלַם I) *sound, capable of restoration to the original strength* or *form.* Ab. Zar. 69ᵃ

דמיינן דח׳ sometimes the disturbed pitching of the stopper resumes its original shape (by melting and hardening again). Ḥull. 123[b] עור ח׳ leather (if split or rent) can be so mended as to regain its original strength. Ib. כי אמרינן דח׳ וכ׳ when do we say, leather can be mended &c., when it is split straight through.—[R. Hash. 28[a], v. חֲלַם I].—[Targ. Prov. IX, 17 חלים some ed., v. חֲלֵי.]

חֲלִים *dreaming*, v. חֲלַם II.

חַלִּים, *Pa.* of חֲלַם I.

חֲלִימָה, v. חֶלְמָה.

חֲלִין, v. חִלִּין.

חֲלֵיף, v. חֲלַף.

חֲלִיף m. (חָלַף) *sharp knife, slaughtering-knife.—Pl.* חֲלִיפוֹת.—בית הח׳ the place in the Temple where the slaughtering knives were kept. Midd. IV, 7 (Talm. ed. פה . . . ., corr. acc.); Yoma 36[a] מן בית הח׳ וכ׳ Ms. M. a. Ar. (ed. מן הח׳) inside of the knives' cell.

חֲלִיפָא pr. n. m. *Hălifa.* B. Bath. 123[a] bot. אבא ח׳ (Ms. M. חלפתא, Var. חילפא, חלפא, סיל׳, v. Rabb. D. S. a. l. note).

חֲלִיפָה f. (b. h. חָלַף) 1) *replacement, substitution.* Y. Ber. II, 5[c] when a scholar dies, מי מביא לנו חֲלִיפָתוֹ who will get us one to take his place?—2) pl. חֲלִיפוֹת *shoots*, v. חֲלַף I.

חֲלִיפִין, חֲלִיפִים m. pl. (חָלַף) 1) *exchange, substitution.* Kidd. I, 6 כיון . . . . זה בַחֲלִיפָיו as soon as one of the parties to the exchange has taken possession, the other takes the risk for its exchange. Y. Ber. II, 5[c], a. e. יש להן ח׳ can be replaced; a. fr.—Esp. *ḥălifin*, a form of possession by handing to the purchaser an object as a symbolical substitute (v. Ruth IV, 7). Kidd. 22[b] אף בח׳ a slave, may be taken possession of also by symbol. B. Mets. 45[b], a. fr. אין מטבע נעשה ח׳ coins cannot be used for symbolical delivery; a. fr.—2) *young shoots* (coming out of a stump). Shebi. I, 8. Tosef. B. Kam. II, 1 (Y. ib. 3[a] top חִילְפִין).

חֲלִיץ m. (חָלַץ) *knot, loop-knot.—Pl.* חֲלִיצִין. Tosef. Neg. V, 10 וח׳ שבבקעת ed. Zuck. (Var. שבפקע׳; some ed. incorr. חליצו) the loops in a skein.

חֲלִיצָה f. (חָלַץ) *taking out; untying, putting off.* Tosef. Neg. VI, 10 בח׳ as regards taking out the leprous stone (Lev. XIV, 40), v. נְתִיצָה. Y. Ber. III, beg. 5[d] בח׳ as regards taking off the T'fillin.—Esp. (=חֲלִיצַת מִנְעָל) *Hălitsah*, the ceremony of taking off the Yabam's shoe (Deut. XXV, 5—11). Yeb. XII, 1 מצות ח׳ וכ׳ the proper way of performing the *H.* is before three men acting as judges. Ib. חֲלִיצָתָהּ פסולה the act &c. is invalid; a. v. fr.

חֲלִיצְתָא ch. same. Yeb. 102[a] ח׳ מעליתא a fully legal *Hălitsah.* Ib. 106[b] גיטא דח׳ a document testifying to the performance of the *Hălitsah.*

חֲלִיק, pl. constr. חֲלִיקֵי, v. חֵילֶק II.

חֲלִיקָה, v. חֵילְקָא II.

חלקוסתא, חליקוסתא, B. Kam. 31[a] Ar., Ms. H., v. סְלִיקוּסְתָא.

חֲלִי קוּפְרִי, חֲלִיקוּפְרִי m. (patron. of Σόλοι Κύπριοι) *one from Soloe* (*Aligora*), a sea-port town of Cyprus. Makhsh. I, 3 Abba José ח׳ איש טבעון Ar. (ed. two words) of Soloe, a citizen of Tibon.

חֲלִישׁ *to be weak*, v. חֲלַשׁ.

חֲלִישׁ, חָלִישׁ m.=h. חַלָּשׁ, *weak, sick.* Targ. Joel IV, 10 (ed. Lag. חַלָּשׁ).—*Fem.* חֲלִישָׁא. Targ. Lam. I, 13 (Var. חָלֵי׳; h. text דָוָה). Targ. I, Sam. IX, 21 חֲלָשָׁא.

חֲלִישׁוּת f. (preced.) *weakening, faintness.* ח׳ דעת *humiliation, defeated pride.* Num. R. s. 6 לא אעשה לחם ח׳ ד׳ I will not make them feel humiliated.

חֲלִישׁוּתָא ch. same. Targ. Hos. VII, 9 (h. text שֵׂיבָה, ed. Lag. חַלָּשׁוּ׳).

חלישתא, v. חֲשִׁילְתָא.

חֲלִיתָא f. *sweet*, v. חֲלֵי.

חלך, Targ. Job XI, 17, v. חֲלַד.

חָלַל (b. h.; v. Ges. H. Dict.[10] s. vv. חלל I, II) 1) (v. חול) *to roll, turn.* Ber. 32[a] (ref. to ויחל, Ex. XXXII, 11) שֶׁחִלֵּל עליהם מדת הדין למדת הרחמים Ms. M. (v. חָלָה) he (Moses) turned justice into mercy in their behalf; Yalk. Ex. 392 הֵחֵל (*Hif.*).—[Tanḥ. Yithro 1 מית חולל, read יְחַלֵּל.]—2) *to bore, hollow, pierce*, v. חָלִיל, חָלַל, חָלַל I.—3) *to surround; to place outside a circle*, v. חוּל III, חִילוֹנִי.

Nif. נֶחֱלַל (v. חָלַל I) *to be cut all around, be severed.* Naz. 54[a] (ref. to Num. XIX, 18) בחלל זה אבר הנ׳ מן החי 'on something severed', that means a limb which has been cut off a living body, and on which there was not flesh enough to have made healing possible; בכית זה אבר הנ׳ וכ׳ 'on something dead', that means a limb severed from a corpse; ib. 53[b].

Nif. נָחוֹל *to become* חוּלִין, *to cease to be sacred.* Shebi. I, 8 עד שֶׁיֵּחוֹלּוּ until the fruits become available for private use; Y. ib. 33[c] top מהו עד שיח׳ עד שיפדו או עד שיעשו חולין וכ׳ what does *ad sheyeḥôllu* mean? Until they are redeemed (in the fourth year), or until they become *ḥullin* of themselves (in the fifth year)?

Hif. הֵחֵל 1) [*to set in motion,*] *to begin.* Sifré Num. 134 (ref. to Deut. III, 24) אתה הַחִלּוֹתָ וכ׳ thou hast begun to open the door &c. Dem. VII, 4 וּמֵחֵל ושותה Y. ed. (v. Rabb. D. S. a. l. note) and he may at once commence drinking (Maim.; v. infra).—2) *to make* חוּלִין; *to break a vow; to profane.* Ber. l. c. (ref. to Num. XXX, 3) הוא אינו מֵיחֵל אבל אחרים מְחַלְּלִין לו he himself cannot break a vow, but others may break it for him (absolve him; Hag. 10[a] מוחל אבל . . . . מיחל . . . מוֹחֲלִין; Ex. R. s. 43 . . . .

חכם מוחֵל, corr. acc.). Dem. l. c. ומיחל ושותה and thus he *redeems*, and he may drink (R. S.); Tosef. ib. VIII, 7 ומ׳ ושותה מיד.—Kidd. 77ª (ref. to Lev. XXI, 15) מֵיחֵל he *produces profanation* (begets degraded priests), v. חָלָל II.—3) *to turn, change*. Yalk. Ex. 392, v. supra.

Pi. חִלֵּל 1) *to break a vow, to profane, to desecrate; to degrade*. Deut. R. s. 2 (play on החלת, Deut. III, 24) חִלַּלְתָּ וכ׳ hast thou not broken the oath? (Sifré Num. 134 הַחִלּוֹתָ, v. supra). Ab. III, 11 הַמְחַלֵּל את הקדשים who treats profanely sacred things (causes them to be carried out and burnt). Ab. Zar. 28ª מְחַלְּלִין עליה וכ׳ you may desecrate the Sabbath for the sake of curing it; a. fr.—Esp. *to cause the loss of the priestly status*. Macc. 2ª הַמְחַלֵּל אינו מִתְחַלֵּל he (the priest marrying a divorced woman) who causes the loss of priestly status (to his issue) does not lose the priestly status himself; הבא לְחַלֵּל ולא חִילֵּל he who intended to cause the loss of priestly status (by false testimony) and did not succeed.—2) (v. Deut. XIV, 24, sq.) *to redeem, to make available for private use*. Maas. Sh. I, 2; a. fr.

Pa. חוּלַּל 1) *to be removed from the priestly status, become a* חָלָל. Kidd. 77ª (ref. to Lev. XXI, 15 'he shall not degrade') לא יְחוּלַּל זה וכ׳ no degradation shall be caused—which can only refer to a person who had a status and now becomes degraded (i. e. his wife).—2) *to be redeemed, to become secular again*. Part. מְחוּלָּל, f. מְחוּלֶּלֶת. Dem. V, 1, a. fr. ומח׳ על המעות and it is redeemed by setting aside its value. Maas. Sh. II, 10 מה ... סלע זו ח׳ עליו (not על זו, v. Rabb. D. S. a. l.) this Sela (which has been set apart as an equivalent for second tithes) shall be redeemed against the wine which the clean (sons of mine) may drink in Jerusalem, i. e. I buy with this Sela only that portion of the wine which the clean may drink. Ib. הרי מעות האלו מְחוּלָּלִים וכ׳ that money (dedicated for purchasing equivalents in Jerusalem) shall be redeemed against thy fruits; a. v. fr.—3) *to be loosely joined, to be a movable link*. Sabb. 52ᵇ בִּמְחוּלָּלִין referring to movable links, (v. חוּלְיָא I). Y. Pes. I, 27ᶜ top בִּמְחוּלָּלוֹת when the vessels can be rolled about, opp. אפיצות close together (v. חָלַחַל).

Hithpa. הִתְחַלֵּל, *Nithpa.* נִתְחַלֵּל 1) [*to be perforated*,] (of bowels) *to be loose*. Esth. R. to I, 8 שיִּתְחַלְּלוּ מעיו.—2) *to be profaned, desecrated, degraded*. Ab. I, 11. Macc. 2ª, v. supra. Yeb. 79ª ואל יִתְחַלֵּל וכ׳ rather than that the name of the Lord be profaned in public; a. fr.

חֲלַל I ch. same, 1) *to perforate*, v. חֲלִיל.—2) *to degrade, profane*. Part. pass. חֲלִיל, f. חֲלִילָא. Targ. O. Lev. XXI, 14.—3) (denom. of חוּלָּא) *to be profaned*. Targ. Ez. XXII, 26 וְחַלֵּת.

Pa. חַלֵּיל 1) *to desecrate, profane, degrade*. Targ. Prov. XXX, 9; a. e.—*Part. pass.* מְחַלַּל, f. מְחַלְּלָא, מְחַלָּא. Targ. O. Lev. XXI, 7 (ed. Berl. מְחַלָּא, Regia מְחָלְלָא).—Y. Kil. IX, 32ᵇ top, a. e. דילמא דִחַלֵּלְנַן וכ׳ did we perhaps desecrate the Sabbath?—Ber. 6ª מְחַלְּלֵי Ms. (ed. מחללין); a. e.—2) *to redeem*. B. Mets. 44ᵇ טבעא אפירא לא מְחַלְּלִינַן we dare not redeem coins with goods.

Af. אַחֵיל, אַחֵיל same, *to desecrate*. Targ. O. Lev. XIX, 8. Targ. Am. II, 7 לְאַחָלָא (ed. Lag. לאפסא); a. fr.—Part. pass. f. מְחַלָּא, v. supra.

Ittaf. אִתְּחַל, אִתְּחַל, אִתְחַל *to be profaned*. Targ. Ez. XXXVI, 23 (not אִתְחַל). Ib. VII, 24; a. fr.—Snh. 51ª הדיכא מיח׳ וקדימא דמִיתְחַלָּא השתא if she degraded herself now; she was degraded before this.

חֲלַל II (cmp. חלחל), (mostly) *Pa.* חַלֵּיל (v. preced.) [*to turn in a hollow space*,] *to wash, rinse*. Targ. II Chr. IV, 6. Targ. Lev. I, 9; a. fr.—Hull. 113ª דחַלְלֵי בי טבחא when they washed the meat in the slaughter house.

Af. אַחְלִיל same. Targ. Ruth III, 3.—Hull. 95ᵇ top מַחְלִיל רישא וכ׳ (or מְחַלֵּיל) Ar. (ed. מחוור) he was washing an animal's head in the river, v. חֲוַר.

חָלָל I m. (b. h.; חָלַל) *cut all around, beheaded*, in gen. *slain*. Sot. 45ᵇ (ref. to Deut. XXI, 1) ח׳ ולא חנוק slain but not strangled, ח׳ ולא מפרפר וכ׳ slain but not rolling in dying agony. Ib. IX, 4 ממקום שנעשה ח׳ מצוארו from the place where he has been cut, that means, (the measurement starts) from his throat, v. חָלָל III. Y. Naz. VII, 56ᶜ (ref. to Num. XIX, 18) בח׳ כל שהוא ח׳ *beḥalal* means whoever is slain, בח׳ זה אבר וכ׳ *beḥalal* means a severed limb ...... without sufficient flesh, v. חָלַל, *Nif.*—Hull. 3ª, a. e. (ref. to Num. XIX, 16) חרב הרי היא כח׳ a sword (with which a person has been killed) has the same levitical status as a slain body. Koh. R. to VIII, 10; Yalk. Ps. 808, a. e. (play on מתחולל Job XV, 20) מת וח׳ (the wicked man even in his life-time) is dead and beheaded; Tanh. Yithro 1 מת חולל (corr. acc.); ib. ed. Bub.; a. fr.—*Pl.* חֲלָלִים. Sot. 45ª; a. e.

חָלָל II (b. h.; חָלַל) [*put outside*,] *halal, one unfit for priesthood on account of his father's illegitimate connection* (Lev. XXI, 7; 14, sq.). Kidd. IV, 6. Snh. 51ª; a. fr.—*Pl.* חֲלָלִין, חֲלָלִים. Kidd. 77ª, v. מִקְוֶה; a. e.—Fem. חֲלָלָה *the female issue of a priest's illegitimate connection*, or *a priest's wife illegitimately married to him*. Ib. ח׳ מזוכרת, v. זָכַר; a. fr.—*Pl.* חֲלָלוֹת. Ib., v. מִקְוֶה; a. e.

חָלָל III m. (חָלַל) 1) *cavity, empty space, hollow; throat; inside*. Ukts. II, 8 ממעך את חֲלָלָהּ you squeeze its cavity (compress it); Y. Yoma VIII, 44ᵈ bot. (v. Löw, Pfl. p. 123). Ab. Zar. 28ª מכה של ח׳ an internal sore (as in the mouth, throat &c.). Y. ib. II, 40ᵈ top; Y. Sabb. XIV, 14ᵈ top כל שהוא מן הח׳ ולפנים וכ׳ whatever is in the throat and farther inside may be cured on the Sabbath, opp. to מן השפה; cmp. Sot. 45ᵇ quot. s. v. חָלָל I. Hull. III, 1 if the heart is perforated לבית חֲלָלוֹ up to its chamber. Ber. 19ᵇ ח׳ טפח a hollow space of one hand-breadth. Hull. 44ᵇ. Pes. 54ª חֲלָלָהּ the formation of its interior; a. fr.—*Pl.* חֲלָלִים. Ber. 60ᵇ, v. חָלוּל.—2) (cmp. חַלְחוֹלִית) *intricacy, devices*. Sabb. 11ª חֲלָלָהּ של רשות the devices of political government.

חֲלָלָא, חֲלָלָה ch. same, 1) *space, cavern, hole*. Targ. Y. Lev. XXIII, 42.—Y. Kil. IX, 32ᶜ bot.; Y. Keth. XII, 35ᵇ יהבון בית ח׳ put them into a cavern. Ab. Zar. 28ᵇ ח׳ דבי צוארא neck-hole of a garment. Y. ib. II, 40ᵈ top עביר עינא כחללה (not כחל לה) considers the eye like an inner organ (for treatment on the Sabbath, v. preced.).—2) pl. חֲלָלֵי, in ח׳ דעלמא the underground treasures of the world. Snh. 97ᵃ; B. Mets. 49ᵃ (חללא, corr. acc., v. Rabb. D. S. a. l. note 6).—3) secrets. Sabb. 77ᵇ if they asked him כל ח׳ עלמא about all the secret processes of nature.

חֲלָלָה f., v. חָלָל II, a preced. w.

חָלַם I (b. h.; cmp. חלב) [to be soft, moist, viscous,] to have good humors, to be well. Part. pass. חָלוּם, f. חֲלוּמָה sane, opp. to שוטה; well, opp. to חולה. Tosef. Ter. I, 3 פעמים . . . . ח׳ if one is at times insane, at times sane; R. Hash. 28ᵃ חָלִים (Ch. form).—Y. Gitt. VII, beg. 48ᶜ.—Pes. 78ᵇ.—Fem. חֲלוּמָה. Y. Yeb. XIV, beg. 14ᵇ.

חֲלַם ch. same, v. חֲלִים.

Pa. חַלֵּים to join closely. Kidd. 25ᵃ זמנין דח׳ שפוותיה Ar. (ed. שפתיה) sometimes a man closes his lips firmly.

חָלַם II (b. h.; v. preced. wds.) [to gather humors, to sleep well (cmp. יָשֵׁן).—Denom. חֲלוֹם (cmp. ἐνύπνιος, somnium) dream; from which חָלַם] to dream. Ber. 55ᵇ חלום חֲלַמְתִּי I had a dream. Ib. חלום שח׳ לו חבירו a dream which his neighbor had about him. Tosef. Sabb. VI (VII), 7 שתחא חולם חלומות that you may have dreams; a. fr.

חֲלַם, חֲלִים ch. same. Targ. Gen. XXXVII, 5. Ib. XLI, 1; a. fr.

Af. אַחְלֵים to consult an interpreter of dreams or a dreamer. Targ. Jer. XXIX, 8, v. חָלְמָא.

חֲלַם, v. חֲלוֹם.

חֶלְמָא, חֵיל׳ m.ch.=h. חֲלוֹם. Targ. Gen. XXXVII, 6; a. fr.—Ber. 56ᵃ חֶלְמַאי my dream. Ib. בְּחֶלְמִין in our dream; a. fr.—*Pl.* חֶלְמַיָּא, חֶלְמִין, חֵיל׳. Targ. Joel III, 1; a. fr.—[Targ. Job VI, 6 מרירי חלמיא, ed. Lag. לחמא, ed. Wil. ריירא דחלמונא.]

חָלְמָא m. (preced., v. P. Sm. 1284) dreamer, or interpreter of dreams.—*Pl.* חָלְמַיָּא, constr. חָלְמֵי. Targ. Jer. XXIX, 8 חָלְמֵי חֶלְמֵיכוֹן וכ׳ (not חֶל׳, חֵיל׳) your dreamers (or interpreters) whom you consult.

חֲלָמָא (חלמה) I f. (חָלַם I) a sort of cement used for making vessels. Kel. XI, 4 (Ar. a. ed. Dehrenb. חלמה); Tosef. ib. B. Mets. I, 4, sq.

חֲלָמָה II f. (v. preced.) joint, seam in leather; cmp. חֲלָבָה. Sabb. 91ᵇ bot. מקום ח׳ the place where the bag is joined (which the thief might rip to take possession of its contents).

חַלְמִית, חֶלְמָה f. (חָלַם I) name of several mucilaginous plants (v. P. Sm. 1284 s. v. חלמתא), prob. mallows. Y. Kil. V, end, 30ᵃ; Y. Ber. VI, 10ᵇ bot. חלמיה (read: חֵיל׳); Tosef. Kil. III, 12 חֵילְמִית ed. Zuck. (Var. חלמית).

חֶלְמוֹן (חֵל׳) m. (v. preced.) yolk, yellow of an egg. Ab. Zar. 40ᵃ: Hull. 64ᵃ (corr. as in Ab. Zar. l. c.). Y. Ter. X, 47ᵇ bot. בלובן חלמין (read: בחלמון, v. Tosaf. to Hull. 64ᵇ, s. v. וחוא); v. חֶלְבּוֹן. [Ar. reads חלמון.]

חֶלְמוֹנָא ch. same. Targ. Job VI, 6 ed. Wil. (v. חֶלְמָא).

חַלָּמִית, חַלָּמוּת f. (b. h.?; v. preced. wds.) mucilaginous juice of mallows, used for the preservation of gourd seed. Kil. I, 8 (Y. ed. a. Ar. ית ...., Mish. a. Babli ed. ות ....).

חלמין, v. חֶלְמוֹן.

חַלָּמִישׁ pr. n. pl. Hallamish (Rock), a place near Naveh (v. נָוֶה III) and inhabited by hostile gentiles. Lev. R. s. 23; Cant. R. to II, 2; Lam. R. to I, 17.

חַלְמִית, v. חֶלְמָה; חַלָּמִית, v. חַלָּמוּת.

חלכונא, v. חִלְזוֹנָא.

חָלַף (b. h.; cmp. חלב, חלם) [to be smooth, glistening, sharp-edged,] 1) to cut. Denom. חֲלִיפָה, חַלְּיָה.—2) (cmp. פוּז) to pass by, be gone. Num. R. s. 10 (ref. to חֲלוֹף, Prov. XXXI, 8) שח׳ וחלך וכ׳ of him who passed away and went &c.—3) to change, exchange. Y. Ber. II, 5ᶜ top נַחֲלִיף את וכ׳ let us change our meeting-place. Dem. III, 5 חשודה לַחֲלוֹף (Y. ed. לחַלֵּף, *Pi.*) suspected of exchanging (the provision in her trust). Ib. 6 לח׳ את המתקלקל to replace what has been spoiled; a. fr.

Pa. חַלֵּף same. Yalk. Gen. 148 מי מְחַלְּפוֹ who will replace him? (v. חֲלִיפִין). Dem. III, 5, v. supra; a. e.

Hif. הֶחֱלִיף 1) to exchange, barter. B. Mets. VIII, 4 המַחֲלִיף פרה בח׳ if one exchanges a cow for an ass.—Dem. l. c. חשודה לְהַחֲלִיף, v. supra; Hull. 6ᵇ חשודה מַחֲלֶפֶת; a. fr.—2) to drive young shoots, to grow again.. Erub. 100ᵇ; a. e., v. גָּזַע. Pesik. R. s. 11 בְּמַחֲלִיף וכ׳, v. גָּזַז.—3) to change; to reverse. Erub. 9ᵃ ובלבד שלא יַחֲלִיפוּ provided they do not change carriers. Sabb. 8ᵇ; a. fr.—Erub. 99ᵃ לעולם לא תַחֲלִיף it is not necessary to reverse (the authorities; Bets. 3ᵇ, a. e. היפוך, v. אָפַךְ).—Part. pass. מוּחְלָף, f. מוּחְלֶפֶת. Ib. מ׳ חשיטה the statement must be reversed (the authorities for the two opinions must be exchanged); Bets. 3ᵃ.—4) to be ambiguous, to equivocate. Snh. 92ᵃ; a. e. כל המחליף וכ׳ he who equivocates in his speech, is like an idolater.

Nif. נֶחֱלַף, *Hithpa.* הִתְחַלֵּף, *Nithpa.* נִתְחַלֵּף 1) to be exchanged, mixed up. Y. Pes. VI, 33ᶜ bot. דבר שאין דרכו לְהֵחָלֵף (לִיתְחַלֵּף) a thing which is not likely to be exchanged (by mistake); ib. לִהִתְחַלֵּף; ib.ᵈ top. Ab. Zar. 17ᵇ מעות . . . נִתְחַלְּפוּ לו וכ׳ money set aside for Purim was mixed up with money &c. Nidd. 52ᵃ ונִתְחַלְּפָה לך וכ׳ and thou madest a mistake between *Iyob* and *oyeb*; B. Bath. 16ᵃ ונתחלף לא נ׳ לי Ib. I make no mistake; a. e.—2) to change (in appearance). Pesik. R. s. 29 (—30—30) נִתְחַלַּפְתֶּם מן הרעב you have changed (beyond recognition) through starvation; יש לכם לְהִתְחַלֵּף וכ׳ you will change through plenty. Yalk. Gen. 133 מאיזה שם אני מִתְחַלֵּף (prob. לאיזה) what name I may be ordered to assume in turn.—3) to be succeeded, relieved, transferred. Lev. R. s. 23, end נתח׳ המלך the king has been succeeded (displaced; Num. R. s. 9, beg. מת וכ׳). Yalk. Deut. 813 כיון שנ׳ וכ׳ when the governor was recalled and another &c. Num. R. s. 5, beg. להִתְחַלֵּף מעבודה וכ׳ to be transferred from one service to another. Y. Taan. II, beg. 65[a] הוו מִתְחַלְּפִין עליה took turns in guarding it.

חֲלַף I, חֲלֵיף ch. same, *to pass by, be gone.* Targ. Cant. II, 11. Targ. Job IX, 11. Ib. 26; a. e.

Pa. חַלֵּיף 1) *to pass repeatedly, promenade.* Kidd. 12[b] ח׳ אבבא וכ׳ went up and down in front of the house of his father-in-law (to attract the attention of his mother-in-law).—2) *to exchange.* Targ. O. Lev. XXVII, 10; a. e. —Ḥull. 6[b] חַלּוּפֵי מבעיא so much the more may she be suspected of exchanging (substituting something of her own). Meg. 7[b] מְחַלְּפֵי וכ׳ (v. Rabb. D. S. a. l. note 8; some ed. מיח׳ *Ithpa.*) used to exchange their meals (on Purim).—*Part. pass.* f. מְחַלְּפָא. Y. Peah IV, 18[d] bot., a. e. מח׳ שיטתיה, v. preced. *Hif.*

Af. אַחֲלֵיף same. Targ. O. l. c.; a. e.

Ithpa. אִתְחַלַּף, אִיחַלַּף, *Ithpe.* אִיחֲלִיף *to be exchanged; to change; to disappear.* Targ. Ps. XC, 5; a. fr.—Gen. R. s. 78, beg. מִתְחַלְּפִין change their names. Ḥull. l. c. ולאִיחַלּוּפֵי לא וכ׳ Rashi (ed. לחַלּוּפֵי) and do we not apprehend an exchange?—Meg. l. c., v. supra.—B. Mets. 59[b], v. חָסֵר II.

חֵלֶף I m. (preced. wds.) 1) *shoot.*—*Pl.* חֲלָפִים, constr. חֶלְפֵי, חִילְ׳. Bets. 3[b]; Yeb. 81[b]; Zeb. 72[b] ח׳ תרדין the young shoots of beet growing out of the root; Orl. III, 7 Ms. M. (ed. חוּלְפוֹת; Y. ed. חִילְפוֹת); Tosef. Ter. V, 10 חֲלִיפוֹת ed. Zuck. (Var. חילפות); Ukts. I, 4 חִלְפוֹת. V. חֲלִיפָה, חֲלִיפִין.—2) *rush,* v. חִילְּה.

חֵלֶף II m. (preced. wds.) *reversion.* Y. Sabb. VII, 9[c] או ח׳ is not perhaps the reverse the case?

חֵלֶף pr. n. pl. (b. h.) *Ḥelef,* a place in Naftali. Y. Meg. I, 70[a] bot. (ref. to Josh. XIX, 33) מחלף ח׳ *me-Ḥelef* is (the present) *Ḥ.* Y. Erub. II, 20[a] top ר׳ . . . בחורי ח׳ וכ׳ R. Jerem. taught at Ḥ. &c.

חֲלַף II, חוּלַף m. st. constr. (חלף) *in place of, instead.* Targ. Ex. XXI, 24; a. fr.—Sabb. 129[a] נפשא ח׳ נפשא life for life (meat is required after bloodletting), סומקא ח׳ סומקא red (wine) for red (blood).—*Pl.* חֲלָפֵי, with suffix חֲלָפוֹי in his place. Targ. Prov. XI, 8 Ms. (ed. תחותוהי, ed. Lag. both words).—חֲלַף סִדְרָא f. (an adaptation of κλεψύδρα) [*change of order,*] *clepsydra,* a water clock used in courts of justice for measuring the time given for argument. Gen. R. s. 49 (not סרדה); Yalk. ib. 83.

חִלְפָא, v. חִילְ׳.

חֲלָפוֹת or **חִלְפוֹת,** v. חֵלֶף I.

חִלְפֵּיו, v. חִילְ׳.

חֲלַפְתָּא pr. n. m. *Ḥălafta,* R. Ḥ., a Tannai, father of R. José. Ab. III, 6. Taan. II, 5. B. Kam. 70[a] אבא ח׳ my father H.; Tosef. B. Bath. II, 10 (read: אבא ח׳); a. fr.—V. חִלְפָא.

חֲלַפְתָּא or **חִלְפְּתָא** f. (v. חִילְפָא II) a species of *willow,* corresp. to h. צַפְצָפָה. Succ. 34[a] ח׳ ערבתא וכ׳ what formerly was called *ḥ.* is now named *ărabta* and vice versa; (Rashi reads חילפא, Ms. M. corrupt vers., v. Rabb. D. S. a. l. note; Sabb. 36[a] ערבה צפצפה וכ׳).

חָלַץ (b. h., v. Ges. H. Dict.[10] s. v. חלץ I, II) 1) *to surround, fortify; to gird, arm.* Yalk. Gen. 133 (fr. Midr. Vayis'u) חָלְצוּ עצמם they armed themselves, v. *Pi.* a. *Hif.*—2) *to untie, loosen, tear out; to strip, lay bare.* M. Kat. 22[b] חוֹלֵץ one bares the shoulder (in mourning). Ib. IV, 7 (24[b]) חוֹלְצִין. B. Mets. 59[b] וח׳ מנעליו and took his shoes off. Y. M. Kat. III, 82[b] חוֹלְצָן he takes them (the T'fillin) off; Ber. 23[a]; Y. ib. II, 4[c].—Pes. 4[a]; M. Kat. 20[b] חֲלוֹץ לי מנעלי take my shoes off. Ḥull. 90[b] חוֹלְצוֹ לתפוח he takes the sinew out and puts it on the pile &c. Tosef. Neg. VI, 10 בזמן שהוא חוֹלֵץ when he has to tear out (a leprous stone), v. נָתַץ.—Y. Ab. Zar. II, end, 42[a]; Tosef. ib. IV (V), 8 כדי שיהו חוֹלְצִין את גלעיניהן in order to loosen the stones (of the olives); a. fr.—Part. pass. חָלוּץ, f. חֲלוּצָה, pl. חֲלוּצִים, f. חֲלוּצוֹת. Y. Sot. I, beg. 16[b] וזרועותיה ח׳ her arms bared.—Sabb. 137[a], a. e. חֲלָצַתּוּ חמה the fever left him.—Esp. *to perform the ceremony of taking off the Yabam's shoe* (v. יָבָם); ח׳ ביבמה *to arrange the Ḥălitsah, to act as judge;* ח׳ ל־ *to have the shoe taken off for refusing the leviratical marriage;* ח׳ מ־ *to take the shoe off.* Yeb. 102[a] כלום ראית שח׳ וכ׳ did you ever see him act as a judge at a *Ḥălitsah?* Ib. IV, 1 החוֹלֵץ ליבמתו וכ׳ if one gave *ḥălitsah* to his sister-in-law, and it was found out afterwards &c. Ib. III, 1 חוֹלְצוֹת ולא מתיבמות they must be released by *ḥăl.*, but must not be married by the *yabam.* Ib. XII, 1 חָלְצָה במנעל if she performed the ceremony with a leather shoe. Ib. 102[a] חוֹלְצִין במנעל you may have the ceremony performed with &c. Ib.[b] שמא חָלְצָה סנדל לאחד וכ׳ perhaps she has performed the ceremony of *ḥal.* on one of the brothers. Ib. החוֹלֶצֶת מן וב׳ if one performed the ceremony on an adult ... Ib. (ref. to Hos. V, 6) מי כתיב ח׳ להם ח׳ מהם וכ׳ is it written, He had his shoe taken off by them (the Lord being the rejecting party)? It is written, He took their shoe off &c., v. next w.; a. v. fr.—חֲלוּצָה *a woman released from leviratical marriage by ḥălitsah.* Ib. VII, 1. Ib. IV, 12 חֲלוּצָתוֹ his rejected sister-in-law; a. fr.

Nif. נֶחֱלַץ *to be peeled off.* Y. Sabb. XX, 17[c] bot. ועורו נ׳ and his skin will peel itself off.

Pi. חִלֵּץ 1) *to extract, loosen, to deliver.*—2) *to gird, strengthen.* Yeb. 102[b] (in a discussion about the meaning of וחלצה, Deut. XXV, 9) והכתיב יְחַלֵּץ עני but do we not read (Job XXXVI, 15), He *girds* the poor? Answ. יְחַלְּצוֹ מדינה וכ׳ It means, He will *deliver him* from the judgment &c. Ib. (after ref. to יחליץ, Is. LVIII, 11) the root חלץ means both (girding and loosening), but here (Deut. l. c.), if it meant *tying on,* it would read וחלצה נעלו ברגלו she shall tie his shoe *on* his foot.

Hif. הֶחֱלִיץ 1) *to loosen, untie;* 2) *to gird, arm;* 3) *to deliver;* 4) *to smoothen, give ease of mind.* Lev. R. s. 34 (ref. to יחליץ, Is. l. c.) יזרין (Ar. ישלוף) ישמוט ישזיב ויניח (which means) He shall *loosen* as in Deut. l. c., *gird* as ib. III, 18, *deliver* as in Ps. CXL, 2, and *give ease* as in the Sabbath prayer after meal רצה והַחֲלִיצֵנוּ be pleased to give us ease of mind. V. חִלּוּץ.

חֲלַץ ch. same, 1) *to take off, undress.* Part. pass. חֲלִיץ. Targ. II Sam. VI, 20.—Lam. R. introd (R. Joh. 1) חֲלִיצֵי מסאני without shoes. M. Kat. 22[b] לְמִיחְלַץ to bare their shoulders.—2) *to withdraw.* Yeb. 102[b] עמא דח׳ ליה . . . מיניה a people from which its lord has withdrawn (with ref. to חלץ מהם, Hos. V, 6).—3) *to perform the rite of ḥălitsah;* v. infra.

Pa. חַלֵּיץ 1) *to perform or arrange the rite of ḥălitsah.* Ib. ואילו יבמה דחַלְּצוּ (or דחלצו) לה אחין וכ׳ suppose brothers would untie the shoe of their sister-in-law, would this be of any legal consequence? Ib.[a] אנא לא הואי חַלֵּיצְנָא וכ׳ I should not have allowed a *ḥălitsah* except &c.; a. fr.—2) *to undress, strip.* Targ. I Sam. XXXI, 9. Ib. 8 (h. text לפשט); Targ. I Kings XI, 15 (h. text לקבר!).

חֲלָצַיִם m. du. (b. h.; חָלַץ 1) *loins.* Ḥag. 14[b] יצא מֵחֲלָצֶיךָ is thy offspring; a. e.

חָלַק (b. h.) 1) *to be smooth, to be viscous.* V. חָלָק.—2) (denom. of חֵלֶק) *to assign, allot.*—ח׳ כבוד *to honor, pay regards.* Ber. 19[b], a. e. כל מקום . . אין חוֹלְקִין וכ׳ wherever the desecration of the name of the Lord is threatened, no regards must be paid to a teacher. Zeb. 102[a]; a. fr.—3) (denom. of חֵלֶק) *to divide (by lot); to part; to take a share.* Peah III, 5 האחין שחָלְקוּ brothers who divided an estate. B. Mets. I, 1, a. fr. יַחֲלוֹקוּ they shall divide the object (equally). Zeb. XII, 1 אינן חוֹלְקִין וכ׳ take no share &c. Ḥull. 65[a] אם חוֹלֵק את רגליו וכ׳ if the birds parts its toes (on the rope) so that there be two on each side &c. Y. Sabb. VII, 9[c] bot. דבר . . . אינו חולק חולק if a prohibition (included in a law) is specified again for a purpose, it does not intimate a division (that each single act of the class must be atoned for singly, v. חֲבָרָה). Tosef. Dem. VI, 1 חוֹלְקָן he divides the fruits with the landlord. [Ib. 2 החולק, read: החוכר.] Y. ib. VI, beg. 25[a] מישראל חולק if the property is farmed from an Israelite, he divides the produces (before separating T'rumah); a. v. fr.—4) (with על) *to differ with, object, oppose.* Y. Sabb. XV, beg. 15[a] מה חוֹלְקִין על וכ׳ how is it? do they differ with &c.?—Ber. 27[b] החולק על ישיבתו וכ׳ וכ׳; Snh. 110[a] הח׳ על רבו (Ar. הֶנֶחְלָק, *Nif.*) he who opposes (the school of) his teacher. Ber. l. c. כלום יש אדם חוֹלֵק בדבר זה is there any one here differing from this opinion?; a. v. fr.—*Part. pass.* חָלוּק, pl. חֲלוּקִים, חֲלוּקִין *divided, interrupted; disputed; of different opinion.* Mikv. VIII, 2 מים ח׳ interrupted flow of urin.—B. Bath. 176[a] ח׳ היה ר׳ וכ׳ R. . . differed &c. Ib. IX, 10 (158[b]) על חֲלוּקִין ואתה בא לַחֲלֹק עלינו וכ׳ . . . we grieve over the divided opinions, and you come to assert a division for us on things on which they (the schools of Shammai and Hillel) agree?; (Y. Shek. III, beg. 47[b] לַחֲלוֹק). Y. Keth. I, end, 26[a] ח׳ על אביו differs with his father; a. fr.—Tosef. Yoma V (IV), 6, a. e. ארבעה חֲלוּקֵי כפרה there are four persons under different categories as to atonement. Arakh. 10[b] דחֲלוּקָה בקרבנותיה which differs (from other days) as regards sacrifices. Ib. חֲלוּקִין וכ׳ the numbers of sacrifices are different each day.

Nif. נֶחְלַק 1) *to be divided, distributed.* Midr. Till. to Ps. XXVII (ref. to אחלק, Ex. XV, 9) אֵיחָלֵק I shall be divided (plundered).—2) *to differ.* Ḥag. 16[b] נֶחְלְקוּ בה גדולי וכ׳ the great men of the age differ about it. Ber. 27[b]; Snh. 110[a], v. supra. Keth. XIII, 1; a. fr.

Hif. הֶחֱלִיק 1) *to smoothen, make even, level; to improve the appearance.* Maasr. I, 8 משיַחֲלִיקֶנּוּ from the moment that he smoothens the cake of figs (by rubbing it with figs or grapes). Ib. הַמַּחֲלִיק בענבים if one uses grapes for smoothening.—Shebi. IV, 4 בְּמַחֲלִיק when one levels a field (by taking out plants); expl. ib. המח׳ ג׳ זה בצד זה *levelling* means taking out (at least) three plants next to each other, contrad. to המדל, taking out one or two plants.—Peah III, 3, v. אָחַד; a. e.—Trnsf. *to close a tune softly* (piano). Arakh. II, 3 (10[a]) ולא היה מַחֲלִיק ולא היה מְחַלֵּק (Talm. ed. אלא . . . . מפני שהוא מחליק יפה . . .) מחליק וכ׳ none but a flute solo was used for closing a tune, because it makes a pleasant finale.—3) *to glide, slip.* Erub. X, 14 בשביל שלא יַחֲלִיקוּ that the priests might not slip. B. Mets. VI, 3 אם הֶחֱלִיקָה if the animal injured herself by slipping.—4) *to be smooth.* Yeb. 80[b] בשרו מַחֲלִיק his flesh is smooth.

Hof. הוּחְלַק 1) *to be injured by slipping.* B. Kam. 47[b] הוּחְלְקָה בהן the animal was injured by tripping over the fruits.—2) *to be smoothed.* Part. מוּחְלָק, pl. מוּחְלָקִין. B. Mets. 103[b] קנים מח׳ smoothed (peeled) poles.—[3) *to be divided up*, v. infra.]

Pi. חִילֵּק *to divide, distribute, part.* Y. Keth. II, beg. 26[a] ביא וחַלֵּק וכ׳ come and divide with me &c. Y. Peah VIII, 20[c] top; Y. Shebi. VI, beg. 36[b] שבע שחִילְּקוּ the seven years during which they distributed the land (among the tribes); Zeb. 118[b].—B. Bath. IX, 7 הַמְחַלֵּק נכסיו וכ׳ if one disposes (wills) . . by word of mouth; a. fr.—Sabb. 70[a], a. e. לְחַלֵּק, v. חֲבָרָה.—[Arakh. II, 3 (10[a]), v. supra.]—*Part. pass.* מְחוּלָּק a) *divided up, plundered.* Yalk. Ex. 249 (ref. to אחלק, Ex. XV, 9) מ׳ אני להם I shall be divided up among them; v. *Nif.*; Mekh. B'shall., Shirah, s. 7 מוחלק.—b) *distinct, separate.* Tanḥ. Ḥuck. 6 והן מְחוּלָּקִין זה מזה and they are different from one another (in the range of their intellects).

Hithpa. הִתְחַלֵּק, *Nithpa.* נִתְחַלֵּק *to be divided, distributed; to part, separate.* Par. III, 11 היה מִתְחַלֵּק וכ׳ was distributed among &c.—Snh. 34[a], v. נִיצוֹץ.—Sifré Num. 132 לְיוֹצאי מצרים נִתְחַלְּקָה וכ׳ the land was divided up according to the census taken at their going out from Egypt. Ib. לא נתח׳ . . . לכל שבט וכ׳ the land was allotted to each tribe (in a lump), according to its population. Ib. לא נתח׳ . . אלא בשמיון it was divided according to value; B. Bath. 122[a] לא נ׳ אלא בכסף.—Midr. Till. to Ps. XVIII, 2 היה מתח׳ מחיילותיו he separated himself from his armies (for prayer). Ib. וכשהיה המחנה שלו מתח׳ and because his camp was thus divided (some praying, others not praying); a. fr.

חָלָק (חָלוּק) m. (preced.) 1) *smooth, blank* (paper); *empty.* Y. Sabb. VIII, 11[b] אם יש בו ח׳ וכ׳ if there is blank space on it enough for &c. Snh. 17[a] ושנים הניח ח׳ and two ballots he left blank; a. fr.—יצא ח׳ (=ריקם) *to go out without having effected anything.* Sifré Num. 131 חלוק

ed.; Yalk. Lev. 631 (Yalk. Ex. 178 ריקם); Yalk. Hos. 517 חלוק.—Gen. R. s. 11 להוציאך ח׳ אי אפשר I cannot dismiss you without an answer; a. e.—Fem. חֲלָקָה. Kel. XXIV, 7 וח׳ and a plain board (without a receptacle). Midd. II, 5; Succ. 51[b] ח׳ היתה בראשונה formerly the compartment was plain (without a guarded balcony), v. בְּצוֹצְרָה.—Pl. חֲלָקוֹת. Tosef. Obol. XV, 1.—*2) division. Kerith. 7[a], a. fr. אַךְ ח׳, v. אַךְ I. [prob. to be read: חַלֵּק, divide!]

חֵלֶק m. (b. h.; preced. wds.) [smooth stone used for casting lots, v. I Sam. XVII, 40 חַלֻּקֵּי; cmp. גורל, גווזא; cmp. Is. XXXIV, 17; Ps. XXII, 19,] lot, share, portion. Snh. X (XI), 1 ח׳ לעו״הב a share in the world to come. Sabb. 118[b] יהא חֶלְקִי מ׳ Oh, that my lot fell among &c.; M. Kat. 18[b] יהא חלקי עם; a. fr.—Sifré Deut. 312 תנו לי חֶלְקִי give me my estate (my title) back, v. נָכַר.—Pl. חֲלָקִים. B. Mets. I, 1 שלשה ח׳ three portions (fourths). Sabb. 34[b] שלשה חֶלְקֵי מיל three parts of a mile, expl. three fourths; ב׳ ח׳ מיל two thirds; a. fr.

חֵלֶק or **חֶלֶק**, a fictitious name, v. חִילְּק.

חֲלַק m. ch. (b. h. חֶלְקָה, v. חֵלֶק) lot, field. Targ. Y. II Gen. XLIX, 21 (Var. חַקְלָא).—Pl. constr. חֲלָקֵי. Targ. I Chr. VIII, 8 Var. (ed. חקלי).

חֵילְ׳, חֶלְקָא f. (preced.) 1) same, lot, field. Targ. Prov. XXIII, 10.—Pl. חֶלְקָתָא. Targ. Mic. II, 4 חֶלְקָתְהוֹן (Var. חַלְקָתְהוֹן, ed. Lag. חַקְלָתְהוֹן; h. text שָׂדֵינוּ).—2) share, portion, ḥelka, a market term for a certain portion of meat; cmp. אוּזְיָא. Bets. 29[a].

חֲלָקָא, v. חוּלַּק.

חַלְקָא m. (cmp. חָלוּק) [shirt,] husk.—Pl. חַלְקַיָּא. M. Kat. 13[b] דשקל חַלְקַיְירוּ (Rashi דשקיל) its husks are taken off; (Ms. M. דַּשְׁוֵי חֵילְקַיְירוּ he made its parts even, divided the grain into two); v. חֵילְקָא II.

חלקוסתא, v. סְלִיקוּסְתָּא.

חִלְקִיָּה (b. h.) pr. n. m. Ḥilkiya, Hilkiah, 1) the high priest in the reign of Josiah. Meg. 14[b]; Yalk. Josh. 9; a. e.—2) father of Jeremiah the prophet. Num. R. s. 8, end. Snh. 95[a], a. fr.—3) name of several Amoraim. Y. B. Bath. III, 14[a]; Bab. ib. 39[b].—Y. Shek. I, 46[b]; a. e. (v. Fr. M'bo p. 85[a]).—Kidd. 83[b].—Yeb. 9[a].—B. Mets. 96[b]; a. e.

חֲלַקְתָא, v. חֶלְקָא.

חָלַשׁ (b. h.) 1) to relax, be weak, prostrated (cmp. חָלָה).—V. חַלָּשׁ.—2) [to round, smoothen, denom. חַלָּשׁ smooth stone; (cmp. חֵלֶק) ballot; fr. which חָלַשׁ] to cast a lot; to assign. Pesik. Zakh., p. 22[a] expl. ויחלש, (Ex. XVIII, 13) הפיל עליהן גורלות he (Joshua) cast lots over them (for their destruction). Arakh. IX, 4 (31[b]) שיהא חוֹלֵשׁ . . ללשכה (Mish. ed. בלשכה) that he might assign his redeeming money to the Temple fund (deposit it there, to assert his privilege of redemption).

חֲלַשׁ, part. **חָלִישׁ** ch. same, 1) to be weak, get sick. Targ. Is. II, 9. Targ. Lam. V, 17; a. e.—Pes. 50[a]; B. Bath. 10[b], v. נְגַד.—R. Hash. 17[a]; a. fr.—Yoma 18[a] חֲלַשָׁא דעתיה he might feel discouraged.—2) to pass away. R. Hash. l. c. חזייה דחליש ליה עלמא (Yalk. Mic. 559 . . חזא דחלש) he saw that his world (life) was passing away (he was sinking rapidly).—3) to be smooth and fine. Ḥull. 48[a] סכינא דח׳ פומיה a knife whose edge is very fine.—*4) to untie, undress. Gen. R. s. 22 דין אמר חֲלוֹשׁ Ar. ed. Koh. (ed., a. Yalk. ib. 38 חֲלוֹץ) the one (Abel) said, Take thy clothes off. Ib. s. 75 ח׳ פורפירא Ar. (ed. שלח) he took off the purple cloak.

Pa. חַלֵּישׁ 1) to weaken, reduce. Targ. Job XII, 21 Ms. (ed. מַחֲלֵשׁ, מְחַלֵּישׁ Af.).—2) to smoothen, polish, forge (armour). Ab. Zar. 16[a] משום דְחַלְשֵׁי וכ׳ (Ms. M. דחשלי; v. infra) because they forge of them their polished armour.

Af. אַחֲלִישׁ 1) to weaken, v. supra.—2) to cut with a sharp and smooth edge, opp. to בזע to tear with a notched knife. Ḥull. 17[b] (Rashi quoting Ab. Zar. l. c. דחשלי, a. Keth. 77[a] חשלי דודי appears to have read מחשיל).—*3) to strip. Targ. Y. II Lev. I, 6 (O. a. Y. I שלח). Targ. Y. II Num. XX, 26 ותחליש (some ed. ותשליח).

חֲלָשׁ m. (v. חֲלַשׁ, cmp. חֵלֶק) lot, ballot. Pesik. Zakh., p. 22[a] (ref. to ויחלש, Ex. XIII, 13) בח׳ לקח וכ׳ Amalek was smitten by ballot (v. חָלַשׁ). Ib. ארבעה שמות נקראו לגורל ח׳ וכ׳ the lot has four names, Ḥelesh, pûr &c.; Yalk. Ex. 265.—Pl. חֲלָשִׁים, חֲלָשִׁין. Ib. (quotation) וכאשר יטילו ח׳ על חמנות; Sabb. XXIII, 2 (148[b]) מטילין ח׳ וכ׳ lots may be cast for shares of sacred meat &c. Ib. 149[b] מאי משמע דהאי ח׳ וכ׳ what evidence is there that ḥălashim means lot? (Answ. ref. to Is. XIV, 12).

חֵלֶשׁ or **חֵלֶשׁ** reed, v. חֵילַשׁ.

חַלָּשׁ m. (b. h.; חָלַשׁ) weak. Sabb. 77[b] אימת ח׳ וכ׳ the fear with which the weak inspires the strong person.—Ex. R. s. 24; Sifré Deut. 309; a. e.—Pl. חַלָּשִׁים, חַלָּשִׁין. Ex. R. l. c.

חֲלָשָׁא, חֲלַשׁ, חַלָּשׁ ch. same, v. חֲלִישׁ. Targ. O. Deut. XXVIII, 44. Targ. I Sam. IX, 21.—Pl. חַלָּשִׁין, חַלָּ׳. Targ. Ex. XXXII, 18.

חַלָּשׁוּתָא, חֲלָשׁוּת f. (preced.) weakness, laxity. Targ. I Kings XII, 10. Targ. Koh. X, 17; a. e.

חַלְתָא f. ch.=h. חַלָּה; esp. the priest's portion. Targ. Num. XV, 20.—Erub. 83[a] איתי ח׳ שדי עליהו he brought the priest's portion in addition to it.

חַלְּתָא f. (חלל, cmp. חילת I) a loose wicker-work used for making bee-hives, strainers, for wine presses, screens &c. Snh. 107[a] תותי ח׳ behind a screen (Rashi: bee-hive; Yalk. Sam. 148 כילתא). Ib. פתקה לח׳ it (the arrow) made an opening in the screen. Sabb. 35[a] ח׳ בת תרי כורי a basket containing two khor. Ib. 74[b] האי מאן דעבד ח׳ he who makes a wicker-work on the Sabbath (going through the whole process of cutting reeds &c.).—Pl. חַלְּאתָא, חַלָּתָא. Ab. Zar. 75[a] חלתא דיקולי וכ׳ Ms. M. (ed. דקולי וחלא׳, Ar. incorr. ח׳ דדיקי) the palm or reed strainers which are twined with ropes of palm-rind.

חלתותא, חֲלְתִית, חֲלְתִיתָא, v. חִילְ׳.

חַם, perf. of חָמַם.

חָם I (b.h.) pr.n.m. *Ham*, the son of Noah. Snh. 69[b] ח׳ גדול וכ׳ H. was the elder of Japheth by one year &c. Ib. 108[b] ח׳ לקה בעורו H. was punished on his skin (was made black); Gen. R. s. 36 יצא ח׳ מפוחם H. came out (of the ark) blackened; a. e.

חַם II m. (b. h.; חָמַם) *warm, hot, boiling*. Pes. 75[b], sq.; a. fr.—Nidd. 43[a] בשרו חם his membrum excited.—*Pl.* חַמִּים, חַמִּין (sub. מים) *hot water*. Sabb. 134[b] ח׳ שהוחמו וכ׳ hot water which was made hot on the Sabbath; a. fr.—חַמֵּי טבריה *the hot springs of Tiberias*, in gen. *natural hot water*, opp. to חמי האור water heated by fire. Hull. 8[a] (Neg. IX, 1 מֵי); a. fr.—*Fem.* חַמָּה. Makhsh. III, 3 פת ח׳ hot bread.

חָם III (b. h.; v. Ges. H. Dict.[10] s. v.) *father-in-law, husband's father, wife's father*. Yeb. XV, 7 חָמִי my husband's father. Ib. I, 1 חָמִיו his (the *yabam's*) father-in-law. Pes. 87[a] כלה בבית חָמִיהָ a bride in the house of her father-in-law (after being conducted to the husband's home); a. v. fr.—*Fem.* חָמוֹת q. v.

חָמָא I ch. same. Targ. Gen. XXXVIII, 13 חֲמוּיִיךְ (ed. Berl. ׳חַ; oth. חֲמוּךְ). Targ. O. ib. 25 חֲמוּהָא. Targ. O. Ex. XVIII, 2 חֲמוּהִי ed. Berl. (oth. ׳חָ, Y. חָמוּי); a.e.—Y. Ber. I, 2[d] bot. חמוי. B. Mets. 74[b] בי חֲמוּהּ in the house of *his daughter's father-in-law*. Kidd. 12[b]; Yeb. 52[a] חמוה his father-in-law. Ib. 117[b] חֲמוּהָ her father-in-law; a. fr.

חָמָא II pr. n. m. *Hama*, name of several Amoraim. Y. Nidd. III, 50[c] bot. R. H., father of R. Hoshaya.—Y. Peah VIII, 21[b] top; Y. Shek. V, 49[a] bot.; a. e. (v. Fr. M'bo, p. 85[b]).—Ib. 49[b]; Y. Sabb. VI, 8[a]; B. Mets. 86[b], a. fr. R. Ḥ. bar Hănina.—B. Kam. 99[b]; Y. Kidd. III, 64[d], a. fr. R. Ḥ. bar Gurya.—Y. Erub. VII, 23[c]; Bab. ib. 65[b] bot. Ms. M. (ed. חנינא, v. Rabb. D. S. a. l. note) R. Ḥ. bar Joseph.—Y. Kil. VIII, 31[c] top, a. fr. R. Ḥ. bar Ukba.

חֲמָא *to see*, v. חמי.

חֲמָא, חֵמָא ch.=h. חֵמָה, *anger*. Dan. III, 13; 19.

חַמָּא m. (חמם; cmp. חַמָּם) *radish*. Ab. Zar. 28[b] bot. ח׳ לחמה Ms. M. a. Ar. (ed. חַמָּה) radishes are good for fever. Pes. 116[a] קפא דחסא ח׳ וכ׳ against the injurious effects of lettuce apply radishes &c.

חֶמְאָה f. (b. h.; v. חמי) [*pressed, thick,*]. *cream* or *butter*. Ber. 63[b] (ref. to Prov. XXX, 33) ח׳ של תורה the cream of the Law (sound knowledge). B. Mets. 86[b] בשכר ח׳ וכ׳ as a reward for the offer of cream and milk (Gen. XVIII, 8).

חֶמְאָתָא ch. same. Targ. Prov. XXX, 33, v. חֶזְוָתָא.

חָמַד (b. h.; cmp. חמם) 1) [*to be hot,*] *to desire, covet; to be carnally excited*. Nidd. 20[b] חֲמַדְתִּיו (or ׳חִמַּ *Pi.*) I had a desire for his embrace. Midr. Till. to Ps. XIX, 11 מי חָמְדָן which (of the two) holds them desirable; Yalk. ib. 676 [read]: מי חוֹמְדִין. Mekh. Yithro, Baḥod. s. 8 שאתה ח׳ חומד וכ׳ that you may desire his daughter for your son; ח׳ בדבור expressing a desire by words (without thinking of means to obtain the object of his desire). [Ib. ed. Weiss, אם תתאוה סופו לַחְמוֹד if one desires (what belongs to his neighbor), he will finally covet it (think of means to obtain it). Ib. אם ח׳ סופו וכ׳ if he covets, he will finally use force and rob. B. Mets. 5[b] לאו דלא תַחְמוֹד, v. לָאו; a. fr.—*Part. pass.* חָמוּד, f. חֲמוּדָה *desirable, precious*. Pesik. R. s. 36 ח׳ ונאה precious and fine (of conduct).—Sabb. 88[b] ח׳ גנוזה ed., v. חֶמְדָּה.—[2) (=חָמַר) *to produce shrivelling* by heat. Snh. VII, 2 (52[a]) Ar. (ref. to Dan. X, 3; Var. חמר).

Nif. נֶחְמַד 1) *to be desired, desirable*. Tanh. Vayera 5 שאתה נֶחְמָד לפני וכ׳ that thou art held desirable before the Lord; a. e.—[2) *to be shrivelled*. Hull. III, 3 Ar., Var. נחמר, v. supra.]

Pi. חִימֵּד *to covet*. Macc. III, 15 שנפשו . . . מתאוה להן וּמְחַמַּדְתָּן which man longs for and covets.

Hithpa. הִתְחַמֵּד, *Nithpa.* נִתְחַמֵּד (with ל) *to be anxious for; to be pleased with*. Tanh. Mishp. 17 ארץ שנִתְחַמְּדוּ לה וכ׳ a land which all the great men were anxious to possess (Yalk. Jer. 271 שֶׁחָמְדוּ). Koh. R. to IX, 7 בוראך מִתְחַמֵּד לָךְ thy Creator is pleased with thee; תורתו מִתְחַמֶּדֶת לָךְ His law is &c.

חֲמִיד, חֲמַד ch. same. Targ. Is. I, 29; a. fr.—Part. f. חֲמִידָא (חֲמִידַת). Targ. Y. Gen. IV, 1.

Pa. חַמֵּד, חַמֵּיד same, *to long*. Targ. O. Gen. XXXI, 30 (Y. מִתְחַמְדָא חַמְדְתָּא).—Nidd. 66[a] bot. מְחַמְּדָא, v. חימוד.

Ithpa. אִתְחַמַּד, *Ithpe.* אִתְחֲמֵד same.—Targ. Y. Gen. l. c.—Ib. XXVIII, 10.—Y. Taan. III, 66[d] top מִתְחַמֵּד וכ׳ being desirous to hear her talk. Y. Sabb. VI, 8[c] bot. הוו מִתְחַמְדִין וכ׳ were anxious to see &c. Koh. R. to IX, 10; a. e.

חֶמְדָא m. (preced.) (*sexual*) *appetite*. Sabb. 152[a] חֶמְדָּה.

חֶמְדָּה f. (b. h.; preced. wds.) 1) same. Sabb. 152[a] (expl. אביונה, Koh. XII, 5) זו ח׳ that means the sexual appetite; (Koh. R. to l. c. תַּאֲוָה).—2) *desirability, desirable object, precious gift*. Tanh. Sh'moth 29, a. e. דבר שהוא ח׳ מתוך ח׳ something which is the most desirable of all desirable things. Y. Taan. II, beg. 65[a] כלי אחד של ח׳ the only precious vessel (the Torah) left to us. Sabb. 88[b] ח׳ גנוזה Ms. M. (ed. חמודה) a reserved treasure (the Law); a. fr.

חַמְדָן, v. חַמְדָן.

חֶמְדְּתָא, חֶמְדְ׳ ch.=h. חֶמְדָּה. Targ Zech. VII, 14; Targ. Jer. III, 19. V. חֲמִידְתָא.

חֲמֵה *to see*, v. חמי.

חֵמָה, חֵי׳ f. (b.h.; חמם or חום) 1) *heat, anger*. Snh. 82[b] משיב ח׳ בן וכ׳ he is an allayer of (divine) anger, the son of &c. Num. R. s. 20 נתמלא עליה ח׳ he became angry at her. Lam. R. to I, 6 חֲמָתוֹ של הב״ה the anger of the Lord; a. fr.—2) *Hemah*, allegorical name of one of the angels of justice. Ex. R. s. 41, end; a. e., v. אַף II.

חַמָּה f. (b. h.; חמם) 1) *sun.* Ber. 59ᵇ ח׳ בתקופתה the sun starting on his new cycle (of twenty eight years). Num. R. s. 14 י״ב חדשים לח׳ the twelve solar months. Ned. III, 7 רואי חח׳ those seeing (or feeling) the sun; שלא נתכוין . . . שחח׳ וכ׳ for he meant him whom the sun sees; a. v. fr.—Yeb. VIII, 4, a. fr. סריס ח׳ a eunuch from the time of seeing the sun, i. e. born without visible testicles; opp. to סריס אדם.—2) *fever.* Sabb. 137ᵃ, a. e., v. חֲלֵץ. Y. Sabb. XIX, end, 17ᵇ, v. אַחוּ. Gen. R. s. 19, a. e., v. אַבְאָבִית. Y. Sabb. I, end, 4ᵇ (prov.) פת חמה חַמָּתָהּ בצדה hot bread has its heat by its side, i. e. eating hot bread causes fever; a. fr.—3) *radish.* Ab. Zar. 28ᵇ bot., v. חַמָּא.—V. חֵמַת.

חֲמוּדָא ch.=h. חֶמְדָּה. Targ. Jud. V, 30 (ed. Lag. חֲמוּדָה).

חָמוֹדָא m. (חמד) *covetous.—Pl.* חֲמוֹדִין, חֲמוֹדַיָּא. Targ. Y. Ex. XX, 14; Deut. V, 18 (ed. Amst. חָמוּ׳).

חֲמוּדָה, v. חֶמְדָּה, חָמַד a. חֲמוּדָא.

חֲמוּתִי, חֲמוּה, חֲמוֹהָ &c., v. חָמָא I.

חֲמוּטְלְיָא, v. חֲמַטְלְיָא.

חמולות, v. חֲמִילָה.

חִמּוּם, v. חִימּוּם a. חָמַם.

חֲמוּם m., **חֲמוּמָה** f. (חמם) *heated, rash.—Pl.* חֲמוּמוֹת. Y. Snh. VI, 23ᵇ bot. חוו ידיו ח׳ his hands were heated, i. e. he was very severe in executing judgment.

חִמּוּץ, חִמּוּצָא, v. חִימ׳.

חַמּוּק m. (b. h.; חמק, cmp. חבק) *rundle.—Pl.* חַמּוּקִים. Yalk. Ex. 370 שתי ידות . . . . ח׳ two handles (pins) of the shape of two rundles, v. חָרִיץ.

חֲמוֹר c. (b. h.; v. חָמַר II a. חֲמִיר I) 1) [*load-carrier,* cmp. גָּמָל.] *ass.* Nidd. 31ᵃ, v. גָּרַם. Sabb. 152ᵃ דעל ח׳ וכ׳ he who rides an ass is a freeman. B. Bath. 143ᵃ את וח׳ thou and the ass (shall own my property, a form of donation implying a rational and an irrational being).—Bekh. I, 2 ח׳ שילדה וכ׳ if an ass gave birth to &c. Snh. 33ᵃ הלכה חֲמוֹרְךָ וכ׳ thy ass is gone, Tarfon! (I shall have to make compensation for erroneous judgment); a. fr.—2) (cmp. various uses of *horse*) *a contrivance for workingmen, rest, jack, stocks* &c. Kel. XIV, 3 ח׳ של נפחין the smiths' ass ('on which the smith sits while using its head as an anvil', Maim.; 'the rest of the bellows', R. S.). Ib. XVIII, 3 וח׳ a stand on which the bedstead is placed. Gen. R. s. 65, end ח׳ של חרשים carpenters' sawing-jack (an instrument for torture); Ib. s. 70 (alluding to Prov. XXVII, 22) אפי׳ . . . בח׳ של חרשים וכ׳ even if you put the wicked man on a carpenter's jack, you cannot make anything useful out of him (sufferings will have no effect on him); Yalk. Kings 201; Yalk. Prov. 961; (Pesik. Shek., p. 15ᵃ במכתש).—*Pl.* חֲמוֹרִים. Sabb. 112ᵇ. Gen. R. s. 75; a. fr.—Denom. חַמָּר, חָמַר, חַמָּר.—*Fem.* חֲמוֹרָה. Tosef. Kil. V, 5.

חָמוּר m., **חֲמוּרָה** f. (חָמַר I) *heavy, weighty, important; strict, severe, stringent, restrictive.* Kel. I, 4 ח׳ שבכולם וכ׳ the most stringent of all are the laws concerning corpses.—איסור ח׳, v. אִיסּוּר.—Snh. 50ᵃ שריפה ח׳ וכ׳ death by burning is a severer punishment than &c. Ib. IX, 4, a. e. נידון בח׳ he suffers the severer penalty of the two. Ab. II, 1 כבחמורה as in the observance of a difficult commandment (requiring self-denial); a. fr.—*Pl.* חֲמוּרִים, חֲמוּרִין, f. חֲמוּרוֹת. Hull. XII, 5; a. fr.—Y. Snh. X, 28ᵇ top חֲמוּרוֹתָיו של וכ׳ (not חומר׳) the heaviest sins that Jeroboam committed.—דורשי חֲמוּרוֹת, v. חוֹמֶר II. קלים וחֲמוּרִים, v. חוֹמֶר I.

חֲמוּרָה, v. חָמוּר.

חֲמוֹרְתָּא f. (חֲמַר) *a drove of asses.* Gen. R. s. 75, v. גַּמַּלְתָּא.

חָמוֹת f. (b. h.; v. חָם III) *mother-in-law.* Yeb. I, 1 חמותו the *yabam's* wife's mother. Ib. XVI, 1 היתה לה ח׳ וכ׳ if the childless widow had a mother-in-law abroad (who may have given birth to a son), she need not take it into consideration (and may marry again); a. fr.

חֲמוֹתָא ch. same. Targ. Deut. XXVII, 23; a. e.; v. חֲמָתָא.

חֲמַט I (cmp. חמץ) 1) *to be dark.*—Denom. חוּמְטָא.—2) *to be bitter, salty,* v. חוּמְטוֹן.

Ithpe. אִיחֲמַט *to be inflamed, become pestered.* Sabb. 54ᵇ Ar., v. next w.

חֲמַט II (cmp. חבט) *to knock down.—Part. pass.* חֲמִיט, חֲמִיט *prostrated, kneeling,* (as verb) *to kneel.* Targ. Is. XLVI, 1. Targ. Ps. XCV, 6 נַחְמוֹט (some ed. נַחְמִיט). Targ. Y. Deut. XXVIII, 35 חֲמִיטְתּוּן . . . עבירתא (some ed. חָמִי׳ incorr.; not עבידתא); cmp. Targ. Job IV, 4 דַּחְמָטָן. [Koh. R. to IV, 9, end חמטת, some ed., read: דִּמְטַת.]

Pa. חַמֵּיט *to prostrate, subdue.* Targ. Ps. XVII, 13. Ib. XVIII, 40 Reg. (ed. תברתא).

Af. אַחְמִיט same. Ib. LXXVIII, 31.

Ithpe. אִיחֲמַט *to knock against, be battered.* Sabb. 54ᵇ דלא לִיחַמְטָן אלויתיהו Ms. M. (ed. incorr.) that their tails may not knock against (the rocks &c., Rashi; Ar.: 'may not ulcerate'; v. Syr. חמטא pustula, ulcus, P. Sm. 1303; v. preced.).

חֲמָטָה, v. חֲמִיטָה.

חֲמִי, חֲמָא, חֲמָה (Arab. *ḥama* tueri) [*to surround, guard,* v. חוֹמָה,] *to observe, see* (in Y. dialect). Targ. Y. Gen. I, 4 (O. חֲזָא); a. v. fr.—Targ. Prov. XXIII, 33 Ms. (ed. ויחוור׳).—Y. Peah III, 17ᵈ bot. אתא חמי (=תא חזי, h. בא וראה) come and see. Gen. R. s. 14 דאת חָמֵי לאפויי וכ׳ (not דאתת׳) that thou shalt see his face in the hereafter; Midr. Till. to Ps. II; Yalk. ib. 621 חמיי (corr. acc.). Ib. חַמְתֵּיה (fr. חמה) he saw him. Pesik. Eth Korb. p. 57ᵇ (v. Bub. note 15) חַמְתֵּיה אכיל חַמְתֵּי שתי did he (Moses) see me (the Lord) eat &c.?; Yalk. Num. 776 חַמְתֵּיה וכ׳ did he see Him &c.?; a. fr.—*Part. pass.* חֲמֵי (v. חֲזִי) *fit, worthy.* Targ. Ps. XV, 1. Ib. LVIII, 2 (ed. חמר); a. fr.—Fem. חֲמִיָא. Targ. Y. Ex. XXII, 16.

Af. אַחְמֵי 1) (followed by מִן, cmp. סור) *to turn* (*the eye) from.* Targ. Prov. XXVIII, 27 (Ar. מחמי, h. text מעלים, v. Syr. חמא P. Sm. 1017).—2) *to cause to see, to show.* Targ. Y. Gen. XLI, 28; a. e.—Lam. R. to I, 1 וְאַחְמְיָן ליה וכ׳ and showed him a measure full of denars. Ib. דכל עמא מַחְמְיָן לי וכ׳ (1 חַד כות׳) רבתי that all people point at me with their fingers.

Pa. חַמֵּי same. Y. Kil. IX, 32[b] bot.; Y. Keth. XII, 35[a] bot. חַמֵּי (לה) לי let me see it (the tooth).

Ithpa. אִתְחַמֵּי, *Ithpe.* אִתְחֲמֵי *to be seen, to appear.* Targ. Y. Gen. VIII, 5; a. fr.—[Targ. Ps. XLII, 3 אִתַּחְמֵי Ms. (*Ittaf.*) *I shall appear before* (h. text אֵרָאֶה, Var. a. ed. אֶחְמֵי)].—M. Kat. 25[b] אִתְחֲמִיאוּ וכ׳ stars were seen in day time. Y. Peah VIII, end, 21[b] דחמי ולא מִתְחֲמֵי He who sees but cannot be seen. Lam. R. introd. (R. Joh. 1) מִתְחַמְּאִין, v. מַשְׁתָּרֵי; a. e.

חָמֵיד, v. חֲמַד.

חֲמִידְתָּא f. ch.=h. חֶמְדָּה. Targ. Am. V, 11 (ed. Wil. חֶמְדָּתָא, ed. Lag. חֶמְדְּאתָא). Targ. Is. XXXII, 12.—Ib. XXVI, 8 חֲמִידַת constr.

חֲמִיטָא, v. אֲמִיתָא.

חֲמִיטָה f. (חמט II, cmp. חָבִיץ, חוּבְטָא) *a batter of which flat cakes are made, batter-cake.* T'bul Yom I, 1. Ib. II, 4; Tosef. ib. II, 2 (ed. Zuck. חמיתה, corr. acc.). Maasr. I, 7 נותן לחמי׳ ed. Y. a. Ms. M. (Bab. ed. a. Mish. לַחֲמָטָה) he may put (the oil) on the cake (Maim.: into the *pan*); Tosef. ib. I, 7; 9 נותן לחם מיטה ed. Zuck. (Var. לחמיתה, corr. acc.)—*Pl.* חֲמִיטוֹת. Y. Ter. X, 47[a] bot. חמטתינו (read: חֲמִיטוֹתֵינוּ or חֲמָ׳).

חמיטליא, v. חֶמְטַלְיָא.

חֲמִילָה f. (חמל; cmp. Syr. חמל, P. Sm. 1303, sq.) *a blanket of thick, coarse stuff.* Ned. VII, 3. Ib. 55[b]; Tosef. Sabb. V (VI), 14 מילא ed. Zuck. (Var. חמלא, חמלא).—*Pl.* חֲמִילוֹת. Tosef. Kel. B. Bath. V, 11. Tosef. Neg. V, 14 חמולות (corr. acc.).

חֲמִים m., **חֲמִימָא** c.=h. חַם II, *warm, hot, fresh.* Targ. I Sam. XXI, 7; a. e.—Y. Shebi. IV, 35[a] bot., a. e. פיתא ח׳ fresh bread. Erub. 3[a]; B. Bath. 24[b] (prov.) קדרא .... לא ח׳ וכ׳ a pot belonging to two partners is neither warm nor cold. Hull. 6[b] בר ... ליכול ח׳ let the scholar eat fresh food, and I shall be contented with cold; a. fr.—*Pl.* חַמִּימִין, חַמִּימֵי *hot water* (v. חַם II). Y. Ab. Zar. IV, 44[b] bot. חמר וח׳ wine mixed with hot water. Hull. 46[b].—Sabb. 55[a] רישך בקרירי .... בח׳ thy chief (I) shall be punished with cold water, but thy chief's chief (the Resh Galutha) with boiling water (he is reponsible); a. e.

חֲמִימוּתָא f. (preced.) *heat, heated state.* Pes. 76[a] מחמת ח׳ דחרס through the heat of the earthen vessel.

חֲמִימְתָא f. pl. (cmp. Arab. *ḥamâm*) [*dark-colored*] *a species of doves, ring-doves* (?). Gitt. 69[b] (oth. opin. *hens*).

חַמִּין m.=חַמִּים. Y. Ber. IV, 7[b] top שמשא ח׳ it is warm in the sun, טולא ח׳ in the shade. [Midr. Till. to Ps. XXIV ויומא דח׳, v. חֲמָיָן.] [ח׳, pl. of חַם II.]

***חֲמִיסִין** m. pl. *those using such words as ḥamis* ἥμισυ, cmp. חומש), a mockery on Talmudic scholars using foreign words. Snh. 14[a] כל מן דין ... לא מסרמיסין ולא מסרמיטין מח׳ וכ׳ Ms. F. a. Ag. Hatt. (v. Rabb. D. S. a. l. note 7; ed. ואמרי לה לא מח׳) such men (as R. Ammi &c.) appoint for us, but do not appoint for us any of those using such words like *sermis* (semis, ἥμισυ) *sermit* (prob. distortion of tremis), *hemis* or *tremis* (cmp. Y. Gitt. IV, 47[b] quot. s. v. טוֹרְדְּרִינֵי). [Oth. opin. v. Rashi, a. Ar. s. v.]

חֲמֵיסַר (=חמיש עסר) *fifteen; the fifteenth.* Targ. Y. Lev. XXIII, 6. Ib. XII, 4; a. e.—Meg. 5[b] בר ח׳ one observing Purim on the fifteenth of Ădar; a. e.

חֲמֵיסְרָאָה m. (preced.) *the fifteenth.* Targ. I Chr. XXIV, 14.

חֲמִיעַ, חֲמִיעָא m. (חמע) 1) *sour.* Lam. R. to III, 40, v. בְּסִימָא.—2) (Targ. Y. חָמִיעַ)=h. חָמֵץ, *leavened (bread).* Targ. Ex. XII, 15; a. fr.—Y. Snh. III, 21[b] הורו מיפי ח׳ וכ׳ they permitted to bake leavened bread on Passover (for the troops).

חֲמֵיץ, v. חֲמַץ.

חֲמִיצ, v. חָמֵץ.

חֲמִיר I m., **חֲמִירָא** f.=h. חָמוּר 1) *loaded.* Targ. Y. Gen. XLIX, 14 ח׳ באורייתא loaded with the (knowledge of the) Law.—2) *grave, strict, stringent.* Targ. Y. Num. XIV, 30.—Hull. 10[a] ח׳ סכנתא וכ׳ regulations concerning health and life are made more stringent than ritual laws; a. fr.—*Pl.* f. חֲמִירָתָא *restrictions, strict measures.* Y. Ab. Zar. II, 41[d] bot. מן ח׳ דרב one of Rab's strict regulations.

חֲמִיר II (**חָמִיר**), **חֲמִירָא** m. (חֲמַר II) *strong leaven* (h. שְׂאֹר); *leavened bread.* Targ. Ex. XII, 15; a. fr.—Pes. 5[b], v. בְּעַר.—Ab. Zar. 66[a] ח׳ דשערי leaven of barley flour. Men. 43[a], v. אַרְבְּסָא; a. fr.

חֲמֵישׁ, v. חֲמֵשׁ.

חֲמִישָׁאֵי, חֲמִישָׁאָה, v. חֲמִישַׁי.

חֲמִישִׁי m. (b. h.; חָמֵשׁ) *fifth;* (sub. יום) *the fifth day of the week.* Meg. I, 2, sq.; a. fr.—*Fem.* חֲמִישִׁית. Ib. III, 4 בח׳ on the fifth Sabbath; a. fr.—Esp. (Lev. V, 24) *the penalty of the fifth part* added to the indemnity. B. Kam. 65[b].—*Pl.* חֲמִישִׁיּוֹת. Ib. (ref. to חֲמִשִׁתָיו, Lev. l. c.) ח׳ הרבה וכ׳ (ed. חֻמְשִׁ׳) repeated penalties connected with one object of indemnity.

שָׁאָה..., שַׁאי, חֲמִישַׁי... ch. same. Targ. Gen. I, 23 (ed. Amst. שָׁאַי...); a. fr.—*Fem.* שִׁיתָא, חֲמִישֵׁיתָא ... Targ. Lev. XIX, 25.—Pesik. R. s. 23 (ed. Fr. p. 115[b]) חֲמִישְׁתָּא; ib. (p. 120[a]) חמשיתא (corr. acc.) the fifth day of the week.—V. חֲמִשִׁיתָא.

תָה, חֲמִיתָא..., v. אֲמִיתָא.

חמיתה, v. חֲמִיטָה.

חָמַל (b. h.) [*to be warm,*] *to have compassion.* Men. 53[b] (play on חמולה, Jer. XI, 16) חָמַלְתִּי עליהם I had mercy on them.

חמלא, v. חֲמִילָה.

חַמַלְתָּא, v. חִימַלְתָּא.

(חִימוּם) חֲמָם m. (v. next w.; cmp. ἄμωμον, v. Sm. Ant. s. v.) *amomum*, an Indian (also Syriac) spice. Ukts. III, 5 (some ed. incorr. חמם); Nidd. 51[b] חימום (corr. acc.); Sifré Deut. 107 חימום; Y. Erub. IX, end, 25[d] חכם (corr. acc.); Y. Ḥag. III, 79[c] חמה (corr. acc.).—Gen. R. s. 45, beg. ח׳ חיא צריכה (חימום, corr. acc.) she needs amomum (as medicine for sterility). Cmp. אֲמִירְתָא, חִימַלְתָּא.

חָמַם (b. h.) *to be warm, hot*; [(of color) *to be dark, red*; (of taste) *to be pungent, sour, bitter*]. *Part.* חָם, q. v.

Pi. חִמֵּם *to heat, warm, boil.* Y. Ned. IV, 38[c] bot. לְחַמֵּם בו את ידיו to warm his hands against it (the bread). Gen. R. s. 14, end מְחַמֶּמֶת הגוף keeps the body warm. Sabb. 40[b] ומְחַמְּמָתָהּ וכ׳ and warms it (her hand) before the fire; a. fr.

Hif. הֵיחֵם same. Bets. II, 5 לא יָחֵם וכ׳ one must not prepare warm water for &c. Sabb. 40[a] התחילו . . לְהָחֵם בשבת the bathers began to heat (the water) on the Sabbath; a. fr.—Part. מֵחֵם, מֵיחֵם, pl. מְחַמִּין. Ib.[b]; Tosef. ib. III (IV), 7 מיחם אדם וכ׳ (ed. Zuck. מייחם, read: מְיַחֵם), v. אַלּוּנְטִית I; [Y. ib. XIX, 17[a] bot. מחמין הוא אדם (read as ib. IX, 12[a] bot. מְחַמֵּם הוא וכ׳].—Ib. אם מפני הסכנה מְחַמִּין לו וכ׳ if it is for the sake of averting danger to life, may we not even boil water on the Sabbath?—Bets. 22[a]; a. v. fr.

Nif. נֶחַם, נֵחוֹם *to be warmed.* Sabb. III, 5 (41[a]) בשביל שיֵחַמּוּ that they become warm; ib. 41[b] שיֵחוֹמּוּ; Tosef. ib. III (IV), 5 שֶׁיֵּיחַמּוּ; a. e.

Hof. הוּחַם same. Sabb. 134[b] שהוּחַמּוּ, v. חַם II. Y. Bets. II, 61[c]; a. fr.—B. Mets. VI, 3 הוּחַמָּה the animal was overtaken by the heat.

Hithpa. הִתְחַמֵּם, *Nithpa.* נִתְחַמֵּם *to warm one's self; to become heated.* Bets. II, 5; Tosef. Sabb. l. c. Tam. I, 1. Ab. II, 10 הוי מִתְחַמֵּם וכ׳ warm thyself by the fire of the scholars (try to associate with them); a. fr.—Y. Sot. I, 16[c] bot. נתח׳ was heated (had pollution). Gen. R. s. 24 מִתְחַמְּמוֹת, מִתְחַמְּמִים *conceived.*

חֲמַם ch. same. Targ. O. Gen. XVIII, 1; a. e.; v. חוּם.

Pa. חַמֵּים *to warm, heat.*—*Part. pass.* מְחַמַּם. Targ. Hos. VII, 7.

Af. 1) אַחֵים *to heat, excite,* v. חוּם.—2) אַחְמֵם *to become hot; to have pollution.* Nidd. 43[a] כל אחמומי והדר א׳ וכ׳ getting heated once and again immediately after.

Ithpa. אִתְחַמַּם, *Ithpe.* אִיחַמֵּם 1) *to warm one's self.* Targ. Y. II Gen. XVIII, 1.—Sabb. 110[b] כד איח׳ ed. (Ms. M. אִתְ׳, v. supra) when he had warmed himself.—*2) *to restrain one's anger.* Targ. II Esth. V, 10 [prob. to be read: וְאִתְחַסַּם, v. חֲסַם; cmp. חֲסַן].

חַמָּן m., pl. **חַמָּנִים** (b. h.; v. חַמָּה) *solar columns,* [prob. *a phallus*, cmp. חֲנִיסְנָסָא]. Sifra B'har ch. IX, end (ref. to לא תקימו, Lev. XXVI, 1) אלו הח׳ וכ׳ that means the *ḥammanim* on roof-tops. Mekh. Bo, s. 11 (ref. to Ex. XII, 21) משכו מִחַמָּנֵיכֶם withdraw from your ḥ. Ib. Yithro, s. 5, end לח׳. Ib. s. 6 מן הח׳ (ed. Weiss a. Fr. everywhere ע״ז).

חמס, Ukts. III, 5, v. חֲמָם.

חָמַס (b. h.; v. Ges. H. Dict.[10] s. v.) [*to be heated, passionate,*] *to insult, do violence, to rob.* Y. Ab. Zar. II, 40[d] bot. לא סוף... אלא חֲמוֹס וכ׳ finally one does not say to another man, Kill that man, but, Attack &c. Gen. R. s. 45 (ref. to חמסי, ib. XVI, 5) חוֹמְסַנִי את בדברים וכ׳ thou provokest me to speak harshly, because thou seest &c. Ib. s. 65, beg. מלכות . . . גוזלת וחוֹמֶסֶת the wicked government (Rome) robs and extorts; a. fr.—Lev. R. s. 26 דור ודור וחוֹמְסָיו each generation with its violent men.—Part. pass. חָמוּס. Ib. s. 30 גזול אני ח׳ אני I have been taken by force, by extortion.

Nif. נֶחְמַס *to be ruined* (cmp. חָבַל). Lam. R. to II, 6 כגנה שנ׳ מעיינה וכ׳ like a garden the spring of which has been ruined, so that its vegetables fade.

Pi. חִימֵּס (of beasts of prey) *to seize with fangs, scratch with nails.* Gen. R. s. 45 (play on חמסי, v. supra) חִימְּסָה פניו Ar. (ed. בפניו, some ed. חימסא, incorr.) she scratched his face; Y'lamd. to Gen. l. c. (quot. in Ar.) וחימסה אותו וחימסה פניו כנמיה she scratched him and marked his face like a marten; Yalk. ib. 79 (not חומסה).

חֲמַס ch. same.—Denom. חוּמְסָא.

Ithpa. אִתְחַמַּס *to do violence to one's self, to restrain one's self.* Targ. II Esth. V, 10, v. חֲמַם. [Targ. Y. Gen. VII, 21 אתחמסי, read: אִתְּמְסִי or אִתְחַמְסִי, v. מְסִי.]

חָמָס m. (b. h.; preced.) *violence, extortion.* Y. B. Mets. IV, 9[c] bot. (ref. to Gen. VI, 13) מה היה חֲמָסָן what was the nature of their violence? Gen. R. s. 31 (distinction between ח׳ a. גָּזֵל); a. e.—*Pl.* חֲמָסִים. Ib. s. 65 . . . שלא ח׳ גזילות that thou wilt not give me to eat what has been obtained by robbery or extortion. Lev. R. s. 2. Koh. R. to III, 9; a. e.

חוּמְסָן, חַמְסָן (preced.) *violent man, extortioner.* B. Kam. 62[a] (defining the difference between the ח׳ and the גַּזְלָן) ח׳ יהיב וכ׳ the *ḥamsan* takes by force and pays.—*Pl.* חַמְסָנִין, חַמְסָנִים. Snh. 25[b] הוסיפו עליהן . . . והח׳ (Ar. והחו׳) they added to them (the class of persons disqualified for judges or witnesses) the robbers and those taking forcibly (and paying); Y. Shebu. VII, 37[d] bot.; Y. R. Hash. I, 57[c] top.

***חָמַע**=חָמֵץ; *Pi.* חַמֵּעַ. Ab. Zar. 68[a] לְחַמֵּעַ, Ms. M. לחמץ.

חֲמַע I ch.=h. חָמֵץ *to be sour; to be leavened.* Targ. O. Ex. XII, 34; a. e.; v. חֲמִיעַ.—Y. Pes. II, end, 29[c] בגין דיחמע that it might turn sour (vinegar).

Pa. חַמֵּעַ *to leaven.* Pes. 41[a] חמוּעֵי מְחַמַּע (not מחמצא; Rashi: אַחְמוּעֵי מַחְמַע *Af.*) (the flour) causes leavening.—*Part. pass.* מְחַמַּע, v. infra.

Af. אַחְמַע 1) *to turn sour, leaven, ferment.* Targ. Y. Ex. l. c.—2) *to cause leavening.* Targ. Y. II Lev. II, 11 דמְחַמְּעַ (Var. דמחמע); v. supra.

חָמַץ (b. h.; cmp. חמס) [*to be hot,*] *to do violence, to wrong.* Snh. 35[a] (ref. to Is. I, 17) אשרו חָמוּץ ולא חוֹמֵץ

right the oppressed, but not the oppressor (listen to the complainant first); Yoma 39[b].

חָמֵץ I (b. h.; v. preced.) [*to be hot,*] *to ferment, be sour.* Ab. Zar. 68[b] מי גרם לה שֶׁתֶּחְמַץ וכ׳ what was the cause that it (the dough) became leavened (rose) in one hour?

Pi. חִמֵּץ *to cause leavening.* Ib.[a] ראויה לְחַמֵּץ וכ׳ Ms. M. (ed. לְחַמֵּע) fit to leaven with it many other doughs. Ib. וְחִימְּצוּ; Orl. II, 11 נצטרפו וְחִמְּצוּ (Y. ed. הצטרפו וְחִימֵּיצוּ) and the two combined produced the required leavening. Ib. 9 וְחִמְּצָה (Y. ed. וְחִימֵּיצָה; Ab. Zar. l. c. וְהֶחְמִיצָה) and it made the dough rise. Orl. II 6 כל הַמְחַמֵּץ whatever is used for producing fermentation; a. fr.—Trnsf. *to mature, to continue a case over night, to reserve judgment.* Snh. 35[a] (ref. to Is I, 17, v. preced.) אשרו דיין שֶׁמְּחַמֵּץ את וכ׳ Ms. K. (ed. אשרי, v. Rabb. D. S. a. l. note 20) praise the judge (in capital cases) who reserves his judgment (over night); Yalk. Is. 257.

Hif הֶחְמִיץ 1) same. Pes. 40[a] מי פירות אינן מַחְמִיצִין juice of fruits produces no leavening (in the ritual sense). Ab. Zar. 68[a] כדי להחמיץ (Orl. II, 8 לְחַמֵּץ) enough to leaven the dough. Mekh. Bo s. 10 שאור שהוא מַחְמִיץ לאחרים leaven which is used for leavening other doughs; a. fr.—Trnsf. *to procrastinate.* Ib. s. 9 (play on הַמַּצּוֹת, Ex. XII, 17) כדרך …… אין מַחְמִיצִין את הַמִּצְוָה as well as you must not allow the *matsah* to become sour, so you must not allow the *mitsvah* (religious act) to become sour by postponement; Yalk. Ex. 201.—2) *to turn sour, to ferment.* Ab. Zar. 68[b] ראויה לְהַחְמִיץ וכ׳ (Ms. M. לחמיע) is likely to ferment in two hours. Nidd. IX, 7 מי רגלים שֶׁהֶחְמִיצוּ urin which ferments.—Trnsf. *to degenerate, become wicked.* R. Hash. 3[b] קודם שה׳ before he (the Persian King) changed for the worse.

Nithpa. נִתְחַמֵּץ *to become sour* (חָמֵץ). Pes. 28[b]; 43[a] נ׳ מאליו became sour of itself (not through a leavening means).

חֲמַץ ch. (preced. wds.) 1) *to be hot,* (of color) *red,* v. חִימּוּצָא, חִימּוּצְתָּא.—2) *to be sour, salty* &c.

Pa. חַמֵּיץ *to put to shame.* Targ. Prov. X, 1 (h. text תוגת), v. חִימּוּצָא.

Af. אַחְמִיץ 1) same. Ib. XXV, 8; XXVIII, 7 (Ms. *Pa.*: h. text הכלים).—2) *to degenerate.* R. Hash. 4[a] מנלן דא׳ what evidence have we that he became wicked?, v. preced.

חָמֵץ II m. (b. h.; preced. wds.) *leavened bread, anything containing leavened substance* (of the five species of grain, v. Ḥall. I, 1, sq.). Pes. I, 1, v. בָּדַק. Ib. II, 2 ח׳ של עכ״ום וכ׳ *ḥamets* belonging to a gentile over which the Passover passed (which existed during the Passover week). Ib. 3 על חֲמֵצוֹ (trad. pronunc. חָמְצוֹ as if fr. חֹמֶץ) on ḥ. belonging to him. Y. Shebi. VIII, 38[b] bot. חֲמֵיצָן של וכ׳ ḥ. belonging to Samaritans; Y. Ab. Zar. V, 44[d] bot. אכל חמצין (read: חֲמֵיצָן) ate their (the Samaritans') ḥ. (immediately after Passover); a. v. fr.—*Pl.* חֲמֵצִים, חֲמֵצִין *salads,* v. חוּמְצָן.

חֲמָץ pr. n. pl. (Gr. Ἔμεσα, Ἔμισσα) *Hămâts, Emesa* (mod. *Hums*) a city of Syria on the Eastern bank of the Orontes. Gen. R. s. 37; Y. Meg. I, 71[b] bot. (expl. צמרי, Gen. X, 18).—Y. Kil. IX, 32[c] bot.; Y. Keth. XII, 35[b] bot. ימא דח׳ the Lake of E. (an artificial bay made under Diocletian); Midr. Till. to Ps. XXIV ימא דחמין (corr. acc.).—Denom. חוּמְצָאֵי, חֲמָצָאֵי m. pl. *inhabitants of Emesa.* Targ. Y. Gen. X, 18; Targ. I Chr. I, 16.

חַמְצָא, v. חִימְ׳.—[חמצין, Y. Ab. Zar. V, 44[d] bot., v. חָמֵץ II.]

חַמְצָן m. (חָמַץ), בן ח׳ *a grasping person.* Yoma 39[a], sq. (Ms. O. omits בן); Kidd. 53[a]; v. חָאפּוּן.

חָמַר I (cmp. חָבַר) 1) *to join; to pile up, to load.* Ukts. II, 5 והבצלים שֶׁחֲמָרָן and the onions which one has piled up; v. אָמַן.—Zeb. 53[a] וחוֹמֵר בגודלו וכ׳ and loads (i. e. supports the index finger) with his thumb on top and the little finger below (like a balanced load, v. חֶבֶר a. אֵבֶר); [Var. סוֹמֵךְ, v. Rabb. D. S. a. l. note 3]; Yalk. Lev. 469.—2) (denom. of חוֹמֶר) *to be weighty, stringent.* Ohol. XIV, 3 אל יַחְמוֹר זה וכ׳ this must not be made more stringent than &c.; [ed. Dehr. יַחְמִיר.]

Hif. הֶחְמִיר [*to put a load on,*] *to pass a restrictive law, to incline to the stricter opinion,* opp. הקל to make easy. Yeb. 88[a] מתוך חומר שֶׁהֶחְמַרְתָּ עליה וכ׳ on account of the restrictions under which the law puts her in the end (if she marries again and her first husband appears), it is made easy for her in the beginning (by allowing her to marry again), i. e. her heavy responsibility will make her cautious; Y. Gitt. I, beg. 43[a] (add: מתוך). Nidd. 66[a], a. fr. הֶחְמִירוּ על עצמן they placed themselves under greater restrictions (than the law requires). Ned. I, 1 לְהַחְמִיר, v. חָבַב II. Eduy. III, 10, a. e. מַחְמִיר כדברי וכ׳ he adopts the stricter opinion of &c.; a. v. fr.

[*Pi.* חִמֵּר, v. חָמַר II.]

חֲמַר ch. same.

Pa. חַמֵּר, *Af.* אַחְמִיר as preced. *Hif.*—Y. Shek. VII, 50[c] bot. [read:] חמיתון מקילין לון וה׳ וכ׳ he saw them to be lax in their practices, and he enjoined strictness on them. Yeb. 88[a] לא לִיחַמֵּיר וכ׳ let one not put her under heavy restrictions (in the end), and not make it too easy for her (in the beginning, v. preced.). Nidd. 66[a] היכא דאַחְמוּר וכ׳ in those cases in which they have placed themselves under greater restrictions (than the law requires, v. preced.), they have done so (and follow the usage like a law), but where they have not &c. (you cannot extend the adopted usage by analogy); a. fr.—*Part. pass.* מְחַמַּר, מִיחַמַּר *piled up, ruins;* v. מַחְמַר a. הִמְתַּמְרָא.

Ithpa. אִתְחַמַּר *to be piled up, to form a pile of ruins* (cmp. תֵּל). Targ. Is. XVII, 9; XXX, 13.

חָמַר II (b. h.) [*to be hot,*] 1) *to glow, to parch* (cmp. כָּבַר). Snh. VII, 2 וחוֹמֶרֶת את וכ׳ and parches his entrails (Ar., v. חָבַד).

Nif. נֶחְמַר *to be parched.* Ḥull. III, 3 נפלה לאור וְנֶחְמְרוּ וכ׳ if the bird fell into fire, and (on examination after slaughtering it was found that) its bowels were affected by inhaling heat (Ar., v. חָמַד). Gen. R. s. 38, end.

חֲמַר ch. same, 1) *to be hot, parched.* Targ. Job XXX, 27 חַמְרוּ (Var. חֲמָרוּ, Ms. חַמָּרוּ *Pa.*; h. text רתחו).—2) *to ferment*, v. next w., a. חֲמִירָא.

חֲמַר III, חַמְרָא I (preced.) *wine* (b. h. חֶמֶר). Targ. Num. VI, 3; a. fr.—Targ. Hos. III, 1 בְּחַמְרֵיה ed. Lag. (ed. בחבריה, corr. acc.) in his wine (intoxication).—Sabb. 77ª, a. e., v. הָדָר II. Hull. 112ª קרי ליה חמר בשר (Ar. חמר) called it (that juice) meat-wine.—Gen. R. s. 91 end ח׳ קטף wine mixed with resin.—Erub. 53ᵇ, v. אִימַר; a. fr.—*Pl.* חַמְרִין. Targ. Y. Gen. L, 1.

חֲמַר, חֲמָרָא, חַמְרָא (II) m. ch.=h. חֲמוֹר, 1) *ass; trnsf. workingman's contrivance, jack* &c. Targ Is. XXI, 7. Targ. Ex. XIII, 13; a. fr.—Sabb. 66ᵇ; Y. ib. VI, 8ᶜ, v. אַנְקְטְמִין; a. v. fr.—*Pl.* חֲמָרִין, חֲמָרַיָּא, חֲמָרֵי. Targ. Gen. XII, 16 (Y. ed. Amst. חַמְרִין). Ib. XXXVI, 24 (Y. ed. Amst. חַמְרַיָּא); a. e.—Gen. R. s. 38 (ref. to בני האדם, Gen. XI, 5) וכי מה נאמר בני ח׳ could we think young asses (built it)?—Y. Dem. I, 21ᵈ bot. Ib. 22ª top; a. fr.—2) ח׳ דמיא *sea-ass*, name of a sea fish, *hake* (v. Sm. Ant. s. v. Onos). Ab. Zar. 39ª.

חֲמָר I m. ch. (v. חֲמַר II; cmp. חֲמַם) *dark; trnsf. mourning.* Targ. Ps. XXXV, 14; XXXVIII, 7 Ms. (ed. חַפִּיר, Lev. חביר; h. text קֹדֵר).

חַמָּר II m. h. (denom. of חֲמוֹר) *ass-driver, attendant of beasts of burden.* Kidd. IV, 14, a. e., v. גַּמָּל. Kel. XXVI, 5 (6) עור החמור ועור הח׳ Maim. (v. comment. ed. Dehr.; Mish. ed. עור הח׳, Talm. ed. עור החמור) the ass' leather cover and the ass-driver's apron; a. fr.—ח׳ גמל, v. גַּמָּל.—*Pl.* חַמָּרִים, חַמָּרִין. Dem. IV, 7. Kidd. l. c. a. fr.—Denom.: חִמֵּר *to direct a loaded beast's motions by walking behind it, to load a beast.* Sabb. 153ᵇ; Ab. Zar. 15ª המחמר אחר וכ׳ he who drives his beast of burden by walking behind it. Sabb. l. c. והלא מחמר but does he not violate the Sabbath as a driver (by placing his money bag on the ass)?—Pes. 66ᵇ מח׳ כלאחר יד הוא it is an act of driving in an unusual way (the lamb usually not being used as a beast of burden); a. fr.

חַמָּר, חַמָּרָא ch. same. Y. Taan. I, 64ᵇ bot. ח׳ אנא I am an ass-driver. Ib. פלן ח׳ יצלי let that certain ass-driver pray. [Ib. חמר עבון החוא גוברא וכ׳, read: חמש עבירן וכ׳, v. margin ed. Krot.]—Y. Snh. VI, beg. 23ᵇ הא שאלתא דח׳ in that form it would be an ass-driver's question.—*Pl.* חַמָּרַיָּא. Y. Taan. IV, 67ᶜ bot.

חֲמְרָא *wine*, v. חֲמַר III.

חֲמָרָא, חַמְרָא *ass*, v. חֲמַר.

חֲמָרָא, v. חֵימָרָא.

חֲמֶרֶת f. (חַמָּר) *a company of ass-drivers, caravan.* Snh. X, 5 (111ᵇ); B. Bath. 8ª. Tosef. Dem. I, 10 (contrad. to חַמָּר אחד); Y. ib. I, 22ª bot. (incorr. version).

חֲמַרְתָּא ch.=h. חֲמוֹרָה. Y. Dem. I, 21ᵈ bot.; Y. Shek. V, 48ᵈ top; Gen. R. s. 60 חֲמָרְתֵּיה דר׳ וכ׳ the she-ass of R. &c. Y. Yeb. IV, 6ª bot. חֲמָרְתִּי my ass. Ib. חֲמָרְתָּה, v. פָּחַת.

חָמֵשׁ f., **חֲמִשָּׁה** m. (b. h.) *five* (numeral letter ה׳). Snh. V, 3 בחמש (sub. שעות) during the fifth hour of the day. Ib. בחמשה (sub. ימים) on the fifth of the month.—Sabb. 77ᵇ חמשה אימות וכ׳ (sub. מִינֵי), v. אֵימָה. B. Mets. IV, 9 תשלומי ארבעה וח׳ fines of the fourfold or fivefold value (Ex. XXI, 37); a. v. fr.—*Pl.* חֲמִשִּׁים (נ׳) *fifty.* R. Hash. 21ᵇ. Ab. V, 21 בן ח׳ at the age of fifty years; a. v. fr.—Denom. חִמֵּשׁ *to divide into five.*—*Part. pass.* מְחוּמָּשׁ; f. מְחוּמֶּשֶׁת, pl. מְחוּמָּשׁוֹת. B. Bath. 150ª ובלבד שיהו מח׳ provided the minimum of wool required is equally divided between the five lambs.—חֲמֵשׁ עֶשְׂרֵה f.; חֲמִשָּׁה עָשָׂר m. (ט״ו) *fifteen.* Y. Sabb. VI, 8ᵇ (ref. to וחמשים, Ex. XIII, 18) בח׳ ע׳ מיני וכ׳ with fifteen kinds of arms. Taan. IV, 8 כח׳ ע׳ באב like the celebration of the fifteenth of Ab; a. fr.—Constr. of חֲמִשָּׁה; חֲמֵשֶׁת. Kidd. 30ª ח׳ אלפים five thousand; a. fr.

חֲמֵשׁ f., **חַמְשָׁא, חַמְשָׁה** m. ch. same. Targ. Gen. XLV, 11. Ib. XLVII, 2; a. fr.—Yoma 84ª ח׳ ומעלי וכ׳ on Thursday and on Friday; a. fr.—*Pl.* חַמְשִׁין *fifty.* Targ. Num. XXXI, 47; a. fr.—B. Mets. 51ª; a. fr.—חֲמֵישַׁת עֲשָׂרָה (חֲמֵישְׁתֵּי) *fifteen.* Targ. O. Lev. XXIII, 6; a. fr.; v. חֲמֵיסַר.

חֲמִשִּׁי, חֲמִשִׁי, v. חֹמֶ׳.

חֲמִשְׁתָּא, חֲמִשִׁיתָא f. (preced. wds.) *a collection of five.* Y. Meg. II, 73ᵇ bot.; Y. Ber. II, 4ᵈ ח׳ קדמייתא the first five (mentioned Ter. I, 1); ח׳ בתרייתא the second five (mentioned ib. 6); (Readings vary חמשתא, חמשתיה).

חֵמֶת f. (b. h.) *the skin of a goat* drawn off the body without opening the belly and sewed up and pitched at the ends where the legs and the tail were cut off (v. Sm. Bible Dict. s. v. *Bottle*), *bottle, bag.* Kel. XIX, 8 חח׳ שבצים וכ׳ a bottle (of a skin of a he-goat) whose scrotum (originally made to receive liquids in connection with the bottle) became defective. Ib. XX, 2 חֵמַת חלילין bag of the bagpipe (ascaula). Ib. XXVIII, 5 ח׳ שעשאה שטיח a closed up pouched skin which (by cutting open) was made a spread skin. Sabb. 152ª a woman is ח׳ מלא דם (!) a bag full of blood (v. vers. Ms. O. in Rabb. D. S. a. l. note 7). Tosef. Kel. B. Kam. VI, 13. Ib. VII, 11 חח׳ מעור הדג a bag made of the skin of a fish. Y. Ab. Zar. IV, end, 44ᵇ bot. בְּחֶמְתּוֹ (not מח׳) in his wine bottle; a. fr.—*Pl.* חֲמָתוֹת. Kel. XXVI, 4 (5) כל ח׳ Mish. ed. (Talm. ed. כלי, corr. acc.); Men. 37ᵇ. Hull. 107ᵇ בבלאי ח׳ with pieces of goat skins wrapt around their hands (like gloves).—Midr. Till. to Ps. CXXXVII חֵמוֹת.

חֲמַת pr. n. *Hammath*, name of a demon (*fever*, cmp. חֵימְתָא). Snh. 101ª זיקא דח׳ וכ׳ the blast (breath; Ms. M. ריקא the spittle) of H. do I see in thy face (an eruption).

חֲמַת, constr. of חֵמָה *heat of*; מֵחֲ׳ *through the heat of, from the effect of, in consequence of.* B. Mets. VI, 3 מח׳ המעלה overcome by heat through the exertion of climbing up the ascent. Hull. 4ᵇ מֵתוּ אחיו מח׳ מילה his brothers had died in consequence of the circumcision.

Nidd. 36^b מח׳ עצמה spontaneously; מח׳ ולד in consequence of travailing; מח׳ אונס from an accidental cause; a. fr.—(Also in Chald. phraseology) Targ. II, Esth. VII, 9 מחמת ד־ (ed. Lag. מֵחֵימַת) because they take &c.— B. Kam. 114^a כל אונסא דאתי מֵחֲמָתֵיה any injury that may arise from his action (of selling). Ab. Zar. 15^a אזל מחמתיה (the animal) moves at his instance; a. fr.

חֲמַת (v. חֲמָתָא) *to get hot, angry.* [חמת־, *to see,* v. חֲמַר.]

Pa. חַמֵּית, *Af.* אַחְמֵית *to make angry.* Targ. Prov. XX, 2 מְחַמֵּית (Var. מַחְמֵית).

חֲמָת pr. n. pl. (b. h.) *Hamtath,* a Syrian city, near the later Antiochia. Targ. O. Num. XIII, 21 (Y. אנטוכיא); ib. XXXIV, 8 (Y. טבריא, v. חַמְּתָא); a. fr.—Num. R. s. 10 (ref. to Am. VI, 2) זו חֲמת אנטוכיא that is H. near Antiochia (Yalk. Am. 545 זה אנט׳).

חַמַּת pr. n. pl. (b. h.) *Hammath,* v. חַמְּתָא.

חֲמָתָא *anger,* v. חֵימְ׳.

חֲמָתָא f. ch.=h. חָמוֹת. Targ. O. XXVII, 23 (Var. חֲמוּתָא).—Gitt. 67^b bot. (Ar. חמותא), v. דִּיסְקָנָא I. Kidd. 12^b חֲמָתֵיה; Yeb. 52^a חימתיה (corr. acc.), v. דּוּם; a. fr.

חַמְּתָה, חַמְּתָא pr. n. pl. (b. h. חַמַּת; חמם) *Ḥamm'tha,* [*Hot Springs*], name of several Jewish places, esp. a) *Ḥ., near Tiberias.* Y. Meg. I, 70^a (expl. חמת, Josh. XIX, 35; Bab. ib. 6^a top חמת זו טבריא). Tosef. Erub. VII (V), 2; Y. ib. V, 22^d bot.; a. e.—b) *Ḥ., near Geder.* [Meg. l. c. (expl. חמת, Josh. l. c.) זו חמת גדר Ms. M. 2 (ed. חמי גרר).] Y. Erub. VI, 23^c bot.; Y. Kidd. III, 64^d top.—c) Y. Shebi. VI, 36^c bot. ח׳ דפחל *Ḥ. near Pella* (v. Neub. Géogr. p. 274).—Lam. R. to I, 16 ח׳ (Neub. l. c. p. 115 חמתן) Emmaus in Judæa.—V. אַמָּאוּס.

חַמְּתָן (v. preced.) pr. n. pl. *Ḥamm'than.* Meg. 2^b כמח׳ לטבריא as far as from Ḥ. to Tiberias (one mile).— Lam. R. to I, 16, v. preced.

חֶמְתָּנָא m. (v. חֵימְתָא) *irascible.* Targ. Prov. XV, 18; a. e.

חַן, v. חָנָה a. חָנַן.

חַן, v. חָנַן.

חֵן, חִין m. (b. h.; חָנַן) *grace, favor; loveliness.* Ab. Zar. 20^a (ref. to תחנם, Deut. VII, 2) לא תתן להם חן ascribe no gracefulness to them (pay no attention to their beauty). Yeb. 63^b (quot. fr. Ben. Sira) אשת חן *coquette.* Keth. 17^a; Snh. 14^a, v. יַעֲלָה. Succ. 49^b אדם שיש עליו חן (Ms. M. לו; Var. חסד) a person that makes a favorable impression on men. Ber. 60^b ותננר . . . לחן וכ׳ and let me find grace and favor &c. Keth. 77^b אם חן מעלה וכ׳ if the Law makes pleasing those who study it, will it not also protect them?—Y. Gitt. V, 46^d top מפני חִינָהּ וכ׳ for the sake of her grace (to raise her estimation in the eyes of men), that people may be anxious to marry her; v. next w.—

Gen. R. s. 34, end שנתן חן וכ׳ who made every place attractive to its inhabitants; a. fr. — *Pl.* חִינִּין, חִינּוֹת. Sot. 47^a ג׳ ח׳ חן וכ׳ there are three remarkable favors, the favor in which the inhabitants hold their place &c.; Y. Yoma IV, beg. 41^b.

חִינָא, חִנָּא ch. same. Targ. Prov. XXXI, 30. Targ. Y. Gen. VI, 8.—Yeb. 38^b (the law is easy in the case of a woman's widowhood) משום ח׳ in order to make her attractive (v. preced.); [oth. opin.: in order that women may be willing to marry; oth. opin.: in order to maintain pleasantness between husband and wife;] Keth. 84^a; a. e.

חֵינָא, חֵנָא m. (חון, cmp. חבן s. v. חֲבִינְנוּתָא) *lap, bosom.* Targ. Is. XL, 11. Targ. II Sam. XII, 3; 8 ed. Lag. (oth. ed. חיק׳; Ar. חֲרָיִ׳). Targ. I Kings XVII, 19.— Cmp. לְחֵינָא.

חַנֵּג, *Pa.* חַנֵּג (denom. of חִינְגָא) *to employ the ḥinga, to dance, play.* Targ. Y. Ex. XV, 20. Ib. XXXII, 19.

חִינְגְּתָא, חִנְגָּא &c., v. sub חִינְגּ׳.

חֲנָה, v. חנו.

חֲנוָאה m. (v. חָנוּת) *a frequenter of taverns, idler* (cmp. הַטְלִים). Pes. 110^b.

חֲנוּגָא, v. חִינְ׳.

חֶנְוָנִי, חֶנְוָוְנִי m. (v. חָנוּת) *shop-keeper, salesman; tavern-keeper.* Shebu. VII, 1 וחח׳ על פנקסו and the storekeeper swears to the correctness of his book account. Kidd. IV, 14 רועה וח׳ the trade of a shepherd or tavern-keeper; Y. ib. 66^c; Treat. Sof'rim XV, 10; a. fr.—*Pl.* חֶנְוָונִים. Y. M. Kat. III, 82^b bot. שני ח׳ two shop-keepers (in the same shop).—*Fem.* חֶנְוָונִית. Keth. IX, 4 המושיב ח׳ . . . if one appoints his wife to be his sales-woman.

חֲנוּיָא pr. n. m. בֶּן ח׳ *Ben-Ḥănoya.* Pesik. Baḥod., p. 105^a; Gen. R. s. 31 a. Yalk. Ps. 876 בר חטיא (corr. acc.).

חֲנוּךְ, חֲנוּכָא, sub חִינ׳.

חֲנוּכָּה f. (b. h. חֲנֻכָּה; חָנַךְ) *inauguration, dedication, festival of dedication;* esp. *Ḥănuckah,* the eight days' feast commemorating the rededication of the Temple after its desecration under Antioch Epiphanes, lasting from the 25th of Kislev to the second (or third) of Tebeth. Sabb. 21^b מאי ח׳ why dedication ceremonies (illumination)? Ib. מצות ח׳ the proper observation of Ḥ. (illumination). Ib. נר ח׳ the lights kindled on Ḥ.—Pesik. R. s. 2 חֲנוּכַּת שמים וארץ the dedication of heaven and earth (by illumination, ref. to Gen. I, 18); ח׳ החומה the dedication of the wall of Jerusalem (Neh. XII, 27); ח׳ הכהנים the dedication (illumination) instituted by the Asmonean priests; a. fr.—*Pl.* חֲנוּכּוֹת. Ib.

חֲנוּכְּתָא, חֲנֻכְּ׳ ch. same. Targ. Num. VII, 84. Targ. Ps. XXX, 1; a. e.—Y. M. Kat. III, end, 83^d. Sabb. 45^a.

חַנּוּן m. (b. h.; חָנַן) *merciful, gracious* Sabb. 133ᵇ.

חֲנוּן, v. חִינ׳.—[בְּנֵי ח׳, or חנון pr. n. pl., v. חִינִי 3).]

חָנוּן I m. 1) part. pass. of חָנַן.—2) (v. next w.) *supplied with an application of Henna;* [oth. opin.: *mercifully protected*]; fem. חֲנוּנָה, pl. חֲנוּנוֹת. Sabb. V, 4 (expl. ib. 54ᵇ *a compress dipped in oil;* Y. ib. 7ᶜ top *a wool-cap;* oth. opin., v. next w.). [Ms. Maim. יַחְנוּנוֹת, quot. Löw Pfl. p. 213.]

חָנוּן II or **חָנוּן (יַחְנוּן)** *Henna, Alcanet,* a plant of the leaves of which a paste is made for dyeing nails, hair &c. Sabb. 54ᵇ (ref. to חנונות, v. preced.) there is a tree in the sea-towns (Cyprus), וח׳ שמו וכ׳ ed. (Ms. M. יחנון) its name is ḥ., and a chip thereof is taken and put into the nostrils (of the sick ewe), that it may sneeze and be released of the worms in the head (v. Löw Pfl. p. 213 a. quotations).—Y. ib. V, 7ᶜ top it is a root ושמיה יַחְנוּנָה its name is *yaḥnunah.*

חָנוּן III pr. n. m., v. חָנָן.

חֶנְוָנִי, v. חֶנְוָנִי.

חֲנוּפָה f. (b. h. חֲנֻפָּה, some ed. חֲנֻפ׳; חָנַף) 1) *hypocrisy, dishonesty, flattery.* Sot. 41ᵇ אדם שיש בו ח׳ a man in whom there is insincerity. Ib. אגרופה של ח׳ the power of flattery (towards Agrippa). Ib. 42ᵃ עדה ... ח׳ a community in which insincerity (flattery to power) prevails. Snh. 52ᵃ בשביל ח׳ שהחניפו לקרח because they flattered Korah. Kidd. 49ᵇ ח׳ וגסות וכ׳ cringing submission (to power) and haughtiness (towards the weak); a. e.—2) *faithlessness to religion, apostasy.* Gen. R. s. 48, beg. כל ח׳ וכ׳ where the root חנף is used in the Bible, it means heresy; Yalk. Is. 304.

חֲנֻפְ׳, חֲנוּפְתָא ch. same. Targ. Jer. XXIII, 15.

חֲנוֹקָא, חֲנוֹקָה, חַנּוֹק m. (חָנַק) *strangler, fighter.* Gen. R. s. 78, beg.; Cant. R. to I, 2, a. e. ח׳ סברת וכ׳ strangler, doest thou mean to choke me, i. e. do you think you can embarrass me with your arguments?

חָנוּת f. (b. h.; חָנָה) *tent,* esp. *tradesman's shop, tavern; meat-market* &c. Tosef. Pes. I (II), 19; Pes. 31ᵇ. Ab. III, 16 החן׳ פתוחה וכ׳ the shop is open, the shopkeeper gives on credit, i. e. man has free volition and Providence is long-suffering &c.—Gitt. 67ᵃ ח׳ מיוזנת well-stocked shop (a man of vast learning and readiness), v. זָיַן. Toh. VI, 3 ח׳ שהיא טמאה ed. Dehr. (ed. שהוא טמא); a. fr.—*Pl.* חֲנֻ׳ חֲנוּיוֹת. Ib.—B. Mets. 88ᵃ, v. חִינִי 3). Ḥull. 95ᵃ תשע ח׳ וכ׳ if there are nine meat-shops (in one market) all of which sell &c.; Pes. 9ᵇ; Nidd. 18ᵃ; Keth. 15ᵃ. Sabb. 35ᵇ שניה להבטיל מלאכה מעיר וַחֲנוּיוֹתֶיהָ Ms. M. (ed. להבטיל עיר וחנויות) the second signal was given to stop work in the town and in its shops. Ib. וננעלו הח׳ and the stores were closed. Ib. 15ᵃ גלתה ... לח בח׳ the Sanhedrin were removed from the Temple and held their meetings in the market; (Ab. Zar. 8ᵇ בחנות); a. fr.

חֲנוּתָא ch. same. B. Mets. 60ᵃ חמרא מח׳ wine from the shop; a. e.—*Pl.* חֲנְוָתָא, חֲנְוָ׳, חֲנָא׳. Targ. Jer. XXXVII, 16; a. e.—Sabb. 32ᵃ, v. בְּזִיוּנָא I. B. Bath. 68ᵃ. Y. Peah I, 16ᵃ a. e. [read:] חֲנְוָ׳ דבותנאי וכ׳ the shops (tradesmen) of Bashan. [Y. Ber. VI, 10ᵃ top בי ח׳, v. חֲרוּתָא.]

חָנַט (b. h.) 1) *to assume shape, form a texture;* (of trees) *to show a distinct shape of fruits, to form fruits;* (of fruits and leaves) *to assume a distinct shape* (v. חֲנָטָה). R. Hash. 14ᵇ אתרוג שֶׁחָנְטוּ פירותיו Ms. M. (ed. פירותיה) an Ethrog-tree whose fruits were formed before the fifteenth of Shebat. Ib. אילן שחנטו וכ׳ a tree whose fruits &c. Y. Shebi. V, beg. 35ᵈ אילן שח׳ a tree which formed fruits. Tosef. ib. IV, 20; a. fr.—2) [*to be handsome;* (Arab.) *to be red,*] *to make handsome,* or *flagrant,* esp. *to embalm.* Gen. R. s. 100.

חֲנַט ch. same, *to embalm.* Targ. O. Gen. L, 2 (Y. בסם); a. e.—Taan. 5ᵇ וכי בכדי . . חֲנָטוּ חנטייא was it for nothing that . . . the embalmers embalmed (Jacob)?

חֶנֶט m., **חֲנָטָה** f. (preced. wds.) *formation of fruits* or *leaves.* Y. Shebi. IV, end 35ᶜ, a. e. שלשולן הוא חֲנָטָן their formation of chains is what in other trees is the formation of fruits. Ib. V, beg. 35ᵈ עקרתה חֲנָטוֹ thou disregardest the time of its formation. Y. Maasr. V, 51ᵈ bot. בח׳ והשרשה as regards the law regulating the tithes according to the time of the formation of fruits and of taking root.—R. Hash. 15ᵇ אחר חנטה לשביעית for the laws concerning the fruits of the Sabbatical year the formation of fruits is the deciding mark. Ib.ᵃ (in Chald. diction) זיל בתר ח׳ be guided by &c. Men. 69ᵃ ח׳ דפירא the formation of the fruit, ח׳ דעלה the formation of the texture of leaves; v. חֲנָצָה.

חַנָּטָא m. (חֲנַט) *embalmer.*—*Pl.* חַנָּטַיָּא. Taan. 5ᵇ, v. חֲנַט.

חִיטְ׳, חִנְטָא=חִיטָּא.—*Pl.* חִנְטַיָּא, חִנְטִין. Targ. Y. Ex. XXIX, 2. Targ. Job XXXI, 40; a. e.

חֲנָטָה, v. חֶנֶט.

חַנְטַיָּא, v. חֲנִיטַיָּא.

חָנָה, חני (b. h.; cmp. גני) [*to be covered, surrounded,*] *to encamp, rest.* Num. R. s. 11 (ref. to ויחנך, Num. VI, 25) יַחֲנֶה ד׳ אצלך the Lord have His tent with thee. Lam. R. introd. (R. Naḥm.) (ref. to Is. XXIX, 1) שח׳ בה וכ׳ where David (lawfully) resided, v. חֲנָיָיא. Ib. (R. Alex. 1) נוסעים . . וחונים וכ׳ they moved in discord and encamped in discord; Mekh. Yithro, Baḥod., s. 1; Lev. R. s. 9; a. fr.—Apocop. form: חָן (as if from חון). Midr. Till. to Ps. LXXVIII, 47 (play on בחנמל ib.) בא חָן מָ׳ל he (the locust) came, encamped, cut; (Tanḥ. Vaëra 14 בא נ״ח מ״ל; Ex. R. s. 12 interpol. from Midr. Till. l. c.: נח).

Hif. הֶחֱנָה *to cause to rest.* Fut. apocop. יַחַן. Y. Taan. III, 66ᶜ (play on יַחְנִיף, Num. XXXV, 33) הדם יחן אף וכ׳ bloodshed causes the anger (of the Lord) to rest upon the ground (rain being withheld); Sifré Num. 161, Yalk. ib. 788 יחון (corr. acc.).

חֲנָיָא, חֲנָיְיָא ch.=h. חֲנִיָּיה. Targ. Y. Num. XIII, 19 חֲנָיְיתְהוֹן their encampment.—Lam. R. introd. (R. Naḥm.) לא ח׳ ליה בה וכ׳ (not לית; some ed. חֲנָיָה h. form) where none but David had a right of encampment.

חֲנִיּוּת, v. חָנוּת.

חֲנִטַּיָּא, חֲנִיטַיָּא m. pl. (b. h. חֲנֻטִים; חָנַט) *embalming*. Targ. O. Gen. L, 3.

חֲנִייָא, v. חֲנָיָא.

חֲנִיָּיה f. (חָנָה) *encampment, rest;* opp. נְסִיעָה. Y. Erub. VI, 22[c] bot. בַּחֲנִיָּיתָן in the order of their encampment. Men. 95[a] בחנייתן Ms. M. (ed. incorr. תו . . .) when they were at rest. Sot. 34[b].—Esp. *right of colonization, acquiring property.* Ab. Zar. 20[a] (ref. to תחנם, Deut. VII, 2, as if תְּחֲנֵם) לא תתן להם ח׳ וכ׳ give them no chance of acquiring property (sell them no trees in the ground); Yalk. Deut. 845.

חֲנִיךְ, v. חָנַךְ.

חַנִּיךְ m. (חָנַךְ) *educator, father.* M. Kat. 25[b] Ms. M., v. next w.

חֲנִיכָה f. (חָנַךְ) [*rubbing the infant's palate with a chewed fig*, v. Fl. to Levy Talm. Dict. II, 206,] *the name given to the child* by the person rubbing is palate; in gen. *surname.* Gitt. IX, 8 כתב חֲנִיכָתוֹ וַחֲנִיכָתָהּ if in the letter of divorce his and her family names are written. Ib. 88[a] חֲנִיכַת אָבוֹת the surname of ancestors. Taan. 20[b]; Meg. 28[a] I never called my neighbor בַּחֲנִיכָתִי וא״ל בַּחֲנִיכָתוֹ (Ar.) by an opprobrious surname given him by myself or, as others relate, by his by-name (which others had given him); ed.: בהכינתו וא״ל בחנוכתו by his *hăkhina* (v. הֲכִינָה); some say, (Rab Ada used the expression) *hănikha.* M. Kat. 25[b] בעת חֲנִיכָתוֹ אבד חַנִּיכוֹ (Ms. M. 2) at the time when he was to receive his name (when his palate was rubbed) died he who was to rear him (his father); (ed., v. חֲנִינָה II). Gen. R. s. 43, beg. (expl. חניכיו, Gen. XIV, 14) בעלי חֲנִיכָתוֹ וכ׳ those bearing his name, their name being Abram, like his own.

חֲנִיכַיִים I m. du. (חָנַךְ; cmp. חִיכְּכֵי) *palate and tongue,* contrad. to teeth. Hull. 103[b] בין חח׳ in the posterior part of the mouth, i. e. if he spit out the forbidden foot just before swallowing.

חַנִּין m. (חָנַן) *he who bestows love, affectionate father.* M. Kat. 25[b], v. חֲנִינָה II.

חַנִּין II pr. n. m. *Ḥannin.* M. Kat. 25[b], a. e., v. חָנַן.

חֲנִינָה, חֲנִינָא I pr. n. m. *Ḥănina,* name of several Tannaim and Amoraim. *Ḥ. b. Antigonos:* Tosef. Arakh. I, 15 (ed. Zuck. חנניא); Arakh. II, 4 (10[a]) Talm. ed. (Mish. חנניא). Tem. VI, 5 חנינא.; Tosef. ib. IV, 10 חנניה. Nidd. 52[a]. Bekh. VI, 3; a. fr. (v. Darkhe Mish. p. 128).—*Ḥ. b. Gamliel:* Macc. III, 15 (23[a]) Ms. M. (ed. חנניא). B. Bath. X, 1. (Tosef. Yoma I, 6 חנניא; Sifra Emor ch. I, Par. 2, a. e. חנניה). Snh. 111[a] ח׳ בן גמלא (v. Rabb. D. S. a. l. note).—Nidd. 8[a] (v. Darkhe Mish. p. 130).—*Ḥ. b. Hăkhinai:* Kil. IV, 8 (Ms. M. a. Y. חנניה, v. Rabb. D. S. a. l. note). Men. 62[a]; a. e. (mostly חנניא, חנניה).—*Ḥ., S'gan hak-Kohanim* (v. סְגַן). Eduy. II, 1; a. fr. (v. Darkhe Mish. p. 59, sq.).—Rabbi Ḥ.: Sabb. 59[b]; a. fr. (v. Frank. M'bo, p. 86[b], sq.).—Other Amoraim by that name, v. Frank. l. c. 87[b], sq.—Snh. 98[b], v. next w.

חֲנִינָה II f. (b. h.; חָנַן) 1) *mercy.* Gen. R. s. 78; s. 92 שמענו ח׳ בי״א וכ׳ we find *grace* applied to the eleven tribes (before Benjamin was born; Gen. XXXIII, 5).—2) *caressing* (of the new-born child). M. Kat. 25[b] (play on Ḥannin) בעת חֲנִינָתוֹ אבד חַנִּינוֹ (v. חֲנִיכָה) at the moment of his receiving caresses died he who was to caress him.—3) (name of fiction, v. preced.) *Hăninah* (Love). Snh. 98[b] דבי ר׳ חנינה אמרי ח׳ שמו the disciples of R. Ḥ. said, the Messiah's name is Ḥ.

חֲנִינִיא, Targ. Y. II Deut. XXXII, 24 some ed., read: תַּנִּינַיָּא.

(חֲנִיסְסַיָּא) חֲנִסְנ׳, חֲנִיסְנְסַיָּא m. pl. 1) *gauzy dresses* or *veils.* Targ. Is. III, 19 (h. text רעל).—2) *obscene statuary devoted to the Sun* (h. חַמָּנִים). Targ. O. Lev. XXVI, 30. Targ. Ezek. VI, 4; 6. Targ. Is. XVII, 8; a. e. [In various ed. our w. is written חניס נ׳ in two words, also חֲנִיסְסַיָּא. Our w. seems to be a derivative of a stem חסס, with anorganic נ, having the meaning of *nakedness, shame.* (cmp חָסִית I, חֶסֶד, חסם).]

חֲנֵיף, v. חָנֵף.

חֲנֵיפָא, v. חֲנִפָּא.

חֲנֵיקָא, v. חֲנָקָא.

חֲנִיקָה f. (חָנַק) *death by strangulation.* Y. Snh. VII, beg. 24[b], v. חֶנֶק.

חֲנִית f. (b. h. חנה *to bend*, v. Ges. Thes. s. v.) *spear.* Yalk. Job. 927.—Pl. חֲנִיתוֹת. Ib. Gen. 133.

חֲנִיתָה, חֲנִיתָא pr. n. pl. *Hănitha,* a place in the district of Tyre. Tosef. Shebi. IV, 9 ח׳ עיליתא וח׳ ארעיתא Upper and Lower Ḥ.; Y. Dem. II, 22[d] top עליתה וח׳ תחתיה (corr. acc.).

חָנַךְ (b. h.; sec. r. of חוך) *to rub, polish, finish;* trnsf. *to train; to dedicate.*

Pi. חִנֵּךְ *to train, initiate* (a child); *to inaugurate, prepare for office; to dedicate.* Y. Yoma I, 38[b] top . . . מה מְחַנְּכִין אותו וכ׳ as the Highpriest's inauguration lasted seven days (Lev. VIII, 33, sq.), so is the Highpriest prepared for the service of the Day of Atonement seven days. Naz. 29[a] כדי לְחַנְּכוֹ במצות in order to initiate his son into the performance of religious duties. Yoma VIII, 4; Tosef. ib. V (IV), 2 מְחַנְּכִין וכ׳ you must train them gradually (to fast on the Day of Atonement) a year or two before religious maturity.—M. Kat. I, 6 מח׳ את הכוכין וכ׳ you may finish up the excavated chambers; v. חִינּוּךְ; a. fr.

Pu. חֻנַּךְ, *Hithpa.* הִתְחַנֵּךְ, *Nithpa.* נִתְחַנֵּךְ *to be inaugurated, to be dedicated.* Yalk. Prov. 964 יצחק ח׳ וכ׳;

Pesik. Bahod., p. 101^{a} יצחק נתח׳ וכ׳ Isaac was initiated into the covenant on his eighth day. Sifra Vayikra, Ḥoba, ch. III, Par. 3 שיִתְחַנֵּךְ המזבח וכ׳ that the altar must be dedicated by offering frankincense. Zeb. 40^{b}; a. e.

חֲנִיךְ, חֲנַךְ ch. same. Targ. O. Deut. XX, 5; a. e. *Pa.* חַנֵּיךְ, *Af.* אַחְנִיךְ same. Ib. חַנְּכֵיה (ed. Berl. חֲנֵכ׳ *Pe.*). Targ. Y. I, II Deut. XXXII, 3 (sanctified his mouth); a. e.

חֲנֻכָּה, v. חֲנוּכָּה.

חִנְכֵי, v. חִירְכֵי.

חַנִּכְּתָא, v. חֲנוּכ׳.

חִנָּם m. (b. h.; חֵן) *gratuitous act, favor*, mostly adv. ח׳, לח׳, בח׳, על ח׳ *gratuitously; for no reason.* Ex. R. s. 41 על ח׳ בראתני וכ׳ hast thou created me for no purpose?— B. Kam. 92^{b}, a. e., v. זַרְזִיר. Ex. R. s. 28, beg. נטלה ח׳ he took it gratuitously. Num. R. s. 1 מה אלו ח׳ וכ׳ as these things (fire, water &c.) are free to all &c.—מַתְּנַת ח׳ *an undeserved gift.* Ib. s. 11; a. fr.—שִׂנְאַת ח׳ *gratuitous hatred, hostility without cause.* Sabb. 32^{b}; a. fr.

חֲנַמְאֵל (b. h.) pr. n. m. *Hanameel*, 1) cousin of Jeremiah. Meg. 14^{b}; a. e.—2) H., the Egyptian, a High-priest. Par. III, 5.

חֲנָמַל m. (b. h.) *beetle*, prob. a species of *locusts.* Yalk. Ex. 185, quot. fr. Tanḥ. (ed. Bub., Vaëra 19) כח׳ חוה הוה יורד the hail came down formed like the *ḥănâmal*, as it says (Ps. LXXVIII, 47) &c.—Midr. Till. to Ps. l. c., v. חָנָה.

חנן, Y. Peah I, 16^{b} מה ח׳ קריימין, read, as Y. Snh. X, beg. 27^{c}, מה נן. [חנן Syr., rare form, v. P. Sm. 250 s. v. אנא.]

חָנַן (חון) (b. h.; cmp. גנן) [*to cover, surround,*] *to caress, grace, favor.* Sabb. 104^{a} (in children's acrostics) זן אותך וחָן אותך sustains and graces thee. Num. R. s. 11 (ref. to Num. VI, 25) יָחוֹן אותך בבנים may He favor thee with (good) children. Ib. (quot. from daily prayers) אתה חונן לאדם דעת thou graciously endowest man with knowledge. Ib. עתיד הקב״ה לָחוֹן עליהם the Lord will in due time protect them. Sifré Num. 41 יָחְנְךָ בתלמוד תורה may He grace thee by enabling thee to study the Law. Pesik. Asser, p. 97^{a} (ref. to מהונך, Prov. III, 9) ממה שחֲנָנְךָ out of what He has endowed thee with; a. fr.—[Midr. Till. to Ps. LXXVIII חָן, v. חָנָה.]—*Part. pass.* חָנוּן, pl. חֲנוּנִים 1) *graced, endowed.* Num. R. l. c. (ב)דעת חֲנוּנֵי endowed with knowledge. Pes. 87^{a} בני חֲנוּנֶיךָ children of thy favored ones, Abraham &c. (Ms., v. בָּחַן).—2) *bandaged.* *Pl.* fem. חֲנוּנוֹת. Sabb. V, 4, v. חָנוּן I, 2.

Nif. נֶחֱנַן *to be shown favor.* Deut. R. s. 7 (ref. to Is. XXVI, 10) אבל אם למד .. אינו נ׳ but if he has learned ..., he will be shown no favor (will not be forgiven).

Hithpa. מִתְחַנֵּן *to bend one's self, to supplicate* (v. תְּחִנָּה). Deut. R. s. 2, beg. מִתְחַנֵּן, v. חָבַט. Ib. התחיל לְהִתְחַנֵּן (התחיל מתחנן) he began to pray; a. fr.

Hithpol. (fr. חָנָה=חון) *to come to rest, to be collected.* Ber. 30^{b} (adopting the expression in conformity with ואתחנן, Deut. III, 23) until his mind be collected again (for prayer), v. חוּל.

חוֹן, חֲנַן ch., pret. חַן same. Targ. O. Gen. XXXIII, 5. —Targ. O. Ex. XXXIII, 19 אֵיחוֹן. Targ. Jud. XXI, 22 חֲנוּנוּן לחון ed. Lag. (oth. ed. חנרנינון) be gracious to them.—Pes. 110^{b} (in an incantation) אדחֲנַנִי וחֲנַנְכִי וכ׳ while He graced me and yourselves, I had not come to that (v. Ar. s. v. חר 8, a. Rabb. D. S. a. l. note for var. lect.).

חָנָן (b. h.) pr. n. m. *Hanan*, name of several Tannaim and of several Amoraim, esp. *H.*, one of the Justices of Peace in Jerusalem, v. אַדְמוֹן. Keth. XIII, 1. Y. ib. 35^{c} a. fr.—*H. the Egyptian:* Snh. 17^{b}; a. e.—H. (interch. with חנין). M. Kat. 25^{b} אסיקו ליה ח׳ וכ׳ (Ms. M. חנין) they gave him the name of H. from his father (Hanin).— Y. Yeb. XI, 12^{a} top (ed. Krot. חָנוּן). Y. Sot. VII, 21^{d} bot. חנין.—Y. Ber. IV, beg. 7^{a} ח׳ בר אבא (ח׳ בר ווא); Y. Pes. IV, 31^{a} חנין; a. oth.—V. Frank. M'bo p. 86^{a}.

חֲנָנָא, חֲנָנָא m. ch.=h. חָנוּן. Targ. Ex. XXII, 26. Targ. Ps. CXI, 4 (ed. Lag. חֲינָנָא); a. e.

חֲנַנְאֵל (b. h.) pr. n. m. *Hananeel.* Y. Keth. XIII, 35^{d} top; a. e.

חֲנַנְיָה, חֲנַנְיָא (b. h. חֲנַנְיָהוּ, חֲנַנְיָה) pr. n. m. *Hanania;* 1) H., one of the Babylonian exiles at the Babylonian court. Sabb. 67^{a} אישתא דח׳ וכ׳ the fire prepared for H., Mishael and Azariah. Snh. 93^{a} כי היכי דח׳ וכ׳ ..... as I tested H. &c.; a. v. fr.—2) several Tannaim and Amoraim (interchanging with חֲנִינָא q. v.); esp. *H. b. ʿAkashia:* Macc. III, 16. Tosef. Shek. III, 18.—*H. b. T'radion*, a martyr of the Adrianic persecution. Tosef. Kel. B. Kam. IV, 17. Ab. Zar. 17^{b}, sq. (חנינא). Taan. 16^{b}; a. fr.—*H. b. 'Akabia:* M. Kat. 21^{a}; (Keth. VIII, 1, a. fr. חנינא); a. e.—*H., 'the Haber of the Rabbis'.* Y. Ter. VIII, 45^{c}; (Y. Ber. I, 2^{c} top. חנינא); a. fr.—Other Amoraim by that name, v. Frank. M'bo, p. 88^{b}, sq.—כְּפַר ח׳ pr. n. pl. *K'far Hanania* in Galilee. Shebi. IX, 2; a. fr.

חנסי, v. חֲנַס.

חֲנַסְנְסִיָּא, v. חֲנִיסְנִי.

חָנֵף, חָנַף (b. h.) [*to bend, decline* from the right path,] *to be insincere, to flatter; to show favor in court; to deceive.* Der. Er. Zuta ch. II אֶחְנוֹף לזה וכ׳ I will flatter (lower myself before) this one that he may give me to eat &c.

Hif. הֶחֱנִיף same. Sot. 41^{b} הֶחֱנִיפוּ לו וכ׳ they flatterec Agrippa (saying to him, 'Thou art our brother'). Ib מותר לְהַחֲנִיף וכ׳ it is permissible to flatter (submit to th power of) the wicked &c. Y. Ber. VII, 11^{c}. Pesik. R. s. 2 (ref. to Is. XXIV, 5) הבריות מַחֲנִיפִים זה לזה men de insincerely with one another; והוא מַחֲנִיפוֹ וכ׳ and he pu him (the priest or Levite) off with deceptive intent, a says &c.; a. fr.

חָנַף, *Pa.* חַנֵּיף ch. same. M.Kat. 17ᵃ ...לא חַנֵּיפִי דאפי׳ ליה not even a man like thee did I flatter. Shebu. 30ᵃ לְחַנּוּפֵי ליה that I should favor him in court?—Keth. 84ᵇ מְחַנְפִיתוּ לְהוּ would you favor them?; ib. 63ᵇ מְחַנְפִיתוּ ליה (*Af.*) would you favor him?—Pesik. Asser, p. 98ᵃ (ref. to Is. XXIV, 5) את סבר מְחַנְּפָא לה והיא מְחַנְּפָה לך thou meanest to deceive it (the land by withholding the tithes, v. preced.), but it will disappoint thee; Tanḥ. R'eeh 14 את כבר מחנף וכ׳ (corr. acc.).

Af. אַחְנִיף same, v. supra.

חָנֵף m. (b. h.; preced. wds.) *hypocrite, flatterer; faithless, arbitrary, fickle.* Esth. R. to I, 1 (ref. to Job XXXIV, 30) בשעה שהמלך ח׳ וכ׳ when a king is arbitrary and rules tyrannically &c. Ib. שהיה ח׳ וכ׳ for he (Ahasverus) was arbitrary, for he put to death &c.—*Pl.* חֲנֵפִים, חֲנֵפִין, חֲנֵי׳. Tosef. Yoma V (IV), 12; Yoma 86ᵇ מפרסמין את החנ׳ וכ׳ you may expose the hypocrites to prevent defamation of the divine Name. Koh. R. to IV, 1 חֲנֵיפֵי תורה pretenders of scholarship. Sot. 42ᵃ; Treat. Der. Er. ch. II. Ib. חֲנֵפוֹת (masc., v. מָסוֹר); a. e.

חַנְפָא, חֲנִיפָא ch. same. Targ. Is. X, 6.—Esth. R. to I, 1 מלכא ח׳ an arbitrary King, v. preced.—*Pl.* חֲנֵפִין, חֲנֵי׳. Targ. Is. IX, 16.

חֲנֻפְתָּא, v. חֲנוּפָ׳.

חָנַק (b. h.; cmp. ענק, אנק, ענק) [*to press,*] *to seize by the throat, to choke.* Tosef. Sabb. III (IV), 6 ואין חוֹנְקִין בשבת you must not press (the jugular veins, to relieve from belly-ache) on the Sabbath; v. infra *Pi.*—B. Bath. X, 8 (175ᵇ) הרי החוֹנֵק את וכ׳ if one seizes a debtor by the throat (threatening violence). Ib. 176ᵃ בְּחָנוּק in the case of one being threatened (and another pledging himself for him). Sabb. 57ᵃ אין אשה חוֹנֶקֶת וכ׳ a woman will not choke herself (will not tie a band around her neck so closely that no water could get under it when bathing); ib.ᵇ אשה ח׳ וכ׳ a woman does tie a chain closely in order to appear fleshy. Gen. R. s. 34 (ref. to דם האדם באדם, Gen. IX, 6) אף החוֹנְקוֹ (the gentile is guilty of bloodshed) even if he only chokes a man ('shedding the blood of man in man'); Y. Kidd. I, 58ᶜ top בחונקו מפני עצמו (read: ממונו) when he merely chokes him to take his money; a. e.—Esp. *to strangle to death.* B. Kam. 47ᵇ ח׳ את עצמו (the ox) strangled himself (by being caught in a rope). Y. Sot. IX, 23ᶜ נמצא חָנוּק if he was found strangled; a. e.—Trnsf. *to produce anguish, agony.* Ḥull. I, 2 מפני שהן חוֹנְקִין because they (a saw &c.) cause agony as if by choking (instead of cutting).—[Kidd. 62ᵃ (ref. to Num. V, 19—20) according to R. Meïr (who says that a condition is not valid unless both the negative and the positive alternatives are stated) חִנָּקִי מיבעי ליה it ought to have been added (to vers 20) 'die in agony'. א״ר תנחום הנקי כתיב said R. T. it says (verse 19) *hnki* (which may be read *hinnaki* for the one alternative and *hinki* for *ḥinki* for the other); Ar. reads חנקי, v. נָקִי.]

Nif. נֶחְנַק 1) *to be strangled.* Snh. XI, 1 (84ᵇ) הַנֶּחְנָקִין those sentenced to death by strangulation. Pes. 112ᵃ לֵיחָנֵק, v. אִילָן.—2) *to feel like choking, to be sorry* (cmp. אָנַק). Cant. R. to IV, 12 ...רואה וכ׳ ...התחיל the seller sees it and grieves (over his loss); Yalk. Ex. 225 Mekh. B'shall. s. 1 לֵיחָנֵק.—[Sabb. 66ᵇ, v. infra.]

Pi. חִינֵּק 1) *to squeeze in, immure.* Pirkê d'R. El. ch. XLVIII; Yalk. Ex. 169 (היו) מְחַנְּקִין את ישראל וכ׳ pressed Israelites between the walls (having mingled their bodies with the clay).—2) *to strangle.* Tosef. M. Kat. I, 5 מְחַנְּקִין וכ׳ (M. Kat. 6ᵇ חונקין) the aunts choke each other to death.—3) *to press the throat, to squeeze the jugular veins* (an operation applied in cases of abdominal affection, Ar. s. v. חנק; *to reset a laryngal muscle or ring,* Rashi; oth. defin., v. Ar. s. v.). Sabb. 66ᵇ לְחַנֵּק to perform the operation (Rashi a. Ar. ed. Koh. לֵיחָנֵק to have the operation performed).

חֲנַק ch. *to strangle.* Targ. II Esth. I, 3.—Keth. 60ᵇ וְחַנְקְתֵּיה she choked her child to death; דלא ... הַחַנְקָן בנייהו for women (of sound mind) will not choke their children (in order to be allowed to marry again before the lapse of a certain time). Y. Taan. IV, 69ᵇ top .. חוה וחוה ח׳ ליה air burst forth out of the bottle and choked him. Y. Ab. Zar. II, 40ᵈ חַנְקַת גרמה she hanged herself. Y. Ber. II, 5ᵃ top בעייא .. מִיחְנְקִינֵיה I would rather choke him; a. e.—Gitt. 67ᵇ דחַנְקָא, v. דִּיסְתְּנָא I.

Ithpa. אִתְחַנֵּק *to hang one's self.* Targ. II Sam. XVII, 23. —Y. Snh. X, 29ᵃ bot. כדון דוד מִתְחַנֵּק now David will die in despair (cmp. preced. *Nif.*). Ib. יהא סופיה מִתְחַנְקָא will end his life by suicide.

חֶנֶק m. (preced. wds.) *execution by strangulation.* Snh. VII, 1; a. fr.

חֲנִיקָא, חֲנָקָא m. (preced. wds.), *pl.* חֲנָקִין, חֲנִיק׳ *ropes* or *chains* around the neck. Targ. Jer. II, 20. Ib. XXVII, 2; a. e.

חַס m. (חוּס) *sparing, forbearance,* only (adverbial) חַס וְשָׁלוֹם *forbearance and peace!, God forfend!, don't say that!* Eduy. V, 6 ח׳ וש׳ שעקביא וכ׳ God forbid (to think) that ʿAkabia was excommunicated! Sabb. 138ᵇ ח׳ וש׳ שתשתכח וכ׳ God forbid (to entertain the idea) that the Law will be forgotten &c. B. Mets. 85ᵇ ח׳ וש׳ אי וכ׳ if, which God forfend, the Law should be forgotten &c.—Y. Pes. VI, 33ᵃ bot. (in Chald. phraseology) ח׳ וש׳ דהוה בעי לה God forbid (to think) that he would have done it!; a. v. fr.

חַס ch. same; חס ל׳ [*God spare him!,*] *far from him!* Targ. Gen. XLIV, 7 (h. text חָלִילָה); a. e..—Kidd. 44ᵇ וחס ליה לזרעיה וכ׳ and far it is from the son of Abba ... (Samuel) to have said so; Ḥull. 111ᵇ. Y. Ḥag. II, 77ᵈ bot. חס ליה לא וכ׳ far from him! He never did &c.

חָסָא, v. חֲסִי.

חַסָּא I m. (prob. fr. חוס *to bend,* cmp. Ber. 56ᵃ quoted below) *lettuce* (h. חֲזֶרֶת). Pes. 39ᵃ, v. חוּס ch. Ib. 116ᵃ, v. חַמָּא. Ber. 56ᵃ (to one who dreamt that he saw lettuce on the wine keg) עיף עיסקך כח׳ thy business will be doubled (thrive) like lettuce; ח׳ ... מרירו, v. מְרִירָ I. Y. Kil. I, 27ᵃ top (expl. וחזרת גלים) חַס דגורין (constr.), v.

דְּגוֹרָא.—*Pl.* חָסִין. Y. Maas. Sh. IV, end, 55[c] top., v. בְּסִין. Gen. R. s. 67 ח׳ רברבין large (old) lettuce plants. Lam. R. to I, 1 (1 חד כות׳) ח׳ מיסרא דח׳ a bundle of &c.

חָסָא II pr. n. m. *Ḥasa.* Yeb. 121[b].

חסאין, Tosef. Kel. B. Mets. V, 13, read: חס׳, v. סוּג II.

חָסַד I (v. next w.) *to be white, pure, charitable, graceful.*—Part. pass. חָסוּד, fem. חֲסוּדָה, *endowed with* חֶסֶד, *graceful.* Keth. 17[a] (in a bridal song) כלה נאה וח׳ handsome and graceful bride. Num. R. s. 12; Cant. R. to III, 10 (not חסידה).

חָסַד II (b. h.; cmp. חסר, חסף); *Pi.* חִסֵּד, חַשֵּׂד [*to scrape off,*] (cmp. גרף, גדף) *to jeer, scoff at, to shame.* Ruth R. to IV, 8 שֶׁחִסְּדָן ברבים (or שֶׁחֲסָדָן; ed. Wil. שחשדן) he scoffed at them publicly (speaking ironically, with ref. to II Chr. XIII, 8); Y. Yeb. XVII, beg. 15[c] שֶׁחִישֵּׁד וכ׳ he jeered at Jeroboam; Gen. R. s. 65; ib. s. 73 שחסדם ed. Wil. (oth. שחש׳); Lev. R. s. 33; Midr. Sam. ch. XVIII שֶׁחִיסְּדָן; Yalk. Kings 205 וּמְחַשֵּׁד.—Ex. R. s. 30 (ref. to Ex. II, 14) שֶׁחִיסְּדוּ וכ׳ when Dathan and Abiram sneered at him. Ib. בזה שֶׁחִיסַּדְתֶּם אותו וכ׳ with the very word (שופט) with which you sneered at him, I shall give him the rulership (משפטים). Pesik. R. s. 42 מְחַסְּדִים את שרה (not מחסרו׳) jeered at Sarah; a. e.—V. חִיסּוּד.

חֲסַד ch. same, 1) *to be put to shame (be whitened).* Targ. Ps. XXXIV, 6 Ms. (ed. עצבו). Ib. XL, 15 (ed. Lag. a. oth. Ithpa.; some ed. ר for ד).—2) *to shame* &c.; v. infra.

Pa. חַסֵּד, *Af.* אַחְסִיד *to jeer, blaspheme, disgrace* (in ed. frequ. *Pe.*). Targ. I Sam. XVII, 36. Targ. Prov. XXV, 10 נַחְסִידָךְ Lev. (ed. נֶחְסְדָךְ); a. fr. [Some ed. ר for ד.]

Ithpa. אִתְחַסַּד *to be reviled, put to shame.* Targ. Ps. LXXI, 24; a. e.; v. supra. Targ. Prov. XX, 4 (v. LXX).

חֶסֶד m. (b. h.; חָסַד I) *grace, kindness, love, charity.* Sifra K'dosh., Par. 4, ch. X (ref. to חסד, Lev. XX, 17) שמא תאמר ... ח׳ הוא if you will object, why did Cain marry his sister? (Answ.) It was an act of kindness (to secure the propagation of the race); Y. Yeb. XI, 11[d] top ח׳ עשיתי וכ׳ I (the Lord) dealt kindly with &c.—חוט של ח׳, v. חוּט. Succ. 49[b] אין צדקה ... לפי ח׳ שבה charity is rewarded only in proportion to the benevolence in it. Ib. תורה של ח׳ a study of love (for its own sake); a. fr.—Ruth R. Par. 3, beg., v. חַסְדָּאָה.—Gen. R. s. 8 ח׳ אומר Charity said &c.—*Pl.* חֲסָדִים *acts of kindness.* Succ. l. c.; a. fr.; v. גָּמַל a. גְּמִילוּת.

חִיס׳ I, חַסְדָּא, חֲסַד ch. same. Targ. Y. Lev. XX, 17 (v. Y. Yeb. XI, 11[d] top, quot. in preced.). Targ. Gen. XXXIX, 21; a. fr.—Y. Ab. Zar. III, 42[c] top; Y. Ḥag. II, 77[d] bot., v. גְּמַל; a. e.—*Pl.* חִסְדִּין, חַסְדַּיָּא, חַס׳; חִיס׳, חַס׳. Targ. O. Gen. XXXII, 11. Targ. Ps. CVII, 43; a. e.

חִי׳ II, חִסְדָּא m. (=b. h. חֶסֶד) *shame, revilement,* interch. with חִיסוּדָא q. v.

חִי׳ III, חִסְדָּא pr. n. m. *Ḥisda,* name of several Amoraim. Ber. 8[a]; Y. ib. IV, 9[a] top.—Ḥull. 10[a].—Y. Ḥall. I, 57[c] top; a. fr. V. Fr. M'bo, p. 89[b], sq.

חִסְדָּאָה m. (denom. of חִסְדָּא I) *kind, pleasing.*—*Pl.* חִסְדָּאִין. Gitt. 7[a] חיסדא שמך וח׳ מילך thy name is Ḥisda (Love), and lovable are thy words; [Ruth R. Par. 3, beg. את חסד ומה לך חסד, read: וּמִילָּךְ].

חִסְדַּאי, חִסְדַּיי pr. n. m. *Ḥisdai* (interch. with חִסְדָּא). Ruth R. Par. 3, beg. חסדאי; (Gitt. 7[a] חיסדא). Y. Snh. I, 18[d] bot.. Y. Erub. IV, end, 22[a]; a. fr.—V. Fr. M'bo, p. 90[a].

חִסְדוּתָא f.=חֲסִידוּתָא. Targ. Cant. VII, 6 (ed. Lag. חֲסִי׳). Targ. Ps. LXIX, 11 Ms. (ed. Lag. חסיד׳, oth. ed. חסודית׳).

חסדיגרון, v. חָסָא I a. דְּגוֹרָא.

חִסּוּדָא, v. חִיס׳.

חֲסוּדָא f. ch.=next w. Targ. II Esth. II, 7; 8.

חֲסוּדָה I f. *amiable,* v. חָסַד I.

חֲסוּדָה II f. (prob. fr. חָסַד II) *the vein opened for blood-letting.* Sabb. 108[b] bot. (old ed. חסורה); (cmp. Taan. 21[b] bot.).

חִסּוּדְתָא, v. חִסְדוּתָא.

חסוח, v. חָסוּת.

חסוסה, v. חֲסִיסָה.

חֲסוֹךְ I m. (חֲסַךְ) *sparing, clemency.* Targ. Jer. XXX, 11; XLVI, 28. Ib. X, 24 ed. Lag. a. Rashi (ed. חֲשׂוֹךְ, not חֲשׂ׳).

חֲסוֹךְ II m. (v. חֲסִיךְ) *diminution; (adv.) less.* Targ. Ez. XVI, 47.

חסולא, חסום, v. sub חִיס׳.

חָסוֹם (חוֹסֶם) m. (חָסַם I; b. h. מַחְסוֹם) *muzzle.* Kel. XVI, 7 (ed. Dehr. חִיסּוּם; Mish. ed. חסים, incorr.). Tosef. Sabb. IV (V), 5 חוסם; Sabb. 53[a].

חֲסוֹמִית, v. מַחְסוֹמִית.

חֲסוּסָה, v. חֲסִיסָה.

חִסּוּר, v. חִיס׳.

חֲסוּרִין, v. חֲסַר ch.

חָסוּת f. (b. h.; חָסָה) *a projecting rock, shady place.* Ex. R. s. 2, beg. (some ed. חָסִית). [Levy Talm. Dict. reads: חסוח, cmp. next wds.]

חסחום, v. next w.

חַסְחוּס m. (חסחס, *Pilp.* of חסם, v. חִיס a. preced. art.) [*projection, protection,*] *the cartilages forming the ear, helix,* &c. Bekh. VI, 1 (37[a]) נפגמה אזני מן החו׳ (ed. חסחום; Mish. ed. a. Ar. חסחוס) if its ear it split (defective) from the cartilages (inward).—*Pl.* חַסְחוּסִים, סִין .... *gristles.* Pes. VII, 11 (84ᵃ) Y. ed. (Mish. a. Bab. ed. חַסְחוּסִין; Ms. M. 2 also חסחיסין, v. Rabb. D. S. a. l. note 30).—Y Snh.VIII, beg.26ᵃ אכלו חסוקים, read: אכל ח׳.—V. חַסְחָסִית.

חַסְחוּס ch. same. Targ. Am. III, 12 (h. text בדיל). Targ. Y. Lev. VIII, 23 (h. text תְּנוּךְ, v. גְּדִירָא); a. e.

חסחף, Targ. Y. II Deut. XXXII, 11 מח׳, read: מחפחף, v. חֲפַף I.

חַסְחָסוּת f. (v. חסחוס) *the system of cartilages of the ear, helix and anti-helix.* Bekh. 40ᵇ אזניו .. בח׳ אחת (Rashi חסחיס, read: חסחוס) double ears with one system of &c.—*Pl.* חַסְחָסִיּוֹת. Ib.—V. חֲסִיסָה.

***חֲסִי, חֲסָא** (cmp. חסר II) *to be scraped.* Denom. חֲסִיָא.

Af. אַחְסֵי *to revile, sneer at.* Targ. I Sam. I, 6 ומרגזה פנינה ארתה ומַחְסָא לה Ar. s. v. מחס (ed. differ. vers.). V. מְחוֹסָא.

חֲסִיָא c. (preced.) *scrubby, lean.—Pl. fem.* חֲסִיָין. Targ. Y. Gen. XLI, 3 (some ed. חסכן; v. 4 חסירן); ib. v. 19.

חָסִיד m. (b. h.; חֶסֶד I) *kind, God-fearing, submissive, pious, abstemious.* Tem. 15ᵇ כל הי‍כא דאמר מעשה בח׳ אחד וכ׳ wherever we read (in Talmudic writings), 'It is reported of a pious man', either R. Juda b. Baba it meant or &c. Sot. III, 4 ח׳ שוטה a foolish saint. Ab. V, 10 שלי ... ח׳ he who says, Mine is thine and thine is thine, is a *ḥasid.* Ib. 11; a. v. fr.—*Pl.* חֲסִידִים. Ber. V, 1 ח׳ הראשונים the pious men of olden days; a. v. fr.

חֲסִיד, חֲסִיד, חֲסִידָא ch. 1) same. Targ. Ps. XVIII, 26; a. fr.—B. Kam. 30ᵃ האי .... למיהוי ח׳ he who desires to be a conscientious man (in business) let him live up to the laws laid down in *N'zikin* (v. נֶזֶק). B. Bath. 7ᵇ; a. fr.—Frequ. as a distinguishing surname. M. Kat. 17ᵃ. Ber. 29ᵇ; a. fr.—*Pl.* חֲסִידִין, חֲסִידַיָּא. Targ. Ps. CXLV, 10; a. e.—Ḥull. 122ᵃ, a. e. ח׳ דבבל the meek men of Babylonia, opp. תקיפי. M. Kat. 17ᵃ למערתא דח׳ to the cave where the pious were buried; a. fr. —*Fem.* חֲסִידָא, חֲסִידְתָא. Sabb. 77ᵇ, v. אֲסִיתָא.—2) *graceful.* Targ. Prov. XI, 16. Ib. XVII, 8.

חֲסִידָה f. 1) fem. of חָסִיד; v. also חֲסוּדָה, s. v. חֶסֶד I.—2) (b. h.) *stork.* Hull. 63ᵃ, v. דַּיָּה; ולמה ... ח׳ שעושה חסידות וכ׳ and she is named 'the kind' because she acts kindly with her kind; Midr. Till. to Ps. CIV, 17. Ex. R. s. 35.

חֲסִידוּת f. (חָסִיד) *piety, scrupulousness, abstemiousness; kindness.* Ḥull. 63ᵃ, v. preced.—B. Mets. 52ᵇ; Ḥull. 130ᵇ, a. fr. מדת ח׳ the conduct of a very scrupulous person. Ab. Zar. 20ᵇ; Y. Sabb. I, 3ᶜ top; a. fr.

חֲסִידוּתָא ch. same. Targ. Cant. III, 6; a. e., v. חִסְדּוּתָא.—Snh. 110ᵇ שַׁבְקָהּ ר״ע לַחֲסִידוּתֵיהּ R. Ak. has abandonned his (usual) kindness, i. e. his harsh opinion does not agree with the liberality shown elsewhere.

חֲסִידְתָא, v. חֲסִיד.

חֲסִיךְ m., **חֲסִיכָא** c. (חסך II, v. חֲסִיךְ II and חֲשִׁיךְ II) *rubbed off, lessened;* (of animals or plants) *stunted, lean.* Men. 29ᵃ ומי ח׳ כולי האי Ar. (ed. חסר; Rashi to Taan. 11ᵃ: חֲסִיכֵי, pl.) is there so much reduction (loss in weight by smelting)?—*Pl.* חֲסִיכֵי; fem. חֲסִיכָן, חֲסִיכָתָא. Targ. Gen. XLI, 19; 20; 27 (interch. with חסיר׳ a. חסיו׳, v. חֲסִיָא).—Pes. 48ᵃ חיטי ח׳ poor wheat.

חֲסִיכָא m. (preced.) *a little less.* Targ. Is. XXVI, 12 ח׳ מחיבנא a little less that our sins deserved (h. text גם, cmp. גמם).

חֲסִיל, v. חֲסַל.

חָסִיל m. (b. h.; חָסַל) [*the peeler,*] name of *a species of locusts.* Snh. 94ᵇ. Y. Taan. III, 66ᵈ, v. חָסַל.

חֲסִילָא, ח׳ m. (חָסַל) *weaned child, infant.* Targ. Is. XI, 8 (h. text גָּמוּל); a. e.

חֲסִים m., v. חָסַם.

חֲסִימָה I f. (חָסַם I) *muzzling, the law forbidding muzzling* (Deut. XXV, 4). B. Mets. 88ᵇ אתה מצווה על חֲסִימָתוֹ thou art warned not to muzzle him. Ib. 89ᵃ כל מילי איתנהו בח׳ all things (animals) are implied in the law &c. Ib. 90ᵇ ח׳ מעלייתא הוא it is a real case of muzzling; a. fr.

חֲסִימָה II f. (חָסַם II) 1) = חִיסּוּם, *steel-edge.* Tosef. Kel. B. Mets. III, 7.—2) *varnish, glaze.* Ib. I, 3 (quot. in R. S. to Kel. XI, 4), v. מַחְסוֹמִית.

חסין, Ex. R. s. 43 קאלא ח׳, v. קאלוחסין.

חֲסִין, חֲסִינָא m., **חֲסִינְתָא** f. (חָסַן I) *strong; hard.* Targ. Ez. XXIII, 31 (32). Targ. Am. II, 9; a. e. —*Pl.* חֲסִינִין, חֲסִינַיָּא; f. חֲסִינָן, חֲסִינָתָא. Targ. O. Deut. XXVIII, 23. Targ. Is. XXVIII, 2. Ib. XXI, 1; Targ. Deut. X, 21 *mighty deeds.*

חֲסִינָה f. (v. חִסְנָא) [*storage,*] *a wicker work* used for purposes of storage. Kel. XVI, 5.

חֲסִיסָא m., pl. **חֲסִיסֵי** (חסס, v. חֲסִיָא) *stunted grains* used for parching, v. אַבְשׁוּנָא. Ned. 49ᵇ. Pes. 40ᵇ.

חֲסִיסָה f. (contr. of חסחיסה) = חַסְחָסוּת. Tosef. Bekh. IV, 13 חסו׳ ed. Zuck. (Var. חסי׳).—*Pl.* חֲסִיסוֹת. Ib.

חֲסִיר, חֲסִירָה, v. חֲסֵר.

חֲסִיר, חַסִּיר m. (חֲסַר) *wanting, less; reduced, lean* (v. חֲסִיָא a. חֲסִיךְ). Targ. Prov. VII, 7; a. fr.—*Fem.* חֲסִירָא, חֲסִי׳. *Pl.* חֲסִירָן, חַסִּ׳. Targ. Gen. XLI, 3; 4; a. e.—V. also חֲסֵר ch.

חֶסְרוּ׳, חֲסִירוּ׳, חַסִּירוּתָא f. (preced.) *want, absence.* Targ. O. Deut. XXVIII, 48; a. e.—V. חוּסְרָנָא.

חֲסִית I f. (= חססית; חסס, cmp. Ar. *ḥassa*) *peeling plants, alliacea, leek plants.* Ter. X, 10 **אלא עם הח׳ (Ms.**

M. חתיסות; Y. ed. חחיסית) except they are combined with leek-plants. Y. ib. 47[b] ח׳ בח׳ מין במינו if the same species of leek plants (of T'rumah and Ḥullin) are pressed together. Lam. R. to II, 11, v. דְּמָעָה.—Pl. חֲסִיּוֹת. Tosef. Ter. IX, 3 אלו הן מיני ח׳ וכ׳ (ed. Zuck. חרסיות, Var. חסיות, חוריות) the following belong to the leek-plants, common leek, garlic, onion and allium porrum, v. קַפְלוֹט.

חֲסִית II f. 1) (חוס) *saving, protection.* Yalk. Ex. 200 אין פסיחה אלא ח׳ passing over (the root פסח) means sparing; (Mekh. Bo, Pisha, s. 11 חַיִּיס).—2) (חָסָה) *shady place*, v. חָסוּת.

חָסַךְ (b. h. חָשַׂךְ) [*to scrape off,*] *to diminish, deduct; to stint, withhold.* Dem. VII, 3 (4) וחוֹסֵךְ גרוגרת וכ׳ Ar. a. ed. Y. (Mish. a. Bab. ed. חוֹשֵׂךְ, Ms. M. repeatedly חוך) and retains one fig (which he does not eat). Ib. לא יַחְסוֹךְ (Var. same).—*Part. pass.* חָסוּךְ *stripped, wanting.* Kel. I, 2 וַחֲסוּכֵי (וחֲשׂוּכֵי) בגדים and to make unclean the persons alone but not their clothes. Erub. 28[a] חֲסוּכֵי בנים Ms. M. a. oth. (ed. חשוכי) those who want children, opp. מרובי בנים.

Pi. חִיסֵּךְ *to spare, be regardful, lenient.* Tosef. Sot. VI, 7 ח׳ עליו הכתוב the Biblical text (the Lord) spared him (did not rebuke him). Ib. מְחַסְּכִין לו they (in heaven) spare him. Zeb. 6[b] חי׳ הכתוב the Biblical law has regard to expenses; v. חִיסָּכוֹן.

חֲסַךְ ch. same, Part. pass. חֲסִיךְ q. v. Targ. Y. Gen. XLI, 3 חַסְכָן, read: חֲסִיכָן.

חֶסְכוֹן, v. חִיסָּ׳.

חָסַל (b. h.; cmp. preced. wds.) *to peel off, to bare.* Y. Taan. III, 66[d] the locust is called *ḥasil* שהוא חוֹסֵל וכ׳ because it bares everything.

חֲסַל, חֲסִיל ch. same, [*to scrape off;* (cmp. חֲנַךְ) *to finish,*] 1) *to cease, have done* (cmp. גְּמַר). Targ. II Chr. IV, 11.—חֲסִיל *to be exhausted, gone.* Targ. Y. II Gen. XLVII, 15. Targ. Y. II Deut. XXXI, 24; a. e.—Targ. Y. II Gen. L, 19 חַסְלַת וכ׳ the evil is paid off (atoned for; cmp. גמל).—Y. R. Hash. II, 58[b] top מן דַחֲסַל . . . מן וכ׳ when R. . . had ceased from praying. Gen. R. s. 17, beg. מן דחַסְלִין (not דמן ח׳) when they had finished their studies; a. fr.—2) *to mature, ripen.* Targ. Y. II Num. XVII, 23 (h. text גמל).—3) *to wean.* Targ. I Sam. I, 24 (h. text גמל); a. fr.

Af. אַחְסִיל, *Pa.* חַסֵּל 1) *to peel off, lay bare.* Targ. O. Deut. XXVIII, 38.—2) *to finish.* Targ. Y. II Gen. XLIV, 18. —Y. Bicc. I, 64[a] מְחַסֵּל לה finished the sentence (by adding a general rule). Cant. R. beg. זימנין מח׳ לה וכ׳ sometimes he goes through the entire alphabet &c.; (Koh. R. to I, 13 חשל); a. fr.

Ithpe. אִתְחֲסִיל *to be weaned.* Targ. O. Gen. XXI, 8 (ed. Berl. אִתְחַ׳); a. e.

חָסַם I (b. h.; cmp. preced. wds., esp. חָסַךְ) [*to withhold, prevent,* v. Ez. XXXIX, 11,] 1) *to muzzle,* esp. *to prevent the animal from eating while at work* (with ref. to Deut. XXV, 4). B. Mets. 90[a] עובר משום בל תַּחְסוֹם he trespasses the law forbidding to muzzle (if he prevents the animal from eating). Ib. חֲסוֹם פרתי muzzle my cow. Ib.[b], a. e. חֲסָמָהּ בקול if he prevents her from eating by shouting at her; a. fr.—Trnsf. (an adaptation of Deut. l. c. which is followed by the law concerning leviratical marriage) *to tie a woman to a man* (*Yabam*) *with whom she cannot live*; [Rashi: *to shut a woman's mouth, ignore her objections*]. Yeb. 4[a] שאין חוֹסְמִין אותה that we do not coërce her (to be the wife of a leper).—2) *to form the rim of basket work or of a leather bag.* Kel. XVI, 2; 3; 4.

Nif. נֶחְסַם *to be muzzled, to be prevented from eating while at work.* B. Mets. 89[a] לאקושי חוֹסֵם לְנֶחְסָם וכ׳ to draw a parallel between the muzzler (human laborer) and the muzzled (laboring brute).

Hithpa. הִתְחַסֵּם, *Nithpa.* נִתְחַסֵּם *to be bent into a rim.* Kel. XX, 2.

חֲסַם ch. same, *to muzzle; trnsf. to silence.* Sot. 35[a] וּחָסְמִין לי and they will silence me. Snh. 32[b].

Ithpe. אִתְחֲסַם, אִיתְ׳ *to be muzzled, silenced.* Targ. Ps. XXXII, 9. Ib. CVII, 42.—Snh. l. c. וּלִיתְחַסְמוּ let them be silenced (intimidated).

חָסַם II (cmp. חסל) *to peel, scrape, to polish, glaze, harden* (*steel*). Tosef. Shebi. VI, 10; Y. ib. VIII, 38[b] bot. אין חוֹסְמִין וכ׳ you must not use it for glazing stoves or ranges. Tosef. Bets. III, 16 כדי לְחוֹסְמָן for the purpose of glazing them; Bets. 34[a] לְחַסְּמָן (*Pi.*).—Y. M. Kat. I, end, 81[a], v. infra.—[Tosef. Dem. IV, 12 משיחסום, read: משיתנם?]

Pi. חִיסֵּם same. Bets. l. c., v. supra. Ib. מפני שצריך לְחַסְּמָן because it is necessary to glaze the tiles (by heating them).

Hithpa. הִתְחַסֵּם *to be glazed.* Y. M. Kat. I, end, 81[a] [read:] ואין מפיגין אותן בצונן כדי שיִתְחַסְּמוּ nor must you cool them off suddenly in order that they may be glazed (hardened). V. חִיסּוּם.

חֲסַם ch. same. *Part. pass.* חֲסִים *bright and hard, flinty.*—*Pl.* חֲסִימִין. Targ. Y. II Deut. VIII, 9; (Y. I שאילן מסימן, read: חֲסִימָן fem. pl.). Targ. Y. ib. XXXIII, 25.

Pa. חַסֵּם [*to scrape,* cmp. גמגם, חָכַךְ II] *to hesitate, be uncertain what to do.* Sabb. 147[a] הוה קא מְחַסֵּם וכ׳ he hesitated to hand it to him. Keth. 20[b]. B. Mets. 23[b]. Ḥull. 50[a]. [Ar. a. some Mss. have חסס; v. Koh. Ar. Compl. s. v. חסם a. Rabb. D. S. to B. Mets. l. c.]

Ithpa. אִתְחַסֵּם 1) *to receive a steel edge;* trnsf. (of the mouth) *to become able to speak.* Lev. R. s. 23; Cant. R. to II, 2 אתח׳ ר׳ וכ׳ R. E. (who on a former occasion was unable to pronounce a blessing) has received a steel edge, and they named him R. E. Ḥisma; [Ar.: הא חֲסִים אלעזר, v. supra].—2) *to rub against,* trnsf. (cmp. גָּרַר) *to seek a quarrel, to vie with* (v. P. Sm. 1333). Targ. Prov. XXIV, 19 (h. text תתחר).

חֲסַן I 1) *to be strong.* [Targ. Is. LXIII, 15, v. *Ithpa.*]— V. חוּסְנָא.—2) (cmp. חזק) *to take possession* (mostly in *Af.*).

Pa. חַסֵּין *to strengthen.* Targ. Is. XXXV, 3 (h. text אמץ).

Af. אַחְסִין 1) same. Targ. O. Gen. XLIX, 24. Targ. Am. II, 14 (h. text אמץ); a. e.—2) *to take possession* (for one's self and heirs). Targ. Ps. XXXVII, 29. Targ. O.

Lev. XXV, 46 (Y. תַּחְסְ׳, *Pe.*); a. fr.—B. Bath. 148[b] bot. אַף יַחְסִין וירית וכ׳ also if he uses the expression *yaḥsin*, he shall take possession, or *yereth*, he shall inherit, referring to an heir.—3) *to give possession, to bequeathe.* Targ. O. Deut. XXXII, 8 באחסנא (Y. בְּאַחְסָנוּת verbal noun, constr.). Targ. Y. I Num. XI, 26.—4) *to hoard up* (v. חִסְנָא). Targ. Am. II, 6; VIII, 6 (h. text נעלים, v. נְעַל).—5) (cmp. חָזַק Hif.) *to hold, have room for.* Y. Snh. X, 29[a] top (ref. to II kings VI, 1) לא א׳ אוכלוסייא וכ׳ (not אסחין) it did no longer hold the masses &c.

Ithpa. אִתְחַסַּן, אִתְחַסֵּין 1) *to strengthen one's self, to betake one's self; to control one's own emotions.* Targ. Jer. III, 8. Targ. Is. LXIII, 15 ed. Lag. (oth. ed. יִתְחַסְ׳).—Targ. O. Gen. XLIII, 31 (v. זְרַז). Targ. I Sam. XIII, 12; a. fr. (h. text התאפק).—2) *to be put in possession.* Targ. Job VII, 3 (h. text הָנְחַלְתִּי).

חֲסַן II (=חֲסַל 1), *Af.* אַחְסֵין *to wean.* Targ. Y. Gen. XXI, 8.

Ithpa. אִתְחַסַּן 1) *to be weaned.* Ib.—2) *to be fully compensated.* Targ. Prov. XI, 31 (h. text יְשֻׁלָּם).

חֹסֶן, v. חוֹסֶן.

חִסְנָא m. (חֲסַן) 1) *strength, power.* Dan. II, 37; v. חוּסְנָא.—2) *stronghold, store-house* (b. h. חֹסֶן).—*Pl.* חִסְנַיָּא. Targ. Joel I, 17 Ar. (ed. Lag. חוּסְנַיָּא; v. אַסְנָא).

חֲסַף I (cmp. חֲסַל) *to peel off;* (neut. verb) *to be scaly, rough.*

Pa. חַסֵּף *to pound grain* &c. Y. Sabb. VII, 10[b] bot. ח׳ פלפלין pounds pepper (cmp. מחספס, Ex. XVI, 14). [Y. B. Mets. II, 8[c] bot. וחספתה, v. חֲפַס.]

Ithpa. אִתְחַסַּף [*to become white*, cmp. כסף,] *to feel ashamed.* Targ. II Esth. VI, 12.

חֲסַף II, **חַסְפָּא** or **ח׳** I m. (preced.) (=h. חֶרֶשׂ) 1) *rough clay,* מאנא דח׳ *clay vessel* (common and easily broken). Targ. O. Lev. XI, 33; a. e.—2) [*something with which to peel or scrape,*] *fragment of a vessel, potsherd.* Targ. Prov. XXVI, 23.—Yeb. 92[b], a. e., v. דְּלֵי. Kidd. 18[a] (prov.) נקיט . . . יהיבנא ליה ח׳ he had a pearl in his hand, and we give him a sherd, i. e. for a valuable object we give him a valueless paper; a. fr.—*Pl.* ח׳, חַסְפִּין. Gen. R. s. 14, v. דְּבַק; Midr. Till. to Ps. II; a. e.

חַסְפָּא, ח׳ II m. (חסף; cmp. כסופא) *shame;* (cmp. b. h. בֹּשֶׁת) *idol.* Y. Ned. I, 37[a] top (in answer to the question, 'Does not *ḥeres* mean a sherd?') לשון אומות . . . קריין לח׳ כספא (*ḥeres* may be used as a substitute for חֵרֶם) for it is a gentile dialect, the Nabatæans say *ḥispa* for *kispa* (כסופא) (which means *shame* or *idol*); Y. Naz. I, beg. 51[a] (corr. acc.); v. Ned. 10[b] top.

חַסְפִּיָה pr. n. pl. *Ḥaspiah* (*Hasbeya*), a border town in Northern Palestine. Y. Dem. II, 22[d] top; Tosef. Shebi. IV, 10 צפיה ed. Zuck. (Var. חצפיא, צפיא).

חַסְפְּנִיתָא f. (חֲסַף) 1) *scaly skin.* Num. R. s. 19; Koh. R. to VII, 23 רגלוי . . . לח׳ דנונא the feet of chickens resemble (as to their covering) the scale-covered skin of the fish, v. חַרְסְפִּיתְּ.—2) *scab, eruption.* Sabb. 133[b], sq. ליה ח׳ . . . האי מאן דמשי (Ms. M. חוספנתא) he who washes his face and does not dry it well, will get a scab. Ab. Zar. 28[b], sq. (Rashi: חוס׳).

חָסַר, חָסֵר, חָסֵר I (b. h.; cmp. חָסַל) [*to scrape off,*] *to diminish, take off; to be diminished, less; to want, miss; to be imperfect.* Snh. 68[a] ולא חָסַרְתִּי מרבותי וכ׳ yet I skimmed of the knowledge of my teachers no more than a dog takes who licks out of the sea. Ib. ולא חֲסֵרוּנִי וכ׳ they skimmed of my knowledge &c.; Cant. R. to I, 3 לא חָסַרְתִּיהָ וכ׳ what wisdom I skimmed of the Law, was no more than &c., v. זִכְרוּת. Ib. רבותי חֲסֵרוּהָ וכ׳ my teachers carried off at least a real smattering of it &c. B. Kam. 20[a] bot. מאי חֲסַרְתִּיךָ what loss have I occasioned to thee?—Ib.[b], a. fr. זה נהנה . . . חָסַר the one profits while the other loses nothing (therefore can claim no damages). Lev. R. s. 1 מה חָסַרְתָּ, v. דֵּעָה. Men. 30[a], a. e. is it possible ס״ת ח׳ אות וכ׳ that the Book of the Law wanted one letter yet (to be written) &c.?—Pesik. R. s. 3 (ref. to מתה עלי, Gen. XLVIII, 7) שֶׁחֲסַרְתִּיהָ for I miss her; a. fr.

Pi. חִיסֵּר *to lessen, omit; to deprive.* Ker. 6[a] חי׳ אחת וכ׳ if he left out one of its ingredients. Erub. 13[a] שמא אחת מְחַסֵּר וכ׳ for if thou omit one letter. Koh. R. to I, 15 (ref. to חסרון, ib.) משאדם מְחַ׳ עצמו וכ׳ as soon as a man deprives himself of the words of the Law (neglecting them); ib. מַחְסִיר (*Hif.*). Y. Snh. XI, beg. 30[a] אפי׳ חַבּוּרָה (v. חַבּוּרָה) he did not create a diminution (open wound); a. fr.—*Part. pass.* מְחוּסָּר, constr. מְחוּסַּר *wanting, requiring.* R. Hash. 6[a] מח׳ זמן wanting time, i. e. too young for sacrifice. Ker. II, 1 מח׳ כפרה requires a ceremony of atonement (before he may partake of a sacred meal). Gen. R. s. 32, a. e. מח׳ אמנה, v. אֻמָּנָה I. Hull. 25[a], v. חֲמִיטָה.—Y. B. Mets. V, 10[c] bot. מח׳ מעשה אחד wanting one action to be available; a. fr.—*Pl.* constr. מְחוּסְּרֵי. Ker. l. c. ארבעה מ׳ וכ׳ there are four persons requiring a ceremony of atonement before being permitted &c., v. supra; a. fr.

Hif. הֶחְסִיר same, v. supra.

חֲסַר, חֲסֵר ch. same. Targ. Y. Ex. XVI, 18 (O. ed. Berl. חַסַּר, oth. ed. חֲסַר, חַסִּיר) had less. Targ. Deut. II, 7; a. fr.—Nidd. 68[a] חַסְ־ת, v. דּוּגָא; a. e.

Pa. חַסַּר 1) same, v. supra.—2) *to lessen, deprive, reduce.* Targ. Ps. VIII, 6. Targ. Koh. IV, 8; a. fr.—Snh. 22[a] חַסְרֵיה וכ׳ v. נְּנָבָא; a. e.—*Part. pass.* מְחַסַּר (v. preced. *Pi.*) *wanting.* Targ. Y. Num. XI, 32.—Bets. 24[a]; Bekh. 39[a], a. fr. חַסּוּרֵי מְחַסְּרָא (or מִיחַסְּרָא *Ithpa.*) the relation is defective (a clause has been omitted).

חָסֵר II m., **חֲסֵרָה, חֲסֵי׳** f. 1) *wanting, defective; less.* Sabb. VII, 2 ארבעים ח׳ אחת forty (labors) less one. B. Bath. VII, 2, v. הֵן. Ib. 89[b] מדה ח׳ וכ׳ a measure too small or too large. Tosef. Taan. I, 2 אם . . השנה ח׳ if the year had a deficiency of rain; Y. ib. I, 64[b]; a. fr.—*Pl.* חֲסֵרִים, חֲסֵרִין . . .; חֲסֵרוֹת. Macc. 23[a] חֲסֵירֵי כח of feeble physics; a. fr.—Esp. a) (calendar) חָסֵר *a defective month* (of 29 days), opp. מלא of thirty days. B. Mets. 59[b] ואיחליף . . . מלא לח׳ and he made a mistake between a full and a defective month (thought it was the thirtieth day of the preceding month). R. Hash. 19[b]; a. fr.—*Pl.* as ab. Ib.—

b) (orthogr.) *a defective writing, omission of the vowel letter*, opp. מלא (plene), e. g. חֹדֶשׁ, plene חוֹדֶשׁ.—*Pl. f.* חֲסֵרוֹת. Erub. 13ª; Kidd. 30ª ח׳ ויתרות the rules concerning *defective* and *plene*; a. fr.—2) *creating a defect.* Ḥag. 3ᵇ (ref. to Koh. XII, 11) אי מה .... ח׳ וכ׳ you **might think,** as the nail (driven in) creates a hole and **not an addition,** אף ד״ת חַסְרִין וכ׳ so do the words of the **Law &c.**; Yalk. Koh. 989 end אף ד״ת מְחַסְּרִין וכ׳.

חָסַר, constr. **חֲסַר** ch. same. Targ. I Kings XI, 22. Targ. I Sam. XXI, 16; a. fr.—Targ. II Esth. III, 8 חד ח׳ one month is defective (of 29 days).—*Pl.* חֲסֵרִין, חֲסֵרֵי. Targ. Prov. XXVII, 12 (ed. Wil. חַסְרִין, v. חֲסַר).—Targ. II Esth. l. c. (ed. Lag. חֲסוּרִין) *starving.*

***חֶסֶר** m. (preced.) *diminution.* Keth. 66ᵇ, v. מֶלַח.

חֶסְרוֹן (b. h.), **חִי׳, חִסָּרוֹן** m. (preced.) 1) *want, loss.*—ח׳ כיס loss of money. Sabb. 157ª, a. fr., v. מוּקְצֶה. Kidd. 32ᵇ שאין בה ח׳ כיס with which no material loss is connected. Lev. R. s. 5 המקום ימלא חֶסְרוֹנְךָ the Lord replace thy deficiency; Ber. 16ᵇ. Tosef. Taan. I, 2 נותנין לה חֶסְרוֹנָהּ the year's deficiency (of rain) will be supplied to him (who prays); Y. ib. I, 64ᵇ חסרונה. Ib.ᵈ top (ref. to Job XXX, 3) אם ראית ח׳ בא וכ׳ when thou seest scarcity &c.; (Gen. R. s. 31; s. 34 חוֹסֶר), v. גַּלְמוּד. Hull. 47ᵇ, a. fr. נקב שיש בו ח׳ a perforation connected with a loss of substance. Ib.; Bekh. 39ª, a. e. ח׳ מבפנים ... ח׳ a deficiency of substance inside of an organ is not considered a defect (in ritual law); a. fr.

חֶסְרוֹנָא, חֶסְרָנָא, v. חוּסְרָנָא.

חָף, חַף, v. חפף, חוף.

חַף m. (cmp. b. h. חוֹף; חפף I) 1) *border, shore.* Num. R. s. 13 (ref. to Num. VII, 26) אין כף אלא חף וכ׳ *Kaf* (bowl) means the same as *ḥaf* (shore), as it is said (Ps. XCVIII, 8) rivers strike the *Kaf.*—2) (cmp. חִיפָא) [*rim, ridge,*] *ward of a lock* (פותחת); *bit of a key* (corresponding to the ward); *pivot of a door* (v. Sm. Ant. s. vv. Cardo, Clavis). Sabb. VIII, 6 כדי ... חף bone large enough to make of it a *ḥaf*; expl. ib. 81ª חַפֵּי פותחת the rims (ward) of a lock; Y. ib. 11ᵇ bot מהו חף סרגיד what *ḥaf* is meant? (Answ.) the key-ward; ib. תמן הוא עביד חף בלוט וכ׳ (not כלוט) there (Kel. XIV, 8) he (R. Judah) uses *ḥaf* in the sense of a key-bit, and here (Sabb. l. c.) in the sense of a key-ward.—3) *the border of a web,* used for starting a new web by fastening the warp to it. Y. ib. VII, 10ᶜ, v. נִיר IV.—*Pl.* חַפִּין, חַפִּים. Kel. XIII, 6 פותחת של עץ וחף וכ׳ if the lock is of wood and its key-bits of metal (ed. Dehr. חָפִין). Ib. XIV, 8 ניטלו ח׳ if the teeth of the bit are broken off (damaged). Sabb. 81ª, v. supra. Y. ib. IV, 7ª top חַפֵּי לסוטה borders used for weaving veils. Cant. R. to III, 10 (expl. פתות, I Kings VII, 50) חפיפות, read: חַפֵּי פותחות the pivots; (Pesik. R. s. 6 בלוטין שבפותחות, v. בָּלוּט).—Kel. XI, 4 חַפִּין = חוחין.

חַפָּא, חֲפָא, v. חפי.

חפאמיקון, v. הִיפְּטִיקוֹס.

חֲפָאִין, חֲפָאִים m. (pl. of חֵפֶה; חָפָה) *covering over burnt clay vessels.* Tosef. Kel. B. Kam. III, 14; ib. Par. V (IV), 2 גילה ח׳ וכ׳ (לח׳) ed. Zuck. (ed. corrupt) if he removes the covering and finds dust on the vessels (proving that none had touched them; v. R. S. to Par. V, 1 for correct version).

חָפַת, v. חֲפַת.

חָפָה, v. חפי.

חִפּוּי, חִי׳ m. (preced.) 1) *covering, wrapping.* Kel. XVI, 8 (הנשוי) לח׳ whatever is intended for wrapping, opp. תיק, casing. Ib. XXVI, 6. Tosef. ib. B. Bath. IV, 11; a. e.—*Pl.* חִפּוּיִים, חִי׳. Ib. XVI, 8 חִפּוּיֵי האלה וכ׳ the wrapping of a lance &c.—2) *upholstered seat.* Ib. XXII, 4 a bridal chair שנטל חִפּוּיוֹ whose seat is missing; (Eduy. I, 11 חִפּוּיָיו, Ms. M. דפניו, Mish. Nap. חופיו, v. Rabad a. l.). Kel. l. c. 6 שנטל חִפּוּיוֹ האמצעי whose middle cushion (of the three forming the seat) is wanting.—*Pl.* as ab. Ib. 5 שלא היו חִפּוּיָיו יוצאין (ed. Dehr. חִפּוּיָיו) whose seats were not movable (v. Rabad to Eduy. l. c.); a. fr.—[Tosef. Sabb. IV (V), 7 כל חיפוי ed. Zuck., read with ed.: כוּר.]

חִפּוּיָא ch., constr. **חִי׳, חִפּוּי** same, *covering, coating, overlaying.* Targ. Ex. XXXVIII, 17; 19 (h. text צִפּוּי). Targ. Is. XXX, 22.

חפופיתא, v. חִיפ׳.

חפופתא, v. חֲפִיפִיתָא II.

חָפוֹר m. (חָפַר) *digger, attendant of earth-work on farms.*—*Pl.* חֲפוֹרוֹת. Tosef. B. Mets. IX, 14 (ed. Zuck. חופורות, corr. acc.; Y. ib. IX, beg. 12ª החוֹפֵר).

חֲפוּרָא m., pl. **חֲפוּרֵי**, v. חֲפוּרָה II.

חֲפוּרָא f., constr. **חֲפוּרַת**, v. חֲפוּרְתָּא.

חֲפוּרָה, חֲפִירָה I f. (חָפַר) *pit.* Yeb. 121ª; Ber. 33ª חפ׳; (Tosef. Yeb. XIV, 4; Y. ib. XVI, 15ᶜ בּוֹר).

חֲפוּרָה, חֲפִ׳ II f. (preced.) *products of the earth gained by digging,* opp. to those gained by cutting; *bulbs, roots* &c. [Also used in Chald. phraseology.] Tosef. Ned. IV, 3 הנודר מן החפו׳ וכ׳ (Var. חפירה) if one vows abstinence from *ḥăfirah*, he is forbidden melons &c.; Y. ib. VII, beg. 40ᵇ האפירה (corr. acc.). Bekh. 52ᵇ ח׳ והוה שובלי (if on the father's death) what was available of the products of the ground was classed under *ḥ.* (vegetable, e. g. green of grains), and now it is *shublê* (ears); B. Bath. 124ª (Ms. M. חֲפוּרֵי והוו). Yeb. 63ª מאה ... מילחא וח׳ invest a hundred Zuz in land, and you will have salt and common vegetable.

חֲפוּרִית f., pl. **חֲפוּרִיּוֹת** (preced.) *fruits belonging to the class of ḥăfurah, inferior produces.* Pesik. Asser, p. 100ª; Tanh. R'eh 18; Yalk. Deut. 897.

חֲפוּרְתָא f., constr. **חֲפוּרַת** (preced. wds.) *digging, mine.*—ח׳ לִבָּא mine of the heart, seat of deep-laid plans. Targ. Ps. LXXIII, 7, v. חוּטְבָא.

***חֲפוּשִׁית** f. (חָפַשׁ) *a grant of emancipation, pardon, liberty.* Gen. R. s. 53, a gloss expl. הוּרְיָיה (some ed. חפושיה; Yalk. Gen. 92 חָפְשִׁיּוּת).

חֲפוּשִׁית, חֲפוּשִׁיתָא, v. חיפ׳.

חָפַז (b. h.) *to be in haste, to hurry.*

Nif. נֶחְפָּז *to be hurried, excited.* Pirke d'R. El. ch. XXVI נבהל ונֶחְפָּז frightened and excited.

חִפָּזוֹן m. (b.h.; preced.) *haste, being hurried.* Ber. 9ª (ref. to Ex. XII, 11) עד שעת ח׳ (which means, you may eat of the Passover lamb) up to the time of leaving in haste. Ib. על שעת ח׳ וכ׳ (they differ) as to the time of *ḥippazon;* R. El. saying ח׳ דמצרים *hipp.* refers to the hastening of the Egyptians (ib. 30, sq., at night), while R. Ak. refers it to ח׳ דישראל the haste of the Israelites (in the morning, Num. XXXIII, 3); Mekh. Bo, s. 7 זה חִפָּזוֹן מצרים this (Ex. XII, 11) refers to &c. Ib. ח׳ שכינה the haste (anxiety) of the Deity. Sifré Deut. 130 (ref. to Deut. XVI, 3) יכול ח׳ לישראל ולמצרים you might think, there was anxiety (fear) on the part of Israel and of Egypt. Pes. IX, 5. Ib. 96ª אותו נאכל בח׳ וכ׳ this was eaten in haste, but no other &c.—Ex. R. s. 19; a. e.

חָפֵי *barefooted,* v. חַפְיָא II.

חָפָה, חָפֵי (b. h.; cmp. חפף I) 1) *to cover, spread over.* Hull. III, 7 וכנפיו חופין וכ׳ and whose wings cover the largest portion of its body. Sot. IX, 15 (49ª) וְחָפוּ ראשם and covered their heads (in shame).—Part. pass. חָפוּי. Esth. R. to VI, 12 וַחֲפוּי ראש וכ׳ and his head covered (in shame) over what had happened to him; Meg. 16ª.—2) *to bend, curve.* Yoma 47ª חוֹפֶה שלש וכ׳ he bends three of his fingers (grasping with them) up to &c.; cmp. חָפַן.

Pi. חִיפָּה 1) *to cover, strew over.* Tosef. Kil. I, 15 הַמְחַפֶּה who covers up (mixed seeds with earth); M. Kat. 2ᵇ; Macc. 21ᵇ. Ib. החופה ed. (Ms. M. המח׳). Y. Kil. VII, 31ᵇ לא במחפה is it not because in plowing over he covers the seeds up? Shebi. IV, 5 לא יְחַפֵּהוּ בעפר he must not cover it (the cut) with loose ground, opp. to (כסה) covering with stones. Y. Taan. II, beg. 65ª אבותינו חִיפּוּ ... חִיפִּינוּ וכ׳ our ancestors covered it (the reader's desk) with gold, and we with dust. Nidd. 16ª ותְחַפֶּה וכ׳ and semen virile may have covered it up; a. e.—2) *to cover over, to protect from justice, to be partial.* Shebu. 39ª מפני שמְחַפִּין עליו because they (the publican's or robber's relations) protect him. Ex. R. s. 30 היו מְחַפִּין אותו tried to protect him; a. e.—3) (cmp. גָּבַב) [*to heap up words,*] *to invent fictions* (v. II Kings XVII, 9). Gen. R. s. 94 (play on חפים, ib. XLVI, 21) שחִיפּוּ עליו דברים וכ׳ about whom they invented a fiction (Gen. XXXVII, 3).

חֲפָא, חֲפֵי ch. same, *to cover, overlay.* Targ. Ex. XXXVI, 34; a. fr.—Targ. Ez. XXVI, 19 וִיחַפּוּנָךְ they shall cover thee up (bury).—Targ. Y. Deut. XXXII, 11 וְחָפָא וכ׳ he spread over them the shade etc.—Ab. Zar. 39ª חַפְיֵיה בדיקולא Ms. M. (ed. חפיא, incorr.) he put a basket over it. Sot. 22ᵇ דְחָפוּ, v. גּוּנְדָּא II.

Pa. חַפֵּי 1) *to cover, overlay.* Targ. Is. XL, 19; a. e.—Part. pass. מְחַפָּא, pl. מְחַפִּין, f. מְחַפְּיָן. Targ. Ex. XXVI, 32.—2) as preced. *Pi.* 2. Targ. Y. Lev. XX, 5 (cmp. Shebu. 39ª).

Af. אַחְפֵּי *to cover, overlay.* Targ. Ex. XXVI, 29; a.e. (ed. Berl. תַּחְפֵּי *Pe.*).

Ithpa. אִתְחַפֵּי, *Ithpe.* אִתְחֲפִי *to be covered.* Targ. I Kings XVIII, 45. Targ. Is. XLII, 22 אִתְחֲ׳ בהתא were covered with shame (h. text הפח); a. e.

חִפְיָא I m. (preced.) 1) *cover, overlaying.*—*Pl.* חִפְיֵי. Targ. Y. Num. XVII, 3, sq.; v. חוּפָאָה.—2) (adj.; cmp. חוס) *bending over, concerned.* Koh. R. to I, 3 ח׳ לגרמיה הוא (some ed. חֲפָיָה) he is concerned about himself (his honor, because he has not been invited.)

חַפְיָא II m. (v. חפף II a. חוּף I; cmp. יָחֵף) *barefooted* (in mourning). Gen. R. s. 100 נפיק ח׳ (some ed. חפי) went out barefooted, opp. לביש סנדלוי.

חֲפָיָה, v. חִפְיָא I.

חֲפִינָה f. (חָפַן) *the priest's taking handfuls of incense* (Lev. XVI, 12). Yoma 19ª top ללמדו ח׳ (they took him to the house of Abtinas) to teach him the manipulation of *ḥăfinah.* Ib. וגמר ח׳ and he learned *ḥăf.* Ib. 49ª בַּחֲפִינָתוֹ with what the dying highpriest had seized with his hands. Men. 11ª והארכא ח׳ is there not *ḥăfinah* among the difficult priestly functions?; a. e.

חֲפִיסָה f. (חפס *to collect,* cmp. Arab. *ḥafaš,* a. *ḥafṣ*) *a small leather bag, valise* (for documents &c.). B. Mets. I, 8, expl. ib. 20ᵇ חמת קטנה; Gitt. III, 3; ib. 28ª. Yoma 75ᵇ כמו שמונח בח׳ Ms. M. (ed. בקופסא) as if lying (pressed) in a valise. [Also in Ch.] Y. B. Mets. II, 8ᶜ top מכסי בח׳ covered up with a bag. Pesik. B'shall. p. 93ª [read:] הדה חֲפִיסְתִּי וכ׳ my valise here and my cloak.

חֲפִיפָה I f. (חָפַף I) *covering.* M. Kat. 12ᵇ.

חֲפִיפָה II f. (חָפַף II) *cleansing the head* with a detergent, comb &c. B. Kam. 82ᵇ top. תיקן ח׳ ordained (for women before bathing) cleansing &c. Nidd. 66ᵇ. Y. Maas. Sh. II, 53ᶜ top; Tosef. ib. II, 1 חֲפִיפָתָהּ when she cleanses her hair.

***חֲפִיפוּת**, Cant. R. to III, 10, v. חָה.

***חֲפִיפוּתָא I** f. (חָפַף I) *being bent;* חֲפִיפוּת לב *humiliation, sorrow.* Targ. Lam. III, 65 Ar. (ed. תבירות, h. text מְגִנַּת).

חֲפִיפוּתָא II (**חֲפוּפְתָא,** Ar.) f. (חפף I) *preparation for the ḥuppah* (v. חוּפָּה). Keth. 17ª מישחא דח׳ קאמר מר do you speak of oil used at bridal arrangements? Ar.; [oth. opin. (חפף II) oil used for curing *sores of the head,* v. חֲפָפִית].

חֲפִיצָה f. (חָפֵץ) *use of the root* חפץ, *finding pleasure.* Gen. R. s. 80; Midr. Till. to Ps. XXII (ref. to Mal. III, 12).

חָפִיר m. (part. pass. of חָפַר) *one for whom a grave is dug.* Koh. R. to X, 7 ח׳ טב וכ׳ a dead man is better off than he; Sabb. 151^b דחפיר וקביר וכ׳ one who is dead and buried.

חֲפִירָה, v. חֲפוּרָה.

חֲפִישָׁה f. (חָפַשׁ) *searching, digging.* Pes. 31^b כמה חֲפִישַׁת הכלב how far does the dog reach in digging?

חֲפִישׁוּתָא, v. חַפְשׁוּשִׁיתָא.

חֲפִיתָא f. (v. חָהּ) *fish remaining on the shore after the water receded, mud-fish.* Cant. R. to I, 4 (ref. to תדוץ דאבה, Job XLI, 14, cmp. דָּאַב) מקרטעא כחדא ח׳ jumping like raked fish. Y. Ab. Zar. II, 42^a חֲפִיתָה; cmp. חִיפוּשָׁא.

חָפַן [*to bend the fingers, form a hollow of the hand,* denom. חוֹפֶן; whence] *to take handfuls.* Maas. Sh. II, 5 אם בלל וח׳ וכ׳ if he mixed the coins up and took by handfuls, you go by the proportion of the coins mixed. Y. ib. 53^c כבולל וחוֹפֵן it is as in the case of him who &c.— Esp. (of the priest) *to take grabs of incense with both hands* (v. חֲפִינָה). Yoma V, 1. Ib. 47^a היה חוֹפֵן וכ׳ used to grab &c.; a. fr.

Nif. נֶחְפַּן *to be grabbed.* Y. Maas. Sh. l. c. הנבללין והנֶחְפָּנִין the coins which were mixed up and then collected by handfuls.

חֲפַן ch. same. Yoma 47^b (ref. to Lev. XVI, 12) כדחָפְנֵי אינשי as people usually grab. Gen. R. s. 5 ההוא דח׳ תרי וכ׳ he who takes a grab takes twice as much as he who fills his fist, v. קמץ; Yalk. Josh. 14.

חֹפֶן, חוֹפֶן m. (b. h.; preced. wds.) *the hollow of the hand* formed by bending the fingers so as to touch the wrist, contrad. to קֹמֶץ; *a handful.* Gen. R. s. 5 חָפְנוֹ של משה the quantity of a handful of Moses' hand. Ex. R. s. 11 מלא ח׳ שלו מלא ח׳ וכ׳ his (Moses') handful and that of Aaron; a. fr.—Du. חוֹפְנַיִם, חָפְנַיִם. Yoma V, 1 מלא חָפְנָיו his two handfuls. Ib. 47^a חוֹפְנָיו. Ex. R. l. c. לקחו חָפְנֵיהֶם . . . both of them took, each his handfuls; a. fr. [Tosef. B. Mets. IX, 14 חפן ed., read סָפָן as ed. Zuck.].

חוֹפְנָא, חָפְנָא ch. same. Targ. Koh. IV, 6 מלא חפני, read: חָפְנֵיה.—*Pl.* חוֹפְ׳, חָפְנֵי, חָפְנִין. Ib. Targ. Ex. IX, 8. Targ. Ez. I, 8; a. e.—Sabb. 62^b מלא ח׳ by handfuls, liberally.

***חֵפָנִי** (v. חֵיפָה I) *of Haifa.* Keth. 103^a (v. Rashi); Y. ib. XII, 35^a top; Y. Kil. IX, 32^b top חפנים; v. חֵיפָנוֹס.

חֲפַס = h. חָפַשׂ 1) *to dig.* Targ. Y. Ex. XXI, 33 (ed. Amst. יַחְפַּס). Targ. Job III, 20.—Y. B. Mets. II, 8^c bot. וחספתה, read: וְחַפְסוּנָהּ and when they were digging it up.—2) (cmp. חֲפִיסָה) *to grab.* Targ. Y. I. Num. XI, 8 (some ed. חַפְּ׳ *Pa.*; h. text שָׁטוּ). Targ. Job III, 21.

Pa. חַפֵּשׁ, חַפֵּס same. Ib. XXXIX, 21 מְחַפְּשִׁין ed. Lag. (oth. ed. מחפרין).

חָפַף I (b. h.; cmp. כפף, גבב) *to bend over, to cover; trnsf. to be anxious, to care.* Meg. 26^a; Zeb. 53^b sq. שנ׳ חוֹפֵף וכ׳ . . מצטער . . . . והיה Benjamin took pains . . . to conquer it, as it says (Deut. XXXIII, 12) he (Benjamin) is bent over it &c. [Rashi: *rubs his head,* v. חָפַף II.]

חָפַף, חוּף, *Polel* חוֹפֵף ch. same. Targ. Y. 1. Deut. XXXII, 11 חָפָא. (Y. II מחסחף, read: מְחַפְחֵף).

Ithpol. אִתְחוֹפֵף same. Targ. O. ib. (h. text ירחף).

Palp. חַפְחֵף, v. supra.

חָפַף II (cmp. חָפַס) *to scrape, rub,* esp. *to cleanse one's head, rub, comb.* Sabb. 31^a והיה הלל חוֹפֵף וכ׳ Ms. M. (ed. והלל חפף) and Hillel was washing his head. Naz. VI, 3 נזיר חופף וכ׳ a Nazir may wash (rub with his hand) his hair. Ib. לא יָחוֹף באדמה he must not use an earth, v. נֶשֶׁר. Yalk. Gen. 150 (play on חפים, Gen. XLVI, 21) לא חָפַפְתִּי וכ׳ I did not wash (my head) or comb. Tosef. Ter. X, 4 שחִיפְּפָה וכ׳ ed. Zuck. which a priest's daughter has used for washing her hair; ib. Maas. Sh. II, 1 שחפה.

חֲפַף ch. same, *to rub.* Targ. Jer. VI, 26 חפו וכ׳ rub your heads with ashes (h. text התפלשו).—Part. pass. חֲפִיף, pl. חֲפִיפִין. Targ. Ez. XXVII, 30.

חֲפָפִית f. (preced. wds., cmp. חִפּוּף) *sore, eruption.* Sabb. 77^b; Y. Ber. IX, 13^c bot. Cmp. חִיפּוּפִיתָא.

חָפֵץ (b. h.; cmp. חָפַף I) 1) *to bend* (v. Job XL, 17); חָפֵץ *to be busy with, to be anxious, desire.*—Pesik. Haḥod. p. 47^b הוא ח׳ לגאול אתכם He is anxious to redeem you; ib. ח׳ בגאולתכם; Pesik. R. s. 15 ח׳ לגאולתכם; Cant. R. to II, 8; a. e.—[2) *to hold in one's hand,* cmp. חָפַן; v. next w.]

חֵפֶץ m. (b. h.; preced.) 1) *thing* (held in hand), *object.* B. Mets. IV, 10 בכמה ח׳ זה how much is this worth? Cant. R. to I, 4 כל ח׳ טוב any good thing; a. fr..—2) *concern, business; desire, desirable object.* Ib.; Pesik. Sos, p. 147^a אין לי ח׳ טוב ממך I have nothing more desirable than thyself. Koh. R. to V, 7 נעשה חֶפְצוֹ his desire was fulfilled. Num. R. s. 19 אל תחזירני מן חֶפְצִי וכ׳ do not turn me off from (refuse) my desire which &c.; a. fr..—*Pl.* חֲפָצִים. M. Kat. 9^b (ref. to Prov. III, 15, a. VIII, 11) הא חֶפְצֵי שמים but heavenly affairs (religious deeds) are equal to it (the study of the Law). Y. Peah I, 15^d bot. (ref. to Prov. I. c.) חפצים וכ׳ 'desirable things', that means jewels and pearls, 'thy desirable things', that means &c. Ib. חֲפָצֶיךָ וַחֲפָצַי וכ׳ thy treasures and my treasures cannot compare to what I sent you; Gen. R. s. 35, end.—Sabb. 113^a (ref. to Is. LVIII, 13) חֲפָצֶיךָ אסורין ח׳ שמים וכ׳ thy pursuits are forbidden (on the Sabbath), but heavenly affairs (consultation about public welfare, education &c.) are permitted; ib. 150^a; a. fr.

חֶפְצָא ch. same, esp. *a sacred object held in hand at the delivery of an oath.* Shebu. 38^b צריך לאתפושי ח׳ בידיה the judge must make him hold an object (Torah) in his hand. Ib. האי דיינא דאשבע . . . ולא תפיס ח׳ בידיה Ms. F. margin (v. Rabb. D. S. a l. note 40) a judge that administers an oath by the Lord . . . ., while the affirmant holds no object &c. Ib. דהא לא נקיט ח׳ (Ms. M. מידעם) for he had nothing in his hand.—B. Kam. 91^a למימד ח׳ וכ׳

to give an opinion on the fact whether or not he has caused that injury.

חִיפְצָא, חֲפִצָא m. a kind *of peas*. *Pl.* חֲפְצֵי (חִיפְ׳ Rashi). Hull. 52ª (Ar. חַפְצֵי, expl. עפצים).

חָפַר (b. h.; cmp. חפש) *to dig, hollow out.* B. Kam. V, 5 החופר בור וכ׳ if one hollows out a pit on private ground, but opens it on public ground; Tosef. ib. VI, 4. B. Mets. 50ª, v. אוּשׁ II. Midr. Sam. ch. XXXII, end לַחְפּוֹר to dig graves, v. חֲפַר; a. fr.

חֲפַר I ch. same, 1) *to dig.* Targ. Ps. VII, 16 (Ms. כרא). Targ. Gen. XXVI, 15; a. fr.—*Part. pass.* חֲפִיר q. v.—2) (trnsf.) *to plan, espy.* Targ. Prov. XVI, 27. Targ. Job XXXIX, 29.

חֲפַר II (b. h. חָפֵר; cmp. חֲוַר) *to be white, be ashamed.* Targ. Prov. XIII, 5.

חֲפַר m. (חָפַר) *grave-digging.* Y. Taan. IV, end, 69ᶜ בטל החי׳ the grave-digging (for the generation of the wilderness) ceased; Lam. R. introd. (R. Z'era). Y. l. c. צאו לח׳ go out for grave-digging; (Lam. R. l. c.; Midr. Sam. ch. XXXII, end לַחְפּוֹר).

חֲפִרִיתָה f. name of *a root* (?) Y. Shebi. III, 34ᶜ bot.

חָפַשׂ (b. h.; cmp. חָפַר), *Pi.* חִיפֵּשׂ *to dig, search.* Pes. II, 3 כל .... לְחַפֵּשׂ אחריו what the dog cannot reach by digging for it. Sabb. 89ª חִיפַּשְׂתִּי וכ׳ I searched all over the world. Cant. R. to I, 1 אם אתה מְחַפֵּשׂ אחר וכ׳ if thou wilt dig after the words of the Law as for secret treasures; a. fr.

חֲפַשׂ, *Pa.* חַפֵּשׂ, v. חֲסַס.

חָפַשׁ (b. h.) [*to be white*, cmp. Arab. *ḥafaš decorticare*, cmp. חֲפַר II,] *to be free* (cmp. חוֹר II). V. next w.

Pi. חִיפֵּשׁ *to deliver.* Pesik. R. s. 8 (ref. to אֲחַפֵּשׂ, Zeph. I, 12) לא תהא קורא סמ״ך אלא שי״ן אֲחַפֵּשׁ וכ׳ read not the word with *Samme* but with *Shin*, 'I shall deliver &c.'; Yalk. Zeph. 567.

Pu. חוּפַּשׁ *to be set free.* Kerith. 11ª (ref. to Lev. XIX, 20) מכלל דהוא ח׳ this implies that he (her betrothed) has been liberated, is a freedman.

חָפְשִׁי (b. h.; preced.) 1) fem. *freedom.* Pesik. R. s. 8 (ref. to Zeph. I, 12) מוציא אני אותה לח׳ I shall lead her out to liberty (v. preced.); a. fr.—2) masc. *free, exempt.* Nidd. 61ᵇ, a. e. (ref. to Ps. LXXXVIII, 6) כיון ..... נעשה ח׳ וכ׳ when one is dead, one is free from religious duties. Tanh. Emor 2 (ref. to ויתחפש, I Sam. XXVIII, 8) נעשה ח׳ מן המלכות divested himself of the (insignia of) government; Lev. R. s. 26 (not למלכות); Midr. Sam. ch. XXIV, v. פַּנְּקְרִקָא; a. fr.

חֲפְשׁוּשִׁיתָא f. (preced. wds.) *scrapings, sediment.* Lam. R. introd. (R. Abbahu 2), (interpreting Ezek. XXIV, 6) דחַפְשׁוּשִׁיתָהּ בגווה whose sediments (lowest classes) remain within her; (Ar. ed. Koh. דחפישותא לגווה); Yalk. Ez. 362.

חֶפֶת or **חֵפֶת** f. (חפת I, v. חִיפָּא) *border* of a garment (*limbus*), a kind of front bosom in which things can be hidden. Sabb. X, 3 (92ª) ובח׳ חלוקו Ms. M. (v. Rabb. D. S. a. l. note, ed. ובשפת) in the bosom of his shirt. Yoma 77ᵇ ובלבד ... מח׳ חלוקו Ms. M. (ed. מתחת ח׳) provided he takes not his hand out of the bosom of his shirt (to throw his cloak over his shoulder). Sabb. 96ᵇ, v. חִיפָּא.—Denom.

חָפַת *to provide with a bosom* or *border.* Part. pass. חָפוּת. Shek. III, 2 אין התורם .... בפרגוד ח׳ he who takes the money out of the Temple cell must not enter with a bordered cloak (in order not to create suspicion; Ms. M. האפות, Mish. Pes. הֶ;זפות, v. Rabb. D. S. a. l.).—*Pl.* חֲפוּתִין. Midr. Sam. ch. XXI נמצאו ח׳ וכ׳ the garments were found (to fit David) forming a bosom, not dragging along &c.; (Lev. R. s. 26, a. e. עשוין לו as if made for him).

Pi. חִיפֵּת *to fold the bosom.* Tosef. Ber. VII, 18 לְחַפּוֹת לו חלוק והוא לא ח׳ וכ׳ ed. Zuck. (Var. חפך) to form the bosom of his shirt, while he never had &c.

חֲפַת ch., v. next w.

חֵי׳, חֶפְתָא ch.=h. חֶפֶת. Gen. R. s. 75 יהיבתי׳ה בחֶפְתִּי (בחי׳) I put him in my pocket, i. e. I outwitted him.—Denom. חֲפַת, part. pass. pl. חֲפִיתִין *bosomed.* Ib. s. 100; Y. Kil. IX, 32ᵇ top ח׳ (מאנין) חיורין white, bosomed garments; Y. Keth. XII, 35ª top חפיתין. Y. M. Kat. III, 83ᶜ top (expl. סנטירית) מאנין דלא ח׳ garments without bosoms; (Gen. R. s. 100 דלא בוידין, v. סִנְטְרָא).

Af. אַחְפַּת *to put in the bosom*, i. e. *to outwit.* Gen. R. s. 80 סברון לְמַחְפַּת ואִתְחַפְתּוּן they intended to outwit (Jacob), and they were outwitted.

Ithpa. אִתְחַפַּת *to be outwitted*, v. supra.

חֵץ (b. h.; חָצַץ I) 1) *wedge, arrow.* Mikv. X, 8 חץ שהוא תחוב באדם an arrow sticking in a person's body; Tosef. ib. VII (VIII), 9. Arakh. 15ᵇ חץ עד מ״ה אמה the range of an arrow is forty five cubits. Ib. אין חץ אלא לשון arrow means (an evil) tongue (ref. to Jer. IX, 7); a. fr. [Y. Keth. II., beg. 26ª שחיצה, read: שֶׁחֶצְיָה]—*Pl.* חִיצִּים, חִצִּין, חִי׳. Lam. R. to III, 12 (expl. כמטרה לחץ ib.) כקורת ח׳ וכ׳ like the post for arrows (for military practice) at which all shoot &c.—Tanh. Nitsab. 1 (ref. to Deut. XXXII, 23) חִצַּי כָּלִין וכ׳ my arrows will be spent, but they (Israel) shall not cease; ib. חִצָּיו כלין וכ׳ his arrows will be spent, but the post will remain; Sot. 9ª. B. Kam. 22ª אשו משום חִצָּיו he is responsible for his fire, because it is his arrows (i. e. his action), opp. משום ממונו because it is his property which caused the damage. Ib. חציו דכלב it is the action of (his) dog; חציו דגמל of his camel; a. fr.—2) *shaft.*—*Pl.* as ab. Succ. 12ᵇ; 15ª ח׳ זכרים plain shafts, opp. נקבות shafts with a hole into which the arrow-head is sat.

חֲצָא, v. חצי.

חָצַב (b. h.; cmp. חטב) *to cut, chisel, hew, shape.* Tosef. Yoma I, 6 כשהוא חוצב engaged in stone-breaking; Sifra Emor ch. I, Par. 2; Tanh. Emor 4 ח׳ אבנים; Lev.

R. s. 26 ח׳ באבנים. Y. M. Kat. I, 80[d] לא יַחְצוֹב one must not cut stones &c. Yalk. Deut. 854 אתה חֲצוֹב וכ׳ chisel thou the tablets &c.; a. fr.—Part. pass. חָצוּב, f. חֲצוּבָה; pl. חֲצוּבִים, חֲצוּבוֹת. Y. M. Kat. l. c. Y. Shek. VI, 49[d] bot.; a. e.

Nif. נֶחְצַב *to be hewn, chiselled.* Y. Yoma III, 40[c] bot. בקודש יֵחָצְבוּ on sacred ground they must be chiselled.—Trnsf. (cmp. גזר) *to be decided, decreed.* Lev. R. s. 5 (ref. to Is. XXII, 16) ממרום נ׳ עליו from on high it has been decreed over him; Yalk. Is. 291 נֶחְצְבָה עליו גזרה.

חֲצַב ch. 1) same.; interch. with חֲצַד q. v.—Part. pass. חֲצִיב, v. חֲצִיבָא. — *2) (used of the Cistus) *to cut through the ground, to grow.* Pes. 111[b], v. חֲצוּבָא II.—[Lev. R. s. 25 ח׳ חצובין, v. חֲצַד I.]

Ithpe. אִתְחֲצַב *to be hewn.* Targ. Is. LI, 1.

חַצָּב m. (preced. wds.) *stone-cutter* in the quarry. B. Mets. 118[b] הח׳ . . . לסתח after the stone-cutter has surrendered (the stone) to the polisher; Y. ib. X, 12[c] bot. החוֹצֵב לגַּמָּל.—*Pl.* חוֹצְבִין. Y. Shek. VI, 48[a] top.

חָצָב m. (preced. wds.) *stone pitcher, earthen jug.*—*Pl.* חֲצָבִים, חֲצָבִין. Men. VIII, 7. Kel. II, 2; Tosef. ib. B. Kam. II, 2.

חָצָב I (חָצָד) a species or variety of *dates* (v. Löw Pfl., p. 109, sq.). Ab. Zar. I, 5 (Y. ed. חצר, with ר). Ib. 14[b], expl. קַשְׁבָּא. Y. ib. I, 39[d] bot. חצד, v. חֲצָדָא II. [Maim.: *sugar cane*, v. Löw l. c.]

חָצָב II, חָצוּב m. (חצב) [*cutter,*] *a shrubby plant*, with deep and straight roots, used for hedges to mark boundaries, prob. *cistus.* B. Bath. 55[a] המצר והח׳ וכ׳ a landmark (stone &c.) and the *hazab* form a legal boundary &c. Ib. 56[a], v. חֲצוּבָא I. Tosef. Sabb. XIV (XV), 8; Y. ib. XVIII, 16[c] bot; Bab. ib. 128[a] מטלטלין את הח׳ וכ׳ you may (on the Sabbath) handle the (cut) *ḥ.*, because it is food for gazelles. Kil. I, 8 חצוב (Ar. חצב).—*Pl.*, v. חֲצוּבָה I.

חַצְבָא ch. v. חֲצוּבָא II.

חַצְבָּא m. ch.=h. חָצָב. Succ. 29[a]. Ber. 22[a] bot. תקן ח׳ בת וכ׳ (Ms. M. חוצבא) ordained that a pitcher containing nine kab must be used for purification. Ib. אתבר חַצְבֵּיהּ וכ׳ R. N.'s pitcher is broken (the rule he laid down is rejected). Bets. 30[a]; a. fr.—*Pl.* חַצְבֵּי, חַצְבִּין. Targ. II Esth. III, 8 מלקטין פישרי טבת ויתיבין בחַצְבֵּי תמוז they collect the thawing snows of the winter and put them in summer pitchers (coolers).—Bets. l. c. מלוין חַצְבַּיְיהוּ ח׳ filled their pitchers with water. Ber. 28[a] ח׳ חוורין וכ׳ white pitchers full of ashes (unworthy students). Ib. 58[a], v. יָא I.

חָצָד m. a species or variety of *dates*, v. חָצָב I.

חֲצַד I (cmp. חצב) *to cut, mow* (corresp. to h. קָצַר). Targ. Deut. XXIV, 19; a. fr.—M. Kat. 9[b] דתזרע ולא תֶחְצַד that you may sow but not cut (that your children may not die in your life time). Taan. 10[a] עתירה בבל דחַצְדָא וכ׳ (Ms. M. דחצרא . . . עתידה) Babylonia is rich because she harvests without rain (independent of rain-fall on account of her canalization). Koh. R. to II, 20; Lev. R. s. 25 קאים וחָצֵיד חצובין וכ׳ (וחָצֵיב, also וחצב, והצד) cutting down cistus shrubs to plant shoots of fig-trees; a. fr. [Y. Dem. III, 23[b] bot. מירחצד, מחצדן, v. חֲצַר.]

חַצָּד II m. (preced.) *cutter.* Targ. Ps. CXXIX, 7; v. חָצוֹדָא.

חַצְדָא (חִצְּדָא) I m. (preced.) *crop, harvest-time.* Targ. Gen. VIII, 22.—Targ. Lev. XIX, 9; a. fr.—M. Kat. 12[b] ח׳ וכ׳ חצדו ליה had his crop cut &c. Ib. ח׳ דחיטי הוה it was the wheat crop; a. e.

חַצְדָּא or **חַצְדָא** II m.=h. חָצָד or חָצָב I. Y. Ab. Zar. I, 39[d] bot. (ref. to חצד, Mish.) מין הוא ושמו ח׳ it is a species (of dates) named Ḥ.

חַצָּדָא, v. חָצוֹדָא.

חַצְדָד pr. n. pl. *Ḥatsdad*, in Babylonia. Yoma 77[b] אמברא דח׳ at the ford of Ḥ. [Var. חצידר, בי ח׳, הצדר, הינדר, חצדר, v. Rabb. D. S. a. l. note 8.]

חָצָה, v. חצי.

חָצוּב, v. חָצָב II.

חֲצוּבָא I, v. חֲצוּבָה II.

חֲצוּבָא II m. ch.=חָצָב II. B. Bath. 56[a] ח׳ שבי תיחם וכ׳ (Ms. O. חצב, Rashi חצובה) it is the *ḥ.* which Joshua introduced as landmarks. Bets. 25[b] ח׳ מקטע וכ׳ (some ed. חצובה) the *h.* cuts the feet of (convicts) the wicked (who remove the boundary lines).—Pes. 111[b] בטולא דחצבא דלא חצב גרמידא (Rashi: דחצובא) in the shade of a *ḥ* that has not cut through (grown) to an arm's length (v. Rabb. D. S. a. l. note); Yalk. Deut. 945.

חֲצוּבָה I h. same, v. חָצָב II, a. preced.—*Pl.* חֲצוּבוֹת. Y. Peah II, beg. 16[d] ח׳ מפסיקין לפיאה cistus shrubs (between two fields) form a boundary line with regard to the poor man's corner. Gen. R. s. 31, end.

חֲצוּבָה II f. (v. חָצָב) *a stand for a pitcher, tripod.*—כח׳ in the shape of a tripod, *triangulary arranged.* B. Mets. 25[a] כח׳ מהו (Ms. H. כחוצבא) if coins are found lying in a triangle; (Y. ib. II, 8[b], sq. מצובה, expl. קרפיפא). B. Bath. 83[b] (also כחצובא) planted in a triangle. Erub. 85[b] דקיימי כח׳ (Ms. M. דעבידת כי חציבא, read: חצובא, v. Rabb. D. S. a. l. note) the three ruins between two buildings stand in a triangle (so as to make only the central ruin equally near to both dwellings).

חָצוֹדָא, חֲצוֹדָא m. (חצד) *mower, harvester.* Targ. Am. IX, 13. Targ. Jer. IX, 21 ed. Lag. חצד׳ (oth. ed. חַצָּדָא).—*Pl.* חָצוֹדַיָּא. Targ. Ruth II, 3, sq.

חֲצוֹצְרָא, v. חֲצוֹצְרְתָא.

חֲצוֹצְרָה, v. next w.

חֲצוֹצֶרֶת f. (b. h. חֲצֹצְרָה;=חצרצר׳, redupl. of חצר) [*closed all around*,] *trumpet.* Y. Sabb. XVII, beg. 16[a] ח׳ תוקע וכ׳ as to the trumpet, he blows for the third time (announcing the Sabbath) and deposits it in the place designated for it (on the roof, v. Bab. ib. 35[b] bot.).—*Pl.* חֲצוֹצְרוֹת. R. Hash. III, 4 שתי ח׳; a. e.

חֲצוֹצַרְתָּא ch. same. Targ. Hos. V, 8 (ed. Lag. חֲצֹצ׳).—Sabb. 36[a]; Succ. 34[a] ח׳ שופרא וכ׳ what (before the destruction of the Temple) was called Shofar is now called *ḥătsotsereth* &c.—*Pl.* חֲצוֹצְרָתָא, חֲצוֹצְרָן. Targ. Num. X, 2; 8; a. e.

חֲצוֹת, constr. **חֲצוֹת** f. (b. h.; חָצָה) *half*, (sub. הלילה) *midnight.* Ber. I, 1; a. fr.

חָצָה, חצי (b. h.; v. חָצַץ) 1) *to split, divide.* B. Bath. 3[a] שרצו לֶחֱצוֹת, v. מְחִיצָה.—2) *to pick one's teeth.* Tosef. Bets. III, 18, v. חָצַץ I.

Hif. הֶחֱצָה *to order a division, to assign half, divide.* B. Kam. 34[a] פחת שפחתתו מיתה מַחֲצִין בחי Ms. M. a. Rashi (ed. שפחתו) half of the loss of value which death has caused, is collected from the living animal; Y. ib. I, end, 2[c] מחצין את הנזק the loss is divided.

חֲצָא, חֲצִי ch. same, *to pick out* (of birds, v. P. Sm. 1349); *to pick one's teeth.* Targ. Prov. XXX, 17.—Y. Hall. IV, end, 60[b] מִיחֲצֵי שיניי (not ניח׳) to pick my teeth with; Y. Dem. III, 23[b] bot. מיחצד, מחצדן (corr. acc.).

חֲצִי, חֵצִי m. (b. h.; preced. wds.) *half.* B. Kam. IV, 9 חֲ׳ נזק half the damage. Gitt. IV, 5 מי שֶׁחֶצְיוֹ עבד וכ׳ he who is half a slave and half a freedman (having been emancipated by one of the partners); a. v. fr.—*Pl.* חֲצָאִין, חֲצָאִים, חֲצָיִין, חֲצָיִים. Sifra Vayikra, N'dab., ch. X, Par. 9 לא יביאנה ח׳ he must not offer it in parts. Ned. 83[a] אין נזירות לח׳ there is no nazaritism by halves, i. e. one cannot vow to be a nazarite by partial abstinence; ואין קרבן לח׳ nor is there a sacrifice for partial nazaritism. Y. Hor. I, 46[b] top אין הפסח לח׳ the Passover offering does not take place in divisions (of clean and unclean parties). Kerith. 5[a] מפטם לח׳ taking only a part of each ingredient; Y. Yoma IV, 41[d] bot. פיטמה ח׳; a. fr.

חֲצִיבָא m. (חֲצַב) *a hewn stone, block.* Targ. Is. LI, 1.—*Pl.* חֲצִיבִין *chiselled stones.* Targ. Y. Ex. XX, 22.

חציבא, Erub. 85[b], Ms. M., v. חֲצוּבָה II.

חֲצִיבָה f. (חָצַב) *chiseling.* Y. Yoma II, 40[c] bot. חֲצִיבָתָן בקדש their chiseling must take place in holiness.—[Y. Peah II, beg. 16[d] חציבות, some ed., v. חֲצוּבָה I.]

חֲצִינָא, חֲצִינָא m. (חצר) *carpenter's adze*, also *pick-axe* or *spade* (v. Sm. Ant. s. v. Dolabra). Targ. Is. XLIV, 12 (h. text מעצד); a. e.—Sabb. 123[b] ח׳ דנגרי carpenters' adze. B. Bath. 73[b] נפל ליה ח׳ וכ׳ Ms. M. a. Ar. (ed. חציצא) a carpenter lost his adze there. Erub. 77[b], v. מָרָא II; a. e.—*Pl.* חֲצִינֵי. B. Kam. 119[b] .... באתרא תרי ח׳ וכ׳ in the place of our Tanna (in the Mishnah) there are two *ḥătsinê* a large one called כשיל (axe), and a small one called מעצד (adze). Yoma 37[b]; Bets. 33[b], v. נַרְגָּא.

חֲצִיפָא, חֲצִיף m. (חֲצַף, sub. אַפִּין) 1) *bare-faced, impudent, impertinent.* Targ. Ps. XVII, 4. Targ. Koh. VIII, 1 חֲצִיף אפין (constr.); a. e.—Ber. 34[b]; Sot. 7[b] ח׳ עלי מאן וכ׳ I consider him impertinent who &c. Kidd. 33[a] כמה ח׳ האי גברא how irreverently behaves this man; a. e.—*Fem.* חֲצִיפָא, חֲצִיפְתָּא. M. Kat. 16[b]. Y. Taan. III, 66[d] top.—Pl. m. חֲצִיפִין, constr. חֲצִיפֵי. Targ. Y. Ex. XXVIII, 37; a. e.—2) *undaunted, persevering, strong.* Yalk. Koh. 989, v. נָכוֹרָא. Pesik. Shub., p. 161[a] ח׳ נצח לבישא וכ׳ the persevering (in prayer) conquers even the bad man, so much the more the Good One of the world; Y. Taan. II, 65[b] חֲצִיפַת .. לכשירא (corr. acc.); Yalk. Jon. 550.

***חֲצִיץ** m. (v. חֲצִיצָה) *intermediate contact, shaking an object between which and the person causing the vibration there is a partition.* Tosef. Ḥag. III, 21 וחֲצִיצוֹ ed. Zuck. (missing in oth. editions). V. חֲצָצוֹת.

חציצא, B. Bath. 73[b], v. חֲצִינָא.

חֲצִיצָא v. חֲצָצָא.

חֲצִיצָה f. (חָצַץ I) *interposition, an intervening object.* B. Kam. 82[a] bot. משום ח׳ to prevent an interposition (to remove anything sticking to the body or in the hair before bathing). Zeb. 19[a] ותיפוק ליה משום ח׳ ought it not to be forbidden as an unlawful interposition between the priest's hand and the object he has to handle?; a. fr.—*Pl.* חֲצִיצִין *the laws concerning interpositions.* Erub. 4[a]; Succ. 5[b].

חֲצִירָ־, v. חָצֵר.

חָצִיר m. (b. h.; חצר *to cut, be small*, cmp. Targ. of חציר, Num. XI, 5) *leek.*—*Pl.* חֲצִירִים, constr. חֲצִירֵי. Kel. XVII, 5; Tosef. ib. B. Mets. VI, 10 (ed. Zuck. חצר, R. S. to Kel. l. c. חצירי); Y. Orl. III, 63[a] bot. חריצי (corr. acc.), v. גֶּבַע. [In b. h. חציר also *grass, moss.*]

חֲצִירָא ch. same, *moss.* Targ. Ps. CXXIX, 6 (ed. Lag. חֲצַר, Var. חֲצַד).

חָצַף (cmp. חָסַף a. P. Sm. 1353 חצפא=ch. חספא) *to peel off, bare*; part. pass. חָצוּף (sub. אפיים); f. חֲצוּפָה 1) *barefaced, impudent, arrogant.* Snh. 3[a] ב״ד ח׳ an arrogant court (two sitting in judgment instead of three). Y. Taan. III, 66[d] top אחת ח׳ ואחת כשירה one was unabashed, the other chaste. Ned. 20[b]; a. e.—2) *undaunted, energetic, strong.* Tanh. Vayera 23 הנפש ח׳ היא the instinct of life is strong. Ex. R. s. 42 ג׳ חֲצוּפִים הם ח׳ בחיה וכ׳ (Bets. 25[b] עז) three (creatures) are persevering (undaunted by failure or opposition), among beasts it is the dog &c. Y. Taan. IV, 69[b] מה חציפה וכ׳ (read: חצו׳) how irrepressible is the Land of Israel that it still is productive (after all devastations).—*Pl.* חֲצוּפִים, f. חֲצוּפוֹת. Ex. R. l. c., v. supra.—Y. Ber. V, 8[d] bot. שעות החו׳ וכ׳ those irresistible, hard and evil times.

Hif. הֶחֱצִיף *to bare* (one's face), *to act irreverently.*

Koh. R. to IX, 18 כל המַחֲצִיף פניו וכ׳ whoever speaks irreverently of &c. Ib. III, 9 מַחֲצִיפִין אתם you embolden yourselves.

חֲצַף ch. same; part. pass. חֲצִיף q. v.
Af. אַחֲצִיף as preced. *Hif.* Targ. Prov. VII, 13. Ib. XXI, 29. Targ. Ez. XIII, 6 מַחְצְפִין וכ׳ (Var. מְחַצְפִין) they boldly insist upon it &c. [Dan. II, 15; III, 22 part. pass. *insisted upon, urgent.*]

חָצַץ I (b. h.; v. חוץ I) 1) *to drive a wedge in* (v. Prov. XXX, 27). —Denom. חֵץ. —2) *to pick one's teeth.* Bets. IV, 6 לַחֲצוֹץ וכ׳; (Tosef. ib. III, 18 לחצות, v. חָצָה).— 3) *to interpose*, v. חוּץ I. Zeb. 19ª מהו שיְּחוֹצוּ (or שִׁיְּחוֹצוּ). Ib. אפי׳ נימא אחת חוֹצֶצֶת even one thread forms an unlawful interposition. Ib. חוֹצְצוֹת; a. fr.
Pi. חִיצֵץ *to pick one's teeth.* Y. Sabb. VIII, end, 11ᶜ; Ḥull. 16ᵇ אין מְחַצְּצִין וכ׳ one must not use it for &c.

חָצַץ II (b. h.) *to cut off, divide; to line a wall so as to leave a space* (חָצִין) *between the two partitions.* Ohol. XV, 4 בית שֶׁחֲצָצוֹ וכ׳ a room which one partitioned off with boards or tapestry on the sides (walls) or on the ceiling. Ib. 5 ח׳ מארצו if he partitioned it off from the floor (laying an additional floor with a vacuum between); Tosef. ib. XV, 4.

חָצָץ m. (preced.) *space between two partitions, vacuum.* Ohol. XV, 4; 5; Tosef. ib. XV, 4. [In b. h. חָצָץ (v. חָצַץ I) *wedge-like objects, gravel, sand.*]

חֲצַץ, *Pa.* חַצֵּץ (denom. of חֵץ, v. חָצַץ) *to sharpen, or to shoot an arrow.* Targ. Jud. V, 8. מְחַצְּצֵי גירריא (missing in ed. Lag.)

חֲצָצָא m. ch. (=b. h. חָצָץ, v. חָצַץ, end) *gravel, sand.* Targ. Prov. XX, 17 (Ms. חֲצִירָא).—*Pl.* חֲצָצֵי. Lam. R. introd. (R. Joh. 1) סגירתון בטורי בח׳ וכ׳ you have to walk over rocks and gravel without shoes &c.

***חֲצָצוֹת** f. pl. (v. חֲצִיצָה) *intermediate contacts, laws concerning the shaking of an object by an unclean person through a partition* (v. חָצִיץ). Y. Ḥag. II, end, 78ᶜ (v. emendation in R. S. to Toh. VII, 5).

חֲצֹצַר (denom. of חצוצר) *to blow the trumpet.* Targ. I Chr. XV, 24 מְחַצְּצְרִין. Targ. II Chr. XIII, 14 מְחַצְּרִין.— V. מְחַצְּרָא.

חֲצֹצְרָא, חֲצֹצְרָה &c., v. חֲצוֹצ׳.

חֲצַצְתָּא f. (v. חָצַץ II, a. חצר; cmp. בָּצַע) *arbitration,* דייני דח׳ untrained judges who arbitrate from ignorance of the law. B. Bath. 133ᵇ, v. מִגְרִזְתָּא II. [R. Ḥan.: ח׳ *cemetery,* from חוץ II=חוּץ לעיר.]

***חֲצַר** (dial. for חֲצַד) *to cut, harvest.* Taan. 10ª עתידה בבל דחָצְרָא וכ׳ Ms. M. (v. חֲצַד) Babylonia shall in the future harvest without rain (on account of the canalization introduced). Cmp. חֲצִיר.—[מְחַצְּרִין, v. חֲצֹצַר.]

חֲצַר *grass, leek,* v. חֲצִיר, חֲצִירָא.

חָצֵר c. (b. h.; חצר, v. preced. wds.; cmp. גָּזַר a. גִּזְרָה &c.) *court, yard,* in gen. *private property.* B. Mets. 11ª חֲצֵרוֹ של אדם וכ׳ the ground belonging to a person takes possession for him (of what is found there) even without his knowledge. Ib. ח׳ המשתמרת a well-guarded ground (fenced-in). B. Kam. 12ª; Gitt. 21ª, a. e. ח׳ מהלכת a moving ground, e. g. the back of a slave. Erub. VI, 1 הדר עם . . . בח׳ if one dwells in the same court yard with a gentile. Ib. 3 אנשי ח׳ the residents of dwellings in one court yard; a. v. fr.—ח׳ הצירית Tyrian yard (with a lodge at the entrance). Maasr. III, 5; Nidd. 47ᵇ.—חֲצַר הקבר the excavated ground to which all the caves of a cemetery open. Ohol. XV, 8; Tosef. ib. XV, 7.—חֲ׳ הכירה *the rim* of the cooking range. Kel. VII, 3; Tosef. ib. B. Kam. V, 5.—חֲ׳ הכבד (=b. h. יֹתֶרֶת) *lobe* of the liver. Yoma VIII, 6; a. e.—חֲ׳ מות *cemetery,* v. supra. Ber. 18ᵇ. —*Pl.* חֲצֵרוֹת, חֲצֵרִ׳. Erub. IV, 6. Ib. VI, 8; a. fr.

חֲצֵרָא, חֵיצְרָא, constr. חֲצַר ch. same.—ח׳ דעל כבדא, חֲצַר כבדא=h. חֲצַר הכבד, v. preced. Targ. Ex. XXIX, 13; a. e. (h. text יותרת). Targ. II Chr. XVIII, 33.

חֵק, חַק, v. חֵקֶק, חֵקֵק.

חֹק, חֻקָּה, v. חוֹק, חוּקָּה.

חֲקָה, v. חקר.

חֲקוּלָא I=חַקְלָא. Y. Dem. IV, 24ª top מן דבר ח׳ וכ׳ when the manager of the estate came out to him.

חֲקוּלָא II, **חֲקוּלַאי** pr. n. m. *Ḥăkula, Ḥăkulai.* Y. Peah I, 16ᶜ bot.; a. e. Y. Gitt. III, 45ª top אר . . . . Ib. VIII, 49ᶜ bot. חֲקוּלָה.

חֲקוּקָא, חֲקוּקָאה, חֲקוּקָה, v. חִיקוּק.

חִקּוּר m. (חָקַר) *ascertainment.*—ח׳ דין judging ability. Ab. VI, beg.

חָקָה, חָקֵי, *Pi.* חִיקָּה (b. h.; denom. of חֹק) 1) *to draw circles, to survey.* Gen. R. s. 39, end (ref. to Gen. XII, 9) מְחַקֶּה והולך וכ׳ surveying as he went along, with the direction towards the Temple.—2) *to imitate a person's customs, to follow a person's footsteps.* Sifra K'dosh. beg. (ref. to Lev. XIX, 2) פמליא של מלך מה עליה להיות מְחַקָּה למלך Rab. (ed. פ׳ למלך ומה וכ׳) what is the duty of the King's retinue?—To follow in the wake of the King; (Yalk. Lev. 604 מְחַקָּה). Ḥull. II, 9 שלא יְחַקֶּה וכ׳ that he may not appear to imitate the customs of the heretics.

חִקִּיין, v. חֵקֵק.

חֲקִיל, חֲקִילָא=חַקְלָא. Targ. Y. Gen. XXVII, 27 (some ed. חֲקַל). Ib. XXIII, 19 חֲקִיל (constr.).—Y. Ab. Zar. II, 41ᵈ top; (Y. Sabb. I, 3ᵈ top בטורא; Y. Ter. VIII, 45ᵈ bot. בחלא, read: בחקלא).

חֲקִיק, v. חֵקֵק.

חֲקִיקָה f. (חָקַק) *digging out, engraving.* Gitt. 20ª ח׳ לאו כתיבה היא engraving is not writing (for legal purposes).

חֲקִירָה f. (חָקַר) *search, speculation, study.* Y. Keth. VII, 31ᶜ bot., a. e. נדר ... חֲקִירַת חכם a vow which requires the study of a scholar (to find out means of absolving).—Esp. *examination of witnesses, cross-examination.* R. Hash. 25ᵇ חקירת העדים the hearing of witnesses (testifying to having seen the first appearance of the new crescent). Snh. IV, 1 בדרישה וח׳ require investigation and examination of witnesses; a. fr.—*Pl.* חֲקִירוֹת *cross-examination referring to date, time and place,* contrad. to בדיקות referring to accompanying circumstances. Ib. V, 1 היו .. בשבע ח׳ (in capital cases) they examined by means of seven questions, what year-week, what year, month, day, hour and place. Ib. 2 מה בין ח׳ לבדיקות what is the difference in point of law between &c.? Ib. 40ᵇ שמונה ח׳ eight questions; a. fr.

חֲקַל, חַקְלָא I m. (חקל, cmp. חקר) [*marked out,*] *field.* Targ. Gen. II, 5. Targ. O. Num. XX, 17; a. fr.—Gen. R. s. 74, v. אִיזְגָּרָא; a. fr.—*Pl.* חַקְלִין, חַקְלַיָּא. Targ. Jer. XXXII, 15. Targ. Joel I, 10; a. fr.

חֲקַל, חַקְלָא II, **חַקְלְתָא** f. (preced.) *estate, farm.* Targ. Is. V, 8.—Y. Snh. II, 20ᵇ bot.; Ruth R. to II, 9; Midr. Sam. ch. XX (translat. of (א)פס דמים, I Sam. XVII, 1, I Chr. XI, 13) חקל סומקתא Red Field.—*Pl.* חַקְלָן, חַקְלָתָא. Targ. Jer. IV, 17. Targ. O. Ex. VIII, 9.—חַקְלָוָון, חַקְלָוָתָא. Y. Keth. X, end, 34ª. Pesik. B'shall. p. 93ª.

חַקְלָאָה, חַקְלָיָיא m. (preced.) *field-laborer, peasant;* trnsf. *boor, ignorant man.* Meg. 7ᵇ, v. הֵיקוּלָא. Keth. 79ª חזי מר נחמן ח׳ see, sir, how this ignoramus Naḥman &c.—*Pl.* חַקְלָאֵי. Ber. 37ᵇ.—Mixed pl. חַקְלָיָיתָא *peasantry.* Sabb. 12ª אבל דח׳ וכ׳ Ms. M. (ed. דבני חַקְלָיָתָא) but the garments of the peasantry are easily distinguishable (as to men's or women's).

חַקְלְתָא, v. חַקְלָא II.

חָקַק (b. h.; cmp. חוּק) *to draw a circle, to limit;* 1) (denom. of חֹק) *to legislate.* Y. Kil. I, 27ᵇ top, a. e. שתְקַקְתִּי, v. חוּק. Num. R. s. 19, beg., v. חוּקָּה; a. fr.—2) *to hollow out, to shape a receptacle.* Y. Bets. I, 60ᵇ bot. קערה שֶׁחֲקָקָהּ קוף a dish which an ape has hollowed out.—Part. pass. חָקוּק, f. חֲקוּקָה. Tosef. B. Bath. III, 1; B. Bath. 65ᵇ, a. e. מכתשת הח׳ the mortar which has been hollowed out (of stone &c.), opp. הקבועה stationary in the ground.—3) *to engrave, write with the stilus.* Tanḥ. Ki Thissa 14, v. חָרַט. Gitt. 20ª וכתב ולא וח׳ 'he writes' (Deut. XXIV, 1) but not 'he engraves' (on tablets &c.). Ib. חָק תוכות he chisels out the surroundings (making the letters come out in relief); חק ירריכות he digs the sides, i. e. he engraves the letters. Gen. R. s. 68; s. 78 שאיקונין שלך חֲקוּקָה וכ׳ whose picture is engraven above (in the heavenly throne). Y. Yoma IV, beg. 41ᵇ חֲקוּקִים היו the inscriptions were engraven (not written with ink). Y. Ned. VI, 40ª top מפני צלמי .. שחקוקים וכ׳ on account of the Chaldean images which were engraven on the walls (Ez. XXIII, 14); a. e.

Nif. נֶחְקַק *to be hollowed out.* Y. Erub. II, 20ª top אם תֵּיחָקֵק if the block be hollowed out. Sot. 36ᵇ שֶׁיֵּחָקֵק על וכ׳ (not שיחקוק) to have his name engraven on the jewels &c.; a. e.

חֲקַק ch. same. Lev. R. s. 6 נטל ... וחַקְקֵיה he took a reed and hollowed it out. Ḥull. 25ª; Sabb. 103ª חַק קפיזא וכ׳ he hollowed out &c., v. חֲטַט I.—Part. pass. חָקִיק, חָקִיק *engraven, marked.* Targ. Y. Ex. XXVIII, 11 (Ar. חקיין). Targ. Y. Lev. XIX, 28 (h. text קעקע). Targ. Cant. II, 9; a. fr.

Ithpa. אִתְחַקַּק *to be engraven, to engrave itself.* Targ. Y. Ex. XX, 2; 3.

חָקַר (b. h.) *to go around, to espy, to examine;* esp. *to cross-examine,* v. חֲקִירָה. Ab. I, 9 הוי מרבה לַחְקוֹר וכ׳ cross-examine witnesses as much as possible. Snh. 40ᵇ מדהוי ליה .... חָקוֹר תַּחְקוֹר the text might have read (for emphasis) thou shalt diligently inquire, or thou shalt diligently investigate (instead of the unusual phrase ודרשת היטב, Deut. XVII, 4); a. e.

Nif. נֶחְקַר *to be investigated, examined.* Koh. R. to I, 16 הלב נ׳ the heart is examined (by the Lord). R. Hash. III, 1 נֶחְקְרוּ העדים when the evidence was closed. Tosef. Snh. VI, 4 עד שֶׁתֵּחָקֵר עדותן וכ׳ until their examination in court has been closed; נֶחְקְרָה עדותן וכ׳ after it has been closed, they cannot retract. Ib. 5; a. fr.

חֲקַר ch. same. Targ. II Sam. X, 3. Targ. Ps. CXXXIX, 23; a. e.

חֵקֶר m. (b. h.; preced.) *search.*—אין (להם) ח׳ *unsearchable, innumerable.* Num. R. s. 19; Tanḥ. Ḥuck. 20.

חַקָּר, constr. חַקַּר m. (preced. wds.) *examiner.* Targ. Jer. XVII, 10.

חַקְרָא m. ch. (preced. wds.) *surrounded place, fortification.* Targ. II Sam. V, 9 (h. text מצדה); a. fr.—Targ. Y. Num. XXXII, 17 קִרְוֵי ח׳ ed. Amst. (some ed. קרוין, incorr.) fortified cities.—*Pl.* חַקְרִין. Ib. XIII, 20.—V. אַקְרָא.

חַקְרָה f. h. same. Arakh. IX, 6 ח׳ של וכ׳ the fort of Giscala.

***חַקְרָן** m. (חָקַר) *overwise, critic. Pl.* חַקְרָנִים. Sifré Num. 131, v. נַקְרָן.

חַר, v. חָרַת.

חַר, חָרָא, חָרִין, pl. חָרִין, v. חוֹר II, חוֹרָא II.

חָרָא *hole,* v. חוֹרָא I.

חָרָא (=אחרא, v. חוֹרִי), יומא ח׳ *next day,* v. יוֹמָחְרָא. Targ. II Chr. XX, 16 (ed. Lag. אחרא).—B. Mets. 17ª למחר ולוּמא ח׳ (Ms. H. a. oth. אוחרא, v. Rabb. D. S. a. l. note 30) to-morrow or the day after.

חָרָא, v. חָרֵי.

חָרֵב I (b. h.) *to be burned, dried up, ruined, waste.* Snh. 22ª כאלו ח׳ בה״מ וכ׳ as if the Temple had been destroyed in his days. Tosef. Men. XIII, 22 מפני מה חָרְבָה וכ׳ why was Shiloh destroyed?; Yoma 9ª. Kil. IV, 1 (expl. קָרַחַת הכרם) כרם שח׳ באמצעו a vineyard the central part of which is laid waste. Ib. V, 1; a. fr. [Num. R. s. 7, end ובבל ח׳ מקדש, read: חחריב. Taan. 29ª כשח׳ טורנוס, read: כשחרש, v. Rabb. D. S. a. l.]

Nif. נֶחֱרַב *to be destroyed.* Erub. 18ᵇ. Yoma 39ᵇ שסופך עתיד לֵיחָרֵב that it is thy final destiny to be destroyed; a. fr.

Hithpa. הִתְחָרֵב, *Nithpa.* נִתְחָרֵב same. Pesik. R. s. 31 שֶׁיִּתְחָרֵב. [Pirkê d'R. El. ch. XXXIII, v. חָרַךְ.]

Hif. הֶחֱרִיב *to destroy, lay waste.* Tosef. M. Kat. I, 5 מַחֲרִיבִין חורי וכ׳ you may destroy ant-stores (during the festive week). Num. R. s. 7, end שֶׁהֶחֱרִיבוּ בה״מ for they (the Romans) destroyed the Temple; a. fr.

**Hof.* הָחֳרַב *to be destroyed.* Pes. 42ᵇ (ref. to Ez. XXVI, 2) אי מלאה זו הָחֳרְבָה זו Ms. M. (ed. חרבה, v. Rabb. D. S. a. l. note 9) when the one (Jerusalem) is populated, the other (Caesarea) is laid waste; Yalk. Gen. 110 חֲרֵיבָה.

חֲרֵב, חָרִיב, חָרוּב, חֲרֵב ch. same. Targ. Ez. XXVI, 2. Targ. Hos. XIII, 15. Targ. Is. XIX, 5; a. fr.—Naz. 32ᵇ דח׳ בה״מ that the Temple has been destroyed. Ib. דִּיחְרוּב that it will be destroyed. Gitt. 56ª דלא לִיחְרוּב וכ׳ that Jerusalem may not be destroyed. Y. Ber. II, 5ª top דברגליה חריב with whose arrival it was destroyed; a. fr.

Af. אַחְרִיב, אַחְרוּב *to destroy, lay waste.* Targ. Is. XLII, 15. Targ. Jud. XVI, 24; a. fr.—Yoma 69ᵇ דְּאַחְרְבֵיה וכ׳ who destroyed the Temple. Taan. 29ª top לְאַחְרוּבֵי Ms. M. a. Rashi (ed. לְחָרוּבֵי); Gitt. 56ª לְחָרוּבֵי; a. fr.

Ithpe. אִיחֲרִיב, אִיחֲרוּב *to be destroyed.* Y. Ber. l. c.

חָרֵב II m., **חֲרֵבָה** , **חֲרֵי׳** f. (b. h.; preced. wds.) 1) *ruined.* Y. Ber. IV, 8ª. Yalk. Gen. 110, p. חָרֵב I; a. fr.—*Pl.* חֲרֵבִים, חֲרֵי׳; f. חֲרֵבוֹת, חֲרֵי׳. Ex. R. s. 31 (ref. to Num. XXIV, 5) ומִשְׁכְּנוֹתֶיךָ כשהם ח׳ thy pledges, when they are in ruins, v. מַשְׁכּוֹן; a. fr.—2) *dry.* Y. Sot. III, beg. 18ᶜ ח׳ של חטין the dry (oil-less) offering of wheat, opp. בלול. Kidd. 62ª top; a. e.

חֲרֵב ch., v. חָרוּב.

חֶרֶב f. (b. h.; cmp. חרה) 1) *sword.* Hull. 3ª, v. חָלַל I. B. Bath. 8ᵇ ח׳ קשה וכ׳ death in war is a greater affliction than natural death. Snh. 116ª מהם הרגו בח׳ some of them they put to death by the sword. Tanh. Balak 8; Num. R. s. 20 אא״כ שלף חַרְבּוֹ without drawing his sword. Ib. בח׳ חייהם live on their sword. Taan. III, 5 על הח׳ on the sword, i. e. when armies are passing the country. Ib. 22ª ח׳ של שלום a friendly army passing; a. fr.—2) *the sword-shaped handle of a plough.* Kel. XXI, 2. Tosef. ib. B. Bath. I, 7.—*Pl.* חֲרָבוֹת. Pesik. R. s. 21 ח׳ מכאן וכ׳ (soldiers with) swords here &c.; a. e.

חַרְבָּא, חֶרֶב I same. Targ. Gen. XXXIV, 26. Ib. III, 24; a. fr.—Sabb. 123ᵇ, v. אוּשְׁפָּא; (Ar. *scraping knife*).

חַרְבָּא, חֲרַב II m. (חרב) *dry eruption.* Targ. Y. Deut. XXVIII, 27 Ar. ed. Koh. חרב (oth. ed. חרבא, חרבטא; Targ. ed. גרבא; h. text גרב).

חֲרָבָא, חַרְבָא, v. חוּרְבָּא a. חָרוּב.

חַרְבָּה f. (v. חֶרֶב) *knife.* Shebi. VIII, 6 קוצץ אותם בח׳ (Ar. ed. Koh. בחורבה, R. S. בחרבא) you may cut them with a knife, opp. to מוקצה the tool especially intended for cutting figs.

חָרְבָּה *ruin*, v. חוּרְבָּה.

חַרְבּוֹנָא, v. חַרְבָּא II.

חַרְבוֹנָה, חַרְבוֹנָא pr. n. m. (b. h.) *Harbona*, one of King Ahasver's eunuchs. Gen. R. s. 49; Treat. Sof'rim XIV, 6 (צ״ל) גם ח׳ זכור לטוב one must say, H., too, be remembered &c. Meg. 16ª; a. e.

חַרְבִּינִין, v. חַרְחֲבִינָה.

חַרְבָּן, v. חוּרְבָּן.

חרבריה, v. חֲבַרְבָּרֵי.

חַרְגָּא f., constr. חַרְגַּת (חרג, v. P. Sm. 1366) [*rough sound, sawing,*] *dying agony.* Targ. Deut. XXXII, 25. Targ. Lam. I, 20 ed. Lag. (oth. ed. חַרְגַּת).

חַרְגָּא, חִיר׳ m. (v. preced.) [*saw-dust,*] *sun-motes* (cmp. נְסָר). Yoma 20ᵇ האי ח׳ דיומא לא וכ׳ those sun-motes are called *la* (Dan. IV, 32).

חַרְגּוֹל m. (b. h. חַרְגֹּל; חגל with ר inserted; cmp. חגב) name of an edible *locust.* Sabb. VI, 10 (67ª) ביצת הח׳ the egg of a *hargol* (carried in the ear for ear-ache).

חַרְגּוֹלָא ch. same. Targ. O. Lev. XI, 22 (ed. Berl. חַרְגְּלָא).

חַרְגִּינִין m. pl. (comp. of חר a. גִּינָּה, v. חַרְחֲבִינָה) *garden-ivy*, the leaves of which may be used for bitter herbs on the Passover night. Pes. 39ª ed. (Ms. M. 1 הרגנין read with Ms. M. 2: הַרְגִּנִין).

חַרְגְּלָא, v. חַרְגּוֹלָא.

חָרַד (b. h.) *to be excited, to tremble.* Gen. R. s. 67 (ref. to מאד, Gen. XXVII, 33) מחרדה שח׳ וכ׳ more than the trembling which he felt on the altar; (Yalk. ib. 115 שֶׁחָרֵיד). Tanh. Tol'd 13 שתי חרדות ח׳ וכ׳ twice did Isaac tremble. Gen. R. l. c. חָרֵיד is he frightened?; Yalk. l. c. חָרֵד; a. e.

Hif. הֶחֱרִיד 1) same, v. supra.—2) *to frighten.* Gen. R. l. c. חרדה שה׳ יעקב וכ׳ the fright which Jacob caused to Isaac; Tanh. l. c.; Ruth R. to III, 8. Ib. חרדה שֶׁהֶחֱרִידָה וכ׳ the alarm which Ruth caused &c. Ib. שהן מַחֲרִידוֹת וכ׳ they (the fowl) excite the man (who tries to catch them); a. e.

חרדא, חרדה, Lev. R. S. 24, v. חֲרָרָא.

חֲרָדָה f. (b. h.; preced. art.) *excitement, anxiety, fear, reverence.* Gen. R. s. 67; Ruth R. to III, 8, a. e., v. חָרֵד. Nidd. IV, 7, a. e. ח׳ מסלקת וכ׳ excitement prevents the regular menstruation. Ber. 30[b] (ref. to Ps. XXIX, 2) א״ת בהדרת קדש אלא בחֶרְדַּת קדש Ms. M. read not 'in the glory' of the sanctuary, but in reverence of &c.; Yalk. Sam. 78; Y. Ber. V, 8[d] bot.—[Tanh. K'dosh. 9 כחרדת דם, v. חֶרְדָּה.]—*Pl.* חֲרָדוֹת. Tanh. Tol'd. 13, v. חָרֵד.

חַרְדּוֹן m. *large Libyan lizard.* Y. Ber. VIII, 12[b]; Gen. R. s. 82, end; (Hull. 127[a] צב).

חַרְדּוֹנָא ch. same. Targ. Y. Lev. XI, 29 ed. pr. (ed. הדרונא, Ar. חרדונא; h. text צב; v. Fl. to Levy Targ. Dict. I, 425[2]). Targ. I Chr. XI, 22 ed. Lag. a. oth. (ed. Beck חרדנא, ed. Wil. חדרונא).—Y. Ber. I, 3[d] top דלא יעביד כחרדין חַרְדּוֹנָה he must not (in bowing at prayers) bend like the *hardon* (with head erect).

חַרְדָּל m. (חד, with ר inserted; cmp. גַּד I) *mustard.* Kil. I, 2 ח׳ וח׳ המצרי common mustard and Egyptian mustard. Ber. 40[a] הרגיל בח׳ וכ׳ he who is used to take mustard once in &c. Ib. 31[a], a. e. כח׳ as large as a grain of mustard; a. fr.—*Pl.* חַרְדְּלִים, חַרְדְּלִין. Cant. R. to VI, 11 כמה ח׳ ever so many grains of &c. B. Bath. 25[b] הרחק דבורך מן חַרְדָּלַיי keep thy bee-hive from my mustard plants; ib. 18[a] חַרְדְּלַאי (Ms. F. a. R. חרדלי).

חַרְדְּלִי m. (preced.; sub. יין) *mustard-colored, red wine.* Gen. R. s. 98. Sabb. 63[a] top יין ח׳ (an obscene disguise for a dark-complected woman), v. גּוּרְדְּלִי.

חַרְדְּלִית f. (preced. wds.; cmp. חד I, 2) *rain water rushing down a slope, torrent.* Eduy. V, 2; Mikv. V, 6; expl. Tosef. ib. IV, 10, v. מִדְרוֹן. Hag. 19[a] ח׳ של גשמים; Tosef. Mikv. III, 4 חַרְדֶּלֶת; a. e.

חַרְדְּנָא, v. חַרְדּוֹנָא.

חָרָה, v. חרי.

חָרֵה, *Pa.* חָרֵה, v. חָרַח.

חֲרוֹב, v. חָרֵב.

חָרוֹב, חָרִיב m., **חֲרוֹבָא, חֲרִיבָא** f. (preced.) *ruined, desolate.* Targ. Hag. I, 4; 9 (Levita חריב). Targ. Ps. LX, 11 (ed. Wil. חָ׳, Ms. חריבא). Targ. Ez. XXVI, 19 חרו׳ ed. Lag. (ed. Ven. I חֲרֵבָא, ed. Wil. חָרְבָא).—*Pl. fem.* חַרְבָתָא, חֲרֵבָ׳, חֲרֵיבָן. Targ. Ez. XXXVI, 38. Ib. 35. Targ. Is. LXI, 4; a. e.

חָרוּב I m. (חרב) [*dry,*] 1) *carob-pod; carob-tree.* B. Bath. IV, 8 ח׳ שאינו מורכב a carob-tree which has not yet been ingrafted (bears no fruit). B. Mets. 59[b]; a. fr.—*Pl.* חֲרוּבִים, חֲרוּבִין. R. Hash. 15[b]. B. Bath. 70[a]. Lev. R. s. 35, a. e. (play on חרב תאכלו, Is. I, 20) ח׳ תֹּאכֵלוּ (some ed. וחרבין, corr. acc.) ye shall eat carobs (live in poverty); a. fr.—2) *a variety of beans,* the pods of which resemble the carob, v. חֲרוּבָא. Kil. I, 2.

חָרוּב II pr. n. pl. *Hărub,* 1) מגדל ח׳ *Tower of H.*, in Northern Palestine. Y. Shebi. VI, 36[c]; Tosef. ib. IV, 11 (v. Hildesh. Beitr. p. 37).—2) כפר ח׳ *K'far (Village of) H.* Y. Dem. II, 22[d] top, כפר וח׳ (corr. acc.); v. חֲרוּבָא II.

חֲרוּבָא, חֲרוּבָה I ch.=h. חָרוּב I, *carob.* Lev. R. s. 35 צריכין ישראל לח׳ וכ׳ Israel needs carob (poverty) to do repentance; Yalk. Is. 256; Lev. R. s. 13 (not לחיר׳). Y. Kil. I, 27[a] (expl. חרוב Mish. ib. I, 2) (פרסי) כמין פול מצרי הוא ... דמיין לח׳ it is a variety of the Egyptian (Persian?) bean, and its pods look like those of the carob. Y. Succ. III, 53[d] top.

חֲרוּבָא, חֲרוּבָה II, **כפר ח׳** pr. n. pl. *K'far Hăruba,* on the lake of Genezareth (v. Hildesh. Beitr. p. 37). Y. Taan. IV, 69[a] כ׳ חריבה; Lam. R. to II, 2 (ed. Wil. חרוכא, corr. acc.); Yalk. Deut. 946 כפר חנניא.

חרובות, חרובתא, v. next wds.

חֲרוּבִית f. (חָרוּב I) *carob-tree.* Num. R. s. 9 (p. 232[b] ed. Amst.); Midr. Sam. ch. XIII כח׳ גדולה היה Absalom was as tall as a large carob-tree; ib. ch. XXVII; Y. Sot. I, 17[b] top (not בות...). Pesik. R. s. 4 פערה הח׳ וכ׳ the carob tree opened itself and swallowed him (Isaiah).

חֲרוּבִיתָא ch. same. Y. Sot. I, 17[b] top (not חרובו׳); Num. R. s. 9; a. e.

חרוד, Treat. S'mah. ch. IX, end, read: יָדִיד.

חרודי, Targ. Y. II, Deut. XVIII, 10, v. חָרוֹרָא.

חֲרָוָתָא, v. חֲרוּתָא a. חָרֵי.

חָרוּז, pl. **חֲרוּזִין**, v. חָרַז.

חָרוֹזָא m. (חָרַז) *a stringer of pearls;* trnsf. *one who combines verses* from various Biblical books for homiletical purposes. Cant. R. to I, 10, v. קָדוֹזָא.

חֲרוּזִיתָא, pl. **חֲרוּזְיָאתָא, חֲרוּזְיָתָא**, v. חַרְזָא.

חרויין, v. חַדוּיִין.

חֲרוֹכָא m. (חָרַךְ) *burned, charred meat.* Bets. 32[b] ואזדהר מח׳ but guard against its becoming charred (by touching a solid object in the oven). Pes. 41[a] דשוייה ח׳ Ms. M. (ed. דשויא) he made (the Passover lamb) charred meat (instead of roast). Zeb. 106[a]; Yoma 68[b] דשויא ח׳ if it has been reduced to lumps of charred flesh (instead of being burnt to ashes), v. נָתַךְ.—B. Mets. 85[a] they surnamed R. Zeira ח׳ קטין שקיה Ms. M. (ed. קטין חֲרִיךְ ש׳) the burnt one with dwarfed legs: Snh. 37[a] חֲרִיכָא (early prints חרו׳); (Ber. 46[a] קטינא חריך שקי).—[Lam. R. to II, 2 כפר חרוכא, some ed., v. חֲרוּבָא II.]

חָרוּל m. (b. h.; חרל *to sting, burn,* cmp. חרר) *thorn, nettle.*—*Pl.* חֲרוּלִים, constr. חֲרוּלֵי. Pirké d'R. El. ch. XXX; Yalk. Gen. 95.

חָרוּם, v. חָרַם.

חָרוּם, v. חֵירוּם.

חָרוֹן m. (b. h.; חָרָה) *anger.* Gen. R. s. 70 (play on מחרן, Gen. XXIX, 4) מֵחֲרוֹנוֹ של וכ׳ we flee from the anger of the Lord; Yalk. ib. 123. Zeb. 102[a] כל חרון אף וכ׳

wherever in the Scriptures the expression 'anger of the Lord' is used, there remains a lasting mark of it; Yalk. Ex. 173.

חֲרוֹסֶת f. (חרס; cmp. הֲרִסְנָא) *a pap made of fruits and spices with wine or vinegar*, used for sweetening the bitter herb on the Passover night. Pes. X, 3. Ib. 116ª (play on חֶרֶס I) זכר לטיט ח׳, v. זֵכֶר. Tosef. ib. X, 9; a. e.

חֲרוּף, חֲרוּפָא, v. חֵיר׳.

חֲרוּפָה f. (חָרַף) *scraper, rake.*—*Pl.* חֲרוּפוֹת. Shebi. V, 4 בח׳ של עץ Ms. M. (ed. בְּמַגְרוֹפוֹת) with wooden rakes.

חֲרוּפָה f. (v. חָרַף) 1) *designated, betrothed.* Kidd. 6ª האומר חֲרוּפָתִי וכ׳ if one says to a woman, Be my *hărufah*, she is betrothed, for in Judæa they call the betrothed (אֲרוּסָה) *hărufah.*—Esp. שפחה ח׳ (v. Lev. XIX, 20) *a handmaid designated to become the wife of one selected by her master.* Gitt. 43ª ארוסה שפחה ח׳ (Ker. II, 5 only שפחה) what is the legal condition meant in the law concerning the designated handmaid?—Tosef. Ker. I, 19 אשם ש׳ ח׳ the sacrifice due for sleeping with an engaged handmaid. Ib. 16; a. fr.—*Pl.* חֲרוּפוֹת. Ker. 9ª; a. e.—2) *defloured*, v. חָרַף.

חֲרוּץ m. (b. h.; חָרַץ) *one having an abnormal incision or cavity on his body* (Lev. XXII, 22). Bekh. 41ª ח׳ במקום עצם having the depression in a bone, ח׳ בשר in a fleshy part. V. חָרִיץ.

חֲרוֹרָא m. (חור, v. חֲוַרְוָרָא; cmp. P. Sm. 1226, sq. s. v. חור) *dazzling the eye, deceiver.*—*Pl.* חֲרוֹרִין, constr. חֲרוֹרֵי (חֲרֵי), with עיינין. Targ. Y. I Deut. XVIII, 10 (Y. II ed. Amst. חֲרוֹרֵי, corr. acc.); ib. 14 (h. text מְעֹנֵן, derived fr. עין, v. Snh. 65ᵇ quot. s. v. זְכוּרוּ). [Targ. Y. Lev. XIX, 26 ולא אחורי סנהדרין עיינין, read: ולא חרורי עיינין, the word סנהדרין being a glossator's reference to Snh. l. c.]

חרורו, Yoma 68ᵇ Ar. ed. Koh., v. חֲדוּרָא.

חֲרוֹרִי m. (חור II) *one belonging to the class, having the status, of freedmen.* Kidd. IV, 1.

חֲרוֹרֵי m. pl. (v. preced.) *claims of liberation from slavery.* Gitt. 86ª (in a formula of sale of a slave) ופטיר ועטיר מן ח׳ וכ׳ and is free and guarded from any claims of liberation.

חֲרוּשְׁתָּא f.=חַרְשׁוּתָא, *witchcraft.* Pes. 110ª bot. נשי דח׳ Ms. M. (ed. v. חָרְשֵׁי) women practicing witchcraft.

חֲרוּת, v. חֵירוּת.

חָרוּת I m. 1) (חרת, sec. r. of חרה, v. חֲרָיָה) *dried up by heat, shrunk.* Succ. 32ª top ח׳ פסול if the palm-branch is dried up, it is unfit for use; דומה לח׳ if it only looks as if dried up (blackish) &c.—*Fem.* חֲרוּתָה. Hull. III, 2 ח׳ בידי שמים if the animal's lungs are shrunk (wood-like) through an accident; ib. 55ᵇ ח׳ בידי אדם by violence done to it. Tosef. ib. III, 12 אי זוהי ח׳ וכ׳ what animal is called *hărutha?*—Answ. whose lungs are shrunk.—2) *engraven*, v. חָרַת. [Y. B. Bath. IV, 14ᶜ bot. חירותך, v. חוּט.]

חָרוּת II, v. חֶרֶת.

חֲרוּתָא f. ch. (preced.)=h. חֲרָיָה, *a dried-up twig, hardened palm-twig*, opp. כפות flexible. Succ. 32ª. B. Bath. 161ᵇ; Gitt. 36, a. e. צייר ח׳ drew a palm-twig (as his signature). [Targ. Is. LX, 21 דחרותי ed. Ven., read: דחדותי, v. חֶדְוָא.]—*Pl.* חֲרְוָן׳, חֲרְוָתָא. B. Bath. 101ᵇ דעביד להו כי ח׳ he makes the burial caves like palm-twigs (in the shape of a fan). Pes. 82ª קני וחרוותא Ms. M. 2 (Ms. M. 1 קני דחרות׳, corr. וח׳, ed. וחרויאתא, read: וְחַרְוָוָתָא; Ar. חֲרִיָתָא, fr. חֲרָיָא) reeds and twigs. Y. Shebi. II, 33ᵈ bot. בכנישתא חדתא וחֲרְוָתָה (read: דח׳) with a new broom of palm-twigs.

חֲרוּתָא, v. חֵיר׳.

חָרוּתָא f. (חרר) *blackness, black sediment.* Nidd. 20ª, v. חֶרֶת. [Kidd. 81ᵇ אנא ח׳, v. חֲדוּתָא.]

חָרַז (b. h.) [*to bore holes, to carry thread through a hole,*] 1) *to squeeze into.* Cant. R. to I, 10 (ref. to בחרוזים ib.) שחוֹרְזִים צואריהם וכ׳ (not שחוזרין) who squeeze their necks (through window holes, open doors &c.) to hear the words of the Law (v. Yoma 35ᵇ; Ber. 6ᵇ; v. הוּחְקָא); Yalk. ib. 983 שהם חוזרים אחרי וכ׳ (read: חוֹרְזִים אחוֹרֵי).—2) *to string.* Ex. R. s. 20 ישב וח׳ וכ׳ he sat down and strung (assorting) the larger pearls separately &c.—Part. pass. חָרוּז, pl. חֲרוּזִים, חֲרוּזִין. Cant. R. l. c. [read:] אלו ע׳ זקנים שהיו חֲרוּזִים אחריהם כליניא וכ׳ (v. Yalk. l. c.) those are the seventy elders who were strung (arranged) behind them (Moses and Aaron) like a string of pearls.—Hull. 95ᵇ בחרוזין (Ar. חֲרִיזִים, noun) if the pieces of meat are strung together. Lam. R. to V, 13 ג׳ מאות ... ח׳ וכ׳ three hundred children were found strung up on the branches of one tree.—Trnsf. *to draw parallels between Biblical passages, to explain one passage by another.* Cant. R. l. c. הייתי יושב וחוֹרֵז וכ׳ I was sitting and comparing verses of the Pentateuch, and Pentateuch with Prophets &c.—Ib. שהיו חוֹרְזִים וכ׳; Yalk. l. c. חוזרים (corr. acc.). Cant. R. l. c. שהן חֲרוּזוֹת וכ׳ which are strung together (illustrate one another).

Hif. הֶחֱרִיז same. Lev. R. s. 16 מַחֲרִיז ד״ת וכ׳ I was comparing &c.

חֲרַז ch. same, 1) *to sting, perforate.* Yeb. 75ᵇ top חַרְזֵיה סילוא וכ׳ a thorn wounded him &c. Ab. Zar. 28ᵇ זיבורא ודחרזיה וכ׳ he who suffers from the sting of a wasp, or of a thorn.—2) *to string beads; trnsf. to compare verses* (v. preced.). Cant. R. to I, 10 אית דידע לְמֵיחְרוֹז וכ׳ some know how to string but not how to bore pearls, i. e. some know how to bring on parallels without having the ability to enter into the depth of a subject.

Af. אַחְרִיז *to cause to sting, to prickle.* Gitt. 84ª מַחְרִיז Ar., v. בְּרַז.

חַרְזָא, v. חִירְזָא.

חַרְזָא m. (preced. wds.) *stinging, spiny.* B. Kam. 80ª (expl. תולדת הסנאים) שרצא הוצא וא״ד ח׳ דקטינר וכ׳ Ms. M. (ed. שרצא חרצא; for oth. var. v. Rabb. D. S. a. l. note 20; marginal vers. שרצא חרצא וא״ד חרצא) a creeping animal (which is) prickly, and some use the word *ḥarza* (spiny), with tiny legs. But why 'creeping'?—Because its legs are low. V. חַרְצָא.—Fem. חַרְזִיתָא, pl. חַרְזְיָיתָא. Erub. 26ᵇ אצוותא ח' Ms. M. (ed. חֲרוּזְיָאתָא, חרוזית'), v. אַצְוָוא.

חַרְזָק, v. חַרְזֵק.

חָרַח, *Pa.* חָרַח (=h. חִרְחֵר) *to inflame.* Targ. Prov. XXVI, 21 מְחָרַח Ms. (ed. Lag. מחרחר, oth. ed. מחרחר, corr. acc.; ed. Wil. מְחַרֵח, fr. חֲרַח).

חַרְחֲבִינָא, חַרְחֲבִינָה m. (a comp. of חרתר=חרח, *to bore, sting,* v. חָרַר II, a. בּוּן, v. בִּינָא III, בִּינְתָא II) *a hair-like creeper, creeper on palm-trees* (cmp. חַרְהוּפְנִין, חַרְגִּינָן). Tosef. Shebi. V, 3 הרחבינה ed. Zuck. (Var. החרוח'). Pes. II, 6, expl. ib. 39ᵃ, v. אַצְוָוא.—*Pl.* חַרְחֲבִינִין. Ib. בחרחלין ובח' ed. (Ms. M. 1 ובחרחבנין; Ms. M. 2 ובחרבנין), v. חַרְחֲלִין. Ib. ובחרגינין ובחַרְבִינִין וכ' ed. (Ms. M. ובהרחבינה, v. Rabb. D. S. a. l. note 200) with palm-ivy, garden-ivy and wall-ivy.

חַרְחוּר m. (reduplic. of חור, v. חָרַר I) [*point of a lance,* v. Maim. to Kel. XIII, 3 ed. Dehr.,] *the coulter,* inserted into the horizontal pole (מַרְדֵּעַ) in front of the ploughshare (דָּרְבָן). Kel. XIII, 3. Ib. XXV, 2, v. חֵיךְ. Tosef. ib. B. Mets. III, 7. Tosef. ib. B. Bath. III, 5.

חַרְחוּר or **חַרְ'** m. (חִרְחֵר) *burnt part of a loaf, burnt crust.* Teb. Yom I, 3, sq. Cmp. חֲרוּבָא.

חַרְחוּרָא m. (preced.; = b. h. חַרְחֻר) 1) *fever.* Targ. O. Deut. XXVIII, 22.—2) (cmp. הרהר) *heated imagination, fantasy, delirium. Pl.* constr. חַרְחוּרֵי. Targ. Y. Deut. l. c. ח' דלוחי (some ed. ה') the frightful fantasies of &c.

חַרְחַלִּין m. pl. (redupl. of חרל, v. חָרוּל) *a prickly plant, thistle,* (v. Sm. Ant. s. v. Carduus). Pes. 39ᵃ בח' ובחרחבינין וכ' (you may use for bitter herb) thistles, palm-ivy &c.

חַרְחַר or **חַר חַר** (onomatop.) *ḥarḥar,* a word in an incantation for choking. Sabb. 67ᵃ ח' נחית בלע Ar. (ed. חד חד, Ms. O. both versions combined, v. Rabb. D. S. a. l. note 90) *ḥ.,* go down swallowed thing.

חִרְחֵר (b. h.; Pilp. of חָרַר III) 1) *to set twigs on fire* for driving out the bees. Ukts. III, 11 משיְּחַרְחֵר from the moment he smokes the bees out; [Maim.: *he heats the honey-comb;* Var. in Ar.: משיְּהַרְהֵר].—2) (sub. ריב) *to stir up strife.* Cant. R. to VIII, 13 ולא תְחַרְחֲרוּ זה עם זה do not quarrel with one another.—3) *to make hot with fever.* Lev. R. s. 17, v. הִרְהֵר. [Y. Kidd. I, 58ᶜ top מחרחרין מוזהרין, a cacography of מוזהרין; in ed. Amst. only מוזהרין.]

חַרְחֵר ch., v. חֲרַר III.

חָרַט (b. h.) *to scrape; to chisel.* Tanḥ. Ki Thissa 14 below the Israelites were sitting חוֹרְטִין את העגל וכ' chiselling the calf . . ., and above the Lord engraving the tablets.

Hif. הֶחֱרִיט *to model.* Pirké d'R. El. ch. III אם איני מַחֲרִיט .. יסודותיו וכ' unless he models ... its foundations and its entrances and exits, he does not begin to build. Ib. הקב"ה ה' לפניו וכ' the Lord modelled before Him the world, but it would not stand.

Hithpa. הִתְחָרֵט [*to scratch one's self,*] *to regret, feel sorry.* Hag. 5ᵃ וּמִתְחָרֵט בו and feels sorry for it. Nidd. 31ᵇ מִתְחָרֶטֶת she regrets (her vow of abstinence); a. fr. V. חֲרָטָה.

חֲרַט ch. same, *to regret.* Targ. Cant. V, 4 לְמֶחְרַט to repent.—Pes. 113ᵃ וְתֶחְרַט, v. זְבַן.

חֲרָטָה f. (preced. wds.) *regret,* esp. *the expression, before a court, of regret for a vow made under misapprehension.* Nidd. 31ᵇ ובח' תליא מילתא and the case is dependent on a formal declaration (and decision by a court). Ned. 8ᵇ שליח לַחֲרָטַת אשתו a deputy to declare his wife's regret (and procure absolution). Ib. 77ᵇ פותחין בח' the court begins with suggesting reasons for regret; a. e.

חַרְטוֹם m. (b. h. pl. חַרְטֻמִּים; חרט; prob. an adapt. of the Egyptian *her-tum*) *charmer, magician.*—*Pl.* חַרְטוּמִּים. Ex. R. s. 10. Num. R. s. 18 כל חַרְטוּמֵּי העולם all the magicians of the world; a. fr.—Tanḥ. Sh'moth. 11 חַרְטוּמִּין (חַרְטֻמִּין, sub. מעשׂי) *deceptions.*

חַרְטוֹם m. (חטם, with ר inserted)=חוֹטֶם, *nose, beak.* Toh. I, 2. Sifra Aḥăré, Par. 8, ch. XII פרט לח' וכ' except the beak, the nails, feathers &c. [Tam. IV, 3 Ar. (ed. חוטמו) the nostrils.]

חַרְטוּמָא ch. same, esp. (v. חוֹטֶם 4) *the knotted straps of the shoe.* Lam. R. to I, 1 (8 חד מאת) רבתי איפסיק ח' דסנדליה Ar. (ed. חד סנד') the straps of his sandal were broken.

חָרֵי *behind;* חֹרִי *another,* v. חוּ'.

חֲרֵי or **חֹרִי**, v. חֲרָרָה.

חָרִי, חָרָה (b. h.) *to be hot, to glow.* Yalk. Sam. 158 ח' אפו וכ' His anger is enkindled &c., v. אַפִּרְלוּן.

Pi. חִרָה *to ignite, stir.* Midr. Till. to Ps. XVIII, 8 מְחָרֶה אפו He stirs up His anger.

חֲרָא, חֲרֵי ch. same. Targ. Ps. LVII, 5 חָרְיָא Lev. (ed. Lag. חָיְירָא, oth. ed. חָרְיָא fr. חור; Ms. הָיְירָא, v. הוּר ch.; ed. Wil. חדיא, corr. acc.). [Targ. Prov. XVII, 24 חָרְיָן, quot. in Luzz. Philox. p. 106, *glowing* (with wisdom).]—[Gitt. 69ᵃ ולירחרו לכלבא, v. נְחַר.]

Pa. חָרֵי *to stir, rake.* Ab. Zar. 38ᵇ ואתא ישראל וחרי חרורי Ar. (prob. חָרוּרֵי; ed. וחתה בה חתויי) and raked the fire. Hag. 5ᵃ top וּמְחָרְיָא תנורא and raked the fire in the oven (Rashi: out of the oven).

חֲרֵי, חֲרָיָא m. pl. (חרר) *excrements.* Taan. 9ᵇ חריא דעיזי excrements of goats (v. Rabb. D. S. a. l. note 7). Pes. 110ᵃ bot. ח' חמימי וכ' hot excrements in broken baskets (words in an incantation). Gitt. 70ᵃ קורטמי דחרי Ar. (ed. דחחר) carthamus growing in dunged fields.

חֲרָיָא, v. חֲרוּתָא.

חָרֵיב, חָרֵיבָא, v. חָרֵב a. חָרוּב.

חָרֵיד, v. חָרֵד.

חרידן, Targ. Y. Ex. XII, 39 some ed., v. חֲרָרָא.

חֲרָיָה f., pl. **חֲרָיוֹת** (b. h. חָרִי, חֲרִי; חָרָה) *dried branches, twigs used for fuel.* Succ. IV, 6, v. חִיבּוּט. Y. Sabb. III, beg. 5ᶜ שיורי ח׳ remnants of twigs (in the stove); a. fr.

חֶרְיוֹנִים m. pl. (b. h. חרייונים, v. חֲרָיָא) *excrements.* Meg. 25ᵇ ח׳ דביונים ed. (expl. in Ar. a. Rashi Ms. חֲרֵי יוֹנִים excrements of doves?) for *heryonim* they substituted &c., v. דִּבְיוֹנִים.

חֲרָיָינָא, חֲרָיָינוּתָא, v. חֲרָנָ׳.

חֲרֵיךְ, חֲרִיךְ, v. חֲרַךְ.

חֲרִיכָא, v. חֲרוּכָא.

חֲרִינָה=אַחֲרִינָא. Y. Ter. II, 41ᶜ top, v. חוֹרָן.

חִירְ׳, חֲרִינָא m. (חרי) *glow (of face), anger.* Targ. Prov. XXX, 33 (ed. Wil. חִר׳). Ib. XXI, 24 (ed. Wil. חדר׳, corr. acc.). Ib. XXII, 8.

חֲרִינוּתָא f. (preced.) *stirring up, fomenting hatred.* Targ. Prov. X, 24 (h. text מגורה, v. גְּרַר).

חֲרִיסִית, v. חַרְסִית.

חֲרִיעַ m. (Syr. חריע *yellowish*, cmp. b. h. חרוץ *gold;* cmp. חרה) *Bastard safron* (Carthamus tinctorius, cmp. κνῆκος a. κνηκός). Kil. II, 8. Tosef. Maas. Sh. I, 13 (Chald. form) בנת חריעא ed. Zuck. (Var. בנות ח׳) the seeds of &c.; חַלּוֹת דח׳ lozenges made of &c. (v. Löw Pfl. p. 218). Y. Kil. II, 28ᵃ (expl. מוריקא); a. fr.

חֲרִיף. (v. חֲרַף) *to be quick, acute.* Hull. 110ᵇ חֲרִיפַת טובא thou art quick of perception.

חֲרִיף, חֲרִיפָא m., **חֲרִיפָא, חֲרִיפְתָּא** f. (preced.) 1) *quick, sharp; pungent; acute.* Targ. Ps. LII, 4. Targ. Is. VII, 20; a. fr.—Hor. 14ᵃ ח׳ ומקשה is acute and inclined to raise questions. Nidd. 45ᵇ דח׳ טפי that she is very bright (for her age). B. Bath. 111ᵇ, a. e. סכינא ח׳ דמפסקא וכ׳ a sharp knife which cuts verses apart (interpreting without regard to syntax). Hull. 77ᵃ דח׳ סכיניה whose knife is sharp (who reasons well); Yeb. 122ᵃ דחריף סכינא. Meg. 7ᵃ, a. e. (prov.) טבא חדא פילפלתא ח׳ וכ׳ one grain of pepper is worth more than a basketful of pumpkins, i. e. a reasoning mind is worth more than learning. Ned. 31ᵇ top זבינא ח׳ goods which sell quickly, v. מִיצְּצָא; a. fr.—*Pl.* חֲרִיפִין, חֲרִיפֵי. Targ. Josh. V, 2. Targ. Hab. I, 8.—Ber. 59ᵇ האי דח׳ בני וכ׳ the reason that the men of Mahuza are acute. Kidd. 39ᵃ, a. e. ח׳ דפומבדיתא the ingenious students of Pumb'ditha (Efa and Abimi); a. e.—2) *current coin, easily passing.* B. Mets. 44ᵃ sq. כספא דח׳ silver coin which is current, is considered coin, gold being less current is considered a produce.—*Pl.* חֲרִיפֵי. Ib. ח׳ טפי וכ׳ are easier passed than &c.

חֲרִיפָא pr. n. m. (preced.) *Hărifa* (the acute). Targ. Y. Gen. XXV, 15 (h. text חֲדַד).

חֲרִיפוּתָא f. (preced. wds.) 1) *early manhood, energy.* Targ. Job XXIX, 4.—2) *rapid current, water-course* in the river. Keth. 85ᵃ מח׳ דנהרא from the current of the river (not near the shore); Kidd. 73ᵇ חֲרִיפְתָּא.

חֲרִיפְתָּא, v. preced., a. חֲרִיף.

חָרִיץ m. (b. h.; חָרַץ) 1) *incision, furrow, trench.* Kil. V, 3. Ib. II, 8. Meg. 14ᵃ top.—Sabb. 22ᵃ לעשות ח׳ to make a rut in the floor; Y. ib. III, 6ᵃ top; Y. Bets. II, end, 61ᵈ חָרֶץ.—Hull. 55ᵇ top מקום ח׳ (Ar. חרץ) at the indentation in the kidneys. Men. 34ᵇ אם אין חֲרִיצָן ניכר (Ar. חֲרָצָן; Ms. M. חוט, v. Rabb. D. S. a. l. note) if the grooves marking the partitions in the T'fillin are not distinguishable; a. fr.—*Pl.* חֲרִיצִים, חֲרִיצִין. B. Kam. V, 5; a. fr.—2) (from the shape) *eye-lids with eye-lashes.* Bekh. VI, 2 (38ᵃ) ח׳ של עין Ar. (Mish. רִיס, Talm. ed. הריס). Gitt. 56ᵃ בח׳ של עין Ar. (ed. בְּרוֹקְין).—3) *an abnormal depression or cavity in the body.* Bekh. 41ᵃ bot. ח׳ במקום בשר, v. חָרוּץ.

חֲרִיצָא ch. same, *channel.*—*Pl.* חֲרִיצִין, constr. חֲרִיצֵי. Targ. Job XXXVIII, 25. Targ. Josh. XI, 8 ח׳ ימא Kimḥi (ed. חַרְצֵי) channels for the manufacture of salt (h. text משרפות).

חֲרִיצָה f. (preced. wds.) *pressing into a channel;* חֲרִיצַת לשון *putting the tongue between the lips, effort in speaking.* Midr. Till. to Ps. LXII, beg. (cmp. Ex. XI, 7). [Gen. R. s. 70 ואינון בחריצה, some ed., read בַּחֲרֵיצָה.]

חריצותא, Targ. Prov. X, 24 some ed., read: חֲרִינוּתָא. [Targ. I Kings III, 6 ובחריצות, read with best editions: ובְתְרִיצוּת.]

חֲרִיקָא (חָ׳ Ar.) m. (חָרַק) *gap;* בַּחֲרִיק־ *in the gap caused by the absence of, in the place of.* Keth. 61ᵃ עיילית לך איתתא בַּחֲרִיקָאי I brought thee a wife in my place (a hand-maid for domestic labors otherwise resting on the wife). Ib. 105ᵃ הבו לי . . . בחריקאי get me a man to irrigate my fields in my stead. Yoma 77ᵃ (in a passage omitted in later eds.) בַּחֲרִיקֵיה (Ms. M. בַּחֲרִיקִי) in his (my) place. Arakh. 27ᵇ bot. בַּחֲרִיקִין in our stead.

חָרִיר m., (חֲרִירָה f.), v. חוֹר I.

חֲרִיר, חֲרִיר, v. חֲרַר.

חֲרִירָא, pl. **חֲרִירָן**, v. חֲרָרָא.

חֲרִישׁ, v. חֲרַשׁ.

חָרִישׁ m. (b. h.; חָרַשׁ I) *ploughing, ploughing season.* Mekh. Vayakhel (ref. to Ex. XXXIV, 21) שבות מח׳ וכ׳ cease from ploughing &c. R. Hash. 9ᵃ ח׳ של ערב וכ׳ a ploughing at the eve of the Sabbatical year (in the sixth year) which enters into (effects the growth of) the Sabbatical year; a. e.

חֲרִישָׁה I f. same, *ploughing.* Sabb. 70ᵃ. Ex.R. s. 6; Koh. R. to VII, 7, a. e. בַּחֲרִישַׁת הקבר concerning a grave which has been ploughed over; a. fr.—Trnsf. *sexual connection.*—*Pl.* חֲרִישוֹת. Y. Yeb. I beg. 2ᵇ. Gen. R. s. 98.

חֲרִישָׁה II f. 1) (חָרַשׁ II, Hif.) *silence, acquiescence.* Sifré Num. 153 sq. (with ref. to Num. XXX, 5; 8; 12); v. שְׁתִיקָה.—2) (חָרַשׁ II *Pi.*) *making deaf, deafening.* B. Kam. 86ᵃ לפי שא״א לח׳ וכ׳ (Ms. M. לְהַחֲרִישׁ) because it is not possible to cause deafness without afflicting a wound, a drop of blood &c.; ib. 98ᵃ.—3) *deafness,* v. חֲרִישׁוּת.

חֲרִישָׁה III f. (v. חוֹרֶשׁ) *thicket,* only in חֲרִישַׁת קנים *a thicket of reeds.* Gen. R. s. 12, beg.; Koh. R. to II, 12; (Cant. R. to I, 1 חורשא של וכ׳); v. חֲישָׁה.

חֵרִישׁוּת f. (denom. of חֵרֵשׁ) *deafness.* Sifra K'dosh. Par. 4, ch. IX שכן חֵרִישׁוּתוֹ גרמה לו where his deafness may be the reason why we must not curse him; Snh. 66ᵃ חֵרְשׁוּתוֹ.

חֲרִישׁוּתָא ch.=h. חֲרִישָׁה III, *dense ramification.* Targ. Y. Gen. XXII, 13.

חָרִית part. pass. of חֲרַת.

חֲרִיתָא, v. חֲרוּתָא.

חָרַךְ (b. h.; cmp. חָרָה) *to roast, parch.*

Pi. חֵרֵךְ, חִירֵךְ *to char, burn bread* so as to make it uneatable; *to prepare a wick by charring.* Pes. 21ᵇ חֵרְכוֹ קודם וכ׳ he charred the leavened bread before the time appointed for the removal of leavened matter. Y. Sabb. II, 5ᵃ top מְחָרְכִין (לִין לן) they char them (the wicks).—Part. pass. מְחוֹרָךְ, fem. מְחוֹרֶכֶת, pl. מְחוֹרָכוֹת, מְחוֹרָכִין. Tosef. Sabb. II, 1 (v. Var. ed. Zuck.); Sabb. 29ᵃ (v. Tosaf. a. l.).

Hithpa. הִתְחָרֵךְ, *Nithpa.* נִתְחָרֵךְ *to be singed, burnt.* Tanh. Noah 13 כ׳ שער וכ׳ the hair of his head and beard was singed. Pirké d'R. El. ch. XXXIII נִתְחָרְכוּ וכ׳ (not ב) his hair was singed. Y. Sabb. XVI, 15ᶜ הדורשה מִתְחָרֵךְ he who preaches it (the Agadah) will burn himself (at the fire of the Law); (Treat. Sof'rim XVI, 2 מתברך, corr. acc.)

חֲרַךְ, חֲרוֹךְ, חֲרֵיךְ ch. same, 1) (neut. verb) *to be burnt, blackened.* Targ. Job XXX, 30 (h. text חרה). Targ. Jer. VI, 29 חֲרֵיךְ. Targ. Is. IX, 18 חֲרוֹכַת (ed. Lag. חרובת).—2) (act. verb) *to burn, roast.* Pes. 40ᵃ לא לֵיחְרוֹךְ וכ׳ one must not roast two ears &c.—Part. pass. חֲרִיךְ. B. Mets. 85ᵃ; Ber. 46ᵃ, a. e., v. חֲרוּבָא.

Pa. חָרֵיךְ *to burn, singe the hair off.* Kidd. 41ᵃ מְחָרֵיךְ רישא he himself singed the hair off the animal's head (in preparing for the Sabbath). Ab. Zar. 38ᵃ.

Ithpe. אִתְחֲרִיךְ, איח׳ *to be burnt* &c. Targ. Y. Gen. XXI, 15 אתח׳ he was parched (with fever). Targ. Y. Ex. XII, 37.—B. Mets. 85ᵃ אִיחֲרְכוּ שקיה (Ar. חרכו) his legs were burnt. B. Bath. 74ᵃ אִיחֲרֵךְ אִיתְחֲרוּכֵי Ms. M. 2 (ed. ... הוה איח׳, v. Rabb. D. S. a. l. note) it (the wool) was singed. Nidd. 28ᵃ איחרך אִיחֲרוּכֵי Rashi (ed. אִיחרכי, corr. acc.) it (the corpse) was charred (not burnt to ashes).

חֶרֶךְ m. [*burn,* v. preced.] *ḥerekh,* a verbal substitute or *ḥerem* (חֵרֶם), v. כִּינּוּי. Ned. I, 2.—*Pl.* חֲרָכִים, v. חֲרָכַיָּא.

חָרָךְ I m. (b. h. חֲרַכִּים; חרך, cmp. חרק a. חרם) *lattice, latticed window.* Pesik. Haḥod., p. 49ᵇ כשם ... בין חלון לח׳ as there is a difference between (the light as it comes through) an open window and a latticed window, so &c.; Num. R. s. 11; Pesik. R. s. 15; Yalk. Cant. 986 בין חלון לחלון (corr. acc.).—*Pl.* חֲרַכִּים, חֲרַכִּין. Gen. R. s. 98.

***חָרָךְ** II m. (חָרַךְ) *parched grain;* תגרי ח׳ vendors of parched grain who sold also spices &c.; *grocers* (κάπηλοι). Pes. 116ᵃ; [oth. opin. vendors sitting behind *lattices,* v. preced.—Var. חֲרָךְ, v. הוּךְ, *pounded spices*].

חֲרַכָּא ch.=h. חָרָךְ I, 1) *breaking through, breaking in.* Targ. Y. Ex. XXII, 1 (h. text בַּמַּחְתֶּרֶת).—2) *window.* Targ. I Chr. XV, 29; Targ. II Sam. VI, 16 (h. text חלון); a. e.—*Pl.* חֲרַכִּין, חֲרַכַּיָּא. Targ. Y. Gen. VIII, 2. Targ. Cant. II, 9; a. e.

חֲרָכַיָּא m. pl. (חָרַךְ) [*burnings,*] *hărakhaya,* a verbal substitute of חֵרֶךְ, q. v. Ned. 10ᵇ, Rashi (ed. חֲרָכִים) v. חֲרָקַיָּא.

חָרַם (b. h.) [*to perforate, break through* (cmp. Arab. *ḥaram,* a. חָרָךְ I),] 1) *to make a net.* Men. 37ᵃ top ר׳ יוסי החורם R. J. the *net-maker* (or *fisher*); [Rashi, reading הַחָרוּם, (v. Rabb. D. S. a. l., note 100), v. infra].—2) *to perforate. Part. pass.* חָרוּם (b. h. חָרֻם) *one whose nose is so flattened as to show its holes, flat-nosed.* Bekh. VII, 3 איזהו ח׳ הכוחל וכ׳ a *ḥarum* is he who can paint both of his eyes with one movement. Ib. 43ᵇ ח׳ שחוטמו שקוע *ḥ.* is one whose nose is sunk.—3) *to cut off, to set outside* (cmp. Arab. *ḥaram*), v. infra, a. חֵרֶם.—[4) *to burn,* cmp. חָרַב, חָרַךְ; v. חוּרְמָן.]

Hif. הֶחֱרִים (denom. of חֵרֶם) [*to set outside, apart,*] 1) *to dedicate for priestly or sacred use* (Lev. XXVII, 28, sq.); *to renounce private use.* Arakh. VIII, 4 מַחֲרִים אדם וכ׳ a man may renounce a portion of his sheep &c.; ואם ה׳ את כולם אינן מוּחְרָמִין but if he renounces all of them, they are not dedicated (his vow is invalid). Ib. מה אם לגבוה לְהַחֲרִים וכ׳ since man is not permitted to renounce all his property even for a sacred purpose &c. Ib. 7 מח׳ אדם את קדשיו וכ׳ one may declare *ḥerem* one's own designated offerings (in which case he has to pay their value to the priest or the sanctuary); a. v. fr.—Part. pass. מוּחֲרָם, pl. מוּחֲרָמִים, מוּחְרָמִין. Ib. 4, sq., v. supra; a. fr.—2) *to excommunicate, to pronounce the higher ban* (which includes the withdrawal of protection of property). M. Kat. 16ᵃ מנדין . ומַחֲרִימִין וכ׳ the smaller ban is pronounced (over one disregarding a legal summons) at once . . ., the great ban after sixty days.

חֲרַם ch. same, *to perforate. Part. pass.* חָרִים, חֲרִים, *flat-nosed,* v. preced. Targ. O. Lev. XXI, 18.

Pa. חָרֵים, *Af.* אַחֲרִים 1) *to declare* חֵרֶם. Targ. Josh. VI, 18 תַּחְרְמוּן (Var. תַחַר׳, read: תְחַר׳). Targ. I Sam. XV, 21 די חַרְמוּן (ed. Lag. a. oth. דיחַרְמוּן).—Targ. O. Lev. XXVII, 28.—Arakh. 28ᵃ כל דאית ליה לא לַחֲרִים . . . לֵיחַרְמֵיה כוליה one must not renounce (for sacred purposes) all his property, but of one kind he may renounce all he has.—2) *to excommunicate.* M. Kat. 16ᵃ מנלן דמַחְרְמִינַן (or דמַחַרְמִי׳) whence is it proven that we (the court) have a right to excommunicate a recreant person?—Y. ib. III, 81ᵈ top אילולא דלא חַרְמִית . . . מְחָרֵם וכ׳ were it not that I never in my life excommunicated a person, I should have excommunicated that man; a. e.—Part. pass. מְחָרַם, pl. מְחָרְמִין. Ib. bot. ייא החוא גברא מ׳ this man (thou) be excommunicated. Ib. לירהון ההיא עמא מח׳ those people (you) be excommunicated.

Ithpe. אִיתְחָרַם *to be declared* חֵרֶם, *to be dedicated.* Targ. O. Lev. XXVII, 29 דיתְּחַ׳ ed. Berl. (oth. דיתָּחַ׳).

חֵרֶם m. (b. h.; preced.) 1) *net.* Kel. XXIII, 5; XXVIII, 9, v. זֶוֶג; a. fr.—Ned. II, 5, v. infra.—2) *a place adapted for catching fish in nets, fishing coast, fishery.* B. Kam. 81ᵇ מלא חבל ח׳ בדרומה a rope's length (district) of fishing coast south of it (the Lake of Tiberias); Tosef. ib. VIII, 18 Var. ed. Zuck.—Erub. 47ᵇ ח׳ שבין וכ׳ a fishpond between two territories.—3) [*cut off, excluded,* cmp. הֶפְקֵר, חוּלִּין,] *herem, property set apart for priest's or Temple use; doomed to destruction.* Ned. II, 4 אם כח׳ של שמים if (he said, This shall be to me) like the *herem* consecrated to the Temple, opp. ח׳ של כהנים assigned to the private use of priests. Ib. 5 נדר בח׳ . . כְּחֶרְמוֹ של ים if he made a vow of abstinence using the word *herem,* and he says, I meant the *herem* of the sea (fisher's net). Ib. I, 2 כינויין לח׳ verbal substitutes for *herem* (effecting prohibition); a. fr.—4) *excommunication.* M. Kat. 17ᵃ.—*Pl.* חֲרָמִין, חֲרָמִים. Snh. 43ᵇ מעל עכן בג׳ ח׳ Akhan committed three sacrileges. Ned. II, 4 סתם ח׳ vows containing the expression *herem* unqualified. Ib. חֶרְמֵי הכהנים the dedications as priestly property. Arakh. VIII, 6 סתם ח׳ לבדק הבית unqualified dedications (this be *herem*) go to the repair of the Temple; a. fr.—[Y. Kil. IX, 32ᵃ top שצבעה בחרם, read: בְּחֶרֶת.]—V. חֵירוּם.

חָרָם m. (preced.) 1) *fisherman.*—*Pl.* חָרָמִים, חָרָמִין, constr. חָרָמֵי. Y. M. Kat. II, end, 81ᵇ; Y. Pes. IV, 30ᵈ top ח׳ טבריה the net-fishers of Tiberias.—2) *confiscator, official oppressor,* v. הָרָג.—Tosef. Ab. Zar. VII (VIII), 6; Ab. Zar. 58ᵃ. Tosef. B. Mets. III, 19; Y. ib. IV, end, 9ᵈ a defective coin must not be given לתגר . . . ולא לח׳ וכ׳ to a travelling merchant, to a highwayman, or to an oppressor, because they will cheat &c.—*Pl.* as ab. Ned. III, 4; B. Kam. 113ᵃ, v. נָדַר.

חַרְמָא m. ch. = h. חֵרֶם, 1) *net.* Targ. Hab. I, 15.—2) = חֵרֶם 3). Targ. O. Lev. XXVII, 21 (ed. Berl. וּזִרְמָא).—Targ. Josh. VI, 17, sq. (ed. Lag. חיר׳; some ed. חָרָ׳); a. fr.

חָרְמָא, חָרְמָה pr. n. pl. (b. h.) *Hormah* (*Destruction,* v. preced.). Targ. Num. XXI, 3 (ed. Berl. חוּרְמָה). Targ. O. ib. XIV, 45 (ed. Berl. חור׳; Y. שֵׁצִיו).

חרמיני, v. הַרְמִינֵי.

חָרְנָה, חָרָן, v. חוּרָ׳.

חַרְנוּגָא m. (cmp. חַנָּג, a. הִירְגֵּי) *thistle.* Sabb. 110ᵇ ח׳ דחירגא וכ׳ (Ar. חַרְנ׳; Ms. M. הרגנא), v. הִיגְתָא.—V. חַרְנוּגָא.

חַרְנְפָּא, v. חוּר׳.

חֶרֶס I m. (b. h. חֶרֶשׂ; חרס *to be rough; to scrape*) 1) *common earthware.* כלי ח׳ earthen vessel. Kel. III, 1 (ed. Dehr. חרש); a. v. fr.—Ib. 4 חיה בה ח׳ if there remained of it a (sound) piece large enough to contain &c.—Tanh. Sh'lah. 1 (ref. to חֶרֶשׂ, Josh. II, 1) קרי ביה ח׳ read it *heres* (**with earthware**, in the disguise of potters); Num. R. s. 16, beg. חרש; a. fr.—Esp. (v. חַסְפָּא) *potsherd.* Y. Ned. I, 37ᵃ top; Y. Naz. I, beg. 51ᵃ והתני . . . . לא חספא did not Bar K. say, *heres* is a substitute for *herem* (חֵרֶם)? now, does not this mean *a sherd* (which has no reference to anything forbidden either as sacred or as doomed to destruction)?; v. next w.—*Pl.* חֲרָסִים, חֲרָסִין. Kel. III, 4. Ib. IX, 5 (Ar. חֲרָשִׁין); a. e.—Hag. 13ᵇ (expl. בזק, Ez. I, 14) כאור . . מבין החח׳ like the flames from between the perforated earthen pieces (used in smelting gold).

חֶרֶס II m. (b. h.; חרס *to glow;* cmp. חַרָה) *the sun.* Men. 110ᵃ (ref. to Is. XIX, 18) מאי עיר החח׳ (late eds. הח׳, v. Rabb. D. S. a. l. note) what is *Ir ha-Heres?* קרתא דבית שמשא the city of Beth-Shemesh; מאי משמע דהאי ח׳ לישנא וכ׳ where is the evidence that *heres* means sun? (Answ. ref. to Job IX, 7). Y. Ned. I, 37ᵃ top; Y. Naz. I, beg. 51ᵃ ח׳ לשון גבוה הוא *heres* (as a substitute for חֵרֶם, v. preced.) has reference to Deity, (as we read) 'who speaks to the sun' (Job l. c.).

חֶרֶס III (b. h.; cmp. preced. a. שְׁחִין) *an eruption of the skin.* Bekh. 41ᵃ גרב זה החח׳ *garab* (v. גָּרָב) is the same as *heres.*

חֲרַס (חֲרֶס) ch. same. Targ. O. Deut. XXVIII, 27 (Y. quot. in Ar. חַרְסוּנָא, v. חִיכּוּכָא).

חַרְסוּם pr. n. m. *Harsum.*—Yoma 9ᵃ; Y. ib. III, 40ᵈ אלעזר בן ח׳ (or אליעזר) El b. H. a highpriest; Tosef. ib. I, 22 חרסות ed. Zuck. (Var. . . סום).—Yoma 35ᵇ R. El b. H. a rich scholar; Lam. R. to II, 2 (some ed. חַרְסָנָה) Treat. S'mahoth ch. IX בימי ח׳ (prob. to be read: בן ח׳) in the days (of persecution) of &c.

חַרְסוּן pr. n. m. *Harsun.* Koh. R. to IV, 8 גבינִי בן ח׳ G. b. H., a rich heir (cmp. preced.).

חַרְסוּנָא, v. חֲרַס.

חרסות, v. חַרְסוּם.

חַרְסִית I (b. h.) pr. n., שער החח׳ *Gate of Harsith,* one of the Jerusalem gates. Y. Erub. V, 22ᶜ (the Eastern gate) was called שער חריסית שהוא מכוון וכ׳ (corr. acc.) Gate of H., because it was facing the East; v. חֶרֶס II.

חַרְסִית II f. (חֶרֶס I) *potter's clay, clay-ground.* Maas. Sh. V, 1 בח׳ must be marked off with burned clay. Hull VI, 7 בח׳; ib. 88ᵃ שחיקת ח׳ powdered burned clay. Kel. III, 7; a. fr.—[Tosef. Ter. IX, 3 חרסיות, v. חָסִית I.]

חַרְסָן m. (preced.) *earthen vessel, bed-chamber.* Tosef. Ter. X, 13; Tosef. Toh. V, 3; Y. Ter. XI, 48ᵃ הרריסן (corr. acc.). [Ar. ed. Koh., s. v. חרסנא, reads חַרְסָן.]

חַרְסָנָה, v. חַרְסוּם.

חרספותייא, v. next w.

חַרְסְפִּיתִין m. pl. (חַסָּה with ר inserted, v. חַסְפְּנִיתָא) *scales.* Targ. Y. Lev. XI, 9, sq. Targ. Y. Deut. XIV, 9 sq.— Pesik. R. s. 14 דמיין לְחַרְסְפּוּתְיָיא דנונר, v. חַסְפְּנִיתָא; Pesik. Par., p. 35ᵃ להחרפותא דיונה (corr. acc.).

חֵרֶף m. (next w.) [*shame,*] *ḥeref,* a phonetic substitute for חֵרֶם. Ned. I, 2.—*Pl.* חֲרָפִים, v. חֲרָפַיָּא.

חָרַף (b. h.) 1) *to scrape, sharpen, grind.*—Part. pass. חָרוּף, f. חֲרוּפָה, pl. חֲרוּפוֹת. Pesik. R. s. 21 פנים ח׳ sharp (severe) countenance (Var. הדופות).—Trnsf. *to deflour,* v. infra.—2) (cmp. חלף) *to change, transform; to change possession. Part. pass.* f. חֲרוּפָה *designated for change of condition,* v. חֲרוּפָה.

Nif. נֶחֱרַף 1) (of grist) *to be ground;* trnsf. *to be defloured, have intercourse.* Y. Kidd. I, 59ᵃ top (expl. Lev. XIX, 20) נֶחֱרֶפֶת .... בכתושה לפני איש ‘*neḥĕrefeth* by a man’ means crushed before a man (with ref. to Prov. XXVII, 22, v. חֲרִיפוֹת).—2) *to change condition.* Kerith. 11ᵃ (ref. to נחרפת explained by בְּעוּלָה) .... דשנויי מאי משמע הוא (Rashi: דשינויא) what proof is there that *neḥĕrefeth* has the meaning of change from natural condition? Answ. ref. to הָרִיפוֹת (II Sam. XVII, 19) and to Prov. l. c.

Pi. חֵירֵף, חֵרֵף (cmp. גָּדַף, גֵּדֵּף) [*to scrape off,*] *to revile, blaspheme, shame.* Lev. R. s. 7, end מְחָרֶפֶת ומגדפת she (Rome) blasphemes and reviles. Num. R. s. 10 מְחָרְפִם, v. גָּדַף. Snh. 94ᵃ, sq. שחר׳ ע״י וכ׳ who blasphemed (the Lord) through a messenger; a. fr.

Hithpa. הִתְחָרֵף, *Nithpa.* נִתְחָרֵף 1) *to be reviled.* Midr. Till. to Ps. LXXIV, end שמִּתְחָרֵף ומתנאץ which is reviled and blasphemed. Ib. to Ps. XVIII, 1 עד שנִתְחָרַפְתִּי until I was reviled; a. e.—2) *to become white, pale.* Tanḥ. B’resh. 12 (play on קרץ וחרף) שתהיו מתקייצין ופניכם מִתְחָרְפִין (some ed. מתחפרין) that you will feel nauseous and your faces become pale.

חֲרַף ch. same; *Pa.* חָרֵף 1) *to sharpen, grind.* Targ. I Sam. XIII, 20, sq. Targ. Job XVI, 9 (not חָרִיף; h. text ילטש).—Part. pass. מְחָרַף. Targ. Jer. IX, 7 ed. Lag. (oth. ed. מְחָרֵיף, corr. acc.). Targ. Is. V, 28.—2) *to blaspheme, revile.* Targ. Y. Lev. XXIV, 11. ; a. fr.—[Ib. 15, sq. יְחָרֵף *Pe.!*]

Af. אַחְרֵיף *to be quick, be early.* Snh. 70ᵇ אַחְרִיפוּ ועולו וכ׳ go in early (before sunset), and leave early, that people may take notice of you. Sabb. 115ᵃ דהוו קא מַחְרְפֵי that they did it earlier (than they were told to).

חֹרֶף, v. חוֹרֶף.

חַרְפָּא or **חֲרָפָא** m. (v. חֲרַף *Af.*) *early.* B. Bath. 90ᵇ הרעא ח׳ וכ׳ the early market (soon after the crop) at the early market price, opp. הרעא אפלא later market.—*Pl.* חֲרָפֵי. Targ. Koh. XI, 2 early seeds.—Taan. 3ᵇ בח׳ concerning early clouds (when rain is gathering). Nidd. 65ᵇ, v. אֲפִילָא.—*Fem. pl.* חֲרָפָתָא. R. Hash. 8ᵃ Ar. (ed. חֲרִפְיָיתָא), v. אֲפִילָא.

חֶרְפָּה f. (b. h.; חָרַף) [*paleness,*] *shame; revilement.* Gen. R. s. 80. Sabb. 88ᵇ, a. e. שומעין חֶרְפָּתָן וכ׳ hear themselves reviled and answer not.

חַרְפּוּפְתָּא, חַרְפּוּפִיתָא f. (חָרַף) *scab,* v. חִירְפּוּפִיתָא.

חֲרָפַיָּיא m. pl. (v. חֵרֶף) *ḥărafaya,* a phonetic substitute of חֵרֶף in place of חֵרֶם. Ned. 10ᵇ, v. חֲרָקַיָּיא.

חֲרָפִיתָא f. *early conceiving, vigorous sheep. Pl.* חֲרָפְיָיתָא, v. חֲרָפָא; cmp. חוּרְפָא.

חַרְפְּתָא ch.=h. חֶרְפָּה. Targ. Ps. XXII, 7 חֶרְפַּת Ms. (ed. חִיסוּדֵי).

חֲרַפְפָּא f. *bat.* Targ. Y. II Deut. XIV, 18 (Y. I ערפדא).

חָרַץ (b. h.) 1) *to dig a cavity, to cut a trench* of even width all through. Y. Kil. VII, 31ᵇ bot. חפר ח׳ נעץ וכ׳ if (on the Sabbath) one dug (a pit), made a trench, and cut a wedge-like ditch (narrow below), he is guilty of one act; Y. Sabb. VII, 9ᵈ bot.; a. fr.—2) *to decree, designate.* Tanḥ. B’huck. 1 (ref. to Job XIV, 5) ח׳ ימיו וכ׳. He designated the duration of life of every creature.—*Part. pass.* חָרוּץ, f. חֲרוּצָה; pl. חֲרוּצִים, חֲרוּצוֹת a) *grooved.* Sabb. 98ᵇ ח׳ היו הקרשים וכ׳ the boards of the Tabernacle were grooved, and the sockets hollowed out correspondingly.—b) *decreed, decided; determined.* Gen. R. s. 67 (ref. to Prov. XII, 27) the blessings שמעיקר העולם חרוצות לו which were designated to him from primeval days. Ib. חרוצה ביד וכ׳ it is a decided fact known to the righteous that they will in this world receive none &c. Deut. R. s. 1 שידיך חדות וח׳ that thy hands are quick and determined.—c) *flat-nosed,* v. חָרוּץ.

Nif. נֶחֱרַץ *to be cut into, dug, ploughed.* Y. Nidd. I, 49ᵃ bot. a soil is called virgin כל שלא נ׳ בה מימיה when it has never been cut into; v. חֶרֶץ.

חֲרַץ ch. same, *to cut into.* Part. pass. חָרִיץ. Gitt. 20ᵃ רושמא מִיחֲרַץ ח׳ וכ׳ is the stamp of a coin dug into (are the devices formed with a loss of substance), or is it pressed into (by compressing the substance)?—Bekh. 41ᵃ מיחרץ ח׳ (a dry scab is) cut into (deeper than the surface).

Ithpe. אִיתְחֲרַץ *to be cut into,* v. supra.

חֶרֶץ m. (preced.) *incision, groove, mark of a seam.* Y. Nidd. I, 49ᵃ bot. כל שאין בה ח׳ (a virgin soil is) such as shows no grooves. Y. Maasr. I, 48ᵈ bot. משיתמלא החי׳ from the time the incision in the growing fruits begins to fill up.—Y. Bets. II, end, 61ᵈ, a. e., v. חָרִיץ.

חֶרֶץ m. ch. *loin,* v. חַרְצָא II.

חַרְצָא I m. (חָרַץ) *digging, a digger.* B. Kam. 80ᵃ (marginal version) שרצא ח׳ וא״ח ח׳ a digging animal, and some use only the word *ḥartsa:* digger; v. חַרְזָא.

חַרְצָא II m. (חָרַץ) 1) *groove, channel,* v. חָרִיצָא.—2) (cmp. כֶּסֶל) [*incision,*] *loins.* Targ. Deut. XXXIII, 11 (Y. II חֶרֶץ).—Targ. Gen. XXXVII, 34 (Y. חַרְצוֹי *pl.*); a. fr.—*Pl.* חַרְצִין, constr. חַרְצֵי. Targ. O. Ex. XXVIII, 42 (some ed. חַרְצָן *their* loins); Y. ib. אתר קטור חַרְצֵיהוֹן

חַרְצֵיהוֹן the place of the knot of their loins (belt). Targ. Y. Gen. L. 11; a. fr.

חַרְצִינִיתָא, חרצינתא, v. חַרְצָנִיתָא.

חַרְצָן m., pl. חַרְצַנִּים (b. h.) *a pomace of kernels or shells of grapes;* v. זָג. Naz. VI, 2. Ib. 35ª; a. fr.—Ib. 38ᵇ אכל חרצן if he ate the shell (or the interior) of one berry. Ḥull. 82ᵇ זרע חטה וח׳ if he sowed a wheat grain and a kernel; a. fr.—V. גּוּחַרְקָא II.

חַרְצָנָה f. (preced.; collect. noun) *kernels.* Y. Maasr. I, 48ᵈ שתהא ח׳ שלהן וכ׳ their kernels must be seen through the berries.

חַרְצָנִיתָא, חַרְצַנְתָּא ch. same, *stones of a fruit.* Tanḥ. Vaëra 14 כהדא פרטתא דרמונא דח׳ מתחמיא מלגאו like the berry of a pome-granate whose stones are seen from within (shining through); Pesik. Vayhi, p. 3ᵇ דחרצנריתא (read: דְחַרְצִינִיתָא); Ex. R. s. 12 דְחַרְצִינִיתֵיה; Num. R. s. 12 דחרצינתה (corr. acc.); Cant. R. to III, 11 דכל הדא פיטרתא (read: . . . חרצנתא); Yalk. Ex. 186 דחרצנתי (read: . . . תֵיה); Yalk. Job 912 (corr. acc.).

חֵרֵק m. (next w.) [*cleft,*] *ḥerek*, a phonetic substitute for *ḥerem* (חֵרֶם). Ned. I, 2.—*Pl.* חֲרָקִים, v. חֲרָקַיָּיא.

חָרַק (b. h.) *to cut a gap; to squeeze into a gap; to prick. Part. pass.* חָרוּק, f. חֲרוּקָה; pl. חֲרוּקִים, חֲרוּקוֹת a) *having incisions, edged, serried.* Ḥull. 59ᵇ ed., v. חָרַק.—b) *wedged in.* Par. XII, 8 החרוקות (Var. הַחֲדוּקוֹת) those handles which are squeezed into holes, opp. הקדוחות bored handles; Tosef. ib. XII (XI), 17 אֶת הרוק וצואה וכ׳ (read: אֶת החרוקות · צואה וכ׳).

Pi. חֵרֵק [*to set at edge,*] (with שֵׁן) *to gnash, grind the teeth.* Pesik. R. s. 37 מְחָרְקִין שיניהם ground their teeth (in sneer). Ex. R. s. 5; Tanḥ. Vaëra 6 התחיל מְחָרֵק עליהם וכ׳ he began to gnash his teeth against them (in rage).

חֲרַק ch. same. Sabb. 67ª לִיחֲרוֹק ביה פורתא let him cut a little notch into it. Part. חָרֵיק. Y. Kil. IX, 32ᶜ bot. וח׳ בשינוי and gnashing his teeth; Y. Keth. XII, 35ᵇ וחרוק (corr. acc.),

Ithpe. אִיחֲרוֹק, אִתְח׳ same. Y. Kil. l. c. הויתא א׳ בשיניך thou wast gnashing thy teeth; Y. Keth. l. c. הוות א׳ בשינוי (corr. acc.).

חִרְקָא, חִירְ׳ m. (preced.) *edge, notch. Pl.* חִרְקֵי, חִירְ׳. Ḥull. 59ᵇ והוא דמיבלע חִירְקֵיהוּ provided the edges of their horns run irregularly into one another. Sabb. 46ª דאית בה חרקי Ar. it has indentations (making the candlestick appear as if composed of movable parts), v. חִדְקָא.

חֲרָקַיָּיא m. pl. (preced.) [*incisions,*] *ḥărakaya*, a Chaldaic substitute of חֵרֵק which is itself a substitute of חֵרֶם. Ned. 10ᵇ what are the substitutes of *ḥerem?* ח׳ חרכייא חרפייא Rashi (Ar. חר׳; ed. חֲרָקִים &c., h. pl. of חֵרֵק &c.).

חָרַר I, *Pi.* חֵרֵר (v. חור I) *to break through, to cave.* Ohol. III, 7; Succ. 20ᵇ חור שֶׁחֲרָרוּהוּ מים (or שֶׁחָרְרוּהוּ) a cavity made by water, by animals &c.

חֲרַר ch. same, *to perforate.—Part. pass.* חֲרִיר *discharging* (v. חַרְיָא). Targ. Y. Lev. XV, 3 ח׳ . . . ית וכ׳ (some ed. חָרֵיר part. act.) his membrum discharges &c.

חָרַר II, *Pi.* חֵרֵר (denom. of חור II) *to set free.—Part. pass.* מְחוֹרָר *freed, free.* Gen. R. s. 14, end (ref. to Gen. II, 7 עבד מח׳ בפני עצמו וכ׳ (נפש חיה (Var. מכודן, v. כָּדַן) a freed slave left to himself for a living.—Keth. 51ᵇ; B. Kam. 95ª (נכסים) הַמְחוֹרָרִין unencumbered property. [Shaf. שַׁחְרֵר.]

חֲרַר ch. same, *to set free.* Targ. Y. Gen. XVI, 2 אֲחָרְרִינָהּ I will liberate her. Ib. 3 חַרְרָתָהּ (not . . . תא). Ib. 5.

Ithpa. אִתְחַרַר, אִיתְחַר *to be set free.* Targ. Lev. XIX, 20.

חָרַר III (b. h.; cmp. גרר) [*to be rough, excited,*] *to glow. Pilp.* חַרְחֵר, q. v.

חֲרַר ch. same, *to burn, to be blackened, charred.* Targ. Ps. II, 12 יֵיחוֹר. Ib. CII, 4. Targ. Ez. XV, 4, sq. חַר; a. e.

[*Pa.* חָרֵיר *to stir the fire.* Ab. Zar. 38ᵇ חרורי, v. חֲרֵי.]
Ithpa. אִתְחַר *to be heated, dried up.* Targ. II Esth. V, 1.
Ithpalp. אִתְחַרְחַר same. Targ. Ps. LXIX, 4.

חָרַר IV (cmp. חרר I) *to heap up, round.* Denom. חוֹרָר, חֲרָרָה.

חֲרַר same.—*Pa.* חָרֵיר *to round, make a* חֲרָרָא. Targ. Ez. IV, 12 (some ed. תַּחַר׳ *Af.*; h. text תעגינה).

חֵרֵר *freedom*, v. חֵירֵר.

חָרָר m. 1) *needle-eye*, v. חור I.—2) *pile*, v. חוֹרָר.—*Pl.* חֲרָרִין, v. חֲרָרָה.

חֲרָרָא, חֲרָר c. = next w., 1) *a cake.* Targ. Jud. VII, 13 (h. text צליל). Targ. I Kings XVII, 13 (h. text עגה); a. fr.—Pesik. R. s. 18 [read:] תמן אמרין עבדין מיניה ח׳ לכלבא ולא טעמיה there (in Babylonia) they say, they made out of it a cake for a dog, but he would not taste it (v. Erub. 81ª); Pesik. Haomer, p. 71ᵇ חֲרָרָה.—*Pl.* חֲרָרָן. Targ. Y. I Num. XI, 8. Targ. Y. Ex. XII, 39 (some ed. חֲרִירָן; חרידן, corr. acc.).—2) *clot.* Lev. R. s. 24 ח׳ דדמא (ed. חרדא, חרדה, corr. acc.) a clot of blood.

חֲרָרָה f. (חרר IV) [*rounded heap,*] 1) *a thick cake baked on coals.* Kidd. 59ª, v. הָפַךְ (v. also Rashi a. l. a. infra). Sabb. I, 10. Tosef. Ḥag. III, 12; Y. ib. III, 79ᵇ, v. חָתַב. B. Kam. II, 3 שנטל ח׳ that took a cake (with live coals sticking to it).—*Pl.* חֲרָרִין. Bets. II, 6 (21ᵇ) גריצין וח׳ Bab. ed., v. גְּרִיצָה (Mish. ed. חוֹרִי,-Y. ed. חֹרִי b. h., collect. noun: *cakes*); Y. ib. 61ᶜ bot. (play on חֲרֵי, Deut. XXIX, 23, a. on חֹרִי, Gen. XL, 16).—2) *pile of sheaves, temporary stack* in the field. Peah V, 8 לח׳ for the purpose of temporary piling, opp. לגוֹרֶן. [Kidd. 59ª

עני המהפך בח׳ a poor man moving about a stack (waiting for its removal to take up eventually a forgotten sheaf); cmp. Peah l. c.; oth. defin. v. חָפַךְ.]—Y. Peah V, end, 19ª, expl. ח׳ with גַּלְגַּל a globular heap.—3) חֲרָרַת דם *a clot of blood.* Bekh. III, 1 (21ᵇ). Nidd. 66ª; a. e.—Tanh. K'dosh. 9 כחרדת (corr. acc.)—4) *a ball of iron ore.* Kel. XI, 3 he who makes vessels מן הח׳ of iron ore (before it is smelted).

חָרֶשׁ, v. חֶרֶס.

חָרַשׁ I (b. h.) 1) *to engrave, draw, design.* Koh. R. to I, 16 הלב חוֹרֵשׁ the heart designs.—2) *to plough.* Macc. III, 9 יש חוֹרֵשׁ תלם וכ׳ one may plough one bed and &c. Taan. 29ª וח׳ את העיר Ms. M. and passed the plough over the city of Jerusalem. Sabb. VII, 2; a. fr.—Trnsf. *to have sexual intercourse.* Y. Yeb. I, 2ᵇ top. Gen. R. s. 98; a. e.

Nif. נֶחְרַשׁ *to be ploughed over.* Taan. IV, 6 נֶחְרְשָׁה העיר the plough was passed over the city of Jerusalem; a. e.

חָרַשׁ II, *Pi.* חֵרֵשׁ, חֵר׳ (denom. of חֵרֵשׁ) *to deafen, make deaf.* B. Kam. 86ª שֶׁחֵרְשׁוֹ וכ׳ when he made him deaf without wounding him. Ib. החוֹרֵשׁ את אביו (Ms. H. a. R. חֵרֵשׁ); ib. 98ª חֵרְשׁוֹ לאביו if one injured his father's hearing; v. חֵרִישָׁה II. Kidd. 24ᵇ.—Sabb. 109ª top. יד מְחָרֶשֶׁת the unwashed hand put to the ear causes deafness.

Hif. הֶחֱרִישׁ 1) same. B. Kam. 86ª לְהַחֲרִישׁ, v. חֲרִישָׁה II.—2) (b. h.) *to be silent.* Y. Pes. IX, end. 37ª (ref. to Prov. XVII, 28) ואין צ״ל חכם מַחֲרִישׁ and it is needless to say the same of a wise man keeping silence. [Usu. שָׁתַק.]

Nithpa. נִתְחָרֵשׁ *to become deaf (and dumb).* Yeb. XIV, 1; Tosef Ter. I, 1 פיקח וכ׳ if he had been well-hearing and became etc.; v. חֵרֵשׁ.

חֲרַשׁ ch. (v. preced. wds.) 1) *to be entangled.* Targ. Job VIII, 17.—2) *to be choked, obstructed, deaf.* Gen. R. s. 81 (prov.) כּהולתך חַרְשָׁה וכ׳ if thy sieve is choked, knock at it (when you are forgetful of your duties, the Lord will remind you through affliction); v. כְּרַשׁ II.—3) *to practice witchcraft.* Ib. s. 86 באתר דחרשין חָרְשִׁין where there are sorcerers witchcraft is practiced.

Pa. חָרֵשׁ *to entangle, inure.* Targ. Ez. XIII, 20 (h. text צדד).

Ithpa. אִתְחָרֵשׁ *to be entangled, confounded.* Y. Hag. II, 77ᶜ top (expl. תאלמנה, Ps. XXXI, 19) יִתְחָרְשָׁן וכ׳ may their lips be confounded, crushed, silenced, cmp. אָלַם a. חָרֵשׁ; Gen. R. s. 1 (corr. acc.)

חָרָשׁ m. (b. h.; חָרַשׁ I) *artist, artisan, carpenter, turner* (faber). Deut. R. s. 2 לח׳ שהיה וכ׳ like an artist that was making an image &c.—*Pl.* חָרָשִׁים. Gen. R. s. 65, end; s. 70, v. חֲמוֹר; Pesik. Shek., p. 15ª.—Trnsf. *scholar.* Gitt. 88ª (ref. to II Kings XXIV, 16) ח׳ שבשעה....כַּחֲרָשִׁין the scholars were named *harash*, for when they opened argument, all were like dumb; Snh. 38ª; Yalk. Dan. 1066; a. e—*Pl.* as above. Hag. 14ª (ref. to Is. III, 3).

חָרָשׁ m. ch. *sorcerer,* v. חָרָשָׁא.

חֶרֶשׁ m. (b. h.; v. חֵרֵשׁ) *silence.* Tanh. Sh'mini 9 (play on חָרָשׁ, II Kings XXIV, 16) אלו...תפלת ח׳ בלחש וכ׳ *harash* means those who hold silent prayers in murmuring, and yet conquer &c.

חֶרֶשׁ or **חֶרֶשׁ** pr. n. m. *Heres* or *Heresh.* Ab. IV, 15. Yoma 4ᵇ; a. e.

חֵרֵשׁ m. (b. h.; cmp. חָרַשׁ) [*closed up,*] *deaf, dumb* (cmp. אִלֵּם); *deaf and dumb.* Ter. I, 2 ח׳ שדברו וכ׳ the *heresh* of which the scholars speak (in a legal sense) means everywhere *deaf and dumb.* Ib. ח׳ המדבר וכ׳ a *heresh* that can talk but not hear. Meg. II, 4 חוץ מח׳ except a deaf person. Sifré Num. 153 (ref. to Num. XXX, 5; 12) להוציא את הח׳ this excludes the case of the father (the husband) being deaf; Ned. 73ª; a. fr.—*Pl.* חֵרְשִׁין, חֵרְשִׁים. Hag. 14ª; Gitt. 88ª, v. חָרָשׁ. Ruth R. s. 2 beg. (ref. to חרש, Josh. II, 1) עשו עצמכם ח׳ pretend to be deaf.—*Fem.* חֵרֶשֶׁת. Gitt. V, 5. Yeb. XIV, 1; a. e.—*Pl.* חֵרְשׁוֹת. Ib. 3.

חֵרְשָׁא, חֵירְשָׁא ch. same. Targ. Ex. IV, 11; a. fr.—*Pl.* חֵרְשַׁיָּא, חֵרְשִׁין. Targ. Is. LVI, 10; a. e.—Y. Ber. IX, end, 14ᵈ כל חרשייא טבין וכ׳ Var. (v. כַּבָּבָא) all dumb (silent) persons are good, but those silent (abstaining) from reciting the Law are bad.

חָרָשׁ, חָרָשָׁא m. (v. חָרַשׁ; cmp. לָחַשׁ) *fascinator, charmer, sorcerer.* Targ. O. Deut XVIII, 10 (some ed. חָרָשׁ); a.e.—Cant. R. to III, 6. Y. Hag. II, 77ᵈ bot. עיסקיה דהדין ח׳ וכ׳ it is the nature of a sorcerer that he can do nothing when lifted from the ground. Ber. 62ª bot. (in an incantation) לא חָרְשֵׁי דח׳ וכ׳ (Var. דחָרָשֵׁי ... pl., v. Rabb. D. S. a. l, note 8) no charm of a sorcerer or of a sorceress.—*Pl.* חָרָשִׁין, חָרָשַׁיָּא, חָרָשֵׁי, חָר׳. Targ. Y. Deut. l. c. (ed. Amst. חָרָשִׁין). Targ. Ps. LVIII, 6; a. e.—Y. Hag. l. c.; Y. Snh. VI, 23ᶜ bot.—*Fem.* חָרְשָׁא, חָרְשְׁתָא,. Targ. O. Ex. XXII, 17.—Ber. l. c. (Var. חַרְשִׁיתָא).—V. חַרְשִׁין.

חַרְשֵׁי (preced.) *sorcery,* v. חַרְשִׁין.

חָרְשִׁיתָא f. same. Targ: Y. Ex. XXII, 17; a. e.—V. חָרוּשְׁתָא.

חַרְשִׁין, חַרְשַׁיָּא, חַרְשֵׁי, חַר׳, m. pl. *sorcery, witchcraft.* Targ. Koh. XI, 4 (ed. Amst. חַר׳); a. fr.—Sabb. 75ª, v. אַמְגּוּשָׁתָא. Ber. 62ª bot., v. חָרָשָׁא. Cant. R. to III, 6 לית ח׳ מצלחין וכ׳ (not חרשין) witchcraft has no effect by night. Gen. R. s. 86 ח׳ במצרים sorcery imported to Egypt!. v. חֲרַשׁ 3.—Hull. 84ᵇ; B. Mets. 29ᵇ כסא דח׳ וכ׳ rather drink a cupfull of witchcraft (charmed drink) than of tepid water. Pes. 110ª, v. next w.

חַרְשִׁיתָא f. (preced.) *sorceress.* Ber. 62ª, v. חָרָשָׁא.—*Pl.* חַרְשִׁיָתָא, חַרְשָׁיָין. Y. Hag. II, 77ᵈ bot. נשיין ח׳ women practicing witchcraft. Pes. 110ª נשי ח׳ Rashi (ed. נשי דחרשייא, Ms. M. דחרושתא), v. חָרוּשְׁתָא.

חַרְשְׁתָּא, v. חָרָשָׁא.

חָרַת (b.h.; cmp. חָרַשׁ) *to engrave.* Part. pass. חָרוּת, v. חֵירוּת.

חֲרַת, ch. same. Part. pass. חָרִית, pl. חֲרִיתִין. Targ. O. Lev. XIX, 28 (ed. Berl. חֲתִיתִ׳). Targ. Jer. XVII, 1.

חֶרֶת f. (חרר III) *soot, sediment of ink, shoe-black.* Nidd. II, 7 כַּח׳; ib. 19ª כְּחָרוּת; Tosef. ib. III, 11 (not בח׳); expl. Nidd. 20ª כי חרותא דריותא, v. דְּיוּתָא.—Y. Sot. VII, 22ᵈ חֲרוּתָהּ אש וכ׳ its ink was black fire. Y. Kil. IX, 32ª top פשתן שצבעו בח׳ (ed. בחרם, corr. acc.) linen dyed with blacking (looking like wool).

חַרְתָּא I ch. same. Sabb. 104ᵇ; Gitt. 19ª, v. אוּשְׁכָּפָא. Lam. R. to IV, 8.

חַרְתָּא II f. (חרר III) [*heat,*] *strife, anger.* Targ. Prov. XV, 18; XVIII, 6 (ed. Lag. חַרְתָּא).

חֲרָתָא, v. חוּר׳.

חֵרְתָּא f. (v. חוֹרָא II) *a free woman.*—*Pl.* חֲרָתָא. Yeb. 118ᵇ בי ח׳ among the women of nobility; Keth. 75ª חֲרָאתָא.

חַרְתְּנָא m. (v. חַרְתָּא II) *querulous man.* Targ. Prov. XVI, 28 (ed. Lag. הַ׳; some ed. דרתנא, incorr.)

חָשׁ, חַשׁ, v. חוּשׁ, חָשַׁשׁ, חֲשַׁשׁ.

חֲשָׁא, v. חֲשִׁי.

חָשָׁא (or חָשָׁא) m. (חוּשׁ, חֲשַׁשׁ; cmp. P. Sm. 1391) *what man has to suffer, predestination, luck.*—*Pl.* חֲשַׁיָּא or חֲשִׁ׳. Lam. R. to I, 16 דְּחָשַׁיָּיה קשיי לינוקי hard fates are in store for my child (Matt. K. quotes a version נחשייה, v. נַחֲשָׁא). Ib. [read:] לא אמרית לך דח׳ קשייא ליה דעל ריגליה חרב בית מקדשא.

חֲשִׁי, חֲשָׁאֵי m. pl. (v. P. Sm. 1391) *thyme.* Sabb. 128ª, expl. קורניתא (v. Löw Pfl. p. 181).

חֲשָׁאי m. (חָשָׁה) *whispering, stillness, secret.* Pes. 56ª להביא בח׳ to offer it to her in secret. Ib. שיהו אומרים ... בח׳ that they say it in a whisper. Arakh. 16ª; Zeb. 88ᵇ; Yoma 44ª דבר שבח׳ something done in secrecy (the offering of frank-incense on the inner altar); מעשה שבח׳ what is committed in secrecy (calumny). Ber. 15ᵇ; a. fr.—*Pl.* חֲשָׁאִים. Shek. V, 6 לשכת ח׳ the Hall of Secret (donations).

חֲשַׁאי, חֲשִׁי, חֲשִׁיי ch. same. Targ. Ps. XLI, 8. Targ. Job IV, 16; a. e.

חָשַׁב (b. h.; cmp. חָשָׁה) 1) *to think, intend, plan.* Ber. 6ª; Kidd. 40ª (ref. to Mal. III, 16) אפי׳ ח׳ אדם וכ׳ even if one only had the intention of doing etc.; Sabb. 63ª חִישֵּׁב (*Pi.*).—Tanḥ. P'kudé 11 וכשהן חוֹשְׁבִין להעמידו וכ׳ and when they thought they had put it up, it fell apart again. Sot. 35ª אני חֲשַׁבְתִּיהָ .. והם חָשְׁבוּ וכ׳ I planned it for their good, but they considered it an evil; a. fr.—2) *to consider, regard; to count.* Ber. 14ª (ref. to Is. II, 22) במה חֲשַׁבְתּוֹ לזה ולא לאלוה with what right didst thou pay thy regard to him and not to God?—Sot. l. c., v. supra. Pesik. R. s. 21, v. סוֹפִּרְסְטָא; a. fr.—3) *to design, trace.* Yoma 72ᵇ (ref. to חשב a. רקם, Ex. XXVI, 31ª 36) רוקמין במיים שחוֹשְׁבִין they embroidered over what they had traced.—*Part. pass.* חָשׁוּב fem. חֲשׁוּבָה a) *counted, regarded*; כ־ ח׳ *equal to.* Lam. R. to I, 5 לא .. מדינה ח׳ כלום the country towns were of no account. Ned. 64ᵇ ח׳ כמת is like dead; ib. חֲשׁוּבִין כמת; Gen. R. s. 71 חֲשׁוּבִים כמתים; a. fr.—b) *valuable; important; respectable, of high standing.* Bets. 3ᵇ ביצה ח׳ an egg is a valuable object. Ber. 19ª, a. fr. אדם ח׳ שאני with a man of high standing it is different. Pes. 108ª אשה ח׳ a woman of rank. Tanḥ. Shmini 9 איש ח׳ שמחשבים וכ׳ a man of standing whom they respected in his place; a. fr.

Pi. חִישֵּׁב same, 1) *to consider, regard; to respect,* v. supra.—2) *to account, calculate, figure.* B. Bath 78ᵇ המְחַשְּׁבִים the thoughtful. Sabb. 150ª. חשבונות... לְחַשְּׁבָן וכ׳ accounts of a religious nature may be figured out on the Sabbath. Ab. II, 1 הוי מְחַשֵּׁב וכ׳ count what you sacrifice in doing good, against what you gain thereby. Snh. 65ᵇ המח׳ עתים וכ׳ he who calculates seasons and hours (which are auspicious and which are not). Ib. 97ᵇ מְחַשְּׁבֵי קיצין those who make calculations (from Biblical verses) as to when the Messiah will come; a. fr.—[Sabb. 150ᵇ top מותר לחוֹשְׁבָן (Kal), Ms. M. לחַשְּׁ׳.]—V. חֶשְׁבּוֹן.—3) (sub. מחשבה זרה) *to have in mind an undue intention in the performance of a sacrificial ceremony.* Yoma 48ª חי׳ בחפינת וכ׳ if he had an undue intention when grasping the frankincense (e. g. to offer it tomorrow). Ib.ᵇ; a. fr.

Hithpa, הִתְחַשֵּׁב, *Nithpa.* נִתְחַשֵּׁב 1) *to be counted.* Ohol. I, 3 אין האהל מִתְחַשֵּׁב the tent is not counted (as a special item). Yalk. Num. 768 מתח׳ לנו will be counted against us (be deducted from our share). Mikv. III, 3 עד שיִּתְחַשֵּׁב וכ׳ until it is calculated that all the original water has run off. Pesik. R. s. 44 the former sins אינן מִתְחַשְּׁבוֹת לו וכ׳ are not counted or remembered to him. —2) *to be considered, believed to be.* Tanḥ. Masé 5, v. כִּבְּבָן.—3) *to occupy a high position.* Shebi. VIII, 11 אם מתחשב הוא (Ms. M. כמ׳, v. Rabb. D. S. a. l. note) if he (is like one who) holds a high position.—4) *to conspire* (with the Romans). Tosef. Ab. Zar. II, 7 ואם מתחשב וכ׳ but when he (the Israelite besieging a city) does it as an ally (in the Roman interest), he is forbidden (to conduct the siege); Ab. Zar. 18ᵇ ובלבד שלא יִתְחַשֵּׁב עמהם provided he does not conspire with them; ואם נתח׳ וכ׳ (Ms. M. יתח׳); Y. ib. I, 40ª מתחשד (corr. acc.).

חֲשַׁב (חֲשִׁיב) חֲשֵׁב ch. same. Targ. Gen. L. 20. Targ. Esth. VIII, 3; a. fr.—Pesik B'shall., p. 82ª (translating Ex. XVIII, 11ᵇ) במחשבה דהֲשִׁבוּן איתחשב לחון what they had planned (against Israel) was planned against them. Sabb. 3ª קא חָשִׁיב he counts in; a. fr.—*Part. pass.* חֲשִׁיב, pl. חֲשִׁיבִין = h. חָשׁוּב, v. preced. Targ. Y. Ex. IV, 19; a. fr.—Keth. 8ᵇ ח׳ את וכ׳ thou hast been found worthy to be seized (to suffer) for etc. Gitt. 56ᵇ מאן ח׳ וכ׳ who is highly esteemed in that world (the hereafter)?; a. fr.

Pa. חַשֵּׁיב same, *to plan, to count, calculate.* Targ. Jer. XXI, 11.—Targ. O. Lev. XXV, 27; a. fr.—Meg. 11ᵇ חַשֵּׁיב ועייל וכ׳ count, and include in their place &c. Pes. 94ª דקא חָשְׁבֵי דקדמא וכ׳ because they also counted the distances which one walks before dawn and after sunset. Sabb. 74[a] ולִיחַשֵׁב וכ׳ let him also count the act of pounding; ib. 6[b]; a.e. וּלְחַשּׁוֹב (Pe.); a. fr. [Y. Pes. IV, end, 31[c] מחשבנא v. חֲשַׁךְ.]

Ithpa. אִתְחַשַּׁב, *Ithpe.* אִתְחֲשֵׁב. אִיחֲשַׁב 1) *to be planned.* Targ. O. Gen. L, 20.—Pesik. l. c., v. supra.—2) *to be considered, valued.* Targ. Lev. XVII, 4. Targ. Ps. L, 23; a. fr. — [Targ. Prov. XXIX, 11 מִיחֲשַׁב Ms. (ed. Lag. מחשב, Var. מאשב) *is respected* (v. Pesh. a. l.; ed. Wil. מאכח v. מְאַךְ).]

חָשָׁבָא (חֲשָׁ׳) m. (preced.) *accountant, calculator.* —*Pl.* חָשְׁבַיָּא (חָשָׁ׳). Targ. Is. XXXIII, 18.

חֶשְׁבּוֹן m. (b. h.; preced. wds.) 1) *account, sum; accountability; punishment and reward.* B. Bath. 9[b] ח׳ גדול sum total. Ib. 78[b] (play on *Ḥeshbon*, Num. XXI, 27; 30) באו ונחשב חֶשְׁבּוֹנוֹ וכ׳ come and let us examine the account of the world (human affairs), the loss etc. Ib. אבד ח׳ וכ׳ the accountability of the world is gone (there is no reward or punishment). Ex. R. s. 51, beg., a. fr. ליתן ח׳ to render an account. Tosef. B. Kam. X, 21 מה ח׳ עשה וכ׳ how our father settled with you; Y. ib. X, 7[b] bot.—Y. Ab. Zar. II, 42[a] top ח׳ מים וכ׳ he understands the calculation of the action of the water. Ib. ח׳ גדול הוא this is a great thing to calculate; a.fr.—2) *promptness in business.* Deut. R. s. 4 איני מכיר חֶשְׁבּוֹנְךָ I do not know your way of settling (whether you are prompt); ib. עשית לי ח׳ טוב you paid me promptly. [Yalk. Deut. 808 חח׳ read בעל חח׳ *market commissioner.*]—*Pl.* חֶשְׁבּוֹנוֹת. Sabb. 150[a], sq., v. חָשַׁב. Bekh. 5[a] בקי בח׳ a good arithmetician.

חֶשְׁבּוֹנָא, v. חוּשְׁבָּנָא.

חָשַׁד, v. חָסַד II.

חָשַׁד (cmp. חָשָׁה) [*to whisper,*] *to suspect* (cmp. דום a. דּוּמָה). Yoma 19[b], a. e. החושד בכשרים he who entertains a suspicion against worthy men. Ib. חֲשָׁדוּהוּ (ב)צדוקי they suspected him of being a Sadducee. Sabb. 127[b] במה חֲשַׁדְתַּנִי whereof did you suspect me?—Ib. 118[b]; M. Kat. 18[b] מי שחוֹשְׁדִין וכ׳ whom people suspect without cause; a. fr. — Part. pass. חָשׁוּד, f. חֲשׁוּדָה; pl. חֲשׁוּדִים, חֲשׁוּדוֹת; חֲשׁוּדִין. Dem. III, 5, v. חָלָה. Erub. 69[a] ח׳ לדבר אחד ח׳ וכ׳ one who is suspected of neglecting one religious law, is suspected of disregarding the whole Law; Bekh. 30[b]. Ib.[a] ח׳ על השביעית suspected of ignoring the laws of the Sabbatical year. Shebu 32[b], a. fr. ח׳ על השבועה suspected of swearing falsely (not admitted to oaths). Y. Taan. III, beg. 66[b] מפני פרנסת ח׳ for the sustenance of those suspected (of neglecting the laws of the Sabbatical year); a. fr.

Nif. נֶחְשַׁד *to be suspected.* Ber. 31[b] (ref. to I Sam. I, 16) מכאן לנ׳ בדבר וכ׳ from this we learn that he who is unjustly suspected, must make it known (clear himself). Bekh. 30[b]; Ab. Zar. 39[a] עד שֶׁיֵּחָשְׁדוּ until there is reason to suspect them of neglecting the observances of the associates (v. חָבֵר); a. fr.—[Y. Ab. Zar. I, 40[a] מתחשד, v. חָשַׁב.]

חֲשַׁד, ch. same. Targ. Y. Deut. XXIV, 9.—Sabb. 118[b] לדידי חַשְׁדָן וכ׳ they suspected me without cause; a. fr.—

Part. pass. חֲשִׁיד. Ber. 5[b] ומי חֲשִׁידְנָא וכ׳ am I suspected by you (of doing wrong)?; ומי ח׳ קב״ה וכ׳ can the Lord be suspected of injustice?, v. דִּינָא. Shebu. 32[b] דח׳ מאן which of the contestants is suspected (of swearing falsely)?; a. fr.

Ithpe. אִתְחֲשַׁד *to be suspected.* Targ. Y. Deut. XXI, 3.

חָשֵׁד m. (preced. wds.) *suspected.*—*Pl.* חֲשֵׁדִים; constr. חֲשֵׁדֵי. Pes. 85[a] ח׳ כהונה the suspected among the priesthood, i. e. priests suspected of wilfully unfitting a sacrifice in order to spite the owner.

חֲשָׁד m. (preced. wds.) *suspicion.* מפני חח׳ *to avoid suspicion.* Sabb. 23[b] מפני חח׳ (Tosef. Peah I, 6 מפני מראית העין) to avoid suspicion (as if he appropriated to himself the poor man's share). Yoma 30[a]; a. fr.

חַשְׁדָא ch. same. Ḥag. 5[a] מייתי לה לידי ח׳ exposes her to suspicion.—משום ח׳ *to avoid suspicion.* Ber. 43[b]; a. fr.—

חָשָׁה, v. חשי.

חָשׁוּ pr. n. m. *Ḥashu.* Keth 84[b] bot. יימר בר ח׳.

חָשׁוּב, v. חָשַׁב.

חָשׁוּךְ m. (b. h.; חָשַׁךְ) 1) *dark, black.* Ab. Zar. 8[a], v. חָשַׁךְ.—*Pl.* ...; כְּגוֹן חֲשׁוּכִים; f. חֲשׁוּכוֹת. Bekh. VII, 5 (expl. מרוח אשך, Lev. XXI, 20) שמראיו ח׳ whose complexion is very dark. Yalk. Ex. 258 פנים ח׳ dark (frowning) countenance; Mekh. B'shall., Vayassa, s. 2 חֲשֵׁכוֹת.—2) *obscured, benighted.* Pesik. R. s. 6, beg. (ref. to Prov. XXII, 29) פרעה חח׳ Pharaoh, the benighted.—*Pl.* as ab. Cant. R. to I, 1 (ref. to Prov. l. c.) לפני ח׳ אלו הרשעים 'before the benighted' that means the wicked.

חֲשׁוֹךְ, חֲשׁוֹכָא I. ch. 1) same, *dark.* Targ. Am. V, 20.—2) (חֲשַׁךְ II) *lean, reduced, poor.* v. חֲשִׁיךְ II.

חֲשׁוֹךְ, חֲשׁוֹכָא II m. (preced.) 1) *darkness.* Targ. Ex. X, 21, sq.; a. fr.—Targ. Ez. XIII, 18, v. קִירְנָא II.—Pes. 34[b] ארעא דח׳ a land of darkness (fogs). Ḥag. 12[b] bot. ומי איכא ח׳ וכ׳ is there darkness before the Lord?; a. fr.—*Pl.* חֲשׁוֹכַיָּא. Targ. Ps. LXXXVIII, 7.—2) *charred wick, snuff.* Bets 32[a] עדווי ח׳ Ar. (ed. חוּשְׁפָא). v. סְחַט.

חשוף, Tanh. P'kudé 3, some ed. (oth. ed. חצוף), read סחוף, v. סָחַף.

חשופא, v. חֲשִׁיפָה.

חַשְׁחַשׁ, v. חֲשַׁשׁ.

חָשָׁה, חשי (b. h.) [*to whisper,*] *be silent, quiet* (cmp. דמם, דום). Part. (fr. חוּשׁ) חָשׁ, f. חָשָׁה, pl. חָשׁוֹת. Hag. 12[b] ... ... אומרות . . . . וחשות ביום וכ׳ say praise by night, and are silent by day. Ib. 13[b] (play on חַשְׁמַל) חיות עתים חשות . . . מְמַלְלוֹת Ms. M. *Ḥayoth* (v. חַיָּה I end) who at times are silent etc.

חֲשָׁא, חֲשִׁי ch. 1) same. Y. Ab. Zar. I, 39[b] top חֲשִׁי דמלכא וכ׳ hush, for the king wants it so (desires to be worshipped in the form of a calf).—2) (=חוּשׁ) *to feel, suffer*, v. חוּשׁ ch.

חָשִׁי v. חָשַׁאי.

חָשֵׁי, v. חָשָׁאֵי.

חָשִׁיב, חֲשֵׁיב, v. חָשַׁב.

חֲשִׁיבָא m. (חָשַׁב) *prominent person, notable. Pl.* חֲשִׁיבֵי. Gitt. 58ª ח׳ דרומאי the Roman notables. Ib. 56ᵇ [read:] ואימנו להו ח׳ דר׳ לאותיבך וכ׳ and the Roman nobility resolved to place thee at their head; Yalk. Prov. 953.

חֲשִׁיבוּתָא f. (preced.) *importance, value.* B. Bath. 146ª ח׳ דא״י ed. (Ms. M. a. F., Rashb. שְׁבָחָא) the valuableness of Palestine (for its fertility).

חֲשִׁיד, v. חֲשַׁד.

חֲשִׁיךְ, v. חֲשַׁךְ.

חֲשִׁיךְ, חֲשִׁיכָא I m. (חֲשַׁךְ I) *dark, black.* Targ. Y. Lev. XXI, 20 ח׳ חזווירה Ar. s. v. חז whose complexion is very dark (v. חָשׁוּךְ; ed. פחדור וכ׳).—*Fem.* חֲשִׁיכָא, pl. חֲשִׁיכָן. Targ. Lam. V, 17.

חֲשִׁיךְ, חֲשִׁיכָא II m. (חֲשַׁךְ II) *lean, poor; luckless* (interch. with: חֲשׁוּכָא ,חֲשׁוּךְ). Targ. Ez. XVIII, 12. Targ. II Sam. XIII, 4. Targ. Ps. LXXII, 13; a. fr.—Lam. R. to I, 5 ולמה ח׳ כן and why is he so reduced?—Ib. to III, 20 (prov.) עד דשמינא חשיך חשיכא מיית Ar. (Var כחיש כחישא; ed... קטין.. דקטינא...) while the fat one becomes lean, the lean one is dead (retribution to the oppressor comes too late). Midr. Till. to Ps. XXII, 7, v. חַי ch.—*Pl.* חֲשִׁיכַיָּא, חֲשׁוּכֵי. Targ. Jer. LII, 15, sq. — Succ. 44ᵇ לחשוכיא (Ms. M. 2 לחסיריא, read לַחְסִרַ׳) to the poor.—*Fem.* חֲשִׁיכָא, חֲשִׁיכְתָא. Targ. Is. LIV, 11.—*Pl.* חֲשִׁיכָן ,חֲשִׁיכָתָא. Targ. Y. Gen. XLI, 19, sq; v. חֲסִיךְ.

חֲשֵׁכָה, חֲשֵׁיכָה f. (b. h.; חָשַׁךְ I) *darkness, nightfall.* Sabb. II, 7 עם ח׳ near nightfall. Ib. ספק ח׳ וכ׳ if it is doubtful whether or not night has set in; a. fr.—*Pl.* חֲשֵׁכוֹת (*adj.*), v. חָשׁוּךְ.

חֲשִׁיכָה f. (v. חָשַׁךְ I *Hif.*) *awaiting the nightfall* (on the Sabbath), *approaching the Sabbath limit in day-time and waiting there for the night for the transaction of business.* Sabb. 151ª רשאי אני בַחֲשִׁיכָתוֹ (Mish. להחשיך עליו) I am permitted to take the preliminary steps for it before nightfall.

חֲשִׁיכְתָא, v. חֲשִׁיךְ II.

חָשִׁיל, v. חָשַׁל.

חֲשִׁילָא c. (חָשַׁל) *mashed.*—*Pl.* fem. חֲשִׁילָתָא. Hull. 93ª bot. ביעי ח׳ mashed testicles (undevelopped).

חֲשִׁילְתָא f. (preced.; v. חוּשְׁלָא) *a brew made of peeled and pounded fruits,* v. טְרִימָא. Ber. 38ª (ח׳ (ודאי קאמרת (Ms. F. ח׳ דתמרי, v. Rabb. D. S. a. l. note; Ar. חלישתא, incorr.) (by *trimma*) you (surely) mean a brew of ground dates.

חֲשִׁיפָה f. (חָשַׂף, v. חָסַף I) 1) *stripping, uncovering.* Y. Ber. IX, 13ª top חֲשִׂיפַת זרועו the baring of His arm (Is. LII, 10).—2) *paring, shavings* used for basket work. Tosef. Kil. III, 14 הח׳ Var. (ed. Zuck. חשופה); Y. ib. V, end, 30ª השיפה. Tosef. Toh. XI, 16 של ח׳ quot. by R. S. to Toh. X, 8 (ed. Zuck. של השיפה) basket work made of shavings; Ab. Zar. 75ª של שיפה (ed. Pes. חש׳). Succ. 20ª מחצלת של ח׳ Ms. M. (ed. שיפה) matting made of etc.; Tosef. ib. I, 10 שירופא ed. Zuck. (Var. חשופא, oth. ed. חשי׳).

חֲשִׁיקָה f. (חָשַׁק) *pleasure, favor, use of the root* חָשַׁק. Gen. R. s. 80, a. e.; v. חֲפִיצָה.

חָשַׂךְ, v. חָסַךְ.

חֲשַׁךְ (v. חָסַךְ) *to spare, withhold.* Targ. Prov. XIII, 24 חֲשֵׁךְ ,חָשִׂיךְ (part.). Ib. XVII, 27.

Af. אַחְשֵׁךְ *to deduct.* Y. Pes. IV, end, 31ᶜ מַחְשְׁכִינָא (not מחשב׳), v. גּוּדְלָנָא.

חָשַׁךְ (b. h.; cmp. חשש) [*to be pressed, thick,*] *to be dark.* Sabb. 34ª; 51ª משתחשכה; ib. IV, 2 משתחשך when it darkens (at nightfall, v. חֲשֵׁיכָה). Snh. 22ª עולם ח׳ בעדו the world around him is dark; Ab. Zar. 8ª (some ed. חָשׁוּךְ). Ber. 16ᵇ אל תֶּחְשְׁכוּ וכ׳ let not our eyes be obscured; a. fr. V. חָשׁוּךְ.

Hif. הֶחְשִׁיךְ 1) *to be overtaken by (the Sabbath) nightfall.* Sabb. XXIV, 1 מי שה׳ בדרך he who is on the road at nightfall (on Friday).—2) *to wait for the nightfall, to make preparations to be ready for work on the exit of the Sabbath,* v. חֲשִׁיכָה. Ib. XXIII, 3 אין מַחְשִׁיכִין על וכ׳ you must not, during the day, walk to the extreme end of the Sabbath limit to await the night there for the purpose of hiring workmen etc.; אבל מַחְשִׁיךְ הוא וכ׳ but one may do so for the purpose of going at nightfall to watch his field, and then he may also take his fruits home. Ib. לְהַחְשִׁיךְ עליו to await the night at the Sabbath limit for the purpose of doing it. Ib. 4; a. fr.—3) *to darken, obscure.* Cant. R. to I, 1 (ref. to חשכים, Prov. XXII, 29) that is Potifar שה׳ הקב״ה וכ׳ whose eyes the Lord darkened etc. Ex. R. s. 51 (ref. to חשכה Gen. XV, 12) that is Media שֶׁהֶחְשִׁיכָה וכ׳ who made Israel's eyes dim (with tears) by her decrees. Pesik R. s. 47 (ref. to Job XXXVIII, 2) הֶחְשַׁכְתָּ וכ׳ (not החשב׳) thou hast obscured the council which I held in heavens (when the Lord vouched for Job's integrity); a. fr.—4) *to become dark.* Midr. Till. to Ps. XVIII, 12 (ref. to the versions חשכת, Ps. l. c., and חשרת II Sam. XXII, 12) when the clouds are laden with the waters, הן מַחְשִׁיכִין מן המים וכ׳ they receive a dark color from the waters, and afterwards they drop them as through a sieve.

חֲשַׁךְ, חֲשׁוֹךְ I ch. same. Targ. Job. XVIII, 6. Targ. Ex. X, 15; a. fr.—Taan. 10ª חָשׁוּךְ ענני וכ׳ when the clouds are dark, they contain much water.

Pa. חַשֵּׁיךְ 1) *to darken, obscure.* Targ. Ps. CV, 28; a. e. —2) *to do something at night, to be late.* Tam. 27[b] חַשֵּׁיךְ תקין נפשך וכ׳ at bed-time attend to thy body, and in the morning etc. Ber. 8[a] מקדמי ומְחַשְּׁכֵי וכ׳ they go to Synagogue early and late. Ib. קדימו וחַשִּׁיכוּ ועיילו וכ׳ (Ms. M. וְאַחְשִׁיכוּ, *Af.*, v. Rabb. D. S. a. l.) go ye early and late to etc. Targ. Y. Deut. XXVIII, 65, v. מַחְשְׁכָן.

Af. אַחְשִׁיךְ 1) *to obscure.* Targ. Job XXXVIII, 2; a. e. —2) *to do something late.* Targ. I Sam. XVII, 16.—Ber. l. c., v. supra.

Ithpe. אִיתְחֲשַׁךְ, אִיחֲשַׁךְ *to grow dark.* Targ. Ps. LXIX, 24; a. e.—Snh. 96[a] עד דאתא אי״ח׳ by the time he came it had grown dark.

חֲשַׁךְ, חֲשוֹךְ II (cmp. חסך) *to be reduced, lean.* Targ. Ps. XXXI, 11 (h. text עששו, v. Rashi a. l.)

Ithpe. אִיתְחֲשַׁךְ same. Targ. Job XXXIII, 21 Ms. (ed. שפיין).

חֲשַׁךְ, חוֹשֶׁךְ m. (b. h.; זֹשֶׁךְ) *darkness.* Ex. R. s. 14. Ḥag. 12[a]; a. v. fr.—הָרֵי ח׳ *Dark Mountains*, behind which the Amazons live (*Amazonici Mountes*, v. Sm. Class. Dict. s. v.). Lev. R. s. 27; Pesik. Shor, p. 74[a]; Tam. 32[a]. [The Jewish legend relating the meeting of Alexander the Great with the Amazons seems to point to Africa, v. קרטגינא).

חֶשְׁכָּא ch. same. Targ. Ps. XVIII, 29 (Ms. חבריא, v. חֲבִירָא); Targ II Sam XXII, 29 (ed. Lag. חֲשׁוֹכָא). Targ. Ps. LXXXVIII, 13 חֲשַׁךְ, constr. (Ms. חֲשׁוֹךְ).—V. חַשְׁכּוּתָא.

חֲשֵׁכָה, v. חֲשֵׁיכָה.

חַשְׁכּוּתָא f. (preced. wds.) *dimness, darkness.* Targ. O. Deut. XXVIII, 65 (ed. Vien. חֲשֵׁכַת).

חֲשֵׁכְתָּא f. same. Targ. O. Deut. XXVIII, 65, v. preced.—*Pl.* חֲשֵׁכָתָא. B. Mets. 30[b] בקדמתא ובח׳ every early morning or every evening after dark.

חַשְׁכְּתָא, v. חֲשִׁיךְ II.

חֲשַׁל = חֲסַל.

חָשַׁל (b. h.; cmp. חָסַל) *to scrape off, polish; to reduce.*

Pi. חִישֵּׁל *to crush, batter.* Koh. R. to I, 6 the Lord מְחַשְּׁלוֹ בהרים breaks it (the vehemence of the wind) through the mountains; (Lev. R. 15; Gen. R. s. 24 מרשלו; Y. Ber. IX, 13[c] bot. מכשלו).

Nif. נֶחְשַׁל *to be crushed.* Sifré Deut. 296 (ref. to נחשלים, Deut. XXV, 18) שנמכו .... ונֶחְשְׁלוּ מתחת וכ׳ who have been crushed out of the ways of the Lord and battered away from under the protection of etc.

חֲשַׁל, חֲשִׁיל ch. same, 1) *to furbish, forge, hammer.* Dan. II, 40.—Ab. Zar. 16[a] דְּחַשְּׁלֵי מינייהו וכ׳ Ms. M., v. חֲלַשׁ.—Trnsf. *to plan, design* (corresp. to b. h. חרש a. חשב). Targ. Ps. XXXVI, 5. Targ. Prov. XIV, 22; a. fr.—2) *to peel, pound grits*, v. חוּשְׁלָא.—V. חֲשִׁילָא.

Pa. חַשֵּׁיל same, esp. *to plan.* Targ. Ps. XXI, 12, a. fr. Ms. (ed. *Pe.*). Targ. Y. Deut. I, 12.

חַשָּׁלָא m. (preced.) *furbisher, smith.*—*Pl.* constr. חַשָּׁלֵי. Keth. 77[a] (expl. מצרף נחשת. Mish.) ח׳ דודי kettle smiths.

חַשְׁמוֹנַאי n. gent. m. *Asmonean, Hasmonean*, family name of Mattathias the priest and his descendants (Maccabean dynasty). Midd. I, 6 בני ח׳ the sons of the Asmonean (Judah and his brothers). Sabb. 21[b] מלכות בית ח׳ the government of the Asmonean house. Midr. Till. to Ps. XCIII, beg. (ed. Bub. plur.). Sot. 49[b]; Men. 64[b]; B. Kam. 82[b] (v. Rabb. D. S. a. l.) מלכי בית ח׳ the kings of the Asmonean house (Hyrcan and Aristobulus).—*Pl.* חַשְׁמוֹנָאִים. B. Kam. l. c. (some ed.).—[*Chald.* Targ. I Sam. II, 4. Targ. Cant. VI, 7 (some ed. ...נָאֵי, pl.).]

חַשְׁמַל m. (b. h.; cmp. חסם II; v. Ges. H. Dict. 10 s. v.) *a glittering substance; amber* or *galena* (?). Ḥag. 13[a] עד הח׳ including the verse in which *hashmal* appears (Ez. I, 27). Ib. היה מבין בח׳ was speculating on the meaning of *hashmal*; ויצאה אש מח׳ and fire came out of the *hashmal.* Ib., sq. מהו חשמל חיות אש ממללות *Hayoth* (v. חַיָּה) speaking fire; v. חָיָה.

חַשְׁמְלָא, חַשְׁמַל ch. same. Targ. Ez. I, 4; a. e.—Ḥag. 13[a].

חֹשֶׁן, v. חוֹשֶׁן.

חָשַׁק (b. h.) *to press, tie, surround.* Ab. Zar. 35[a] (ref. to Cant. I, 2) חֲשׁוֹק שפתותיך זו בזו press thy lips together and be not too hasty in replying.—2) (cmp. חָפֵץ) *to be attached to, in love with; to elect.* Tosef. Yeb. VIII, 4 חָשְׁקָה .. בתורה my soul has chosen the Law (as bride); Yeb. 63[b]. Ḥull. 89[a] (ref. to Deut. VII, 7) חוֹשְׁקַנִי בכם I elected you.

חֲשַׁק ch. same, *to bandage, saddle, harness.* Targ. II Sam. XIX, 27.—Part. pass. חֲשִׁיק, pl. חֲשִׁיקִין, f. חֲשִׁיקָן. Targ. Jud. XIX, 10. Ib. V, 10.

חָשַׁר [(cmp. חֲשַׁךְ II a. חָשַׁל) *to peel*, whence חֲשָׁרָה *an implement for removing peels, sieve*, from which חָשַׁר] *to sift, distil drops as if through a sieve.* Midr. Till. to Ps. XVIII, 12, v. חָשַׁךְ. Ib. .... אדם נוטל כברה וחוֹשֵׁר אצבעות וכ׳ a man takes a sieve and lets (a liquid) down a height of two or three fingers; before it comes down to the ground, the drops will be mixed up; Yalk. Sam. 160. —Gen. R. s. 13 וחוֹשְׁרִים אותו כמין כברה and they (the clouds) distil it (the rain) as if from a sieve; Yalk. Gen. 20; Yalk. Koh. 967.

Pi. חִישֵּׁר same. Taan. 9[b] מנוקבות .... ומְחַשְּׁרוֹת they (the clouds) are perforated like a sieve and distil water to the ground.

חֲשַׁר ch. same, *to sift.* Y. Sabb. VII, 10[b] bot. הן דח׳ וכ׳ he who (on the Sabbath) sifts powder of gypsum &c. Y. Meg. I, 71[b] top מכיון שהוא מרחיק ואת ח׳ וכ׳ because its meshes are wide and you may sift flour through it; Y. Ned. IV, beg. 38[c], v. זוֹסְמָא.

חָשַׁשׁ (v. חוּשׁ) 1) *to feel heavy, feel pain.* Y. Sabb. IV,

8[c] top החוֹשֵׁשׁ אזנו he who has ear-ache. Esth. R. to I, 1 (play on אחשורוש) who ever thinks of him חוֹשֵׁשׁ את ראשו gets a head-ache; a. e. — (Mostly with ב). Cant. R. to V, 2 אם חושש ... בראשו if one of the twins has a head-ache; a. fr.—2) *to apprehend, take into consideration.* Pes. I, 2 אין חוֹשְׁשִׁין שמא וכ׳ we do not take into consideration that perhaps a weasel &c. Tosef. Ḥull. III, 24 ואין ח׳ שמא של וכ׳ and we need not hesitate to use them for fear that they may be eggs of &c.; Ḥull. 63[b] אין ח׳ לא משום וכ׳. Sabb. XVI, 7; XXII, 3 חוֹשְׁשַׁנִי לו מחטאת I am afraid he has committed a sin which requires a sin-offering to atone for; a. fr.

חֲשַׁשׁ ch. same, 1) *to suffer.* Y. M. Kat. III, 82[d] top פומיה הוא ח׳ he has an ailing on his mouth (and therefore ties it up). Cant. R. to II, 16 ועבד ח׳ וכ׳ and continued suffering with fever for three years; a. fr.—2) *to be affected, troubled; to care, apprehend.* Targ. Prov. XXVIII, 17 דחָשֵׁישׁ וכ׳ he who is troubled (feels compunction) about blood-guiltiness (h. text עשק); a. e. —Y. M. Kat. III, 81[d] bot. צריך את חשש על נפשך thou must mind the excommunication for thy soul's sake. Ib. חַשׁ על נפשיה he minded the excommunication. Ib. וחַשּׁוּן אילין על אילין they minded each the other's excommunication. Keth. 26[b] בְּמֵיחַשׁ לזילותא וכ׳ they differ as to providing against the disregard of the court; a. fr. (interch. with חוש).—[3) (=חֲשָׁא) *to whisper, hiss.* Targ. Jer. VI, 29 חַשׁ (ed. Wil. חֲשָׁא).]

Ithpa. אִיתְחֲשֵׁשׁ, אִיתְחַ׳ *to become sick.* Cant. R. l. c. אתחו׳ ר׳ זעירא (Var. אִתְחַ׳; ed. Wil. אחשש, corr. acc.).

Palp. חַשְׁחֵשׁ 1) *to feel.* Targ. Y. Num. XI, 12.—2) *to care for.* Targ. Ps. CXLI, 1 Regia (ed. חִישׁ).

חֲשָׁשָׁא m. (preced.) *anxiety, fear, suspicion.* Targ. Koh. II, 25. —Yoma 83[b] אימר דאמרי אנא ח׳ וכ׳ (Ms. M. לְמֵיחַשׁ, v. preced.) what I said (that a name was an omen) was meant only as an apprehension, but I did not mean it as a certainty. Bekh. 36[a] אימר דאמר ר״מ לח׳ what R. M. said, was meant as an apprehension (worth investigating), but not to make one legally disqualified. Ib. ח׳ הוא it is merely a suspicion, ובמקום ח׳ וכ׳ and against such a doubt, we may argue that he had no reason to tell a falsehood. Nidd. 17[b] אי בתר ח׳ וכ׳ if you are guided by a doubt, opp. חֲזָקָה; a. fr.

חָתָא, חֲתָא, חֲתָה, v. חתי.

חִתּוּי m. (v. חָתַת) *breaking, killing.* Ḥull. 27[a] זב ע״י ח׳ בעינן the flow must have been caused by the action which kills (cutting).

חִתּוּךְ, חִתּוּכָא, v. חִית׳.

חָתוּל m. (v. Fl. to Levy Targ. Dict. I, p. 426[1]) *cat.* B. Kam. 80[b]. Hor. 13[a]. Bekh. 8[a]; a. fr.—*Pl.* חֲתוּלִים, ־לִין...; f. חֲתוּלוֹת. B. Kam. 80[a], sq.; Tosef. ib. VIII, 17. Hor. l. c. מפני מה ח׳ .. בעכברים Ms. M. a. Ar. (v. Rabb. D. S. a. l. note; ed. חכל) why have the cats been given power over the mice?—Koh. R. to VI, 11. Cant. R. to VII, 2 ומצא חח׳ מקורעות לפניהם and found the cats lying torn in front of the chickens; Y. Peah III, 17[d] top.

חֲתוּל, חֲתוּלָא ch. same. Ḥull. 52[b].—*Pl.* חֲתוּלַיָּא, חֲתוּלִין. Targ. Is. XIII, 22; XXXIV, 14 (h. text איים) wild cats. [Hos. IX, 6 חתולין, read: חֲרוּלִין.]

חִתּוּם, v. חיתום.

חַתּוֹמָא m. (חָתַם) *signer, witness.*—*Pl.* חַתּוֹמַיָּא. Y. Gitt. IX, 50[c] bot. יהב רשו ... ולח׳ וכ׳ (not ולחתימייא) gave permission to the scribe to write and to the witnesses to sign.

חִתּוּן, חִתּוּנָא, v. חית׳.

חֲתוּנָּה f. (b. h. חֲתֻנָּה; חָתַן) *wedding.* Num. R. s. 12; a. e., v. חיתון.

חִתּוּת, חִתִּית, v. חיתית.

חָתָא, חֲתֵי, (v. נחת); *Hif.* (א)הַחֲתִי *to put down, rest.* Y. Yoma V, 42[b] bot. יחליף ... ויַחֲתִי let him change hands ....and set (the pan) down. Ib. אם ח׳ מימינו וכ׳ if he set it down from his right towards his left side.

חֲתָא, חֲתֵי I ch. *Af.* אַחֲתֵי same. Yoma 47[a] ונַחֲתִיָּה למחתה וכ׳ (v. Rabb. D. S. a. l. notes 3, 4) and let him put the pan on top of it. V. נְחַת.

חָתָה, חתי (b. h.) *to dig,* esp. *to take coals out with a pan.* Yoma IV, 4 בכל יום היה חוֹתֶה וכ׳ every other day the priest used to take coals out in a silver pan &c. Sabb. VIII, 7 כדי לַחְתּוֹת בו את האור large enough to take fire out in it. Zeb. 64[a]; a. fr.—Y. Yoma IV, 41[c] bot. צריך לחות (read לחתות) he must take coals out as before.

Pi. חִיתָּה *to stir embers, rake.* Sabb. 34[b] שמא יְחַתֶּה בגחלים he might rake the coals under the ashes. [Ḥull. 27[a], v. חָתַת.]

חֲתָא, חֲתֵי II ch. same. Targ. Is. XXX, 14.—Part. חָאתֵי. Targ. Prov. XXV, 22 ed. Lag. (oth. ed. חָתֵי).—

Pa. חַתֵּי *to stir.* Ab. Zar. 38[b] וחַתֶּה בה חַתּוּיֵי ed. (v. Rabb. D. S. a. l. note 8), v. חָרֵי.

חֲתָיָיה f. (preced. wds.) *taking coals out in a pan.* Y. Yoma IV, 41[c] bot. Bab. ib. 48[b] חישב בחֲתָיַית וכ׳ if he entertained an undue thought on taking coals from the altar.

חֲתִיכָה f. (חָתַךְ) 1) *cutting.* Erub. 103[a], v. בְּבֵלָת. Ḥull. 31[b], v. זְבִיחָה.—2) *a piece (of meat), portion* (cmp. מָנָה, נֵתַח). Ib. VII, 5 ח׳ של דג וכ׳ a portion of an unclean fish. Ib. 100[a] שאני ח׳ הואיל וכ׳ with an entire piece the case is different, because it is fit to be offered to guests; a. fr.—*Pl.* חֲתִיכוֹת. Ib. VII, 5. Kerith. 17[b] חתיכה משתי ח׳ a doubt as to one piece out of two (of which one was forbidden and one allowed, and it is unknown which he ate); a. fr.

חֲתִים, v. חָתַם.

חֲתִימָה f. (חָתַם) 1) *signature, stamp, mark.* Gitt. 87[a] bot. וידעינן בהא ח׳ וכ׳ when we know about that signature that it is not Jacob's. Ib. II, 4 עד .. וחֲתִימָתוֹ בתלוש unless it was written and signed on a movable material (v. חָבַר). Y. Keth. II, 26[c] top על חֲתִימַת העד וכ׳ to identify the signature of the second witness. B. Bath. 89[b] עד דחזי ח׳ כיון דלא חזי ח׳ Ms. M. (ed. אי לא חזי ח׳, Ms. H. חתמא) since he does not see the official stamp on the measure; a. fr.—Trnsf. חֲתִימַת זָקָן *the mature manly expression which the beard gives, full manhood.* B. Mets. 39[b]; Yeb. 88[a]; Gen. R. s. 91; a. e.—[Targ. Cant. III, 8 חֲתִימַת מִילָה the seal of the covenant.]—*Pl.* חֲתִימוֹת. Keth. 21[b] ח׳ ידי העדים the signatures (handwritings) of the witnesses; a. e.—2) (v. חִיתּוּם) *the concluding clause of a prayer.* Pes. 104[a] צריך ... ח׳ סמוך לַחֲתִימָתוֹ he must use expressions corresponding to the closing formula immediately before the latter.—3) *locking up, obstruction.* Nidd. 43[b], a. fr. (with ref. to Lev. XV, 3) חֲתִימַת פי האמה the filling up of the aperture of the membrum (with mucus).

חֲתִימְתָּא, חַתְמוּתָא, חֲתִימוּתָא same. Keth. 21[a] אסהד אַחֲתִימוּת ידיה וכ׳ he testified to (identified) his own signature &c.—B. Bath. 167[a] חַתְמוּת ידא (Ms. M. חֲתִימַת). Gitt. 66[b], v. חָתַם.—*Pl.* חֲתִימָתָא. Keth. 21[b] חֲתִימַת ידייהו.

חתימויא, Y. Gitt. IX, 50[c] bot., v. חִיתּוּמָא.

חֲתִימְתָּא, v. חֲתִימוּתָא.

חֲתִירְאָ, v. חֲתִירְתָּא.

חֲתִירָה f. (חָתַר) *breach, opening made by digging.* Gen. R. s. 76 וחתר לו הקב״ה ח׳ וכ׳ and the Lord created an opening for him etc. Ruth R. to II, 14; Y. Snh., X, 28[c] bot., v. חָתַר. Ruth R. l. c. צווחין לח׳ עתירה, v. next w.

חֲתִירְתָּא (חֲתִירָא) ch. same. Lev. R. s. 30; Gen. R. s. 63 (ref. to II Chr. XXXIII, 13; Gen. XXV, 21) בערביא קירין לח׳ עתירתא in Arabia they say for *ḥăthirta* (breach) *ʿăthirta*; Y. Snh. X, 28[c] bot. לַחֲתִירְתָּה עתירתה...; Ruth R. to II, 14, v. preced.—*Pl.* חֲתִירָן. Y. Maas. Sh. V, 55[d] bot. אתעביד ... ח׳ בתים (strike out בתים) three hundred robberies by breaking in were committed; Gen. R. s. 27 חוֹתְרִין m. pl.; Yalk. Job 909 (corr. acc.).

חָתִית, v. חִיתִּית.

חָתַךְ (b. h.) 1) *to cut, dissect; to sever.* Hull. 33[a] חוֹתֵךְ כזית וכ׳ cuts out flesh of the size of an olive. Ib. 32[a] ח׳ דלעת וכ׳ if in slaughtering he cut a pumpkin at the same time. Ib. 48[b] a. e. חוֹתְכָהּ מכאן וכ׳ he amputates on one place and the animal survives &c. Bets. 32[b] חוֹתְכָהּ באור he may sever the wick over the light. Y. Meg. IV, 75[a] חותך the reader cuts one verse into two (reading Gen. I, 5, a. I, 8 as two verses severally); a. fr.—[Lev. R. s. 10 לחתוך את אביו וכ׳, v. חָתַר.]—*Part. pass.* חָתוּךְ *cut into, having the incisions of limbs &c., outlined.* Nidd. 24[b] גוף שאינו ח׳ a shapeless body (not articulated); ראש שאינו ח׳ a shapeless head (without indications of the nose &c.) Ib. 24[a] יד חֲתוּכָה a well-shaped hand (of an embryo); a. fr.—2) (cmp. פָּסַק, גָּזַר) *to decide, sentence.* Lev. R. s. 4, beg. (ref. to חתוך, Jer. XXXIX, 3) ששם חוֹתְכִין את ההלכה for there they decide the practice. Ib. וחוֹתֶכֶת דיניהם וכ׳ and decides the cases &c. Shebu. 30[b] bot. אֶחְתְּכֶנּוּ I will decide the case (in accordance with the testimony).—Part. pass. as ab. Y. Snh. IV, beg. 22[a] אילו ... התורה חתוכה if the Law had been given in the form of clear decisions (leaving no room for differences of opinion, discretion &c.)

Nif. נֶחְתַּךְ 1) *to be cut off, severed; to be cut into.* Hull. IV, 6 שנֶּחְתְּכוּ רגליה whose feet have been amputated. Ib. 32[a] נֶחְתְּכָה דלעת וכ׳ if by accident a pumpkin has been cut simultaneously with the animal (opp. to חָתַךְ, v. supra); a. fr.—2) *to be decided, decreed.* Meg. 15[a] (play on התך, Esth. IV, 5) שכל ... נֶחְתָּכִין על יפיו all the government affairs were decided upon his opinion.

Pi. חִיתֵּךְ 1) *to cut.* Hull. IV, 2 מְחַתֵּךְ אבר אבר he may cut off limb after limb. Ib. 98[b] מחתך לה וכ׳ he carves the foreleg and then boils it.—*Part. pass.* מְחוּתָּךְ *piecemeal, limbwise.* Y. Nidd. III, 50[c] יצא מח׳ if the embryo came out by pieces.—2) *to decide.* Snh. 7[b] צדק...חַתְּכֵהוּ make the case clear and then decide it. Ber. 61[a] לשון מְחַתֵּךְ וכ׳ the tongue forms the sentence, the mouth closes (the case, makes it irreversible).—3) *to dig ore (in lumps).* Keth. 77[a] (expl. מצרף) מעיקרו ... הַמְחַתֵּךְ he who digs copper in the shaft. [Tosef. Ohol. IV, 3 וחתכו, וחיתכו, read: והִתִּיכוּ or והִתְּכוּ, v. נָתַךְ a. התך.]

חֲתַךְ ch. same. *Pa.* חַתֵּיךְ *to cut off.* Hull. 11[a] ח׳ ליה לגמרי he severed it entirely, v. לוּף.—*Part. pass.* מְחַתַּךְ *in pieces.* Targ. Y. Lev. VII, 30 (ed. Amst. מְחַתֵּךְ, incorr.). Targ. Y. I Num. XII, 12 כד מח׳ (not מְחַתֵּיךְ).

Ithpa. אִתְחַתַּךְ *to be cut, to be decided.* Targ. Esth. IV, 5 (v. Meg. 15[a], quot. in preced.).

חֶתֶךְ m. (preced.) *cut, wound.* Tosef. Mikv. VII (VIII), 3 מפני הח׳ on account of the place where the handle is intended to be lopped off (v. Mikv. X, 5).—Erub. 18[a]. Hull. 32[b] שחט במקום ח׳ he slaughtered by setting the knife into the wound (and continued the cut).

חָתַם (b. h.; cmp. b. h. חָתַל) 1), *to tie up, close, lock.* Tanh. B'resh. 1 ח׳את הים וכ׳ he locked the Ocean up, that it might not go forth &c.—2) *to seal.* Y. Ab. Zar. III, 42[c] bot. טבעת שחוֹתֵם בה the ring with which he seals. Ib. אסור לַחְתּוֹם בה you dare not use it for a seal; Tosef. ib. V (VI), 2; a. fr.—2) *to sign, subscribe* (as witness, judge &c.) Gitt. VI, 7 אחד ... חוֹתְמִין one writes the document and two sign it as witnesses. Ib. 66[b] ח׳ סופר if the scribe signed as one of the witnesses. Ib. 67[a] ואתם חֲתוֹמוּ and sign you. Shebi. X, 4 הדיינים חותמין וכ׳ the judges sign under it; a. fr.—Part. pass. חָתוּם, f. חֲתוּמָה; pl. חֲתוּמִים, חֲתוּמוֹת; חֲתוּמִין. Yeb. 25[b], a. e. עדים הח׳ וכ׳ if witnesses are signed &c.; a. fr.—3) *to close* a benediction (v. חֲתִימָה). Pes. X, 6 וחותם בגאולה and he closes with redemption (Blessed be the Lord who redeemed Israel). Ib. לא היה חותם he did not close with a benediction. Ber. I, 4 מקום שאמרו לַחְתּוֹם where the Rabbis ordained to close a benediction with Barukh &c.; a. fr.—Part. pass. as ab. Gitt. 60[a] תורה ח׳ ניתנה the Law was given as one complete book, opp. מגילה מגילה in single sheets. [Cant. R. to I, 11, v. next w.]

Pi. חִיתֵּם *to provide with signatures.* Y. Gitt. I, beg.43[a], a. e. מְחַתְּמוֹ בעדים וכ׳ he may have provided it with the signatures of unfit witnesses. Ib. חִתְּמוֹ וכ׳.—*Part. pass.* מְחוּתָּם. Y. Keth. II, 26[c]; Y. Shebu IV, 35[c] מח׳ בארבע וכ׳ provided with four signatures.

Nif. נֶחְתַּם, *Hithpa.* הִתְחַתֵּם, *Nithpa.* נִתְחַתֵּם 1) *to be signed, sealed.* Gitt. I, 1 בפני נח׳ (Y. ed. נתח׳) in my presence has it been signed; a. fr.— 2) *to be finally sentenced* (by attaching the seal or signature). R. Hash. 16[b] נכתבין ונֶחְתָּמִין וכ׳ their verdict is written and sealed at once; Y. ib. I, 57[a] מִתְחַתְּמִין. Gen. R. s. 31, beg. נתח׳ גזר דינם their decree was sealed; a. e.

חֲתַם, ch. same. 1) *to close up.* Ber. 6[a] ולִיחְתּוּם פומיה and let him close up its opening. Part. pass. חֲתִים. Targ. O. Lev. XV, 3.—2) *to seal, sign.* Targ. Jer. XXXII, 44; a. fr.—Gitt. 66[b] מְחַתֵּם וכ׳ to draw their signatures.—*Part. pass.* as ab. Targ. l. c. 11.—B. Bath 89[b] דלא חֲתִימֵי where they do not stamp measures officially.—3) *to close a benediction.* Meg. 22[b] ח׳ ולא בריך he closed his prayer without saying *Barukh* &c. Cant. R. to I, 11 [read:] מלה חֲתִימָה ... מסיימה a closed and finished word (complete in itself).

Pa. חַתֵּים *to lock up.* Targ. Job XXIV, 16 (some ed. *Ithpa.*).

Ithpa. אִתְחַתֵּים 1) *to lock one's self up.* V. supra.—2) *to be sealed, stamped.* Targ. Esth. IV, 1. Targ. Is. VIII, 21; a. fr.— 3) *to be closed up.* Targ. Y. Lev. XV, 3 ed. pr. (ed. אתסתם).

חֲתָמָא, חֲתְמוּתָא, v. חֲתִימָה a. חֲתִימוּתָא.

חָתַן (b. h., cmp. preced.) *to tie, connect, to covenant* (Assyr. *ḫatânu, to protect.* Friedr. Del. Proleg. p. 91).

Hithpa. הִתְחַתֵּן, *Nithpa.* נִתְחַתֵּן *to become connected, to enter into the family, to intermarry.* Snh. 82[a] כאלו מִתְחַתֵּן בע״א as if he connected himself with idols. Gen. R. s. 82, beg. שנ׳ ביהודית וכ׳ who married Judith &c. Sifré Deut. 52, a. e. שנ׳ ... עם וכ׳ when Solomon married the daughter of Pharaoh; a. fr.

חֲתַן ch. same. Y. Sot. IX, end, 24[c] [read:] חוון בעון מְחַתְּנְתֵיה לנסיותא, they desired to ally him to the Nasi family; Y. Ab. Zar. III, 42[c] bot הוון אילין .. בעון מהוֹחנתיה (read: מְיחַתּ׳) members of the Nasi family desired to take him into the family.

Ithpa. אִתְחַתַּן *to become connected.* Targ. I Sam. XVIII, 22, sq.; a. fr.—Y. Sabb. XII, 13[c] bot. אִיתְחַתְּנוּן וכ׳, v. נְשִׂיאוּתָא.

חָתָן m. (b. h.; preced.) *connection, son-in-law; bridegroom;* (metaph., with ref. to the covenant of circumcision, v. בְּרִית) *the infant fit for circumcision.* B. Bath. 98[b] ח׳ הדר וכ׳ a son-in-law who lives in the house of his father-in-law. Pes. 113[a] הוי זהיר... מַחֲתַנְךָ הראשון guard thy wife against her former affianced. Y. Ned. III, end, 38[b] (ref. to Ex. IV, 24 sq) משה קרוי ח׳ Moses is called the *ḥathan* ... (and she said) ח׳ דמים מתבקשין ממך (ed. מתבקש) husband, blood (circumcision) is asked of thee; תינוק קרוי ח׳ the infant is called the *ḥathan*, (and she said) ח׳ בדמים אתה עומד לי child of the covenant, a high price I pay for thee; Bab. ib 32[a]; Ex. R. s. 5 חֲתָנִי תהיה את וכ׳ thou shalt be my affianced by covenant, thou art given to me &c. Nidd. V, 3 an infant one day old . . . is לאביו . . כח׳ שלם (as regards mourning ceremonies) like a perfect circumcised child to his parents &c. — Ber. II, 5 ח׳ פטור וכ׳ a bride-groom in the first night is exempt &c. Keth. 8[a] (in wedding benedictions) משמח ח׳ עם הכלה who causest the bridegroom to rejoice with the bride; a. fr.—Trnsf. (cmp. בַּעְלָא) *the fructifying rain.* Ber. 59[b]; Taan. 6[b] משיצא ח׳ לקראת כלה when the bridegroom goes forth to meet the bride, i. e. when the falling rain-drops meet the water on the ground and bubble; [oth. opin.; when the rivulets formed by the rain meet each other in gutters.]—*Pl.* חֲתָנִים. Keth. l. c. Ib.[b], v. בְּרָכָה; a. fr.—

חַתְנָא, חֲתָנָא ch. same. Targ. Ex. IV, 25, sq. (Targ. Y. II ib. 26 חתנת, corr. acc.).—Targ. I Sam. XVIII, 18.— Targ. Is. LXII, 5; a. fr.—Yeb. 52[a] ח׳ דדאיר a son-in-law who resides &c., v. הוּר. Hull. 83[a] בי ח׳ in the bridegroom's family; a. fr.—*Pl.* חַתְנִין. Targ. Jer. VII, 34; a. e. —Sabb. 23[b] חַתְנֵי Ms. O. sons-in-law, v. חַתְנוּתָא.

חֲתָנוּת f. (preced. wds.) *marital relation, intermarriage, wedlock* (connubium). Ab. Zar. 31[b], a. e. משום ח׳ as a guard against intermarriage (between Jews and gentiles). Ib. 36[b], v. אִישּׁוּת. Yeb. 76[a] לית להו ח׳ they have no connubium (a marriage with them is not legally recognized); a. e.—בית ח׳ *additional rooms for the young couple* in the bridegroom's paternal house. B. Bath. VI, 4 (98[b]). Taan. 14[b].

חַתְנוּתָא ch. same. Targ. G. I Deut. XXXII, 50.—*Pl.* חַתְנְוָתָא *connections through marriage, sons-in-law* &c. Sabb. 23[b] הוו ליה ח׳ רבנן (Ms. O. חַתְנֵי) will have scholars in the family through intermarriage.

חתנת, v. חָתָן.

חֲתַף=חֲטַף. Targ. Job. IX, 12 ed. Lag. (ed. חטף).

חָתַר (b. h.; cmp. חָתַת) *to dig, break in, make an opening.* Kidd. 24[b] לַחְתּוֹר לי שיני Ar. (ed. לַחְתּוֹר לו שינו) scrape my tooth (to clean it). Deut. R. s. 2 (ref. to וַיֵּעָתֵר, II Chr. XXXIII, 13) וַיַּחְתֹּר לו וכ׳ the Lord made an opening for his prayer; ח׳ את הרקיע He broke through the heavens; Y. Snh. X, 28[c] bot.; Ruth R. to II, 14 ח׳ לו חתירה וכ׳ (v. Snh. 103[a]).—Ex. R. s. 37 נטל את הצפורן לַחְתּוֹר וכ׳ (Ar. s. v. צפורן: לחפור) he took the digging tool to undermine his father's house; Lev. R. s. 10 (לחתך, לחתוך את אביו אחתוך) (corr. acc.). Gen. R. s. 63 (ref. to וַיֶּעְתַּר, Gen. XXV, 21, v. supra) like a prince שהיה חוֹתֵר על אביו ליטרא וכ׳ who undertook a siege (for military practice) against his father for a *litra* of gold (for the winner) והיה זה ח׳ מבפנים וכ׳ and so the one did mine from within &c. (the father assisting his son's efforts).—Snh. 109[a] וחוֹתְרִים שם and broke in there; Gen. R. s. 27; a. fr.—Part. pass. חָתוּר, f. חֲתוּרָה, pl. חֲתוּרִים, חֲתוּרוֹת. B. Kam. 114[b] היתה מחתרת ח׳ וכ׳ his house was broken into. Ib. 23[a] סתם דלתות ח׳ הן וכ׳ with reference to dogs, ordinary doors are subject to being broken in, i. e. the owner of a dog is responsible for damages done by breaking in.

חֲתַר ch. same. Targ. Ez. VIII, 8; a. e.

Ithpa. אִתְחַתַּר, *Ithpe.* אִתְחֲתַר, אִיתְ׳, 1) *to be broken into.* M. Kat. 25^b אִיתְחַתְּרוּ שבעין מחתרתא וכ׳ Ms. M. (ed. אִיתְחַתְּרוּ) seventy robberies were committed in Tiberias (ed. in N'hardea). Snh. 109^a אִתְחַתְּרִין ..... מחתרתא וכ׳ (Ms. O. אִיתְחַתְּרוּ וכ׳) that night three hundred robberies were committed in S.—2) *to break in for one's self.* Targ. Ez. XII, 7.

חֲתַרְתָּה, תְּרְתָּא, v. חֲתִירְתָּא.

חתת (b. h.) *to break, shatter.* Hull. 27^a (play on וזבחת Deut. XII, 21) ממקום שזב חַתֵּהוּ from where the blood flows, break it (the animal's life); ממאי דהאי חתהו לישנא דמתבר הוא what proof have you, that this *hottehu* has the meaning of breaking? (Answ. ref. to תחת, Deut. I, 21). [Ib. חִתּוּי formed fr. חִתָּה *Pi.*, sec. r. of חתת.]

ט

ט *Teth,* the ninth letter of the Alphabet. It interchanges dialectically with צ, as טביא a. צבי, with ת, as חתך a. חתח; with ד, as דפק a. טפק.

ט׳, as a numeral, *nine,* v. א׳.—Maas. Sh. IV, 11, v. ט״ת.

טא, v. טַאטֵא.

טְאֵב, טָאִיב, טְאֵב (=h. טוב) *to be bright, good, well.*— ט׳ ל־, ט׳ על *to feel well, be happy.* Dan. VI, 24.—Targ. I Sam. XVI, 23 (ed. Wil. טַב).

טָאבָא m. (preced.) *good (thing).*—*Pl.* טָאבֵי. Targ. Prov. XIV, 22 (ed. Wil. טָבֵי).

טאוי, Tosef B. Kam. X, 2, v. טְוִי.

טַאטֵא (Palp. of טא, cmp. טהר) [*to brighten,*] *to sweep.* R. Hash. 26^b; Meg. 18^a שקולי טאטיתא וטַאטֵי ביתא (Ms. M. 2 טאטיך וכ׳) take the (thy) broom and sweep the house (from which the Rabbis learned the meaning of Is. XIV, 23).

טַאטְאָ m., **טַאטִיתָא** f. (preced.) *broom.* R. Hash. 26^b; Meg. 18^a, v. preced.

טָאִיב, טָאִיב, v. טְאֵב.

טָאִיס, v. טוּס ch.

טָאִיף, v. טוּף ch.

טאירין, read: טְאָרִין, v. טְיַיר.

***טאל,** Y. Sabb. VII, 9^a top מטאלין מילריא, read: מן אילרן מ׳; cmp. Bab. ib. 70^a.

טָנִיס, טָאנִיס, טְאָנִיס pr. n. pl. (h. צֹעַן) *Tanis* (*Zoan*) in Lower Egypt. Targ. Num. XIII, 22. Targ. Y. Gen. XLI, 50 (h. text און). Targ. Y. Ex. I, 11 (h. text פתם); a. e.

טָאֵס, v. טוּס ch.

טָאֵף, v. טוּף ch.

***טארגא,** Midr. Till. to Ps. I (ed. Bub. איסקוטא), a gloss to תְּרִיס, (Ital. *targa*) *buckler,* v. Yalk. Ps. 833.

***טאריקי,** Ex. R. s. 11 בט׳, read: קְטָאדִיקִי.

טַב I (contr. of טאב) = h. טוֹב, *to be good, well.*— טב ל־ *to feel well, be satisfied, fare well.* Targ. Deut. XV, 16; a. e.

Af. אָטִיב *to do good.* Targ. Zech. XII, 4 לְאָטָבָא (ed. Lag. לאוט׳). V. טוֹב, a. יְטַב.

טַב II m., **טָבָא** c., **טַבְתָּא** f. (preced.) 1) *good, precious.* Targ. Gen. II, 9.—Targ. II, Esth. I, 19 דטבא ed. Lag. (oth. ed. דְּטַבַת)—Targ. Jud. V, 26 (missing in ed. Lag.); a. v. fr.—Gen. R. s. 22; Lev. R. s. 22, v. בְּרִישׁ. Ber. 60^b כל מאי דעביד ... לטב (v. Rabb. D. S. a. l. note) whatever God does is for a good purpose. Tam. 32^a דידי טבא מינה וכ׳ my advice is better than yours.—Lev. R. s. 33, beg. ט׳ וכ׳ from it (the tongue) comes what is good &c.; a. v. fr.— 2) *worth, valued.* Y. Keth. IV, end, 29^b חד בית בטב וכ׳ (ed. Krot. חד ביתא טב) read: בדב, a house worth &c. Ib. מכיין דלית ביתא טב וכ׳ as the house is not worth more than &c.— Y. Peah I, 15^d bot. מילא דט׳ דכוותה something of equal value; Gen. R. s. 35, end (corr. acc.); a. fr.—3) *best man, elder, officer.* Y. Taan. IV, 68^d top טב קרתא an officer of the town.—*Pl.* טָבִין, טָבַיָּא, טָבֵי; fem. טָבָן, טָבָאתָא, טָבְתָא. Targ. Mic. VII, 1. Targ. Ps. CXXV, 4; a. fr.—B. Mets. 44^b שלים לה ט׳ וכ׳ pay her in good and full-weight coin. Y. Snh. X, 28^b bot. כל טָבָן וכ׳, v. נְחֲמְתָא. Lam. R. to I, 1 רבתי (1 חד מאת) טבאתא the good fruits; a. fr.—4) (adv.) *much, more.* Targ. Prov. XVII, 10.—Gitt. 14^b טב טב רמו ליה Ar. (ed. only one טב) strike him more (or, *it is right,* v. Rashi a. l.)—Y. Shek. IV, 48^a top, v. טַבָּאוּת.

טַב III, עֵין טַב pr. n. pl. *En Tab,* a place where the New Moon was proclaimed in the days of Rabbi (v. Neub. Géogr. p. 272). R. Hash. 25^a; Y. ib. II, 58^a bot.; Y. Taan. II, 66^a bot. עיינר טב; Pesik. R. s. 41 עֵיןטַב.

טָבָא, v. טַב II.

טָבָא (טְבָא) *rumor,* v. טִיב II.

טִבָא, v. טְבַע.

***טַבָּאג** m. *tabag,* name of a jewel in the High-priest's breastplate. Targ. Cant. V, 14 (Fl., to Levy Targ. Dict. I, 426^2, suggests טבאז = *topaz*).

טָבָאוֹת, טַבְוָואוֹת) טָבָאוֹת (טַבְוָואוֹת), טָבוּת f. (v. טַב a. טַבְוָא) (*in a*) *good manner, well, properly* (h. הֵיטֵב). Targ. Y. Deut. IX, 21; a. e.—Y. Ber. V, 9ᶜ top לא עבדין ט׳ do not do right. Cant. R. to I, 1 מאן דקרי ט׳ וכ׳ I will go to whosoever explains the Bible well etc. — Y. Shebu. VII, 38ᵃ bot. אין אתא הא ט׳ if he appears, it is well. Y. Shek. IV, 48ᵃ top וטבות כן Bab. ed. (Y. ed. וטבא) and so it is right. Y. Maas. Sh. I, 52ᵈ top וטבבו כן (corr. acc.)—Hebr. form: טָבִית. Meïl. 17ᵃ ט׳ אמר he spoke well (he is right).

טַבַּאי, pr. n. m. *Tabbai*. Ab. I, 8; a. fr.

טָבְאַל (Is. VII, 6) pr. n. place (!) *Tobal*. Y. Ab. Zar. I, beg. 39ᵃ חיזרנו .... מקום ששמו ט׳ we searched the whole Bible and could not find a place by the name of Tobal.

טבב, Y. Maas. Sh. I, 52ᵈ top וטבבו, read: וְטָבוּת.

טַבְהַק m., pl. טַבְהֲקֵי (Pers. tâbah, tâvah, tapak, Lag. Ges. Abh. p. 49) (*pieces of*) *roasted meat*. Erub. 29ᵇ bot. (Ar. sing.; ed. Ven. ט׳ ט׳ pieces after pieces &c.).

טַבְוָא, טֵבְוָא, טַבְוָות, טַבְוַת f. constr. טַבְוַת, (טבי, sec. r. of טב) *beneficence, good deed.* Targ. Mic. VII, 20 (perh. pl.). — *Pl.* טַבְוָון, טַבְוָן, טַבְוָתָא. Ib. (ed. Lag. טַבְוָן). Targ. Gen. XXXII, 11; a. e.

טַבְוָאוֹת, טַבְוָו׳, v. טָבָאוֹת.

טָבוֹחַ m. (infin. of טָבַח) 1) *slaughtering and preparing the pilgrim's offering.* Ḥag. II, 4 (17ᵃ) יום ט׳ וכ׳ the slaughtering day is observed after the Sabbath. Y. ib. 78ᵃ bot. יומה הוא טְבוֹחָהּ its day (the festive day itself) is its slaughtering day.—2) *Taboah*, name of a windstorm (demon). Sabb. 129ᵇ.

טִבּוּלָא, טִבּוּל, v. טִיב׳.

טבוסה, Y. Sabb. VI, 7ᵈ (P'nê Mosh. סכוסה), read סְבָכָה or שְׂבָכָה, v. סָבוּל; cmp. Bab. ib. 57ᵇ.

טִבּוּעִין, v. טִיבּוּעִין.

טִבּוּר, טַבּוּר, v. טִיבּוּר.

טָבוּת I, v. טָבָאוֹת.

טָבוּת II pr. n. m. *Tabuth*. Snh. 97ᵃ, v. טַבְיוֹמִי; B. Mets. 49ᵃ (Ms. Alf. טָאבוּת, v. Rabb. D. S. a. l. note 6).

טַבּוּתָא, v. טִיבוּ.

טַבְזָא, v. טַפְזָא.

טָבַח, (b. h.) *to prepare a feast*, esp. *to slaughter and dress meat, to cook.* Keth. 4ᵃ טִבְחוֹ טָבוּחַ his meat for the feast is ready (for cooking).—Bets. 25ᵃ (expl. בית טביחה) מקום שטּוֹבַחַת וכ׳ the place where the animal cooks (digests) its food.

טְבַח ch. same. Ber. 56ᵃ טַבְחַתְּ ולא אכלת thou shalt prepare and not eat. Sabb. 129ᵇ הוה ט׳ להו וכ׳ it (the wind or demon טָבוֹחַ) would have feasted on them (the Israelites), on their flesh and their blood; a.e.—V. בִּטְבִּיזְיָא.

Pa. טַבַּח same. Gen. R. s. 57, end טבח טַבְּחוּן Tebah (Gen. XXII, 24) means, 'Slaughter them' v. בַּחְמוּן.

טֶבַח m. (b. h.; preced. wds.) 1) *the meat for a feast.* Keth. 4ᵃ, v. טָבַח.—2) *feast*, trnsf. *onslaught.* Gen. R. s. 83 (ref. to Is. XXXIV, 6) אעפ״כ ט׳ גדול וכ׳ nevertheless the main onslaught will be in the land of Edom (Rome); Pesik. R. s. 14, end; s. 15; Yalk. Num. 759.

טַבָּח m. (preced.) *meat-dresser, butcher, cook.* Bets. 28ᵃ ט׳ אומן a professional butcher; a. fr. — *Pl.* טַבָּחִים. Kidd. IV, 14; a. e.

טַבָּחָא ch. same. Targ. Y. Lev. I, 5.— Targ. I Sam. IX, 23, sq. — Ḥull. 18ᵃ; a. e. — *Pl.* fem. טַבָּחָן. Targ. I Sam. VIII, 13.

טִבְחָא, טַבְחָא ch.=h. טֶבַח. Targ. Prov. VII, 22.— Gen. R. s. 65 לקבל תורא ט׳ according to the size of the ox is the feast (as you call Esau (Rome) great, so will his punishment be great, ref. to Is. XXXIV, 6); Pesik. Haḥod. p. 56ᵇ; Pesik. R. s. 15 (read לפום for נפיל); Cant. R. to II, 15 טבחיא (corr. acc.).

***טַבְּחוֹן**, v. טְבַח.

טָבִי I pr. n. m. (cmp. טַבְיָא) *Tabi.* 1) a slave. Ber. II, 7; a fr.—2) name of several Amoraim. R. Hash. 22ᵃ. Meg. 6ᵇ; a. e.—3) *T. Rishba* (*the hunter*, Rashi). Sabb. 17ᵇ top.

טָבִי II, כְּפַר ט׳ pr. n. pl. *K'far Tabi*, near Lydda. Bets. 5ᵃ; R. Hash. 31ᵇ. Tosef. Ohol. IV, 2 כ׳ טַבְיָא (Var. טמא).

טַבְיָא m. (=h. צְבִי) *deer, gazelle.* Targ. Deut. XII, 15; a. fr. — Snh. 95ᵃ. Ḥull. 59ᵇ, v. קֶרֶשׁ II; a. e. — Ib. 59ᵃ בר ט׳ a young deer. — *Pl.* טַבְיֵי, טַבַיָּא. Targ. II Sam. II, 18; a. e. — Keth. 103ᵇ וצידנא טביא (Rashi: וצדיינא טביי) and I caught deer. — Fem. pl. טַבְיָן, טָבְיָן. Targ. I Kings V, 3. Targ. Y. Deut. XIV, 5. — Y. Snh. VII, end, 25ᵈ.—[Y. Ter. IX, end, 48ᵇ מה טביה, v. טִיב I ch.]

טַבְיוֹמִי pr. n. m. *Tabyomi*. Snh. 97ᵃ ... רב טבות וא״ל רב ט׳ his name was R. Tabuth, some say, R. Tabyomi. Kidd. 14ᵇ. Men. 70ᵃ ט׳ בר קיסנא (Ms. M. טובי, v. Rabb. D. S. a. l. note).—Gen. R. s. 4. Ex. R. s. 93, end.

טְבִיחָה f. (טָבַח) 1) *slaughtering;* 2) *digestion.* Bets. III, 3 בית טְבִיחָתָהּ the place where it is cut (neck); ib. 25ᵃ מאי לאו מבית ט׳ ממש וכ׳ does this not mean actually from the place etc.? No, במקום שטובחת וכ׳ v. טָבַח.

טְבִילָה f. (טָבַל I) 1) *dipping.* Mekh. Bo, Pisha, s. 11 (ref. to Ex. XII, 22) על כל הגיעה ט׳ you must dip the hyssop into the blood for each time you strike. Sifra Vayikra, Ḥobah, ch. III, Par. 3. — Zeb. 93ᵇ; a. fr. — 2) *immersion, purification.* Yoma 88ᵃ, a. fr. ט׳ בזמנה

מצוה 'ט the immersion in due time is obligatory (must not be postponed). Kerith. 9ᵃ; a. v. fr.—*Pl.* טְבִילוֹת. Men. 7ᵇ שיעור ט' enough for all dippings.—Yoma l. c.; a. fr. חייבי ט' those bound to take an immersion. Nidd. 29ᵇ ומטבילין אותה.....ט' and we make her take immersions at intervals during ninety five days; a. fr.

טְבִילוּתָא ch. same. Snh. 39ᵃ ומי סלקא ט' בנורא is the law requiring immersion (for levitical purification) complied with by putting the object in fire? Ib. עיקר ט' וכ' the true purification is by fire (ref. to Num. XXXI, 23).

טְבִילְתָא f. same. Nidd. 30ᵃ ט' יתירתא (Rashi טבילה) an additional immersion.

טְבִיעָה I f. (טָבַע I) *being drowned.* Num. R. s. 14, beg. שהסרתי אותו מן חט' וכ' whom I saved from drowning through the intervention of &c. [Y. Ber. V, 9ᵇ תשנו מטביעה, v. מְטְבֵּעַ.]

טְבִיעָה II, v. next w.

טְבִיעוּת f. (טָבַע II) *impression;* ט' עַיִן *identification of an object from a general impression of its form* without stating particular marks. Sabb. 114ᵃ... שמחזירין בט' העין to whom a lost object is restored on his identification etc. [Some ed. טְבִיעַת.]

טְבִיעוּתָא ch., טְבִיעוּת עֵינָא same. Gitt. 27ᵇ; B. Mets. 19ᵃ אי סימנא... או ט'ע' וכ if you require a special mark, I have one on it, if you require identification on general impression, I have it (I recognize it). Ib. 23ᵇ... להדורי מרבנן בט' ע' as to restoring it to a scholar on his identification &c., v. preced.—Hull. 96ᵃ אית לן ט' ע' בגויה we know him by his general impression (not by special marks). Ib. ט' ע' דקלא identification by one's voice; a. fr.

טְבִירְיוֹס, טְבִירְיָא, v. sub טבר'.

טָבִיתָה pr. n. f. (v. טָבִי I) *Tabitha,* name of a handmaid. Y. Nidd. II, beg. 49ᵈ.

טָבַל I (b. h.; cmp. טָבַע I) 1) *to dip.* Zeb. 93ᵇ, a. e. וט' ולא מספג, v. סָפַג.—2) *to immerse, to bathe for purification.* Yoma VII, 4 ירד וט' went down to the bath and took an immersion. Ber. 2ᵇ שהכהנים טוֹבְלִין וכ' when the priests (that have been unclean) bathe in order to be permitted to partake of their priestly share; a. v. fr.—Ib. 22ᵃ טוֹבְלֵי שחרין those taking a bath in the morning (after emission of semen virile); Y. ib. III, 6ᶜ top ט' שחרית.—Tosef. Yad. II, 20 טובלי שחרין (Var. טוֹבְלָנֵי) morning bathers (Essenes, v. Graetz Gesch. d. Jud. III², p. 468, a. for correct vers. R. S. to Yad. IV, 8).—*Part. pass.* טָבוּל.—טְבוּל יום (one who has bathed in day-time,) *one who has bathed but must wait for sunset to be perfectly clean* (Lev. XXII, 7). T'bul Yom I, 1; a. fr.—Nidd. 30ᵃ טְבוּלַת יום ארוך a woman after bathing whose day is adjourned (having to wait a long time for perfect levitical purity).—טְבוּל יוֹם *T'bul Yom,* name of a treatise of Mishnah and Tosefta of the order of *Tahăroth.*

Pi. טִיבֵּל 1) *to dip into vinegar, salt &c., to make tasty;* esp. *to take a luncheon, to take the first course of a meal consisting of relishes; to take the antepast.* Maasr. IV, 1 הַמְטַבֵּל בשדה he who makes a luncheon (of fruits) in the field. Pes. X, 3 מטבל בחזרת he takes lettuce as antepast. Tosef. ib. X, 9 לא טי' וכ' if he has eaten as antepast only &c. Pes. 107ᵇ אבל מטבל וכ' Ms. M. a. comment. (ed. מטביל) but he may make a luncheon of &c. Ib. חשמש מטבל בבני וכ' comment. (ed. מטביל; Tosef. ib. X, 5 מכביש, v. כָּבַשׁ); a. fr.—2) (cmp. תבל) *to season with spices.* *Part. pass.* מְטוּבָּל. Y. Shek. III, 47ᶜ top מבושל כמ' boiled (wine) is (in ritual law) like spiced wine; v. infra.

Hif. הִטְבִּיל 1) *to immerse* vessels for purification, *to order immersion.* Ter. II, 3 הַמַּטְבִּיל כלים וכ' he who immerses vessels on the Sabbath. Bets. II, 2 מַטְבִּילִין את הכל וכ' you must immerse whatever needs immersion (both persons and vessels) before &c.—Ib. 3 (17ᵇ), v. גַּב.—Nidd. 29ᵇ, v. טְבִילָה; a. fr.—2) *to take luncheon,* v. supra.—3) *to season.* Erub. 28ᵇ מטבילין בו וכ' they used to season the roast with it (in place of pepper).

Hof. הוּטְבַּל *to be immersed, to be made clean.* Mikv. V, 6 לא הוּטְבָּלוּ are not considered as clean through immersion; Tosef. ib. IV, 10.

טְבַל (טְבִיל) ch. same. Targ. Lev. IX, 9; a. fr.—*Part pass.* טְבִיל, f. טְבִילָא. Targ. Josh. III, 15 (טְבִילָן?).—Snh. 39ᵃ במאי טביל wherewith did he purify himself (after contact with a corpse)?; בנורא טביל he did it by means of fire, v. טְבִילָה. Nidd. 30ᵃ לִיטְבְּלָהּ let her bathe; a. fr.—

Af. אַטְבֵּיל as preced. *Hif.* 1) *to immerse, order immersion.* Nidd. l. c. אַטְבְּלִינַן לה we make her bathe. Bets. 19ᵃ לְאַטְבּוּלֵיה to immerse it; a. fr.—2) as preced. *Pi.* 1, *to take an antepast.* Pes. 114ᵇ למיהדר לְאַטְבּוּלֵי must take the bitter herb a second time; a. e.

טָבַל II (denom. of טֶבֶל) *to create Tebel, to make obligatory the setting aside of tithes &c.* Y. Maasr. IV, beg. 51ᵃ אור טוֹבֵל fire (roasting) makes subject to sacred gifts; מלח טוֹבֶלֶת salting makes subject &c.; a. fr.—*Part. part.* טָבוּל *that which is subject to sacred gifts, forbidden as Tebel.* Ber. 47ᵇ טבל ט' מדרבנן *Tebel* declared to be such by rabbinical enactment; a. e.—*Pl.* טְבוּלִים, טְבוּלִין. Y. Dem. VI, 25ᶜ bot., opp. מְתוּקָנִים. Ib. VII, 26ᵇ top פירות ט' fruits of which the sacred gifts have not been set aside.

Nif. נִטְבַּל *to become,* or *to be declared Tebel.* Y. Maasr. I, end, 49ᵇ טבל שנ' מדבריהן *Tebel* which is declared to be such by rabbinical law, v. supra. Ib. IV, beg. 51ᵃ נִטְבְּלוּ the roasted ears became subject to tithes; a. fr.

טְבַל ch. same. Men. 70ᵃ טַבְלָהּ לה (not טבלא) he made it subject to tithes. Bets. 13ᵃ טַבְלִנְהוּ ביומיה Ms. M. (ed. טבלא, corr. acc.) he made them *Tebel* on that day (by designating them for immediate use); a. e.

טֶבֶל m. (טָבַל I, v. *Pi.* a. *Hif.*) *fruits of which you are permitted to make a luncheon or improvised meal in the field without separating the priestly or levitical shares.* Ber. 35ᵇ אין הט' מתחייב וכ' the *tebel* is not subject to tithes, until it is brought home (for consumption or storage).—Esp. *Tebel, produces in* *that stage in which the separation of levitical and priestly shares respectively is required, before you may partake of them; eatables forbidden pending the separation of sacred gifts.* Ter. X, 6 חבילי תלתן של ט׳ bundles of fenugrec subject to T'rumah; expl. Bets. 13ᵃ. ט׳ טבול של תרומה (Rashi: לתרומה) *Tebel* considered as such, because it is subject to T'rumah (Deut. XVIII, 4; Ms. M. של ת׳ גדולה to the general gifts of T'rumah and tithes); ט׳ טבול של תרומת מעשר *Tebel* (in the possession of a Levite who received it for tithes, and) considered *Tebel*, because it is subject to the T'rumah from tithes (Num. XVIII, 26). Ter. IX, 6 הט׳ גדוליו וכ׳ the growth of seeds that had been subject to sacred gifts the separation of which had been omitted &c. Ib. 7 אע״פ שפירותיו ט׳ although its growth is considered *Tebel* (because the seeds were not tithed) &c. Kidd. 58ᵇ טִיבְלוֹ של וכ׳ his neighbor's *Tebel;* a. fr.—[Erub. 86ᵃ יש לו ט׳, read: טַבְלָא I.].—*Pl.* טְבָלִים. Ib.—Ned. 20ᵃ סופך להאכילך ט׳ he will finally give thee to eat things from which the tithes have not been given. Hull. 132ᵇ; a. e.

טִבְלָא ch. same. Nidd. 46ᵇ ט׳ דאורייתא *Tebel* by Biblical law (lacking the separation of T'rumah). Bets. 13ᵃ אסורייתא טובלא (some ed., corr. acc.), v. אֲסוּרְיְיתָא. Ib. התם לא ט׳ וכ׳ there (in the case of ears, ib.) it was not subject to T'rumah &c.; a. e.

טַבְלָא I (טבל, cmp. Aeth. טבלל *to tie around*, v. Ges. H. Dict.[10] s. v. טְבוּלִים; cmp. טבעת, טבור) *a bell or collection of bells,* an instrument especially used at public processions (in Arab. *drum*, Gr. ταβαλά; v. Sm. Ant. s. v. Tintinnabulum as to forms and uses of bells). Targ. Koh. VII, 5 קל ט׳ וכ׳ the music of the fools. Targ. Cant. I, 1.—Sot. 49ᵇ (expl. אִרוּס) ט׳ דחד פומא a *tabla* with one mouth (a single bell). Ber. 57ᵃ תלאי ט׳ וכ׳ (I dreamt) I suspended a *tabla* and shouted into it (differ. in Rashi). Sabb. 110ᵃ בט׳ to the sound of a *tabla* (at a wedding). M. Kat. 9ᵇ (prov.) בת שיתין . . . לקל ט׳ רהטא a woman of sixty years, like one of six, runs at the sound of the *tabla* (to see the procession). Y. Erub. VIII, 25ᵃ bot. אפי׳ ט׳ if even he has there a *t.* (which he dare not move on the Sabbath); Bab. ib. 86ᵃ יש לו טבל.—In gen. *musical instrument.* Arakh. 10ᵇ, v. גּוּרְגְּנָא.

טַבְלָא II, **טַבְלָה** f. (tabula, tabella, τάβλα) *plank, board, tablet for writing; book of accounts, list; will.* Erub. IV, 8 (49ᵇ) כטבלה מרובעת (Talm. ed. כטבלא) like a square tablet. R. Hash. II, 8 (24ᵃ) כל הט׳ בכותל Ms. M. (ed. בט׳ ובכותל, v. Rabb. D. S. a. l. note) (drawings of the phases of the moon) on a tablet on the wall. Gitt. 20ᵃ כתב שע״ג ט׳ ופינקס writing (of manumission) on a tablet or on a board (account book or will, v. Treat. 'Ăbadim, ed. Kirchh. ch. III, Rev. des Etudes Juives 1883, p. 150). Y. Snh. I, 18ᵈ bot. ט׳ של רפואות list of (superstitious) remedies (Pes. 56ᵃ ספר וכ׳); a. fr.—[Y. Bets. I, 60ᶜ bot. טבלה ברוריתא וכ׳ (read טַבְלָתָה *pl.*) the outside stone plates of the colonnade of Asi.]—*Pl.* טַבְלָוֹת, טַבְלָאוֹת. Y. B. Bath. VI, 14ᶜ bot. ט׳ של שיש וכ׳ polished marble plates for walls. Yalk. Ex. 426 ונראין ט׳ ט׳ וכ׳ and they appeared like marked off squares surrounding &c. Pes. 57ᵃ ט׳ של זהב gold plates.—Chald. pl. טַבְלָתָה, v. supra.

טַבְלָא III pr. n. m. *Tabla*, an Amora. Hull. 132ᵇ Y. Gitt. IV, 46ᵃ; a. e; v. next w.

טַבְלַאי, טַבְלֵיי pr. n. m. *Tablai*, an Amora. Y. Erub. V, 25ᵃ bot.; (Sabb. 101ᵃ טַבְלָא).—Y. Sabb. VI, 8ᵃ bot.; a. e.

טַבְלָה, v. טַבְלָא II.

טַבְלֵיי, v. טַבְלַאי.

*__טַבְלָר__ m. (tabellarius) *courier.*—*Pl.* טַבְלָרִין. Pesik. R. s. 21 [read:] ט׳ שלו ושמו חקוק על לבם כהדין איספרגים the angels are His couriers, and His name is engraven upon their hearts like a seal (v. Pesik. Bahod, p. 108ᵇ, note 161); Midr. Till. to Ps. XVII ed. Bub. (corr. acc.).

טַבְלָרָא ch. same. Targ. Prov. XXIV, 34 (h. text איש מגן).

טָבַע I (b. h.; cmp. טָבַל I) 1) (act. verb) *to sink, drown.* Gitt. 56ᵇ לטוֹבְעוֹ to drown him (sink his ship). Ib. טְבָעוֹ He drowned him; a. fr.—2) (neut. verb) *to sink, be drowned.* Ber. 16ᵇ טָבְעָה ספינתו וכ׳ if his ship went down &c. Meg. 10ᵇ; Snh. 39ᵇ מעשה ידי טוֹבְעִין וכ׳ my creatures (Egyptians) are perishing in the sea, and you want to sing?; a. e.

Hif. הִטְבִּיעַ *to sink.* Yalk. Gen. 120 ה׳ האבן He made the stone sink down to the depth &c.; (Pirké d'R. El. ch. XXXV, וְטָבְעָה האבן; Midr. Till. to Ps. XCI, end וטבע אותה). Yalk. Ex. 241 לְהַטְבִּיעַ את מצרים to drown the Egyptians; a. e.

טְבַע ch. same. Targ. Y. Gen. IV, 8.—Targ. I Sam. XVII, 49; a. e.—Pes. 40ᵇ דְטָבְעָא . . ארבא וכ׳ a ship with wheat sank &c. Sabb. 108ᵇ מעולם לא ט׳ וכ׳ never was yet a man drowned in the Lake of Sodom. B. Bath. 153ᵃ אמרה ליטְבַּע ארביה (Ms. H. אמרה ליה טבאר וכ׳, Ar. אמרה לו טבאר) said she, May his (thy) ship go under; a. e.—[Targ. Y. Deut. XXVIII, 29 טבריק some ed., read. חב׳, v. חֲבַע.]

Pa. טַבַּע *to sink.* B. Bath. 73ᵃ גלא דמְטַבַּע וכ׳ the wave which threatens to sink the ship. Hull. 60ᵃ אתא מיטרא טַבְּעֵיה בימא there came a rain and sank the provision into the sea.

Ithpa. אִיטַּבַּע *to be sunk.* Targ. O. Ex. XV, 4.

טָבַע II [*to round, shape,* denom. טֶבַע, fr. which טָבַע] 1) *to coin.* Snh. IV, 5 (37ᵃ) אדם טוֹבֵעַ כמה מטבעות בחותם וכ׳, v. חוֹתָם; Y. ib. VI, 22ᵇ bot.; a. e.—Trnsf. *to formulate.* Gitt. 5ᵇ, a. e. כל המשנה ממטבע שֶׁטָּבְעוּ וכ׳ he who deviates from the formula of the deed of divorce which the scholars have fixed. Ber. 40ᵇ כל המשנה... שט׳... בברכות he who changes the formula of benedictions which &c.; a. fr.—2) *to specify, mention explicitly.* Num. R. s. 20 (ref. to Deut. XXVII, 12, sq.) . . . . בברכות היה מזכירן לא היה טוֹבְעָן in ordering blessings He mentioned them (the people) . . ., but in ordering curses He did not mention them explicitly; (Tanḥ. Balak 12 לא היה מזכירם; ed. Bub. 18 תובען, Yalk. Num. 766 תובעין, incorr.).

טְבַע ch. same, *to assume shape.* Targ. Prov. VIII, 25 נִטְבְּעוּן.

טֶבַע m. (v. טָבַע II) 1) *coin, medal.* טִבְעוֹ של פ׳ יצא one's coin passes, i. e. one's authority is recognized. Shebu. 6^b^ זו רומי חייבת שטִּיבְעָהּ וכ׳ Ms. M. (ed. פרס) that is wicked Rome whose government is recognized all over the world. Meg. 14^b^ לא יצא טִבְעֲךָ בעולם thou art not yet the legitimate king; cmp. מוֹנִיטָא. [Y. Ber. V, 9^b^ מטבעה של תפלה ed. Lehm., oth. ed. מטבריעה, v. מַטְבֵּעַ.]—2) *Teb'a*, a coin equal to half a Sela. Y. Shek. II, 46^d^ top (the ten brothers) sold Rachel's first-born for twenty silver pieces (denars) ונפל לכל א׳ וא׳ מהם ט׳ so that a Teb'a came upon each (Bab. ed. טבעה, טיבעה, Ms. M. טובע).—*Pl.* טְבָעִים, טְבָעִין (טוֹבְעִין, fr. טוֹבַע). Shek. II, 4. Y. l. c. טו׳ פלגי סלעין (Bab. טבעין) *tib'in* i. e. half-Shekels. — 3) *that which is to be shaped, substance, element.*—*Pl.* as ab. Num. R. s. 14 כנגד ארבעה ט׳ וכ׳ corresponding to the four elements of which the Lord created &c. [In later Hebr.: *nature, character; Nature.*]

טְבַע II, **טִבְעָא**, **טִיב׳** I ch. same, *coin; Teb'a.* Targ. Y. Gen. XXIV, 22 Levita (ed. דרכמונא; v. Y. Shek. II, 46^d^ top, quot. in preced.). Targ. Y. Ex. XXX, 13 (ed. Amst. טַבְעָא). Targ. II Esth. VI, 10 טִבְעִי וטִבְעָךְ אזיל וכ׳, v. preced.—B. Mets. 46^a^ דליכא עלייהו ט׳ which have no stamp. Ib. 44^b^ הוי ט׳ is considered as coin (money), opp. to פירא merchandise. Shebu. 6^b^ ט׳ דמאן וכ׳ the coin of which goes farther (whose power is greater)? — Nidd. 20^b^ ט׳ דבבל וכ׳ the Babylonian coin (which I could not understand) was the cause &c.; a. fr. —*Pl.* טִבְעֵי. B. Mets. 25^a^ ט׳ מכריז Ms. H. a. R. (ed. sing.). he publishes that he has found 'coins'.

טִבְעָא, **טִיבְעָא** II m. = h. טְבִיעָה, *shipwreck.* B. Bath. 153^a^ לא איפרק מט׳ (Ms. M. מטונשרה) did not escape the loss through shipwreck (which the woman had wished him.)

(טִבְעִים) טִי׳, **טִבְעִין**, **טִבְעוֹן** pr. n. pl. *Tibon* or *Tibin* (prob. *Tubun*, west of Sepphoris, Neub. Géogr. p. 196). Makhsh. I, 3, v. חֲלִיקוּפְרֵי.—Tosef. Meg. II, 5; Y. ib. IV, beg. 74^c^ בה״כ של טיבעין the synagogue of T.—Sifré Deut. 323 איש טיבעים; Yalk. Deut. 946 כפר טיבעין.—[Erub. 29^a^ bot. לטיבעין (Var. טבעים, v. Rabb. D. S. a. l. note 6), missing in Tosef. ib. IX (VI), 4, v. עֲרָדִיסְקוֹס.]

טִבְעוֹנִי m. (preced.) *of Tibon, Tibonite.* — *Pl.* טִבְעוֹנִין, טִי׳. Y. Ber. II, 4^d^ bot.; Meg. 24^b^ אנשי טבעונין (prob. to be read: טִבְעוֹן).

טִבְעִין, **טִבְעִים**, v. טִבְעוֹן.

טַבַּעַת f. (b. h.; טָבַע II) *round band, ring.* Tosef. Kel. B. Mets. II, 1 ט׳ שהוא חוגר וכ׳ a ring which one puts around his loins; ט׳ של אצבע finger ring; Sabb. 52^b^. Ib.; Kel. XII, 1 ט׳ אדם ornamental ring; ט׳ בהמה והכלים a ring used for beasts or for garments (for fastening); a. fr.—Esp. *seal-ring.* Sabb. 59^b^. Deut. R. s. 2; a. fr.—הֲסָרַת ט׳ the authority given by transfer of the ring. Meg. 14^a^; Lam. R. to IV, 22. — *Pl.* טַבָּעוֹת. Sabb. l. c.; a. fr.—Ab. d'R. N. ch. XVIII ט׳ ט׳, v. מַטְבֵּעַ.—Trnsf. (פי הט׳) *anus, end of the rectum.* B. Kam. 92^a^. Sabb. 108^b^ bot.; a. fr. —Y. ib. VIII, end, 11^c^ לטבעות, read לטבעת, v. אַמְבָּטִיתָא.

טברטי, v. טבריטי.

(טְבֵירְיָא) טִיבְ׳, **טְבֶרְיָה**, **טְבַרְיָא** pr. n. pl. *Tiberias* in Galilee. Targ. Y. I Num. XXXIV, 8, v. חַמַּת. Targ. Y. I Deut. III, 17 (?). Ib. XXXIII, 23.—Gen. R. s. 23, beg. ט׳ ע״ש טיבירייאוס Tiberias is named after Tiberius; Yalk. Ps. 758 (corr. acc.). Gen. R. s. 31, v. בִּטְרִיָּא. Meg. 6^a^; a. fr.—Y. Taan. IV, 69^b^ bot. טיברי (corr. acc.).—Denom. טִבְרָנִי, f. טִבְרָנִית. Y. Hall. II, 58^c^ bot. Y. Pes. X, 37^c^ bot. ט׳ ישנה old Tiberian measure.—*Pl.* טִבְרָנִיּוֹת. Y. Keth. I, 25^b^ top סבירינות (corr. acc.), v. חָנָן. — *Ch.* טִבְרָיָאָה, pl. טִבְרָיָאֵי. Y. Taan. l. c. Y. Bets. II, 61^b^ top טיבראי (corr. acc.)

טִבֵּר׳, **טִבְרִיוֹס** pr. n. m. *Tiberius*, the Roman emperor. Yalk. Ps. 758 (not ת . . . .); Gen. R. s. 23 טיברייאוס, טיבירייאוס, v. preced.

טברירי, **טברטי**, **טבריטי**, Pesik. Hashsh'mini, p. 191^b^ Ms. O. (ed. טוב בעי); Pesik. R., addit. (ed. Fr., p. 201, v. Var. lect. notes a. l.),— a corruption, prob. to be read: טִיָּטְרוֹן or תֵּיאַטְרוֹן (q. v.) *theatre, spectators*, opp. קנגיא (κυνήγιον) the participants in the fights of the arena; cmp. בלטוורא.

טִבֵּר (denom. of טיבור) [*to measure the length from shoulder to belly*, v. Macc. III, 13, a. Bart. a. l.; Tosef. ib. V (IV), 15,] *to lash a transgressor* with a strap commensurate to his size (v. מַלְקוּת). Y. Yoma V, 42^c^ (expl. מצליף, Mish. V, 5) כמְטַבֵּיר Ar. s. v. צלף (ed. כמטוורד, read כִּמְצַוֵּיר, cmp. צַיּוֹרָא) like the movement of the lasher in court; (cmp. Bab. ib. 55^a^ top כמנגדנא).

טֵבֵת (b. h.); *Tebeth*, the tenth month of the Hebrew calendar, containing twenty nine days, varying between the second of December and the twenty ninth of January. Targ. Esth. II, 16. Targ. II Esth. III, 7. Ib. 8 מלקטין פשרי דט׳ store up the melting snows of Tebeth (in their cisterns).—Taan. 6^b^ טבא . . . . דט׳ מנוולתא auspicious is the year whose Tebeth is ugly (muddy from heavy rains); דט׳ ארמלתא whose Tebeth is a widow (without rain, v. בַּצָּלָא).

***טַבַּת** f. (v. טָבְאוּת) (*in a*) *good condition, right.* Gen. R. s. 26 (ref. to טֹבֹת, Gen. VI, 2) טבת כתיב משהיו מטיבין וכ׳ you may read *tabbath* (that they were all right); when people had made the bride ready &c.

טַבְתָּא, v. טַב.

טגיות, Sifré Deut. 234 quot. in Ar. (ed. ריגא), v. טוֹגָא.

טגים, Pesik R. s. 43, v. טִיגָן, s. v. טִיגָּן.

טָגֵן, *Pi.* טִיגֵּן, v. טִיגֵּן.

טִיגְרִס, טִיגְרוֹס m. (tigris, v. Sm. Ant. s. v.) *tiger.* Hull. 59[b] ט׳ אריה וכ׳ the tiger is the lion of Be-Ilai (the mountains of interior Asia), i. e. what the lion is in other regions.

טָדִי pr. n. m. *Tadi,* ט׳ (שַׁעַר), name of a northern gate of the Temple. Midd. I, 3; 9; II, 3 (Var. טרי).

טָהוֹר, טְהוֹרָה m., f. (b. h.; next w.) 1) *clean, pure; not subject to levitical uncleanness.* B. Mets. 86[a] שגופך ט׳... נשמתך בט׳ (Ms. בטהרה) thy body is pure, and thy soul expired with (the word) 'pure'; Snh. 68[a].—Kidd. 70[b] וסימניך טמא טמא ט׳ ט׳ and the sign (by which to remember which of the two families is of unblemished descent) is, that with the name of an unclean animal (raven) is unclean, that with the name of a clean animal (dove) is clean; B. Bath. 91[a]. Kel. III, 7 ובחרסית ט׳ and the person that touches the clay is clean (not affected by levitical uncleanness). Ib. IV, 1 ט׳ is not subject to levitical uncleanness; a. v. fr.—בהמה טהורה ,עוף, דג ט׳ a fish, a bird, a domestic animal *permitted to eat.* Hull. XII, 2. Ib. IV, 3 בטהורה טהור if it occurs with an animal of the clean class, the person is levitically clean; a. v. fr.—*Pl.* טְהוֹרִים, טְהוֹרִין; טְהוֹרוֹת. Kel. II, 1 פשוטיהן ט׳ the flat-surfaced among them are not subject to uncleanness.—Ber. 2[b] שהכהנים ט׳ וכ׳ Ms. M. (ed. מטוהרים) when the purified priests enter &c. B. Mets. 61[b]; a. v. fr.

טָהַר, טָהֵר (b. h.; cmp. צהר, זהר) [*to be bright, to glitter,*] 1) *to be clean, pure,* esp. *to be levitically clean; to be unsusceptible of levitical uncleanness.* Neg. X, 8 שט׳ שעה אחת which has been declared clean once. Mikv. II, 2 עד שיודע שט׳ until it is ascertained that it has become clean. Ib. III, 2 ויִטְהֲרוּ העליונים מן וכ׳ so that the waters coming from above become cleansed from the impurity of the lower waters. Neg. VII, 4 ויִטְהַר ממנו and is declared clean from it (the last scall); a. fr.—2) *to be cleared, removed.* Ber. 2[b], v. next w.

Pi. טִיהֵר 1) *to purify, make (levitically) clean; to absolve from sin.* Yoma VIII, 9 מי מְטַהֵר וכ׳ who is it that absolves you? Ib. (ref. to Jer. XVII, 13) מה מקוה מט׳ וכ׳ as the ritual bath (v. מִקְוֶה) cleanses the unclean, so does the Lord &c.; a. fr.—2) *to keep clean, guard against contact with unclean things.* R. Hash. 16[b] חייב לְטַהֵר את עצמו וכ׳.. one is bound to keep one's self clean for the festive days.—3) *to declare* טָהוֹר, *to decide in favor of cleanness.* Snh. 17[a] bot. מי שיודע לטַ׳ וכ׳ one who knows how to prove a creeping thing to be clean. Ib. אני אדון ואֲטַהֲרֶנּוּ I will argue and prove it to be clean. Eduy. VIII, 7 לטמא ולטַ׳ to decide on unclean and clean; a. v. fr.—*Part. pass.* מְטוֹהָר, pl. מְטוֹהָרִים. Ber. 2[b], v. preced.—4) *to become clean.* Snh. 94[b] מיד ט׳ it becomes clean at once. Hull. 60[b] טִיהֲרוּ; Gitt. 38[a] טהרו, v. סִיחוֹן.

Nif. נִטְהַר *to become clean.* Tanh. Metsora 7 נִטְהֲרָה וכ׳ she became clean on the eighth day. Ib. ונִטְהֶרֶת and becomes clean; a. fr.

Hithpa. הִטַּהֵר *to be cleansed, to cleanse one's self; to amend.* Yoma 38[b] בא לִטַּהֵר מסייעים אותו (Ms. M. 2 לְהִטַּהֵר) if one is willing to do good, he will be assisted; Sabb. 104[a]; Yalk. Prov. 935 לִיטַּהֵר; a. e.—Yoma VIII, 9 (85[b]) לפני מי אתם מִיטַּהֲרִים Mish. a. Y. ed. (Bab. ed. מִטַּ׳) before whom do you cleanse yourselves (from sin)?; a. e.

טְהַר, טְהַר ch. same, 1) *to be clean* (usually דכי). Ber. 2[b] וט׳ גברא, v. infra.—2) *to be cleared away, be gone.* Ib. 2[a], sq. (ref. to Lev. XXII, 7 ובא השמש וטהר) ממאי דהאי... והאי וטהר ט׳ יומא דלמא ... ט׳ גברא how do you know that this *uba hash-shemesh* means his sunset (the finished sunset of the seventh day, v. Ms. M. in Rabb. D. S. a. l.), and *v'taher* means, the day is gone; may be *uba* &c. means the approach of his evening (beginning sunset. Tosaf. a. l.; Rashi: the arrival of his (eighth) morning), and *v'taher* (referring to the man) means, the man becomes clean (by means of his sacrifice, Rashi).—3) (denom. of טִיהֲרָא) *to be noon-time.* Yoma 59[a], a. e., v. טִיהֲרָא a. next w.

Pa. טַהֵר *to declare clean.* B. Mets. 84[b] טַהֲרִינְהוּ he declared them clean.

טוֹהַר or **טֹהַר** m. (b. h.; preced. wds.) 1) *the pure, real surface* (of gold). Yoma V, 6 על טָהֳרוֹ של מזבח (or טְהָרוֹ) immediately on the top of the golden altar (free from coals or ashes, v. גִּילּוּיָא). Men. 97[a] על טהרו של שולחן (Ms. M. על השל׳) immediately on the golden table.—2) (cmp. חָזֶה) *the centre of the front.* Yoma 59[a] (one opinion explain. טהרו של מזבח, v. supra) פלגיה דמזבח the centre of the altar front, as people say, טהר טיהרא והוי פלגא דיומא 'the noon-light shines' meaning by *tihara* the middle of the day; ib. 15[a]; Zeb. 38[b].

טְהַרְרֵי, טְהִירִירֵי, טְהַרֵי, טְהָרָא, טְהַר v. sub טִיה׳.

טָהֳרָה or **טַהֲרָה** f. (b. h. טָ׳; preced. wds.) 1) *clearness* of the sky after the rainy season. Ber. 59[a] הרואה רקיע בְּטָהֳרָתָהּ (or בטַהֲ׳) he who sees the sky in its restored brightness (Ms. F. בטיהרו, v. טִיהַר). Ib. נראית רקיע בטהרתה (Ms. M. נראו שמים בטהרה; Yalk. Is. 335 נראה שמים בטָהֳרוֹ, corr. acc.).—2) *pureness, condition of levitical cleanness; purification.* Sabb. 152[b] תנה לו כמו שנתנה לך מה היא בט׳ אף אתה בט׳ Ms. M. (v. Rabb. D. S. a. l. note) give her (the soul) to Him as He has given her to thee, as He (has given her) in pureness, so give thou &c. Snh. 68[a], v. טָהוֹר.—Ber. 16[a] (ref. to Num. XXIV, 6) מה נחלים ... מטומאה לט׳ וכ׳ as the rivers raise man from a condition of uncleanness to one of cleanness, so do the tents (schools) &c. Ab. Zar. 8[a] עובדי ע״ז בט׳ encouraging idolatry, though from no impure motives. Yoma 72[b]; Men. 110[a] הלומד תורה בט׳ he who studies the Law in (sexual) purity.—Snh. l. c. וטָהֳרָתָן במה שהן and their purification (immersion) is performed in whatever condition they are (whole or torn); a. v. fr.—Esp. ט׳ or טָהֳרַת הקודש *observance of levitical rules originally prescribed for the handling of sacred food;* also (mostly in pl.) *secular food so prepared* or *pretended to be so prepared;* v. חָבֵר.—Gitt. 62[a] אין עושין חלת ע״ה בט׳ you must not separate the priest's share under levitical precautions for a non-observant (because it might mislead the priest); Tosef. Dem. III, 1. Sabb. 13a עד היכן פרצה ט׳ וכ׳ how far the custom of observing the rules of levitical cleanness for secular food has spread &c. Ḥag. II, 7 היה אוכל על ט׳ הקודש used to eat his ordinary meals with the observance required for sacred food; a. fr.— *Pl.* טַהֲרוֹת, טָהֳרוֹת. Tosef. Dem. l. c. אין עושין ט׳ לכ״ה one must not prepare food with observance of levitical precautions for &c., v. supra. Ber. 19a; B. Mets. 59b כל ט׳ שטיהר וכ׳ all objects which R.... had declared clean. Tosef. Dem. II, 20 אין משלחין ט׳ וכ׳ you must not send food levitically prepared through a non-observant; a. v. fr.— *Tohŏroth*, or *Tahăroth*, (euphem. for טומאות), name of the sixth order of the Mishnah and Tosefta (סדר ט׳), and of one treatise of that order.

טְוָא, v. טוי.

טוּב I (b. h.) *to be good, fit, handsome, valuable.*

Hif. הֵטִיב 1) *to prepare, outfit, dress, adorn.* Gen. R. s. 26, v. טֶבֶת. Ib. s. 83 (play on מהיטבאל, Gen. XXXVI, 39) שהיו מְטִיבֵי אלוהות היו they were dressers of idols; שהיו מֵטִיבִין עצמן וכ׳ they adorned themselves in honor of the idols. Ib. מטיבי נשים וכ׳ they dressed women for their wedding; a. e.—Esp. (את הנרות) ה׳ *to trim, cleanse the lamps.* Yoma III, 4 ולְהֵטִיב. Ib. I, 2. Ib. 14b יֵיטִיב; a. fr.—V. הֲטָבָה.—2) *to turn a dream unto good* (saying, 'I have dreamt a good dream'). Ber. 55b יְטִיבֶנּוּ בפני וכ׳ he shall turn it in the presence of three persons, and say &c.—3) *to do good, be beneficent.* Ib. IX, 2 הטוב והמטיב who is good and beneficent. Taan. 31a .. תקנו הטוב והמ׳ they introduced in Jabneh the benediction 'who is good &c.' (in the grace after meal).—Kidd. I, 10 מטיבין לו good will be done to him; a. fr.— *Part. Hof.* מוּטָב, q. v.

Pi. טִיֵּיב *to improve a field, to till oftener than usual.* Y. Shebi. IV, 35b top טִיְּיבָהּ וכ׳ if, after he improved a field, he died &c.

Nithpa. נִיטַּיֵּיב *to be improved.* Shebi. IV, 2; Tosef. ib. III, 10; a. e.—Denom. טִיּוּב.

טוּב, טוֹב ch., *Pa.* טַיֵּיב, *Af.* אָטִיב *to do good, to favor.* Targ. Y. I Ex. XXIII, 2 לְמֵיטְיָיבָא; Y. II לְמֵיטְבָא. V. יְטַב.

טוֹב II m., **טוֹבָה** f. (b. h.) 1) *good; a good thing.* Ber. 5a (ref. to Ps. XXXIX, 3) אין ט׳ אלא וכ׳ under *good* the Torah is meant. Ib. 60b זו מדה ט׳ this refers to a good dispensation; a. v. fr.—יום טוב (abbr. י״ט) *festival.* Bets. I, 1; a. fr.—כי טוב (ref. to Gen. I, 4) *day-time.* Pes. 2a.—Ber. V, 3 (33b) על טוב וכ׳ thy name be praised for the good (thou doest).—זכיר לְטוֹב, v. זָכַר.—עין טובה, v. עַיִן.—*Pl.* טוֹבִים, f. טוֹבוֹת. Ber. l. c. (34a, omitt. in Mish.) האומר יברכוך ט׳ he who says in prayer, The good praise thee. Ib. IX, 2 בשורות ט׳, v. בְּשׂוֹרָה; a. v. fr.—V. טוֹבָה.—2) *noble, elder.*—*Pl.* טוֹבִים. Tosef. Shek. II, 16 בני ט׳ of noble descent; a. fr.—טוֹבֵי העיר *representatives* of the town. Meg. 27a.

טוּב m. (b. h.; preced.) *goodness, good.* Ber. 44a לשבוע מטּוּבָהּ to be satisfied out of its (the land's) riches; a. e.

טוּבָא m. ch. same, *good, goodness, mercy.* Targ. Is. I, 19. Targ. Ps. XXXIII, 22; a. fr.—2) (mostly in pl. constr. טוּבֵי) *happines*, used like אַשְׁרֵי, *happy!, blessed!* Targ. I Kings X, 8. Targ. II Kings V, 3 (h. text אחלי). With personal suffix טוּבֵיה, טוּבוֹי, טוּבוֹהִי. Targ. Prov. XXVIII, 14. Targ. Ps. I, 1; a. fr.—Snh. 7a v. הוּש ch.—Y. Yoma IV, 41d top טובוי ... טיבוי, v. לְוָוְיָתָא; a. fr.—3) *much; many; very.* Snh. 41b ט׳ אמריתו בה you said much (had many reasons to offer). Ber. 30b מרירת ליבא ט׳ very bitter at heart.—Ib. 18b אבא ט׳ many by the name of Abba. Ib. 52b ט׳ נהורי many lights (colors); a. fr.—*Pl.* fem. טוּבָן *more.* Y. Peah I, 15c; Y. Kidd. I, 61b top ט׳ פריטין a higher price.

טוֹבָה f. (b. h., v. טוֹב) 1) *good, goodness.* Y. Shek. I, beg. 45d לט׳ כל נדיב לב for a good purpose—every liberal-hearted &c. Sot. 47b ופסקה ט׳ and blessing (plenty) has departed. Yeb. 47a, sq. אינם .... לא רוב ט׳ וכ׳ they cannot stand either too much prosperity or &c.; a. fr.— *Pl.* טוֹבוֹת. Kidd. 40b ט׳ הרבה the effect of many good deeds; a. fr.—2) *favor.* Sot. 47b משרבו מקבלני טוֹבָתְךָ ומחזקני טובוֹתֶיךָ (read: ומחזיקני) when those became numerous who say, 'I accept thy favor' and 'I shall appreciate thy favors' (in official life); Tosef. ib. XIV, 7 טוֹבֹתֶיךָ ומחזיקני טוֹבָתְךָ ....; a. fr.—בְּט׳ *as a favor*, i. e. *expected to be reciprocated*, שלא בט׳ *not expected* &c. Shebi. IV, 1; 2; a. e.—טוֹבַת הֲנָאָה the benefit of a pleasure, i. e. *the satisfaction which one feels in obliging somebody.* Pes. 46b, a. e. ט׳ ה׳ ממון the benefit of putting a person under obligation is equal to a consideration in money; a. fr.—4) *inclination, good will.* Gen. R. s. 86 בע״כ ברחה שלא בטוֹבָתָהּ by force, against her will; Tanh. Vayesh. 4. Y. Ab. Zar. I, 40a bot חביט בה שלא בטובתו he looked at her involuntarily; a. fr.—טוֹבַת עַיִן (v. עַיִן) *liberality.* Ned. 38a נהג בה ט׳ ע׳ וכ׳ was liberal with the Law (that had been given to him), and he gave it to Israel.

טוֹבִי (v. next w.) pr. n. m. *Tobi.* M. Kat. 16a רב ט׳ בר מתנה.

טוֹבִיָּה (b. h.) pr. n. m. *Tobijah, Tobias.* Kidd. 70b בטי בר ט׳, a slave. Keth. 85b שני ט׳ two by the name of T.— Pes. 113b, a. e., v. זִיגֵּד.— Lev. R. s. 1, beg.; Sot. 12a (one of the names of Moses).

טוֹבִינָא, v. טוֹבְיָנָא.

טוּבְיָנָא m. (v. טוּבָא) *happy, blessed.* Gitt. 26b; Keth. 40a; Kerith. 13b ט׳ דחכימי happiest of all scholars.

טוּבְלָא, Bets. 13a, read: טִבְלָא.

טוּבְלָן m. (טְבַל I) *bather.*—*Pl.* טוּבְלָנִים, constr. טוּבְלָנֵי. Tosef. Yad. I, 20 Var., v. טָבַל I.

טוֹבַנְיָא (טוֹבְיָנָא) pr. n. pl. *Tobanya (Tobyana).* Tosef. Shebi. VII, 14 Pes. 53a; Erub. 28b טובי׳.

טוּבְעִין, v. טֶבַע 2.

טוּבְעָנָא m. (טְבַע I) *flood.* Targ. Y. Gen. VI, 17; a. fr. (O. טוֹפָנָא).

טוּבְעָנִי I m. (preced.) *land submerged by a flood.* Taan. 10ª ט׳ ולא יובשני better flooded land than rainless land.

טוּבְעָנִי II = טְבְעוֹנִי.

טוּבְתָא f. ch.=h. טוֹבָה, *blessing.* Targ. Y. I Deut. XXXII, 50. [Targ. Jud. V, 26 some ed., read טַבְתָא.]

***טוֹגָא** f. (*toga*) *toga, Roman gown.* Sifré Deut. 234 פרט לרגא; Yalk. Deut. 933 לרגא; Treat. Tsitsith (ed. Kirchheim p. 22) הטריגון (corr. acc.).—*Pl.* טוֹגִיוֹת. Sifré l. c. quot. in Ar., s. v. טג: טגיות אינן וכ׳ (read: טוג׳) *togae* are exempt from *tsitsith.*

טוֹהַר, v. טֹהַר.

טְוָוא, טְוָוה, v. טוי.

טַוְזָא, v. טַפְזָא (a. next w.)

***טַוְז׳, טְוָוזִיג** m. (=טַב זִיג, v. זוֹגָא) *merry company, picnic of young men.* Ab. Zar. 14ª בט׳ (Ms. M. בטוויזא) 'the son's feast' of which R. Judah speaks (Tosef. ib. I, 21) means a picnic (not a wedding). [Perles Et. St. p. 11 refers to Pers. *ṭûzi. ṭus'i*, Arab. תוזיע.]

טוֹוַח, טְוָוח, טְוָח m. (טוּחַ II) *pressing the bow, shot, shooting distance.*—*Pl.* טְוָחִ׳, טְוָוחִים. Gen. R. s. 53 (ref. to כמטחוי, Gen. XXI, 16) שני ט׳ בקשת מיל ('Rashi' a. l. מיחות) two shooting distances with the bow are a mile (מִיל); Yalk. Gen. 94.

טָווּי, part. pass. of טְוָה.

טְוִיָה, טְוִיָא, טְוָוי, v. sub טוי׳.

טַוָּוס m. (טוּס; cmp. ταώς, Pers. tavus, v. Lydd. Gr. Dict. s. v.) *peacock.* Gen. R. s. 7, end. Tosef. Kil. I, 8 תרנגול ט׳ וכ׳ Var. (ed. Zuck. טווח, corr. acc.) the cock, the peacock and the pheasant, although resembling each other, &c.; Y. ib. I, 27ª bot.; B. Kam. 55ª (Ms. H. טָאוּס); Y. ib. V, end, 5ª טַוּוֹסֶת(?).—*Pl.* טַוָּוסִים, טַוְּוסִין. Pesik. R. addit. s. 1 (ed. Fr. p. 193ᵇ). Yalk. Esth. 104ᵇ ט׳ של שן peacocks made of ivory.

טַוָּוסָא, טַוְוסָא ch. same. Targ. II Esth. I, 2.— Y. Ab. Zar. III, 42ᵈ top (expl. Adrammelech and Anammelech, II Kings XVII, 31) ט׳ וכ׳ peacock and pheasant. Sabb. 130ª רישא דט׳ וכ׳ Ms. M. (Ms. O. טַאוּסָא, ed. incorr. טוותא) the head of a peacock cooked in milk.— *Pl.* טַוְוסִין, טַוָּוסִין, טַוָּס׳. Targ. Ez. XXVII, 15 (h. text הובנים). Targ. I Kings X, 22 (h. text תכיים).

טַוְפָא, v. טְיָפָא.

טוּרָא, טְוּוּרָא, טַוּוָר, v. טוּרָא.

טַוּרוֹס, ט׳ אוּמָנוֹס (מָנוֹס, אוּמָנִיס) pr. n. (Ταῦρος) *Taurus Amanus* (v. אֲמָנָה II, 2) corresp. to *Hor-Hahar.* Targ. Y. Num. XXXIV, 7, sq. (O. הר טורא).— Targ. Y. ib. XX, 22; 25; Targ. Y. I Deut. XXXII, 50 (!) (Y. II a. O. הור טורא).

טְוָת, טְוָות, טוֹוָת f. (stem טו, טח, cmp. טחח; cmp. Arab. *ṭavi*) [*clearness, emptiness,*] (adv.) *with an empty stomach, without meal, fasting.* Dan. VI, 19.—Pes. 107ª, v. בִּית.— Ber. 55ª כל חלום בלא ט׳ Ms. M. (ed. ולא) no dream is to be feared in which fasting plays no part; [Ar.: every dream has some reality, except that which one dreams while fasting].

טוות, טוותא, v. טַוָּוסָא, טַוָּוס.

טוּחַ I (b. h.) 1) *to cover with a cohesive substance, to plaster.* Part. טָח. M. Kat. 7ª ואינו טָח בטיט but puts no clay on. Cant. R. to VIII, 6 טָחֵי גגות roof-plasterers. Neg. XIII, 1 וטח and plasters the spot over; a. fr.— *Part. pass.* טוּחַ *coated, covered with viscid or glittering matter.*—Midd. IV, 1 ט׳ בזהב coated with gold; (Num. R. s. 12 נְטוּחַ).—Nidd. 24ª בפניו טוחות (Rashi טְחוּת) when the face of the embryo is covered over (no features distinguishable).

Nif. נִיטוֹחַ *to be pasted on, to stick.* Y. Kil. VI, 30ᶜ top והיא נִיטוֹחָה and it (the fig) stuck (against the wall); Y. Sabb. XI, 13ª bot. והיה נ׳ (corr. acc.). Tosef. Kel. B. Mets. II, 17 לִיטוֹחַ some ed. (ed. Zuck. לִיטוּל, corr. acc.), v. infra.

Hif. הֵטִיחַ 1) *to plaster, to polish.* Hull. 25ª . . . עתיד לְהָטִיחַ (לְהַטִיחוֹ) וכ׳ (Tosef. Kel. l. c. ליטיח, v. supra) which wants polishing, v. אֲטוּנָס. Bets. 9ª להָטִיחַ גגו וכ׳ he needs the ladder for plastering his roof. [Tosef. Kel. B. Kam. IV, 19, sq. [read:] אם יכול הטיח, v. טִיחַ.]—2) *to cast mud,* trnsf. (with or without דברים) *to speak rebelliously, to reproach* (with נגד or כלפי). Taan. 25ª; Meg. 22ᵇ, a. e. לעולם אל יָטִיחַ וכ׳ one must, in his prayer, never reproach the Lord. Ber. 31ᵇ, sq.—Gen. R. s. 53 (ref. to כמטחוי, Gen. XXI, 16) כִּמְטַחַת וכ׳ as if thrusting reproaches against the Lord; Tanh. Vayetse 5. Ex. R. s. 3. B. Bath. 134ª ה׳ עלי וכ׳ Ben U. insulted me.

טוּחַ ch. same, *to plaster, smear.* Pes. 30ª, v. טִיהְיָא.

Af. אַטַח 1) same. Zeb. 95ᵇ אַטְחוּ (Ms. R. 2 דטחו), v. טִיהְיָא.—2) (with מִלִּין) *to talk rebelliously.* Targ. Y. Gen. XV, 6.

טוּחַ II (v. טחי) *to press, squeeze.* Hull. 109ᵇ טָחוֹ בכותל presses it against the wall (to make the milk flow out).—*Part. pass.* טוּחַ *squeezed in.* Num. R. s. 10 (ref. to Job XXXVIII, 36) אלו הכליות שהן טוחות וכ׳ that means the kidneys which are wedged into the body.

Hif. הֵטִיחַ 1) *to press, squeeze, knock against.* Ber. 34ᵇ אלמלי ה׳ וכ׳ (Ms. M. הניח, v. Rabb. D. S. a. l. note) if Ben. Z. (myself) had squeezed his head between his (the son's) knees (praying for his recovery). Gen. R. s. 20 התחיל מֵטִיחַ וכ׳ he knocked his head against the wall; Yalk. ib. 30 לְהָטִיחַ. Ohol. XVII, 2 ה׳ בסלע struck (with the plough) against a rock. B. Kam. 28ᵇ ה׳ צלוחיתו וכ׳ he struck (with) his bottle against the stone; Y. ib. III, 3ᶜ top, v. הֲטָחָה.—Tanh. P'kudé 11 כיון שהטיחו פניהם וכ׳

when they had squeezed their faces from all sides (had in vain tried in all directions).—2) *to press the bow-string, to shoot;* (euphem.) *to emit semen virile.* Yeb. 54[a]. Snh. 46[a] ה׳ באשתו Ms. M. (ed. את אשתו).

טוֹחֵן m. (טְחַן) *miller.*—*Pl.* טוֹחֲנִים. Tanh. Mishp. 19 כגון חמורים של ט׳ like the mask over the faces of the millers' asses.

טוֹחֲנוֹת f. pl. (preced.) *millstones,* v. טַחֲנָה.

טוֹט m. (onomatop.) *blow on the horn.* M. Kat. 16[a] ט׳ אסר וכ׳ a blow binds (proclaiming excommunication), and a blow unbinds.

טוֹטַלְוָותָא f. pl. (= טלטל׳; טְלַל) *branches of the vine, arbor.* Targ. Y. Lev. XIX, 10; Targ. Y. II Deut. XXIV, 21 טוֹטְלָיַית׳.

טוֹטְפָא f., pl. **טוֹטְפָן,** v. טוֹטֶפְתָּא.

טוֹטַפְרָאוֹת, v. טַטְפְּר׳.

טוֹטֶפֶת f. (b. h. in pl.; = טפטפ׳, v. טִיפְטֵף 2) [*something glistening,*] *beads* used as *charms, ornament* worn on the forehead, *frontlet.* Sabb. VI, 1, expl. ib. 57[b], v. חוּמַרְתָּא a. אֱפּוּזְיְינֵי; Y. ib. VI, 7[d] דבר שהוא נותן במקום הט׳ (read נָתוּן) something which is put on by women in the place of the *totafoth* (by men, v. infra).—*Pl.* טוֹטָפוֹת. Tosef. ib. IV (V), 6.—Esp. pl. טוֹטָפוֹת *phylacteries,* (corresp. to אות, Deut. VI, 8, a. e.) slips of parchment containing inscriptions and put in the casings of the T'fillin (v. תְּפִלִּין). Mekh. Bo. s. 17 מה בראש ארבע ט׳ אף ביד ארבע ט׳ as the T'fillin on the head contain four inscriptions, so those on the hand. Snh. XI, 3 (88[b]); a. e.

טוֹטַפְתָּא ch. same, *charm, ornament.* Targ. II Sam. I, 10 ט׳ דעל ידא *bracelet* (h. text אצעדה).—*Pl.* טוֹטְפָתָא, טוֹטְפָן *phylacteries,* v. preced. Targ. Esth. VIII, 15 (cmp. Men. 35[b]). Targ. Ez. XXIV, 17; 23 (h. text פאר, cmp. M. Kat. 15[a]; Keth. 6[b]).

טוֹטְרְפְלִיוֹת, v. טִיטְרַפְּלִיּוֹת.

טָוָה, טָוָה, טְוִי (b. h.) [*to go to and back,* cmp. אָזַל, זול,] *to spin.* Keth. VII, 6 טוֹוָה בשוק she spins in the street. Ib. 72[b], v. וֶרֶד II.—Tosef. Toh. IV, 11; Zeb. 79[b] פשתן שטְוָואָתוֹ וכ׳ linen which a menstruant spun.—*Part. pass.* טָווּי. Kil. IX, 8 ט׳ או ארוג spun or woven, v. שַׁעַטְנֵז. Sabb. 79[a]; a. e.—V. טְוִי.

טְוִי I ch. same. Denom. מַטְווּיאָתָא.

טְוִי II, **טְוָא** (v. preced. wds.) [*to turn,*] *to roast.* Targ. Is. XLIV, 16 (ed. Wil. טְוָה); a. fr.—Part. pass. טְוֵי, constr. טְוֵי. Targ. Ex. XII, 8, sq.—Gitt. 69[b] נִיטְווֹיֵיה וכ׳ let him roast it in a smithy; a. fr.

Af. אַטְוִי same. Bets. 4[a] מהו לאַטְווּינְהוּ וכ׳ is it permitted to roast them to-day &c.

Ithpe. אִיטְּוִי *to be roasted.* Pes. 76[b] דאִיטְּוָוא וכ׳ which was roasted together with meat. B. Kam. 19[b] דמְטַווּר (Ar. בְּטָווּר) it means that it was roasted. Ber. 44[b] משיתא מְטַוְויָתָא than six (eggs) roasted.

טְווִי or **טְוָוי, טְוִי,** m. (טְוָה) *spinning, that which is spun.* Meg. 26[b]; Snh. 48[a], v. אָרִיג. Tosef. B. Kam. X, 2 טאור (read טְוָאר, Var. טְוָור).

טוּוִי, טְוַיָא, טִיוּי, טְוִי m. (טְוִי II) *roast, roasted meat.* B. Kam. 19[a] Ar. (v. טְוִי II).—Sabb. 109[a] שריקא ט׳ a roast glaired, Rashi (differ. in Tosaf.) Y. Ter. X, 47[b] top טְווּיָה.

***טְוָיָא** m. pl. (טְוִי) *spinning animals, spiders.* Lev. R. s. 25 (expl. בטחות, Job XXXVIII, 36) בט׳ (Ar. בטיטוריא; cmp. LXX Job. l. c.); v., however, בְּטוֹנְיָא.

טְווִיָּה, טְוִיָּה טְוִיָה f. (טָוָה) *spinning.* Sabb. 74[b]. Ib. 79[a]; a. fr.

טְוִיָה, v. טְוָיָא.

טוויסין, v. טיוסין.

טוֹל, טוּל, imperat. of נְטַל, נָטַל.

טוּל I *Pi.* טַיֵּיל 1) *to walk about, to be at leisure, to enjoy one's self.* Snh. 102[a] נְטַיֵּיל בג״ע we shall walk about in paradise. Succ. 28[b] ומְטַיֵּיל בסוכה and enjoys himself &c. Tosef. Sabb. XVI (XVII), 18; Tosef. Bets. II, 10, v. טְרִיקְלִין. Tanh. Ki Thissa 3; a. fr.—2) *to make walk.* Ib. טִיַּילְתַּנִי עמך thou madest me walk by thy side.

טוּל ch. same, *to walk about, stride.* Targ. Jer. L, 11 (h. text צהל; cmp. Targ. ib. VIII, 16).

Pa. טַיֵּיל 1) *to walk, travel.* Targ. Y. Gen. XXIV, 61. Targ. Y. Num. XXII, 20. Targ. Ps. LXVIII, 8 טַיָּילְתָּא (ed. Wil. טְיָיָל׳; h. text צעד); a. fr.—2) as preced. *Pi.*—Targ. Y. Gen. III, 8 (h. text מתהלך).—Y. Ber. III, 6[a], a. fr. הוו מְטַיְּילִין וכ׳ were walking about &c. B. Bath. 91[b] כד הוו מְטַיְּילָן וכ׳ when boys and girls used to play &c. Succ. 53[a] הוה מט׳ קמיה וכ׳ (Ar. מטלל) was sporting before &c., v. טָלַל; a. fr.—3) *to drive off, send away.* Targ. Y. Deut. XXIV, 1; 3 (ed. pr. ישיל, corr. acc.).

Af. אַטֵּיל *to cause to travel.* Targ. Ps. LXXVIII, 52 Ms. (ed. אַשִּׁיל).

טוּל II, **טוּלָא** m. (טלל) = h. צֵל, *shade, shadow.* Targ. Jud. IX, 36; a. fr.—Yoma 74[b] תוב בט׳ sit in the shade.—Gitt. 17[a] או בטוּלָּךְ וכ׳ either let us live in thy shadow (protection) or in the shadow of the son of Esau (Rome). Snh. 18[b] בט׳ תאינה in the shade of a figtree; Y. R. Hash. II, 58[b] top בְּטַל תינתא; Y. Snh. I, 18[c] bot. בטיל תינתא (corr. acc.); a. fr.—*Pl.* טוּלַיָּא, טוּלֵי. Targ. Jer. VI, 4; a. e.—Targ. Is. IX, 1 בארע טולי מותא ed. Lag (oth. ed. טוּלְמוּתָא in one word, h. text צלמות).—Pes. 111[b] חמשה ט׳ וכ׳ there are five shades (where demons dwell); a. e.—V. טְלָלָא.

טוֹלָא m. (cmp. טְלָאי) *rag* tied around the finger. Meïl. 18[a] עומד לט׳ Ar. (ed. לנולה; v. R. S. to Kel. XXVII, 4) fit for tying &c.

טוֹלִימוֹתָא, v. טוּלָא.

טוּלְמָא I m., **טוּלְמְתָא** f., constr. טוּלְמַת (טְלַם) [panis aqueus ac mollis, P. Sm. 1477] *cake, loaf.* Targ. Job. XXXI, 17 ט׳ דלחמי Ms. (ed. only טולמי); a. e.—Targ. Esth. III, 2 ט׳ דלחם ed. Lag.; Yalk. ib. 105b ט׳ דנחמא.—[Y. Snh. II, 20c bot. מנחם טלמא, v. טַלְמָיָא.]—*Pl.* טוּלְמִין, טוּלְמֵי. Targ. I Kings XIV, 3; a. e.—Meg. 15b בטולמי דנחמא Ms. M. 2 (ed. only בִּטְלָמֵי) for loaves of bread. [Ar. s. v. זיף quotes, in Hebr. diction, (play on Josh. XV, 24) כל המוזיף טולמיין וכ׳ ed. Koh. (oth. ed. טולמין, טולמון) he who lends bread to the poor, will be raised.]

טוּלְמָא II *oppression*, v. טְלוּמָא.

טולמוסין, v. next w.

טוֹלְמִיסִין (ἐτόλμησεν, fr. τολμάω) *he dared.* Gen. R. s. 41, beg.; s. 52 (ref. to Gen. XII, 17) [read:] על דו ט׳ למקרב למסנא וכ׳ because he dared to come near the shoe of that matron; Y. Keth. VII, end, 31d על דטלמסן למגע בסמה (corr. acc.); Yalk. Gen. 69.

טולר, Yalk. Josh. 31, read פּוֹלֵר.

טוּלְשָׁא m. *crab-apple* (cmp. Syr. טלש, P. Sm. 1482).—*Pl.* טוּלְשֵׁי. Ber. 40b (expl. עוזרדין of Dem. I, 1).

טוּם (v. טָמַם) *to fill up.* B. Kam. 51b טָם טפח if one filled up again one hand-breadth (of the depth of the pit).

טוּם ch. same. Targ. II Kings III, 19, v. טְמַם.—B. Kam. 50a עד דטָאֵים ליה (Ms. M. אָטֵים *Af.*, v. Rabb. D. S. a. l. note) until he fills it up.

Ithpa. אִיטַּיֵּים *to be filled up.* Erub. 79a למיטַיְימֵיה קאי the intention is that it be filled up (with the pebbles).

טוּמְאָה f. (b. h. טֻמְאָה; טָמֵא) *uncleanness, esp. levitical uncleanness*, v. טָהֳרָה. Pes. 19a טוּמְאַת ידים uncleanness of hands by touch. Eduy. II, 1, v. אָב. M. Kat. 5a ט׳ קורא וכ׳ the uncleanness (the unclean spot being marked) calls unto him warning &c.; a. v. fr.—*Pl.* טוּמְאוֹת Kel. I, 1; a. v. fr.

טוּמְאָה f. ch. (hebraism; preced.) *unclean woman, menstruant.* Targ. Ez. XXII, 10.—*Pl.* טוּמְאָתָא. Targ. Is. XXX, 22.

טוֹמוֹס (טִימוֹס) m. (τόμος) 1) *scroll, roll, tome.* Tosef. B. Kam. IX, 31 בט׳ של וכ׳ with a roll of papers in his hand; Y. ib. VIII, beg. 6b; Sifra Emor Par. 14, ch. XX טימסמירות, טִימִיסִמ׳ (read: ט׳ של נירדות or שטרות); Yalk. Lev. 658; a. e.—2) *document, record.* Y. Hor. III, 48a bot. ראש טו׳ at the head of the list; Lev. R. s. 5 בראש ט׳ Ar. (ed. only בראש). Gen. R. s. 25 beg. בתוך טִימוֹסָן וכ׳ in the record of the righteous; Yalk. ib. 42; Yalk. Chr. 1072 טִימוֹסִין pl.—*Pl.* טוֹמוֹסִין, טוֹמוֹסוֹת, טִי׳. Pesik. Zakh. p. 27a [read:] ונטל כ׳ וכ׳ (or טִימוֹסָן) he took the lists of the tribes &c.; Tanḥ. Ki Thetse 9. Y. Snh. X, 28a top אף שמותיהם . . . טִמְסוֹתֵיהֶם even their names disappeared from their books of records. Ex. R. s. 15 הוציא הנמוסין וכ׳ (corr. acc.; Tanḥ. Vaëra 5 הִפִּתְקָא) he brought out the lists of the deities.—3) *census.* Lam. R. to II, 2 היה טִימוס . . . בעגלה their census had to be carried to Jerusalem on a wagon; [Y. Taan. IV. 69a bot. קטמי׳ read הטומוס or קִינְסוֹס].

טוּמְטוּם m. (redupl. of טָמַם) *a person whose genitals are hidden, or undevelopped; one whose sex is unknown.* B. Bath. 126b ט׳ שנקרע וכ׳ a *tumtum* who was operated upon and was found to be a male. Bicc. IV, 5 (Talm. ed.); a. e.—[Midr. Till. to Ps. I; Yalk. Prov. 953 ט׳ הוא העולם, v. אַבְטוּמְטוּס.]—*Pl.* טוּמְטוּמִין. Yeb. 64a bot. (not טומטמין).

***טוּמַיָּיא** m. pl. (טוּם; cmp. סָתַר, סָתַם) *secret, hidden place.* Targ. Y. II Deut. XXVII, 15 (later ed. טוּמְרַיָּא).

טומיות, v. טוּרְמִיּוֹת.

טומיקון, v. טַמְיָקוֹן.

טוּמְעָא m. (טְמַע) 1) *secret place.* Targ. Job. XL, 13.—2) *hidden treasure.*—*Pl.* טוּמְעַיָּא. Ib. III, 20.

טוּמְרָא m. (טְמַר, cmp. preced.) *secret, hiding place.* Targ. Y. Deut. XIII, 9. Targ. Y. I, ib. XXVII, 15; a. fr.—*Pl.* טוּמְרַיָּא. Targ. Ps. X, 8; a. e.; v. טוּמַיָּא.

טון, v. טָנַן.

טוּנָא I (=טְעוּנָא; טְעַן) 1) *burden, load; bag.* Targ. Y. Gen. XLIV, 1, sq. (h. text אמתחת). Targ. Y. Ex. XXIII, 5; a. e.—Ber. 61a דלא דרי ט׳ Ms. M. (ed. מידי) when he is not carrying a load. Sabb. 92a דכל ט׳ דמידלי וכ׳ every load which is lifted on poles &c.; a. fr.—2) (v. טַעֲנָה) *argument.* Zeb. 32b מטוּנָךְ I borrow thine own argument; R. Hash. 4a; Ḥull. 132a top (Rashi derives fr. מְטֵי: 'we have reached thee').—*Pl.* טוּנִין. Targ. Y. Gen. XLIII, 23.

***טוּנָא** II m.=טוּלָא (?), *shade, shadow.* Ber. 56b (v. vers. in Rabb. D. S. a. l. Ms. M. a. note).

טונוס, Y. Ber. IX, 14b bot. ט׳ רופוס, v. טוּרְנוּס.

טוּנֵס pr. n. pl. (Tunes) *Tunis* in Northern Africa. Sifré Deut. 320, v. בַּרְבַּרְיָא.—*Targ. Y. Ex. II, 3 חיבותא דט׳ (prob. meaning טָנִיס; some ed. . . . נַס) a Tunesian box (h. text גמא).

טוּס (b. h. טוּשׂ) [1) *to glisten.* Denom. טַוָּס.—2) (cmp. חָלַף)] *to fly swiftly.*—Y. Taan. IV, 69b לא נראה עוף טָס וכ׳ no bird has been seen flying in all Palestine; Lam. R. introd. end.—Deut. R. s. 6 קושט . . וטס כעוף goes straight like an arrow, and swift like a bird. Midr. Till. to Ps. XC, 10 גוזין חשין וטָסִין they pass, hasten and fly; a. fr.

Pi. טִיּוּס same. Koh. R. to IX, 7 ט׳ וחזר וט׳ he flew to and back.

Hif. הֵטִיס *to cause to fly, to bring on by flight.* Ruth R. to IV, 1 הטיסו וכ׳ the Lord would have made him fly and brought him (to the place). Gen. R. s. 59, end. Cant. R. to I, 9 הֲטִיסָן; Ex. R. s. 23 end הסיטן (corr. acc.).—Lev. R. s. 16 'חסיט, (read as) Yalk. Kings 232. Lev. R. s. 11, beg. הסיטן (corr. acc.) he winged them; a. fr.

טוּס ch. same. Targ. Job V, 7 (Ms. טוּשׁ); a. fr.—Part. טָאֵס, טָאֵיס, טָיֵס, טָיֵיס. Ib. XXXIX, 18.—Targ. II Esth. I, 2 שׁוּרִין טַיְיסִין (read: נִשְׁרִין).—Targ. Is. XVIII, 1 (ed. Lag. דטאס); a. fr.—Y. Yeb. XVI, 15[c] bot. נפשא טָיְיסָא 'וכ the soul hovers over the body; Y. M. Kat. III, 82[b] bot.; Lev. R. s. 18; (Gen. R. s. 100 תייבא).

Pa. טַיֵּיס 1) same. Targ. II Esth. l. c. טַיְּיסִית I flew.—2) *to cause to fly.* Targ. Y. Deut. XXVIII, 49. [Ib. טַיֵּיס נישרא, read: טָיֵיס, v. supra.]

טְוָסָא, טַוָּס, v. sub 'טוּ.

טוֹעֵי f. (טְעֵי) *thoughtlessness.* Targ. Prov. I, 32 (ed. Lag. טוּעיי, Var. טוער).

(טְעוֹן) טֹעַן, טוֹעַן m. (טָעַן I) *requirement.* Sifra introd., v. טָעַן I.

טוּעְנָא m. (טְעַן II) *burden, load, bag.* Targ. O. Ex. XXIII, 5; a. fr.; v. טוּנָא I.—V. טְעוֹנָא.

טוּף ch.=h. צוּף, 1) [*to shine,*] *to come to the surface, float, bubble up.* Part. טָאֵיף, טָיֵיף. Targ. Y. Deut. XXI, 1. Targ. Y. Gen. XXVIII, 10; a. e.—Koh. R. to V, 8 (mixed diction) 'וטָפַת בארה של וכ Miriam's well came up.—Ab. II, 6; Succ. 53[a], v. infra.—Y. Shebi. IX, 38[d]; Pesik. B'shall. p. 89[b] הוה טָיֵיף the corpse came up to the surface. Gen. R. s. 81 (in Hebr. dict.) וטָפַת רוחי 'וכ and my mind in me was swimming (I became proud, v. טָפַח); a. fr.—2) (denom. of טִיף) *to drip; to be inundated.* Targ. O. Gen. XLIX, 12; a. e.—Keth. 111[b] חלבא 'טייף וכ milk was dripping &c. Y. Taan. III, end, 67[a] 'הוה עלמא טָ the world would have been flooded. Gen. R. s. 32; Yalk. ib. 57 'דלא טָף וכ' it (the mount Gerizim) was not flooded by the waters of the flood; a. e.—[Targ. Y. Deut. XXI, 23 תטופון, v. נְטַף a. נְטַף.]

Pa. טָאֵף, טַיֵּיף 1) *to direct the overflow, to assign channels.* Targ. Job XXXVIII, 24, v. טַיָּפָא.—Gitt. 69[b] top 'וניטַיְּיפֵיה וכ and let it (the milk) run over &c.—2) *to cause to glisten, to turn in all directions.* Keth. 60[b] מְטַיְּפֵי עינא Ar. (ed. מצייצי, v. infra) with restless eyes.—3) *to cause to float,* v. infra.

Af. אַטִּיף, אָטֵיף (נְטַף ·) 1) *to make flow.* Targ. Deut. XI, 4.—[Keth. l. c. מְטִיפֵי עינא Ar. s. v. נְטַף I 'with dripping eyes', v. supra.]—2) *to cause to float.* Ab. II, 6 על דאַטֵּפְתְּ אֲטִיפוּךְ וסוף מְטִיפָךְ יְטוּפוּן ed. Strack (oth. eds. אַטְפוּךְ. Strack reads מְטַיְּפָךְ *Pa.;* oth. pointed eds. מְטִיפָיִךְ h. form) because thou (the person whose skull was seen to float) hast caused (a corpse) to float, they made thee float, and those who made thee float, shall also float.

Ithpa. אִיטַּיַּיף *to be glittering, to be turned in all directions.* B. Kam. 92[b]; Meg. 14[b] ועיניה מְשַׁיְּיפֵי and its eyes look all around (for food).

טוּפָא, Koh. R. to V, 10 'ליה טָ דהדא, read: סוּפָא.

טוּפָא, pl. טוּפֵי, v. טְרָפָא.

טוּפוּס, v. טָפוּס a. טוּפֶס.

טוֹפַח m. (טָפַח II) *irrigating engine.* Peah V, 3 אין 'מגלגלין בט (Y. ed. טוּפִיחַ) one must not irrigate (a field) with an irrigator (before the poor have collected their share; v. Tosef. ib. II, 20); Y. ib. V, 19[a] top. [Maim. identifying our w. with next w. explains: you must not *sow the tofah* in conjunction with other seeds.]

טוֹפַח m. (v. preced.) an *aquatic plant* like the Colocasia; *bean, tofah;* [Maim. קרטמאן Arab., defining it 'a seed similar to barley.'] Kil. I, 1. T'bul Yom I, 2; Tosef. ib. I, 1, sq. טפיח (R. S. to T'bul Yom l. c. quotes טופח). Tosef. Makhsh. III, 6 טוּפִּיחַ. Tosef. T'rum. VI, 11 טפיח ed. Zuck. (Var. טופח, טופיח). Peah VI, 7 'אפי היא 'של ט even if the barley in the field have the size of *tofah* (R. S.; Maim.: "even if it be a field of the inferior kind of barley named *t.*").—V. טְפִיחַ II.

טוּפִיחַ, v. preced. wds.

טוֹפְיָינָא m. (טְפֵי III) *additional amount, surplus.* B. Mets. 63[b] 'ואשכח ביה ט (Var. טפיאתא, טפיתא, טפייתא, v. Rabb. D. S. a l. note 9) and he (the borrower) finds in the bundle more money than the loan agreed upon. V. טִיפוֹנָא a. טְפִיתָא.

טופיסטוס, טופיסוס, Pesik. R. s. 21, read: סוֹפִיסְטֵיס.

טופיתא, Targ. Job XXVIII, 7 ed. Lag., v. טַרְפִיתָא.

טוּפִיתָא, pl. טוּפְיָיתָא, טוּפְיָאתָא, v. טְפִיתָא.

טוּפְלָא, v. טַפְלָא.

טוֹפָנָא, 'טוֹ m. (טוּף) *flood.* Targ. O. Gen. VI, 17 (Y. טוּבְעָנָא); a. fr.

טוֹפֶס m. (v. טָפַס; cmp. דְּפוּס, טִפּוּס) *frame;* trnsf. (influenced by Greek τύπος) *formula* (to be filled out according to occasion). Y. Ber. I, 3[d] 'ט' ברכות וכ such is the formula of the benedictions; Lev. R. s. 34, end; Y. Sabb. XV, end, 15[b] טופס.—Esp. *the formula* or *blank of documents,* opp. תּוֹרֶף containing names, dates &c. Y. Gitt. III, beg. 44[c] 'כתב תרפו בט (also בתופס) if the writer filled out a blank. B. Mets. 7[b]; a. fr.—*Pl.* טוֹפְסִין, constr. טוֹפְסֵי. Y. Gitt. II, beg. 44[a] 'פוסל בט declares illegal deeds of divorce written into ready-made blanks. Gitt. III, 2 'הכותב ט' גיטין וכ he who writes formulas of letters of divorce must leave blanks for the name &c.; a. fr.

טוֹפְסָא, ch. same, = h. טָפוּס, דְּפוּס, *frame, mould, cast.* Targ. Y. Num. XXV, 1 (cmp. Sabb. 64[a] s. v. דְּפוּס). Targ. Y. Ex. XXXII, 4 בְּטַפְסָא Ar. a Levita (ed. בטופרא, corr. acc.) in a mould.—[B. Bath. 103[b] טופסא Ar., v. טַפְתָּא.]

טוּפְרָא, טְפַר m. = h. צִפֹּרֶן, 1) *nail* of the human finger; *claw; hoof;* trnsf. *pencil.* Targ. Jer. XVII, 1.—Ḥull. 17[b] the knife must be examined, אבישרא ואט׳ וכ׳ on the fleshy top of the finger and on the nail &c.; a. fr.—*Pl.* טוּפְרִין, טְפַ׳, טוּפְרַיָּיא. Targ. Jud. V, 22 (h. text עקבות) Targ. O. Deut. XXI, 12 טוּפְרָהָא ed. Berl. (ed. Vien. טוּפְרְנָהָא; Y. טוּפְרַיָּיהָא).—M. Kat. 18[a] חזנהו לטופריה וכ׳ (not לטופרי) saw that his nails were long; a. e.—Midr. Sam. ch. XI, v. אִסְטְלִי.—2) *onycha* (*unguis odoratus*) a spice. Targ. O. Ex. XXX, 34.—[Targ. Y. Gen. III, 7 לבוש טופרא, read: שׁוּפְרָא.—Lev. R. s. 33 טופרין ושער ועצמות, read: טפוסין של צלמים, v. Yalk. Dan. 1061.—Targ. Y. Ex. XXXII, 4, v. טוּפְסָא.]—V. next w.

טוּפְרְנָא m., collect. noun (preced.) *nails.* Targ. O. Deut. XXI, 2.—[Y. Snh. I, 18[c] bot. טופרני, read: טוּפְרוֹי; Y. R. Hash. II, 58[b] top טפרוי; v. דְּקָקָה.]

***בקעת בית ט׳, טוֹפֶת** pr. n. *Valley of Beth-Tofeth* Koh. R. to V, 8; v., however, נְטוֹפָה II.

***טוּק**, Y. Sabb. VI, 7[d] bot. פרוש טוק טקלין ed., Ar. פרוסטוקטולין, פרסטקולין, prob. a corruption of כְּרוּסוֹקַסְטֵלוֹן (χρυσοκαστέλλιον) *a golden castle,* name of *a head-dress* (עיר הזהב; v. Sm. Ant. s. v. Corona).

טוּר I, *Pa.* טַיֵּיר (cmp. תור) *to espy, to augur.* Targ. Y. Gen. XLIV, 8; 15 (h. text נחש).

Af אַטִּיר (denom. of טַיָּיר) *to consult divination.* Ib. XXX, 27.

טוּר II, **טוּרָא** I, **טַוְרָא** m. (preced., cmp. b. h. צוּר) *mount, mountain.* Targ. O. Ex. III, 12 (Y. טוורא). Targ. Y. Gen. XXIII, 2; a. fr.—Ḥull. 7[b], v. גְּבַהּ. Sabb. 152[a] ט׳ תלג a mountain of snow (my head is white). Gen. R. s. 32, v. בְּרַךְ; a. fr.—*Pl.* טוּרִין, טוּרַיָּא, טוּרֵי, טְוָרֵי, טַוֵּי. Targ. Job. IX, 5. Targ. Deut. XI, 11; a. fr.—Gen. R. l. c. אי מט׳ רמיא if it belongs among the high mountains; a. e.—[Sabb. 98[b] כי טורין, v. טְרָיז.]—טור מלכא (h. הר המלך) *King's Mountain,* ט׳ שמעון *Mount Simeon.* Gitt. 55[b]. Y. Taan. IV, 69[a]; Lam. R. to II, 2 (v. Neub. Géogr. p. 41; p. 267).—ט׳ פרזלא *Iron Mount.* Targ. Y. Num. XXXIV, 3. —For other compounds, v. respective determinants.

טוּרָא II m. (cmp. נְהַר, v. preced.) *clearness, sky.* Gen. R. s. 99 (ref. to המסדרונה, Jud. III, 23) [read:] ערפלי ט׳ וכ׳ the clouds of brightness, where the angels are seated in order.

***טוּרָא** III m. *tura,* name of a bitter herb. Pes. 39[a] (Ms. M. סורא).

טוּרְבֵּל, טוּרְבִּיל (tribulum, τρίβολος) only in מִטָּה של ט׳ *threshing sledge* (couch) consisting of a wooden platform studded underneath with sharp pieces of flint or with iron teeth. Ab. Zar. 24[b] (Ar. a. Yalk. Sam. 122 טרבן); Zeb. 116[b]; Men. 22[a] Ms. M. (ed. טרבל), v. דִּיָּשָׁה. Par. XII, 9 טְרָבֵל.

טוּרְגִינוֹס, v. טְרְיָינוֹס.

***טוּרוֹס** (sub. מִיטָּה) f. (torus) *bolster, couch, sofa.* Pirke d'R. El. ch. XLI כטנדס שהיא פרוסה Ar. (ed. only כטנדס, corr acc., and add בתוך האהל: v. Mekh. Yithro, Baḥod. s. 4 כאדם שהוא מציע את הכר על ראש המטה) like a couch which is spread in a tent. [Ar. refers טנדס to the late Latin *tenta,* Gr. τέντα (τένδα), Italian *tenda.*]

טוּרְזַיָּא m. pl. (טרז=טרד II; cmp. טְרוּזָא) [*locked up things,* cmp. אוֹצָר,] *royal wardrobe, armory.* Ber. 56[a] ריש ט׳ וכ׳ (some ed. טורזינא, Ar. טרזיא) the chief of the royal wardrobe dreamt. Ib. אתייה לריש ט׳ וכ׳ (Ms. M. אמר קיסר אייתיה לריש טריא) they brought the chief.... up, and he was put do death. [For Var. lect., v. Rabb. D. S. a. l. notes 1, 2.]

טוּרְזִינָא, טַרְ׳ (preced.) 1) *treasury-office, armory.* Ber. 56[a] אפתחא דריש ט׳ (Ar. טרזיא, v. preced.) at the entrance of the chief treasury; [prob. to be read: דבי ט׳, דריש having come in by tautography from the suceeding ריש טורזיא.]—B. Bath. 8[a] לשורא . . . ולטר׳ וכ׳ (Ms. F. טורדינא, Alf. Ms. טורדיתא) for the maintenance of the town-wall, the horse-guard and the armory even orphans must contribute.—2) (sub. ריש) *superintendent of the armory* or *treasury.* Erub. 80[a] ההוא ט׳ וכ׳ (ed. Sonc. טורזיינא) there was a (gentile) superintendent that lived in the neighborhood &c.

טוֹרַח (b. h. טֹרַח; טָרַח) *toil, labor, trouble, painstaking preparations.* Sabb. 153[a] כלום . . . . בלא ט׳ is there a banquet without visible preparation?; (Koh. R. to IX, 8 הֶטְרֵחַ). M. Kat. 8[b] מפני הט׳ on account of the labor (connected with preparing the wedding). Y. Pes. X, 37[d] top מה הט׳ . . מטריחים וכ׳ what is all that trouble for to which you put us &c.?; a. fr.—*Pl.* טְרָחוֹת. Ber. 58[a] כמה ט׳ טרח וכ׳ to how much trouble did the host go &c.; (Y. ib. IX, 13[c] כמה טורח טרח). Lev. R. s. 1 משה עסוק בט׳ וכ׳ Moses (like an *agoranomos*) was engaged in the (dietary) affairs of Israel. Gen. R. s. 94 ט׳ נפש אחת the troubles of providing for one soul.—V. טַרְחוּת a. טִרְחָא.

טוֹרְחָא, טָרְחָא ch. same. Targ. O. Deut. I, 12. Targ. Koh. II, 21; a. fr.—Ib. 11 טוֹרְחָתִי.—B. Mets. 40[b] טִרְחֵיה, v. בִּרְזְנַיְיתָא.—V. טִרְחָא.

טוֹרְחָן, טוֹרְחוּתָא, v. sub טרח׳.

טוּרְחָנָא m. (preced. wds.) *trouble, care.* Targ. Y. I Num. XI, 12.

טוֹרְחָתָא f., v. טִרְחָא.

טוּרְטוּר, pl. טוּרְטוּרִין, v. next w.

טְרִיטְנֵי, טְרוּטִינֵי, טוּרְטָנֵי, טוּרְטִינֵי, f. (trutina, τρυτάνη, prob. of Semit. origin, cmp. טְרָא) *balance, steel-yard.* Sifra K'dosh. Par. 3, ch. VIII במשקל זו טרו׳ 'in weight' (Lev. XIX, 35) that means the trutina. Sabb. 81[a] וכי ט׳ יכניס shall a (gold) balance be brought in (to weigh accurately)?; Men. 87[b]. B. Kam. 119[a]. B. Bath. 89[a] ט׳ (for weighing gold), contrad. to באזנים. Tosef. Kel. B. Mets. II, 5.—Y. Shek. VI, end, 50[b] כבין ט׳ arranged like a steel-yard. Sot. 34[a] (ref. to מוֹט, Num. XIII, 23) ט׳ וט׳ דט׳ a combination of balancing poles (for four couples of carriers); Y. ib. VII, 21[d] bot. טרטורין several poles (each carried by two); ט׳ וטוּרְטוּרֵי טרוטורין a combination &c.—*Pl.* טוּרְנְיָן. B. Kam. l. c. Ms. R. 2 (v. Rabb. D. S. a. l. note 400).

טוּרְיוֹת, v. טִירָא.

טוּרְיָיא pr. n. pl., v. דְּרָיָיא.

טוּרְיָינוּס, טוּרְיָינָא, v. טְרָיָינָא, טְרָיָינוּס.

טוּרִיסְקִי, v. טורייסקי.

טוּרְמוּטָא, v. טְרוֹמִיטָא.

טוּרְמִי f., pl. טוּרְמִיּוֹת, טוּרְמִיאוֹת (turma, τούρμη) *turma, a squadron of horse;* in gen. *division of an army.* Y. Sot. VIII, beg. 22[b] (ref. to Ps. XVIII, 13) כנגד טומיות שלהם (corr. acc.) corresponding to their (the enemy's) squadrons. Yalk. Sam. 160; Mekh. B'shall s. 2 תּוּרְמִיּוֹת. Ib. ת׳ ת׳ של מה״ש troops of angels. Ib. (ref. to סַעֲ: Ex. XIV, 10) נעשו . . . ת׳ ת׳ כאיש אחד they all formed squadrons marching like one man; Yalk. Ex. 230 ט׳ ט׳. Ib. מכאן . . . מתנהגות ת׳ from here (the Egyptian warfare) the governments learned to form squadrons; Yalk. Ex. 230 ט׳.

טוּרְמִיטָא, v. טְרוֹמִיטָא.

טוּרְמִיסִין, v. חֲמִיסִין.

טוּרְמְנְטִין m. pl. (tormenta) *engines for hurling missiles; missiles, shots from the engine.* Y. Sot. VIII, beg. 22[b] (ref. to גחלי, Ps. XVIII, 13) כנגד טרמנטן וכ׳ (corr. acc.) corresponding to their (the enemy's) tormenta (v. טוּרְמִי); Yalk. Sam. 160 תרמצה; Mekh. B'shall. s. 2 טרמנסנה (corr. acc.). Midr. Till. to Ps. XVIII סימנטרא (read: טוּרְמִינְטָא). Sifré Deut. 204 מיני מטראאות; Yalk. ib. 923 מיני מטרסאות (read: טוּרְמִינְטָאוֹת).

טוּרָנָא m. (טוּר, נְטַר) *officer,* less than שׁוּלְטָן.—*Pl.* טוּרָנַיָּא, טוּרָנִין. Targ. Is. X, 17 (h. text שמיר!). Ib. XXXIV, 7; a. e.—Esp. *Philistean magistrates.* Targ. Jud. III, 3 (h. text סרני); a. fr.

***טוֹרְנוֹס** m. (τόρνος, tornus) *turner's wheel, lathe.* Pesik. R. s. 21 למורנס הזה (read: כט׳, v. Friedm. a. l. note 29) like the lathe which shows a front wherever you turn it.

טוּרְנוֹס, ט׳ רוּפוּס (also in one word) pr. n. m. *Turnus Rufus* (supposed to be a corruption of *T. Annius Rufus*), a Roman commander in the days of the Hadrianic persecutions. Taan. 29[a] טורנסרופוס ed. (Ms. M. טורנוסרופוס, or טורנוסט׳, v. Rabb. D. S. a. l. note). Y. Ber. IX, 14[b] bot. טונוס טר׳ (Tosaf. to Sot. 31[a] טורנוסר׳). Koh. R. to III, 17. Snh. 65[b]. Ned. 50[b] top; Ab. Zar. 20[a]. Pesik. R. s. 23.

טוּרְנוֹסְרוּפוּס, v. preced.

טוּרְסוֹס, v. טַרְסִים.

טוּרְסִי, v. טַרְסִי.

טוּרְפִי, Targ. Ps. I, 3 ed. Lag., v. טַרְפָא.

טוּרְקוֹס, Sifré Num. 89, v. נוֹטָרִיקוֹן.

טוֹרְתוּק, Ar. s. v. ברנט; v. לַבְרָטִין a. נַרְתֵּק.

טוּשׁ, v. טוּס.

טוּשׁ I (cmp. טוּחַ I) *to cover with a cohesive substance, to polish* (with a fatty matter); *to besmear, soil, pollute.* Pes. 30[b]; Zeb. 95[b], a. e. אין טָשִׁין וכ׳ one must not polish the stove with &c. Tosef. B. Kam. IX, 31 [in a misplaced passage, belonging after שבידיו; read:] חרק כנגד פני חבירו וטש פניו (ref. to Is. L, 6[b]) who spat into or besmeared his neighbor's face; (cmp. Mish. ib. VIII, 6; Sifra Emor Par. 14, ch. XX).

Pilpel טִשְׁטֵשׁ (fr. טְשַׁשׁ) 1) *to make viscid, soften.* Taan. 22[b] מְטַשְׁטְשִׁין את הארץ (the heavy rains) make the soil muddy and it yields no fruit; Yalk. Lev. 671.—2) *to smear over, besmear.* Part. pass. מְטוּשְׁטָשׁ, pl. מְטוּשְׁטָשִׁין. Pes. 65[b] היו בגדיו מט׳ if his (the priest's) garments were besmeared (with blood &c.); Zeb. 18[a], sq.; ib. 35[a].—Meg. 18[b] אותיות מְטוּשְׁטָשׁוֹת letters made illegible by being smeared over.

Nithpalp. נִיטַשְׁטֵשׁ, *Hithpa.* הִיטַשְׁטֵשׁ *to be smeared over, be dirty.* B. Bath. 168[b] נמחק או נט׳ if the writing was blotted out or blurred. Tosef. Kel. B. Mets. IV, 13 נִטַּשְׁטְשָׁה a metal mirror which became blurred (blind). Sabb. 81[a] נִיטַשְׁטְשׁוּ Ms. M. (ed. נשטש׳, corr. acc.) the spots were washed away (became indistinct). Cant. R. to VIII, 9 a picture on a wall אע״פ שֶׁנִּטַשְׁטֶשֶׁת (prob. שֶׁמְּטוּשְׁטֶשֶׁת, v. supra) even if it be smeared over.

טוּשׁ ch. same. Targ. Y. Deut. XXVIII, 40 תטושון Ar. (ed. תשוטון, corr. acc. or תשוצון, v. שׁוּעַ) you will oint yourselves. Targ. Y. II Lev. XIV, 42 ויטשון (read וִיטוּשׁוּן) shall plaster over; (Targ. Y. I ויתטש *Ithpa.*).—Gen. R. s. 34, end טָשִׁין מוחיה (not וטושין) and paste the plaster on its scull.

Ithpa. אִיתְּטַשׁ *to be plastered.* Targ. Y. Lev. XIV, 43; 48; v. supra.

Palp. טַשְׁטֵשׁ *to smear over, to make muddy.* Part. pass. מְטַשְׁטַשׁ; v. infra.

Ithpalp. אִיטַּשְׁטַשׁ *to be smeared over, to be made muddy.* Targ. Job. XVI, 16 מט׳ Ms. (ed. כְּטַ׳; h. text חמרמר׳); Targ. Ps. XLVI, 4 (h. text חמר; cmp. חֲבָרָא).

טוּשׁ II (v. טְשַׁר), *Af.* אַטִּישׁ *to hide, reserve* (corresp. to h. צָפַן). Targ. Ps. XXXI, 20 אַטֵּשְׁתָּא Ms. (ed. אַטְשִׁירְתָּא, v. טְשַׁר). Ib. CXIX, 11 (some ed. אטיש׳, corr. acc.). Targ. Job X, 13. Ib. XXIII, 12.

Ithpe. אִתְטִישׁ, אִתְטְשׁ *to be hidden.* Ib. XV, 20. Ib. XXIV, 1.—V. טְשַׁר, נטש.

טְזוּת, v. טְווּת.

טְחָא, v. כחי.

טְחָאֵי, v. טְחָיֵי.

***טַחַב**, m. *dew, moist grass* (Ar.: *cold*). Sifra Aḥăré beg.; Yalk. Lev. 571.

***טַחֲבוּת** f. (preced.) *dew, vapor.* Targ. Job XXXVII, 11 Regia (ed. ברירותא, h. text בריר).

טְחוֹל m. (cmp. טוּחַ II) *spleen, milt.* Hull. III, 2. Snh. 21b; Ab. Zar. 44a נטולי ט׳ having had their milt cut out (as fast runners); a. fr.

טְחוֹלָא ch. same. *Pl.* טְחוֹלִין. Targ. Esth. VIII, 10; v. טַחֲלָא.

טְחוֹן, v. טְחִינָה.

טְחוֹנָא m. (טְחַן) *miller.—Pl.* טְחוֹנִין, טְחוֹנַיָּא. Y. Peah I, 15c bot.; Y. Kidd. I, 61b bot. אתת ... ט׳ an ordinance was issued for millers (for government work); Pesik. R. s. 23-24 טחונים (read יא ...). Y. Pes. III, 30a top; a. fr.

טָחוֹר* m. (v. טָחַר) *sufferer from piles.* Midr. Sam. ch. X היה יושב כט׳ when one sat straining himself like &c.

טְחוֹרִין, טְחוֹרַיָּא m. pl. (b. h. *k'ri* טְחֹרִים; v. טחר) *piles, hemorrhoids.* Targ. Deut. XXVIII, 27; a. e.—Targ. Ps. LXXVIII, 66 (h. text אחור).

טְחָא, טְחִי (v. טוּחַ II) *to squeeze into, fasten to.* Gitt. 69b נִיטַחְיֵיהּ בתנורא (not חייא ...) let him squeeze it (the milt) into (the cracks of) an oven; ניט׳ ביני אורבי let him squeeze it in between bricks &c.

טְחָיָא, v. טִיחְיָא.

טַחְיֵי, טַחְאֵי, טַחְיָא m. pl. (טחא, cmp. טוּחַ I) *cakes smeared with oil.* Sabb. 119a; Hull. 111a תלת סאיי ט׳ three S'ah of flour made into glistening cakes.

טְחִין, v. טְחַן.

טְחִינָה f. (טָחַן) *grinding.* Pes. 11a; a. fr.—Men. XI, 3 (96a) טְחִינָתָן (Mish. ed. טְחוֹנָן); Tosef. ib. XI, 4 טִחְנָן.—Trnsf. *sexual contact.* Sot. 10a; Num. R. s. 9 (ref. to Jud. XVI, 21, a. Job XXXI, 10).

טְחִינִין m. pl. (preced.) *grist, meal,* v. פַּרְשִׁינָה. Tosef. Dem. I, 24; Hull. 6a; Y. Dem. I, 22a סח׳ (corr. acc.)

טַחֲלָא ch.=h. טְחוֹל. Gitt. 69b לט׳ for pain in the milt. Hull. 93a; a. fr.—*Pl.* טַחֲלֵי. Ib. רט׳ וכ׳ the veins (sinews) of milts must be removed as fat; v. חוּטְא. Ib. 111a תבשילא דט׳ a dish of pieces of milt.

טָחַן (b. h.; cmp. טְחַר) 1) *to mill, grind.* Sabb. VII, 2 הטוחן he who grinds (on the Sabbath). Ex. R. s. 36, beg. טוֹחֲנִין אותם (the olives) are crushed. Sot. 9b .. ועקרן וטְחָנָן וכ׳ and Samson uprooted them (the mountains) and ground them against one another; Snh. 24a; a. fr.—Trnsf. *to have sexual intercourse* (cmp. μύλλω). Gen. R. s. 48, end.—*2) *to force* to menial labor. Pesik. R. s. 23-24 (ed. Fr. p. 122b) טְחָנוּ ברחיים, v. infra, a. פָּדַן.

Hif. הִטְחִין *to cause to grind.* Kidd. 31a bot. וייש מַטְחִינוֹ ברחיים and some one may make his father grind in the mill (v. supra, a. פָּדַן). Keth. 59b (ref. to ib. V, 5) טוֹחֶנֶת ס״ד .. מַטְחֶנֶת you cannot mean that she must do the grinding? ... she must attend to the grinding.

טְחַן, טְחִין, טַחֵן ch. same. Targ. Jud. XVI, 21; a. e.—Pesik. R. s. 23-24; Y. Kidd. I, 61b bot.; Y. Peah I, 15c bot. חוּט תחותי טְחוֹן grind thou in my place. Ib. חוה אִיטְחִין, read: חוה טָחֵין as Y. Kidd. l. c.—Snh. 96a טָחֲנֵי קשייתא were grinding date-stones; a. fr.—*Part. pass.* טְחִין, טְחִינָא. Ib.b קמחא ט׳ טְחִינַת thou groundest ground flour (you conquered Israel because it was doomed to destruction). Ber. 43a bot. משחא ט׳ oil perfumed with ground ingredients, contrad. to כבישא.—Y. Ned. VI, end, 40a קלִיין וטְחִינָן וכ׳ roasted and ground &c. [Cant. R. to I, 16 לא מטחנא, read: מְטַמְּנָא (?), v. נְצַב.]

טַחַן m.=טְחִינָה q. v.

טַחֲנָה f. (b. h.; preced. wds.) *mill.* Koh. R. to XII, 7 נמשלו ד״ת כט׳ וכ׳ the study of the Law is allegorized as a mill, as the mill does not stop &c.—*Pl.* טוֹחֲנוֹת (fr. טוֹחֲנָה) *millstones.* Lam. R. introd. (R. Josh. 2) נמשלו ישראל כט׳ Israel is compared to millstones (never resting), v. supra. Ib. הט׳ אלו משניות וכ׳ 'the millstones' (Koh. XII, 3), that means the study of the great Mishnayoth of &c.

טָחַף* (cmp. טחב) *to be moist, soiled.—Part. pass.* טָחוּף; fem. טְחוּפָה, pl. טְחוּפוֹת (of wool) *dirty-white, gray,* opp. לבנה bright-white. Hull. XI, 2; ib. 136b Ar. (ed. שחופות). [Cmp. Arab. ṭaḥf moeror, nubes.]

טָחַר (=תחר, denom. of אחר; cmp. טְרַגַן) *to press, to strain the rectum.* Sabb. 82a לא לִיטְחַר טפי Ar. (ed. ליטרח; Ms. M. לִיתְחַר, v. Rabb. D. S. a. l. note) one must not strain himself too much.—V. טְחוֹרַיָּא.

טַט* or **טָט** *two* (in the language of כתפי, כתפי or גדפי). Snh. 4b; Zeb. 37b; Men. 34b.

טַטְלַפוּשׁ* pr. n. pl. *Tatlafush* (?). Hull. 110a (in R. Gershon Ms. טלטל לפוש, v. Koh. Ar. Compl. s. v.;—perh. a perversion of בלשפט).

טוֹט׳, טַטְפְּרָאוֹת f. pl., a corruption of טֶרְפּוּלָאוֹת, v. טֶטְרַפְּלִוּת.

טֹטֶפֶת, טוֹטַפְתָּא, v. טוֹט.

טֶטְרָאמוּלִי, טֶטְרָאמוּלִין m. (τετράμουλος) *a chariot with four animals (mules) abreast,* (Lat.) *quadriga;* [a compound not recorded in Greek dictionaries]. Ex. R. s. 3 I shall come down בט׳ שלי with my *quadriga* (ref. to Ez. I, 5); ib. s. 42 מילין ... (corr. acc.); Tanh. Ki Thissa 21. Ex. R. s. 43 והם שומטים אחד כן ט׳ וכ׳ and they will unhitch one of the four animals of my chariot.

טֶטְרָאפִילוֹת, v. טֶטְרַפְּלִוּת.

טַטְרַג* (=טרטרג, reduplic. of טרג, cmp. טְרִיף, טַרְפְּנוּתָא) *to molest, provoke.* Erub. 61a טַטְרוּגֵי מְטַטְרְגֵי לחי וכ׳ the residents of G. used to molest those of H. (visiting their place; v. Ms. M. a. Rabb. D. S. a. l. notes).

טֶטְרָגוֹן m. 1) (τετράγωνος) *four-cornered, in a quadrangle, in a square.* Naz. 8b; B. Bath. 164b (בית) ט׳ a house of four corners. Cant. R. to IV, 4 (expl. תלפיות) טֶטְרָגוֹנִין (τετραγώνιος) in a square. Pesik. R. s. 10

בוטרגונין (corr. acc.), v. אַסְטְרוֹנְגִּילוֹן.—2) (τετράγονος, v. הֵיגוֹן) *for the fourth time.* Tosef. Naz. I, 2 הריני נזיר ט׳ וכ׳ 'I will be a Nazir tetragon', means four times; Naz. l. c.; B. Bath. l. c.—3) *fourfold, four combined.* Midr. Till. to Ps. LXXVIII, 49 מט׳ היה (corr. acc.) each plague was fourfold; ed. Bub. טֶטְרָאגוֹן.

טֶטְרָגוֹנָה, טֶטְרָגוֹנָא ch. same. Y. Sot. VIII, 22[d] top (ref. to Ex. XXXII, 15) ט׳ the engraving on the tablets was in a square (containing the Ten Commandments four times on each side, and readable whichever way you turned it); Cant. R. to V, 14 טטרוגא (corr. acc.).

טטרוגא, v. preced.

טַטְרוּגֵי, infin. of טַטְרֵג.

טטרומולין, v. טֶטְרָאמ׳.

טטרטין; טִטַרְטוֹן, v. טִיטַ׳.

טטרפאות, v. טִיטְרַפְלִיּוֹת.

טטרפלין, Tosef. Ohol. XVIII, 13, v. טִיטְרַפְּלוֹן.

טיאוניס, Y. Gitt. IV, 45[d] bot., הרנירק ט׳, v. אנדכתרי.

טיאמרון, Cant. R. beg., some ed. טיארון, read: תֵּיאַטְרוֹן.

טְיָארִין, v. טְיָיר.

טִיב I m. (טוב, cmp. טֶבַע) *form, nature, character, peculiarity.* Y. Ber. VII, 11[b] ט׳ ברכה the form of a benediction. Kidd. 13[a] ט׳ גטין וכ׳ the legal form of deeds of divorce and of betrothals. Gen. R. s. 17 אדם זה מה טִיבוֹ this man (whom thou art going to create)—what will his nature (distinction) be?—Keth. I, 8 מה טיבו של זה what is that man? Ib. 9 מה ט׳ של עובר זה what is this expected child (who is its father)?—Snh. 108[b] מה טִיבָם וכ׳ what is the nature of these seven days?—Sifra Emor ch. XVIII, Par. 14 מה טִיבְךָ ליטע וכ׳ what art thou (what right hast thou) to put up thy tent &c.?; a. fr.

טִיב, טִיבָא ch. 1) same. Targ. Cant. VII, 1 מה טִיבְכוֹן what right have you?—Y. Sabb. II, 4[d] top מה טִיבֵיה והוה what sort of a man was he?; Y. Ter. XI, end, 48[b] מה טבייה (corr. acc.).—*2) *seal, sign of recognition.* Targ. I Sam. XVII, 18 טִיבְהוֹן ed. Lag. (oth. ed. טִיבֵיהוֹן, h. text עֲרֻבָּה). [Targ. Am. IX, 4 לטיבא, some ed., read לְטָבָא. Targ. Is. IX, 9 טיבין, some ed., read טָבִין.]

טִיב II, **טִיבָא, (טִיבָא)** m. (טבב, cmp. דָּבַב, דִּבָּה) *murmuring, rumor, (evil) report.* Targ. O. Gen. XXXVII, 2 טִיבְהוֹן ed. Berl. (oth. ed. דִּבְ׳; Y. טִיבֵיהוֹן). Targ. Prov. X, 18 טיבא ed. Lag. (some ed. טָבָא, read טִבָ׳); a. fr.—[Targ. Y. Gen. XXXIV, 30 טיבי, Var. שִׁבִי, read טִיבִי.]

טִיב, *Pi.* טִיֵּיב, *Pa.* טַיֵּיב, v. טוּב.

טִיבָה f. = טִיב I.—*Pl.* טִיבוֹת. Snh. 61[b] מטִיבוֹתָן וכ׳ from the qualities of the near deities &c., [Ms. F. טוּבוֹתָן, v. Rabb. D. S. a. l. note 90].

טִיבוּ, טֵיבוּ, טֵיבוּתָא f. ch. = h. טוֹבָה, *goodness, good deed; profit, enjoyment, pleasure.* Targ. Gen. XXIII, 13. Targ. Koh. IV, 8; a. fr.—Y. Ḥag. II, 77[d] bot. חדא ט׳ one good deed. Tam. 32[a] יעביד ט׳ עם וכ׳ let him act kindly towards &c. Taan. 23[b] ולא נחזיק ט׳ וכ׳ without having credit given to us. Y. Ber. II, 5[a] bot., v. חֲזַק. Lam. R. to I, 5; a. fr.—Men. 52[a] מטֵיבוּתָךְ לא אמרי Ms. M. (ed. מטֵבוּתִין) of our good teachings they do not speak. Ib. הני נמי מטיבותן היא Ms. M. (ed. טבותין) this is also one of our good things.

טִיבּוּל, טִבּ׳ m. 1) (טָבַל I) *dipping; luncheon, antepast.* Pes. 115[a] כל שטִיבּוּלוֹ במשקה וכ׳ whatever eatable is dipped into a liquid, requires hand-washing (before partaking of it). Gitt. 70[a] יהא רגיל בט׳ וכ׳ let him make it a habit to eat relishes dipped (in vinegar &c.) in the summer as well as &c. Bets. 18[b]; Sabb. 111[a] קודם ט׳ before the antepast. Pes. 115[b] בט׳ ראשון when dipping the first time; a. e.—2) (טָבַל II) *the act which makes food subject to priestly gifts* (טֶבֶל). Y. Ḥall. III, 59[b] top גילגולה טִיבּוּלָהּ the rolling of the dough makes it *Tebel.*

טִיבּוּלָא, טִבּ׳ ch. same, *dipping, immersion, bathing.* Targ. Y. Num. XIX, 4. Ib. 7, sq.; a. e.—*Pl.* טִיבּוּלֵי. Pes. 114[b] תרי ט׳ dipping twice.

טִיבּוּעִין m. pl. (טָבַע I) *sinking;* לט׳ *for being sunk, at the risk of receiving no consideration.* Keth. 76[b] קידושין לט׳ ניתנו the object of value given at betrothal is made a present even at the risk of death before the consummation of marriage; B. Bath. 145[a].

טִבּוּר, טִיבּוּר (b. h. טַבּוּר; טבר, cmp. טַבְלָא I) *[rounded, arched,] navel, umbilicus.* Sabb. XVIII, 3 (128[b]) את הט׳ the infant's navel string. Nidd. 13[b] על טבּוּרוֹ (Ar. טיב׳) above his navel. Yoma 85[a] מטיבורו the formation of the embryo begins from the navel. Midr. Till. to Ps. XIX; a. fr.—Trnsf. *centre* or *highest part.* Meg. 6[a] (homiletic etymol. of טבריה) שיושבת בטִיבּוּרָהּ של א״י it is situated on the height of Palestine.

טִיבּוּרְיָא, טִיבּוּרָא ch. same. Sabb. 66[b] סחופי כסא אטיבורא Ms. M. (ed. אטיבורי, אטבורי, corr. acc.) to put a dry cup on the navel.—Y. Kil. VIII, 31[c] bot. חייי מן טִיבּוּרְיֵיה it draws nourishment through its navel string; איפסיק טיבורייה when its navel string is cut.

טֵיבוּתָא, v. טִיבוּ.

טִיבִירְיָאוּס, טִיבִירְיָא, v. sub טבר׳.

טִיבְלָא, v. טַבְלָא.

טִיבַרְיוּס, טִיבַרְיָה, טִיבִרְיָאוּס, טִיבַרְיָאה, v. sub טבר׳.

טִיבְרָנִי, v. טַבַרְיָא.

טִיגוּן, v. next w.

טִיגָן, טִיגְנוֹן, טִגְנָן m. (τήγανον, τάγηνον, also

ἤγανον, v. Lydd.-Scott Gr. Dict. s. v.; prob. of Semitic origin=חגן, denom. of אגן; as for ט=ח cmp. Syr. טגר P. Sm. 1432 with Chald. חגרא) 1) *frying pan; also* (interch. with טִיגּוּן) *a flour-dish prepared with oil.* Snh. 21ᵃ (ref. to ותצק, II Sam. XIII, 9) עשתה לו מיני ט׳ she made for him oil-dishes. Men. 104ᵇ ה׳ מיני טיגון (most eds.) five sorts of oil-dishes (ref. to Lev. II, 1; 4; 5; 7; 14—15).—*Pl.* טִיגָּנִין. Tosef. Ab. Zar. V (VI), 1; VIII (IX), 2 חט׳ the frying pans.—2) (cmp. Syr. טוגנא, P. Sm. 1431) *an engine of torture and execution.* Pesik. R. s. 43 נתנוהו בתוך חטיגנו (read: חטיגנן or חטיגנון) they put him into the *teganon.*—Denom. טָגַן, *Pi.* טִיגֵּן 1) *to fry, roast.* Men. 50ᵇ (expl. תפיני, Lev. VI, 14; 21) אופה ואח״כ מְטַגְּנָהּ one baked it and then fried it with oil; a. fr.—Part. pass. מְטוּגָּן. Y. Ned. VI, beg. 39ᶜ. [Ib. VI, end, 40ᵃ, v. next w.]—2) *to torture, put to death.* Pesik. R. l. c. וטיגס אותו (Var. וטגים), read: וטִיגְּנוּ אותו or וטִיגְּנוּהוּ.—Trnsf. *to torture, agonize.* Tanḥ. Vayiggash 9 אתה טִגַּנְתָּה אבא וכ׳ thou causedst agony to thy father &c.

טִיגְנָא I ch. same. Kidd. 44ᵃ כמן ימא לט׳ הוא (some ed. לטִיגְנֵי) (his report of the proceedings of the college is) as direct as catching a fish from the lake and throwing it into the frying pan. Y. Ber. III, 6ᵈ מן ימא לט׳ from the lake into the pan, i. e. this is an immediate application of the lesson learned.—Y. Kidd. II, 62ᵇ top וחות מן ימא לט׳ it was a fresh report, v. supra; Y. Gitt. VI, 48ᵃ לטִיגְנֵי....—Denom. טַגֵּן *to fry with oil.* Part. pass. מְטַגַּן, מְטַגְּנָא. Targ. Y. Lev. VI, 14; VII, 12.—*Pl.* מְטַגְּנָן. Y. Ned. VI, end, 40ᵃ (not מטוגן).

***טִיגָּנָא** II m. (τήγανον=πήγανον, v. Löw Pfl. p. 372) *rue.* Ab. Zar. 28ᵃ bot.

טִיגְנוֹ, טִיגְנוֹן, טִיגְנֵי, טִיגַס, v. טִיגֵּן, טִיגָּנָא.

טִיגְרוֹס, v. טִגְ׳.

טִידְוִינָא, v. טִירְוָנָא.

טִיהַר, טִיהֲר, טִהַר m. (v. טָהֳרָה) *bright sky* after rain. Ber. 59ᵃ Ms. F.; Y. ib. IX, 13ᵈ; Yalk. Is. 335 נראה שמים בטִהֲרוֹ (read: רקיע).

טִהֲ׳, טִיהֲרָא ch. 1) same. Ber. 59ᵃ bot. אימת מתחזי בטִיהֲרֵיהּ Ms. M. (ed. only אימתי) when is the sky seen in its brightness?—*Pl.* טִיהֲרִין, טִהֲ׳. Targ. Jer. IV, 11 רוח ט׳ a clearing, sweeping wind (h. text צח).—2) (cmp. Targ. Jer. l. c.) *cold wind, cold* (cmp. אִסְתְּנָא). Lam. R. introd. (R. Joh. 1) בט׳ ובקייטא in cold weather and in summer heat.—3) (cmp. צהרים) *midday.* Targ. O. Deut. XXVIII, 29; a. fr.—Yoma 59ᵃ, a. e., v. טְהַר. Sabb. 63ᵃ שרגא בט׳ a lamp at noon (useless thing); Ḥull. 60ᵇ; a. fr.—*Pl.* טִיהֲרַיָּא. Targ. Ps. XCI, 6 Ms. (ed. sing.), Ib. XXXVII, 6 Ms. (ed. sing.).

טִהֲ׳, טִיהֲרְרֵי, טִיהֲרִירֵי, טִיהֲרֵי m. pl. (preced.; v. Ps. XCI, 6) *midday-demons* during the summer. Targ. Cant. IV, 6 טהרי ed. Lag.—Targ. Y. I Deut. XXXII, 24 (some ed. incorr. טיהרירי).

טִיוּוּטָא m. (טַיֵּיט) *blotting, filling a blank with dots or blots.* B. Bath. 163ᵃ (commentaries use h. form טיאוט a. טיוט). [Targ. Prov. IX, 17 Ar. ed. Koh., s. v. טיטוירא v. טִימוּרָא.]

טִיוּל, טִיוּלָא m. (טול) *walking, going errands.* Targ. Job XXIX, 15 ט׳ רגליא Ms. (ed. only ט׳; ed. Lag. טיוּל), v. טַיָּיל.

***טִיוֹסִין** m. pl. (טוס; v. P. Sm. 1443) *high-flying, proud.* Ex. R. s. 15 (some ed. טויסין).—V. טַיְיסָן.

טִיוּפָא, v. טְיָפָא.

טִיוּפָא, v. טִירָפָה.

טִיחַ m. (b. h.; טוּחַ I) *plaster, lining of vessels.* Tosef. Kel. B. Kam. IV, 19, sq. [read, as R. S. to Kel. V, 11:] אם יכול הט׳ לעמוד בפני עצמו if the lining can stand by itself (form a vessel of itself); v. חֲשַׁה.

טִיחָה f. (preced.) *plastering.* Neg. XII, 6; Sifra Metsora, Neg., Par. 6, ch. IV.

טִיחָ׳, טִיחְיָא m. (preced.) *smearing with a fatty substance, glazing.* M. Kat. 17ᵃ ימהניא ביה כי ט׳ בתנורא and (the excommunication) retains its effect on him as does the glazing on the tiles of the oven. Pes. 30ᵃ חחוא תנורא דטחו ביה ט׳ an oven which they smeared with fat for glazing purposes; Zeb. 95ᵇ דאטחו בה טיחייה (Ms. R. 2 טחו . . טחויי; Ms. K. טָחֲיֵי 'in which they baked cakes smeared with fat', Rashi; v. טְחָיֵי).

טִיט c. (b. h.;=טנטן, v. טָנַן; cmp. גִּגּ; Assyr. ṭîṭu) [*moist, viscid substance,*] *plaster, clay, mud.* Pes. 55ᵃ, v. גְּרִיד. M. Kat. 7ᵃ; v. טוּחַ I. Mikv. VII, 1 חט׳ הנרוק, v. רָקָק. Ib. 7 ט׳ העבה thick clay; a. fr.—[Sabb. 67ᵃ בר ט׳ *son of mud,* a demon, prob. a Var. lect. of בר טינא.]

טִיטוּיא, Targ. Prov. IX, 17 Ar. (Var. טיוטא, טיטורא) a. some ed., a corrupt. of טִימוּרָא.

טִיטוּס pr. n. m. *Titus* (Flavius Sabinus Vespasianus), Roman general, later emperor, captor of Jerusalem. Targ. Lam. I, 19.—Gitt. 56ᵇ; a. fr. (mostly with the by-name 'the wicked').—[Sot. IX, 14 (49ᵇ) פולמוס של ט׳, v. Frankel Monatssch. 1852, p. 393 sq.]

טִיטוּרא, v. טיטויא.

טִיטְיוֹן, Esth. R., to I, 2, v. טַמְיָקוֹן, a. טַמְיוֹן.

טִיטָס pr. n. m. (v. טִיטוּס) *Titas.* Y. Ber. III, 6ᶜ; Y. Bicc. III, 65ᵈ יודה בר ט׳.—Y. Ter. VIII, 45ᶜ bot. חייה בר ט׳.

***טִיטְרוֹס** m. (= טרטרוס, טרטר׳, v. טְרֵי, with format. ס; cmp. אַטְלֵס) *a perforated vessel, sprinkler, strainer.* Kel. II, 6 (Var. סיטרוס).

טִיטַרְטוֹן m. (τέταρτον) *tetarton* (*quart*), a liquid measure, about one quart of a pint. Y. Sabb. VIII, beg. 11ᵃ; Y. Shek. III, 47ᵇ bot.; Y. Pes. X, 37ᶜ top ט׳

וּרבִיע (not טַ'טִרטִין ,טִטְרטִן) one and one fourth of a *t.* (is a ritual cup). Ib. III, 30ª top ט׳ דמיר בגו מודייה (not טרטון) one *t.* of water for a modius of wheat.

טִיטְרַפְּלוֹן m. (v. next w.) *tetrapylon,* (*Mansion-house*), name of a prominent building in Caesarea Palestinae. Tosef. Ohol. XVIII, 13 טטרפלין ed. Zuck. (corr. acc., Var. מטרפלון).

טִיטְרַפְּלִיּוֹת f. pl. (τετράπυλον) *buildings with four gates, prominent mansions.* Y. Succ. I, 52ª bot. טר׳ שבכרכים the *tetrapyla* (mansions) in fortified cities; Y. Kil. IV, 29ᵇ bot. טר׳ שבכרמים (corr. acc.).—Midr. Till. to Ps. XLVIII טִטְרַאפִּילוֹת Ar. (ed. טטפראות); Yalk. Ps. 756; טטרפאות; Yalk. Zech. 568; B. Bath. 75ᵇ טוטפראות (v. Rabb. D. S. a. l. note 50).

טִיּוּב m. (טוּב I) *improvement, industrious tilling.* Y. Shebi. IV, beg. 35ª איזהו הט׳ wherein consists the improvement (spoken of in the Mishnah)?

*__טַיְיזָן__ m. (dialect. for טַיְיסָן q. v.) *proud fool.* Ab. Zar. 26ª גרדנא דלא ט׳ שתא בצירּ מְשַׁנֵּי (Ms. M. ... טיידזאן, מַשְׁנָיה, read: טַיְיזָאן) a year (of) scarce earning will change (better) a weaver, if he be no proud fool. [Var. in Ar. s. v. ג׳ דִּלְטִירא : גרדנא or דלטיריה; Yalk. Gen. 133 ... שמתא בצרא ....] [The supposed meaning of our w. of *humble* seems to have risen from a misunderstanding of a running commentary embodied in Rashi a. Tosafoth, where דלא ט׳ is interpreted ענוו.]

טַיֵּיט (denom. of טִיט) *to smear over, blot, soil.* B. Bath. 163ª דמְטַיֵּיט ליה he marks the blank space with blots (Ar. מְדַיֵּית, v. דִּיוּתָא).

טַיֵּיל, טְיֵיל, v. טוּל.

טַיָּיל m. (preced.) *one at leisure,* opp. to פועל. Keth. 62ª bot.—*Pl.* טַיָּלִים, ...לִין. Ib. V, 6 (61ᵇ). Ib. 62ª מאי ט׳ who are meant by *tayyalin*?

טַיָּל, טַיּוֹל ch. (v. preced.) *walker, errand-man.* Targ. Job XXIX, 15 Var., v. טִיּוּלָא.

טיינון, v. אלטינון.

טַיִּיס, טָיִיס, v. טוּס ch.

טַיָּיסָא m. (preced.) *a bird swooping for prey, bird of prey.* Y. II Gen. XV, 11 (h. text עיט).

טַיְיסָא m. (preced.) *flight.* Targ. Y. Gen. I, 20.

*__טַיְיסָן__ m. (טוס, cmp. טַיְיסָן) *proud.* Y. Ber. III, 6ᵈ bot.; (Y. Naz. VII, 56ª top סריסן; comment.: סריטן *flighty, restless*).

טַיָּיעָא, טַיְיעָא m. (טוע, cmp. טער) *traveller,* esp. *Arabian caravan merchant.* B. Bath. 73ᵇ. Ber. 56ᵇ ט׳ בעלמא dreaming of an Arab in general (not of Ishmael, the son of Abraham). Men. 69ᵇ כדיכדי ט׳ (Ms. M. בר עדי) as in the case of Adi the merchant; Ab. Zar. 33ª בר עדי ט׳. Yeb. 102ª סנדלא דט׳ וכ׳ a traveller's sandal which fits closely.—*Pl.* טַיָּיעֵי. Sabb. 112ª, v. אוּשְׁכָּפָא. Ab. Zar. 34ᵇ, v. אַבְטָא. B. Bath. 36ª בנהרדעא ט׳ שכיחי in N. Arabs (stealing cattle) are frequent.

טַיָּיעוּת f. (preced.) *travellers' custom;* (adv.) *in the manner of travellers.* Pes. 65ᵇ (v. Rabb. D. S. a. l. note 60).

טַיְיעָתָא f. (preced. wds.) *Arabian woman.* Gitt. 45ᵇ (Ar. ed. pr. טיירתא).

טַיָּפָא, v. טְרָפָא.

ט׳ סַמּוֹקָה ,(טוֹפָה) טַיְיפָה pr. n. m. *Tayfa Sammoka* (dyer of red colors?). Y. Dem. III, 23ᶜ; Y. Yeb. VIII, beg. 8ᶜ טיו׳ סמוקר.

טַיָּיר, v. טוּר.

טַיָּיר or **טַיִּיר** m. (preced.) *divination from birds, augury.* Pesik. Par. p. 33ᵇ שהיו יודעים במזל וערומים בט׳ they understood astrology and were shrewd in augury; (Pesik. R. s. 14, v. אַסְטְרוֹלוֹגְיָא); Tanḥ. Huck. 6; ed. Bub. 11; Koh. R. to VII, 23 קוסמין בעופות יבקיאין בט׳ divined from birds and were experts in divination.—*Pl.* טַיָּרִין (בַּיְאוּרִין ,בְּיָארִין); חכמת הט׳ the art of divination. Ib. to X, 20 (ref. to עוף ib.) זה היא העורב בח׳ ט׳ Ar. (ed. חכמת טיארין, read ...(בח׳ ,ין) that means, the raven (carries the sound) through the art of divination; Midr. Till. to Ps. VII, beg. וח׳ טיארין; Yalk. Koh. 979 העורב ח׳ .. וח׳ טייארין (read בח׳); Lev. R. s. 32 טיאורין.

טַיָּר m. (טוּר) *spy,* v. תַּיָּיר.

טיותא, v. טַיְיעָתָא.

*__טִיכּוּס__ m. (טְכַס) [*stamping,*] *rampart, earth-dam.* Pesik. R. s. 14 the sand stands before the Ocean כט׳ וכחומה like a dam and a wall (cmp. טִיכְסָא). [It is not likely that our w. is the Greek τεῖχος, which is identical in meaning with חומה.]

טִיכוֹסָא, טִיכּוּסָא m. (טְכַס) *fastening with rings.* Targ. Y. Ex. XXVIII, 8; XXXIX, 5 (h. text אֲפֻדָּה).

טִיכְנִי f. (τέχνη) *art, cunning.* Y'lamd. Shᵉlaḥ, quot. in Ar. (v. Koh. Ar. Compl. s. v.).

טִיכְסָא, טִכ׳, (מַטְכְּסָא) m.=h. טִיכּוּס. Gen. R. s. 63 על טי׳ דמדינ׳ Ar. (ed. מכבסא) on the rampart of the fortress (in spite of the gates being closed); Yalk. Gen. 110.—*Pl.* טִיכְסַיָּיא, טִכ׳. Lam. R. to I, 5 פליג ד׳ ט׳ וכ׳ he assigned the demolition of the four ramparts of the Temple mount to the four generals, and the western gate came under the command of Pangar.

טִיל, v. טוּל.

טִילָא I m. (טוּל) *travel.* Targ. Y. Gen. XXIX, 1 לְטִילָא (perh. to be read לְטַיָּלָא).

טִילָא II (טִילְיָא) m. *tila* or *tilia,* name of an inferior austere wine. Ab. Zar. 28ª bot. (Rashi: טילייא).

Ib. 30ª bot. (by יין חד is meant) ט׳ חריפא וכ׳ the austere *tila* which bursts the bag. Gitt. 70ª the worst of all is טיליא וכ׳ white *t*.

*טִילְוָא m. (טלר, v. טְלָאר) *patch, rag;* trnsf. *insignificant person.*—*Pl.* טִילְוִי. Koh. R. to XI, 10 כל ט׳ סירוי טפשן . . . all rags are 'ill-smells' (paltry persons are quarrelsome), and all 'ill-smells' are foolish.

טִילוּלַיָּא, v. טִלְטוּלַיָּרא.

טִילְמוּלָא, טִילְמוּל &c., v. sub טְלְט׳.

טִילְיָא, טִילְיָיא, v. טִלָּא.

טִילְמָא, v. טְלוּמָא.

טִילְפָא, v. טִלְפָא.

טִימְהוֹן, טִימְהָא, v. טִימִי I.

טִימוּס, v. טוּמוֹס.

טימוק, Y. Dem. II, beg. 22ᵇ, read: סִימּוֹק (v. R. S. to Dem. II, 1).

טִימוּרָא, טְמוּ׳ m. (טְמַר) 1) *secrecy.* Targ. Prov. IX, 17 ed. Lag. a. oth. (some ed. טיטורא, טיטוריא; corr. acc.).—[Targ. Ps. XI, 4 טמורוי ed. Lag., v. תְּדִמְרָא.]—Targ. Job XL, 21 טְמוּר constr.—2) *hiding, turning away.* Ib. XXIV, 15.

טִימוּרְתָּא, טְמוּ׳ f. same. Targ. Koh. X, 20 (ed. Amst. טְמוּ׳).

טִימְטוּם m. (next w.) *becoming a cohesive shapeless mass.* Y. Ḥall. III, beg. 59ª, contrad. to גִּלְגּוּל.

טִימְטֵם (Pilp. of טָמַם) 1) *to knead into a cohesive shapeless mass,* contrad. to גלגל to roll and shape the dough. Ḥall. III, 1 טִימְטְמָהּ בשעורים after one has formed a lump of barley flour; Tosef. ib. I, 11; a. e.—2) *to thicken, obstruct,* esp. *to blunt the understanding.* Pes. 42ª מְטַמְטֵם את חלב obstructs the heart (makes a person dull). Yoma 39ª עבירה מְטַמְטֶמֶת . . . ונטמתם Ms. (ed. ונטמטם, corr. acc.) sin dulls the heart of man, read not (Lev. XI, 43) *v'nitmethem* (you will be defiled) but *un'tammothem* (from טָמַם) (you will become dull-hearted); Yalk. Lev. 545.—Ch. טַמְטֵם.

Hithpalp. הִיטַּמְטֵם *to become a shapeless mass.* Ḥall. l. c. ותִּטַּמְטֵם; Tosef. ib. l. c. ותִיטַּמְטֵים.

טִימִי I f. (τιμή, inflected like a native word; cmp. אוֹנִי I) 1) *valuation, value, consideration.* Targ. Esth. III, 8. Targ. Y. Num. XX, 19 טִימְהוֹן. Targ. Prov. XXXI, 10 טִימְהָא (missing in some eds.) her value.—Y. Peah I, 15ᵈ bot., a. fr. דלית לה ט׳ invaluable (cmp. אֲטִימִיטוֹן). Gen. R. s. 2, beg., v. אוֹנִי I. Koh. R. to XI, 9 אייתי ט׳ מה דאכלת make payment for what thou hast eaten; a. fr.—Y. Shek. V, end, 49ᵇ [read:] הא לך טִימִיתָהּ וזבין קופד here is its price and buy a piece of meat for it. Y. Taan. I, 64ᵇ bot. טִימִיתֵיה (not תי . . .) the money received for it; a. fr.—Also: טִימִין (accus. of τιμή). Targ. Y. Gen. XXIII, 15. Targ. Esth. VII, 4.—2) *dignity, object of worship.* Y. Ab. Zar. III, 42ᵈ ט׳ דרומי the figure of a Roman deity. [Targ. Y. Gen. XXXIV, 30, v. טִיב II.]

*טִימִי II pr. n. m. *Timi.* Koh. R. to IX, 7 ר׳ יהושע בריה דר׳ ט׳ (Yalk. Koh 979 only ר׳ שמלאר).

טִימְיוֹן, v. טַמְיוֹן.

טִימַיָּיא, v. טַמְיָא.

טִימִין I m. pl., constr. טִימֵי (Chaldaism, v. טַמְיָא) *bones.* Tanḥ. Mick. 2 (play on חרטמים, Dan. II, 2) אלו בטִימֵי מתים . . . those who consult the bones of the dead.

טִימִין II *price,* v. טִימִי I.

טימיסמירות, v. טוּמוֹס.

טִימְיָקוֹן, v. טַמְיָקוֹן.

טִימִיתָא, v. טִימִי I.

טימסמירות, טימס, v. טוּמוֹס.

טִין *to moisten,* v. טָנַן.

טִינָא, טִין m. ch. (v. next w.) *mud, clay.* Targ. Ez. XIII, 11. Targ. Zech. X, 5 (ed. Lag. סִין; h. text טִיט). Targ. Ex. I, 14 (h. text חֹמֶר); a. fr.—Ab. Zar. 39ª דלא מרבי ט׳ וכ׳ (not מרבה) the muddy soil of the river suffers no unclean fish to live in it; Succ. 18ª Ms. M. 2 (ed. טינריהו, v. Rabb. D. S. a. l. note 40). Yoma 29ª ט׳ בר ט׳ cement made out of cement (that has before been used, is hard to make). B. Bath. 3ª בט׳ when clay has been used as cement, contrad. to ריכסא. Ib. 73ᵇ, v. אַכְלָה I; a. fr.—Sabb. 67ª, v. טִיט.

טִינָּא, טִינָּה f. (טנן) 1) *moist muddy ground, clay.* Y. Kil. II, 27ᵈ top, a. e., v. גְּרִיד. Y. Shebi. II, 33ᵈ עפר עושה לה ט׳ by covering it with earth he prepares for the plant a muddy ground. Y. Kidd. III, end, 65ª (prov). מוליכין ט׳ אצל ט׳ וכ׳ mud is carried to mud, and thorns to thorns. Deut. R. s. 5, beg.; Yalk. Prov. 938 מפני הט׳ on account of the moist soil.—2) (cmp. זִימָּה a. בְּנָנָא) *impure thought, lust.* Ḥag. 15ᵇ ט׳ היתה בלבם there was impurity in their hearts (heathen sensuality). Snh. 75ª העלה לבו ט׳ a vehement passion seized him (which threatened his health).

מינדיסין, טִנ׳, Targ. Y. Lev. XXV, 31, בט׳ דפריסן, read כִּטִינָּרֵי דפריסין, v. טִינָּרָא.

טִינָּה, v. טִינָּא.

טינון, v. טיינון.

טִינּוּף, טִנּ׳ m. (טָנַף) *filth, impurity, defilement.* Cant. R. to V, 3. Ex. R. s. 5 לשון ט׳ *nirpim* (Ex. V, 8) has the meaning of uncleanliness (in secretory functions, v. רפי), opp. קדושים. Bekh. III, 1 ט׳ *a discharge from the womb* indicating abortion; Nidd. 25ª; a. e.

טִינּוּפָא, טִנּ׳ ch. same. Sabb. 125ª.

טִינּוֹפֶת, טִנּ׳ f. 1) same. Meg. 3ª (in Chald. dict.)

במקום הט׳ at a place soiled with secretion. Gen. R. s. 50 ט׳ עבודת וכ׳ the defilement by idolatry; a. fr.—2) *worthless admixture in grain, refuse.* B. Bath. VI, 2 (93[b]) the buyer must accept רובע ט׳ לסאה one fourth of a Kab of refuse in a S'ah; Tosef. ib. VI, 2; a. e.—*Pl.* טִינוּפוֹת, טִנ׳ *worthless grains.* Num. R. s. 4, beg.; Tanh. B'midbar 19; ed. Bub. 22.

טִינְנָא, v. טַנְנָא.

טִינַץ, Y. Snh. I, 18[c] bot., read מֵינַץ or רֵינַץ, v. נוּץ ch.

טִינָר, טִינֵר m. (Chaldaism, v. next w.) *rock, flint.*—*Pl.* טִינָרִין. Ex. R. s. 23 שני ט׳ two pieces of flint (Sot. 11[b] (עגולין).

טִינָרָא, טִינָר ch. (enlargement of טוּר;=h. צור) same. Targ. Job. XXXIX, 28. Targ. O. Ex. IV, 25 טִינָ׳ ed. Berl. (ed. Amst. a. Y. טִינְרָא); a. fr.—Gitt. 68[a] ומכסיא בט׳ and covered it up with a stone.—*Pl.* טִינָרַיָּא, טִינָרִין, טִינָרֵי, טִנָ׳. Targ. Y. I. Num. XXIV, 21 (ed. Amst. טִינָר׳). Targ. Ps. LXXVIII, 15 Ms. (ed. Lag. a. oth. טוּרִין). [Targ. Job. XXVII, 16 טינרין Ms., ed. טינא.] — Trnsf. *large, hard tubercles.* Hull. 48[b] דקיימא ט׳ ט׳ lungs covered with &c.

טִינְתָא f.=טִינָא *moist, muddy soil.* Targ. Jud. XV, 15 בט׳ in the mud (h. text בריה).

טִיסְבְּרָא, v. טַס׳.

טִיסָה f. (טוּס) *flight.* Yalk. Ex. 243 טס . . . ט׳ אחת flew to Egypt in one flight.

טִיסְנִי, טִסְנִי f. (πτισάνη, ptisana, also tisana) *barley-groats, pearl-barley.* Makhsh. VI, 2. Tosef. Bets. I, 18 ed. Zuck. (ed. סיטני, corr. acc.); a. fr.

טִיסְקָא, v. טַסְקָא.

טִיעָא, v. טַיְיעָא.

טִיף I, pl. טִיפִּין, v. טִיפָּה.

***טִיף** II m. (cmp. next w.) *receptacle of overflow, a stand for a portable stove.* Tosef. Kel. B. Kam. V, 4.

טִיף III m. ch. (v. טִיפָּה) *dripping;* ט׳ ט׳ *constant dripping.* Pes. 111[b] מאן דשתי ט׳ ט׳ one who drinks the drippings of wine. Ab. Zar. 30[b] מי ט׳ ט׳ ארץ וכ׳ (Ms. M. omits מי) to liquids which drip into a vessel the rule concerning uncovered liquids does not apply; והוא דעביד ט׳ ט׳ בהדרי ט׳ ט׳ Ms. M. (ed. ט׳ לחדרי ט׳ ט׳ . . . ., v. Rabb. D. S. a. l. note) provided the drops follow each other without intermission.

טִייפָא, טִיפָא, טִיפָּא m.; pl. טִיפַּיָּא, טִיפֵּי, טִיפִּין (טוּף (טְיָף) טְיָף׳), cmp. preced. wrds.) 1) *duct of overflow, channels.*—Targ. Prov. V, 16 (ed. Lag. טופי). Targ. Ps. I, 3 טְוָפֵי ed. Wil. (ed. Lag. טורפי, some ed. טרופי, read טוו׳). Ib. CXIX, 136. Targ. Job XXIX, 6 (h. text everywhere פלגי). Ib. XX, 17 (h. text פלגות).—2) *drops.* Ib. XXXVI, 27 טִיופֵי ed. Lag. (oth. ed. טייפי, Ms. טופי, h. text נטפי).

טִיפָּא c. ch.=next w. Arakh. 7[a] ט׳ דמ״ה the venomous drop (on the sword) of the angel of death, v. next w.—*Pl.* טִיפַּיָּא. Y. Hag. II, 78[a] top [read:] בינו ט׳ חוינא מהלכין we walked between the rain drops (so that we did not get wet).

טִיפָּה, טִפָּה f. (טָפַף II, cmp. נטף) *drop.* Taan. 6[b] על כל ט׳ וט׳ וכ׳ for every drop of rain which thou hast caused to come down for us. Toh. III, 3. Kerith. 13[a] ט׳ מלובלבת וכ׳ the drop mixing with the moisture of the nibble. Ab. Zar. 20[b] וט׳ של מרה וכ׳ and a drop of poison hangs on it (the sword of the angel of death); a. fr. — Y. Nidd. III, 50[d] כט׳ של זבוב like the dripping of a fly (v. infra).—*Pl.* טִיפּוֹת, טִפ׳, טִיפִּין. Mikv. VIII, 3. Cant. R. to I, 2 מה מים יורדין ט׳ ט׳ וכ׳ as waters come down in drops and form rivers . ., so does learning &c. Y. Nidd. l. c.; Bab. ib. 25[a] כשתי ט׳ like two drippings of a fly (Rashi: like the two *eye-balls*). Hor. 10[a] כמה טפות וכ׳ (Ms. M. טפין, v. Rabb. D. S. a. l. note) how many drops there are in the sea; a. fr.

טִיפּוּחַ m. (טָפַח 1) *clapping* of hands (in mourning or rejoicing). Y. Bets. V, 63[a] ט׳ שהוא לרצונו *tippuah* means a clapping which is done purposely, opp. סיפוק spontaneous clapping; M. Kat. 27[b] ט׳ ביד *tippuah* is done with the hands, opp. קילוס, striking of feet.—

טִיפּוּל m. (טָפַל) 1) *nursing, attendance, care.* Tosef. Nidd. II, 4 חייבת . . בט׳ וכ׳ a woman is bound to nurse her child twenty four months (during which she must not remarry), whether her own &c. B. Mets. 69[a] טִיפּוּלָה מרובה the care-taking of small cattle is more troublesome; Bekh. 26[b] טִפ׳; a. e.—2) *toilet-paste,* v. טְפַל. Pes. 42[b] טִיפּוּלָן של וכ׳ the paste used by the daughters of rich men.—*Pl.* טִיפּוּלִין, constr. טִיפּוּלֵי. Y. ib. II, beg. 29[d] אית תניי תני ט׳ some read in the Mishnah *tippulê* (in place of תכשיטי).

טִיפוּנָא m. (v. טוּפְרָנָא) *surplus, excess.* Tem. 30[a] טִיפוּנָה דכלב the excess of the value of the dog over that of any single lamb taken in exchange.

טִיפּוּס, pl. טִיפּוּסִים, v. טָפוּס.

***טִיפַּח** m. constr. (v. טָפַח II), ט׳ רוחא *conceitedness.* Y. Yeb. XVI, 15[d] פלוני אינו בעולם ט׳ רוח׳ה עליה 'the man—is not in this world', is not a clear testimony of death, as it may be interpreted, 'his conceit came over him'.—V. תִּיפַּח.

טִיפְטֵף, v. טָפַף II.

טִיפִּיטִין, טִיפִּיטִיוֹת, טִיפִּיטִיאוֹת, v. טִפִּיטָא.

טִיפְסְרָא, v. טִפְ׳.

טִיפֵּשׁ, טִיפְשָׁא, טִיפְשׁוּת, &c., v. sub. טפש׳.

טִיפְתָא, טִפְ׳ ch.=h. טִיפָּה. Nidd. 20[b] ט׳ קמייתא the first dripping of menstruation. B. Kam. 98[a] דט׳ דדמא וכ׳ an extravasation of a drop of blood took place in his ear.

טִיקוּסָא, טִיק׳ m. (טְקַס) 1) = טִיכּוּס, *rampart, embankment.* Targ. II Kings XVI, 18 (h. text מיסך).—2) *arrangement, measurement, proportions.* Targ. Jer. I, 13 טיקוס משירויתיה (v. טְקַס). Targ. Ez. XLIII, 10 (h. text תכנית). Ib. 13 (h. text גב); a. e.

טִיקְסָא m., constr. טִיקַס, טֶקֶס, (preced.) *banner, arrangement of troops, standard, division belonging to one standard* (corresp. to h. דֶּגֶל). Targ. Num. II, 2; 3; a. fr. Y. ib. וטִיקְסֵיה וכ׳ and its banner was made of wool &c. —*Pl.* טִיקְסִין, טִיקְסַיָּא, טִיק׳. Ib. 17; a. fr.—Targ. Cant. VI, 4 ארבע טִקְסַיִךְ וכ׳ thy four divisions in the desert.—[Lam. R. to I. 5 טִיקְסָה Ar., ed. טכס׳, v. טִיכְסָא].

טִיר m. (טור or נטר) *castle.*—*Pl.* טִירִים, טִירִין. Macc. 10[a]; Yalk. Deut. 921.

טירא, Y. M. Kat. III, 83[c] bot., בר ט׳, v. נְזִירָא II.

טִירָא f., pl. טִירָאוֹת (v. טִירָה) *places for augury, (templum).* Gen. R. s. 83 (play on מגדיאל, Gen. XXXVI, 39) שהיו מעמידין טיראות וכ׳ 'Rashi' (in ed. Wil. 1878; text טוּרִיוֹת) they put up auguries for idolatry, v. טוּר I; Yalk. ib. 140 טירוין (read: טִירָיוֹת.).

טירבוס, Pesik. R. s. 10 באים עליהם ט׳, read: באים לעסק טירונין, v. טִירוֹן I.

טִירְדָא v. טִרְדָא.

טִירָה f. (b. h., v. Ez. XLVI, 23; טור or נטר) *guard,* trnsf. *surrounding of an oven, brick-work.* Kel. V, 3 טִירַת התנור. Tosef. ib., B. Kam. IV, 3 חפר ... להן ט׳ if he made a guard around them by digging in the ground. Ib. טִירַת כירה (Kel. l. c. עֲטָרַת), v. פִּירָה. Ib. הרי הן כט׳.. (Var. corrupt קטירה) are in ritual law like &c.

טירודא, v. next w.

טֵירוּדִין, טֵר׳ m. pl. (טְרַד) *banishment.* Lev. R. s. 18, end בו״ד גוזר ט׳ וכ׳ (not טירודא) a human authority decrees banishment, so does the Lord (to the leper). Gen. R. s. 2, beg.; Yalk. ib. 4. [Num. R. s. 7, v. טָרַד.]

טִירוֹן I m. (tiro, τίρων) *young soldier,* trnsf. *beginner, novice.* Ex. R. s. 3, beg. ט׳ היה וכ׳ Moses was a novice in prophecy. Y. Erub. V, beg. 22[b] (ref. to I Kings XVII, 1, where Elijah is for the first time mentioned as a prophet and yet says, 'the Lord before whom I stood') והלא אלי׳ ט׳ לנבואה היה (not טירונין לנביאים) was not Elijah at that time a novice &c.?—*Pl.* טִירוֹנִין. Tanḥ. Ki Thissa 1 לעסק ט׳ Ar. (ed. טרופין, corr. acc.) for the levy of soldiers; Pesik. R. s. 10 עליהם טירבוס (corr. acc.).

***טִירוֹן** II m., pl. טִירוֹנִין (טור or נטר, cmp. טוּרָנָא, v. טִיר) *guards of observation.* Lam. R. introd. (R. Josh. 2) ט׳ (expl. כרים על שערים, Ez. XXI, 27; Koh. R. to XII, 8 כרקומין).

***טִירוֹנָא** ch. same, pl. טִירוֹנִין. Targ. Y. Num. XXXI, 10 טִירוֹנֵיהוֹן (h. text טִירֹתָם).

***טִירוּנָא, טרונא** m. (τύραννος) *imperial, powerful.*—*Pl.* טִירוּנִין. Targ. Y. Deut. XX, 1 (synonym. with גִּיוְתָנִין).

***טִירוֹנְיָא** f. (tironia, a denom. of tiron, not otherwise recorded) *levy of soldiers.* Cant. R. to II, 8; Gen. R. s. 42; s. 70 שמכתבת ט׳ וכ׳ which writes out a levy from all nations. [Ib. s. 88 שכותבת ט׳ Ar., ed. שמכתבת טרימוסיאה; Yalk. ib. 147 טירני׳, prob. a corrupt. of טְרִיבוּטָא (tributa) *tributes*]

טִירוּנְיָא, טִירוּנְיָיא, טִר׳ f. (τυραννία) *sovereignty, absolute rule, usurpation* (corresp. to h. זְרוֹעַ). Y. Yeb. VIII, 9[d] top; Y. Kidd. IV, 65[d] bot. עיקר ט׳ וכ׳ the principal designation of their (the priests') usurpation lies in the words (Hos. IV, 4). Pesik. R. s. 15; Pesik. Haḥod. p. 52[b]; Lev. R. s. 23, beg. (ref. to בזרוע, Ps. LXXVII, 16) בטר׳ with imperial power. Y. Maas. Sh. V, end, 56[d] אלו שהן באין בט׳ לפני וכ׳ those who come before the Lord with power (interch. with בזרוע). Ab. Zar. 3[a] אין הקב״ה בא בט׳ וכ׳ the Lord does not deal despotically with his creatures. Yalk. Deut. 945 היה עולה אצל אביו בט׳ (Ruth R. introd. במרוצה) came to his father with arrogance.

טֵירוּף, טֵרוּף m. (טָרַף) 1) (sub. הדעת) *confusion, distraction; trouble.* Ber. V, 4 (34[a]) מפני הטר׳ because he might become confused (and be unable to resume his prayers); Deut. R. s. 7, beg.—Cant. R. to VIII, 13 בט׳ הדעת in confusion (not in concert).—Tanḥ. Mick. 2 נטרף טרוף אחד had only one trouble (about the interpretation of his dream).—*Pl.* טֵירוּפִין, טֵר׳. Ib. נטרף שני ט׳ had two troubles (not knowing even the dream).—Sifré Deut. 296 (ref. to בדרך, Deut. XXV, 17) בשעת טֵירוּפֵיכֶם when you were in a state of disorder.—2) *ejection, banishment* (cmp. טֵירוּדִין). Gen. R. s. 15; Midr. Till. to Ps. CXXXIX (omitt. in ed. Bub.); Yalk. ib. 887 טֵירוּפִי מתוכה my banishment from Eden.

טִירְהָא, v. טִרְ׳.

טִירְחוּת, v. טַרְחוּת.

טִירְיָא, טִירְיָיא, טִרְ׳ m. (טרי) *the shaking movement* of the mill. B. Bath. 18[a] (v. Rabb. D. S. a. l. note 50). Ib. 20[b].—V. טַרְיִיתָא.

טִירְיוֹן m. (cmp. preced.) *trouble, excitement.* Sifré Num. 157; Yalk. ib. 785 (play on טירתם, Num. XXXI, 10) מקום שהיו בט׳ the place where they were in trouble (fear of the enemy).—[Yalk. Gen. 140, v. טִירָא.—Y. Taan. II, 66[a] יום ט׳, v. טְרָיְינוֹס.]

טִירָיוֹת, v. טִירָא.

טִירְיָיא, v. טִירָא.

טִירְיְינָא, v. טִרְיְינָא.

טִירְיַסְקֵי, טִירְיַיסְקֵי, טוּרְיַסְקֵי m. pl. name of a *Persian festival.* Ab. Zar. 11[b] (v. Rabb. D. S. a. l. note); Y. ib. I, 39[c] טִירְיַיסְקֵי a *Median festival.*

***טִירְיָנָא, טִירְיָנָא** m. (Pers. tiryân, Lag.; v. P. Sm. 1508) *basket.* Pes. 88ᵃ (Ms. M. טרדיר׳, read טיר׳; v. Rabb. D. S. a. l. note; Taan. 9ᵇ צנא).

טִירְכִי, Esth. R. to I, 2 כטירכי מרכבתו, a corrupt tautography; read: כמרכבתו, v. מֶרְכָּבָה.

טִירם, v. טרים.

***טִירְנָאָה** m. *Tirnaah,* surname of one R. Ḥănina. Kerith. 9ᵃ; (Ned. 57ᵇ תִּירְתָאָה; ib. 59ᵇ תִּירְתָאָה; Y. Peah II, 17ᵈ תורתייה; Y. Kidd. I, 60ᶜ bot. תִּרְתָּיָה; Y. Ber. III, 6ᵈ תִּרְתָּיָה).

טִירְסָאִי, v. טַרְסָאָה.

טִירְפָּא m. (טְרַף) *document conferring the right of seizure of a debtor's property sold after the loan,* v. אַדְרַכְתָּא. B. Bath. 169ᵃ כל ט׳ וכ׳ a *tirpa* which fails to contain the words, 'We have torn the note of indebtedness' &c. B. Kam. 9ᵃ אחוי טִירְפָּךְ וכ׳ show thy *t.,* and I shall pay thee. Keth. 95ᵃ top.

טִירְפֵּס v. טַפָּס.

טִירְקְסוֹן, v. טְרַקְסִין.

טִישָׁא m. (טוש II) *secrecy.* Targ. Prov. XXI, 14.

טִישְׁמוּשָׁא, טִשְׁ׳ m. (טוש I) *mire.* Targ. Ps. XL, 3.

טי״ת *Teth,* name of the ninth letter of the Alphabet. Maas. Sh. IV, 11 טי״ת טבל Y. ed. (Mish. a. Bab. ed. ט׳) if the vessel is marked *Teth,* it means *Tebel* (טֶבֶל). V. ט׳.

טכמכא, v. תַּכְתְּקָא.

טִכְנִי, v. טִיכְנִי.

טָכַס (cmp. דָּכַס) *to stamp, tread upon, press.* Cant. R. to III, 7 [read:] היו רואין שבע מחיצות של אש טוֹכְסוֹת וכ׳ they saw seven partitions of fire one pressing the other; Midr. Sam. ch. XVII טונסות (corr. acc.); (Yalk. Ex. 362; Yalk. Ps. 795 נוצצות; Num. R. s. 11, Pesik. R. s. 15, Pesik. Hahod., p. 45ᵃ, v. כָּסַס).

Pi. טִיכֵּס 1) same.—Part. pass. מְטוּכָּס *filled up.* Midr. Till. to Ps. XC, 2 מקום מט׳ a filled up place, *mound* (v. טִיכְסָא, טִיכּוּס).—2) (v. next w.) *to equip,* v. טָקַס.

טְכַס ch. same, *Pa.* טַכֵּיס 1) *to press, squeeze, fit on.* Targ. Y. Lev. XVI, 4 [read:] יְטַכֵּיס.—2) (corresp. to b. h. אָסַר) *to fasten, to harness and load.* Targ. Y. Ex. XXVIII, 28. Targ. Y. I Deut. XXXIV, 8 (ed. Amst. טַכִּיס *Pe.*).—Part. pass. מְטַכַּס *harnessed, equipped.* Targ. Y. II Gen. XLIX, 19. Targ. II Esth. VI, 10 (some ed. מִיט׳ *Ithpa.*), v. טְקַס.—V. טִיכּוּסָא.

טִכְסָא, v. טִיכְ׳.

***טכסמסיס,** Lev. R. s. 12, beg., quot. in Ar., expl. תקנה, prob. meant for next w.; missing in eds.

טִכְסִין, טכסים, v. next w.

טַקְסִיס, טַכְסִיס m. (τάξις; inflected like a native word, formed like קַצִּיץ, as if fr. טכס) *order, array, order of battle; arrangement.* Pesik. Vayhi, p. 66ᵇ בט׳ מלכים Ar. (ed. . . בטכסיסר של, read: בְּטַכְסִיסִין, pl.) in the order in which kings go to war; Tanh. Bo. 4 כטכסין של וכ׳; ed. Bub. ib. 4 בטכסים מלך וכ׳; Pesik R. s. 17 בְּטַכְסִיסֵי מלכים (pl. constr.). Cant. R. to IV, 12 בטק׳ המלכים in the order of a royal (regular) army. Ex. R. s. 8, end בט׳ הזה הבא וכ׳ in this consecutive order bring &c.; Tanh. Vaëra 9 בטקסין הזה הביא (corr. acc.). Midr. Till. to Ps. XC בט׳ של נבואה under the order of prophecy. Num. R. s. 15 בט׳ גְּדוּלָּה (not בטקסים) in the array of power (arrogating power to themselves); Tanh. B'haăl. 14 בטקסים גדולים (corr. acc.). Ib. B'midb. 12 יש להם טכסין מן יעקב אביהן they have a traditional order from the way their father Jacob arranged his funeral escort; ed. Bub. ib. 12 יש בידן טכסים אביהן. Cant. R. to II, 4 טקסים של מעלה (read ס . . . .) the heavenly array; a. v. fr.—2) (fem.) *garrison.* Y. Ab. Zar. I 39ᶜ, הדא טק׳ דקסרין the garrison of Caesarea, v. הוּקִים.—*Pl.* טַכְסִיסִין, טַק׳, constr. טַכְסִיסֵי, טַק׳. Sabb. 31ᵃ ט׳ מלכות court ceremonial. Pesik. R. s. 17, a. e., v. supra.

טִכְסַת, v. סִטְפַּת.

טַל (טלל) טַל m. (b. h.; טָלַל) [*hanging drop,* cmp. טְלַטוּלָא,] *dew.* Taan. 3ᵃ בטל וברוחות וכ׳ as to mentioning dew and winds in the prayer &c.—Ib.ᵇ טל דברכה a fructifying dew; a. fr.—*Pl.* טְלָלִים, טְלָלִין. Ḥag. 12ᵇ עליית ט׳ the upper chamber (store) of dews, v. אֲגָלִים. Lev. R. s. 28 ט׳ קשים injurious dews; a. fr.

טַלָּא, טַל ch. same. Targ. Is. XVIII, 4. Targ. O. Gen. XXVII, 28; a. fr.—*Pl.* טַלִּין. Targ. Y. Gen. l. c.; a. e.

טַלָּא, טְלָא, v. טלי.—[Targ. Y. Lev. XVI, 27, v. טַלְיָא.]

טְלָאי m. (טְלָא) 1) *a piece of cloth* used as blanket. Succ. 17ᵇ ראוי לט׳ על וכ׳ Ms. M. a. Ar. (ed. לטלית) fit for a blanket over an ass.—2) *patch.* Ber. 43ᵇ ט׳ על גבי ט׳ patch upon patch. V. טְלָיוֹת.

טְלָאֵי I m. pl. *young,* v. טְלֵי.

***טְלָאֵי** II m. pl. *inhabitants* or *descendants of Tela.* Kidd. 70ᵇ (prob. a nickname, v. בַּלָּאֵי).

טָלֶה m. (b. h.; טְלָא) [*tender,*] *lamb.* Hag. 9ᵇ בקרו ט׳ examine the lamb, v. בָּקַר; a. e.—*Pl.* טְלָאִים, טְלָיִים. Y. Ber. IV, 7ᵇ top ט׳ מבוקרים, v. בָּקַר. Ib.; Tam. III, 3 לשכת הט׳ the (Temple) store for daily offerings; a. e.

***טָלֵה (טְלֵה)** m. = טְלֵי. Targ. Y. Gen. XXXVII, 2 (ed. Amst. טלה, corr. acc.)

***טָלוּי** m. (preced. wds.) *brood.* Targ. Y. Deut. VII, 14 (prob. to be read טַלְיֵי).

***טְלוּי,** Targ. Y. Num. VI, 24. read טְלָנֵי.

טָלוּל *moist,* v. טָלַל I.

טְלוּכָא m. *jest*, v. אִטְלוּלָא. [טְלוּלַיָא, v. טַלְטוּלָיָא.]

טְלוּמָא, טְלוֹ׳, טוּלְ׳ m. (טְלַם) 1) *oppression*. Targ. Ps. VII, 4 (Ms. טוּל׳). Ib. LXII, 11 (Var. טִילְ׳, טְלַ׳); a. fr.— Pl. טְלוּמַיָא. Targ. Prov. XXVIII, 16 (ed. Wil. טוּל׳).— 2) *wronged*, v. טְלַם.

טַלוֹמָא, טְלוֹ׳ m. (preced.) *oppressor*. Targ. Ps. X, 3 (some ed. incorr. טְלוֹ׳); a. fr.—Pl. טְלוֹמַיָא, טַלוֹ׳. Ib. XVIII, 5.

טְלוּמְיָא* f. (preced.) *wrong-doing*. Targ. Prov. XXIX, 25 (v. Pesh., h. text חרדת!).

טְלוּפְחָא, טְלָפְ׳ m., pl. טְלוּפְחִין, טְלוּפְחֵי, טְלָפְ׳ (cmp. טופח) 1) *lentils*. Targ. Gen. XXV, 34; a. e.—Ab. Zar. 38[b] ט׳ דמיא, ט׳ דחלא lentils boiled in vinegar, ... in water. Yeb. 63[b]; Yalk. Koh. 976 טַפְלוּחָאי; a. fr.—2) (cmp. Lat. lenticula) *a trough* in the wine or oil press (h. עדשה). B. Bath. 67[b], expl. יָם (v. עֲדָשָׁה).

טלותה, Targ. II Esth. II, 7 ט׳ some ed., read: בִטְלִיוּתָהּ, v. טַלְיוּ.

טְלַח*, Af. אַטְלַח (=טלע) *to halt*. Targ. Y. Gen. XXXII, 32 (some ed. אטלע). [Targ. Y. ib. XXXVII, 2, v. טְלַח.]

טִלְטוּל, טִילְ׳ m. (טִלְטֵל) 1) *moving, handling*. Sabb. 43[b] ט׳ מן הצד moving a thing sideways (in an unusual manner); a. fr.—2) *migration, exile*. Lev. R. s. 5 (ref. to Is. XXII, 17) ט׳ אחר ט׳ repeated migration from land to land. Gen. R. s. 39 (expl. נָדִד, B. LV, 8), v. נִדְנוּד.

טִלְטוּל, טַלְטוּלָא, טִילְ׳ ch. same. 1) *moving, trembling*. Targ. Job XVI, 5 (h. text ניד).—2) *migration, exile*. Targ. Is. XXII, 17. Targ. Ps. XVIII, 19 (h. text איד).—Ib. LVI, 9 (some ed. pl.; h. text נֹד); a. fr.—טַלְטוּלִין, טִלְטוּלֵי, טִילְ׳. Keth. 28[a] (ref. to Is. XXII, 17) ט׳ דגברא קשין וכ׳ the sufferings of homelessness are harder on man than on woman; (Snh. 26[a]; Yalk. Is. 280 *sing.*).

טַלְטוּלָא m. (preced.) *an exile, homeless man*.—Pl. טַלְטוּלִין. Targ. Lam. III, 45 (h. text סחי).

טַלְטוּלַיָא, טַלְ׳, טִילְ׳ m. pl. (preced. wds.) *hangings, drops, female ornaments*. Targ. Is. III, 21 (Ar. טִילְטוּלְ׳, טְלוּלַיָא; h. text נזמי האף).

טִלְטֵל (b. h.; Pilp. of טלל, cmp. דלדל) 1) *to move, carry, handle*. Sabb. III, 6 מְטַלְטְלִין וכ׳ you may handle (on the Sabbath) a new lamp; a. v. fr.—2) *to make unsteady, to exile*; (with דעת) *to confound*. Gen. R. s. 39 טַלְטֵל עצמך וכ׳ banish thyself (travel) from place to place. Ib. s. 38 (expl. הניעמו, Ps. LIX, 12) טַלְטְלֵימוֹ make them exiles. Y. Peah I, 15[d] top (expl. נעו, Prov. V, 6) טי׳ הקב״ה מתן וכ׳ the Lord made unsteady (irregular) the reward of the observants, that they might observe the commands in faith. Num. R. s. 10 (ed. Amst. p. 238[a]) שהן מְטַלְטְלִין דעתו וכ׳ they (carnal pleasures) confound man's judgment (cmp. טָרַף).—Part. pass. מְטוּלְטָל, f. מְטוּלְטֶלֶת. Tanh. ed. Bub., Sh'mini 7 והדעת מט׳ and the mind becomes confused.—

Hithpa. הִתְטַלְטֵל, הִיטַ׳, *Nithpa.* נִתְטַלְטֵל, נִיטַ׳ 1) *to be moved, handled; to be made restless*. Sabb. l. c. כל הנרות מִטַּלְטְלִין all lamps may be handled. Ib. 35[a] מעיין הַמִּיטַּלְטֵל a travelling spring (changing its place). Gen. R. s. 39. Sifra Sh'mini ch. VII, Par. 6 מִטַּלְטְלִין במלואם are carried with their contents; Kel. XV, 1 עשויין לִיטַּלְטֵל וכ׳. Yalk. Prov. 964; Midr. Prov. to XXX, 27 Alexander the Macedonian שנ׳ בכל וכ׳ who in his unrest drove all over the world like a locust &c.; a. fr.—V. מְטַלְטְלִין.—2) (with דעת) *to be confounded*. Tanh. Sh'mini 5 נִתְטַלְטְלָה דעתו וכ׳ his mind is confused, and he knows not what he is talking &c. Ib. כדי שלא תִּטַּלְטֵל דעתו in order that he may not get mixed up; a. e.

טַלְטֵל ch. same, 1) *to move, shake*. Targ. Ps. XXII, 8; CIX, 25; a. fr.—2) *to exile*, Targ. Deut. XXIX, 27; a. fr. Part. pass. מְטַלְטַל. Targ. Gen. IV, 12; 14; a. fr.—3) *to move, handle, carry, lift*. Targ. Y. Ex. XVI, 29 (cmp. Erub. 17[b]).—Sabb. 45[a] לְטַלְטוּלֵי שרגא וכ׳ to remove the light of Hanuckah, v. חַבְרָא. Pes. 69[a] טלטולי בעלמא הוא it is merely a moving (no creative labor). Sabb. 49[a] לא מְטַלְטְלִינַן להו we must not handle them.—Y. Snh. VI, 23[c] bot.; Y. Hag. II, 77[d] bot. וִיטַלְטְלִינָהּ מן וכ׳ and shall lift her off the ground. Ib., sq. טַלְטַלְתְּנֵיהּ וכ׳ as soon as thou liftest him off &c., he can do nothing; a. fr.

Ithpalp. אִיתְטַלְטֵל, אִיטַ׳ 1) *to be exiled, to wander*. Targ. Lam. IV, 14. Targ. Ps. LXVIII, 13.—2) *to be unsteady, to be moved, to be movable*. Targ. Prov. V, 6.—Y. Lev. XXV, 14 עסקא דמִיטַּלְטְלָא *movable chattel*.—B. Bath. 150[a] כל דְּמִטַּלְטֵל (or הַמִּ׳) whatever is movable; a. fr.

טָלָה, טָלָא, טלי (b. h.; cmp. דָּלָה, תָּלָה) *to hang on, to patch, line*. Kel. XXVI, 2 טלא עליו וכ׳ Ar. (Mish. ed. טלה, Talm. ed. טִילָּה), v. מַטְלִית. Ib. XXVII, 6 שֶׁטְלָיָיה וכ׳ which he put on &c. Y. Meg. I, 71[d] top וטוֹלִין, v. מַטְלִית. Hull. 122[b] שֶׁטְלָאָהּ לקופתו which he hanged over his basket. Gitt. 45[b] ט׳ עליהן עור covered them with a leather casing.

Pi. טִילָּה, טִילָּא same, v. supra. Part. pass. מְטוּלָּא, pl. מְטוּלָּאִים. Ber. 43[b], a. fr. מנעלים המט׳ patched shoes; v. טְלַאי.

טְלָא, טְלִי ch. (preced.) 1) *to lift up*. Koh. R. to IX, 5 טְלִי טליתיך lift up thy cloak (Ber. 18[a] דלי־).— [2) *to sport*, v. טְלַל II.]

טְלִי, טָלִי m. (preced. wds.) *hanging, covering*, esp. *table outfit, linen*.—Pl. טְלִים, constr. טְלֵי. Keth. 68[a] top, will you dine בט׳ כסף או בט׳ זהב with the silver outfit, i. e. with the outfit used in connection with silver vessels, or with the gold outfit?—B. Mets. 78[b] has the worm come בט׳ כסף או בט׳ זהב in the silver outfit (white linen) &c.?; cmp. הִימוּנְיָא, אוֹלָרִין.

טַלְיָא, טַלְיָא, טְלֵי, טָלֵי m. (טלי, cmp. טָלֶה) 1) *tender, young; young man, servant*. Targ. Y. Lev. XV, 2. Targ. Ps. XXXVII, 25. Targ. Y. Gen. XLI, 12; a. fr.—Targ. Y. Lev. XVI, 27 טַלְיָא.—B. Bath. 142[b], v.

חוּלָּק. Y. Yeb. XII, 12[d] bot. הוא ט׳ וכ׳ if he is young and she old. Lam. R. to I, 16 בגין דאית לי ט׳ וכ׳ (not טלאר) since I have a young slave &.; a. fr.— Yeb. 114[a] top טלי וטליא *boys and girls.*—*Pl.* טַלְיָא, טַלְיָיא, טַלְיִין, טַלְאֵי. Targ. Joel II, 16. Targ. II Esth. I, 2 טַלְיָן וְטַלְיָין ed. Lag. boys and girls, v. supra.—Targ. Prov. I, 4; a. fr.— Sot. 33[a] נצחו ט׳ the boys (sons of the Highpriest) have won the battle; Y. ib. IX, 24[b]. Y. Meg. III, 74[a] bot. טַלְיָיה. Y. Ter. VIII, 46[b] bot. טַלְיֵי דבי וכ׳ the boys of the Nasi's house; a. fr.—*Fem.* v. טַלְיְתָא.—2) = h. טָלֶה *lamb.* Targ. Y. Ex. I, 15.—*Pl.* as ab. Targ. Y. Gen. XXX, 40. Targ. Ps. CXVIII, 27.—3) pr. n. m. *Tali.* Snh. 52[b], v. אִימַּרְתָּא.

טַלְיוּ, טַלְיוּת, טַלְיוּתָא f. (preced.) *childhood, youth.* Targ. Ps. LXXXVIII, 16 טליו Ms. (Levita טליותא, ed. טליא, incorr.). Targ. Job XXXVI, 14; a. fr.—Lev. R. s. 18, beg. Midr. Till. to Ps. IX מן ט׳ עד וכ׳ from childhood to old age. — Lam. R. to I, 16 *young woman,* v. טַלְיְתָא.

טַלְיוֹת, v. טַלִּית.

טַלְיוּתָא, v. טַלְיוּ.

טְלִיוּתָא f. (v. טְלַל II) *pleasure, enjoyment.* Targ. Y. II Gen. XLIX, 1 (Y. I טְלָנִיתָא).

טַלְיְתָא, v. טַלְיְתָא.

טְלִימָא, v. טְלוּמָא.

טְלִימוֹן pr. n., מערת ט׳ *the Cave of T'limon,* near the sea-shore of Judaea. Y. Dem. II, 22[c] (Hildesh. Beitr. p. 10 suggests סלימון).

***טְלִיקָא** m. (טְרַק=טְלַק) *box* for papers, documents. Gitt. 28[a]; B. Mets. 20[b] (Ms. F. טלוקא, Ms. R. 1 טלרסקא, v. Rabb. D. S. a. l. note 400), v. גְּלוּסְקְמָא.

טַלִּית f. (טלל) *cover, sheet, cloak* (similar to the Roman pallium, Gr. φᾶρος). Sabb. 147[a] ט׳ מקופלת a cloak folded up and thrown over the shoulder. Men. 41[a] ט׳ כפולה a double-sized sheet worn by doubling it. Sabb. 138[a] ט׳ כפולה וכ׳ one must not make a tent on the Sabbath by spreading a double-sized sheet on poles so that the ends hang down. Kidd. 18[a] sq. (ref. to בבגדו, Ex. XXI, 8) כיון שפרש טַלִּיתוֹ עליה since he spread his (bed-) sheet over her (v. בֶּגֶד).—Esp. *Tallith, the cloak of honor, the scholar's or officer's distinction* (adorned with fringes according to Num. XV, 38 sq.); *the cloak of the leader in prayer.* Num. R. s. 8, end שמלה זו ט׳ *simlah* (Deut. X, 18), that means the cloak to which the show-fringes are attached. Gen. R. s. 36 (ref. to השמלה, Gen. IX, 23) לפיכך זכה שם לט׳ וכ׳ therefore was Shem privileged to wear the Tallith &c. Ex. R. s. 27 נתמנה.... ונטל ט׳ וכ׳ when one has been appointed to an office and has taken the *T.*, he must not &c.; a. fr.—*Pl.* טַלִּיּוֹת, טַלֵּיתוֹת. Sabb. 147[a] ed. (Ms. M. sing.). Tanh. Korah 2; Num. R. s. 18, beg. ט׳ תכלת cloaks all of purple blue; Y. Snh. X, 27[d] bot. טליות, ed. Krot. טלור׳ (corr. acc. or טַלִּיוֹת). Zab. IV, 5 עשר טליות וכ׳ if ten sheets are placed above one another. Ib. 7; Sabb. 93[a].

טַלִּיתָא, טַלִּית ch. same. 1) *sheet.* Targ. Y. Ex. XXII, 26 (ed. Amst. טַלִּית, Var. טַלָּה).—2) *the Tallith.* Koh. R. to IX, 5 טַלִּיתֵיה (Ber. 18[a] תכלתיה). Ib. טלי טַלִּיתָךְ, v. טְלֵי.

טַלְיָא, טַלְיוּ׳, טַלְיְתָא f. (v. טַלְיָא) *young; girl.* Targ. Y. Gen. XXXIV, 4 (ed. Amst. טַלְיָ׳); a. fr.—Yeb. 114[a], v. טְלֵי.—Y. ib. XII, 12[d] bot. היא ט׳ וכ׳ if she is young and he old. Lam. R. to I, 16 (v. טַלְיוּ).—*Pl.* טַלְיָתָא, טַלְיָין, טַלְיָיר׳. Targ. II, Esth. I, 2 טליותא ed. (ed. Lag. טליין). Targ. Prov. IX, 3 טלייתהא ed. Lag. (ed. Wil. טַלְיָת׳, corr. acc.). Ib. XXXI, 15; a. fr.

טְלָל, pl. טְלָלִים, v. טַל.

טָלַל (b. h.; cmp. דלל, תלל) 1) *to hang over,* (of liquids) *to form drops;* v. טַל.—*Part. pass.* טָלוּל, f. טְלוּלָה a) *hanging.* Y. Ab. Zar. IV, 44[a] bot. [read:] שלא היתה שם טיפה אחת ט׳ that there should not have been there (in the vat) one drop hanging (which drops down on being touched or shaken). b) (with שנה, denom. of טַל) *blessed with dew.* Taan. 24[b]; Y. Yoma V, 42[c] top.; Lev. R. s. 20; Tanh. Ahăre 3; ed. Bub. ib. 4, v. גֶּשֶׁם.—2) *to be movable,* v. טִלְטֵל.—3) *to cover,* v. טְלִית.

טְלַל I ch. same, *Pa.* טַלֵּיל *to make a* טְלָלָא; *to cover, screen.* Targ. I Kings VI, 9 (h. text ספן). Targ. Y. Ex. XL, 21 (O. *Af.*; h. text ויסך). Ib. XXV, 20 מְטַלְּלִין (O. מַטְלִין); a. fr.—Succ. 31[a] (a beam) דגזולה ומְטַלֵּל עלה Ms. M. (ed. דגזולה only) which one stole and put upon it the covering of the Succah, v. מְטַלַּלְתָּא.—*Part. pass.* מְטַלַּל, f. מְטַלְּלָא. B. Kam. 50[b] משום דמט׳ because the cave is roofed. Ib. דלא מְטַלְּלֵי which are uncovered.—Trnsf. *to obscure.* Sabb. 78[a] מסו ומְטַלְּלֵי they heal (the eye-sore) but dim the eye-sight.

Af. אַטֵּיל, אַטְלֵל 1) same, *to cover,* v. supra. Targ. Is. IV, 5, sq.; a. fr.—2) *to find shelter.* Dan. IV, 9.

Ithpa. אִיטַּלַּל *to be covered.* Targ. Ps. LXVIII, 14 מיט׳ (some ed. מט׳, v. supra). Targ. I Chr. II, 55.

טְלַל II (v. טול I), *Pa.* טַלֵּיל, *Af.* אַטְלֵיל *to play, sport.* Succ. 53[a] לוי הוה מְטַלֵּל וכ׳ Ar. (ed. מְטַיֵּיל, v. Rabb. D. S. a. l. note 200) L. was sporting .... with eight knives. B. Bath. 91[b] נהירנא.. מְטַלְּלִין וכ׳ Ar. (ed. מטיילין, Var. מְטַלְּלִין, מְטַיְּילִין or מְטַלְּלִין, v. Rabb. D. S. a. l. note 40) I remember that boys and girls enjoyed themselves &c.

Ithpe. אִיטְּלֵיל same. Kidd. 21[b] אִיטַּלְלִיתוּ, v. אִיסְקוּנְדְּרֵי.

טְלַל III, טְלָלָא m. (טְלַל I) 1) (=h. צֵל) *shade, shadow.* Targ. Koh. VIII, 13 (some ed. טול). Ib. VI, 12. Targ. Ps. XCI, 1; a. fr.—2) (cmp. סְכָךְ, סֻכָּה, סכך) *cover of twigs, reeds* &c.; in gen. *ceiling, cover, screen.* Targ. Ps. XXVII, 5; a. fr.—Ber. 19[a] נפל קניא מט׳ (Ms. M. משמי ט׳) a reed fell down from the ceiling. Ib. 48[a] אחוי לשמי ט׳ pointed up to the ceiling. B. Kam. 66[b] מעיקרא כשורא והשתא ט׳ formerly it was named *beam,* now *ceiling,* v. מְרִישׁ.—*Pl.* טְלָלַיָּא. Targ. Job XL, 21, sq. (h. text צאלים).

טְלַם *to bend, press,* esp. (corresp. to h. עָשַׁק) *to take undue advantage of, to oppress.* Targ. Y. Lev. V, 21. Targ.

Ps. CXIX, 122; a. fr.—Part. pass. טְלִים, (טְלוּם). Targ. Y. Deut. XXVIII, 33. Targ. Ps. CIII, 6 (some ed. incorr. טְלוֹ׳); a. e.—Lev. R. s. 12 (ref. to Prov. XXIII, 35) טָלְמִין ליה וכ׳ they overcharge him (in his drunkenness), and he knows it not &c.

Pa. טַלֵּים same. Targ. I Chr. XVI, 21.

טְלָמָא, v. טוּלְמָא I.

***טַלְמָיָא** m. (v. טוּלְמָא I) *cake-baker.* Koh. R. to V, 10. [Y. Snh. II, 20ᶜ bot. מנחם טלמא, perh. מנחם טלמיא.]

טלמסן, v. טוּלְמִיסִין.

טְלָנֵי m. pl. (טְלַל II) [*sporters,*] *night demons, urchins.* Targ. Cant. III, 8. Ib. IV, 6. Targ. Koh. II, 5. Targ. Y. Num. VI, 24 טְלוּי (corr. acc.)

טְלָנֵיתָא, v. טְלָיוּתָא.

***טלנס**, Cant. R. to VII, 8 כמין ט׳, read: כמי נִילוּס like the inundation of the Nile (so did the fire spread from the furnace when it was broken through); v. אוקירי. [The entire passage from כיצד to אוקירי belongs to VII, 9, after the words: מכאן שנפרץ הכבשן; v. פַּלְטְרָא.]

טְלַע I (b. h. צלע; cmp. טלל) [*to hang over, incline,*] *to halt.*

Af. אַטְלַע same. Targ. Gen. XXXII, 32, v. טְלַח. [Yeb. 39ᵇ אַטְלַע לה רגליך וכ׳ turn thy right foot towards her ואטלע לה וכ׳ and he did so, Rashi; v. next w.]

Ithpe. אִיטְּלַע *to become lame.*. Meg. 22ᵇ; Taan 25ᵃ; Succ. 53ᵃ.

טְלַע II (cmp. preced.) *to loosen, untie.* Targ. Ruth IV, 7; 8 (h. text שלף). Targ. Lam. IV, 3 (h. text חלץ).

Ithpe. אִיטְּלַע *to be untied, taken off.* Targ. Y. Deut. XXIX, 4.—Yeb. 39ᵇ אִיטְּלַע לה וכ׳ ed. (Ar. לך) have the shoe of thy right food untied (for her); ואַטְלַע ליה וכ׳ Ar. and he loosened the shoe of . . ., and she took it off (ed. ואיט׳ לה) and he had his shoe . . . loosened &c.); [other interpret., v. preced.].

Af. אַטְלַע *to untie,* v. supra.

טֶלֶף c. (cmp. צלף) [*glittering, pealing,*] *hoof,* esp. (b. h. פרסה) *cloven foot.* Ex. R. s. 18 beg. B. Bath 75ᵇ; Kidd. 22ᵇ אחזה בטַלְפָּהּ if he seized the animal by its hoof.—*Du.* טְלָפַיִם, טְלָפַיִם, טְלָפִין, pl. טְלָפִים (?), טְלָפוֹת. Bekh. 44ᵃ; Tosef. Par. II (I), 2.—Par. II, 2 שקרניה וטְלָפֶיהָ וכ׳; Bekh. l. c. שקרנים וטלפים (corr. acc.). Nidd. VI, 9 יש לו ט׳ has cloven feet. Ruth R. to III, 13 מטַּלְפֵי סוסי by the hoofs of my horse (counting his steps, I know the distance); Koh. R. to VII, 8 (v. next w.).—Y. Snh. X, 28ᵈ bot. ואין טְלָפֶיהָ סדוקות and are not her feet cloven (is she not clean for you, fit to be your wife)?—Midr. Till. to Ps. XVIII, 11 טַלְפוֹת סוסיהן וכ׳ the hoofs of their horses fell off; a. e. [Tosef. Ukts. II, 10 טלפין Var., v. מרלפפון.]

טְלַף, טַלְפָא, טִילְ׳ ch. 1) same. *Pl.* טַלְפִין, טַלְפַיָּא, טַלְפֵי, טִילְ׳. Targ. Lev. XI, 3; a. fr.—Y. Ḥag. II, 77ᵇ bot. מן ט׳ דסוסיי וכ׳ by counting the steps of my horse &c., v. preced.—Denom. מְטַלַּף, מְטַלַּף, מְיטַלַּף, מְטַלַּף (מְטַלְפָא) *with cloven foot, cloven.* Targ. Lev. l. c.—Targ. O. Deut. XIV, 6; a. fr. (v. Berl. Targ. O. II, p. 34).—2) (dial. for טלופחא) *beans.* Ned. 66ᵇ a Babylonian asked his Palestinean wife בשילי לי תרי טלפי cook for me two (a few) beans, בשילה ליה תרי טלפי and she cooked two feet (Rashi); [anoth. interpret.: she cooked for him just *two beans* and no more; marginal emendation בשילה ליה תרי טלפחי.]

טַלְפְּחָא, v. טְלוּפְחָא.

טלפירא, Y. Shek. VIII, beg. 51ᵃ לט׳, read אַפְלַיְרָא.

טְלַק (cmp. טלל) *to cast, throw.* Targ. Ps. LV, 23; Targ. Lam. II, 1; a. fr. (h. text השליך).—Gen. R. s. 75 שלח . . . וטַלְקֵיה וכ׳ he took off the purple cloak and threw it down before him. Y. Yeb. XII, 12ᵈ top; Y. Sabb. VI, 8ᵃ bot. [read:] טלקיה לחנותא דחליטרא pitched it into a confectioner's shop. [Targ. Y. II, Ex. XXI, 18, v. *Ithpa.*]

Pa. טַלֵּיק same, also *to cast away, reject.* Targ. Ps. LI, 13 (ed. Lag. *Pe.*).—Y. Sabb. l. c. מְטַלֵּק לה; (Y. Yeb. l. c. מסלק). Y. Keth. XII, 35ᵃ טליק גרמיה threw himself down; (Y. Kil. IX, 32ᵇ top טְלַק); a. e.—Part. pass. מְטַלַּק. Targ. Y. Lev. XVII, 15.—Y. Snh. VII, end, 25ᵈ דאינון מְטַלְּקִין בימא they have been thrown into the sea. Lam. R. to I, 1 רבתי (חד מאת׳ 3) מְטַלְּקָא, v. מְדוּכָא.

Ithpa. אִיטַּלַּק, *Ithpe.* אִיטְּלִיק *to be thrown, to be cast away.* Targ. Job III, 4, v. אַטְלְקוּתָא. Targ. Y. II Ex. XXI, 18 [read:] ויִטַּלַּק, or ויטליק (h. text נפל). Targ. Ps. XXII, 11.—Y. Sot. V, 20ᵇ bot. א׳ עלוי it was thrown upon him, i. e. a penalty was imposed &c.

***טְלָרִיתָא** f. (prob. dial. for טלל, טלל׳, cmp. Syr. טלרא P. Sm. 1482) *soldier's iron shoe.* Targ. I Kings II, 5 (h. text מנעל).

טְלֵת, v. טַלִּית ch.

טַמָא or **טָמָא** m. (=טעמא, v. M. Kat. 18ᵃ quot. s. v. טַעֲמָא, a. T'shuboth G'onim ed. Cassel, p. 22ᵃ) *reason, argument* (on the cause of grief), *consolation.* - *Pl.* טַמַּיָּא, or בֵּי ט׳—טַמַּיָא *gathering of comforters around the mourner* in his house or at the place of worship. Ber. 6ᵇ אגרא דבי ט׳ וכ׳ (Ar. טמא, Tshub. G'onim l. c. טעמא) the merit of attending the mourner's gathering lies in the silence (which must be observed until the mourner begins to speak). Snh. 113ᵃ [read:] למשאל ביה ט׳ (v. Rabb. D. S. a. l. note), v. טַעֲמָא.

טָמָא I (**טָמָה**) (b. h.; cmp. טמם) [*to be filled up, inaccesible,*] *to be unclean*; v. טְמָא II.

Pi. טִימֵּא (טִימָּה) 1) *to make unclean, to soil, defile.* Yoma 39ᵃ אדם מְטַמֵּא עצמו מעט מְטַמְּאִין וכ׳ if a man begins to defile himself a little (through sin), he will soon be defiled largely. Yad. III, 5, a. fr. מט׳ את הידים their handling makes the hands unclean (washing the hands is required after handling them). Kel. I, 1; a. v. fr.—2) *to declare unclean.* Toh. VI, 2. Eduy I, 11; a. v. fr.—Makhsh. VI, 2 טִימְּאוּ; Y. Dem. V, 24ᵈ טִימּוּ.

Nif. נִטְמָא, *Hithpa.* הִיטַּמֵּא, הִתְטַמֵּא 1) *to become unclean, to be made unclean.* Ukts. I, 1 מְטַמֵּא וּמִיטַּמֵּא eventually makes unclean and becomes unclean. Kel. II, 1 מִיתְטַמְּאִין וכ׳ (ed. Dehr. מִיטַ׳) are fit to become unclean and to make unclean. Ib. ומיט׳ מאחוריהן ואינן מיט׳ וכ׳ Mish. ed. (Talm. ed. מְטַ׳) may be made unclean through their backs (touching uncleanness), &c. Ib. VI, 4 וְנִטְמְאוּ and which became unclean; a. v. fr.—Yoma 38ᵇ [read:] בא לִטַּמֵּא פְּתָחִין לו (v. Rabb. D. S. a. l. note) to him who is willing to defile himself, doors are open; Sabb. 104ᵃ; Ab. Zar. 55ᵃ; Men. 29ᵇ.—2) *to make one's self unclean* by handling a corpse &c. (v. Lev. XXI, 1, sq.). Yeb. 60ᵃ מִטַּמֵּא לה he (the priest) may attend to her burial; a. fr.

טְמָא ch. same, v. טְמֵי.

טָמֵא II m., **טְמֵאָה** f. (b. h., v. preced. art.) *unclean, levitically impure, forbidden.* Kel. XII, 2 המחובר לט׳ ט׳ whatever is attached to an object which is fit to become unclean, may become unclean. Ib. 1 טבעת אדם ט׳ a ring used by man may eventually become unclean; a. v. fr.—Hull. VII, 5 דג ט׳ a fish forbidden to eat. Ib. 6 (בהמה) ט׳ a forbidden animal; a. v. fr.—Ab. Zar. 39ᵃ (referring to 'the ass of the sea', v. חֲמָר, a. 'the ox of the sea', v. תּוֹרָא) ט׳ טהור טהור ט׳ what is unclean (on land) is clean (in water) &c.—טְמֵא מֵת = b. h. טָ׳ לְמֵת, *one made unclean through a corpse.* Pes. 19ᵇ; a. fr.—*Pl.* טְמֵאִים, טְמֵאִין; f. טְמֵאוֹת. Hull. VIII, 6. Pes. 17ᵃ. Kel. XI, 8; a. v. fr.—טְמֵאֵי מתים, v. supra. Pes. 66ᵇ; a. fr.

טְמֵא ch. same, v. טְמֵי.

טַמְאָשָׁא m. (טְמַשׁ) *putting in ashes.* Esth. R. to I, 4, v. גְּרָאפָּא.

***טַמְדּוּרְיָא** pr. n. pl. *Tamduria,* in Babylonia (?). Ab. Zar. 39ᵃ (Ms. M. טמו ביריא, v. Neub. Géogr. p. 392).

טמו ביריא, ט׳ בִּירִיא, v. preced.

טִמוֹס, v. טוֹמוֹס.

טְמוֹעָא m. (טְמַע) *sinking, sun-set.* Targ. Ps. CIV, 19 טְמוֹעֵיה (Ms. טְמוּ׳).

טְמוֹר m. (טְמַר, v. טִימוּרָא) *hiding place, refuge.* Targ. Ps. XXXII, 7. Targ. Job XXII, 14 ed. Lag. (ed. טְמִיר, טַמִּיר). [Targ. Ps. XIX, 13 טמורות ed. Lag., v. טְמִיר.]

טְמוֹר, טְמוּרְתָא, טְמוּר, v. sub טִימ׳.

טמורה, v. טְמִיר.

טִמְטֵם, v. טִימ׳.

טִמְטֵם, v. טָמַם.

טְמָא, טְמֵי = h. טָמֵא, *to be, become unclean.* Targ. Ps. CVI, 39 טְמִיאוּ (some ed. incorr. טְמִי׳).

Pa. טַמֵּי, טַמֵּא *to make unclean.* Targ. Y. II Num. XII, 12.—Targ. Mic. II, 10 בדיל לְטַמְּיוּתָהּ ed. Lag. (ed. בדיל ט׳ corr. acc.) in order to defile her.—Hull. 3ᵃ לְטַמְּיֵיהּ וטַמְּיֵתִיה לבשר ... the person will make the knife unclean and then the knife will make the flesh unclean. Pes. 79ᵃ דבשר הוא דְּמִטַּמְּיָא ליה וכ׳ which affects only the flesh, but not the person. (Ms. M. דמִיטַּמֵּי ... מִיטַּמְאֵי, *Ithpe.*). Ib. 67ᵇ טַמּוּיֵי מְטַמֵּי makes unclean; a. fr.

Ithpe. אִיטְּמֵי, אִיטְּמָא, אִיתְטְמָא *to be made unclean.* Hull. 2ᵇ; a. e.

טְמֵא, טְמֵי m., constr. (preced.) *unclean.* Targ. Num. V, 2, a. fr. ט׳ נפשא, v. טָמֵא II.—Pl. f. טַמְיָין. Targ. Y. Deut. XIV, 4 [read:] עִיבּוּרֵי ט׳ (v. Bekh. 7ᵃ) offsprings of unclean mothers.

טַמְיָא m. (טמי, cmp. טמם, אָטוּם) [*substantial,*] *bone.*—*Pl.* טַמַּיָּא, (טִימַיָּא). v. אוֹב, אובא ט׳ ch.—שחיק ט׳ (an imprecation) whose bones be ground to dust. Lev. R. s. 25; a. fr.—[Tosef. Ohol. XVII, 3 מלוא טימיא, v. לָטוֹמְיָא.]—שׁוּם טַמְיָא pr. n. pl. *Shum T'mayya,* in Babylonia. B. Bath. 153ᵃ (Ms. M. שוטמי׳; oth. Verss. v. Rabb. D. S. a. l. note).

טַמַּיָּא, טַמ׳, v. טַמָּא.

טַמְיאוֹן, v. next w.

טִימְיוֹן, טַמְיוֹן m. (ταμεῖον) *treasury,* esp. *Roman aurarium, fiscus.* Lev. R. s. 19 מכניס ממונם לט׳ confiscated their property for the fiscus. Ib. s. 11, a. e. גבאי ט׳ tax collector; Ruth R. introd. end טַמְיאוֹן (insert גבאי). Gen. R. s. 61 עד שנמצאת ארץ מצרים לט׳ until it was found by calculation that the entire land of Egypt would be forfeited to the treasury (for its indebtedness to the Jews); Yalk. ib. 110; (Meg. Taan. ch. III עד שהיתה מצרים שלהם). Gen. R. s. 51 תשרף מן ט׳ shall be set on fire at public expense; a. fr.—Esth. R. to I, 2 טירון, read טימ׳, v. טַמְיָקוֹן.

טַמְיוּתָא, טַמָּיוּתָא, v. טְמֵי *Pa.*

טְמִינָה f. (טָמַן) *a place for chafing dishes,* contrad. to כירה cooking stove. Y. Sabb. IV, end, 7ᵃ.

טִימְיָ׳, טַמְיָקָא m. (ταμιακός, tamiacus) *belonging to the imperial treasury, tamiaca (praedia), crown-lands, imperial domains.* Esth. R. introd. אתם ט׳ אתם you are crown property (God's own people); הלוקח לו עבד מן הט׳ שוב וכ׳ (read של בשר ודם, abbr. של ב״ו, for שוב) does not he who takes to himself a slave from the crown lands forfeit his life? Ib. (ref. to Esth. VIII, 7) על דפשט ידיה בט׳ because he stretched forth his hand against crown property (the Jews).

טַמְיָקוֹן m. (variously corrupted) same. Pesik. Vayhi, p. 7ᵇ הן דמלכא שרי ט׳ where the king resides (in the seventh heaven) there is the crown property (which must not be desecrated by symbolical representations); Num. R. s. 12; Cant. R. to VI, 4; [Esth. R. to I, 2 טירון, v. טַמְיוֹן.]

טְמִיר, טמיר, טְמִיר m., **טְמִירָא** c. (טְמַר, v. טָמוֹר) *hidden, secret;* (also as noun) *secrecy.* Targ. I Sam. X, 22. Ib. XXI, 3 (h. text אלמני); a. fr.—עבד ט׳ *to live hidden.* Y.

Shebi. VIII, 38[b] top. Y. Dem. I, 21[d] bot. עבדת טמירה **גבן** (not טמו׳), was hidden with them; Y. Shek. V, 48[d] top טמירא.—*Pl.* טְמִירִין, f. טְמִירָן, טְמִירָתָא. Targ. Josh. VII, 21. Targ. Ps. XLIV, 22. Ib. XIX, 13 (ed. Lag. טמורות). Targ. Gen. XLI, 45 (v. Berl. Targ. O. II, p. 15).

טָמַם (v. טָמָא I) *to fill up, stop.* Sabb. 73[b]; 81[b] טְמָמָהּ filled it up. V. טום.

טְמַם ch. same. Targ. O. Gen. XXVI, 15; 18 טַמוּנוּן (ed. Berl. טַמּוּנִין; Y. טמונינון, corr. acc.). Targ. II Kings III, 19.—Gitt. 68[a] וטַמְּרִינְהוּ and filled the pits up. Yeb. 63[a] טום וכ׳ fill up a hole in the wall (in time) &c.—Part. pass. טְמִים, טְמִימָא. M. Kat. 4[b] למיכרא נהרא ט׳ to dig up a channel the source of which is choked up.

Ithpe. אִיטּוֹם *to be covered up, buried.* Meg. 27[b] דתיטום בשיראי that thou be buried in silk. Ib. עד דא׳ וכ׳ until he was covered up with the silk garments (put upon him while he was asleep).

Palp. טַמְטֵם *to close around, to close.* Targ. Jud. III, 22 (h. text סגר). Targ. Y. Deut. XXIX, 3. Targ. Is. VI, 10 טמטם ed. Lag. (ed. עמעם, corr. acc.); a. e.—Part. pass. מְטַמְטַם. Ib. XLIV, 18.

Ithpalp. אִיטַּמְטַם *to be closed.* Ib. XXXII, 3. Targ. Ps. CXIX, 70 Regia (ed. איטפש).

טָמַן (b. h.; cmp. preced.) *to hide, store away, preserve,* esp. *to keep dishes warm* for the Sabbath. Sabb. II, 7 טוֹמְנִין את החמין you may put warm dishes in the chafing stove &c. Ib. IV, 1; a. fr.—Makhsh. I, 6 הטומן פירותיו וכ׳ if one hides his fruits in water against thieves.—Koh. R. to X, 8 שהוא ט׳ וכ׳ that he buried it there; a. e.—Part. pass. טָמוּן. B. Kam. 5[b], a. e. נזקי ט׳ באש damage caused to things hidden in a pile to which fire was set. Gen. R. s. 68 היה ט׳ וכ׳ he (Jacob) was hiding (before Esau) in the house of Eber; Meg. 17[a] מוּטְמָן (Ms. M. נטמן, v. Rabb. D. S. a. l. note); a. fr.

Nif. נִטְמַן *to be hidden, to hide one's self, to be stored up.* Ib. שנ׳ בבית עבר, v. supra. Lev. R. s. 3 ויִטָּמְנוּ ד״ת בפיך and the words of the Law shall be stored up in thy mouth. Pesik. R. s. 4 נ׳ במערה sought protection in a cave; a. e.

Hif. הִטְמִין 1) *to hide, keep.* B. Kam. 61[b] שדרכם להַטְמִין וכ׳ which it is customary to hide in the stack. B. Mets. 61[b] לא יַטְמִין... במלח he must not keep his weights in salt (by which they gain in weight); a. fr.—Part. pass. מוּטְמָן, v. supra.—2) *to hide one's self, lie in wait.* B. Kam. 79[b] ראוהו שה׳ וכ׳ if he has been seen hiding himself in the woods (waiting for a chance to steal).

טְמַן ch. same. Targ. Job XIV, 13 Ms. (ed. טשא). [Targ. Esth. V, 14 נטמון, Buxt., some ed. נטמא, נדמון, read with ed. Lag.: נרמי, נרמון.—Targ. Y. Gen. XXVI, 15; 18, v. טְמַם.]

טמן, Y. Dem. II, end, 23[a], read: נוּמִּין, v. לוּמָא.

טָמַע, (cmp. טָמַן) *to hide, sink* (cmp. טָבַע I).

Nif. נִטְמַע *to be hidden, sunk, to be mixed up beyond recognition.* Kidd. 70[b] וכולן נִטְמְעוּ בכהונה and all of them have been lost among the priesthood (can no longer be distinguished from original priests). Ib. 71[a] a family שנִיטַּמְעָה נ׳ (or שנִיטְמְעָה *Nithpa.*) once mixed with Israelites beyond traces of genealogical disabilities, shall remain so (shall not be traced up). Keth. 14[b], v. עִיסָּה; a. e.

טְמַע ch. same, 1) *to sink, be covered up.* Targ. Lam. II, 9 (h. text טבע). Targ. Y. Num. XXVI, 11. Targ. Ps. LXIX, 3; a. e.—2) (of the sun) *to set.* Targ. Y. Gen. XV, 17; a. fr.—3) *to cover up, bury.* Targ. Y. Ex. XV, 4; 12. Targ. Job XXXI, 33; a. e.—*Part. pass.* טְמִיעַ a) *hidden, buried.* Ib. III, 16 (h. text טמון); a. e.—b) *darkened, obscured.* ט׳ מזלא one whose planet is obscured, *hapless fellow.* Koh. R. to VII, 15. Ib. XI, 9; a. e.—4) (cmp. טמם) *to be inaccessible to argument, to be dull.* Targ. Job XVIII, 3 טְמַעְנָא (not ט׳; Ms. Var. אִיטַּנַּפְנָא, v. טְנַף; h. text נטמינו).

Pa. טַמַּע *to sink, bury.* Ib. XL, 13 Ms. (ed. *Pe.*)

Ithpa. אִיטַּמַּע *to be sunk.* Targ. Job XXXVIII, 6 Ms. (ed. טְמִיעָן).

טְמַר (v. preced.) *to hide, preserve, guard.* Targ. Gen. XXXV, 4 (h. text טמן); a. fr.—Part. pass. טָמִיר q. v.

Pa. טַמַּר, *Af.* אַטְמַר *to hide, withhold, keep removed.* Targ. Is. XXIX, 10. Targ. Ex. II, 2; a. e.—Part. pass. מְטַמַּר, v. infra.

Ithpa. אִיטַּמַּר, *Ithpe.* אִיטְּמַר, אִיטְּמִיר *to be hidden, hide one's self.* Targ. Gen. III, 8; a. fr.—B. Kam. 57[a] כיון דמִיטְּמַר וכ׳ when he hides himself from people; ib. 79[b] דקא מִטַּמַּר מינייהו Ms. M. (ed. מטמרי, incorr.; Ms. H. מיטמר). Ib. מִטַּמְּרֵי אִיטַּמּוּרֵי; a. e.—Gitt. 56[b] מילי דמִטַּמְּרָן (or דמִטְמְרָן, v. supra). hidden treasures.—[Tosef. Sabb. XVII (XVIII), 19 ואין מטמרין אותו, ed. Zuck., a corrupt tautography of אין משמרין אותו.]

טְמַשׁ (cmp. preced.; corresp. to h. טבל) *to dip, immerse.* Targ. Y. Ex. XII, 22; a. fr.—Part. pass. טְמִישׁ. Targ. Ps. LXXX, 6 (not טְמַ׳).

Pa. טַמֵּשׁ same. Targ. Ruth II, 14 (ed. Amst. *Pe.*); a. fr.—Snh. 110[a] bot. וטַמְּשֵׁיה במיא Ar. (ed. ואמשייה מיירא) and dipped it in water. B. Bath. 74[a] וטמשיה Ar. (ed. אמשינה, v. Rabb. D. S. a. l. note 6). Gitt. 69[a] וניטַמֵּישׁ וכ׳ (or וניִטְמְשׁ) and let him dip them &c.; a. e.—*Part. pass.* מְטַמְטַשׁ *bathed, washed.* Targ. Job XXIV, 8 (ed. Wil. מְטַ׳ Ithpa.).

Ithpa. אִיטַּמַּשׁ, *Ithpe.* אִיטְּמִישׁ *to be dipped, to sink.* Targ. Ps. LX, 10.—Succ. 10[b] אִיטְּמִישָׁא ליה וכ׳ (Ms. M. אשתמיטא, cler. error for אִתְּטְמִישָׁא) his garment became soaked with water.

טמשא*, Lam. R. to I, 17, read טרשא, v. טְרַשׁ II.

טַן, v. טַנְּדוּ.

טְנָא, v. טְנִי.

טְנָאנָא, טִנָאנָא, v. טְנָנָא.

טַנְבּוּרָא m. (טבר, v. טִיבּוּר, cmp. טַבְלָא I) *tamburine, taborin.* Sot. 49[b].

טַן דּוּ, טַנְדּוּ (=טַעַן דּוּ, v. דְּוִיו; cmp. טוּנָא I) adv. *with a load of grief, in trouble.* Targ. Job XVII, 16 (Regia טַנְדִּוּ;

h. text כַּהֵי).—Kidd. 7ª, a. fr. טב למיתב ט׳ מלמיתב ארמלא Ar. led. (טַן דו) it is better to dwell in grief than to dwell in widowhood, i. e. a woman prefers an unhappy married life to singleness.

טנדיסין, v. טרנדיסין.

***טנדס**, Pirkê d'R. El. ch. XLI טב׳, v. טורוס.

טִנוּף, טִנּוּפָא, טִנּוֹפֶת, v. טִינ׳.

טְנֵז *the second element of the word* שַׁעַטְנֵז, phonetically representing טוּי, the act of *spinning*, and נוֹז, the act of *weaving*. Y. Kel. IX, end, 32ᵈ, v. שַׁעַטְנֵז.

טְנִי m. (b. h. טֶנֶא, cmp. טוּנָא I) [*traveller's load,*] 1) *T'ni*, a certain dry measure. Tam. III, 6, v. תַּרְקַב. Ib. 9.—2) *travelling box, basket*. Kel. XII, 3 כסוי ט׳ וכ׳ the metal cover of a box; של רופאים physicians' medicine box. Ib. XIV, 6; XVI, 7; Tosef. ib., B. Mets. II, 9 כסיטנא (corr. acc.); ib. IV, 11.—Y. Sot. IX, 24ᵇ bot. לתוך ט׳ וכ׳; Bab. ib. 48ᵇ בט׳ Ar. (ed. אִיטְנֵי q. v.) into a box made of lead and filled with barley husks.

טָנִיס, v. טַאֲנִיס.

טניף, v. טָנַף.

טנכי, Y. Kil. IX, 32ᶜ top, read: מנכר, v. נְכַר.

טָנַן (cmp. טִין) *to be moistened and softened*, (of grains) *to be easily pealed in grinding*. Makhsh. III, 4 וטָנְנוּ and the wheat grew prepared for grinding. [Tanḥ. Vayiggash 9 טנותה some ed., read טִנּ׳.]

Pi. טִינֵּן *to prepare for grinding*. Makhsh. l. c. הַמְטַנֵּן בחול if one prepares wheat by mixing with sand; ib. 5 חטי׳ בטיט וכ׳ with dried clay.—Part. pass. מְטוּנָּן, f. מְטוּנֶּנֶת. M. Kat. 6ᵇ שדה מ׳ moist and fat soil, opp. גריד.

Hif. הֵטֵן same. Makhsh. l. c. מְטִינִּים בחול (or מַטִּינ׳ fr. טִין). Ib. 5 לְהָטֵן Mish. ed. (Talm. ed. לְהָטֵל fr. טָלַל). Tosef. ib. II, 2 להטיח ed. Zuck. (Var. לְהָטִין). Tosef. Shebi V, 16 (twice) להטיל (Var. להטין), (once) להטין; Y. ib. VII, beg., 37ᵇ מהו לחטן בחוטין (read: לְהָטֵן בו חטין); ib. (repeatedly) לחטן (corr. acc.).

טְנַן ch. same, 1) *to moisten*. Targ. Job III, 5 (h. text גאל, Regia יטנפ׳).—2) (cmp. our *to drivel*, Germ. *geifern*) *to be jealous, zealous, agitated* (corresp. to h. קנא). Targ. Ps. LXXIII, 3. Targ. Prov. III, 31; a. fr.

Pa. טַנֵּין 1) *to moisten*. Y. Pes. VII, 30ª top מְטַנְּנָה אסור to mix the wheat with moist sand is forbidden, v. preced.—2) *to be jealous* &c. Targ. Ps. XXXVII, 1 תְּטַנֵּין Ms. (ed. *Pe.*, תִּטְנִין *Af.*). Targ. Job XXXVI, 33 מְטַנְּנִין וכ׳ (Ms. מְטַנִּין) attacking each other in the heat of discussion (cmp. קנאת סופרים, s. v. קִנְאָה).

Af. אַטְנִין, v. supra.

טִינָנָא, טְנָנָא f. (preced.) *jealousy, zeal, agitation* (corresp. to h. קִנְאָה). Targ. Ps. LXIX, 10. Targ. Job V, 2. Targ. II Esth. V, 8 (Var. טִנְאָנָא, טְנָאנָא). Ib. VII, 4 (h. text נֵזֶק!); a. fr.

טְנָנוּתָא f. same. Targ. Ps. LXXIX, 5.

טָנַף (b. h.; cmp. טנו) *to be soiled*.

Pi. טִינֵּף *to soil* with excrements, secretions &c.; *to secrete* (blood or mucus from the womb). Pesik. Par., p. 40ᵇ שטי׳ בפלטין וכ׳ that made a nuisance in the palace &c. Bekh. 20ª, a. e. מְטַנֶּפֶת an animal secreting from the vagina (an evidence of birth or abortion). B. Kam. 3ª טִינְּפָה פירות the animal soiled fruits (by rolling in them). Tosef. Joma V (IV), 5 כדי שלא יְטַנְּפוּ וכ׳ that his feet may not soil his garments; a. fr.—*Part. pass.* מְטוּנָּף, f. מְטוּנֶּפֶת; pl. מְטוּנָּפִין, מְטוּנָּפוֹת *soiled, filthy, defiled, polluted*. Y. Snh. X, 27ᵈ top. Cant. R. to II, 8; a. fr.

Nithpa. נִיטַּנֵּף, *Nif.* נִטְנַף *to be soiled, defiled*. Y. Yoma VIII, 44ᵈ נִיטַּנְּפוּ רגליו (or נִיטְנְפוּ) if his feet became muddy.—*Y. Ber. I, 3ᶜ bot. ראה כפים הללו שלא נִיטַנְּפוּ בבנין וכ׳ ed. Lehm. (ed. Ven. נטפו, ed. Krot. חטפו, v. חָטַף) see these hands which have not been in the least soiled by misappropriating the Temple funds.

טְנַף ch. same. Part. pass. טְנִיף. Sabb. 57ª טְנִיפָן they were soiled with dirt (Rashi: מִיטַּנְּפֵי *Ithpa.*).

Pa. טַנֵּף *to soil, pollute*. Targ. Cant. V, 3 (ed. Lag. אטופ׳, read: אֲטַנְּפִנּ׳). Targ. Job III, 5 (v. טְנַן). Targ. Y. Num. XXXV, 33. [Ib. יְטוֹף; Targ. Y. Deut. XXI, 23 תְּטוּפוּן, prob. to be read: יְטַנֵּף, תְּטַנְּפוּן.]—Bekh. 20ª ודאי לא ט׳ it has certainly not had any secretion indicative of birth, v. preced.

Ithpa. אִיטַּנֵּף *to be soiled, defiled*. Targ. Lam. IV, 14. Targ. Job. XVIII, 3 (v. טְמַע). Targ. Ps. CVI, 38; a. e.—Sabb. 57ª, v. supra. B. Bath. 82ᵇ קמִיטַּנְּפֵי פירי the fruits are soiled (will rot, when falling on moist plants).

טִנָּר, טְנָרָא, v. טִינָ׳.

טָס, v. טוּס.

טַס m. (טסס, sec. r. of טוּס) [*glittering, flying*] *foil, plate*. Gitt. 20ᵇ כתב . . . על טס וכ׳ if he wrote to her a letter of divorce on gold foil; Y. ib. II, 44ᵇ. Kel. XIII, 6 חשן שבטס a key-ward fastened to a thin plate. Sabb. 60ª ט׳ של זהב וכ׳ the pin has on one end a gold plate.—*Pl.* טַסִּין, טַסִּים. Kel. XI, 3 מן הט׳ וכ׳ of (tin) foil or other plating material; Tosef. ib. B. Bath. V, 16. Sabb. 103ª טַסֵּי משכן the foils used for the Tabernacle (Ex. XXXIX, 3).

טַסָּא, טַסָּא I ch. same. Targ. Prov. XXVI, 8 (Var. כיפא, h. text אבן); v. נִיקְצָא.—*Pl.* טַסִּין, טַסַּ׳. Targ. Num. XVII, 3. Targ. Ex. XXXIX, 3.

***טַסָּא** II collect. noun (v. preced.) *soldiers with glittering armor* (?). Targ. Nah. III, 17 (h. text מנזריך).

טסבלאות, Sifré Num. 42, read אִסְטַבְלָאוֹת=סְטַ׳ *stables*.

טִיס׳, טְסִבְרָא m. (Ispe. noun of סבר II, cmp. צְדָקָא) *treasure, store, store-house*.—*Pl.* טְסִבְרִין, טִיס׳. Targ. Koh II, 8. Targ. Esth. VIII, 1.—Targ. Ps. LXVIII, 14 (h. text אברות!).—V. תִּסְבְּרָא.

טסורא, Y. Keth. XI, 34ᵇ bot., v. סַנְטֵירָא.

מסים, v. דמסים.

טְסָנִי, v. טִיסָנִי.

טַסְקָא f. (v. Freit. Arab. Dict. s.v. ṭask) 1) *a basket, as a measure.* Gitt. 78ª לאיתויי ט׳ דאכלא בה וכ׳ (Tosaf. to Ab. Zar. 14ᵇ quotes ...בית) to include the measure in which she measures (or eats) figs (destined) for her particular use. Meg. 7ᵇ מלא ט׳ וכ׳ (Ms. O. טיסקא, v. Rabb. D. S. a. l., Var. צנא) a *taska* full of &c.—2) name of a Persian *land-tax* (a certain measure for each certain quantity of produces). B. Mets. 73ᵇ ארעא לט׳ וכ׳ the land is pledged to the *taska*, and the king has decreed that he who pays the *taska* shall have the usufruct of the land; B. Bath. 54ᵇ. B. Mets. 110ª תקינו ... יהיב ט׳ the Rabbis have given him a remedy in hand in ordering that the mortgagee shall pay the taxes (and thus secure his ownership against the mortgager's eventual claims). Gitt. 58ᵇ קב׳ ל ארעא בט׳ rented a piece of land for the taxes on it; Ned. 46ᵇ. B. Bath. 55ª, v. זִיהֲרוּרָא.—Kidd. 70ᵇ, v. הַסְקָא.

טְעָא, טְעָה, v. טעי.

טְעוּ f. (preced.) 1) *going astray.* Targ. Jer. III, 8 (ed. Wil. טְעוֹ). Targ. Is. XIX, 14. Targ. Ps. CXXXIX, 24 אורח דט׳ Regia (ed. דְטָעֲיָן; h. text עצב); a. fr.—*Pl.* טַעֲוָותָא. Targ. Nah. III, 4; a. e.—2) (cacophem.), also טַעֲוָא, טַעֲוָוא m. *idol.* Targ. Y. Deut. IV, 16. Targ. II Chr. XXXII, 15. Ib. XXXV, 21 טָעֲוָתִי (or טַעֲוָתִי) my deity. — *Pl.* טַעֲוָן, טַעֲוָתָא, טַעֲוָן, טַעֲוָנ׳. Targ. Is. I, 29. Targ. Deut. XXVIII, 36; a. fr.

טְעוּן, v. טְעַן a. טְעֵן. [Constr. of טְעוּנָא q. v.]

טָעוּן 1) part. pass. of טָעַן; 2) *requirement*, v. טוֹעַן.

טְעוּנָא m., constr. טְעוּן (טְעַן II, v. טוּנָא I) 1) *load.* Targ. I Sam. XVI, 20 ט׳ חמרא ט׳ דלחמא ed. Lag. (oth. ed. טעין דלחמא) an ass-load consisting of a load (or *bag*, v. infra) of bread and &c. Targ. II Kings V, 17; a. e.—Sot. 34ª, v. הִלֵּךְ. B. Mets. 97ª; a. e.—*Pl.* טְעוּנֵי, טְעוּנַיָּיא. Ib. 32ª .. דרמי וטעונייהו וכ׳ when they themselves and their loads lie on the road.—2) *bag.*—*Pl.* as ab. Targ. Josh. II, 6 ט׳ כיתנא bags of flax.—Y. Dem. II, 22ᵈ, contrad. to אַשְׁפָּלָה. Lam. R. introd. (R. Joh. 1) מובלי ט׳ דחלא loads of bags of sand.

טָעוּת f. (טָעָה) 1) *error, mistake.* B. Mets. 15ᵇ; Keth. 51ª, a. fr. ט׳ סופר, v. אַחֲרָיוּת. Gen. R. s. 99, v. סוּתָה.—B. Kam. 113ᵇ וּבְטָעוּתוֹ (v. Rabb. D. S. a. l.) and a gain through his (the gentile's) mistake; a. fr.—*Pl.* טָעֻיוֹת Macc. 12ª. Men. 29ᵇ; a. e.—2) (v. טְעוּ) *idol.* Sifré Num. 131 אוי לכם ולְטָעוּתְכֶם woe is unto you and your idol; Y. Snh. X, 28ᵈ אוי לכם וכ׳ (corr. acc.).

טְעוּתָא, טַעֲוָתָא, v. טְעוּ.

טָעָה, טעי (b. h.) 1) (cmp. תָּעָה) *to err, be mistaken.* Ber. II, 3 קרא וט׳ יחזור למקום שט׳ if in reading the Sh'ma one made a mistake, he must go back to the passage in which he made a mistake. B. Mets. 63ᵇ בכדי שהדעת טועה within the limits of a reasonable mistake in counting. Snh. 33ᵇ ט׳ בדבר שהצדוקין וכ׳ if the judge made a mistake in a case in which there is no difference of opinion between the Sadducees and Pharisees. Ib. 6ª, a. e. ט׳ בדבר משנה if the judge gave a wrong decision against an explicit law in the Mishnah; ט׳ בשיקול הדעת, v. דַּעַת; a. fr.—2) *to seek, to miss* (cmp. טְעַן I). Taan. III, 8 אבן הטועים; B. Mets. 28ᵇ אבן טוֹעִין Ms. M. (ed. טוֹעַן, v. Rabb. D. S. a. l. note), v. אֶבֶן.—Lev. R. s. 13, beg. אני טָעִיתִי אי׳ החלכה I had *forgotten* the law in the case.

Hif. הִטְעָה *to lead astray, to deceive, disappoint.* B. Mets. VI, 1 הִטְעוּ זה את זה they deceived one another, i. e. the agent employed to engage laborers did not act according to instruction, v. next w. — M. Kat. II, 1 הִטְעוּהוּ פועלים hired men disappointed him. Gen. R. s. 19 end (interpret. *hishshiani*, Gen. III, 13) הִטְעַנִי he deceived me with false promises; a. e.

Hof. הוּטְעָה *to be led astray, be deceived.* Tanh. Balak 5 כמו שהטעה ה׳ as he led astray, so was he led astray.—Part. מוּטְעָה, f. מוּטְעֵית, מוּטְעַת *misled, brought about by mistake, under false premises.* Yeb. 106ª חליצה מ׳ a *ḥalitsah* to which the *yabam* consented in consequence of a deception (a promise not kept); Tosef. ib. XII, 13; Keth. 74ª.—R. Hash. 25ª אתם אפי׳ מוּטְעִין 'ye' (shall appoint), even if deceived by witnesses (your decision stands). Sabb. 101ᵇ מוטעין (mattings fastened, or spread) by mistake; a. e.

טְעָא, טְעֵי ch. same, 1) (corresp. to b. h. תָּעָה) *to wander, be lost; to reel.* Targ. Y. Gen. XXI, 14 טְעַת (O. ed. Berl. טָעַת, ed. Vien. תְּעַת). Targ. Is. XXVIII, 7. Ib. XIX, 13; a. fr.—Gitt. 68ᵇ רויא דהוה קא טָעֵי באורחא a drunken man that was lost on the road; a. e.—2) (corresp. to b. h. זָנָה) *to go astray, worship idols, to be licentious* &c. Targ. Am. VII, 17. Targ. Ex. XXXIV, 15 ויטעון (ed. Amst. O. וִיטְעוֹן). Ib. 16 וִיטְעָן ed. Berl. (ed. Amst. וִיטְעֵיָן, Y. I וכד טָעֲיָין, Y. II וְיִטְעָיָן); a. fr.—Gen. R. s. 87, beg. (expl. סררת Prov. VII, 11) טָעְיָא running about, prostitute, v. טָעִיתָא.—3) *to err, be mistaken.* Targ. Ps. LXXVIII, 9 טְעוֹ miscalculated the term of redemption (v. Ex. R. s. 20).—Yeb. 121ª מיטעא טְעִינָא I was mistaken; a. e.—4) *to forget.* Targ. Prov. II, 17. Ib. XXXI, 5; 7. Ib. VI, 20 (ed. Vien. תטעי מנימוסא *deviate from*).

Af. אַטְעֵי 1) *to lead astray, to deceive.* Targ. Deut. XXVII, 18 יַטְעֵי (not יט׳). Targ. Ex. XXXIV, 16; a. fr.—B. Mets. 76ª אַטְעוּ פועלים וכ׳ the hired men deceived (the one engaging the others deceived them as to their wages, v. preced.); (Var. איטעו וכ׳ they were deceived by one of their own).—Hull. 94ᵇ מַטְעוּ נפשייהו they deceive themselves; a. fr.—2) *to prostitute.* Targ. O. Lev. XIX, 29.—3) (denom. of טַעֲוָא) *to deify, worship as deity.* Targ. II Chr. XXIV, 17 (v. Ex. R. s. 8).—[4) *to cause to be forgotten, to ignore.* Targ. Prov. XVII, 14 אַטְעֵי (ed. Lag. מטעי, prob. to be read: אַנְשֵׁי, h. text נְטוֹשׁ.]

Ithpe. אִיטְּעָא, אִיטְּעֵי 1) *to be deceived.* B. Mets. 76ª, v. supra.—2) *to be forgotten.* Targ. Prov. VI, 33 (h. text תמחה).

טְעַיִם, v. טְעַם.

טְעִימָה f. (טְעַם) *tasting*, transf. *testing, the quantity used for testing* the color. Men. 42ᵇ ט׳ פסולה the quantity taken out of the kettle for testing is unfit for sacred use; ט׳ פסלה that quantity, if put back, disqualifies the entire contents of the kettle. Ib. 40ᵃ גזירה משום ט׳ (not דטעימא or טעימא) it is to be feared lest the quantity used for testing may be put back again.

טְעִין, v. טְעַן.

טְעִין (טְעוּן) טְעִין m., **טְעִינָא** f. (טְעַן II) *laden, carrying.* [Targ. I Sam. XVI, 20, v. טְעוּנָא.] Targ. Esth. II, 15 טְעִינַת טיבו (h. text נשאת חן).—Gen. R. s. 70 ממון אתית ט׳ וכ׳ that I came laden with money; I bring only words.—*Pl.* טְעִינִין (טְעוּ׳); f. טְעִינָן. Targ. Gen. XXXVII, 25 (Y. ed. Amst. טְעוּ׳). Ib. XLV, 23; a. e.

טְעִינָה f. (טְעַן II) 1) *loading, assistance rendered in loading up*, opp. פְּרִיקָה. B. Mets. 31ᵃ. Ib. 32ᵃ ט׳ בשכר for assistance in loading one may claim wages; a. e.—2) *carrying.* Num. R. s. 6 לשם טְעִינַת הארון for the office of carrying the Ark.

טַעְיָא, טְעִיתָא f. (טְעֵי) *prostitute.* Targ. Nah. III, 4; a. e.—Yalk. Prov. 940 (expl. סררת, Prov. VII, 11); (Gen. R. s. 87 טעייא), v. טְעֵי.

טָעַם (b. h.) [*to be bright, wise* (v. Ps. XXXIV, 9),] *to examine, to taste, test, try, experience.* Yoma 22ᵇ לא ט׳ טַעַם חטא never tasted the taste of sin (was innocent). Y. Succ. V, 55ᵇ לא היו טוֹעֲמִין טעם וכ׳ had not even a taste of sleep. Ber. 35ᵃ אסור.. שיטעום וכ׳ one must not taste food without a blessing. Ib. 14ᵃ מהו שיטעום dare he (who fasts) taste food when cooking? Num. R. s. 7 כל מי .. היה טוֹעֲמוֹ whoever desired to eat meat felt its taste (in the mannah); a. v. fr.

Hif. הִטְעִים 1) *to give to taste.* Ned. 66ᵇ עד שתַּטְעִימִי לרב וכ׳ ... until thou makest R. J. taste of thy dish. B. Mets. 75ᵃ כדי לְהַטְעִימָן וכ׳ in order to give them a taste of usury (that they might feel its oppressiveness). Cant. R. to VII, 2 תהא ... ומטעמני (read וּמַטְעִימֵנִי or וּמְטַעֲמֵנִי *Pi.*) thou shalt bring some of them before me and let me taste them; a. fr.—2) *to make tasteful, to explain.* Sot. 21ᵇ המַטְעִים דבריו וכ׳ who explains his case to the judge (trying to preoccupy him), before his adversary appears; Tanh. Mishp. 6; a. e.—V. מַטְעֶמֶת.

טְעֵם, טְעִים (טְעָים) טְעַם ch. same. Targ. I Sam. XIV, 24; a. fr.—Targ. Y. Deut. XXXII, 1 דלא טַעֲמִין מיתותא which taste no death (heaven and earth).—Ber. 44ᵃ דלא ט׳ זדינא that he tasted no food. Sabb. 11ᵃ ליטעום מר מידי take some refreshment, Sir!—Hor. 11ᵃ אִטְעוֹם טעם דאיסורא I wish to try how a forbidden thing tastes; a. fr.

Af. אַטְעֵים *to give to taste.* Targ. Y. Gen. XXIV, 17.—Koh. R. to I, 3 לית את מַטְעַם לי מתבשילי wilt thou not let me taste what I have cooked (for thee?); Lev. R. s. 28; Pesik. R. s. 18; Pesik. Haomer, p. 70ᵃ .. מַטְעִים.. מתבשילך of the dish prepared for thee?

Pa. טַעֵם *to taste.* Part. pass. מְטַעַם *tasted, touched.* Lev. R. l. c. why do the dishes come out ולא מְטַעֲמִין without being touched?; (Koh. R. l. c. ולא טעמין and they taste them not).

טַעַם m. (b. h.; preced.) [*pleasure, will* (Jonah III, 7),] 1) *sense, wisdom, sound reasoning; reason, cause, ground.* Ab. Zar. 18ᵃ דברים של ט׳ sensible argument. Hull. 6ᵃ להחזיר לו ט׳ to give him a clear answer.—Sabb. 83ᵇ ולא נתגלה טַעֲמָהּ the reason of it has not been made known. Hull. 101ᵇ מאיזה ט׳ וכ׳ for what reason it has been forbidden to them; a. fr.—*Pl.* טְעָמִים, טַעֲמִין. Snh. 34ᵃ מקרא אחד יוצא לכמה ט׳ ואין טעם אחד וכ׳ one biblical expression may be used for many arguments, but one and the same argument must not be deduced from different biblical expressions. Erub. 13ᵇ טַעֲמֵי טומאה arguments in favor of uncleanness; a. fr.—פִּסְקֵי טְעָמִים *the incisions, in the Bible verse, according to sense; punctuation signs, accents.* Meg. 3ᵃ (ref. to ויבינו במקרא, Neh. VIII, 8) אלו פ׳ ט׳ that means the punctuation signs; Y. ib. IV, 74ᵈ bot.; Gen. R. s. 36 (ref. to ושום שכל, Neh. l. c.) אלו חט׳ (sub. פסקי).—Esp. *taste.* Yoma 22ᵇ, v. טָעַם. Hull. 98ᵇ ט׳ כעיקר the taste of a forbidden thing is as forbidden as the substance itself. Pes. 44ᵇ top ליתן ט׳ כעיקר to intimate that the taste (of grapes soaked in water) is equally forbidden as the substance (of grapes). Hull. 108ᵃ טַעֲמוֹ ולא ממשו וכ׳ the taste of a thing without the substance (after removing the forbidden substance) is in all cases biblically forbidden. Ib. VII, 4 אם יש בה בנותן ט׳ if there is enough of it to give a taste to the entire mixture. Ib. בזמן שמכירו בנותן ט׳ as long as it can be recognized (and removed), it depends on its giving a taste (whether or not the mixture is forbidden). Ib. 111ᵇ נותן ט׳ בר נותן ט׳ an object forbidden for its having absorbed the taste of a forbidden thing, and which (through mixture) has again given taste to another thing, a taste-giver in the second degree. Ab. Zar. 39ᵇ, a. fr. נותן טעם לפגם (abbr. נ״ט) imparting a deteriorating taste, נ״ט לשבח giving an improving taste; a. v. fr.—

טַעֲמָא, טַעַם, טְעֵים, טְעֵם ch. same, 1) *pleasure, will.* Dan. III, 10; a. e.—2) *good cheer.* Ib. V, 2.—3) *reason, argument, sense* &c. Targ. Job XII, 20; a. e.—B. Bath. 173ᵇ דלא יהבי ט׳ וכ׳ who give no reason for their decisions (judge arbitrarily). Ib., a. fr. מאי ט׳ (abbr. מ״ט) what is the reason (of the law of the Mishnah)?—Kidd. 68ᵇ, a. fr. דריש ט׳ דקרא interprets the biblical law on its reason and accordingly modifies it, extending or limiting, e. g. (B. Mets. 115ᵃ) applying the law Deut. XXIV, 17 only to poor widows. Ib. אלא לרבנן מאי טַעֲמַיְיהוּ but according to the Rabbis (who do not interpret the law on its reason), where is the argument for it? (prob. to be read: טַעֲמַיְיהוּ; Yeb. 23ᵃ מנא לן). Ber. 7ᵇ מ״ט לא אתי מר וכ׳ why do you not come to synagogue for prayer?—Ib. 11ᵃ קא מפרשי טַעֲמַיְיהוּ וט׳ וכ׳ they give their reason for their own opinion and for differing with Beth-Sh.—Keth. 83ᵇ הלכה כר׳... ולא מִטַּעֲמֵיהּ the rule (practice) is in agreement with R. S.'s opinion, but not for the reason he had for it. Ib. 84ᵃ כטעמיה וכהלכתיה in agreement both with his argument and his legal opinion; a. fr.—Pes. 21ᵇ, a. fr. ט׳ דכתב וכ׳ the reason (of this) is, because &c., i. e. this is so only because

&c.—וּלְטַעֲמֵיךְ now, according to your argument (assuming it to be correct, — what then?). Ber. 43ª; a. v. fr.— 4) *argument on the cause of bereavement, consolation* (v. טַעֲמָא). M. Kat. 18ª למישאל ט׳ מיניה (Ms. M.; second time, לשיולי ביה ט׳) to get his permission to argue (with him), i. e. to console him. Snh. 113ª [read:] למשאל ביה ט׳ (or טמא, v. Rabb. D. S. a. l. note 7) to console him.—בַּר טַעֲמָא, v. טַעֲמָא.—5) *taste.* Targ. Num. XI, 8; a. e.—Yoma 78ᵇ ט׳ דמיתותא a foretaste of death. Hor. 11ª, v. טַעַם. Hull. 97ª בט׳ it depends on the taste (whether a mixture be forbidden), v. preced. Ib.ᵇ מין בשאינו מינו .. בט׳ in case of a mixture of heterogeneous things which are permitted, we decide by the taste; a. fr.—*Pl.* טַעֲמִין. Targ. Cant. V, 11; 13.

טַעֲמָא m. (preced.) *pleader. Pl.* טַעֲמַיָּא. Esth. R. to I, 3 בני ט׳ ובני סגניא דיליה his young pleaders and counsellors. Ib. בני ט׳ . . . דיליה *pleaders* means his counsellors.

טָעַן I (cmp. טָעָה) [*to seek, ask,* (cmp. בְּעָא),] 1) *to claim* before court, *to sue, to plead.* Keth. XIII, 4 הטוען את חבירו כדי וכ׳ if one claims from his neighbor a certain number of jugs of oil. Ib. 108ᵇ, a. e. טְעָנוֹ חטין וכ׳ if one claims wheat and barley (two different things), and defendant admits barley. Shebu. 43ª עד שיטְעָנֶנּוּ בדבר וכ׳ until he sues him for something weighable or countable. Gitt. 58ᵇ טוֹעֲנִין ליורש וכ׳ the court pleads in behalf of the heir &c.; a. v. fr.—Part. pass. טָעוּן, f. טְעוּנָה *is required for, requires.* Zeb. V, 7 דמן ט׳ הזייה their blood is required for sprinkling (must be sprinkled). Bicc. II, 1 טְעוּנִים רחיצת וכ׳ require washing of hands; a. v. fr.—Denom. טוֹעַן, טַעַן *requirement, obligation,* fr. which ט׳ בָ׳ *to require.* Sifra introd. ויצא מן הכלל לִיטְעוֹן ט׳ אחר שהוא וכ׳ and is specified for another requirement in keeping with the general subject.—2) *to seek after, to suspect,* v. infra.

Nif. נִטְעַן 1) *to be sued, to be respondent, defendant.* Y. B. Kam. X, beg. 7ᵇ אפי׳ קטנים נִטְעָנִין להן בב״ד even for minors defense is made in court (prob. to be read: טוֹעֲנִין, cmp. Gitt. 58ᵇ, quoted supra). [In later literature טוֹעֵן *claimant,* נִטְעָן *defendant.*]—2) *to be inquired after, suspected, to be summoned on suspicion.* Yeb. II, 8 הנ׳ על א״א וכ׳ if one was suspected of intercourse with a married woman, and the court caused her to be sent away from him (her husband) on his account; ib. 24ᵇ; Tosef. ib. IV, 5 הנט׳ מא״א. Y. ib. II, 4ª bot. בנ׳ בעדים when the suspicion has been corroborated by witnesses.

טְעֵין, טְעַן ch. same, *to plead.* Keth. 105ᵇ אי בעי טָעֵין וכ׳ if he chooses, he may plead thus. Gitt. 58ᵇ אי דקא טען וכ׳ is it that he pleads (demurs) and says &c.?; a. fr.

טָעַן II (b. h.; cmp. טָעָה, טְעִיָא, a. Ges. H. Dict.¹⁰ s. v. צען) [*to move, make ready for travelling,*] 1) (cmp. נָשָׂא) *to load, pack up.* Num. R. s. 6 וטוֹעֲנִים על העגלות and pack (them) upon wagons; a. fr.—Part. pass. טָעוּן (interch. with טוֹעֵן) *laden, carrying.* Ib. s. 5 מי שהוא ט׳ בקרשים some had a share in carrying (moving) the boards. Ib. טוענין כל כלי האריגה had to carry all woven materials. Ib. s. 6 היה מִטּוֹעֲנֵי וכ׳ was one of those carrying the ark. B. Mets. 32ᵇ טְעוּנָה יין אסור carrying forbidden wine.— Midr. Till. to Ps. XVIII בשעה . . . טְעוּנִין את המים when the clouds are charged with water; Yalk. Sam. 160 טוענין מן המים (corr. acc.), v. חָשַׁךְ. Ib. אלו טוענין חרבות וכ׳ those carrying swords, others lances &c.; a. fr.—3) Esp. *to help one broken down on the road to load again,* contrad. to פרק to help in unloading. B. Mets. II, 10 מצוה . . . . לִטְעוֹן the biblical law requires man to help in unloading, but not in loading (without remuneration); אף לט׳ loading, too, must be done gratuitously, v. טְעִינָה; a. fr.

Nif. נִטְעַן 1) *to be laden.* Gen. R. s. 82 נ׳ ברכות was laden with blessings; a. e.—Trnsf. (cmp. כָּבֵד) *to be very ill.* Treat. S'maḥ. ch. VIII אמר לו נ׳ he said to him, He (thy son) is very ill.—2) *to be carried.* Midr. Till. to Ps. LXXXVII [read:] אינן יכולין לְהִטָּעֵן . . . וטוֹעֲנִין וכ׳ who cannot be carried (on wagons &c.) . . . and they carry them on their hands (in a chair); (v. next w. a. Yalk. Ps. 838).

Hif. הִטְעִין 1) *to lade, put on.* Lev. R. s. 13 ה׳ לחמורו וכ׳ he put on his ass five S'ah &c. Sabb. 5ª הִטְעִינוֹ חבירו his neighbor placed something in his hand to carry, ה׳ שמים the heavens placed &c. (when he put his hand forth to collect and carry rain water); a. e.—2) *to carry goods for sale.* Y. Peah I, 16ª top (ref. to Lev. XIX, 16) שלא תהא כרוכל הזה מַטְעִין דבריו וכ׳ be not like the peddler carrying the talk of this one to the other &c.

טְעֵין, טְעַן ch. same, 1) *to be laden; to carry, bear* (h. נשא). Targ. Y. II Num. XIII, 23 (ed. Amst. טַעֲנוּהִי *Pa.*). Targ. O. Gen. XLIV, 1. Targ. Joel II, 22; a. fr.—B. Mets. 40ᵇ כיון דטָעֲנָן טְעוּן when they are once impregnated (with the fluid), they resorb no more.—Trnsf. *to suffer, bear.* Targ. Prov. IX, 12; a. e.—2) *to lade, to harness.* Targ. O. Gen. XLV, 17 טְעוּנוּ ed. Berl. (oth ed. a. Y. טְעִינוּ). Targ. Y. ib. XLIV, 13.—Esp. *to help carrying,* opp. פרק, v. preced. Gen. R. s. 96 משל הדיוט . . . טעון וכ׳ the common adage says, if thy friend's son is dead, help carrying; if thy friend is dead, throw off (common people show no favor where no return can be expected). Y. Hag. II, 77ᵇ top מִיטְעוֹן תרי וכ׳ that two carry one load; a. fr.

Pa. טַעֵין same. Ib. הוון מְטַעֲנִין להון they made them carry &c.—Part. pass. מְטַעַן *carried, moved.* Cant. R. to IV, 8 דלית אינון . . מְטַעֲנִין וכ׳ who are too feeble to be carried in a *lectica,* and whom they carry in a *cathedra.*

Af. אַטְעֵין 1) *to carry.* Ib. מַטְעִינִין. Y. Hag. l. c. אַטְעוּנִנוּן יחידאין carry them singly, אַטְעוֹנִינוּן וכ׳ they did so; אטעונונן צלוחיין carry straight through (without resting). —א׳ חינא = h. נשא חן *to find grace.* Targ. Esth. II, 17 (ed. Lag. אִיטְ׳, *Ithpe.*); a. e.

Ithpe. אִיטְעַן 1) *to be laden.* Targ. Lam. V, 5. Targ. Esth. l. c., v. supra.—2) *to be carried* (in a chair). Y. Bets. I, 60ᶜ bot. מִיטְעַן מערס וכ׳ allowed himself to be carried from one seat (where he lectured) to another. Ib., v. סְדִינָא.—3) (v. preced. *Nif.*) *to become severely ill.* Targ. II Sam. XII, 15 (h. text ויאנש).

טַעַן III *to move to and back, to swing* a whip &c. Num. R. s. 12 דלא יהוון טָעֲנִין וכ׳ that they should not swing the rod over the children (Midr. Till. to Ps. XCI מחון . .; Yalk. Ps. 842 מחיין).

Pa., part. pass. מְטַעַּן *swung upon, struck* with a spear &c., *wounded.* Targ. Is. XIV, 19 מְטַעֲנֵי חרב (h. text מְטֹעֲנֵי). Targ. Jer. XXXVII, 10 מְטַעֲנִין (h. text מְדקרים); a. e.

טְעַן m. (טְעַן I) 1) *requirement,* v. טוֹעַן a. טָעַן I.— 2) *search, claim.* B. Mets. 28[b] אבן ט׳, v. טָעַח.

טַעֲנָה f. (טָעַן I) 1) *plea, suit, claim.* Shebu. VI, 1 חט׳ . . . והחודאה וכ׳ if the claim is for two M'ah silver, and the defendant admits the value of a P'rutah. Ib. אם אין ההודאה ממין חט׳ if the defendant's admission is not homogeneous with the claim (e. g. one sues for wheat and the defendant alleges to owe barley). Ib. 39[b] כפירת ט׳ שתי וכ׳ the claim of two M'ah in the Mishnah means that amount of the claim which is disputed; ט׳ עצמה וכ׳ it means that the original claim was for two &c. Keth. I, 1 טַעֲנַת בתולים, v. בְּתוּלִים.—B. Kam. 57[a] ט׳ גנב, v. גַּנָּב. Ib. ט׳ לסטים, v. לִסְטֵיס; a. fr.—*Pl.* טַעֲנוֹת. Y. Snh. III, 21[b] bot. צריך . . לשנות טַעֲנוֹתֵיהֶן the judge must repeat the pleas of the contesting parties; Midr. Till. to Ps. LXXII לשקול ט׳ בפני שניהם; Yalk. Kings 175 לשקול ט׳ weigh their pleas in the presence of both parties; a. e.— 2) *suspicion, talk, fault-finding.* Num. R. s. 10 (ed. Amst. p. 240[a]) מפני טענת הבריות not to give rise to people's talk; Ab. d'R. N. ch. II. Y. Ber. I, 3[c] מפני ט׳ המינין not to give support to the talk of the heretics (Bab. ib. 12[a] תרעומת).

טַעֲנְתָא ch. same, *plea.* Kidd. 28[a] האי ט׳ מעלייתא היא is not this a good plea?—*Pl.* טַעֲנָתָא. Keth. 18[a] כולהו ט׳ טענת וכ׳ all pleas consist of the claim of other people and one's own admission (replique).

***טְעַק** (עוק, ט for ח; cmp. טְרַגְּ) *to be narrow.* Targ. Prov. IV, 12 תִּטְעַק ed. Lag. (Levita תִּטְעַק; ed. Wil. תתעיק).

Ithpa. אִיטְעַּק, אִיתְטְעֵיק, *Ithpe.* אִיטְּעֵיק *to be pressed, troubled.* Targ. Ps. XXXI, 10 אִיטְעַק Ms. (ed. אִיטְעַק, ed. Wil. אִתְעַק; ed. Lag. איטלק). Targ. Prov. XXIV, 10 מִתְטְעֵיק Ms. a. Lev. (ed. Lag. a. oth. מתהעיק). V. חֲעַק.

טַף m. collect. pl. (b. h.; טָפַף I; cmp. טפל) [*joined to, dependent,*] *children.* Ḥag. 3[a] (ref. to Deut. XXXI, 12) טַף למה באין why must the children come?; Tosef. Sot. VII, 9 טַף למה בא (Var. טַפְלִין . . באין); Ab. d'R. N. ch. XVIII. Mekh. Bo. s. 16 וכי טַף היה יודע וכ׳ would children have known to distinguish &c.?

טַפָּא, v. טְפֵי.

טִפָּה, טִפָּא, v. sub טִיפ׳.

טפו, Y. Ber. I, 2[c] bot., read: נופו, v. נוֹף II.—Targ. Cant. II, 8, v. טְפַו.

טִפּוּח, v. טִיפּוּח.

טְפוּחַ, v. טָפַח II a. טְפִיחָה II.

***טְפוּחָא** f. (טְפַח I) *rapping* (at the door). — *Pl.* טְפוּחִין. Targ. Y. Gen. XXVII, 30 כתרתין ט׳ about the time needed for two raps.

***טַפּוּחָא** m. (v. preced.) *knocker, one who by rapping at the wall discovers hidden treasures.*—*Pl.* טַפּוּחָאֵי. B. Mets. 42[a]; cmp. גַּשּׁוֹשָׁא.

טפוטין, v. טַפִּיטָא.

טִפּוּיִין m. pl. *tippuyin,* name of certain small insects. Sabb. 107[b] חט׳ Ms. M. a. Rashi (ed. טַפּוּיֵי; Ms. O. טִיפּוּיִין); cmp. טִיפָּה.

טָפוּס m. (טָפַף, v. דְּפוּס) *frame, mould.* Kel. XVI, 7 ט׳ של תפלה the block on which the case of the phylacteries is shaped. Y. Snh. X, 28[d] top ט׳ של פעור a cast of the idol P'or; (Sifré Num. 131 דפוס; Snh. 106[a] יראתה). Y. Sabb. IV, 8[b] bot. ט׳ של דדים, v. דְּפוּס. Dem. V, 4 (ed. Y. טִיפּוּס). Y. ib. 24[d] top נחתום עושה ט׳ אחד if the baker makes only one form of loaves. Ib. (once) טופוס אחד (corr. acc.); a. e —*Pl.* טְפוּסִין. Dem. V, 3 (Ar. דפ׳). Y. ib. l. c. נחתום . . כמה ט׳ if the baker makes several forms of loaves. Ib. שני טפסין (corr. acc.). — Cant. R. to VI, 4 טִיפּוּסִים של פעור, v. supra.

טְפַז (corresp. to h. קפץ) [*to join, contract,*] 1) *to close.* Targ. Job V, 16 טָפְזַת ed. Lag. (some ed. טַפְזַת).— 2) *to leap.* Targ. Y. Num. XXI, 35.—Targ. Cant. II, 8 וט׳ על קיצא (ed. Lag. וטפו, ed. Vien. וטפז, corr. acc.) leaped over (redeemed them before) the destined end of the captivity. Targ. Ps. LXVIII, 17; a. fr.

Pa. טַפֵּז same. Ib. CXIV, 6 דאתון מְטַפְּזִין Ms. (ed. טפזו incorr.). Targ. Job XXI, 11; a. fr.—V. טְפֵי IV.

טַפְזָא (טַוְזָא) m. (preced.) *cony* or *rabbit.* Targ. O. Lev. XI, 5 (ed. Berl. טַב׳, v. Berl. Massor. p. 86; Y. טַוְי׳); Targ. Deut. XIV, 7. Gen. R. s. 12 הדין ט׳ מיגין וכ׳ the rabbit seeks protection under a projecting rock from the bird of prey &c.; Yalk. Ps. 862. — *Pl.* טַפְזַיָּא. Targ. Ps. CIV, 18.

טָפַח I (b. h.; cmp. נפח I) [*to join closely,* whence טֶפַח (cmp. קוֹמֶץ) *joined fingers, hand-breadth,*] *to come in close contact;* (cmp. נָקַשׁ) *to strike, knock.* B. Kam. 32[b] ניתזה בקעת וְטָפְחָה לו על פניו Ms. M. a chip flew off and struck him in the face. Ib. ניתוז . . . וְטָפְחוּ לו וכ׳ Ms. M. sparks flew off and hit him &c.; a. fr.—Esp. (denom. of טֶפַח) טָפַח, a.

Pi. טִיפַּח 1) *to strike with the flat hand, to slap.* Gen. R. s. 22, end התחיל אדה״ר מְטַפֵּחַ על פניו Adam slapped his own face; Lev. R. s. 10 טוֹפֵחַ. Kidd. 31[a] טִפְּחָה לו על ראשו slapped him on his head. Gen. R. s. 45 טִפְּחָתָהּ וכ׳ (Yalk. ib. 79 קפחתה) she slapped her face with her shoe. Y. Kil. VIII, 31[c] top טי׳ כנגד וכ׳ (Kidd. 24[b] הכהו) if he struck him over his eye and blinded him. Ab. Zar. IV, 10 היה מְטַפֵּחַ על וכ׳ (Bab. ed. 60[b] מְטַפְּחָהּ, Y. ed. מהפח) he slapped upon the fermenting barrel (to check fermentation). Toh. III, 8 שדרך התינוק לְטַפֵּחַ a child likes to slap (dough &c., to dabble); a. e.—2) *to clap hands* to a certain tune in rejoicing or mourning, v. טִיפּוּחַ. Bets. V, 2 לֹא מְטַפְּחִין וכ׳ we must not clap hands, or strike upon the knees, or stamp on the Holy Day. M. Kat. III, 8 מענות אבל לא מְטַפְּחוֹת may sing the dirge but must not clap. Ib. 9. Num. R. s. 4 . . . שחיה מקיש וטוֹפֵחַ he knocked his hands against each other and clapped; ib. וטפח. Cant. R. to II, 14 מְטַפַּחַת באגפיה clapped her wings.—3) *to collect the contents of a broken vessel by palming, to wipe with the palm.* Ter. XI, 7. Sabb. 143ᵇ ולא יְטַפֵּחַ בשמן must not use the palm for collecting oil in the broken vessel.

Hif. הִטְפִּיחַ same. Ab. Zar. 60ᵇ, v. supra.

טְפַח, *Pa.* טַפַּח ch. same, 1) *to close carefully.* B. Kam. 23ᵃ לא ט׳ באפיה (Ms. H. טפא, v. טְפֵי IV) he did not carefully close (the stable) before him.—2) *to slap, strike with hand, stamp with foot.* Targ. II Kings XIX, 24; Is. XXXVII, 25. Targ. Ez. XXI, 17; 19; a. fr.—Targ. Jon. IV, 8 ט׳ שמשא וכ׳ the sun beat upon &c.—B. Kam. 32ᵇ ט׳ ליה רבא בסנדליה Raba struck him upon his (R. Shimi's) sandal (to silence him); M. Kat. 25ᵃ; B. Bath. 22ᵃ; a. e.—3) *to clap hands.* Y. Snh. II, beg. 19ᵈ; Y. Hor. III, beg. 47ᵃ שרי ט׳ בחדא וכ׳ he made the motion of clapping with one hand; ובחדא טַפְּחִין do people clap with one hand?; a. e.—4) *to strike, forge.* Targ. Ps. CXLI, 5; Targ. Is. XLI, 7 (h. text חלם).

טָפַח II (cmp. טָפַף II) *to drip, be moist.* Sabb. 17ᵃ עדיין משקה טוֹפֵחַ וכ׳ moisture is still dripping on them. Yoma 78ᵃ טוֹפֵחַ ע״מ לְהַטְפִּיחַ moist enough to moisten other objects. Ab. Zar. 60ᵇ טופח ע״מ לְהטפיח Ms. M. (ed. ט׳ לחט׳). Toh. VIII, 9; a. fr.—2) (cmp. דוב, דאב) *to melt, decay, ferment* (of a running and fermenting dough). B. Mets. 59ᵇ אַף בצק . . ט׳ (Ms. R. 2 תפח, v. תָּפַח) even the dough under the hands of the kneading women fermented.—Y. Yeb. XII, end, 13ᵈ וטפח רוחי עלי; Yalk. Prov. 964 טָפְחָה וכ׳ my mind in me became fermenting, i. e. I felt proud (v. טוּחַ).—*Part. pass.* טָפוּחַ *decaying, languishing* (from starvation). Sifra B'ḥuck. Par. 2, ch. VI טְפוּחֵי רעב (v. תָּפַח).

Hif. הִטְפִּיחַ *to moisten, wet.* Yoma 78ᵃ טינא מַטְפַּחַת clay which makes wet (those sitting on it). Ib.; Ab. Zar. 60ᵇ לְהַטְפִּיחַ, v. supra. Ber. 25ᵃ כל זמן שֶׁמַּטְפִּיחִין as long as the spot is wet enough to moisten.

טֶפַח m. (b. h.; v. טָפַח I) *hand-breadth, breadth of four fingers joined.* Succ. 4ᵇ, a. fr. ארון תשעה וכפרת ט׳ the Ark was nine handbreadths high, and the lid one. Ib. 7ᵃ ט׳ שוחק a liberal hand-breadth (four fingers not closely joined). v. אַמָּה.—Yoma 55ᵃ top טִיפְחָהּ של כפורת Ar. a. Ms. M. 2 a. Ms. O. (v. Rabb. D. S. a. l. note 9, ed. עוביה) the hand-breadth, i. e. the hight, of the lid, v. supra.; a. v. fr.—*Pl.* טְפָחִים, *Du.* טְפָחַיִים. Taan. 25ᵇ; a. v. fr. [טְפָחִין, or טְפָחִין, v. טְפִיחַ II.]

טפטיות, טפטיאות, v. טַפִּיטָא.

טְפָטֵף, v. טָפַף II.

טְפָא, טְפֵי I (cmp. טָפַח II) 1) *to grow faint, to die out, be extinguished.* Targ. I Sam. III, 3. Targ. Job XVIII, 5, sq.; a. e.—Y. Sabb. I, 3ᵇ bot. אילין בעיין דיִטְפֵי וכ׳ they (the children) desire that the lamp grow dim (so that they need not study, and therefore will not snuff it). Lev. R. s. 9 אשכחא בוצינא טָפֵי she found the lamp gone out; (Y. Sot. I, 16ᵈ bot. מִיטְפֵי *Ithpe*); a. e.—2) *to put out, extinguish.* Targ. Cant. VIII, 7. Targ. II Sam. XXI, 17; a. e. —Y. Yoma VIII, 45ᵇ בעי מִטְפְּתָה wanted to put it out; Y. Ned. IV, 38ᵈ מיטפירה (read: מִיטְפִּינָהּ). Ib. אפי׳ ר׳ אימר יִטְפֵי (or *Af.*) even R. I. would have been permitted to extinguish the fire on the Sabbath.

Af. אַטְפֵּי same. Tanḥ. Vayigg. 5 נורא דתמר כלתך אנא מַטְפֵּי I will put out the fire intended for Tamar &c. (I will curb thy passion; Yalk. Gen. 150 אנן מנהרין we shall light for thee).

Ithpe. אִיטְּפֵי, אִיתְטְפֵי *to be extinguished, grow dim.* Y. Sabb. VI, 8ᶜ bot. [read:] איטפי בוצינא אמרה לה לא׳איתטפי אמרי לא מיטפי בוצינא וכ׳ is the light out? Said she, it is not out. Upon which they said (this means) the light of Israel is not extinguished (R. A. is not dead). Y. Sot. I, 16ᵈ bot., v. supra. Y. Ḥag. II, 77ᶜ top ואִיטְפִּיַת and the fire over the grave was extinguished (v. חֲמַם).

טְפָא, טְפֵי II (=h. צָפָה, v. טוּף) 1) *to float.* Targ. Y. Ex. XXVI, 28 והוה טָפֵי (not ויהות). — 2) *to flood.* Y. Snh. X, 29ᵃ bot. ובעי מִטְפָא עלמא and wanted to inundate the world.

******Af.* אַטְפֵּי (denom. of טִיפָא) *to drop.* Targ. Job XV, 8 some ed. (v. טָפַף II).

טְפָא, טְפֵי III (v. טָפַף I) 1) *to join, add, increase.* Taan. 24ᵃ אי טָפוּ לה וכ׳ when they put on too much or too little. Ab. Zar. 9ᵃ ונִיטְפֵי עלוידהו וכ׳ and let him add thereto twenty years. Yoma 35ᵃ אי בציר מחנו וט׳ אחנו if he makes the ones less in value and adds to the value of the others; a. fr.—Part. טָפֵי, f. טָפְיָא *more.* Sabb. 19ᵃ אי ט׳ if it is more in measure (than before washing). —Ab. Zar. 9ᵇ דמתניתא ט׳ וכ׳ the calculation of the Boraitha is three years more.—Adv. טְפֵי *more.* Gitt. 44ᵃ, a. e., v. חַד II.—R. Hash. 26ᵇ bot. כמה . . . . . ט׳ מעלי the more . . . . the better it is. B. Bath. 144ᵇ חריף ט׳ he is smarter (than his brother); a. fr.

***טְפָא, טְפֵי** IV (v. P. Sm. 1502) = טָפַח I, *to close,* Targ. Job V, 16 טְפִיַת (some ed. טַפְּרַת *Pa.*), v. טְפָא.—B. Kam. 23ᵃ, v. טְפַח. [Targ. Cant. II, 8, v. טְפַז.]

טָפֵי m. (= טְפִיחַ I, v. טְפֵי II) [*dripper,*] *vessel with a narrow neck.* Kel. II, 3 ט׳ שהתקינו לענבים a pitcher which was made with the intention of using it for grapes. Ib. III, 2. Neg. XII, 5 טְפָיו (R. S. a. l. תְּפָיו) man's oil vessels.

טִפְיָא f., v. טְפֵי III.—[טַפְיָא m., v. next w.]

טְפִיחַ I m. (טָפַח II, v. טְפֵי) 1) *pitcher* for drawing water for drinking or hand-washing. Sabb. XVII, 6 (125ᵇ), v. זְמוֹרָה. Ib. XXIV, 5, v. פָּקַק. B. Bath. 63ᵃ 'give him a share in my well לט׳ Ms. M. a. Rashb. (ed.

לטפיחר, corr. acc.; Ms. F. לַטְּפָךְא, cmp. טְפַי) for the pitcher', i. e. for drinking purposes. Tosef. Ber. IV, 11 [read as] Yoma 30[a] ומחזיר הט׳ על האורחים (v. Rashi a. l.; Ms. M. והט׳ חוזר וכ׳) and passes the pitcher (which he had used for washing his hands) around the guests.—2) *a pitcher-shaped vessel* put up in walls and cornices as bird's nest.—*Pl.* טְפִיחִין, טְפִיחִים. Bets. 24[a]; 25[a]; Tosef. Sabb. XII (XIII), 4; ib. XVIII, 4 ed. Zuck. (Var. טפחין); ib. Bets. I, 10; Hull. 139[b].—3) *muddy soil, ground on which water subsided*, opp. to גריד. Gen. R. s. 33, end (Yalk. ib. 56 מקפה).

טְפִיחַ II m., (v. טָפַח II,2) 1) pl. טְפִיחִין, טְפִיחִים *stinted, poor grains*; [another opinion: (v. טָפַח I, a. cmp. סְפִיחַ) *growth between grass*]. Shebi. IX, 4. Y. ib. 39[a] top טפחין; Tosef. ib. VII, 15 רחיפין ed. Zuck. (Var. ספיחין, רפיחין). [Tosef T'bul Yom. I, 1, sq., v. טוֹפַח.]—2) (sub. רעב) *one looking like those who suffer from the effects of famine, yellowish-black.* Bekh. 45[b] שָׁחוּר . . . . יצא מהן טְפוּחַ ed. (Rashi טפיח) a very dark-complected man must not marry an equally complected woman, lest their offspring may be a *t'fiah*; [Rashi: *black as a pitcher*, v. טְפִיחַ I].

טְפִיחָה f. (טָפַח I) *hammering* for the purpose of *polishing*. Tosef. Sabb. XI (XII), 2.

טַפִּיטָא m. (τάπης, ητος) *carpet, rug.* Lev. R. s. 30 (Ar. דיופוטא).—*Pl.* טַפִּיטִין. Koh. R. to III, 9 טפו׳ (corr. acc.). Gen. R. s. 33 saw in Rome עמודים מכוסין בט׳ וכ׳ (not בטפיסין) statues covered with rugs, in winter &c., Yalk. Ps. 727 בטיפיטין (corr. acc.); Lev. R. s. 27 בטיפטיאות (read: טַפִּיטִיאוֹת). Lam. R. to I, 16; ib. introd. (R. Joh. 2) טפטיות (read: טַפִּיטִיּוֹת).

טַפִּיטָן m. (tapeta, acc. -tam) same, ט׳ של סוס *horse-cloth, housing.* Kel. XXIII, 2.

טַפְיָין, Targ. Y. Lev. XI, 35 Bxt., v. תַּפְיָא.

טְפֵילָה טְפֵילָא, v. טְפַל.

טְפִילָה f. (טָפַל) *care, sustenance.* Y. Keth. VIII, 32[b] top כדי טְפִילָתָן as much as their sustenance costs. Y. Orl. I, 60[d] top כדי טְפִילָתָהּ worth the labor given to its (the grape-vine's) cultivation (R. S. to Orl. I, 2 נפילתה).

טפיסין, v. טַפִּיטָא.

***טְפִיפִית** f. (טָפַף I) *circular enclosure, circumvallation.*—*Pl.* טְפִיפִיּוֹת. Bekh. 22[a] מִשֶּׁיֵּרָאוּ ט׳ from the time travailing has reached that stage when the ringlike formations at the mouth of the vagina are visible (indicating the passage of the embryo's head); [Ar. reads: קְפִיפִים, Var. קְפִיפִיּוֹת; Tosef. Ohol. VIII, 8 קְפִיפִים.]—Cmp. טֶפֶף.

טְפִישׁ, v. טְפַשׁ.

טְפִיתָא f. (טְפֵי III)=טוֹפִירְנָא, *surplus, liberal measure.* B. Mets. 73[b] ושפכו ליה טפי כופיתא (Ms. M. ושפכו כופיתא, read טפיתא; Alf. טְפִיְיתָא *pl.*; Ms. H. טפי טוּפְיָאתָא; Ms. R. טפי טופיתא, v. Rabb. D. S. a. l. note) and they (in delivering the wine) poured a liberal addition to the stipulated quantity.

טָפַל (b. h.; cmp. טָפַח I) [*to join, add,*] 1) *to paste, line.* Kel. III, 4 וּטְפָלָן בגללין and lined them (the cracked vessels) with a paste of ordure. Ib. 5 הטופל וכ׳ if one covers with paste a sound vessel. Bets. 34[a] אין טוֹפְלִין וכ׳ you must not cover (the fowls) with potter's clay (to get the feathers off); Tosef. ib. III, 19 וטובלין ed. Zuck. (corr. acc.). Sabb. 80[b]; Pes. 43[a]; M. Kat. 9[b] טוֹפְלוֹת אותן בסיד dress their skins with lime (to keep them hairless). Y. Ab. Zar. II, 40[d] (in Chald. diction) שחוק וטפול grind it to powder and apply it (as a remedy); a. fr.—2) *to add, join.* Hag. 8[a] טוֹפְלִין בטופל when he combines two different funds. Ib. בהמה לבהמה וכ׳ you may use the second tithe money for buying an additional animal to that designated for the pilgrim's offering (חֲגִיגָה), but you must not join the two funds (in order to buy a larger animal). Ab. Zar. 25[b] טוֹפְלוֹ לימינו lets the gentile walk to his right side, v. זָמַן; (Tosef. ib. III, 4 נותנו); Hull. 91[a].—*Part. pass.* טָפוּל a) *affixed, attached.* Y. Sabb. XVI, 15[c] bot. (ref. to Mish. ib. 2) בשאינו ט׳ לו וכ׳ when the casing is not attached to the book, but if it is &c.—b) *dependent on, supported by.* Y. Dem. II, 23[a] top; Y. Peah IV, 18[b] bot. טְפוּלִין לאביהן dependent on (living with) their parents (cmp. B. Mets. 12[b], s. v. סָמַךְ).

Nif. נִטְפַּל 1) *to be attached, affixed.* Lev. R. s. 6; s. 15; Yalk. Is. 281 וְנִטְפְּלוּ בישעיה and they were embodied in the Book of Isaiah. Tanh. Vayhi 17 נִטְפַּלְתֶּם בעצמי you will be attached to myself (be called sons of Jacob); Yalk. Gen. 161; (Gen. R. s. 100 זכיתם בעצמי you will have a share in me).—2) (cmp. זָוַג) *to meet, join.* Hull. 91[a] וישראל שנ׳ וכ׳, v. זָמַן. Men. 65[a] נט׳ להם וכ׳ R. J. joined their discussions. Snh. 9[a] הנ׳ לעוברי עבירה he who is an accessory to sin. Y. B. Kam. X, 7[c] top, שלא . . . נִטְפָּלִין לגנבים that citizens may not be in conspiracy with thieves (and sell the stolen goods to their owner under the pretence of having bought them).—3) *to attend to, to nurse, tend.* Y. Keth. XII, 35[a] top מי שנט׳ . . . יִטָּפֵל בי וכ׳ those who attended to me (nursed me) in life, shall attend to me in death; Y. Kil. IX, 32[b] top; Gen. R. s. 100; Tanh. Vayhi 3. Ib. a. e. לְהִטָּפֵל בקבורתו to attend to his funeral; a. fr.

Hithpa. היטפל 1) same. B. Kam. 10[b], a. e. הבעלים מִטַּפְּלִין וכ׳ the owner has to attend to the disposal of the carcass. B. Mets. 28[b] מִטַּפֵּל בהן must take care of them. Ex. R. s. 20; Deut. R. s. 11 אני בעצמי מט׳ וכ׳ I myself shall attend to thy burial; a. fr.—2) (of lower animals) *to breed, increase* (v. טַפֵּל). Kidd. 80[a] ושרצים . . . מִיטַּפְּלִין שם vermin and frogs breed in the house.

Pu., part. מְטוּפָּל (denom. of טַפֵּל) *burdened with a large family.* Taan. 16[a], sq. מט׳ ואין לו one having a large family with no means of support.

טְפַל ch. same, *to paste, plaster* &c. Pes. 74[b] טַפְלֵיהּ החוא וכ׳ put a dough paste over a pigeon. M. Kat. 9[b] טַפְלָהּ אבר אבר put a paste on her (for improving her complexion) limb-wise; Sabb. 80[b].—Trnsf. (with שקרא) *to charge false-*

ly, calumniate (cmp. טוּחַ I, v. Ps. CXIX, 69).—Targ.Y. I Deut. I, 1.

Ithpa. אִיטַּפַּל, *Ithpe.* אִיטְּפֵיל *to be put on.* Part. מִיטַּפַּל, מִיטַּפְּלָא, מַשׁ׳ (not מְ׳) *forming a scab* (h. מִסְפַּחַת). Targ. Y. Lev. XIII, 6; 7; 8; 19.—2) *to attend, care.* Y. Taan. IV, 68[d] top עד דהוון מִיטַּפְּלִין ביה while they were engaged in burying him.—3) *to join, attach one's self.* Keth. 23[a] אִיטַּפַּל בקריבותיך marry one of thy relations. Snh. 26[a] א׳ בהדיהו joined them. Y. Kil. IX, 32[c] bot.; Y. Keth. XII, 35[b] אזל וא׳ בהון מן תמן (not זמן) he went and remained in their company from thence.

טְפֵל m. (b. h.; preced.) 1) *attachment, of secondary import,* opp. עיקר. Gen. R. s. 39 ולוט ט׳ לו (Var. נטפל) and Lot was merely an attachment to Abraham. Ber. 12[b] ט׳ לו.. ויציאת and the exodus from Egypt will be considered of secondary import to it (the redemption from the powers). Ib. 13[a] ויעקב ט׳ the name *Jacob* will be secondary to *Israel;* a. fr.—2) *pl.* טְפֵלִים, טְפֵלִין *dependants, children, minors.* Kidd. 34[b] (ref. to Deut. XXXI, 12) ט׳ חייבין minors are obliged to appear; v. טַף. B. Bath. 117[a]; a. fr.—Y. Shebi. VII, beg. 37[b] הַפִּילִין, v. אֲלוּנְבִּית II.—V. טְפֵלָה.

טַפְלָא ch. (preced.) *children, family, household.* Targ. O. Gen. XXXIV, 29 (Y. *pl.*); a. fr.—*Pl.* טַפְלִין, טַפְלַיָּא, טַפְלֵי. Targ. Y. Gen. XLVII, 12. Targ. Y. I Ex. XIII, 18; a. e.—Hull. 18[a] חלו ביה ט׳ (Ar. טוּפְלֵי) children are dependent on him.

טְפֵלָא, טְפֵי׳ m. ch. (v. next w.) *paste, plaster, coating.* Targ. Jer. XLIII, 9 טְפֵיל constr. (h. text מֶלֶט).—Pes. 74[b] אי מעלי טַפְלֵיה if its dough-paste is good. M. Kat. 9[b], a. e. דשתי... בעיין בנתיה ט׳ because he drinks beer, his daughters need paste (to improve their complexion), v. טַפַּל.

טְפֵי׳, טְפֵלָה f. (טָפַל) 1) *paste, plaster.* Kel. V, 7 גורר את הט׳ scrapes the plastering off. Ib. 8; 11. Tosef. ib. B. Kam. IV, 18; a. e.—2) *attachment, dependence,* opp. עיקר. Ber. VI, 7 כל שהוא עיקר ועמו ט׳ whatever food is the chief dish and something is offered to be eaten with it.—Tanh. Ki Thissa 27; Ex. R. s. 45, end, v. אָתַר.—Y. M. Kat. III, 82[c] bot. ט׳ לט׳ (not בט׳) distant relations, grand-children.—*Pl.* טְפֵילוֹת. Y. Meg. I, 71[d] bot. טְפֵילוֹתֵיהֶם their affixes (prefixes and suffixes).

טַפְלוּחָאֵי, v. טְלוּפְחָא.

טָפַס (cmp. טָפַח I) *to join;* part. טוֹפֵס q. v.

Hithpa. הִטַּפֵּס (cmp. טָפֵּז) *to seize with hands or feet, to climb.* Tosef. Toh. VII, 10 הרבים מִטַּפְּסִין וכ׳ many climb (over the fences) and walk therein. Erub. 21[a] אדם מִטַּפֵּס ועולה מט׳ וכ׳ a human being may climb up and down; Y. ib. IX, beg. 25[c] כמִטַּרְפֵּס וכ׳ (fr. טְרַפֵּס) it is as in the case of accessibility by climbing &c. B. Bath. 11[b] מטפס וכ׳ Ms. M. a. oth. (ed. מטפיס, corr. acc., v. Rabb. D. S. a. l. note) the chicken climbs &c. Cmp. חָפַס.

טְפַס ch. (v. preced.) [*to join hands,*] *to agree, make a covenant.* Targ. O. Gen. XXXIV, 15; 22; 23 (Y. אתפייס, h. text נֵאוֹת). Targ. Prov. I, 10 ed. Lag. תטפס (ed. תתפייס); [prob. everywhere *Ithpe.*].

Ithpe. אִיטַּפַּס same, *to be won, bribed.* Targ. II Kings XII, 9. Targ. Is. XIII, 17, ed. Lag. (ed. מתקסין, corr. acc.).

***טַפְסָא** m. (v. טַפָּס; cmp. טוּפְסָא) *chest.*—ט׳ דמלכא *royal chest, treasury, archive.* Yeb. 46[a]; B. Mets. 73[b] (Ms. M. טפט׳, Ms. H. a. F. ספתא, ed. Ven. טפסרא, Ar. s. v. מחרק: ספטא, ספתא, v. סִיפְטָא).

טַפְסָא or **טְפ׳** v. טוּפְסָא.—טפסין. Y. Dem. V, 24[d] top, v. טָפוּס.

***טַפְסָן** f. pl. (τάπης, cmp. Syr. טפסתא, P. Sm. 1505) *carpets, horse-cloths.* Targ. Jer. XXXVIII, 11; sq.

טִפְסָר, טַ׳ m. (b. h., Assyr. *dupsarru,* Schr. KAT[2] p. 424) *scribe, royal dignitary.* Ex. R. s. 43 (some ed. מלך as Num. R. s. 2). Gen. R. s. 90 (ref. to Jer. LI, 27) נבוכדנ׳ טִפְסַר ושׂר וכ׳.. טִפֵּשׁ dull as to wisdom though prince in years, v. אַבְרֵךְ.

טַפְסְרָא ch. same. Targ. Y. Deut. XXVIII, 12 (divine key-keeper). [B. Mets. 73[b] ed. Ven., v. טַפְסָא.]—*Pl.* טַפְסְרַיָּא. Nah. III, 17 טַפְסְרַיִךְ (ed. Lag. טפסרך).

טָפַף I (b. h.) *to touch closely,* (b. h. *to mince*); *to join, add.* Part. pass. טָפוּף, f. טְפוּפָה (cmp. טְפֵי III) *added to, liberally measured,* contrad. to מחוק levelled, a. גדוש heaped. Men. 7[a] לביסא ט׳ to a basin brimful, with something added on top.—*Pl.* טְפוּפוֹת. Yoma 48[a].

טָפַף II (v. טוּף 1) *to float; to drip.*

Pilp. טִפְטֵף 1) *to drip, drop.* Midr. Till. to Ps. LXXVIII, beg. טִיפְטְפָה דם issued drops of blood. Y. Ter. VIII, 46[a] top הגשמים מְטַפְטְפִין ווורדין the rain dripped into it. Sabb. 44[a] שמן המְטַפְטֵף oil dripping from the lamp.—2) *to glisten.* Y. Ber. I, 3[a] sq. החמה מְטַפְטֶפֶת וכ׳ the sun glistens on the tops of the mountains.

טְפַף ch. same.

Ithpa. אִיטַּפַּף *to be dripped.* Targ. Job XV, 8 ואיטַּפַּת (some ed. אִטְפֵי, h. text תגרע, v. גָּרַע II).

***טְפַף** m. (טָפַף I) *addition to city limits, suburb;* pr. n. pl. *Tefef.* B. Bath. 75[b] עתיד... אלף ט׳ גינואות in the future the Lord shall add to Jerusalem one thousand times the area of Tefef for gardens; Yalk. Zech. 568 (for Var. lect., v. Rabb. D. S. to B. Bath. l. c. note 40. Comment. takes טפ״ף as numerals = 169).

***טַפְקָא** m. *tile;* מעשה ט׳ *cake baked on heated tiles.* Sabb. 125[a] (Syr. טפקא panis tenuis in sartagine coctus, P. Sm. 1505).

טִפְרָא, טְפַר, v. טוּפְרָא.

טְפָרִי pr. n. pl. *T'fari.* Gen. R. s. 37, end (expl. סְפָר, Gen. X, 30, v. Sm. Bibl. Dict. s. v. Sephar).

טָפַשׁ (b. h.) *to be covered with fat; to be inaccessible, dull, obdurate, stupid* (cmp. Lat. pinguis).

Hithpa. הִטַּפֵּשׁ *to grow dull.* Ber. 63[b] מִטַּפְּשִׁים they become dull; Taan. 7[a]; Macc. 10[a].

Pu. טוּפַּשׁ, part. מְטוּפָּשׁ (denom. of טְפֵשׁ) *decried as a fool, made sport of.* Sifré Deut. 309; Yalk. ib. 942 (corresp. to נבל a. לא חכם, Deut. XXXII, 6) מנוולים ומְטוּפָּשִׁים disgraced and ridiculed as fools.

טְפֵשׁ, טְפִישׁ ch. same, v. infra.

Pa. טַפֵּשׁ *to make dull, obdurate.* Targ. Is. VI, 10. Targ. Y. Deut. XXVIII, 28, v. סוֹקְרָא II.

Ithpa. אִיטַּפַּשׁ *to become* or *to be dull, foolish; to act foolishly.* Targ. Prov. XXX, 32 (some ed. תִּטְפַּשׁ *Pe.*). Targ. I Sam. XXVI, 21. Targ. Num. XII, 11. Targ. I Kings VIII, 47 (some ed. אַטְפֵּ׳ *Af.*).; a. e.

טִיפֵּשׁ, טִפֵּשׁ m. (preced.) *obdurate, dull, stupid.* Tem. 16ª. Y. Pes. X, 37ᵈ (Mekh. Bo., s. 18 תם). Cant. R. to I, 1 חכם ט׳ וכ׳ first wise, then foolish &c.; a. fr.—*Pl.* טִפְּשִׁים, טִיפְּ׳, טִפְּשִׁין. Sabb. 152ᵇ. Y. Pes. IX, end, 37ª; a. fr.—*Fem.* טִפֶּשֶׁת. Num. R. s. 20 שזו הט׳ שבבהמה for this (the ass), the stupidest of animals; Tanḥ. Balak 9 הטִּפְּשִׁית.

טִפְּשָׁא, טַפְשָׁא, טִיפְּ׳, טְפֵשׁ ch. same. Targ. O. Lev. XXVI, 41 (h. text ערל). Targ. Koh. II, 19; a. fr.—Koh. R. to X, 3 ט׳ .. עמא טפשין וכ׳ the fool thinks all people are fools &c. Lam. R. to I, 1, ט׳ דלבא (חד כות׳) רבתי dull of understanding; a. fr.—*Pl.* טִפְּשִׁין, טִפְּשַׁיָּא, טִיפְּ׳, טִפְּשָׁאֵי. Targ. Jer. IV, 22. Targ. Koh. V, 3; a. fr.—Ber. 17ᵇ (expl. אבירי לב, Is. XLVI, 12), v. גּוּבַיָּא. Yoma 57ª; a. fr.

טִפְּשׁוּת, טִיפְּ׳ f. (preced.) *obduracy, folly, stupidity.* Ned. 22ᵇ מוסיף ט׳ gets more and more foolish. Sabb. 152ª טִפְּשׁוּתָן מתוספת בהן Ms. M. (ed. טפשות ניתוסף) their stupidity increases. Yalk. Num. 742 (expl. כסלם, Ps. LXXVIII, 7) טיפשותן; a. e.

טִפְּשׁוּתָא, טִפְּ׳, טִיפְּ׳ ch. same. Targ. Deut. X, 16 (h. text ערלת).

טִפֶּשֶׁת, טִפְּשִׁית, v. טִפֵּשׁ.

טַפְתָּא f. (טְפַר III, cmp. טְפַח) *additional, second layer* of a clay dam. B. Mets. 103ᵇ (Ms. F. טוּפְתָא; Ar. s. v. ארבבתא : טופסא, corr. acc.; v. Koh. Ar. Compl. s. v.), v. אַרְבַּבְתָּא.

טִפְתָּא, v. טִיפְ׳.

***טַצְדְּקָא** I m., pl. טַצְדְּקֵי (= אִצְטַ׳; צדק, v. Pesik. Zutr. to Gen. XLIV, 16) *excuse, subterfuge.* Men. 41ª ט׳ למיפטר וכ׳ you want excuses to free yourself from the duty of wearing show-fringes. [For the phonetic inflection of our and the following wds., cmp. Nöld. Mand. Gramm. § 49.]

***טַצְדְּקָא** II m. (=אִסְטַ׳; סדק) *split, break, damage.* B. Kam. 56ª כל ט׳ וכ׳ (Ar. a. Ms. F. טַצְדְּקֵי, pl.) whatever damage there is in the power of the animal (left in the scorching sun) to do, it will do in order to get out.

טַצְהָר m. (צָהַר, cmp. preced. wds.) *white spot, indication of leprosy.* Gitt. 86ª (in a formula of sale of a slave) free from any organic defect ומן שחין דנפק עד ט׳ חדת וכ׳ and from any eruption that has come out, down to 'white spot', recent or old. [Alf. ומן כל שחין עד צהר; Asheri מן ט׳. The misconception of our w. by commentators, as if denoting a foreign numeral (2 or 4 years) arose from a tradition concerning the definition of עתיק.]

טְקוֹסָא, טְקוּס, v. טִיק׳.

טַקְלִין, Y. Sabb. VI, 7ᵈ bot., v. טוּק.

טָקַס, *Pi.* טִיקֵּס (v. טכס) [*to stuff, press,*] *to harness, equip.*—Part. pass. מְטוּקָּס, f. מְטוּקֶּסֶת, pl. מְטוּקָּסִין, מְטוּקָּסוֹת. Num. R. s. 12 אין צב אלא מט׳ וכ׳ wagons of *tsab* (Num. VII, 3) means fully equipped, nothing wanting; Sifré Num. 45; Yalk. ib. 713; Cant. R. to VI, 4 מְטוּכָּס; Yalk. Is. 372 מטוכ׳.—V. next w. end.

טְקַס ch., *Pa.*, טַקֵּיס, *Af.* אַטְקֵיס same, 1) (corresp. to b. h. אסר) *to harness* for war, *to prepare battle.* Targ. I Kings XX, 14. Targ. Ex. XIV, 6. Targ. I Sam. XV, 5 וט׳ וכ׳ he arranged his camp (h. text וירב); a. fr.—2) *to arrange coins, to count, collect.* Targ. II Kings XXII, 4 (*Af.*); ib. 9 (ed. Wil. טְקִיסוּ *Pe.*).—Ib. XXIII, 35 (h. text נגש).—Part. pass. מְטַקַּס *arranged, fitted, joined.* Ib. XII, 12. Targ. I Kings VI, 31 (h. text חמשית). Targ. II Esth. V, 1 מט׳ *trimmed.*

Ithpa. אִיטַּקַּס, *Ithpe.* אִיטְּקַס *to be equipped, arranged.* Targ. Ps. XX, 6 נִיטְקַס Ms. (ed. Ven. a. Levita נִיטַּקַּס; Bxt. a. oth. נִטַּקַּס, read ניט׳; h. text נדגל). [Targ. Is. XIII, 17, v. טְפַס.] Targ. I Kings VI, 7 מט׳ Levita, *closely fitted* stones (ed. מַטְקַס noun; h. text מסע); cmp. מַטְכְּסָא. [Some of the meanings of טקס a. of טכס are influenced by the Greek τάσσω, τάξις.]

טַקְסִיוּוּט, read:

טַקְסִיוֹטֵי m. pl. (ταξιῶται=ταξᾶτοι, S.) *garrison.* Y. Erub. III, 21ᵇ פרהגבן באילין ט׳ Ar. s. v. (ed. טקסיווט) concerning those troops which come as a garrison (whom one likes to meet), opp. רומאי Roman (hostile) troops.

טַקְסִיס, טַקְסִין, טקסים v. טַכְסִיס.

טַר imper. of נְטַר.

טְרָא, v. טְרֵי.

טַרְדָקָא v. טְרַקָא.

טַרְבַל, טרבן, v. טוּרְבִּיל.

טרגול, Y. B. Bath. I, 15ª, read: פַּרְגּוֹל.

טַרְגּוֹנָא, v. טְרָכוֹנָא.

טְרָגוֹס m. (tragos, τράγος) *a mess of groats* of wheat, barley &c., *groats* used for a mess. Makhsh. VI, 2 טרגים. Ber. 37ª טרגים (Ms. F. טרגוס); Ib. Ms. M. (missing in ed.) טרגוס, also טירגוס (v. Rabb. D. S. a. l. notes 20, 30). M. Kat. 13ᵇ טרגים חדא לתלתא (Ms. M. also טירגים) it is called *tragos,* when each grain is broken in three parts, v. חִילְקָא II.

טַרְגִּיא, v. לטרגיה.

טרגיאנוס, v. טְרָיָינוֹס.

טרגידה, v. לטרגיה.—Tosef. Neg. VI, 3, v. טְרִיגוֹן.

טְרוֹגִימָא, טְרָגִימָא m. (τράγημα, τρῶγμα) *sweetmeats, dessert* (dried fuits &c.). Pes. 107ᵇ .... מטביל במיני ט׳ Ar. (ed. תרג׳) he may make a luncheon of various sweetmeats. Yoma 79ᵇ; Succ. 27ᵃ ת׳. Tosef. Ber. IV, 4 תרגי׳ (Var. תרגומה).

טרגים, v. טְרָגוֹס.—[Tosef. Erub. III (II), 9 טרגים ed. Zuck., read בּוּרְגָּין.]

טָרַד (b. h.; cmp. ט״י) [*to move, shake,*] 1) *to be running, to drip.* Nidd. 49ᵇ היה טוֹרֵד וכ׳ if the liquid drips drop after drop. Bekh. 44ᵃ (עיניו) טוֹרְדוֹת running eyes (more than דֶּלֶף); [Ar.: *restless, constantly twinkling;* oth. opin.: *shutting with great trouble,* v. infra).—2) (of waves) *to carry.* Tosef. Yeb. XIV, 5 שמא גל טורד אותו וכ׳ (v. ed. Zuck. note) perhaps a wave carries and lands him. Ib. טְרָדַנִי גל לחבירו one wave carried me to the other; (Y. ib. XVI, 15ᵈ top טרפני).—3) *to make homeless, banish* (cmp. טִלְטֵל). Lam. R. to I, 21 טְרָדָהּ חוץ וכ׳ he sent her out of the palace. Gen. R. s. 83 (play on מהוטבאל בת מטרד) שהיו מטרבין ... ואח״כ טוֹרְדִין וכ׳ they dressed her for her husband and then led her away from her husband. Kidd. 31ᵃ וטוֹרְדוֹ מן העולם and drives him (his father) out of the world (makes him desperate). Midr. Till. to Ps. XXXI, beg. וט׳ אותם מן העולם and drove them into despair, a. fr.—3) *to weary, make unsteady.* Snh. 22ᵇ; Erub. 64ᵇ דרך טוֹרַדְתּוֹ (Taan. 17ᵇ מַטְרִידָתוֹ *Hif.*, Ms. M. everywhere מַטְרַחְתּוֹ, v. טָרַח) walking makes him unsteady (feel the wine).—4) *to stir up* (dregs), *trouble.* Sabb. 139ᵇ. Nidd. 25ᵃ, sq. מים ... וטוֹרְדִין וכ׳ water is strong (is in commotion) and stirs the mass up, opp. מצחצחו makes it clear.—*Part. pass.* טָרוּד, f. טְרוּדָה; pl. טְרוּדִים ,טְרוּדִין ..., טְרוּדוֹת a) *busily engaged, troubled, anxious.* Gen. R. l. c. (play on מטרד, v. supra) ט׳ היו וכ׳ they were anxious for a living. Y. Ber. IX, 13ᶜ bot. טרודין Asheri to Ber. IX, 13 (ed. Krot. טוֹרדין) uninterrupted lightnings; a. fr.—b) *banished.* Num. R. s. 7, v. מַטְלוֹן.

Nif. נִטְרַד 1) *to be troubled, agitated, confused.* Num. R. s. 20; Tanh. Balak 11, end היה נִטְרַד he became confused, opp. שפוי.—2) *to be banished.* Deut. R. s. 2 יִטָּרֵד למטלון he shall be sent into exile. Ib. s. 6 תִּיטָּרֵד וכ׳; a. fr.

Hif. הִטְרִיד *to weary.* Taan. 17ᵇ, v. supra.

טְרַד I ch. same, 1) *to trouble, stir up, keep in commotion.* B. Bath. 168ᵇ הוו קא טָרְדֵי ליה they were troubling him (begging persistently).—Part. pass. טְרִיד, f. טְרִידָא; pl. טְרִידִין, טְרִידָן. Targ. Is. LVII, 20 (h. text נגרש). Targ. Nah. II, 5 ט׳ ברקין, v. preced.—Ber. 16ᵇ הכא ט׳ in the one case his mind is preoccupied. Erub. 68ᵃ טְרִידְנָא בגירסאי I am engrossed in my studies. Snh. 108ᵇ [read:] דהוית טריד (or דִטְרִידַתְּ; Ms. F., טְרִיחַתְּ, v. Rabb. D. S. a. l. note 9) that thou wert troubled (in my behalf); Yalk. Job 917 [read:] חַמִּית דטרידת וכ׳; a. fr.—2) *to banish, expel.* Targ. Y. Gen. III, 24; a. fr.—

Ithpe. אִיטְּרִיד, אִתְּטְרִיד 1) *to be banished.* Targ. Prov. XXV, 5. Targ. Y. Gen. XXVII, 45; a. e.—2) *to be troubled.* Ber. 35ᵇ; Yalk. Deut. 863 דלא תִיטַּרְדוּ וכ׳ that you may not be troubled about support &c.—3) *to quarrel.* Arakh. 16ᵇ אתי לאִיטְּרוּדֵי he may get into a quarrel.

טְרַד II (cmp. טרק a. נְטַר) *to guard, lock up, bolt.* Targ. Y. Gen. XIX, 6 Ar. a. Levita (ed. אחד). Targ. Y. Ex. XIV, 3; a. e.—Lam. R. to I, 1 ט׳ תרעא (חד מירד׳) רבתי locked the door. Ib. to I, 18 טְרוּדוּ תרעין shut the doors closely.—Y. Keth. VII, 31ᶜ תרעה טְרִיד if her door is found locked, contrad. to מוּגָף, v. גּוּף I.

Ithpe. אִיטְּרַד *to be locked.* Targ. Y. II Gen. XLIX, 1.

טִירְדָא, טִירָ׳ m. (טְרַד I) *anxiety, excitement.* Ber. 16ᵇ אי משום ט׳ if anxiety be a cause for omitting to pray. Ib. ט׳ דרשות anxiety about a secular affair, ט׳ דמצוה about a religious matter; Succ. 25ᵃ.

טרדימר, v. טַרְטִימַר.

טַרְדִּין=תַּרְדִּין, Tosef. Ter. IV, 5 והט׳ ed. Zuck. Var.

טרוגינוס, v. טְרָיָינוֹס.

טְרוֹגִימָא, v. טְרָגִימָא.

טָרוּד, v. טָרַד.

טָרוֹדָא m. (טְרַד I) 1) *a troublesome person, bore.* Snh. 26ᵃ. [2) = h. טָרוּד *busy, restless.* Targ. Y. Gen. XXXVI, 30 quoted in 'Rashi' to Gen. R. s. 83, end, v. מַטְרְדָה.]

***נחל ט׳, טְרַוְיָא** pr. n. *Valley of Tarvaya* (h. נחל זרד). Targ. Y. Deut. II, 13; 14.

טְרוּזָא or **טְרִיזָא** m. (טרד = טרז I, cmp. טרוזא P. Sm. 1512) [*moist, cool,*] a kind of *cucumber* or *melon* eaten for medicinal purposes. Sabb. 109ᵃ (Ar. טרי׳, ed. Sonc. טריד).

טָרוּט m., **טְרוּטָה** f. 1) (cmp. טָרַד) *bleared, dripping and dim;* [oth. opin. *half-closed;* Rashi: *round.*]—*Pl.* טְרוּטוֹת. Tosef. Bekh. V, 3 עיניו ט׳ Var. (ed. Zuck. ת׳); Bekh. 44ᵃ (expl. הצירקן, cmp. Targ. Y. I Gen. XXIX, 17) עיניו ט׳ Ar. (ed. ת׳). Taan. 24ᵃ עיניה ט׳, opp. יפות. Sabb. 31ᵃ ת׳. Snh. 107ᵇ (in a passage omitted in later eds.) עיניה ט׳.—2) (v. טְרַטֵּט) *straight-lined, abruptly ending,* v. תָּרוּט.

טְרוֹקְסִימוֹן, v. טְרוֹקְסִימוֹן.

***טְרוֹמִיטָא, טַרְמִיטָא, טַרְמִיטָן** m. (τρῆμα, ατος, τρηματιον) *perforation,* also *eye of a needle;* only in בֵּיצַת ט׳ (בֵּיצָה) *an egg boiled down to the size of a pill* which, on being swallowed by the patient, passes the body unchanged, carrying with it matter which serves the physician for diagnosis. Ned. VI, 1 ביצת טרמיטא Mish. (Bab. ed. ביצה מורמוט׳; Y. ed. טרמיטן); ib. 50ᵃ ביצה טורמיטא; Y. ib. VI, 39ᶜ bot. ביצה טרומיטא, expl. רופיטן.

***טרון** adv. (נְטַר) *waiting, looking out for business, idle.* Lam. R. introd. (R. Isaac 3) קאים ט׳ וכ׳ one stands idly waiting a whole day and is not tired, but for prayer one is tired; (Yalk. Is. 318 קאי וטרי; Esth. R. to I, 9 יתיב ומשתעיר).

***טְרוּן** (a contr. of טרי אנא, v. טְרִי) *I throw.* Lam. R. to II, 1 הא לכון ט׳ באפיכון here, you have it, I throw it in your face.

טְרוֹנְיָא, טְרוּנְא, v. טִיר׳.

טרונוס, v. תְּרוֹנוֹס.

טָרוּף m. 1) (denom. of טָרָף) *covered with leaves.* Tosef. Neg. VIII, 2, v. טָרֵף.—2) (part. pass. of טָרַף, cmp. *Pi.*) *disfigured by irregular spots;* (oth. opin.) *chopped, full of incisions;* (oth. opin.) *planed, smooth.* Ned. 25ª; Shebu. 29ᵇ (ref. to one swearing that he had seen a serpent 'like the beam of an oil press') בט׳ he meant 'spotted' like a beam &c. Ib. (in answer to the argument כולהו נחשי מיטרף טריפין (or טריפי, not טרפי) that all serpents are 'spotted') בשגבו ט׳ (Ms. M. שבגבו) he meant a serpent spotted on the back (and not only around the neck). Ned. l. c. קורת... גבו ט׳ (read גבה) the back of a press beam may be spotted (i. e. no objection of the purchaser is valid based on the spotted condition of the beam); according to the opinion: ט׳=*planed,* all beams must be planed, (otherwise the purchaser has a right to reject).—[Other meanings, v. טָרַף.]

טְרוּף, v. טֵירוּף.

טְרוֹפָאָה m., pl. טְרוֹפָאֵי (denom. of טְרֵפָה) 1) *those deciding on defects of animals* for ritual purposes, *meat-supervisors.* Hull. 55ᵇ.—2) *those who decided in favor of t'refah,* Ib. 48ᵇ. Ib. 49ª שקילו... דט׳ seize the cloak of those who decided &c. (make them pay damages).

טרופי, Targ. Ps. I, 3 some ed., v. טַרְפָּא.

טרופין, Tanh. Ki Thissa 1, לעסק ט׳, v. טִירוֹן I.

טְרוֹקְטֵי f. (τρωκτή, sub. σταφυλή) *dessert grapes, yielding no wine.* Yalk. Num. 709 טריק׳ (corr. acc.)—Trnsf. *a woman that has no menstruation.* Y. Keth. I, 25ª bot.; Nidd. IX, 11 Var. in Hai Gaon, v. הוֹרְקְטֵי.

טרוקי, Yoma 10ª Ms. M., v. תרייקי.

***טרוקיתקא**, Targ. Ps. XXXV, 3 ed. Lag. a. oth., for h. text סְגֹר, read: טְרוֹק יָתִי וזמן וכ׳ guard me, and meet &c. [Ed. Bxt. a. oth. only טרוק.]

טרוקנין, Ber. 37ᵇ, v. טְרִיקְטָא.

טְרוֹכְסִימוֹן, טְרוֹקְסִימוֹן, טְרוֹקְסִימָא, (טרק׳, טרכ׳) m. (τρώξιμον, τὰ τρώξιμα) 1) *whatever can be eaten raw,* applied to *kitchen vegetables,* esp. *endive* &c. Lev. R. s. 3 אגודה אחת של טרוקסימא (some ed. מון...) a bunch of vegetables. Y. Pes. IV, 31ᵇ, sq. Y. Sabb. VII, 10ª טריקס׳ ed. Krot. (corr. acc.).—Y. Pes. II, 29ᶜ top (expl. עולשין); Y. Kil. I, 27ª top (some ed. מין..., pl.)—Tosef. Ter. IV, 5 טרקסמן ed. Zuck. (Var. טְרָכְסְמִין, pl.) Tosef. Makhsh. III, 10 טרכ׳, contrad. to יָרָק.—2) (sub. κῆπος) *kitchen-garden.* Ber. 35ᵇ הוו.... דרך ט׳ וכ׳ (Ms. M. טרסק׳; Ms. F. טריבסמון, corr. acc.) used to bring their fruits home (from the field to the barn) by the way of the kitchen-garden (in sight of the house) in order to make them subject to tithes; Gitt. 81ª; Yalk. Deut. 938.

טְרַז, v. טְרִיז.

טַרְזְיָנָא, טַרְזָנָא, v. טוּר׳.

טָרַח (b. h.; cmp. טָרַד) *to run about, be busy, to take pains, prepare.* Ab. Zar. 3ª מי שט׳ וכ׳ he who has made preparations on Friday has food for the Sabbath (he who does good in this world can expect reward in the hereafter). Keth. 10ª; Kidd. 45ᵇ חזקה אין.. טוֹרֵחַ וכ׳ the presumption is that one will not go to the trouble of preparing a (wedding) feast and let it go to ruin, i. e. one must have weighty reasons for a divorce immediately after marriage; Yeb. 107ª. Ber. 58ª, v. טוֹרַח; a. fr.—[Y. M. Kat. I, 80ª bot. דבר שאינו ט׳, v. טָרֵיחַ.]

Hif. הִטְרִיחַ 1) *to put to trouble, put a task on.* Taan. 24ª אתה הִטְרַחְתָּ וכ׳ thou hast put thy Creator to the trouble of &c. Snh. 8ª מַטְרִיחִין אותי they (the wicked) put me to &c. Lev. R. s. 27 לא הִטְרַחְתִּי עליכם I did not tax you too heavily; a. fr.—2) *to weary.* Snh. 22ᵇ; Erub. 64ᵇ, a. e., v. טָרַד.—3) *to trouble, beg persistently.* Yalk. Ex. 244 ה׳ עליו he begged him instantly.

טְרַח I ch. same. Targ. Koh. II, 11. Ib. IX, 9; a. fr. —B. Kam. 11ª בדנפשיה ט׳ he takes pains with what belongs to himself (for his own benefit). Hull. 83ª דאורח ארעא לְמִטְרַח וכ׳ in the bridegroom's family they generally take more trouble in preparing the wedding feast &c.; a. fr. [Sot. 7ᵇ ומטרח, v. טְרִי.]—*Part. pass.* טְרִיחַ, f. טְרִיחָא *giving trouble, troublesome.* Ned. 25ª מילתא דלא ט׳ an easily intelligible expression. Hull. 51ª, a next w.— B. Mets. 112ᵇ ט׳ להו מילתא (Ms. M. ליה) it is too troublesome for them (for him); a. e.—[Sabb. 82ª, v. טְחַר.]— B. Kam. 80ᵇ Ar., v. תְּרַח.

Af. אַטְרַח 1) *to make ready for moving, to load* (cmp. טְעַן II) Targ. Job XXXVII, 11 (h. text יַטְרִיחַ).—2) *to trouble.* Meg. 22ᵇ לא מַטְרַח צִיבורא Ms. M. (ed. לא בעי למִיטְרַח, read לְמַטְרַח, v. Rashi, a. Rabb. D. S. a. l. note) he would not trouble the congregation (to rise before him); Yalk. Lev. 669; a. fr.—3) *to beg persistently.* Lev. R. s. 16 א׳ עליה he insisted upon his telling him.—Y. Peah I, 16ᵇ bot. אין מַטְרְחַת עלוי if you strain the chord too much.

Ithpe. אִיטְּרַח 1) *to be wearied.* Targ. Y. Num. XIX, 2 אִיטְּרְחָא (not אִט׳).—2) *to be troublesome, difficult.* Taan. 24ᵇ מי ארכא דמִיטְּרַח וכ׳ is it so hard a labor to the Lord?

טֹרַח, v. טוֹרַח.

טְרַח II m. = טוּרְחָא, *painstaking, trouble.* Hull. 51ª ט׳ טְרִיחַ לההוא גברא what trouble has been taken by that man (myself)!—[Oth. version: ט׳ טְרִיחָה וכ׳ weariness (of travel) made me shaky.]

טַרְחָא, v. טוּרְחָא.

טַרְחָא, טִירְ׳ f. (preced. wds.) *trouble, labor, discomfort.* Tem. 24ª דקא טרח טר׳ וכ׳ because he would undertake a labor unfit for him (on the Holy Day). B.Mets. 93ᵇ לט׳ יתירתא with reference to special painstaking. Shebu. 45ª bot. טר׳ ליה מלתא, v. טְרַח I. M.Kat. 13ª מועד משום ט׳ ולא ט׳ Ms. M. (ed. only משום ט׳) in the festive week it is forbidden only for being a labor to some extent; a. fr.

טִירְ׳, טַרְחוּת f. 1) same. Y. Ber. II, 5ª bot. טַרְחוּתָם מרובה the trouble of climbing them down is very great. Pesik. Bayom, p. 193ª ט׳ הדרכים the trouble of travelling. Cant. R. to VIII, 6 שהגשמים .. סימן טיר׳ for there are those rains which betoken trouble &c.—Pesik. Shek. p. 20ᵇ; Pesik. R. s. 16 end; Ex. R. s. 34 אין הק״בה בא בט׳ וכ׳ the Lord comes not with burdensome laws to be imposed upon &c.—2) *necessaries of life, living.* Lev. R. s. 1 משה עסוק בט׳ וכ׳ Moses occupied himself with arranging the living of Israel (ordaining dietary laws). Gen. R. s. 94 ט׳ נפש אחת provision for one soul. Pesik. R. s. 3 (ref. to מתה עלי, Gen. XLVIII, 7) עלי היתה טַרְחוּתָהּ mine was the care for her.

טְרִיחוּתָא, טוּרְחוּ׳, טַרְחוּתָא ch. same. Targ. Koh. II, 10; a. e.—Sabb. 10ª טריח׳ למיסר וכ׳ (Ar. פְּרִיהוּתָא) is it such a trouble to tie on a belt?—Pesik. Haḥod. p. 50ª, a. e. עיקר ט׳ מטרא the real discomfort of the winter season is the rain; a. e.

טרטא, טרטס, Lev. R. s. 7 ר׳ יוסי בן ט׳, read, as Yalk. Ps. 766: פִּיטְרָס.

טרטון, v. טִיטַרְטוֹן a. טְרָטִין.

טַרְטֵט (רטרט=טרט, cmp. צִבְצֵב; v. טְרוּט 2) *to plait straps, to strap.* Tosef. Kel. B. Mets. VI, 1 משיְּטַרְטֵט ed. Zuck. (Var. משיִּרְטֵט) until the leather for the strap-mattress is plaited; (cmp. Kel. XVI, 4).

טַרְטְיָאוֹת, טַרְטָרָאוֹת f. pl. (cacophem. perversions of תֵּיאַטְרָאוֹת; cmp. meanings of טרט in טְרוּט, טַרְטֵט, a. of טרי, a. similar perversions in אִצְטְדָיָא &c.) *theatres, shows.* Lam. R. to III, 5 ומכניסין את הגמל לבתי ט׳ they bring a camel on their stage (ib. also תֵּיאַטְרוֹן a. תַּרְטֵיאוֹת). Yalk. II Sam. 158; Midr. Till. to Ps. XVIII טַרְטְרָאוֹת (ed. Bub. טרטרא׳). Keth. 5ª; Sabb. 150ª (Ms. O. טַרְטַסְיָ׳, early eds. טַרְטְרָאוֹת); a. e. [Various forms in eds. a. Mss.: טַרְטִסָאוֹת, טַרְטִיוֹת &c.]—[Ab. Zar. 42ª דרכים וט׳ ed., Ms. M. סרטיאות, v. סְרַטְיָא a. אִסְרַטְיָא.]

טרטיוטין, Ex. R. s. 36, read: סְרַטְיוֹטִין or סַטְרַטְיוֹטִין.

טַרְטִימַר (טַרְטֵ׳, טַרְתְּ׳, תַּרְטֵ׳) m. (τριτημόριον, S.) *triens, one third of an as,* a *coin* and a *weight* (about three ounces). Snh. VIII, 2 ט׳ בשר (Bab. ed. 70ª ת׳; Ms. F. ט׳, in Gemarah טרדימר; Y. Mish. טרת׳, Gemarah 26ª טרט׳) a triens (worth?) of meat. Ib. 70ª ט׳ זה וכ׳ (ת׳) I do not know what this *ṭarṭemar* means, but judging from R. José doubling the standard for wine, it may be inferred that *ṭ.* is half a Manah; Y. l. c. ט׳ חצי ליטרא *ṭ.* is half a Litra. (V. Zuckerm. Talm. Münzen p. 8).

***טַרְטֵין** (denom. of טוּרְטִינֵי) *to balance,* i. e. *to ride with one foot on each side of the animal.* Nidd. 14ª דמְטַרְטֵין when he rides like a man on horseback, דלא מט׳ when he rides like a woman.

טרטין, Sifré Num. 86 לשאר חט׳, read הֶדְיוֹטִין, v. Yalk. Num. 732, end.

טְרָטִין m. pl. (=טורטורין, cmp. Arab. *ṭarṭur* in Dozy Dict. des noms des vêtem., p. 262 sq., Lat. *turritum* capitis ornamentum &c.) *t'ratin, a head cover.* Kel. XXIX, 1; Tosef. ib. B. Bath. VII, 5 טְרָטוֹן ed. Zuck. (Var. טרסי).

***טרטיס**, Koh. R. to VII, 11 ואתי מן ט׳ ואמר ליה טליא (emended in later eds. טרסים) a corrupt passage to be restored by collation with Y. Ber. III, 6ᶜ bot.; perhaps: ואתי חד טליא ואמר ליה.

טרטיסאות, טרטיראות, טרטסאות, v. טַרְטְיָאוֹת.

***טַרְטֵף** (reduplic. of טְרַף) *to cut out edges, to pink, scallop* (a leather garment). Tosef. Kel. B. Mets. VI, 1 משיְּטַרְטֵף ed. Vien. (ed. Zuck. a. oth. משישטרטף, ed. Zolk. משישוטף) (cmp. Kel. XVI, 4 משיחסום וכ׳ &c.).

טַרְטְקָל m. (transpos. of craticulum, v. P. Sm. 1516) [*net-work,* esp.] *a small gridiron.* Targ. Prov. XXVI, 21 (h. text פחם).

טרטר, Midr. Till. to Ps. XCIII, 3 היה מטרטר, v מִיטַטוֹר.

טְרָא, טְרֵי [*to set in motion,*] 1) *to shake.* Hull. 45ᵇ טָרֵיהּ לרישיה shook his head constantly; [Ar.: he *bumped* his head, *shocked* his brain]. Ib. 51ª, v. טְרַח II.—2) *to throw, cast; to squirt, drip.* Tam. 32ᵇ ט׳ באפיה sprinkled his face (with that water). Sabb. 108ᵇ מהו למִטְרָא וכ׳ Ar. (ed. למימשר, Ms. O. למישרא, v. Rabb. D. S. a. l. note 8) is it permitted to drop some of this water into the eye?—Lev. R. s. 25 יהוי טָרֵי וכ׳ (not טרו) shall cast one fig in his face; Koh. R. to II, 20 יהא טריה (read: יהא טרי חד). Taan. 24ª bot. טַרְיוּהוּ מן גודא וכ׳ Ms. M. 2 (ed. חבוטו) throw him down from the elevation; a. fr.—3) Trnsf. שקיל וטרי [*to take up and throw back* a ball &c.,] *to hear and reply, to argue; to negotiate* (corresp. to h. נשא ונתן). Targ. Ruth IV, 7. Targ. Cant. III, 8 וטָרָן (not ומירן; ed. Lag. וטָאְרָן).—B. Mets. 64ª דלא ט׳ וט׳ בהדיה with whom he was not accustomed to deal. Sot. 7ᵇ למישקל ולמִיטְרָא וכ׳ Ar. (ed. ומטרח, corr. acc.) to argue with &c.; a. fr.—V. טָרוֹן.

טְרִי f., v. טְרִיתָא.

טרי, pr. n., v. טָדִי.

טַרְיָא, or **טִרְ׳** m. *shaking,* v. טִירְיָא.—[In later literature שקלא וטַרְיָא *argument,* v. טְרִי.]

***טַרְיָא** m. (טְרִי) *dripping;* מי ט׳ a sort of *ink,* prob. from wine-lees (v. Löw Graph. Requisiten, p. 158, p. 161). Gitt. 19ª; Sabb. 104ᵇ (early eds. מיטריא in one w.; Rashi: 'juice of a certain fruit', oth. opin. 'rain water').

טריא, Ber. 56ᵃ Ms. M., v. טוּרְזָא; [cmp., however, טַרְיָיתָא.]

טְרָיָא pr. n. pl., v. טְרָיָיא.

***טְרִיבָא** m. (טרב, cmp. צרב) *an eruption, inflammation.* Targ. Y. Ex. II, 5, constr. טְרִיב בשרא.

טְרִיגוֹן m. 1) (τρίγωνος) *triangular.* Neg. XII, 1; Naz. 8ᵇ; B. Bath. 164ᵇ (בית ט׳) a triangularly built house; Tosef. Neg. VI, 3 טריגון ed. Zuck. (Var. טריגיה, corr. acc.); —2) (τρίγονος) *for the third time.* Naz. l. c.; Y. ib. I, 51ᵇ top; Tosef. ib. I, 2 דרגון ed. Zuck. (Var. דיגון, corr. acc.); v. דִּיגוֹן.

טריגון, Treat. Tsitsith, ed. Kirchh. p. 22, v. טוֹגָא.— Ib. p. 23 מכסה כמין ט׳, prob. to be read: טְרִיבוֹן (τρίβων) *coarse cloak.*

טריגין, v. טְרִיגוֹן.

טְרִיד, v. טְרַד, a. טְרוּזָא.

***טריון**, Gen. R. s. 79; Yalk. Gen. 133 בטרו, read טַרְטִין; emend the entire passage as follows: קו״ף ק׳ מיליא סמ״ך ס״ס ט״ית טרטין the *Kuf* (of קשיטה, Gen. XXXIV, 19) means one hundred millia, the *Sammekh—ses,* the *Teth—tertin,* i. e. *one hundred millia Sestertium* (v. Sm. Ant. s. v. Sestertius), v. דִּנְקְנְתִּין.

טריון, Y. Taan. II, 66ᵃ top, v. טְרָיָינוֹס.

טריונין, Tosef. Ab. Zar. II, 7 Var., v. אִצְטְרִין.

***טְרִיז** m. (supposed to be a Persian word, expl. by R. Ḥananel by Arabic *banîke*) *gusset, gore.* Sabb. 98ᵇ עד דט׳ .. שפי Ar. (read כי ט׳, v. Koh. Ar. Compl. s. v., ed. כי טורין) they planed the boards (so as to be gradually decreasing in thickness) like a gusset; Yalk. Ex. 370 כי טורין.

טְרִיזָא, v. טְרוּזָא.

טְרַח, טְרִיחַ m. (טְרַח) *troublesome, laborious.* Y. M. Kat. I, beg., 80ᵃ דבר שאינו ט׳ (Y. Shebi. II, end, 34ᵇ טוֹרַח).

טְרִיחַ, טְרִיחָא, v. טְרַח.

טְרִיחוּתָא, v. טַרְחוּתָא.

טְרִימָא, Bets. 29ᵃ top Ar., v. תְּרָטָא.

טְרִימָנִי, v. טוּרְמִינִי.

טְרִיי pr. n. m. *Taryi.* Cant. R. to IV, 1; I, 15 (Gen. R. s. 33 בִּיבִי; Lev. R. s. 31 ברכיה, Yalk. Gen. 59 בִּיבִי).

טְרָיָיא, טְרָיָיה, טוּר׳ pr. n. pl. (?) *Traya, Turya;* אִישׁ ט׳ surname of Abba Hoshaya. Y. B. Kam. X, end, 7ᶜ. Gen. R. s. 58, beg.; a. fr. (V. Neub. Géogr. p. 267).

טְרִיָיא, ט׳ קוֹנְטָא read:

טְרִיָיאקוֹנְטָא (τριάκοντα) *thirty.* Y. B. Bath. X, 17ᶜ, v. אִיגְדוֹרִיקוֹנְטָא.

טְרָיָינָא m. (v. next w.) *Trajanic.* Ab. Zar. 52ᵇ דינרא ט׳ והדריינא שיפא Ms. M. (ed. הדרייאנא טורייגא) the Trajanic and Hadrianic denars which were rubbed off; Bekh. 50ᵃ bot. הדריינא טרייאנא שייאפא; ib. top ד׳ טרינא שייפא (Tosaf. טרינא).

טְרָיָינוֹס, טוּר׳ (variously corrupted, the *j* sound being rendered by ג or כ) pr. n. m. *Trajanus,* the Roman emperor. Taan. 18ᵇ (טר׳ a. טור׳); Treat. S'maḥoth ch. VIII טרגיא׳; Sifra Emor Par. 8, ch. IX מריינוס (corr. acc.); Y. Taan. II, 66ᵃ top טריון. Y. Succ. V, 55ᵇ top טרוגינוס; Lam. R. to I, 16; ib. to IV, 19, a. e. טרכינוס. Ib. to III, 2; 4; a. e. (v. Joel, Blicke in die Religionsgesch. I, p. 17, sq.).—טְרָיָינִי (genitive of Trajanus) *Trajan's (followers).* Ib. to I, 17 טרכיני, v. אִסְפַּסְיָינִי.

***טְרָיוּתָא** f. pl. (נטר) *guarded things, property.* Targ. Y. Deut. XI, 6 (h. text יקום).

טְרֵיךְ m. (טרך, cmp. טרח a. טְרַק I) *troublesome, provoking.* Targ. Prov. XIX, 7 (ed. Wil. טָרֵךְ; ed. Lag. טַרְכָן). V. טַרְכָנוּתָא.

טריכונוס, Esth. R. to III, 1, read: טְרִיבוּנוֹס, v. ארטיגוס.

טריכסון, v. טְרַקְסִין.

***טרים**, Y. Sabb. III, 6ᵃ, מיסחי .... בטרים בר יטסם ed., Ar. ed. Koh. בטרים בטרים, oth. ed. בט׳ טירים read: במי טבריא ביו״ט bathing . . . in the waters of Tiberias on a Holy Day.

טְרִימָא m. (τρῖμμα) *a drink* or *brew prepared of pounded groats and spices, a spiced drink.* Ber. 38ᵃ תמרי מחן ט׳ . . . you are permitted to make *trimma* of dates &c., v. חֲשִׁילְתָא; Tosef. Maas. Sh. II, 2 ed. Zuck. (some ed. תרומה, corr. acc.).

***טרימומטה**, read: טְרִימִיטְרָא.

טרימוסיאה, Gen. R. s. 88, v. טְרוֹנְיָא.

טְרִימִיטְרָא m. (τρίμετρος) *trimeter, a verse* (or *tune*) *of three iambic meters.* Y. R. Hash. IV, 59ᶜ bot. (defining הַרְעָה) [read:] כאהן ט׳ like the trimeter (short-long, short-long &c.), contrad. to הלת דקיקן three small (short) notes.

טְרִימִיסָא m. (tremis) *Tremis,* a Roman coin, one third of an Aureus. Lam. R. to I, 1 רבתי (חד מאת׳ 8). Y. Gitt. III, 47ᵇ סרימיסין (read: טְרִימִיסִין tremissis), v. גּוּרְדְּיָינִי.

טְרִינָא, v. טְרָיי׳.

טריסים, v. טריסיס.

טריסין, Tosef. Erub. XI (VIII), 17 Var., v. סָרִיג.

טְרִיסִיס, טְרִיסִין (incorrect טריסית) m. *tressis,* a coin worth *three ases.* Shebu. VI, 3 טריסית (Y. ed.

קטריסי׳, a corrupt. of quadrussis, *four ases*). Ib. 40ª top. B. Mets. 46ª ...יוּן, a. יח ... Tosef. Maas. Sh. IV, 2; 13; a. e.

טריסיס, טריסים, Pesik. R. s. 15 בט׳, a gloss to בר סימאר, corrupted from בש״ר סימ׳; v. Pesik. Haḥod., p. 55ᵇ. [Neub. Géogr., citing fr. Ms. Bodl. בטרסוס, refers to *Tarsus*.]

טְרִיסִית, v. טְרִיסִין.

טְרֵיפָא, v. טְרֵיפְתָא.—[B. Kam. 16ᵇ, v. next w.]

טְרִיפָה f. (טָרַף) 1) *tearing* (by beasts of prey). B. Kam. 16ᵇ למימרא דט׳ לאו וכ׳ (some ed. דטריפא, Ms. M. דְטָרַף, ref. to the preceding טרף ואכל) does that mean to say that tearing is not his (the lion's) habit?—2) *being carried away by waves, being cast ashore.* Y. Yeb. XVI, 15ᵈ top נותנין ... כדי ט׳ the court allows a reasonable time sufficient for the discovery of an eventual escape of the husband by being cast ashore.—3) (denom. of טְרָף) *covering with leaves, night cover in open air.* Yalk. Gen. 119, v. רְטִיבָה.

טְרֵפָה, טְרֵיפָה f. (b. h.; טָרַף) 1) *an animal torn by a beast of prey.* Midr. Till. to Ps. VII, v. טָרַף.—2) (ritual law) *an animal afflicted with a (fatal) organic disease,* the discovery of which, after slaughtering, makes it forbidden, *t'refah,* (of persons, m.) *one having a fatal organic disease* (the killing of whom would not be considered murder before the law). Ḥull. 42ª ט׳ אינה חיה a *t'refa* animal cannot survive (a year); a. fr.—Snh. 78ª ההורג את הט׳ if one kills a person afflicted with a fatal organic disease; וט׳ שהרג and if such a person committed a murder. Ib. עדיו ט׳ witnesses afflicted &c.; a. fr.—3) *organic disease.* Lev. R. s. 13 (ref. to החיה, Lev. XI, 2) החיה מטְּרֵיפָתָהּ וכ׳ that which can recover from its disease, you may eat.—*Pl.* טְרֵפוֹת, טְרֵיפוֹת. Ḥull. III, 1; a. fr.—Esp. *cases of t'refah, ritual law concerning t'refah.* Ib. 48ᵇ; a. fr.

טְרִיפוֹלָאֵי m. pl. (denom. of Tripolis) *Tripolitans, residents of Tripolis* on the Phoenician coast. Targ. Y. II Gen. X, 17 (h. text חוי).

טְרִיפוֹן pr. n. m. *T'rifon.* Y. Bicc. II, beg. 64ᶜ.

***טְרִיפְתָא** f. (טְרַד) *vagrancy, irregular life.* Pesik. B'shall., p. 93ª כל הדא ט׳ להן לך whither will all this irregular life lead thee?

טְרֵיפָא, טְרֵיפְתָא f. ch. = h. טְרֵיפָה. Ḥull. 94ᵇ.—*Pl.* טְרֵיפְתָא, טְרֵיפָן. Targ. Y. Lev. XI, 1; Targ. Y. Num. XIX, 3 (some ed. טְרִיפָן, v. Ḥull. 42ª ר״ח טרפות).

טְרִיקָא m. (טְרַק II) *enclosure, prison.* Targ. Lam. III, 7.

טְרַקְטָה, טְרִיקְטָא f. (tracta) *a long piece of dough pulled out in making pastry* (*tracta* or *tractum*). Y. Ḥall. I, 57ᵈ ר׳ יוחנן אמר טריק׳ חייבת וכ׳ R. J. says, *tracta* is subject to *Ḥallah;* Ber. 37ᵇ כי אתא ... אמר ר׳ יוחנן טרקנין חייבת וכ׳ Ms. M. (corr. acc.; v. Rabb. D. S. a. l. note 6; ed. טרוקנין פטורין) when R.... came to Babylonia from Palestine, he related in behalf of R. J. &c. Y. Pes. III, 30ª טרקטה הורי וכ׳ as to *tracta* (on Passover) R.... permitted to make only one at a time, but two &c.

טְרִיקְטֵי, v. טְרוֹקְטֵי.

טְרִיקַיָּא m. pl. (טְרַק I *to sting*) a sort of *wasps.* Targ. Y. Deut. VII, 20 (a gloss to אורעייתא, h text צרעה).

טְרִיקְלוֹנָא, v. טְרִקְלִינָא.

טְרִיקְלִילִין, v. טְרַקְלִילָא.

טְרַקְלִין, טְרִיקְלִין m. (τρικλίνιον, triclinium) 1) *dining couch.* Y. Ḥag. II, 77ª bot. הט׳ מוצע לכם the banqueting couch is spread for you (your reward in the hereafter is prepared).—2) *dining room, reception room.* Y. R. Hash. IV, 59ᵇ bot. אפי׳ מט׳ לקיטון even if they adjourned from the tricl. to the sleeping room. Y. Keth. IV, 28ᵈ; Y. Snh. XI, end, 30ᶜ [read:] בציא הדא אומנתא ט׳ וקיטון חופה וקיטון וכ׳ the following construction is required (in order to make the reception of the bride in the triclinium a legal consummation of marriage) a tricl. and a marriage chamber, and that chamber communicating with the tricl.—Ab. IV, 16, v. פְּרוֹזְדוֹר.—Tosef. Sabb. XVI (XVII), 18 ט׳ שהסיקה .... בה in a banqueting room (triclinium hibernum) which has been heated a day before..., you may entertain company on the Sabbath. Tosef. Bets. II, 10 ט׳ שהסיקוהו וכ׳; a. e.—3) (τρίκλινος = ὅρριον, S.) *granary.* Y. Sot. V, 20ᵇ bot. ארטלק עלוי חד ט׳ וכ׳ he was fined to fill a granary of forty by forty &c.

טְרַק׳, טְרִיקְלִינָא ch. same. Targ. II Esth. VII, 8 טרקלו׳ (corr. acc.)—Lev. R. s. 16 בטְרִיקְלִינֵיה (some ed. בתורק׳, corr. acc.) in his reception room.—*Pl.* טְרִיקְלִינִין, טְרַק׳. Targ. Y. I Num. XXXI, 50.

טריקסימון, v. טְרוֹק׳.

טְרִיקְסִין, v. טְרַקְסִין.

טָרִית f. (נטר, cmp. אִטְּרִי) *preserve, pickle,* esp. *salted* or *pickled fish.* Meg. 6ª טמוני זו ט׳ 'stored things' (Deut. XXXIII, 19) refers to *tarith* (as a valuable article of commerce); Sifré Deut. 354; Num. R. s. 13.—Ab. Zar. II, 6 ט׳ טרופה brine containing hashed *tarith* (when you cannot recognize the clean and unclean fish). Ib. ט׳ שאינה טרופה in which the fish can be recognized. Ned. VI, 4 he who vows abstinence from 'fish' מותר בט׳ טרופה is permitted to partake of hashed *t.* Ber. 44ª.

טָרִי, טָרִיתָא ch. 1) same. Y. Ned. VI, 39ᵈ top זבון לי טרי וכ׳ (not ליטרי) sell me *tari,* and he sells him *tsaḥăna* (v. צַחֲנָא). Ib. תמן...לט׳ וכ׳ (not ליט׳) there they call *taritha tsaḥăna.*—2) (cmp. אִטְּרִי) *a sort of pastry, fritters* &c. Ber. 37ᵇ, v. הַדְּקָא a. גְּבִיל.

טֶרֶךְ m. (טרך, cmp. טְרַק II), pl. טְרָכִים, constr. טַרְכֵי *binders, preservers* (cmp. Syr. טרק a. derivatives P. Sm. 1528). Tosef. Sot. XV, 9, v. טְרַכְסִיד.

טָרֵף, v. טָרֵיף.

טַרְכוֹנָא pr. n. *Trachona, Trachonitis*, town and district east of the Jordan. Targ. O. Deut. III, 4; 13; 14 (Y. טַרְגוֹנָא; h. text ארגב). Targ. Y. II Num. XXXIV, 15 טְרָכוֹן זמרא; Sifré Deut. 51 טרכונא דנימרא; Yalk. ib. 874 ט׳ דזימר׳ (not טרנינא); Tosef. Shebi. IV, 11 ט׳ דבתחום בצרה ed. Zuck. (Var. טרכתא, incorr.); Y. Shebi. VI, 36ᶜ ט׳ דמתחם לבוצרה (v. Hildesh. Beitr. p. 55, sq.).

טַרְכוּנְתָא, v. טַרְכְנוּתָא.

טרכוס, v. טַרְקַשׁ.

טרכינוס, טרכיני, v. טְרָקִינוּס.

טַרְכָן, v. טָרֵיף.

טַרְכָנוּתָא f. (v. preced.) *trouble, anger*. Targ. Prov. XXVI, 28 Ar. a. Lev. (Var. טַרְפוּנְתָא; ed. תַּרְפוּנְתָא; Ms. סרכונא).

טְרַכְסִיד m. (a comp. of טֶרֶה a. סִיד) *binding cement*. Tosef. Sot. XV, 9 if one put sand in the lime, חרי זה ט׳ ואסור ed. (ed. Zuck. טרכיו סיד הוא, Var. טְרָכֵי סיד) it is cement and therefore forbidden; B. Bath. 60ᵇ חרי זה ט׳ (Ms. O. טַרְכְּסָאוֹ the binding of it (the lime), cmp. טְרַקְסִין); Sabb. 80ᵇ (Ms. M. תר׳). [Treat. S'maḥ. VIII טרכסי׳, in a corrupt passage, prob. to be read: כרכים.]

טְרַכְסִימוֹן, v. טְרוֹקְסִ.

טַרְקוּשׁ, טַרְכֵּשׁ m. (enlargement of טרך or טרק, v. טָרֵיף, a. טְרַק I) [*a wine-stirrer*,] *a board on which drinks for the table are mixed, side-board* (abacus, mensa delphica), *a plain board attached to the wall with hinges, to be put up and down* (cmp. הַלְפְּקִי, Kel. XXV, 1). Tosef. Kel. B. Bath. III, 3 ט׳ חלק (R. S. to Kel. XXV, 1 טרכוס וחלק) a plain tray (without rims). Ib. I, 12 ט׳ שעשה וכ׳ a side-board under which they placed a piece of wood, formed like a spear (as an improvised support) for eating at it. Tosef. Sabb. XIV (XV), 2 תרקוש ed. Zuck. (Var. ט׳, by cler. error מרקוש).

טַרְלוֹסָה pr. n. pl. *Tarlosa, Talluza*, near Samaria. Y. Taan. IV, 68ᵈ top מעברתא דט׳ the ford of T.

טרמוסיא, Midr. Till. to Ps. XIII, 5 באיזה ט׳ וכ׳; ed. Bub. תלמוסא, Ms. Vien. טל׳; Yalk. Ps. 660 תלמידא, prob. to be read: באיזו טולְמִירְיָא וכ׳ (τολμηρία) with what *hardihood* do you speak such words (of bad omen)?

טרמיות, v. טוּרְמִי.

טַרְמִיטָא, טַרְמִיטָן, v. טְרוֹמִיטָא.

טרמנסנה, טרמנמן, v. טוּרְמְנְטִין.

טרמסין, Snh. 14ᵃ Ms. M., v. טוּרְמִיסְך.

*__טְרַס__ *to search*. Lev. R. s. 37 טְרָסִין וכ׳ Ar. (Var. a. ed. פשפשין) they searched every ship &c.—[B. Kam. 98ᵃ, v. טְרַשׁ I.]

טֶרֶס m., pl. טְרָסִין, v. טֶרֶשׁ.

טַרְסָאָה m. nom. gent. *of Tarsus*.—*Pl.* טַרְסָאֵי. Targ. Esth. II, 21 (ed. Lag. טיר׳), v. טַרְסִי II.

טַרְסוֹס pr. n. pl., v. טַרְסִיס.

טַרְסִי I m. (v. next w.) [*a Tarsian*,] 1) *weaver of metallic thread, artistic weaver*, differ. fr. גַּרְדִּי.—*Pl.* טַרְסִיִּים. Ab. Zar. 17ᵇ Ar. a. Ms. Pes. (ed. תרס׳, v. Rabb. D. S. a. l. note 40). Succ. 51ᵇ וט׳ בפ״ע וכ׳ (v. Rabb. D. S. a. l. note 400) artistic weavers apart and common weavers apart; Tosef. ib. IV, 6.—Sabb. 47ᵃ מטה של ט׳ the weavers' horizontal loom or frame for embroidery (differ. in Rashi).—2) *worker in copper, bronze* &c. Ḥull. 57ᵇ מטלית של ט׳ the bronzers' apron.

טַרְסִי II, טוּרְסִי m. nom. gent. of *Tarsus, Tarsian*.—*Pl.* טוּר׳, טַרְסִיִּים. Meg. 7ᵃ בגתן .. שני ט׳ היו והיו מספרים Ms. M. (only בגתן .. שני טרשיים היו בלשון טרסי) Bigthan and Teresh were two Tarsians and conversed in the Tarsian language; ib. 13ᵇ שני ט׳ ... טורסי (Ms. M. ... תרסיים תרסי). Ib. 26ᵃ בה״כ של ט׳ Ms. M. (ed. טור׳; Tosef. ib. III (II), 6 אלכסנדרים) the synagogue of the Tarsians in Jerusalem (Rashi: of the bronze-workers, v. preced.). Y. Shek. II, 47ᵃ בח״כ של ט׳ (Yeb. 96ᵇ טבריא).

טרסיאות, read: סְרַטְיָאוֹת.

טַרְסִיי ch.=h. טַרְסִי I. Y. Gitt. VII, beg. 48ᶜ; Y. Ter. I, 40ᵇ (perh. proper noun).—*Pl.* טַרְסִיָּא, טַרְסִיִּיה. Y. Kil. IX, end, 32ᵈ.—Lev. R. s. 35, end כנישתא דט׳ וכ׳ the synagogue of the weavers in Lydda (or bronze-workers, or Tarsians), v. טַרְסִי II.

טַרְסִיס pr. n. pl.=h. תַּרְשִׁישׁ *Tarsis* (*Tarentum*). Targ. Y. I Gen. X, 4 טַרְסָס ed. Amst. (oth. eds. טרסים, v. אַלָּס); Targ. I Chr. I, 7 טרסוס ed. Lag.—2) (prob.) *Tartessus, in Spain*. Targ. Ps. XLVIII, 8. Ib. LXXII, 10. [V. טריסים.]

טְרַסְקָל m. (τρισκελής, τρισκέλλιον, sub. כסא) *a chair on three legs*, esp. *a camp-chair*. Num. R. s. 12; Tanḥ. Naso 19; (Tanḥ. T'rumah 9; Gen. R. s. 68 תְּרוֹנוֹס). Sabb. 138ᵃ כסא ט׳ (Ms. O. כסא וט׳).

טְרַסְקָל m. (a corrupt. of κάρταλλος, v. קרסטל) *basket*. Lev. R. s. 19; (Midr. Sam. ch. V קרסטל). Sabb. 5ᵃ. Ib. 53ᵃ תולין ט׳ לבהמה you may hang a basket with fodder around the neck of an animal.—V. next w.

טְרַסְקְלִין m. (κάρταλον, v. preced.) *a basket* (fiscellus) containing fodder, used *for muzzling*. Sabb. 53ᵃ bot.; (Tosef. ib. IV (V) 5 קרסטלין, Var. קרטלין). B. Mets. 90ᵃ (Ms. M. קרסטילין, oth. Mss. קרסטלין, קסרטל, v. Rabb. D. S. a. l. note).

טרסקמון, v. טְרוֹקְסִימוֹן.

טַרְעֲפִיקָא, v. טַרְפְּעִיקָא.

טָרַף (b. h.; cmp. טָרַד) [*to move with vehemence*,] 1) *to tear, prey*. Lev. R. s. 26 טוֹרֵף ואוכל tears in order to satisfy his appetite. Koh. R. to X, 11 'הארי ט the lion goes out for prey. Sot. 47[b] טוֹרְפֵי בֶּרֶךְ those robbing (the poor). Zeb. 53[b] חלקו של טוֹרֵף the territory of the tearer (wolf=Benjamin, Gen. XLIX, 27). B. Kam. 116[b] לְטוֹרְפָהּ to plunder it; a. fr.—2) *to cast with force, knock, strike against; to throw away, reject, eject.* Hull. III, 3 טְרָפָהּ בכותל he cast or knocked the bird against the wall. Pesik. R. s. 11; Num. R. s. 2 מגרשה אני טוֹרְפָהּ אני I will divorce her, I will cast her out (cmp. טָרַד).—Ber. 5[b] 'טוֹרְפִין לו וכ his prayer is thrown in his face (refused). Y. Yeb. XVI, 15[d] top טְרָפְנִי, v. טָרַד.—3) *to seize forcibly.* Yoma IV, 1 'ט בקלפי he took the ballot out with haste.—Esp. *to seize for a debt.* B. Mets. 15[a] ובא ב"ח וְטָרְפָהּ and a creditor of the previous owner came and seized it, v. טִירְפָא.—4) *to chop, hash, to beat, mix.* Sabb. XIX, 2 'ט יין ושמן beat wine and oil; a. e.—Part. pass. טָרוּף, f. טְרוּפָה. Ib. 38[a] 'בשר ט chopped meat. Ab. Zar. II, 6, v. טְרִית. Y. Nidd. IV, 51[a] (of a foetus). Sabb. VIII, 5 (80[b]) 'ביצה ט an egg beaten and mixed with oil; a. fr. V. טָרוּף.—5) *to hackle, comb* (flax or wool). Kil. IX, 1. Y. Orl. III, 63[a]; Y. Keth. VI, end, 31[a] צמר בכור שטְּרָפוֹ wool of a first-born that has been hackled (and mixed up with other wool).—6) *to scrape, scour, to plane.* Makhsh. II, 4 הטוֹרֵף את גגו (Var. הממחר) if one scrubs his roof; Tosef. ib. I, 8.—7) *to make* טְרֵפָה, *to inflict an organic defect.* Hull. 85[b], sq. צא טְרוֹף go and maim the animal (before slaughtering it).

Nif. נִטְרַף 1) *to become t'refah.* Ib. 9[a], a. e. במה נִטְרְפָה from what cause it became *t'refah.*—2) *to be in disorder,* a) (with דעה, or לב) *to be confused, bewildered, not fully conscious.* Y. Sabb. II, 5[b] bot. נִטְרְפָה דעתו של אבא my father's mind is unclear; Snh. 68[a]. Ib. 43[a] כדי שתִּטָּרֵף דעתו (not שתטרוף) that his (the culprit's) consciousness may be benumbed; Num. R. s. 10.—Ib. 'נ לבו his mind becomes confused (from drinking); a. fr.—b) (with שעה, of political disturbances) *to be troubled.* Snh. 11[a]; Sot. 48[b]; Tosef. ib. XIII, 5 נטרפה (ה)שעה the political condition was too much troubled (persecutions prevailing). Y. Dem. V, 24[d] bot.; a. e.

Pi. טֵרֵף 1) *to shake vehemently, constantly.* Succ. III, 9 כל העם מְטָרְפִין בלולביהן ed. Y. (Mish. ed. Pes. 'מט'את לול; ed. מנענעין) all the people shook their branches constantly (during the recitation at Hallel, contrad. to נענע).—2) *to unbalance* (the mind, cmp. טִלְטֵל).—Part. pass. מְטוֹרָף. Num. R. s. 10 'לבו מ' וכ his mind is disturbed and he talks improper things, v. supra.—3) *to reject one's petition, to refuse.* Part. pass. מְטוֹרָף. Ber. V, 5 'שהוא מ that he (the patient for whom prayer is said) is rejected (bound to die), opp. מקובל accepted.—4) *to disfigure, to make ungainly* by spots, incisions &c., v. טָרוּף). Part. pass. as ab. Koh. R. to X, 11 the serpent is asked 'מפני מה גופך מט why has thy body been disfigured (v. Gen. III, 14)?—5) *to cast about* (a ship on high sea), v. Hithpa.—Part. pass. as ab.; *pl.* מְטוֹרָפִים, מְטוֹרָפִין. Yeb. 47[a], v. סָחַף.

Hif. הִטְרִיף 1) *to become t'refah, to be afflicted with a fatal organic disease.* Num. R. s. 12, end; Cant. R. to VI, 4; Pesik. Vayhi p. 10[a], a. e. לא הִטְרִיפוּ the animals were found to be free from an organic disease.—[2) (in later liter.) *to declare t'refah.*]—3) (denom. of טֶרֶף) a) *to cover with foliage.* Yalk. Gen. 119, v. רָטַב.—b) *to sprout with moisture, be sappy.* Gen. R. s. 69 'ה' מצות וכ (Yalk. Jud. 38 הפריח) sprouted with good deeds &c., v. רָטַב.—[4) *to distribute food,* v. טָרַף.]

Hithpa. הִיטָּרֵף, *Nithpa.* נִיטָּרֵף *to be tossed about, to be in a storm* near the shore. Taan. III, 7 (19[a]) על הספינה 'הַמִּיטָּרֶפֶת וכ for a ship which is seen from the coast to be tossed about; ib. 14[a] הַמְּטוֹרֶפֶת (v. supra; Ar. ed. Koh. נִטְרֶפֶת *Nif.*). Tosef. Sabb. XIII (XIV), 11 נִיטָּרְפָה 'ספינה וכ the ship has been thrown back several times (was prevented from landing by the breakers).

טְרֵיף I, טְרַף ch. same, 1) *to take by force, seize.* B. Mets. 14[a] אתי . . . וטַרְפָהּ מינה (not וטרפא) the creditor came and took it from him (by legal seizure); ib. וקא טָרֵיף ליה מינה (Ms. H. וטַרְפָה מינה)—'ט לקוחות to seize property sold by the debtor, v. לָקוּחוֹת. Ib. 19[a]; a. fr.—2) *to throw, strike, knock down.* Y. Snh. X, 29[a] וּטְרִיף לון לארעא and let them fall down. Lam. R. to I, 5 וִיטְרוֹף גרמיה and let him throw himself down. Ib. to IV, 2 'טְרוֹף קולתיך וכ cast down thy pitcher before me; a. fr.—3) *to knock at, shake, rap.* Ber. 28[a] 'ט אבבא knocked at the door. Snh. 97[a].—Ib. 67[b] 'ט ליה בטבלא he struck the *tabla* before him; a. v. fr.—Trnsf. *to carp at, to contest the validity of a decision.* Y. Snh. I, beg. 18[a] בעי מִיטְרוֹף wanted to protest (against R. Isaac's decision because he acted as a single judge).—5) *to declare t'refah.* Hull. 10[b]. Ib. 48[b] סבר . . . לְמִיטְרְפָה Mar. . . . wanted to declare it *t'refah;* a. fr.—*Part. pass.* טְרִיף a) *struck down* (in the agony of death). Targ. Jud. III, 25; IV, 22 (h. text נֹפֵל). Lam. R. to IV, 5 טְרִיפִין בקיקלא (not טריפון) lying on dunghills.—b) *thrown away.* Y. Snh. X, 29[a] top הא טריפין לך they are thrown down before thee (cmp. טְרוּף).—c) (denom. of טרפא, v. טָרוּף) *spotted, full of incisions; planed.* Ned. 25[a]; Shebu. 29[b], v. טָרוּף.—[Y. Shebi. I, end, 33[c] א"ר יודן כד טריפן לעוביה, read with R. S. to Shebi. I, 8: א"ר יודן בר טרפון or טריפון, לעוביה being a corrupt tautography of לִיעֶזֶר בן יעקב=ליעז' ב"ר.]

Pa. טָרֵיף 1) *to knock, strike, dash.* Targ. II Kings VIII, 12 (h. text רטש). Targ. Nah. II, 8 (h. text תפף).—2) *to prey, wait for prey.* Targ. Prov. XXIII, 28 מְטָרְפָא.—3) *to drive about.* Part. pass. מְטָרַף. Targ. Y. I Ex. XIV, 3 (ed. Amst. 'מט *Ithpa.*). Targ. Y. II Num. XII, 12 מְטָרְפָא.—Trnsf. *to agitate, trouble,* v. infra.

Ithpa. אִיטְּרֵיף, *Ithpe.* אִיטְרִיף 1) *to be knocked about, dashed; to be tossed about; to be in spasms.* Targ. Is. XIII, 16. Ib. LI, 20; a. e.—Lev. R. s. 12 beg. בהד' אילפא 'דמִיטָּרְפָא וכ like the ship that is tossed about in the breakers &c. Snh. 95[a] אתו יונה אי' קמיה a dove came down and rolled before him in spasms.—Trnsf. *to be agitated, troubled.* Targ. Gen. XLI, 8 (some ed. 'מְטַר Part. pass. *Pa.*, v. supra). Targ. Ps. LXXVII, 5; a. fr.—Y. Taan. I, 64[b] bot. למה אִיטָּרְפִין . . להכא why did the rabbis (you) take the trouble of coming hither.—2) *to be spotted, full of incisions* &c., v. supra a. טָרוּף.—3) *to become,* or *be t'refah.* Hull. 57[b] במידי דמִיטָּרְפָה בה in the same limb through the mutilation of which the animal became *t'refah.* Ib. 48[a] דלאו מיניה מִיטָּרְפָא where the cause of its being *t'refah* lies not in the mutilated limb itself.

טְרַף II m., v. טַרְפָּא.

טֶרֶף m. (b. h.; preced.) 1) *prey.* Sot. 47[b], v. טָרַף.— Gen. R. s. 99 (ref. to מטרף, Gen. XLIX, 9) מִטַּרְפּוֹ של יוסף from making Joseph a prey, i. e. saving Joseph; מִטַּרְפָּהּ של תמר saving Tamar. Yalk. Ps. 637; Midr. Till. to Ps. VII, ed. Bub. יושב על טַרְפּוֹ (oth. ed. טְרֶפְתּוֹ) sits over his prey.—2) *food.* Snh. 108[b], v. next w.—3) (v. next w.) *foliage, green.* Sifra Metsora, beg. ובראשה ט׳ with green foliage on its top, v. next w.; Y. Sot. II, 18[a] top וראשה ט׳ (corr. acc., or read as Tosef. Neg. VIII, 2 טרוף).

טָרָף m. (b. h., preced.) *plucked, fresh*; (homilet., v. preced.) *nourishment.* Snh. 108[b] (ref. to Gen. VIII, 11) מאי משמע דהאי ט׳ לישנא דמזוני הוא what evidence is there that *taraf* has the meaning of food? Answ. ref. to הטריפני (Prov. XXX, 8); Erub. 18[b] (v. Rabb. D. S. a. l. note).

טַרְפָּא I, **טְרַף** ch. same, 1) *leaf.* Targ. Gen. VIII, 11. Targ. Is. XXXIV, 4; a. fr.—Hull. 47[b] ט׳ דאסא leaf of a myrtle; a. fr.—Nidd. 20[a] ט׳ מצירתא fem. (Rashi: מצירא), v. infra.—Trnsf. ט׳ דנחירי *wing of the nose.* Ber. 55[b].— *Pl.* טַרְפִּין, טַרְפַיָּא. Targ. Gen. III, 7; a. fr.—Succ. 37[b] נתרי ט׳ leaves may fall off. Sabb. 129[a] חמרא בר תלתא ט׳ Rashi (ed. בת) wine of a vine that has changed foliage three times, i. e. wine in its third year. Nidd. l. c. טַרְפָּן fem., v. הִדְרָא I.—2) *a piece torn off, fragment.* Ber. 59[a] top, and it looks כט׳ דטריף like an irregular piece that has been torn off (from the star); Rashi: like a battered piece that has been mended by hammering; (Ms. F. ומתחזי דמיטרפא מיטרף you can see that it has been torn off, Vers. in Rashi: כדטרפא מטרף, prob. to be read כטרפא דמִטַּרַף).

טַרְפָּא II f., constr. טַרְפַת (טְרַף) *rapping.* Targ. Jud. V, 11 (in a passage missing in ed. Lag.).

טרפא, Gen. R. s. 10 בקעת בר ט׳, v. נְטוֹפָא.

טְרָפָא, v. טִירְ׳.

טְרֵפָא, טְרֵפָה, v. טְרֵיפ׳.

טַרְפוֹן pr. n. m. *Tarfon,* a Tannai (v. Fr. Darkhé Mish., p. 101 sq.). Pes. X, 6; a. v. fr.—V. טְרִיפוֹן.

טרפונימיס, v. טְרַפִּיזִיטֵיס.

טרפזין, read: טְרַפִּיזִין.

טַרְפַּחַת f. (טפח, with ר inserted; cmp. טִפִּיחַ I) [*pitcher,* cmp. אָכוּז,] *mouth of the womb.* Hull. 55[b] = אֵם =שַׁלְפּוּחִית. Ib. 56[b].

טרפידא (טרפירא), Targ. Y. Lev. XI, 19, v. צַרְפְּדָא.

טְרַפִּיזָא m. (τράπεζα) *table, counter.*—*Pl.* טְרַפִּיזִין. Gen. R. s. 64, end ('Rashi': טְרַפִּיזוֹת).—V. טְרַפִּיזִין.

טְרַפִּיזִיטֵיס m. (τραπεζίτης) *money-changer, banker.* Y. B. Mets. IV, beg. 9[c] טרפוניטים (corr. acc.). Num. R. s. 4 טְרַפְּסִיטִים (cmp. τράπεσα for τράπεζα, S.).

טְרַפִּיזִין m. (τραπέζιον) *table, trencher.* Gen. R. s. 11 Ar., v. הִיסְקוֹס I.

טרפירא, v. טרפידא.

טַרְפִּישָׁא, v. טַרְפְּשָׁא.

טַרְפִּיתָא, f. (טְרַף) *hawk.* Targ. O. Lev. XI, 14; Deut. XIV, 13 (h. text איה).

טַרְפִיתָא f. adj. (preced.) *tearing.* Targ. Y. Lev. XI, 14 ט׳ הַיְיתָא (not דחיא); cmp. הַיָּה.

טְרַפֵּס, *Hithpa.* הִשְׁתַּרְפֵּס *to climb,* v. טָפַס.

טְרַפֵּס, *Ithpa.* אִשְׁתַּרְפֵּס (v. preced., cmp. טְפַז) *to leap, take exercise.* Y. Kidd. II, 62[c] bot. בעייא הוינא מִשְׁתַּרְפְּסָא אזלה מט׳ וכ׳ I expected to have exercise in going to and coming from the bath.

טְרַפְּסִיטֵיס, v. טְרַפִּיזִיטֵיס.

טַרְפֵּעִיק, טַרְפֵּעִיקָא (טרעפ׳) m. (corresp. to τροπαϊκός = Victoriatus) *Victoriatus* = Quinarius, half a denar (v. Zuck. Talm. Münz. p. 30). Yoma 35[b]. Gitt. 45[b]; Keth. 64[a] מאי ט׳ (not טרפעיקין) how much is a *T.?* Sifré Deut. 294; Yalk. ib. 938.—*Pl.* טַרְפְּעִיקִין. Keth. V, 7; Tosef. ib. V, 7 (missing in ed. Zuck., Var. טרפקעי; oth. ed. טַרְפְּעִיקִים).

טרפקעי, v. preced.

טַרְפְּשָׁא m. (טרף, with formative ש, as in טַרְעַשׁ; v. P. Sm. 1527 s. v. טרפשתא) *a rag-like, irregularly shaped organ, membrane &c.* Hull. 49[b] ט׳ דליבא pericardium with the fat attached to it.—*Pl.* טַרְפְּשִׁין *shreds.* Ib. 46[a] (in Hebr. dict.) נדלדלה כבד ומעורה בט׳ if the liver is detached and disarranged in shreds.

טָרַק (cmp. טָרַד, טָרַף) *to shake, stir.* B. Kam. 115[b] לא טְרָקוֹ nobody stirred, or mixed it.

טְרַק I ch. same, 1) *to stir, mix.* Sabb. 110[a] ולִטְרוֹקִינְהוּ בהדי הדדי let him mix them together.—2) *to stir up.* Taan. 25[a], v. אִסְקוּטְלָא I.—3) (prob. only in) *Pa.* טָרֵק *to sting, bite.* Sabb. 109[b] דְּטָרְקֵיהּ חיויא whom a serpent has stung. Ib. 110[a], v. חִוְיָא; a. fr.—[Yoma 77[a], v. מִטְרְקָא.]

טְרַק II (cmp. טְרַד II) *to bolt, tie, gird; to guard.* Targ. Ps. XXXV, 3, v. טרוקיתקא.—Ber. 28[a] טְרוֹקוּ גלי; Snh. 113[a] וּטְרַקֵיהּ לבבא וכ׳, דטרקיה, v. גַּלָּא. B. Mets. 83[a] and bolted the door before him. Erub. 102[a] דין לא נִטְרוֹק this must not bolt, i. e. with this bolt as it is you dare not bolt or unbolt. *Part. pass.* טָרִיק *locked up.* Targ. Job XXVI, 13 (h. text בָּרִחַ).

טַרְקָא m. (preced.; cmp. Syr. טרק, P. Sm. 1528) *a castle, palace.* Targ. Prov. XXV, 24 וביתא ט׳ though the house be a palace (h. text ובית חבר).

טְרָקָא m. (טְרַק I) *stirring up, disturbance.* Targ. Koh. X, 11 לט׳ ולנזקא (ed. Amst. a. oth. לִטְרָאְקָא) for disturbance and injury.

טרקאריך, טרקאירין, v. טְרַקְלִין.

טרקווינוס, Esth. R. beg. 'בימי ט; read: בימי חֵוְונִים.

טַרְקוּש, v. טַרְפַּשׂ.

טְרַקְמָה, טְרַקְמָא, v. טְרִיקְמָא.

טרקי, Yoma 10ª Ar., v. תרייקי.

טַרְקִיָא, טַרְקִין m. (Ar. s. v. בלס: תַּרְקְיָא; cmp. *anthracias*, ἀνθράκιον) name of a *gem*. Targ. O. Ex. XXVIII, 19 (Y. ערקין, corr. acc.); ib. XXXIX, 12. Targ. Y. Num. II, 18.

טרקילין, read: טְרִיקְלִין.

אִסְטַרְקְלִילָא, טַרְקְלִילָא m. (comp. of טְרַק II a. קלילא) *the runner's strapping, leggin, greave*. Targ. Esth. V, 9 אִסְטַרְקְלִילֵיה his leggin.—*Pl.* טַרְקְלִילִין. Targ. I Sam. XVII, 6 (ed. Lag. 'טְרִיקְל; Kimḥi Vers. טרקלין). [טרקלילין, Tosef. Sabb. XVI (XVII), 18; Tosef. Bets. II, 10 Ar., v. טְרִיקְלִין.]

טַרְקְלִינָא, טַרְקְלִין, v. 'טְרִיקְל. [V. preced. w.]

טַרְקְלָרִין m. (torcularium) *store-room for oil and wine*. Y'lamd. to Num. XX, 8 (quot, in Ar.) 'אם יהיה ט ביד אדם if a man possesses a torcularium; Yalk. ib. 763 (our w. omitted); Ex. R. s. 25, beg. טרקארין, טרקאררין (read: טַרְקְלָארִין).

טרקנין, v. טְרִיקְמָא.

טְרַקְסָאוֹת f. pl. (enlargement of טְרַק II, cmp. טְרַכְסִיד) *lath- and plaster-wall, partition in the interior of houses*. Tosef. Ohol. V, 5 'כלים שבט R. S. to Ohol. IV, 1 (ed. רסטקאות, Var. 'רטסק) vessels lying in niches or closets of partition walls.

טְרִיקְ׳, טְרַקְסִין m. pl. same, esp. 'אַמָּה ט *the two cedar-covered partitions*, with a vacant space between, which separated the Holy of Holies from the Holy and occupied the space of *one cubit*, the text (I Kings VI, 16) leaving it undecided from which of the two sacred areas that cubit's space was deducted. In the second Temple that partition was replaced by two curtains with a space between. Midd. IV, 7 'אמה ט one cubit for the partition. Yoma 51ᵇ 'אבל ... אמה ט' וכ but in the second Temple, where there was no partition wall, ... they made two curtains. B. Bath. 3ª; a. fr.—Y. Kil. VIII, 31ᶜ bot. (among doubtful things) 'ואמה ט (add to the above six things) the *ammah traksîn*. 'מהו ואמה ט why is it called *a. tr.?* (Answ., taking our w. for τάραξιν, acc. of τάραξις, confusion) טריכסון מהו מבפנים מבחוץ (ἐτάραξεν, cmp. ברבסון) it created confusion: what is it? inside? outside?; Y. Yoma V, 42ᵇ bot. טירקסון.

טרקסמון, v. טְרוֹקְסִימוֹן.

טְרַשׁ I (cmp. טרף) *to batter*. B. Kam. 98ª מחייה ..וטַרְשֵׁיה (Var. טרסיה, v. Rabb. D. S. a. l. note 300) he struck upon the coin with the hammer and battered it (so that the stamp was effaced).

Pa. טָרֵישׁ (denom. of טֶרֶשׁ) *to harden, make brittle*. Ḥull. 46ᵇ בקרירי לא דמְטָרְשֵׁי you must not put the lungs in cold water, because it makes the coat of the lungs brittle (so as to crack when you blow them up; [Ar. ed. Koh. 'בחמימי לא דמט not in hot water because 'it makes strong']; v. פְּנַן.

טְרַשׁ II (cmp. טְרַק II) *to lock up, obstruct*; (neut. v.) *to be stopped up*, (trnsf.) *to be deaf, silent*. Tanh. Vayishl. 8 'מחולתך טַרְשָׁא וכ, v. חָרֵשׁ; Y'lamd. to Lev. XXVII, end and to Num. XXI, 1 (quot. in Ar.).—Lam. R. to I, 17 [read:] 'ט' סלקית וט נחתית (not טמשא) silent do I go up (to Jerusalem) and silent do I go down.

טֶרֶשׁ m., pl. טְרָשִׁים, טְרָשִׁין (טרש I) *rugged, stony ground; crags, clefts; quarry*. B. Bath. 103ª 'ט' צאמרי the crags of which they speak (נקעים a. סלעים ib. Mish. VII, 1). Y. Kil. I, 27ᵇ bot. Arakh. 14ᵇ; Yalk. Lev. 677 טְרָשִׁין. Gen. R. s. 23 'נעשו ט became craggy (unarable). Lev. R. s. 36 'ט' גדולים large stony clods, v. בָּלַשׁ. Sot. 34ᵇ. Y. B. Bath. IV, 14ᶜ bot. 'חט' המוקצין וכ the rocks which are cut from it (the quarry).

טַרְשָׁא m. (טְרַשׁ II) [*deafness*,] (sub. רִבִּית) *deaf or silent usury, tarsha, a sale on time at a price higher than the seller would take if he sold for cash*, e. g. one sells beer in Tishri (when it is cheap), to be paid for in Nisan (when beer is higher) at the Nisan price. B. Mets. 65ª 'ט' שרי *tarsha* is permitted (is no usury). Ib. 'ט' דידי my (R. Papa's) *tarsha* (sale of date beer on time &c., v. supra). Ib. 'ט' דידי ודאי וכ my (R. Ḥama's) *tarsha* (selling goods to be carried at his risk to the dearer market, the money to be paid on returning) &c. Y. ib. V, 10ᶜ bot. 'אין זו רביתא אלא ט (not חטרשא) this is not direct usury, but it is *tarsha*.—*Pl.* טַרְשֵׁי. Bab. ib. 68ª 'ט' פפונאי, expl. 'כט' דרב פפא like the sales of R. Papa, v. supra.

טַרְשִׁי, v. טַרְסִי.

טַשׁ, טַשׁ, v. טוּשׁ.

טִשְׁטוּשָׁא, v. 'טִישׁ.

טַשְׁמַקְ׳* m. pl. [or טַשְׁמְקָא f. sing.] (= שקי תַּשְׁתִּ׳; cmp. מַצִּיקְקָא) *troughs*, or *bucket arrangement* for pumping water for the boiler. Nidd. 68ª 'אטו . . . ט' חסרת וכ Ar. (ed. omit אטו) dost thou want boilers? dost thou want buckets? dost thou want slaves? [Rashi: *bathing chairs*; Tosaf. to Nidd. 66ᵇ, a. v. אם, identifies our w. with טכטכא; Saadia: *combs*.]

טִשְׁטֵשׁ, טִשְׁטֵשׁ, v. טוּשׁ I.

טְשָׁא, טְשֵׁי (v. טוּשׁ II) 1) *to hide, protect; to reserve*. Targ. Ps. XXVII, 5. Targ. Prov. II, 1; a. e.—2) *to be hidden, lie in wait*. Targ. Ps. LVI, 7 יִטְשׁוּן בכמנא (ed. Lag. 'כמנא ר; h. text יצפינו, K'ri יצפונו). Targ. Prov. I, 11; a. e.—Taan. 24ª (הוו) טְשׁוּ מינרה they hid themselves before him. Ib. 29ª טשא מינידהו hid himself before the Romans. Ab. Zar. 70ª 'כי היכי דטְשֵׁינָא אנא אִיטְשֵׁי וכ as well as I hide myself here, an Israelite may have hidden himself &c.; a. e.

Ithpe. אִיתְּמְשֵׁי, אִתְמְשֵׁי *to hide one's self, to be hidden* Targ. Prov. XXVIII, 28. Ib. XXVII, 5 מְטַשְּׁיָא hidden. Targ. Ps. LXXXIII, 4 מִתְמַשְׁיִן (some ed. מִטַּמְּשִׁין).—Ab. Zar. 70ª, v. supra.

Af. אַמְשֵׁי *to hide.* Targ. Prov. XXV, 2. Ib. XXVI, 15.

מַשְׁיוּתָא f. (preced.) *that which is reserved, future compensation.* Targ. Ps. XVII, 14. Targ. Job. XX, 26.

י

י *Yod,* the tenth letter of the Alphabet. It interchanges with ו, e. g. יָדַע a. וְדַאי; with א as יבד a. אבד; with ה, v. letter ה.—י is frequently a *mater lectionis* for ē, ĕ, and ī, ĭ, e. g. לֵישֵׁב, לֵילֵךְ (for b. h. לָשֶׁבֶת, לָלֶכֶת); דִיבּוּר=דִּבּוּר, הֵיסֵב=הֵסֵב.—יי is frequently used to indicate the consonantal value of י, as הִתְיַירָא=הִתְיָרֵא.

י׳ as a numeral, *ten,* v. א׳.

יָא, יֵיא I=b. h. אַיֵּה. *where?*—לְיָא, לְיֵיא *whither?* Ber. 58ª, v. בְּאַנְגְּנָא. [V. לְיָיא.]

יָא, יֵיא II=וְהָא, v. הֲוֵי.

יָאֶה, יָאָה, v. יָאֵי.

יָאוּ, יָאֵי, יָי׳ pr. n. pl. *Yau, Yai.* Ḥull. 6ª פונדקא דיויאו Ar. (ed. דיאי, prob. to be read: דיאי) the inn of Yau (*I,* v. אִיתּוֹי II).

יָאוֹן, יָאֵין, v. יָאֵי.

יְאוֹר m. (b. h.; v. אֲרִיתָא) *channel, river,* esp. *the Nile.* Cant. R. to III, 4 (ref. to מיער with suspended ע, Ps. LXXX, 14) אם זכיתם מן הי׳.... מן היער if you will do good, the enemy attacking you will be (powerless like an animal) coming from the river, if not, he will be like a beast of the forest; Midr. Till. to Ps. l. c.; Yalk. Ps. 830; Ab. d'R. N. ch. XXXIV כחזיר של י׳ like a water swine (pork-fish, silurus). Ex. R. s. 1. Ib. s. 9 המים ששמרוך... לי׳ וכ׳ the waters which saved thee (Moses) when thou wast thrown into the Nile, must not be smitten through thee; a. fr.

יְאוֹרָא ch. same, *channel, dyke.*—*Pl.* יְאוֹרֵי. B. Mets. 103ᵇ אריסא בי י׳ (Ar. ביה), v. אַוְורָא.

יֵאוּשׁ, יֵיאוּשׁ m. (יָאַשׁ) *despairing of recovering a lost object, resignation.* B. Kam. 66ª י׳ אינו קונה the owner's resignation gives the robber no right of possession (and he must restore the object itself, not its equivalent). Ib.ᵇ ואי ס״ד י׳ קנה וכ׳ and if we should assume that resignation gives a right of possession, how could the robber say, Here is thy property before thee (since in the meantime it has become valueless)?—B. Mets. 21ᵇ top י׳ שלא מדעת unconscious resignation, i. e. a thing which, if missed, is usually given up, but which has as yet not been missed. Ib. הוי י׳ is considered as given up. Y. B. Kam. IV, end, 4ᶜ י׳ טעות a resignation under a false presumption; a. fr.

יְאוּשָׁא ch. same, *despair.* Targ. Job VI, 26.

יָאוּת f. h. a. ch. (יאי) *propriety;* adv., (cmp. כְּבָאוּת) *right; properly; it is right.* Targ. Ps. CXXVII, 2 על י׳ in propriety (honestly). Targ. Y. Gen. XXII, 10 כפוס. . י׳ tie me well. Targ. O. Deut. XIII, 15 (Y. טבאות, h. text היטב); a. fr.—Y. Ḥag. I, 76ᵈ top וי׳ הרי וכ׳ and it is right so; for there is the case &c.; Y. Peah II, 17ª וי׳ היא (corr. acc.). Y. Dem. I, 21ᶜ bot. י׳ הוא מקשי he asks a proper question; a. fr.

יָאוּתָא, v. יָאֵיוּתָא.

יָאֵי, יָאָה m. (h. נָאָה; v. אָוָה I, אוּת) *fitting, right, nice.* Targ. I Chr. XI, 11; Targ. II Sam. XXIII, 8; a. fr.—Men. 53ª; Yalk. Ex. 166 י׳ it is good; י׳ וי׳ (v. Rabb. D. S. to Men. l. c. note 40) so much the better. Tam. 32ª בימא י׳ למידר וכ׳ is it better to dwell on the water or on land?—Ib. לא י׳ למלכא כזב falsehood would not become a king. B. Bath. 111ª הוא י׳ וגולתיה יאיא Ar. (ed. וג׳ יאי) he looks nobly and so does his cloak; a. e.—*Pl.* יָאֵיִן, יָאֵין, יָאִין, יָאֵן. Targ. Cant. III, 7. Ib. IV, 1 sq. Targ. II Sam. XV, 3; a. fr.—*Fem.* יָאָה, יָאֲיָה, יָאֲיָא, יָאֲתָא. Targ. Y. II Num. XII, 1. Targ. Gen. XXIX, 17 (ed. Berl. יָאֲיָה; Y. II יָיָא). Targ. Jer. VI, 2 יאתא (ed. Lag. יָאֲיְתָא; h. text נוה). Targ. Prov. XIII, 19 (h. text נהיה); a. fr.—B. Bath. 111ª, v. supra.—*Pl.* יָאֲיָן, יָאֲיָין, יָאֲתָא. Targ. O. Gen. XXIX, 17 (ed. Berl. יָאֲיָן). Targ. Y. Num. XXXI, 50; a. e.—

יָאֵיוּתָא, יָאֵייתָא f. (preced.) *beauty, grace.* Targ. Prov. I, 9 ed. Lag. (oth. ed. יָאוּתָא). Ib. IV, 9. Targ. Job VIII, 6 יָאֵית constr. ed. Lag. (oth. ed. יָאֲיַת; h. text נְוַת).—Pesik. Baḥod. p. 109ª (ref. to אָנֹכִי, Ex. XX, 2) אנא נהורך כלילך יָאוּתָךְ I am thy light, thy crown, thy grace; Pesik. R. s. 21 יונתי (corr. acc.)

יָאִיָּא, יָאִיתָא, v. יָאֵי.

יָאִיר (b. h.) pr. n. m. *Jair,* 1) son of Manasseh. B. Bath. 121ᵇ. Num. R. s. 14; a. e.—2) J. the Gileadite. B. Bath. 113ª.—Denom. יָאִירִי, ch. יָאִירָאָה m. *Jairite.* Targ. II Sam. XX, 26 (missing in ed. Lag.).—Cant. R. to I, 2ᵇ; Erub. 63ª; a. e.

יָאֲיתָא, v. יָאֵיוּתָא.—יָאֲיתָא, v. יָאֵי.

יָאֵל=יָעֵל, v. הוֹאִיל.

יָאנָא, Y. Kidd. IV, 66ᵇ top את חמי מפייס י׳, read: אהחמי מפייסי ואנא וכ׳ act as if you did appease me, and I will allow him to get up.—Y. Kil. III, beg. 28ᶜ וי׳, read: כל הן דאנא משכח לה וי״ו אנא וכ׳ wherever I shall find it (*zeruëha*) with a *Vav,* I shall erase it; Y. Sabb. IX, 12ª top (corr. acc.), v. זֵרוּעַ.

יָאנִיבָא, v. יָנִיבָא.

יָאסִין, יָסִיאָן, יָאסִיין pr. n. m. *Yasyan.* Koh. R. to VII, 11 R. José b. Y.; Ab. Zar. 42ª; Bets. 8ᵇ יאסיין Ms. M. (ed. יאסניא׳ v. Rabb. D. S. a. l. note); Men. 6ᵇ (Ms. K.

a. R. 2 אסרין); Tosef. ib. I, 15; (Y. Succ. IV, 54c bot. יוסי בר אשיאן).

יָארוֹד, v. יָרוֹד.

יָאַשׁ (b. h.; cmp. אִישׁ a. יֵשׁ) [*to exist, be strong.*]

Pi. יִאֵשׁ (privat., cmp. דִּשֵּׁן) *to consider undone, to give up;* v. יֵאוּשׁ.

Hithpa. הִתְיָאֵשׁ, הִתְיַי׳; *Nithpa.* נִתְיָאֵשׁ, נִתְיַי׳ 1) *to lose energy, relax.* Y. Ber. IX, end, 14d שנתיָאֲשׁוּ ידיהם וכ׳ whose hands have grown lax concerning the Law (who do not care to uphold the Law; Midr. Till. to Ps. CXIX, 126 רפו ידיהם).—2) (with מן) *to give up hope, to discard from the mind.* Ab. I, 7 אל תִּתְיָאֵשׁ וכ׳ do not give up the idea of divine retribution (when you see sinners prosper).—Esp. (of lost things) *to despair of recovery, to resign possession* (by which the finder acquires the right of keeping what he has found, and the robber obtains possession of the stolen object and must make restoration in value). B. Kam. 68b, a. e. גזל ולא נִתְיָאֲשׁוּ הבעלים if one has robbed, and the owner has not yet given the hope of recovery. B. Mets. 21b מפני שהבעלים מִתְיָאֲשִׁין מהן because the owners (who dropped the coins) have given them up; a. v. fr.

יְאַשׁ, *Pa.* יָאֵשׁ ch. same, *to relax.* Targ. Koh. II, 20 לְיָאָשָׁא ית לבי על וכ׳ to relax my mind concerning (to give up thinking of) the trouble &c.

Ithpa. אִתְיָאֵשׁ 1) *to become careless.* Targ. Y. Deut. XXIX, 18.—2) contr. אִיָּאֵשׁ, אִיאָשׁ, *Ithpe.* אִיאַשׁ (איאוש) *to resign possession, give up.* B. Kam. 68b ודילמא לא איי׳ but may it not be that he has not resigned? Ib. שמעינהו דאיאוש they heard him say that he gave it up; B. Mets. 21b דמֵיאַשׁ (Ms. F. דאיאש). Ib. מְיָאֲשִׁי (Ms. F. a. R. מְיַי׳) they give it up. Ib. איאושי מיאוש (better: יָאוּשֵׁי מְיָאֲשָׁר, v. Rabb. D. S. a. l. note 8). Ib. 22a; a. fr.

יֹאשִׁיָּה, יֹאשִׁיָּהוּ pr. n. m. (b. h.) *Josiah,* 1) King of Judah. M. Kat. 25b (ref. to Am. VIII, 9) זה יומו של י׳ that is the day when J. was killed. Ib. 28b כמספד דר׳ וכ׳ like the lamentation over J. &c.; Meg. 3a; a. fr.—2) R. J. a Tannai. Men. 57b. Snh. 66a (v. Fr. Darkhé, p. 146, sq.).—3) R. J. name of two Amoraim (v. Fr. M'bo, p. 90b sq.). Y. Shebi. IX, 39a top. Y. Snh. III, 21d; a. fr.—Kidd. 36b, v. הָדָא I.

יָאתָא, v. יָאֵי.

יַב, v. יְהַב.

יָבָא, יֵיבָא (=יְהָא בָא) י׳ כי (=ch. אתיא כי, v. אֲתָא) *it agrees with, corresponds to.* Y. Sabb. III, 6b top י׳ כיי דמר ר׳ וכ׳ it agrees with what R. Z. said. Ib. XVI, 15c bot. יי׳ וכ׳. Y. Erub. VI, 23c top יי׳ כי וכ׳ (read כיי). Y. Pes. I, 27b top [read:] יי׳ כהדא דתני כ׳ זכריה; a. fr.—Y. Ber. I, 3a top יֵיבָה כיי דר׳ זעירא ed. Lehm. (oth. ed. יְהָא בָא כיי דמר וכ׳, ed. Krot. יהא בה).—Y. B. Kam. II, end, 3a יי׳ בתפלוגתה וכ׳ it enters into (depends upon) the difference of opinions between &c.; ib. IV, 4b top יי׳ כפלוגתא (read: כפ׳).

יָבַב (b. h.) [*to break forth,* cmp. רעע.]

Pi. יִבֵּב *to speak in a trembling voice, to lament.* Y. Yeb. XVI, 15d מְיַבְּבֵתוֹ בין המתים calling his name, in lamentation, among those of deceased persons; (Tosef. ib. XIV, 7 מַזְכִּירָתוֹ).

יַבֵּב ch. same; *Pa.* יַבֵּב 1) (=h. ריע) *to sound an alarm.* Targ. Num. X, 7; 9; a. fr.—*2) (=h. רעע) *to dash* waves against one another. Targ. Job XXXIV, 24 מְיַבֵּב Ms. Var. (ed. יתבר; h. text יָרֹעַ).

Ithpa. אִתְיַבַּב (=h. התרועע) *to shout.* Targ. Ps. LXV, 14. Ib. CVIII, 10.

יבבא, Targ. Y. Lev. XV, 19 some ed., read: יַתְבָא, v. יְתֵב.

יַבָּבָא, יַבָּבוּתָא, יַבַּבְתָּא f. (preced. art.) *sounding an alarm, alarm.* Targ. Num. XXIX, 1, quoted R. Hash. 33b. Targ. O. Num. X, 5 sq. יַבַּבְתָּא ed. Berl. (oth. ed. יבבא, Y. ed. יַבֶּבְתָּא). Y. ib. 10 יַבָּבוּ׳; a. fr.

יְבָבָה f. h. same, esp. *trembling, disconnected note (staccato).*—*Pl.* יְבָבוֹת. R. Hash. IV, 9 the value of a *T'ruah* (תרועה) כשלש י׳ is equal to three disconnected short notes. Pirké d'R. El. ch. XXXII; Yalk. Gen. 102.

יַבָּבוּתָא, v. יַבָּבָא.

יבבי, Targ. Y. Lev. XI, 20 דִּיבְבֵי, read: דִּיבְבֵי, v. דִּיבָבָא.

יַבֶּבְתָּא, יַבַּבְתָּא, v. יַבָּבָא.

יְבַד=**אֲבַד**. Y. Shebi. IX, 38d אפי׳ צפור ... לא יָבְדָא even a bird perishes not without the will of God; [Gen. R. s. 79, a. e. מתצדא, מצדיא, v. צדי; Midr. Till. to Ps. XVII אתיא (ed. Bub. אתאר); read: אתציד;] Esth. R. to I, 9; Koh. R. to X, 8 יברח (corr. יָבְדָה).

Pa. יַבֵּד *to ruin.* Targ. Prov. XII, 4 מְיַבְּדָא (ed. Wil. מְיבְדָא).

Af. יוֹבֵד, v. אֲבַד.

יְבוּל m. (b. h.; יָבַל) *growth, produce.* Ex. R. s. 12 י׳ הארץ the produce of the ground; a. e.

יבום, v. יִיבּוּם.

יַבּוֹלֶת, v. יַבֶּלֶת.

יַבְחוּשׁ m. (v. בָּחַשׁ) a sort of *gnat, a (red) insect* found in liquids. Tosef. Yad. (T'bul Yom) II, 3 י׳ שבריתו וכ׳ a *yabhush* which originates in the water.—*Pl.* יַבְחוּשִׁים, יַבְחוּשִׁין. Tosef. Ter. VII, 11; Hull. 67a. Nidd. III, 2 כמין י׳ אדומים looking like a mass of red insects; Tosef. ib. IV, 2. Zeb. 22a.

יְבִימָה, יְבִימָא, v. יָבָם ch.

יְבִימְתָּא, v. יְבַמ׳.

יָבִישׁ, v. יָבֵשׁ.

יַבִּישׁ, v. יָבֵשׁ ch.

יְבִישָׁה, v. יָבֵשׁ I.

יַבִּישְׁתָּא, יְבִישְׁתָּא, v. יַבֶּשְׁתָּא, a. יָבֵשׁ ch.

יָבַל I (b. h.) [*to break through, come forth, run, flow.*— V. יְבוּל, יִבְלָא &c.]

Hif. הוֹבִיל *to lead; to carry, bring.* Sifrê Deut. 43 (ref. to יבולה, Deut. XI, 17) אף לא מה שאתה מוביל לה not even as much as thou carriest to it (as seed); Yalk. ib. 869. R. Hash. 9ᵇ, v. הוּר ch.—*Part. pass.* מוּבָל *one carried, unable to move, feetless* &c. Toh. VII, 5 אפי׳ מ׳ אפי׳ כפות even if he is unable to move, even if he is tied; Tosef. ib. VIII, 7 והלה מוּבָל או כפות ed. Zuck. (ed. ממלאו, read: מוּבָל או); Y. Hag. II, end, 78ᶜ אפי׳ מאכל ואפי׳ כסות (corr. acc.). [For הוֹבִיל *to study,* v. בִּיל h.]

יְבַל, Af. אוֹבִיל, אֵיבִיל (הֵיבֵל), אַיְיבֵל ch. same. Targ. Ps. LXVI, 6. Targ. Is. X, 32 (v. infra); a. fr.—Erub. 27ᵇ, a. e. מוֹבִילְנָא מאניה וכ׳ I will carry his clothes after him to the bath-house. Snh. 95ᵃ (ref. to ינפף, Is. l. c.) מוֹבִיל ומייתי וכ׳ moving his hand to and back (= h. מוליך ומביא, v. בּוֹא); a. fr.—[Ezra V, 14; VI, 5.]—Y. Meg. IV, 75ᵇ bot. כד דאנן הרתרייתי מַיְבֵל וכ׳ when two scrolls are used, he carries one away and brings another in; Y. Sot. VII, end, 22ᵃ תרתיר תו מַיְיבֵל (corr. acc.); Y. Yoma VII, 44ᵇ top מייכל (corr. acc.). Y. Sot. l. c. מַיְיבְלִין, v. אוֹרַיְיא. Y. Taan. III, 66ᵈ bot. הוה מַיְיבְלָה וכ׳ (not מייבללה) brought it thither.—[Y. Ab. Zar. III, 43ᵃ ניבל, v. בִּיל ch.

Ithpe. אִיתּוֹבִיל *to be carried.* Targ. Is. XXXIX, 6.

יָבַל II, *Pi.* יִיבֵּל (denom. of יַבֶּלֶת) *to cut off dry twigs, warts* &c., *to trim.* Shebi. II, 2 מְיַבְּלִין מפרקין (Ms. M. a. Y. ed. מְזַבְּלִין, incorr.); expl. Y. ib. 33ᵈ top, v. יַבֶּלֶת.

יִבְלָא I m. (יבל I) = h. יָבָל, *cut, brook.*—*Pl.* יִבְלִין. Targ. Lam. III, 48 (Levita sing.)

יִבְלָא* II m. (נבל) *withered piece.*—*Pl.* constr. יִבְלֵי. Targ. Is. XLIV, 19, v. בְּלֵי II.

יַבְלָא m. (v. preced., a. יַבֶּלֶת) *a species of grass, Cynodon* (*Agrostis,* v. Sm. Ant. s.v., a. Löw Pfl. p. 183). Gitt. 68ᵇ bot. Ab. Zar. 28ᵃ bot., v. גִּירְדָּא I.—*Pl.* יַבְלֵי. Sot. 10ᵃ (quot. Rashi to Ab. Zar. l. c., ed. דובלא, read: דְּדִי׳); Num. R. s. 9 (sing.), v. גִּירְדָּא I. Hull. 105ᵇ כרך ריפתא אַיִּ׳ (not לריפתא) ate his meal so that the crumbs fell among the *yablé.* Ib. עקרינהו לְיַ׳ וכ׳ he tore the plants out and cast them &c.—Yoma 78ᵃ בְּדִיַ׳ in shoes made of *yablé* [Ar. בדיקולי, v. דִּיקוּלָא).

יבלונה, Y. Shebi. VI, 36ᵈ top, read: גּוּבְלָנָא.

יַבְלִית f. (v. יַבְלָא) *a pulp made of Cynodon leaves* and used for lining large water vessels. Kel. III, 6 (ed. Dehr. יִבְלִית); Tosef. ib. B. Kam. III, 2 יַבְלוּת (v. Löw Pfl. p. 186).

יַבְלָן m. (v. next w.) *one afflicted with warts.* Targ. O. Lev. XXII, 22 (ed. Berl. יַבְלָן).

יַבֶּלֶת f. (b. h.; נָבַל) *withered excrescence;* 1) *wart* on the skin. Erub. X, 13 (103ᵃ) חותכין י׳ וכ׳ (Rashi in ed. Sonc. יַבּוֹלֶת, v. Rabb. D. S. a. l. note) you may cut off (on the Sabbath) a wart of an animal in the Temple. Ib.; Pes. VI, 1 חתיכת יַבַּלְתּוֹ the cutting of its (the sacrifice's) warts; ib. 68ᵇ לחה (י׳) a moist wart, יבשה whose neck is dried up; a. e.—*Pl.* יַבָּלוֹת. Neg. VI, 7; Tosef. ib. II, 12 יוֹבלת (corr. acc.); Sifra Thazr., Neg., Par. 1, ch. II יַבּוּלוֹת, distinguished fr. תלתלים or דלדולים, v. דִּלְדּוּל.—2) *parasitic excrescences on trees,* or *withered twigs.* Y. Shebi. II, 33ᵈ top (expl. מיבלין, not מזבלין, Mish.) מעבירין את היַבּוֹלֶת to remove excrescences; v. יָבַל II.

יָבָם m. (b. h.) *husband's brother, brother-in-law* who in the case of his brother dying without issue enters his estate and marries his wife (Deut. XXV, 5, sq.). Lev. R. s. 20; Zeb. 102ᵃ יְבָמָהּ מלך her brother-in-law (Moses) was a ruler.—Yeb. IV, 3, a. fr. שומרת י׳ a widow waiting for the *yabam* to marry or reject her. Ib. III, 9 שעליה זיקת י׳ אחד who is tied to one *yabam,* v. זָקַק; a. fr.—*Pl.* יְבָמִין. Ib. שעליה זיקת שני י׳ who is tied to two *yabamim* (one *yabam* having died after having engaged to marry her, the surviving brother combines in his person the original duty of the *yabam* to his first deceased brother, and the subsequent duty falling upon him on his second brother's death). Ib. IX, 1 אסורות לִיבָמֵיהֶן are forbidden in marriage to their brothers-in-law. Ib. 52ᵃ שטר כתובת י׳ the deed of marriage for *yabamim.* Ib.ᵇ התקדשי לו במאמר י׳ be betrothed unto me by dint of the promise arranged for *yabamin;* v. מַאֲמָר. B. Bath. 119ᵇ פרשת י׳ the chapter relating to the duties of *the yabam* and *y'bamah*; a. fr.—Denom.

יִבֵּם, יִיבֵּם (b. h.) *to marry the wife of a brother who died without issue.* Yeb. II, 1 ואח״כ י׳ וכ׳ and afterwards the second brother married &c. Ib. 6 ואחד מְיַבֵּם and one of the brothers may marry her. Ib. IV, 5 או חלוץ או יַבֵּם either discharge (v. חָלַץ) or marry (her). Ib. מצוה בגדול לְיַבֵּם on the eldest brother the duty devolves (in the first order) to marry the deceased's widow. Ib. II, 7 לא יְיַבְּמוּ וכ׳ the other brothers must not both marry, but one discharges one, and the other &c.; a. fr.

Hithpa. הִתְיַבְּמָה, *Nithpa.* נִתְיַבְּמָה *to be married by the yabam.* Ib. I, 2 חולצת ולא מִתְיַבֶּמֶת she must take off the *yabam's* shoe, but cannot be married to him. Ib. 4 נִתְיַבְּמוּ if they have been married &c. Ib. 20ᵇ לא תִתְיַבְּמְנָה ought not to be &c. Num. R. s. 21 ואם לאו תִּתְיַבֵּם אמנו and if daughters are not considered as legal heirs, let our mother be taken in marriage by the *yabam;* a. fr.

יַבֵּם, יַיבֵּם ch. same. Targ. Gen. XXXVIII, 8. Targ. Deut. XXV, 7; a. e.—Yeb. 39ᵇ אי בעית יַיבֵּם if thou so desirest, marry her. Ib. אי צבית לְיַבֵּם יַבֵּם if thou consentest to marry, marry. Ib. 40ᵃ יַבּוּמֵי מְיַיבְּמֵי they must marry &c.—Ib. 31ᵇ וְנַיַיבֵּם לחדא וכ׳ let him marry one and &c.; a. e.

Ithpa. אִתְיַיבֵּם, contr. אִיַּיבֵּם as preced. *Hithpa.* Ib. 30ᵇ לְיִיבּוּמֵי (=לְאִתַּיַ׳) to be taken in marriage by the *yabam.* Ib. 32ᵃ תִּתְיַיבֵּם יַבּוּמֵי let her be taken &c.; a. e.

יְבָם, יְבִימָא, יְבָמָא, יֵי׳ ch. = h. יָבָם. Targ. Y. Num. XXVII, 4 נטרא י׳ (=h. שומרת יבם), v. יָבָם h.—Targ. Deut. XXV, 5. Y. ib. 9 יְבִימְתֵּהּ (יְבִימָא); a. e.

יְבָמָה f. (b. h.; v. יָבָם) *sister-in-law,* esp. *y'bamah,* *the widow of a brother who died without issue.* Yeb. IV, 10 הד׳ לא וכ׳ a widow must be neither discharged nor married before three months after her husband's death. Ib. 1 החולץ לִיבִמְתּוֹ he who discharges his sister-in-law. Ib. 2 הכונס את יבמתו he who marries &c.; a. fr.—*Pl.* יְבָמוֹת. Ib. V, 3; 5; a. fr.—*Y'bamoth* (the legal relations between Yabam and Y'bamah), name of a treatise of Mishnah, Tosefta, Talmud Babli and Y'rushalmi, of the Order of Nashim.

יְבָמוּת f. (preced. wds.) *the marriage of the yabam.* Yeb. 52[b] קידשה לשום י׳ if he betrothed her with the intention of complying with the law concerning the *yabam,* v. אִישׁוּת.

יְבִימְ׳, יְבִמְ׳, יְבִמְתָּא ch.=h. יְבָמָה. Targ. Ruth I, 15.—Targ. Deut. XXV, 7; a. e.

יַבְנֶה (b. h.) pr. n. pl. *Jabneh, Jamnia,* north of west of Jerusalem, seat of the Sanhedrin after the destruction of Jerusalem. R. Hash. 31[a], sq. Gitt. 56[b] תן לי י׳ וכ׳ give me (promise to spare) J. and her scholars; Ab. d'R. N. ch. IV.—Keth. IV, 6, a. fr. בכרם בי׳ in the college of R. Johanan b. Zackai in J., v. כֶּרֶם. Y. Sot. VII, end, 22[a].—Tosef. Dem. I, 13 אוצר י׳ וכ׳ the store of provision in J., inside of the fortification. Ib. 14; Tosef. Makhsh. III, 15; Y. Dem. III, 23[c] bot.; v. נָזָה.

יַבְקָא, v. יוּבְקָא.

יַבְרוּחַ m. *mandragora, mandrake* (v. Löw Pfl., p. 188).—*Pl.* יַבְרוּחִין. Gen. R. s. 72 (expl. דודאים, Gen. XXX, 14).

יַבְרוּחָה, יַבְרוּחָא ch. same. Y. Sabb. VI, 8[b] top; Y. Erub X, 26[c] וחהן דקרא על י׳ וכ׳ to read a Bible verse over mandrake is forbidden (as a superstitious practice).—*Pl.* יַבְרוּחֵי, יַבְרוּחִין. Targ. Gen. XXX, 14, sq.—Snh. 99[b].

יָבֵשׁ I m. (b. h.; cmp. בָּאַשׁ, בְּאוּשָׁה, אוּבְשִׁין, אַבְשׁוּנָא) *parched, dry, withered,* opp. לח moist, green. Dem. II, 3 לח וי׳ fresh or dried fruits. Ib. 5 בי׳ שלשת קבין wholesale dealing in dried fruits means three Kab. Y. ib. II, end, 23[a] לי׳ נתנו שיעור for dried fruit they make quantity the standard; a. fr.—*Pl.* יְבֵשִׁים, יְבֵשִׁין; יְבֵ׳. Sabb. IV, 1. Pes. II, 6; a. fr.—*Fem.* יְבֵשָׁה, יְבֵ׳. Ukts. I, 2; a. fr.—Tosef. Ter. VII, 16 נעשית י׳ the date became dry (so as to be called יְבֵישָׁה).—*Pl.* יְבֵ׳, יְבֵשׁוֹת. T'bul Yom III, 6 חמרים י׳, opp. רטובות; a. fr.

יְבֵישׁ, יָבֵשׁ ch. same. Targ. Josh. IX, 5; 12. Targ. Job. XIII, 25 (ed. Wil. יָבֵשׁ); a. e.—*Pl.* יְבֵ׳, יְבֵשַׁיָּא, יְבֵשִׁין. Targ. Ez. XXXVII, 2; 4.—*Fem.* יְבֶשְׁתָּא, יְבֶ׳שׁ׳. Gitt. 69[b]. Bets. 33[a]; a. e.—[V. יַבַּשְׁתָּא.]

יָבֵשׁ II (b. h.; preced.) *to be dry, to wither.* Bets. 26[b] מוקצה שי׳ stored fruits (v. מוקצה) which were dry (on Friday), though the owner did not find it out until the Sabbath day; Y. ib. I, beg. 60[a].

Pi. יִיבֵּשׁ *to dry up.* Gen. R. s. 33 עתיד . . . ולייבש וכ׳ in the future a righteous man (Elijah) will come and lay the world dry (through want of rain).

יְבִישׁ, יְבֵשׁ ch. same. Targ. O. Gen. VIII, 14 יְבֵישַׁת (ed. Berl. (oth. ed. יְבִישַׁת).—Y. Taan. III, 66[d] יְבֵשַׁת ידיה his hand withered. Gitt. 69[b] כי היכי דיביש הדא ידא וכ׳ (read דִּיבְישַׁת) as this hand (of the dead man) is withered, so may the milt of ..... dry (shrink to its normal size); a. e.

Pa. יַבֵּשׁ, יַי׳ *to dry.* Targ. Josh. II, 10.—Targ. Prov. XVII, 22; a. e.—Gitt. l. c. וְנִיַּבְּשִׁינְהוּ בטולא and let him dry them (the leeches) in the shade; a. e.

Ithpa. אִתְיַבַּשׁ, אִיַּיבַּשׁ *to be dried up, withered.* Targ. Ps. CII, 5 Ms. (missing in ed.). Targ. Y. Gen. VIII, 14; a. e.—Targ. Job XXXVIII, 11 Ms. (ed. חשור).—Gitt. l. c. נִיַּיבֵּשׁ ההיא טוחלא, v. supra.

יַבָּשָׁה f. (b. h.; preced. wds.) *dry land, shore.* Gitt. 56[b] עלה לַיַּ׳ he went ashore. Yeb. 121[a] וכשעליתי בי׳ and when I landed. Ber. 61[b]; a. fr.

יַבֶּשֶׁת f. (preced.) *dry fruits, dried vegetables.* Tosef. Shebi. IV, 16, contrad. to כַּבֶּשֶׁת.

יַבְשׁ׳, יַבִּישׁ׳, יַבַּשְׁתָּא f. ch.=h. יַבָּשָׁה. Targ. Gen. I, 9 (some ed. יַבֶּשְׁ׳).—Targ. Ps. XCV, 5; a. e.—Tam. 32[a], v. יָאַר.

יגא, Sifré Deut. 233, v. טוּגָא.

יַגְדִּי, v. יַגְרִי.

יָגָה, v. הָגָה.

יגוד, v. יָגַר.

יְגוּדְיָא pr. n. pl. *Y'gudya,* near Ascalon. Tosef. Ohol. XVIII, 15 ed. Zuck. (R. S. to Ohol. XVIII, 9 יְגוּר).

יָגוֹן m. (b. h.; יָגָה) *pain, grief.* Midr. Till. to Ps. CXLVII, end.—Tanh. Sh'mini 11 כי היין . . . והי׳ בא בלבו for when the wine leaves his body, grief enters his (the drunkard's) heart; a. fr.

יְגוּר, v. יָגַר, a. יְגוּדְיָא.

יְגַר״ל, v. יג״ל.

יְגִרַע v. יָגַע.

יְגִיעַ m. (b. h.; יָגַע) *painstaking, labor.* Ber. 8[a] הנהנה מִיגִיעוֹ he who enjoys the fruits of his own labor. Koh. R. to I, 3 כמה צער וכמה י׳ וכ׳ how much trouble and how much weariness does he experience. Midr. Till. to Ps. II וכל יְגִיעָן וכ׳ and all their toil is in vain; a. fr.

יְגִיעָה f. (b. h.) same. Gen. R. s. 10, end; ib. s. 3, a. e. לא בעמל ולא בי׳ וכ׳ (some ed. בְּיֶגַע) not with trouble and wearisome labor did the Lord create &c.—Y. Snh. X, 28[a] top לי׳; Koh. R. to XII, 12 לִיגִיעַת בשר for painful study, v. הִגָּיוֹן. Taan. 16[a] ויש לו י׳ בשדה has his labor invested in the field.—Lev. R. s. 19; Midr. Sam. ch. V לא שכר י׳ וכ׳ does not the Lord reward the work of studying?; a. fr.—*Pl.* יְגִיעוֹת. Ber. 58[a]; Y. ib. IX, 13[c] top כמה י׳ יגע וכ׳ how many labors did Adam have to go through &c.; (Tosef. ib. VII (VI), 2 כמה יגע). Lev. R. s. 28, beg. כמה י׳ הוא יגע; a. fr.

יג״ל, *Yagel*, a mnemotechnical acrostic, for יחיד offering of an *individual*, בגלל עצמה, being offered *by itself* (not as an attachment), לבונה requiring frankincense. Men. 51ᵃ Ms. K. (v. Rabb. D. S. a. l. note; ed. יגי״ל, the second י meaning יין requiring libation of *wine*, incorrect).

יָגַע (b. h.; cmp. יָגָה) [*to feel pain*,] *to take pains, to labor; to be tired.* Ber. 58ᵃ, v. יְגִיעָה. Y. ib. V, 5ᶜ אנו יָגַעְנוּ וכ׳ we have been busy at work for an entire day. Ib. זה י׳ לשתי וכ׳ this one has worked (accomplished) more in two hours &c.; Ib. כך י׳ .. בתורה וכ׳ so has R. Bun accomplished in studies in the twenty eight years (of his life) &c.; Cant. R. to VI, 2; Koh. R. to V, 11. Meg. 6ᵇ אם יאמר ... יָגַעְתִּי וכ׳ if one tells thee, 'I have toiled (studied) and achieved nothing', do not believe; 'I have not toiled and have achieved', do not believe &c.—Y. Ber. IX, end, 14ᵈ צריך לִיגַע בתורה must study the Law. Midr. Till. to Ps. XII, beg. חדלו מליגע בתורה they ceased from studying the Law; a. fr.

Pi. יִיגַּע, יִגַּע *to put to trouble, to weary.* Sot. II, 1 (14ᵃ) כדי לְיַגְּעָהּ (Rashi: לְיָרֵי) in order to wear her out (so that she may be induced to confess). Sifra Vayikra, Hobah, Par. 5, ch. VII אבל אם היה מְיַגְּעָן וכ׳ but if after having troubled them (the judges) an entire day, he says finally &c.; Yalk. Lev. 469 היה מוגע (corr. acc.); Tosef. Toh. VI, 14 ומשהגיע (read ומשהִגִּיעָן *Hif.*). Y. Bets. II, 61ᶜ bot. מתוך שאתה מְיַגְּעוֹ וכ׳ because you put him to special trouble (by ordering a special form of cakes) &c.—Ex. R. s. 41 התלמיד ... יִגַּעְתִּיךָ the pupil says to the teacher, I have wearied thee; Yalk. Sam. 161; a. fr.—Part. pass. מְיוּגָּע, pl. מְיוּגָּעִין, מְיוּגָּעִים. Keth. 8ᵇ ואתם אחינו המ׳ המדוכאין וכ׳ and you, our brethren, who are worn out and crushed by this bereavement.

Hif. הוֹגִיעַ (הִגִּיעַ) same. Tosef. Toh. VI, 14, v. supra. Midr. Till. to Ps. XXXIX, beg. (ref. to Mal. II, 17) הוֹגַעְתֶּם לי במעשיכם וכ׳ (ed. Bub., differ.) it does not say, you wore me out with your doings, but with your words. Ib. to Ps. XVIII, 36 והרב .... רב לך כי הוֹגַעְתִּיךָ and the teacher will say to the pupil, thou hast enough now, for I have wearied thee?; a. e.

Hithpa. הִתְיַיגֵּעַ, *Nithpa.* נִתְיַיגֵּעַ *to be tired, to take pains.* Gitt. 70ᵃ הבא בדרך וכ׳ who has been travelling and is tired. Pesik. Shub., p. 164ᵃ שלא תִתְיַיגֵּעַ בחזירה that you may not get tired on your way back. Pesik. R. s. 14 אני נִתְיַיגַּעְתִּי בה וכ׳ I took pains with her and smote her &c.; a. fr.

יָגֵעַ, יָגִיעַ, יָרֵ׳ m. (b. h.; preced.) *wearied, painstaking.* Ex. R. s. 13, beg. במה אני יג׳ of whom am I wearied?—Y. Hag. II, 77ᵇ bot. זה הוא הלשון שהיה י׳ וכ׳ is this the tongue which was wearing itself out with teaching the Law?; a. fr.—*Pl.* יְגֵעִין, יְגֵעִים, יְגֵי׳. Midr. Till. to Ps. XII, beg. י׳ בתורה studying the Law. Y. Peah I, 15ᵇ bot. ref. to Deut. XXXII, 47) ואם רק הוא מכם למה שאין אתם י׳ בו and if it (the word of the Law) seems to you empty, it is your fault, ... because you do not study it carefully; אימתי בשעה שאתם י׳ בו when (is it your life)? When you are busy studying it; Y. Succ. IV, beg. 54ᵇ; a. fr.

יְגָע m. (b. h.)=יְגִיעָה. Gen. R. s. 10, end, v. יְגִיעָה.

יְגַר m., constr. יְגַר ch.=h. אָגוֹר, *hill, heap of stones.* Targ. O. Gen. XXXI, 47 (Y. אוֹגַר).—*Pl.* יַגְרִין. Targ. Jer. IX, 10. Ib. XXVI, 18 (ed. Wil. יָגְרִין); a. fr.—Targ. Job XV, 28 יְגַר שַׂהֲדוּתָא.—יְגוּרִין pr. n. pl. (bibl.) *Y'gar Sahădutha* (Hill of Testimony). Tosef. Shebi. IV, 11 Var. (ed. Zuck. יגור סיכותא, read יְגוּר v. סְכוּתָא); Y. ib. VI, 36ᶜ (v. Hildesh. Beitr. p. 57, sq.).

יַגְרִי pr. n. pl. *Yagri*, in the district of Nivay (v. נִוַּאי). Tosef. Shebi. IV, 8; Y. Dem. II, 22ᵈ top יגדי.

יָד f. (rarely m.) (b. h.; יָדָה) 1) *hand; forefoot; handle.* Ex. R. s. 42, end מיד ליד from hand to hand, directly, opp. ע״י שלוחו through his messenger.—י׳ רחבה a wide hand, *liberality.* Y. Hag. I, 76ᶜ top עני וידו ר׳ a poor man who is liberal, opp. י׳ מעוטה stingy.—Hull. 58ᵇ, a. fr. בְּיָד on the forefoot (of a quadruped).—Ukts. I, 1 כל שהוא יד ולא שומר whatever part of a fruit serves as a handle (as the stem) and not as a protector (as the shell of a nut &c.). Kel. XXIX, 4 יַד הקורדום the handle of an ax; a. v. fr.—Cant. R. to I, 4 לא חלתה יד ליד hand does not fit hand, i. e. the two cases are incongruous.—Trnsf. *an intimation, an incomplete statement intelligible from context, surroundings* &c. Y. Ned. I, 36ᵈ top תופסין אותו משום יד לקרבן we make him responsible because what he said is suggestive of the word *korban* (as a vow); a. fr.—*Du.* יָדַיִם; *pl.* יָדוֹת. Yad. I, 1 נותנין לי׳ is required for pouring on the hands. Ib. II, 3 הי׳ מטמאות וכ׳ hands (when being washed) become unclean or clean up to the wrist; a. v. fr.—י׳ יפות, v. יָפֶה.—Ned. 2ᵇ ידות נדרים (or ידות) suggestions of vows, contrad. to כינויים, v. כִּינּוּי. Ib. 5ᵇ, a. fr. י׳ שאין מוכיחות לא הויין י׳ suggestions which are not beyond doubt, are no (binding) suggestions; a. fr.—2) *power, authority, possession, share.* B. Mets. 70ᵇ, v. אֶצְבַּע. Kidd. 3ᵇ קטנה דלית לה יד וכ׳ a minor who cannot accept a betrothal for herself. Ned. 88ᵇ יד אשה כיד בעלה the wife's possession is her husband's possession. Kidd. 23ᵃ גיטו וידו באים כאחד his letter of manumission and his right of self-disposal come simultaneously. Yeb. 39ᵃ; Keth. 83ᵃ ידו כְּיָדָהּ the husband's right of disposal is as great as the wife's (concerning what belongs to her); ידו עדיפא מידה his rights are stronger than hers. B. Mets. VI, 2 יָדָן על התחתונה their rights are the lowest, i. e. they are responsible for losses but can derive no benefits from favorable chances; ib. כל המשנה ידו על התחתונה וכ׳ whichever side changes the agreement is at a disadvantage, and whichever side breaks the agreement &c.; a. v. fr.—*Du.* יָדַיִם, constr. יְדֵי. Ab. Zar. 41ᵇ, a. e. מִידֵי וראי, v. וַדַּאי.—יְדֵי חובתו, v. יָצָא.—3) *portion, part.*—*Pl.* יָדוֹת. Tosef. Men. IX, 10 שתי י׳ two thirds; a. fr.—מִיָּד (=מיד ליד) *at once, directly, immediately.* Tosef. Dem. VIII, 7, v. חָלַל *Hif.*—Y. Pes. VI, 33ᵃ מיד כל מי וכ׳ presently, every one whose Passover offering was a lamb &c.; a. v. fr.—

על יְדֵי, עַל יַד (abbr. ע״י) *through, by means of.* Gitt. 40[b] שמא זיכה לו ע״י אחר he may have benefitted him (given him his liberty) through the agency of another person (without the slave's knowledge). Nidd. I, 1 מעת לעת ממעטת ע״ו וכ׳ the period of twenty four hours is modified by the interval between one examination and the other (if that interval is less than twenty four hours); a. v. fr.— על ידי ש־ *because.* Lev. R. s. 32 ע״י שגדרו וכ׳ because the Israelites guarded themselves against unchastity, they were redeemed; a. v. fr.—עַל יַד עַל יַד *gradually, little by little.* B. Kam. 80[a] (opp. מיד); Tosef. ib. VIII, 15. Par. VIII, 7 Hai G. (ed. only once ע״י).—כלאחר יד, v. אַחַר.—יָדַיִם *Yadayim*, name of a treatise of the Mishnah and Tosefta, of the Order of Toh'roth, containing the laws of levitical cleanness or uncleanness of the hands.

יְדָא, יַד ch. same. Targ. Num. XXXV, 17; a. fr.— V. אִידָא.—Kidd. 30[a] top אַדִּיָּדָךְ על וכ׳ while thy hand yet rests on thy son's neck (as long as you have control over him). Ab. Zar. 15[a] אִיָּדָא דספסירא (=h. על ידי) through an agent; a. fr.—*Pl.* יְדַיָּא, יְדִין. Targ. Ez. XXI, 12 (ed. Wil. יְדִין). Targ. Is. XIII, 7; a. fr.—עַל יְדֵי, עַל יַד, v. preced. Targ. Ps. LXXXIX, 20. Targ. Y. Num. XXXIII, 1; a. fr.— על יְדֵי ד־=h. ע״י ש־. Targ. Y. II Gen. XLIV, 18.—מִן יַד, מִיַּד, v. preced. Targ. Y. Gen. I, 3. Targ. Ps. LIX, 12; a. e.

***יְדַד** pr. n. pl. *Y'dad*, Y. M. Kat. III, 82[a].

יְדָה, v. ידי.

יַדּוּעַ, (b. h.) pr. n. m. *Jaddua.* B. Mets. VII, 9 J. the Babylonian.

יְדוּעַ m. name of *a bird* (Maim.) or *a beast* (Rashi), a bone of which is used for witchcraft. Targ. Y. Lev. XIX, 31 (ed. Amst. יָדוּעַ); a. e.—Snh. 65[b]; (Tosef. ib. X, 6 ידעוני).

יָדוּעַ, v. יָדַע.

יָדָה, ידי (b. h.) *to point, move* (cmp. b. h. הָדָה).—Denom. יַד.

Hif. הוֹדָה [*to raise hands,*] 1) *to thank, acknowledge; to give praise.* Taan. 6[b] מוֹדִים ... לָךְ we offer thanks unto thee. Ber. V, 3 he who says in public prayer מודים מודים...אותו 'we thank, we thank' (as if pointing in different directions and acknowledging two divinities) must be silenced. Ib. IX, 5 (play on מְאֹדֶךָ, Deut. VI, 5) בכל מִדָּה ומדה ... הוי מוֹדֶה לו for whatever measure He metes out to thee, give thanks to Him. Ib. 54[b] ארבעה צריכין להודות four persons are bound to offer public thanks; a. v. fr.—2) *to admit, consent, to confess.* Pes. IV, 9 (56[a]); Ber. 10[a] על ג׳ הודו לו concerning three of his acts they agreed with him. B. Mets. 3[a], a. fr. מוֹדֶה במקצת הטענה he who admits part of his opponent's claim. Shebu. VI, 3; Keth. 108[b], a. e. טָעֲנוֹ...והוֹ׳ לו בשעורים, v. טָעַן I. B. Mets. 12[b] בשחייב מודה when the debtor admits his indebtedness; a. v. fr. [Tosef. Par. IX (VIII), 6 שהן מודין, v. מוּרִיר.]

Hithpa. הִתְוַדָּה, *Nithpa.* נִתְוַדָּה, (denom. of הוֹדָה, cmp. Josh. VII, 19) *to confess* one's sins before God. Yoma III, 8 ומִתְוַדֶּה and confesses in public. Ib. 40[a] להגריל ולהִתְוַדּוֹת to cast lots and to make confession (on the head of the scapegoat). Y. ib. VIII, end, 45[c] אע״פ שנ׳ בערבית צריך להתוודות וכ׳ although he has made confession in the evening prayer, he must again confess &c.; a. fr.—V. וִידּוּי.

יְדֵי, *Pa.* וַדֵּי, *Ithpa.* אִתְוַדֵּי ch. same, *to confess.* Targ. O. Lev. V, 5 (Y. יוֹדֵי *Af.*). Targ. Y. II Deut. III, 29 מִתְוַדְּיִן; a. e.

Af. אוֹדִי, הוֹדִי as preced. *Hif.* Targ. Prov. XXVIII, 13.— Targ. Gen. XLIX, 8; a. fr.—Yoma 7[a] מוֹדֵינָא I admit (agree). Keth. 85[a] ומוֹדְיָא and she may admit her debt.—Ber. 54[b] צריך לאוֹדוּיֵי וכ׳ he must offer thanks in the presence of &c.—Shebu. 39[b] כפר במקצת וא׳ במקצת if he denies part and admits part of the claim; a. fr.

יְדִיד m. (b. h.; redupl. of ידי; cmp. הוֹד) [*pointed out,*] *chosen, beloved; chosen spot.* Men. 53[a] יבא י׳ בן י׳ ויבנה י׳ ... ויתכפרו בו ידידים ... the beloved (Solomon), son of the beloved (Abraham), shall rise and build a chosen structure (Temple) to the beloved (the Lord) in the lot of the beloved (Benjamin), that in it the chosen ones (Israel) be atoned for. Y. Ber. IX, 14[a] bot.; Sabb. 137[b] (benediction on circumcision) אשר קידש י׳ מבטן who sanctified the chosen one (Abraham, Is. XLI, 8; others: Isaac, with ref. to Gen. XXII, 2) from the womb.—*Pl.* יְדִידִים, v. supra.

יְדִידוּת f. (b. h.; preced.) *choice; the chosen people.* Y. Ber. IX, 14[a] bot.; Sabb. 137[b] י׳ (זרע קודש) שארנו the chosen (of the holy seed) of our blood (race).

יְדִיעָה f. (יָדַע) *knowledge,* esp. (Lev. IV, 14; 23; 28) *finding out, discovery, consciousness.* Shebu. 5[a], a. e. יְדִיעַת בית רבו שמה י׳ the knowledge acquired in the teacher's house (a theoretical knowledge that one who touches an unclean thing becomes unclean &c.) is also called a knowledge (as regards the applicability of the verb נעלם). Ker. IV, 2 אם היתה י׳ בנתיים if there was consciousness between the two acts (if he found out his first transgression before committing the second). Shebu. I, 2 י׳ בתחלה וי׳ בסוף והעלם בנתיים original consciousness (knowing that he became unclean) and final consciousness (finding out that he had eaten sacred things in uncleanness) but forgetfulness between. Hor. 2[a], a. fr. השב מִידִיעָתוֹ he who regrets when he finds out his transgression; a. fr.—*Pl.* יְדִיעוֹת. Sheb. I, 1 י׳ הטומאה the laws concerning the discovery of having sinned through uncleanness; ib. II, 1; a. fr.

יְדִיעֲתָא ch. same, *knowledge.* Targ. Prov. I, 4. Ib. XXII, 17; a. fr.

יָדַע (b. h.; cmp. יָדָה) [*to point out, select, love,*] 1) *to recognize, know; to find out.* Pes. 87[b] כיון שי׳ שחטא when he was convinced that he had done wrong. Ib. ואין אתה יוֹדֵעַ אם וכ׳ and thou knowest not whether &c. Ib. יודע הקב״ה את ישראל וכ׳ the Lord knows that Israel cannot endure the cruel persecutions of Rome (v. Rabb. D. S. a. l. note); Yalk. Hos. 529. Shebu. 4[b]; ib. 5[a] ונעלם מכלל שי׳ it says, 'and it escaped his memory' (Lev. V, 3)—this proves that there was a time when he knew (the nature of his act, v. יְדִיעָה). Zeb. 115[b] דבר זה ... ולא יְדָעוֹ וכ׳ this word (Ex. XXIX, 43) the Lord had said to Moses, but he did not understand it, until the sons of Aaron died. Ib. כיון שי׳ ... יְדוּעֵי מקום הן when Aaron learned that his sons were the chosen of the Lord (Lev. X, 3); a. v. fr.—*Part. pass.* יָדוּעַ a) *chosen. Pl.* יְדוּעִים, constr. יְדוּעֵי, v. supra.—b) *known, special, certain.* Sifra Vayikra, Ḥobah, Par. 6, ch. VIII חטא י׳ a known (discovered) sin, v. יְדִיעָה. Y. Sot. I, 16ᶜ טומאה יְדוּעָה (not ידוע) an ascertained levitical uncleanness, opp. ספק; a. fr.—בְּיָדוּעַ *it is sure.* R. Hash. 20ᵇ בי׳ שנראה וכ׳ the moon must have been visible &c. Succ. 49ᵇ כל אדם . . . בי׳ שהוא וכ׳ a popular man (v. חֵן) is, you may be sure, a God-fearing man; a. fr.—2)(euphem.) *to have sexual intercourse with.* Yeb. 57ᵃ בלא יְדָעָהּ when he never had connection with her. Esth. R. to III, 7 שלא יְדָעָהּ איש וכ׳ whom no man except her husband touched; a. e.

Hif. הוֹדִיעַ *to make known, inform.* Gen. R. s. 22, beg. (ref. to Gen. IV, 1, reading יָדַע for homiletical purposes) ה׳ דרך ארץ לכל he showed to all the way of the land (propagation, v. דֶּרֶךְ). Hull. V, 3 צריך להוֹדִיעַ must inform (the purchaser). Ab. IV, 22 לֵידַע להודיע ולְהִוָּדַע to learn, to proclaim and to be made to feel (be thoroughly convinced). Sabb. 10ᵇ צריך להוֹדִיעוֹ must inform him. Ib. לך והוֹדִיעֵם go and tell them. Ib. הנותן . . . צריך לה׳ לאמו he who gives bread to a child must inform his mother; a. fr.

Hof. הוּדַע *to be informed, become conscious; to be made known.* Shebu. I, 6 ה׳ ולא ה׳ whether he became conscious (of his transgression) or not. Sifra Vayikra, Ḥobah, ch. XX, Par. 12 (ref. to Lev. IV, 23; 28) את ה׳ שלהם when they become known; a. fr.—B. Bath. 113ᵇ הוּדְעָה Ms. M. (v. אֲרַע II).

Nif. נוֹדַע same. Hor. III, 3. Ab. IV, 22, v. supra. Shebu. 9ᵇ שסופו לִיוָּדַע of which he is likely to be informed. Hull. 9ᵃ עד שיִוָּדַע לך, v. חֲזָקָה. Nidd. IX, 5, v. infra; a. fr.

Hithpa. הִתְוַודַּע, *Nithpa.* נִתְוַודַּע 1) same. Bekh. 25ᵇ עד שיִתְוַודַּע הטומאה (Nidd. l. c. עד שיודע לך וכ׳) until he ascertains the exact place of uncleanness; Pes. 10ᵃ עד שתִּוָּדַע לך Ms. M. (v. Rabb. D. S. a. l.). Y. Sabb. III, 6ᵇ ניתודע לו וכ׳ he found it out after sunset; a. fr.—2) (v. מוֹדַע) *to force one's self upon the notice of, to pretend friendship for.* Ab. I, 10 אל תִּתְוַדַּע לרשות do not make thyself a partisan of the (foreign) government.

יְדַע ch. same. Targ. Gen. IV, 1; a. fr.—Ib. XXX, 26; a. fr.—Fut. יִדַּע, יִנְדַּע (fr. נדע). Targ. Ps. XXXIX, 5 אִידַּע Ms. (ed. אֵידַע). Targ. Ex. VIII, 6; a. fr.—Ber. 33ᵇ אנא לא הא׳ יָדַעְנָא I learned nothing either about this &c. Snh. 103ᵃ (prov.—of one who derives no lesson from adversity or success) בכיר ליה למר ולא י׳ וכ׳ Ms. M. (ed. דלא, v. Rabb. D. S. a. l.) they lament to you and you understand it not, they laugh to you and you understand it not; וי ליה למאן דלא י׳ וכ׳ (not למר) woe to him who knows not the difference between good and evil; a. fr.

Af. אוֹדַע, הוֹדַע as preced. *Hif.* Targ. Ex. XXXIII, 13. Targ. Ps. CVI, 8 לאוֹדָעָה (Ms. לְאַנְהָ׳, v. supra); a. fr.—Snh. 11ᵇ מְהוֹדְעִין אנחנא וכ׳ we (the Sanhedrin) notify you &c.; Y. ib. I, 18ᵈ top מוֹדְעִנָא. Tosef. ib. II, 6 מְהוֹדְעִנָא (Var. מְהוֹדְעֵי אנחנא). Sabb. 33ᵇ מאן לוֹדְעֵיה לבר וכ׳ (Ms. M. מוֹדְעֵיה) Oh, that some one would inform the son of Yoḥai &c. Ned. 62ᵃ לאוֹדוּעֵי נפשיה to make one's self known (as a scholar). Gen. R. s. 11 מנאן את מוֹדַע לי (some ed. מְיַדַּע) how will you prove it to me?; a. fr.

Pa. יַדַּע same. Cant. R. to III, 6 לינא מְיַדַּע לדין וכ׳ shall I not let him know with whom he is dealing?. Gen. R. s. 11, v. supra.—*Part. pass.* מְיַדַּע *friend.* Targ. Ps. LXXXVIII, 9 מְיַדְּעַי Ms. (ed. מיודעי, hebraism).

Ithpe. אִתְיְדַע, *Ithpa.* אִתְיַדַּע *to be made known, to make one's self known.* Targ. O. Gen. XLV, 1. Ib. XLI, 21; a. fr.—[Targ. Y. Deut. XXI, 11 תתידעון, read: תיתרעון, as in v. 14.]—Hor. 2ᵃ כי מִתְיַדַּע להו לבי דינא if the court were made aware of it. Sabb. 71ᵇ א׳ ליה קודם וכ׳ he became aware of it before setting the sacrifice aside; a. e.

יִדְּעוֹנִי m. (b. h.; יָדַע) *sooth-sayer, charmer.* Snh. 65ᵇ; Tosef. ib. X, 6, v. יָדוּעַ; a. e.

יְדַעְיָה (b. h.) pr. n. m. *Jedaiah,* 1) a priestly division, named after its head. Taan. 27ᵃ, sq.; Arakh. 12ᵇ. Y. Taan. IV, 68ᵈ.—2) poetic name of *Sepphoris* in Galilee whither the division of J. was exiled (v. Y. l. c.). Koh. R. to VII, 11; IX, 10 בני י׳ sons of J. (inhabitants of Sepph.).

יְדֻפַּת, v. יוֹדְפַת.

יְדֻקֶרֶת, v. יוֹדְקֶרֶת.

יָהּ (b. h.) *Yah,* abbreviation of the Tetragrammaton. Succ. IV, 5 (45ᵃ, missing in Ms. M., v. marginal note to ed.); Tosef. ib. III, 1 לְיָהּ ולך מזבח unto Yah and unto thee, O altar (do we give praise); Succ. 45ᵇ ליה אנחנו מודים ולך וכ׳ to Yah we offer thanks and thee (altar) we praise. Ib. V, 4 (51ᵇ) אנו ליה וליה עינינו we are Yah's and to Y. we lift up your eyes. Gen. R. s. 79, end, v. דְּקִינְתִּין; a. e.

יָהּ II (interj.) *Oh!* exclamation of distress. Gen. R. s. 92 (play on יה, Ps. XCIV, 12).

יְהַב (h. יָהַב) *to give.* Targ. Gen. III, 12. Targ. Job III, 19 יִיהַב Ms. (ed. יְהִיב, ed. Wil. יְהִיב); a. fr.—Part. pass. יְהִיב. Targ. Num. III, 9; a. fr.—Imperative הַב. Targ. Gen. XXX, 26; a. fr.—Y. Ber. VIII, 11ᵇ bot., a. fr. י׳ ליה מילא gave him assurance of safety. Ib. יהב את פלגא (read as:) Y. Naz. V, end, 54ᵇ הב וכ׳ give thou half of it. Ib. [read:] אמר דייבין ליה יְהָבוּ ליה ואכל he ordered that they give him (to eat); they gave him, and he ate. Kidd. 9ᵃ אי יהבינא לך וכ׳ (read: יָהֲבִינָה) if I give it to thee, wilt thou be betrothed unto me? Said she הָבָה מֵיהֲבָה give it; כל הבה מיהבה וכ׳ all such phrases as 'give it', mean nothing (do not mean assent to the proposal); a. v. fr.—וי׳ נסב (h. = נשא ונתן) *to deal.* Cant. R. to III, 6. Y. Shebi. VII, 37ᶜ top; a. e.—Lev. R. s. 19, v. infra.—2) *to put, place.* Targ. Ex. XVI, 33; a. fr.—Y. Keth. XII, 35ᵃ bot. אין אנן יָהֲבִין ליה נִיהֲבִיה וכ׳ if we put him (his coffin) anywhere, we must put him with R. &c.; a. fr.

Ithpa. אִתְיְהַב, *Ithpe.* אִתְיְהִיב *to be given.* Targ. Is. IX, 5. Targ. Ex. V, 16; a. fr.—Kidd. 7ᵃ משום דא׳ למחילה because it (money or money's worth) may be given away without consideration; v. נְתַן.—[Lev. R. s. 19 ... תתיהב דיהבת וכ׳, read: תִּתְיְהַב .. דִּיהַבְתְּ, v. יָהַב I.]

יְהָבָא m. (= b. h. יְהָב; preced.) [*that which is put on,*] *bundle, load* on the back. R. Hash. 26ᵇ; Meg. 18ᵃ (as an analogy to יהב, Ps. LV, 23) the Arab said, שקול יְהָבִיךְ

וכ׳ take off thy bundle and put it on my camel; Gen. R. s. 79, end תלי הדין ר׳ עלי help me to put my load on; שמעון מינה ר׳ משור from this they learned that *y'haba* means *load.*

יְהָבַת, יְהָבִית f. constr. (preced. wds.) *giving; share, dispensation.* Targ. Koh. V, 10 יהבית אגרהא=h. מַתַּן שָׂכָר. Targ. Ps. XI, 6 (h. text מנת).

יַהֲדוּת f. (v. יְהוּדִי) *Jewish religion, monotheism.* Esth. R. to III, 7 והחזיקו בִּיַהֲדוּתָן (not ביהודתן) and clung to their creed.

יֵהוּא (b. h.) pr. n. m. *Jehu,* King of Israel. Meg. 14ᵃ. Hor. 11ᵇ אַף ר׳.. לא נמשח וכ׳ Jehu, too, would not have been anointed, but for the opposition to Joram; a. e.

יְהוּד pr. n. *Judaea.* Dan. II, 25; a. e.—Lam. R. to I, 2 ר׳ מדינתא the province of J.

יְהוּדָא=יְהוּדָה.

יְהוּדַיי, יְהוּדַאי, יְהוּדָאָה m. ch.=h. יְהוּדִי. Targ. Esth. V, 13; a. e.—Y. Shebi. IV, 35ᵇ top, v. אֲרַמַּאי.—*Pl.* יְהוּדָאֵי, יְהוּדָאֵי, יְהוּדָאִין. Targ. Esth. IV, 16; a. e.—Gen. R. s. 63 רברבני דר׳ the leaders of the Jews (of Tiberias); a. fr.—*Fem.* יְהוּדָאִיתָא. Targ. II Esth. IV, 1.—Lam. R. to I, 11 חזיין אפיך כר׳ (not כיהודייאתא) thou lookest like a Jewess.—V. יוּדַאי.

***יְהוּדָאִיקִי** f. (Ἰουδαϊκή, sub. συναγωγή or ἀγωρά) *Jewish court-house.* Y. Gitt. I, 43ᵇ top במקום ר׳ in the Jewish meeting place (where Jews have their own jurisdiction); אם אין שם ר׳ וכ׳ if there is no Jewish court-house there, it must be done in the synagogue.

יְהוּדָאוּת, v. יְהוּדָאָה.

יְהוּדָה (b. h.) pr. n. *Judah,* 1) son of Jacob; *tribe of Judah.* Pes. 50ᵃ. Yoma 12ᵃ, a. e. מחלקו של ר׳ from the area of Judah.—Gen. R. s. 85; a. v. fr.—2) name of several Tannaim; a) R. J. b. B'thera in Babylonia Ber. 22ᵃ; a. fr.—b) J. b. Tabbai, chief of the Sanhedrin in the days of queen Salome. Ab. I, 8. Ḥag. II, 2; a. fr.—c) R. J. the priest. Eduy. VIII, 3.—d) R. J. b. Baba. Ib. 2. Sabb. 62ᵇ; a. fr.—e) R. J. b. Ilai, usu. mentioned in the Mishnah as R. J. only. Ber. 63ᵇ; Sabb. 33ᵇ. Men. 103ᵇ; a. v. fr.—f) R. J. b. Tema. Ab. V, 20. Erub. 17ᵃ; Tosef. ib. III (II), 6 (ed. Zuck. בתירה). Tosef. Gitt. VII (V), 8; a. fr.; a. others (v. Fr. Darkhé, p. 42; p. 137).—Esp. R. J. han-Nasi I a. II, surnamed Rabbi, v. רַבִּי.—3) name of several Amoraim, the most renowned of whom is R. J. (b. Ezekiel), a Babylonian. Keth. 110ᵇ bot.—Y. Taan. I, 64ᵇ top; a. fr.—V. Fr. M'bo p. 91ᵃ.—4) *Judaea,* the southern province of Palestine. Keth. I, 5 (12ᵃ); Tosef. ib. I, 4. Kidd. 6ᵃ; a. v. fr.

יְהוּדִי m. (b. h.) *Judaean, Jew* (mostly in a religious sense), *worshipper of one God.* Meg. 12ᵇ קרי ליה ר׳ אלמא מיהודה וכ׳ he is called Y'hudi (Esth. II, 5), which would indicate that he belongs to the tribe of Judah, and yet he is called *ish y'mini* &c.?, v. יְמִינִי. Ib. 13ᵃ ... ואמאי ר׳ ... שכל הכופר בע״ז נקרא ר׳ but why is he designated as Y'hudi? Because he disowned idolatry; for whosoever disowns idolatry, is called a Jew (ref. to Dan. III, 12); Esth. R. to II, 5 לפי שייחד ... נקרא ר׳ לומר ר׳ יחידי because he professed the unity of God, he was called Y'hudi, meaning to say, a Y'hudi, a believer in One God. Ex. R. s. 42 אתה סבור ... או ר׳ או צלוב thou thinkest that calling Israel 'persistent' is meant for blame; it is meant for their praise, either a Jew or hanged. Meg. l. c. מאכל ר׳ Jewish food (in accordance with the Jewish dietary laws); a. e.—[Pes. 113ᵇ ר׳, read with Mss. a. early ed. מי; Yeb. 63ᵃ כל ר׳, read אדם.]—*Pl.* יְהוּדִים. Esth. R. to III, 9. Ib. to VIII, 8 שונאי הר׳ the enemies of the Jews. Ib. 15 ... מלך על הר׳ Mardecai was made king of the Jews; a. fr.—*Fem.* יְהוּדִית, יְהוּדִיָּה. Meg. l. c. (v. Rabb. D. S. a. l. note 7); Yalk. Esth. 1052 (ref. to I Chr. IV, 18) אמאי קרי לה ר׳ why is she (Bithya, the daughter of Pharaoh) called Y'hudiyah (a Jewess)?—Esth. R. to III, I אם אסתר ר׳ היא וכ׳ if Esther is a Jewess &c., opp. גוידה.—Keth. VII, 6 (72ᵃ, sq.) דת ר׳, v. דַּת.

יְהוּדִיָּה, v. preced.

***יְהוּדִינַיי**, pr. n. f. *Y'hudinyi,* sister of R. Judah han-Nasi. Y. Naz. VII, 56ᵃ top; (Y. Ber. III, 6ᵃ bot. נהוראי).

יְהוּדִית, v. יְהוּדִי.

יהודת, v. יַהֲדוּת.

יְהוֹיָדָע (b. h.) pr. n. m. *Jehoiada,* the high-priest. Num. R. s. 23; a. e.

יְהוֹיָקִים (b. h.) pr. n. m. *Jehoiakim,* king of Judah. M. Kat. 26ᵃ. Snh. 103ᵃ, sq. Lev. R. s. 19; a. fr.

יְהוֹיָרִיב (b. h.) pr. n. m. *Joiarib,* head of a priestly division named after him; *(fem.) the division J.* Y. Taan. IV, 68ᵈ.

יְהוֹנָתָן, v. יוֹנָתָן.

יְהוֹרָם, יוֹרָם (b. h.) pr. n. m. *Jehoram, Joram,* 1) son of Ahab, king of Israel. Ber. 10ᵃ. Ex. R. s. 31; a. e.—2) son of Joshafat, king of Judah. Hor. 11ᵇ, v. יֵהוּא.

יְהוֹשֻׁעַ, יְהוֹשֻׁעַ (b. h.) pr. n. m. *Joshua,* 1) *J. bin Nun,* the successor of Moses. Ab. I, 1. Ber. 4ᵃ bot. B. Kam. 80ᵇ, sq. עשרה ... התנה ר׳ וכ׳ J., on conquering the promised land, laid down ten conditions (regulations) &c.; Erub. 17ᵃ; a. v. fr.—Meg. I, 1, a. fr. מימות ר׳ בן נון *dating from the days of the conquest or before.*—2) the high-priest of the returning Babylonian exiles. Snh. 93ᵃ; a. e.—3) name of several Tannaim; a) J. b. Praḥya. Ab. I, 6; a. fr.—b) R. J. b. Ḥănania, mostly quoted as R. J. only. Maas. Sh. V, 9. Erub. IV, 1; 2. Ḥag. 5ᵇ; a. v. fr.; and others (v. Fr. Darkhé pp. 97; 134; 178; 189).—4) name of several Amoraim, esp. R. J. b. Levi. Ber. 3ᵇ; a. v. fr.—R. J. of Sikhnin. Y. ib. IV, 7ᵇ bot.; a. fr.; and others (v. Fr. M'bo p. 91ᵃ, sq.).—(ספר) ר׳ *the Book of Joshua.* B. Bath. 14ᵇ; a. e.

יְהוֹשַׁעְיָא, v. הוֹשַׁעְיָא.

יְהוֹשָׁפָט (b. h.) pr. n. m. *Joshafat*, king of Judah. Sabb. 56[b]. Gen. R. s. 33; a. fr.

יהט, v. יָהַט.

יְהִי, v. יְחִי.

יָהִיר m. (b. h.; יָהַר) [*glittering*,] *showy, proud, aristocratic*.—*Pl.* יְהִירִים. Sot. 47[b], v. מָשַׁךְ; Tosef. ib. XIV, 8 (ed. Zuck. יְהָרִים).

יָהִיר ch. same. Targ. Hab. II, 5 י׳ ברשע boastful of his wickedness.—Ḥull. 111[b] top כמה י׳ וכ׳ how assuming is this scholar!; cmp. יוּהֲרָא.—[Meg. 29[a] האי מאן די׳ וכ׳ he who is proud, has a certain blemish (missing in Mss., v. Rabb. D. S. a. l. note).]—B. Bath. 98[a], v. יְהַר.—*Pl.* יְהִירֵי. Snh. 98[a], v. אַמְגּוּשָׁא.—*Fem. pl.* יְהִירָן. Meg. 14[b] תרתי נשי י׳ וכ׳ there were two proud women (Deborah and Huldah), and their names are invidious.

יְהִירוּתָא f. (preced.) *haughtiness*. Meg. 14[b] לא יאה י׳ וכ׳ pride is unbecoming to women.—V. יוּהֲרָא.

יְהַר, v. יָהִיר.

יָהַר (cmp. נהר, אור) *to be shining, showy, proud*, v. יָהִיר. *Hithpa.* הִתְיַהֵר (denom. of יָהִיר) *to assume airs, to be boastful*. Pes. 66[b] כל המִתְיַהֵר וכ׳ whoever is boastful, if he is wise, his wisdom will desert him &c. B. Bath. 10[b] שאין עושין אלא לְהִתְיַהֵר בו they do good only to boast themselves thereof; וכל המתיהר וכ׳ and whoever boasts, falls a prey to Gehenna.

יְהַר ch., *Ithpa.* אִיַּהַר, *Ithpe.* אִיהַר same. Sot. 47[b] האי מאן דמִיהַר וכ׳ an overbearing man is unpopular even with his own household; B. Bath. 98[a]; Yalk. Hab. 562 דיָהִיר.

יוֹאָב (b. h.) pr. n. m. *Joab*, general of king David. B. Bath. 116[a]. Snh. 48[b]; a. fr.

יוֹאֵל (b. h.) pr. n. m. *Joel*, the prophet. Taan. 5[a]. Succ. 52[a]; a. e.

יואני, v. וָאנֵי.

יוֹאָשׁ (b. h.) pr. n. m. *Joash*, king of Judah. Tosef., Snh. IV, 11; Y. Hor. III, 47[c] bot.; Bab. ib. 11[b] ואת י׳ מפני עתלי׳ and they anointed J. on account of his opposition to Athalia; cmp. יֵהוּא. Snh. 95[b]; a. e.

יוּבְדָנָא m. (יבד) *perdition*. Targ. Prov. XI, 10 (Ms. מוֹבְדָנָא).

יוֹבֵילָא, v. יוּבְלָא.

יוֹבֵל m. (b. h.; יָבַל) 1) (cmp. נְגוֹדָא, בַּרְחָא) *leader, bell-wether, ram*. Y. Ber. IX, 13[c] top (ref. to קרן יובל, Josh. VI, 5) בערביא . . יובלא in Arabia they call a ram *yubla*; R. Hash. 26[a].—2) (ellipt. for קֶרֶן הַי׳) *ram's horn*. Mekh. Yithro, Baḥod., s. 3 (ref. to Ex. XIX, 14) בשימשוך הי׳ את קולו when the horn prolongs its sound; Yalk. Ex. 281.—3) c. (ellipt. for שְׁנַת הַי׳) *Jubilee, Yobel-year, the fiftieth year, the year following the succession of seven Sabbatical years* (Lev. XXV, 8—16; 23—24). R. Hash. III, 5 שוה הי׳ לר״ה the proclamation of the Jubilee resembles that of the New Year as to blowing &c.—Arakh. 12[b] בתחלת הי׳ at the beginning of the Jubilee cycle; a. fr.—*Pl.* יוֹבְלוֹת. R. Hash. l. c. Arakh. l. c. י״ז י׳ מנו וכ׳ the Israelites counted seventeen jubilee cycles from their entrance into the Holy Land to their leaving it.

יוּבְלָא ch. same, 1) *ram*. Y. Ber. IX, 13[c] top; R. Hash. 26[a], v. preced. (cmp. Targ. Josh. VI, 4, sq.).—2) *Jubilee*. Targ. O. Lev. XXV, 10 יוּבְלָא (ed. Berl. יוּבֵילָא, ed. Amst. יוּבָלָא; Y. יוּבְּלָא); a. fr.—*Pl.* יוּבְלֵי. Arakh. 12[b] תמניא י׳ eight jubilee cycles; a. e.

יוֹבֶלֶת, v. יַבֶּלֶת.

יוּבְקָא pr. n. (h. יַבֹּק) *Yubka*, name of a brook, a valley and a border place. Targ. O. Gen. XXXII, 23 ed. Berl. (oth. ed. a. Y. יוּבְ׳). Targ. O. Deut. III, 16 יוּבְ׳ נחלא ed. Berl. (oth. ed. a. Y. יוּבְ׳ דנ׳); a. e.—Y. Shebi. VI, 36[c] חשבון ויבקא; Sifré Deut. 51 משקא וחשבון; Yalk. ib. 874 יוסקא וח׳ (corr. acc.); Tosef. Shebi. IV, 11 יוקפא ed. Zuck. (Var. יבקא).

יוּבְשָׁא, יוּבַשׁ m. (יְבֵשׁ) *dry matter, dry condition*. Targ. II Chr. IV, 5 בי׳ in dry measure. Targ. Jud. VI, 37, 39, sq.

יוּבְשָׁנִי m. (v. preced.) *rainless land*. Taan. 10[a], v. טוּבְעָנִי I.

יו״ד *Yod*, the tenth letter of the Alphabet. Y. Shebi. I, 33[b] bot.; Sabb. 103[b]; Taan. 2[b] הרי מ״ם יו״ד מ״ם הרי מים the Mem of ונסכיהם (Num. XXIX, 19), the Yod of ונסכיה (ib. 31), and the Mem of כמשפטם (ib. 33) intimate *water* as libation. Gen. R. s. 47, beg.; Num. R. s. 18. Y. Snh. II, 20[c] bot., a. e. יו״ד שבירבה וכ׳ the Yod in *yarbeh* (Deut. XVII, 16, sq.) denounced him (Solomon); a. e.—*Pl.* יוּדִים, יוּדִין. Sifré Deut. 36 לווים י׳ ולי׳ וכ׳ if he made the Vav like Yod or vice versa; Sabb. l. c.

יוּד pr. n. m. *Yud*. Taan. 22[b] רמי בר רב י׳ ed. (Ms. M. רב יהודה אמר רב; v. Rabb. D. S. a. l. notes 1, 2). Ib. 9[a] רמי בר רב י׳ Ms. M. 2 (v. Rabb. D. S. a. l. note 60); Sabb. 32[b] Ms. M.; (Macc. 23[b] רמי בר רב only); Zeb. 55[b] Ms. M. (ed. יודא).

יוּדָא pr. n. m. *Yuda*, an Amora. Y. Ned. VII, beg. 40[b]. Zeb. 55[b], v. preced.

***יוּדָאי** m. = יְהוּדָאָה. Y. Ab. Zar. II, 41[a] top וחוה י׳ אזיל וכ׳ and when a Jew came to have his hair cut &c.

יודאפא, read: יוֹדְפָאָה.

יְהוּדָה = יוּדָה. Y. Ber. III, 6[a] bot.; a. fr.—V. Frank. M'bo, p. 92[a], sq. V. יוּדָן.

יודייה, Y. Succ. IV, 54[c] top, read: וְיוֹדְיָיה, v. יְדָאי.

יודיקי, v. יודקי.

יְהוּדָה = יוּדָן q. v. Y. Ber. III, 6[a] bot., a. fr. ר׳ י׳ נשיאה R. J. (II), the Nasi; (V. Fr. M'bo p. 92[a], sq.).—Pesik. R.

s. 14 ר׳ י׳.—Gen. R. s. 10 אבא י׳ (abbr. אַבְּדָן q. v.).—Y. Ber. II, 5ª top. Ib. IX, 14ª top; a. v. fr.

יוּדָן (=הוּ דֵן) *is this.* Targ. II Esth. VII, 5 (h. text הוא זה, הוא זה).

יוּדָנָה, יוּדָנִי pr. n. f. (v. יוּדָן) *Yudanah, Yudani.* Y. Ab. Zar. II, 41ª בר יודנה; Y. Ter. VIII, 45ᶜ bot. בר... י׳ Bar. Y.; cmp. יְהוּדִינִי.

יוֹדְפָאָה, v. next w.

יוֹדְפַת, יָדְפַת, יָטְבַת pr. n. pl. *Yodfath, Yotapata,* a fortress in Galilee (v. Jos. B. J. III, 7, 6, sq.; cmp. יָטְבָה II Kings XXI, 19). Arakh. IX, 6 י׳ הישנה the old fort of J.—Tosef. Nidd. III, 11 בקעת יטבת the valley of J.; Nidd. 20ª יודפ׳.—Denom. יוֹדְפָאָה m. *of J.* Zeb. 110ᵇ; Meil. 13ᵇ יודאפה (corr. acc.); Y. Succ. IV, 54ᶜ bot. יוֹתְפָרִיה.

ארכי ר׳, יודיקי, יודקי, יודקו, read: יוּדִיקָן m. pl. (judices) *judges;* א׳ ר׳ *chief justice*, v. אַרְכֵי III. Gen. R. s. 50, beg. Ar.—[Mus. in Ar. ed. Koh. s. v. ארכידיקי, Var. אַרְכִיקְרִיטִיס (ἀρχικρίτης); ed. א׳ הדיינים.]

יוֹדְקֶרֶת, יְד׳ pr. n. pl. *Yodkereth* (a disguised translation of *Diospolis=Lydda*). Taan. 23ᵇ, sq. ר׳ יוסי דמן יודק׳ Ar. (ed. יוֹקֶרֶת, Ms. M. יוקדת, Ms. M. 2 ידקרת) R. J. of Yodkereth (cmp. ר׳ יוסי דרומיא, Fr. M'bo, p. 5ᵇ, sq.).—*Kidd. 16ᵇ ר׳ קא חזינא הכא Ar. (ed. יו״ד קרת) I see here the influence of the Yodk. school; (for other explan., v. Rashi a. l., a. Koh. Ar. Compl. s. v. ידקרת).

יוֹהֲרָא m. (יְהַר) 1) *a sparkling gem.* Targ. Y. Gen. VI, 16.—*Pl.* יוֹהֲרִין. Targ. Esth. I, 4; Targ. Lam. IV, 7 (Var. זְהוֹרִין); Targ. Cant. VII, 2 (ed. Lag. גּוּהֲרִין.).—2) (=יְהִירוּתָא) *haughtiness, assumption.* Ber. 17ᵇ מחזי כי׳ it looks like an assumption (to appear more observant than others). Ib. חייש לי׳ cares for the appearance of assumption (and therefore forbids); Pes. 55ª. Succ. 26ᵇ לית ביה משום י׳ there is no appearance of presumption to be apprehended in doing so.

יָוָן, יָוָנָאָה, יָוָנִי, v. יָוָן, יְוָנ׳.

יוּזִיף m. (יְזַף) *debtor.* Targ. Prov. XXII, 7; v. יָזְפָא.

יוֹחַי, יוֹחָאי pr. n. m. *Yohai*, esp. known Y. the father of R. Simeon. Sabb. 33ᵇ; a. v. fr.

יוֹחָנָה, יוֹחָנָא I, *Yohana.* 1) pr. n. m. Hull. 133ª מר י׳; Ab. Zar. 16ᵇ מר יוֹחָנִי.—2) pr. n. pl. Gen. R. s. 40, beg.; ib. s. 25, end; ib. s. 64, beg.; Midr. Sam. ch. XXVIII, a. e. (prov.) שילה חטיא וי׳ משתלמא (not חטא) Shilo sinned a. Y. is punished (i. e. the later generation pays for the sins of ancestors).—V. יוֹחָנִי.

יוֹחָנָא II f. *Yohana*, name of a species of *locusts.* Sifra Sh'mini, Par. 3, ch. V; Hull. 65ª י׳ ירושלמית the Jerusalem Y.

יוֹחָנִי pr. n. *Yohani;* 1) pr. n. m. Ab. Zar. 16ᵇ, v. יוֹחָנָא I.—Men. 85ª י׳ וממרא (some ed. יוחנא) Y. and Mamre (two Egyptian sorcerers); v. יַנִּיס.—Esth. R. to I, 4 בר י׳ (some ed. יוחני) Bar-Y.—2) pr. n. f.—Zeb. 62ᵇ (a fictitious name).—Sot. 22ª י׳ ברת רטיבי (a hypocritical sorceress, v. Rashi a. l.).

יוֹחָנָן (b. h.) pr. n. m. *Johanan, John;* 1) J. ben Kareah, a follower of the Babylonian governor of Judaea (Jer. XL, 8 sq.). Esth. R. introd., beg.; Y. Succ. V, 55ᵇ top; Mekh. B'shall., Vayhi, s. 2.—2) John Hyrcan, the Asmonean highpriest and king (י׳ כהן גדול). Maash. Sh. V, 15; Sot. IX, 10; a. fr.—3) name of several Tannaim, esp. a) Rabban J. b. Zaccai. Ab. II, 8. R. Hash. IV, 3. Mekh. Yithro, Bahod., s. 11. Sot. IX, 9; 15. Gitt. 56ª, sq.; a. v. fr.—b) R. J. b. Bag-Bag (usu. only Ben-Bag-Bag). Y. Keth. V, 29ᵈ bot. B. Kam. 27ᵇ; a. fr.—c) R. J. b. B'roka. B. Kam. X, 2; a. fr.—d) R. J. b. Godgada. Eduy. VII, 9; a. e.—e) R. J. has-Sandlar. Ab. IV, 11; a. fr.—f) R. J. b. Nuri. Erub. IV, 5; Gitt. 67ª; a. fr.; 4) name of several Amoraim, esp. R. J. han-Nappah or Bar Nafha (the Smith). Y. R. Hash. II, 58ᵇ top. Hull. 137ᵇ; a. v. fr. (as R. J. only); v. Fr. M'bo p. 95ᵇ, sq.—V. חִיקוֹק.

יוֹחָס m., pl. יוֹחֲסִין, יוֹחֲסִים (יְחַס) *genealogical records, traced genealogy.* Kidd. IV, 1 עשרה י׳ עלו וכ׳ ten classes of Jews of traced genealogy went up from Babylonian captivity. Y. Taan. IV, 68ª bot.; Gen. R. s. 98 מגילת י׳ מצאו וכ׳ a roll containing genealogical records was found &c. Yeb. IV, 13; ib. 49ᵇ.—Y. Succ. V, end, 55ᵈ; Cant. R. to V, 5 שלשלת (ה)י׳ the genealogical chain; Gen. R. s. 82. Ib. בכורת י׳ the genealogical privileges of the first-born, opp. to בכורת ממון the material privileges (double-share). Ruth R., end מה אתם יש לכם י׳ what records have you to show?—Pes. 62ᵇ מיום שנגנז ספר י׳ since the Book of Genealogy (a commentary to Chronicles) was suppressed (or disappeared, in the Roman days). Ib. ניתנו לי מר ספר י׳ teach me the book of records (Chronicles); a. e.—V. יִחוּס.

יוֹכֶבֶד (b. h.) pr. n. f. *Jochebed*, the mother of Moses and Aaron. Sot. 12ª; B. Bath. 120ª; Ex. R. s. 1; Gen. R. s. 94; a. fr.

יוּכְלָא f. ch.=h. יְכוֹלֶת, *power, ability.* Targ. Y. Gen. IV, 13. Targ. Num. XIV, 16; a. e.; v. יְכוּלְתָּא.

בַּר י׳, יוֹכְנִי, m. *Bar-Yokhani*, name of a fabulous bird. Bekh. 57ᵇ. Yoma 80ª (Ms. M. 2 בריכני, v. Rabb. D. S. a. l. note 9); Succ. 5ᵇ top.—[Koh. Ar. Compl. s. v. בר (vol. II, p. 176) refers to *Varaghna* (Bactrian) *ostrich*.]

יְוַל, v. יָבַל Hif.

יוּלַד, v. יָלַד.

יוֹלֵד m. pl. יוֹלְדִים (b. h.; יָלַד) *parents.* Keth. VII, 6 המקללת יוֹלְדָיו בפניו she who curses his (her husband's) parents in his presence; quot. ib. 72ᵇ יוֹלְידָיו (an emphatic form), and interpreted במקללת יוֹלְדָיו בפני מוֹלְדָיו (v. מוֹלָד) also when she curses his parents before any one of his begotten; Y. ib. VII, 31ᵇ bot. וולדיו בפני יולדיו, v. יָלַד.

יוֹלֶדֶת, יוֹלֵדָה f. (b. h.; preced.) *a woman in confinement; a mother.* Ab. II, 8 אשרי יוֹלַדְתּוֹ blessed is his mother.—*Pl.* יוֹלְדוֹת. Sabb. 32ª נשים מתות י׳ women die in confinement (v. לֵידָה); Y. ib. II, 5ᵇ top; v. יָלְדָה.—Sot. I, 5 את הי׳ (not יולדת) the women appearing in the Temple after confinement.

יוֹלַדְתָּא, *midwife*, v. יָלַדְתָּא.

יוֹלִיד, v. יוֹלֵד.

***יוֹלִימְנָא** pr. n. m. *Yolimna*, an Amora. Pesik. R. s. 7, beg.

יוֹלִין, Pes. 39ª, חזרת י׳, v. חֲוֹרוּלִין.

יוּלְפָנָא m. (יְלַף)=אוּלְפָנָא, *instruction.* Targ. Prov. IV, 2.

יוֹם (b. h.) *light, day* (opp. night); (*astronomical*) *day*; trnsf. *day of life; time.* Gen. R. s. 6 הי׳ והגשמים וכ׳ the noise of the moving light (Yoma 20ᵇ קול גלגל חמה) and the rains &c.; Midr. Sam. ch. IX. Gen. R. l. c. (ref. to Mal. III, 19) י׳ שהוא מלהט וכ׳ it is the day light which will glow the wicked (cmp. נְהַק). M. Kat. 25ᵇ (ref. to Am. VIII, 9) זה יוֹמוֹ של וכ׳ that means the day of life of Josiah (who was slain in the bloom of manhood). Gen. R. s. 3 (ref. to ib. I, 5) י׳ אחד . . . ואיזה זה יוה״כ 'one (distinguished) day' . . . that is the Day of Atonement. Hull. V, 5 (83ª) הי׳ הוֹלֵךְ וכ׳ the day follows the night, i. e. the beginning of the night is the beginning of the new day. Taan. 29ª, v. זַכַּאי; a. v. fr.—י׳ טוב (abbr. יו״ט) *Holy Day; festival.* R. Hash. IV, 1; a. fr.—Yoma VII, 4 ויו״ט היה וכ׳ and the Highpriest gave a festival to his friends; a. fr.—*Yom Tob*, name of a treatise of the Tosefta (v. בֵּיצָה).—י׳ הכפורים (abbr. יוה״כ, יו״כ) Day of Atonement. Yoma I, 1; a. v. fr.—בֶּן יוֹמוֹ *of the same day, not quite one day old, used on the same day.* Sabb. 151ᵇ. B. Kam. 65ᵇ; a. fr.—Tanḥ. Kor. 3; ed. Bub. 6; Num. R. s. 18 תינוקות בְּנֵי יוֹמָן (not בן) children just born; a. fr.—*Du.* יוֹמַיִם. Mekh. Mishp., N'zikin, s. 7; B. Kam. 90ª ישנו בדין יום או י׳ comes under the law of 'one or two days' (Ex. XXI, 21); B. Bath. 50ª.—Mekh. l. c. יום שהוא כי׳ וי׳ שהוא כיום a time which counts like two days, and two days which count like a day, which is twenty four hours (from the time of the accident, including part of this and part of the next day).—Snh. 65ᵇ מה יום מיומים (Ms. M. a. Rashi מה היום וכ׳) what difference is there between to-day (Sabbath) and the next day?; Gen. R. s. 11; Yalk. Deut. 918; Yalk. Lev. 617.—*Pl.* יָמִים; constr. יְמֵי, יְמוֹת. Erub. III, 6 לשני י׳ for both days. Zeb. V, 7 לשני י׳ during two days and one night. Pes. 52ª, a. fr. שני י׳ טובים של גליות, v. גָּלוּת. Taan. IV, 8 לא היו י׳ ט׳ וכ׳ Israel had no days as merry as &c.; a. fr.—Ab. I, 17, a. fr. כל יָמַי all my lifetime.—Esp. יְמוֹת *season, period of.* י׳ הגשמים, v. גֶּשֶׁם I.—י׳ החמה a) *summer season.* Toh. VI, 7; a. fr.—b) *the solar year.* Gen. R. s. 33, end; a. fr.—י׳ הלבנה *the lunar year.* Ib.; a. fr.—י׳ נערות, י׳ בגרות, v. בַּגְרוּת &c.

יוֹמָא, יוֹם ch. same. Targ. Gen. I, 5. Ib. XXXIX, 11; a. fr.—Targ. Prov. XII, 16 בר יוֹמֵיה (ed. Wil. incorr. כד) on the same day, *at once.*—Kidd. 39ᵇ דעבדין ליה י׳ טב וי׳ בריש they prepare for him (the righteous man) a good day, and (for the bad man) a bad day (v. Rashi a. Tosaf. a. l.).—Sabb. 134ª; Hull. 60ª top להדי י׳ towards the sunlight. Ib. י׳ דחד וכ׳ the sun which is only one of the ministering powers &c. Keth. 106ª וכסי ליה לי׳ and obscured the sun.—Yeb. 72ª י׳ דעיבא a cloudy day; י׳ דשותא a day when a southern wind blows. Erub. 40ᵇ במעלי י׳ דריש וכ׳ on the eve of the New Year's day.—R. Hash. 21ª י׳ רבה the Great Day, Day of Atonement (also only יומא, v. infra); a. v. fr.—בַּר י׳, בַּת י׳ *of the same day, one day old, used the same day.* Bets. 4ᵇ, v. בֵּיעָא. Hull. 58ᵇ, v. בִּקָּא.—Sabb. 134ª גבינה בת י׳ fresh-made cheese. Ab. Zar. 67ᵇ, a. fr. קדירה בת י׳ a pot used the same day.—Sabb. 49ᵇ bot. החוא מרבנן בר יוֹמֵיה (omitted in Ms. M.) a student that had just come to college; [oth. opin.: allusion to R. Idi, dubbed בר בי רב דחד י׳ the one day's student of the college, Hag. 5ᵇ].—י׳ חרא, י׳ מחרא, יום מחרא, מחרן, v. next w.—*Pl.* יוֹמִין, יוֹמַיָּא, יוֹמֵי. Targ. Gen. VIII, 10. Targ. Esth. I, 2; a. v. fr.—Bets. 4ᵇ עבדינן תרי י׳ we observe two days (as Holy Days). Erub. 65ª חשתא...י׳ דאריכי וכ׳ soon will come the days which are long (of duration) and short (of action), when we shall sleep much; a. v. fr.—יוֹמָא (sub רבה, v. supra) *Yoma*, name of a treatise of the Mishnah, Tosefta (where it is named יום כפורים), Talmud Babli a. Y'rushalmi. Yoma 14ᵇ כדר י׳ the treatise on the order of exercises of the Day of Atonement.—V. יְמָמָא, יוֹמָנָא.

יוֹמְחָרָן, יוֹמְחְרָא m. (=יומא אוחרא, י׳ אוחרן) *to-morrow, next day.* Targ. Y. Ex. XIX, 10 (ed. Amst. יום מחרא). Targ. Esth. III, 4 ed. Lag. (ed. Amst. יומא). Targ. Y. Lev. VII, 16 (ed. Amst. יום מחרן); a. e. [Targ. II Chr. XX, 16 יומא חרא, ed. Lag. יומא אחרא.]—V. חֲרָא.

יוֹמָנָא (contr. of יוֹמָא דְנָא) *this day, this life.* Targ. Y. Deut. XXVII, 1.—Targ. Y. I Deut. XXVI, 17 (Y. II יומא דין); ib. 18. Targ. Prov. VII, 14. [Ib. v. 20 ולירמנא Ms., ed. ולירמא דעידא.] Targ. Ps. XXIII, 6 נגדא די׳ (h. text ארך ימים).

יָוֵן m. (b. h.; יון to be thick, dark, cmp. יַיִן) *thickness,* טיט הי׳ *thick, heavy clay*, opp. to טיט טופח (v. טָפַח II). Mikv. IX, 2. Tosef. ib. VI (VII), 12; 13 אם היה טיט (ה)י׳ וחיברו if it was a thick massive clay and he attached it.—Denom. יְוֵנִי m. *muddy, thick.* Mikv. l. c., v. גֵּץ 2.

יָוָן, יָוָן (b. h.) 1) pr. n. m. *Javan*, son of Japheth, progenitor of the Grecian tribes, in gen. *Greek, Greece;* —2) fem. (sub. מלכות) *Greek (Syrian) Government.* Targ. Gen. X, 2; a. e.—Targ. Y. Gen. XV, 12.—Gen. R. s. 44 (ref. to אַיִל משלש, Gen. XV, 9) זו י׳ this alludes to the Greek government (founded by Alexander the Great). Ib. כל רוחות כבשו בני י׳ וכ׳ in all directions did the Greeks conquer, except in the East. Esth. R. introd. בבקרה של י׳ when Greece (Syria) is in the ascendancy, v. בֹּקֶר; a. fr. —Denom. יְוָנִי, יְוָנָאָה.

יוֹן, יוֹנָא, v. יוֹנְתָא.

יְוָנָאָה, יְוָנִי m. ch.=h. יְוָנִי.—*Pl.* יְוָנָאֵי. Targ. I Sam. II, 4 (ed. Lag. יְוָנֵי, ed. Wil. מְקַדּוּנָאֵי). Targ. Y. I Deut. XXXII, 24 (ed. Amst. יוני, ed. Vien. יוֹנֵי; corr. acc.).

יוֹנָה I (b.h.) pr. n. m. *Jonah,* 1) the prophet. Y.Erub. X, beg. 26ª; Bab. ib. 96ª. Snh. 89ª, sq Gen. R. s. 21; a.fr. —2) name of several Amoraim. a) R. J. father of R. Mana. Taan. 23ᵇ. Y. Shebi IV, 35ª bot.; a.v.fr.—b) R. J. of Bozra. Y. Kil. IX, beg. 31ᵈ; a. fr.—[Hull. 43ᵇ ר׳ אמר ר׳ זירא Jonah said in behalf of R. Z.; oth. opin.: as to the gullet of a *dove,* &c., v. next w.]

יוֹנָה II f. (b.h.) *dove.* Hull. 6ª דמות ר׳ וכ׳ the effigy of a dove was found on Mount Gerizim which they (the Samaritans) worshipped. Gen. R. s. 39 הד׳ הזו בשעה שהיא פורחת וכ׳ the dove when flying and tired, flaps one wing and flies with the other. Ib. s. 44 (expl. גוזל, Gen. XV, 9) בר ר׳ a young dove, (v. infra, a. Targ. Gen. l. c.).—בֶּן ר׳, pl. בְּנֵי ר׳ *pigeons.* Hull. I, 5 כשר בתורין פסול בבני ר׳ what is fit for offering in doves (large size), is a defect in pigeons; a. fr.—[Sabb. 129ª פתורא דיונה, v. יוֹנָס.].—*Pl.* יוֹנִים, יוֹנִין. Snh. III, 3 מפריחי ר׳ those who let doves fly (betting on them), v. יוֹנְתָא. B. Bath. V, 3, v. שׁוֹבָךְ. Ib. 79ª; a. e.

יונוס, v. יַנִּיס.

יוֹנִי, v. יָוָן.

יְוָנִי, יְוָנִית, יְוָנִי, יוֹנִי m., **יְוָנִית, יְוָנִי** f. (יָוָן) *Grecian, Greek.* B. Kam. 82ᵇ חָכְמַת ר׳ the principle of Greek culture (philosophy, ethics, religion &c.). Ib. 83ª לשון ר׳ Greek language, distinguished fr. חכמת ר׳. Meg. 9ª התירו יונית permitted the use of a Greek translation. Y. ib. I, 71ᶜ top, v. בָּדָא; a. fr.—V. לָשׁוֹן.—*Pl.* יְוָנִים, יְוָנִי *Greeks* (mostly of the Syrian government). Meg. 11ª בימי ר׳ in the days of the Greeks (of Antiochus Epiphanes and successors); Esth. R., beg. טרקווינוס (corr. acc.).

***יוֹנָס** m. (prob. a corrupt. of juniperus) *Juniper-tree* (v. Sm. Ant. s. v. Cedrus). Sabb. 129ª פתורא די׳ old ed. (later ed. דיונה, Ms. M. דיינס, v. Rabb. D. S. a. l. note; Ar. דינוס, expl.: *cypress*) a table made of &c.

יוֹנֵק m. (b. h.; יָנַק) *child.*—*Pl.* יוֹנְקִים. Cant. R. to I, 4 הי׳ the school children. V. יָנוּקָא.

יוֹנְקָא, v. יָנוּקָא.

יוֹנֶקֶת f. (b. h.; יָנַק) *sucker, sprout* (of hyssop).—*Pl.* יוֹנְקוֹת. Par. XI, 7, v. גָּמַל; Tosef. ib. XI (X), 7 (one opin.) ר׳ שלא הנצו וכ׳ *yon'koth* are such as have not yet begun to blossom.

יוֹנָה, יוֹנָא, יוֹנְתָא f. (יון c.) ch.=h. יוֹנָה II. Targ. Gen. VIII, 8, sq. Targ. Ps. LVI, 1; a. e.—Snh. 25ª (expl. מפריחי יונים, v. יוֹנָה II) אי תקדמיה יוֹנָךְ ליון if thy dove shall overtake the cock-pigeon (thou shalt win &c.). Ib. חולה בדעת יוני v. דַּעַת. Y. Ab. Zar. V, 44ᵈ bot. כמין יון וכ׳ they (the Samaritans) have an image resembling a cock-pigeon to which they offer libations (cmp. יוֹנָה II). Snh. 95ª אתא יונה וכ׳ (masc.) a dove came down &c., v. טְרַף I. —*Pl.* יוֹנְתָא, יוֹנִין, יוֹנֵי, יוֹנְיָא, יוֹנָן. Targ. Is. LIX, 11. Targ. Y. Lev. V, 7; 11 בני יוניא (O. בני יונה, v. יוֹנָה II). Ib. XII, 6 בר יונן (O. יונה). Targ. Cant. I, 15.—Ber. 56ª חזאי תרתי יוני דפרחן I saw (in my dream) two doves fly off. Ib.ᵇ תרי יוני.

יְהוֹנָתָן, יוֹנָתָן (b. h.) pr. n. m. *Jonathan,* 1) J. b. Gershom (Jud. XVIII, 30), a priest of idolatry, supposed to be a descendant of Moses. B. Bath. 109ᵇ רי׳ Ms. M. (ed. יהו׳). Cant. R. to II, 5; Ab. d'R. N. ch. XXXIV; Y. Ber. IX, 13ᵈ top; a. e.—2) J. son of Saul. Ab. V, 16 אהבת דוד וי׳ the friendship between David and J. Hull. 95ᵇ כי׳ בן וכ׳ like the omen of J. &c. (I Sam. XIV, 8 sq.). Cant. R. to VIII, 6; a. e.—3) J. b. Uziel, author of the Chaldaic version of the Prophets (v. Zunz, Gottesd. Vortr. p. 66, sq.). Succ. 28ª; B. Bath. 134ª. Meg. 3ª תרגום של נביאים ר׳ וכ׳ the version of the Prophets has been composed by J. b. U. at the dictation of Haggai &c. Y. Ned. V, end, 39ᵇ גדול שבהן ר׳ ב׳ ע׳ the greatest among the disciples of R. Joh. b. Zaccai, was J. &c.—4) R. J., a Tannai. Sot. 24ª. Pes. 24ª. Hull. 70ᵇ; a. v. fr.—[Erub. 96ª ר׳ הקיטוני.]—[Ab. IV, 9, v. Frank. Darkhé, p. 147, note.]—5) name of several Amoraim (v. Fr. M'bo, p. 99ª, sq.). Gitt. 78ᵇ. Y. Maas. Sh. III, 54ᵇ top. Ber. 18ª; Y. ib. II, 4ᶜ bot.; a. fr.—Y. Yoma VII, 44ᵇ bot. R. J. of Beth Gubrin.—Y. Peah V, beg. 18ᵈ (R. S. to Peah V, 1 quotes R. Johanan); Y. Shek. I, 46ª bot. R. J. son of R. Isaac bar Aha.—Y. Ter. XI, end, 48ᵇ J. b. ʿAkhmai; a. e.

יוֹסָה, יוֹסָא, abbrev. of יוֹסֵף, v. יוֹסֵי.

יוּסְטַי, יוּסְטָא pr. n. m. (abbrev. of Justus or Justinus) *Yusta, Yusti.* 1) Cant. R. to VI, 12 ר׳ חייטא Yusta, the tailor.—2) name of several Amoraim. Y. Erub. VI, 23ᶜ bot. ר׳ יוסטי; Y. Shek. II, beg. 46ᶜ ר׳ יוסטא.—Y. Ter. XI, 48ª; Y. Maas. Sh. V, 55ᵈ bot. יוסטי בר שונם; Y. Shebi. VI, 36ᵈ יוסטא בר ש׳.

יוּסְטִינִי, יוּסְטִינָה pr. n. m. (cmp. preced.; abbrev. of Justinus or Justinianus) *Yustinah, Yustini,* an Amora. Y. Keth. IX, 32ᵈ bot. (not יוסטתה); Y. B. Bath. VIII, 16ᵇ יוסטיני.

יוסטתה, v. preced.

יוֹסֵי pr. n. m. (abbrev. of Joseph, interch. with יוֹסֵף, אִיסִי, אַסִּי, יַסָּה, יַסָּא, יוֹסָה, יוֹסָא) *José* 1) name of several Tannaim, esp. J. b. Joezer, and J. b. Johanan. Ab. I, 4, sq. Eduy. VIII, 4; a. fr.—B. Bath. 133ᵇ יוסף (Ms. H. a. R. יוסי). —R. J. hak-Kohen, or only R. J. Ab. II, 8; 12. Hag. 14ᵇ; Y. ib. II, 77ª bot. יוֹסֵף; a. v. fr.—R. J. b. Halafta, or only R. J. B. Kam. 70ª; Tosef. B. Bath. II, 10 (v. Fr. Darkhé, p. 132). Erub. 46ᵇ. Maas. Sh. IV, 7; a. v. fr. (v. Fr. ib. p. 164, sq.).—R. J., the Galilean. Zeb. 57ª. Ab. Zar. III, 5. Tosef. Mikv. VII (VIII), 11; a. fr. (v. Fr. ib., p. 125).—2) name of several Amoraim, esp. R. J. (in Babli אַסִּי, in Y. also יוֹסָה, יַסָּא). Y. Ber. II, 5ᶜ bot. Y. Kil. IX, 29ᵇ bot.; Y. Erub. I, 19ᶜ; a. v. fr.—R. J. bar Zabda, mate of R. Jonah. Y. Shek. VII, 50ᶜ bot. Men. 70ᵇ; a. v. fr.—3) יוסי or יוסה a disguise of one of the Divine Names. Snh. VII, 5 (56ª) בכל יום . . . יכה ר׳ את ר׳ (v. Rabb. D. S. a. l. note) during the proceedings against the blasphemer the witnesses are requested to make their statements in disguise (v. כִּינּוּי), e. g.: "the defendant said, 'May J. strike J.'" (meaning, I curse Jehovah Elohim, J. Zebaoth &c.; cmp. ib. עד שיברך שם בשם).—4) one *J. M'shitha,* a repentant Hellenist. Gen. R. s. 65 (some ed. יוֹסֵף); Yalk. ib. 115.

יוֹסִינָא, יוֹסִינָה, יוֹסִינָא pr. n. m. *Josina.* Y. Meg. IV, 75[b] bot.; Y. Yeb. XIII, 13[c] top; ib. X, 10[d] top. Cant. R. to V, 1 יוֹסָנָה; Pesik. R. s. 5 יוֹסֵי; Num. R. s. 13 יוֹסְנָיָה.

יוֹסֵף (b. h.) pr. n. m. *Joseph,* 1) son of Jacob. B. Bath. 123[a], v. בְּכוֹרָה. Sot. I, 9. Gen. R. s. 30; a. v. fr.—2) name of several Tannaim and Amoraim, v. יוֹסֵי.—3) Sabb. 119[a] י׳ מוקיר שבי Joseph, the honorer of the Sabbaths.—Ib. 130[a] J. Rishba (the fowler).—Gen. R. s. 65, v. יוֹסֵי.

יוסטניא, יוסתניא, v. וַסְתַּנְיָא.

יוֹעֶזֶר (b. h.) 1) pr. n. m. *Joezer.* Orlah II, 12 a disciple of Shammai's school.—Ab. I, 4; a. fr., v. יוֹסֵי.—2) name of *a plant.* Sabb. XIV, 3, expl. Y. ib. 14[c] פוליטרריכון *polytrichon, Maiden-hair*; Bab. ib. 109[b] פותנק.

יוֹפִי m. (b. h.; יָפִי; v. יָפֶה) *fine build, beauty; propriety.* Taan. 31[a] (the fair maiden said) תנו עיניכם לי׳ ed. (Ms. M. בי׳) put your eyes on (give your choice to) beauty. Succ. 45[b] Ms. M. (ed. in Mish. 45[a], v. Rabb. D. S. a. l.) י׳ לך מזבח thine, altar, is the beauty (of forgiveness). Ex. R. s. 25 אני מראה לך י׳ פנים אל פנים I shall let thee see the beauty of a revelation of face to face (as granted to Moses). Yoma 54[b] מוכלל (יָפְיוֹ) יוֹפְיוֹ של וכ׳ the perfection of the beauty (harmony) of the universe. Kidd. 49[b] עשרה קבים י׳ וכ׳ ten measures of beauty have come down to the world, nine of which Jerusalem has taken; Esth. R. to I, 3. B. Mets. 87[a] וחזר י׳ למקומו and (her) beauty came back again; a. fr.—Peah VI, 6 י׳ כח, v. יָפֶה.

יוֹפִיאֵל pr. n. (preced.) *Yofiël,* name of an angel. Targ. Y. I Deut. XXXIV, 6.

יוֹפִיוּת, v. יָפְיוּת.

יוֹצְאָנִית f. (יָצָא) *loving to go out, restless.* Tanh. Vayishl. 7.—*Pl.* יוֹצְאָנִיּוֹת. Gen. R. s. 45.

יוֹצֵאת f. constr., י׳ החוץ (preced.) *running about, prostitute.* Kel. XXVIII, 9; Tosef. ib. B. Bath. V, 14, v. חוּץ II.—*Pl.* יוֹצְאוֹת. Ib. some ed.

יוֹצְפָא, v. יָצַף.

יוֹצֵר m. (b. h.; יָצַר) 1) *Creator.* Lev. R. s. 23, end (ref. to Deut. XXXII, 18) רפו ידיו של י׳ the Creator's hands become lax (undecided). [Ib. השוי ידיו של י׳, read: צַיָּיר.]—Mekh. Bo. s. 13; Tanh. Bo. 7 (ref. to Ex. XII, 29) יוצרו חלקו He who created it (the night) divided it (exactly into two halves); Gen. R. s. 43. Ber. 61[a] (play on וייצר, Gen. II, 7, v. יְצִירָה) אוי לי מִיּוֹצְרִי אוי לי מִיִּצְרִי woe is to me from (my responsibility to) my Creator, woe to me from (my struggle with) my inclination; a. fr.—2) [*turner,*] *potter.* Gen. R. s. 55 (ref. to Ps. XI, 5) הי׳ הזה וכ׳ the potter when examining his batch, will not try the defective vessels &c. Lev. R. l. c. תלמידו של י׳ a potter's apprentice; a. fr.; —*Pl.* יוֹצְרִים. Maasr. III, 7; Succ. 8[b], a. fr., v. סוּכָּה.—Par. V, 6, v. בֵּיצָה.—Lev. R. l. c. שגנב ביצת י׳ who stole a lump of potters' clay; Pesik. R. s. 24 שגנב יָצְרִים (corr. acc.).

יוצרה, Y. B. Mets. VIII, end, 11[d], v. יְצִירָה 2.

יוֹקִידְתָא, v. יְקֵדָא.

יוֹקִינָוּס, דְּיוֹ׳=אוֹקְיָינוּס(?). Targ. Y. II. Num. XXXIV, 15; [the entire verse is corrupt].

יוקפא, v. יוּבְקָא.

יוֹקֶר m. (יָקַר) [*weight, importance,*] 1) *high price* (opp. זול); *dearth, scarcity.* Maas. Sh. IV, 1 מקום י׳ where fruits are dear; B. Mets. 73[a]. Sabb. 32[b] והי׳ הוה and scarcity is permanent. Y. Hor. III, 48[c] top יין בי׳ wine is dear; a. fr.—2) *nobility, aristocracy.* Sot. IX, 15, a. e.; v. אָמַר II.

יוֹקְרָא ch. same, 1) *high price.* Targ. Job XXVIII, 17.—2) *weight.* Men. 94[b] אגב י׳ דלחם on account of the heavy pressure of the bread.—3) *feeling of heaviness;* י׳ דִלְבָּא *asthma.* Sabb. 140[a].

יוֹקֶרֶת, v. יוֹדְקֶרֶת.

יורדא, Targ. Ez. XXVII, 24 דיו׳ ed. Lag., read: דִּי וַרְדָּא v. וֶרֶד. [Targ. Y. Gen. VI, 16 ed. pr., read: יוֹהֲרָא.]

יוֹרְדָנָא, v. יַרְדְּנָא.

יוֹרֶדֶת f. (יָרַד) *rivulet* (cmp. מוֹרָד). Tosef. Par. IX (VIII), 2 י׳ הצלמון the rivulet coming down from Mount Zalmon.

יוֹרֶה I m. (b. h.; יָרָה) *a soaking rain, early rain.* Sifré Deut. 42 (ref. to Deut. XI, 14) י׳ במרחשון וכ׳ *yoreh* (early rain) is the rain of Marḥeshvan, the late rain (*malkosh*) in Nisan; Taan. 5[a]. Ib. (ref. to Mish. I, 2) י׳ בניסן וכ׳ is the *yoreh* in Nisan? is it not in Marḥeshvan? Ib. 6[a]; a. e. —Trnsf. *early season, spring.* Tanh. Ḥayé 6 (ref. to Koh. XI, 6) אם זרעת בי׳ וכ׳ if thou hast sown in the spring &c.; cmp. בָּכִּיר.—

יוֹרָה II m., **יוֹרֶה** f. (denom. of אוּר, cmp. Syr. אירא P. Sm. 167) *boiler, kettle.* Hull. 108[a] י׳ של חלב a kettle of milk. Ib.[b] י׳ רותחת a boiling kettle. Ab. Zar. 76[a] י׳ קטנה בתוך י׳ גדולה put a small boiler into a large one filled with water, v. גָּעַל; a. fr.—Esp. *the dyer's kettle, dye.* B. Kam. 99[a] top הקדיחתו י׳ (Ms. H. הקדיחתו) the dye burnt it (the wool); ib. IX, 4 (100[b]) הקדיחתו י׳ (v. Rabb. D. S. a. l. note 30); Y. ib. IX, 6[d] bot. הקדיחה י׳.—Ḥag. 15[b] (in Chald. dict.) כל עמר דנחית לי׳ סליק does the wool that goes into the kettle always come out sound?, i. e. does every student of mystic philosophy escape death or scepticism?—Sabb. I, 6; a. e.—*Pl.* יוֹרוֹת; י׳ הערביים *improvised fire places of the Arabs, a cavity in the ground laid out with clay.* Kel. V, 10 (ed. Dehr. יוֹרַת). Men. V, 9 (63[a]).

יוריה, Yalk. Gen. 133 Koh. Ar. Compl., v. יְרִיָּה.

יורכין, Targ. Y. Deut. XXXIV, 6, read: יוֹהֲרִין (cmp. Targ. Esth. I, 4); v. יוֹהֲרָא.

יוֹרָם v. יְהוֹרָם.

יורם, Targ. Prov. XVIII, 11 some ed., read ירום, v. רוּם. —Ib. XXIII, 29 יורם קנצן עינוי ed. Lag., Ms. Var. יודמקנען, יודענען, a corrupt. of סמקנות עיינין, v. סְמַקְתָא.

יוּרְקָא, v. יָרוֹקָא a. יְרַקָא.

יוּרְקְמִי* (יורקמו, Ar. ירוקמי) pr. n. *Yurkami*, name of an angel. Pes. 118ª י׳ שר הברד Y. the chief of the hail storms; Yalk. Ps. 873; Midr. Till. to Ps. CXVII.

יוּרְקָנָא, v. יַרְקוֹנָא.

יוֹרֵשׁ m. (b. h.; יָרַשׁ) *heir, successor, heir-at-law*. B. Bath. IX, 2 אם אין שם י׳ וכ׳ if there is no other heir besides. Ib. 139ª שויוה רבנן כי׳...כלוקח the Rabbis gave him the privileges of an heir (to his wife's property) and those of a purchaser; a. v. fr.—*Pl.* יוֹרְשִׁים, יוֹרְשִׁין. Ib. 140ª. Ib. IX, 9 יוֹרְשֵׁי האשה וכ׳ the wife's heirs-at-law claim that the husband died first; a. v. fr.—*Fem.* יוֹרֶשֶׁת, *pl.* יוֹרְשׁוֹת. Ib. 119ª יודע . . . י׳ חן Moses knew that the daughters of Z. were legal heirs.

יוֹשֶׁן m. (יָשָׁן) *former condition, original usage* (cmp. אֵיתָן). Snh. 19ª החזיר...הדבר ליוֹשְׁנוֹ restored the usage to its original state; Y. ib. II, 20ª bot.; Y. Ber. III, 6ᵇ החזרו הדברים ליוֹשְׁנָן; Keth. 8ᵇ החזירו הדבר ליוֹשְׁנוֹ (not לירושנה). Kidd. 66ª עד שבא . . . והחזיר את התורה ליוֹשְׁנָהּ until Simon b. Sh. came and restored the Law to its former authority. Yoma 69ᵇ, v. עֲטָרָה; Y. Ber. VII, 11ᶜ; a. e.

יוֹשֶׁר m. (b. h. יָשֵׁר; יָשַׁר) *straightness, equity*. Ruth R. introd. במדת י׳ in equity, v. יְשָׁרוּת.

יוֹתָא, v. אָתָא III.

יוֹתָם (b. h.) pr. n. m. *Jotham*, king of Judah. Succ. 45ᵇ.

יוֹתָן, כִּי י׳, v. נָתַן.

יוֹתְפָאָה, v. יוֹדְפַת.

יוֹתֵר m. (b. h.; יָתַר) *much*; (followed by מִ־, or מִ־ implied) *more*. Y. Ber. IV, 7ᵈ top בן תורה י׳ ממני a greater scholar than I am. Keth. 86ª, a. e. י׳ ממה שהאיש וכ׳ more than man desires to marry, does woman desire to be married. Pes. 112ª י׳ ממה שהעגל וכ׳ more anxious than the calf is to suck, is the cow to nurse, i. e. the teacher is more anxious to teach than the pupil to learn. M. Kat. 27ᵇ י׳ מדאי more than enough, י׳ מכשיעור more than the proper measure, *too much*; a. v. fr.—בי׳ a) *in a higher degree, especially*. Sifré Deut. 31 עלינו הוחל שמו בי׳ upon us especially has His name been made to rest. Lev. R. s. 14 ובי׳ אם היה זכר and especially so when it is a male; a. e.—b) *for a higher price, above market value*. Ned. III, 11; a. e.—V. יֶתֶר.

יוֹתֵר ch. same. Targ. Ruth I, 13. Ib. III, 12 (ed. Lag. יַתִּיר).

יוֹתְרָן, יוֹתְרָנָא m.=h. יִתְרוֹן, *advantage, profit*. Targ. Prov. XXVIII, 3 (ed. Wil. יַתְרָן). Ib. XIV, 23. Ib. XXI, 5.

יוֹתֶרֶת f. (b. h. יֹתֶרֶת; יָתַר) 1) *the large lobe of the liver*. Sifra Vayikra, N'dabah, ch. XVII, Par. 14; Yalk. Lev. 462; a. e.—2) *an additional limb* or *lobe*, v. יַתֶּרֶת.

יְזִיפְ׳, יְזוּפְתָא f. (יְזַף) *a loan*. M. Kat. 28ᵇ (Ms. M. יְזִיפְ׳, v. Rabb. D. S. a. l. note); v. אַזוּרָא.

יְזִיף, v. יְזַף.

יָזַן, *Pi.* יִזֵּן (denom. of זַן) *to supply with all kinds and assort*.—Part. pass. f. מְיוּזֶּנֶת *well supplied and assorted*. Gitt. 67ª, v. חָנוּת.

יָזַע, *Hif.* הִזִּיעַ *to sweat*, v. זוּעַ.

יָזַף* (v. זוף) [*to join*; cmp. לָוָה,] *to borrow*.

Hif. הוזיף *to lend*. Sot. 48ᵇ המוזיף Ar. (not found in ed.), v. טוּלְמָא I.

יְזַף, יְזִיף, (זוּף) ch. same 1) *to borrow*. Targ. O. Deut. XV, 6; ib. XXVIII, 12 תְּזִיף (some ed. תְּזוּף); Y. ib. לְמִיזוּף.—Part. יָזֵיף. Targ. II Kings IV, 1 (ed. Lag. מוֹזִיף *Af.*).—B. Mets. 64ª כי יָזִיף וכ׳ if this man shall borrow money of thee. Kidd. 20ª ולא נֵיזִיף וכ׳ (some ed. נוֹזִיף, v. infra) rather than borrow on interest. Erub. 65ª הוה י׳ ופרע Ms. M. (v. Rabb. D. S. a. l.) borrowed and paid off (made up by night for neglect of study by day). Taan. 12ᵇ ליְזוּף מר וכ׳ Ms. M. (ed. לוזיף) borrow and pay back (postpone your fast for another day); a. fr.—2) *to lend*. Targ. Y. Deut. XV, 2 לְשַׁבּ׳ ב־ דִּיזוּף.—Sabb. 119ª מאן דיזיף שבתא וכ׳ (Ms. M. לשב׳, Buxt. דיוזיף) him who lends to the Sabbath (incurring an additional expense in honoring the Sabbath), the Sabbath will repay; Yalk. Gen. 16; Yalk. Is. 356.

Af. אוֹזִיף 1) *to borrow*. Targ. Ps. XXXVII, 21.—B. Bath. 32ᵇ הדרת אוֹזְפְתִּינְהוּ מינאי (Rashb. הדר יזפתינהו, Ms. M. שקלתינהו) thou hast borrowed it again of me. B. Mets. 63ᵇ האי מאן דאו׳ וכ׳ (Ms. H. דיזיף) if one borrowed &c. Kidd. 20ª; Taan. 12ᵇ, v. supra.—Lam. R. to I, 2 אוֹזְפִיתוּן, v. חוֹבָא.—Lev. R. s. 3 beg. דיוזיף וכ׳ some ed. he who borrows on interests.—2) *to lend*. Targ. O. Deut. XV, 6. Ib. 8 אוֹזָפָא תוֹזְפִינֵּיהּ (Y. מוֹזָפָא תוז׳). Ib. XXVIII, 12; a. e.—Targ. Prov. XIX, 17 מְיוֹזִיף Ms. (ed. מְזֵיף).—Bekh. 8ᵇ גברא דאו׳ וטרף ...דהדר מוזיף he who once lent money and had to resort to seizing (v. טְרַף I), why does he lend again?; a. e.

יָזְפָא m. (preced.) *debtor*. Targ. Is. XXIV, 2.—V. יוֹזִיף.

יָזֵק pr. n. 1) *Yazek*, name of a Babylonian river or channel. Y. Kidd. IV, 65ᵈ top; Bab. ib. 71ᵇ עֲזֵק; Y. Yeb. I, 3ᵇ top זרוק.—2) בית י׳, v. יַעֲזֵק.

יְחָא, v. יְחִי.

יָחַד, *Pi.* יִחֵד, יִיחֵד (b. h.; v. אָחַד) 1) *to unite, concentrate*. Y. Ber. IV, 7ᵈ bot. ותְיַיחֵד לבבינו וכ׳ and concentrate our hearts (inclinations) to fear thy Name.—2) (with על) *to confer a distinction, name* &c. Gen. R. s. 68 אברהם י׳ . . שמו עליו on Abraham did the Lord confer His Name (Gen. XXVI, 24, a. e.). Ib. ידע שהקב״ה מְיַחֵד שמו עליו he inferred that the Lord would confer His Name upon him (to be called 'the God of Jacob'). Mekh. Mishp. s. 20 על ישראל י׳ שמו ביותר (although the Lord of the universe) He conferred His Name particularly on Israel (v. יוֹתֵר); a. fr.—3) *to declare the unity of God, to recite*

Sh'ma (Deut. VI, 4). Gen. R. s. 20 אנו.. וּמְיַחֲדִים שמו וכ׳ we trust in Him and profess His unity &c. Cant. R. to II, 16 ואני מְיַחֶדֶת שמו וכ׳ and I (Israel) profess the unity of His name twice every day, (saying) Hear, O Israel &c.; a. fr.—4) *to single out, select, designate.* Snh. 57ª שיי׳ שפחה לעבדו who designated a handmaid (as a wife) for his slave. Lev. R. s. 12 ויי׳ אליו הדבור וכ׳ addressed the command to him exclusively (Lev. X, 8); a. e.—Yoma 11ᵇ (ref. to Lev. XIV, 35) מי שמְיַיחֵד ביתו לו וכ׳ he who devotes his household exclusively to himself, and is unwilling to lend his vessels &c.; Arakh. 16ª שמיוחד (v. infra); Yalk. Lev. 564.—5) *to leave persons alone in a special room, to arrange a private meeting for.* Keth. 12ª; Tosef. ib. I, 4; Y. ib. I, 25ª bot. היו מְיַיחֲדִין וכ׳ they used to leave bride and groom in a private room alone for a while.—*Part. pass.* מְיוּחָד, f. מְיוּחֶדֶת; pl. מְיוּחָדִים, מְיוּחָדִין, מְיוּחָדוֹת a) *especial, particular, designated; chosen, distinguished* (v. יָחִיד). Snh. 60ª, a. e. שם המי׳ the proper Name of the Lord (Jehovah).—Yoma 11ª ביתך ביתך המי׳ לך '*thy* house' (Deut. VI, 9; XI, 20), thy house which is designated for thy personal use. Ib.ᵇ מה בית מ׳ לדירה *bayith* means a room designated for a dwelling, יצאו אלו שאינן מי׳ לדירה to the exclusion of those rooms (gate lodge &c.) which are not designated for dwellings. Arakh. l. c. מי׳ לו devoted to his own exclusive use, v. supra; a. fr.—Gen. R. s. 99, end (ref. to כאחד, Gen. XLIX, 16) כמי׳ שבשבטים like the most distinguished among the tribes. Yeb. 62ª אני שמ׳ לדבור בכל וכ׳ I (Moses) who am singled out (must be prepared) for divine communication every hour; Ab. d'R. N., II Vers., ch. II (ed. Schechter, p. 10) שאני כלי מי׳ who am a special vessel (of revelation). Meil. 15ª קדשים המי׳ לה׳ sanctified things which are exclusively dedicated to the Lord; Sifra Vayikra, Ḥobah, Par. 11, ch. XX.—Ib. Sh'mini, ch. II, Par. 2 כבשים ועזים המי׳ lambs and goats which are specified (Deut. XIV, 4); a. fr.—b) *locked up with.* Num. R. s. 9 בזמן שהאשה מי׳ עם וכ׳ when a wife is locked up with her husband.

Hithpa. הִתְיַיחֵד, *Nithpa.* נִתְיַיחֵד 1) *to be conferred* (with על); *to be especially addressed* (with אל). Ex. R. s. 7 היה ראוי... לְהִתְיַיחֵד עליו וכ׳ the divine communication was to bear his name alone. Lev. R. s. 12 נתי׳ אליו הדבור the divine communication was addressed to him especially; a. e.—2) *to be alone with, to be closeted with.* Kidd. IV, 12 לא יִתְיַיחֵד אדם וכ׳ a man must not be alone (even) with two women, but one woman מִתְיַיחֶדֶת וכ׳ may be alone with two men. Ab. Zar. II, 1. Tosef. Gitt. VII (V), 4; a. fr.—V. יִחוּד.

יַחֵד, *Pa.* יַחֵד ch. same, 1) *to concentrate.* Targ. Ps. LXXXVI, 11.—*Part. pass.* מְיַחַד *united, harmonious.* Targ. Y. Ex. XIX, 2 (cmp. הוֹמוֹנְיָא).—2) *to specify, single out, designate.* Macc. 18ª לְיַחוּדֵי לאוי וכ׳ Ms. M. (ed. לי׳ להו) to forbid each of these acts singly (as if each were prohibited by a special prohibitory law, v. לָאו).—*Part. pass.* מְיַחַד = h. מְיוּחָד (v. preced.). Targ. O. Gen. XXVI, 10 דמי׳ בעמא ed. Berl. (oth. ed. מְיָחִיד; Y. מלכא דמיחד) a distinguished person of the people. Targ. Y. Lev. XV, 20; 22 מְיַיחַד designated; a. e.

Ithpa. אִתְיַיחֵד, contr. אִיַּיחֵד *to be joined; to be locked up.* Targ. Y. I Gen. XLIX, 6. Targ. Job. III, 6.—Targ. Y. II Num. XXXI, 50.—Snh. 37ª שרי לְיִיחוּדֵי וכ׳ is permitted to be closeted up with her husband.

יִחוּד, יִיחוּד m. (preced. wds.) 1) *private meeting, esp. privacy between man and woman.* Y. Keth. XI, beg. 34ª דברים של יי׳ private attendance, e. g. assistance at washing and ointing. Y. Sot. I, 16ᶜ top אין זה י׳ this is no ascertained private meeting (with her former husband, on account of which a second letter of divorce would be required). Snh. 21ª, sq. גזרו על הי׳ ועל וכ׳ they forbade privacy (with a married woman) and with a single woman. Ib. י׳ דאורייתא הוא is not privacy with a married woman biblically interdicted?—Kidd. 81ª משום.. מלקין על הי׳ הי׳ we punish private meetings between a man and a woman, but we do not prohibit the wife to her husband on account of her private meeting with a man. Ib. בעלה בעיר אין חוששין משום י׳ if her husband is in town, we do not consider her private meeting with a man a suspicious act; a. fr.—בְּי׳ a) *privately.* Bets. 22ᵇ; Pes. 37ª שאילית את רבי בי׳ I asked my teacher privately.—b) *particularly, exactly; by a special sign.* Shek. VI, 2; Yoma 54ª.—2) (later Hebr.) י׳ השם *declaration of the unity of God.* Pesik. Zutr., Nitsabim, end.—[Gen. R. s. 99, end כיחודו של עולם, read: כיחידו, v. יָחִיד.]

יְחוּד, יְחוּדָא, יי׳ ch. same, esp. *profession of the unity of God, Jewish religion.* Targ. Lam. III, 28. Targ. Cant. VIII, 9 למקני י׳ וכ׳ to buy the permission to profess the Jewish religion.

יְחוּל, יי׳ m. (יָחַל) *hope.* Ber. 16ᵇ; Y. ib. IV, 7ᵈ bot. ונמצא י׳ לבבינו that we may obtain what our heart longs for.

יִחוּס, יי׳ m. (יָחַס) *genealogy, pedigree* (v. יוּחָס). Num. R. s. 13 לכן הוא מונה שם יִחוּסָם therefore the Scripture records there (Ex. VI, 14 sq.) their genealogy; a. e.—[Y. Gitt. VIII, 49ᶜ bot. כהונה יי׳, v. זִיהוּם.—Y. Yeb. II, 4ª top, v. יָחַס.]—*Pl.* יִחוּסִין, יי׳. Num. R. l. c. שמרו יִחוּסֵיהֶם they preserved their genealogical records; Cant. R. to IV, 7. Gen. R. s. 37 הראשונים... יִיחוּסֵיהֶם וכ׳ as regards former generations whose genealogies were known, their names were published in connection with historical events; אנו... יִיחוּסֵינוּ וכ׳ but with us who do not know our records, our names are defined by those of our fathers; (Yalk. Gen. 62 יִחוּסֵנוּ, יִחוּסֵהֶן sing.); Yalk. Chr. 1074.

יְחוּס, יְחוּסָא, יי׳ ch. same; also *family (gens).* Targ. Y. Gen. V, 1. Ib. XXIV, 38; 40, sq. Ib. XLIII, 7; a. e.—Kidd. 71ᵇ שתיקותיה דבבל היינו יי׳ (v. marginal vers.) silence of a Babylonian (in case of an offered insult) is a sign of good descent; v. יַחֲסוּתָא.—*Pl.* יי׳, יְחוּסִין, יְחוּסַיָּא. Targ. Y. Gen. VI, 9. Targ. Y. Ex. VI, 14. Targ. Job. XXXI, 34 Ms. Var. (ed. גְּנִיסְתָא).

יְחוּסָא m. (preced.) *noble.*—*Pl.* constr. יְחוּסֵי. Targ. Ps. XCVI, 7 (some ed. יַחוּ׳, v. preced.)

יְחוּף, יי׳ m. (יָחַף) *bare-footedness, homelessness.* Yoma 77ª (ref. to Jer. II, 25) מנער...... לידי י׳ keep off from sin, in order that thy foot may not be reduced to bareness (exile); Yalk. Jer. 266 לידי יָחֵף.

יְחוּפָה m. (preced.) *bare-footed, homeless.* Lam. R.

to I, 7 .כד ר׳ ברא וכ׳ (some ed. יְחֵיפָה) when the son is homeless (foot-sore), he remembers the comforts of his paternal home.

יִיחוּר, יְחוּר (יחר, cmp. אחר, a. חֲלִיפִין) *a young shoot*, esp. of a fig-tree. Kil. I, 8. Ukts. III, 8; Ḥull. 128[b]. Y. Maasr. II, 49[d] top כיי׳ שהוא נוטה וכ׳ like a shoot (of a fig-tree) hanging over into a court (ref. to Mish. ib. III, 10); a. e.—*Pl.* יְחוּרִים, יִי׳. Gen. R. s. 31, end ... הכניס עמו ר׳ לתאנים he (Noah) took with him ..... shoots for the preservation of fig-trees; ib. s. 36 ר׳ של תאנה. Y. B. Kam. VI, 5[b] bot. יִיחוּרֵי תאנים; Bab. ib. 59[a] יח׳.

יְחֶזְקֵאל (b. h.) pr. n. m. *Ezekiel*, 1) the prophet. Snh. 39[a], v. יָסַר. Hag. 13[b] למה ר׳ דומה לבן וכ׳ to whom is Ez. to be compared? To a villager that saw the king; a. fr.—ספר ר׳ the Book of Ezekiel. Ib.[a]; Sabb. 13[b], v. גָּנַז; Men. 45[a]; a. e.—2) Ez., the father of R. Judah, v. יְהוּדָה. Kidd. 70[a].

יָחַט (cmp. חטא); *Hif.* הוֹחִיט *to fail, miscarry.* Y'lamd. to B'resh., (quot. in Ar. s. v. מחט) לא חיתה... מוֹחֶטֶת none of them miscarried.

יַחַט m. (preced.) *abortion.* Targ. Is. XIV, 19 כיחט ed. Lag. (oth. ed. כי חט, corr. acc.; Var. כיחט).—*Pl.* יַחְטַיָּיא. Y. Nidd. III, 51[a] אילין להטיירה וכ׳ (corr. acc.) the abortions come out first.

יַחְטָא or **יַחֲטָא** m. (preced. wds.) *searcher of sin, accuser.* Targ. Zech. III, 1; ib. 2 (ed. Lag. חטא, v. ib. p. XLII[3]), v. חֲטָאָה.

יְחִי (cmp. חיי), *Af.* אוֹחִי *to hurry, press on.* Targ. Ex. X, 16. Targ. Esth. VI, 10. Targ. O. Gen. XVIII, 6 אוֹחָאִי ed. Berl. (ed. אוֹחִי, Y. אוֹחָא). Targ. Ex. XII, 33. לאוֹחָאָה; a. fr.—Part. מוֹחִי, מְוֹחֵי; f. מוֹחֲיָא. Targ. Prov. XXII, 29 (ed. Wil. מְוֹחֵי). Targ. Zeph. III, 1; a. fr.

יָחִיד m. (b. h.; יָחַד) 1) *only, single, individual.* Gen. R. s. 99, end (ref. to כאחד, Gen. XLIX, 16) כִּיחִידוֹ של וכ׳ (not כיחודו) like the Only One of the world, as He needs no help &c.; ib. s. 21 (ref. to כאחד, ib. III, 22). Ib. s. 55 זה ר׳ לאמו וכ׳ this one (Ishmael) is the only son of his mother, and the other (Isaac) is &c.—Taan. 9[a] בשביל ר׳ for an individual's sake, opp. רבים. Ber. 9[a], a. fr. ר׳ ורבים הלכה וכ׳ where a single opinion is opposed to the opinion of more than one, the law follows the latter. Bets. V, 5 בור של ר׳ a well belonging to an individual. Erub. 46[a] ר׳ במקום ר׳ an individual opinion opposed to an individual opinion; a. v. fr.—Y. Keth. VII, 31[b] bot. בְּיִ׳ (=בְּיִחוּד) *privately.*—*Pl.* יְחִידִים, יְחִידִין. R. Hash. 17[b] כי׳ דמי are to be considered as individuals (in prayer); a. fr.—*Fem.* יְחִידָה. Num. R. s. 12 בת ר׳ an only daughter; a. fr.—Deut. R. s. 2, end מה הקב״ה .... כך הנפש ר׳ בגוף as the Lord is matchless in his world, so is the soul in the body; Midr. Till. to Ps. CIII; Gen. R. s. 14, end שכל האברים ... והיא ר׳ בגוף all limbs are paired, but she (the soul) is unmatched in the body.—As a noun (b. h.) יְחִידָה *soul.* Ib. Deut. R. l. c.; a. e.—2) *select*, esp. *one devoted to a particularly scrupulous life.* Taan. 10[b] איזהו ר׳ who is called a *yaḥid*? Ans. כל שראוי וכ׳ ר׳ whoever is worthy to be appointed manager of a community. Ib. אל יאמר אדם ... להיות ר׳ one must not say, I am only a student, I am not fit to lead the life of a *yaḥid* (it would be an assumption, v. יוֹהֲרָא); Tosef. ib. I, 7 (v. Var. in ed. Zuck. a. Rabb. D. S. to Taan. l. c.); Y. Ber. II, end, 5[d] כל דבר של צער ... ר׳ עושה in all matters of self-abnegation, whoever desires to make himself a *yaḥid*, may do so.—*Pl.* as ab. Taan. I, 4; a. fr. V. יְחִידִי.

יְחִיד, יְחִידָא, ר׳ ch. same. Targ. Gen. XXII, 2. Targ. Prov. IV, 3; a. e.—*Fem.* יְחִידְתָא, יְחִידָאָה. Targ. Jud. XI, 34 (ed. Lag. יְחִדָא, some ed. יְחִידָה).—Ned. 51[a] תספרתא ר׳ a particular kind of hair-dressing.

יְחִידָאָה f., v. preced.—ר׳ m., v. יְחִידִי ch.

יְחִידִי m. (v. preced. wds.) 1) *singular, single, lonely.* Macc. 23[b] בלשון ר׳ in the singular number, opp. ל׳ רבים.—Kidd. 20[a] (expl. בגפו, Ex. XXI, 3) ר׳ נכנס וכ׳ single (unmarried) he entered &c. Ab. III, 4 המהלך בדרך ר׳ who travels alone. Ib. IV, 8 אל תהי דן ר׳ וכ׳ do not hold court as a single judge, for there is only One who judges singly; a. fr.—*Fem.* יְחִידִית. Y. Kil. II, 28[a] bot. גפן ר׳ a single (isolated) vine tree. Y. Ab. Zar. IV, 44[a] top מצבה כל שהיא ר׳ it is called *matsebah* when consisting of one piece (v. בימוס); a. e.—*Pl.* יְחִידִיּוֹת. Y. Kil. V, beg. 29[d] בר׳ in the case of isolated vine trees. Y. Sot. IX, 23[c] top ר׳ isolated tombstones.—2) *believer in One God.* Esth. R. to II, 5, v. יְהוּדִי.

יְחִידִי (דִּי...), יְחִידָאָה, דָאִי... יְחִידָיָא ch. same, 1) *lonely; only one.* Targ. Ps. XXV, 16 (ed. Lag. יְחִידָאִי).—Targ. Y. Deut. XXXII, 50 (ed. Amst. ... דָאִי incorr.). Targ. Job XIV, 4 Ms. (ed. חד).—2) *single authority, opinion of one.* Pes. 103[b] לא יחידאה אנא (v. Rabb. D. S. a. l.) I do not report the opinion of one man. Y. Ter. VI, beg. 44[a] אתיא דר׳ דהכא כסתמא דתמן וכ׳ the opinion of the single authority here agrees with the anonymous (editorially adopted) one there &c.; Y. Ned. VII, beg. 40[b]. Y. Sabb. III, 6[a] bot. לית אנן ... לר׳ we need not consider the opinion of a single authority; a. fr.—*Pl.* יְחִידָיִין, יְחִידָאֵי, יְחִידָאִין. Targ. Y. Gen. XXII, 10 (v. יָחִיד 2).—B. Kam. 81[b] bot. בר׳ לא אמרינן we do not speak of single authorities. Y. Ḥag. II, 77[b] top ר׳ single-handed, each for himself, v. טְעַן II.

יְחִידְתָא, v. יָחִיד ch.

יְחִיף, יְחֵיף, v. יָחֵף, יָחֵף.

יְחֵיפָה m. ch., v. יָחוֹפָה.

***יַחְכִּים**=חַכִּים. Targ. I Chr. IV, 9 ed. Beck, Var. ed. Rahmer ויח׳ (ed. וח׳).

יָחַל (b. h.; v. חול) *to hover around, rest on.*

Pi. יִחֵל, יִי׳ 1) (with על) *to cause to rest upon.* Pesik. R. s. 47 מְיַיחֵל אני ... כשם שיִיחַלְתִּי וכ׳ I shall cause my Name to rest upon him (Job) as I did upon &c.—2) (b. h.; with אל) *to wait for the turn, to wait, trust; to inspire trust*; v. יִחוּל.

Hof. הוּחַל *to be made to rest.* Sifré Deut. 31, v. יוֹתֵר.

***יָחַם** (b. h.; v. חום) *to be warm, hot*; *Pi.* יִחֵם *to heat.*

Tosef. Sabb. III (IV), 7 מְיַיחֵם, v. חָמַם.— Pesik. Zutr. (ed. Bub.), Vayetsé 39 לְיַחֲמֶנָּה to heat it (the flock). Ib. 41 לְיַחֵם.

יחם ch. same. Targ. O. Gen. XVIII, 1; Targ. II Sam. IV, 5 מֵיחַם (perh. fr. חֲמַם).

Pa. יַחֵם *to heat.* Targ. O. Gen. XXX, 41 לְיַחֲמוּתְהֶין ed. Berl. (ed. לְיַחֲמוּתְהֶן; Y. לְיַחֲמוּת׳).

Ithpa. אִתְיַחֵם *to be heated, to conceive.* Ib. 38, sq.

***יַחֲמָא** m. (preced.) *heating, exciting ingredient of drinks.* Targ. Hab. II, 15 (ed. Lag. חמא; h. text חמתך).

יַחְמוּר m. (b. h.; v. Ges. H. Dict. s. v.) *yaḥmur,* a species of *deer,* prob. *fallow-deer.* Pesik. Eth Korb., p. 57[a] (ref. to Deut. XIV, 4, sq.) וז׳ אינן ברשותך... וי׳ and seven are not in thy possession (must be hunted) as the hart, the roebuck, the fallow-deer &c.; Lev. R. s. 27; a. e.

יַחְמוּרָא ch. same. Targ. O. Deut. XIV, 5.—*Pl.* יַחְמוּרִין. Targ. Y. l. c.—Targ. I Kings V, 3.—*Fem.* יַחְמוּרְתָּא. Bekh. 7[b], v. חַלָּא.

יַחַן, v. חָנָה.

יַחְנִינָה, יַחְנוּנָה, יַחְנוּן, v. חָנוּן II.

יחס (b. h. יָחַשׂ; v. חוּס 2) *to connect, be connected.*— Denom. יַחַס.

Pi. יִחֵס, יִי׳ (denom. of יַחַס) 1) *to trace the connection* (יַחַס) *of events or descent.* Meg. 17[a] כדי לְיַיחֵס בהן שנותיו וכ׳ (Rashi: לְהִתְיַיחֵס) in order to trace through them the years of Jacob (in which the principal events of his life occurred); Yeb. 64[a]; Yalk. Gen. 110. Ib.; Gen. R. s. 62 (ref. to Gen. XXV, 12 sq.) מה ראה הכתוב לייחס תולדותיו וכ׳ what reason was there for the Bible to insert here the genealogy of that &c.?—Snh. 82[b] בא הכתוב ויִחֲסוֹ the Scripture comes and records his genealogy (Num. XXV, 11). Sabb. 55[b] אפשר.... והכתוב מְיַחֲסוֹ is it possible that he was a sinner and the Scripture would state his genealogy?; a. fr.—2) *to nobilize, distinguish, invest with prerogatives.* Num. R. s. 13 יִיחֲסוֹ הכתוב על שם שבטו the Scripture distinguished him (giving him the privilege of the first offering) for the sake of his tribe (Num. VII, 12). Gen. R. s. 82 אין מְיַיחֲסִין ליוסף וכ׳ not Joseph is ranked in the records as the first-born; a. e.— *Part. pass.* מְיוּחָס, f. מְיוּחֶסֶת. pl. מְיוּחָסִין, מְיוּחָסִים; מְיוּחָסוֹת *of traceable genealogy, of legitimate descent; of distinguished birth, well-connected.* Hor. 13[a] שזה מי׳ וזה אינו מי׳ for this one (the Israelite) is of legitimate birth, and the other (the bastard) is not. Kidd. 70[b] משפחות מי׳ וכ׳ families in Israel of traceable descent. Ib. 71[b] האי מי׳ טפי this one (who first ceased quarreling) is of nobler birth; a. fr.

Hithpa. הִתְיַיחֵס, *Nithpa.* נִתְיַיחֵס 1) *to claim a pedigree.* Tosef. Peah IV, 11 היתה מִתְיַיחֶסֶת עם וכ׳ ed. Zuck. (Var. על) claimed to be connected with Arnon, the Jebusite; Y. ib. VIII, 21[a] bot. היתה מתי׳ של וכ׳ boasted to be descendants of &c.—2) *to be enrolled in genealogical lists, be recorded.* Num. R. l. c. זכו להִתְי׳ וכ׳ they were privileged to have their genealogy recorded by the side of Moses. Cant. R. to I, 1 כ׳ ראש לשלשלת יוחסין (not לשלשת) he was recorded as the starter of a chain of genealogy (I Kings XIV, 21). Gen. R. l. c. (expl. I Chr. V, I) לא לראובן להתייחס not to Ruben was genealogical priority to be given; a. fr.

יַחַס, *Pa.* יַחֵס same, 1) *to nobilize, distinguish.* Targ. Y. Num. XXV, 13.—2) *to trace, to record.* Meg. 12[b] [read:] אי לְיַחוּסֵיה קאתי לְיַחֲסֵיה וליזיל וכ׳ (v. Rabb. D. S. a. l. note) if the text (Esth. II, 5) were intended to give Mordecai's genealogy, it ought to trace him back to Benjamin. Yeb. 62[a] יַחֲסִינְהוּ בשמייהו וכ׳ he recorded them by their names and those of their fathers &c.

Ithpa. אִתְיַיחֵס *to be enrolled, recorded.* Targ. Num. I, 18 (h. text ויתילדו). Targ. Y. Gen. XXI, 12. Targ. I Chr. V, 1; a. e.

יַחַס m. (b. h. יַחַשׂ; יַחַס) *connection, family relation,* v. חַיִיס I. B. Kam. 15[a] משום דאין לו י׳ (Ms. M. חייס) because the slave has no legal relationship. Y. Yeb. II, 4[a] top ועבדים יש להם ייחוס (read יַיחַס) have slaves legal pedigrees?—*Pl.* יְחָסִין, יְחָסִים. Ib. Y. Kidd. II, 62[c] bot. אם הטעה לשבח י׳ if he deceived her inasmuch as he proved of higher birth than he had presented to her.

יַחְסוּתָא f. (preced. wds.) *tracing the pedigree, searches.* Kidd. 71[b] בי׳ by searching &c.; v. יְחוּסָא.

יָחֵף I m. (b. h.; v. חָפַף II) *rubbed off, bare,* esp. *barefooted, foot-sore.* Y. Snh. X, 28[b] bot (expl. אט I Kings XXI, 27) היה מהלך י׳ he walked bare-footed (in penance); Cant. R. to I, 5.—Yoma 77[a] (ref. to II Sam. XV, 30) י׳ ממאי וכ׳ 'bare' of what?—Does it not mean bare of sandals?; v. מְטַרְקָא.—Sabb. 114[a] (ref. to Is. XX, 3) י׳ במנעלים וכ׳ 'bare' means in patched shoes; a. fr.—*Pl.* יְחֵפִין, יְחֵפִים, יְחֵי׳. Num. R. s. 5; a. fr.—Fem. יְחֵפָה, יְחֵי׳. Ruth R. to I, 19; a. e.—*Pl.* יְחֵיפוֹת. Yalk. Ruth 601 (Ruth R. to I, 7 בְּיַיחֵף); a. e.

יָחֵף, יְחֵיף ch. same. Targ. II Sam. XV, 30. Targ. Is. XX, 2, sq.—*Pl.* יְחֵיפִין. Ib. 4.

יחף II (preced. wds.) *to be bare.*—*Hithpa.* הִתְיַיחֵף, *Nithpa.* נִתְיַי׳ *to be exposed, to take cold.* Lam. R. introd. (R. Joh. 2) כדי שלא יִתְיַיחֲפוּ רגליהם that their feet might not be exposed (that they might not take cold); אע״פ כן נִתְיַיחֲפוּ וכ׳ and yet they did take cold. Ib. to I, 16.

יְחֵף, יְחֵיף ch. same, *to be rubbed, sore, worn out.* Targ. O. Deut. VIII, 4.

Pa. יַחֵף, part. pass. מְיַחַף *sore.* Targ. Y. ib.

יַחַף, יי׳ m. (preced. wds.) 1) *barefootedness.* Ruth R. to I, 7, v. יָחֵף I. Yalk. Jer. 266, v. יִחוּף.—2) *footsoreness.* Makhsh. III, 8 בשעת הי׳ והדיש in the season of footsores (of animals) or of threshing (when moistening the animal's foot is welcome to the owner); Var. lect. האף, v. אַף II.

יַטָא, v. יְטַר.

יָמַב (v. next w.), *part. Hof.* מוּטָב, q. v.

יְמַב ch. (cmp. טוב) *to be good, well.* Impf. יִיטַב. Targ. O. Gen. XII, 13 ed. Berl. (ed. יוֹטַב, Y. יִיטַב). Targ. O. Deut. IV, 40 (Y. יוֹטִיב); a. fr.

Af. אוֹטִיב, אֵיטִיב 1) same, v. supra.—2) *to do good, be kind.* Targ. Gen. XXXII, 10; a. fr.—3) *to do a thing well.* Targ. I Sam. XVI, 17 מוֹטִיב לנגנא who plays well. Targ. Gen. IV, 7; a. e.

יָמְבַת, v. יוֹדְפַת.

***יְטוּר** I pr.n. (b. h.) *Ituraea*, a district along the base of Mount Hermon. Y. Ber. III, 6ª bot. אפי׳ לי׳ יוצא וכ׳ even to Ituraea he must go and reclaim Jewish property.

יְטוּרָא, יְטוּר II, m. (v. טור II; cmp. יְקוּם) *rising pillar* (of smoke). Targ. Jud. XX, 38; 40 (ed. Lag. וידטור). Targ. Ez. VIII, 11.—*Pl.* יְטוּרִין. Targ. Joel III, 3.

יְטָא, יְטֵי (cmp. מְטָא, נְטָא, v. P. Sm. 1591), *to incline, turn.*

**Pa.* יַטֵּי *to adduce, prefer.* Y. Ber. II, 4ᵇ top לית אפשר דלא י׳ מילה it was impossible that he should not have brought on (in his lecture) a word (alluding to the exodus from Egypt); cmp. Bab. ib. 13ᵇ מהדר רבי אשמעתא וכ׳. [Vers. in Fr. Ahăb. Zion: יְטִיק; ed. Lehm. יִרְתֵי, v. אֲתָא.]

Af. אַיְטֵי *to hand, reach over.* Gen R. s. 38 א׳ לי כולבא Ar. s. v. כלב (ed. אייתי .. קולב׳; Yalk. Gen. 62 אמטי) hand me a pair of tongs (an axe). Gen. R. s. 15, end דאייטיאת Ar. s. v. ברת (ed. אמטיית), v. אַלְּיְתָא. Koh. R. to III, 9 כל . . . יַיְטֵי ליה מה וכ׳ every one shall bring for himself something whereon to recline.

יטסס, Y. Sabb. III, 6ª, v. טרים.

יט״ת *yetath*, substitute for מנא (Dan. V, 25), by permutation of letters called אתב״ש. Snh. 22ª; Cant. R. to III, 4; v. אד״ך.

יְיָ m. (abbrev. of the Tetragrammaton) *Adonai, the Lord.* Targ. Ps. I, 2 (ed. Lag. יהוה); a. fr.—Y. Snh. X, 28ª top; a. fr. (interch. in eds. with ה׳).

וַי. (interj.) O!, oh!, *woe!* Targ. Prov. XXXI, 2 ed. Lag. (oth. eds. וַי). Ib. IV, 4 וַי some eds. (ed. Lag. יהוה, corr. acc.). Targ. Ps. XLIX, 7 וי לחיביא Ms. (ed. Lag. וַוי, ed. Wil. omitted).

—יי, —כִּי = כְּחִיי; לְחִיי = לִיי; v. כְּיי, לְיי.

וַיָא (v. וַי) *woe!* Targ. Y. I, Num. XXI, 29

ויא, v. יָא.

וַיָא, v. יָאֵי.

וַיְבָא, v. יָבָא.

וַיאבַק = וְהָא בַק. Y. B. Kam. VIII, beg. 6ᵇ.

—ויְרָא, v. הִירְדָא a. לִירְדָא.

וירח, v. יְרַח.

ויטור, v. יְטוּר.

וִיכא, B. Bath. 146ª Ar., v. בְּרִיכָא.

יָאלָא, יָלָא, יְלָא m. *hedge-hog*, believed to suck and injure the udders of cattle. Targ. O. Lev. XI, 30 יְלָא ed. Berl. (Var. יָלָא, יְלָא; Y. מינקת חויא; h. text אנקה).—*Pl.* יָלֵי &c. Sabb. 54ᵇ כי .. לימצוה יי׳ Ar. (ed. יָאלֵי) to prevent hedge-hogs from sucking them. B. Bath. 4ª top Herod put around Baba's head כלילא דיי׳ (Ms. M. דיא׳, v. Rabb. S. a. l. note) a garland made of skins of hedge-hogs which pricked his eyes out.

וילעו, Y. Kil. IX, 32ᵇ bot. כמו יבא עלי וילעו עלי, read: כמו יבא עלי (v. עול), ויעול עלי being a gloss to יי׳ עלי.

וימם חֲמִים, v. sub יֵמ׳.

ויְמַר pr. n. m. *Yemar*, an Amora. Hull. 56ª bot.; a. fr.

יַיִן m. (b. h.; יון; cmp. יָוֵן) [*thick, fermenting,*] *wine.* Snh. 70ª חי י׳, v. חַי. Sifré Num. 23 (ref. to Num. VI, 3) זה מזוג וכ׳ *yayin* means mixed wine, *shekhar* unmixed. Ab. Zar. V, 1, a. fr. יֵין נסך, v. נֶסֶךְ.—Hull. 4ᵇ, a. e. סתם יֵינָן, v. סְתָם. Ib. יינן של נכרים wine prepared or handled by gentiles; a. v. fr.—*Pl.* יֵינוֹת. Tosef. Ab. Zar. IV (V), 1 sq. Keth. 65ª, v. פָּסַק; a. e.

יינוּבְרִיס pr. n. m. *Januarius*, name of a legendary Roman general who sacrificed his life to save his country. Y. Ab. Zar. I, 39ᶜ הוה תמן . . . . . שמיה י׳ וכ׳ there was there (in Rome) an old man whose name was J., and who had twelve sons. Ib. בגין כן . . . . קלנדס י׳ therefore they name it (that day) calendae Januariae. Cmp. יַמְבְּרִיס.

יינוּמְלִין, יינוּמְלִים, v. אִינוּמִילִין.

אינון = ינון, יינוּן. Y. Peah VII, 20ᵇ. Ib. VIII, 21ª top הירדן ויינון (corr. acc.) what are those?—Y. Ber. I, 3ᵈ bot. וְאינון = יינון. V. ארהו a. דֵינוּן.

יינס, v. יַנְּס.

ייס, v. זוּ. Y. Ber. VI, 10ᵈ top (ed. Lehm. וייסו).

ייסוּרא, ייסור, v. יִס׳.

***ייסי**, Y. Kil. VIII, 31ᶜ bot. ר׳ ערקי, read: ר׳ יוסי אומר (v. R. S. to Kil. VIII, 5).

ייעָא, v. יְעָא.

ייעוּד, v. יְעוּד.

ייצְפָא, v. יִצְפָא.

ייקונְמִין, v. דִּיקְרוּתִין.

יירוּנוֹן, Y. Dem. I, 22ᵇ top שמן וורד ויי׳; Tosef. ib. I, 27 (ed. Zuck. only שמן וורד ודנין) שמן וורד ודירנון, read: ש׳ ור׳ ורודינון rose-oil and (ῥόδινον, sub. μύρον) *rose-unguent.*

יירַךְ, v. יְרֵךְ.

יִירְעָנִין, יִירְעִין, v. יַרְעָנָה.

יִישׁוּב, v. יְשׁוּב.

יִישׁוּעַ, v. יֵשׁוּעַ.

יִישַׁר, v. יָשַׁר.

יִיתּוּר, v. יִתּוּר.

יִיתֵי. v. אֲתָא.

יִיתִיק, v. יַתִּיק.

יִיתַם, v. יָתַם.

יָכֹל, יָכוֹל (b. h.; יכל, cmp. כּוּל, כָּלַל, כַּלְכֵּל) 1) (adj.) m., יְכוֹלָה f. *capable, able to sustain, enduring;* 2) (verb), impf. יוּכַל, *to be capable, able; one can, may; it is possible.* Cant. R. to III, 6 לארי יָכָלְתִּי .. אִינִי י׳ I overpowered the lion, and I should not overpower the dog? Ib. שר שלכם לא י׳ . . . . ואתם יְכוֹלִים להם your guardian angel could not stand against their father (Jacob), and (you think) you could master them?—י׳ אני = יְכוֹלְנִי I can. Ḥag. 15ᵃ top Ms. M. (ed. יכול אני); Nidd. 64ᵇ.—Keth. 95ᵃ יְכוֹלָה היא מפני שר׳ לומר וכ׳ because he may plead &c. Ib. י׳ שתאמר she may plead. Ib. 43ᵃ, a. e. י׳ הרב לומר וכ׳ the master may (has a right to) say to his slave &c. Ber. 6ᵃ אין כל בריה י׳ לעמוד וכ׳ no creature could stand up (exist) before the demons. Taan. 30ᵇ בִּיָכוֹל of an able-bodied person.—Yalk. Esth. 1048 שמא תוּכַל להשיאה וכ׳ canst thou give her in marriage to both of them?—Midr. Till. to Ps. XLV לא יָכְלוּ להתודות וכ׳ they could not confess their sins with their mouth; a. v. fr.—Esp. יָכוֹל (=יכול אני לומר or י׳ אתה לומר) *I (you) might think, argue, conclude.* Sabb. 64ᵃ י׳ שאני מרבה וכ׳ from the Bible text (Lev. XI, 32) I might infer that ropes and cords are included; Sifra Sh'mini Par. 6, ch. VIII; a. v. fr.—כִּבְיָכוֹל *as though it were possible, as it were* (ref. to an allegorical or anthropomorphous expression with reference to the Lord). Mekh. Bo, Pisḥa, s. 14 כל זמן . . . כ׳ שכינה עמהם whenever Israel is enslaved, the Divine Majesty, as it were, is with them in slavery. Ib. כ׳ אמרו ישראל וכ׳ the Israelites said, thou, as it were, hast redeemed thyself. Ib. B'shall., Shirah, s. 6 כ׳ כלפי מעלה as if referring to the Lord's eye. B. Kam. 79ᵇ, v. מַשָּׁה; a. fr.—Ch. יְכִיל.

יְכוֹלְנִי, v. preced.

יכולני, Esth. R. to I, 3, v. בִּרְקוּדְיָאנִי.

יְכֹלֶת, יְכוֹלֶת f. (b. h.; infin. of יָכוֹל) *power, ability.* Num. R. s. 16 (not להוסיף) מפני שלא היה לו י׳ להספיק וכ׳ because he had no power to sustain him, אין לשון י׳ אלא מזונות the word י׳ refers to sustenance (ref. to מכלת, I Kings V, 25, cmp. כִּלְכֵּל).

יְכוּלְתָּא ch. same. Targ. II Chr. XX, 6, v. יוּכְלָא.

יָכַח (b. h.; v. כֹּחַ) *to be firm, stand, be right.*—Denom. נֹכַח.

Hif. הוֹכִיחַ [*to place opposite,*] 1) *to admonish, reprove.* Ber. 31ᵃ sq. (ref. to I Sam. I, 14) מכאן ... שצריך להוֹכִיחוֹ from here we learn that he who sees in his neighbor something unbecoming, is bound to admonish him; Arakh. 16ᵇ. Ib. הוֹכִיחוֹ .... ויוֹכִיחֶנּוּ if he did admonish him and he did not heed it, he must do it again. Ib. . . . . תמיהני שיודע להוכיח I wonder whether there is in this generation one who knows how to admonish; a. fr.—2) *to prove, to serve as an analogy.* B. Kam. 6ᵃ אש תּוֹכִיחַ let the law concerning incendiary (Ex. XXII, 5) be taken as a standard (it being the result of human action); בור תוכיח let the law about a pit (ib. XXI, 33) decide (it being stationary). Kidd. 7ᵃ; a. v. fr.—3) *to be evidence, to show.* M. Kat. 4ᵇ זיבלו מוֹכִיחַ עליו his dung shows what he is about doing; a. fr.

Hithpa. הִתְוַכֵּחַ, *Nithpa.* נִתְוַכֵּחַ *to argue, be justified.* Lev. R. s. 27 בא הקב״ה לה׳ וכ׳ the Lord came to argue with Israel; ib. כלום אינון יכולין לה׳ עם בוראן can they argue (successfully) with their Creator?; Num. R. s. 10, beg.; a. fr.

Nif. נוֹכַח same. Cant. R. to V, 16 מי יוכל לִיוָּכַח וכ׳ (not לִיו׳) who dares to argue with &c.

יְכִיל, יְכֵיל ch. = h. יָכוֹל. Targ. Gen. XLV, 1. Targ. O. Ex. II, 3. Targ. O. Gen. XXXII, 26.—Targ. O. Ex. XXXIII, 20 תִּיכּוּל ed. Berl. (ed. Amst. תִּכוֹל). Targ. Job IV, 2 יְכוֹל Ms. (ed. יְכוֹל, יִיכוֹל).—Ib. XXXIII, 5 תִּיכּוּל Ms. (ed. תּוֹכַל); a. fr.

יְכֹלֶת, יָכֹל, v. יְכוֹלֶת, יָכוֹל.

יכרותה, Y. Sabb. XIV, 14ᵈ bot., v. זִכְרוּתָא.

יָלָא, יָלָא, v. יִילָא.

יָלַד (b. h.; v. בָּלַע) *to bear, bring forth; to beget,* v. וָלַד. Yeb. VII, 5 יָלְדָה הימנו בן she had a son from him. Ib. י׳ תאכל וכ׳ after she has given birth, she may eat (T'rumah). Snh. 52ᵃ ארור שזו י׳ cursed he who begot this woman. Yalk. Sam. 146 והיא ילדה מהם and she was with child from them (the male demons); והיו יוֹלְדוֹת ממנו and they (the female demons) were with child from him (Adam); Gen. R. s. 20 מולידות (corr. acc., or מוּלָּדוֹת *Hof.*). Sot. 11ᵇ בשעה שכורעת לֵילֵד when she kneels down to give birth; a. v. fr.—*Part. pass.* יָלוּד *born;* יְלוּד אשה born of woman, *human being.* Sabb. 88ᵇ; a. fr.—V. יוֹלֵד, יוֹלֶדֶת, יוֹלֵדָה.

Nif. נוֹלַד *to be born, to originate.* Bets. I, 1 ביצה שנוֹלְדָה כ׳ an egg which was laid on a Holy Day. Bekh. II, 3 להם כ׳ מום וכ׳ a permanent blemish appeared on them. Ib. V, 3 כשיִוָּלֵד לו וכ׳ when another blemish shall have appeared. Tosef. Keth. VII, 10 [read:] שדרכן לִיוָּלֵד which ordinarily appear; Y. ib. VII, end, 31ᵈ לְהִיוָּלֵד. Sabb. 137ᵃ יום הִוָּלְדוֹ his day of birth; a. v. fr.—Pesik. R. s. 15 כל חדש שלא נ׳, v. מוֹלָד.—*Part.* נוֹלָד *forthcoming, future event, result.* Ab. II, 9 הרואה את הנ׳ he who considers what may result (from his actions); Tam. 32ᵃ. Ned. III, 9 הנודר מן הַיִּלּוֹדִים מותר בנוֹלָדִים if one foreswears enjoyment of the *yillodim* (those born), he is permitted to derive benefits from those born after his vow (v. Gem. ib. 30ᵇ).—Esp. a) (in festive ritual) *nolad, an object which became available for use on a Holy Day.* Bets. 2ᵃ אית ליה נ׳ holds to the opinion that *nolad* is forbidden to be used on the Holy Day,

v. מוּקְצָה. Sabb. 29ᵃ מעיקרא כלי ... והוה ליה כ׳ ואסור before it was broken, it was a vessel (and not designated for fuel), and now it is a broken vessel and, therefore, is a *nolad* and must not be used as fuel. Erub. 46ᵃ top כ״ש דהוו להו כ׳ וכ׳ so much the more they must be considered as *nolad* &c.; a. fr.—b) (in votive law) *nolad, a novel incident* which changes the aspects of a vow and eventually nullifies it. Ned. IX, 2 פותחין בנ׳ the court in trying to absolve him may open the questions by pointing out a circumstance since occurred. Ib. 3 יש..שהן כנ׳ ואינן כנ׳ there are incidents which are and yet are not like *nolad*, i. e. incidents which may have been anticipated by the vowing person; a. fr.

Hif. הוֹלִיד 1) *to beget.* Tosef. Yeb. X, 4 מפני שמוליד because he is capable of begetting children. Cant. R. beg. את מוצא צדיק מוליד וכ׳ you will find cases of a righteous man having a righteous son &c. Ex. R. s. 1 ולריק ישראל מולידים shall Israelites beget in vain?; a. v. fr.—[Gen. R. s. 20 מולידות, v. supra. Keth. 72ᵇ מולדיו, v. יוֹלֵד.]—2) *to bear living brood*, opp. to laying eggs. Bekh. 7ᵇ, v. רָבַץ.

Pi. יִילֵּד, יַלֵּד 1) *to assist in birth, to deliver.* Sabb. XVIII, 3 מְיַלְּדִין את האשה וכ׳ you may deliver a woman on the Sabbath; ib. 129ᵇ מְיַלְּדִים את החיה Ms. M. (ed. מיי׳ את הולד you may take the child). Ab. Zar. II, 1 (26ᵃ) לא תְיַלֵּד וכ׳ must not deliver a gentile woman; a. fr.—2) *to rear.* Ib. מפני שמְיַלֶּדֶת וכ׳ because she rears a child for idolatry; a. e.

יְלִיד, יְלֵיד, יְלַד ch. same, *to bear; to beget.* Targ. Gen. IV, 1. Ib. 2 לְמֵילַד. Targ. Jer. XXXI, 7 יָלְדָן women giving birth (h. text יֹלֶדֶת). Targ. Prov. XXIII, 22 יְלָדָךְ who begot thee. Targ. Gen. XVII, 19 תְּלִיד; usu. תֵּילִד, תֵּלֵד. Targ. Ps. XXII, 32 לְמֵילַד to create; a. v. fr.—B. Bath. 91ᵃ (prov.) בחייך דיַלְדַּת שיתין למה לך דילַדַּת Ms. M. (v. Rabb. D. S. a. l. note) by thy life, the sixty (weaklings) thou begottest, what didst thou beget them for? איכפיל ואוליד וכ׳ (v. infra) marry again and beget one as strong as sixty; Yalk. Jud. 66. Macc. 17ᵇ דִּילִידָא אימיה כר״ש תֵּילוֹד whose mother soever is with child may she bear a son like R. S.; Yalk. Deut. כל דילַדָה אימה כר״ש תְּלִיד; a. v. fr.

Af. אוֹלִיד 1) *to beget, produce.* Targ. Gen. IV, 18; a. fr. —Yeb. 76ᵃ בר אוֹלוּדֵי capable of begetting; ib. בני אולודי. Erub. 104ᵃ is it not because דקמוליד קלא וכל אולודי וכ׳ he produces a sound, and every production of sound is forbidden (on the Sabbath)?; a. fr. — 2) as preced. *Pi.* Targ. Ex. I, 16.—Sot. 11ᵇ לאוֹלוֹדָהּ to deliver her.

Pa. יַלֵּד 1) *to act as midwife.* Y. Keth. V, 30ᵃ bot. [read:] דמְיַלְּדָא, v. חָכַם.—2) *to give birth.* Targ. Ps. CXLIV, 13.

Ithpa. אִתְיַלַּד, *Ithpe.* אִתְיְלִיד 1) *to be born, to grow, to come forth.* Targ. Ps. LXXVIII, 6. Targ. Gen. IV, 26; a. fr. — Sabb. 136ᵃ א׳ ליה וכ׳ a child was born to him. Bets. 2ᵇ כל ביצה דמִתְיַילְדָא האידנא וכ׳ (some ed. דמִתְיְלִידָא) an egg laid to-day was fully developed yesterday. Ib. הנך דמִתְיַלְדָן וכ׳ those laid on the same day. Hull. 9ᵃ אִתְיְלִידָא בה ריעותא (not אתיליד) an accident occurred to it which made the case suspicious. Ned. 30ᵇ (ref. to נולדים, Mish. ib. III, 9, v. preced.) למימרא ... דמִתְיַילְדָן משמע does this mean to say that *noladim* means 'things which will be forthcoming'?; אלא מעתה .. ה״נ דמִתְיַילְדִין הוא (v. marginal note) if this be so, does *hannoladim* in Gen. XLVIII, 5 also mean 'those to be born'? ואלא מאר דְּאִילִידוּ משמע (=דְּאִתְיְלִידוּ, *Ithpe.* contr.) but what else? Does it (always) mean 'those that have been born'?—2) *to multiply, grow populous.* Targ. O. Ex. I, 7 אִתְיַלָּדוּ ed. Berl. (Y. אִתְיְלִי׳). Targ. Gen. VIII, 17. Ib. IX, 7; a. e.

יֶלֶד m. (b. h.; preced.) *child, young man.* Nidd. 60ᵇ י׳ וזקן וכ׳ a young man and an old man travelling. Ex. R. s. 1; Sot. 12ᵇ הוא י׳ וקולו כנער he (Moses) was an infant, but his voice was that of a lad.—Y. Meg. III, 74ᵃ bot., v. אֶבְדוֹקוֹס; a. fr.—*Pl.* יְלָדִים. Ex. R. 1 c. קיימו את הי׳ (החיו) they spared the lives of the new-born. Kidd. 76ᵇ, a. e. ד׳ מאות י׳ וכ׳ David had four hundred young men in his suite; a. fr.—*Fem.* יַלְדָּה *girl, young woman.* B. Kam. 60ᵇ אחת י׳ ואחת זקינה one wife was young, the other old. Yeb. 101ᵇ; a. fr. — *Pl.* יְלָדוֹת. Sabb. 32ᵃ ר״א ... מתות י׳ ... R. El. reports, 'for three sins women die young' (in place of יוֹלְדוֹת, v. יוֹלֶדֶת); Y. ib. II, 5ᵇ top.—Trnsf. יַלְדָּה *a young plant.* Men. 69ᵇ; Sot. 43ᵇ, a. e. י׳ שסבכה בזקנה a young shoot (subject to the law of *Orlah*, v. עָרְלָה) which was grafted on an old tree. Ib. י׳ בי׳ a young shoot grafted on a young tree.

יַלְדוּת f. (b. h.; preced. wds.) *childhood, youth; waywardness.* Hull. 24ᵇ בְּיַלְדוּתִי in my childhood. Ab. Zar. 52ᵇ שנית לנו ביַלְדוּתְךָ וכ׳ in thy earlier days thou didst teach us &c.; B. Mets. 44ᵃ (not בילדותיך). Succ. 53ᵃ, v. בּוּשׁ.— B. Bath. 131ᵃ י׳ הויתה בי וכ׳ I was wayward and set my face against &c.; a. e.

יַלְדוּתָא ch. 1) same. B. Mets. 44ᵃ ביַלְדוּתֵיה מאר וכ׳ what was his view in his early years? (Ab. Zar. 52ᵇ בילדותו, v. preced.).—2) v. next w.

יַלְדוּתָא f. (preced. wds.) =h. מוֹלֶדֶת *birth, birthplace, family.* Targ. O. Gen. XI, 28 ed. Berl. (Y. יַלְדּוּ׳). Ib. XII, 1; a. fr.

יוֹלַדְתָּא, יַלְדְּתָא f. (preced. wds.) *midwife.* — *Pl.* יוֹלַדְתָא, יַלְדָתָא. Targ. Y. II Ex. I, 15 [read:] יו׳ עִבְרָיָיתָא. Ib. 19 יָלְדָתֵי (corr. acc.).

יַלְדְּתָא, v. יָלֵידְתָא.

יְלוּד, constr. יְלוּד, v. יָלַד.

יְלוּד ch., constr. יְלוּד same. Targ. Job XV, 14 י׳ אתתא (Ms. יְלִיד) born of woman.

יִלּוֹד m. (b. h.; preced. wds.) *born, existing.*—*Pl.* יִלּוֹדִים. Ned. III, 9; ib. 30ᵇ, v. יָלַד *Nif.*—Ab. IV, 22 הי׳ למות the living are destined to die.

יְלוּלָא m. (יָלַל) *howler, monster.* — *Pl.* יְלוּלִין. Targ. Job XXX, 29 Ms. Var. (ed. ירודין, ed. Lag. ירורין; h. text תנים).

יְלִיד, יְלֵיד, v. יְלַד.

יְלִיד m. (b. h.; יָלַד) *born;* יְלִיד בַּיִת *a slave born in the owner's house; child of a slave,* contrad. to מקנת כסף an acquired slave. Sabb. 135ᵇ.

יְלִיד ch. same. Targ. O. Gen. XVII, 12, sq.—Targ. Job XV, 14; v. יָלוּד ch.—*Fem.* יְלִידָא. Targ. O. Lev. XVIII, 9.

יְלִידְתָּא, יְלֵיד׳ f. ch. = h. יוֹלֶדֶת. Targ. Lev. XII, 7 (O. ed. Amst. יָלְדָ׳). Targ. Is. XXI, 3; a. fr.—Lam. R. to I, 1 ירחי ביטנתא דר׳ (6 חד מאת׳) רבתי (not דילדיתא), v. ביטְנָתָא.—*Pl.* יְלֵידְתָא, יְלֵדָ׳. Targ. Is. XIII, 8 כִּילְ׳ (ed. Wil. כְּלְ׳; h. text sing.)

יַלִּיל, *Pa.* of יְלַל.

יְלִיל (dial. for אֲלִיל, v. אֲלַל) *to espy.* Targ. Y. II Deut. I, 24.

Pa. יַלֵּיל same. Y. Taan. IV, 68[d] top הוון מְיַלְּלִין וכ׳ they went through the town espying and left again.—V. יְלַל I.

יְלִילָא m. (preced.) *spy.*—*Pl.* יְלִילַיָּא. Targ. Y. II Num. XXI, 1.

יְלֵילָא, v. יְלָלָא.

יְלֵין = אִילֵּין. Y. B. Bath. VIII, 16[b] bot. יְאִילֵּין = וְיִלֵּין.—Y. Ber. II, 5[b] אי ילין ed. Lehm. (oth. ed. אִילֵּין).

יְלִיף, יְלֵיף (v. אֲלַף) *to get accustomed, to learn.* Targ. Prov. XXX, 3. Targ. Jer. XII, 16 מֵילַף יֵלְפוּן. Targ. Prov. XI, 25; a. fr.—Ab. I, 13 ודלא יָלֵיף he who does not study (the Law). Yeb. 57[a], a. fr. יַלְפִינַן we derive; a. v. fr.—Part. pass. יְלִיף, f. יְלִיפָא *accustomed, used to.* Y. Sot. I, 16[d] bot. הוה ר׳ דריש וכ׳ used to preach &c. Ib... והוה יְלִיפָה שמעה קליה and there was there a certain woman who made it a habit to listen to him; (Lev. R. s. 9 רציבא, corr. acc.); a. fr.—[B. Mets. 100[b], בדיילפר, v. לוּף.]

Pa. יַלֵּיף *to teach.* Targ. Job XV, 3; a. e.—Y. Hag. II, 78[a] top מֵילִיף וּמֵילַפָה to learn (from you) and to teach (you).

Af. אוֹלֵיף same, v. אֲלַף.—Y. Shebi. V, end, 36[a] ולא כך אוֹלְפַן רבי did you not teach us thus?; Y. Dem. I, 22[a] top אִילְפַן (corr. acc.).

יְלַךְ, Hif. הוֹלִיךְ, v. הָלַךְ.

יָלַל I, *Pi.* יִלֵּל (= אִילֵּל, אָלַל) *to espy.* Yalk. Prov. 955 אחר ד״ת יִלַּלְתְּ, v. אָלַל.—Cant. R. to I, 10 (play on תורים, ib., v. תּוּר, תַּיִּיר) בשעה שמְיַלְּלִין ההלכה וכ׳ when they go out together (like spies) to espy the true decision.—Ch. v. יְלִיל.

יָלַל II (b. h.), *Pi.* יִלֵּל *to howl, hollow.* Gen. R. s. 19; 20 (מְיַלֶּלֶת) התחילה מְיַלֶּלֶת וכ׳ she began to cry after him with her full voice. Pirké d'R. El. ch. XXXII; a. e.

יְלַל ch. same. Targ. Jer. XLVII, 2.

Af. אַיְלֵיל, אֵילֵיל same. Targ. Ez. XXVII, 32. Targ. Is. XXIII, 1; a. e.

Pa. יַלֵּיל same. Ib. XV, 4; a. e.—Lam. R. to I, 1 שריית מְיַלְּלָא (חדא אתתא) רבתי she began to lament. R. Hash. 33[b], sq. יַלּוֹלֵי יַלֵּיל, v. גְּנַח I.

יְלָלָא f. ch. = next w. Targ. Zeph. I, 10. Targ. Jer. XXV, 36 יְלָלַת constr.—Targ. Y. II Deut. XXXII, 10 הִילִיל = דְּלֵיל.

יְלָלָה f. (b. h.; preced. wds.) *lamentation, howling.* Yoma 76[b] יין... ר׳ לעולם wine is called *yayin* (cmp. יַיִן), because it brings lamentation into the world (cmp. אַלְלַי a. וַיְנַיָא); Snh. 70[b] top.—*Pl.* יְלָלוֹת. Pirké d'R. El. ch. XXXII; Yalk. Gen. 102.

יְלָלְתָא, constr. יְלָלַת, v. יְלָלָא.

***ילע**, Y. Kil. IX, 32[b] bot., v. וילעו.

יְלַף, v. יְלִיף.

יַלְפָא = אִילְפָא, *ship.* Targ. Prov. XXIII, 34 בִּילְפָא Ms. (ed. Lag. a. oth. באל׳, some ed. כולפא, corr. acc.).—*Pl.* יַלְפֵי. Ib. XXXI, 14 (ed. Lag. אלפיה; ed. Wil. ארלפת, some ed. זולפיה, corr. acc.)

יַלֶּפֶת f. (b. h.; ילה, cmp. לָפַת) *lichen,* a cutaneous disease. Bekh. 41[a] ר׳ זו חזזית וכ׳ *yallefeth* is the Egyptian lichen, v. חֲזָזִית.

יֶלֶק m. (b. h.; cmp. לָקַק) *yelek,* a species of locusts (LXX: βροῦχος). Pesik. Zakh., p. 26[b] (play on עֲמָלֵק) עַם ילק פרח כהדין זחלא Ar. (ed. לק) a people of locusts, quick as the *zahal* (v. זַחֲלָא); Yalk. Deut. 938; Tanh. Ki Tetsé 9; ed. Bub. 12 לק (v. לָק).

יְלַקְ, Y. Maas. Sh. IV, beg. 54[d], v. לקן.

יַלְתָּא pr. n. f. (= אִילְתָּא) *Yalta,* wife of R. Nahman, daughter of a Resh G'lutha. Gitt. 67[b]. Ber. 51[b]. Sabb. 54[b] עשיתה ר׳ thou treatest that animal as if she were Yalta.

יָם m. (b. h.) *sea, lake, reservoir.* Ber. 54[b] יורדי הים seafarers (on landing). B. Bath. 74[b] יַמָּה של טבריא the Lake of Tiberias; ים הגדול the Mediterranean Ocean. Gitt. 8[a] ים אוקיינוס; (Tosef. Ter. II, 14; a. e. only אוק׳).—Bekh. 13[b], a. fr. ים המלח the Dead Sea; a. fr.—*Pl.* יַמִּים, B. Bath. l. c.; a. fr.—Esp. a) *the cosmetic paint bottle.* Cant. R. to I, 3, v. זִכְרוּת.—b) ים נפה *the receiver of flour* at sifting or in the mill. Kel. XV, 3; (Tosef. ib. B. Mets. V, 5 only נפה). Zab. IV, 2 (only הים).—c) *the receptacle in the wine or oil press, tank.* B. Bath. IV, 5.—d) *the water reservoir in the Solomonic Temple.* Zeb. 62[b]; Yoma 58[b]; a. e.—Fem. form: יַמָּה. Y. Shek. V, 48[d] לְיַמָּתִי (I offer a sacrifice) for my *yammah,* סברין מימר שופעת כים they thought she meant that she had a hemorrhage (flowing like a sea), אמר לון בימה סכנת said he to us, she was in danger on sea; Men. 64[b], v. זִיבָה).

יַמָּא ch. same. Targ. Gen. IX, 2.—Targ. I Kings VII, 23; a. v. fr.—Tam. 32[a], a. fr. נחותי ר׳ = יורדי הים, v. preced.; a. fr.—*Pl.* יַמֵּי, יַמַּיָּא, יַמְמֵי, יַמְמַיָּא. Targ. Gen. I, 10. Targ. Ps. XXIV, 2 ed. Lag. (ed. ימיא); a. e.—Gitt. 57[a] ומבדרי אשב ר׳ (not ומבדרו) and they scatter (his ashes) over seven seas; a. fr.—Erub. 12[a]; R. Hash. 35[a] כי סליק... מִיַּמֵּי when R.... came up from 'the waters' (prob. channels of the Euphrates; Ar.: יַמֵּי pr. n. pl. *Yammé*).

יַמְבְּרִיס (יַמְבְּרֵס) pr. n. (corrupt. of Januarius; cmp. יָינוּבְרִיס) *Yambris,* legendary name of an Egyptian sorcerer, always in connection with יַנִּים. Targ. Y. Ex. I, 15; VII, 11; Num. XXII, 22 (יַמְרִיס).—Tanh. Ki Thissa 19 יונו״ס וימוברו״ס.—V. יוֹחָנֵי.

יַמָּה, v. יָם.

יָמוֹת, v. יוֹם.

יָמֵי, v. יְמָא.

יְמָא, יְמֵי 1) *to speak*; impf. יֵימֵי, יֵימָא, v. אֲמָא.—2) (cmp. אֲמַר I, 2, a. Ps. CXXXIX, 20 with Targ. a. l.) *to swear*. Targ. O. Ex. XX, 7 (h. text נשא). Targ. Jer. V, 2 יֵימְּן ed. Lag. (oth. ed. יָמַן, יֵמוּן, h. text אמר); a. fr.—Pes. 113ᵇ וכי יָמְיָין וכ׳ Ar. s. v. מם (Ms. M. 2 a. Ar. Ms. Koh. מְיַימָן וכ׳; Ms. M. 1 ומוֹמִי קרו להון; ed. ומומתיותי הכי, v. Rabb. D. S. a. l. note) and when they swear, they swear, 'by the life &c.'

Af. אוֹמֵי, אַיְימֵי 1) same. Targ. Jud. XVII, 2 (ed. Lag. יֵימַת); a. fr.—Gen. R. s. 26 מוֹמֵי, v. אֲלָה.—Pes. l. c., v. supra; a. fr.—2) *to cause to swear*. Targ. I Kings VIII, 31. Targ. O. Ex. XIII, 19 אוֹמָאָה אוֹמֵי; a. fr.—V. מוֹמָתָא, מוֹמֵי, אוֹמָתָא.

יָמִים, v. יוֹם.

***יֵמִים, יֵ׳** m. pl. (b. h.; חמה) *mules* (v. Targ. Y. to Gen. XXXVI, 24). Y. Ber. VIII, 12ᵇ; Gen. R. s. 82, end, v. הֶמְיוֹנָס. Hull. 7ᵇ (v. Pes. 54ᵃ).

יָמִין (sub. יָד) f. (b. h.; v. אָמַן) [*firm*,] *right hand*. Men. 37ᵃ מה כתיבה בְּי׳ as the writing is done with the right hand, so is the binding to be done with the right hand (on the left). Ib. אִטֵּר . . . בִּימִינוֹ וכ׳ a left-handed man ties the T'fillin on his right hand, because this is his left (weak) hand. Lam. R. to II, 3 (ref. to קץ הימין, Dan. XII, 13) קץ נתתי לִימִינִי וכ׳ I have fixed a term to (the servitude of) my right hand (power); when I redeem my children, I vindicate my right hand. Zeb. 62ᵇ, a. fr. דרך י׳ towards the right; a. fr.—Denom. יְמָנִי, f. יְמָנִית.

יְמִינָא, יַמִּינָא ch. same. Targ. Gen. XLVIII, 18; a. fr.—[ימינא, Pesik. R. s. 1, אבא בן י׳, read: זְמִינָא II.]

יְמִינִי m. (b. h.) *Benjamite*. Meg. 12ᵇ (ref. to Esth. II, 5) וקרי ליה י׳ וכ׳ and the text calls him (Mardecai) a Y'mini which means that he is a descendant of Benjamin. Ib., sq. ומה שילם לי י׳ and how the Benjamite (Saul) repaid me.

יְמָם, יֵימָם ch. = h. יוֹמָם, *day-time*; (adv.) *by day*. Targ. Is. XXXIV, 10; a. e. Targ. Job V, 14 בִּימָם (Ms. בִּיְימָם). Targ. Ps. XLII, 9; a. e.

יְמָמָא m. (preced.) *day-time, day-light*. Targ. Ex. XIII, 21, sq.; a. fr.—Ber. 3ᵃ י׳ הוא there is the day-light (to indicate the end of the night-watch); a. fr.—*Pl.* יְמָמִין, יְמָמֵי. Targ. Gen. VII, 4; a. e.—Hor. 4ᵃ בִּימָמֵי in day-time.

יְמָמֵי, יְמָמְיָא, v. יְמָא.

יממיא, a word in a charm formula. Tosef. Sabb. VII (VIII), 1 י׳ ובוצציא ed. Zuck. (Var. ימיא ומצריא, י׳ ובוצציא).

יָמַן, *Pi.* יַמֵּן (denom. of יָמִין; cmp. אָמַן) *to endow with skill, strength, distinction*. Part. pass. מְיוּמָּן, f. מְיוּמֶּנֶת. Hull. 91ᵃ הירך המ׳ שבירך it says '*the* hip' (Gen. XXXII, 33) that means the strongest of the hips (the right); ib. 134ᵇ הכא נמי הזרוע המ׳ וכ׳ here, too, we read '*the* arm' (Deut. XVIII, 3), that means the right arm; Hor. 12ᵃ ה״נ המשיח המ׳וכ׳ here, too, we read '*the* anointed' (Lev. IV, 3), the distinguished among the anointed (the Highpriest). Sifra Vayikra, Hoba, ch. III, Par. 3 מה . . . חימנית המ׳ שבימין וכ׳ as the finger mentioned there (Lev. XIV, 16) is '*the* right' which means the most skilled (the index) finger of the right hand &c.; [Zeb. 40ᵃ sq. לא נצרכא אלא להכשיר אָמוּן שבאצבע Ms. M. (ed. אמין, omitting אלא; v. Rabb. D. S. a. l. note) the את (Lev. IV, 6 את אצבעו) would not have been required, were it not to indicate, as the fittest for the ceremony, the most skilled of the fingers. —Rashi: אמין *blister*.]

Hif. [*to go to the right*, b. h.;] *to do the right thing*, opp. השמאיל. Sabb. 63ᵃ (ref. to Prov. III, 16) לַמַּיְמִינִין בה וכ׳ to those who make the right use of it &c.; Yalk. Prov. 934.—Cant. R. to I, 9 אלו מַיְמִינִים וכ׳ the ones stand on the right side (pleading in favor of the accused) &c. —Sabb. 88ᵇ, v. next w.

יְמַן ch., *Af.* אַיְימִין same. Sabb. 88ᵇ דאַיְימִין ליה Ms. M. (ed. מיימינים) he who uses it in the right way (v. preced.); Yoma 72ᵇ דאוֹמַן לה (Ms. M. דאַימִין).

יְמָנִי m., **יְמָנִית** f. (denom. of יָמִין) *right*. Neg. II, 4 יד הי׳ the right hand. Sifra Vayikra, Hoba, ch. III, Par. 3, v. יָמַן; a. e.

יְמַס (=מְסִי, מְסַס) *to melt, waste*.

Ithpa. אִתְיַמַּס same. Targ. Is. XXXIV, 3 (ed. Lag. יתמסון). Targ. Y. I Gen. XLIX, 10. Targ. Y. Lev. XXVI, 39 (O. יתמסון).

יָמַר, יְמַר, v. מוּר.

יַמְרִיס, v. יַמְבְּרִיס.

יָנָא, v. יְנֵי.

יַנַּאי, יַנַּי pr. n. m. (abbrev. of יוֹחָנָן) *Yannai* (*Jannaeus*), 1) King of Judaea. Kidd. 66ᵃ י׳ המלך (for *John Hyrcan*). Ber. 29ᵃ הוא י׳ הוא יוחנן Y. a. Johanan are the same; (another opin.) י׳ לחוד וכ׳ Y. a. Joh. are different persons.—Snh. 19ᵃ י׳ המלך, י׳ מלכא (ref. to Hyrcan II).—Ber. 44ᵃ. Ib. 48ᵃ; Lev. R. s. 9 (Alexander Jannaeus). Sot. 22ᵇ (Alex. J.); a. e.—2) name of several Amoraim. Meg. 32ᵃ.—Y. Ber. III, 6ᵃ.—Lev. R. s. 16; a. fr.

יָנָה, v. ינה.

יְנוּבְּרִיס, v. יַיִן.

יָנוֹן, v. יִינוּן.

יִנּוֹן pr. n. m. *Yinnon*, symbolical name of the Messiah (with ref. to י׳ שמו Ps. LXXII, 17). Snh. 98ᵇ. Midr. Till. to Ps. XCIII; Pirké d'R. El. ch. XXXII, v. יָנַן.

יָנוּקָא I m. (יְנַק) *suckling, infant; child; school-boy.* Targ. Y. Gen. XLVIII, 20.—Gitt. 57ª כי הוה מתיליד י׳ ... ינוקתא וכ׳ whenever a male child was born, they used to plant a cedar, when a female, they planted &c. Sabb. 134ª האי י׳ דלית ליה וכ׳ an infant (to be circumcised on the Sabbath) for which no bandage has been prepared, v. חָלוּק I.—Succ. 56ᵇ (prov.) שותא דר׳ וכ׳ the child's talk in the street is either the father's or the mother's (talk at home). Snh. 110ᵇ (ref. to פתאים, Ps. CXVI, 6) ... שכן קורין לי׳ פתיא for in the sea towns they call a child *pathia.* B. Bath. 21ª כד מחית לי׳ וכ׳ when thou (as teacher) strikest a child, strike it only with a shoe-strap. Ib. לא ממטינן י׳ וכ׳ we must not let a child go to school from one place to another (but must provide a school for each place).—Gen. R. s. 36, a. e. יַנּוּקָא; a. fr.—*Pl.* יָנוּקֵי. B. Bath. l. c. מקרי י׳ primary school teacher, v. מַקְרְקָא; a. fr.—*Fem.* יָנוּקְתָא. Gitt. l. c., v. supra.—B. Bath. 3ᵇ האי י׳ that maiden (of Hasmonean descent, Mariamne).

יָנוּקָא II, מר י׳ pr. n. m. *Mar Yanuka,* son of R. Hisda. B. Bath. 7ᵇ top.

יַנּוּקָא m., pl. יַנּוּקַיָּא (יְנַק) *breasts.* Tanḥ. Ki Thissa 27 [read:] טוביי לי׳ דהדין ינקין happy the breast that nursed such a child.

יָנוּקְתָא, v. יָנוּקָא I.

יָנַח, יְנַח, v. נוּחַ.

יָנָה, יָנַח, יני, *Hif.* הוֹנָה (b. h.; v. אָנָה) *to oppress, treat overbearingly, vex, taunt.* Gen. R. s. 88, beg. שלא יהו מוֹנִים את וכ׳ that they might not taunt Israel saying &c. Cant. R. to I, 6. Tanḥ. Vayera 14 כל מי שיוֹנֶה להבירו whoever aggrieves his neighbor. Ib. הוֹנַת את עצמה humbled herself; a. fr.—V. הוֹנָאָה, אוֹנָאָה.

יְנִי I ch., *Af.* אוֹנִי same. Targ. Ez. XVIII, 12. Targ. O. Ex. XXII, 20. Targ. Y. Lev. XXV, 14 לאוֹנָיָא (not נַיָּא...); a. fr.—Gen. R. s. 53 דלא יהו מוֹנִין לה וכ׳ that they might not taunt her, calling her a barren woman.

יְנִי II (cmp. b. h. נוא, a. נוּץ) *to be undecided, waver.*

Af. אוֹנִי *to cause to waver, discourage.* Targ. O. Num. XXXII, 7; 9.

יְנִיבָא, יְאָנִיבָא, m. (cmp. אֶנְבָּא II) name of *an insect in flax.* Ḥull. 85ᵇ נפל ליה י׳ בכיתניה Ar. (ed. יאנ׳) the *yaniba* came into his flax crop. Ib. 28ª בעי ... לי׳ Ar. (ed. יניכא, corr. acc.) he needs its blood for killing the flax worm.

יניכא, v. preced.

יַנִּיס pr. n. m. *Yannis* (Janus), v. יַמְבְּרִיס; cmp. יוֹחָנָר.

יַנִּיק, יְנִיק, יְנִיקָא m. (v. יָנוּקָא) 1) *suckling, child; young.* Targ. I Sam. XV, 3. Targ. Jud. VIII, 20 (h. text נער). Targ. Is. LXV, 20 י׳ יומין (h. text עול ימים); a. fr.—Kidd. 32ᵇ י׳ וחכים young but wise; a. fr.—*Pl.* יַנִּיקַיָּא. Lev. R. s. 5, beg. (translating עויליהם, Job XXI, 11) יַנִּיקֵיהוֹן their young ones (v. Gen. R. s. 36; Yalk. Job. 908).—2) (v. יוֹנֶקֶת) *branch, twig.*—*Pl.* as ab. Targ. Ps. LXXX, 12 יַנִּיקָהָא (Ms. ינקיהא; h. text יוֹנְקוֹתֶיהָ).

***יָנַן** (b. h.; cmp. נענע a. יְנִי II) 1) (neut. verb) *to move quickly; to glisten, be bright.*—2) (act. verb), v. infra.

Pi. יִינֵּן (=נענע) *to shake, awaken, stir up.* Pirké d'R. El. ch. XXXII the Messiah is named *Yinnon* (v. יִנּוֹן) שהוא עתיד לְיַינֵּן ישני עפר (Mus. quotes לִינוֹן *Kal,* cmp. לִישוֹן fr. ישן, Koh. V, 11) for he will awaken those sleeping in the dust; Midr. Till. to Ps. XCIII לִינוֹן (missing in ed. Bub.); Yalk. Kings 200 עתיד ליינן רשעי ארץ he will stir up the wicked of the earth; Yalk. Gen. 45 לְיָאנֵן לעכו״ם.

יָנַץ, v. נָרץ.

יָנַק (b. h.; cmp. אנק) [*to press,*] (cmp. מָצַץ) *to suck.* Sot. 12ᵇ ולא י׳ and he (Moses) would not suck; פה.. יִנַק דבר טמא shall the mouth destined to speak with Divinity suck in an unclean substance?—Ber. 10ª; a. fr.—Trnsf. *to draw sap, absorb.* B. Bath. 71ᵇ יוֹנְקִין משדה וכ׳ they (the plants) are nurtured from the consecrated field. Y. Erub. III, 21ᵇ איברים יונקין זה מזה the limbs of an animal draw nourishment from one another, i. e. in either portion of a slaughtered animal to be divided between two partners there are substances absorbed from the other; a. fr.

Hif. הֵינִיק, הֶינִיק *to give suck, feed.* Pes. 112ª ... יותר לִינֹק ... לְהָנִיק more than the calf desires to suck, does the cow desire to give suck, i. e. the teacher is more anxious to teach than the pupil to learn. Bekh. 7ᵇ כל המוליד מֵנִיק every viviparous animal is a mammal. Keth. V, 5 וּמֵינִקָה את בנה וכ׳ (Y. ed. ומיני׳) and she is bound to nurse her child herself. Nidd. I, 4 נתנה בנה לַמֵּינִקָה (Y. למיני׳) if she gave her child out to a wet-nurse. Ib. 5 ומניקה and while she nurses a child. Tosef. ib. II, 2; Keth. 60ª מֵינֶקֶת שמת וכ׳ a woman whose husband died during her nursing period. Ib. 65ᵇ סתם מֵנִיקוֹת וכ׳ as a rule nursing women are of delicate health. Taan. 27ᵇ מניקות שיְנִיקוּ וכ׳ in behalf of the nursing women (they prayed) that they might be able to nurse &c.; a. fr.

יְנַק ch. same. Targ. Job III, 11 אֵינִיק (Ms. אֵינַק; ed. Lag. אוֹנִיק); a. fr.—Y. Ned. I, 37ª; Gen. R. s. 56 אימר דלא י׳ וכ׳ the lamb that never sucked (the ram offered in Isaac's place). Ber. 40ᵇ [read:] מירבא ... מֵינַק לא יַנְקֵי וכ׳ they grow out of the ground, but draw no nurture from it. B. Bath. 71ᵇ מדנפשיה קא ינקי they draw from the ground which belongs to himself. Bets. 37ᵇ החומין מהדדי י׳ the parts of an animal whose partners are bound by opposite Sabbath limits draw substances one from the other (v. Y. Erub. III, 21ª quoted in preced.); a. fr.

Af. אוֹנִיק, אֵינִיק as preced. *Hif.*—Targ. Ex. II, 9. Targ. Y. Deut. XXXII, 13; a. fr.—Gen. R. s. 98, end דהכן אוֹנִיקוּ which nursed such a child; Y. Kil. I, 27ᵇ top אֵינִיק; Gen. R. s. 5 end מנרק (corr. acc.), v. בִּרְזָא III; a. fr.—מֵינִיקְתָא *nurse.* Targ. Ex. II, 7; a. e.—*Pl.* מֵינִיקָתָא, v. infra.

Pa. יַנֵּק same. Targ. Y. II Ex. XV, 2 (Y. I מוֹנִיק). Targ. I Sam. VI, 7; 10 (ed. Lag. מְנִיקָן); Targ. Ps. LXXVIII, 71 מְיַנְּקָן (Targ. Is. XL, 11 מֵינִיקָתָא) animals giving suck (h. text עלות).—Tanḥ. Ki Thissa 27 יַנְּקִין v. יַנּוּקָא.

יַנְקָא I, **יוֹנְקָא** m. (preced.) *suckling, child.* Targ. Cant. VIII, 1; a. fr.—Num. R. s. 4, end (ref. to Ps. CXXXI,

2) כְּהָן ר׳ וכ׳ like the infant leaving the mother's womb &c.; Y. Snh. II, 20^b bot.—*Pl.* רוֹנְ׳ יַנְקַיָּא, Targ. Ps. VIII, 3 יַנְ׳ Ms. (ed. רוֹנְ׳); a.e.—Targ. Is. III, 4 (some ed. יַנְקָנַיָּא) childish men.

יַנְקָא II f. (preced.) = h. אֲנָקָה, נְאָקָה, *young camel.* Targ. Jer. II, 23 (h. text בכרה).

יַנְקוּתָא f. (preced. wds.) *childhood, youth.* Targ. Jer. XIII, 27; a. e.—Sabb. 152^a, v. יְרַד. **Taan.** 20^b בינקותיה לא דכירנא of his earlier days I remember nothing. Sabb. 21^b, v. גִּירְסָא I; a. e.

יַנְקְנָא m., pl. יַנְקָנַיָּא, v. יַנְקָא I.

יַסָּא, v. יוֹסֵי.

יָסַד (b. h.; v. סד) [*to join, fasten*; denom. יְסוֹד, whence יָסַד] *to found, establish.* Tanḥ. B'resh. 1 ובה ... ור׳ ארץ and with it (the Torah) he stretched the heavens and established the earth. Meg. 3^a; Sabb. 104^a; Succ. 44^a וחזרו ויסדום and they reintroduced them. Ib. 20^a, v. עֶזְרָא; a. fr.

Pi. יִיסֵּד, יַסֵּד 1) *to establish; to join in between.* Y. Erub. V, 22^c שער היסוד ששם היו מְיַסְּדִין וכ׳ the Eastern Gate was named the Foundation Gate, because there they (in their meetings) established the decisions of the Law; a. e.—Part. pass. מְיוּסָּד. Ib. שער התווך שהוא מי׳ בין וכ׳ it was named the Middle Gate because it was fastened in between two gates; a. e.—2) *to rebuild* (a ruin). Tosef. B. Mets. XI, 4 לא יאמר לו הריני מייסד עמך מכנגד וכ׳ (not עמו) he has no right to say, I will help thee rebuild the party wall from where my (higher situated) ground commences and upward, אלא מייסד עמו וכ׳ but he must help him build from the bottom (of the neighbor's ground) &c.; Y. ib. X, beg. 12^c; (B. Bath. 6^b מסייע מלמטה). [Cant. R. to I, 2 שהרי חבירו בא לְיַסֵּד עליו כן the next following sentence comes to found upon it a base (thus proving that the reading is דּוֹדֶיךָ and not דּוֹדַיִךְ). Some eds. read לימד; Ab. Zar. II, 5 חבירו מלמד; Yalk. Cant. 981 מוכיח.]

Nithpa. נִתְיַסֵּד *to be established.* Tanḥ. l. c. העולם לא נ׳ וכ׳ the world has been founded on nothing but the Law.

יְסַד, ch. same. Targ. Ps. LXXVIII, 69; a. e.

Pa. יַסֵּד same. Ib. CIV, 5.

Ithpa. אִתְיַיסַּד, *Ittof.* אִתּוֹסַד *to be fastened, supported, founded.* Targ. Job. XLI, 15, sq.—Targ. Ps. LXXXVII, 1.—Targ. II Chr. XXXI, 7 לְאִתּוֹסָדָא (ed. Lag. לְאִתְיַסָּדָא).

יַסָּה, v. יוֹסֵי.

יִסּוּד m. (יָסַד) *institution, confirmation; reestablishment.* Men. 99^a sq., v. בִּיטּוּל. Succ. 44^a ערבה י׳ נביאים the use of the willow-branch (on Hoshanah Rabbah) is an institution of the prophets, opp. מנהג נביאים a custom arisen in the days of the prophets; Y. Shebi. I, 33^b bot. מִי׳ נביאים וכ׳ belong to the institutions of the early prophets; Y. Succ. IV, beg. 54^b.

יְסוֹד m. (b. h.; v. יָסַד) *foundation.* Y. Erub. V, 22^c שער הי׳, v. יָסַד.—Esp. (sub. המזבח) *the base of the altar, y'sod.* Midd. III, 1. Zeb. V, 1, a. fr. י׳ מערבי the western side of the *y'sod.* Ib. 3 (53^a) י׳ דרומית (read דרומי, v. Rabb. D. S. a. l. note 200) the southern side &c.; a. fr.—*Pl.* יְסוֹדוֹת. Cant. R. to I, 1 אביו בנה את הי׳ Solomon's father laid the foundations of the Temple; a. e.

יְסוֹדָא ch. 1) same. Targ. Ex. XXIX, 12; a. fr.—*Pl.* יְסוֹדַיָּא, constr. יְסוֹדֵי. Targ. O. Num. V, 17 (ed. Berl. אֱיסוֹדֵי; h. text קרקע).—Y. B. Mets. X, beg. 12^c תרוויהו אילין י׳ both (the upper and the lower portions) are foundations (v. יָסַד).—2) *pl. rest, head-rest* (cmp. אִיסְדָא). Targ. Y. II Gen. XXVIII, 10 תחות י׳ רישיה in place of his head-rest.

יְסוֹף*, Targ. Y. II Deut. XXVIII, 65, read: וסִיוּף עיינין.

יִיסּוּר, יִסּוּר m. (יָסַר) *correction by example, warning example.* Snh. 45^a (ref. to Ez. XXIII, 48) אין לך י׳ גדול מזה there is no severer warning than this (capital punishment, and therefore disgrace by exposure would be an unnecessary hardship).—2) *Pl.* יִסּוּרִין, יִסּוּרִים, יי׳ *corrections by suffering, suffering, trials, visitation.* Sifré Deut. 32 חביבים י׳ לפני .... על מי שרי׳ באים עליו trials are precious in the sight of the Lord, for the glory of the Lord rests upon him who is visited with trials (ref. to Deut. VIII, 5). Ib. הי׳ מרצים וכ׳ sufferings atone more than sacrifices. Ber. 5^a י׳ של אהבה visitations of (divine) love (ref. to Prov. III, 12). Ib.^b חביבין עליך י׳ are the sufferings welcome to thee (as trials)?—Cant. R. to II, 16 מה קשין הן הי׳ how hard to bear are sufferings!; a. v. fr.

יִיסּוּ׳, יְסוּ׳, יְסוּרָא ch. 1) (v. אִיסוּרָא) *chain; prison.* Targ. II Esth. I, 2 end לבושי יִיסּוּרֵיהּ his prison clothes; (Targ. Jer. LII, 33 איסוריה).—*Pl.* יְסוּרִין, יִיס׳, יִיסּוּרֵי, יְסוּ׳. Targ. Lam. III, 6.—Targ. Is. XXVIII, 22 (ed. Wil. יְסוּ׳).—2) *chastisement, suffering.* Targ. Jer. XXX, 14.—*Pl.* as ab. Ib. 11 (v. אִיסוּרָא II). Targ. Y. Lev. XX, 5; a. fr.—Ber. 60^a י׳ בעי וכ׳ Ms. M. (ed. יסורים h. form) that man desires to bring suffering upon himself. B. Mets. 84^b קביל עליה י׳ he submitted patiently to sufferings. Ib. 85^a; a. fr. Lam. R. introd. end למימר ליה יִיסּוּרַיָּא חשיבין וכ׳ as if saying, sufferings count to me for nothing.

יְסַט, יָסַט, v. סוּט.

יסמיכס, יסטיבס, v. סְטִיבָס.

***יַסֵּי׳ חֳלִי, יי׳** m. [*healer of sickness,*] *yassé ḥŏli,* name of a bitter herb. Y. Kil. II, 27^a top (not יסיח לי, expl. חזרת גלים); Y. Pes. II, 29^c (expl. חרחבינה).

י׳ לי יסיח, v. preced.

יִסְכָּה f. (b. h.) pr. n. f. *Jiscah.* Snh. 69^b; Yalk. Gen. 62 (identified with Sarah). Gen. R. s. 38, end.

יָסַם (v. סוּמָא, סָמָא, סָמַם) *to close* or *to be closed.*

Nithpa. נִתְיַיסֵּם (with בעיניו) *to become blind.* Tanḥ. Tol'doth 7.

יַסְמִין m. pl. (?) (cmp. ἰάσμη) *Jasmine flowers.* Sabb. 50^b, v. בּוּסְפָּא.

יָסַף (b. h.; cmp. אָסַף), *Hif.* הוֹסִיף *to heap up, to add* (with עַל). Snh. XI, 3 להוֹסִיף על דברי וכ׳ thus adding to the words of the Scribes (against Deut. IV, 2). Ib. 88[b] ויש בו להו׳ when there is a possibility to add. Ib. ואם ה׳ גורע and if he did add, he diminishes (violates the law). Ib. 29[a] המוסיף, v. גָּרַע I. Tosef. Sabb. VI (VII), 17 והאומר הוֹסִיפוּ על השולחן (not ואומר) and who (from superstition) says, Add (put one more) to the table; a. fr.—Yalk. Lev. 559 מוֹסְפַנִי על וכ׳ (Sifra Metsora beg. מוסיף אני) I will add to what thou saidst.

Nithpa. נִתּוֹסַף, נִית׳, *Hithpa.* הִתּוֹסַף *to be added; to be added to, increase, wax.* Mekh. Bo. s. 16; Yalk. Ex. 217 והשני נ׳ לו and the second name was added to the first (without abrogating the first). Ex. R. s. 7, beg. נ׳ לו עוד וכ׳ two additional years (of imprisonment) were given him. Sabb. 152[a] ת״ח... חכמתן מִתּוֹסֶפֶת עליהן Ms. M. (ed. חכמה נִיתּוֹסֶפֶת בהן) when scholars grow old, their wisdom grows with their age; ib. טפשותן מתוספת וכ׳, v. טִפְּשׁוּת.

יְסַף ch., *Af.* אוֹסֵף, אוֹסִיף same, *to add, increase; to do again.* Targ. Deut. I, 11.—Targ. Gen. VIII, 10; a. fr.—Sabb. 116[b] אנא... אלא לאוֹסֻפֵי וכ׳ Ms. M. (v. Rabb. D. S. a. l. note) I have not come to diminish from but to add to the law of Moses. Y. Ber. IV, 7[c] אוֹסְפוּן עליה add thereto.—Part. pass. מוֹסַף, f. מוֹסְפָא. Kidd. 20[a] והא מ׳ ואזלא but this (the debt on interest) is continually growing; a. fr.

Ittaf. אִתּוֹסַף *to be added.* Targ. Gen. XLIX, 26; a. fr.—Ber. 28[a] אִתּוֹסְפוּ כמה ספסלי many forms had to be added (to accommodate the hearers). Ib. א׳ ד׳ מאה וכ׳ four hundred forms were added; a. e.

יָסַר (b. h.; cmp. אָסַר) [*to tie up*; cmp. חוב.]

Pi. יִסֵּר, יִיסֵּר *to chastise, chasten, try.* Snh. 39[a]... מְיַיסֵּר בִיסוּרִין he (the king) punishes the prominent among them (the rebellious citizens); כך הקב״ה מי׳ וכ׳ so did the Lord visit Ezekiel in order to wash away the sins of Israel. Ab. Zar. 4[a] אֲיַסְּרֵם ביסורין וכ׳ I would visit them with afflictions in this world, in order that their arms be strengthened &c. Ex. R. s. 3, end המטה שתְּיַיסְּרֶנּוּ בו the staff wherewith to strike him (Pharaoh); a. fr.

Hithpa. הִתְיַסֵּר, *Nithpa.* נִתְיַסֵּר *to be chastened, tried.* Gen. R. s. 62 היו מִתְיַיסְּרִין בחולי וכ׳ used to be visited with bowel diseases for ten days &c. (prior to their death), to indicate that the disease purifies (from sin); Treat. S'maḥ. ch. III.. Y. Snh. X, 27[d] נתי׳ בבנו הבכור he was punished with the death of his first-born son. Tanḥ. Noah 14 נתי׳ בבנו he was visited with trials through his son (being asked to sacrifice him). Ib. Vayigg. 6 נתי׳ בבנו was tried by his son (Joseph being sold); a. e.

יְסַר ch. same, 1) *to tie, put on.* Targ. Is. XV, 3 יַיסְרוּן וכ׳ ed. Lag. (ed. יַסְרוּן; h. text חגרו); a. e.—2) *to bind one's self, to vow.* Targ. Num. XXX, 3, sq.—Y. Taan. II, 66[a] top (quot. fr. Meg. Taan. ch. XII) יֵיסַר בצלו (Meg. Taan. l. c. יאסר) may vow (a fast) in his prayer; Bab. ib. 12[a] (v. corr. vers. Ms. M. in Rabb. D. S. a. l. notes); v. אֲסַר.

Ithpa. אִתְיַיסַּר *to be tried.* Cant. R. to II, 16 ר׳ י׳ א׳ ועבד וכ׳ R. J. was tried and suffered with fever &c.

יָסַת* (cmp. אָסַר a. עָשָׂה) *to do habitually.*—Denom. הֵיסֵת, וֶסֶת.

Hif. הֵסִית, הִסִּית [b. h., by way of syncope, forms resembling Kal of סית, as וַיָּסֶת=וַיָּסֶת, יַיסִר=יְסִיתְךָ &c.] *to cause to do, stir up, instigate.* Sot. 35[a] (expl. ויהס.. אל, Num. XIII, 30) הִסִּיתָן בדברים (he quieted them, because) he (apparently) instigated them (against Moses). Ḥag. 5[a] עבד שמְּסִיתִין עליו רבו וניסת וכ׳ Ms. M. (ed. שרבו מסיתין לו) a slave against whom they incite his master and he (the master) is influenced by the instigation (ed.: a slave whose master, when they incite him, yields &c.), what help is there for him?—B. Bath. 16[a] (ref. to Job II, 3) כביכול כאדם שמסיתין וכ׳ (v. Rabb. D. S. a. l.) like a human being, as it were, that is influenced by instigation. Ib. יורד ומֵסִית Ms. R. (ed. ומתעה) Satan comes down and incites (to sin). Y. Snh. VII, 25[d] top יַסִּית עצמו וכ׳ he will stir himself up (become bold) and incite others; a. fr.—Esp. מֵסִית or מַסִּית (with ref. to Deut. XIII, 7, sq.) *he who stirs people up to worship idols.* Snh. VII, 10. Y. ib. l. c. מ׳... בלשון גבוה וכ׳ the *massith* speaks in a loud voice, the *maddiaḥ* (v. נָדַח) in a low voice; a. fr.—*Pl.* מְסִיתִים, מְסִיתִין. Ab. d'R. N. ch. XVI, end האפיקורסין והמ׳ ומדיחין (ed. Schechter... המינין והמשומדים.... המסורות).

Nif. נִיסַּת, נִיסִית *to be stirred up, give way to instigation; to be impassioned.* Ḥag. 5[a], v. supra. B. Bath. 16[a], v. supra. Sifré Deut. 89 מצוה ביד הנ׳ וכ׳ he who was to be incited to idolatry must first lay his hand on &c.—Y. Snh. l. c.; Y. Yeb. XVI, 15[d] bot. מכיון שהוא ניסית וכ׳ since he is prevailed upon (to worship idols), he is no longer a wise man. Yalk. Gen. 127 (play on נפתלי) [read:] נִיסֵּיתִי פּוּתֵּיתִי תְּלִיתִי וכ׳ I was prevailed upon, I was persuaded, I gave my sister the preference over myself; Gen. R. s. 71 (corr. acc.). [For נִיסֵּית *she was married,* v. נָשָׂא.]

יְעָא, יְיעָא *to burst forth, bloom.* Targ. O. Num. XVII, 23 ed. Berl. (ed. נְעָא; Y. I יְיעָא; h. text פרח). Ib. 20 יְנְעֵי ed. Berl. (ed. יְנְעֵי, ר׳). Targ. Ps. CIII, 15 ינעי Regia (ed. a. Ms. יָנְיץ).

Af. אֲוֹעֵי *to let burst forth, to utter.* Targ. Prov. X, 31 מוֹעֵי ed. Lag. (oth. ed. מבער; h. text ינוב). Targ. Ps. XIX, 3 מוועי Ar. a. Ms. (ed. מבער a. מַבִּיעַ). [Cmp. בוע, בער a. נבע.]

יָעָא m., pl. יָעֵי (=h. יָעִים; cmp יָעָה Is. XXVIII, 17) *'scraper, sweeper.* Targ. Y. II Ex. XXVII, 3 (usu. מגרופיתא).

יַעְבֵּץ (b. h.) pr. n. m. *Jabez,* 1) Tem. 16[a], homiletically identified with Othniel.—2) R. J., an Amora. Y. Ḥag. II, beg. 77[a].

יָעַד, וָעַד (b. h.; v. עוד) *to appoint;* denom. מוֹעֵד.

Pi. 1) יִיעֵד, יִעֵד *to designate,* esp. *to designate a Hebrew handmaid to be a freeman's wife* (Ex. XXI, 8, sq.). Kidd. 19[a] צריך לְיַעֲדָהּ he must express to her her designation, i. e. בקדושי יעוד by betrothal through designation, v. יִעוּד. Ib. מהו שמְּיַיעֵד אדם וכ׳ may a man designate (a handmaid) for his minor son? Ib.[b] אם רצה לייעד מייעד if he chooses to betroth her, he may do so. Mekh. Mishp. s. 3 לבנו יְיַעֵד וכ׳ he may give her to his son, but not to his brother. Ib. יַעֵד לך או לבנך וכ׳ betroth her to thyself or to thy son or redeem her; a. fr.—*Part. pass. f.* מְיוּעֶדֶת *designated, betrothed.* Y. Kidd. I, 59[b] bot. he tells her in the presence of witnesses הרי את מי׳ לי thou art designated for me (as my wife). Bab. ib. 6[a] מי׳ לי מהו if one says to a free woman, Thou art &c. (using מיועדת for מקודשת), is it a valid betrothal?

Pi. 2) יִיעֵד *to make an appointment, to meet.* Lam. R. to II, 13, a. e., v. יִיעוּד.

Hif. הוֹעִיד *to appoint*; part. pass. מוּעָד *designated, invited.* Ex. R. s. 19 מ׳ לדיבור appointed to receive the revelation; ib. מוּעָדִין לדבור (Yeb. 62[a] מיוחד, v. יָחַד; Ab. d'R. N. ch. II מזומן).—[V. מוּעָד *forewarned.*]

Hithpa. הִתְוַעֵד, *Nithpa.* הִתְוַעֵד *to be appointed, engaged; to meet.* Num. R. s. 14, end שלא נִתְוַעֲדוּ בדבור עם משה who were not invited with Moses for the reception of the revealed word. Ib. עתיד אני לְהִתְוַעֵד להם I shall meet them (appear to them); Sifra Vayikra Par. I, ch. II להיות ועד (corr. acc.); Yalk. Lev. 430 להתוו׳ בהם (corr. acc.).

יְעַד ch., *Pa.* יַעֵד 1) as preced. *Pi.*, *to designate.* Kidd. 18[b] הא יַעוּדֵי מְיַעֵד לַהּ but betroth her he may?—2) (v. מוּעָד, עוּד) *to forewarn* the owner of a noxious beast. B. Kam. 84[b] וְיַעֲדוּהָ and declared the beast noxious. Ib. 24[a] שלשה . . . לְיַיעוּדֵי תורא וכ׳ the three days mentioned —are they required for declaring the ox noxious (making the owner responsible, if the ox gored three days in succession) or for warning the owner (i. e. that the owner must have three notices in three consecutive days)?; ib. 41[a]; a. e.

Ithpa. אִיַּיעֵד *to be forewarned, to be declared noxious* (מוּעָד). Ib. 84[b] דא׳ התם וכ׳ he was declared noxious there (in Palestine) and was brought to Babylonia. Ib. 24[a] מְיַיעַד he stands forewarned. Ib. 37[b] לשוורים הוא דא׳ he stands forewarned with reference to damage done to oxen only; א׳ ליה לכולהו מיני he stands forewarned with reference to all kinds (oxen, asses and camels); a. e.

יַעְדָה, v. יְעִידָה.

יַעֲדוּט (?) pr. n. pl. *Yaădut.* Y. Dem. II, 22[d] top עיון וי׳; Tosef. Shebi. IV, 10 עין יעריט ed. Zuck. (ed. עין יערים).

יִיעוּד, יְעוּד m. (יָעַד) *designation*, esp. *betrothal of a Hebrew handmaid* to the owner or his son. Kidd. 18[b] י׳ נישואין וכ׳ does *yiud* have the effect of marriage or of betrothal? Ib. י׳ קידושי, v. יָעַד. Ib. 19[a] אין י׳ אלא בגדול *yiud* is legal only when he for whom the handmaid is designated is of age. Ib. אין י׳ אלא מדעת *yiud* is legal only when consented to (by the son), מדעת דידה by her; a. fr.—*Pl.* יִעוּדִים, יִעוּדִין, יִי׳. Y. ib. I, 59[b] bot. בסוף נותן לה כסף י׳ towards the end of her term of servitude he gives her an object of value as a consideration for her betrothal; יִי׳ . . . משעה ראשונה from the first hour (at the time of the purchase the money turns out to have been given (to her father) for the purpose of betrothal; a. e.

בֵּית י׳, יַעֲזֵק pr. n. *Beth-Yazek*, name of a court in Jerusalem where the witnesses for ascertaining the New Moon were heard. R. Hash. II, 5. Ib. 23[b] question as to יעזק (as a denom. of עזק) or יָזֵק (as a denom. of זקק).

יְעַט, יְעֵט (=יְעַץ) *to counsel.* Targ. Y. Gen. XLII, 24. *Ithpa.* אִתְיְעֵט *to take counsel, to deliberate, plan.* Dan. VI, 8.—Targ. I Chr. XIII, 1. Targ. Y. Gen. XXVII, 42; a. e.

יְעִידָה f. (יָעַד) 1) =יִיעוּד. Arakh. 25[b] the son stands in the place of his father לי׳ ולעבד וכ׳ (Rashi: לִיעָדָה) with reference to acquiring his father's handmaid as his wife and taking possession of the Hebrew slave for the ensuing term; Kidd. 17[b] לִיעד׳ Ar. (ed. לִיעָ׳); B. Bath. 108[b] ליעד׳ Ms. M. (ed. לִיעָ׳); Sifra B'huck. Par. 4, ch. X; Yalk. Lev. 677 לִיעָ׳.—2) (ref. to Ex. XXIX, 42 אִוָּעֵד) *appointment, divine call.* Num. R. s. 14, end; Sifra Vayikra Par. I, ch. II.—3) (=הוֹדָאָה) *statement of facts, testimony.* Ib. ch. II, Par. 2 יְעִידַת עד אחד the statement of one witness (opinion of one expert; v. Tem. 28[a]); י׳ שני עדים the statement of two witnesses.

יְעִילָא, v. יַעֲלָא.

***יָעַל** (b. h.; cmp. עָלָה) *to go up.*

Hif. הוֹעִיל *to bring up, effect; to profit, accomplish.* Y. Sot. VIII, 21[c] ולא הוֹעַלְתֶּם לעצמיכם כלום and you have profited nothing for yourselves; (Snh. 90[b] העליתם בידכם); v. זוּז I. Erub. 24[b] לחי מוֹעִיל וכ׳ a post helps (has the effect of making the moving about on the Sabbath permitted) for all vineyard paths. Ib. 25[a] ה׳ it does good (it serves its purpose). Yoma 47[a] ולא הוֹעִילוּ and did not succeed (in obtaining distinction). Meg. 6[a] אינו מועיל ופ׳ will not succeed in business. Keth. 10[a] מה הועילו חכמים וכ׳ what have the scholars accomplished with their measure?; Gitt. 17[b], sq. Ib. 32[b] (if one said) גט זה לא יועיל this letter of divorce *shall* have no effect, contrad. to אינו מועיל *has* no effect. Ib. 57[b] תפלה שמוֹעֶלֶת a prayer which was efficacious. Ib. 65[b] (if he said, Write ye a letter of divorce and) הוֹעִילוּ לה make it of avail to her. B. Bath. 100[a] אין הילוך מועיל walking through the field (as a symbol of possession) has no legal effect. Ḥull. 70[b]; a. fr.

יָעֵל I (b. h.; v. next w.) pr. n. f. *Jael*, the wife of Heber the Kenite. Meg. 15[a], v. זָנָה. Lev. R. s. 23; a. e.

יָעֵל II (b. h.; v. יָעַל, cmp. אַיָּל) *mountain-goat, wild goat.* R. Hash. III, 3.—*Pl.* יְעֵלִים. Ib. 5 (26[b]). Kil. I, 6. Gen. R. s. 12.—V. יַעֲלָה.

יְעִילָא, יַעֲלָא ch. same. Targ. O. Deut. XIV, 5 (ed. Berl. יַעְלָא, read: יְעָ׳; h. text אקו).—Y. Ned. III, 37[d] bot. ארכובה די׳ the leg of the wild goat; (Y. Shebu. III, 34[d] bot.; Y. Maasr. V, end, 52[a] דפילא, v. אַרְכּוּבְתָא).—*Pl.* יַעֲלִין, יְעִילַיָּא. Targ. Y. Deut. l. c. Targ. Ps. CIV, 18 Ms. (ed. יַעְלֵי). Targ. Ez. XXVII, 15 (ed. Wil. יַעֲלִין).

יַעֲלָה (or **יְעֵלָה**) f. (b. h.; v. יָעֵל II) *gazelle.* Gen. R. s. 12; Yalk. Ps. 862 (ref. to Ps. CIV, 18) [read:] . . . הזו הי׳ הוא והיא מתייראה וכ׳ the gazelle is of tender build and she is afraid of the wild beasts &c.; (Midr. Sam. ch. IX אַיֶּלֶת).—יַעֲלַת חן 'graceful gazelle', an expression used in praise of a bride and also of a scholar on his ordination (v., however, עָלָה). Keth. 17[a]; Snh. 14[a].

יַעַן m. (b. h.; v. עָנָה) *corresponding*; (conj.) *because.*

Sifra B'huck. Par. 2, ch. VIII (ref. to יען וביען, Lev. XXVI, 43) וכי ראש בראש וכ׳ have I indeed paid them item for item (for all their sins)?—Ruth R. to II, 19; Lev. R. s. 34 ר׳ וב׳ הוא יען הוא כנ׳ 'because and because' (Lev. l. c.) *ya'an* and *'ani* have the same letters (intimating, 'because they have rejected my statutes concerning the poor').

יַעֲנָה f. (b. h.; cmp. עָנָה) *ostrich*; also בַּת הַי׳ (v. Ges. H. Dict.[10] s. v.). Hull. 64[b] (argument about the meaning of בת הי׳ concluded) כתיב י׳ וכתיב בת י׳ the Bible uses *y.* a. *bath y.* indiscriminately. Y. Sabb. I, 3[d], v. נַעֲמִית.

***יָעַף** (b. h.; cmp. עוּף) *to be bent, to be tired.*

Pi. יִיעֵף *to tire, annoy.* Tanh. Vayera 22 ... אל תשגיח לְיָעֵף לנו do not mind him (Satan), for he came only to annoy us; v., however, יָצַף.

יָעַץ (b. h.; v. עוּץ, cmp. אוּץ) [*to press,*] *to encourage, plan; to advise.* Ber. 61[a] כליות יוֹעֲצוֹת the kidneys are the seat of deliberation. Ib. אחת יוֹעַצְתּוֹ לטובה וכ׳ one (kidney) urges him to do good etc.—Snh. 76[b] הוֹעֲצְךָ וכ׳, v. זָהִיר. Ber. 8[b] וכשיוֹעֲצִים אין יועצים וכ׳ and when they (the Medians) hold council, they meet in open air. Snh. 87[a] ממך זה יוֹעֵץ 'hidden from thee' (Deut. XVII, 8) that means (the need of) a counselor (Sifré Deut. 152 זו עצה). Hull. 11[a] (expl. לעמת הָעֵצָה, Lev. III, 9) ממקום שהכליות יועצות from where the deliberating kidneys are seated, v. supra.—Tem. 16[a] (play on יַעְבֵּץ, I Chr. IV, 9) שיִּעֵץ וריבץ וכ׳ he advised and advanced the study of the Law &c. Snh. 106[a], a. e. בלעם שי׳ Balaam who gave his advice (encouraging the oppression of the Israelites); a. fr. — [Ber. 3[b]; Snh. 16[a], v. infra.]

Hithpa. הִתְיָיעֵץ, *Nithpa.* נִתְיָעֵץ *to ask advice; to consult with* (with ב). Yalk. Ps. 776 מִתְיָעֲצִים באחיתופל (Ber. 3[b]; Snh. 16[a] יועצין, read: נוֹעָצִין, *Nif.*) they deliberated with Ah.—Erub. 53[b] (in enigmatic speech) נת׳ במכתיר took counsel of the Nasi (v. כֶּתֶר). Sifré Num. 157 שהיו מתייעצים על וכ׳ they were planning against Israel; Yalk. Num. 785 מִיָּעֲצִים.

יְעַץ ch. same. Targ. Prov. XII, 20.

Pa. יַיעֵץ same. Meg. 15[b] עצה קא מְיַיעֲצֵי עילויה וכ׳ Ms. M. (ed. שקלי) they plan against this man (me).

Ithpa. אִתְיַיעֵץ *to take counsel.* Targ. Jud. XIX, 30.—V. עוּץ.

***יָעַק** (v. עוק ch.) *to press.*

Ithpa. אִתְיָיעֵק *to be narrowed in, to be troubled.* Targ. Y. Ex. I, 12 (O. עקתל׳; h. text ויקצו). Targ. Y. Num. XXII, 3. Targ. Job XVIII, 7 Ms. (ed. יתעייקן).

יַעֲקֹב (b. h.) pr. n. m. *Jacob,* 1) J. the patriarch. Ber. 13[a] לא שיעקר י׳ וכ׳ not that the name Jacob should be entirely abandoned, but &c., v. טָפֵל. Gen. R. s. 1; a. v. fr.—2) R. J., name of a Tannai (or of several Tannaim, v. Fr. Darkhe Mish. p. 202). Ab. IV, 16. Pes. 84[a]; Snh. 63[b], a. e., v. שֵׁם. Hull. 45[b].—Hor. 13[b] ר׳ י׳ בן קרשי; Y. Pes. X, beg. 37[b] ר׳ י׳ בן קורשי.—3) R. J., name of many Amoraim, esp. a) R. J. of K'far Nibburaya. Y. Bicc. III, 65[d] top, a. fr., v. נִבּוּרַיָא.—b) R. J. b. Idi. Y. Ber. II, 4[b]; Y. Shek. II, 47[a] top; Y. M. Kat. III, 83[c] bot.; Midr. Sam. ch. XIX; Yeb. 96[b]; a. fr.—V. Fr. M'bo p. 104[a], sq.—4) J. the bathing master (?). Y. Ber. II, 4[c] top עד י׳ הרמוסרא הוה לובשן until he came to the station of J. &c. he kept the T'fillin on; Pesik. R. s. 22 עד יעקר תורמוסא.—5) J. of K'far Sikhnaya, a disciple of Jesus of Nazareth. Ab. Zar. 17[a]; a. e.; v. סִכְנַיָא.

יַעַר m. (b. h.) *forest.* B. Kam. 32[b] (ref. to Deut. XIX, 5) ומה י׳ וכ׳ when in the case of unintentional homicide in the forest where each entered of his own accord &c.; Sifré Deut. 182 מה י׳ רשות וכ׳ as in the case .... in the forest, both had a right to enter. Cant. R. to III, 4, v. יְאוֹר; a. fr. —[יער, יאר=עור, עור, *to break forth,* applied to vegetation, water-course and light (cmp. נָהָר a. נְהוֹרָא); cmp. יְאוֹר a. Sam. יאר Gen. I, 11 for h. דשא.]

יַעְרָא I ch. same, *forest, thicket* (of reeds). Targ. O. Ex. II, 3; 5 (h. text סוּף). Targ. II Chr. IX, 16 ed. Beck י׳ דכרמלא (eth. Lag. a. oth. מקרת כלביא as I Kings X, 17). —*Pl.* יַעְרֵי. Targ. Prov. XXIV, 31 (h. text קמשונים).

יַעְרָא II or **יַעְרְתָא** f., constr. יַעְרַת (b. h. constr. יַעֲרַת, v. יַעַר) *flow* of honey. Targ. Cant. IV, 11.

יָפֶה m., **יָפָה** f.; pl. יָפִין, יָפוֹת (b. h.; יפי *to join,* cmp. אוֹף I, a. יפע) [*well-joined,* cmp. נָאֶה, כָּשֵׁר a. Arab. *wafa,*] 1) *appropriate; strong, healthy; handsome, beautiful, fine* (of build); *auspicious;* (adv.) *well, right.* Ned. 66[b] (an ambiguous expression, v. מוּם) עד שתראי מום י׳ שביך וכ׳ until thou showest to R. ... 'an appropriate blemish' (or 'something handsome') in thee; י׳ קורין וכ׳ it was nice (appropriate) that they named her *lakhlukhith* (aversion). Ber. 4[a] י׳ חייבתי׳ דנתי have I well argued (was I right)?; י׳ חייבתי was I right in convicting?—Ib. 34[a], a. e. רובן קשה ומיעוטן י׳ a large dose of them is injurious, a small one wholesome (or becoming). Ib. 39[a] י׳ ללב וטוב וכ׳ wholesome for the heart, and good &c. Ib. 56[b] י׳ לו or י׳ is an auspicious dream; a. v. fr.—יָדַיִם יָפוֹת, v. דֵּעָה—דעת יָפָה *skilled hands* for grabbing. Pes. 89[b] members of a Passover party שהיו ידיו של אחד מהן י׳ one of whom is extremely quick (in taking and eating); Tosef. ib. VII, 10 רפית ed. Zuck. (corr. acc.). Sifra K'dosh. Par. 1, ch. III אפי׳ בריא אפי׳ ידיו י׳ even if (among the poor coming for their share in the harvest) he (who insists on grabbing instead of distributing) is very strong, very skillful.—כֹּחַ יָפֶה *a strong legal right, privilege, prerogative.* Kidd. 21[a] י׳ כחו ליגאל לעולם the privilege of its redemption remains unimpaired forever (up to the jubilee year); י׳ ... בשנה שניה the privilege of redemption in the second year is unimpaired; opp. הורע כחו. Shebu. 48[a] י׳ כח הבן וכ׳ the son's prerogative is stronger (more extended) than that of his deceased father was; Hull. 49[b]; a. fr.—Ohol. XVIII, 6; Zab. III, 1, v. כֹּחַ.—יְפַת תֹּאַר *handsome woman,* esp. (ref. to Deut. XXI, 10 sq.) *a gentile captive* with whom the captor has had intercourse before deciding on converting and making her his legitimate wife. Kidd. 21[b] כהן מהו בי׳ ת׳ is a priest permitted to marry a gentile captive?—Snh. 21[a]. Ib. 107[a] כל הנושא י׳ ת׳ וכ׳ he who marries a gentile captive will have a rebellious son (ref. to Deut. l. c. a. ib. 18 sq.);

a. fr.—2) (cmp. טוֹב) *worth, valued.* Keth. VIII, 3 (79[b]) שמין אותה כמה היא יָפָה וכ׳ (Mish. ...הן יָפִין ... אותן...) we assess the land how much it is worth with the fruits and how much without. Ib. III, 7; a. fr.—Denom.

יִפָּה, יוֹפָּה 1) *to beautify; to make pleasant, popular.* Gen. R. s. 39, beg. (ref. to Ps. XLV, 12) לְיַפּוֹתֵךְ בעולם to make thee popular in the world. Ned. IX, 10 יִיפּוּהָ they improved her appearance. Ber. 43[b] (ref. to Koh. III, 11) שי׳ הקב״ה אומנתו בפני כל וא׳ א׳ Ms. M. (differ. in ed.), v. אוּמָנוּת.—*Part. pass.* מְיוּפֶּה *adorned, elaborate.* Cant. R. to I, 1 נמצא מי׳ ומרובה וכ׳ was Solomon's palace more elaborate and extensive than the Temple?—2) *to improve* (land). Y. Sabb. VII, 10[a] top קצר לְיַיפּוֹת וכ׳ he cut the grass for the sake of improving the land. Ib. חייב משום מְיַיפֶּה וכ׳ he is guilty of the offence of improving the land on the Sabbath. Pesik. S'lihoth, p. 166[a] יַפֵּה כחך improve thy strength (by practicing).—3) (with כח) *to strengthen one's rights, to confer prerogatives.* B. Bath. VII, 2 לְיַיפּוֹת כחו של מוכר to give the seller the prerogative. Y. ib. VIII, 16[a] top יִיפִּיתָה כחה בנכסי האם thou hast (the Law has) given her a prerogative with reference to her mother's property; a. fr.

***Pu.* יוּפָּה, with כח, *to be made stronger.* Peah VI, 6 [read:] יופה כחו של וכ׳ (Ms. M. ייפיה, ed. יופי) the prerogative of the owner has been made firmer, opp. הורע.—*Part.* מְיוּפֶּה (v. supra). Y. Gitt. II, beg. 44[a] כחו .. חתימה מי׳ by two persons testifying to the signature her case is improved.

Hithpa. הִתְיַפֶּה, *Nithpa.* נִתְיַפֶּה 1) *to become handsome.* Taan. 23[b] תִּתְיַיפִּי חנה Hannah, grow handsome, ונִתְיַיפָּתָה Ms. M. (ed. ...פת) and she did &c.—2) *to be praised.* Gen. R. s. 59 נִתְיַיפִּיתָ וכ׳ thou (Abraham) hast been praised among the angels &c.

יָפוֹ (b. h.) pr. n. pl. *Japho (Joppa),* the harbor of Jerusalem. Pirkê d'R. El. ch. X. Yalk. Is. 334 עד שיחיה די׳ to the excavations of the harbor of J.; Cant. R. to VII, 5 ריפע (corr. acc.); v. יָקָב. Ex. R. s. 43 ...ר׳ חייא... די׳ (some ed. דיָפוֹא) R. H... of J.

יִפּוּר, יִפּוּר m. (יָפֶה) *excellence, distinction.* Tanh. Hayé 1 (ref. to יפיפית, Ps. XLV, 3) אי זה הי׳ שלי where is my prerogative (of age)?

***יַפַּח** m. (נפח) *blowing up* (of cheeks). Snh. 18[b] (as a rule for appointing the Spring month, v. אָבִיב) אם קידום... ר׳ בלועך נפיק לקיבליה וכ׳ (Ms. M. רפח מלועך, corr. acc.; oth. Var. v. Rabb. D. S. a. l. note) when the East wind is ever so strong, and a blow out of thy cheek goes out to meet it (i. e. if a person feels the warmth of thy breath blown against the East wind),—such is Adar (and no Adar Sheni is to be intercalated); Y. ib. I, 18[c] bot. פח בלועה יפיק וכ׳ (read: פח בלועך); Y. R. Hash. I, 58[b] top פוח לוחיך ופוק וכ׳ blow up thy cheek &c.

יְפִיוּת f. (יָפֶה) *beauty, excellence.* Meg. 9[b] (ref. to Gen. IX, 27) יְפִיוּתוֹ של יפת תהא וכ׳ (not יהא, v. Rabb. D. S. a. l. note) the beauty of Japheth (Greek language) shall reside in the tents of Shem (ref. to the Greek Bible translation); Yalk. Gen. 61 יוֹפְיוּ.

יְפֵיפָה (b. h.; Pealal of יפה) *to be beautiful, distinguished.* Y. Meg. I, 71[c] top יָפְיָפִיתָ מבני אדם (Ps. XLV, 3, applied to Aquila, the translator of the Bible into Greek; cmp. preced.) thou art distinguished among the sons of man.

יְפֵיפוּת f. (v. preced.) *beauty, distinction.* Cant. R. to IV, 4 (play on תַּלְפִּיּוֹת, ib.) אני הוא שעשיתיו תל...ר׳ וכ׳ I made it (the Temple) a ruin in this world, and I shall make it a beauty in the future (some ed. יְפָיָפִיה).

יְפֵיפֵי m., **יְפֵיפִיָּה** f. (b. h. יְפֵה־פִיָּה; preced. wds.) *very fine, choice.* Pes. 6[b] גְּלוּסְקָא י׳ Ms. M. a. Ar. (ed. יפה), v. גְּלוּסְקָא.

יְפֵיפְיָה pr. n. (v. preced.) *Yefifyah, (Divine Beauty),* name of an angel. Targ. Y. Deut. XXXIV, 6 (cmp. יוֹפִיאֵל).

יָפֵק, v. אָפֵק.

יָפַע (b. h.; cmp. יָפָה), *Hif.* הוֹפִיעַ 1) *to join, arrive* (cmp. אָתָא), *to come forth, appear.* Gen. R. s. 12 כל א׳ וא׳ ה׳ בזמנו each (part of creation) came forth in its due time (though all were created at once).—2) *to bring, transfer.* B. Kam. 38[a] (ref. to Deut. XXXIII, 2) מפארן ה׳ ממונם וכ׳ from (what occurred at) Paran (the gentiles refusing to receive the Law) he (the Lord) transferred their wealth to Israel.—3) *to bring about, bring to light, reveal.* Gen. R. s. 90; Yalk. ib. 148 (play on צָפְנַת פַּעְנֵחַ) צפונות הופיע ונוחות וכ׳ he reveals secrets, and it is easy to him to tell them; צפונות הופיע בדעת מניח וכ׳ he brings secret things to light through his intelligence; with them he sets mankind at ease. Macc. 23[b]; Gen. R. s. 85 בג׳ מקומות ה׳ רוה״ק on three occasions did the holy spirit reveal (the true state of affairs); (oth. opin. v. פּוּעַ). Koh. R. to VII, 1 (play on פּוּעָה, Ex. I, 15) שהוֹפִיעָה את מעשה אחיה she (Miriam) brought about what happened to her brother (she was the cause of Moses' peculiar career).—4) *to lift up, raise.* Ex. R. s. 1 (play on פועה, v. supra) שהופיעה את ישראל לה׳ וכ׳ she (Miriam) lifted Israel up to God.—ה׳ פנים כנגד *to lift one's face up against, to have the courage to rebuke.* Ib. שהופיעה פ׳.. וזקפה וכ׳ she lifted her face up against Pharaoh and turned her nose up against him (in angry rebuke). Ib. שה׳ פ׳ כנגד אביה she dared to reprove her father. Y. B. Kam. IV, 4[b] top.

יְפַע ch. same, *to appear, rise.* Targ. Job III, 4 תֵּפַע (תְּפִיעַ; h. text תּוֹפַע).

Af. אוֹפַע 1) same. Ib. X, 3 אוֹפַעְתְּ thou appearest (approving, h. text הופעת). Targ. Ps. LXXX, 2. Ib. XCIV, 1.—2) *to send forth.* Targ. Job XXXVII, 15.

יֶפֶת (b. h.) pr. n. m. *Japheth,* one of the sons of Noah, progenitor of the Aryan races (Greeks, Persians &c.). Gen. R. s. 36 (ref. to Gen. IX, 27) זה כורש that is Cyrus (the Persians). Ib. יהיו... בלשונו של י׳ the words of the Law shall be recited in the language of J. (Greek). Pesik. R. s. 35 כורש... שהוא מזרעו של י׳ Cyrus ... who is a descendant of J. Meg. 9[b], v. יְפִיוּת; a. fr.

יִפְתָּח (b.h.) pr. n. m. *Jephthah*, the Judge. R. Hash. 25[b] יִ׳ בדורו כשמואל וכ׳ the authority of a J. in his days must be respected as that of a Samuel in his; Tosef. ib. II (I), 3 בית דינו של יִ׳. Gen. R. s. 60; a. fr.

יָצָא (b. h.) 1) *to go forth; to rise* (of the sun); *to go out.* Gen. R. s. 39 אֵצֵא והדיו וכ׳ I shall leave (my father's house), and they may desecrate &c. Ib. יָ׳ לו מונטון a medal was issued in his memory, v. מוֹנִיטוֹן. Ib. s. 6 בשעה שהוא יוצא when he (the sun) rises; בשעה שהיא יוֹצֵאת when she (the moon) rises. Snh. 52[a] ארור שֶׁיָּצָאת זו מחלציו (v. Rabb. D. S. a. l. note) cursed is he from whose loins this woman went forth.—Sabb. V, 1 במה ... יוֹצְאָה what is an animal permitted to wear on going out (on the Sabbath)? Ib. VI, 1 לא תֵּצֵא וכ׳ a woman must not wear on going out &c.; a. v. fr.—2) *to end; to go to the end of, to live through.* Y. Ber. VIII, 12[b] bot. כיון שֶׁיָּצְאָה שבת when the Sabbath ended. Y. Shebi. VI, 36[c] top אינו יוצא שבתו ולא יָ׳ וכ׳ he shall not live to the end of this week, and he did not arrive at the end of the week before he was dead; (Erub. 63[a] הוציא שנתו, v. infra); a. e.—3) *to be expended.* Num. R. s. 14, end, v. הוֹצָאָה.—4) *to be excluded; exempt;* (rarely) *to exclude, deduct.* Y. Ned. II, beg. 37[b] יָ׳ דבר של איסור this is to exclude a vow concerning a forbidden act; Bab. ib. 17[a] יָ׳ נשבע לבטל וכ׳ this excludes the case of one who makes oath that he will disregard a law. Y. Yeb. I, 2[c] top אשר תלד יָצְתָה זו וכ׳ 'whom she may bear' (Deut. XXV, 6), herewith is excluded she (the אַיְילוֹנִית) who &c.; a. v. fr.—Y. Ḥag. I, 76[c] top צֵא מהם שני ימים deduct from them two days; ib. צא שבת מהם deduct the Sabbath day.—Esp. idiomatic uses: a) יָ׳ לחירות, יָ׳ בן חורין, or only יָ׳ *to be freed.* Peah III, 8; Gitt. 42[a]. Kidd. 24[a] יוצא בשן וכ׳ he is freed, when his master caused his loss of a tooth or an eye; a. v. fr.—b) (of a wife) *to be sent away, to be divorced.* Keth. VII, 6 ואלו יוֹצְאוֹת שלא בכתובה the following wives have to leave without receiving their K'thubah. Ib. 7 תֵּצֵא she must leave. Ib. X, 5; a. v. fr.—c) יָ׳ ידי (or מִידֵי) *to go out of the power of; to be released; to do justice to, be justified before.* Shek. III, 2 ... לפי שאדם צריך לָצֵאת ידי הבריות לָצֵאת ידי המקום because man must appear justified before men as well as before God; Ex. R. s. 51; a. fr.— יָ׳ ידי חובתו, or יָ׳ *to comply with the requirements of the law.* Ber. 8[b]. Ib. II, 1 אם כיון לבו יָ׳ if he read with attention, he has done his duty (which requires the reading of the Sh'ma). Y. Shek. III, 47[b] bot. מהו לצאת וכ׳ is the law complied with when one uses wine &c.?—Mekh. Bo, Pisha, s. 6; a. v. fr.—Gen. R. s. 39 לא יָצָאתָ ידי השבועה thou hast not redeemed thy oath; ib. s. 49; Lev. R. s. 10, beg.—Makhsh. VI, 5; Tosef. Toh. X, 3 יָ׳ מידי שמן, v. מִקְרָא, v. יָ׳ מידי פשוטו.—מוּחָל—d) יָ׳ מן הכלל or יָ׳ *to be taken out of the general rule, to be specified* (although being implied in the general rule). Sifra, introd. כל דבר שהיה בכלל ויָ׳ ... לא ללמד על עצמו יָ׳ וכ׳ whatever would have been implied in the general law and yet is specified again (in the Biblical text) in order to teach (something not mentioned before), has been specified not only to teach something new concerning the specific case, but to teach it concerning the whole class. Ib. יָ׳ לִטְעוֹן, v. טָעַן I. Tem. I, 6 ולמה יָ׳ and for what purpose are tithes especially mentioned (Lev. XXVII, 30, sq.)?; a. fr.—e) כַּיּוֹצֵא בּ־ *like that which passes with it* (in the same class), *similar; in a similar way.* Pes. III, 2 אם יש כי׳ בו שהחמיץ if there is a similar dough (started simultaneously with the one in question) which has begun to ferment. Ber. 59[b], sq. ואין לו כי׳ בו when he has no house like it; כי׳ בהם garments like them. Zeb. V, 6 המורם מהם כי׳ בהם what is taken of them for the priest, is like them (subject to the same laws). M. Kat. 16[b] כי׳ בדבר אחה אומר וכ׳ in a similar way (as something coming under the same category) you read &c. Sifré Num. 32; a. v. fr.—f) יָ׳ שכרו בהפסדו its benefit *is lost* in its disadvantage; i. e. benefit and disadvantage are counterbalanced. Ab. V, 11, sq.—g) (euphem.) *to retire for human needs* (v. Toh. X, 2). Ber. 62[a] השכם וצא וכ׳ go out early in the morning &c. Ex. R. s. 9 ואינו יוצא and has no human needs. Ib. לא היה יוצא אלא וכ׳ לנקביו he used to go out only to the water (to make believe he was a superhuman being); a. fr.—h) *to be proved, identified.* Keth. II, 3 היה כתב ידם יוצא ממקום אחר if their signature can be identified otherwise (than by their own declaration); a. e.

Hif. הוֹצִיא 1) *to take out, to lead forth, bring forth; to release, discharge, send off.* Ber. VI, 1 before eating bread one says, המוציא לחם וכ׳ (blessed be thou, O Lord) who hast brought forth bread out of the earth (v. ib. 38[a] as to המוציא or מוציא); ib. 37[b]; a. fr.—Ab. Zar. 41[b], a. fr. אין ספק מוציא וכ׳, v. וַדַּאי. B. Mets. 37[b] לא זו הדרך מוֹצִיאָתוֹ מידי עבירה עד וכ׳ this is not the way that relieves him from sin (this is no full atonement), (he is not relieved) until he pays &c.; Yeb. XV, 7. Ib. 6, sq. אין זו דרך מוֹצִיאָתָהּ וכ׳ she is not relieved from the possibility of sin, unless she is not permitted to marry again and forbidden to partake of T'rumah.—Ib. 36[b] יוֹצִיא (יוֹצִיאֶהָ) בגט he dismisses her with a letter of divorce. Ib. ואם נשא יוציא and if he married her (against the law), he must dismiss her (divorce her); a. fr.—Ab. II, 11, a. fr. מוֹצִיאִין את האדם מן העולם take a man out of the world, i. e. cause him to lose the true enjoyment of life.—2) *to exclude.* Y. Yeb. I, 2[c] top איילונית מטעם אחר הוֹצֵאתָהּ the *aylonith* thou dost (the law does) exclude for another reason (v. supra). Num. R. s. 14, end אוֹצִיא את ישראל let me exclude the Israelites, א׳ את הזקנים the elders; a. fr.—להוֹצִיא (= ch. לאפוקי, v. אֲפַק, or למעוטי, v. מעט) *to the exclusion of.* Succ. 28[a]; Kidd. 34[a] האזרח לה׳ את הנשים '*the* native' (Lev. XXIII, 42) intimates the exemption of women (from the duty of dwelling in booths); a. v. fr.—3) *to lead to the end, to live through.* Erub. 63[a], v. supra.—4) *to produce, present.* Keth. XIII, 8 המוציא שטר חוב ... והלה ה׳ וכ׳ if one produces a note of indebtedness against his neighbor, and the latter produces evidence that the claimant sold him a field (and paid him, which he would not have done, if he had a claim). Ib. 9. Ib. IX, 9 הוֹצִיאָה גט if she produces a letter of divorce; a. v. fr.—5) *to spend, lay out.* Ib. VIII, 5, v. הוֹצָאָה; a. fr.—Esp. idiomatic uses: a) ה׳ ידי חוב־ or ה׳ (v. supra) *to be the instrument of a person's complying with the law,* e. g. to read a prayer and thus cause the listener to perform his duty as though he read it himself; *to act in another's behalf effectively.* R. Hash. III, 5 אין מוֹצִיאִין את הרבים ידי חובתן they cannot act (blow the Shofar) in behalf of the assembled congregation. Ib. 29ª אע״פ שיצא מוציא although he has done his duty (has read the prayer for himself), he may act in behalf of others. Ib. ולעצמו מוציא and can he (the half-slave and half-freedman) act in his own behalf?; a. fr.—b) *to collect, to claim.* Keth. VIII, 1 הבעל מוציא מיד הלקוחות the husband can reclaim the property from those who bought it. B. Kam. III, 11 המוציא מחבירו עליו הראיה the claimant must produce evidence; a. v. fr. —c) *to utter.* Arakh. 5ª, a. fr. אין אדם מוציא דבריו לבטלה no man utters his words for no purpose (he must have meant something). — ה׳ לעז *to slander, discredit.* Sabb. 97ª, a. fr., v. לַעַז.—d) *to carry an object* (on the Sabbath) *out of a private to a public place,* or *from one private place to another,* v. רְשׁוּת. Sabb. VII, 2, sq.; a. fr.—e) *to secrete.* Sifré Num. 88 יש לך... שאין מוציא וכ׳ is there a woman-born being that does not discharge the food he eats?; a. e.—f) ה׳ שבת *to dismiss the Sabbath with prayer,* opp. הכניס. Sabb. 118ᵇ מוֹצִיאֵי שבת וכ׳ those who dismiss the Sabbath at Sepphoris.

יְצָא ch. *to end,* only in *Shaf.* שֵׁיצֵא q. v.

יצאה, B. Kam. 100ᵇ Mish.; ib. 102ª הר׳ read: הַיְצִיאָה or הַהוֹצָאָה. Gen. R. s. 98 דביה ר׳, v. יָצָה.

יָצַב (b.h.) *to stand, be erect.*—Denom. יְצִיבָה.—V. נָצַב. *Hithpa.* הִתְיַצֵּב *to place one's self; to be firm.* Cant. R. to I, 1 (ref. to Prov. XXII, 29) מִתְיַצְּבִים בתורה they are firm in the Law. Pesik. R. s. 6 (ref. to Prov. l. c.) בל יִתְיַצֵּב לפני פרעה וכ׳ he will not place himself (praying) before Pharaoh, the benighted (v. חָשׁוּךְ); Cant. R. l. c. לפני מלכי תורה יתיצב he will be placed before (ranked as the foremost of) the kings of the Law; Koh. R. to I, 1 לפני מלאכים יתי׳ he will be ranked before angels; a. e.

יְצַב ch. same; Pa. יַצֵּב *to establish.* [Dan. VII, 19 *to ascertain.*] Targ. I Chr. IV, 23.—V. נְצַב.

יִצְהָר I m. (b. h.; צהר) *oil.* Sifré Deut. 42. Snh. 24ª (ref. to Zech. IV, 14) ר׳ אלו ת״ח שמשמינים וכ׳ Ms. M. (ed. כשמן... שנוחים) 'sons of oil', those are the Palestinean scholars who oil (smoothe) one another in their discussions; Yalk. Zech. 579.

יִצְהָר II (b. h.) pr. n. m. *Izhar,* father of Korah. Snh. 109ᵇ בן י׳ שהרתיח... כצהרים 'the son of I.', for he made the world as hot to himself as noon-heat.

***יָצוּל** m. (יצל; cmp. אֵצֶל; v. Wetzst. in Levy Talm. Dict. s. v. כורך) *the cross-piece* or *handle* of a plough. Kel. XXI, 2.

יָצוּעַ m. (b. h.; יָצַע) *spreading, bed-mattress, couch.* Gen. R. s. 98 (play on פַּחַז, Gen. XLIX, 4) פּרקת עול חִלַּלְתָּ יְצוּעַי זע וכ׳ thou hast thrown off the yoke (restraint), thou hast desecrated my couch, thy passion within thee was agitated. Sabb. 55ᵇ (ref. to Gen. l. c.) א״ת יְצוּעִי אלא יְצוּעָיו (missing in Ms. M., v. Rabb. D. S. a. l. note) read not 'my couch' but 'my couches'.—*Pl.* יְצוּעִים, יְצוּעִין. Gen. R. l. c. קלקל את הי׳ he disgraced his father's couches. Tosef. B. Bath. III, 1 הַיְצוּעִין ed. Zuck. (Var. הַיְּצָעִים); Y. ib. IV, 14ᶜ bot. יְצוּ׳ the mattresses in the press (for the laborers or watchmen). Tosef. ib. IV, 1 יְצוּ׳; Y. ib. V, beg. 15ᶜ יְצוּ׳ the mattresses on board of ships.

יָצוּק, v. יָצַק.

יָצוּר, v. יָצִיר.

יִצְחָק (b. h.) pr. n. m. *Isaac,* 1) son of Abraham. Ber. 26ᵇ; Num. R. s. 2 ר׳ קבע וכ׳ I. introduced the afternoon prayer (Minḥah). Gen. R. s. 19; a. v. fr.—R. Hash. 16ª, a. fr. עקידת י׳ the intended offering up of Isaac.—אפרו של י׳, v. אֵפֶר.—2) R. I., a. Tannai. Succ. 25ᵇ; Sifré Num. 68. Macc. 13ᵇ; a. fr. (v. Fr. Darkhé Mish. p. 203).—3) name of many Amoraim, esp. a) R. I. Roba or Rabbah (the Elder). Y. Maas. Sh. V, beg. 55ᵈ. Y. Ber. V, 9ᵇ bot. Bab. ib. 33ᵇ ר׳ י׳ בר אבדימי; a. fr.—b) mate of R. Imi. Y. Kil. III, beg. 28ᶜ; a. fr.—Taan. 5ᵇ; Meg. 15ª; a. fr.—c) R. I. of Magdala. B. Mets. 25ª. Sabb. 139ª. Yoma 81ᵇ.—4) I. Saḥora (the merchant). Y. Ber. IV, 7ᶜ bot.; Y. Taan. IV, 67ᶜ bot.—V. Fr. M'bo, p. 105ᵇ sq.

יְצִיאָה f. (יָצָא) 1) *going out, departure; separation.* Midd. I, 3 משמשין כניס׳ וי׳ used for entrance and exit. Ber. IX, 4. Ib. I, 5 מזכירין יְצִיאַת מצרים we must recite (the section alluding to) the exodus from Egypt (Num. XV, 37—41). Ib. 12ᵇ; a. fr.—Kidd. 5ª, v. הֲוָיָה.—יציאת נשמה the separation of the soul from the body, *death.* M. Kat. 25ª. Ib. 28ᵇ bot.; a. fr.—B. Mets. 107ª יְצִיאָתְךָ מן העולם thy departure from this world.—Pesik. R. s. 26 יְצִיאָתוֹ... לעולם when Jeremiah was born; a. v. fr.—*Pl.* יְצִיאוֹת. Ex. R. s. 1 שתי י׳ יצא וכ׳ twice did Moses go out &c.; a. e.— 2) *expense, ready money for expense.* Gen. R. s. 11 ברכו בי׳ He blessed the Sabbath day by providing for its additional expense; Yalk. Gen. 16 בִּיצִיאָתוֹ. Gen. R. l. c. מפני הי׳ (he blessed the Sabbath) on account of its expensiveness (Yalk. l. c. מפני הוצאה). Ib. s. 39 ממעטת את הי׳ (travelling) reduces a person's means; Num. R. s. 11. Ib. שלא תמעט... את הי׳ that travelling may not reduce thy means; Midr. Till. to Ps. XXIII. B. Kam. IX, 4 (100ᵇ); ib. 102ᵇ היצאה (corr. acc.), v. הוֹצָאָה; a. fr.—*Pl.* as ab. Cant. R. to VII, 3 משמוציא יְצִיאוֹתָיו after having made all his expenses (for the wedding); Midr. Till. to Ps. II. Lam. R. to IV, 2 עושה שלחנות יותר מן הי׳ made the outfit of the tables for the wedding feast more expensive than the costs (of the domestic arrangements). Ex. R. s. 9; Esth. R. to I, 4, a. e. מיני י׳ הראה להם he showed them various expensive dishes; a. fr.—3) *rise of the sun.* Y. Ber. I, 2ᶜ top; a. e.—4) *the carrying* (on the Sabbath) *of an object from private to public ground* &c.—*Pl.* as ab. Sabb. I, 1; a. fr., v. הוֹצָאָה.—5) *discharge of the bowels.* Ber. 62ᵇ; a. e.

יַצִּיב m. (יָצַב) *firm, irrefutable.*—אמת וי׳ *true and irrefutable,* name of a prayer after Sh'ma in the morning and evening prayers. Ber. II, 2 בין ויאמר לאמת וי׳ between *vayomer* (Num. XV, 37—41) and *ĕmeth v'yatsib.* Y. ib. I, 2ᵈ bot. א׳ וי׳ של שחרית the *ĕmeth v'yatsib* of the morning prayer, contrad. to אמת וי׳ of the night prayer (which, in the Babylonian liturgy, begins אמת ואמונה, Ber. 12ª).

יַצִּיב, יַצִּיבָא ch. same, 1) *firmly planted,* v. נְצַב.

Targ. Ps. XXXVII, 35 (h. text אזרח). Targ. Zech. XIV, 9. —2) (cmp. אֶזְרָח) *native, citizen.* Targ. Ps. LXXXVIII, 1 (h. text אזרחי). Targ. O. Ex. XII, 19 (ed. Berl. *pl.*); a. fr. —Yoma 47ª, a. e. ר׳ בארעא, v. גִּיּוֹר.—[Lev. R. s. 9 יציבא, read: ילדפא, v. יְלֵיף.]—*Pl.* יְצִיבַיָּא, יַצִּיבֵי. Targ. O. Lev. XVI, 29. Targ. Y. Ex. l. c.; a. e.

יְצִיבָה f. (יָצַב) *standing, use of the verb* יצב. Mekh. B'shall., Shirah, s. 10 אין ר׳ אלא נבואה the verb יצב expresses (readiness for) prophecy; v. הֲצָבָה.

יְצִידִין, v. יְצִירִין.

יָצִיעַ I m. *mattress*, v. יָצוּעַ.

יָצִיעַ II f. (b. h. יצוע K'ri; יָצַע) *extension, wing* of a building. B. Bath. IV, 1 (61ª), v. אַצְּפְּתָא II, a. בַּרְקָא III. Pes. 8ª. Erub. 102ᵇ ושל ר׳ and the door-pin of an extension. Tosef. Neg. VI, 5.

יָצִיף, v. יְצַף.

יציצין, יציציין, Targ. Ps. CXXXIX, 9 some ed., v. צִיצִיתָא.

יְצִיקָה f. (יָצַק) *casting* (metal), *pouring* (oil). Y. Ber. I, 2ᵈ top; Yalk. Gen. 19 נראין כבשעת יְצִיקָתָן they (the heavens) look (as bright) as at the time they were cast. Men. VI, 3 (74ᵇ) ר׳ ובלילה the pouring of oil (on the flour, Lev. II, 1) and the mixing. Hor. 12ª; Kerith 5ᵇ, contrad. to מְשִׁיחָה; a. fr.—*Pl.* יְצִיקוֹת. Tosef. Dem. II, 7; Men. 18ᵇ; Hull. 132ᵇ.

יְצִיר (יְצוּר) m. (יָצַר) 1) *creature, creation.* Gen. R. s. 9 (ref. to I Chr. XXVIII, 9) קודם עד שלא נולד יצור וכ׳ ere yet a human creature is formed, his thought is revealed before thee; Midr. Sam. ch. V; Yalk. Chr. 1080 יציר. Pesik. R. s. 47 האדם ר׳ כפיי Adam, the formation of my hands; Koh. R. to III, 11 ר׳ כפי. Keth. 8ª כשמחך יְצִירָךְ וכ׳ as thou didst rejoice thy creature (Adam) in the garden &c.—*Pl.* יְצִירִים, (יְצוּ׳). Pesik. R. s. 26 אחד מארבעה יצו׳ ... one of the four persons that are called divine creations (concerning whom the verb יצר is used in the Scriptures); Yalk. Jer. 262 יצי׳.—2) v. יְצִירִין.

יְצִירָה f. (preced.) 1) *formation, creation; nature.* Yoma 85ª לענין ר׳ as regards the stages of embryonic formation. Lev. R. s. 14, beg. כשם שיְּצִירָתוֹ של אדם וכ׳ as well as the creation of man took place after that of the animals, so is the law concerning man (Lev. XII—XV) issued after that concerning animals (ib. XI). Ib. יְצִירַת הוולד the formation (development) of the embryo.—Sot. 2ª; Snh. 22ª ארבעים יום קודם ר׳ הוו׳ וכ׳ forty days before the embryo is formed, a divine voice goes forth &c. Nidd. 22ᵇ דנין ר׳ מי׳ we may draw an analogy between animals concerning whose formation the verb יצר is used (contrad. to ברא). Keth. 8ª חדא ר׳ הואי there was one act of formation for Adam und Eve (male and female persons combined, v. Erub. 18ª); a. fr.—*Pl.* יְצִירוֹת. Ib. שתי ר׳ הואי there were two different formations. Gen. R. s. 14 (ref. to וייצר with two י, Gen. II, 7) שתי ר׳ וכ׳ two formations, one referring to Adam, the other to Eve; יצירה לשבעה וכ׳ there is a viable birth at seven months, and one at nine months. Ib. שתי ר׳ יצירה מן התחתונים וכ׳ two creations, one partaking of the nature of earthly creatures, the other of heavenly beings. Y. Yeb. II, 5ᶜ bot.—2) ר׳ or בית הי׳ (v. יוֹצֵר) *potter's workshop.* Tosef. Kel. B. Kam. III, 8.—Y. B. Mets. VIII, end, 11ᵈ בית הרוצרה (corr. acc.); Tosef. ib. VIII, 27 ור׳ אין פחות וכ׳ ed. Zuck. (Var. וצירה) a pottery is rented on no less than twelve months' notice.

***יְצִירִין** m. pl. (יָצַר) (probably) *moulds* for pressed raisins or olives. Tosef. B. Bath. III, 2 יצירי׳ ed. Zuck. (Var. יציר׳, quot. in comment. to B. Bath. 67ᵇ (יְצָרִים); B. Bath. l. c. נסרים (v. Rabb. D. S. a. l. note 8); Y. ib. IV, 14ᶜ אֲסוּרִין.

יָצַע (b. h.; cmp. יָצָא) *to spread, unfold.* Denom. יָצוּעַ, יָצִיעַ.

Hif. הִצִּיעַ *to spread, to prepare the* יָצוּעַ, *lay out the mattresses* &c.; *to unfold, to arrange.* Sabb. XV, 3 ומַצִּיעִין את המטות וכ׳ and one is permitted to rearrange the couches, after being used on the Sabbath night, for use during the Sabbath day. Keth. 67ᵇ מציעין לו מטה they (the guardians of the poor) procure for him the requirements for a couch. Men. 44ª הִצִּיעָה לו ז׳ וכ׳ she arranged for him seven couches. Gitt. 56ᵇ ה׳ ס״ת he spread a scroll of the Law (to lie upon it); Num. R. s. 18, end; Tanh. Huck. 1; a. fr.—Mekh. B'shall., Vayhi, s. 1 ומציעין בהמתם לצאת and putting spreadings upon (saddling) their animals &c.—Tosef. Ber. II, 12 ובלבד שלא יַצִּיעַ את המשנה but he must not arrange (lay before them the full text of) the Mishnah; Y. ib. III, 6ᶜ bot.; Bab. ib. 22ª.—Part. pass. מוּצָע, f. מוּצַעַת. Y. Hag. II, 77ª bot., v. טְרִיקְלִין. Arakh. VI, 3 מטה מו׳ a spread couch (supplied with all necessaries). Pesik. Ekhah, p. 122ᵇ ומצאה מוצעת וכ׳ and found it (the garment) spread over his couch; Yalk. Is. 258 ומצאו מוצע (corr. acc.).

יְצַע ch., *Af.* אַצַּע, *Pa.* יַצַּע same. Targ. Y. Deut. XXXIV, 6.—Part. pass. מְיַיצַּע. Targ. Y. Ex. XXIV, 10 (ed. Amst. מְיַיצַּע; of a folding stool). Targ. Y. Num. XXIV, 5 (of the Tabernacle.

יְצָעִין, יְצָעִים, v. יָצוּעַ.

***יָצָף** pr. n. m. *Yatsaf.* Y. Taan. IV, 68ª bot. בן י׳ מן דאסף Ben Y. is of the family of Asaph; Gen. R. s. 98 דבית יצצה וכ׳ those of the house of Y. &c.

יָצַף (v. צוּף) [*to flow, melt,*] *to be troubled, afraid* (cmp. דאג, דאב).

Pi. יִצֵּף *to trouble, discourage.* Tanh. ed. Bub. Vayera 48 (quoted in 'Rashi' to Gen. R. s. 56) [read:] הוא בא לְיַצֵּף אותך אבל הקב״ה יִיצַּף לנו וכ׳ he (Satan) comes to discourage thee, but the Lord will look out (v. צָפָה) for us, as it is said, God will see &c. (Gen. XXII, 8); (Tanh. Vayera 22 אל תשגיח עליו שאינו בא אלא לירכך לנו, prob. to be read: לְיַצֵּף); Pesik. R. s. 40 לְיַ׳ לך.

יְצַף, יְצִיף ch. same, *to be afraid* (h. דָּאַג). Targ. Is. LVII, 11 ית מן יְצִיפַתְּ (Buxt. יְצַפְתְּ) of whom wast thou afraid?—Targ. I Sam. IX, 5 ויִיצִיף ed. Lag. (some ed. ויִצַּף); ib. X, 2. Targ. Jer. XLII, 16. Ib. XXXVIII, 19.

Pa. יַצֵּף, יָצֵף same. Targ. Jer. XXXI, 11 (h. text דאב).—Y. Taan. II, 65[b] top נפח צפונה יַצֵּף לבניך (read לבנירך or לבנינך) when the northern wind blows, be anxious for thy bricks (thy buildings). Gen. R. s. 56 יצף להחוא גברא וכ׳ beware of that man (Satan), v. גְּעַר.

Ithpe. אִתְּיְצִיף to trouble one's self. Targ. Ps. XXXVIII, 19 (ed. Lag. אִתְיַצַּף; h. text אדאג).

יִיצַף, יוּצַף, יַצְפָּא, יַצָּף m. (preced.; cmp. אַצְפָּא) *care, trouble.*—Targ. Josh. XXII, 24 מיוי ed. Lag. (oth. ed. מיו׳; h. text מדאגה). Targ. Jer. XLIX, 23; Ib. XXXI, 24 נַפְשׁ י׳ troubled soul (h. text דאבה). Targ. I Sam. XXV, 31 (ed. Wil. יַצְפָּא) *regret* (h. text פוקה). Targ. Ez. IV, 16.

יָצַק (b. h.; cmp. זקק) *to pour, cast.* Zeb. 112[b]; Snh. 82[b] הזוצק a non-priest who pours oil, v. יְצִיקָה. Ib. 83[a] אזהרה ליוצק וכ׳ where in the Scriptures is the warning for the non-priest not to pour oil &c.?—Men. III, 2; a. fr.—*Part. pass.* יָצוּק (or מוּצָק, fr. מָצַק) *cast,* a poetic expression for *mortal,* opp. to angel.—*Pl.* יְצוּקִים (מְצוּקִים). Y. Kil. IX, 32[b] top; Y. Keth. XII, 35[a] י׳; Keth. 104[a] מ׳, a. e., v. אֶרְאֵל.

Hif. הֵצִיק same. Hor. 12[a] מַצִּיקִין לו על ראשו Ms. M. (ed. מוּצָקִין שמן, v. מָצַק) they pour oil upon his head; Kerith. 5[b] מַצִּיק לו שמן וכ׳. Yalk. Gen. 19 בו״ד מֵצִיק וכ׳ (Gen. R. s. 12 מוּצָק) a human being casts a lens, v. בּוּלָס.

Hof. הוּצַק *to be poured, cast.* Snh. 92[b] יוּצַק זהב רותח וכ׳ may hot gold be poured into the mouth &c.; Yalk. Dan. 1062 י׳ סיד רותח.—*Part.* מוּצָק a) *cast (metal), bright.* Y. Ber. I, 2[d] top (ref. to כראי מוצק, Job XXXVII, 18) כראי מ׳ בכל שעה וכ׳ 'like a cast metal mirror', at all times the heavens look as bright &c., v. יְצִיקָה; Yalk. Gen. 19; Gen. R. s. 12, end.—b) (cmp. זקק) *well-joined, firm* (cmp. II Sam. XV, 24; =מוצג). Yalk. Kings 185 (ref. to I Kings VII, 23) זה העולם שהוא מ׳ the basin is typical of the world which is called *mutsak* (firm), as we read &c. (Job XXXVIII, 38). Y. Ber. I, 2[c] bot. (ref. to Job XXXVII, 18, v. supra) you might think that the heavens become lax, . . . ת״ל כראי מוּצָקִים therefore it is said . . . ., at all times they appear firmly joined.

Nif. נִיצּוֹק, נִצּוֹק q. v.

יָצַר (b. h.; cmp. צרר) *to turn, shape, form.* Keth. 8[a] (marriage benediction) אשר י׳ את וכ׳ who hast formed man in thine image. Ber. 58[b] (prayer in a burial place) אשר י׳ אתכם וכ׳ who created you in justice &c.; a. fr.—Part. יוֹצֵר (as noun, v. יוֹצֵר). Ib. 11[b] (in the morning prayer) י׳ אור בורא וכ׳ who didst form light and create darkness.—יוֹצֵר אוֹר or יוֹצֵר name of one of the benedictions preceding the reading of the morning Sh'ma. Ib.; ib. 12[a]; a. fr.

Nif. נוֹצַר *to be formed, created; to be fully developed.* Gen. R. s. 9 קודם עד שלא נוֹצְרָה מחשבה וכ׳ ere yet a thought is formed in the heart of man &c. Ib. קודם . . . . נ׳ יצור, v. יְצִיר. Ab. II, 8 לכך נוֹצַרְתָּ for that purpose (of studying) thou hast been created. Ib. IV, 22. Gen. R. s. 14, beg.; Y. Yeb. IV, 5[d] top נ׳ לשבעה if the embryo was fully developed at seven months, contrad. to סלד, v. יָלַד. Yoma 85[a]; Sot. 45[b] מהיכן הולד נ׳ from where does the formation of the embryo start? a. fr.—V. צור.

יְצַר ch. same. Targ. Am. IV, 13 דִּיצַר (some ed. דְּצַר), v. צוּר.

Ithpa. אִיתְּצַר *to be created, formed.* Yoma 85[a]; Sot. 45[b] ממציעתיה מִיתְּצַר the formation of the embryo starts from the central portion of the body.

יֵצֶר m. (b. h.; preced.) [*shape, formation,* whence] (v. Gen. VI, 5) =י׳ מחשבות *the formation of thoughts, bent of mind, inclination, desire.*—י׳ טוב or י׳ הטוב (abbr. יה״ט or י״ט) *the good nature* of man, *the inclination to do good;* (personified) *the good genius;* י׳ הרע (abbrev. יצה״ר), also only י׳ *the evil inclination, worldly desires;* (personified) *the tempter.* Ber. 61[a] מִיצְרִי, v. יוֹצֵר. Gen. R. s. 9; Koh. R. to III, 11 אילולי יצה״ר לא בנה וכ׳ but for the worldly desires of man, none would build a house &c. Ab. II, 11 עין הרע ויצה״ר וכ׳ greed, sensual passion and hatred &c. Snh. 103[a]; Yalk. Ps. 842 שלא ישלוט בך יצה״ר that temptation may have no power over thee. Succ. 52[a] . . . לעתיד מביאו ליצה״ר וכ׳ in the days to come the Lord shall bring the Tempter and slaughter him &c. Gen. R. s. 22 מפנק את יִצְרוֹ who indulges the senses. Ib. אם בא יִצְרְךָ להשחיקך when thy inclination (Tempter) comes to lead thee to amusement. Cant. R. to VII, 8 י׳ ע״ז the passion for idolatry, י׳ זנות the passion of lust. Ab. IV, 1 הכובש את יצרו who conquers his inclination; a. v. fr. [Yoma 69[b] כובש את יצרו, read with Ms. M. כעסו.]—*Pl.* יְצָרִים. Ber. 61[a] (ref. to וייצר, Gen. II, 7, v. יְצִירָה) שני י׳ וכ׳ two natures, the good and the evil. Cant. R. l. c. שני י׳ ברא וכ׳ two passions did God create in this world, v. supra. Snh. 105[a] יסרו יצריכם chasten your passions; Yalk. Is. 302.—[יְצָרִים *moulds,* v. יְצִירִין.]

יִצְרָא, יֵצֶר ch. same. Targ. Gen. VI, 5. Targ. Ps. XIII, 5; a. fr.—Sabb. 156[b] אלמיה יִצְרֵיה, v. אֲלַם. Hag. 16[a] דמצי כייף ליה ליצריה when he can conquer his passion. Kidd. 81[b]; Keth. 51[b] יצר אלבשה, v. לְבַשׁ. Snh. 64[a] היינו י׳ דע״ז this (lion of fire) is the passion for (tempter to) idolatry. Ib. ניבעי רחמי אַיְ׳ דעבירה let us pray against the sensual desire (the tempter to sexual indulgence); a. fr.

יָצַת (b. h., cmp. יָצָא) [*to break through, spread,*] *to kindle.*

Hif. הִצִּית *to kindle, cause to spread.* Yoma VI, 7 (67[b]) משהִצִּית האור ברובן ed. from the time that he (the officiating priest) causes the fire to spread over the major portion of them; [Ms. M. משתַּצִּית את האור from the time that thou (whoever it may be) causest &c.; Ms. M. 2 משתיצת האור (Kal, אור fem.) that the fire seizes &c.; Y. ed. משיצת; Ms. L. משוצת (*Hof.*) when fire has been set; v. Rabb. D. S. a. l. note]. Ib. 68[b] המַצִּית את האור he who kindles (stirs) the fire, contrad. to השורף who attends to the burning of the pieces. Men. 26[b] משתצית בו את האור (Ms. M. משיצית האור, Ms. R. 1 משתיצת); Sot. 15[a] משתיצת האור. Men. l. c. bot. לא משכחת לה שתצית האור וכ׳ (Ms. R. 1 שתיצת; Ms. M. שיצית, v. Rabb. D. S. a. l. note) it is impossible that the fire should have seized the major portion of it (at sunset). Tam. II, 4 שהיו מַצִּיתִין וכ׳ where they set the kindling wood on fire, v. אֲלִיתָא. Ab. Zar. 38[a], v. אֲגַם. Y. B. Kam. II, 3[a] במַצִּית את האור וכ׳ setting fire to each ear f corn separately. Bab. ib. 22[b] בשה׳ בגופו וכ׳ when he et fire to the body of the slave; a. fr.

Hof. הוּצַּת *to be set to, to be made to spread.* Yoma l. c., supra.—Part. מוּצָּת. B. Mets. 59[a] (ref. to Gen. XXXVIII, 5) א״ת מוצאת אלא מוּצָּת Ar. s. v. א״ת (=מוצתה, missing ed. a. Mss.; cmp. Gen. R. s. 85 a. 'Rashi' a. l. מוצת קרי) ead not, 'she was carried out', but 'she was about to be urnt'. Num. R. s. 12 (expl. זהב מופז, I Kings X, 18) דומה לגפרית מוּצֶּתֶת בא׳ it looks like sulphur when fire is set o it; Cant. R. to III, 10 מוצצת (corr. acc.).

***יַקָּא** pr. n. m.. *Yaka.* Y. Sabb. VII, 10[b] ר׳ חנינא בן ר׳; Y. Keth. VII, 31[c] top אִיקָּא). V. יָקֶה.

יָקַב (cmp. נקב) *to hollow out.* Cant. R. to VII, 5 (ref. o Zech. XIV, 10) עד היקבים שיְּקָבָן מלך מ״ה up to the ollows which the king of kings has caved out; Yalk. s. 334; v. יָפוֹ.

יֶקֶב m. (b. h.; preced.) *excavation, tank.—Pl.* יְקָבִים, יִקְבֵי. B. Bath. 67[b]; Tosef. ib. III, 2; Y. ib. IV, 14[c] bot. tanks f the press. Cant. R. to VII, 5, a. e., v. preced.

יָקַד (b. h.; cmp. נָקַד I) [*to penetrate,*] *to burn; to be n fire.* Yalk. Deut. 808 אתמול יָקְדוּ גְדִישָׁיו (not גרישר) he other day their stacks were on fire.—V. מוֹקֵד.

Hof. הוּקַד *to be kept burning; to be burnt into.* Hull. 15[a]; Kidd. 56[b]; Y. Pes. II, beg. 28[c] (ref. to Deut. XXII, 9) פן תקדש פן תּוּקַד א׳ 'lest it may become sacred (forbidden) property', lest a fire must be lighted (for burning it). Part. מוּקָד. Tanh. Tsav. 14 האש המ׳ על המזבח וכ׳ the fire entertained on the altar will atone for him. Yalk. Lev. 479, end, v. infra.

Nithpa. נִתּוֹקֵד *to burn itself into.* Lev. R. s. 7 (ref. to Lev. VI, 2) it does not say 'the fire of the altar shall be kept burning *on* it, but *in* it, האש היתה מִתּוֹקֶדֶת בו the fire was burning itself into it (the altar); Yalk. l. c. המזבח היה מוּקָד באש the altar was burned into by the fire. Lev. R. l. c. קרוב ... היתה האש מִתּוֹקֶדֶת בו וכ׳ for nearly one hundred and sixteen years was the fire burning itself into it, (and yet) its wood was not consumed &c.

יְקַד, יְקֵיד ch. same; also *to set on fire.* Targ. Is. X, 16. Targ. Y. Ex. III, 2 יָקֵיד (Var. יָקִיד) being burnt into. Targ. Y. II ib. 3.—Y. Yeb. XV, 15[a] [read:] ערקתא יקְדַת וספסלה יקד the strap is on fire (heated) and the bench is on fire. Ib. לא ערקתא יקדת וכ׳ the strap was not heated &c. Cant. R. to III, 4, v. infra. Snh. 33[b], v. מוֹקְדָא I.

Af. אוֹקֵד, אוֹקִיד *to set on fire, burn.* Targ. Lev. VIII, 17. Targ. II Sam. V, 21 (h. text וישאם, v. יְקוֹד); a. fr.—Pesik. Dibré, p. 112[b] וא׳ היכלי he set my Temple on fire. Lam. R. introd., end סליק עפרא יקידא ואוקיד דרעיה glowing dust came up and burnt his arm; Pesik. l. c. p. 114[a]; Y. Taan. IV, 69[b] וא׳ זרעא and burnt the seed. Lam. R. to I, 13 קרתא יקידא אוֹקִידְתָּא thou hast set on fire a burning city (v. טְחַן); Cant. R. to III, 4 דרא יקידא יַקְּדַת (*Pa.*), v. דָּרָא I.

Ittaf. אִתּוֹקַד *to be burnt.* Targ. Lev. X, 16. Targ. II Sam. XXIII, 7; a. fr.

Ithpa. אִיַּיקַּד *to be on fire.* Y. Hag. II, 77[c] top קבריה דרבך א׳ thy teacher's (Elisha's) grave is on fire.

יָקְדָא, יָקְדְתָּא, v. יְקֵיד׳.

יָקֶה (יָקָא) (b. h.) pr. n. m., בן י׳ *Ben Yakeh,* an homiletical surname of king Solomon. Num. R. s. 10 בן י׳ שהקיא וכ׳ Solomon is named Ben Yakeh (a son of discharge) for he discharged (abandoned) the words of the Law, like a vessel which is filled in its time and emptied in its time; Koh. R. to I, 1; Cant. R. to I, 1.

***יְקוֹד** m. (infin. of יָקַד) *burning, setting on fire.* R. Hash. 22[b] מאי משמע דהאי משיאין לישנא די׳ הוא what evidence is there that the word *massiin* (Mish. ib. II, 2) has the meaning of burning (a signal fire)? Answ.: ref. to Targ. II Sam. V, 21, v. יְקַד. [The passage is missing in Mss.; v. Rabb. D. S. a. l. note.]

יָקוּם, v. יְקִים.

יְקוּם m. (b. h.; v. קוּם) *existence, substance, being.* Koh. R. to VI, 3 מהו הי׳ קיומא what is *hayy'kum* (Gen. VII, 23)? Existence; R. B. says: the inhabited world (v. אִיקוּמֵינֵי); R. El. says, י׳ זה הממון וכ׳ *y'kum* means property (substance) which makes firm &c.; Gen. R. s. 32. Num. R. s. 18; Pes. 119[a]; Snh. 110[a] (ref. to Deut. XI, 6).—*Pl.* יְקוּמִים. Yalk. Gen. 56 נמחו כל הי׳ (Pirké d'R. El. ch. XXIII היקום collective noun) all beings were swept away.

יְקוּמָא ch. same. Targ. O. Gen. VII, 4; 23. Targ. O. Deut. XI, 6.

יקומוני, יקומיניה, v. אִיקוּמֵינֵי.

יָקוּשׁ m. (b. h.; יקש) *fowler.* Midr. Prov. to VI, 2 (play on יָקוּשׁ, ib. 5) כדי שלא תעשו קַשׁ וכ׳ (not יעשו) that you might not become straw (fuel) for the fire of Gehenna.

יָקִיד, v. יְקַד.

יָקִיד, יַקִּיד m., **יְקִידָא, יְקִידְתָּא** f. *burning,* v. יְקַד.

יְקִידָא, יְקִידְתָּא, יְקֵד׳ f. (יְקַד) *fireplace, fire; conflagration.* Targ. Am. IV, 11 (ed. Lag. יקידה; some ed. קידא, incorr.). Ib. VI, 10 (h. text מסרפו). Targ. Lev. X, 6 (O. ed. Amst. יוּקִידְתָּא); a. fr.

יְקִידָה f. h. same. Sabb. 82[a] לחתות אש כי׳ גדולה to take coals out of a large fire (on the fireplace).

יְקִידוּתָא, יְקִי׳ f. (preced. wds.) *burning, consumption.* Targ. Is. XXXIII, 14 יְקִידוּת constr. (ed. Lag. יְקִידַת, constr. of יְקִידְתָּא). Targ. Jer. XXXIV, 5 (ed. Lag. יקידה).

יְקִידְתָּא, יָקְדְתָּא, v. יָקִיד a. יְקִידָא.

יָקִים (יָקוּם) (b. h.) *Jakim.* Gen. R. s. 65 end; Midr. Till. to Ps. XI י׳ איש צרורות J. (Alkimos) of Seroroth, a Hellenist, nephew of R. Jose ben Joezer.

יְקִינְתִּין, יְקִינְבִּינוֹן, יְקִינְתִּין, v. הַיָּקִנְ׳.

יַקִּיר m. (b. h.; יָקַר) *weighty, honorable.—Pl.* יַקִּירִים. Yoma VI, 4 מִיַּקִּירֵי ירושלים some of the nobility of Jerusalem.

יַקִּיר, יַקִּירָא ch. same, 1) *heavy.* Targ. Ps. XXXVIII, 5 (some ed. יקר). Targ. Prov. XXVII, 3.—Targ. O. Ex. IV, 10; VI, 12 ממלל י׳ heavy of speech.—Sabb. 59ª דר׳ when the shoe is too heavy for running.—2) *dear, precious.* Targ. Ps. XXXVI, 8 (ed. Lag. יקר); a. fr.—Y. Kidd. I, 58ᵈ כספא זליל כספא י׳ silver falls or rises in price (copper being the standard) נחשא י׳ וכ׳ it is copper that falls or rises (silver being the standard). Y. Ab. Zar. V, 44ᵈ אין הוה עלוויה י׳ if the higher price (paid for Jewish wine) is very great; a. e.—3) *honored, worthy.* Targ. Deut. XXVIII, 58.—Koh. R. to XI, 1 וי׳ מאומתך and worthier than the rest of thy people; a. e.—*Pl.* יַקִּירֵי, יַקִּירִין. Targ. Is. XXIII, 8, sq. Targ. Ez. III, 5. Targ. Num. XXII, 15; a. e.—B. Mets. 21ᵇ אגב די׳ because they are weighty; a. fr.—*Fem.* יַקִּירְתָא, יַקִּירָא. Targ. Prov. III, 15. Ib. VI, 26; a. e.—*Pl.* יַקִּירָתָא. Targ. II Chr. XXXII, 27 (ed. Lag. יקרתא). Targ. Is. III, 17 יַקִּירָת וכ׳ ed. Lag. (oth. ed. יְקָרַת) the nobles of the daughters &c.

יַקִּירוּ f. (preced.) *dignity.* Koh. R. to XI, 1 את חכים בי׳ דברייתא (some ed. יקרי) thou knowest what human dignity means.

יקירן, Tosef. Kel. B. Kam. III, 2, v. יָקַר.

***יָקָם** m., pl. יְקָמִים, יָקְמִין (v. יקום) *restoratives,* esp. *towels put on the bather's head in the sudatory.* [Oth. opin., based on the version יקבים (v. infra): *tanks.* V. Koh. Ar. Compl. s. v.] Tosef. B. Bath. III, 3 he who sells a bathing house, sells with it implicitly ... בית הדקמין וכ׳ ed. Zuck. (Var. הַקָּמִין) the compartment for restoratives, but has not sold .... את הד׳ the implements themselves; B. Bath. 67ᵇ בית הד׳ ... ולא י׳ עצמן ed. (Ms. M. יקבים, v. Rabb. D. S. a. l. note); [Y. ib. IV, 14ᶜ bot. (defective passage) בסלקר וקמין read: (פַּלְּבּוּס וִיק׳). V. קָמִין.

יַקְנָאוֹת, v. דִּיוּקָן.

יָקַר (b. h.) *to be heavy;* (cmp. חוּמְרָא, כָּבֵד &c.) *to be weighty, important, honored;* [*to be dear, precious; to hold dear,* v. infra.] Tanh. B'shall. 27 יָקְרוּ ידיו של משה וכ׳ Moses' hands grew as heavy as &c.; Mekh. B'shall., Amalek, s. 1. Ib. י׳ חטא על וכ׳ sin weighed heavily on Moses' hands.

Pi. יִיקֵּר *to hold dear, honor.* Deut. R. s. 7, end אני מגדיל ומְיַיקֵּר אתכם וכ׳ I shall make you great and honored &c. Num. R. s. 23, end (ref. to a citation כי חנני משלחך כגבירה, found nowhere in the Bible—probably a reference to Jer. XXII, 26 a. XXIX, 2) מה הגבירה חזו אדם מְיַקֵּר אותה וכ׳ (or מֵיקַר *Kal*) as one (surely) holds in honor the *g'birah* (king's mother), so did he (Nebucadnezar) to him (Jehoiachin); Tanh. Massé 13; ib. ed. Bub. 10 אדם מיקר לה. (Gen. R. s. 18 מיקרת ראשה she bears her head proudly; Yalk. Gen. 24; Yalk. Is. 265 מקלת, v. קָלַל).—Part. pass. מְיוּקָּר. Num. R. l. c. קשר אותו בקורכין שלו מי׳ he tied (and seated) him in his most honored (state) carriage; Tanh. l. c. בקורנין וכ׳ ....; ib. ed. Bub. l. c. קשר אותו בקרובין ומוקר לו (Ms. M. בקרונין) he tied ... and paid him honor.

Hif. הוֹקִיר 1) *to grow dear, scarce; to rise in value.* Y. Keth. XI, 34ᵇ bot. ה׳ המקח the price of the field was higher (than the amount due her for alimentation). Ib. XII, beg. 34ᵈ חזרו בזול והוקירו, v. זוֹל. B. Mets. V, 9 שמא יוקירו חטים wheat may rise in value; a. fr.—2) *to honor.* Tanh. ed. Bub. l. c., v. supra.

Hof. הוּקַר as *Hif.* 1.—B. Bath. V, 8 והוּקְרוּ; B. Mets. V, 9 הוקרו (Y. ed. הוקירו). Gen. R. s. 35 ה׳ השמן oil became scarce (Yalk. Kings 228 הוקיר); a. fr.

יְקַר ch. same. 1) *to be heavy.* Targ. Ps. XXXVIII, 5 יְקִירוּ (Ms. יקירו). Targ. Job XXXIII, 7 (some ed. אֵיקַר Af.). Targ. Gen. XLVIII, 10; Targ. O. Ex. XVII, 12 יְקָרָן, ed. Berl. יְקָרָא, v. Berl. Targ. O. II, p. 17); a. e.—2) *to be dear, precious.* Targ. I Sam. XXVI, 21. Targ. II Kings I, 13, sq.; a. fr.—B. Mets. 64ª אי יַקְרָא וכ׳, v. זוֹל I, ch.

Pa. יַקַּר 1) *to make heavy.* Targ. Lam. III, 7 (ed. Amst. יְקַר, corr. acc.). Targ. Zech. VII, 11; a. fr.—2) *to honor, hold dear.* Targ. Is. V, 2. Ib. LVIII, 13; a. fr. Targ. Prov. XXV, 27 מילי מְיַקְּרָתָא honoring words (flatteries).—Koh. R. to II, 20; Lev. R. s. 25 תְּיַקְּרִינֵיה, v. מוֹקְרָא I; a. e.—[Gen. R. s. 17 מיקרך, v. יְקָרָא.]—3) *to offer, present.* Targ. Is. XLIII, 23 (not יְקָרְתָּא). Targ. Prov. III, 9; a. e.

Af. אוֹקִיר, אֵיקַר 1) *to honor, treat with regard.* Targ. Ps. XV, 4. Targ I Sam. II, 30; a. e.—B. Mets. 59ª אוקירו לנשייכו וכ׳ honor your wives (in dress &c.), in order that you may be blessed with wealth. Ber. 48ª לא את קא מוֹקְרַת לי ... קא מוֹקְרָא לי .. Ms. M. (ed. היא דמְיַקְּרָא ...) it is not thou that honorest me, but it is the Law that honors me. Y. Kidd. I, 61ᵇ הלואי ... דאוֹקְרִינוּן ואירות ג״ע Oh, that I had father and mother (alive) that I might honor them and inherit paradise; Y. Peah I, 15ᶜ bot. דאוֹקְרִינְהוֹן ונירות וכ׳; a. fr.—2) *to offer.* Y. Bets. V, end 63ᵇ אוֹקְרֵיה חד סרקיי כמהין a Saracen sent him mushrooms as a present (on a Holy Day). Y. B. Bath. II, end, 13ᶜ אוֹקְרַת תאנין וכ׳ brought R ... figs as a present; a. fr.—[3) *to be heavy.* Targ. Job XXXIII, 17, v. supra.]

Ithpa. אִתְיַיקַּר, אִיַּיקַּר 1) *to become heavy, burdensome.* Targ. Lam. I, 14. Targ. O. Ex. VII, 14 (h. text כבד); a. e.—[Ab. Zar. 46ᵇ אייקר ליה תלמודא ed., Ms. M. ארעקר גמריה, v. עֲקַר.]—2) *to be honored, to honor one's self.* Targ. II Sam. VI, 20. Targ. Ex. XIV, 17, sq.; a. fr.—Snh. 46ᵇ כי הרכי דמִיַּיקַּר וכ׳ (Ms. M. מִתְיַקַּר, לִיתְיַקַּר &c.) that Abraham be honored through her (at her funeral). Ib. לִיקְרוּ בך ... דמִתְיַיקְּרֵי וכ׳ Israel will be honored through thee (at thy funeral), as they were honored at the funerals of thy ancestors. Meg. 28ª אִתְיַיקּוּרֵי דמתיקרי בי they desire to be honored by me (by inviting me); a. e.—3) *to rise in value.* B. Kam. 103ª איי׳ כיתנא flax grew dearer. Ber. 5ᵇ; a. e.

יָקָר m. (b. h.; preced. wds.) 1) *heavy; dear, precious, worthy; honored.* Tosef. B. Kam. IX, 12 המתבייש מן הי׳ who is put to shame by a person of high dignity (opp. פגום).—*Pl.* יְקָרִים, יְקָרִין. B. Bath. 100ᵇ; Meg. 23ᵇ (address to mourners) עמדו י׳ עמודו וכ׳ stand up, dear friends, stand up &c. Men. 44ª דמיו י׳ its price is high; a. fr.—Tosef. Kel. B. Kam. III, 2 הַיְקָרִין R. S. to Kel. III, 5 (ed. היקירן, הייקרין) the heavy earthen vessels used for boiling pitch.—*Fem.* יְקָרָה, *pl.* יְקָרוֹת. Keth. 106ª; Snh. 43ª נשים י׳ וכ׳ worthy women in Jerusalem.—V. יַקִּיר.—2) (noun) *precious object, prize; choice.* Gen. R. s. 67 (ref. to Prov. XII, 27) כדי ... שהוא יְקָרוֹ של עולם וכ׳ in order that Jacob might come who is the choice of the world &c.; ib. שארנם נוטלים מן יְקָרָם שלעתיד לבוא וכ׳ that they shall receive in this world nothing of their prize reserved for the hereafter; Yalk. ib. 115, v. חָרַץ.—*Pl.* יְקָרוֹת. Ib. כדי ... ויטול את הברכות שהן י׳ של עולם חרוצות לו in order that Jacob might come and take the blessings, which are the choice of the world, decreed to him (Gen. R. l. c. שמעיקר העולם חרוצות לו).

יְקָר m. (b. h.; preced. wds.) 1) *gravity, dignity, honor.* Meg. 16[b] (ref. to Esth. VIII, 17) וי׳ אלו תפלין 'and dignity (distinction)' that means the T'fillin.—2) *heavy fog, mist.* Yalk. Ps. 730 כי׳ של מדבר (ref. to כִּיקַר, Ps. XXXVII, 20) like the mist of the desert.—*Pl.* יְקָרִים Ib.

יְקָרָא, יְקָר ch. same, 1) *honor, dignity.* Targ. Ex. XVI, 7. Targ. Ps. LXXXVII, 3. Ib. VIII, 6 Ms. (ed. אִיקְרָא, v. אִיקָר); a. fr.—Ber. 28[a] top מָן י׳ Ms. M. (ed. כסא דמוקרא, Ms. F. דִיקְרָא) a vessel of honor (precious vessel). Snh. 46[b] הספידא י׳ וכ׳ are funeral ceremonies (eulogies, wailings &c.) for the honor of the deceased or of the survivors? Ib. הנהו בני י׳ ניהוו were those (the survivors of the house of Jeroboam) worthy of honors?—Lev. R. s. 34 לית היא עבדא לִיקָרָךְ she acts (treats thee) not according to thy dignity; Gen. R. s. 17 לִיקָרְתָּךְ. Ib. דליתה מִיקָּרָךְ for she is not (part) of thy dignity, i. e. not worthy of thee; Yalk. Lev. 665 דלית היא יקרך, a. דיקרך; Yalk. Is. 352 דיק׳; Y. Keth. XI, 34[b] bot. דאִיקָרָךְ.—Ber. 19[a] הקב״ה תבע בִּיקָרֵיה the Lord takes up the cause of his offended dignity; a. fr. —*Pl.* יְקָרַיָּא. B. Kam. 102[b] bot. יְקָרַיְיכוּ, v. זִילוּתָא.—2) *value, price.* Targ. Ps. XLIX, 9 אילו יהיב יקר וכ׳ Ms. (ed. Lag. ויהיב יקר; ed. ויהי יקיר) were he to pay the price for their redemption.—Y. Sabb. VI, 8[a] bot. (in a prob. corrupted sentence) וי׳ אוף צבחר הוה סדרה יקיר though the value (of the sandal) was but a trifle, yet order (consistency in decisions) is precious; Y. Yeb. XII, 12[d] top (corr. acc.).

יַקְרָא, יְקָרָא, יַקָר, v. יַקִּיר ch.

יַקְרוּת f. (preced. wds.) *dignity, dignified demeanor.* Lam. R. to IV, 2 (ref. to היקרים ib.) ומה היתה יַקְרוּתָן wherein did their dignity manifest itself?

יקרי, v. יַקִּירוּ.

יְקָרְתָא f. *dignity*, v. יְקָר ch.

יָקַשׁ (b. h.; cmp. נקש) *to clap, catch in a trap.*

Nif. נוֹקַשׁ *to be entrapped.* Midr. Prov. to VI, 2 [read:] נוֹקַשְׁתֶּם באמרי פיכם וכ׳ you have been entrapped through your own words (Ex. XXIV, 7), you have been caught (taken captives) through (neglecting) them.

יַקְשָׁן, v. קַיְשָׁן.

יָרֵא (b. h.) *to tremble, fear; to revere; to shun.* Sabb. 88[a] (ref. to Ps. LXXVI, 9) אם יָרְאָה וכ׳ if she (the earth) trembled, how could she be at rest, &c.?—Ber. 16[b] לְיִרְאָה את שמך so as to fear thy name.—(Usu. as participle or adjective) יָרֵא m. Ned. 8[b] (ref. to Mal. III, 20) ... אלו שהן יְרֵאִין להוציא וכ׳ who are afraid to utter the name of the Lord in vain.—יְרֵא חֵטְא *shunning sin, of careful conduct, conscientious.* Ab. II, 5. Ib. 8; a. fr.—יְרֵא שָׁמַיִם *God-fearing, pious.* Ber. 8[a] גדול ... יותר מי׳ ש׳ he who lives on the (honest) labor of his hand, stands higher than the pious man. Succ. 49[b], v. יָדַע; a. fr.—*Fem.* יְרֵאָה, constr. יִרְאַת. Lam. R. to II, 13 (play on ירושלם) הבת שיראה ומשולמת לי the daughter that fears (me) and is at peace with me. Ib. כשאת יְרֵיאָה את מושלמת לי Ar. (missing in ed.) when thou art God-fearing, thou art at peace with me. Yeb. 62[b].—Part. pass. יָרוּאי. Ber. 33[b]; Meg. 25[a] Ms. M. (v. Rabb. D. S. a. l. note).

Nif. נוֹרָא, fut. יִוָּרֵא *to be feared.* Koh. R. to IX, 7; Pesik. Ul'kah., p. 183[b], a. e. למען תִּוָּרֵא וכ׳ (Ps. CXXX, 4) 'in order that thou mayest be feared', that the fear of thee be put on mankind.—Part. נוֹרָא *fearful, awe-inspiring.* Ber. l. c. Yoma 69[b] לא אמר נ׳ Jeremiah did not say *nora* (only *gadol* a. *gibbor*, Jer. XXXII, 18).—*Fem. pl.* נוֹרָאוֹת *awe-inspiring deeds.* Ib. אתא ... נכרים ... איה נוֹרְאוֹתָיו came Jeremiah and said, Strangers dance on His temple ruins, where are His awful deeds?; Y. Ber. VII, 11[c]. Ib. לזה נאה לקרות נורא בנ׳ וכ׳ (Daniel said) Him it is becoming to call awe-inspiring for the awful deeds He performed for us &c.; Midr. Till. to Ps. XIX; a. fr.

Hithpa. הִתְיָירֵא, *Nithpa.* נִתְיָירֵא 1) *to be feared, revered.* Zeb. 115[b] (ref. to Ps. LXVIII, 36) בשעה ... מִתְיָירֵא ומתעלה וכ׳ when the Lord executes judgment on His saints, He is feared and praised &c.; Yalk. Lev. 525.—2) *to be afraid.* Ber. 61[b] אי אתה מתי׳ מפני וכ׳ art thou not afraid of the (Roman) government?—Midr. Till. l. c. שנכנסו ... ולא נִתְיָירְאוּ the enemy entered His house and were not afraid (of the Lord). Ex. R. s. 29 אם המטרונה מִתְיָירֵאת וכ׳ if the queen is afraid, what shall the servants ... do?; a. fr.

יִרְאָה f. (b. h.; preced.) 1) infin. of יָרֵא q. v.—2) *fear.* Ber. 17[a] יִרְאָתִי the fear of me. Ib. ערום בי׳ cautious in religious affairs. Koh. R. to IX, 7 שתהא יִרְאָתְךָ וכ׳, v. preced.—עשה מי׳ (or עבד) to do good (to worship) from motives of fear, opp. מאהבה. Sot. 31[a]; a. fr., v. אַהֲבָה.—Y. Sot. V, 20[c] bot. פרוש י׳, v. פָּרוּשׁ; a. v. fr.—יִרְאַת שמים fear of the Lord; יִרְאַת חטא fear of sin (v. preced.). Ber. 6[b]. Ib. 16[b]; a. fr.—3) *object of fear, idol.* Snh. 106[a] הוציאה יִרְאָתָהּ וכ׳ she took her idol out of her bosom. Pesik. Vayhi. p. 65[b]; Mekh. Bo. s. 13 יִרְאָתֵנוּ our (Egyptian) deity; a. fr.—*Pl.* יִרְאוֹת. Ib. B'shall., Vayhi, s. 1; Yalk. Ex. 230 מכל הי׳ שלהם of all their (the Egyptians') gods.

יָראוּי, v. יָרֵא.

יַרְבּוּז m. *strawberry-blite* (v. Löw Pfl. p. 189 sq.); [oth. opin. *asparagus.*] Tosef. Kil. I, 11; Y. ib. I, 27[a] bot. דרבון (Ar. s. v. שוק: דרקון; R. S. to Kil. I, 4 ירבון; corr. acc.).—*Pl.* יַרְבּוּזִין. Shebi. IX, 1 הי׳ השוטים wild *yarbuz* (with large leaves); Ms. M. הי׳ והשוטין (v. comment.); Succ. 39[b] הי׳ והשיטין (Ms. M. 2 והשוטין, v. Rabb. D. S. a. l.).

יַרְבּוּזָא, יַרְבּוּזָה ch. same. Y. Kil. V, 30[a] (R. S. to Kil. V, 6 ירבוזאי, read זא ...).—*Pl.* יַרְבּוּזִין. Y. Maasr. V, end, 52[a] (R. S. to Maasr. V, 8 זרבונין, corr. acc.).

יָרָבְעָם (b. h.) pr. n. m. *Jeroboam*, 1) J. ben Nebat, the first king of Israel. Ber. 35[b]. Snh. X, 2 (90[a]); a. fr.— 2) J. ben Joash king of Israel. Pes. 87[b]. Yeb. 98[a].

יָרַד (b. h.) *to move about, run;* esp. *to go down;* ־י׳ ל *to enter;* ־י׳ מ *to leave.* Tanh. B'huck. 5 (ref. to וירדתי, Jud. XI, 37) וכי... יוֹרֵד על ההרים... עולים להרים does one *go down* on the mountains, do not men go up to &c.?; ib. הניחני ואֵרֵד אצל ב״ד (ed. Bub. 7 ואלך) give me leave that I may go down to the court-house; Yalk. Jud. 67. Men. 109[b] מה זה שלא י׳ לה כך when this one (Shimei) who was not permitted to enter into it (the office) became so jealous, היוֹרֵד לה וכ׳ how much more so is he who once has entered it (and is to be ousted). Ib. כל האומר לי לֵירֵד ממנה וכ׳ whoever would ask me to resign it (the office), I would throw at him &c.—Taan. 8[b] יָרְדוּ גשמים it rains. Ib.[a] אין גשמים יוֹרְדִים וכ׳ the rain falls only for the sake of the men of faith. Cant. R. to I, 2[b] מה מים יורדין וכ׳ as the water (rain) comes down in drops. —י׳ לנכסי *to take possession of, seize, administer property.* B. Mets. 38[b] היוֹרֵד לנ׳ שבוים he who takes possession of the property of captives. Tosef. Keth. VIII, 2, sq.; a. fr.— י׳ מנכסיו *to be compelled to leave an estate, to become poor* (cmp. הִדַּלְדֵּל). Gen. R. s. 71; Lam. R. to III, 4; Ned. 64[b]; a. fr.— (קרבן) עוֹלֶה ויוֹרֵד *a sacrifice of higher or lesser value* according to pecuniary conditions (Lev. V, 6—11). Shebu. 21[a]. Hor. II, 7 (9[a]); a. fr.—[For other idiomatic uses, v. עָלָה.]—Part. pass. יָרוּד q. v.

Hif. הוֹרִיד *to let down, bring down; to lower.* Taan. 8[a] בשעה שהשמים... מִלְּהוֹרִיד וכ׳ ed. (Ms. M., v. Rabb. D. S. a. l.) when the heavens are locked up so as not to let down rain. Lev. R. s. 1 ירד שה׳ את התורה Moses is surnamed *Yered* (I Chr. IV, 18) because he brought down the Law; שה׳ את השכינה וכ׳ he caused the Divine Presence to come down &c. Y. Ber. IV, 7[d] top לא הוֹרִידוּ אותו מגדולתו they did not remove him from his position. Sot. 13[b] (ref. to Gen. XXXIX, 1) א״ת הוּרַד אלא הוֹרִיד שה׳ וכ׳ read not 'he was brought down', but 'he did bring down', for he (Joseph) was the cause of the removal of the astronomers of Pharaoh from their positions.—Y. B. Kam. IV, 4[b] top הוֹרִידָן מנכסיהן he drove them out of their estates (cmp. Bab. ib. 38[a]); a. v. fr.— ה׳ לנכסי (v. supra) *to appoint as administrator.* B. Mets. 38[b] מוֹרִידִין קרוב לנ׳ שבוי we may appoint a relative (presumptive heir) an administrator of the estate of a captive; a. fr.—לא מעלה ולא מוריד neither raises nor lowers, i. e. *has no effect* or *influence.* Hull. 45[b]. Gitt. 52[a], a. e. דברי חלומות לא מעלין ולא מוֹרִידִין dreams must not be regarded. Men. V, 6, a. e. מעלה ומוריד moves upward and downward.—[Tosef. Par. IX (VIII), 6 שהוא מוריד, v. מוֹרִיד.]—ולא מורידין... מעלין, v. עָלָה.

ירדינון, Ex. R. s. 23, corrupt. of הַרְהוּפַּנְין, v. הַרְהַפְנֵי. —[Y. Dem. I, 22[b] top some ed., v. יירינון.]

יַרְדֵּן (b. h.) pr. n. *Jordan*, the river of Palestine. Tosef. Bekh. VII, 4; Bekh. 55[a], v. יְרַח; a. fr.—Y. Sabb. IV, end, 7[a] עריבת הי׳; Bab. ib. 83[b] ספינת הי׳ Jordan boats which are loaded on dry land and let down into the river.— כיפת הי׳, v. כִּיפָּה.

יוֹרְדְּנָא, יַרְדְּנָא ch. same. Targ. Gen. XIII, 10. Ib. XXXII, 11; a. fr.—Bekh. 55[a], v. זִכְרוּתָא.

יְרַח, v. ירוי.

***יְרוֹאַר** m. *ferule* (v. Löw Pfl. p. 190). Pes. 39[a] מר י׳ ed. (Ms. M. מר ואלאר). Ib. מר זה הוא י׳ (Ms. M. אלאר) *mar*, that is *y'roar*; [for Var. lect. v. Rabb. D. S. a. l. note.] [Syr. ירורא, P. Sm. 1630.]

יָרוּד m., **יְרוּדָה** f. (יָרַד) *low, common, of little value.* Cant. R. to I, 2[b] י׳ שבכלים the commonest of vessels (earthen); (Taan. 7[a] פחות, Sifré Deut. 48 גרוע). Y. B. Mets. V, beg. 9[c] כל הי׳ מחבירו וכ׳ the less valuable metal is in exchange considered the coin, the more valuable is the merchandise. Pesik. R. s. 13 י׳ מכל השבטים the lowest of the tribes (Joseph, being a slave). Lam. R. to IV, 2 (אשה) י׳ ממנו a wife of a lower position than himself. Ex. R. s. 30 לי׳ שבאומות וכ׳ do you desire to connect yourself with the lowest of all nations (Israel)?; a. fr.—*Pl.* יְרוּדִים, יְרוּדִין; יְרוּדוֹת. Pesik. R. l. c.

***יָרוּד I, יָארוּד, יר׳** m. [prob. to be read: יָרוֹד; v. חֲוַרְוָר a. יָרִיר] *white spot in the eye (leucoma).* Sabb. 78[a] יא׳ ed. (Ar. יר׳; Ms. O. ־יר׳); Tosef. ib. VIII (IX), 8 חֲוַרְוָאר ed. Zuck., Var. חוורד, חרוד, Rashi to Sabb. l. c. quotes חֲוַרְוָר).

יָרוֹד II (יָרוֹר) c. (v. next w.) *yarod*, a bird of solitary habits, mentioned in connection with the ostrich (as in b. h. תנים ובנות יענה).—*Pl.* יְרוֹדִין, יְרוֹדוֹת (יְרוֹר׳). Tosef. Kil. V, 8 הי׳ והנכמיות וכ׳ (Var. הירורין והנעמית) the *y.* and the ostrich are considered as birds in every respect (opposing the popular belief that the ostrich is a cross-breed between a camel and a bird, v. Sm. Ant. s. v. Strouthos); Y. ib. VIII, 31[c] bot. הירודות והנעמית (some ed. הירור׳).— [Ab. Zar. 11[b] ירוד, Ms. M., v. יָרִיד.]

יָרוֹד, יָרוֹדָא (יְרוֹדָא) ch. (v. P. Sm. 1630) 1) same. —*Pl.* יְרוֹדִין, יְרוֹדֵי. Targ. Mic. I, 8, a. fr. (ed. Lag. everywhere ירורין; h. text תַּנִּים).—Targ. Job. XXX, 29 ירודין ed. Lag. (Var. יַלּוֹלִין). Targ. Ps. LXXIV, 14 לירודי (ed. Lag. לירורי, h. text לצִיים).—2) (= עָרוֹד, עֲרוֹדָא) *wild ass.* Targ. Jer. II, 24 כירודא (ed. Lag. כירורא, h. text תאנתה, v. Rashi a. l.). Keth. 49[b] יארוד ילדה ואבני וכ׳ ed. (Ar. יר׳) a *yarod* gives birth and casts (her young) upon the people of the town, i. e. a parent must support his minor children. Snh. 59[b] י׳ נאלא thou howling *y.* (talking out of the way; Yalk. Gen. 14 תנין שוטה h.).—*Pl.* as ab. Targ. Jer. XIV, 6 (ed. Lag. ירור׳; h. text תנים). Targ. Y. I Deut. XXXII, 10 שידין וי׳ (ed. Amst. יְרוּדִין, corr. acc.). Targ. Is. XIII, 22 וי׳ (in connection with תתולין, ed. Lag. וירורין; h. text וְתַנִּים).—*Fem. pl.* יְרוֹדָאתָא. Lam. R. to IV, 3 (ref. to גם תנין וכ׳) אילין י׳ כמין מסוון פריסן וכ׳ (Ar. איח, ib.) אילין (לחון כמין וכ׳) those *yaruds* (knowing their ferocious instincts) have a sort of mask spread over their faces when sucking their young &c.; [diff. interpret. of the verse in Tanh. B'huck. 3, ed. Bub. 5.]

ירוית, v. יְרִיָּה.

יָרוֹק m. (b. h.; יָרָק II) *light-colored, yellow* or *greenish*. Eduy. V, 6 דם הי׳; Nidd. II, 6 הי׳ the greenish secretion (menstruation). Ib. 19[b] כתם י׳ וכ׳ a greenish stain on the garment; a. fr.—Succ. III, 6 הי׳ ככרתי an Ethrog green like leek.—*Pl.* יְרוֹקִים *green colors.* Neg. XI, 4, a. e., v. יְרַקְרַק.—*Fem.* יְרוֹקָה. Num. R. s. 9 מאדמת עושין אותה י׳ if she was of a ruddy complexion, the test waters make her pale.

יָרוֹקָא, יָרוֹק ch. 1) same. Targ. Ex. X, 15; a. fr.—Targ. Lev. XIII, 49 (h. text ירקרק).—Hull. 62[a] בדירוק׳ כרסה as regards the bird whose belly is green.—Pes. 30[b] בין חיורא בין אוכמא ובין י׳ Ms. M. (ed. יורקי) whether white, dark or green (glazed).—*Pl.* יְרוֹקִין, יְרוֹקֵי. Ib. בעו מיניה י׳ Ms. M. (ed. יורקא).—2) *green, foliage, grass.* Targ. Gen. IX, 3, a. e. יְרוֹק עסבא.—B. Kam. 44[a]. Arakh. 31[b] אנא קדים אכיל י׳ וכ׳ I ate grass before thee (am older); a. e.—*Pl.* constr. יְרוֹקֵי. Targ. Y. Gen. I, 30 י׳ עסבין.—3) = יַרְקוֹנָא, q. v.—4) (v. יֶרֶק) name of a species of *fish* (green fish). Y. Kil. I, 27[a], bot., v. אַסְפְּרוֹן.

יְרוֹקָה f. (preced.) 1) י׳ שעל פני המים *grass upon the water*, a sort of *sea-weed* or *moss* used for wicks. Sabb. II, 1, expl. ib. 20[b] אוכמתא דארבא, v. אוֹצָם.; Y. ib. II beg. 4[c], v. פִּיתָן.—2) *jaundice.* Ib. XIV, 3 שהן לי׳ they are used as a remedy for jaundice.

ירוקמי, v. יוּרְקְמִי.

יְרוֹקָנָא (יַרְקוֹנָא) m.; *pl.* יַרְקוֹנִין, יְרוֹקָנִין (preced. arts.) *various herbs.* Targ. II Kings IV, 39 (ed. Lag. ירקונין, some ed. יַרְקָנִין).—Y. Meg. IV, 74[d] חד מחזר פטירין עם ירקונין one scholar made a translator read over again who translated (Ex. XII, 8) 'unleavened bread with herbs' (in place of מרורין bitter herbs); Y. Bicc. III, end, 65[d] (corr. in accord. with Y. Meg. l. c.).

יְרוֹקֶת, v. יֶרֶק.

יְרוּקְתָא, v. יַרְקָן.

יָרוֹר, יָרוֹדָא, v. יָרוֹד, יָרוֹדָא. [Ab. Zar. 11[b] ירור Ms. M., v. יָרִיד.]

יְרוּשָּׁה f. (b. h. יְרֻשָּׁה; יָרַשׁ) 1) *conquest, taking possession.* Sifré Num. 107 (ref. to Num. XV, 18) אחר י׳ וישיבה וכ׳ the text means after conquering and settling in the land (proving from Deut. XI, 31); Kidd. 37[b]. Ib.[a] מושב לאחר י׳ וישיבה משמע the word *dwelling* (e. g. Lev. XXIII, 14) means after conquest &c. Ib. 38[a]; a. fr.—2) *inheritance, heirloom.* Ab. II, 12 שאינה י׳ לך for it (the knowledge of the Law) does not come to thee by inheritance (without toil). Ned. 81[a] that it may not be said י׳ הוא להם scholarship comes to them by inheritance. Sifré Deut. 345 (ref. to Deut. XXXIII, 4) שומע אני י׳ לבני מלכים וכ׳ I might understand, it is an inheritance of the sons of the nobles &c. Ib. לִירוּשָּׁתִי אני חוזר I am returning to my own heirloom; Ex. R. s. 33 לִירוּשַּׁת אבותי to my paternal heirloom. B. Bath. 110[b] בת י׳ having the right of inheritance. Ib. 113[b] י׳ ראשונה the first succession (direct heirs, children &c.); י׳ שניה indirect heirs (brothers &c.); a. v. fr.

יְרוּשָׁלַיִם, יְרוּשָׁלֵם (b. h.) pr. n. pl. *Jerusalem.* Succ. 51[b] מי ... י׳ בתפארתה וכ׳ he who has not seen J. in her glory, has never seen &c. Gen. R. s. 43 (interpret. מַלְכִּי־צֶדֶק, Gen. XIV, 18) צדק נקראת י׳ Jerusalem is called by the name of *Tsedek* (Righteousness; ref. to Is. I, 26). Num. R. s. 10; Meg. 15[a] שמו .... בידוע שהוא מי׳ (a prophet) whose name is mentioned without the name of his home, is, to be sure, from Jerusalem (v. יְרוּשַׁלְמִי); a. v. fr.

יְרוּשְׁלֵם ch. same. Targ. Gen. XIV, 18 (h. text שלם). Targ. Josh. XII, 10; a. fr.—Ned. 50[a] י׳ דדהבא a golden head-band with the picture of Jerusalem on it; Sabb. 59[a] (expl. עיר של זהב).—Lam. R. to I, 1 רבתי (J. compared with Athens); a. fr.

יְרוּשַׁלְמִי m. (preced.) *of Jerusalem, Jerusalemite.* Lam. R. introd. (R. Joh. 1) כל נביא...י׳ הוה every prophet whose home is not mentioned was a citizen of Jerusalem (v. יְרוּשָׁלַיִם). Ib. to I, 1 רבתי (8 חד מאת׳) אזל י׳ לאתינס the Jerusalemite went to Athens. Tosef. Keth. XIII (XII), 3 איזהו כסף צורי זה י׳ what does Tyrian currency mean? It means the Jerusalem standard. Num. R. s. 14 לשון י׳ Jerusalem (Palestinean) dialect, v. פִּיסוּפָא.—תלמוד י׳ *Jer. Talmud*, the Palestinean collection of Mishnah and Gemarah, contrad. to the Babylonian (תלמוד בַּבְלִי).—תרגום י׳ (abbr. ת״י, misnamed Targ. Jonathan) *Targum Y'rushalmi*, name of a Chaldaic version of the Pentateuch, contrad. to Targ. Onkelos (v. Berliner Targ. O. II, p. 100, a. Sm. Dict. of the Bible s. v. *Versions*).—Fem. יְרוּשַׁלְמִית. Hull. 65[a], v. יוֹחֲנָא II. Erub. 83[a], v. סְאָה.—*Pl.* יְרוּשַׁלְמִיּוֹת. Y. Keth. I, 25[b] top, v. חָנַן. Yoma 44[b]; a. e.

יָרְתָא, יָרוֹתָא m. (יְרַת) = h. יוֹרֵשׁ, *conqueror; heir.* Targ. II Sam. XIV, 7.—Gen. R. s. 56 שנאיה דביתא י׳ the enemy of the house (Ishmael) will be the heir.—*Pl.* יָרוֹתִין, יָרְתִין; יָרוֹ׳. Targ. Jud. XVIII, 7. Targ. Jer. VIII, 10. Targ. Y. II Num. XXIV, 18.—Y. Snh. III, end, 21[d] כתב .. לְיָרְתוֹי R. L. wrote to his (Kahana's) heirs.

יְרוּתָא, יְרוּתְּתָא, יְרֻתָּא f. ch. (preced.) = h. יְרוּשָּׁה, 1) *a conquered land.* Targ. O. Num. XXIV, 18 (h. text יְרֵשָׁה; Y. I תריכין).—2) *conquest; possession, heirloom.* Targ. Deut. II, 5; 9, a. fr. (ed. Berl. יְרוּתָ׳; oth. ed. a. Y. יְרוּתָ׳).—Targ. Prov. XX, 21 יְרוּתְתָ׳ ed. Lag.; a. e.—Lev. R. s. 9 יְרוּתְתִי גבך וכ׳ my heirloom (the Law) is with thee, and thou wouldst withhold it (refuse to teach me)?; ומה יְרוּתְתָךְ גבי (not ירותותן) and what heirloom of thine do I hold?; a. e.

יָרֵחַ f. (b. h.; ירח, cmp. ארח) [*traveller,*] *moon.* Hull. 60[b] אמרה י׳ וכ׳ said the Moon to the Lord; Yalk. Gen. 8. Ib. מיעטתי את הי׳. v. מָעַט. Ber. 56[b] Ms. M. (ed. סיהרא).

יֶרַח m. 1) (b. h.; preced.; Assyr. *arḥu*) *month.* R. Hash. 11[a], v. זִיוְתָן. Tanh. Noah 11, v. בּוּל III; a. e.—2) pr. n. pl. *Yeraḥ*, at the southernmost point of Lake Tiberias; בית י׳ *Beth-Yeraḥ*, near Yeraḥ, a twin-town of Sennabris (v. סִנַּבְרַאי). Gen. R. s. 98 (expl. כנרת, Deut. III, 17) R. El. says י׳; R. Samuel ... בית י׳; R. Judah ... Sennabris *and* Beth Yeraḥ. Y. Meg. I, 70[a] two autonomies כגון בית י׳ וכ׳ like B. Y. and Sennabris. Midr. Sam. ch. XXX,

XXXII, expl. חדשי, II Sam. XXIV, 6 בית י׳.—Tosef. Bekh. VII, 4 איזהו ירדן מבית יְרֵחוֹ ולמטה (ed. Zuck. ירחו) the real Jordan is from B. Y'reḥo and down; Bekh. 55ᵃ אין ירדן אלא מבית ירחו וכ׳.

יְרַח, יַרְחָא ch. (=h. יָרֵחַ a. יֶרַח) *moon; month.*—יומא די׳ or י׳ (sub. ריש) the *first day of the month, New-Moon-Day.* Targ. Is. XLVII, 13. Ib. LXVI, 23. Targ. I Sam. XX, 18. Targ. Ez. XLVI, 1; a. fr.—Targ. O. Deut. XXI, 13 יְרַח יומין ed. Berl. (oth. ed. יְרַח; Y. תלתא יַרְחִין).—Lev. R. s. 29; Pesik. R. s. 40 (ref. to בחדש השביעי, Lev. XXIII, 24) בי׳ דשבועתא in the month of oaths (Gen. XXII, 16). Sabb. 86ᵇ בחד בשבא איקבע י׳ the New-Moon was declared on the first day of the week. Ib. פליגי בקביע די׳ they differ as to the day on which the New Moon was declared. Bets. 4ᵇ והשתא דידעינן בקביעא די׳ and now that we know the time of the New Moon (by fixed calendar); a. fr.—*Pl.* יַרְחִין, יַרְחַיָּא, יַרְחֵי. Targ. Y. Gen. I, 14. Targ. Ex. II, 2; a. fr.—R. Hash. 20ᵃ בשאר י׳ as to the other months (than Nisan and Tishri). Y. ib. II, 57ᵈ bot. Macc. 23ᵇ; a. fr.—תריסר ירחי שתא twelve months (forming) a year, twelve months from date. B. Mets. 16ᵇ; 35ᵃ. Ab. Zar. 8ᵇ; a. e.

יְרֵחוֹ, v. יְרִיחוֹ a. יְרַח.

יַרְחִינָאָה m. (denom. of יַרְחָא) *versed in the regulation of the lunar year, Yarḥinaah,* surname of Samuel, the Babylonian scholar (v. R. Hash. 20ᵇ top). B. Mets. 85ᵇ שמואל י׳ אסייה וכ׳ Samuel Yarḥinaah was the physician of Rabbi.

יָרָה, ירי (b. h.; cmp. אָרֵי I) *to permeate, penetrate; to shoot forth.* Nidd. 43ᵃ; Ḥag. 15ᵃ [read:] כל ... שאינו יוֹרֶה כחץ אינה מזרעת (Ms. M. אינו מוליד; Ms. M. 2 שאינה יוֹרֶה, v. Rabb. D. S. a. l. note) a spermatic emission which does not permeate (shoot forth) like an arrow, cannot fructify; Yeb. 65ᵃ היא קיימא לה בי׳ כחץ she can feel it whether the emission is permeating &c. Sifré Deut. 42 יוֹרֶה שמתכון...יורד וכ׳ the rain is called *yoreh* (shooting), for it is aimed at the earth with deliberation, and does not come down in a storm; Taan. 6ᵃ יורה שיורד בנחת.—2) *to throw, shoot.* Yalk. Gen. 133 לִירוֹת בב׳ ידיו to throw spears with both hands; v. infra.

Hif. הוֹרָה 1) *to permeate.* Sifré l. c. שמוֹרָה ומרוה הארץ וכ׳ for it (the *yoreh,* v. supra) pervades and satisfies the earth and gives her drink down to the deep (Taan. l. c., Yalk. Deut. 863 only שמַּרְוֶה).—[Y. Maasr. I, 49ᵃ top משרורו וכ׳, read: משרוּוּ, v. רָוָה a. מַרְוִית.]—2) *to point, aim at, shoot, cast.* Lam. R. to I, 18 שלש...הורו בו three hundred arrows did they shoot into his body; Y. Kidd. I, 61ᵃ bot. יורו במשיח וכ׳ (read: הורו or יָרוּ, *Kal*). Yalk. Gen. l. c. (fr. Midr. Vayisu) היה מוֹרֶה חניתות וכ׳ he threw spears with both hands &c. Ex. R. s. 3 (ref. to והוריתיך, Ex. IV, 12) מורה אני וכ׳ I shall shoot my words into thy mouth like an arrow; a. fr.—3) *to point out, to direct, teach, instruct; to decide.* Hor. I, 1 הוֹרוּ ב״ד וכ׳ if a court has (through error) directed to transgress one of the commands &c. Ib. 2 ה׳ ב״ד וידעו וכ׳ if a court has given a decision and finding out its mistake reversed it. Yeb. X, 2 הוֹרוּהָ ב״ד לינשא if a court instructed her that she may marry again. Ber. 31ᵇ; Erub. 63ᵃ כל המוֹרֶה הלכה בפני וכ׳ whoever decides a law-point in the presence of his teacher. Ab. V, 8 המוֹרִים בתורה וכ׳ who decide in religious matters against the law (by means of sophistry). Sabb. 19ᵇ ה׳...כר׳ וכ׳ R... decided in agreement with the opinion of &c.; a. fr. [Erub. 65ᵃ (a citation, from Sirach X, 26?; v., however, Rabb. D. S. a. l. note 70) בצר אל יוֹרֶה he who is in trouble, should give no opinion—applied by analogy to prayer in an unsettled condition of mind.]

ירי, *Af.* אוֹרִי, הוֹרִי same, *to teach.* Targ. Y. Num. XVI, 2. Targ. Mic. VI, 4.—Sabb. 19ᵇ ההוא תלמידא דא׳ וכ׳ there was a student who decided ... in favor of R. S.'s opinion. Y. Maasr. I, 49ᵃ (ה׳; a. fr.—אֲיָרֵי, v. אֲרֵי I.

יָרֵי, a word in a charm formula, beginning with שַׁבְרִירִי q. v.

יְרִיאָה, v. יְרָא.

יָרִיד m. (יָרַד) *meeting-place, market, annual fair* generally dedicated to a deity. Ab. Zar. 11ᵇ י׳ שבעין בכי, י׳ שבעכו (Ms. M. ירוד, ירור) a market-place (with the idol) at Baalbek, at Acco (v. נְדַבְּכָה). Ib. 13ᵃ הנושא ונותן בי׳ של גוים (Ms. M. ed. בשוק של עכ״ום) one who deals at a fair of gentiles. Ib. הולכין לי׳ של עכ״ום וכ׳ one may go to an idolatrous fair and buy there &c.; Y. ib. I, 39ᵇ; ᶜbot. (only) הולכין ליריד; Gen. R. s. 47; a. fr.—*Pl.* יְרִידִים, יְרִידִין. Y. l. c. 39ᵈ top ג׳ י׳ הן וכ׳ there are three (Palestinean) fairs, that of Gaza &c.; Gen. R. l. c.—Ib. s. 67; Yalk. Gen. 115 [read:] את לך י׳ והוא יש לו שווקים thou (Esau-Rome) hast fairs, and he (Israel) has markets (i. e. you compete in commerce); a. e.

יְרִידָה I m. ch. same. Y. Ab. Zar. I, 39ᵈ top י׳ דצור the market place of Tyre. [Ib. יְרִידָה של בוטנה, v. preced.]

יְרִידָה II f. (יָרַד) *going down, fall, decline, degradation.* יְרִידַת גשמים rain-fall. Y. Ber. IX, 14ᵃ top; a. fr.—Zeb. 53ᵃ יְרִידָתוֹ מן הכבש his descent from the inclined plane (v. כֶּבֶשׁ). Y. Hor. III, beg. 47ᵃ עלייתו י׳ היא לו his elevation (to office) would rather be a degradation to him (placing him under legal disadvantages). Ex. R. s. 42 שהיה לו י׳ מצד אחיו degradation (excommunication) came to him from his brothers' side. Lev. R. s. 29 כשם שלאלו י׳ as for these (nations) decline is in store; a. fr.—*Pl.* יְרִידוֹת. Cant. R. to I, 1 ג׳ י׳ ירד שלמה Solomon had three declining periods of his power.

יְרִיָּה f. (יָרָה) *shooting.* Yalk. Gen. 133 (fr. Midr. Vayisu) יְרִיַּית חצים וכ׳ (not ירוית) shooting of arrows and stones from catapults.

יָרִיךְ, v. יָרֵךְ.

יְרִיכוּנָא, v. יַרְכוּנָא.

ירינון, v. יירינון.

יְרִיעָה f. (b. h.; ירע to shake, cmp. יָרֵא) *tent-cloth, curtain.* Ohol. VIII, 1; a. fr.—*Pl.* יְרִיעוֹת. Ib. XV, 4 בית שחצצו

אוֹ בי׳ . . . a room which has been divided off by boards or curtains. Tanḥ. T'rumah 9. Ex. R. s. 50; a. fr.—Trnsf. *a writing sheet* containing several columns of writing and being part of a scroll. Treat. Sof'rim II, 6 אין פותחין בי׳ וכ׳ a sheet of a Torah scroll must have no less than three and no more than eight columns. Ib. 5 עושה אותו י׳ קטנה he may have for that column a special small sheet. Men: 30ᵃ. Tosef. Sabb. VIII (IX), 13; a. fr.—*Pl.* as ab. Sabb. 11ᵃ אם . . . ושמים י׳ וכ׳ if all waters were ink . . . ., and the heavens sheets &c., v. חָלָל III. Tosef. Yad. II, 10; a. fr.

יְרִיעְתָא, יְרִיעָא ch. same, *curtain, hanging.* Targ. Ex. XXVI, 2; a. fr.—*Pl.* יְרִיעָתָא, יְרִיעָן. Ib. 1, sq.; a. fr.

יְרִיקָה, v. יָרֵק.

יְרִית, v. יְרַת.

יָרֵךְ, constr. יֶרֶךְ f. (b. h.; cmp. ארך) [*length-side,*] 1) *haunch, thigh,* i. e. "the thick and fleshy member which commences at the bottom of the spine and extends to the lower leg (שׁוֹק)" (Ges. H. Dict. s. v.). Ḥull. VII, 1 נוהג בי׳ של ימין applies to the right leg. Ib. 2 שולח אדם י׳ וכ׳ one may send to a gentile a haunch with the nervus ischiadicus (v. גִּיד) in it. Sot. 11ᵇ; Ex. R. s. 1 י׳ מכאן וי׳ מכאן וכ׳ a leg on one side, and a leg on the other, and the potter's mould between; a. fr.—Y. Pes. VII, beg. 34ᵃ כִּירֵךְ עבה עבד וכ׳ R. J... wants the Passover lamb roasted like a thick (stuffed) thigh.—יוצאי י׳ *descendants.* B. Bath. VIII, 2 כל יוצאי יְרֵיכוֹ של בן וכ׳ all direct descendants of the (deceased) son (male heir) have the precedence to the daughter (the decedent's sister); a. fr.—*Du.* יְרֵכַיִם. Tosef. Ohol. III, 4, sq. —*Pl.* יְרֵיכוֹת. Sot. l. c.; Ex. R. l. c. (expl. אָבְנַיִם, Ex. I, 16) בשעה...יְרֵכוֹתֶיהָ...כאבנים when a woman is about to give birth, her thighs grow cold like stones.—2) *side.* Gen. R. s. 69, v. חָדַר. Meg. 13ᵃ אין אשה . . . . בי׳ של חבירתה a woman is made jealous only by the side of another woman (rival). 3) *the perpendicular stroke of a letter, leg.* Y. Meg. I, 71ᶜ top יְרֵיכוֹ של ה״א the leg (stroke on the left side) of the *He*; ib. י׳ קטנה a small indication of it. Ib. אם גורדו . . . י׳ קטנה if he erases the (blotted letter *Gimmel*) and there remains a slight leg (indication of the vertical stroke connecting the head of the *Gimmel* with its foot).—*Pl.* as ab. Gitt. 20ᵃ, v. חָקַק. Sabb. 138ᵇ כירה . . . אחת מִיְּרֵכוֹתֶיהָ a portable stove one of whose legs is off.

יְרַךְ, יַרְכָא, יִירְךְ ch. same. Targ. O. Num. V, 22 יירך ed. Berl. (Mss. יַרְכָא, יְרֵךְ; ed. יַרְכִּין pl.). Ib. 21. Targ. Ex. I, 5; a. fr.—Gen. R. s. 78 מטלע על יַרְכֵיה (not ירריכה) limping on his thigh; a. e.—*Pl.* יַרְכָּן, יַרְכִין, (יַרְכִּין). Targ. Ex. XXVIII, 42; a. e.—[B. Bath. 4ᵇ, v. הֶדֵר.]

יַרְכוּנָא m. same.—*Pl.* יַרְכוּנִין. Targ. Y. Num. V, 22 (some ed. יַרְכֵ׳). Ib. 21 יַרְכּוּנִיךְ (ed. Amst. יְרֵיכוּנָךְ).

יַרְמוּךְ pr. n. *Yarmukh, Hieromax,* a river emptying into the Jordan below Lake Tiberias. Par. VIII, 10.

יַרְמַטְיָא, יַרְמְטִיָּה pr. n. f. *Yarmatia.* Arakh. V, 1 (19ᵃ); Tosef. ib. III, 1 רימטיא.

יִרְמְיָה, יִרְמְיָהוּ (b. h.) pr. n. m. *Jeremiah,* 1) J. the prophet. Pesik. Dibrê, p. 114ᵇ י׳ רם יה he is named J., because in his days the Lord (Shekhinah) moved from place to place; Yalk. Jer. 257 י׳ ירום יה. Ib. . . . שבימיו י׳ ארימין he is called J., because in his days the Temple became deserted; Koh. R. beg., v. אֲרֵימִיאָה. Meg. 14ᵇ. Snh. 95ᵃ; a. v. fr.—(ספר) י׳ the Book of Jeremiah. B. Bath. 14ᵇ.—2) name of several Amoraim, esp. R. J., pupil of R. Zera. Ib. 23ᵇ ועל דא אפקוה לר׳ י׳ וכ׳ for this (burlesque question) they ejected R. J. from college. Ib. 135ᵇ עיילוה לר׳ י׳ וכ׳ upon this (reply) they reinstated R. J.—Y. M. Kat. III, 81ᵈ bot.; a. fr.—V. Fr. M'bo p. 108ᵃ; 118ᵇ.

ירנקא, Ab. Zar. 30ᵃ, v. יַרְקוּנָא.

יַרְסָא, Targ. Ps. LVIII, 5 Ms.=אֵירְסָא, v. אֶרֶס ch.

יָרַע, *Hif.* הוֹרִיעַ; *Hof.* הוּרַע, v. רָעַע.

יְרַע, *Pa.* יְרַע, *Ithpa.* אִתְיְרַע, v. רְעַע.

***יַרְעֲנָה** m. *an alkaline plant,* used as soap. Tosef. Shebi. V, 6 (El. Fuld: יירעין).—*Pl.* יַרְעָנִין. Y. ib. VII, beg. 37ᵇ הַיּרע׳; (Sabb. 90ᵃ; Nidd. 62ᵃ לעינין, לעוניך; El. Fuld. to Tosef. l. c. לוענין).

יָרַק I (b. h.) *to spit,* v. רָקַק, רוּק.

יְרַק ch. same. Targ. Y. Deut. XXV, 9 תירוק.—Yeb. 39ᵇ וירקת וכ׳ and she spat before him &c. (Y. ib. XII, 13ᵃ top ורקת).—V. רְקַק, רוּק.

ירק II (b. h.) *to be light-colored, pale, green, yellow.* *Hif.* הוריק 1) *to become green, pallid, pale.* Sot. III, 4 פניה מוריקות her face grew pale (sickly); Sifré Num. 8; Tosef. Sot. III, 3; a. fr.—2) *to make pale, cause to fade.* Ber. 44ᵇ כל ירק חי מוריק vegetable eaten raw makes pale. Gen. R. s. 13 (ref. to ארקא, Jer. X, 11) כנגד...שהיא מוֹרֶקֶת וכ׳ the earth is called *arka,* corresponding to the season of Tebeth which causes her fruits to fade.—3) *to make shine* (like gold, bronze &c.; cmp. ירקרק Ps. LXVIII, 14). Ib. s. 43; Yalk. Gen. 73 (ref. to וירק, Gen. XIV, 14) בכלי זיין הוריקן he made them glisten with armor; באבנים . . . ה׳ with jewels; בפרשת שוטרים הוריקן he made them bright (courageous) by reading the section (Deut. XX, 1—9); Ned. 32ᵃ הוריקן בתורה; הוריקן בזהב (Var. הֵרִיקָן מן התורה v. ריק).—ה׳ פנים כנגד (cmp. פָּרֵכֶם) *to turn a brazen face against, to defy, oppose.* Gen. R. l. c.; Yalk. l. c. הן הוריקו פ׳ וכ׳ they opposed Abraham. Ib. אברהם ה׳ פ׳ וכ׳ Abraham defied them.

יְרַק, *Af.* אוֹרִיק same, *to become pale* &c. Targ. Y. Num. XXXI, 18 אפהא מוריקן her face grew pale. Targ. Ps. CXIII, 9 מוֹרִיקָא looking pale (with envy; Ms. מוֹרִיקָא, v. הוּק).

יֶרֶק m. (b. h.; preced. wds.) *green, herb.* Peah III, 4, v. מְלַבֵּן. Maasr. IV, 5, v. זֵירָא. Ib. יַרְקָהּ פטור its herb (foliage) is exempt from tithes. Ber. 36ᵃ מין י׳ הוא it is a species of herb, opp. אילן; a. fr.—*Pl.* יְרָקוֹת. Ib. VI, 1. Pes. II, 6 ואלו י׳ וכ׳ and these are the (bitter) herbs which may be used as *maror.* R. Hash. I, 1 ר״ה . . . לנטיעה ולי׳

a new year as regards . . . the planting (of trees) and (the tithes from) herbs; a. fr.—יַרְקוֹת חמור (Var. יְרוֹקֶת, יְרִיקַת) *ass-herbs*, the large-leaved *cucumis agrestis* (v. Löw Pfl. p. 333). Ohol. VIII, 1 (cmp. Tosef. ib. XIII, 5).—2) *name of a species of green-fish.* Y. B. Mets. II, beg. 8[b], opp. to כּבִיס (v. יָרוֹקָא).

יַרְקָא ch. 1) same, *herb.* Targ. Deut. XI, 10. Targ. I Kings XXI, 2; a. e.—Men. 85[a] (prov.) לבית י׳ ירקא שקול Ms. M. (Ms. L. לְמַת, ed. לִמתא) to Herbtown carry herbs.—*Pl.* יַרְקִין, יַרְקֵי, יַרְקַיָּא. Targ. Y. Ex. XV, 19 (ed. Amst. יַרְקֵי). Targ. Y. Deut. XXVIII, 23.—R. Hash. 20[a] משום י׳ on account of the herbs (which would spoil by lying over two days, if the Day of Atonement would immediately precede or follow the Sabbath).—2) (adj.) *green.* Targ. Job XXVIII, 19 מרגלא י׳ (h. text פִּטְדָה, v. יַרְקָן).—*Pl.* יַרְקִין, *fem.* יַרְקָן. Targ. Esth. I, 6.— Targ. O. Lev. XIV, 37 (Y. יְרוֹקַן), v. יְרוֹקָא.

ירקומי, v. יְרוּקְמֵי.

יֵרָקוֹן m. (b. h.; preced. wds.) 1) *jaundice.* Ber. 25[a]. . . מביא לידי י׳ causes jaundice. Sabb. 33[a] סימן לשנאת חנם י׳ a type of (punishment for) gratuitous hatred is jaundice; a. fr.— 2) *a disease of the grain, mildew.* Taan. III, 5 (some comment.: 'a human disease'). Keth. 8[b].

יֵרָקוֹנָא, יֵרָקָנָא ch. same, 1) *jaundice.* Targ. Jer. XXX, 6.—2) *mildew.* Targ. Deut. XXVIII, 22 (?). Targ. I Kings VIII, 37; Targ. II Chr. VI, 28 יוּרְקָנָא; a. e.

יַרְקוֹנָא m. (v. יָרֵק) 1) (sub. חמר) *a wine flavored with herbs.* Ab. Zar. 30[a] מר י׳ Ms. M. (ed. ירנקא) bitter wine, that is *y'rakona.*—2) pl. יַרְקוֹנִין, v. יַרוֹקָנָא.

יַרְקָן m. (preced. wds.) *a greenish jewel.* Targ. O. Ex. XXVIII, 17 (ed. Berl. יַ׳); XXXIX, 10; Targ. Ez. XXVIII, 13 (h. text פִּטְדָה).—Fem. form. יַרְקָתָא, יְרוּקְתָּא. Targ. Y. Ex. l. c.

יַרְקָנָא m. 1) *mildew,* v. יַרְקוֹנָא.—2) *pl.* יַרְקָנִין, *herbs.* v. יְרוֹקָנָא.

יְרַקְרוֹקֶת, v. יְרַקְרַק.

יַרְקְרִיקָא m. (v. next w.) name of an *unclean bird,* supposed to be the *gier-eagle.* Targ. O. Lev. XI, 18; Deut. XIV, 17 (h. text רחם, רחמה; Y. שרקרקא).

יְרַקְרַק m. (b. h.; preced. wds.) *pale-colored, greenish.* Tosef. Neg. I, 5; Y. Succ. III, 53[d] איזהו י׳ שבירוקים which of the green colors is called *y'rakrak?* Answ. . . the color of wax &c.—Sifra Thazr. Par. 5, ch. XIV (ref. to Lev. XIII, 49; XIV, 37) י׳ ירוק שבירוקים *y.* means the palest of the pale (green) colors. Neg. XI, 4; Tosef. ib. l. c. י׳ שבירוקים the palest of &c. Tosef. ib. V, 5; a. fr.—Fem. יְרַקְרוֹקֶת. Meg. 13[a] אסתר י׳ היתה (Ms. O. ירקרקות היתה כהדסה) Esther was of a greenish complexion (like a myrtle).

יַרְקְתָא, v. יַרְקָן.

יָרַשׁ (b. h.) [*to enter into, take the place of,*] *to conquer; to take possession, to succeed, inherit.* Gen. R. s. 11, end י׳ את העולם במדה had his worldly share assigned to him with limitation. Ib. s. 44 לִירָשֵׁנִי to be my heir. B. Bath. VIII, 5 איש . . . . לא יירש וכ׳ this man, my son, shall not be an heir with the rest of his brothers. Ib. בתי תִּירָשֵׁנִי my daughter shall be my heiress. Ib. ראוי לִירוֹשׁוֹ entitled to succeed him. Ib. IX, 1 (139[b]) חבנים יִירְשׁוּ (Bab. ed. יִרְשׁוּ) the sons take possession of the estate; a. fr.—V. יוֹרֵשׁ.

Hif. הוֹרִישׁ 1) *to cause to inherit, to leave* by will or by the law of succession; *to transmit.* Ib. 119[b] מוֹרִישִׁין ואינן יוֹרשין they shall leave (the Holy Land to their children) but shall not take possession themselves. Shebu. 47[a] אין אדם מוריש שבועה לבניו a man cannot transmit an oath to his sons, *i. e.* property to be obtained only by the claimant's oath cannot be claimed by his heirs. Keth. 43[a]; Kidd. 16[b] אין אדם מוריש זכות בתו וכ׳ a man cannot bequeathe his daughter's privileges to his sons. B. Bath. IX, 8 if the house fell עליו ועל מוֹרִישָׁיו over himself (the heir) and his ancestors; a. fr.—2) *to drive out, dispossess.* Sifré Deut. 51 סמוך . . . לא הוֹרַשְׁתָּ (the Jebusite) who is near thy palace thou hast not driven out; a. e.

יְרֵית, יְרֵת ch. same. Targ. Gen. XV, 4. Targ. Deut. IX, 1; a. fr.—Keth. IV, 10 (in a marriage contract) יֵרְתוּן וכ׳ they shall succeed to thy dowry (כְּתוּבָּה); B. Bath. 131[a]. Yoma 72[b] לא תֵּירְתוּן, v. גֵּיהִינָּם. Cant. R. to VII, 7 מן דיירות, v. בְּזַז I. Gen. R. s. 44 יְרֵית, v. לוּט I. Y. Kidd. I, 61[b] יְאִירְתָה, v. יְקַר; a. fr.

Af. אוֹרִית *to bequeathe, leave, give possession.* Targ. Prov. VIII, 21. Ib. XIII, 22; a. e.—B. Bath. 131[a] בר אוֹרוּתֵי one likely to make a will (a sick person). B. Mets. 16[a] אוֹרְתָהּ if he willed it away; a. e.

יַרְתָא, v. יְרוּתָא.

יַרְתָּא, יְרוּתְתָא, v. יְרוּת׳.

יַרְתּוּ f. (preced. wds.) *heirloom, legacy.* Targ. Y. Num. XXVII, 7.—Y. Snh. III, 21[d] שבק י׳ וכ׳ left a legacy to &c.

יֵשׁ m. (b. h.; cmp. אִישׁ) 1) *being, substance, wealth* (of knowledge &c.). Y. Ned. V, end, 39[b]; Succ. 28[a]; B. Bath. 134[a] (Prov. VIII, 21, applied to R. Joh. b. Zaccai).—2) *there is, there are,* v. אִית. Ber. VI, 4 אם יש ביניהם וכ׳ if there is among them one species &c. Peah VIII, 8 מי שיש לו וכ׳ he who possesses &c. Ḥag. 14[b] יש נאה דורש וכ׳ many a one preaches well but does not act well; a. v. fr.—יש אוֹמְרִים (abbr. י״א) some say (anonymous authority). Hor. 13[b] אסיקו . . . ולר׳ נתן י״א the editors introduced 'others say' for R. M. and 'some say' for R. Nathan. B. Bath. 93[b] וי״א אף הוצאה and some say, he must indemnify him also for carrying the seed out; כאן י״א who is meant by 'some say'? (v. Tosaf. a. l.). Ab. V, 6; a. v. fr.—יֶשְׁנוֹ *he is, it is.* Kidd. I, 10 כל שי׳ במקרא וכ׳ whosoever is (engaged) in the study of the Bible &c. Ḥag. 4[b] כל שי׳ בביאה י׳ וכ׳ whosoever is bound to visit the Temple, is also bound &c., v. הֲבָאָה; a. fr.—יֶשְׁנָהּ *she is, it is.* Kidd. 48[a], a. fr. י׳ לשכירות וכ׳ the relation of employment exists from beginning to end, i. e. the employer is under obligation for every portion of the contracted labor, opp. אינה ל׳ . . . . אלא בסוף the obligation takes effect only when the work is finished; a. fr.

יָשַׁב (b. h.) 1) *to sit down, rest; to dwell, remain; to be inactive.* Macc. III, 15 כל היוֹשֵׁב ולא עבר וכ׳ whoever is inactive and commits no sin, i. e. omits to do wrong; Kidd. 39[b].—Erub. 100[a] שֵׁב ואל תעשה עדיף 'sit and do nothing', i. e. not to act in doubtful cases, is better, opp. קום ועשה. Ber. 20[a] שב ואל תעשה שאני with an omission it is different. Tosef. Snh. VII, 8 ולא יֵשְׁבוּ .. להם שֵׁבוּ and they must not sit down until he says to them, Be seated; Hor. 13[b]; Y. Bicc. III, 65[c] bot.—Y. Dem. II, 23[a] top שר׳ בישיבה who has a seat in the scholars' meetings. Snh. 10[b]; Tosef. ib. II, 1 אחד אומר לֵישֵׁב if one is in favor of sitting (holding deliberation in court). Zeb. II, 1 יוֹשֵׁב in a sitting position. Ber. 28[b] מיוֹשְׁבֵי בה״מ one of the attendants at college, יושבי קרנות those placed at street corners (traders, idlers). Gen. R. s. 75 יושבי קרנות (corr. קרוניות) sitting in chariots; a. v. fr.—2) *to be settled* (v. יִישּׁוּב), *be inhabited.* Num. R. s. 4 הגבעה ... יוֹשְׁבִים Gibeah and Kiryath Jearim were settled at the same time.—Erub. 86[a] (ref. to Ps. LXI, 8) אימתי יושב עולם לפני וכ׳ (Rashi a. Ar. יֵשֵׁב) when is the world settled (evenly balanced) before God? When kindness and truth are appointed to guard it (differ. in Rashi; v. infra).

Pi. יִישֵּׁב, יֵשֵּׁב 1) *to settle, put in place, to arrange evenly.* Y. Sabb. XII, beg. 13[c] חבנאי ר׳ את האבן וכ׳ the builder that placed a stone on top of the row (v. דימוס I). Ib.[d] top; Y. Pes. VIII, 33[b] top מפני שהוא כמְיַישֵּׁב בידו because it is like settling the web with one's own hand. Lev. R. s. 37 [read:] יָשַׁב וִי׳ להם סבלותם וכ׳ he sat down (as a judge) and arranged their burdens in proper proportions between man and woman. Ib. אתה עתיד לְיַישֵּׁב וכ׳ thou art designated to settle and explain to my children their vows &c. Ex. R. s. 31 (ref. to Ps. LXI, 8, v. supra) יַשֵּׁב עולמך make thy world evenly balanced (as to property); Tanh. Mishp. 9 תיישר עולמך בשוה (read: תְּיַישֵּׁב). Ex. R. s. 52 לא היו יודעין לְיַישְּׁבוֹ they knew not how to put its parts together; a. fr.—Trnsf. *to set the mind at ease, to quiet.* Sabb. 87[a] דברים שמְיַישְּׁבִין לבו וכ׳ Ms. M. (ed. שמושכין) words which quiet the mind of man &c.; Gen. R. s. 80 דברים שמְיַישְּׁבִים את הלב. Y. Pes. V, end, 32[d] (expl. וישב, II Sam. VII, 18) וַיְיַשֵּׁב עצמו לתפלה he quieted his mind for prayer; a. e.—2) *to settle, cultivate, populate.* Ber. 58[b] ... עתיד לחוזרו ולְיַישְּׁבוֹ Ms. M. (ed. לְיַישּׁוּבוֹ) the Lord will again people it. Sot. 22[a] מְיַישְּׁבֵי עולם cultivators of the world. —*Part. pass.* מְיוּשָּׁב, f. מְיוּשֶּׁבֶת a) *seated.* Meg. 21[a]. Y. Gitt. VII, 48[d] top; a. fr.—b) *sedate, at ease.* Y. Ber. IV, 8[b] bot. לבו מי׳ his mind is at ease (about his animal); Bab. ib. 30[a] לפי שאין דעתו מי׳ עליו because his mind is not at ease without it. Sifré Num. 131 ... בקי ומי׳, חיה the polemarch was experienced and cool-headed; a. fr.

Hif. הוֹשִׁיב *to seat, place, appoint; to settle.* Yoma 38[a] sq.; Tosef. ib. II, 7 במקומך יוֹשִׁיבוּךָ people will finally seat thee in the place which thou deservest. Tosef. Sabb. VI (VII), 17 (among superstitious practices) המוֹשֶׁבֶת אפרוחים (ו)אמרה איני מוֹשִׁיבָתָן וכ׳ a woman who sets hens to brood and says I will not set them except in pairs (v. ed. Zuck. note). Snh. IV, 4 מוֹשִׁיבִין אותו וכ׳ a seat is assigned to him in the third row. Macc. 10[a] ואין מוֹשִׁיבִין אותם וכ׳ and we must not lay them out except on a river; (Tosef. ib. III (II), 8 בונין וכ׳).—Tosef. l. c. ומושיבין ... מביאין other people are imported and settled in their place. B. Kam. 16[b] bot. הוֹשִׁיבוּ ישיבה וכ׳ they held scholars' meetings by his grave. Snh. 17[a] אין מושיבין בסנהדרי וכ׳ none can be appointed members of the Sanhedrin except &c.; a. v. fr.

Nif. נוֹשַׁב *to be inhabited.* Pirké d'R. El. ch. XLIII ארץ נוֹשֶׁבֶת an inhabited land, settlement; (Koh. R. to I, 15 יישוב).

Hithpa. הִתְיַישֵּׁב, *Nithpa.* נִתְיַישֵּׁב 1) *to be settled, colonized.* Ber. 31[a] כל ארץ שגזר ... לישוב נִתְיַישְּׁבָה every land which Adam designated for settlement, has been settled. —2) *to be at ease, to be refreshed, to come to.* Yoma 82[a] אם נִתְיַשְּׁבָה דעתה if she feels that her craving has been gratified. Lam. R. to I, 11 (ref. to להשיב נפש, ib.) עד כמה מִתְיַישֶּׁבֶת נפש how much is required for one fainting from hunger (v. בולימוס) to come to himself again?—Hag. 3[b] לאחר שנתיישבה דעתו after his excitement had subsided. Erub. 65[a] כל המתיישב ביינו he who remains clear-minded when drinking wine. Kinnim III, 6 כל זמן ... דעתם מתישבת עליהם the older they grow, the more clear-minded do they become, opp. מיטרפת; a. fr.

יְתֵב ch., *Ithpa.* אִתְיַישַּׁב, contr. אִיַּישַּׁב as preced. *Hithpa.* 2. Ber. 58[b] חזייה דלא מִיַּישְּׁבָא דעתיה ed. (Ms. מִתְיַישְּׁבָא) he saw that he was not comforted.—V. יְתֵב.

יֶשֶׁבְאָב (b. h.) *Jeshebab,* name of a priestly division. Tosef. Succ. IV, 28 ed. Zuck. (Var. יֶשֶׁבָב); Succ. 56[b] ישבב. V. next w.

יְשֵׁבָב (v. preced.) pr. n. m. *Jeshebab, Y'shebab,* 1) brother and substitute of the Highpriest Ishmael b. Kimhith. Yoma 47[a] (Ms. M. 2 ישובאב).—2) name of a priestly division, v. preced.—3) a Tannai, contemporary of R. Akiba. Keth. 29[b]. Ib. 50[a]. Hull. II, 4.

יִשְׁבִּי (b. h.) pr. n. m. *Jishbi,* a Philistine. Snh. 95[a]; Gen. R. s. 59.

יֵשׁוּ (abbrev. of יֵשׁוּעַ) pr. n. m. *Jesus* of Nazareth. Snh. 43[a] י׳ הנוצרי Ms. M. (ed. only י׳). Ib. 107[b] (represented as a disciple of R. Joshua b. P'rahia, with whom he fled to Egypt); Sot. 47[a]. Ab. Zar. 17[a] מצאתי אדם אחד מתלמידי י׳ הנוצרי ויעקב וכ׳ I met one of the disciples of J. the Nazarean whose name was Jacob (v. יַעֲקֹב 5); Tosef. Hull. II, 24 יֵשׁוּעַ בן פנטירי (Var. פנטרי); Ib. 22 ובא ... ישוע בן פנטרא and Jacob ... came to cure him with the name of J. the son of Pantera; Ab. Zar. 27[b] (v. Rabb. D. S. a. l. note 300); Y. ib. II, 40[d] bot. נימא לך בשם י׳ בן פנדרא shall I speak a charm to thee in the name of J. the son of Pandera; Y. Sabb. XIV, 14[d] bot. .... משם של ישו פנדירא Ib. ולחש ליה משמיה די׳ פ׳ and he whispered to him a charm, in behalf of J. P.; [In Babli editions published unter censorial restrictions all the above quoted passages are omitted or changed; in Koh. R. to I, 8 פלוני is substituted.]

יִישּׁוּב, יְשׁוּב m. (יָשַׁב) 1) *settlement, inhabited land,* opp. מדבר or ים; *cultivation, social world, civilization; public welfare.* Koh. R. to I, 15; Ruth. R. to I, 17 אם אין

אדם מתקן ביי' וכ' if man does not prepare provision in the inhabited settlement (this world), what will he have to eat in the desert (the hereafter)?—Y. B. Kam. V, end, 5ª, v. אָוַוז. Ber. 31ª, v. יָשַׁב. Ib. 58ᵇ הרואה בתי ... בְּיִשּׁוּבָן he who sees Israelitish places in their inhabitable condition (restoration), opp. בחורבנן. Ib. עתיד הקב״ה להחזירו לְיִשּׁוּבוֹ the Lord will restore it again. Tam. 29ᵇ; B. Kam. 80ᵇ כְּשׁוּם י' א״י in order to maintain the cultivation of Palestine. Y. B. Bath. II, end, 13ᶜ י' עולם בבורות social welfare depends on wells; באילנות on trees. Kidd. I, 10 אינו מן הי' does not belong to the civilized world. Gen. R. s. 35 בני אדם של י' civilized (polite) people; a. fr.—2) (with or without דעת) *ease of mind, calmness.* Ib. s. 19 בי' הדעת באת עליו she came to him with deliberation (logical arguments). Y. Ned. I, 36ᵈ bot.; Num. R. s. 10 (הדעת) מתוך י' in a calm state of mind, opp. אקפדה; a. fr.

יְשׁוּין, v. יְשִׁירִין.

יִשּׁוּן m. (יָשַׁן) *allowing to dry up, leaving unused.* Tosef. Ab. Zar. VIII (IX), 3 וכמה יִשּׁוּנָן (ib. Toh. XI, 16 כמה היא מְיַשְּׁנָן) how long must they remain unused?

יֵשׁוּעַ (b. h.) pr. n. m. *Jeshua,* 1) name of several persons. Yad. III, 5 Bab. ed. (Mish. יהושע). Y. M. Kat. III, 82ᶜ יֵישׁ'.—Tosef. Ḥull. II, 22; 25; v. יֵשׁוּ.—2) (sub מִשְׁמָר) *the priestly division of Jeshua* which was the ninth in the order of divisions on duty each week (I Chr. XXIV, 7—18). Pesik. Haomer, p. 69ᵇ; Pesik. R. s. 18; Koh. R. to I, 3; Yalk. Lev. 643 [read:] אימתי הן תמימות בזמן שיש י' ושכניה ביניהם when are the seven weeks between Passover and Pentecost 'complete' (Lev. XXIII, 15), i. e. beginning and ending with the week? When the divisions of J. and Shekhania are between them, i. e. when there are ten Sabbaths between the first of the month of Nisan on the first Sabbath of which the turn commences, and the sixth of Sivan.—3) *Jeshua* (redemption), a disguise for פִּדְיוֹן; v. בֵּן. B. Kam. 80ª.

יְשׁוּעָה f. (b. h.; יָשַׁע) *redemption, help.* Midr. Till. to Ps. XIV; Lev. R. s. 24. M. Kat. 5ª יְשׁוּעָתוֹ של הקב״ה the salvation by the Lord; a. fr.

***יָשַׁט** (b. h.; cmp. שוט) *to spread, stretch.*—V. וֶשֶׁט.

Hif. הוֹשִׁיט *to stretch forth, to hand, reach.* Ḥull. 140ᵇ ה' ידו לקן וכ' if one put his hand forth into a nest and cut there. Ab. Zar. 6ᵇ לא יוֹשִׁיט וכ' one must not hand a cup of wine to a nazarite &c. Ib. קתני לא יושיט .... לא יתן it says, 'he shall not reach over' and not 'he shall not give' (which means that the object is beyond the reach of the other person). Pesik. S'lih. p. 167ᵇ; Yalk. Num. 744 ה' הדסים offered myrtles, i. e. *asked pardon;* a. e.

יְשַׁט ch., *Af.* אוֹשִׁיט same. Targ. Jud. VI, 21. Targ. Ex. XXII, 7; a. fr.—Y. Meg. IV, 74ᵈ top מוֹשֵׁט תרגומא מן גו סיפרא reaching forth for a Chaldaic version from between the (Hebrew) book.

יִשַׁי (b. h.) pr. n. m. *Jesse,* father of king David. Ber. 58ª. Pes. 119ª; a. fr.

יְשִׁיבָה f. (יָשַׁב) 1) *sitting, rest.* Ḥag. 15ª למעלה . . . לא עמידה ולא י' וכ' Ms. M. (v. Rabb. D. S. a. l.) on high there is no standing up and no sitting down (effort and rest), no emulation &c. Yoma 69ᵇ, a. fr. אין י' בעזרה none were allowed to sit down in the Temple court. Gen. R. s. 38, a. fr. כל מקום שאתה מוצא י' וכ' wherever you find sitting (retirement, use of the word ישב) recorded in the Bible, there Satan leaps forth (trouble arises). Yeb. 106ª יְשִׁיבָתָהּ זו היא עמידתה this her sitting is to her a getting up (sitting up is to her a great effort; oth. expl.: her being left seated, is her erection, i. e. her failure to be married to the *yabam* is a benefit to her); a. fr.—2) *settlement, dwelling.* Kidd. 37ª, a. e., v. יְרוּשָׁה. Keth. 110ᵇ יְשִׁיבַת כרכים קשה living in large cities is a hardship. Sabb. 10ᵇ עיר שֶׁיְּשִׁיבָתָהּ קרובה a town of recent settlement; a. fr.—3) *scholars' session, council, academy; court.* Yoma 28ᵇ זקן ויושב בי' an elder and member of council. Ib. לא פרשה י' מהם they (our early ancestors) were never without council (a representative body). Pes. 119ª top המכיר ... בי' who knows his colleague's place in meetings; ... המקבל בי' who greets his colleague in meetings with kindness. Ber. 57ª ראש י' presiding officer. Y. Ber. IV, 7ᵈ top ומינו את ר״א ... בי' they elected R. El.... (president) in regular session. Ib. הושיבו ... בי' they installed him as president. B. Bath. 120ª בי' הלך וכ' in court or college give the preference to learning, in social entertainment to age; a. fr.—י' של מעלה divine court. B. Mets. 86ª נתבקש בי' של מ' has been summoned before divine justice (is dead); a. fr.—*Pl.* יְשִׁיבוֹת. Koh. R. to I, 8 אפשר שהי' הללו טועות וכ' is it possible that those colleges be lost in such futile errors; Tosef. Ḥull. II, 24 שהסיבו הללו טועים (corr. acc.; v., however, סִיבוּ). Y. Sabb. X, 12ᶜ bot. שימשתי את אבא עומדות מה שלא שמשת י' I have served my father at more 'standing meetings' (standing up as an Amora) than you have served at college sessions; Y. Ḥag. III, beg. 78ᵈ; a. fr.

***יְשִׁירִין** m. pl. (שָׁוָה; cmp. הוֹגְיִן) [*balance-holders,*] *anchor, ballast-stones.* Tosef. B. Bath. IV, 1 ed. Zuck. (Var. יְשׁוּין, disagreeing with Mish. B. Bath. V, 1, v. הוֹגְיִן; Y. ib. V, beg. 15ª עיבין, read עוגין).

בַּר י', יְשִׁיטָא pr. n. m. *Bar-Y'shita.* Y. Meg. IV, 75ᶜ top.

יְשִׁיכ-, v. יָשֵׁן.

יָשִׁישׁ m. (b. h.; cmp. יֵשׁ) [*substantial,*] *old, venerable.*—*Pl.* יְשִׁישִׁים. M. Kat. 25ᵇ, v. גָּזַע.

יִשְׁמָעֵאל (b. h.) pr. n. m. *Ishmael,* 1) son of Abraham; also (as patron.) *the people of I., Arabs, Bedouins.* [Targ. Job XV, 20, Var. in ed. Lag.]—Gen. R. s. 45 אף י' באומות I., too, among the nations (was named before he was born, Gen. XVI, 11). B. Bath. 16ᵇ; Gen. R. s. 59 שעשה י' תשובה וכ' in as much as I. repented of his evil deeds in his (Abraham's) life-time; a. fr.—Sabb. 11ª תחת י' ולא וכ' (v. Rabb. D. S. a. l. note 80 a. Rashi a. l.) rather under I. (Arabic dominion) than under Byzantium; a. fr. [Pes. 118ᵇ מלכות י' (Ms. M. a. older eds. הרשעה) a censorial change for רומי, Roman government.]—2) I. ben Nathaniah, the murderer of governor Gedaliah. R. Hash. 18[b]. Nidd. 61[a]; a. e.—3) I. b. Kimhith, a high priest. Yoma 47[a]; Tosef. ib. IV (III), 20, v. יָשֵׁבָב.—4) I. b. Piabi or Pâbi, a priest. Tosef. ib. I, 21; Y. ib. III, 40[d] top; Bab. ib. 35[b]. Sot. IX, 15; a. e.—5) name of several Tannaim, esp. a) I. b. Elisha, redeemed from Roman captivity. Gitt. 58[a]. [Ber. 7[a] top, prob. his grandfather, a high priest.]—Shebu. II, 5; a. fr.—V. Fr. Darkhé, p. 105 sq.—6) I. son of R. Johanan b. B'roka. B. Kam. X, 2. Tosef. Eduy. II, 4; a. fr.—V. Fr. ib., p. 185 sq.—7) name of several Amoraim. Y. Gitt. I, 43[c] top; a. fr.—Y. Yoma III, 40[d] bot.—V. Fr. M'bo, p. 108[b], sq.

יִשְׁמְעֵאלִי m. (b. h.; preced.) *Ishmaelite, Arab, Bedouin.—Pl.* יִשְׁמְעֵאלִים. Ex. R. s. 23 (ref. to אהלי קדר Cant. I, 5) אהליהם של י׳ the tents of the Bedouins. Gen. R. s. 84; a. fr.

יָשֵׁן I (b. h.; cmp. אָשַׁן) [*to recover strength*, cmp. חָלַם,] *to sleep*, trnsf. *to be idle, lazy*. Shebu. III, 5 (I swear) שאִישַׁן that I will sleep, שֶׁיָּשַׁנְתִּי that I have slept. Num. R. s. 20 בא לִישַׁן going to sleep.—Cant. R. to III, 1 ישנתי לי מן התורה וכ׳ I (Israel) have been lazy in the study of the Law and the performance of good deeds; a. fr.

יָשֵׁן II (b. h.; preced.) *asleep, inactive*. Midr. Till. to Ps. LIX הקב״ה עושה עצמו כביכול י׳ the Lord sometimes pretends, if it were permitted to say so, to be asleep; a. fr. —*Pl.* יְשֵׁנִים, יְשֵׁנִין, יְשֵׁי׳. Num. R. s. 20 הרי הן י׳ מן וכ׳ they are sluggish in study &c., v. preced. Cant. R. to VII, 10 י׳ במערת וכ׳ sleeping in the cave of Makhpelah. Ex. R. s. 1; a. fr.—Fem. יְשֵׁנָה, יְשֵׁי׳. Midr. Till. to Ps. CX, beg. (ref. to Is. XLI, 2) הצדקה היתה י׳ וכ׳ Righteousness was asleep and Abraham waked her up. Cant. R. to V, 2 אני י׳ מן וכ׳ I (Israel) was lazy &c., v. supra; a. fr.

יָשַׁן (b. h.; cmp. preced. wds. a. אֵיתָן) *to be strong, hard, old* (cmp. קשיש).—V. יוֹשֶׁן a. next w.

Pi. יִישֵּׁן *to let grow old (strong), keep, reserve*. B. Bath. 91[b] דברים שדרכן לְיַישְּׁנָן things which it is customary to keep (to store, as wine &c.). Deut. R. s. 9, beg. מן היין הזה אני מְיַישֵּׁן וכ׳ of this wine I will store away a portion for my son's wedding. Tosef. Ab. Zar. VIII (IX), 3 צריך לְיַשְּׁנָן he must store them away (leave them unused); Tosef. Toh. XI, 16. Ib. כמה הוא מְיַשְּׁנָן, v. יָשׁוּן; Y. Ab. Zar. V, end 45[b] מְיַישְּׁנָן כל י״ב וכ׳ he must leave them unused for the whole twelve-month; Bab. ib. 75[a].—Part. pass. מְיוּשָּׁן *stored up*, v. infra. Y. B. Bath. VII, end, 15[c]. Y. Gitt. III, end, 45[b] 'old' means last year's crop, מי׳ של וכ׳ 'stored' means three years old.

Hithpa. הִתְיַשֵּׁן *to be stored up, to improve with age*. Sifra B'huck. ch. III; Yalk. Lev. 672 (ref. to ישן נושן, Lev. XXVI, 10) כל המִּתְיַשֵּׁן יפה מחבירו the sort which is stored up is the better of its kind; B. Bath. l. c. [read with Ms. R.: כל המְיוּשָּׁן יפה מחבירו]. Y. Gitt. l. c. הדא אמרה דאי מתישן וכ׳ this intimates that if wine is sold as *mithyashshen* (fit for storage) the seller is responsible for three years. Sifra l. c. לרבות כל המִתְיַישְּׁנִים including all produces fit for storage (besides wine); Yalk. l. c. לרבות כל הדבר המיושן.

Nif. נוֹשַׁן same. B. Bath. l. c.; a e., v. next w.

יָשָׁן m. (b. h.; preced.) *hard, dry; old, of last year*, opp. חָדָשׁ. Dem. IV, 7. B. Bath. 91[b], a. e. expl. י׳ נוֹשָׁן (Lev. XXVI, 10), v. preced. Ab. IV, 20 קנקן חדש מלא י׳ a new vessel full of old wine (a young man but learned). Ab. Zar. III, 9 ואם י׳ וכ׳ and if the oven is old (dried) &c.; a. fr. —*Pl.* יְשָׁנִים. Ib. 33[a] י׳ ומזופפין old or pitched wine vessels. Yoma II, 4, v. חָדָשׁ. Lev. R. s. 2, v. חָדָשׁ; a. fr.—*Fem.* יְשָׁנָה. Kidd. IV, 5, Num. R. s. 9, v. אַרְכִּי I.—*Pl.* יְשָׁנוֹת. Tosef. Ab. Zar. IV (V), 10 י׳ זפופות, v. supra; a. fr.

יָשַׁע (b. h.; cmp. preced. wds.) [*to be strong, to recover.*] *Hif.* הוֹשִׁיעַ *to assist, help, deliver*. Sot. 34[b] (ref. to יהושע, Num. XIII, 17) יה יוֹשִׁיעֲךָ וכ׳ Yah save thee from &c. Meg. 14[a] עתידה .. שיוֹשִׁיעַ וכ׳ my mother shall bear a son who will deliver Israel; Sot. 11[b] שמוֹשִׁיעַ. Midr. Till. to Ps. XVIII, 4 כשתוֹשִׁיעֵנִי מאויבי when thou shalt have saved me from my enemies. Snh. 73[a], v. מוֹשִׁיעַ. Ber. IV, 4 הוֹשַׁע וכ׳ help, O Lord &c.; a. fr.—V. הוֹשַׁעְנָא.

Nif. נוֹשַׁע *to be saved, released*. Midr. Till. l. c. אִוָּשַׁע מן וכ׳ let me be delivered from my enemies, and I shall call the Lord the praised One. Tanh. Aḥăré 12 (ref. to ויושע, Ex. XIV, 30) וַיִּוָּשַׁע כתיב כביכול הוא נ׳ it may be read *vayivvasha* (and he was saved), He, as if it were, was delivered. Ib. בעוה״ז הייתם נוֹשָׁעִים ע״י ב״א in this world (the past) you were delivered through human agencies.

***יְשַׁף** (= נשף), *Af.* אוֹשִׁיף *to blow, kindle*. Sabb. 119[a] מוֹשִׁיף נורא fanning the fire.

יָשְׁפֵה f. (b. h.) *Jaspis*, Benjamin's jewel in the high-priest's breast-plate. Ex. R. s. 38, end. Y. Kidd. I, 61[b] top.

יָשַׁר (b. h.; cmp. אָשַׁר) *to be firm, strong, healthy; to be straight, right*. יִישַׁר כֹּחֲךָ or חֵילָךְ 'may thy strength (health) be firm', a phrase of approval and thanks. Sabb. 87[a], a. fr. (play on אֲשֶׁר, Ex. XXXIV, 1) י׳ כ׳ ששברת, be thanked for having broken (the tablets). Gen. R. s. 54 (play on וישרנה, I Sam. VI, 12) י׳ חילכם; a. e.—(יָשַׁר) יִישַׁר (sub. כחך) *thanks! right!* Ber. 42[b]; Sabb. 53[a]; Erub. 32[b]; a. fr.—Cmp. אִישַׁר.

Pi. יִשֵּׁר, יִישַּׁר, יִשְּׁ׳ *to straighten, direct, to make firm*. Ex. R. s. 1 (ref. to יֵשֶׁר, I Chr. II, 18) זה כלב שיי׳ את עצמו that is Caleb who kept himself straight (did not yield to the rest of the spies). Num. R. s. 8 (ref. to Ps. L, 23 ושם דרך) המְיַישֵּׁר אורחותיו וכ׳ he who directs his ways straight (pays regard to his doings).—Part. pass. מְיוּשָּׁר, f. מְיוּשֶּׁרֶת. Pirké d'R. El. ch. X דרכי מי׳ לפני my way is levelled before me.—Meg. 18[b] (ref. to יישרו, Prov. IV, 25) מְיוּשָּׁרִין הן אצל וכ׳ they remain firm with (in the memory of) &c.

יְשַׁר ch. same. Targ. II Esth. VII, 9 יישר חילך (Var. יִשַּׁר). [Cant. R. to I, 4 ישרירך, v. next w.]

Ithpa. אִתְיַשַּׁר, *Ithpe.* אִתְיְשַׁר *to be strengthened*. Targ. Y. Deut. X, 2, v. אֲשַׁר.

יָשָׁר m. (b. h.; preced.) *firm, sound; straight, right, upright*. Gen. R. s. 49 אברהם זה י׳ מן הַיְשָׁרִים this Abraham is firmer than all the firm (angels); Yalk. ib. 82 אברהם זה י׳; Midr. Till. to Ps. XI, 7 קודם לִישָׁרוֹ של עולם וכ׳ before they see the Right One of the world, they (the pious) shall behold the faces of the firm (believers); a. fr.—*Pl.* יַשְׁרִין, יְשָׁרִים. Cant. R. to I, 4 מה ישריין רחמיך, [read as:] Yalk. ib. 982 מה ישרים וכ׳) מה תקיפין וכ׳, expl.) how strong are thy mercies. Midr. Till. l. c. איזו כת ... זו כת ר׳ which is the highest class among those who will greet the countenance of the Divine Presence (in the hereafter)? The class of the firm believers. Ib. to Ps. XXV, 14 ... בתחלה ואח"כ נתן לר׳ first the secret of the Lord is communicated to those who fear him (human beings), and then to the firm ones (the angels, cmp. יְצוּקִים s. v. יָצַק), Gen. R. s. 49; a. e.—*Fem.* יְשָׁרָה, *pl.* יְשָׁרוֹת (sub בעיניו; with ref. to Deut. XII, 8) [*right in the eyes of the offerer,*] *free-will offerings* (opp. חוֹבָה). Zeb. 114a ר׳ תקריבו וכ׳ free-will sacrifices you may offer (on the *bamoth*, v. בָּמָה), but no obligatory offerings; ib. 117b. Ib. ר׳ נינהו they belong to the class of free-will offerings. Ib. 118a; a. fr.—סֵפֶר הַיָּשָׁר *the Book Yashar*, a lost book (Josh. X, 13; II Sam. I, 18). Ab. Zar. 25a. Y. Sot. I, end, 17c.

ישְׁרָא ch. same, *firm believer, upright man.* Y. Taan. II, 65b (ref. to Mic. VII, 4) ר׳ דבהון וכ׳ the upright man among them is like thorns.

יִשְׂרָאֵל (b. h.) pr. n. *Israel,* 1) I. (Jacob), the patriarch. Gen. R. s. 68 ר׳ סבא the patriarch I. (not the people); a. fr.—2) I., the people. Ber. 6a; a. fr.—שונאי ר׳ the enemies of Israel, often euphem. for *Israel.* Ib. 32a נתמוטטו .. של ש׳ ר׳ the feet of Israel would totter (in judgment); a. fr. —V. כְּנֶסֶת.—3) ר׳ (=בן ר׳) *an Israelite,* a) one not belonging to the priestly or levitic tribe; b) *a Jew,* opp. נכרי, גוי. Gitt. V, 8. Tosef. Kidd. V, 3; a. fr.—Tosef. Ab. Zar. III, 5, sq. Ab. Zar. II, 6; a. fr.—בַּת ר׳ *an Israelitish woman.* Tosef. l. c. 1; 3; a. fr.—*Pl.* יִשְׂרְאֵלוֹת (opp. to כֹּהֲנוֹת, לְוִיּוֹת). Tosef. Snh. IV, 2.

יִשְׂרְאֵלִי m. (preced.) *one belonging to a common Israelitish family,* contrad. to כֹּהֵן, a. לֵוִי. Kidd. IV, 1; Yeb. 37a (collective noun).—*Pl.* יִשְׂרְאֵלִים. Ib. 85a. Tosef. Ber. V, 14.—*Fem.* יִשְׂרְאֵלִית *an Israelitish (Jewish) woman.* Nidd. IV, 2 (33b) (collective noun, opp. to כותיות).

יַשְׁרוּת f. (v. יָשַׁר a. יוֹשֶׁר) *firmness, faith, right conduct, equity.* Y. Meg. I, 72c top (ref. to Deut. XII, 8, cmp. יָשָׁר) ומה תעשו שם דבר שהוא בא לידי ר׳ וכ׳ and what dare you do there (on the *bamoh*)? An act by which one is led towards faith, which is burnt-offerings and peace-offerings. Midr. Till. to Ps. XCIX, 4 (ref. to מישרים ib.) אתה כוננת ר׳ של עולם (ed. Bub. ר׳ בעולמך) thou hast established the firmness of thy world (through courts of justice); Yalk. Ps. 852 ר׳ בעולמך.—Gen. R. s. 54 (ref. to וישרנה, I Sam. VI, 12) מהלכות בי׳ they walked with propriety (paying reverence to the Ark; Midr. Sam. ch. XII ביופי). Ruth R. introd. 3 (ref. to ישר, Prov. XXI, 8) במדת ר׳ in fairness; ib. בי׳; Yalk. Prov. 959. Deut. R. s. 8 היא וכל כלי אומנתה ניתנה ... יַשְׁרוּתָהּ she (the Torah) and all her implements have been given to man, her humility, her righteousness and her fairness.—Sot. 9b, v. next w.

יַשְׁרוּתָא f. ch. (v. preced.) *that which seems right, arbitrary will.* Sot. 9b (ref. to Jud. XIV, 3 וישרה בעיני) כי אזל מיהא בתר יַשְׁרוּתֵיה אזל when he (Samson) went out (to marry), he, at all events, followed only his own liking (not the will of the Lord); [marginal version יַשְׁרוּת עיניו]; Yalk. Jud. 69.

יַת (v. אית) [*being, existence,*] a particle 1) indicating the objective case (=h. אֶת). Targ. Gen. I, 1; a. v. fr.—With pronominal suffixes: יָתִי *me,* יָתָךְ, יָתִיךְ, יָתָךְ *thee* &c. Targ. Deut. IV, 14. Targ. Gen. XII, 12. Ib. L, 21; a. v. fr.—2) (with pronominal suffix of the third person) *he himself, this one* &c. Y. Bicc. III, 65d top אמר יָתֵיהּ דמן רבנן said he (who was before mentioned as) one of the scholars. Gen. R. s. 9, beg.; Koh. R. to III, 11, a. e. יָתְהוֹן those (opp. to דין), v. חֲנִי.—With prepositional prefix: לְוָת, v. לְוַת, כְּוַת.

יְתֵיב, יְתַב I ch.=h. יָשַׁב, *to sit, dwell* &c.; *to be inhabited, settled.* Targ. O. Gen. XXXVI, 7 מִיתַּב ed. Berl. (oth. ed. a. Y. מֵיתַב). Targ. O. Ex. XVI, 35 יָתֵיבְתָּא (Y. מִיתְיְבָא) *inhabited*; a. v. fr.—Imper. תִּיב, תִּיבִי, תִּיבוּ. Targ. Gen. XX, 15. Targ. Is. LII, 2 (ed. Wil. תִּבִי); a. fr.—Yeb. 109a יָתְבָא תותיה she lives under (with) him. Ber. 6a עד דיָתְבֵי when they are seated. Ib. 48a ורחמנא היכא ר׳ and where does the Lord reside?—M. Kat. 9b ליחרוב ביתך וליתוב אושפיזך may thy house (grave) be vacant, and thy inn (temporary home on earth) be inhabited; Tanh. B'resh. 13; a fr.—ר׳ .. וקאמר N. N. sat down (lecturing) and said &c. Bets. 20a; a. fr.

Pa. יַתֵּיב 1) *to set down, place.* Y. Kil. IX, 32c top; Y. Keth. XII, 35b top ר׳ ליה ולא וכ׳ he set him down (let his coffin down) and would not take him back again (v. תּוּב); a. e.—2) *to settle, establish.* Targ. Is. XLIII, 20 אֲיַתֵּיב (ed. Wil. אַיְתֵב *Af.*).—Targ. Ps. XXII, 4; a. e.—3) *to quiet, set at rest.* Targ. Ps. XXIII, 3 יְיַתֵּיב (ed. Wil. יְתִיב, v. תּוּב).—Ber. 28a לְיַתּוּבֵי דעתיה to set his mind at ease. Yoma 81a יַתּוּבֵי דעתא making one come to. B. Bath. 3b לְיַתּוּבֵיה לִיצריה in order to gratify his passion. Lev. R. s. 19 [read:] תִּתְיַתַּב ליך נפשיך היך כמה דיַתֶּבְת לנפשי may thy soul be restored to thee as thou hast restored my soul; a. e.—*Part. pass.* מְיַתַּב, מְיַתְּבָא, מִיַּתְּבָא a) *inhabited.* Targ. Ps. CVII, 4.—b) *quieted.* Tam. 32a נחותי ימא לא מְיַי׳ דעתידהון וכ׳ (or מִיַּתְּבָא, v. infra) sea-farers do not feel at ease until they reach land.

Af. אוֹתֵיב, אַיְתֵב *to place, seat, settle* (v. יָשַׁב *Hif.*). Targ. I Kings XXI, 9. Targ. Gen. XLVII, 6; a. fr.—Y. Kidd. I, 58d אַיְיתִיבוּנִי על גיף וכ׳ bury, me at the bank of the river; Y. Keth. VI, end, 31a אייחבון (corr. acc.). Hull. 59a יַיְתְבֵיה בתנורא .. אוֹתְבֵיה let it be put in the oven; ... he put it in. Yoma 69b אוֹתִיבוּ בתעניתא וכ׳ they made (people) sit fasting, they ordered a fast of three days &c.; a. fr. [אוֹתִיב for אָתִיב, v. תּוּב.]

Ithpa. אִתְיַתַּב, *Ithpe.* אִתְיְתֵיב, אִיתְּתִיב, אִיתְּתֵיב; *Ittaf.* איתותב 1) *to be allowed to dwell, to sojourn* (h. גּוּר). Targ. O. Gen. XX, 1 (Y. אתותב, corr. acc.). Targ. Jer. XLIX, 33; a. fr.—Sabb. 33b אִיתְּתִיבוּ תריסר וכ׳ they dwelt in the cave twelve years.—2) *to be inhabited.* Targ. Is. XLIV, 26. Targ. Jer. L, 13; a. fr.—3) *to be set at ease, be gratified.* Targ. Is. LXII, 5.—B. Mets. 83b bot. לא מִיתְּתְבָא דעתיה he was not satisfied. Yoma 80b; מי׳ דעתיה he will come to again.—Sabb. 51b, sq. כי היכי דתיתותב דעתיה Ms. O. (Ms. M. דתיתיב, ed. דאיתותב, v. Rabb. D. S. a. l. note) that he may be reconciled. Lev. R. s. 19, v. supra; a. fr. [אִתּוֹתַב for אִתְּתַב, v. תּוּב.]

יָתֵב II (v. preced.; cmp. יהב *to give* and *to place*) *to give* (not used in perf. tense). Sabb. 19ª במשחא נִיתֵיב ליה וכ׳ (Ms. M. נמשח וכ׳) let him measure when giving (the goods to wash) and when receiving it back. Kidd. 78ᵇ אי בעי מֵיתְּבָא . . . לא יהיב ליה (not יהבי) if he desired to give it to him as a donation, could he not do it? Keth. 106ᵇ ולינא למיתבא ליה and he will have nothing to give him. B. Kam. 83ᵇ; a. e.—B. Bath. 13ᵇ למיהב Ms. M. (ed. לְמִיתַּן).

יָתֵב, יָתִיב m. (יָתֵב I) *inhabitant*. Targ. O. Gen. XXXIV, 30 יָתִיב ed. Berl. (ed. יָתְבֵי *pl.*). Targ. O. Num. XIV, 14. Targ. Is. VI, 11; a. fr.— *Pl.* יָתְבֵי, יָתְבַיָּא. Targ. Y. Num l. c.; a. fr.

יָתְבָא m., pl. יָתְבִין *dwelling places*, v. יָתוּבָא.

יָתֵד f. (b. h.; cmp. עתד) [*something fastened, driven in,*] *peg, nail; handle of a tool* &c. Y. Taan. IV, 67ᵈ אשרי אדם . . . י׳ לְהִיתָלוֹת בה (cmp. Is. XXII, 23, sq.) happy the man who has a peg to hang on, i. e. who has a renowned ancestry; ומה היתה יְתֵידָתוֹ וכ׳ and what was R. E.'s. peg?; Y. Ber. IV, 7ᵈ top. Gitt. 17ª י׳ היא שלא תמוט (my last opinion) is an immovable peg. Meg. 6ª והיא היתה י׳ תקועה וכ׳ and she (Cæsarea) was a peg driven into Israel, i. e. an obnoxious foreign element.—י׳ של מחרישה the pin of the plough. Sabb. XVII, 4; a. e, v. מַחֲרֵישָׁה.—י׳ האהל *tent-pin*, v. infra.—י׳ הדרכים *a way-mark of hardened clay pegs*, v. גַּיִץ; v. infra.—*Pl.* יְתֵידוֹת, יְתֵדוֹת. Gen. R. s. 43 שלשה י׳ גדולות three great pegs (Abraham, Isaac and Jacob). Ib. s. 62 נתגרו בהן י׳ הארץ the pegs of the land (the remnants of the seven nations, cmp. Num. XXXIII, 55) arose against them. Kel. XIV, 3 י׳ אהלים י׳ המשוחות Mish. ed. (Bab. ed. ידות) the (metal) pegs of tents and those of the land measurers. Tosef. ib. B. Bath. I, 7 החרב שפרשה עם י׳ המחרישה the knife (coulter) which has been taken out with the handle of the plough. Mikv. IX, 2 י׳ הדרכים, expl. גיץ יוני. Tosef. ib. VI (VII), 14. B. Kam. 81ª מסתלקין . . . מפני י׳ הד׳ you may (in walking) turn out from the highway towards the private sidewalk in order to avoid the road-pegs; Y. Ber. II, end, 5ᵈ top.

יָתוּבָא m. (יָתֵב I) *dweller, sojourner*, opp. בן מתא citizen.—*Pl.* יָתוּבֵי, יָתוּבִין. B. Bath. 8ª.

יָתוּבָא m. (preced.) *dwelling place*. Targ. Job. XVIII, 19.—*Pl.* יָתוּבַיָּא. Targ. Ps. LXXXIX, 13 Ms. (ed. יָתְבִין).

יָתוּךְ, v. יַתִּיךְ.

יָתוֹם m., **יְתוֹמָה** f. (b. h.) [*by one's self*, cmp. גּוּף, גַּף I,] *single, alone, forsaken*. Ḥag. 3ᵇ; Mekh. Bo s. 16, a. e. אין הדור י׳ וכ׳ that generation is not forsaken in which &c.—י׳ אָמֵן, v. אָמֵן.—Esp. 1) *fatherless, orphan, public charge*. Meg. 13ª המגדל י׳ וי׳ בתוך ביתו וכ׳ he who rears a male or female orphan in his house, is regarded as the parent. Tosef. Keth. VI, 8 י׳ וי׳ צריכין פרנסה מפרנסין את היתומה וכ׳ if an orphan boy and an orphan girl need public support, we must support the girl first &c.; Keth. 67ᵃ. Taan. 24ª בי׳ וי׳ we were engaged in collecting for an orphaned couple to be married; a. v. fr.—יתומה בחיי האב self-depending in her father's life-time, i. e. *a minor over whom her father has no control*, e. g. when he has given her away in marriage, and she being divorced or widowed returns to her paternal home. Yeb. XIII, 6. Keth. 73ᵇ; a. fr.—2) *an animal whose mother died during or soon after childbirth*. Bekh. IX, 4. Hull. 38ᵇ.—3) (Law) *a minor heir* whom the authorities must protect by appointing a guardian to plead his cause &c.; in gen. *heir* (mostly in the plural).—*Pl.* יְתוֹמִים, יְתוֹמִין; f. יְתוֹמוֹת. B. Mets. 70ª מעות של י׳ minor heirs' funds. B. Bath. 124ª שבח שהשביחו י׳ לאחר וכ׳ improvements which the heirs made after their father's death (before division). Arakh. VI, 1 (21ᵇ) שום הי׳ the assessment for public sale of minors' (heirs') property which the court sells to satisfy the decedent's creditors. Gitt. V, 1; a. fr.—Yeb. XIII, 7 שתי אחיות י׳ two orphan sisters; a. fr.

יָתוֹם, יְתוֹמָא ch. same. Targ. Y. Ex. XXII, 21 (O. יַתַּם).—*Pl.* יְתוֹמֵי. Targ. Job XXII, 9.—*Fem.* יְתוֹמְתָּא. Lev. R. s. 37 (some ed. יְתִימְתָּא).—V. יַתַּם.

יִתּוּר, יִיתּוּר m. (יָתַר) *addition*. י׳ בגדים putting on more than the prescribed number of priestly garments (v. Yoma VII, 5). Zeb. 19ª; Erub. 103ᵇ.

יְתוּרָא ch. same, *superfluousness*.—*Pl.* constr. יְתוּרֵי. Hull. 36ª מי׳ קראי קאמר he derives it from the superfluous verses.

יַתּוּשׁ m. (fr. חָשַׁשׁ ?) 1) *mosquito* or *gnat*. Gitt. 56ᵇ בא י׳ ונכנס וכ׳ a mosquito came and entered his (Titus') nose; Gen. R. s. 10; Lev. R. s. 22. Sabb. 77ᵇ י׳ לְנָחָשׁ the mosquito (an application of a pulp made of mosquitos) is a remedy for a serpent's bite. Ib. אימת י׳ על הפיל the fear which the elephant has of the *yattush*, v. אֵימָה. Snh. 38ª; Lev. R. s. 14, beg. י׳ קדמך וכ׳ the *y.* has been created before thee (man); a. e.—*Pl.* יַתּוּשִׁים, יַתּוּשִׁין. Gen. R. s. 5 (ref. to Gen. III, 17) דברים ארורים כגון י׳ ופרעושין וכ׳ cursed things like gnats, fleas and flies; a. fr.—Tosef. Sabb. XII (XIII), 4 זבובין וי׳; Y. ib. XIV, beg. 14ᵇ ותושין (corr. acc.), v. חָגָז.—2) *a bug (on a fruit)*. Sifra Sh'mini Par. 10, ch. XII; Hull. 67ᵇ; a. e., v. פְּלִים.

יַתּוּשָׁא, יַתּוּשָׁה ch. same. Gen. R. s. 10; Lev. R. s. 22.—*Pl.* יַתּוּשַׁיָּא, יַתּוּשִׁין. Ib. s. 19, beg. וצואה עבדה י׳ and the excrements produced gnats. Gen. R. s. 34, end, דלא יכלוניה י׳ (some ed. יַתּוּשַׁיָּה) lest the mosquitos bite it (on the head).

יָתֵי, v. אֲתָא.

יָתִיב, v. יָתֵב.

יָתִיב, v. יָתֵב.

יָתִיבְתָּא, י׳ f. *inhabited*, v. יָתֵב.

יְתֵידָה f., v. יָתֵד.

יָתֵין, v. אֲתָא.

יַתִּיךְ, יָתוּךְ m. (נְתַךְ) a sort of *thongs* used for seizing a hot pot; (oth. opin.) *a strainer* (cmp. Targ. Job X, 10). —*Pl.* יַתּוּ׳, יַתִּיבְן. Kel. XII, 3 ed. Dehr. יִיתּוֹ׳ (ed. יַתּוּ׳); Tosef. ib. B. Mets. II, 10, v. נָעַר II.

יְתִימְתָּא, v. יָתוֹם ch.

יַתִּין, v. אֲתָא.

יַתִּינָיא, v. וְתִינָיא.

יָתִיר, v. יָתַר.

יַתִּיר I, יַתִּירָא m., **יַתִּירָא, יַתִּירְתָּא, יְתִירָ׳** f. (יְתַר) *remaining over, too much, too many; extraordinary, especial.* Targ. O. Ex. XXVI, 12 (Y. מותרא). Ib. דיַתִּירָא (ed. Berl. דִיתְרָא, Y. יְתִירָא). Ib. 13.—Hull. 47ª חסיר או י׳ one lobe wanting or one too many. B. Mets. 93ᵇ, v. בִּרְתָא. Ib. נטירותא י׳ ed. (Ms. M. מעלייתא) a special watchfulness. M. Kat. 4ª טירחא יתירה איכא (read יתירא, v. Rabb. D. S. a.l. note 400) it requires great labor. Ib. 21ª מילתא י׳ something more than duty requires. B. Mets. 104ᵇ מילתא י׳ a disproportionate amount. Gitt. 64ᵇ ידא י׳ an additional hand (her own and her father's power of accepting the letter of divorce). B. Bath. 104ᵇ top [read: ואי איכא יתירא and if there is a surplus, v. מְלִיתָא.—B. Kam. 94ª תעזוב י׳ the superfluous verse containing תעזוב (Lev. XIX, 10, repeated ib. XXIII, 22); a. fr.—Esp. יתירתא *an additional lobe of the lungs.* Hull. 47ª.—*Pl.* יַתִּירִין, יַתִּירַיָּא, יַתִּירֵי; f. יַתִּירָתָא, יַתִּירָ׳. Targ. O. Num. III, 46.—B. Mets. 51ª בדמי י׳ at an extremely high price. Ruth R. to II, 14; Cant. R. to II, 9 ארבעין י׳ those forty five days more (Dan. XII, 11; 12). Ab. Zar. 9ᵇ sq. שית שנין י׳ .... ההוא שטרא a document which contained six years too many (was postdated by six years); a. fr.—*Adv.* יַתִּיר *more.* Targ. Ps. XIX, 11; a. e.—בְּיַתִּירְתָּא (=h. יותר מדאי) *beyond measure.* M. Kat. 27ᵇ הוה קא בכיא בי׳ (Ms. M. בתדירותא) she mourned unreasonably.

יַתִּיר II pr. n. pl. *Yattir,* v. מְחַרְתָּא.

יְתִירָא m. *cord,* v. יִתְרָא I.

יְתִירָה f. (יָתַר) *superfluity.* Gen. R. s. 10 שהן י׳ בעולם (better: יְתֵירִין, v. יָתַר a. יֶתֶר).

יְתֵירְתָּא, יַתִּירְתָּא, v. יַתִּיר.

***יתך**, Y. Ab. Zar. III, 43ᵇ, המיותכו׳, read: המתיך כוס (a tautography), v. נָתַךְ.

יָתַם, *Pi.* יִיתֵּם (denom. of יָתוֹם) *to make orphans, to cause bereavement.* Pes. 49ª מְיַיתֵּם את בניו Ms. M. (ed. גוזלין) will be forced to leave his children uprovided for; Yalk. Am. 545; v. אַלְמֵן. Yalk. Gen. 95.

Nithpa. נִתְיַיתֵּם *to become an orphan.* Keth. 44ᵇ נִתְיַיתְּמָה she lost her father.

יָתֵם, יַיתָּם, יַתְמָא ch.=h. יָתוֹם, Targ. O. Ex. XXII, 21 (ed. Amst. יִיתָּם; Y. יתום); a. e.—Y. Ab. Zar. II, 41ᵈ bot. דין די׳ וכ׳ the case of an orphan or a widow; Y. Sabb. I, 3ᶜ sq. דיינין די׳ (read דין). Keth. 54ª י׳ an orphan (figuratively for a hired laborer whom the employer provides with clothes, v. לָקִיט I); a. fr.—Ab. Zar. 24ᵇ מזמורא י׳ an *anonymous* or *titleless* psalm.—Trnsf. (as a friendly rebuke) *ignorant child!* Keth. 17ᵇ; Ab. Zar. 13ᵇ; Hull. 111ᵇ.—*Pl.* יַתְמִין, יַתְמֵי, יַתְמַיָּא. Targ. Ex. XXII, 23; a. fr.—Ber. 18ᵇ זוזי די׳ heirs' fund. Y. Shek. IV, 48ª bot., a. e., מדל די׳, v. מְדַל. B. Mets. 108ª; B. Bath. 8ª אפי׳ מְיַ׳ even orphans' funds must be taxed, v. אַגְלָא. Y. Sot. III, 19ª אתון י׳ וכ׳ the heirs came complaining; a. v. fr.—Keth. 106ª קרו לנפשיהו י׳ they (the surviving scholars) called themselves orphans; י׳ די׳ orphans of orphans (few survivors).

יתניא, v. וְתִינָיא.

יָתַר (b. h.; cmp. עתר, אשר) [*to be strong;* denom. יֶתֶר *cord,* v. יִתְרָא I,] *to be rich, plentiful.*

Nif. נוֹתַר *to be left over.*—Part. נוֹתָר m. *portions of sacrifices left over beyond the legal time and bound to be burnt.* Kerith. III, 4 והיה נ׳ מן וכ׳ and it was an overdue remnant of sacrifices. Ib. I, 1 דם נ׳ blood of overdue sacrifices. Meil. I, 3, a. fr. משום נ׳ as coming under the law of *nothar;* a. v. fr.—*Pl.* נוֹתָרִים, נוֹתָרוֹת. Sifré Aḥaré Par. 5, ch. VII.—Cant. R. to V, 14 כמה נ׳ how many laws about *nothar.* Num. R. s. 11 שלא לפסול...בנ׳ not to unfit any of the sacrifices by allowing them to become overdue.

Hif. a) הוֹתִיר *to leave over; to go beyond; to be more.* Mekh. Bo s. 6 אם ה׳ if he left a part of the Passover lamb over until morning. Sifra Tsav, Par. 7, ch. XII אם ה׳ ה׳ if he has left over, he has left over (and it may be eaten). Ib. אם הותירו כולו if they left the whole of it over (for the second day); a. fr.—Ber. 34ᵇ לא חסרתם ולא הוֹתַרְתֶּם you stated the time neither too early nor too late. B. Bath. VII, 2 ה׳ כל שהוא if it was somewhat more (than the stated measure).—b) הִתִּיר (cmp. הִצִּיק fr. יָצַק), v. infra.

Pi. יִיתֵּר (denom. of יֶתֶר) *to add; to do too much.* Erub. 13ª שמא אתה ... מְיַיתֵּר for if thou omit one letter or write one too many; Sot. 20ª הַתִּיר *Hif.* (v. supra). Ex. R. s. 27; Tanh. Yithro 4 his name was Jether (Jethro) שֶׁיִּ׳ פרשה וכ׳ because he gave rise to an additional chapter (about judges) in the Law; Mekh. ib., Amalek, s. 1 שהותיר.—Ib. שיי׳ במעשים טובים because he did more (than ordinary men, was liberal in) good deeds. [Y. Keth. IV, end, 29ᵇ ויותר, v. וָתַר.]—*Part. pass.* מְיוּתָּר, *pl.* מְיוּתָּרִין *added, superfluous.* Koh. R. to V, 8 (ref. to ויתרון, ib.) דברים שתראה (ש)הן מי׳ לתורה (not בתורה) things which thou wouldst regard as additions to the Law. Ib. אפי׳ דברים...מי׳ בעולם even things in nature which thou wouldst believe to be superfluous (useless); Ex. R. s. 10; (Gen. R. s. 10 יְתֵירָה); a. e.

Nittaf. נִתּוֹתַר *to be left over.* Yoma 46ª איברי עולה שנתותרו parts of a burnt-offering which remained over (failed to be entirely burnt). Pes. 59ᵇ כשנִיתּוֹתְרוּ when they were left over (unoffered).

יְתַר ch. same. [Targ. Ruth II, 16, a. e. מיתר, v. נְתַר.]

Af. אַיְיתַר, אוֹתִיר 1) *to leave over.* Targ. II Kings IV, 43; a. e.—Y. Peah VII, 20ª bot. ואַיְיתְרוּן.—2) *to bless with plenty.* Targ. O. Deut. XXVIII, 11; XXX, 9.

Pa. יַיתַּר, as preced. *Pi.*—*Part. pass.* מְיַיתַּר, f. מְיַיתְּרָא *larger.* Meg. 19ª מחסרא או מיי׳ smaller in size or larger.

Ithpa. אִיתַּר, אִיַּיתַּר 1) *to be left over;* (in legal interpret.) *to be superfluous* in the Bible text and **therefore** *available for interpretation.* Targ. O. Ex. XXXVI, 7 וְיִתְּרַת (=ואית׳, ed. Berl. וְיִתְּרַת, corr. acc.).—Ber. 35ᵃ, v. הִילּוּל. Men. 93ᵃ אַיְיתְּרוּ ליה תרי קראי two verses remain for interpretation; Arakh. 2ᵇ אייתרי לחו תרי (v. Rabb. D. S. to Men. l. c. note).—*2) *to be added, included.* Sabb. 64ᵃ אִיַּיתּוּר ליה (some ed. אייתר) they are now included (Ms. M. אייתי they include it, v. אָתָא).

יָתִיר, יַתִּיר m. (preced. wds.) 1) *additional, a person having an additional limb.* Bekh. VII, 6 י׳ בידיו וכ׳ if one has an additional finger (or toe) on each of his hands and feet. Ib. 45ᵇ.—Ib. 40ᵃ חסר וי׳ ביד having one toe less or one too many on the forefoot. Ib. כל יתיר כנטול דמי every addition is considered equal to the entire absence of the respective limb; Hull. 58ᵇ כל יתר וכ׳. B. Bath. VII, 2, sq. חן י׳ (יתיר a. יתר interchanging), v. חֵן; a. fr.—*Fem.* יְתֵירָה, יְתֵרָה; (as noun also) יְתֶרֶת, יֹתֶרֶת. Bekh. VII, 6 (45ᵃ) היתה (בה) בו יתרת וכ׳ (Rashi יתירה; Gem. יתירת) if there has been an additional limb and he had it cut off. Ib. 40ᵃ י׳ על של משה וכ׳ (a cubit measure) larger than the Mosaic by &c. Hull. III, 6 (as a sign of clean birds) כל שיש לו אצבע י׳ that which has an additional toe (on top of those in a line). Keth. 76ᵃ יתירת a woman having an additional limb. Erub. 83ᵃ י׳ על מדבריה וכ׳ one sixth larger than &c.; a. fr. [V. יְתֵירָה.]—*Pl.* יַתִּירִין, יְתֵרִים, יַתִּירֵי; f. יְתֵירוֹת. Macc. 23ᵃ יַתִּירֵי מדע men of more than ordinary knowledge; י׳ כח of more than common physical strength.—[Gen. R. s. 98 הניחו יתירות left remants of the conquered nations, prob. to be read: יְתֵידוֹת, v. יָתֵד.]—Esp. יֹתֶרֶת *an additional lobe of the lungs.* Hull. 47ᵃ (not יות׳).—2) *a word written plene, with vowel letters.*—*Pl.* יְתֵירוֹת. Erub. 13ᵃ, a. e., v. חָסֵר II.

יֶתֶר I m. (b. h., v. יָתַר) 1) *cord, bow-string.* Lev. R. s. 5 (ref. to Ps. XI, 2), v. מִיתְּתָא.—2) =יוֹתֵר *addition,* (adv.) *more.* Bekh. VII, 1 (43ᵃ) וי׳ עליהן וכ׳ Bab. ed. (Mish. ויותר עליהן באדם וכ׳) to these must be added, with reference to blemishes of human beings, the wedge-shaped head &c. Erub. 83ᵇ י׳ על כן more than that. Gitt. III, 1 י׳ מכן nay, even more; a. fr.

יֶתֶר II (b. h.) pr. n. m. *Jether,* v. יִתְרוֹ a. יִתְרָא II.

יַתְרָא, יִת׳ I m. ch. = h. יֶתֶר I, 1, *strong cord,* esp. 1) *the cord of the bow.* Snh. 42ᵃ למיהוי כי י׳ (some ed. יְתִירָא) until the shape of the moon is like that of the cord (with the bent bow, semicircular).—*Pl.* יַתְרֵי (יַתִּירֵי). M. Kat. 26ᵃ לקל י׳ דמזיגת וכ׳ from the sound of the cords (of the catapults) at M. (v. מְגִיזָה) the wall of Laodicea burst.—2) *rope.*—*Pl.* יַתְרַיָּא, יַתְרִין. Targ. Jud. XVI, 7; 8; 9. 3) *the straight side of the stomach,* opp. to קשתא the curved side, v. הֵימְצָא. Hull. 50ᵃ דְּאַיְּיתְרָא the fat covering &c. Pes. 51ᵃ אכל דאיי׳ (Ms. M. דיי׳) ate the fat &c.—[Targ. Prov. XXV, 20 יתרא Ms. (Var. ed. Lag.), ed. נִתְרָא.]

יִתְרָא II (b. h.) pr. n. m. *Ithra* (*Jether*) the Israelite (the Ishmaelite), father of Amasa. Ruth. R. to I, 21; Y. Yeb. VIII, 9ᶜ top (ואליתר הישמעאלי); Midr. Till. to Ps. IX.

יִתְרָה, יֹתֶרֶת, v. יָתֵר.

יִתְרוֹ (b. h.) pr. n. m. *Jethro,* the father-in-law of Moses. Ber. 63ᵇ. Ex. R. s. 27 יֶתֶר כשהוא גוי . . . . ונקרא י׳ as a heathen he was named Jether, and when he was converted . . . he was named J.—Zeb. 116ᵃ י׳ קודם מ״ת וכ׳ the arrival of J. (Ex. XVIII) took place before the giving of the Law; Ab. Zar. 24ᵃ; a. v. fr.

יִתְרוֹן m. (b. h.; יָתַר) 1) *surplus, difference.* Koh. R. to II, 13 כשם שיש י׳ בין וכ׳ as there is a difference between light &c.—2) *addition.* Lev. R. s. 22 (ref. to Koh. V, 8) אפי׳ דברים . . . . י׳ למ״ת even what thou deemest to be an addition to the original Law (Koh. R. to V, 8, a. e. מיותרין).—3) *superfluity, useless thing.* Ib. אפי׳ . . י׳ בעולם even what thou mightest deem to be mere useless creatures (Koh. R. to V, 8, a. e. מיותרין), v. יָתַר.

יִתְרָן, v. יוֹתְרָן.

יַתֶּרֶת, v. יָרֵד.

כ

כ, ך *Kaf,* the eleventh letter of the Alphabet. It interchanges with ג q. v.; with ק, e. g. כּוֹבַע a. קוֹבַע; with ח, cmp. כבש a. חבש a. derivatives.

כ׳, as a numeral letter, *twenty.*

כְּ־, כִּי־, כִּי־ prefix, h. a. ch. (v. כֵּן) 1) *as, like.* Targ. Gen. IX, 3. Targ. Hos. IV, 9; a. v. fr.—Ber. I, 2 כאדם וכ׳ like one reading in the Torah. Ib. 3 כדרכו as usual; a. v. fr.—*2) *whereas.* Tosef. Snh. II, 6 כגוזליא . . . וכאימריא וכ׳ ed. Zuck. (Var. דגוזליא . . . ואמריא, as Snh. 11ᵃ, Y. ib. I, 18ᵈ top) whereas the spring pigeons are yet tender &c.—[Ib. 5 בגוזליא וכ׳.]—[Compound particles כְּדֵי, כְּבָת &c., v. s. vv. or second component.—ך as affix, frequ. indicating place (כ *locale*) or instrument, as בְּנָך, דוּך, אוּשְׁפִּיזְכָּא &c.]

כָּא, כָּה ch. (b. h. כֹּה, v. preced.) adverb of place: *here,* v. הָכָא; of time: *now.* Targ. Gen. XXII, 5. Targ. Job XXXVIII, 11; a. fr.—Y. Ber. IV, 7ᶜ top וכא אמר הכין and here he says so? Ib. וכה; a. v. fr.—לְכָא *hither;* מִיכָּא *from here.* Targ. Josh. VIII, 20. Targ. Ex. XVII, 12; a. fr.—Y. Bets. V, 63ᵃ פצל . . לכא ולכא skimmed the water in both directions. Y. B. Mets. VI, 11ᵃ top מיכא ללוד from here to Lydda; a. fr.—V. אִיכָּא, לִיכָּא &c.; כָּאן, כַּן &c.

כָּאֵב (b. h.) *to be heavy, to feel pain.* Y. Sabb. IX, 12ª ib. XIX, 17ª bot. (ref. to Gen. XXXIV, 25) בהיותו כּוֹאֵב ... כל איבריהם כּוֹאֲבִים עליהם it does not say, 'when it (the wound) was painful', but ...., which intimates that all their limbs pained them.

Hif. הִכְאִיב *to cause pain, grief.* Ex. R. s. 3 (ref. to Ex. III, 7) ידעתי ... לְהַכְאִיבֵנִי וכ׳ I know how much they will grieve me &c. Pirké d'R. El. ch. XII שלא לְהַכְאִיבוֹ so as to make him feel no pain. Midr. Till. to Ps. XCIV (ref. to Prov. III, 12) שמַּכְאִיבוֹ ... א״ת וּכְאָב אלא וּכְאֵב read not *ukh'ab* (and like a father) but *ukh'eb* (and pain), when He sends him pain.

כְּאֵב I, **כְּאֵיב**, **כֵּיב** ch. same. Targ. Prov. XIV, 13. —Part. כָּאֵב, כָּאֵיב, כָּיֵיב. Targ. Job XIV, 22. Targ. Ps. LXIX, 30; a. fr. — Targ. Jer. IV, 19 כֵּיבִין (ed. Lag. כָּיְיבָן). — B. Kam. 46ᵇ מאן דכאיב ליה כאיבא וכ׳ Ms. F. (v. Rabb. D. S. a. l. note, Ms. H. כיבא) he who feels sick, goes to the physician. Ib. 85ᵇ הוה כ׳ ליה מידי וסליק ואיתיב וכ׳ Ms. M. (ed. ואייתי) he had a sore and it was going away, and one put on a corrodent drug for him &c., v. חֲוַר. Gitt. 68ᵇ כָּיֵיב; a. fr.—B. Kam. 35ª כיבין, v. חִיוְרֵי.

Pa. כַּיֵּיב, כָּאֵב *to cause pain, wound, grieve.* Lam. R. to II, 1 translating יעיב, ib.) איך כ׳ וכ׳ how did the Lord wound &c., v. כֵּיבָא.

כְּאֵב II m. (b. h.; preced.) 1) *heaviness, pain.* Ber. 55ª כ׳ לב heaviness of heart (fretfulness). Gen. R. s. 67, end כ׳ על כ׳ grief added to grief; a. e. — 2) *grievous offence.* Deut. R. s. 3 (ref. to מכאביו, Ex. III, 7) יודע אני מה כ׳ וכ׳ I know what grievous offence they are going to commit, v. כְּאַב.

כְּאֵיבָא, **כְּאֵבָא** ch. 1) same. Targ. Prov. X, 10. Targ. Is. LXV, 14.—[Targ. Job XXXI, 18 כְּאֵבָא Ms. (ed. הֵיךְ כְּאַבָּא.] —B. Kam. 46ᵇ, v. כְּאֵב I; a. e.—2) *sick, sufferer.* Targ. Ps. LXIX, 30; a. fr.—*Pl.* כְּאֵבִין, כְּאֵבַיָּא, כְּאֵבַיָּא, כֵּי׳, כְּאֵי׳. Targ. Ez. XXXIV, 4. [Targ. Jer. IV, 19, v. כְּאֵב I.]—V. כֵּיבָא.

כאגני, v. בְּאַגְנָא.

כְּאַוְותָא, v. כַּתָּא.

כָּאוּר, v. כָּעַר.

לִכְאוֹ׳, כְּאוֹרָה, v. אוֹרָה I.

כְּאוֹרֶת, v. כְּוֹרֶת.

כְּ׳ צַד, כְּאִי, v. כֵּיצַד.

כְּאֵיבָא, v. כְּאֵבָא.

כָּאִיל, part. of כִּיל.

כָּאִיף, part. of כּוּף.

כְּאֵיצַד, v. כֵּיצַד.

כָּאלֵי, כָּאלָא, part. of כְּלָא, כְּלֵי I.

כאלירקין, Sifré Deut. 317, some ed., read: כְּלִיאַרְקִין, v. כלורכין.

כאמי, v. באמי.

כָּאן (v. כָּא) *here; now.* Y. Ber. IV, 7ᶜ bot., a. e. כ׳ נתפלל וכ׳ here (in this inn) did my father say the prayer of &c. Bets. IV, 7 מִכָּ׳ ועד כ׳ from here to there (will I use). Ber. I, 2, a. fr. מכ׳ ואילך, v. אֵילָךְ. Snh. IX, 1 ולאחר מכ׳ and subsequently; a. fr. — (חכמים) מכ׳ אמרו from this originates what the scholars said. Ab. I, 5; a. fr.—מִכָּ׳ ל־, מִכָּ׳ ש־ from this is derived, do we learn. Ber. 64ª מכ׳ לבעל וכ׳ from this (that Jacob is mentioned and not his ancestors) we learn that the owner of the beam must carry the heaviest side of it. B. Mets. 87ª מכ׳ שצדיקים אומרים וכ׳ from this we see that the righteous promise little &c.; a. fr.—כ׳ ... כ׳ here (in this case) ..., there (in another place, in that case). Succ. 44ᵇ; a. v. fr.—Contr. כַּן, with pref. מ׳, מִיכַּן. Y. Ber. IV, 7ᶜ top [read:] כן ליחיד כן לציבור in this case (when Levi disfavored many prayers), it is meant for individuals, in the other case, it is meant for congregations. — Y. Erub. VII, 24ᵇ bot. מ׳ ומ׳ on both sides; a. fr.

כָּאר m. (Pers. *khar*, *ḥar*) *ass.* Snh. 98ª, v. חֲזָר.

כָּאַר, v. כָּעַר.

כַּבָּא, m. (v. כָּבַב) *ball, excrement* (cmp. גָּלָל). Zeb. 113ᵇ, v. כפותא.

כַּבָּא, v. כּוּבָּא.

כבאי, כביי, v. כַּבַּי.

כְּבָאסָא, v. כְּבָסָא.

***כָּבַב** *to be thick, hollow, arched.*— Denom. כַּבָּא, כּוּבָּא.

Pa. כַּבֵּיב (denom. of כּוּבָּא, v. Fl. to Levy Targ. Dict. I, 427ᵇ) *to burn thorns, to char.* Erub. 29ᵇ וניכַבְּבֵיה and let him char it (the meat; Rashi: let him *roast it over the charred thorns*; v. כּוּבָּא).

כַּבְּבָא m. (preced.) *burning to coals, charring.* Zeb. 46ᵇ לאפוקי כ׳ (Ms. M. בטבא, some ed. חטבא) to exclude charring the meat (instead of burning it to ashes); Yalk. Lev. 445 כבתה (corr. acc.).—V. כּוּבָּא.

כָּבֵד I (b. h.) *to be heavy, weighty, important*; cmp. יָקַר.

Pi. כִּבֵּד, כִּיבֵּ׳ 1) *to honor, hold precious; to show honor.* Ab. IV, 1 איזהו מכובד המְכַבֵּד וכ׳ who will be honored? He who honors men. Sabb. 113ᵇ ר״י קרי למאניה מְכַבְּדוֹתַי Rabbi Joh. called his garments 'my honorers'; B. Kam. 91ᵇ; Snh. 94ª; a. fr. — Ber. 46ᵇ bot. אין מְכַבְּדִין וכ׳ we must not show honors (saying, 'you go first') on high-roads &c. Part. pass. מְכוּבָּד, *pl.* מְכוּבָּדִים, מְכוּבָּדִין. Ab. l. c., v. supra. Ib. 6 כל המכבד ... גופו מ׳ על וכ׳ he who honors the Law, will himself be honored of men. Ber. 60ᵇ, v. infra. Ab. Zar. III, 3, v. בָּזָה; a. fr. — 2) (cmp. יְקַר, אִיקְרָא) *to offer a gift.* Tanḥ. Vayḥi 13 שמְכַבְּדִין מפירותיהם וכ׳ they offer of their fruits to kings; Gen. R. s. 99, end והם מכברין (corr. acc.); a. e. — 3) [*to make look respectable,*] *to sweep, adjust the room.* Ber. VIII, 4 מכבדין את הבית וכ׳ (after meal) the room is put in order (the crumbs swept), and then &c. Bets. II, 7 (22ᵇ) מכבדין בין המטות (Bab. ed. בית המטות) (on Holy Days) you may sweep between the dining couches (the dining room); Y.

b. II, 61[c] bot. Tam. V, 5 היה מְכַבְּדָן לאמה one swept them (the coals) into the duct; a. fr.—Mikv. VIII, 4 כִּיבְּדָה את, הבית, v. בַּיִת 6.—[Ruth R. end וכבר some ed., read: וְכָבֵר.]

Hithpa. הִתְכַּבֵּד, *Nithpa.* נִתְכַּבֵּד *to be honored; to pride, exalt one's self.* Gen. R. s. 1 כל המִתְכַּבֵּד בקלון וכ׳ whoever elevates himself at the expense of his neighbor's degradation, has no share in the world to come; Y. Hag. II, 77[c]. Meg. 28[a] מימי לא נִתְכַּבַּדְתִּי וכ׳ I never elevated myself &c. Ber. 60[b] הִתְכַּבְּדוּ מְכּוּבָּדִים be in honor dismissed, you honored ones (angels); a. e.—2) *to be cleaned, swept; to be dressed, adorned.* Pes. 7[a] שוקי . . . עשויין לִהתכ׳ וכ׳ the streets of Jerusalem used to be swept every day. Y. Nidd. I, beg. 48[d] כמבוי שהוא מתכבד וכ׳ like an alley which is regularly swept and flushed. Bab. ib. 56[a] חזקתו מתכבד it is presumed to be clean. Num. R. s. 13 לאכול ולשתות ולהתכבד to eat and drink and dress. [Tosef. Ter. X, 15 ליכבד, read with ed. Zuck. ליכבר, v. כָּבַר.]

Hif. הִכְבִּיד 1) *to be heavy.* Naz. I, 2 ה׳ שערו if his hair is too heavy on him.—2) *to make heavy.* Ex. R. s. 9; Tanh. Vaera 12 (play on כָּבֵד, Ex. VII, 14, a. הִכְבַּדְתִּי XIV, 18) בלשון (כבד) שהִכְבַּדְתָּ בו בלשון אני מתכבד with the same expression with which thou didst make heavy (Israel's yoke), I shall be honored; Tanh. ed. Bub. ib. 14 שהכבדת את לבך wherewith thou didst harden thy heart.—3) *to grow worse, be very sick* (cmp. בָּיַן II), opp. הֵיקֵל. Snh. IX, 1 ה׳ ומת grew worse and died; ib. 78[b]; a. e.—4) *to sweep.* Num. R. s. 23; Tanh. Mas'ê 13 הִכְבִּידָן he swept (drove) them out, v. כַּבֵּד a. חָמַם.

כְּבַד ch. same; *Pa.* כַּבֵּיד *to clean, sweep.* Nidd. 56[a] bot. (כַּבְּדִי=) כַּבֵּיד ולא בדיק I swept (the alley) but did not search (for unclean objects).

Ithpa. אִתְכַּבַּד *to be swept.* Ib. 56[b] גומה לא מתכבדא a cavity is not swept (the broom does not strike it).

Af. אַכְבֵּיד (v. כָּבֵד III) *to irritate, grieve.* Targ. Prov. XVII, 25 ed. Lag. (ed. Ven. מכביר, Ms. מַכְבִּיר, h. text כעס).

כֹּבֵד, v. כּוֹבֶד.

כָּבֵד II m. (preced. wds.) 1) *weight, pressure.* Hag. 21[a] כְּבִידוֹ של כלי the pressure of the (inner) vessel. Snh. 63[b]; Meg. 25[b] (sarcasm on כבודו, Hos. X, 5) א״ת כְּבוֹדוֹ אלא כְּבֵידוֹ (Ms. M. כּוֹבְדוֹ) read not 'his dignity' but 'his weight' for it is gone, i. e. the idol's weight is reduced; Yalk. Is. 326 כְּבֵדוֹ.—2) *importance,* v. כָּבוֹד.

כָּבֵד III c. (b. h.; preced. wds.) [*heaviness, seat of anger and melancholy.*] *liver.* Ber. 61[b] top כ׳ כועס ומרה וכ׳ the liver is excited, and the gall pours a drop over it and quiets it. Hull. III, 1 ניטל הכ׳; ib. 2 ניטלה הכ׳ if the liver of an animal is gone. Arakh. V, 2 (20[a]) ערך כְּבֵדִי עלי (Bab. ed. כְּבֵדִי) I vow the value of my liver (being a vital organ); a. fr.

כַּבְדָא ch. same. Targ. Ex. XXIX, 13; 22. Targ. Lam. II, 11; a. e.—Hull. 109[b]; a. fr.—Koh. R. to XII, 7; Lam. R. introd. (R. Josh. 2) וחמי בכבדיה, v. אִימַר.

כָּבָה, v. כבי.

כָּבוֹד m. (b. h.; כָּבֵד) 1) *importance.* Arakh. 18[a] ולידון בִּכְבוֹדוֹ (Ar. בכבידו) and that the value of a limb be judged according to its importance (vitality); ib. 4[b]; B. Mets. 114[a].—2) *honor, respect; dignity.* Ber. 19[b], a. e., v. חֵלֶק. Ib. משום כְּבוֹד מלכים on account of the respect due to royalty. Ib.; Men. 37[b] גדול כְּ׳ הבריות וכ׳ human dignity (in proper appearance) is very important, for it may even suspend a Biblical law. Ber. l. c. ואינו לפי כְּבוֹדוֹ and it is not becoming his dignity (to drive an ass). Sot. 13[a] הניחו לו כְּבוֹדוֹ במלכים יותר וכ׳ let him alone, the honor shown to him (Jacob) by princes is higher than that by private men. Ib. נהגו בהן כ׳ they treated them with respect. Ned. 39[b] בִּכְבוֹדִי לא מחיתם בכ׳ וכ׳ as long as My honor was concerned, you did not interfere, and when the honor of a human being is at stake &c. Ab. IV, 12 יהי כְּ׳ תלמידך וכ׳ let the honor of thy pupil be as dear to thee as thine own, and thy fellow student's honor as that of thy teacher; a. v. fr.—כסא הכ׳, v. כִּסֵּא. מחל על כבודו *to forego due honors,* v. מָחַל.

כִּבּוּר, כִּבּוּד, v. sub כִּיב׳.

כְּבוּיָא* m. (כבי, v. כָּבָא) *heap, excrement.*—*Pl.* כְּבוּיֵי. Erub. 29[b] bot. כ׳ דרעיתא דניסן (Ms. M. כְּפוּיֵי דרעיא) excrements of cattle cast in Nisan. V. כְּבוּתָא.

כָּבוּל I (b. h.) pr. n. *Cabul,* 1) אֶרֶץ כ׳ a district in Northern Palestine presented by Solomon to Hiram, king of Tyre. Sabb. 54[a], v. כַּבְלָא, כָּבַל, כֶּבֶל.—2) *Cabul, (Kābūl,)* a place south-east of Accho. Tosef. M. Kat. II, 15; Tosef. Sabb. VII (VIII), 17; Y. Pes. IV, 30[d] top; Bab. ib. 51[a].

כָּבוּל II m. (כָּבַל) 1) (cmp. אִיסְטְמָא) *hair-net,* a cap worn under the head-dress. Sabb. VI, 1; 5.—Y. ib. 7[d] ולא בכבולה נבוסה, read: ולא בכ׳ שבכה 'and not in a *Kabul*' (Mish. l. c.), that is a hair-net. Bab. ib. 57[b] כ׳ זה איני יודע אי וכ׳ this *Kabul* (Mish. l. c.) I do not know whether it means a slave's chain &c.—2) *chain.*—*Pl.* כְּבוּלִין *chain-works* for drawing water. Tosef. Mikv. IV, 2.

כְּבוּנָא, v. כְּבִינָא.

כִּבּוּס, v. כִּיבּוּס.

כְּבוּסָה, v. כְּבִיסָה.

כבוסין, Targ. Ps. LVIII, 10 Ms., read: כְּבוּסְרִין, v. בּוּסְרָא.

כִּבּוּשׁ, v. כִּיבּוּשׁ.

כָּבָה, כבי (כָּבָא) (b. h.; cmp. כאב) *to grow dim, to be extinguished, go out.* Sabb. 21[a] כָּבְתָה זקוק לה if the Hănuckah light went out, he is bound to attend to it. Y. Yoma II, 39[d] קטורת שֶׁכָּבְתָה frankincense which went out (was not entirely burnt). Sabb. 30[b] טוב תִּכְבֶּה נר וכ׳ it is better that a human light (candle) be extinguished, than that God's light (life) be extinguished; a. fr.

Pi. כִּיבָּה, כִּבָּה (כִּיבָא) *to extinguish.* Ib.[a] לא יְכַבֶּה ואם כִּבָּה פטור he must not put it out, but if he did &c. Ib. II, 5

הַמְכַבֶּה את הנר he who puts the (Sabbath) lamp out. Gen. R. s. 68 (play on כי בא, Gen. XXVIII, 11) כִּיבָּא השמש (some ed. כיבה) He extinguished the sun (made the sun set earlier). Tosef. Sabb. XIII (XIV), 9 נכרי שבא לְכַבּוֹת אין אומ׳ לו כַּבֵּה ואל תְּכַבֶּה if a gentile comes (on the Sabbath) to extinguish (a fire), we say to him neither 'extinguish' nor 'do not'. Gen. R. l. c. אמר המלך כַּבּוּ וכ׳ (not כיבו) said the king, put out &c.; a. fr.

כְּבָא, כְּבִי ch. same. [Sabb. 21^b כבתה; ib. 30^a לִכבות, h. forms.]

Pa. כַּבֵּי *to extinguish.* Ber. 58^a וְכַבְּיִנְהוּ לעיניה Ar. (Ms. M. וכבינהו, corr. acc.; ed. חברוהי כחלינהו וכ׳) dimmed his eye-sight, v. בּוֹטְנָא. Ib. 60^b bot. אתא.. כַּבְּיֵיה לשרגיה there came a wind and put out his lamp. Sabb. 44^a אתי לְכַבּוּיֵי he may be induced to extinguish the fire; Yoma 85^a.

כְּבֵיד, v. כָּבֵד I, II.

כְּבִינָא (Ar. כְּבוּנָא) f. (part. pass. of כבן)=h. רחל הכבונה (v. כָּבַן) *a sheep wearing a wrap, fine sheep.* Targ. Ez. XXVII, 18 (cmp. Shebu. 6^b, s. v. כָּבַן).

כְּבִינָה f. (כָּבַן) *brooch* or *buckle.* B. Bath. IX, 7 תנו כְּבִינָתִי וכ׳ give my brooch to my daughter.

כְּבִינְתָא f., pl. כְּבִינָתָא (Ar. כברינתיא) (v. preced. wds.) *a garment pinned or buckled on.* Targ. Is. III, 23 (h. text רדידים; cmp. περόνημα).

כְּבִיסָה f. (כָּבַס) 1) *washing.* Y. Shebi. VIII, 38^b, top כְּבִיסָתָן וחיי אחרים וכ׳ as between the use of the spring for their (the inhabitants') washing purposes and for strangers' living (drinking purposes); a. fr.—[Mikv. VIII, 1, v. כְּבִישָׁה.]—2) (also כְּבוּסָה) *water mixed with alkaline substances, lye-water* &c. Tosef. Shebi. VI, 25 פירות שביעית . . . המשרה ולא לתוך הכ׳ produces of the Sabbath year must not be used for an infusion nor for preparing lye-water; Succ. 40^a; B. Kam. 102^a; Y. Shebi. l. c.—*Pl.* כְּבִיסוֹת. Ib. VII, beg. 37^b מיני כ׳ (ed. Krot. כנרס׳, corr. acc.) alkaline plants.

כְּבִישׁ, v. כָּבַשׁ.

כְּבִישׁ m., **כְּבִישָׁא**, **כְּבִישְׁתָּא** f. (כְּבַשׁ) 1) *stepping stool* (scamnum). Targ. Ps. CX, 1 (h. text הֲדֹם), v. כְּבַשׁ II. —2) *paved path.* Ib. LXXVIII, 50 (h. text נתיב).—Targ. I Sam. VI, 12, a. e. (h. text מסלה), v. כְּבַשׁ II. Targ. II Sam. XX, 12 כבישתא ed. Lag. (oth. ed. כְּבִשָּׁא).—*Pl.* כְּבִישִׁין. Targ. Is. XL, 3 ed. Lag. (oth. ed. כְּבָשִׁין); a. e.—3) *recess, secret.* Targ. Lam. III, 10 (h. text מסתרים).—*Pl.* כְּבִישֵׁי. Ber. 10^a bot. בהדי כ׳ דרחמנא וכ׳ Ar. (ed. כִּבְשֵׁי) what hast thou to do with the secret ways of the Lord?

כְּבִישָׁה f. (כָּבַשׁ) *making a path, side-path.* Mikv. VIII, 1 מפני הכ׳ Ar. on account of the passing by (of travellers that leave the highway for some cause). [Ed. מפני הכְּבִיסָה on account of the ponds being used for washing clothes, v. comment.]

כבישן, Gen. R. s. 66, v. כִּיבּוּשׁ h.

כְּבִישְׁתָּא, v. כְּבִישׁ.

כַּבְכָּב (כַּפְכָּף) m. (reduplic. of כבב or כפף, v. כָּבַב) *an arched round vessel.* Kel. II, 3 כ׳ שעשאו לסל הפת a *kabkab* which was intended for a cover for the bread-basket (and not as a receptacle). Tosef. ib. B. Kam. II, 5 כסוי כ׳ וכסוי אלפס ed. Zuck. (ed. only כסוי אלפס) the lid of a *k.* and that of a pot. Ib. 8 העשוי לכך ולכך כגון הכ׳ וכ׳ R. S. to Kel. III, 1 (ed. Zuck. a. oth. כוכב) a vessel made for both purposes (for liquids and for solid food), e. g. the *k.*, the stew-pot &c.

כָּבַל [*to press, to impede,* whence כֶּבֶל *the foot-chain;* denom. כָּבַל] *to chain.* Gen. R. s. 87 כּוֹבַלְתָּךְ אני I have the power to put thee in chains. Tanh. Thazr. 8 מביא . . . . וכובלו he orders chains and chains him.—*Part. pass.* כָּבוּל, f. כְּבוּלָה, pl. כְּבוּלוֹת *tied, prevented,* esp. *sheep prevented from conceiving by having their tails tied down.* Sabb. V, 2 רחלות יוצאות . . . . כ׳ ewes may be led out (on the Sabbath) . . . tied up; Tosef. ib. IV (V), 1 כ׳ שלא יעלה עליהן זכר. Sabb. 54^a מאי כ׳ שכּוֹבְלִין אליה וכ׳ Ms. M. (ed. שמְכַבְּלִין) what is *k'buloth*? They tie their tails downward &c. Ib. מאי משמע דהאי כבול וכ׳ where is the evidence that *kabul* has the meaning of sterility? (Answ. ref. to I Kings IX, 13, v. next w.); Y. ib. V, 7^b bot.

Pi. כִּיבֵּל same, v. supra.—*Part. pass.* מְכוּבָּל. Sabb. l. c. the district was called Cabul, שהיו בה ב״א שמְכוּבָּלִין בכסף וכ׳ because there were people there who were chained with silver and gold.

כְּבַל ch. same, part. pass. כְּבִיל, f. כְּבִילָא *impeded, detained.* Targ. Koh. XII, 4 ריגלך כְּבִילָן וכ׳ thy feet are detained from going out &c. (h. text סגרו).

Pa. כַּבֵּל same; part. pass. מְכַבַּל, f. מְכַבְּלָא *tied up,* (cmp. עצר) *sterile.* Sabb. 54^a (ref. to I Kings IX, 13, v. preced.; v. חוּמְרָן) ואמרי אינשי ארעא כ׳ דלא עבדא פרי (Ms. O. מְכַבַּלְתָּא) and people say, it is a tied up land, which bears no fruits.

כֶּבֶל m. (b. h.; preced. wds.), pl. כְּבָלִים, כְּבָלִין *foot-chains, irons.* Gen. R. s. 91 ליתן עליהם כ׳ to put them in chains. Tanh. Thazr. 8, v. כָּבַל. Deut. R. s. 4 כ׳ של ברזל iron chains, opp. בוּנְיִיק של זהב. Tosef. Ab. Zar. II, 4 אין מוכרין . . . . ולא כ׳ (ed. Zuck. כִּיבְלִין) we must not sell them torturing blocks or irons.—Sabb. VI, 4 כ׳ טמאין וכ׳ a woman's *ankle-chains* are fit for levitical uncleanness &c. (contrad. to בירית). Y. ib. VI, 8^b, v. בִּירִית; Bab. ib. 63^b. Ib. עשו להן כ׳ וכ׳ they made for them ankle-bands and put a chain between, that their steps may not be wide; a. e.

כַּבְלָא ch. same. Sabb. 57^b כ׳ דעבדא a slave's neck-chain, v. כָּבוּל II. Ib. 58^a כ׳ דעבדא תנן the *Kabul* of the Mishnah means &c. Ib. 54^a (v. כָּבוּל I) it was named Cabul דמשתרגא בה כרעא עד כ׳ ed. (Ar. דמשתקעא) because the foot is entangled in (sinks into) the sandy soil up to the ankle-band; [oth. vers. in Ar. דמשתקעא כרעא בגווה כר כ׳ (read דמשתרגא) because the foot is entangled in it as if in a foot-chain.]—*Pl.* כַּבְלֵי, כַּבְלִין. Targ. Lam. III, 7. Targ. Ps. CXLIX, 8 (Ms. *sing*).

כָּבַן (cmp. כָּבַל) *to clasp, fasten.* Part. pass. כָּבוּן, f. כְּבוּנָה,

pl. כְּבוּנוֹת *clasped*, esp. *sheep wearing a clasped cover* (v. כְּבִינְתָא) for the protection of their wool. Sabb. V, 2; Tosef. ib. IV (V), 1 כ׳ למילת covered for the sake of the fine wool. Bab. ib. 54ª שמְּכַבְּנִין אותן למילת (not אותו).—V. כְּבִינָא.

Pi. כִּבֵּן *to clasp a wrap; to wrap up.* Sabb. l. c., v. supra. Ib. (defining צמר לבן נקי .... שמְּכַבְּנִין אותו (צמר לבן) למילת like the wool of a new-born lamb which they wrap up for the sake of the wool; Shebu. 6ᵇ שמכבנין אותו Ms. M. (ed. incorr. בו).

כְּבַן ch. same, *Pa.* כַּבֵּין *to fasten; to put on a* כְּבִינְתָא. Targ. Job XXIII, 9 (h. text יעטף). Ib. XXXI, 36 אֲכַבְּנִינֵיה Ms. Var. (ed. Lag. אֲכַרְפִּינֵיה, v. כְּרַף; oth. ed. אֲכַרְכְּנֵיה, v. כרב I; ed. Wil. אֲרַכְּבְנֵיה, v. רְכַב; h. text ענד).

כִּבְנָה, v. כְּבִינָה.

כָּבַס (b. h.) *to press, tread.*

Pi. כִּבֵּס *to wash* (clothes). M. Kat. III, 1 ואלו מְכַבְּסִין במועד and these are permitted to wash their clothes during the festive week. Taan. 29ᵇ; M. Kat. 18ª, a. e. מותר לְכַבְּסוֹ וכ׳ is permitted to wash it; a. fr.—Pesik. Eth Korb., p. 61ᵇ; Pesik. R. s. 16 (play on כבשים, Num. XXVIII, 3) שהם מְכַבְּסִים וכ׳ for they (as sacrifices) wash (cleanse) the sins of Israel.—Part. pass. מְכוּבָּס, f. מְכוּבֶּסֶת; pl. מְכוּבָּסִין, מְכוּבָּסוֹת. Mikv. X, 4 בגדים שהטבילן מכ׳ garments immersed while still wet from washing.

Hithpa. הִתְכַּבֵּס *to be washed.* Cant. R. to I, 5 (play on שלמה) [read:] מה שַׂלְמָה זו מתלכלכת ומִתְכַּבֶּסֶת וכ׳ as a garment is soiled and washed again &c.; Yalk. ib. 982. Tanh. Vayhi 10 (ref. to Gen. XLIX, 11) אם יטעו בהלכה תהא מתכבסת בתחומו וכ׳ when they err in a decision, it shall be cleansed (atoned for) in his (Judah's) dominion (the Temple); Gen. R. s. 99 (not מתכבסים).

כְּבַס, Targ. I Chr. XI, 5, sq., ed. Lag. a. oth., v. כְּבַשׁ.

***כֶּבֶס**, m. (preced.) *cleansing material.*—*Pl.* כְּבָסִים. Y'lamd. to Num. XXVIII, 3 quot. in Ar. s. v. כבשים (ref. to כבשים, ib.) אע״פ שכתוב כבשים אנו קורין כ׳ וכ׳ though it is written *K'basim* (with *Sin*, sheep), we read *K'basim* (with *Sammekh*), for they cleanse Israel's sins.

כּוּבְסָא, כַּבְסָא m. (כבס) *something pressed, ball, lump*, esp. 1) *cluster of dates.* Sabb. 67ª כמאן תלינן כבסא בדיקלא Ar. (ed. כּוּבְסֵי, Ms. O. כַּבְסֵי pl., v. Rabb. D. S. a. l. note 70) by what authority dare we suspend a cluster of dates on a sterile date-tree (and not consider it a forbidden superstitious practice)? Macc. 8ª ומחיוה לכ׳ (ed. לְכַבְּאסָא, Ms. M. a. Rashi לכיבסא) and it (the struck twig) struck the cluster.—2) (trnsf.) *testicles.* Shebu. 41ª האי לגלימיה הוא ... נקטיה בכּוּבְסֵיה that is "hold him by his testicles that he may give up his cloak', i. e. this is force worse than laying distress on his property; B. Mets. 101ᵇ.

כְּבָר I (b. h.) pr. n., נְהַר כ׳ *river* (or *channel*) *K'bar* (*Chebar*) in Babylonia. Gen. R. s. 16 הוא פרת הוא נ׳ כ׳ Euphrates and K. are the same. Ib. כ׳ בפני עצמו וכ׳ K. and Euphrates are different rivers. Ib. כ׳ שמימיו כלין it is called K'bar (v. next w.), because its waters give out; שפירותיו גסין ואינן יורדין בכברה because its fruits are large and go not into the basket; (Yalk. Gen. 22 שמימיו קָלִין).

כְּבָר II m. (b. h.; = זמן כבר; כבר *to be thick, strong, round*) *a long time since; long ago, already; once.* Sabb. 51ª, a. e. כ׳ הורה זקן it has already been decided by an authority. Ber. 63ª bot. כ׳ בנית וכ׳ you have once built and can no more tear down, (having once praised me, you cannot now censure me). Y. Sabb. XIV, 14ᶜ bot. וכ׳ חלה וכ׳ and once when he was taken sick, and &c. Num. R. s. 3, end כ׳ נקדתי עליהם have I not put dots upon them (to mark that the words are spurious)? [Ib. כ׳ אמחוק וכ׳, read: אוֹמַר I shall say, I will erase &c.]—Y. Gitt. VII, end, 49ª מִכּ׳ (*retroactively*) *at once*; a. fr.

כְּבַר I ch. same. Targ. Koh. I, 10. Targ. Jer. XXXVIII, 9 כ׳ מית he would have been dead by this time; a. fr.—B. Bath. 167ª, a. e. כ׳ קדמוך רבנן our rabbis have long preceded thee (have warned us before this); a. fr.

כָּבַר (denom. of כְּבָרָה) *to sift.* Gen. R. s. 4 אדם כּוֹבֵר בכברה . . . if one sifts wheat or straw in a sieve. Ohol. XVIII, 2 וכוֹברוֹ בשתי כברות and sifts it twice. Maasr. I, 6 הקיטניות משיִכְבּוֹר peas are subject to tithes from the time he sifts them. Ruth R., end וכ׳ את הצבר וכ׳ (not וכבד) and sifted one pile. Y. Ab. Zar. IV, 44ᵇ top .... טוחנין כוללין, read כּוֹבְרִין; a. fr.—Part. pass. כָּבוּר. Y. Maasr. I, 49ª bot. מן הכ׳ וכ׳ from the portion which has been sifted in behalf of that which has not.

Nif. נִכְבַּר *to be sifted.* Tosef. Ter. X, 15 שדרכו לִיכָּבֵר (not ליכבד) which it is customary to sift.

כַּבַּר II, *Pa.* כַּבֵּיר (denom. of כַּבְּרִיתָא) *to fumigate with sulphur, to bleach.* Ber. 27ᵇ לְכַבְרוּיֵי סלי to fumigate baskets. B. Kam. 93ᵇ דכַּבְּרֵיה כברויי when he (in addition) bleached the wool with sulphur.

***כְּבַר** III *to be heavy, to grieve*; *Af.* אַכְבִּיר *to irritate, grieve*, v. כְּבַר.

כְּבָרָה f. (b. h.; v. כְּבָר II) 1) *a large round vessel* (cmp. כְּוֶורֶת). Sabb. 35ª כמין כ׳ בים a rock in the sea of the shape (and size) of a *K'barah*; Tosef. Succ. III, 11 סלע מלא כ׳ a rock of the size &c.; Tanh., ed. Bub., B'midb. 2 סלע כמין כ׳ Ms. R. (v. ib. note 21); v. כְּוֶורֶת.—2) *basket* used as a *sieve* (v. Sm. Ant. s. v. Vannus). Kel. XV, 4 כ׳ של בעה״ב a household sieve, contrad. to כְּבָרַת גרנות the large sieve of the threshing floor. Tosef. Bets. I, 20, contrad. to נפה. Taan. 22ᵇ עשו כל גופו ככ׳ they made his body (perforated with arrows) like a sieve; M. Kat. 28ᵇ עשאוהו ככ׳; Y. Kidd. I, 61ª; a. fr.—*Pl.* כְּבָרוֹת. Ohol. XVIII, 2, v. כָּבַר. Deut. R. s. 6 כְּבָרוֹתָיו his sieves. Par. III, 11 כ׳ של אבן perforated stone vessels for sifting ashes.

כּוּב׳, כַּבְרִיתָא, כַּבְּרִיתָא f. (cmp. preced.)=h. גָּפְרִית; [*a thick porous lump*,] *sulphur.* Targ. Ps. XI, 6 כַּבְ׳ Ms. (ed. Wil. כָּבְ׳; ed. Lag. כּוּפְרִיתָא). Targ. Y. I Gen. XIX, 24 כַּבְרִיתָא (O. a. Y. II גופריתא). Targ. Y. Deut. XXIX, 22 כּוּבְרִיתָא.—Gitt. 86ª. Nidd. 62ª; Sabb. 90ª (expl. בורית) כ׳ sulphur used for whitening clothes.

כַּבְרִיתָא I (Ms. כַּבְּרִיתָא) f. (v. preced. wds.; cmp. נוֹפֶת) [*the sieve*,] *honey-comb.* Targ. Prov. V, 3 (ed. Lag. כב׳, Var. כב׳). Ib. XVI, 24 (ed. Lag. כב׳). Targ. Ps. XIX, 11 (Ms. כוורית׳א). V. כַּפְּרִיתָא.

כַּבְרִיתָא II, כַּבְרָתָה pr. n. pl. (preced.; cmp. נפת, Targ. פלכין, Josh. XII, 23; XVII, 11; I Kings IV, 11) *Kabritha, K'bartha* (*el-Kabîre*, v. Hildesh. Beitr. p. 15), a border town of northern Palestine. Tosef. Shebi. IV, 11 כברי׳ ed. Zuck. (Var. כברתא); Y. ib. VI, 36ᶜ כברתה; Sifré Deut. 51 סברתה; Yalk. Deut. 874 נברת׳ (corr. acc.).

כָּבַשׁ (b. h.; cmp. כָּבַס) 1) *to press, squeeze.* Ohol. VIII, 5 כ׳ את האבן וכ׳ if one pressed a stone on (weighted) the sheet. Bets. 23ᵇ שהיא כּוֹבֶשֶׁת because it (the wagon) presses (the ground) down. Sabb. XX, 5 לא כּוֹבְשִׁין you must not screw down, v. מַכְבֵּשׁ; a. fr.—*Part. pass.* כָּבוּשׁ, f. כְּבוּשָׁה *pressed, compressed; pressing.* Ib. 135ᵃ; Tosef. ib. XV (XVI), 9; a. e. ערלה כ׳ היא the foreskin (which seems to be wanting) is pressed (to the membrum). Tosef. Ohol. IX, 4 כאילו אבנים כְּבוּשׁוֹת וכ׳ as if stones were placed tightly upon them. Ex. R. s. 15 ...החר כְּבוּשִׁין על וכ׳ a mountain on each side pressing upon (preventing the run of) the springs; a. fr.—2) (כ׳ פנים (בקרקע *to press the face* into the ground, *to hide one's self* in fear or shame. Snh. 19ᵇ כָּבְשׁוּ פניהם בקרקע they cast their looks down (were afraid to give an opinion). Y. ib. X, 27ᵈ (ref. to Is. VII, 3) א״ת כובס אלא כּוֹבֵשׁ שהיה כיבש פניו וכ׳ read not *kobes*, but *kobesh*, for he hid his face and fled before him; (Bab. ib. 104ᵃ דכבשינהו לאפר Chald.).—3) *to press vegetables, meat* &c.; *to preserve, pickle.* Toh. II, 1 ....האשה כּוֹבֶשֶׁת וכ׳ if a woman was pressing vegetables in a pot. Ukts. II, 1 זתים שֶׁכְּבָשָׁן וכ׳ olives which one pressed with their leaves; a. fr.—Part. pass. כָּבוּשׁ *preserved substance, pickle.* Hull. 97ᵇ, a. fr. כ׳ הרי הוא כמבושל preserved substances are in ritual law like cooked.—*Pl.* כְּבוּשִׁין. Pes. II, 6. Y. Sabb. I, 3ᶜ bot. כְּבוּשֵׁיהֶן preserves made by gentiles; a. fr.—4) Trnsf. *to store, hide.* Hag. 13ᵃ (ref. to Prov. XXVII, 26) א״ת כבשים אלא כְּבוּשִׁים Ms. M. (missing in ed.; v. Rabb. D. S. a. l. note) read not *K'basim* (sheep) but *K'bushim* (hidden things), v. כִּבְשָׁן; Yalk. Prov. 961.—Sot. 10ᵇ; Macc. 23ᵇ (ref. to Gen. XXXVIII, 25) ...יצאה ממני יצאו כבושים a divine voice went forth and said, 'from me went forth the secret things' (I declare that Judah is the father of Tamar's children; Ar.: ממני היו הדברים כ׳, v. Rabb. D. S. a. l. note 6); Yalk. Gen. 145; Yalk. I Sam. 112.—5) *to detain* (cmp. עצר). Pesik. Bayom, p. 193ᵇ; כָּבְשָׁה אותם מטרונא וכ׳ the matron detained them one day longer; כבשה אותן התורה וכ׳ the Law detained them one day longer (before the Lord); ib. 195ᵃ, sq.; Pesik. R. suppl., s. 4. Gen. R. s. 8, end האיש כּוֹבֵשׁ וכ׳ the man detains his wife from going out; a. e.—6) *to suppress, restrain, conquer.* Snh. XI, 5 (89ᵃ) הַכּוֹבֵשׁ את נבואתו (a prophet) who suppresses his prophecy (being afraid to proclaim it). Ab. IV, 1 הכובש את יצרו who conquers his passion. Lam. R. to V, 1 כיבש את הגדול (not כביש), v. זַרְזִיר I. Y. Succ. V, 55ᵇ top עד ...שאתה מְכַבֵּשׁ בוא וכבוש וכ׳ instead of conquering the barbarians, come and subdue the Jews; Lam. R. to I, 16; ib. to IV, 19. Ex. R. s. 25 הוא כּוֹבְשׁוֹ וכ׳ he suppresses (withholds the evidence) and does not produce it.—כ׳ עון *to suppress guilt, to forgive, cause forgiveness.* Pesik. Eth Korb., p. 61ᵇ; Pesik. R. s. 16, v. כֶּבֶשׂ; a. fr.—7) *to violate.* Esth. R. to VII, 7 [read:] הרי הוא כּוֹבְשֵׁנִי וכ׳ behold, he is attacking me in thy presence.—8) *to pave, grade a road.*—Part. pass. כָּבוּשׁ, f. כְּבוּשָׁה. Tanh. Huck. 20 דרך כ׳ a graded road; ib. ed. Bub. 47; Yalk. Num. 764. [Pirké d'R. El. ch. LII כובשים במזלות, read with Yalk. Josh. 22: חושבים; Yalk. Gen. 77 רוגשים.]

Pi. כִּיבֵּשׁ 1) *to press, squeeze.*—Part. pass. מְכוּבָּשׁ, pl. מְכוּבָּשִׁים. Tosef. Mikv. VI (VII), 17 לכלוכי צואה..המ׳ (ed. Zuck. והמכושים, corr. acc.) secretory substances... which are compressed, i. e. dried up by being sat upon.—2) (cmp. סָלַל II) *to press down, make even, grade.* Bets. IV, 5 מְכַבְּשִׁין you may press the ashes down (make a graded surface for baking); a. e.—Trnsf. *to level, make plain.* Cant. R. to I, 2 (play on כבשים, Prov. XXVIII, 26, v. כֶּבֶשׂ) ...כְּבָשִׁים תהי׳ מְכַבֵּשׁ לפניהם וכ׳ it may be read *K'bashim* (*grades*), as long as thy pupils are young, make the words of the Law plain before them; when they are older reveal to them the secrets (reasons) of the Law; Yalk. ib. 985 הֱיֵה כּוֹבֵשׁ לפניהם (another expl., v. infra).—כ׳ את הריחיים [*to carve steps for the grain,*] *to put the millstones in working order.* M. Kat. I, 9; expl. ib. 10ᵃ to sharpen the millstones (v. נָקַר I), (oth. opin.) to cut the hole out for the hopper.—3) (interch. with *Kal*) *to conquer, defeat.* Y. Peah VII, 20ᶜ top שבע שֶׁכִּיבְּשׁוּ seven years during which they were engaged in conquering the land; Hull. 17ᵃ שכבשו. Sifré Deut. 51 לְכַבֵּשׁ ח״ל עד שלא יְכַבְּשׁוּ וכ׳ to conquer foreign land before they shall have conquered Palestine. Pes. 5ᵇ נכרי שֶׁכִּיבַּשְׁתּוֹ a gentile who is in thy power. Yeb. 65ᵇ (ref. to וכבשה, Gen. I, 28) איש דרכו לְכַבֵּשׁ וכ׳ it is man who conquers (the earth) but not woman; Kidd. 35ᵃ; a. fr. —4) *to suppress, withhold.* Cant. R. l. c. תהי׳ מכבש לפניהם וכ׳ withhold from them, i. e. teach them merely the words of the Law without arguments; (another expl., v. supra). —5) (denom. of כֶּבֶשׁ) *to storm, climb over.* Tosef. Sot. VI, 6 מכבש את הגנות וכ׳ climbing over the garden fences and violating the women; Gen. R. s. 53; Yalk. Gen. 94 מַכְבִּישׁ *Hif.*

Nif. נִכְבַּשׁ 1) *to be pressed down, suppressed.* Pesik. Eth Korb. p. 61ᵇ כל דבר שהוא נ׳ סופו לצוף whatever is pressed down, is liable to come to the surface again; Pesik. R. s. 16.—2) *to be submissive.* Midr. Till. to Ps. XXX, end when scholars sit down וְנִכְבָּשִׁין אלו לאלו and are submissive (respectful) to one another; (Sabb. 63ᵃ ונוחין).—3) *to have surreptitious intercourse.* Sifra Emor, Par. 6, ch. V נ׳ עם; Yeb. VII, 5 נ׳ על.

Hif. הִכְבִּישׁ *to climb*, v. supra.

Hithpa. הִתְכַּבֵּשׁ, *Nithpa.* נִתְכַּבֵּשׁ *to be conquered, be taken.* Y. Shebi. VI, 36ᶜ bot. כמי שֶׁנִּתְכַּבְּשׁוּ they are to be treated as if they had been subdued (in the days of Joshua). Ib. שמא נִתְכַּבְּשָׁה מד״ת perhaps it was to be taken by the command of the Law; Y. Yeb. VII, 8ᵃ bot. (corr. acc.). Ex. R. s. 18 ...עכשיו מִתְכַּבֶּשֶׁת בידו just now Jerusalem may be taken by him (Sennacherib). [Pesik. Zutr., Ekeb, ed. Bub. p. 30 מתכבשות, מתכבשים, v. כָּחַשׁ.]

כְּבִישׁ, כְּבַשׁ ch. same, 1) *to press, grade, make a path.* Targ. Job XIX, 12 (h. text סלל). Targ. Is. XL, 3; a. e.—

Part. pass. כְּבִישׁ, f. כְּבִישָׁא. Targ. O. Num. XX, 19 (not כְּבָשָׁא). Targ. Is. XI, 16; a. e.—*Pl.* כְּבִישִׁין *dams.* Ib. XIX, 10.—Erub. 34b כְּבוּשׁוּ כבשי וכ׳ make a dam (or embankment) in the reed-marshes.—2) *to press on, to put on* (*the head*). Targ. Y. Lev. VIII, 13 (h. text חבש).—3) *to bind, fillet; to inlay.* Targ. Y. Ex. XXXVIII, 28 (h. text חשק; O. *Pa.*). Targ. Is. LIV, 11.—Part. pass. as ab.; pl. f. כְּבִישָׁן.—4) (with על) *to tread upon, to stamp out.* Targ. Mic. VII, 19. Targ. Esth. I, 5.—5) (interch. with *Pa.*) *to suppress, oppress; to conquer, force; to violate.* Targ. Josh. VIII, 21. Targ. Ps. IV, 6. Targ. II Esth. VII, 8; a. fr.—Part. pass. as ab. Targ. Hos. V, 11.—Zeb. 73b, נִיכְבְּשִׁינְהוּ, v. נוּד ch. Y. Sabb. IV, end, 7a דילמא לא כ׳ צינתה will it (the band around the head) not overcome (counter-act the effect of) the cold?—6) *to withhold, detain.* Targ. Y. II Gen. XXIX, 22.—Nidd. 39b a hen that laid one day וכַבְשָׁה יומא וכ׳ and held back (failed to lay) one day &c.—7) *to hide* (the face); *to close* (the eyes). Targ. Ex. III, 6. Targ. Lev. XX, 4; a. fr.—Targ. O. Deut. XXII, 1 ed. Berl. (ed. *Ithpe.*); ib. 4 (sub. עינין).—B. Bath. 40b כְּבִשְׁנָא לשטר וכ׳ I shall hide the deed of mortgage.

Pa. כַּבֵּישׁ same. Targ. Prov. XVI, 32 מְכַבֵּישׁ Ms. (ed. מַכְבֵּישׁ *Af.*) who conquers. Targ. Josh. VIII, 19.—Targ. O. Ex. XXXVIII, 28 (v. supra). Targ. Lam. III, 34; a. fr.—Snh. 95a דכַבְּשִׁית בתקוף ידי which I conquered with the strength of my hand; [ib. כבשית כל מדינתי, read כנשית;] Yalk. Is. 284.—Part. pass. מְכַבַּשׁ, f. מְכַבְּשָׁא; pl. מְכַבְּשִׁין; מְכַבְּשָׁן. Targ. Ex. XXXVIII, 17 (h. text מחשקים). Ib. XXVII, 17 (not מְכָבְשִׁין, v. O. ed. Berl.). Targ. Am. VI, 4.—Targ. Jer. XVIII, 15 (h. text סלולה); a. e.

Af. אַכְבֵּישׁ, v. supra.

Ithpe. אִתְכְּבִישׁ 1) *to be conquered; to be subdued, oppressed.* Targ. Num. XXXII, 22. Targ. Y. Gen. XVI, 9 (some ed. אתכנער); a. e.—2) (of the face) *to be sunk* (in fear, shame), *to grieve.* Targ. Gen. IV, 5; 6 (h. text נפל).—3) *to withdraw one's self.* Targ. O. Deut. XXII, 1, v. supra.

כֶּבֶשׂ m. (b. h.; prob. fr. כבשׂ *to be thick, strong*; cmp. Arab. *kabš,* a. v. אִימַּר) *sheep* (at least one year old). Men. XIII, 7, sq.; a. fr.—*Pl.* כְּבָשִׂים. Ib. 9 אחד מִכְּבָשַׂי one of my sheep. Zeb. IX, 5; a. fr.—*Fem.* כִּבְשָׂה or כַּבְשָׂה. Gen. R. s. 44 כ׳ של יחיד the sheep which is offered as an individual's sacrifice. Tosef. Yeb. III, 4; Yoma 66b (v. Tosaf. a. l.)—Lev. R. s. 37; Tanh. Vayishl. 8 מביא (אדם) כִּבְשָׂתוֹ וכ׳ let man bring his sheep directly to the Temple court (without previous dedication by a vow); Y. Ned. I, 36d כִּשְׂבָּתוֹ. Tanh. Tol'd. 5; Esth. R. to IX, 2 גדולה היא חכ׳ וכ׳ great is the sheep (Israel) that lives among seventy wolves (nations). Tanh. Ki Thissa 4 אדם ששבה את חכ׳ וכ׳ a man who captured the lamb (Bathsheba, v. II Sam. XII, 3, sq.) and killed the shepherd (Uriah); a. fr.

כֶּבֶשׁ m (b. h.; כָּבַשׁ) 1) *press.*—*Pl.* כִּבְשִׁין, כְּבָשִׁים. Pesik. Eth. Korb., p. 61b (play on כבשים, Num. XXVIII, 3) כ׳ שהן כובשין וכ׳ (the sacrifices are) presses, for they suppress the sins &c.; Pesik. R. s. 16.—2) *ascent, grade, landing bridge.* Zab. III, 1; 3. Sabb. XVI, 8; a. e.—Esp. *the inclined plane leading to the altar.* Midd. III, 3. Zeb. V, 3; a. fr.—*Pl.* as ab. Ib. 62b. Ib. 63a כל כִּבְשֵׁי כבשים ... חוץ של מזבח וכ׳ all grades of ascents (in the Temple) were at the rate of three cubits per one cubit (of vertical elevation), except the ascent of the altar which was at the rate of three cubits and a half and &c.; (for Var. lect. v. Rabb. D. S. a. l., and Tosaf. a. l. a. Men. 41b s. v. ארבעה); Y. Erub. II 24b bot., v. כִּיבּוּשׁ h.—Lam. R. introd. (R. Josh. 2); Koh. R. to XII, 7 (expl. דָּיֵק, Ez. XXI, 27) כ׳ *embankments* round a besieged city (Lat. agger, v. כּוֹבֵשׁ).—3) *preserving fruit.* Ter. II, 6 זיתי כ׳ olives good for preserves, opp. זיתי שמן.—*Pl.* as ab. *pressed, preserved vegetables* &c. Shebi. IX, 5 הכובש שלשה כ׳ וכ׳ if one puts three sorts of pressed vegetables into one vessel. Sabb. 108b; a. e.—[Gen. R. s. 66 כבשיהן some ed., v. כִּיבּוּשׁ h.]

כֵּבַשׁ I, v. כִּיבּוּשׁ ch.

כֵּבַשׁ II, כִּבְשָׁא, כִּיבְשָׁא ch.=h. כֶּבֶשׁ, 1) *ascent* (scamnum), *stepping stool.* Targ. I Chr. XXVI, 16 (h. text מסלה). Ib. XXVIII, 2 כבש (constr.); Targ. Ps. CXXXII, 7 (h. text הדם). Targ. Is. LXVI, 1 כְּבַשׁ (ed. Lag. כֵּיבַשׁ).—2) *press-board and loading stone.*—*Pl.* כִּבְשֵׁי, כִּבְ׳. B. Bath. 67b (expl. עבירים, Mish. ib.) כִּי׳ Ms. M. (ed. כב׳).—3) *grade;* בֵּי כ׳ *a graded field* which requires no artificial irrigation, opp. בי שקיא. Kidd. 62b.—4) *dam or embankment. Pl.* as ab. Erub. 34b, v. כְּבַשׁ.—5) *the hot ashes* (*pressed and levelled*) *in the oven* (v. Bets. IV, 5 quot. s. v. כָּבַשׁ *Pi.*). Hull. 93b רישא בכ׳ a head put in ashes (for removing the hair before boiling).—6) *path.* Targ. II Sam. XX, 12, sq. כי׳ ed. Lag. (ed. Wil. כִּבְ׳). Targ. I Sam. IV, 13 כִּבַשׁ constr., v. כְּבִישׁ.—6) (archit.) *recess, enceinte.* Targ. Ez. XLV, 4; ib. XLVIII, 21 constr. כִּיבַשׁ ed. Wil. (h. text מקדש).

כַּבְשָׁה, כַּבְשָׁא f. ch.=h. כֶּבֶשׁ 3. Y. B. Kam. IV, 5b bot.; Y. B. Bath. V, end, 15b, v. אֲחִינָא.

כִּבְשָׁה, v. כֶּבֶשׁ. [Y. Ned. VII, beg. 40b הנודר מן כבשה, read פירות שנה as Tosef. ib. IV, 1.]

כִּבְשׁוֹן, v. כִּבְשָׁן.

כַּבְשִׁישִׁין m. pl. (כָּבַשׁ) *compresses,* v. פְּתִית 4.

כִּבְשָׁן m. (b. h.; כָּבַשׁ) 1) *kiln, furnace.* Kel. VIII, 9 כ׳ של סיידין וכ׳ the furnace of lime burners, glass-makers and potters. Succ. 7b עשויה ככ׳ shaped like a furnace (round). Gen. R. s. 44 כִּבְשַׁן האש the heated furnace. Cant. R. to II, 16 היוצר ... בודק כִּבְשָׁנוֹ when the potter examines a batch of his kiln; a. fr.—*Pl.* כִּבְשׁוֹנוֹת. B. Kam. 82b אין עושין בה כ׳ no furnaces were erected in Jerusalem; Hag. 26a; Zeb. 96a. Ib. יהדרינהו לכ׳ Ms. M. (ed. אהדר׳) let them be put back into the furnaces (to be baked over). Tosef. B. Bath. I, 10 מרחיקין את הכ׳ וכ׳ (ed. Zuck. כבשניה, corr. acc.) furnaces must be removed from the town fifty cubits.—*2) *that which is withheld, secret.* Hag. 13a (play on כבשים, Prov. XXVII, 26) א״ת כבשים אלא כְּבוּשִׁים דברים שהם כִּבְשׁוֹנוֹ של עולם וכ׳ Ms. M. read not *K'basim* but *K'bushim,* things which are the secret of the world (esoteric doctrines) must be kept under one's garment (in one's bosom).

כבשנית, v. preced.

כַּבֶּשֶׁת (כּוּבּ׳) f. (כָּבַשׁ) *pressed vegetables.* Tosef. Shebi. IV, 16, contrad. to יַבֶּשֶׁת.

כבתה, Yalk. Lev. 445, v. כַּבְּבָא.

כבתותא, v. בַּתְּיָא.

כְּגוֹן, v. גּוּן.

כגני, v. בְּאַגְנָא.

כַּד I, כַּד, כִּיד, כִּדֵי, כִּידִי (a comp. of כ a. ד, corresp. to h. כַּאֲשֶׁר or כְּשֶׁ־) *when, as, as though.* Targ. Ex. XVII, 11. Targ. Ps. CXIX, 109 כיד על גב Ms. (ed. only ע״ג) as though (carried) on &c.; a. v. fr.—Targ. Is. XXIX, 15 כִּדְבְקַבְלָא (ed. Lag. כיד בק׳) as though in darkness. Targ. O. Num. XXIX, 18 כדחזי, v. חֲזִי, as it is proper; a. fr.—Y. Ab. Zar. III, 42[c] top. Y. Yoma VII, 44[b] top כד דהיא וכ׳ when there is &c. Y. Taan. I, 64[a] bot. כד הוינן; Y. Meg. III, 74[b] bot. כדי דהוינן, v. נְהַר I. B. Kam. 52[a] (prov.) כד רגיז וכ׳ when the shepherd is angry with his flock, he makes a blind sheep the leader. Ib. 64[b], a. fr. כִּדְאָמְרֵי וכ׳ as they say &c. Ib.[b] כִּדְתָנָא דבי וכ׳ as (that which) the scholars of the school of ... said. Ib. מיבעי ליה לִכְדְתָנֵי it is needed for (something like) what has been taught. Ib. לִכְדְרָבָא for what Raba said. B. Mets. 99[b] כדרבא agreeably to what R. said; a. v. fr.—[Num. R. s. 14 א״ת כדרבונות אלא כִּדְרַבָּנוּת read not (Koh. XII, 11) *kaddarbonoth*, but *kidd'rabbanuth*, like a command of authority.]

כַּד II m. (כרר, cmp. כָּדַר, *to be rounded*) 1) (adj.) *arched*, opp. חד pointed. Ab. Zar. 40[a]; Hull. 64[a], v. חַד I.—*Pl.* כַּדִּין, Ib.—2) c. (b. h.) *an arched, pouched vessel, jug* &c.; cmp. חָבִית. Num. R. s. 12 מִתגלגל ככד rolling like a jug. B. Kam. III, 1 (identical with חבית). Tosef. Kel. B. Mets. X, 1 כַּדּוֹ ריקנית (fem.) one's vessel when empty; a. fr.—*Pl.* כַּדִּים, כַּדִּין. Tanh. Vayigg. 11 (ref. to Ps. XVI, 7) נעשו ... כשתי כ׳ של מים וכ׳ his two kidneys became like two water pitchers and they were giving forth a flow of religious wisdom; ib. ed. Bub. 12 שלמים (corr. acc.); Gen. R. s. 61 כמין שני רבנים (corr. acc.); Midr. Till. to Ps. I כעין שני כדים ed. Bub. (oth. ed. כשני רבנן, corr. acc.); Ab. d'R. Nath. ch. XXXIII חכמים (corr. acc.).—Keth. XIII, 4 כַּדֵּי שמן vessels with oil, opp. קִנְקַנִּים empty vessels; a. fr.

כַּדָּא ch. same. B. Kam. 27[a] באתרא דכ׳ לא קרו וכ׳ in a place where they distinguish between *kadda* a. *habitha* (v. preced.). B. Mets. 59[a] (prov.) כמשלם שערי מכ׳ וכ׳ (v. Rabb. D. S. a. l.) when the barley is gone from the pitcher, strife knocks and enters; Yalk. Ps. 888 כַּדָּה.—Hull. 58[b] top חני חמרי דכ׳ (Var. דכרים, v. כְּרוּם ch.) dates kept in a vessel (which became worm-eaten); a. fr.—*Pl.* כַּדִּין, כַּדַּיָּא. Targ. I Kings XVIII, 34. Targ. Jud. VII, 20; a. e.—Trnsf. כַּדָּא *a big figure, important personage.* Yeb. 70[a] בן בתר כ׳ my grandson, the big vessel (high-priest), opp. כוזא the little jug (bastard).

כְּדָא *like this*, v. דָּא.

כַּדַּאי, v. כְּדַיי.

כְּדַב (v. כזב) *to be false.* Targ. Hos. IV, 2.

Pa. כַּדֵּיב 1) *to lie, give false evidence; to be faithless; to deny.* Targ. O. Gen. XVIII, 15. Targ. Job XXXI, 28 (Ms. כַּדְּבִיב׳); a. fr.—2) *to give the lie, to refute.* Ib. XXIV, 25.—3) *to flatter.* Targ. Ps. XVIII, 45; a. e.

Ithpa. אִתְכַּדֵּיב 1) *to be proved false.* Targ. II Kings IV, 16. Targ. Prov. XXX, 6.—2) *to flatter, be submissive.* Targ. II Sam. XXII, 45. Targ. O. Deut. XXXIII, 29 יִתְכַּדְּבוּן (Y. יִתְכַּ׳).

כִּדְבָא, כִּיד׳, כַּד׳, כַּדְבָא m. (preced.) 1) *falsehood, lie.* Targ. Ps. V, 7 כיד׳ Ms. (ed. כדבותא). Ber. 59[a] ... אובא כיד׳ ומילֵיה כיד׳ Ms. M. (ed. כַּדִּיבִין ... כַּדִּיב ...), v. אוב ch.—*Pl.* כַּדְבִין, כַּדּ׳, כִּיד׳, כִּדְ׳. Targ. Hos. VII, 13 כדב׳ ed. Lag. (ed. Wil. כִּדְּבִ׳). Targ. Jud. XVI, 10; a. fr.—2) *fiction, story.*—*Pl.* כִּדִיבֵי. Bekh. 8[b] מילי דכ׳ En Yaăk. (ed. דבדיאי; Ar. דכדי).

כַּדָּבָא, כַּדִּיב, כַּדְּבָא m. (preced.) 1) *liar; false.* Targ. Prov. XIX, 22 (Ms. כַּדָּבָא).—Ber. 59[a], v. preced.—*Pl.* כַּדָּבִין, כַּדָּבַיָּא, כַּדּ׳. Targ. Is. XXX, 9; a. e.—2) *fiction-teller, story-teller.*—*Pl.* as ab. Y. Ber. IX, end, 14[d] כל כ׳ טבין וכ׳ all fiction-tellers are good, but those who tell their own inventions concerning the Law are bad; (Var. חרשיא, v. חַרְשָׁא; anoth. Var. ברביא corr. acc.);—[perh. to be read: כִּדְבַיָּא *fictions*, v. preced.].

כַּדְבֵב, *Palel* of כְּדַב q. v.

כַּדְבוּבָא, כַּד׳ m. (preced.) *falsehood, lie; fiction.* Targ. Job XVI, 8.—*Pl.* כַּדְבוּבִין. Ib. XI, 3.

כַּדְבוּתָא, כַּדְבוּ׳, כִּדִיבוּ׳ f. same. Targ. Ps. IV, 3 כדי׳ ed. (Ms. כדב׳). Ib. V, 7 (v. כַּדְבָא). Targ. Prov. XXX, 8 מילתא כ׳ (read: דכ׳); a. e.

כָּדַד *to be rounded*, v. כָּדַר.

כַּדָּד m. (denom. of כַּד II) *potter.* M. Kat. 13[b]; Pes. 55[b] Ms. M. (ed. כדר). [Tosef. Kel. B. Mets. X, 6 כדדין, some ed., v. גַּרְדּוּם.]

כַּדָּה, v. כַּדָּא.—[Y. Yoma VIII, 44[d] top; Y. Taan. I, 64[c] חתות כ׳, read: כָּרִיָּה, v. כָּרָא.]

כִּדוּ, (כְּדוֹ), כִּידוּ (comp. of כַּד הוּ, v. כַּד I, cmp. הוּ) 1) *when it (happens that), whenever, when.* Targ. Lam. III, 50 עד כ׳די until what time he &c.—Y. Peah I, 15[c] bot. כ׳ נפיק וכ׳ (ed. Krot. כד) whenever he comes from school. Y. Hall. I, end, 58[a] כידו אתי וכ׳ (not בידו) whenever he went to take (bread) into his hand.—2) *as it is* (כִּדְהוּ), *now.* Targ. Y. Gen. XXVI, 28 כ׳ נפקת now that thou hast gone away. Targ. Jud. V, 9. Targ. Jer. XXXI, 18. Targ. Is. XXXII, 14.—Succ. 44[b] כ׳ הוית דייר וכ׳ (v. Rabb. D. S. a. l. note) I have now been in this country &c.; a. fr.—[Gen. R. s. 44 כִּין כ׳, v. מַלְכְּיָא.]—V. כְּדַי.

כדוכסין, Y. B. Mets. II, 8[c] bot. Var., v. פַּרְכְּסִין.

*__כִּדּוּם__ m. (denom. of כַּד II) *a sort of lever* with which a pitcher is fished out of the well; oth. opin.: *a pitcher-stand, watercooler.*—*Pl.* כִּדּוּמִים, כִּדּוּמִין. Kel. XIII, 7; T'bul Yom. IV, 6, v. אֲשְׁקְלוֹן.

עינבין דכ׳, כדום, v. כְּרוּם ch.

כְּדוֹן, כְּדוֹן, (כְּהוֹן Ms.) (contr. of כְּעִידָּן, v. כְּעַן; cmp. הָאִידָּנָא) *now, at that time.* Targ. Y. Num. XXII, 4; 6 (O. כְּעַן; h. text עתה). Targ. Y. Gen. XIII, 7 עד כ׳ as yet; a. fr. —Y. Ber. I, 2^d bot. דעד כ׳ וכ׳ for up to that time people are awake. Y. Hall. II, beg. 58^b עד כ׳ לחה thus far (so much about) fresh flour. Y. Sot. V, 20^b bot. כ׳ right now, opp. בתר זמן. Gen. R. s. 22, beg. (ref. to Ps. XXV, 6) לא מן דכ׳ וכ׳ not from this day, but from eternity; Yalk. Ps. 702 מן הדין (read: מן כ׳). — Y. Ber. I, 2^c מאי כ׳ how is it now? (what is the result, the law &c.?); Y. Peah IV, 18^b bot. מיה כ׳; a. fr. — Y. Ter. VI, 44^a bot. ולית אתון אמרין מְהָן כ׳ ונתן וכ׳ (not מהו) and you did not say whence it was derived. Now (I will tell you, We read,) 'and he shall give' &c.—Ib. ולית אתון מינרהון מהו כ׳ (corr. acc.).

כדופסלא, כר׳, Y. Sabb. VI, 8^b bot., read: פּוּדוֹפְסִילָא.

כַּדּוּר c. (b. h.; כַּדַּר) *ball, globe.* Tosef. Sabb. IX (X), 6 כדי ליתן לתוך כ׳ וכ׳ as much as is required to stuff a small ball. Ib. X (XI), 10 המשחקין בכ׳ who play at ball. Koh. R. to XII, 11 (play on בדרבנות, ib.) ככ׳ של בנות like the girls' ball; מה כ׳ זה וכ׳ as the ball &c., v. כָּדַר; Num. R. s. 14; s. 15 (corr. acc.); Tanh. B'haal. 15; Pesik. R. s. 3. Lev. R. s. 23 לבנה בִּכְדּוּרָהּ the moon on re-entering her periodical orbit (after nineteen years); (Y. Ber. IX, 13^d בתקופתה, Bab. ib. 59^b בגבורתה). Ab. Zar. III, 1 כל שיש בידו . . . או כ׳ a statue holding in its hand . . . a ball (globe); ib. 41^a כ׳ שתיפש את עצמו . . . וכב׳ the ball (means symbolically) that he causes himself to be caught like a ball in behalf of the entire world (vicarious sacrifice); Num. R. s. 13; Y. Ab. Zar. III, 42^c bot. כ׳ שהעולם עשוי ככ׳ the ball symbolizes the world which has the shape of a ball; a. e.

כַּדּוּרָא ch. same. Y. Ab. Zar. III, 42^c bot. [read:] בגין כן . . . . ליה בכ׳ בידיה therefore he (Alexander the Macedonian) is represented in statuary with a ball in his hand; Num. R. s. 13.

כַּדּוּרִית, כַּדּוּרֶת f. same. Tanh. B'midb. 2 סלע כמין כוורת או כ׳ (the well moving with the Israelites in the desert was) a rock in the shape of a bee-hive or a globe (v. Tanh. ed. Bub. ib. note 21). — *Pl.* כַּדּוּרִיּוֹת. Pesik. B'shall., p. 87^a (description of Roman tortures) שהיו נותנים כ׳ של אש וכ׳ they put glowing iron balls under their armpits; Cant. R. to II, 7; Midr. Till. to Ps. XVI; Yalk. Ps. 667 ברודיות (corr. acc.).

כְּדִי I, (כַּדִּי, כְּדֵי) (= כַּד הִי, v. כְּדוּ) *when; now (that).* Targ. Y. Gen. XXVII, 34. Ib. XXXIX, 10; a. e. — Y. Ab. Zar. II, 40^d top כ׳ טבא when it (the eye-paint) is good. Y. Dem. VI, 25^c bot. כ׳ יהב ליה וכ׳ when he gives him the whole of it. Y. Meg. III, 74^b bot. כ׳ דהוינן, v. כַּד I.— 2) [*as it is,*] *incidentally, without special reason, not meaning it exactly.* R. Hash. 5^a פסח כ׳ נסבה the writer uses the word Pesah (ib. 4^a, quot. fr. Tosef. Arakh. III, 17) incidentally (cmp. אַשְׁגָּרָה); Zeb. 99^b. Kidd. 5^b סיפא כ׳ נסבה the second proposition was incidentally asserted (is not to be pressed), opp. דַּוְקָא.—3) *as such, alone, merely.* Keth. 36^b bot. מעיד בה כ׳ if he merely testifies in her favor (without having been instrumental in redeeming her from captivity). Gitt. 55^a יאוש כ׳ וכ׳ the mere giving up of robbed property (without a change of hands after the renunciation) gives the robber no rights. — מילי דכ׳ *words spoken merely for saying something, for fun.* Snh. 29^b כל מילי דכ׳ וכ׳ people do not remember words thrown out in a jocular way. — [Bekh. 8^b מילי דכ׳ Ar. *fictions, stories;* v. כַּדְבָא). — בְּכ׳ *for whatever it be, for a trifle; for no cause.* Yeb. 39^b בכ׳ תיפוק can she be dismissed without any formality (with his mere refusal to marry her)?—Taan. 5^b, v. בְּקָא. Keth. l. c. לא שדי . . . . בכ׳ one does not throw away one's money at random (unless sure that there is no legal impediment to marrying the woman whom he is about to redeem). Ned. 22^a בכ׳ לא אדרתה for a paltry reason she would surely not have forbidden her, v. נֶדֶר. Ib. 29^a פקעה בכ׳ ceases without any formality; a. e.—מִכ׳ *from such (a condition) as it is, now, well, you know.* Gitt. 68^b מ׳ כי מירת וכ׳ now when you die, you will have &c. Sabb. 78^a מ׳ כל מילתא וכ׳ you know, whenever there is an ordinary and an extraordinary way of using an object, &c. Hull. 109^b; a. e.—Esp. (introducing an argument) *now, is it not so?* Ib. 29^a מ׳ על עוף קאי וכ׳ does not the writer of the Mishnah treat of birds? Well then, if he meant sacrificial fowls he ought to have said *hammolek!* B. Kam. 3^a מ׳ שקולין וכ׳ now that they are alike, let both be included, for which will you exclude? —Bets. 2^b מ׳ מאן סתמה וכ׳ now, who is it that states that proposition in the Mishnah anonymously? Of course, Rabbi. Now, why &c.; a. fr.

***כְּדִי II** pr. n. m. *K'di* (?). B. Mets. 2^a; Yoma 44^a; 72^b, a. fr. ואמרי לה כ׳ and some say. It was K. [Prob. meaning: *as the case may be,* i. e. and some introduce respectively other persons, v. preced.]

כְּדֵי, v. כְּדָיֵיר.

כְּדֵי, v. דַּי.

כְּדִיב, כַּדִּיב, כְּדִיבָא, v. כַּדְבָא, כַּדְבָא.

כְּדִידִית f. (dimin. of כַּד) *round small vessel.*—*Pl.* כְּדִידִיּוֹת. Tosef. Men. IX, 10 כ׳ בינוניות middle-sized vessels of the sort called *K'didith;* Men. 87^a חביות כְּדִיּוֹת לודיות בינוניות Ms. M. middle-sized round Lydda vessels.

כְּדִיּוֹת, v. preced.

כְּדָיֵיר, כְּדָי, כְּדַאי I m. (formed from כְּדֵי, v. דַּי) *adequate, worthy, competent, deserving.* Gen. R. s. 76 (ref. to Gen. XXXII, 11) איני כ׳ I am not deserving (of any of all the mercies); כ׳ אני אבל וכ׳ I am worthy (of some) but too small for all &c. B. Bath. 165^b אני איני כ׳ שאתם וכ׳ I do not deserve the honor of having that question put to me by you. Gitt. 90^b; Tosef. Sot. V, 9 כ׳ הוא במיתה he deserves death. Ber. 9^a, a. fr. the authority of כ׳ הוא וכ׳ R . . . is sufficient to be relied upon &c.; a. fr.—*Pl.* כְּדָאִים, כְּדָאִין, כְּדָיִין. Mekh. Yithro, Amalek, s. 1 אין אנו כ׳ שישמשנו (ed. Weiss כְּדַיִן) we are not worthy to be served by him; a. e.—*Fem.* כְּדָאִית. Cant. R. to I, 2 איני כ׳ לשפחתו I am not worthy to be his handmaid.

כְּדֵיי, כְּדֵי, כְּדַאי II, m. (preced.) *sufficiency, worthiness.* Tosef. Sot. III, 19 'אין כְּדֵיי באר העולם וכ human beings are not worthy for me to live among them; (Num. R. s. 9 אין באר.. כְּדָאִין, a. כְּדַאי, v. preced.).—Gen. R. s. 46, v. אֱלָהוּת.

כְּדֵין, v. כְּדֵיי I.

כְּדֵין, v. הֵן.

כַּדְכֹּד m. (b. h.; v. כַּדְכְּדוֹן) *chalcedony*, a gem. Pesik. R. s. 32 'אלו אבני כ these are the gems of *kadkod*. [Y. Shek. IV, 48[b] bot., v. 'שבטא דכ, Bab. ed. דכדכדא, v. כַּרְכָּר).

כַּדְכְּדָא ch. same. [Y. Shek. IV, 48[b] bot., v. preced.]—*Pl.* כַּדְכְּדַיָּא, v. next w.

כַּדְכְּדוֹן or **כַּרְכְּדוֹן**; ch. form **כַּרְכְּדָנָא** m. (χαλκηδών, v. Fl. to Levy Talm. Dict. II, p. 449[b]) *chalcedony*, Judah's gem in the high priest's breastplate. Targ. Y. I Ex. XXVIII, 18 כדכודי (incorr. a. misplaced); Y. II כדכדנא (h. text נפך). Ex. R. s. 38, end ברדינין, ברדינך (corr. acc.).—*Pl.* כַּדְכְּדוֹנִין. Pesik. Aniya p. 136[a] כדכריינון, כדכדיינון (corr. acc.). Ib. אבני כַּדְכְּדַיָּיה Ar. (ed. כודכייא, corr. acc.); Yalk. Is. 339 כַּדְכּוֹדַיָּיה; Pesik. R. s. 32 אבני כרכדנא Chalcedonian stones; v. כַּדְכֹּד. Targ. II Esth. I, 2 כַּדְכּוֹדָנִין

כדכדיינון, v. preced.

כַּדְכּוֹדָא, pl. כַּדְכּוֹדַיָּיא, v. כַּדְכְּדוֹן.

כדכודי, כדכודנין, v. כַּדְכְּדוֹן.

***כַּדְכּוֹר**, Targ. Y. Num. XXIV, 8, read: כַּרְכּוֹי, v. כְּרָכָא.

כדכיאות, Sifré Deut. 204 'תקון וכ, Yalk. Deut. 923 תיקון ודוגיאות, a corrupt., read: תִּיקּוּנֵי כַּרְכּוֹמִין *preparations for sieges;* cmp. Targ. Deut. XX, 20 a. Pesik. Zutr. a. l. (Deut. p. 67).

כדכריינון, v. כַּדְכְּדוֹן.

כדמת, v. כַּרְמֶת.

כָּדַן, (cmp. Assyr. *kidînu* servant, Friedr. Del. Proleg. p. 200 note 7) [*to bend,*] *to yoke, put to work.* Y. Peah I, 15[c] bot.; Y. Kidd. I, 61[b] (בריחיים) כּוֹדְנוֹ לריחיים he puts his father to treading the mill (Bab. ib. 31[a] bot. מטחינו, v. טְחַן). Y. Pes. IV, 31[a] top לכשיזקין הוא כודנו בריחיים when the horse grows old, he puts him &c.

Pi. כִּידֵּן same.—Part. pass. מְכוּדָּן. Lam. R. to I, 14 (ref. to נפש חיה, Gen. II, 7, as if meaning *self-supporting*) עשאו 'עבד מ' בפני עצמו וכ the Lord made man a slave put to work for himself, for if he does not work, he has nothing to eat; Gen. R. s. 14 מחורר, מכורן; Koh. R. to II, 17 מכורן עבד (corr. acc.).—*Pl. fem.* מְכוּדָּנוֹת. Lev. R. s. 16 (play on יְשַׂפַּח, Is. III, 17) 'עשאן שְׁפָחוֹת מכ the enemies made them handmaids, forced to hard labor; ib. מהו מ' אמהן משעבדן; Lam. R. to IV, 15 מכודניות (corr. acc.).—V. כּוּדְנָא.

***כַּדְנָא** f. *jug.* Targ. II Esth. I, 2 (prob. כַּדְתָא fem. form of כַּדָּא).

כְּדָנָא, כְּדֵנָא *thus*, v. הֵן.

כָּדְנִין, pl. of כּוּדְנָא.

כָּדַר (v. כַּר II) *to be arched, rounded.* Ab. Zar. 40[a]; Ḥull. 64[a] (sign of eggs of clean birds) כל שכּוֹדֶרֶת ועגולגולת (Var. קוֹדֶרֶת, כּוֹדֶרֶת, כּוֹדֶרֶת) that which is arched (on top not pointed) and rounded (rolling); Tosef. ib. III (IV), 23.

Hithpa. הִתְכַּדֵּר (v. כַּדּוּר) *to be thrown around in a circle of players.* Koh. R. to XII, 11 'מה הכדור הזה מִתְכַּדֵּר וכ as the ball is thrown around from hand to hand.

כַּדַּר, v. כַּדַּד.

כֹּה (b. h.) *here; thus.* Gen. R. s. 56 (ref. to עד־כה, Gen. XXII, 5) נלך . . . בסופו של כה we shall go and see what will be the outcome of *koh* (the promise, '*thus* shall be thy seed', Gen. XV, 5); Tanḥ. Vayera 23.

כָּה ch., v. כָּא.

כָּהָא, כָּהָה, כְּהָה, v. כחי.

כֵּהֶה, כֵּה', כֵּהָה m., **כֵּ'** f. (b. h.; preced.) 1) (of light) *dim.* Gen. R. s. 31 'בשעה שהיא כ when it (the jewel) shone faintly.—*Pl.* כֵּהִים, כֵּהוֹת, כֵּ'. Ib.; Y. Pes. I, beg. 27[a] בשעה 'שהיו כ' וכ when the lights burned dimly, we knew it was day-time. Ib.[b] top בשעה שהיו כיהות when the jewels were dim.—Pesik. Kumi, p. 145[b] (ref. to כחחלנות Ez. XL, 25) חלונות כ' היו the windows were dim (stained glass). Ḥag. 16[a] 'עיניו כ his eyes will grow dim; a. e.—2) (of leprosy) *faint, dull,* opp. עזה. Neg. II, 1, v. בַּהֶרֶת. Ib. לפי שהכ'נראית עזה because (in the early morning &c.) the faint spot appears bright; Sifra Thazr., Neg., Par. II, ch. II.—Y. Shebu. I, 32[d] 'כֵּהָה טמא הכ' מן הכ' מן כהוו if it grows one shade fainter, it is unclean, but when it grows fainter than the next fainter shade, it is clean; Sifra l. c. ed. Ven.; Yalk. Lev. 551 'כֵּיהָה מן הכ; Y. l. c.; a. fr.—*3) (trnsf.) *doubtful.* Nidd. 19[a]; Naz. 65[b]; Snh. 87[b]; Keth. 75[b] ר' ר' אומר 'כ R. Josh. says, It is doubtful; (Neg. IV, 11 ר' ר' קֵיהָה or כֵּיהָה, v. כחר, קהי).

כְּהוּנָּה f. (b. h. כְּהֻנָּה; v. כֹּהֵן) *priesthood, priestly privileges; priestly community.* Ab. IV, 13. Sot. 11[b] בתי 'כ priestly families. Midd. I, 8, a. fr. 'פרחי כ young priests (novices). Y. Ber. III, 6[a] bot.; Y. Naz. VII, 56[a] top 'אין כ היום there is no priesthood to-day (the laws for priests are suspended on the day of Rabbi's funeral). Tosef. Ḥall. II, 7, a. fr. 'כ"ד מתנות כ twenty-four gifts of priesthood (priestly prerogatives). Keth. 14[a] 'כשרה לכ fit to marry into the priesthood; a. v. fr.

כְּהוּנְּתָא, כהונתא ch. same. Targ. Ex. XXIX, 9. Targ. Num. XVI, 10 'כ' רבתא high-priesthood; a. fr.—Targ. O. Ex. XL, 15 כהונת ed. Berl. (ed. כְּהֻנּוּת).—Y. Keth. I, 25[c] 'סליקא לכ she rose to priesthood (as a priest's wife); נחיתא 'מן כ went down from priesthood (ceased to enjoy priestly privileges as a priest's wife).

כֵּהוּת f. (כָּהָה) *dimness.* Meg. 28[a] (ref. to Gen. XX, 16) 'א"ת כסות . . אלא כ' עינים Ms. M. (ed. כסיות) read not 'cover of the eyes' but 'dimness of eye-sight'; Yalk. Gen. 91.

כְּהוּתָא f. (כְּהִי) *worriment, trouble.* Targ. Prov. XXVI, 21, v. בְּהוּתָא (ed. Lag. הַרְתָא).

כָּהָה, כחי (b. h.; cmp. כָּוָה) 1) *to be dim* (of sight, light). Gen. R. s. 65 כָּהוּ עיניו his eyes grew dim. Ib. שיִּכְהוּ עיניו that his eye-sight shall fail. Kidd. 24b.. הכהו וכָהֲתָה if the master struck him on his eye, and it grew dim; a. fr.—Part. pass. כָּהוּי, f. כְּהוּיָה. Ib. הרי שהיתה עינו כ׳ וכ׳ if his eye-sight was dim, and he (the master) made him perfectly blind.—2) (of color) *to be dull*, v. כֵּהֶה. [Tosef. Erub. XI (VIII), 8; Tanḥ. Noah 9, v. כָּהַח.]

Pi. כִּהָה, כֵּהָה *to grow duller, to be shaded.* Sifra Thazr., Neg., Par. 2, ch. II אם חזו וכ׳ if the spot grew brighter and grew duller again; a. fr.—2) *to declare doubtful.* Neg. IV, 11 ר׳ י׳ כ׳, v. כֵּהֶה.

Hif. הִכְהָה 1) same. Y. Shebu. I, 32d, v. כֵּהֶה. Neg. XI, 5 ה׳ בתחלה if the suspicious spot grew fainter at once (before the ordered isolation was begun); ה׳ בראשון if it grew faint in the first week; Tosef. ib. V, 6 quot. in R. S. to Neg. l. c. (ed. Zuck. כהה כתחלה, oth. ed. only כתחלה, corr. acc.); a. fr.—2) *to make dim.* Gen. R. l. c. הריני מַכְהֶה וכ׳ I will make his eye-sight dim. Yalk. Ruth 601 יסורין ... מַכְהִין וכ׳ ... sufferings of poverty dim men's eyes. Pesik. R. s. 14 מכהה גלגל חמה dimmed (outshone) the sun in brightness; Pesik. Parah, p. 37a שיַּכְהֶה; a. e.

כְּהָא, כְּהֵי ch. same. Targ. Gen. XXVII, 1. Targ. I Kings XIV, 4; a. e.—Y. Ned. IX, 41b bot. עיני כַּהֲיָיא my eye-sight is failing.

Pa. כַּהֵה, כַּהֵי 1) *to dim, make blind.* Yoma 69b; Snh. 64a כַּהֲיִינְהוּ לעיניה Ar. (ed. כחלינהו, cmp. כְּבַר) they made his eye-sight dim. Ib. 27a ליכַהֲיוּהוּ לעיניה (v. Rabb. D. S. a. l. note 80) he shall be blinded.—2) (sub. לִבֵּיה) *to be angry;* (with ב־ of person) *to rebuke.* Targ. I Sam. III, 13.

Af. אַכְהֵי 1) *to dim.* Targ. Ez. XXXII, 7 באַכְהָיוּתִי when I make dim (h. text בכבותך).—2) *to make the heart faint, to annoy, reproach (falsely).* Ib. XIII, 22 אַכְהֵיתִין לב וכ׳ ye denounced the heart of the righteous to be false (h. text הכאות).

Ithpe. אִתְכְּהֵי *to be reproached.* Ib. (h. text הכאבתיו).

כַּהֲיוֹן m. (preced. wds.) *dimness, fainter color.* Tosef. Neg. V, 6 חזר לכ׳ if the suspicious spot again turned fainter.

כַּהֲיוּתָא f. (preced. wds.) *blindness.* Bekh. 44a, contrad. to מחסורייתא defective eye-sight.

*כַּהֲיֵי pr. n. m. *Kahăyi.* Y. Pes. II, end, 29c ed. Krot. (oth. ed. בחיי).

כַּהֲיל, v. כְּהֵל.

כַּהֲין, v. כָּהֵן I.

כֹּהֵן m. (b. h.; כהן, v. כּוּן; cmp. b. h. כֵּן) [*standing, stationed,*] *officer,* esp. *priest.* Yoma 6a, a. fr. כ׳ גדול (abbr. כ״ג) high priest, כ׳ הדיוט ordinary priest. Meg. I, 9 כ׳ משוח an anointed high priest, contrad. to מרובה בגדים a high priest distinguished only by his robes (but not anointed, as in the days of the Second Temple). Ib. כ׳ משמש officiating highpriest, כ׳ שעבר a substitute of the high priest no longer required, ex-substitute. Hor. III, 8 ממזר.. קודם לכ״ג ע״ה a bastard who is a scholar has the precedence of an ignorant high priest; a. v. fr.—*Pl.* כֹּהֲנִים. Yeb. 86b, a. e. בכ״ד מקומות נקראו הכ׳ וכ׳ in twenty four Biblical passages the priests are designated as Levites; a. v. fr.—תּוֹרַת כֹּהֲנִים (abbr. ת״כ) *Torath Kohănim,* a) name of *the third book of Moses, Leviticus.* Kidd. 33a. Lev. R. s. 7 מפני מה.. בת״כ why do we, in teaching children, commence with Leviticus? a. e.—b) name of *an halachic commentary to Leviticus,* also named *Sifra.* Yeb. 72b; a. fr.—Fem. כֹּהֶנֶת, כּוֹהֶ׳ *a priest's daughter* or *wife.* Hull. 131b, sq.—Keth. IV, 8 ובכ׳ and in the case of a priest's wife. Ib. VII, 1, sq. (70a) ובכ׳ Mish. a. Y. ed. (Bab. ed. ובכהן). Ib. 71a; a. fr. —*Pl.* כֹּהֲנוֹת, כּוֹהֲ׳. Ber. 44a. Yeb. III, 10 אם היו כ׳ (Y. ed. כוה׳) if they are daughters of priests; a. e.

כָּהַן, (b. h.), *Nithpa.* נִתְכַּהֵן (denom. of כֹּהֵן) *to be appointed priest, to act as priest.* Zeb. 101b לא נ׳ פנחס וכ׳ Phineas was not appointed high priest until &c. Ib. 102a לא נ׳ משה וכ׳ Moses acted as priest only during &c.

כָּהֵן, כָּהֵין, כָּהֲנָא I ch.=h. כֹּהֵן. Targ. Jer. XIV, 18. Targ. Mal. II, 7. Targ. Lev. I, 7; a. v. fr.—Snh. 110a, a. fr. כ׳ רבא high priest. Hull. 49a ישמעאל כ׳ מסייע כהני Ishmael, being a priest, favors the priests. Gitt. 59b קרי בכ׳ read from the Torah in the priest's place, i. e. was called up the first; Meg. 22a Ms. O. (ed. בכהני pl.); a. fr.—*Pl.* כָּהֲנִין, כָּהֲנֵי, כָּהֲנַיָּא. Targ. Ex. XIX, 6. Targ. O. Lev. I, 5; a. fr. —Gitt. l. c. כ׳ חשיבי דא״י highly esteemed Palestinean priests; a. fr.—*Fem.* כָּהַנְתָּא (כֹּהֶנֶת). Hull. 131b .... יהיב לכ׳ gave priestly gifts to a priest's daughter (married to an Israelite). Pes. 49a נסיב כ׳ married a priest's daughter. —*Pl.* כָּהֲנָתָא. Ber. 44a.

כָּהֵן (or כֹּהֵן), כָּהֲנָא II pr. n. m. *Kahen, Kahăna,* name of several Amoraim. Y. Ber. III, 6a, a. fr. ר׳ כהן.— B. Kam. 117a. Y. R. Hash. IV, beg. 59b; a. fr.—Erub. 8b רב כ׳ רביה דרב (v., however, Ms. M. a. Rabb. D. S. a. l. notes); a. fr.—V. Fr. M'bo, p. 109b, sq.

כַּהֲנוּתָא, v. כְּהוּנְתָא.

כֹּהֲנִי m. (denom. of כֹּהֵן) *one proving priestly descent, belonging to the priestly caste.* Kidd. IV, 1; Yeb. 37a (collective noun).—*Pl.* כֹּהֲנִים. Ib. 85a; v. יִשְׂרְאֵלִי.

*כַּהֲנִכָא or כַּהֲנִכְתָא f. (כהן, with format. כ; v. letter כ) *the attendant's* or *priest's lustral basin* (v. Sm. Ant. s. v. Chernips).—*Pl.* כַּהֲנִכְתָא. Targ. Y. Num. XXXI, 23; cmp. כַּרְנִיבָאוֹת.

כֹּהֶנֶת, v. כֹּהֵן.

כַּהַנְתָּא, v. כָּהֵן I.

כַּו, pl. כַּוִּין, v. כַּוְּוָא, end.

כְּוָא, v. כְּוִי.

כַּוָא, v. כַּוְּוא.

כְּוָאָה f. ch.=h. כְּוִיָּה, *burn, searing, cautery.* Targ. O. Ex. XXI, 25. Targ. O. Lev. XIII, 24 (Y. ed. Amst. כַּוְּוָאָה). —Sabb. 62b, v. כֵּיבָא.

*כְּוָאנָא m. (Pers. Arab. ḫiwân) *dining table.* Yalk. Ms. to II Kings ch. XVI (from Taan. 25a) אבואנא (read אַכְּ׳)

a ta table; (Taan. l. c. פתורא, Ms. M. אתְּבָא, v. Rabb. D. S. l. c. note). Comp. next w.

כְּרַאנְגַּר, v. אַכְוָנְגַּר.

כְּוָארָא, v. כְּוְרָא.

כּוּב m. (כָּבַב, v. כְּבַב) 1) [*ball,*] *thorn, a prickly salt-plant.*—*Pl.* כּוּבִּים, כּוּבִּין. Gen. R. s. 49 למגל כוסחת כ׳ like a sickle mowing thorns; Yalk. Prov. 950 כֹּוב. Ex. R. s. 42 נעשו כובים (corr. acc.), v. סְרָיוּת.—2) מדבר כ׳ pr. n. *Desert of Kub* (cmp. Ez. XXX, 5)=Biblical שׁוּר. Ib. s. 24; Yalk. ib. 255; (Tanh. B'shall. 18; Mekh. ib., Vayassa 1; Yalk. Jer. 266 כזב).

כּוּבָא I, **כָּבָא** ch. same. Targ. Prov. XXVI, 9 (h. text חוח).—Gen. R. s. 44; Yalk. Jer. 285 (prov.) עד דסנדלך... כ׳ while the sandal is on thy foot, tread the thorn down; Pesik. Asser, p. 99[b] כבוש כופה (corr. acc.); Yalk. Deut. 892.—*Pl.* כַּבֵּ׳, כּוּבֵּי, כּוּבַּיָּא, כּוּבִּין. Targ. Gen. III, 18 (some ed. כּוּבְּין, incorr.). Targ. II Sam. XXIII, 6. Targ. Hos. II, 8.—Lam. R. to I, 1 רבתי (חד כות׳ 1), v. גָּבַב.—Y. Ab. Zar. V, 44[d] לאילין כ׳, v. סְדַר. Ib. bot. סייגין כ׳ (read דכ׳) hedges of thornbushes. Gen. R. s. 2 (ref. to Gen. I, 2) עד דהיא פנה אפיקת כ׳ while she (the earth) was yet in her incipiency, she produced thorns; Yalk. Gen. 4 כובה (corr. acc.); Yalk. Jer. 274 כובי; Yalk. Prov. 959.

כּוּבָּא II m. (v. preced.; cmp. כַּד II) 1) *wine cask* (h. קנקן). Sabb. 48[a]. Ab. Zar. 60[a] נכרי אדנא וישראל אכ׳ the gentile attending to the barrel (emptying it) and the Israelite to the cask (receiving the wine). Ib. כ׳ מליא (if the gentile carries) a cask which is brimful. Sabb. 141[a] [read:] לא ליצדד... כ׳ בארעא (v. Rabb. D. S. a. l. note) one must not (on the Sabbath) bend sideways a cask which rests in the ground; a. e.—*Pl.* כּוּבֵּי. Ab. Zar. 33[b] אנס הנך כ׳ וכ׳ carried casks away from Pumbeditha by force. B. Mets. 25[b].—בי כ׳ *the retailer's wine shop.* B. Kam. 86[a]; B. Mets. 64[b] מרקיד בי כ׳ he dances in the wine house.—2) (cmp. כּוּבָּא, אַקִינְבֵּי), *pl.* כּוּבֵּי *turrets* of a fort. Yoma 11[a] חזוק אקרא דכ׳ a support for the Fort of Turrets (of M'ḥuza); [Ms. L. ליוקרא דכ׳ for the weight of &c.; v. Rabb. D. S. a. l. note 400.]—Kidd. 70[b] בי כ׳ דפומבדיתא the fort of P.—[Meg. 6[a] בי כ׳ ed. (Ms. M. כסי, Ms. O. מְכְסֵי); Keth. 112[a] בִּירְכְסֵי.]

כּוּבָּא III m. (v. כָּבַב *Pa.*) *roasted* or *charred dough,* כ׳ דארעא *roasted* (*over coals*) *in a cavity of the ground,* name of *a pastry baked in a cavity made in the stove.* Ber. 37[b], expl. טרוקנין. Ib. 38[a]. [Ar. s. v. כבא, reads כוכא.] [Gitt. 68[a] bot., v. כּוּכָא.]

כובאי, v. כִּיבְי.

כּוֹבֶד m. (b. h. כֹּבֶד; כָּבֵד) 1) *weight, heaviness, pressure.* Snh. 63[b] א״ת כבודו אלא כּוֹבְדוֹ Ms. M., v. כָּבֵד II. Yoma 41[b] בעי כ׳ it requires weight (must be heavy so as to sink into the fire). Ib. כדי שיהא בהן כ׳ (they are tied together) in order that they may be heavy. Y. Ḥag. II, 77[d] צריך לכבוש את כּוֹבְדוֹ (in putting his hands on the sacrifice) he must press his weight on it; (Bab. ib. 16[b] סמיכה בכל כחו). Naz. 5[a] כ׳ the feeling of heaviness (of the hair).—כ׳ ראש *bending down the head; humble, solemn disposition,* opp. קלות ראש. Ber. V, 1 אין עומדין.... כ׳ ראש we must not rise for prayer in any other than a humble &c. Y. Ab. Zar. I, 39[d] top; Tosef. ib. I, 2 שואל בשלומו בכ׳ר׳ greet him with a bent head (without ostentation). M. Kat. 21[b] בשפה רפה ובכ׳ ר׳ in an undertone and with solemnity.—2) *roller* or *beam of a loom;* כ׳ העליון the upper beam from which the warp depends; כ׳ התחתון the lower beam, the roller on which the web is wound as it advances. Kel. XXI, 1 (Talm. ed. כֹּבֶד). Neg. XI, 9 (*fem.*). Sabb. 113[a]; Y. ib. XVII, 16[a] bot.

כובדים, כובדין, v. כוברים.

כּוּבְיָא m. *frying pan,* v. בּוּבְיָא I.

***כּוּבִיתָא** f. (כָּבַב, cmp. כּוּב) *a little globe.* R. Hash. 24[a] כ׳ דעיבא וכ׳ ed. (Ms. M. 1 כּוֹכְבִיתָא, Ms. M. 2 a. Ar. כוכיתא) they saw merely a globe-shaped cloudlet (which, they thought, was the moon).

כובליאר, v. כּוּכְלִיאָר.

כּוֹבְלִין, v. כֶּבֶל.

כּוּבֶלֶת, v. כּוֹבֶלֶת.

כּוֹבֵס m. (b. h.; כָּבַס) *washer, fuller.* Ber. 28[a]; Keth. 103[b]; a. e.—*Pl.* כּוֹבְסִין. Tosef. Kel. B. Mets. III, 14 (ed. Zuck. כובשין), v. מְלַקֵּט II.

כּוּבְסָא, v. כִּבְסָא.

כּוֹבַע m. (b. h.; כבע, cmp. גבע a. denominatives) *helmet, turban.* Ber. 24[a] מניחן בכ׳ וכ׳ let him put them (the T'fillin) into the turban under his pillow. Gitt. 14[b] (of the Persians) כּוֹבְעָן אמה their turban is one cubit high; a. e.—*Pl.* כּוֹבָעִין, כּוֹבָעִים. Gen. R. s. 99 לובשי כ׳ wearing helmets. Y. Gitt. I, end, 43[d]; Y. Kidd. III, 64[a] bot. כּוֹבְעֵיהֶן אמה (v. supra).—Trnsf. *the thyroid cartilage, Adam's apple.* Hull. 19[a] משיפור כ׳ וכ׳ from where the thyroid cartilage begins to protrude and downward.

כּוֹבְעָא ch. same, esp. *the priest's turban.*—*Pl.* כּוֹבְעִין, כּוֹבְעַיָּא. Targ. Ex. XXVIII, 40; XXXIX, 28; a. e. (ed. Berl. ק׳; h. text מגבעות).—Trnsf. חודא דכובעא the highest point of the *thyroid cartilage,* v. preced. Hull. 18[b].

כּוֹבָעָה f., *pl.* כּוֹבָעוֹת (preced. wds.) the *tops of stalks of sheaves.* Peah V, 8 המעמר לכ׳ he who binds sheaves for covering the stalks; expl. Y. ib. V, end, 19[a] מן לעיל sheaves to be put on top, opp. לכומסות; v. כּוֹמְסָה.

כובד׳, כוברים, Pesik. R. s. 14 לולייאנר בר׳ כ׳, Pesik. Par., p. 39[a] שוורי׳, read: צַבְּרְנֵי, as Tanh., ed. Bub., B'resh. 4 (v. Pesik. l. c. note 167).

כּוּבְרִיתָא, v. כַּבְרִיתָא.

כּוֹבֵשׁ m., *pl.* כּוֹבְשִׁים, כּוֹבְשִׁין (כָּבַשׁ) *troops of siege, stormers.* Pesik. Vayhi p. 67[a] העמיד עליהן כ׳ כנגן הארבה he orders against them the storming troops which corresponds to the plague of locusts; Pesik. R. s. 17.—[Y. Erub. II, 24[b] bot. כובשי כבשים, read: כַּבּוּשֵׁי]. [Tosef. Kel. B. Mets. III, 14 ed. Zuck., v. כּוֹבֵס.]

כּוּבְשָׁנָא, v. זוּפְשָׁנָא.

כּוּבֶשֶׁת, v. כֶּבֶשֶׁת.

כּוּד, v. כִּיר.

***כּוּדָא** or **כֻּדָּא** m. (=כבדא, cmp. Syr. כודא, כודתא, P. Sm. 1690 sq., a. קָשָׁה) *suffering in child-birth*. Ab. Zar. 29ᵃ לכ׳ בשיכרא for a woman in child-birth the mixture is made with beer.

כּוּדְנָא c. (כדן) [*working beast*,] *mule*. Targ. Ps. XXXII, 9 (Ms. כּוּנדא).—Sabb. 110ᵇ כפותא דכ׳ חיורא (Rashi חיוורתא) excrements of a white mule.—B. Bath. 91ᵃ כ׳ עקרה במאי פרע לי Ms. M. (ed. פרעא, Ar. כודניא) the mule (Manoah) being barren, how will he pay me back?—*Pl.* כּוּדְנַיָּא. Targ. Zech. XIV, 15.—*Fem.* כּוּדַנְתָּא, כּוּדַנְיָא. Targ. II Sam. XIII, 29; a. e.—Bekh. 8ᵇ.—*Pl.* כּוּדְנְיָתָא, כּוּדַנְיָן, כּוּדַנְוָן. Targ. I Kings X, 25; Targ. II Chr. IX, 24. Targ. Y. Gen. XXXVI, 24 (not כּוּדְנַיְיתָא). Targ. Is. LXVI, 20 כודנון ed. Lag. (ed. Wil. כּוּדְנָן); a. e.—Hull. 7ᵇ כ׳ חיוורתא white mules. [B. Mets. 97ᵃ כודנייתא, Ms. M. כונדתיה, read כּוּדַנְתֵּיה his mule.]

כָּוָה, v. כוי.

כּוֹהֵן, כּוֹהֶנֶת, v. כֹּהֵן.

כַּוָּא, כַּוָּא m., **כַּוְּתָא, כַּוּוּתָא** f. (√ כו, v. כבב, *to be arched, hollow*)= h. חַלּוֹן, *aperture, window*. Targ. Zeph. II, 14 (ed. Lag. כַּוָּה). Targ. Prov. VII, 6 ed. Lag. (oth. ed. כַּוַּיָּא *pl.*). Targ. Hos. XIII, 3 כַּוַּת נורא smoke-hole; a. e.—M. Kat. 11ᵃ כוותא דדשא Ar. a. Rashi Ms. (ed. קבותא, Ms. M. קבוותא, v. Rabb. D. S. a. l. note) the arch of the door, upper door-post. Y. Yeb. IV, 6ᵇ bot. אודיק ר׳ מן כ׳ Rabbi looked out of the window. Sabb. 35ᵃ וסימניך כ׳ (or כַּוָּתָא *pl.*) thy sign by which to remember be 'window' (which reflects the light of the setting sun); a. fr.—*Pl.* כַּוָּתָא, כַּוַּיָּא, כַּוִּין, כַּוֵּי &c. Targ. I Kings VI, 4. Targ. Y. II Gen. XLIX, 22. Targ. Cant. II, 9.—B. Bath. 6ᵃ בֵּי כַּוֵּי לא וכ׳ apertures in the party wall (for beam-rests) are no evidence of the neighbor's share in the wall. Ib. 75ᵃ כ׳ דבי זיקא (Ms. O. כַּוֵּי זיקא) apertures for the air (windows, contrad. to openings for doors).—*Hebr. pl.* כַּוִּין. Sifré Deut. 309 (play on ויכוננך, Deut. XXXII, 6) עשאך כ׳ כ׳ he made thy body full of cavities (v. Pesik. Zutr. ed. Bub., Deut. p. 111); Yalk. ib. 942 כיון כיון (corr. acc.).

כַּוָּאָה, v. כְּוָאָה.

כַּוָּוה, v. כוי.

כַּוֵּי f. (v. כַּוָּא) *aperture*. Yalk. Jer. 276 (ref. to כַּוָּנִים, Jer. VII, 18) היה חופר בתוך ביתו כ׳ קטנה והיו מכוונים וכ׳ used to make in his house a small aperture which was directed exactly towards the east, so that when the morning star rose, he might rise and worship it; Pesik. R. s. 31 קטה כמין ניכוי (corr. acc.); v. כּוֹכֶבֶת.

***כַּוָּן** m. (b. h. כַּוָּן; v. next w.) *exactly determined place* (for worship).—*Pl.* כַּוָּנִים. Pesik. R. s. 31; Yalk. Jer. 276 (ref. to Jer. VII, 18) מהו כ׳ what is *kavvanim?*, v. preced. [In b. h. our w. seems to mean certain *cakes* placed due east.]

כִּוּוּן m. (כּוּן, cmp. כַּוָּנָה) *exact selection of place*. Gen. R. s. 15, beg. צריכה כ׳ (planting) requires exact selection; ib. צריך לְכַוֵּן את רוחותיה one must determine its position with reference to the cardinal points.

כַּוָּנָא, v. כִּיוָּנָא.

כַּוָּנָה, כַּוּנוּתָא, כַּוָּנְתָּא, v. sub כונ׳.

כַּוָּנִיתָא, כַּוַּנְתָּא, v. כִּיוָנ׳.

כְּוָרֶץ, v. כְּוִיץ.

כַּוְרָא, כַּוָּרָא m. (v. כְּוֶורֶת) [*basket, cauf*, cmp. נְדִיל,] *fish in the cauf*, in gen. *fish*. M. Kat. 11ᵃ [read:] כ׳ טווייה באחוה וכ׳ (v. Rabb. D. S. a. l.) roast the fish with its brother (salt) &c. Y. Sabb. VII, 10ᵃ החן דצייד כ׳ he who catches fish (on the Sabbath). Gitt. 36ᵃ, a. e. צייר כ׳ drew the figure of a fish (in place of his signature); a. fr.—*Pl.* כַּוְּ׳, כַּוּוּרֵי, כַּוּוּרַיָּא. Targ. Y. Gen. I, 26, a. fr. (only in Targ. Y.).—[Targ. Job. XLI, 26 בני כוורי, Ms. כונדי, Regia טורי; h. text בני שחץ.]—Taan. 24ᵃ פירא דכ׳ *the fish-pond*. Kidd. 72ᵃ.—M. Kat. l. c. לבאי כ׳ (Var. כַּוָּארֵי), v. בְּדִירָתָא; a. e.

כוורדקי, v. אַכְוַנְגַּר.

כַּוְּוֵרִיתָא f. *honey-comb*, v. כַּבְרִיתָא I.

כְּוַרְדְּנָקִי, כַּוּרְנָק, v. אַכְוַרְנְקָא.

כְּוֶורֶת f. (כור, cmp. כְּבָרָה; v. Fl. to Levy Targ. Dict. I, p. 428ᵃ) 1) *a large round vessel, receptacle* of grain, water &c.; כ׳ דבורים *bee-hive*. Num. R. s. 1; Tanh. B'midb. 2, v. כַּוּוֹרֶת. Shebi. X, 7. Kel. XV, 1 כ׳ חקש וכ׳ הקנים a receptacle made of straw or reeds. Ib. VIII, 1; Tosef. ib. B. Kam. VI, 3 כ׳ פחותה וכ׳ a defective *k'vereth* which was repaired with a stuffing of straw. Ib. V, 8 [read:] כְּאוֹרֶת של מתכת וכ׳ (ed. Zuck. כיארת, corr. acc.) a metal *k*. used in the household. Men. 95ᵃ כמין כ׳ a kind of bee-hive (honeycombed plate in the stove); Tosef. ib. XI, 2 מורת, מורת (corr. acc.); a. e.—*Pl.* כְּוָורוֹת. Tosef. Ohol. X, 5 שתי כ׳ (כוורת ed. Zuck., Var. כיארת, corr. acc.).—2) the *ramifications of the vine, espalier, the widest extent of branches*. Tosef. Kil. III, 4; Y. ib. V, 29ᵈ הכ׳ מְכוּוֶּנֶת והגוף וכ׳ (sub בית) if the espalier is in a certain direction, but the body of the vine is not in the line. Y. Erub. III, 21ᵃ top בשהיתה כְּוֶורְתוֹ ארבעה when its ramifications had a circumference of four cubits; Y. Succ. II, 52ᵈ bot. כברתו (corr. acc. or כְּבָרָתוֹ). Y. Ber. I, 2ᶜ bot., v. נוֹף I; a. e.—Midr. Sam. ch. XIII קוֹרָתוֹ של חרוב (= כְּוְ׳), v. next w.—*Pl.* m. כְּוָורְתִים, כְּוָורְתִין. Y. Kil. IV, 29ᵇ top הכוור׳ R. S. to Kil. IV, 3 (ed. כְּרָתִים contr., cmp. הֶרְבֵּן). Ib. VI, beg. 30ᵇ כרתין. Ib. IV, 29ᶜ כרתין; ib. V, 30ᵃ top כרתין (corr. acc.).

כּוּרְתָּא (כּוּרְתָּא) כְּוֹרֶת, כְּוֶורְתָּא ch. same, 1) *bee-hive*. Targ. Jer. V, 27 ככ׳ דמליא זיבורייתא Vers. in ed. Lag. (v. preface to Proph. XXXIV, 13) like a hive full of bees.—2) *ramification*. Num. R. s. 9 כ׳ דחרוביתא the circumference of a carob-tree; Y. Sot. I, 17ᵇ top ed. Amst. (ed. Krot. אורתא, corr. acc.); Y. Peah VII, 20ᵃ bot. בירתא (corr. acc.); (Midr. Sam. ch. XIII, v. preced.).

כְּוָות, v. כְּוֵת.

כַּוְּותָא I f. *window*, v. כַּוָּא.

כַּוְּותָא II f. (כְּוִי) *searing, blister* from a burn. Snh. 84ᵇ ed., v. בּוּעְתָא I.

כּוּז m. (cmp. כַּד II) *an oil vessel*, used in the Temple. Tam. III, 6 והכ׳ דומה וכ׳ the *kuz* had the shape of a large wine cup. Ib. 9.

כּוּזָא f. ch. same, *wine pitcher, jug*. Targ. II Esth. II, 21.—Sabb. 77ᵇ (playful etymology) כּוּזָה כָּזֶה ed. (Rashi כוזא) it is named *kuza*—'like this' (give us to drink from). Ḥull. 107ᵃ כ׳ בת רביעתא a *Kuza* must contain one fourth of a Log. Sabb. 33ᵇ. Taan. 20ᵇ (Ms. M. אֲכוּזָא); a. fr.—Yeb. 70ᵃ, v. כַּדָּא.

כּוֹזָב, v. next w.

כּוֹזִיבָא, כּוֹזְבָה, כּוֹזְבָא 1) (בַּר) בֶּן כ׳ pr. n. m. *Ben-(Bar-)Koz'ba*, name of the leader of the Jewish uprising against Hadrian, usually named בר כוכבא *Bar-Kokhba*. Y. Taan. IV, 68ᵈ bot. עקיבא ... דרך כוכב ... דרך כ׳ Akiba, my teacher, preached, 'A star goes forth from Jacob' (Num. XXIV, 17) Koz'ba went forth; Lam. R. to II, 2 א״ת כוכב אלא כּוֹזָב read not *Kokhab* but *Kozab*. Y. Taan. l. c. בן (בר) כוזבה. Ib. 69ᵃ top כוזבה (corr. acc.). Lam. R. l. c. בן (בר) כוזיבא; Yalk. Deut. 946.—Denom. כּוֹזְבִי; f. כּוֹזְבִית, pl. כּוֹזְבִיּוֹת. Tosef. Maas. Sh. I, 6; B. Kam. 97ᵇ מעות כ׳ coins issued by Bar-K.—*2) בֵּית כ׳ pr. n. *Beth-Koz'ba*, name of a valley. Tanḥ. Ḥuck. 1; (ed. Bub. ib. טופח; Num. R. s. 18 תופח; Gen. R. s. 10 בר טרפא; Lev. R. s. 22 בית שופרי; Koh. R. to V, 8 טופח; Yalk. Koh. 972 נטופא).

כּוּזָה, v. כּוּזָא.

כּוֹזִיבָא, v. כּוֹזְבָא.

כּוּזִית pr. n. m. *Kuzith*, surname of one R. Samuel. Gen. R. s. 23; s. 51 Ar. (absent in eds.).

כּוֹזְנִי, v. next w.

כּוּזַנְתָּא f.=כּוּזָא, *jug*. Ab. Zar. 71ᵇ. M. Kat. 12ᵃ quot. in Rashi to Ab. Zar. l. c. (ed. כּוּזְתָא, Ms. M. כּוּזָא). Sabb. 139ᵇ אפומא דכוזנתא Rashi Ms. (ed. בפומיה דכוזני דחביתא; Ms. O. בפומא דכוזתא, v. Rabb. D. S. a. l. note) on the mouth of the jug (used for taking wine out of the larger vessel).

כּוּזְתָא, v. preced.

כּוּחַ *to cough*, v. כָּחַח.

כּוּחַ, כּוּחָא, v. כֹּחַ, כָּחָא.

כּוֹחִילְנָא m. (v. next w.) *koḥilna*, name of a bird. Ḥull. 62ᵇ (Ar. גְּחִילְנָא).

כּוֹחָל (כְּחוֹל) m. (cmp. גחל, v. Lane Customs, 1837, p. 51 sq.) *koḥl, a powder used for painting the eye-lids, stibium*. Sabb. VIII, 3 (78ᵇ) כּוֹ׳ Ar. (ed. כְּחָ׳); Y. ib. 11ᵇ bot. כּוֹ׳. Ḥull. 88ᵇ השחור והכ׳ powdered coal and stibium. Snh. 14ᵃ; Keth. 17ᵃ (in a song) לא כֹּחָל here is no paint (no showiness). [Tosef. Nidd. VI, 4 כוחל, read: בּוֹחַל.]

כּוֹחֲלָא ch. 1) same. Targ. II Esth. I, 3 (2); Ber. 18ᵇ, v. גּוּבְתָא.—Ḥull. 47ᵇ ככ׳ as black as stibium. Gitt. 69ᵃ top תרתי מנתא כ׳ וכ׳ two portions of stibium and one of &c.—2) אבנא דכ׳ a species of *black marble* (b. h. פּוּךְ, v. Sm. Ant. s. v. Carbunculus). Kidd. 12ᵃ אקדיש בא׳ דכ׳ betrothed a woman by giving her a piece of black marble (of little value). B. Bath. 4ᵃ; Succ. 51ᵇ, v. מַרְמָרָא.

כּוֹחֲלִי, v. כּוֹחֲלִית.

כּוֹחֲלִין m. pl. (used as sing.; v. preced. wds.; cmp. b. h. פּוּךְ a. נֹפֶךְ) *carbuncle*, name of a jewel. Ex. R. s. 38, end (corresp. to לשם, Ex. XXVIII, 19). [V., however, כַּחְלִי.]

כּוֹחֲלִית pr. n. *Koḥălith*, a district conquered by John Hyrcan, [perh.=נֹפַח, Num. XXI, 30, cmp. preced. wds. a. פֶּחָם]. Kidd. 66ᵃ כ׳ שבמדבר K. in the desert.—אזוב כ׳ a species of *hyssop* named after that district. Neg. XIV, 6 כּוֹחֲלִי; Succ. 13ᵃ לית ... Ms. M. (ed. לי ...). Par. XI, 7; Ḥull. 62ᵇ; Sifré Num. 129.

כּוֹי, כָּוָה, כָּוָא (b. h.; cmp. כחח) [*to cause discoloring*,] *to sear, cauterize; to scald*. B. Kam. VIII, 1 כְּוָאוֹ בשפוד וכ׳ if a person hurt another with a hot spit &c.; Y. ib. 6ᵃ, ᵇ (Mish. a. Gem.) כְּוָיוֹ, כְּוָיוֹ; a. e.—*Part. pass.* כָּווּי *burn-marked, flame-spotted*. Lev. R. s. 15 ... חמורה ונכוית ויצא בנה כ׳ a she-ass was sick and was cauterized, and her child was born with a flame-mark; (Num. R. s. 9 מרושם).

Hif. הִכְוָה same. Neg. VII, 4 וה׳ את המחיה if one cauterized the cicatrizing spot.

Pi. כִּיוָּה same. Num. R. l. c. הוליכה ... וכי׳ אותה he took her to the veterinary surgeon, and he cauterized her.

Nif. נִכְוָה *to be burnt; to be cauterized*. B. Bath. 75ᵃ כל אחד וא׳ נִכְוָה חופתו מחופת וכ׳ Ms. M. (v. Rabb. D. S. a. l. note) each man's tent will be stained by fire from his neighbor's tent. Lev. R. l. c. נִכְוֵית, v. supra. Num. R. l. c. ממה שנִכְוֵת אמו because his mother had been cauterized. Sabb. 30ᵇ; Pes. 117ᵃ תִּכָּוֶינָה (his lips) be burnt. Tosef. Ḥag. II, 6 היטה לכאן וניכ׳ באור . . ונכווה בשלג if he deviates this way, he will be burnt by the fire, if that way, he will be frost-bitten; (Ab. d'R. N. ch. XXVIII לוקה בצינה). Tosef. Ḥull. III, 6 יכולה לִיכָּווֹת וכ׳ she may be cauterized and recover.—Y. Sabb. III, 6ᵇ top והיא נכוית and it (the hand) is scalded (v. סָלַד). Y. Ber. II, 5ᵇ bot. כמדומה ... שאתם נִיכְוִין בפושרין וכ׳ I thought you would be scalded with tepid water (understand a slight hint), but you do not feel even hot water (distinct intimation); Bab. ib. 16ᵇ.—Y. Nidd. III, 50ᵈ [read:] רישיה דרישך יִכָּוֶה בפושרין ואתה לא תִיכָּוֶה אפי׳ ברותחין thy head's head (thy teacher's teacher) feels tepid water, but thou &c., i. e. you must not claim superiority to your predecessors (cmp. Sabb. 55ᵃ); a. fr.

כְּוָא, כְּוִי ch. same. Y. Bets. II, 61ᶜ top; Y. Maas. Sh. V, 56ᶜ top, a. e. (כָּוְיָה) כָּוְיָא, v. גּוּמְרָא.

Ithpa. אִתְכַּוֵּי *to be burnt*. Targ. Prov. VI, 28 מִתְכַּוְיָין Ms. (ed. כְּוַיִין ..., corr. acc.).

כּוֹי m. *Koy*, (prob.) a kind of *bearded dear* or *antelope* (τραγέλαφος). [The rabbis leave it undecided whether K. belongs to the genus of cattle (בְּהֵמָה) or beasts of chase (חַיָּה).] Y. Bicc. II, end, 65ᵇ, v. כְּוִי. Hull. 80ᵃ (various opinions). Tosef. ib. VI (V), 1. Tosef. Bekh. II, 9; a. fr.

כֻּרֵיץ, v. כְּוִיץ.

כּוּךְ m. (= כוכו, v. כְּוָא) *cavity, cave*, esp. *sepulchral chamber*. [Taan. 25ᵇ כ׳ המחרישה R. Gersh. (Ms. M. כון, v. Rabb. D. S. a. l. note, ed. בֶּרֶךְ) the cavity made by the plough.]—Y. B. Bath. III, beg. 13ᵈ המוכר ... בכ׳ חזקה לכל הכ׳ if one sells a burial place (קבר) to his neighbor, as soon as the latter has buried one dead in the chamber, he has the possession of the entire chamber; a. e.—*Pl.* כּוּכִין. Ib. קבר ... בג׳ כ׳ וכ׳ when he buried three dead in three different chambers &c. Tosef. Ohol. XVII, 11 [read:] שדה .. בתוכה היא כשדה כ׳ ואיזו היא שדה כ׳ כל ... הכ׳ לצדדין a field in which a grave (known to have been there) has disappeared, is like a field of sepulchral chambers. And what is a field &c.? Where you dig out (a square) in the ground, and make chambers in the walls. B. Bath. VI, 8; a. e.

כּוּכָא, כּוּךְ ch. 1) same. Targ. Job XXX, 2; ib. V, 26 (h. text כלח).—2) *an improvised subterranean dwelling*. Taan. 22ᵃ כי דציידי Rashi (ed. כַּכּוּבֵי, pl., Ar. s. v. ככי: לא נצרכה אלא לבי כ׳ דאגמא) like the hunters' cave. Gitt. 68ᵃ bot. מטא גבי כ׳ דההיא וכ׳ Ar. (ed. כובא, corr. acc.) he came to the hut of a certain widow. [Ber. 37ᵇ כ׳ דארעא Ar., v. כּוּבָא III.]

כּוֹכָב, כֹּכָב m. (b. h.; = כבכב, v. כבב) [*rounded, globe,*] *star, planet*. Y. Ber. I, 2ᵇ כ׳ אחד ודאי יום as long as one star only is visible, it is surely day-time. Hor. 10ᵃ כ׳ אחד יש ועולה וכ׳ Ms. M. (v. Rabb. D. S. a. l. note) there is a certain star (comet) which appears once in seventy years. Gen. R. s. 100 עשרה כוכבים בקשו לאבד כ׳ אחד ten stars (sons of Jacob) desired to destroy one star (Joseph); a. fr. —*Pl.* כּוֹכָבִים, כֹּכָ׳. Ib.—Ber. 10ᵃ כ׳ ומזלות stars and planets; a. fr.—עבודת כ׳ (עכו״ם, עו״כ abbr.) עובד כ׳ ומזלות, עובד כ׳, v. עֲבוֹדָה, עָבַד. Succ. 22ᵇ; Y. ib. II, beg. 22ᵈ כּוֹכְבֵי חמה scintillations of the sun as seen through the covering of the festive booth. Yalk. Esth. 1053 כ׳ חנגה, v. next w.

כּוֹכַב, כּוֹכְבָא, כֹּכ׳ ch. same. Targ. Am. V, 26.—Y. Maas. Sh. IV, 55ᵇ bot.; a. fr.—Esp. *the planet Mercury*. Sabb. 156ᵃ האי מאן דבכ׳ he who was born under Mercury. —כ׳ נוגהא, כ׳ נוגה *Venus*. Targ. II Esth. II, 7 (v. אִיסְתְּהַר); Yalk. Esth. 1053 (hebr.), v. אִסְתְּהַר.—Sabb. l. c.; a. e.—כ׳ דשביט *comet*. Ber. 58ᵇ.—*Pl.* כֹּכ׳, כּוֹכְבֵי, כּוֹכְבַיָּא. Targ. Gen. I, 16; a. fr.—Snh. 39ᵃ מצינא למימני כ׳ I can count the stars. Ib. מני לי כ׳ the number of the stars is known to me. Ab. Zar. 29ᵃ דתלי לה בי כ׳ which he suspended under the stars (in open air over night); a. fr.—[B. Mets. 86ᵃ כֹּכְבִין דנרדא Ar. balls of nardus, ed. כְּבְרִין.]

כּוֹכְבִיתָא f. *a little globe*, v. כּוּבִיתָא.

כּוֹכֶבֶת f. (preced. wds.) *the planet Venus, morning star, evening star*. Yalk. Jer. 276 (ref. to Jer. VII, 18) שהיו עובדים למלכת השמים זו היא הכ׳ (not מְלֶאכֶת) they worshipped the queen of the heavens, that is Venus; Pesik. R. s. 31 חכוכבים (corr. acc.). Ib. היו בני ירושלם עובדים לכ׳ וכ׳ (not לכוכבים) the Jerusalemites worshipped Venus openly &c. Ib. שכשתעלה הכ׳ (not חכוכבים), v. כְּוִי.

כּוֹכַבְתָּא ch. same. Targ. Jer. VII, 18, a. e. כּוֹכַבַת שמיא, v. preced.—Y. Ber. I, 2ᵇ בר מן הדא כ׳ ... ובלחוד provided three stars are seen besides the evening star.—Ib.ᶜ מאן דאמר כ׳ וכ׳ he who says *ăyalta d'shahra* is the morning star, is mistaken; Y. Yoma III, beg. 40ᵇ; Gen. R. s. 50 כ׳ דצפרא.

***כּוּכְיָא** m. (cmp. כָּבָר) *spiderweb*, v. בּוּכְיָא.

כוכיתא, v. כּוּבִיתָא.

כּוּכְלִיאר, כּוּכְלְייר m. (cochlear) [*a kind of spoon pointed on one end for drawing snails out of their shells,*] *a pin of the shape of a cochlear*. Sabb. VI, 3 כוכליר Y. ed., Ms. O. כוכליאר (Mish. a. Bab. ed. 62ᵃ כוליאר, Ms. M. in Gem. כובליאר, corr. acc., v. Rabb. D. S. a. l. notes 20 a. 70); expl. ib. 62ᵃ מַכְבֶּנְתָּא. V. next w.

כּוּכְלִיאס, כּוּכְלְייס, קוכ׳ m. (χοχλίας, cochlea) *any thing spiral, a spiral stair-case, screw* &c. (v. Gr. a. Lat. Dict. s. v.). Tosef. Succ. IV, 16 מקיפין ועומדין כקבולין ed. Zuck. (Var. ככוליִיר, בכוליִיס, read בכוכליִיס) stood around in a spiral figure; Tosef. Yoma I, 10 בקבילין ed. Zuck. (Var. בכלאים, ככוליוּר); Yoma 25ᵃ כמין בכוליאר (Ms. M. כוליִיר, O. a. L. ככוליִיר, v. Rabb. D. S. a. l. note). Y. Shek. VII, beg. 50ᶜ כמין כובלין היו עשוין (corr. acc.) the boxes in the Temple for contributions were put up so as to form a spiral figure; (Bab. ed. קובליים, בוכלייאר, כובליי׳, corr. acc.).

***כּוּכֶלֶת** f. (= כלכלת, cmp. גוּגְלְתָא; כַּלְכֵּל) [*refreshing bottle,*] *a charm containing a perfume*. Sabb. VI, 3. Ib. v. 62ᵃ, חוּמְרְתָא; [Ed. a several Mss. read: כּוּבֶלֶת (כֶּבֶל) *chain*, v. Rabb. D. S. a. l., a. Koh. Ar. Compl. s. v.]; Tosef. ib. IV (V), 11.

כּוּל (b. h.) [*to enclose,*] *to measure*. Ter. X, 8 וכָל גרב Ms. (ed. כל), v. גָּרָב I.—

Pilp. כִּלְכֵּל q. v.

כּוּל, כִּיל ch. same. Perf. כָּל; part. כָּאֵיל, כָּיֵיל. Targ. O. Ex. XVI, 18 (Y. אֲכִילוּ *Af.*). Targ. Ruth. III, 15. Targ. Is. XXVII, 8.—Men. 53ᵇ כי קא כייל וכ׳ when he measures, he measures by &c. Ab. Zar. 71ᵇ קא כ׳ ודמי וכ׳ he measures and pours (the wine) into &c. Ned. 51ᵃ, v. אֲבַל II. —Hull. 12ᵃ, a. e. לכי תֵיכוּל עלה כורא דמילחא (I will tell you,) if you will measure out for it a *kor* of salt (a jesting remark). Kidd. 79ᵇ כולי עלמא בְּכֵילָה ליה וכ׳ to all the world (wisdom) has been measured in a small *kab*, and to this scholar in a large *kab*, i. e. he wants to be wiser than all the world.

Af. אֲכִיל same. Targ. Y. Ex. XVI, 18, v. supra. Targ. Y. II Gen. XXXVIII, 26 מְכִיל (not מְ׳).

Pa. כַּיֵּיל (denom. of כְּלָלָא) *to generalize; lay down a rule*. Keth. 60ᵃ, v. כְּלָלָא.

Ithpe. אִתְכַּל, אִתְכִּיל *to be measured*. Targ. Y. II Gen. l. c. Targ. Is. XL, 12; a. e.

כּוּל־ h., v. כֹּל.

כּוּל, כּוּלָא, כּוּלָּא ch.=h. כֹּל 1) *all, every one; any.* Constr. כָּל (frequ. used absolutely). Targ. O. Gen. XVI, 12, sq. Targ. Ex. XX, 9. Targ. Y. Deut. XXXII, 49 לא כל חיאך not at all as (thou sayest); a. fr.—Y. Yoma VIII, 45[b] bot. לא כולא מן הדין וכ׳ all does not depend upon this man (it is not at all within his power) to say to the king, Thou art no king, i. e. his saying that the Day of Atonement has no atoning power, cannot affect its power; Y. Shebu. II, 33[b] bot.—Snh. 46[b], a. fr. (לאו) לא כל כמיניה all is not as if dependent on him, i. e. he has no power to &c. Gen. R. s. 79, beg. (expl. בכלח, Job V, 26) תבא בכולא אלי וכ׳ (some ed. בכולה) thou shalt enter the grave in fulness, full, wanting nothing.—כָּל קְבֵל=h. כָּל עֻמַּת, v. כֹּל. Targ. Job IV, 19; a. fr.—Nidd. 51[a]; a. fr.—כָּל עלמא, v. infra.—With suffix כּוּלָּךְ, כּוּלֵּיה &c. (Buxt. כָּלָּךְ &c.) *all of thee, of him* &c., *entire.* Targ. Gen. XXV, 25; a. fr.—Yoma 14[b] כוליה יומא the entire day; ib. 19[a] (not כולי). Ib. 26[a] כּוּלְהוּ מצפרא אתו (v. Rabb. D. S. a. l. note 10) all of them come in (for their share) by the lots cast in the morning; a. fr.—*Pl.* constr. כּוּלֵּי *all of.* Targ. Esth. VI, 1 כ׳ ליליא (ed. Lag. כוליה). Targ. Koh. X, 12 כ׳ עלמא (ed. Lag. כוליה).—Y. Ber. II, 4[b] כ׳ עלמא ידעין ed. Lehm. (ed. כל) all the world, *all people* know (abbr. כ״ע); Y. M. Kat. III, 83[c] bot. כל עמא; v. עָלְמָא. Kidd. 79[b], v. כּוּל ch. —כ׳ האי all of that, *to that extent.* Erub. 61[a]. B. Mets. 84[b] כ׳ ה׳ ודאי וכ׳ after it has come to all this (it being so well known), it is surely not proper. Ab. Zar. 24[a]; a. v. fr.—Ḥag. 4[b] כ׳ ה׳ ואולי all this (is required of us) and yet only 'perhaps' (Zeph. II, 3)! Taan. 25[a] כ׳ ה׳ ואפשר all this (trouble) and 'only perhaps'!—*2) *capacity, power* (cmp. יכל). Y. Peah VIII, 20[d] bot. לא כָּלָּן מסתור וכ׳ our (my) strength consists not in tearing down but &c.

כּוּלָב, כּוּלְבָא, כּוּלְבָה m. (v. כָּלַב; cmp. פֶּה, στόμα for edge) *a sharp instrument, axe.* Targ. I Sam. XIII, 20 (some ed. כולב׳, Ar. כולבא; h. text קרדם).—Gen. R. s. 38 איתוי לי כולב Ar. (ed. איתי לי קולב), v. יְתַר.—Lev. R. s. 4 הן דרי זיינא כּוּלְבֵיה וכ׳ . . (not זייניה כולבא) where the owner of arms (warrior) hangs up his battle axe, the shepherd hangs up his bag, i. e. in the place of justice sits wickedness; Koh. R. to III, 16 קולביה; (Yalk. Koh. 969 באתרא זייניה . . . where the lord hangs up his armor). Y. Naz. I, 51[b] כולבה a. כולבא; Y. Ned. I, 36[d] top כולבה, v. קִנְתָּא.—*Pl.* כּוּלְבַיָּא. Targ. I Sam. XIII, 21. Targ. Jud. IX, 48 (Ar. כולב׳). Targ. Ps. LXXIV, 5.—V. כָּלוּב.

כּוּלְבּוּס, v. כַּלְבּוּס.

כּוּלְבְּסִין or כּוּלְכ׳, Y. Dem. II, 22[c] bot., v. כּוּלְבּוּס.

כּוּלָה, *a measure,* v. כִּלָה.

כּוּלָּה, v. כּוּלָּא.

כּוּלוּנִיס, Tosef. Kel. B. Mets. IV, 7, v. כָּלִינוּס.

כּוּלֵי, v. כּוּלֵי I, II.—כּוּלֵּי pl. constr. of כּוּלָּא.

כּוּלְיָא, כּוּלְיָיא (כָּל׳, כּוּל׳) f. ch. (v. כִּלְיָה) [*rounded,*] 1) *testicle.* Targ. Y. II Lev. XXI, 20. Targ. Y. ib. XXII, 23.—2) *kidney.* Hull. 97[a].—*Pl.* כּוּלְיָתָא, כּוּלְיָין, כּוּלְיָן (כּוּל׳) (כָּל׳). Targ. Lev. III, 4; a. fr. Targ. Job XXXVIII, 36 כולרין ed. Lag. (oth. כָּלְיָן, Ms. Var. כוליתא). Targ. Is. XXXIV, 6 כָּלְיַת constr.—Sabb. 119[b].—[כּוּלְיָא h., v. כִּלְיָה.]

כּוּלִיאר, v. כּוּבְלְיָיר.

כּוּלְיָה, v. כִּלְיָה.

כּוֹלִיקוֹס m. (χολικός, in the sense of μελαγχολικός) *one afflicted with melancholy.* Y. Ter. I, 40[b] המקרע את כסותו כ׳ if one tears his clothes, I may say, he is melancholy (but not insane); Y. Gitt. VII, beg. 48[c] המקרע קינוקיס . . . . (corr. acc.).

כּוּלָךְ, v. כָּלָךְ.

כּוּלְכָא m. ch.=h. כָּלָךְ, *cissaros-blossom* (v. אִגְבִּין). Sabb. 20[b]; Y. ib. II, beg. 4[d], expl. כָּלָךְ. Y. Kil. IX, 32[a] top כָּלְכָה שמו its name is *kall'kha.* [כולכה, כולכא, for כולבא, v. כּוּלְבָא.]

כּוּלְכְּסִין, v. כּוּלְבְּסִין.

כּוּלָם, Ex. R. s. 15 וכן דימוס וכן כ׳ (some ed. כולו), read: כּוּלֵי II.

כּוּלְמָתָא, v. next w.

כַּלְנִיתָא, כּוּלְנִיתָא f. (v. Löw Pfl. p. 200 sq.) [*Little Bride,*] *Papaver Spinosum.*—*Pl.* כּוּלְנְיָיתָא. Pes. 35[a] Ar. (ed. כַּלְנִיתָא; Ms. O. כַּלְנְיָיתָא; Ms. M. 1 כולמתא; Ms. M. 2 כולניתא); v. קִרְמִית.

כּוּלְסָא, Sabb. 154[b], v. בּוּלְסָא.

כּוּלָף m. (כלה, cmp. קלף, גלב). *plane.* Tosef. Kel. B. Bath. VII, 3 יד הכ׳ וּבֶן כ׳ (not וּבֵין) the handle of a large or of a small plane (some ed. הכילוף וכן הכילוף, corr. acc.).

כּוּלְפְּסוֹן, Tosef. Kil. III, 12 ed. Zuck., read: כּוּלְבְּסִין, v. כּוּלְבּוּס.

כּוּלְקוֹס, v. כַּלְקִיס.

***כּוּלְקְטָר** m. (collectarius), *pl.* כּוּלְקְטָרִין *cashiers.* Pesik. Haḥod. p. 56[a] מי פורע . . . שני דלקטירין וכ׳ (corr. acc.) who will collect for you the debt from them (bring about their punishment)? Two collectors, Mordecai and Esther; Pesik. R. s. 15 בלקטירים; Yalk. Ex. 191 סלקטירין (corr. acc.).

כּוּלְתָא *wrath,* v. כְּלוּ.

כּוּמָז m. (b. h.; cmp. כּוּמְצָא) an opprobrious name for *an ornament* bearing the impress of the female breast or pudenda. Y. Sabb. V, 8[b] bot.; Bab. ib. 64[a].

***כּוּמְנֵי** f. (prob. a corrupt. of χαμεύνη, *a pallet-bed*) *mattress* used as a seat for travelling women. Tosef. B. Bath. IV, 2; B. Bath. 78[a], expl. מרכבתא דנשי.

כּוּמְסָה, כּוּמְסֵי f., *pl.* כּוּמְסָאוֹת, כּוּמְסוֹת (כָּמַס) *sheaves put at the bottom of a stack* as foundation, contrad. to כּוּבְעָה. Peah V, 8; Y. ib. V, end, 19[a], expl. מן לרע (with ref. to Deut. XXXII, 34).

כּוּמְצָא m. (כמץ, cmp. כמן) *trap, pit.* Targ. Is. XXIV, 17, sq.; Targ. Jer. XLVIII, 43, sq. (h. text פחת). V. קוּמְצָא II, cmp. גּוּמְצָא.

כּוּמֶר I m. (כָּמַר) *a mass of olives or grapes shrunk* from exposure to the sun or from being put in the ground, prior to being placed in the press. B. Mets. 74ᵃ. Y. Ber. II, 4ᵇ bot. כב׳ הוה של ענבים וכ׳ like the mass of heated grapes that drips of itself; Cant. R. to VII, 10 כבמריזה וכ׳ some ed. (read כִּכּמֶר הזה); Yeb. 97ᵃ; Bekh. 31ᵇ; Y. Shek. II, end, 47ᵃ כֹּמֶר.

כּוֹמֶר II or **כּוּמָר** m. (b. h. כְּמָרִים; כָּמַר *to guard*, cmp. כֹּהֵן. In Syriac כומרא interchanges with כהנא, v. P. Sm. 1757 s. v.) *attendant, priest*, always used of idolaters. Kidd. 20ᵇ נעשה כ׳ לע״ז (Arakh. 30ᵇ משרת) became an attendant of an idolatrous temple. Y. Ab. Zar. I, 39ᵈ. Pesik. R. s. 35 יתרו לא כ׳ וכ׳ was not Jethro an idolatrous priest?; a. fr. —*Pl.* כּוּמָרִין, כּוּמָרִים. Ab. Zar. 51ᵇ בטובת כ׳ for the benefit of the idolatrous priests, opp. עובדיה worshippers; Y. ib. IV, 43ᵈ bot. Erub. 79ᵇ bot. Ms. M. (ed. משרתי ע״ז). Gen. R. s. 65, beg.; a. fr.

כּוּמְרָא, כּוּמָרָא I ch. same. Targ. Jud. XVII, 5; 13 (interch. with כהין ib. 10; 12; h. text כֹּהֵן); a. e.—Lam. R. to I, 9 ההוא כ׳ (Yalk. Ez. 356 ההיא אפיקודוס).—*Pl.* כּוּמְרַיָּא, כּוּמְרִין, כּוּמְ׳. Targ. Jud. XVIII, 30. Targ. II Kings XXIII, 5; a. fr.—Gen. R. s. 26, v. אֱלָהּ. Ex. R. s. 9 (prov.) מחי אלהיא ויבעתין כ׳ strike the gods, and the priests will be frightened.

כּוּמְרָא II m. (v. כּוּמֶר I) *withering.* Ber. 40ᵇ בושלי כ׳ Ms. M. a. oth. (ed. כמרא, expl. נובלות) dates ripened through withering.

כּוּמְרָנָא = כּוּמְרָא.—*Pl.* כּוּמְרָנַיָּא (כּוּמְרָנַיָּא). Targ. Y. Gen. XXXIX, 20; a. e. (in Y.).

כּוּמְתָא f. (כמם, v. כּוּן; cmp. Arab. *kummath*, Fl. to Levy Talm. Dict. II, 450ᵇ) *skull-cap*, worn under the turban (סוּדָרָא). Erub. 84ᵇ דילמא כשהרבים ... בכ׳ וסודרא perhaps the public use of them (the low roofs) refers to people putting their cap and turban on them? Ib. 91ᵃ bot. בכ׳ וס׳ it may be possible with cap &c. (by putting them on in the house and taking them off in the court). M. Kat. 15ᵃ אכ׳ וס׳ it refers to (the mourner's) cap and turban. Gitt. 39ᵇ שקל כּוּמְתֵיהּ וכ׳ he took his cap and threw it at her. Sabb. 147ᵃ הב לי כּוּמְתָאִי hand me my cap.

כּוּן (b. h.) *to stand, exist, be firm.*

Pi. כִּוֵּין 1) *to straighten.* Sifré Deut. 308 מְכַוְּונוֹ במעגילה he tries to straighten the wood in a press; Yalk. Deut. 942 (not מכונן); Pesik. Zutr. Haäz. (ed. Bub. V, p. 111) נתנו לאומן שיְּכַוְּונוֹ he gave it to a mechanic to straighten it.—2) *to place in a line, direct.* Macc. II, 5 (9ᵇ) מְכַוְּונִין להן דרך וכ׳ Ms. M. (ed. ומְכוּוָּנוֹת להן דרכים, v. infra) we make for them direct roads from one place of refuge to the other.—3) *to determine exactly* (place, time &c.). Y. Erub. V, 22ᶜ לְכַוֵּין את הרוחות how to determine exactly the four cardinal points (v. רֶבַע). Ib. bot. הארון היה מְכַוֵּין וכ׳ the Ark indicated for them the points of the compass. Gen. R. s. 15, beg., v. כִּוּוּן. M. Kat. 10ᵃ אין יכול לְכַוֵּין אימרא וכ׳ is unable to sew the fringe accurately on the bosom of the shirt. Ber. 7ᵃ לְכַוֵּין אותה שעה to seize the opportunity of just that moment; a. fr.—4) (with לב or sub. לב) *to direct or prepare one's mind, to pay attention, to do a thing with an intention.* Ber. II, 1 אם כ׳ לבו if he (while reading in the Law) had his mind directed (to the Sh'ma); ib. 13ᵃ אם כ׳ לבו לקרות it means, he read with attention (to the sense, not merely like one going over the text for correction). R. Hash. 28ᵇ כ׳ לבו לצאת he had the intention of complying with the law (v. יָצָא); opp. (כ׳) לשמוע he directed his attention to listening, i. e. heard the sound with consciousness (but without devotion); v. כַּוָּונָה. Ber. V, 1 היו שוהין ... כדי שיְּכַוְּונוּ לבם וכ׳ tarried a while before prayer, in order to direct their hearts to their Father in heaven. Y. ib. II, 5ᵃ חזקה כִּוֵּין the presumption is that he read with attention; a. fr.—*Part. pass.* מְכוּוָּן, f. מְכוּוֶּנֶת, מְכוּוָּנָה; pl. מְכוּוָּנִים, ־נִין . . .; מְכוּוָּנוֹת a) *in a line, corresponding.* Y. Kil. V, beg. 30ᵇ מכ׳ הן ערוס המכ׳ a straight bed of vines, opp. מעוקם. Ib. they (the vines) are in a straight line. Y. Ber. IV, 8ᶜ top בית ... מ׳ כנגד .. של מעלן the situation of the earthly Holy of Holies corresponds with that of the heavenly &c. Macc. II, 5 ומכוונות להן דרכים (not נת ...), v. supra. Ib. 9ᵇ ומכוונות היו כמין וכ׳ (Ms. M. ומכוונין הן) and they (the three towns on this side and those on the other side of the Jordan respectively) were in straight parallel lines like two rows in a vineyard; a. fr.—b) *exact, precise.* Toh. III, 1 sq. כביצה מ׳ exactly the quantity of an egg. Mikv. VII, 6; Hag. 19ᵃ; Gitt. 16ᵃ.

Hif. הֵכִין *to put in proper position, to prepare; to hold ready, to designate.* Bets. 2ᵇ (ref. to Ex. XVI, 5) חול מֵכִין לשבת וכ׳ a week day prepares for the Sabbath (that which has become ready for use on a week day may be used on the Sabbath), but a Holy Day does not prepare for the succeeding Sabbath, ואין שבת מְכִינָה ליו״ט nor can the Sabbath prepare for a succeeding Holy Day, v. הֲכָנָה.—Meg. 12ᵇ (play on ממוכן, Esth. I, 14) כלום הֵכִינוּ וכ׳ have they (the Persians) arranged a table before thee?; Esth. R. to l. c. מי מֵכִין וכ׳ who arranges an altar &c.?; a. fr.—[Tosef. Maasr. I, 4 משירכינו ed. Zuck., Var. משיירכינו, read: משירציו.]—*Part. pass.* מוּכָן *prepared, designated, ready.* Bets. I, 2 עפר מ׳ מבעוד יום dust (for covering the blood) made ready a day before. Ib. אפר כירה מ׳ הוא ashes of the stove are considered ready (destined to be used for the purpose). Ib. III, 4 אין זה מן המ׳ this is not among the things designated for use on the Holy Day. Ib. IV, 6.—Meg. l. c. (play on ממוכן, v. supra) שמ׳ לפורענות he was ready for evil; a. fr.

Hithpa. הִתְכַּוֵּין, הִתְכַּוֵּן, *Nithpa.* נִתְכַּוֵּין 1) *to be made straight, to be remedied* (cmp. תכן). Pesik. Zutr. l. c. אין אתם מִתְכַּוְּונִים אלא באור you (your crookedness) can be remedied only through fire; Sifré Deut. l. c. אין אתם הולכים אלא לאור; Yalk. Deut. l. c. הולכין אלא לאחור (corr. acc.).—2) *to prepare one's self.* Y. Meg. I, 71ᶜ (ref. to הִכּוֹן, Am. IV, 12) הִתְכַּוֵּין לקראת וכ׳ put thyself in proper condition to meet thy God.—3) *to intend, propose.* B. Kam. VIII, 1 עד שיהא מִתְכַּוֵּין unless he did it with malicious intent. Tosef. Naz. III, 10 לא נִתְכַּוַּנְתִּי אלא כמותה my intention was to be exactly like her (as to her vow). Ib. 14 מי שנ׳ לעלות וכ׳ if he who had the intention to eat the flesh of swine &c.; v. עָלָה. Sabb. 22ª ובלבד שלא יִתְכַּוֵּין וכ׳ provided he has not the intention of making a groove. —Bets. 23ª, a. fr. דבר שאינו מִתְכַּ׳ a forbidden act which was produced without intent, i. e. an unintended but unavoidable effect of a permitted act. R. Hash. 28ᵇ. Pes. 53ᵇ, a. fr. שניהם ... נִתְכַּוְּנוּ both meant the same thing; a. fr.

Polel כּוֹנֵן *to establish, base firmly.* Ex. R. s. 15 מבקש לְכוֹנֵן עולמים wanted to establish worlds. Ib. על אלו אני מְכוֹנֵן וכ׳ upon those (the patriarchs) I will establish the world.—Part. pass. מְכוֹנָן, f. מְכוֹנֶנֶת. Midr. Sam. ch. XVI (ref. to הכינני, I Kings II, 24) בזכות התורה המ׳ בארון (the world exists) for the sake of the Law that is put up straight in the holy Ark.

כּוּן ch. same; *Pa.* כַּוֵּין 1) *to direct, aim, draw a direct line.* Targ. Y. Num. XXII, 23. Targ. Num. XXXIV, 7, sq. (h. text תאה). Targ. Y. Deut. X, 5 וכוונית (h. text פנה). Ib. XIX, 3 (h. text תכין, v. preced.); a. e.—2) *to draw a parallel, compare.* Targ. Is. XLVI, 5 (h. text תמשילני).—3) (with דעתא, or sub. דעתא) *to direct the mind, to pay attention; to do a thing intentionally.* Targ. Y. Num. XI, 1 מכ׳ והגיאן ביש intentionally speaking evil.—Ber. 17ᵇ לא מצי לְכַוּוּנֵי דעתיה he cannot collect his mind (for prayer). Ib. 30ᵇ מעיקרא לא כ׳ וכ׳ the first time he read without attention. Ḥull. 31ª דלא קָמְכַוֵּין (or קָמִכַּוֵּין *Ithpa.*) when he had no intention whatever (to cut); a. fr.—*Part. pass.* מְכַוֵּין a) *directed towards, corresponding.* Targ. Ez. I, 9. Targ. Ex. XXVI, 5; a. fr.—b) *straight, firm, upright.* Targ. Job XXI, 8 מְכַוְּונִין Bxt. (Ms. מְכַוְּונָן; ed. מכוין, מְכַוּון, corr. acc.; h. text נכון). Targ. Ps. LI, 12. Ib. LVII, 8 (ed. Wil. מְכַוָּן, corr. acc.); a. fr.—Yoma 28ᵇ לא מְכַוְּונֵי Ms. M. (ed. לא מ׳ טובא) the Temple walls were not exactly straight (the lower portions being thicker than the upper); [Ms. M. 2 משום דמכווני because the walls were exactly built in correspondence with the points of the compass]. Y. Snh. IV, beg. 22ª; III, 21ᶜ top [read:] כד הוא חמי סהדו מְכַוְּונָא ... חבן והבן מְכַוֵּין when he found evidences (of two) exactly corresponding, he cross-examined; but when he found them turning hither and thither (differing in details), he tried to harmonize (allowing for errors in time &c., v. חֲקִירָה).

Ithpa. אִיתְכַּוֵּין, אִיכַּ׳, כַּוֵּין ... 1) *to place one's self, to stand.* Targ. Ps. CI, 7.—2) *to be precise in doing.* Ib. XC, 12 מן יִתְכַּ׳ להודע ed. Lag. (oth. ed. כן, corr. acc.) who can exactly make known? (h. text כן הודע). Targ. Y. Lev. XIII, 12.—3) *to be trained, to be in the habit of.* Targ. Y. Num. XXII, 30 (h. text הסכן).—4) *to intend, mean.* Ib. XXX, 5 ויתכ׳ וישתוק and keeps silence intentionally. Targ. Y. Deut. XIX, 4; a. e.—Ḥull. 95ª דאיכ׳ לצעורי׳ וכ׳ who meant to vex his neighbor. Ib. 31ª מִיכַּוֵּין לשום חתיכה had the intention merely to cut (not to slaughter according to the ritual, v. זְבִיחָה). Ib. מה כלים דלא מִיכַּוְּונֵי וכ׳ as vessels (lifeless things) which have no thought &c.; a. e.

Ithpe. אִיתְכַּן *to be prepared, ready* (מוּכָן, v. preced.). Ib. 14ª כיון דלא א׳ וכ׳ because it was not prepared (designated for use) yesterday.—V. חכן.

כַּוָּנָא, כַּוָּן, v. sub כַּוֵּין׳.

כַּוְנָא, or **כּוּנָא** m. (v. כַּפְּוָא; cmp. כַּף חוּפָן a. כַּף) *the hollow of the hand, handful* (as a measure), *spoonful* (mostly in medicine; cmp. Lat. coclear). [Editions, except ed. Sonc., have ב׳, Ar. a. Mss. כ׳, v. Rabb. D. S. a. l. c. infra.] Sabb. 110ᵇ כ׳ דכמונא וכ׳ (Ms. M. כו׳) one handful of cumin-seed, and one of &c. Gitt. 70ª כ׳ דחמרא וכ׳ a spoonful of old wine.—*Pl.* כַּוְנֵי or כּוּנֵי. Erub. 29ᵇ (ed. Sonc. כַּוְונֵי, v. Rabb. R. S. a. l. note). Gitt. 69ª ed. כ׳. Ib.ᵇ (ed. ב׳).

כּוּנְדָּא, v. כּוּדְנָא.

כונדקא, v. אַכְוַנְּתָּר.

כונדת׳, v, כּוּדְנָא.

כַּוָּנָה, כַּוָּ׳ f. (כּוּן, *Pi.* a. *Hithpa.*) *intention; attention; devotion.* Ber. 13ª ש״מ מצות צריכות כ׳ shall we derive fom this (Mish. II, 1 אם כיון לבו וכ׳) that religious exercises require the intention (of complying with the law, and must be repeated if performed without such intention)? R. Hash. 28ᵇ, a. fr. מצות אין צריכות כ׳ the intention of compliance is not indispensable; Erub. 95ᵇ לצאת בעי כ׳ (v. Rabb. D. S. a. l. notes 90 a. 100) in order to have complied with the law, intention of compliance is required. Ber. 13ᵇ כ׳ בלא קריאה meditating (on the Biblical passage to be recited) without audible recitation. Ib. עד כאן צריכה כַּוָּנַת הלב up to this (*sh'ma* to *eḥad*) attention to the meaning is indispensable. Meg. 20ª (ref. to Deut. VI, 6) אחר כ׳ הלב הן הן הדברים the value of 'the words' (the recitation) depends on the attention of the mind (devotion). -Ḥull. 31ª כ׳ לשחיטה the intention to slaughter according to the ritual; opp. לחתיכה; a. fr.

כַּוָּנְתָּא, כַּוָּ׳, כַּוְּנוּתָא, ch. same. Targ. Y. Num. XXXV, 20 בכַוָּונוּת לבא with premeditation (h. text בצדיה). Targ. Ps. VII, 4.

כַּוָּנִים, v. כַּוָּון.

כּוּנִישְׁרָא, v. כּוּנְשְׁרָא.

כּוֹנָן, pl. כּוֹנָנִים, כּוֹנָנִין, v. next w.

כּוֹנָנִית f., pl. כּוֹנָנִיּוֹת (כון, cmp. כַּוֵּין) [*arrangements,*] *chambers,* applied to the entrails arranged above each other. Ḥull. 56ᵇ (ref. to ויכננך, Deut. XXXII, 6) שברא הקב״ה כ׳ באדם וכ׳ the Lord has created carefully arranged chambers in man, one of which being disturbed man cannot live; Sifré Deut. 309 עשאך כנונים כנונים מבפנים וכ׳ (prob. to be read כּוֹנָנִים); (Yalk. ib. 942 בסיסים, v. בָּסִיס; cmp. כַּן II). Yalk. Lev. 547 כּוֹנָנִין (Lev. R. s. 14 קִינִּין).

כּוֹנֵס m. (כָּנַס) *receiver, the lower part of the winnowing shovel.* B. Mets. 105ª.—כ׳ משקה, v. כָּנַס.—B. Bath. 68ª v. כּוּנוּס.

כּוֹנָסָה, v. כְּנִיסָה.

כּוּנְשְׁרָא m. (כשר, with inserted נ, cmp. גּוּנְדְּרָא) 1) (=h. כִּישׁוֹר) *distaff* with the ball of flax. Targ. Prov. XXXI, 19 (ed. Lag. כּוּשְׁרָא, cmp. כְּשׁוּרָא).—2) (cmp. קשר) *navel.*

Ib. III, 8 (ed. Lag. 'פּוּנִישְׁ; Levita Var. פּוּשְׁרָא; h. text 'שָׁה).

כִּנְתָּא, v. פּוּנְתָּא.

כּוּנְתָּא (כּוּנְתָּא) m. (כתת, with inserted נ, cmp. פּוּנִישְׁרָא) [*that which is pounded,*] *spelt.* M. Kat. 13ᵇ כי .. אמר כ׳ when Rab Dimi came (to Babylonia) he defined *ḥelka* (v. חִילְקָא II) as *kunta.*—*Pl.* פּוּנְתְיָא, פּוּנְתִּין (פּוּנְתָיָא). Targ. Ex. IX, 32 'פּוּנְ ed. Berl. (ed. Amst. 'כּוּנְ; Y. 'פּוּנְתַּ, Var. 'כֻּנְתַּ, 'כֻּנְתַ). Targ. Is. XXVIII, 25; Targ. Ez. IV, 9 (ed. Wil. פּוּנְתִּין, oth. ed. 'כונת).

כּוֹס I c. (b. h.; כוס or כנס, v. Ges. Thes., a. Hebr. Dict.[10] s. v.) 1) *cup,* also *a drink.* Tam. III, 4. Erub. 65ᵇ בג׳ . . . בכיסו בכוסו בכעסו man's character is found out in three things, in his money bag, in his cup (when drinking) and in his anger; Der. Er. Zutta ch. V.—Keth. 75ᵇ, sq., v. בָּדַק. Pes. 105ᵃ קדושה על הכ׳ sanctification (of the Sabbath or Holy Day) over a cup of wine. Ib. אם אין לו אלא כ׳ אחד if he has only enough wine for one cup. Sabb. XIV, 3 כ׳ עיקרים, v. עִיקָּר; a. fr.—*Pl.* כּוֹסוֹת. Kel. XXII, 1; Y. Ab. Zar. II, end, 42ᵃ, v. הֲנָחָה. Men. 28ᵇ, v. אֲלֶכְּסַנְדְּרִי. Pes. X, 1, a. fr. ארבע כ׳ four cups of wine to be drunk on the Passover night; a. fr.—2) *cavity.* Par. II, 5 (two black or white hairs) בתוך כ׳ אחד in one follicle (v. גּוּמָּא).—*Pl.* as ab. Ib. Y. Ab. Zar. l. c. הן כ׳ הן גומות *kosoth* and *gummoth* mean the same things.—בֵּית הַכּוֹסוֹת *the second stomach* of ruminants. Hull. III, 1 (42ᵃ), v. comment. a. הַבְלִילָא. Ib. 49ᵃ; 50ᵇ עובי בית הכ׳ the folds (thick walls) of the etc.; a. fr.

***כּוֹס II** m. (כסס, v. כִּיסָא) *thorn.*—*Pl.* כּוֹסִים. Pesik. B'shall. p. 92ᵃ (Y. Maasr. III, 50ᵈ bot. קוצין), v. כָּסַח.

כּוּס III, כּוֹס, v. כּוּס, נְכַס a. כָּסַס.

כּוּסָא *night-bird, owl,* v. בָּאיְת.

כּוּסָא *cup,* v. כָּסָא.

כּוּסָאתָא, v. כּוּסְתָּא.

כּוּסְבָּר m., **כּוּסְבָּרָה, כּוּסְבֶּרֶת** f. (v. Löw Pfl. p. 209) *coriander* (v. Sm. Ant. s. v. Coriandrum). Kil. I, 2 ׳כ׳ וכוסבר שדה וכו (garden) coriander and field (wild) coriander . . . . are not heterogeneous plants. Shebi. IX, 1. Dem. I, 1. Y. ed. 'כוס (Mish. a. Bab. ed. 'כס); a. fr.—Y. ib. 21ᵈ top, v. next w.—Tosef. B. Bath. V, 6 כיסברת בפלפלין ed. Zuck. (Var. כסבורא; corr. acc.) he who adulterates pepper by admixing coriander; Koh. R. to VI, 1 כרשנים (corr. acc.).

כּוּסְבַּר, כּוּסְבָּרָה m., **כּוּסְבַּרְתָּא** f. ch. same. Targ. Y. Ex. XVI, 31; Targ. Y. Num. XI, 7 (h. text גד).—Y. Dem. I, 21ᵈ top כוסבר(ה) כוסברתא *kusbar* (of the Mish.) is *kusbarta.* Ib. (derisive play on the word) [read:] כּוּס בְּרָה כּוּס בְּרַתָּה וכ׳ 'chew the son, chew the daughter', who classed thee among the spices?—Ab. Zar. 10ᵇ (expressing an advice symbolically = כוס ברתא put the daughter to death, v. נְכַס; v. גַּרְגִּילָא).

כּוּסְטְרִיוִינוּס, Cant. R. to VI, 11; קוסטרינוס Lev. R. s. 35, a corrupt. of *quaestionarius, executioner*; v. קוּסְטִינָר.

כּוּסְיָא, Targ. Y. Ex. XXII, 8, a. e., v. כַּסְיָא.

כּוּסִיוֹת, Tosef. Kel. B. Mets. X, 6, read: כִּיסִיּוֹת, v. כִּסָּא.

כּוּסִילְתָּא f. (כסל, v. כֶּסֶל; cmp. P. Sm. s. v. 1786, sq.) 1) *the space between the shoulders* (interscapilium), *shoulder-blade.* Taan. 21ᵇ [read:] לבושא דיתיב ביה קרנא והוה בזיעא בי כ׳ (v. Var. in Rabb. D. S. a. l. note) a garment in which there was placed (fastened) a cup (for receiving the blood) which (garment) was cut in at the shoulder (so that the operator could let blood standing behind the female patient); [Ar. לבושא דאית ליה ביזעי ביזעי באפי כ׳ a garment in which there were several incisions to correspond to the shoulder-blade.]—2) *the lancet for blood-letting.* ריבדא דכ׳ the puncture made by the lancet. Sabb. 129ᵃ עד דנפיק מר׳ דכ׳ until the puncture was healed up. Snh. 93ᵇ. Macc. 21ᵃ. Keth. 39ᵇ כר׳ דכ׳ as much pain as is caused by the puncture of the lancet. Nidd. 67ᵃ הני רבדי דכ׳ the marks of the punctures &c.

כּוּסְכּוּס, v. נְכַס.

כּוּסְלָא, v. כִּסְלָא.

כּוּסְמִין, כּוּסְמִים m. pl. (b. h. כֻּסְּמִים, כֻּסֶּמֶת; כסם, cmp. כסס; v. כּוּנְתָּא) *spelt.* Hall. I, 1. Pes. II, 5. Ib. 35ᵃ כ׳ מין חטים הוא *Kuss'min* is a species of wheat. Y. Ḥall. I, 57ᵇ top (ref. to Is. XXVIII, 25) כּוּסֶּמֶת זה הכ׳ *kussemeth is spelt*; a. fr.

כּוּסֶּמֶת f., v. preced.

כּוּסְפָא m. (כְּסַף) *paring, husk*; כ׳ דתמרי *substance of ground dates* after the juice is pressed out. Taan. 24ᵇ אכ׳ דת׳ קיימי דקא מזדבן they stand around a mass of ground dates which is to be sold (there being a famine). Sabb. 50ᵇ כ׳ דיסמין puppy pomace flavored with jasmin (used for a lotion).

כּוּסְפָּן m. h. same (collect. noun). Ab. Zar. 38ᵇ הכ׳ של נכרים וכ׳ (Rashi: הכּוּסְפָּן) pomace of dates belonging to gentiles which was boiled (brewed a second time) in a large caldron.

***כּוּסְתָּא** m. (an adapt. of ξέστης, by confusion with כּוּס, כָּסָא) *kusta,* a liquid measure. Sabb. 109ᵇ חד כ׳ דשיכרא (Ms. O. כִּיסְתָא) one *k.* of beer.—*Pl.* כּוּסְיָתָא (fem.). Ib. חמש עשר כ׳ Ms. M. (ed. חמשא כוסתא, Ms. O. כסתתא; Rashi כּוּסָאתָא, v. Rabb. D. S. a. l. note). [Oth. opin. כּוּסְתָא fem. form of כּוּסָא, v. כָּסָא.]

כּוּף I *to bend, force,* v. כָּפָה a. כָּפַף.

כּוּף ch. same, *to bend* (act. a. neuter verb).—Part. כָּיֵיף, כָּיִף, כָּאִיף. Targ. Ps. LVII, 7. Targ. Job XL, 17 Ms. (ed. Lag. כפיף; ed. Wil. כָּפַף, Var. כפין).—Snh. 36ᵃ מִיכַף הוה כָּיֵיף ליה לרב וכ׳ he bent (yielded preference) to R. A.; Gitt. 59ᵇ מיכף הוו כָּיְיפֵי ליה. Pes. 51ᵃ אנן כָּיְיפִינַן להו we pay reverence to them. Sabb. 77ᵇ, v. כְּפַף.—Hag. 16ᵃ, v. אי...לְמִיכְפְּיֵיה...הוה כָּיְיפִינָא יִצְרָא. Snh. 107ᵃ; Yalk. Ps. 765 ליה if I had desired to bend my passion, I should have succeeded. B. Bath. 4ᵃ דכייף ליה וכ׳ Ms. M. (ed. אכפר,

(מיכפר) he bends the pegs of the wall inside, . . . outside, v. חָזִית.

כוף II m. (כְּפַף) *cover, basket.* Y. Erub. VII, beg. 24[b] למיכבש עלור כ׳ to press a cover over it.

כוּפָּה, v. כִּיפָּה. [Pesik. Asser, p. 99[b] כבוש כ׳, v. כּוּבָּא I.]

כוּפָּח (כָּפַח) [*a pouched receptacle,*] *a small stove, brazier.* Sabb. III, 2. Ib. 38[b] כ׳ מקום שפיתת וכ׳ a *kuppah* is a stove which has room only for one pot. Men. V, 9 מאפה כ׳ what is baked in a brazier. Kel. V, 2 הכ׳ עשאו לאפייה לבישול . . . a *k.* made for baking, . . . for cooking.

כוּפְיָא m. *Kufia,* name of *a fish,* supposed to be identical with *colias,* v. אִסְפָּנִי. Pes. 39[a] מרירתא דכ׳ the gall of &c.

כופיח, Y. Keth. VII, end, 31[d], read: כִּיפֵּחַ.

כופיתא, B. Mets. 73[b], v. כְּפִיתָא.—[Snh. 98[b], v. כִּיפְתָא; B. Bath. 73[b], v. כַּפּוּתָא.]

כוּפְלָא, v. כִּיפְלָא.

כּוּפְנִי, כּוּפְנִיתָא, v. כַּפְנִיתָא.

כּוּפֵר, v. כָּפַר.

כֹּפֶר, כּוֹפֶר I m. (b. h.) *cyprus flower* (v. Löw Pfl. p. 212). Shebi. VII, 6 והכו׳ Ms. M. (ed. והכפ׳); Nidd. 8[a].—Chald. כְּפוּרָא.

כּוֹפֶר II m. (b. h. כֹּפֶר; כָּפַר) *indemnity, fine;* [*atonement.*] B. Kam. IV, 5 משלם כ׳ must pay indemnity for a life lost. Ib. 40[a] חצי כ׳ half the assessed fine. Ib. כ׳ שלם אמר רחמנא וכ׳ the law (Ex. XXI, 30) speaks of a full indemnity (as an atonement) &c., v. next w.; a. fr.—Treat. Sof'rim XXI, 4 לשם כ׳ as an obligatory ransom, opp. לשם נדבה.—*Pl.* כּוֹפְרִין. B. Kam. l. c. חייבי כ׳ מאי how is it about seizing the property of those bound to pay indemnities?; a. fr.

כּוּפְרָא I ch. same. B. Kam. 40[a] כ׳ כפרה the fine is intended for an atonement (like a sacrifice); כ׳ ממונא it is an indemnification; a. fr.

כּוּפְרָא II m. (b. h. כֹּפֶר; כפר, cmp. כַּבְרִיתָא) *pitch.* Targ. O. Gen. VI, 14.—Arakh. 19[a] באתרא דתקלי כ׳ where they sell pitch by the weight. Gitt. 69[b] משחא דכ׳ oil of pitch (tar). Sabb. 74[b] האי מאן דארתח כ׳ he who heats pitch (on the Sabbath). B. Mets. 23[b]. Ib. 70[a] top בני כ׳ *sailors* ('tars').—*Pl.* כּוּפְרֵי. Sabb. 67[a] ז׳ כ׳ מז׳ ארבי seven kinds of pitch taken from seven ships. [B. Kam. 101[a] top. v. כַּפְרָא.]

כּוּפְרָא III m. (כפר) *the inflorescence of palms, a spike covered with numerous flowers, and enveloped by one or more sheathing bracts called spathes* (v. Cyclop. Brit. s. v. Palm, a. Löw Pfl. p. 118); *the date-berry in its early stage.* Pes. 56[a] מנחי כ׳ דיכרא וכ׳ (for fertilization) they put the male flower (scatter the pollen) over the female tree. B. Kam. 59[b] האי מאן דקיץ כ׳ וכ׳ if one cuts a date flower what damages has he to pay?—Succ. 32[a] וארכא כ׳ perhaps (Lev. XXIII, 40) the spike is meant?—Ber. 36[b] בכ׳ in the early stage of the berry.—*Pl.* כּוּפְרֵי. Pes. 52[b] (Ms. M. sing.), v. כָּפְנֵי.—Keth. 10[a] אסבוהו כ׳, v. סְבָא. [Y. Shebi. II, 34[a] bot. כופריא, v. next w.]

כּוּפְרָאה ch. = h. כּוּפְרִי.—*Pl.* כּוּפְרָאֵי. Y. Shebi. II, 34[a] bot. בצליא כ׳ R. S. to ib. II, 9 (ed. כופריא, corr. acc.) wild onions, v. כּוּפְרִי.

כּוּפְרָה pr. n. pl. *Kufra.* Y. Shek. V, 48[d] bot.; Y. Peah VIII, 21[a] כַּפְרָה.—Y. Meg. I, 70[a] bot. כִּיפְרָא (near Tiberias); a. e.

כּוּפְרִי I m., **כּוּפְרִית** f. (denom. of כָּפָר) *belonging to the village, wild.*—כלב כ׳ *village dog, ferocious dog.* Tosef. Kil. V, 8 כלב כ׳ וכ׳ a *Kuf'ri* dog is a species of wild beasts (not a domestic animal). Kil. I, 6 כלב הכ׳ והשועל וכ׳ the wild dog and the jackal . . . . are heterogeneous (כלאים). Y. ib. I, 27[a] bot. (not כופרין). Lam. R. to I, 4; a. e.—בצל כ׳ wild onion, opp. to בני המדינה ב׳ townsmen's (garden) onion. Ned. 26[b]; 66[a] הכ׳ יפה וכ׳ (Ar. הכּוּפְרִים יפין) the wild onion is good for the heart (stomach); Tosef. ib. V, 1 הכופרין יפה (corr. acc.), opp. בני בצלים (Var. שאר) small onions.—*Pl.* כּוּפְרִין, כּוּפְרִים, כּוּפְרִיִּים. Ter. II, 5, v. פּוֹליטִיקִין. Tosef. B. Kam. VIII, 17. Tosef. Ab. Zar. II, 3. Tosef. Ned. l. c.; Ned. l. c., v. supra; a. e.

כּוּפְרִי II, pr. n. pl., 1) prob. *Cyprus,* v. זְפִירִין. Yalk. Num. 701.—2) v. כַּפְרִי.

כּוּפְרִיתָא, v. כַּבְרִיתָא.

כּוּפְרָנָא, v. כַּפְרָנָא.

***כּוּפֶשׁ** m. (v. כְּפִישָׁה) *basket* in which olives are kept for softening. Toh. IX, 5 Var. (ed. כּוּתֵשׁ); Tosef. ib. X, 10 כיפש (R. S. to Toh. l. c. כותש).

כּוּפְשָׁנָא m., pl. כּוּפְשָׁנֵי (v. preced.) a species of *tamed doves (kept in coops).* Ḥull. 62[b] כ׳ צוצריני ed. K. of Zeizûn (?); Ar. דצ׳ כּוּבְשָׁנֵי (v. כְּבַשׁ).

כּוּפָּת c. (כָּפָת, cmp. מנח כפויה s. v. כָּפָה) [*an inverted vessel,*] *a low seat, a block with a concave top to sit upon; bolster, stool.* Kel. XXII, 9. Tosef. Sabb. XIII (XIV), 17 כ׳ בין חקוק וכ׳ (ed. Zuck. כפ׳, Var. כיפ׳, corr. acc.) a block whether caved out &c. Kel. XX, 5 כ׳ שקבעו וכ׳ if one put a stool in the rubble of a wall (v. נִדְבָּךְ; Tosef. ib. B. Mets. XI, 6 כסא . . . בבנין). Tosef. ib. B. Bath. II, 1 [read:] כ׳ חלקה שאין בה וכ׳ (v. R. S. to Kel. XXII, 9; ed. Zuck. כיפת חלק) a plain (not shaped) block which has not the height of &c. Y. Pes. VII, 28[d] bot. בצק שעשאו כ׳ a mass of hardened dough which one made into a seating block. Ohol. XI, 3 כ׳ וכ׳ עבה a thick carpet-cover of a seating block (cmp. Tosef. Kel. B. Mets. XI, 10). Y. Erub. VII, 24[b] bot. כ׳ שהדריגוה a seating block into which steps were cut. Tosef. Ohol. XII, 2 שתי..וכ׳ ע״ג האבן R. S. to ib. XI, 3 (ed. Zuck. a. oth. וכו׳) two stones above one another and a seating block on top &c.; a. e.—*Pl.* כּוּפָּתִין. Ib. in R. S. to Ohol l. c. (ed. Zuck. a. oth. כָּפִיתִין).

כּוּפְתָא I ch. 1) same. Sabb. 77[b] (phon. etymol.) כ׳ כּוֹף וְתִיב invert and sit on it.—2) *prisoner's stocks.*

Targ. Jer. XX, 2 Ar. (h. text מַהְפֶּכֶת), v. כִּיפְתָא. [B. Bath. 73[b], v. כַּפּוּתָא.]

כּוּפְתָּא II f.=h. כְּפִיפָה, *basket*. Gitt. 32[a] קניא בכ׳ the reed in the basket.

כּוּפְתָּא III m. (כְּפַת) *being tied* on the altar (= h. עֲקֵדָה). Targ. Job. III, 18 (19).

כְּוַוץ, כָּוֵיץ, כָּוֵץ (cmp. קָוַץ, קָוַע) *to curl, shrink*. Sabb. 20[b] עמר מכוויץ כָּוֵיץ wool (if used as a wick) curls. Nidd. 3[a] מוך . . מכוין כווץ the lint . . shrinks (and leaves room for the blood to pass). Succ. 23[b] כיון דמייתא כָּוִוצָא when the animal is dead, the body shrinks. Ḥull. 43[b] כל שחותכו וכוויץ that portion of the gullet which shrinks when you cut it. Ib. 46[b], v. infra.

Pa. כַּוֵּיץ *to cause to shrink*. Sabb. 19[a] דכַוּוצָה for he made it shrink (by using too hot water). Ḥull. 46[b]; 47[b] [read:] בחמימי לא דמכַווצי not in boiling water, for it causes the lungs to shrink (Ar. ed. Koh. בקרירי לא דכווצא not in cold water, for it will contract, v. טְרַשׁ I).

כּוֹר m. (b. h.; כּוּר, כרר, v. כְּרָה) [*a heap*,] *Khor*, a measure of capacity, בֵּית כ׳ (or כ׳, sub. בית) *an area requiring a Khor of seed*. B. Mets. 105[b] כ׳ זרע a field requiring a *Khor* of seed; כ׳ תבואה a field yielding a *Khor* of grain. Ib. ד׳ סאין לכ׳ four S'ah of seed for a Beth Khor of land, v. נְפִלָּה. B. Bath. VII, 1; 2 בית כ׳. Ib. 104[a] נותן . . . לכל כ׳ וכ׳ we allow a surplus or deficit of seven Kab and a half for each Beth Khor; a. fr.—*Du.* כּוֹרַיִם, כּוֹרַיִים. Ib.[b]—Ohol. VIII, 3; Kel. XV, 1 ארבעים סאה בלח שהן כ׳ ביבש forty S'ah in liquid measure which is equal to two Khor in dry measure.

כּוֹרָא, כּוֹר ch. same. Targ. Lev. XXVII, 16 (h. text חֹמֶר); a. fr.—B. Mets. 105[a], v. אַלְלָא.—*Pl.* כּוֹרִין, כּוֹרֵי. [Targ. Y. Ex. VIII, 10 כירין Ar. *heaps*; ed. כְּרוֹוִין, v. כְּרָיָא.]—Targ. I Kings V, 25; a. fr. — B. Mets. l. c. — Y. ib. IV, 10[c] bot. Sabb. 35[a], v. חַלְתָא; a. fr.—[Ḥull. 62[b] בי כורי Ar., Var. כירי, between *heaps* (ed. כַּרְבֵי).]—V. כּוֹרִיתָא.

כּוּר I pr. n. pl. מִכְלְתָא דְכ׳ *Fort of Khur*, a northern Palestinean border-town. Tosef. Shebi. IV, 11 Var. (ed. Zuck. מימחא דבור); Y. ib. VI, 36[c] מילתא דביר; Sifré Deut. 51 (במותה דבירייין) כמותה דכריין; Yalk. Deut. 874 במתא דבירריין; Targ. Y. I Num. XXXIV, 9 כּוֹרַיָּיא דבית סכל (v. כּוּרָייר). V. Hildesh. Beitr. p. 20, sq.

כּוּר II m. (b. h.; כור, cmp. כְּבָרָה a. כְּוֶורֶת) *smelting pot, smelting furnace*. Tosef. Kel. B. Kam. VI, 16. Kel. VIII, 9 כ׳ . . . של עושה זכוכית (Var. בור) the glassmaker's pot. Sabb. VIII, 4 כ׳ של צורפי זהב the gold refiners' pot. Midr. Till. to Ps. CXIV כאדם . . . מתוך הכ׳ וכ׳ like a man that takes gold out of the smelting pot without tongs &c. Pirké d'R. El. ch. XLVIII כ׳ של אש a burning furnace; a. e.

כּוּרָא I ch. same. Targ. O. Deut. IV, 20 (Y. כּוּר); a. e.

***כּוּרָא II** (v. preced.) (supposed to be a disguise for) *female pudenda*. Sabb. 140[b]; v., however, בּוּרָא.

כּוֹרָא, v. כּוֹר ch.

כּוּרָא, v. בּוּרָא.

כּוֹרַבְלִין m. pl. (χοραύληç) *flute-players accompanying the chorus of dancers*. Gen. R. s. 23; s. 50 (variously corrupted), v. אַדְרַבְלָא.

כורדקי, v. אַכְוְנַּר.

כּוֹרְהֲנָא, v. כְּרַה׳.

כּוֹרְוָון, v. כְּרָיָא.

***כורוסתי**, a corrupt. for כְּרִיזַסְתִּי (χαρίζεσθαι) *to do a favor*. Y. Ned. III, 38[a], v. בְּיָיא II.

כּוֹרֵז, v. כָּרוֹז.

כּוֹרְזִילָא, v. כַּרְזִילָא.

כּוֹרֵחַ, כּוֹרְחָא, v. sub כּר׳.

כּוּרָייר pr. n. pl. כ׳ רבתא *Great Khuray*, a northern Palestinean border town. Tosef. Shebi. IV, 11 Var. (ed. Zuck. note כּוּרָיָן, v. כּוּר I); Y. ib. VI, 36[c] בִּירַיִי. (V. Hildesh. Beitr. p. 21).

כּוֹרִים, Kel. XII, 8 some ed., v. כְּרִים.

כּוֹרִיתָא f. (v. כּוֹר) *a Khor-ful*. Lam. R. to I, 1 (העיר) כ׳ דדינרין (some ed. כּוֹרְיָיתָא *pl.*) a Khor-ful (Khor-fuls) of Denars.

***כּוֹרֵךְ** m. (כָּרַךְ; cmp. כְּרוּכָא) *part of a plough containing a receptacle out of which the seed falls during the ploughing*. Kel. XXI, 2 R. Hai G.; v., however, בֶּרֶךְ.

כּוֹרְכָא = כַּרְכָא *fort*. Tosef. Shebi. IV, 8 כּ׳ דבית חרב Fort Beth Hereb, in the district of Nivay; Y. Dem. II, 22[d] top כרכה דבר הזרג.

כּוּרְכְּיָא m. (onomatop.; cmp. אַקְרוּקְתָא) *crane*. Targ. Jer. VIII, 7 (h. text סוּס).—Kidd. 44[a] צווח ר״ל כר כ׳ Ar. (ed. כְּרוּכְיָא) Resh Lakish cried like a crane. [Y. Dem. II, 22[c] top כחדא כ׳, v. סִידְקִי.]

כּוּרְכָּם m. *saffron*, v. כַּרְכּוֹם I.

כּוּרְכְּמָא, כּוּרְקְמָא ch. same. Targ. Prov. VII, 17 Levita (ed. כורק׳, h. text אהלים).—Sabb. 110[a] כ׳ רישקא garden crocus (Rashi; v. Löw Pfl. p. 216).

כּוֹרֵם (b. h. כֹּרֵם; denom. of כֶּרֶם) *vintager, gardener*.—*Pl.* כּוֹרְמִים. Tanh. Bo 4; Yalk. Ex. 182 המה . . . כּוֹרְמֵיהֶן they (the Egyptians) planned that they (the Israelites) should be their gardeners.

כּוּרְמֵיזָא m. (כמז with inserted ר; cmp. h. קֹמֶץ) *fist*. Targ. O. Ex. XXI, 18. Targ. Is. LVIII, 4.—Midr. Prov. to XXII, 6 (prov.) לחכימא ברמיזא ולשטיא בכ׳ to the wise man a hint, to the fool a fist.

כּוּרְנַק, כְּוַרְנְקִי, v. אַכְוַרְנְקָא.

כּוּרְסָא, v. כּוּרְסְיָא.

כּוּרְסָאֵי m. pl. (prob.) *people of Karsa* or *Karsana* (v. כַּרְסָנָא). Y. M. Kat. III, 82c.

כורסגניות, Cant. R. to II, 2 some ed., read: כְּרִיסַגְוְנִיּוֹת, v. כְּרִיסוֹ.

כורסון, אולון כ׳, אולו כ׳, v. אוֹלוֹכְרוּסוֹן.

כּוּרְסְיָא, כּוּרְסְיָה, כּוּרְסַיָּא m. pl. (used as sing.), constr. כּוּרְסֵי, כָּרְסָא (כרס; cmp. כַּר) *divan, upholstered chair, throne.* Dan. V, 20; VII, 9.—Targ. I Kings X, 19. Targ. Ex. XVII, 16; a. fr.—Ḥull. 59b [read:] נפל מִכּוּרְסְיֵהּ וכ׳ he fell from his throne to the ground. Yeb. 118b; Keth. 75a רמי לה כּוּרְסְיָהּ .. דשומשנא גברא if her husband be (as small as) an ant, put up her seat among the women of nobility, i. e. a woman feels elevated by marriage. Yeb. 83b אותבוה אבי כורסי׳ they put him on an operator's chair. Ib. 110a אותבוה אבי כ׳ ואהדרוה Ar. (ed. omit ואהדרוה) they put her on a bridal chair (v. אַפִּרְיוֹן) and carried her around in procession. Lev. R. s. 27 תחות כ׳ דאמהון under their mothers' chair (of delivery); Midr. Till. to Ps. II; Yalk. Ex. 165; Yalk. Esth. 1055 (only תחות כורסי). Gitt. 35a הפכוה לכורסְיֵהּ (*fem.*) turn his judicial chair over; הפכוה לכ׳ ותרצוה (Rashi: הפכו) they turned his chair over and set it up again; a. fr.—*Pl.* כּוּרְסָוָתָא, כָּרְסָוָן, כּוּרְסָוָן. Dan. VII, 9 (cited Ḥag. 14a; Snh. 38b). Targ. Ps. CXXII, 5. —Koh. R. to III, 9 אית דאייתי כ׳ some brought divans (for the banquet). Ib. to I, 8 (in Hebr. Dict.) יעשו כ׳ לרבים (sub. בתי) let them be made into *privies* for the public.

כורסין, Tosef. Neg. V, 14 ed., read: בורסין, v. בִּרְסִין.

כּוּרְעֲתָא, v. כַּרְעָא.

כּוּרְקְמָא, v. כּוּרְכְּמָא.

כּוּרַתָּא, כּוּרֶת, v. sub כוור׳.

כּוּשׁ I m. (cmp. כּוֹס, כִּיס) [*something hollow,*] *reed,* esp. reed used as *spindle* (v. Ar. s. v.); also as *fork.* Yoma 82a תּוֹחבין לה כ׳ ברוטב we put for her a reed into the juice (and let her suck it); Tosef. ib. V (IV), 4 (corr. acc.). Sabb. 123a; Y. ib. XVII, 16b top, v. כַּרְכָּר. Y. Erub. III, 20d bot. לתחוב בכ׳ ובקיסם to stick it on a reed or a chip. Kel. IX, 8 מלא כ׳ the size of a reed. Tosef. ib. B. Mets. VI, 12 בכ׳ בכ׳ הבינוני wherever the size of a reed (or spindle) is mentioned, a middle-sized reed is meant. Kel. IX, 7 כ׳ שבלע את הצנורא a reed in which the iron hook has disappeared. Par. XII, 8; Tosef. ib. XII (XI), 16, v. אַרְבָּן; a. fr.—*Pl.* כּוּשִׁין. Y. Yeb. XII, 12d bot. (in Chald. diction, in a disguised answer to a ritual question propounded to R. Akiba by a pretended street vendor) אית לך כ׳ אית לך כשר hast thou spindles? hast thou '*Kasher*'? (play on כִּישּׁוֹר, v. כּוּנְשְׁרָא; intimating 'It is legal').

כּוּשׁ II (b. h.) pr. n. *Cush,* 1) son of Ham. Targ. Gen. X, 6; a. e.—2) *the land of Cush, Aethiopia.* Targ. II Kings XIX, 9. Targ. Y. Num. XII, 1; a. e.—Yalk. Ex. 168. Pes. 94a; Taan. 10a בכ׳ .. מצרים Egypt is one sixtieth as large as Aethiopia. Y. Ber. I, 2c bot. חמצית כ׳ וכ׳ the juice (moisture) of Aeth. is absorbed by Egypt; a. e.

כּוּשָׁא *bunch,* v. כִּישָׁא.

כּוּשָׁאָה, v. כּוּשָׁיָא.

כּוּשִׁי m., **כּוּשִׁית** f. (b. h.; כּוּשׁ II) *Cushite, negro; Aethiopian.* Gen. R. s. 60, beg.; Cant. R. to II, 8 (not כותי), v. בַּרְבָּרִי. Gen. R. s. 73, end; a. fr. [B. Kam. 113b, a. e. in later ed. כושי for גוי or נָכְרִי.]—Succ. III, 6 אתרוג הכ׳, expl. ib. 36a דומה לכ׳ a Palestinean Ethrog resembling an Aethiopian one; (oth. opin.) a real importation from Aethiopia. Y. ib. 53d אתרוג הכ׳ פסול the Aeth. Ethrog is ritually unfit; הבא מן הכ׳ כשר one of Palestinean growth descended from an Aethiopian Ethrog is available for ritualistic use.—Trnsf. *abnormally dark-complexioned.* Bekh. VII, 6. Ber. 58b; Tosef. ib. VII (VI), 3; a. e.—עֵין כּוּשִׁי pr. n. pl. *En Kushi.* Ab. Zar. 31a; Y. ib. V, 44d ע׳ כושי׳; Y. Shebi. V, 36a top ע׳ כּוּשִׁין.

כּוּשָׁאָה, כּוּשָׁיָא ch. same. Targ. Y. II Num. XII, 1. *Pl.* כּוּשָׁאֵי. Targ. Y. I Num. l. c.—Succ. 53a.—*Fem.* כּוּשִׁיתָא, כּוּשַׁיְתָא. Targ. I, II, Num. l. c.

כּוּשִׁית, v. כּוּשִׁי.

כּוּשְׁפָּא* m. (כשף, cmp. חשב) *embroidery, design.* *Pl.* כּוּשְׁפִּין. Targ. Ez. XXVII, 24 כ׳ דוורדא וכ׳ Ar. (ed. Lag. דיורדא, ed. אריזא) designs of roses (cedars) on purple cloaks (h. text רקמה).

כּוּשְׁפָן m. (כִּשֵּׁף) *a believer in sorcery or omens.* Y. R. Hash. III, end, 59a.

כּוּשֶׁר m. (כָּשֵׁר) *fitness, legitimacy, being* כָּשֵׁר. Pes. 83a היתה לו שעת הכ׳ was at one time fit for use. Y. Yeb. VIII, 9d top כל ... חחמה בכ׳ וכ׳ whom the light of the sun has never seen in a condition of sexual fitness, v. סָרִיס. Y. Bets. III, 62a top חזקת בני מעיים לכ׳ the presumption in the case of entrails is in favor of their being כָּשֵׁר, v. חֲזָקָה; Y. Ter. VIII, 46a top (corr. acc.). Y. Succ. V, 55b bot. (in Chald. dict.) עבדין בכ׳ behaving with propriety (during worship), opp. בפחז irreverently; a. fr.

כּוּשְׁרָא I (כְּשַׁר) *attachment.* B. Mets. 93b כ׳ דה׳ the attachment which one has for one's animal.

כּוּשְׁרָא II, v. כּוּנְשְׁרָא.

כּוּשָׁרוֹת, v. כַּשְׁרוּת.

כּוּשְׁתְּ m. *putchuck,* v. קוֹשְׁטְ.

כְּוָת, כְּוָות, constr. כְּוַת, כְּוָות (v. יַת) [*likeness,*] *like, in agreement with.* Targ. Y. II Gen. XLIV, 18. Targ. Y. II Num. XII, 7; a. e.—With pron. suffix: כְּוָתִי, כְּוָתָךְ, כְּוָתֵיהּ, כְּוָתֵיהּ &c. *like me* &c. Targ. Ps. CXIII, 5. Targ. Y. Ex. XV, 11; a. v. fr.—With prefix דְּ, v. דִּכְוָת־.—Ber. 36a, a. fr. הלכתא כותיה ד׳ the practice is in agreement with the opinion of—(v. הֲלָכָה). Ib. קיימי כותיה agree with him. Ib. מסתברא כותך reason agrees with thee. Ib.b כותיה דרב כהנא וכ׳ reason is in favor of R. Kahana's opinion. B. Bath. 65a הילכתא כְּוָתֵיכוּ ... אוֹ כְּוָתִין must the rule be adopted agreeably to our opinion or to yours? (Ms. M.... כְּוָתֵיךְ; (כְּוָתֵיךְ); ib. 142b. Y. Ber. I, 3a top עבד עובדא כוותיה acted in accordance with his own opinion; a. fr.

כּוּת, כּוּתָה pr. n. pl. *Cuth, Cuthah*, a Babylonian town whence Assyrian colonists were introduced into Samaria (v. Schr. KAT², p. 278). Targ. II Kings XVII, 24; 30. [Targ. Is. XXXIV, 9 דכות some ed. (ed. Lag. דרומי; missing in ed. Wil.)—an inserted gloss, v. Lag. Prophetae I, p. XXX33.]—V. כּוּתִי.

כּוּתָא, v. כּוּתִי I.

כּוּתָא, v. כּוּתְחָא.

כּוּתָא f. *owl*, v. בָּאוּת.

כּוּתָאָה, v. כּוּתִיי.

כּוּתָב m. (כְּתַב) 1) *writing, writer*, v. כָּתַב.—2) *the pointed end* of the writing instrument (stilus), contrad. to מוחק the flat end for erasing. Kel. XIII, 2; Tosef. ib. B. Mets. III, 4; Y. Sabb. VIII, 11b bot.

כּוּתְבָן m. (v. preced.) *writer, calligrapher*.—*Pl.* כּוּתְבָנִים. Y. Meg. I, 71d bot. כ׳ אומנים professional writers of Biblical books.

כּוֹתֶבֶת f. (cmp. קְשִׁבָּא) *date* of a certain species, *kothebeth*, used as a measure of size כַּכּ׳ (cmp. זַיִת). Yoma VIII, 2. Bets. I, 1 חמץ בְּכַכּ׳ the standard for leavened bread (on Passover, as for being guilty of a transgression) is the size of a *kothebeth* (less than an olive); a. fr.—*Pl.* כּוֹתָבוֹת. Succ. II, 5 (26b) ש׳ כ׳ Ms. M. (ed. שני) two dates.

כּוּתָה, v. כּוּת.

כּוּתָּח m. (Pers. *katah*, v. Perl. Et. St. p. 85, note; Fl. to Levy Talm. Dict. II, p. 459b) *a preserve consisting of sour milk, bread-crusts and salt*. Pes. III, 1 כ׳ הבבלי the Babylonian *k.*, described ib. 42a, v. אוּמָא a. נַסְיוּבֵי.

כּוּתָּח, כּוּתְּחָא ch. same. Keth. 60b; Erub. 62b אפי׳ ביעתא בכ׳ וכ׳ even as plain a case as the question about an egg that fell into *k.*, a student must not decide in the presence of his teacher. Kerith. 6a מכ׳ דרמי כיפי than a *k.* which is hard enough to break rocks; Hor. 12a (Ms. M. ככּכא, v. Rabb. D. S. a. l. note). Erub. 65a קריב לי כ׳ (Ar. כּוּתְּחָא) hand me the *k.* Sabb. 145b רייק מכ׳ דבבלאי (Ar. מכותא) spat out when thinking of the *k.* of the Babylonians.

כּוּתִי I pr. n. pl. (v. כּוּת) *Kuthi*, a Babylonian town. B. Bath. 91a Abraham was imprisoned שלש בכ׳וכ׳ (v. Rabb. D. S. a. l. note, a. Koh. Ar. Compl. s. v. כרדו) three years in Kuthi &c.; Pirké d'R. El. ch. XXVI כותא.

כּוּתִי II m. (כּוּת) *Cuthean, a member of the sect of Samaritans.* [In editions published under censorial influences our w. frequently takes the place of גוי, עכו״ם, מין &c., a. vice versa.] Hull. 3b. Tosef. Ab. Zar. III, 5 (distinction between כ׳ a. גוי). Ib. 13a. Y. Keth. III, beg. 27a; a. fr. —*Pl.* כּוּתִים, כּוּתִיִּים, כּוּתִין. Y. Yeb. VII, 8b bot. Hull. 3b Sot. 33b ספרי כ׳ the books of the Samaritans, v. זִיּוּף I; Snh. 90b צדוקים ed. (Ms. M. כ׳, v. Rabb. D. S. a. l. note); a. fr.—*Fem.* כּוּתִית. Keth. III, 1. Tosef. Oh. XVIII, 6; a. fr. —*Pl.* כּוּתִיּוֹת. Nidd. IV, 2; Tosef. ib. V, 2; a. e.

כּוּתָאָה, כּוּתָיָא, כּוּתִיי ch.=h. כּוּתִי II. Y. M. Kat. III, 83b. Y. Taan. IV, 68d bot.; a. e.—*Pl.* כּוּתָאֵי, כּוּתָיֵיא. Y. Ab. Zar. V, 44d. Hull. 6a; a. fr.

כְּוָתִירִין (?) pr. n. pl. *K'vathirin*, Targ. Y. Deut. IV, 43 (h. text בֶּצֶר).

כּוֹתֶל, (כֹּתֶל) m. (b. h. כֹּתֶל; כתל *to press together*, cmp. כתת) [*something solid*, cmp. אִיטָם, אָטוּם,] *wall*. Gen. R. s. 68 (ref. to Gen. XXVIII, 11 'he struck') נעשה... כמין כ׳ וכ׳ the whole world was before him blocked as by a wall. Ohol. VI, 3 כ׳ שהוא לאויר a wall which faces the air (which is continued above the roofing, or faces the court yard). Ib. כ׳ המשמש את הבית a wall made for forming an enclosure, contrad. to ib. 6 בית המשמש את הכ׳ a wall formed by digging two cavities next to each other. B. Bath. I, 1; a. fr.—*Pl.* כְּתָלִ׳, כּוֹתָלִין, כּוֹתָלִים. Y. Shek. IV, 48a bot. כתלין (Bab. ed. כתלים, Ms. M. כותל). Gen. R. s. 18, beg. כ׳ של זהב golden partitions (of Adam's tent). B. Mets. 59b כּוֹתְלֵי בה״מ וכ׳ let the walls of the school house decide. Nidd. 3a כותלי בית הרחם the enclosures of the womb; a. fr.

כּוּתְלָא, כֻּתְלָא ch. same. Targ. I Sam. XX, 25. Targ. II Kings IV, 10; a. fr.—Sabb. 80b. Y. Kil. I, 27a top; a. e. —[Ber. 58b נפל כתלא Ar., ed. בתלא, v. תֵּלָּא.]—*Pl.* כּוּתְלִין, כּוּתְלַיָּא, כּוּתְלֵי, כֻּתְ׳. [Esra V, 8 כֻּתְלַיָּ׳.] Targ. Lev. XIV, 37; a. fr.—Yoma 28b מכי משחרי כ׳ from the time the walls throw a shadow (in the afternoon); a. fr.—כותלי דחזירי (כת׳) *bacon* (cmp. אַטְמָא). Hull. 17a כת׳ (Ar. כות׳). Meg. 13a Ms. M. a. Rashi (ed. קדלי).

כּוּתְנָאר, Y. Peah I, 16a, read: כּוּתְנָאֵר, v. כּוּתְנַיָּא. [Comment. כּוּתְנָאֵר *dealers in linen*, v. כִּיתָּן.]

כּוּתָנִיאָס, כּוּתָנְיָיס, כּוּת׳, v. כּוּתְנִיאָס.

כּוּתְנִיין, Y. Maas. Sh. IV, beg. 54d, read: כּוּתְנִיִּין.

כּוּתָנְיָיס, v. כּוּתְנִיאָס.

כּוּתְרָא, v. כִּתְרָא.

כּוּתְרָן, v. כּוּתַרְתָּא.

כּוֹתֶרֶת f. (b. h. כֹּתֶ׳; כתר) *crown, capital*. Tanh. B'har 1 כ׳ מלמעלן ובסיס וכ׳ a capital above and a pedestal beneath; Yalk. Cant. 990; (Cant. R. to V, 15 קיפלורוסים).

כּוֹתַרְתָּא ch. same. Targ. Ez. XLI, 18, sq. (h. text תמרה).—*Pl.* כּוֹתַרְתָּא, כּוֹתָרָן. Ib. 20. Ib. XL, 16; 22 (ed. Wil. sing.); a. e.

כּוֹתֶשׁ m. (כָּתַשׁ) *a vessel for olives*, v. כּוּפְשׁ. [שער כותש, v. כָּתַשׁ.]

כָּזַב (b. h.; cmp. כזז) [*to shrink*, cmp. כָּחַשׁ,] *to fail, dry up* (of watercourses); *to be false, to lie; to flatter*. Tosef. Par.

IX (VIII), 2 מפני שֶׁכָּזְבָה וכ׳ because it gave out during the war.—Snh. 82[b] (play on כזבי, Num. XXV, 15) כזבה באביה she was false to her father (in disobeying his instructions). Tanh. Sh'lah 5 לא כָזַבְתִּי לך I did not tell thee a falsehood; a. e.

Pi. כִּיזֵּב same. Par. VIII, 9 המים המְכַזְּבִים waters which fail at certain times. Y. Taan. II, 65[b] bot. (ref. to Num. XXIII, 19) אם יאמר ... מְכַזֵּב הוא if a man says, I am a God, he is a deceiver. Num. R. s. 23 (ref. to Num. l. c.) איש עושה לאל שיְכַזֵּב a man (through his prayer) may cause God to fail (to execute his evil decrees); Tanh. Masé 7 לא איש עושה לאל שיכ׳ does not a man cause God &c.?—Yoma 69[b] לא כִיזְּבוּ לו Ms. M. (ed. בו) they would not be false in His praise (flatter); a. fr.—*Part. pass.* מְכוּזָּב, *pl.* מְכוּזָּבִים *reduced.* Ruth. R. to I, 1 (play on כזבה, I Chr. IV, 22) אלו בניו שהיו מכ׳ that refers to his (Elimelech's) sons who were reduced (died).

כְּזַב, *Pa.* כַּזֵּב same. Targ. Job VI, 28 (Ms. כד׳). Targ. Prov. XIV, 5 (ed. Lag. מכדב); v. כְּדַב.

כָּזָב m. (b. h.; preced.) *falsehood.*—*Pl.* כְּזָבִים. Pesik. Bahod., p. 154[a]; Lev. R. s. 29 הבלים וכ׳ vain and false things. Cant. R. to II, 13 (play on סתו, ib. 11) that is the wicked (Roman) government שמסיתה ... בִּכְזָבֶיהָ which entices the world and leads it astray with its falsehoods. Pesik. R. s. 40 כ׳ שישראל מכזבים וכ׳ the falsehoods which the Israelites commit during the whole year.—[Ex. R. s. 42 כזבים, v. כּוּב.]—[מדבר כזב, v. כּוּב.]

כַּזְּבָן m. (preced.) *liar.* Tanh. Masé 5 אתחשב כ׳ I shall be considered a liar; Num. R. s. 23.

כַּזְּבָנָא ch. same. Gen. R. s. 47.

***כָּזַז** (v. P. Sm. 1691 s. v. כוז), [*to shrink,*] *to be shy, bashful.* Part. כָּזִיז. Pes. 72[b] כ׳ מינה Ar. a. Ms. O. (v. Rabb. D. S. a. l. note, ed. בזיז) he is reserved towards her (not yet intimate). Yeb. 26[a] דכ׳ בניה מיניה Ar. (ed. דב׳) before him his son is shy. Ib. 112[a] top מִיכְזַז כ׳ מינה Ar. (ed. מיב׳ ב׳), opp. גִּיס, v. גִּיס I. Nidd. 15[b] ילדה דכְזִיזָא למיטבל (ed. דב׳) a young woman who is ashamed to go to the bath-house.

כְּזִיב (b. h.) pr. n. pl. *Chezib,* v. אַכְזִיב. Hall. IV, 8 (Y. ed. כְּזִיב). Dem. I, 3 (Y. ed. ג׳, Ms. M. גויב, corr. acc.); a. fr.

כַּזַּיִת, v. זַיִת.

כזניתא, Y. Kidd. I, 60[b] top, v. זַנִּיתָא.

כָּזַר (cmp. כזז) *to shrink; to be hard* (v. אַכְזָר a. denom.). *Ithpe.* אִתְכְּזַר *to loathe.* Targ. Job. X, 1 אִתְכַּזְרִית וכ׳ Ms. (Var. אתבזיית, ed. אתגזרת) I myself loathe my life.

כַּח, v. כָּחַח.

כֹּחַ, כּוֹחַ m. (b. h.; v. כָּחַח) *firmness, strength, power.* Hor. 9[a] בנוי בכ׳ וכ׳ in beauty, in physical strength, &c. Hag. 12[a]. Snh. 96[a] תשש כֹּחוֹ his strength failed him. Ber. 63[a] כל ... אין בו כח וכ׳ he who is careless about the study of the Law, will have no strength to endure on the day of trouble; a. v. fr.—Bets. 2[b], a. fr. (mixed diction) להודיעך כֹּחָן .. to show the power of ..., i. e. how far-reaching are the consequences of the opinion of ..... Ib., a. fr. כח דהיתרא עדיף showing the power of the more lenient opinion is preferred (as an evidence of courage of conviction, while the more rigid opinion may be the outcome of doubt).—כח כֹּחוֹ *indirect action,* opp. כֹּחוֹ direct action. B. Kam. 18[a] שאני ... בין נזק כחו לכח כחו S. distinguishes between direct and indirect injury. Ib. 19[a]. Macc. 8[a].—Ab. Zar. 60[a] כ׳ כ׳ pressing wine by turning a wheel. B. Kam. 10[b], v. לָאו.—Snh. 77[b] כ׳ ראשון direct agency, כ׳ שני indirect agency.—Shebu. 48[a], a. fr. יָפֶה כ׳, v. יָפֶה.—Ohol. XVIII, 6 שֶׁכֹּחַן יפה who (which) can endure pressure without shaking, opp. כחן רע; Zab. III, 1; B. Mets. 105[b]; a. e.—Gen. R. s. 98, v. לִיבְדְּקוֹס. Y. Pes. I, 27[c] bot. ל״ת שבא מכח עשה a prohibition derived from a positive law, v. לָאו; a. fr.—Trnsf. *coition.* Yeb. 34[a].

כֹּחַ, כּוֹחָא, כּ׳ ch. 1) same. Targ. Lam. I, 6.—Bets. 2[b], a. fr. (mostly in Hebrew form), v. supra.—2) name of a *lizzard.* Targ. Lev. XI, 30 (h. text כח).—3) בַּר כּוֹחָא pr. n. m. *Bar-Koha.* Y. Sabb. XIV, 14[d] bot.

כָּחַד (b. h.; cmp. כחש) *to diminish.*

Pi. כִּיחֵד *to withhold, deny.* Num. R. s. 13 לא כ׳ מיעקב did not withhold (the truth) from &c.

Hif. הִכְחִיד *to destroy.* Ib. s. 20 לקללן ולהַכְחִידָן to curse and destroy them. Ex. R. s. 12; a. e.

Nif. נִכְחַד *to be destroyed.* Ib. הייתה כ׳ מן וכ׳ thou wouldst have been wiped out from the earth.

כְּחַד ch. same. [Y. Sabb. VII, 10[a] bot. מכחד, v. בְּחַר.] *Ithpa.* אִתְכַּחַד *to be destroyed.* Targ. Job IV, 7.

כְּחַד m. constr. (preced.) *missing, being missed.* Targ. Ps. CXXXIX, 16 (ed. Lag. a. oth. בחד, Var. כ׳).

כַּחֲדָא, v. חֲדָא I.

כָּחָה, v. כָּחַח.

כָּחוֹל, v. כּוֹחָל.

כָּחוּשׁ m., כְּחוּשָׁה f. *lean, weak,* v. כָּחַשׁ.

כָּחַח (onomatop., cmp. חָכַךְ II) [*to scratch,*] *to cough, to bring up mucus.* Erub. 99[a] כָּח בפני רבו (not כיח, v. Rabb. D. S. a. l. note 16) he who coughs in sight of his teacher, expl. ib. כח ורק (not כיח) when he coughs and spits out. Tosef. ib. XI (VIII), 8 הכּוֹחֶה וכ׳ (fr. כָּחָה) he who coughs (brings mucus up in his mouth) in the street. Tanh. Noah 9 גונח וכוֹחֶה דם coughing and spitting blood; (Tanh. ed. Bub. ib. 14 גונח מלבו), v. גָּנַח.

כְּחִישׁ, כְּחִישָׁא, כְּחִישְׁתָּא m., **כְּחִישְׁתָּא** f. (כָּחַשׁ) *lean, weak.* Kidd. 24[b] נהורא כ׳ feeble eye-sight, opp. בריא normal. B. Bath. 155[b] אי כ׳ .. לבריר if he is lean, we let him be fattened. B. Mets. 105[b] הוה כ׳ ארעא the soil was exhausted, opp. שמינא.—*Pl.* כְּחִישִׁין, f. כְּחִישָׁתָא. Targ. Y. Gen. XLI, 27.—B. Kam. 118[b], opp. ברייתא.

כְּחִישׁוּתָא f. (preced.) *reduction, weakness, leanness.* Targ. Koh. XII, 5.—Yeb. 79[b] כ׳ דאתחילא ביה it was weakness that befell him (but no organic defect). Bekh. 45[b] כ׳ אתחלא וכ׳ it is a weakness of the right hand, v. בְּרִיאוּתָא. B. Bath. 155[b]; a. e.

כָּחַל, v. כּוֹחַל.

כָּחַל (b. h.; denom. of כּוֹחַל) *to paint the eyelids* (for [m]edical or for cosmetic purposes). Sabb. VIII, 3 (78[b]) [כ]די לִכְחוֹל [ע]ין a quantity sufficient for painting one eye. [Keth]. 80[a] צנועות כּוֹחֲלוֹת וכ׳ chaste (veiled) women paint only [o]ne eye. Ib. X, 6 הכּוֹחֶלֶת she who paints her eyes (on the [S]abbath); a. fr.—Part. pass. כָּחוּל; f. כְּחוּלָה, pl. כְּחוּלוֹת. Gen. [R]. s. 98 (play on חַכְלִילִי, Gen. XLIX, 12) שעיניהם כחולות [ו]כחם יפה whose eyes are bright as if painted, and [t]hose abilities for study are fine. [Y. Sabb. VII, 10[a] top [ל]הכחי, מכחיל, v. כְּחַל II.]

כְּחַל I ch. 1) same. Targ. II Kings IX, 30; a. e.—Sabb. [8]0[a] ... הא לא כָּחֲלָי עין but people never paint one eye [o]nly!—2) (ironically, v. infra) *to blind the eyes.* Ber. 58[a] [ו]כ׳ חבריהו כַּחֲלִינְהוּ his associates put his eyes out, v. כְּבַר. —[Y. Ab. Zar. II, 40[d] top כחל לה, read in one w., v. חֲלָלָא.]

Ithpe. אִיתְכְּחַל *to be painted.* Nidd. 55[b] if one desires to [b]ecome blind, (מכב״ום) לִיתְכְּחוֹל מארמאי let him have his [e]yes painted by gentiles; Y. Ab. Zar. l. c. מִיתְכְּחִיל מינהון.

כְּחַל (tradit. pronunc. כְּחָל) m. (prob. from its reddish [c]olor, v. כְּחָלִי) *udder, bag.* Hull. VIII, 3. Tosef. ib. VIII, 8 [כ]׳ של מניקה the bag of a milk-cow; a. fr.

כַּחֲלָא, כַּחַל II, ch. same. [Targ. Ps. LXXIV, 6 some [e]d., read כַּחְדָא.]—Hull. 110[a] תבשילא דכחלא Ar. (ed. דכחל) [a] dish made of udder.—*Pl.* כַּחְלֵי. Ib. ... כ׳ בסורא in Sura [t]hey do not eat udders. Ib. אפקינהו כ״ע לִכַחְלַיְיהוּ (not [ל]כחלינה) all of them brought out the udders they were [a]bout to cook.

כַּחְלֵי m. pl. = h. כּוֹחֲלִין, *carbuncle.* Targ. Cant. V, 14 corresp. to נֹפֶךְ, Ex. XXVIII, 18).

כחלינהו, Hull. 110[a], v. כְּחַל II.

כָּחַשׁ (b. h.; cmp. כחד; cmp. חסר, חַסְיָא &c.) 1) *to fail, be reduced, be lean,* opp. בריא, שמן. B. Kam. 34[a] כ׳ כשעת [ה]נזק וכ׳ if the injured ox became reduced after being wounded, damage is assessed according to the value at the time of standing before court; Y. ib. III, end, 3[d] הִכְחִישׁ. Gen. R. s. 53 (ref. to Hab. III, 17) כּוֹחֲשִׁים היו (Sarah's face) was haggard (and the announcement of the angels made it shine like olive oil); Yalk. Hab. 565 כְּחוּשִׁים; [oth. interpret., v. infra].—*Part. pass.* כָּחוּשׁ, f. כְּחוּשָׁה; pl. כְּחוּשִׁים, כחושות *lean, reduced, weak.* Snh. 78[a] כח כ׳ a weak force. Hull. 97[a] (in Chald. diction). B. Kam. 6[b] אכל כ׳ if he ate fruits of a garden-bed with scanty fruits; Gitt. 48[b]; a. fr. —2) (cmp. כָּזַב) *to be false.* Gen. R. l. c. כּוֹחֲשִׁים היו were they (the angels) false (deceiving)?—

Hif. הִכְחִישׁ 1) *to be reduced, fail, deteriorate.* Y. B. Kam. l. c., v. supra.—Meil. 17[a] מי שיש . . יַכְחִישׁ וכ׳ if you have an enemy, do you desire him to be weak or strong? Ib. ימולו . . ויַכְחִישׁוּ let their children be circumcised . . ., and they will become weak. Yeb. 34[b] ויַכְחִישׁ יופיה her beauty may be ruined. Y. M. Kat. I, beg. 80[a] עמדה מִלְּהַכְחִישׁ if the field ceased to deteriorate; a. e.—2) *to lessen, reduce, ruin, weaken.* Gitt. 70[a] ג׳ . . . מַכְחִישִׁים כחו וכ׳ three things lessen a man's energies. Snh. 84[b] הִכְחִישָׁהּ באבנים he ruined the animal by loading stones upon her (without causing a wound). Y. B. Kam. l. c. הִכְחִישׁוֹ חמשים וכ׳ he lessened his (the ox's) value by fifty Zuz. Esth. R. to I, 1 (play on אחשורוש) שהכחיש ראשן וכ׳ he caused haggardness to the heads of &c. Sabb. 22[a] מַכְחִישׁ מצוה he impairs the religious act (lessens the brightness of the Ḥanuckah lights). Snh. 67[b]; Hull. 7[b], v. כְּשָׁפִים; a. fr.—[Yalk. Ps. 627 אַכְחִישׁ, v. כָּבַס.]—3) *to declare false, deny, contradict,* v. הַכְחָשָׁה. Keth. 20[a] כשם שאין מזימין . . . אין מַכְחִישִׁין וכ׳ as an evidence of alibi cannot be taken up except by confrontation, so cannot contradictory evidence &c. Ber. 27[b] יכול החי לְהַכְחִישׁ וכ׳ can the living contradict the living? Gen. R. s. 48, beg. מפני מה אתה מַכְחִישֵׁנִי וכ׳ why dost thou contradict me (declare me wrong) in the presence of my servant?—Sifra introd., v. כְּרַע; a. fr.

Pi. כִּיחֵשׁ *to be false; to flatter.* Sifré Deut. 356 בשעה . . . . מְכַחֲשִׁים להם when the Israelites prosper, the nations flatter them; Yalk. Deut. 967.

Hof. הוּכְחַשׁ *to be contradicted, rebutted.* B. Kam. 74[b] כדים שהוּכְחֲשׁוּ בנפש witnesses that have been contradicted in a capital case.—Ib. מוּכְחָשִׁין witnesses whose evidence has been contradicted (but not rebutted through an alibi). Keth. l. c. עדות מוּכְחֶשֶׁת a rebutted evidence; a. fr.

Hithpa. הִתְכַּחֵשׁ *to contradict each other.* Sifré Deut. 37 מִתְכַּחֲשׁוֹת; v., however, כָּתַשׁ.

כְּחַשׁ ch. same, *to be lean, weak;* v. כַּחִישׁ.—Snh. 95[a] כ׳ חיליה his strength failed him. B. Mets. 104[b] (prov.) תִּכְחוּשׁ ארעא ולא לִיכְחוּשׁ מרהּ Ms. M. (ed. כחשא) let the land deteriorate (exhausted by strong seeds) rather than that its owner become reduced (by reduced income); a. e.

Af. אַכְחֵשׁ 1) *to reduce, weaken, impair.* Nidd. 47[b]; Yeb. 97[a] אַכְחֲשׁוּהוּ reduce him (by scanty food); B. Bath. 155[b] אכחשיה Ms. M. (corr. acc., ed. ליכחוש, v. infra). B. Kam. 34[a] את מַכְחֲשָׁה ואנא וכ׳ thou didst ruin her (by neglect), and I should pay for it?—2) *to contradict.* Gen. R. s. 48, beg. אַכְחֲשָׁהּ קדמה he contradicted her (his wife) in her (the servant's) presence.

Ithpe. אִיכְּחוּשׁ, אִתְכְּחִישׁ 1) *to reduce one's self, to be reduced.* B. Bath. l. c. לִיכְּחוּשׁ let him reduce himself. B. Mets. l. c., v. supra.—2) *to be contradicted, rebutted.* B. Kam. 74[a] מִתְכַּחֲשֵׁי are contradicted, contrad. to מיתזמי, v. זָמַם I.—Snh. 81[b] אִתְכַּחוּשׁ בבדיקות they contradicted each other in cross-examinations, v. בְּדִיקָה.

כַּחְשָׁא m. (preced.) *reduction, deterioration.* B. Kam. 59[a] כַּחַשׁ גופנא the weakening of the vine (by allowing the grapes to remain on it until they are ripe). B. Mets. 101[b] משום כ׳ דארעא because he exhausted the soil by planting trees. Ib. 104[b] מנכי ליה כ׳ דארעא he must allow him a reduction of his rent in consideration of the lesser exhaustion of the soil (by having planted wheat in place of poppy).

כטספטייס, Ab. Zar. 39[a] ed., Ms. M. כספטייס, Hull. 66[b]; Tosef. ib. III (IV), 27 כספתיאס, a corrupt. of קְסִיפְיָיס, קְסִיפְיָאס (ξίφιας) *sword-fish,* v. אכספטיאס.

כי, כ״י *the Greek letter Chi* (χ). Men. VI, 3 כמין כי, expl. ib. 75[a] כמין כי יוני (Ar. יונית) drawing the figure of a Greek Chi; Tosef. ib. VIII, 8; 10; Ker. 5[b]; Hor. 12[a], expl. כמין כָּף יוני ed. (Ms. M. כי). Kel. XX, 7.

כַּי (=כַּאִי, v. אִי III) *like which?*; כַּיזה צד, כַּי זֶה צַד *how?, in what manner?* Tosef. B. Kam. III, 4. Tosef. Ter. I, 5; a. fr. ed. Zuck. (ed. usu. כֵּיצַד).

כִּי (b. h.; v. כִּי־) 1) *like.* Sot. 35[b] כי סיד like lime. Y. Yeb. XVI, end, 16[a] כי חיה like a lying-in woman; a. fr.— 2) *when.* Ex. R. s. 9, beg. (ref. to Ex. VII, 9) . . . אם ידבר אלא כי וכ׳ it does not read, '*if* Pharaoh . . ., but *when*...; he *will* say so. R. Hash. 3[a], v. אִי II.— 3) *so, thus.* Y. Ḥag. III, 77[b] וכי היה הבעשה and thus it came to pass. Yeb. VIII, 3 לא כי הלכה וכ׳ (some ed. לא כי אלא וכ׳) it is not so; I am reciting a Halakhah. Shek. I, 4 לא כי אלא וכ׳ it is not so, but &c. B. Kam. 25[b]; a. fr.—4) *for.* Yoma 87[b] (quoting from a prayer) כי עונותינו וכ׳ for our iniquities are &c.—5) וְכִי (introducing a question to which a negative answer is expected) *is it really so that?* R. Hash. 9[a] וכי בתשעה . . . . והלא וכ׳ do we fast on the ninth? Is it not the tenth &c.? Sabb. 4[a] וכי אומרים וכ׳ dare we say to a man &c.?; Men. 48[a]. Yoma 7[a]; a. v. fr.

כִּי ch. same, 1) *as, like.* Targ. Is. XIV, 19, v. יָהֵב; a. fr., v. כִּי־.—M. Kat. 28[b] מותא כי מותא וכ׳ death like death, i. e. death must naturally ensue, v. חֲבוּלְיָא. Sabb. 140[b]. v. אוּרְפָּא.—Kidd. 81[a] יומא כי האידנא on a day like this.— כי הא ד־ as that which is told of &c. Pes. 117[a]; a. fr.—Ḥag. 2[a], a. fr. דלא כי האי תנא which is not in agreement with the opinion of &c.—B. Kam. 46[a] לְכִי הא דאיתמר for a case like the one that is told.—Ned. 49[a], a. fr. כי אתריה, v. אֲתַר. —Hor. 13[b] נתקין . . כי לדידן let us institute something like that which has been done concerning ourselves; a. fr.— 2) *when.* Targ. Y. II Lev. XXVI, 44; a. fr.—Ḥull. 110[a]; B. Bath. 87[a] כי סליק וכ׳ when R. El. went to Palestine. Snh. 74[a], a. fr. כי אתא וכ׳ when R . . . . came (from Palestine).—וכי תימא (abbr. וכ״ת), v. אֲמָא II.—Y. Snh. VII, end, 25[d] כי יתבון וכ׳ (not כיי) when they sat down to eat; a. v. fr.—כי היכי a) *in order that,* v. הֵיכִי.—b) *as well as, in the same way as.* Taan. 9[b] כי ה׳ . . . הכי וכ׳ as the Babylonians are deceitful, so are their rains; a. fr.—[כַּי, v. כַּיי.]

***כִּיאוּרָא** (v. כָּאַר) *ugliness.* Sabb. 62[b] Ms. M., v. כֵּיבָא.

כיארי, Y. Dem. II, beg. 22[b] (R. S. to ib. II, 1 בראר׳) prob. to be read: בְּאַרְיֵי or בֵּירַאִי.

כֵּיב, v. כְּאֵב I.

כֵּיבָא m. (preced.) *pain, sore,* v. כְּאֵבָא. Targ. Job V, 18; a. e.—B. Kam. 46[b], v. כְּאֵב I. Lam. R. to II, 1 איח . . . לכ׳ עייבא there is a place where they call a sore *'ayba* (heaviness), v. כְּאֵב I *Pa.*—Esp. *ulcer, ulceration* (mostly as a collective noun). Sabb. 62[b] (ref. to Is. III, 24) חלף שופרי כ׳ instead of beauty ulcers; [Kimḥi quotes כְּיָאָה; Ms. M. כיבא כיאורא, combining two versions]. Kidd. 39[b] שיחנא וכ׳ scabs and ulcers. Ib. 81[a] [read:] יתיב עליה מלא נפשיה שיחנא וכ׳ he sat down before it (the tray), his body being full of &c.—Sabb. 67[a] לכ׳ לימא הכי Ar. (ed. כיפא, Ar. s. v. כס: כיסא) against ulcers say the following charm.—*Pl.* כֵּיבִין. Ib. שיחנין וכ׳ Ms. M. (ed. שחיני כְּאִיבִין, read ש׳ וכ׳). —[Koh. R. to I, 2, v. כִּיב.]

כִּיבָא m. (כָּבַב) *roast over thorn-fire.* Snh. 70[a] בשר כ׳ וכ׳ (Ar. כִּיבֵּי *pl.*) like the meat roasted over a thorn fire which thieves eat.

כִּיבּוּד m. (כָּבַד) 1) *doing honor to; respect, reverence.* Peah I, 1 כ׳ אב ואם filial respect. Sifra K'dosh. beg. Kidd. 31[b], a. e. (ref. to Lev. XIX, 3, a. Ex. XX, 12) איזהו מורא ואיזהו כ׳ what constitutes filial fear (reverence), and what filial respect?—Pesik. R. s. 23—24; Y. Kidd. I, 61 top אדיין לחצי הכ׳ וכ׳ he has not come up yet to half of the filial duties which the Law implies; a. fr.—2) *sweeping, cleansing.* Nidd. VII, 2 (56[a]) עד שעת כִּבּוּד up to the time of sweeping; ib. 3[a] עד שעת הכי׳. Treat. S'maḥ. ch. XI; a. e.—*Pl.* כִּיבּוּדִים, כִּב׳. Nidd. 56[b] בשעת כִּבּוּדֵיהֶם when they are being swept.

כִּיבּוּי m. (כָּבָה) *extinguishing.* Sabb. 120[b] גרם כ׳ causing extinction indirectly. Y. ib. XVII, end, 15[d] [read:] יש לו צורך בכ׳ he has use for (profits by) the extinction

כיבוי, Targ. Prov. XXX. 14, some ed., read: גִּיבּוֹר, v. גִּיבָּא.

כִּיבּוּס, כִּבּוּס m. (כָּבַס) *washing.* Zeb. XI, 3. Ib. 94[b], v. כִּסְכּוּס; a. fr.—*Pl.* כִּיבּוּסִים, כִּב׳. Nidd. 56[b] בשעת כִּבּוּסֵיהֶן when they are being washed.

כִּיבּוּשׁ m. (כָּבַשׁ) 1) *conquest, dominion.* Y. Hor. III, 48[c] top בכ׳ הארץ for the conquest of Palestine. Gitt. 8[b] (ref. to Syria) כ׳ יחיד . . . כ׳ the conquest of an individual (David) is not called a (national) conquest (so as to give the land the sacred character of Palestine); ib. 47[a], a. fr.— [Gen. R. s. 17 לכבוש, v. כִּיבּוּס.]—2) =כֶּבֶשׁ 2, *ascent, grade.* Y. Erub. II, 24[b] bot. [read:] כל כִּיבּוּשֵׁי כבשים . . מכִּיבּוּשׁוֹ וכ׳ all grades of ascents in the Temple . . . . ., with the exception of the grade of the altar-bridge which was at the rate of about ten handbreadths to three handbreadths and one third of a finger's width (of vertical height; i.e. 10 to 3 1/12), v. כֶּבֶשׁ.—*Pl.* כִּיבּוּשִׁים, כִּיבּוּשִׁין, constr. כִּיבּוּשֵׁי, v. supra.—3) (only in *pl.*) *means of subduing one's pride; reproof; evil prediction, penitence.* Pesik. V'zoth, p. 197[a] הן וכִיבּוּשֵׁיהֶן they (the blessings) but also the reproofs connected therewith (Deut. ch. XXXII); Yalk. Deut. 550. Gen. R. s. 66 (ref. to Gen. XXVII, 28) [read:] יתן לך ברכות ויתן לך כיבושין הראויות לך; Yalk. Gen. 115 כיבושיהן may He give thee blessings, but also such means of preventing overbearing as may be proper for thee.—דברי כ׳ *admonitions to penitence.* Taan. II, 1 (15[a]); Tosef. ib. I, 8.

כִּיבּוּשׁ, כְּבַשׁ, כִּיבְשׁ m. ch. (v. כָּבַשׁ 3) *fastening, connection, hammering in, welding.* Targ. I Kings VII, 29 עובד כ׳ welding work (h. text מוֹרָד). Ib. 30 כִּבְשֵׁי constr. (h. text מִעֶבֶר!). Ib. 36 (כ״) כִּבְשׁ חד one connected body (h. text כמער איש). — *Pl.* כִּיבּוּשִׁין. Targ. Ex. XXVII, 10, a. e. *sockets* for the hooks (h. text וָוֵיהֶם). Targ. I Kings VII, 33 *naves* (h. text חִשֻּׁרֵי).

כִּיבְשָׁא, כִּיבְשׁ, v. כֶּבֶשׁ II a. preced.

כִּיד, *Pi.* כִּייד, v. כִּיר.

כִּיד, כִּידֵי, v. כַּד I.

כִּידְבָא, v. כַּדְבָא.

כִּידוּ, v. כְּדוּ.

כידום, v. כידוס.

כִּידוֹן I m. (b. h.) name of *a tree*, trnsf. *light spear, javelin.* Kel. XI, 8. Num. R. s. 9 יכול כב׳ you might think (Absalom with his head of hair was slender, looking) like a *kidon*, opp. כוזרובית; Y. Sot. I, 17[b] בכ׳ (corr. acc.); Midr. Sam. ch. XIII; ib. XXVII; a. e.—*Pl.* כִּידוֹנִים. Yalk. Gen. 133.

כִּידוֹן II (b. h.) pr. n. m. *Kidon*; גורן כ׳ the threshing floor of K. (I Chr. XIII, 9), in place of נָכוֹן (II Sam. VI, 6). Sot. 35[b]; Num. R. s. 4 בתחלה כ׳ וכ׳ at first (the Ark was shaking like) a javelin (v. preced.), but afterwards (it was) firmly established; [oth. interpret., v. Rashi to Sot. l. c.]

כידוס, כידום, Tosef. Meg. IV (III), 30, read: בִּירוֹס.

כִּידוֹר pr. n. pl. *Kidor*. Yoma 83[b] (as an ominous name, with ref. to כי דור, Deut. XXXII, 20); Y. R. Hash. III, end, 59[a].

כידי, Pesik. Shub., p. 162[a] כ׳ ומנקייה, v. פִּירוֹמָנִיקְיָא.

כידים, כידין, v. פִּירִים.

כִּיהוּן m. (denom. of כֹּהֵן) *priestly outfit.* Yoma 43[a] הכהן בכיהונו 'the priest' (as such) in his priestly garments (v. Rabb. D. S. a. l. note 7); Yalk. Num. 760.

כִּיוּד, v. כִּיּוּר.

כִּיווּן, v. כְּוּוּן, a. כִּיוּן.

כִּיוּן, כִּיוּנְתָּא, כִּיוּוּנִיתָא, כִּיהֲנְתָּא, v. כִּיוּן, כִּיוּנ׳.

כִּיּוּן m. (b. h.) *Kiyyun*, name of an idol. Targ. Am. V, 26 (some ed. כִּיווּן).

כִּיוָן m. (כון) [*firmness, directness, fitness*;] 1) (adv.) *directly, exactly.* Pes. 37[a] אפשר ... וּיקבענה כ׳ he may form the dough in a mould and attach it to the cake directly (well fitting, without loss of time). Tam. III, 6 אחד ... ואחד פותח כ׳ (with one key) a priest puts his hand through an opening in the door (v. אַמָּה), and another priest opens (with the other key) directly; (Talm. ed. 30[b] ואחד שהוא פותח כ׳ and another key which opens directly). —2) (conj. followed by ש־) *as soon as, since.* Macc. 3[a], a. fr. כ׳ שהגיד וכ׳ as soon as a witness has finished his evidence, he is not permitted to testify again (retract or modify). Keth. 11[a] כ׳ שהגדילה וכ׳ as soon as she was of age for one while without protesting &c. Erub. 93[b] כ׳ שהותרה הותרה being once permitted (for one part of the Sabbath), it remains permitted; a. v. fr.

כִּיוָן, כֵּיוָן ch. same, 1) *firmly established, true, straightforward.* Targ. Deut. XIII, 15 (h. text נָכוֹן). Targ. Hab. I, 4 לא כ׳ (h. text מעוקל).—*Pl.* כֵּיוָנֵי *honest men.* Targ. O. Gen. XLII, 11; 19; a. e.—2) (conj. followed by ד־) *as soon as, when, since* (also כִּיוָן). Targ. Y. Gen. XXI, 15. Targ. Y. II Gen. XXVIII, 10; a. fr.—Ber. 8[a] כ׳ דאמרי ליה when they told him. Ib. כ׳ דשמענא להא וכ׳ when we heard that which &c.; a. v. fr.

כִּיוָנָא I c. (preced.) *straight, proper.* Targ. II Sam. XXII, 31 (ed. Lag. כִּיוָנָא).—*Pl.* f. כֵּיוָנָן. Targ. Ps. XVIII, 31 (ed. Lag. כֵּוָן׳); a. e.

כִּיוָנָא II, כֵּיוָנְתָּא f. (preced.) *propriety, proper thing* (h. יְשָׁרָה, נְכֹחָה). Targ. Job XLII, 7 (ed. Wil. כֵּוָן׳); ib. 8 (ed. Lag. כִּיוֹן׳). Targ. Mic. III, 9 (ed. Lag. כְּיָוֹנִיתָא). Targ. Am. V, 10 (ed. Lag. כְּיָוֹנִיתָא; h. text תמים).—*Pl.* כֵּיוָנָן. Targ. Is. XXXIII, 15; XLV, 19 (h. text מישרים).—[Targ. Ps. XXXII, 9 כיונא, some ed., read: בִּיוּנָא.]

כיונותא, Targ. Ps. CIII, 2, in an interpolation, read: בִּיוּנְתָא.

כֵּיוָנְתָּא, כֵּיוָנִיתָא, v. כִּיוָנָא II.

כִּיּוּר (כִּיוּד) m. (כִּיר, כִּיר) *paneling work, panel* (abacus). B. Bath. 53[b] וסד בהן סיוד אחד או כ׳ אחד and added one piece of stucco or one panel. Midd. IV, 6 אמה כ׳ one cubit for the paneling work (tablature of the ceiling in the Temple). Zeb. 62[a], v. כַּרְכֹּב.

כִּיּוֹר m. (b. h.; cmp. כּוּר II) *basin*, esp. the *laver* for the priests in the Temple court. Midd. III, 6. Tosef. Yoma II, 2; a. e.

כִּיּוֹרָא (כִּיוֹרָא) ch. same. Targ. Ex. XXX, 18; a. fr. —*Pl.* כִּיּוֹרַיָּא, כִּיּוֹרִין. Targ. II Chr. IV, 6. Targ. I Kings VII, 40; a. e.

כִּיּוּרָא (כִּיוּרָא) ch.=h. כִּיּוּר *panel-work.* Targ. II Chr. VI, 13 (h. text כִּיּוֹר).—*Pl.* constr. כִּיּוּרֵי; כ׳ ארזיא *cedar panels* in ceilings. Targ. II Sam. VII, 2; 7; Targ. I Chr. XVII, 1 (ed. Rahm. כיוורי).—Targ. Jer. XXII, 14. Targ. Ḥag. I, 4 (ed. Wil. נִסְרֵי).

כִּיזְבָא* m. (supposed to be) *a measure of length*, v. נִזְבָא.

כִּיזָה, כִּיזְצַד, v. כֵּי, a. כֵּיצַד.

כִּיחַ m. (כָּחַח) *coughing, phlegm* of the lungs. Erub. 99[a] בכיחו it refers to the phlegm in his mouth. Ib. כיחו שנתלש phlegm which is loose in the mouth. [Ib. כ׳ בפני כיח ורק, v. כָּחַח.]—B. Kam. 3[b] כיחו וניעו the phlegm brought out by coughing or hawking. Nidd. 55[b]. Ib. 56[a] כיחו וניעו ורוקו phlegm, mucus and spittle (prob. to be read כרוקו). Kidd. 81[b] (in Chald. dict.) כיחו, v. אַבְמַר.

כִּיר, v. חִיר.

כִּייד, v. כִּיר.

כִּיוּרָא, v. כִּיּוּרָא.

כַּיִּיל, כַּיִּל, v. כּוּל.

כַּיָּיל m. (כּוּל) *measurer*, a rural officer. Y. B. Mets. IX, beg. 12[a].—*Pl.* כַּיָּלִין. Tosef. ib. IX, 14 חבירי (corr. acc.).

כַּיְלָא, כַּיִּילָא m. (preced.) *measure.* B. Mets. 40[a] (Ms. H. בכילתא, v. Rabb. D. S. a l. note 6). Bets. 38[b] כיי׳ חסריה

Ms. M. (ed. 'כי) he lessened the measure (quantity) of his wheat by taking out the pebbles. Ib. 29ª מנא דכ' a vessel used for measuring.

כַּיְיפָא m. (כוף) *pressure, necessity.* Targ. Prov. XVI, 26 ed. Lag. (oth. כִּיפָא).

כְּיִיר, v. כִּיר.

כייר, Y. B. Mets. IX, beg., 12ª, v. בָּיִיר.

***כִּיכְלֵי** m. pl. (=כלכלי, Assyr. Kulukuku, Kaku-ullu, v. Del. Assyr. Thiernamen, p. 103) *partridges.* Yoma 75ᵇ ד' מיני שליו .. וכ' Ar. (ed. קיבלי; Ms. M. 1 קיפלי, 2 קיבלי, v. Rabb. D. S. a. l. note) there are four kinds of *s'lav* &c. (v. Winer Realwörterbuch s. v. Wachtel); Yalk. Ex. 260 קיבלי. [Mus.: κίχλη, *thrush.*]

כִּילָא, v. כִּירָלָא.

כִּילָאוֹת, v. כִּילָה.

כִּילְבִית, כִּלְ', v. כִּילְבִּית.

כילדין, Y. Pes. III, beg. 29ᵈ והוא עביד כ' (?)—prob. a corrupt. to be restored after Bab. ib. 42ᵇ שואבת הזוהמא.

כִּילָה f. (כול or כָּלַל) [*enclosure,*] *curtain, curtained bed, canopy.* Gen. R. s. 36, beg. כדיין שמותחין כ' על פניו like a judge before whom they spread the curtain (that he may be undisturbed; Lev. R. s. 5 את הוילון). Y. Sabb. XX, beg. 17ᶜ (in Chald. dict.) ההן כ' דעל וכ' that curtain before the ark. Succ. 10ᵇ מותר לישן בכ' וכ' it is permitted to sleep in the Succah in a tester-bed though it has a top cover. Ib. 11ª כִּילַת חתנים a bridal bed (without cover overhead). Num. R. s. 12 (ref. to Cant. III, 9, v. אַפִּרְיוֹן) 'the king... made for himself a bridal litter', that is the world שהוא עשוי כמין כ' which is formed like a canopy (v. Ps. CIV, 2, sq.). Ib. s. 13; a. fr.—*Pl.* כִּילְיוֹת, כִּילָאוֹת (fr. כִּילֵי or כִּילָא). Gen. R. s. 28 (Yalk. ib. 47 וִילָאוֹת, some ed. פלאות, read: 'כִּיל).

כילה, Yalk. Esth. 1056, v. קִילָא.

כִּילוּ=כְּאִילוּ, v. אִילוּ.

כִּילוּ, Targ. Ps. LIX, 14 Ms., v. כְּלוֹ.

כִּילְוָות, v. כִּילְוָא II.

כִּילוֹזָא, v. כְּלוֹזָא.

כִּילּוּי m. (כָּלָה) 1) *finishing.* Sifra K'dosh. ch. I; Y. Peah IV, 18ᵇ בשעת הכ' at the time when the end of the field is cut (with ref. to תכלה, Lev. XIX, 9); a. e.—2) *extinction, destruction.* Lev. R. s. 7, beg. (ref. to שמד, Deut. IX, 20) כ' בנים וכ' the extinction of his family; ib. s. 10. Mekh. Bo s. 8 מצות כִּילּוּיוֹ בכל דבר it (the leavened bread) may be destroyed in any manner, opp. מצות כ' בשריפה it must be destroyed by fire.

כִּילּוּיָא ch. same, *destruction.*—*כִּילּוּי סִילְוֵי (or סִילְוֵי) *destruction of thistles,* name of an insect, prob. *caterpillar* (or *bruchus* (?), v. Sm. Ant. s. v.). Gen. R. s. 51, beg. (expl. שבלול, Ps. LVIII, 9) [read:] כחדין כ' סילוי כשלשול וכ' [לימצא is a gloss borrowed from a comment. to Ps. l. c. and absent in Yalk. Ps. 776] like the caterpillar, like the abdominal secretion &c. Y. Shek. VI, 50ª top בקרני סילוי וכילוי (Bab. ed. to VI, 2 Ms. M. סילוי וכילוי, early ed. only ס') the water coming forth from the Temple (Zech. XIV, 8) will be ... as minute as the horns (feelers) of the caterpillar (thinner than those of חגבים).

כִּילּוּלָא m. (כלל) *crowning, finishing;* כִּילּוּל בַּתֵּי *house-finishing,* the reception given on the finishing of a house. Tanh. B'resh. 2 (Sh'ilt. 1 הילול בתי).

כִּילוֹן (בִּילוֹן) m. (v. אוּבְלָא II) *one whose head has the shape of a basket* (calathus), *wedge-shaped.* Bekh. VII, 1, expl. ib. 43ᵇ. [Mus. refers to Lat. cilo.]

כילוס, Y. Sabb. VII, 10ᵇ bot., v. בילוס.

כילוף, v. כּוּלָּה.

***כילסופיס, כילופיס**, Pesik. R. s. 23 כשהן כ', read: כשהוא פִּילוֹטִימוֹס (φιλότιμος) when he is *liberal* (v. פילוטמיא).

כִּילִי (χιλι-) *one thousand-.* Pesik. Baḥod., p. 107ᵇ; Pesik. R. s. 21; Yalk. Ps. 796 [read:] כילי כיליאדין מירי מיריאדין (χιλι-χιλιάδες, μυρι-μυριάδες) a thousand times thousand, a myriad of myriads.

כִּילְיָה, כִּילְיָא, v. כִּלְיָה.

כִּילְיָאדִין m. pl. (χιλιάδες) *thousands,* v. כִּילִי.

כִּילְיוֹן m. =כִּילָה, *enclosure, partition, curtain.* Y. Ber. III, 6ᵈ.

כיליונין, Lam. R. to I, 4 quot. in Ar., prob. a corrupt. of בִּירְיוֹנִין (v. בִּירְיוֹן); ed. בולוטין, v. בּוּלְבְּטֵס.

כילוי, Gen. R. s. 51, beg. כ' סילוי; Y. Shek. VI, 50ª top סילוי וכ', v. כִּילּוּיָא.

כילוונא, Yalk. Lam. 1042, v. בֶּלְיוֹנָא.

כִּילְכּוּל, v. כַּלְ'.

כילכיד, v. כַּלְכִּיד.

כִּילְבִּית (כִּילְבִית), כִּלְ' f. (=כילכלית, v. כלכל; or denom. of כלב, cmp. כּוּלָב) name of a *small fish,* supposed to be *stickleback.* Tosef. Ab. Zar. IV (V), 11 כל שכילב' אחת או שתי כּוּלְבִּיּוֹת וכ' ed. Zuck. (Var. כלכלה.. כלכלוית, כלבת .. כלביות) when one or two *k.* swim in it (the brine); Ab. Zar. 39ᵇ bot. כילבית .. כילבוית ed. (Ms. M. מלבי, read 'כי as ib. 40ª; Alf. ed. Cost. כלכלית, v. Rabb. D. S. a. l. note). Sabb. 77ᵇ אימת כילב' וכ' ed. (Ms. M. כּוּלְבִית, Ms. O. כילב') the fear which the Leviathan has of the *k.*—Hull. 97ª.

כִּילַן m. ch.=h. כִּילָה, *curtain, cover.* Targ. Y. I Gen.

XXV, 25 (Y. II כִּבְלַן read: כְּבָלַן, q. v.).—Y. Meg. III, 73ᵈ bot. [read:] תחתוי דחהן כ׳ under the curtain or wrapper (for the chest containing the Book of the Law).

כִּילְרִין, v. בּוּלְרִין.

כִּילְתָא I f. same, *enclosure; bridal canopy, curtained bed.* Targ. Job XV, 32 כִּילְתֵיה Ms. (ed. כְּלָתֵיה, h. text כִּפָּה). Targ. Y. Ex. II, 1. Targ. Y. Gen. XLVI, 21 כִּילַּת חֻפָּה (to h. text חֻפִּים, v. חוּפָּה).—Snh. 29ᵇ בְּכִילְתֵיה הילולא behind the curtain of his bed-room. Succ. 26ᵃ למיגגא בכ׳ וכ׳ to sleep in the Succah under a canopy.

***כִּילְתָא** II f. (v. כִּירְכָּא) *measure, vessel.*—B. Mets. 40ᵃ Ms. H., v. כִּירְכָּא.—*Pl.* constr. כִּילְוָות. Targ. Job XXXVIII, 37 (Ms. כִּילְוָות?; h. text נִבְלֵי).

כִּימָא, v. next wds.

כִּימָה f. (b. h.; כים or כמם, cmp. Assyr. *Kimmut*, Rawl. Five Gr. Mon. ch. VII; *Kimtu* family, Schr. KAT² p. 557) *Kimah (gathering)*, a constellation, prob. *Draco* (not Pleiades). Ber. 58ᵇ (etymol. play) כְּמֵאָה ככבי as bright as a hundred stars. Ib. 59ᵃ; Yalk. Gen. 56 נטל ... מכ׳ וכ׳ the Lord took two stars away from *K.* and brought the flood &c.; R. Hash. 11ᵇ, sq. B. Mets. 106ᵇ. Y. Taan. I, 64ᵃ bot. Num. R. s. 10 הדעת ... ככ׳ knowledge is compared to the *K.* ... מה כ׳ מבשלת וכ׳ as the Kimah causes the ripening of the fruits and gives them taste, so does knowledge &c. Gen. R. s. 10 כ׳ מעדנת וכ׳, v. עָדַן; a. e.

כִּימָא, כִּימְתָא ch. same. Targ. Am. V, 8 (ed. Lag. כימה). Targ. Job IX, 9 כימא (Ms. כימתא). Ib. XXXVIII, 31. Targ. II Esth. III, 3 כימה.

כִּין, v. כֵּן.

כִּינָּא (כִּינָּה) ch.=h. כִּינָּה, *louse, vermin.* Sabb. 82ᵃ (Ms. M. a. some ed. כינה). Erub. 65ᵃ כינה.

כִּינָאֵי=חֲבִינָאֵי. Tosef. Shebu. III, 6 ed. Zuck.

כִּינָּה, כִּנָּה f. (כנן, cmp. קנן) 1) *nest, cavity, chamber.*—*Pl.* כִּנִּין, כִּינִּין, כִּינִּים. Lev. R. s. 14 Ar. (ed. קינין); Yalk. Job 905; cmp. פּוֹנְנִית.—2) (b. h. pl. כִּנִּים, collect. כִּנָּם) *vermin, louse* (also collect.). Par. IX, 2 הכ׳ שבתבואה the vermin in grain. Ḥag. 5ᵃ; a. e.—*Pl.* as above. B. Kam. 82ᵃ הורג כ׳ שבבני מעיים (Var. in Ms. הכינה) (garlic) kills the parasites in entrails. Pes. 112ᵇ. Kidd. 49ᵇ; Esth. R. to I, 3; a. fr.—Sabb. 107ᵇ בּיצי כ׳ *nits*, or a species of vermin called *lice-nits*; Ab. Zar. 3ᵇ.

כִּנּוּי, כִּינּוּי m. (כָּנָה) *by-name, surname; attribute, substituted word.* Snh. VII, 5 בכ׳ ... דנין the witnesses are examined by using a substitute for the Divine Name (v. יוֹסֵי). Sot. VII, 6 במקדש ... ובמדינה בכינויו in the Temple the Divine Name is pronounced as it is written, in the country (outside the Temple) by its substitute (Ădonai). Ib. 38ᵃ בכ׳, opp. שם המפורש; a. e.—*Pl.* כִּינּוּיִים, כִּנּ׳, כִּינּוּיִין. Ned. I, 1 כִּינּוּיֵי נדרים words used as substitutes for vows (נדר); ib. 2 כ׳ לחרם substitutes for *ḥerem* (v. חֵרֶם); a. fr.—כִּינּוּיֵי כִינּוּיִין secondary substitutes, e. g. the use of *g'rog'roth* for *tirosh* and this for *eshkol*, v. גְּרוֹגֶרֶת. Tosef. Naz. II, 1; Y. ib. II, beg. 51ᵈ.

כִּינּוּיָא, כִּנּ׳ ch. same. Targ. Y. Lev. XXIV, 15 constr. כִּינּוּי.

כִּינּוּס, כִּנּ׳ m. (כָּנַס) 1) *gathering, piling up.* Kel. XV, 5 העשוי לכ׳ a vessel used for piling up (shovel &c.), opp. לקבלה as a receptacle. Nidd. 49ᵇ כ׳ ע״י הדחק receiving (absorbing) liquids under pressure (through pores, perforations &c.) B. Bath. 68ᵃ בית כ׳ העצים (Ms. O. כּוֹנֵס; Tosef. ib. III, 3 כְּנִיסַת) store-room for wood. Snh. VIII, 5 כ׳ לרשעים כו׳ gathering (living together) of the wicked is bad &c., opp. פִּיזּוּר. Y. Kidd. I, 59ᵈ top מקום כ׳ שיער a spot of the body where hair grows in quantities. Gen. R. s. 32 (ref. to Gen. VII, 5) זה שיכון לכ׳ וכ׳ this is the execution of the command to gather in the animals. Midr. Till. to Ps. VIII (ref. to ויצר, Gen. II, 19) לשון כ׳ it means the gathering (the animals before Adam); Gen. R. s. 17 וכאן לבבוש (corr. acc.); a. fr.—2) (cmp. כְּנֵסֶת) *retirement for prayer.* Ib. s. 84, beg. (ref. to קִבּוּצַיִךְ, Is. LVII, 13) כִּינּוּסוֹ וכ׳ בניו וכ׳ his (Jacob's) and his sons' prayers saved him &c.; Yalk. Gen. 140; Yalk. Is. 349.

כִּינּוּפְיָא, v. כְּנוּפְיָא.

כִּינּוֹר, כִּינּוֹרָא v. sub כִּנּ׳.

כִּינֵי, v. כֵּן.

כִּינִּים, כִּינִּין, v. כִּינָּה.

כִּינַּר, כִּינָּרָא, כִּינֶּרֶת, v. sub כִּנ׳.

כִּינָרִיס, Tosef. Kil. III, 12 ed. Zuck., v. קִינָרַס.

כִּינְשָׁא, כִּינְתָא v. sub כִּנ׳.

כִּיס (b. h.; cmp. כּוֹס I) *receptacle, pouch, bag; purse, fund.* Bekh. 39ᵇ; Tosef. ib. IV, 6, v. זוּבָן. B. Kam. X, 1 כ׳ של גבאין the collection fund of (royal) collectors. Erub. 65ᵇ בְּכִיסוֹ, v. כּוֹס I. Keth. X, 4 שהטילו לכ׳ who formed a partnership for business. Y. Hor. III, 48ᶜ (ref. to Prov. XVI, 11) כולהם ... מכ׳ אחד all of them receive their wages out of the same fund (of divine rewards).—חסרון כ׳, v. חֶסְרוֹן.—Sabb. 53ᵃ הזב בכ׳ שלו the gonorrhoist with his bag (for his genitals); העזים בכ׳ וכ׳ the goats with the bag over their teats; Tosef. ib. IV (V), 5 בכיסין. Lev. R. s. 12 (ref. to כיס, K'ri כוס, Prov. XXIII, 31) הוא נותן עינו בכוס וחנוני..בכ׳ he (the drunkard) sets his eye on the cup, the shopkeeper—on the money bag. Ib. בכיס כתיב לשון נקי הוא it is written (Prov. l. c.) 'on the bag' which is a euphemism (for illicit intercourse) as in (Prov. I, 14) &c. Tanḥ. Sh'mini 11; a. fr.—*Pl.* כִּיסִים, כִּיסִין. Y. Ab. Zar. III, 42ᵈ bot.—Tosef. l. c.; a. e.

כִּיס, כִּיסָא ch. same. Targ. XLVI, 3. Targ. Prov. I, 14; a. e.—Ber. 58ᵇ לא שקל ידא מן כ׳ never took his hand out of his pocket (always prepared for charity). Pes. 113ᵃ שרי כִּיסָךְ וכ׳ untie thy purse, open thy sack, i. e. sell only for cash (Var. lect., v. Rabb. D. S. a. l. note). [Sabb. 67ᵃ לכ׳ לימא חכי Ar. for a bag (*ulcer*), v. כִּיבָא.]—*Pl.* כִּיסַיָּא, כִּיסֵי. Y. Kidd. I, 60ᵈ, v. גְּרַד. Ab. Zar. 70ᵃ כמה כ׳ וכ׳ how many money-bags ought to be found on the street! Sabb.

147ª כִּיסֵי בבליירתא pouches (a sort of *cape* or *hood*) worn by the Babylonian women; (Ar.: כישר, Ms. M. כושר, v. מַרְזֵב a. כִּישָׁא).—V. כִּיסְתָא.

כִּיסָא or **כִּיסָא** m. (כָּסַס) 1) *thorn* (cmp. קִיסָא).—*Pl.* כִּיסִין, כִּיסֵי, כִּיס׳. Y. Sabb. VI, 8ᶜ bot. מקטע כ׳ to cut thorns. Sabb. 77ᵇ אכל כ׳ (Ms. M. בוצר, בינר, Ar. ביסי) (the camel) eats thorns. B. Mets. 42ᵇ, sq. בכ׳ . . . דמי כ׳ (Ms. H. ב׳, v. Rabb. D. S. a. l. note 6) when what he gave him in trust was thorns (on which the cuscuta was hanging), and he pays him the value of thorns.—2) *fodder*, v. כִּיסְתָא II.

כִּיסָאנֵי, כִּיסָאנִין, v. כִּיסְנִין, כִּיסָנִין.

כִּיסּוּחַ, כִּס׳ m. (כָּסַח) *cutting down, clearing.* M. Kat. 3ª. Gen. R. s. 12; Cant. R. to I, 1; Koh. R. to II, 12 דרך הכ׳ in the path made by clearing the thicket; a. e.

כִּיסּוּי, כִּס׳ m. (כָּסָה II) 1) *act of covering.* Hull. VI, 1 כ׳ חדם the law concerning the covering with ashes of the blood of killed animals (Lev. XVII, 13). Ib. 4 כ׳ אחד לכולן for all of them one covering up is sufficient.—Koh. R. to IV, 6 (ref. to וכסה, Lev. XVI, 13) חכ׳ הזה וכ׳ what this expression 'to cover' meant &c.—2) *cover, lid, roofing.* Num. R. s. 4 כי׳ interch. with כסוי (b. h. כְּסוּי constr.). Gen. R. s. 1 וכיסוין, v. אִלְפַּס. Pes. 94ª ככ׳ קדירה like the lid of a pot. Kel. XII, 3, v. בִּיבָר. Tosef. ib. B. Mets. IV, 11 כ׳ קביא, v. קַבְיָא; a. fr.—[Pesik. R. s. 39 בחדש שהוא כי׳, read: כָּסוּי, v. כָּסָה I.]—*Pl.* כִּיסּוּיִין, כִּס׳. Tosef. l. c.; a. e.—[Y. Ter. VIII, 45ᵈ חכיסוין, read: הַכְּסוּיִין, v. כָּסַח II.]

כִּיסּוּיָא, כִּס׳ ch. same, 1) *covering, roofing.* Taan. 22ᵇ ככ׳ דתנורא (Ms. M. כי כיסתא, corr. acc.) as high up as the arch of the oven.—2) *cover, cloak.* Keth. 68ª לבושא וכ׳ garment and wrap.—*Pl.* כִּיסּוּיִין. Targ. II Esth. VI, 10 [read:] מן כִּיסּוּיֵי.—*3) *secret.*—*Pl.* fem. כִּיסּוּיָין, כִּס׳. Targ. Job XI, 6.

כִּיסּוּפָא, כִּס׳ m. (כְּסַף) *putting to shame; disgrace, shame.* Targ. Y. Gen. III, 10 (nakedness). Targ. Ps. LXIX, 8 (*fem.*); a. fr.—Hor. 13ᵇ אתיא מילתא לידי כ׳ this may lead to putting (R. S.) to shame. Taan. 9ᵇ רחמנא . . . מכ׳ דשימי the Lord save us from being put to shame through Shimi (by his questions). Snh. 11ª מחמת כ׳ in order to save the man from shame. Taan. 25ª top משום כ׳ to avoid exposure, v. אַקְטַרְתָא. B. Kam. 86ᵇ כ׳ feeling of shame, contrad. to זילותא disgrace though not felt. Num. R. s. 14 כס׳ . . . . בלשון ירושלמי in the Jerusalem dialect (of the Chaldaic) they say for *ḥerpah, kissufa.* [כיסופין Targ. Prov. II, 22 some ed., read: נסופין, v. סוּף II ch.]

כִּיסּוּת, v. כְּסוּת.

כִּיסִיתָא f. (dimin. of כִּיס) *a little bag.* Meg. 26ᵇ bot. לספרא כ׳ ... מיעבדיה Ms. M. (Ms. M. 2 כְּסָיָאתָא *pl.* of כִּסְיָא; Ms. O. כִּיסְתָא; ed. פריסא, v. Rabb. D. S. a. l. note) to alter it into a bag for a book of the Law.

כִּיסְכּוּס m. (כִּסְכֵּס) *rubbing* (clothes, in washing). Zeb. 94ᵇ כ׳ . . . כיבוס washing without rubbing.

כִּיסְלָא, v. כִּסְלָא.

כִּיסְנָא, v. כִּסָן.—[Sabb. 138ᵇ בכיסנא, v. כֶּסֶף.]

כִּיסְנֵי, v. כִּיסְנִין.

(כִּסָאנִין, כִּיסָאנִין) כִּסְנִין, כִּיסָנִין m. pl. (כסס, adopt. fr. Chald.; cmp. כְּלִילָה) *nibblings, dessert.* Tosef. Ber. IV, 4 כסאנ׳ ed. Zuck. (Var. כיסאנ׳, כיסנ׳). Ber. 41ᵇ פת הבאה בכ׳ bread offered as dessert. Y. Snh. X, 28ᵈ top נשים . . . . מיני כ׳ women selling all kinds of sweetmeats (Sifré Num. 131 בשמים). Y. Pes. X, beg. 37ᵇ מיני כִּיסָנִית nibblings.

(כִּסָא׳, כִּיסָא׳) כִּס׳, כִּיסְנֵי, כִּיסָנִין ch. same. Targ. Y. Num. XXIV, 25 (v. Y. Snh. quot. in preced.). Targ. I Kings XIV, 3 (h. text נקדים). Targ. Josh. IX, 5; 12 *crumbling* (h. text נקדים).—Erub. 29ᵇ כיסא׳, כסא׳ ed. (Ar. ed. Koh. כוסאני, oth. ed. כי׳). Keth. 17ᵇ ארמלתא לית לה כ׳ at the wedding of a widow no nibblings (roasted ears) are distributed.

כִּיסָנִית, v. כִּיסָנִין.

כִּיסְתָא I f. = כִּיסָא, *bag.* Ber. 24ª bot. בכ׳ (Ms. F. בכִּיסְתֵּיה) in the bag (of the T'fillin). Sabb. 105ᵇ top דעבדה כי׳ Ms. M. (ed. כי כסתא, Rashi כי כי׳, v. Rabb. D. S. a. l.) when he shapes the garment so as to form (a kind of) a pocket. Pes. 72ª ודמי ליה כמאן דמנחא בכִּיסְתֵּיה and it was to him as if lying in his pocket (ever ready to recite it); Keth. 50ª; Meg. 7ᵇ בכִּיסֵיה. [Keth. 98ª, v. כְּסִיתָא.]

כִּיסְתָא II, כִּיס׳ f. (כָּסַס) *fodder.* Targ. O. Gen. XXIV, 25; 32 (v. Berl. Targ. O. II, p. 9; Targ. Y. אספסתא, Ar. כִּסָּא). Targ. Jud. XIX, 19; 21 (some ed. כִּסְתָא); a. e.—B. Mets. 85ª כדהוה רמי כ׳ וכ׳ when casting fodder for the animal.

כִּיעוּר m. (כָּעַר) *hideousness.* Hull. 44ᵇ (prov.) הרחק מן הכ׳ וכ׳ keep aloof from everything hideous and from whatever seems hideous; Ab. d'R. N. ch. II; Tosef. Yeb. IV, 7; a. e.

כִּיף *to bend*, v. כּוּף.

כִּיף, pl. כִּיפִין, v. כִּיפָה.

כֵּף, כִּיף f. (b. h.; כֵּפָה) 1) [*ball*,] *rock.*—*Pl.* כֵּיפִים, constr. כֵּפֵי, כֵּיפֵי. Y. Shek. VI, 50ª; Gen. R. s. 23, v. בַּרְבַּרְיָא.—2) (v. כִּיפָּה) *arch, tuft, umbel.* Tosef. Kel. B. Bath. V, 5 כ׳ של נייר a tuft of papyrus; כ׳ של סיב of hemp.—*Pl.* כִּיפִּין, כֵּפ׳. Ib., sq.; v. כִּיפָּה.

כֵּיפָא, כִּיף I ch. same, *rock, stone, ball.* Targ. Is. XXXII, 2. Targ. Prov. XVII, 8; a. fr.—Y. Shek. V, 48ᵈ חייו דין כ׳ מקורר וכ׳ which rock (when bored) will give forth water, and which &c., v. שַׁרְבְּרוּבֵי.—*Pl.* כֵּיפִין, כֵּיפַּיָא, כֵּיפֵי. Targ. Y. I Deut. XXXII, 13. Targ. I Kings XIX, 11. Targ. Ps. CIV, 18; a. fr.—כיפי טבתא *pearls, jewels.* Targ. Prov. III, 15; a. e.—M. Kat. 25ᵇ כ׳ דנורא (Ms. M. טיפי) fire-balls; כ׳ דברדא hail-stones. Y. Ab. Zar. IV, 43ᵈ דאת ... אילין כ׳ thou must remove these stones. Keth. 112ª bot. מנשק כ׳ דעכו kissed the rocks (Rashi: *corals*) of the shore of Ptolemais (as sacred ground); Y. Shebi. IV, end, 35[c] לְכֵיפַּתָא. Ib. מתקל כֵּיפֵי weighed the stones (to demonstrate his appreciation of the sacred ground); a. fr. — Esp. כֵּיפֵי (v. supra) *precious stones, jewelry* (prob. *amber*, v. כֵּיפָה). Erub. 96[b]; Keth. 81[b] כ׳ תלא לה has he jewelry suspended on it (his opinion)?, i. e. must his opinion absolutely be accepted?—B. Bath. 52[a], B. Mets. 35[a] אפקיד כ׳ וכ׳ gave jewelry in trust &c. Ib. הב לי כֵּיפַי (Ms. M. כֵּיפַאי) give me my jewelry back; a. e.—3) also כֵּפָא (cmp. כֵּף, גִּיף &c.) *shore, border*. Targ. Jud. VII, 12. Targ. Is. XIX, 7 כְּכֵיפֵיה (ed. Lag. כְּכֵפֵיה; ed. Wil. בכיפי, corr. acc.) like its shore.—Pes. 4[a], v. אֶסְיָסָא. Ned. 40[a] bot. נהרא מִכֵּיפֵיה וכ׳ the Euphrates grows from (the waters coming down) its shores (not from rain); Sabb. 65[b]; Bekh. 55[b]. Koh. R. to XI, 1 הוה מיטמר בכיף ימא (some ed. בְּכֵף) was hiding himself at the sea-shore; a. e.—*Pl.* as ab. Targ. Is. VIII, 7 כֵּיפוֹהִי; Targ. Josh. III, 15 (some ed. כֵּפּוֹהִי).—Sabb. 65[b] מִכֵּיפֵי some ed. (v. supra).—M. Kat. l. c. נשוק כ׳ אהדדי .... the shores of .... touched each other (the waters rising to the level of the shores; Rashi: *the arches* of the ruined bridges, v. infra).—4) *arch, vault*, v. כִּיפְּתָא.—5) *cap*, v. כִּיפָּה.—6) *bundle, sheaf*, v. כֵּפָא. [כיפא, Tosef. Mikv. IV, 5, v. כִּיפָּה, end.]

כֵּיפָא II m. *pressure, necessity*, v. כְּרִיפָא.

כֵּפָה, כֵּיפָה f. (v. כֵּיף) 1) *ball, stone.* Ohol. VIII, 5 כֵּיפַת הברד hail-stone.—2) *resin* (or something similar) *found in balls.* Tosef. Dem. I, 29 כֵּפַת המרחץ ed. Zuck. (Var. כפת, emend. by El. Wil. קופה) resin used (with oil) in the bath-room.—כֵּיפַת הירדן *Jordan-resin, amber* (an adapt. of Eridanus, v. Sm. Ant. s. v. Electrum, Lübker's Reallex. s. v. Electron). Kerith. 6[a] (one of the ingredients of frankincense).—3) *ball, lump.* Y. Sabb. V, 7[b] bot. (in Chald. dict.), v. גְּבִינְתָּא.

כִּיפָה f. = כְּפִיפָה, *bending.* Y. Succ. III, 54[a] top (in mixed dict.) כ׳ קומוי (not קומי) bending is due before Him; Y. Meg. I, 72[a] top כפה קומך (corr. acc.).

כִּפָּה, כִּיפָּה f. (b. h.; כָּפַף) 1) *arch, doorway, bow.* Yeb. 80[b] עושה כ׳ forms a bow (when urinating). Yoma 11[b]; Erub. 11[b] כ׳ ר״מ וכ׳ as to an arched doorway R. M. says, it requires a M'zuzah. Tosef. ib. VII (V), 2 עד מקום הכי׳ (ed. Zuck. הקופא) to the site of the (now ruined) arch (of Tiberias); Y. ib. V, 22[d] bot. עד הכ׳. Y. Naz. VII, 56[a] top הגיעו לכ׳ when they arrived at the arch (or arcade). Ab. Zar. I, 7 (16[a]) כ׳ שמעמידין וכ׳ the arched chamber in the bath where they put up idolatrous statues. Pesik. R. s. 41 כ׳ של חשבונות .... אותה כ׳ an arcade named Arch of Accounts (a sort of Exchange) existed outside of Jerusalem, and they used to go out and settle their accounts under this arcade &c. Tanh. B'shall. 17 (ref. to קפאו, Ex. XV, 8) כמין כפה (Mekh. ib., Shir. s. 6 קיפה) like a vault; a. e.— Esp. כִּיפַּת הרקיע, or כִּיפָּה *the heavenly arch, sky* (believed to be a solid mass). Gen. R. s. 48, beg. Ib. s. 4 הרקיע ... ולמעלה .. כ׳ וכ׳ the firmament is like a lake, and above the lake is the arch, and owing to the heat of the lake the arch exudes drops &c. B. Bath. 25[b] אחורי כ׳ back of (above) the sky. Meg. 11[a] ג׳ מלכו תחת הכ׳ Ms. M. 2 (ed. בכ׳, Ms. M. 1 בקופה) three persons ruled over the whole world; a. e.—2) *a vaulted chamber, prison.* Snh. IX, 3 כונסין אותן לכ׳ they put them in prison (for life). Ib. 5.—3) *skull-cap, cap.* Y. Gitt. IV, 45[d] bot.; Bab. ib. 20[a]; v. אנדכתרי; Treat. 'Abadim ch. III (ed. Kirchh.) קיפה. Sabb. 57[b] כ׳ של צמר a woolen cap, v. כָּבוּל II. Y. ib. V, end, 7[c] כ׳ של צמר a woolen cap on the head of a lamb, v. חָנוּן I; a. e.—Tosef. Mikv. IV, 5, v. infra.—4) (cmp. קוּפָּה) *heap, pile.* Y. Snh. X, 27[d] bot.; Y. M. Kat. III, 83[c] top כ׳ של אבנים a heap of stones; Gen. R. s. 100 כִּיפַּת אבנים. Hull. 129[a] כִּיפַּת שאור וכ׳ a heap (lump) of leavened dough which one intended to use as a block to sit on; Pes. 45[b] כורית some ed. (corr. acc.; Ms. M. 2 כר׳; v. Rabb. D. S. a. l. note 90); v. כִּיפְּתָא.—*Pl.* כִּפִּים, כִּיפִּין (or כִּיפִּ׳ fr. כִּיף) a) *top-branches (arches) of palm-trees.* Tosef. Shebi., VII, 16 על (של) בין הכיפ׳ ed. Zuck. (Var. שבכופין, על מה שבכר׳); Pes. 53[a] כל של בין הכ׳ as long as there are fruits in the tops. Tosef. Kel. B. Bath. II, 1 שכיפה שתי כ׳ של תמרה וכ׳ (R. S. to Kel. XXII, 9 כופית) who tied together two palm branches and sat upon them. Sabb. XXIV, 2 מפספסין את הכ׳ you may spread the bunches of branches (for fodder), contrad. to זִירִין a. פְּקִיעִין. Ib. 155[a] כ׳ תלתא bunches are called *kippin* when tied with three bands.—b) *billow-crests, surf.* Sot. 34[a]. Hag. 19[a]; Hull. 31[b] אין מטבילין בכ׳ you must not immerse vessels in the surf (caps of waves), contrad. to ראשין; Tosef. Mikv. IV, 5 בכיפא ed. Zuck. (oth. ed. בכיפה).

כִּיפּוּר, v. כִּפּוּר.

כִּיפֵּחַ (כִּיפֵּיחַ), קִיפֵּ׳, קְפֵּ׳ m. (כּוּפַּח, קִפֵּחַ, כָּפַח, v. כּוּפַּח) 1) (sub. שוקים) *one having high and arched shoulders, hump-backed.* Y. Keth. VII, end, 31[d] עובדא .... בכ׳ (not בכופיח) a case (petition for divorce) came before R. J. against a husband who had become hump-backed (after marriage), and he forced him (to a divorce).—2) (v. גִּבֵּחַ, גִּיבֵּחַ) *an extremely tall and unshapely person.* Bekh. VII, 6 (45[b]) כ׳ Ar. (ed. קפ׳), v. גִּבֵּחַ. Y. Ber. IX, 13[b] bot. כ׳; Bab. ib. 58[b] קפח ed. (Ms. M. קי׳; Ms. F. כופח, corr. acc.); Tosef. ib. VII (VI), 3 כ׳ (Var. קפח, כִּיפִּיחַ); Tanh. Pinh. 10; ed. Bub. 1 ק׳. V. הַדְרָנִיקוֹס.

בֵּי כ׳, כִּיפֵּי pr. n. pl. *Be-Khefé* in Babylonia. Ber. 31[a] (Ms. M. קופאר, v. Rabb. D. S. a. l. note).

כִּיפְלָא, כּוּפְלָא, כְּפֵ׳ m. (כָּפַל) *duplication*; בכ׳ *double.* Targ. Y. II Gen. XLIII, 12. Targ. Job XLII, 10; a. fr.—Y. Pes. 30[d] bot. [read:] וקנסיה בכיפלה and he fined him double the amount. Y. Peah VII, 20[b] top בכפ׳ הוות מעביד it would have yielded twice the quantity. Gen. R. s. 91 יהבון לי בכ׳ give me double the amount. Lam. R. to I, 5 אוכלוסין בכ׳ twice as many troops; a. e.—V. כְּפֵילָא.

כִּיפְלָה, v. preced.

כִּיפְלִיסִין, Y. Peah VII, 20[a] top דיעבי׳ ד׳ כ׳, read: דיעביד כְּלוּפְסִין.

כִּיפַּר pr. n. m. *Kippar.* Gitt. 14[b]; Y. ib. I, end, 43[d]; Y. Kidd. III, 64[a] ר׳ יוסי (בר) בן כ׳; Tosef. Shebi. II, 5; a. fr.

כִּיפְרָא, v. כּוּפְרָה.

כִּיפֵּשׁ, v. כּוּפֵּשׁ.

כִּיפַּת, constr. of כִּיפָּה; כֵּיפַּת, constr. of כֵּיפָּה.—[Tosef. Ohol. XII, 2, a. e. כיפת ed. Zuck., v. כּוּפֶּת].

כִּיפָא, כֵּיפָא, כִּיפְּתָא f. ch.=h. כִּיפָּה 1) *vault, vaulted chamber; arcade.* Y. Snh. VII, 25[d] top חפשיתון כיפ׳ the vaulted chamber (in the bath) seized them (kept them spell-bound). Y. Naz. VII, 56[a] top כ׳ דקסרין the arcade of the gate of Caesarea (considered unclean); Y. Ber. III, 6[a] כִּפְּתָה דק׳.—*Pl.* כִּיפִּין. Targ. II Esth. I, 5, v. כְּפַּת.—2) *bow, curve.* Targ. Job XLI, 12 דעביד כיפא which forms a bow (in boiling over; h. text ואגמן); cmp. כִּיפָּה beg.

כִּפְתָא, כִּיפְתָא f. (כְּפַת) 1) *stocks,* an instrument of torture in the shape of a wooden *collar.* Targ. Jer. XX, 2, sq.; ib. XXIX, 26 (h. text מהפכת, which Rashi explains by כיפה).—2) (v. כְּפִיפָה) *muzzle* with fodder basket. Snh. 98[b] בטולא דכי׳ דחמריה Ms. M. (ed. דכופיתא, v. כַּפִּיתָא) in the shadow of the basket of the Messiah's ass.—*Pl.* כִּיפָּתָא, כְּפִ׳. Midr. Sam. ch. XXI (expl. ירומו, Ps. CXL, 9, v. זָמַם) רומם כְּפָּתוֹר (some ed. כְּפָּתוֹר) lift high his muzzle (strengthen his enemies); Lev. R. s. 21; Yalk. Sam. 126 חזק כתפיו (corr. acc.) tighten his muzzle.—[Y. Shebi. IV, end, 35[c] כִּיפָּתָא, v. כֵּיפָא I.]

כֵּיצַד (contr. of כֵּאֵי זֶה צַד, v. כֵּי) *how?, in what manner?, in what respect?* B. Kam. II, 1 כ׳ הרגל וכ׳ in what respect is the foot of an animal a constant danger (no fore-warning being required to make the owner responsible)? Ib. V, 4 כ׳ משלם וכ׳ how is the value of the embryo assessed? Zeb. V, 3 כ׳ in what manner (is the sprinkling performed)?—B. Mets. III, 12; a. v. fr.—Tosef. B. Kam. IX, 2, a. fr. ed. Zuck. כֵּיזְצַד.—Num. R. s. 4 הא כְּאֵר צַד וכ׳ (some ed. כיצד) how now &c.?

כִּיר (כִּיד) כִּיר, *Pi.* כִּיֵּיר (כִּיֵּיד) (denom. of כִּירָה II or of כַּד II) [*to do the work of the stove-setter* or *of the potter* (כַּיָּיר or כַּיָּיד, v. בִּרְכַּיָּיר),] *to cement; to lay out with tiles, panels* &c. [Ar. reads ר, editions mostly ד.] B. Kam. 51[a] bot. אחד ... וסייד וכ׳ (Ms. F. וסייר וכייר) if one dug a pit ten handbreadths deep, and another came and lined it with plaster and cemented it; Mekh. Mishp., N'zik., s. 11. Ab. Zar. III, 7 (47[b]) סיידו וכִיְּירוּ לאליל Mish. (Bab. ed. וכיידו לע״ז) he plastered the room and put tiles on (v. Sm. Ant. s. v. Abacus) designing it for idolatrous purposes. Ib. סיידה וכִיְּירָהּ וכ׳ (Ms. M. וציירה) if one plastered and stuccoed a stone (slab) for an idolatrous purpose. Gen. R. s. 28 סיידה וכיירה וציירה he plastered and panelled and painted the wedding chamber; Lam. R. to IV, 11 וכיידה. Tosef. Sot. VIII, 7 כִּיְּירוּהוּ וסיידוהו וכ׳ (Var. כִּיְּירוּהָ, כִּיְּדוּהָ) they panelled the stone and stuccoed it and wrote upon it. B. Bath. 60[b] אין מסיידין ואין מְכַיְּירִין וכ׳ we must not decorate our rooms with plaster, panels and paintings in these days (after the destruction of the Temple); Tosef. ib. II, 17.—Part. pass. מְכוּיָּיר, f. מְכוּיֶּירֶת. Ib.

כירבי, Y. Kil. I, 27[a] bot. כ׳ לבנון, read: כְּרִיסוֹלָכְנוֹן.

כִּירָה, כֵּרָה f. (b. h.; כרר) *a circle,* esp. *banquet.* B. Bath. 75[a] (expl. יכרו Job XL, 30, with ref. to II Kings VI, 23) אין כ׳ אלא סעודה *kerah* means banquet.

כִּירָה I f. (כָּרָה) 1) *digging, making a pit.* Mekh. Mishp., N'zik., s. 11 (prob. to be read: כְּרִיָּה).—2) [*selecting,*] *buying, sale.* R. Hash. 26[a] הוו קירין למכירה כ׳ (in the sea-towns) I heard them call a sale *kirah* (which accounts for כריתי, Gen. L, 5); Sot. 13[a].

כִּירָה II f. (b. h. כִּירַיִם; cmp. כּוּר II) *a portable stove on feet,* with caves for two pots, v. כּוּפָּה. Sabb. 38[b]. Ib. III, 1. Ib. 138[b], v. יָרֵךְ. Kel. VI, 1 העושה שתי ... כ׳ if one improvises a stove by means of two stones; Tosef. ib. B. Kam. V, 3 כרה ed. Zuck. (R. S. to Kel. VI, 4 כירה). Kel. VI, 2 כִּירַת המבחים the butchers' stove (improvised with several stones). Y. Bets. II, 61[c] top בשעה שכִּירָתְךָ סתומה at a time when thine own (private) stove is closed (when you are not permitted to cook), opp. כירת רבך thy Master's stove (the altar); Bab. ib. 20[b]; Tosef. Hag. II, 10; a. fr.—*Pl.* כִּירִים. Kel. VI, 3 שתי כ׳ two fire-places.—Dual form: כִּירַיִם, כִּירַיִים. Sabb. III, 2. B. Mets. VIII, 7. Sifra Sh'mini Mill. לא ... אלא מן הכ׳ they brought the fire in from the (private) stove; Lev. R. s. 20; Tanh. Aharé 6; ed. Bub. 7 מבית (ה)כ׳ from the kitchen. Ab. d'R. N. ch. XII כ׳ זה טמא (Var. כ׳ זו טמאה; v. II Vers., ed. Schechter, ch. XXVIII) this stove is unclean.

כִּירְווּתָא, כִּירָוֹן, v. כִּרְיָא.

כִּירוֹמָנִיקְיָא m. pl. (χειρομάνικα=μανίκια, S.) [*tight sleeves,*] *handcuffs, manacles* (cmp. Lat. manicae). Targ. II Chr. XXXVI, 6 (a gloss to שושלון דנחשא). Ib. XXXIII, 11 כירומנק׳ ed. Lag. (h. text חחים);—Y. Snh. X, 28[c] bot.; Ruth. R. to II, 14 כירומניקאה; Pesik. Shub. p. 162[a] כרדי ומנקייה (corr. acc.). Cant. R. to IV, 8 (ref. to זקים, Is. XLV, 14) קרקומניקיא, Bxt. כרקומ׳ (corr. acc.).

כִּירְחָא, v. כְּרַחְנָא.

כִּירִי (χαῖρε, imper. of χαίρω) *hail!* Gen. R. s. 89 (play on כר, Is. XXX, 23) (when thy cattle has pasture) כ׳ כ׳ מרובה בעולם Ar. 'hail! hail!' is largely heard in the world (good-will prevails); [ed. כ׳ עבד קירי אדון; 'Rashi': כ׳ קירי מרובה בעולם (χαῖρε κύριε, hail, O Lord &c.), misinterpreting: כ׳ עבד קירי אדון (v. next w.), which gloss came into the text of the ed. in place of the original passage]. Tanh. Mikk. 9 א״ל קירי כ׳ Mus. (ed. ברא; ed. Bub. 11 בדא; corr. acc.), he said to him, hail mylord!

כִּירִי I m. (χείριε, vocat. of χείριος=ὑποχείριος) *in the control of, captive.* Erub. 53[b] (of a Galilean woman who wished to say קירי, κύριε, O Lord) מרי כ׳.—Hull. 139[b] (of doves which uttered a sound like קירי קירי) .... אמרה קירי בירי (corr. acc.) said she, blind one, say rather κύριε χείριε lord slave (an allusion to Herod the Great, v. הֵרְדְּסִיאוֹת).—[Gen. R. s. 89 כ׳ עבד קירי אדון, v. preced. w.

*__כִּירִי II__, כ׳ רָם *Kiri Ram,* an imitation of a musical sound for beating time for dancers. Num. R. s. 4 (expl. מכרכר, II Sam. VI, 14) שהיה מקיש . . . ואומר כ׳ רם he clapped his hands and kalled *kiri ram*.

כִּירִי, Hull. 62[b] Ar., v. כּוֹרָא.

כ׳ דבית סכל ,כִּירְיָא pr. n. pl. *Kiraya near Beth Sekhel*. Targ. Y. I Num. XXXIV, 9 (v. Hildesh. Beitr., p. 46, sq.).

כִּירְיוֹן ,כִּירְיוֹן, v. כְּרִי.

כִּירַיִם, v. כִּירָה II.

***כִּירִים ,כִּירִין** m. pl. *iron tools for crowding olives into the vat* (Maim.; cmp. כְּרִי). Kel. XII, 8 (some ed. כורים, ed. Dehr. כידרים; Ar. כידין, Var. כיד׳, expl. = עֲבִירִים q. v. —R. Hai Gaon quotes a Var. כידון); [Tosef. ib. B. Bath. VII, 12 עתידין, some ed. עמידין, עבירים].

כִּירְכּוּר, v. כִּרְכּוּר.

כִּירְכֵּר ,כִּירְכֵּם, v. sub כִּרְכֵּ׳.

כִּירְצָא, v. כִּרְצָא.

כִּישׁ (cmp. בְּשְׁבֵּשׁ) *kish*, an imitation of a clapping sound. B. Mets. 85[b] (prov.) אסתירא . . . כ׳ כ׳ קריא Ms. H. a. Ar. (ed. קִישׁ) a coin in a bottle cries *kish kish* (clappers, i. e. an ignorant man boasts of what little knowledge he has).

כִּישָׁא m. (כוש or כנש, בנש, cmp. כיס) 1) *bunch*. B. Bath. 146[b] כ׳ דירקא a bunch of vegetables. Kidd. 45[b]. Hull. 105[b] כ׳ דאסר וכ׳ out of a bunch which the gardener has tied. Sabb. 140[b] כ׳ כ׳ כ׳ (Ms. M. ב׳, incorr.) a bunch is a bunch, v. אִירְכָּא. Ib. כִּישְׁתָּא fem. (Ms. M. בישא, corr. acc.; Ar. הוצא).—*2) *a pouch* (of a garment).—*Pl.* כִּישֵׁי. Ib. 147[a] Ar. (Ms. M. כושי), v. כִּיסָא a. מְרֻזֵּב.—[Ib. 108[b], v. כְּשׁוּרָא.]

כִּשּׁ׳ ,כִּישׁוּף m. (כָּשַׁף) *sorcery, witchcraft*. Snh. 56[b] אף על הכ׳ the prohibition of sorcery is also included in the Noachidic laws (v. נֹחַ). Ib. פרשת כ׳ (Ms. M. a. Rashi מכשף) the passage referring to sorcery (Deut. XVIII, 10. sq.). Pesik. R. s. 14 לא כ׳ ולא כשפים וכ׳ I applied neither sorcery nor witchcraft; a. e.

כִּישׁוּת, v. כְּשׁוּת.

כִּישְׁרָא, v. כְּשׁוּרָא.

כִּשּׁ׳ ,כִּישְׁרוֹן m. (b. h. כִּשְׁרוֹן; כָּשֵׁר) *virtue, fitness*. Num. R. s. 3 (ref. to בכושרות, Ps. LXVIII, 7) בכ׳ אין כתיב כאן וכ׳ it is not written here 'in fitness' but *bakkosharoth*, that means through the merits of noble and worthy women.

כִּישְׁתָּא, v. כִּישָׁא.

כִּיתָּא I m. (כתת) *beating* (*of flax*). Sabb. 140[b], v. כִּיתּוּנִיתָא.

כִּיתָּא II *band*, v. כִּתָּא.

כִּיתָּה f. same, v. כַּת.

כִּת׳ ,כִּיתּוּנָא m. ch. (v. כִּיתָּן) =h. כְּתֹנֶת, *linen coat*, in gen. *undergarment, shirt*. Targ. O. Gen. XXXVII, 3; a. fr.—R. Hash. 27[b] דהפכיה ככ׳ that he turned it like a shirt (the inside outside). Ned. 55[b] כ׳ דצלא a leather coat (v. אִיסְקוֹרְטְיָא). Hull. 46[a], v. וְרַד; a. e.—*Pl.* כִּיתּוּנַיָּא, כִּיתּוּנִין, כִּת׳. Targ. Ex. XXVIII, 40. Targ. Is. III, 22; a. fr.

כִּיתּוּנִיתָא f. (diminut. of preced.) *fine linen shirt*. Sabb. 140[b] דזבן כ׳ וכ׳ he who wishes to buy &c. Ib. מאי כ׳ כיתנא נאה Ms. O. (not כיתניתא) what is a *k.*?—Fine flax; ed. כיתא נאה 'fine beating', v. כִּיתָּא I.—*Pl.* כִּיתּוּנְיָיתָא. Ib.[a] bot. Ms. M. (ed. כִּיתְּנִיתָא q. v.).

כִּיתּוּנָתָא, v. כִּיתְּנִיתָא.

כִּיתִּים ,כִּיתּוֹת, v. כַּת.

כִּיתְמָא, v. כִּתְמָא.

כִּת׳ ,כִּיתָּנָא (כִּיתְנָא ,כִּיתָּן) כִּיתָּן m. (כתן, cmp. כתת, a. כּוּתְנָא) [*beaten*,] *flax*. Targ. Deut. XXII, 11. Targ. Ex. IX, 31; a. fr.—Y. Snh. X, 29[a] bot. (in Hebr. dict.) זרעו חטים וכ׳ sow wheat and flax. Yoma 71[b] מאי . . . כ׳ הוא what proof is there that *shesh* means flax?; ib. כ׳ אגב לקויהיה וכ׳ flax splits into branches only when beaten (while it grows in plain stalks); Zeb. 18[b]. B. Mets. 29[b] bot. כ׳ רומיתא (fem.; Ar. a. M. R. רומאה) Roman (fine and expensive) linen; Hull. 84[b]. Ib. 51[b] כ׳ דעביד בטוני flax-stalks in bundles. Ib. כ׳ דדייק וכ׳ flax which has been pounded &c., v. נְפַץ. Y. Sabb. II, beg. 4[c] (expl. ירוקה) כ׳ דמיי 'water-flax' (a sort of lichen); a. fr.—*Pl.* כִּיתְּנַיָּא. Ib. VII, 10[a] bot. ההן כ׳ (insert דעבד) he who works in flax-stalks &c., v. אֲפַסְטִיתָה.

כִּיתְנַאי, Y. Peah I, 16[a], v. כּוּתְנַאי.

כִּית׳ ,כִּיתְּנִיתָא f. collect. noun (preced. wds.) *washed linen clothes, underwear*. Sabb. 140[a] בסכוסי כ׳ ed. (Or Zar. Sabb.,' end כיתונא, R. H. quot. ib. כִּתְּנָאתָא *pl.*, Ms. M. כִּיתוּנְיָיתָא, pl. of כִּיתּוּנִיתָא; Alf. a. Ash. כִּיתּוּנְתָּא ,כִּתּוּ׳) to rub the starch out of linen underwear; לרכוכי כ׳ וכ׳ he intends only to soften the linen &c. Ib. bot. האי כ׳ וכ׳ (Or Zer. l. c. a. Ash. כיתונא, v. Rabb. D. S. a. l. for Var. lect.). Y. Snh. II, 20[c] bot. אותניתיה read: כִּיתְּנִיתֵיה (= חלוקא דכיתנא ib.) his linen garments.

כִּיתְרָא, v. כֶּתֶר II.

כָּךְ (b. h. כָּכָה) *thus, so*. Ab. IV, 5 וכך היה הלל וכ׳ and even so (in the same sense) did Hillel say. B. Kam. 61[a] כך מקובלני וכ׳ such is my tradition from &c. Tosef. Keth. V, 9 כך תתנו וכ׳ even so much (and no more) may you have wherewith to endow your daughters; Bab. ib. 66[b]; ib. 65[a] כך תפסקו; Y. ib. V, end, 30[c] כָּכָה; a. fr.—כך וכך *so and so many, a certain number, date* &c. R. Hash. 18[b] בשנת כך וכך ליוחנן וכ׳ in the year—of John &c.; a. fr.—אחר כך, v. אַחַר.—לְכָךְ (cmp. b. h. לָכֵן) *for such a purpose, therefore*. Ab. II, 8, v. יָצַר. Num. R. s. 4, beg. ל׳ דקדק וכ׳ therefore be exact in recording the numbers &c.; a. fr.—V. חִילְּכָךְ, לְפִיכָךְ.

כַּבָּא m. (collect. noun), *pl.* כַּבֵּי (אכך or חכך, dropped guttural; cmp. אַכְּבָא) *molars*, in gen. *teeth*. Targ. Jud. XV, 19 ed. Lag., a. Kimḥi Var. (ed. כֵּיפָא, h. text מכתש). Targ. Y. Num. XXI, 35 כַּבֵּיה ושיניה his molars and his (front) teeth. Ib. XI, 33; a. fr.—Pes. 113ᵃ לא תעקר כ׳ never have a molar tooth extracted. Gitt. 69ᵃ לכ׳ for pain of the molars. B. Kam. 92ᵇ (prov.) שיתין . . . לכ׳ דקל וכ׳ sixty pains befall the teeth of him who hears his neighbor's sounds (at meals) and is himself not permitted to eat (not being invited). Ab. Zar. 28ᵃ; a. e.—כ׳ דאקלידא, v. אַקְלִידָא. —B. Bath. 167ᵃ כַּבֵּיה דבי״ת Ar., Ms. H. (Ms. M. בבי, v. Rabb. D. S. a. l. note; ed. פֵּיה דבי״ת וכרעיה) the teeth, the upper and the lower horizontal lines of the letter Beth.—[כַּבֵּי *cakes*, v. כַּבְּבָא.]

כְּבָּבָא, כְּבָב, v. sub כּוֹכ׳.

ככדיתא, v. כַּבְּרִיתָא.

כָּבָה, v. כָּךְ.

כָּבֵי, כְּבָרִי f. (=כּוֹכֵי, √כו, cmp. כַּוָּא) [*small apertures, meshes*,] *spiderweb*; trnsf. *the web-like marrow of reeds*. Ohol. XIII, 5 כ׳ שיש בה ממש substantial spiderweb; [oth. opin.:] substantial reed marrow. Kel. XVII, 17 עד שיוציא את כל הכ׳ (Var. כבאר, read כִּבָּאר) until he has taken out the entire marrow; Tosef. ib. B. Mets. VII, 12 כ׳ quoted by R. s. to Kel. l. c. (ed. זָבָר).

***כַּכְלָא** m. (κόχλος) *purple-fish* (murex); trnsf. *purple*, esp. *the purple stripe on the tunica, a badge of nobility*. Y'lamd. to Gen. XXV, 23; 25, quot. in Ar., corresp. to ציצית on the Jewish garment.

***כַּכְלָן**, m. (preced.) *purple cloak*. Targ. O. Gen. XXV, 25 ed. Berl. (oth. ed. כַּגְלִים, codices כַּגְלַם, v. Berl. Targ. O. II, p. 9); Targ. Y. II ib. כְּבָלֵן (corr. acc., or כַּכְלָן).

ככר, Targ. Prov. XVII, 25 מככור Ms., v. כְּבַד *Af*.

כִּכָּר c. (b. h.; =כרכר, v. כִּרְכֵּר) [*circle*,] 1) *district*. Gen. R. s. 41 כל ערי הכ׳ all the towns of the (Jordan) district.—2) *loaf*. Erub. VIII, 2; Kel. XVII, 11 מכ׳ בפונדיון וכ׳ bread for two meals consists of a loaf bought for a *dupondium* when four S'ah of wheat are worth one Sela; ib. משתי ידות לכ׳ וכ׳ of two thirds of a loaf three of which represent a Kab of grain. Sifré Deut. 40 כ׳ ומקל ירדו וכ׳ bread and stick (reward and punishment) came down from heaven tied together; a. v. fr.—*Pl.* כִּכָּרִים, כִּכָּרוֹת. Toh. V, 6 שני כ׳. Ber. 39ᵇ שתי כ׳; a. fr.—3) *Kikkar*, a weight of silver or gold, *talent* (=3000 Shekel, v. Zuckerm. Talm. Münz. p. 7). Ab. Zar. 44ᵃ שוה כִּכַּר זהב worth a gold talent; a. fr.—*Pl.* כִּכָּרִים, constr. כִּכְּרֵי. Y. Shek. VI, 50ᵇ top.

כַּכְּרָא, כַּ׳ ch. same, 1) *talent*. Targ. O. Ex. XXV, 39; a. e.—*Pl.* כַּכְּרֵי, כַּכְּרִין, כַּ׳. Ib. XXXVIII, 27; a. e.—Bekh. 5ᵃ כללי קחשיב בכ׳ וכ׳ large round sums the Bible counts by Kikkars, units of Kikkars it does not (but counts by Shekels).—2) *ball*.—*Pl.* as ab. B. Mets. 86ᵃ, v. כּוּבָּא.

***כַּכְּרִיתָא** f. (preced.) [*loaf*,] *honey-comb*. Targ. Prov. V, 3 ed. Lag. (Ar. a. Lev. ככדיתא, v. Koh. Ar. Compl. II, p. 221); a. e., v. כַּבְרִיתָא I.

ככרתו, Y. Succ. II, 52ᵈ bot., v. כְּוֶרֶת.

כֹּל, constr. כָּל (b. h.; כָּלַל) *all, every one*. Sot. 5ᵃ הקב״ה הניח כל הרים וכ׳ the Lord passed over all mountains and hills and caused his Presence to rest on Sinai. Ib. (ref. to Job XXIV, 24) ככל כאברהם . . . בַּכֹּל מִכֹּל כֹּל like Abraham, Isaac and Jacob of whom is written 'with everything' &c. (Gen. XXIV, 1; XXVII, 33; XXXIII, 11).—Ḥull. I, 1 הַכֹּל שוחטין וכ׳ all persons are competent to slaughter &c.; וכוּלָּן וכ׳ but all those (mentioned as unfit), if they &c. Ib. 2 ובכֹל שוחטין וכ׳ and you may slaughter with any cutting tool except &c. Tem. I, 1; a. v. fr.—דברי הכל the words of all, (*it is*) *the unanimous opinion, all agree*. Bets. 9ᵃ ד׳ ה׳ מותר all agree that it is permitted; a. fr.—אין . . . כל עיקר *not at all*. Y. Dem. I, 21ᵈ אינו מפריש כל עיקר he does not set aside at all; a. fr.—Y. Shebi. VIII, beg. 37ᵈ, a. e. לא הכל ממנו it is not in his power to do so, v. חֵימָה.—כָּל העולם כולו the whole world. Ber. 17ᵇ; a. fr.—כל, כל ה־ ש־ *whosoever, whatsoever*. Gitt. 11ᵇ כל האומר תנו וכ׳ whoever says, 'Give you' (a letter of emancipation &c.), is considered as having said, Take possession (in behalf of the person concerned). Kidd. 43ᵇ כל שאין יכולה וכ׳ whatever woman is incapable of guarding her letter of divorce, is incapable of being divorced. Ḥag. 4ᵇ, v. יֵשׁ; a. v. fr.—כָּל שֶׁהוּא whatever it be, i. e. *the smallest quantity*. Macc. 17ᵃ, a. e. כ׳ ש׳ למכות for punishment with lashes, the partaking of any quantity is sufficient, opp. כזית, v. זַיִת. Shebu. III, 1 ואכל כ׳ ש׳ and ate the least thing; a. v. fr.—כָּל שֶׁכֵּן (abbr. כ״ש) there is every reason that it is even so, i. e. *so much the more, a matter of course*. Sabb. 63ᵃ . . . אורך וכ״ש וכ׳ there is length of life promised and, as a matter of course, wealth and honor; a. fr.—לא כ״ש, v. הַשְׁתָּא.

כָּל, כֹּלָא ch., v. כּוֹל.

כָּלָא, כְּלָא, v. כְּלִי.

כִּלְאָב (b. h.) pr. n. m. *Chileab*, son of David. Tanḥ. Tol'doth 6 כלאב שהיה כולו אב Kilab, he was entirely (like) his father; Y'lamd. to Gen. XXV, 19 כאילו אביו.

כְּלָאָה f. ch.=h. כְּלָיָה, *extinction*. Lam. R., introd. (R. Joh. i) לא תשוון כ׳ גמירא do not exterminate (them) entirely.

כִּלְאֵי m. pl. (כְּלָא I), כ׳ בבא *guard-house at the gate* (cmp. הַרְזִיקֵי). Ned. 91ᵇ איתיב בכ׳ ב׳ he was placed in the guard-house &c. [Ar. s. v. בב: בלאי, ed. Koh. כלאי.]

כִּלְאַיִם m. du. (b. h.; כלא, v. Ges. H. Dict. s. v.) *junction of two*, esp. *Kilayim, the forbidden junction of heterogeneous plants in the same field, of heterogeneous animals by hybridization or by harnessing together, of wool and linen in the same web* (Lev. XIX, 19; Deut. XXII, 9 to 11). Gen. R. s. 82; Y. Ber. VIII, 12ᵇ top האש והכ׳ וכ׳ fire and hybrids (mules) although not having been created in the six days &c. Kil. VIII, 1 כִּלְאֵי הכרם mixed seeds in the vineyard. Ib. I, 1 אינם כ׳ זה בזה are no forbidden junction. Ib. 9 משום כ׳ as coming under the law of K.—Tosef. ib. III, 16 כשות אינו כ׳ *cuscuta* is not forbidden (in the vineyard); Sabb. 139ª; a. v. fr.—*Kilayim*, name of a treatise of the Mishnah and Tosefta, of the Order of Z'raïm.

כִּלְאַמִּין *chlamys*, v. כְּלָמִיס.

כָּלַב (cmp. כָּלַל) *to seize.*—Denom. כָּלֶב.

Pi. כִּלֵּב, *Hif.* הִכְלִיב (denom. of כֶּלֶב) [*to make stitches resembling dog-bites* (cmp. our 'cat-stitching'),] *to stitch*, opp. to תָּפַר to sew in a workmanlike manner. M. Kat. I, 8 (8ᵇ) האומן מְכַלֵּב Ms. M. a. Y. ed. (Mish. a. Babli מַכְלִיב) the professional tailor is permitted (during the festive week) to stitch (but not to sew); expl. ib. 10ª מפסיע he makes wide steps (cross-stitches); (another opin.) שִׁינֵּי כלבתא (Ms. M. only כַּלְבָּתָא q. v.) dog's teeth, i. e. irregular stitches; Y. ib. 80ᵈ bot. מפסיע; (oth. opin.) אחת אחת each stitch singly. Ib. הרוצענין מְכַלְּבִין the saddlers are permitted to do dog-stitching.

כֶּלֶב m. (b. h.; preced.) *dog.* Snh. 63ᵇ (expl. נִבְחַן, II Kings XVII, 31) כ׳ they worshipped a dog. Yoma VIII, 6, a. e. כ׳ שוטה a mad dog. Kil. I, 6, v. כּוֹפְרִי. Kel. XVII, 13 כ׳ המים sea-dog. Gen. R. s. 77, v. אַגְרִיאוֹן. Y. Snh. VII, 23ᶜ top (ref. to Ps. XXII, 21) מִכַּלְבּוֹ של וכ׳ from the dog (the vicious accuser) of that pious man, v. ib. 23ᵇ bot., sq.); a. fr. *Pl.* כְּלָבִים. Ber. 3ª. Tosef. B. Kam. VIII, 17. Ex. R. s. 20 עשו . . כ׳ של וכ׳ the Egyptians made golden dogs by sorcery that they should bark &c.; a. fr.

כַּלְבָּא, כַּלַב, כְּלֵב I ch. same. Targ. Ps. LIX, 7. Targ. Prov. VII, 22 (Ms. כְּלִיבָא; h. text עכס); a. fr.—Y. Ab. Zar. III, 42ᵈ top, expl. נִבְחַן, v. preced.—Erub. 61ª (prov.) כ׳ בלא נתיה וכ׳ a dog away from home barks not for seven years, i. e. however quarrelsome a man may be, he will not fight in a strange place; a. fr.—Trnsf. *a mean person.* Lev. R. s. 9.—*Pl.* כַּלְבֵי, כַּלְבַיָּא, כַּלְבִין. Targ. Ps. XXII, 17. Targ. Is. LVI, 10; a. e.—Y. Peah I, 15ᶜ bot.; Y. Kidd. I, 61ᵇ, v. הדיוֹשׁ ch.—Sabb. 152ª כַּלְבּוֹהִי לא וכ׳ his (euphem. for *my*) dogs no longer bark, i. e. my voice is weak from old age. B. Mets. 94ª top כך וכך כ׳ איכא וכ׳ so and so many dogs have we with us. Pesik. B'shall., p. 86ª תרין כלבי חרשין (not כלבא) two dogs (of gold) made by the sorcerers (v. preced.). Ib., sq. כ׳ דקושטא the real (natural) dogs do not bark at us (ref. to Ex. XI, 7); a. e.—[Targ. Koh. IV, 6 כלב גוזלא, some ed., read כלא ג׳.—Lam. R. to I, 4 כלבא, read: כַּלְבָּה.]

כַּלְבָּא II, pr. n. m. בֶּן כ׳ שְׂבוּעַ *Ben Kalba S'bu'a*, name of a wealthy citizen of Jerusalem. Gitt. 56ª.

כַּלְבָּא III or **כַּלְבָּא**, Var. of אַכְלְבָא. V. Ar. Compl. ed. Koh. IV, 235.

כַּלְבָּה f. (v. כֶּלֶב) 1) *she-dog.* Lam. R. to I, 4 (not כלבא). Y. Snh. VI, 23ᵇ bot. נִזְקָקִין לכ׳ having connection with a dog. Koh. R. to VII, 26.—2) *tongs, pinchers.* Tosef. Kel. B. Mets. III, 11 כ׳ של ספרין וכ׳ the barbers' tongs, the physicians' &c.; v. כַּלְבּוּס.

כלבודא, v. כַּלְבִּיד.

כַּלְבּוּס m. (enlarg. of כלב, v. כַּלְבָּה 2) 1) *tongs, pinchers,* Sot. 19ᵇ כ׳ של ברזל (Alf. ק׳) iron tongs (to force her mouth open; Tosef. ib. II, 3 צבת). Tosef. Kel. B. Mets. III, 11 some ed., v. כַּלְבָּה. Men. 63ª כמין כ׳ עמוק (Ar. כיל׳) a baking form in the shape of forceps with cavities (which clapped together give the dough the shape of an apple &c.).—2) (v. כֶּלֶב) *shape of cross-stitches, zigzag* of nails in the sole. Sabb. 60ᵇ עשאו כמין כ׳ (Ms. M. כלכוס, Alf. ק׳) if he drove the nails in in the shape of &c. Koh. R. to XII, 11 כ׳ הכ׳ אינו וכ׳, v. כַּלֶּבֶת.—[B. Kam. 100ᵇ כ׳, v. כַּלְבּוּס.—Tanh. Balak 13, read: כְּלִינוּס.]

***כַּלְבִיָּא** f. (an assumed word for כַּלְבָּה, after the form of לְבִיָּא) *she-dog, bitch.* Midr. Till. to Ps. XXXIX (in an allegorical contest of the limbs) הא לך חלב כ׳ here is dog-milk for thee, ed. Bub. כלבא; Yalk. Ps. 721 כלבתא (corr. acc.). Ib. הבאת חלב כ׳ (read with Yalk. l. c. כַּלְבָּא; ed. Bub. כלבתא) thou hast brought dog-(instead of lion-) milk. Ib. ועוד ג״כ כי לבריא קורין אותה כ׳ (differ. in Yalk; ed. Bub. ועיד ללבריא . . . כלבתא) and furthermore a lioness may likewise be called a bitch.

כַּלְבִית, v. כִּילְבִית.

כַּלֶּבֶת f. (כָּלַב, v. כַּלְבּוּס) *dog-stitch, the shoemaker's pegging* of the sandal. Y. Snh. X, 28ª כ׳ אינה עולה וכ׳ the *kallebeth* does not count among the number of nails to be driven into shoes; Y. Sabb. VI, 8ª כלי בית (corr. acc., or כִּלְיבִית); Koh. R. to XII, 11 הכלבוס אינו וכ׳.

כַּלְבְּתָא (tradit. pronunc. כַּלְבָתָא) f. ch. = h. כַּלְבָּה, *bitch.* R. Hash. 4ª. Yalk. Ps. 721, v. כַּלְבִיָּא; a. e.—שִׁינֵּי כ׳ (cmp. preced. w.) *dog-stitch.* M. Kat. 10ª, v. כָּלַב.

כַּלְדָּאָה m. ch., *pl.* כַּלְדָּאֵי *Chaldeans, soothsayers.* Sabb. 119ª. Yeb. 21ᵇ; a. e.

כַּלְדִּי m. h. same. *Pl.* כַּלְדִּיִּים. Pes. 113ᵇ אין שואלין בכ׳ (Ar. כַּלְדָּאִין) we must not consult soothsayers.

***כְּלָה** m. (v. עוּכְלָא, אוּכְלָא) *K'lah*, a measure for spices. Y. Bets. III, end, 62ᵇ תן לי כ׳ וכ׳ give me a *k'lah* of spices, for housekeepers are in the habit of putting a *k.* of spices &c. Y. Peah VIII, 20ᵈ bot. כולה תבלין a K. is the ordinary quantity for spices; (Erub. 29ª; R. S. to Peah VIII, 5 עוכלא).

כַּלָּה f. (b. h.; כָּלַל) 1) [*crown, ornament*, v. Is. XLIX, 18,] (sub. בעלת or בת, cmp. בֶּן חוֹרִים a. חוֹרִים ,אִיתוּ) *bride; daughter-in-law.* Yeb. I, 1 וְכַלָּתוֹ and his (deceased) son's wife. Sot. IX, 14 שתצא הכ׳ וכ׳ that the bride on her wedding day may be taken around in procession, v. אַפִּרְיוֹן. Keth. 71ᵇ; Pes. 87ª ככ׳ שנמצאת וכ׳ like a bride (daughter-in-law) found perfect in the house of her father-in-law. Ib. כ׳ בבית אביה a bride in her father's house (not yet taken to her husband's paternal house). Ex. R. s. 41 (play on כִּכַלֹּתוֹ, Ex. XXXI, 18, cmp. כָּלַל *Pa.*) מה כ׳ זו מקושטת וכ׳ as the bride is adorned &c.; a. fr. [Tanh. Ki Thissa 18 כ׳ נופר, read with ed. Bub. ib. 9 כְּלִי נִיגּפּר.]—*Pl.* כַּלּוֹת. Sot. l. c. עטרות כ׳ (Talm. ed. *sing.*) the bridal wreaths. Ib. 49ᵇ; a.

fr.—2) *general assembly*, esp. *Kallah, the assembly of Babylonian students in the months of Elul and Adar*. Ber. 8[b] פרשייתא דכ׳ Ar. (Ms. Paris דְּכַלָּא, v. Rabb. D. S., Vol. I, p. 384; ed. דכולא שתא) the weekly Scripture lessons of the Kallah weeks (during which R. Bibi could not find time to peruse the section of each week). Ib. 6[a], v. הוּתְקָא. Ib. 57[a] ראש לבני כ׳; B. Bath. 22[a] ריש כ׳ the president of the Kallah.—*Pl.* (of כַּלָּא) כַּלֵּי. Hull. 49[a] רישי כ׳.—מסכת כלה, מסכתא דכ׳ a (small) treatise of the Talmud named *Kallah* (from its first word). Sabb. 114[a]; Kidd. 49[b]; Taan. 10[b]; [oth. opin.: a subject which has been discussed in the general assembly].

כָּלָה, v. כלי.

כָּלוֹ, constr. **כְּלוֹ** f. (כְּלִי I, sub. חֵימְתָא) *finishing, venting full wrath*. Targ. Y. Deut. XXIX, 27. Targ. Ps. LIX, 14 בכ׳ (Ms. בכְלוֹ). Targ. Y. II Gen. XXVII, 44 כילתיה (read: כְּלוֹתֵיה). Targ. Y. Deut. XXIX, 22 כְּלֵיתֵיה.

כְּלוּב m. (b. h.; כָּלַב) [*twisted together, united by tenons,*] *shed, coop*. Bets. 24[a] באין לִכְלוּבָן בערב enter their coop in the evening.

כְּלוּב* m. (כָּלַב, cmp. כּוּלָב) *axe*.—*Pl.* כְּלוּבִין. Pesik. Zakh., p. 22[b].

כְּלוּבָא ch. same, v. כּוּלְבָא.

כלודי, Yalk. Gen. 147, v. כְּלִי.

כְּלוּזָא=אוּכְלוּזָא. B. Bath. 8[a] Ms. H. (Ar. s. v. כר 11 quotes כילוזא).

בֵּי כ׳, כְּלוּחִית pr. n. pl. *Be-K'luḥith*. Bets. 5[b] מבי כ׳ (Ms. M. מכ׳). Keth. 40[b].

כלוט, v. כְּלוּט.

כלוכסין, v. כְּלוּפְסִין.

כָּלוּל m. 1)=כְּלִיל; 2) part. pass. of כָּלַל. [Tanh. Bo 5 כ׳ לדברות; Mekh. Bo, beg. כלל לדברות, read: כְּלִי (v. Levy, Catal. of Rabb. Semin. of Breslau 1889, p. 38, note).]

כְּלוּם m. (=כל מ, cmp. מְאוּם) 1) *anything, something, somebody* (Lat. ullus). Targ. Koh. I, 9 לית כ׳ (h. text אין כל).—Yalk. Num. 730 (ref. to Num. X, 35) ואין... מפניך אנו כ׳ לפניהם before thee they flee, and are we nothing before them? אלא כשפניך אתנו אנו כ׳ לפניהם וכשאין פניך אתנו אין אנו כ׳ לפניהם but (it means) when thy countenance is with us we are *something* before them &c.; Sifré Num. 84 (corr. acc.).—Kel. XXIV, 1 טהורה מכ׳ is clean from any (of the aforementioned impurities). Ber. 22[b], a. fr. פטור מכ׳ is entirely exempt. Ned. I, 1, a. fr. לא אמר כ׳ he has said nothing, i. e. what he said is void.—לא כ׳ *not the least, nothing at all*. Erub. 11[a] לא עשה ולא כ׳ (Rashi לא עשה כ׳) he has done nothing at all, i. e. what he has done has no legal consequences. Ib.[b] הכל מודין ... לא כ׳ הוא Ms. M. all agree that if . . . , there is nothing at all (to consider; ed. ולא כ׳=לא כ׳) פטורה ולא כ׳ it is exempt, and there is nothing &c.); Yoma 11[b] לא כ׳ הוא (ולאו) (v. Rabb. D. S. a. l. Ms. M. and note).—Koh. R to IX, 10 כאן הוא דכ׳ ודבר בגרמיה כ׳ וכ׳ if a person i somebody and comports himself as somebody (is proud of his value), it were better he had not been born; a. fr.—2) (interrog.) introducing a question to which a negative answer is expected, *is there any? has any?* &c. Snh 105[a] כ׳ יש לזה על זה כ׳ has the one still any claim on the other? Sabb. 31[a] כ׳ מעמידין וכ׳ is there ever a king appointed except &c.? Ned. VIII, 7 כ׳ אמרת וכ׳ wouldst thou have said it, but for thy wish to honor me?; a. fr.—[Tosef. Men. XIII, 19; Tosef. B. Kam. VII, 8, v. הֲלֹם.]

כְּלוֹמַר (=כְּאִילּוּ אָמַר) *as though one said, that is to say, this means*. Naz. II, 3 (11[a]) לא נתכוונה זו אלא כ׳ וכ׳ (Mish. ed. לומר) she had no intention except that of one who says, 'This be unto me a sacrifice', i. e. she meant only to forbid herself this cup (cmp. ib. כבאן דאמר). Snh. VI, 4 (interpret. כִּי קללת וכ׳, Deut. XXI, 23) כ׳ מפני מה וכ׳ which means as much as, (people will say,) Why has this man been hanged? &c.—Ib. 6 כ׳ שאינו וכ׳ as if saying (intimating), we bear no grudge &c. Ex. R. s. 41 היא מגלה פניה כ׳ וכ׳ she uncovers her face, as if saying &c.; a. v. fr.

כלונוס, Ab. d'R. N. ch. XLIV, ed. Schechter, v. כְּלִינוֹס.

כלונייס, כלוניא, v. לִינְיָא.

כלוניס, Tosef. Kel. B. Mets. IV, 7, v. כְּלִינוֹס.

כְּלוֹנָס m. (a sing. of κελεύοντες, as if κελέονς) *beam of the loom*, in gen. *beam, pole*. Kel. XX, 3 קבעו בכ׳ if he inserted the transverse staff of the loom in the beam; כסא שקבעו בכ׳ if one fixes a chair on the top of a beam; Tosef. ib. B. Mets. XI, 5. Zab. III, 3 על הכ׳ Ar. (ed. האכ׳) was seated on a beam. Tosef. Kel. B. Bath. II, 2 כלינים ed. Zuck. (corr. acc.). Ib. VII, 2 כלונים ed. Zuck. (ed. כלינוס, corr. acc.). [Ab. d'R. N. ch. XXIV, v. כְּלִינוֹס.]—*Pl.* כְּלוֹנָסוֹת, כְּלוֹנְסִיּוֹת, כְּלוֹנָסָאוֹת. B. Bath. 67[b] (expl. בתולות) כ׳ של ארז וכ׳ cedar beams supporting the transverse press beam. R. Hash. II, 3 (22[b]) כלונסא׳ (Ms. M. 2 קְלוֹנָסוֹת). Sifré Num. 160. Tosef. Kel. B. Bath. II, 2; a. e.

כְּלוֹנְסָא ch. same. Targ. I Kings VI, 4; VII, 5 Ar., Rashi a. Kimhi (ed. כְּלִינְסָא, כְּלַנְ׳, Levita Var. קלונסא; h. text שְׁקֻפִים) beam used for arches (v. Sm. Ant. s. v. Camara). Ib. 4.—*Pl.* כְּלוֹנְסַן. Targ. Y. II Num. XXXV, 20 (v. Sifré Num. 160).

כלוסין, v. next w. a. כְּלִיס.

כְּלוּפְסִין, גְּלוּפ׳, קְלוּפ׳, לַבְסִים, לַבְסִין m. pl. (Lesbii; v. גְּלוּסְקָא a. גְּלוּגְרְקָא) *Lesbians*, 1) a species of *figs*. Ned. 50[b] (quoting Maasr. II, 8) היה עושה בכ׳ if one is doing hired labor among Lesbian figs; Maasr. l. c. לבסים; Mish. Y. ed. לבסים; Y. ib. II, 50[a] כלוסין. Ned. l. c. מאי כ׳ what is K.? Answ. מינא דתאיני וכ׳ a species of figs used for cooking purposes. Ib. 49[b] (in Chald. dict.) כלוספרין, read כְּלוּסְפִּירִין (or ...פְּרִין); [Ar. reads בלופסין; Mus. refers to φιβαλέως, a species of *early figs*.]—2) (cmp. גְּלוּסְקָא) a species of *table-olives*, opp. זיתי שמן. Tosef. Ter. IV, 3 קלופסין ed. Zuck. (Var. גלופ׳; Ter. II, 6 זיתי כבש). Ib.

III, 15 ק׳ (Var. קולפ׳, קלפין); Y. ib. I, end, 41ᵃ כלוכסין (read: כלופ׳ or כלוב׳).

כלורכין, v. כלירכין.

כְּלוּתָא, v. כְּלוּ.

כְּלִי, כֶּלִי m. (b. h.; next w.) 1) *vessel, receptacle; bag* &c. B. Bath. 85ᵃ כֵּלָיו של אדם וכ׳ a man's vessel takes possession for him (of its contents). Ber. 23ᵃ כ׳ שהוא כֵלְיָין a receptacle which is intended for them (the T'fillin). Ib. כ׳ בתוך כ׳ one wrapper within the other. Y. Sabb. VII, 10ᵈ top הגודל כְּלִי צורה he who shapes an earthen vessel; הנופח כ׳ זכוכית who shapes a glass vessel by blowing; העושה כ׳ בדפוס who makes a vessel in a mould. Y. Ḥag. III, 79ᵃ top, a. fr. נזקקו לִכְלְיָין they are tied to their vessel, i. e. the vessel in which they are offered makes them to be considered one mass, though they are otherwise disconnected; Ḥag. III, 2 חכ׳ מצרף וכ׳. Mekh. Yithro, Amalek, 2 (ref. to Ex. XVIII, 19) היה להם ככ׳ מלא דברות be unto them like a vessel filled with divine revelations. Ab. d'R. N., II vers., ch. II, v. יָחַד. Mekh. Bo., beg. כלל לדברות; Tanḥ. Bo. 5 כלול לד׳ (read כלי) a vessel of revelation; a. fr.—*Pl.* כֵּלִים, constr. כְּלֵי. Ḥag. III, 1 כ׳ בתוך כ׳ vessels put into larger vessels. Kel. I, 1. Ib. II, 1; a. fr.—2) *outfit, apparel, garment, tool, weapon. Pl.* as ab. Keth. 59ᵇ כ׳ פשתן linen garments. Sabb. 114ᵃ כ׳ לבנים white garments; a. v. fr.—Gen. R. s. 90 (expl. Gen. XLI, 44) כ׳ ידים official badge of the hands (bracelets, rings &c.), כ׳ רגלים greaves &c.; (Ar. a. Rashi כלידו״ם, כלידרין, corrupt. of כלי ידים). Ib. s. 89 שאין עבד ... כ׳ ידים (some ed. כלידים, Ar. כלידרין; Yalk. ib. 147 כלודי׳, corr. acc.) that no servant was to hold office or wear rings &c. (v. Sm. Ant. s. v. Annulus).—כלי זיין, v. זַיִין.—B. Mets. IX, 13 חייב משום שני כ׳ he is guilty of having seized two implements (the upper and the lower millstone). Ib. שני כ׳ two objects of use (a mattress and a plough). B. Bath. V, 2 כֵּלָיו the outfit of the ass (saddle &c.); a. fr.

כָּלָה, כָּלָא, כלי (b. h.; v. כָּלַל) 1) *to enclose; to restrain, keep back.* Midr. Till. to Ps. CXIII לִכְלוֹת את המכה וכ׳ to ward this plague off from thee. Midd. IV, 6 כַּלֵּה עֹרֵב 'keeping off the raven', an arrangement of *iron points* on the roof of the Temple; Sabb. 90ᵃ כולי עורב (*pl.*) Ms. M. (ed. כַּלְיָא ch.; v. Rabb. D. S. a. l. note); Men. 107ᵃ כולי Ms. M. (ed. כַּלְיָה); M. Kat. 9ᵃ כילי Ms. M. (ed. כלייא); Arakh. 6ᵃ כלוה.—Part. pass. כָּלוּי. Y. Naz. II, beg. 51ᵈ כ׳ אני ממנו I will be restrained from it (for 'I will abstain').—2) (cmp. שלם) *to be full, to be finished, to cease.* Ber. 39ᵃ צריך שתִּכְלֶה ברכה וכ׳ the benediction must be finished simultaneously with breaking the bread. Tanḥ. Ki Thissa 5 כבר כָּלוּ ישראל וכ׳ Israel would have ceased to exist; (Pesik. Shek., p. 13ᵇ חיו .. מְכוּלָּין, v. infra). Snh. 97ᵇ כָּלוּ כל הקצין all the predicted terms of redemption are ended (have passed by); a. fr.—[Pesik. R. s. 12 מת וכלה בקבר, read: ובלה.]—Part. (fr. כּוּל, cmp. חול, part. חולות a. חלות) כָּל. Snh. 17ᵃ (ref. to כלאם, Num. XI, 28) חטל ... והן כָּלִין מאליהם throw upon them the care for the public, and they will cease (to prophesy) of themselves; a. fr.

Pi. כִּלָּה 1) *to finish, cease.* Yoma 60ᵇ (ref to Lev. XVI, 20) אם כפר כ׳ when he has atoned (for the sanctuary &c.), he has finished (his task). Ib. אם כ׳ כפר when he has done all (the prescribed ritual), he has achieved atonement; Sifra Aḥăré ch. IV, Par. 4; a. e.—Tanḥ. Vayetse 2 מְכַלִּין את שדותיהן they reap their fields entirely (leaving no corners for the poor). Snh. 67ᵇ כַּלֵּה מִדְּבָרוֹתֶיךָ ולך וכ׳ (some ed. כלך, v. Rab. D. S. a. l. note) cease from thy homiletical interpretations, and turn to &c.; Midr. Till. to Ps. CIV, 6; Ex. R. s. 10, v. כַּלָּךְ.—2) *to finish, destroy.* Y. Shek. VI, 50ᵇ top (ref. to מכלות, II Chr. IV, 21) הן כִּילוּ וכ׳ they (these vessels) consumed all the gold (of the country); Men. 29ᵃ שכִּילָּתוֹ וכ׳ it consumed &c. Pesik. R. s. 2 שכ׳ אותה וכ׳ whom the Lord destroyed. Num. R. s. 3 היה הארון מְכַלֶּה בבני וכ׳ the Ark made havoc among the sons of Kehath (who had charge of it; cmp. II Sam. VI, 7). Mekh. B'shall., Amalek, s. 2 לְכַלָּן to destroy them. Y. Ḥag. II, 78ᵃ bot. (cited in Tosaf. to Ḥag. 17ᵇ a. v. אלא) ובלבד שיְּכַלֶּה עיסתו (ed. שיבלים) provided he has used up all his dough for the day; a. fr.—Part. pass. מְכוּלֶּה, pl. מְכוּלִּין. Pesik. Shek., p. 13ᵇ כבר היו ישראל מ׳ וכ׳ Israel would then have been destroyed; a. e.

Hithpa. הִתְכַּלֶּה, *Nithpa.* נִתְכַּלֶּה *to be destroyed, visited by death.* Num. R. s. 5 היו מִתְכַּלִּין they were diminished. Ib. שלא יִתְכַּלּוּ מן וכ׳ that they may not be destroyed from the world. Ib. s. 3 לא כ׳ וכ׳ not one of them was missing on being counted &c.; a. e.

כְּלָא, כְּלֵי I ch. same, 1) *to keep enclosed, to withhold, restrain.* Targ. I Sam. VI, 10. Targ. Ps. XXI, 3. Targ. Is. XXXIII, 15 כָּלֵי (ed. Wil. כָּל) restrains his eyes. Targ. Prov. XI, 26 כָּאלֵא ed. Lag.; ib. XVII, 28 כָּאלֵי ed. Lag. —Part. pass. כְּלֵי. Targ. Jer. XXXII, 2; (Targ. Ps. LXXXVIII, 9 כְּלִיא, h. form).—Sabb. 57ᵇ כְּלִילָא פריחי v. בִּזְיוֹנָא I; [Var. Ar. כְּלִיָא עִירב, v. בַּאלֵי.]—דידבר, reminiscence fr. Nidd. 17ᵃ, v. preced.—2) *to be finished, gone.* Ber. 39ᵃ כַּלְיָא ברכה the benediction is finished &c., v. preced. B. Mets. 79ᵃ וקא כליא קרנא and the capital itself is used up (v. infra). Yoma 69ᵇ כ׳ עלמא the world would come to an end; a. fr.— 3) (cmp. שלם) [*to be entirely with,*] *to trust.* Targ. Ps. XXXI, 7. Ib. 25 כָּלְיָין (ed. Lag. a. oth. כיילין, corr. acc.). Ib. XXXII, 10; a. e.; v. אֲכַל. [Differ. fr. b. h. כָּלָה *to be consumed* by anxiety, *to long, die for.*]

Af. אַכְלֵי *to lock up, restrain.* Targ. II Chr. VII, 13.— Kidd. 81ᵇ מַכְלֵי לְהוּ בִּכְלִּיתָה וכ׳ Ar. a. Tosaf. (ed. מכלליה, read: מכלי ליה) kept the cattle off from the entire field (in which he walked); (ed.: kept himself aloof from the entire pasture ground). B. Bath. 5ᵃ, v. next w.

Pa. כַּלֵּי *to destroy, use up, diminish.* B. Mets. l. c. מְכַלִּינַן קרנא (when hiring the usufruct of an object,) we are permitted to use up the stock itself, e. g. if you hired an ass for travelling, and it died on the road, you may sell its carcass, and hire another ass for the money; ib. לא מכ׳ קרנא we must not use up the stock, i. e. you may *buy* another ass for the carcass, but not hire one. Ib. Ms. M. לְכַלּוּיֵי קרנא לא חיישינן (v. Rabb. D. S. a. l. note 8) and as for using up the stock, we need not take that into consideration. B. Kam. 3ᵃ דמְכַלְיָא קרנא when the obnoxious subject destroys the object itself (not only the fruits).

Ithpe. אִתְכְּלֵי *to be closed up, withheld; to refrain.* Targ. O. Gen. VIII, 2. Targ. Prov. III, 27; a. fr.

כְּלָא, כְּלִי II, *Af.* אַכְלִי (v. preced.) [*to assemble, call together* (cmp. אוֹכְלוֹסָא),] 1) *to call, give a signal.* Targ. Jer. I, 15. Targ. Zeph. II, 15; a. e.—2) (of the lion) *to roar; to shout, thunder* &c. Targ. Ps. CIV, 21, v. אַכְלִי. Ib. XXIX, 3. Ib. LXXIV, 4; a. e.—B. Bath. 5ª עיזא בעלמא לאו לאכלויי מַכְלִינַן בה v. Ar. s. v. כל; (incorr. in eds. בעיא) as to a goat, we need only shout at her (to drive her off). Ib. ולאו גברא בעי לאכלויי Rashi (ed. דמיכלי, read דמַכְלֵי) and need you not a man to shout at her?; [oth. opin. we need only *keep* her *off*, v. preced.]

כִּלְיָא, v. כִּלְיָה.

כַּלְּיָא, v. כַּלָּיִיה.

כְּלָיָא, v. כְּלִי I.

כְּלִיבָא, v. next w.

כְּלִיבָה f. (v. כְּלוּב) *box, consisting of movable tenoned links.* Tosef. Kel. B. Mets. IX, 1 כ׳ של חייטין the tailors' box.—Pesik. Anokhi, p. 138ª ונתנום בכ׳ and put them (the Cherubs of the Temple) in a box; a. e.—Esp. *coffin* with *bier.* M. Kat. 27ª, sq. ועניים בכ׳ (not בכליכה) and the poor were carried out on a common bier; opp. דרגש; Tosef. Nidd. IX, 16 בִּכְלִיבָא. Par. XII, 9 קרן של כ׳ the movable support of the bier, Maim.; (oth. opin.: the ring for keeping the corpse in position). Lam. R. to III, 16 כליבא.

כְּלִיד, כְּלִידָא m. (χάλις, -ιδος, only in χαλιδοφόρος; κύλιξ, κάλιξ, calix) 1) *cup.* Targ. II Chr. IV, 5. Targ. O. Gen. XLIV, 12, a. e. (Var. ק׳, v. Berl. Targ. O. II, p. 16). Targ. Ps. XI, 6; a. e.—*Pl.* כְּלִידִין. Targ. Jer. XXXV, 5.—2) *calyx* of flowers. *Pl.* as ab. Targ. Ex. XXV, 33, sq. (Ms. I ק׳).

כלידרין, כלידרים, כלידים, כלידו, corrupt. of כלי ידרים, v. כְּלִי.

כִּלְיָה, כּוּלְיָה, ...יָא f. (b. h. כִּלְיָה; כלי, v. כּוּלְיָא) 1) *kidney.* Y. B. Mets. II, beg. 8ᵇ. Hull. 55ª כוליא; a. fr.—*Pl.* כְּלָיוֹת, constr. כִּלְיוֹת. Ib. III, 2. Ber. 61ª, a. e., v. יָעַץ. Tanh. Vayigg. 11, a. e. כִּלְיוֹתָיו, v. כַּד II; a. fr.—2) *the belly* of a stove. B. Bath. II, 11 כליא (Ms. F. a. H. כיליא). Ib. 20ᵇ כ׳ דתנור טפח the protuberance of the belly of the stove is one hand-breadth beyond the rim; Tosef. ib. I, 3 כירלא ed. Zuck. (Var. כּוּלְיָיה, כִּלְיָיה). [R. Hănanel: כירליא=κοιλία.]

כְּלָיָה, v. כְּלָיָיה.

כליונים, Tosef. Kel. B. Bath. VII, 2, v. כְּלוֹנָס.

כְּלִיוּתָא f. (כְּלִי I 3) *cheer, trust.* Targ. Ps. CXIX, 116 Ms. (ed. כְּלִי; h. text שבר).

כַּלָּיִיה, כַּלָּיָא m. pl. (v. כַּלָּה) [*crowns, ornaments,*] *brides.* Y. Ab. Zar. III, 42ᶜ top; Y. Peah I, 15ᵈ.—Targ. Y. Deut. XXIV, 6 חתנין וכַלִּין (h. text רחים ורכב).—[Targ. Y. II Gen. XVIII, 21 כַּלָּיִיה, v. כְּלָיָיה.]

כְּלָיִית, v. כְּלָיָה.

כְּלָיָיה f. (כְּלָה) *destruction, diminution, extinction.* Ab. V, 8 רעב של כ׳ a destructive famine (general miscrop). Y. Ber. II, 5ᶜ bot. Snh. 63ª נתחייבו שונאיהם... כ׳ the enemies of Israel (censorial change רשעיהם, euphem. for *Israel*) would have been condemned to destruction. Gen. R. s. 10 ויכלו ... אין ויכלו לשון כ׳ *vaykhullu* (Gen. II, 1) has the meaning of affliction, of diminution (ref. to the reduction of the planetary courses after Adam's sin). Ib. s. 49 (expl. כלה, Gen. XVIII, 21) הן חייבין כ׳ they deserve extinction; [Targ. Y. II Gen. l. c. כַּלָּיִיה עבדו גמירא, read: עבדו כְּלָיָיה גמירא]. Mekh. B'shall., Shirah, s. 5 גמרת ... כ׳ thou hast passed the verdict of destruction &c.; a. fr.

כליכה, v. כְּלִיבָה.

כָּלִיל (כָּלוּל) m. (b. h.; כָּלַל) *entire,* esp. *Kalil, a sacrifice burnt entirely.* Sifra Tsav, Par. 3, ch. V; Men. 51ᵇ בכ׳ תקטר shall be burned as a *Kalil.* Y. Sot. III, 19ᵇ top קריבה בכלול is offered as a *K.*—Men. 74ª; a. e.—Tosef. Par. I, 2; Zeb. V, 4 כ׳ לאישים, v. אִשֶּׁה.

כְּלִיל, כְּלִילָא c. (כְּלַל) 1) *circle, wreath, crown.* Targ. Y. II Ex. XXV, 11. Targ. Num. VI, 7 (h. text נֵזֶר). Targ. Y. I Deut. XIV, 1 כ׳ דיסער (cmp. כַּלְכּוּל). Ib. XXXIV, 5 fem. (also כְּלִילַת constr.). Targ. Is. XXVIII, 5; a. fr.—Sabb. 152ª, v. חִילְפָא II. Gen. R. s. 98, end (ref. to נזיר, Gen. XLIX, 26) כְּלִילֵיהוֹן דאחוך the crown of thy brothers. Gitt. 7ª כ׳ לברתיה a bridal wreath for his daughter. B. Bath. 4ª, v. יָרְלָא; a. e.—*Pl.* כְּלִילֵי, כְּלִילִין, כְּלִילַיָּא. Targ. Y. Deut. l. c. Targ. Job XXXI, 36. Targ. Jud. VIII, 26 ed. Lag. (oth. ed. *sing.*); a. e.—B. Bath. 16ᵇ כלילי הוו להו Ms. M. (ed. *sing.*) they had wreaths (each dedicated to a friend).—2) דמי כ׳ or כ׳ *coronation tax* (aurum coronarium, v. Sm. Ant. s. v.). Ib. 8ª כהחוא דמי כ׳ וכ׳ as in the case of a coronation tax which they put on the city of Tiberias. Ib. פקע כ׳ (Ms. M. בטל) the tax was repealed.—3) כ׳ מלכא or כ׳ *melilot.* Keth. 77ᵇ. Sabb. 109ᵇ חד כ׳ one dose of melilot.—*Pl.* כְּלִילֵי. Ib. חמשא כ׳ five parts of melilot (Rashi: roses). [Y. M. Kat. II, 81ᵈ bot. וגנבון מנחין כליליא, read: כל לילא.]

כְּלִילָאֵי m. pl. (v. preced.) *coronation tax.* Meg. Taan. II אתנטילו כ׳ the coronation tax was remitted (v. I Macc. XIII, 39); [Scholion to Meg. Taan.: *wreaths,* an idolatrous rite forced upon the Jews by the Syrians.]

כְּלִילְתָּא, constr. כְּלִילַת, v. כְּלִיל.

כְּלִימָּה f. (b. h. כְּלִמָּה; כָּלַם) *disgrace,* usu. with בּוּשָׁה. B. Bath. 75ª; a. fr.

כלימך, Ex. R. s. 15 Mus., read: כל הימך, v. הֵימ־.

כַּלִּין, v. כַּלָּיִיה.

כְּלִינוֹס m. (χαλινός) *bridle.* Tanh. Balak 13 כלבוס (corr. acc.); Num. R. s. 20 בכלינוס; Y'lamd. to Num. XXIII, 5 quot. in Ar., v. פָּקַם.—Ab. d'R. N. ch. XXIV לסוס שיש לו כלינס Ar. (ed. כלים נאים, Var. כלונס, corr. acc.) like a horse which is bridled. Tosef. Kel. B. Mets. IV, 7 כלינס, כלונים, כולונים (corr. acc.). Pesik. R. s. 42 בכ׳ (corr. acc.)

כְּלִינִדִּין m. (χλανίδιον meant for χλαμύδιον, cmp.

Cast. Lex. Syr. s. v.) *a fine mantle*, an officer's distinction. Y. Snh. X, 29[a] top, v. זוֹנָרָא.

כלינס, v. קְלִינוֹס.

כְּלִינְסָא, v. כלוּנְסָא.

כְּלִיס m., pl. כְּלִיסִין, כְּלִיסִים (כלס, enlarg. of כל; cmp. Ges. H. Dict.[10] s. v. כרש) *bags*. Tosef. Kil. V, 26 אחולין והכ׳ כ׳ הגרגים וכ׳ ed. Zuck. tents and bags, filters &c., v. אבסלר.—Trnsf. *pods, a dehiscent fruit*, similar to carob. Ter. XI, 4 כ׳ והרובים *k'lisin* and carobs; Ukts. I, 6 כְּלוֹס (Maim.: a species of *figs*, v. כְּלוּפְסִין).—Hull. 67[b] (a species of *peas*, Rashi); Sifra Sh'mini, Par. 10, ch. XII, a. e. יתושין שבכ׳ the bugs found in &c.; Y. Ter. VIII, 45[b] bot. Tosef. Ter. V, 7; Y. Bicc. III, beg. 65[c]; a. e.—[Ukts. III, 2, v. בולבוס. Y. Maasr. II, 50[a], v. כְּלוּפְסִין.]

כליסריקים, v. next w.

כלירכין, read: כִּילִירְכִין m. pl. (χιλίαρχοι, chiliarchi) *chiliarchs*, commanders of one thousand soldiers. Koh. R. to XII, 7 (expl. לשום כרים, Ez. XXI, 27[a]) (כלור׳) כלירכין to appoint chiliarchs; [Lam. R., introd. (R. Josh. 2) פלימרכים, v. פּוֹלִימַרְכוֹס.]—Sifré Deut. 317 (expl. כרים, Deut. XXXII, 14) אלו כאלירקין שלהם (ed. Fr. כליסריקים, corr. acc.) this refers to their (the Roman) chiliarchs; Yalk. Deut. 944 כלירקין.

כלירקין, v. preced.

כְּלֵיתָא, v. כְּלוֹ.

כַּלָּךְ m. (v. כּוּלְכָא) *cissaros-blossoms*, a woolly substance, v. אַגְבִּין. Kil. IX, 2, expl. Y. ib. 32[a] top אגבין קיסריר. Sabb. II, 1. Ib. 20[b] הדינו כ׳ this (metaxa) is *kallakh*. Ib.; Men. 39[b] השיראים והכ׳ וכ׳ (garments of) silk, *K.* &c. (v. סְרִיקִין). Sabb. 27[a]. Tosef. ib. IX (X), 3 צמר כ׳ *Kallakh* wool. Tosef. Kel. B. Bath. V, 11 כולך ed. Zuck. (R. S. to Kel. XXVIII, 8 כלך).

כַּלֵּךְ (contr. of כַּלֵּה וְלֵךְ, v. כָּלָה) *cease and turn!*, *go!* Yeb. 44[a] כ׳ אצל שכמותך turn towards one corresponding to thine own age. B. Mets. 22[a] כ׳ אצל יפות go to better fruits (to take T'rumah from); Erub. 71[a]. B. Bath. 164[b] כ׳ מלשון וכ׳ turn away from this kind of slander. Sifra Thazr., Neg., Par. 2, ch. II או כ׳ לדרך זו or turn this way, i. e. I may argue thus; (ib. Emor, Par. 12, ch. XVII או לכה וכ׳). Ib. Vayikra, Hobah, Par. 7, ch. XI או כ׳ לך (corr. acc.); a. e.

כִּלְכֵּל, כְּלָל, כִּיל׳, כִּלְכּוּל m. (כִּלְכֵּל) 1) *hair-crown* (cmp. כְּלִילָא), *front hair* from temple to temple. Sabb. VIII, 4 (78[b]) כדי לעשות כ׳ (Bab. ed. כלכל; Ms. M. כדי לסוד כר׳, v. Rabb. D. S. a. l. note) enough to produce a crown by depilation of undergrowth. Ib. 80[b], v. אַנְדִּיפֵי. Naz. 3[a] (ref. to Mish. I, 1 הריני מכלכל) how do we know דהאי כ׳ שערי הוא that this vow refers to letting the hair grow?—Nidd. 52[b]; Tosef. ib. VI, 6 (ref. to the hair around the pudenda as evidence of maturity) (מחו) כ׳ זה איני יודע about this *kilkul* I know nothing.—2) *support*, *sustenance*. Naz. l. c. אימא מיזן עניי I may say that the *kilkul* (of the Mishnah, v. supra) means supporting the poor.

***כַּלְכּוּס** m. (χαλκός) *a copper, caldron*. B. Kam. 100[b] (ref. to Mish. IX, 4 צבעו כעור) [read:] מאי כעור... שצבעו כ׳ (v. Rabb. D. S. a. l. note 50) what does, 'he dyed it *kâur*' mean? ... the copper dyed it (cmp. הקדירה הירוה ib.); מאי שצבעו כ׳ כפרא דודי (Ms. H.) what does it mean &c.? The sediment of kettles. [Editions a. Mss. have קלבוס, כלבוס with ב].—*Pl.* כַּלְקִין. Y. B. Bath. IV, 14[c] bot. בסלקי, (read: בית כלקין, corresp. to בית הירורות Tosef. ib. III, 3) the copper room.

כַּלְכִּידָא, כַּלְכִּיד f. (χαλκίς, -ίδος) *chalkis*, a small fish resembling sardines (v. Sm. Ant. s. v.). Y. Ned. VI, 39[c] bot. if one says, I will taste no דָּגָה, אינו... אלא בכ׳ he is forbidden ony *ch.* (small fish). Ib.[d] top כ״ל׳ אנא טעים I feel as if I were eating *ch.*—Ib. לית... והוא זבין ליה כ׳ is it not often the case when a man says to his neighbor, buy me a fish, that he will buy *ch.* for him?—Y. Erub. III, 20[d] top כלבודא (corr. acc.); Y. Peah VIII, 21[a] top (סלק׳) כלקורא, read: כַּלְקִידָא.

כַּלְכִּית, v. כִּיל׳.

כִּלְכֵּל (b. h.; כול, כלל) [*to surround*,] 1) *to provide with everything; to sustain*. Naz. 3[a], v. כִּלְכּוּל. Ber. 58[b] וכ׳ אתכם בדין וכ׳ and provided for you (while alive) in justice, and gathered you in justice.—2) (cmp. כְּלִילָא) *to raise a crown of hair, to be a nazir*. Naz. I, 1 הריני מְכַלְכֵּל I will grow a crown (as a substitute for, 'I will be a *nazir*', v. כִּינּוּי). Y. ib. 51[b] top כאומר הריני מן המְכַלְכְּלִין as if he said, I will be one of those who wear a crown of hair.—Tosef. Nidd. VI, 6; Nidd. 52[b] עד שתְּכַלְכֵּל (euphem.) until she has a full growth of hair (around the pudenda).—*3) denom. of כְּלִי) *to arm, fit out*. Midr. Till. to Ps. VII א״ל הקב״ה ולא אני כלכלתי בה (read: כִּלְכַּלְתִּיו) said the Lord to him (Doëg), is it not I that fitted him (David) out with it (the sword of Goliath deposited in the Sanctuary)?—[The entire sentence is missing in ed. Bub.; note 69 a. l. quotes fr. mss. קלקלתי.]

Nithpalp. נִתְכַּלְכֵּל *to be supported*. Pesik. R. s. 4 אליהו (not נתכלכל) כ׳ וכ׳ Elijah was supported by the woman of Zarephath.

כַּלְכֵּל, v. כִּלְכּוּל.

כַּלְכָּלָה f. (preced. art.) 1) *support, provision*. Ber. 44[a] על המחיה ועל הכ׳ (be blessed &c.) for sustenance and support.—2) *supply*, esp. *basket containing chosen fruits* designated for use. Eduy. IV, 10 (9); Maasr. IV, 2 כַּלְכָּלַת שבת supply of fruits for the Sabbath (not for sale). Ib. הלוקט תאנים וכ׳ he who selects figs to send as a present. Y. ib. IV, 51[b] כ׳ שבת אינה וכ׳ Sabbath supply must not be sold. Y. Ter. II, end, 41[d] תאינים שבכ׳ figs in the provision basket, opp. מוּקְצֶה. Y. Dem. I, 21[c] bot. כ׳ אחת וכ׳ there is only one basketful (of the late fruits) which I reserve &c. Lev. R. s. 33, beg. כ׳ של תאנים a basket of figs for use (subject to tithes even for luncheon, v. טֶבֶל); a. fr.—*Pl.* כַּלְכָּלוֹת. Dem. VII, 6; a. fr.

כָּלַל (b. h.; v. כּוּל) 1) *to surround, comprise, include*. Gen. R. s. 4 חזר וּכְלָלָן כולן וכ׳ (not וכללו כולו) he again included them all in the praise (Gen. I, 31). Shebu. 23[b]

בכולל המותרים וכ׳ when he (in his vow) includes permitted things as well as forbidden things. Ib. 24ª, a. fr. איסור כולל, v. אִיסּוּר. R. Hash. IV, 5 וכולל מלכיות עמהן and inserts that section of prayers concerning the divine rulership, v. מַלְכוּת; a. fr.—*Part. pass.* כָּלוּל, כְּלוּלָה f. a) *included.* Y. Pes. V, 32ᶜ bot. ירידת גשמים כ׳ וכ׳ the praise for the rain-fall is included therein (Ps. CXXXV, 7); Y. Taan. III, 67ª, end.—Y. Ber. I, 3ᶜ top עשרת הדברות כְּלוּלִין בהן the Ten Commandments are contained therein.—b) *entire,* v. כָּלִיל.—2) *to generalize* (v. כְּלָל). B. Kam. 63ª חזר (הדר) וכ׳ the text generalizes again.—[Y. Ab. Zar. IV, 44ᵇ top כוללין . . . טוחנין, read: כּוֹבְרִין, v. כָּבַר.]

Nif. נִכְלַל *to be implied, to be stated in general terms,* opp. נִפְרַט. Y. Sot. VII, 21ᵈ top דברים שנִכְלְלוּ ונפרטו things which have been stated both implicitly and specifically.

Pi. כִּילֵּל 1) *to crown.* Tanh. R'eh 7 אם נוצחין...ומְכַלְּלִין אותו when they (the legions) are victorious, they come and make a wreath, and crown him (the king).—2) *to include, imply. Part. pass.* מְכוּלָּל, *pl.* מְכוּלָּלִים *enclosed* (as a germ), *potential.* Gen. R. s. 10 (ref. to ויכלו, Gen. II, 1) מ׳ היו המעשים things had been created potentially, and then they developed more and more.—[Y. Ber. VI, 10ª top יכללו, read: יְכַלְּלוּ, v. כָּלַל.]

Hif. הִכְלִיל *to crown, finish, perfect.* Part. pass. מוּכְלָל. Yoma 54ᵇ (expl. מכלל, Ps. L, 2) מציון מ׳ יופיו וכ׳ from Zion the beauty of the world was perfected (by religion). [Cant. R. to V, 11, end מוכללה, read: מוּכְלֶלֶת, v. כָּלַל.]

כְּלַל ch. same, 1) *to surround, crown.* Targ. Cant. III, 11.—2) (denom. of כּוֹלָּא) *to make whole, combine.* Y. Meg. IV, 75ᵇ bot. לינן חזרין וְכָלְלִין לון do we not again combine them (the separated portions)?

Pa. כַּלֵּיל 1) *to surround, crown.* Targ. Ps. V, 13.—2) (v. כִּילְּתָא, כִּילָּה I) *to prepare a bridal room.* B. Mets. 101ᵇ כַּלְּלֵיהּ לבריה if the owner of the rented dwelling gave it to his son as a bridal room (Rashi: if he was making preparations for his son's wedding, and needed the dwelling for the young couple). Gen. R. s. 70; Yalk. Gen. 125 כולי יומא הוו מְכַלְּלִין (ביה) ליה the whole day they were helping him to prepare the bridal chamber (decorating it).

Af. אַכְלֵיל *to crown, surround.* Targ. Ps. LXV, 12. Ib. CIII, 4; a. e.—[Kidd. 81ᵇ מכללית, read: מְכַלֵּי להו, v. כְּלֵי I.]

Ithpa. אִיכַּלַּל, אִיתְכַּלַּל, *Ithpe.* אִיכְּלִיל 1) *to be crowned, to adorn one's self.* Gen. R. s. 34, beg. (expl. Ps. CXLII, 8) יִתְכַּלְּלוּן בי וכ׳ the righteous shall adorn themselves with me.—2) *to be led into the bridal room, be married.* Meg. 27ᵇ כי איכ׳ רבה וכ׳ when his son R. was to marry.

כְּלָל m. (preced. wds.) 1) *general rule, principle.* Sifra K'dosh., Par. 2, ch. IV (ref. to Lev. XIX, 18) זה כ׳ גדול וכ׳ this ('love thy neighbor as thyself') is the most important principle in the Law. Sabb. VII, 1. Hull. III, 1 זה הכ׳ this is the general rule; a. v. fr.—Trnsf. לִכְלַל, בִּכְלַל *under the influence of.* Sifré Num. 157 לפי שהיה בכ׳ כעס בא לכ׳ טעות because he was under the influence of anger, he came under the influence of mistaken judgment; Yalk. ib. 786; a. fr.—2) *community.* Ber. 49ᵇ לעולם אל...מן הכ׳ a person must never exclude himself from the community (by saying, 'Praise ye', instead of 'Let us praise'). Mekh. Bo., Pisha, s. 18 ולפי שהוציא.... מן הכ׳ וכ׳ and as he excluded himself from the community (by saying 'you') &c.; a. e.—3) *total, sum.* B. Bath. 123ª בִּכְלָלָן אתה וכ׳ as their sum total you find seventy (Gen. XLVI, 27), whereas the detailed record counts only sixty nine.—4) *generalization, statement by implication,* opp. פרט specification; *inclusion, comprehension under a class.* Ber. 26ᵇ, a. fr. עד ועד בכ׳, v. עַד.—Sifra introd. מכ׳ ופרט מפרט וכ׳ וכ׳ interpretation based upon a general law followed by specification, or specification followed by generalization. Ib. כל דבר שהיה בכ׳ וכ׳ when a law is once laid down in general, and in another place a specification is given (e. g. Lev. VII, 37, a. ib. 20), it is stated specifically not for its own sake alone, but as applicable to the whole class. Ib. beg. מכ׳ ופרט וכ׳ אי אתה דן וכ׳ if a general rule is followed by a specification and this again by a generalization, you must be guided by the specification (e. g. Deut. XIV, 26). Tosef. Sot. VIII, 10; Sot. 37ª ברוך בכ׳ . . ארור בכ׳ וכ׳ 'blessed be' was pronounced on Mount Gerizim in general (corresp. to the general curse, Deut. XXVII, 26) and was specified (corresp. to ib. 15—25); 'cursed be' was pronounced on Mount Ebal in general (ib. 26) &c.; a. fr.—מִכְּ׳ *by implication.* Ned. 11ª, a. fr. מכ׳ לאו אתה שומע הן from *no* you understand *yes,* v. הֵן.—Pes. 16ᵇ שהותרה מִכְּלָלָהּ וכ׳ which was permitted (dispensed with), by implication, for a community (if unclean, derived fr. Num. IX, 2, v. Pes. 77ª). Hull. 37ᵇ מכ׳ דטרפה וכ׳ this proves by implication that *t'refah* is not the same as &c.; a. v. fr.—לאו . . . כ׳ *not at all* (cmp. כְּלוּם). Ib. 20ᵇ; a. fr.—[Mekh. Bo, beg. כ׳ לדברות, read: כְּלַי.]—*Pl.* כְּלָלוֹת (*fem.*). Naz. 48ᵇ. Sot. 37ᵇ. Erub. 27ª אין למדין מן הכ׳ וכ׳ from general rules (the use of the word כל, as ib. III, 1) we must not derive anything, not even when an exception is stated (as there may be other exceptions); a. fr.—Ex. R. s. 32, beg. כְּלָלִים.

כְּלָלָא ch. same. Targ. Y. Deut. XXVII, 26 ברכתא בכ׳ וכ׳ blessings in general &c. (v. Sot. 37ª quot. in preced.).—Sabb. 147ª, a. fr. נקוט האי כ׳ בידך take this as a rule. B. Mets. 103ᵇ, a. e. כ׳ דמילתא the general rule is &c. Hull. 95ª הא דרב לא בפירוש איתמר אלא מכ׳ איתמר this opinion of Rab has not been delivered explicitly but only arrived at by implication; Ber. 9ª; a. fr.—Yeb. 21ᵇ וכ׳ הוא is this rule without exceptions?—Shebu. 26ª אהני כ׳ לאתויי וכ׳ the generalization (after specification) has the effect of including &c.; a. v. fr.—*Pl.* כְּלָלֵי, כְּלָלַיָּא, כְּלָלִין. Y. Ter. I, 40ᶜ לית (כללי) כְּלָלוֹי דרבי כ׳ the general rules of Rabbi (in the Mishnah; expressions like זה הכלל or כל הכל, &c.) are not without exceptions. Keth. 60ª לא..להני כ׳ דביריל וכ׳ do not heed those rules which my brother... laid down. Gen. R. s. 33 [read:] אליף . . . כל כ׳ דאורייתא ואילין אינון הלכתא דבבלאי (v. 'Rashi' a. l.) he taught Rab . . . all the general rules (of interpretation) of the Law, and these became the guiding laws of the Babylonians.

כָּלַם (b. h.; cmp. כָּלָא) *to be restrained, to be retired.*

Nif. נִכְלַם *to be retired,* (cmp. בּוּז) *to be put to shame, be rebuked.* Ab. d'R. N. ch. IX (ref. to Num. XII, 14) שתִּכָּלֵם ז׳ ימים that she should live in retirement for seven days (and not appear before the king); (Sifré Num. 106 שתהא מוּכְלֶמֶת). Ber. 16[b] שלא נבוש ולא נִכָּלֵם מאבותינו (v. Rabb. D. S. a. l. note 4) that we may not be put to shame and not be abashed when compared with our fathers (Y. ib. IV, 7[d] bot. שלא נבוש מאבותינו לעו״הב). Cant. R. to I, 14 בְּהִכָּלְמוֹ in his shyness.

Hif. הִכְלִים *to cause to retire, to rebuke, shame.* Kidd. 31[a] bot. ולא הִכְלִימָהּ and he did not scold her. Ib.[b] כלום ... ולא הִכְלַמְתָּהּ did she (thy mother) throw a bag of money into the sea in thy presence, and thou didst not reproach her?—Midr. Till. to Ps. IV, 3 עד מתי אתם מַכְלִימִין וכ׳ how long will you slander me and my dignity?; a. e.—Part. Hof. מוּכְלָם, f. מוּכְלֶמֶת, v. supra.

כְּלַם ch. same. [Targ. Y. Deut. XXIX, 4 כלמו, Var. בלמו, read: בְּלַת or בְּלֵיאוּ, v. בְּלֵי I.]

Af. אַכְלֵם as preced. *Hif.* Targ. I Sam. XX, 34. Ib. I, 16; a. e.—B. Kam. 86[a] bot. דמַכְלְמוּ ליה ומִיכְּלֵם when you rebuke the child and he shrinks back in shame; ib.[b] (not דמיכלמו).—Part. pass. מְכַלַּם. Y. Yeb. XII, 12[d] bot. והיא מְכַלְמָה עלך and she (the young woman) will be put to shame on account of thee (the old man); ib. והוא מכלמה וכ׳ (read: מְכַלַּם).

Ithpa. אִיתְכַּלַּם, *Ithpe.* אִיתְכְּלֵם, אִיכְּלַם as preced. *Nif.* Targ. O. Num. XII, 14. Targ. II Sam. X, 5; a. e.—B. Kam. l. c., v. supra.

***כְּלוּמָא, כְּלָמָא** m. (preced.) *refraining, warding off.*—*Pl.* כְּלָמֵי. B. Mets. 103[b] Ar. (Ms. כלומ׳, ed. בְּלָמָא q. v.).

כַּלְמָא, *pl.* כַּלְמֵי *vermin*, v. כַּלְמְתָא.

כְּלָמוּס m. (χλαμύς) *chlamys, officer's cloak* (v. Sm. Ant. s. v.). Y'lamd. to Gen. XXV, 23; 25, quot. in Ar., corresp. to the Jewish garment טַלִּית, v. כִּבְלָא.—Tanh. Vayera, ed. Bub., 21 [read:] כל הימים ... היה מהלך בסגון כיון שנכנס הלביש הכלמוס שלו (v. ib. notes 124; 125) as long as he was on the road, he travelled in a *sagum* (common soldier's cloak), when he entered to take office, he put on the chlamys; Gen. R. s. 50, beg. כפגן.. כקאלמין; Lev. R. s. 26 כבגן ... כקלאמין; Yalk. Gen. 84 כגפ׳ ... כקאלמין (read: בסגון .. בִקְלָאמִין or בִּקְלָאמִין).

קַלְ׳, כַּלְמְתָא f. (collect. noun; a dialect. adapt. of h. כִּנָּם, v. כִּינָּה) [*nesting*, cmp. כלם,] *vermin.* Targ. O. Ex. VIII, 12 sq. ק׳ (cod. 10 כ׳, v. Berl. Targ. O. II, p. 21).—ק׳, כַּלְמֵי. Targ. Y. ib. ק׳.—Ber. 51[b] ממהדורי .... כ׳ from peddlers comes gossip, from rags—vermin. Nidd. 20[b] כ׳ (Ar. s. v. סרק: קלמי).

כָּלָן, Y. Peah VIII, 20[d] bot., v. כּוֹל.

כַּלָּן, v. כַּלְּתָא.

כלנוס, v. כְּלִינוֹס.

כְּלַנְדִּיָּיא m. pl. (χλανίδιον,—ια) *fine cloaks* for women. Y. Sabb. VI, 8[b] bot. כ׳ (expl. הרעלות, Is. III, 19; not ב׳).

כַּלְנִיתָא, v. כּוּלְנ׳.

כַּלְנְסָא, v. כְּלוּנְסָא.

כלעס, Y. Ter. VIII, 46[a] ואיתכ׳, v. בְּלַס.

כְּלַפֵּי h. a. ch. (=כּוּן) לאפי (כְּ, v. אַפָּא, אַף, a. כּוּן) *directed towards, opposite, against.* Targ. Job XXIV, 15; a. e.—Snh. VI, 4 פניו כ׳ העם his (the culprit's) face towards the people; כ׳ העץ towards the cross. Ib. 105[a], v. חוּצְפָּא. Pes. 8[b] כ׳ שאמרה תורה in the face of what (considering that) the Law says; Y. Macc. II, 31[d] top כ׳ שנאמר; a. fr.—כ׳ לייא, אליה, v. אֵלָיָה.

כַּלְקְדִיקָה, v. גְּלוּגְדְּקָא.

כלקורא, v. כַּלְפִּיד.

כלקטורין, כלקטורים read:

כַּלְקְטִירִין (m. pl. χαρακτῆρες) *features* of the face. Lev. R. s. 23 הריני צר את כל קטורין וכ׳ (corr. acc.) I will shape his features in resemblance to &c.; Pesik. R. s. 24 יושב וצר בל׳ וכ׳ (corr. acc.). Ib. בלקטירים, בלקטרים (corr. acc.) was painting the picture of the ruler (Lev. R. l. c. איקונין). [Ar. s. v. קנכתר: קנכתירין.]—V. also כּוּלְקָטֶר.

כַּלְקִידָא, v. כַּלְפִּיד.

כַּלְקִיס pr. n. pl. (Χαλκίς) *Chalkis*, a town of Cœlesyria. Y. Meg. I, 70[c] bot. פליטת ... במדינת כ׳ וכ׳ refugee scholars in the city of Ch. and in Beth Zibdin; Y. Taan. II, 66[a] בולקוס (כול׳); Meg. Taan. XII בליקו׳ (corr. acc.). [Schol. to Meg. Taan. defining our w.: במדינת קוסליקוּס, prob. a corrupt. of Cœlesyria.]

כלקירא, v. כַּלְפִּיד.

כלרויה, Tosef. B. Kam. VII, 4 את הכ׳ some ed., read: את הכל, דויה.

כַּלְּ׳, כַּלְּ׳, כַּלְּתָא f. ch.=h. כַּלָּה, *bride; daughter-in-law.* Targ. Is. LXI, 10 (ed. Wil. כַּלְּתָא). Targ. Gen. XI, 31; a. fr.—Gitt. 57[a] כי הוו מפקי חתנא וכ׳ when they led forth bride and groom in procession. B. Bath. 143[b] כַּלְּתֵיהּ his daughter-in-law. Meïl. 19[a] דהבא דכלתיה דנון the gold ware of the daughter-in-law of Nun (which was found to have lost in weight); a. fr.—[Targ. Job XV, 32 וכַלְּתֵיהּ, v. כִּילְּתָא I.]—*Pl.* כַּלָּן, כַּלָּתָא, כַּלָּתָה. Targ. Ruth I, 6. Targ. Jer. VII, 34.—Meïl. l. c. דהבא דרמיין כַּלָּתָיךְ the gold ware which thy daughters-in-law cast carelessly about (by which they wear off). Keth. 17[a] משרי קמי כ׳ they sang before (the processions of) brides. Yeb. 21[b] כלתה ... דבי the daughters-in-law of the house of ... (where there were wives of his daughter's sons and wives of his son's sons).—V. כַּלִּירָה, כַּלִּין.

כלתין, Y. R. Hash. II, 58[a] top, read: כַּלְּתִין.

כְּמָא, כְּמָה (v. כְּ a. מָא, דִּי) 1) (followed by ד׳) *like that which.* Targ. Jud. XI, 39 a. fr. [Usu.: הֵיךְ מָא, הֵיכְמָא.]—

2) (mostly כמה) *how! how many!, how much!, how long!*; (also interrog.) *how much?* &c. Targ. Ps. CXXXIX, 17. Ib. XXXV, 17; a. fr.—Gen. R. s. 6 כ׳ נפשיה וכ׳ how the soul of this man's (my) brother is now chopping cedars and sawing &c. (is in the agony of death)! (Midr. Sam. ch. IX; Yalk. Ps. 743, only נפשיה וכ׳). Yoma 22ᵇ, v. חֲלַר. Ber. 14ᵇ כ׳ מעליא וכ׳ how excellent &c. B. Mets. 86ᵃ כ׳ כברין וכ׳ how many cakes of nardus do we owe to &c.!—M. Kat. 16ᵇ כל כ׳ דהוה וכ׳ as long as &c.; a. fr.—Y. Ab. Zar. II, 41ᵃ top כַּמָּן קטל how many of them did he kill?

כַּמְאר (v. preced.) *as much as.* Yoma 43ᵇ כ׳ דמסיק וכ׳ (Var. כמה) as much as a fox carries (on its feet) from a ploughed field; (Nidd. 65ᵇ כדמסיק).

כַּמָּה, v. כַּמָּא.

כַּמָּה, כַּמֶּה h. (preced. wds.) 1) *how much?, how many?* Kidd. 9ᵇ כ׳ אתה נותן וכ׳ how much (dowry) wilt thou give &c.? Ber. 14ᵃ עד כ׳ up to how much? Ib. 30ᵇ כ׳ ישהה וכ׳ how long must he pause between &c.?; a. fr.—2) *how!, how many!, how much!* Sabb. 12ᵇ כ׳ גדולים דברי וכ׳ how grand are the words of &c.; a. fr.—על אחת כ׳ וכ׳, v. אֶחָד.—3) (I don't know) *how many, many.* M. Kat. 16ᵇ איבדתי כ׳ דוד מפניו I should have destroyed many Davids for his sake. Y. Keth. V, 30ᵃ bot. לאחר כ׳ ימים after ever so many days. Ib. אפי׳ כ׳ even much longer; a. fr.—[Y. Succ. I, 51ᵈ top גבוה מכמה, prob. to be read: מכ׳ אמה= מעשרים ib.]

כְּמֵהוֹת, כְּמֵהִים, כְּמֵהִין, כְּמֵי׳ c. pl. (כָּמַהּ *to be hot, to thirst, long for*) a kind of *mushroom, morils.* Gen. R. s. 69, beg. (ref. to כמה, Ps. LXIII, 2) ככ׳ הללו שהן מצפין וכ׳ like those morils which look out for water; Yalk. Gen. 119 כִּכְּמֵהִיוֹת (not כמ׳); Yalk. Ps. 786 כאמבטאות (corr. acc.). Ned. 55ᵇ; Y. Maasr. I, 48ᵈ top, כ׳ ופטריות morils and truffles which are not planted; Ber. 40ᵇ; a. fr.

כְּמֵהִין ch. same. Y. Bets. V, end, 63ᵇ.

כְּמוֹ (b. h.; v. כַּמָּה) *as, like.* Yalk. Ex. 246 הקשו לבם כ׳ אבן they made their hearts hard like stones (Mekh. B'shall., Shirah, s. 5 כאבן). With suffixes: כָּמוֹנִי, כָּמוֹךָ &c. *like me, like thee* &c. Ned. 9ᵇ, v. כְּמוֹת. Mekh. l. c., s. 8; a. fr.—V. כְּמוֹת.

כמון, a word in a charm formula. Sabb. 67ᵃ (v. next wds.).

כַּמּוֹן m. (b. h. כַּמֹּן, v. כָּמַן, cmp. חָמַם) *cumin.* Dem. II, 1. Ter. X, 4 בכ׳ של וכ׳ with cumin stalks of T'rumah.

כַּמּוֹנָא, כְּמוֹנָא ch. same. Targ. Is. XXVIII, 25; 27.—Ab. Zar. 29ᵃ, v. כְּרוּיָא.—*Pl.* כְּמוֹנֵי, כְּמוֹנַיָּא. Sabb. 67ᵃ כמונרא (Rashi: כמוני; Ms. M. sing.), v. בְּרִינְתָא I.

כְּמוֹנָא m. (כְּמַן) *insidiousness, crafty plan.* Targ. Y. II Ex. XXI, 14 (h. text ערמה).—V. כְּמָנָא.

כְּמוֹת (=כְּמוֹ את, cmp. כְּוָת) *like, as.* Y. Maas. Sh. IV, 54ᵈ כ׳ שהוא מוכר according to the selling price. Sabb. 51ᵃ, a. fr. (כ׳ שהוא (חי in its natural condition (raw). Keth. 17ᵃ כלה כ׳ שהיא the bride at weddings must be praised according to her perfections (without exaggeration); a. fr.—With suffixes: כְּמוֹתִי, כְּמוֹתְךָ &c. *like myself, like thyself* &c. B. Mets. 59ᵇ אם הלכה כ׳ if the law is in accordance with my opinion, v. כְּוָת. Y. Ned. I, 36ᵈ bot. כ׳ ירבו וכ׳ may there be many like thee &c.; (Bab. ib. 9ᵇ כָּמוֹךָ). Ber. V, 5, a. fr. שלוחו של אדם כמותו a man's messenger is like himself, i. e. action by proxy is legal; a. fr.

כְּמֵיהוֹת, ־יהִים, ־יהִין, v. sub כָּמַהּ.

כמין, a word in a charm formula. Sabb. 67ᵃ.

כְּמִין, v. כְּמַן.

כְּמִינָא, v. כְּמָנָא.

כְּמֵיסַת, v. כְּמֵסַת.

כְּמִישׁ, v. כְּמַשׁ.

כָּמָךְ, m. (Pers. Kâmakh, Arab. Kâmah, Fl. to Levy Talm. Dict. II, 452²) *Kamakh, a Persian sauce* of milk, curdled milk &c.; cmp. כּוּתָּח. Nidd. 51ᵇ שבת העשויה לכ׳ dill intended to be put into the *k.*

כַּמְכָא ch. same. Pes. 30ᵃ Ar. (ed. כותחא). Ib. 76ᵇ Ar. (ed. כותחא). Hor. 12ᵃ Ms. M. (ed. כות׳). Hull. 112ᵃ; a. e.

כְּמָן, v. כַּמָּא.

כָּמַן (cmp. כָּמַר) [*to be heated* in the ground,] *to be hidden, lie in wait.*

**Pi.* כִּמֵּן *to hide fruits* in the ground. Maasr. IV, 1 המכמן Mish. a. Bab. ed. (Ms. M. המכמיר, Y. ed. המכמר, v. כָּמַר).

Hif. הִכְמִין *to keep witnesses hidden,* a proceeding applied only against seducers to idolatry (v. מֵסִית). Snh. VII, 10 מַכְמִינִין לו עדים וכ׳ the court puts witnesses in wait for him behind an enclosure. Y. Yeb. XVI, 15ᵈ bot.; a. e.—Y. Snh. VIII, 21ᶜ top המכמין עדיו וכ׳ he who keeps witnesses hidden (while eliciting a confession of indebtedness from his debtor), has done nothing, i. e. the confession has no legal consequences.

כְּמַן ch. same. Targ. O. Ex. XXI, 13; a. fr.—Part. כָּמֵין, f. כָּמְנָא (כָּמֵינָא). Targ. Jer. IX, 3 כ׳ מִכְמַן (h. text עקב יעקב). Targ. Prov. VII, 12.—Koh. R. to IV, 14; Midr. Till. to Ps. IX, v. כַּשְׁכֵּשׁ.

Pa. כַּמֵּין *to hide, cover.* Targ. Prov. X, 18 מְכַמֵּין Ms. (ed. מַכְמִין *Hif.*).—Part. pass. מְכַמַּן *lurking.* Targ. Lam. III, 10 (ed. Amst. מְכַמַּן; h. text אֹרֵב).

Af. אַכְמִין 1) same, v. supra.—2) as preced. *Hif.* Snh. 29ᵇ.

כַּמָּן, v. כַּמּוֹן.

כְּמָנָא f. (preced. wds.) *ambush, trap; insidiousness.* Targ. Jud. IX, 35. Targ. II Sam. XIII, 32 (ed. Lag. כְּמִינָא; h. text שימה); a. e.—*Pl.* כְּמָנַיָּא, constr. כְּמָנֵי. Targ. I Chr. I, 20 (ed. Lag. כמרנא). Targ. Ps. X, 8; 10.—V. כְּמוֹנָא.

כַּמָּנָה f. h. same.—*Pl.* כַּמָּנוֹת. Yalk. Deut. 804 . . . אין שאין בה כ׳ there is no road on which ambushes are not to be apprehended; Sifré ib. 20 מקומות (corr. acc.).

כַּמְנוֹן m. (preced. wds.) *craft, artfulness.* Koh. R. to IX, 14 (expl. מצודים ib.) כ׳ ועקמון Craft and Trap (allegorical names of towers); Yalk. ib. 989 כַּמָּן; Gen. R. s. 33 עַקְמָן וּכַמְנָן Tricky and Wily.

כָּמַס (b. h.; cmp. כָּמַן) *to hide, store away.* Part. pass. כָּמוּס. Yalk. Ex. 165 היא כ׳ מעינינו he is hidden from our sight; Pirkê d'R. El. ch. XLVIII.—V. כּוֹמְסָה.

כָּמַס m. (preced.) *subterranean prison* (carcer). Yalk. Hos. 532 בתחלה קורא ארלוגין . . . . . נותן לו כ׳ וכ׳ first he reads the charge, then he strikes him (to extort confession), and then he assigns to him a prison &c.; Pesik. Shub., p. 159[b] (corr. acc.).

כָּמַס ch. (v. preced.) *store-room, cellar* (Assyr. כמס, Schr. KAT² p. 559). B. Bath. 145[b] עתיר כ׳ rich of stores.

כְּמֵיסַת, כְּמֵסַת c. (v. מִסְּתָא; a phrase borrowed fr. Deut. XVI, 10; 17, v. Targ. Y.; =h. כְּדֵי) *adequate, able, worthy.* Targ. Y. II Lev. XXIII, 29 דכ׳ וכ׳ that is able (or of adequate age) to fast. Targ. Y. Gen. XX, 16. Targ. II Sam. VII, 18; Targ. I Chr. XVII, 16 לית אנא כ׳ I am not worthy (h. text מי אנכי).

כָּמַר (b. h., v. כָּמַס, כָּמַן, כָּמָה) 1) [*to heat,*] *to make* כּוֹמֶר (v. כּוֹמֶר I), *to produce shrinking and maturing of fruits by underground storage* or *by exposure to the sun.* Tosef. Men. IX, 10 לא היו . . וכוֹמְרִין אותן (Var. וכורמין) they did not cut the grapes and let them shrink (before putting them in the press), but cut and immediately pressed them. B. Mets. 89[b] ולא יִכְמוֹר באדמה וכ׳ (Ar. יִכְמַר *Pi.*, v. Rabb. D. S. a. l. note 90) the laborer must not hide grapes in the ground (to eat them afterwards).—2) (trnsf.) *to watch, guard.*—Denom. כּוֹמֶר II.—3) *to lay a trap,* v. infra.

Pi. כִּימֵּר, *Hif.* הִכְמִיר 1) *to hide in the ground, heat.* Maasr. IV, 1, v. כָּמַן. B. Mets. l. c., v. supra.—2) (denom. of מִכְמָר) *to lay a trap, net.* Tosef. Yeb. XIV, 6 שהיו מְכַמְּרִין מכמרות that were laying nets; Yeb. 121[a] מְכַ׳ מכמורין; Y. ib. XVI, 15[d] top לִכְמוֹר מ׳.

Nif. נִכְמַר 1) *to shrink, fall in by the effect of the heat, to tumble inward.* Y. B. Mets. X, beg. 12[c] נ׳ כתנור if the house fell in like a furnace, opp. נפל לחוץ.—2) (trnsf.) with רחמים, *to be bent over, to feel compassion* (cmp. גָּלַל). Yalk. Gen. 150 נִכְמְרוּ רחמיו של יוסף Joseph was moved to compassion; (Tanh. Vayigg. 4 נתגלגלו ר׳).

כְּמַר ch. same, 1) *to hide, keep warm* (corresp. to h. כָּמַן). Y. Sabb. IV, beg. 6[d] (read:) כַּמְרָא׳ גו גיפתא, v. גִּיפְתָּא. Ib. כַּמְּרָהּ גו וכ׳ put it in &c. B. Mets. 74[a] מחוסר מִכְמַר ועיולי וכ׳ requiring heating (of grapes) and carrying to the press. —2) *to shrink, be wrinkled.* Pes. 58[a] מכמר בישרא the shrinking and drying up of the meat (from lying over too long).—3) (with רחמין as object) *to feel compassion.* Targ. Y. Deut. XIII, 18. Targ. Ps. LXXVII, 10.—[Kidd. 81[b], v. אִכְמַר.]

כּוּמֶר, כּוּמְרָא, v. כּוֹמֶר, כּוֹמְרָא.

כַּמְרִיָּתָא f. pl. (preced. wds.) *withered, black fruits.* Lam. R. to V, 10 (expl. נכמרו ib.) כאילין כ׳ wrinkled like withered fruits.

כמרוסא, Num. R. s. 12, v. קָמְרוֹסָא.

כָּמַשׁ (cmp. כָּמַר) *to wrinkle, wither.* Y. Maas. Sh. IV, 54[d] bot. עד שִׁיִּכְמוֹשׁוּ until they are withered.—Part. pass. כָּמוּשׁ, f. כְּמוּשָׁה; pl. כְּמוּשִׁין, כְּמוּשׁוֹת. Lev. R. s. 23; Cant. R. to II, 2 מה שושנה . . והיא כ׳ וכ׳ as the lily, when the heat comes upon it, is withered, but blooms again when the dew falls . . . נראין כ׳ וכ׳ so does Israel . . . seem to be withered &c. Succ. 31[a] bot. כמושין withered fruits, contrad. to יבשין dried up; a. fr.

Nif. נִכְמַשׁ same. Cant. R. to II, 1 נוחה לְהִכָּמֵשׁ withers easily.

כְּמַשׁ ch. same. B. Bath. 16[b] וכיון דִּכְמִשֵׁי וכ׳ and when they withered, they knew (that an accident had befallen their friend).—Part. כָּמִישׁ, pl. כָּמִישִׁין. Y. Pes. IV, end, 31[c]; Esth. R. to I, 4, v. זְלִיל.

כְּמָתִ־ (v. כְּמָא a. דִּכְמָא) *like.*—Targ. Ps. LXXIII, 15 דִּמְכַמְּתְהוֹן ed. Lag. (oth. ed. דכמתהון) (something) which is of the nature of their speeches.

כַּן *here,* v. כָּאן.

כֵּן I (b. h.; v. כִּי, כָּךְ) *so, thus.* Ber. 11[b] כֵּן הוא אומר and so we read; a. v. fr.—אם כן, אלא אם כן, v. אִם.—לְכֵן *for such a purpose.* Y. Maas. Sh. II, 53[b] bot. דרכו ל׳ it is usually employed for such a purpose. Y. Erub. VII, beg. 24[b] ייחדו ל׳ he devoted it to such &c.—יתר על כן, יתר מִכֵּן, v. יָתֵר I.

כֵּין, כֵּן, ch. same. Targ. Is. LI, 6. Targ. O. Ex. I, 12; a. fr. —Ber. 11[b] וכן אורי ליה וכ׳ and so taught R. El. &c.; a. v. fr.—בָּתַר כן, contr. בָּבֵן, *after this; therefore.* Targ. II Sam. II, 1; a. fr.—Ib. XXII, 47; a. e.—מִבְּכֵין וּלְהָלָּה, מִבְּכֵן וּלְהָלְאָה from now and further on=h. מכאן ואילך. Targ. I Kings XIV, 14.—Y. Sabb. XIV, 14[d] ר״י מטתיה כן such (disease) befell R. J.; Y. Ab. Zar. II, 40[d] ימות ולא כן. Ib. bot. הוה ליה כן let him rather die than do this (idolatrous cure); a. fr.— Y. Ber. III, 6[b] top לְכֵן דאתינן (v. preced.) it is for this purpose that we came here (to be reminded of death).—הָל כֵּן, הָלְכֵן, v. הָל.—כל דכן, v. כּוֹל.—כין הוי=כֵּינִי *it is so*; (interrog.) *is it so, indeed?* Y. Peah II, 17[a] bot. כ׳ אלא כ׳ וכ׳ is that so? (No,) but it is thus. Ib. III, 17[c] top כ׳ (insert מתניתא); ib. II, beg. 16[d] כ׳ מתניתא (not ב׳) so is the Mishnah to be read. Y. B. Mets. III, beg. 9[a] וְאִין כ׳ but if this be so; a. fr.

כֵּן II, with suff. כַּנּ־, m. (b. h.; כּוּן or כָּנַן) 1) *base, stand, rest.* Cant. R. to I, 1 (ref. to ויחנה חלום, I Kings III, 15) על כַּנּוֹ . . . החלום the dream (after he awoke) remained standing on its firm stand (was realized); Yalk. Kings 175. Yoma V, 3, sq. הניחו על כ׳ וכ׳ he set it down on the stand. Tosef. Kel. B. Mets. II, 17 מחוסרין כן vessels that have lost their rest; a. fr.—*Pl.* כַּנִּים, constr. כַּנֵּי. Kel. XI, 3.—

Trnsf. *social status.* Yeb. 77[b] גיורת מִכַּנָּהּ a proselyte of her own status, i. e. born after the conversion of her parents both of whom were of the same nation.—2) (cmp. כּוּן Pi.) *ruler.* Ib. XII, 8; Tosef. ib. B. Bath. VII, 12 הכן והכַּנָּה (Var. והכַּפָּא) the ruler and that which is ruled (the writing material); oth. opin.: the ruled material and the ruler; [oth. opin.: (cmp. σταθμός) the *base* of the scales and the *scales*; oth. opin. *the strike* and *the measure.*]

כַּנָּא ch. same, 1) *base, fixed place, line.*—*Pl.* כַּנַּיָּא. Ber. 57[b] בכַנַּיְיהוּ חזי (Ms. M. בכ׳) he saw them (in his dream) in the regular places (as planted in the field). V. כַּנְדָּא.—2) *kanna,* a small measure (v. preced.). Keth. 99[b]; Meïl. 21[b] כ׳ כ׳ בפרוטה each *k.* for a P'rutah (no reduction for larger quantities).—*Pl.* כַּנֵּי. Ib.

כִּנָּא *louse,* v. כִּינָּא. [Targ. Y. II Gen. XXXVIII, 26 בכנא some ed., read: בדינא.]

***כַּנְגַּד** m. (prob.=גִּנְגִּידְרִין) a kind of *chervil.* Sabb. 109[b] אניגרון כ׳ וכ׳ Ms. M. (ed. אבנגר, Ar. כנגר; Rashi ed. Sonc. כנגדר, v. Rabb. D. S. a. l.) elaiogaron, *kangad* and theriacon are good for &c., v. פִּילְּרָא. [Ar.:=ḥantal, *cucumis colocynthis*; Löw Pfl. p. 294: =Κανάρα *artichoke.*]

כַּנְדָּא I m. (κάνδυς, Pers.) *a gown* with wide sleeves. —*Pl.* כַּנְדֵּי. M. Kat. 24[a] תליסר כ׳ מאני Ar. (ed. תריסר מני; Ms. M. חל׳ בגדי מני, מני being a gloss to our w.).

כַּנְדָּא II m. (dial. for כַּדָּא, cmp. גּוּנְדְּרָא) *pitcher, pot.* [Pes. 111[b], v. כַּנְּרָא.]—*Pl.* כַּנְדֵּי. Pes. 30[a] מזבני כ׳ sellers of earthen ware. Ib. אשוו זבינו אכַּנְדַּיְיכוּ (not דיכי..; Ms. M. אשוו זבינייכו) set a fair price on your pots.—Ḥull. 48[b] דקיימו כ׳ כ׳ lungs upon which there are pot-like excrescences.—[Ber. 40[b], v. כַּנְּרָא.]

כַּנְדּוֹקָא m. *Kandoka,* surname of one Minyomin. Ḥull. 49[b]. [Rashi: *dealer in pottery,* cmp. Syr. כנדוקא, P. Sm. 1764; v. Fl. to Levy Talm. Dict. II, 452[b].]

כִּנָּה, v. כִּינָּה.

כַּנָּה f. (v. כֵּן II) 1) *base, stand.* Kel. VII, 6 נותן את הכ׳ וכ׳ he places the base of a stove between them; [oth. opin. he puts *a ruler* between, measuring a straight line.] —2) *ruler* or *ruled material.* Ib. XII, 8, v. כֵּן II.

כִּנָּה, *Pi.* כִּינָּה, v. כני.

***כְּנָהָא** (v. כני; cmp. Ezra IV, 9; 17) *of the same class, rank.*—*Pl.* כְּנָהַיָּא. Kerith. 3[b] תנא יתהון בכְנָהֵיהוֹן Ar. (ed. בינכיהון, אבינכיהון, v. כִּינְּבָא) the redactor specifies them among their classes.

***כְּנָווֹתָה** (preced.) *K'navatha,* an adaptation of the name of a Babylonian festive time and fair. Y. Ab. Zar. I, 39[c] מוחרו וכנוני וכ׳; cmp. אַקְנִיָּיתָא.

כִּנּוֹר, כִּנּוֹרָא, v. כִּינ׳.

כִּנּוֹן, pl. כִּנּוֹנִים, v. כִּינָּנִית.

כָּנוּנָא m. (כנן) *a (fire) stand, a portable brazier,* v. כַּנָּה. Bets. 21[b]; Sabb. 47[a].

כְּנוֹנֵי (preced.) an adaptation of a *Babylonian festive season* and fair., v. כְּנָווֹתָה.

כִּנּוּס, v. כִּינּוּס.

כִּינּוּפְיָא, כְּנוּפְיָא m. (כְּנַף 1) *crowd, assembly* (cmp. הוּתְקָא). Targ. Y. Num. XXXIII, 25 (transl. מקהלות) אתר כ׳.—Sabb. 60[b] איכא כי׳ there is a large gathering (in synagogues &c.). Ib. כי׳ דאיסורא gathering on a day when labor is not permitted. R. Hash. 27[a] כל כי׳ דבכסף הוא all signals for assemblies were blown on silver horns. Yoma 51[a] אתי בכ׳ is offered by large crowds. Gitt. 11[a] כ׳ דארמאי Ar. a. Rashi (ed. כְּנוּפְיָאתָא *pl.*) popular assemblies of gentiles, opp. ערכאות, v. עַרְכִּי. B. Kam. 113[a] וכי לדידכו כְּנוּפְיַכוּ is your gathering (v. כִּפָּה) held for your individual benefit? (Var. v. כִּנָּה I).—*Pl.* כְּנוּפְיָאתָא, v. supra.

כִּינּוֹר, כִּנּוֹר m. (b. h.; prob. fr. כרר with נ inserted, v. כִּרְכֵּר, cmp. תִּיבְגָּא) *lute, cithern.* Arakh. 13[b] כ׳ של מקדש וכ׳ the *kinnor* of the Temple was seven-stringed. Ber. 3[b]; Y. ib. I, 2[d] כ׳ היה תלוי וכ׳ David had a lute suspended &c. Snh. 101[a] עשאוני בניך כב׳ וכ׳ thy children made me (the Law) like an instrument upon which the scorners play; a. fr.—*Pl.* כִּי׳, כִּנּוֹרִים, כִּנּוֹרוֹת. Arakh. II, 5. Shebu. 15[b]. Kinnim III, 6 בני מעיו לכ׳ its small bowels are used for strings for the cithern; Ab. Zar. 47[a] מהו לכ׳ Ms. M. (ed. לפארות). Pesik. R. s. 26; a. e.

כִּנְּרָא, כִּינּוֹ׳, כִּנּוֹרָא ch. same. Targ. Gen. IV, 21 (v. Berl. Targ. O. II, p. 3). Targ. Job XXX, 31 כִּינּ׳ (ed. Wil. כִּנ׳); a. fr.—*Pl.* כִּנָּרַיָּא, כִּנָּרִין, כִּנָּ׳, כִּי׳. Targ. Ps. XCII, 4. Targ. Y. Gen. XXXI, 27 (O. חִנְגִּין, v. Berl. l. c. p. 12). Targ. Is. XVI, 11 (ed. Lag. sing.); a. fr.

כְּנוּשָׁאָה m. (כְּנַשׁ) *sweeper.*—*Pl.* כְּנוּשָׁאֵי. Ḥull. 60[a], v. זְלוּחָאָה.

כִּנָּה, כני, *Pi.* כִּינָּה, כִּנָּה (b. h., v. כֵּן I) 1) *to qualify, define; to surname, to nickname; to modify an expression, circumscribe; to compare.* B. Mets. 58[b] המְכַנֶּה שם רעו וכ׳ he who calls his neighbor by a nickname. Shebu. 36[a] כִּנָּה circumscribe (use the third person as euphemism). Sifré Num. 84, a. fr. כי׳ הכתוב the Bible modifies the expression (to avoid anthropomorphism, e. g. Zech. II, 12 עינו for עיני). Meg. IV, 9 המכנה בעריות he who modifies (symbolizes) in translating the laws of incest (e. g. Lev. XVIII, 7, 'uncover not thy parents' weakness or disgrace'). Yalk. Num. 771, v. פּוֹלְיְטוֹן; a. fr. Part. pass. מְכוּנֶּה. Tanḥ. Ki Thissa 17 (ref. to באדם, Ps. LXVIII, 19) מכ׳ משה באדם (not לאדם) the name of Moses is here disguised by the substitute *Adam.* —[Yalk. Ps. 832 מכונה, v. כָּנַן.]

כני, *Pa.* כַּנֵּי ch. same. Targ. Y. Gen. IV, 26.—Shebu. 36[a] לא מְכַנִּינַן we must not modify the (Biblical) expression (to avoid cacophemism).—[Bets. 33[b] מכניא, read: מכניק, v. כְּנַק I.]

Ithpa. אִתְכַּנֵּי, *Ithpe.* אִתְכְּנֵי 1) *to be surnamed.* Targ. Is. I, 4.—*2) *to associate one's self* (v. כְּנָהָא). Targ. Ez. XXIX, 7 באִתְכְּנָיוּתְהוֹן וכ׳ when they form an alliance with thee (h. text בתפשם; Kimḥi quotes a Var. באתכנעותהון, v. כְּנַע).

כ׳ פַּרְוָא, כַּנְיָא m. *Kanya Parva,* name of an unclean bird. Ḥull. 62[b] כ׳ פ׳ אסיר Ar. (ed. בונא שרי פ׳ אסיר).

כְּנִימָה f. (denom. of כִּנָּם; cmp. כַּלְמְתָא) *vermin, moth.* Sifré Deut. 40. Y. B. Kam. IX, beg. 6[d] הרקיבו מן הכ׳ if the grain became ruined by moths, contrad. to תולעים. Makhsh. VI, 1; Tosef. ib. III, 1 מפני הכ׳ in order to prevent the grain from getting mothy.—*Pl.* כְּנִימוֹת. Midr. Till. to Ps. XXIII ולא היו עושין כ׳ (ed. Bub. עושין בהם כְּמָמִיּוֹת..; v. note a.l.) but did they not get vermin?; Cant. R. to IV, 11 כִּנָּמִיּוֹת; (Yalk. Ps. 691 בלאות; Deut. R. s. 7 מאבולת)

כְּנִיסָא, v. כְּנִישָׁא.

כְּנִיסָה f. (כָּנַס) 1) *gathering, assembly.* Meg. I, 1 מקדימין ליום הכ׳ read the M'gillah in advance on the gathering (market) day before Purim. Ib. 4[b]; a. e.—2) *entering,* opp. יציאה. Y. Erub. V, 22[c]; Midd. I, 3, v. יְצִיאָה.—B. Mets. 104[a] בשעת כְּנִיסָתָן לחופה when they were being led to the wedding chamber. Keth. 12[a]. Ber. IV, 2 בכניסתו לבה״מ on his entering college (for teaching and judging). B. Mets. 83[b] בכניסתו the time consumed in going home, v. פּוֹעֵל; a. fr.—3) *keeping in, detention.* Yalk. Num. 782, v. עֲצִירָה.—[Y. Shebi. VII, beg. 37[b] כניסות, v. כְּבִיסָה.]—4) *recess, settle.* Men. 97[b], interch. with כּוֹנֶסֶת a. כְּנֶסֶת.

כניסתא, Targ. Prov. XXV, 23 some ed., read בְּנִיסְתָא, v. בְּנִיסָא.

כְּנִישׁ m. (כְּנַשׁ) *festive gathering.* Targ. O. Deut. XVI, 8. Targ. II Chr. VII, 9 (h. text עצרת).

כְּנִישְׁתָא ,כְּנִישָׁא ,כְּנֵשׁ׳ f. (preced.) 1) *gathering; assembly.* Targ. O. Gen. I, 10 בית כְּנִישַׁת מיא (h. text מקוה). Targ. Ex. XXXV, 1 (ed. Amst. כְּנִישׁ׳). Targ. Joel I, 14. Targ. Ps. XLVIII, 12 (some ed. כְּנִישְׁתָא *pl.*, h. text בנות); a. fr.—Y. Peah I, 15[d] איזיל צור כ׳ עליה shall I call a meeting against him?; a. e.—2) כ׳ or (בי״) בית כ׳ *synagogue, school-house.* Targ. Ez. XI, 16; a. fr.—Y. M. Kat. III, 81[d] bot. קומי חדא כ׳ before a certain synagogue. Ber. 7[b]; a. fr.—כ׳ רבתא *the Great Synagogue, Synagoga Magna,* v. כְּנֶסֶת. Targ. Cant. VI, 5; a. e.—*Pl.* כְּנִישָׁתָא, v. supra; כְּנִיסָן, כְּנִישָׁן. Y. Kil. IX, 32[b] top אשרוניה תמני עסרי כ׳ they stopped the funeral procession eighteen times for mourning assemblies; Y. Keth. XII, 35[a] בניסן (corr. acc.).—[B. Mets. 21[a] כ׳ דבי דרי Ar., v. מְכַנַּשְׁתָּא.]

כַּנְכָב, v. כַּבְכָּב.

כָּנַן (cmp. כּוּן a. כּוֹנָנִית) *to nest.*—Denom. כִּינָּה.

Pi. כִּנֵּן *to form circles, to wind around.* Par. VII, 7 המכנן.... על יד על יד (Talm. ed. only once על יד) he who winds the rope (for drawing the bucket up) around his hand until a sufficient length is wound up; ואם כִּנְּנוֹ באחרונה but if he winds it after he has finished drawing; Tosef. ib. VII (VI), 4 יחזר ויבואר ed. Zuck. (Var. יכר, read: וכיננו as R. S. to Par. l. c.).—*Part. pass.* מְכוּנָּן a) *wound around.* Makhsh. IV, 1 בחבל שהוא מכ׳ וכ׳ with the rope which is wound around the neck of the vessel.—2) *nested.* Gen. R. s. 37 מכ׳ כביצה shut up in the nest like an egg, i. e. selfish; Yalk. Ps. 832 מכונה (corr. acc.).

כָּנַס (b. h.; v. כּוּס I) 1) *to collect, gather; to cover, shelter, bring home.* B. Kam. VI, 1 הכונס צאן לדיר he who takes the flock into the stall; a. fr.—כ׳ משקה *to absorb* liquids through pores, opp. to הוציא to let liquids escape through pores. Nidd. 49[a] יביא... אם כָּנְסָה וכ׳ get a tub full of water and put the pot in, if it draws water &c. Kel. X, 8 היו כונס משקה (sub. נקובין) if the vessels were so porous as to be called absorbers of liquids. Nidd. l. c. כיצד.. לידע אם ניקב בכונס משקה how do we examine to find out whether a vessel is porous to the extent of absorbing liquids? (v. supra); a. fr.—Esp. *to take a woman home, to consummate a marriage by conducting a woman to one's house, to wed,* v. נִשּׂוּאִין a. אֵירוּסִין. Keth. 3[b] וברביעי כּוֹנְסָהּ and on the fourth day of the week he weds her. Ib. ומסכנה ואילך נהגו... לִכְנוֹס וכ׳ and from the days of persecution .. the people adopted the custom to wed on the third day; .. ובשני לא יִכְנוֹס but on the second day one must not marry. Y. Yeb. IV, 6[b] כְּנָסָהּ ולא וכ׳ he took her to his home but did not touch her &c.; a. fr.—Part. pass. כְּנוּסָה. Y. Sot. II, 18[b] top שומרת יבם וכ׳ neither while waiting for the *yabam* nor after having been taken to his house.—2) (of a sore) [*to gather,*] *to grow smaller, to contract,* opp. פשה. Neg. IV, 7; Tosef. ib. II, 6; Sifra Thazr., Neg., Par. 2, ch. II; a. e.—3) (archit.) *to recede, to form a settle* or *recess* in a wall. Midd. III, 1 עלה אמה וכ׳ אמה (the altar) rose one cubit and then receded one cubit; Men. 97[b].—Y. Erub. VII, 24[b] bot. (of an inclined plane) עולה אמה וכונס שלש it rises vertically one cubit, while the incline measures three cubits, v. כִּיבּוּשׁ.—Part. pass. כָּנוּס, f. כְּנוּסָה. Tosef. Erub. I, 10 כותל שצידו אחד כ׳ מחבירו וכ׳ a wall which is more receding on one side than on the other, either the inner wall being even &c.; Erub. 9[b]; 15[a]; (Y. ib. 19[b] top כותל הנכנס). Y. Succ. I, 52[a] אפי׳ כנוסה כמה even if the reduction be ever so large.

Nif. נִכְנַס 1) *to be brought in, to enter,* opp. יצא; *to assemble, meet.* Erub. 65[a], v. סוֹד. Ib. 15[b] נ׳ ויוצא is easily passed in and out. Kel. IX, 7 מלא... נ׳ when a piece of the size .... can be passed, לא נ׳ when it cannot pass (exactly fitting in). Y. Erub. I, 18[c] bot. אין... לִיכָּנֵס וכ׳ it is not the habit of man to enter through one door and leave through another.—Hull. 3[a], a. fr. יוצא ונ׳ superintending by going in and out. Sabb. 137[b] כשם שנ׳... יִכָּנֵס וכ׳ as he (the child) has been entered into the covenant, so may he be introduced to the study of the Law &c. Snh. 101[a] נִכְנְסוּ תלמידיו וכ׳ his pupils came together to visit him. Tosef. Ber. VII (VI), 19, a. e. לא יִכָּנֵס אדם להר וכ׳ one must not enter the Temple mount &c.—Meg. I, 3 מקום שנִכְנָסִין וכ׳ a place where the country people are in the habit of assembling on Mondays &c.; a. fr.—2) *to form a recess* or *settle.* Y. Erub. I, 19[b] top, v. supra.—3) *to be married,* v. supra. Y. Yeb. IV, 6[b] הִיכָּנְסִי וכ׳ be my wife and raise thy sister's children; Koh. R. to IX, 9; a. fr.

Pi. כִּינֵּס *to gather, collect.* Tosef. Ber. VII (VI), 24 בשעת המְכַנְּסִין... כַּנֵּס when people collect (learning), scatter, when they scatter (are indifferent), gather in (withdraw); v. בָּדַר; Ber. 63[a] המכניסים (read: המְכַנְּ׳, v. Rabb. D. S. a. l. note 9). Ex. R. s. 17, beg. שכִּינְּסָן מעל הארץ which (waters) he gathered from upon the land. Deut. R. s. 3 כִּינְּסָה את בניה she assembled her children; a. fr.—Part. pass. מְכוּנָּס, f. מְכוּנֶּסֶת; pl. מְכוּנָּסִין, מְכוּנָּסוֹת. Erub. 21[a] (מים) מ׳ collected water, opp. מים חיים. Midr. Till. to Ps. LXX הרי

הצאן מכ' the flock is gathered again. Neg. IV, 3 'במ when the hairs on the leprous spot are close together, opp.מפוזר; a. fr.

Hif. הִכְנִיס *to bring in, to lay in, store up; to introduce, pass; to initiate.* Lev. R. s. 9 הִכְנִיסוֹ לביתו he invited him to his house. Ex. R. s. 20 אם אני מַכְנִיסָן וכ' if I lead them now into the land. Ib. 'ה' יינו וכ he stored his wine in the cellar. Men. 97ᵃ ומכניס קנה וכ' and passes a tube under it. Sabb. 118ᵇ 'ה' ידו וכ put his hand under his belt. Ib. מַכְנִיסֵי שבת who usher the Sabbath in (with prayer). Ib. 137ᵇ 'לְהַכְנִיסוֹ בבריתו וכ to initiate him into the covenant &c. (v. supra). Y. Yeb. I, 3ᵃ bot. 'הרי אתם מַכְנִיסִין ראשי וכ you want me to put my head between two great mountains. Mekh. B'shall., Shir., s. 6 לא מוציא ולא מַכְנִיס neither lets escape nor receives, v. נוד; a. fr.

Hithpa. הִתְכַּנֵּס, *Nithpa.* נִתְכַּנֵּס 1) *to assemble, meet, be reunited.* Taan. 27ᵇ מִתְכַּנְּסִין לבה"כ meet at the synagogue. Gen. R. s. 39, a. e. 'אם מתכנסין כל וכ if all human beings were to join for creating &c.; Cant. R. to I, 3 מִתְכַּנְּסִין. Mekh. B'shall. s. 6 'אין הגליות מִתְכַּנְּסוֹת וכ the diaspora will be reunited only as a reward for faith; a. fr.—Gen. R. s. 12, beg. מתכנסין ויוצאין; (Koh. R. to II, 12 נכנסין) they go in and out.—2) *to gather, become closer* (v. supra). Neg. I, 6 נִתְכַּנְּסָה the sore gathered.

כְּנַס ch. same, 1) *to gather, receive.* Targ. Ps. XLI, 7 Ms. (ed. כנכ, h. text יקבץ). Targ. Esth. IV, 16 (Targ. II Esth. ib. כנוש). Targ. Y. Gen. XVIII, 3 'אֶכְנוֹס וכ I shall receive the passers-by.—V. כְּנַשׁ.—2) *to marry.* Y. Erub. III, 21ᵇ top ומִיכְנְסִינָךְ ליום פלן and to marry thee before such a date; Y. Gitt. VII, end, 49ᵃ ומנכסיך (corr. acc.). Ib. ולא כְנַסְתִּיךְ and I shall not have married thee. Y. Keth. I, beg. 24ᵈ 'אילין דִּכְנְסִין וכ those who marry widows; a. fr. —3) *to enter.* Y. Snh. VI, 23ᶜ bot. 'כיון דכ when he had entered; a. e.—[Targ. Esth. II, 21; IV, 17, v. בְּנַס.]

Pa. כַּנֵּס *to gather, heap.* Targ. Ps. XXXIII, 7 Ms. (ed. מַכְנִיס *Af.*). Ib. CXLVII, 2 (Ms. *Pe.*).

Ithpe. אִתְכְּנֵס *to be gathered, to assemble.* Targ. I Chr. XI, 1 (ed. Lag. a. Rahmer 'אתכנש). Targ. Ps. XLVII, 10 Ms. (ed. 'אתכנש).

כנסא, Targ. Job XVI, 10 Ms., v. בְּנָסָא.

כְּנָסָה, v. כְּנִיסָה end.

כְּנֵסִיָּה f. (preced. wds.) *gathering, union.* Ab. IV, 11 'כל כ' וכ every union for a sacred purpose. Ex. R. s. 21; Midr. Till. to Ps. XIX; ib. to Ps. LXXXVIII, end כ' האחרונה the latest gathering (for prayers); Yalk. ib. 840 כנסת; a. e.—[Num. R. s. 1 'אני בונה כ, read: אַבְסַנְיָא, v. Tanḥ. B'midb. 2.]—*Pl.* כְּנֵסִיּוֹת, v. next w.

כְּנֶסֶת f. (preced.) 1) *gathering, storage.* Y. B. Bath. IV, 14ᶜ bot. בית כ' של עצים a store-house for wood (=אוצר). —2) *assembly, community, congregation,* esp. *congregation of worshippers.* Ex. R. s. 21 (interch. with preced. w.); Yalk. Ps. 840, v. preced.—בית כ' (abbr. בה"כ) *synagogue.* Ber. 6ᵃ. Meg. III, 1 (25ᵇ); a. fr.—Sot. VII, 7 'חזן כ the sexton of the synagogue within the Temple precincts; Succ. 51ᵇ of the synagogue of Alexandria, v. חַזָּן; a. fr. —כ' ישראל (abbrev. כ"י) the congregation of Israel, *the Ecclesia,* (often personified as a woman betrothed to the Lord). Cant. R. to I, 4; a. fr.—כ' הגדולה (abbr. כה"ג) *the Great Assembly, Ecclesia* or *Synagoga Magna,* a supreme authority established under Ezra and Nehemiah. Ab. I, 1, a. fr. 'אנשי כ' הג the men of the original Great Synagogue. Ib. 2 שירי כה"ג the last members of the Great Synagogue.—*Pl.* כְּנֵסִיּוֹת, כְּנֵסִי׳. Lam. R. introd. (R. Yitsh. 3) בני כְּנֵסִיּוֹתָיו his fellow-members in the royal council; (Yalk. Is. 318 בני המלך).—בתי כ' synagogues. Meg. 6ᵃ. Y. ib. III, beg. 73ᵈ 'ארבע . . . ב' כ' וכ there were four hundred and eighty synagogues in Jerusalem, and each had a school &c. Hull. 51ᵃ 'כפניר כ janitor at meetings of scholars in college. Pes. 49ᵇ 'ראשי כ chiefs of congregations or synagogues.

כָּנַע (b. h. כָּנַע) *to press, oppress.*—Part. pass. כָּנוּעַ, pl. כְּנוּעִין *depressed, mournful.* Y. Ter. XI, end, 48ᵇ בי"ר דאינון כ' because they are low-spirited.

Ithpa. אִתְכַּנַּע, *Ithpe.* אִיכְּנַע *to lower one's self, be humble.* Targ. Y. Gen. XVI, 9 (h. text התעני). Targ. I Kings XXI, 29. Targ. Is. XLI, 11 (h. text יכלמו); a. fr.—Targ. Ez. XXIX, 7 באִתְכְּנָעוּתְהוֹן Var., v. כני ch.—Y. Taan. III, 66ᶜ bot. מִתְכַּנְּעִין they humble themselves (in penitence).—Esp. *to bow to a superior, to salute.* Gen. R. s. 33 ולא א' מיניה and he did not salute him. M. Kat. 16ᵇ ולא אִיכְנְעָא מקמיה and she did not bow to him; a. e.

כנעה, Y. Ned. III, 37ᵈ bot., read: נִנְעָה.

כְּנַעַן (b. h.) pr. n. *Canaan,* 1) son of Ham. Gen. R. s. 36 'חם חטא וכ' וכ Ham sinned and C. was cursed?; Tanḥ. Noah 15; a. e.—2) *the land of Canaan.* R. Hash. 3ᵃ כ' על שם מלכותו (Sihon is named) C. from his kingdom; a. fr.

כְּנַעֲנָאָה m. ch.=next w. Targ. O. Gen. XII, 6.—*Pl.* כְּנַעֲנָאֵי, כְּנַעֲנָאִין. Targ. Y. ib. Targ. Gen. X, 18; a. fr.

כְּנַעֲנִי m. (b. h.) 1) *Canaanite.* Tosef. B. Kam. VIII, 19. Mekh. Mishp., Nzikin, s. 7 (ref. to Ex. XXI, 26) 'בכ' וכ the text speaks of a Canaanite slave, opp. to עבד עברי. Kidd. I, 3 'עבד כ' נקנה וכ a Canaanite slave is taken possession of &c.; a. fr.—*Pl.* כְּנַעֲנִים. Tosef. B. Kam. IX, 10. Mekh. l. c. s. 3 'כדרך שהכ' וכ as the Canaanite slaves go free. Sot. 35ᵇ כ' שבח"ל Canaanites outside of Palestine.—2) *Phœnician, merchant.* Sifré Deut. 306; Yalk. ib. 942 (ref. to יערף, Deut. XXXII, 2) 'לְשׁוֹן כ' וכ it is a merchant's expression, f. i., a man says not to his neighbor, 'change for me &c.,' but 'break &c.' (ערוף).

כָּנָה (b. h.) *to bend; to cover.*

Nif. נִכְנָה *to be covered, hidden.* Pesik. Zachor, p. 29ᵃ, a. e., v. כָּנָה.

כְּנַף I ch. same, *to press, crowd; to gather.* Targ. Ps. XLI, 7 (v. כְּנַס).—Taan. 23ᵇ ניתי לִיכְנוֹף גברי הדדי Ms. M. (ed. נִיכְנוֹף הדדי) let us go and crowd together (for prayer). Ab. Zar. 19ᵇ 'כְּנִיף ואתי וכ all the world crowded about him.—Part. pass. כְּנִיף. Snh. 29ᵇ כְּנִיפֵי ויתבי if they (before whom he made the admission, v. אודיתא) were assembled (for some other business), opp. to כַּנְפִינְהוּ איהו if he himself called them to a meeting.

Pa. כַּנֵּיף 1) *to collect, grab* (corresp. to כָּבַב). Sabb. 73ᵇ האי מאן דכ׳ וכ׳ he who grabs (skims with his palm) salt out of the salina. Bets. 33ᵇ מחזי כמאן דמְכַנֵּיף וכ׳ Ms. M. (ed. מכנזא, corr. acc.) it looks as though he raked together for the next day.—2) *to assemble, call a meeting.* Targ. Y. I Deut. I, 1.—Snh. l. c., v. supra. B. Kam. 113ᵃ לדידכו כַּנֵּיפִינְהוּ Ms. M. (ed. v. כְּנוּפְיָא) have we assembled them for your individual benefit?—Part. pass. מְכַנַּף. Ber. 58ᵇ כמאה ... דמְכַנְּפֵי like one hundred stars ... collected in one spot, opp. מבדרי. Gitt. 20ᵃ, v. infra.—3) (corresp. to קְפַל) *to fold, crease.* Sabb. 147ᵃ אדעתא דלכַנּוּפֵי with the intention of creasing.

Ithpa. אִתְכַּנַּף, *Ithpe.* אִתְכְּנֵיף, אִיכְּנֵיף 1) *to be assembled, to meet, join.* Targ. Cant. VIII, 7.—Taan. 23ᵇ, v. supra.—2) *to be compressed.* Gitt. 20ᵃ כַּנּוּפֵי מְכַנֵּיף (ed. Rashi מִכַּנַּף), v. חֲרַץ.

כָּנָף (mostly) m. (b. h.; preced. wds.; cmp. גַּף II) [*bend,*] 1) *wing, wing-feather.* Kel. XVII, 14 כְּנַף הנוז things made of feathers of the sea-eagle; a. e.—*Du.* כְּנָפַיִם, *pl.* כְּנָפִים, כְּנָפוֹת. Ib. Toh. I, 2. Ḥull. III, 4 נמרטו כְּנָפֶיהָ if the wing-feathers are plucked out, v. נוֹצָה. Ib. 7 כל שיש לו ארבע ... כ׳ ... וּכְנָפָיו וכ׳ that (locust) which has four feet and four wings ..., and whose wings cover the larger portion of its body (is clean); a. fr.—2) *border, lap.* Sifrê Num. 115 בְּן הכ׳, v. גְּדִילָה II. Ib. מצות כ׳ the law concerning the borders of garments (Num. XV, 38).—*Pl.* as ab. Lev. R. s. 18; Koh. R. to XII, 3 (ref. to הרואות ib.) אלו כַּנְפֵי הריאה those are the laps (extreme ends) of the lungs. Ḥull. 45ᵃ עד כנפי ריאה התחתונה to the borders of the lowest lung (of the animal suspended by its feet).—Euphem. for *a woman's lap (pudenda).* Yeb. 4ᵃ; 49ᵃ (expl. Deut. XXIII, 1) כ׳ שראה אביו the lap which his father has seen, i. e. any woman with whom his father has had sexual connection.—3) *cover.* Pesik. Zakh., p. 29ᵃ; Pesik. R. s. 12; Tanḥ. Ki Thetsé 11 (ref. to יִכָּנֵף, Is. XXX, 20) ... כל זמן כ׳ מכסה וכ׳ as long as the seed of Amalek survives, it is as if a cover hid the face (of Divinity) &c.—4) (*pl.*) *hands, arms;* (of animals) *shoulders, fore-legs.* Pes. VII, 11 (84ᵃ) ראשי כ׳ the cartilaginous tops of the fore-legs. Y. Naz. VI, 55ᶜ bot. (ref. to Num. VI, 19) בין שיש לו כ׳ וכ׳ whether or not he has hands (to receive the offerings; Bab. ib. 46ᵇ כַּפַּיִם). Tosef. Dem. II, 11 מקבלין לכ׳ we accept a *ḥaber* (v. חָבֵר), if he promises to observe levitical cleanness of hands; Bekh. 30ᵇ. Y. Dem. II, 23ᵃ top מקריבין לכ׳. Ib. כ׳ מדפות וכ׳ the laws concerning hands, &c., v. מִדָּף.—אלישע בעל כ׳ one Elisha, a *ḥaber* observing cleanness of hands. Y. Ber. I, 4ᶜ bot.; Sabb. 49ᵃ; 130ᵃ (legendary origin of the surname).—Lev. R. s. 32 בעל כ׳ the winged angel.—5) *curved attachments, handles* &c. Kel. XI, 6; Tosef. ib. B. Mets. I, 7, v. סִימְפּוֹנְיָא. Kel. XIV, 4 הכ׳ המקבלות וכ׳ the curves on the harness for holding the reins; ib. 5 כ׳ העשוים לנוי for ornament.—Trnsf. כנפי השכינה or כ׳ *divine protection;* תחת כ׳ הש׳ under the wings of divine Majesty, i. e. *belief and faith in God, Jewish religion.* Lev. R. s. 2 פושטין ... להכניסו תחת כ׳ הש׳ we must reach out a hand to him (the proselyte) in order to take him in &c. Mekh. B'shall., Amalek, s. 2 לאבד .. מתחת כְּנָפֶיךָ to lead thy people away from the faith in thee.—Ruth R. to II, 12; a. fr.

כְּנַף II, כַּנְפָא ch. same, 1) *wing, lap.* Targ. I Kings VI, 24; a. fr.—Targ. Zech. VIII, 23; a. fr.—B. Mets. 85ᵃ בכַנְפֵיה דרבו in the lap of Rabbi's garment. Sabb. 5ᵃ פשיט כנפיה וכ׳ he spread the lap of his garment and received it. B. Bath. 12ᵇ בכנפיה דאבוה on her father's lap. Ib. 58ᵃ בכַנְפַּהּ דשרה in Sarah's lap; a. fr.—[Euphem. Targ. Deut. XXIII, 1, v. preced.]—Trnsf. *protection.* Targ. II Esth. IX, 14.—*Pl.* כַּנְפֵּי, כַּנְפַיָּא, כַּנְפִין. Ib. Targ. Ez. XVII, 3. Targ. O. Num. XV, 38; a. fr.—[כַּנְפָּתָא, constr. כַּנְפַּת. Targ. Y. II ib., emend. by Bxt., ed. צִיצַּת.]—2) בַּת כַּנְפָא name of an unclean *bird.* Targ. O. Deut. XIV, 13 (h. text הראה).

כָּפָר m., pl. כְּפָרִים, כפ׳=next w. Y. Meg. I, 70ᵃ bot., v. next w.

כְּנָרָא, כי׳ I m. ch. name of *a shrubby tree, Christ's-thorn* or *lote* (Greek adapt. κόνναρος, v. Löw, Pfl., p. 283 sq.). Meg. 6ᵃ Kinnereth is Ginnosar (Gennesareth) and why is it called Kinnereth משום דמתיקי פירהא כב׳ Ar. (v. Rabb. D. S. note 3) because its fruits are as sweet as those of the Kinnara; [Var. quot. in Ar. כי קלא דכ׳ as sweet as the sound of the *lute*; Ms. O. בקוליא דכ׳]. Y. ib. I, 70ᵃ bot. (hebr.) שהן מגדלות כִּינָּרִים because they produce *Kinnars.* Pes. 111ᵇ טולא דכנירא Ms. M. (ed. דכמיא, Ms. M. 2 דכנארא; Ms. O. דכנרא, v. Rabb. D. S. a. l. note) the shade of a *K.* B. Bath. 48ᵇ תלא לפאפי אכר׳ Tabi suspended P. on a Kinnara (to force him to sell a field of his; for oth. opin., v. comment.).—*Pl.* כִּינָּרֵי, כי׳. Ber. 40ᵇ רימין כ׳ Ar. a. Ms. F. (v. Rabb. D. S. a. l. note 30; ed. כנדי) *Rimin* (Dem. I, 1) means *K.*

כִּנָּרָא, כְּנָרָא II, *lute,* v. כִּנּוֹרָא.

כנריות, Gen. R. s. 45 Ar., v. כְּנֵרִיּוֹת.

כִּנֶּרֶת, כִּינֶ׳ (b. h.) pr. n. *Kinnereth* (Gennesareth), name of a town and of a lake in Galilee. Meg. 6ᵃ; Y. ib. I, 70ᵃ bot., v. כִּנָּרָא.

כָּנַשׁ=כָּנַס, *Hithpa.* הִתְכַּנֵּשׁ. Cant. R. to I, 3 מִתְכַּנְּשִׁין, v. כָּנַס.

כְּנַשׁ ch. (v. preced.) 1) *to gather, collect; to gather in.* Targ. Ex. XXXV, 1 (ed. Amst. כְּנַשׁ). Targ. Koh. II, 8. Targ. Is. XXIV, 22; a. fr.—Y. Maas. Sh. IV, end, 55ᶜ ליה את כ׳ thou shalt not harvest; a. fr.—2) (cmp. גבב) *to rake together, to sweep.* B. Mets. 85ᵃ קא כָּנְשָׁא ביתא Ms. M. (v. Rabb. D. S. a. l. note) was sweeping the house. Ḥull. 60ᵃ אתא ... כַּנְשֵׁיה לימא a blast of wind came and swept it (the store of provision) into the sea.

Pa. כַּנֵּישׁ same. Targ. Mic. II, 12; a. e.—Lev. R. s. 25 היא מְכַנְּשָׁא להון she calls the chickens together. Y. Ber. IX, end, 14ᵈ דִּמְכַנְּשִׁין, v. בְּדַר; a. e.

Af. אַכְנֵישׁ same. Targ. Ez. XI, 17 (ed. Lag. אַרְכֵּינֵשׁ *Pe.*); a. e.

Ithpa. אִתְכַּנַּשׁ, *Ithpe.* אִתְכְּנֵישׁ, אִתְכְּנֵשׁ *to be gathered, to be called in; to retire.* Targ. Jud. XII, 1 (ed. Wil. כ...) Targ. Gen. XXV, 8. Targ. Jer. XLVII, 6; a. fr.—Koh. R. to IX, 10 אִתְכַּנְּשׁוּן כל קרייתא וכ׳ all the towns (people) met to mourn for him. Tanḥ. Ki Thetsé 4 טב ליה לצדיקא דאי׳ בשלם (not לצדיקיא) it is better for the righteous man to be gathered in (die) in peace; Pesik. Zakh., p. 23ᵃ טב ליה לצדיקא דמִתְכְּנֵישׁ בשלם; Yalk. Ps. 868 טב ליה לתורא סבא דמִתְכְּנֵישׁ וכ׳.

כְּנִשָׁא, כְּ׳ f. (preced.) *gathering, people.*—*Pl.* כִּנְשָׁן, כְּ׳. Targ. O. Gen. XVII, 16 (Y. כְּנִשִׁין m.; h. text גוים).

כְּנִשְׁתָּא, v. כְּנִישְׁתָּא.

כַּנְתָּא f. (כנן) *winding, convolution,* 1) (sub. דמעיא) *ileum,* the third division of the small intestines. Hull. 48[b]; 113[a], v. הֲדוּרָא. Gitt. 69[a] כ׳ פּבירתא the ileum of a first-born.—Yalk. Koh. 976 (counting ten stations of the digestive process) מכרובא עבה לִכְנַת מעיא from the large winding (jejunum) to the ileum (corresp. to סני(א) דיבי, Lev. R. s. 3, a. Koh. R. to VII, 19). [Koh. R. l. c. בְּנַת מעיא some ed., read בנת.]—2) (cmp. אַמְבּוּרְקְלוֹן ,כָּרַךְ) *wrapper* of loosely woven matting. Succ. 20[b] חזו לכ׳ דפירי Ar. (ed. לכיני, Ms. M. לכני; v. Rabb. D.S. a.l. note) are fit for baling fruits. Keth. 105[b] כ׳ דפירי a bale of fruits, כ׳ דגלדני of small fish.

כנתי, a word in a charm formula. Yoma 84[a] כ׳ כ׳ קלירוס (Ms. M. קנגר קנדי קלירויס).

כס, Num. R. s. 1 כס נאה, read אַכְסַנְיָא, v. Tanh. B'midb. 2. —Sabb. 67[a], v. כַּסְכְּסֵירָה.

כַּס, כָּס, v. כְּסַס, כָּסַס a. נְכַס.

כֹּס, כָּס, *cup*, v. כּוֹס, כַּסָּא.

כְּסָא I *to cover*, v. כְּסִי II.

כְּסָא II *to reprehend*, v. כְּסַס a. כְּסַן.

כַּסָּא I, כָּסָא, כַּס m. ch.=h. כּוֹס, *cup, calyx.* Targ. Gen. XL, 11; a. fr.—Targ. I Kings VII, 26; a. fr.—Targ. II Sam. XII, 3 כָּסֵיהּ ed. Lag. (oth. כּוֹסֵיהּ).—Ber. 28[a], v. יְקָרָא. Ib. 51[b], v. בִּרְכְתָא. Y. Hag. II, 78[a] bot., v. בְּשׁוּרוּתָא. Ib. כ׳ דקיסא וכ׳ out of a cup of sharp-edged glass drink quickly (ere it cut your lip); [Y. Bets. II, 61[c] top סמא; Y. Maas. Sh. V, 56[c] top סבא, Meïri to Bets. 20[b] ססא]; a. fr.—*Pl.* כַּסִּין ,כַּסַּיָּיא ,כַּסֵּי, כָּס׳. Targ. Jer. XXXV, 5.—Y. Nidd. II, end, 50[b] כ׳ טיברייאי (not אה . . .) Tiberian glass cups (transparent). Pes. 110[a]; a. fr.—בֵּי (בית) כַּסַּיָּא=h. בית הכוסות, v. כּוֹס. Lev. R. s. 3; [Koh. R. to VII, 19 (of the human body) בית כסא, by mistake borrowed from Lev. R. l. c.; v. Yalk. Koh. 976].

כַּסָּא II m. (כָּסַס) 1) *fodder*, v. כִּיסְתָּא II.—2) *hash.* כ׳ דהרסנא, v. הַרְסָנָא.—*Pl.* כַּסֵּי. Ab. Zar. 38[a] ed.

כִּסֵּא m. (b. h.; an adapt. and contr. of כּוּרְסַיָּא) *bolsters, chair, throne.* Tosef. Bets. III, 11. Ib. 17 אין יוצאין בכִּסֵּא ed. Zuck. (Var. בכסא) you must not be carried out on a sedan chair (on Holy Days); Bets. 25[b]. Ib. כ׳ מה אתון ביה what is your opinion about carrying a person on a chair &c.?—Kel. XXII, 3 הכ׳ שלפני קתידרא the bolster in front of the cathedra (a kind of footstool). Ib. 4, v. חִפּוּי; a. fr. —כ׳ הכבוד the throne of Divine Majesty. Hag. 13[a]; a. fr.—כ׳ הדין the throne of Divine judgment; כ׳ רחמים mercy-seat. Lev. R. s. 29 אני עומד מכ׳ הדין וכ׳ I rise from the throne of judgment and seat myself on the throne of mercy; a. fr.—Euphem. בית הכ׳ *privy.* Tam. I, 1 בית הכ׳ של כבוד a chaste privy. Ber. 25[a]; a. fr.—*Pl.* כִּסְאוֹת, כִּסְּאוֹת, כִּסּ׳; with suff. כִּסְאֵי. Ex. R. s. 31; a. fr.—Tosef. Kel. B. Mets. X, 6 הכיסיות שבבסיכה (not הכ׳) the (stationary) seats in public courts. Pesik. R. s. 23-24 עמדו מִכִּסְאֵיהֶם arose from their thrones.—[Zab. IV, 4 כסאות, v. כֶּסֶת.]

כֶּסֶה, כֶּסֶא m. (כָּסָה I) *mark, distinction; marked, appointed time.* Lev. R. s. 29; Pesik. Bahod., p. 153[a] (ref. to Ps. LXXXI, 4) וכי כל החדשים אינן חדש אלא בכ׳ 'on the New Moon', are all other new moons no New Moons (festive days)?; but (therefore is added) *bakkesé*, on the distinguished (month), v. כָּסָה I. [Pirké d'R. El. ch. VII, end, a. Bets. 16[a] our w. is taken in the sense of *cover.*]

כְּסָאן, v. כְּסָן.

כְּסָאנִין, v. כִּיסְנִין ,כִּיסָנִין.

כְּסַבַּר, v. כּוּסְבַּר.

כַּסְדָּאָה, v. כַּשְׂדָּ׳.

כָּסָה, v. כֵּסֵא.

כֶּסֶה, v. כֶּסֶא.

כָּסָה, v. כסי.

כְּסוּ, v. כְּסוּתָא.

כִּסּוּחַ, v. כִּיס׳.

כְּסוּי, v. כְּסוּתָא.

כְּסוּיָא, כִּסּוּי, v. sub כִּיס׳.

כָּסוּל m. (denom. of כֶּסֶל) *an animal with a deformed hip.* Bekh. VI, 7 (40[a]) כ׳ שאחת מירכותיו גבוהה (Talm. ed. גבוהות, corr. acc.) a *kasul* is one whose one hip is higher than the other. Ib. 40[a] כ׳ שרגלו אחד וכ׳ a *k.* is he whose one foot is seated in the loin and the other over the loin; Tosef. ib. IV, 10 איזהו פסול (corr. acc.).

כְּסוּסְמָא, v. כִּיסְסְמָא.

כְּסוּסְטְרָא f. *balcony*, v. בְּצוֹצְרָה a. גְּזוּזְטְרָא.

כְּסוּפָא, v. כִּיס׳.

כסוריא, v. אַכְסוֹרְיָה.

כְּסוּת f. (b. h.; כָּסָה II) *cover, clothing.* B. Bath. 9[a] אין בודקין לכ׳ we must not investigate in the case of a poor man asking for clothes; Y. Peah VIII, 21[a], v. דָּקְדֵּק. Tam. I, 1 ומתכסין בכ׳ עצמן and covered themselves with their own (private) garments; a. fr.—[Y. Hag. II, end, 78[c] ואפר כ׳, read כְּפוּת, v. יָבַל.]

כְּסוּתָא, כְּסוּ, כְּסוּי f. ch. same. Targ. O. Ex. XXII, 8 כסו ed. Berl. (oth. ed. a. Y. כִּסּוּי *m.*). Ib. 25; a. fr.

כָּסַח (b. h.; cmp. כסס) *to cut down, clear* (of thorns, bushes &c.); *to trim.* Cant. R. to I, 1; Gen. R. s. 12; (Koh. R. to II, 12 כיסח *Pi.*). Gen. R. s. 49 למגל כּוֹסַחַת וכ׳ like a scythe cutting thorns and not being satisfied &c.; a. fr.—Part. pass. כָּסוּחַ, pl. כְּסוּחִים, כְּסוּחִין. Y. Maasr. III, 50[d] bot. קוֹצִין כ׳ כָּסַחְתִּי (not כסיחין) I cut mowed thorns, i. e. I only put to death doomed culprits; Pesik. B'shall., p. 92[a] כיסים כוסחים (corr. acc.), v. כּוֹס II.

Pi. כִּיסֵּחַ same. Kil. II, 5 אם נכש או כ׳ if he weeded or cut. Shebi. II, 10 אין מְכַסְּחִין you must not cut (trim) rice plants (in the Sabbath year). Y. Shek. V, beg. 48[c] הראשונים כִּיסְּחוּ וכ׳ . . . our predecessors sowed . . ., cleared . . ., yet we have nothing to eat, i. e. they did their utmost for the Law, but we do not profit by their labors. Sifra B'huck. Par. 2, ch. V כיסה, כיסח ed. Weiss (corr. acc.); a. e.

כְּסַח ch. same. Targ. O. Lev. XXV, 3, sq.; a. e.—Snh. 26[a]. [Y. Sabb. VI, end, 8[d] קריב למכסח, v. מוֹכְסָא.]

Pa. כַּסַּח same. Targ. Ps. LXXX, 13.

כָּסָה, כסי I (cmp. כסח) *to make incisions, mark, count.* *Part. pass.* כָּסוּי *marked, distinguished.* Pesik. R. s. 39 (ref. to Ps. LXXXI, 4, v. כֶּסֶא) מהו בכסא בחדש שהוא כ׳ (not כיסוי) what is *bakkesé?* In the month which is marked (v. infra).

Nif. נִכְסָה, *Nithpa.* נִתְכַּסֶּה *to be marked, distinguished.* Lev. R. s. 29 (ref. to Ps. l. c.) וכל החדשים אינן נִכְסִין אלא ליום חגנו are all other months (or New Moon Days) not marked?—But (it must be marked by) 'a festive day'; [read:] והלא ניסן חדש נִכְסָה ויש לו חג: חגו בפני עצמו (Ar. חדש ונתכסה . . .) but is not Nisan a marked month with a festival? (Answ.) Its festival is separate from it (not coinciding with the New Moon Day); אלא איזהו חדש כ׳ ויש לו חג וכ׳ but what month is there that is marked and has a festival, and that on the same day?; Pesik. Bahod., p. 153[a].

כֶּסֶא, כְּסֵי, v. כְּסַן.

כָּסָה, כסי II (b. h.) *to cover.*—Part. pass. כָּסוּי, f. כְּסוּיָה; pl. כְּסוּיִים, כְּסוּיִין; כְּסוּיוֹת. Gen. R. s. 52 אתם כְּסִיתֶם . . . . . . כְּסוּי עינים you have concealed from me the sight (of truth), therefore the son that you will raise will be of covered eyes (blind); Yalk. Gen. 91 כסות (corr. acc.); B. Kam. 93[a] הואיל וכִיסִּית . . . בנים כְּסוּיֵי עינים (v. Rabb. D. S. a. l. note). Y. Ter. VIII, 45[d] הַכְּסוּיִין (not הכיסוין) the covered liquids.

Pi. כִּסָּה, כִּיסָּה *to cover, hide.* Hull. VI, 4 שחט ולא כ׳ . . לְכַסּוֹת if one slaughters and fails to cover the blood, and another person sees it, he is bound to cover it. Pes. 119[a] (ref. to Is. XXIII, 18) זהו הַמְכַסֶּה דברים וכ׳ he who keeps secret the things which the Old of Days has covered (mysteries). B. Kam. l. c.; Gen. R. l. c., v. supra. Pesik. R. s. 26 מְכַסֶּה אני ממך shall I conceal it from thee?—Gen. R. s. 87 כִּסְּתָה פניה she covered her (the idol's) face. Ib. לא כ׳ עליהם הכתוב the Bible did not cover their guilt (v. חָפָה); a. fr.—Part. pass. מְכוּסֶּה, f. מְכוּסָּה; *pl.* מְכוּסִּים, מְכוּסִּין; מְכוּסּוֹת. Ib. s. 52 (ref. to Gen. XX, 16 [read:] עשאה מטרונה כסות עינים שהיא מכ׳ מן העין) he (Abimelech) made a matron of her (Sarah) (giving her) 'a cover of the eyes', by which she was protected from the gaze (of men). Pes. 54[b] שבעה . . . מכ׳ וכ׳ seven things are hidden from man; a. fr.—[Gen. R. s. 79, end מה את מכסה בי, read: מב׳, v. בְּסָא.—Sifra B'huck., Par. 2, ch. V כיסה, v. כָּסַח.]

Nif. נִכְסָה *to be covered, hidden.* Snh. II, 1 (18[a]; 19[a]) הן נִכְסִין...והוא נ׳ when they (who form the funeral cortege) are hidden from his view (when entering an alley), he (the high priest) appears; when they emerge, he disappears (in the alley). Cant. R. to II, 9 נראה וחוזר ונ׳ is visible and disappears again; Ruth. R. to II, 14; Pesik. Hahod., p. 49[b]. Num. R. s. 22 (play on נִכְסִים) נ׳ מזה וכ׳ they disappear from one and appear to the other; a. fr.

Hithpa. הִתְכַּסֶּה *to be covered, clothed.* Bets. 16[a] (ref. to בַּכֶּסֶה, Ps. LXXXI, 4) איזהו חג שהחדש מִתְכַּסֶּה בו what festival is that on which the new moon is hidden (seen only by a few)?; Pirké d'R. El. ch. VII, end ביום שמ׳ כולו on the day when the moon is entirely covered. Deut. R. s. 3 מתכ׳ משלו clothed himself at his (the fosterfather's) expense. Ib. כל . . . אוכל ומתכ׳ וכ׳ all that is spent on you for eating and clothing &c. Keth. V, 8 מִתְכַּסָּה, v. בְּלָאוֹת. Tam. I, 1 מִתְכַּסִּין, v. כְּסוּת; a. fr.

כְּסָא, כְּסֵי ch. same, *Part. pass.* כְּסֵי, f. כְּסָיָא *hidden.* Targ. I Sam. III, 1 כְּסֵי Bxt. (ed. כַּסֵּי, כְּסֵי; h. text יקר). Targ. II Kings VI, 8 (h. text פלני). Targ. Job XXVIII, 21. Targ. II Kings VI, 9 כְּסַן (h. text נְחִתִּים).

Pa. כַּסֵּי *to cover, hide, conceal.* Targ. O. Gen. XXXVIII, 15 (Y. כעיסה). Ib. XLVII, 18; a. fr.—*Part. pass.* מְכַסָּא *unknown, remote.* Targ. II Kings XIX, 2. Targ. O. Lev. IV, 13. Targ. II Sam. XIII, 2 (h. text ויפלא); a. e.—Sabb. 156[b] כַּסֵּי רישיך וכ׳ keep thy head covered in order that the fear of the Lord may rest upon thee. Ib. 125[a] לְכַסּוּיֵי בהו וכ׳ to cover a nuisance with it. Gen. R. s. 52, [read as:] Yalk. ib. 91 וכסי עיניך מינאי and close thine eye from upon me, i. e. take the indulgence money. Taan. 25[a] רקיע . . כסי פניך ולא אִיכַּסִּי 'cover thy face, O sky,' but the sky was not covered. Hull. 87[a] אפשר . . ומְכַסֵּי בחדא he may kill with one hand and cover (the blood) with the other; a. fr.

Ithpa. אִיכַּסֵּי, אִיתְכַּסֵּי *to be covered, hidden; to cover one's self; to conceal one's self, withdraw.* Targ. Y. Gen. XX, 16. Targ. Y. Lev. IV, 13. Targ. Gen. XVIII, 14 (h. text יפלא, v. supra); a. fr.—Targ. Ps. CXXXIX, 6 מִכַּסְיָא.—Taan. l. c., v. supra. Ib. 23[a] א׳ מעינא ונים וכ׳ he disappeared and slept seventy years. Keth. 63[a] שאילי . . . ואִיכַּסַּאי borrow some garments and dress thyself; a. fr.

כְּסָיָא, כַּסֵּי *hidden*, v. preced.—[כסי, Tosef. Kel. B. Mets. II, 9, v. כִּיסּוּי.]

כְּסַיָּאן, v. כְּסַן.

כסידא, Targ. Y. Ex. IX, 31, read: בְּסִירָא, v. בְּסַר II.

כְּסִימְנָא=כִּיסּוּי מָנָא, v. כִּיסּוּי.

כְּסִיָּיה f. (כָּסָה II) *covering*; כְּסִיַּית עינים *blindness.* Meg. 28[a] א״ת כסות אלא כ׳ ע׳ ed., v. כְּהוּת.

כְּסִיל m. (b. h.) 1) (a denom. of כֶּסֶל q. v.) [*one with thick loins, stout,*] 1) (cmp. טִפֵּשׁ) *fool, foolish, overbearing.* Y. Peah I, 15[b] bot.; Yalk. Ex. 415 (ref. to Prov. III, 26) דברים שאתה כ׳ בהם וכ׳ in things in which thou art foolish (ignorant), He will guard thy foot &c.—*Pl.* כְּסִילִים. Num. R. s. 16 (ref. to Prov. XXVI, 6) עשו עצמן כ׳ they (the spies) made fools of themselves.—2) *K'sil*, the constellation *Orion* (v. Winer, Reallex. s. v. Nimrod). Ber. 58b.

כְּסִילָא ch. same, 1) *fool.*—*Pl.* כְּסִילַיָּיא. Targ. Ps. XLIX, 11 (Bxt. *sing.*). Ib. XCIV, 8 (some ed. כְּסִילַי). [In Targ. mostly סכלא.]—2) *Orion.* Targ. Am. V, 8 (v. נִיפְלָא).—Ber. 58b כְּסָלָא (Ms. M. כּוּסְלָא, Ms. F. כִּיס׳).

כְּסִיסְטָא, כְּסוּס׳ (ξέστης, v. Sm. Ant. s. v.) *xestes, sextarius*, a dry and liquid measure (nearly a pint).—*Pl.* כְּסִיסְטָאוֹת, כְּסוּ׳. Gen. R. s. 4; Yalk. ib. 5. ['Rashi' reads גְּזוּזְטְרָאוֹת.]

כסיפא, v. כְּסְפְּיָא.

כְּסִיפוּתָא f. = כִּיסוּפָא. B. Mets. 22a משום כ׳ (Ms. M. מחמת כסופא, v. Kidd. 52b).

כְּסִיפְתָא, v. כְּסַפְתָּא.

כְּסִיקְבְיָא=כִּיסוּי קְבְיָא. Tosef. Kel. B. Mets. II, 9 some ed. (ed. Zuck. כסי קמיא).

כסירא, Targ. Y. Ex. IX, 31, v. כְּסַר II.

כְּסִיתָא f. (כְּסִי II) [*the covered, rare,*] 1) *coral*; 2) *coral-wood.* B. Bath. 80b, sq.; R. Hash. 23a, v. אַלְמוּג; Yalk. Is. 314 סכסיתא (corr. acc.). R. Hash. l. c. דבי ארמאי מסקן כ׳ the light ships (v. בּוּרְנִי) of the Romans are employed for fishing corals. Ib. (describing the diving process) .. וקטר בכ׳ and flax ropes are tied to the coral plants &c. Keth. 98a כ׳ דיתמי Var. in Rashi (ed. כיסתא) corals belonging to minor orphans.

***כְּסִיתָא** f. a phonetic rendition of קְשִׁיטָה q. v. Gen. R. s. 79 (corr. vers. after Ar. s. v. קשיטה) (they heard one woman say to another) אשאלי לי כְּסִיתְתָךְ (for קשיטתך, meaning to say מרגליתיך); (and furthermore) אפיק הדא כ׳ לִמְרִיעָא lead this *K'sitta* out to pasture (meaning to say אִימַּרְתָּא); [Ar. reads קשיט׳].

כְּסְכַּס, כֶּסֶךְ m. (transpos. of סכסך q. v.; cmp. גַּבְגַּב), *pl.* כַּסְכַּסִּים, כְּסָכִים *leather thongs* for crosswise fastening (cmp. b. h. עֹרוֹךְ a. נַעַל שָׂרֹךְ). Sabb. 138b הגוד בכְסָכָיו Ar. (Ms. O. בכַסְכַּסָּיו; ed. בכיסנא, read: בכיסכא; Ms. M. חגור בנסבא, read: הגוד בכסכא, v. Rabb. D. S. a. l.) it is permitted to stretch the milk (or wine) bag by its thongs, v. גּוֹד. Ib. 139b בכילה ובכְסָכֶיהָ Ar. (ed. ובכַסְכַּסֶּיהָ) wrapt in a bed-curtain with the thongs attached.

כִּסְכּוּס m. (next w.) *rubbing.* Zeb. 94b כיבוס דלית ליה כ׳ וכ׳ washing without rubbing is not called *kibbus*.

כִּסְכֵּס (v. כָּסַס) 1) *to rub, scour.* Nidd. IX, 7 וצריך לְכַסְכֵּס וכ׳ one must scour with these substances three times. Sabb. 141a מְכַסְכְּסוֹ מבפנים he may rub the mud off from the inside. Y. ib. VII, 10a bot. ובלבד שלא יְכַסְכֵּס provided that he does not rub.—2) *to chew, gnaw*, v. כָּסַס.

כַּסְכֵּס ch. same, *to rub, to polish.* Sabb. 140a כַּסְכּוּסֵי, v. כִּיתָּנִיתָא. M. Kat. 10b לְכַסְכּוּסֵי קירמי to gloss fine clothes by rubbing with a substance. Zeb. 94b top שכשוכי אין כסכוסי לא (quot. in Sh'ilt. d'R. Aḥai s. 86; ed. . . . שכשוך . . כיבוס) cleansing by rinsing is permitted, by rubbing is forbidden. [Sabb. 147a כגון כסכוסי מאנא דמחזר כמרזב Ms. M. a. Ar., a gloss, interpreting כיסי בבלייתא.]

כַּסְכַּס, v. כֶּסֶךְ.

כַּסְכְּסָיָיה m. pl. (v. preced.) *makers of confusion, of strife* (cmp. Is. XIX, 2), allegorical name of messengers from Sodom (Edom), v. בְּזִבְזִירָה. Sabb. 67a Ms. M. (ed. כס כסיא, read: כַּסְכְּסָיָא).

כסכסייך, a word in a charm formula (v. preced.). Sabb. 67a Ms. M. (missing in ed.).

כֶּסֶל c. (b. h.; כסס, cmp. חַרְצָא) 1) [*incision,*] *groin, loin.*—Bekh. 40a, v. כָּסוּל. Yalk. Gen. 133 (quot. fr. Midr. Vayisu) בכסא ימנית (corr. acc.) in the right loin.—*Pl.* כְּסָלִין, כְּסָלִים. Tosef. Bekh. IV, 10 [read:] כל שֶׁכְּסָלָיו יוצאין a *kasul* is one whose loins protrude. Sabb. 31b וי״ט להם חלב על הכ׳ Ar. (ed. כִּסְלָם) and yet have fat on the groins (are careless).—Trnsf. 2) (cmp. כּפש) *laziness, inactivity*; 3) *trust*; 4) *thought.* Yalk. Num. 742; Yalk. Ps. 819 quot. fr. Y'lamd. (v. Ar. s. v. כסל) מחשבתם וכ׳ . . . כִּסְלָם *kislam* (Ps. LXXVIII, 7) means their thought, as we read (Lev. III, 4, cmp. כִּלְיָה) 'that which is by the loins'; (oth. opin.) כיפשותן it means their inactivity, as it is said (Koh. IV, 5) &c.; (oth. opin.) בטחונן their trust as we read (Job XXXI, 24) &c.

כִּסְלָא I ch. same, 1) *ridge.* Ber. 6a (Ar. כִּסְלֵי *pl.*), v. אוּגְיָא.—2) *loin.*—*Pl.* כִּסְלִין. Targ. Ps. XXXVIII, 8 כִּסְלַי (Regia כַּפְלַי).

כִּסְלָא II, v. כְּסִילָא.

כִּסְלֵיו, כִּסְלֵו (b. h.; v. Schr. KAT[2], p. 380) *Kislev*, the ninth month of the Jewish calendar, of thirty or twenty-nine days, beginning between the third of November and the first of December, and ending between the third of December and the second of January. Targ. Zech. VII, 1; a. e.—Sabb. 21b. Meg. Taan. ch. IX.

כִּסְמָה, v. כּוּסֶ׳.

כְּסַן (cmp. כָּסַס) [*to scrape*, cmp. חסד II,] *to rebuke, chastise.* Targ. Y. Deut. XXI, 18; a. e., v. infra.

Pa. כַּסֵּן, כַּסֵּין same. Targ. Ps. XXXVIII, 2; a. fr.

Af. אַכְסֵין same. Ib. XVII, 4. Ib. CXVIII, 18 מִכְסְנָא אַכְסְנַנִי (some ed. מִכְסָא); a. fr.

כִּיסְנָא, כְּסָאן, כֶּסֶן m. (preced.; cmp. חרס I) *mud, mire* (from its white and glistening surface). Targ. Ps. XL, 3 ed. Lag. (ed. סיין, סאין, סכן; Regia כַּסְיָאן). Targ. Job VIII, 11 כיסנא ed. Lag. (ed. בּיסנא, בִּצָּא). Ib. XLI, 22 כְּסָאן Ms. (ed. כַּסָּאן, סָאן), v. סִין.

כִּסְנִין, כְּסָנִין, v. פִּיסְנִין, פִּיסְנִין.

כָּסַס 1) *to cut, grind, chew, nibble.* Tosef. Ber. IV, 6 הכּוֹסֵס חטים he who chews wheat grains; Ber. 37ª; a. fr. —Num. R. s. 11 (ref. to אש אכלת, Ex. XXIV, 17) ... שבע היו כּוֹסְסוֹת זו בזו seven partitions (strata) of fire were eating into one another; Pesik. Haḥod. p. 45ª; Pesik. R. s. 15 בוכסות (corr. acc.); v. כָּבַס.—2) (b. h.) *to make incisions, to mark, count.* Mekh. Bo. s. 3; Pes. 61ª; Y. ib. V, 32ª bot., v. נָכַס.

Pilp. כִּסְכֵּס *to chew* &c. Tanḥ. Vayigg. 3 מְכַסְכֵּס בשיניו cut (the bronze peas) with his teeth.—V. סַכְסֵךְ II.

Nithpa. נִתְכַּסְכֵּס, נִיכ׳ *to be gnawed at* (by fire), *be charred.* Y. Bets. IV, 62ᶜ bot. בשביל שלא תִּכַּסְכֵּס (prob. to be read תתכ׳) that it (the log) may not catch fire.

כְּסַס ch. same, 1) *to cut, chew.* Yoma 81ᵇ; Ber. 36ᵇ כַּס פילפלי וכ׳ if one chewed pepper on the Day of Atonement. Meg. 7ᵇ בעאי לְמִיכַס וכ׳ I should have liked to chew the plate after it; Yalk. Esth. 1059 דאִיכְסִיסָה (not דאיב׳). —2) [*to cut* or *scratch off, peel, diminish,* (v. P. Sm. 1777),] *to rebuke, chastise* (v. כְּסַן). Targ. Prov. IX, 8 תְּכוּס (ed. Lag. תְּכִיס *Af.*).

Af. אֲכִיס, אַכֵּס 1) *to give to chew.* Keth. 77ª אַכְסוּהוּ שערי וכ׳ give El. barley to chew (as to an animal, i. e. he is an ignoramus). Ib. על דא אכסוה וכ׳ on account of this (opinion), they gave El. barley to eat in Babylonia.—2) *to rebuke, chastise.* Targ. Prov. l. c., v. supra. Ib. XXVIII, 23.

כָּסַף (b. h.) *to peel, whiten* (cmp. חָסַף).—Part. pass. כָּסוּף, pl. כְּסוּפִים *bright.* Sifré Deut. 13 וותיקים כ׳ distinguished (of position), bright of intellect; ib. Num. 92 וכסופים.

Hif. הִכְסִיף 1) *to grow pale, fade, wither.* Pes. III, 5 (expl. שיאור) כל שהִכְסִיפוּ פניו כאדם וכ׳ a dough the surface of which becomes pale and wrinkled, like (the sight of) a man whose hair (שֵׂעָר) stands up from fright. Nidd. 47ª משיַּכְסִיף ראש וכ׳ when the centre of the oblate portion of the breast begins to be wrinkled; Tosef. ib. VI, 4 משיִּכָּסֵף (*Nif.*). Sabb. 34ᵇ ה׳ התחתון when the lower horizon becomes pale (is no longer red); Y. Ber. I, 2ᵇ bot.—Pes. 39ª פניו מַכְסִיפִין the leaves look faded (and curled); a. e.—2) *to deteriorate, fall in value,* opp. השביח (cmp. חָסַר). Arakh. 30ª וה׳ ועמד על מנה and fell until it was worth only one Manah. Keth. 80ᵇ שמא תַּכְסִיף the soil may deteriorate (through neglect); a. e.—3) *to put to shame; to frighten, to alarm.* Ex. R. s. 35 (play on כֶּסֶף, I Chr. XXIX, 4) שהיה מַכְסִיף כל הזהבים it alarmed all gold-workers (emptying their shops); Cant. R. to III, 10; Y. Yoma IV, 41ᵈ top שהיה מ׳ בעד וכ׳ spread alarm among all the shops of &c.

Nif. נִכְסַף *to grow pale* &c., v. supra.

כְּסַף I, **כְּסִיף** ch. same, *to feel ashamed, frightened.* Targ. Y. Num. XII, 14 (h. text חכלם); a. e.—Arakh. 16ᵇ דלִיכְסוֹף זרעיה וכ׳ that the seed of Rab should be put to shame through me. Taan. 22ª וּכְסִיפָא להו מילתא וכ׳ Ms. M. 2 a. Rashi (Ms. M. 1 only וכסיפא להו, ed. ואִכְּסִיפוּ *Ithpe.*) and the gentlemen (you) felt abashed to tell us; a. fr.—[Targ. Ps. XLI, 7 יכסף some ed., read: יִכְנַף, v. כְּנַף I.]

Pa. כַּסֵּיף, *Af.* אַכְסֵיף 1) *to frighten; to put to shame.* Targ. Ps. XLIV, 10; a. fr.—Kidd. 81ª כַּסִּיפְתִּינָן (כַּסְפָּ׳) thou didst frighten us (by a false alarm). Ḥag. 5ª וכַסְּפְתֵּיה and thou didst put him to shame; Koh. R. end וכַסִּיפְתֵּיה. Sabb. 3ᵇ דאי לאו... כספתיה וכ׳ for if he were not a great man, thou mightst have put him to shame, for he might have given thee an inappropriate reply. Hor. 13ᵇ מַכְסְפִיתוּ לי Ms. M. (ed. כסיפיתנך, corr. כַּסִּיפְתּוּנַן) you might have put me to shame; a. e.—2) *to reduce in value, to cause deterioration.* Keth. 104ᵇ מְכַסְפִי (or מַכְסְפִי) they (the heirs) will neglect it (instead of improving).—[3) *to feel ashamed.* Targ. Ps. LXXIV, 21 מְכַסְפָא (prob. to be read: מְכַסְפָא or מְכַסְּפָא, part. pass.).]

Ithpa. אִתְכַּסַּף, אִיכַּ׳, *Ithpe.* אִתְכְּסַף, אִיכְּסִיף *to be made pale, to be frightened, to be put to shame.* Targ. Job VI, 20; a. e.—Kidd. l. c. טוטב תִּיכַּסְפוּ . . . . ולא תיכספו מינך וכ׳ it is better that you of the house of Amram be frightened through me in this world, than that you should be ashamed of me (as a sinner) in the world to come. B. Bath. 111ª; Ab. Zar. 36ª איכ׳ he felt alarmed. Taan. 25ª איכַּסְפָא ועיילא וכ׳ (missing in Ms. M.) she felt abashed and went &c.; a. fr.

כֶּסֶף m. (b. h.; preced. wds.) *silver*; (sub. מעה) *a silver piece, M'ah* (one sixth of a Denar, v. Zuckerm. Jüd. Münz. p. 15; p. 33, note 203); in gen. *money, value.* Kidd. I, 1 בכ׳ by (handing to her) an object of value. Yeb. 63ᵇ שמזונותיו תלויין בכַסְפּוֹ whose livelihood depends on his money (a money-lender). Shebu. VI, 1 הטענה שתי כ׳ the claim must amount to no less than two M'ah. Tosef. Keth. XIII (XII), 3 כ׳ בבל the Babylonian silver standard; כ׳ א״י the Palestinean &c. Ib. כ׳ שדיברה... זו היא כ׳ צורי זה ירושלמי wherever the Torah speaks of *Kesef* (as fines), it must be paid according to the Tyrian standard ... that is the Jerusalem *kesef* (eight times the provincial *kesef* כ׳ מדינה, v. Zuckerm. l. c.); a. v. fr.—*Pl.* כְּסָפִים. B. Mets. 42ª; Pes. 31ᵇ כ׳ אין להם שמירה וכ׳ coins given in trust are not duly guarded unless they are buried in the ground. Y. Yoma IV, beg. 41ᵇ בשלשה . . . . ובכ׳ by three methods was the land of Israel divided, by lots, by the Urim and Tummim, and according to the value of property; a. e.

כְּסַף II, **כַּסְפָּא** I ch. same. Targ. Gen. XX, 16. Ib XLIV, 8; a. fr.—Y. Kidd. I, 58ᵈ יַקִּירָא. Y. Bicc. III, 65ᵈ top מיתמני בכ׳ appointed to office for money. B. Kam. 87ª אפחתה מכַסְפַּהּ Ms. M. he lessened her value; a. fr.—*Pl.* כַּסְפַּיָּא. Targ. Gen. XLII, 25; 35.—Y. Bicc. l. c. לא בכ׳ אתמני was it not through gifts of money that he was appointed?

כַּסְפָּא II (in Nabatean dialect)=חַסְפָּא. Y. Ned. I, 37ª a. e., v. חַסְפָּא II.

כַּסָּף or **כַּסְפִי** m. (denom. of כֶּסֶף) *silver-smith.*—*Pl.* כַּסָּפִין, כַּסָּפִים. Succ. 51ᵇ. Cant. R. to V, 5.

כָּסִפְיָא (b. h.) pr. n. pl. *Casifia.* Lev. R. s. 5 (ref. to ארץ רחבת ידים, Is. XXII, 18) זו כ׳ (some ed. כסיפא, v. Rashi to Is. l. c.) that means the exile to C.

כְּסִיפְ׳, כִּסְפְּתָא f. (denom. of כַּסְפָּא) *money-chest.* B. Kam. 62ª. Hull. 133ᵇ.

כספתיאס, v. אכספטיאס.

כסרא, Targ. Job XVIII, 13 ed. Lag., read: בִּסְרָא or כִּבְסְרָא *as meat*, a gloss to חִקּוּק משכיה.

כֶּסֶת f. (b. h.; denom. of כִּיס) 1) *bag, bolster, cushion.* Mikv. X, 2 הכר והכ׳ של עור mattress and pillow cases of leather; כ׳ עגולה a round cushion (closed all around). Ber. VIII, 3; Tosef. ib. VI (V), 3 על הכ׳ on the cushion (whereon the diner reclines); a. fr.—*Pl.* כְּסָתוֹת. Gitt. 56^a. Kil. IX, 2; a. fr.—כִּיס׳, כְּסִיּוֹת. Tosef. Zab. IV, 4 מוטל על ה׳ כ׳ stretched on five (separated) bolsters; Zab. IV, 4 (Talm. ed. כסאות, ed. Dehr. כסיות).—2) (trnsf.) *thick flesh.*—*Pl.* כְּסָתוֹת. Bekh. 45^a כ׳ calves. Gen. R. s. 17; Koh. R. to III, 19 כ׳ לתחתיתו thick flesh of the ischium; Yalk. Koh. 969 כסות (corr. acc.).—3) חכ׳, *Hakkeseth*, surname of one Ben Tsitsith. Gitt. l. c. [כסת, Sifra B'ḥuck. Par. 2, ch. V, v. כָּסַת.]

כעבים, כעבן, v. כַּעַךְ.

כָּעוּס m. (part. pass. of כָּעַס) *an excited serpent.* Sabb. 62^b (play on תעכסנה, Is. III, 16) ומכניסות ... כארס בכ׳ they caused lust to seize their (the men's) hearts (as hot as) as the venom of the excited serpent; (older eds. כארס נחש כעוס; Ms. O. כא׳ של עכנה, Ms. M. כאש בנעורת); Yoma 9^b; Yalk. Is. 264.—V. כָּעַס.

כְּעִירוּת f. (כָּעַר) *ugliness, repulsiveness.* Y. Gitt. IX, end, 50^d אוּף היא עצמה מביאה לידי כ׳ even this very thing (neglect of toilet) will make her repulsive (in her husband's eyes); Sifra M'tsora, end (נכנס הדבר לידי איבה). Esth. R. to I, 3 (opp. נוֹי).

כַּעַךְ m., *pl.* כַּעֲכִים, כַּעְכִין (=כעבע, transpos. of עכבך, formed like כֶּסֶף; cmp. כַּבָּא) [*teeth,*] *pronged and lengthy unleavened cakes.* Tosef. Ḥall. I, 7 עשאה כ׳ if he shaped 'the dogs' dough' into prongs, opp. לימודין; Y. ib. I, end, 58^a כעבין (corr. acc.); Ber. 38^a top כעכים a. לימודין Ms. M. (ed. כעב׳ a. כלימודין). Pes. 48^b.

כַּעֲכָא, pl. כַּעֲכֵי same. Ber. 42^a top ריפתא כ׳ Ar. (ed. only ריפתא, Ms. F. כעכי ריפתא; Var. in Ar. כַּכֵּי).

כעכע, v. כַּעְכַּע.

כְּעַן (contr. of כְּעִידָּן, v. כְּדוּן) *now.* Targ. O. Num. XXIV, 4; 6 (Y. כדון, h. text עתה). Targ. II Sam. III, 8 מכ׳ (h. text היום); a. fr.—Cant. R. to I, 1 הוינה כד הוינא ברם כ׳ וכ׳ I was (king) when I was, but now I am no more.

כְּעֶנֶת adv. (עִנֵּי) *correspondingly,* וכ׳ *and so forth,* i. e. and as the corresponding titles may be. Ezra IV, 10; a. e.—Ib. 17 וּכְעֶת.

כָּעַס (b. h.) [*to be dark, hot,* cmp. חמץ,] 1) *to be angry, displeased.* Ber. 61^b top, v. כָּבֵד III. Tem. 16^a (play on עַכְסָה) כל ... כּוֹעֵס על וכ׳ whoever saw her became displeased with his own wife. Ned. 22^a, a. fr. כל הכועס whoever allows himself to be carried away by his wrath. Ex. R. s. 45 מטרונה שֶׁכָּעֲסָה על וכ׳ a matron (queen) that was angry with the king's daughter; a. fr.—Part. pass. כָּעוּס, f. כְּעוּסָה; *pl.* כְּעוּסִים, כְּעוּסוֹת. Ib. כשיהיו פניך כ׳ וכ׳ when thou shalt be angry, I shall conciliate thee &c.; (Tanḥ. Ki Thissa 27 כשאהיה אני בכעס); a. e.—V. כָּעוּס.—*2) *to grow hot* in the stomach, *to ferment, swell.* Gitt. 70^a לכשתִּכְעוֹס תעמוד על מלואה Ar. (ed. מילואך) when it (the food) swells, it will just fill the capacity of thy stomach.

Hif. הִכְעִיס *to provoke to anger.* Deut. R. s. 3. שהם עתידים לְהַכְעִיס אותי that they are going to provoke me (through idolatry). Ab. V, 2 היו מַכְעִיסִין וכ׳ were constantly provoking (the Lord). Snh. 27^a, a. fr. לְהַכְעִיס in a spirit of defiance, v. מוּמָר; a. fr.—Imper. אַכְעִיס (for הכעיס). Ruth R. end (ref. to Ps. IV, 5) ארגיז יצרך ... א׳ יצרך ולא תחטא let thy tempter rage, but sin not; but the Rabbis say, arouse thy (good) inclination to indignation, and thou shalt not sin. [Midr. Till. to Ps. l. c. אַכְחִישׁ ... ואל יחטיאך weaken thy tempter (by ascetics) &c.; Yalk. Ps. 627;—Pesik. Shubah, p. 158^a אכופס, corr. acc.]

כְּעֵיס, כְּעַס ch. same. Targ. Ps. CXII, 10.—Y. Ber. VII, 11^b bot. שמע .. מלכא וכ׳ King Jannai heard of it and became angry; Gen. R. s. 91; a. fr.—[Targ. Y. Gen. XXXVIII, 15 כְּעִיסַת אפין angry-looking, morose (h. text כסתה פניה); prob. a. corrupt. of כְּסִיאַת, and רחים, at the end of the sentence, to be read חכים; cmp. Gen. R. s. 85].

Af. אַכְעֵס *to provoke to anger;* א׳ (עובדא) קדם *to act provokingly, defiantly against.* Targ. Y. II Deut. XXXII, 19. Ib. 21.—Esth. R. introd. עובדיהון וכ׳ ... מַאַכְעֲסוּ when the beloved children (Israel) defied &c.; (Yalk. Esth. 1044; Yalk. Job 920 ארגיזו).

כַּעַס m. (b. h.; preced.) *anger, grief.* Tosef. Yeb. VI, 6 היה לה כ׳ מבעלה if she had been living on bad terms with her husband; Yeb. 42^b; Keth. 60^b בבית בעלה; Erub. 47^a עם כ׳. Ex. R. s. 45 כשאהיה בכ׳ וכ׳, v. כָּעַס. Ab. IV, 18 אל ... בשעת כַּעְסוֹ do not try to pacify thy neighbor while he is excited. Sifré Num. 157, v. כְּלָל; a. fr.

כַּעְסָא ch. same. Targ. Y. II Deut. XXXII, 19. Ib. 27.

כָּאַר, כָּעַר (cmp. כָּעַס) *to be dark, ugly, repulsive* (cmp. אוּכְמָא).—Part. pass. כָּאוּר, כָּעוּר; f. כְּעוּרָה; *pl.* כְּעוּרִים, כְּעוּרִין; כְּעוּרוֹת, כְּא׳ a) *ugly, ungainly.* Gen. R. s. 36 לפיכך ... כ׳ ומפוחם therefore shall this man (thou) be ugly and black. B. Kam. IX, 4 (100^b) צבעו כ׳, v. כְּלְכּוּס. Esth. R. to I, 12 אם רואין אותי כ׳ if they find me ungainly. Cant. R. to V, 11; a. fr.—b) *unbecoming, indecent.* Y. Keth. VII, 31^c top כא׳ הדבר תצא that is indecent conduct, and cause for divorce; (Yeb. 24^b, sq. מכוער). Gen. R. s. 60 שכ׳ לאיש וכ׳ for it is unbecoming for a man to walk behind a woman.—c) (cmp. חָוַר) *not evident, strange, implausible.* Hull. 115^b; 117^a; Kidd. 9^b כעורה זו ששנה וכ׳ is what R... taught to be rejected?—Tosef. Kel. B. Bath. II, 2 כ׳ מזו נימא וכ׳ something more strange than this (or more inappropriate to be used as a seat) did R . . . declare unclean.

Pi. כִּיעֵר *to make* or *declare repulsive.*—Part. pass. מְכוֹעָר, f. מְכוֹעֶרֶת; *pl.* מְכוֹעָרִין, מְכוֹעָרוֹת=כָּעוּר &c. Keth. 105^a מ׳ הדיין וכ׳ contemptible is the judge who receives fees for giving judgment. Yeb. 24^b, sq., v. supra. Yoma 86^a כמה מכ׳ דרכיו how mean are his ways!; a. fr.

Hithpa. הִתְכָּעֵר *to appear ugly, become ungainly.* Gen. R. s. 17 הִתְכָּעַרְתִּי בעיניו I appeared repulsive to him. Ib. s. 45 מִתְכָּעֶרֶת ומתעזבת she becomes ungainly and is neglected. Cant. R. to II, 14 מתכ׳ ומתעזבת, v. הָעַב.

כְּעַר ch. same; *Pa.* כַּעֵר, part. pass. מְכַעַר, f. מְכַעֲרָא *repulsive, ugly.* Nah. III, 6 (h. text כראי).—Keth. 60ᵇ bot. בנר מְכַעֲרֵי (not מכוערי) ugly children (differ. from אוכמי).

כְּעַת, v. כְּעֶנֶת.

כ״ף *Kaf,* the eleventh letter of the Alphabet. Lev. R. s. 19, v. בר״ח; a. e.—*Pl.* כָּפִין. Sabb. 103ᵇ, v. בר״ח.

כַּף, כַּף־, v. כָּפַף, כְּפַף.

כַּף, v. כֵּיף.

כַּף c. (b. h.; כָּפַף) [*something arched, hollow,*] 1) *palm of the hand, hand.*—*Du.* כַּפַּיִם. Y. Ber. I, 3ᶜ bot., v. חָטַף. Naz. 46ᵇ, v. כָּנַף; a. fr.—נשא כ׳ *to raise the hands, to pronounce the priestly benediction.* Ber. V, 4 לא ישא את כַּפָּיו must not pronounce &c.; a. fr.—2) *sole of the foot. Du.* as ab. Hull. 70ᵇ מהלכי כ׳ animals walking on soles (having no split hoofs, Lev. XI, 27).—Trnsf. *glove; sole of the shoe.* Kel. XXVI, 3 כַּף לוקטי(ם) קוצים (R. S. כפלוקטי) the thorn-pickers' glove. Tosef. ib. B. Bath. IV, 5 רוב כַּף אחת, the larger portion of one sole; כל כַּף אחת the whole of &c.—3) *the crest* (fleshy elevation) *over the genitals.* Tosef. Nidd. VI, 4, sq. עד שתפשט את הכף (Var. משתתפשט) when the crest (of the girl) begins to flatten; Y. Yeb. I, 2ᵈ bot. עד שתתפשט הכַּף; Y. Snh. VIII, beg. 26ᵃ משתפשט הכ׳ (of a male); Nidd. 47ᵃ, sq. נתמעך הכ׳ the crest grows lower. Ib. 52ᵇ אחת על הכ׳ one hair on the crest; a. e.—4) *pan, censer.* Tam. V, 4 (containing the בָּזִךְ). Ib. VII, 2 כף וכסויה the censer and its lid; a. fr.—*Pl.* כַּפּוֹת. Num. R. s. 14; a. e.—5) *spoon, mason's trowel* &c. Kel. XIII, 2; 4; a. fr. Sabb. VIII, 5 כ׳ סיד, expl. ib. 80ᵇ כ׳ של סיידין the plasterers' trowel.—*Pl.* כַּפִּין, כַּפִּים. Midd. III, 4 כפין של ברזל Ar. (ed. כפים, Var. כפים) iron trowels.—6) (with, or without מאזנים) *scale of the balance.* Ab. II, 8. Pesik. Aḥărê, p. 167ᵃ כ׳ עונות וכ׳ the scale of sins on the one side, and that of merits on the other; והקב״ה מטה לכ׳ זכות and the Lord bends (the balance) towards the scale of merits. Ab. I, 6, v. זכות; a. fr.—*Du.* כַּפַּיִין, כַּפַּיִים. Tosef. Kel. B. Mets. II, 5 (ed. Zuck. כיפין, read: כפיין).—7) *shore, banks* (v. כֵּיפָא). Num. R. s. 13, v. חַף.—*Pl.* כַּפִּים, constr. כַּפֵּי. Lam. R. introd. (R. Hăn. 3) (transl. גיא המלח, II Chr. XXV, 11) כ׳ המלח the salt shores.

כַּף, כַּפָּא I ch. same, 1) *palm, hand.* Targ. Y. Gen. III, 19.—*Pl.* כַּפַּיָא. Targ. Ps. XCVIII, 8 (v., however, Num. R. s. 13, s. v. חַף).—2) *border, shore,* v. כֵּיפָא.—3) *bundle, sheaf.* Snh. 26ᵇ bot. חד גנב כ׳ Ar. (v. Rabb. D. S. a. l. note 6, Var. in Ar. חומת כ׳, v. חומת; ed. קבא דשערי) one stole a sheaf.—*Pl.* כַּפִּין (כיפי). Y. Sabb. III, 5ᵈ bot. מיתן תלתא כ׳ וכ׳ to bring three bunches (of twigs) and put dishes upon them. Gitt. 86ᵇ דבינר כיפי, v. דִּידְבָא. Pes. 40ᵃ, v. חֲפַף. Ned. 48ᵇ top כר׳ דכיתנא flax bunches, v. שְׁמַט; a. e.—Ib. bot. דשדיא בכיפי, v. כְּפִילָא.—4) *top branch* of palm trees (v. כִּיפָּה).—*Pl.* כַּפֵּי. Succ. 32ᵃ ואימא תרתי כ׳ דתמרי perhaps *kappoth* (Lev. XXIII, 40) means two tops of palm trees?—5) *pan, spoon* &c. Pes. 28ᵃ, v. חֲטַט I. Sabb. 142ᵇ מנח כ׳ אכיפי (Ms. M. כיפא) placed a ladle on a pile of sheaves. Hull. 54ᵃ מאי כ׳ what *kappa* do you mean?—כ׳ דידא pan of the fore foot (shoulder), כ׳ דמוחא *scull.*—6) *shoulder* (also of human beings). B. Bath. 96ᵇ top אכ׳ Ms. M. a. Ar. (ed. אעַבתפא); Sot. 34ᵃ bot. בכ׳ Ar. (ed. לכתפיה); Taan. 23ᵇ אחד כַּפֵּיה Ar. (ed. כתפיה), v. כַּתְפָא.—Sot. 6ᵇ . . . אטו בכַפָּה תלי לה Ar. (ed. בכיפה) do the young priests (that guard the woman) suspend her by her shoulder (Rashi: by her cap), i. e. can they watch all her movements?

כַּפָּא II (Κάππα) *the Greek letter Kappa,* as a numeral (κ′) *twenty.* Lam. R. to I, 1 רבתי (חד בר נש), v. הוּקְיָא.

כַּפָּא, v. כֵּיפָא.

כְּפָא, כְּפָא, v. כפר h. a. ch.

כְּפָאתִין, v. כְּפָתָא.

כְּפָה, v. כִּיפָּה.

כֻּפָּה, v. כֵּיפָה.

כְּפוּר, v. כָּפָה.

כְּפוּרֵי, v. כְּבוּרָא a. כְּפוּתָא.

כְּפוּלוֹת *folding doors,* v. כְּפִילָה, a. כָּפַל.

כפוני, v. כְּפְנִיתָא.

כִּפּוּר, כִּיפּ׳ m. (b. h. כִּפֶּר; כִּפֻּרִים) *redemption, atonement;* mostly *pl.* כִּפּוּרִים, כִּפ׳. Meïl. II, 1 מחוסר כ׳ one wanting the ceremony of atonement for full restoration to cleanness; a. fr.—יוֹם כִּפּוּר, mostly יוֹם הַכִּפּוּרִים (abbr. יוה״כ, י״ה יה״כ) *Day of Atonement,* the tenth day of Tishri. Yoma 85ᵇ יום כפור ed. (Ms. M. יום הכפורים). Y. Shebu. I, 32ᵈ bot. י״ה a. יום הכפ׳. Zeb. V, 1. Yoma I, 1. Ib. 4 ערב יוה״כ on the eve of the Day of Atonement (the ninth of Tishri). Ib. VIII, 9 אחטא...אין יה״כ מכפר if one says, I will sin, and repent, the Day of At. will bring him no atonement. Y. ib. VII, 45ᵇ bot., v. אֶפֶשׁ; a fr.—Sifré Num. 24 ומה כפורים (=יה״כ) וכ׳ the institution of the Day of Atonement being a strict one &c.—יה״כ *Yom hak-Kippurim,* name of a treatise of the Tosefta, v. יוֹמָא.

כִּפּוּר, כִּפּוּרָא, כִּיפּ׳ ch. same. Targ. Hos. III, 2.—Targ. Y. II Lev. XXIII, 29 יום צום כִּפּוּרַיָּא.—*Pl.* כִּפּוּרַיָּא, כִּפּוּרֵי, כִּפ׳.—Targ. Ex. XXIX, 36; a. fr.—יומא דכפורא, י׳ דכפוריא, י׳ דכפורי *Day of Atonement.* Targ. Lev. XXIII, 27; a. fr.—Yoma 20ᵃ; a. fr.—Keth. 67ᵇ מעלי יומא דכ׳ = ערב יה״כ, v. preced.

כְּפוֹר I m. (b. h.; כָּפַר) [*crust,*] *hoar-frost,* cmp. גְּלִיד. Ohol. VIII, 5; Tosef. ib. XIV, 6. Mikv. VII, 1.

כְּפוֹר II m. (b. h.; v. preced.) (prob.) *plated vessel.*—*Pl.* כְּפוֹרִים, constr. כְּפוֹרֵי. Zeb. 25ᵃ; 93ᵇ; Men. 7ᵇ (ref. to Ezra I, 10, etymol. fr. כפר *to wipe off*).

כִּפּוּרָא, v. כִּפּוּר ch.

כְּפוֹרָא I ch.=h. כְּפוֹר I. Targ. Y. II Ex. XVI, 14.

כְּפוֹרָא II ch.=h. כְּפוֹר II. Targ. I Chr. XXVIII, 17.—*Pl.* constr. כְּפוֹרֵי. Ib.

כְּפוֹרָא III ch.=h. כּוֹפֶר I, *cyprus flower.—Pl.* כְּפוֹרִין. Targ. Cant. IV, 13.

כַּפּוּרֵי m. pl. (v. כַּפּוּרָא) *atonement*; בית כ׳ *the place of atonement*, v. next w.—Targ. Lev. XVI, 2 (some ed. O. כַּפּוּרְתָּא). Targ. I Chr. XXVIII, 11 (h. text בית הכפרת). Targ. I Kings VI, 5 (h. text דביר); a. e.

כַּפֹּרֶת, כַּפּוֹרֶת f. (b. h.; v. preced.) [*cover*; in symbolical language *place of atonement*,] 1) *cover of the Holy Ark.* Sifra Vayikra, N'dabah, Par. 1, ch. II. Men. 27b אל פני הכ׳ up to the very front of the *kapporeth*, contrad. to מבית לכ׳ the room occupied by the *k.*, Holy of Holies. Ib. מקדש שני דלא הוו ארון וכ׳ during the Second Temple when ark and cover no longer existed. Yoma 55a; a. e.—2) (=בית הכ׳) *the innermost of the Temple, the Holy of Holies* (מקדש הקדש). Shek. VI, 5; Tosef. ib. III, 1 זהב לַכַּ׳ (inscription on one of the offering boxes) 'Gold for the *k.*,' expl. ib. 6 עושין... ציפוי לבית קה״ק of these offerings were made gold foils for the inside of the Holy of Holies. Tosef. Tem. IV, 8 אין... אפי׳ לאחורי בית הכ׳ we dare not use it for gold foils even for the back wall of &c.; [Ar.: כַּפּוֹרֶת *plating for the Temple roof*; comment. כְּפ׳ (collect. noun) *vessels*, v. כְּפוֹר II.]

כַּפֹּרְתָּא (כַּפּ׳, כַּפּ׳, כְּפ׳) כַּפּוּרְתָּא ch. same. Targ. Ex. XXV, 17; a. fr.—בית כ׳, v. כַּפּוּרֵי.

כְּפוּשָׁה, v. כְּפִישָׁה.

כָּפוּת m. 1) part. pass. of כָּפַת.—2) *bandage.—Pl.* כְּפוּתִים. Pesik. R. s. 31 כְּפוּתֵינוּ חזקים וכ׳ our bandages were as strong as iron.—[כְּפוּתִין, Tosef. Kel. B. Kam. VII, 7, v. קְבוּת.]

כְּפוּתָא f. (כָּפַה, cmp. כֵּיפָא I, כְּבוּרָא) *ball, excrement.* B. Bath. 73b אפיק כ׳ וכ׳ Ar. (ed. רמא כופתא, Ms. H. רמא כפו׳, v. Rabb. D. S. a. l. note 2; Rashi to Snh. 98b רמי כופיתא) it cast a ball of excrement with which it obstructed the Jordan; Zeb. 113b כַּפָּא (Ms. M. קלא, v. Rabb. D. S. a. l. note). Sabb. 110b.—[Snh. 98b, v. כֵּיפָרָא; Rashi: *excrement.*—Ib. 110a כי כופתא ed., Ms. M. כפותא, Ar. מלפפונא].

כָּפַח, v. קָפַח.

כְּפֵחַ, v. כִּיפֵחַ.

כָּפָה, כָּפָא, כְּפָא, כפי (b. h.; v. כָּפַף) 1) *to bend over, invert, turn upside down.* Tam. V, 5 היה כּוֹפֶה עליהן וכ׳ he inverts a large vessel and puts it over them (the coals). Ib. כּוֹפִין אותה וכ׳ they invert it over &c. Pesik. Ekhah, p. 123a כ׳ סיח את המנורה the ass (of gold, given as a bribe to the judge) has upset the lamp (offered on the other side; whence a proverbial expression for litigants outbidding each other in bribery); Y. Yoma I, 38c bot.; Lev. R. s. 21; Pesik. Ahăré, p. 177a.—Esp. כ׳ את המטה *to upset the couch, to place the mattresses on or near the floor*, as a sign of mourning, opp. to זָקַף. M. Kat. 15b top [euphemistic version, read with Ms. M.:] דמות... בכם ובעונותיכם כְּפוּ מיטותיכן וכ׳ . . . . I (the Lord) had placed my image among you, and for your sins I upset it (decreed death), upset now your beds; Y. Ber. III, 6a top; Y. M. Kat. III, 83a top כְּפָה מיטתך. Ib. כבר כְּפִינוּם we have already lowered them (the couches); Y. Ber. III, 5d bot. כפינם (corr. acc.). Keth. 4b כּוֹפֶה מיטתו he lowers his couch (when his wife is in mourning); כּוֹפָה מיטתה she lowers &c. (when her husband is in mourning); a. fr.—Part. pass. כָּפוּי, f. כְּפוּיָה, pl. כְּפוּיִים, כְּפוּיוֹת. Tosef. Ohol. XII, 2 סאה כ׳ על פיה a dry measure turned upside down. Lam. R. introd. (R. Hăn. 3) (play on כְּפֵי המלחמה, v. כַּף) כְּפוּיֵי מלחמה those upset by war. Y. Ber. III, 6a top מטה כ׳ a lowered couch; a. fr.—Esp. כְּפוּי טובה *one on whom kindness is upset, ungrateful, unappreciative.* Ab. Zar. 5a כפויי טובה בני וכ׳ you ungrateful ones, sons of ungrateful ones. Lev. R. s. 4; a. fr.—2) *to press, force.* Keth. V, 5 כּוֹפָהּ לעשות וכ׳ he may compel her to work in wool. Yeb. 106a, a. fr. כּוֹפִין אותו עד וכ׳ the court uses means of coercion, until he says 'I will', opp. to בעל כרחו. Sot. 46b כ׳ ללויה we force a host to escort (protect) his guest on parting. B. Bath. 12b כגון זו כ׳ על מדת סדום in such a case we apply force on the ground of the law of equity (v. סְדוֹם). Y. Peah I, 15d; Y. Kidd. I, 61c top וכוֹפִין do we compel (a son to support his father)? Ib. כופין את חבן we do compel &c.—R. Hash. 28a כְּפָאוֹ ואכל וכ׳ if somebody forced him, and he ate Matsah (on the first Passover night). Ib. כ׳ שד a demon possessed him. Ib. כְּפָאוּהוּ פרסיים Persians (gentiles) forced him; a. fr.—[Snh. 70b כפאתו, v. כָּפַת.]—V. כּוּף I a. כָּפַף.

Nif. נִכְפָּה 1) *to be inverted, upset; to be forced.* Y. M. Kat. l. c. וְיִכָּפֶה הסרסור let the agent (of sin, the evil inclination) be overpowered (by mourning ceremonies); Y. Ber. l. c. ויכ׳ כפה (corr. acc.). Ib. 5d bot.; Y. M. Kat. l. c. אינה נִכְפֵּית need not be upturned, v. הַרְגֵּשׁ; a. fr.—2) *to be overtaken by a demon*, esp. *to be epileptic.* Lev. R. s. 26 ישראל..שנכפו an Israelite and a priest that were afflicted &c.—Pes. 112b אותו תינוק נִכְפֶּה that child will become epileptic. Ib. בנים נִכְפִּין epileptic children; Keth. 60b (Chald. form) בני נִכְפֵּי. Tosef. B. Bath. IV, 5 נִכְפֵּית היא she is subject to epileptic attacks; B. Mets. 80a. Yeb. 64b משפחת נִכְפִּין a family subject to epilepsy.

כְּפָא, כְּפִי ch. same, 1) *to bend, upturn, invert.* Gitt. 68b top כפא לקומתיה מיניה he bent his body away from it (the wall of the hut). Y. Hag. II, 77d bot. וּכְפוּנוּן על רישיהון and they inverted the pots and put them over their heads; a. e.—2) *to force.* Targ. Esth. I, 22.—Y. Gitt. I, 43b כְּפוּנֵיה ויהב לה חורן the court compelled him to give her another letter of divorce. Snh. 107a, v. כּוּף I ch. B. Bath. 8b רבא כַּפְיֵיה וכ׳ Ms. M. (ed. אַכְפִּיה *Af.*) Raba forced R. N. Kidd. 45b כַּפְתֵיה עד וכ׳ she forced him, until &c.

Af. אַכְפֵּי same. B. Bath. 4a, v. כּוּף I ch. Ber. 56a וְאַכְפָּה לך וכ׳ (Beth Nathan וְאַכְפַּת) and she shall finally make thee yield, and thou shalt give them (thy daughters) away to her relatives; a. e.

Ithpe. אִיתְכְּפֵי *to be upset.* Y. Ab. Zar. III, 42c top איתְכְּפוּן, v. אַנְדְּרְטָא.

כְּפִיזָא, v. קְפִיזָא.

כְּפִיָּה f. (כָּפָה) *inverting*, כְּפִיַּית חמטה the lowering of the couch in mourning. M. Kat. 15ᵃ bot. אבל חייב בכ׳ הח׳ a mourner is bound to have his couch lowered. Tosef. ib. II, 9 מי שקיים כ׳ חמ׳ וכ׳ he who has been observing the lowering of the couch for three days &c., needs not invert it &c. Y. ib. III, 83ᵃ; a. fr.

כְּפֵיל, v. כְּפַל.

כְּפֵיל־, v. כֶּפֶל.

כְּפִילָא m. ch. 1) = h. כֶּפֶל. B. Kam. 65ᵇ כ׳ ד׳ וחומשא זוזא the thief's fine amounts to four Zuz and the one-fifth-fine (v. חוּמְשָׁא) to one Zuz; a. e. — 2) *twofold condition*. Ned. 48ᵇ לאהוויי מילתא דשדיא בכ׳ Ar. (marg. vers. כפילה) to include that case (mentioned before) which was decided on the basis of a twofold eventuality (either the son or the grandson becoming a scholar); [ed. הא..דשדיא בכיפי that case which came up in consequence of the son's roaming about (stealing) sheaves of flax].

כְּפֵלָה, כְּפֵילָה f. (preced. wds.) 1) *the double share of the first-born*. Y. B. Bath. VIII, 16ᵇ top, opp. פשוטה the single share. Ib. כְּפֵילַת אביו the double share to which his (deceased) father would have been entitled. — 2) *folding door*. — *Pl.* כְּפֵילוֹת, כְּפֵל׳. Lev. R. s. 16 כפו׳ (corr. acc.); Yalk. Lev. 557, v. כָּפַל. — 3) *twofold condition*, v. preced.

כְּפֵלְתָּא, כְּפֵילְתָּא f. (preced.), מערת כ׳ *the double cave, Makhpelah*. Targ. Gen. XXIII, 19; a. fr. [Var. כָּפֵר׳, כְּפֵר׳, כְּפֵר׳.]

כְּפִין m., **כְּפִינָא** f. (כְּפַן) *hungry, starving*. Targ. Ps. CVII, 9; a. e. — V. כְּפַן I. — Meg. 7ᵇ (prov.) כ׳ עניא ולא ידע the poor man is hungry and knows it not (until food is placed before him). Koh. R. to V, 12 'an evil disease' מסכן ותשיש ערטיל וכ׳ one poor and feeble (unable to work), naked (unfit to go out) and hungry (v. דגלוס). — Ber. 58ᵇ; a. fr. — *Pl.* כְּפִינֵי, כְּפִינִין. Targ. Job V, 5. Targ. Ps. CVII, 5. Ib. 36 כפינין Ms. (ed. Lag. כפינים, oth. כְּפָפִים).

כְּפִינֵי m. pl. constr. (preced.) *want, need, desire*. Targ. Y. Gen. XLII, 19; 33 (h. text רעבון).

כְּפִיס m. (b. h.; v. כָּפַס) *girder, bond-lath*. [Midd. III, 4 שבכ׳ של ברזל, read כפים, v. כַּף. — Y. Bets. III, 62ᵃ top שבכ׳, read: שבכפים, v. שֵׁירָץ.] — *Pl.* כְּפִיסִים, כְּפִיסִין. B. Bath. I, 1, v. אַרִיחָא. B. Mets. 117ᵇ תחתון שבא לשנות .. בכ׳ when the owner of the lower story desires to make an alteration ... in the girders. Tosef. Erub. XI (VIII), 2 כפיס׳ (Ar. כפיתים). Tosef. Kel. B. Bath. II, 3 שני כ׳ R. S. to Kel. XXII, 9 (ed. כתפין, כתיפין, corr. acc.).

כְּפִיפָה f. (כָּפַף) 1) *bending, being bent*. Y. Ber. I, 3ᵈ top לך כ׳ unto thee is bending due. Ib. חזקפנו מכפיפתינו erect us from our humiliation. Snh. 65ᵃ כְּפִיפַת קומתו bending one's body (before the idol). Sabb. 104ᵃ (ref. to the shape of certain letters, v. כָּפַף) הוסיף .... כ׳ על כְּפִיפָתוֹ the Lord has given thee repeated admonitions to humility, v. מָנוֹד. — 2) (v. קְפִיפָה; cmp. Assyr. *kuppu*, Schr. KAT², p. 582) *cage, prison*. Keth. 72ᵃ, a. fr. אין אדם דר עם נחש בכ׳ nobody can be expected to dwell in a cage with a serpent, i. e. no man or woman can be compelled to live with an obnoxious consort. Tosef. Dem. III, 9; Y. ib. II, 22ᵈ bot. — 3) [*muzzle*, in gen.] *a basket of osier*, v. זְמָמָא. Kel. XXVI, 1 כ׳ מצרית a basket made of palm twigs; Sot. II, 1; a. fr. — Y. Yoma VIII, end, 45ᶜ אין..מתוך כ׳ וכ׳ an ass brays only when a basket of carobs is before him, i. e. living in plenty makes haughty, cmp. Ber. 32ᵃ. — Tosef. Kel. B. Kam. V, 8 Var., v. כְּפִישָׁה; a. fr. — *Pl.* כְּפִיפוֹת. Ter. IX, 3 תולה כ׳ וכ׳ we may muzzle beasts by hanging baskets with fodder &c.; Y. ib. IX, 46ᵈ top תולה כ׳ .. בדישו you may hang a basket over the neck of a beast in threshing.

כְּפִירָה f. (כָּפַר) *denial*. B. Mets. 4ᵃ טענה וכ׳ claim and denial. Shebu. 39ᵇ כְּפִירַת טענה, v. טַעֲנָה. B. Mets. 36ᵃ כ׳ ממון, v. פִּיטוּר. Ib. 4ᵇ, a. e. כ׳ שעבוד קרקעות a disputed hypothecary obligation; a. fr.

כְּפִישָׁא, v. next w.

כְּפִישָׁה f. (כָּפַשׁ) 1) *an inverted vessel*, usu. *a vessel divided into two compartments by the bottom between*. T'bul Yom IV, 2 בכ׳ מצרית או וכ׳ on an inverted basket of twigs or on a tray (which have no distinct receptacles, בית קבול); Tosef. ib. II, 14; Nidd. 7ᵃ; Tosef. Dem. III, 1 לפי כפישא ed. Zuck. (Var. לתוך) on the rim of an inverted vessel; Gitt. 62ᵃ בכפישא או באנחותא. Tosef. Kel. B. Kam. V, 8 עשויה כב׳ ed. Zuck. (Var. בכפיפה, read כב׳) formed like a *k'fisha*, i. e. resting on the projecting sides, not on pegs. Ohol. V, 6 וכ׳ נתונה עליה and an inverted vessel put on it as a tight lid. Ib. 7 כ׳ שהיא ... שבתוך הכ׳ וכ׳ if a *k'fisha* is put on pegs ... with an unclean object beneath, the things which lie in the (upper compartment of the) *k*. are clean. Ib. XI, 8 וכ׳ נתונה ... וכ׳ עומדת an inverted vessel is so put over it, that it would remain in position if you removed &c. Ib. 9 בין שפתי הכ׳ לבין וכ׳ between the sides (the hollow space) of the inverted vessel over the cistern and the sides of the cistern; a. fr. — Y. Shebi. VIII, 38ᵃ זה שהוא מודד בכ׳ וכ׳ one who measures fruits in a *k*. whose capacities he has found out by using it twice or three times. — Trnsf. מדד בכ׳ *to deal unfairly*. Y. Yeb. XIII, 13ᶜ, v. כָּפַשׁ. Tanḥ. Thazr. 6 Var.; ed. Bub. 8 אין הקב״ה מודד בכ׳ (not בנפישה) the Lord has not two measures for man. — 2) (colloquial expression) כְּפִי׳ or כְּפוּשָׁה *an ungainly woman*. Midr. Till. to Ps. XXIV [read as] Yalk. Job 917 אבוד חבחור חזה על הכ׳ חזו this fine young man has thrown himself away on this &c. [Midr. Till. l. c. באפריון כב׳ הזאת, ed. Bub. דכ׳, strike out דכ׳ or כ׳ הזאת, v. Yalk. l. c.]

כָּפִית, pl. **כְּפִיתִין**, v. כּוּפֶת. [כפיתים, Tosef. Erub. XI (VIII), 2, v. כְּפִיס.]

כְּפִיתָה f. (כָּפַת) *binding, collar-band* for animals. Kel. XII, 1.

כִּפְכֵּף, v. כַּבְכַּב.

כָּפַל (b. h.; cmp. כפת) *to bend over, fold, double*. Ber. 63ᵃ כופלין לו וכ׳ his means of support will be doubled to him. Gen. R. s. 95, end כל מי שכ׳ שמו וכ׳ every one whose name the Scripture mentions twice in the blessings of Moses;

(B. Kam. 92ª אותן שהוּכְפְּלוּ בשמות). Succ. III, 11 ... מקום לִכְפּוֹל יִכְפּוֹל where it is customary to recite twice (each verse of Ps. CXVIII, 21—29), let one do so. Tosef. Pes. X, 9 רבי היה כּוֹפֵל בה דברים Rabbi used to repeat certain words (in singing the Hallel); Pes. 119ᵇ; Succ. 39ª מוסיף לכפול מאודך וכ׳ adds (to Rabbi's repetitions) by doubling the verses from *Od'kha* (Ps. l. c.). Sifra Vayikra, N'dabah, Par. 10, ch. XII; Men. VI, 4 (75ᵇ) כופל אחד וכ׳ (Bab. ed. קופל) he folds it twice over and breaks it (into four parts). Ned. 61ᵇ יכפלו, v. קָפַל. Gitt. 62ª כּוֹפְלִין שלום וכ׳ we must double the greeting (say twice *shalom*) &c. B. Mets. 104ᵇ לכפול וכ׳ where it is costumary to write out the *K'thubah* for double the amount of the dowry, half the amount is collected; a. fr. — Part. pass. כָּפוּל, f. כְּפוּלָה; pl. כְּפוּלִים; כְּפוּלוֹת, כְּפוּלִין. Kel. XXVII, 5 נמדד כ׳ is measured as it is doubled (folded). Ib. 6. — Ohol. XI, 3 כ׳ Var. in R. S. a. l. (ed. ק׳) folded up one above the other. Ned. 66ᵇ כ׳ הן her ears are bent over (deformed).—Treat. Sof'rim II, 11 אותיות הכ׳ letters which have two forms (מנצפך); a. fr.— תנאי כ׳, v. תְּנַאי.

Nif. נִכְפַּל *to be doubled.* Y. Kil. IX, 32ᶜ top נִכְפְּלוּ לו שנין his years of life were doubled to him. Gen. R. s. 30, beg.; Tanh. Sh'moth 18, a. e. כל מי שנ׳ שמו every one whose name appears twice in immediate succession (as Noah Noah, Gen. VI, 9); a. fr.

Hif. הִכְפִּיל *to double, fold up.* Ned. 61ᵇ, sq., v. קָפַל.

Hof. הוּכְפַּל *to be doubled, bent.* Ib., v. קָפַל. M. Kat. 25ᵇ (in a poetic eulogy) קאת ... הוּכְפְּלוּ לראות וכ׳ pelican and owl were bent upon looking (took pains to see, cmp. next w. Ithp.).—B. Kam. 92ª, v. supra.—Part. pass. מוּכְפָּל (*Pu.* מְכוּפָּל) *doubly guarded, surrounded.* Yalk. Lev. 557 מוכ׳ כמה כְּפָלוֹת; Lev. R. s. 16 מכו׳ בכמה כפולות (the tongue) is guarded by several folding doors (teeth, lips).

Pi. כִּיפֵּל *to fold.* Sifra l. c.; Men. l. c. לא היה מְכַפְּלָהּ (Bab. ed. מק׳) he did not fold it (in four parts, v. supra).

כְּפַל ch. same. Part. pass. כְּפִיל *double.* Targ. Cant. VIII, 7.—Gitt. 62ª דִכְפִלִינָן שלמא וכ׳, v. preced.

Ithpe. אִיכְּפִיל, אִתְכְּפִיל 1) *to be folded up, doubled.* Targ. Is. XXXVIII, 12 (ed. Lag. אתק׳). Targ. Ez. XXI, 19.—B. Mets. 104ᵇ אי מקנא לא מִיכְּפַל if formal obligation is to be entered into (v. קִנְיָן), the document must not be made out for double the amount, v. preced.; a. fr.—2) *to be bent upon, take pains.* Sabb. 5ª איכ׳ תנא וכ׳ was it necessary for the Tannai to take pains to let us hear all this (to be so explicit)?—B. Mets. 46ª ואי׳ תנא וכ׳ should the Tannai have taken the trouble to speak of such an exceptional case as that of a naked man &c.?—B. Bath. 91ª אִיכְּפַל ואוליד וכ׳ apply thyself (Rashi: *marry again*), and beget &c. Shebu. 48ᵇ אִיכְּפַלִי ואתאי וכ׳ have I taken the trouble to come all this distance for the sake of upsetting &c.?; a. e.—[Y. Ter. VIII, 46ª top אכפלן ed. Zyt., v. אֲפַךְ.]

כֶּפֶל m. (b. h.; preced. wds.) *doubling, double amount,* esp. כ׳ (תשלומי) *the additional amount to be paid as fine on restoring stolen goods* (Ex. XXII, 3; 6—8). Snh. I, 1. B. Kam. VII, 1; a. fr. — Ib. 65ª עולה לו בִּכְפֵילוֹ (fr. כְּפַל; Rashi: בתוך הכפל) is credited to him as the thief's fine; Tosef. ib. VIII, 8 ...מתוך כפילו is deducted from &c. Y. Sot. III, end, 19ᵇ; Kidd. 18ª ולא בכפילו cannot be sold for the fine; a. fr.—*Du.* כִּפְלַיִם, כְּפָלַיִם. Succ. 51ᵇ; Tosef. ib. IV, 6 כ׳ כיוצאי מצרים twice as many as those who went out of Egypt; a. e.—*Pl.* כְּפָלִים *even numbers.* Pes. 110ª השותה כ׳ Ms. M. he who drinks even numbers of cups, v. זוּגָא.— כְּפָלוֹת *folding doors,* v. כָּפַל.

כִּפְלָא (or כּ׳) m. (preced. wds.) 1) *curve, winding road.* Targ. Is. XL, 4 (h. text עָקֹב). Ib. XLII, 16 (h. text מַעֲקַשִּׁים).—2) (cmp. כֶּסֶל) *groin, loin.* Targ. Job XV, 27.—Hull. 93ª חמשא . . . ביה בכ׳ (Ar. בחו בִּכְפְלֵי) there are five veins (of forbidden fat) in the loin.—*Pl.* כִּפְלֵי. Targ. Y. Lev. III, 4 (ed. pr. כּ׳); a. e.—Targ. Ps. XXXVIII, 8, v. כִּסְלָא.—Hull. 8ᵇ. Ib. 93ª; a. e.—3) = h. כֶּפֶל, v. כְּפֵילָא.

כפלון, Gen. R. s. 59 בא בכ׳ מפולש, read as Yalk. ib. 103 a. Ar. s. v. פלן: בְּפִילוֹן.

***קִיפְלָאוֹת, כְּפָלִיוֹת** f. pl. (κέφαλος) a species of *mullet,* a delicious fish (v. Sm. Ant. s. v. Cephalus). Gen. R. s. 98 (expl. מעדני מלך, Gen. XLIX, 20), כ׳ ואנפקינון (not ...טן) mullets and oil of unripe olives. Sifré Deut. 355 (ref. to Deut. XXXIII, 24) שהיה.. בשמן אנפיקין ובקר׳ וכ׳ (corr. acc) Asher made himself agreeable to his brother tribes by furnishing them oil ... and mullets, while they supplied him with grain; Yalk. ib. 962 (comment.: *fine fruits*).

כפליין, Y. Nidd. II, 50ª bot. כפ׳ של ראש וכ׳, read: כפִילְיוֹן like the color of a felt cap &c.; v. אַפִּילְיוֹן III.

כָּפַן (b. h.; cmp. כפף) *to bend*; part. pass. כָּפוּן *bent upon, eager for.* Gen. R. s. 79, beg. (ref. to Job V, 22) זה לבן שבא כ׳ וכ׳ that refers to Laban who rushed with eagerness at his (Jacob's) money to plunder it.

כְּפַן I, כְּפֵין same 1) *to bend.*—Part. pass. כְּפִין. Targ. Job XL, 17 (ed. Lag. כפיף, ed. Wil. כפף, Ms. כאיף; h. text יחפץ).—2) *to pine* (for food), *to starve.* Targ. Ps. XXXIV, 11. Targ. Gen. XLI, 55; a. fr.—Ber. 62ᵇ (prov.) עד דכפנת אכול eat while thou art hungry (delay nothing). Pes. 107ᵇ bot. כי היכי דאגרר׳ ואכפן אמצה וכ׳ Ms. M. (read: דאיגרר, v. Rabb. D. S. a. l. note; ed. דניגרריה לליביה) that I may get an appetite and be eager for the *Matsah* in the evening. B. Mets. 83ª וּכְפִינַן and we are hungry; a. fr.—[Esth. R. to I, 4 כְּפְנָאי I am hungry (?).]

Af. אַכְפִּין *to cause to hunger.* Targ. Deut. VIII, 3; a. e.—Sabb. 33ª מַכְפִּין נפשיה he starved himself (and grew sick in consequence).

כַּפְנָא, כְּפַן II m. (preced.) *hunger, famine.* Targ. Ruth I, 1. Targ. Gen. XII, 10; a. fr.—Sabb. 33ª נפיחי כ׳ swelling (and lying) from starvation.—Taan. 19ᵇ top, v. בִּצּוֹרְתָא. Ib. 8ᵇ כ׳ ומותנא famine and pestilence; a. fr.—*Pl.* כַּפְנִין. Targ. Ruth l. c.—V. כַּפְנֵי.

כַּפְנֵי, v. כַּפְנִיתָא.

כְּפָנִים, v. כָּפוּן.

כְּפָנִית f. (כָּפַן, cmp. כּוּפְרָא III a. גפן) *the inflorescence of palms, date-berry in its early stage.*—*Pl.* כְּפָנִיּוֹת. Orl.

I,9. Tosef. Maas. Sh. I, 14 כ׳ הרי הן כפרי וכ׳ *Kofniyoth* are in every respect to be considered as fruits, excep &c.; a. fr.

כּוּפְנִי, כַּפְנִי, כּוּפ׳, כַּפְנִיתָא, ch. same. Y. B. Kam. VI, 5^{b} bot. גנב חדא כפוני (corr. acc.) stole one palm-flower (cmp. Bab. ib. 59^{b} s. v. כּוּפְּרָא III).—*Pl.* כּוּפ׳, כַּפְנִייָתָא. Bekh. 18^{a}; B. Bath. 107^{b} עד דאכלת כ׳ וכ׳ while thou wert yet eating date-berries in Babylonia, did we expound &c. Pes. 52^{b} (identified with כופרי).—Y. Shebi. IX, end, 39^{a} [read:] מייבלא כופנין לאשקלון to export date-berries to A. (in the Sabbatical year).

כָּפַס (cmp. כפת) *to tie, fasten.*—Part. pass. כָּפִיס, f. כְּפִיסָא, *pl.* כְּפִיסָן. Targ. Esth. I, 6.

***כָּפַע** (v. כָּפָה), *Hif.* הִכְפִּיעַ *to upset, make havoc.* Gen. R. s. 28 מַכְפִּיעַ Ar. (ed. מפקיע), v. חִיצָא.

כְּפַע ch. *Ithpe.* אִתְכְּפַע, Targ. II Chr. XXXIII, 13, v. גְּפַע.

כָּפַף (b. h.) 1) *to bend, curve.* Gen. R. s. 87, end כּוֹפֶפֶת אני את קומתך ... כְּפוּפִים (Potiphar's wife said to Joseph) I shall bend thy proud stature (humiliate thee with slave labor); said he, The Lord erects those who are bowed down. B. Kam. 55^{b} הַכּוֹפֵף ... בפני וכ׳ he who bends his neighbor's grain stalks before the fire (so as to make them catch fire). Num. R. s. 6, beg. נביא כופף ידיו וכ׳ the prophet must bend his hands and feet to sit before (surrender his power to) the high priest; (Y. Hor. III, 48^{b} bot. מְכַפֵּף). Cant. R. beg. לָכוֹף אזניך וכ׳ to bend thy ear and listen; a. fr.—Part. pass. כָּפוּף, f. כְּפוּפָה, *pl.* כְּפוּפִים, כְּפוּפוֹת; כְּפוּפִין. Sabb. 17^{a} היה הלל כ׳ ויושב וכ׳ Hillel sat bent (in submission) before Shammai. Gen. R. l. c., v. supra. R. Hash. III, 4 בשל זכרים כ׳ with bent horns of rams. Yalk. Ex. 276 דווים וכ׳ suffering and humbled (v. סָחַף, סָגַף); a. fr.—Esp. the *curved letters* כ, נ, פ, צ, opp. פשוט the straight-lined, the shape of the final letters. Sabb. 104^{a} (symbolization of letters) נו״ן כ׳ ... נאמן כ׳ וכ׳ *Nun* bent, *Nun* straightened, faithful when bent (in distress), faithful when straightened (raised up) &c. Ib. 103^{b} כ׳ פשוטין וכ׳ that one must not write the curved letters straightened &c.—2) *to bend, force, conquer.* Y. Snh. I, 18^{a} bot. מומחה שכ׳ ודן an authorized judge that forced (the law requiring three judges) and judged singly. Y. Yeb. XII, 12^{c} ר׳ יצחק כ׳ R. J. forced (the law requiring three judges for *ḥălitsah*); ib. הא רבן כ׳ it was our teacher who did it. Keth. 4^{b} אין ... לָכוֹף וכ׳ no husband dares force his wife (in mourning) to paint &c. Num. R. s. 14 (play on כַּף) זה אברהם שכָּפַף את יצרו וכ׳ (some ed. שכבש) that refers to Abraham who conquered his inclinations &c.—3) *to invert, upset.* Y. Ber. III, 6^{a} top גרמתני לכופפה thou didst cause me to upset it (the divine image), v. כָּפָה; (M. Kat. 15^{b} ובעונותיכם הפכתיה). Y. l. c. כְּפוּיוֹת=מטות כְּפוּפוֹת, v. כָּפָה; a. fr.—[Num. R. s. 10 הסיט כפוף כפפתו אימו, read כפתתו, v. כָּפַת.—Sabb. 106^{a} Ar., ed. כָּפוּל, v. סיט.]—4) *to bend one's self upon, to take pains* (cmp. כָּפַל). Cant. R. to I, 17 כפפתי לעקור וכ׳ I took pains to destroy the passion for idolatry.

Nif. נִכְפַּף *to be bent.* Pesik. R. s. 28 [read:] עד שנִכְפְּפָה קומתם וכ׳ so that their statures were bent under their load. Arakh. 19^{a} שרביט שאינו נכפף a staff (of gold or silver) which cannot be bent. Num. R. s. 5, end נִכְפְּפָה הריעה וכ׳ the curtain around the Ark was bent aside (prob. to be read נכפלה). B. Kam. 61^{a} בנִכְפֶּפֶת when the fire is diverted from its course through the wind; (oth. opin.: when the fire is subdued (low) and creeping over the plants on the ground), opp. קולחת or קודחת. Cant. R. to I, 17. Pesik. R. s. 14 שתי השערות נִכְפָּפוֹת (not ...פים) the two hairs (on the neck) are bent, opp. נִזקפות; a. e.

כְּפַף, כְּפֵיף, ch. same, 1) *to bend.* Targ. Job XL, 17, v. כְּפַן I. Targ. Ez. XVII, 7 כָּפַת (h. text כפנה, v. כְּפַן). Targ. II Esth. I, 5 כַּף אילנא וכ׳ bent tree to tree and made arches. Targ. Is. LVIII, 5; a. e.—Part. pass. כָּפִיף, f. כְּפִיפָא, pl. כְּפִיפִין. Ib.—Targ. II Esth. V, 1. Targ. Is. LX, 14.—2) *to invert.* M. Kat. 25^{a} כף כדא וכ׳ inverted a pitcher on the ground and placed thereon &c.

Pa. כַּפֵּף same. Targ. Ezek. XVII, 6. Ib. 7 כַּפֵּת some ed., v. supra.

כְּפֵפְתָא f. ch.=h. כְּפִיפָה, *muzzle, basket.*—*Pl.* כְּפֵפָתָא. Midr. Sam. ch. XXI, v. כֵּיפְתָא.

כָּפַר (b. h.; cmp. כפף) 1) *to bend, arch over, cover*; v. כּוֹפֶר, כְּפוֹר &c.—2) [*to pass over with one's palm* &c., *to wipe out, rub* (cmp. חפף),] *to deny, withhold the truth by claiming ignorance; to ignore* (mostly with ב of the object). B. Mets. 4^{a} הכּוֹפֵר במלוה he who denied having received a loan (and was refuted before being sworn, v. הֶיסֵּת). Ib. על מה שכ׳ וכ׳ he is sworn on what he denied. Shebu. IV, 1 עד שיִכְפְּרוּ בהן בב״ד until they declare their ignorance (of the testimony) before court. Ib. 4 כָּפְרוּ שניהן וכ׳ if both witnesses pleaded ignorance at the same time. Ib. כָּפְרָה הראשונה if the first set of witnesses pleaded ignorance. Ib. VI, 3 והודה ... וכ׳ בקרקעות and defendant admits the debt concerning vessels, but denies it as to landed estate. Sabb. 116^{a} מכירין וכוֹפְרִין they know (true religion) and yet are disbelievers. Cant. R. to I, 14 (play on הכפר, ib.) שכ׳ באו״ה He disowned the gentiles (did not assist them), opp. הודה; a. v. fr.—כ׳ בעיקר *to deny the principle of religion* (unity of God &c.). B. Bath. 16^{b}; a. fr.—Snh. 39^{a} א״ל כּוֹפֵר ed. (Ms. M. קיסר) an infidel said &c.

Hif. הִכְפִּיר (v. כַּפָּרָה) *to say of a person, 'May his death be an atonement for his sins!'* euphem. for *to be angry at.* Pes. 69^{a} אל תַּכְפִּירֵנִי בשעת הדין ed. (Ms. M. a. Ar. תְּכַפְּרֵנִי) do not make me an atonement (saying תהא מיתתו כפרה) at the time of judgment (differ. in comm.); Ab. Zar. 46^{b} (some eds. תכפרינני).

Pi. כִּיפֵּר, כִּפֵּר [*to wipe out,*] *to forgive, atone; to procure forgiveness.* Yoma 5^{a} כאילו לא כ׳ וכפר as if he (the priest) had not procured atonement (in the proper manner), although he has procured atonement (for the person concerned); Neg. XIV, 10 כ׳ ומעלין עליו כאילו לא כ׳ he has brought atonement, but it is accounted to the officiating priest as if he had not done so. Ber. 55^{a} כל זמן ... מזבח מְכַפֵּר על וכ׳ as long as the Temple existed, the altar was the means of atonement for Israel, but now each man's table must be the means of atonement (ref. to Ez. XLI, 22). Tanḥ. Vayishl. 6 כשם ... מְכַפֶּרֶת וכ׳ as the altar brings atonement, so does she (the chaste wife) atone for her household. Kidd. 57^{a}, a. e. מכשיר ומכפר, v. כָּשַׁר I; a. v. fr.—[Ab. Zar. 46^{b}, v. supra].

Hithpa. הִתְכַּפֵּר, *Nithpa.* נִתְכַּפֵּר *to be expiated; to be forgiven.* R. Hash. 18ª; Yeb. 105ª (ref. to I Sam. III, 14) בזבח ... מִתְכַּפֵּר וכ׳ through sacrifice .. it will not be expiated, but it may be so by the study of the Law. Shebu. 12ª אשם .. שנִתְכַּפְּרוּ בעליו an animal dedicated for a guilt-offering... whose owner has otherwise obtained atonement; (Tem. III, 3 שֶׁכִּפְּרוּ וכ׳ whose owner has procured atonement &c.). Yoma 50ᵇ, a. e. המִתְכַּפֵּר he for whose atonement the animal is dedicated. Ib. 51ᵇ שאין הצבור מִתְכַּפְּרִין בו as the community is not to obtain forgiveness through it (the bullock); a.fr.—Y. Macc. II, 31ᵈ bot. יעשה...וְיִתְכַּפֵּר לו let him repent and he shall be forgiven; Pesik. Shub. p. 158ᵇ; Yalk. Ez. 358; Yalk. Ps. 702. Tanh. T'rum. 8 נתכ׳ לחם they were forgiven; a. fr.

כְּפַר ch. same, *to deny, renounce.* Targ. Jer. II, 27. Targ. Y. Lev. V, 21, sq.; a. fr.—B. Kam. 107ª בכוליה בעי דנִכְפְּרֵיה ed. (Ms. M. דנכפר ליה, v. Rabb. D. S. a. l.) he would have liked to deny the whole of his indebtedness, והאי דלא כָּפְרֵיה and the reason why he did not do so. Ib. 105ᵇ ממונא קא כ׳ ליה through his denial he withholds from him value. M. Kat. 18ᵇ כָּפְרַת בה Ms. M. thou growest a disbeliever through it (when thy prayer is not answered; ed. כ׳ בה׳ thou renouncest the Lord); a. fr.

Pa. כַּפֵּר 1) *to wipe out, efface.* Targ. Prov. XXX, 20.—B. Bath. 167ª כ׳ ליה וכ׳ Ms. M. (ed. מחקיה) he erased the horizontal lines of the Beth (v. כַּפָּא). Hull. 8ᵇ למִיכַפְּרֵיה with which to wipe the knife off. Yeb. 115ᵇ מיכַפַּר הוה כַּפֵּר he would have obliterated the mark. Gitt. 56ª ואתי לכַפּוּרֵי וכ׳ and wants to wipe his hands off on this man (me), i. e. desires to put the responsibility on me; a. e.—2) *to forgive, atone, procure forgiveness.* Targ. Lev. XVI, 17; a. fr.—Zeb. 6ª מקיבעא לא מְכַפְּרָא וכ׳ as a specially appointed offering it has no atoning effect, by implication it has; a. fr.

Ithpe. אִתְכַּפַּר, אִיכַּ׳ 1) *to be wiped out, obliterated.* Targ. II Esth. III, 8.—2) *to be forgiven, to be expiated.* Ib. Targ. Deut. XXI, 8; a. fr.—Yoma 50ᵇ בקביעותא מִתְכַּפְּרֵי וכ׳ (Ms. M. 2 מִיכַּ׳) do they (the high priest's kindred and fellow priests) obtain forgiveness by special appointment (so as to be considered fellow owners of the sacrifice) or by implication? Kerith. 24ª מִיכַּפְּרָנָא באידך חבריה my atonement shall be effected through the other animal; a. e.

כֹּפֶר, v. כּוֹפֶר.

כְּפָר m. (b. h.; כפר *to be round,* cmp. כִּכָּרָה, כְּבִירָה) [*circle,*] *village, country town.* Meg. I, 3 פחות מכאן הרי זה כ׳ if a place has less (than ten persons of leisure), it is considered a country place, opp. עיר גדולה. Hag. 13ᵇ v. יְחֶזְקֵאל. Eduy. II, 3; a. fr.—*Pl.* כְּפָרִים. Meg. I, 1, sq.; a. fr. [In compounds: ... כְּפַר pr. n. pl., v. respective determinants.]

***כַּפְרָא** m. (כָּפַר) *wipings,* or *covering,* כ׳ דודיי (read: דרודיי) sediments of dye (or rust) of the kettles. B. Kam. 101ª top (Rashi כּוּפ׳), v. כַּלְכּוּס.

כַּפְרָה, כַּפְרָא, pr. n. pl., v. כּוּפְרָה.

כַּפָּרָה f. (כָּפַר) *atonement, expiation, expiatory service.* Zeb. 8ª שתהא כ׳ וכ׳ that the act of expiation (sprinkling) be performed with the understanding that the sacrifice is a sin-offering. Tosef. Yoma V (IV), 6, a. e. חלוקי כ׳, v. חֵלֶק.—Neg. II, 1 אני כַּפָּרָתָן my life be an expiatory sacrifice for them (an expression of love); Esth. R. to I, 11 א״ר איבו [אני] כ׳ של ישראל. Kidd. 31ᵇ (one reporting an opinion of his deceased father must say) כך ... הריני כַּפָּרַת משכבו so said my lord my father, may I be an expiation for his rest. Yoma 40ᵇ כפרת דמים atonement through blood; כ׳ דברים atonement by confession; a. fr.—*Pl.* כַּפָּרוֹת. Zeb. 52ª (expl. Lev. XVI, 20) שלמו כל הכ׳ with this are all the acts of expiation (of the Day of Atonement) finished. Y. Shebu. I, 33ª מחלוקי כ׳ about the classes of atonements (v. חֵלֶק). Gen. R. s. 44 כל הכ׳ הראה לו he showed him all expiatory sacrifices; Lev. R. s. 3; a. fr.

כַּפְרוֹנָיָא, v. כַּפְרָנָא.

כַּפְרוּסָאֵי m. pl., nom. gent. *Kafruseans.* Targ. Y. II Gen. X, 17 (h. text סיני), v. אַרְהוּסְיָיה.

כַּפְרִי pr. n. pl. *Kafri* in Babylonia. Kidd. 44ᵇ. Snh. 5ª. B. Bath. 153ª כופרי (Ms. M. בי כפרי׳). B. Mets. 73ª (Ms. H. כופרי); v. Berl. Geogr. p. 37, sq.

כַּפְרָן m. (כָּפַר) *denier, liar.* Shebu. 41ᵇ הוחזק כ׳ he is presumed to be a liar (and cannot be sworn). Ib. 42ª; a. fr.

כּוּפ׳, כַּפְרָנָא m. ch. = h. כָּפָר, *village.*—*Pl.* כַּפְרָנַיָּא, כַּפְרָנִין, כּוּפ׳. Targ. Num. XXXII, 41, sq. (h. text חוות).—Y. Ber. I, 2ª, v. דַּקִּיק. Cant. R. to I, 5 (expl. בנות, Ez. XVI, 61) כופרנין country towns.—Targ. II Esth. IX, 19 כַּפְרוֹנַיָּא (Var. כּוּפְרָנָאִין).

כַּפְרָנוּת f. (v. כַּפְרָן) *an obligation decreed in court over the defendant's denial.* Y. Gitt. V, 46ᶜ bot. מלוה שנעשית בו כ׳ אינה נשמטת (strike out בו) a loan which has been passed in court over the debtor's denial, does not fall under the law of prescription in the Sabbatical year; כ׳ שנעשית מלוה נשמטת a decreed obligation which has been converted into a loan (the defendant giving his note in settlement) is subject to prescription. Ib. [read:] מלוה שנעשית כ׳ גובה בעידית כ׳ וכ׳ a loan which has been passed &c. is collectible from the best class of landed property; a decreed obligation which has been converted into a loan is collectible from the middle class &c.; Y. Shebi. X, 39ᶜ כַּפְרָנִית; ib. מלוה שהיא נעשית מלוה (read: כ׳ שהיא וכ׳).

כַּפֹּרְתָּא, כַּפֹּרֶת, v. sub כַּפּוֹר.

כָּפַשׁ (cmp. כפה) *to invert.* מִדָּה כְּפוּשָׁה *an invertible measure,* a measure containing two uneven compartments separated by the bottom; מדר במדה כ׳ *to deal unfairly,* v. כְּפִישָׁה. Yeb. 107ᵇ פישון...במ׳ כ׳ מדד לפיכך וכ׳ Pishon .. acted unfairly towards his wife, therefore the court dealt with him unfairly (against the rule).—כפושה (sub. אשה) *an ungainly woman,* v. כְּפִישָׁה. [Tosef. Ohol. VI, 3 היתה כפושה, read: כְּפִישָׁה, v. R. S. to Ohol. V, 7.]

כָּפַת (cmp. preced.) *to twist, tie.* Tam. IV, 1 לא היו כוֹפְתִין וכ׳ they did not twist (tie together the four feet of) the lamb, opp. העקיד, v. עָקַד. Snh. 70ᵇ (ref. to Prov. XXXI, 1) שֶׁכְּפָתָתוּ אמו וכ׳ Ms. M. (ed. שכפאתו) his mother tied him to a post; Num. R. s. 10 כפפתו (corr. acc.). Par. III, 9 כְּפָתוּהָ וכ׳ they tied her (the red heifer) with a rope

&c. Gen. R. s. 56 כל מה.. עוקד... כופת וכ׳ (some ed. כובש) as much as Abraham bound Isaac..., the Lord tied (held in check) the genii of the gentiles; Yalk. Gen. 101; Yalk. Nah. 561. Gen. R. l. c. כְּפָתֵנִי וכ׳ tie me well. Macc. III, 12 כופת שתי ידיו וכ׳ (some ed. כופח) one puts both his hands in stocks on the pole. Gitt. 14[b] אומרין כְּפוֹתוּ כּוֹפְתִין when they (the officers) say, put him in stocks, they put him &c. Succ. 32[a] (ref. to כפת, Lev. XXIII, 40) כָּפוּת אם היה פרוד יִכְפְּתֶנּוּ (Ms. M. omits כפות) it must be tied; if the branch is spread, one must tie it closely. Ib. כָּפוּת מכלל וכ׳ 'tied' implies that it is sometimes spread, while this (the stalk) is always tied (closely pressed together). Toh. VII, 5 אפי׳ כפות, v. יָבַל. Y. Gitt. I, end, 43[d]; Y. Kidd. III, 64[a] bot. ורוסי אחי כ׳ וכ׳ and (I saw) my brother J. in stocks and the lash passing over him. Midr. Till. to Ps. II, 3 (ref. to 'their bands', ib.) אלו שבע מצות שֶׁהֵן כְּפוּתִין בהן (not כתופין, כתים, v. ed. Bub. note) those are the seven (Noachidic) laws by which they (the gentiles) are tied (restrained); a. e.

Pi. כִּיפֵּת same. Tosef. Kel. B. Bath. II, 1. Y. Hor. III, 48[b] bot. מְכַפֵּת, v. כָּפַף.—Part. pass. מְכוּפָּת, pl. מְכוּפָּתִין. Esth. R. to I, 6, v. כְּפָתָא.

Nif. נִכְפַּת *to be tied.* Cant. R. to. I, 14.

כְּפַת ch. same. Targ. Y. Gen. XXII, 9. Targ. Ps. CXVIII, 27; a. e.—Part. pass. pl. כְּפוּתִין (hebr.) *put in stocks.* Targ. Y. II Num. XXI, 29.—Tam. 31[b] דכַפְּתֵיה בשיראי if one tied the sacrifice (hands and feet) with silk ropes. B. Bath. 167[a] כפתיה ואודי he put him in stocks (or in prison), and he confessed. Gitt. 14[a] דכָפְתֵי ושקלי וכ׳ who use force (have him arrested) and collect their due immediately (allowing no time). Y. Gitt. I, end, 43[d]; Y. Kidd. III, 64[a] כַּפְתוּן ואפקון מיניה they put him in stocks and forced him to pay; a. e.—[Gitt. 62[a] מְכַפַּת וכ׳, v. אִכְפַּת.]

Pa. כַּפִּית 1) same. Targ. Cant. VII, 5.—Y. Kil. IX, end, 32[d] דהוא מְכַפֵּת ביה he (the weaver) uses it for tying (or *knotting*, v. infra).—2) (v. P. Sm. 1803) *to produce knots, to mature fruits.* Targ. O. Num. XVII, 23 ed. Berl. (Var. כְּפִית, כָּפִית; h. text גמל); cmp. כַּפְתּוֹר.

כָּפֵת, v. כִּיפָּח.

כֵּפַת, כֵּפְתָא, v. כֵּיפָּח, כֵּיפְתָא.

כִּפְתָא m. (כפת) *tie, knot.*—*Pl.* כִּפְתִּין, כִּפְתַּיָּא. Gen. R. s. 56; Yalk. Gen. 101; Yalk. Nah. 561 אילין כ׳ those bonds (with which the genii of the nations were tied, v. כָּפַת).— Esth. R. to I, 6 (in Hebr. dict.) היו מכופתין בכִפְּאתִין של כסף the couches were tied with silver straps.

כְּפָתָה f. h. (v. preced.) *travelling implements tied up, bundle.*—*Pl.* כְּפָתוֹת. Gen. R. s. 100 קשרי כְּפְתוֹתֵיהֶן התירו (some ed. קשרות) they (the Canaanites) untied the knots of their (the pall-bearers') bundles (assisted them in their preparations for camping); Yalk. Gen. 161 בחרי כתפותיהם; Y. Sot. I, 17[b] bot. קשרי כתפיהן (corr. acc.).

כַּפְתּוֹר m. (b. h.; כפת with format. ר; v. כָּפַת Pa. 2, a. preced. wds.) *ball*, esp. *an ornament* of the candlestick in the shape of *a pomegranate.* Gen. R. s. 91 end כ׳ ופרח pomegranate and blossom!, i. e. well and nicely said!— Men. 28[b].—*Pl.* כַּפְתּוֹרִים, כַּפְתּוֹרִין. Ib.

כַּפְתּוֹרִים (b. h. כפתרים) pr. n. gent. *Kaftoreans.* Gen. R. s. 37; Yalk. ib. 62; Yalk. Chr. 1074 כ׳ ננסין Kaft. were dwarfs.

כֵּצַד, v. כֵּיצַד.

כצוצרה, כצוצטרה, v. חֲצוֹצְרָה a. גְּזוּזְטְרָא.

כַּר m. (b. h.; כרר, v. כָּרָה) 1) *bolster, mattress.* Mikv. X, 2. Kel. XXVI, 5, v. כֶּסֶת; a. fr.—*Pl.* כָּרִים. Kil. IX, 2; a. fr.—Meg. 12[a] (expl. כרפס, Esth. I, 6) כ׳ של פסים mattresses of striped goods.—2) *rounded*; (cmp. כֶּבֶשׂ) *fat lamb.* Men. 66[b], a. e., v. כַּרְמֶל.—Esth. R. to I, 14 (play on כַּרְשְׁנָא). מי כר בן שנה (not פר) who offers unto thee a lamb one year old?—*Pl.* as ab. Meg. 12[b] כ׳ בני שנה; Yalk. Esth. 1051 פרים (corr. acc.). [Y. Sabb. V, 7[b] bot. כ׳ יוצאין לבובין ed. Krot., read: זכרים.]—Trnsf. *commander.*—*Pl.* as ab. Koh. R. to XII, 7, a. e., v. כלירכין.—4) *runner, roller.*—*Pl.* as ab. Gen. R. s. 69 מעבירין כ׳ עליהם pass the paving rollers over them; (ib. s. 41 רדיה; Yalk. Is. 337 דדין).

כַּר, כָּרָא ch. same, *bolster.* Gitt. 47[a] כריסי כָּרִי my fat belly is my bolster. Y. Yoma VIII, 44[d] top; Y. Taan. I, 64[c] [read:] (תותי) תחות כָּרֵיה under his bolster.—*Pl.* כָּרִין. Targ. Lam. II, 21.

כָּרָא, v. כְּרֵה a. כְּרֵי.

כְּרָזָא, v. כְּרָזָא.

כְּרָאכָא, v. כְּרָכָא.

***כְּרַב** I (cmp. כָּרַח), *Af.* אַכְרֵב *to surround, crown.* Targ. Job XXXI, 36, v. כְּבַן.

כְּרַב II (preced.) [*to dig around*, denom. כְּרוֹבָא, fr. which כְּרַב] *to plough.* B. Kam. 96[b] כ׳ בהו כרבא (Ms. M. omits כרבא) he ploughed with them. Sabb. 33[b] ... חזו מכדי כָּרְבִי וזרעי they saw people plough and sow. Ib. 73[b] מְכְרַב כרבי ברישא do not people first plough (and then sow)? Ib. ... באי״ ... והדר כרבי the Mishnah speaks of Palestine where they first sow and then plough. B. Mets. 105[a] כָּרֵיבְנָא לה I shall plough it over. Ib. 107[a] כָּרֵיב ותני he ploughs twice (after harvesting and before seed-time); a. e.

כַּרְבָא I m. (preced.) *ploughing.* B. Kam. 96[a], v. preced. —B. Bath. 12[a] יומא כ׳ one day's ploughing (Rashi: at ploughing season, opp. to the second ploughing before seed-time).—בי כ׳ a ploughed field. Yoma 43[b]; Nidd. 65[b], v. כְּמַאר.

כַּרְבָא II or **כַּרְבָּא** m. ch.=h. כְּרוּב II, *cabbage.* Macc. 16[a], v. כְּרִיתָא; [Tosaf. a. l. *a ploughed field*, v. preced.]. B. Kam. 92[a], v. חוּצָא I. Sabb. 115[a]; a. e.—*Pl.* כַּרְבֵּי. Hull. 62[b] דבי כ׳ (Rashi sing.; Ar. כּוֹרֵי) those (locusts) found among cabbage.

כרבוניי, v. כַּרְפּוּמָא II.

כַּרְבַּיָּא, Targ. Job IV, 10, v. כְּרַכָּא.

כרבין, כרביז, v. כַּרְפּוּז.

***כַּרְבִּיתָא** f. (denom. of כַּרְבָא I) *like a ploughed field, of rough surface.* B. Kam. 85[a] (expl. כְּרְוּיתְנִי) נאתא כ׳ Ms. M. (v. Rabb. D. S. a. l. note; ed. כריכתא; Yalk. Ex. 332 כרכית) a rough seam (of the wound), *scar.*

כִּרְבֵּל (v. כְּרַב I) *to turn around, shake a sieve* (cmp. חֲזַר). Y'lamd. to Gen. XXII, 21, quot. in Ar. מְכַרְבֵּל.

כרבלין, v. כּוּרְבְּלִין.

כַּרְבֶּלֶת f. (v. כִּרְבֵּל, cmp. הדר), *crown, crest.* Sabb. 110[b] יִטּוֹל כַּרְבַּלְתּוֹ let him cut off his (the cock's) crest.

כַּרְבַּלְתָּא ch. same, 1) *helmet, crest.* Ber. 7[a]; Ab. Zar. 4[b] כי חוורא כ׳ דתרנגולא when the crest of the cock is white. Erub. 100[b] [read:] שונרא לישמטיה לכַרְבַּלְתֵּיה דהדוא תרנגולא וכ׳ (v. Rabb. D. S. a. l. note) may the cat tear off this cock's (my) crest, if I have (wherewith to buy) and do not buy for thee.—*Pl.* כַּרְבַּלָּתָא. Y'lamd. to Gen. III, 22, quot. in Ar. (expl. כרבלתהון, Dan. III, 22) קסידין *cassides* (v. Koh. Ar. Compl. s. v.).—2) (cmp. אַדֶּרֶת) *a certain kind of cloak.* Ber. 20[a] חזיה . . דהות לבישא כ׳ saw a Samaritan woman (whom he believed to be a Jewess) wearing a *karbalta* (which was considered improper for a Jewish woman).—*Pl.* as ab. Y'lamd. l. c., (another opin.) expl. כרבלתהון (v. supra) טלוות, v. טַלִּית.

***כַּרְבֵּק** (Parel of בבק, dial.=קְוַק) *to call, give a signal.* Targ. Job XXVII, 23 ed. Ven. (oth. ed. שרק, ed. Lag. Var. ברבק, Bxt. s. v. quotes Var. ברכק).

כַּרְגָּא (כְּרָגָא) m. (cmp. חֲרִיקָא, a. Arab. ḫarag) *capitation tax, tax, tribute.* Targ. Lam. I, 1; a. e.—B. Bath. 55[a] כ׳ אקרקף וכ׳ *karga* rests on the head of man, i. e. is a personal liability, opp. to טַסְקָא. Ib. אפי׳ . . . משתעבדי לכ׳ even the barley in the pot is seizable for *k.*—B. Mets. 73[b] דיהבי זוזי אַכ׳ דארנשי וכ׳ who pay the taxes for other people and force them to unreasonable services. Keth. 87[a], v. אַכְרְזְתָּא.

כַּרְדּוּ, v. קַרְדּוּ.

כַּרְדּוּט m. (chiridota, χειριδωτός) *a tunic with sleeves.* Targ. I Sam. II, 18; a. e. (h. text אפוד).—*Pl.* כַּרְדּוּטִין. Targ. II Sam. XIII, 18 (h. text מעילים).—V. next art.

כרדוכאות, v. כַּרְנִיבָאוֹת.

כַּרְדִּיטִין (כְּרְדּוּ׳) m. pl. (a corrupt. of כונדריטין χονδρῖται) *bread made of groats.* Targ. Jer. VII, 18; XLIV, 19 (h. text כַּוָּנִים).

כרדכאות, v. כַּרְנִיבָאוֹת.

כָּרָה, v. כרי.

כְּרָה, v. כִּירָה.

כְּרֵה (v. כרח) *to shrink, be narrow,* (with or sub. רוחא) *to be ill-tempered.*—Part. כְּרֵי, f. כַּרְיָא (=כריהא, כריהא); *pl.* כְּרַיִין. Targ. Prov. XIV, 17; 29 דכ׳ רוחיה (h. text קצר רוח, קצר אפים).—ענבי דְּכַרְיָין grapes which shrunk, undeveloped (blackish) grapes. Naz. 34[b], a. e., v. כְּרוּם ch.

Ithpe. אִיכְּרַה *to be ill.* Targ. Prov. XXIII, 35.

כַּרְהָא m. (preced.) *distress, illness.* Targ. Y. Deut. VII, 15 Ar. (Levita כרחא, ed. מרעין, v. Koh. Ar. Compl. s. v.).

כּוּר׳, כַּרְהָנָא m. same. Targ. Prov. XVIII, 14 (Levita כִּירְחֵיה).

כרו, Pes. 111[b] כ׳ משא, v. כְּרוּמְשָׁא.

כְּרוּב I m. (b. h.; cmp. כְּרַב I; v., however, Schr. KAT[2] p. 39; p. 609) *[head,] Cherub.* Succ. 5[b]; Hag. 13[b] . . . מאי כ׳ כרביא וכ׳ what is K'rub?—. . 'Childlike', for in Babylonia they call a child *rabia.* Ib. והפכו לכ׳ and he changed it (the face of the ox, Ez. I, 10) into that of a Cherub. Ib. היינו פני כ׳ וכ׳ the face of the Ch. is the same as that of man, the one being large, the other small. Yoma 77[a]. Lev. R. s. 32; a. e.—*Pl.* כְּרוּבִים. Tanh. ed. Bub. B'resh. 25 לפיכך נקראו כ׳ שהן רבים (read: רוֹבִים, v. רוֹבֶה) they are called Ch., because they are young (childlike), v. supra. Yoma 54[b] ראה הכ׳ מעורים וכ׳ saw the figures of the cherubs twined around each other. Ib.[a] כ׳ דצורתא וכ׳ painted cherubs were in the Second Temple; a. e.

כְּרוּב II m. (v. preced.) *[rounded,] cabbage.* Ter. X, 11 כ׳ של שקייא cabbage from an irrigated field, opp. כ׳ של בעל, v. בַּעַל 3.—Ber. 44[b] קלח של כ׳ cabbage stalk. Ib. כ׳ למזון cabbage is good for a satisfying meal. Ned. VI, 10, v. אִיסְפַּרְגּוֹס; a. fr.

כְּרוּבָה, כְּרוּבָא ch. same, v. כְּרָבָא II. Ber. 38[b] Ar. ed. pr. (ed. Koh. a. Talm. ed. כרבא).—Y. R. Hash. I, 57[b] bot.; Y. Hall. I, 57[c] top [read:] צם . . אַפְסֵק כרובה (v. פְּסַקָא) fasted two days in succession on a last meal of cabbage, and died.—*Pl.* כְּרוּבָּתָא *various species of cabbage,* cmp. אִיסְפַּרְגּוֹס. Y. Ned. VII, beg. 40[b].

כְּרוּבָא ch.=h. כְּרוּב I. Targ. Ex. XXV, 19; a. e.—*Pl.* כְּרוּבַיָּא, כְּרוּבִין. Ib. 18, sq.; a. e.

כְּרוּבָא (כְּרוּ׳) m. (כְּרַב II) *dug around, marked off*; כרוב ארעא (cmp. חַקְלָא) *a certain measure of land.* Targ. O. Gen. XXXV, 16; XLVIII, 7; Targ. II Kings V, 19 (h. text כברת ארץ).

כְּהוּבָה, v. כְּרוּבָא.

כְּרוּבְתָא f. (כְּרַב I, cmp. כַּרְבַּלְתָּא) *wrap, blanket.*—*Pl.* כְּרוּבָתָא, constr. כְּרוּבַת. Targ. Zech. XIV, 20 (ed. Wil. כְּרוּבַת, ed. Lag. כרורת, Var. כרובת, בדורת; h. text מְצִלּוֹת).

כַּרְוָן, v. כַּרְיָא.

כָּרוֹז m. *a vessel.* Lev. R. s. 10 כי כ׳ Ar. (ed. כַּבְּדִין; Pesik. Shub. p. 163[a]; Yalk. Jer. 303 כְּבלִי), v. קָרוֹז.

כְּרוֹז m. (כְּרַז) *public announcement.* Lev. R. s. 6 הוציא כ׳ he issued a proclamation. Snh. VI, 1 (43[a]) והכ׳ יוצא וכ׳ Ms. M. (ed. וכ׳) and it is cried out before him (the delinquent). Ib. 43[a] (missing in later ed.) והכ׳ יוצא לפניו וכ׳ and forty days before his (Jesus') execution, it was published &c.; a. fr.

כָּרוֹז m. (preced.) *public crier.* Y. Succ. V, 55[b] bot. גבינר כ׳ (not גבר) G. the Temple crier. Pesik. R. s. 5 שילח את הכ׳ he sent the crier forth. Esth. R. to VI, 12 כּוֹרֵז, v. גּוֹלְיָיר.—*Pl.* כָּרוֹזוֹת. Deut. R. s. 4.

כְּרוֹזָא, כָּרוֹז ch.=h. כָּרוֹז. Targ. O. Ex. XXXVI, 6 כָּרוֹז (Y. כְּרוֹזָא, some ed. כְּרוֹ׳).—Y. Sabb. XVI, 15ᵈ; Y. Ned. IV, 38ᵈ top אפיק... כ׳ R. I. issued a proclamation; a. fr.

כָּרוֹזָא ch.=h. כָּרוֹז. Dan. III, 4.—Targ. Y. Lev. XIII, 45 וּכְרוֹ׳ (read: וְכָרוֹ׳).—Y. Shek. V, 48ᵈ bot. (transl. קרא הגבר) אכריז כ׳ the Temple crier has announced the morning; Y. Succ. V, 55ᶜ.

כְּרַוְיָא, כְּרַוְיָא m. (careum, sub. cuminum, v. Sm. Ant. s. v.) כַּמּוֹנָא כ׳ caraway. Ab. Zar. 29ᵃ (a remedy for nausea, v. אוּנְקְלָי I) מייתי כ׳ כ׳ (Ar. כרויא כמונא, v. Koh. Ar. Compl. s. v. כמן, IV, p. 247, note 15) let him take caraway &c. [Rashi: כמין כַּק אגרוּן (כמון), obviously a corruption of a Provençal word.]

כְּרוֹזָה, v. כְּרָה v.

כָּרוֹךְ to tie around, v. כָּרַךְ I.

כְּרוֹךְ m. (preced.) band, priestly division. Targ. Y. Deut. XVIII, 6 (cmp. Y. Yeb. XI, 12ᵃ bot. בכל משמר שירצה).

כְּרוֹכָא, כְּרוֹכַת f. (כָּרַךְ) winding, intestines; כ׳ קטנא small winding (duodenum), כ׳ עביא the large winding (jejunum). Koh. R. to VII, 19; Yalk. Koh. 976; Lev. R. s. 3, v. כַּנְתָא. [Targ. Y. Lev. XI, 22 כרוכא Ar. a. Levita, v. כַּרְזְבָא.—Y. R. Hash. I, 57ᵇ bot. כרוכה, v. כְּרוּבָא.]

כְּרוּכְיָא, v. כּוּרְכְיָא.

כרוכין, Y. Shebu. III, 34ᵈ Ar., v. קְרוּבִין.

כרוכסין, Y. B. Mets. II, 8ᶜ bot., Var. in ed. פרוכ׳, כרוכ׳, v. פַּרְכְסִין.

כְּרוֹכַת, v. כְּרוֹכָא.

כְּרוּם m. (כָּרַם) 1) [coating,] color, esp. yellow or green. Cant. R. to I, 14 (play on בכרמי, ib.) זה יעקב... בכ׳ פניו וכ׳ that alludes to Jacob who went in to his father with paleness of face, trembling in his shame &c.—2) K'rum, name of a bird changing colors in the sun. Ber. 6ᵇ.

כְּרוּם, כְּרוּמָא ch. same, color, v. אַכְרוּם.—כ׳ יַמָּא sea-green, name of a beryll (aqua marina). Targ. Ex. XXVIII, 20; a. e.—* עִינְבֵי דכ׳ [green berries,] undeveloped grapes, worm-eaten grapes. B. Mets. 106ᵇ ע׳ דכרום ed. a. Ar. (Ms. H. a. Rome 2, Alf. דקרום; v. Rabb. D. S. a. l. note 50). Naz. 34ᵇ (38ᵇ) ע׳ דכרין (Ar. דכרום, Rashi frequ. ענבין דיכרין), v. כְּרַם. Hull. 58ᵇ top Var. דכרים.

כְּרוּמְשָׁא m. service-tree. Pes. 111ᵇ כרו משא ed. (Ms. M. כרכמושא, emend. כרמ׳); v. Löw Pfl. p. 287.

כרוסא, v. אוֹלוֹכְרוּסוֹן.

כְּרוּסְפְּדָא m. (κράσπεδον, mostly pl. κράσπεδα) edge, border, fringe. Targ. O. Num. XV, 38 כְּרוּסְפַּד כנפא ed. Berl. (Mss. a. ed. כרוספדא דכ׳).—Pl. כְּרוּסְפְּדִין. Ib., sq. Targ. O. Deut. XXII, 12.

כְּרוּסְפְּדַאי pr. n. m. Crusp'day. Snh. 69ᵃ (v. קרוספדאי, a. כְּרִיסְפָּא).

כְּרוּפְיָיתָא m. pl. (prob. fr. כְּרוּךְ, dial.=כרוב, cmp. כְּרַךְ) dealers in vegetables, greens &c. M. Kat. 13ᵇ כ׳ דפומבדיתא (Alf. קְרוּפְיָאתָא).

כרופסלה, Y. Sabb. VI, 8ᵇ bot. some ed., v. פּוּדוֹפְסִילָא.

כְּרוּשְׁיָיתָא f. pl. (כרש, cmp. כרס) balls, cakes. Gitt. 69ᵇ כ׳ דשערי Ar. (ed. ברושייאתא; Ar. s. v. כמך: קְרוּשְׁיָתָא) barley cakes; כ׳ דחיטי wheat cakes.

כְּרוּשְׁתִּינָא f. (=כרושת עינא; v. preced.) [with large eye-balls,] name of a species of bats. Sabb. 78ᵃ ed. (Ms. M. כרושתנא, Ms. O. ברושטינא; Ar. ed. Koh. כרשתינא).

כְּרוּת, v. כְּרַת.

כָּרוֹת, v. כָּרַת.

כָּרַז to call together (cmp. כְּלִי II); to call out, announce. Tanh. Mishp. 19 וכשהמלאך כּוֹרֵז האדם בשלום as long as the angel cries out ('give honor to the image of God'), man is safe. Ib. (ref. to Job XXXIII, 23) אם יהא מן אותן אלף כורז וכ׳ if there be one out of the thousand (angels) crying out before him, to proclaim a man's righteousness. Esth. R. to VI, 12 כּוֹרֵז, v. כָּרוֹז. Deut. R. s. 4 והכרוזות כּוֹרְזִין וכ׳ and the criers (angels) call out before him, Give room &c., v. infra.

Hif. הִכְרִיז same. Tanh. l. c. ואחד מהם מַכְרִיז...תנו וכ׳ and one of them (the angels) cries out before him, saying, Give honor &c.; Midr. Till. to Ps. XVII; Yalk. Ps. 670 מַכְרִיזִין, v. אִירְקוֹנְיָא. B. Mets. II, 1, sq. אלו חייב לְהַכְרִיז the following finds one must publish. Ib. 28ᵇ אבידתא מַכְרִיז the crier announces that something has been found (not defining the object), opp. to גלימא מכריז 'a cloak' (or whatever the object may be).—Pes. 113ᵃ שלשה הקב״ה מכריז עליהם וכ׳ Ms. M. there are three persons for whose sake the Lord sends out the crier every day (to announce their praise); a. fr.

כְּרַז, *Af.* אַכְרֵיז same. Targ. Jon. III, 7 (h. text ויזעק); a. fr.—Targ. Ps. CV, 16 Ms. (ed. ואכלי, v. כְּלִי II). Targ. Y. Deut. XXIV, 3 אַכְרִיזוּ וכ׳ it has been announced (decreed) in heaven.—Kidd. 81ᵃ מר זוטרא מלקי ומַכְרִיז M. Z. punished (a woman for being closeted with a man) and published the fact (in order to protect her children's legitimacy). Ib. אי לאו דקא מַכְרְזִי (מַכְרְזֵי) וכ׳ if it had not been called out in heaven, Beware of R. M. &c. Yoma 72ᵇ, a. fr.

כַּרְזָא m., pl. כַּרְזֵי name of two species of winged locusts. Hull. 62ᵇ כ׳ דבי חילפי וכ׳ (Ar. כְּרָאזֵי) those living in rushes are permitted, דבי כורי וכ׳ Ar. (ed. כרבי, v. כְּרָבָא II) those among heaps are forbidden (v. Tosaf. a. l.).

כרזג, v. בַּרְזַג.

כַּרְזְבָא, כַּרְזוּבָא a species of locusts. Targ. Y. Lev. XI, 22 (Ar. a. Levita כרוכא; h. text חגב). Targ. Ps. LXXVIII, 47 (h. text חנמל). Cmp. אַרְזְבוֹנִית.

כַּרְזִיִּים, v. כַּרְזִים.

כַּרְזִילָא m. (כְּרַז, with format. ל) 1) the shepherd's as-

sistant that gathers the scattered flock. B. Kam. 56ᵇ מסרו לרועה לכַּרְזִילֵיהּ Ar. (ed. לב׳, corr. acc.) 'he surrendered it to the shepherd' (in Mish.) means to his assistant.—2) *he who calls to, and leads in prayer.*—*Pl.* כַּרְזִילִין. Targ. Cant. I, 8 כַּרְזִילָהָא (not פ׳, v. ed. Lag. II, p. XIV) her (the congregation's) leaders. Targ. Koh. X, 10.

כַּרְזַיִם, כַּרְזַוִים pr. n. pl. *Karzayim*, near Jerusalem. Men. 85ᵃ חיטי כ׳ (Ms. M. כרוים, Ms. R. 2 a. Ms. K. כ׳, v. Rabb. D. S. a. l. note) wheat of K.

כַּרְזִימִין, v. כַּרְזִימֵי.

כַּרְזַנְיָיתָא f. pl. (כְּרוּז) *calling out.* B. Mets. 40ᵇ, v. כַּרְזָנִיתָא.

כָּרַח (v. כָּרָה a. כָּרַךְ) *to be tied, narrowed in.*—Denom. פֹּרַח.

Hif. הִכְרִיחַ *to force, subdue.* Gen. R. s. 75, beg. (ref. to הכריעהו, Ps. XVII, 13) הַכְרִיחֵהוּ וכ׳ force him down on the scale of guilt, break his resistance; (Yalk. Gen. 130 הכריעהו). Cant. R. to IV, 12 אם בנפשותן חן מַכְרִיחִין וכ׳ (not בעשותן) if they did violence to their souls, how much more &c.; (Pesik. B'shall. p. 82ᵇ שלוטין).

כְּרַח ch., v. כְּרָה.

כֹּרַח, פּוֹרַח m. (preced.) *force, unwillingness, necessity.* על כרח־ (or בעל) *against* or *without one's will.* Ab. IV, 22 על כָּרְחֲךָ וכ׳ without thy will thou hast been created &c. Gitt. 21ᵃ בעל כּוֹרְחָהּ against her will, opp. מדעתה, v. דַּעַת; a. fr.

כּוּרְחָא, כ׳ ch. same. Targ. Y. II Gen. XLIV, 18. Targ. I Sam. II, 16 (h. text בחזקה).—[Targ. Y. Deut. VII, 15, v. כַּרְהָא.]

כרטוסה, v. next w.

כַּרְטֵיס m. (χάρτης) *document.* Y. Keth. IX, end, 33ᶜ כהן (not ...סן) דמר אבד כַּרְטֵיסוֹ וכ׳ in accordance with the opinion of him who says, if one's document (of indebtedness) is lost, write a duplicate for him. Ib. לבר מן כרטוסה קדמייא (read: כַּרְטֵיסָהּ or כַּרְטֵיסַיָּה *pl.*) וכ׳ irrespective of a previous document (or previous documents, against me) which may be in thy possession. Ib. [read:] אלא כי אורחא דבר נשא מימר אבד כַּרְטֵיסִי עבד חורן but is it a usual matter for a man to say (to his debtor), my document has been lost, write another for me?—V. קַרְטֵיס.

כָּרָה, כרי (b. h.) [*to round, heap, cave,*] 1) *to dig.* Mekh. Mishp., N'zikin, s. 11 כּוֹרֶה מנין how am I to know that he who digs a pit is responsible?—B. Kam. 51ᵃ כורה אחר כורה one who digs after another one, i. e. who completes the pit to its legal size. Succ. 53ᵃ; Macc. 11ᵃ בשעה שכ׳ דוד וכ׳ when David dug for the foundations; a. fr.—Part. pass. כָּרוּי, f. כְּרוּיָה *hollowed out.* Kel. III, 5, a. e., v. הִירוּק a. כָּרַךְ.—2) *to sit in a circle*, v. infra.

Hif. הִכְרָה 1) *to heap, pile.* Gen. R. s. 100 (ref. to כריתי, Gen. L, 5) הרבה ממון תַּכְרֶה עליה much money shalt thou pile up (give me) for it (the grave); (some ed. הכרה Jacob piled up in settling with Esau). Ib. הִכְרִיתִי (corr. הִכְרֵיתִי); v. כְּרִי; Pesik. R. s. 1 וכל ממון שהיה לו ה׳ וכ׳ (not מסר לו) and he (Jacob) piled up whatever money he had to place it before Esau &c.—2) *to invite to a banquet*; 3) (with play on כרת) *to excise, to destroy.* Snh. 20ᵃ; Yalk. Sam. 142 (ref. to לחברות, II Sam. III, 35, where Raba had before him a K'thib. להכרות) כתיב להכרות . . . . בתחלה לְהַכְרוֹתוֹ וכ׳ it is written *l'hakhroth* (to entertain) and read *l'habroth* (v. בָּרָה): originally they came with the intention of destroying him (for the murder of Abner), and finally (when convinced of his innocence) they came to comfort him; [Yalk. Ms. to Sam. l. c., quoted in Rabb. D. S. Snh. l. c. note 9: כתיב לִבְרוֹת וקרינן לְהַבְרוֹת בתחלה לברות וכ׳ it is written *libroth* (*to pierce*, cmp. Ez. XXIII, 47), and we read *l'habroth* &c.].

כְּרָא, כְּרֵי ch. same, *to dig, bore.* Targ. O. Ex. XXI, 33 יִכְרֵי ed. Berl. (oth. ed. יִכְרֵה). Targ. Ps. XL, 7; a. e.—B. Kam. 51ᵃ אמרי ליה זיל כְּרֵי לן ואזל כְּרָא לחו (some ed. כָּרָה hebr.) they said to him, go and dig for us, and he went and dug &c. Ib. 48ᵃ כמאן דִכְרָיֵיהּ דמי he is as responsible as if he had dug it. Succ. 53ᵇ כָּרֵינַן פורתא וכ׳ we bore only a little and there comes water; a. e.—*Taan. 24ᵃ דהוה כָּרְיָא בחוצא that he was boring a hole in the fence (v. Rabb. D. S. a. l. note for Var. lect.).—[כרי *to be narrow, distressed*, part. כְּרִי, כְּרִיָא, כַּרְיָא, *pl.* כְּרִין, v. כְּרָה]

כְּרִי m. (preced.) *heap, pile.* Ex. R. s. 31 (ref. to כריתי, Gen. L, 5, v. כָּרָה) נטל . . . ועשה אותו כ׳ he (Jacob) took all the money he possessed and made a pile of it; כ׳ של דינרין וכ׳ a pile of denars have I given to Esau. Tosef. Ter. III, 17. Ter. III, 5. Y. ib. I, 40ᵇ bot. חבקיר כְּרְיוֹ (not כריר) if a man renounced possession of his pile (store) of grain. Ib. IV, 42ᵈ top לפטור את כְּרְיוֹ to discharge the duty of T'rumah for his entire store. Y. Gitt. VII, 48ᶜ bot. תרם את כְּרְיוֹ if he gave T'rumah for his store; a. fr.—*Pl.* כְּרָיִים. Y. Shek. III, end, 47ᶜ אילו שני כ׳ וכ׳ if it were a case of two piles for which a person had discharged T'rumah &c.

כַּרְיָא I, כְּרִיָּה ch. 1) same. B. Mets. 105ᵃ (in a tenant's contract) ואוקים כ׳ וכ׳ and I will place the pile (of my crop) before thee. Y. Maasr. I, 49ᵃ bot. (expl. משיחמרח) מן דו ישפר אפוי דכ׳ from the time he gives shape to the pile; a. e.—*Pl.* כְּרְיָיתָא, כְּרְיָוָון, כְּרְיָון. Targ. Y. Ex. VIII, 10, v. כּוֹרָא. Targ. II Chr. XXXI, 6, 7, sq. (h. text ערמות).—2) *digging, ditch; well.* B. Bath. 8ᵃ רמו כ׳ חדתא וכ׳ (v. Rabb. D. S. a. l. note 80) put on orphans (heirs) the obligation of contributing towards a new ditch. Ib. (הכל) לכ׳ (ד)פתיא׳ (Ms. F. כְּרְיָא, v. Rabb. D. S. a. l. note) even scholars must lend their services in digging a street-well; B. Mets. 108ᵃ (v. Rabb. D. S. a. l. note 60). Ib. 110ᵃ וכרי כ׳ and must do what digging may be required (ditch, well), v. כַּסְקָא. Ib. לכ׳ דנהרא for dredging the river (or channel).—*בית כ׳ *House of Heaps* (Ruins), a cacophemistic change of the name בֵּית גַּלְיָא, v. גַּלְיָא II. Ab. Zar. 46ᵃ; Tem. 28ᵇ (Var. כַּלְיָיא *destruction*).—[V., however, גַּדָּא a. גַּלָּא.]—Meg. 6ᵃ בית כ׳ שלחן Ms. M. (ed. במיא, v. Rabb. D. S. a. l. note).

כַּרְיָא II m. (cmp. כָּרָה) *a worm in poppy*, v. קַרְיָא.

כְּרִיָּה, כְּרִייָה f. (כָּרָה) *digging*, esp. *digging a pit* through which an animal was injured (Ex. XXI, 33). Mekh. Mishp., N'zikin, s. 11; Tosef. B. Kam. VI, 13 נפל לפניו מקול כ׳ if the animal fell forward (into the pit) frightened by the sound of digging (within the pit), נפל לאחריו מקול הכ׳ if it tumbled backward &c. B. Kam. 49ᵇ על עסקי כ׳ for the act of digging a pit (although not on his own soil). Ib. 50ᵃ ה״א כ׳ הוא דבעי כיסוי I might have thought only when he dug the pit he is bound to cover it up; a. e.

כְּרִיחָא, כְּרִיחָא m. (v. כְּרַח) *sufferer*.—*Pl.* כְּרִיחֵי, כְּרִיחַי. Sabb. 21ᵃ כל כ׳ דמערבא Ar. (ed. בריחי, corr. acc.) all sufferers of Palestine, v. קִיקָיוֹן. Ib. 145ᵇ כריחי ed. Sonc. (ed. ב׳; Ms. Rashi כְּרִיכֵי, v. Rabb. D. S. a. l. note).

כְּרִיחוּתָא f. (preced.) *distress, misfortune*. Sabb. 10ᵃ כ׳ וכ׳ Ar. is it such a misfortune &c., v. טִרְחוּתָא.

כְּרִיוּתָא f. (preced.) *pain*. Targ. Prov. XXV, 20, v. בְּרִיוּתָא.

כְּרִיָּיה, v. כְּרִיָּה.

כְּרֵיךְ, v. כְּרַךְ.

***כְּרִיךְ** m., *pl.* כְּרִיכִין (כְּרַךְ) *parasites, lichens, moss*. Lev. R. s. 15 כל זמן . . . היא עושה כ׳ as long as the well empties into the garden, it will grow lichens (compared to leprous spots on the body, v. חֲזָזִית; Yalk. Lev. 554 היא כשויה בִּיצִין).

כְּרִיכָא I m. (כְּרַךְ) *winding; rounded*. B. Kam. 50ᵇ (v. Rabb. D. S. a. l. note 6); Yalk. Ex. 341.

כְּרִיכָא II f. ch.=h. כְּרִיכָה, *sheaf*.—*Pl.* כְּרִיכָן. Targ. Y. Gen. XXXVII, 7 מכרכן כ׳ Ar. (quoted in Rashi to B. Mets. II, 1; ed. מפרכן פירוכין).

כְּרִיכָא III m. (preced.) *bundle* or *band*.—*Pl.* כְּרִיכֵי. Snh. 67ᵇ (of a juggler) שדי כ׳ וכ׳ cast ribbons (or bundles) of silk out of his nose.—V. כְּרָכָא.

כְּרִיכָה f. (כָּרַךְ) 1) *winding around*. Tanh. Vaëra 4 (ref. to Ber. V, 1) מה . . . כְּרִיכַת נחש למלכות what led the scholars to place the serpent winding itself around a person side by side with the (Roman) government?; Ex. R. s. 9.—2) *bundle, bunch, small sheaf*, contrad. to אֲלוּמָּה.—*Pl.* כְּרִיכוֹת. B. Mets. II, 1. Ib. 22ᵇ; a. e.—[Ib. 37ᵇ כְּרֵיכוֹת, v. כְּרַךְ.]

***כְּרִיכְתָא** f. (v. כְּרִיךְ) *lichen-like, scabby*. B. Kam. 85ᵃ נאתא כ׳ (Yalk. Ex. 332 כְּרִיכְתָא), v. פַּרְבִּיתָא.

כרים, כְּרִין, v. כְּרָה.

כְּרִיסָא, כְּרִיס־, v. כְּרֵס, כַּרְסָא.

כ׳ אַרְגִּירָא, כְּרִיסַר m. (χρυσάργυρον, usu. χρυσάργυρον) *gold and silver tax* levied by Constantine the Great (v. Sachs Beitr. II, 140; Rapap. Er. Mill. p. 193, a. authors there quoted). Y. B. Kam. III, 3ᶜ top אתן כ׳ א׳ וכ׳ as to the chrysargyron: before that tax is arranged, it is permitted to say (to the officers), 'this man is my fellow-trader'; when it has been arranged (and is being collected), it is not permitted (because it would injure the person omitted in the list without alleviating the burden of others); cmp. אכסניי.—*Pl.* כְּרִיסַרְגּוּרִיּוֹת. Cant. R. II, 2 (variously corrupted).—Midr. Till. to Ps. XII מרגזאות, ed. Bub. מזה נמסאות; Yalk. ib. 656 מדגראות, read: כְּרִיזַרְגְּרָאוֹת (ascribed to Hadrian).

כְּרִיסוֹלָכָנוֹן m. (χρυσολάχανον) *orach*. Y. Kil. I, 27ᵃ bot. כירבי לבנון (corr. acc.).

כְּרִיסְמִיוֹנָא m. (χαριστίων) *charistion*, an instrument for weighing or lifting (Lidd. et Scott. Gr. Dict.); *scales for minute weights* (P. Sm. s. v. כרסטונא, p. 1836). Lam. R. to I, 5 כרסטיריתא Ar. (corr. acc.; ed. קַרְצְבִּיוֹנָא).

כְּרִיסִית f. (denom. of כֶּרֶס) *a leather bag*, (as a measure) *K'resith* containing one S'ah. Kel. XX, I Talm. ed. (Mish. ed. a. ed. Dehr. כריתית, Ar. ed. Koh. כרתית, denom. of כַּר).

כְּרִיסְפָּא, ק׳ pr. n. m. (Crispus) *Crispa*, name of an Amora. Pesik. Shubah, p. 157ᵇ; (R. Hash. 16ᵇ כרוספדאי); Y. ib. I, 57ᵃ bot. קרוספא ed. Krot.—Ib. II, 58ᵇ top קריספא; Y. Snh. I, 18ᶜ bot. קריספדא. Pesik. R. s. 15 קריספא.

כְּרִיעָה f. (כָּרַע) *kneeling*. Ber. 34ᵇ; Meg. 22ᵇ, contrad. to קִידָּה. Y. Ber. I, 3ᶜ bot., a. e., v. בְּרִיכָה. Ib.ᵈ top לך כ׳ unto thee is kneeling due.—*Pl.* כְּרִיעוֹת. Ber. 31ᵃ, v. הִשְׁתַּחֲוָאָה.

כְּרֵישָׁא, כְּרֵישׁ I (כרש, cmp. כְּרוֹשְׁיָיתָא) name of a *fish*, prob. *shark*. B. Bath. 74ᵃ bot. כרויש Ms. M. (ed. כרישא, Ar. כרשא).

כְּרֵישָׁא II, כְּרֵישָׁה m. (v. preced.; cmp. כַּרְשִׁינָה) *leek*. Sabb. VIII, 5 (80ᵇ) כדי לזבל כ׳ as much manure as is required for one leek plant. Y. ib. VII, 9ᵈ bot. כדי ליטע כרישה as much space as is required for planting one leek. Makhsh. I, 5; Tosef. ib. I, 5.—*Pl.* כְּרֵישִׁים, כְּרֵישִׁין. Kil. I, 2 כ׳ וּכְרֵישֵׁי שדה וכ׳ (garden) leek and field-leek . . . are not heterogeneous, v. כִּלְאַיִם. Tosef. Sabb. XV (XVI), 14 גוזזין לו כ׳ ed. Zuck. (Var. כרשינן) we may cut leek for him (on the Sabbath, as a remedy for a serpent's bite). Ned. VI, 9; Tosef. ib. III, 6; Y. ib. VI, 39ᵈ bot., v. קַפְלוֹט; a. fr.—V. כַּרְתֵּי.

כְּרִית f. (כָּרָה) 1) *the groove* in the mountain slopes made by running water. Y. M. Kat. I, 80ᵇ top עד כדי שתפרח הכ׳ (ed. הב׳, corr. acc.) until the grooves bloom (are covered with vegetation). Ib. פרחה כ׳ ולא פסקו if the grooves have bloomed, but the rains have not ceased (set in again); Y. Ter. VIII, 46ᵃ top עד כדי שתפוח הכ׳ (corr. acc.).—2) (b. h.) *K'rith*, name of a brook. Targ. I Kings XVII, 3.

כְּרֵית pr. n. *K'reth*, a district near Philistia. Targ. I Sam. XXX, 14 (ed. Lag. כרת; h. text הכרתי).

כְּרִית־, v. כְּרַת.

כְּרִיתָה f. (כְּרַת) 1) *cutting of genitals, mutilation*. Yeb.

75^b, v. שְׁפַךְ.—2) *divorce by means of a deed* (סֵפֶר כְּרִיתוּת). Gitt. 10^b והא לאו בני כ׳ נינהו but they (the gentiles) are not subject to the Jewish mode of divorce (how, then, can they act as judges in divorce cases)?—3) (sub. ברית) *the making of a covenant.*—*Pl.* כְּרִיתוֹת. Tosef. Sot. VIII, 10; 11 ed. Zuck., v. בְּרִית.—4) = כָּרֵת *excision.* Macc. III, 15, v. כָּרֵת.—*Pl.* כְּרִיתוֹת, v. כָּרֵת.—5) *decision.* Pl. as ab. Midr. Till. to Ps. III (ref. to כרתי, II Sam. XV, 18) כורתי כ׳ (ed. Bub. כריתות) those who pass (final) decisions.

כְּרִיתוּת f. (b. h. כְּרִיתֻת; preced.) *final divorce.* Sifré Deut. 269 (ref. to Deut. XXIV, 1) שיהא כורת מכאן .... אין זה כ׳ he must make the thing final, from this we derive that if a man says, this is thy letter of divorce under the condition that thou wilt never go ...., this is no final (valid) divorce; Gitt. 83^b. Tosef. ib. IX (VII), 1; a. fr.—Gitt. l. c.; ib. 21^b; Succ. 24^b, a. e. כרת כ׳ the legal deduction from the use of the word כריתות (Deut. l. c.) where the word כָּרֵת might have been used.

כְּרִיתִינוֹן, v. כְּרֵתִינוֹן.

כְּרֵיתִית, v. כְּרֵיסִית.

כָּרַךְ (cmp. כָּרָה) *to encircle, twine around, embrace, wrap.* Men. 39^a תכלת שכ׳ רובה a fringe the larger portion of which he twined together (v. תְּכֵלֶת). Ib. כדי שיִכְרוֹךְ וישנה וכ׳ enough to twine around three times. Yoma 38^a כְּרָכָהּ embraced it (clung to the bronze door). Sabb. 133^b וְכָרְכֵהוּ בשיראין נאין Ms. M. (ed. וכורכו) and twine handsome ribbons around it. Pes. 115^a; Zeb. 79^a היה כּוֹרְכָן וכ׳ used to wrap them together (insert the Passover meat and the bitter herb between the Matsah). Ab. Zar. 18^a כְּרָכוּהוּ בס״ת וכ׳ they wrapped him in a scroll of the Law and burned him. Tosef. Meg. IV (III), 20 כּוֹרְכִין תורה וכ׳ you may wrap the Pentateuch in covers intended for &c.; (Meg. 27^a גוללין); a. fr.—Pes. IV, 8; Tosef. ib. II (III), 19 כּוֹרְכִין את שמע they recited the confession of faith (Deut. VI, 4 sq.) in one כֶּרֶךְ, without the proper pauses (or without inserting 'Blessed be the Name of His glorious kingdom &c.' between verses 4 and 5), v. Pes. 56^a, a. Y. ib. IV, 31^b.—Part. pass. כָּרוּךְ, f. כְּרוּכָה; pl. כְּרוּכִין, כְּרוּכִים, כְּרוּכוֹת; *twined around, wrapped up*; trnsf. (with אחר) *clinging to, running after.* Ber. V, 1 אפי׳ נחש כ׳ וכ׳ even if a serpent is wound around his heel, he must not interrupt his prayer, v. כְּרִיכָה. Kidd. 66^a הרי כ׳ ומונחת וכ׳ behold it (the Law) is wrapped up and lies in the corner, whoever wishes may study it. Gen. R. s. 78 בפנים כ׳ אני מהלך I shall walk with my face wrapped up (in humility).—Hull. 78^b (expl. Lev. XXII, 28) מי שבנו כ׳ אחריו that animal to whom the young clings (the mother). Sabb. 52^a כרוכין with the chain or halter twined around them, opp. נמשכין led by the chain &c. Hull. 59^b (קרנים) כרוכות horns the layers of which encircle one another. Ex. R. s. 33 הרי כ׳ זה בזה their bodies were twisted around each other; a. e.

Nif. נִכְרַךְ *to be twined around; to be wrapped up.* Y. Ter. VII, 46^b bot. יִכָּרֵךְ המת בסדינו shall the dead be wrapped up in his sheet?, i. e. shall that man be abandoned to his fate?—Yoma 69^a שמא תִכָּרֵךְ וכ׳ lest one thread wind itself around (stick to) his body.

Pi. כֵּרֵךְ, כִּר׳; *Hif.* הִכְרִיךְ *to wind around, wrap.* Ab. d'R. N. ch. III, beg. הַמְכָרֵךְ סמרטוטין וכ׳ he who ties a bandage over his eyes (pretending blindness) &c. Men. 39^a אפי׳ לא כי׳ בה וכ׳ even if he formed only one link by winding the twine around. Y. Hag. III, 79^a top וִיכַרְכֶינָּה בסיב ויטבילה let him wrap bast around it and so immerse it; ib. II, end, 78^c (corr. acc.). Tosef. Kel. B. Mets. IX, 6 שהוא מְכָרֵךְ בו וכ׳ which one twines around the couch. Ib. מַכְרִיךְ.—Part. pass. מְכוֹרָךְ, *pl.* מְכוֹרָכִין. Lev. R. s. 35 הסייף ... ניתנו מכ׳ וכ׳ (Sifré Deut. 40 כְּרוּכִים) the sword and the book have been handed from heaven wrapped up together; a. e.—[Tosef. Kel. B. Mets. VI, 1, v. כָּרְכֵּם.]

כְּרַךְ I, כְּרֵיךְ, כְּרוֹךְ ch. 1) same. Targ. Job XXXI, 36, v. כְּבַן. Targ. Prov. VI, 21. Targ. I Kings XIX, 13; a. fr. (interch. in ed. with *Pa.*).—Taan. 22^a top לצפרא כַּרְכִינְהוּ וכ׳ (v. Rabb. D. S. a. l. note) in the morning they rolled the mattresses up and carried them off. Yoma 78^b; Yeb. 102^b כריך סודרא וכ׳ tied a cloth around his legs. Sabb. 110^a האי מאן דכַרְכֵיה וכ׳ he around whom a serpent has twined itself. B. Bath. 14^b רב׳ ביה פורתא ומנח ליה לכַרְכֵיה לעיל Ms. H. (ed. פורתא וכַרְכֵיה לעיל ..., v. Rabb. D. S. a. l. note 40) he rolled up a small portion (of the scroll) and placed that rolled portion on top (of the scroll). Ab. Zar. 18^b כַּרְכְתֵּיה she embraced him; a. fr.—Part. pass. כְּרִיךְ. Y. Ter. VIII, 45^d top כ׳ עליה wound around it.—Esp. כ׳ ריפתא *to double the bread,* placing salt, herbs &c. between (v. preced.), in gen. כ׳ ר׳ (or sub. ר׳) *to begin a meal, to dine.* Targ. Y. I Deut. XXXII, 50 ובעו .. לְמִכְרַךְ ר׳ and the guests were about beginning to eat.—Ber. 22^b כָּרוּכוּ ר׳ sat down to dine together. Taan. 23^b יתיב וכ׳ ר׳ ... איתו כְרוּכוּ he sat down to eat and did not say to the scholars, come eat with us; Y. ib. I, 64^b bot., sq. אתון כריכין (corr. acc.).—Trnsf. כְּרוֹךְ ותני combine the two versions into one. Sabb. 34^b. Men. 87^a.—2) *to surround, fortify.* Targ. Jer. LI, 53.—Part. pass. כְּרִיךְ, f. כְּרִיכָא, כְּרִיכְתָא; pl. כְּרִיכִין, כְּרִיכָן, כְּרִיכְתָא; כְּרִיכָיָא. Targ. Is. II, 15. Ib. XXVII, 10. Targ. Ps. XXXI, 3; 22. Targ. O. Deut. III, 5; a. fr.—[V. כְּרִיכָא.]

Pa. כָּרֵיךְ 1) same, v. supra.—2) *to turn around.* Targ. Prov. XXVI, 14 (h. text סבב).—Sabb. 129^a, v. זִרְקָא I.

Ithpe. אִכְּרִיךְ 1) *to be wrapped up.* Targ. Esth. VIII, 15 מִיכְּרִיךְ וכ׳ clothed in &c. (h. text תכריך). Koh. R. to VIII, 11; IX, 10 ורישיה מִיכְּרַךְ with his head wrapped up (in mourning). Sabb. 110^b איכְּרַךְ גלא ביה he wrapped himself up in the cloak and slept in it.—Trnsf. *to attach one's self.* Keth. 77^b מי אִיכַּרְכַת וכ׳ hast thou mingled with gonorrhoeists &c.? Ib. א׳ בהו mingled with them.

כֶּרֶךְ m. (preced. wds.) 1) *twining.* Men. 39^a חוט של כ׳ the thread which is used for twining (v. תְּכֵלֶת).—2) *roll, volume* (of a book). B. Mets. 29^b ולא יהיו ג׳ קורין בכ׳ אחד Ms. M. (differ. in ed.) three persons must not read together in one volume (of a book held in trust by the finder).—3) *bundle*; trnsf. *a combined action*; בכ׳ אחד *simultaneously; without intermission.* Ib. 37^a כמי שהפקידו לו בכ׳ א׳ as if they had entrusted their money to him by one act (v. Rabb. D. S. a. l. note 50), opp. to שני כְּרִיכוֹת.

—Y. Shek. III, 47[b] bot. בכ׳ א׳ (drinking four cups) in immediate succession (Pes. 108[b] בבת אחת), opp. בפיסקין (v. פָּרַךְ).—Tosef. Maas. Sh. IV, 11 [read:] נתנן כולן בכ׳ וכ׳ if he put all of them into one fund, he takes the money realized from their sale out of the common fund. Tosef. Meg. IV (III), 17, sq. ג׳ פסוקים בכ׳ אחד three verses without intermission (for the expositor, v. מְתוּרְגְּמָן).—*Pl.* (fr. כְּרַךְ) כְּרֵיכוֹת, v. supra; B. Mets. 37[b] שתי כ׳.

כְּרַךְ c. (v. כָּרַךְ 2) *fortified place*, in gen. *city, capital.* Meg. 3[b] כ׳ שישב ולבסוף הוקף a place which was first settled and then fortified. Hag. 13[b] בן כ׳ an inhabitant of a city, a refined person, opp. בן כפר. Succ. 51[b] he who has not seen Jerusalem in her glory, לא ראה כ׳ וכ׳ has never seen a beautiful city; a. fr.—כ׳ גדול (של רומי) *Rome.* Snh. 21[b] כ׳ ג׳ שברומי ed. (Ms. ר׳ של); Sabb. 56[b]. Pes. 118[b] בכ׳ ג׳ ed. (Ms. M. של רומי). Yalk. Num. 759 לדחוק את שרה של כ׳ ג׳ וכ׳ to drive out the genius of Rome &c.; Pesik. R. s. 14 (corr. acc.); Pesik. Par., p. 41[a] (corr. acc.); a. fr. —*Pl.* כְּרַכִּין, כְּרַכִּים. Erub. 21[b] judge me not כיושבי כ׳ like the dwellers in large cities (where there are many vices). Meg. I, 1. Keth. 110[b] ישיבת כ׳ קשה living in large cities is a hardship. Sifré Deut. 52 Remus and Romulus arose ובנו ב׳ כ׳ ברומי and built two forts in Rome (Cant. R. to I, 6; Y. Ab. Zar. I, 39[c] צריפים); a. fr.—כְּרַכֵּי הים *sea-towns, mercantile ports* (Tyre &c.). R. Hash. 26[a]. Cant. R. to I, 4; a. fr. —[Ruth. R. to II, 4 בין הכרכים, read: באַרְכָּיִים, v. אַרְכִּי I.]—כְּרַךְ *Fort . . .*, v. respective determinants.

כְּרַךְ II, **כְּרַכָּא**, ch. same. Targ. II Sam. XX, 19. Targ. Jer. LI, 25 (h. text הר); a. fr.—Yoma 53[b] דתרום רישך אכולה כ׳ that thy head be raised over the whole city (that thou become the leader of the Jewish community). Taan. 22[a] מגינית אכולה כ׳ thou art the protector of the whole community. Hull. 56[b] כ׳ דכולה ביה a community in which everything (all classes) can be found; a. fr.—*Pl.* כְּרַכִּין, כְּרַכַּיָּא, כְּרַכ׳. Targ. Num. XIII, 19 (O. ed. Berl. כְּרַכִּין, Var. כְּרַכִּין, כְּרָכִין). Targ. Job IV, 10 ed. Lag. מרתיתין כרכיא (ed. מרתיתין כריכא, corr. acc.).—[כְּרַכָּה די, כְּרַכָּא ד־ *Fort . . .*, v. respective determinants.—Targ. Y. Num. XXXIV, 8 כְּרַכּוֹי דבר סניגירא the forts of &c. Ib. כדכור דבר זעמה or כדכור, read: כְּרַכּוֹי.]

כִּרְכָא m. (כְּרַךְ) 1) *roll.* B. Bath. 14[b] כְּרִכֵיה, v. כְּרַךְ I.—2) *pl.* כִּרְכֵי *matting* which can be rolled up. Sabb. 19[b] (Ms. O. כְּרָאבֵי); ib. 156[b] (Ms. O. כְּרִיכֵי), v. זָוָוא I.

כִּרְכֵּב (redupl. of כרב, v. כֵּרוּב) *to round off, to make a rim by hollowing out the centre* (as on a mechanic's stool, a pot-lid &c.). Hull. 25[a] bot. unfinished wooden vessels שעתיד . . . לְכַרְכֵּב which require polishing . . . . or caving out; Tosef. Kel. B. Mets. II, 17 כרכב (read לכ׳). Ib. 10 (of metal ware) לכרכב; Hull. 25[b] לְכַרְכֵּר (Ar. לכרכם).

כרכד, v. כַּרְכָּר.

כרכדיונון, כַּרְכְּדַיָּא, כַּרְכְּדוֹן, v. כַּרְכְּדוֹן.

כְּרָכָה, v. כְּרַכָּא.

כַּרְכּוֹב m. (b. h. כַּרְכֹּב, v. כִּרְכֵּב) *a rim* around the altar. Zeb. 62[a] איזהו כ׳ . . זה כיור what is meant by *Karkob* Rabbi says, a panel work; R. J. says, the rim (סוֹבֵב) Ib. כ׳ בין קרן לקרן (another) rim between one horn and the other; Tosef. Shek. III, 19; Y. ib. VIII, end, 51[b] (ref. to Shek. VIII, 8; Tosef. ib. III, 18).

***כַּרְכּוֹז, כ׳(ד)עִיזָּא**, name of a goat-like animal, *Carcuz-goat.* Hull. 59[b] ed. עיזא כ׳ ed. (Ar. עיזא דכרבין goat of *Carbin* (a place); Var. כרביז, כרבין, v. Ar. Compl. s. v.).

כַּרְכּוֹם I, כַּרְקוֹם, m. (b. h. כַּרְכֹּם; v. כַּרְכֵּם a. כַּרְכֵּם I) [*paint*,] *crocus, saffron.* Kerith. 6[a]; Y. Yoma IV, 41[d] (one of the ingredients of frankincense).—Nidd. II, 6 כקרן כ׳ of the color of the bright-colored crocus; expl. ib. 7 ברור שבו like the choicest of all (expl. ib. 20[a] as the middle leaf of the middle row); Y. ib. 50[b] top; Tosef. ib. III, 11; a. e.—Tosef. Kil. I, 1 כרקם ed. Zuck. (oth. ed. כרפס, corr. acc.).—[Ib. III, 12 ed. Zuck., v. כַּרְפַּס II.]—[Targ. Cant. II, 1 כרקום some ed., read: נַרְקִיס.]—*Pl.* כַּרְכְּמִין. Y. Maasr. V, end, 52[a]. Y. B. Bath. IX, end, 17[b] כּוּרְכְּמִין (Chald. form).

כַּרְכּוֹם II, (כּוּרְכ׳, כַּרְקוֹם) m. (v. כָּרַם, cmp. כָּרַךְ) [*encircling*,] 1) *troop of siege, stage of siege.* Keth. II, 9; Ab. Zar. 71[a] עיר שכבשוה כ׳ (v. Rabb. D. S. a. l. note 80) a town which troops of siege have taken. Gitt. III, 4 על עיר שהקיפה כ׳ concerning a husband living in a town during a siege (that he is legally presumed to be alive), opp. to עיר שכבשה כ׳. Y. Keth. II, 26[d]; Y. Gitt. III, 45[a] top איזהו כ׳ what is called a stage of siege (for legal purposes); Ib. כ׳ של אותה מלכות a siege by the government troops of the country, opp. to a siege by the enemy.—2) *camp of besiegers, the Roman castra.* Ab. Zar. 18[b] ההולך . . . ולכ׳ whosoever goes to the arena or the camp; Tosef. ib. II, 6 ולכַּרְקוּמִין (*pl.*). Ib. 7 ולכ׳ (מותר) מפני וכ׳ and going to the camp is permitted for the sake of maintaining the political order, v. חָשַׁב *Hithpa.*—*Pl.* כַּרְכּוֹמִין (כַּרְק׳). Koh. R. to XII, 7 (ref. to לשום כרים על שערים, Ez. XXI, 27) עשה כ׳ he erected camps of siege (Lam. R. introd., R. Josh. 2 כירונין, v. כִּירוֹן II). Tosef. l. c., v. supra.

כַּרְכּוֹם, כַּרְכּוֹמָא I (כַּרְק׳) ch. same, mostly *pl.* כַּרְכּוֹמִין (כַּרְק׳) *works of siege.* Targ. O. Deut. XX, 20 כרכ׳ (ed. Berl. כרק׳; Targ. Y. קַרְקוֹמִין). Targ. Lam. I, 19. Targ. Is. XXIX, 3 כרקום (ed. Lag. קַרְקוֹם; h. text מֻצָּב). Targ. I Sam. XXVI, 5; 7 כרכומא (ed. Lag. כרק׳, h. text מעגל).

כַּרְכּוֹמָא II m. (v. כרכום I, cmp. כְּרוֹם) *bronze, brazen* (cmp. יָרָק II). Targ. Job XX, 24 (some ed. כרבוניר, corr. acc.). Ib. XL, 18 Ms. (ed. נחשא). Targ. Ps. XVIII, 35 (ed. Lag. כרכומיא, Targ. II Sam. XXII, 35 נחשא).

כרכוס, Ab. Zar. 18[b] some ed., read: כַּרְכּוֹם.

כַּרְכּוֹר, כִּרְכ׳ m. (כִּרְכֵּר) 1) *circle, circuit, round about way.*—*Pl.* כִּרְכ׳, . . . רִין, כַּרְכּוּרִים. Gen. R. s. 20; s. 45, end; s. 63; Yalk. Gen. 80; 82 כמה כ׳ כרכר בשביל להסיח וכ׳ how many circuits did the Lord make before he addressed Sarah directly (ref. to Gen. XVIII, 13 to 15, and interpreting ויאמר, verse 15, 'and the Lord said'); Y. Sot. VII, beg. 21[b] [read:] כמה כִּירְכּוּרֵי כ׳ חקב״ה מתאוה בשביל להשיח

כ׳ עם אותה צדקנית how many circles around circles did the Lord draw in order &c.—2) *whirl*, v. כַּרְכַּר.

כַּרְכּוּשְׁתָּא f. (v. כַּרְכֵּשׁ I) *weasel*. Targ. Y. Lev. XI, 29 (h. text חלד).—B. Mets. 85ª בני כ׳ young weasels (v. Rabb. D. S. a. l. for correct vers.). Snh. 105ª (prov.) כ׳ ושונרא וכ׳ weasel and cat (making peace) feast on the fat of the luckless. Meg. 14ᵇ (translation of Huldah), v. חוּלְדָּה III.—[B. Kam. 52ª, v. כַּרְכַּשְׁתָּא I.]

כַּרְכִּימִישָׁא, v. כַּרְכְּמִשָׁא.

כרכין, v. כַּרְכּוּז.

כַּרְכֵּישׁ, v. כַּרְכֵּשׁ.

כַּרְכִיתָא, v. כְּרִיכְתָּא.

כִּרְכֵּם (reduplic. of כרם) 1) *to draw a circle*; denom. כַּרְכּוֹם II. 2) (cmp. כְּרוּם) *to paint, varnish; to polish, bronze*. Kel. XV, 2 סירקן או כִּרְכְּמָן if he painted or varnished the boards. Ib. XXII, 9 כופת שסירקו או כִּרְכְּמוֹ וכ׳ a block which one painted or varnished so as to give it a distinguishable surface. Ḥull. 25ᵇ לְכַרְכֵּם Ar. to polish or bronze (metal vessels), v. כַּרְכֵּב. Tosef. Kel. B. Mets. VI, 1 ואם.. לכרכם עד שֶׁיְּכַרְכֵּם if he intends to varnish (the leather goods), they cannot become unclean until he has varnished them. Cant. R. beg. סיתתה וכִרְכְּמָהּ he chiseled and polished the stone, v. מְרַק.—כ׳ פנים [*to braze the face,*] *to be bold, defiant* (cmp. יָרַק). Y'lamd. to Num. XX, 8 quot. in Ar. והוא מְכַרְכֵּם פניו כנגדן (some ed. Ar. מכרכס, (v. Koh. Ar. Compl. s. v.) and he (Moses) defied them; Yalk. Num. 763 נִתְכַּרְכְּמוּ פניו, v. infra.—Part. pass. מְכוּרְכָּם; פנים מְכוּרְכָּמוֹת *green, pale face*. Gen. R. s. 99 יצאו ופניהם מכ׳ they went out pale-faced (abashed).—Denom. כַּרְכּוֹם I.

Nithpa. נִתְכַּרְכֵּם (denom. of כַּרְכּוֹם I, cmp. יָרַק), with פנים 1) *to look saffron-like, pale, abashed, grieved*. Ib. s. 20 נִתְכַּרְכְּמוּ פניו he turned pale. Y. Snh. I, 19ª bot. Pesik. Par. p. 38ª; Num. R. s. 19 (some ed. נתכרמו, corr. acc.).—Midr. Till. to Ps. XVIII, 35 ופניו מִתְכַּרְכְּמִין and his (Abraham's) face turned pale (from jealousy); Yalk. Sam. 162 ופני אברהם מִתְכַּרְכְּמוֹת.—2) *to become bronze-colored*. Cant. R. to I, 6 נתכ׳ פניו his face was tanned (from exposure to the sun; Yalk. ib. 982 נפחם).—3) *to become angry, defiant*. Yalk. Num. 763, v. supra.

כרכמא, Sabb. 139ª כשותא בכ׳ Ar., v. כַּרְמָא.

כרכמושא, v. כְּרוּמְשָׁא.

כַּרְכְּמִין, v. כַּרְכּוֹם I.

כַּרְכִּימ׳, כַּרְכְּמִישָׁא m. (prob. a. denomin. of כַּרְכְּמִישׁ) *lead* (plumbum). Targ. Job XIX, 24. Targ. Y. I Num. XXXI, 22.

כּוּר׳, כַּרְכְּמִית pr. n. f. *Kark'mith*, a freed woman. Eduy. V, 6; Ber. 19ª; Sifré Num. 7;—Yalk. Num. 706; Num. R. s. 9 כור׳. Y. Sot. II, end, 18ᵇ תוכיח כור׳ let the case of K. come in as evidence.

כרכס, v. כַּרְכַּס.

כַּרְכַּס (b. h.) pr. n. m. *Carcas*, one of the seven attendants of King Ahasuerus. Esth. R. to I, 10 (interpret. by way of acrostics) [read:] זתר וכ׳ כס זנות רְאֵה של אותו רשע וְכַרְכֵּם (the Lord said to the angel) see the profligacy of this wicked man, and tie them (like sheaves for threshing; v. Matt. K. a. l.); v. כרכסון.

כַּרְכָּסָא ch. form of preced. Esth. R. to I, 10 (an objection to the interpretation וְכַרְכֵּם (v. preced.), because of ignoring the ס) כ׳ כתיב but it is written *Carcasa* (and not *Carcam*).

כרכסון, read: כְּרוּכְסִין (ἐκήρυξεν, sub. ὁ κῆρυξ; cmp. בריכסון) *it has been announced*. Esth. to I, 10 (ref. to זתר וכרכס, v. כַּרְכַּס) לשון יוני הוא היך מה דאת אמר כ׳ Carcas it a Greek expression ('see the profligacy . . . and *publish* it', κήρυσσε) as you say ἐκήρυξεν, proclamation has been made.

כִּרְכֵּר (Pilp. of כרר, v. כָּרָה) 1) *to go around, go about*; [b. h. *to dance*]. Gen. R. s. 20, a. e., v. כִּרְכּוּר.—2) *to finish by designing circles, emblazon*. Ḥull. 25ᵇ, v. כַּרְכֵּב.—3) *to form a circle in order to make an announcement*. Pesik. R. s. 21 למלך שהיה עומד וּמְכַרְכֵּר כל וכ׳ like a king standing and gathering a circle around him at the entrance of his palace; כך . . . כשעמד ומכ׳ על הר סיני so the Lord when he stood addressing a meeting on Mount Sinai.

כַּרְכָּר (כרכד) m. (preced.) 1) *whorl* of the spindle (vorticulus), also *shuttle* (v. Sm. Ant. s. v. Tela). Sabb. VIII, 6 (81ª) ראש הכ׳ (Y. ed. a. Mish. Pes. הכרכד, v. Rabb. D. S. a. l. note) the top of the whorl; Y. ib. XVII, 16ᵇ. Bab. ib. 123ª תוחבין בכוש או בכ׳ (Ms. M. בכַרְכִּיר) you stick it up with a reed or a whorl; Y. l. c. top. Tosef. ib. IX (X) 10; Sabb. 92ᵇ; Sifra Vayikra, Ḥobah, ch. IX, Par. 7, v. לָנֶה. Sifré Deut. 96; Ab. Zar. III, 9 (49ᵇ) נטל הימנה כ׳ Ms. M. (ed. כַּרְכּוֹר, Var. כַּרְכּוּר, v. Rabb. D. S. a. l. note) if one took from it (the Asherah) a piece to use it as a shuttle; a. fr.—2) [*turner,*] *a rod used for shaking olives down*. Y. Peah VII, 20ª ברכרה, ברכר, read: כַּרְכָּרָה, כַּרְכָּר (f.), v. מַחְבֵּא a. מַחְבוֹא.

***כַּרְכָּרָא, כַּרְכַּר** ch. as preced. 1. Y. Shek. IV, 48ᵇ bot. שבטא דכרכר ביניהן (Bab. ed. דכרכרא, corr. acc.) the staff of the shuttle (the cane which brings the threads of the web into their place [arundo]), is between them, i. e. there is a great difference between them (cmp. 'stamen secernit arundo', Ovid M. 6, 55).

כִּרְכָּרָן f. pl. (v. כִּרְכֵּר) *dances, rejoicing*. Targ. Is. LXVI, 20 בכ׳ ותושבחן (missing in ed. Lag.; h. text בכרכרות, cmp. Targ. II Sam. VI, 14 שבח for h. כרכר) with dances and songs of praise.

כַּרְכֵּישׁ, כַּרְכֵּשׁ I (reduplic. of כרש, v. כְּרוּשִׁיְיתָא a. כֶּרֶס) 1) *to hollow out*, v. כַּרְכּוּשְׁתָּא, כַּרְכֶּשֶׁא.—2) (cmp. b. h. קרס) *to bend, bow.*—כ׳ (ב)רישא *to nod assent*. Erub. 65ᵇ רישיה . . . . כ׳ R. nodded &c. Nidd. 42ª כ׳ ליה ברישיה showed his approval of it by nodding; B. Bath. 143ª top.

כַּרְכֵּישׁ, כַּרְכֵּשׁ II=כַּשְׁכֵּשׁ *to knock, strike*. Sabb. 77ᵇ ed. (Ms. M. לְכַשְׁכּוּשֵׁי) לְכַרְכּוּשֵׁי, v. כַּשְׁכֵּשׁ.

כַּרְכְּשָׁא m. (כַּרְכֵּשׁ I) *large intestines, great-gut and rectum*. Sabb. 82ª [read with Rashi:] האר כ׳... יתיב (or with Ms. O. יתבא ... כַּרְכַּשְׁתָּא, v. Rabb. D. S. a. l. note) the rectum is supported by three teeth-like glands. Ib. שיני שמטיה דכרכשתא the glands of &c. Gitt. 57ª; Ber. 62ᵇ חיטי לְכַרְכַּשֵׁיה he dropped his gut (from fright). Hull. 49ᵇ חיטי דכ׳ the fat glands surrounding the large intestines. Ib. 113ª כ׳ ומעייא great-gut and (small) intestines.

קַרְקַשְׁתָּא I, כַּרְכַּשְׁתָּא f. (כַּרְכֵּשׁ II) *the shepherd's bell*. B. Kam. 52ª (expl. משכוכית) כ׳ Ms. M. (Ms. R. כרכוש׳, v. Rabb. D. S. a. l. note; ed. קרק׳).

כַּרְכַּשְׁתָּא II f. (כַּרְכֵּשׁ I) 1) = כַּרְכְּשָׁא q. v.—2) (cmp. פְּרוּשְׁיָיתָא) *tufts, tassels* (v. Sm. Ant. s. v. Fimbriae). B. Mets. 7ª דתפיסי בכ׳ (Ms. R. 2 בכרשתא, corrected into בכרדשתא, v. Rabb. D. S. a. l. note 60) both taking hold of the fringes of the cloth (which they claim as finders).

כַּרְכָתָא f. (כְּרַךְ) *a plantation fenced in from all sides*. B. Mets. 22ᵇ (Ms. R. 1 כַּרְכָאָתָא *pl.*; Ms. M. כראכת׳, corr. acc., v. Rabb. D. S. a. l. note).

כָּרַם (v. כָּרָה) 1) *to surround, cut off*. Denom. כֶּרֶם, כַּרְכּוֹם, כַּרְמְלִית II.—2) *to pile up*. Kel. XXIII, 4 the washer's chair שהוא כּוֹרֵם עליו את הכלים (ed. Dehr. כּוֹרֵס) upon which he piles the clothes (to press them); Tosef. ib. B. Bath. II, 9 שמוברין ed. Zuck. (oth. ed. שמוברים, read: שכּוֹרְמִ׳); Sabb. 88ᵇ (play on כרמי עין גדי Cant. I, 14) עון גדי שֶׁכָּרַמְתִּי לי וכ׳ the guilt of the kid (= golden calf; oth. opin. גְּדִי the idol Gad) which I piled (stored up) for me (for future punishment). Ib. מאי ... כרמי לישנא דמבניש הוא (Ms. M. דמכבש ,כרם.., Ms. O. דמכמש, v. Rabb. D. S. a. l. note) what evidence is there that the word *Kerem* has the meaning of gathering (or of *pressing, preserving*)?—Answ. (by ref. to Kel. l. c.) שכּוֹרְמִים עליו את הכלים.—3) *to cover, paint*, v. כַּרְכּוֹם, כָּרוּם I.—[Tosef. Men. IX, 10 וכורמין Var., v. כָּמַר.]

כֶּרֶם m. (b. h.; preced.) [*enclosure*,] *plantation*, esp. *vineyard*. Ber. 35ª, a. e. כ׳ זית איקרי כ׳ סתמא לא אקרי an orchard of olive trees is called *kerem zayith*, but not plain *kerem*. Ib. (ref. to Maas. Sh. V, 1 sq., a. fr.) חד תני כ׳ רבע ... נטע רבעי ... one authority reads everywhere a *kerem* of the fourth year's crop, the other *n'ṭa* (plantation) &c. Lev. R. s. 32 (play on כֶּרֶם, Ps. XII, 9) כַּרְמָן של ממזרים the plantation (genealogy, cmp. יחוס) of the bastards. Peah VII, 6. Kil. IV, 1, v. קָרַחַת; a. v. fr.—Trnsf. *circle of scholars, college*, esp. כ׳ ביבנה the college of R. Johanan b. Zaccai in Jamnia (v. יַבְנֶה). Keth. IV, 6; B. Bath. 131ᵇ; Y. Ber. IV, 7ᵈ top; a. fr.—[Ber. 63ᵇ כ׳ ביבנה for which Cant. R. to II, 5: אוּשָׁא.]—*Pl.* כְּרָמִים. Men. VIII, 6 (86ᵇ) כ׳ העבודים carefully cultivated vineyards (dug over twice a year); a. e.—בֵּית כֶּרֶם pr. n. pl. *Beth-Kerem*. Nidd. II, 7 בקעת ב׳ כ׳ the valley of Beth K. (whose soil was red); Tosef. ib. III, 11.

כַּרְמָא, כֶּרֶם ch. same. Targ. Ex. XXII, 4; a. fr.—B. Mets. 104ª; B. Bath. 7ª if one says (כרם) כרמא אני מוכר לךוכ׳ 'I sell thee a vineyard', although there are no vines in it &c.; והוא דמתקרי כ׳ provided the property goes by the name of vineyard (*Karma*); a. fr.—Yeb. 42ᵇ ממתניתן דכ׳ וכ׳ he changed his opinion on account of what had been taught in the college (at Jamnia), v. preced.—[Yeb. 121ª בכרמא, v. כַּרְמֵי.]—*Pl.* כַּרְמֵי, כַּרְמַיָּא, כַּרְמִין. Targ. Deut. VI, 11. Targ. Jud. XV, 5. Targ. Koh. II, 4 כ׳ ביבנה *schools*, (v. preced.); a. fr.—Y. Kil. IV, beg. 29ª, v. next w.—Succ. 44ᵇ, v. קַשְׁקֵשׁ.

***כַּרְמוֹן** m. (preced.) *a row of vines in a vineyard*. Y. Kil. IV, beg. 29ª נסב חד כ׳ if the owner took away one of the five rows.—*Pl.* כַּרְמִין (prob. to be read: כַּרְמוֹנִין). Ib. תלתא כ׳ ותרי בינייין three rows and two intervals.

כַּרְמֵי pr. n. pl. *Carmi* in Babylonia. Yeb. 121ª דאטבע בכ׳ וכ׳ (Ar. בכרמא) a man that was drowned at *C.* and whose body was found &c.

כַּרְמֶל m. (b. h.; v. כֶּרֶם) 1) *a well-cultivated plot*; whence (sub. גֶּרֶשׂ) (*grist of*) *early ripened and tender barley*. Men. 66ᵇ; Sifra Vayikra, N'dabah, ch. XIV, Par. 13 (ref. to Lev. II, 14). כַּרְמֶל רַךְ וּמַל soft yet brittle; Y. Sabb. I, 2ᵈ bot. [read:] רך מל לא לח וכ׳ soft yet brittle, neither green nor dry, but between the two. Sifra l. c.; Men. l. c. (another explan.) כַּר מָלֵא rounded and full.—2) pr. n. *Carmel*; (prob. everywhere) *Mount Carmel*. Y. Succ. III, 53ᵈ כשעוה וכשושנת כ׳ of the color of wax or of the lily of Carmel (v. יְרַקְרַק); (Tosef. Neg. I, 5 כשעוה וכקורטל, Var. וכקורמן; R. S. to Neg. XI, 4 וכקורמין).—Y. Ber. I, 2ᵇ bot. ראש הר הכ׳; Sabb. 35ª ראש הכ׳ (Ms. M. ראש הר הכ׳) the summit of M. C. Gen. R. s. 99; Mekh. Yithro, Bahod., s. 5 (alluding to Jer. XLVI, 18) תבור ... וכ׳ מאספמיא Tabor came (to the desert for the law-giving) from Beth-Elim and C. from Ispamia; Meg. 29ª.

כַּרְמְלִי m. (sub. יַיִן; v. preced.) *Carmel wine*. Tosef. Nidd. III, 11 [read:] היין השרוני הדומה לכ׳ חי ולא מזוג חדש ולא ישן Sharon wine (mixed) which resembles in color the Carmel wine pure but not mixed, new &c.; Nidd. 21ª.

כַּרְמְלִית f. (v. כָּרַם) *a marked off plot in a public thoroughfare*, in gen. *an area which cannot be classified either as private ground* (רשות היחיד) *or as public ground* (רשות הרבים). Y. Sabb. XI, 13ª כל המעכב.. נקרא כ׳ whatever obstructs the public road is called *karm'lith*. Tosef. ib. I, 1; Sabb. 6ª, v. רְשׁוּת. Ib. אבל .. ואיסטוונית והכ׳ but the sea, the valley, the colonnade and the *carm'lith*; expl. ib. 7ª קרן זוית הסמוכה לרה״ר a corner plot adjoining the public road; a. fr.—*Pl.* כַּרְמְלִיּוֹת. Y. ib. XI, end, 13ᵇ.

כַּרְמַת f. (denom. of כֶּרֶם) *vines trained over the wall of the vineyard*. Tosef. Men. IX, 10 לא מן הכ׳ וכ׳ (Var. הכדמת) neither from vines trained over the wall nor from those trained on espaliers, v. דָּלִית.

כָּרֵן m., constr. כָּרֵן (v. כרי, cmp. קרן) *roundness, fullness, essence*; כ׳ יומא *the very day* (h. עצם היום). Targ. Ez. XXIV, 2. Targ. Lev. XXIII, 28; a. fr. [Nahm. to Lev. l. c. quotes a version קֶרֶן.]

כַּרְנְבָאוֹת, v. כְּרִינְבָ׳.

כַּרְנְבוֹ pr. n. f. *Carn'bo* (*Lamb of Nebo*), legendary name of Abraham's grandmother. B. Bath. 91[a].

***כְּרַנְבִּי** f. (κράμβη) *cabbage*. Lam. R. to III, 42 (not כרנכי), v. כְּסִמָּא.

***כַּרְנִיבָאוֹת** f. pl. (χέρνιψ, -βος) *vessels containing lustral water*, placed at the doors of Greek and Roman temples (v. Sm. Ant. s. v.). Sifré Num. 158 כרדוכאות (corr. acc.; Ar. כַּרְנְבָאוֹת).

כרנכי, v. כְּרַנְבִּי.

***כרס**, *Af.* אַכְרִיס, v. ברס.

כֶּרֶס f. (b. h. כֶּרֶשׂ in כְּרֵשׂוֹ; cmp. כְּרִכְּשָׁא (כַּרְכָּשָׁא) [*bag*,] *stomach, belly*. Taan. 26[a] top על נפש..וכ׳ מלאה when the appetite is satisfied and the stomach filled. Sabb. 151[b] (ref. to Koh. XII, 6) זה הכ׳ 'the pitcher is broken', that means the stomach. Ib. לאחר שלשה..כְּרֵיסוֹ נבקעת וכ׳ three days after burial one's stomach bursts open . . . saying (to the mouth), Take what thou hast put into me; Koh. R. to l. c.; Y. Yeb. XVI, 15[c] bot.; Gen. R. s. 100. Keth. 16[a], a. fr. כְּרֵיסָהּ בין שיניה her belly extends to her teeth, i. e. she cannot deny her pregnancy. Koh. R. to VII, 8 [read:] היה מפעפע בִכְרֵיסָהּ כארסה וכ׳ burned in her stomach like the venom of &c.; [Y. Snh. X, 28[d] top ככריסה, v. חֲכִינָה]; a. fr.—Esp. *the stomach of ruminants, maw*. Hull. III, 1 הכ׳ הפנימית the inner stomach, expl. ib. 50[b] כל הכ׳ כולו . . . ואיזהו כ׳ החיצון וכ׳ (masc.!) the whole maw is called the inner stomach, and the outer stomach is the flesh (muscle) which covers the largest portion of the stomach; ib. (another opinion) טפח בכ׳ סמוך לכ׳ וכ׳ ,טפח בוושט corrected; טפח בכ׳ סמוך לוושט one handbreadth of the stomach where it joins the gullet is called the inner stomach; [oth. defin., v. מִילַּת a. הִירָבָא ,אִסְתּוּמְכָא a.].—*Pl.* כְּרֵיסוֹת. Succ. 21[b] שֶׁכְּרֵיסוֹתֵיהֶן רחבות whose bellies are broad (projecting further than the rider's body; Tosef. Par. III (II), 2 שֶׁכְּרֵיסָן רחבה).

כְּרֵיסָא, כַּרְסָא ch. same, also *womb*. Targ. Y. Num. V, 21. Targ. Y. Lev. IV, 8 (O. גַּוָּא; h. text קֶרֶב). Targ. Job XXXI, 18; a. fr.—Hull. 50[b], v. אִסְתּוּמְכָא. Ib. נפל כ׳ בב״א the stomach fell into the well, i. e. your definition of the 'inner stomach' is of no value. Gen. R. s. 70 (prov.) כ׳ טענא רגליא the stomach carries the feet, i. e. cheerful prospects lend physical energy; Yalk. ib. 123. Gitt. 12[a] דנהום כְּרֵסֵיה לא שוי (Ar. דנהם כריסא) (who is not worth the bread he eats; B. Kam. 97[a]. Koh. R. to XI, 9 כְּרֵיסֵיה דהאי גברא קומך בוצה this man's (my) stomach is before thee, cut it open (I cannot pay for my meal); Pesik. Shub., p. 164[b] בוציה . . . הא כ׳ (masc.); a. fr.—Yeb. 65[b] bot. איכו ילדת לי חדא כ׳ אחריתי Oh that you would bear unto me one more issue of the womb!—Gen. R. s. 68 מני . . . בכ׳ דביתך (=h. בקרב ביתך) count twenty beams in the inner chamber of thy house; (Y. Maas. Sh. IV, 55[b] bot. גו בייתיך).—*Pl.* כְּרֵיסַיָּא (m.); כְּרֵיסָן, כַּרְסָתָא. Targ. Y. Num. V, 22 (not כְּרִיסָן). Targ. Ps. XVII, 14.—Keth. 103[a] תרתי כ׳ לית לה she has not two stomachs (double alimentation is of no use to her).

כָּרְסֵא, *chair, pl.* כָּרְסָוָן, v. כּוּרְסְיָא.

כָּרְסָוֹן, f. pl. (v. preced.) *upholstered seats*, satirical expression for *stoutness*. Lev. R. s. 34 חמי כ׳ see (that beggar's) fat body! (Yalk. Lev. 665 ערפין).

כרסום, v. כִּרְסֵם.

כרסטיותא, v. כְּרִיסְטִיוֹנָא.

כרסין, Tosef. Neg. V, 14 some ed., read: בִּרְסִין.

כרסלא, Snh. 5[a], read: בַּר סַלָּא (v. Rabb. D. S. a. l. note).

כרסם, v. כִּרְסֵם.

כַּרְסָנָא pr. n. m. *Carsana*. Y. Shebi. IX, 39[a] אילין דבית ברסנה (corr. acc.) those of the family (or school) of C.—Y. Erub. III, 21[a] bot.; V, 22[d], a. e., ר׳ שמעון בר כ׳. Y. Dem. III, 23[b] bot. בר בר סנא (corr. acc.). [Fr. M'bo, p. 129[b]: *Carsana*, pr. n. pl., fr. which כּוּרְסָאֵי.]

כרסס, v. כִּרְסֵם.

כַּרְסְפַּת f. (cmp. כְּרִיבָא (כַּ) a species of *locusts*. Hull. 65[b] (Var. in Ar. כַּרְפֶּסֶת, כרסנית).

כַּרְסְתָן m. (denom. of כַּרְסָא) *large-bellied, stout*. Hull. 60[a] שור כ׳ וכ׳ an ox (in order to fetch a high price) must be stout, have large hoofs &c.

כָּרַע (b. h.; denom. of כֶּרַע) *to bow, bend the knee*. Ber. 12[a] כשהוא כּוֹרֵעַ וכ׳ when bowing in prayer, one must bow at the word *barukh*, opp. זָקַף. Ib. 34[b]; Y. ib. I, 3[c] bot. (interch. with שחה); a. v. fr.

Hif. הִכְרִיעַ 1) *to cause to kneel; to subdue; to humiliate, sadden*. Gen. R. s. 65; Yalk. Gen. 114 אני מַכְרִיעַ את אוהבי I shall sadden my friend. Gen. R. s. 75, beg., v. כָּרָה. Ib. s. 67 מה אני מכריע וכ׳ (Yalk. ib. 116 מַעֲבִיר) why shall I sadden my father?—2) *to put the knee of the balance down; to overbalance; to outweigh*. Y. Peah I, 16[b] bot. הזכיות מַכְרִיעוֹת the good deeds overbalance (the sins). Ab. II, 8 מַכְרִיעַ את כלם outweighs them all. B. Bath. V, 11 חייב לְהַכְרִיעַ לו טפח (weighing a litra of meat or more) he must allow the scale (which contains the meat) to sink one handbreadth lower than the scale of weights, i. e. he must give overweight, opp. עיין to weigh exactly. Ib. 89[a] שקול לי . . . וְהַכְרִיעָה weigh for me each litra for itself and give me the legal overweight on it; a. fr.—Y. Sabb. I, 3[c] bot. הִכְרִיעַ עליו כסף put money to it in the balance (bribe him). Gen. R. s. 80 כמה ממון ה׳ how much money he put in the balance (paid for it).—Trnsf. *to cast the deciding vote, to decide*. Tosef. Hull. VII, 1; Hull. 90[b]; Pes. 83[b] הדעת מַכְרַעַת reason decides, v. דַּעַת. Y. Keth. II, 26[b]; Y. Yeb. X, 10[d] bot. הדעת מכרעת בעידי מיתה (not לידדי) reason decides in favor of trusting the witnesses testifying to the death of a person.—3) *to keep the balance*; trnsf. *to harmonize two contrary opinions, to compromise*. Sifra introd. שני כתובים המכחישים . . . וְיַכְרִיעַ ביניהם when two Biblical verses contradict each other, you must not draw any conclusions until a third verse is found which harmonizes them. Ib. end (ref. to Ex.

XIX, 20 a. Deut. IV, 36) הכ׳ השלישי a third passage (Ex. XX, 22) harmonizes (that the Lord lowered the heavens so as to make them rest on Mount Sinai); Mekh. Yithro, Bahod. s. 9. Sifré Num. 58.—Kidd. 24ᵇ הַמַּכְרִיעִים לפני חכמים the harmonizers arguing before the scholars. Sabb. 39ᵇ כל מקום ... ואחד מכריע הלכה כדברי המכ׳ whenever you find two scholars differing and one compromising, the practice follows the opinion of the compromiser; a. fr.—V. הֶכְרֵעַ, הַכְרָעָה.

כְּרַע ch. same, 1) *to bow, bend the knee.* Targ. O. Gen. XXIV, 26 (Y. גחן). Targ. II Esth. III, 2; a. e.—Y. Ber. II, 5ᵃ bot. הוא כ׳ מגרמיה it (the head) bowed spontaneously. 2) (of the balance) *to sink, outweigh.* Targ. Y. Ex. I, 15.— —3) *to decide by majority.* Targ. Y. Deut. XXV, 1 (v. Snh. 10ᵃ).

Af. אַכְרַע 1) *to sadden.* Targ. Jud. XI, 35.—2) *to weigh.* Pesik. B'shall., p. 82ᵃ באכרעתא דאַכְרְעוּן וכ׳, v. אַכְרָעְתָּא.

Ithpe. אִתְכְּרַע *to be weighed.* Ib.

כֶּרַע c. (b. h.; cmp. כָּרָה) [*hollow*, cmp. בֶּרֶךְ.] *knee, leg.* Zeb. VIII, 5 כַּרְעוֹ של וכ׳ the leg of one of them (Talm. ed. 77ᵇ כרעים *du.*). Kel. XVIII, 7 כ׳ שהיתה וכ׳ a knee-shaped piece of wood which became unclean ... and which one fastened to a bedstead; Tosef. ib. B. Mets. IX, 3. Ib. VIII, 8 כ׳ שפרש וכ׳ a leg of a bedstead which was taken off with the long side &c.; a. e.—*Du.* כְּרָעַיִם, כַּרְעַיִם; *pl.* כְּרָעִים, כְּרָעִין. Tam. IV, 2. Zeb. VIII, 5. Succ. 15ᵇ, v. אֲרוּבָּה. Cant. R. to VII, 3 מה כרס ... והכ׳ וכ׳ as the belly is bounded by the heart (chest) on the one, and the legs on the other. Kel. XVIII, 5; Tosef. ib. B. Mets. VIII, 5; a. fr.

כַּרְעָא ch. same. Ber. 7ᵃ קאי אחד כ׳ stands on one leg. Men. 34ᵃ; Yoma 11ᵇ כי עקר אינש כַּרְעֵיה וכ׳ when a person starts to walk, he moves his right leg first. Ib. 78ᵃ הוה כאיב לי כַּרְעַאי my leg was hurting me. Ib. גבא דכ׳ הוה מסאנא דרב I mean the upper portion of the leg. Kidd. 49ᵃ מִכַּרְעַאי וכ׳ I want no shoe larger than my foot, i. e. I want no husband too high in rank.—Sabb. 104ᵃ כַּרְעֵיה דדל״ת, דגימ״ל the foot of the letter Gimmel, ... Daleth; a. fr.—*Pl.* כַּרְעִין, כַּרְעַיָּא. Targ. O. Lev. I, 13 (Y. ריגלי). Ib. 9 חמון כַּרְעוֹהִי. Targ. Am. III, 12; a. e.—Y. Shek. V, 49ᵃ bot. כ׳ look at these legs (how fat); Y. Bicc. III, 65ᶜ bot.; Lev. R. s. 34; Yalk. ib. 665; Koh. R. to V, 13.—Ab. Zar. 38ᵇ עד טופרי דכַרְעַיְיהוּ to the nails of their feet; a. fr.—Y. Maas. Sh. IV, end, 55ᶜ כַּרְעָתָא דערסא legs of the bed.

***כָּרַף** (cmp. כָּרוּב), *Ithpe.* אִיכְּרַף *to become round* (of the nipple of the breast), *to develop.* Nidd. 48ᵇ top (ref. to Ez. XXIII, 21) אִיכְּרְפוּ דדיך ... אישתדו וכ׳ thy breasts began to develop, yet thou didst not repent, thy breasts were fully developped, yet &c.; [other interpret. in Rashi: איכ׳ *to be swollen*, אישת׳ *to dry up*; Ar.: איכרפית, v. Koh. Ar. Compl. s. v.].

כרפונה, כרפוזנה, Y. Kil. I, 27ᵃ top (ref. to פול הלבן Mish. I, 1; Ar. ספרווה, R. S. to Kil. l. c. מרשיא) corrupt. of a probably Greek name for *white beans.*

כַּרְפַּס I m. (b. h.; cmp. κάρπασος, carbasus, Sanscrit carpâsa *cotton*) *fine linen.* Esth. R. to I, 6, expl. קִרְפַּסִּינוֹן. Meg. 12ᵃ, v. כַּר.

כַּרְפַּס II m. (cmp. כָּרוּב II, כָּרַף) *an umbelliferous plant, celery, parsley.* Shebi. IX, 1 כ׳ שבנהרות (Y. ed. Krot. כוסבר, corr. acc.) water-parsley, expl. Y. ib. 38ᶜ פיטרוסילינון (πε-τροσέλινον), contrad. to garden-parsley; Succ. 39ᵇ (Rashi: *cress*, or 'apium', *parsley*). Y. Sabb. VII, 10ᵃ; a. e.—[Tosef. Kil. I, 1 הכוסבר והכ׳ (ed. Zuck. והכרקם, v. כַּרְכּוֹם I.].

כַּרְפְּסָא I ch.=h. כַּרְפַּס I. Targ. Esth. VIII, 15.

כַּרְפְּסָא II ch.=h. כַּרְפַּס II. Ab. Zar. 28ᵃ כ׳ בטילא parsley put in strong wine. Ib. 38ᵇ בִּיזרא דכ׳ parsley-seed. Keth. 61ᵃ.—[Tosef. Kil. III, 12 והכרפסא ed. Zuck., Var. והרַכְפָא.]

כרפת, Tosef. Sabb. XIII (XIV), 17 ed. Zuck., read: כּוֹפֶת.

כַּרְצָא, כּוּרְצָא m. (קרץ, cmp. ברץ) *intestinal worms.* Gitt. 69ᵇ לכ׳ Ar. (ed. לכרי) a remedy for &c. Ib. לכ׳ חיורא for white worms.

כַּרְקוֹם, כַּרְקוּמָא, v. sub כַּרְכּ׳.

כרקומניקיא, v. פִּירוּמָנִיקְיָא.

כַּרְקֹם, v. כַּרְכּוֹם.

***כָּרָר** m. (v. כַּר) *upholsterer.* M. Kat. 13ᵇ quot. in Kimḥi Shorash. s. v.; v. כַּבָּד.

כַּרְשָׁא, v. כְּרֵיש.

כַּרְשִׁינָא I f. ch. (v. כְּרֵיש) *ball, pebble.*—*Pl.* כַּרְשִׁינֵי. Sabb. 81ᵃ כ׳ בבלייתא Babylonian pebbles (cloddy and brittle).

כַּרְשִׁינָה, (כַּרְשִׁינָא) II f. (cmp. כְּרֵישָׁה) *a porraceous plant.*—בורית כ׳ an alkaline solution of *carshina.* Ker. 6ᵃ; Y. Yoma IV, 41ᵈ.—*Pl.* כַּרְשִׁינִים, כַּרְשִׁינִין. Sabb. I, 5 (17ᵇ) אין שורין...כ׳ אלא וכ׳ (shortly before Sabbath) we must not lay in ink-material, ... or alkaline plants; [comment. refer to next w.].

כַּרְשִׁינָה II (כַּרְשִׁינָא III) f. (cmp. כַּרְשִׁינָא I) a species of *vetch*, prob. *horse-bean*, rarely used as human food. Bekh. VI, 1 (37ᵃ) ניקבה מלא כ׳ if there is a hole in the ear lap of the size of a *carshinah*; ib. 37ᵇ, expl. הינדא; Tosef. ib. IV, 1. Y. Kidd. I, 59ᵈ top פחות מן הכ׳ less than the size of &c.; a. e.—*Pl.* כַּרְשִׁינִים, כַּרְשִׁינִין. B. Mets. 90ᵃ. Hall. IV, 9, a. fr. כַּרְשִׁינֵי תרומה beans set aside for the priest's share. Maas. Sh. II, 4; Tosef. ib. II, 1. Y. Hall. IV, 60ᵇ אימתי גזרו על הכ׳ (contrad. to בִּיקְיָא) when was the law declaring *carshinah* subject to T'rumah enacted?— Answ. בימי רעבון in days of famine (when it served as human food). Esth. R. to I, 14 (play on כַּרְשְׁנָא, ib.) אני בוזק לפניהם כרשינין ומשירן מן העולם I shall crush vetch (to be placed) before them (send a famine compelling them to eat vetch) and make them fall off (fade away) from the world. Y. Maas. Sh. II, 53ᶜ קל ... בכרשיני (read: בכרשינין) they made the law concerning *carsh*. less stringent. Ib. עיסה של כ׳ a dough made of *c*.—Meïl. III, 6 כרשיני חקדש; Tosef. ib. I, 21 כַּרְשָׁנֵי ed. Zuck. (some ed. כר שני, corr. acc.), v. הֶקְדֵּשׁ; a. fr.—Koh. R. to VI, 1 כַּרְשָׁנִים בפלפלין he who puts vetch into pepper; (Tosef. B. Bath. V, 6 כּוּסְבֶּרֶת).

כַּרְשָׁנִים, כַּרְשָׁנֵי, v. preced.

כרשתנא, כרשתינא, v. כְּרוּשְׁתֵּינָא.

כָּרֵת, v. כְּרֵית.

כָּרַת (b. h.; cmp. כָּרָה) 1) *to cut*. Num. R. s. 16 ונקרא אשכול ... לִכְרוֹת וכ׳ and he (Abraham's ally) was named Eshkol (Cluster), on account of the cluster of grapes which the Israelites were destined to cut in his home. —Esp. *to cut genitals, mutilate*. Bekh. 33ᵇ ניתק אחר כורת, v. נָתַק.—Part. pass. כָּרוּת. Ib.; a. fr.—כ׳ שפכה one that is mutilated at his membrum, v. שָׁפָךְ. Tosef. Yeb. XI, 2. Yeb. VIII, 2; a. fr.—2) [*to draw a circle, place outside*, cmp. meanings of ברי, חרם,] *to cut off, excommunicate*, v. כָּרֵת. Y. Bicc. II, beg. 64ᶜ; Y. Snh. XI, 30ᵇ צא .. עונשין וכוֹרְתִים deduct twenty years up to which age the divine court neither punishes nor decrees excision.—3) *to separate, divorce; to make final*. Gitt. 21ᵇ; Succ. 24ᵇ (ref. to Deut. XXIV, 3) ספר כּוֹרְתָהּ וכ׳ the delivery of the deed divorces her and nothing else does. Ib. דבר הכּוֹרֵת ביני לבינה something (a condition) which (if fulfilled) severs definitely the connection between him and her (e. g. a condition that she will drink no wine for the next thirty days, after the lapse of which time the letter of divorce takes its effect retroactively, opp. to a condition that she will abstain from wine all the rest of her life in which case the letter of divorce cannot take effect).—Part. pass. כָּרוּת *definite*. Y. Gitt. VII, 48ᵈ כגט כ׳ הוא it is like a final divorce (taking effect immediately); Y. B. Bath. VIII, 16ᶜ top כ׳ הוא. Y. Gitt. III, 44ᵈ top; IX, 50ᵇ bot. זה כ׳ לשמה וזה כ׳ לשמה (not וו) this letter was definitely made out for this woman, and so was the other for the other woman. Ib. III, beg. 44ᶜ אלא שלא הי׳ לה כ׳ ... ראשונה (strike out לה); a. fr.—3) *to decide, make final*. Ber. 4ᵃ; Snh. 16ᵇ (ref. to כְּרֵתִי as a symbolical name for the Urim and Tummim, or for the Sanhedrin) שכּוֹרְתִים את דבריהם they give definite and precise decisions; Midr. Till. to Ps. III כּוֹרְתֵי, כריתות. v. כְּרִיתָה; a. e.—כ׳ בְּרִית (v. בְּרִית) *to covenant, make a firm promise*. Gen. R. s. 44 כָּרַתָּ ב׳ עם וכ׳ thou hast promised to Noah that thou wilt not destroy his descendants; Yalk. Gen. 76 כָּרַתָּה.—Part. pass. כָּרוּת, f. כְּרוּתָה. M. Kat. 18ᵃ, a. fr. ברית כ׳ לשפתים, v. בְּרִית. R. Hash. 17ᵇ ב׳ כ׳ לי״ג מדות וכ׳ there is a solemn insurance given that the invocation of the thirteen divine attributes (Ex. XXXIV, 6, sq.) will never be without effect (ref. to Ex. ib. 10).—Trnsf. ב׳ כ׳ *it is a necessity, unavoidable*. Nidd. 58ᵇ ב׳ כ׳ לו שכל וכ׳ whoever crushes it cannot help smelling it.

Nif. נִכְרַת 1) *to be cut, mutilated*. Yeb. VIII, 2 (expl. כרות שפכה, Deut. XXIII, 2) כל שני׳ הגיד when the membrum is mutilated. Ib. 75ᵇ נִכְרְתוּ ביצים when the testicles are cut out; a. fr.—2) *to be covenanted*. Sot. 37ᵇ שלא נִכְרְתוּ עליה וכ׳ upon which were not closed forty eight covenants; Tosef. ib. VIII, 11; a. fr.—3) *to be cut off, destroyed*. Y. Peah I, 15ᵈ bot. (ref. to Num. XV, 31) מלמד שהנפש נִכְרֶתֶת ועונה בה which intimates that (the idolator's) soul is cut off (through premature death, כָּרֵת), while her guilt remains with her (unexpiated by death); Snh. 64ᵇ (ref. to the emphasized expression הכרת תכ׳, Num. l. c.) הִכָּרֵת בעו״הז וכ׳ *hiccareth* refers to this world &c.; a. fr.—Verbal noun הִיכָּרֵת, v. כָּרֵת.

Hif. הִכְרִית *to destroy, exterminate*. Tanh. R'eh 7 והִכְרַתָּם and exterminate them. Ib. כשיַּכְרִית וכ׳ when the Lord ... shall have destroyed ..., you will enter. Tosef. Snh. IV, 5 לְהַכְרִית זרעו וכ׳ to exterminate the seed of Amalek; a. fr.

Pi. כֵּרֵת *to doom to destruction*. Arakh. 15ᵇ שכבר כֵּרְתוֹ וכ׳ for David has doomed him &c. (ref. to Ps. XII, 4); Yalk. Lev. 559.

כְּרַת ch. same, esp. *to separate, divorce*. Gitt. 21ᵇ, a. fr. עידי מסירה כָּרְתֵי it is the witnesses of delivery (in whose presence the deed of divorce is handed to the wife) that effect the divorce (and the signature of the witnesses is unessential); opp. to עידי חתימה כרתי it is the signing witnesses &c.—Imper. כְּרוֹת (only in) כ׳ גיטא *make the divorce final, definite* (v. preced.). Ib. 9ᵃ היינו טעמא משום דלאו כ׳ ג׳ ה״א the reason (that the manumission of the slave is not lawful) is because the form was not in compliance with the rule, 'make the divorce definite'; B. Bath. 150ᵇ.

כָּרֵת f. (= הִכָּרֵת, v. כָּרַת *Nif*.) *excommunication, extermination*; (in Talm. law) *divine punishment* through premature or sudden death, opp. to מיתה בידי אדם capital punishment. Snh. 60ᵇ זובח .. כ׳ הוא is not slaughtering consecrated animals outside of the Temple punishable with extinction?, opp. קטלא death by execution. M. Kat. 28ᵃ מת בחמשים שנה זו היא מיתת כ׳ if one dies at the age of fifty, that is death of divine visitation; Y. Bicc. II, beg. 64ᶜ בהִיכָּרֵת; Treat. S'mah. III, 8 בהִכָּרֵת. Ib. 10 וכי מה מודיענו שמיתתם בהכרת what is there to indicate that they died by divine visitation?; Y. l. c. 64ᵈ top שהוא בהיכרת.—M. Kat. l. c. נפקי לי מכ׳ I have escaped the punishment of *kareth* (being sixty years old). Ib. כ׳ דשני the *kareth* of years, premature death; כ׳ דיומי the *k*. of days, sudden death. Hull. 31ᵃ עון כ׳ a transgression punishable with *k*., opp. איסור מיתה. Macc. III, 15 (23ᵃ) נפטרו מידי כְּרִיתָן Ms. M. (ed. ידי כְּרִיתָתָם) are released from *k*. (which would otherwise await them). Ib. 13ᵇ ולמה יצאת כ׳ באחותו why is the punishment of *k*. specifically mentioned with reference to incest with a sister (Lev. XX, 17, being included in Lev. XVIII, 29)?—Gen. R. s. 28 (ref. to כְּרֵתִים, Zeph. II, 5, v. Targ. a. l.) גוי שהוא ראוי כ׳ a nation deserving extermination; (Yalk. Zeph. 567 ראוי לִיכָּרֵת); a. v. fr.—*Pl*. כְּרִיתוֹת (fr. כְּרִיתָה). Ker. I, 1 שלשים ושש כ׳ בתורה there are thirty six transgressions mentioned in the Torah as (eventually) punishable with *kareth*. Macc. III, 15, a. fr. חייבי כ׳ those on whose transgressions the penalty of *k*. is pronounced; a. fr.—K'rithoth, a treatise of the Mishnah, Tosefta, and Talmud Babli, of the Order of Kodashim.

כַּרְתָּא, כַּרְתָּה, v. כַּרְתֵּי.

כרתון, Y. Kil. V, 30ᵃ top, read: כרתין, v. כְּוֶורֶת.

כְּרֵתִי m. (b. h.) gent. n. *K'rethi, Cherethi*; (collect.) *the body-guard of David*; (homilet.) *the Sanhedrin* (or *Urim and Tummim*). Ber. 4ᵃ, v. כָּרַת. Midr. Till. to Ps. III, v. כְּרֵיתָה; a. e.—*Pl.* כְּרֵתִיִּים. Men. 28ᵇ כמין תפוחי הכ׳ ed. (ed. Ven., a. oth., and Ar. חכרתיים) the shape of the apples of the *K'rethiim* (Cretans?); ib. 63ᵃ הכ׳ Ms. R. 2 (ed. הכריתים), v. כְּרֵיתָה.

כַּרְתִּי (כְּרָתִי) m. (Hebr. denom. of Ch. כַּרְתָּא, v. next w.) *porraceous* (of color), *leek-green stuff*. Ber. I, 2 (משיכיר) בין תכלת לכ׳ when one can distinguish between blue and green; (Y. ed. כְּרָתָן; Ar. Var. כרתה, כרתא). Succ. III, 6 ירוק ככ׳ (Y. ed. ככרתן) an Ethrog green like a porraceous plant (v. כַּרְתִּינוֹן).—Gitt. 31ᵇ סרבלא דכ׳ a cloak of green wool.

כַּרְתֵּי, כַּרְתִּיָא, כַּרְתִּין m. pl. ch.=h. כְּרֵישִׁין (v. כְּרֵישָׁה) *leek*. Targ. Num. XI, 5 ed. Berl. כ׳ (oth. ed. כ׳; Yarg. Y. II כַּרְתָּיָא, some ed. כַּרְתָּא; h. text חָצִיר).—Ab. Zar. 10ᵇ שדר ליה כ׳ he (the emperor) sent him leek (symbolically alluding to כרת, 'my progeny will be cut off', Rashi). Ker. 6ᵃ; Hor. 12ᵃ. Y. Kil. IV, end, 29ᶜ זרע כרמיה כרתין planted leek in his vineyard. Y. Sabb. VII, 10ᵃ החן דגזז ... כ׳ וכ׳ he who cuts (on the Sabbath) coriander ...., leek &c. Bab. ib. 110ᵇ, v. כַּתְוָא a. כְּתָא; a. fr.

כְּרָתִים, כְּרָתִין, *ramifications*, v. כְּוֶורֶת.

כְּרָתָן, v. כַּרְתֵּי.

כַּרְתִּינוֹן, כְּרֵתִי m. (a denom. of כַּרְתֵּי, כְּרָתָן, formed after the Greek πράσινος) *leek-colored, green*. Y'lamd. to Gen. XLIX, 1 quot. in Ar. בין תכלת לצבע כ׳ (Ber. I, 2 לכרתי), v. כַּרְתֵּי. Y. Succ. III, 53ᵈ (ref. to Mish. ירוק ככרתן, v. כַּרְתֵּי) כהן כ׳ או דדמי לחן כרתינין (corr. acc.) does the Mishnah mean exactly as green as leek, or any shade like leek?

כרתית, Kel. XX, 1 Ar., v. כְּרֵיסִית.

כְּרָתָן, v. כַּרְתֵּי.

כַּרְתְּנִין m. pl. (denom. of כַּרְתֵּי) *green material*. Targ. Esth. I, 6 (h. text כַּרְפַּס, v. כַּרְפַּס II).

כַּשׁ, *Ithpa.* אִתְכַּשַּׁשׁ, v. כְּשַׁשׁ.

כְּשָׁאמָא, v. גְּשָׁמָה.

כְּשַׁב, כִּשְׁבָּה, v. כֶּבֶשׂ.

כַּשְׂדָּאָה, כַּסְ׳ m. ch.=next w.—*Pl.* כַּשְׂדָּאֵי, כַּסְ׳. Targ. Gen. XI, 28; a. fr.

כַּשְׂדִּי, כַּשְׂדִּיי m. (b. h. כַּשְׂדִּים, *pl.*) *Chaldean*. Meg. 12ᵇ כלי ..... כשדיי the vessel which I use (my wife) is neither ..., but a Chaldean.—*Pl.* כַּשְׂדִּיִּים, כַּשְׂדִּים. Succ. 52ᵇ. Pesik. R. s. 37 כשנפרע מן הכ׳ when the Lord punished the Chaldeans (Babylonia, v. Midr. Till. to Ps. XCIII, 1).—B. Bath. 15ᵇ. Lam. R. to I, 14 קשה כ׳ the Chaldean government was tyrannical (contrad. to בבל); a. e.—*Fem.* כַּשְׂדִּית, *pl.* כַּשְׂדִּיּוֹת. Snh. 92ᵇ.

כַּשּׁוּף, v. כִּישּׁוּף.

כְּשׁוּרָא, כְּשׁוּ׳ f. (כשר; cmp. גְּשׁוּרָא) *joist, beam, post*. Targ. Y. Gen. XIX, 8 (O. שְׁרִיתָא; h. text קֹרָה). Targ. II Kings VI, 2 (ed. Lag. שדי, Var. שרי, כ׳); a. e.—B. Kam. 66ᵇ, v. טַלְלָא. Ib. 11ᵃ, v. זוזא I. Hor. 3ᵇ כי היכי דניטעון שיבא מכ׳ in order that each of us may carry off a chip of the beam (that you may share the responsibility with me). Keth. 17ᵃ אין דמיין עלייכו ככ׳ if they (the brides you carry in procession) are on your shoulders like a beam (awaking no sensual desire). Ib. 86ᵇ; B. Kam. 98ᵇ כי כ׳ לצלמי like a beam fit for decorative mouldings (proverbial expression for *straight and exact*), v. גְּבַר. Kidd. 80ᵇ ... מיחברי כ׳ וכ׳ ten persons combine to steal a beam and are not ashamed of one another; a. e.—*Pl.* כְּשׁוּרֵי, כְּשׁוּרִין. Targ. II Chr. XXXIV, 11. Targ. Cant. I, 17 כְּשׁוּרוֹהִי (some ed. כַּשִּׁירוֹהִי); a. e.—Sabb. 67ᵃ ז׳ ציבי מז׳ כ׳ seven chips from seven beams. B. Kam. 96ᵃ גיבי ועבדינהו כ׳ if one stole trunks and made them into joists (by trimming). Gitt. 67ᵇ איעסק בכ׳ busied himself with carrying (or trimming) beams; a. e.—Trnsf. *lengthy slices of a radish*. Sabb. 108ᵇ במערבא מלחי כ׳ כ׳ Ms. M. (ed. כְּשׁוּרֵי, Ar. כַּשְׁרֵי, Var. פִּישֵׁי; Alf. פישרי) in Palestine they salt them (on the Sabbath) each slice by itself (just as they are eaten).

כְּשׁוּרְתָא f. same. Y. Bets. II, 61ᶜ top quot. in Ḥidd. Meiri, v. מוֹלְיֵי.

כְּשׁוּת f. (cmp. כִּישָׁא) 1) *tuft, pubescence, fine hairs or fibres*. Ukts. II, 1. Mikv. IX, 4 כ׳ של קטן the downy hair growth of a youth before puberty; Tosef. ib. VI, 10 כ׳ של גדול וכ׳ quot. by R. S. to Mikv. l. c. (ed. כתות) the hair growth of one entering on puberty, about which he cares not.—Esp. (also masc. sub. שער) *cuscuta*, a parasite growing on shrubs (v. Löw Pfl. p. 230, sq.). Tosef. Kil. I, 11 (Var. קשות), v. חִיזְמָא. Ib. III, 16 כ׳ אינו וכ׳ ed. Zuck. (oth. ed. אין); Sabb. 139ᵃ Ms. M. (ed. כישות), v. כִּלְאַיִם.—2) (collect. noun, sub. מינין) *cucumbers or melons in an early stage when they are pubescent*. Ib. 109ᵃ כ׳ אין בהם משום רפואה pubescent cucumbers or melons are not considered medicinal (in Sabbath law). Ib. כל מיני כ׳ שרו וכ׳ (Ms. O. כישות, Ar. s. v. טרז: קישות or קִישּׁוּת q. v.) all kinds of downy plants are permitted (on the Sabbath as not medicinal), except *t'ruza*, v. טְרוּזָא.

כְּשׁוּת, כְּשׁוּתָא ch. same, esp. *cuscuta*. Erub. 28ᵇ כ׳ נמי מארעא קא רבי וכ׳ cuscuta, too, draws its nourishment from the ground, for behold, as soon as you cut the shrub, the cuscuta on it dies. Sabb. 107ᵇ האי מאן דתלש כ׳ וכ׳ he who tears c. loose from the shrubs &c. Sabb. 139ᵃ כ׳ בכרמא עירבובא cuscuta in a vineyard is a forbidden mixture (v. כִּלְאַיִם). Ib. 109ᵇ bot. איכליה כ׳ וכ׳ ordered him to eat c. with salt and to run &c. Gitt. 69ᵃ, v. חוּמְרְתָא.—Hull. 47ᵇ כ׳ דדמיא looking like c. (yellowish).—V. כַּשְׁרְתָא.

כְּשַׁט* (v. קשט), *Af.* אַכְשֵׁט *to do well, prosper*. Targ. Josh. I, 8 תַּכְשֵׁט (ed. Lag. תַּכְשְׁטוּן; h. text תשכיל, Pesh. תכשר).

כַּשִּׁיל m. (b. h.; כָּשַׁל) *a carpenter's tool for chipping, axe*. B. Kam. X, 10 ובכ׳ של בעה״ב when working with the axe, the chips belong to the owner, contrad. to מעצד. Ib.

119^b, v. חֲצִינָא.—*Pl.* כַּשִּׁילִים, כַּשִּׁילִין. Sot. VIII, 6 כ׳ של ברזל iron axes (as a weapon in war). Sifré Deut. 337 כשלים (corr. acc.).

כַּשִּׁילָא ch. same.—*Pl.* כַּשִּׁילִין. Targ. Jer. XLVI, 22 (h. text קרדמות).

כשיר־, v. sub כשר׳.

כִּשְׁכּוּשׁ m. (כִּשְׁכֵּשׁ) *striking* (with the tail). B. Kam. 19^b כ׳ יתירא a more than ordinary habit of knocking about. Ib. כ׳ באמתא Ms. M. (ed. כשכשה באמתה, v. Rabb. D. S. a. l. note), v. כִּשְׁכֵּשׁ.

(בַּשְׁכָּר)כַּשְׁכָּר pr. n. pl. *Cashkar, Cascara* (v. P. Sm. 1843) in Babylonia. Yoma 10^a אכד זה כ׳ Ms. M. 2 a. Ms. L. (ed. ב׳; v. Rabb. D. S. a. l. note 10) Accad is C. Sabb. 139^a בני כ׳. Gitt. 80^b אסטנדרא דכ׳, v. אִסְטַנְדְּרָא. [V. Schr. KAT², p. 346 ⁵ Arku, Nipur, Kiš.]

כִּשְׁכֵּשׁ 1) (כשש; cmp. נִשְׁנֵשׁ) *to knock, strike, move to and fro, shake.* Bets. 20^a כ׳ לחם בזנבה (Ms. M. כ׳ לה) he made for them (in their presence) striking movements with the animal's tail (making believe it was a female); Y. ib. II, 61^c top התחיל מְכַשְׁכֵּשׁ בזנבה; Y. Ḥag. II, 78^a bot.—Ḥull. II, 6 עד שֶׁיְּכַשְׁכֵּשׁ בזנבה unless the animal strikes about with its tail (an evidence of vitality). Ib. 38^a top כִּשְׁכְּשָׁה באזנה if it shook its ears (with vital force). Y. B. Kam. II, beg. 2^d; Bab. ib. 19^b כ׳ בזנבה if the beast struck (and did damage) with its tail. Ib. כ׳ באמתה (v. preced.) if she struck (and did damage) with her fore-leg.—V. שִׁכְשֵׁךְ II.—[2) (=שִׁכְשֵׁךְ; cmp. נִעְנַע) *to soothe, pat.* Pesik. Zakh. p. 24^b (את) מְכַשְׁכְּשׁוֹ, v. שִׁכְשֵׁךְ I.]

כַּשְׁכֵּשׁ ch. same, *to shake, knock about* &c. Yoma 84^b וּמְכַשְׁכְּשִׁין ליה באמגוזי Ms. M. (ed. משבּיש, Var. in Ar. s. v. שבש: מְקַשְׁקֵשׁ) he may rattle nuts for it (to entertain the child). Sabb. 77^b לְכַשְׁכּוּשֵׁי בקי Ms. M. (ed. לִכְרְכּוּשֵׁי) to chase off gnats by striking (with the tail).

כַּשְׁכֵּשׁ* (transpos. of שכשך, v. סַכְסֵךְ I) *to entangle, catch, confound.* Koh. R. to IV, 14 (ref. to בית הסורים ib.) דהוא מְכַשְׁכֵּשׁ לברייתא כמן בוני סריאתא he (the seducer) catches the people like one coming forth from between the bushes; Midr. Till. to Ps. IX.

כָּשַׁל (b. h.; cmp. כִּשְׁכֵּשׁ) *to strike against, stumble.* Lev. R. s. 19 (ref. to Is. XXXV, 3) שהן נראות כאילו כּוֹשְׁלוֹת knees which have the appearance of stumbling (threaten to stumble). Ib. שֶׁכְּשַׁלְתֶּם וכ׳ for you have really stumbled (sinned) through your evil deeds. Num. R. s. 16 כְּשַׁלְתֶּם you have stumbled (were discouraged; Tanḥ. Shlaḥ 2 נתרשלתם); a. e.—כּוֹשֵׁל (law) *weak, under legal disadvantages* (in adapt. of Is. l. c. a. Job IV, 4). Keth. IX, 2 ינתנו לַכּ׳ שבהן let it be given him who is under the greatest disadvantage of all (the claimants being the deceased man's widow, his creditor and his heirs); expl. ib. 84^a לכ׳ שבראיה to him who is under disadvantage for evidence (whose document is of the latest date); [oth. opin.] לכתובת אשה to the widow, v. חִינָּא; Y. ib. IX, 33^a top לכ׳ שבראיותיו וכ׳ to him who is the weakest as to evidence, e. g. he who loaned without witnesses as against him who has witnesses. Ib. לכ׳ בגופו to him who is in feeble health (and poor).

Nif. נִכְשַׁל 1) *to be struck, meet with an accident.* Mekh. B'shall. s. 2 לא נ׳ אחד וכ׳ not one of them (the Egyptians) met with an accident (was detained) on the road. Y. Sabb. VI, 8^c bot. נ׳ באצבעו got a sore finger; ib. XVI, 15^c top; Lam. R. to IV, 20; a. e.—2) *to stumble, fall; to be led to sin.* Pesik. Shub., p. 165^a והוו . . . . נִכְשָׁלִין בו and people stumbled over it (the rock); Yalk. Hos. 533. Ib. אדם נ׳ בעבירה if man becomes a victim of sin. Gitt. 43^a אין אדם . . . אא״כ נ׳ בהן one never gets at the true sense of the words of the Law, except after mistakes; Ḥag. 14^a; Sabb. 120^a.—Ber. 28^b ולא אֶכָּשֵׁל בדבר הלכה and that I may not err against a *hălakhah*; ולא יִכָּשְׁלוּ וכ׳ nor may my colleagues &c. Midr. Till. to Ps. XXII בשביל.. איני נִכְשֶׁלֶת because I am a queen, I shall not come to grief; a. fr.

Hif. הִכְשִׁיל *to cause to stumble, to be an obstruction; to weaken; to cause sin.* Y. Shebi. III, end, 34^d a breach in the fence מַכְשֶׁלֶת את הרבים annoying the public (an obstruction to traffic). R. Hash. I, 6 נמצאת מַכְשִׁילָן לע״ל thou wilt make them sin in future cases (by their refraining from going to court); Yoma 77^b שלא תהא מַכְשִׁילָן וכ׳ that thou mayest not cause them to sin (by staying away from college); Kidd. 33^a; Ḥull. 54^b מְכַשְּׁלָן (*Pi.*).—Ab. Zar. 11^b פיהם הִכְשִׁילָן לרשעים Ms. M. (ed. ה׳ פיהם) their own (ominous) words brought these wicked men to fall; Num. R. s. 18. B. Kam. 16^b; B. Bath. 9^b (ref. to מכשלים, Jer. XVIII, 23) הַכְשִׁילֵם וכ׳ make them stumble by sending them unworthy subjects of charity. Midr. Till. to Ps. XC לעצמי הייתי מַכְשִׁיל I should have injured myself.

Pi. כִּישֵּׁל 1) same, v. supra.—2) *to weaken, break the force of.* Y. Ber. IX, 13^c bot. מְכַשְּׁלוֹ בגבעות (Gen. R. s. 24 מרשלו), v. חָשַׁל.

כְּשַׁל ch. same, *Af.* אַכְשֵׁל *to bring to fall.* Gitt. 57^a אַכְשְׁלֵיה פומיה לבר וכ׳ his own mouth (his presumptuous prayer) caused Bar-Daroma's downfall.

כִּשָּׁלוֹן m. (b. h.; preced.) *downfall, stumbling, weakness.* Ḥag. 14^a; Sabb. 119^b אפי׳ בשעת כִּשָּׁלוֹנָהּ וכ׳ even at the period of Jerusalem's downfall (moral decay) the men of faith did not fail her. Midr. Till. to Ps. XXII (ref. to Prov. XXIV, 16) תכף לכ׳ רעה the evil immediately follows their stumbling (leaving no time to rise). Yalk. Job 897 (ref. to Job IV, 4) היית מנחם כל בעלי כ׳ thou didst console all the afflicted (Tanḥ. Vayishl., ed. Bub. 8 יסורין).

כשלים, v. כַּשִּׁיל.

כָּשַׁף (b. h.; cmp. חָשַׁב) [*to whisper*, v. Fl. to Levy Talm. Dict. II, p. 459,] *to think, devise*, v. כּוּשְׁפָּא.

Pi. כִּישֵּׁף *to charm, practice sorcery* (cmp. לָחַשׁ). Snh. 43^a (suppressed in later eds., v. יֵשׁוּ) על שכ׳ והסית וכ׳ because he practiced sorcery and enticed &c. Ib. VII, 4 הַמְכַשֵּׁף he who practices witchcraft, expl. ib. 11 המכ׳ העושה מעשה וכ׳ he who produces a real effect is guilty, not he who produces an optical delusion, v. אָחַז; a. fr.—V. מְכַשֵּׁף, מְכַשֵּׁפָה.

כֶּשֶׁף, m., *pl.* כְּשָׁפִים (b. h.; preced.) *sorcery.* Ḥull. 7^b (ref. to Deut. IV, 35) אין עוד מלבדו ואפי׳ כ׳ 'there is none (no power) besides Him', ... not even sorcery (can do anything without the will of God); Snh. 67[b] (ed. ואפי׳ לדבר כ׳; v. Rabb. D. S. a. l. note 2); Yalk. Deut. 828.— Ber. 53[a] בנות ישראל מקטרות לכ׳ daughters of Israel (in large places) are suspected of letting incense rise for sorcerous practices. Erub. 64[b] בדורות אחרונים.. פרוצות בכ׳ in these latter days when daughters of Israel are unrestrained in practicing sorcery. Snh. 67[a] מצוירות בכ׳ habitually inclined to sorcery, v. כַּשְׁפָנִית. Y. Kidd. IV. end, 66[c] בעלת כ׳ sorceress; a. fr.

כַּשָּׁף m. (b. h.; preced.) *sorcerer.*—*Pl.* כַּשָּׁפִים, כַּשָּׁפִין. Hull. 7[b]; Snh. 67[b] למה . . . כשפים (Ms. M. מכשפים) why are they called *kashshafim*? מפני שמכחישין פמליא של מעלה because they lessen the power of divine agencies. Midr. Till. to Ps. LXXX, end כשפין (ed. Bub. כַּשְׁפָנִין; oth. ed. מְכַשְּׁפִין); a. e.—V. כְּכַשָּׁף.

***כְּשָׁף** m. (supposed to mean) *wild plum-tree.* Sabb. 23[a] שרף כ׳ וכ׳ Ms. M. a. Ar.; copyist's correction in Ms. M. כנף; ed. קטף) resin of the plum-tree is the best for making ink.

כַּשְׁפָּא m. *design, embroidery,* v. כּוּשְׁפָּא.

כַּשְׁפָן m., *pl.* כַּשְׁפָנִין, v. כַּשָּׁף.

כַּשְׁפָנִית f. (כַּשָּׁף) *engaged in, inclined to sorcery. Pl.* כַּשְׁפָנִיּוֹת. Y. Snh. VII, 25[d] top (ref. to Ex. XXII, 17) (the text speaks only of females) מפני שרוב הנשים כ׳ because most women are inclined to sorcery (Bab. ib. 67[a] מצויות בכשפים, v. כֶּשֶׁף). Yoma 83[b] נשים כ׳ women engaged in sorcery. Pes. 110[a], v. דִּשְׁתְּיָתָה.

כָּשֵׁר I (b. h.; cmp. גשר) [*to be well-joined,* (cmp. יָפֶה, אָרִיךְ II),] *to be proper, fit, right; to turn out well, to succeed.* Y. Hall. I, 57[b] top החטים שֶׁכָּשְׁרוּ לשאר וכ׳ wheats which are fit for all other meat offerings; ib. 57[c]; Sifra Vayikra, N'dabah, ch. XIV, Par. 13; a. fr.—V. כָּשֵׁר II.

Hif. הִכְשִׁיר 1) (ritual, v. כָּשֵׁר II) *to pronounce kasher, to permit.* Hull. III, 2 ר׳ . . . מַכְשִׁיר R. pronounces it fit to be eaten, opp. פוסל; a. v. fr.—2) *to make fit, to prepare.* Ab. VI, 1 מַכְשַׁרְתּוֹ להיות וכ׳ enables him to be righteous &c. Hull. 140[a] מַכְשִׁיר an offering which makes fit for admission to the Temple or eating sacred food, contrad. to מכפר an offering which procures atonement; Kidd. 57[a], a. e.— Snh. 42[b] היצא . . . מכשיר ומכפר 'the carrying outside of the camp' (Lev. IV, 12; 21) makes the act legal and procures atonement; ib. מכשיר ממכשיר עדיף ליה the analogy between one fitting act and another is preferred.—B. Kam. I, 2 הִכְשַׁרְתִּי את נזקו I have prepared (am responsible for) the damage, v. חִיֵּב. Ib. הכשרתי (ב)מקצת נזקו וכ׳ wherever I am the partial cause of a damage (e. g. by completing a pit to its legally indictable depth), I am as responsible as if I had been the entire author. Gen. R. s. 56 the slaughtering knife is called מַאֲכֶלֶת (causing the eating) (not שמכשר) לפי שֶׁמַּכְשֶׁרֶת את האוכלים because it makes the food fit for eating.—Esp. (with or without לקבל טומאה) *to make an object fit for levitical uncleanness* (v. Lev. XI, 34; 38). Hull. 35[b] וכי הדם מַכְשִׁיר . . . מַכְשֶׁרֶת is it the blood (as a liquid) which fits the meat for uncleanness?; is it not rather the slaughtering (because it makes it 'an eatable')?—Ib. 33[a] חיבת הקדש מַכְשַׁרְתָּן, v. חִבָּה; ib. 36[b] מַכְשַׁרְתָּהּ. Makhsh. VI, 6. Y. Gitt. I, 43[c] על מי בצים שאינן מַכְשִׁירִין that the liquid of eggs does not fit for uncleanness; Y. Shebi. VI, 36[c] top שאין כשירין (corr. acc.); a. v. fr.—V. הֶכְשֵׁר, מַכְשִׁירִין.

Hof. הוּכְשַׁר *to be made fit; to be pronounced fit; to be prepared; to be fitted for levitical uncleanness.* Yoma 50[a] במה ה׳ אהרן וכ׳ through what act is Aaron (a high priest) made fit to enter &c.?—Sabb. 76[a] כל שאינו כשר.. וה׳ לזה וכ׳ that which is not fit for preservation but appeared fit to this man, and he did preserve it. Hull. 22[b] הוּכְשְׁרוּ are pronounced fit for sacrifices. Ib. II, 5 הוכשרו בדם they became fit for uncleanness through the blood (flowing out at killing); ה׳ בשחיטה they became fit through the act of slaughtering (v. supra); a. v. fr.—[Y. Keth. XII, 35[a] מכושר, read: מכ׳, v. כָּשֵׁר.]

Hithpa. הִתְכַּשֵּׁר *to adapt one's self, to work with zeal and conscientiousness.* Koh. R. to V, 11 מִתְכַּשֵּׁר במלאכתו וכ׳ more skilled and zealous in his work than &c. (cmp. זָרִיז). Gen. R. s. 9; a. e.

כְּשַׁר ch. same, *to be right, pleasing, fit.* Targ. I Sam. XVIII, 20. Targ. Jud. XIV, 3. Targ. Ez. XV, 4; a. fr.

Ithpa. אִתְכַּשַּׁר, *Ithpe.* אִתְכְּשַׁר, אִיכְּשַׁר *to be (made) fit* &c. (v. preced. *Hof.*). Targ. Y. Deut. XXIX, 22. Targ. Y. Lev. XI, 2; a. fr.—Gitt. 87[a] לִיתְכַּשַּׁר האי וכ׳ let the one deed be declared valid through the signature 'Reuben ben' &c. —Hull. 36[b] איתכ׳ במשקי וכ׳ it was made fit for uncleanness through the fluids &c.; ib. אתכ׳ בחבת הקדש, v. חִבָּה; a. e.

Af. אַכְשַׁר 1) as preced. *Hif.* Targ. I Sam. XVII, 8. Targ. Ruth II, 13.—B. Mets. 89[b] top לְאַכְשׁוּרֵי גברא וכ׳ as to making the man fitter, i. e. as to the laborer in fruits being permitted to use means for increasing his appetite, there is no question, opp. to לאכשורי פירא using means for making the fruits more appetizing.—Zeb. 25[a] בשמאל אכשורי מַכְשַׁר he (R. S.) declares it permissible to use the left hand (for קְמִיצָה). Sabb. 154[a]; Yeb. 45[b] אַכְשְׁרֵיהּ וכ׳ pronounced R. Mari . . . to be legally a Jew. Hull. 58[b] סבר . . . לאַכְשׁוּרֵיהּ R . . . wanted to pronounce it *kasher*; a. fr.—2) *to grow better, improve.* Ib. 39[b]; Yeb. 39[b], v. בָּרָא I.

כָּשֵׁר II m. (b. h.; preced.) 1) *fit,* esp. *kasher, ritually permitted, legal,* opp. טרפה, פסול. *Fem.* כְּשֵׁרָה, כְּשֵׁירָה. Hull. I, 4 כ׳ בשחיטה פסול במליקה what is legal in slaughtering (cutting the throat) is illegal in pinching (the neck). Ib. שְׁחִיטָתוֹ כ׳ his act of slaughtering has been properly executed. Kidd. IV, 6 בתו כ׳ לכהונה his daughter is fit to marry a priest. Gitt. IX, 4 הולד כ׳ the issue is legitimate, is under no religious or civil disabilities; a. v. fr.—*Pl.* כְּשֵׁרִים, כְּשֵׁרִין, כְּשֵׁרִ׳; f. כְּשֵׁרוֹת. Hull. III, 2 אלו כ׳ בבהמה the following defects in a domestic animal are *kasher*, i e. do not make the animals unfit for eating. Ib. 3 אם אדומים כ׳ if they (the entrails) are red (have their natural color) they are (the animal is) *kasher*; a. v. fr.— 2) *worthy, honest, of noble conduct.* Ber. II, 7 כ׳ היה he was a worthy man. Kidd. IV, 14 הכ׳ שבטבחים the best of butchers; a. fr.—*Pl.* as ab. Ib. רובן כ׳ are mostly honest men, opp. רשעים. Y. Yoma III, end, 41[b] כְּשֵׁירֵי כל דור ודור the worthiest of every generation; Y. Shek. V, beg. 48[c]. Y. Dem. VI, 25[d] top (ref. to Mish. ib. 6 מהו (צנועי בית הלל צנועי כְּשֵׁירֵי in what sense is צנועי here used? In the sense of K'sheré (the worthies of the house of Hillel). Yoma 19[b], v. חָשַׁד; a. fr.—[Y. Shebi. VI, 36[c] top שאין כשירין, read: מַכְשִׁירִין, v. כָּשֵׁר I.]—3) *apt, convenient.* Mekh. Bo, s. 16; Tanḥ. Bo 11 חדש שהוא כ׳ לכ׳ a month convenient to you, when it is not too warm &c.

כָּשֵׁר, כְּשַׁרָא, כַּשִּׁירָא m., **כְּשֵׁירָא, כְּשֵׁירְתָא** f. same, 1) *fit, adapted, proper.* Targ. Num. XX, 5 ed. Berl. כָּ׳ (oth. ed. כְּ׳; Y. כָּשֵׁר). Targ. Jud. XVII, 6. Targ. Zech. III, 5; a. fr.—2) (cmp. זָרִיז, חָרִיץ) *well-equipped; quick, zealous, industrious, worthy.* Targ. Prov. VI, 11 (h. text איש מגן).—Koh. R. to III, 9 וכ׳ בכשרותיה and what has the industrious profited by his industry? (v. אוּמְנוּתָא); a. fr. [Y. Taan. II, 65[b], v. חֲצִיף.]—*Pl.* כַּשִּׁירִין, כְּשֵׁירִין; f. כַּשְׁרָן. Targ. Lev. IV, 2. Targ. Zech. III, 3, sq.; a. fr.

כִּשְׁרָא, *beam,* v. כָּשׁוּרָא.

כַּשְׁרוּת f. (כָּשֵׁר) *fitness, worthiness, legitimacy.* Yeb. 57[a] (in Chald. diction) כ׳ מיתוסֿסא בה וכ׳ (by her mother being a native Jewess) has her fitness been increased (so that a priest may marry her) . . . or has her sanctity also been increased (so as to be subject to the restrictions placed upon a native Jewess, acc. to Deut. XXIII, 2) and she may not eat T'rumah (when married to an impotent); [oth. opin.: כ׳ *legal status,* Jewish citizenship; קדושה *fitness to marry a priest,* v. Rashi a. l.].—Kidd. 72[b] כל ארצות בחזקת כ׳ וכ׳ the Jewish inhabitants of all countries (outside of Babylonia) are presumed to be of legitimate descent, opp. עִיסָּה. Num. R. s. 20 בתחלה הבריות נוהגות בכ׳ formerly people conducted themselves morally, opp. בַּעֲרָיוֹת. Koh. R. to V, 11 יגע זה . . . . בְּכַשְׁרוּתוֹ (not בכושרות) this man in his zeal has accomplished more &c., v. יָגַע.

כַּשְׁרוּתָא ch. same. Koh. R. to III, 9 בְּכַשְׁרוּתֵיה (some ed. בִּכְשֵׁירוּתֵיה), v. כָּשֵׁר.

כְּשֵׁרְתָא, v. כָּשֵׁר.

כַּשְׁרְתָא f. *a fragrant root* (same as קוֹשְׁטְ, the Latin *costum,* v. Löw Pfl. p. 357), *putchuck.* Ber. 43[a].

כָּשַׁשׁ (v. כִּשְׁכֵּשׁ) *to knock, strike.*—Denom. מַכּוֹשֶׁת.

Af. אַכֵּישׁ *to strike, chase away by knocking.* Gen. R. s. 44 נסב . . . וחוה מַכֵּישׁ לחון . . . מִתְכַּשִּׁין Ar. (ed. מכתשין) Abraham took a knocker and tried to frighten them away by knocking, but they minded it not; Yalk. ib. 77 וחוה מכיש לחון ולא חוו מתכתשין . . . .

Ithpe. אִתְכַּשֵּׁשׁ, אִתְכַּשׁ *to be frightened off by knocking,* v. supra.

כּשְׁתְּ, v. קוֹשְׁטְ.

כֻּשְׁת m. ch.=h. קוֹשְׁטְ, (*costum*), *putchuck* (v. כַּשְׁרְתָא). Targ. Y. I Ex. XXX, 34 (h. text שחלת).

כַּת c. (כָּתַת) *band, party, class.* Pes. V, 7 כת ראשונה the first division. Ib. של כ׳ שלישית those of the third division; a. v. fr.—Kel. XXV, 4 של כת קודמין היא וכ׳ this belongs to the class of things of which you cannot tell which was first; may be the one-quart measure is the lower side of the half-quart measure (Maim.; for oth. explan., v. comment.); [ed. Dehr. של בת, Ar. שלוֹחת, Var. שלבה, Mus. שלבב, Bart. שלוֹת].—*Pl.* כִּתּוֹת, כִּתִּין, כִּתִּים. כִּי׳. Y. Taan. II, 65[d] top ארבע כ׳ נעשו וכ׳ our ancestors at the Red Sea were divided into four parties (opinions); Mekh. B'shall. s. 2. Gen. R. s. 8 נעשו מה״ש כ׳ כ׳ the ministering angels formed parties (of divided opinions concerning the creation of man). Shebu. 47[b]; B. Bath. 31[b] שתי כִּיתֵּי עדים two sets of witnesses. Lev. R. s. 9 כ׳ כ׳ של לִיסְטִים bands of (captured) robbers (rebels). Midr. Till. to Ps. XI, 7; Yalk. ib. 656 שבע כ׳ הן וכ׳ there are seven classes of people who will (after death) be admitted into the presence of the Ever-living. Ib. אלו שבע כ׳ של צדיקים these are the seven classes of righteous men. Sabb. 104[a] (v. א״ל) כ״ה כ״ה ר״ש כ׳ כ׳ וכ׳ נר יש לי כ׳ כ׳ וכ׳ wait, I have many classes of gentiles &c.; a. fr.

כִּיתָּא, כִּתָּא ch. same. Targ. Y. I a. II Ex. XIV, 13, sq. (v. Y. Taan. II, 65[d] top, cited in preced).—[Sabb. 140[b], v. כִּיתָּא I.]—*Pl.* כִּתִּין, כִּיתִּין, כִּתֵּי. Targ. Y. l. c. Targ. Ps. XXIX, 1 כִּתֵּי constr.; a. e.—B. Kam. 24[a] תלתא כִּיתֵּי סהדי three sets of witnesses; a. e.

כַּתָּא, כְּתָא m. (כָּתַת)=h. סְפִיחַ, 1) *concretion, glebe, or alluvial mound.*—*Pl.* כְּתִין, כַּתִּין, with suffix כְּתָהָא (כַּתְּהָא). Targ. Job XIV, 19.—2) *after-crop.*—*Pl.* as ab. Targ. Is. XXXVII, 30; Targ. II Kings XIX, 29. Targ. Lev. XXV, 5 (some ed. O. sing., v. Berl. Targ. O. II, p. 38). Ib. 11 כְּתָהָא ed. Berl. (oth. כְּתָ׳; Y. כְּאֲוֵיהָא, some ed. כָּ׳, perh. to be read: כְּתְוָתְהָא).—[Sabb. 110[b] מכבתיתא דמישרי, perh. מִכַּתְוָתָא of the after-crop of valleys, v. כַּתְוָא.]—כְּתַכְּתִין, כְּתַכְּתִין *third crop.* Targ. Is. l. c.; Targ. II Kings l. c. (h. text סחיש, שחיס).

כָּתַב b. h.; v. Ges. H. Dict. s. v.) [*to join sign to sign,*] *to compose, write; to promise in writing, to will, assign, consign.* Gitt. 20[a] וכ׳ ולא חקק it says (Deut. XXIV, 1) 'and he shall write' but not engrave; Y. ib. II, 44[b] top, v. כְּתִיבָה. Macc. III, 6 (ref. to Lev. XIX, 28) עד שֶׁיִּכְתּוֹב וכ׳ unless he writes (designs) and etches with ink, stibium or anything that marks; Sifra K'doshim, Par. 3, ch. VI, v. כְּתוֹבֶת.—Meg. 9[a] כִּתְבוּ לִי תורת וכ׳ write (translate) for me the Law &c. Ib. 7[a] כִּתְבוּנִי בספר Ms. M. (ed. לדורות) write me down (record my deeds) in a book (Book of Esther). Ex. R. s. 47, beg. כְּתוֹב אתה write thou thyself. Sabb. XII, 3 הַכּוֹתֵב וכ׳ he who writes two letters (on the Sabbath). Ib. 5 נתכוין לִכְתּוֹב ח״ית if he intended to write a Ḥeth.—Keth. IX, 1 הַכּוֹתֵב לאשתו וכ׳ he who declares to his wife &c.; ib. 83[a] תנו ר׳ חייא האומר R. H. interpreted it, 'he who says' (verbally). Ib. 102[b] מאי כּוֹתְבִין אומרים 'they write' (in the Mishnah) means merely they declare. Ib. V, 1 והיא כּוֹתֶבֶת וכ׳ and she may write (a receipt), I have received &c.—Pes. 50[b] כּוֹתְבֵי ספרים וכ׳ copyists of sacred books, or T'fillin &c. B. Bath. 14[b] משה כ׳ ספרו וכ׳ Moses is the author of his book, the chapter of Balaam, and the Book of Job; a. v. fr.—Part. pass. כָּתוּב, f. כְּתוּבָה; pl. כְּתוּבִים, כְּתוּבִין; כְּתוּבוֹת. Meg. 31ª דבר זה כ׳ בתורה וכ׳ this is written in the Law, and repeated in the Prophets &c. Ib. 7ª כבר כ׳ אני וכ׳ I am already recorded in the chronicles of &c. Y. Shek. VI, 49ᵈ bot. כיצד היו הלוחות כ׳ how was the writing on the tablets arranged?—Gitt. 54ᵇ כל ס״ת... כ׳ לשמן any scroll of the Law in which the Divine names are not written with full consciousness, v. שֵׁם; a. fr.—V. כְּתוּב.

Nif. נִכְתַּב *to be written, be reduced to writing; to be written upon.* Meg. I, 8 הספרים נִכְתָּבִים בכל לשון the Biblical books may be written in (translated into) any language (v. ib. 9ª); ib. לא התירו שֶׁיִּכָּתְבוּ וכ׳ they permitted them to be translated only into Greek. Ib. 7ª נאמרה לִיכָּתֵב was indited (by the divine spirit) for the purpose of being written (as a book); Yoma 29ª נתנה ליכתב (some ed. לְכָתוֹב); a. v. fr.

Hif. הִכְתִּיב 1) *to cause to be written* or *recorded, to dictate, indite.* Gen. R. s. 22 כבר הִכְתַּבְתִּי לך וכ׳ I have already ordered to be written in the Law &c. Ruth R. to II, 14 אילו היה ראובן יודע שהקב״ה מַכְתִּיב עליו וכ׳ if R. had known that the Lord would cause to be written about him (Gen. XXXVII, 21) &c.; a. fr.—Lev. R. s. 24 ג׳ פרשיות ה׳ לנו וכ׳ (Pesik. R. s. 15; Yalk. Ex. 307 כתב) there are three sections that Moses indited for us in the Law.—2) *to consign, enlist in the army, levy.* Ex. R. s. 15 (מלך) ב״וד מַכְתִּיב לו וכ׳ a human king levies soldiers for himself, strong &c.; Tanh. Ḥayé 3 מסביב (corr. acc.). Cant. R. to II, 8, a. e. מַכְתֶּבֶת, v. טִירוֹנְיָא.—Part. pass. מוּכְתָּב *recorded; levied.* Kidd. IV, 5, v. אִסְטְרַטְיָא II.—Tosef. B. Bath. IV, 7; B. Bath. 92ᵇ; Keth. 58ª מ׳ למלכות levied for royal service (comment.: *sentenced to death*); Kidd. 11ª נִכְתַּב.—Gen. R. s. 89 (Yalk. ib. 147 כתיב), v. סַקְרָרִין.

כְּתַב I, כְּתוֹב ch. same. Targ. Deut. VI, 9 (v. Berl. Targ. O. II, p. 51). Ib. XXXI, 24. Targ. Josh. XVIII, 4; a. v. fr.—Part. pass. כְּתִיב (כְּתוּב). Targ. Ex. XXXI, 18. Targ. O. Num. XI, 26 (Y. כתוביא); a. fr.—B. Kam. 88ª bot. כַּתְבִינְהוּ לנכסי וכ׳ she willed her property to &c. Gitt. 20ª איהו קא כָּתְבָה ליה she (the wife) had it written (at her expense). B. Bath. 168ᵇ וּלִכְתּוֹב לן מר וכ׳ write for us another document (copy) in addition to this; a. v. fr.—Sabb. 115ᵇ היכא דִּכְתִיבִי תרגים וכ׳ when the books are written in Chaldaic or any other tongue (than Hebrew); a. fr.—Esp. (in arguments on Biblical texts) כ׳ רחמנא or כ׳ the Lord has written, *the text reads.* Pes. 21ᵇ טעמא דכ׳ רחמנא לא יֵאָכֵל וכ׳ this is so because the text reads לא יֵאָכֵל (passive voice), but if it did not read so &c. Ib. לִכְתּוֹב רחמנא וכ׳ it ought to read &c. Ber. 3ᵇ א״ה לכתוב מהנשף וכ׳ if this were so (that נֶשֶׁף invariably means *evening*), it ought to read (I Sam. XXX, 17) מהנשף ועד הנשף; a. v. fr.—כְּתִיב *it is written, it reads* (used also in Hebr. diction). Ib. 13ᵇ דִּכְ׳ לדבר בם for it says (Deut. XI, 19) 'to *speak* thereof'; ה״נ הא כ׳ ודברת בם here, too, (in the first part of the Sh'ma) it says (VI, 7), 'and thou shalt *speak* thereof'!—Meg. 10ᵇ כ׳ הכא ויהי ... וכ׳ התם ויהי here (Lev. IX, 1) *vayhi* is used, and there (Gen. I, 5) *vayhi* is used. Ib. והא כ׳ וְהָיָ׳ but does it not also read &c.?—Gen. R. s. 1 ומאי כ׳ אחריו and what do we read after this?—הדא הוא דכ׳, v. הָא I.—Snh. 71ª, a. e. בעינן קרא כִּדִכְ׳ we must construe the Biblical text as it is written (literally, e. g. Mish. ib. VIII, 4 as an interpretation of Deut. XXI, 19); a. v. fr.—B. Kam. 66ª שינוי קונה כְּתִיבָה ותנינא כ׳ that a change of form of a stolen object gives possession (compelling the thief to restore in value) is written (intimated in the Biblical text) and has been taught in the Mishnah.—V. כְּתִיב.

Ithpe. אִיכְּתִיב, אִתְכְּתִיב *to be written, recorded* &c. Targ. Esth. I, 19. Targ. Ps. XL, 8. Ib. LXXXVII, 6 דמִתְכַּתְבִין Ms. (ed. דמְכַתְּבִין *Pa.*); a. fr.—Meg. 7ª דאיבעי אִיכְּתִיב וכ׳ (Ms. M. מאי דבעי כתיב, v. Rabb. D. S. a. l. note; Rashi: דאי בעי כתב) that which was liked was written down &c.; a. fr.

כְּתָב m. (b. h.; preced.) *writing, writ; character.* Ab. V, 6; Pes. 54ª; Sifré Deut. 355 (of things created in the last hour of the sixth day) הכתב והמִּכְתָּב the art of writing and the writing on the tablets (Ex. XXXII, 16; Rashi to Pes. l. c. והמַּכְתֵּב and the pencil); Mekh. B'shall., Vayassa, s. 5 only כתב. Ab. Zar. 10ª אין להם לא כ׳ ולא לשון they (the Romans) have neither (original) types nor language; Gitt. 80ª (of פרסיים). Y. Meg. I, 71ᵇ bot., v. לִיבּוֹנָאָה; Snh. 21ᵇ; Meg. 8ᵇ (ה) כ׳ עברי, v. אַשּׁוּרִי. [Ib. עד שיכתבנו בכתב אשורית, strike out בכתב, v. Rabb. D. S. a. l., a. Meg. 9ª.]—תורה שֶׁבִּכְ׳ written Law, opp. שבעל פה. Yoma 28ᵇ; a. fr.—Meg. 18ᵇ שלא מן הכ׳ without a written copy, from memory.—Pes. 21ᵇ, a. e. דברים כִּכְתָבָן וכ׳ וכ׳ construe the Biblical words as they are written (Deut. XIV, 21), to the resident stranger give it as a present, to the foreigner sell it.—כְּתַב יד *signature.* Keth. II, 3 sq.; a. fr.—Tosef. B. Kam. VII, 4 כ׳ חיבר יד שלו.—Gen. R. s. 48 בכל מקום... הכ׳ רבה על הנקודה אתה דורש את הכ׳ וכ׳ wherever you find in the Biblical text the plain writing, i. e. the number of undotted letters in a word, prevailing over the number of the dotted, you must interpret the undotted (ignoring the dotted); where the dotted prevail, you must interpret the dotted, e. g. אֵלָיו (Gen. XVIII, 9) read אַיּוֹ, where is he (Abraham)?; ib. s. 78; Cant. R. to VII, 5.—Tosef. Meg. IV (III), 41 (ref. to II Kings X, 27 קורין אותו כִּכְתָבוֹ (מחראות) we read it as it is written (not as emended in the K'ri); a. fr.—*Pl.* כְּתָבִין, כְּתָבִים. Tanh. Masé 1; Num. R. s. 23, beg. כ׳ רעים מן המלכות government papers containing orders of hard measures against the Jews. Esth. R. introd. כְּתָבָיו של מלך royal decrees. Ex. R. s. 20 עד שילמוד בני כ׳ (some ed. כתובין) until my son shall have studied documents; a. e.

כְּתַב II, כְּתָבָא, כְּתָ׳ ch. same. Targ. Y. Lev. XIX, 28 (h. text כְּתֹבֶת).—Targ. Y. Gen. XLVIII, 9 (marriage contract, v. כְּתוּבָּה). Targ. Ex. XXXII, 16 (h. text מכתב); a. fr.—Lev. R. s. 28, end מה דאמר כְּתָבְכוֹן what your sacred writ says.—*Pl.* כְּתָבֵי, כְּתָבִין (כְּתָבִין), כְּתָבַיָּא. Targ. II Esth. IV, 12. Ib. VII, 10; a. e.—Gen. R. s. 10; Lev. R. s. 22 כ׳ בישין וכ׳ evil decrees against the Jews of Caesarea (v. preced.); Tanh. Huck. 1.

כַּתְבָן, v. כְּתִיב.

כַּתְבָן m. ch. = h. כּוֹתְבָן, *writer, copyist* (of Biblical books). Koh. R. to II, 18 R. Meïr was כ׳ טב מובחר an exceedingly skillful copyist, v. לַבְלָר.

כְּתֹבֶת, v. כְּתוּבֶת.

כְּתוֹב, v. כְּתַב I.

כָּתוּב m. (כָּתַב) *Biblical verse, passage*; הַכָּ׳ *the Bible text.* Hag. 18[a], a. fr. במה הכ׳ מדבר of what does the text speak? Ib. הא לא מסרן הכ׳ אלא וכ׳ this proves that the Law intended to leave it to the discretion of the scholars to decide &c.—Pes. 3[a] עקם הכ׳ שמנה וכ׳ the text made a circumlocution of eight letters (more than would have been required). Sifra introd., beg. בנין אב מכ׳ אחד a standard rule derived from one verse. Ib. end כ׳ אחד אומר וכ׳ one verse reads . . ., and another reads &c.; a. fr.—*Pl.* כְּתוּבִים, כְּתוּבִין. Sifra l. c. Snh. 45[b]; Meïl. 11[b], v. לְמַד; a. fr.—[Ex. R. s. 20, v. כְּתַב.]—Esp. *K'thubim, Hagiographa,* the third part of the Bible. Keth. 50[a] תורה נביאים וכ׳ (abbrev. תנ״ך) Pentateuch, Prophets and Hagiographa. B. Bath. 14[b] סידרן של כ׳ וכ׳ the order of the books of the Hagiographa is: Ruth &c. Meg. 31[a] ומשולש בכ׳ and for the third time intimated in the Hag.; a. fr.

כְּתוּבָא ch. same.—*Pl.* כְּתוּבֵי, כְּתוּבַיָּא. Y. Ned. I, end, 37[a] בקדושת כ׳ as sacred as the Biblical writings.—Esp. כְּתוּבֵי *the Hagiographa.*— Taan. 9[a] מי איכא מידי דכתיבא בכ׳ וכ׳ is there anything written in the Hagiographa that is not intimated in the Law? B. Bath. 8[a] עברת אדאורייתא . . ואדכ׳ thou didst act against what is written in the Law, the Prophets and the Hagiographa. Keth. 106[b] דאקרייך כ׳ לא וכ׳ he who taught thee the Hagiographa has not taught thee the Prophets; a. e.

כְּתוּבָא, כְּתוּבָה m. =כָּתְבָן, *writer, notary.* Y. Gitt. IX, 50[c] bot. Y. Snh. II, beg. 19[d]; Y. Hor. III, beg. 47[a] ר׳ חנינא כ׳ R. Ḥ., the notary.

כְּתוּבָּה f. (preced. wds.) *writ, deed,* esp. *marriage contract,* containing, among other things, the settlement of a certain amount due do the wife on her husband's death or on being divorced; *K'thubah, the wife's settlement, widowhood.* [For the formula of the marriage contract, v. Keth. IV, 7—12.] Y. Yeb. XV, 14[d] ב״ש עבדו כ׳ מדרש the Shammaites made the wording of the marriage contract the text for legal interpretation; מספר כְּתוּבָּתָהּ נלמוד וכ׳ from her marriage contract we learn (that she must receive her widowhood), for he writes to her &c. Ib. ר׳ מאיר עבד כ׳ וכ׳ R. M. made the formula of the deed of sale the text &c. (v. B. Mets. IX, 3).—Keth. I, 2 בתולה כְּתוּבָּתָהּ מאתים the widowhood of one marrying as a virgin is two hundred Zuz. Sabb. 14[b]; 16[b] שמעון...תיקן כ׳ לאשה Simon b. Shetah introduced the written marriage contract (with the promise of a widowhood, in place of a deposit of the widowhood in securities); Keth. 82[b] תיקן כל נכסיו אחראין לכתובתה ordained that the contract must contain a clause making all his landed estate a mortgage for her widowhood; Y. ib. VIII, 32[b], sq. Bab. ib. 10[a] כְּתוּבַּת אשה מן התורה the widowhood endowment is intimated in the Torah. Ib. כתובת אלמנה אינה וכ׳ the endowment of one that married as a widow is not Biblical. Ib. 56[a] כ׳ דרבנן the widowhood is a Rabbinical institution. Ib. IV, 2 כְּתוּבָּתָהּ שלו her widowhood belongs to him (her father). Ib. IX, 8 הפוגמת כתובתה, v. פָּגַם. Ib. 9 הוציאה גט ... גובה כתובתה if she produces evidence of divorce but has no contract to show, she is entitled to her settlement; a. v. fr.—*Pl.* כְּתוּבּוֹת. Ib. שני...כ׳ גובה שתי כ׳ if she produces two letters of divorce (evidence of having been divorced and remarried to her former husband and again divorced) and two contracts, she is entitled to two widowhoods; a. fr. — כְּתוּבּוֹת *K'thuboth,* name of a treatise of Mishnah, Tosefta, Talmud Babli and Y'rushalmi, of the Order of Nashim.

כְּתוֹבֶת f. (b. h. כְּתֹבֶת; preced. wds.) *writing, inscription;* כ׳ קעקע *etched-in inscription* on the skin (Lev. XIX, 28). Macc. III, 6. Lev. R. s. 19 שנמצאת כ׳ ק׳ חקוקה וכ׳ an etched-in writing was found on his (Jojakim's) body. Gitt. 20[b] בכ׳ ק׳ in the case of the slave's emancipation being etched in on his hand (so as to be indelible).

כְּתוּבְתָּא ch.=h. כְּתוּבָּה. Targ. Y. II Gen. XXXIV, 12 (h. text מֹהַר).—Keth. IV, 7 (in a Chald. formula of the marriage contract) אחראין לִכְתוּבְּתִיךְ security for thy widowhood. Ib. 10 אינון ירתון כסף כתובתיך they shall inherit the amount of widowhood stated in thy K'thubah. Ib. 87[a] ושקילנא מִכְּתוּבְתָּאִי and I may take it in advance as partial payment of my widowhood; a. e.—*Pl.* כְּתוּבָתָא. Targ. Y. II Gen. XXXI, 15 לחוד כְּתוּבָתָן except our settlements (deposited with our father).—Kidd. 70[b] אקרען כמה כ׳ וכ׳ many marriage contracts were torn (marriages cancelled) in Nehardea.

כְּתוּנָא, v. כִּיתּוּנָא.

כְּתֹנֶת, כְּתוֹנֶת, כִּתּוֹנֶת f. (b. h.; v. כִּיתָּן, כִּיתּוּנָא) [*linen,*] *shirt, undergarment,* esp. *the priest's undercoat.* Yoma VII, 5. Ib. 35[b]; Tosef. ib. I, 21. Zeb. 88[b]. Gen. R. s. 84, v. פַּרְגּוֹד; a. e.—*Pl.* כָּתְנוֹת. Ib. s. 20, v. אוֹר II, 3. [Post-biblical חָלוּק.]

כְּתוּשָׁא, v. כְּתִישָׁא.

כָּתוּת, v. כָּתִית.

כְּתִיב m., **כְּתִיבָא** f. (כְּתַב I) 1) *written; it is written,* v. כְּתַב I.—[Targ. II Esth. VII, 10 כְּתִיבֵי some ed., read כְּתִיבֵי, v. כְּתַב II].—2) (Massorah) כְּתִיב *K'thib,* the traditional spelling of Biblical words, opp. to קרי, K'ri, the Massoretic instruction for reading, e. g. Gen. VIII, 17: K'thib הוצא (הוֹצֵא), K'ri הַיְצֵא; v. Treat. Sof'rim VI, 5; VII, 4. Ab. Zar. 24[b] (ref. to I Sam. VI, 9) ויעלה כ׳ the K'thib allows the reading וַיַּעֲלֶה (with feminine suffix). Snh. 20[a], v. פָּרָה; a. v. fr.—*Pl.* כְּתִיבָן. Ned. 37[b] קריין ולא כ׳ וכ׳ ולא קריין וכ׳ the rules about reading words not written (omitted in the text) and such as are written but not read (marked as superfluous) are a Mosaic (ancient, traditional) *halakhah* (v. הֲלָכָה). Ib. הלין קריין ולא כְּתִיבָן those (quoted) are those read but not written; וּכְתִיבָן ולא קריין וכ׳ and those written but not read are &c.; v. Treat. Sof'rim VI, 8—9.

כְּתִיבָה f. (כָּתַב) 1) *writing*. Sabb. 104^b כ׳ היא אלא וכ׳ it is a writing, and what is needed to make it one word is bringing the two ends of the papers close together. Men. 34^a כ׳ הנוהגת לדורות a mode of writing used at all times (not stone inscriptions). Sabb. 103^a אין דרך כ׳ בכך this (using the left hand) is not the way of writing. Ib.^{b} (ref. to וּכְתַבְתָּם, Deut. VI, 9) שתהא כתיבה תמה that the writing must be perfect. Ib. 105^a (expl. אנכי, Ex. XX, 2, v. אָנֹכִי) אמירה נעימה כ׳ יהיבה a sweet proclamation, a writing, a gift; Yalk. Gen. 81. Gitt. 17^b משעת כ׳ ועד וכ׳ from the time the letter of divorce was written to the time of its delivery. Ib. 45^b (ref. to Deut. VI, 8—9) כל שישנו בקשירה ישנו בכ׳ only he who is under the obligation of binding (the T'fillin on his arm), is fit for writing (the scrolls of the Law &c.). Keth. 102^b וקרי ליה לאמירה כ׳ and is 'saying' (verbal declaration) called 'writing' (consignment)?; a. fr.—2) *the word* כתב *in Biblical texts*. Ber. 16^a בין כ׳ לכ׳ וכ׳ if a person in reading the Sh'ma is in doubt as to whether he is at וכתבתם (of Deut. VI, 9) or at וכתבתם (of ib. XI, 20), he must go back to the first וכתבתם; Y. ib. II, 5^a כתיבת (corr. acc.).

כתיבת, v. preced.

כתליקין, כתלקין, v. קָתוֹלִיקוֹס.

כְּתִיפ׳, v. כְּתַף.

כְּתִישׁ, v. כְּתַשׁ.

כְּתִישָׁא, כְּתוּ׳ m. (כְּתַשׁ) *a scab* on a camel's back. B. Mets. 38^b דבש לכ׳ דגמלא spoiled honey is fit for a liniment for a camel's sore back, v. כְּתִיתָא.

כְּתִישָׁה f. (כָּתַשׁ) *crushing, pounding*. Sabb. 74^a עני ... בלא כ׳ a poor man eats his bread without pounding the grain before grinding (to remove the husks), v. כָּתַשׁ. Bets. 7^b והא קא עביד כ׳ but (by crushing the clods of earth) does he not do the (forbidden) act of pounding? Cant. R. to I, 3 מה השמן ... אלא ע״י כ׳ וכ׳ as the oil cannot be improved except by pounding (the olives), so can Israel only by suffering; Men. 53^b מה זית ... ע״י כ׳ Ms. M. (ed. כתית, corr. acc.) as the olive gives forth its oil only through pounding &c.; Yalk. Jer. 289.

כָּתִית m. (b. h.; כָּתַת) 1) *oil gained from pounded olives*. Men. VIII, 5. Ib. 86^b אין כ׳ אלא כָּתוּשׁ the Biblical *kathith* means *pounded*. [Ib. 53^b, v. preced.].—2) *pl*. כְּתִיתִין (sub. פַּת, v. preced.) *bread or pastry made of pounded wheat, delicacies*. Midr. Till. to Ps. XV, 1; Yalk. Ps. 664 שמוכרין מיני כ׳ וכל דבר [טוב] who had for sale various fine pastries and all sorts of [good]things.—3) (cmp. b. h. ספחת) *scab* on an animal's back from friction. Sabb. VIII, 1 (76^b) דבש כדי ליתן על פי כ׳ (v. Rabb. D. S. a. l. note) honey, as much as required for putting on a scab (v. כְּתִישָׁא); ib. 77^b, v. מוֹרְשָׁא a. הוֹרְדְנָא. Ib. ב״א שבלול לכ׳ He created the snail as a remedy for a scab; Y. Ber. IX, 13^c bot. שבלון לכ׳ ed. Lehm. (ed. לחזוית, v. חֲזָזִית).—4) (also כָּתוּת) *compress of rags* (cmp. בְּלָיוֹת, שְׁחָקִים); *pad*. [Tosef. Mikv. VI, 10 כתות של גדיל, v. כְּשׁוּת.]—*Pl*. כְּתִיתִין, כְּתִיתִים, כְּתוּ׳. Tosef. Sabb. XII (XIII), 14; Sabb. 134^b יבשין כ׳ dry compresses. Ib. 53^a כ׳ ע״ג השבר Ms. M. (ed. קשישין, Ms. O. כבשושין) pads upon a fractured limb. Ib. VI, 8 (66^a); Yoma 78^b אם יש לו בית קבול כתי׳ Ms. M. (ed. כתו׳) if the wooden leg has a cavity for the reception of pads, v. next w.

כְּתִיתָא ch. same, 1) *scab*. Sabb. 154^b לכ׳ דגמלי (Rashi: לכתותי דגמלא); B. Mets. 38^b (quot. in Rashi to Sabb. 76^b a. v. הכתית) כתותא, v. כְּתִישָׁא.—2) *pad*.—*Pl*. כְּתִיתִין, כְּתִיתֵי. Sabb. 134^b, v. נְקָרָא 2. Yoma 78^b דאית ביה כ׳ when the wooden leg has pads. Ib. כ׳ משוי ליה מנא (omitted in Ms. M., v. Rabb. D. S. a. l. notes 20, 30, 50) do the pads make it a garment? Yeb. 102^b דאית ביה כ׳ when the felt-shoe has pads inside.

כְּתַכְתִּין, v. כְּתָא.

כְּתַל, כְּתָלָא, v. כּוֹת׳.

כתליקין, v. כתלקין.

כָּתַם (b. h.) *to be compressed, dark, hidden* (cmp. אטם, טמן, טמא).

Nif. נִכְתַּם *to be stained, marked*. R. Hash. 18^a; Yeb. 105^a (ref. to Jer. II, 22) taken as equivalent with נחתם.—*Part. Pu*. מְכוּתָּם *stained*. Midr. Till. to Ps. XVI (play on מכתם) David said to the Lord מכ׳ אני ed. Bub. (oth. ed. מכתם, corr. acc.) I am stained (with sin).

כְּתַם ch. same.—Part. pass. כְּתִים *dark, red*. *Pl*. כְּתִימִין. Targ. Is. I, 18.

כֶּתֶם m. (b. h.; preced.) 1) *dark-red stain*, esp. *stain on a woman's clothes* or *body*, as an indication of uncleanness (v. נִדָּה). Nidd. 4^b כִּתְמָהּ טמא למפרע a stain found on her makes her unclean retrospectively (up to the time when she last washed herself). Ib. 5^a יש לה כ׳ is subject to the law concerning *kethem*. Ib. VIII, 1. Y. ib. I, 49^c אין לה כ׳ is not subject to the law &c., v. supra; a. fr.—*Pl*. כְּתָמִים, כְּתָמִין. Ib. VII, 3, sq. Tosef. ib. VIII, 12; a. fr.—2) *gold*. Ex. R. s. 8; Tanh. Vaëra 8, v. פָּז. R. Hash. 4^a (ref. to Ps. XLV, 10) זכיתם לכ׳ אופיר you are rewarded with gold of Ophir.

כִּתְמָא, כִּי׳ ch. same, *blood-stain*. Targ. Jer. II, 22.—*Pl*. כִּתְמִין, כִּתְמֵי, כִּי׳. Nidd. 5^a. [Snh. 95^a חזינהו כתמי דבא, a corrupt., v. Rabb. D. S. a. l. Ms. M. a. note, a. Yalk. Sam. 155.]

כָּתַן, v. כִּיתָּן.

כַּתָּן m. (v. preced.) *flax-beater*. Kel. XXVI, 5; Tosef. ib. B. Bath. IV, 8 הפתן ed. Zuck. (Var. הכ׳).

כְּתֹנֶת, v. כְּתוֹנֶת.

כָּתַף (cmp. כָּתַת) *to join*; denom. כָּתֵף.—[Midr. Till. to Ps. II, 3 כתופין, ed. Bub. כתיפין, read: כפיתין, v. כָּפַת.]

Pi. כִּיתֵּף (denom. of כָּתֵף) *to carry; to shoulder*. Y. Shebi. VIII, 38^b מְכַתְּפֵי פירות carriers of fruits (in the Sabbatical year). Y. Nidd. II, beg. 49^d דהוה מְכַתֶּפֶת יינות וכ׳ carried vessels with wine for libations; (Bab. ib. 6^b גפה, v. גַּפָּה).—B. Kam. 31^a עמד לְכַתֵּף he halted for the sake of shifting the burden on his shoulder; Keth. 31^a, sq.; Sabb. 5^b. Ib. 8^a; Erub. 33^a רבים מְכַתְּפִין עליו people rest and rearrange their burdens on it. [Bets. 25[b] ובלבד שלא יְכַתֵּף provided one allows not the chair to be carried on shoulders, v. אֲלְנְקִי; perhaps to be read: יִכָּתֵף *Nif.*]

כָּתַף, *Pa.* כַּתֵּף same. Sabb. 8[a] ולא כְּתוּפֵי מְכַתְּפֵי עלויה Ms. M. nor do they not use it for rearranging burdens; ודאי מְכַתְּפִין עילויה people surely use it &c. Ib. 119[a] מְכַתֵּף ועייל כ׳ carried things in and out. Ib. מי לא מְכַתֵּיפְנָא קמיירהו וכ׳ should I not carry things in and out for their reception? —Esp. *to carry a person* (*in a chair*) *on shoulders*, v. אֲלְנְקִי. Yoma 87[a]; Snh. 7[b]. Bets. 25[b] חוו מְכַתְּפֵי להו (v. Rabb. D. S. a. l. note 8) they carried them; (ed. מִכַּתְּפוּ להו *Ithpa.* allowed themselves to be carried).

Ithpa. אִיכַּתֵּף *to be carried on shoulders*, v. supra.

כַּתָּף m. (preced.) *carrier, porter.* Tosef. Ber. II, 7. Kel. XXVI, 5 עור הכ׳ the hide which the porter uses to protect his clothes. Y. Kidd. II, beg. 62[a] ע״י הכ׳ on the testimony of the carrier (that delivered the goods); a. e.—*Pl.* כַּתָּפִים, כַּתָּפִין. Y. M. Kat. III, 82[b] bot.; Y. Ber. III, 6[a] top נמסר לכ׳ when the corpse has been given over to the pall-bearers. Y. Shebi. VIII, 38[b] [read:] החמרין הכ׳ וכל הנושין בשביעית שכרן וכ׳ the drivers and porters and all employees in the Sabbatical year take their wages in fruits of that year (v. Tosef. ib. VI, 26); a. e.—שבח המגיע לכ׳ an improvement touching the carriers, i. e. an increase of the value of the crop, opp. to an increase of the value of the land. B. Kam. 95[b]; B. Mets. 15[b]; a. e.

כַּתָּף, כַּתָּפָא ch. same.—*Pl.* כַּתָּפַיָּא, כַּתָּפִין. Y. Shebu. VII, 38[a] top סמכון כ׳ גבי וכ׳ paid the porters with orders drawn on the retailers (sellers of provision &c.).

כָּתֵף m. (b. h.; v. כָּתַף) 1) *joint, shoulder.* Shebi. III, 9 אבני כ׳ באין וכ׳ heavy stones may be taken in the Sabbatical year from any place (their size showing their designation for building purposes); כל שהן נטלות... על הכ׳ those which are carried, two or three at a time, on the shoulder. B. Mets. 68[b]; Tosef. ib. V, 6 מקום שנהגו להעלות שכר כ׳ למעות where it is customary to add a remuneration for carriage to the money (to be paid to the partner on settling). Gen. R. s. 56 (ref. to Gen. XXII, 6) כזה שהוא טוען.. על כְּתֵפוֹ like him (the culprit) who carries his cross on his shoulders; a. fr.—2) *grapes on an arm of a vine which branches off into twigs*, contrad. to נטף grapes hanging down from the trunk. Peah VII, 4 what is gleaning (belonging to the poor, Lev. XIX, 10)? כל שאין לה כ׳ וכ׳ the grapes remaining on a stalk which has no arm (its grapes having been collected) &c.; expl. Tosef. ib. III, 11; Y. ib. VII, 20[a] bot., v. סְרִיגָה.—*Pl.* כְּתֵפִים, כְּתֵיפִים, constr. כִּתְפוֹת. Pesik. R. s. 20 נאה להרכיבה על כ׳ it is proper to carry her on (human) shoulders; a. e.—[Yalk. Gen. 161; Y. Sot. I, 17[b] bot., v. כְּפָתָה.—Tosef. Kel. B. Bath. II, 4, v. כְּפִיס.]

כְּתַף, כִּתְפָא ch. same. Targ. Zeph. III, 9. Targ. Job XXXI. 22 כִּתְפִי; a. fr.—Kidd. 81[a] מותיב... על כִּתְפֵיה placed a halter over his shoulder. Y. Kidd. I, 61[a] bot. מסתמיך אַכִּתְפֵיה וכ׳ leaning on the shoulder of &c.; Y. Sabb. I, 3[a] כִּתְפְתֵיה.—*Pl.* כִּתְפִין, כִּתְפֵי. Targ. Ex. XXVIII, 12; a. fr.—B. Mets. 107[b]

כמלא כ׳ נגדי וכ׳ as much space along the riverside as is occupied by those dragging the tow.—[Lev. R. s. 21; Yalk. Sam. 126 חזק כתפיו, v. כִּיפְתָא.]

כַּתְפָא, v. כְּתַף.

כַּתְפִי m. (sub לשון) *Coptic language* (?). Snh. 4[b]; Zeb. 37[b]; Men. 34[b] (Ar. s. v. טט, some ed. גדפי, cmp. גִּיפְטִי).

כִּתְפְתָא f. = כִּתְפָא, v. כְּתַף.

כָּתַר (b. h.) *to knot, tie, join closely.*—Denom. כֶּתֶר, כּוֹתֶרֶת.

Hif. הִכְתִּיר (denom. of כֶּתֶר) *to tie a wreath, to offer a crown.* Lev. R. s. 24 העליונים מַכְתִּירִין להקב״ה וכ׳ the angels wreathe three 'holies' to the Lord (Is. VI, 3); Yalk. ib. 603 העליונים מַכְתִּירִים לפני וכ׳; Yalk. Is. 272 מה״ש מכתירין ג׳ קדושות.—Erub. 53[b] (in enigmatic speech) נתייעץ בְּמַכְתִּיר he took counsel with the crown-maker (him who ordains the scholars, the Nasi).—[Tanh. Ki Thissa 6 שהכתיר, read: שהבחיר, as Pesik. Shek., p. 15[b].]—*Part. pass.* מוּכְתָּר *adorned, distinguished.* Meg. 12[b] (in being called *Jehudi*, Esth. II, 5) מרדכי מ׳ בנימוסו היה (כעדי) (v. Rabb. D. S. a. l. note 300) Mordecai was intended to be described as adorned with his faith (as with an ornament), i. e. *Jehudi* is meant not as a gentile noun but as an epithet of religious devotion (than whom no better Jew was found).

כַּתַּר ch., *Pa.* כַּתַּר (preced.) [*to turn around*, cmp. יָחַל,] *to wait upon, hope for.* Targ. Job XXXVI, 2 Bxt. (ed. אמתין). Targ. Is. XLII, 4 (h. text יחל). Ib. LI, 5 יְכַתְּרוּן ed. Wil. (oth. ed. יְכַתְּ׳, *Af.*).

Af. אַכְתִּיר same, v. supra.—Part. pass. מְכַתַּר *made to wait, dependent upon.* Targ. Mic. V, 6 (h. text יְיַחֵל).

כֶּתֶר m. (b. h.; preced.) *garland, crown.* Hull. 60[b] the Moon said אפשר.. בכ׳ אחד is it possible for two kings to use the same crown (to occupy an equal rank)? Ex. R. s. 1 כִּתְרוֹ של פרעה Pharaoh's crown. Sabb. 104[a] (play on letters כ ל) וקושר לך כ׳ לעוה״ב and he will wreathe a crown for thee in the world to come; a. fr.—*Pl.* כְּתָרִים. Ab. IV, 13 שלשה כ׳ הן... על גביהן there are three crowns, the crown of the Law (learning) . . ., but the crown of a good name rises above all of them. Sabb. 88[a]; a. fr.—Ib. 89[a]; Men. 29[b] קושר כ׳ לאותיות providing certain letters with crownlets (v. זִיּוּן).

כְּתַר, כִּתְרָא, כִּי׳, כּוֹ׳ ch. same. Targ. Is. LXII, 3. Targ. Jer. XLVIII, 9; a. e.—*Pl.* כִּתְרַיָּא. Targ. Is. III, 23 (ed. Wil. כִּתְרַיָּא).

כֹּתֶרֶת, כֹּתַרְתָּא, v. sub כּוֹת׳.

כָּתַשׁ (b. h.; v. כָּתַת) 1) *to crush* (olives), *to pound, beat* Shebi. IV, 9 כּוֹתֵשׁ וסך וכ׳ he may crush olives and use the oil for ointment in the field. Sabb. 74[a] וליחשוב נמי כותש let the Mishnah (VII, 2) count (among the forbidden labors) also *pounding* (grain), v. כְּתִישָׁה. Men. VIII, 4 (86[a]). Tanh. Huck. 8; Pesik. Par., p. 40[a] וכוֹתְשִׁין אותה and pound it (the burnt body). Koh. R. to VII, 2 ולמה כותשין על הלב

why do mourners beat their hearts?; a. e.—Part. pass. כָּתוּשׁ, f. כְּתוּשָׁה crushed. Men. 86[b], v. כָּתִית.—Trnsf. defloured. Y. Kidd. I, 59[d] top, v. חָרַךְ.—2) *to press, to be closely joined, grouped*; שער כּוֹתֵשׁ *a thick hair crown*, i. e. *ramifications forming a sort of arbor*. Peah II, 3 אם היה ש׳ כ׳ if the ramifications are intertwined; Y. ib. 17[a] top [read:] מה כ׳ כעלי במכתש וכ׳ (v. R. S. to Kil. V, 3) what does this כותש mean? Does it mean, like the pestle in the mortar (i. e. the partition is formed by a depression in the ground between the two fields, out of which the fence rises), or does it mean, pressing upon (overgrowing) the fence? Answ. מן מה דתנינן סער כותש ואין הגדר כותש וכ׳ reading as we do 'the hair (ramification) presses', and not 'the fence presses', it is evident that it means 'overgrowing the fence.'

Nif. נִכְתַּשׁ *to be crushed, pounded.* Tanh. Ki Thabo 3 מה השמן הזה נ׳ וכ׳ as oil is pounded, and the more it is pounded, the better it becomes, v. כְּתִישָׁה. Ter. I, 8 זתים הנִכְתָּשִׁין crushed olives. Tosef. ib. III, 14 עתידין לִיכָּתֵשׁ designated for pounding; a. fr.

Pi. כִּיתֵּשׁ *to crush to powder.*—Part. pass. מְכוּתָּשׁ, f. מְכוּתֶּשֶׁת. Tosef. Ohol. II, 5 some ed. (oth. מְכוּתֶּתֶת, ed. Zuck. מכתתת; Y. Naz. VIII, 56[c] מְכוּתָּתִין).

Hithpa. הִתְכַּתֵּשׁ [*to come in contact with,*] *to wrestle, fight* (cmp. נָגַשׁ). Y. Peah IV, 18[b] top שנים שהיו מִתְכַּתְּשִׁין וכ׳ if two persons were fighting about a (forgotten) sheaf; Tosef. Peah II, 2 מִכַּתְּשִׁין ed. Zuck. (Var. מתכשין, corr. acc.). Sifré Deut. 37 ד׳ מלכיות מִתְכַּתְּשׁוֹת וכ׳ (ed. Fr. מתכחשות) four governments disputed about it (each naming it differently); Yalk. Num. 743 מתרחשות (corr. acc.); Pesik. Zutr. Deut. ed. Bub. p. 9 מלכים מִתְכַּתְּשִׁין . . . .; ib. p. 30 מתכבש׳ (corr. acc.).

כְּתַשׁ ch. same, 1) *to crush.* Targ. Y. Ex. XXX, 36.—Part. pass. כְּתִישׁ, f. כְּתִישָׁא; pl. כְּתִישִׁין; כְּתִישָׁן. Targ. Ex. XXVII, 20. Targ. Y. Lev. XXII, 24 (h. text כָּתוּת).—2) (=h. נגע) *to touch, strike, afflict.* Part. pass. as ab. Targ. Ps. LXXIII, 14 (ed. Wil. כְּתִישׁ). Targ. Is. XXVIII, 1 (h. text הלומי). Ib. LIV, 4; a. e.—Den. מַכְתֵּשׁ.

Ithpa. אִתְכַּתַּשׁ, אִכַּתַּשׁ 1) *to wrestle, fight.* Targ. Y. Gen. XXXII, 25, sq.—Gen. R. s. 48, beg. הות מִכַּתְּשָׁא וכ׳ was quarrelling with her maid. Lev. R. s. 9 ולא חמית . . . מִתְכַּתְּשִׁין וכ׳ and I never saw two quarrel with one another without making peace between them. Ib. s. 22 פשושין מכתשין Ar. ed. Koh. (ed. ציפרין מתנצירין).—2) mostly *Ithpe.* אִתְכְּתֵשׁ *to be smitten, afflicted* (with leprosy). Targ. Ps. LXXIII, 5. Targ. Y. Ex. II, 23 (cmp. Ex. R. s. 1). Targ. Y. Gen. XVI, 1.—[Gen. R. s. 44; Yalk. ib. 77, v. כְּבַשׁ.]

**Pa.* כַּתֵּשׁ *to press, beg persistently.* Shebu. 30[b]; Hull. 7[b], v. כְּתַשׁ.

כָּתַת (b. h.) [*to join closely* (in a friendly or hostile sense);—Denom. כַּת;] *to press, crush.* Part. pass. כָּתוּת, *one whose parts are crushed.* Sifra Emor Par. 7, ch. VII; Kidd. 25[b]; Bekh. 39[b].

Pi. כִּיתֵּת 1) *to strike.* Gen. R. s. 22 (with ref. to Ps. LXXXIX, 24) התחיל מְכַתְּתוֹ he began to strike him; Yalk. ib. 36; Yalk. Ps. 840. Midr. Till. to Ps. XXIII היה מה״מ מְכַתֵּת וכ׳ the angel of death smote fifteen thousand and some of them. Ber. 63[b] (play on הַסְכֵּת, Deut. XXVII, 9) כַּתְּתוּ עצמיכם וכ׳ expose yourselves to being smitten (by death) over the study of the Law.—2) *to pound, pulverize.* Ab. Zar. 44[a] כִּיתְּתוֹ ground it (the bronze serpent) to powder.—Trnsf. (cmp. גרס) *to discuss, argue.* Ber. l. c. הס ואח״כ כַּתֵּת first listen (and receive) and then discuss.—Part. pass. מְכוּתָּת, f. מְכוּתֶּתֶת, *pl.* מְכוּתָּתִין, v. כָּתַשׁ.

כְּתַת ch. same, 1) *to join closely, be grouped.* Targ. Job XXX, 7 בתתין Ms. Var., read: כְּתִתִין (ed. מתחברין, h. text יְסֻפָּחוּ).—Denom. כִּתָּא, כְּתָא.—2) *to strike*, v. infra.

Pa. כַּתֵּת 1) *to pound, crush.* Ab. Zar. 44[a] בדין הוא דכַתּוֹתֵי לא וכ׳ by law it was necessary to grind it (the bronze serpent) to powder, v. preced.—2) *to ally, form into factions.* Targ. Y. I Num. XXIV, 23 (play on כִּתִּים, ib. 24) מְכַתֵּת וכ׳ causes nations . . . . . to form alliances and incites them against one another.—Part. pass. מְכַתַּת, v. infra.

Ithpa. אִיכַּתַּת 1) *to be powdered, crushed.* Succ. 31[b] כַּתּוֹתֵי מִיכַּתַּת שיעוריה the size which the Lulab must have, is (in the eyes of the law) crushed to powder (as an object of idolatry); Hull. 89[b] כתותי מִכַּתַּת שיעורא (or מְכַתַּת, v. supra). Ib. כל מה דמכ׳ וכ׳ the more it is crushed to powder, the better it is fitted (for covering the blood). Yeb. 103[b] בִּדְמִכַּתַּת דמי (or בִּדְמְכַתַּת) the house doomed to destruction (Lev. XIV, 45) is to be considered as crushed to powder.—2) *to come in contact* (hostile or friendly, cmp. זווג). Gen. R. s. 78 (ref. to פגש, Gen. XXXIII, 8) א״ל מִיכַּתַּת אנא גבירהון א״ל וכ׳ said he (Esau), I had a meeting with them. Said he (Jacob) they came to find grace &c. Said he, I have had enough blows; Yalk. ib. 133.

End of Volume I.